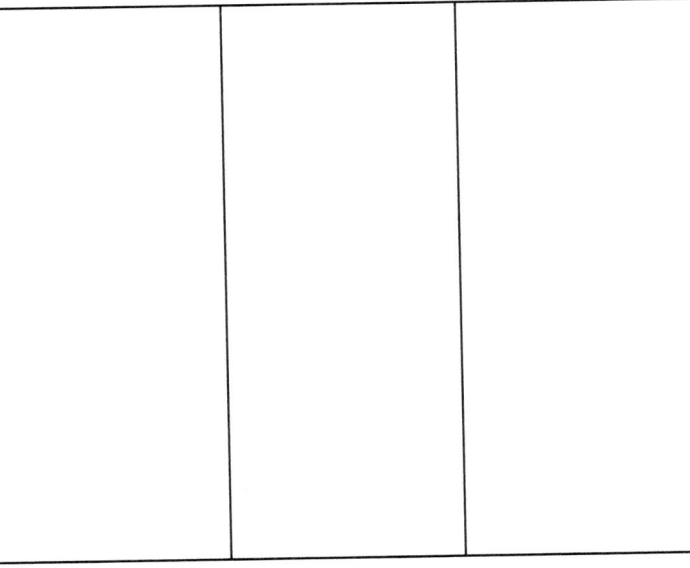

High Risk Pregnancy
Management Options

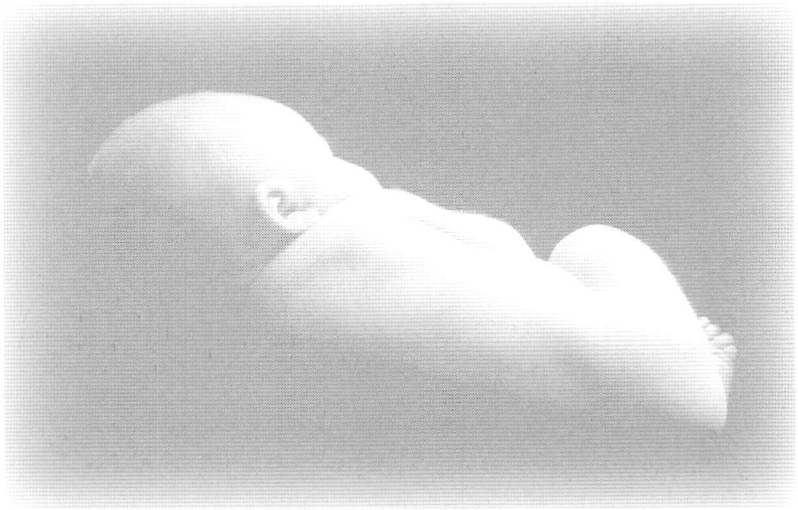

High Risk Pregnancy
Management Options

FOURTH EDITION

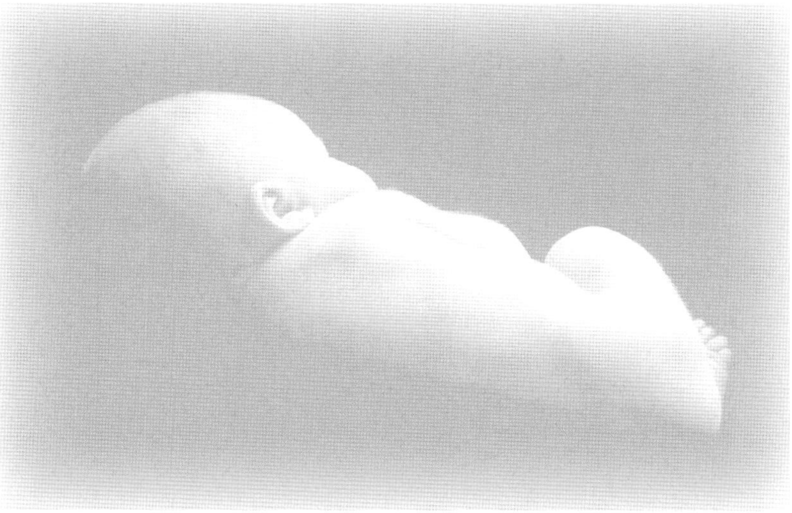

Senior Editor
David James, MA, MD, FRCOG, DCH
Emeritus Professor of Fetomaternal Medicine, Foundation Director of Medical Education
Queen's Medical Centre, Nottingham, United Kingdom

Editors
Philip J. Steer, BSc, MD, FRCOG, FCOGSA (hon)
Emeritus Professor
Faculty of Medicine
Imperial College London
Chelsea and Westminster Hospital
London, United Kingdom

Carl P. Weiner, MD, MBA, FACOG
K.E. Krantz Professor and Chair
Department of Obstetrics and Gynecology
University of Kansas School of Medicine
Kansas City, Kansas

Bernard Gonik, MD, FACOG
Professor and Fann Srere Chair of Perinatal Medicine
Department of Obstetrics and Gynecology
Wayne State University School of Medicine
Detroit, Michigan

Associate Editors
Caroline A. Crowther, MD, FRANZCOG, FRCOG, Cert MFM
Professor
Discipline of Obstetrics and Gynaecology
The University of Adelaide
Women's and Children's Hospital
North Adelaide, South Australia, Australia

Stephen C. Robson, MD, MRCOG, MBBS
Professor of Fetal Medicine
Institute of Cellular Medicine
University of Newcastle upon Tyne
Newcastle upon Tyne, United Kingdom

ELSEVIER
SAUNDERS

ELSEVIER
SAUNDERS

3251 Riverport Lane
St. Louis, MO 63403

HIGH RISK PREGNANCY: MANAGEMENT OPTIONS ISBN: 978-1-4160-5908-0

Library of Congress Cataloging-in-Publication Data

High risk pregnancy : management options / senior editor, David K. James; associate editors, Philip J. Steer ... [et al.]. – 4th ed.
p. ; cm.
Includes bibliographical references and index.
ISBN 978-1-4160-5908-0
1. Pregnancy–Complications. I. James, D. K. (David K.)
[DNLM: 1. Pregnancy, High-Risk. 2. Pregnancy Complications. WQ 240 H6377 2011]
RG571.H46 2011
618.3—dc22 2010012490

Acquisitions Editor: Stefanie Jewell-Thomas
Senior Developmental Editor: Dee Simpson
Design Direction: Steven Stave
Publishing Services Manager: Pat Joiner-Myers
Project Manager: Marlene Weeks

Printed in China

Last digit is the print number: 9 8 7 6 5 4 3 2 1

INTERNATIONAL ADVISORY BOARD

Ahmad M. Abdel Wahed
Department of Obstetrics and Gynaecology
Jabal al-zaiton Hospital
Zarka, Jordan

Gustaaf Dekker, MD
Professor, Obstetrics and Gynaecology
The University of Adelaide
Adelaide, South Australia, Australia

Tao Duan, MD, PhD
Professor, Obstetrics and Gynecology
Tongji University
Professor and Chief of the Hospital
Department of Obstetrics and Gynecology
Shanghai 1st Maternity and Infant Hospital
Shanghai, China

J. Ravichandran R. Jeganathan, MD
Associate Professor, Obstetrics and Gynaecology
Monash Malaysia School of Medicine, Monash University
Johor Bahru, Malaysia

Tze Kin Lau, MD
Professor, Obstetrics and Gynaecology
Faculty of Medicine
The Chinese University of Hong Kong
Hong Kong, SAR

Keun-Young Lee, MD
Professor, Obstetrics and Gynecology
College of Medicine, Hallym University
Seoul, Korea

Kunihiro Okamura, MD
Professor Emeritus, Obstetrics and Gynecology
Tohoku University Graduate School of Medicine
Sendai, Japan

Friday E. Okonofua, MD
Professor, Obstetrics and Gynecology
College of Medical Sciences, University of Benin
Benin City, Nigeria

Robert C. Pattinson, MD
Professor, Obstetrics and Gynaecology
University of Pretoria
Pretoria, Gauteng, South Africa

Shantala Vadeyar, MD
Consultant, Obstetrics and Feto-Maternal Medicine
Kokilaben Dhirubhai Ambani Hospital
Mumbai, India

Jose Villar, MD
Professor, Nuffield Department of Obstetrics and Gynaecology
University of Oxford
Oxfordshire, United Kingdom

CONTRIBUTORS

Anthony Ambrose, MD
Associate Professor, Maternal-Fetal Medicine, Penn State University College of Medicine; Staff Physician, The Milton S. Hershey Medical Center, Hershey, Pennsylvania
Puerperal Problems

Janet I. Andrews, MD
Assistant Professor, University of Iowa, Iowa City, Iowa
Hepatitis Virus Infections

John Anthony, MB, ChB, FCOG, MPhil
Professor, Department of Obstetrics and Gynaecology, University of Cape Town; Groote Schuur Hospital, Cape Town, South Africa
Major Obstetric Hemorrhage and Disseminated Intravascular Coagulation; Critical Care of the Obstetric Patient

Domenico Arduini
Professor and Chairman, Department of Obstetrics and Gynecology, Università Roma Tor Vergata; Department of Obstetrics and Gynecology, Ospedale Fatebenefratelli Isola Tiberina, Rome, Italy
Fetal Cardiac Anomalies

Vincent T. Armenti, MD, PhD
Administrative Course Director, Human Form and Development, Professor of Pathology, Anatomy and Cell Biology, and Professor of Surgery, Jefferson Medical College, Philadelphia, Pennsylvania; Thomas Jefferson University, Philadelphia, Pennsylvania
Pregnancy after Transplantation

George Attilakos, MD, MRCOG
Consultant in Obstetrics and Fetal Medicine, St. Michael's Hospital, University Hospitals Bristol NHS Foundation Trust, Bristol, United Kingdom
Invasive Procedures for Antenatal Diagnosis

Marie-Cécile Aubry, MD
Department of Obstetrics and Gynaecology, Port Royal Hospital, Paris; Department of Obstetrics and Gynaecology, Antoine Beclere Hospital, Clamart, France
Fetal Genitourinary Abnormalities

Loraine J. Bacchus, PhD, MA, BSc
Lecturer, Gender Violence and Health Centre, Department of Public Health and Policy, London School of Hygiene & Tropical Medicine, London, United Kingdom
Domestic Violence

May Backos, MBChB, MRCOG
Consultant in Obstetrics and Gynaecology, West Middlesex University Hospital, Isleworth, Middlesex, United Kingdom
Recurrent Miscarriage

Mert O. Bahtiyar, MD
Assistant Professor, Department of Obstetrics and Gynecology, Yale University School of Medicine, New Haven, Connecticut
Fetal Cardiac Arrhythmias: Diagnosis and Therapy

David Allan Baker, MD
Professor, Department of Obstetrics, Gynecology and Reproductive Medicine, Health Sciences Center, Stony Brook University Medical Center, Stony Brook, New York; Director, Division of Infectious Diseases, Department of Obstetrics and Gynecology, Kantonsspital Schaffhausen, Schaffhausen, Switzerland
Cytomegalovirus, Herpes Simplex Virus, Adenovirus, Coxsackievirus, and Human Papillomavirus

Imelda Balchin, BSc, MBChB, MSc, MFFP, MRCOG
Academic Clinical Fellow, University College London Institute for Women's Health; Honorary Research Fellow, CEMACH, London, United Kingdom
Prolonged Pregnancy

Ahmet Alexander Baschat, MD, MB, BCh, BAO
Professor, University of Maryland School of Medicine, Baltimore, Maryland
Fetal Growth Disorders

Marie H. Beall, MD
Clinical Professor of Obstetrics and Gynecology, David Geffen School of Medicine at UCLA, Los Angeles; Vice Chair, Harbor-UCLA Medical Center, Torrance, California
Abnormalities of Amniotic Fluid Volume

Michael A. Belfort, MD, PhD
Professor (tenured), Department of Obstetrics and Gynecology, University of Utah, Salt Lake City, Utah; Director of Perinatal Research, Director, HCA Fetal Therapy Program, and Director, HCA Obstetric Telemedicine Program, Hospital Corporation of America, Mountain Star Division, Nashville, Tennessee
Postpartum Hemorrhage and Other Problems of the Third Stage

Ron Beloosesky, MD
Faculty of Medicine, Technion Israel Institute of Technology; Rambam Medical Center, Haifa, Israel
Abnormalities of Amniotic Fluid Volume

Susan Bewley, MD, FRCOG, MA
Honorary Senior Lecturer, Kings College London; Consultant Obstetrician, Kings Health Partners, London, United Kingdom
Domestic Violence

Joseph R. Biggio, Jr., MD
Director, Division of Maternal Fetal Medicine, Medical Director, Obstetric Services, and Associate Professor, Department of Obstetrics and Gynecology and Department of Genetics, University of Alabama at Birmingham, Birmingham, Alabama
Fetal Tumors

Ralph B. Blasier, MD, JD
Professor of Orthopaedic Surgery, Wayne State University; Residency Program Director, Detroit Medical Center, Detroit, Michigan
Spine and Joint Disorders

Renee A. Bobrowski, MD
Director of Maternal Fetal Medicine and Women and Children's Services, Saint Alphonsus Regional Medical Center, Boise, Idaho
Trauma

D. Ware Branch, MD
H.A. and Edna Benning Research Chair, and Professor, Obstetrics and Gynecology, University of Utah Health Sciences Center; Medical Director, Women and Newborns Clinical Program, Intermountain Healthcare, Salt Lake City, Utah
Autoimmune Diseases

Anneke Brand, PhD, MD
Professor, Department of Immunohaematology and Blood Transfusion, and Specialist, Hematology – Internal Medicine, Leiden University Medical Center, Leiden, The Netherlands
Fetal Thrombocytopenia

Christopher S. Bryant, MD
Fellow, Division of Gynecologic Oncology, Wayne State University/Karmanos Cancer Center, Wayne State University School of Medicine, Detroit, Michigan
Malignant Disease

Catalin S. Buhimschi, MD
Director, Perinatal Research, Yale University, New Haven, Connecticut
Medication

David J. Cahill, MD, MRCPI, FRCOG
Reader in Reproductive Medicine, and Head of the Academic Unit of Obstetrics and Gynaecology, University of Bristol, St. Michael's Hospital, Bristol, United Kingdom
Bleeding and Pain in Early Pregnancy

J. Ricardo Carhuapoma, MD
Assistant Professor, Department of Neurology, Neurosurgery and Anesthesiology and Critical Care Medicine, Johns Hopkins University School of Medicine; Faculty, Department of Neurology, Neurosurgery and Anesthesiology and Critical Care Medicine, The Johns Hopkins Hospital, Baltimore, Maryland
Neurologic Complications

Frank A. Chervenak, MD, MMM
Given Foundation Professor and Chairman, Weill Cornell Medical Center, New York, New York
Fetal Craniospinal and Facial Abnormalities

Lyn S. Chitty, BSc, PhD, MROCG
Professor of Genetics and Fetal Medicine, UCL Institute of Child Health; Consultant in Genetics and Fetal Medicine, University College London Hospitals NHS Foundation Trust, London, United Kingdom
Fetal Skeletal Abnormalities

Joshua A. Copel, MD
Professor, Obstetrics, Gynecology and Reproductive Sciences and Pediatrics, Yale University School of Medicine, New Haven, Connecticut
Fetal Cardiac Arrhythmias: Diagnosis and Therapy

Caroline A. Crowther, MD, FRANZCOG, FRCOG, Cert MFM
Professor, Discipline of Obstetrics and Gynaecology, The University of Adelaide, Women's and Children's Hospital, North Adelaide, South Australia, Australia
Multiple Pregnancy

Peter Danielian, MA, MD, FRCOG
Honorary Senior Lecturer, Department of Obstetrics and Gynaecology, Aberdeen University Medical School; Consultant Obstetrician, Aberdeen Maternity Hospital, NHS Grampian, Aberdeen, United Kingdom
Fetal Distress in Labor

John Maelor Davies, MA, MD, FRCP, FRCPath
Consultant Haematologist, Western General Hospital, Edinburgh, United Kingdom
Malignancies of the Hematologic and Immunologic Systems

John M. Davison, BSc, MD, MSc, FRCOG
Professor, Newcastle University, Newcastle upon Tyne, United Kingdom
Pregnancy after Transplantation

Gustaaf Dekker, MD, PhD, DCOG, FRANZCOG
Professor, Obstetrics and Gynaecology, The University of Adelaide; Director, Women's and Children's Division, Lyell McEwin Hospital, Adelaide, South Australia, Australia
Hypertension

Isaac Delke, MD
Professor, Department of Obstetrics and Gynecology, University of Florida College of Medicine; Chief, Division of Maternal-Fetal Medicine, and Medical Director, Obstetric Services, Shands Jacksonville Medical Center, Jacksonville, Florida
Induction of Labor and Termination of the Previable Pregnancy

Jeff M. Denney, MD
Clinical Instructor, Division of Maternal-Fetal Medicine, Department of Obstetrics and Gynecology, University of Wisconsin, Madison, Wisconsin; Physician/Research Consultant, Division of Adolescent Medicine, Department of Pediatrics, Children's Hospital of Philadelphia, Philadelphia, Pennsylvania
Autoimmune Diseases

Jan Deprest, MD, PhD
University Hospitals Leuven, Leuven, Belgium
Fetal Problems in Multiple Pregnancy

Jan E. Dickinson, MD, FRANZCOG, DDU, CMFM
Professor, Maternal Fetal Medicine, School of Women's and Infants' Health, The University of Western Australia, Perth; Maternal Fetal Medicine Specialist, King Edward Memorial Hospital, Subiaco, Western Australia, Australia
Cesarean Section

Gary A. Dildy III, MD
Clinical Professor, Department of Obstetrics and Gynecology, Louisiana State University School of Medicine, New Orleans, Louisiana; Director of Maternal-Fetal Medicine, Hospital Corporation of America, Mountain Star Division, Nashville, Tennessee
Postpartum Hemorrhage and Other Problems of the Third Stage

Jodie M. Dodd, MBBS, FRANZCOG, Cert MFM
Professor, Discipline of Obstetrics and Gynaecology, The University of Adelaide, Women's and Children's Hospital, North Adelaide, South Australia, Australia
Multiple Pregnancy; Threatened and Actual Preterm Labor Including Mode of Delivery; Prelabor Rupture of the Membranes

Marc Dommergues, MD
Professor, Groupe Hospitalier Pitié Salpêtrière; Université Pierre et Marie Curie, Paris, France
Fetal Genitourinary Abnormalities

Tim Draycott, MD, MRCOG
Senior Clinical Lecturer in Obstetrics, University of Bristol; Consultant Obstetrician, Southmead Hospital, Bristol, United Kingdom
Training for Obstetric Emergencies

Joseph M. Ernest, MD
Clinical Professor, Department of Obstetrics and Gynecology, University of North Carolina, Chapel Hill; Chair, Department of Obstetrics and Gynecology, Carolinas Medical Center, Charlotte, North Carolina
Parasitic Infections

Peter A. Farndon, MSc, MB BS, MD, FRCP, DCH
Professor of Clinical Genetics, University of Birmingham; Consultant Clinical Geneticist, West Midlands Regional Genetics Service, Birmingham, United Kingdom
Genetics, Risks of Recurrence, and Genetic Counseling

Roy G. Farquharson, MD, FRCOG
Consultant Gynaecologist, Liverpool Women's Hospital NHS Foundation Trust, Liverpool, United Kingdom
Recurrent Miscarriage; Thromboembolic Disease

Tom Farrell, MBChB, MD, FRCOG
Consultant Obstetrician and Gynaecologist, Jessop Wing, Royal Hallamshire Hospital, Sheffield, United Kingdom
Diabetes

Albert Franco, MD
Assistant Clinical Professor, Department of Obstetrics and Gynecology, University of North Carolina, Chapel Hill; Assistant Director, Division of Maternal Fetal Medicine, Carolinas Medical Center, Charlotte, North Carolina
Parasitic Infections

Robert Fraser, MBChB, MD (Sheffield), FRCOG, DCH
Reader in Obstetrics and Gynaecology, University of Sheffield; Honorary Consultant in Obstetrics and Gynaecology, Jessop Wing, Royal Hallamshire Hospital, Sheffield, United Kingdom
Diabetes

Harry Gee, MD, FRCOG
Consultant Obstetrician, and Retired Head of West Midlands Postgraduate School of Obstetrics and Gynaecology, Birmingham Women's Hospital, Birmingham, West Midlands, United Kingdom
Dysfunctional Labor

Robert B. Gherman, MD
Head, Division of Maternal/Fetal, Prince George's Hospital Center, Cheverly, Maryland
Shoulder Dystocia

Paul S. Gibson, MD
Associate Professor, University of Calgary, Calgary, Alberta, Canada
Respiratory Disease

Joanna Girling, MA, MRCP, FRCOG
Consultant Obstretrician and Gynaecologist, West Middlesex University Hospital, Isleworth, Surrey, United Kingdom
Hepatic and Gastrointestinal Disease

Francesca Gotsch, MD
Research Fellow, Perinatology Research Branch, NICHD, NIH, DHHS, Bethesda, Maryland, and Detroit, Michigan
Intrauterine Infection, Preterm Parturition, and the Fetal Inflammatory Response Syndrome

Michael Greaves, MBChB, MD, FRCP, FRCPath
Professor of Haematology, and Head of School of Medicine and Dentistry, University of Aberdeen, Aberdeen, United Kingdom
Thromboembolic Disease

David R. Griffin, MD, FRCOG
Consultant Obstetrician and Gynaecologist, West Herts Hospital HMS Trust, Waterford, Hertferdshire, United Kingdom
Fetal Skeletal Abnormalities

Rosalie M. Grivell, BSc, BMBS, FRANZCOG
Senior Lecturer, Discipline of Obstetrics and Gynaecology, The University of Adelaide, Women's and Children's Hospital, North Adelaide, South Australia, Australia
Multiple Pregnancy

A. Metin Gülmezoglu, MD, PhD
Coordinating Editor of the World Health Organization Reproductive Health Library, Department of Reproductive Health and Research, World Health Organization, Geneva, Switzerland
Global Maternal and Perinatal Health Issues

Christina S. Han, MD
Clinical Instructor, Department of Obstetrics, Gynecology and Reproductive Sciences, Yale University School of Medicine; Clinical Instructor, Yale-New Haven Hospital, New Haven, Connecticut
Clotting Disorders

Roger F. Haskett, MD
Professor of Psychiatry, University of Pittsburgh School of Medicine; Psychiatrist, Western Psychiatric Institute and Clinic of UPMC Presbyterian, Pittsburgh, Pennsylvania
Psychiatric Illness

Robert Hayashi, MD
J. Robert Wilson Professor Emeritus, University of Michigan, Ann Arbor, Michigan
Assisted Vaginal Delivery

Darren Travis Herzog, MD
Orthopaedic Surgery Resident, Detroit Medical Center, St. John's Providence Hospital, Detroit, Michigan
Spine and Joint Disorders

G. Justus Hofmeyr, MRCOG
Consultant, East London Hospital Complex, East London, Eastern Cape, South Africa
Global Maternal and Perinatal Health Issues

Elizabeth Helen Horn, MD, FRCP, FRCPath
Royal Infirmary of Edinburgh, Edinburgh, United Kingdom
Thrombocytopenia and Bleeding Disorders

Jonathon Hyett, MBBS, MSc, MD, MRCOG, FRANZCOG
Clinical Professor, Faculty of Obstetrics and Gynaecology, Central Clinical School, University of Sydney; Clinical Professor, RPA Women and Babies, Royal Prince Alfred Hospital, Sydney, New South Wales, Australia
Screening for Spontaneous Preterm Labor and Delivery

Robin B. Kalish, MD
Associate Professor, Weill Cornell Medical College; Attending Physician, New York Presbyterian Hospital, New York, New York
Fetal Craniospinal and Facial Abnormalities

Humphrey H. H. Kanhai, MD, PhD
Leiden University Medical Center, Leiden, The Netherlands
Fetal Thrombocytopenia

Lucy H. Kean, BM, BCh, DM, FRCOG
Consultant in Fetal and Maternal Medicine, Nottingham University Hospitals NHS Trust, Nottingham, United Kingdom
Malignancies of the Hematologic and Immunologic Systems; Thrombocytopenia and Bleeding Disorders

Rohna Kearney, MD, MRCOG, MRCPI
Consultant Gynaecologist, Subspecialist in Urogynaecology, Addenbrooke's Hospital, Cambridge University Hospitals Trust, Cambridge, United Kingdom
Perineal Repair and Pelvic Floor Injury

Anna P. Kenyon, MBChB, MD, MRCOG
Clinical Training Fellow, Elizabeth Garrett Anderson Institute for Women's Health, University College London, London, United Kingdom
Thyroid Disease

Mark D. Kilby, MD, FRCOG
Professor of Fetal Medicine, Head of Reproduction, Genes and Development/Deputy Head of School of Clinical and Experimental Medicine, College of Medical and Dental Sciences, University of Birmingham; Head of Fetal Medicine Centre, Birmingham Women's Foundation Trust, Edgbaston, Birmingham, United Kingdom
Genetics, Risks of Recurrence, and Genetic Counseling

Justin C. Konje, MD, FWACS, FMCOG (NIG), FRCOG
Professor of Obstetrics and Gynaecology, Reproductive Sciences Section, Department of Cancer Studies and Molecular Medicine, University of Leicester and University Hospitals of Leicester, Leicester, United Kingdom
Bleeding in Late Pregnancy

George Kroumpouzos, MD, PhD, FAAD
Clinical Assistant Professor of Dermatology, Brown Medical School, Providence, Rhode Island
Skin Disease

Juan Pedro Kusanovic, MD
Assistant Professor, Department of Obstetrics and Gynecology, Wayne State University, Detroit, Michigan; Perinatology Research Branch, NICHD, NIH, DHHS, Bethesda, Maryland, and Detroit, Michigan
Intrauterine Infection, Preterm Parturition, and the Fetal Inflammatory Response Syndrome

Mark B. Landon, MD
Professor and Interim Chair, College of Medicine, and Director, Division of Maternal Fetal Medicine, Department of Obstetrics and Gynecology, The Ohio State University, Columbus, Ohio
Pituitary and Adrenal Disease

Tze Kin Lau, MD
Professor, Department of Obstetrics and Gynaecology, Faculty of Medicine, The Chinese University of Hong Kong, Hong Kong, SAR
Prenatal Fetal Surveillance

Steven R. Levine, MD
Professor and Vice Chair, Neurology, and Associate Dean for Clinical Research and Faculty Development, The State University of New York Health Science Center - Brooklyn; Chief of Neurology, University Hospital of Brooklyn, Brooklyn, New York
Neurologic Complications

Liesbeth Lewi, MD, PhD
Professor, School of Medicine, Catholic University; Consultant, University Hospitals Leuven, Department of Obstetrics and Gynecology, Leuven, Belgium
Fetal Problems in Multiple Pregnancy

Stephen W. Lindow, MB, ChB, MMed (O&G), MD, FCOG (SA), FRCOG
Senior Lecturer in Perinatology, University of Hull, Hull, East Yorkshire, United Kingdom; Honorary Associate Professor of Obstetrics and Gynaecology, University of Cape Town, Cape Town, South Africa; Honorary Consultant in Obstetrics and Gynaecology, Women and Childrens' Hospital, Hull Royal Infirmary, Hull, East Yorkshire, United Kingdom
Assisted Vaginal Delivery; Major Obstetric Hemorrhage and Disseminated Intravascular Coagulation

Charles J. Lockwood, MD
Anita O'Keefe Young Professor and Chair, Department of Obstetrics, Gynecology and Reproductive Sciences, Yale University School of Medicine; Director of Obstetrics and Gynecology, Yale-New Haven Hospital, New Haven, Connecticut
Clotting Disorders

Pisake Lumbiganon, MD, MS
Professor, Khon Kaen University, Khon Kaen, Thailand
Global Maternal and Perinatal Health Issues

Ian Z. Mackenzie, MD, FRCOG, DSc
Reader in Obstetrics and Gynaecology, University of Oxford; Honorary Consultant Obstetrician and Gynaecologist, John Radcliffe Hospital, Oxford, United Kingdom
Unstable Lie, Malpresentations, and Malpositions

Kassam Mahomed, MD (Bristol), FRCOG (UK), FRANZCOG
Associate Professor, Department of Obstetrics and Gynaecology, University of Queensland; Senior Staff Specialist, Department of Obstetrics and Gynaecology, Ipswich Hospital, Ipswich, Queensland, Australia
Abdominal Pain; Nonmalignant Gynecology

Melissa S. Mancuso
Instructor/Fellow, Maternal-Fetal Medicine and Medical Genetics, University of Alabama at Birmingham School of Medicine, Birmingham, Alabama
Fetal Tumors

Neil Marlow, DM, FMedSci
Professor of Neonatal Medicine, UCL Elizabeth Garrett Anderson Institute for Women's Health, University College London; Honorary Consultant Neonatologist, University College London Hospitals NHS Foundation Trust, London, United Kingdom
Resuscitation and Immediate Care of the Newborn

Anthony J. Marren, BMed (Hons), MMed (R. H. & H. G.)
Registrar, Department of Obstetrics and Gynaecology, Royal Prince Alfred Hospital for Women and Babies, Sydney, New South Wales, Australia
Screening for Spontaneous Preterm Labor and Delivery

Alec McEwan, BA, BM, BCh, MRCOG
Consultant in Obstetrics and Fetal Medicine, Department of Obstetrics and Gynaecology, Nottingham University Hospitals NHS Trust, Nottingham, United Kingdom
Video Editor

Michael J. Moritz, MD
Professor of Surgery, Penn State College of Medicine, Hershey; Chief, Transplantation Services, Lehigh Valley Health Network, Allentown, Pennsylvania
Pregnancy after Transplantation

Adnan R. Munkarah, MD
Professor, Wayne State University School of Medicine; Chairman, Women's Health, Henry Ford Health System, Detroit, Michigan
Malignant Disease

Kimta Nanhornguè, MD
University of Padova; Medical Resident in Gynecology, Department of Gynecological Sciences and the Human Reproduction, University of Padua School of Medicine, Padova, Italy
First-Trimester Screening for Fetal Abnormalities

Osric B. Navti, MBBS, MRCOG
Consultant in Fetal and Maternal Medicine, University Hospitals of Leicester NHS Trust, Leicester, United Kingdom
Bleeding in Late Pregnancy

Catherine Nelson-Piercy, MA, FRCP, FRCOG
Consultant Obstetric Physician, Guy's and St. Thomas Foundation, Queen Charlotte's and Chelsea Hospital, Imperial College Healthcare Trust, London, United Kingdom
Thyroid Disease

Robert Ogle, FRANZCOG, FHGSA
Director, Royal Prince Alfred Hospital, Sydney, Australia
Screening for Spontaneous Preterm Labor and Delivery

Colm O'Herlihy, MD, FRCPI, FRCOG
Professor, University College Dublin; Consultant Obstetrician/Gynaecologist, National Maternity Hospital, Dublin, Ireland
Perineal Repair and Pelvic Floor Injury

Michael J. Paidas, MD
Associate Professor, Co-Director, Yale Women and Children's Center for Blood Disorders, and Co-Director, National Hemophilia Foundation - Baxter Clinical Fellowship at Yale, Yale University School of Medicine; Attending Physician, Yale-New Haven Hospital, New Haven, Connecticut
Clotting Disorders

Robert C. Pattinson, MD, FRCOG, FCOG (SA), MMed (O&G)
Professor, Obstetrics and Gynaecology, University of Pretoria, Pretoria, Gauteng, South Africa
Global Maternal and Perinatal Health Issues

Zoë Penn, MD, FRCOG
Consultant Obstetrician, Chelsea and Westminster Hospital, London, United Kingdom
Breech Presentation

Troy Flint Porter, MD, MPH
Director, Maternal-Fetal Medicine, Intermountain Healthcare; Associate Professor, University of Utah Health Sciences, Salt Lake City, Utah
Autoimmune Diseases

Raymond O. Powrie, MD
Senior Vice President, Quality and Clinical Effectiveness, Women & Infants Hospital of Rhode Island; Associate Professor of Medicine and Obstetrics and Gynecology, The Warren Alpert Medical School of Brown University, Providence, Rhode Island
Respiratory Disease

Susan M. Ramin, MD
Professor and Chair, Department of Obstetrics, Gynecology and Reproductive Sciences, University of Texas Health Science Center at Houston, Houston, Texas
Renal Disorders

Margaret Ramsay, MB, BChir, MA, MD, MRCP, FRCOG
Consultant in Fetomaternal Medicine, Nottingham University Hospitals, Queen's Medical Centre Campus, Nottingham, United Kingdom
Appendix: Normal Values

Lesley Regan, MD
Professor, Consultant Obstetrician and Gynaecologist, Imperial College London, St. Mary's Hospital, London, United Kingdom
Recurrent Miscarriage

John T. Repke, MD
University Professor and Chairman, Department of Obstetrics and Gynecology, Penn State University College of Medicine; Obstetrician-Gynecologist-in-Chief, The Milton S. Hershey Medical Center, Hershey, Pennsylvania
Puerperal Problems

Laura E. Riley, MD
Assistant Professor, Obstetrics and Gynecology and Reproductive Biology, Harvard Medical School, Cambridge; Medical Director of Labor and Delivery, Massachusetts General Hospital, Boston, Massachusetts
Rubella, Measles, Mumps, Varicella, and Parvovirus

Giuseppe Rizzo, MD
Professor, Università Roma Tor Vergata; Department of Obstetrics and Gynecology, Ospedale Fatebenefratelli Isola Tiberina, Rome, Italy
Fetal Cardiac Anomalies

Jeffrey S. Robinson, BSc (Hons), MB ChB, BAO (Hons), FRCOG, FRANZCOG
Emeritus Professor, Discipline of Obstetrics and Gynaecology, School of Paediatrics and Reproductive Medicine, Faculty of Health Sciences, The University of Adelaide, Adelaide, South Australia, Australia
Threatened and Actual Preterm Labor Including Mode of Delivery; Prelabor Rupture of the Membranes

Stephen C. Robson, MD, MRCOG, MBBS
Professor of Fetal Medicine, Institute of Cellular Medicine, University of Newcastle upon Tyne, Newcastle upon Tyne, United Kingdom
Fetal Thyroid and Adrenal Disease

Roberto Romero, MD
Department of Obstetrics and Gynecology and Center for Molecular Medicine and Genetics, Wayne State University, Detroit, Michigan; Chief, Perinatology Research Branch, and Program Director for Obstetrics and Perinatology, *Eunice Kennedy Shriver* National Institute of Child Health and Human Development, National Institutes of Health, Bethesda, Maryland, and Detroit, Michigan
Intrauterine Infection, Preterm Parturition, and the Fetal Inflammatory Response Syndrome

Thomas Roos, MD
Assistant Professor, University of Regensburg Medical School, Regensburg, Germany; Chief, Section of Obstetrics, Department of Obstetrics and Gynecology, Kantonsspital Schaffhausen, Schaffhausen, Switzerland
Cytomegalovirus, Herpes Simplex Virus, Adenovirus, Coxsackievirus, and Human Papillomavirus

Michael G. Ross, MD, MPH
Professor of Obstetrics and Gynecology, David Geffen School of Medicine at UCLA, Los Angeles; Professor of Public Health; UCLA School of Public Health; Los Angeles,Perinatologist, Harbor-UCLA Medical Center, Torrance, California
Abnormalities of Amniotic Fluid Volume

Rodrigo Ruano, MD
Research Fellow, Université Paris V; Consultant, Hôpital Necker Enfants Molades, Paris, France
Fetal Genitourinary Abnormalities

Jane M. Rutherford, MBChB, DM, MRCOG
Consultant in Fetomaternal Medicine, Nottingham University Hospitals, Nottingham, United Kingdom
Anemia and White Blood Cell Disorders

Luis Sanchez-Ramos, MD
Professor, Division of Maternal-Fetal Medicine, Department of Obstetrics and Gynecology, University of Florida College of Medicine, Jacksonville, Florida
Induction of Labor and Termination of the Previable Pregnancy

Veronica L. Schimp, DO
Associate Professor, M.D. Anderson Cancer Center Orlando, University of Central Florida College of Medicine, Orlando, Florida
Malignant Disease

Dimitrios Siassakos, MBBS, MRCOG, MSc, DLSHTM
Clinical Lecturer in Medical Education, University of Bristol; Research Fellow in Obstetrics, Southmead Hospital, Bristol, United Kingdom
Training for Obstetric Emergencies

Gordon C. S. Smith, MD, PhD
Professor and Head, Department of Obstetrics and Gynaecology, University of Cambridge; Honorary Consultant in Maternal Fetal Medicine, Addenbrooke's Hospital, Cambridge, United Kingdom
Delivery after Previous Cesarean Section

John S. Smoleniec, MD, FRCOG, FMS, FRANZCOG, CMFM, DDU
Associate Professor, University of New South Wales, Sydney; Director, Maternal Fetal Medicine, Liverpool Hospital, Sydney South West Area Health Service, New South Wales, Australia
Fetal Hydrops

Peter W. Soothill, BSc, MD, MBBS, FRCOG
Emeritus Professor of Maternal and Fetal Medicine, Medical School, University of Bristol; Consultant in Fetal Medicine, Fetal Medicine Unit, St. Michael's Hospital, University Hospitals Bristol NHS Foundation Trust, Bristol, United Kingdom
Invasive Procedures for Antenatal Diagnosis

Philip J. Steer, BSc, MD, FRCOG, FCOGSA (hon)
Emeritus Professor, Faculty of Medicine, Imperial College London, Chelsea and Westminster Hospital, London, United Kingdom
Prolonged Pregnancy; Fetal Distress in Labor

Peter Stone, BSc, MBChB, MD (Bristol), FRCOG, FRANZCOG, DDU, CMFM
Professor of Maternal Fetal Medicine, Department of Obstetrics and Gynecology, University of Auckland; Professor of Maternal Fetal Medicine, National Women's Hospital, Auckland Hospital, Auckland, New Zealand
Fetal Gastrointestinal Abnormalities

Jane Strong, MBChB, MRCP, FRCPath
Consultant Pathologist (Haematology), Leicester Royal Infirmary, Leicester, United Kingdom
Anemia and White Blood Cell Disorders

John M. Svigos, MB BS, DRCOG, FRCOG, FRANZCOG
Associate Professor, Discipline of Obstetrics and Gynaecology, School of Paediatrics and Reproductive Medicine, Faculty of Health Sciences, The University of Adelaide, Adelaide; Senior Visiting Medical Specialist, Maternal Fetal Medicine Unit, Women's and Children's Hospital, North Adelaide, South Australia, Australia
Threatened and Actual Preterm Labor Including Mode of Delivery; Prelabor Rupture of the Membranes

Rebecca Swingler, MSc, MRCOG
Academic Clinical Lecturer, University of Bristol, St. Michael's Hospital; Senior Registrar in Obstetrics and Gynaecology, St. Michael's Hospital, Bristol, United Kingdom
Bleeding and Pain in Early Pregnancy

Mark W. Tomlinson, MD
Regional Director of Obstetrics, Providence Health System, Providence St. Vincent's Hospital, Portland, Oregon
Cardiac Disease; Neurologic Complications

Lawrence C. Tsen, MD
Associate Professor in Anaesthesia, Harvard Medical School; Co-Editor in Chief, International Journal of Obstetric Anesthesia; Director of Anesthesia, Center for Reproductive Medicine, Brigham and Women's Hospital, Boston, Massachusetts
Neuraxial Analgesia and Anesthesia in Obstetrics

Frank P. H. A. Vandenbussche, MD, PhD
Professor of Obstetrics and Fetal Medicine, Radboud University Medical Center, Nijmegen, The Netherlands
Fetal Thrombocytopenia

Alex C. Vidaeff, MD, MPH
Professor of Obstetrics and Gynecology, Department of Obstetrics, Gynecology and Reproductive Sciences, Maternal-Fetal Medicine Division, University of Texas Health Science Center at Houston, Houston, Texas
Renal Disorders

Yves Ville, MD
Professor, Descartes University, GHU Necker-Enfants-Malades, Paris, France
First-Trimester Screening for Fetal Abnormalities

Anthony M. Vintzileos, MD
Professor of Obstetrics, Gynecology and Reproductive Medicine, Stony Brook University School of Medicine, Stony Brook; Chairman, Department of Obstetrics and Gynecology, Winthrop-University Hospital, Mineola, New York
Second-Trimester Screening for Fetal Abnormalities

Ann M. Walker, MBChB
Prescribing Doctor for Pregnancy and Parenting Team, Leeds Partnership NHS Foundation Trust, Leeds, West Yorkshire, United Kingdom
Substance Abuse

James J. Walker, MBChB, MD, FRCP (Edin), FRCPS (Glas), FRCOG
Professor of Obstetrics and Gynaecology, University of Leeds; Consultant, Obstetrics and Gynaecology, St. James University Hospital; Chairman of Perinatal Research Group, Leeds Institute of Molecular Medicine, Leeds, West Yorkshire, United Kingdom
Substance Abuse

Peter G. Wardle, MD, FRCS, FRCOG
Honorary Senior Lecturer, University of Bristol; Consultant Gynaecologist and Subspecialist in Reproductive Medicine, and Lead Consultant for Fertility Services, North Bristol NHS Trust, Southmead Hospital, Bristol, United Kingdom
Bleeding and Pain in Early Pregnancy

Stephen P. Wardle, MB, ChB, FRCPCH, MD
Consultant Neonatologist, Nottingham University Hospitals, Nottingham, United Kingdom
Resuscitation and Immediate Care of the Newborn

D. Heather Watts, MD
Medical Officer, Pediatric, Adolescent, and Maternal AIDS Branch, Center for Research on Mothers and Children, Eunice Kennedy Shriver National Institute of Child Health and Human Development, Bethesda, Maryland
Human Immunodeficiency Virus

Bevin Weeks, MD
Assistant Professor of Pediatrics, Yale University School of Medicine; Director for Pediatrics, Yale Fetal Cardiovascular Center, New Haven, Connecticut
Fetal Cardiac Arrhythmias: Diagnosis and Therapy

Carl P. Weiner, MD, MBA, FACOG
K.E. Krantz Professor and Chair, Department of Obstetrics and Gynecology, University of Kansas School of Medicine, Kansas City, Kansas
Fetal Hemolytic Disease; Fetal Death; Medication

Hajo I. J. Wildschut, MD
Consultant in Obstetrics and Gynecology, Erasmus University Medical Center, Rotterdam, The Netherlands
Constitutional and Environmental Factors Leading to a High Risk Pregnancy

Catherine Williamson, MD, FRCP
Professor, Imperial College London, London, United Kingdom
Hepatic and Gastrointestinal Disease

Lami Yeo, MD
Associate Professor, Department of Obstetrics and Gynecology, Wayne State University School of Medicine, Detroit, Michigan; Director of Fetal and Maternal Imaging, Perinatology Research Branch, NICHD, NIH, DHHS, Bethesda, Maryland, and Detroit, Michigan
Second-Trimester Screening for Fetal Abnormalities

Mark H. Yudin, MD, MSc, FRCSC
Assistant Professor, University of Toronto; Attending Physician, Department of Obstetrics and Gynecology, St. Michael's Hospital, Toronto, Ontario, Canada
Other Infectious Conditions

EVIDENCE BASED SUMMARY OF MANAGEMENT OPTIONS BOXES

One of the most popular features of the first thee editions of *High Risk Pregnancy—Management Options* were the 'Summary of Management Options' (SOMO) Boxes. The SOMO Box was placed at the end of each chapter or section within a chapter and presented the reader with an *aide memoire* of the main points regarding the management options for a specific condition discussed in detail in the preceding chapter. For the third edition, we included an evidence based approach in the SOMO Boxes.

We continued this approach for the fourth edition. The following is the evidence based scoring system for the SOMO Boxes that we asked contributors to use.

SCORING SYSTEM FOR SUMMARY OF MANAGEMENT OPTIONS BOXES

Quality (level) of Evidence

Ia	Evidence obtained from meta-analysis of randomized controlled trials
Ib	Evidence obtained from at least one randomized controlled trial
IIa	Evidence obtained from at least one well-designed controlled study without randomization
IIb	Evidence obtained from at least one other type of well-designed quasi-experimental study
III	Evidence obtained from well-designed non-experimental descriptive studies, such as comparative studies, correlation studies and case studies
IV	Evidence obtained from expert committee reports or opinions and/or clinical experience of respected authorities

Strength (grade) of Recommendation

A	At least one randomized controlled trial as part of a body of literature of overall good quality and consistency addressing the specific recommendation (Evidence Levels Ia or Ib)
B	Well-controlled clinical studies available but no randomized clinical trials on the topic of the recommendations (Evidence Levels IIa, IIb or III)
C	Evidence obtained from expert committee reports or opinions and/or clinical experiences of respected authorities. Indicates an absence of directly applicable clinical studies of good quality (Evidence Level IV)
GPP	Good Practice Point: recommended best practice based on the clinical experience of the chapter authors and editors

PREFACE TO THE FOURTH EDITION

The fourth edition of *High Risk Pregnancy: Management Options* brings growth and change while remaining true to the original vision of an evidence-based user friendly text. Good clinical practice should be a universal goal, and we have sought to produce a truly International Postgraduate Textbook. There are over 150 contributors who reflect expertise from around the world with 20 countries represented. The third edition was sold in over 80 countries in four different versions—English, Chinese, Turkish and an English language adaptation for the Indian market. It is now a standard text used in the qualifying examinations of many countries. The book continues to grow in popularity with the third edition being the best-seller yet.

As the complexity of medicine continues to increase, so has the burden on the editors to review and process the material so it remains relevant to the reader. To that end, we are delighted that Caroline Crowther, an international leader in clinical design, performance and analysis of clinical trials, and Stephen Robson, a world recognized perinatologist have joined the original editorial team. In addition, we are most grateful to our contributors for their enormous efforts (and often those of their secretaries). We are especially indebted to Dee Simpson from Elsevier who has kept the project on course.

Each chapter in the fourth edition has been revised and where indicated, new ones added to reflect new developments. As reassuring as the traditional textbook is to hold, the fourth edition is published with a greatly expanded electronic version providing easy access to references and expanded figures. In addition, the website not only includes these electronic features, but also has video clips (edited by Alec McEwan), each making learning dynamic. Other changes to the fourth edition include:

- A major overhaul and revision of the book's appearance to further enhance readability including the transfer of the full reference list for each chapter to the accompanying complementary electronic publication so that only 10 key references ('Suggested Reading') are retained in the printed text.
- A clearer presentation of the text while keeping to the original layout style of
  - "Introduction"
  - "Risks (Maternal and Fetal)"
  - "Management Options (Prepregnancy, Prenatal, Labor and Delivery, Postnatal)"
  - "Summary of Management Options" Box
- The Summary of Management Options Box includes a simplified evidence-based scoring system for each management strategy proposed. It illustrates how strong the evidence is for each option.
- All chapters were written or updated to reflect the current management options and to incorporate changes in practice since the last edition. Twelve chapters are either new or rewritten by new authors to bring a fresh view [1, 2, 6, 10, 12, 35, 44, 49, 65, 67, 75, 77].
- One feature that deserves special mention in the Preface is Margaret Ramsay's popular and valuable Appendix on 'Normal Values'. This section has had its own separate publication (both written and electronic) in the past and these publications will be updated in the future.

As in prior editions, we have appreciated the comments of readers and reviewers and sought to respond to them wherever possible in this edition.

Previous editions of *High Risk Pregnancy: Management Options* were popular because readers have found them relevant to their daily clinical practice; in other words the book is a manual for the management of problem pregnancies. We hope that the fourth edition will uphold and enhance that reputation and will prove even more valuable to busy clinicians.

David James
Philip J. Steer
Carl P. Weiner
Bernard Gonik
Caroline A. Crowther
Stephen C. Robson

PREFACE TO THE FIRST EDITION

This new international textbook in obstetrics will, we believe, be of major value to all practicing clinicians, be they trainees or established in practice.

It aims to assist with the questions: How do I manage this patient? or How do I perform this procedure?

It presents a wide range of reputable management options. Unlike many traditional texts, based on a single individual's experience and view, all the contributors to each section were asked to give their preferred management in all areas of their section. Each resulting chapter reflects that wide range of acceptable practice. This means you will have a *choice* about which option or combination of options suits you and your patient.

This book is designated to be practical. It addresses those difficult questions which arise in practice, which often stem not only from the medical facts, but from the constraints of time, facilities, finance, and patient acceptability. Moreover, we have standardized the presentation of each topic as far as possible (while still allowing the personality of the original authors to shine through!) to enable the reader to become familiar with the format.

We have deliberately chosen a panel of contributors who are both leaders in their field and who can represent practice in the USA, Europe, and Australasia and this we feel gives the text a unique universality.

Finally it is our intention that the book is comprehensive. We hope that we will have something to say on all the important problems you come across. If you find any exceptions, please let us know, with your comments, in time for the next edition.

CONTENTS

VIDEO CONTENTS

VIDEO EDITOR: Alec McEwan

CHAPTER 1

Global Maternal and Perinatal Health Issues*

A. METIN GÜLMEZOGLU, ROBERT C. PATTINSON, G. JUSTUS HOFMEYR, and PISAKE LUMBIGANON

INTRODUCTION

In 2000, 189 member states of the United Nations signed up to the Millennium Development Declaration committing themselves to ambitious health and development goals to be achieved by 2015. Agreement on these important goals within the Declaration was later translated into a structured framework of Millennium Development Goals (MDGs) with measurable targets and indicators. This MDG framework is the most significant global public health event since the 1990s. It has encouraged many donors to prioritize their funding on specific areas linked to the MDGs. Three of the eight MDGs (4, 5, and 6) relate directly to maternal and perinatal health (Table 1–1).

The MDG process has had several positive effects so far. By highlighting the areas of largest disease burden, the MDGs have not only improved resource flows to low- and middle-income countries toward effective practices such as antiretroviral treatments in sub-Saharan Africa but also led to better ascertainment of the causes of morbidity and mortality and improved evaluation of interventions likely to have an impact on health outcomes.

Since 2000, there has been an increase in the number of analytical studies of the global burden of sexual and reproductive ill health, including the monitoring and evaluation of care, and these have improved our understanding of the barriers to improvement. For example, in 2003, a group of scientists initiated the "Countdown to 2015 Initiative," tracking coverage levels for health interventions that have been shown to reduce maternal, newborn, and child mortality (http://www.countdown2015mnch.org/). In 2008, this group reported the coverage, equity, financing, and policy progress on those interventions.[1] These analyses represent important advances on our ability to measure and report key global maternal and perinatal health markers.

THE MEASUREMENT CHALLENGES

In the past, data on maternal and perinatal mortality and morbidity have been lacking in many parts of the world.[2] However, since 2000, the number of studies on maternal and perinatal mortality and morbidity has increased significantly, in terms both of primary studies such as Demographic and Health Surveys (DHS) collecting representative data at the national level and the number of systematic reviews synthesizing such data to assess current status and monitor trends.

Confidential inquiries into maternal deaths are accepted as the relevant gold standard audit tool. In the United Kingdom, implementation of the confidential inquiry methodology and the consequent uptake of the recommendations from it are thought to have been a driver of the reduction in maternal deaths in this country over the past 50 years.[3] More recently, India, Jamaica, Sri Lanka, South Africa, and Tunisia have all successfully implemented either confidential inquiries into maternal deaths or specific surveillance systems to capture the number and causes of maternal deaths.[4–8] The 2005 Maternal Mortality estimates developed by the World Health Organization (WHO), United Nations Children's Fund (UNICEF), United Nations Population Fund (UNFPA), and the World Bank represent a methodologic advance in an area that has often been controversial. Maternal mortality estimates for countries are sometimes contentious because of adjustments for underreporting, and modeling estimates for countries that do not have data from methodologically sound studies. However, the results of such studies are a big improvement on having no data at all, and more recent estimates have used improved methodology, including an analysis of trends. A systematic review of the global causes of maternal death was published in 2006, presenting for the first time a synthesis of population-based representative data on studies reporting the major causes of maternal death,[9] and our current picture is much more robust compared to the 1990s.

MATERNAL MORTALITY AND SEVERE MORBIDITY

About 99% of all maternal deaths occur in developing countries, and current estimates suggest that 536,000 women die every year during pregnancy or within the 42 days following completion of the pregnancy. Deaths in sub-Saharan Africa and southern Asia accounted for 86% of global maternal deaths. The trend analysis indicates a global reduction of less than 1% annually, which is way behind the 5.5% required to reach MDG 5.[10]

The majority of maternal deaths in Africa and Asia are due to obstetric hemorrhage (Fig. 1–1).[9] In Latin America and the Caribbean, hypertensive disorders are responsible for the largest proportion of direct obstetric deaths (26%). Unsafe abortion is an important cause of maternal death and probably one of the most preventable.

In developed countries, the most common causes of death are direct causes such as thromboembolism and indirect causes such as cardiac disease. Maternal deaths in these countries are now rare, and the events that lead to death are often multifactorial, but this does not mean that pregnancy is entirely safe. Waterstone and coworkers[11] reported that in the 1990s in the South East Thames region of the United Kingdom, there was a severe obstetric morbidity rate of 12.0 per 1000 births, and a "severe morbidity to mortality" ratio of 118 : 1. Say and colleagues[12] conducted a systematic review of reports of severe acute morbidity worldwide up to 2004, using organ system–based criteria and unselected groups of women, and concluded that its incidence varied between 0.3% and 1.08%. Recently, the concept of maternal morbidity as a continuum ranging between healthy pregnancy and death has attracted much interest (Fig. 1–2). "Maternal severe morbidity" and "near-miss" are terms often used to identify women who experience a severe event during pregnancy, labor, or the postpartum period. Although there are currently no internationally agreed criteria, maternal near-miss can usefully be defined as "a woman who nearly died from a complication but survived." The WHO Working Group on Maternal Mortality and Morbidity Classifications has recently proposed clinical, laboratory, and management criteria based on earlier studies and audit data from Brazil, Canada, and South Africa (Table 1–2).[13]

Maternal near-miss estimates can be regarded as a valid proxy for maternal death and have practical value. In an individual facility, the number of maternal deaths will usually be too few to be useful for monitoring progress and highlighting areas that require action. Maternal near-misses occur more frequently than mortality and allow identification of inadequate care in a way similar to confidential inquiries into maternal death. The criteria proposed by the WHO Working Group have been developed taking into consideration the lack of resources in low- and middle-income countries. The criteria have been validated in Latin American countries but still require validation in other parts of the world.[14]

It is widely acknowledged that poor and socially disadvantaged sections of our communities share the highest burden of ill health. The equity analysis conducted by the Countdown 2008 Equity Analysis Group[15] found that the poorer quintiles of the communities are less likely to receive effective, guideline-recommended interventions. As expected, the equity gap has large variations within and between countries. Maternal and newborn health interventions represented an area of greater than average inequity, with a mean difference of 27.5% between the wealthiest and the poorest quintiles.

TABLE 1–1

United Nations Millennium Development Goals

Goal 1: Eradicate extreme poverty and hunger
Goal 2: Achieve universal primary education
Goal 3: Promote gender equality and empower women
Goal 4: Reduce child mortality
Goal 5: Improve maternal health
Goal 6: Combat HIV/AIDS, malaria and other diseases
Goal 7: Ensure environmental sustainability
Goal 8: Develop a Global Partnership for Development

PERINATAL MORTALITY

The MDGs identified a reduction in the mortality of children younger than 5 years of age as a priority (MDG 4), and within that group, reducing early neonatal deaths (~40% of the total) is a priority. It is estimated that around 4 million newborn babies die every year.[16] In addition, stillbirths occur in about 1% to 3% of all births, amounting to more than 3 million perinatal deaths annually at a global level.[17,18]

Measuring and classifying perinatal deaths is not easy. Several classification systems exist, suggesting that no classification system is optimal.[19–22] Kramer and associates[23] suggest that antepartum, intrapartum, and early neonatal deaths should be reported separately.

Global modeling estimates based on data from 45 countries suggest that preterm birth (28%), severe infections (36%, including pneumonia [26%], tetanus [7%], and diarrhea [3%]), and complications of asphyxia (23%) account

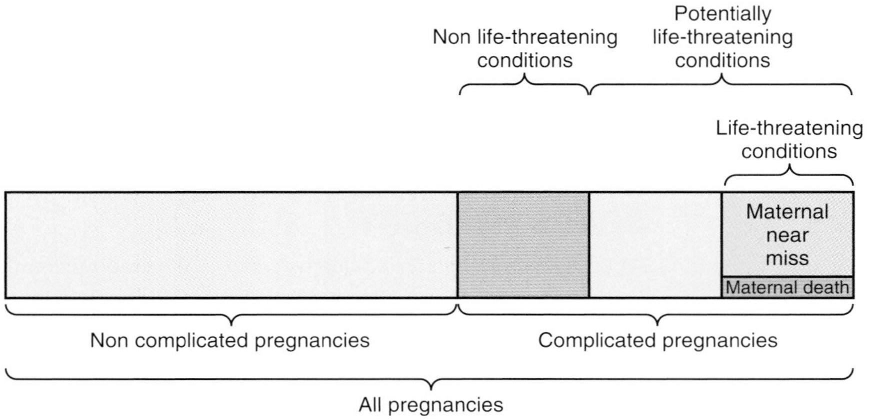

FIGURE 1–1
Pregnancy morbidities as a continuum.

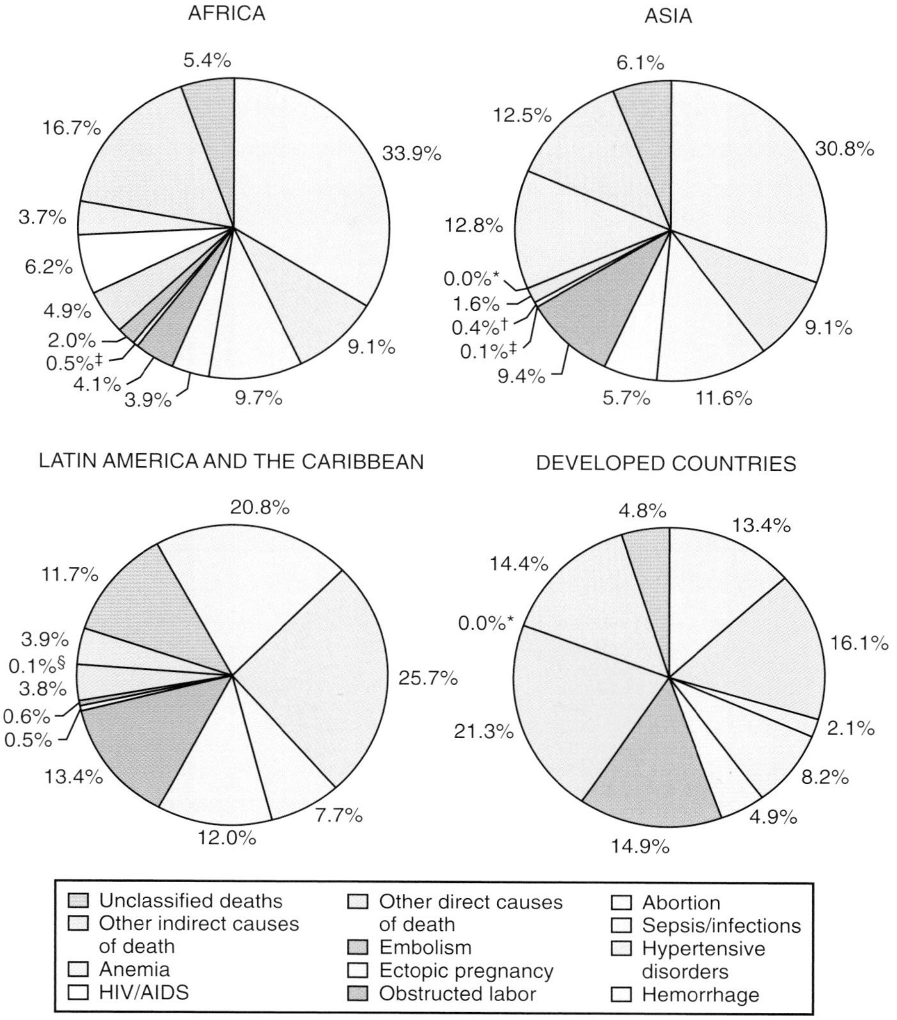

FIGURE 1–2
Regional distribution of causes of maternal death.

for most neonatal deaths.[24] In sub-Saharan Africa, 1.16 million babies die in the neonatal period, and another million babies are stillborn every year. In South Africa, in-depth analyses of perinatal deaths have been conducted since 1999 through the "Perinatal Problem Identification Programme" (PPIP) (http://www.ppip.co.za/savbab.htm). Each year about 22,000 babies die in South Africa. The Sixth Perinatal Care Survey of South Africa is a comprehensive report on causes of perinatal deaths, avoidable factors, and recommendations.[25] Unexplained stillbirths and preterm-related deaths constitute the largest groups (Table 1–3). The top three causes of perinatal deaths in all birth weight categories were unexplained stillbirth, spontaneous preterm labor, and intrapartum asphyxia and birth trauma.

Perinatal death rates in industrialized countries are generally much lower than in developing countries, and preterm births and congenital abnormalities tend to play a more prominent role.[26] In 2006, in England, Wales, and Northern Ireland, the stillbirth rate was 5.3 (95% confidence interval [CI] 5.1, 5.5] per 1000 total births, the neonatal mortality rate was 3.4 (CI 3.3, 3.6) per 1000 live births, and the perinatal mortality rate was 7.9 (CI 7.7, 8.1) per 1000 total births. However, in the United Kingdom, the perinatal mortality rate is rising in the growing numbers of births to immigrant mothers, and immigration is increasing rapidly in many developed countries because of the need to rebalance the age pyramid (the indigenous population is aging owing to low birth rates).

STRATEGIES TO IMPROVE MATERNAL AND PERINATAL HEALTH

Public Health and Political Context

A comprehensive evaluation of global, regional, and national strategies to reduce maternal and perinatal mortality and morbidity is beyond the scope of this book. Broad population-level strategies have been summarized by the World Bank (Table 1–4).[27]

TABLE 1–2

The WHO Near-Miss Criteria

A woman presenting any of the following life-threatening conditions and surviving a complication during pregnancy, childbirth, or within 42 days of termination of pregnancy should be considered a near-miss case.

DYSFUNCTIONAL SYSTEM	CLINICAL CRITERIA	LABORATORY MARKERS	MANAGEMENT-BASED PROXIES
Cardiovascular	Shock[a] Cardiac arrest[b]	pH <7.1 Lactate >5 mEq/mL	Use of continuous vasoactive drugs[i] Cardiopulmonary resuscitation
Respiratory	Acute cyanosis Gasping[c] Respiratory rate >40 or <6 bpm	Oxygen saturation <90% for ≥60 min Pao_2/Fio_2 <200 mm Hg	Intubation and ventilation not related to anesthesia
Renal	Oliguria nonresponsive to fluids or diuretics[d]	Creatinine 300 μmol/L or ≥3.5 mg/dL	Dialysis for acute renal failure
Hematologic/coagulation	Failure to form clots[e]	Acute severe thrombocytopenia (<50,000 platelets/mL)	Transfusion of ≥5 units of blood/red cells
Hepatic	Jaundice in the presence of preeclampsia[f]	Bilirubin >100 μmol/L or >6.0 mg/dL	
Neurologic	Any loss of consciousness[g] lasting >12 hr Stroke[h] Uncontrollable fit/status epilepticus Total paralysis		
Alternative severity proxy			Hysterectomy following infection or hemorrhage

[a] Shock is a persistent severe hypotension, defined as a systolic blood pressure < 90 mm Hg for ≥ 60 min with a pulse rate at least 120 despite aggressive fluid replacement (>2 L).
[b] Cardiac arrest refers to the loss of consciousness AND absence of pulse/heartbeat.
[c] Gasping is a terminal respiratory pattern and the breath is convulsively and audibly caught.
[d] Oliguria is defined as an urinary output <30 mL/hr for 4 hr or <400 mL/24 hr.
[e] Clotting failure can be assessed by the bedside clotting test or absence of clotting from the intravenous site after 7–10 min.
[f] Preeclampsia is defined as the presence of hypertension associated with proteinuria. Hypertension is defined as a blood pressure of at least 140 mm Hg (systolic) or at least 90 mm Hg (diastolic) on at least two occasions and at least 4–6 hr apart after the 20th week of gestation in women known to be normotensive beforehand. Proteinuria is defined as excretion of 300 mg or more of protein every 24 hr. If 24-hr urine samples are not available, proteinuria is defined as a protein concentration of 300 mg/L or more (≥1 + on dipstick) in at least two random urine samples taken at least 4–6 hr apart.
[g] Loss of consciousness is a profound alteration of mental state that involves complete or near-complete lack of responsiveness to external stimuli. It is defined as a Coma Glasgow Scale <10 (moderate or severe coma).
[h] Stroke is a neurologic deficit of cerebrovascular cause that persists beyond 24 hr or is interrupted by death within 24 hr.
[i] For instance, continuous use of any dose of dopamine, epinephrine, or norepinephrine.
Fio_2, fractional concentration of oxygen in inspired gas; Pao_2, arterial oxygen pressure.
Adapted from Say L, Souza JP, Pattinson RC: Maternal near miss—Towards a standard tool for monitoring quality of maternal health care. Best Pract Res Clin Obstet Gynaecol 2009;23:287–296.

TABLE 1–3

Most Common Causes of Perinatal Death Greater than 500 g in South Africa

CAUSE	%	PERINATAL MORTALITY/ 1000 BIRTHS
Unexplained stillbirths	24	9.2
Spontaneous preterm birth	22	8.3
Intrapartum asphyxia and trauma	16	6.2
Hypertensive disorders	12	4.7
Antepartum hemorrhage	10	3.8
Infections	5	2.0*
Fetal abnormality	4	1.4
Intrauterine growth restriction	2	0.74

* Underestimate, because late neonatal deaths not captured in the Perinatal Problem Identification Programme (PPIP) dataset.
Saving Babies 2006–2007: Sixth Perinatal Care Survey of South Africa. Pretoria, South Africa, Tshepesa, 2009.

Maternal mortality reduction should be taken as a national priority and actions planned accordingly. There is a need to act on various levels at the same time. The confidential inquiry system is useful to concentrate efforts on avoidable causes of deaths and assess new interventions. Such strategies are inevitably context-specific.

TABLE 1–4

Strategies to Reduce Maternal Mortality

1. Strengthening outreach services and community-based approaches
2. Improving education for girls and women
3. Targeting public sector subsidies to poor families and disadvantaged areas
4. Developing effective “poor-friendly” referral systems
5. Improving quality and availability of essential and emergency obstetric care services (EOC) for the poor
6. Promoting affordable maternal health services. Scale up adolescent sexual and reproductive health information and services
7. Strengthening monitoring and evaluation

From World Bank. Successful approaches to improving maternal health outcomes. http://web.worldbank.org/WBSITE/EXTERNAL/TOPICS/EXTHEALTHNUTRITIONANDPOPULATION/EXTPRH/0,,contentMDK:20200260~menuPK:645470~pagePK:148956~piPK:216618~theSitePK:376855,00.html (Accessed March 8, 2010).

Prerequisites for Saving Lives

Saving lives is mainly dependent on two aspects of health care: whether effective interventions are available to all and the quality of care with which that intervention is implemented. Without patients having access to the specific interventions, lives cannot be saved, and providing the intervention in an inadequate way also inhibits the effect of that intervention (Fig. 1–3). Full access in turn requires that the community has a basic knowledge of when to use the

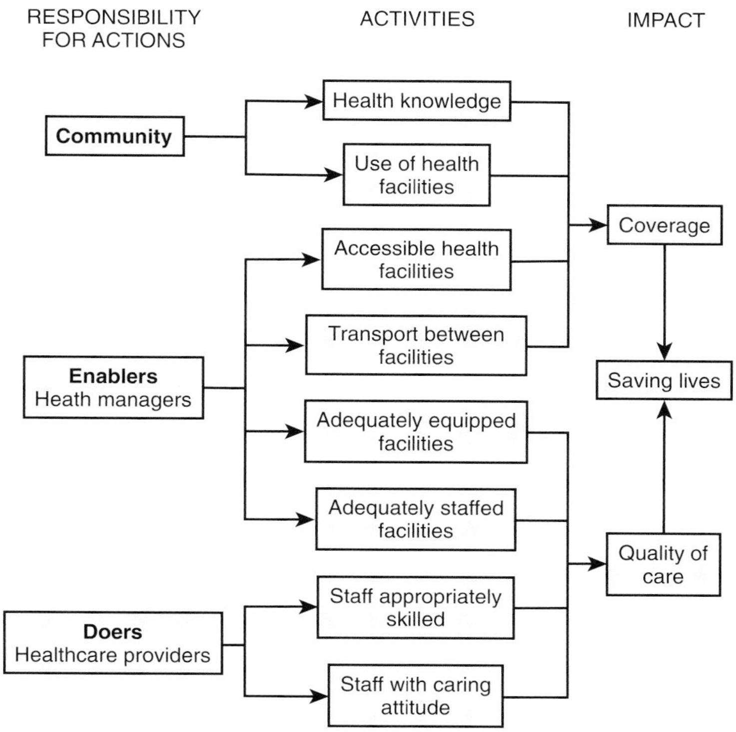

FIGURE 1–3
Factors associated with and the relationship between coverage and quality of care in saving lives.

health care facilities, and health care managers/planners must ensure that health facilities are accessible to the community. Such facilities must have the equipment, drugs, and staff to provide the intervention effectively and the staff must have the appropriate skills.

Community-Based versus Facility-Based Care

There is an ongoing debate internationally regarding which are the most effective strategies to reduce maternal deaths and that, therefore, deserve promotion at a national or provincial level. Some suggest that ensuring that skilled attendants are at all births within central facilities should be the priority, whereas others advocate embarking on community-level interventions because most births currently occur outside such facilities. In our opinion, a one-size-fits-all approach will not work and will be difficult to implement if the context is not appropriate. It is likely that a combination of strategies, including those at community level, utilizing best evidence on antenatal, intrapartum, and postpartum care, will be needed in many countries for the foreseeable future. Complete access to facility-based obstetric care may be the best practice but is likely to be many years away, and even then, it will not be acceptable or accessible to all.[28] It is plausible that community-level interventions could improve outcomes either by increasing the standard of out-of-facility care through training or education or by improving care-seeking behavior and access to facility-level care.

In a systematic review of community-based interventions, two important large randomized controlled trials implemented in Nepal and Pakistan were identified.[29] These trials have produced valid policy-relevant evidence to show that neonatal and perinatal mortality can be reduced by community-level interventions to improve perinatal care practices. Such interventions, directed at improving maternity services, are likely to influence both maternal and perinatal outcomes. Since this review was completed, two other trials on the topic have been published. Baqui and coworkers[30] evaluated the effects of antenatal and postnatal home visits by female community health workers in rural Bangladesh. In this study, the home visit package was significantly more effective than community-level group sessions and resulted in a 34% reduction in neonatal mortality (95% CI 7–53). The second trial was conducted in rural India, in the Shivgarh district of Uttar Pradesh state.[31] The intervention was a package of basic newborn care interventions consisting of birth preparedness, clean delivery, cord care, thermal care, breast-feeding promotion, and danger sign recognition. The neonatal mortality risk was reduced by 54% (95% CI 40–65) in this trial.

All these community-level trials have used the same strategic approach but delivered carefully constructed and contextualized interventions that are different in each trial. Unfortunately, these impressive improvements in perinatal outcome were not reflected in maternal outcomes; although the Pakistan trial showed a reduction in maternal mortality, it was not statistically significant. In another study, a community-based nutritional supplementation of vitamin A suggested an impressive reduction in maternal mortality, but those findings have not been replicated to date.[32]

The presence of such high-quality community-based studies with consistent results is encouraging to those wishing to pursue such activities both as research projects and as program implementation where appropriate.

Community strategies, however, need to be backed up by facility-based care as much as possible, and the presence of one does not mean the other is not needed. Even minor obstetric life-saving interventions, such as manual removal of a retained placenta, are best delivered in a health facility. Internationally, WHO, UNICEF, and UNFPA recommend that there should be at least four facilities offering basic emergency obstetric care (EmOC) for every 500,000 people. Basic EmOC includes the administration of uterotonics, parenteral antibiotics, and magnesium sulfate and provision of manual removal of the placenta.

Clinical Interventions

Appropriate clinical interventions are presented and discussed in detail in specific chapters of this book. The effects of clinical interventions to reduce maternal and perinatal mortality and morbidity have been evaluated through systematic reviews published in the *Cochrane Library* and other journals. Although we know of some interventions that address the main causes of mortality and morbidity, we badly need innovation and new technologies relevant to resource poor as well as rich countries. Tsu and colleagues[33,34] reported on some new and underused technologies to reduce maternal mortality in 2003 and in 2008. Some emerging promising technologies in obstetrics and gynecology have recently been described by Papageorghiou and El-Toukhy.[35] Unfortunately, some well-established effective practices such as magnesium sulfate for preeclampsia and eclampsia and oxytocin or misoprostol to limit postpartum hemorrhage are not implemented as widely as they should be.

SUMMARY OF MANAGEMENT OPTIONS

Some Recommended Practices for Improved Maternal and Perinatal Survival

	Evidence Quality and Recommendation	Reference
Maternal		
Postpartum hemorrhage		
• Active management of the third stage of labor, including administration of uterotonic agents.	Ia/A	39
Hypertensive disorders		
• Magnesium sulfate for women with eclampsia	Ia/A	40
• Calcium supplementation for women with low dietary calcium intake	Ia/A	41
• Labor induction using extra-amniotic saline infusion or very low dose misoprostol for severe cases	Ia/A	42
Obstetric sepsis		
• Clean birth practices	GPP	
HIV		
• Primary prevention (lifestyle changes, condom use)	III/B	43
• Antiretroviral treatment for immunocompromised women	Ia/A	44
Perinatal		
Unexplained intrauterine death		
• Community education on monitoring fetal movements in developing countries	GPP	
Preterm birth		
• Steroids for women at risk of preterm birth	Ia/A	45
• Kangaroo mother care	Ia/A	46
• Nasal continuous positive airway pressure (in settings with no access to mechanical ventilation)	IV/C	47
Intrapartum asphyxia and trauma		
• External cephalic version for breech presentation	Ia/A	48
• Cesarean section for breech delivery	Ia/A	49
• Vacuum extraction	Ia/A	50
• Access to cesarean section	IIb/B	51
• Symphysiotomy	III/B	52
HIV		
• Antiretroviral prophylaxis for mother-to-child transmission of HIV	Ia/A	53
Childhood infections and malnutrition		
• Exclusive breastfeeding for 6 months	Ia/A	54
General		
Prevention of unplanned pregnancy	GPP	

GPP, good practice point.

There are currently no new drugs in the offing that are likely to have an impact on maternal and perinatal survival in the near future, and the pharmaceutical industry has not brought a new effective drug into use since the 1980s.[36]

Some clinical interventions that should be achievable in many resource-poor settings and are likely to reduce the important causes of maternal and perinatal mortality are listed and evidenced in the Summary of Management Options box. These recommendations are based on critical incident audits conducted in South Africa and have been shown to be effective. A tool has been developed to prioritize the interventions for implementation. Choice of the most appropriate interventions for a particular setting can be calculated by estimating the number of lives saved by the introduction or expansion of the intervention to cover 95% of the population using the Lives Saved Tool (LiST).[24,37] Although these methods may not be very precise, they could nevertheless be useful in prioritizing and focusing policy and program decisions.

Reducing the Know-Do Gap: Implementing Best Practices

Reducing maternal mortality and morbidity is complex and involves political commitment and organized persistent action at the health systems and community services levels. In recent years, it is increasingly acknowledged that the implementation of effective practices is often patchy and interventions that are ineffective and harmful remain entrenched in practice. A major cause of this so-called know-do gap is the lack of access to reliable information, although even when this is available, traditional practices can be difficult to change. Since the late 1980s, systematic reviews of effects of maternal and perinatal interventions have greatly increased our knowledge about practices that are more likely to be beneficial than harmful. There is however, a great need to transfer this knowledge widely and in formats that are accessible and user-friendly. Since 1997, WHO has published *The WHO Reproductive Health Library* (RHL)[38] including selected *Cochrane* reviews with commentaries on the relevance of the review results to underresourced country settings. RHL provides access to information from the *Cochrane* reviews and their interpretation to more than 30,000 health workers every year. It is published in Chinese, French, Spanish, and Vietnamese as well as English, which enhances its reach to many settings in which most health workers do not speak English. *The Cochrane Library* is available in English and partially in Spanish. Access to the *Cochrane Library* and more than 2000 periodicals from low- and middle-income country institutions has been made possible through the WHO Access to Research Initiative (HINARI) project (http://www.who.int/hinari/en/).

CONCLUSIONS

At a clinical level, there are many important interventions likely to reduce maternal and newborn mortality. However, many of these interventions are not implemented in the places where they are needed most. The implementation of effective practices varies substantially between and within countries. Since 2000, our knowledge about the effectiveness of implementation strategies has increased substantially. Many strategies such as educational outreach, audit, and feedback, active dissemination through seminars and interactive workshops, have only modest to moderate positive effects. Barriers to the adoption of evidence-based practices exist at multiple levels; tradition is often a major stumbling block. Although there is no single intervention or strategy that can be recommended for every situation, several have been shown to have positive effects. What is clear is that waiting passively for the best practices to be brought into use will be inadequate and active implementation strategies are usually needed.

Reducing maternal mortality and morbidity is possible as several countries have shown. However, for this to happen, all the various stakeholders (politicians, health care workers, and the community at large) need to agree on a concerted plan of action.

Acknowledgments

We acknowledge the assistance of Dr. Lale Say and Dr. João Paulo Souza for information on confidential inquiries and maternal near-miss sections.

SUGGESTED READINGS

Horton R: Countdown to 2015: A report card on maternal, newborn, and child survival. Lancet 2008;371:1217–1219.

Khan KS, Wojdyla D, Say L, et al: WHO analysis of causes of maternal death: A systematic review. Lancet 2006;367:1066–1074.

Kidney E, Winter HR, Khan KS, et al: Systematic review of effect of community-level interventions to reduce maternal mortality. BMC Pregnancy Childbirth 2009;9:2.

Lawn JE, Cousens S, Zupan J: 4 Million neonatal deaths: When? Where? Why? Lancet 2005;365:891–900.

Maternal Mortality in 2005: Estimates Developed by WHO, UNICEF, UNFPA and The World Bank. Geneva, World Health Organization, 2007.

Saving Babies 2006–2007: Sixth Perinatal Care Survey of South Africa. Pretoria, South Africa, Tshepesa, 2009.

Say L, Souza JP, Pattinson RC: Maternal near miss—Towards a standard tool for monitoring quality of maternal health care. Best Pract Res Clin Obstet Gynaecol 2009;23:287–296.

REFERENCES

For a complete list of references, log onto www.expertconsult.com.

SECTION ONE

Prepregnancy

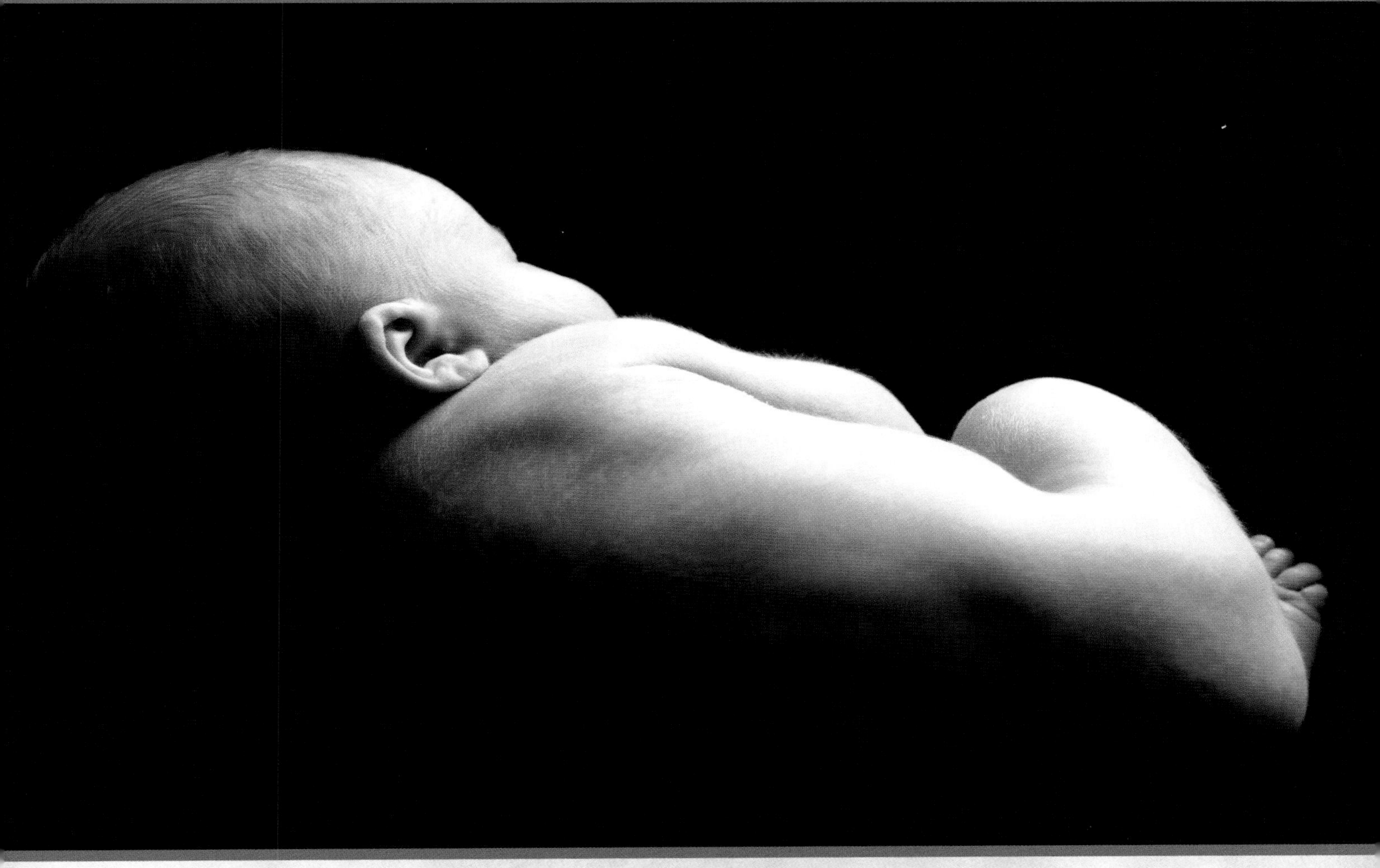

CHAPTER 2

Constitutional and Environmental Factors Leading to a High Risk Pregnancy

HAJO I. J. WILDSCHUT

DEFINITION OF A HIGH RISK PREGNANCY

Pregnancy should be considered a unique, physiologically normal episode in a woman's life. However, preexisting disease or unexpected illness of the mother or fetus can complicate the pregnancy. *Risk* is defined as the probability of an adverse outcome or a factor that increases this probability. A pregnancy is defined as *high risk* when the probability of an adverse outcome for the mother or child is increased over and above the baseline risk of that outcome among the general pregnant population (or reference population) by the presence of one or more ascertainable risk factors, or indicators. This classification does not take into consideration the magnitude of risk or the importance of the risk to the health outcome of the pregnant population at large.

CONSTITUTIONAL RISK

Ethnicity

Race and ethnicity are complex, controversial sociologic issues that are difficult to measure accurately. Race and ethnicity are often considered surrogate measures for standard of living and lifestyle. However, both between and within ethnic populations, marked variations occur in cultural beliefs and practices, language, household structure, sexual behavior, contraceptive patterns, general health, perception of illness and disease, childbirth and child-rearing practices, postnatal customs, dietary habits, housing, education, employment, economic status, level of assimilation, stress, and access to health care services. Some of these attributes have little to do with health or disease, whereas others may be important factors. In clinical research, the terms *race* and *ethnicity* are often defined inadequately, if at all. Therefore, epidemiologic associations with health problems should be interpreted cautiously.

Risks

Ethnicity is one of the factors that is most strongly associated with low birth weight.[1–6] Low birth weight is closely related to infant mortality and childhood morbidity rates.[7] In the United States, preterm birth rather than growth restriction is implicated as the most important cause of low birth weight in black women. Given the high rates of preterm delivery, crude survival rates for black infants are less favorable than those for white infants.[5,8,9] The biologic explanation for the high preterm delivery rate among black women is unclear. The excess birth weight–specific mortality in black infants may be compounded by a failure to seek or receive optimal medical care.[10]

Many diseases and problems that occur during pregnancy have both ethnic and geographic distributions. The risks are summarized in Table 2–1. Uterine fibroids occur more often in black women than in white women.[11] Nonengagement of the fetal head late in pregnancy is not uncommon in black primigravidae.[12] The available data on ethnic differences in the frequency of dysfunctional labor are inconclusive.

MANAGEMENT OPTIONS

Information, screening, and appropriate counseling services should be made available for communities that are considered at risk for specific diseases (see Table 2–1 and other relevant chapters).

PRENATAL

Communication is often a problem because of language barriers. Video displays and informative pamphlets or brochures written in several languages should be made available.[13] Standard information should include guidelines for lifestyle and nutrition as well as preparation for parturition and parenthood, preferably in keeping with sociocultural features of the relevant ethnic communities. The use of interpreters, either in person or by telephone, is advisable for dealing with specific problems.[13]

Once prenatal care has been initiated, women at risk for specific diseases, such as hemoglobinopathies, may be selected for further testing or treatment.[14,15] In parous women, it is important to obtain all necessary information about the course and outcome of previous pregnancies.

TABLE 2–1
Risks in Pregnancy Associated with Certain Ethnic Groups

ETHNIC GROUP	RISKS
Mediterranean islands, parts of the Middle East, Southeast Asia, and parts of the Indian subcontinent	Beta-thalassemias: Minor: Anemia in pregnancy, treated with oral iron and folate, but not parental iron Major: Rare to survive to reproductive age, but those who do often have pelvic bony deformities and problems with labor and delivery; also iron overload with subsequent hepatic, endocrinologic, and myocardial damage Major/minor: Possible risk of inheriting the disease, requiring prenatal counseling and diagnosis
	Alpha-thalassemias: Minor: Usually asymptomatic Major: Rare, but a spectrum of presentation: in adults, usually manifests as a hemolytic anemia of variable severity Major/minor: Possible risk of inheriting the disease, requiring prenatal counseling and diagnosis; homozygous alpha-thalassemias in the fetus can manifest as hydrops fetalis and associated severe preeclampsia in the mother
Afro-Caribbean, Mediterranean, Middle East, India	Sickling disorders (especially HbSS, HbSC): Maternal: Infection, sickling crises, preeclampsia, renal compromise, jaundice; although HbSC tends to be a milder disease (Hb levels usually within normal limits), it can cause massive sickling crises if the diagnosis has not been made; HbAS (carrier state) mothers are rarely at risk for sickling crises with, for example, anoxia, dehydration, or acidosis Fetus: Possible risk of inheriting the disease, requiring prenatal counseling and diagnosis; growth restriction is a risk with HbSS and HbSC
Mediterranean, American Blacks	Glucose-6-phosphate dehydrogenase deficiency: Mother: Hemolytic anemia Fetus: Risk of inheriting the disease, requiring prenatal counseling and diagnosis; fetal hydrops
Far East	Hepatitis B (chronic carriers): Risk of transmission to the fetus or neonate and health care workers
Africa, Caribbean, Hawaii	HIV infection: Risk to the mother of symptomatic infection; risk to the fetus and health care workers of acquiring the infection
Africa (especially Horn of Africa), developing countries	Female circumcision: Problems with vaginal delivery (dystocia, trauma, hemorrhage) Varied effects of endemic infection on the mother or fetus

Hb, hemoglobin; HbAS, hemoglobin AS; HbSC, hemoglobin SC; HbSS, hemoglobin SS.

Immunization status should be checked, and fetal growth should be monitored.

LABOR AND DELIVERY

The continuous presence of a supportive female companion during labor and delivery benefits maternal well-being by improving her emotional status, shortening labor, and decreasing the need for medical intervention.[16] Psychosocial support may also improve mother-infant bonding. It is unlikely that ethnicity in itself affects the duration of labor and delivery.

POSTNATAL

Breastfeeding should be encouraged.[17] Contraceptive advice should take into account individual sociocultural norms and values.[18,19]

Socioeconomic Status

The importance of maternal social factors on the health and well-being of the offspring is well known. However, caution should be exercised in interpreting studies of the effect of social conditions on pregnancy outcome because of variations in definitions and practices in time and geographic area, availability of reliable data, and interpretation of the findings.[21–23]

Various measures of social status are used, some of which tend to be crude and meaningless. In England and Wales, for example, the maternal social class index is traditionally derived from the Registrar General's Classification, which is based on the occupation of the father of the child (Table 2–2). Other criteria of categorization include educational attainment, income, type of health care, employment, legitimacy, family affluence, and household characteristics.[23] Although there is a strong association between social class, however defined, and infant mortality, this observation does not explain why some infants die and others do not.

Social adversity probably represents a wide range of behavioral, environmental, medical, and psychological factors that are causally related to pregnancy outcome, some of which are more amenable to intervention than others. In scientific research, correlations with socioeconomic status should be the impetus for further investigation, rather than the endpoint of an analysis.[24]

Risks

Lower socioeconomic status is associated with an increased risk of various adverse pregnancy outcomes, including perinatal mortality, preterm birth, and low birth weight. Smoking has been suggested as the key factor underlying socioeconomic differences in low birth weight and infant mortality.[6,23,25–27] Differences in care along the social strata may

SUMMARY OF MANAGEMENT OPTIONS

Pregnancy in Women from Different Ethnic Backgrounds

Management Options	Evidence Quality and Recommendation	References
Prepregnancy		
The integration of preconception care services within a larger continuum of women's health care should be promoted.	III/B	20
Provide education, screening, and counseling for communities at specific risk.	Ia/A	14,15
Prenatal		
Overcome language and cultural barriers.	IV/C	13
Offer screening and counseling where specific risk exists.	III/B	14,15
Offer prenatal diagnosis if appropriate.	III/B	14,15
Provide maternal and fetal surveillance for any specific risk.	IIa/B	1,3–5
Labor and Delivery		
Offer the continuous presence of a supportive companion during labor and delivery.	Ia/A	16
Postnatal		
Encourage breast-feeding.	IV/C	17
Offer contraceptive advice, taking account of individual sociocultural norms and values.	III/B	18,19

TABLE 2–2

Social Class by Occupation of the Father

CATEGORY	OCCUPATION
I	Higher professionals
II	Other professionals, including those in managerial positions
IIIa	Skilled workers, nonmanual
IIIb	Skilled workers, manual
IV	Semiskilled workers
V	Unskilled workers

also account for some of the extra risks. The contribution of poor nutrition is discussed in the next section.

Management Options

PRENATAL

Socially disadvantaged women are less likely to seek prenatal care and also have more pregnancy complications. Some claim that apart from recognizing the increased risk associated with socioeconomic disadvantage, there is little to do in terms of prevention. Social support, however, benefits women psychologically, although the effect of social intervention on mean birth weight, low birth weight, and preterm delivery is limited.[16]

LABOR AND DELIVERY

Intrapartum management need not be substantially modified if no other risk factors are present.

POSTNATAL

Women of higher socioeconomic status tend to breast-feed more often and longer than women of lower socioeconomic status. Breast-feeding should be encouraged and social support provided, when indicated.[28] Contraception must be discussed.[19]

Parity

Incidence

In western societies, nulliparous women constitute approximately half of all pregnant women.

Definitions

Parity is the number of times a woman has given birth to an infant, dead or alive. However, the gestational threshold may vary between countries (e.g., 23 completed weeks' gestation vs. 27 completed weeks' gestation).

Risks

Parity is closely correlated with maternal age and with socioeconomic status to a certain extent. On the whole, the risk of adverse outcome with parity does not show a consistent pattern. Mean birth weight for infants born to nulliparous women is consistently lower than that for infants born to multiparous women, and this accounts for most of the differences in mortality risk in the offspring of nulliparous and multiparous women.[32,33] Differences in the mean birth weight of infants born to women of different parity are partially explained by differences in maternal weight. Nulliparity is associated with an increased risk of pregnancy-induced hypertension, which in turn is strongly related to low birth

SUMMARY OF MANAGEMENT OPTIONS

Pregnancy in Women of Low Socioeconomic Background

Management Options	Evidence Quality and Recommendation	References
Prepregnancy		
Recommend health education measures specifically directed at smoking cessation and family planning.	Ib/A	29
Prenatal		
Encourage patients to seek preconception care.	III/B	30
Provide specific and directed social support.	Ia/A	16
Look for clinical evidence of poor fetal growth.	III/B	25
Labor and Delivery		
No additional measures are needed on the basis of adverse socioeconomic factors alone.	—/—	—
Postnatal		
Encourage breast-feeding.	Ib/A	28
Provide specific and directed social support.	Ib/A	31
Discuss contraception.	III/B	19

weight. Further, in nulliparous women, there is an increased risk of perineal trauma as a result of either episiotomy or spontaneous tear.

Women of high parity tend to receive inadequate obstetric care owing to delays in seeking care and poor attendance. Moreover, it is assumed that women with a history of rapid or precipitated childbirth have an increased risk of unattended out-of-hospital delivery. High parity is associated with an increased likelihood of abnormal fetal presentation and obstetric hemorrhage.[34] Parity, however, does not have a significant effect on the incidence of Down syndrome when the effect of maternal age is taken into account.[35]

Management Options

PRENATAL

Nulliparity is a nonspecific risk factor and no specific precautions need to be taken.

In parous women, it is of fundamental importance to obtain all clinically relevant details of previous pregnancies, which will guide patient specific care. Provision of child care facilities may facilitate prenatal care.

LABOR AND DELIVERY

There is a difference in the normal labor patterns of nulliparous and multiparous women. In practice, however, the duration of the second stage of labor is highly variable. In both nulliparous and multiparous women, policies for imposing limits on the length of the second stage of labor tend to be subjective and are usually based on uncontrolled observational data. If the maternal and fetal condition are satisfactory and progress is occurring, with descent of the presenting part, obstetric intervention is not warranted. Cephalopelvic disproportion, however, must be considered when progress in labor is slow. For women with a history of rapid or precipitated delivery, timely admission to the hospital and elective induction of labor are often considered, although there is no evidence that this approach is beneficial.

POSTNATAL

Discussion of long-term contraception is recommended.[36,37]

Age

Adolescent Pregnancy

DEFINITIONS

Epidemiologically, a distinction is often made between pregnancy rates among adolescents aged 15 to 19 years and those among adolescents aged 10 to 14 years.[38–42] *Reproductive age* is the interval from the age of menarche to the chronologic age at conception, whereas *gynecologic age* is the time span from the age of menarche to the chronologic age at delivery. With the improvement of socioeconomic conditions, the median age of menarche has shown a downward trend. The median age of menarche in developed countries is currently 12.5 years.[38] Conception or delivery within 2 years after the onset of menarche represents the lower

SUMMARY OF MANAGEMENT OPTIONS

Women at the Extremes of Parity

Management Options	Evidence Quality and Recommendation	References
Prepregnancy		
Discuss the risks, with emphasis on the effects of parity alone and nulliparity or high multiparity (≥5).	III/B	34,35
Prenatal		
Encourage regular attendance for care in those of high parity.	III/B	34
Look for pregnancy-induced hypertension in those of nulliparity.	III/B	34
Look for abnormal presentation from 36 weeks' gestation in those of high parity.	III/B	34
Labor and Delivery		
No specific recommendations are needed on the grounds of parity alone.	III/B	34
Postpartum hemorrhage is more likely with increasing parity.	III/B	34
Postnatal		
Discuss long-term contraception.	III/B	36,37

extreme of the distribution of both reproductive and gynecologic age.

INCIDENCE

The incidence of teenage pregnancy varies by country. In England and Wales, the teenage (15–19 yr) pregnancy rate is 45/1000, the abortion rate is 19/1000, and the birth rate is 26/1000.[38] In the United States in the mid-1990s, the comparable figures were 84/1000, 29/1000, and 54/1000.[43]

RISKS

Teenage pregnancy is associated with both social and medical problems.[44] Many teenage mothers originate from working-class families and ethnic minorities. Many are themselves the children of teenage or very young parents.[45] Many teenage pregnancies are unplanned and unwanted. Consequently, in western societies, abortion rates among adolescents range from 30% to 60%.[46]

Reports on adolescent pregnancy complications are contradictory because of the confounding effects of adverse social circumstances and poor attendance for prenatal care. However, one risk factor for poor outcomes in adolescent pregnancy is a maternal history of adverse childhood experiences (e.g., emotional, physical, or sexual abuse; living with someone with substance abuse or mental illness or involvement in criminal activity; divorced or separated parents). These experiences are associated with subsequent sexual risk behaviors, smoking, alcohol consumption, and mental health problems such as depression.[47]

Medical complications associated with adolescent pregnancy include preterm birth and low birth weight, perinatal mortality, short interval to next pregnancy, and sudden infant death syndrome. Adolescents who become pregnant are at particular risk for nutritional deficiencies, anemia, HIV infection, and other sexually transmitted diseases.[38] The increased incidence of pregnancy-induced hypertension is largely explained by nulliparity.[39] It has been suggested that competition for nutrients between the fetus and the mother could affect pregnancy outcome in adolescents by interrupting the normal growth process.[48] However, biologic "immaturity" does not affect reproductive performance in terms of length of labor and route and mode of delivery.[38]

MANAGEMENT OPTIONS

Prevention and Prepregnancy Management

Primary prevention includes sexual education in schools and includes information about values, responsibilities, and the right to say "no."[49–51] Teenagers should be encouraged to discuss the realities of pregnancy and parenthood openly.[52] Secondary prevention is directed at sexually active women through a flexible approach to the use and provision of contraceptives for both males and females.[50] Teenagers require different but sensitive approaches.[51] Tertiary prevention involves adolescents who become pregnant. They are encouraged to seek early adequate prenatal care and to discuss options for the resolution of pregnancy.[53–55]

Prenatal

Compliance with prenatal care can be poor, especially among teenagers in their second pregnancy. Strategies for intervention should be focused on individual medical and social risk factors, in particular, poor nutritional status, adverse health habits, and perceived isolation. Pregnant adolescents should be offered social support when feasible, preferably in close cooperation with the family physician, an empathetic midwife, or a social worker.[16,47] Information on pregnancy, delivery, and child-rearing should be made available.

SUMMARY OF MANAGEMENT OPTIONS

Pregnancy in Adolescence

Management Options	Evidence Quality and Recommendation	References
Prepregnancy		
Education and advertising directed toward sexual behavior and family planning.	IIa/B	49,50
Emphasize self-referral for care when pregnant.	III/B	53–55
Prenatal		
Encourage early referral for routine prenatal care and regular attendance.	III/B	53,54
Confirm gestation with early ultrasonography.	III/B	53
Provide advice about diet and adverse habits (e.g., smoking).	III/B	56
Mobilize social support.	III/B	55
Labor and Delivery		
Ensure adequate psychological support.	Ia/A	16
Schedule delivery in a special unit if dystocia is anticipated.	III/B	58
Postnatal		
Provide advice and support for maternal and child care.	III/B	57
Discuss contraception.	III/B	50,51

Labor and Delivery

Continuous emotional support during labor should be provided by a professional (e.g., nurse, midwife) or nonprofessional caregiver (e.g., spouse, friend, relative).[16]

Postnatal

Infant feeding practices, infant growth, and infant safety should be reviewed. Social and financial concerns should be discussed.[55] Teenage girls should be encouraged to continue secondary education.[52] Effective contraception should be implemented. A large percentage of teenagers who give birth before the age of 17 years have a repeat pregnancy before they are 19 years old.[56,57] Home visitation programs by public health nurses can have a positive effect on the health of the adolescent mother and her child.[56,57]

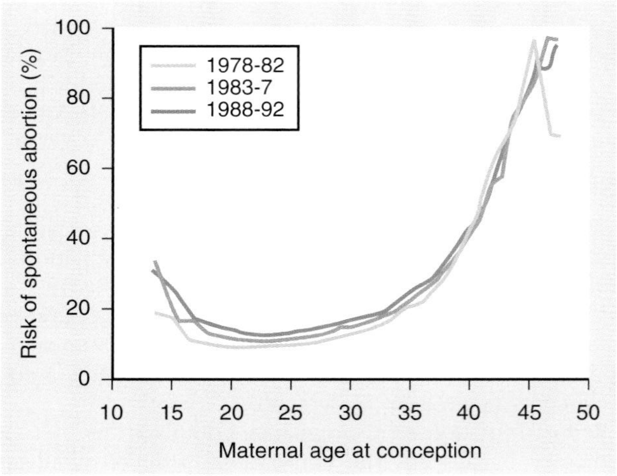

FIGURE 2–1
Risk of spontaneous abortion according to maternal age at conception, stratified according to calendar period, based on Danish civil registry data from 1978-1992. During this period, a total of 634,272 women had 1,221,546 pregnancies, of which 126,673 ended in fetal loss, 285,022 in an induced abortion, and 809,762 in a live birth.
(From Andersen A-MN, Wohlfahrt J, Christens P, et al: Maternal age and fetal loss: Population-based register linkage study. BMJ 2000;320:1708-1712, with permission.)

Advanced Maternal Age

INCIDENCE

In the last decades, there has been a trend toward deferred childbearing, especially among healthy, well-educated women with career opportunities, although the proportion of pregnant women aged 35 years and older varies from country to country. Formerly, pregnant women aged 35 years and older tended to have several unplanned children, whereas today, the proportion of first births to such women is growing.[59–63]

RISKS

Advanced maternal age is a risk indicator for several pregnancy complications, including spontaneous miscarriage (Fig. 2–1)[64]; ectopic pregnancy; stillbirth; chromosomal abnormalities (see Chapter 4); twins; uterine fibroids; hypertensive disorders; gestational diabetes; prolonged labor; cephalopelvic disproportion necessitating operative delivery; bleeding disorders, including placenta previa; low birth weight; antepartum and intrapartum fetal loss; and neonatal mortality.[62–65] However, most reports of pregnancy outcome in elderly nulliparous women have not taken into account effects other than age, such as details of general health, smoking habits, and reproductive history (including a history of miscarriage or infertility and its treatment).[61] Information about whether the first pregnancy was postponed deliberately is often lacking.

Maternal age has no effect on the incidence of birth defects of unknown etiology.[66] Advanced paternal age has little or no independent effect on the risk of autosomal trisomies.[67]

MANAGEMENT OPTIONS

Preconception and Prenatal

The main focus for discussion is the risk of chromosomal abnormalities. This should include careful distinction of the risks at different stages of pregnancy, the options for screening, and the risks of miscarriage from invasive procedures and advanced maternal age itself.[67–71] These issues are also discussed in Chapters 4, 7, 8, and 9.

Although medical and obstetric complications tend to be more common in women aged 35 years and older, in practice, normal prenatal care is not modified unless another specific risk factor or complication is identified.

Labor and Delivery

Elderly women are usually advised to be delivered in a specialized unit because of the risk of dystocia during labor. However, there is no evidence that intrapartum care should be modified because of the extremes of maternal age. Nonetheless, the woman's age often contributes strongly to decisions to intervene.[63]

Postnatal

Discussion of long-term contraception is recommended.[36,37]

Nutrition

Risks

GENERAL

Nutritional conditions in pregnancy are a major determinant of health in later life.[72,73] Conditions such as type 2 diabetes, hypertension, and coronary heart disease are considered to be the result of fetal programming of physiology and metabolism.[72,74] Studies of the Dutch famine of 1944–1945 showed a relative increase in placental weight in infants whose mother's nutrition was compromised around conception or in the first trimester.[74] The increase in the placenta weight–to–birth weight ratio is interpreted as a compensatory mechanism after reduced caloric intake in early pregnancy.[75,76] An increased ratio is also seen with maternal anemia, tobacco use in pregnancy, and births at high altitude.[75] Fetal cardiovascular adaptations are a recognized feature of intrauterine growth restriction and divert nutrient-rich, highly oxygenated blood to spare the growth of the brain and other critical organs. Furthermore, reduced availability of micronutrients may affect fetal body composition. The relative amounts of fetal bone and lean and fat mass influence the risk of adult obesity and type 2 diabetes.[72] When undernutrition during early development is followed by improved nutrition, many animals and plants have accelerated compensatory growth.[72] However, in animals, this compensatory growth may reduce life span.[73]

SUMMARY OF MANAGEMENT OPTIONS

Advanced Maternal Age

Management Options	Evidence Quality and Recommendation	References
Prepregnancy		
Discuss risks, but they should be put into perspective.	III/B	62,63
Spontaneous miscarriage risk increased.	III/B	64
Discuss prenatal diagnosis of chromosomal abnormalities.	III/B	69,71
Advanced paternal age has little or no independent effect on the risk of autosomal trisomies.	III/B	71
Multiple pregnancy risk increased.	III/B	65
Prenatal		
Discuss options for aneuploidy screening and prenatal diagnosis with invasive procedures.	III/B	70
Labor and Delivery		
Delivery in a unit that can manage dystocia and other complications.	III/B	62
Postnatal		
Discuss long-term contraception.	III/B	36,37

CAFFEINE

Caffeine consumption in pregnancy is a controversial topic. Reports of teratogenicity from animal studies led the U.S. Food and Drug Administration (FDA) to advise pregnant women to eliminate caffeine from their diets.[77] Subsequent epidemiologic studies showed inconsistent results. Moreover, cigarette smoking may confound the association of caffeine consumption with pregnancy outcomes.[77]

VITAMINS

The current reference daily intakes (RDIs) for vitamins are summarized in Table 2–3.[78] Pregnancy may increase vitamin requirements. Mechanisms underlying vitamin deficiency include inadequate dietary intake and abnormal metabolism.

FOLATE

Folate is a water-soluble vitamin and is found mainly in polyglutamated form. Folic acid (folacin) is the synthetic form present as a monoglutamate in vitamin tablets and fortified foods. Folate is important for the biosynthesis of DNA and RNA. It also plays an important role in the conversion of homocysteine to methionine, an essential amino acid. An adequate level of folate should be established before conception and maintained during the first trimester to reduce the risk of neural tube defects. Fruits, green vegetables, beans, nuts, and bread are the primary sources of folate. Cooking may destroy some forms of dietary folate. In pregnancy, folate requirements are usually increased. A low-folate plasma concentration could be caused by inadequate dietary intake or the use of anticonvulsant drugs, such as phenytoin, phenobarbital, and carbamazepine, which are known folate antagonists. Moreover, folate deficiency could be the result of inherited metabolic disorders, associated, for instance, with methylenetetrahydrofolate reductase (MTHFR) gene polymorphism. MTHFR is a key enzyme in homocysteine metabolism.[79] The homocysteine plasma concentration is considered a sensitive biomarker of the levels of folate and vitamins B_6 and B_{12}. In pregnancies complicated by a fetal neural tube defect, maternal plasma homocysteine levels are elevated and plasma folate concentration is decreased, suggesting a defect in the folate-dependent homocysteine metabolism. Hyperhomocystinemia is also associated with various conditions characterized by placental vasculopathy, such as preeclampsia and abruption, and with recurrent pregnancy loss.[80]

TABLE 2–3

Current Reference Daily Intakes for Vitamins

VITAMIN	DAILY VALUE
Vitamin A	1500 μg (5000 IU)
Vitamin C	60 mg
Vitamin D	10 μ (400 IU)
Vitamin E	20 mg (30 IU)
Vitamin K	80 μg
Vitamin B_6	2 mg
Vitamin B_{12}	6 μg
Folate	400 μg
Thiamin	1.5 mg
Riboflavin	1.7 mg
Niacin	20 mg

From Fairfield KM, Fletcher RH: Vitamins for chronic disease prevention in adults: Scientific review. JAMA 2002;287:3116–3126.

OTHER VITAMINS

Vitamin A is a member of the family of fat-soluble *retinoids*.[78] Isotretinoin, a derivative of vitamin A, is a powerful prescription drug for the treatment of severe recalcitrant nodular acne. Doses of vitamin A at three times the daily allowance can cause birth defects (e.g., heart defects, craniofacial anomalies). Thus, isotretinoin has been labeled as pregnancy category X, meaning it should not be used during pregnancy. Another derivative of vitamin A, etretinate, is a prescription drug for the treatment of psoriasis. This drug is also contraindicated in pregnant women. In adults, vitamin A toxicity results in hepatotoxicity and visual changes.[78] Xerophthalmia, night blindness, and increased susceptibility to disease characterize vitamin A deficiency.

Vitamin B_6 (pyridoxine, pyridoxal, and pyridoxamine) is water-soluble and found in various plant and animal products. Vitamin B_6 is involved in many enzymatic reactions. Deficiency is uncommon.

Vitamin B_{12} (cyanocobalamin) is water-soluble and found in animal products only. Cyanocobalamin must be converted to a biologically active form (methylcobalamin or adenosylcobalamin). Methylcobalamin is an essential cofactor in the conversion of homocysteine to methionine.[79] When this reaction is impaired, hyperhomocysteinemia occurs and folate metabolism is deranged. The cobalamins are involved in fat and carbohydrate metabolism, protein synthesis, and hematopoiesis. Deficiency can result from poor intake, including strict veganism, malabsorption from the absence of intrinsic factor, and rare enzyme deficiencies. Vitamin B_{12} deficiency results in macrocytic anemia and neurologic abnormalities. There are no consistent reports of adverse effects from high intake.[78]

Vitamin C (ascorbic acid) is water-soluble and a cofactor in hydroxylation reactions required for collagen synthesis. It is also a strong antioxidant. Vitamin C deficiency leads to bruising and easy bleeding (scurvy). Large doses (≤2000 mg) of vitamin C are generally well tolerated.

Vitamin D (calciferol) is not a true vitamin because humans can synthesize it with adequate sunlight exposure. Vitamin D deficiency is associated with rickets in children. In adults, vitamin D deficiency leads to secondary hyperparathyroidism, with subsequent bone loss and increased fracture risk. There is evidence that genetic polymorphisms strongly affect fracture risk.[78] Inadequate vitamin D intake is more common than previously believed, particularly among housebound women of specific ethnic minority groups.[78] There is no documented evidence of vitamin D deficiency and adverse pregnancy outcome, apart from neonatal hypocalcemia. Given the relatively high prevalence of vitamin D deficiency in certain communities, vitamin D supplementation at a dosage of 0.01 mg (400 IU) is advocated. High intake of vitamin D (>0.05 mg or 2000 IU) results in hypercalcemia and soft tissue calcification.[78]

Vitamin E is a family of eight related compounds, the tocopherols and the tocotrienols. The only reported perinatal effect of dietary vitamin E deficiency has been hemolytic anemia and retinopathy in preterm infants, However, genetic deficiencies in apolipoprotein B or α-tocopherol transfer protein lead to severe vitamin E deficiency syndromes, with symptoms including hemolytic anemia, muscle weakness, and brain dysfunction.[78] With doses of 800 to 1200 mg/day, antiplatelet effects and bleeding may occur.[78] Because of its antioxidative properties, vitamin E is believed to prevent diseases associated with oxidative stress, such as cardiovascular diseases, cancer, chronic inflammation, and neurologic disorders. It is assumed, but not proved, that vitamin E requirements increase during pregnancy. It is uncertain whether supplementation with vitamins C and E help prevent preeclampsia (see Chapter 35).[81]

Vitamin K is fat-soluble and essential for normal clotting, especially for the production of prothrombin, factors VII, IX, and X, and protein C and S. Vitamin K has two subtypes, vitamin K_1 and K_2. Vitamin K_1, or phylloquinone, is found in most vegetables and dairy products. Vitamin K_2, or menaquinone, is synthesized by the intestinal flora and absorbed only in small amounts.[82] Vitamin K deficiency occurs when dietary intake is inadequate or intestinal bacteria, which synthesize vitamin K, are altered. Newborn infants are at risk for vitamin K deficiency because of poor placental transfer, lack of intestinal bacteria, and low content in breast milk.[82] The risk of vitamin K deficiency is higher in the breast-fed infant because breast milk contains lower amounts of vitamin K than modern formula or cow's milk.[82] A single dose of either oral or intramuscular vitamin K, 1 mg, to all infants is advocated to prevent hemorrhagic disease of the newborn in the first week after birth.[82] Pregnancy women using antiepileptic drugs, including phenytoin, carbamazepine, and phenobarbital, are particularly at risk for vitamin K deficiency in their offspring. They are advised to take oral vitamin K, 10 mg daily, from 36 weeks to prevent neonatal hemorrhagic disease.[83]

SUMMARY OF MANAGEMENT OPTIONS

Nutritional Preparation for Pregnancy

Management Options	Evidence Quality and Recommendation	References
Prepregnancy		
Offer counseling to women at risk for nutritional deficiency.	III/B	88,89
Recommend folate supplements (0.4 mg/day) for all women contemplating pregnancy.	Ia/A	90
Offer continuing folate supplementation (0.4 mg/day) to all women at increased risk for neural tube defects in pregnancy.	Ia/A	90
Prenatal		
The decision to recommend supplements is based on individual requirements.	Ia/A	91
Routine iron supplementation is warranted in populations in which iron deficiency is common.	Ia/A	92
Avoid excess vitamin A (i.e., more than the daily allowance).	III/B	78
Advise supplemental vitamin K (10 mg/day from 36 weeks' gestation) to women who take antiepileptic drugs to prevent neonatal hemorrhagic disease.	IIa/A	83
Advise women to avoid large amounts of caffeine (>600 mg daily, which is equivalent to six 10-oz cups of coffee).	III/B	73
Labor and Delivery Postnatal		
Give a single dose (1 mg) of either intramuscular or oral vitamin K to the newborn to prevent classic hemorrhagic disease. Vitamin K prophylaxis improves biochemical indices of coagulation status at 1–7 days.	Ib/A	82

IODINE AND ZINC

Trace minerals, such as iodine and zinc, are needed in greater quantities during pregnancy. Deficiencies have been implicated in low birth weight, perinatal mortality, mental retardation, childhood hearing and speech disorders, and birth defects.[84]

IRON

In Europe, iron deficiency is an important nutritional disorder, affecting large fractions of the population, particularly children, menstruating women, and pregnant women. Moreover, vegetarians, vegans, and patients with malabsorption are at increased risk for iron deficiency. A reduction in body iron is associated with a decrease in the level of functional compounds, such as hemoglobin (see also Chapter 38).

Management Options

GENERAL

From an overview of randomized controlled trials, no firm conclusions could be drawn about the implications of nutritional advice to prevent or treat impaired fetal growth.[76] Most physicians agree that RDIs, except those for iron and folic acid, can be obtained through a proper diet. Pregnant teenagers, smokers, drug users, alcohol drinkers, and strict vegetarians tend to be deficient in various vitamins.[85–87] Multivitamin supplements can be of value.

To reduce the incidence of neural tube defects, most countries advocate folic acid supplementation in a dosage of 0.4 mg/day to all women from at least 4 weeks before until 8 weeks after conception.[77]

Large quantities of caffeine consumption should be avoided.

Maternal Weight and Weight Gain

Body mass index (BMI), also known as Quetelet's index (weight [kg]/height [m]^2), is the most commonly used measure. Naeye[90] classified pregnant women into four BMI categories: "thin," less than 20; "normal," 20 to 24; "overweight," 25 to 30; and "obese," greater than 30. In clinical practice, however, these can be difficult to apply because prepregnancy weight is usually unavailable at the first prenatal visit.[93]

Underweight Women

Nutritional deprivation may arise as a result of starvation, dieting, or chronic eating disorders, such as anorexia nervosa and bulimia. Eating disorders are a public health concern in affluent societies.[85]

Anorexia nervosa is a syndrome characterized by severe weight loss, a distorted body image, and an intense fear of becoming obese.[85,94] Anorexia nervosa is not synonymous with bulimia, although bulimic symptoms may occur in women with anorexia nervosa. *Bulimia* is characterized by recurrent episodes of secretive binge eating followed by self-induced vomiting, fasting, or the use of laxatives or diuretics.[85] Depression and alcohol and drug abuse are also prominent features of this disorder.[95] Patients show frequent weight fluctuations but are not likely to have significant weight loss, as seen in women with anorexia nervosa. Both syndromes, which primarily affect adolescents and young adults from middle-class and upper-middle-class families, are often associated with oligomenorrhea and amenorrhea.[85] Despite menstrual irregularities, women with chronic eating disorders may become pregnant.

SUMMARY OF MANAGEMENT OPTIONS

Underweight Women

Management Options	Evidence Quality and Recommendation	References
Prepregnancy		
Advise women with an eating disorder wishing to become pregnant to wait until the disorder is in remission.	III/B	89
Use a multidisciplinary approach for eating disorders.	III/B	85
Prenatal		
Check for fetal growth restriction.	III/B	89,97
Provide multidisciplinary treatment for women with eating disorders not yet in remission.	III/B	94,97
Labor and Delivery		
Provide continuous electronic fetal heart rate monitoring if the fetus is small.	IIa/B	98
Postnatal		
Monitor signs of maternal depression, and provide treatment if indicated.	III/B	94

RISKS

Underweight women are more likely than women of normal weight to give birth to infants who are small for gestational age.[90,96,97] Poor fetal growth may result in birth asphyxia and complications, such as neonatal hypoglycemia and hypothermia.[98] Underweight women my be more susceptible to anemia. In "thin" women (Quetelet's index < 20), the perinatal mortality rate is increased.[90]

The outcome of pregnancy in women with anorexia and bulimia varies. If the eating disorder is in remission, then an uneventful pregnancy and outcome can be anticipated. However, expectant women with active anorexia nervosa or bulimia at the time of conception may have a number of severe health problems, including electrolyte imbalances, dehydration, depression, social problems, and poor fetal growth. Appropriate psychiatric treatment is warranted.[89,94]

MANAGEMENT OPTIONS

Prepregnancy

Women who have anorexia or bulimia and wish to become pregnant are advised to wait until the eating disorder is in remission.[89] The treatment of underweight women with anovulatory infertility should be focused on restoration of weight by an integrated multidisciplinary approach rather than on ovulation induction.[85]

Prenatal

Prenatal care should focus on early detection of impaired fetal growth.[94] However, the beneficial effects of dietary advice, with or without specific food supplements, are controversial.[76,85,99]

Labor and Delivery

If fetal growth restriction is suspected, the patient should be admitted to a specialist unit. Continuous electronic fetal heart rate monitoring is advised.[97] Emergency neonatal services should be readily available for resuscitation.

Postnatal

Approximately 40% of women with eating disorders have a history of affective disorders, which also puts them at risk for postpartum depression.[94] No additional specific management strategies need to be considered. Treatment with antidepressant drugs may be warranted.

Overweight Women

According to the World Health Organization, "overweight" is defined as a BMI between 25 and 30 kg/m^2 and "obesity" is defined as a BMI of 30 kg/m^2 or greater.[100] The degree of obesity is classified into three categories: class I (BMI 30.0–34.9 kg/m^2), class II (BMI 35.0–39.9 kg/m^2), and class III (BMI > 40 kg/m^2; "morbidly obese"). For an online BMI calculator, see www.nhlbisupport.com/bmi. There are also BMI percentiles, which are age-, gender-, and population-specific.[101] The prevalence of obesity in industrialized countries is increasing rapidly.[102]

RISKS

Hypertensive disorders, including preexisting hypertension and pregnancy-induced hypertension, are more common in women with excess weight, although reported prevalence varies widely (7%–46%).[102,103] Gestational diabetes is also more frequent, affecting 7% to 17% of obese women.[103] Other problems associated with obesity include gallbladder disease, shortness of breath, fatigue, hiatus hernia, raised cholesterol levels, urinary tract infections, postnatal hemorrhage, and possibly thrombophlebitis.[102,104,105] Controversy exists regarding the association between obesity and congenital malformations. Watkins and coworkers[106] explored the association between several birth defects and obesity in a population-based case-control study. They concluded that obese women (BMI ≥ 30) were more likely than average-weight women (BMI 18.5–24.9) to have an infant with spina bifida (unadjusted odds ratio [OR] 3.5; 95% confidence interval [CI] 1.2–10.3), omphalocele (OR 3.3; 95% CI 1.0–10.3), heart defects (OR 2.0; 95% CI 1.2–3.4), and multiple anomalies (OR 2.0; 95% CI 1.0–3.8). The biologic mechanism behind obesity and birth defects is unknown.

There is conflicting evidence about the effect of obesity on perinatal mortality. Obese women are more likely to give birth to large-for-gestational-age infants. Increased maternal weight is independently associated with poor labor progression and increased risk of cesarean delivery.[102,104,105] Overall, the increased need for abdominal delivery in obese women can be attributed mainly to the relatively high rates of prenatal complications and to factors such as advanced age and high parity. When surgical delivery is required, obese women are more prone to wound infection than nonobese women.[103,107]

The risks of anesthesia are increased in obese women including failed epidural, difficult intubation, inability to identify landmarks, difficulty in placing the regional block, and erratic spread of anesthetic solution.[102] Management of the airway in morbidly obese patients can be extremely difficult. They have an increased risk of aspiration because of a larger volume of gastric fluid and increased intra-abdominal pressure with a higher incidence of gastroesophageal reflux.[108] The anesthetic problems can be compounded by coexistent cardiovascular and respiratory problems. Finally, transportation of the grossly obese patient can be extremely difficult.

MANAGEMENT OPTIONS

Prepregnancy

Ideally, an obese woman should be encouraged to lose weight before or after pregnancy. However, data on the efficacy of numerous dietary programs are limited [109–111] Dietary manipulation should not be advocated during pregnancy because it is difficult to achieve, offers no benefit to the mother, and may have ill effects on fetal weight and health after birth.[112,113] Behavior modification including daily exercise programs is probably the key to weight loss[100,109,114] (see "Physical Activity," later). However, if a woman insists on severe caloric restriction for weight reduction, the problem of maintaining reduced weight for prolonged periods should also be addressed. The recurrence rate of obesity after weight reduction is high.[114]

Bariatric surgery encompasses the various surgical procedures performed to treat obesity by modification of the gastrointestinal tract to reduce nutrient intake and/or absorption. It is considered with morbid obesity when all other treatments have failed.[115] The majority of patients are women.[116] The three most common surgical procedures currently performed worldwide are laparoscopic gastric bypass, laparoscopic adjustable gastric banding and open gastric bypass. Sixty-three percent of bariatric surgery is now performed laparoscopically.[117] A recent *Cochrane* review concluded that bariatric surgery resulted in greater weight loss than conventional treatment and led to improvements in quality of life and obesity-related diseases such as hypertension and diabetes. However, the comparative safety and effectiveness of the surgical procedures remain unclear.[118] A systematic review concluded that women who had bariatric surgery before pregnancy had lower rates of a number of adverse maternal and neonatal outcomes when compared with rates in pregnant women who did not have surgery for morbid obesity.[119] Most pregnancies after bariatric surgery appear to have a benign course.

Prenatal

Prepregnancy weight and maternal height should be documented routinely at the first visit. Weight is usually recorded at each prenatal visit, using calibrated scales, although the value of this is uncertain. Blood pressure should also be monitored with an appropriately sized cuff to minimize the artificially high recordings that might result when a standard cuff is used.[120]

In obese women, it can be difficult to assess fetal growth and presentation clinically. Ultrasonography is helpful in resolving problems of presentation. However, poor ultrasound visualization in obese women lessens the accuracy of measurements and assessment of fetal anatomy.[121] Tissue harmonic imaging improves the quality of ultrasound images of the fetal heart.[122] Anesthetic consultation is advisable. This has greater urgency if patient has medical problems

SUMMARY OF MANAGEMENT OPTIONS
Overweight Women

Management Options	Evidence Quality and Recommendation	References
Prepregnancy		
Provide advice on interventions for weight reduction.	Ia/A	110
Explain the risks of hypertension, diabetes, urinary infections, large fetal size, and postpartum hemorrhage.	III/B	104–107, 123
In the selected group of women, pregnancy following bariatric surgery is associated with a better outcome than being pregnant and morbidly obese.	Ia/A	119
Prenatal		
Avoid attempts to manipulate the diet during pregnancy.	Ib/A	109,111,114
Screen for hypertension, diabetes, and bacteriuria.	III/B	105
Monitor the blood pressure with an appropriately sized cuff.	III/B	120
Monitor fetal growth with ultrasound.	III/B	123,124
Labor and Delivery		
Maintain vigilance for cephalopelvic disproportion and shoulder dystocia.	III/B	123
Cesarean Section		
Use regional rather than general anesthesia.	IIa/B	133
Give prophylactic antibiotics.	Ia/A	125
Use thromboprophylaxis.	IV/C	102
There is no evidence for the best incision.	Ia/A	127
Subcutaneous fat closure decreases the incidence of wound dehiscence.	Ia/A	130,131
Subcutaneous drains do not prevent wound complications.	Ia/A	131
Postnatal		
Following cesarean section give subcutaneous heparin until the patient is fully ambulatory.	IV/C	126
Recommend early mobilization.	IV/C	126
Continue with measures to lose weight.	IV/C	100
Breast-feeding has a small protective effect against childhood obesity.	I/A	134

such as hypertension, diabetes mellitus, or pulmonary dysfunction. Obese women should be evaluated for gestational diabetes at the first prenatal visit and at the start of the third trimester (see Chapter 44).

Ultrasound screening for fetal macrosomia is commonly undertaken in pregnancy.

Labor and Delivery

Fetal macrosomia is strongly associated with problems in labor, including poor progress as a result of cephalopelvic disproportion, shoulder dystocia, and birth asphyxia.[123] Attempts to derive a prediction score to identify large-for-gestational-age infants have been unsuccessful because of unacceptably high false-positive rates.[124]

Cesarean section in obese women requires specific considerations. Regional anesthesia has advantages over general anesthesia.[104,125] As with all cesarean sections, obese patients should receive prophylactic antibiotics and thromboprophylactic measures.[125,126] Evidence about the most appropriate surgical technique is limited[127] (see also Chapter 74). Gross[128] reviewed the benefits and risks of the two common operative approaches (Pfannenstiel and midline vertical) in obese women. He concluded that the favorable aspects of the Pfannenstiel incision are (1) less postoperative pain and early ambulation; (2) a more secure closure; (3) less adipose tissue to incise; and (4) better cosmetic results. However, the potential adverse effects of the Pfannenstiel incision are (1) greater likelihood of wound infection; (2) potentially restricted access to the infant; and (3) more difficult exposure of the upper abdomen. Exteriorization of the uterus is of no proven benefit.[129] Naumann and colleagues[130] tested the hypothesis that closure of the subcutaneous fat decreases the incidence of wound disruption after cesarean section. There was no significant difference in the incidence of wound infections between the two study groups. However, there was a significantly lower incidence of wound disruption in the subcutaneous closure group (relative risk [RR] 0.5; 95% CI 0.3–0.9). A recent multicenter randomized trial concluded that the additional use of a subcutaneous drain does not prevent of wound complications in obese women being delivered by cesarean section.[131] There is no conclusive evidence about how the skin should be closed after cesarean section.[132]

Postnatal

Prophylactic administration of anticoagulants should be continued until the patient is fully mobilized. Early mobilization appears to improve maternal outcome.

In newborn infants born to grossly obese women, especially those that are large for gestational age, the blood glucose levels should be monitored during the first hours of life. From a systematic review, it was concluded that breastfeeding seems to have a small but consistent protective effect against obesity in children.[133]

Weight Gain in Pregnancy

The total weight gain of a healthy nulliparous woman eating normally is approximately 12.5 kg (27.5 lb).[92] However, large variations in weight gain are seen with normal outcomes.[92,135] In western societies, average total weight gain ranges from 10 to 16 kg (22–35 lb).[136] In healthy, well-nourished women with uncomplicated pregnancies, the proportional weight gain (i.e., total weight gain at term expressed as a proportion of prepregnancy weight) is 17% to 20%.[88] The increase is mainly due to an increase in total body water (~7.5 kg [16.4 lb] when no edema is present) and body fat mass (~2.2–3.5 kg [5.0–7.7 lb]).[92,136,137] The remainder (~0.9 kg [2 lb]) is caused by an increase in protein content, half of which is fetal. Mean weight gain in pregnancy, from conception to birth, does not show a linear trend. In the normal, lean nulliparous woman, weight gain during the first trimester is 0.65 to 1.1 kg (1.4–2.4 lb).[90,137] In the second trimester, average weekly weight gain is 0.45 kg (1 lb), and 0.36 kg (0.8 lb) thereafter.[92] Weight loss or failure to gain weight over a 2-week interval in the third trimester is not uncommon in both nulliparous and parous women. The maximum rate of weight gain occurs between 17 and 24 weeks.[135]

After delivery, the most rapid weight loss, mainly as fluid, occurs between 4 and 10 days. Subsequently, weight loss is more gradual, at 0.25 kg (0.55 lb) per week due to mobilization of fat stores.[138] The average woman eventually loses most of the weight she gained during pregnancy.[92,139] Breastfeeding for longer than 60 days has a favorable effect on the rate of postpartum weight loss.[140]

RISKS

Inadequate weight gain during pregnancy is associated with low–birth weight and small-for-gestational-age infants. Excessive weight gain during pregnancy does not necessarily enhance fetal growth and has been consistently found to contribute to postpartum weight retention and later obesity.[141] The magnitude of the association between inadequate maternal weight gain and low birth weight depends on prepregnancy weight. Thus, women of low prepregnancy weight with little weight gain during pregnancy are more likely to give birth to a low–birth-weight infant than overweight women with a similar overall weight gain. Net weight gain in underweight women is strongly related to birth weight. In overweight women, net weight gain is only marginally related to birth weight.[141,142] The optimum weight gain in terms of minimum perinatal mortality is 7.3 kg (16 lb) for overweight women, 9.1 kg (20 lb) for women of normal weight, and 13.6 kg (30 lb) for underweight women.[112] The possibility of an eating disorder should be considered in women who do not gain appropriate weight or who have intractable vomiting.[89]

MANAGEMENT OPTIONS

Prenatal

Despite the risks previously discussed, evidence that interventions based on poor weight gain improve outcome is lacking and many units no longer weigh pregnant women regularly through pregnancy. Those that do often check for abnormal fetal growth in such women, consider physical and organic causes, and if the abnormal weight gain is thought to be dietary, offer advice about improving diet and lifestyle.[113,124,138,142–144] Advice on reducing weight is not helpful.

Labor and Delivery

Important considerations were discussed in the previous sections.

SUMMARY OF MANAGEMENT OPTIONS

Abnormal Weight Gain

Management Options	Evidence Quality and Recommendation	References
Prenatal		
Check for abnormal fetal growth.	Ib/A	113
Consider physical and organic causes.	IIb/B	143
Offer advice on improving diet and lifestyle.	Ia/A	124,138,144
Advice on reducing weight is not useful.		
Labor and Delivery		
See the recommendations for "Overweight Women."	—/—	—

Physical Activity

Definition

Physical activity can be

- Daily activities (domestic, occupational, and commuting).
- Leisure activities (sports and exercise).

It accounts for 15% to 40% of total energy expenditure. The magnitude of the physiologic response is determined by age, fitness, body weight, body position, concurrent physical adaptations to pregnancy, and psychological factors.[145]

Risks

GENERAL HEALTH

Physical activity, diet, and health are linked, especially through obesity.[100] However, physical inactivity is an independent risk factor for type 2 diabetes, hypertension, cardiovascular disease, and stroke.[100]

PREGNANCY

Physically and emotionally demanding work during pregnancy is associated with an increased risk of hypertension, low birth weight, and preterm birth[146] (see "Occupational Factors"). Regular recreational exercise in pregnancy, including aerobics and competitive sports, improves the outcome for both mother and fetus, in terms of maternal cardiovascular reserve, placental growth, and functional capacity.[145–150] Activities with a high risk of abdominal trauma should be avoided.[147] Scuba diving should be discouraged throughout pregnancy, because the fetus is not protected from decompression problems and is at risk for malformation and gas embolism after decompression disease.[147,149]

Management Options

A woman's overall health, including obstetric and medical risks, should be evaluated before an exercise program is prescribed. The American College of Obstetricians and Gynecologists (ACOG) recommends that healthy pregnant women engage in 30 minutes or more of moderate exercise daily, provided there are neither medical nor obstetric complications.[147] Healthy pregnant women are allowed to exercise vigorously or take part in competitive sports, provided there are no noticeable health hazards to themselves or their infants.[147,149,150]

SUMMARY OF MANAGEMENT OPTIONS

Exercise in Pregnancy

Management Options	Evidence Quality and Recommendation	References
Healthy pregnant women may engage in daily exercise if there are no medical or obstetric complications.	Ia/A	147,149
Women should avoid activities with a high risk of abdominal trauma.	IV/C	147
Discourage scuba diving in pregnancy.	IIb/B	151
Regular aerobic exercise during pregnancy appears to improve or maintain physical fitness	Ia/A	150
Regular exercise carries no demonstrable harm to the mother or fetus.	Ia/A	149

ENVIRONMENTAL RISK

General

Some environmental risk (such as infection, prescribed drugs, drugs of abuse) is covered in other chapters.

It is difficult to ascertain the clinical importance of each of these environmental influences on reproductive health because of lack of evidence and the existence of confounding variables.

Chemicals

Polychlorinated Biphenyls

Polychlorinated biphenyls (PCBs) have been used in pesticides, surface coatings, inks, adhesives, flame retardants, paints, and old electrical equipment.[152] Many countries have severely restricted or banned the production of PCBs.

Highly chlorinated PCB congeners persist in the environment, the air, drinking water, and food, particularly meat, fish, and poultry. They are rapidly absorbed from the intestinal tract and distribute to and accumulate in the liver. They also cross the placenta and are excreted in breast milk. Formula milk is free of PCBs. Much concern exists that PCBs transferred to the fetus across the placenta may induce long-lasting neurologic damage.[153] The beneficial effects of breast-feeding, however, outweigh the potentially adverse effects of PCB exposure from breast milk.

Dioxins

Dioxins are a heterogeneous mixture of chlorinated dibenzo-*p*-dioxin and dibenzofuran congeners. Dioxins are emissions of industrial incineration processes. They accumulate in the food chain to result in human exposure.[154] Few data are available on the effects of dioxins on female reproductive health. In animal models, dioxin has an antiestrogenic effect. Environmental chemicals have been implicated in the temporal decline in the age of onset of puberty, the development of polycystic ovarian syndrome, and shortened lactation. Reports of cryptorchism and hypospadias need more careful study, particularly because they are linked to testicular cancer. The effects of environmental chemicals on sperm quality are inconsistent. Because of methodologic shortcomings in epidemiologic studies, it is unknown whether dioxins affect spontaneous abortion rates or fetal growth restriction.

Pesticides

Pesticides (e.g., fungicides, herbicides, insecticides, and rodenticides), often found in commercially available food products, are a reproductive health concern in many countries. However, the almost universal exposure to low concentrations of these compounds makes it very difficult to determine the effect of pesticides on the incidence of fetal abnormalities. Occupational exposure to pesticides has been implicated in increased birth defect rates.[155,156]

Occupational Risk

Risks

With the rising number of women in paid employment in both developing and developed countries,[157] exposures to unsafe and unhealthy conditions, such as toxic chemicals, radiation, and physically or mentally demanding work, have become more common. Because women's occupations are multidimensional and risk exposure perhaps subtle, a simple guide for establishing specific health risks is not always possible.[156,158] However, the adverse effects of poor working environment can be magnified by problems of isolation, stress, tiredness, and depression. Physical violence is a major contributor to women's health risks, either in the home or in the formal workplace (see Chapter 3).

Occupational exposure to risk can be specific such as anesthetic agents, laboratory chemicals, organic solvents, and pesticides (see earlier).[159,160] A meta-analysis of studies of working conditions in pregnancy concluded that physically demanding work is significantly associated with preterm birth (OR 1.22; 95% CI 1.16–1.29), fetal growth restriction (OR 1.37; 95% CI 1.30–1.44), and hypertension or preeclampsia (OR 1.60; 95% CI 1.30–1.96). Other occupational exposures significantly associated with preterm birth include prolonged standing (OR 1.26; 95% CI 1.13–1.40) and shift and night work (OR 1.24; 95% CI 1.06–1.46).[161] It appears that interventions to reduce physical exertion among pregnant women could improve birth outcomes.[161–164] Exposure to magnetic fields emitted by video display

SUMMARY OF MANAGEMENT OPTIONS

Work and Pregnancy

Management Options	Evidence Quality and Recommendation	References
Precautions to protect women against specific occupational risks (e.g., toxic chemicals or radiation).	IV/C	157
Avoid long hours of standing and walking.	Ia/B	157
Avoid excess lifting and exercise.	Ia/B	161
Patients can continue to work if they wish and are not unduly tired.	Ia/B	161,163
There is no evidence that video display units (VDUs) are associated with adverse pregnancy outcome.	III/B	165,166

SUMMARY OF MANAGEMENT OPTIONS
Air Travel in Pregnancy

Management Options	Evidence Quality and Recommendation	References
Long-distance air travel is safe in normal pregnancy.	IV/C	167,171
Long-distance flights are not recommended for women <36 weeks' gestation with singleton pregnancies and <32 weeks' gestation with multiple pregnancies.	IV/C	171
Air travel is not recommended for infants younger than 7 days.	IV/C	167
Update travelers on routine immunizations, including tetanus, diphtheria, polio, measles, mumps, rubella, hepatitis A and B, and influenza vaccines. Other immunizations are based on geographic risk.	IV/C	180
Travel is not recommended during pregnancy for women with medical or obstetric problems that could result in emergencies.	IV/C	171
Preventive measures (e.g., supportive stockings, periodic movement of lower extremities) minimize thromboembolic risk. Additional prophylaxis is advised in those with increased thromboembolic risk (see Chapter 42).	Ib/A	171,177
Travelers should take steps to prevent mosquito bites in malarial endemic areas.	Ia/A	182
Antimalaria prophylaxis in pregnancy significantly reduces the likelihood of severe maternal anemia and low birth weight.	Ia/A	183
Malaria should be suspected in all patients who have symptoms after traveling to an area where malaria is endemic.	III/B	184
See also Chapter 32 for Malaria.		

terminals is not a risk to the reproductive health of women or their children.[165,166]

Management Options

A careful workplace history should be taken, including level of activity, hazardous exposures, and ease of workplace modification.[162] Precautions should be taken to protect women from specific occupational health risks, such as exposure to toxic chemicals or radiation.[157] Women whose work is physically or emotionally demanding should be monitored carefully throughout pregnancy for evidence of hypertension, intrauterine growth restriction, and symptoms of preterm labor.[161] It is important for health care professionals, family members, and employers to recognize the potential negative effect of adverse working conditions on pregnancy outcome.

The ultimate decision on continuation of employment during pregnancy should be made by the pregnant woman after careful counseling by her physician, involving the company medical officer and the employer, when indicated.

Air Travel in Pregnancy

General

Little evidence exists on this topic, and recommendations are typically based on common sense rather than scientific evidence.[167]

Risks

RADIATION EXPOSURE

The annual exposure dose limit for a member of the general public is 1 millisievert (mSv). The occupational limit is 5 mSv. Cosmic radiation exposure during high-altitude flight is less than 0.005 mSv/hr.[168] Thus, it takes about 200 flight hours to reach the annual dose limit for the general public. There is less exposure with shorter flights and lower altitudes. Airlines usually restrict commercial airline crew members from long-haul flights once pregnancy is diagnosed.

FETAL AND MATERNAL HYPOXIA

On long-distance commercial high-altitude flights (~32,000 ft), cabin pressure is set at the equivalent to an altitude of 6000 feet.[167] Acute ascent to 6000 feet produces transient cardiovascular and pulmonary adaptations (decreased heart rate, increased blood pressure, decreased aerobic capacity and partial oxygen pressure).[169,170] These changes should not affect women with uneventful pregnancies, but it may affect those with oxygen-dependent conditions. Such pregnant women either should not travel or should receive supplemental oxygen during air travel.[167,171]

VENOUS THROMBOSIS

There is a link between long-distance air travel and deep venous thrombosis and the risk is not confined to those

TABLE 2–4
Vaccination in Pregnancy

VACCINE	USE IN PREGNANCY	COMMENTS
Bacille Calmette-Guérin	No	
Cholera	Yes, administer if indicated	Avoid unless high risk
Hepatitis A	Yes, administer if indicated	Safety not determined
Hepatitis B	Yes, administer if indicated	Safety not determined
Influenza	Yes, administer if indicated	Consult a physician
Japanese encephalitis	Yes, administer if indicated	Avoid unless high risk
Measles	No	
Meningococcal disease	Yes, administer if indicated	
Mumps	No	
Poliomyelitis	Yes, administer if indicated	Normally avoided
Rubella	No	
Tetanus and diphtheria	Yes, administer if indicated	
Rabies	Yes, administer if indicated	
Typhoid	Yes, administer if indicated	Avoid unless high risk
Varicella	No	
Yellow fever	Yes, administer if indicated	Avoid unless high risk

From World Health Organization: International travel and health. Vaccine-preventable diseases. Available at www.who.int/ith/chapter06_16.html; and Thomas RE: Preparing patients to travel abroad safely: Part 2. Updating vaccinations. Can Fam Physician 2000;46:646–652, 655–656.

traveling in economy. The risk, however, appears small and is largely confined to those with additional risk factors.[172–176] There are insufficient scientific data on which to base specific recommendations for prevention, other than leg exercise and the use of elastic compression stockings.[177]

PRETERM LABOR

Air travel does not increase the risk of preterm labor, however, ACOG recommendations suggest that pregnant women with evidence of preterm labor or who are at increased risk for preterm birth should avoid long-distance air travel on empirical grounds.[171]

SEAT BELTS

Advice for airline seat belt use is the same as that for cars. One study showed that the likelihood of adverse pregnancy outcome among belted pregnant women who were involved in a passenger car accident is comparable with that of those who were not pregnant.[178] Because air turbulence cannot be predicted and this risk of trauma is not trivial, pregnant women are advised to use their seat belts continuously while seated.[171]

VACCINES

Live vaccines carry the greatest fetal risk. The World Health Organization advises that administration of live attenuated measles, mumps, rubella, bacillus Calmette-Guérin, and yellow fever virus vaccines should be avoided in pregnancy (Table 2–4).[179,180] Otherwise, the risks and benefits of vaccination should be examined in each case.[181]

MALARIA PROPHYLAXIS

This is addressed in Chapter 32.

SUGGESTED READINGS

Barker DJP, Eriksson JG, Forsén T, Osmonda C: Fetal origins of adult disease: Strength of effects and biological basis. Int J Epidemiol 2002;31:1235–1239.

Dodd JM, Anderson ER, Gates S: Surgical techniques for uterine incision and uterine closure at the time of caesarean section. Cochrane Database Syst Rev 2008;3:CD004732.

Eichholzer M, Tönz O, Zimmermann R: Folic acid: A public-health challenge. Lancet 2006;367:1352–1361.

Figà-Talamanca I: Reproductive health and occupational hazards among women workers. In Kane P (ed): Women and Occupational Health: Issues and Policy Paper for the Global Commission of Women's Health. Geneva, WHO Press, 2003, pp 65–73. Available at http://www.who.int/oeh/OCHweb/OCHweb/OSHpages/OSHDocuments/Women/WomenOccupHealth.pdf

Harvey EL, Glenny A-M, Kirk SFL, Summerbell CD: Improving health professionals' management and the organisation of care for overweight and obese people: Cochrane review. In Cochrane Library. Oxford, UK, Update Software, Issue 2, 2003.

Heijmans BT, Tobi EW, Stein AD, et al: Persistent epigenetic differences associated with prenatal exposure to famine in humans. Proc Natl Acad Sci U S A 2008;105:17046–17049.

Kramer MS, Séguin L, Lydon J, Goulet L: Socio-economic disparities in pregnancy outcome: Why do the poor fare so poorly? Paediatr Perinat Epidemiol 2000;14:194–210.

Schlüssel MM, de Souza EB, Reichenheim ME, Kac G: Physical activity during pregnancy and maternal-child health outcomes: A systematic literature review. Cad Saude Publica. 2008;24(Suppl 4):s531–s544.

World Health Organization: Pregnancy, Childbirth, Postpartum and Newborn Care: A Guide for Essential Practice. Geneva, WHO

Press, 2006. Available at http://whqlibdoc.who.int/publications/2006/924159084X_eng.pdf

World Health Organization: International Travel and Health. Situation as of 1 January 2009. Geneva, WHO Press, 2009. Available at http://www.who.int/ith/ITH_2009.pdf

REFERENCES

For a complete list of references, log onto www.expertconsult.com.

CHAPTER 3

Domestic Violence

LORAINE J. BACCHUS and SUSAN BEWLEY

INTRODUCTION

Since the late 1990s there has been growing awareness of the importance of domestic violence as a public health issue. Obstetricians, gynecologists, and midwives have a key role in identifying women who are experiencing domestic violence; documenting the abuse; and ensuring that appropriate advice, support, and interventions are offered. Domestic violence is one part of a spectrum of human rights abuses against women and girls. It includes rape and sexual abuse, sexual harassment and intimidation at work, "honor killings," female genital mutilation, trafficking of children and women for prostitution, and systematic rape as a tool of war. Gender-based violence is predominantly inflicted by men upon women and girls. It reflects and reinforces inequalities between men and women and adversely affects the health, dignity, safety, and autonomy of those affected.

"Domestic abuse" is defined by the U.K. Home Office as "Any incident of threatening behaviour, violence or abuse (psychological, physical, sexual, financial or emotional) between adults who are or have been intimate partners or family members, regardless of gender or sexuality."[1] Throughout this chapter. the terms *domestic violence* and *domestic abuse* are used interchangeably on pragmatic grounds. Both terms have been used by academics and health professionals in their work on the topic both inside and outside the United Kingdom.

Domestic violence is rarely an isolated incident and the abusive behavior often begins insidiously, growing more oppressive and harmful with time.[2] In most cases, violence is directed toward a woman by her male partner.[3] Women are more likely than men to sustain physical injuries, experience repeated assaults, report fear and emotional distress, and seek medical attention as a result of the violence.[4] This chapter deals with violence by men against female partners in pregnancy.

PREVALENCE

The 2006/2007 British Crime Survey reported that 28% of women had experienced domestic abuse at some point in their lives, with 21% threats or force and 24% sexual assault. The prevalence of any partner abuse in the past year was 5.9%.[5] Similar rates have been reported in surveys from Canada[6] and the United States.[7] Higher rates of domestic violence (≤40%) have been reported in clinical settings.[8,9]

In most cases of domestic violence that are identified in pregnancy, there is preexisting violence that continues throughout the pregnancy and following the baby's birth.[10] However, domestic violence may also begin pregnancy.[11] The prevalence of domestic violence in pregnancy is reported to be between 3%[12] and 33.7%,[13] with the greatest risk occurring during the postpartum period.[14,15] Higher rates of violence during pregnancy have been found among pregnant teenagers.[16,17] Thus, domestic violence is more common than many obstetric complications such as preeclampsia.

Domestic violence also contributes to maternal mortality—either directly or indirectly, for example, by impeding access to care. The 2003–2005 Confidential Enquiries into Maternal Deaths in the United Kingdom[18] reported the deaths of 19 pregnant or recently delivered women who were murdered. Seventy of 295 women who died from all causes (i.e., 14% of all maternal deaths) had documented features of domestic abuse, including 4 women with genital mutiliation or cutting.

RECOGNITION

Significant associations with domestic violence include:

Psychosocial Factors

- Mental health issues such as depression, suicidal ideation, self-harming, post-traumatic stress disorder, and anxiety.[19–24]
- Alcohol and substance misuse is associated with both the experience and the perpetration of domestic violence.[14,25,26]

Behavioral Factors

- Unwanted pregnancy or rapid repeat pregnancy (within 24 months).[27,28]
- Increased parity and younger age at first pregnancy.[29,30]

Contact with Health Services

- Frequent use of health care services, requiring treatment for injuries and symptoms resulting from the violence.[31–33]
- Late initiation of antenatal care.[34]

Interactions with Partner Indicative of a Controlling Relationship

- The partner may accompany the woman to all her antenatal appointments, taking a keen interest, holding the maternity notes, or answering questions directed at her, or may appear reluctant to leave the woman alone with a health professional.[35]
- Noncompliance with treatment regimens, lack of independent transportation, and difficulties in communicating by telephone.[35]
- Where domiciliary care is available, health professionals can experience difficulties in gaining access.[36–38]

Clinical Presentations

- The woman's explanation for how an injury occurred seems implausible.
- Forced sex that can lead to infection of perineal sutures and delay the healing process.[39]
- Difficulties occurring while conducting pelvic examinations prenatally or during labor, with the woman becoming distressed, withdrawn, or even hostile. This may be significant when a woman requests a female health professional for such examinations.

Although the presence of these risk factors and indicators may raise a health professional's index of suspicion, no single factor will accurately identify which women are likely to be affected by domestic violence. Abused women may present with a range of these symptoms and behaviors or none at all (Table 3–1).

RISKS

Maternal Risks

Women who experience domestic violence have significantly poorer health outcomes than nonabused women including

- Chronic pain[40] (e.g., headaches, backaches, pelvic pain), hearing or vision problems,[41] sleep disturbance, poor appetite,[42] and gastrointestinal disorders such as irritable bowel syndrome.[43] These effects may be caused directly by recurrent physical or sexual injury or indirectly from underlying stress.[44]
- Gynecologic problems (e.g., sexually transmitted infections, urinary tract infections, pelvic inflammatory disease, vaginal bleeding, menstrual irregularities, genital irritation, and pain during intercourse).[44,45]
- Depression,[46] especially after delivery when domestic violence may get worse.[14,15,47]

Fetal and Neonatal Risks

These include

- Low birth weight babies.[48,49]
- Trauma to the abdomen may result in placental abruption, premature rupture of membranes, preterm labor, miscarriage, and fetal death.[50–52]
- Bruising, fractures, hemorrhaging, and deformity.[53]

MANAGEMENT OPTIONS

General

In recognition of the serious health implications of domestic violence, in the United Kingdom, the Royal College of Midwives[35] and the Royal College of Obstetricians and Gynaecologists[54] have published guidelines for the identification and support of women affected by domestic violence. The Department of Health[55] has also produced a domestic abuse handbook for health care professionals in which they recommend that "all Trusts should be working towards routine enquiry and providing women with information on domestic abuse support services. It is important to take the initiative and be proactive." Similarly, the American Medical Association[36] and the American College of Obstetricians and Gynecologists[56] have developed guidelines for health practitioners in North America. The 2003–2005 Confidential Enquiries into Maternal Deaths in the United Kingdom recommend that "once multi-agency support services are in place ... routine enquiries should be made about domestic abuse, either when taking a social history at booking, or at another opportune point during a woman's antenatal period."[18]

TABLE 3–1
Physical Signs and Injuries Associated with Domestic Violence

Head, neck, or facial injuries	Multiple bruises or lacerations in various stages of healing
Back, chest, or abdominal pain or tenderness	Patterned injuries that show the imprint of the object used
Injuries to the breasts, abdomen, or genitals	Burns from cigarettes, appliances, rope, or friction
Vaginal bleeding or discharge, sexually transmitted infections, genital injuries	Scalding from boiling water
Dizziness, black outs	Strangulation marks
Numbness	Fractures
Injuries to the extremities	Broken bones
Delay in seeking treatment	Knife wounds
Premature removal of and infection of perineal sutures	Dental injuries (e.g., broken or lost teeth)
Distress, aggression, or withdrawn behavior during pelvic examinations, labor, and delivery	Hair loss consistent with hair pulling
Partial loss of hearing or vision	Bite marks or scratches

SUMMARY OF MANAGEMENT OPTIONS

Domestic Violence

Management Options (Any Stage of Pregnancy or the Postpartum)	Evidence Quality and Recommendation	References
Stage 1: Awareness and Recognition		
Increase awareness and recognition of domestic violence and its health effects through training and education.	III/B	70,72,73
Develop guidelines for identifying and supporting women affected by domestic violence, in conjunction with other health professionals and community groups.	IV/C	55,73
Stage 2: Provision of Safe Environment		
Provide the woman with a safe and private environment away from partners, family, or friends.	IV/C	35,55,73
Stage 3: Identification and Aiding Disclosure		
When language translation is required, arrange for independent professional interpreters, preferably female.	IV/C	35,55
Ask direct questions about domestic violence, routinely.	III/B	61,74,75
Adopt a supportive and nonjudgmental response.	IV/C	35,55,73
Stage 4: Documenting the Abuse		
Document the abuse and any interventions offered in the confidential maternity record.	IV/C	35,55,73
Stage 5: Safety Assessment, Information Giving, and Ongoing Support		
Offer referral information about advocacy organizations that provide immediate and long-term support to women and children affected by domestic violence.*	Ib/A	62,63*
Assess the immediate safety of the woman and any children.	IV/C	35,55
Provide ongoing support and monitoring at subsequent appointments, ensuring continuity of care wherever possible.	IV/C	35,55
Display and disseminate information about local and national domestic violence organizations and other helpful agencies so that it is accessible to users and providers of maternity services.	IV/C	35,55
Work in partnership with local multiagency domestic violence initiatives.	IV/C	35,73

* Little experimental work on interventions in health care settings, but one community-based randomized controlled trial in a nonpregnant population showed a reduction in violence, decreased difficulty in obtaining community resources, and a higher quality of life at 2 years in the intervention group that received advocacy compared with the control group.[62,63]

Five key stages to the clinical management of domestic violence are applicable to any stage of the pregnancy and postpartum period[35,55]:

- Awareness and recognition of domestic violence.
- Provision of a safe and quiet environment.
- Identification and aiding disclosure.
- Documenting the abuse.
- Safety assessment, information giving, and ongoing support.

Stage 1: Awareness and Recognition of Domestic Violence

All health professionals providing care for pregnant women should be aware of the potential indicators (see earlier) of domestic violence and the maternal and fetal risks. Women may present with a range of physical and emotional indicators or none at all. Although these indicators may increase the index of suspicion, if abuse is suspected, inquiry about domestic violence should be made using stages 2 and 3.

Stage 2: Provision of a Safe and Quiet Environment

The woman should be provided with a safe and quiet environment before any inquiry about domestic violence takes place. Maternity services must have management policies and guidelines that ensure women will have confidential time with health professionals, both at booking and during other stages of pregnancy. Strategies for creating individual private consulting time may include requesting to see the woman alone as a routine procedure, asking the partner to wait outside at the end of the appointment to conduct a physical examination, or taking the woman to another part of the clinic for a urine sample, blood test, or weight check. In suspicious cases, for example, a "check up" after "a fall" with an overbearing accompanying partner, admission for observation might be suggested to ensure private time. Issues of safety and confidentiality should be paramount when working with women experiencing domestic violence. Anecdotally, children as young as 2 years may report back to the partner or family members that abuse was discussed. The woman should be reassured that any information she provides will not be shared with her partner, family members, or friends. However, the woman must be advised about the limitations of confidentiality with regards to sharing information with other professionals involved in her care. If the woman does not feel safe discussing the violence in depth with her partner waiting nearby, it may be preferable to make another appointment at a time when the partner is unable to attend. Health professionals working in the community could offer to meet women at the clinic or at the home of a trusted friend or family member. If a woman has hearing difficulties or her first language is not English, arrange for an independent professional interpreter, preferably female, to be present. Family or friends should never be asked to translate when discussing domestic violence.

Occasionally, a health professional may become aware that a child or other vulnerable person living with the abused woman is also at risk of harm. Child protection procedures should be followed. The other exceptional circumstance in which confidentiality may be breached is when the health professional becomes aware that a victim of domestic violence is at risk of serious harm or death from a violent partner (see "Safety Assessment, Information Giving, and Ongoing Support," later). Any referrals to social services should be discussed with the mother and her consent and cooperation sought.[57] Much more is likely to be achieved by working openly with the woman and reassuring her that social services are able to support her in protecting herself and her children. Any information disclosed to a third party without consent should be the minimum necessary to secure the best interests of the woman and her children.[57]

Stage 3: Identification and Aiding Disclosure

Studies conducted in a range of health care settings have shown that the use of direct questions about domestic violence, asked routinely of all patients, increases the rate of detection.[58] Evidence shows that the majority of women find routine inquiry for domestic violence during health care appointments acceptable.[8,9]

A woman's willingness to discuss the abuse will partly depend on the approach of the health professional, and disclosure is more likely if a sensitive and nonjudgmental manner is adopted. Simply asking about domestic violence can be an important intervention in itself, by reducing the stigma attached to it and directing women to sources of help.[59,60] Important principles are to listen and offer validation of the woman's experiences, to acknowledge the seriousness of the situation, and to emphasize that she does not have to deal with it by herself.

It is recommended that the health professional begin by asking a few open-ended questions before following up with specific questions about abuse. For example:

"How are things at home?"

"Are you getting the support you need?"

"Is there anything you are unhappy about?"

This will help to establish some degree of rapport with the woman.[35,54] Women often talk tangentially around the issue of domestic violence, for example, referring to feeling "stressed," overwhelmed, not coping, financial worries, or housing problems. When asking directly about domestic violence, the question should be framed in a way that conveys you recognize domestic violence is an important health issue and difficult to talk about. For example:

"Many women I see experience some form of emotional or physical abuse from their partner, but find it difficult to bring the subject up themselves, so I ask everyone about it."

This can be followed up with one or more direct questions appropriate to the situation. For example:

"Do you ever feel afraid of your partner?"

"Do you and your partner argue or fight? Do the arguments get physical?"

"I've noticed a number of bruises/cuts/scratches; has someone at home hurt you?"

"Some women tell me that their partners are cruel, sometimes emotionally and sometimes physically hurting them—is this happening to you?"

"Does your partner ever treat you badly such as shout at you, constantly call you names, push you around, or threaten you?"

If a woman makes a disclosure of abuse, stages 4 and 5 should be followed. If a woman tells you that she has not been abused, it is important to accept her response even if you suspect otherwise because this conveys respect. However, it is important to allow the opportunity for future disclosure by reminding her that she can talk to you about any concerns or problems at home at any time. It has been demonstrated that repeated inquiry about domestic violence increases the detection rate and can facilitate detection of violence that begins later in pregnancy.[61]

Robust evidence regarding the potential benefits and harmful outcomes of interventions based in health care settings is limited and what evidence does exist originates from North America. One U.S. randomized controlled trial found that domestic violence advocacy intervention can reduce the levels of violence up to 2 years postintervention[62] and lead to improvements in social support and quality of life[63] up to 3 years postintervention. However, with the exception of a few studies conducted in antenatal settings,[64–66] most of the evidence is based on samples of women who had already disclosed partner violence and were actively seeking help from professional services.[67,68] In a recent systematic review of the evidence for screening interventions, the authors state that although there is enough evidence to justify access to advocacy services for survivors of partner violence in general, the evidence is weakest for women who are identified through screening by health professionals.[67]

Health professionals have a key role in providing women with information about services and options available to them, assessing current and future risk, and documenting the abuse. Maternity services can raise public awareness of domestic violence as an important health issue and convey the message that violence of any kind is unacceptable. Posters and leaflets about domestic violence and support services should be placed in clinic waiting rooms and areas where women will be able to access the information safely (e.g., the toilets, baby-changing rooms). These should be available in a range of languages that reflect the local community.

Stage 4: Documenting the Abuse

The medical records of treatment for any injuries or symptoms resulting from the violence are important documents. Women experiencing domestic violence are often required to provide evidence of the abuse when seeking help from agencies (e.g., housing, divorce proceedings, obtaining injunctions, or prosecution of the perpetrator), and medical evidence can be important to support her statement. Documentation is also important to ensuring the flow of information to other health professionals involved in the woman's care, which will facilitate ongoing support and monitoring. Inform the woman of the benefits of documentation, even if she does not wish to take immediate action.[35,54] To maintain the woman's safety and confidentiality, domestic violence should never be recorded in places accessible to her partner (e.g., in hand-held maternity records) but placed in a separate record that is kept in the clinic or hospital.[35,55] An agreed plan of action that can be followed up by the midwife or doctor at a later date may also be useful. Without a follow-up plan, the woman may feel that she has not been listened to.[35] Clear and accurate notes are important, including

- Date and time that the abuse took place.
- Where the incident occurred.
- Name and relationship of the perpetrator to the woman.
- Any new or old injuries sustained including psychological symptoms; information, advice, or treatment offered; and whether the woman accepted this.
- A body map picture can be used to indicate the location of any injuries sustained.[69] Alternatively offer the services of medical photography in the hospital.

Injuries consistent with domestic violence that are explained implausibly should also be documented in the confidential records. Records should be signed and dated by the health professional. Remember to check and gain the woman's permission to share the information with other relevant health professionals, emphasizing that information will be shared only on a "need to know" basis.

Stage 5: Safety Assessment, Information Giving, and Ongoing Support

The immediate safety of the mother and her children should be assessed by asking whether it is safe for her to return home. Inform the woman of her options and of the specialist domestic violence services in and out of her area that can provide emergency help and long-term support.[55] Provide written information about domestic violence organizations and other support services, after confirming that it is safe for her to take the information away with her. Discreet credit-sized cards may be preferable. The woman may prefer to use a telephone in a private room to contact the agencies herself, if she cannot do this at home. It is always best to encourage the woman to talk to the agencies herself so that she is in control of her sources of help and gains confidence in explaining her situation and asking for help. Health professionals can best facilitate the woman's exploration of her options by maintaining a supportive position but avoiding personal and emotional investment in the choices she makes.

A variety of emotional and situational factors make leaving an abusive relationship difficult, and women often return to their partners several times before terminating the relationship. Isolation from friends and family, lack of self-esteem, self-blame, financial hardship, inappropriate accommodation, and living in constant fear of retaliation by the partner are just some of the challenges women encounter when ending an abusive relationship. Other factors that may undermine the woman's capacity to initiate change or increase her dependence on her partner include alcohol and substance misuse, mental health issues, pregnancy, having dependent children, and cultural or religious values that emphasize family and marriage over the woman's well-being.[27]

It is suggested that each woman is provided with a mutually agreed safety plan that can be modified over time.[35,55] However, each item on the safety plan should be achievable. This may include

- Making a list of important phone numbers, including emergency numbers that can be called at any time of the day or night (e.g., emergency housing, National Domestic Violence Helpline).
- Identifying a trusted friend or family member that the woman can stay with in an emergency.
- Leaving a bag packed with clothes, medicines, other essential items with a trusted friend or family member.
- Having money for bus, train, cab fares.
- Getting an extra set of house and car keys.
- Taking original copies or photocopies of any important legal and financial papers (e.g., passport, birth and marriage certificate, bank book, rent book, credit cards).

If the woman agrees to being referred to a specialized domestic violence service, the health professional can offer to speak to someone from the organization to make an introduction, give basic details of the situation, and identify any needs. It is good practice to ensure that, wherever possible, the woman is given the option of seeing the same health professional at subsequent appointments.[35] Reconciliation work with the couple should not be attempted, because this may jeopardize the safety of both the woman and the health professional.

CONCLUSION

Domestic violence is a complex issue, and health professionals should not work in isolation because many local and national initiatives offer expertise on the subject. Therefore, health professionals should equip themselves with the skills and knowledge necessary to provide an informed response to women affected by violence by requesting and accessing opportunities for training and education.

SUGGESTED READINGS

Bacchus L, Aston G, Torres Vitolas C, et al: A Theory-Based Evaluation of a Multi-Agency Domestic Violence Service Based in Maternity and Genitourinary Medicine Services at Guy's & St. Thomas' NHS Foundation Trust. London, Kings College London, 2009. Available at http://www.kcl.ac.uk/schools/nursing/research/themes/women/projects/maternal/domesticviolence.html

Bewley S, Friend J, Mezey G (eds): Violence Against Women. London, Royal College of Obstetricians and Gynaecologists Press, 1997.

British Medical Association: Domestic Violence: A Health Care Issue? London, British Medical Association Science. London, Department and the Board of Science and Education, 1998, pp 51–52.

Bybee DI, Sullivan CM: Predicting re-victimisation of battered women 3 years after exiting a shelter program. Am J Community Psychol 2005;36:85–96.

Department of Health: Responding to Domestic Abuse. A Handbook for Health Professionals. London, DOH, 2006.

Feder G, Ramsay J, Dunne D, et al: How far does screening women for domestic (partner) violence in different health-care settings meet criteria for a screening programme? Systematic reviews of nine UK National Screening Committee criteria. London, UK Health Technology Assessment Programme, 2009. Available at: http://www.hta.ac.uk/1501

Lewis G, Clutton-Brock T, Cooper G, et al: Saving Mother's Lives: Reviewing Maternal Deaths to Make Motherhood Safer—2003 to 2005. The Seventh Report of the Confidential Enquiries into Maternal Deaths in the United Kingdom. London, CEMACH, 2007, pp 173–179.

Ramsay J, Rivas C, Feder G: Interventions to reduce violence and promote the physical and psychological well-being of women who experience partner violence: A systematic review of controlled evaluations. London, Department of Health, 2005, p 43.

Royal College of Midwives: Domestic Abuse: Pregnancy, Birth and the Puerperium. Guidance Paper No. 5. London, RCM, 2006.

Sheridan DJ: Forensic documentation of battered pregnant women. J Nurse Midwifery 1996;41:467–472.

REFERENCES

For a complete list of references, log onto www.expertconsult.com.

CHAPTER 4

Genetics, Risks of Recurrence, and Genetic Counseling

PETER A. FARNDON and MARK D. KILBY

INTRODUCTION

An abnormal fetal phenotype can be caused by environmental factors, chromosomal anomalies, specific genes, or more complex genetic mechanisms.

Because families with single-gene disorders or parental chromosomal anomalies are at the greatest risk, it is important to identify couples from such families before they undertake pregnancy. An assessment of a couple's probability can often be made by a combination of pedigree analysis, precise clinical diagnosis, and genetic testing, which is available for a large number of conditions.

Particular pointers that might suggest that a couple is at increased probability of having a child with an anomaly include

- A previous child affected with a single-gene disorder.
- A family history of a single-gene disorder.
- A parent with a chromosomal anomaly.
- Structural anomalies found on ultrasound examination.

DETERMINING THE GENETIC BASIS OF A CONDITION

To ensure that a family receives accurate genetic information, it is recommended that the following steps are undertaken:

- Record and examine the family tree to detect a pattern of inheritance.
- Refine and confirm the diagnosis by clinical examination and testing.
- Perform karyotype analysis or DNA testing, as appropriate.
- Assess the genetic risks to family members.
- Explain the genetic information to the family (*genetic counseling*).
- Discuss the available options.
- Support the family while they make decisions appropriate to their situation.

IDENTIFYING FAMILIES WITH AN INCREASED PROBABILITY OF A GENETIC CONDITION

The couple may have realized that the family tree suggests a genetic condition and volunteer this information. In other cases, a high risk is appreciated only when a formal history is taken.

The best and easiest way to record genetic information is to draw a pedigree. The standard notation is shown in Figure 4–1. Guidelines include

- Create the tree from the "bottom," starting with the affected child and siblings, including the names of the children and their dates of birth, in order of age.
- Choose one parent (usually the mother) and ask about her siblings and their children, and then her parents, moving from generation to generation.
- Add information about the paternal side of the family.
- Use clear symbols (e.g., circles for females, squares for males). Fill in the symbol if the person is affected.
- Put a sloping line through the symbol (from the bottom left to the top right corner) if the person has died.
- Record all names, dates of birth, and maiden names.
- Ask about miscarriages, stillbirths, or deaths in each partnership: "How many children have you had?" "Have you lost any children?" "Have you had any previous partners?"
- Note parental occupations, medical and drug history, and pregnancy and birth history, especially when a child has a dysmorphic syndrome.
- Record at least basic details for both sides of the family, even when it appears that a condition is segregating on one side.
- Ask about consanguinity: "Are you and your partner related?" "Are there any surnames in common in the family?"
- Date and sign the pedigree.

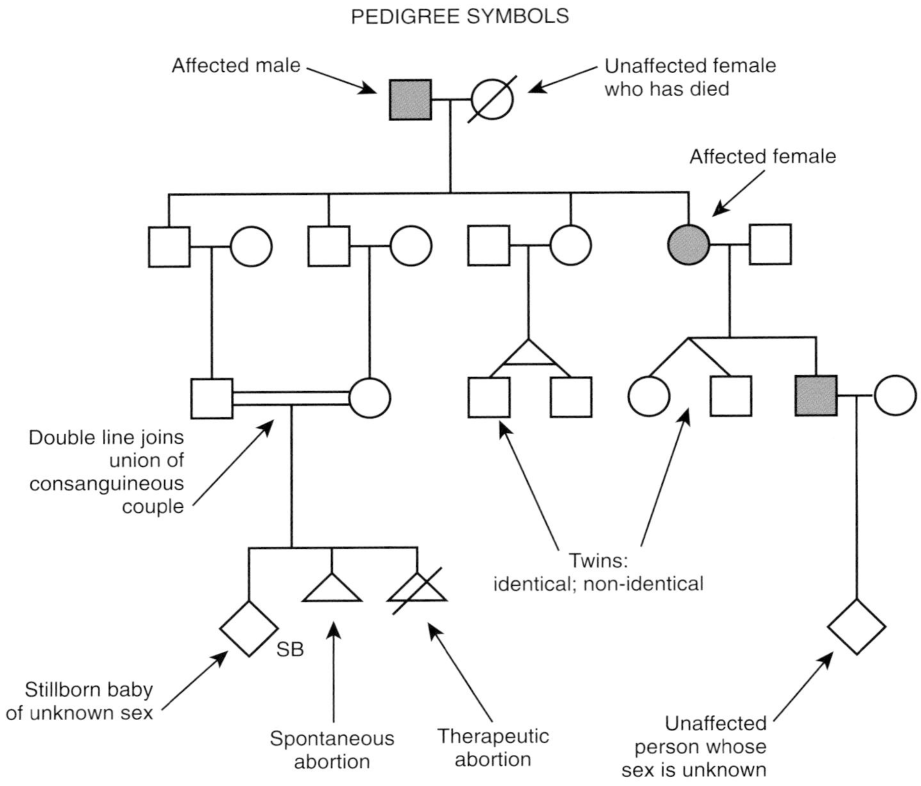

FIGURE 4–1
Symbols used in drawing a pedigree.

When the mode of inheritance is certain from the diagnosis (e.g., a known autosomal recessive condition), it may not be necessary to record personal details about all family members in as much detail as would be required for an unknown condition.

It is strongly recommended that the couple's consent is obtained and documented to share their medical information and test results with professionals and family members, should this be helpful for other family members in the future.

Interpretation of the Genetic Family History

The precise pattern of members with the condition may suggest dominant, recessive, or X-linked inheritance, as discussed later. Inherited chromosomal anomalies may show a pattern of unaffected members having children with multiple anomalies and/or several pregnancy losses (Table 4–1).

Although consanguinity in a family may support the likelihood of an autosomal recessive mode of inheritance, care must be taken to consider and exclude the other modes of inheritance. Sometimes, there may be no family history, but the person who appears to be an isolated case can still have a genetic cause.

Confirmation of the Diagnosis

Accurate genetic information requires a precise diagnosis, which may need to be confirmed by a specialist, who may be able to identify clinical subtypes with different modes of inheritance. Confirmatory documents, such as specialists' letters and laboratory or necropsy results, may also be required. Apparently unaffected individuals may need to be assessed to exclude mild or early disease, especially in autosomal dominant conditions, such as neurofibromatosis, tuberous sclerosis, myotonic dystrophy, retinitis pigmentosa, and adult polycystic kidney disease.

Genetic Counseling

Harper[1] defined genetic counseling as "the process by which patients or relatives at risk of a disorder that may be hereditary are given information about the consequences of the disorder, the probability of developing and transmitting it and the ways in which it may be prevented or ameliorated."

Providing Genetic Counseling

The provision of clinical genetic services varies between countries. In the United Kingdom, medically trained clinical geneticists, supported by a team of genetic counselors, are usually based in tertiary referral centers, but most have clinics in district hospitals.

As part of clinical care, most obstetricians give genetic information about common chromosomal trisomies found at prenatal diagnosis, for instance, but seek advice from a clinical geneticist for DNA diagnosis, familial chromosomal conditions, single-gene disorders, and malformation syndromes.

Giving Genetic Information

Genetic information should be given in a nondirective manner, presenting facts, discussing options, and helping

TABLE 4-1

Establishing the Mode of Inheritance

Autosomal Dominant Inheritance

Males and females affected in equal proportions.
Transmitted from one generation to next ("vertical transmission").
All forms of transmission are observed (i.e., male to male, female to female, male to female, and female to male).

Autosomal Recessive Inheritance

Males and females affected in equal proportions.
Individuals affected in a single sibship in one generation.
Consanguinity in the parents may provide further support.

X-Linked Recessive Inheritance

Males affected almost exclusively.
Transmitted through carrier females to their sons ("knight's move" pattern).
Affected males cannot transmit the condition to their sons.

X-Linked Dominant Inheritance

Males and females are affected but affected females occur more frequently than affected males.
Females are usually less severely affected than males.
Affected females can transmit the condition to male and female children, but affected males transmit the condition only to their daughters, all of whom are affected.

Inherited Chromosomal Anomalies

May give a pattern of unaffected family members having children with multiple anomalies with growth and developmental retardation.
The hallmarks of chromosome anomalies are multiple organ systems affected at different stages in embryogenesis.
May give a pattern of multiple pregnancy losses.

Mitochondrial Inheritance

If all the children of affected mothers are affected, but no children of affected fathers, consider the possibility of mitochondrial inheritance.

An Apparently Isolated Case

Could be caused by a

- Phenocopy (caused solely by environmental factors).
- New dominant mutation.
- More severe expression in a child of a dominant condition in a parent.
- Recessive condition.
- X-linked condition (if a male).
- Chromosome anomaly (either inherited or spontaneous).
- A combination of environmental influences acting on a genetic predisposition.

couples and families to reach their own decisions. It may not be easy to be completely nondirective because the professional's views can affect the tone and manner of presentation of the information. There is no "right" or "wrong" decision; a couple must make a decision that they believe is right for them. Whenever possible, the partners should be seen together when discussing genetic information or anomalies found at prenatal diagnosis.

Timing

Couples who consider themselves to be at potentially high risk for a genetic condition and who have sought genetic information before embarking on a pregnancy have time to decide which option is the most appropriate.

The diagnosis of a serious genetic condition or malformation syndrome during pregnancy may require difficult management decisions to be made relatively quickly. The family may have little time to understand the severity and consequences of the condition, identify the options (including available treatments), and discuss the genetic implications. Families want to know whether the condition is lethal or severely disabling, whether there is a high risk that a future pregnancy will be affected, and whether specific prenatal diagnosis would be available.

Genetic information may play an important role in the consideration of options for future pregnancies and clinical management of the current pregnancy. Options include

- Having no further children.
- Accepting the risk.
- Undertaking prenatal diagnosis, if available.
- Seeking adoption.
- Accepting gamete donation.
- Seeking preimplantation diagnosis.

A couple's choice will depend on many factors, but social, economic, moral, and practical factors appear particularly important.

DETERMINING THE PROBABILITY OF RECURRENCE

The mathematical *risk of recurrence* can usually be derived with certainty for a single-gene (mendelian) condition. For other conditions, empirical figures must be used (see later).

Genetic Risk: Burden and Probability

A genetic *risk* figure has two components: the probability that the condition will occur and the burden of the

SUMMARY OF MANAGEMENT OPTIONS

Genetics, Recurrence Risks, and Genetic Counseling

Management Options	Evidence Quality and Recommendation	References
Population Genetic Screening		
Policies vary on the basis of • Financial constraints. • Prevalence and health burden of the conditions. • Political issues.	IV/C	2,3
If screening is implemented, patients should be given the following information: • Nature of the medical condition. • Mode of inheritance. • Reliability of the screening test. • Procedures for giving results. • Implications for their future, their existing children, and their family members if the screening test result is positive. • Possibility that genetic screening may result in unexpected information being revealed.	IV/C	2,3
General (Prepregnancy, Prenatal, and Postnatal)		
Families with single-gene disorders and parental chromosomal anomalies have the highest risks and may often be detected by taking a family pedigree.	IV/C	1
Adequate time should be made available in a quiet setting that is free from interruptions.	IIa/B	40
Both partners should be seen together whenever possible.	IIb/B	41
Obtain accurate and comprehensive information to make a secure diagnosis, including taking a family pedigree.	IIa/B	40
Provide nondirective and supportive counseling.	III/B	42,43
Ensure that stated probabilities are accurate and up-to-date.	IIa/B	40
What constitutes an "acceptable" probability to an individual varies with the condition because the figure has two components: the probability of occurrence and the burden of disease.	III/B	43
Consider referring complex cases to a clinical geneticist.	III/B	42

condition. Families may view the same mathematical figure entirely differently. For example, for autosomal dominant conditions with a "1 in 2" risk, the family may view the effect of the condition as mild (e.g., brachydactyly) or very severe (e.g., Huntington's disease). Their view may also be affected by whether screening and treatment are available (e.g., bilateral retinoblastoma, adenomatous polyposis coli). Families usually want to discuss such issues during the genetic consultation.

Explaining Risks (See also Chapter 2)

Although some people perceive probabilities only as "high" or "low," most wish to understand how a figure has been reached, and so a discussion about modes of inheritance and mechanisms of genetic disease may be helpful. Expressing a risk figure as a fraction (e.g., 1 in 2, 1/2), as odds (50:50), or as a percentage (50%) is less likely to lead to confusion. The perception of what constitutes a "high" or "low" probability varies with the individual. Some families find it easier to understand probabilities when they are presented as odds, whereas others prefer to discuss these figures as percentages. Most clinical geneticists use both odds and percentages during a consultation, concentrating on the one that the patients find easiest to understand. The decision as to what constitutes an "acceptable" risk varies with the condition and the individual. However, providing some reference points (Table 4–2) may be helpful.

TYPES OF GENETIC CONDITIONS: MECHANISMS AND PROBABILITIES

Humans have approximately 23,000 genes arranged on 23 pairs of chromosomes that allow their physical transmission from cell to cell and generation to generation. Generally, alteration of gene function is the underlying mechanism for single-gene disorders, and alteration of copy number underlies chromosomal conditions. Many isolated congenital anomalies are the result of multifactorial inheritance in

TABLE 4–2

Examples of Approximate Reproductive Risks in Developed Countries

REPRODUCTIVE OUTCOME	RISK ODDS	RISK %
Infertility	1 in 10	10.0
Pregnancy ending in a spontaneous miscarriage	1 in 8	12.5
Perinatal death	1 in 30 to 1 in 100	1.0
Birth of a baby with a congenital abnormality (major and minor)	1 in 30	3.3
Birth of a baby with a serious physical or mental handicap	1 in 50	2.0
Death of a child in the first year after the first week	1 in 150	0.7

which the condition occurs in individuals with a liability above a particular threshold. The liability is composed of *environmental* components that act with a genetic predisposition caused by the summation of the effects of several genes.

CONDITIONS WITH MENDELIAN INHERITANCE: SINGLE-GENE DISORDERS

General

Single-gene (mendelian) disorders behave as though they are under the control of only one pair of genes. They have high probabilities of recurrence. Mendelian inheritance is usually recognized by a combination of clinical diagnosis and the pattern of affected people in the family.

Probabilities of recurrence can usually be determined from knowledge of the mode of inheritance of a particular condition. However, some conditions, such as retinitis pigmentosa, have dominant, recessive, and X-linked forms, so care is needed.

For many mendelian conditions, DNA tests are available for presymptomatic diagnosis, carrier detection, and prenatal diagnosis. Up-to-date information should be sought from a clinical genetics department because advances are too rapid for published literature to remain current. In addition, access to online databases is helpful (see Appendix). Prenatal diagnostic possibilities may have changed by the time a couple is considering having another child.

Autosomal Dominant Inheritance (Fig. 4–2)

A dominant trait manifests in a heterozygote (a person with both the altered and the usual alleles) and is usually transmitted from one generation to the next (*vertical transmission*). Each offspring of a parent with an autosomal dominant condition has a 1 in 2 chance of inheriting the altered allele. Because autosomal dominant traits can exhibit variable expressivity, reduced penetrance, and sex limitation, it may be more difficult to predict the clinical severity in a fetus than would be suggested by the simple probability of 1 in 2 of inheriting the altered allele.

In dominant conditions with variable expression, careful physical examination may be needed to detect the minute

FIGURE 4–2
Single-gene disorders: examples of pedigrees and modes of inheritance. *A*, Autosomal dominant inheritance. Three generations are affected, and male-to-male transmission is shown. *B*, Autosomal dominant inheritance. If one parent has a dominant condition, each offspring has a 50% (1 in 2) probability of inheriting the altered gene.

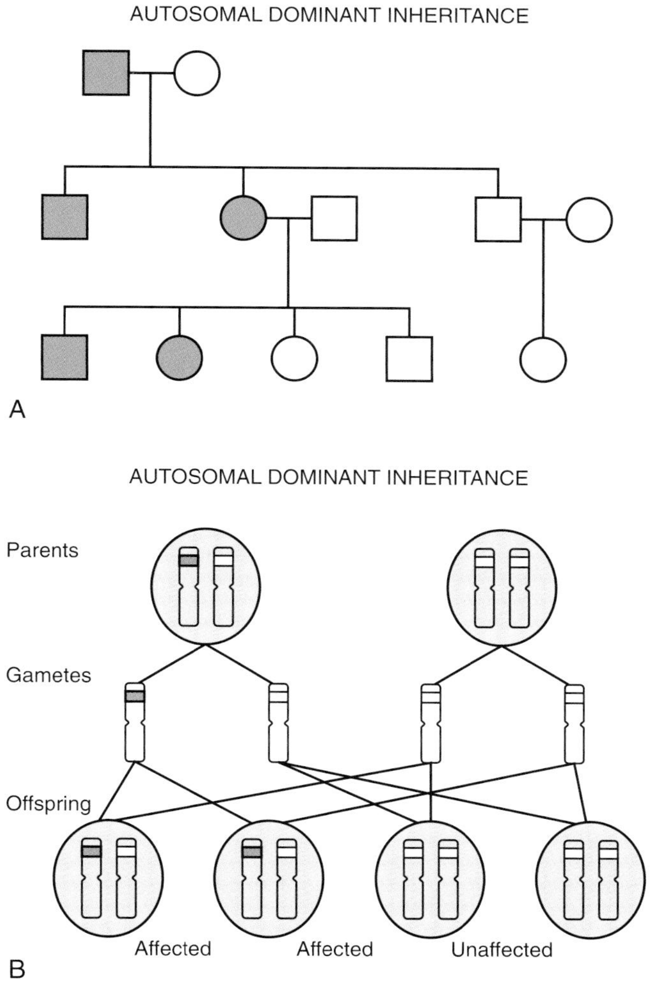

signs that a parent has the altered gene. For example, axillary freckling may be the only sign of neurofibromatosis. Variable expression can also result in a fetus having more severe manifestations of the condition than the affected parent. For example, in myotonic dystrophy, a mother with mild signs can have a child with the severe congenital form of myotonic dystrophy due to an increase in size during maternal transmission of the trinucleotide repeat associated with the condition. In contrast, some dominant conditions show no variation in expression, resulting in all people with the condition having the same phenotype (e.g., achondroplasia).

Very rarely, a person who carries an altered gene for an autosomal dominant condition (with an affected parent and an affected child) has no physical signs of the condition. The allele is said to be *nonpenetrant* in the person who has no clinical signs of the condition.

Some autosomal dominant conditions appear to occur sporadically. If both parents are found to be unaffected after appropriate examinations and investigations, then the child's condition is likely to be the result of a new mutation causing the dominant condition. The probability of recurrence in further children of the parents is low, but not zero, because there is a small probability that a parent of a child with an apparently new dominant mutation has gonadal mosaicism. Gonadal mosaicism—in which a parent has two populations of gonadal cells, one population containing the mutation and one with the normal gene—can explain the rare cases in which unaffected parents have two children with the same autosomal dominant condition.

Autosomal Recessive Conditions (Fig. 4–3)

Autosomal recessive conditions are manifest only in the homozygous state: the affected person has two copies of the altered gene. Heterozygotes (carriers) are healthy. When both parents are heterozygous for the same autosomal recessive condition, each child has a 1 in 4 chance of inheriting the condition. An unaffected sibling of an affected person has a 2 in 3 chance of being a carrier. When someone with an autosomal recessive condition has children, offspring will be at risk of inheriting the condition only if the partner is a carrier for the same autosomal recessive condition.

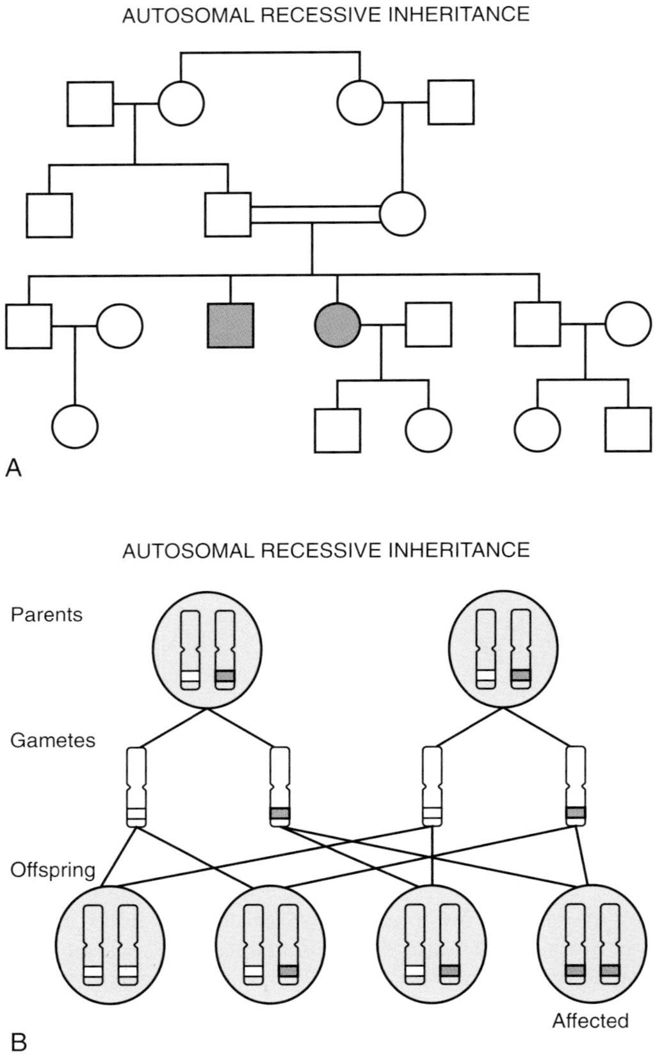

FIGURE 4–3
Single-gene disorders: examples of pedigrees and modes of inheritance. *A*, Autosomal recessive inheritance. Siblings in only one generation are affected. In this family, the parents are first cousins. *B*, Autosomal recessive inheritance. If both parents carry the same altered gene for a recessive condition, each offspring has 25% (1 in 4) probability of inheriting the altered gene from both parents and, therefore, of having the condition.

Carriers for some inborn errors of metabolism can be identified by biochemical tests. Unfortunately, for many conditions, the range of results for carriers overlaps with the range of results for noncarriers; test results generate a probability of being a carrier rather than giving a definitive answer. DNA techniques allow diagnosis of the carrier state for some autosomal recessive conditions in some families. This *genetic testing* is offered when other evidence (usually being closely related to an affected person or a known carrier) suggests that the prior probability is increased.

For some conditions, genetic testing can be offered to populations in which there is a high incidence of carriers, particularly where there are a few common mutations. This *genetic screening* may detect carriers with no known family history and is discussed in more detail later.

Unless the condition is very common or unless consanguinity is present, the probabilities for half-siblings, children of affected individuals, and especially children of unaffected siblings are minimally increased over those of the general population. The precise probability depends on the frequency of heterozygotes in the population and can be calculated using mendelian principles.

If a couple requests sterilization after the birth of a child with a very severe autosomal recessive condition, it is important to discuss sensitively that other forms of contraception are available. This is because, if in the future, either parent were to have children with a new, unrelated partner, the probability of recurrence would likely be very low.

X-Linked Recessive Inheritance (Fig. 4–4)

Although males and females have similar sets of the 22 pairs of autosomes, the sex chromosome pair is different. Females have two X chromosomes, whereas males have one X chromosome and a Y chromosome. X–Linked recessive traits usually manifest only in males because males have a single copy of the genes on the X chromosome. Although females have two copies of the X chromosome, one is inactivated at random early in gestation to ensure equal amounts of gene products from the X chromosome in males and females. In an individual female cell, the genes on either the paternal or the maternal X chromosome are active and most of the genes on the other X chromosome are silenced. Therefore, a female who is heterozygous for an X-linked condition will be a mosaic of cells in which the normal or the altered gene is active, the numbers of each type in a given tissue related to the chance pattern of X inactivation. Carrier detection in X-linked recessive conditions may, therefore, be difficult. For example, approximately 30% of known carriers of Duchenne muscular dystrophy have biochemical carrier test results within the normal range, because, by chance, relatively few of their muscle cells express the altered gene. Reliable techniques for carrier detection are particularly important to determine whether apparently isolated cases of

FIGURE 4–4
Single-gene disorders: examples of pedigrees and modes of inheritance. *A*, X-Linked inheritance. In this family, the grandfather has a nonlethal X-linked condition (e.g., hemophilia). Males affected in several generations are linked through unaffected females. Daughters of affected men are obligatory carriers. *B*, X-Linked recessive inheritance in which a father is affected. If a father has an X-linked condition, all of his daughters will be carriers, but none of his sons will be affected. (Sons inherit his Y chromosome; that is why they are male!) *C*, X-Linked recessive inheritance in which a mother is a carrier. If a woman carries a gene for a recessive condition on one of her X chromosomes, each of her sons has a 1 in 2 probability of being affected and each of her daughters has a 1 in 2 probability of being a carrier.

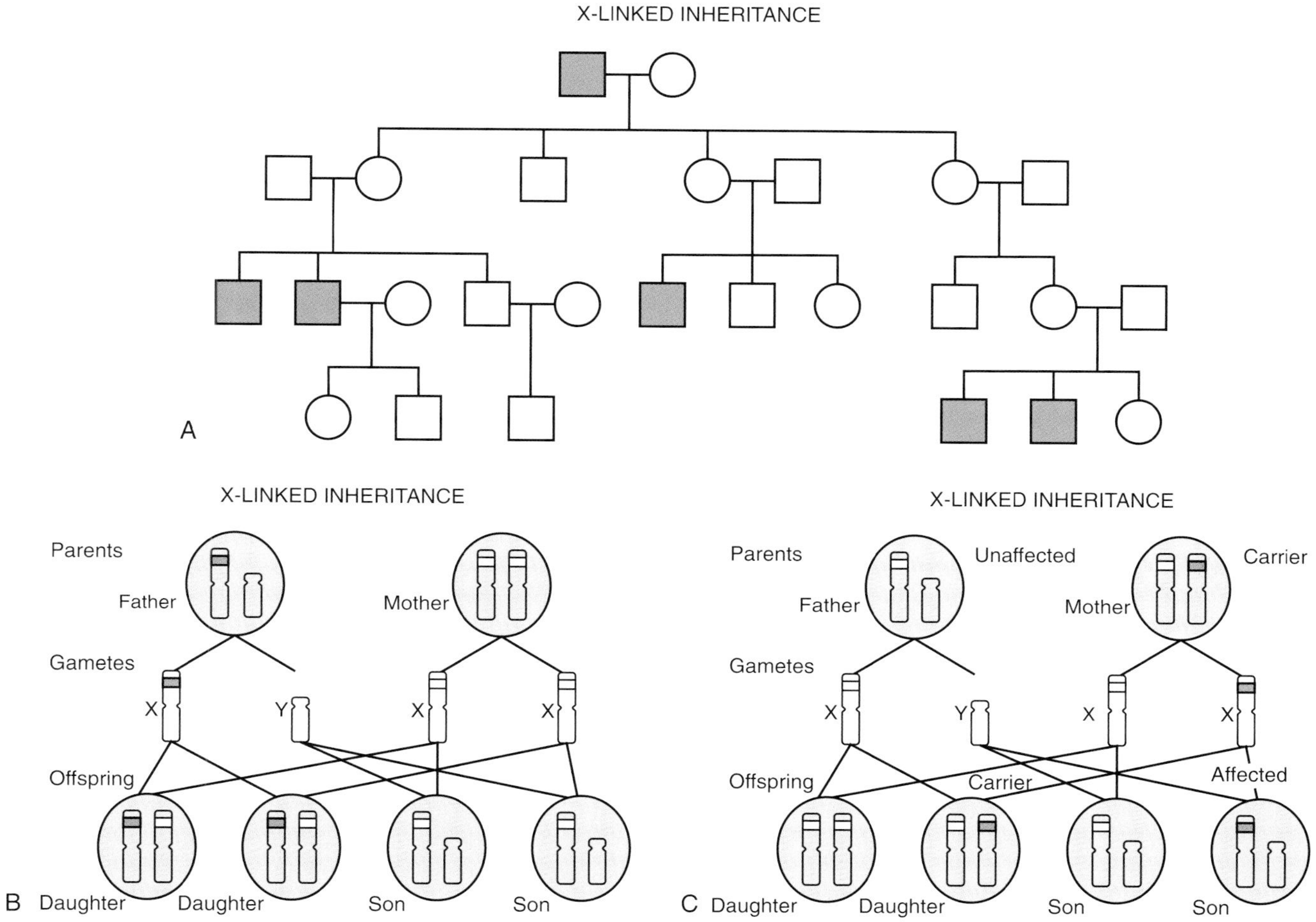

X-linked recessive conditions are the result of a new mutation or whether the mother is a carrier. Fortunately, DNA techniques may be able to answer these questions, either by direct detection of a mutation or by gene tracking (discussed later).

Each son of a woman who is heterozygous for an X-linked recessive condition has a 1 in 2 chance of inheriting the altered allele from his mother and of being affected (see Fig. 4–4*C*). Each daughter has a 1 in 2 chance of inheriting the altered allele, and so of being a carrier, but would be expected to be unaffected. (Women who are carriers for the fragile X mental retardation syndrome can have daughters who are mentally handicapped; because of the complexities involved, patients should be referred for genetic counseling.)

As daughters of males with an X-linked condition inherit their father's X chromosome, they are obligate carriers (see Fig. 4–4*B*).

Rarely, females show signs of an X-linked recessive trait or condition because they are homozygous for the allele (e.g., color blindness), have a single X chromosome (Turner syndrome), have a structural rearrangement of an X chromosome, or are heterozygous with skewed or nonrandom X inactivation.

If male-to-male transmission is observed in a family, then X linkage is excluded.

Unusual Patterns of Inheritance

Unusual inheritance patterns can be explained by phenomena such as genetic heterogeneity, mosaicism, anticipation (i.e., an earlier age at onset in successive generations), imprinting, uniparental disomy (UPD), mitochondrial mutations, and on occasion, mistaken paternity.

GENETIC SCREENING AND TESTING

Genetic screening is a term used when members of a particular population are offered a test for a condition or carrier status when there is no prior evidence of its presence in an individual.

The potential benefits of genetic screening include identifying treatable genetic conditions at an early stage and allowing couples to make informed choices about parenthood. Potential disadvantages include whether or not to communicate information to the family and, when screening is performed in pregnancy, the urgency of deciding about prenatal diagnosis and considering the options available. In the future, it may be possible to identify people who have a genetic susceptibility to common complex conditions, but the advantages of early identification will need to be weighed against possible adverse effects.

Guidelines for genetic screening programs have been recommended by several organizations.[2–5] These are helpful in determining the aims, limitations, scope, and ethical aspects of a genetic screening program as well as considerations for the storage and registration of data or material, the need for follow-up (including social consequences), and the risk of side effects.

People undergoing genetic investigations are entitled to receive sufficient information about what is proposed and about substantial risks in a way they can understand. They should be given time to decide whether or not to agree to what is proposed. They must be free to withdraw at any time.

Specifically, they should receive information about the following:

- Nature of the medical condition.
- Mode of inheritance.
- Reliability of the screening test.
- Procedures for giving results.
- Implications for their future, their existing children, and family members if the result is positive.
- Possibility that genetic screening may result in unexpected information being revealed (e.g., nonpaternity).

The debate in the United Kingdom over population screening for carriers for the autosomal recessive condition cystic fibrosis (CF) illustrates many of these points. The condition is common, with 1 in 25 of the white population in the United Kingdom being a carrier. Routine DNA tests can identify approximately 85% of carriers; these people have the common mutations. A "negative" result for commonly tested mutations does not exclude a member of the population from being a carrier, but greatly reduces the probability. This is in contrast to DNA testing for sickle cell disease which detects all carriers of the altered sickle cell hemoglobin (HbS) allele.

The current program for screening newborns for CF in England focuses on identifying affected individuals. Positive results from screening based on serum immunoreactive trypsinogen measurement are followed by direct gene analysis; the combination of tests has proved to be highly effective.[6] *Cascade genetic testing* for the mutations identified in the family can then be offered to the relatives of people with CF. Compared with other methods, offering testing to relatives of an affected person produces a high ratio of positive test results.

Cascade screening is up to 10 times more powerful than unfocused population screening in detecting carriers.[7] The uptake of CF carrier tests when offered to anyone interested in the general population has been shown to be low, but a high uptake (>70%) did follow an invitation by an interested health professional to be screened during pregnancy. However, screening during pregnancy might not allow people to be fully informed or couples at high risk to have the choice of all options.[8] A "two-step" approach in pregnancy has been studied,[9] in which the woman was tested first and then testing offered to those men whose partner was found to be a carrier. However, considerable anxiety may occur when the woman is shown to be a carrier and the man is not. An alternative procedure is to regard the couple as the screened unit and to provide information on carrier status only when both partners are carriers.[10]

As illustrated in the CF example earlier, the term *genetic testing* is used when an individual is tested for a condition or genetic status that other evidence suggests may be present. This may be to confirm a diagnosis or to test for carrier status within a family. Although the same laboratory procedure is likely to be used for both genetic screening and genetic testing, there are important clinical conceptual differences. Those undergoing genetic testing are likely to have more knowledge about the genetic implications because of their family history. This is unlikely to be the case in a genetic screening program, in which education and information have been shown to be key factors in successful programs (e.g., a carrier screening program for thalassemia in Cyprus, screening for Tay-Sachs disease in Montreal).

Experience shows that the optimal timing of the testing procedure changes as a community becomes more informed. For example, a screening program designed to detect newborns with a recessive condition so that treatment may be instituted might have the effect of encouraging relatives to undergo carrier testing. This can increase awareness of the benefits of antenatal screening and may lead to an offer of testing to couples or individuals in the general population[4] before pregnancy. Some communities encourage individuals leaving school to be tested.[5]

It is widely accepted that genetic testing of children may be offered to confirm a diagnosis or assist treatment in childhood, but that children should not be tested for adult-onset genetic conditions (unless specific preventive measures are available) nor for carrier status until they are old enough to decide whether to undergo testing.[11]

DNA TECHNIQUES AND CLINICAL PRACTICE

Online databases that list DNA tests provided by genetic laboratories are increasingly available. To ensure clinical reliability and validity, it is important to confirm that laboratories that offer testing are part of recognized quality control programs and to ask about the experience of the laboratory with the particular test.

Although recent advantages in DNA sequencing offer the possibility of determining the mutation responsible for a single-gene condition in a family, it is important to tailor the ordering of DNA tests to those clinical situations in which the result is likely to influence management. Such situations include

- Confirmation of the diagnosis, especially when the clinical features can be equivocal.
- Confirmation that a family member has not inherited the condition.
- Carrier testing, especially when biochemical testing is not available or the results are equivocal.

- Presymptomatic diagnosis so that surveillance can be instituted (e.g., familial adenomatous polyposis coli, some types of breast cancer).
- Prenatal diagnosis, especially for conditions for which biochemical or hematologic testing or ultrasound detection of associated structural anomalies were formerly the only possibilities.

DNA diagnosis for some conditions still relies on family studies to "track" the allele for the disease through the family. This may be necessary where the chromosomal location of the gene responsible for the condition is known but the gene itself has not yet been identified. Some genes have a structure that makes direct DNA sequencing more difficult, and until technological difficulties are overcome for these genes, gene tracking may be useful for families. "Gene tracking" is discussed later.

Identifying Families Who May Benefit from DNA Diagnosis

Families are often identified from the pattern of affected members or when a precise diagnosis is made. Each family must be assessed individually because some techniques rely on the family structure and availability of the necessary DNA samples. Therefore, DNA diagnosis may require considerable time. Families are best referred to a clinical genetics unit before pregnancy for completion of the steps outlined in Table 4–3.

The Principles of Diagnosis Using DNA

The Regional Clinical Genetics Service will be able to advise whether gene tracking or sequencing is available for particular conditions.

TABLE 4–3

Practice Points* for Prenatal Diagnosis by DNA Techniques for Single-Gene Conditions

Identify families through:
- Previously affected child
- Carrier screening programs for autosomal recessive conditions
- Family history

Do they wish to proceed to further testing?
Consider the techniques available for prenatal diagnosis:
- Biochemical assays
- Ultrasound
- DNA diagnosis

Is DNA diagnosis possible? Consult the regional Genetics Services. Check before each pregnancy because of the rate of advances.
- Is the clinical diagnosis secure?
- Has the gene been localized or cloned?
- Is the family structure suitable, and are samples available for testing?
- Is sufficient time available for testing?

Explain procedures and the accuracy of results to family.
Collect appropriate samples.
Order laboratory testing:
- Gene tracking
- Direct mutation detection

Explain the results and options.
Proceed with diagnostic testing

* A clinical genetics unit can advise and arrange for much of these. The genetics of some single-gene conditions may be complicated (e.g., retinitis pigmentosa can be inherited as autosomal dominant and autosomal and X-linked recessive).

Following the Inheritance of Genes in a Family to Predict Genetic Status (Gene Tracking)

The aim of gene tracking is to follow the inheritance through a family of a "marker" piece of DNA which is known (from research studies) to be in close physical proximity to the gene causing the condition. These marker sequences of DNA vary naturally in the population (polymorphisms). Markers used include those which vary at one base position (single-nucleotide polymorphisms) and those with a set of alleles each of which varies in length (CA repeat markers). The latter are detected by their different positions on a gel after electrophoresis, as shown in Figure 4–5.

Figure 4–6 shows an example of gene tracking for an autosomal recessive condition. It should be noted that for gene tracking, DNA from the affected person and family studies are required. The fragment "tracking" with the disease allele can be identified by observing which fragment pattern is common to affected family members. There is an error rate associated with the use of linked markers because recombination may occur between the DNA marker and the disease gene. To minimize the risk of misdiagnosis, markers that show no more than 1% recombination with the disease gene are used whenever possible.

Detection of Mutations and Copy Number Variants

The definitive diagnostic test is to show a change in DNA that is predicted to disrupt gene function, and thus cause disease. When a mutation is predicted to cause truncation of the protein product (usually through a frameshift mutation or the introduction of a stop codon), this is strong evidence that the mutation is pathogenic. Other sequence changes may be more difficult to interpret, especially missense mutations that result in replacement of one amino acid by another. Additional genetic studies may be needed to determine the likelihood of pathogenicity. These may include testing members of the population to determine whether this is a polymorphism or performing a family study to determine whether the DNA change is being inherited with the condition.

In some conditions, certain mutations occur at a high frequency (e.g., δ-F508 mutation in CF, G380R mutation in achondroplasia). For most conditions, however, the precise mutation must first be identified in an affected person in the family. This may take months, depending on the structure of the gene and the laboratory techniques used. DNA sequencing is used to detect variants in the coding sequence, but other techniques need to be used to detect deletions or large rearrangements. After the mutation is identified, other family members can be offered definitive diagnosis. Even when the DNA sequence of a gene is known, gene tracking may have to be used if technical constraints make direct mutation testing impractical.

Microarrays and Their Use in Prenatal Diagnosis

Clinical cytogenetics is being transformed by widespread implementation of array comparative genomic hybridization (array CGH). This technique represents arguably the most

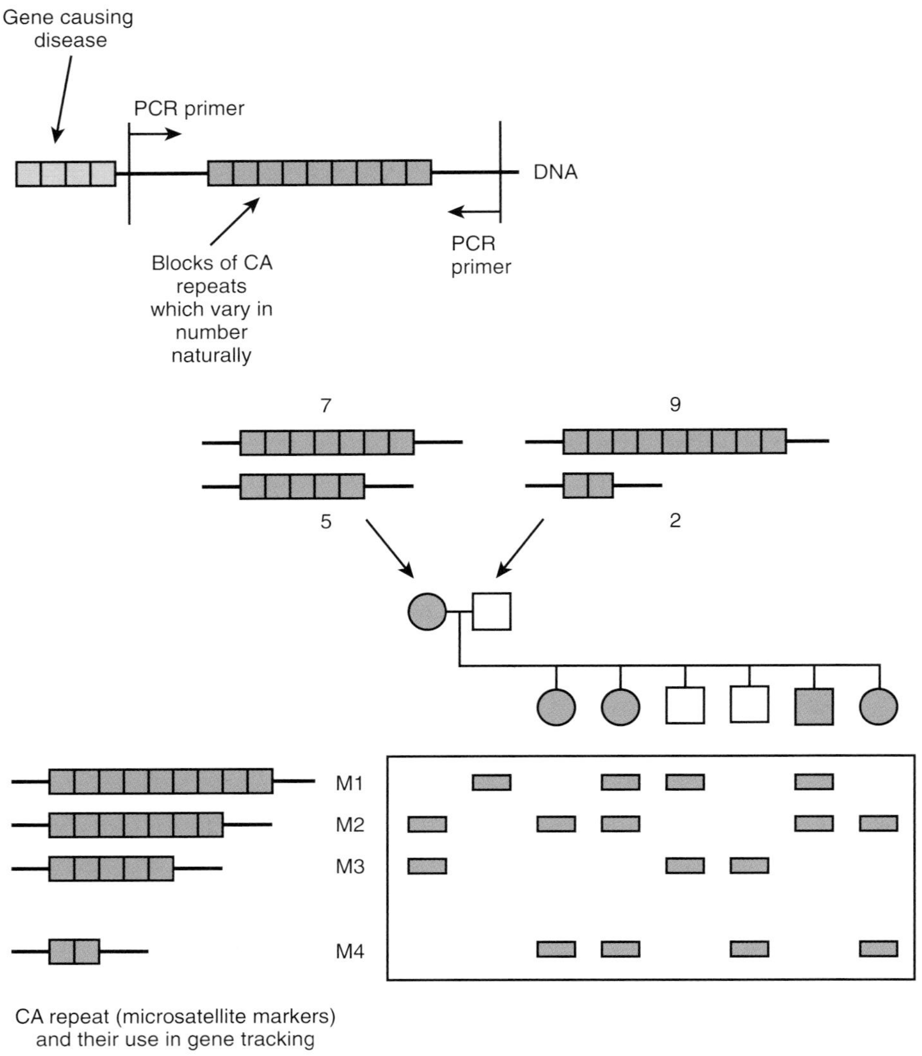

FIGURE 4–5
Principles of gene tracking with CA repeat markers. A variable DNA sequence (consisting of two DNA bases, CA, repeated several times) is fortuitously situated immediately in front of a gene that is known to cause a particular condition. The length of the $CA_{(n)}$ sequence varies naturally from individual to individual and is usually of no significance. Variation in its length is used as a marker tracking the gene of interest in a family. Members of this family whose symbols are blocked in are affected with an autosomal dominant condition. DNA is extracted from lymphocytes, and the DNA segment containing the CA repeat is amplified by polymerase chain reaction (PCR) so that there are sufficient copies to be visualized. The different $CA_{(n)}$ lengths are separated by electrophoresis. In this family, the father has CA repeats of lengths 9 and 2, and the mother with the dominant condition has repeats of lengths 7 and 5. Because the CA repeat sequence is acting as a marker of the parental disease gene alleles, all affected children have inherited the same maternal $CA_{(n)}$ allele. This marker allele could be used for diagnosis in other family members. In other families with the same condition, however, the condition will be associated with this CA marker system, but the altered allele that causes the condition could be tracking with a different length of CA repeat. When using gene tracking, a study of each family is needed to determine which allele is associated with the disease gene.

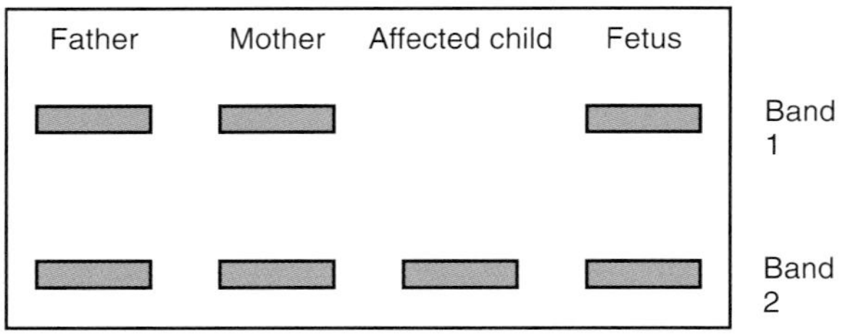

FIGURE 4–6
DNA diagnosis of an autosomal recessive condition by gene tracking. In this family, both parents have two detectable fragments (*1* and *2*) but their son, who is affected with an autosomal recessive condition, shows only one (*2*). Therefore, the altered alleles must be located on the parental chromosomes that give the fragment labeled *2*. In the next pregnancy, the fetus had two fragments, *1* and *2*, and therefore is predicted to be a carrier, but is not affected with the condition.

powerful direct application of the human genome mapping project in medicine today, both in terms of design of microarrays to interrogate the human genome in one assay (at previously unthinkable resolution) and in terms of establishing very accurate phenotype-genotype correlations from the results obtained.

The technique involves differentially labeling patient and reference DNA with fluorochromes and co-hybridizing the samples onto a glass slide or chip that is spotted either with genomic clones (bacterial artificial chromosome [BAC] probes) or, increasingly, synthetic oligonucleotide probes. Hybridization occurs relative to the amount of patient and reference DNA competing for any individual spot or feature. After hybridization and washing, the microarrays are scanned with a laser scanner and the resulting raw data are then extracted using sophisticated software that plots fluorescent ratio relative to each feature's position in the genome and calls regions as potentially aberrant via user-defined thresholds. In this way, copy number imbalances (loss or gain) can be detected in patient DNA relative to normal copy number DNA. Array CGH has substantial advantages over conventional chromosome analysis.

Conventional cytogenetics at highest resolution can detect imbalances of 3 to 5 to 10 Mb. Array CGH using the highest resolution oligonucleotide arrays is capable of detecting changes in the order of 1 Kb, which is significantly smaller than the average gene. Resolution at this level is not in routine clinical use and not yet appropriate for prenatal diagnosis. Current applications in clinical use typically aim for a resolution of between 200 Kb and 1 Mb, and this has led to a major step change in detection rate over conventional cytogenetics. Of particular note, studies of children with learning difficulties and congenital malformation with previously normal cytogenetics have revealed pathogenic copy number imbalances in 10% to 20% of cases, which represents a fourfold increase in detection rate over conventional cytogenetics. International collaborations with the pooling of results from microarray analysis and phenotypic data through initiatives such as the DECIPHER consortium (https://decipher.sanger.ac.uk/) has led to the rapid establishment of several new microdeletion syndromes, such as the 17q23.1 microdeletion syndrome.

One of the current challenges to the application of microarrays in the clinical setting is determining whether a given copy number imbalance is de novo and likely to be causative or inherited and likely to be benign. Up to 12% of any individual's genome is likely to exhibit normal copy number variation (CNV), and there is emerging evidence of a huge degree of structural complexity within these CNV regions. In addition, limited data exist on the prevalence of CNVs between different ethnic populations. High-resolution studies using 500 K single nucleotide polymorphism (SNP) arrays analysis of patient-parent trios have showed previously unreported or "private" inherited CNVs in up to 30% of individuals. Interpretation of data at this resolution in the setting of prenatal diagnosis would be challenging, given the necessity for parental samples for rapid follow-up by microarray analysis and demands for unambiguous and robust reporting. In addition, reporting a novel CNV as benign, even if inherited from a phenotypically normal parent, would not be recommended, because some causative CNVs have been well documented to exhibit highly variable penetrance between generations. On a technical level, DNA yield from prenatal samples (amniotic fluid and chorionic villous) is usually lower than that from blood samples, and array design and protocols need to reflect the importance of this. Fundamental array design can be adapted to meet these criteria. There is little doubt that this cytogenetic technological advance may lead to the identification of subtle differences in DNA in fetuses that appear both phenotypically normal and abnormal. This raises a host of ethical considerations that need discussion and consensus view before such technology is applied widely.

CHROMOSOMAL ANOMALIES

The Karyotype Report: Nomenclature

Karyotyping is labor-intensive because high-resolution (extended) chromosome preparations reveal more than 850 bands. These bands are usually analyzed by light microscopy, although computer imaging is beginning to have a major effect. Occasionally, only limited analysis may be possible because of poor elongation of the chromosomes.

The human chromosome composition is reported in an internationally agreed format that gives a precise description of an anomaly. The format has three parts that are separated by a comma: the total number of chromosomes seen, the sex chromosome constitution, and normal variants or anomalies.

- The first figure gives the total number of chromosomes (e.g., 46, 45, 47).
- The second part gives the sex chromosome complement (e.g., XX, XY, X, XXY).
- The third part describes normal variants or anomalies affecting the following:
  - Whole chromosomes.
  - Arms of chromosomes.

The short arm of a chromosome is designated "p" (for *petit*), and the long arm is designated "q" (the next letter in the alphabet). Each arm is further subdivided into bands and subbands.

Breakpoints involved in structural rearrangements are described according to the arm involved, the region of the arm, and then by band and subbands within that region. For example, the location Xq27.3 is found on the long arm of the X chromosome, in region 2, band 7, and subband 3. Further examples are given in Table 4–4.

Molecular Cytogenetic Techniques

Some syndromes are caused by submicroscopic deletions of chromosomal material. Molecular techniques (usually

TABLE 4–4
Examples of Cytogenetic Nomenclature

Normal	
46,XX	Normal female
Sex Chromosome Aneuploidies	
45,X	Monosomy X (Turner syndrome)
47,XXY	Klinefelter syndrome
45,X/46,XX	Mosaic Turner syndrome
Autosomal Aneuploidies	
47,XY, +21	Male with trisomy 21 (Down syndrome)
47,XX, +13	Female with trisomy 13 (Patau syndrome)
Polyploidy	
69,XXY	Triploidy
Deletions	
46,XX,del(18)(q21)	Deletion of part of the long arm of one chromosome 18 from band q21 to the end of the long arm (qter)
46,XX,del(17)(p13)	Female karyotype with a deletion of part of the short arm of chromosome 17, from band p13 to the end of the short arm (pter)
Translocations	
46,XY,t(2;12)(p14;p13)	Male with a balanced reciprocal translocation between chromosomes 2 and 12, with breakpoints on the short arms, at p14 on chromosome 2 and at p13 on chromosome 12
46,XX,der(2)t(2;12)(p14;p13)mat	Female with an unbalanced complement, having received the derivative chromosome 2 from her mother, who carries a translocation between chromosomes 2 and 12; this child would have too little material from chromosome 2 (from p14 to pter) and an additional copy of material from chromosome 12 (from p13 to pter), making her effectively monosomic for 2p and trisomic for 12p
45,XY,rob(14;21)(q10q10)	Carrier of a robertsonian translocation between one chromosome 14 and one chromosome 21
Other	
46,XY,inv(5)(p14;q15)	Pericentric inversion of one chromosome 5
46,XX,r(15)	Female with one normal and one ring chromosome 15
46,XY,fra(X)(q27.3)	Male with a fragile site in subband 27.3 on the X long arm
46,XX,add(20)(p13)	Additional material of unknown origin attached to band p13 on one chromosome 20

fluorescence in situ hybridization [FISH]) can be used for diagnosis when the loss or gain of material is beyond the limit of light microscopy. This technique is also helpful for determining the origin of chromosomal material.

This method can also be applied to interphase nuclei to determine the numbers of copies of specific chromosomes, particularly as a rapid screening test for common trisomies (array CGH).

A Parent with a Chromosome Anomaly

Chromosomal Translocations

During the formation of a translocation during cell division, breaks will have occurred in chromosomes from different pairs with rejoining in an unusual pattern. Chromosomal material normally found on a particular chromosome will now be placed on a different chromosome. If the exchange results in no loss or gain of DNA, the individual is clinically normal and is said to have a "balanced translocation." A translocation carrier is, however, at risk of producing chromosomally unbalanced gametes, which may result in a baby with multiple congenital anomalies, miscarriages, stillbirth, or infertility depending on the origin and amount of chromosome material involved. It may be possible to determine the relative probabilities of each of these outcomes, depending on the particular translocation involved, by consulting the cytogenetic literature of previous cases, and by using special formulas—both of which require consultation with clinical genetics or cytogenetics services.

For most couples, however, understanding the precise probability is not the overriding consideration because they choose to undertake fetal karyotyping in future pregnancies. It is important to offer carrier testing to other family members because of the potentially high risks of having offspring with unbalanced forms of the translocation. Referral to a clinical genetics service is recommended for contacting and counseling family members.

There are two types of translocations: reciprocal and robertsonian.

RECIPROCAL TRANSLATIONS

Reciprocal translocations are characterized by the exchange of chromosomal material distal to (i.e., beyond) the breaks in two chromosomes. The long or short arms of any pair of chromosomes may be involved. Approximately 1 in 500 people is a carrier of a reciprocal translocation.

When a fetus has inherited an apparently balanced reciprocal translocation from a clinically normal parent, there appears to be no increased incidence of phenotypic abnormality in the child, especially if the translocation is present without effect in several family members. A cryptic unbalanced complement is more likely if a translocation is de novo (see later).

ROBERTSONIAN TRANLOCATION ("CENTRIC FUSION")

A *robertsonian translocation* ("centric fusion") is one in which effectively all of one chromosome is joined end-to-end to another. Robertsonian translocations involve the acrocentric chromosomes (13, 14, 15, 21, and 22) and are among the most common balanced structural rearrangements in the general population, with a frequency in newborn surveys of approximately 1 in 1000.

Centric fusion may arise from breaks at or near the centromere in two acrocentric chromosomes, with the two products fusing together. This usually results in the production of a single chromosome and most frequently involves chromosomes 13 and 14. Next in frequency are chromosomes 14 and 21. Clinically, the most important fusions are those involving chromosome 21, which give rise to familial Down syndrome.

For female carriers of a robertsonian 14;21 translocation, the observed probability of having a liveborn infant with Down syndrome is approximately 10%. The risk is approximately 1% for a male carrier. A robertsonian translocation involving both copies of chromosome 21 is rare, but all children of a carrier will have Down syndrome.

Where a robertsonian translocation involves chromosome 15 and a balanced translocation karyotype is detected at prenatal diagnosis, it is appropriate to test for UPD. This is to exclude Angelman's syndrome or Prader-Willi syndrome in the fetus caused by UPD for chromosome 15. This can occur by postzygotic "correction" of trisomy 15 when one parental chromosome 15 that is not involved in the robertsonian translocation is lost during mitosis.

Deletions and Duplications of Chromosomal Material

When a person with partial autosomal monosomy or trisomy has children, the probability that a child will inherit the parental chromosomal anomaly is theoretically 50%, because the parent passes on either the normal homologue or the chromosome with the deletion or duplication.

Inversions

An inversion (inv) affects just one chromosome, with a segment between two breaks inverted and reinserted. A pericentric inversion has one break in the short arm and one in the long arm. A paracentric inversion has both breaks in the same chromosome arm.

A carrier of a pericentric inversion is usually phenotypically normal, but the inversion may cause chromosomally unbalanced gametes. For the normal and inverted chromosomes to pair at meiosis, they have to adopt an unusual physical configuration so that if a crossover occurs in the inverted segment, unbalanced products will result. In theory, the larger the inverted segment, the greater the likelihood of recombination occurring and liveborn children with congenital anomalies and developmental problems. In practice, this is uncommon when the inverted segment is less than one third the length of the chromosome.

The overall probability of having a child with problems is approximately 1% when there is no family history of the recombinant form, but the individual probability depends on the precise inversion. For instance, there are also common pericentric inversion variants of chromosomes 1, 9, 16, and Y that are not associated with an increased risk. If, however, a family is identified through the birth of an individual with problems due to a recombinant chromosome, then the probability of having a liveborn child with problems increases to 5% to 10%.

A carrier of a paracentric inversion (involving only one chromosome arm and not the centromer) is usually phenotypically normal, and empirical data suggest a very low risk of having a child with an unbalanced form of the inversion.

A Parent with Trisomy 21

Few data are available, but a literature review of about 30 pregnancies gives an empirical figure of approximately 1 in 3 of a woman with trisomy 21 having a child with trisomy 21. In addition, the probability of a chromosomally normal fetus having a congenital anomaly or mental handicap could be as high as 30%.[12]

Fetal Chromosomal Anomaly Found on Karyotyping during Pregnancy

Aneuploidies

Most structural chromosomal anomalies are aneuploidy, numeric abnormalities that involve the loss or gain of one or two chromosomes, or even the gain of a whole set. These anomalies are most commonly caused by nondisjunction, a process that is more common with increased maternal age. Fraser and Mitchell[13] noted a lack of hereditary factors but an association with advanced maternal age in cases of Down syndrome. Subsequently, in a study of 350 cases, Shuttleworth[14] reported a considerable proportion of affected infants born to women approaching the climacteric. Bleyer[15] proposed an association with degeneration of the ovum. Antonarakis and associates[16] examined DNA polymorphisms in infants with Down syndrome and showed that 95% of nondisjunction trisomy 21 is maternal in origin.

In the late 1970s and early 1980s, when prenatal diagnosis was in its infancy, eight large studies were carried out to assess the age-specific prevalence of trisomy 21 in live births.[17–24] Some of these studies had incomplete ascertainment and little information about the distribution of maternal age and the effect of selective abortion after prenatal diagnosis.

However, two studies[19,22] had nearly complete ascertainment. Cuckle and colleagues[25] combined the data from these eight surveys on a total of 3,289,114 births to determine the prevalence of trisomy 21 at each maternal age. Regression analysis was applied to smooth out fluctuations in the observed data.

In the 1970s and 1980s, genetic amniocentesis at 16 to 20 weeks was offered to women 35 years of age or older. This group was considered to be at increased risk for aneuploidy. Similarly, these groups were targeted for chorionic villus sampling between 9 and 14 weeks.

Data from these prenatal studies confirmed that the prevalence of trisomy 21 increased with maternal age and that the prevalence was higher during pregnancy than at birth.

Combined data from two multicenter studies of amniocentesis (one in the United States and one in Europe) showed that the prevalence of trisomies 13, 18, and 21 was approximately 30% higher at 16 to 20 weeks than at birth.[26,27] Similarly, data from fetal karyotyping by chorionic villus sampling showed that the prevalence of these aneuploidies was approximately 50% higher between 9 and 14 weeks than at birth (Fig. 4–7).[28]

Ultrasound studies have demonstrated that major chromosomal defects are often associated with multiple fetal

FIGURE 4–7
The prevalence of trisomy 21 (*A*), trisomy 18 (*B*), and trisomy 13 (*C*) at 9 to 14 weeks' gestation (*triangles*) and the prevalence of these trisomies at 16 to 20 weeks (*squares*) compared with the prevalence of live births affected with trisomy 21 (*dashed line*) in women 35 to 42 years old.
(From Snijders RJM, Nicolaides KH: Assessment of risk in ultrasound markers for fetal chromosome defects. In Nicolaides KH [ed]: Frontiers in Fetal Medicine. London, Parthenon, 1996.)

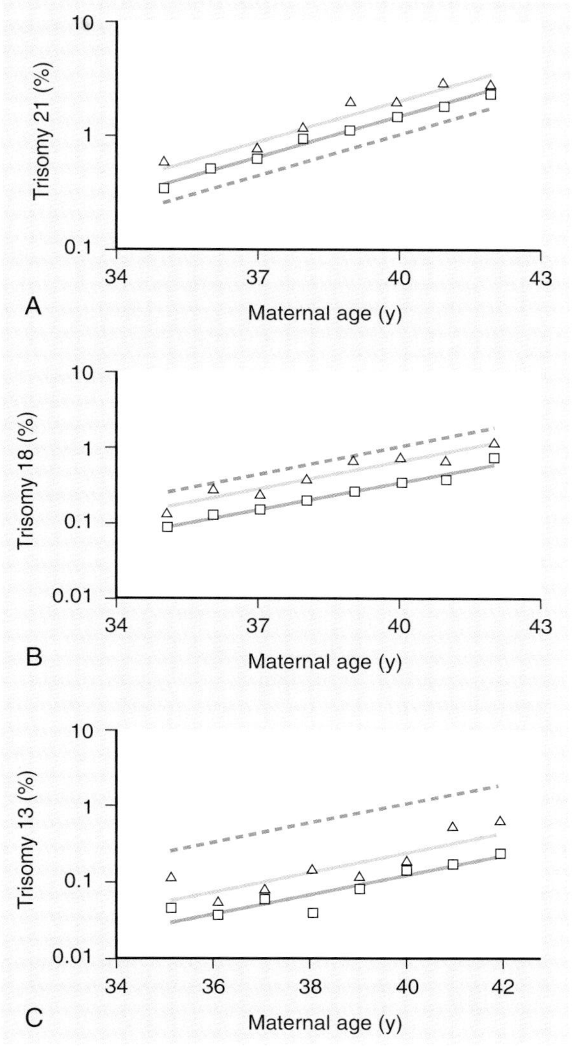

abnormalities. Conversely, in a fetus with multiple abnormalities, the frequency of chromosomal defects is high and the relative risk increases with the number of anomalies identified. However, prenatal karyotyping is often performed because the prognosis for the baby may be dictated not only by the combination of structural anomalies identified but also by marked neurodevelopmental morbidity associated with aneuploidy. The frequency of chromosomal defects, such as aneuploidy, increases with maternal age. Traditionally, counseling of patients about the risk of fetal chromosomal defects depends on the provision of live birth indices of trisomy 21. However, with ultrasound screening, the prevalence must be established for all chromosomal defects that are associated with structural and biometric anomalies.

Chromosome anomalies differ in the rate of intrauterine attrition, and it is important to establish maternal and gestational age–specific risks for each of the common aneuploidies. Data from a subgroup of women 35 to 42 years old have been used to examine the radiance of regression lines that describe the relationship between maternal age and the prevalence of aneuploidy. For trisomy 21 (see Fig. 4–7*A*), trisomy 18 (see Fig. 4–7*B*), and trisomy 13 (see Fig. 4–7*C*), the increase in frequency is nearly parallel, suggesting that there are no maternal age–related differences in the rate of intrauterine loss. If the prevalence of each of the common trisomies in live births is considered to be 1, then the relative prevalence of other gestational ages can be calculated and relative prevalence curves calculated.

The identification of fetal structural abnormalities leads to a stepwise increase in prevalence risk with each additional abnormality. A detailed discussion is beyond the scope of this chapter, but may be found elsewhere (see Snijders and Nicolaides, listed in Suggested Readings). Since the late 1990s, the use of first-trimester scanning to measure nuchal translucency (as related to fetal crown–rump length), combined with maternal serum free β-human chorionic gonadotropin (β-hCG) and pregnancy-associated plasma protein A, has been used to screen for aneuploidy (see Chapter 7).

Triploidy

Survival to term of fetuses with triploidy is rare, and those born alive die shortly after birth. Most have partial hydatidiform mole, and the rest are nonmolar, with a normal or hypoplastic trophoblast. It is reasonable to offer prenatal karyotyping in future pregnancies. The phenotypes of the fetus and placenta depend on whether the additional set of chromosomes is paternally or maternally derived. The overall recurrence risk is usually low, but diandric triploidy associated with partial hydatidiform mole has a 1% to 1.5% risk of recurrence, and some women appear to have a predisposition for digynic triploidy.

Structurally Abnormal Chromosomes

When an unexpected structural chromosomal anomaly is found, the first step should be to examine the parental chromosomes. If the structural anomaly is present in a parent who is otherwise normal, it is unlikely that a similar chromosome anomaly in the child will cause severe problems. Exceptions may occur when chromosomes known to be imprinted are involved, principally chromosome 15, and genetic advice should be sought. If neither parent has the chromosomal anomaly, it is likely to have occurred during gamete formation. If chromosomal material has been duplicated or deleted during its production, this may cause severe clinical effects (Fig. 4–8).

De Novo Apparently Balanced Structural Rearrangements

The concern is that there could be a submicroscopic abnormality, either deletion, duplication, or gene disruption, involving the breakpoints. Molecular techniques, such as comparative genomic hybridization or the use of arrays, may be able help to determine whether there is cryptic gain or loss of material in apparently de novo rearrangements found at prenatal diagnosis.

FIGURE 4–8
A flow chart to assist in determining risks and the appropriate type of presymptomatic or prenatal diagnosis.

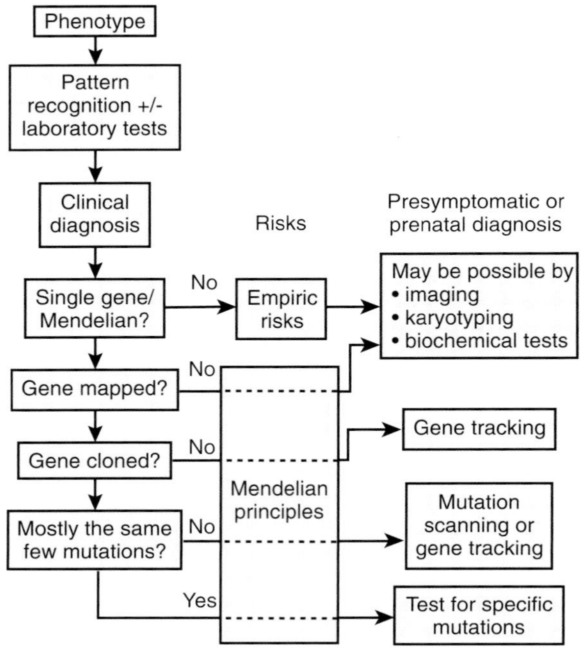

De Novo Apparently Balanced Reciprocal Translocation

In a very large study, Warburton[29] found that serious malformations were detected in 6.1% of pregnancies at elective termination or in liveborn infants, which is approximately 3% greater than the background risk of malformation that applies to all pregnancies. No prospective data on the risks of cognitive impairment or mental retardation are available, but an overall figure of 5% to 10% is often used to include not only malformations but also neurologic and developmental deficiencies. Whereas a detailed scan may give reassurance about the absence of malformations, there remains a risk of an adverse cognitive outcome. If, however, malformations are found on ultrasound, this is a strong indication that chromosomal imbalance is likely to be present.

De Novo Robertsonian Translocation

Because the formation of robertsonian translocations does not disrupt coding sequences, the risk of phenotypic abnormalities is low. When a robertsonian translocation involves chromosome 14 or 15, fetal UPD studies may be indicated to exclude the small probability that the fetus has inherited both copies of chromosome 14 or 15 from the same parent, resulting in dysmorphic and developmental features because of imprinting effects (see later).

De Novo Apparently Balanced Inversions

The risk of phenotypic anomaly is increased if the inversion is de novo. Empirically, the risk appears to be approximately 9%. Figures for cognitive impairment are not available.

Structurally Abnormal Additional Chromosomes ("Marker Chromosomes")

If a structurally abnormal extra chromosome (marker, supernumerary, accessory chromosome) or a ring chromosome is discovered, parental karyotyping should be performed urgently. Further advice should be sought because specialized genetic tests (e.g., painting with chromosome-specific fluorescent probes, array technology) may be able to determine whether the fetus is at high or low risk by determining the chromosomal origin and nature. Mosaicism (discussed later) with a normal cell line often accompanies the finding of a cell line with a marker chromosome and can make clinical interpretation even more difficult. The size of the marker and the ratio of cell lines in tissue used for prenatal diagnosis cannot be used prognostically. There is no accurate information relating to the residual risk of mental handicap when ultrasound examination shows no fetal anomalies.

De Novo Duplications and Deletions

During meiosis, the two chromosomes of a particular pair naturally swap genetic material between themselves, by breaking and rejoining, thereby producing different combinations of genes to pass on to offspring. Sometimes, repair of the breaks can be faulty or unusual pairing of chromosomes can occur. This may result in deletion or duplication of genetic material in the gamete. When fertilization occurs with a normal gamete, the fetus will have half the usual amount of gene products from that segment where a deletion is present, and one and a half times the normal amounts in duplications. The altered amounts of gene products affect development, resulting in congenital malformations and mental retardation. The precise features depend on the amount of chromosomal material involved and the chromosome from which it was derived.

Duplications are more common than deletions and generally result in a less severe phenotype. Specific syndromes are associated with certain deletions, but fewer phenotypes associated with duplications have been given names.

Further information about the likely clinical effects may be available from similar cases reported in the literature, or from online databases (such as DECIPHER) which are attempting to catalogue information from array studies in patients with structural chromosome anomalies.

The recurrence risk for a de novo deletion or duplication is very low, but not zero. Rare recurrences are likely to be caused by parental mosaicism, which is not usually detected by routine karyotyping. Although recurrence is extremely rare, many couples request prenatal diagnosis for reassurance. When the deletion/duplication is caused by an unbalanced product from a familial translocation, the risk of recurrence can be high.

Fragile Sites

Hereditary fragile sites can occur on several chromosomes, giving the appearance of breakage at a specific point. On autosomes, they appear to be harmless. However, a fragile site near the end of the long arm of the X chromosome at Xq27.3 is a marker for fragile X syndrome, an X-linked mental retardation syndrome. Because of the high risks and complex genetics of this single-gene disorder, families should be referred to the clinical genetics department.

Mosaicism

Mosaicism occurs when an individual's tissues or organs contain more than one genetic line of cells. One line of cells may contain a chromosomal anomaly or sometimes a single gene containing a mutation. The phenotype can be difficult to predict: depending on the number and disposition of cells with the genetic anomaly, the clinical effects will lie between those of the full condition and those of a normal individual. Testing other tissues (chorionic villi, amniotic cells, fetal blood) might be helpful. Even so, the proportion of cells with the genetic anomaly in one tissue might not be the same as the proportion elsewhere.

As mosaicism occurs postzygotically, the probability of recurrence in another pregnancy of normal parents is low.

A parent who is known to have mosaicism can have a child with the full features of the chromosome or single-gene condition, if the gamete making the child contains the anomaly, which will then be present in all the child's cells. It is not possible to give an exact figure for the child inheriting the condition because this depends on the numbers and disposition of cells in the gonads. Most parents, therefore, request prenatal diagnosis.

Although placental mosaicism with a chromosomally normal fetus is a well-recognized phenomenon (see Chapter 9), mosaicism involving chromosomes 13, 18, and 21 often predicts fetal abnormality and especially so when mosaic trisomy 9 or mosaic trisomy 22 is found. Mosaicism for a structurally abnormal additional chromosome appears to carry a greater risk than autosomal trisomy mosaicism. However, another concern when autosomal trisomy mosaicism is found at prenatal diagnosis is that a trisomic fetus may have "lost" one of the three copies of the chromosome in some cells to "correct" the imbalance. If both remaining copies of the chromosome originated from the same parent (UPD), this too could give an abnormal phenotype (see next section).

OTHER MECHANISMS OF GENETIC ANOMALY: UNIPARENTAL DISOMY AND GENOMIC IMPRINTING

Uniparental Disomy

The genomic stimulus for fetal growth is affected by the constant constraints of maternal size, placental function, and nutritional sufficiency. However, the expression of certain genes in both the fetus and the placenta is probably crucial to growth potential. It is probable that the placenta can control not only its own size but also, through a variety of mechanisms, that of the fetus. Few studies of the genetic control of fetal and placental growth have been done. However, UPD may be a cause of abnormal fetal growth, especially when it occurs without classic risk factors.

Abnormal growth in utero predisposes the fetus to increased perinatal and neonatal morbidity and mortality. In mammals, reproduction requires the fusion of two haploid chromosome sets, one paternal and the other maternal. The fertilized egg then contains two copies of each chromosome. It is usual, and previously has been assumed invariable, for one member of each chromosome pair to be derived from each parent. However, in UPD, one homologous chromosome pair comes from the same parent (in isodisomy, the chromosomes are identical, but in heterodisomy, the two different maternal or paternal chromosomes are inherited). Catanach and Kirk in 1985[30] showed UPD in mice that resulted in specific abnormal phenotypes associated with growth disturbance. The progeny of mice with maternal disomy of chromosome 11 were smaller than their normal litter mates. Those with paternal disomy 11 were considerably larger than their litter mates.

Cases have been described in human pregnancies in which UPD for specific chromosomes has caused a clinical condition. The first example was an individual with maternal isodisomy 7 and homozygosity for the CF gene.[31] A similar case was subsequently described by Vosse,[32] the progeny showing phenotypically short stature.

Other conditions may be associated with UPD and show the following characteristics:

- Occurrence that is usually sporadic.
- No consistent cytogenetic abnormalities.
- Abnormal growth patterns and rates of growth.

Three separate mechanisms have been postulated for UPD:

- Chromosomal duplication in a monosomic somatic cell after postzygotic loss of a homologous chromosome.
- Fertilization of a nullisomic gamete by a disomic gamete.
- Loss of a supernumerary chromosome from a trisomic cell, leaving two homologues from the same gamete (trisomic rescue).[33]

Supporting the evidence for this has been provided in several publications.[34,35] The paper by Purves-Smith reported a confined placental mosaicism for trisomy 15, but an apparently normal karyotype on amniotic fluid cytogenetic and postnatal blood analysis.[35] However, at the age of 2 years, Prader-Willi syndrome was diagnosed clinically and maternal disomy 15 confirmed on molecular studies. The second study reported confined placental mosaicism for trisomy 16 in four fetuses with severe intrauterine growth restriction.[36] Subsequent skin karyotyping and molecular studies showed a normal karyotype with maternal disomy of chromosome 16.

Alternatively, postzygotic mitotic recombination could result in "mosaic" UPD. This phenomenon was recently identified in four patients with Beckwith-Wiedemann syndrome.[33]

Further mechanisms for UPD include gamete complementation or monosomic zygote correction; the latter has supporting evidence from some isodisomy cases of Angelman's syndrome when no evidence of recombination between chromosome 15 was found.[37] Whatever the mechanism, UPD may play an important role in unresolved genetic syndromes that affect growth.

Similarly, we carried out pilot chromosomal studies of 11 babies born with idiopathic growth restriction. The fetuses had prenatal diagnosis performed before 26 weeks' gestation. In the 11 cases, we showed 5 instances of placental chromosomal mosaicism. The chromosomal abnormalities identified varied from trisomies for chromosomes 7 and 8 to structural abnormalities and deletions. In a further 6 pregnancies in which chromosomal mosaicism was detected prenatally after first-trimester chorionic villus sampling, 3 cases occurred involving chromosome 7, 1 chromosome 8, and 2 chromosome 15 for uteroplacental disomy. In 1 of these 6 cases, UPD was found and this was for chromosome 15. Maternal heterodisomy was detected and would have resulted in Prader-Willi syndrome if the pregnancy continued.[37]

About 100 well-documented pregnancies have been reported as having intrauterine growth restriction or fetal death associated with confined placental mosaicism. To date, only 12 chromosomes have been involved: 2, 3, 7, 8, 9, 13, 14, 15, 16, 18, 22, and X.[35] Trisomy 16 is the most common trisomy associated with pregnancy loss and confined placental mosaicism in intrauterine growth restriction. A prospective study investigated the incidence of UPD associated with growth restriction in 35 infants born between 25 and 40 weeks.[38] However, only 2 fetuses were born before 28 weeks, and both had chromosomal UPD of chromosome 16 plus confirmed placental mosaicism. No other UPD was found for the 12 chromosomes tested. It was concluded that UPD for the chromosomes tested did not explain the etiology of most cases of intrauterine growth restriction. However, many of these cases occurred after 32 weeks, and a higher detection rate is likely in fetuses with severe intrauterine growth restriction before 28 weeks.

Genomic Imprinting

The concept that male and female genomes do not contribute equally to mammalian development derives from observations made in mice in the late 1980s.[39] In those experiments, the development of uniparental diploid embryos was severely disrupted. Pathogenetic conceptuses developed embryos up to the 25-cell stage but showed only very rudimentary extraembryonic tissues. Androgenic conceptuses were characterized by relatively well-developed extraembryonic membranes and severely perturbed embryos. These reciprocal uniparental phenotypes probably resulted from disruption of the normal parental-specific expression patterns of a subset of imprinted genes. A detailed discussion is outside the scope of this chapter (see Suggested Readings, Georgiades and coworkers, 2001).

MALFORMATION SYNDROMES

The Pathogenesis of Malformation Syndromes

The term *dysmorphology* has been applied to the study of birth defects occurring in recognizable syndromic combinations. The cellular pathways involved in the pathogenesis of some malformation syndromes are being delineated and key genes identified. An increasing number of syndromes is being shown to be associated with mutations in specific genes, raising the possibility of prenatal diagnosis by DNA analysis.

Structural Malformations Found at Ultrasound Examination

A detailed screening fetal ultrasound examination may reveal a pattern of major anomalies that suggests a specific diagnosis (see Chapters 7 and 8). Recognizable patterns are most likely to be caused by chromosomal anomalies, but rare single-gene or dysmorphic syndromes may be diagnosed in utero in the absence of a history of the syndrome. In addition to major structural anomalies, careful evaluation of the fetus may show other dysmorphic features that are not commonly sought in a routine "screening" ultrasound examination. These include micrognathia and anomalies of eye spacing and of the hands (e.g., clinodactyly) or feet (e.g., sandal gap of the toe). Careful evaluation of the fetal posture or attitude when the fetus is stationary and moving may also give important diagnostic information.

Evaluation of the features with a clinical geneticist or perinatologist with a special interest in fetal dysmorphology may aid in the prospective diagnosis of a dysmorphic syndrome. The use of computer databases (see Suggested Readings) may be helpful, but it is important to compare the features of patients with a suspected diagnosis with photographs in original reports. A written description of dysmorphic features may suggest a match, but comparing photographs may be needed to confirm or refute the diagnosis.

As with all aspects of genetic counseling, accuracy of the diagnosis is paramount. Information obtained prenatally should be supplemented by information from postnatal examination or from a detailed examination by a perinatal pathologist if the couple wishes to end the pregnancy or if the fetus is stillborn. Photographs of the main features are helpful when seeking the diagnostic advice of a clinical geneticist.

Probability of Recurrence of a Syndrome

For many common conditions, empirical risk tables are available (see Suggested Readings and especially Harper, 2004). If the diagnosis is not clear or no accurate data on which to base a recurrence risk are available, it is advisable to refer the case to a clinical geneticist.

ISOLATED ORGAN AND SYSTEM ANOMALIES

Many conditions involving a single organ system appear to have a genetic or inherited component but show no clear pattern of mendelian inheritance or identifiable chromosomal abnormality. The term *multifactorial* has been used to describe this group. In some cases (e.g., Hirschsprung's disease, congenital heart disease), the condition is not a single entity but a heterogeneous group of indistinguishable conditions. Some of these may be inherited in a mendelian fashion, others may result from interplay of an inherited component and environmental factors, and others may be "acquired" in the sense that environmental factors are largely influential. Empirical risk data, obtained from observing recurrences in population studies, are available for many of these conditions (see Suggested Readings), but a clinical geneticist should be consulted.

SUMMARY OF MANAGEMENT OPTIONS

Counseling Points for Common Conditions

Management Options	Evidence Quality and Recommendation	References
Mendelian Inheritance		
High recurrence risks.	IV/C	1
Establish an accurate diagnosis and the mode of inheritance before counseling.	IV/C	1
Seek the latest information about carrier detection tests.	IV/C	1
Plan invasive procedures requiring DNA methods in consultation with the laboratory.	IV/C	1
Autosomal Dominant Conditions		
Each offspring of an affected parent has a 50% probability of inheriting the condition	IV/C	1
Potential pitfalls in conditions with variable expression	IV/C	1
Autosomal Recessive Conditions		
Each offspring of a couple in which both parents are carriers has a 25% probability of being affected with the condition.	IV/C	1
Prenatal diagnosis is possible for some.	IV/C	1
Donor gametes may be an acceptable therapeutic option for some; much discussion is required.	IV/C	1

SUMMARY OF MANAGEMENT OPTIONS

Counseling Points for Common Conditions—cont'd

Management Options	Evidence Quality and Recommendation	References
X-Linked Recessive Conditions		
Male-to-male transmission does not occur.	IV/C	1
All daughters of an affected male are carriers.	IV/C	1
For female carriers, each son has a 1 in 2 risk of being affected and each daughter has a 1 in 2 risk of being a carrier; affected homozygous females are rare.	IV/C	1
Chromosome Anomalies		
Refer families with translocations to a clinical geneticist so that family studies can be performed and to quantify the risk of an unbalanced karyotype (which may lead to miscarriage or a child with anomalies).	IV/C	1
With an unexpected structural chromosome abnormality, examine the parents' chromosomes.	IV/C	1
Duplication or deletion of chromosomal material can result in congenital anomalies or mental retardation.	IV/C	1
Predicting the clinical effects of mosaicism is difficult; karyotyping of other tissues may be required.	IV/C	1
De novo chromosomal conditions have a low probability of recurrence; offer fetal karyotyping for reassurance.	IV/C	1
Check karyotype reports with a laboratory if the meaning is in doubt.	IV/C	1
Clarify whether probabilities quoted in laboratory reports relate to "at amniocentesis" or "at delivery."	IV/C	1
Specific Syndromes		
Ensure the accuracy of diagnosis and recurrence risks.	IV/C	1
Empirical risk figures are available for some conditions (see "Suggested Readings").	IV/C	1
Prenatal diagnosis is available for some conditions with a biochemical basis, in which the gene responsible has been identified, or in which a microdeletion or duplication is the cause.	IV/C	1
If the diagnosis or probabilities are in doubt, refer the patient to a clinical geneticist.	IV/C	1
Organ and System Anomalies		
For many conditions, obtain information from a clinical geneticist.	IV/C	1
Empirical risk figures for siblings and children are available for some conditions (see "Suggested Readings").	IV/C	1

SUGGESTED READINGS

Cassidy SB, Allanson JE (eds): Management of Genetic Syndromes, 2nd ed. New York, John Wiley and Sons, 2005.

Donnai D, Winter RM (eds): Congenital Malformation Syndromes. London, Chapman and Hall, 1995.

Farndon P: Fetal anomalies—The geneticist's approach. In Twinning P, McHugo JM, Pilling DW (eds): Textbook of Fetal Abnormalities, 2nd ed Churchill Livingstone, 2006.

Gardner RJM, Sutherland GR (eds): Chromosome Abnormalities and Genetic Counseling, 3rd ed. Oxford, Oxford University Press, 2003.

Georgiades P, Watkins M, Baxton GJ, Ferguson-Smith AC: Roles of genomic imprinting and the zygotic genome in placental development. Proc Natl Acad Sci U S A 2001;98:4522–4527.

Harper PS (ed): Practical Genetic Counselling, 6th ed. London, Hodder Arnold, 2004.

Jones KL (ed): Smith's Recognizable Patterns of Human Malformation, 6th ed. Philadelphia, Saunders, 2005.

Rimoin DL, Connor JM, Pyeritz RE, et al (eds): Emery and Rimoin's Principles and Practice of Medical Genetics, 5th ed. London, Churchill Livingstone, 2006.

Scriver CR, Beaudet AL, Sly WS, Valle D (eds): The Metabolic and Molecular Basis of Inherited Disease, 8th ed. New York, McGraw-Hill, 2002.

Shashidhar Pai G, Lewandowski RC, Borgaonkar DS (eds): Handbook of Chromosomal Syndromes. New York, Wiley-Liss, 2002.

Snijders RJM, Nicolaides KH: Assessment of risk in ultrasound markers for fetal chromosome defects. In Nicolaides KH (ed): Frontiers in Fetal Medicine. London, Parthenon, 1996.

Dysmorphology Databases:

The Winter-Baraitser Dysmorphology Database (www.lmdatabases.com).

POSSUM (Pictures of Standard Syndromes and Undiagnosed Malformations) (www.possum.net.au).

REFERENCES

For a complete list of references, log onto www.expertconsult.com.

SECTION TWO

Early Prenatal

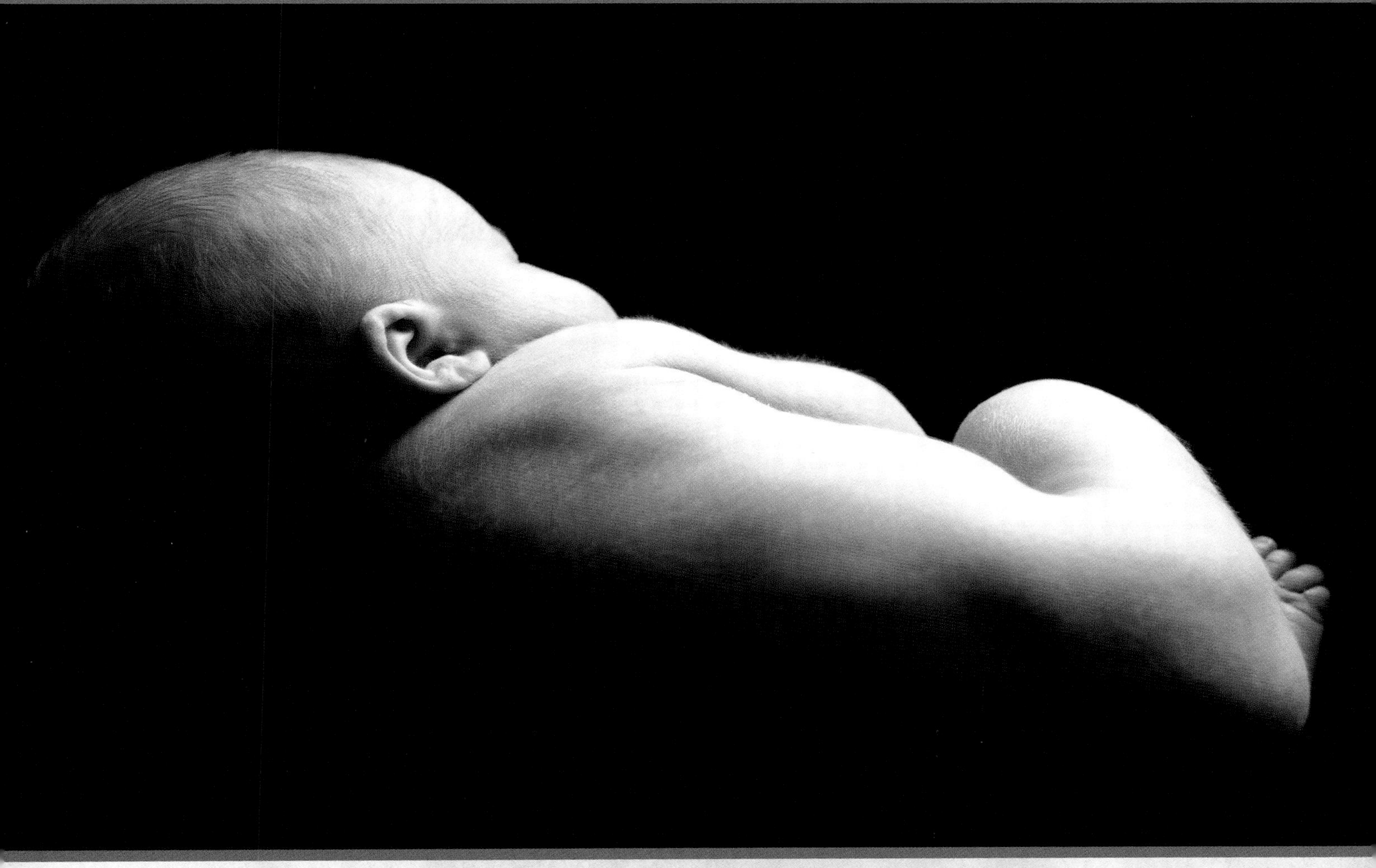

CHAPTER 5

Bleeding and Pain in Early Pregnancy

DAVID J. CAHILL, REBECCA SWINGLER, and PETER G. WARDLE

INTRODUCTION

Complications arise more frequently during the first trimester than at any other stage of pregnancy. Most present with bleeding, pain, or both. Vaginal bleeding occurs in about 20% of clinically diagnosed pregnancies.[1] It causes considerable anxiety for the woman and her partner. In the vast majority of cases, no intervention alters the outcome. The main aim of clinical management is a prompt and accurate diagnosis, with reassurance if the pregnancy is appropriately developed and viable, or appropriate intervention if not. The differential diagnoses are shown in Table 5–1.

Approximately 15% to 20% of clinically recognized pregnancies miscarry.[2] When bleeding occurs in the first trimester, about 30% of pregnancies will miscarry, 10% to 15% will be an ectopic pregnancy, approximately 0.2% will be a hydatidiform mole (HM), and about 5% of women will have a termination of pregnancy. The remaining 50% will continue beyond 20 weeks.[3]

Ectopic pregnancy is the most important cause of maternal mortality in the first trimester of pregnancy in the United Kingdom[4] and other western countries[5] and is the single largest cause of death in pregnancy among blacks. The most recent U.K. Confidential Enquiry into Maternal Mortality reported 11 deaths due to ectopic pregnancies (in contrast to 1 women who died following spontaneous miscarriage and none from sepsis).[4]

Understanding the psychological effects of early pregnancy loss has lagged behind that of perinatal bereavement.[6] However, there is now greater recognition of the psychological and psychiatric sequelae and the consequent need for support that should be part of the management of couples who suffer early pregnancy loss.[7]

INITIAL MANAGEMENT

Resuscitation and Triage

Heavy bleeding in early pregnancy should be assessed urgently. The rate and amount of blood loss should be assessed as accurately as possible, including a speculum examination to estimate any additional concealed loss from intravaginal blood and clot. Most women with first-trimester bleeding will be young and fit and will be able to maintain their blood pressure even after substantial blood loss. When the woman's initial blood pressure is low, it is important to visualize the cervix carefully and remove any products of pregnancy, which may be lying within the cervical canal. It is important to differentiate between

- "Cervical shock," which will respond rapidly to this removal of retained products of conception, and
- Vascular decompensation, due to catastrophic hemorrhage requiring rapid resuscitation.

If the patient is clinically shocked and there are no products of conception in the cervical canal, she should be managed as if there has been a major blood loss, irrespective of the amount of revealed bleeding.

When severe blood loss is evident or suspected, adequate staff should be available for resuscitation. Pulse and blood pressure should be recorded frequently and a large-bore intravenous access should be established. Blood should be taken for a full blood count, a clotting screen, and blood grouping and to cross-match blood. A minimum of 4 units of blood would be required for a patient who is clinically shocked. The woman should be rapidly assessed from her clinical history and examination while resuscitation is proceeding. If this assessment suggests a catastrophic intraperitoneal hemorrhage from a ruptured ectopic pregnancy, it is unlikely that resuscitation will render her clinically stable. Under those circumstances, an emergency laparotomy should be arranged.

If the woman responds promptly to appropriate resuscitation, or if she is not clinically shocked (the vast majority of patients), a careful history and examination should be undertaken and investigations arranged.

Diagnosis (see Table 5–1)

History

The date of the woman's last menstrual period, her usual menstrual cycle length, and any variation of this and the date of her first positive urinary pregnancy test should define her likely gestational age. The severity of any early pregnancy symptoms, particularly nausea and breast discomfort, may be of diagnostic value. Nausea and vomiting in the first trimester are more frequently associated with a positive pregnancy outcome,[8] even among women presenting with a threatened miscarriage.[9] The loss of early pregnancy symptoms around the time of any vaginal bleeding is a

TABLE 5-1

Differential Diagnosis of First-Trimester Pain and/or Bleeding

Pregnancy Related
Miscarriage (threatened, inevitable, incomplete, complete, missed, or septic)
Ectopic pregnancy
Hydatidiform mole
Bleeding from cervical ectropion
Coincidental to the Pregnancy—Gynecologic
Ruptured corpus luteum of pregnancy
Ovarian cyst accident
Torsion/degeneration of a pedunculated fibroid
Bleeding from cervical malignancy
Coincidental to the Pregnancy—Nongynecologic
Appendicitis
Renal colic
Intestinal obstruction
Cholecystitis
Pelvic inflammatory disease
Dysfunctional uterine bleeding
Endometriosis

bad prognostic sign. Increased early pregnancy symptoms are associated with molar pregnancies and multiple pregnancies.

The outcome of previous pregnancies should be noted and is an important indicator of the risk of miscarriage, ectopic pregnancy, or gestational trophoblastic disease. Primigravidae and women with previous live births have a lower risk of miscarriage. Miscarriage risk increases cumulatively according to the number of previous miscarriages.[10,11] Similarly, women with a previous ectopic pregnancy are at substantially increased risk of a further ectopic pregnancy.[12] There is about a 10-fold increased risk of repeat HM in women with a history of a previously affected pregnancy.[13]

The nature and distribution of any associated pain can be helpful. Unilateral pelvic pain is not necessarily related to an ectopic pregnancy and may simply be due to ovarian capsule distention from a corpus luteum of pregnancy, particularly if the pain radiates to the anterior thigh from irritation of the adjacent cutaneous nerves. Shoulder tip pain suggests diaphragmatic irritation from intra-abdominal bleeding. Although more likely with an ectopic pregnancy, this can also occur with retrograde bleeding from a miscarriage. The extent of first-trimester vaginal bleeding gives a useful prognostic guide. Pregnancy is rarely successful if the loss is equivalent to, or greater than, a woman's normal menstrual blood loss.[14] One of the more common exceptions to this is when there is loss of one of a twin pregnancy, although spontaneous reduction to a single pregnancy is often not accompanied by bleeding; the so-called vanishing twin phenomenon.[15]

Examination

The aims of examination should be to differentiate between an early pregnancy complication and a coincidental abdominal pathology and to identify women who need surgical intervention promptly. The woman's pulse and blood pressure should be monitored frequently to identify early any developing clinical shock. On inspection, the abdomen may be distended because of intraperitoneal bleeding or bowel dilation. Rarely, Cullen's sign (a bluish tinge of the periumbilical skin or an umbilical "black eye") may be present in cases of ruptured ectopic pregnancy. Generalized lower abdominal guarding or rebound tenderness on abdominal palpation may suggest intraperitoneal bleeding. Localized unilateral iliac fossa tenderness may be present with an unruptured ectopic pregnancy but can also be caused by a physiologic corpus luteum cyst of pregnancy.

A vaginal examination with a Cusco speculum should identify any local cause of bleeding due to trauma or any cervical cause due to a polyp or physiological ectropion (in which bleeding can frequently be related to coitus). An open cervical os suggests either an incomplete or an inevitable miscarriage. Blood loss through the cervical os and whether this is fresh or "old" should be noted. If products of conception are extruding through the cervix, these can be removed with sponge forceps, which may relieve pain and correct any reflex shock due to cervical distention. In general, removed products of conception should be sent for histologic assessment.

Bimanual examination should assess any cervical dilation and identify whether cervical excitation tenderness is present (see later) as a clinical sign of an ectopic pregnancy. The size and shape of the uterus should be assessed. If larger than expected from the menstrual dates, this may suggest a multiple pregnancy, an HM, or coincidental uterine pathology, most frequently fibroids. Adnexal palpation may identify a tender mass, which might be either an ectopic pregnancy or a normal corpus luteum cyst.

Special Investigations

A urinary β-human chorionic gonadotropin (β-hCG) pregnancy test should always be done, if not previously checked. Currently available commercial tests are now very sensitive and specific and can be expected to yield a positive result even 2 or 3 days before a missed period. If positive, the critical and complementary diagnostic investigations are a transvaginal pelvic ultrasound scan (TVUS) and quantitative serum β-hCG measurements.

The Role of Ultrasound, β-Human Chorionic Gonadotropin, and Progesterone Levels in the Investigation of Early Pregnancy Problems

The key purpose of an ultrasound scan and/or measuring hormones is to predict or differentiate an ectopic pregnancy from a normal intrauterine pregnancy. The ultrasound scan findings that predict an ectopic pregnancy include a living extrauterine pregnancy, an extrauterine gestational sac containing a yolk sac or embryo, an empty "tubal ring," or any adnexal mass other than a simple cyst. In both pooled retrospective data and prospective cohort data, the criterion that performed best in sensitivity, specificity, and predictive value was the presence of any adnexal mass other than a simple cyst.[16,17]

Transvaginal Ultrasonography

This generally provides more immediate information than hCG levels but is unhelpful in women who are less than 7 days past their missed period (conventionally taken to be 4 weeks after the first day of the last period). Rapid changes occur in appearance between 4 and 7 weeks of amenorrhea (Table 5–2). At 5 weeks' gestation from the woman's last menstrual period (assuming a regular 28-day cycle), a gestation sac of 2- to 5-mm diameter should be visible. However, this can often be difficult to differentiate from a pseudogestational sac associated with an ectopic pregnancy, in which there is simply a small collection of fluid secretions within the uterine cavity, or a decidual cast, in which the pregnancy has failed and decidual separation from the basal endometrium has occurred. A genuine intrauterine gestation sac should have two recognizable concentric decidual rings surrounding it, whereas a decidual cast or pseudogestational sac will have only one.

Confirmation of an intrauterine sac can be secure when the yolk sac or fetus becomes visible. The yolk sac is the first structure that becomes identifiable within the gestation sac, usually by 5½ weeks (Fig. 5–1). It will usually measure 2 to 5 mm in diameter. Initially, up to about 6 weeks, it will be larger than the fetus. However, an excessively large yolk sac (>5.6-mm diameter) is often an early sign of impending miscarriage.[18] Other early indicators of an almost certain miscarriage are when the gestation sac diameter exceeds 20 mm without any visible yolk sac or exceeds 25 mm without a visible fetus.

When an intrauterine pregnancy is clearly visible, a useful formula to calculate approximate gestational age (in days from the last menstrual period) is

Gestational age (days) = mean sac diameter (mm) + 30[19]

This formula is valid up to 9 weeks. A second, more accurate but more complex, formula and that is valid to at least 12 weeks is

Mean sac diameter (mm) =
0.986 (days after ovulation/conception) − 17.1[20]

The presence of an intrauterine pregnancy with a live fetus is a good prognostic finding. When a live embryo or

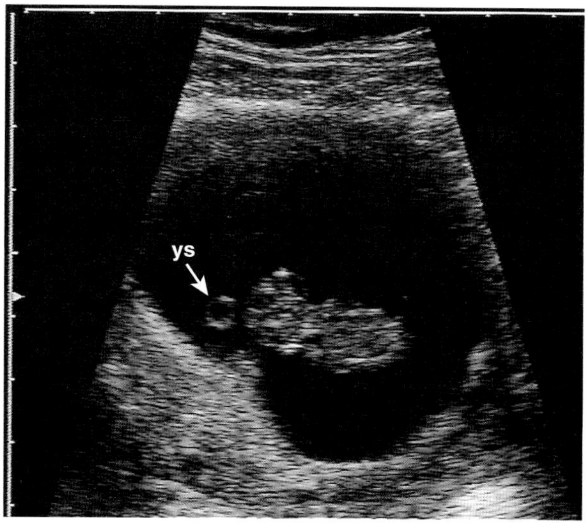

FIGURE 5–1
Pregnancy with yolk sac (ys) at eight weeks' gestation.

TABLE 5–2

Ultrasound Findings and β-hCG Concentrations for a Singleton Intrauterine Pregnancy at Particular Gestational Age Points in Early Fetal Life*

	TRANSVAGINAL ULTRASOUND FINDINGS					
WEEKS (DAYS) FROM THE LAST MENSTRUAL PERIOD (ASSUMING A 28-30-DAY CYCLE)	ENDOMETRIUM	GESTATIONAL SAC (AFTER HOLLANDER, 1972,[32] AND MILLS, 1992[20])	YOLK SAC (AFTER MILLS, 1992[20])	CROWN-RUMP LENGTH (AFTER HOLLANDER, 1972,[32] AND MILLS, 1992[20])	FETAL HEART (RATE) (AFTER MERCHIERS ET AL, 1991,[23] AND ROBINSON AND SHAW-DUNN, 1973[33])	SERUM HCG (IU/L; 3RD IRP) (MEAN 95% CI VALUES FOR IMMULITE HCG ASSAY) (AFTER NEPOMNASCHY ET AL, 2008,[168] AND BARNHART ET AL, 2004[26])
4 weeks (28 days)	10-15 mm	–	–	–	–	88 73-105
5 weeks (35 days)	15-20 mm	3 mm	2 mm	–	–	600
5½ weeks (38-39 days)	20 mm	7-8 mm	3 mm	3-4 mm	–	1000 500-1500
6 weeks (42 days)	20 mm	10-12 mm	4 mm	4 mm	85-100	1500 900-2900
6½ weeks (45-46 days)	–	14-15 mm	4.5 mm	7 mm	–	6000 3500-14000
7 weeks (48-49 days)	–	17-18 mm	5 mm	10 mm	125	15000 6500->25000

* For optimal interpretation, data are presented for half weeks where possible and from more than one source, leading to a range of values in some cells and no data in other cells.
β-hCG, β-human chorionic gonadotropin; CI, confidence interval; hCG, human chorionic gonadotropin.

fetus is seen on ultrasound, the pregnancy is likely to continue in over 95% of cases.[21,22] As well as ultrasound structures, fetal circulation becomes evident at 5½ weeks and is visible in all viable pregnancies by 6 weeks.[20] Initially, the fetal heart rate is slower than normal, but it increases over time, from 85 to 90 beats/min at 6 weeks to levels of up to 180 beats/min at 9 weeks.[23] Rates persistently slower than 100 are more likely to be associated with a poor outcome.[23]

Measurement of Human Chorionic Gonadotropin

Serum β-hCG concentrations complement the information available from TVUS in assessing early pregnancy problems. For this chapter, β-hCG values and ranges relate to the Third International Reference Preparation (3rd IRP). Absolute levels may be helpful in recognizing when a normal intrauterine pregnancy should be seen at TVUS. Levels of β-hCG greater than 1500 to 2000 IU/L (depending on local laboratory variations) should almost always be associated with the finding of a gestational sac in the uterus if the pregnancy is intrauterine.[24] If it cannot be seen in the uterus, it should be assumed there is a pregnancy elsewhere (Fig. 5–2). However, caution should be exercised when women have had assisted conception treatment (by in vitro fertilization or ovulation induction). In these situations, more than one embryo might be present and, therefore, an intrauterine and extrauterine pregnancy might coexist (i.e., a heterotopic pregnancy) or two intrauterine pregnancies might exist, giving rise to higher β-hCG levels (≤20 times normal) without a pregnancy yet being visible on TVUS. Excessively high serum β-hCG levels are also found with gestational trophoblastic disease and levels up to twice normal can be found in pregnancies affected by Down syndrome. Generally, β-hCG levels will be lower at any given gestational age with ectopic pregnancies than with normal intrauterine pregnancies. However, the overlap in values between the two clinical conditions is too great for this to be a diagnostic criterion.

Changes in β-hCG levels are more useful clinically. Usually, β-hCG values are best tested at intervals of 48 hours or longer. A falling β-hCG concentration in the first few weeks identifies a pregnancy as abnormal. If the β-hCG falls by more than more than half within 48 hours, it suggests that residual trophoblastic activity has ceased and that the pregnancy is likely to resolve without intervention. With a viable intrauterine pregnancy, previous data supported the view that β-hCG values should increase by at least 66% in 48 hours.[25] However, more recent and more accurate data for viable pregnancies support a view that the slowest rise at 1 day was 24% and 53% at 2 days; median increases in hCG at 1 day and 2 days were 50% and 124% (considerably

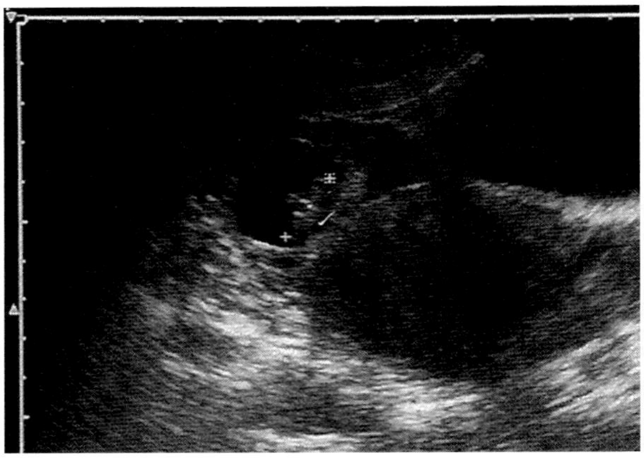

FIGURE 5–2
Uterus with an ectopic pregnancy (crown-rump length [CRL] = 19 mm) shows fetal heart activity at 7 weeks' gestation.

SUMMARY OF MANAGEMENT OPTIONS

Initial/General Management

Management Option	Evidence Quality and Recommendation	References
Identify cause by combination of history, examination, β-hCG assay, progesterone measurement, and transvaginal ultrasound	Ia/A III/B	28 9,11–14,20–23,25,27,29–33
The presence of an extrauterine mass is the most accurate predictor of an ectopic pregnancy	III/B	16,17
Assess amount and rate of blood loss	III/B	14
Regular recordings of pulse and blood pressure	IV/C	—
Intravenous access if actual or risk of hemodynamic instability	IV/C	—
FBC for all; clotting screening if coagulopathy suspected or excess blood loss; cross-match blood if excessive blood loss	IV/C	—

β-hCG, β-human chorionic gonadotropin; FBC, full blood count.

lower than previously thought).[26] In addition, a β-hCG doubling time of more than 7 days is never found in a normal pregnancy.[25]

Measurement of Progesterone

In both natural conceptions and in pregnancies arising from assisted conception, progesterone has been assessed in its role to determine the health of a pregnancy, particularly with reference to the site of that pregnancy. Levels of 30 to 45 nmol/L (10–15 ng/mL) suggest a healthy ongoing pregnancy. However, low levels are poor at differentiating miscarriages from ectopics (though combining with hCG measurements may help).[27–29]

SPONTANEOUS ABORTION OR MISCARRIAGE

Definition

Now used synonymously, the terms *spontaneous abortion* and *miscarriage* imply the natural loss of a pregnancy before independent viability of the fetus. Until recently, the term "abortion" was generally used in professional communication and "miscarriage" was used in discussion with patients. However, because this was not an exclusive definition, and as the term "abortion" (which many patients find offensive) has pejorative connotations of "elective termination of pregnancy," there has been an overall shift away from using "abortion" to describe the spontaneous loss of a pregnancy.[34] *Viability* implies the ability of the fetus to survive extrauterine life. This is generally taken to be around 24 weeks, and rarely, fetuses born before that will survive for a short while or at least show some signs of life. The cutoff point for the use of the term "miscarriage" might lie at 22 weeks (154 days), therefore, as recommended by the World Health Organization (WHO).[35] The WHO also includes in this a baby's weight (the value being < 500 g). In the United Kingdom, the legal definition changed in 1992 to 24 weeks (168 days) whereas in North America, the gestational age limit for a miscarriage is 20 weeks.[36]

In addition to these changes in terminology, there has been a marked alteration in the way in which early pregnancy problems of bleeding and pain are managed. Much of this is attributable to the

- Availability of rapid access to serum β-hCG estimations.
- High-resolution TVUS.
- Introduction of fast-track referrals to early pregnancy assessment units/clinics (EPU/EPC).

In EPCs, access to integrated evaluation by ultrasonography, serum sampling for β-hCG, and the presence of experienced timetabled medical and nursing staff has permitted women to be managed more as outpatients or in the office, providing a more streamlined service.

A summary of requirements for an EPC service is provided in Table 5–3. EPCs have improved the quality of care and produced savings in financial and staff resources. However, as a tool in patient management, EPC services have not yet been fully evaluated.[37] Management of women through an EPC service is not without its drawbacks. Inappropriate delays in diagnosis of true ectopic pregnancies and overmanagement by laparoscopy of suspected ectopic pregnancies both occur, despite rigid adherence to protocols.

TABLE 5–3
Requirements for an Early Pregnancy Assessment Clinic

- Appropriate resources for rostering of ultrasonographic, medical, and nursing staff (exact calculation of time required is not evidence-based; experience suggests that for a hospital with a delivery rate of 5000 deliveries/yr, 3 hours of patient contact time for all disciplines and 1 hour of telephone contact time later in the day is reasonable).
- Dedicated clinic space with rooms for ultrasonography, clinical assessment and investigation, counseling, and a waiting area.
- Good quality ultrasound machines with transvaginal facility.
- Availability of same-day hCG estimation.
- Responsibility for development of guidelines and resolution of conflicts and problems should be the responsibility of a designated senior member of the clinical staff.

hCG, human chorionic gonadotropin.

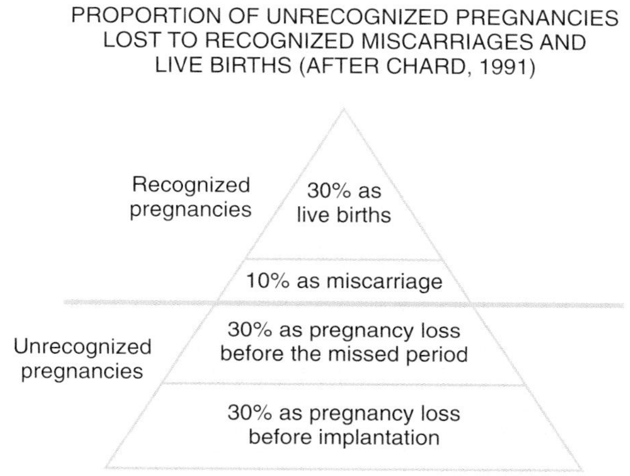

FIGURE 5–3
Proportion of unrecognized pregnancies lost to recognized miscarriages and live births.
(From Chard T: Frequency of implantation and early pregnancy loss in natural cycles. Baillieres Clin Obstet Gynecol 1991;5:179–189.)

A pregnancy loss may be clinically evident, following presentation with bleeding or pain, or be clinically silent, identified at routine ultrasound scan. The introduction of almost routine scanning to confirm gestational age has had a dramatic effect of the management of early pregnancy loss. Bleeding occurs in a fifth of recognized pregnancies before 20 weeks. It is likely, however, that a far greater unrecognized pregnancy loss is present in the background, with more pregnancies being lost before the pregnancy has been suspected, recognized, or confirmed (giving rise to the term "pregnancy loss iceberg"; Fig. 5–3).[38,39] In one study, 12% of pregnancies in which bleeding occurred went on to miscarry.[40] Other studies have reported higher rates (≤16%),[40] but these studies do not include those women who did not know they were pregnant (≤22%)[41] or those who did not seek medical advice about their bleeding, knowing they were pregnant (~12%).[40]

Risks

The maternal risks are blood loss, infection, and the psychological effects of the loss of the pregnancy.

Presentation and Diagnosis

Most women will present to a hospital, family doctor, or EPC in a number of ways:

- Bleeding without pain,
- Bleeding with pain (with possible passage of pregnancy tissue vaginally).
- Bleeding with pain with symptoms and signs of blood loss.
- Absence of bleeding with pregnancy symptoms diminishing.

The amount of bleeding can vary and has some prognostic value. Bleeding without pain is more likely to be associated with a threatened miscarriage. Presentations to an EPC service will frequently be for painless bleeding. Once the pregnancy is confirmed on ultrasound to be ongoing, this situation can be dealt with by reassurance. Most of these cases will be due to bleeding from local causes such as physiologic changes in the cervix. The additional presence of pain is often associated with cervical opening or distention as a result of tissue or blood clot passing through and is a painful process. Blood loss can give rise to symptoms in itself, and the passage of tissue through the cervical os can promote a vagal response causing shock, which is rapidly relieved if the products are removed from the os.

Management Options

Threatened miscarriages are managed expectantly. If the bleeding is slight and not associated with pain, then the woman can be reassured that the pregnancy is likely to continue. For all pregnancies in which bleeding occurs, more than 50% will continue.[3] If the bleeding occurs at 10 weeks more than 90% will continue; at 13 weeks, 99% will continue.[42] If the menstrual/gestational age is 6 weeks or older, then ultrasound may show a healthy ongoing pregnancy. In such cases, the likelihood of pregnancy loss is less than 3%.[22] Ultrasonography before 6 weeks is less likely to be helpful. If a patient needs the reassurance of an ongoing pregnancy by ultrasound scan, then this should be undertaken after 6 weeks.

The management options for the loss of an early intrauterine pregnancy are

- Expectant.
- Medical.
- Surgical.

Cases of complete spontaneous miscarriage can be managed expectantly. Most difficulty in the management of early pregnancy bleeding concerns cases of missed or incomplete miscarriage.

In most western countries, historically, the surgical approach ("evacuation of retained products of conception" [ERPC]) has been the most common emergency gynecologic procedure. The procedure was traditionally carried out with ovum forceps and curettage and evolved to vacuum aspiration. Vacuum aspiration is associated with less blood loss and pain and a shorter procedure than surgical curettage.[43]

Expectant management avoids a surgical procedure and allows the woman to continue in her normal daily routine. It is more acceptable to women and has less impact on quality of life.[44] It is an approach that has been adopted readily in primary care without hospital admission.[45]

Many reported studies compare two of the three modalities of treatment (expectant, medical, and surgical). Some are included in the Summary of Management Options at the end of this section. However, current management of miscarriage should now be based on published meta-analysis and randomized, controlled trial (RCT) papers, together with both economic and quality of life data, which these studies have also produced. The advice from these is not entirely in harmony. This is partly because the meta-analysis attempted to synthesize data from disparate studies comparing two modalities of treatment, whereas the RCTs compared all three modalities in a randomized approach. The RCTs were published after the meta-analysis.

In their meta-analysis, Sotiriadis and colleagues[46] suggest that surgical management appears most likely to achieve success and expectant management least so. The largest RCT combining all three modalities (the miscarriage treatment [MIST] trial) recruited 1200 women in approximately equal proportions to the three modalities of treatment.[47] In that study, there were no differences in rates of infection, hemoglobin or hematocrit levels, incidence in surgical complications, sick leave, or scores in hospital anxiety and depression questionnaires between the three modalities. Compared with expectant and medical management, those patients managed surgically had fewer unplanned admissions and unplanned surgical curettages, no blood transfusion (compared with 1%–2%), and less analgesia.

A second much smaller RCT (40 patients) had broadly similar results but was stopped early because of failure to recruit to randomization.[48] Data from the MIST study on women's preferences for treatment suggested that women particularly value alternatives being offered to expectant management[49]—clearly an important consideration when planning service provision. The level of pain experienced appeared to be the most important determinant for preference for an alterative treatment, and to a lesser extent, time to return to normal activity, number of days of bleeding, and likelihood of complications. When costs are analyzed, expectant management was least expensive and medical treatment was 40% and surgical treatment 50% more expensive.[50] One other large study analyzed medical and surgical modalities for quality of life and acceptability, finding no differences.[51]

For practical purposes, expectant management is well tolerated, cost-efficient, and safe and should be used for women in the first instance, providing that they are hemodynamically stable. It appears difficult to predict for which women expectant management will be effective.[52] Patients need to understand that they will bleed for slightly longer[53] and have a risk of needing surgical evacuation[47] so they need to have ready access to hospital services if needed. Medical management is not much more effective than expectant, but it is more expensive and, therefore, its role is less clear as a management option. Expectant and surgical seem to be the practical options—no intervention if possible, and then surgical if required.

Vacuum aspiration is preferable to surgical curettage, being safer, less painful, and quicker to undertake.[43] Whether any women should electively have surgical treatment rather

SUMMARY OF MANAGEMENT OPTIONS

Spontaneous Miscarriage

Management Options	Evidence Quality and Recommendation	References
Expectant, medical, and surgical all compared	Ia/A	46–48
Expectant management	Ia/A	46–48,55,61,62
Medical evacuation	Ia/A	46–48
	Ib	55,61,63–65
Surgical evacuation	Ia/A	46–48,61,63
Adequately resourced; Early Pregnancy Clinic is key to management of early pregnancy problems	III/B	37
Many cases do not need hospital admission	Ia/A	45
Expectant and surgical managements are equally effective	Ia/A	62
Expectant management does not affect future fertility	Ib/A	62,66
Medical management before recourse to surgical management	Ib/A	63,67
Vacuum aspiration should be used in preference to surgical evacuation	Ia/A	43
Couples require no more psychological support and women no more time off work following expectant, medical, or surgical management of miscarriage	Ia/A	47
	Ib	68
Patient preference should play a dominant role	Ia/A	46–48

than any other is not clear, though in terminations, women of high parity (>para 3) are more likely to have a complete abortion following surgical management.[54]

Ideally, tissue should be sent from all miscarriages for histologic examination. However, there are obvious practical problems in achieving that goal if medical and expectant management are undertaken. It certainly should be requested on all those having surgical curettage. Ultrasound findings suspicious of trophoblastic disease are an indication for surgical rather than medical management.

Some have suggested that the optimum management option can be determined on the basis of ultrasound and biochemical evaluation. The volume of tissue remaining in the uterine cavity on ultrasound may be a useful guide in management. No intervention is required in the absence of tissue or if products of conception are present with a mean diameter less than 15 mm. Medical or expectant management may be considered if the tissue mass is between 15 and 50 mm, and an ERPC is probably required if tissue diameter is greater than 50 mm.[55] More complications (37% vs. 3%) occurred when women with significant intrauterine tissue (an intrauterine sac >10 mm in diameter) were managed expectantly compared with surgically.[56] Tissue volume has not been used in the evaluation of the data in the three-modality RCTs[47,48] or the meta-analysis,[46] so further clarification is still awaited.

Evidence regarding the value of serum β-hCG levels[56,57] or progesterone[58] to determine the need for surgical intervention is insufficient. When color Doppler imaging of uterine blood flow and of the intervillous space was examined in missed miscarriages,[59] uterine blood flow could not differentiate between those women whose miscarriage resolved spontaneously and those who required an ERPC. Intervillous space blood flow was associated with an 80% chance of spontaneous resolution compared with 23% in those for whom flow was absent.[59] Although this technique shows promise, it requires validation. At present, these adjuvant techniques are of little value in determining which women should be managed expectantly or otherwise.

Should women undergoing surgical evacuation of uterus have *Chlamydia* screening in line with other invasive interventions in the uterine cavity? One inadequately powered randomized trial showed no benefit, but because the intervention reduces infection in induced abortion, it is probably worth continuing until evidence suggests otherwise.[60]

Much of the management of early pregnancy bleeding may remain within the remit of general practitioners[45] or midwives,[1] but accurate diagnosis of ectopic pregnancies[56] and molar pregnancies[52] remain particular concerns. Rapid access to ultrasound and β-hCG assays should remain as a fundamental part of the management of early pregnancy bleeding.

ECTOPIC PREGNANCY

The management of ectopic pregnancy has changed over the past 20 years because of several important developments:

- Recognition of high risk individuals (Table 5–4).
- Increased sensitivity of home pregnancy tests.
- Early referral to dedicated EPCs in hospital settings.
- Development and refinement of high-resolution TVUS.
- Accurate and rapid estimation of serum β-hCG.
- Laboratory techniques allowing 24-hour access to automated sample processing.

However, there is no room for complacency with regard to ectopic pregnancy management. The most recent report on maternal deaths in the United Kingdom shows an increase in ectopic pregnancy rates over the previous 20 years, from 8.6/1000 pregnancies in 1985 to 1987, to 11.1/1000 pregnancies in 2003 to 2005.[69] Deaths from ectopic pregnancies in that report are no better than 20 years previously: 4.7 compared with 4.8 deaths/1,000,000 maternities. Although the death rate expressed as a proportion of ectopic pregnancies in that time span (6.1 compared with 3.5 /1000 ectopic pregnancies) is an apparent fall, in real terms, there have been about 10 deaths in each triennium from 1985 to 2005.

A major recommendation from the most recent report on maternal deaths suggests that every unit should have clear guidelines for the management of pain and bleeding in early pregnancy because "there are persisting failures to recognise these conditions [ectopic pregnancies] promptly."[69]

Definition

An *ectopic pregnancy* is one that occurs in a site outside the uterine cavity, but usually in an adjacent site. In over 98% of ectopic pregnancies, the primary site is in the fallopian tube and the remainder will be in the abdominal cavity, the ovary, or the cervix. In the fallopian tube, about 80% of the pregnancies will occur in the ampullary region. Given these relative frequencies, this chapter deals largely with sites in the extrauterine fallopian tubes.

Risks

These are blood loss and its consequences, implications for future reproductive performance (see later), and psychological effects of the loss of the pregnancy.

Diagnosis

Symptoms

Diagnosis of an ectopic pregnancy can be difficult. Some, all, or none of the following symptoms may be elicited in a woman presenting with an ectopic pregnancy:

- Amenorrhea.
- Abdominal pain.
- Vaginal bleeding.
- Fainting.
- Shoulder tip pain.

Signs

At presentation to an EPC, many women with an ectopic pregnancy may have few or no signs. Unilateral iliac fossa pain is more in keeping with ectopic pregnancy, but bilateral pain is not uncommon. Guarding, rigidity, and signs of peritonism may be elicited on abdominal palpation. Guarding may be reduced if the knees are drawn up to relax the abdominal muscles.

On vaginal examination, it may be possible to elicit tenderness on the affected adnexal side by manipulating the cervix laterally ("cervical excitation") or by direct adnexal palpation. Because the uterus moves in the opposite direction owing to rotation around the fulcrum of the transverse cervical ligaments, there is increased tension on the side where the ectopic pregnancy is sited. The uterus may be softer and even enlarged slightly in the presence of an ectopic pregnancy owing to the softening effect of increased levels of progesterone on the endometrium and myometrium.

It is now rare in U.K. practice for women with an ectopic pregnancy to present with hypovolemic shock or in severe pain. The practical implications of this change in practice means that greater clinical acumen is required in managing those women presenting with pain and bleeding in early pregnancy.

Investigations

The diagnosis of ectopic pregnancy needs to be differentiated from other causes of lower abdominal pain in a woman of reproductive years (see Table 5–1).

Critical to the diagnosis of ectopic pregnancy are TVUS, and serum β-hCG, and to a lesser extent, serum progesterone. Confirmation of the diagnosis by laparoscopy is not always necessary. Laparoscopy is indeed not even the absolute answer, having a false-negative rate of 3% to 4% (being done too early) and a false-positive rate of 5% (owing to retrograde uterine bleeding).[70]

The complementary roles of TVUS and β-hCG measurements were discussed earlier. Serum progesterone is also considered to have a role in the differentiation of an ectopic pregnancy. Its use is not as widespread as β-hCG and TVUS. Serum progesterone concentrations well into the normal range for early pregnancy (>80 nmol/L) are associated with a high probability of the pregnancy being normal and intrauterine in site.[31] Conversely, values lower than 15 nmol/L are highly likely (98%) to be associated with a nonviable pregnancy.[71] Most ectopic pregnancies have progesterone concentrations between these values, making the test of little value at present for routine clinical practice. Algorithms have been devised with and without the use of serum progesterone and can be referred to and integrated into local practice guidelines if considered appropriate.[24,72] Figure 5–4 shows an example of such a practical algorithm.

The patient presenting acutely with obvious intra-abdominal bleeding will be diagnosed without difficulty. The less acute clinical scenario in which a women presents

TABLE 5–4
Particular Risk Factors Associated with Ectopic Pregnancy

Peak age-specific incidence 25-34 years
Infertility (fourfold increased risk)
Sexually transmitted disease (especially chlamydia)
Raised *Chlamydia* antibody titer
Tubal sterilization and reconstruction
Intrauterine contraceptive device
Endometriosis

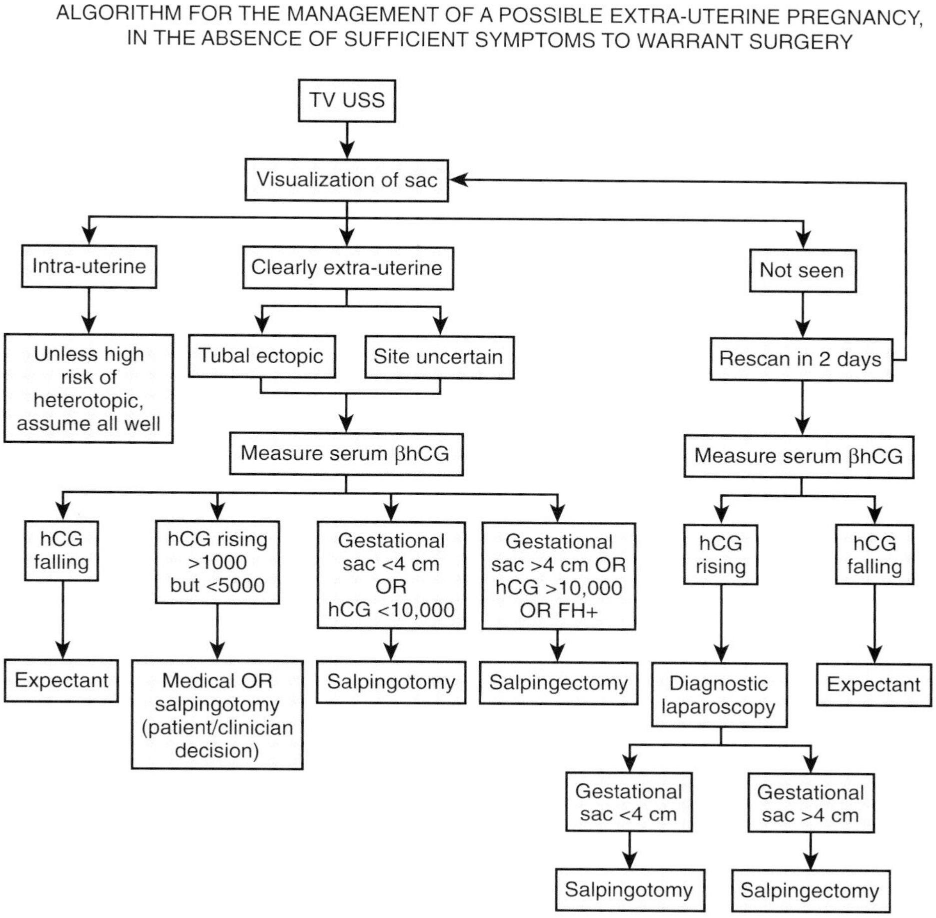

FIGURE 5–4
Algorithm for the management of a possible extrauterine pregnancy, in the absence of sufficient symptoms to warrant surgery. βhCG, β-human chorionic gonadotropin; TV USS, transvaginal pelvic ultrasound scan.

with little or no pain, vague symptoms, slowing rising β-hCG levels, and nonspecific findings on ultrasound is more challenging.

Management Options

Management of the acutely ill woman differs from the more common presentation of a woman who is clinically stable, in which situation there are a number of treatment options.

The acute presentation with hypotension, tachycardia, pain, and other signs of shock, usually, though not always, associated with amenorrhea is generally dealt with by laparotomy. The acute symptoms are usually due to fallopian tube rupture and/or significant intraperitoneal bleeding. Surgical treatment usually requires partial or total salpingectomy, securing hemostasis and removing blood and products of conception from the abdominal cavity.

In the less acute situation, there are several treatment options, which include expectant, medical, and surgical (conservative and radical) management. The gradation of quality of evidence is presented in the Summary of Management Options box (later). The algorithm in Figure 5–4 shows the critical criteria that influence appropriate management, namely, the trend in serum β-hCG level and the findings on TVUS. Serum β-hCG rising above a critical threshold in the absence of an intrauterine gestation sac will usually be an indication for surgical intervention. Whether by laparoscopy or laparotomy will depend on the patient's past surgical history, the TVUS findings, and the absolute level of β-hCG and its rate of rise.

Expectant Management

As shown in Figure 5–4, this management is most appropriate when the woman is hemodynamically stable, with no symptoms of pain. Some authors have suggested that this approach should not be undertaken with a gestational sac size greater than 4 cm and/or the presence of a fetal heartbeat on TVUS.[73] Certainly, expectant management is more likely to be effective if the initial serum β-hCG concentration is less than 1000 IU/Ll and falls thereafter and if a gestational sac is not seen on TVUS.[73] The serum β-hCG level, both the initial level and the trend, is generally the most important predictor of successful expectant management.[73] Some publications suggest that of vaginal bleeding, endometrial thickness, serum β-hCG, and serum progesterone, the most useful modality to predict spontaneous resolution was serum progesterone with a cutoff level of less than 20 nmol/L.[74]

In practice, expectant management involves establishing a reliable diagnosis of early extrauterine pregnancy failure, informing the patient of other treatment options, and obtaining consent that this method of management is acceptable. Having done so, serum β-hCG levels should be monitored every 3 to 4 days until they fall to less than 10 to 15 IU/L.[71]

Success rates for this approach range from 70% to 75% for β-hCG levels of less than 1000 IU/L[73,74] falling to 25% with levels greater than 2000 IU/L.[75]

Medical Management

Current methods of medical management focus on the use of methotrexate, generally as a single dose, although multiple-dose regimens are less commonly used. Adjunctive mifepristone is only of additional benefit in improving success rates when the serum progesterone is greater than 10 nmol/L.[76]

Methotrexate is a folic acid antagonist (inactivating dihydrofolate reductase and depleting tetrahydrofolate, required for RNA and DNA synthesis) and, as a chemotherapeutic agent, is active against rapidly dividing tissues such as those in the placental trophoblast. Methotrexate can produce side effects through its actions on other tissues in the body such as the gastrointestinal tract (stomatitis, gastritis, diarrhea, transient liver enzyme disorders), and rarely, the hematologic system (bone marrow suppression).[77] A single dose can produce symptoms, though less than multiple doses (daily or alternate-day), including gastrointestinal symptoms (31% single vs. 41% multiple [$P < .04$]), abdominal pain (22% vs. 26% [nonsignificant]).[77] Folinic acid (leucovorin) is given to counteract this (0.1 mg/kg). Folinic acid is not required when doses are given at more than weekly intervals.[78] Medical management is particularly appropriate when surgical intervention would be difficult (e.g., cervical and interstitial pregnancies). Medical treatment has been available since the mid 1980s[79] but has not been adopted extensively. This is lamentable because studies involving large series of women show success rates around 90%.[80] Predictors of success of medical treatment include sac size, presence of fetal cardiac activity, and serum β-hCG concentration. β-hCG is the most important of these.[80] For values of 2000 to 5000 IU/L, the likelihood of success is 92% (86%–97% 95% confidence interval [CI]), but higher when less than 1000 IU/L (98%, 96%–100% 95% CI).[80] Compared with conservative laparoscopic surgery, methotrexate use is associated with a shorter in-hospital stay but a longer return to normal β-hCG levels.[81] Given that in U.K. practice, one might expect most women to attend an outpatient EPC for diagnosis, this is not a particular advantage. Opinions vary on the effect of medical therapy on quality of life: one study found higher well-being scores in women managed medically[82]; another failed to confirm this.[83] However, future reproductive expectations are better with methotrexate, with higher intrauterine pregnancy and lower ectopic rates subsequently.

The dose of methotrexate used in clinical practice varies. Given systemically, and usually intramuscularly, the dose is either 1 mg/kg or 50 mg/m^2. These doses seem to be equally effective, and most favor the easier dose calculation of the former with a minimum total dose of 50 mg.[84] When single-dose therapy is planned, most women will only require one dose (85%). When multiple-dose therapy is planned, most (90%) will have at least two doses, and 54% will have four.[77]

Surgical Management

Salpingectomy has long been considered the gold standard treatment for ectopic pregnancy. In situations of emergency care and rupture of the fallopian tube, this may still be unavoidable. However, considerable recent emphasis has been placed on conservation of the fallopian tubes where possible and debate now focuses on:

- When is it appropriate to conserve a fallopian tube?
- Does fallopian tube conservation significantly affect subsequent fertility rates?

WHEN IS IT APPROPRIATE TO CONSERVE A FALLOPIAN TUBE?

The Royal College of Obstetricians and Gynaecologists recommends that surgical treatment by laparoscopic salpingectomy is the preferred method of treatment for an ectopic pregnancy when the fallopian tube on the other side is normal.[85] However, the majority of women in the United Kingdom were having open surgery, not laparoscopic surgery, for the management of their ectopic pregnancy until recently.[86] Furthermore, open surgery may be the more appropriate route as concluded by a meta-analysis, based on the combined results of three studies, involving women with unruptured tubal pregnancies, which showed laparoscopic conservative surgery had more failures (defined as persistence of trophoblastic tissue and raised hCG levels) than an open surgical approach (odds ratio [OR] 0.28; 95% CI 0.09–0.86).[87] Laparoscopic salpingotomy is, however, less costly.[87]

There is insufficient evidence from RCTs to answer the questions raised in the salpingectomy/salpingotomy debate and opinions vary. In the management of an ectopic pregnancy, removal of the fallopian tube (salpingectomy) is considered to be the safest,[88] most clinically effective,[89] and most cost-effective technique.[90] A meta-analysis of nine well-designed comparative studies showed similar intrauterine pregnancy rates whether salpingectomy (49%) or salpingotomy (53%) was used.[84] That paper and a separate meta-analysis showed higher subsequent ectopic pregnancy rates after salpingotomy (15% vs. 10%).[84,91] There is general agreement that salpingectomy would be appropriate if a women desired no further children, if a second ectopic occurred in the same fallopian tube, if bleeding could not be controlled, or if the tube was severely damaged by the ectopic pregnancy. If salpingotomy is undertaken, further quantitative β-hCG monitoring is required to confirm successful treatment because persistence of the ectopic pregnancy occurs in 8% to 19% of cases.[84,92] We would expect that the ongoing multicenter randomized, controlled ESEP (salpingostomy versus salpingectomy for tubal ectopic pregnancy) trial will address whether the advantages of salpingostomy outweigh the disadvantages when compared with salpingectomy.[93]

In the woman with a solitary fallopian tube who has a salpingostomy in her single remaining tube, it has been reported that 54% of women achieved a subsequent intrauterine pregnancy but 21% of the remainder had a further ectopic pregnancy.[84]

The details of the techniques used to undertake these surgical techniques are beyond the scope of this chapter. Salpingectomy may be undertaken laparoscopically or by open surgery. Open surgery is more likely to be undertaken if the woman is shocked or otherwise showing signs of being hemodynamically unstable. Laparoscopic salpingectomy techniques include resection using diathermy and scissors, loop ligatures, or single-use proprietary stapling instruments. Conservative surgery generally involves a linear incision along the antimesenteric border of the fallopian tube over the site of the ectopic pregnancy. The pregnancy is removed by flushing with high-pressure hydrodissection, and hemostasis is achieved by (bipolar) diathermy. In two small studies, prophylactic vasopressin was used in 40 hemodynamically stable women with a small unruptured ectopic pregnancy[94] and diluted oxytocin in 25 similar women.[95] These interventions reduced the need for electrocoagulation for hemostasis (relative risk [RR] 0.36; 95% CI 0.14–0.95) without side effects, resulting in a significantly shorter operation time, reduced intra- and postoperative blood loss, and easier removal of the tubal pregnancy without side effects. However, neither study showed any benefit in reducing the likelihood of persistent trophoblastic disease. Suturing of the incision in linear salpingostomy had no benefit in reducing adhesion formation or subsequent pregnancy rate.[96]

FERTILITY AFTER SURGERY

After salpingectomy, in the presence of a normal fallopian tube on the contralateral side, the likelihood of an intrauterine pregnancy is greater than 50%.[97] After salpingotomy, the likelihood of an intrauterine pregnancy is approximately 65%.[84,98]

Any study that looks at fertility after radical or conservative treatment must take account of the fact that there is a higher chance of salpingectomy if the initial ectopic had ruptured. In studies that took this factor into account, no appreciable difference was found in the subsequent intrauterine pregnancy rates.[99] Factors that did alter the likelihood of conception included the woman's age, previous tubal damage, and infertility.[99] This holds true even if the previous ectopic pregnancy had ruptured.[100] The reported likelihood of a future ectopic pregnancy after 3 years is 18% to 23% after conservative treatment and 28% after radical treatment.[99,101]

On economic and fertility outcome grounds, there is no clear indication whether salpingectomy or salpingostomy is more appropriate for women who have both fallopian tubes.

Future Advice and Appropriate Treatment

The likelihood of a further ectopic pregnancy varies little with the management of the index case. Previous tubal rupture does not appear to have a detrimental effect on future fertility. Smoking is an independent risk factor for fertility and the likelihood of a future intrauterine pregnancy appears to be increased by stopping smoking.[99] Future

SUMMARY OF MANAGEMENT OPTIONS

Ectopic Pregnancy

Management Options	Evidence Quality and Recommendation	References
Diagnosis		
Accurate and rapid β-hCG estimation and high-resolution transvaginal ultrasound are key to the management	III/B	24
Expectant		
Suitable for some ectopic pregnancies if β-hCG levels are low and falling (<1000 IU/L)	Ib/A	102–104
Medical		
Valid option with no fetal heartbeat, β-hCG < 5000 IU/L, patient is asymptomatic and willing to have serial β-hCG estimations	III/B	80
Methotrexate local	Ib/A	102
Methotrexate systemic	Ib/A	102,105
Hyperosmolar glucose	Ib/A	102
Prostaglandins and methotrexate	Ib/A	102
Methotrexate and mifepristone	Ib/A	76
Single and multiple doses of methotrexate	Ia/A	77
Surgery—General		
Laparotomy has higher success rates	Ib/A	102
Salpingectomy is marginally better than salpingotomy; subsequent fertility rates are no different	III/B	84,101
Use agents preoperatively to reduce bleeding	Ib/A	94,95
Surgical—Laparoscopy		
Salpingotomy/salpingectomy	Ib/A	87
Surgical—Laparotomy		
Salpingotomy/salpingectomy	Ib/A	87
Surgical—Laparoscopy		
Suturing salpingostomy edges does not improve subsequent fertility	Ib/A	96

β-hCG, β-human chorionic gonadotropin.

fertility also decreases if the women is older (>35 yr)[100] or has had previous tubal damage or infertility.[99] For these women, perhaps, assisted conception may offer a better chance of an intrauterine conception. The risk for a further ectopic is strongly increased (three to four times) if the woman was previously nulliparous, if this was not her first ectopic, if she has had previous tubal surgery,[101] or if there are adhesions around either fallopian tube.[99]

If a woman has had a previous ectopic, any subsequent pregnancy is more likely to be ectopic again. Under these circumstances, early review by high-resolution TVUS in a specialist EPC is advisable so evaluation can be made of the site and viability of the pregnancy as soon as possible. This will provide reassurance if appropriate or allow timely intervention if not.

GESTATIONAL TROPHOBLASTIC DISEASE AND NEOPLASIA

Gestational trophoblastic disease (GTD) is an uncommon cause of vaginal bleeding in the first half of pregnancy. The disease encompasses a wide range of conditions that vary in their clinical presentation; their propensity for spontaneous resolution, local invasion, and metastasis; and their overall prognosis. These conditions include complete hydatidiform mole (CHM) or partial hydatidiform mole (PHM) and the malignant conditions invasive mole, choriocarcinoma, and placental site trophoblastic tumors.[106–109] The worldwide incidence of GTD is approximately 0.6 to 2.3/1000 pregnancies. Most cases are CHMs or PHMs.[110–112] The most invasive form of GTD, choriocarcinoma, has an incidence of 0.2 to 2.0/10,000 pregnancies.[113]

The incidence of all types of GTD in Asia and Africa is reported to be higher than that in Europe.[113,114] However, these regional differences may in part be due to differences in histologic classification of GTD, methodologic difficulties in the studies, or possibly, dietary differences.[115] The woman's age is a consistently demonstrated risk factor for HM. Compared with women aged 25 to 30 years, there is approximately a 6-fold excess risk in women who become pregnant before 15 years of age and approximately a 300-fold excess risk in women who become pregnant after 45 years of age.[110,116] This age association is much greater for CHM, rather than PHM.[116–118] However, because women at these extremes of reproductive age represent such a small proportion of all pregnancies, more than 90% of molar pregnancies still occur in women aged 18 to 40 years. A history of a previous molar pregnancy is also a risk factor. Women with a history of one HM have at least a 10-fold greater risk of a repeat molar pregnancy, usually the same type of mole as in the preceding pregnancy, which equates to an incidence of approximately 18/1000 pregnancies.[114,119] This risk appears to be independent of chemotherapy exposure. Although maternal A and AB blood groups are associated with an increased risk of a woman developing GTD, no plausible explanation for this association has been proposed yet.

HM is classified as a CHM or a PHM on the basis of histopathologic features and karyotype. A CHM is usually diploid and entirely androgenetic in origin. Most have a 46XX karyotype; a few have a 46XY karyotype. There is a rare form of CHM in which a haploid set of maternal and paternal chromosomes are present but failure of maternal imprinting causes only the paternal genome to be expressed.[120] It appears to be inherited as an autosomal recessive trait and women can present with recurrent molar pregnancies.[121,122] A mutation of a gene (NALP7/NLRP7) on chromosome 19 is thought to be the cause of the disease.[123,124] A complete molar pregnancy consists of diffuse hydropic chorionic villi with trophoblastic hyperplasia, forming a mass of multiple vesicles. There is usually no evidence of a fetus and minimal embryonic development.

A PHM is usually triploid, with one maternal and two paternal haploid sets, either from dispermic fertilization or from fertilization with an unreduced diploid sperm. There is usually a fetus and a large placenta. The hydropic villi show a less florid appearance than is seen with a CHM and are interspersed with normal chorionic villi. The fetus usually dies within a few weeks of conception, and a review by Petignat and coworkers[125] did not identify any case in which a fetus of paternal (diandric) origin survived to term. Occasionally, a PHM pregnancy develops with two maternal and one paternal haploid set (digynic). In these cases, the placenta is small, the villi show minimal hydropic changes, and the fetus is growth-restricted.[126] Some of these pregnancies have been reported to result in live births, with subsequent early neonatal death.[127] One study suggested that diandric PHM pregnancies have a greater malignant potential than digynic PHM pregnancies. Of 3000 women with PHMs, 0.1% had a choriocarcinoma. All were genetically diandric.[128]

The term GTD generally refers to the premalignant forms of trophoblastic disease. When the term *gestational trophoblastic neoplasia (GTN)* is used, it refers to persistent GTD and to the malignant forms of trophoblastic disease (invasive moles, gestational choriocarcinomata, placental site trophoblastic tumors). Further details on the histologic classification and macroscopic appearance of these subgroups is beyond the scope of this chapter but available from the Trophoblastic Tumour Screening and Treatment Centre website (Charing Cross Hospital, London, UK).[158] GTN is much more common with a CHM pregnancy than with a PHM. The incidence of these complications is approximately 15% and 0.5%, respectively, compared with a risk of approximately 1:50,000 after a full-term pregnancy.[128]

Diagnosis

Presentation and Clinical Features

Historically, women with molar pregnancy presented in the second trimester with an enlarged uterus, vaginal bleeding, passing vesicles per vagina, and systemic symptoms such as hyperthyroidism, anemia, and respiratory distress (Table 5–5). However, the advent and accessibility of routine TVUS in the first trimester has changed the clinical presentation of molar pregnancy,[129,130] with most women in the developed world presenting before 12 weeks as early pregnancy failure with or without vaginal bleeding.[131] A recent large retrospective study demonstrated that pre-evacuation ultrasound identifies 44% of HMs (80% of CHMs and 30% PHMs).[132] The ease with which CHMs are detected increases after 14 weeks when the characteristic "snowstorm"

TABLE 5–5

Presenting Symptoms and Signs Suggestive of Gestational Trophoblastic Disease (and Their Approximate Frequency)

Irregular first-trimester vaginal bleeding (70%)
Uterus large for dates (20%)
Pain from large benign theca-lutein cysts (15%)
Exaggerated pregnancy symptoms:
Hyperemesis (10%)
Hyperthyroidism (<1%)
Early preeclampsia (1%)

From Seckl MJ, Fisher RA, Salerno G, et al: Choriocarcinoma and partial hydatidiform moles. Lancet 2000;356:36–39; and Niemann I, Petersen LK, Hansen ES, Sunde L: Differences in current clinical features of diploid and triploid hydatidiform mole. BJOG 2007;114:1273–1277.

FIGURE 5–5
Ultrasound image of a hydatidiform mole in the first trimester shows mixed echogenic "snowstorm" appearance in uterine cavity.

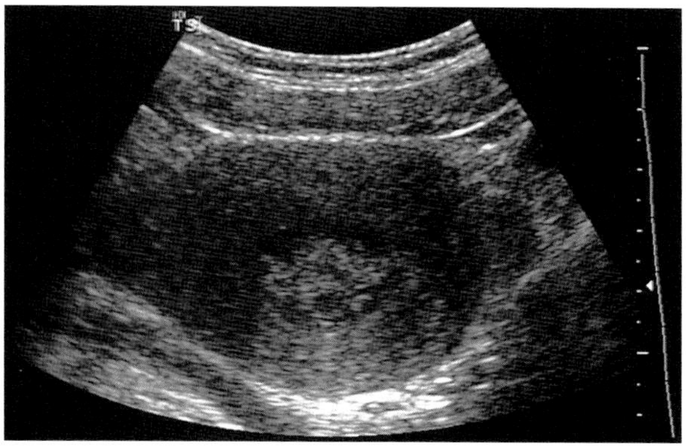

TABLE 5–6

Clinical and Pathologic Differences between Complete and Partial Hydatidiform Moles

	COMPLETE MOLE	PARTIAL MOLE
Clinical		
Features	Often severe and early.	Often mild, similar to miscarriage, fetal tissue may be passed.
Diagnosis	Usually suspected from clinical and ultrasound features.	Often missed clinically and on ultrasound, diagnosed from histology of conception products.
Persistent trophoblastic disease/tumor	15% of cases.	0.5% of cases.
Pathologic		
Macroscopic appearance	"Grapelike" vesicles often recognized. No fetal tissues.	Often normal or suspected hydropic miscarriage. Fetal tissue may be seen.
Microscopic appearance	Diffuse hydropic villi. Trophoblastic proliferation.	Focal hydropic villi. Variable mild trophoblastic proliferation. Often focal. Microscopic diagnosis sometimes difficult.
Karyotype	Usually diploid. Paternal chromosomes only.	Usually triploid. Diploid paternal and haploid maternal contribution.

From Seckl MJ, Fisher RA, Salerno G, et al: Choriocarcinoma and partial hydatidiform moles. Lancet 2000;356:36–39.

appearance of mixed echogenicity, representing hydropic villi and intrauterine hemorrhage, is seen (Fig. 5–5).[132] At earlier gestations, a mole often shows a fine vesicular or honeycomb appearance on scan. The ovaries often contain multiple large theca-lutein cysts as a result of increased ovarian stimulation by excessive hCG. Ultrasound diagnosis of a PHM is more difficult. The fetus may still be viable but may show signs consistent with triploidy, such as unusually early growth restriction or developmental abnormalities. There may be only scattered cystic spaces within the placenta, and ovarian cystic changes are usually much less pronounced. When there is diagnostic doubt, the scan should be repeated after 1 to 2 weeks.

The quantitative serum β-hCG level is higher than expected in women with a CHM, often exceeding 100,000 IU/L. This is much less likely in women with a PHM; in these women, the level is often within the wide range associated with normal pregnancy. Partly as a result of the elevated β-hCG, early pregnancy symptoms are usually more severe and present earlier in a CHM than in a PHM in which the symptoms and signs can be mild enough to be missed. These women more often have a missed miscarriage or a spontaneous miscarriage, with the passage of a recognized fetus. Consequently, the gold standard for detection of a molar pregnancy remains at present histologic examination of the products of conception from early pregnancy failures. The clinical and pathologic differences between CHMs and PHMs are summarized in Table 5–6.

Investigations

Investigations directed at disease assessment include a complete blood count, measurement of creatinine and electrolytes, liver function tests, thyroid function tests, and a baseline quantitative β-hCG measurement. A careful pelvic and abdominal ultrasound scan should be undertaken to look for evidence of an invasive mole, exclude a coexisting pregnancy, and look for possible metastatic disease. Computed tomography (CT) or magnetic resonance imaging (MRI) of the thorax, abdomen, and pelvis may provide supplementary information. Chest radiography or CT should be considered if there are symptoms that suggest pulmonary metastases. CT or MRI of the brain should also be considered. If cerebrospinal metastases are suspected despite normal findings on imaging, a lumbar puncture may be done to measure β-hCG levels in the cerebrospinal fluid. A plasma–to–cerebrospinal fluid ratio for β-hCG of greater than 1:60 is strongly suggestive of occult cerebral metastases.[133,134]

Risks

Risks include hemorrhage, persistent trophoblastic disease, malignant changes, psychological problems related to the loss of pregnancy, and the risks and need for follow-up of persistent or malignant disease.

Management Options

An algorithm for the management of GTD is shown in Figure 5–6.

Evacuation of Molar Pregnancy

CHM and PHM pregnancies are managed differently. For CHM pregnancies, suction curettage is the method of choice for uterine evacuation. A suction catheter of up to 12 mm in diameter is usually sufficient because of the absence of fetal parts. It is best to avoid prior cervical preparation, the routine use of oxytocic drugs and sharp curettage, or medical evacuation with a CHM to minimize the risk of dissemination of tissue leading to metastatic disease.[135,136] Oxytocic agents and prostaglandin analogues are best used only after uterine evacuation when there is significant hemorrhage. Data for the use of mifepristone are limited. Evacuation of CHM pregnancy with this agent should be avoided because it increases the sensitivity of the uterus to prostaglandin.

In PHM pregnancies that are recognized before uterine evacuation, again suction curettage is the method of choice. However, when pregnancy is more advanced and the size of any fetal parts may reduce the chance of complete suction evacuation, medical termination can be used.

Total abdominal hysterectomy, with the molar pregnancy in situ, can be considered for older women whose families are complete. This approach reduces the risk of persistent trophoblastic disease by up to 50%.[137]

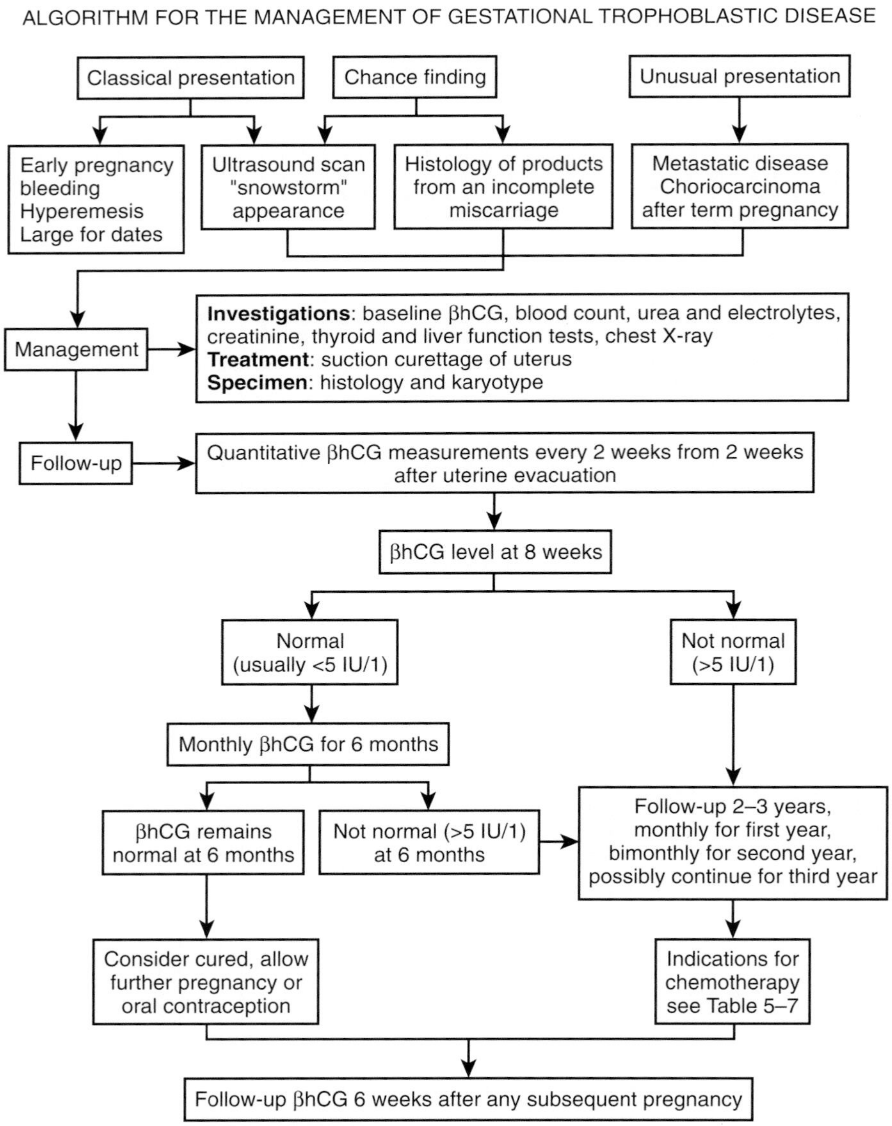

FIGURE 5–6
Algorithm for the management of gestational trophoblastic disease. βhCG, β-human chorionic gonadotropin.

Follow-up after Uterine Evacuation

The aims of follow-up are to confirm successful treatment and to identify women with GTN. GTN can occur after molar pregnancy or nonmolar pregnancy irrespective of the site and gestational age. GTN begins as a molar pregnancy or an abortus that fails to completely regress. Proliferation of the residual trophoblast results in an enlarging uterine mass that may embolize and spread to the vagina, lungs, liver, or brain. Continued vaginal bleeding, an enlarged uterus, and rising β-hCG are the most common clinical features.[138] Continued elevation of serum hCG, measured using an assay that detects all the different forms of the hormone seen in cancer, has a sensitivity and specificity of virtually 100% for malignant GTD.[139,140] The approach to follow-up and the criteria for initiating chemotherapy vary around the world. The most effective systems are based on regional or national registries that involve experienced specialist oncologists.

Clinical follow-up and β-hCG surveillance after uterine evacuation of a molar pregnancy also vary according to the different prognosis for GTN between CHMs and PHMs with chromosome analysis predicting prognosis more precisely than histology.[141] The clinical course for women who have had a PHM is almost always benign after uterine evacuation. Persistent disease occurs in 1.2% to 6% of cases; metastatic disease occurs in only 0.1% of cases.[131,142,143] In CHMs, these risks are approximately five times greater after treatment with uterine evacuation and two to three times greater after treatment with hysterectomy.[137,144] The risk of persistent or recurrent GTN is greatest in the first 12 months after evacuation, with most cases evident within 6 months.

In North America, current recommendations for surveillance after uterine evacuation of a molar pregnancy are for β-hCG monitoring 48 hours after surgery and then weekly until three normal levels (<5 IU/L) have been obtained. Levels of β-hCG are monitored at 2-week intervals for 3 months and monthly for 6 and 12 months for PHM and CHM pregnancies, respectively.

In the United Kingdom, there is a central registry for patients with molar pregnancies. Monitoring is supervised by a small number of screening centers. Monitoring of β-hCG levels usually begins 2 weeks after uterine evacuation. The frequency and duration of monitoring are dependent on serum or urinary β-hCG levels. If the β-hCG falls to normal (<5 IU/L) within 8 weeks of evacuation, the monitoring can be stopped at 6 months postevacuation. If the β-hCG falls more slowly, monitoring can stop at 6 months after the first normal value. After normalization of the serum β-hCG, monitoring is done by urinary β-hCG monthly. If β-hCG levels remain normal for 6 months, the risk of malignant GTD is very small (~1:300) and the woman can consider a further pregnancy from that point.[145]

There is a debate about the use of a combined oral contraceptive pill (OCP) after treatment. Limited data from the United Kingdom suggest that it slows the rate of decrease of the β-hCG level and may increase the risk of persistent GTD, and the advice is to avoid the OCP until β-hCG levels have returned to normal. However, data from other countries suggest the combined OCP is safe,[146] and because the risk associated with an unplanned early pregnancy is greater, the use of oral contraception is considered acceptable by some North American clinicians.[131,144]

Adjuvant chemotherapy may be required in approximately 10% of women after uterine evacuation. The indications for chemotherapy are shown in Table 5–7. In 2002, the International Society for the Study of Trophoblastic Diseases adopted the revised WHO/FIGO (International Federation of Gynecologists and Obstetricians) scoring system for GTN (Table 5–8).[147] It differentiates women with low risk disease from those with high risk disease. Women with low risk disease are usually treated with a single agent, most commonly methotrexate and folinic acid rescue.[148] This is still the recommended approach, although a recent systematic review concluded that "pulsed" dactinomycin is superior to weekly parenteral methotrexate in achieving primary cure, without significantly increasing toxicity.[138] Single-agent chemotherapy will cure only 31% of patients classified as high risk.[149] These women are best given multiagent chemotherapy with etoposide, methotrexate, and actinomycin D [EMA], alternating with cyclophosphamide and vincristine [CO]). The remission rate with this regimen is reported to be 80% to 95%.[150]

After chemotherapy is completed, serial β-hCG measurements are usually assessed twice-weekly for 1 year, monthly for a second year, with decreasing frequency over the next 3 years, and then a 6-monthly urinary β-hCG for life. Cure rates are high, sometimes with the need for additional salvage surgery, and women with a history of GTN can anticipate normal reproductive outcomes, with no increase in the risk of fetal abnormalities, miscarriage, ectopic pregnancy, premature delivery, or stillbirth, compared with the normal population.[151–155] Monitoring of β-hCG is advisable after any subsequent pregnancy, regardless of gestational age or outcome, to exclude recurrent GTD.

In a subsequent pregnancy after chemotherapy for GTN, an ultrasound scan should be performed at 8 weeks' and 14 weeks' gestation. The risk of further GTN is 1.4% to 2.4%.[154] Monitoring of β-hCG levels should be performed 6 weeks and 3 months after delivery.

Although there is a very high cure rate with GTN, it is not surprising that many women experience psychosocial sequelae, such as depression, marital and sexual dysfunction, and concerns about future pregnancy.[156] It is, therefore, important to offer support and counseling to these women.

TABLE 5–7

Indications for Adjuvant Chemotherapy in Gestational Trophoblastic Disease[158]

Serum hGC levels > 20,000 IU/L more than 4 weeks after uterine evacuation
Static or rising hCG levels at any time after uterine evacuation
Raised hCG level 6 months after uterine evacuation
Metastases in liver, lung, brain, or gastrointestinal tract
Histologic diagnosis of choriocarcinoma
Pulmonary, vulval, or vaginal metastases unless hCG concentrations are falling
Heavy vaginal bleeding or evidence of gastrointestinal or intraperitoneal hemorrhage

hCG, human chorionic gonadotropin.

From Gestational Trophoblastic Disease Screening Service Unit. Information for Clinicians (cited 2009 April 14). Available at http://www.hmole-chorio.org.uk/clinicians_info.html

TABLE 5–8

Modified World Health Organization Prognostic Scoring System, as Adapted by FIGO, by Which Women Whose Score Is 0–6 Are Considered Low Risk (Requiring Single-Agent Chemotherapy) and Score of 7 or More, High Risk (Requiring Multiagent Combination Chemotherapy)

SCORES	0	1	2	3
Age	<40	≥40	–	–
Antecedent pregnancy	Mole	Abortion	Term	–
Interval months from index pregnancy	<4	4–6	7–13	≥13
Pretreatment serum hCG	<1000	1000–10,000	10,000–100,000	>100,000
Largest tumor size	–	3–5 cm	≥5 cm	–
Site of metastases	Lung	Spleen, liver	Gastrointestinal	Liver, brain
No. of metastases	–	1–4	5–8	>8
Previous failed chemotherapy	–	–	Single drug	≥2 Drugs

FIGO, International Federation of Gynecologists and Obstetricians; hCG, human chorionic gonadotropin.
From FIGO staging for gestational trophoblastic neoplasia 2000. FIGO Oncology Committee. Int J Gynaecol Obstet 2002;77:285–287.

SUMMARY OF MANAGEMENT OPTIONS

Gestational Trophoblastic Disease and Neoplasia

Management Options	Evidence Quality and Recommendation	References
Presentation		
Complete moles cause more exaggerated symptoms and signs than partial moles	III/B	157,158
Partial moles are often missed clinically and by ultrasound scan and are often diagnosed histologically after uterine evacuation of an incomplete miscarriage	IV/C	159
Surgical Evacuation		
Primary treatment of choice for all moles	III/B	160
Suction curettage for uterine evacuation is safer (lower risk of metastasis) than sharp curettage, particularly for evacuation of complete moles	IIb/B	161
Oxytocics, cervical preparation, and medical termination are better avoided, particularly for evacuation of complete moles	IV/C	145
Medical (for Partial Moles)		
Methotrexate	III/B	148
Actinomycin-D	III/B	148
Combination therapy	III/B	162,163
Follow-up		
If β-hCG levels remain normal 8 weeks to 6 months after evacuation, a woman can be considered cured and further pregnancy allowed	—/GPP	—
β-hCG should be measured 6 weeks after any subsequent pregnancy because of the risk of further trophoblastic disease	—/GPP	—
Gestational Trophoblastic Neoplasia		
(See Table 5–8 for categorization of risk)		
Low risk disease management: methotrexate or actinomycin-D	III/B	148
High risk disease management: multiagent chemotherapy (EMA alternating with CO) and if recurrent disease (cisplatin and etoposide with EMA)	III/B	145,159

β-hCG, β-human chorionic gonadotropin; CO, cyclophosphamide and vincristine; EMA, etoposide, methotrexate, and actinomycin-D; GPP, good practice point.

SUMMARY OF MANAGEMENT OPTIONS

Rhesus Prophylaxis

Management Options	Evidence Quality and Recommendation	References
Bleeding associated with threatened miscarriage before 12 weeks' gestation does not require anti-D	IV/C	164
Anti-D is required for an incomplete miscarriage only when surgical evacuation is required	III/B	165
Anti-D Ig should be given to all nonsensitized RhD-negative women who have an ectopic pregnancy	IV/C	165
Trophoblastic cells express RhD factor, so RhD-negative women should receive anti-D at the time of evacuation	IV/C	169,170

RHESUS PROPHYLAXIS

Guidelines from the Royal College of Obstetricians and Gynaecologists and the British Blood Transfusion Society[164,165] recommend that women who have a miscarriage after 12 weeks' gestation should be given anti-D. Between 12 and 20 weeks' gestation, a Kleihauer test to quantify fetomaternal hemorrhage is not required. Treatment with 250 IU anti-D immunoglobulin is adequate.

For miscarriages and ectopic pregnancies earlier than 12 weeks' gestation, the evidence to guide decision-making is poor. There is general consensus that complete spontaneous miscarriages without surgical intervention do not require anti-D prophylaxis.[164] When surgical evacuation of the uterus is required, even before 12 weeks' gestation, it is associated with a higher chance of transfer of fetal cells to the maternal circulation.[166] Under these circumstances, 250 IU anti-D immunoglobulin should be given to all Rhesus-negative women.[165]

With a threatened miscarriage before 12 weeks' gestation, anti-D is generally not required. However, Rhesus prophylaxis may be prudent empirically if the patient has very heavy bleeding or considerable abdominal pain. If a threatened miscarriage occurs later than 12 weeks, anti-D (≥ 250 IU) should be given. If bleeding is persistent, this may be repeated at intervals of no more than 6 weeks. The half-life of anti-D is 2 weeks. Prophylaxis may be needed at 2-week intervals if bleeding is heavy or if it is indicated by the results of a Kleihauer test.[164]

Most religious groups who have concerns about the use of blood products do not object to the use of anti-D prophylaxis.

If it is indicated, anti-D prophylaxis should be given within 72 hours of the sensitizing episode.[167] A 250-IU dose is sufficient for fetomaternal hemorrhage before 12 weeks. The use of anti-D immunoglobulin in Rhesus-negative women in later pregnancy is addressed in Chapter 58. For Rhesus negative women with trophoblastic disease, Anti-D should be given at the time of evacuation or as soon as possible afterwards. Even though fetal red blood cells ought not to be present in a complete mole, nonetheless the consensus view is that it is more prudent to give Anti-D (P. Savage, Imperial College, personal communication).[169,170]

SUGGESTED READINGS

Barnhart KT, Sammel MD, Rinaudo PF, et al: Symptomatic patients with an early viable intrauterine pregnancy: HCG curves redefined. Obstet Gynecol 2004;104:50–55.

Drife J, Lewis G (eds): Why Mothers Die. Confidential Enquiry into Maternal Deaths in the United Kingdom. Norwich, UK, HMSO, 2001.

FIGO staging for gestational trophoblastic neoplasia 2000. FIGO Oncology Committee. Int J Gynaecol Obstet 2002;77:285–287.

Hajenius PJ, Mol F, Mol BW, et al: Interventions for tubal ectopic pregnancy. Cochrane Database Syst Rev 2007;1:CD000324.

Regan L, Braude PB, Trembath PL: Influence of past reproductive performance on risk of spontaneous abortion. BMJ 1989;299:541–545.

Royal College of Obstetricians and Gynaecologists: The Management of Gestational Trophoblastic Disease. Guideline No. 38. London, RCOG, 2004.

Saving Mothers' Lives: Reviewing Maternal Deaths to Make Motherhood Safer—2003–2005. London, CEMACH, 2007.

Sebire NJ, Fisher RA, Fockett M, et al: Risk of recurrent hydatidiform mole and subsequent pregnancy outcome following complete or partial hydatidiform molar pregnancy. BJOG 2003;110:22–26.

Trinder J, Brocklehurst P, Porter R, et al: Management of miscarriage: expectant, medical, or surgical? Results of randomised controlled trial (miscarriage treatment [MIST] trial). BMJ Clin Res Ed 2006;332:1235–1240.

Wilcox AJ, Weinberg CR, O'Connor JF, et al: Incidence of early loss of pregnancy. N Engl J Med 1988;319:189–194.

REFERENCES

For a complete list of references, log onto www.expertconsult.com.

CHAPTER 6

Recurrent Miscarriage

LESLEY REGAN, MAY BACKOS, and ROY G. FARQUHARSON

INTRODUCTION

A *miscarriage* is the spontaneous loss of a pregnancy before the fetus has reached viability. In the United Kingdom, viability was historically taken to occur at 28 weeks, but with improvements in neonatal care, the transition was changed to 24 weeks. In developing countries, where gestation at birth is often uncertain, the World Health Organization (WHO)[1] recommends that the criterion of viability should be a birthweight of 500 g or more. In the United Kingdom, therefore, miscarriages include all pregnancy losses from the time of conception until 23 completed weeks of gestation. Miscarriage is the most common complication of pregnancy, and epidemiologic data have demonstrated that the fate of a fertilized egg is "precarious." Approximately 50% of all conceptions are lost, the majority of which are unrecognized clinically. Furthermore, 15% (almost one in six) of all clinically recognized pregnancies end in miscarriage.[2–4]

There are two distinct types of miscarriage—sporadic and recurrent. The lifetime chance of a woman having a sporadic miscarriage (each pregnancy has a risk of miscarriage that is unrelated to the previous pregnancy history) will depend on the number of pregnancies she has. If each clinically apparent pregnancy carries a one in six (16.7%) risk of miscarrying, then the chance of a woman experiencing at least one miscarriage with two pregnancies is 31%, 42.5% with three pregnancies, 52.1% with four pregnancies, 60.1% with five pregnancies, 67% with six pregnancies, and so on. The chance of two consecutive sporadic miscarriages is 1 in 36 and of three is 1 in 216.

In the majority of cases, the pregnancy loss is due to a random fetal chromosomal abnormality,[5,6] the risk of which rises with increasing maternal age.[7] The vast majority of miscarriages occur early in pregnancy, before 12 completed weeks of gestation (first trimester). The incidence of late miscarriage (second-trimester pregnancy loss, from 13 to 23 completed weeks) is estimated at 2%.[8]

Recurrent miscarriage (RM), the accepted definition of which is three or more consecutive pregnancy losses, affects 1% of couples.[9] As can be seen from the previous calculation of the likelihood of sporadic miscarriages, this is about twice the incidence that would be expected by chance and, therefore, indicates the likelihood of additional pathology. However, some clinicians argue that couples who have had two or more losses should be included in the definition, to avoid the trauma of a third loss before undergoing diagnostic evaluation, in which case, the scale of the problem increases from 1% to 5% of all couples trying to achieve a successful pregnancy.[10] Such a reduction in the stringency of diagnosis will inevitably have large resource implications because of the cost of investigations.

As explained earlier, the incidence of RM is higher than that expected by chance alone (0.34%)[11,12]; hence, a proportion of couples must have a persistent underlying cause for their recurring pregnancy losses. Several additional strands of evidence support the view that RM may be a distinct clinical entity rather than one that occurs by chance alone:

- A woman's risk of miscarriage is not the same with each successive pregnancy, but is related to the outcome of her previous pregnancies.[13–16]
- Women with a history of RM are more likely to have reproductive characteristics (demographics, physical attributes) associated with a poor prognosis for future pregnancy outcome than women suffering sporadic miscarriage.[17–20]
- In contrast to women with sporadic miscarriage, those with RM are more likely to lose pregnancies with a normal chromosome complement[5,21]; in observational terms, fewer of their miscarried fetuses are chromosomally abnormal.

EPIDEMIOLOGY

Maternal Age

The risk of miscarriage increases with advancing maternal age, secondary to an increase in chromosomally abnormal conceptions[22] together with a decline in uterine and ovarian function. Previous miscarriages and multigravidity are also well-recognized risk factors that are strongly correlated with maternal age. A large prospective register linkage study has demonstrated that maternal age at conception is a strong and independent risk factor for miscarriage, irrespective of previous pregnancy outcome. The overall incidence of miscarriage in this study was 13.5%, but the risk of fetal loss classified by maternal age at conception increased steeply with age, rising from 9% at 20 to 24 years to over 70% at 45 years[16] (Table 6–1). The rate of increase in risk escalates

TABLE 6–1

Miscarriage Rates Stratified by Maternal Age at Conception

AGE (YR)	TOTAL NO. OF PREGNANCIES	MISCARRIAGE RATE (%)
20-24	350,395	9
25-29	414,149	11
30-34	235,049	15
35-39	93,940	25
40-44	25,132	51
≥45	1865	75
Overall risk of miscarriage for 634,272 women = 13.5%		
	@ 22 yr = 8.7%	
	@ 35 yr = 23.5%	
	@ 42 yr = 54.5%	
	@ 48 yr = 84.1%	

After Nybo Andersen AM, Wohlfahrt J, Christens P, et al: Maternal age and fetal loss: Population based register linkage study. BMJ 2000;320: 1708–1712.

sharply after 35 years of age, and the chance of a successful pregnancy in women aged 40 years or more is poor. The risks of ectopic pregnancy and stillbirth show similar increases.

Significant changes in reproductive behavior have occurred in our society during recent decades. Many women delay childbearing for social and professional reasons. According to U.K. census data, the number of babies born to mothers aged 35 years or older doubled between 1985 and 2001 from 8% to 16%, and more recent data show a continuing rise. The wider availability of assisted fertility treatments and donor gametes will undoubtedly accelerate this trend. Although no comparable miscarriage figures are available, it is logical to conclude that the incidence of miscarriage has also increased owing to the increase in maternal age at conception. Advanced paternal age has also been identified as a risk factor for miscarriage. A large multicenter European study reported that the risk of miscarriage is highest for couples in which the woman is 35 years of age or older and the man is 40 years of age or older.[23]

Reproductive History

Reproductive history is an independent predictor of future pregnancy outcome. One prospective study reported that a woman's risk of miscarriage is affected by her obstetric history, the single most important factor being a previous miscarriage.[14] Primigravidae and women with a history of a live birth in the immediately previous pregnancy have a significantly lower (5%) risk of miscarriage than women whose last pregnancy ended in miscarriage (19%).[14] Both retrospective[15] and prospective[14,16] studies have reported that the risk of a further miscarriage increases after each successive pregnancy loss, reaching 45% after three and 54% after four consecutive pregnancy losses. These observations are partly explained by reproductive compensation because women who miscarry tend to embark on further pregnancies at progressively later ages, until they achieve their desired family size and partly because they tend to get pregnant again very quickly (an interpregnancy interval of less than 18 months increases the risk of a miscarriage). However, it is important to be aware that a previous live birth does not preclude women from experiencing RM in the future.[18,24]

It is not just first-trimester miscarriage that increases the risk of subsequent early pregnancy loss. In a large study of 500 consecutive couples attending a specialist RM clinic, a previous stillbirth or neonatal death was noted in 6%, termination of pregnancy for fetal abnormality in 2%, an episode of second-trimester (late) miscarriage in 25%, and an ectopic gestation in 5%. Among the 45% of couples with a living child, obstetric complications such as premature delivery and low–birth weight infants were common. In addition, one third of this population had a history of conception delays and previous subfertility investigations.[20]

RISK FACTORS FOR RECURRENT MISCARRIAGE

RM is a heterogeneous condition. Historically, the causes have been grouped into genetic, anatomic, infective, endocrine, immune, environmental, and unexplained categories. Our recent understanding that thrombophilic disorders play an important part in the etiology of recurrent pregnancy loss at various gestations has widened the scope of investigations and management options for this distressing condition.

Genetic Factors

Fetal aneuploidy is the most important cause of miscarriage before 10 weeks' gestation.[25] Chromosomal abnormalities of the embryo account for at least 50% of first-trimester sporadic miscarriages[26] and 29% to 57% of further miscarriages in couples with RM.[16,27] However, most published studies have used conventional cytogenetic analysis, which can identify only gross chromosomal aberrations and depends on tissue culture before karyotyping can be performed. Consequently, the results are limited by external contamination, potential culture failure, and selective growth of maternal cells.[28] When miscarriage tissues are analyzed by comparative genomic hybridization, it appears that the contribution of chromosomal abnormalities to first-trimester miscarriage is almost 70%.[29] Knowledge of the karyotype of a miscarriage may help to predict future pregnancy outcome and informs clinical investigation. Women who miscarry a euploid (normal chromosome complement) embryo have a greater risk of RMs than women whose lost pregnancy is aneuploid.[9,30]

Parental Chromosomal Rearrangement

In approximately 3% to 5% of couples with RM, one partner carries either a balanced reciprocal translocation, in which there is an exchange of two terminal segments from different chromosomes, or a robertsonion translocation, in which there is centric fusion of two acrocentric chromosomes (Fig. 6–1).[20,31,32] Although carriers of a balanced translocation are usually phenotypically normal, abnormal segregation at meiosis leads to 50% to 70% of their gametes, and hence embryos, being unbalanced. These pregnancies are at increased risk for miscarriage and may result in a live birth

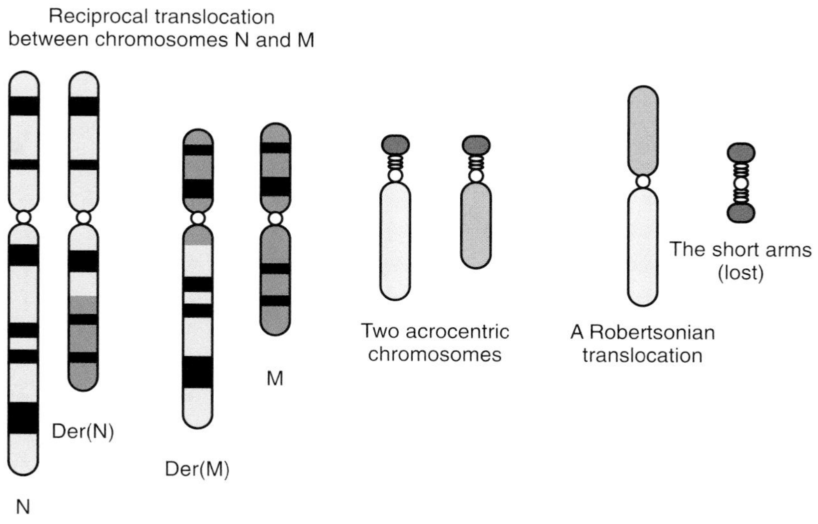

FIGURE 6–1
Parental chromosomal reciprocal and robertsonian translocations.
(Courtesy of Dr. Jonathan Wolfe, Department of Biology, Galton Laboratory, University College, London.)

of a child with multiple congenital malformations or mental handicap. This justifies offering chorionic villus sampling (CVS) or amniocentesis to assess the chromosomal status of the fetus.[32] (The reproductive risks conferred by chromosome rearrangements differ both according to the type of rearrangement[33] and whether the rearrangement is carried by the female or the male partner.[34]) Until recently, little could be offered to such couples other than referral to a genetic counselor for advice regarding the prognosis for a future pregnancy and the offer of CVS or amniocentesis for established pregnancies. This has changed with the introduction of in vitro fertilization and preimplantation genetic screening (PGS), in which fluorescent in situ hybridization (FISH) is used to infer the genetic status of an embryo from a single cell biopsied 3 days after fertilization.[35,36] However, the live birth rate among couples with a structural chromosome abnormality who conceive spontaneously is significantly higher (50%–65%)[33,37] than that currently achieved after IVF + PGS (38% per embryo transfer[38]), and so couples may still prefer to go down the CVS/amniocentesis route, with the option of termination of pregnancy if the baby is found to be abnormal.

Fetal Aneuploidy and Polyploidy

The vast majority of human aneuploidies arise from errors in the first meiotic division of the oocyte, which is initiated prenatally and is not complete until ovulation. In contrast to females who are born with their complete complement of oocytes, meiosis in males begins only at the time of puberty, new spermatazooa being produced continuously with an average life span of 70 days. Although an increased incidence of sperm chromosome abnormalities in couples with RM has been reported,[39,40] only 7% of fetal trisomies arise from paternal meiotic errors.[41]

The meiotic error may lead to an extra chromosome (trisomy) or the deletion of a chromosome (monosomy). Triploidy, in which there is a complete set of extra chromosomes, usually arises from fertilization of the oocyte by two spermatozoa, whereas tetraploidy (four times the haploid number) is usually caused by failure to complete the first zygotic division. In couples with RM, conventional cytogenetic analysis reports the incidence of trisomy, polyploidy, and monosomy X in miscarriage tissue as 30%, 9%, and 4%, respectively.[5,6] Most trisomies are the result of meiotic error associated with advanced maternal age.[42] In one study from the United States, the rate of trisomy in miscarriages rose from 22% to 42% from the 1980s to the early 2000s as mean maternal age rose from 29 to 34 years.[43] However, gonadal mosaicism and sperm aneuploidies also increase the risk of trisomic conceptions. The risk of sex chromosome monosomy and polyploidy conceptions does not increase with maternal age.[22] Some couples with a history of RM are at risk for recurrent aneuploidy and may be prone to heterotrisomy, a recurrence of trisomy involving different chromosomes.[44]

Single-gene mutations leading to abnormalities of embryonic development (particularly placental and cardiac lesions) together with skewed X chromosome inactivation (preferential expression of maternal or paternal X chromosome in maternal cells) are more common in women with RM than in controls.[45] Transcervical embryoscopy has demonstrated that the disordered growth and development seen in aneuploid embryos may also be present in some 18% of euploid pregnancies that have ended in miscarriage.[46]

Anatomic Disorders

Congenital Uterine Malformations

Congenital uterine malformations (Fig. 6–2) are the result of disturbances in müllerian duct development, fusion, canalization, and septal reabsorption. In the most extreme form, the uterus is duplicated in its entirety (uterus didelphus), and in the least severe form, it is only slightly indented at the fundus (arcuate uterus). The contribution of congenital uterine anomalies to recurrent pregnancy loss is unclear because the true prevalence and reproductive implications of uterine anomalies in the general population are unknown. In patients with RM, the reported frequency of uterine anomalies varies widely, from 1.8% to 37.6%.[47–49] This variability is due to differences in the criteria and imaging techniques used for diagnosis and the fact that women with a history of two, three, or more miscarriages at both early and

FIGURE 6–2
The American Society for Reproductive Medicine classification of mullerian anomalies.
(Reprinted by permission of the American Society for Reproductive Medicine, Birmingham, Alabama.)

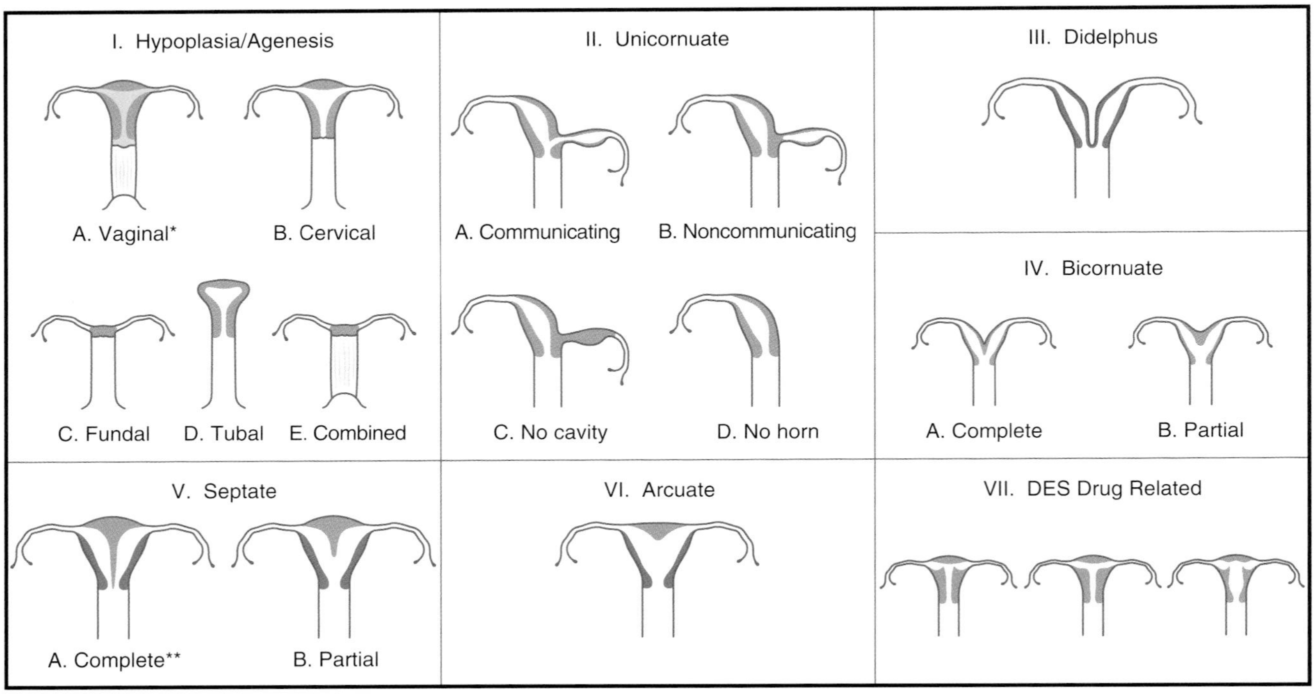

* Uterus may be normal or take a variety of abnormal forms.
** May have two distinct cervices.

late stages of pregnancy have been included in the studies. The prevalence of uterine anomalies appears to be highest in women with a history of late miscarriages, which probably reflects the greater prevalence of cervical incompetence in women with uterine malformation.[50] However, a large prospective study that employed three-dimensional ultrasound as a diagnostic tool reported that the frequency of uterine anomalies was 23.8% in women with first-trimester RM (three or more consecutive pregnancy losses) compared with a frequency of 5.3% in low risk women who were referred for ultrasound for a variety of reasons unrelated to reproductive outcome.[49] By contrast, a recent literature review of uterine anomalies in early and late RM patients reported a prevalence of 16.7% (96% confidence interval [CI] 14.8–18.6).[51] A retrospective review of reproductive performance in patients with untreated uterine anomalies suggested that these women have high rates of miscarriage and preterm delivery and a term delivery rate of only 50%.[47] Open uterine surgery is associated with postoperative infertility and carries a significant risk of scar rupture during pregnancy.[52] These complications are probably less likely to occur after hysteroscopic surgery,[53] but no randomized trial assessing the benefits of open or hysteroscopic surgical correction of uterine abnormalities on pregnancy outcome has been performed.

Cervical Incompetence (Insufficiency or Dysfunction)

Cervical incompetence is defined as the inability of the cervix to retain a pregnancy, owing to a functional or structural defect, in the absence of contractions or labor. The term is outdated and is probably better described as cervical insufficiency or dysfunction. It is a well-recognized cause of late miscarriage and the diagnosis is often made retrospectively after a woman has had a second-trimester loss. Cervical incompetence occurs along a spectrum of severity, severe incompetence leading to mid-trimester miscarriage, lesser degrees underlying some cases of preterm delivery.[54] The true incidence of cervical incompetence is unknown because the diagnosis is essentially clinical and there are no objective tests to reliably identify women with cervical weakness in the nonpregnant state.

Epidemiologic studies suggest an approximate incidence of 0.5% in the general obstetric population[55] and 8% in women with a history of previous mid-trimester miscarriages.[8] Although some cases involve mechanical incompetence (e.g., congenital hypoplastic cervix, previous cervical surgery, or extensive trauma), many women with a clinical diagnosis of cervical incompetence have normal cervical anatomy. When considered as a continuum, premature cervical ripening may represent a final common pathway of a variety of pathophysiologic processes, such as infection, immunologically mediated inflammatory stimuli, and subclinical abruptio placentae together with a hormonal or genetic predisposition.[56,57] The cervix is the main mechanical barrier separating the pregnancy from the vaginal bacterial flora, and many patients who have asymptomatic mid-trimester cervical dilation also have evidence of subclinical intrauterine infection.[58] It is unclear whether this high rate of microbial invasion is the result or the cause of premature cervical dilation. When cervical incompetence is associated with mechanical weakness, supportive measures such as cerclage may prevent ascending infection and, hence, may prolong pregnancy. In contrast, if cervical changes result from nonmechanical processes, then cerclage would be less effective, and even harmful in some cases, because of possible inflammatory, prothrombotic, and infectious complications. Some surgical approaches, for example, the use of double sutures (one suture at the internal os and another to close the external os [occlusion suture]), are not primarily mechanical but aim to trap cervical mucus and thus improve the barrier against ascending infection.[59] The efficacy of this approach is unknown and is currently being assessed by a large multicenter prospective, randomized controlled trial.[60]

Fibroids

Uterine fibroids have long been associated with a variety of reproductive problems, including pregnancy loss. Although the exact mechanisms are unclear, the presumed theories of pathophysiology include mechanical distortion of the uterine cavity, abnormal vascularization, abnormal endometrial development, endometrial inflammation, abnormal endocrine milieu, and structural and contractile myometrial abnormalities,[61] any or all of which may impede embryonic implantation. The expression of HOX10, a gene that controls differentiation and is involved in implantation, has been shown to be lower in uteri with fibroids.[62] Evidence of the association between uterine fibroids and RM is retrospective[63] and insufficient to determine differences in pregnancy outcome or assess the effect of the size and location of the fibroids. Data from patients with infertility suggest that only fibroids with a submucosal or an intracavitary component are associated with a reduced implantation rate and an increased rate of miscarriage.[64] Subserous fibroids have no deleterious effect, and the role of intramural fibroids that do not distort the cavity is controversial.[65]

Intrauterine Adhesions

Intrauterine adhesions (Asherman's syndrome, an acquired uterine defect of varying severity) result from intrauterine trauma after vigorous endometrial curettage or evacuation of retained products of conception. Intrauterine adhesions have been associated with RM. The presumed mechanisms are decreased uterine cavity volume and fibrosis and inflammation of the endometrium that predispose the patient to defective implantation, abnormal placentation, and pregnancy loss. However, evidence of the association is mostly retrospective[66] and conflicting,[67] with no robust prospective evidence to confirm a causal relationship. Despite the advances in hysteroscopic surgery, pregnancies following surgical treatment remain at high risk of complications.[68]

Endocrine Factors

Historically, a variety of endocrine disorders have been suggested as causal in RM, but few have withstood critical scrutiny.

Systemic Endocrine Factors

Diabetes mellitus and thyroid disease have been associated with sporadic miscarriage, but there is no direct evidence that they contribute to RM. The prevalence of both endocrinopathies in women with RM is similar to that expected in the general population.[20] Women with diabetes who have high hemoglobin A1c levels in the first trimester are at risk for miscarriage and fetal malformation.[69] In contrast, well-controlled diabetes mellitus is not a risk factor for RM,[70] nor is treated thyroid dysfunction.[71] A meta-analysis has reported an association between the presence of thyroid autoantibodies, a history of one or two miscarriages, and outcome of the next pregnancy.[72] Women with RM are no more likely than fertile control subjects to have circulating thyroid antibodies.[73] The presence of thyroid antibodies in euthyroid women with a history of RM did not affect future pregnancy outcome in a prospective observational study.[74] However, thyroxine therapy for euthyroid women with antithyroid antibodies was reported to improve pregnancy outcome in a general population, including a reduction in pregnancy loss.[75]

Prolactin is involved in both ovulation and endometrial maturation. It has been reported that hyperprolactinemia is a cause of RM and that treatment with bromocriptine, which suppresses prolactin secretion by the anterior pituitary, significantly reduces the miscarriage rate.[76] Lack of expression of endometrial prolactin during the luteal phase of the menstrual cycle has also been reported to be associated with RM in one small study.[77]

Luteal Phase Defect and Progesterone Deficiency

A functional corpus luteum is essential for the implantation and maintenance of early pregnancy, primarily through the production of progesterone, which is responsible for the conversion of a proliferative endometrium to a secretory endometrium suitable for embryonic implantation. Luteal phase defect, in which insufficient progesterone production results in retarded endometrial development, has long been associated with RM. However, standard diagnostic criteria required to assess the true incidence and effect of luteal phase defects are lacking.[78] Diurnal variations and pulsatile secretion make serum progesterone measurements unreliable, and the interpretation of the results of endometrial biopsy is susceptible to sampling and interobserver variation.[79] In addition, serum progesterone levels are not predictive of pregnancy outcome; low progesterone levels in early pregnancy appear to reflect a pregnancy that has already failed. Moreover, no convincing studies show that treatment of luteal phase defect improves pregnancy outcome in women with RM,[80,81] although a Cochrane meta-analysis suggested that progesterone supplementation in early pregnancy may be of benefit for some women.[82] A recent review of the literature suggests that progesterone has an important immunoregulatory role in altering maternal cytokine production and natural killer (NK) cell activity and regulating human leukocyte antigen (HLA)-G gene expression in pregnancy, prompting a call for further therapeutic intervention studies.[83] The Medical Research Council (MRC) recently funded a multicenter randomized placebo-controlled trial of progesterone treatment in early pregnancy for women with a history of unexplained RM (the PROMISE trial). The results of this are eagerly awaited and will inform clinical practice.

Polycystic Ovary Syndrome, Hypersecretion of Luteinizing Hormone, and Hyperandrogenemia

Polycystic ovaries and the various endocrinopathies associated with polycystic ovary syndrome (PCOS), high luteinizing hormone (LH) levels and hyperandrogenemia, have been linked to infertility and miscarriage for several decades. Although polycystic ovaries are found significantly more often among women with RM than among parous control subjects, polycystic ovaries themselves do not appear to predict future pregnancy outcome in ovulatory women with RM.[84] A high level of LH or testosterone does not correlate with pregnancy outcome in ovulatory women with RM.[85] Further, a prospective, randomized placebo-controlled trial[86] reported that prepregnancy suppression of high LH did not improve the live birth rate—the outcome of pregnancy in women in the placebo group was similar to that of women with a normal LH level.

More recently, the association between PCOS and insulin resistance leading to compensatory hyperinsulinemia has come under scrutiny as a risk factor for RM. The mechanism underlying this relationship may be through impairment of the fibrinolytic response, which is important in the tissue remodeling that accompanies embryonic implantation. The 4G/5G polymorphism in the plasminogen activator inhibitor-1 (PAI-1) gene promoter influences plasma concentrations of fibrin. Homozygosity for the 4G/4G polymorphism, which is associated with hypofibrinolysis, is found significantly more often among women with PCOS and a history of RM than among those with normal ovarian morphology. Of particular interest is the fact that there is an insulin response element in the promoter region of the PAI-1 gene. Hence, hyperinsulinemia is associated with impairment of fibrinoylyis, which in turn, is associated with miscarriage.

Insulin resistance is associated with a higher rate of miscarriage among women with PCOS undergoing ovulation induction than among those who are not insulin resistant,[87] and the prevalence of insulin resistance is increased among women with RM.[88] Metformin treatment for women with PCOS during induction of ovulation and early pregnancy may improve endometrial receptivity and implantation, thereby reducing the risk of future miscarriage.[89,90] However, the role of insulin resistance and the efficacy and safety of metformin in women with polycystic ovaries and RM remain to be established in prospective controlled trials.

Infective Factors

The evidence for a role of infection in recurrent early miscarriage is weak. Any severe infection that leads to bacteremia or viremia can cause an early sporadic miscarriage. However, for an infective agent to be implicated in the etiology of repeated early pregnancy losses, it must persist in the genital tract and avoid detection or cause insufficient symptoms to disturb the woman. Toxoplasmosis, rubella, cytomegalovirus, herpes, and *Listeria* infections do not fulfill these criteria, and routine screening for these disorders has been abandoned.[91] A recent study has reported that positive immunoglobulin G (IgG) serology for *Chlamydia trachomatis* is associated with early but not late miscarriage.[92] The authors suggest that even in the absence of a detectable organism, previous *Chlamydia* infection increases the miscarriage risk, possibly by triggering chronic inflammation.

The evidence of an association between endometritis and first-trimester miscarriage is inconsistent.[93,94] However, the presence of bacterial vaginosis in the first trimester has repeatedly been reported as a risk factor for second-trimester miscarriage and preterm delivery.[95,96] Two randomized controlled trials conducted in low risk obstetric populations found that the incidence of late miscarriage and preterm birth was reduced by screening and treating women for bacterial vaginosis in early pregnancy with oral clindamycin[97] or alternatively with a combination of oral erythromycin and metronidazol.[98] However, the results from another eight randomized trials concluded that there is no benefit in screening and treating all pregnant women for bacterial vaginosis in order to prevent preterm birth and its consequences.[99] By contrast, a Cochrane review suggested that detection and treatment of bacterial vaginosis early in pregnancy may reduce the risk of preterm delivery, but only in women with a history of mid-trimester miscarriage or preterm birth.[100] These findings, coupled with the recent report of long-term outcomes from the ORACLE II study that observed an increase in the incidence of cerebral palsy in the children of women in threatened preterm labor given erythromycin, co-amoxyclav, or both,[101] suggest that the empirical use of antibiotics in pregnancy should be avoided.

Thrombophilic Factors

The hemostatic system plays a crucial role in both the establishment and the maintenance of pregnancy. The fibrinolytic pathways are intimately involved in ovulation and the implantation of the fertilized egg into the uterine decidua. Once pregnancy has been established, an intact placental circulation is maintained by a dynamic balance between the coagulation and the fibrinolytic systems. Pregnancy is a hypercoagulable state secondary to an increase in the levels of some coagulation factors, a decrease in the levels of anticoagulant proteins, and an increase in fibrinolysis.[102]

A thrombophilic defect is an abnormality in the coagulation system that predisposes an individual to thrombosis. The first studies of the prevalence of coagulation abnormalities in women with adverse pregnancy outcome appeared in the mid 1990s.[103,104] Numerous studies of the prevalence of individual coagulation defects in women with RM have since reported very variable findings, but the role of antiphospholipid syndrome (APS), an acquired thrombophilic defect, has become an established and treatable cause of RM and the potential role of other thrombophilic defects (acquired or inherited) has been extensively explored. The presumed hypothesis is that some cases of RM and later pregnancy complications are caused by an exaggerated hemostatic response during pregnancy, leading to thrombosis of the uteroplacental vasculature and subsequent fetal demise.

Antiphospholipid Syndrome

APS is now recognized to be the most important treatable cause of RM.[9] Antiphospholipid antibodies (aPLs) are a family of heterogeneous autoantibodies (numbering approximately 20) directed against phospholipids-binding plasma proteins. In the etiology of pregnancy morbidity, the two most clinically important aPLs are lupus anticoagulant (LA) and anticardiolipin antibodies (aCLs) of the IgG and IgM subclass. APS, as originally defined, refers to the association between aPLs and either RM, thrombosis, or thrombocytopenia.[105] "Primary APS" affects patients with no identifiable underlying systemic connective tissue disease, whereas APS in patients with chronic inflammatory diseases, such as systemic lupus erythematosus, is referred to as "secondary APS." APS is associated with fetal loss in every trimester of pregnancy, and the clinical criteria thought to suggest it have now been extended to include (1) three or more consecutive unexplained miscarriages before the 10th week of gestation, (2) one or more deaths of morphologically normal fetuses after the 10th week of gestation, and (3) one or more preterm births before the 34th week of gestation as a result of severe preeclampsia, eclampsia, or placental insufficiency.[106]

APS can be associated with pregnancy loss in any trimester, but because the vast majority of miscarriages occur early, numerically it has the greatest impact before 12 weeks.[107] It is generally accepted that the prevalence of APS in women with RM is about 15%[108] and the fetal loss rate in untreated future pregnancies is as high as 90%.[109] However, the prevalence of APS in a highly selected cohort of late miscarriage sufferers has been reported to be over 40%.[110] By comparison, the prevalence of APS in women with a low risk obstetric history is less than 2%.[111] The mechanisms by which aPLs are thought to cause adverse pregnancy outcome are varied, reflecting in part their heterogeneity. Historically, the suggested pathogenesis of aPL-related pregnancy loss focused on placental thrombosis and infarction,[112,113] but it is important to note that these findings are neither specific nor universal.[114,115] Advances in our understanding of early pregnancy development and the biology of aPLs have provided new insights into the mechanisms of aPL-related pregnancy failure. In vitro studies report that aPLs.

- Impair signal transduction mechanisms controlling endometrial cell decidualization.[116]
- Increase trophoblast apoptosis.[117]
- Decrease trophoblast fusion.[117,118]
- Impair trophoblast invasion.[115,119]

Interestingly, the effects of aPLs on trophoblast function are reversed, at least in vitro, by low-molecular-weight heparin (LMWH).[117,119–121] Elegant experiments in mice have highlighted the pivotal role that complement plays in the pathogenesis of aPL-induced fetal damage. aPLs activate the classical complement pathway, generating the potent anaphylotoxin C5a, which in turn, recruits and activates inflammatory cells leading to tissue damage in the placenta and fetal death or growth restriction.[122,123] Heparin prevents aPL-induced fetal loss by inhibiting complement activation,[124] which raises the possibility that complement inhibitory therapies targeted to the placenta might be a useful treatment option for prevention of miscarriage in the future.

Inherited Thrombophilic Defects

Inherited thrombophilic defects are a well-established cause of systemic thrombosis, but their association with obstetric morbidity is more recent and less clearly understood. The publication of retrospective prevalence studies of thrombophilic disorders such as activated protein C resistance, protein C, protein S, and antithrombin III deficiencies in women with a history of fetal loss and later pregnancy complications was followed swiftly by the identification of three common thrombophilic mutations—factor V Leiden (FVL) G1691A, factor II prothrombin G20210A, and methylene tetrahydrofolate reductase C667T.

Since then, a plethora of studies have reported that individual defects are as or more frequent in women with RM as they are in control subjects. However, these prevalence data are compromised by the small sample size of individual studies, ascertainment bias, and poor matching of cases and controls owing to racial heterogeneity. Nonetheless, two meta-analyses have confirmed an association between RM and both the FVL and the prothrombin gene mutations.[125,126] The meta-analysis by Rey and coworkers[126] using pooled data from 31 retrospective studies suggested that carrying the FVL mutation (which gives rise to the inherited form of activated protein C resistance) is associated with a history of both early and late recurrent fetal loss and late nonrecurrent fetal loss. Carrying the prothrombin gene mutation is associated with early recurrent and late nonrecurrent fetal loss, whereas protein S deficiency is associated with late nonrecurrent fetal loss only. Methylenetetrahydrofolate mutation, protein C, and antithrombin III deficiencies are not significantly associated with fetal loss. Regrettably, there are little prospective data on the outcome of untreated pregnancies among women with genetic thrombophilic defects. One small prospective study showed that women with unexplained first-trimester RM who carry the FVL mutation are at significantly increased risk for further miscarriage compared with those with a normal factor V genotype (live birth rates 37.5% vs. 69.5%: odds ratio 3.75, 95% CI 1.3–10.9).[127] An equally important finding from this study was that carrying the FVL mutation did not preclude an uncomplicated pregnancy delivered at term, but at the present time, we have no means of reliably predicting those women with FVL mutation who are destined to miscarry and those who will have a successful outcome.

It may well be that "multiple hits"are necessary to substantially increase the likelihood of adverse pregnancy outcome in carriers of weakly prothrombotic genotypes. Indeed, one European cohort study identified a 14-fold increased risk of stillbirth in patients with combined thrombophilic defects.[103]

Global Markers of Hemostatic Function

The limitations of individual genetic thrombophilic defects in predicting pregnancy outcome has led to the introduction of "global tests" of hemostatic function in the assessment of women with RM. Using such tests, it has been reported that these women are in a prothrombotic state outside pregnancy.[128–130] This may result not only in an exaggerated hemostatic response during pregnancy, leading to thrombosis of the uteroplacental vasculature and subsequent fetal loss[131,132] but also confer an increased risk of ischemic heart disease in later life.[133]

Vincent and colleagues[130] reported that the levels of thrombin-antithrombin (TAT) complexes, a marker of thrombin generation, were significantly higher among women with a history of RM compared with age-matched fertile parous controls. This finding was independent of the gestation at previous miscarriage and unaffected by the woman's aPL status. Using alternative global markers, it has also been reported that women with RM suffer from a chronic state of endothelial activation,[134] and abnormally high levels of procoagulant particles have been reported in the circulation of women with a history of hitherto unexplained early and late pregnancy miscarriage.[128,135] In addition to their direct effect on the coagulation cascade, these circulating microparticles may be exerting a proinflammatory or proapoptotic action resulting in a disturbance in the implantation process and subsequent impairment of fetal growth.

Further evidence for an inherent prothrombotic state outside of pregnancy in women with RM has been demonstrated using thromboelastography. The thromboelastogram (TEG) is a cheap but effective tool that assesses the kinetics, strength, and stability of whole blood coagulation.[136] A variety of parameters scoring different stages of clot formation are registered, ranging from the initial platelet-fibrin interaction, through platelet aggregation, clot strengthening, and fibrin cross-linkage to clot lysis. Among women with RM, the maximal clot amplitude (MA)—a measure of the absolute strength of the fibrin clot formed—is significantly greater than among parous controls.[129] Moreover, the prepregnancy MA has also been found to be predictive of future pregnancy outcome, being significantly higher in those RM women whose next pregnancy ends in a further miscarriage than in those having a live birth. Once pregnancy is confirmed, serial TEG testing during the first trimester is capable of identifying increases in the MA that predate the clinical evidence of impending miscarriage by several weeks.[129]

Immunologic Factors

Maternofetal Alloimmune Disorders

The hypothesis that successful pregnancy depends on maternal immunologic tolerance of the semiallogeneic fetus suggests that fetal survival is dependent on suppression of the maternal immune response that would normally be expected against paternal antigens expressed by the fetus. However, the hypothesis that some cases of RM result from failure of maternal alloimmune recognition of the pregnancy has never been substantiated. No alloimmune mechanisms have been shown unequivocally to cause RM in humans. Further, there is no clear evidence to support the hypothesis that HLA incompatibility between couples, the absence of maternal leukocytotoxic antibodies, or the absence of maternal blocking antibodies is related to RM. Tests of such parameters should not be offered routinely to women with RM. Although it is clear that lymphocyte function does indeed change during pregnancy, there is no generalized suppression of the maternal immune response. Indeed, the concept that maternal immunization with paternal white blood cells, third-party donor leukocytes, trophoblast membranes, and intravenous immune globulin (IVIG), in order that she may mount a protective immune response to prevent rejection of the genetically dissimilar fetus and improve the live birth rate, has been refuted repeatedly by randomized therapeutic studies, summarized in two Cochrane systematic reviews.[137–140]

Furthermore, immunotherapy is expensive and has potentially serious side effects, including transfusion reaction, anaphylactic shock, and hepatitis. U.K. and U.S. current recommendations are that immunotherapy should no longer be offered to women with unexplained RM outside the context of approved clinical research projects.[141]

Contemporary concepts in reproductive immunology are now focused on the cooperative nature of the interaction between individual cells and molecules of the immune system with the fetus in determining pregnancy outcome.[142] In particular, interest is currently focused on the relationship between natural killer (NK) cells and reproductive failure. NK cells are lymphocytes that form part of the innate immune system and are found in both peripheral blood and the endometrium. There are, however, important phenotypic and functional differences between NK cells present at the two sites.[143] Microarray analysis combined with flow cytometric and reverse transcriptase polymerase chain reaction (RT-PCR) studies have demonstrated that the phenotype of uterine natural killer (uNK) cells ($CD56^{bright}$ $CD16^{-}$) is different from that of peripheral blood NK cells (PBNK) ($CD56^{dim}$ $CD16^{+}$).[142] In addition, uNK cells have an immunoregulatory potential that PBNK cells do not demonstrate.[143] More recently, it has been demonstrated that there is no relationship between PBNK and uNK cell levels and that PBNK cell levels are not predictive of pregnancy outcome among women with unexplained RM. The value of peripheral blood NK cell testing in the evaluation of women with RM is, therefore, questionable.[144]

The temporal and spatial distribution of uNK cells suggest that they play a role in controlling trophoblast invasion. Increased numbers of CD56+ NK cells have been documented in preconceptual decidual biopsies from women with RM compared with controls and those women with the highest levels of CD56+ cells had a higher rate of miscarriage in future untreated pregnancies.[145,146] However, although a recent study confirmed an increase in peri-implantation uterine NK cells in women with a history of RM, this did not have any useful prognostic value for the outcome of a subsequent pregnancy.[147] At the present time, there is no justification for the measurement of uNK cells in routine clinical practice. Furthermore, the use of systemic immunomodulatory drugs to suppress NK cell numbers in an attempt to improve pregnancy outcome has no logical basis.

The cytokine response at the maternofetal interface, to which uNK cells contribute, is currently under investigation. In general terms, the cytokine response may be divided into either a predominantly T helper-1 (Th-1) type (characterized by the production of interleukin 2 [Il-2], interferon, and tumor necrosis factor-α [TNF-α]) or a Th-2 type response (characterized by the production of Il-4, -6, and -10). It has been suggested that normal pregnancy is the result of a Th-2 type cytokine response that allows the production of blocking antibodies to mask fetal trophoblast antigens from immunologic recognition by a maternal Th-1 cell-mediated cytotoxic response.[148] In contrast, women who recurrently miscarry tend to produce a predominantly Th-1 type response both in the period of embryonic implantation and during pregnancy.[149–151]

These observations support the view that disturbances of immune tolerance of the fetus may account for some cases of RM. Future studies should be aimed at (1) identifying the subgroup of women with RM who produce a dominant Th-1 cytokine profile at the maternofetal interface during pregnancy and (2) the effect of immunomodulatory interventions aimed at shifting the balance toward Th-2 dominance.

Autoimmune

The prevalence of a variety of autoantibodies is reported to be increased among women with RM,[152,153] but this association is inconsistent and depends on which tests are employed and the population studied. Prospective data on the outcome of untreated pregnancies of autoantibody-positive compared with antibody-negative women is also conflicting, but the majority of studies demonstrate no association.[74,73,154,155] Furthermore, a placebo-controlled randomized study has reported that the use of steroids to suppress autoantibody titers does not improve the live birth rate but is associated with an increased risk of preterm delivery.[156]

Environmental Factors

Most data on environmental risk factors have concentrated on sporadic miscarriage rather than RM. The results have been conflicting and are undoubtedly biased by difficulties in controlling for confounding factors, the inaccuracy of exposure data, and the measurement of toxin dose. However, some environmental factors have been shown to affect pregnancy outcomes. Cigarette smoking has an adverse effect on trophoblast invasion and proliferation and is associated with a dose-dependent increased risk of miscarriage,[157] although these findings have been challenged.[158] Alcohol has adverse effects on fertility and fetal development and even moderate consumption of 5 or more units per week appears to increase the risk of sporadic miscarriage.[159] (In the UK, a unit of alcohol is defined as 10 ml [or approximately 8 g] of ethanol [ethyl alcohol].) Caffeine consumption is associated with a dose-dependent increased risk of miscarriage with the risk becoming significant when intake exceeds 300 mg (3 cups of coffee) daily.[158,160] Some forms of occupational exposure, such as working with or using video display terminals, does not appear to increase the risk of miscarriage,[161] and evidence of an adverse effect of anesthetic gases among surgical workers is contradictory.[162,163] Obesity has become a major health problem worldwide and in the United Kingdom affects 25% of the female population. Compelling evidence is accumulating that obesity is a risk factor for infertility, sporadic miscarriage and RM,[164,165] late pregnancy complications, and perinatal morbidity.[166] A recent review has highlighted the adverse impact that obesity exerts on every aspect of obstetric practice and outcome.[167] Concerns have also arisen that an increased risk of miscarriage is associated with the use of nonsteroidal anti-inflammatory drugs and some antidepressants during the periconceptual period.[168]

Psychological Factors

Miscarriage is a stressful life event: depression, anxiety, denial, anger, sense of loss, inadequacy, and marital disruption have all been reported in female and male members of couples experiencing pregnancy loss. RM may seriously affect a woman's mental health.[169] One study indicated that a third of women with RM were clinically depressed and 21% had levels of anxiety that were equal to or higher than those in typical psychiatric outpatient populations.[170] Animal data indicate that stress may induce miscarriage.[171] A small prospective study indicated that among 14 psychological parameters studied, only a high depression scale affected the miscarriage rate in women with a history of two previous miscarriages.[172] Larger prospective studies are needed to address the scope of psychological disorders and their contribution to RM.

MANAGEMENT OPTIONS

"Prepregnancy" When the Third Miscarriage Occurs

A detailed history of the previous miscarriages is essential. When the third miscarriage occurs, it is important to consider the following factors:

- The underlying causes of first-trimester miscarriage are different from those responsible for mid-trimester loss. Therefore, it is important to accurately determine gestational age, confirmed by ultrasound whenever possible, at the time of the miscarriage.
- In cases of first-trimester miscarriage, one should determine whether the loss was at a very early stage (biochemical evidence of pregnancy only), anembryonic (blighted ovum), embryonic (6–8 wk), or fetal (>8 wk). Different pathologic factors affect the various stages of early pregnancy. For example, biochemical and anembryonic losses are more likely to be associated with chromosomally abnormal embryos.
- Note whether fetal heart activity was detected before the miscarriage. Many first-trimester miscarriages associated with APS occur after the establishment of fetal heart activity.
- When surgical evacuation of the products of conception is performed, it is important to document suspected uterine abnormalities, such as a bicornuate or subseptate uterus or fibroids. Tissue should be collected and sent for both histologic examination (to confirm pregnancy and exclude trophoblastic disease) and fetal karyotyping (Table 6–2).
- In the event of a second-trimester miscarriage, note whether the pregnancy loss was preceded by intrauterine fetal death, spontaneous rupture of the membranes, vaginal bleeding, painful uterine contractions, or painless cervical dilation. This information is particularly useful in identifying or excluding a presumed diagnosis of cervical incompetence. The couple should be encouraged to consent to a full fetal postmortem examination, fetal karyotyping, and placental histologic examination.
- Coexisting pathology is a frequent finding in cases of second-trimester miscarriage. If the fetal karyotype and morphology are normal, the search for evidence of anatomic problems (including cervical weakness) should always be accompanied by a detailed thrombophilia and infection screen.
- Ensure that a follow-up appointment is scheduled for the couple.

Prepregnancy Assessment and Counseling after the Third Miscarriage

The loss of a pregnancy at any stage is a tragic event, and sensitivity is required in assessing and counseling couples with RM. A specialist miscarriage clinic is a better environment in which to provide this care than a busy postnatal or general gynecology clinic. Ideally, the couple should be seen together and offered information to facilitate decision-making about future pregnancies (see "Risk Factors for Recurrent Miscarriage"). Wherever possible, the couple should be given written information to take home.

TABLE 6–2
Chromosome Analysis of the Products of Conception—Tissue Collection

General	It is good practice, and in some countries a legal requirement, to obtain patient consent prior to tissue collection for diagnostic testing. Ensure aseptic technique in tissue handling.
Collection–first-trimester miscarriage	Collect all fetal tissues and placental villi.
Collection–second-trimester miscarriage	Obtain a small piece of full-thickness fetal skin samples with subepidermal layers. In cases of intrauterine fetal death and macerated fetus, it is particularly important to send a placental biopsy in addition to a fetal sample, because fetal karyotyping is often unsuccessful. Placental biopsies should be a wedge from the cord insertion site and include membranes.
Container	Sterile universal container containing sterile saline or transport media provided by the cytogenetics laboratory. **DO NOT ADD FORMALIN.** Transport media should be regularly renewed.
Labeling	Patient's details including name, date of birth, and hospital number should be recorded on the sample container label and accompanied by a completed referral form. Samples should be prebooked with the laboratory.
Transport and storage	Send samples immediately after collection to the laboratory; transport at room temperature. Sample can be refrigerated at 4°C if not sent until the following day. **DO NOT FREEZE.**
Causes for rejection	Gross contamination, necrotic tissue, specimen in formalin fixative.
Limitations	Some products of conception may contain only maternal tissues. Trophoblast cells may contain mosaicisms or aneuploidy not present in the fetus.

History

A comprehensive history should be obtained from both partners, noting their ages and obstetric, gynecologic, medical, surgical, social, psychological, and family histories. Seeking the cooperation of the patient's family doctor and other physicians may be necessary to obtain relevant information.

Physical Examination

The physical examination should include height, weight, blood pressure, and a general assessment for signs of endocrine disease. Pelvic examination should assess signs of previous cervical trauma or surgery, genital tract anomalies, and uterine size.

Investigation of Recurrent Miscarriage (Table 6–3)

Testing should include

- Parental karyotyping of both partners to determine abnormal chromosome rearrangements, translocations, or inversions.
- Two-dimensional pelvic ultrasound to identify polycystic ovaries and assess the uterine anatomy. Suspected uterine anomalies may require further studies using hysterosalpingography (HSG), hysteroscopy, laparoscopy, or three-dimensional pelvic ultrasound.
- Early follicular phase (days 2–4 of menstrual cycle) LH, FSH, and testosterone levels are measured to exclude LH hypersecretion, hyperandrogenemia, and possible high FSH levels.
- All women with RM should be screened for aPLs before pregnancy. A diagnosis of APS requires at least two positive test results for either LA or aCLs IgG or IgM antibodies in samples obtained 6 weeks apart. Women with one positive test result and a second negative test result should have a third aPL test to confirm or refute the APS diagnosis. The detection of aPL is subject to considerable variation between laboratories because of temporal fluctuation of aPL titers in individual patients, transient positivity as a result of infection, suboptimal methods of sample collection and preparation, and lack of standardization of laboratory tests for their detection.[173] Therefore, laboratory assays should be performed according to international guidelines.[174] Because maternal aPLs might be down-regulated during pregnancy,[175] tests are best performed preconceptually. Testing for aPLs other than LA or aCLs is uninformative.[174] The dilute

TABLE 6–3
Investigation of Recurrent Miscarriage

All patients	Karyotype
	  Parental
	  Miscarried tissues **[NB Consent issues - see earlier]**
	Pelvic ultrasound
	Early follicular phase LH, FSH, testosterone
	aPLs
	  Lupus anticoagulant and
	  aCLs IgG and IgM
	Activated protein C resistance
	Factor V Leiden gene mutation
	Prothrombin gene mutation
	Serology for rubella
	Blood group and rhesus type

Selected patients	HSG/hysteroscopy/laparoscopy
	Three-dimensional pelvic ultrasound
	Full thrombophilia screening:
	  In addition to those taken in all patients—see earlier
	  Protein C, protein S, antithrombin III, MTHFR, factors XII and VIII
	Thromboelastography—where available
	Glucose tolerance test
	Thyroid function tests
	Cervical length screening in pregnancy
	Vaginal swab culture for bacterial vaginosis

aCLs, anticardiolipin antibodies; aPLs, antiphospholipid antibodies; FSH, follicle-stimulating hormone; HSG, hysterosalpinography; Ig, immunoglobulin; LH, luteinizing hormone; MTHFR, methylenetetrahydrofolate reductase.

Russell viper venom time test, together with platelet neutralization procedure, is a more sensitive and specific test for the detection of a LA than either the activated partial thromboplastin time or the kaolin clotting time test.[107] aCLs are detected with a standardized enzyme-linked immunosorbent assay.[175]

- Screening for APC resistance should include coagulation tests for both unmodified and modified APC resistance and factor V genotyping. Factor II (prothrombin) genotyping should also be undertaken. Additional thrombophilia tests may be requested on the basis of positive findings on history, examination, and laboratory tests. Table 6–3 shows a complete list of possible tests. In the majority of cases of RM, an underlying systematic cause will not be identified.[176]
- Thromboelastography is not widely available. However, this method of assessing whole blood hemostasis is a useful tool for identifying evidence of prothrombotic and impaired fibrinolytic parameters among women with RM in whom the more conventional hemostasis tests are normal.[129] It has the great advantage of being cheap and reproducible with results that are available within a few hours. Because pregnancy may trigger proinflammatory hemostatic changes, it is helpful to repeat TEG testing in early pregnancy. Abnormal results may help to inform decisions regarding the use of variable-dose aspirin.

Prepregnancy Treatment Options

General Considerations

Couples should be treated sensitively and sympathetically. The management of couples with RM has traditionally been based on anecdotal evidence, personal bias, and the results of small uncontrolled studies.[136] As our knowledge of early pregnancy development increases, it is incumbent upon us to reject such customs and embrace evidence-based practice. It is important to avoid recommending unproven treatments.

Epidemiologic Factors

Advanced maternal age and the number of previous miscarriages are two important independent risk factors for further miscarriage that should be considered (see Table 6–1).

Genetic Factors

When a parent carries a balanced chromosome rearrangement, the risk of producing chromosomally unbalanced offspring depends on the specific chromosomes involved, the size of the segments involved in the rearrangement, and the sex of the transmitting parent. The risk of miscarriage in couples with reciprocal translocation is approximately 50%, whereas in robertsonian translocation, the risk is approximately 25%.[177] Most couples with balanced chromosome rearrangements have healthy children; however, homologous robertsonian translocations always result in fetal aneuploidy. The finding of an abnormal parental karyotype warrants genetic counseling. Genetic counseling offers the couple a prognosis for future pregnancies, prenatal diagnostic options, and the opportunity to perform familial chromosomal studies if desired.

If a subsequent miscarriage occurs, karyotyping of the products of conception is essential, regardless of the parental karyotype. Table 6–2 summarizes the procedure for collecting the products of conception for chromosome analysis. Traditionally, reproductive options in couples with chromosomal abnormality have included proceeding to a further natural pregnancy, with or without prenatal diagnostic tests, CVS, or amniocentesis; gamete donation[178]; and adoption. Preimplantation genetic diagnosis has been explored as a treatment option for translocation carriers[179,180] and couples with unexplained RM.[181,182] Preimplantation genetic diagnosis is a technically demanding procedure and requires the couple to undergo in vitro fertilization to produce embryos. Therefore, couples with proven fertility must be made aware of the high financial cost and low implantation and live birth rates per cycle after in vitro fertilization. In summary, aneuploidy screening does not improve the live birth rate for couples with RM,[182] and in women aged between 35 and 41 years, it significantly lowers the live birth rate.[183]

Anatomic Considerations

As a screening test for uterine anomalies, noninvasive two-dimensional pelvic ultrasound assessment of the uterine cavity, with or without sonohysterography,[20,184] when performed by skilled and experienced staff, is as informative as invasive HSG. Three-dimensional ultrasound offers additional accuracy in the diagnosis and classification of uterine malformations[185,186]; hence, its use might obviate the need for hysteroscopy and laparoscopy. Minor defects rarely warrant surgical correction. Historically, abdominal metroplasty was advocated for a uterine septum. However, open uterine surgery has not been assessed in prospective trials, is associated with postoperative infertility, and carries a significant risk of scar rupture during pregnancy.[52] These complications are less likely to occur after transcervical hysteroscopic resection of uterine septa, and experience from case series appears promising.[187] These procedures must be performed by clinicians with appropriate training and experience in hysteroscopic surgery. Metroplasty has been traditionally advocated for bicornuate uterus and uterus didelphys, even though it is of unproven benefit and carries a significant risk of morbidity. Unicornuate uterus is rare and has limited treatment options. Cervical cerclage has been proposed, but is of uncertain value.[188] Uterine anomalies resulting from in utero diethylstilbestrol exposure are rarely amenable to surgical correction, but prophylactic cervical cerclage has been advocated.[189] Intrauterine adhesions can be corrected by hysteroscopic lysis, placement of an intrauterine device, and administration of cyclic estrogen and progesterone after surgery.[68] Occasionally, abdominal or hysteroscopic myomectomy is warranted for RM associated with significant submucous fibroids that distort the uterine cavity or occupy a large subendometrial area. A 3-month course of a GnRH analogue preoperatively facilitates surgery by reducing the size and vascularity of the fibroids. More recently, percutaneous thermal ablation of uterine fibroids under real-time magnetic resonance control has been pioneered and appears to be a safe and effective therapy that offers the advantage of preserving fertility.[190–192]

Traditionally, the diagnosis of cervical incompetence has relied on a clinical history of late miscarriage preceded by spontaneous rupture of the membranes or painless cervical dilation. This clinical diagnosis has not been evaluated in terms of its ability to predict future pregnancy outcome. Although HSG and painless passage of an 8 Hegar dilator have been used to make the diagnosis before pregnancy, neither procedure has been studied prospectively. There is no satisfactory objective test to identify nonpregnant women with cervical incompetence.

Experience with prepregnancy abdominal cerclage is limited and of unproven value. It has been advocated in women with a history of mid-trimester loss and previous failed cervical vaginal cerclage and for those with a very short or scarred cervix in which the transvaginal approach would be difficult. Transabdominal cerclage has been associated with a lower rate of perinatal death or delivery at less than 24 weeks' gestation, but is accompanied by a higher risk of operative complications, particularly hemorrhage and damage to the bladder or bowel.[193,194] Necessarily, the procedure commits the woman to two major operations: (1) a laparotomy for placement of the suture either before or in early pregnancy and (2) cesarean delivery.

Endocrine Factors

There is no value in performing glucose tolerance tests in women with RM who have no history suggestive of diabetes mellitus. In women with established diabetes, poor glycemic control increases the risk of pregnancy loss. Consequently, these women require prepregnancy counseling with the aim of obtaining optimal periconceptual glycemic control.[195] The contribution of luteal phase defect to RM is controversial, and a review of pregnancy rates after hormonal treatments for luteal phase deficiency concluded that the benefits are uncertain[81] and that standardized diagnostic criteria are lacking.[76] A multicenter placebo-controlled study of human chorionic gonadotropin (hCG) supplementation in early pregnancy showed no benefit in pregnancy outcome.[196] Subsequently, a small placebo-controlled study suggested that the benefit of hCG is confined to a small subgroup of patients with RM and oligomenorrhea.[197] One meta-analysis based on three small studies reported that progesterone support for pregnancy in women with RM may have a beneficial effect.[80] This could be explained by the immunomodulatory action of progesterone in shifting the proinflammatory Th-1 cytokine response to a more favorable Th-2 response. Prepregnancy suppression of high LH levels with an LH-releasing hormone analogue followed by low-dose ovulation induction in ovulatory women with RM does not improve pregnancy outcome.[86] Further, the live birth rate without pituitary suppression is excellent. The role of insulin resistance and the safety and effectiveness of metformin treatment in women with RM and polycystic ovaries require further study. Metformin should be used only in the context of prospective controlled trials.

Infections

All women with RM should be screened routinely to establish their rubella antibody status and be offered immunization if not immune before the next pregnancy. The empirical use of antimicrobial drugs in the treatment of women with recurrent pregnancy loss cannot be justified and might increase the risk of neonatal neurologic problems, according to the results of a recently published long-term follow-up study.[101]

Antiphospholipid Antibodies

aPLs are associated with a wide spectrum of pregnancy complications, including RM, late fetal loss, fetal growth restriction, preeclampsia, placental abruption, preterm birth, and maternal thromboembolic disease.[107,198,199] Several treatment modalities including aspirin, steroids, IVIG, and heparin have been used in an attempt to improve the pregnancy outcome of these women. However, a meta-analysis shows that only a combination of low-dose aspirin and low-dose (i.e., prophylactic rather than therapeutic) heparin significantly improves the live birth rate in women with RM and APS (Fig. 6–3).[200] This treatment enhances pregnancy outcome by 54%, to achieve a live birth rate of 70% or more in women with the syndrome.[108,201] Since this meta-analysis was published, two small trials have suggested that aspirin alone is sufficient to improve pregnancy outcome in women with APS.[194,202] In one study, 25% of the participants switched treatment group.[194] The use of steroids during pregnancy leads to significant rates of maternal and fetal morbidity and does not improve pregnancy outcome compared with other treatment modalities.[203,204] Further, a randomized trial found that aspirin plus heparin is superior to IVIG,[205] and a recent systematic review of IVIG[140] concluded that this treatment has no place in the management of women with aPL-related pregnancy loss. Because heparin does not cross the placental barrier, it is not teratogenic and does not cause fetal hemorrhage. Unfortunately, heparin is associated with significant maternal complications, including bleeding, hypersensitivity reactions, heparin-induced thrombocytopenia, and when used long term, osteopenia and vertebral bone fractures. However, two prospective studies showed that the loss in

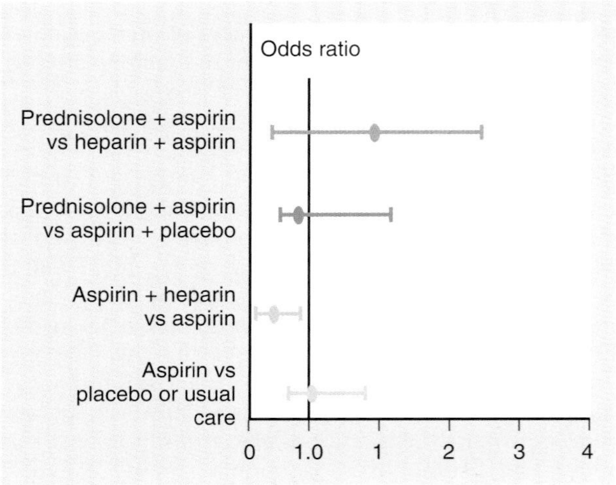

FIGURE 6–3
Meta-analysis of treatments for antiphospholipid antibody (aPL)–associated pregnancy loss.
(Modified from Empson M, Lassere M, Craig JC, Scott JR: Recurrent pregnancy loss with antiphospholipid antibody: A systematic review of therapeutic trials. Obstet Gynecol 2002;99:135–144.)

bone mineral density at the lumbar spine associated with long-term, low-dose heparin therapy is similar to the loss that occurs physiologically during normal pregnancy,[206,207] although whether it is equally reversible has not been established. A combination of these two effects might be more serious than either alone, and it is probably wise to warn women of the possible sequelae of osteopenia. Nonetheless, risk-benefit assessment of aspirin plus heparin treatment supports its use in women with APS. After the diagnosis of APS is made, women should be advised to start aspirin and heparin treatment after confirmation of their next pregnancy (at 4–5 wk). No evidence suggests that preconceptual treatment of APS improves pregnancy outcome.

Hereditary Thrombophilia

The pregnancy outcome for women with a history of RM associated with FVL mutation is poor if no pharmacologic treatment is offered during pregnancy.[127] The efficacy of thromboprophylaxis during pregnancy in women with RM and inherited thrombophilic defects, who are otherwise asymptomatic, has not been assessed in prospective, randomized controlled trials, but uncontrolled studies suggest that heparin therapy may improve the live birth rate in these women.[208,209] Until further evidence becomes available, the poor pregnancy outcome associated with FVL mutation, coupled with the maternal risks during pregnancy, probably justifies routine screening for FVL and antenatal thromboprophylaxis for those with the FVL mutation or evidence of placental thrombosis. Full anticoagulation may be required throughout pregnancy and puerperium in some patients with a personal or family history of thromboembolism (see Chapter 42).

Maternofetal Alloimmune Disorders

None of the proposed alloimmune theories have been substantiated, and no immunologic tests have been identified to predict pregnancy outcome. It is of concern that some women with RM are being treated with a variety of agents—IVIG, anti-TNF-α drugs, and/or glucocorticoids—in order to dampen an "excessive immune response." Not only is there no evidence base for these interventions, they are also potentially associated with significant morbidity.

IVIG is a pooled blood product and is associated with anaphylactic reactions, fever, flushing, muscle pains, nausea, and headache.[210] Anti-TNF-α agents have been reported to be associated with the development of lymphoma, granulomatous diseases such as tuberculosis, systemic lupus erythematosus–like syndromes, demyelinating disease, and congestive cardiac failure.[211] Of equal concern is that whereas TNF-α has traditionally been viewed as a cytokine involved in triggering immunologically mediated pregnancy loss, it is also involved in antiapoptotic signaling pathways and has a regulatory role in cell proliferation. Indeed, studies in TNF-α knock-out mice suggest that this cytokine may play an important role in embryo development and the prevention of structural abnormalities.[212] These abnormalities might not, of course, be unmasked until later in life. Glucocorticoids during pregnancy are associated with an increased risk of preterm delivery secondary to rupture of membranes and the development of preeclampsia and gestational diabetes.[156] Immunotherapy should be offered to women with RM only in the context of prospective controlled trials.

Unexplained Recurrent Miscarriage

Despite extensive testing, in approximately 50% of couples with RM no cause is identified.[20] Although the mechanism is unclear, several nonrandomized studies suggest the benefit of supportive care and attendance at a dedicated early pregnancy clinic. The prognosis for a successful future pregnancy in women with unexplained RM who receive supportive care alone is in the region of 60% to 70%; this figure is lower with increasing maternal age and number of previous miscarriages. Two studies have reported that aspirin does not improve the live birth rate in women with unexplained RM.[213,214] The use of aspirin and other nonsteroidal anti-inflammatory agents has been associated with an increased rate of miscarriage[215,216] and both a case-controlled study[217] and a meta-analysis[218] have reported a two- to threefold increased risk of gastroschisis in mothers taking aspirin during the first trimester of pregnancy. These data suggest that empirical treatment in women with unexplained RM is unnecessary and should be avoided. A prospective placebo-controlled trial would be needed to establish the efficacy of heparin in the treatment of women with unexplained RM.[219] General advice about stopping smoking, avoiding excessive alcohol and caffeine intake, dietary balance, and weight loss for obese women is important. Taking folic acid (400 µg/day) for at least 2 months before attempting conception should be advised to prevent neural tube defects.

Management during Subsequent Pregnancy, Delivery, and Puerperium

Strategies for management during a pregnancy following a miscarriage differ according to the underlying cause of miscarriage. The risk of repeated miscarriage increases with each successive pregnancy loss and with advancing maternal age. Even when the pregnancy progresses beyond 24 weeks' gestation, evidence suggests that women with RM are at risk for late pregnancy complications such as preeclampsia, intrauterine fetal growth restriction, preterm delivery, perinatal loss, and operative delivery.[19,198,201] Close antenatal surveillance and delivery in a unit with specialized obstetric and neonatal intensive care facilities are indicated.

First Trimester

Couples with RM are understandably anxious and need support and reassurance throughout the first trimester. Ultrasound is valuable in the management of early pregnancy to confirm viability and, after fetal heart activity has been detected, to provide ongoing maternal reassurance. Using transvaginal ultrasound, an intrauterine gestation sac will be visible at 5 weeks, a yolk sac at approximately 5.5 weeks, and fetal heart activity at 6 weeks. Thereafter, a scan to check fetal heart activity may be obtained every week or every 2 weeks until the end of the first trimester. The demonstration of normal sequential fetal growth and activity is very reassuring for many couples.

Women with APS should be offered aspirin and heparin treatment. Low-dose aspirin (75 mg/day) should be commenced as soon as the patient has a positive urinary pregnancy test result. Subcutaneous low-dose heparin therapy in the form of LMWH (enoxaparin [Clexane] [Lovenox]

20 mg/day or dalteparin [Fragmin] 2500 units/day) or unfractionated heparin ([Calciparine] 5000 IU twice daily) should be started as soon as an intrauterine pregnancy is confirmed by ultrasound scan (gestational sac and a yolk sac within the uterine cavity). Some clinicians prefer to commence the heparin therapy as soon as the pregnancy test is positive. Although unfractionated heparin is equally beneficial, LMWH offers the advantage of once-daily injection owing to its longer half-life and increased bioavailability. A platelet count should be done at the start of treatment and repeated 2 weeks later to exclude the rare complication of heparin-induced thrombocytopenia. Despite significant improvement in live birth rates, pregnant women who have APS and are treated with aspirin plus heparin until 34 completed weeks of gestation remain at risk for later pregnancy complications, including preeclampsia, intrauterine growth restriction, placental abruption, and preterm delivery.[199] Some clinicians prefer to continue treatment until the time of delivery in the belief that this reduces the risk of these late pregnancy complications, but there is no hard evidence to support this view. Indeed, the randomized controlled trial by Rai and associates[108] emphasized that the main benefit of combination therapy with aspirin and heparin is to improve the quality and depth of embryonic implantation during the first trimester of pregnancy. After 13 weeks' gestation, the number of pregnancies ending in live births did not differ significantly by treatment group.

Second Trimester

When cervical incompetence is suspected in pregnancy, transvaginal ultrasonic assessment of the cervix is a noninvasive and objective means of assessing cervical length and shape and predicting preterm birth in high-risk populations.[220–222] The three ultrasound signs that suggest cervical incompetence are shortening of the endocervical canal, funneling of the internal os, and sacculation or prolapse of the membranes into the cervix, either spontaneously or as a result of fundal pressure (Fig. 6–4). A short cervix (<25 mm)

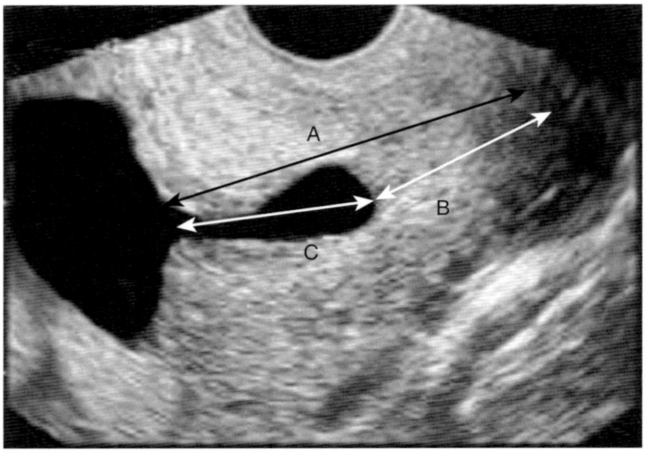

FIGURE 6–4
Transvaginal ultrasound scan of the cervix shows cervical shortening and funnelling. *A*, Total cervical length. *B*, Length of distal cervical segment. *C*, Depth of cervical funnel.

is the best independent predictor of spontaneous preterm birth before 34 weeks' gestation. Cervical cerclage is a recognized treatment for cervical incompetence. However, a meta-analysis of four randomized controlled trials found no conclusive evidence that prophylactic cervical cerclage reduces the risk of pregnancy loss and preterm delivery in women at risk for preterm birth or mid-trimester loss because of cervical factors.[223] Further, the procedure was associated with an increased risk of minor morbidity, but no serious morbidity. A small decrease in the number of deliveries before 33 weeks' gestation was noted in the largest trial.[224] The benefit was greatest in women with three or more second-trimester miscarriages or preterm births. There was no significant improvement in neonatal survival. The same meta-analysis assessed the role of therapeutic cerclage in women with a short cervix seen on ultrasound.[223] The pooled results from two small randomized controlled trials showed no reduction in mid-trimester pregnancy loss and preterm delivery before 28 and 34 weeks in women assigned to undergo ultrasound-indicated cerclage.[57,225] However, the numbers of women randomized were too small to allow firm conclusions to be drawn. A recent trial of elective cerclage inserted on the basis of historical risk factors versus cerclage inserted after detection of cervical length shortening using ultrasound showed no difference in pregnancy outcome, but a higher rate of cerclage (32% vs. 19%, relative risk 1.66; 95% CI 1.07–2.47) and its associated morbidity in the ultrasound-monitored group.[226] This suggests either that cerclage made no difference in either group or that ultrasound monitoring overdiagnoses women at risk of preterm labor. Based on this evidence, it would seem reasonable to divide women with a history of mid-trimester miscarriage that suggests cervical incompetence into two groups, with the therapeutic approach tailored accordingly.

The first group includes women at high risk for second-trimester miscarriage, including those with two or more second-trimester miscarriages without bleeding or clear signs of labor preceding the miscarriage. These women may benefit from prophylactic cervical cerclage at 13 to 16 weeks, with removal at 37 to 38 weeks. Several adjuvant measures may be considered to minimize the risk of infection or other complications at the time of suture insertion including a short course of antibiotics and bed rest for 24 hours (although there is no randomized controlled trial evidence to suggest that either of these precautions is necessary). Before prophylactic cerclage, women should be offered ultrasound examination to assess fetal viability and exclude apparent fetal anomalies. This will avoid inserting a suture in a pregnancy in which there is no possibility of improving the outcome.

The second group, considered at medium risk, includes women with a history of one second-trimester miscarriage and those with evidence of other factors predisposing to preterm delivery such as infection and thrombophilic disorders, both of which should be treated aggressively. These women can be offered serial transvaginal cervical ultrasound scanning beginning at 12 weeks and performed every 2 weeks until 23 weeks to measure cervical length and exclude funneling of the upper cervical canal. Therapeutic cervical cerclage may be offered to women with ultrasound signs of cervical shortening (<25 mm) or with progressive funneling in the absence of uterine activity or signs of chorioamnionitis, although it must be emphasized that currently there is no randomized controlled trial evidence that such "rescue cerclage" is beneficial.[227]

CERVICAL CERCLAGE FOR RECURRENT MID-TRIMESTER PREGNANCY LOSS

There is a lack of good epidemiologic data on the incidence of mid-trimester loss; however, a commonly quoted figure is 2%. It is important to remember that many cases are multifactorial, and demonstration of cervical weakness does not exclude the coexistence of other causes. Thus, screening for causes such as APS or thrombophilia should also be carried out, in addition to planned cerclage.

Factors in the history suggestive of cervical incompetence include a painless mid-trimester delivery (characteristically the mother presents fully dilated, not having realized she was in labor), previous major cervical surgery (e.g., conization, including large loop excision), documented trauma to the cervix in a previous birth, in utero exposure to diethylstilbestrol (taken by the woman's mother to try to prevent miscarriage—this was still in clinical use as recently as the mid-1970s), or prelabor preterm rupture of the membranes.

As stated by the Euro-Team Early Pregnancy Protocol,[228] there is no agreed definition of cervical weakness by absolute measurable and reproducible criteria. It is important that before cervical weakness is diagnosed, appropriate diagnostic criteria are applied and other causes excluded, because management is invasive and carries a significant risk of an adverse outcome. The diagnosis is made in the absence of other causes of preterm delivery such as uterine anomaly, fibroids, or infection, and in which only singleton pregnancies are included.[229] As has been written as the premise for a randomized controlled trial, "the overuse of prophylactic cerclage is a manifestation of our inability to diagnose cervical incompetence with any degree of reliability on the basis of historical criteria alone."[230] More recently, this message has been underlined and it has been emphasized that "prophylactic and reactive interventions remain largely unevaluated or ineffective."[231]

McDonald Suture

As explained previously, there is currently no good evidence for the effectiveness of rescue cerclage, and thus whenever possible, if cerclage is indicated by the history, it should be planned at the end of the first trimester, following a reassuring scan. The most common suture employed is that first described by McDonald.[232] This is a simple purse-string suture placed around the cervix at the vault of the vagina, just below the reflection of the vaginal skin onto the cervix. Mersilene tape or nylon can be used. Knots are usually tied anteriorly to make removal easier at about 37 weeks' gestation (the uterus anteverts as pregnancy progresses, making access to the posterior aspect of the cervix difficult). The anterior knot is easily visualized with a speculum, grasped with a tenaculum, and the suture cut at the side of the knot, allowing it to slide out. With a good light and the correct instruments (e.g., long-handled scissors), this can be done in the clinic or office, with the woman lying in the left lateral position. There is no need to leave large loops of suture material in the vagina; indeed, these can cause maternal discomfort and excessive discharge. There is no evidence that tocolysis or an overnight stay is necessary, provided the insertion is straightforward. Some advocate use of a sharp needle, taking multiple small bites to encircle the cervix, whereas others use a large-diameter curved needle passed in the subcutaneous tissues, a plane that can be found by its relative lack of resistance.

Despite the attraction of the McDonald suture as a simple procedure, initial, prospective, randomized controlled trials failed to demonstrate benefit.[233,234] However, a much larger trial (including > 1200 subjects), carried out under the auspices of the Medical Research Council (United Kingdom) and the Royal College of Obstetricians and Gynaecologists and reported in 1993, recruited women with borderline indications for cerclage. Results showed that after cerclage, delivery prior to 32 weeks' gestation occurred in 13% of women as opposed to 17% in the control group ($P < .03$). This can either be taken to mean that the procedure needs to be performed 25 times to prevent one case of very preterm birth or that it reduces preterm labor by 25%, depending on whether one is an enthusiast or a skeptic.[224]

Shirodkar Suture

Often, the cervix is short, making it difficult to insert a McDonald suture containing a significant amount of cervix. In such cases, it is necessary to incise the skin over the anterior cervix and dissect under the skin in order to push the bladder up and allow access to the upper part of the cervix. The bladder is most easily pushed up using a gauze swab over a gloved finger. Defining the position of the bladder and the internal os is made much easier by the use of simultaneous ultrasound visualization. This is most conveniently done via a suprapubic transducer because a vaginal probe makes it difficult to insert the suture. The basics of the technique were first described by Shirodkar in 1955[235] and so the procedure is usually called a "Shirodkar suture." There have been no randomized controlled trials of this technique, but if it is thought that a suture is justified, then it is necessary to use this approach if the cervix is too short for a McDonald suture. Some authorities recommend opening the posterior fornix, but if a large-diameter blunt needle is used, it can often be passed high behind the cervix without colpotomy, provided care is taken to ensure the needle stays in contact with the cervix and does not enter the peritoneal cavity. One important attribute of the Shirodkar suture is that the knot is buried, which means much less vaginal discharge than with the McDonald. However, this also means it needs to be removed using an anesthetic.

Transabdominal Cervicoisthmic Cerclage (Fig. 6–5)

The concept of placing a suture at the internal os via an abdominal approach was introduced by Benson and Durfee in 1965.[236]

FIGURE 6–5
Transabdominal cervicoisthmic cerclage. *A*, Lateral view. *B*, Anterior view.

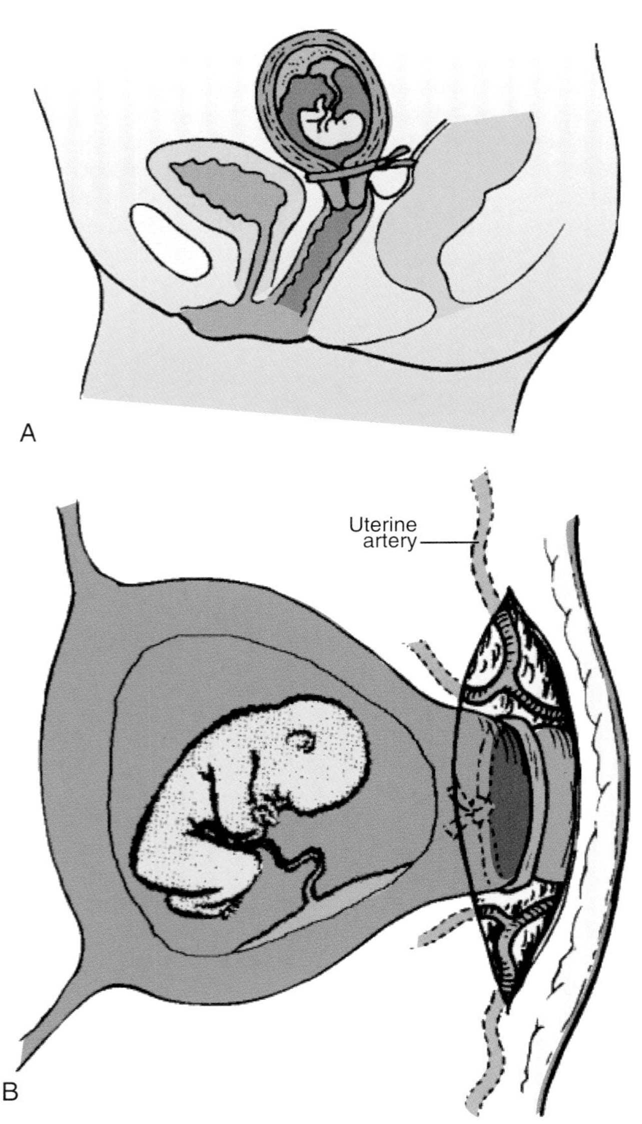

The indications for a transabdominal suture are[237]

- Previous failed vaginal suture.
- Traumatic or surgical damage making a vaginal approach difficult.
- Severe scarring or chronic cervicitis.
- Cervicovaginal fistula.

A preconceptual interview is ideal, allowing full disclosure and explanation regarding risks of failure and complications of insertion following previous surgery (e.g., classic cesarean delivery); damage to the cervix and adjacent major vessels, bowel, or bladder; and the need for two major operations (insertion of the suture and subsequently delivery by cesarean section). All these factors need to be addressed, ideally by a second counseling interview when consent can be obtained. The patient has by then received all the relevant information before conception and understands that abdominal cerclage should be seen as a last resort.

The technique is ideally carried out at 12 weeks' gestation, with prior ultrasound screening for fetal anomaly as previously described. It can be carried out earlier, but this increases the risk that there will be fetal demise or abnormality diagnosed subsequently. It can also be carried out later, up to 24 weeks, but the increasing size of the uterus makes it technically more difficult and there is a requirement for a larger abdominal incision. At 12 weeks, a Pfannenstiel incision is usually appropriate. Placement of abdominal sutures using minimal access techniques (laparoscopic transabdominal cervicoisthmic cerclage) has been described, but the series are small and it is not yet a generally used technique.[238,239] The use of the technique may be accelerated by the use of robotic surgery.[240]

The procedure is performed under general anesthesia. The bladder should be emptied and the catheter left in situ during the operation. Packing the vagina before laparotomy can elevate the uterus with improved access to the cervicoisthmic region. The patient is placed in the Trendelenburg position. A low transverse abdominal incision is made and packs used to keep bowel away from the operative field.

Scanning directly onto the uterus using an ultrasound probe covered in a sterile sleeve enables precise visualization of the internal os, which can then be identified externally using an opposed finger and thumb on either side (fore and aft) of the broad ligament. The finger and thumb can also be used to identify the ascending branch of the uterine artery by feeling it pulsate and drawing it laterally, forming an avascular space of about 2 mm^2 in the broad ligament just lateral to the cervix and about 2 mm below the internal os through which to pass the needle mounted with the encircling tape. The suture is traditionally passed from anterior to posterior using a blunt needle. Mersilene tape and double-stranded nylon are both commonly used. It is traditional to tie the knot posteriorly to avoid the knot irritating the bladder (which may need to be dissected clear of the lower segment and pushed down before the suture is inserted; again, its location can be determined using ultrasound). A posterior knot allows removal of the suture via a posterior colpotomy in the event of fetal demise, so that vaginal birth can be achieved. However, it is easier to tie the knot anteriorly, and some recommend this as routine as it avoids intraperitoneal exposure of the surgical knot and prevents adhesion formation to bowel and its attendant complications.[241]

Scanning also allows the confirmation of fetal life, and intact membranes, before closure of the abdomen. A single dose of intraoperative antibiotics is commonly given. Nonsteroidal anti-inflammatory agents (diclofenac sodium suppositories 100 mg) may be prescribed for pain relief and uterine quiescence over the following 72 hours. Preoperative thromboprophylaxis is recommended, using LMWH.

Delivery by cesarean section is necessary, usually carried out at 38 weeks' gestation. The suture is commonly left in place in case of a further pregnancy. Whether it should eventually be removed once childbearing is complete is uncertain.

As explained previously, there are no randomized trials of transabdominal cerclage. However, 13 individual series have been published, reporting the results of 332 pregnancies, with 279 resulting in a live birth (84%). These encouraging figures may result from a positive reporting bias (series with lower success rates are less likely to be submitted for publication). However, the personal series of the authors and the editor are consistent with a favorable outcome in 85% of pregnancies (Table 6–4).

TABLE 6–4

Results of Published Series of Transabdominal Cervicoisthmic Cerclage

FIRST AUTHOR	YEAR OF PUBLICATION	NUMBER OF PATIENTS	NUMBER OF PREGNANCIES	LIVE BABIES	SUCCESS PER PREGNANCY (%)
Benson[236]	1965	10	13	9	69
Mahran[246]	1978	7	10	7	70
Novy[247]	1982	16	22	19	86
Olsen[248]	1982	29	35	32	91
Wallenburg[249]	1987	14	16	15	94
Herron[250]	1988	8	13	8	85
Borruto[251]	1990	54	54	43	80
Novy[252]	1991	20	21	18	90
Van Dongen[253]	1991	16	16	15	94
Cammarano[237]	1995	23	24	22	92
Gibb[254]	1995	50	61	52	85
Anthony[255]	1997	13	13	11	85
Craig[256]	1997	12	10	7	70
Cho[257]	2003	20	22	21	95
Farquharson[241]	2005	40	40	36	90
Steer*		31	36	31	86
Total		**363**	**406**	**346**	**85**

* Steer is the only unpublished series.

Insertion of Transabdominal Cerclage prior to Pregnancy

Insertion of a transabdominal cervicoisthmis cerclage is technically much easier when it it done before the woman is pregnant, and it is therefore probably less dangerous, but difficulties with the technique include difficulty in the precise identification of the internal os and accidental inclusion of the uterine artery, which may restrict blood flow in a later pregnancy. In addition, it is an unnecessary procedure if the woman never subsequently conceives, and it can complicate evacuation of the uterus in the event of early pregnancy failure. The personal experience of the authors and editor is limited to a few cases in which prepregnancy laparotomy was indicated for other reasons. Published series are very small. Prepregnancy screening for thrombophilia and bacterial vaginosis is increasingly used as the presence of either may double the risk of preterm delivery before 34 weeks.[241]

Further Pregnancy Management

Uterine artery Doppler ultrasonography at 22 to 24 weeks may be useful in predicting preeclampsia and intrauterine growth restriction in APS pregnancies. Women with circulating LA or high titers of IgG anticardiolipin antibodies are at increased risk for these complications.[242] A glucose tolerance test at 28 weeks may be prudent for women with PCOS because of the increased risk of gestational diabetes. Although the 2008 National Institute for Clinical Excellence (NICE) guidelines[243] recommended that there was no evidence that management of gestational diabetes improved outcomes for the mother and fetus, this has been challenged because the Australian Carbohydrate Intolerance Study in Pregnant Women (ACHOIS) trial[244] reported that treatment of gestational diabetes mellitus reduces serious perinatal morbidity and may also improve the woman's health-related quality of life.

Third Trimester

During the third trimester, serial fetal growth scans and umbilical artery Doppler recordings are advisable. The risk of intrauterine growth restriction is increased in women with a history of RM, particularly those with APS or inherited thrombophilia (see Chapters 41–43). Those women with a cervical suture in situ will need to be admitted for removal of suture under regional anesthesia between 37 and 38 weeks' gestation.

Delivery and Puerperium

If the pregnancy is progressing well, a history of RM is not an indication for any specific interventions. However, many women with a history of RM will become anxious toward the end of the pregnancy and request early delivery, either by induction of labor or by elective cesarean section. The obstetrician will wish to consider this sympathetically, but needs to bear in mind the increase in iatrogenic morbidity for the child, ranging from an increased incidence of respiratory distress (especially at < 39 wk) to the long-term increases in the risk of asthma and diabetes (among other problems) associated with elective cesarean section. In women receiving heparin, it is important to plan regional anesthesia to minimize the risk of epidural hematoma, and coordination with the anesthetist is required. Current guidelines[245] recommend that regional techniques should not be used until at least 12 hours after the previous prophylactic dose of LMWH and 6 hours after a dose of unfractionated heparin. Heparin should not be given for at least 4 hours after the epidural catheter is removed. There are no prospective data on the risk of systemic thrombosis to determine the optimal management of asymptomatic women with inherited thrombophilia. Current Royal College of Obstetricians and Gynaecologists guidelines based on expert opinion recommend that postnatal thromboprophylaxis is indicated for women with known inherited thrombophilias (e.g., FVL and prothrombin gene mutations), but individual assessment will be guided by the type of thrombophilia and the presence of other thrombotic risk factors. Similarly, in women with APS and no symptoms other than RM, there is no evidence to justify routine postnatal thromboprophylaxis. In women with APS without additional thrombotic risk factors, postnatal thromboprophylaxis is not recommended.

SUMMARY

The management of RM requires a combination of sensitivity and a systematic approach to care. The goal is to identify a cause and implement appropriate treatment whenever possible. Of the many risk factors, parental karyotype abnormalities, APS, activated protein C resistance, and cervical incompetence are the only established causes of RM. Of the many treatment options for couples with RM, only aspirin plus heparin treatment in women with APS has proven benefit. Despite detailed studies, in more than 50% of couples with RM, no cause is found. However, even without pharmacologic treatment, the prognosis is good and supportive care appears to play an important role. Empirical treatments for women with RM should be avoided, and new treatments should be introduced only after their benefit has been assured through properly designed prospective controlled trials.

SUMMARY OF MANAGEMENT OPTIONS
Recurrent Miscarriage

Management Options	Evidence Quality and Recommendation	References
Prepregnancy Assessment Options		
At the Time of the Third Miscarriage		
Document pattern and trimester of the pregnancy loss and whether a live embryo or a fetus was present. Clinical and ultrasound features.	III/B	14
Carefully document any suspected uterine abnormality at surgical evacuation.	—/GPP	—
Send products of conception for histology or autopsy and karyotype with consent of patient as appropriate (see Table 6–2).	II/B	5
General approach is important (e.g., see couple together, sympathy, sensitivity).	II/B	5
Offer follow-up assessment and counseling.	IV/C	9,20
Prepregnancy Assessment and Counseling after the Third Miscarriage		
History and Examination for Causative and Associated Factors		
Obstetric history to confirm true diagnosis of "recurrent miscarriage" (pattern of losses, gestation of former losses, previous confirmation of pregnancy: biochemical, ultrasonographic and/or histologic).	III/B	14
General medical history: • Features associated with autoimmune disease (e.g., joint pains, skin rash, allergy). • Features related to APS (e.g., migraine, epilepsy, vascular thrombosis, joint pain, Raynaud's). • Features related to thrombophilic disorders (e.g., personal or family history of vascular thrombosis). • Exposure to environmental toxins or drugs. • Surgery to cervix, uterus, ovary.	—/GPP	—
Family history of recurrent miscarriage, PCOS, diabetes, genetic disorders, thrombophilia, early-onset cardiovascular disease or stroke (<50 yr).	—/GPP	—

Management Options	Evidence Quality and Recommendation	References
Physical examination: identify signs of endocrine or gynecologic disease, opportunistic screening (BP, cervical cytology, breast palpation), assess any specific risk factors raised by history.	—/GPP	—
Routine Investigations on All Cases (see Table 6–3)		
Karyotype		
• Both partners.	III/B	5,7,20,27,29,31,32
• Miscarried tissue (with consent as appropriate).	III/B	
Pelvic ultrasound.	III/B	20,48,49,50,184–186
Anticardiolipin antibodies (IgG and IgM).	III/B	106,107
Lupus anticoagulant	III/B	106,107
Early-follicular phase LH, FSH, testosterone	III/B	20,84
Thrombophilia screening:	IIa/B	126,127
• Activated protein C resistance/factor V Leiden and factor II (prothrombin) gene mutation only indicated in all cases.	III/B	126
• Antithrombin III, factor XII, factor VIII, protein C, protein S, MTHFR reserved for cases with high personal or family history of thrombophilia.		
• Thromboelastography—if available.	III/B	129
Prepregnancy opportunistic screening:	—/GPP	—
• Serology for rubella status.		
• Blood group and rhesus type.		
Others determined by positive features in history or examination (see Table 6–3).	—/GPP	
Counseling with the Following Key Principles/Guidelines		
See couple together, dedicated miscarriage clinic, sympathetic approach.	—/GPP	—
The true rate of recurrent miscarriage is affected by a reproductive compensation effect.	IV/C	14–16
After three consecutive losses, intensive investigation will identify a probable cause in less than 50% of couples.	III/B	9,20
The majority of cases are due to repeated fetal chromosome abnormalities occurring consecutively by chance.	III/B	5,21,27
Advanced maternal and paternal age and previous reproductive history are important risk factors for a further miscarriage.	III/B	9,14–16,23
Parental chromosomal rearrangements, anatomic defects of the uterine fundus and cervix, phospholipid antibodies, activated protein C resistance, factors V and II gene mutations also play a role.	III/B	20,37,41,51,67,103, 107,126,127,131
Progesterone deficiency, hypersecretion of LH, infective agents, and immune rejection are not currently considered causes of recurrent miscarriage. Empirical treatment with progesterone, high LH suppression, or immunotherapies are of no proven benefit.	Ia/A	80,81,84–86, 137–141
Subclinical thyroid disorders or diabetes mellitus are rare.	III/B	20,73

SUMMARY OF MANAGEMENT OPTIONS
Recurrent Miscarriage—cont'd

Management Options	Evidence Quality and Recommendation	References
Recurrent miscarriage is associated with significant psychological morbidity.	III/B	9,169–172
Role of psychological stress is unclear.	IV/C	9,171
Even after three miscarriages, the chance of success without treatment is approximately 60%, except for women with antiphospholipid syndrome and those with activated protein C resistance in which success rates are lower.	III/B IIa/B	9,14,15,24 109,127
Prepregnancy Treatment Options		
Do not advocate "unproven" treatments.	—/GPP	—
Parental translocations:		
• Genetic counseling couple and relatives.	IV/C	20,37
• Proceed to a further pregnancy with or without prenatal diagnosis (amniocentesis or chorionic villous biopsy).	III/B	38,177–181,183,184
• Gamete donation.		
• Artificial insemination by donor sperm.		
• In vitro fertilization by donor egg.		
• Preimplantation genetic diagnosis with in vitro fertilization.		
• Adoption.		
Uterine abnormalities:		
• Uterine septum: GnRH analogue and hysteroscopic septal resection and temporary intrauterine device.	III/B	47,52,53
• Intrauterine adhesions: hysteroscopic division and temporary intrauterine device; postoperative course of cyclic estrogen and progesterone therapy.	III/B	66
• Fibroids: GnRH analogue and myomectomy.	III/B	63,191
Management during Subsequent Pregnancy, Delivery and Puerperium		
Psychological support, reassurance, and the like.	III/B	18,24
Do not advocate "unproven" treatments.	—/GPP	—
There is no evidence that any immunologic therapy is of benefit.	Ia/A	138
Offer low-dose aspirin and heparin to women with APS.	Ib/A	108,200,205
Offer low-dose heparin to women with activated protein C resistance (or other thrombophilia).	IIb/B	127,208,209
Patients with diabetes mellitus: good metabolic control.	IIb/B	61,195
First trimester:		
• Transvaginal USS to confirm fetal viability.	—/GPP	—
• Serial scans for reassurance.	—/GPP	—

Management Options	Evidence Quality and Recommendation	References
Second trimester:		
• Options with suspected cervical incompetence:		
• Serial cervical ultrasonography with insertion of cervical suture with evidence of shortening/funneling.	Ib/A	225,226
• Primary cervical cerclage.	Ib/A	224
• Serial vaginal swabs for pathogens.	—/GPP	—
• Uterine artery Doppler studies in selected cases.	III/B	241
• Consider prophylactic maternal steroids at 28 wk in selected cases.	—/GPP	—
• Consider formal GTT at 28 wk in selected cases	—/GPP	—
Third trimester:		
• Vigilance for fetal growth restriction, preeclampsia and preterm labor in selected cases.	III/B	198,199
Labor/delivery:		
• Consider elective LSCS/IOL at term in some cases.	III/B	199
Puerperium:	—/GPP	
• Consider postnatal thromboprophylaxis in selected cases.		

APS, antiphospholipid syndrome; BP, blood pressure; FSH, follicle-stimulating hormone; GnRH, gonadotropin-releasing hormone; GTT, glucose tolerance test; Ig, immunoglobulin; LH, luteinizing hormone; LSCS/IOL, lower segment cesarean section/induction of labor; MTHFR, methylenetetrahydrofolate reductase; PCOS, polycystic ovary syndrome.

SUGGESTED READINGS

Althuisius SM, Dekker GA, Hummel P, et al: Final results of the Cervical Incompetence Prevention Randomized Cerclage Trial (CIPRACT): Therapeutic cerclage with bed rest versus bed rest alone. Am J Obstet Gynecol 2001;185:1106–1112.

Clifford K, Rai R, Watson H, Regan L: An informative protocol for the investigation of recurrent miscarriage: Preliminary experience of 500 consecutive cases. Hum Reprod 1994;9:1328–1332.

Drakeley AJ, Quenby S, Farquharson RG: Mid trimester loss—Appraisal of a screening protocol. Hum Reprod 1998;13:1975–1980.

Empson M, Lassere M, Craig JC, Scott JR: Recurrent pregnancy loss with antiphospholipid antibody: A systematic review of therapeutic trials. Obstet Gynecol 2002;99:135–144.

Goddijn M, Leschot NJ: Genetic aspects of miscarriage. Baillieres Best Pract Res Clin Obstet Gynaecol 2000;14:855–865.

Nybo Anderson AM, Wohlfahrt J, Christens P, et al: Maternal age and fetal loss: Population based register linkage study. BMJ 2000;320:1708–1712.

Porter TF, LaCoursiere Y, Scott JR: Immunotherapy for recurrent miscarriage. Cochrane Database Syst Rev 2006;2:CD000112.

Rai R, Regan L: Recurrent miscarriage seminar. Lancet 2006;368:601–611.

Rai R, Cohen H, Dave M, Regan L: Randomised controlled trial of aspirin and aspirin plus heparin in pregnant women with recurrent miscarriage associated with phospholipid antibodies (or antiphospholipid antibodies). BMJ 1997;314:253–257.

Rey E, Kahn SR, David M, Shrier I: Thrombophilic disorders and fetal loss: A meta-analysis. Lancet 2003;361:901–908.

Saravelos SH, Cocksedge KA, Li TC: Prevalence and diagnosis of congenital uterine anomalies in women with reproductive failure: A critical appraisal. Hum Reprod Update 2008;14:415–429.

REFERENCES

For a complete list of references, log onto www.expertconsult.com.

CHAPTER 7

First-Trimester Screening for Fetal Abnormalities

KIMTA NANHORNGUÈ and YVES VILLE

Videos corresponding to this chapter are available online at www.expertconsult.com.

INTRODUCTION

The screening for and diagnosis of fetal abnormalities in the first trimester are characterized by the confidentiality surrounding parental decisions. Early termination of pregnancy has proven medical and psychological benefits for women compared with late termination. The early first-trimester ultrasound examination is also an opportunity to identify a family history of genetic syndromes or anomalies that warrant more frequent or detailed ultrasound assessments (see Chapter 4).

The goals of first-trimester screening were until the mid-1980s limited to localization of the pregnancy, assessment of viability and diagnosis of miscarriage, determination of gestational age (GA), and identification and typing of multiple pregnancies. However, prenatal diagnosis has rapidly shifted over the last two decades from the second to the first trimester owing to the development of high-resolution abdominal and transvaginal ultrasound. As a result, a significant amount of information can be garnered about the fetus as well as the obstetric management.[1] The 11- to 14-week window of GA is the best compromise to assess GA, to screen for fetal aneuploidy based on the measurement of nuchal translucency (NT), and to obtain a potentially detailed anatomic survey.

ULTRASOUND EXAMINATION AT 11 + 0 TO 13 + 6 WEEKS

Localization of the Pregnancy

The evaluation of an intrauterine pregnancy requires the exclusion of ectopic pregnancy, bearing in mind the incidence of heterotopic pregnancy is about 1 in 4000 spontaneously and as high as 1 in 100 after assisted conception. For gestations greater than 5½ weeks, a transvaginal ultrasound examination should identify an intrauterine pregnancy with a close to 100% accuracy.[2] Because of the inaccuracies of pregnancy dating, β-human chorionic gonadotropin (β-hCG) is often used as a surrogate for GA. Sequentially, structures become visible by transvaginal ultrasonography, including a gestational sac ("double decidual sign" at 4½–5 wk after the last menstrual period [LMP]), yolk sac (at 5 wk), and fetal pole with later cardiac motion (at 5½–6 wk). A pseudosac is a collection of fluid within the endometrial cavity that results from bleeding of the decidualized endometrium when an extrauterine gestation is present. Although it may sometimes be mistaken for a gestational sac, it can be distinguished by its central location, filling the endometrial cavity itself.[3] However, the identification of a presumed pseudosac on ultrasonography is not diagnostic of ectopic pregnancy because it has a high false-positive rate.[4]

Critical to the diagnosis and management of suspected ectopic pregnancy is the concept of the *discriminatory cutoff* of β-hCG, defined as that level of β-hCG at which a normal intrauterine pregnancy can be reliably visualized by ultrasonography.[5] It is now accepted that a normal intrauterine pregnancy should always be visualized above the discriminatory cutoff of 1500 to 2500 IU/L using transvaginal ultrasonography, and its absence implies an abnormal gestation.[6] The discriminatory cutoff should be set by each institution based on that hospital's success in identifying ectopic pregnancies, based mostly on the equipment used and the expertise of the sonographers. Varying the discriminatory cutoff will affect the sensitivity (positively identifying an ectopic gestation) and specificity (correctly excluding an ectopic when none exists). A decrease in the cutoff will increase the risk of misclassifying a developing intrauterine pregnancy as an abnormal gestation, and increasing the value provides "extra" reassurance that lack of visualization of an intrauterine pregnancy did not miss an early viable gestation, but may delay the diagnosis of an ectopic pregnancy leading to tubal rupture.[3]

Identifying a Viable Pregnancy, Predictors of Adverse Outcome, and the Diagnosis of Miscarriage

An ultrasound examination between 11 to 13 + 6 weeks is often the first opportunity to diagnose early pregnancy failure (Fig. 7–1). The prevalence of early pregnancy failure (EPF) in one screening study of 17,870 women 10 to 13 weeks was 2.8% (501 cases), including 313 (62.5%) embryonic deaths and 188 (37.5%) anembryonic pregnancies.[7] The accurate diagnosis of EPF is paramount in being able to counsel patients appropriately about their pregnancy management options.[8] There are key chronologic landmarks in

FIGURE 7–1
Risk of spontaneous miscarriage.

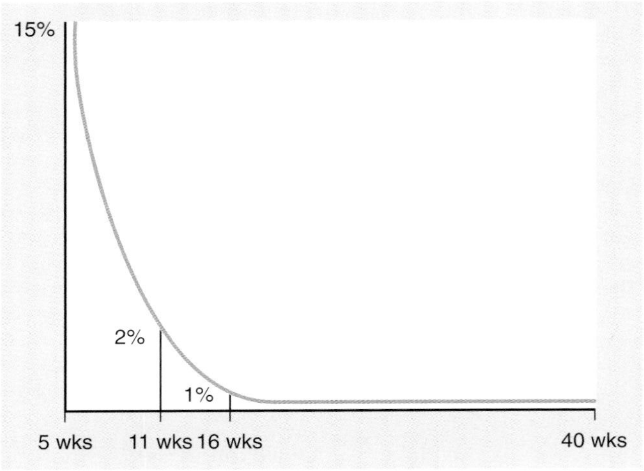

the normal development of an embryo that can be identified by transvaginal ultrasound scan, facilitating the distinction between normal and abnormal pregnancy. Stringent diagnostic criteria are required to avoid an incorrect diagnosis in those women who have irregular cycles, who are unsure of their dates, or whose initial ultrasound findings do not correspond with the expected gestation.[9] An intrauterine pregnancy can first be diagnosed sonographically by visualization of a gestational sac. GA can be estimated either by measurement of the mean sac diameter (MSD) or the embryonic pole/crown-rump length (CRL). A true "crown" and "rump" should be visible with a MSD greater than 18 mm; before then, only an embryonic pole (the long axis of the embryo) can be seen.[10] A yolk sac should be visible transvaginally when the MSD is greater than 8 mm and an embryonic pole should be visualized with a MSD greater than 16 mm.[11] A gestation sac with a MSD of 20 mm and no evidence of a yolk sac is highly suggestive of early embryonic demise.[12,13] If the gestation sac is greater than 15 mm, a second scan should be performed at least 7 days later. If an embryo of more than 6 mm is present and heart activity is not observed, the scan should be repeated again in another 7 days.[13] The diagnosis of early fetal demise can be made with certainty if cardiac activity is still not seen. Some authors advocate the use of a 10-mm cutoff [12] when looking for cardiac activity in the embryo, because approximately one third of embryos with a CRL of less than 5 mm have no demonstrable cardiac activity at the time of initial scan.[13] A recent study suggests that the improved sonographic technology allows for the detection of embryonic demise with a CRL less than 5 mm. In particular, the absence of cardiac activity with a CRL of 3.5 mm or greater had, under ideal conditions, 100% positive predictive value and specificity.[14] If the gestational sac is smaller than expected, the possibility of incorrect dates should be considered and caution exercised, especially if there has been no pain or bleeding. However, in cases of a normal CRL, if the gestational sac volume is 2 or more standard deviations (SDs) below normal, the prediction of subsequent miscarriage can be made with a high sensitivity.[15] Likewise, early embryonic demise may be signified by absent cardiac activity, a CRL greater than 6 mm, and an excessively large gestation sac compared with the CRL.[15,16]

A fetal heart rate less than 120 beats/min in the first trimester is associated with pregnancy loss (sensitivity 54%, specificity 95%). The specificity rises to 100% when the fetal heart rate is greater than 85 beats/min.[17] However, caution is recommended before diagnosing impending early embryonic demise based on a bradycardia, especially a single recording. A continued reduction in heart rate over a few days is more likely to be associated with miscarriage.[18]

Dating the Pregnancy

First-trimester aneuploidy screening using NT and maternal biochemistry depends upon the reliable pregnancy dating. As consequence, ultrasound dating in the first trimester is now recommended for all women with spontaneous pregnancies, even those with certain menstrual dates owing to misclassification bias that occurs because of both incorrect memory of the LMP and oligo- and polyovulation. An increasing number of pregnancies are now dated in the late first trimester during aneuploidy risk assessment, which is typically performed at 11 to 13 + 6 weeks' gestation.[19] Dating a pregnancy by menstrual history can be unreliable. Up to 40% of women are uncertain of their menstrual dates, and even when they are certain, GA is often overestimated compared with ultrasound findings.[20] Although early ultrasound systematically underestimates the GA of smaller fetuses by approximately 1 to 2 days, this bias is relatively small compared with the large error introduced by LMP estimates of gestation, as evidenced by the number of implausible birth weight-for-gestation.[21] In one study of 165,908 women comparing LMP with ultrasound estimates, the prevalences of preterm birth were 8.7% versus 7.9% (<37 wk), 81.2% versus 91.0% for term (37–41 wk) birth, and 10.1% versus 1.1% for post-term (≥42 wk birth). The sensitivity of the LMP-based preterm birth estimate was 64.3%, and the positive predictive value was 58.7%. Overall, 17.2% of the records had estimates with an absolute difference of greater than 14 days.[21] Early GA dating is more accurate and affects pregnancy management. There seems little logic to support routine dating in the mid to late second trimester.

The maximum embryonic length and the fetal CRL can be used to accurately determine GA in a normal first-trimester pregnancy to within 3 to 5 days. The CRL is measured excluding the inferior limbs and without correction for body flexion. Transvaginal ultrasound can be used for measurements earlier than transabdominal ultrasound. The original Robinson[22] curve used for dating pregnancies is still valid in most cases.[23]

The gestation sac is always visible by 4 weeks. The yolk sac is the first sonographically evident embryonic structure within the gestational sac. Its size correlates to GA and is usually visible between the 5th and the 12th weeks as a round anechoic area. Rarely, it can be seen until the end of pregnancy. Before 6 weeks, dating is done by description and measurement of the gestation sac.[24,25] In 95% of cases, the yolk sac is present by 5 weeks, and in all cases, it is present by 6 weeks. The fetal heart is seen beating in 86% of cases by 6 weeks, and always by 7 weeks.

Of all of the available measurements, the maximum embryo length between 6 and 10 weeks and the CRL up to 14 weeks are the most accurate for determining GA. The random error is 4 to 8 days at the 95th percentile.[22,26–28] The largest study using a strict dating method is that of Wisser and Dirscheld,[28] who highlighted potential pitfalls of earlier studies and reported a predictive interval of 4.7 days (SD) in 160 patients who underwent in vitro fertilization, including 21 with multiple pregnancies.[28] All charts are concordant before 60 mm (predictive interval 3 days [SD]), but differ significantly thereafter.

Another recent study suggests that gestational sac and amniotic sac volumes assessed during the first trimester by transvaginal three-dimensional ultrasonography (3DUS) also have excellent correlation with the GA and CRL and hence may be used for determining GA.[29] Though this result was not confirmed,[30] larger studies are needed to determine the importance of these volumes in predicting normal pregnancy outcomes and whether these volumes can be used in the management of pregnancies at risk for spontaneous abortion.

When the CRL is greater than 60 mm, other biometric parameters are more useful for dating the pregnancy up to 20 weeks.[31] These parameters include the biparietal diameter, head circumference, femur length, and abdominal circumference. First-trimester fetal biometry is underused to diagnose or characterize abnormal fetal development. Fetal growth during the first trimester was previously considered relatively uniform, but increasing evidence shows that anthropometric differences and other growth abnormalities are expressed in the first trimester. Maternal factors (multiparity, diabetes, small stature, and high pre-pregnancy body mass index [BMI]) and fetal factors (chromosomal abnormality and female fetus) have been reported to be associated with a greater difference between expected and observed fetal size in 46,514 women with both early ultrasound and menstrual estimations of GA.[32] One study of 464 women undergoing 1063 ultrasound assessments between 5 and 14 weeks' gestation observed that embryonic and fetal growth rates increased with maternal age and was higher in fetuses of black than of white or Asian women.[33] Fetal gender has also been suggested to influence fetal growth, with male fetuses being larger than female in two series at 7 weeks.[34]

Detecting Multiple Pregnancies and Determining Chorionicity (See also Chapters 23 and 59)

Twin pregnancies constitute 2% of all pregnancies (Table 7–1).[35] Two thirds of these are dizygotic, and one third are monozygotic. An important task of the first-trimester scan is to diagnose twin pregnancy and determine chorionicity. For obstetricians, the management of multiple pregnancies relies mainly on chorionicity owing to the fact that the prevalence of prenatal and perinatal complications differs by chorionicity. It is estimated that monochorionic twins have a three- to sixfold increase in perinatal morbidity compared with dichorionic twins.

The relationship between chorionicity and zygosity can be kept simple. Two thirds of dichorionic pregnancies (two placentas) are dizygotic, but one third of them are monozygotic. The only way to determine zygosity is through invasive testing, with chorionic villus sampling, amniocentesis, or cordocentesis to analyze the fetal DNA. In 2% of cases, monozygotic twins share organs (Siamese, or conjoined, twins).

The first trimester is the best time to determine chorionicity. Dichorionic twins have two placentas, but in most cases, the placentas are adjacent, making the diagnosis of chorionicity difficult. Sonographic determination of chorionicity and amnionicity carried out at 11 to 14 weeks is based on the number of placental sites, the visualization of and the characteristics of an intertwin membrane, and the identification of the "lambda" (Fig. 7–2)[36] or "twin-peak" sign on the one hand or the "T" sign on the other enables accurate categorization compared with placental histology.[37,38] The lambda sign is formed by the triangular tissue projection at the base of the intertwin membrane. It is an extension of the two chorion layers within the intertwin membrane that is present only in dichorionic pregnancy. In monochorionic pregnancies, there is no layer of chorion between the two

TABLE 7–1

Types of Monozygotic Twins and Time of Division after Fertilization

CHORION	AMNION	TIME OF DIVISION (DAY)	FREQUENCY (%)
Dichorionic	Diamniotic	0–3	33%
Monochorionic	Diamniotic	4–8	65%
Monochorionic	Monoamniotic	>8	2%
Monochorionic	Monoamniotic (Siamese)	>13	Rare

From Wigglesworth JS, Singer DB: Textbook of Fetal and Perinatal Pathology. Amsterdam, Blackwell, 1991, p 131.

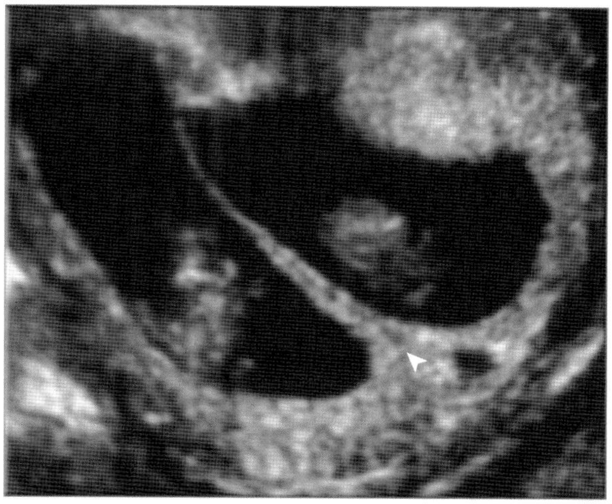

FIGURE 7–2
Dichorionic diamniotic twin pregnancy and the lambda sign.

layers of amnion, and the lambda sign is absent. This sign can be seen during transvaginal ultrasound examination as early as 7 to 9 weeks and has high agreement with the 11- to 14-week scan.[39] Note that the chorion disappears with advancing gestation, and the lambda sign becomes progressively more difficult to identify. By 16 weeks and 20 weeks, respectively, the lambda sign, or twin-peak sign, is present in 98% and 87% of cases.[40]

Although the twin-peak sign is the current standard of care in ultrasound assessment of chorionicity, other methods have been proposed. Carroll and coworkers[37] used a combination of signs (number of placental sites, lambda and T sign, thickness of intertwin membrane) in 150 twin pregnancies scanned between 10 and 14 weeks' gestation to demonstrate that the most reliable indicator for dichorionicity was two separate placentae, and when there was a single placental mass, the presence of the lambda sign (sensitivity 97.4%, specificity 100%). For monochorionicity, of the single best marker was the T sign (sensitivity 100%, specificity of 98.2%). This study supports the observation of others that whereas the presence of the lambda sign indicates dichorionicity, its absence does not rule it out. Shetty and Smith[41] suggested a monochorionic placenta that appears to be two separate placentas is bilobed or has a succenturiate lobe in 97.7%. Moon and colleaguesl[42] sought chorionicity in first trimester of 306 diamniotic twin pregnancies directly by depiction of the amnion and chorion, describing three patterns of intertwin membranes (Fig. 7–3): pattern 1, two relatively thin layers of even thickness, which indicate no layer of the chorion and two layers of the amnion; pattern 2, one relatively thick and two relatively thin intertwin membranes, which indicate one layer of the chorion and two layers of the amnions; pattern 3, one relatively thick and one relatively thin intertwin membrane, which indicate one layer of the chorion and one layer of the amnion. The twin pregnancies with pattern 1 were considered monochorionic diamniotic twin pregnancies, and pattern 2 and 3 were considered dichorionic diamniotic twin pregnancies. They concluded it was possible to determine the chorionicity in the majority of the twin pregnancies between 11 and 14 weeks' gestation (92.9%) and all of the determined chorionicities corresponded correctly with the ultimate chorionicity confirmed postnatally on histologic evaluation (a predictive accuracy of 100%).

Identifying Normal Sonographic Features in the First Trimester

Prenatal diagnosis of fetal structural malformations during either the first or the second trimester has helped reduced perinatal morbidity and mortality by decreasing the prevalence of congenital anomalies at birth. Although many major fetal defects are diagnosable in the first trimester, the diagnostic accuracy is significantly higher in the mid-second trimester owing to the larger size and more advanced development of the fetus. Conversely, the second trimester scan is generally considered less reliable as a screening tool.

Several studies have assessed the ability of sonographers and sonologists to detect fetal structural malformations by first-trimester ultrasound. It is widely accepted that the measurement of NT to screen for aneuploidies should be combined with a search for detectable malformations. This approach requires standardization and quality control. Most fetal structures can be visualized in the first trimester using either vaginal or abdominal ultrasound (Table 7–2).[43] Whereas some structures such the posterior fossa, cerebellum, genitalia, and sacral spine are less reliably seen in the first trimester[44] than in the second and third trimesters (see also Chapter 8), other findings are characteristic of the first trimester. Visualization of normal fetal anatomy in the first trimester provides the patient reassurance and reduces anxiety. Earlier detection of fetal structural malformations also allows for timely referral to a tertiary care facility and coordination of care among appropriate subspecialists. Some may argue, however, that the first-trimester anatomic survey adds cost and burden to the health care system. It is, however, feasible to continue to perform a single ultrasound examination at 11 to 14 weeks of gestation to measure the fetal NT and assess the fetal anatomy. There are additional costs that will accompany widespread use of the first-trimester anatomic survey just as there are for later screening. Though aneuploidy screening is now accepted in most industrialized countries, the benefit of first-trimester anatomic screening needs to be demonstrated in the research arena before performing a cost-benefit analysis of first-trimester screening in clinical practice.[44]

The fetus should be sonographically evaluated in three planes:

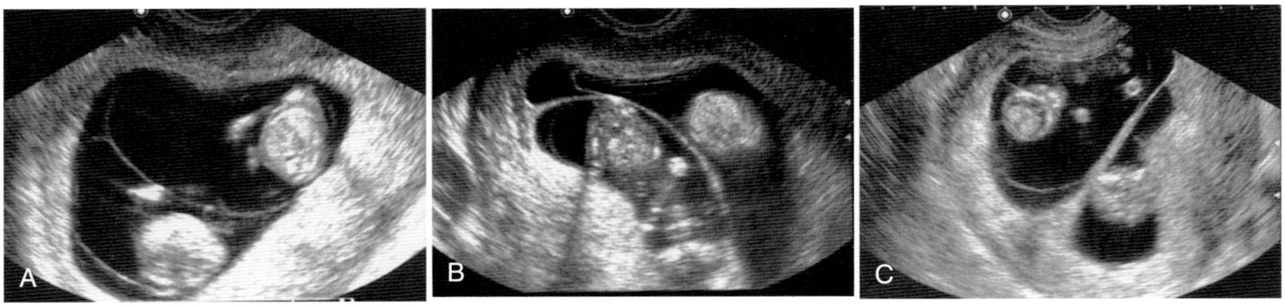

FIGURE 7–3
The chorionicities determined by depiction of the amnion and chorion: *A*, Monochorionic diamniotic twin pregnancy. *B* and *C*, Dichorionic diamniotic twin pregnancy.
(*A–C*, From Moon MH, Park SY, Song MJ, et al: Diamniotic twin pregnancies with a single placental mass: Prediction of chorionicity at 11 to 14 weeks of gestation. Prenat Diagn 2008;28:1011-1105.)

TABLE 7–2

Visualization of Fetal Anatomic Structures According to Crown-Rump Length

		SUCCESSFUL VISUALIZATION (*N* (%))										
CRL (MM)	*N*	ANATOMY CHECK I*	ANATOMY CHECK II†	HEAD/BRAIN	FACE	SPINE	HEART	ABDOMEN	STOMACH	KIDNEYS	BLADDER	EXTREMITIES
45-54	174	113 (64.94)	38 (21.83)	174 (100)	171 (98.27)	172 (98.85)	44 (25.28)	172 (98.85)	166 (95.40)	123 (70.68)	170 (97.70)	174 (100)
55-64	400	337 (84.25)	173 (43.25)	400 (100)	398 (99.5)	399 (99.75)	183 (45.75)	400 (100)	398 (99.50)	341 (85.25)	397 (99.25)	400 (100)
65-74	413	386 (93.46)	233 (56.41)	413 (100)	409 (99.03)	413 (100)	238 (57.62)	413 (100)	412 (99.75)	388 (93.94)	412 (99.75)	413 (100)
75-82	157	150 (95.54)	105 (66.87)	157 (100)	157 (100)	157 (100)	105 (66.87)	157 (100)	157 (100)	150 (95.54)	157 (100)	157 (100)
Total	1144	986 (86.18)	549 (47.98)	1144 (100)	1135 (99.21)	1141 (99.73)	570 (49.82)	1142 (99.82)	1133 (99.03)	1002 (87.58)	1136 (99.30)	1144 (100)

CRL, crown-rump length.
* Anatomy check I includes all organs except the heart.
† Anatomy check II includes all organs including the heart.
From Souka AP, Pilalis A, Kavalakis Y, et al: Assessment of fetal anatomy at the 11–14-week ultrasound examination. Ultrasound Obstet Gynecol 2004;24:730–734.

- A strict midsagittal plane for measurement of CRL and examination of the abdominal wall and cranial and caudal fetal extremities. The NT measurement is performed in this plane.
- An axial view of the skull to identify the cranial contour, the midline of the brain, and the posterior fossa.
- A cross-section of the abdomen to identify the abdominal cord insertion site and the intra-abdominal position of the stomach. The presence of four limbs with three segments is also verified.

Fetal anatomy should be examined as previously described[43]:

- Skull and brain: completeness of the skull, the presence of the falx, and the butterfly shape of the choroid plexuses.
- Face: presence of orbits and lenses and the view of the fetal profile.
- Spine: alignment of the vertebrae and the skin covering the spine from the cervical to the sacral regions.
- Heart: four-chamber view (visualization of the two atria and ventricles, the crux, and the atrioventricular valves) and the three-vessel view of the great vessels (visualization of the cross-sectional view of the pulmonary artery, aorta, and superior vena cava).
- Stomach: visualization of the stomach as a hypoechoic structure in the left upper abdomen.
- Abdomen: examination of the abdominal wall and the umbilical cord insertion.
- Kidneys: visualization of the kidneys as hyperechoic structures with a hypoechoic center lateral to the spine.
- Bladder: visualization of the bladder as a hypoechoic structure in the fetal pelvis; add color flow to demonstrate arterial flow on both sides indicative of a two-vessel cord.
- Extremities: examination of the long bones and fingers.

External Features

- Ossification begins at approximately 11 weeks with the occipital bone. The skull appears regular and hyperechogenic compared with the underlying tissues.[45]

Central Nervous System

From 9 weeks onward, the outline of the lateral ventricles, the echogenic choroid plexus, and the midline echo are visible. By 10 to 11 weeks, the third and fourth ventricles become visible, and from 14 weeks onward, the cerebellum and thalami are seen. The ventricles occupy most of the cerebral hemispheres. The choroids plexus should fill the lateral ventricles completely. Choroid plexus cysts are more common in the first trimester than in the second (incidence 5.7% vs. 1.4%)[46,47] and are not associated with fetal abnormalities.

The width of the third ventricle becomes narrow toward the end of the first trimester. The corpus callosum is not visible at the end of the first trimester, though the area where it will develop can be identified. The cerebellar hemispheres seem to meet in the midline during weeks 11 to 12. At the end of the first trimester, the choroid plexuses lie close to the caudal border of the cerebellum. Successively, the ossification of the spine appears.[48]

3DUS imaging has made it possible to obtain images of the developing embryonic brain in planes not previously available.[49] The lack of skull ossification allows visualization of the brain in any plane, which is not the case during the second and third trimesters. 3DUS is particularly helpful because volumes acquired with a transvaginal transducer can be easily rotated to evaluate the anatomy, which is not possible with the limited motion of a transvaginal transducer.[50] Geometric visualization of brain cavities including the choroid plexuses by manual segmentation shows the form and shape and enables volume calculation that has provided new insights into embryonic development not obtainable from aborted specimens.[49] Recently, a study using the "inversion-rendering" mode revealed 3-dimensional development of the ventricles of the brain in early pregnancy, from 6 to 13 weeks, providing a reference for early diagnosis of central nervous system anomalies such as hydrocephalus and holoprosencephaly.[51]

Heart

Abnormalities of the heart and great arteries are the most common congenital defects and account for about 20% of all stillbirths and 30% of neonatal deaths due to congenital defects. The position, axis, four-chamber view, and symmetry of the heart can be seen in the first trimester. Smrecek and associates[52] found it was impossible evaluate the fetal heart at 10 weeks. The success rates rose to 45% at 11 weeks and 90% between 12 and 14 weeks' gestation. Huggon and coworkers[53] found that a highly trained cardiologist could obtain transabdominally informative images under 14 weeks in 84% of cases. With less specialized operators, the four-chamber view was imaged successfully in 76% and 95% of cases transabdominally and transvaginally, respectively, at 12 to 13 weeks' gestation.[54] Whitlow and Economides[55] observed that the four-chamber view was seen in 83% at 11 weeks and in 98% from 13 weeks onward. Souka and colleagues[43] reported the visualization of heart anatomy according to CRL measurement (Table 7–3).

Interest in early examination of fetal heart is related to the significant clinical impact of early detection of cardiac problems. Early cardiac scanning should be offered to high risk

TABLE 7–3

Visualization of the Four-Chamber View and the Three-Vessel View of the Fetal Heart According to Crown-Rump Length

		SUCCESSFUL VISUALIZATION (*N* (%))		
CRL (MM)	*N*	HEART	FOUR-CHAMBER VIEW	THREE-VESSEL VIEW
45-54	174	44 (25.28)	117 (67.24)	44 (25.28)
55-64	400	183 (45.75)	344 (86)	184 (46)
65-74	413	238 (57.62)	386 (93.46)	238 (57.62)
75-82	157	105 (66.87)	153 (97.45)	105 (66.87)
Total	1144	570 (49.82)	1000 (87.41)	571 (49.91)

CRL, crown-rump length.

From Souka AP, Pilalis A, Kavalakis Y, et al: Assessment of fetal anatomy at the 11–14-week ultrasound examination. Ultrasound Obstet Gynecol 2004;24:730–734.

pregnancies in specialized centers because fetal echocardiography in the first trimester has been proved to be accurate in defining major cardiac anomalies when performed by a specialist, but the degree of assessment of the early cardiovascular system that is possible and the lack of operators who are trained specifically makes its application questionable for routine scanning of the fetal heart in the first trimester of low risk patients by the first-level operator.[56] This could produce apparent contradictions in light of prevalence[57] of cardiac defects, the association with both chromosomal anomalies and genetic syndromes,[58] and the assessment of cardiac anatomy at this stage of gestation.[59,60] Because the prevalence of congenital heart disease (CHD) in fetuses with increased NT thickness (discussed later) is between 5% and 10%,[61–63] a detailed fetal cardiac examination should be recommended only in these cases (see later).

Stomach

The stomach bubble is seen as a small, sonolucent cystic structure in the upper left quadrant of the abdomen, below the heart by 8 weeks in 31%[64] and in all cases by 12 to 13 weeks. Fluid production by the intestinal epithelium is the most likely explanation for visualization of a stomach because fetal swallowing movements are not seen until 11 weeks onward.[64,65] The relationship of this structure to the diaphragm should be noted.

Abdominal Wall

Physiologic hernia of the midgut into the umbilical cord is part of embryonic intestinal development.[64] It is a large, hyperechogenic mass that retracts into the abdominal cavity between 10 weeks and 4 days and 11 weeks and 5 days. Fetuses older than 11 weeks and 5 days should not show herniation.[64] At that point, a differential diagnosis of omphalocele and gastroschisis should be considered.

Bladder and Kidneys

The fetal kidneys are visible in most cases at 12 to 13 weeks and appear more echogenic than the rest of the intra-abdominal contents. Renal echogenicity decreases as excretory function develops.[55] As a result, the fetal bladder is seen in 80% of fetuses[66] by 11 weeks and in more than 90% by 13 weeks. The sagittal long axis of the bladder is less than 6 mm in the first trimester. In one study of 300 pregnancies between 10 to 14 weeks' gestation, the fetal bladder was always visualized when the CRL was greater than 67 mm. The fetal bladder was visualized in 90% of fetuses with a CRL of 38 to 67 mm.[67]

Skeleton

All three parts of the long bones are consistently seen from 11 weeks onward, although measurement of the long bones before 14 weeks seems clinically irrelevant. All long bones are similar in size at 11 to 14 weeks, ranging from approximately 6 mm at 11 weeks to 13 mm at 14 weeks.[68] Body and limb movements are seen from 9 and 11 weeks onward, respectively.

Fetal Gender

Fetal gender assessment should not be considered part of a screening ultrasound during the first trimester and care should be taken not to communicate gender impressions. However, an ultrasound determination of the fetal sex can benefit decision-making regarding invasive testing in pregnancies at risk for sex-linked genetic abnormalities, and several techniques have been proposed.

In one, the angle of the genital tubercle to a horizontal line extending through the lumbosacral skin surface is measured (accomplished in 99.6% of males and 97.4% of females). The fetus is assigned male gender if the angle is greater than 30 degrees, and female if the angle is parallel or convergent (<10 degrees) to the horizontal line. Gender cannot be determined if intermediate (10–30 degrees). The accuracy of male assignment is unaffected by the CRL,[69] whereas the accuracy of female assignment increases with increasing CRL.

In another technique, a "caudal acute angle" between the axis of the ventral surface of the fetus and the long axis of the clitoris is interpreted to mean female genitalia, whereas a "cranial acute angle" between the axis of ventral surface of the fetus and the long axis of the penis indicates male genitalia.[70] Other proposed methods either combine the sagittal and transverse views of the genitalia[71] or use only the transverse plane in order to assign sex with better accuracy. These techniques indicate that males are recognizable by the presence of a third echogenic point in addition to two echogenic points or lines that are present in both sexes on this plane.[72] 3DUS is also used for first-trimester fetal gender determination. Michailidis and associates[73] reported that a correct prediction of fetal gender can be achieved in 85% of cases. Mazza and coworkers[70] found gender could be correctly assigned in 95% to 99% with a biparietal diameter (BPD) of 20 mm and 99% to 100% with a BPD of 22 mm. They concluded fetal sex assignment should not be undertaken below a BPD of 22 mm, especially in cases in which fetal sex is not relevant.

Uterine Artery Doppler Ultrasound

As first-trimester ultrasound became more popular for aneuploidy screening, attention turned to the development of a risk profile predictive of other adverse pregnancy outcomes. The concept underlying uterine artery Doppler measured flow is that it reflects impedance of uterine artery blood flow, which normally decreases with increasing gestation. A high vascular resistance continues in pregnancy disorders associated with suboptimal placental function.[74] The high resistance is thought to promote endothelial cell injury, disruption of vascular integrity, vessel occlusion, and placental ischemia.[75] Women with first-trimester uterine artery resistance indices above the 75th percentile are 5.5 times more likely to experience this outcome.[76] It also appears that first-trimester uterine artery Doppler resistance measurements can aid the identification of women at risk for early, severe preeclampsia or growth restriction.[77,78] Currently, uterine artery Doppler interrogation in the first trimester does not perform well as a screening test despite documented associations. The role of Doppler studies in the first trimester for adverse pregnancy risk outcome assessment is being studied in conjunction with biomarkers including pregnancy-associated plasma protein A (PAPP-A), free β-hCG, and placental protein 13 (PP13).[74]

Nuchal Translucency

Definition

Nuchal translucency (NT) is the ultrasound term for the physiologic collection of fluid underneath the nuchal skin extending for a variable distance over the fetal head and back at 11 to 14 weeks. For unclear reasons, the amount of fluid at this gestation is highly sensitive to fetal problems. An anteroposterior measurement of this layer of fluid with the fetus in a longitudinal view provides an accurate and reproducible measurement, provided it is done in a standardized fashion. NT thickness normally increases with CRL between 44 and 85 mm.[79–81] Therefore, GA can influence the risk calculation significantly (Fig. 7–4). The 50th percentile values for NT thickness are 1.2 mm and 1.9 mm for a CRL of 45 mm (11 wk) and 85 mm (13 wk and 6 days), respectively, and the 95th percentile values are 2 mm and 2.8 mm, respectively.

Because of the need to standardize the measurement process, initial attempts to differentiate the NT from cystic hygroma have been abandoned. However, cystic hygroma can be clearly differentiated from an increased simple NT, and further efforts to assess the prognosis of these fetuses are needed. When the NT thickness is greater than 3.5 mm, thin septations are typically seen. The typical ultrasonographic appearance of cystic hygroma is that of two dilated jugular lymphatic sacs seen on a transverse scan at the level of the neck and separate from the NT (Fig. 7–5).

Measurement

Standardization and quality control in NT measurement is best served by the Fetal Medicine Foundation initiative. This initiative established a process for certification in the 11- to 14-week scan to ensure those performing the examination are adequately trained and maintain an appropriate level of performance through continuing education and audit (www.fetalmedicine.com).[82] Local branches for certification have been established in numerous countries to enhance efficiency.

To obtain a reliable measurement of fetal NT, the following steps are needed (Fig. 7–6):

- All sonographers who perform fetal scans must be appropriately trained. The ability to measure NT reproducibly improves with training; good results are typically achieved after approximately 100 scans. Intraobserver and interobserver differences in measurements are less than 0.5 mm in 95% of examinations.[83,84]
- The ultrasound equipment must be of good quality, with a video-loop function. The calipers should be able to provide measurements to 0.1 mm.
- NT can be measured successfully by transabdominal ultrasound in approximately 95% of pregnancies; in the rest, transvaginal sonography is required.
- The minimum fetal CRL should be 45 mm and the maximum, 84 mm, because the optimal GA for the measurement of NT is 11 weeks to 13 weeks and 6 days.
- Gestation must be taken into account when determining whether a given NT increases risk because the fetal NT thickness increases with CRL.
- A good sagittal section with the fetus in the neutral position is needed for accurate measurement of the CRL and NT.
- The magnification should be such that each increment in distance between calipers is 0.1 mm.
- Care must be taken to distinguish between the fetal skin and the amnion. Both structures appear as thin membranes at this gestation. This distinction is made by waiting for spontaneous fetal movement away from the amniotic membrane or by "bouncing" the fetus off of the amnion with a maternal cough or by tapping the maternal abdomen.
- More than one measurement is taken and the maximum technically acceptable measurement is recorded.
- A nuchal umbilical cord (Fig. 7–7) may falsely increase the NT measurement and is present in approximately 5% of scans. In such cases, the NT measurements above and below the umbilical cord are different. It is more appropriate to use the average of the two measurements in the calculation of risk.[84]

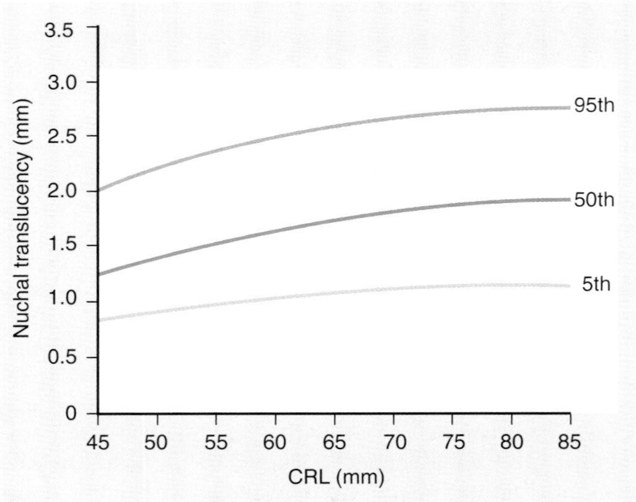

FIGURE 7–4
Changes in nuchal translucency with gestational age, as expressed by crown-rump length (CRL).
(Adapted from Pandya PP, Snijders RJM, Johnson SJ, et al: Screening for fetal trisomies by maternal age and fetal nuchal translucency thickness at 10 to 14 weeks of gestation. Br J Obstet Gynaecol 1995;102:957–962.)

Screening for Fetal Aneuploidies

FETAL NUCHAL TRANSLUCENCY AND TRISOMY 21

Down syndrome is the most common chromosomal abnormality in liveborn children, and every woman is at risk for having an affected fetus. This pervasive risk justifies the screening programs that have been established worldwide. A woman's risk of having a fetus with Down syndrome depends on her age, the GA, and her history of chromosomal defects. These three factors establish the background risk or a priori risk. A 33-year-old woman at 10 weeks' gestation has a 1 in 352 risk of having a fetus with trisomy 21. Because the risk decreases with advancing gestation as a result of the spontaneous death of fetuses with chromosomal abnormalities, the risk decreases to 1 in 547 at 40 weeks. NT measurement at 11 to 14 weeks, combined with maternal age, provides an effective method of screening for trisomy 21.

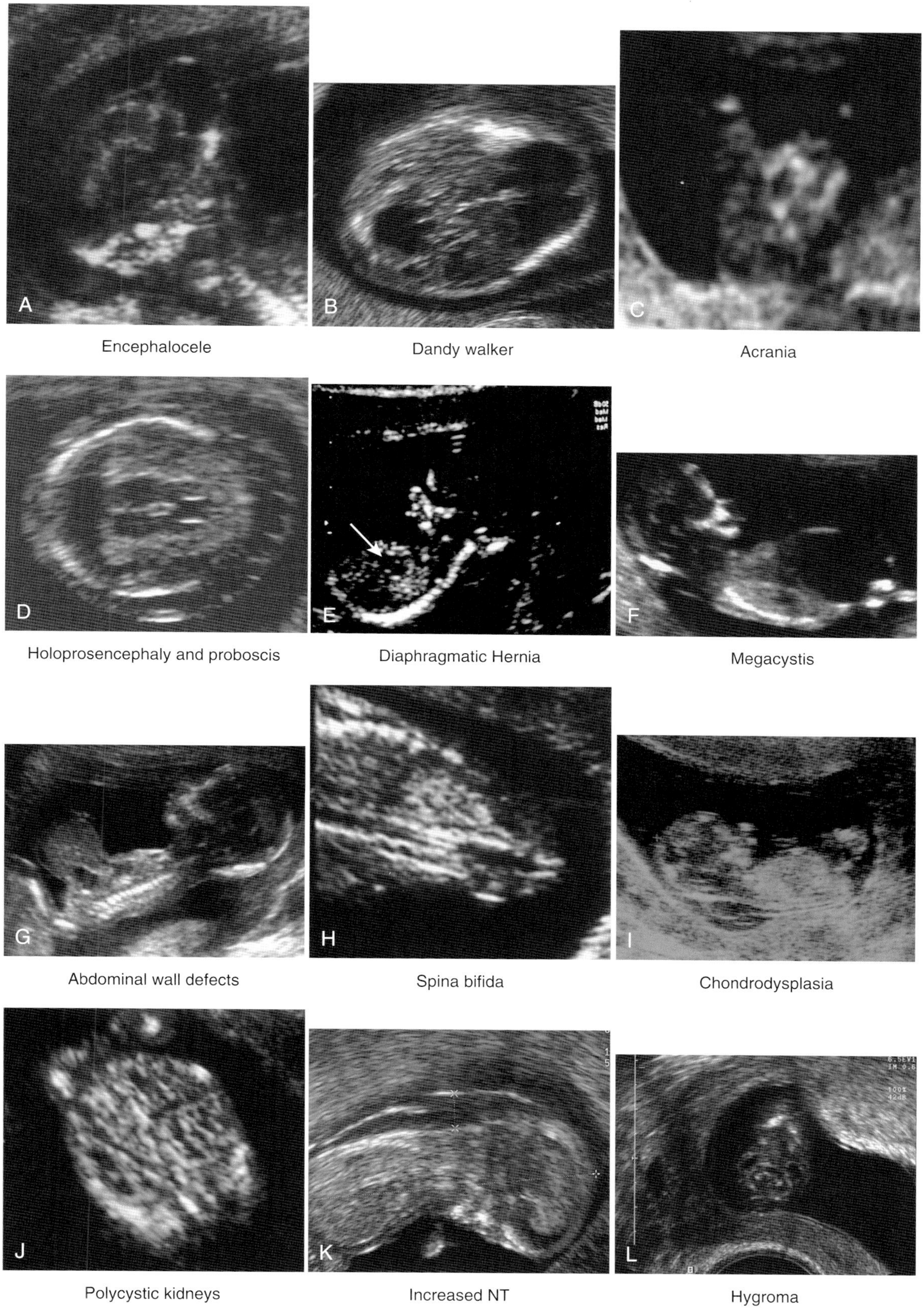

FIGURE 7–5
The most common structural defects diagnosed during screening at 11 to 14 weeks. *A*, Encephalocele. *B*, Dandy-Walker syndrome. *C*, Acrania. *D*, Holoprosencephaly and proboscis. *E*, Diaphragmatic hernia. *F*, Megacystis. *G*, Abdominal wall defects. *H*, Spina bifida. *I*, Chondrodysplasia. *J*, Polycystic kidney. *K*, Increased nuchal translucency. *L*, Hygroma.

FIGURE 7–6
Measurement of nuchal translucency. A strict sagittal view is appropriate for measuring crown-rump length. Appropriate magnification is greater than 70%. The view should be obtained away from the amnion. The fetal head should be in a neutral position. The largest of three to five measurements is recorded.

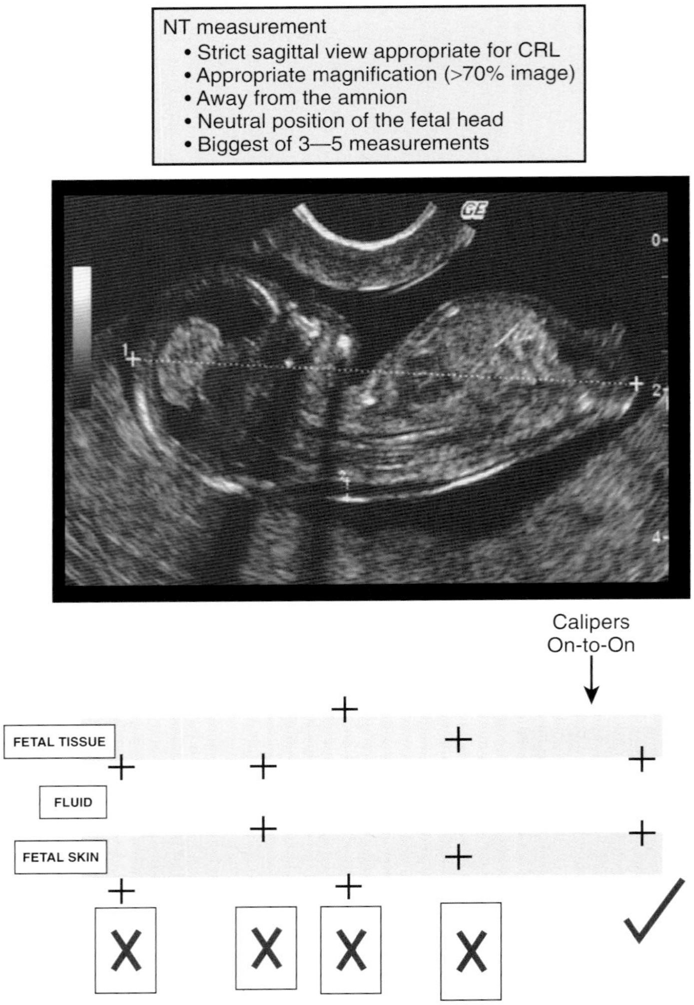

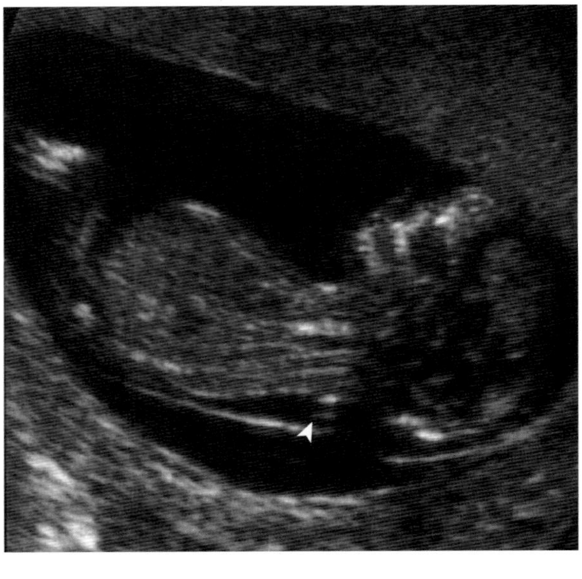

FIGURE 7–7
Umbilical cord around the neck (*arrow*).

FIGURE 7–8
Likelihood ratios for trisomy 21 in relation to the deviation in fetal nuchal translucency thickness from the expected normal median for crown-rump length. (From Snijders RJM, Nicolaides KH: Assessment of risks. In Ultrasound Markers for Fetal Chromosomal Defects. Carnforth, UK, Parthenon, 1996, pp 63–120.)

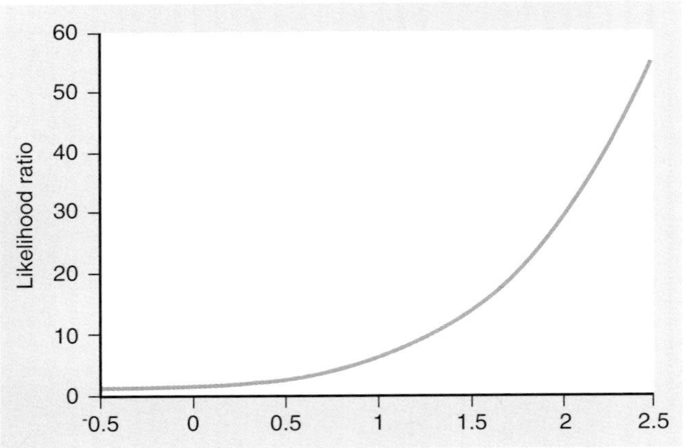

An association between NT thickness and chromosomal abnormalities has been recognized since the early 1990s.[79,83–97] The average reported detection rate with NT measurement is 77%, for a false-positive rate of 4.7%. The false-positive rate is the percentage of karyotypes potentially performed because of a positive screening test result. This detection rate represents the combined results of 14 prospective studies on NT measurement for chromosomal abnormalities involving 174,473 patients, including 728 with trisomy 21 (Table 7–4).[79,83–98] In comparison, screening by maternal age only using a cutoff age of 37 years has a detection rate of 30%, for a false-positive rate of 5%, The detection rate is approximately 60% with second-trimester maternal serum markers using the same false-positive rate.[99]

Whenever a screening test is performed, the background risk is multiplied by the test factor to calculate a new risk. Thus, the NT measurement in a fetus with a given CRL is converted to a likelihood ratio that is multiplied by the background risk to provide a new risk (Fig. 7–8).[79,100,101] A woman's risk of having a fetus with trisomy 21 is higher if the NT measurement is large and lower if it is small (Figs. 7–9 and 7–10).[36,100] The median NT thickness is approximately 2.0 mm in fetuses with trisomy 21. However, because NT thickness increases with gestation, the use of a cutoff value rather than a continuous assessment with CRL and maternal age leads to a 5% loss in sensitivity.[102]

NUCHAL TRANSLUCENCY AND CHROMOSOMAL DEFECTS OTHER THAN TRISOMY 21

Less prevalent chromosomal abnormalities are also associated with an increased NT thickness. In these fetuses, other characteristic sonographic findings are associated with increased NT measurements.

In trisomy 18, early-onset intrauterine growth restriction (IUGR) often occurs and may cause an error in dating the pregnancy. In approximately 30% of these cases, other anomalies, such as omphalocoele, are seen after 11 weeks.[103]

TABLE 7-4

Studies Examining the Implementation of Fetal Nuchal Translucency Screening for Trisomy 21

STUDY	*N*	GESTATION (WK)	CUTOFF	FALSE-POSITIVE RATE (%)	DETECTION RATE
Pandya et al, 1995[83]	1763	10-14	≥2.5 mm	3.6	3/4 (75%)
Szabo et al, 1995[86]	3380	9-12	≥3.0 mm	1.6	28/31 (90%)
Taipale et al, 1997[87]	6939	10-14	≥3.0 mm	0.8	4/6 (67%)
Hafner et al, 1998[88]	4371	10-14	≥2.5 mm	1.7	4/7 (57%)
Pajkrt et al, 1998[89]	1547	10-14	≥3.0 mm	2.2	6/9 (67%)
Snijders et al., 1998[79]	96,127	10-14	≥95th percentile	4.4	234/327 (72%)
Economides et al, 1998[90]	2281	11-14	≥99th percentile	0.4	6/8 (75%)
Schwarzler et al, 1999[91]	4523	10-14	NT > 2.5 mm	2.7	8/12 (67%)
Theodoropoulos et al, 1998[92]	3550	10-14	≥95th percentile	2.3	10/11 (91%)
Zoppi et al, 2001[93]	12,311	10-14	≥95th percentile	5.0	52/64 (81%)
Gasiorek-Wiens et al, 2001[94]	23,805	10-14	≥95th percentile	8.0	174/210 (83%)
Brizot et al, 2001[95]	2996	10-14	≥95th percentile	5.3	7/10 (70%)
Audibert et al, 2001[96]	4130	10-14	≥95th percentile	4.3	9/12 (75%)
Wayda et al, 2001[97]	6750	10-12	≥2.5 mm	4.3	17/17 (100%)
Total	174,473			4.7	562/728 (77%)

NT, nuchal translucency.
Adapted from Nicolaides KH: Screening for chromosomal defects. Ultrasound Obstet Gynecol 2003;21:313–321.

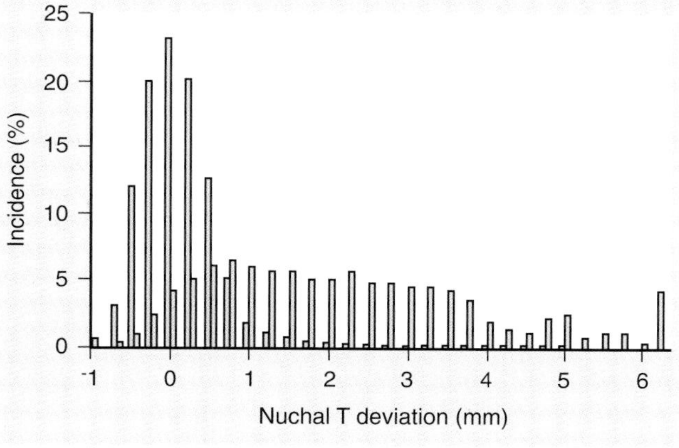

FIGURE 7-9
Distribution of fetal nuchal translucency thickness expressed as deviation from the expected normal value for crown-rump length in chromosomally normal fetuses (*open bars*) and 326 fetuses with trisomy 21 (*solid bars*).
(From Snijders RJM, Noble P, Sebire N, et al: UK multicentre project on assessment of risk of trisomy 21 by maternal age and fetal nuchal translucency thickness at 10-14 weeks of gestation. Lancet 1998;351:343-346.)

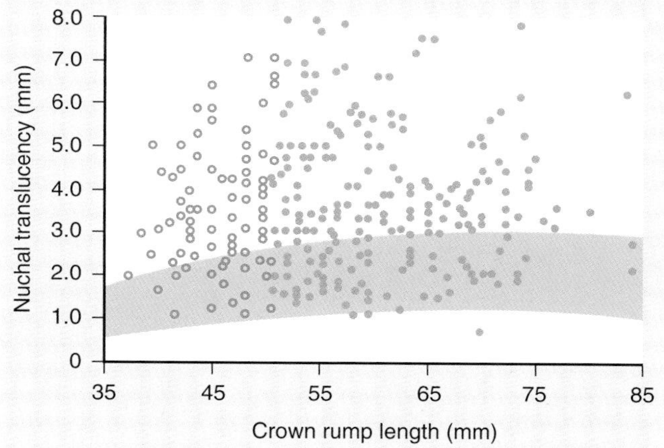

FIGURE 7-10
Nuchal translucency measurements in 326 fetuses with trisomy 21 plotted against the normal range for crown-rump length (95th and 5th percentiles).
(From Snijders RJM, Noble P, Sebire N, et al: UK multicentre project on assessment of risk of trisomy 21 by maternal age and fetal nuchal translucency thickness at 10-14 weeks of gestation. Lancet 1998;351:343-346.)

Trisomy 13 may also cause early-onset IUGR and severe brain anomalies, mainly holoprosencephaly, in up to 30% of cases at 11 to 14 weeks.[104]

Turner's syndrome is characterized by fetal tachycardia in approximately 50% of cases. These fetuses often have large cystic hygromas.[105]

In triploidy, there is early-onset, but asymmetrical IUGR, with an almost normal-sized head. Other severe anomalies are present in approximately 40% of cases, and molar changes in the placenta are seen in approximately one third of cases.[106]

INCREASED NUCHAL TRANSLUCENCY AND NORMAL KARYOTYPE

By definition, 5% of fetuses screened at 11 to 14 weeks have an NT measurement greater than the 95th percentile. Most of these fetuses are chromosomally and anatomically normal antenatally and at birth.[79,107,108] Fetuses with increased NT thickness but a normal karyotype are at increased risk for major cardiac defects as well as other structural anomalies, rare genetic syndromes, and other unfavorable outcomes (Table 7-5).[109–113] Because an increase in the amount of this

TABLE 7–5

Anomalies Associated with Increased Nuchal Translucency

Chromosomal abnormalities
Cardiac defects
Diaphragmatic hernia
Exomphalos
Achondrogenesis type II
Asphyxiating thoracic dystrophy
Beckwith-Wiedemann syndrome
Blomstrand's osteochondrodysplasia
Body stalk anomaly
Campomelic dysplasia
Congenital adrenal hyperplasia
Ectrodactyly-ectodermal dysplasia-cleft palate syndrome
Fetal akinesia deformation sequence
Fryns' syndrome
GM
Sotos syndrome
Hydrolethalus syndrome
Jarcho-Levin syndrome
Joubert's syndrome
Meckel-Gruber syndrome
Nance-Sweeney syndrome
Noonan's syndrome
Osteogenesis imperfecta type II
Perlman's syndrome
Robert's syndrome
Short-rib polydactyly syndrome
Smith-Lemli-Opitz syndrome
Spinal muscular atrophy type 1
Thanatophoric dysplasia
Trigonocephaly C syndrome
VACTERL association
Zellweger's syndrome

GM, gangliosidosis; VACTERL, vertebral abnormalities, anal atresia, cardiac abnormalities, tracheoesophageal fistula and/or esophageal atresia, renal agenesis or dysplasia, and limb defects.
Adapted from Souka AP, Snidjers RJM, Novakov A, et al: Defects and syndromes in chromosomally normal fetuses with increased nuchal translucency thickness at 10–14 weeks of gestation. Ultrasound Obstet Gynecol 1988;11:391–400.

fluid is associated with a number of apparently unrelated fetal problems, it is safe to assume there are multiple mechanisms underlying the increased thickness. It is also likely that more than one mechanism is involved in some circumstances. These include cardiac dysfunction, abnormalities of the heart and great arteries, venous congestion of the head and neck, altered composition of the extracellular matrix, failure of lymphatic drainage due to abnormal or delayed development of the lymphatic system or impaired fetal movements, fetal anemia, and congenital infection.[114]

Souka and colleagues[109] looked at pregnancy outcome in 1320 chromosomally normal fetuses with NT thickness greater than 3.5 mm in the first trimester. The chance of a live birth and no structural defects was 86% when the NT thickness was 3.5 to 4.4 mm, 77% when the NT thickness was 4.5 to 5.4 mm, 67% when the NT thickness was 5.5 to 6.4 mm, and 31% when the NT thickness was greater than 6.5 mm. Thus, parents should be counseled that even if the NT thickness exceeds 6.5 mm, there is a one in three chance that the pregnancy will end with the live birth of an infant with no major defects.[109]

CARDIAC DEFECTS

Increased NT in a fetus with a normal karyotype is associated with a greater risk of CHD.[61–63,115] The prevalence of congenital cardiac defects in fetuses with increased NT thickness is between 5% and 10%.[116] Moreover, although NT may be increased in fetuses with CHD and a normal karyotype, the median NT is significantly higher when the karyotype is abnormal for almost any given diagnosis of CHD. A meta-analysis of studies examining the screening performance of NT thickness for the detection of cardiac defects in fetuses with normal karyotype concluded the detection rates were about 37% and 31% for the respective NT cutoffs of the 95th and 99th percentiles[62] Some 60% of CHD in the chromosomally abnormal group and 23% of CHD in the chromosomally normal fetuses will be identified by applying the 99th percentile.[63] The policy regarding referral for NT between the 95th and the 99th percentiles is much less consistent, and probably only a portion in this group gets to see a fetal cardiologist specifically because of the increased NT. Another recent meta-analysis concluded that about half the cases of CHD could be prenatally identified with an NT cutoff of 1.7 multiple of the median (MoM) and a 5% false-positive rate.[117] Fetal echocardiography is recommended as early as the first trimester because it would identify one major cardiac defect in every 16 patients examined for all chromosomally normal fetuses with NT above the 99th percentile.[62]

The performance of screening by increased NT does not vary with the type of cardiac defect. The NT is increased in all types of heart defects: left as well as right heart l esions, septal defects, outflow tract disorders, laterality disorders, and complex heart lesions.[63] Other first-trimester sonographic markers of trisomy 21 have been proposed as part of a two-stage assessment of risk.[118] With the exception of the nasal bone (NB), these markers are related to the cardiovascular system, and include tricuspid regurgitation (TR) and increased impedance to flow in the ductus venosus (DV). These may be explained in part by the theory of dysfunctional or abnormal angiogenesis in aneuploidy.[119]

DIAPHRAGMATIC HERNIA

In a study of 19 fetuses with diaphragmatic hernia, NT thickness was increased in 37%, including 83% of those who died in the neonatal period as a result of pulmonary hypoplasia. Only 22% of the survivors had an increased NT measurement. Increased NT thickness may reflect venous congestion in the head and neck as a result of mediastinal shift or compression and impaired venous return.[120]

OMPHALOCOELE

The prevalence of omphalocoele is approximately 10 times higher in fetuses with a normal karyotype and an increased

NT measurement compared with the general population.[108,121] Other structural defects are associated with increased NT thickness and a normal karyotype.[108]

Miscellanous Associations

An increased NT measurement (>3.5 mm) with a normal karyotype is an indication for detailed, follow-up ultrasound examinations.[122] An anomaly scan should be performed at 14 to 16 weeks to determine the evolution of the NT to nuchal edema and to diagnose or exclude most fetal defects.[109] Nuchal edema is diagnosed when subcutaneous edema is noted in the midaxial plane of the neck and tremors occur if the uterine wall is tapped or if the edema measures more than 6 mm.[123] If no obvious abnormalities are seen during the 14- to 16-week scan, echocardiogram should be performed at 20 to 22 weeks, when further genetic testing may be indicated (Fig. 7–11).[109]

An adverse outcome may be expected in about one out of five fetuses with persistent, unexplained nuchal edema at 20 to 22 weeks,[109] including progression to hydrops, genetic syndromes detected at birth, and cardiac defects (one third) that could have been detected, but were missed antenatally.

Based on combined data from two studies that included 4540 chromosomally normal fetuses with increased NT and no obvious structural defects, the incidence of miscarriage or fetal death increased from 1.3% in those with NT between the 95th and the 99th percentiles to about 20% for NT of 6.5 mm or greater.[108,109] Another study of 6650 pregnancies undergoing NT screening reported that in chromosomally normal fetuses, the incidence of miscarriage or fetal death was 1.3% in those with NT below the 95th percentile, 1.2% for NT between the 95th and the 99th percentiles, and 12.3% for NT above the 99th percentile (3.5 mm).[124] The authors concluded that once aneuploidy is ruled out, the risk of fetal mortality does not statistically increase until the NT reached 3.5 mm or above. The majority of fetuses that die do so by 20 weeks, progressing from the increased NT to severe hydrops fetalis. Chromosomally and structurally normal fetuses with history of thickened NT found to be alive and well at 20 weeks with no evidence of nuchal fold thickening or nonimmune hydrops are no longer considered at an increased risk for perinatal or long-term morbidity and mortality.

The prevalence of neurodevelopmental delay in the group with normal findings on follow-up scans is 0.4%, but rises to 1.2% in those with persistent nuchal edema. Other studies report a 3.2% to 5.6% prevalence of residual neurodevelopmental delay in fetuses with increased NT thickness.[125,126] Methodologic issues make it difficult to compare the prevalence of mental retardation in infants with increased NT measurements with the general population, which ranges from 0.5% to 2%.[127] Etiologies include chromosomal abnormalities in 25% of cases and genetic syndromes in 7% to 10% of cases. Mental retardation is unexplained in 30% to 50% of cases,[127] or less than 1% of the population. Children with an isolated NT measurement in utero of greater than 3.5 mm should be followed jointly by pediatricians and geneticists to allow enhanced prenatal counseling (Table 7–6).[107,109,128,129] Elucidation and integration of these data are essential if the counseling is to be balanced. Otherwise, counseling may resemble this confusing statement: "The good news is that the karyotype is normal, and the bad news is the karyotype is normal."[128,129] Such uncertainty is potentially lethal, particularly when announced in the first trimester in countries in which pregnancy termination is an option at 14 weeks, but is challenged or forbidden at a later GA.

The association between increased NT thickness and a wide range of structural abnormalities and genetic syndromes indicates the need for long-term follow-up of these children, even when they appear normal at birth. Hiippala and associates[122] followed 50 chromosomally normal children 2.4 to 7.1 years of age who had NT thickness greater than 3 mm at 13 to 15 weeks' gestation. Their growth was within normal limits, but 1 in 12 had a previously unrecognized cardiac defect. One child had Noonan's syndrome, 1 had cleidocranial dysplasia, and a third had developmental delays and an undefined syndrome. Webbing was seen in the neck region of 2 children who were otherwise free of associated pathology.

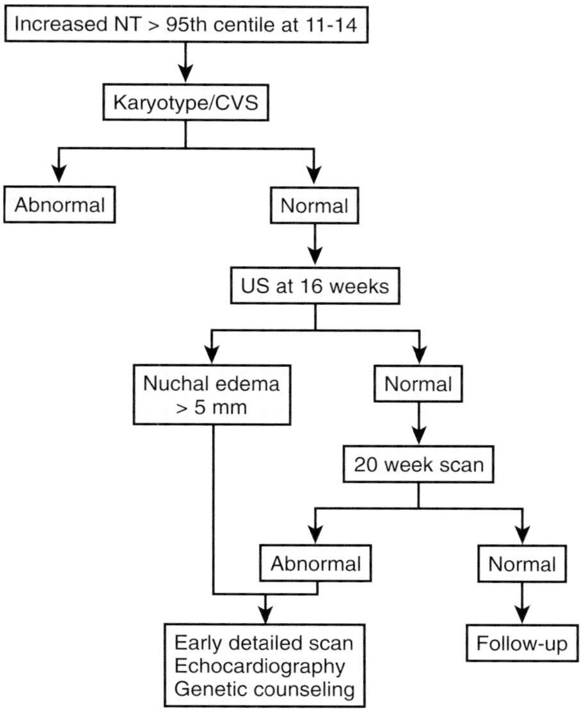

FIGURE 7–11
Follow-up of fetuses with increased nuchal translucency and normal karyotype. CVS, chorionic villus sampling.
(From Senat MV, De Keersmaecker B, Audibert F, et al: Pregnancy outcome in fetuses with increased nuchal translucency and normal karyotype. Prenat Diagn 2002;22:345-349.)

Nuchal Translucency in Multiple Pregnancies

First-trimester NT thickness measurement in combination with maternal age is an efficient technique for trisomy 21 screening in multiple gestation. Sebire and coworkers[130,131] reported that it has a performance comparable with that in singletons, although with a slightly higher false-positive

TABLE 7–6

Outcome of Fetuses with Nuchal Translucency Greater than the 95th Percentile, Normal Karyotype, and Normal Findings on Examination at Birth

STUDY	NO. OF FETUSES	MEAN NT AT 11–14 WK (MM)	MEAN POSTNATAL FOLLOW-UP (RANGE)	LOST TO FOLLOW-UP (%)	ADVERSE OUTCOME (*N*)
Cha'ban et al, 1996[129]	19	4.6	18 mo (4–32 mo)	0	0
Van Vugt et al, 1998[125]	50	3.6	33.5 mo (7–75 mo)	32	Various minor health problems, 5 (5/50; 10%)
Adekunle et al, 1999[126]	31	NA	23 mo (12–38 mo)	26	Developmental delay, 2; Noonan's syndrome, 1 (3/23; 13%)
Souka et al, 2001[109]	980	4.5	NA	0	22 adverse outcomes including 4 with developmental delay (22/980; 2%)
Hiippala et al, 2001[122]	59	4.0	56 mo (29–85 mo)	15	Noonan's syndrome, 1; cleidocranial dysplasia, 1; unknown syndrome, 1; delayed speech and visuomotor disturbances, 2 (5/50; 10%)
Senat et al, 2002[107]	58	4.6	39 mo (12–72 mo)	7	Developmental delay, 2; delay in walking, 1; stuttering, 1; torticolis, 1 (6/54; 11%)

NA, not applicable; NT, nuchal translucency.
Adapted from Senat MV, De Keersmaecker B, Audibert F, et al: Pregnancy outcome in fetuses with increased nuchal translucency and normal karyotype. Prenat Diagn 2002;22:345–349.

rate. Fetus-specific risk estimation helps select the best invasive technique for diagnostic testing.

In dichorionic multiples, the risk of aneuploidy depends on the number of fetuses, because each additional fetus proportionally increases the risk of aneuploidy per pregnancy. In monochorionic multiples, which are always monozygotic, the maternal age–related risk for chromosomal abnormalities is the same as in singleton pregnancies, and in the vast majority of cases, both fetuses are affected. The findings of a retrospective study of 769 monochorionic twin pregnancies suggests that effective screening for trisomy 21 is best provided by using the average of NT measured in the two fetuses. If the fetus with the smaller NT is considered, the detection rate of trisomy 21, for any given false-positive rate or risk cutoff, is substantially lower than using the average NT measured in the two fetuses.[132] Moreover the false-positive rate of NT screening (13% per pregnancy) is higher than in dichorionic twins, because increased NT in at least one of the fetuses is an early manifestation of twin-twin transfusion syndrome (TTTS; see next section for additional details).[132]

Increased Nuchal Translucency Measurement and Twin-Twin Transfusion Syndrome

A NT measurement above the 95th percentile for CRL between 11 to 14 weeks is associated with a fourfold increase in the risk of severe TTTS in a study of 132 monochorionic twin pregnancies[133] (see also Chapters 23 and 59). Another study of 287 monochorionic twin pregnancies, including 43 that developed severe TTTS at 16 to 24 weeks, reported that the NT was above the 95th percentile in at least one of the fetuses in 28% of the TTTS group at 11 to 13 + 6 weeks compared with 10% in the non-TTTS group.[134] Although the positive predictive value of this screening test is low, it is important to follow these pregnancies closely for the early diagnosis of TTTS. A recent evaluation of 512 monochoronic twin pregnancies revealed that a NT discordance of 20% or more was found in about 25% of cases and that in this group, the risk of developing TTTS was more than 30%.[135]

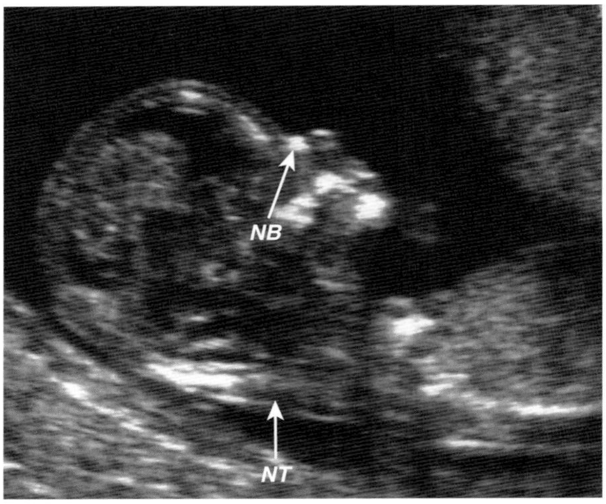

FIGURE 7–12
Ultrasound picture of a 12-week chromosomal fetus with normal nuchal translucency thickness and a present nasal bone.
(From Nicolaides KH: Nuchal translucency and other first-trimester sonographic markers of chromosomal abnormalities. Am J Obstet Gynecol 2004;191:45–67.)

Other Fetal Measurements as Markers for Fetal Aneuploidy

Nasal Bones

In the combined data from nine studies, the NB was absent in 176 of 12,652 (1.4%) chromosomally normal fetuses and in 274 of 397 (69.0%) fetuses with trisomy 21, yielding a likelihood ratio for absent NB of 49.3.[136–144] The prevalence of absent NB (Fig. 7–12) reflects ethnicity (it is highest in individuals of African origin), NT thickness (it increases as the NT measurement increases), and the CRL measurement (it decreases with GA). Therefore, likelihood ratios for trisomy 21 must also be adjusted to account for these factors.[137,138] Methodologic problems surrounding that part of the first-trimester scan can generate a high false-positive rate, together with significant interoperator and intraoperator variability.[139]

Ductal Blood Flow

A high proportion of fetuses with trisomy 21 and other chromosomal abnormalities have increased impedance to flow in the DV at 11–13 weeks' gestation (Fig. 7–13). In combined data from seven studies, ductal blood flow with an absent or reversed a-wave was observed in 5.2% of euploid fetuses, and 70.8%, 89.3%, 81.8%, and 76.9% of fetuses with trisomies 21, 18, and 13 and Turner's syndrome, respectively.[145] In combined data from six studies, abnormal ductal flow was observed in 273 of 5462 (5.0%) chromosomally normal fetuses and in 108 of 131 (82.4%) fetuses with trisomy 21, and therefore the likelihood ratio for abnormal ductal flow was 16.5.[146–151] There may be an association between increased fetal NT and the presence of abnormal ductal flow, but it appears weak. These findings suggest that Doppler evaluation of the DV flow can be combined with NT screening.[149–151] Ductal flow measurement requires skilled operators because the interference from adjacent vessels is commonly encountered.

Blood Flow across the Tricuspid Valve

Regurgitant flow across the tricuspid valve (TR), determined by pulsed wave Doppler, is a common finding in trisomy 21 fetuses at 11 + 0 to 13 + 6 weeks' gestation (Fig. 7–14).[152,153]

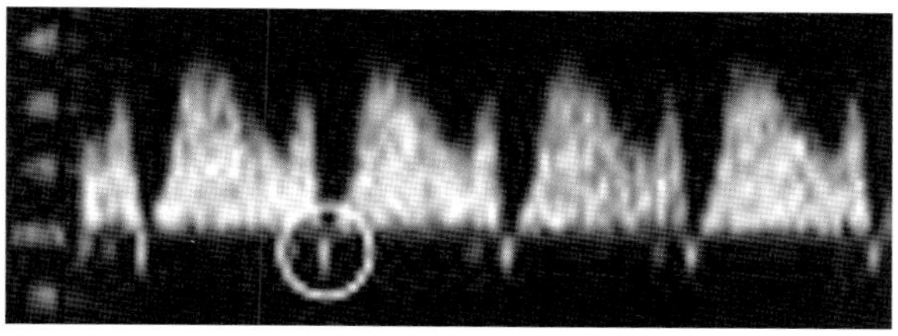

FIGURE 7–13
Reversed a-wave in the ductus venosus in a fetus with trisomy 21 at 12 weeks of gestation.
(From Maiz N, Valencia C, Kagan KO, et al: Ductus venosus Doppler in screening for trisomies 21, 18 and 13 and Turner syndrome at 11–13 weeks of gestation. Ultrasound Obstet Gynecol 2009;33:512–517.)

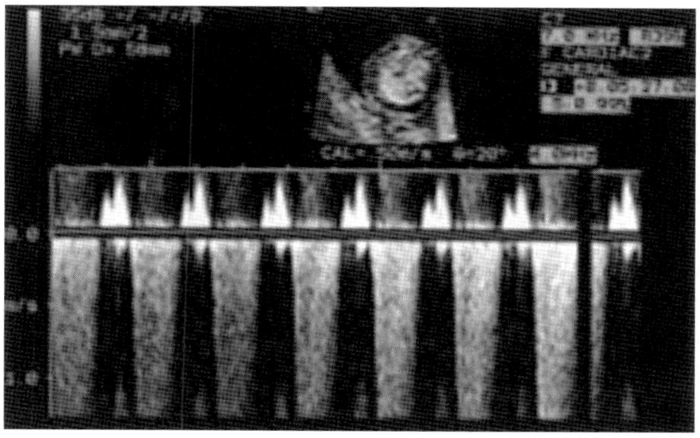

FIGURE 7–14
Holosystolic regurgitation on pulsed Doppler examination of the tricuspid valve in a fetus at 12 weeks' gestation.
(From Huggon IC, DeFigueiredo DB, Allan LD: Tricuspid regurgitation in the diagnosis of chromosomal anomalies in the fetus at 11–14 weeks of gestation. Heart 2003;89:1071–1073.)

A study performed by experienced fetal cardiologists revealed that the prevalence of TR in fetuses with trisomy 21 at this GA approximates 74% whereas only 7% of chromosomally normal fetuses have this finding.[153] The prevalence of TR decreases with CRL in both normal and trisomic fetuses. In studies performed by the Fetal Medicine Foundation Center, TR was present in 72 of 1394 (5.2%) chromosomally normal fetuses and in 109 of 162 (67.3%) fetuses with trisomy 21.[118] An additional benefit of this measurement is a high association between TR and cardiac defects, suggesting that the high prevalence of TR in the chromosomally abnormal fetuses can be partly attributed to the coincidence of cardiac defects.[152] Like the DV examination, the assessment of tricuspid flow necessitates specialist training.

It is questionable whether NB, abnormal ductal blood flow, and TR can be routinely combined with the other first-trimester sonographic and biochemical markers of chromosomal abnormalities to improve the performance of first-trimester screening. The complexity of the assessment of these procedures and the rigor required to maintain the skills, together with the potential for a subjective assessment, are limitations for their implementation as a one-step risk procedure performed at the time of NT measurement. However, these markers have the characteristics to be a second-line screening that can be performed in early pregnancy, resulting in a major reduction in the need for invasive testing. It is likely their use will grow in fetal medicine laboratories with added experience.

Other Markers of Aneuploidy

Several other measurements in the first trimester are more common in chromosomally abnormal fetuses than in the chromosomally normal population.

A novel method for evaluating the relative position of the fetal maxilla with respect to the forehead was introduced in the first trimester to investigate the location of the front of the maxilla in relation to the forehead in fetuses with trisomy 21.[154] A three-dimensional volume of the fetal head was obtained before karyotyping in 100 fetuses with trisomy 21 and 300 euploid fetuses. The *frontomaxillary facial (FMF) angle* (Fig. 7–15), defined as the angle between the upper surface of the upper palate and the frontal bone in a midsagittal view of the fetal face, was measured. The FMF angle was significantly larger in the trisomy 21 (mean 88.7 degrees, range 75.4–104 degrees) than in the euploid fetuses (mean 78.1 degrees, range 66.6–89.5 degrees). The FMF angle was more than 85 degrees in 69% of the trisomy 21 fetuses and in 5% of the euploid fetuses. There was no significant association between the FMF angle and the NT measurement. The authors postulate that measurement of FMF angle will be a useful adjunct in screening for trisomy 21. Unfortunately, it is more cumbersome to measure than all other sonographic markers.

Other fetal measurements potentially affected in chromosomally abnormal fetuses include the fetal heart rate,[155] maxillary length,[156] ear length,[157] femur length,[158] and humeral length,[158] and in general, fetal growth (see later). Even though statistical differences between trisomy 21 and euploid fetuses exist, the differences are small, limiting their clinical utility.[1]

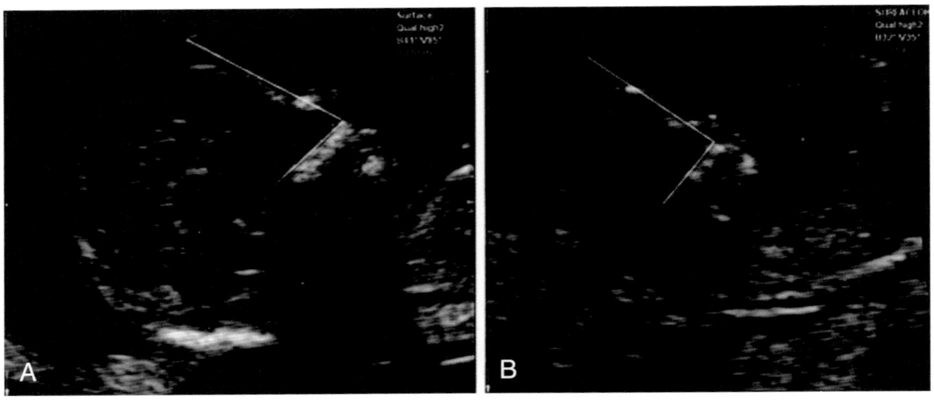

FIGURE 7–15
A, Frontomaxillary facial (FMF) angle in a chromosomally normal fetus. *B*, FMF angle in a trisomy 21 fetus.
(*A* and *B*, From Sonek J: First trimester ultrasonography in screening and detection of fetal anomalies [review]. Am J Med Genet C Semin Med Genet 2007;145C:45–61.)

TABLE 7–7
Most Common Structural Defects Diagnosed Prenatally during Screening at 11 to 14 Weeks

Atrioventricular septal defects and hypoplastic left heart syndrome
Acrania and alobar holoprosencephaly
Omphalocele and gastroschisis
Megacystis
Lethal skeletal defects

Ultrasound Diagnosis of Fetal Abnormalities

The majority (80%) of common fetal malformations develop before 12 weeks' gestation; therefore, a good visualization of the fetus at this stage should be able to detect these malformations. Most fetal structures can be seen at 12 to 13 weeks, and this GA offers the earliest opportunity for screening for fetal abnormalities. Though the available reports of detection rates in the first trimester for fetal structural defects other than those associated with increased NT thickness are confined mostly to high risk or selected populations (Table 7–7),[159–162] there is increasing evidence that early detailed ultrasonography is technically feasible as a screening test for fetal structural defects in low risk pregnancies.[162] The most frequently detected first-trimester anomalies involve the central nervous system, such as anencephaly, encephalocele, and holoprosencephaly.[163]

Lethal, incurable, or curable severe abnormalities with a high risk of residual handicap are defined as *major structural abnormalities*. The diagnosis of spina bifida is a challenge because the indirect sonographic signs that are characteristic later in gestation are usually missing prior to 14 weeks.[89] Omphalocoele, gastroschisis, and megacystis are also commonly diagnosed in the first trimester. There are case reports of the first-trimester diagnosis of a wide range of severe skeletal defects (see Fig. 7–5). The remaining cases of less severe or benign abnormalities, of no cosmetic or functional significance, constitute the group of minor structural abnormalities. A review[44] analyzed several studies reporting first-trimester detection rates that are comparable with those achieved in the routine second-trimester anatomic survey at 18 to 22 weeks (Table 7–8).[159,162,164–183]

Central Nervous System Defects

The development of the fetal central nervous system is not completed at the end of the first trimester and the anomalies reported differ from those described later in pregnancy. In first-trimester studies, the vast majority of defects described are lethal or severe major structural anomalies. Empty or enlarged brain cavities or abnormal contours of the head and spine are important diagnostic markers for the detection of central nervous system anomalies in the very early pregnancy.[48]

ACRANIA, EXENCEPHALY, AND ANENCEPHALY

Anencephaly can be diagnosed reliably on routine 11- to 14-week ultrasound examination. Acrania is the main feature of anencephaly in the first trimester. Fetuses with acrania may have a normal brain or one that shows varying degrees of disruption.[184,185] In one large, multicenter study, screening for fetal abnormalities was performed in 53,435 singleton and 901 twin pregnancies. Eight of the 47 fetuses with anencephaly were missed.[185] The sonographers were then instructed to look specifically for the cranial vault and at brain organization. All subsequent cases of anencephaly were identified at the 11- to 14-week scan.

ENCEPHALOCELE

Encephalocele appears as a bony defect in the skull, with brain tissue protruding. It is associated with Meckel-Gruber syndrome.[186,187] In most cases, the lesion arises midline in the occipital area. The main alternative diagnosis is cystic hygroma. Once the diagnosis is suspected, the prognosis usually cannot be ascertained before the late second trimester.

HOLOPROSENCEPHALY

Holoprosencephaly results from incomplete cleavage of the forebrain. The most severe forms, alobar and semilobar, are amenable to first-trimester ultrasound diagnosis. They are characterized by a monoventricular cavity and fusion of the thalami. One study suggests that failure to identify both choroid plexuses (the "butterfly" sign) is a first-trimester warning sign of holoprosencephaly.[188] These forms are often associated with facial abnormalities.[189,190] The most common related chromosome abnormality is trisomy 13.

TABLE 7-8

Detection Rates of First-Trimester and Second-Trimester Ultrasound Screening for Fetal Structural Malformations

AUTHOR	YEAR	BASELINE RISK OF STUDY POPULATION	ULTRASOUND MODALITY (TAS/TVS)	GESTATIONAL AGE (WK)	*N*	*N* (%) OF MAJOR MALFORMATIONS	FIRST-TRIMESTER SENSITIVITY (%)	SECOND-TRIMESTER SENSITIVITY (%)
Achiron and Tadmor[164]	1991	Low	Both	9-13	800	15 (1.9)	57	93
Yagel et al[159]	1995	High	TVS	13-16	536	50 (9.3)	84	89
Hernandi and Töröcsik[165]	1997	Low	Both	11 0/7-14 6/7	3991	64 (1.6)	55	69
Economides and Braithwaite[166]	1998	Low	Both	12 0/7-13 6/7	1632	17 (1.0)	65	82
D'Ottavio et al[167]	1997	Low	TVS	14	4078	88 (2.2)	61	89
Whitlow et al[168]	1999	Low	Both	11 0/7-14 6/7	6634	92 (1.4)	59	81
Guariglia and Rosati[169]	2000	Low	TVS	10-16	3478	64 (1.8)	52	84
Drysdale et al[170]	2002	Low	NR	12 0/7-13 6/7	984	31 (3.1)	16	NR
Den Hollander et al[171]	2002	High	Both	11-14	101	11 (11)	82	100
Carvalho et al[172]	2002	Low	Both	11-14	2853	66 (2.3)	38	79
Taipale et al[162]	2003	Low	Both	13-14	20,465	307 (1.5)	52	NR
Chen et al[173]	2004	High	Both	12 0/7-14 6/7	1609	26 (1.6)	54	77
Taipale et al[174]	2004	Low	TVS	13-14	4855	33 (0.7)	18	48
Markov et al[175]	2004	N/A	NR	11 0/7-14 6/7	1135	53 (4.6)	22	69
McAuliffe et al[176]	2005	Low	Both	11 0/7-13 6/7	325	6 (1.8)	17	83
Becker and Wegner[177]	2006	Medium	Both	11 0/7-13 6/7	3094	86 (2.8)	84	91
Souka et al[178]	2006	Low	Both	11 0/7-14 6/7	1148	14 (1.2)	50	93
Saltvedt et al[179]	2006	Low	TAS	11-14	39,572	1,252 (3.5)	38	47
Cedergan and Selbing[180]	2006	Low	TAS	11-14	2708	32 (1.2)	40	NR
Weiner et al[181]	2007	Low	Both	10 2/7-13 4/7	1723	22 (1.3)	41	100
Dane et al[182]	2007	Low	Both	11-14	1290	24 (1.9)	71	95
Chen et al[183]	2008	Low	Both	10-14 6/7	4282	63 (1.5)	48	66

N/A, not applicable; NR, data not available; TAS, transabdominal scan; TVS, transvaginal scan.
From Timor-Tritsch IE, Fuchs KM, Monteagudo A, D'Alton ME: Performing a fetal anatomy scan at the time of first-trimester screening. Obstet Gynecol 2009;113:402–407.

Different authors have used the 3DUS "inversion rendering" mode to described abnormal brains.[51] Inversion rendering of early fetal brain ventricles is feasible and should be attempted if additional information is needed.[191]

SPINA BIFIDA

The sonographic diagnosis of spina bifida aperta is difficult prior to 14 weeks. The diagnosis of hydrocephaly is also difficult to establish in the first trimester because of the large relative proportions of the lateral ventricles to the calvarium. Therefore, in the absence of cranial signs in the first trimester, the sensitivity of detection of spina bifida is unlikely to be as high as in second-trimester scanning. At this early gestation, indirect signs, such as sacral irregularities, the lemon (frontal bone scalloping) and banana signs (abnormal curvature of the cerebellar hemispheres), are usually absent.[163,192] Other signs, such as a flattened occiput, parallel peduncles, a straight metencephalon, and the acorn sign (frontal bone narrowing), are not consistently present.[163,192] Blaas and colleagues[193] studied high risk pregnancies prospectively and identified three first-trimester fetuses with lumbosacral myelomeningocele characterized by an irregularity in the caudal part of the spine before 10 weeks. 3DUS examination might be helpful but is not necessary to make the diagnosis.

Heart Defects

See the detailed discussion of NT thickness of greater than 3.5 mm and heart defects, earlier. The prevalence of major cardiac defects increases with NT thickness, from 5.4 per 1000 with an NT measurement of 2.5 to 3.4 mm, to 233 per 1000 with an NT measurement of greater than 5.5 mm. The sensitivity of NT is 15% to 56% for the diagnosis of major cardiac defects.[102,110–112] Early fetal echocardiography is recommended and can be performed reliably by trained operators from 14 weeks onward.[58,59,194] Care should be taken not to extrapolate the results of these studies to low risk populations.

Omphalocoele

Reduction of the physiologic midgut hernia ends by 11 weeks and 5 days.[195] An abdominal defect, especially omphalocoele, should be suspected if the herniation continues after 12 weeks. This defect is sporadic, having a birth prevalence of approximately 1 in 4000. Omphalocele is commonly associated with other abnormalities such as aneuploidy, most commonly trisomy 18.[196] Because trisomy 18 has such a high rate of mortality, its association with an omphalocele decreases significantly with GA: 61% at 11 to 13 + 6 weeks' gestation, 30% in the second trimester, and 15% at term.[197] There are many reports of first-trimester ultrasound diagnosis of omphalocele,[196,198] gastroschisis as well as body stalk anomaly, pentalogy of Cantrell, and ectopia cordis.[44]

Megacystis

Megacystis is defined as a bladder with a longitudinal diameter of 7 mm or more at 10 to 14 weeks' gestation. It is found in approximately 1 in 1500 pregnancies.[67] One study of 145 fetuses with megacystis observed a 25% aneuploidy rate, mainly trisomies 13 and 18.[199] In 75% of fetuses with chromosomal abnormalities, the NT was also increased, possibly the result of thoracic compression. Ninety percent of chromosomally normal fetuses had spontaneous resolution, with no obvious adverse effects on the development of the urinary system. The risk of a chromosomal abnormality when the longitudinal diameter is more than 15 mm is actually lower, approximately 11%.[200] Here, there is a strong association with progressive obstructive uropathy.[199] Favre and associates[200] reported a high prevalence of aneuploidy in fetuses with megacystis and a longitudinal diameter of 9 to 15 mm. Parents can usually be reassured when the megacystis is between 7 and 15 mm and the karyotype is normal that 90% of abnormalities will resolve and renal function will be normal. Vesicoamniotic shunting in midgestation has no benefit and there is no experience with first-trimester decompression.[201] It is interesting to note that megacystis is associated with an increased NT regardless of the karyotype.[199]

Renal Anomalies

Bilateral renal agenesis, hydronephrosis, and multicystic dysplastic kidney have been diagnosed by ultrasound in the first trimester.[165,202,203]

Skeletal Defects

Skeletal dysplasias complicate approximately 1 in 4000 births. Twenty-five percent of affected fetuses are stillborn, and 30% die in the neonatal period. In some skeletal dysplasias, growth impairment is not apparent until later in gestation. However, first-trimester diagnosis of isolated cases has been reported, mainly because they were associated with an increased NT.[204,205]

Two-Vessel Cord

The finding of a two-vessel cord in the first trimester is not associated with an increased prevalence of trisomy 21, but it increases the risk of trisomy 18 approximately sevenfold.[206]

Variation in First-Trimester Growth

First-trimester growth in normal pregnancy is influenced by maternal and fetal factors. Early fetal growth restriction is demonstrable in many pregnancies that subsequently end as a first-trimester loss. However, slow growth occurs prior to miscarriage in both chromosomally normal and abnormal pregnancies. Serial growth assessment of ongoing viable pregnancies and those that subsequently fail suggests that whereas they have significantly different growth rates, those that miscarry also fall broadly into two groups: those that have antecedent growth restriction and those that do not.[33] It is potentially easy to overlook early growth delay by misdating an abnormal pregnancy.[207] The assessment of growth restriction in the first trimester using the cross-sectional studies described relies on an accurate recall of menstrual age and a regular menstrual cycle so that expected fetal size can be calculated. Functional linear discriminant analysis (FLDA) using serial measurements of CRL or MSD was found to differentiate normal from abnormal early pregnancy growth, predicting a spontaneous loss with a sensitivity of 60.7% and a specificity of 93.1%.[32] In contrast, a single CRL more than 2 SD below expected has a sensitivity of only 53.6% and a specificity of 72.2%.[33]

In pregnancies that continue, various studies have shown some chromosomal abnormalities such as trisomy 18 as well as triploidies,[207] but not trisomy 21, trisomy 13, monosomy X (Turner's syndrome), or sex chromosome triploidies[208] are associated with poor growth. The spectrum of aneuploidy associated with growth restriction and first-trimester miscarriage includes a wider range of trisomies, commonly 7, 16, and 22.[209]

Several studies document that slow growth in the first trimester (absent chromosomal abnormality or miscarriage) is associated with adverse late pregnancy outcomes.[23] Smith and coworkers[210] reviewed 30,000 pregnancies and concluded that a CRL 2 to 6 days smaller than expected is associated with an increased risk (compared with a normal or slightly larger than expected CRL) of a birth weight less than 2500 g (relative risk [RR] 1.8), a birth weight less than 2500 g at term (RR 2.3), a birth weight below the 5th percentile for GA (RR 3.0), and delivery between 24 and 32 weeks' gestation (RR 2.1). In a prospective study of 976 assisted reproduction pregnancies, increased size for gestation in the first trimester was associated with higher birth weight, with the risk of of a small-for-GA newborn diminishing with increasing first-trimester embryonic/fetal size.[34] Thus, adverse outcomes in late pregnancy may at least in part be predicted by early pregnancy growth assessment using ultrasound.[23]

Variation in Growth in Twin Pregnancies

Twins provide a particularly useful model for assessing first-trimester growth. In cases in which there is a discrepancy in size between the two embryos or fetuses, the normally growing twin can be used as a control for the other. The incidence and significance of early intertwin growth discrepancy are controversial. In a study of 182 twin pregnancies (20 monochorionic and 162 dichorionic),[207] the authors observed that up to 95% of twins show discordance in CRL of up to 9.8 mm at 11 to 14 weeks, but there was no indication for further investigation should the fetal anatomy appear normal. In such cases, it may be more appropriate to date the pregnancy based on the smaller twin. Moreover, the risk of significant weight difference or poor outcome is not increased and discrepancy may simply reflect different growth patterns of two normal fetuses. In contrast, a discrepancy in the CRL greatly exceeding the 95th percentile is likely to reflect major growth delay in one twin, which is often aneuploid, and thus has the same significance as that in singletons.[207] In another large study of 200 monochorionic diamniotic twin gestations, the authors concluded that those who ultimately develop TTTS (see also Chapters 23 and 59) can exhibit intertwin differences in growth as early as 11 to 14 weeks.[211] The earlier the discordance, the earlier the manifestation of TTTS.[211]

Three-Dimensional Ultrasound

3DUS is increasingly being used in obstetric practice. The method offers several advantages during the first trimester because it allows visualization of planes that are otherwise difficult to obtain with two-dimensional scanning (2DUS). It could potentially minimize scan time and provides an excellent way to store scanned data for later study. However, no randomized controlled trials of 3DUS versus 2DUS have been published, and the benefits of 3DUS scanning remain speculative. If the 2DUS images are of poor quality, the resulting 3DUS images will be of little clinical use. As shown by Michailidis and colleagues,[124] 2DUS seems the best way to examine the first-trimester fetal anatomy. In some 94% of cases, a complete anatomic survey can be achieved with 2DUS. However, the examination was adequate in only 81% of cases with 3DUS ($P < .001$).

Several feasibility studies of NT measurement with 3DUS have been conducted.[212–215] Theoretically, an NT measurement could be performed regardless of the fetal position, significantly shortening examination time. Moreover, tomographic examination of the three-orthogonal sectional images should make it easy to distinguish fetal skin from the amnion. Paul and associates[212] concluded that reslicing of stored 3D volumes can be used to replicate NT measurements, but only if the nuchal skin is clearly seen on the 2DUS. When the fetus is lying in a position that precludes clear visualization of the nuchal area, 3DUS is unlikely to help.[212] Whereas Paul and associates[212] could repeat the NT measurement in only 60% using a 3D random volume, a number of other studies using 2D and 3D sonography for the measurement of NT show a good correlation between these two techniques at any position. Moreover, several investigators have observed benefit combining 3D with 2D scanning in the form of decreased acquisition time and an improvement in image resolution.[124,213–218] As a result, some authors have suggested 3DUS may be useful in scanning fetuses in a suboptimal position.[218,219] Chung and coworkers[215] and, more recently, Shaw and colleagues[219] demonstrated in pilot studies that the acquisition of 3D volumes can be a most effective and reproducible method of measuring NT. 3DUS also minimized scanning time and provided views not easily obtained using the strict NT guidelines.[219]

MATERNAL SERUM MARKERS AT 11 TO 14 WEEKS

Median serum concentrations of α-fetoprotein, estriol, and β-hCG (total and free) are independent of maternal age and can be combined in the second trimester to refine the risk of trisomy 21. This testing allows for the identification of approximately 60% of fetuses with trisomy 21 (compared with 30% based on maternal age alone) with a 5% invasive testing rate.[99,220]

Free β-hCG is even more discriminant in the first trimester (11–14 wk), and when combined with PAPP-A and maternal age, it provides an estimated detection rate of 60%, with a 5% invasive testing rate.[221]

Free β-Human Chorionic Gonadotropin

The maternal serum concentration of free β-hCG is higher in fetuses with trisomy 21 than in chromosomally normal fetuses. The MoM in pregnacies affected with trisomy 21 is approximately 2. First-trimester measurement of free β-hCG alone allows for the detection of 35% of fetuses with trisomy 21, with a 5% invasive testing rate. The detection rate is increased to 45% if the findings are integrated with maternal age.[221] The maternal serum free β-hCG level is decreased if the fetus has trisomy 13 or 18.[222,223] It is usually normal in women whose fetus has a sex chromosomal abnormality.[224]

Pregnancy-Associated Plasma Protein A

The PAPP-A level increases with gestation and is lower in pregnancies in which the fetus is affected with trisomy 21. The median value in trisomy 21 is approximately 0.5 MoM. When used alone in the first trimester, PAPP-A allows for the detection of 40% of fetuses with trisomy 21, with a 5% invasive testing rate. The detection rate increases to 50% when the findings are integrated with maternal age.[221] The maternal serum PAPP-A level is also decreased if the fetus has trisomy 13 or 18 or sex chromosomal abnormalities.[222–224]

Free β-Human Chorionic Gonadotropin and Pregnancy-Associated Plasma Protein A

When maternal age is combined with first-trimester maternal serum PAPP-A and free β-hCG levels, the estimated detection rate for trisomy 21 approximates 60%, with a 5% invasive testing rate.[221,225,226] These rates are similar to those obtained in the second trimester. Screening with a combination of fetal NT measurement and maternal levels of serum PAPP-A and free β-hCG allows the detection of approximately 90% of these chromosomal abnormalities, with a 5% invasive testing rate (Table 7–9).[1,227–235]

TABLE 7–9

Detection and False-Positive Rates of Screening Tests for Trisomy 21

SCREENING TEST	DETECTION RATE (%)	FALSE-POSITIVE RATE (%)
MA	30 (or 50)	5 (or 15)
MA + serum β-hCG + PAPP-A at 11–14 wk	60	5
MA + fetal NT at 11–14 wk	75 (or 70)	5 (or 2)
MA + fetal NT + NB at 11–14 wk	90	5
MA + fetal NT + serum β-hCG + PAPP-A at 11–14 wk	90 (or 80)	5 (or 2)
MA + fetal NT + NB + serum β-hCG + PAPP-A at 11–14 wk	97 (or 95)	5 (or 2)
MA + serum biochemistry at 15–18 wk	60–70	5
Ultrasound for fetal defects and markers at 16–23 wk	75	10–15
MA + serum β-hCG + PAPP-A at 11–14 wk ± DV, TR, NB (individual risk-oriented two-stage)	90	2–3

β-hCG, β-human chorionic gonadotropin; DV, ductus venosus; MA, maternal age; NB, nasal bone; NT, nuchal translucency; PAPP-A, pregnancy-associated plasma protein-A; TR, tricuspid regurgitation.

Logistic and Organizational Issues

There is no significant relationship between the NT measurement and the maternal serum free β-hCG or PAPP-A levels whether or not the pregnancy is affected by aneuploidy. Therefore, ultrasonographic and biochemical markers can be combined in the first trimester to provide more effective screening than either method individually. The same is true for NT measurement and second-trimester biochemical markers.[236] Many European countries have adopted first-trimester screening for chromosomal abnormalities with a combination of ultrasound NT measurement and maternal serum testing.[237,238]

In 1997, the 32nd Study Group of the Royal College of Obstetricians and Gynaecologists concluded that the evidence in favor of first-trimester screening for trisomy 21 by NT measurement or biochemical testing was sufficiently well developed to justify moving out of the research phase and into routine practice. They also concluded that ultrasound in early pregnancy is superior to biochemical screening in the second trimester. Several large studies support these conclusions.[98,237–241] Spencer and associates[242] studied 12,339 women with singleton pregnancies who were screened by the measurement of NT and maternal serum markers at 11 to 14 weeks in a one-stop clinic for assessment of risk (OSCAR).[242] These authors too concluded it was time to shift the screening for trisomy 21 from the second to the first trimester.[242]

Fetal Nuchal Translucency Measurement and Maternal Serum Free β-Human Chorionic Gonadotropin and Pregnancy-Associated Plasma Protein A (Combined Screening Test)

Spencer and coworkers[235] concluded that the most effective method of screening for trisomy 21 was achieved by a combination of maternal age, fetal NT, and maternal serum free β-hCG and PAPP-A concentrations at 11 + 0 to 13 + 6 weeks' gestation. The detection rate for trisomy 21 was 92% (23 of 25) for a 5% screen-positive rate, a rate far superior to that achieved with maternal age alone (30%) or by maternal age and second-trimester serum biochemistry (65%). This combined method for first-trimester screening also identified 94% of all other major chromosomal defects, such as trisomies 13 and 18, triploidy, and Turner's syndrome, and 60% of other chromosomal defects, such as deletions, partial trisomies, unbalanced translocations, and sex chromosomal aneuploidy other than Turner's syndrome.[98] Wapner and colleagues[240] achieved similar results in a prospective study of 8514 patients (detection rate 78.7%, 5% screen-positive rate) (Table 7–10).

In twin pregnancies, the combination of first-trimester NT and maternal serum biochemistry is less effective than in singleton pregnancies because placental products from the normal twin can mask the abnormal levels of the affected twin. Further, an abnormal result cannot distinguish which twin is affected.[243] As consequence, the combination of first-trimester NT and maternal serum biochemistry is less effective than in singleton pregnancies and not at present recommended. NT screening alone, however, provides similar detection and false-positive rates in multiples as in singleton pregnancies. There may be new options in the future. The authors of one large study concluded that twin pregnancy screening requires an adjustment of the calculated MoM to account for the presence of two fetuses. In general, this should be by dividing the observed corrected MoM by 2.023 for free β-HCG. Two different correction factors are required for PAPP-A, 2.192 in dichorionic twins and 1.788 in monochorionic twins.[244] Further, the distribuition of PAPP-A in monochorionic twins is lower than in dichorionic twins, as previously suggested.[245] Such corrections require an accurate diagnosis of chorionicity. Alternative strategies have been proposed[246] that use estimated distributions of markers in twins rather than making correction for twins and the calculation of a singleton equivalent or pseudorisk. The problem with this approach is the sparse data available to determine the distribution of markers in twins concordant or discordant for trisomy 21.

TABLE 7–10

Major Prospective and Retrospective Studies that Used a Combination of Maternal Age, Fetal Nuchal Translucency, Maternal Serum Pregnancy-Associated Plasma Protein A, and Free β-Human Chorionic Gonadotropin to Detect Down Syndrome

STUDY	N	PREVALENCE OF TRISOMY 21 (%)	GESTATION (WK)	FALSE-POSITIVE RATE (%)	DETECTION RATE FOR TRISOMY 21 (%)
Orlandi et al, 1997[227]	744	0.9	9–13.4	5	87
De Biasio et al, 1999[231]	1467	0.9	10–13+6	3.3	85
Spencer et al, 1999[221]	1156	18	10–14	5	89
Krantz et al, 2000[228]	5809	0.8	9–13+6	5	91
Hafner et al, 2001[232]	3316	0.3	10–13	4.1	90
Niemimaa et al, 2001[230]	1602	0.3		5	80
Bindra et al, 2002[234]	15,030	0.5	11–14	5	90.2
Von Kaisenberg et al, 2002[229]	3864	0.5	11–14	6.6	84.2
Crossley et al, 2002[233]	12,560	0.2	10–14	5	82
Spencer et al, 2003[235]	12,339	0.2	10–14	5.2	92

Individual Risk-Oriented Two-Stage First-Trimester Screening

Studies from fetal medicine centers demonstrate that in addition to NT, other highly sensitive and specific first-trimester sonographic markers of trisomy 21 can be used to enhance screening. They include the absence of the NB and increased impedance to flow in the DV and TR.[136,143,152] The addition of these new ultrasound markers to the combined screen (NT and free β-hCG and PAPP-A) requires a sufficient degree of independence among the markers, and this has been shown for NB,[137] TR,[147] and DV.[151] A prospective study of more than 75,000 pregnancies examined the potential impact of a new individual risk-oriented two-stage approach to screening.[118] After undergoing combined fetal NT and maternal serum free β-hCG and PAPP-A screening, patients were assigned to either a high risk category with a risk estimate of 1 in 100 or more, a low-risk category with a risk estimate of less than 1 in 1000, or an intermediate-risk category with a risk estimate of between 1 in 101 and 1 in 1000. Those in the intermediate-risk category had further assessment of risk by first-trimester ultrasound to determine the presence/absence of the NB, normal/abnormal Doppler velocity waveform in the DV, or the presence/absence of TR. Chorionic villus sampling was offered if their adjusted risk became 1 in 100 or more.[118] The results of this study demonstrate that individual risk-oriented two-stage screening for trisomy 21 can potentially identify in the first trimester of pregnancy more than 90% of affected fetuses with a screen-positive rate of 2% to 3%. However, the accurate examination for these markers is time-consuming and requires skilled operators. Although it is unlikely this assessment will be incorporated into the routine first-trimester scan, it is likely to be used in fetal medicine centers across the board or to evaluate the risk in patients with intermediate risk after screening by fetal NT and maternal serum biochemistry.

FETAL NUCHAL TRANSLUCENCY MEASUREMENT AND MATERNAL SERUM MARKERS AT 14 TO 17 WEEKS

Sonographic and biochemical screening methods evolved independently. As a result, many women undergo sequential two-stage screening, even if the NT screen result is negative. Each method is designed to generate a 5% invasive testing rate, and the two-stage screening paradigm has a cumulative rate. Thus, the proportion of patients undergoing invasive prenatal diagnostic testing can be as high as 10%, or even higher in countries that offer invasive prenatal diagnosis to women older than 35 years, regardless of the screening result. This illogical approach increases the iatrogenic loss rate of normal pregnancies and all related costs. The rate of invasive testing for fetal karyotyping is indeed an important public health issue that must be controlled. When the combined first-trimester test is not available, one approach is to combine NT measurement and second-trimester maternal serum screening into a single risk assessment and not to consider the results independently (integrated screening) (Table 7–11).[236] At least in that instance, the screen-positive rate remains around 5%.

TABLE 7–11

Definitions

TERM	DEFINITION
Combined screening	Nuchal translucency measurement + first-trimester serum markers
Fully integrated screening	Nuchal translucency measurement + first-trimester serum markers + second-trimester serum markers
Serum integrated screening	Pregnancy-associated plasma protein-A + second-trimester serum markers
Sequential screening	Successive independent risk assessments, leading to cumulative false-positive rates
Individual risk-oriented two-stage first-trimester screening	Nuchal translucency measurement + first-trimester serum markers ± NB, DV, TR

DV, ductus venosus; NB, nasal bone; TR, tricuspid regurgitation.

In women undergoing second-trimester biochemical testing after first-trimester NT screening (with or without maternal serum testing), the background risk must be adjusted to take into account the first-trimester screening results. Otherwise, it should not be done. For example, a 41-year-old woman whose age-related background risk of having a fetus with trisomy 21 is 1 in 50 has reduced risk (e.g., 1 in 200) after a thin NT. If the risk then after second-trimester screening with serum markers is 1 in 100, this woman has an integrated risk of 1 in 400 because the NT measurement allowed a fourfold reduction of the background risk and maternal serum testing has done so by twofold. Use of both tests, therefore, divided the background risk by 8. Because first-trimester combined screen can identify almost 90% of pregnancies affected by trisomy 21, second-trimester serum testing identifies, at best, an additional 6% of affected pregnancies (60% of the residual 10%), but doubles the overall invasive testing rate from 5% to 10%. It is theoretically possible to use various statistical techniques to combine NT measurement with different components of first- and second-trimester serum testing.[133] One hypothetical model combines the first-trimester NT measurement and PAPP-A testing with second-trimester free β-hCG, estriol, and inhibin A testing (fully integrated test), claiming a potential sensitivity of 90%, for a 5% false-positive rate.[241] This offers no advantage over comprehensive first-trimester screening.

In a multicenter interventional study,[236] NT was measured at 12 to 14 weeks' gestation in 9444 women. Maternal serum markers were measured between 14 weeks and 1 day and 17 weeks' gestation. Karyotyping was delayed until after maternal blood was obtained. A combined risk for NT measurement and maternal serum markers was estimated retrospectively. The invasive testing rate generated by sequential two-stage screening was 8.6%, which means that 8.6% of patients underwent amniocentesis because of an increased risk generated by any of these tests. Twenty-one fetuses (0.22%) had trisomy 21. Adjusting for a 5% invasive testing rate, the detection rates would have been 55% and 80% for NT measurement alone and NT measurement combined with second-trimester serum marker testing, respectively. The results of the study suggest a 25% increase in the detection rate with a combination of NT measurement at 12 to 14 weeks and serum marker studies between 14 weeks and 1 day and 17 weeks, with a 5% invasive testing rate and a modest increase in cost. Four other studies reported screening with a combination of fetal NT measurement in the first trimester and maternal serum marker testing in the second trimester, with similar results.[236–239]

Sequential (but not integrated) screening programs also increase the invasive procedure–related pregnancy loss rate. This increased rate is an important issue in populations in which the prevalence of Down syndrome is less than 1 in 1000 births. In these populations, an invasive testing rate of 8.6% might be considered unacceptably high in women who are at relatively low risk,[236] compared with the 5% rate generated by a single-test screening program. A single risk assessment that integrates the results of NT measurement, free β-hCG levels, and α-fetoprotein levels with maternal age is possible. Here, it would be possible to keep the sensitivity as high as that obtained with combined screening while maintaining an invasive testing rate as low as 5%. However, the cost is also significant because the 25% increase in the detection rate would delay risk calculation and invasive testing by 2 to 4 weeks. Such information should be included in genetic counseling, especially when termination for fetal abnormality is an issue. Further, screening strategies in the first trimester are cost-effective compared with the use of second-trimester biochemical markers.[236]

SUMMARY OF MANAGEMENT OPTIONS
First-Trimester Screening for Fetal Abnormalities

Management Options	Evidence Quality and Recommendation	References
General Approach		
Prerequisites:	See also Chapter 4	
• Details of the history, examination, and routine tests completed and known relevant risk factors identified		
• Prescan interview, discussions, and counseling		
Screening is performed ideally between 11 and 14 wk.	III/B	235
Ultrasound is considered safe in both the short and the long terms.	Ib/A	243
First-Trimester Screening—Benefits		
Confirm viability.	III/B	7,10
Dating the pregnancy by crown-rump length before 14 wk is the most accurate method and decreases the risk of post-term pregnancy.	III	22,24–28, 207
Screening for fetal aneuploidy:		
• NT measurement, combined with maternal age and maternal serum markers for trisomy 21, has a detection rate of 80%–90%, for a 5% false-positive rate.	IIa/B	235,236
• Other chromosomal abnormalities are also more likely with increased NT thickness.	III/B	103–106
Detection of structural abnormalities:		
• Some major structural anomalies are detectable as early as 12 wk. These include anencephaly, holoprosencephaly, abdominal wall defects, and major limb defects.	IIb/B	71,109,113
• Detection rates are dependent on sonographer experience.	III/B	162
Multiple pregnancy:		
• Chorionicity is optimally determined by either visualization or absence of the lambda sign.	III/B	40
• Twin–twin transfusion syndrome is more likely in monochorionic pregnancies with increased NT thickness.	III/B	133
Examine the uterus and adnexal structures.	GPP	

GPP, good practice point; NT, nuchal translucency.

SUGGESTED READINGS

Bottomley C, Bourne T: Dating and growth in the first trimester. Best Pract Res Clin Obstet Gynaecol 2009;23:439–452.

Cicero S, Rembouskos G, Vandecruys H, et al: Likelihood ratio for trisomy 21 in fetuses with absent nasal bone at the 11–14-week scan. Ultrasound Obstet Gynecol 2004;23:218–223.

Nicolaides KH: Screening for chromosomal defects. Ultrasound Obstet Gynecol 2003;21:313–321.

Nicolaides KH, Spencer K, Avgidou K, et al: Multicenter study of first trimester screening for trisomy 21 in 75,821 pregnancies: Results and estimation of the potential impact of individual risk-orientated two-stage first-trimester screening. Ultrasound Obstet Gynecol 2005;25:221–226.

Senat MV, De Keersmaecker B, Audibert F, et al: Pregnancy outcome in fetuses with increased nuchal translucency and normal karyotype. Prenat Diagn 2002;22:345–349.

Snijders RJM, Noble P, Sebire N, et al: UK multicentre project on assessment of risk of trisomy 21 by maternal age and fetal nuchal translucency thickness at 10–14 weeks of gestation. Lancet 1998;351:343–346.

Spencer K, Spencer CE, Power M, et al: Screening for chromosomal abnormalities in the first trimester using ultrasound and maternal serum biochemistry in a one-stop clinic: A review of three years prospective experience. BJOG 2003;110:281–286.

Timor-Tritsch IE, Fuchs KM, Monteagudo A, D'Alton ME: Performing a fetal anatomy scan at the time of first-trimester screening. Obstet Gynecol 2009;113:402–407.

REFERENCES

For a complete list of references, log onto www.expertconsult.com.

CHAPTER 8

Second-Trimester Screening for Fetal Abnormalities

LAMI YEO and ANTHONY M. VINTZILEOS

Videos corresponding to this chapter are available online at www.expertconsult.com.

INTRODUCTION

Every pregnant woman desires a healthy child who is free of anomalies. In the general population, the overall risk of having a child with a major malformation is 3% to 5%. As a greater proportion of women delay childbirth, the shortened reproductive window has increased the pressure on all for a successful outcome and rendered the increasing sophistication of ultrasonography and biochemical testing for fetal abnormalities of growing importance to obstetricians and their patients. We find that genetic sonography is a patient-driven service. This chapter focuses on noninvasive modalities of screening for fetal abnormalities in the second trimester.

In the early 1970s, the only method available to screen for fetal Down syndrome was based on maternal age; amniocentesis was offered to all women above a certain age, typically 35 years or older. However, maternal age proved a very inefficient screening tool with less than one third of fetuses with trisomy 21 identified by this means. In the 1980s, a new screening method incorporated second-trimester maternal serum biochemical markers in addition to maternal age. In the 1990s, screening for Down syndrome by combining maternal age and fetal nuchal translucency (NT) thickness in the first trimester was introduced (see Chapter 7). Subsequently, maternal serum biochemical markers of value in the first trimester were identified. In the recent past, three-dimensional sonography entered the arena of screening.

Invasive tests, such as amniocentesis, chorionic villus sampling, and cordocentesis, are diagnostic tools and not screening tests. They allow for essentially 100% accuracy in the diagnosis of fetal aneuploidy but carry a real risk of pregnancy loss. Thus, many women choose biochemical and ultrasound screening modalities for aneuploidy detection because the test efficiency (percentage of abnormal fetuses identified) is so much higher than that based on maternal age alone, even though they have a relatively high invasive testing rate (the so-called false-positive rate), typically set at 5%. Based on the result of the screening test, a decision is made as to whether an invasive test for diagnosis is indicated and acceptable to the patient. The combination of screening and diagnostic tests allows the maximum number of women to gain accurate information about their individual risk status.

SECOND-TRIMESTER BIOCHEMICAL SERUM MARKER SCREENING

Maternal serum testing in the second trimester for the screening of women at low risk for fetal aneuploidy, neural tube defects, and other fetal anomalies remains a standard of care in many countries. Screening for trisomy 21 in low risk patients (women < 35 yr) was initiated in the mid-1980s with the observation that the mean maternal serum concentration of α-fetoprotein was 0.7 multiple of the median (MoM) in affected pregnancies.[1–3] Subsequently, it was recognized that human chorionic gonadotropin (hCG) levels were higher (2.04 MoM) and unconjugated estriol levels were lower (0.79 MoM) in pregnancies with trisomy 21.[4–7] By using the relative risks derived from maternal serum levels, the maternal age–related risk can be modified and a "triple-screen" risk can be derived for each woman.

Triple-marker screening has been the preferred screening modality in some locales for the detection of fetal trisomy 21 in women younger than 35 years.[7–10] In this group, the triple-marker screen identifies approximately 60% of pregnancies affected by trisomy 21 as being at risk, with a 5% screen-positive rate (Table 8–1). In the population of women 35 years and older, the triple-marker screen identifies 75% or more of pregnancies affected by trisomy 21 and some other aneuploidies.[11] Because the maternal age–related risk of trisomy 21 is the basis of the serum screening protocol, both the trisomy 21 detection rate and the screen-positive rate increase with maternal age.[12] Different laboratories use different screen-positive cutoffs. For example, some use the midtrimester risk of trisomy 21 in a 35-year-old woman (1 in 270). Others apply a screen-positive cutoff that provides an acceptable balance between the detection rate and the screen-positive rate (usually 1 in 190 or 1 in 200).

Maternal serum screening can be performed between 15 and 20 weeks but is most accurate between 16 and 18 weeks. Similarly to first-trimester screening, the pregnancy must be dated accurately because an error will affect the assigned risk, causing false-negative and false-positive results. It is important to recalculate the results if the dates are found to be in error or to have a new sample drawn if the original sample was obtained before 15 weeks. Other factors that are

TABLE 8-1

Various Sensitivities for Fetal Down Syndrome (False-Positive Rate of 5%) with Various Screening Tests in Combination

SCREENING TEST	SENSITIVITY FOR FETAL DOWN SYNDROME (%)
Age	30
Age, first-trimester biochemistry results	63
Age, NT	75
Age, first-trimester biochemistry results, NT	85-90
NT, nasal bone	90
Age, first-trimester biochemistry results, NT, nasal bone	97
Age, second-trimester triple-screen results	60-70
Age, second-trimester quadruple-screen results	67-75

NT, nuchal translucency.

incorporated into the risk calculation include the number of fetuses, maternal weight, race, and diabetes.

Serum screening is used primarily to detect trisomy 21, and it does not efficiently detect other fetal aneuploidies, except for possibly trisomy 18. Thus, serum screening misses both lethal (e.g., trisomy 13) and sex chromosomal abnormalities that are not associated with severe physical or developmental limitations or profound mental retardation.

During the first trimester, the free beta subunit of hCG (β-hCG) is superior as a marker to the intact hCG molecule, but this has not been proved in the second trimester. In 1992, the potential use of a fourth analyte (inhibin) in second-trimester screening for Down syndrome was first suggested by Van Lith and coworkers.[13] The median value of the maternal inhibin A level is increased at 1.77 MoM in Down syndrome pregnancies. However, inhibin A is not used in the calculation of risk for trisomy 18.[14] Dimeric inhibin A has emerged as the most promising analyte and is used by many commercial laboratories in combination with the three traditional analytes. This four-analyte combination ("quad screen") detects 67% to 76% cases of fetal trisomy 21 in women younger than 35 years, with a screen-positive rate of 5% or less.[15,16] In 2003, Benn and colleagues[17] screened over 23,000 women for Down syndrome using the quadruple test. They found the sensitivity to be 85.8% for an initial false-positive rate of 9% (which was further reduced to 8.2% after correction for major gestational age errors).

Diagnostic options are limited for screening multiple gestations in the second trimester. In dizygotic twins, the risk of trisomy 21 is calculated by considering the maternal age–related risk and the probability that one or both fetuses will be affected. Thus, the midtrimester risk of trisomy 21 in at least one fetus of a twin gestation in a 33-year-old woman approximates the risk in a singleton pregnancy of a 35-year-old woman.[18]

FETAL ANATOMIC SURVEY ON SECOND-TRIMESTER SONOGRAPHY

The introduction of two-dimensional (2D) static scanning in the early 1970s allowed physicians to view the fetus for the first time. In the late 1970s and early 1980s, real-time B-mode imaging emerged as a widespread clinical tool. The major advantage of ultrasound is the lack of a demonstrable adverse fetal effect[19] because the image is generated with sound waves and not ionizing radiation. It quickly became the preferred method during pregnancy. Despite its apparent safety, some believe fetal sonography should be used only when there is a clear indication. However, most complicated pregnancies are unexpected and occur in low risk women, and ultrasound examinations are routine throughout pregnancy in many countries. We agree that all pregnant women should have access to expert obstetric sonography given that 90% of infants with congenital anomalies are born to women with no risk factors.[20] Ultrasound resolution has improved dramatically, and a detailed examination of the fetus for both structural anomalies and markers of aneuploidy is possible. The diagnosis and management of specific congenital fetal abnormalities are discussed in other chapters. We focus here on the elements of a complete sonographic fetal anatomic survey.

The sonographic examination should be systematic and thorough. Normal findings provide reassurance to patients, and the examination should detect most fetal malformations, along with abnormalities in fetal growth, the placenta, amniotic fluid, and the cervix. We also examined the value, from a patient's perspective, of a targeted ultrasound examination performed after an abnormal karyotype was discovered.[21] All women valued the scan because it helped them to visualize the fetal anomalies and accept the diagnosis of aneuploidy, which, in turn, affected their plans for pregnancy management. All patients considered the effect of the ultrasound greater than that of the chromosomal diagnosis alone, and all believed that ultrasound should be used for patients in similar clinical situations.

The American Institute of Ultrasound in Medicine (AIUM) first published standards for the performance of obstetric ultrasound in 1994.[22] The most recent AIUM *Practice Guideline for the Performance of Obstetric Ultrasound Examinations* was published in 2007.[23] Although it describes indications for second- and third-trimester ultrasound examinations, it notes that the list is by no means inclusive. Imaging parameters for a standard fetal examination in the second and third trimester include (1) fetal cardiac activity, number, presentation (multiple gestations require additional documentation); (2) qualitative or semiquantitative estimate of amniotic fluid volume; (3) placental location, appearance, and relationship to the internal cervical os; (4) imaging of the umbilical cord, and the number of vessels in the cord should be evaluated when possible; (5) gestational (menstrual) age (via biparietal diameter, head circumference, femoral diaphysis length, abdominal circumference, or average abdominal diameter); (6) fetal weight estimation; (7) maternal anatomy (uterus, adnexal structures, cervix); (8) and fetal anatomic survey.[23] The fetal anatomic survey, as described by the AIUM, involves the following areas of assessment: head, face, and neck, chest (including four-chamber view of the fetal heart), abdomen, stomach, kidneys, bladder, abdominal cord insertion site, spine, extremities, and sex.[23] They note that the basic cardiac examination includes a four-chamber view of the fetal heart; however, if technically feasible, views of the outflow tracts should be attempted as part of the cardiac screening examination.[23]

TABLE 8–2

Content of Fetal Anatomic Survey on Second-Trimester Sonography

ORGAN STRUCTURES
Head
Cranial shape, mineralization
Cerebral hemispheres, thalami, cerebral peduncles, lateral ventricles and choroid plexus, third and fourth ventricles, cerebellum and vermis, cisterna magna, cavum septum pellucidum
Face and Neck
Profile, orbits, lips and palate, nasal bone, nuchal fold, ear
Thoracic Cavity
Lungs
Configuration of the bony thorax
Heart
Four-chamber views (apical and subcostal), outflow tracts, longitudinal parasternal arches, inferior and superior vena cava, valves, atria and ventricular septa
Abdomen
Situs
Stomach
Liver, gallbladder, spleen
Bowel
Wall and cord insertion site
Genitourinary System
Kidneys
Bladder
Genitalia
Spine
Extremities
Upper, including both hands
Lower, including both feet
Cord
Number of vessels
Biometric Measurements
Biparietal diameter
Head circumference
Atria of lateral ventricles, cisterna magna, nuchal fold (when applicable)
Cerebellum
Thoracic circumference (when applicable)
Abdominal circumference
Femur length, humerus length, radius and ulna lengths, tibia and fibula lengths
Foot length
Nasal bone length
Orbital diameters
Other
Number of fetuses, position
Placenta
Amniotic fluid
Cervix and lower uterine segment

This was a compromise document, and we suggest the current state of the art requires a more detailed examination than that described by the AIUM for optimal diagnostic accuracy of fetal abnormalities (Table 8–2). Moreover, sonographer training must be focused and audited to ensure these detailed examinations are done appropriately. The sonographer must be familiar with normal fetal anatomy, sonographic landmarks, and normal variants. An adequate examination requires proper equipment. The highest-frequency transducer should be used to maximize the resolution of the fetal anatomy.

The entire uterus is scanned transversely and longitudinally to determine the fetal position, amniotic fluid volume, and placental location. Accurate determination of the right and left sides of the fetus is crucial. Factors that may limit visualization (Table 8–3) include equipment quality, fluid abnormalities, maternal body habitus (discussed later) or tissue density, and other scanning characteristics. Techniques to improve visualization include changing the maternal position (to effectively change the fetal position) and using different scanning probes (including transvaginal). The timing of the second-trimester ultrasound varies with the center and physician preference. Repeating the examination later may aid the resolution of anatomic detail of some structures (e.g., heart) but hinder visualization of others (e.g., extremities). This is not to infer that scanning, even late in pregnancy, cannot provide important information and be highly sensitive for fetal anomalies whose diagnosis will alter pregnancy management. We recommend that the fetal anatomy survey be performed at 18 to 22 weeks to optimize the assessment of anatomy while leaving an adequate window for invasive testing, if necessary. Scans performed during this window are less likely than earlier scans to end incompletely and trigger the need for a repeat examination. In addition to evaluating the fetal anatomy, the number and position of fetuses should be determined. The placental appearance, thickness, echogenicity, and location are important to document, along with amniotic fluid volume. Amniotic fluid abnormalities may indicate an

TABLE 8–3

Factors That May Limit Sonographic Examination of the Fetal Anatomy

Equipment quality
Sonographer expertise
Length of time spent scanning
Quality of sonographic examination performed
Frequency of sonographic examinations
Maternal habitus, tissue density, and scanning characteristics
Incomplete filling or overfilling of the bladder
Fetal positioning
Type of congenital anomaly
Fluid abnormalities (increased or decreased)
Gestational age (early or late)
Timing of the exam (scan done *before* the development of detectable abnormalities or lesions *resolve* over time)
Ossification of fetal bony structures (later in gestation)
Fetal death in utero
Fetal movement

anomalous fetus (e.g., anhydramnios is associated with renal agenesis and polyhydramnios with esophageal atresia). The fetal echocardiogram is best performed between 22 and 24 weeks, when the cardiac structures are larger.

Content of the Fetal Anatomic Survey

The examination begins with the fetal head and proceeds caudally. Imaging the fetal intracranial anatomy is extremely important because central nervous system anomalies can have a devastating effect on perinatal morbidity and mortality. The calvarium can be identified from the late first trimester onward. It should be well mineralized (hypomineralization may indicate a skeletal dysplasia) and elliptical in shape by the second trimester. Brachycephaly (anteroposterior shortening) suggests fetal trisomy 21 or 18 ("strawberry" head). A "lemon"-shaped head suggests a neural tube defect. Tangential imaging shows cranial sutures (hypoechoic spaces between bones) that are best visualized early in gestation. Premature closure of the sutures occurs in many syndromes (e.g., craniosynostosis) and with several skeletal dysplasias.

The transthalamic view is an axial view through the brain at the level of the thalami (Fig. 8–1). It is here that the biparietal diameter and head circumference measurements are obtained. Biparietal diameter is measured from the outer margin of the near calvarium to the inner margin of the far calvarium (with cranial bones perpendicular to the ultrasound beam). The head circumference is measured circumferentially at the outer margin of the calvarium (see Fig. 8–1). Other structures that are visualized in the transthalamic view include the cavum septum pellucidum (a fluid-filled midline structure anterior to the thalami), midline falx, third ventricle (between the thalami), and frontal horns of the lateral ventricles. A normal cavum suggests proper midline brain formation; its absence may signal abnormalities, such as holoprosencephaly, septo-optic dysplasia, or agenesis of the corpus callosum. The transventricular view is just superior to the transthalamic view and includes the lateral ventricles that contain sonolucent cerebrospinal fluid. Within this lies the echogenic choroid plexus that normally fills the atrium and may contain cysts (a potential marker for trisomy 18) (Figs. 8–2 and 8–3). The cerebral ventricle is measured through the atrium in an axial plane and is normally less than 10 mm. The transcerebellar view contains the cerebellum and vermis, cisterna magna (between the dorsum of the cerebellar hemispheres and inner calvarium), and nuchal fold (Fig. 8–4). Visualization of this area is important to exclude spina bifida; obliteration of the cisterna magna and a banana-shaped cerebellum typically occur with this disorder. This view is also used to exclude Dandy-Walker malformation or variant, occipital encephalocele, and cerebellar agenesis or hypoplasia. The nuchal fold should be less than 6 mm, although with a breech presentation, an extended head onto the neck, or increased pressure by the transducer over the fetal head, this may create a false-positive thickening. The transcerebellar diameter provides a useful estimate of gestational age because it is relatively spared by fetal growth disturbances, including intrauterine growth restriction.[24] Sometimes, the fetal head is low in the pelvis, blocking access to the intracranial structures; in this case, transvaginal scanning is often useful.

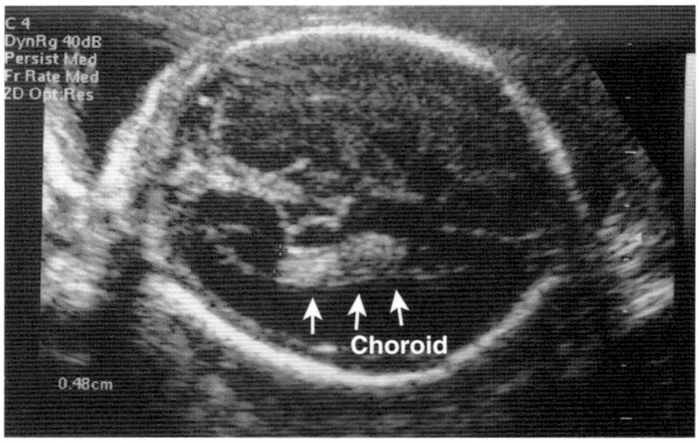

FIGURE 8–2
Transventricular view of the fetal head shows measurement of the atria of the lateral ventricle (0.48 cm) and the echogenic choroid plexus (*arrows*).

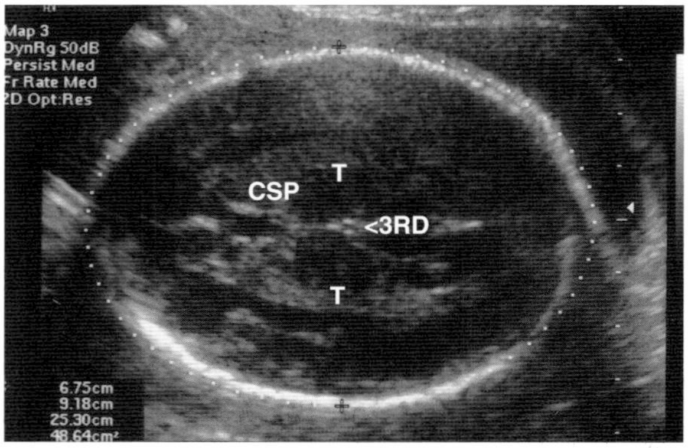

FIGURE 8–1
Axial view through the fetal head shows the thalami (T), falx, third ventricle (3rd) between the thalami, and cavum septum pellucidum (CSP). The calipers also show measurement of the head circumference.

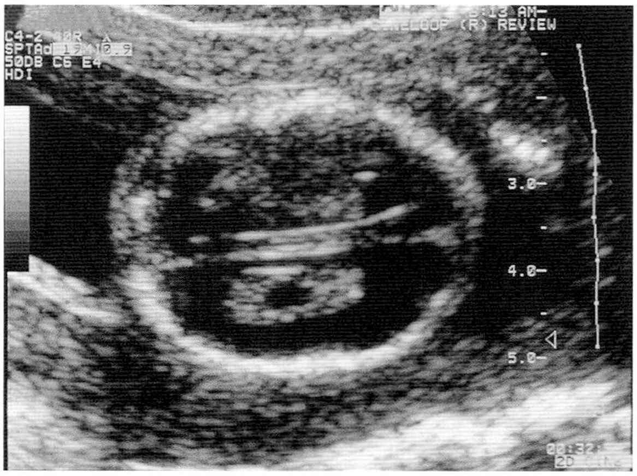

FIGURE 8–3
A single sonolucent choroid plexus cyst in the far lateral ventricle.

FIGURE 8–4
Transcerebellar view shows the cerebellar hemispheres, cisterna magna and a normal nuchal fold measurement (0.34 cm).

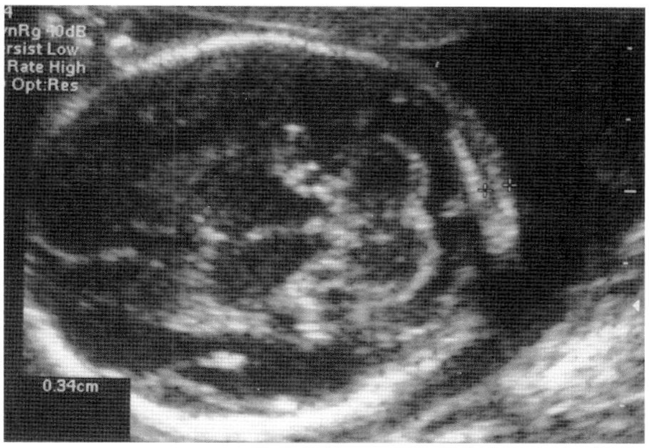

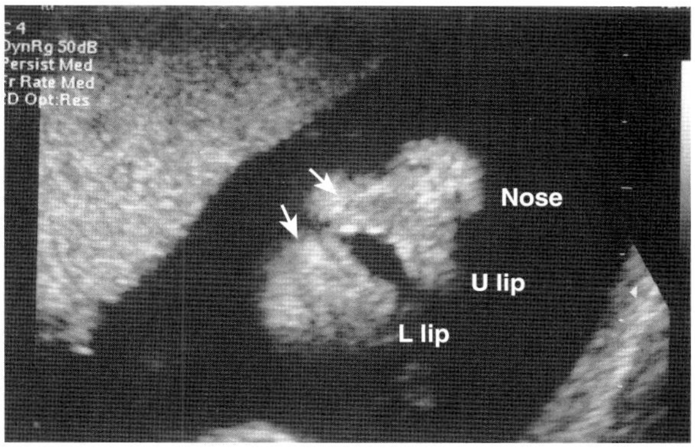

FIGURE 8–5
Coronal view of the fetal face shows the nose, and upper and lower lips (*arrows*).

FIGURE 8–6
Sagittal facial profile of a third-trimester fetus with Down syndrome shows the tongue protruding between the upper and the lower lips.

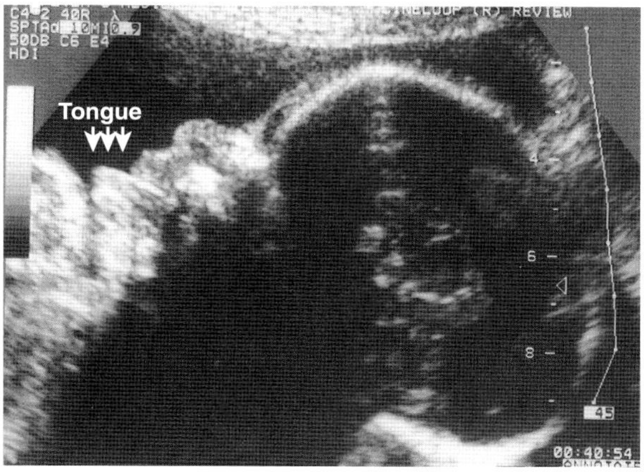

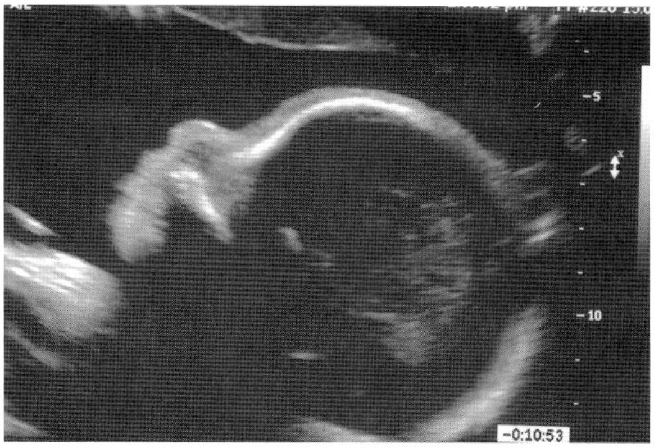

FIGURE 8–7
Profile of a fetus with Down syndrome shows frontal bone, but absent nasal bone.

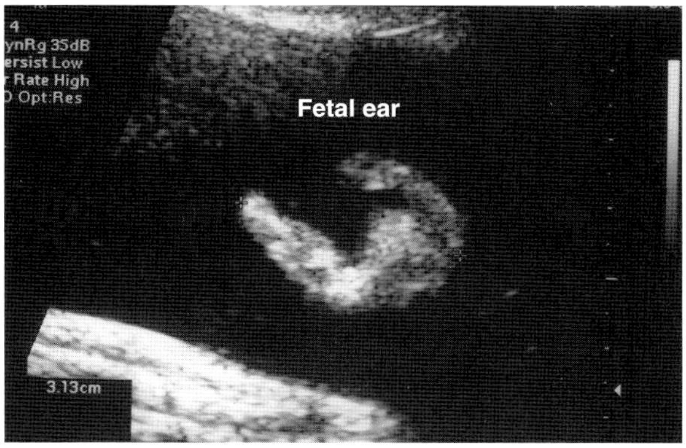

FIGURE 8–8
Frontal view of the fetal ear showing caliper placement.

The facial structures should be examined routinely because they are especially important for the diagnosis of genetic disorders or syndromes. This is accomplished with coronal (Fig. 8–5), sagittal (profile) (Fig. 8–6), and axial views. A combination of these planes is often optimal. Structures important to image include the chin (for micrognathia), nasal bone (NB; absent or shortened) (Fig. 8–7), nose, lips, anterior palate (to exclude cleft lip or palate), orbits (and diameters, if necessary, to exclude hypertelorism or hypotelorism), and ear (which may be shortened in aneuploid and nonaneuploid fetuses) (Fig. 8–8).

Next, the fetal spine is imaged in sagittal (Fig. 8–9), transverse, and coronal views, when possible. The overlying skin should be intact to exclude open spina bifida and masses or tumors. Each normal vertebral segment consists of three echogenic ossification centers (two located posteriorly and one located anteriorly that is the vertebral body) lying in a symmetrical, triangular configuration. In the transverse plane, the posterior processes appear angled in the same way as the roof of a house; if they are splayed, a neural tube defect should be sought (Fig. 8–10). Sagittal and coronal views are useful to observe how well the ossification centers align to exclude hemivertebrae that cause disorganization or absence of ossification centers. The sacrum should curve gently upward.

The ribs, clavicles, and scapulae are examined next. A normal appearance excludes some types of skeletal dysplasia.

FIGURE 8–9
Normal sagittal view of the fetal spine. The overlying skin is intact, and the features of the spinal centers are parallel.

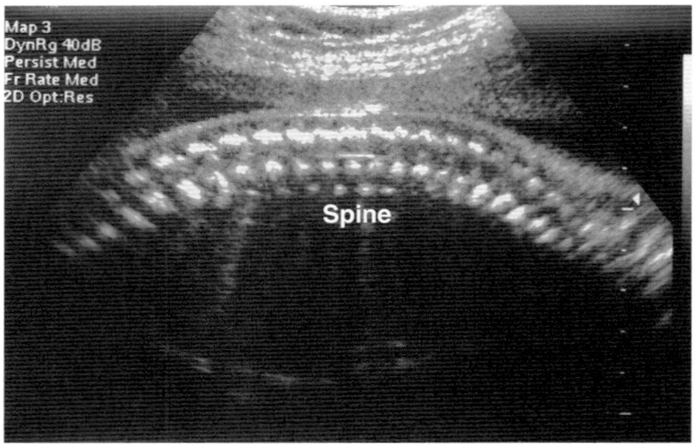

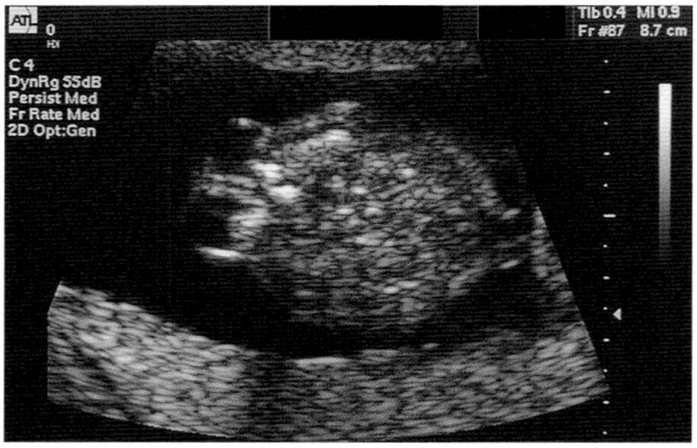

FIGURE 8–10
Transverse view of the fetal spine shows a large neural tube defect with splaying of the posterior processes.

FIGURE 8–11
Apical four-chamber view of the fetal heart shows the left atrium (LA) and ventricle (LV) and right atrium (RA) and ventricle (RV).

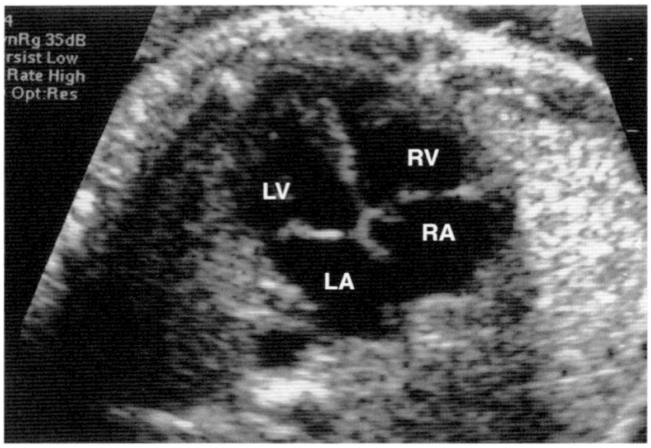

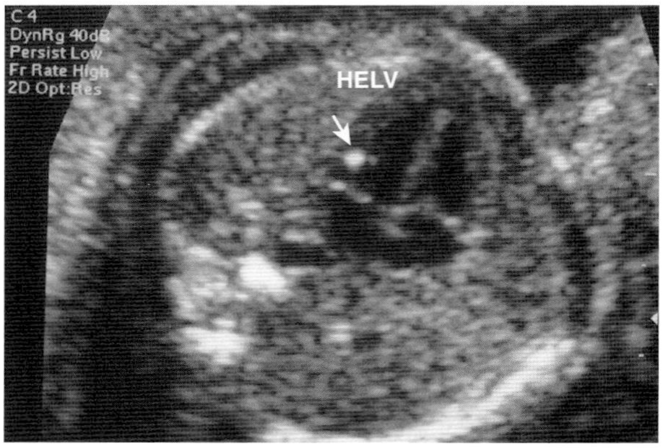

FIGURE 8–12
Apical four-chamber view of the fetal heart shows a single, bright, echogenic focus in the left ventricle (HELV).

Abnormal lung tissue or echogenicity (e.g., cystic adenomatoid malformation) or pleural effusions may be seen. The thoracic circumference is measured to exclude pulmonary hypoplasia, and the diaphragm is examined for evidence of a hernia.

A detailed fetal cardiac examination is perhaps the most challenging task for the sonographer. The cardiac rate and rhythm (normally 120–150 beats/min and regular), size (one third of the fetal thorax), axis and position (apex points to the left at an angle of 45 ± 20 degrees relative to the midline), and situs should be established (liver on the right, stomach on the left). Alterations in position, axis, or both suggest malposition or an intrathoracic mass causing mediastinal shift. Multiple planes and views are used in real time to exclude cardiac defects. Routine imaging of the outflow tracts increases detection sensitivity and should be part of the standard fetal cardiac examination. When screening for cardiac defects, the examination should include, minimally, the four-chamber apical (Fig. 8–11) and subcostal views, outflow tracts, longitudinal parasternal arches (aortic and ductal), inferior and superior venae cava, valves, and atria and ventricular septa. The chambers are roughly equal in size. The pulmonary veins should enter the left atrium; the two atrioventricular valves and septa should be visualized in their entirety, and the rate and rhythm documented as well as the axis, position, and size of the heart. The great vessels should cross each other, and there should be no dependent pericardial fluid. Some recommend routine color, M-mode, or pulsed Doppler sonography to assist in the visualization of the heart and great vessels and to exclude significant valvular stenosis or regurgitation (see Chapter 16 for a discussion of specific cardiac abnormalities). An echogenic focus is commonly seen, typically in the left ventricle. It is caused by specular reflection from the papillary muscles and chordae tendineae (Fig. 8–12).[25]

Identifiable intra-abdominal organs include the liver (occupying most of the upper abdomen), spleen (solid organ posterior to the stomach), gallbladder (teardrop-shaped organ in the right upper quadrant, at the inferior edge of the liver), stomach, bowel, umbilical vein, and umbilical cord insertion site. The abdominal circumference is the single most sensitive fetal growth parameter. It is measured at the transverse level, where the umbilical vein joins the right portal venous system (Fig. 8–13), which should "curve" away from the stomach. If the curve is toward the stomach, persistence of the right umbilical vein is suspected. The stomach and spine should be imaged in this axial plane; the stomach should always be located below the diaphragm. An absent

FIGURE 8–13
Correct method for measuring the abdominal circumference. P, portal vein; ST, stomach; U, umbilical vein.

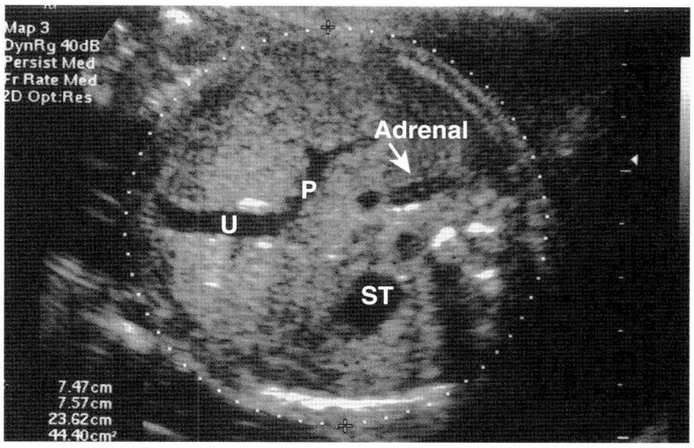

FIGURE 8–14
Fetal hand shows echogenic phalanges of four fingers, including the fifth digit. The thumb is not visible in this image.

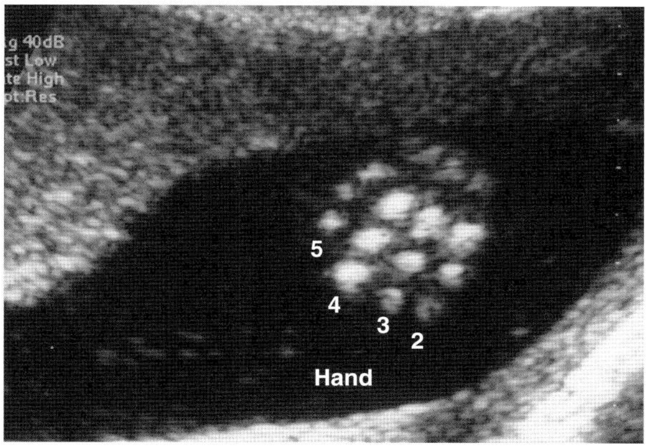

or small stomach, despite prolonged scanning to allow for filling, suggests esophageal atresia, with or without tracheoesophageal fistula, or a diaphragmatic hernia (stomach located within the chest). Most of the abdomen is bowel-filled, and the appearance varies with gestational age. In the second trimester, the bowel appears as midlevel to increased echogenicity filling the abdomen. Hyperechoic bowel is associated with aneuploidy, infection, cystic fibrosis, and bowel abnormalities, and may also be seen with intrauterine growth restriction. In the third trimester, prominent hypoechoic loops of colon may be seen. More dilated loops of bowel may reflect atresia or another cause of obstruction. The umbilical cord insertion and the adjacent ventral abdominal wall should be visualized to exclude ventral wall defects (e.g., omphalocele, gastroschisis). There should be no fetal ascites.

Next visualized is the genitourinary tract, which is a common site for fetal anomalies. The kidneys are bilateral, hypoechoic, paraspinal structures that include the urine-containing renal pelvis. Abnormal findings include dilation of the renal pelvis, calix, or ureter; renal masses; cysts within the parenchyma; hyperechogenicity; and enlargement or absence of the kidneys. Color or power Doppler imaging is useful to identify the renal arteries, especially when the kidneys cannot be seen in their usual location. It is important to distinguish between pyelectasis (dilated renal pelvis) and hydronephrosis (pyelectasis plus upper tract dilation). The bladder is a urine-filled structure located midline, anterior, and low in the fetal pelvis. Absence of the fetal bladder (bladder exstrophy) or a very enlarged bladder (lower obstructive uropathy) should be excluded. The sonographer should confirm that the two umbilical arteries course around the fetal bladder. This image all but excludes a two-vessel cord. Gender is assigned by imaging the genitalia, and not by the lack of an image. Ambiguous genitalia should be excluded. The fetus is male if both the penis and scrotum are seen. The testicles are echogenic and usually descend into the scrotum around 28 weeks. The labia appear as several parallel linear echoes.

All extremities (including hands and feet) should be surveyed because they might provide important diagnostic information. The five fingers should extend fully (Fig. 8–14). Movement and tone should be normal, and the middle

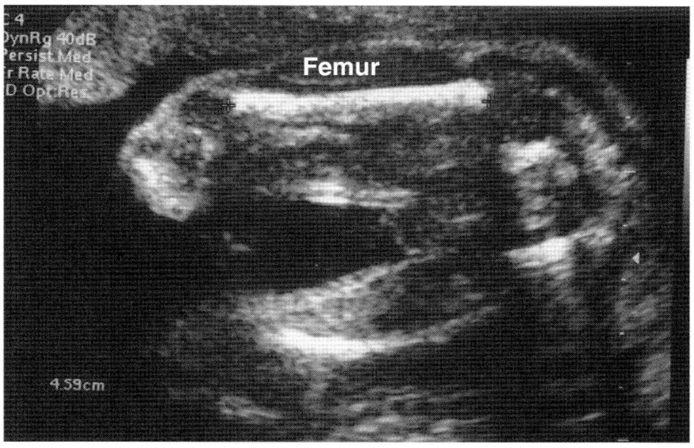

FIGURE 8–15
Femur length measured from the proximal end to the distal metaphysis.

phalanx of the fifth digit should be visualized. Persistently clenched hands with overlapping digits are a highly sensitive (95%) sonographic feature for trisomy 18.[26] The long bones (femur, humerus, radius and ulna, tibia and fibula) should be well mineralized and of normal length. Absence, fractures, contractures, or bowing of these bones is abnormal. The ulna extends farther into the elbow than the radius, and the tibia extends farther into the patella than the fibula. The length of each long bone is measured. Images are obtained with the diaphysis located horizontally in the image (Fig. 8–15) because vertical measurements can falsely "shorten" the length. Multiple images are measured and the longest technically adequate image is the optimal measurement. The lower extremities should not be clubbed, nor should the plantar surface appear "rocker-bottom." There should be five toes (Fig. 8–16), and they should not appear dysplastic. The foot length can also be measured.

Finally, the umbilical cord is examined. There should be two arteries and one vein. Once the umbilical vein enters the fetal abdomen, it should turn superiorly, enter the liver, and communicate with the portal vein. The umbilical vein continues into the ductus venosus and then into the inferior vena cava and right atrium.

FIGURE 8–16
Third-trimester fetal foot shows five toes present.

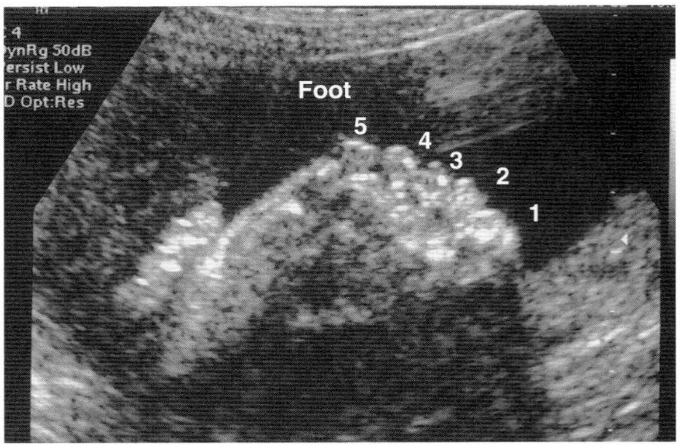

Second-Trimester Ultrasound Screening for Structural Abnormalities

There are many accepted indications for ultrasound examination during pregnancy, and 60% to 70% of all pregnant women in the United States undergo an examination at some stage during pregnancy.[27] The rate is much higher in most other industrialized countries. One of the first studies to quantify the diagnostic accuracy of ultrasound in high risk pregnancies was performed in the United Kingdom in the late 1970s and early 1980s; 95% of malformations were correctly diagnosed.[28] Subsequently, many studies examined the efficacy of routine screening ultrasound. Published sensitivities range from 13.3% to 82.4%,[29] with the collaborative world experience approximating 50%.[30] We suggest that much of the variation reflects differences in the quality of training because there are huge differences among countries in the skill level of accredited sonographers. In light of the wide variations in detection rates, it is understandable why the reliability and utility of sonographic screening for fetal malformations have been challenged. Even among those who recommend routine ultrasound screening, the number and timing of scans are debated. Because 75% of patients with abnormal fetuses are considered low risk, it is important we review the literature to assess the effect of routine sonography.[29]

The antenatal diagnosis of a fetal abnormality has many advantages. It may trigger additional testing to refine the diagnosis or prognosis, alter pregnancy management (e.g., termination, intrauterine therapy, early delivery, and delivery in a tertiary care center), prepare the parents for an adverse pregnancy outcome, and alert the clinician to the possibility of other malformations. For many patients, the benefits of sparing social and psychological costs are also very important. However, the fact that no one contests is that sonographic screening performed by inexperienced individuals increases the costs of health care and generates high false-negative and false-positive rates, with serious consequences, such as termination of an actually normal fetus.

Many biases and problems explain much of the variation in sensitivity.[29] They include technical issues (e.g., fetal positioning, obesity), lesions that resolve over time, and the undetectability of certain anomalies by ultrasound. Selection bias may play an important role, depending on whether the patient population served is derived from a hospital or an office practice. The most important bias is the variation in sonographic skills, capability, and experience of individuals performing the ultrasound examination. In the Helsinki study, which incorporated patient populations from two hospitals, the sonographic sensitivity for detecting anomalies was twofold higher in the university hospital than in the city hospital (77% vs. 36%).[31] A systematic and almost compulsive approach to each examination is necessary, with attention paid to all structures. Each center has different criteria as to what constitutes a detailed ultrasound examination. The less detailed the examination, the lower the sensitivity. Patient selection is also important. Screening high risk women (e.g., those with a prior ultrasound suggestive of congenital anomalies, positive family history, or teratogen exposure) is likely to be more effective because sonographers tend to be more focused, expecting to find an anomaly. One group noted an average sensitivity of 55% in a low risk population and 92% in a high risk population.[29]

Gestational age at screening also affects sensitivity because various anomalies may appear at different gestational weeks. Some are seen only later in gestation (e.g., duodenal atresia). The more scans a patient undergoes, the greater the anomaly detection rate. Levi[29] reported that the average sensitivity of studies that included only scans performed once before 20 weeks was 45%. The sensitivity increased to 60% if the scanning was performed several times during the pregnancy. The type of congenital anomaly plays a role in the detection rate of congenital abnormalities on sonography. For example, a complex cardiac defect is more likely to be detected than a small atrial septal defect.

The prevalence of specific malformations within a population can significantly affect the sensitivity of ultrasound screening. Studies that exclude certain anomalies because they are considered either minor or undetectable can dramatically alter the sensitivity compared with a calculation that includes all anomalies. A 1996 study found that the sensitivity of ultrasound for diagnosing both minor and major anomalies was only 8.7%; however, if only major anomalies detectable by ultrasound were included, the sensitivity rose to 75%.[30]

Finally, other factors may affect the reported fetal anomaly detection rates, such as a lack of autopsies (the gold standard), suboptimal neonatal evaluation, and inadequate length of neonatal follow-up (some anomalies may not express themselves immediately after birth).[29]

Obesity is a global health problem of increasing prevalence. The World Health organization (WHO) characterizes obesity as a pandemic issue, with a higher prevalence in females than in males.[32] Accordingly, many pregnant patients have a high body mass index (BMI), and the examination is compromised by sound attenuation (Video 8–1). This can lead to repeat sonographic examination attempts throughout gestation in order to improve visualization. One group observed that repeated ultrasound examinations for suboptimal visualization of the fetal heart at a later gestational age dramatically reduced suboptimal visualization; however, obese patients continued to have much higher rates of persistent suboptimal visualization.[33] In another study, Hendler and associates[34] found that maternal obesity increased the rate of suboptimal visualization of fetal cardiac structures by 49.8% and of the craniospinal structures by

31%. They reported that the optimal gestational age for visualization of these areas in obese patients was after 18 to 20 weeks. Increased maternal BMI may also affect the accuracy of the sonographic estimate of fetal weight. A recent study in 2009 found that the proportion of estimated fetal weights within ±10% and within ±20% of the birth weight significantly decreased with increasing BMI categories.[35] One strategy we use to optimize sonographic visualization is to perform the ultrasound examination in the early second trimester transvaginally, with a repeat sonogram several weeks later, if necessary.

Unfortunately, obesity confers a higher rate of early miscarriage and congenital anomalies, including neural tube defects.[32] In 2009, a systematic review and meta-analysis was performed examining maternal obesity and the risk of congenital anomalies.[36] Compared with women of recommended BMI, obese women were at increased odds of pregnancies affected by neural tube defects, hydrocephaly, cardiovascular anomalies, cleft lip and palate, anorectal atresia, and limb reduction anomalies. The authors noted that further studies are needed to confirm whether being overweight rather than obese confers the same risks.

The Routine Antenatal Diagnostic Imaging with Ultrasound (RADIUS) trial was the first randomized clinical trial of second-trimester ultrasound in the United States conducted in the 1980s.[37] The trial recruited patients from 109 practices (81 private, 15 academic, and 13 health maintenance organizations). The content of the examinations consisted of the following: identification of the number of fetuses, presentation, placental location, amniotic fluid volume, biparietal diameter, head circumference, abdominal circumference, femur length, and an anatomic survey, including intracranial anatomy, four-chamber view of the heart, demonstration of the spine in transverse and coronal planes, stomach, kidneys, bladder, umbilical cord insertion, and all extremities. More than 15,000 pregnant women were randomly allocated to either routine scanning or an ultrasound examination only when indicated. An additional scan was performed in the study group early in the third trimester. The goal of the trial was to determine the benefits, if any, of routine ultrasound among pregnant women at low risk. Although the identification rate of anomalies in this study was three times better with routine versus indicated ultrasound (35% vs. 11%, respectively), the sensitivity of 17% for anomalies detected between 15 and 22 weeks was extremely low.

The findings of the trial underwent intense scrutiny. One potential source of bias was that practice-based patients were used, which may have created an inadvertent selection bias (vs. a community- or hospital-based population). Others criticized the simplicity of the scans performed. The investigators reported a relative detection rate of 2.7 (95% confidence interval [CI] 1.3–5.8) for tertiary compared with nontertiary ultrasound units.[37] The detection rate of anomalous fetuses was 35% versus 13% in nontertiary centers. Sonographic screening did not significantly affect the management or outcome of pregnancies complicated by congenital malformations. This was to be expected because there was no standardized response to the sonographic findings. Diagnostic ultrasound is not a therapeutic instrument.

In 1998, Van Dorsten and coworkers[38] reported that the sensitivity of ultrasound for anomaly detection at a tertiary care center (in women at risk for anomalies) was 89.7%. Although the sensitivity was decreased (47.6%) in the lower risk population (screening group), it was sufficient to ensure cost-effectiveness for the patients.[38] In 1999, the Eurofetus group[39] reported the results of a study designed to evaluate the sensitivity of routine ultrasound screening for fetal malformations. Nearly 200,000 pregnant women (the largest group among screening studies) were enrolled and evaluated in 60 hospital laboratories in 14 countries. The sensitivity rate was 64% (2363 of 3685), a rate much higher than that in the RADIUS study. However, the two trials may not be comparable. Women in the RADIUS trial were at very low risk because strict exclusion criteria were applied before patient recruitment occurred. Further, the criteria used to designate major fetal anomalies (gold standard) were very liberal. Both of these factors could have lowered sensitivity. In contrast, all women in the Eurofetus trial were studied, regardless of risk status, and only "truly" major abnormalities were considered as endpoints; this classification may have artificially raised the sensitivity of the ultrasound screening.

Women in the Helsinki trial[40] underwent one screening examination in the second trimester; 40% of major fetal anomalies were detected, including most anomalies of the central nervous system or genitourinary system and cases with multiple anomalies. In this trial, screening was less effective in detecting cardiac and gastrointestinal tract anomalies. This finding is logical because many bowel abnormalities are sonographically "silent." In addition, cardiac morphology changes in response to malformations and might not be seen when first imaged, unless flow abnormalities are sought. In the 1991 Belgian Multicentric Study,[41] 154 of 381 structurally abnormal fetuses were correctly detected by ultrasound (sensitivity 40%). The specificity and positive and negative predictive values were 99.9%, 95%, and 98.6%, respectively.

We examined the efficacy of a complete sonographic survey (as described in this chapter) for the detection of fetal abnormalities and correlated the findings with perinatal autopsy results.[42] Of 88 abnormal autopsy findings, 85 fetuses had one or more abnormal structural sonographic findings, giving a sensitivity of 97% for anomalous fetuses. The low sensitivities reported in the past may be, in great part, the result of a failure to look for specific abnormalities. On autopsy, 372 separate abnormalities were found. Antenatal sonography detected 75% and 18%, respectively, of the 299 major and 73 of the minor abnormalities. Thus, the sensitivity for minor abnormalities was poor, even when a complete sonographic survey was performed. In 65% of cases, there was either complete agreement or only minor differences between sonographic and autopsy findings.[42]

Because sensitivity for the antenatal sonographic detection of fetal anomalies is highly dependent on the clinical setting and the expertise of the sonographer, there is insufficient evidence to list a single estimate of the sensitivity of routine ultrasound as a screening tool for fetal anomalies. However, the specificity of a fetal anatomic survey exceeds 99% in many studies.[37,43–45] Specificity measures the proportion of negatives that are correctly identified (i.e., the percentage of truly normal fetuses who are identified as normal on ultrasound) and is related inversely to the rate of false-positive diagnoses. Therefore, in low risk patients, ultrasound is helpful in excluding anomalies and detecting normal features but may not be equally reliable in detecting anomalies. The sensitivity of screening programs should continue to improve because of technological advances (e.g., three-dimensional sonography) and uniform and detailed training of practitioners.[29]

Antenatal detection of an anomalous fetus, especially one with a life-threatening defect, allows the delivery of these infants in a tertiary care center that can provide immediate and appropriate care, maximizing survival. Is this statement supported by evidence in the literature? In the 1994 RADIUS study,[37] screening did not affect the detection, management, or outcome of fetuses with anomalies. However, of the infants with life-threatening anomalies, 75% (21 of 28) survived in the routinely screened group, compared with 52% (11 of 21) in the nonscreened group.[37] The study may have been inadequately powered to address this specific question, and although many fetal medicine practitioners are convinced, additional studies are required.

Another important question is whether routine ultrasound improves overall perinatal morbidity and mortality rates. For example, routine sonography increases the accurate detection of multiple gestations, gestational age, and placental abnormalities. Table 8–4 summarizes three trials that investigated the perinatal morbidity and mortality rates of pregnancies in which routine ultrasonography was performed.[27,31,46] The perinatal mortality rates were similar in the routine sonography and control groups in both the RADIUS[27] and the Stockholm[46] trials. However, the perinatal mortality rate in the Helsinki trial[31] was significantly lower in the routine ultrasound group (4.6 of 1000 vs. 9.0 of 1000). This difference was attributable mainly to improved early detection of major malformations, leading to pregnancy termination.[31] There were no differences in perinatal morbidity rates between the study and the control groups in these three trials (see Table 8–4).[27,31,46] Although two trials had a similar distribution of birth weights between study groups,[27,31] the third trial had fewer births less than 2500 g in the routine ultrasound group.[46] The mean birth weight was also higher in the routine ultrasound group in women who smoked, and the authors speculate that this difference may be attributable to healthier maternal behaviors after these women saw their fetuses on ultrasound.[46] Although the authors of the RADIUS trial concluded that the adoption of sonographic screening in the United States would increase health care costs without improving perinatal outcome or providing measurable benefit from early detection of fetal anomalies, another study concluded that routine screening for anomalies improves perinatal outcome by leading to termination of pregnancy for certain anomalies and delivery at tertiary care centers for life-threatening malformations.[38] The prospective trials also showed that twin gestations are diagnosed earlier with routine sonography. In the Helsinki trial,[31] 100% of twins were detected before 21 weeks in the routine ultrasound group, compared with 76% in the control group. Furthermore, the perinatal mortality rate was reduced (27.8 of 1000 vs. 65.8 of 1000).

A subgroup analysis was also performed in the RADIUS study[27] for infants who were small for gestational age and neonates born at 42 weeks or later. There was no improvement in overall outcome for these conditions when routine ultrasound was performed. The available evidence indicates that routine sonography will, at a minimum, improve perinatal outcome in low risk pregnancies by decreasing perinatal mortality rates following induced abortions after the detection of fetal abnormalities.

Sonographic screening for anomalies may also provide value to both patients and physicians that are not quantifiable in terms of psychological reassurance, antepartum management, referral, genetic counseling, or preparation of families and health care providers. The benefits discussed earlier may outweigh the "risks" of ultrasound (e.g., false-positive diagnosis). Most patients will choose anomaly screening if given a choice and counseled on the current diagnostic capability of sonography. Pregnant women usually do not perceive ultrasound as a "test," but rather as a tool to evaluate the fetus as a patient. We agree with this philosophy and argue that examination of the fetus as a

TABLE 8–4

Three Trials Comparing Perinatal Morbidity and Mortality Rates in Patients Undergoing Routine Ultrasonography (vs. Control Groups)

TRIAL	PERINATAL MORBIDITY	PERINATAL MORTALITY	*P*	MEAN BIRTH WEIGHT AND NO. OF INFANTS WITH LOW BIRTH WEIGHT (<2500 G)	*P*
Ewigman et al, 1993[27] (RADIUS)	Similar*	Similar	NS	Similar birth weight	NS
Saari-Kemppainen et al, 1990[31] (Helsinki)	Similar†	Improved (4.6/1000 vs. 9.0/1000)‡	<.05	Similar birth weight	NS
Waldenstrom et al, 1988[46] (Stockholm)	Similar†	Similar	NS	Fewer low-birth weight infants (2.5% vs. 4%)	.005
				Smokers: higher mean birth weight (3413 vs. 3354 g)	.047
				Nonsmokers: higher mean birth weight	NS

NS, not significant.
* Moderate morbidity defined as neonatal sepsis, grade I or II intraventricular hemorrhage, or stay of >5 days in neonatal unit; severe morbidity defined as ventilation >48 hr or stay of >30 days in neonatal unit.
† Defined as admission to neonatal unit.
‡ Attributable to early detection of malformations, leading to termination of anomalous fetuses.

patient should be a routine practice, as it is in all aspects of adult medicine.

The last screening issue to address is the cost-benefit analysis of routine second-trimester sonography. We performed a cost-benefit analysis based on the RADIUS trial, comparing routine second-trimester sonography in low risk pregnant women with a policy of not offering screening. Routine second-trimester sonographic screening is associated with net benefits only if the sonogram is performed at a tertiary care center.[47] Another study showed that a one-stage second-trimester screening ultrasound was both cost-effective and associated with fewer perinatal deaths.[48] Finally, Van Dorsten and coworkers[38] assessed the cost-effectiveness of anomaly screening in their patient population and concluded that routine screening was cost-effective. There seems to be little doubt that the cost-effectiveness of routine sonographic screening for fetal anomalies rests not on the tool but on the caliber of the sonographer. The costs of poor sonography cannot continue to be tolerated in an already stressed health care system. The cure is not to deny women access to valuable screening techniques; the cure is to require proof of the sonographer's skill.

Sonographic Aneuploidy Markers and Genetic Sonography

The most common autosomal trisomy in liveborn infants is Down syndrome, or trisomy 21, which was first described by John Langdon Down in 1866. Autosomal trisomies are primarily the result of meiotic nondisjunction, the risk of which increases with maternal age. The first screening method for fetal trisomy 21 was introduced in the early 1970s and was based on maternal age. Amniocentesis was offered to women 35 years or older, based on the findings of an early study that stated that the risk of a procedure-related loss approximated the likelihood that a midtrimester fetus of a 35-year-old woman would have trisomy 21 (1 in 270). There has been a fundamental shift in birth trends since the 1970s, with more births occurring to women older than 35 years.[49] In 1974, women 35 to 49 years old accounted for just 4.7% of live births compared with 12.6% in 1997.[49] As a result, the prevalence of fetal trisomy 21 during the second trimester has increased from 1 in 740 in 1974 to 1 in 504 in 1997. However, the fact remains that most infants with trisomy 21 are born to women younger than 35 years. Fetuses with aneuploidy account for 6% to 11% of stillbirths and neonatal deaths,[50] whereas chromosomal defects that are compatible with life, but associated with significant morbidity, occur in 0.65% of newborns.[51]

In January 2007, the American College of Obstetricians and Gynecologists (ACOG) in their *Practice Bulletin*[52] raised the issue of whether invasive diagnostic testing for aneuploidy should be available to *all* women. They stated that the decision to offer invasive testing should not be solely age-based, and that a maternal age of 35 years alone "should no longer be used as a cutoff to determine who is offered screening versus who is offered invasive testing." Therefore, all women (regardless of age) should have the option of invasive testing.[52]

Nevertheless, among high risk women while some will choose to have invasive testing as a first option, others will instead first undergo either first-trimester screening or second-trimester genetic sonography (± biochemistry) and use the information derived from ultrasound to obtain an adjusted risk for Down syndrome to guide their decision about genetic amniocentesis. Accordingly, the genetic sonogram evolved from a patient's perspective, with the purpose of possibly avoiding invasive testing.

A large body of literature attests to the specific use of second-trimester genetic ultrasonography for antenatal detection of trisomy 21 by seeking aneuploidy markers. We offer genetic sonography as an option to all (and only) high risk patients (i.e., advanced maternal age at the time of delivery, abnormal serum marker screen results, or both). The information derived from this sonogram is used to generate an adjusted risk of Down syndrome to guide a woman's decision about genetic amniocentesis. When the findings on genetic sonogram are normal in high risk patients, the amniocentesis rate is only 3%.[53] The amniocentesis rate increases in direct proportion to the number of abnormal sonographic markers identified, with almost 100% of women selecting invasive testing when four or more markers are seen. Since the initiation of our genetic sonography service in 1992, over a 10-year period, more than 5000 women have avoided amniocentesis based on normal findings on genetic sonogram. If the fetal loss rate related directly to amniocentesis is between 1 in 100 and 1 in 300, then more than 17 to 50 fetal lives were saved, attesting to the power of genetic sonography.

Screening based on maternal age identifies at most 47% of fetuses with trisomy 21, with a false-positive rate of 13% to 14% (a rate that has increased in recent years).[49] Based on advanced maternal age, 140 amniocentesis procedures are required to detect one fetus with trisomy 21,[54] implying that one healthy fetus will be lost for every two to three affected fetuses identified. Although the combination of maternal age and second-trimester biochemical screening results increases the detection rate to 60% to 65%,[12] 60 to 70 amniocentesis procedures are required to detect one fetus with trisomy 21.[54] Thus, one healthy fetus will be lost for every three to five fetuses in which trisomy 21 is detected. As a result, some have challenged the practice of offering invasive testing to all high risk pregnant women (based on age or second-trimester biochemical screening results).[12] Reducing the screen-positive rate is beneficial, regardless of an individual's personal opinion on testing. Genetic sonography reduces the invasive testing rate by refining the selection of candidates for invasive testing without significantly decreasing detection rates.

Ideally, genetic sonography is performed between 18 and 20 weeks. The window may be shifted higher to 20 to 22 weeks if the option of pregnancy termination is not lost by the delay because visualization might improve. It is a targeted examination for fetal aneuploidy (predominantly trisomy 21) during which the sonographer searches for abnormal fetal biometry, fetal structural anomalies, and other markers of aneuploidy.[53] Because only 25% of fetuses with trisomy 21 have a sonographically detectable major anomaly in the second trimester,[54] the examination must include other markers to increase sensitivity (Table 8–5). Markers of aneuploidy that are detectable on ultrasound include shortened long bones, increased nuchal fold thickness (Fig. 8–17), pyelectasis (Fig. 8–18), choroid plexus cysts (see Fig. 8–3), short ear length, wide iliac wing angle,

TABLE 8–5
Aneuploidy Markers of the Genetic Sonogram

Structural anomalies, including cardiac (four-chamber and outflow tracts)
Short femur (observed to expected < 10th percentile)
Short humerus (observed to expected < 10th percentile)
Pyelectasis (anteroposterior diameter of renal pelvis ≥ 4 mm)
Nuchal fold thickening (≥6 mm)
Echogenic bowel (similar to echogenicity of iliac bones)
Choroid plexus cysts (>10 mm)
Hypoplastic middle phalanx of the fifth digit
Wide space between the first and the second toes (sandal gap)
Two-vessel umbilical cord
Echogenic intracardiac focus, short tibia, short fibula, short ear (since October 1997)
Absent nasal bone (since 2003)

FIGURE 8–19
Sandal gap (wide space between the first and the second toes) in a fetus with Down syndrome.

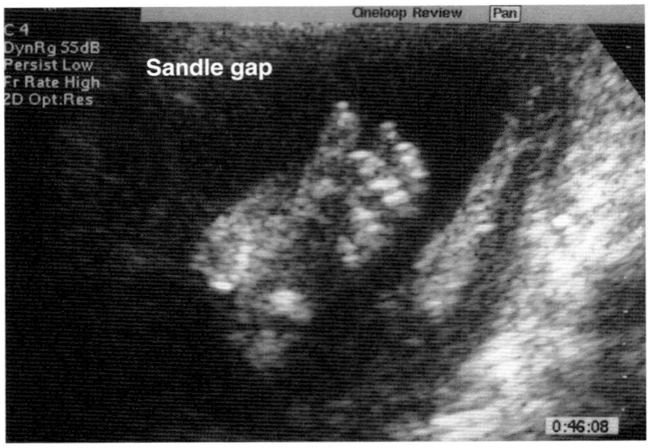

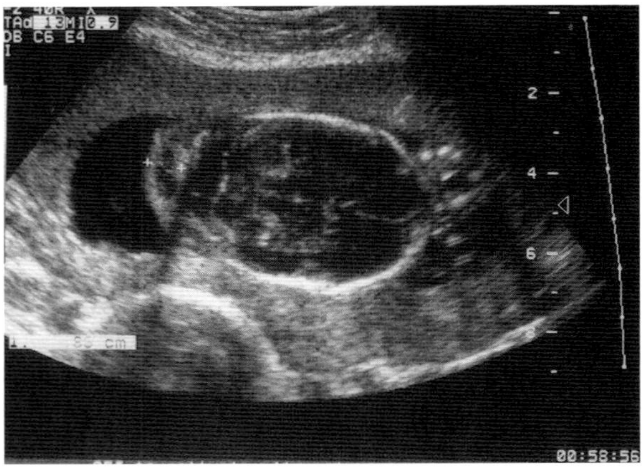
FIGURE 8–17
Thickened nuchal fold (0.86 cm) in a second trimester fetus with Down syndrome.

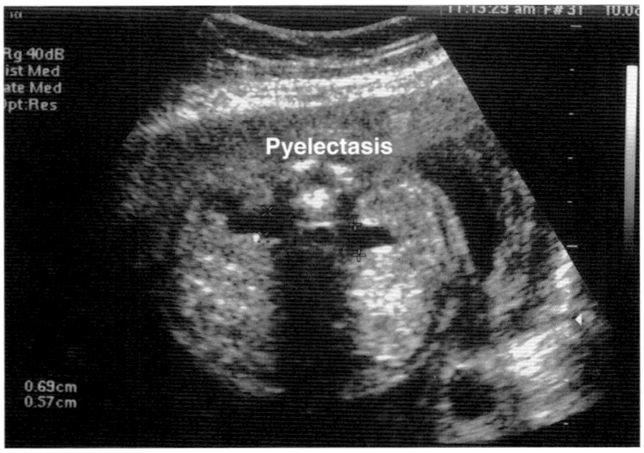

FIGURE 8–18
Bilateral pyelectasis in a second-trimester fetus.

hyperechoic bowel, echogenic intracardiac focus (see Fig. 8–12), sandal gap toes (Fig. 8–19), hypoplastic midphalanx of the fifth digit, clinodactyly, and absent NB (see Fig. 8–7). The risk of fetal trisomy 21 increases with the number of markers present. Each marker alone (except thickened nuchal fold or absent NB) has low to moderate sensitivity for trisomy 21 and does not necessarily increase the risk of aneuploidy when found in isolation in low risk patients. However, the risk of fetal aneuploidy may increase when thickened nuchal fold, absent NB, or multiple sonographic abnormalities or markers are detected in low risk patients or when any isolated markers are seen in high risk patients.

A thickened nuchal fold (sensitivity 40%; false-positive rate 0.1%)[55] along with absent NB (41% sensitivity and 100% specificity for fetal trisomy 21) are among the most sensitive and specific markers for Down syndrome and involve straightforward training.[56] Importantly, when we added absent NB to the other sonographic markers of aneuploidy, the sensitivity of genetic sonography increased from 83% (24 of 29) to 90% (26 of 29).[56] Absence of the NB was noted in two fetuses with trisomy 21 with no other ultrasound markers for aneuploidy.

There is a large overlap in bone measurements between affected and normal fetuses. A short femur length (measurement-to-expected length ≤ 0.91) is found in 24%,[57] and a short humerus (measurement-to-expected length < 0.90) in 50% of affected fetuses, with a false-positive rate of 6.25%.[58] The sensitivity of pyelectasis (anteroposterior diameter of the renal pelvis ≥ 4 mm in the second trimester) for trisomy 21 is 25%.[58] Echogenic bowel has a reported sensitivity of 7% to 12.5%, whereas an echogenic intracardiac focus (see Fig. 8–12) has a reported sensitivity of 18%.[58] We examined the sensitivity of a short sonographic ear length for trisomy 21.[59] Forty-one percent (21 of 51) had an ear length at or below the 10th percentile. However, a short ear length was not as sensitive a marker for trisomy 21 as it was for trisomy 13 (100%) or trisomy 18 (96%). The association between trisomy 21 and choroid plexus cyst(s) is controversial.

In 2008, Molina and colleagues[60] examined the frontomaxillary facial (FMF) angle in normal (n = 150) and trisomy 21 fetuses (n = 23) at 16 to 24 weeks of gestation using three-dimensional ultrasound. In the normal group, there was no significant association between the FMF angle and gestational age. The mean FMF angle was 83.9 degrees (range 76.9–90.2 degrees), and the 95th percentile was 88.5 degrees. In 65.2% (n = 15) of the Down syndrome fetuses, the FMF angle was greater than 88.5 degrees. Therefore, they concluded that in the majority of second-trimester fetuses with trisomy 21, the FMF angle is increased.

Several studies have reported the accuracy of genetic sonography to detect trisomy 21 in high risk populations.[53] When "abnormal" is defined as the finding of at least one marker on ultrasound, the overall sensitivity was 77% (range 50%–93%), and the false-positive rate was 13% (range 7%–17%).[53] Thus, whereas it is clear that the use of multiple sonographic markers improves the sensitivity of sonography for detecting trisomy 21, it also results in a higher false-positive rate. In 1998, an 11-center collaborative study examined the sensitivity of sonography for the detection of trisomy 21.[61] Eighty-five percent of fetuses with trisomy 21 (n = 241) had at least one abnormal finding on ultrasound. In 2003, an eight-center study evaluated the utility of second-trimester genetic sonography in high risk women, including 176 fetuses with trisomy 21.[62] The sensitivity for the detection of trisomy 21 was 72% (center range 64%–80%). Approximately half (47%) of the fetuses with trisomy 21 had a thickened nuchal fold of 5 mm or more.

In 1996, our group[63] was the first to publish findings on the use of second-trimester genetic sonography to guide clinical management of pregnancies in women at high risk for trisomy 21. In 1999, we began to counsel women that the likelihood of trisomy 21, in the absence of abnormalities or markers, was reduced by at least 80% from the a priori risk (second-trimester biochemical screening results or, if unavailable, maternal age).[53] Our experience was reassuring. Over almost a 10-year period (November 1992–August 2002), we evaluated 5299 fetuses with genetic sonography. The findings were normal in 85% (no markers seen); 12% had one marker, and 3% had two or more markers. When at least one marker was present, the sensitivity, specificity, and positive and negative predictive values for trisomy 21 were 87% (52 of 60), 91% (4395 of 4831), 11% (52 of 488), and 99.8% (4395 of 4403), respectively. Approximately two thirds of fetuses with trisomy 21 had two or more abnormal sonographic markers.

Over the years, we have found that more and more high risk women prefer genetic sonography as their first option, rather than amniocentesis (Table 8–6). Since 1998, more than 70% of women chose to begin with genetic sonography. Accordingly, the number of amniocenteses performed has decreased. The total amniocentesis rate (the sum of amniocentesis procedures as the first option plus amniocentesis procedures performed after genetic sonography) decreased from 99.6% in 1993 to 32% in 2002. Several years ago, we examined the accuracy of genetic sonography for the detection of fetal trisomy 21 according to the indication for testing (advanced maternal age, abnormal second-trimester biochemical screening results, abnormal second-trimester biochemical screening results in women younger than 35 years, and abnormal second-trimester biochemical screening results in women 35 years and older). We also examined the risk of trisomy 21 after normal findings on genetic sonography.[64] We found that the magnitude of the risk adjustment after normal findings on a genetic scan was independent of the testing indication and there were no significant indication-specific variations in the accuracy of genetic sonography.

TABLE 8–6

Annual Utilization Rates of Genetic Sonography for Detection of Fetal Trisomy 21 at Robert Wood Johnson Medical School

YEAR	CANDIDATES FOR PRENATAL DIAGNOSIS*	GENETIC ULTRASOUND (N (%))	TOTAL AMNIOCENTESES† N (%)
1993‡	477	2 (0.4)	475 (99.6)
1994	495	82 (17)	423 (85)
1995	523	251 (48)	292 (56)
1996	594	328 (55)	279 (47)
1997	793	510 (64)	315 (40)
1998	856	662 (77)	215 (25)
1999	1285	956 (74)	405 (31)
2000	1537	1114 (73)	468 (30)
2001	1497	1062 (71)	488 (32)
2002	1526	1110 (73)	493 (32)

* Includes advanced maternal age (≥35 yr) with or without abnormal serum biochemistry results, abnormal serum biochemistry results in women younger than 35 years, or family history of chromosome abnormality.

† Includes women who underwent genetic amniocentesis only as their first option and women who underwent amniocentesis after genetic sonography.

‡ The genetic sonogram service was available for only 2 months in 1993 (November and December).

Although some advocate second-trimester genetic sonography for screening of the general population, we believe that it should be reserved only for the high risk population for several reasons. First, a high degree of expertise is required to exclude sonographic fetal malformations (especially subtle cardiac defects), and this expertise is not widely available in many countries including the United States. Second, the application of genetic sonography to low risk women may be inappropriate and perhaps dangerous, in light of the high screen false-positive rate (12%–15% in the high risk population), which is likely even higher in a low risk population. In low risk women, the a priori risk of trisomy 21 may be so low that the presence of one aneuploidy marker (e.g., pyelectasis) would not elevate the risk enough to justify amniocentesis. Therefore, with this approach, the positive predictive value and perhaps even the sensitivity of genetic ultrasound for fetal trisomy 21 are likely to be decreased in low risk patients. Third, the accuracy of second-trimester aneuploidy markers has been studied mainly in high risk populations. Extrapolation of such accuracy to low risk women may not be appropriate. Some have concluded that an isolated marker (other than increased nuchal fold thickness, absent NB, or structural anomalies) should not be used as an indication for amniocentesis testing in the low risk population.[53] Others argue that if it is applied to the low risk population, any risk adjustment must reflect both the a priori risk of trisomy 21 and the sensitivity of the specific marker identified.

Clinicians should not recommend amniocentesis to low risk patients who have an isolated marker identified because the sensitivity is low, with the possible exception of increased nuchal fold thickness[65] and/or absent/hypoplastic NB. However, the incidental finding of an organ or structural anomaly (with few exceptions), nuchal fold thickening, absent/hypoplastic NB, or two or more aneuploidy markers in a low risk patient should trigger counseling and informed consent with the patient. The patient should be informed that if the accuracy of genetic ultrasound is extrapolated from high risk to low risk women, then the risk of trisomy 21 is likely high enough to justify offering genetic amniocentesis. In these patients, the risk of trisomy 21 is higher than the risk of amniocentesis-related fetal loss, regardless of maternal age or second-trimester biochemical screening results (unless the a priori risk < 1 in 10,000). Certain isolated sonographic fetal abnormalities (e.g., gastroschisis) are not usually associated with aneuploidy and do not require further invasive testing.

The following description is the approach that we have used successfully with high risk patients. Genetic sonography is an adjunct to maternal age and serum screening (triple or quadruple, whichever is available) to adjust the risk of fetal trisomy 21 for each patient, based on our accuracy. The a priori risk is based on serum screening results. If serum screening results are not available or if testing was not performed, the risk is based on maternal age. We then multiply the a priori risk with various likelihood ratios (LRs), depending on the presence or absence of aneuploidy markers. For example, if the a priori risk of fetal trisomy 21 is 1 in 274 and the results of genetic sonography are normal, the adjusted risk of fetal trisomy 21 is (1 in 274 × 0.20 [1/5 residual risk]), or 1 in 1370, a reduction of at least 80%. The degree of risk reduction depends on several factors, such as the sensitivity of the ultrasound and the criteria and number of aneuploidy markers sought. Most recent studies utilize a negative LR that ranges somewhere between 0.2 and 0.4 after a normal genetic scan, corresponding to a 60% to 80% reduction in risk. The revised risk is then discussed with the patient. The patient should be told that the genetic scan can never reduce her risk to 0%. In our experience, the presence of only one of the following markers increases the risk of trisomy 21 minimally or not at all: short femur length, short humerus length, pyelectasis, echogenic bowel, hyperechoic focus in the left ventricle, short tibia length, short fibula length, short ear length, choroid plexus cyst greater than 10 mm, a hypoplastic middle phalanx of the fifth digit, a sandal gap toe, and a two-vessel cord. Therefore, the risk of fetal trisomy 21 remains the same (1 in 274). Once two or more markers are visualized, or a thickened nuchal fold, or absent NB, no matter what the a priori risk is, the adjusted risk for trisomy 21 is almost always higher than the risk of amniocentesis. An adjusted risk of trisomy 21, based on the genetic sonogram, is given, even for high risk patients. For example, based on age alone, a 44-year-old patient is at high risk for fetal trisomy 21. However, if second-trimester biochemical screening results are 1 in 798 (a priori risk) and the findings on genetic sonogram are normal, the adjusted risk for trisomy 21 is 1 in 3990. If the same patient has one soft marker, the adjusted risk for Down syndrome remains the same, or is slightly higher than 1 in 798 (LR 1.00).

Although it would intuitively seem that certain markers (e.g., nuchal fold thickening, absent NB, or cardiac defects) in isolation are very "strong" and would increase the risk for trisomy 21, we have found these markers most frequently in combination with other markers. Either a triple or a quadruple screen risk is acceptable as an a priori risk, because most of our findings are based on high risk patients who underwent serum testing.

If the results of genetic sonography are normal, we still reduce the risk of fetal trisomy 21 by 80%, and the revised risk is then discussed with the patient. However, in the presence of aneuploidy marker(s), we no longer multiply the a priori risk with various LRs to give an actual adjusted risk. Instead, we counsel the patient that her risk for fetal Down syndrome is "increased," and we offer and discuss genetic amniocentesis. In other words, if only one marker is present (with the exception of structural anomaly, thickened nuchal fold, or absent NB), we recommend invasive testing *only* if the patient is high risk based on the a priori risk. Conversely, once two or more markers are visualized, or isolated thickened nuchal fold or absent NB, we offer invasive testing, regardless of a priori risk status.

Ideally, it would be optimal to establish an individual LR for each aneuploidy marker so that risk adjustments may be made when a marker(s) is sonographically present. LRs of isolated markers have been reported in several studies.[66–69] By using LRs, the post priori risk is then estimated. However, if one examines the LRs reported for a specific marker (such as short humerus), these values can vary widely. Thus, for this reason, we believe that in general the presence of isolated sonographic markers should not be used to adjust the a priori risk for fetal Down syndrome. We also do not utilize LRs of isolated markers because, in our experience, the overwhelming majority of Down syndrome fetuses have multiple markers in combination, rather than in isolation. In fact, based on our own data, approximately two thirds of fetuses with Down syndrome will have two or more abnormal sonographic markers. Therefore, we have been unable to generate stable and reliable positive LRs of isolated markers. Accordingly, until individualized LRs can be reliably established, we do not provide actual adjusted risks for fetal Down syndrome in the presence of aneuploidy marker(s).

A different method that has been utilized is to integrate the risk of sonographic markers with the a priori risk based on maternal age.[70] This is called AAURA (age-adjusted ultrasound risk adjustment) for fetal Down syndrome and is used for women of all ages. With this method, sonographic markers are "weighted" by the strength of individual findings, expressed as LRs. The authors base the individual risk assessment of fetal Down syndrome on maternal age and the presence or absence of each of the sonographic markers, in terms of LRs. Investigators using AAURA report that both the sensitivity of fetal Down syndrome detection and the false-positive rate increase with maternal age. This is felt to be appropriate because older women desire a high sensitivity, and the clinical alternative is amniocentesis for all women age 35 years or older (100% false-positive rate).[71] AAURA also minimizes the false-positive rate for younger women (4%) with a satisfactory sensitivity (61.5%).[71]

Recently, we have also altered our clinical management to reflect the emergence of first-trimester screening. First-trimester screening is discussed in detail in Chapter 7. Studies performed in the 1990s revealed a strong association between the size of the fluid collection at the back of the fetal neck in the first trimester (NT) and the risk of Down syndrome.[72]

An increased NT thickness is now widely recognized to be an early presenting feature of a wide range of fetal genetic, chromosomal, and structural anomalies. Subsequently, an important achievement in first-trimester screening for Down syndrome occurred when large studies in the United States and United Kingdom demonstrated that NT could be combined with two first-trimester maternal serum analytes (free β-hCG and pregnancy-associated plasma protein A [PAPP-A]). The mean level of free β-hCG in first-trimester Down syndrome pregnancies is elevated to 1.98 MoM,[73] and the mean level of PAPP-A is reduced to approximately 0.43 MoM.[74] When serum analytes are combined with NT (or combined first-trimester screening), the result is higher detection rates for Down syndrome. In looking at prospective first-trimester screening studies, when fetal NT (along with maternal age) is combined with free β-hCG and PAPP-A, the detection rate for Down syndrome is 87%, for a false-positive rate of 5%.[75] Another recent paper examining prospective studies of combined first-trimester screening found that for a total of more than 160,000 pregnancies screened (>600 Down syndrome fetuses), the overall sensitivity for Down syndrome was 87% (95% CI 84.0%–89.4%), for a 5% false-positive rate.[76] Therefore, it is evident that for a 5% false-positive rate, the sensitivity for Down syndrome by utilizing combined first-trimester screening is far superior to that of maternal age (30%) and second-trimester triple screen (60%–70%).

Because of the current availability of both first- and second-trimester screening tests, several approaches to Down syndrome screening have been evaluated. However, it is important to point out that not all strategies include NT measurement because this screening approach is not available in all regions and this measurement may not be successfully obtained in all patients. Nevertheless, when women have undergone first-trimester screening for aneuploidy, they should not undergo independent second-trimester serum screening in the same pregnancy[52] because the false-positive rates are additive, resulting in many more unnecessary invasive procedures (11%–17%).[77,78] Instead, women who desire a higher detection rate for Down syndrome can have either an integrated or a sequential screening test, which *combines* both first- and second-trimester screening results, or seek an ultrasound laboratory that is certified to perform comprehensive first-trimester screening (PAPP-A, hCG, NT, NB, ductus venosus, tricuspid valve). At present, patients undergo combined first-trimester screening, with a subsequent maternal serum concentration of α-fetoprotein (MSAFP) only in the second trimester. We then utilize the combined first-trimester screen risk as the a priori risk for genetic sonography. If the patient does not have first-trimester screening performed (but, rather, quadruple screening), then these results are used as the a priori risk, as has been done traditionally in the past.

Others have evaluated second-trimester genetic sonography after first-trimester Down syndrome screening. In 2005, members of the FASTER (First and Second Trimester Evaluation of Risk) trial in the United States[79] examined the role of second-trimester genetic sonography in a population that already underwent first-trimester combined screening and second-trimester quadruple screening. There were 8533 patients who underwent genetic sonography, including 62 cases of Down syndrome. Although there were 3 Down syndrome cases undetected by either first- or second-trimester or combined screening, genetic sonography detected all these cases, so that no Down syndrome fetus was missed by the overall screening program. The sensitivity of combined first-trimester screening was 84% (false-positive rate 6.6%); however, by using the genetic sonogram to modify the risk, this resulted in higher sensitivity (92%), with a reduction in the false-positive rate to 5.6%. Similarly, the sensitivity of quadruple screening was 88% (false-positive rate 11%); however, by again using the genetic sonogram to modify the risk, this resulted in higher sensitivity (93%) with a reduction in the false-positive rate to 7.4%.[79] Thus, second-trimester genetic sonography improved the performance of both first- and second-trimester screens by significantly reducing the false-positive rates, with simultaneous increases in sensitivity.

Krantz and associates[80] used previously published data in 2007 to mathematically model the effect of second-trimester sonography after combined screening. In this model, when genetic sonography was used as the second part of a stepwise sequential screen, Down syndrome detection increased to 94.6% from 88.5% by combined screening alone, with an accompanying increase in the screen-positive rate from 4.2% to 5.4%. When genetic sonography was used as the second part of a contingent sequential test for intermediate-risk combined screen results, Down syndrome detection and screen-positive rates were 93.3% and 4.9%, respectively. The authors concluded that second-trimester genetic sonography could serve as an effective screening test after first-trimester combined screening.[80] In 2009, a retrospective cohort study was performed to evaluate Down syndrome screening performance of the first-trimester combined test followed by second-trimester genetic sonography.[81] Sonography was evaluated as the second part of (1) a stepwise sequential test applied to combined screen-negative pregnancies and (2) an integrated test applied to all combined screen patients, regardless of the latter results. The authors found that second-trimester genetic sonography after first-trimester combined screening may improve Down syndrome detection, but at the expense of increasing screen-positive rates, which they deemed unacceptably high.

Risk adjustment for trisomy 21 is institution-specific and the published experience from one center does not necessarily apply to another.[82] Each center performing genetic sonography must monitor their sensitivity for the detection of trisomy 21 to provide patients accurate, detailed, and updated counseling about their degree of risk reduction when ultrasound findings are normal. Considering the range of expertise available in many countries, it is reasonable to suggest limiting genetic sonography to specialized centers.[11] In 2007, ACOG stated in their *Practice Bulletin*[52] that risk adjustment based on second-trimester ultrasonographic markers should be limited to centers with ultrasonographic expertise and centers engaged in clinical research, to develop a standardized approach to evaluating these markers.

We analyzed the cost of universal amniocentesis and genetic sonography and concluded that genetic sonography was cost-effective when the sensitivity for the detection of trisomy 21 was greater than 74%.[64] We observed that genetic sonography saved the health care system 9% and reduced the loss rate of normal fetuses as a result of amniocentesis by 87%.[83] Genetic sonography is also cost-effective in women younger than 35 years who are at moderate risk for Down syndrome based on their second-trimester biochemical screening results as well as in patients with advanced maternal age who decline amniocentesis after second-trimester genetic counseling.[84] Offering genetic sonography to these patients is associated with cost savings for most acceptable genetic ultrasound accuracies. Finally, another study indicated that the combination of second-trimester genetic sonography with traditional serum markers may further improve diagnostic accuracy.[85] Various integrated algorithms combining serum analytes and sonographic markers have been reported (e.g., nuchal thickness, humerus length, serum α-fetoprotein, hCG) but have not been validated prospectively.

THREE-DIMENSIONAL SONOGRAPHY

Three-dimensional ultrasound (3DUS) was first introduced in the late 1980s. 2D ultrasound (2DUS) acquires a single plane of image information with traditional transducers. 3DUS, however, acquires *volume* data utilizing one of several techniques. The resulting data can be viewed in single or multiple planes or in combination with a rendered image that conveys the information from the entire volume (the "classic" 3D appearance).[86] The initial machines were somewhat slow, but display times have decreased dramatically with the evolution of computer processors. With the current generation, 3D reconstruction is fast with high resolution, providing not only a 3D image in real time but also a display generated using standardized protocols. The image quality is directly related to the image quality of the 2D scan used to acquire volumes. In some cases, multiplanar imaging in a standard orientation allows the sonographer to be more confident of a finding compared with conventional 2D imaging.

This technology has the potential to provide both the physician and the patient with more accurate and additional information about the fetus (e.g., extent or size of anomalies) than is possible with traditional 2DUS. Other advantages of 3DUS include rapid acquisition of volume data, use of new orientations and planes (not obtainable with 2D scanning), earlier maternal-fetal bonding, and improved comprehension of the fetal anatomy by the patient and family.[86] Another important role of 3DUS relates to the ability to store volume data that can be manipulated long after the patient has left the examination room.[87] Sonographic volumes can also be transmitted electronically from a remote site for full interpretation and evaluation elsewhere, making teleradiology ultrasound image interpretation easier and less operator-dependent.[88] This capability has the potential to increase the use of sonography in remote locations, where a sonographic expert is not present.

3DUS may be more useful than conventional 2DUS for the evaluation of malformations. Merz and colleagues[89] studied 204 anomalous fetuses and concluded that 3DUS ultrasound was advantageous compared with 2DUS in 62%, equivalent in 36%, and disadvantageous in 2%. In a similar study of 63 fetuses with 103 anomalies, 3DUS was advantageous in 51%, equivalent in 45%, and disadvantageous in 4%.[90] Several anomalies, such as cleft lip and abnormal facies, were seen only with 3DUS. Most anomalies were better visualized with 3D than with 2D imaging.[89,90] Not only was patient management altered in 1 out of 20 patients, but the improved visualization helped physician and family understand the anomalies. In 2005, Gonçalves and coworkers reviewed the published literature on 3DUS and four-dimensional ultrasound (4DUS) in obstetrics, to determine whether 3DUS adds diagnostic information to that currently provided by 2DUS.[91] They concluded that 3DUS provides additional diagnostic information for the diagnosis of facial anomalies, especially facial clefts. Moreover, they found evidence that 3DUS provides additional diagnostic information for neural tube defects and skeletal malformations. However, large studies comparing 2DUS and 3DUS for the diagnosis of congenital anomalies have not provided conclusive results.[91]

Second- and Third-Trimesters

3D imaging is useful in the second and third trimesters for anomalies of the skull, brain, face, heart, spine, limbs, urinary tract, umbilical cord, and placenta.[86] Other applications under study include evaluations of the placenta, umbilical cord, cervix, fetal weight, and uterine anomalies (e.g., bicornuate, septate). 3DUS can improve the accuracy of length, area, and volume measurements as well.[88] Various strategies have been utilized, ranging from manual outlining of structures to semiautomatic and fully automatic algorithms that segment organs and structures for analysis.[88]

One of the most valuable features of 3DUS is the ability to rotate the face so that it can be viewed directly in an upright position. Surface-rendered displays are successfully obtained in 70%.[86] The fetal face can be rotated into a standard symmetrical orientation and reviewed millimeter by millimeter by scrolling through the volumes.[92] Several studies have concluded that 3DUS was beneficial for the detection of facial anomalies, such as cleft lip or palate, midface hypoplasia, asymmetrical facies, micrognathia, facial masses, hypotelorism or hypertelorism, facial dysmorphia (sloping forehead, flat facies, flat nose), holoprosencephaly, and deformed ears.[86] 3DUS is particularly valuable when seeking a cleft lip or palate, especially the primary, or hard, palate. Some anomalies detectable on 3DUS were missed on 2DUS, including cleft lip or palate, micrognathia, flat facies, unilateral orbital hypoplasia, and cranial ossification defect.[86] In one series, 2DUS identified only 45% of fetuses with cleft palate, whereas 3DUS enabled the detection of 86%.[93] Artifacts produced from 3D volumes can imitate "clefting" of lips that are actually normal. These artifacts include shadowing by an adjacent umbilical cord, motion during image acquisition, NB shadowing, and misidentifying a nostril as a cleft.[86]

It is almost always possible to obtain a fetal profile, a crucial part of the examination. In addition, rotation of the volume allows consistent and accurate depiction of the midsagittal plane. 3D imaging of the face may be difficult early in gestation, if there is oligohydramnios, if limbs obscure the face, or when the face is close to the uterine wall or placenta.[86]

3D imaging is valuable in the examination for fetal skull defects, intracranial pathology and symmetry, and abnormal sutures or fontanelles. The "three-horn view" contains the anterior, inferior, and posterior horns of the lateral ventricles in a single slice.[94] Fluid in the inferior horn is abnormal and is an early sign of ventriculomegaly. By placing the "marker dot" in the volume, the sonographer can "navigate" through ventricles, parenchyma, and cystic structures and along vascular structures.[86] These images may be useful for consulting pediatric neurologists and neurosurgeons. The fetal spine is often imaged more clearly with 3DUS. Image quality is improved with rendering techniques that optimize the appearance of bone for the diagnosis of scoliosis, hemivertebrae, and neural tube defects. Studies suggest that 3D evaluation allows for an accurate determination of the level of a neural tube defect because the transverse and coronal images are viewed simultaneously with the rendered image.[95]

In the past, cardiac 3DUS was compromised by the rapid motion. However, recent technological developments of motion-gated cardiac scanning allow almost real-time 3D/4D fetal heart scans. Spatiotemporal image correlation (STIC) acquisition is an indirect motion-gated offline scanning mode.[96] Consecutive volumes can then be used to reconstruct a complete heart cycle that displays in an endless loop. Accordingly, this cine-like file of a beating fetal heart can then be manipulated to display any acquired scanning plane at any stage in the cardiac cycle.[97] 3D/4D sonography has been used to estimate fetal cardiac ventricular volume, calculate ejection fraction and stroke volume,[98] and diagnose or facilitate the diagnosis of congenital cardiovascular malformations.[99,100]

Abnormalities of the fetal abdomen and pelvis (and, in some cases, their volume) can be imaged with 3DUS (e.g., gastroschisis, omphalocele, bowel obstruction, hydronephrosis, multicystic dysplastic kidney). However, it is not clear whether additional information is obtained compared with 2D. Abnormalities of the genitalia may also be assessed with 3DUS.

The fetal extremities can usually be imaged with 3DUS because of the rapid acquisition. If the limb moves during an acquisition, the volume should be discarded and another one acquired. With conventional 2D, motion often obscures limb anatomy or makes assessment difficult. However, once a 3D volume is obtained, the structure can be studied carefully without motion, and the limb can be "rotated" to various orientations for full evaluation. Rendered images can be used to evaluate surface and bony features and the number and position of digits. In evaluating the lower extremities for clubfeet, it is often difficult to determine whether this is a "transient" (false-positive) or "fixed" (true-positive) event. 3DUS may help in some cases.

3DUS offers several advantages over conventional 2D imaging in fetuses with skeletal dysplasia. Abnormal bone shapes, shortened ribs, and abnormal facies are more accurately identified with volume acquisition.[86] Garjan and associates[101] reported that 3DUS allowed for the identification of abnormalities that were not seen on 2D in three out of seven fetuses with skeletal dysplasias. Specific bones may be imaged with 3DUS to narrow the normally wide differential diagnosis of skeletal dysplasias (see Chapter 20). A recent study concluded that 3D/4D technology was a useful sonographic tool for evaluating the fetal thorax, in that it enhanced diagnostic precision and provided superior spatial visualization of the anomalies.[102]

3DUS has been used to estimate fetal weight using volume data for the abdomen and extremities because it is impossible to obtain an entire fetal volume.[86] Some studies suggest that 3DUS may be more accurate than 2DUS for weight prediction.[103] Others, however, have found that fetal weight in prolonged pregnancies can be estimated using 2D sonography with the same accuracy as with 3D.[104] Birth weight prediction has also been investigated using 3DUS and fractional limb volume.[105] A 2009 prospective study compared inter- and intraobserver variation of fetal biometric measurements using 2D- and 3D-derived images.[106] The authors observed that the use of 3DUS significantly reduced intraobserver variation for head circumference, abdominal circumference, and femur length and reduced the interobserver variation for femur length. Fetal liver and lung volumes have also been reported.[107,108] Chang and associates[107] concluded that measurements made with 2DUS underestimated the fetal liver volume compared with 3DUS.

The cervix can be imaged with 3DUS, along with the entire cerclage, if present. Vascular structures and their distribution and extent (e.g., umbilical cord, vasa previa, placenta accreta, velamentous insertions, aneurysm of the vein of Galen) have all been evaluated with 3DUS.[86] Image acquisition can be difficult and time-consuming at times because of motion, flash artifacts, and the longer time volume acquisition with color and power Doppler techniques.

A great advantage of 3DUS is the potential for enhanced early maternal bonding with the fetus. Among patients who undergo 3DUS for reassurance, those women with a history of fetal or neonatal demise, those with a history of a fetus with congenital anomalies, those carrying fetuses with lethal anomalies, those treated for infertility, and couples who have a surrogate carrying their pregnancy seem to derive the most benefit.[86]

In summary, the world is three-dimensional and 3DUS provides anatomic images that are more easily understood by both physicians and patients. It offers women and their care team an improved understanding of the anomalies found on 2DUS, clarifies the extent of the anomaly, and provides visual confirmation of the reality of the abnormality. It also facilitates bonding with the fetus.

SCREENING FOR TRISOMY 18 AND OTHER ANEUPLOIDIES

Trisomy 18 (Edwards' syndrome) is the second most common autosomal trisomy and has a uniformly poor prognosis. Second-trimester serum triple-marker screening can identify 60% to 75% of fetuses with trisomy 18 when a separate analysis is performed seeking low levels of all three analytes, with or without consideration of maternal age.[109,110]

Sonography has high but variable sensitivity for detecting trisomy 18 (64%–100%), particularly when the search is part of a thorough anatomic survey.[26] We found that all fetuses with trisomy 18 had four or more sonographic anomalies (one fetus had 19 separate detectable anomalies).[26] Shortened ear length was present in 96%, bilateral clenched or closed hands or overlapping digits in 95%, and central nervous system abnormalities in 87%. In another study, we observed shortened ear length (≤10th percentile) in 100% of fetuses with trisomy 13, 96% of fetuses with trisomy 18, 75% of those with Turner's syndrome, and 91% of those with other various aneuploidies.[59] Many investigators have confirmed that abnormal hands are seen in most fetuses with trisomy 18.[26] Other sonographic abnormalities that are common in trisomy 18 include growth restriction, abnormal feet, choroid plexus cysts, and structural cardiac defects. We observed intrauterine growth restriction in 63% of fetuses with trisomy 18.[26]

In a large retrospective review of 98 second-trimester fetuses with trisomy 18, the authors were able to identify abnormal fetal anatomy or abnormal biometry in 97% of these fetuses.[111] In 2008, Zheng and coworkers[112] observed in a population of 26 trisomy 18 fetuses, that 3D/4D sonography enabled the identification of additional diagnostic information in 84 and influenced the obstetric management in 4.

Choroid plexus cysts are visualized in 1% (range 0.3%–3.6%) of normal fetuses in the second trimester (see Fig. 8–3). These cysts may be associated with trisomy 18,[113] and in the past, genetic amniocentesis was considered even if they were isolated. *However, a cyst can be considered "isolated" only after a detailed fetal survey shows no other structural abnormalities or markers.* In our study, half of the fetuses with trisomy 18 had a choroid plexus cyst, but these were always associated with multiple other sonographic abnormalities (i.e., never isolated).[26] In another study, none of 98 fetuses with an isolated choroid plexus cyst had aneuploidy, whereas 100% of the 13 fetuses with a choroid plexus cyst and major anatomic abnormalities had trisomy 18.[114] In our experience, the risk of aneuploidy is very low and does not justify amniocentesis if no other anomalies are found (especially if the hands are open and the ear length is normal). Many investigators concur that if the choroid plexus cyst is isolated and the patient is at low risk for fetal aneuploidy, the presence of these cysts should not affect management. In fact, the authors of a 2004 editorial recommended that when a choroid plexus cyst is the only detected abnormality (an isolated marker on a second- or third-trimester sonogram that meets the most recently adopted AIUM performance guidelines), the sonographic report emphasizes that as an isolated finding in a patient considered low risk for fetal aneuploidy, a choroid plexus cyst is not clinically significant and does not change her from low to high risk status.[115]

Similarly to genetic sonography for fetal trisomy 21 screening, normal findings on a complete anatomic survey in experienced hands should "decrease" a patient's risk of trisomy 18 (regardless of the presence of choroid plexus cysts or abnormal second-trimester biochemical screening results) to a low level sufficient to avoid genetic amniocentesis after appropriate patient counseling.[26] A 2009 study of 8763 pregnancies at increased risk of trisomy 18 based on serum screening including 56 whose fetuses had trisomy 18 noted sonographic anomalies in 89% of trisomy 18 fetuses compared with 14% of normal.[116] They reported that if the genetic sonogram was normal (no structural anomaly or soft marker), the risk was reduced by approximately 90%.[116] Therefore, the authors concluded that if the genetic sonogram is used as a sequential test following serum biochemistry, a normal ultrasound study reduces the likelihood of trisomy 18 substantially, even if a woman has abnormal serum biochemistry.

Trisomy 13 (Patau's syndrome) has an extremely poor prognosis. Its phenotype is so characteristic that a diagnosis can often be based on clinical features alone. Because fetuses with trisomy 13 usually have severe abnormalities, it follows that the sensitivity of prenatal sonography for the detection is very high, with most studies reporting sensitivities above 90%.[117–119] Watson and colleagues[120] achieved a 95% detection rate (36 out of 38) after 17 weeks based on either the presence of an anomaly or abnormal fetal biometry. Early-onset growth restriction is common in trisomy 13 and triploidy. In particular, triploidy is associated with a characteristically small body relative to the head.

CRITICAL REVIEW OF THE EVIDENCE ON SECOND-TRIMESTER SCREENING FOR FETAL ABNORMALITY

There is no uniform population-based screening for trisomy 21 in the United States. In fact, there are even laboratory-dependent variations in the specific second-trimester serum markers used. Moreover, the emergence and availability of first-trimester screening has complicated screening strategies and choices even further for frontline clinicians. Whereas some centers now use an approach that involves both first- and second-trimester screening, others use second-trimester serum marker screening only, and some couple serum screening with an ultrasound for sonographic markers by unsupervised practitioners; only a small minority attempt to derive individual risks for fetal trisomy 21 (Table 8–7). In short, the current system in the United States is inconsistent with overall high quality and high value and should not be sustained. The addition of more screening tests (especially when additive or sequential) increases false-positive rates, patient anxiety, invasive testing rates, and procedure-related pregnancy losses. However, it may be possible to decrease the invasive testing rates while maintaining high sensitivity if sequential tests are interpreted in light of the results of earlier tests.[121] Another variable to consider is that if 80% to 95% of fetuses with trisomy 21 are detected by first-trimester screening, the predictive values of second-trimester screening (ultrasonography and biochemical screening) will be dramatically reduced.[121] In theory, second-trimester biochemistry will probably identify at best-only 6% (60% of the residual 10%) of affected pregnancies screened by NT alone plus first trimester biochemistry while doubling the overall invasive testing rate (from 5% to 10%).

There is also no uniformity in screening for fetal malformations. Table 8–7 lists several approaches that are used clinically. Examples include A and C (then J or K), B (then J or K), F (then J), H only, J only, and so on. We prefer A and C (then J or K), but believe that regardless of the first- and/or second-trimester screening tests performed, and even if the patient undergoes invasive testing, a second-trimester sonogram to evaluate the fetal anatomy is the standard.

It is clear the plethora of trisomy 21 screening options has proved a source of confusion for patients and physicians. The type of test to offer also depends on several circumstances, such as when the patient presents for prenatal care, number of fetuses, the availability of chorionic villus sampling (CVS), prior obstetric history, family history, desire for early test results, and the availability of registered providers in the region of practice. Not every provider who does ultrasound is qualified; not every laboratory will provide up-to-date options. For example, not all strategies will include NT measurement because this screening approach requires specialized training on an annual basis to have

TABLE 8–7

Various Approaches Used Clinically in Screening for Fetal Malformations and/or Aneuploidy

APPROACH	DESCRIPTION	NOTES
A	First-trimester risk adjustment (age, NT, biochemistry results), with or without other markers (e.g., nasal bone, tricuspid regurgitation).	Might not be available in all regions, and NT measurement might not be obtained successfully in all patients.
B	Second-trimester serum screening (triple or quadruple).	Quadruple screening has higher sensitivity and should be utilized.
C	MSAFP.	Performed in the second trimester for those who had only first-trimester screening for aneuploidy or who have normal results from CVS.
D	Integrated (first plus second trimester).	NT, PAPP-A, quadruple screening. Results reported only after *both* first- and second-trimester screening tests are completed.
E	Serum integrated (first plus second trimester).	PAPP-A, quadruple screening. For patients without access to NT measurement or when reliable measurement cannot be obtained.
F	Stepwise sequential (first plus second trimester).	First-trimester test result: a. Positive: diagnostic test offered. b. Negative: second trimester test offered. c. Final: risk assessment incorporates first and second results.
G	Contingent sequential (first plus second trimester).	First-trimester test result: a. Positive: diagnostic test offered. b. Negative: no further testing. c. Intermediate: second-trimester test offered. d. Final: risk assessment incorporates first and second results.
H	Invasive testing (CVS, amnio) offered automatically to patients with AMA or abnormal screening results.	Discuss risks and benefits of invasive testing. Genetic sonogram not performed.
I	Invasive testing (CVS, amnio) offered to all women, regardless of age.	Discussed in ACOG Practice Bulletin: Screening for Fetal Chromosomal Abnormalities (January 2007)*
J	Sonographic fetal anatomy survey in second trimester; offer amnio, depending on results.	Not AMA or has normal screening results. No calculated adjusted risk for aneuploidy given.
K	Genetic sonogram (only high-risk patients); offer amnio if risk adjustment using negative LR is still abnormal or if marker(s) present.	A priori risk: first-trimester combined screening (if not done, then second-trimester serum screening or maternal age) Based on absence or presence of aneuploidy markers, structural anomalies, and abnormal biometry on ultrasound.
L	No testing performed.	Patient declines testing.

AMA, advanced maternal age; amnio, amniocentesis; CVS, chorionic villus sampling; LR, likelihood ratio; MASFP, maternal serum α-fetoprotein; NT, nuchal translucency; PAPP-A, pregnancy-associated plasma protein A.

* American College of Obstetricians and Gynecologists (ACOG): Screening for fetal chromosomal abnormalities. ACOG Practice Bulletin No. 77. Obstet Gynecol 2007;109:217–227.

access to the calculation algorithms, and this measurement may not be successfully obtained in a given subject. It is not practical to have the patient choose from among the large array of screening strategies that might be used.[52] It is important that providers review the evidence, identify which tests are available in the practice area, and determine which strategy or strategies will best meet the needs of these patients before deciding which strategy to offer.[52] The goal is to offer screening tests with high detection rates and low false-positive rates that also provide patients with the diagnostic options they prefer.[52] It is important but often overlooked that discussions about sensitivity and false-positive rates, disadvantages and advantages, limitations, and risks/benefits of screening tests and invasive procedures be conducted with patients.

One reasonable approach is to offer those patients seen in early pregnancy aneuploidy screening that combines first- and second-trimester testing in some fashion (*integrated, sequential*, or *contingency*).[52] The *integrated* approach to screening uses both first- and second-trimester markers (NT, PAPP-A, quadruple screen) to adjust a woman's age-related risk of having a child with Down syndrome.[122] However, the results are reported only after *both* first- and second-trimester screening tests are completed. In the FASTER trial, the detection rate was 94% to 96% (5% screen-positive rate).[77] Whereas some patients value early first-trimester screening, others are willing to wait several weeks if this will result in a higher detection rate and decreased chance of an invasive test.[123] The disadvantages of integrated screening are many and include (1) patient anxiety generated by having to wait 3 to 4 weeks between start and completion of the screening; (2) the loss of opportunity to consider CVS if the first-trimester screening indicates a high risk for aneuploidy[124]; and (3) patients may fail to complete the second-trimester portion of the screening test (after performing the first-trimester component) and, as a result, be left with no screening results. If comprehensive first-trimester screening (biochemistry, NT, NB, ductus venosus, tricuspid valve) is available, there is little benefit to integrated screening for all women. Whether a patient chooses first-trimester screening or waits for an integrated screen will vary depending on personal preferences, the types of invasive tests available, the risks they present, the patient's plans for termination, and the patient's previous experiences. If NT cannot be performed for various reasons, an alternative is to perform *serum integrated* screening (PAPP-A, quadruple screen, no incorporation of NT measurement). In the FASTER trial, the serum integrated screen resulted in an 85% to 88% detection rate.[77] Under these circumstance, the delay is acceptable to most women.[125]

Sequential screening may be more advantageous because the patient is *informed* of the first-trimester screening result. Those patients who are at highest risk may decide to have a diagnostic test, whereas those at lower risk can still take advantage of the higher detection rate achieved with additional second-trimester screening. There are two proposed strategies: *stepwise sequential* screening, and *contingent sequential* screening. In the *stepwise sequential* strategy, women determined to be at high risk (Down syndrome risk above a predetermined cutoff) after the first-trimester screen are offered genetic counseling and the option of invasive testing, whereas women below the cutoff are offered second-trimester screening. For a 5% false-positive rate, the detection rate using the stepwise sequential strategy is 95%.[77] In the *contingent sequential* strategy, patients are classified as high, intermediate, or low on the basis of first-trimester screen results. Women at high risk are offered CVS, and those at low risk have no further screening or testing. Only those women at intermediate risk are offered second-trimester screening. Contingent sequential screening has been proposed as a model (88%–94% predicted detection rate; 5% false-positive rate),[126] but large clinical trials using this approach have not yet been published. Therefore, this approach maintains high detection rates with low false-positive rates, while reducing the number of second-trimester tests performed. For both the stepwise and the contingent strategies, patients at highest risk identified by first-trimester screening are offered an early invasive procedure. Both first- and second-trimester results are used to calculate a final risk for aneuploidy in patients at lower risk.

As previously discussed, the performance of first- and second-trimester screening tests *independently* yields a high sensitivity for Down syndrome (94%–98%), but the screen-positive rates are additive, leading to many more unnecessary invasive procedures (11%–17%).[77,78] Therefore, it has been recommended that women who have had first-trimester screening for aneuploidy not undergo *independent* second-trimester serum screening in the same pregnancy.[52] Women who desire the highest sensitivity can have either an integrated or a sequential screening test, which *combines* both first- and second-trimester screening results. Many still recommend maternal serum α-fetoprotein for neural tube defect detection; others argue that an examination by a skilled sonographer has an even higher yield.

Ultimately, the screening strategy chosen will depend on the availability of CVS and sonologists who are appropriately trained in obtaining first-trimester sonographic markers. For instance, when CVS and comprehensive first-trimester screening are not available, one can offer: (1) integrated screening to patients who present in the first trimester, in order to take advantage of the improved detection rate and low-false positive rate and (2) second-trimester screening to those patients presenting after the first trimester.[52] It is suboptimal to offer patients first-trimester screening but to have no physician available who can perform CVS if that is what the patient desires. If NT measurement is unavailable or cannot be obtained in a patient, a reasonable approach is to offer: (1) serum integrated screening to patients who present early and (2) second-trimester screening to those who present later.[52] If one practices in an area where every possible screening strategy is available, it is reasonable to choose two screening strategies for the practice. For example, one can offer: (1) either comprehensive first-trimester screening or sequential screening for patients presenting for prenatal care prior to 14 weeks and (2) second-trimester serum screening for patients presenting after 13.6 weeks of gestation.[52]

A relatively new Down syndrome screening protocol is one that combines quadruple screening with nuchal fold and long bone measurements in the second trimester.[127] It has been shown to be a feasible method (90% sensitivity; 3.1% false-positive rate) to improve Down syndrome screening performance over either sonography or second-trimester serum markers by themselves. The authors suggest that efficacy may be comparable with that reported for combined first- and second-trimester (integrated) screening.[127]

Another approach is to provide all women the option of invasive testing, regardless of age. As discussed previously, in January 2007, ACOG[52] raised the issue in their *Practice Bulletin* that *all* women (regardless of age) should have the option of *invasive* diagnostic testing for aneuploidy. However, it is important to discuss the differences between screening and diagnostic testing with all women. Certainly, it would be ideal if all women were offered aneuploidy *screening* before 20 weeks' gestation, regardless of maternal age.[52]

The significance of sonographic markers identified by a second-trimester ultrasound examination in a patient who has had a negative first-trimester screening test result is unknown.[52] We believe that if the patient is otherwise low risk, the presence of only one marker (with the exception of structural anomaly, thickened nuchal fold, or absent NB) after a thorough, targeted survey will not significantly increase the risk of Down syndrome. However, if the patient is otherwise high risk, we would consider her a candidate for genetic sonography and, in the presence of marker(s), would counsel the patient that her risk for fetal Down syndrome is increased and offer and discuss genetic amniocentesis.

We anticipate that, with growing expertise, more genetic sonograms will be offered as a first choice to high risk patients and will become the standard of care in this group, with targeted fetal scans reserved for the low risk patient. Some patients may prefer first-trimester screening, second-trimester screening, or a combination of both, just as some may prefer CVS to second-trimester amniocentesis. High sensitivity is important for high risk women, whereas low false-positive rates are most desirable among low risk women.

SUMMARY OF MANAGEMENT OPTIONS

Second Trimester Screening for Fetal Abnormalities

Management Options	Evidence Quality and Recommendation	References
General		
Discuss the screening options in the first and second trimesters and decide on an individual pregnancy management plan (e.g., serum testing, ultrasound, invasive testing)	—/GPP	—
Invasive diagnostic testing (CVS, amniocentesis) for aneuploidy offered to all women, regardless of maternal age	IV/C	52
Second-Trimester Serum Screening		
Use quadruple screen testing for greater sensitivity	IIa/B	15,16
Combine with detailed sonography to screen for aneuploidy	III/B	53
	IIa/B	64
Neural tube defect screening should be offered in the second trimester to women who elect only first-trimester screening for aneuploidy or who have had a normal result from CVS	IV/C	52
After first-trimester screening, subsequent second-trimester Down syndrome screening is not indicated, unless it is being performed as a component of the integrated test, stepwise sequential, or contingent sequential test	IV/C	52
Second-Trimester Sonography		
Perform a detailed survey to increase sensitivity, and screen all patients with this test	—/GPP	—
Genetic sonography should be offered only to high risk patients and performed by experienced laboratories	III/B	53
Use three-dimensional sonography to add more information to two-dimensional sonography, if available	IV/C	86
	III/B	89,90
Authors' Practice		
For all patients, perform combined first-trimester screening (age, nuchal translucency, biochemistry)	IIa/B	75
For all patients, perform MSAFP only in the second trimester	IV/C	52
For all patients, perform fetal anatomy survey or genetic sonogram in second trimester (both detailed examinations), depending on circumstances	III/B	53
	IIa/B	64
Invasive testing also discussed as an option, when applicable	—/GPP	—
Perform three-dimensional ultrasound, if necessary	IV/C	86
	III/B	89,90

CVS, chorionic villus sampling; GPP, good practice point; MSAFP, maternal serum α-fetoprotein.

SUGGESTED READINGS

American College of Obstetricians and Gynecologists: Screening for fetal chromosomal abnormalities. ACOG Practice Bulletin No. 77. Obstet Gynecol 2007;109:217–227.

American Institute of Ultrasound in Medicine (AIUM): Practice Guideline for the Performance of Obstetric Ultrasound Examinations. Laurel, Md, AIUM, 2007.

Benacerraf BR, Benson CB, Abuhamad AZ, et al: Three- and 4-dimensional ultrasound in obstetrics and gynecology. Proceedings of the American Institute of Ultrasound in Medicine Consensus Conference. J Ultrasound Med 2005;24:1587–1597.

Ewigman BG, Crane JP, Frigoletto FD, et al: Effect of prenatal ultrasound screening on perinatal outcome: RADIUS Study Group. N Engl J Med 1993;329:821–827.

Filly RA, Benacerraf BR, Nyberg DA, et al: Choroid plexus cyst and echogenic intracardiac focus in women at low risk for chromosomal anomalies. J Ultrasound Med 2004;23:447–449.

Malone F, Canick JA, Ball RH, et al: First-trimester or second-trimester screening, or both, for Down's syndrome. First- and Second-Trimester Evaluation of Risk (FASTER) Research Consortium. N Engl J Med 2005;353:2001–2011.

Vintzileos AM, Campbell WA, Rodis JF, et al: The use of second-trimester genetic sonogram in guiding clinical management of patients at increased risk for fetal trisomy 21. Obstet Gynecol 1996;87:948–952.

Yeo L, Vintzileos AM: The use of genetic sonography to reduce the need for amniocentesis in women at high-risk for Down syndrome. Semin Perinatol 2003;27:152–159.

REFERENCES

For a complete list of references, log onto www.expertconsult.com.

CHAPTER 9

Invasive Procedures for Antenatal Diagnosis

GEORGE ATTILAKOS and PETER W. SOOTHILL

Videos corresponding to this chapter are available online at www.expertconsult.com.

INTRODUCTION

Obstetric ultrasound fostered the development of invasive techniques to assist in antenatal diagnosis. Methods such as chorionic villus sampling (CVS), amniocentesis, fetal blood sampling (FBS), and fetal tissue biopsy allow testing of fetal materials for chromosomal, genetic, and biochemical abnormalities. The type of procedure selected depends on many factors, including the indication, the gestational age, and how soon the result is needed. Possible applications are increasing rapidly with advances in human genetics and the evolution of molecular tools, but all invasive in utero diagnostic techniques carry a risk of fetal injury or death. These risks must be properly explained to the parents during the informed consent process. Noninvasive approaches, such as measuring free fetal DNA in the mother's blood, show great promise but, are at present, used clinically only in specific areas, such as fetal blood group or sex prediction.[1] Although the use of free fetal DNA and the introduction of effective screening strategies have led to fewer invasive procedures being performed,[2,3] the latter are required for the definitive diagnosis of most fetal genetic problems.

This chapter summarizes the indications, methods, and complications of the most common invasive diagnostic methods.

ISSUES COMMON TO ALL INVASIVE DIAGNOSTIC TECHNIQUES

All of the techniques described in this chapter share certain features.

Guidelines for Training

The Royal College of Obstetricians and Gynaecologists (RCOG) published guidelines for amniocentesis and CVS, including guidance on training in antenatal invasive diagnostic methods.[4] They are praised for their efforts to seek standards. They suggest that practitioners who perform invasive procedures must have a high level of training in obstetric ultrasound and that training with clinical skills models be considered. Because training is now competency-based, they do not specify a minimum number of supervised procedures before practitioners can act independently. However, they suggest that trainers perform at least 50 ultrasound-guided invasive procedures annually. After completing training, physicians should perform at least 10 invasive procedures per year in order to retain their skills, although it is emphasized that there is no evidence on the subject. It is also recommended that amniocentesis for multiple gestation be performed in a tertiary fetal medicine unit.

Training in CVS and FBS is not part of general obstetric training and is usually limited to trainees who specialize in fetal and maternal medicine. Units that perform more complex fetal procedures should perform enough procedures each year to maintain skills. They should periodically audit the results and make these available to patients and colleagues. A reasonable minimum number of complex procedures is 12 per year.

Consent

The procedure, its goals, and likely or significant complications must be explained in language that is understandable to the patient so that written informed consent can be obtained. The specific considerations for each procedure are discussed later.

Audit of Practice

It is important that the rate of complications for individual operators is monitored through robust mechanisms. Because the incidence of complications is small, it is proposed that the 95% confidence interval (CI) be used as a monitoring tool.[4] For example, the miscarriage rate for amniocentesis should not be more than 3 out of 50 or 4 out of 100 consecutive procedures. If these values are triggered, a change may be necessary. A method of prospective performance monitoring by statistical process control charts has been described.[5] The complication studied was multiple needle insertion for amniocentesis, and the authors used the 90% CI as a "warning" line and the 95% CI as an "action" line. An individual with poor performance would have triggered the action line after 55 procedures.

Sampling Site

Ultrasound is used to determine the best site to obtain the sample, considering the target size, needle length, needle path, and potential injury to structures in the path. The skin site for needle insertion is planned, but the position chosen reflects the ultrasound-guided technique used.

Ultrasound-Guided Needling Technique

Two approaches to ultrasound-guided needling are used: needle guide and freehand.

Needle Guide

The needle guide technique uses a sector or curvilinear ultrasound transducer with a guide that has an attached needle channel. Lines on the ultrasound screen indicate the path of the needle when inserted down the guide. The transducer is moved until these lines cross the intended target. This approach allows the use of thinner needles (i.e., 22–26 gauge) than those needed for a freehand procedure (i.e., 20–22 gauge). Despite the use of a thinner needle and the fact that the entire length of the needle is not usually seen, the tip is visible as a bright dot. Some have suggested that the complication rate may be lower than with the freehand technique, perhaps because the needle is thin and its movement confined to a single plane, though data on this are limited.[6] The guide does not seem to increase the need to remove and reinsert the needle, nor is there a relationship between the number of insertions and the complication rate.

Freehand

The freehand technique uses a curvilinear or linear ultrasound transducer. The ultrasound transducer is moved until the intended sampling site is identified and appears on one side of the ultrasound screen, with the skin insertion point on the other. The intended needle path is nearly perpendicular to the ultrasound beam, allowing the length of the needle to be adequately imaged (Fig. 9–1). The freehand technique allows the operator to adjust to changes during the procedure (such as contractions or fetal movements) and is the preferred approach of the authors.

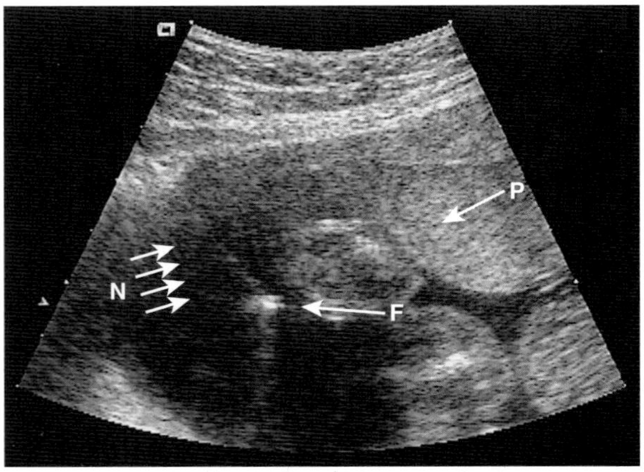

FIGURE 9–1
Ultrasound view of an amniocentesis needle (N) entering a pool of amniotic fluid. F, fluid; P, placenta.

Some operators prefer to have an assistant control the scanning transducer, but then the operator forfeits control of the intended needle path. Others prefer a single-operator technique in which one hand holds the needle and the other holds the ultrasound transducer. An assistant is required to withdraw the needle stylet, fix a syringe, aspirate at the right time, and place the sample in appropriate containers without spillage, contamination, or mislabeling.

Preparation

Regardless of technique, the atmosphere should be informal, and any additional staff required should be present for the procedure and introduced to the patient. Anything that gives the patient an image of an "operation" (e.g., surgical masks, hats, drapes) should be minimized or replaced by a scrupulous "no-touch" technique. The length of the needle required depends on abdominal wall thickness, amniotic fluid volume, and fetal and placental positions. An 8- to 12-cm needle is usually sufficient, but if in doubt, the distance should be measured on the screen before the procedure. Detailed ultrasound examination of the fetus is performed before the procedure because the discovery of structural defects, impaired growth, or other problems may alter the physician's and patient's choice. New ultrasound findings may make the procedure unnecessary, or help subsequently, when there is an unusual chromosomal finding such as mosaicism.

Needle Path Selection

If using the freehand technique, the target is visualized on screen, and the transducer is rotated through 180 degrees until a path that avoids fetal parts and maternal vessels is identified. The transducer is adjusted until the sampling site and the skin insertion point are on opposite sides of the screen. With the freehand technique, the best skin insertion point is determined by observing sonographically the effect of digital pressure on the maternal abdomen. When a needle guide is used, simply line up the needle track with the target.

Antiseptic and Anesthetic

The skin insertion site is scrupulously cleaned with antiseptic solution (e.g., chlorhexidine). Procedures that require larger than a 22-gauge needle may be helped by local anesthetic, which is injected first into the skin and then into the abdominal and uterine peritoneum. When using the freehand technique, the anesthetic injection may help confirm the needle angle required to follow the intended path and may decrease the need to change the direction of the sampling needle during the procedure. When a needle guide is used, simply line up the needle track with the target and inject the local anesthetic with a shorter needle. Patients who have undergone amniocentesis with a 22-gauge needle with and without local anesthesia reported similar pain scores and certainly lower pain scores than outpatient gynecologic procedures.[7–9]

Viral Infections

Consideration should be given to the possibility of fetal infection by maternal-fetal transmission during the procedure. It appears the risk of fetal infection by hepatitis B is low and the hepatitis B e-antigen status can help guide counseling.[10] Similarly the risk of hepatitis C transmission appears low, but such data are limited.[10] Vertical transmission of HIV is rare, and the virus is not detectable in amniotic fluid even if it is detectable in the maternal blood.[11] However, the risk of vertical transmission may be increased by amniocentesis, particularly if the mother is not on antiretroviral therapy[12] and if a fetal "needle-stick" occurs. It is recommended that all screening options are considered in the case of mothers with HIV before invasive procedures are offered.[10] The use of antiretroviral therapy is likely to reduce the risk of infection.[12,13]

Postprocedure Considerations

The patient should be shown both the fetus and the motion of the fetal heart on the ultrasound monitor after the procedure. The sample is carefully labeled, and the details are confirmed by the woman before the sample is taken to the laboratory. The information submitted to the laboratory must be sufficient for testing to be done and diagnosis to be made. It should include information about consent, including permission to store DNA and maintain cells lines, if applicable.

Alloimmunization

An invasive procedure associated with placental bleeding has a risk of Rhesus sensitization.[14–16] After an invasive intrauterine procedure, 500 IU rather than 250 IU anti-D immunoglobulin can be given intramuscularly to an at-risk Rhesus-negative woman, and indeed, the Society of Obstetricians and Gynaecologists of Canada recommends a dose of 1500 IU (300 μg) following amniocentesis, CVS, or cordocentesis.[17]

Multiple Pregnancies

Invasive procedures should be performed in women with multiple pregnancies only in a fetal medicine unit.[4] In the first trimester, the chorionicity of each sac should be carefully determined and the placental implantation site mapped.[18] In monochorionic pregnancies, a single amniotic fluid sample may be reasonable, unless ultrasound shows discordance for fetal abnormalities when both fetuses should be sampled. In dichorionic pregnancies, both sacs should be sampled separately, either with a single needle through the intertwin septum[19–21] or with two separate maternal abdominal punctures.[22] The operator should be able and willing to perform a selective feticide if an abnormal result is discordant or refer the patient to an appropriate center. The fetal loss rate after amniocentesis in twin pregnancies appears slightly higher than in singleton pregnancies.[23] The excess risk of miscarriage in various studies has been calculated between 1.2% and 1.8%,[22,24]

Ultrasound guidance eliminates the need for any dye injection, and if used, potentially harmful dyes such as methylene blue should not be used.[25] Instead of using a dye, some operators inject 2 to 3 mL of amniotic fluid mixed with air back in the amniotic sac after the first amniocentesis. This creates intense echogenicity in the first amniotic sac for 30 to 60 seconds, which allows adequate time for the second amniocentesis to be performed. If an injection of dye seems prudent, indigo carmine is preferred. Fetal zygosity can be determined from DNA when clinically indicated or when the fetuses are at risk for inheritable syndromes.[26]

Complications

The loss rate after an invasive diagnostic procedure is a combination of the procedure-related loss rate and the background loss rate. The background loss rate is much higher if the fetus has an anomaly (e.g., chromosomal abnormality, intrauterine growth restriction, fetal hydrops).[27] The procedure-related loss rate is the product of many factors, including maternal age, operator experience, type of procedure, technique used, and the difficulties experienced during the procedure.[6,28] The gestational age at the time of the procedure is also relevant. In one study, the rate of fetal loss in older women after transabdominal and transcervical CVS was 5.8% and 6.2%, respectively, if done before 12 weeks, but 2.4% thereafter.[29] Some portion of the excess loss early in gestation reflects losses destined to occur whether the procedure was done or not. Early CVS and diagnosis of aneuploidy may result in termination, with all of the physical and psychological implications for the parents, whereas delayed CVS or amniocentesis may, by virtue of the later gestation, allow time for spontaneous loss to precede the planned procedure. Several multicenter studies failed to show consistent procedure-related differences with regard to the safety of CVS compared with other methods.[30,31]

The procedure-related loss rate for CVS, amniocentesis, and FBS is reported in many studies, including those listed in Table 9–1.[6,14,30,32–60] No standard criteria are used to determine background loss rates. Postprocedural loss rates generally include all up to 28 weeks and up to term in some studies.[14,48] Others suggest that most procedure-related losses occur within 2 weeks of the procedure (Table 9–2).[27] Procedures should be confined to centers with volumes large enough to calculate their own loss rates rather than to quote the rates of other units.

SPECIFIC PROCEDURES

Chorionic Villus Sampling

Introduction

CVS, or placental biopsy, is performed from 11 weeks onward for the diagnosis of many chromosomal and genetic conditions. Amniocentesis used to be the most common invasive diagnostic test, but over the last few years, CVS use has grown in some countries to more than 50% of the invasive diagnostic procedures,[3] and the procedure is associated with more than 50% of diagnoses of chromosomal abnormality,[61] probably because of first-trimester screening. CVS is usually performed by transabdominal needle aspiration, although some practitioners still use a transcervical

TABLE 9–1

Reported Outcomes after Invasive Prenatal Diagnostic Procedures

SERIES	PROCEDURE	STUDY TYPE	REPORTING OF OUTCOMES
MRC, 1978[14]	Amnio	Controlled	Reported outcome until the end of the neonatal period
Tabor et al, 1986[58]	Amnio	RCT	Reported outcome as SA (<16 wk and >16 wk), induced abortion, SB (<36 wk and >36 wk)
Canadian trial, 1989[57]	Amnio, CVS	RCT	Reported outcome as induced abortion, loss ≤ 140 days, between 141–196 days postprocedure
Smidt-Jensen et al, 1992[55]	Amnio, CVS	RCT	Reported outcome until the neonatal period; classified as spontaneous loss before the procedure, elective abortion postprocedure, and unintentional loss
Johnson et al, 1996[53]	Amnio	RCT	Reported outcome as postprocedure total fetal loss rate until term
Nicolaides et al, 1996[54]	Amnio, CVS	Observational	Outcomes classified as total loss (spontaneous and induced) and spontaneous loss (IUD/NND)
Sundberg et al, 1997[52]	Amnio, CVS	Observational	Reported outcome as total fetal loss rate and neonatal morbidity
Hanson et al, 1987[56]	Amnio, CVS	Observational	Reported outcomes < 2 wk, > 2 wk, and 28 wk postprocedure
Eiben et al, 1997[42]	Amnio	Observational	Reported outcomes < 28 wk
CEMAT, 1998[59]	Amnio	RT	Reported loss as preprocedure abortion, postprocedure abortion (20 wk), SB, LB, and NND
Borrell et al, 1999[60]	Amnio, CVS	RT	Reported loss as preprocedure, <2 wk, and ≤1 wk after birth
Roper et al, 1999[45]	Amnio	Observational	Reported fetal loss < 24 wk, SB < 36 wk, preterm labor < 36 wk
Papantoniou et al, 2001[43]	Amnio	Observational	Reported fetal loss < 2 wk, < 28 wk, and > 28 wk
Blessed et al, 2001[44]	Amnio	Observational	Reported fetal loss within 30 days
Salvador et al, 2002[39]	Amnio	Observational	Reported outcomes as second-trimester abortions
Corrado et al, 2002[38]	Amnio	RCT	Reported fetal loss < 25 wk
Blackwell et al, 2002[40]	Amnio	Observational	Reported total fetal loss
Muller et al, 2002[37]	Amnio	Observational	Reported fetal loss < 24 wk and preterm delivery 24–28 wk
Eddleman et al, 2006[41]	Amnio	Observational	Reported fetal loss < 24 wk
Caughey et al, 2006[36]	Amnio, CVS	Observational	Reported fetal loss < 24 wk
Rhoads et al, 1989[30]	CVS	Observational	Reported outcome until the end of the neonatal period
MRC European Trial, 1991[50]	CVS	RCT	Reported outcome as spontaneous fetal death < 28 wk, termination, SB, and NND
Wapner, 1997[48]	CVS	Observational	Reported outcomes until 28 wk
Papp et al, 2002[35]	CVS	Observational	Reported fetal loss < 24 wk, SB, and loss for 1–10 wk after procedure
Brambati et al, 2002[34]	CVS	Observational	Reported fetal loss < 24 wk, IUD > 24 wk and NND
Brun et al, 2003[32]	CVS	Observational	Reported fetal loss < 28 wk and > 28 wk
Lau et al, 2005[33]	CVS	Observational	Reported SA < 24 wk, SB > 24 wk, and NND
Maxwell et al, 1991[47]	FBS	Observational	Reported losses in pregnancies with normal fetal anatomy, fetal abnormalities, fetal physiologic assessment, nonimmune hydrops; 2-wk cutoff for procedure-related loss
Anandakumar et al, 1993[49]	FBS	Observational	Reported loss when FBS was done for fetal abnormality on scan, normal fetuses, nonimmune hydrops, advanced maternal age; 2-wk cutoff for procedure-related loss
Ghidini et al, 1993[46]	FBS	Observational	Reported outcomes in low-risk groups as total fetal losses < 28 wk and > 28 wk
Wilson et al, 1994[51]	FBS	Observational	Reported procedure-related loss in cases with normal fetal growth and anatomy, fetal abnormality, or IUGR; 1-wk cutoff for procedure-related loss
Weiner and Okumura, 1996[6]	FBS	Observational	Reported outcomes until term; 2-wk cutoff for procedure-related loss

Amnio, amniocentesis; CVS, chorionic villus sampling; FBS, fetal blood sample; IUD, intrauterine death; IUGR, intrauterine growth restriction; LB, liveborn; NND, neonatal death; RCT, randomized controlled trial; RT, randomized trial; SA, spontaneous abortion; SB, stillbirth.

TABLE 9–2

Overview of Pregnancy Losses after Amniocentesis, Chorionic Villus Sampling, and Fetal Blood Sampling as Classified

TEST	TOTAL (%)	MINUS	KNOWN LETHAL CONDITION	MINUS	>2/52	= PROCEDURE-RELATED (%)
Amniocentesis	10 (1.8)		3		3	4 (0.7)
Chorionic villus sampling	18 (4.1)		14		3	1 (0.23)
Fetal blood sampling	18 (10.7)		16		0	2 (1.19)

From Nanal RKP, Soothill PW: A classification of pregnancy loss after invasive prenatal diagnostic procedures: An approach to allow comparison of units with a different case mix. Prenat Diagn 2003;23:488–492.

technique, with catheter aspiration or biopsy. Many consider transcervical CVS an obsolete technique because of the higher procedure pregnancy loss rates.[55]

Indications

Fetal trophoblast cells, especially from the mesenchymal core of the villi, divide rapidly. The advantage of first-trimester CVS is rapid diagnosis at an early gestation. If an abnormality is detected, surgical termination, rather than medical induction, can be offered. Early detection of chromosomal disorders is the most common indication for CVS. The introduction and growing availability of first-trimester screening for Down syndrome (e.g., nuchal translucency, β-human chorionic gonadotropin [β-HCG] and pregnancy-associated plasma protein A [PAPP-A] measurement)[62] have increased the importance of CVS. Noninvasive approaches, such as measuring maternal plasma free fetal DNA, have made invasive testing for sex-related disease unnecessary in 50% of the cases because it is required only when the fetus is the at-risk sex.[2,63] Because of the increasing number of diagnosable monogenic disorders, couples with a family history of a genetic disorder should be offered genetic counseling, either before conception or early in pregnancy. Rapid direct preparation of the fetal karyotype or fluorescent in situ hybridization (FISH) have largely been replaced with quantitative fluorescent polymerase chain reaction (QF-PCR) of chromosomes 13, 18, 21, and Y, if requested. Fetal cells are also cultured for karyotype analysis, but it is very likely that this will be replaced by molecular whole genome approaches such as array comparative genome hybridization (CGH). CVS can be used at any time in gestation, and placental biopsy is a very successful way to obtain a karyotype after delivery when the fetus has died.

PROCEDURE

CHORIONIC VILLUS SAMPLING

Consent

The procedure should be described to the patient. Counseling must include the aims of the CVS (i.e., karyotype, DNA analysis), and the risk of a serious complication (often described as 1%), including miscarriage, either procedure-related or background, should be quoted. The possible risk of limb defects is mentioned by some, but the risk is minimal after 10 weeks. The limitations of a karyotype and the risks of unrelated abnormalities that are not detected by a karyotype should be explained. Patients should also be informed of the small chance that testing will show confined placental mosaicism or sex chromosome abnormality and the small possibility of a further invasive technique such as amniocentesis or fetal blood sampling to confirm a diagnosis. Alternative diagnostic techniques may be discussed. Only after the counseling process is complete is the patient asked to provide written consent.

Sampling Site

The ideal target is a thick part of the placenta that can be sampled at an angle that allows a long needle path through the placenta and avoids a perpendicular path toward the chorionic plate. Very rarely, at approximately 11 weeks, transabdominal CVS is difficult if the uterus is retroverted, the placenta is posterior, and a lateral approach is not possible. Some operators switch to a transcervical approach, but we would ask the patient to return in a week, when sampling may be easier.

Target Puncture

Transabdominal CVS can be done either freehand or with a needle guide. With the "double-needle" technique (Fig. 9–2), after a local anesthetic has been administered, the first needle is advanced through the maternal skin, through the uterine wall, and into the placenta. The stylet is removed, and a second needle is passed into the placenta and attached to a syringe that contains normal saline. The placental villi are then aspirated.[64,65] By drawing the finer needle into the outer needle during aspiration, the sharp bevel of the first needle seems to cut the villi, reducing the need for needle movement and presumably reducing placental trauma.[66] A placental biopsy forceps may also be used through an outer guide needle. With the double-needle technique, if the tip is inserted correctly into the placenta, maternal contamination cannot occur. If a single needle is used, the aspirated tissue can be examined with a dissection microscope to exclude maternal contamination, but the risk of contamination should be considered. Whatever technique is selected, the sample is placed in a suitable CVS medium before it is transferred to the cytogenetics laboratory.

Maternal contamination of chorionic cell cultures may lead to a false-negative diagnosis, particularly when polymerase chain reaction (PCR) amplification is used and in some biochemical examinations. Operator experience reduces the risk of maternal cell contamination.

Transcervical CVS

This approach is less common now because of an apparent increased risk of fetal loss and an increased

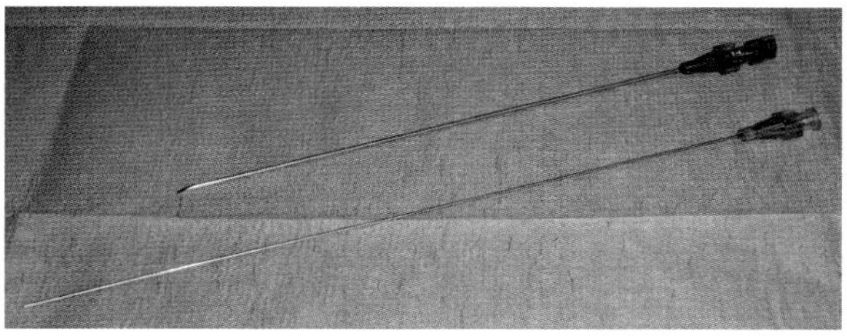

FIGURE 9–2
An 18- to 21-g double needle for chorionic villus sampling (CVS). The stylet of the 18-g (pink) needle is removed and the thinner 21-g (green) needle is passed into the placenta for the aspiration of the villi.

likelihood of failure.[67–69] Only 2%, and now probably less, of fetal medicine consultants in the United Kingdom perform transcervical CVS.[70] Some practitioners consider this approach useful in high risk patients who require early diagnosis or when the uterus is retroverted and the placenta is posterior or when an anterior wall leiomyoma makes an abdominal approach difficult. A bendable polyethylene catheter with a metal obturator is introduced through the cervix and advanced into the placenta under ultrasound guidance. A syringe that is partially filled with saline is attached to the hub and a vacuum created to aspirate 10 to 50 mg of tissue, which is then rinsed into a Petri dish. Some units prefer curved biopsy forceps.[71]

Complications

CVS should be performed only under continuous ultrasound guidance. Canadian[57] and Danish[55] trials found no significant difference in procedure-related loss rates between the first and the second trimesters. Only the Danish study[55] allowed a randomized comparison of transabdominal CVS and second-trimester amniocentesis and the fetal loss rates were similar. A 1% excess fetal loss rate is usually quoted for amniocentesis and CVS.

Some reports suggest that first-trimester CVS (including those performed as early as 6–7 wk) may be associated with severe limb defects.[72–74] These defects were not observed in CVS performed after 11 weeks' gestation. The World Health Organization (WHO) International Registry for Limb Defects found no difference in the prevalence of limb defects after CVS compared with the background population.[75,76] Therefore, during counseling, it is standard practice to indicate that there is no increased incidence of limb defects after 10 weeks.

Placental Mosaicism

Confined placental mosaicism occurs in approximately 1% of samples,[77–80] but this rate may be lower with experienced laboratories. Analyzing several cultures makes it easier to detect in vitro changes because they are usually present in a single culture (pseudomosaicism). However, the same finding in several or all of the cultures increases the likelihood of true mosaicism, either confined to the placenta or present in both placenta and fetus. In this case, another fetal tissue, such as blood or amniotic fluid, should be tested depending in part on the particular chromosome involved. The finding of structural abnormality on ultrasound is very important and makes it much less likely that the results are caused by confined placental mosaicism.

Late Placental Biopsy

Several small series indicate that late placental biopsy is both safe and reliable for diagnosis. The loss rate is similar to that of first-trimester CVS.[81,82]

Conclusion

CVS provides a rich source of fetal cells or DNA for analysis of karyotypic and genetic disorders. It is usually performed after 11 weeks, typically by a transabdominal route. One advantage of first-trimester CVS is that an abnormal result allows surgical termination, if desired. Mosaicism is a rare complication in about 1% of samples; the rate is lower with amniocentesis.

SUMMARY OF MANAGEMENT OPTIONS

Chorionic Villus Sampling and Placental Biopsy

Management Options	Evidence Quality and Recommendation	References
Indications		
Genetic	III/C	61
QF-PCR/fluorescent in situ hybridization, karyotype, DNA		
Procedural Options		
Transabdominal is the route of choice	Ia/A	67
Complications		
Fetal loss rate has been reported to be similar to amniocentesis, though this remains controversial	Ib/A	67
Fear of limb-reduction defects (gestation-dependent)	IIb/B	75,76
Placental mosaicism	III/B	79,80
Alloimmunization	III/B	17
Maternal contamination	III/B	86

QF-PCR, quantitative fluorescent polymerase chain reaction.

Amniocentesis

Introduction

Amniotic fluid contains amniocytes in addition to fetal cells from the skin, genitourinary system, and gut, along with biochemical products that may be removed for analysis. Amniocentesis should be performed only under continuous ultrasound guidance.[4]

Indications

GENETIC

Amniocentesis is usually performed to determine fetal karyotype. Indications for fetal karyotyping include an abnormal screening test result for trisomy 21, advanced maternal age, a sonographically detected structural abnormality, previous aneuploidy, and known chromosomal translocation in either partner. With the advance of genetics and molecular biology, more genetic diseases can be diagnosed by amniocentesis rather than other more "direct" methods: for example, harlequin ichthyosis can now be diagnosed with DNA-based testing on amniotic fluid rather than fetal skin biopsy.[83,84]

The amniotic fluid container is labeled and examined by the patient for accuracy, and the sample is sent promptly to the cytogenetics laboratory for analysis. The amniocytes are studied during the metaphase stage of cell division. Although standard culture techniques require 2 to 3 weeks, newer methods, with the cells grown on a cover slip, allow a complete analysis in 7 to 10 days,[85] and it is likely karyotyping will be replaced by molecular approaches in the next few years. Approximately 0.5% of cultures are unsuccessful; less often, maternal contamination complicates the diagnosis.[86] Less than 0.4% of cultures show evidence of pseudomosaicism or true mosaicism.[87,88] FBS may be helpful, but a normal result does not guarantee that all is well.

Direct DNA probing of interphase chromosomes by FISH can be used to detect known deletions, such as 22q in at-risk pregnancies, in addition to rapid diagnosis of trisomy 13, 18, and 21,[89,90] but the latter has been replaced by QF-PCR. Although a positive test result is reliable, detecting 90% or more of chromosomal abnormalities, some problems detectable by karyotyping will not be found on rapid testing. Currently, rapid aneuploidy screening is usually performed with QF-PCR whose detection rate for the common aneuploidies (chromosomes 13, 18, 21, X, and Y) is 98.6%.[91] QF-PCR has some advantages over FISH, which is why it is used more widely. It has been argued that QF-RCR could be used as a "stand-alone" test (no karyotype performed), but this could result in a small proportion of abnormalities not being diagnosed.[92] PCR-based primers are now used with DNA from amniotic fluid samples to determine almost all potentially relevant fetal red blood cell and platelet genotypes.[93,94] Methods using free fetal DNA in maternal blood are likely to further reduce the need for amniocentesis. In some countries, it is already used to detect fetal D status, when indicated, as part of routine prenatal care,[63] and high throughput testing is being introduced to reduce the administration of the blood product anti-D in routine antenatal prophylaxis.[95]

BIOCHEMISTRY

Molecular DNA analysis has largely replaced amniocentesis to diagnose inborn errors of metabolism and cystic fibrosis by measuring fetal enzymes activity and their products or substrates. Likewise, amniocentesis to measure α-fetoprotein and acetylcholinesterase to diagnose a neural tube defect are rarely necessary because of the reliability of ultrasonography.[96]

FETAL INFECTION

Although cytomegalovirus is excreted in fetal urine and fetal infection is reliably detected by culture of amniotic fluid,[97,98] PCR technology is the method of choice for the antenatal diagnosis of fetal viral infection because many viruses grow poorly in clinical laboratories (also see Chapters 27–31). PCR has replaced the traditional mouse inoculation test for toxoplasmosis because it can be used earlier in pregnancy and has greater sensitivity (also see Chapter 32).[99] As with traditional methods, a false-negative result may occur if there has been insufficient time for transplacental passage to occur. Therefore, in cases of suspected toxoplasmosis, a negative amniocentesis result does not provide complete reassurance and ultrasound follow-up is recommended.[100]

CHORIOAMNIONITIS

Successful amniocentesis is possible in 49% to 98% of women with preterm premature rupture of the membranes (PPROM).[101] The likelihood of successful sampling is higher in more recent publications.[102] The specimen can be assessed by direct microscopy, Gram stain, culture, and a series of new proteomic tools. It is unclear whether management based on the information gained in women with PPROM changes the clinical outcome. No randomized trial supports the use of routine amniocentesis to diagnose chorioamnionitis in women with either preterm labor or PPROM, although a small study showed an increased hospital stay for babies in the "no amniocentesis" group.[103] A recent feasibility study concluded that a randomized study of amniocentesis versus no amniocentesis in women with PPROM would be feasible.[104] Amniocentesis may be useful when the woman is asymptomatic and fetal infection is suspected. Between 17% and 34% of asymptomatic women with PPROM have positive culture findings,[101] which may allow for earlier diagnosis and treatment.[105] However, most women with positive culture findings deliver within 48 hours, and there is inadequate information to guide antibiotic selection to ensure therapeutic concentrations at the site of infection.

FETAL LUNG MATURITY

Improved gestational dating, appropriate use of corticosteroids, and a growing understanding of the timing of iatrogenic premature delivery have nearly eliminated the need for amniotic fluid analysis to assess fetal lung maturity.[106]

Early Amniocentesis

Some had hoped that early amniocentesis (<15 wk) would be an alternative to CVS.[53,107,108] However, the risks of early amniocentesis, including spontaneous abortion, stillbirth, and neonatal death, are greater than those of CVS.[54] The

Canadian Early and Mid-trimester Amniocentesis Trial (CEMAT) group concluded that early amniocentesis should be performed only in special circumstances because of the higher fetal loss rate and incidence of talipes with early versus second-trimester amniocentesis.[59] The risk of membrane rupture is particularly high when performed before 13 completed weeks, possibly because, at this stage, the amnion is not adherent to the chorion and so is more likely to rupture and persistent amnion chorion separation may be a risk factor even later in pregnancy. Several other studies found an increased risk of oligohydramnios and associated orthopedic abnormalities, including talipes equinovarus.[52,54] Tenting of the amniotic membrane and the smaller amount of fluid in the amniotic sac before 15 weeks increase the incidence of a "dry" tap.[109] The sample volume is smaller and there are fewer cells per milliliter, although the percentage of cells dividing is higher. Djalali and colleagues[110] reported that longer culture times were required after early amniocentesis.

PROCEDURE

AMNIOCENTESIS

Amniocentesis is performed under ultrasound guidance after 15 weeks' gestation. A typical karyotypic study requires the removal of 15 to 20 mL of amniotic fluid.[4] Removal of larger volumes should be avoided unless necessary for specific tests.

Consent

The indication and risks of the procedure should be fully explained to the woman. Serious or frequently occurring risks of amniocentesis that should be quoted to patients.[111] These include miscarriage (≤1% excess risk), failure to obtain the sample, fetal injury, maternal bowel injury, amniotic fluid leakage, severe sepsis (<1/1000), and failure of cell culture. Preprocedure counseling by a midwife-practitioner has been successfully introduced in some hospitals.[112]

Antiseptic and Anesthetic

The skin is scrupulously cleaned with antiseptic solution (e.g., chlorhexidine). Local anesthetic is not normally required for diagnostic amniocentesis, because it does not decrease the pain perception.[7,8]

Target Puncture

Under ultrasound guidance, the needle is advanced into the targeted pool of amniotic fluid, with care taken to avoid the fetus, placenta, and cord (see Fig. 9–1). A 22-gauge needle is usually used.[70] If the freehand technique is used, the ultrasound beam is directed so that the length of the needle is visualized, allowing the operator to alter the course in response to fetal movements and contractions. When the tip of the needle reaches the targeted location, a very small volume of amniotic fluid is aspirated and discarded to avoid maternal contamination. Approximately 15 to 20 mL of fluid is aspirated and sent for analysis. To prevent maternal contamination, the syringe is removed from the hub before the needle is withdrawn from the patient.

Complications

Early studies, including CEMAT, reported a total loss rate of 3.2% after amniocentesis.[59,113] These losses are believed to reflect, at least in part, the large needles used (>19 gauge) as well as unsuccessful attempts. The British Working Party on Amniocentesis reported a 2.4% total fetal loss rate before 28 weeks (stillbirth rate of 1.2% vs. 0.8% in control subjects) and neonatal death (0.5% control subjects), but concluded that the loss rate attributed directly to amniocentesis was 1.5%.[14] The only randomized trial of low-risk women suggested a 1% risk of spontaneous abortion after amniocentesis.[58] Interestingly, a secondary analysis of the patients enrolled in the FASTER (First and Second Trimester Evaluation of Risk) trial[114] showed no difference in the fetal loss rates before 24 weeks between the amniocentesis and the control groups.[41] It would be premature to adopt this conclusion, because recent literature reviews suggest an excess fetal loss after amniocentesis of 0.6%.[115,116] It is possible that the control group had a higher loss rate because of undiagnosed chromosomal abnormality cases still being included while not being present in the amniocentesis group. Our study of fetal loss after amniocentesis (defined as the total loss rate minus known lethal condition minus losses beyond 2 weeks postprocedure) was 0.7%.[27] The RCOG advises that a 1% risk should be quoted to patients, and if lower risks are quoted, they should be supported by robust local data.[4] Perforating the placenta increases the relative risk of loss 2.6 times and increases the maternal serum α-fetoprotein level 8.3 times. The transplacental route should, therefore, be avoided unless no other option is available.

Although no randomized controlled trials assessed the procedure-related loss rate from amniocentesis in multiple pregnancies, case-control studies suggest that the loss rate is only slightly higher than the background rate (1.15%–1.8%).[22–24,27,117]

OLIGOHYDRAMNIOS

Up to 2% of amniocenteses are associated with chronic leakage of amniotic fluid. It is plausible that the risk is smaller with the use of smaller needles. There are variable reports of an increased prevalence of neonatal respiratory morbidity after amniocentesis; the small risk of oligohydramnios after amniocentesis may contribute to this complication.[14,118,119] Similarly, talipes equinovarus is rarely attributable to amniocentesis, and probably only secondary to oligohydramnios.

FETAL TRAUMA

Inadvertent puncture of the fetus during amniocentesis has not been not reported in a large series when the procedure was performed under continuous ultrasound guidance by experienced operators.[58] Several case reports suggest an association between amniocentesis and skin dimpling, fistulas, cord hematoma, and corneal perforation.[120–123] Because intended fetal puncture rarely leaves a mark and similar findings occur in neonates who did not undergo amniocentesis, the association is dubious. However, this is obviously to be avoided, partly because of possible risks of viral transmission such as HIV.

Conclusion

Amniocentesis after 15 weeks is the most widely performed antenatal diagnostic technique. It is relatively simple to perform, and although a fetal karyotype is the most common indication, the procedure has many uses. The application of PCR has steadily reduced the amount of amniotic fluid needed for testing and the time required for at least an initial result.

SUMMARY OF MANAGEMENT OPTIONS

Amniocentesis

Management Options	Evidence Quality and Recommendation	References
Indications		
Chromosome analysis: fluorescent in situ hybridization, PCR, karyotype	III/B	89–92
DNA diagnosis: single-gene disorders (e.g., Huntingdon's), X-linked disorders	—/GPP	—
Biochemistry: α-fetoprotein, acetylcholinesterase	III/B	96
Fetal infection: toxoplasmosis, cytomegalovirus	III/B	97–100
Chorioamnionitis	III/B	101–103
Lung maturity	III/B	106
Procedural Options		
Local anesthesia not necessary	Ib/A	7
Continuous ultrasound control	III/B	4
Complications		
Fetal Loss		
Related to experience of operator	III/B	4
Increased with early amniocentesis	Ib/A	54,59,67
Chorioamnionitis	III/B	111
Preterm premature rupture of the membranes, oligohydramnios	IIa/B	111
Alloimmunization	III/B	17
Maternal contamination	III/B	58

GPP, good practice point; PCR, polymerase chain reaction.

Fetal Blood Sampling

Introduction

Fetal blood was first obtained during labor from the capillary circulation of the presenting part.[124] FBS in a continuing pregnancy was first undertaken transabdominally by fetoscopy to diagnose severe inherited diseases, with termination planned if the fetus was affected. Cordocentesis was first reported in the 1980s.[125] The development of medical approaches to fetal disease has made the role of fetal phlebotomy (typically by cordocentesis) comparable with that in postnatal medicine.

Indications

Indications for FBS may be grouped into diagnostic and therapeutic areas. Here we focus on the diagnostic indications. FBS is indicated when the potential benefit of a change in management outweighs the procedure-related risks.

Diagnostic Uses

CHROMOSOMAL ABNORMALITIES

The rapid rate at which white blood cells divide allows a high-quality karyotype with good chromosome banding within 48 to 72 hours. The most common indications for a rapid karyotype are fetal malformation or severe early-onset fetal growth restriction detected by ultrasonography. However the value of the speed of the result is falling with the routine use of amniotic fluid PCR or FISH. Other problems that can be investigated by fetal blood cytogenetic analysis include possible mosaicism and culture failure after either amniocentesis or placental biopsy. For many indications, QF-PCR has replaced FBS.

SINGLE-GENE DEFECTS

FBS can diagnose hemoglobinopathies, coagulopathies, severe combined immunodeficiency, chronic granulomatous disease, and some metabolic disorders.[126] FBS is performed less often for antenatal diagnosis of single-gene disorders than previously because many can be diagnosed earlier in gestation by applying DNA techniques to amniocytes. FBS remains an option for at-risk patients who seek care late and when DNA analysis is not possible.

ANEMIA

Although various indirect methods are used to assess fetal anemia (also see Chapter 13), the definitive test before and after birth is measurement of the hemoglobin concentration. This may be required in maternal red cell alloimmunization[126] and some cases of nonimmune hydrops.[127] The reliability of the use of middle cerebral artery Doppler peak velocity to diagnose anemia has greatly reduced the role of FBS to detect anemia.[18]

THROMBOCYTOPENIA

Severe fetal thrombocytopenia as a result of alloimmune thrombocytopenia may lead to cerebral hemorrhage before, during, or after birth and might cause mental handicap or death (also see Chapter 14). The fetal platelet count can be measured to guide diagnosis and treatment, but this is used much less than previously because of the effectiveness of intravenous immunoglobulin, which is now often used without FBS.[128]

HYPOXIA AND ACIDOSIS

Fetal acidemia may be excluded by Doppler studies of the fetal vasculature (also see Chapters 10 and 11). Suspected fetal hypoxia or acidemia can be confirmed or refuted by fetal blood gas analysis.[129] Increasing evidence shows that chronic fetal acidemia is associated with impaired long-term neurodevelopment.[130] However, there is no convincing evidence that the benefits of fetal acid-base status outweigh the risks of FBS, and therefore, it is rarely indicated.

INFECTION

Appropriate fetal blood tests (e.g., infection-specific fetal immunoglobulin M or detection of specific genomic material by PCR) can determine whether maternal infection has led to fetal infection. However, the difference between being "infected" and "affected" (i.e., damaged) must not be forgotten. Fetal blood tests are almost never used because the reliability of amniotic fluid PCR has become established and the importance of ultrasound findings is clear.

MONITORING OF TRANSPLACENTAL THERAPY

Some fetal diseases are treated by drugs that are given to the mother, cross the placenta, and achieve therapeutic concentrations in the fetus. Examples include antiarrhythmic agents (e.g., flecainide or digoxin) to correct fetal tachyarrhythmias and gammaglobulin to improve low fetal platelet counts. FBS can be used to measure fetal drug levels.[131,132]

Procedure Options

The operator chooses the intended sampling site and guide technique from several options, described earlier.

SAMPLING SITE

Umbilical Cord Vessels (Cordocentesis)

FBS was first performed under fetoscopic guidance[133] and entailed a 2% to 5% risk of serious complication.[134] In addition, the maternal sedation used to facilitate the procedure affected the fetal blood gas measurements.[135] Ultrasound-guided needling is considered safer and the preferred technique.[125,136]

The placental origin of the umbilical cord is often the easiest site to puncture. Many prefer this site because of its fixed location, which prevents movement of the needle. Others accept free loop puncture, but use pancuronium to minimize subsequent fetal movement. Some use free loop puncture without fetal paralysis and suggest no obvious increase in fetal loss rate.[137] A relevant consideration is not the location, but the ease of access. The fetal origin of the umbilical cord is problematic because there is no length to buffer the effect of fetal movement after puncture and the potential for bradycardia may be increased. Although cordocentesis is usually done after 18 weeks, success is reported as early as 12 weeks, at the cost of an increased fetal loss rate.[138,139]

Fetal Intrahepatic Vessels

Blood can also be obtained from the intrahepatic portion of the umbilical vein (Fig. 9–3).[131,140] This procedure is useful when the umbilical cord insertion is not accessible. It can be made easier by administration of vecuronium or pancuronium into the vein[141] for fetal paralysis. This is especially useful when a lengthy transfusion is anticipated. The complication

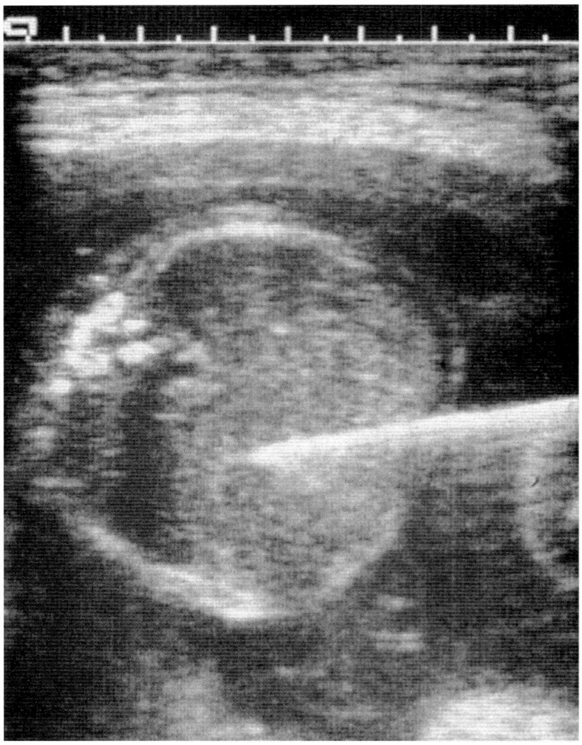

FIGURE 9–3
Fetal blood sampling by ultrasound-guided needling of the intrahepatic vein.

FIGURE 9–4
Fetal blood sampling by ultrasound-guided needling of the heart.

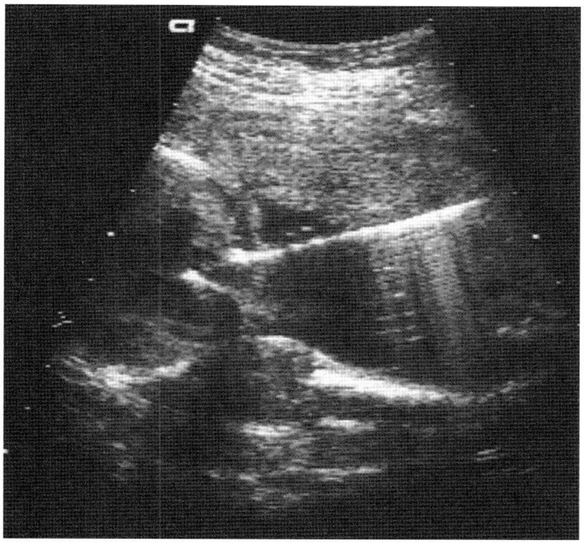

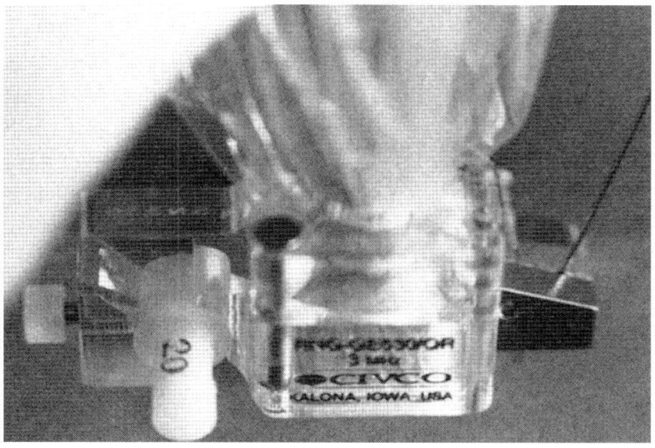

FIGURE 9–5
A typical needle guide used to perform cordocentesis. The small footprint allows the needle to enter the sonographic plane shortly after it penetrates the skin.

rates of this approach are comparable with those of cordocentesis, and this seems applicable to intravascular transfusion as well.[142] There is possibly a smaller likelihood of bleeding after this procedure, which may make it more suitable for use when severe fetal thrombocytopenia is suspected.[143]

Fetal Heart

The heart is larger than the umbilical cord, and puncture of the heart is relatively simple (Fig. 9–4). Despite fear of damage, cardiac puncture is relatively safe.[144] The heart can be used in the unusual event that the umbilical cord or hepatic vein cannot be punctured and fetal blood must be obtained. It can also be useful if an emergency blood transfusion is required (e.g., to treat procedure-related bleeding) or for feticide. Because the fetal heart contains blood from different circulatory origins, it may not be suitable for blood gas assessment.[145]

FIGURE 9–6
Cordocentesis with the freehand technique.

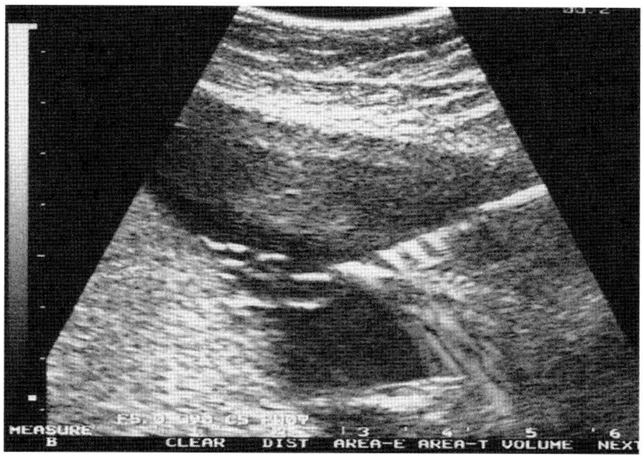

NEEDLING TECHNIQUE

A needle guide or freehand technique may be used (Figs. 9–5 and 9–6). A combined technique, in which the needle guide is used for the approach to the cord and a freehand technique for the vessel puncture, has also been described.[146]

PROCEDURE

FETAL BLOOD SAMPLING

The following elements are shared, regardless of whether FBS is performed freehand or with a needle guide. FBS should be performed only by physicians who have extensive experience with other obstetric, ultrasound-guided needle procedures (e.g., amniocentesis, transabdominal CVS). Units that offer this service must perform enough cases to maintain expertise; 20 procedures per year is a reasonable minimum. This typically requires a center with many referrals.[147]

Preparation

An urgent delivery may be required if the pregnancy is at a potentially viable gestation, and if the indication for the procedure has not led the patient to request a conservative approach in the event of complications (e.g., a major brain malformation). Otherwise, the procedure must be performed at a site with easy and rapid access to an operative delivery room with an anesthetist immediately available in viable pregnancies. The mother should be positioned to avoid supine hypotension; hyperventilation and sedation should be avoided. An 8- to 12-cm needle is usually sufficient depending on several factors including amniotic fluid volume and maternal obesity, and the distance should be measured on the ultrasound screen before starting if there is any doubt.

Needle Path Selection

A transplacental approach usually provides the easiest route to the placental cord origin, unless the placenta is entirely posterior. However, in women with red cell alloimmunization, transplacental puncture boosts the

FIGURE 9–7
Transplacental (*A*) and transamniotic (*B*) fetal blood sampling from the placental insertion of the umbilical cord (cordocentesis). PL, placenta.

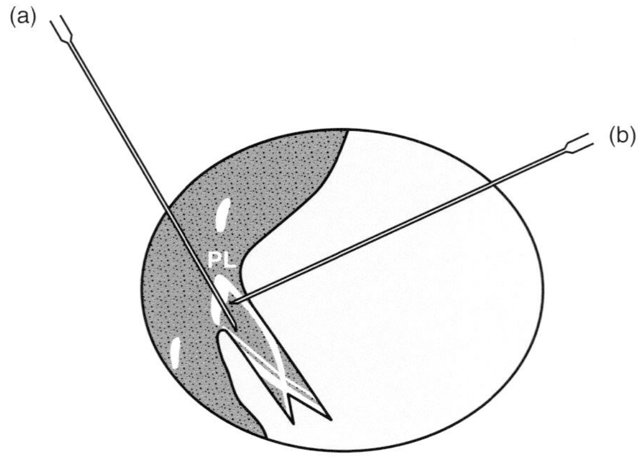

maternal antibody titer as a result of fetal-maternal hemorrhage.[148] Therefore, it is best to avoid the placenta, unless transfusion is anticipated in an alloimmunized woman (Fig. 9–7).

Target Puncture

Cordocentesis

Many operators prefer the placental origin of the umbilical cord, approximately 1 cm from the placenta, because the blood obtained from this site must be fetal. A closer puncture can lead to confusion. The needle is brought close to or even touching the umbilical vein, and then sharply advanced the remaining distance. A slow advance may push the tissue away, even at this relatively fixed site. After the needle tip is visualized within the lumen of the umbilical cord, the stylet is removed. If the needle is ideally sited, blood will fill the hub. A 1-mL syringe is applied tightly to the hub, and blood is withdrawn. After 20 weeks, 7 mL may be sampled, but before 20 weeks, the volume removed should be the minimum necessary for the specific tests. Often, no blood is obtained initially and the operator must assess whether the needle tip has passed through the vessel lumen or perhaps is located in Wharton's jelly. The needle is sharply advanced or gently withdrawn, and the shaft is rotated 180 degrees between the operator's finger and thumb while suction is maintained.

Occasionally, amniotic fluid is obtained when the needle tip appears intraluminal. With the freehand technique, the needle is moved side-to-side in search of cord movement. With a needle guide, an up-and-down movement of the needle produces the same result. Cord movement indicates that the needle has passed through the cord. It is withdrawn until no more amniotic fluid is aspirated, the syringe is changed (because even a small amount of amniotic fluid is a very powerful coagulant), and the procedure is continued. If the needle has passed through the side of the cord without entering a vessel lumen, it is withdrawn slightly and its path adjusted. If the tip is lateral to the umbilical cord, it is withdrawn and the needle used to touch the vein before the puncture attempt is repeated.

It is essential to identify the vessel that has been entered if blood gas results are to be interpretable. If the puncture is performed at either the placental or the fetal origin of the umbilical cord, the vessel can usually be identified by the direction of turbulence after rapid injection of up to 1 mL of normal saline.[136] If fetal paralysis is desired, intravascular administration of pancuronium (0.2–0.3 mg/kg estimated fetal weight) serves the same purpose as saline for identification.

Intrahepatic or Heart

If the intrahepatic vein or the heart is the intended sampling site, fetal paralysis with intramuscular pancuronium (0.2–0.3 mg/kg estimated fetal weight) may be used. The effect is rapid (within minutes) and lasts for 90 to 120 minutes. The techniques for needle path selection and guidance are similar to those described for the umbilical cord. However, the fetal chest or abdomen is entered first, the direction is checked, and the needle is advanced into the sampling site as a separate movement. The heart is best entered through the anterior chest, through the thick muscle of the ventricles to reduce blood leakage and avoid damage to the valves or electrical conduction system.

A double-needle technique has also been described.[149] The first needle is used to puncture the fetal body cavity and a second, finer needle is passed within the first to puncture the target. This technique offers the theoretical advantage of the stiffness of the first needle and the small caliper of the sampling needle.

Postprocedure Monitoring

The puncture site is observed ultrasonically for bleeding after the needle is removed. Bleeding is common after transamniotic cordocentesis, but is usually brief and without clinical significance. After bleeding has stopped, the fetal heart rate is measured. Bradycardia is the most common complication of cordocentesis, but it is usually transient. If the fetus is previable, the woman should wait in the hospital until she feels well and then return home. There are no special precautions or restrictions. If a local anesthetic is used, she should be warned to expect a bruised sensation in a few hours. Cramping is noted in about 10% of women. Acetaminophen (paracetamol) or another nonprescription analgesic can be used safely. If the fetus is viable, the heart rate pattern is assessed by cardiotocography for at least 30 minutes before discharge. Pancuronium causes a nonreactive tracing, with mild fetal tachycardia. The mother should be warned that perceptible movement might not return for several hours.

In the rare event that bleeding from the puncture site is prolonged and heavy, maternal blood may be collected into heparinized syringes for an emergency fetal transfusion. This is most likely with alloimmune thrombocytopenia when the fetus is profoundly thrombocytopenic.

Laboratory Testing

Several laboratory techniques are available to rapidly confirm that the blood sample is fetal and pure. However, they may be unnecessary if the technique described previously is used. Further, they may be unusable if the fetal blood has been replaced with adult blood by transfusion. It is prudent to send a small sample of blood for a hematology profile to confirm that the mean cell volume is increased and that the hemoglobin concentration, white blood cell count, and platelet count are normal.

Complications and Risks

FETAL

The principal complications of FBS that threaten fetal well-being are, in order of frequency, fetal bradycardia (probably as a result of smooth muscle spasm after inadvertent puncture of the umbilical artery), hemorrhage or an obstructing hematoma at the puncture site,[150] and intrauterine infection.[151] Chorioamnionitis is often caused by *Staphylococcus epidermidis*. It typically causes myalgia, arthralgia, and a low fever 4 to 10 days after the procedure. There is no evidence to support prophylactic antibiotic administration, and most of the antibiotic agents used achieve poor amniotic fluid levels so prophylaxis is unnecessary. Placental abruption shortly after cordocentesis has been reported,[152] and PPROM has a frequency similar to that of amniocentesis. There is a risk of transmitting infection from the mother's blood (e.g., hepatitis, HIV) to the fetus, but this risk is probably low and possibly lower with the use of antiretroviral treatment in patients with HIV.[10–13] It has not yet been documented. Nevertheless, invasive procedures should be avoided when a mother has a life-threatening viral illness, unless the fetal indication warrants the additional risk.[153] A case of fetal hepatic necrosis in a growth-restricted fetus within 24 hours of intrahepatic vein blood sampling has been reported.[154]

POSTPROCEDURE LOSS RATES

Several well-recognized factors affect postprocedure loss rates. Loss and complication rates are clearly related to the indication for sampling and the final fetal diagnosis.[6,46,47,49,51,155] The background risk of intrauterine death is high when there is a severe structural malformation or a major chromosomal abnormality. The risk of profound bradycardia is significantly increased by fetal hypoxemia and arterial puncture. There does not appear to be an increased risk after cordocentesis in fetuses with a single umbilical artery.[156] Gestational age at sampling is also an important determinant because a viable fetus can be delivered if a complication arises. Emergency cesarean section may prevent fetal death, but by the time the problem is recognized and delivery is accomplished, the neonate may survive permanently damaged or die in the neonatal period. Performing the procedure near the delivery suite minimizes these risks, if delivery can be accomplished within 15 minutes.

The literature must be interpreted carefully because postprocedure loss rates are described after the application of qualifiers. It is essential to control for the indication or final diagnosis when comparing loss rates. It is only by doing so and by limiting the comparison to healthy fetuses that the risk of the technique is shown. Reports of procedures performed freehand show a total procedure loss rate of approximately 1% to 2%, depending on the mix of indications. In one study of 202 pregnancies, the loss rate was 1 of 76 (1.5%) fetuses sampled for antenatal diagnosis, 5 of 76 (7%) sampled for an anomaly, 4 of 29 (14%) sampled for fetal assessment, and 9 of 35 (25%) sampled for nonimmune hydrops.[47] The fetal loss rate was similarly low in more recent studies.[137,143] Transfusion carries a considerably higher procedure-related risk than FBS.

MATERNAL

The main maternal risk associated with FBS is red cell alloimmunization. The fetal blood type should be tested in at-risk women, and anti-D immunoglobulin should be given if the fetus is Rhesus-positive. Chorioamnionitis or emergency cesarean section can create secondary maternal risks. When FBS or transfusion is undertaken and the fetus is considered viable, maternal aspects of emergency delivery should be considered. Needle injury to the maternal intra-abdominal organs, such as intestines, or vessels may be more common than recognized, but significant morbidity has not been reported after FBS. Maternal intra-abdominal infection and bleeding would be expected to occur at the same rate as that for amniocentesis.

Conclusion

FBS is indicated when the potential benefits of a change outweigh the procedure-related risks. The risks and benefits to both the fetus and the mother should be considered. Most prefer FBS by ultrasound-guided needling of the umbilical cord (cordocentesis). The fetal heart and intrahepatic vein are alternative sampling sites. None of these techniques should be attempted unless the operator has considerable experience with related procedures. The most important determinant of the fetal loss rate is the indication for sampling.

SUMMARY OF MANAGEMENT OPTIONS

Fetal Blood Sampling

Management Options	Evidence Quality and Recommendation	References
Indications: Diagnostic		
Chromosomal abnormalities	—/GPP	—
DNA abnormality or single-gene defects	—/GPP	—
Fetal anemia	—/GPP	—
Fetal thrombocytopenia	—/GPP	—

SUMMARY OF MANAGEMENT OPTIONS

Fetal Blood Sampling—cont'd

Management Options	Evidence Quality and Recommendation	References
Fetal hypoxia or acidosis	—/GPP	—
Fetal infection	—/GPP	—
Monitoring the effects of fetal therapy	—/GPP	—
Procedural Options		
Umbilical cord (cordocentesis)	—/GPP	—
Intrahepatic vessels	—/GPP	—
Fetal heart	—/GPP	—
Complications		
Fetal loss rate related to		
• Gestational age	III/B	138,139,151
• Operator experience	III/B	138,139
• Number of needle insertions	III/B	138,139,151
• Indication (e.g., intrauterine growth restriction, chromosomal abnormality)	III/B	138,139,151

GPP, good practice point.

Fetal Tissue Biopsy

Although progress in molecular biology allows more diseases to be diagnosed from fetal DNA, some conditions still require testing of fetal tissue, such as skin, liver, and muscle. These tests are rarely indicated because the diseases are rare. Only experienced fetal medicine specialists should perform them. Rapid advances in the field mandate close contact with a clinical geneticist to stay abreast of new developments.

Skin Biopsy

INDICATION

Histologic examination of a fetal skin biopsy specimen is useful for the diagnosis of some bullous disorders (congenital bullous epidermolysis, epidermolysis bullosa dystrophica, epidermolysis bullosa lethalis),[134,157–159] hyperkeratotic disorders (congenital ichthyosiform erythroderma, epidermolytic hyperkeratosis, Harlequin ichthyosis)[159–162] (Figs. 9–8 and 9–9), or oculocutaneous albinism.[159] A molecular understanding of these diseases has made early diagnosis by CVS possible, and therefore, the number of skin biopsies performed has decreased since the early 1990s.[159] Occasionally, fetal skin biopsy can confirm true fetal mosacism.[163]

PROCEDURE

Fetoscopy is rarely performed diagnostically, but the development of new fiberoptic scopes has decreased the pregnancy loss rate to less than the rate of 2% to 5% associated with classic fetoscopic methods.[157]

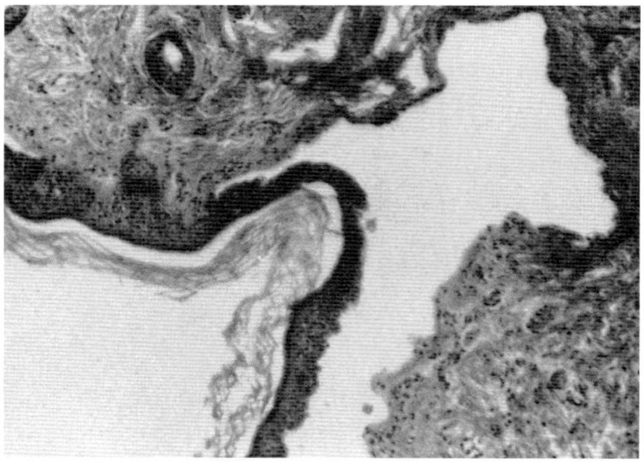

FIGURE 9–8
Histologic features of skin from a fetus with harlequin ichthyosis.

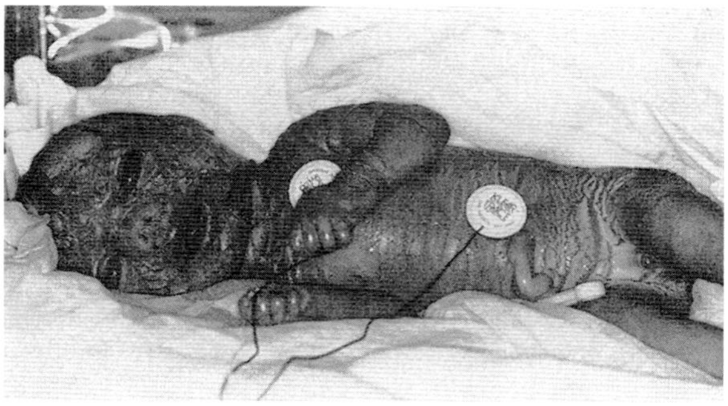

FIGURE 9–9
An infant with harlequin ichthyosis.

These scopes are popular aids for some therapeutic fetal procedures (e.g., laser ablation). For skin sampling, this technique has been replaced by ultrasound-guided biopsy, commonly performed with a 20-gauge biopsy forceps introduced through a 16- to 18-gauge needle. Obtaining multiple small biopsy specimens of skin from the scalp over the occiput or from the buttocks is recommended.[164,165] The fetal skin heals well after biopsy.

LABORATORY TECHNIQUES

Histologic and biochemical tools like electron microscopy and immunohistochemistry[159] are used to diagnose skin conditions. Several ichthyoses and genetic conditions associated with ichthyoses are diagnosable with fetal cells obtained from CVS, amniocentesis, or FBS.[162]

Fetal Liver Biopsy

Amniotic fluid cells and placental tissue may be used to diagnose most fetal metabolic diseases.[166] However, some inheritable inborn errors of metabolism show defects in enzyme activity confined to the liver and require a fetal liver biopsy.[167,168]

PROCEDURE

Fetoscopic[157] and ultrasound-guided[168] procedures are used (Fig. 9–10). Either a hollow needle or a Tru-Cut biopsy needle is inserted through the skin, over the right upper quadrant of the fetal abdomen, and into the liver (Fig. 9–11). The biopsy specimen is sent to a laboratory. Normal overall activity of a number of enzymes but low activity of a specific enzyme is considered evidence of disease.

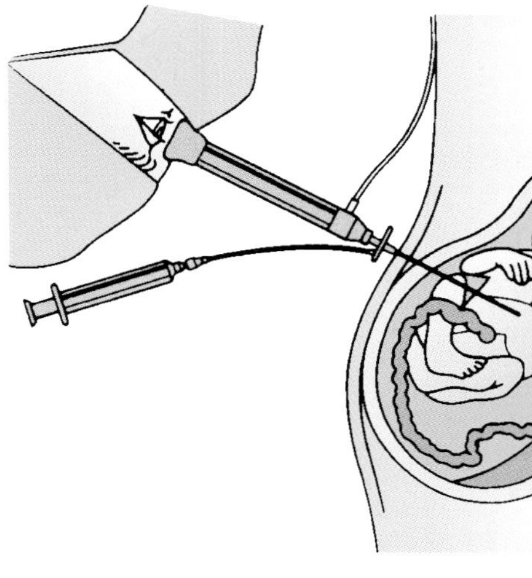

FIGURE 9–10
Fetal liver biopsy performed with a fetoscope.

Fetal Muscle Biopsy

The most common inheritable major muscular dystrophy is Duchenne's muscular dystrophy, which is caused by a defect in the gene for dystrophin.[169] Although it is often diagnosable antenatally from fetal DNA obtained by CVS, with molecular analysis seeking either a deletion mutation or a linkage analysis, the gene is large, with many possible defect sites.[170] In some cases, no deletion is found and biopsy is the only recourse.[171,172] Other myopathies can also be diagnosed.[173]

LABORATORY TECHNIQUES

A wide range of studies is possible. For Duchenne's muscular dystrophy, the biopsy specimen is examined to confirm the presence of muscle and treated with an immunofluorescent antibody for dystrophin protein (Fig. 9–12).[174]

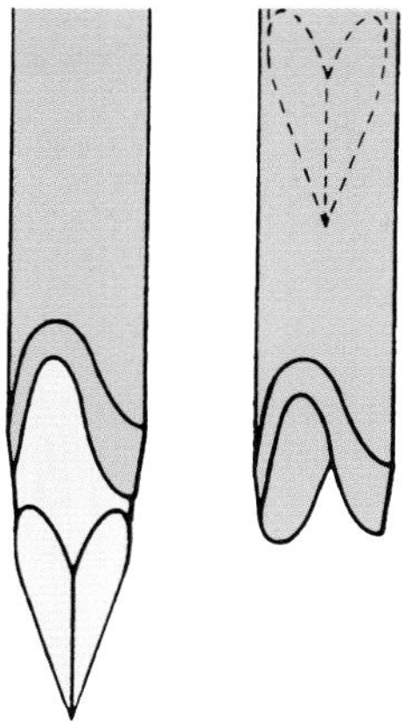

FIGURE 9–11
A cutting needle with an aspiration trocar.

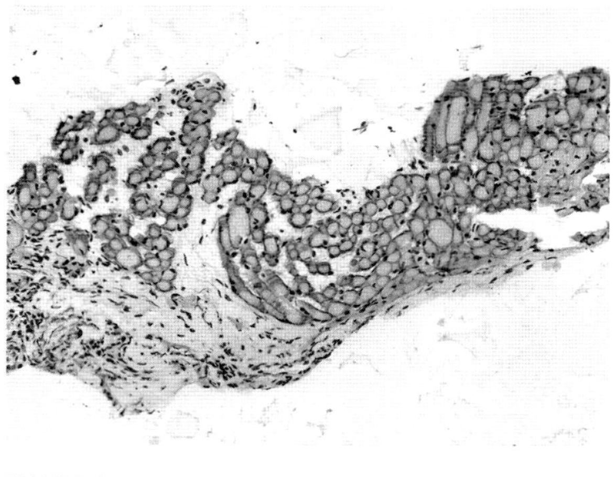

FIGURE 9–12
A fetal muscle biopsy specimen obtained at 22 weeks' gestation. The immunofluorescence of dystrophin indicates that the fetus is normal; this finding was confirmed at birth.
(Courtesy of Prof. S. Love, Department of Neuropathology, Bristol, UK.)

PROCEDURE

These uncommon procedures should be performed only by experienced fetal medicine specialists.[175] The maternal abdominal skin is anesthetized, and a small nick is made with a scalpel to facilitate the entry of a Tru-Cut biopsy gun[171] (Fig. 9–13). Under ultrasound guidance, the tip is advanced into the fetal buttock or thigh in a down-and-out direction. The coring guide is extended, and the trigger is pulled to cut the biopsy specimen. Risks of the procedure include fetal bleeding, nerve damage, and pregnancy loss. There are reports of maternal contamination,[176] but this can be prevented with a double-needle technique.

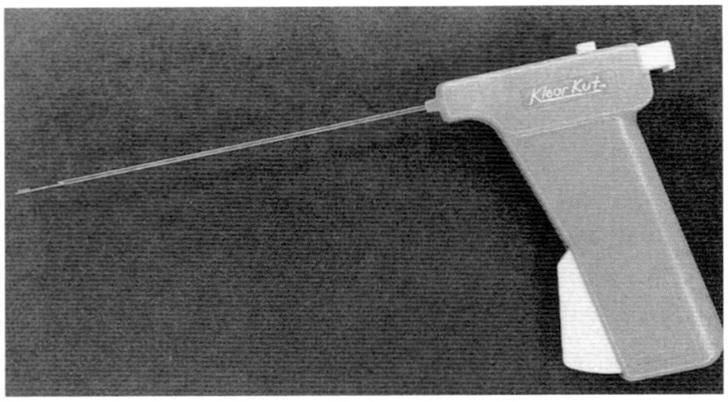

FIGURE 9–13
KlearKut biopsy gun.

Other Organ Biopsy

Histologic diagnosis of fetal tumors would be helpful in many cases, and there are reports of biopsy of fetal mediastinal and renal tumors.[177] However, biopsy of any tumor can cause uncontrollable bleeding, leading to severe fetal damage or death. In many cases, the histologic features vary in different locations. As a result, biopsy of a fetal mass is rarely advised.

Conclusion

Most antenatal fetal diagnoses are based on fetal DNA obtained by CVS, amniocentesis, or FBS. However, fetal skin, liver, and muscle biopsy specimens are required for some lethal or severely disabling conditions. These are complex procedures, with significant risk to the pregnancy, and they should be performed only in tertiary fetal medicine centers by experienced clinicians.

SUMMARY OF MANAGEMENT OPTIONS

Fetal Tissue Biopsy

Management Options	Evidence Quality and Recommendation	References
Indications		
Possible or potential life-threatening disease in the fetal skin, liver, and muscle	—/GPP	—
Procedural Options		
Fetoscopy and biopsy	—/GPP	—
Ultrasound-guided aspiration	—/GPP	—
Ultrasound-guided Tru-Cut biopsy	—/GPP	—
Complication		
Fetal loss	—/GPP	—
Fetal injury (scarring)	—/GPP	—
Preterm rupture of the membranes and/or oligohydramnios	—/GPP	—
Chorioamnionitis	—/GPP	—

GPP, good practice point.

SUGGESTED READINGS

Amniocentesis. RCOG Consent Advice 6. London, Royal College of Obstetricians and Gynaecologists, 2006.

Amniocentesis and Chorionic Villus Sampling. RCOG Green Top Guideline 8. London, Royal College of Obstetricians and Gynaecologists, 2005.

Eddleman KA, Malone FD, Sullivan L, et al: Pregnancy loss rates after midtrimester amniocentesis. Obstet Gynecol 2006;108:1067–1072.

Ekelund CK, Jorgensen FS, Petersen OB, et al: Danish Fetal Medicine Research Group: Impact of a new national screening policy for Down's syndrome in Denmark: Population based cohort study. BMJ 2008;337:a2547.

Finning KM, Martin PG, Soothill PW, Avent ND: Prediction of fetal D status from maternal plasma: Introduction of a new noninvasive fetal RHD genotyping service. Transfusion 2002;42:1079–1085.

Ghidini A, Sepulveda W, Lockwood CJ, Romero R: Complications of fetal blood sampling. Am J Obstet Gynecol 1993;168:1339–1344.

Nanal R, Kyle P, Soothill PW: A classification of pregnancy losses after invasive prenatal diagnostic procedures: An approach to allow comparison of units with a different case mix. Prenat Diagn 2003;23:488–492.

National Collaborating Centre for Women's and Children's Health: Antenatal care. In Routine Care for the Healthy Pregnant Woman, 2nd ed. London, Royal College of Obstetricians and Gynaecologists Press, 2008, pp 154–176.

Smidt-Jensen S, Philip J, Lundsteen C, et al: Randomised comparison of amniocentesis and transabdominal and transcervical chorionic villus sampling. Lancet 1992;340:1237–1244.

Weiner CP, Grose C: Prenatal diagnosis of congenital cytomegalovirus infection by virus isolation from amniotic fluid. Am J Obstet Gynecol 1990;163:1253–1255.

REFERENCES

For a complete list of references, log onto www.expertconsult.com.

SECTION THREE

Late Prenatal-Fetal

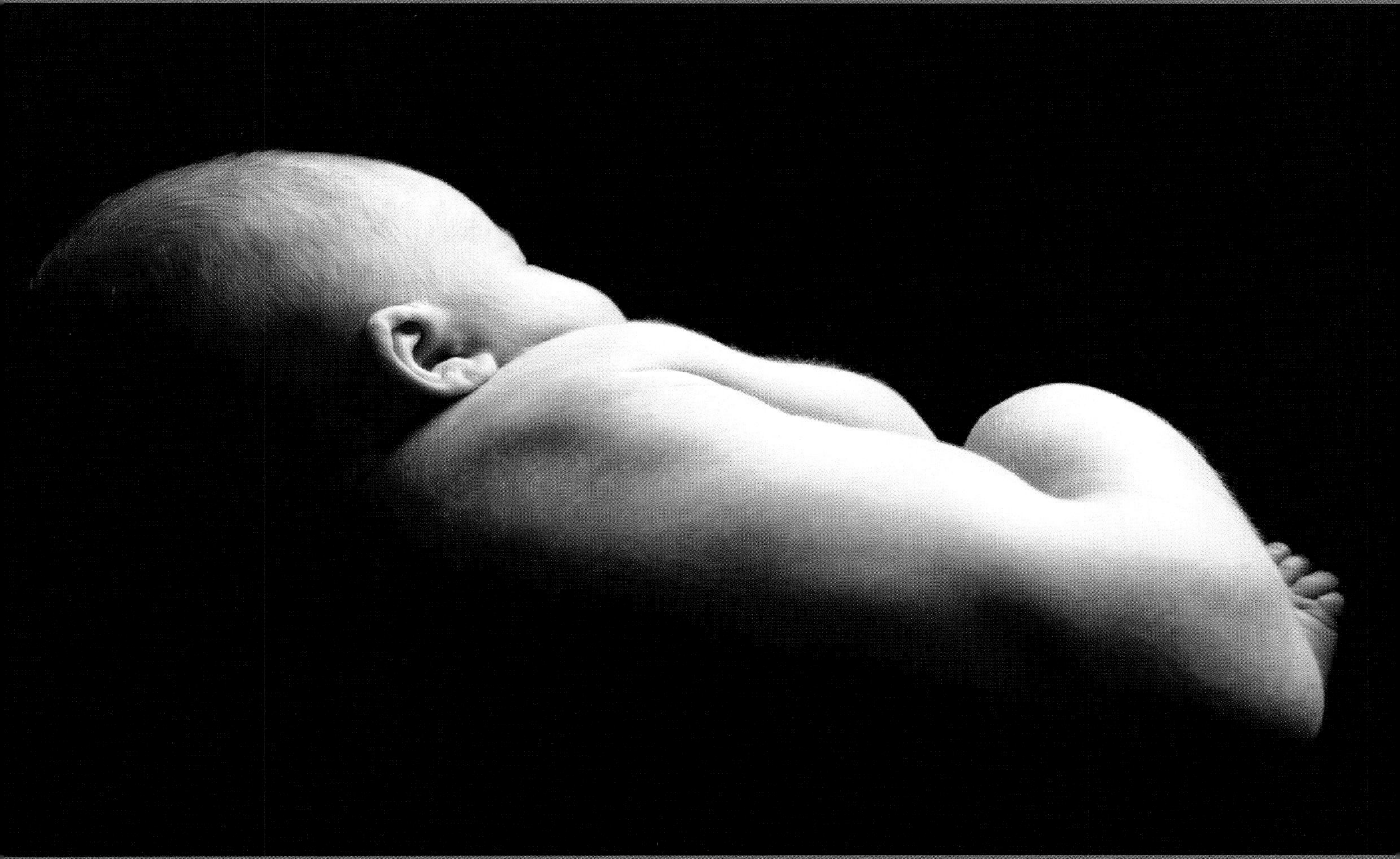

CHAPTER 10

Prenatal Fetal Surveillance

TZE KIN LAU

Videos corresponding to this chapter are available online at www.expertconsult.com.

INTRODUCTION

The purpose of obstetric care is to optimize maternal and fetal safety. The clinical decisions are always a balance between the risks to the fetus if delivered and the risks to the mother and fetus if the pregnancy continues. In an attempt to stratify risk, a variety of screening tests are performed during the prenatal and intrapartum periods to identify the high risk population. These tests include the patient history, physical examination, laboratory tests, and sonographic assessments. In this chapter, we focus on what additional tests are available to monitor those pregnancies identified by one means or another as high risk of chronic hypoxia and determine the optimal timing for intervention or delivery.

Fetal surveillance for specific conditions is addressed in detail in the relevant chapters in this book, including fetal abnormality (see Chapters 7–9, 15–20, and 24), fetal infection (see Chapters 26–32), fetal anemia (see Chapter 13), fetal endocrine problems (see Chapter 21), fetal tumors (see Chapter 22), and multiple pregnancy (see Chapter 23) and are not dealt with in this chapter. Intrapartum fetal surveillance is covered in Chapter 69. This chapter provides a more general discussion on the various tests for suspected or actual chronic fetal hypoxia that are available and their applications and limitations. Specific conditions related to chronic hypoxia are also dealt with in detail in the relevant chapters including growth restriction (see Chapter 11) and amniotic fluid abnormalities (see Chapter 12). In general, most fetal surveillance tests have a single goal—the detection of chronic fetal hypoxia. The theory is that by identifying the hypoxia-associated physiological changes before the fetus has suffered from long-term irreversible damages, preventive measures can be implemented. A corollary is that fetal compromise follows a relatively predictable pattern, allowing the surveillance tests to be repeated in defined intervals. These surveillance tests are not useful for the prediction or prevention of fetal damage due to acute events, such as major abruption or cord accidents.

NORMAL FETAL PHYSIOLOGY AND ADAPTIVE RESPONSES TO HYPOXIA AND METABOLIC ACIDOSIS

In normal pregnancies, the fetus lives in a relatively low-oxygen environment compared with that after birth. Several mechanisms ensure effective delivery of more than adequate oxygen to the growing fetus. First is the high blood flow rate, the consequence of a high cardiac output (estimated to be ~2.5 mL/min and 200 mL/min at 12 and 30 weeks, respectively, corresponding to ~170 mL/kg/min).[1] This is about double the cardiac output of about 75 mL/kg/min in a normal resting adult. In addition, placental exchange surface area continues to grow with advancing gestation. Second is the presence of a central shunting mechanism. Oxygenated fetal blood returning from the placenta through the umbilical vein bypasses the fetal liver via the ductus venosus (DV) to reach the fetal heart directly, and then through the formen ovale or the ductus arteriosus to reach the aortic outflow. These intrauterine shunts ensure that the most oxygenated blood is channeled with shortest delay to the most important organs including fetal brain and heart. Third is the well-known fact that the fetal hemoglobin has a higher affinity for oxygen, assisting the extraction of oxygen from maternal hemoglobin. The higher affinity works synergistically with the higher fetal hemoglobin level, which also increases its oxygen-carrying capacity.

Acute and chronic hypoxia induces different fetal responses.[2] Chronic hypoxia induces many adaptive responses in an effort to compensate for the reduction in oxygen concentration in the environment. However, it is unknown presently what causes cell damage during chronic hypoxia. Organ damages may occur with more severe degree of hypoxia, or perhaps when hypoxia is complicated by metabolic acidosis. Recent study also suggests chronic hypoxia induces a fetal inflammatory response syndrome in the absence of infection.[3]

One of the more important effects of chronic hypoxemia as it relates to monitoring is the redistribution of blood flow so that there is preferential flow to the essential organs including the brain, heart, and adrenal glands,[4] a process referred to as "centralization." Blood flow to other organs tends to remain normal or decreased (the trunk), but further decreases with worsening hypoxemia.[2] Plasma hemoglobin level also increases in association with an increase in erythropoietin. Initially, fetal hypoxemia leads to an increase in fetal cardiac output. But with progression to severe hypoxia, cardiac dysfunction causes a reduction in cardiac output and failure of the normal cerebral vascular protective mechanism, leading to loss of cerebral vascular variability and increase in cerebral vascular resistance, in particular in the presence of metabolic acidosis.[5] Many of the early adaptive changes would seem to favor fetal survival. Many of these adaptations can be detected clinically by sonographic examinations and, therefore, can be useful in assessment of fetal well-being to assist the decision of timing for intervention before irreversible fetal damages occur. Their presence was thought in the past to be suggestive of fetal hypoxia, but not necessarily fetal damage. Recent study suggests that chronic hypoxia induces fetal inflammation, which might explain why randomized trials to date have failed to show improvement in long-term neurodevelopmental status after early intervention.

Conversely, chronic hypoxia alone usually will not induce significant changes in fetal movement or heart rate pattern until it is complicated by metabolic acidosis. Fetal movement and breathing movement are significantly reduced with acute hypoxia, but are usually normalized when the hypoxia is prolonged.[6] Reduction in fetal movement or breathing movement usually does not occur in chronic hypoxia until the fetus develops acidosis.[5] Similarly, fetal heart rate patterns are usually normal in case of mild chronic hypoxia, and abnormalities such as absence of acceleration or deceleration occur only with more severe hypoxia especially when acidosis is also present.[5–7] Because changes in fetal behavioral parameters are late signs of severe hypoxia with acidosis, the observation of normal fetal movement or fetal heart rate pattern does not exclude fetal hypoxia. Frank late decelerations do not usually occur in chronically hypoxemic fetuses until hypoxia-mediated cardiac dysfunction occurs.

INDICATIONS

The aims of fetal surveillance are to

- Reduce the incidence of fetal death.
- Minimize morbidity by optimizing the timing of delivery.
- Identify more clearly those fetuses genuinely at risk of chronic hypoxia and avoid unnecessary intervention in those that are not.
- Identify those fetuses at greater risk of acute hypoxia in labor.

The indications are maternal and/or fetal conditions known to be associated with chronic fetal hypoxia.

Common indications include

- Hypertensive disorders of pregnancy.
- Chronic renal disease.
- Maternal diabetes.
- Antiphospholipid syndrome and related autoimmune diseases.
- Cyanotic heart disease.
- Specific perinatal infections.

Common fetal indications are

- Intrauterine growth restriction (IUGR).
- Abnormal amniotic fluid volume.
- Reduced fetal movements.
- Vaginal bleeding.
- Abdominal pain without a clear explanation of its cause.
- Postdate pregnancy.

Tests of fetal surveillance are also initiated for less clear indications including a history of a previous stillbirth or growth-restricted fetus and raised maternal serum α-fetoprotein.[8] In many of these situations, a statistical association with poor perinatal outcome has been reported, but underlying chronic fetal hypoxia has not been proved. The dangers in instituting fetal surveillance in pregnancies without clear evidence of a risk of chronic hypoxia are unnecessary interventions.

Even for conditions with well-defined fetal risks, strong and clear scientific proof that a particular fetal surveillance test improves perinatal outcome is generally lacking owing to the difficulty in conducting good randomized trials.

For those with an indication for fetal surveillance, the gestation at which these tests should be initiated depends largely on the prognosis for neonatal survival should intervention be required owing to an abnormal test result—"practical fetal viability." If delivery is not considered to be a viable management option, for example, at a gestation of 24 weeks, there seems little ground for initiating fetal surveillance testing. Although the lower threshold for practical fetal viability obviously depends on the ability and performance of the local neonatal intensive care unit, the initiation of fetal surveillance testing cannot be justified under 24 weeks in the best circumstances, and more often not until 26 weeks' gestation.

FETAL MOVEMENT COUNTING

It has been known for decades that women with intrauterine fetal death often note a reduction in the quantity or quality of fetal movement prior to the loss being documented. This led to the introduction of fetal movement counting as a mean to monitor fetal health. However, most trainees in this specialty will quickly realize in their early years of training that many women who present with reduction in fetal movement have perfectly normal pregnancy with normal fetal outcome, and many who had incidental diagnosis of intrauterine fetal death during routine follow-up report normal fetal movement the day before or even at the time of diagnosis. There has been much controversy as to the validity and usefulness of using fetal movement counting as a fetal surveillance tool.

The perception of fetal movement is subjective. Previous studies have shown wide variation in the proportion of fetal movements documented on real-time ultrasound that were perceived by the woman, ranging from 16% to 80%.[9,10] In a recent multicenter study in Norway, 51% of the pregnant subjects reported they were concerned about perceived reduced fetal movement, of which 42% were concerned that her child was sick and 26% that her child would die.[11]

The most obvious question in using fetal movement counting as a fetal surveillance tool is when a reduction in fetal movements becomes significant. There are many methods of fetal movement surveillance, but perhaps the most commonly used is the Cardiff method in which fewer than 10 movements in 12 hours is considered abnormal. However, the period of absent fetal movements in healthy fetuses is only 15.5 and 37 minutes at 32 and 40 weeks, respectively,[12] although this could be up to 75 minutes in term fetuses.[13] The average number of movements per hour is 31 during the last 10 weeks of pregnancy,[6] and the mean time required to appreciate 10 fetal movements is 20.9 ± 18.1 minutes.[14] Therefore, the Cardiff count-to-10 method is too conservative and will not allow early detection of fetal complications. It appears logical to shorten the time during which a reduction is considered significant. Moore and Piacquadio,[14] in their prospective study, instructed their subjects to report to the delivery suit if they had fewer than 10 fetal movement counts within a 2-hour period. When compared with historical data, such a strict protocol was shown to have reduced the perinatal mortality rate by a quarter, with a 13% increase in antepartum tests and tripling of interventions for fetal compromise. Such a strict protocol, although not impossible to accomplish, is not practical in most societies, and the findings have yet to be replicated. However, using a strict protocol of 2 hours to define abnormal fetal movement will undoubtedly increase the false-positive rate into an unacceptable range and impose significant stress to the pregnant women.

In the largest available randomized trial comparing formal fetal movement counting versus no instruction to monitor fetal movements involving 68,654 women, there was a trend to more antenatal admission, increased use of other fetal testing methods in the fetal movement counting group, but no difference in any of the measured fetal outcome variables.[15] The authors acknowledged that maternal reporting of reduced fetal movements did identify fetuses at increased risk of fetal death; however, those deaths were not prevented because of false reassurance provided by the subsequent fetal surveillance (largely nonstress test [NST]). The study could not rule out a small beneficial effect of fetal movement counting, but at best, the policy would have to be used by some 1250 women to prevent one unexplained antepartum late fetal death. In point, decreased/absent fetal movement is a late sign of chronic fetal hypoxia with acidosis. In theory, therefore, compromised fetuses presenting with this sign may be too late for any useful intervention other than to deliver a damaged baby. Furthermore, excessive fetal movement that sometimes accompanies acute events may be incorrectly interpreted by the woman as reassuring.

The Cochrane Database of Systematic Review of the use of fetal movement counting for the assessment of fetal wellbeing reported four studies, involving 71,370 women with 68,654 of these being in one cluster-randomized trial. There were no clinically relevant significant differences. The authors' conclusions were that "the review does not provide enough evidence to influence practice. In particular, no trials compared fetal movement counting with no fetal movement counting. Robust research is needed in this area."[16]

The use of fetal movement counting as a form of fetal surveillance was also not supported by the U.K. National Institute for Clinical Excellence (NICE) guideline on antenatal care for the National Health Service in England published in 2003. It concluded that "routine formal fetal-movement counting should not be offered" as a grade A evidence, and the same recommendation was reconfirmed in the updated version in 2008.[17]

Although formal fetal movement counting should not be offered, there will be times when pregnant women recognize and present themselves because of absent or reduced fetal movement. Abnormal fetal movement has been linked to a long list of possible causes including fetal growth restriction (FGR), oligohydramnios, and congenital malformation,[18] but the false-positive rate is very high. Therefore, the principles of management of this group of women are to exclude imminent fetal jeopardy, to identify possible underlying causes, and to avoid unnecessary intervention. High-level evidence on the appropriate management scheme for this group of women is lacking. A variety of options have been suggested ranging from using simple symphysis–fundal height measurement alone,[19] ultrasound assessment of fetal size/growth, NST or cardiotocogram (NST/CTG), NST with amniotic fluid assessment, or full biophysical profile study to Doppler study.[20] In practice, many advocate a comprehensive approach to assessment of the "at-risk fetus" using several methods in combination rather than relying on a single test alone. This is discussed in more detail later. In general, the simple detection of fetal heart activity may be sufficient in women who present with reduced fetal movement before the gestation of practical fetal viability because of the difficulty in interpreting the CTG at this gestation and the potential risks of unnecessary intervention outweigh the potential benefits.[21] For those who presented with reduced fetal movement late in the third trimester, an NST/CTG should be performed to exclude immediate fetal jeopardy. A sonogram should be performed if the CTG is abnormal unless immediate delivery is considered. If the CTG is normal, the role of routine sonogram is uncertain. The use of fetal Doppler examination in the absence of CTG or sonographic abnormalities late in the third trimester does not seem to provide useful additional information.[21]

BIOPHYSICAL PROFILE OR BIOPHYSICAL SCORE

The biophysical score (BPS) was introduced in 1980 by Manning and coworkers.[23] It assigns a maximum of 2 points to each of five variables including fetal breathing movement, fetal movements, fetal tone, qualitative amniotic fluid volume, and the NST. The first four variables were assessed by ultrasound examination, which was also useful for the detection of fetal anomalies. A normal BPS was defined as a score of 8 or 10 with normal amniotic fluid and indicative of a healthy fetus that is unlikely to die within the subsequent 7 days. A fetus with a score of 8 due to reduced amniotic fluid is considered as high risk for chronic compensated hypoxia and, therefore, either should be delivered or should repeat the BPS not less than twice a week. A BPS of 6 is considered equivocal and has to be individualized. If immediate delivery is not considered possible, the test should be repeated on same day or in the following morning. A BPS of 4 or less is abnormal and delivery should be seriously considered. This team subsequently recommended the BPS be initiated at a frequency of once per week in most high risk cases and at least twice per week at or beyond 42 weeks' gestation.[22]

In their initial study of 216 subjects, the perinatal mortality rate was found to be 0 to 600 when all five variables were normal and abnormal, respectively.[23] Based on a review of more than 54,000 BPS tests, they estimated that the false-negative rate, that is, fetal death despite a normal BPS, was only 0.6 per 1000.[22] The largest experience was subsequently reported by Manning and colleagues,[23] but the false-positive rate was little discussed. The false-positive rate for the BPS has been reported in only small case series and has been estimated to be about 75%.[22,24] Such a high figure was probably due to the incorrect interpretation of the primary data. The latest meta-analysis included five trials, involving 2974 women. Most trials were not of high quality. Although the overall incidence of adverse outcomes was low, available evidence from randomized controlled trials does not support the use of the biophysical profile (BPP) as a test of fetal well-being in high risk pregnancies. There were no significant differences between the groups in perinatal deaths or in Apgar score less than 7 at 5 minutes. Combined data from the two high-quality trials suggest an increased risk of cesarean section in the BPP group (relative risk [RR] 1.60, 95% confidence interval [CI] 1.05–2.44). However, the number of participating women was relatively small ($n = 280$). The authors concluded that additional evidence was required to be definitive regarding the efficacy of this test in high risk pregnancies.[25]

Given the labor-intensiveness of the standard BPS, and the realization that NST and amniotic fluid volume are probably the most important elements of BPS, a modified BPP using just the NST and amniotic fluid assessment was proposed as a fetal surveillance method,[26] reserving the complete BPS or other testing for those with abnormal modified BPP. Miller and colleagues[27] reported the use of modified BPP in more than 15,000 subjects and achieved a false-negative rate of 0.8/1000. It had a lower false-positive rate than the contraction stress test (CST) and was noninvasive.

Overall, the BPS test demands a higher level of technical skill, is more time-consuming, and requires more resources for equipment when compared with other tests. Furthermore, abnormalities of the biophysical parameters used in the BPS are generally late signs of hypoxia likely complicated with acidosis.[28] Intensive monitoring using BPS may be useful in identifying those with impending death, but might not be able to allow the detection of early fetal compromise. Together with the high false-positive rate and lack of supportive evidence of its superiority over other surveillance tests available, BPS does not appear to be a logical choice as a routine or first-line fetal surveillance test. At best, there is only fair evidence to justify their use as recommended in high risk pregnancies.[29]

NONSTRESS TEST

The observed association between gross fetal movements and transient fetal heart rate (FHR) accelerations in normal fetuses formed the basis of NST. It is a simple and noninvasive test that can be repeated as often as necessary. The assumption of the NST is that if FHR accelerations are absent for a prolonged period of time, there is a high likelihood of fetal hypoxemia. However, a clear understanding of the underlying physiologic basis is needed to realize the many limitations of this test.

Physiology

The baseline FHR falls gradually during the last half of gestation up to 30 weeks, and then remains stable at 142 beats/min over the last 10 weeks of pregnancy when all FHR data are analyzed.[30] In general, a baseline FHR between 110 and 160 beats/min in late pregnancy is considered normal, though it is suggested that a baseline rate above 150 beats/min is a potential sign of fetal hypoxemia and should be investigated further.[31,32] At the same time, an increase in variability and frequency of accelerations is observed with rising gestation.[30,33] FHR accelerations are strongly related to gross fetal movement: 85% of all FHR accelerations are associated with gross fetal movements, and 92% of all gross body movements are associated with FHR accelerations.[34] It is thus not surprising that accelerations are absent during fetal quiescence or the quiet phase of fetal sleep. In fetal sleep, neuromuscular blockade abolishes only one third of the FHR accelerations, indicating that the majority of accelerations in the fetus occur with movements as a result of central neuronal output affecting both the cardioaccelerator fibers and the motor neurons, rather than being a direct result of the movement.[35]

A healthy fetus exhibits an average of 34 accelerations per hour in late pregnancy.[36] In one small study, the longest time between successive FHR accelerations was 37 minutes, but it is likely the absence of an acceleration for up to 80 minutes could still be normal.[37] These accelerations require intact and mature neurologic control between the fetal central nervous system and the fetal heart. However, the occurrence of normal FHR accelerations in the presence of significant cerebral anomalies suggested that the NST is dependent only upon the fetal brainstem and NST predicts oxygenation and function at that site rather than normality of the entire central nervous system.[37]

The sympathetic and parasympathetic systems have important roles in the regulation of the FHR. Previous studies, mostly on animals, reveal that the sympathetic system develops early in fetal life, whereas the parasympathetic system develops more slowly[38] and exerts very little influence on the tone of resting fetal cardiovascular function until the third trimester.[39] It is generally believed that the FHR variability is caused in part by the opposing influence of the sympathetic and parasympathetic stimuli to the fetal heart. It is, therefore, not surprising that FHR variability is in general lower in the second and early third trimesters.

Owing to the immaturity of the fetal nervous system, a significant proportion of NSTs performed in the preterm fetuses are nonreactive, estimated to be 50% between 24 and 28 weeks[40] and 25% between 28 and 32 weeks.[41,42] However, once a tracing becomes reactive, it is not correct to attribute a nonreactive tracing to early gestational age. Beyond 32 weeks, the incidence of nonreactive NSTs is no different from that at term.

Fetal bradycardia occurs promptly with acute hypoxia, followed by fetal death if the hypoxia is severe and prolonged. Otherwise, the fetal heart rate will gradually return to normal followed by tachycardia.[6] Mild chronic hypoxia does not usually cause heart rate abnormalities. Moderate to severe chronic hypoxia, in particular those complicated by acidosis, is associated with a reduction in FHR variability and at times an absence of accelerations.

Technique

The NST is a simple test that can be performed in the outpatient setting. A transabdominal Doppler ultrasonic transducer is used to record the FHR, while a tocodynamometer is applied to detect uterine contractions. In principle, the use of tocodynamometer is unnecessary if the woman is not in labor or does not present with uterine contractions. The recording is continued for 20 minutes, although some may stop recording at 10 to 15 minutes when there are already an adequate number of FHR accelerations present. The woman is usually asked to press a button whenever she feels a fetal movement, leaving a mark on the recording to indicate the presence of fetal movement.

Interpretation

There are extensive studies and professional guidelines on the interpretation of intrapartum cardiotocogram. Antenatal NST is usually interpreted using criteria described for intrapartum cardiotocogram (see Chapter 69). The NST is generally considered normal (or reactive) when there are two or more accelerations of FHR of 15 beats/min for at least 15 seconds' duration over a 20-minute recording after 32 weeks. Although by definition each acceleration should be accompanied by fetal movement, the presence of such a marking of fetal movement on the recording at the time of acceleration is usually not considered essential because (1) the majority of FHR accelerations are known to be associated with fetal movements and (2) women are able to detect only 16% to 80% of fetal movements. When the criteria for reactivity are not met, the test is considered nonreactive. A reactive strip is reassuring that the fetus will not die within the next 7 days.

To reduce the incidence of false-positive nonreactive rates when the NST is performed in preterm fetuses, it has been suggested that an acceleration be defined as FHR increase of 10 beats/min or more above the baseline lasting 10 seconds or longer in pregnancies of fewer than 32 weeks.[43]

Implications

A reactive tracing is generally considered a strong indicator of a healthy well-oxygenated fetus; this opinion, though, is inaccurate because fetuses with acidemia typically have reactive tracings until cardiac deterioration begins. About 85% of NSTs are reactive in the initial assessment. The perinatal mortality rate during the subsequent week in this group is low, 0.3% to 0.5%, compared with 3% to 4% in those with nonreactive NST.[44,45] Therefore, if the indication of the NST is ill-defined and there was no other underlying risk factor of worry, there may not be any need for further NST or monitoring. However, if the indication persisted, for example, FGR, the NST may be repeated at weekly intervals. In very high risk pregnancies, the false-negative rate associated with a weekly NST will be higher, and many advocate increasing the frequency of NST from weekly to twice-weekly, which has been shown to be associated with a reduction in the perinatal mortality rate from 6.1 to 1.9/1000.[46] In general, one should interpret a reactive NST to mean only that the fetus is okay at the time of assessment but not necessarily completely normal. How long after the test the fetus will remain okay depends on the rate of deterioration of the underlying pathology. If a rapid deterioration is not considered to be likely, weekly testing is adequate. If a very rapid deterioration is expected, it is appropriate to repeat testing daily or several times a day depending on the disorder.

A normal NST should not be equated to a normal baby. There is good evidence that a fetus who survived after an acute insult may have a normal NST, although the nervous system could have been severely damaged by that insult. The same may be said for chronically hypoxemic fetuses who have for the moment "adapted" to their adverse environment.

Fetal activity is strongly associated with the fetal wake-sleep cycle, with the most movement occurring during rapid eye movement sleep and the least during quiet sleep. The most common cause of a nonreactive NST is fetal inactivity (sleep cycle). Therefore, the test may be continued for an extended period if the initial part is nonreactive with the goal of differentiating a nonreactive NST due to fetal quiescence or to significant fetal hypoxia. The longer the nonreactive pattern persists, the greater the likelihood the fetus is hypoxic. There is no consensus as to how long one should continue with the NST. However, a nonreactive pattern for more than 80 minutes would be very unusual. A prolonged nonreactive pattern for up to 120 minutes is associated with high perinatal mortality and morbidity,[47,48] and such fetuses probably should be delivered if mature, recognizing that significant neurologic damages might have already occurred, and delivery prevents only a perinatal death and not necessarily a handicap. This is an important consideration during counseling of women for delivery in the presence of prolonged nonreactive NST.

The second most common cause of a nonreactive NST is prematurity. This is particularly true for those who are less than 32 weeks' gestation. In this group, the height of accelerations does not normally exceed 10 beats/min. In high risk preterm pregnancies, one should carefully consider what to do in case of a nonreactive pattern before prescribing surveillance with an NST. In this group, the use of the BPS may offer an advantage (see earlier).

Mild variable decelerations are commonly seen in antenatal NST and they are generally not associated with poor perinatal outcome. In fact, it is a normal finding in preterm pregnancies if not associated with oligohydramnios. There is no good evidence to support or refute whether the occurrence of nonuniform decelerations in an antenatal NST is predictive of poor fetal outcome.

The most recent update of the meta-analysis of CTG for antepartum fetal assessment in high risk pregnancies included only four studies involving 1627 pregnancies.[49] Antenatal CTG appeared to have no significant effect on perinatal mortality or morbidity. In fact, there was a trend to an increase in perinatal deaths in the CTG group (risk ratio [RR] 2.05, 95% CI 0.95–4.42, 2.3% versus 1.1%). However, the total number of women studied was too small for meaningful interpretation of the value of this assessment. Furthermore, all the trials were quite old and might be difficult to relate to current practice.

Variation of Techniques

There was a burst of enthusiasm for the application of vibroacoustic stimulation to the fetus who showed a nonreactive pattern during the late 1980s and early 1990s. The technique involved a brief exposure of the fetus to a vibroacoustic signal applied through the maternal abdomen (often using the "electronic artificial larynx") to evoke a response from the fetus, typically in the form of accelerations.

The latest meta-analysis of nine trials including 4838 participants demonstrated that fetal vibroacoustic stimulation reduced the incidence of nonreactive antenatal CTG (reported in seven trials; RR 0.62, 95% CI 0.52–0.74) and reduced the overall mean CTG testing time (reported in three trials; weighted mean difference −9.94 min, 95% CI −9.37 min to −10.50 min).[50] However, it is unclear whether the use of such a strong stimulus will have long-term adverse effects on the unborn fetus, and therefore, this device should be used with caution. It is also unclear whether the fetus with significant acidemia will be more likely to have a reactive tracing, increasing the chance of a false-negative result.

Limitations

Although those pregnancies with nonreactive NST are at higher risk of perinatal mortality and morbidity, the great majority are still normal if delivered at that point, that is, a false-positive result. This high false-positive rate and low positive predictive value can lead to a very high intervention rate without significant improvement in the overall perinatal outcome. The only way to avoid this dilemma is to use this test carefully, in particular to avoid using it in a low risk population. One should resist the temptation to prescribe testing to a woman on a "just in case" basis. Limiting the use of NST to well-defined high risk cases will maximize the positive predictive value.

CONTRACTION STRESS TEST

This CST is included here for completeness, because it is now only rarely performed. The CST was probably the first specific test available for fetal surveillance and based on the understanding that hypoxic fetuses poorly tolerate regular uterine contractions, leading to progressive myocardial dysfunction with bradycardia. The setup for the CST begins with an NST. After confirming a normal fetal heart pattern without strong uterine contractions, intravenous infusion of oxytocin or maternal nipple simulation is initiated to induce uterine contractions, until three contractions in every 10 minutes are obtained for 10 to 30 minutes. The test is considered negative if there are no late or significant variable decelerations, positive if late decelerations are present in at least 50% of the contractions, suspicious or equivocal if there is intermittent late or variable decelerations, and unsatisfactory if adequate uterine contraction cannot be induced. This test is time-consuming and usually takes 1 to 2 hours to complete.

The negative test is highly predictive of a good outcome, and the risk of antenatal death is 0 to 0.4/1000.[51] A positive test is predictive of fetal hypoxia, with a corrected perinatal mortality rate of 176.5/1000. The false-positive rate is usually quoted as high, ranging from 8% to 57%,[51] which is wrong because the definition used by the original studies was the number of unaffected infants delivered after a positive CST.[29] The denominator used was not the total number of true negative, but the total number of test positives.[52]

As with many other fetal surveillance tests, strong scientific proof of clear clinical benefit of CST is lacking. Since the 1990s, the CST has been largely replaced by other alternative methods thath are easier to administer, less invasive, and lack the possibility of precipitating fetal compromise.

DOPPLER STUDIES

The application of Doppler assessment of the unborn fetus as a method of fetal surveillance is relatively new. But research since the early 2000s has demonstrated that Doppler is probably the best available tool for fetal surveillance, providing a physiologic approach to the management of high risk pregnancies. At present, there are two major roles for antenatal Doppler testing as it relates to fetal surveillance: (1) monitoring of pregnancies complicated by uteroplacental dysfunction and FGR and (2) monitoring the fetus at risk for anemia.

Principle of Doppler Studies

All Doppler tests are based on the Doppler principle, which states that sound reflected from a moving target will shift its frequency in proportion to the velocity of the target. This Doppler shift can be measured directly by ultrasound, equipment that then calculates the corresponding velocity of the original target object. In obstetrics, Doppler is typically used for the study of vascular blood flow. A number of display modes exist, but all Doppler examinations discussed herein are limited to pulsed-wave spectral Doppler unless specified. Because the Doppler shift is dependent on the angle of insonation, being highest when they are in parallel, the estimated velocity will not be the true velocity unless this angle of insonation is zero.

To facilitate the Doppler examination, various angle-independent indices have been derived, including the pulsatility index (PI) and resistance index (RI). Under standard conditions, both PI and RI correlate with downstream vascular resistance. Thus, a high PI or RI represents high peripheral resistance, ande a low PI or RI represents a reduction in peripheral resistance and possibly increased blood flow. One must keep in mind that the value of PI or RI is also affected by other determinants such as FHR or blood viscosity.

Pathophysiology of Placental Dysfunction and Fetal Growth Restriction (See also Chapter 11)

Some studies reveal that changes in the Doppler waveforms of different uteroplacental and fetal vessels follow a relatively predictable pattern in pregnancies complicated by placental dysfunction and FGR.[7,53] The early changes may be first manifest in the uterine artery, followed by umbilical artery and middle cerebral artery (MCA). Often, the uterine artery waveform remains normal and the umbilical artery first shows increased resistance. Sequentially, fetal hypoxia leads to decreased resistance in the MCA and, with the onset of hypoxia-mediated cardiac dysfunction, abnormal flow in the DV reflecting decreased cardiac compliance. If the fetus remains undelivered and continues to deteriorate, terminal signs will occur, including a reduction in fetal movement, decelerations in the fetal heart, and evidence of fetal cardiac failure.

Doppler flow pattern and indices of the uterine artery reflect the impedance or resistance of the maternal circulation of the uterus and placental bed. In the nonpregnant state, Doppler waveform of the uterine artery is a high resistance pattern with a notch. During normal pregnancy, trophoblastic invasion and remodeling of the spiral arteries lead to a substantial reduction in resistance and the disappearance of notching. Conversely, persistence of high uterine artery Doppler PI is a typical early feature of abnormal placentation, representing a defective or delayed trophoblastic invasion. There is increasing evidence that the measurement of uterine artery Doppler indices may be a useful screening test in the early or mid trimester for the identification of at-risk pregnancies.[54,55] However, it is not a useful test for fetal surveillance.

Doppler indices of the umbilical artery normally decrease with advancing gestation because of the physiologic reduction in placental vascular resistance. In FGR due to uteroplacental dysfunction, placental vascular resistance remains high and, as a consequence, the PI of the umbilical artery is higher than normal. The umbilical artery gives information only on placental blood flow, and not the fetal adaptation to hypoxia nor the consequences of this adaptation.[56] In other words, a normal umbilical artery waveform is inconsistent with chronic fetal hypoxia due to placental insufficiency unless there has been an acute placental abruption or the mother is herself hypoxemic. In association with fetal hypoxemia, there is a reduction in MCA PI, indicating a reduction in cerebral resistance and an increase in cerebral blood flow, a phenomenon called the "brain-sparing effect."[57] These early changes in Doppler indices of the umbilical artery or the MCA or their ratio may be useful in assisting the diagnosis or early detection of uteroplacental dysfunction.[7]

Progressive placental pathology (thrombosis, fibrosis, inflammation) further increases resistance to umbilical artery blood flow, occasionally demonstrating absence or reversal of end-diastolic flow. These are late signs, associated with a significant increase in perinatal mortality: 20% when there is absent end-diastolic flow and 68% when there is reverse end-diastolic flow.[58] Deterioration of cardiac function leads to disappearance of the brain-sparing effect and the MCA indices become "normal."

Venous Doppler provides valuable information about fetal cardiovascular and respiratory responses to hypoxia. Abnormalities of venous Doppler waveforms are in general late signs of uteroplacental dysfunction, indicating advanced stage of fetal hypoxemia and decompensation.

The DV is the most extensively studied venous vessel. With worsening fetal condition, there will be progressive increase in the PI of DV, and eventually the absence or the reversal of the a-wave.[59] Among all Doppler tools and other fetal surveillance methods, the DV Doppler study is the best single predictor of perinatal outcome.[60] It also appears that deterioration in DV precedes an abnormal CTG, and therefore, DV may be a better parameter than CTG to determine the optimal time of elective delivery of the very premature fetus with growth restriction.[61]

The Use of Doppler Studies in the Diagnosis of Uteroplacental Dysfunction and Intrauterine Growth Restriction

The diagnosis of IUGR depends on the demonstration of small–for–gestational age fetal parameters or flattening of the growth curve. However, size is less important than the mechanism. The diagnosis of IUGR secondary to chronic hypoxia can be accomplished only through Doppler studies. If all these Doppler studies are normal, the fetus is small because of some other mechanism (e.g., genetics, viral infection) and does not require intensive monitoring because intervention has no chance to alter outcome. However, if the Doppler studies demonstrate a high resistance pattern of the uterine artery and the umbilical artery with corresponding changes in the MCA, the fetus is likely to have IUGR secondary to chronic hypoxia and requires close monitoring.

Use of Doppler to Monitor Intrauterine Growth Restriction (See also Chapter 11)

Once IUGR or uteroplacental dysfunction has been diagnosed, the pregnancy should be closely monitored if delivery is not considered the most appropriate action. In general, if the arterial Doppler shows early changes only, that is, raised resistance, the fetus is still in a compensated stage and the risk of immediate intrauterine death is low. Repeating the Doppler studies periodically every 1 to 3 weeks (depending on findings) is usually adequate. If the umbilical artery Doppler shows absence or reversed diastolic flow, the MCA resistance will be reduced and the DV may be abnormal. Under these conditions, a pulsatile waveform may also be seen in the umbilical vein. The risk of perinatal mortality is substantially increased. The fetus should be either delivered or monitored more frequently. Overall, in cases of IUGR, the presence of abnormal Doppler is the best predictor of adverse perinatal outcome, and Doppler wave analysis should be included in the surveillance of these fetuses.[62,63]

The value of Doppler ultrasound in surveillance of the high risk fetus is supported by the latest meta-analysis of 16 studies involving 10,225 fetuses.[64] Compared with no Doppler ultrasound, the use of Doppler ultrasound in high risk pregnancy (especially those complicated by hypertension or presumed impaired fetal growth) was associated with a reduction in perinatal deaths (RR 0.71, 95% CI 0.52–0.98, 1.2% versus 1.7%). The use of Doppler ultrasound was also associated with fewer inductions of labor (RR 0.89, 95% CI 0.80–0.99) and fewer cesarean sections (RR 0.90, 95% CI 0.84–0.97), without reports of adverse effects. The authors' conclusions were that "the use of Doppler ultrasound in high risk pregnancies reduced the risk of perinatal deaths and resulted in less obstetric interventions."

In term pregnancies complicated by uteroplacental dysfunction and IUGR, one should seriously consider delivery if the umbilical artery already shows minimal end-diastolic flow. Although the risk of immediate perinatal mortality and morbidity due to hypoxia is low, the perinatal complications are significant higher if these pregnancies are allowed to go on.

In preterm pregnancies, less than 34 weeks, the risk of prematurity outweighs the benefit of delivery if the venous Doppler is still normal. (Refer to the management paradigm in Chapter 11.) One must remember that, although IUGR due to placental dysfunction usually follows a predictable sequence of cardiovascular changes detectable by Doppler examination, the sequence is less predictable in IUGR associated with other causes such as preeclampsia, perhaps because of the speed with which the pathology evolves.[65] Therefore, the optimal frequency of fetal surveillance has to be considered individually.

Fetal Anemia (See also Chapter 13)

Other than placental dysfunction, Doppler ultrasound plays a central role in the management of fetal anemia. Many sonographic and Doppler measurements have been associated with the degree of fetal anemia secondary to alloimmunization, including placental thickness, umbilical vein diameter, and liver or spleen size.[66] However, most of these parameters are either difficult to measure with precision or the association is not strong enough to have clinical utility. Among them all, the peak systolic velocity (PSV) of the MCA is the most predictive of fetal anemia.[67] The increase in MCA PSV in the anemic fetus is probably the combined result of increased cardiac output and decreased blood viscosity, all of which increase the PSV.

In normal pregnancy, the MCA PSV increases with gestational age. Mari and associates[68] pioneered its application in a study of 111 fetuses at risk of anemia due to red blood cell alloimmunization. Using a cutoff of PSV of 1.5 multiple of median, they observed that MCA PSV predicted all cases of moderate to severe anemia with a 12% false-positive rate.[68] These findings have been confirmed by subsequent investigators with minor discrepancies. It is also possible to predict which fetus is likely to deteriorate and require in utero therapy later because the rate of increase in MCA PSV per week is highest among those who subsequently become moderately to severely anemic.[69]

The assessment of MCA PSV requires meticulous attention to ensure that the measurement is reproducible. It is usually measured in an axial section of the fetal head below the plane for measurement of biparietal diameter. Using color Doppler to aid identification of the MCA, the Doppler gate is placed at the proximal point close to the origin of the MCA, taking care that the angle between the ultrasound beam and the vessel is 0 degrees.[70] The use of MCA PSV assessment enables repeated, noninvasive fetal monitoring to determine the presence and degree of anemia and to determine whether and when in utero therapy is likely necessary.

After in utero transfusion, the immediate fetal MCA response to the increased hematocrit is a reduction in PSV.[71] However, adult red cells have very different characteristics from fetal red cells, and a large amount of adult red cells could affect the reliability of using the MCA PSV to time the next transfusion.[72] The MCA PSV should be used as an adjunct to clinical experience rather than the absolute yardstick upon which to determine the timing of the next procedure.

There is increasing evidence that an elevated MCA PSV reflects anemia and not necessarily a singular cause of anemia. An elevated MCA PSV has been described in cases of fetal parvovirus infection, Kell sensitization, massive fetomaternal hemorrhage, homozygous alpha-thalassemia, or placental chorioangioma.[73–77] Therefore, the assessment of MCV PSV is an important diagnostic tool in the evaluation of pregnancies complicated by fetal hydrops or cardiac failure.

OTHER TESTS

The most recent Cochrane review reported that the use of biochemical tests of placental function led to no obvious differences in perinatal mortality.[78] The available trial data do not support the use of estriol estimation in high risk pregnancies. Unfortunately, the review included only one eligible trial of poor quality. In summary, there is no evidence to support the use of biochemical testing as part of fetal assessment. Furthermore, there is likely to be little enthusiasm for conducting such trials because biochemical testing has been superseded by biophysical testing in antepartum fetal assessment.

Placental grading enjoyed popularity in the 1980s and early 1990s but is now not used widely in clinical practice. However, there has been only one randomized controlled trial of routine placental grading as a screening tool in a low risk population.[79] It showed an improved perinatal outcome in the scanned group compared with those who were not scanned. However, there are several important points about that study. The numbers in the study were smaller than would normally be expected to show a significant difference in fetal outcome measures, the group that did not have placental grading had a higher incidence of adverse fetal outcome than would normally be expected for a low risk population, and the improvement in outcome did not exclusively occur in those with abnormal placental grading. Further research regarding placental grading in high risk pregnancies is needed.[80]

COMPREHENSIVE APPROACH TO PRENATAL FETAL ASSESSMENT AND MANAGEMENT

It is clear that no one test is sufficient for the management of fetuses at high risk of chronic hypoxia and that a comprehensive approach is more appropriate and relevant in practice.[81,82] In studies that have attempted to document the sequence of deterioration in chronic fetal asphyxia, the general conclusions are that abnormalities in the umbilical artery waveform tend to appear first followed by cerebral redistribution, early venous changes, and reduced breathing movements. Amniotic fluid volume starts to fall and FHR short-term variability to reduce next. Abnormal umbilical venous pulsation, reversed umbilical artery pulsation, abnormal fetal movements and tone, and fetal bradycardia tend to be late events. These concepts are graphically displayed in Figure 11–6 in Chapter 11.

Thus, although there is no agreed standard of practice for surveillance and management of high risk fetuses, many centers use a combination of fetal growth and umbilical artery Doppler recordings together with CTG, BPP, other Doppler studies and give the mother steroids if preterm delivery is contemplated. The optimum timing of delivery remains an unanswered question, although most would not continue the pregnancy beyond 34 weeks if there is a persistent abnormality of the umbilical artery Doppler recordings. Chapter 11 discusses these issues in more detail and an example of a management algorithm is shown in Figure 11–9.

SUMMARY OF MANAGEMENT OPTIONS

Prenatal Fetal Surveillance (in the normally formed fetus)

Management Options	Evidence Quality and Recommendation	References
Indications		
High risk patients—where there is a risk of chronic fetal hypoxia	III/B	2,3,5–7
• **Maternal:** cyanotic heart disease; diabetes; autoimmune disease; chronic renal disease; hypertensive disease; inadequate nutrition; smoking (often synergistic with other factors); alcohol and other drug abuse		
• **Placental/fetal:** IUGR; recurrent abruption; preeclampsia; abnormal amniotic fluid volume; reduced fetal movements; abdominal pain without a clear cause; postdates pregnancy; previous stillbirth/IUGR		
• **Combined:** raised serum α-fetoprotein	III/B	8
Principles		
Select test appropriate for pathology/problem if possible/known	—/GPP	—
Comprehensive assessment of mother and fetus	III/B	81,82
Multiple and repeated fetal assessment methods are more likely to be informative than any single test	III/B	81,82
Methods—Maternal		
Clinical (e.g., evaluation of hypertension, cardiac disease)	—/GPP	—
Laboratory (e.g., diabetes, Kleihauer, renal and liver function)	—/GPP	—
Biochemical testing		
No evidence to support use in high risk pregnancies	Ia/A	78
Methods—Fetal		
Ultrasound measurement of fetal growth, see Chapter 11		
Amniotic fluid volume, see Chapters 11 and 12		
Umbilical artery Doppler velocimetry	Ia/A	64
• Only test shown in randomized trials to reduce perinatal morbidity and mortality		
• No information about optimum frequency of use		
Regional recordings of fetal blood flow		
Indicate degree of fetal compromise in		
• Chronic fetal hypoxia	III/B	28,65,81,82
• Anemia	III/B	68,69,71
Uterine artery blood flow before 24 wk	III/B	54,55
Identifies those pregnancies at risk of IUGR and preeclampsia and use may improve outcome		
CTG/NST		
• Predicts short term outcome	III/B	45,46,48
• Computerized assessment is more accurate		30
• No evidence that use improves outcome	Ia/A	49
• Probably best in combination with other methods	III/B	81,82

SUMMARY OF MANAGEMENT OPTIONS

Prenatal Fetal Surveillance (in the normally formed fetus)—cont'd

Management Options	Evidence Quality and Recommendation	References
BPS		
• Gives best indication of both acute and chronic fetal compromise	III/B	28,29
• No grade A evidence that use improves outcome	Ia/A	25
• Probably best in combination with other methods	III/B	28,29,81,82
Placental grading		
• Only one study to support use in low risk population screening; no data in high risk	(Ib)/(A)	(79)
• More research needed	Ia/A	80

BPS, biophysical profile; CTG, cardiotocogram; GPP, good practice point; IUGR, intrauterine growth restriction; NST, nonstress test.

SUGGESTED READINGS

Baschat AA: Pathophysiology of fetal growth restriction: Implications for diagnosis and surveillance. Obstet Gynecol Surv 2004;59:617–627.

Brennand J, Cameron A: Fetal anaemia: Diagnosis and management. Best Pract Res Clin Obstet Gynaecol 2008;22:15–29.

Cosmi E, Ambrosini G, D'Antona D, et al: Doppler, cardiotocography, and biophysical profile changes in growth-restricted fetuses. Obstet Gynecol 2005;106:1240–1245.

Devoe LD: Antenatal fetal assessment: Contraction stress test, nonstress test, vibroacoustic stimulation, amniotic fluid volume, biophysical profile, and modified biophysical profile—An overview. Semin Perinatol 2008;32:247–252.

Mari G, Deter RL, Carpenter RL, et al: Noninvasive diagnosis by Doppler ultrasonography of fetal anemia due to maternal red-cell alloimmunization. Collaborative Group for Doppler Assessment of the Blood Velocity in Anemic Fetuses. N Engl J Med 2000;342:9–14.

Martin CB Jr: Normal fetal physiology and behavior, and adaptive responses with hypoxemia. Semin Perinatol 2008;32:239–242.

Pearce W: Hypoxic regulation of the fetal cerebral circulation. J Appl Physiol 2006;100:731–738.

Robinson B, Nelson L: A review of the Proceedings from the 2008 NICHD Workshop on Standardized Nomenclature for Cardiotocography: Update on definitions, interpretative systems with management strategies, and research priorities in relation to intrapartum electronic fetal monitoring. Rev Obstet Gynecol 2008;1:186–192.

REFERENCES

For a complete list of references, log onto www.expertconsult.com.

CHAPTER 11

Fetal Growth Disorders

AHMET ALEXANDER BASCHAT

INTRODUCTION

Disturbance of normal fetal growth can result in abnormal weight, body mass, or body proportion at birth. The two principal fetal growth disorders are intrauterine growth restriction (IUGR) and macrosomia, both of which are associated with increased perinatal mortality and short- and long-term morbidity. Perinatal detection of fetal growth disorders has evolved dramatically since the late 1960s. Before antenatal ultrasound assessment of fetal growth was clinically available, fetal growth was defined by birth weight. The absolute birth weight was classified as either macrosomia (>4000 g), low birth weight, very low birth weight, or extremely low birth weight (<2500 g, <1500 g, and <1000 g, respectively). The landmark observations of Lubchenco and colleagues[1] in 1963 showed that the classification of neonates by birth weight percentile had a significant prognostic advantage because it improved the detection of neonates with IUGR and who are at increased risk for adverse health events throughout life.[2–4] Neonates are now classified as very small for gestational age (<3rd percentile), small for gestational age (<10th percentile), appropriate for gestational age (10th–90th percentile), or large for gestational age (>90th percentile).[5] With the development of reference ranges for fetal measurements and the study of their growth rates with advancing gestation, it became possible to apply the concept of growth percentiles prenatally. Subsequently, it became possible to relate absolute and serial fetal measurements to their gestational age–specific percentiles in order to diagnose abnormal fetal size and growth velocity. The detection of a fetal growth disorder is further enhanced if the reference ranges for fetal biometric data and birth weight account for maternal height and race and fetal birth order and sex[6] (growth potential). A neonate may be of normal weight but still significantly lighter than its growth potential. Growth potential percentiles are superior to conventional reference ranges for the prediction of adverse perinatal outcome.[7,8]

The detection of abnormal body mass or proportions is based on anthropometric measurements and ratios that are relatively independent of sex, race, and to a certain extent, gestational age. The ponderal index [(birth weight (g)/crown-heel length^3) × 100][9] is one tool that has high accuracy for the identification of IUGR[10] and macrosomia,[11] independent of the birth weight percentile.[12] In one study, 40% of neonates with a birth weight below the 10th percentile did not have growth restriction based on the ponderal index.[10] From a clinical perspective, the ponderal index correlates more closely with perinatal morbidity and mortality than traditional birth weight percentiles, but might miss proportionally small and lean neonates with growth restriction.[13,14] Inappropriate fetal growth is also suggested by abnormal symmetry between head and abdominal measurements. Again, a different subset of neonates is identified with this descriptive approach.[15]

A gold standard for birth weight criteria that distinguishes between abnormal and physiologic growth patterns is highly desirable for any study of the relationship between neonatal size and outcome. Although the immediate effect of disturbed fetal growth is an abnormal expression of the growth potential, the effect on outcome and fetal programming is determined predominantly by the underlying condition.

REGULATION OF FETAL GROWTH

Fetal growth is regulated at multiple levels, and successful placentation is required for the coordination of key components within the maternal, placental, and fetal compartments. The key elements required for successful placentation are the normal development of maternal and fetal vascular supply, synthetic activity of the placenta, establishment of transplacental carrier proteins for substrates that require active transport, a decrease in the maternal-fetal diffusion distance to facilitate passive transport, and a matched increase in maternal-fetal perfusion and surface area with advancing gestational age. First-trimester blastocyst adherence and implantation initiate placental vascular development, which is necessary for the delivery of nutrients and oxygen to the growing trophoblast beyond simple diffusion. Successful adherence permits differentiation of placental transport mechanisms and the activation of paracrine and endocrine signaling pathways between the mother, the placenta, and the fetus by the second trimester. Trophoblast invasion into the maternal spiral arteries and fetal villous sprouting decrease the blood flow resistance in both vascular compartments of the placenta. These developments together with the marked increase in villous vascular surface area are essential for efficient and coordinated nutrient transfer and waste and gas exchange that ensure normal fetal growth and development.

After fertilization, the cytotrophoblast migrates to form anchoring villi between the decidua and the uterus through controlled breakdown of the extracellular matrix by metalloproteinases and localized expression of adhesion molecules, including integrins and collagen IV. Simultaneously, hypoxia-stimulated angiogenesis initiates vascular connections between the maternal circulation and the intervillous space. Angiopoietins, placental growth factor, and placental protein 13 (PP-13) are three important regulatory substances expressed in increasing concentrations during this early critical phase of placental vasculogenesis.[16–18] Once the maternal blood supply to the intervillous space is established, increasing quantities of placental secretory products appear in the maternal circulation. Concurrently, extravillous cytotrophoblasts infiltrate the maternal spiral arteries, progressively remodeling the vessel walls so that the musculoelastic media is lost.[19,20] This decrease in uterine artery blood flow resistance can be documented by Doppler interrogation of the uterine artery waveform, first by the disappearance of the early diastolic notch, then by a progressive increase in diastolic blood flow toward term (see later).

In the fetal compartment, villous proliferation of the trophoblastic trabeculae is initiated by the 18th day after conception. By the 5th week of gestation, all villi contain extraembryonic mesenchyme and capillaries in the villous stroma. These mesenchymal villi form the originating pool for all subsequent villous types. The differentiation into stem villi is critical for establishing distinct arterial and venous circulation in the villous vascular tree. Further differentiation into villous subtypes and continuous villous vascular branching results in an increase in the vascular exchange area, thinning of the cytotrophoblast, and a decrease in blood flow resistance in the umbilical arterial circulation.[21,22] In addition to the angiopoietins, basic fibroblast growth factor and its low-affinity heparin sulfate reception and the vascular endothelial factor system may be involved in the regulation of villous angiogeneis and sprouting.[22]

These vascular maturation processes result in low-resistance, high-capacitance vascular beds that allow increasing and matched perfusion of the maternal and fetal placental compartments. Intervillous blood flow is regulated mainly through paracrine factors, such as nitric oxide, endothelin, adenosine, released cyclic guanosine monophosphate, and fetal atrial natriuretic peptide.[21] After successful placentation, approximately 600 mL/min maternal cardiac output[23,24] is matched to 400 mL/kg/min fetal flow distributed over a term placental exchange area of 12 m^2.[25]

Once the blood supply to the trophoblast and fetal circulation is established, placental transport capacity is the major determinant of maternal-fetal nutrient transport. All substances that traverse between the maternal and the fetal circulation must pass through the villous trophoblast, a syncytial bilayer 4-μm thick that consists of a maternal microvillus and a fetal basal layer.[26] Its capacity for transport is enhanced by a growing membrane surface area and increased density and affinity of carrier proteins for glucose, amino acids (mainly), and fatty acids.[27–30] The sodium/hydrogen (Na/H^+) family of transport proteins maintains syncytiotrophoblast intracellular pH and cell volume homeostasis, ensuring proper function of the transplacental substrate carrier proteins.[31] By the second trimester, these placental activities consume 40% of the O_2 and 70% of the glucose entering the uterus, leaving the rest for fetal use.[32–34] This proportion decreases progressively until term.

With the establishment of placental transport systems, endocrine signaling between maternal, placental, and fetal compartments helps to coordinate placental and fetal growth. Maternal metabolic changes include postprandial hyperglycemia, lipolysis, and increased fasting levels of free fatty acids, triglycerides, and cholesterol. All of these enhance substrate availability to the placenta and fetus and are at least partly mediated by increases in placental levels of lactogen and leptin. Similarly, maternal intravascular volume expansion and its relative refractoriness to vasoactive agents promote steady nutrient delivery to the placenta.[35]

Placental and fetal growth is regulated by a combination of factors including substrate availability, placental perfusion in the maternal compartment, endocrine or paracrine signaling, and perfusion and nutrient exchange area in the fetal compartment of the placenta. In addition, the design of the fetal circulation is unique because it allows for preferential streaming of nutrients via three principal shunts. Nutrients that enter the circulation through the umbilical vein first reach the ductus venosus. Here 70% to 80% of the umbilical venous nutrients returning continue on to the liver first and reach the heart through the hepatic veins. The remainder of umbilical venous blood is distributed directly to the heart through the ductus venosus.[36] Glucose and amino acids thus preferentially reach the liver for glycogen storage and stimulate insulin release from the fetal pancreas. The subsequent release of insulin-like growth factors I and II provides the major stimulus for fetal growth and differentiation.[37] Leptin stimulates fetal pancreatic growth and transplacental amino acid transport and affects fatty acid transport. Therefore, it may be an important modulator of fetal body fat content and body proportions.[38,39]

At the level of the right atrium, the directionality of incoming bloodstreams ensures nutrient-rich blood from the ductus venosus is distributed to the myocardium and brain, whereas venous return from the body is distributed to the descending aorta and ultimately to the placenta for reoxygenation and nutrient and waste exchange.[27,40] Blood leaving the ventricles reaches the brain through branches arising from the preductal aorta. An increase in right ventricular afterload redistributes blood toward the left ventricle and, therefore, the myocardium and brain. At the level of the ductus venosus and aortic isthmus, however, the same changes promote the distribution of blood from the descending aorta toward the cerebral circulation. Therefore, shunting at the level of the ductus venosus affects the whole body whereas changes at the level of the foramen ovale and the aortic isthmus affect the right-left balance of nutrient flux.[41] In addition to the preferential distribution of left- and right-sided cardiac output, several organs can modify local flow by autoregulation to meet oxygen and nutrient demands.[42]

Normal placental and fetal growth across pregnancy is characterized by sequential cellular hyperplasia, hyperplasia plus hypertrophy, and finally, hypertrophy alone.[43] Placental growth follows a sigmoid curve, plateauing earlier in gestation than does the fetal growth curve. Between 16 weeks and term, human fetal weight increases 20-fold.[43] The fetal growth curve is exponential, with maximal growth occurring in the third trimester when significant body mass and particularly adipose tissue are accumulated.

FETAL GROWTH RESTRICTION

Etiology and Risk Factors

Several conditions may interfere with normal placentation and culminate in either pregnancy loss or IUGR. Broadly categorized into maternal, uterine, placental, and fetal disorders, these conditions affect either nutrient and oxygen delivery to the placenta, nutrient and oxygen transfer across the placenta, fetal uptake, or regulation of growth processes. When they are sufficiently abnormal, they produce growth restriction characterized by a reduction in fetal cell size, and when they are early and severe enough, they reduce cell number and thus growth potential postnatally (Fig. 11–1). In clinical practice, considerable overlap occurs between conditions that determine the manifestation, progression, and outcome of growth restriction.

Maternal causes of placental dysfunction such as chronic renal disease, collagen vascular disease, hypertension, and some thrombophilias typically affect placental vascular development. Uterine abnormalities can also interfere with placentation and affect nutrient delivery to the fetus. Abnormal placental vascular development (either primary or secondary to maternal conditions and fetal abnormalities, both chromosomal and anatomic) account for the vast majority of cases of IUGR in singleton pregnancies.[44–48] Usually, the earlier the onset of the disease process, the more likely the fetus is to be symmetrically small, with a reduced cell number, and the more likely the etiology is to be either a severe maternal vascular disorder, a fetal infection, or a chromosome disorder.[49]

In addition to primary factors that initiate placental dysfunction, aggravating circumstances with additional impact include smoking, malnutrition, and drug use. Many risk factors act synergistically. For example, the adverse effect of smoking is doubled in thin, white women and further potentiated by poor maternal weight gain.[50] Similarly, the possible benefits of low-dose aspirin therapy and the detrimental effects of excessive blood pressure reduction are also more apparent in this group of women.[51,52]

Pathophysiology

Interference with the placental nutrient supply can affect all aspects of placental function. The gestational age at onset, the magnitude of injury, and the success of adaptive mechanisms determine the ultimate severity. Mild placental disease is more likely to affect organ function and maturation at the cellular level, with little perceivable growth delay perinatally, but may affect adult health (fetal programming), often through epigenetic modifications. With more severe placental disease, fetal growth delay and adaptive organ responses become evident in utero. Exhaustion of the placental and fetal adaptive potential leads to decompensation, with variable progression and manifestations in the fetal organ systems. Adaptive responses that are intended to enhance fetal survival in a hypoxic environment may become destructive under conditions such as acute ischemia-reperfusion. Much of the long-term effect of growth restriction is unclear, as are the effects of obstetric intervention. As a result, severe disturbances of fetal growth pose a challenge to even the most experienced multidisciplinary team.

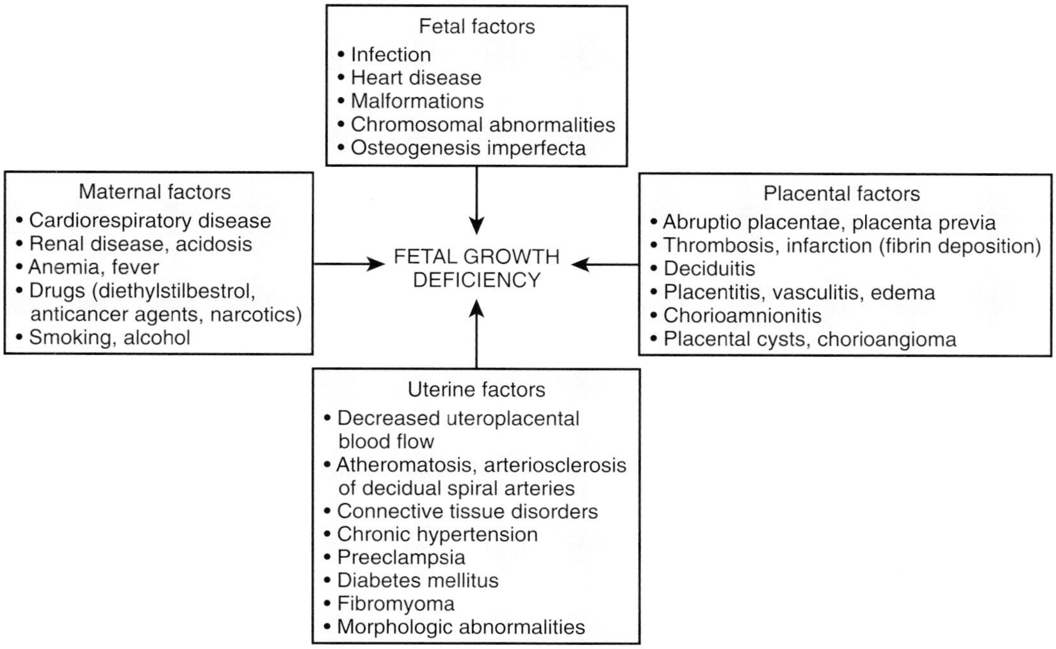

FIGURE 11–1
Causes of growth restriction by compartment.

Mechanisms of Placental Dysfunction

The efficiency of maternal-fetal exchange of nutrients, fluid, and waste can become suboptimal when there is a decrease in substrate transporters, an increase in the diffusion distance between the maternal and the fetal compartments, a decrease in the exchange area or increased impedance to blood flow in the maternal and fetal compartments in the placenta. It is important to recognize that not all of these mechanisms become clinically detectable unless they reach a certain threshold of severity. Typically, earlier-onset placental dysfunction produces a more severe clinical picture with marked manifestations, whereas late-onset growth delay first manifest in the third trimester may produce few clinically detectable findings. Diffusion may be adequate to meet embryonic nutrient needs, but compromises fetal survival and growth potential. Typically, trophoblastic invasion is confined to the decidual portion of the myometrium, and the spiral and radial arteries do not transform into low-resistance vessels.[19,53,54] Altered expression of vasoactive substances increases vascular reactivity, and if hypoxia-stimulated angiogenesis is inadequate, placental autoregulation becomes deficient. Maternal placental floor infarcts and fetal villous obliteration and fibrosis increase placental blood flow resistance, producing a maternal-fetal placental perfusion mismatch that decreases the effective exchange area.[21,41,55,56] With progressive vascular occlusion, fetoplacental flow resistance is increased throughout the vascular bed, which is the metabolically active placental mass, and nutrient exchange decreases or is outgrown.

The severity of placental vascular dysfunction is clinically assessed in the maternal and fetal compartments of the placenta with Doppler ultrasound. An early diastolic notch in the uterine arteries at 12 to 14 weeks (Fig. 11–2) suggests delayed trophoblast invasion,[57] whereas persistence of "notching" beyond 24 weeks provides confirmatory evidence.[19,56,58] A reduction of umbilical venous blood flow volume may be the earliest Doppler sign of subtle decreases in fetal villous perfusion.[59] Umbilical artery waveforms correlate with both the tertiary villous architecture and the blood flow resistance. If villous damage is minimal, elevated blood flow resistance may be seen only with sophisticated Doppler techniques.[60] At least 30% of the fetal villous vasculature is abnormal when the umbilical artery end-diastolic velocities are low and Doppler resistance indices are elevated.[61] Absence or reversal of umbilical artery end-diastolic velocity suggests that 60% to 70% of the villous vascular tree is damaged (Fig. 11–3).[61,62] Abnormal flow patterns in the uterine arteries are consistent with abnormal implantation and indicate an increased risk of preeclampsia, placental abruption, and early-onset IUGR.[63] Abnormal umbilical flow patterns indicate an increased risk of hypoxemia and acidemia proportional to the severity of Doppler abnormality.[21,64–66] It is important to note that mild placental vascular abnormalities leading to fetal growth restriction may not produce umbilical artery Doppler abnormalities but rather may be reflected in isolated abnormalities in cerebral artery Doppler waveforms.[67,68]

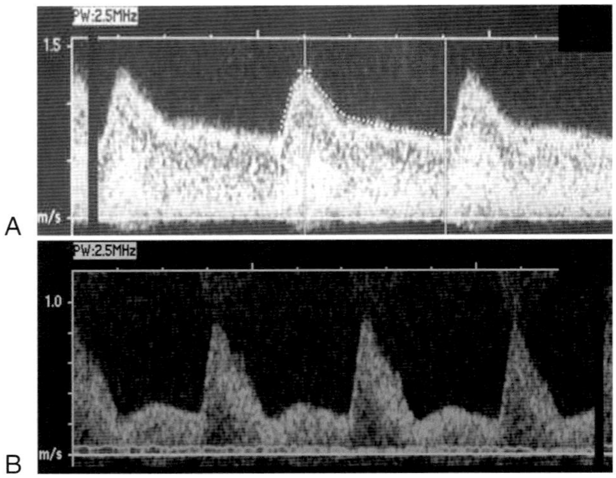

FIGURE 11–2
Flow velocity waveforms obtained from the uterine artery beyond 24 weeks' gestation. *A*, High-volume diastolic flow is established, indicating successful trophoblast invasion. *B*, Impaired trophoblast invasion of the spiral arteries is associated with elevated placental vascular resistance and persistence of an early diastolic notch in the uterine artery flow velocity waveform.

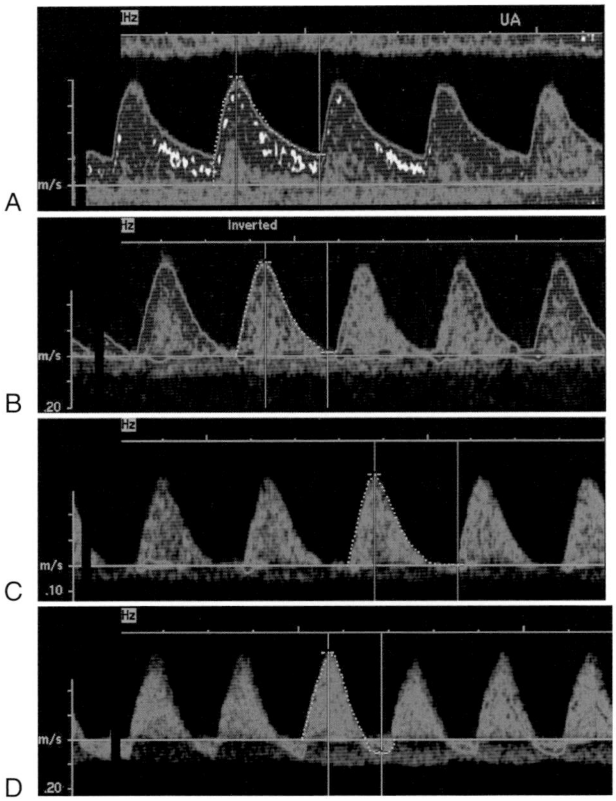

FIGURE 11–3
A, The normal umbilical artery flow velocity waveform has marked positive end-diastolic velocity that increases in proportion to systole toward term. *B*, Moderate abnormalities in the villous vascular structure increase blood flow resistance and are associated with a decrease in end-diastolic velocity. When a significant proportion of the villous vascular tree is abnormal, end-diastolic velocities may be absent (*C*) or even reversed (*D*).

Metabolic and Cellular Effects of Placental Dysfunction

Oxygen and glucose consumption by the placenta is unaffected when nutrient delivery to the uterus is only mildly restricted and fetal demands can be met by increased fractional extraction. Fetal hypoglycemia occurs when uterine oxygen delivery (and likely substrate delivery) is less than a critical value (0.6 mmol/min/kg fetal body weight in sheep) and fetal oxygen uptake is reduced.[32,34,69] Insulin is an important fetal growth factor. Fetal pancreatic insulin responses are blunted by mild hypoglycemia, allowing gluconeogenesis from hepatic glycogen stores.[70–73] At this stage, fetal glucose stores and lactate are preferentially diverted to the placenta to maintain placental metabolic, endocrine, and nutrient transfer function.[27,30,32]

As the nutrient supply worsens, fetal hypoglycemia intensifies and secondary energy sources are required. Proteins are catabolized to gluconeogenic amino acids. However, limitations in placental amino acid transfer eventually result in hypoaminoacidemia.[28] Decreased transfer leads to relative deficiencies of circulating long-chain polyunsaturated fatty acids, whereas metabolic limitation leads to hypertriglyceridemia and the inability to estabish essential adipose stores. Even if provided adequate substrate, inadequate oxygen is available to maintain oxidative metabolism. Hypoglycemia, hyperlactic acidemia, and a growing base deficit correlate with the degree of fetal hypoxemia and protein energy malnutrition.[27,74–78] Down-regulation of several cellular transporters and the Na/H^+ pump affects placental cellular function and aggravates the condition further.[28,29,31,33] In this setting, the fetal brain and heart switch primary nutrients from glucose to lactate and ketones.[79] Cardiac metabolism may consume as much as 80% of the circulating lactate.[80,81]

Simultaneously, the principal endocrine growth axis (insulin and insulin-like growth factors I and II) as well as leptin-coordinated fat deposition is down-regulated.[82] As a result, the placenta and fetus do not reach their size potential. The combination of fetal starvation, a modified endocrine milieu, and deficient tissue stores limits fetal growth and affects cellular and functional differentiation in many target organs.

Fetal Response in Major Organ Systems

Vascular and metabolic disturbances within the placenta lead to alterations in many fetal organ systems. Cardiovascular and central nervous system functions are best studied and provide the most practicable clinical means to document the progression of disease and assess the fetal condition.

Changes in fetal blood flow are related to placental resistance, fetal oxygenation, organ autoregulation, and vascular reactivity. Because of the parallel arrangement of the fetal circulation, placental dysfunction has specific effects on the relative distribution of right and left ventricular output. An increase in the right or a decrease in the left ventricular afterload shifts cardiac output toward the left ventricle, supplying well-oxygenated umbilical venous blood to downstream organs. In the compensated hypoxemic state, fetal cardiac output is increased and organ autoregulation maintained.[83,84] The responses of the fetal trunk and cerebral circulation to hypoxemia differ from each other. The peripheral arteries constrict and truncal resistance increases, as evidenced by the elevated umbilical, thoracic, and descending aorta Doppler resistance indices ("hind limb reflex") that account for most of the increase in right ventricular afterload.[85–88] The fetal cerebral circulation dilates in response to hypoxemia. Fetal cerebral vasodilation is reflected in decreased Doppler indices (poorly described as "brain-sparing")[89,90] and reduces left ventricular afterload. This changing balance between right and left ventricular afterload decreases the cerebroplacental Doppler index ratio[91] and redistributes well-oxygenated left ventricular output to the heart and brain.[85,86,92,93]

Enhanced blood flow to individual organs is documented in the myocardium,[94] adrenal glands,[95] spleen,[96] and liver.[97] Conversely, blood flow resistance in the peripheral pulmonary arteries,[98] celiac axis,[99] mesenteric vessels,[100,101] kidneys,[102,103] and femoral and iliac arteries[104] increases. The overall effect is an improved distribution of well-oxygenated blood to vital organs, with preferential streaming of descending aorta blood flow to the placenta for reoxygenation. In contrast, blood flow to organs that are not vital for fetal survival is decreased. These Doppler-determined parameters are corroborated by direct measurements of cardiac output,[85] increases in umbilical venous volume flow,[59,105] and progressive decreases in amniotic fluid volume after long-standing redistribution.[103] Further, there are increased circulating levels of endothelin, arginine vasopressin, norepinephrine, epinephrine, vasoactive intestinal peptide, and atrial natriuretic peptide[106–108] that are related directly to the severity of the acid-base disturbance. These adaptations are likely responsible for the enhanced vascular reactivity that may aggravate the patient's clinical status and increase the complication rate during cordocentesis.

Mild placental dysfunction results in the delayed maturation of several fetal behaviors. The normal behavioral sequence of development for the fetus proceeds from the appearance of movement, to coupling and cyclicity of behavior, and finally, to integration of movement patterns into stable behavioral states. Likewise, the development of autonomic reflexes superimposed on intrinsic cardiac activity determines the characteristics of the fetal heart rate. These reflexes originate in the brainstem and are modulated by the ambient oxygen tension, signals from higher brain centers, the reticular activating system, and peripheral sensory inputs. Variations of heart rate and episodic accelerations coupled with fetal movement indicate normal functioning of these regulatory sites. Once organized, behavioral states are established (typically by 28 weeks' gestation), diurnal and responsive cyclicity (e.g., to maternal glucose) and their coupling to heart rate variables (heart rate reactivity) are usually achieved.[109]

A delay occurs in all aspects of central nervous system maturation in fetuses with IUGR and chronic hypoxemia.[110–114] There is also a progressive decline in global fetal activity.[115] The combination of delayed central integration of fetal heart rate control, decreased fetal activity, and chronic hypoxemia results in a higher baseline heart rate, with lower short- and long-term variation (on computerized analysis) and delayed development of heart rate reactivity.[113,114,116–119] Computerized heart rate analyses show that the changes in characteristics are particularly evident between 28 and 32 weeks. Progressive fetal hypoxemia is associated with a gradual decline in amniotic fluid volume, fetal breathing, gross body movement, tone, and computerized read and traditional fetal heart rate variability. This decline is determined by the central effects of hypoxemia or acidemia, independent of cardiovascular status.[120–124]

Placental dysfunction affects many other fetal organ systems. Hypoxemia-stimulated erythropoietin release increases red blood cells through both medullary and extramedullary hematopoiesis.[65,74,125–127] More complex interactions are observed with persistent hypoxemia and progressive degrees of placental vascular damage. Nucleated red blood cell precursors enter the peripheral circulation independent of erythropoietin levels.[128,129] Placental platelet aggregation and consumption increases the risk of thrombocytopenia.[130,131] Other organ-specific alterations of note include thyroid dysfunction, increased cortisol level, vitamin deficiency, and immune deficiency. The effect of these fetal manifestations on short- and long-term outcome is unknown.

Fetal Decompensation

If placental dysfunction is progressive or sustained, the adaptive mechanisms become exhausted and decompensation begins. Multiple-organ failure as a result of placental dysfunction is caused by the metabolic milieu and the regulatory loss of cardiovascular homeostasis. Metabolic abnormalities are exaggerated, acidemia worsens, and the risks of intrauterine damage or perinatal death increase dramatically.

Forward blood flow in the venous system is determined by cardiac compliance, contractility, and afterload. The normal venous flow velocity waveform is triphasic and, therefore, more complex than the arterial waveform. It consists of systolic and diastolic peaks (S-wave and D-wave) that are generated by the descent of the artrial-ventricular ring during ventricular systole and passive diastolic ventricular filling, respectively. The sudden increase in right atrial pressure with atrial contraction in late diastole causes a variable amount of reverse flow, producing a second trough after the D-wave (A-wave) (Fig. 11–4). A decrease in forward cardiac function marks the onset of cardiovascular decompensation[83–85,132] and causes decreased forward velocity during atrial systole (A-wave). Impaired preload handling, as evidenced by increased venous Doppler indices (discussed subsequently),[133,134] is documented in the precordial veins (ductus venosus, inferior vena cava,[135] and superior vena cava[136]), hepatic veins (right, middle, and left hepatic[137,138]), and head and neck veins (jugular veins[139] and cerebral transverse sinus[140]). If the failure to accommodate preload is progressive, umbilical venous pulsations may develop as the ultimate reflection of increased central venous pressure (Fig. 11–5).[141] This finding is consistent with umbilical venous pressure measurements obtained at the time of cordocentesis in profoundly growth-restricted fetuses. Simultaneously, autoregulation may be exaggerated in the coronary circulation[84,85] or may become dysfunctional in the cerebral and placental circulation.[142–144]

Progressive metabolic acidemia is associated with oligohydramnios and loss of fetal breathing, movement, and tone.[145,146] Abnormal fetal heart rate patterns, including overt late decelerations or a decrease in the short-term variability on computerized analysis, develop and appear to be related to metabolic status and concurrent worsening of cardiac function.[118,120,123,132,143,147] In the final stages of compromise,

FIGURE 11–4
Arterial and venous flow velocity waveforms. Absolute measurements for arteries include peak systolic and end-diastolic velocities, acceleration time, and heart rate. The venous flow velocity waveform has a triphasic profile. During ventricular systole and diastole, blood flows toward the heart, with a slight decrease after systole as the arteriovenous ring ascends. With the opening of the arteriovenous valves in diastole, antegrade flow increases again and produces the second peak (D-wave). Atrial contraction is associated with a sharp increase in atrial pressure, which is transmitted retrograde to the venous system and may be associated with brief retrograde flow (A-wave).

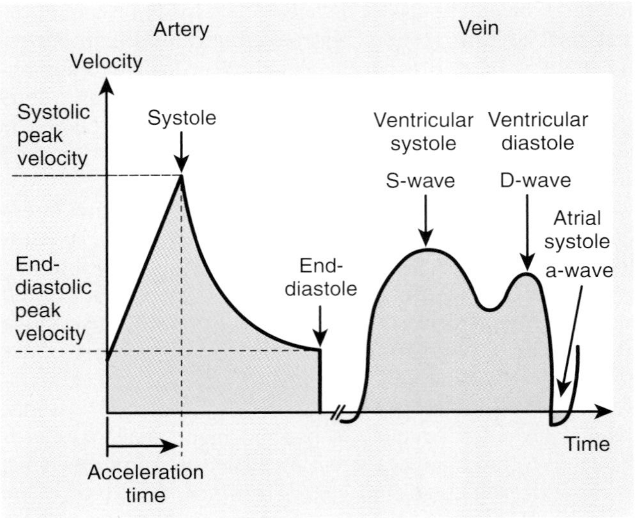

cardiac dilation with holosystolic tricuspid insufficiency, complete fetal inactivity, and spontaneous late decelerations may be seen before fetal death.[148]

The sequence of deteriorating cardiovascular, biophysical, and heart rate parameters is reasonably predictable in 70% to 80% of fetuses with IUGR before 34 weeks.[121,149] Flow abnormalities confined to the umbilical or cerebral circulation are typically early changes.[150–152] The progressive decline in (computerized) heart rate variability and increasing venous Doppler indices are closely related.[140,153] Oligohydramnios, loss of fetal tone and/or movement, abnormal venous flow, and overt heart rate decelerations are typically "late" changes.[152,153] Closer to term, the relationship between cardiovascular and biophysical deterioration is weaker, largely because of less prominent Doppler abnormalities.[154–156] In contrast, the correlation (but not necessarily the slope of the regression) between the deterioration of biophysical parameters and the acid-base status is relatively independent of gestational age (Fig. 11–6).[109,118]

Increasing evidence indicates there are significant differences in the rate and severity of clinical progression in IUGR fetuses based on the gestational age at onset and the degree of umbilical artery Doppler abnormality. Two patterns of progression in venous Doppler abnormalities occur in pregnancies diagnosed prior to 34 weeks. First, there may be a rapid loss of umbilical artery end-diastolic velocity typically leading to venous Doppler abnormalities within 4 weeks of the clinical diagnosis. A slower progression of placental Doppler abnormalities may allow a latency interval of 6 weeks until delivery. In contrast, late-onset IUGR is associated with little change in umbilical artery Dopper but rather

FIGURE 11–5
Progression of abnormal venous flow patterns. *Left*, Normal flow in the ductus venosus, with antegrade flow throughout the cardiac cycle. The umbilical vein equally shows constant flow. An increase in the retrograde flow component during atrial contraction is believed to be the hallmark of decreased cardiac function and reflects increased cardiac end-diastolic pressures. *Center*, Flow in the umbilical vein may show a monophasic pulsatile pattern, with nadirs corresponding to atrial contraction. *Right*, In the most severe form of cardiac dysfunction, reverse flow occurs during atrial contraction in the ductus venosus. Pulsations in the umbilical vein may show a biphasic profile, with systolic and diastolic peaks or even retrograde flow during atrial contraction (triphasic).

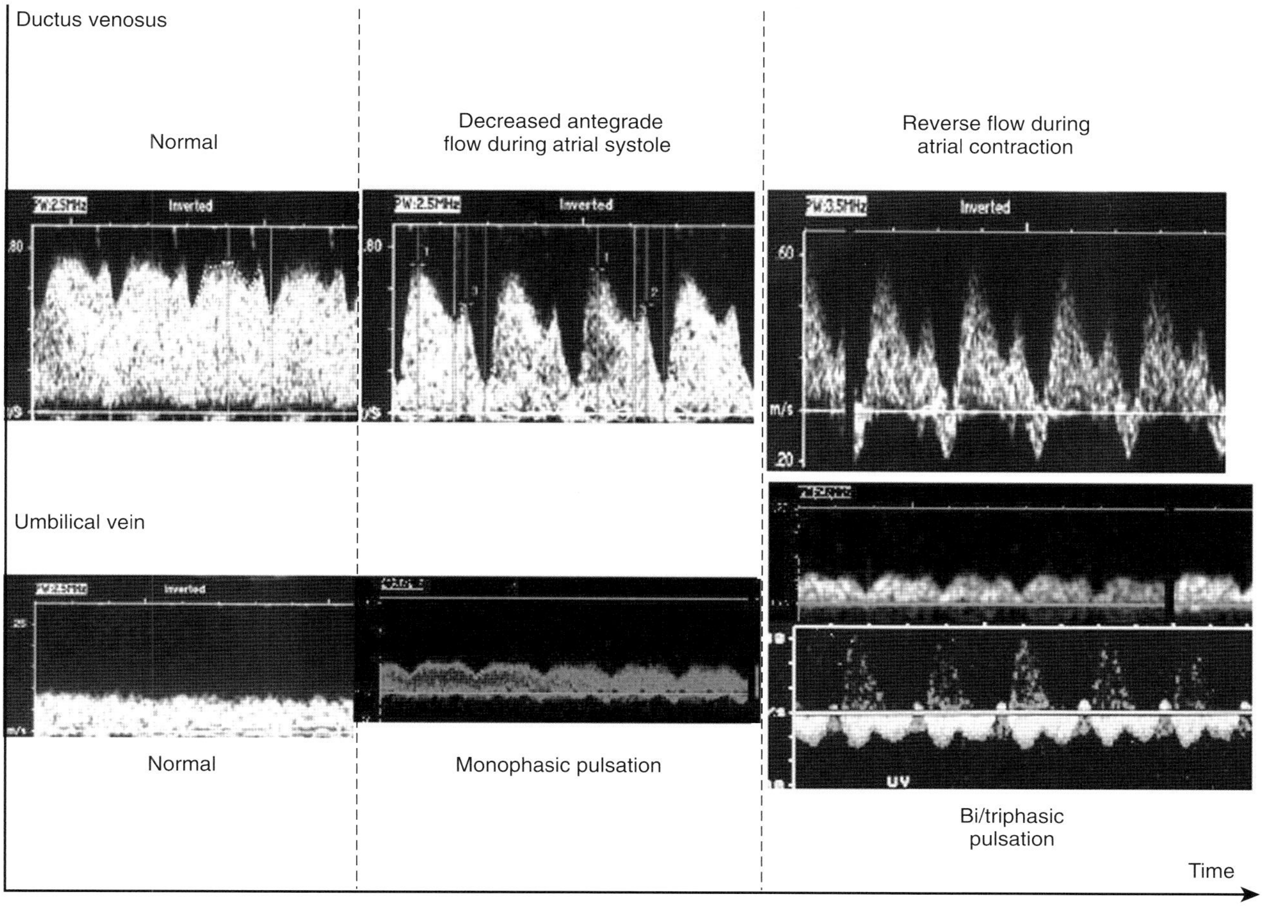

a decline in the cerebroplacental Doppler ratio and/or isolated new onset of brain sparing.[62] These differences in progression between early-onset (<34 wk) and late-onset IUGR have important implications for surveillance (see later).

Screening Options for Growth Restriction

Clinical

The maternal uterine fundus is objectively measured and charted during each antenatal visit. After 20 weeks' gestation, the normal symphyseal fundal height in centimeters approximates the number of weeks' gestation after appropriate allowances for maternal height and the fetal station. The reported sensitivity of fundal height for the detection of IUGR ranges from 60% to 85%, and the positive predictive values are 20% to 80%. Although measurement of the symphyseal fundal height is a poor screening tool for the detection of IUGR, the accuracy of subsequent ultrasound prediction of IUGR is enhanced if there is clinical suspicion of IUGR based on lagging fundal height.

Biochemical

At least four hormone or protein markers measured in the maternal sera early in the second trimester are associated with subsequent IUGR. These include estriol, human placental lactogen (hPL), human chorionic gonadotropin (hCG), and α-fetoprotein (AFP) (see Chapters 7 and 8). Clinically, maternal serum AFP is the most useful as a marker of abnormal placentation. Most studies conclude that a single, unexplained elevated value increases the risk of growth restriction 5- to 10-fold, proportional to the magnitude of the elevation. As a result, some argue that AFP measurement is clinically useful, even after earlier aneuploidy screening by nuchal translucency measurement.

Uterine Artery Doppler Studies

Deficient placentation is highly associated with gestational hypertensive disorders, IUGR, and fetal demise.[157,158] A uterine artery Doppler resistance profile that is high, persistently notched, or both, identifies women at high risk for preeclampsia and IUGR. The sensitivity is up to 85% when performed between 22 and 23 weeks' gestation.[159,160] Because

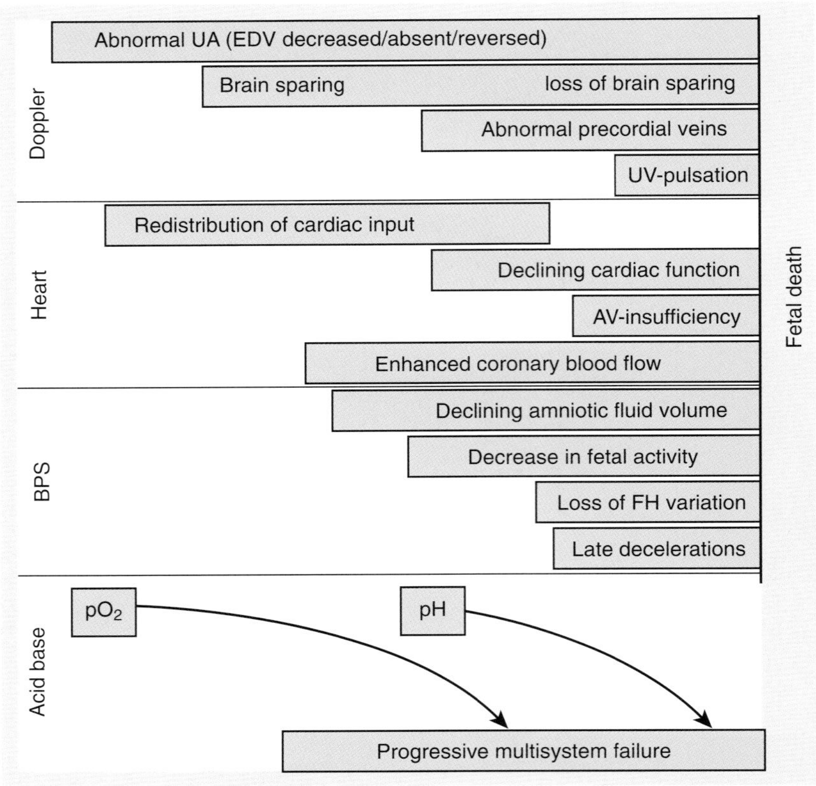

FIGURE 11–6
Progressive deterioration in fetal cardiovascular and behavioral variables seen with declining metabolic status. In most fetuses with intrauterine growth restriction, Doppler abnormalities progress from the arterial to the venous side of the circulation. Although cardiac adaptations and alterations in coronary blood flow dynamics may be operational for a variable period, overt abnormalities of cardiac function and evidence of markedly enhanced coronary blood flow usually are not seen until the late stages of disease. The decline in biophysical variables shows a reproducible relationship with the acid-base status. If adaptation mechanisms fail, stillbirth ensues. AV, atrioventricular; EDV, end-diastolic velocity; FH, fetal heart rate; UV, umbilical vein.

low-dose aspirin treatment initiated this late in pregnancy improves neither placental function nor long-term outcome,[161] first-trimester screening tests are under investigation. However, they cannot be recommended for clinical use at this time. The utility of first-trimester uterine artery screening appears to be profoundly affected by the target population. Although low risk patients derive little benefit, high risk patients (those with thrombophilia, hypertension, or a history of preeclampsia or a fetus with IUGR) who are given low-dose aspirin because of bilateral uterine artery notching at 12 to 14 weeks have an 80% reduction of placental disease compared with matched control subjects given placebo.[162] Although low-dose aspirin therapy initiated beyond the first trimester may have benefit in a highly select group of patients, uterine artery Doppler studies provide diagnostic and prognostic information beyond this point. The risk of complicating preeclampsia or HELLP (hemolysis, elevated liver enzymes, and low platelets) affecting fetal outcome is increased more than 10-fold when abnormal umbilical artery Doppler findings are associated with bilateral uterine artery notching.[163] The response to an abnormal uterine artery Doppler waveform after 24 weeks should be monitoring of blood pressure and not serial Doppler studies.

First-Trimester Integration of Maternal Physical Characteristics, Biochemistry, and Uterine Artery Doppler Studies

Because the most severe forms of placental dysfunction originate during the first trimester and interventional strategies appear most effective at this point, there is increasing focus of late to identify early markers of placental failure. Integration of maternal history, physical characteristics, uterine artery Doppler, and biomarkers of early placental development are considered most promising. Maternal risk factors alone yield a sensitivity of only 45% for the prediction of preeclampsia and/or fetal growth restriction.[164] The addiition of first-trimester mean arterial blood pressure (MAP) increases the detection rate to 62.5% and reduces the false-positive rate.[165] Further integration of uterine artery Doppler indices with serum markers such as placental growth factor (PLGF) and placental protein 13 (PP-13) holds promise in identifying over 90% of pregnancies that will be complicated by early-onset preeclapmsia with a 10% false-positive rate.[166,167] However, performance of these integrated screening models appears to vary among populations and further research is necessary to identify optimal predictive algorithms and determine the best management strategies for patients identified as high risk.[168]

Ultrasound Assessment
(See also Chapter 10 and Appendix)

The first step in the management of IUGR is the identification of fetuses that are truly at risk for an adverse outcome. This requires the exclusion of small, but normally grown fetuses and those normoxic fetuses with IUGR caused by a condition that cannot be altered by obstetric management (e.g., aneuploidy, nonaneuploid syndromes, viral infection). The diagnosis of placenta-based fetal growth restriction relies on the presence of small fetal measurments in association with other ultrasound signs that are consistent with placental dysfunction. Ultrasound biometry is thus the primary diagnostic tool for the documentation of fetal growth disorders, whereas the assessment of amniotic fluid volume and placental, cerebral, and venous Doppler studies provide the supporting evidence for placenta-dependent hypoxia.

Because almost all fetal measurements change with gestation, the accurate assessment of gestational age is a necessary first step so that percentile ranks of the absolute measurements can be derived. Once gestational age is assigned, the interpretation of an ultrasound growth study is based on the fetal anatomic survey, amniotic fluid volume, percentile rank of fetal size measurements, interval growth since the last study, and functional assessment of the fetoplacental unit with Doppler ultrasound (umbilical and uterine arteries). It is not appropriate to describe growth abnormalities in terms of the difference beween the measured "week" size and the expected.

The adequacy of fetal growth cannot be determined by a single sonographic examination without a preexisting estimate of gestational age. Even after several examinations, fetal growth assessment is facilitated by knowledge of the likely gestational age because the rate of growth for many parameters also varies with gestation. The traditional assessment of gestational age is based on the first day of the last menstrual period (LMP). Yet, gestational age is uncertain in 20% to 40% of pregnant women who keep a written menstrual calendar.[169,170] This fact reflects both normal physiologic variation in the timing of ovulation and misinterpretation of implantation bleeding as menses by either the patient or the caregiver. Other potential and common variables that may explain an apparent discrepancy between sonographic and LMP-based gestational age include oral contraceptive use, increased cycle length, breast-feeding, and a limited number of coital exposures. Because all commonly used ultrasound tables are based on women with a known LMP rather than a known ovulation or conception date, they share the inaccuracy of menstrual dates (±3 wk). Because normal variation among fetuses also increases with advancing gestational age, the accuracy of the sonographic estimate of age diminishes. An estimated date of confinement (EDC) is based on the LMP when the sonographic estimate of gestational age is within the predictive error (7 days in the first semester, 10–11 days in the second trimester, and 21 days in the third trimester). Once the EDC is set by this method or a first-trimester ultrasound, it does not change, even if subsequent measurements deviate from the expected values. Repeated reassignments of the EDC are confusing to the physician and patient, and interfere with the ability to diagnose fetal growth abnormalities.

After establishment of the best obstetric estimate of gestational age, the next critical step is the selection of appropriate reference ranges. Because the goal is to identify poorly growing fetuses, the reference tables for ultrasound measurements should not be population-based, but rather based on uncomplicated pregnancies delivered at term. Individualized reference ranges of growth potential that account for maternal, ethnic, and fetal variables provide the most accurate reference.[6]

Because fetal growth restriction has many underlying etiologies that affect the timing of onset and fetal features, no single sonographic method is adequate for diagnosis. Only a complete evaluation that includes the maternal history and fetal, placental, and amniotic fluid characteristics can direct an appropriate diagnostic workup and perinatal management.

Direct Measurements

BIPARIETAL DIAMETER (See also Appendix)

Although biparietal diameter is easy to measure, it is a poor tool for the detection of IUGR. The physiologic variation inherent with advancing gestation is high, cranial growth delay as a result of insufficient nutrition is relatively late, and the shape of the cranium is readily altered by external forces (e.g., oligohydramnios, breech presentation).[171] Further, a technically adequate biparietal diameter may be hard to determine if the fetal head is oriented in a direct anterior or posterior position.

HEAD CIRCUMFERENCE (Table 11-1) (See also Appendix)

Head circumference is not subject to the same extrinsic variability as biparietal diameter. The measurement technique is important because calculated head circumference

TABLE 11-1

Normal Head Circumference Measurements across Gestation

	PERCENTILE RANKS OF HEAD CIRCUMFERENCE (cm)*				
WEEK†	10	25	50	75	90
18	14.0	16.5	16.0	17.0	17.5
19	15.0	16.0	17.0	17.5	18.0
20	16.0	17.0	18.0	18.5	19.0
21	17.0	18.0	19.0	19.5	20.0
22	18.0	19.0	20.0	20.5	21.0
23	19.5	20.0	21.0	21.5	22.0
24	21.0	21.5	22.0	22.5	23.0
25	22.0	22.5	23.0	23.5	24.0
26	23.0	23.5	24.0	24.5	25.0
27	24.0	26.0	26.0	26.5	27.0
28	25.5	26.0	27.0	27.5	28.0
29	26.5	27.0	28.0	29.0	29.5
30	27.0	27.5	28.5	29.0	30.5
31	27.0	28.0	29.0	30.0	31.0
32	27.5	28.0	29.0	30.0	31.5
33	28.0	28.5	29.5	30.5	32.0
34	28.5	29.0	30.5	31.5	32.5
35	29.5	30.0	31.5	32.0	33.0
36	30.0	31.0	32.0	33.0	34.0
37	30.5	31.5	32.5	33.5	35.0
38	30.5	31.5	32.5	34.0	35.0
39	31.0	32.0	33.0	34.5	35.0
40	31.5	32.5	33.5	34.5	35.5
41	32.0	33.0	34.0	34.5	36.0

* Measured directly from tracings in the screen of ultrasound machines or, alternatively, by digitizer from photographs.

† Menstrual weeks of pregnancy.

Adapted from Sabbagha RE: Intrauterine growth retardation. In Sabbagha RE (ed): Diagnostic Ultrasound Applied to Obstetrics and Gynecology, 2nd ed. Philadelphia, Lippincott, 1987, pp 112–131.

measurements are systematically smaller than those directly measured. Thus, the table selected should be based on measurements obtained with the same method as your laboratory used.

ABDOMINAL CIRCUMFERENCE (Table 11-2) (See also Appendix)

Abdominal circumference is the single best measurement for the detection of IUGR because it is related to liver size, which is a reflection of fetal glycogen storage.[172–174] The abdominal circumference percentile has the highest sensitivity and greatest negative predictive value for the sonographic diagnosis of IUGR, whether defined postnatally by birth weight percentile or by Ponderal index.[10] Its sensitivity is further enhanced by serial measurements obtained at least 14 days apart.[175] Because of its high sensitivity, some type of abdominal measurement should be part of every sonographic growth evaluation. Because abdominal circumference reflects fetal nutrition, it should be excluded from the calculation of the composite gestational age after the early second trimester.

The most accurate abdominal circumference is the smallest value obtained at the level of the hepatic vein between fetal respirations because the smallest perimeter most closely approximates the plane perpendicular to the spine. The practice of averaging several measurements only increases the measurement error. A measured circumference is superior to either a calculated circumference or the sum of several diameters because the shape of the fetal abdomen is typically irregular.[176] As with bony measurements, the circumference of a healthy fetus grows within a fixed percentile range. An abrupt change in the percentile, especially an increase, suggests that the current measurement results from an oblique cut and should be repeated.

If a normal table based exclusively on healthy women delivering appropriately nourished neonates at term is used (see Table 11–2), an abdominal circumference above the percentile 2.5 for gestational age is inconsistent with IUGR.[10] If a table based on a cross-sectional population is used (i.e., including small for gestational age, appropriate for gestational age, preterm, and term newborns), the 10th percentile is more appropriate. The positive predictive value of a low abdominal circumference percentile for IUGR is approximately 50% in any given population. It is best not to label a fetus "growth-restricted" and trigger expensive fetal surveillance unless the circumference is far below normal or other ultrasound variables support the suspicion.

TRANSVERSE CEREBELLAR DIAMETER (See also Appendix)

Transverse cerebellar diameter is one of the few soft tissue measurements that correlates well with gestational age[177] in

TABLE 11–2
Normal Abdominal Circumference Measurements across Gestation

	PERCENTILE								
GESTATION (WK)	2.5	5	10	25	50	75	90	95	97.5
18	9.8	10.3	10.6	11.8	13.1	14.2	14.5	15.9	16.4
19	11.1	11.6	12.3	13.3	14.4	15.6	15.9	17.2	17.8
20	12.1	12.6	13.3	14.3	15.4	16.6	16.9	18.2	18.8
21	13.7	14.2	14.8	15.9	17.0	18.1	18.4	19.8	20.3
22	14.7	15.2	15.8	16.9	18.0	19.1	19.4	20.8	21.3
23	16.0	16.5	17.1	18.2	19.3	20.4	20.7	22.1	22.6
24	17.2	17.7	18.3	19.4	20.5	21.6	21.9	23.3	23.8
25	18.0	18.5	19.1	20.2	21.3	22.4	22.7	24.1	24.6
26	18.8	19.3	19.9	21.0	22.1	23.2	23.5	24.9	25.4
27	25.4	20.9	21.5	22.6	23.7	24.8	25.1	26.5	27.0
28	22.0	22.5	23.1	24.2	25.3	26.4	26.7	28.1	28.6
29	23.6	24.1	24.7	25.8	26.9	28.0	28.3	29.7	30.2
30	24.1	24.6	25.2	26.3	27.4	28.5	28.8	30.2	30.7
31	24.7	26.2	25.8	26.8	28.0	28.1	29.4	30.0	31.3
32	25.4	25.9	20.0	27.0	28.7	30.8	30.1	31.5	32.0
33	25.7	20.2	20.0	27.0	20.0	30.1	30.4	31.8	32.3
34	26.8	27.3	27.9	29.0	30.1	31.2	31.5	32.0	33.1
35	28.9	29.4	30.0	31.1	32.2	33.3	33.3	35.0	36.5
36	30.0	30.5	31.1	32.2	33.3	34.4	34.7	36.1	36.6
37	31.1	31.6	32.2	33.3	34.4	35.5	35.8	37.2	37.7
38	32.4	32.9	33.5	34.6	35.7	36.8	37.1	38.5	39.0
39	32.6	33.1	33.7	34.8	35.9	37.0	37.3	38.7	39.2
40	32.8	33.3	33.9	35.0	36.1	37.2	37.5	38.9	39.4

From Tamura RK, Sabbagha RE: Percentile ranks of sonar fetal abdominal circumference measurements. Am J Obstet Gynecol 1980;138:475.

the IUGR fetus. This structure is relatively spared the effects of mild to moderate uteroplacental dysfunction. Whether its measurement offers an advantage over bony measurements in the assessment of compromised fetal growth is controversial.[178,179]

Measurement Ratios

Approximately 70% of neonates with asymmetrical growth restriction have a head circumference–to–abdominal circumference ratio 2 standard deviations (SDs) above the norm.[180] However, both the sensitivity and the positive predictive value of this ratio for growth restriction are worse than that of either abdominal circumference percentile or sonographically estimated fetal weight (discussed later).[10,181]

The cephalic index is the ratio of the biparietal diameter to the occipitofrontal diameter. Proposed as an age-independent aid to identify dolichocephaly and brachycephaly,[182] it is of limited value. Dolichocephaly is rare before the third trimester, and the ability to measure head circumference easily eliminated the need to recognize mild degrees of either dolichocephaly or brachicephaly as it relates to the prediction of gestational age. This ratio has also been proposed as an aid for the diagnosis of trisomy 21. The sonographic signs of aneuploidy are reviewed in Chapters 7 and 8.

The femur length (FL)–to–head circumference ratio was proposed as a tool to identify short-limbed dwarfism, hydrocephaly, or microcephaly.[183] However, the greatly improved resolution of modern ultrasound equipment makes this measurement unnecessary for the diagnosis of hydrocephaly (see Chapter 17); dwarfism, because the length of the fetal limbs is well below the 10th percentile for gestation (see Chapter 20); or microcephaly, which is diagnosed when head circumference is more than 3 SDs below the mean.

It would be attractive if the sonographic FL could be used to generate an index of fetal mass because it correlates with neonatal crown-heel length. Unfortunately, no clinically useful formula has been obtained. The FL–to–abdominal circumference ratio has lower sensitivity, specificity, and positive and negative predictive values for the diagnosis of IUGR than either the abdominal circumference percentile or the sonographic estimate of fetal weight.[10,184,185]

Sonographic Estimate of Fetal Weight

Many general purpose and special application formulas have been devised; several are listed in Table 11–3.[186–188] The accuracy of most (±2 SDs) is 10% or greater, and none has proved superior to the first devised by Warsof and reported by Sheppard.[186] Although an estimate of fetal weight does not routinely add to the abdominal circumference percentile for the diagnosis of IUGR, it adds a graphic image that is easy for both patient and referring physician to conceptualize. Although its sensitivity is considerably lower than that of the abdominal circumference percentile, the positive predictive value of a fetal weight estimate below the 10th percentile is greater.

TABLE 11–3

Sample Formulas Validated Prospectively for Sonographic Estimates of Fetal Weight

PARAMETER	FORMULA	REFERENCE
BPD, AC	Log_{10} BW = -1.7492 + (0.166/[BPD]) + 0.46(AC) - 2 - 646(AC × BPD)/1000	186
AC, FL	Log_{10} BW = 1.3598 + 0.051(AC) + 0.1844(FL) - 0.0037(AC × FL)	187
HC, AC, FL	Log_{10} BW = 1.5662 - 0.0108(HC) + 0.0468(AC) + 0.171(FL) + 0.00034(HC)^2 - 0.003685(AC × FL)	186
HC, AC, FL	Log_{10} BW = 1.6961 + 0.02253(HC) + 0.01645(AC) + 0.06439(FL)	188

AC, abdominal circumference; BPD, biparietal diameter; BW, birth weight; FL, femur length; HC, head circumference.

Amniotic Fluid Measurement

The ultrasound estimation of amniotic fluid volume is a poor screening tool for IUGR or fetal academia.[189] However, in clinical practice, it is an important diagnostic and prognostic tool. Oligohydramnios may be a first incidental finding noticed in pregnancies with fetal growth restriction. If this is noticed, a complete ultrasound assessment of fetal growth should be performed, because up to 96% of fetuses with fluid pockets less than 1 cm may be growth-restricted.[190] In patients with suspected growth delay, amniotic fluid volume can be an important differential diagnostic pointer. In the setting of small fetal size, excess amniotic fluid volume suggests aneuploidy, or fetal infection,[191] whereas normal or decreased amniotic fluid is compatible with placental insufficiency.

Placental and Fetal Doppler Studies

The quantification of blood flow volume with Doppler studies is prone to error because of variations in insonation angle and the measurement of vessel diameter. Consequently, Doppler waveform analysis with angle-independent Doppler indices is preferred for fetal surveillance. The most widely used arterial indices are the systolic-to-diastolic ratio,[192] resistance index,[193] and pulsatility index (Table 11–4).[194] A relative decrease in end-diastolic velocities elevates each of the indices and usually reflects increased downstream resistance. When end-diastolic flow is lost, the systolic-to-diastolic ratio approaches infinity and the resistance index becomes 1. The pulsatility index offers the advantage of a smaller measurement error, narrower reference limits, and the theoretical advantage of ongoing numeric analysis, even when end-diastolic velocity is lost.[195]

In the diagnosis and management of fetal growth restriction, several vascular territories provide information about specific aspects of the disease. The Doppler findings that suggest placental dysfunction are a decrease in absolute umbilical venous volume flow[196] and elevated blood flow resistance in the umbilical arteries and uterine arteries. Findings that suggest fetal hypoxia include a decrease in blood flow resistance in the fetal cerebral circulation.[90] Beyond the early adaptive responses in the cerebral circulation (see later), examination of the venous system provides information about forward cardiac function and the impacts of advanced placental disease and progressive hypoxemia.

TABLE 11–4

Doppler Indices for Arterial and Venous Flow Velocity Waveforms

DOPPLER INDICES	CALCULATION
Arterial Flow	
Pulsatility index	$\frac{\text{Systolic-end-diastolic peak velocity}}{\text{Time-averaged maximum velocity}}$
Resistance index	$\frac{\text{Systolic-end-diastolic peak velocity}}{\text{Systolic peak velocity}}$
Systolic-to-diastolic ratio	$\frac{\text{Systolic peak velocity}}{\text{Diastolic peak velocity}}$
Venous Flow	
Preload index	$\frac{\text{Peak velocity during atrial contraction}}{\text{Systolic peak velocity}}$
Pulsatility index for veins	$\frac{\text{Systolic-diastolic peak velocity}}{\text{Time-averaged maximum velocity}}$
Peak velocity index for veins	$\frac{\text{Systolic-atrial contraction peak velocity}}{\text{Diastolic peak velocity}}$
Percentage reverse flow	$\frac{\text{Systolic time-averaged velocity}}{\text{Diastolic time-averaged velocity}} \times 100$
Ductus venosus preload index	$\frac{\text{Systolic-diastolic peak velocity}}{\text{Diastolic peak velocity}}$

In the venous system, the magnitude of flow reversal during atrial contraction varies considerably in individual veins. Reverse flow may occur during atrial contraction in the inferior vena cava and hepatic veins. In contrast, normal blood flow in the ductus venosus is forward throughout the cardiac cycle. Because of the complex nature of the venous flow velocity waveform, several venous Doppler indices are described (see Table 11–4).[135,152,197–200] No venous Doppler index appears to offer a significant advantage over the others.[201] Except for the descending aorta pulsatility index, all fetal arterial and venous indices change with gestational age. Thus, interpretation of Doppler findings requires accurate knowledge of gestational age.

It is standard practice in many locales to perform ultrasound twice during pregnancy to enhance the identification of fetuses with IUGR and improve outcome,[181] though the cost-benefit ratio of this practice remains unclear.[202,203] The combination of fetal biometry and umbilical artery Doppler is the best available tool for the identification of a small fetus at risk for adverse outcome.[68,204–206] Randomized trials and meta-analyses confirm that the use of umbilical artery Doppler in this setting is associated with a significant reduction in perinatal mortality rates and less iatrogenic intervention, despite the lack of a standardized response in those trials.[207–209] Before 34 weeks, small fetal size associated with an elevated umbilical artery Doppler index is likely to reflect placental dysfunction. Near term, when umbilical artery Doppler findings may be subtler, a decrease in the middle cerebral artery Doppler index or the cerebroplacental ratio increases suspicion for fetal growth restriction, even if the umbilical artery blood flow resistance index remains within the normal range.[156,206]

Although the umbilical artery flow velocity waveform is primarily determined by the architecture of the villous vascular tree (and therefore placental blood flow resistance), study of other fetal arterial vessels is required to determine the effect on the fetus. Changes in Doppler measured flow profiles of numerous arteries are described in association with IUGR. However, it seems logical to use vessels that represent a single vascular bed, are easy to sample at a low insonation angle, and provide the most information about the fetal response to hypoxemia. For example, flow in the fetal descending aorta is affected by changes in the placenta as well as by the peripheral fetal vasculature, and these changes may be difficult to detect at a small insonation angle. In contrast, the middle cerebral artery is easily identified and examined at a favorable angle. The scanning technique and reference ranges also require standardization because measurements may vary significantly in different portions of the same vessel. Similarly, measurements of the cerebroplacental ratio are affected by the indices used in calculation, and a standardized approach with gestational reference ranges rather than single cutoff values should be used.[210]

With continued compromise, there is little further change in the middle cerebral artery Doppler waveform save the notable exception of "normalization" of Doppler indices. Therefore, the next step after identifying evidence of fetal hypoxemia is to monitor cardiac function through study of the venous system. The inferior vena cava and ductus venosus Doppler indices and umbilical venous pulsations correctly predict acid-base status in a significant proportion of neonates with IUGR. This combination, rather than single-vessel assessment, provides the best predictive accuracy. Although the choice of Doppler index is guided by operator preference, familiarity with the examination technique for all three vessels is encouraged to offer the greatest flexibility in clinical practice.[201]

Biophysical Profile Score

The biophysical profile score (BPS) applies categorical cutoffs for a composite of dynamic variables, such as fetal tone, breathing, gross body movement, and amniotic fluid volume, as well as traditional fetal heart rate analysis. The cutoffs were chosen to account for biologic variation and maturational differences; therefore, they produce a reliable relationship with fetal acid-base status, regardless of gestational age and underlying pathology.[146,211] Although a gradual decrease in all of these parameters precedes an overtly abnormal BPS, an analysis of the percent change in these variables offers no advantage for the prediction of acidemia.[115] A normal score is usually achieved within the first 10 minutes of study. One notable disadvantage of the BPS is that apart from amniotic fluid volume, it lacks variables that allow useful longitudinal prediction of compromise in pregnancies affected by IUGR.[124] This limitation must be considered if BPS is selected as the sole monitoring tool (discussed later).

Diagnosis and Evaluation of Fetal Growth Restriction

The diagnosis of fetal growth restriction is based on the measurement of objective fetal parameters and requires

TABLE 11–5

Causes of Severe Intrauterine Growth Restriction, University of Iowa, 1984–1992

DIAGNOSIS	N	%
Placental dysfunction	62	54.9
Chromosomal abnormality	22	19.5
Associated structural malformations	13	11.5
Congenital infection		
Proven	7	6.2
Likely	2	1.8
Miscellaneous	7	6.2
Total	**113**	

knowledge of normal and abnormal growth as well as the basis for these standards. Ideally, the estimate of gestational age is not based solely on a recent sonographic estimate.

The postnatal definition of IUGR is of pragmatic concern because it affects the stated accuracy of antenatal diagnosis. For example, a thin fetus whose estimated weight is normal might be classified postnatally as growth-restricted by the Ponderal index. Practitioners must understand the diagnostic criteria used in their hospitals, and neonatal caregivers should not rely solely on birth weight percentiles.

"Asymmetrical" and "symmetrical" growth restriction are descriptive terms and not diagnoses. More relevant than symmetry is the timing of onset. Late-onset growth restriction of structurally normal fetuses after 32 weeks' gestation usually results from placental dysfunction. These fetuses are slender, with normal head circumference and body length. In contrast, early-onset growth restriction is often associated with aneuploidy, congenital infection, or more severe forms of placental dysfunction (Table 11–5). Although these fetuses may be symmetrically small when delivered weeks or months after the initial diagnosis, they are often asymmetrical when first identified. Although the significant differences in clinical progression between early- and late-onset IUGR are being increasingly recognized, effective incorporation into clinical management has not yet been accomplished. Undiagnosed IUGR continues to account for approximately 60% of unexplained stillbirths at term.[212,213]

Maternal History and Examination

In view of the many maternal disorders that affect placental development, thorough maternal medical, medication, and obstetric histories should be obtained. A family history of unexpected thromboembolic events or a history of a previous pregnancy affected by early-onset IUGR or fetal demise should be sought. Maternal studies for antiphospholipid antibodies and thrombophilia are more likely to have a diagnostic yield with such a history.[214]

Two-Dimensional Ultrasound Assessment of Fetal Size

The most accurate prediction of fetal growth delay can be achieved if fetal growth parameters are related to customized growth curves.[6] When reference ranges based on normally grown fetuses are used, a fetus is considered "at risk" for growth restriction when the abdominal circumference percentile is less than percentile 2.5 (or the 10th percentile if a population-based table is selected) but the estimated fetal weight is above the 10th percentile. Suspicion is strengthened when both the abdominal circumference percentile and the estimated weight are abnormally low or when progressive growth delay occurs. Serial ultrasound examinations at least 14 days apart allow assessment of growth patterns and may provide additional diagnostic clues. Fetuses that are constitutionally small are more likely to show normal interval growth.[175] In contrast, fetuses with aneuploidy or placental dysfunction are more likely to show progressive growth delay and to "fall off" the growth curve.[44,175,215] Because fetuses with "suspected" and "diagnosed" IUGR are managed similarly and because the accuracy of the diagnosis based on a small abdominal circumference alone is only approximately 50%, there is no need to worry the parents unnecessarily by basing the diagnosis on a single parameter. Once the suspicion of IUGR is raised, an evaluation of fetoplacental blood flow and anatomy is required.

Two-Dimensional Ultrasound of Fetal Anatomy and Possible Invasive Testing

A thorough ultrasound examination to detect major anomalies and markers of aneuploidy is mandatory in all fetuses with IUGR. Fetal echocardiography to detect major cardiac anomalies (e.g., atrioventricular canal defect) and evaluate cardiac function should be part of that examination. Echogenic bowel or liver or increased amniotic fluid volume suggest an increased risk of either aneuploidy or viral infection,[216,217] particularly in patients with normal umbilical and uterine artery Doppler findings.[44] A chromosomal abnormality is associated with 20% of cases of severe, early-onset IUGR. Although half of these abnormalities are lethal, a fetus with trisomy 21 may pose philosophical problems for both the physician and the patient. Knowledge of a major anomaly, such as atrioventricular canal defect, can lead the parents in one direction or another in terms of pregnancy termination or cesarean delivery for fetal distress.

Doppler Velocimetry of Arterial and Venous Circulation

The fetal vascular responses to placental dysfunction were discussed earlier. There is now considerable knowledge about the relationship between Doppler findings and perinatal outcome that allows for an accurate, noninvasive assessment of the presence and severity of fetal hypoxemia. Until recently, the clinical role of Doppler ultrasound in the overall evaluation of fetal growth disturbance was unclear. Part of the problem was the diverse nature of the published studies. Investigators sought to predict a variety of neonatal outcomes with disparate etiologies using a single parameter, such as umbilical artery index. Not surprisingly, the positive and negative predictive values were, as a whole, unsatisfactory.

Based on the current level of knowledge, we have designed a clinical evaluation algorithm that uses "progressive" Doppler studies of fetal vasculature. Although Doppler findings in each of the examined vascular beds correlate with fetal acid-base status, there is a wide variation in fetal pH with abnormal results (Fig. 11–7). However, as with most

FIGURE 11–7
Deviation in pH from the gestational age mean (ΔpH) with abnormal results on various antenatal tests. These include fetal heart rate (FHR) analysis with traditional nonstress testing (NST) and computerized cardiotocogram (cCTG). The same relationships are expressed for umbilical artery absent end-diastolic velocity (AEDV) and deviation of the arterial or venous Doppler index more than 2 standard deviations from the gestational age mean for the thoracic aorta (TAO), descending aorta (DAO), middle cerebral artery (MCA), cerebroplacental ratio (CPR), and ductus venosus (DV). + acc., accelerations present; + dec., obvious decelerations present; –react, nonreactive; AFV, amniotic fluid volume; FBM, fetal body movement; FGM, fetal gross movement.
(From Baschat AA: Integrated fetal testing in growth restriction: Combining multivessel Doppler and biophysical parameters. Ultrasound Obstet Gynecol 2003;21:1-8.)

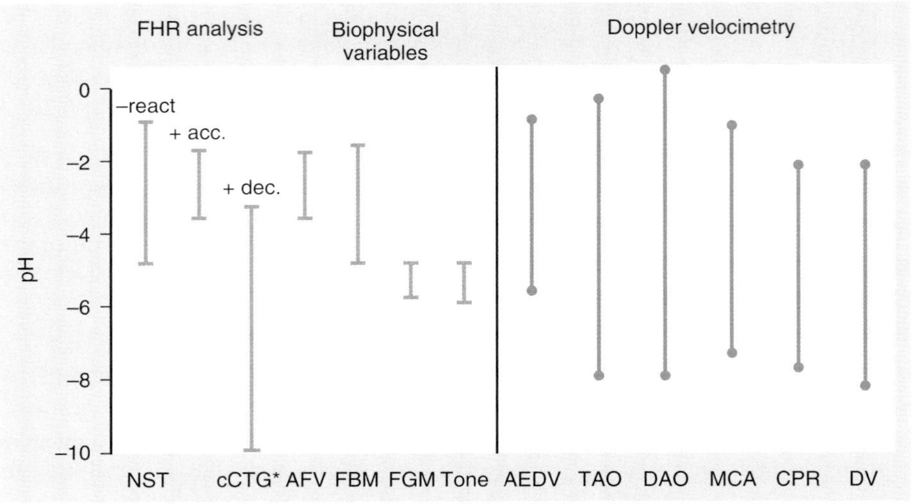

obstetric tests, the negative predictive values are superb. A normal umbilical artery Doppler index is inconsistent with fetal acidemia as a result of uteroplacental dysfunction. Absence of umbilical artery end-diastolic velocity indicates significant villous abnormality; however, the relationship between placental pathology and fetal acidemia is inconsistent both at cordocentesis and at birth.[64,66,218–220] This inconsistency may occur because the oxygen demands of the fetus vary with gestational age. A 23-week fetus can withstand a much higher degree of placental dysfunction than a 32-week fetus. Thus, further evaluation of other fetal organs is necessary to determine the fetal response to the hypoxemia present and to refine the prediction of fetal acid-base balance. Brain-sparing (cephalization, or centralization), elevation of the thoracic and abdominal aortic pulsatility index, and an abnormal cerebroplacental ratio are each associated with fetal hypoxemia and a decrease in pH of at least 2 SDs.[66,88,221] Elevation of the precordial venous Doppler indices (inferior vena cava and ductus venosus) provides the most consistent relationship to a significant decrease in umbilical venous pH (~4 SDs) in fetuses with IUGR.[135,221,222] Because not all fetuses with IUGR have abnormal venous flow, venous Doppler has a sensitivity of approximately 70% and a specificity of 60% to 70% for the identification of significant fetal acidemia typically defined by postnatal norms.[201,221,222] Umbilical venous pulsations occur at a late stage of compromise, and if they are observed concurrently with an elevated venous Doppler index, they improve sensitivity in the prediction of birth pH of less than 7.20.[201] Normal fetal arterial pH in the absence of labor should be greater than 7.32 at term and even higher preterm (Fig. 11–8).

In preterm fetuses with IUGR, Doppler findings of progressive abnormality are associated with increased perinatal mortality and morbidity rates.[94,132,133,154] Although neonatal morbidity is determined primarily by the gestational age, the risks of stillbirth and acidemia are significantly related to the extent of venous Doppler abnormality.[133,154] Therefore, multivessel Doppler studies of the arterial and venous systems are required for the best prediction of critical outcomes in preterm infants with IUGR.[223]

Although our understanding of the relationships between Doppler-derived flow measurements and short-term outcomes has greatly improved, there is relatively little information on the relationships between Doppler measurements and outcome parameters in infancy and adult life. Elevation of fetal aortic blood flow resistance and associated increases in reversal of blood flow in the aortic isthmus are associated with neurodevelopmental delay in early childhood.[224–226] In early-onset growth restriction, early gestational age at delivery, lower birth weight, and absent/reversed umbilical artery end-diastolic velocity are the stronger predictors of adverse neurodevelopment even when biophysical variables are considered.[227,228] Similarly, adverse long-term neurologic development at school age appears most closely related to reversal of umbilical artery end-diastolic velocity.[229] In late-onset fetal growth restriction, evidence of brain sparing has an independent adverse impact on neurodevelopment even in small fetuses with normal umbilical artery blood flow resistance.[230,231] Although initial studies suggested a

FIGURE 11–8
Normal umbilical venous (UV) pH (*A*), pO_2 (*B*), pCO_2 (*C*), and base excess (*D*) shown as the 95% prediction interval across gestation.
(From Weiner CP, Sipes SL, Wenstrom K: The effect of fetal age upon normal fetal laboratory values and venous pressure. Obstet Gynecol 1992;79:71.)

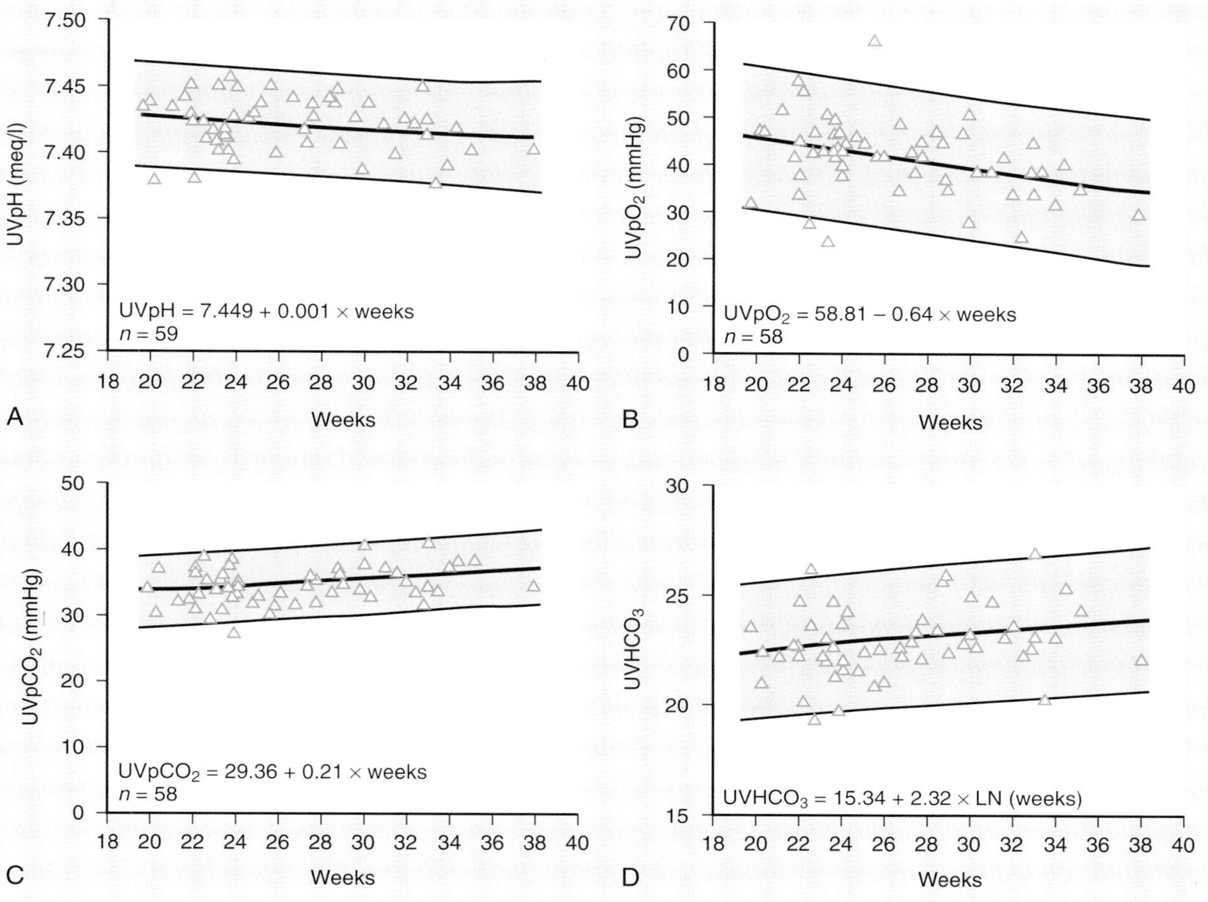

protective effect of brain-sparing on cognitive outcome, 5-year follow-up showed no sustained benefit.[232] This time-worn phrase seems a misnomer.

Computerized Cardiotocography and Biophysical Profile Score

Like the observations made with Doppler measurements, a progressive decline in acid-base status can be identified by fetal heart rate analyses and the assessment of fetal breathing, tone, gross body movement, and amniotic fluid volume. Each component of the BPS relates to fetal oxygenation, but the five-component BPS most effectively predicts fetal acid-base status. Although a reactive cardiotocogram (CTG), even by criteria graded for gestational age, virtually excludes hypoxemia, a nonreactive CTG is associated with a wide range of pH values.[145,211] The prediction of acidemia is improved by computerized fetal heart rate analysis. All computerized variables (e.g., short-term, long-term, and mean minute variations) and episodic or periodic changes are related to a range of normal and abnormal fetal pH values.[116,118,119] In fetuses with IUGR, short-term variation below 3.5 msec as a result of prolonged episodes of low variation appears the best predictor of an umbilical artery pH of less than 7.20.[147] Although it is clearly abnormal in a nonlaboring patient, the clinical relevance of this pH value after labor is not clear. Loss of fetal breathing movements is associated with moderate hypoxemia and a wide range of pH values at the time of either cordocentesis or birth. In contrast, the absence of fetal tone and gross body movement is almost always associated with acidemia (see Fig. 11–7). By accounting for physiologic variability, the BPS maintains its relationship with fetal pH in fetuses with IUGR, independent of gestational age. However, the BPS has limited utility in the prediction of longitudinal deterioration in these fetuses.[124,149]

The relationships between the BPS parameters and long-term outcome were studied in large cohorts of patients. A low BPS was associated with neonatal complications, cerebral palsy, cortical blindness, and attention deficit disorder.[233] Although randomized testing was not performed, the application of the BPS management algorithm was associated with a significant decrease in the frequency of cerebral palsy in the tested population. Our current understanding of the mechanisms underlying cerebral palsy are inadequate to accept or reject the likelihood this association is real or spurious.

Integrated Fetal Testing

The combined use of multiple testing modalities to monitor fetuses with IUGR has several advantages because of the wide clinical spectrum and the variance in the relationship between testing and outcome variables.[234] The information gained by combining them may be additive because deterioration of cardiovascular and biophysical parameters is initially independent. The Doppler studies enable longitudinal assessment, and the BPS helps refine the relationship with fetal pH. This combined approach provides the most accurate fetal assessment, particularly in preterm fetuses with growth restriction even when the computerized CTG is taken into consideration.[235–240] The management details are described later.

Prenatal Management Options

Diagnostic and therapeutic interventions often go hand in hand when IUGR is suspected, and management options may need to be reevaluated as gestation advances. The goal of the initial evaluation is to make a presumptive diagnosis of IUGR and then to use the clinical presentation to direct additional diagnostic workup. Subsequently, antenatal surveillance is instituted and tailored to the severity of the fetal condition and gestational age, considering the strengths and weaknesses of the available tests. Therapeutic interventions are dictated by the maternal and fetal condition as well as by gestational age, while respecting the wishes of the parents.

Presumptive Diagnosis of Intrauterine Growth Restriction

Fetuses with a small abdominal circumference percentile are at risk for IUGR. A flattening growth curve on two consecutive examinations at least 14 days apart (in the third trimester, preferably 21 days apart) heightens diagnostic suspicion. Individualized reference ranges based on normal pregnancies and maternal characteristics are probably the most accurate.[6] Beyond 24 weeks, an elevated umbilical artery Doppler index is strong corroborating evidence for IUGR as a result of placental dysfunction. A false-positive diagnosis of IUGR is likely in a sonographically small fetus with a normal umbilical artery Doppler examination, and the risk of fetal distress in labor as a result of chronic hypoxia is low. After 34 weeks, the umbilical artery Doppler index may be within the normal range, and a decreased cerebroplacental ratio or middle cerebral artery Doppler index the only supporting evidence of placental-based IUGR.[68,156,241,242] After completion of the anatomic survey and assessment of amniotic fluid volume, the fetus is categorized as either likely or unlikely to have IUGR. Based on the combination of findings, the fetus may have evidence of one of four diagnoses: aneuploidy, viral infection, placental dysfunction, or nonaneuploid fetal syndromes.

Diagnostic Workup

It is important to determine the specific etiology of IUGR before delivery when possible. Figure 11–9 illustrates a

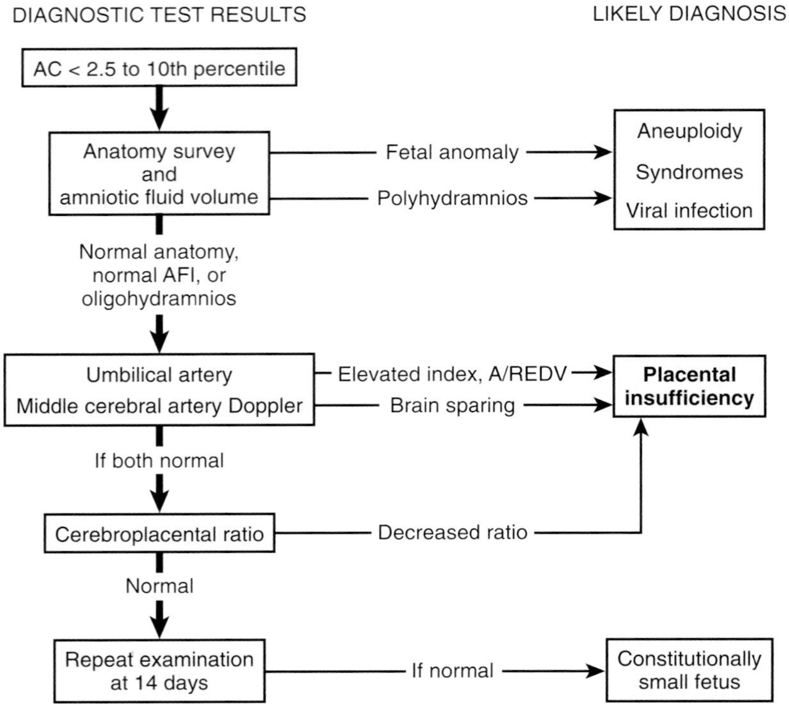

FIGURE 11–9
A decision tree following the evaluation of fetal anatomy, amniotic fluid volume, and umbilical and middle cerebral artery Doppler. The most likely clinical diagnosis is presented on the righthand side. A high index of suspicion for aneuploidy and viral and nonaneuploid syndrome needs to be maintained.

decision tree following the evaluation of fetal anatomy, amniotic fluid volume, umbilical and middle cerebral artery Doppler in cases of suspected IUGR and the most likely clinical diagnosis for a specific combination of parameters.

The wide availability of fluorescent in situ hybridization for fetal karyotyping for major chromosomal abnormalities from amniocytes offers the possibility of a result within 48 to 72 hours in many centers. Polymerase chain reaction of amniotic fluid samples can provide accurate and reproducible detection of the viral genome (see Chapter 30). Thus, amniocentesis should be offered to all patients with early-onset IUGR (<32 wk) and those with symmetrical IUGR detected later in gestation. In addition, women with known familial syndromes may be tested for single-gene mutations if appropriate gene probes are available. The relative ease of amniocentesis and the advances in antenatal surveillance that allow for an accurate assessment of the fetal acid-base status have largely obviated the need for cordocentesis.

However, cordocentesis is the technique of choice if more in-depth diagnostic information is needed. For example, fetal blood sampling provides direct measurement of fetal acid-base status (of value, especially at the threshold of viability, where the variance of Doppler methods is much greater), hepatic transaminases, a complete blood count, serology, and polymerase chain reaction for evidence of fetal viremia, all of which increase the diagnostic yield. For example, although traditional serologic and culture techniques identify an infectious etiology in 5% of fetuses with IUGR,[243] the yield roughly doubles when polymerase chain reaction is employed.[216] Although specific treatments for fetal infection are not available, antenatal diagnosis is important. First, the fetal response to infection is often transient; therefore, the opportunity for diagnosis is lost and the neonate inappropriately excluded from specific follow-up when the diagnostic efforts are delayed until delivery. Further, infected neonates typically shed virus. They should be isolated for the protection of pregnant staff and susceptible nursing mothers of other newborns. Finally, fetuses with IUGR caused by congenital infection are well oxygenated in the absence of placentitis. Extensive antenatal testing geared toward the detection of hypoxemia is unnecessary, and the need for iatrogenic intervention low in the absence of oligohydramnios.

The measurement of hematologic parameters can also shed light on the etiology while final karyotyping is pending and provide additional information about the severity of disease. Fetuses with IUGR and chronic hypoxemia are more likely to have elevated erythropoietin levels and polycythemia. Macrocytosis is more typical of trisomic and triploid fetuses.[244,245] In addition to an elevated nucleated red blood cell count, fetal thrombocytopenia and anemia are signs of chronic compromise associated with poor perinatal outcome.[74,125,128,129,246,247]

The diagnostic benefits of cordocentesis must be weighed against the risks on a case-by-case basis. Early-onset growth restriction increases the risk of reactive fetal bradycardia after cordocentesis in proportion to the severity of fetal hypoxemia.[248] There is roughly a 1 in 5 risk that a fetus with severe IUGR will have bradycardia after cordocentesis. The higher the umbilical artery Doppler resistance index, the greater the likelihood a bradycardia will occur. The mother of a fetus of borderline viability should decide in advance whether emergency cesarean delivery is to be performed in the event of sustained bradycardia. Cordocentesis must be performed in close proximity to a delivery suite and only by individuals trained in surgical delivery.

Once the diagnostic workup is initiated, management and outcome are largely determined by the underlying condition and the decisions made by the parents. If aneuploidy is the explanation, the cause and risk of recurrence are known. This knowledge may help to reduce the inevitable parental soul-searching and guilt feelings that accompany any perinatal loss. The diagnosis of a structural anomaly that is incompatible with survival eliminates both the need for extensive (and expensive) antenatal monitoring and the high likelihood of cesarean delivery for fetal indications. Documentation of infection allows precautions to be taken to minimize the risks of infection in the nursery as a result of viral shedding. Management is difficult in fetuses with early-onset IUGR as a result of placental dysfunction. In these otherwise normal fetuses, outcome is determined by the condition at birth and the degree of prematurity.[133,154,249]

Maternal and Fetal Therapy

Intrauterine therapeutic options are limited in pregnancies complicated by IUGR. The first step is to reduce or eliminate potential external contributors, such as stress or smoking, and to encourage maternal rest daily in a lateral position. Although the efficacy of these maneuvers is unproved, these simple steps should maximize maternal uterine blood flow. In addition, bedrest in the hospital may be considered because it has theoretical advantages over rest at home. First, even the most motivated patient rests less and less as time passes. The family support structure may be poor, and the patient may not have any real opportunity to rest. Second, hospitalization facilitates daily fetal testing. The choice of inpatient versus outpatient management is based on the severity of the maternal or fetal condition and the local standard of care.

Although low-dose aspirin therapy (81 mg/day) does not help severe early-onset IUGR, it may help patients with mild placental dysfunction.[250,251] In view of its documented safety,[252,253] we typically consider low-dose aspirin therapy after the diagnosis of placental-based mild IUGR.

IUGR as a result of placental dysfunction is the most common fetal disorder that is potentially amenable to direct fetal therapy. To be a candidate for this therapy, the fetus must show a proportionate increase in fetal oxygen and substrate delivery. Techniques to achieve these goals are available. Maternal hyperoxygenation,[254,255] intravascular volume expansion,[256] and hyperalimentation[257] are reported. Many issues, such as the effect of therapy on outcome, patient selection, efficacy, and the requisite testing required to monitor the fetus during therapy, remain to be resolved. Until these issues are clarified, this therapy is experimental.

Universally available therapeutic options that may improve outcome include antenatal administration of corticosteroids to hasten fetal lung maturity in the preterm fetus and delivery at an institution with a neonatal care unit that can carry out the complex management of the neonate with

IUGR. Antenatal corticosteroids should be administered to any fetus with IUGR when delivery is anticipated before 34 weeks. The long-held belief that the "stress" of the intrauterine condition enhances maturation and protects against prematurity is not supported by large population studies of neonates with IUGR.[3,258]

Timing and Mode of Delivery

Because of the limited intrauterine treatment options and the possibility of continued fetal damage as a result of progressive metabolic deterioration, the timing of intervention is critical. Only recently have survival statistics for growth-restricted neonates that are prenatally diagnosed become known.[259] Below 26 weeks, less than 50% of IUGR neonates survive, and intact survival in a similar proportion cannot be expected until 28 weeks' gestation. The effect of birth weight and gestational age on these statistics is so strong that deterioration of venous Doppler parameters does not produce an independent impact until 28 weeks. Between 24 and 32 weeks, each day gained in utero may increase the neonatal survival rate by 1% to 2% and earlier delivery without clear indication is likely to increase to result in iatrogenic mortality.[124,249,259] Although chronic in utero acidemia rather than chronic hypoxemia alone appears to be most strongly associated with intellectual impairment postnatally, prematurity and neonatal complications have an independent impact on neurodevelopment.[227,228,260,261] In preterm IUGR pregnancies, the current emphasis lies on modifying monitoring intervals based on clinical signs of disease acceleration in order to achieve safe prolongation of pregnancy to gain gestational age. The delivery threshold can be progressively lowered with advancing gestation. In IUGR pregnancies presenting after 34 weeks' gestation, the timing of delivery is straightforward.[262] Delivery takes place either at term, when fetal lung maturity is documented, if fetal distress occurs, or if the maternal condition dictates delivery. Between the age of viability and 32 weeks, however, the risks of perinatal damage from fetal deterioration compete with the risks of iatrogenic prematurity.

Prenatal Surveillance Tests (See also Chapter 10)

In euploid fetuses with presumed uteroplacental dysfunction, the patterns of deterioration are characteristic, but variable, and place specific demands on antenatal surveillance. In addition to acute assessments of fetal well-being, the likelihood of clinical progression necessitates a plan for longitudinal surveillance. At each examination, signs of disease acceleration should be sought because they require shortening of the montoring interval. Traditional fetal heart rate analysis, assessment of fetal activity (tone, movement, breathing), and evaluation of fetoplacental blood flow (arterial and venous Doppler) allow the most precise assessment of fetal well-being. Computerized fetal heart rate analysis, serial amniotic fluid volume measurement, and knowledge of arterial and venous Doppler status allow a reasonably accurate prediction of longitudinal progression.[140,149,152,153,242]

Management of Intrauterine Growth Restriction with Integrated Fetal Testing

At the University of Maryland, we use an approach that combines fetal heart rate analysis with Doppler and biophysical assessment initiated at 24 weeks' gestation. The management algorithm is guided by the severity of the maternal and fetal condition and by gestational age. It includes arterial and venous Doppler studies and determination of the BPS (Fig. 11–10).

Integrated fetal testing has three core elements: correct diagnosis of IUGR, assessment of fetal well-being, and prediction of fetal deterioration to time delivery. Delivery is indicated when the results of fetal testing are grossly abnormal, when fetal lung maturity is documented, or when maternal disease poses a serious risk to the mother. Before 34 weeks, a single course of betamethasone should be completed over 48 hours, when delivery is anticipated, to ameliorate neonatal respiratory disease and reduce the risk of intraventricular hemorrhage.

Although local preferences for antenatal surveillance and management vary, several guiding principles apply. First, the limits of viability and intervention dictated by the accepted standard of care must be discussed with the patient when management is initiated. Second, because cardiovascular deterioration is such a prominent feature of IUGR, Doppler assessment must be an integral part of antenatal surveillance. No other method effectively predicts deterioration prospectively. Third, the management of IUGR is too complex to rely on a single surveillance modality. If alternative surveillance methods are used, longitudinal monitoring should be tailored to the limitations of the surveillance test. For example, traditional nonstress testing analysis lacks the sensitivity and interobserver agreement needed to facilitate longitudinal monitoring. For this purpose, computerized heart rate monitoring offers superior accuracy. Similarly, if the BPS is the sole method of surveillance in severe IUGR, daily testing may be necessary to provide longitudinal assessment.[263]

Delivery Management Options

The premature neonate with IUGR requires the highest level of neonatal intensive care, and intrauterine transport to an appropriate institution is recommended in all cases of early-onset IUGR. The route of delivery is dictated by the severity of the fetal and maternal condition, along with other obstetric factors. Cesarean section without a trial of labor is indicated when the risks of vaginal delivery are unacceptable. These circumstances include prelabor evidence of fetal acidemia, spontaneous late decelerations, or late decelerations with minimal uterine activity. When fetal testing shows less serious conditions and gestational age is more advanced, the delivery route is tailored to the cervical Bishop score and preinduction oxytocin challenge testing might be required. Pharmacologic or mechanical ripening of the cervix, placement of the woman in the left lateral decubitus position, and the use of supplemental oxygen increase the likelihood of successful vaginal delivery.

FIGURE 11–10
Management algorithm for pregnancies complicated by intrauterine growth restriction (IUGR) based on the ability to perform arterial and venous Doppler as well as a full five-component biophysical profile score (BPS). AC, abdominal circumference; AFV, amniotic fluid volume; A/REDV, absent/reversed end-diastolic velocity; CPR, cerebroplacental ratio; DV, ductus venosus; HC, head circumference; MCA, middle cerebral artery; NICU, neonatal intensive care unit; tid, three times daily; UA, umbilical artery.
(From Baschat AA, Hecher K: Fetal growth restriction in placental disease. Semin Perinatol 2004;28:67–80.)

	IUGR UNLIKELY	
Normal AC, AC growth rat and HC/AC ratio UA, MCA Doppler, BPS and AFV normal	Asphyxia extremely rare Low risk for intrapartum distress	Deliver for obstetric, or maternal factors only, follow growth

	IUGR	
AC < 5th, low AC growth rate, high HC/AC ratio, abnormal UA and/or CPR; normal MCA and veins BPS 8/10, AFV normal	Asphyxia extremely rare Increased risk for intrapartum distress	Deliver for obstetric, or maternal factors only, fortnightly Doppler Weekly BPS
	With blood flow redistribution	
IGUR diagnosed based on above criteria, low MCA, normal veins BPS 8/10, AFV normal	Hypoxemia possible, asphyxia rare Increased risk for intrapartum distress	Deliver for obstetric, or maternal factors only, weekly Doppler BPS 2 times/week
	With significant blood flow redistribution	
UA A/REDV Normal veins BPS 6/10, oligohydramnios	Hypoxemia common, acidemia or asphyxia possible Onset of fetal compromise	> 34 weeks later: deliver < 32 weeks: antenatal steroids repeat all testing daily
	With proven fetal compromise	
Significant redistribution present Increased DV pulsatility BPS 6/10, oligohydramnios	Hypoxemia common, acidemia or asphyxia likely	> 34 weeks later: deliver < 32 weeks: admit, steroids, individualized testing daily vs. tid.
	With fetal decompensation	
Compromise by above criteria Absent or reversed DV a-wave, pulsatile UV BPS < 6/10, oligohydramnios	Cardiovascular instability, metabolic compromise, stillbirth imminent, high perinatal mortality irrespective of intervention	Deliver at tertiary care center with the highest level of NICU care

SUMMARY OF MANAGEMENT OPTIONS
Intrauterine Growth Restriction

Management Options (See also Chapter 10)	**Evidence Quality and Recommendation**	**References**
Prenatal		
First-Trimester Screening		
Uterine artery Doppler in patients with thrombophilia, previous midtrimester loss, or previous IUGR. Give low-dose aspirin (75–100 mg/day) if bilateral notching occurs.	Ib/A	162

SUMMARY OF MANAGEMENT OPTIONS

Intrauterine Growth Restriction—cont'd

Management Options (See also Chapter 10)	**Evidence Quality and Recommendation**	**References**
Second-Trimester Screening		
If bilateral uterine artery notching persists until 24 wk, there is only a marginal benefit of low-dose aspirin in selected patients. There is no evidence of a harmful effect.	Ib/A	161,250–253
On Clinical Suspicion of IUGR		
Two abdominal circumference measurements are obtained at least 14 days apart, with umbilical and middle cerebral arteries, to distinguish between normally grown small and growth-restricted fetuses.	Ib,IIa/A,B	68,156,174,175, 207,208,241
Follow for IUGR if: • Abdominal circumference < 5th percentile or growth rate <11 mm in 2 wk. • Umbilical artery Doppler index is elevated. • Cerebroplacental ratio is decreased. • Middle cerebral Doppler index is decreased (centralization) even if uterine artery Doppler is normal (especially after 34 wk).		
With a Diagnosis of IUGR		
If the sole monitoring tool is biophysical profile scoring, up to daily testing is required. In the preterm fetus with IUGR <37 wk, multivessel Doppler, including arterial and venous Doppler, provides the best assessment of disease severity.	IIa/B III/B	251 133,152,154,223
The most accurate assessment of fetal status is obtained with combined Doppler and biophysical assessment.	III/B,C	124,236,238,239
The timing of delivery is still guided by local standards of care and expert opinion; clear indicators for delivery timing have not been tested in a randomized fashion.	Ib/A	249
Administer betamethasone when delivery is anticipated before 34 wk.	III/B	3,249,258
Labor and Delivery		
Route of delivery is determined by fetal status before the onset of labor as well as maternal and obstetric factors. Oxytocin challenge test may be useful before induction. The left lateral decubitus position is used during labor.	III/B	133,137,149,174

IUGR, intrauterine growth restriction.

FETAL MACROSOMIA

Fetal macrosomia is the result of excessive fetal growth, which is the opposite of fetal growth restriction. Two terms are used to identify such growth: *large for gestational age* (discussed earlier) and *fetal macrosomia*, implying a birth weight above 4000 or 4500 g, regardless of gestational age. Unlike in IUGR, the morbidity and mortality rates for macrosomic fetuses are more closely related to absolute birth weight than to birth weight percentile. Although an estimated fetal weight above the 90th percentile might predict macrosomia, the sharp increase in adverse perinatal outcome with birth weight greater than 4500 g makes this a more suitable diagnostic cutoff.[264–267] In the United States, 10% of neonates have a birth weight greater than 4000 g, and in 1.5%, it is more than 4500 g.[268] Macrosomia is associated with significant fetal, neonatal, and maternal risks that emphasize the need for antepartum detection and modified intrapartum management. Maternal diabetes mellitus is the most common identifiable cause of excessive fetal growth (see Chapter 44).

Etiology and Risk Factors

Genetic factors, such as parental height and race, and the level of maternal hyperglycemia during pregnancy are important determinants of birth weight. In decreasing order of importance, recognized risk factors for macrosomia include a previous macrosomic infant, prepregnancy maternal obesity or excessive maternal weight gain, multiparity,[269] a male fetus, post-term gestation, Hispanic race,[270] present maternal height and weight at birth, and maternal age younger than 20 years.[271]

The positive relationship between maternal height, weight, and body mass index and neonatal birth weight is likely the expression of genetically predetermined growth potential[6] as well as maternal glycemic status.[272,273] Women who previously delivered a child larger than 4000 g are 5 to 10 times more likely than negative control subjects to deliver an infant larger than 4500 g in a subsequent pregnancy.[271,274] Women who themselves had a birth weight greater than 3600 g are twice as likely to deliver a neonate larger than 4000 g.[275] Male infants are typically heavier than females at any gestational age, and more males than females have a birth weight greater than 4500 g.[267] As fetal growth continues, the proportion of infants larger than 4500 g increases from 1.5% at 40 weeks to 2.5% at 42 weeks.[268]

Environmental and genetic interactions are complex. Much birth weight variation is unexplained, and most infants with macrosomia have no identifiable risk factor.[264] Further, no risk factor predicts macrosomia accurately. Several inheritable syndromes associated with fetal macrosomia are listed in Table 11–6.

Pathophysiology

Excessive fetal growth may result from optimal placentation and excess substrate availability or overstimulation of the fetal insulin–insulin-like growth factor–leptin axis. Maternal glucose is freely transported across the placenta whereas maternal insulin is not. Increased fetal blood glucose concentration therefore stimulates endogenous fetal insulin production, which is anabolic in nature and in the presence of sufficient glucose can lead to excess growth. Maternal diabetes mellitus is the primary example of excess substrate availability and subsequent fetal hyperinsulinemia. Maternal obesity and excessive maternal weight gain are also associated with intermittent periods of hyperglycemia and thus may act by the same mechanism. Mean glucose concentration in women with impaired glucose tolerance and increased fetal blood insulin are strongly associated with birth weight and macrosomia.[276,277] Recent results from the Hyperglycemia and Adverse Pregnancy Outcome (HAPO) study revealed a continuum between impaired glucose tolerance and increasing risk for adverse perinatal outcome.[278] Progressive immune recognition and improved placentation with successive pregnancies could explain the increasing birth weight observed in subsequent pregnancies. Overexpression of placental substrate transporters has not been evaluated systematically as a cause of otherwise unexplained macrosomia.

The fetal growth pattern and type of tissue overgrowth reflects the underlying etiology. Insulin-sensitive tissues, such as the heart, liver and spleen, thymus, adrenal gland, subcutaneous fat, and shoulder girdle, display differential glycogen and fat deposition when insulin levels are high. As a result, total body fat, shoulder and upper extremity circumference, upper extremity skinfold thickness, and liver size

TABLE 11–6
Genetic Causes of Macrosomia

SYNDROME	CLINICAL FEATURES	INHERITANCE
Perlman's syndrome	Fetal macrosomia with visceromegaly, ascites, and polyhydramnios; bilateral renal hamartomas; Wilms' tumor; cryptorchidism; facial abnormalities; micrognathia; volvulus; ileal atresia; diaphragmatic hernia; interrupted aortic arch; corpus callosum agenesis	Autosomal recessive
Lethal macrosomia with microphthalmia	Macrosomia, microphthalmia, median cleft palate; associated with respiratory infection in early life and early infant death	Autosomal recessive
Macrosomia adipose congenita	Macrosomia, voracious appetite, precocious skeletal development; death in first year common	Autosomal recessive
MOMO syndrome	Macrocephaly, retinal coloboma, nystagmus, mental retardation, delayed bone maturation	Autosomal dominant
Cleft lip or palate, characteristic facies, intestinal malrotation, congenital heart disease	Macrosomia, bilateral cleft lip or palate, flat facial profile, lethal complex congenital heart defect, bifid thumbs	Autosomal recessive
ABCD syndrome	Macrosomia, defective intestinal innervation, neonatal fatal intestinal dysfunction	Autosomal recessive
Simpson-Golabi-Behmel syndrome	Macrosomia, macrocephaly, coarse facies, hypertelorism, cleft palate, ventricular septal defect, pulmonic stenosis, transposition of great vessels, patent ductus arteriosus, lung segmentation defects, cervical ribs, pectus excavatum, 13 pairs of thoracic ribs, diaphragmatic hernia, polysplenia, duplication of renal pelvis, postaxial polydactyly, syndactyly of the 2nd–3rd fingers, clubfoot, corpus callosum agenesis, cerebellar vermis hypoplasia, hydrocephalus, embryonal tumors, Wilms' tumor	X-linked recessive
Weaver-Smith syndrome	Macrosomia with predominant developmental features	Autosomal dominant
CHIME syndrome	Early-onset migratory ichthyosiform dermatosis, seizures, mental retardation, cleft palate, tetralogy of Fallot, transposition of the great vessels	Autosomal recessive
CANTU syndrome	Generalized congenital hypertrichosis, narrow thorax, cardiomegaly	Autosomal recessive
Marfan's syndrome	Macrosomia, micrognathia, enophthalmos, predominant features postdelivery	Autosomal dominant
Beckwith-Wiedemann syndrome	Macrosomia, macroglossia, cardiomegaly, omphalocele, Wilms' tumor	Autosomal dominant

ABCD, autosomal-recessive neural crest syndrome with albinism, black lock, cell migration disorder of the neurocytes of the gut, deafness; CANTU, congenital hypertrichosis, osteochondrodysplasia, cardiomegaly; CHIME, coloboma, heart anomaly, ichthyosis, mental retardation, ear abnormality; MOMO, macrosomia, obesity, macrocephaly, ocular abnormalities.

are disproportionately greater in macrosomic fetuses of diabetic women compared with those fetuses of women without diabetes.[279,280] These differences in growth patterns are at least partially responsible for the associated fetal, neonatal, and maternal risks. The function of the liver as the primary fetal glycogen storage organ makes preferentially accelerated abdominal circumference growth an important physical characteristic of significant macrosomia.

Fetal and Neonatal Risks

Macrosomia is associated with increased perinatal mortality; intrapartum risks, including shoulder dystocia; brachial plexus injury; skeletal injuries; meconium aspiration; perinatal asphyxia; and postpartum complications, including respiratory distress syndrome and neonatal hypoglycemia.[264,265,281,282] The complication rates reflect the absolute birth weight. Perinatal morbidity rates are increased in infants larger than 4500 g, and mortality rates are increased in infants larger than 5000 g.[283] Rates of shoulder dystocia and associated clavicular fracture increase 10-fold.[284] Yet, only a small percentage of macrosomic fetuses have complicated deliveries. The risk of shoulder dystocia is significantly affected by the underlying cause of macrosomia. In women without diabetes, shoulder dystocia occurs in 9.8% to 24% of deliveries with a fetus weighing more than 4500 g. The prevalence is doubled in women with diabetes.[266,285,286] The additive impact of birth weight and maternal diabetes was recently reaffirmed for neonates with a birth weight above 4000 g. When macrosomia was associated with gestational diabetes, the risk of shoulder dystocia was increased 8 times and the associated risk for brachial plexus injury was increased 12 times.[287] Clavicular fracture and brachial plexus injuries, including Erb-Duchenne palsy, are most frequently associated with shoulder dystocia.[284,288] However, the risk of brachial plexus injury is increased independent of the mode of delivery or the clinical diagnosis of shoulder dystocia. This finding suggests an in utero origin for at least some brachial plexus injuries.[289] When birth weight exceeds 4500 g, the risk of shoulder dystocia is 18- to 21-fold higher than that in neonates with lower birth weight.[267,280,290]

Maternal Risks

Maternal complications of macrosomia are also related to neonatal birth weight. The incidences of cephalopelvic disproportion and prolonged labor increase at birth weights above 4500 g, and as a result, the cesarean delivery rate doubles.[265,290] The incidence of postpartum hemorrhage greater than 1000 mL increases with birth weights above 4000 g.[291] The rate of third- and fourth-degree laceration is especially increased when shoulder dystocia is diagnosed.[292] Thromboembolic events and anesthetic complications are increased in great part because of the increased need for operative intervention.

Diagnosis

There are no useful, general-purpose screening tools for the detection of macrosomia. A history of obstetric and maternal risk factors (discussed earlier) heightens the clinical index of suspicion. In addition, an unexplained very low serum maternal serum AFP level is associated with increased birth weight and an increased prevalence of obstetric complications.[293]

Clinical Examination

Mothers of infants with birth weight greater than 4500 g have greater symphyseal fundal height than expected.[294] However, several variables, including amniotic fluid volume and maternal body habitus, limit the usefulness of this measurement unless it is combined with clinical palpation or Leopold's maneuvers.[295] Prospective studies of fundal height measurement combined with Leopold's maneuvers report sensitivity of 10% to 43%, specificity of 99.0% to 99.8%, and positive predictive values of 28% to 53% for the detection of macrosomia.[296,297] The mother's subjective assessment of fetal weight in comparison with an earlier pregnancy can be as accurate as the clinical assessment by Leopold's maneuvers.[298]

Ultrasound

Ultrasound prediction of fetal weight loses accuracy above 4000 g and does not exceed the diagnostic accuracy of clinical estimates.[298–300] Only 50% of fetuses larger than 4500 g weigh within 10% of the predicted weight.[301] In women without diabetes mellitus, the sensitivity of ultrasound for the detection of macrosomia (birth weight > 4500 g) is 22% to 44%, with specificity of 99% and positive predictive values of 30% to 44%.[302,303] There are several reasons for these inaccuracies. First, even at lower weights, the typical error associated with sonographic estimates is 10%, a large error in a macrosomic fetus. Second, the accuracy of these formulas, when confined to macrosomic fetuses, is even lower, up to 13%.[304] Because the birth weight of macrosomic infants is largely determined by organ size and fat deposition, formulas that include abdominal circumference and exclude bony measurements perform better than those that do not.[302] Ultrasound methods that account for skin thickness[305] or incorporate algorithms to calculate fetal volume might have a role in the future.[306] Ultrasound can provide diagnostic information on fetal anatomy, organ size, and fat deposition. Further, ultrasound allows an objective assessment of amniotic fluid volume that may prompt further evaluation for underlying syndromes (see Table 11–6) or recommendation for diabetes testing when hydramnios is suspected. In women with diabetes mellitus, macrosomia may be a biologic indicator of suboptimal maternal metabolic control. Because hyperglycemia can be a cause of hydramnios and macrosomia, the combined observation of increased amniotic fluid volume and accelerated fetal abdominal girth should prompt repeat ultrasound assessment for the confirmation of accelerated growth and the risk for macrosomia.

Management Options

Accelerated fetal growth is a sign of suboptimal glycemic control in maternal diabetes mellitus. In this setting, increased surveillance and strict glucose monitoring and glycemic control significantly reduce the risk for macrosomia.[307] In the absence of maternal diabetes mellitus, the management of suspected macrosomia focuses on the timing and type of delivery and intrapartum management. Evidence suggests that labor induction for suspected macrosomia, defined as estimated fetal weight of 4000 to 4500 g,[308] increases the cesarean delivery rate without improving perinatal outcome.[309] Although seemingly logical, labor induction should not be undertaken in the absence of a high cervical Bishop's score.

Because perinatal and maternal risks increase with birth weight, and cesarean section reportedly decreases the risks of birth trauma and brachial plexus injury,[265,280,284] it is logical to conclude that elective cesarean delivery should be offered beyond a certain estimated fetal weight. However, there is insufficient study to support this practice. No clinical studies demonstrate a significant reduction in the birth injury rate by adopting such a practice, although arguably, a much larger sample size is needed. Cohort and case-control studies do confirm that a trial of labor is safe and cost-effective at estimated fetal weights of 5000 g or less.[310] For suspected fetal macrosomia less than 5000 g, prophylactic cesarean section does not appear to reduce birth trauma significantly in the absence of maternal diabetes mellitus. In these women and those with other risk factors, such as a history of shoulder dystocia in a macrosomic infant, estimated weight is important when planning the delivery route. In addition, although the predictive accuracy of fetal weight estimates is poor above 5000 g, most authors agree that prophylactic cesarean section should be offered.[265,290]

During labor, special attention is given to the progress of labor and the uterine contraction pattern. Cesarean delivery is indicated when the estimated fetal weight exceeds 4500 g; the second stage is greater than 2 hours with documented adequate uterine contractions (>200 Montevideo units), or there is an arrest of descent. The risk of shoulder dystocia is increased by assisted vaginal delivery. A trial of vaginal delivery after a previous cesarean delivery appears safe for both infant and mother, with success rates of 58% when birth weight is less than 4500 g and 43% when birth weight is higher.[311]

SUMMARY OF MANAGEMENT OPTIONS
Fetal Macrosomia

Management Options	Evidence Quality and Recommendation	References
Prenatal		
On Clinical Suspicion of Macrosomia		
• Abdominal circumference 95th percentile, particularly if associated with increased amniotic fluid volume.	III/B	186
• Exclude gestational diabetes.	—/GPP	—
• Family history of inheritable disorders (see Table 11–6).	—/GPP	—
With Diagnosis of Macrosomia		
• Maternal glycemic control, if indicated.	See Chapter 44	
Labor and Delivery		
Delivery indicated for maternal factors; induction vs. expectant management is associated with increased cesarean rate without improved outcome.	IIb/B	308
Delivery Route	III/B	310,311
• For estimated fetal weight < 4500 g, offer vaginal delivery and vaginal birth after cesarean section.		
• For estimated fetal weight > 4500 g in a diabetic patient, offer elective cesarean delivery.		
• For estimated fetal weight > 5000 g in nondiabetic patient, offer cesarean delivery.		
Early detection of protraction disorder is made by failure to progress over 3 hr with > 200 Montevideo units.	III/B,C	284–286,310

GPP, good practice point.

SUGGESTED READINGS

Baschat AA, Cosmi E, Bilardo CM, et al: Predictors of neonatal outcome in early-onset placental dysfunction. Obstet Gynecol 2007;109:253–261.

Baschat AA, Gembruch U, Harman CR: The sequence of changes in Doppler and biophysical parameters as severe fetal growth restriction worsens. Ultrasound Obstet Gynecol 2001;18:571–577.

Baschat AA, Viscardi RM, Hussey-Gardner B, et al: Infant neurodevelopment following fetal growth restriction: Relationship with antepartum surveillance parameters. Ultrasound Obstet Gynecol 2009;33:44–50.

Froen JF, Gardosi JO, Thurmann A, et al: Restricted fetal growth in sudden intrauterine unexplained death. Acta Obstet Gynecol Scand 2004;83:801–807.

GRIT Study Group: A randomized trial of timed delivery for the compromised pre-term fetus: Short term outcomes and Bayesian interpretation. BJOG 2003;110:27–32.

HAPO Study Cooperative Research Group: Hyperglycemia and adverse pregnancy outcome. N Engl J Med 2008;358:1991–2002.

Poon L, Kametas NA, Maiz A, et al: First trimester prediction of hypertensive disorders in pregnancy. Hypertension 2009;53:812–818.

Thornton JG, Hornbuckle J, Vail A, et al, GRIT Study Group: Infant wellbeing at 2 years of age in the Growth Restriction Intervention Trial (GRIT): Multicentred randomised controlled trial. Lancet 2004;364:513–520.

Vainio M, Kujansuu E, Iso-Mustajarvi M, Maenpaa J: Low dose acetylsalicylic acid in prevention of pregnancy-induced hypertension and intrauterine growth retardation in women with bilateral uterine artery notches. BJOG 2002;109:161–167.

Vintzileos AM, Fleming AD, Scorza WE, et al: Relationship between fetal biophysical activities and umbilical cord blood gas values. Am J Obstet Gynecol 1991;165:707–713.

REFERENCES

For a complete list of references, log onto www.expertconsult.com.

CHAPTER 12

Abnormalities of Amniotic Fluid Volume

MARIE H. BEALL, RON BELOOSESKY, and MICHAEL G. ROSS

INTRODUCTION

Amniotic fluid (AF) surrounds the fetus after the first few weeks of gestation. AF serves to protect the fetus and umbilical cord from compression, has antibacterial properties that may protect the fetus, and serves as a reservoir of water and nutrients. Perhaps most important, it provides the necessary conditions for normal development of the fetal lungs and musculoskeletal and gastrointestinal systems.[1]

Aberrations in AF volume, both low (oligohydramnios) and high (polyhydramnios), are associated with a multitude of pregnancy-related problems. An understanding of the basic physiologic mechanisms that regulate both AF volume and composition is required to devise effective management strategies for pregnancies complicated by disorders of fluid volume.

Sources and Volume of Amniotic Fluid

AF derives from a number of fetal and nonfetal sources, with the relative contribution from each source changing across gestation. Early in gestation, AF is thought to be derived from the mother directly across the amnion and the fetal surface of the placenta and the fetal body surface.[2] In midgestation, fetal urine begins to enter the amniotic sac[3] and the fetus begins to swallow AF, although the daily volume flows are quite small. The fetal lungs also begin to secrete liquid into the AF at this time.

Abundant human and animal data are available regarding the source and composition of AF during the latter half of gestation. The developing human fetus becomes sufficiently large near term to allow noninvasive methods (e.g., ultrasound) to estimate volumes and flows; in addition, direct measurements in chronically catheterized ovine fetuses can be conducted at this time. Near term, the major sources of AF production are fetal urine and lung liquid; the major routes for resorption of fluid are fetal swallowing and the intramembranous pathway (from AF to fetal circulation). The known minor sources of AF production and clearance include secretions from the fetal oral-nasal cavities and the transmembranous pathway (from AF to maternal circulation).

Despite large variances in current estimates of human fetal urine production,[4,5] we feel the best estimates of daily amniotic volume flows in the near-term fetus are[6]

- Flow into the amniotic sac
  - Fetal urine production—800 to 1200 mL/day.
  - Fetal lung liquid secretion—170 mL/day.
  - Oral-nasal secretions—25 mL/day.
- Flow out of the amniotic sac
  - Fetal swallowing—500 to 1000 mL/day.
  - Intramembranous flow—200 to 400 mL/day.
  - Transmembranous flow—10 mL/day.

These values are experimentally derived, primarily using animal models, and likely to be refined as more studies are reported.

In human pregnancy, AF volume increases dramatically during the first two trimesters, from 20 mL at 10 weeks to an average of 770 mL at 28 weeks. After 28 weeks, the AF volume changes little until 39 weeks, after which it decreases dramatically (see Figure 65 in Appendix of Normal Values).[7] Although the average AF volume in the third trimester is 700 to 800 mL, the range of normal is very wide and a normal fetus at 32 weeks may have more than 2000 mL, or less than 500 mL of AF. This wide range of normal compounds the problem of assessing the AF volume in a pregnancy.

Evaluation of Amniotic Fluid Volume

A diagnosis of an AF volume abnormality may be suspected by physical examination (size/dates variance), but the diagnosis is generally made by examination of the fluid compartment. Although AF volume can be assessed by invasive means, such as dye dilution, these are not used in clinical practice. The amount of AF is most commonly evaluated using ultrasound, although the ultrasound estimation of AF does not correlate well with either actual AF volumes[8] or fetal outcomes.[9–11] The amniotic fluid index (AFI)[12,13] or the single deepest pocket (SDP)[14] of AF are both used as semiquantitative measures of fluid volume. In assessing the AFI, the sonographer measures the deepest AF pocket in each of the four quadrants of the abdomen (as defined by the umbilicus and the linea nigra). Pockets are measured perpendicular to the floor with the patient supine and should not contain small parts or umbilical cord. The AFI is the sum of the four measurements. The SDP is the single largest measurement so obtained. Commonly used definitions of AF abnormalities include an AFI of 25 cm or greater or less than 5, or a SDP of 8 cm or more or less than 2. These AFI values are considerably outside of the 5th or 95th percentile (see

Figure 66 in Appendix of Normal Values),[15] leading some centers to adopt different cutoffs. Using the 5th and 95th percentiles, however, greatly increases the number of patients labeled as having an AF abnormality, though many of these fetuses will have no significant pathology[9] supporting the use of the values just discussed. In addition, evidence suggests that the SDP is more specific than the AFI, without sacrificing sensitivity, suggesting that SDP may be a preferable test for AF abnormalities.[16,17] SDP may also be a more satisfactory test for certain special circumstances, such a multiple gestation,[18] when the AFI is undefined.

OLIGOHYDRAMNIOS

Oligohydramnios is a decreased amount of AF, affecting 3% to 5% of pregnancies.[19] The expected amount of AF varies during and between pregnancies, making the absolute definition of "normal" problematic; however, an AF volume of less than 250 to 300 mL appears to be abnormal at any time during the second half of human pregnancy (see Figure 65 in Appendix of Normal Values). Assessing AF volumes is also problematic. In most protocols, a pregnancy lacking a single pocket of 2 cm, or one with an AFI less than 5 cm, is deemed to demonstrate oligohydramnios. Many centers regard AFIs of 5 to 8 cm as being "borderline normal," following the findings of Phelan and coworkers,[12,20] and "severe" oligohydramnios describes a situation in which there is no measurable AF.[21] Unfortunately, two-dimensional estimates of AF volume correlate poorly with actual volume, and in particular, the measurements discussed earlier demonstrate poor specificity for the diagnosis of oligohydramnios, as measured by tracer dilution.[22] When the two measures were compared, a recent meta-analysis suggests that the SDP method yields a similar perinatal outcome with increased specificity for the diagnosis of oligohydramnios when compared with AFI.[16,23,24] Some authors have also suggested that the subjective impression of diminished AF on ultrasound examination is at least as accurate as the various measurement scenarios.[25,26]

Etiology

Conditions associated with ologhydramnios are shown in Table 12–1. The most likely etiology of oligohydramnios varies depending on gestational age (Fig. 12–1). The etiologies and relative frequencies of midtrimester oligohydramnios were illustrated in a series of 128 fetuses first noted to have severe oligohydramnios at 13 to 24 weeks' gestation.[21] The following etiologies were observed: fetal anomaly (51%), preterm premature rupture of membranes (PPROM) (34%), placental abruption (7%), intrauterine growth restriction (IUGF) (5%), and unknown (4%). Six of the 65 anomalous fetuses were aneuploid. The pregnancy outcome was generally poor owing to fetal or neonatal death or pregnancy termination. In the third trimester, the distribution of abnormalities is different. One recent study of patients greater than 28 weeks[27] described a 28% rate of fetal growth restriction, a 9% rate of abruption, and a 4% rate of congenital anomalies. Although this study excluded patients with preexisting ruptured membranes, 14% of patients with oligohydramnios ruptured membranes after the diagnosis had been made. The perinatal mortality was higher in pregnancies complicated by oligohydramnios than in the overall population.

TABLE 12–1
Conditions Associated with Oligohydramnios

Obstetric Complications
Premature rupture of the membranes
Fetal growth restriction
Postmaturity
Maternal Complications
Dehydration
Fetal Anomalies
Renal agenesis
Bilateral multicystic kidneys
Polycystic kidney disease
Chromosomal anomalies
Collecting system abnormalities or obstruction
Rare Complications
Maternal diabetes insipidus
Tubular dysgenesis
Meckel-Gruber syndrome
Perlman's syndrome

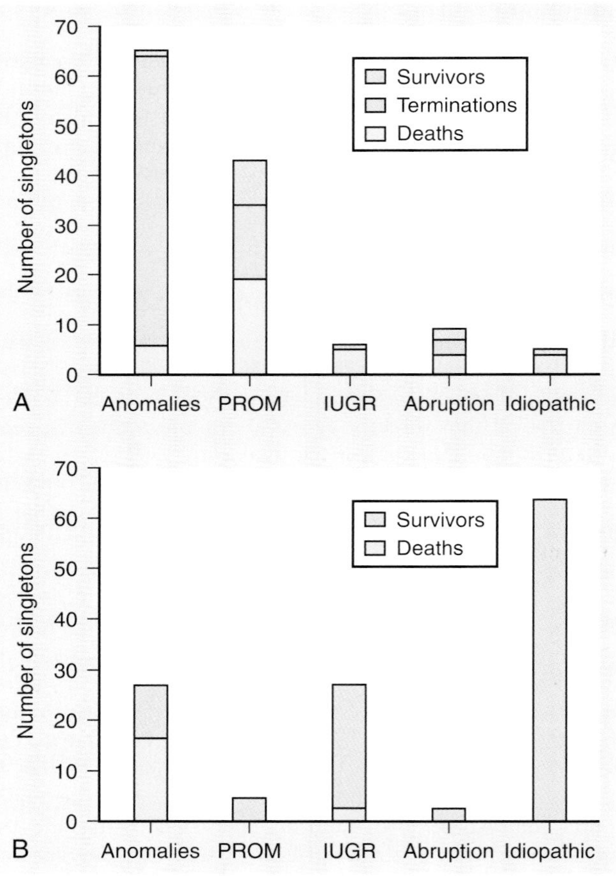

FIGURE 12–1
Etiology of oligohydramnios in fetuses with severe oligohydramnios, defined as no visible amniotic fluid (AF) on ultrasound, diagnosed in the second (*A*) and third (*B*) trimesters.
(*A* and *B*, Redrawn from Shipp TD, Bromley B, Pauker S, et al: Outcome of singleton pregnancies with severe oligohydramnios in the second and third trimesters. Ultrasound Obstet Gynecol 1996;7:108–113.)

Excluding membrane rupture, oligohydramnios may be a consequence of a reduction of urine flow from the fetal kidney to the amniotic cavity. Defective urine production by the fetal kidney may be due to reduced renal perfusion. Maternal dehydration may be associated with oligohydramnios[28,29]; this is thought due to reduced flow of water from the maternal to the fetal compartment decreasing fetal intravascular volume and enhancing fetal plasma hypertonicity and fetal vasopressin-induced urinary antidiuresis. The donor twin in the setting of twin-twin transfusion syndrome (TTTS) will also demonstrate oligohydramnios due to reduced intravascular volume.[30,31] A number of authors have also described alterations in fetal renal artery flow associated with oligohydramnios, both preterm and posterm,[32–34] consistent with the theory that with marginal placental function, fetal blood flow is redirected to vital organs, including the brain. The fetal kidneys are less well perfused, reducing fetal urine volume. Flow in the fetal renal artery also may be reduced by maternal use of certain drugs. Indomethacin has been reported to cause oligohydramnios by this mechanism, although this has been debated.[35] The mechanism of action of indomethacin involves its antagonism of prostaglandins.

Fetal renal function may also be impaired as a consequence of renal disease. Maternal use of angiotensin-converting enzyme (ACE) inhibitors has been associated with fetal renal damage, including renal tubular dysgenesis and renal failure (see also Chapter 35).[36,37] Infantile polycystic kidney disease is an autosomally inherited disease (usually recessive) characterized by fetal kidneys that acquire a characteristic sonographic hyperechoic appearance, and impaired function and is associated with oligohydramnios.[38,39] In addition, there are fetuses with multicystic dysplastic kidneys, a developmental abnormality that may progress during gestation.[39] The pregnancy may also be complicated by fetal renal agenesis, which is associated with profound oligohydramnios. Renal agenesis is occasionally found with many chromosomal abnormalities, and with a variety of other syndromes, as well as an isolated finding.[40]

Finally, fetal urine output may be reduced owing to an obstruction in the urinary tract downstream from the kidney, especially bladder outlet obstructions. Posterior uretheral valves, prune belly syndrome, and uretheral atresia are common diagnoses in these pregnancies.[39,41] These obstructions are generally amenable to diagnosis by antenatal ultrasound, because there is an associated dilation of the bladder and/or renal collecting system above the lesion.

FIGURE 12–2
Posterior urethral valve visualized by magnetic resonance imaging. Note enlarged bladder with "keyhole" appearance of the proximal urethra (*arrow*).

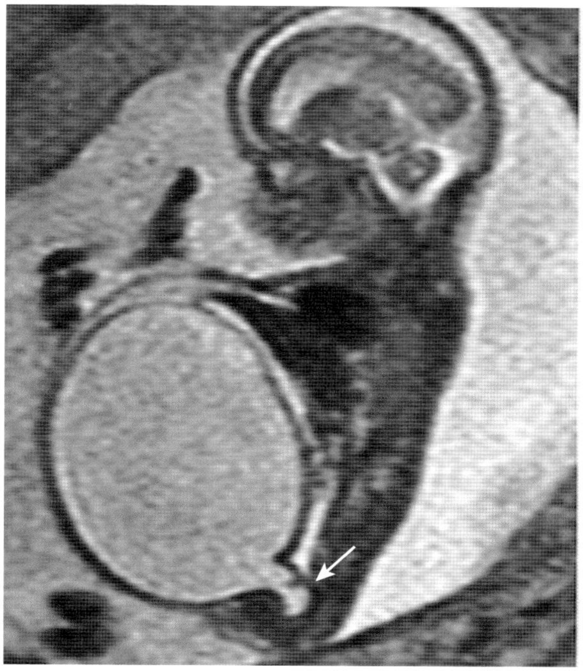

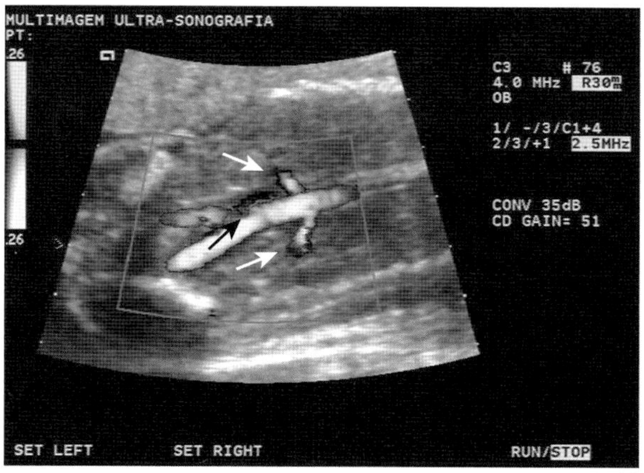

FIGURE 12–3
Normal renal arteries at ultrasound (*arrows*).

Diagnostic Workup

The diagnostic workup of oligohydramnios flows from a knowledge of etiologies. In the second trimester, fetal anomalies are an important cause of oligohydramnios. Ultrasound may be of use in the diagnosis of fetal abnormalities such as renal agenesis or polycystic kidneys[42] or of an obstructive lesion, and magnetic resonance imaging (MRI) may be helpful in confirming these findings (Fig. 12–2). When visualization of the fetus is limited by the oligohydramnios, Doppler ultrasound of the renal arteries (Fig. 12–3) may be helpful in making the diagnosis of renal agenesis[43]; absence of a fetal renal artery signal is reliable evidence of either renal agenesis or a severely dysplastic, nonfunctioning kidney. In some cases, transabdominal amnioinfusion (see later) may be of benefit in allowing a thorough evaluation of the fetus by ultrasound.[43,44] Fetal karyotype may be advisable in order to exclude a fetus with a lethal chromosomal abnormality. With severe oligohydramnios, the karyotype may be obtained by a placental biopsy[45,46] or after amnioinfusion followed by removal of fluid for karyotype.[47] In the face of a fetal urinary obstruction, it has been common to obtain fetal urine for electrolytes or for β-microglobulin in order to predict residual fetal renal function. Such predictive tests have performed poorly, and some authors now consider oligohydramnios as a sufficient indicator of poor fetal renal function (see also Chapter 18).[41,48,49]

In the second or third trimester, ruptured membranes are diagnosed using a combination of history, physical examination, including a sterile speculum examination for pooling of fluid, and confirmatory laboratory tests. Confirmatory tests include vaginal pH, examination of dried secretions for ferning, and ultrasound estimation of AF volume.[50] Used in combination, this testing scheme is more than 90% accurate in the diagnosis of ruptured membranes. Recently developed tools include the measurement of cervical/vaginal placental α-microglobulin-1 (PAMG-1), which is at least as accurate as traditional tools, but is positive in at least a third of women in labor at term despite traditional evidence of intact membranes. Thus, its strength would appear to be its negative predictive value. Others have suggested that a negative fetal fibronectin swab also excludes rupture. If a question persists, a dye such as indigo carmine can be instilled into the amniotic sac and the patient observed for the leakage of blue-stained fluid vaginally. In addition to ruptured membranes, maternal dehydration is a consideration. Dehydration can be suspected by history and physical examination. Although the diagnosis can be confirmed by the finding of increased maternal serum osmolality, in practice, most mothers are offered oral hydration as the remainder of the workup proceeds.

When it develops near term, oligohydramnios should prompt an evaluation of the fetus for evidence of growth restriction and fetal compromise. Although oligohydramnios as diagnosed clinically is associated with fetal growth restriction,[51] it is poorly predictive of abnormal pregnancy outcomes.[51,52]

Risks and Prognosis

Maternal Risks

Oligohydramnios may be associated with an increase in maternal complications. Premature rupture of the membranes, which is one of the main causes of oligohydramnios, is associated with increase risk of chorioamnionitis and maternal morbidity. Among obstetric risks, a meta-analysis of over 10,000 oligohydramnios cases observed an increased risk for cesarean delivery.[53] Others have described an increased risk for labor induction[27] and for small–for–gestational age birth weight.[54]

Fetal Risks

Reduced AF in the first trimester is an ominous finding; the pregnancy often aborts. In one series, 15 of 16 patients (94%) with a normal fetal heart rate and small sac noted on first-trimester sonogram went on to spontaneously abort compared with only 4 of 52 control patients (8%) with normal sac size.[55]

In the second trimester, the prognosis depends on the underlying etiology and severity of the oligohydramnios: Pregnancies with isolated mild or moderate idiopathic oligohydramnios have a good prognosis.[14,56,57] Serial sonographic examinations are helpful for following the natural history of the process, which may remain stable, resolve, or progress to development of severe oligohydramnios and/or fetal growth restriction. In contrast, severe second-trimester oligohydramnios often ends in fetal or neonatal death. In a series of 128 infants,[21] survival occurred in 35/43 (81%) fetuses with PPROM, 2/9 (22%) fetuses with abruption, 1/5 (20%) fetuses with idiopathic oligohydramnios, 1/65 (1.5%) fetuses with congenital anomalies, and 0/6 fetuses with fetal growth restriction. It should, however, be noted that many of these women chose pregnancy termination because of the poor prognosis. In particular, severe oligohydramnios due to PPROM in the second trimester has been reported to have a 90% mortality rate when the duration of the latency period was more than 14 days,[58] leading to a sense of futility regarding these pregnancies. A more recent report,[59] however, describes 23 pregnancies complicated by PPROM and severe oligohydramnios prior to 24 weeks who were delivered between 2006 and 2008. Six pregnancies (26%) were stillborn prior to 24 weeks, and 2 pregnancies were delivered of live (surviving) infants with latency periods less than 14 days. Of the 15 patients delivered after 24 weeks with at least 14 days of PPROM, 1 was not resuscitated and died at delivery, 2 died of pulmonary hypoplasia, and 1 died of necrotizing enterocolitis. The survival of all patients with PPROM prior to 24 weeks was 43%, and the survival of those remaining pregnant to 24 weeks was 76%. Sixty percent of those delivering after 24 weeks with at least 14 days of PPROM had pulmonary hypoplasia, but only 22% of these infants died in the neonatal period. It appears the key element for survival is the presence of at least some amniotic fluid between 18 and 23 weeks' gestation. Absence of amniotic fluid during this interval regardless of the mechanism is highly associated with perinatal death.

Surviving infants may have significant morbidities. Preterm delivery, either spontaneous or indicated by maternal or fetal complications, occurs in more than 50% of pregnancies with severe second-trimester oligohydramnios.[56,57,60,61] Infants may have anatomic and functional abnormalities consistent with the Potter sequence, such as skeletal deformations, contractures, and pulmonary hypoplasia. Pulmonary hypoplasia, in particular, presents a threat to the survival of the fetus with severe second-trimester oligohydramnios, although newer interventions, such as inhaled nitric oxide and high-frequency ventilation, have improved survival in this condition.[59] Various techniques have been suggested to identify fetuses at risk for this complication,[62–66] with the most successful one at present the ultrasound-determined lung volume and pulmonary blood flow.[67] Kohl and colleagues[68] have performed fetoscopic tracheal occlusion to improve pulmonary outcomes in fetuses with ultrasound findings suggestive of pulmonary hypoplasia (see later), though this remains an investigational therapy.

The prognosis of third-trimester oligohydramnios is not as dire as oligohydramnios found in the second trimester. For example, one series included 122 cases of severe oligohydramnios initially diagnosed in the third trimester and 128 initially diagnosed in the second trimester. Perinatal survival was 85% and 10%, respectively.[21] Most cases of severe oligohydramnios in the third trimester occurred at or near term; they were not associated with Potter-like effects, although they were often associated with fetal growth restriction. Some,[69,70] but not all,[71] studies have shown an inverse relationship between AF volume in the third trimester and the incidence of adverse pregnancy outcome. Small sample size likely affected the results of negative studies. Adverse outcomes are related to umbilical cord compression, uteroplacental dysfunction, and meconium aspiration. In particular, uteroplacental dysfunction and cord compression are associated with fetal heart rate abnormalities that may lead to cesarean delivery and low Apgar scores.[21,53,72]

Management Options

Standard Management

Maternal hydration is commonly used in an attempt to increase AF volume in patients without fetal urinary tract abnormalities, and several studies report an increase in amniotic fluid volumes after maternal hydration. In one study, four groups of oligohydramnios patients were randomized to intravenous hypotonic fluid, intravenous isotonic fluid, oral water, or control. Only the intravenous hypotonic fluid and oral water groups had an increased AFI compared with the controls (2.3 and 3.3 cm, respectively), emphasizing that maternal plasma osmolality reduction rather than maternal plasma volume expansion is etiologic in increasing the AFI.[73] In a recent randomized clinical trial comparing the effect of maternal intravenous hydration with 0.5 normal saline versus placebo on the AFI in patients with oligohydramnios, no difference was demonstrated between the two groups,[74] whereas an observational study of hydration with 5% dextrose in water did find an increase in AFI,[75] confirming the importance of hypotonic replacement. In a blinded trial of oral hydration versus control, women with both decreased and normal AFIs increased their AFI in response to consumption of an additional 2 L of water daily.[76,77] Similarly, a trial of oral hydration with water in 10 women with oligohydramnios found an increase in AFI and an improvement in measures of uteroplacental perfusion.[78] These data were sufficient for the Cochrane collaboration to note that maternal hydration "may be beneficial in the management of oligohydramnios."[79] We consider that in cases of oligohydramnios in which immediate delivery is not indicated, oral hydration with water may have benefit, particularly in patients with evidence of maternal dehydration. By contrast, there is no evidence for a benefit from maternal isotonic volume expansion or the use of diuretics to increase fetal urine flow.[80] Although there appears little doubt that maternal fluid status affects the fetus, the clinical utility is weak.

Experimental Management

As a decrease in maternal osmolality appears to improve AF volumes, we examined the effect of reducing maternal osmolality by combining maternal hypotonic hydration with 1-deamino-[8-D-arginine] vasopressin (DDAVP).[81] There was indeed an increase AFI in women with oligohydramnios compared with untreated controls. However, there was no comparison with hydration alone, and this treatment regimen remains experimental.

Procedures

Amnioinfusion, or the instillation of fluid into the amniotic cavity, might be expected to prevent the pulmonary and orthopedic consequences to the fetus and to allow visualization of the fetus by ultrasound. However, multiple procedures are needed because of the natural circulation of the fluid or leakage because of membrane rupture. A few reports describe multiple amnioinfusions being performed to replace AF in pregnancies complicated by fetal renal abnormalities,[82–84] the majority in patients with early membrane rupture in which it was associated with improved perinatal survival,[85–88] an increased latency period,[87,89–91] and a reduced need for cesarean delivery.[86] However, the procedure was more successful in patients who retained the infused fluid,[92] and some authors performed a test infusion to determine those patients who would benefit from the procedure.[93] There was no reported association of amnioinfusion with chorioamnionitis.[87,91] It is difficult, however, to advocate for this procedure after 23 to 24 weeks when fetal lung development should be completed.

PROCEDURE

TRANSABDOMINAL AMNIOINFUSION

1. Some authors pretreat the patient with antibiotics, especially if the procedure is being done for ruptured membranes.[87] Others include antibiotics in the infusion. There is no evidence to objectively support this practice.
2. After informed consent and sterile preparation, a 20-g needle is advanced into the gestational sac:
   - The placenta is avoided if possible.
   - The needle is aimed for an existing fluid pocket or for an area between the limbs.
3. Correct needle placement is identified
   - If fluid is present, fluid may be aspirated.
   - If no fluid is present, a small amount of saline may be injected to confirm intra-amniotic needle placement.
4. Sterile tubing attached to a stopcock, large syringe, and saline intravenous line is attached to the needle.
   - Prime the tubing to avoid injecting air into the amniotic sac, because this greatly interferes with visualization by ultrasound.
5. Fluid is injected with continuous ultrasound guidance.
   - Saline is used in nearly all trials and appears to be effective. An argument has been made that lactated Ringer's solution more closely resembles the composition of natural amniotic fluid.[94]
   - Many authors warm the saline to 37°C,[87] though there are no published studies on the difference between room temperature and warmed saline for preterm amnioinfusion.
   - Fetal heart motion may be observed by ultrasound.
   - For therapeutic amnioinfusion, the aim is to achieve a normal AFI.
6. After the procedure, the patient is monitored for 24 hours for leakage, fever, or uterine contractions.
7. Anti-D globulin is administered to Rh-negative mothers.

Other than amnioinfusion, a variety of interventions have been proposed for the patient with oligohydramnios remote from term, especially for the patient with early gestation and PPROM. O'Brien and associates[95] used a gelatin sponge to plug the cervix, in addition to cervical cerclage and amnioinfusion, in 15 women who suffered rupture of the membranes at or before 21 weeks. Six of the 15 fetuses survived to hospital discharge, though several of these had orthopedic sequelae of oligohydramnios. Human platelets and cryoprecipitate (Amniopatch) have been injected into the amniotic sac in cases of membrane rupture after amniocentesis. Although individual reports have suggested good outcomes with this technique,[96–99] a full comparison of risks and benefits is needed. A number of case reports have examined the injection of fibrin "glue" through the cervix.[100] Here too, a full examination of this technique is lacking.

Fetal Surgery (See also Chapters 18 and 19)

Fetal surgical approaches to the management of oligohydramnios fall into two areas: bladder drainage and tracheal occlusion. In the case of urinary collecting system obstruction, there have been a large number of reports of shunt placement into the fetal bladder. More recently, there have been reports of the ablation of posterior uretheral valves by fetoscopy. Vesicoamniotic shunts may reduce the prevalence of pulmonary hypoplasia, but they have no confirmed value in preserving renal function despite the use of fetal urinary electrolytes to select patients with functioning kidneys for treatment. Among 14 patients who underwent procedures for posterior uretheral valve (average gestational age 22.5 wk), all fetuses had urinary electrolyte values believed to be consistent with adequate renal function. Of the 8 born alive and surviving the neonatal period, 5 had chronic renal disease, including 3 who required renal transplantation.[49] Similarly, a report from Egypt describes 12 patients who had vesicoamniotic shunts placed for posterior uretheral valves. Of the 8 survivors, 4 had normal renal function, a rate similar to that achieved when treatment is postnatal.[101] Another report describes 20 male fetuses treated for a variety of lower urinary tract obstructions.[41] Ninety percent of the treated children survived for 1 year. Of the survivors, 8 had normal renal function, and 6 of 10 with impaired renal function were candidates for renal transplant.

Fetoscopic therapy has been undertaken for some anomalies, but data upon which to judge effectiveness are currently limited.[102–104] Fetoscopic tracheal occlusion has been employed to prevent or alleviate the pulmonary hypoplasia associated with second-trimester oligohydramnios.[68,105] These innovative approaches are exciting but clearly remain experimental.

SUMMARY OF MANAGEMENT OPTIONS
Oligohydramnios

Management Options	Evidence Quality and Recommendation	References
Identify Cause (If Possible)		
Detailed history to include drug exposure, maternal medical illnesses, prior prenatal screening for aneuploidy, prior ultrasound findings, symptoms of membrane rupture.	—/GPP	—
Rupture of the membranes is ruled out by physical examination.	—/GPP	—
Ultrasonography to assess: • Degree of oligohydramnios (AFI). • Presence of growth deficiency. • Presence of fetal anomalies. • Presence and appearance of the kidneys. • Presence of fetal renal arteries. • Fetal and uterine blood flow studies. • Fetal well-being.	III/B	42
Amnioinfusion may have a role in diagnosing or confirming suspected PPROM or fetal anomaly.	III/B	44
Patient Counseling		
Prognosis depends on gestational age, severity of oligohydramnios and diagnosis.	III/B	21
• Severe oligohydramnios in the second trimester is often associated with fetal death and congenital abnormalities. The patient may wish to consider pregnancy termination.	—/GPP	—
• Third-trimester oligohydramnios is more often associated with PPROM and IUGR. Delivery may be indicated.	—/GPP	—

Management Options	Evidence Quality and Recommendation	References
Management (Depends on Etiology)		
PPROM (see Chapter 62).		
Growth deficiency (see Chapter 11).		
Prolonged pregnancy (see Chapter 65).		
Fetal renal anomalies (see Chapter 18).		
Treatments to increase AF volume:		
• Maternal hydration with hypotonic solution	Ib/A	73,76,77
• Serial transabdominal therapeutic amnioinfusions with PPROM remote from term, selected patients (not in labor, retain fluid after infusion).	Ib/A	85–88
• Vesicoamniotic shunting in obstructive uropathies may be of value in preventing pulmonary sequelae (see Chapter 18).	III/B	41,49
• Sealing of membrane leak: investigational	III/B	96–99
• DDAVP: investigational.	III/B	81

AF, amniotic fluid; AFI, amniotic fluid index; DDAVP, 1-deamino-[8-d-arginine] vasopressin; GPP, good practice point; IUGR, intrauterine growth restriction; PPROM, prenatal premature rupture of membranes.

POLYHYDRAMNIOS

Polyhydramnios is the condition of excessive AF. Clinically detectable polyhydramnios occurs in 1% to 3% of pregnancies.[19,106] The 95th percentile for the maximum AF volumes in normal pregnancy is about 2200 mL (see Figure 65 in Appendix of Normal Values); however, abnormal pregnancies can have AF volumes of many liters.[107] At Harbor-UCLA, an AFI of 25 cm or greater is used as the clinical definition of polyhydramnios.[108] Other definitions commonly used include an AFI of 24 cm or greater, or a SDP of greater than 8 cm.[108] The 95th percentile AFI at maximum fluid volumes for normal gestations is between 18 and 20 cm (see Figure 66 in Appendix of Normal Values), leading some centers to use lower cutoff figures. But as with the diagnosis of oligohydramnios, such thresholds greatly increase the number of patients labeled as having an AF abnormality without an association with adverse outcome. The higher AFI cutoff selects the majority of fetuses with an abnormal outcome, while avoiding the need to perform an extensive workup on a number of normal fetuses.[109] Polyhydramnios is often categorized as mild, moderate, or severe; although these terms are not strictly defined, they correspond roughly to AFIs of 25 to 30, 30 to 35, and greater than 35 cm,[110] or SDPs of 8 to 11, 11 to 15, and greater than 15 cm.[42]

TABLE 12–2
Conditions Associated with Polyhydramnios

Obstetric Complications	
	Twin-twin transfusion syndrome
	Maternal diabetes
Fetal Anemias	
	Maternal alloimmunization
	Maternal syphilis/parvovirus infection
Fetal Anomalies	
	Central nervous system abnormalities
	Myotonic dystrophy
	Esophageal blockage
	High gut obstruction
	Thoracic tumors
Rare Complications	
	Inherited disorders of renal function
	Fetal or placental tumors

Etiology

Conditions associated with polyhydramnios are shown in Table 12–2. As for oligohydramnios, knowledge of AF dynamics aids our understanding of the underlying etiology of polyhydramnios. In general, polyhydramnios may be caused either by excess fetal urine or lung fluid or by a defect in AF resorption. Because there are no known conditions characterized by a defect in intramembranous flow, resorptive defects reflect deficiencies in fetal swallowing or upper gastrointestinal tract obstructions that prevent AF resorption.

Inherited disorders causing increased urine production in utero are rare. The Bartter syndromes are autosomal recessive defects in various components of the salt resorption system in the thick ascending limb of the nephron,[111] characterized by polyuria. In some instances, the polyuria may extend to fetal life, creating polyhydramnios.[112] Perlman's syndrome[40,113] and Beckwith-Weideman syndrome[114] are inherited disorders of renal development also associated with polyhydramnios. However, these are overgrowth syndromes, with large fetal kidneys and increased urine output.

More commonly, excess urine flow is due to fetal volume overload. Volume overload is likely the cause of polyhydramnios in the amniotic sac of the recipient in a twin-twin transfusion[31,115]; atrial natriuetic peptide has been implicated in the increased urination.[116] Fetuses with tachyarrhythmias may present with polyhydramnios[42] that resolves with reversion of the cardiac rhythm. Fetuses with severe anemia from red blood cell alloimmunization[117,118] may also present with polyhydramnios. Polyhydramnios due to anemia or tachyarrhythmia may reflect increased cardiac output. Increased cardiac output is responsible for the polyhydramnios associated with placental chorioangioma and other tumors.[119] Fetal infections such parvovirus B19 may result in polyhydramnios in association with hydrops,[120,121] though parvovirus infection is rarely associated with polyhydramnios alone. Polyhydramnios and fetal hydrops may also occur with congenital syphilis infection.[122]

Fetuses of diabetic mothers may demonstrate increased AF, and the likelihood is correlated with glycemic control.[123] Here, excess AF likely reflects increased fetal urine output due to an osmotic (glucose) diuresis. One study using a two-dimensional ultrasound estimate of fetal urine output reported normal fetal urine output in diabetic pregnancies.[124] Three-dimensional methods appear more reliable and may become useful for routine estimation of bladder output in pregnancies with polyhydramnios.[125,126]

Polyhydramnios may also be a consequence of fetal anomalies leading to disruptions in fetal swallowing or resorption of fluid. Fetuses with severe central nervous system abnormalities, such as anencephaly, can have polyhydramnios caused by poor swallowing effort,[42] as may fetuses with disorders characterized by muscle weakness (e.g., myotonic dystrophy).[127,128] In addition, fetuses with obstructions of the mouth or oropharynx,[129–132] esophageal atresia,[133,134] or duodenal atresia[135] are often identified after the development of polyhydramnios. Fetuses with thoracic abnormalities such as diaphragmatic hernia[136,137] or cystic adenomatoid malformation of the lung[138] may also present with polyhydramnios due to esophageal compression,[139] alterations in hemodynamics,[140] or perhaps increased lung fluid production. In many cases, these structural anomalies are associated with chromosomal abnormalities.[141] A lack of fetal swallowing does not lead to polyhydramnios in all cases. Only 26% of anencephalic fetuses developed polyhydramnios in one study,[142] and in animals, the inability to swallow fluid may or may not result in polyhydramnios, depending on changes in intramembranous absorption.[143]

Risks and Prognosis

Some of the more common complications of polyhydramnios are listed in Table 12–3.

Maternal Complications

Mild-to-moderate polyhydramnios creates minimal maternal symptoms, generally consisting of abdominal discomfort and slight dyspnea.[144] In moderate-to-severe polyhydramnios, there may be maternal respiratory distress and often edema of the lower extremities. Severe polyhydramnios increase is associated with an increased prevalence of preeclampsia in association with the "mirror" syndrome.[145] Marked polyhydramnios may increase the incidence of preterm birth due to uterine overdistention[146,147] (see later).

TABLE 12–3
Pregnancy Complications Associated with Polyhydramnios

CONDITION	RELATIVE RISK
Pregnancy-induced hypertension	2.7
Urinary tract infection	2.8
Premature delivery	2.7
Premature rupture of the membranes	3.0
Abnormal fetal presentation	2.5
Cesarean section	4.0
Intrauterine demise	7.7
Neonatal death	7.7
Nuchal cord	3.3

Data from Golan A, Wolman I, Sagi J, et al: Persistence of polyhydramnios during pregnancy—Its significance and correlation with maternal and fetal complications. Gynecol Obstet Invest 1994;37:18–20.

The increased AF volume and overstretched myometrium place the patient with polyhydramnios at risk of labor complications. Spontaneous labor with intact membranes often produces contractions that are of poor quality.[148] There is an increased incidence of fetal malpresentation,[106,149,150] which further increases the likelihood of cesarean delivery.[106,147,151] Rapid decompression following rupture of the membranes has been linked to abruptio placentae[152,153] and amniotic fluid embolus (see also Chapters 58 and 78). Similarly, there appears an increased risk after delivery of uterine atony and postpartum hemorrhage.[42]

Fetal Complications

Most cases of mild polyhydramnios are idiopathic and carry a low risk of undiagnosed anomalies, and abnormalities present may not amenable to antenatal diagnosis.[107] Often, it is associated with fetal macrosomia.[108,147,154] It is, however, associated with an increased risk of delivery complications such as preterm labor and fetal malpresentation (see Table 12–3). In one report,[108] polyhydramnios with a normal fetus carried a 10% to 20% risk of preterm birth and a 3% to 5% risk of fetal death. Severe polyhydramnios has a higher risk of perinatal mortality (Table 12–4).[155,156] Potentially, increased intra-amniotic pressure could interfer with placental blood flow and thus compromise fetal oxygenation.[157,158] Polyhydramnios is also associated with a variety of fetal anomalies and other conditions, such as severe anemia and TTTS. In these cases, the outcome of the pregnancy depends more on the etiology than the polyhydramnios.

Diagnostic Workup

The mainstay of diagnosis in polyhydramnios is targeted ultrasound. Goals of the examination are to define fetal number and chorionicity (if multiple gestation), quantitate the fluid, and evaluate the fetus for structural abnormalities, fetal heart rate, and evidence of fetal hydrops. Fetal activity, bladder volume, and voiding can also be assessed. Amniocentesis for a karyotype (especially when significant congenital anomalies are detected) and a search for fetal infection may be indicated. In one large representative series, the prevalence of aneuploidy in anomalous fetuses with

TABLE 12–4
Severity of Polyhydramnios and Fetal Outcome

DEGREE	SDP	AFI	FREQUENCY (%)	PERINATAL MORTALITY (PER 1000)	ANOMALIES (%)
Mild	>8	>24	68	50	≤6
Moderate	>11	>32	19	190	≤45
Severe	>15	>44	13	540	≤65

AFI, amniotic fluid index; SDP, single deep pocket.
From Harman CR: Amniotic fluid abnormalities. Semin Perinatol 2008;32:288–294.

polyhydramnios was 10%.[159] Whether a karyotype should be obtained in the absence of anomalies or growth restriction is more controversial because the likelihood of aneuploidy is much lower in the setting of a normal sonogram. In this same series, the prevalence of aneuploidy was 1%,[159] a range consistent with that reported in prior series.[109,160–163] We recommend karyotype in cases of severe polyhydramnios because of the increased risk of aneuploidy in most series, the possibility that anomalies escaped detection during the sonographic examination, and the low risk of the procedure, especially if fluid is being withdrawn for therapeutic reasons (see later).

In addition to the fetal examination, maternal testing for diabetes and isoimmunization may be useful if not previously performed. Maternal history may suggest testing for other etiologies such as infections or drug exposures.

Management Options

Standard

The most effective treatments for polyhydramnios address the specific diagnosis, such as diabetes control and fetal TTTS. These treatments are described elsewhere in this text. The goal of nonspecific treatment in polyhydramnios is to relieve intolerable maternal symptoms and to avert preterm delivery. Mild and moderate polyhydramnios are usually managed expectantly, and treatment is reserved for symptomatic patients and for those with severe polyhydramnios. Many authors will treat severe polyhydramnios regardless of maternal symptoms due to the increase in intra-amniotic pressure found in these pregnancies.[157]

One possible treatment paradigm is to reduce maternal to fetal water flow. Although maternal dehydration should reduce transplacental water flow, manipulations of the maternal plasma volume or osmolality, as with diuretics, are not used because they may reduce placental blood flow and impair fetal oxygenation.[164] Fetal urine flow in polyhydramnios has been manipulated with maternally administered prostaglandin synthase inhibitors with good results. Several series and case reports document the use of indomethacin to treat polyhydramnios,[165–171] although there are no randomized trials for this indication. Indomethacin may also act through an effect on the fetal membranes,[106] but most likely, it increases the resorption of water in the renal tubule by inhibition of prostaglandins.[42,106] The most commonly used dose of indomethacin is 25 mg every 6 hours,[106] although some report doses up to 200 mg/day.[150,168,171] In most reports, the dose is reduced or stopped if there is oligohydramnios or signs of fetal ductal constriction. Otherwise, the indomethacin may be continued if effective in reducing the AF volume until 32 to 34 weeks when the risk of ductal constriction begins to rise. It may be possible to taper the dose and discontinue indomethacin treatment earlier if severe polyhydramnios does not recur. Indomethacin is not used in TTTS, because there are serious concerns of exacerbating the condition of the donor fetus.

Indomethacin has a variety of undesirable fetal effects, including closure or constriction of the ductus arteriosus,[170] the development of oligohydramnios,[172] and fetal renal damage,[173,174] although not all reports support these associations.[175] We obtain serial fetal echocardiographic evaluation at weekly intervals if the treatment exceeds 48 hours. Sonographic signs of ductal constriction include tricuspid regurgitation and right ventricular dysfunction. We also monitor the AF volume and reduce or discontinue indomethacin if the AFI is less than 8 cm.

Experimental

SULINDAC

Sulindac is a nonsteroidal anti-inflammatory agent that also results in reduction of the AF volume, but may have less potential than indomethacin to constrict the fetal ductus arteriosus[106,176–178] when used as a tocolytic. One study concluded that sulindac has less effect than indomethacin on fetal urine production, a negative for this indication.[106]

OTHER THERAPIES

In the ovine pregnancy, intra-amniotic DDAVP is rapidly absorbed by the fetus and causes a marked decrease in fetal urine flow.[179] Modulation of the amniotic membrane water channels (aquaporins)[180] may also represent a potential future therapeutic intervention to normalize AF volume.

Procedures

Removal of large amounts of AF by amniocentesis (therapeutic amniocentesis, or amnioreduction) is used to manage the maternal symptoms of polyhydramnios. The procedure has also been used to avert preterm delivery and claimed to improve fetal oxygenation by reducing intra-amniotic pressure,[181] though there is no good evidence of efficacy for fetal indications[182] other than in TTTS.[183–187] The role of amnioreduction in TTTS has diminished after studies showing improved outcome with fetoscopic laser therapy prior to viability.[188]

Two protocols are used for amnioreduction: standard amnioreduction, in which fluid is removed at a rate of 45 to 90 mL/min, and aggressive amnioreduction, in which fluid is removed more rapidly.[189] Both techniques are associated with similar complications rates (4%–15%) including PPROM, infection, placental abruption, and fetal death.[183,189,190] It is uncertain whether some or all of these complications occur as a part of the natural history of polyhydramnios because none of the studies included an untreated control arm. On average, two procedures are needed to reduce AF volume chronically, although some patients, particularly those with TTTS, require many more.[189–191] One case report described 12 amnioreductions removing a total of 21,600 mL of fluid; the infant was diagnosed with West's syndrome at follow-up 16 months after delivery.[107]

PROCEDURE

THERAPEUTIC AMNIOREDUCTION

1. Prior to the procedure, a decision should be made as to the possibility of delivery in the case of fetal distress. If emergency cesarean delivery is a consideration, the procedure is best done in or near the surgical suite.
2. After informed consent and sterile preparation, an 18- to 20-g needle is advanced into the gestational sac, avoiding the placenta if possible. The needle may be angled slightly to allow for a decrease in uterine size with amnioreduction.
3. Once the cavity is entered, a stopcock and tubing are attached to the needle hub, and a large syringe is used to remove fluid one syringe at a time. Wall suction,[192] vacuum bottles,[193,194] and wound suction systems[190] are all described to allow for more rapid fluid removal. The goal is a normal AFI of 10 to 20 cm (some are even more aggressive, aiming for an AFI <10 cm[190] or relative oligohydramnios[189]).
4. There is no evidence identifying the best monitoring protocol after amnioreduction. We monitor uterine activity for 12 to 24 hours, and follow AF volume every 1 to 3 weeks as indicated by the severity of the process. Amnioreduction can be repeated if severe polyhydramnios recurs.

Fetal Surgery

No fetal surgical intervention is specifically targeted to polyhydramnios, with the exception of fetal laser ablation of vascular anastomoses in patients with TTTS. Several reports describe indirect therapy such as shunting of intrathoracic cystic lesions[195] or fetal surgery for thoracic lesions or teratomas.[196,197]

SUMMARY OF MANAGEMENT OPTIONS
Polyhydramnios

Management Options	Evidence Quality and Recommendation	References
Identify Cause (If Possible)		
Detailed history to include drug exposure, maternal diabetes, prior prenatal screening for aneuploidy, family history of myotonic dystrophy or past history of skeletal dysplasia/arthrogryposis, history of red cell alloimmunization.	—/GPP	—
Maternal blood sugar series/glucose tolerance test and blood type/antibody screen if not previously done.		
Ultrasonography to assess:		
• Degree of polyhydramnios (AFI). • Presence of fetal anomalies, especially those that would impede swallowing. • Evidence of fetal anemia. • Evidence of fetal tachyarrhythmia. • Evidence of TTTS.	III/B	161,198,199
Offer karyotope for anomalous fetus or severe polyhydramnios.	III/B	107,159
Karyotyping for isolated mild polyhydramnios controversial—only offer if increased a priori risk. Consider assessment of viral infection.	III/B	120,160
Patient Counseling		
Prognosis depends on severity and etiology. Best prognosis with mild, idiopathic.	—/GPP	—
All pregnancies with severe polyhydramnios have an increased risk for preterm delivery and perinatal mortality. Other risks depend on etiology.	III/B	107,108,147,154

Management Options	Evidence Quality and Recommendation	References
Treatment (to Relieve Maternal Symptoms; Prolong Gestation)		
If mildly asymptomatic, manage expectantly; no evidence to suggest diuretics and salt or fluid restriction are of value.	—/GPP	—
Specific treatment depends on underlying cause (see relevant chapters).	—/GPP	—
Consider amnioreduction (see text) for severe polyhydramnios or earlier if patient is symptomatic and prolongation of pregnancy indicated.	IV/C	106,189
Indomethacin may decrease AFI, but there may be significant fetal side effects.	IIb/B	165–171
Sulindac may be helpful; studies on its use with polyhydramnios are needed.	III/B	106
Alert pediatricians (e.g., need to assess upper gastrointestinal patency, risk of neonatal milk aspiration).	—/GPP	—

AFI, amniotic fluid index; GPP, good practice point; TTTS, twin-twin transfusion syndrome.

SUGGESTED READINGS

Brace RA, Ross MG: Amniotic fluid volume regulation. In Brace RA, Hansen MA, Rodeck CH (eds): Body Fluids and Kidney Function, vol. 4. In Fetus and Neonate. Cambridge, Cambridge University Press, 1998, pp 88–105.

Brace RA, Wolf EJ: Normal amniotic fluid volume changes throughout pregnancy. Am J Obstet Gynecol 1989;161:382–388.

Deshpande C, Hennekam RC: Genetic syndromes and prenatally detected renal anomalies. Semin Fetal Neonatal Med 2008;13:171–180.

Harman CR: Amniotic fluid abnormalities. Semin Perinatol 2008;32:288–294.

Leung WC, Jouannic JM, Hyett J, et al: Procedure-related complications of rapid amniodrainage in the treatment of polyhydramnios. Ultrasound Obstet Gynecol 2004;23:154–158.

Magann EF, Chauhan SP, Doherty DA, et al: A review of idiopathic hydramnios and pregnancy outcomes. Obstet Gynecol Surv 2007;62:795–802.

Nabhan AF, Abdelmoula YA: Amniotic fluid index versus single deepest vertical pocket as a screening test for preventing adverse pregnancy outcome. Cochrane Database Syst Rev 2008;3:CD006593.

Piantelli G, Bedocchi L, Cavicchioni O, et al: Amnioreduction for treatment of severe polyhydramnios. Acta Biomed 2004;75(Suppl 1):56–58.

Shipp TD, Bromley B, Pauker S, et al: Outcome of singleton pregnancies with severe oligohydramnios in the second and third trimesters. Ultrasound Obstet Gynecol 1996;7:108–113.

Williams O, Hutchings G, Debieve F, Debauche C: Contemporary neonatal outcome following rupture of membranes prior to 25 weeks with prolonged oligohydramnios. Early Hum Dev 2008;85:273–277.

REFERENCES

For a complete list of references, log onto www.expertconsult.com.

CHAPTER 13

Fetal Hemolytic Disease

CARL P. WEINER

Videos corresponding to this chapter are available online at www.expertconsult.com.

INTRODUCTION

It is now almost 80 years since neonatal hydrops, anemia, and jaundice were first recognized as a single disease characterized by perinatal hepatosplenomegaly, extramedullary hematopoiesis, and nucleated red blood cells (RBCs) on the peripheral smear.[1] What followed is a fetal success story. Levine and coworkers[2] identified a decade later that the rhesus (Rh) antibodies on the RBCs of affected but not unaffected neonates was cause of the anemia. The basic "story" was 60% completed 7 years later when Chown[3] proved transplacental fetal to maternal hemorrhage was a cause of maternal isoimmunization. In 1961, hemolytic anemia became the first treatable fetal disease after Liley[4,5] characterized its natural history and then successfully transfused affected fetuses intraperitoneally with adult RBCs. Freda and colleagues[6] completed the basic story when they demonstrated in 1964 that passive immunization of Rh-negative individuals with Rh-positive antibodies prior to purposeful exposure to Rh-positive RBCs prevented immunization.

Since then, we have learned progressively more about the intricacies of this complex disease, and incremental progress on the clinical side has rendered fetal hemolytic disease a rare cause of perinatal morbidity and mortality in the industrialized world. Rodeck and associates[7] achieved the first high survival rate for hydropic fetuses using fetoscopic intravascular transfusion in 1981. In 2000, Mari and coworkers[8] demonstrated that the majority of moderately to severely anemic fetuses were noninvasively identifiable by the measurement of the fetal middle cerebral artery peak velocity, essentially ending the need for amniocentesis and reducing that for fetal blood sampling. Lastly, the discovery of fetal free DNA in the maternal circulation by Holzgrieve and colleagues[9] in response to Lo and associates'[10] determination of fetal sex in a maternal blood led to the noninvasive genotyping of fetal Rh genes in many countries.

INCIDENCE

Though antibodies to D antigen remain most common, the development of immunoprophylaxis has diminished its relative importance and enhanced that of the other antigen groups (Table 13–1). Yet, anti-D antibody remains the prototype for maternal RBC alloimmunization and is used for illustration throughout this chapter.

The incidence of Rh-negative individuals varies by race, with a low of 1% in Chinese and Japanese to a high of 100% in the Basques, in whom the mutation likely originated.[11] In North American whites, the incidence of Rh-negative genotype is 15%, and in blacks, it is 7% to 8%. Thus, the incidence of alloimmunization varies greatly among populations. The overall incidence of alloimmunization has declined dramatically since the late 1990s owing in part to immunoprophylaxis and smaller families.[12]

PATHOPHYSIOLOGY AND RISKS

Maternal RBC alloimmunization results from exposure and response to a foreign RBC antigen. Transplacental fetal to maternal hemorrhage is the most common cause of alloimmunization. Heterologous blood transfusion is the second most common cause overall, but the most common cause of sensitization to uncommon antigens (see Table 13–1). Some 75% of women have fetal RBCs identified on a Kleihauer-stained peripheral smear during either pregnancy or delivery.[13] Both the frequency and the size of the bleed increase with advancing gestation: from 3% and 0.03 mL, respectively, in the first trimester up to 45% and 25 mL in the third trimester. Spontaneous abortion, too, is associated with fetal to maternal hemorrhage, but the incidence is less than 1% and the volume usually under 0.1 mL. In contrast, surgically induced abortion has a 20% to 25% risk of transplacental hemorrhage of a significantly greater volume.

The Rh system has long been known to be one of the most complex blood group systems; over 50 different Rh antigens have been identified.[14] The arrangement and configuration of the Rh locus result in gene conversion events that produce hybrid proteins, which represent additional Rh antigens. In most patients, three pairs of closely linked Rh antigens—Cc, Dd, and Ee—are inherited, one from each parent, as two sets of three alleles. An individual may be homozygous or heterozygous for each of the three alleles. The presence, absence, or silence of the D antigen site determines whether an individual is Rh-positive or Rh-negative. Genetic testing for Rh can now be used to detect a recessive D-negative allele or to determine the inheritance of Rh genes carrying mutations that encode altered Rh proteins. The latter is especially relevant for sickle cell disease patients who, because of genetic disparity with white donors, are at high risk for becoming alloimmunized.

The Rh protein complex is critical to cell membrane structure. Rh-null erythrocytes, which lack Rh proteins, are stomatocytic and spherocytic, and affected individuals have hemolytic anemia.[15] Rh proteins appear to mediate key interactions with the underlying cytoskeleton through protein 4.2 and ankyrin.[16–18] Several functional studies and structural modeling reveal that the Rh blood group proteins are members of an ancient family of proteins involved in ammonia transport,[19–21] and nonerythroid Rh proteins have been found in brain, kidney, liver, and skin,[22–24] each sites of ammonia production and elimination.

Because certain combinations are more common than others, the D genotype can be predicted from the phenotype obtained using antibody specific sera for D, C, c, E, and e (Table 13–2). The d antigen has never been detected, and its existence is questionable. The genes for all other Rh alleles are sequenced, and the genotype can be determined directly using polymerase chain reaction (PCR) technology.

There are more than 16 recognized epitopes. The first (and most common) is the Du-positive variant in which the patient is actually Rh-positive, but D expression is weakened by the presence of a C allele on the complementary chromosome (e.g., Cde/cDe). These women are not at risk for D alloimmunization. The second type is sometimes termed Du-negative. Here, part of the D antigen is missing. These women are at risk for D alloimmunization and should receive immunoprophylaxis when otherwise indicated.[25]

The primary immune response to the D antigen occurs over 6 weeks to 12 months. It is usually weak, consisting predominantly of immunoglobulin M (IgM) that does not cross the placenta. As a result, the first pregnancy is not typically at great risk. Fifteen percent of Rh-negative volunteers will become sensitized after a 1-mL exposure of Rh-positive erythrocytes. The proportion increases to 30% after 40 mL and 65% after 250 mL. Three percent of women with uncomplicated pregnancies become sensitized at delivery after a small fetal to maternal hemorrhage (0.1 mL). A second antigen challenge generates an amnestic response that is both rapid and almost exclusively IgG. Bowman[26] observed that the longer the interval between challenges, the greater the increase in both the quantity of antibody and the avidity that it binds the RBC. These features increase the risk of severe fetal disease.

Fetal hematopoiesis consists of three overlapping phases corresponding to the major hematopoietic organ: mesoblastic, hepatic, and myeloid. Erythropoiesis begins in the fetal yolk sac by day 21, then moves to the liver, and finally reaches the bone marrow by 16 weeks' gestation.[27] The decreasing contribution of the liver is characterized by an exponential decrease in the number of circulating

TABLE 13–1

Antigens Causing Fetal Hemolytic Disease Requiring Treatment

Common

Rhesus family: D, C, E, c, e
Kell

Uncommon

JK^a (Kidd)
Fy^a (Duffy)
Kp^a or ^{b}
S

Rare

Do^a Di^a or ^{b}, Fy Hutch, Jk^b Lu^a M, N, s, U, yt

Never

Le^a or ^{b}, p

TABLE 13–2

Prediction of RhD Zygosity Based on Phenotype

		FREQUENCY (%)		WHITES–ZYGOSITY (%)		BLACKS–ZYGOSITY (%)	
PHENOTYPE CDE	GENOTYPE CDE	WHITES	BLACKS	HOMO-	HETERO-	HOMO-	HETERO-
CcDe	*CDe/cde*	31.1	8.8	10	90	59	41
	CDe/cDe	3.4	15.0				
	CDe/cDe	0.2	1.8				
CDe	*CDe/CDe*	17.6	2.9	91	9	81	19
	CDe/Cde	1.7	0.7				
cDEe	*cDe/cde*	10.4	5.7	10	90	63	37
	cDe/cDe	1.1	9.7				
cDe	*CDE/cDE*	2.0	1.2	87	13	99	1
	cDE/cdE	0.3	<0.1				
CcDEe	*CDe/cDE*	11.8	3.7	89	11	90	10
	CDe/cdE	0.8	<0.1				
	Cde/cDE	0.6	0.4				
cDe	*cDe/cde*	3.0	22.9	6	94	46	54
	cDe/cDe	0.2	19.4				

Modified from Mourant AE, Kopec AC, Domaniewska-Sobazak K: The Distribution of Human Blood Groups and Other Polymorphisms, 2nd ed. London, Oxford University Press, 1976, pp 351–505.

erythroblasts. Whereas ABO antigens are weakly expressed on fetal erythrocytes, the Rh antigens are well developed by day 30 of gestation. Anti-D antibody-triggered hemolysis is not complement mediated. Rather, the anti-D–coated fetal RBCs are destroyed extravascularly by the reticuloendothelial system at an increased rate. The response of the affected fetus reflects the quantity and subclass of IgG antibody, the efficiency of placental passage, the avidity at which the antibody binds the antigen site, the maternal HLA makeup, and the maturity and efficiency of the reticuloendothelial system. For example, IgG1 and IgG3 appear to be the important subclasses for fetal hemolytic disease, and the maternal to fetal placental transport of IgG3 is significantly greater in pregnancies at risk for hemolytic disease.[28] Further, there is a strong correlation between human leukocyte antigen (HLA)-DQB1 allele *0201 and both an indirect Coombs titer greater than 512 and fetal anemia.[29]

Hemolytic anemia occurs when the erythrocyte life span declines below 70 to 90 days and the hematopoietic system can no longer meet demands. Anemia may develop slowly over several months in association with a gestationally low reticulocyte count and a gestationally normal bilirubin, or within a week in association with reticulocytosis and hyperbilirubinemia.[30,31] Significant fetal anemia is associated with increased erythropoietin, but in the absence of labor, the concentrations are lower than those observed in adults with the same hemoglobin deficit. Erythropoiesis may occur anywhere in the fetal-placental unit. Both the fetal liver and spleen are enlarged secondary to extramedullary hematopoiesis and congestion. Nucleated RBC precursors (erythroblasts) are released into the peripheral circulation, hence the term *erythroblastosis fetalis*. The greater the number of erythroblasts, the greater the likelihood an antenatal transfusion therapy will be necessary.

All direct fetal sequelae of hemolytic disease relate to the development of anemia. In general, the fetus tolerates mild to moderate anemia well. However, metabolic complications develop as the anemia worsens. Because the RBC is the principal fetal buffer, a metabolic acidemia with hyperlactatemia develops in fetuses with severe anemia.[32]

The precise mechanism leading to the development of hydrops is uncertain, but the elements are clear. First, the hemoglobin deficit for gestation must be extreme.[33] Because the normal hemoglobin concentration rises with advancing gestation, hydrops occurs at higher absolute hemoglobin levels during late compared with early pregnancy and is rare before 20 weeks. Second, though hepatomegaly could potentially hinder cardiac return or cause portal hypertension, it cannot be a major factor in light of the findings listed subsequently. Nor is hypoalbuminemia secondary to liver failure a contributor, as once thought based on postnatal studies,[34] because the albumin concentration is normal for gestation in all but premoribund, hydropic fetuses.[30,31] Finally, cardiac dysfunction, probably secondary to insufficient oxygen-carrying capacity, occurs in at least 90% of hydropic fetuses. This dysfunction is detectable immediately prior to the development of hydrops and resolves rapidly after transfusion with an increase in the fetal oxygen-carrying capacity. It is characterized by an increase in the biventricular cardiac diameter, systolic atrioventricular valve regurgitation, and an elevated umbilical pressure for gestation[35] (Fig. 13–1*A*). Consistent with ventricular

FIGURE 13–1

A, Normal umbilical venous pressure (UVP) (corrected for amniotic fluid pressure) across gestational age (GA) illustrated as the 95% prediction interval. *B*, Normal fetal serum albumin concentration across gestation illustrated as the 95% prediction interval. *C*, Normal fetal serum total bilirubin (TB) across gestation illustrated as the 95% prediction interval.

(*A* and *B*, From Weiner CP, Heilskov J, Pelzer G, et al: Normal values for human umbilical venous and amniotic fluid pressures and their alteration by fetal disease. Am J Obstet Gynecol 1989;161:714-717, with permission.)

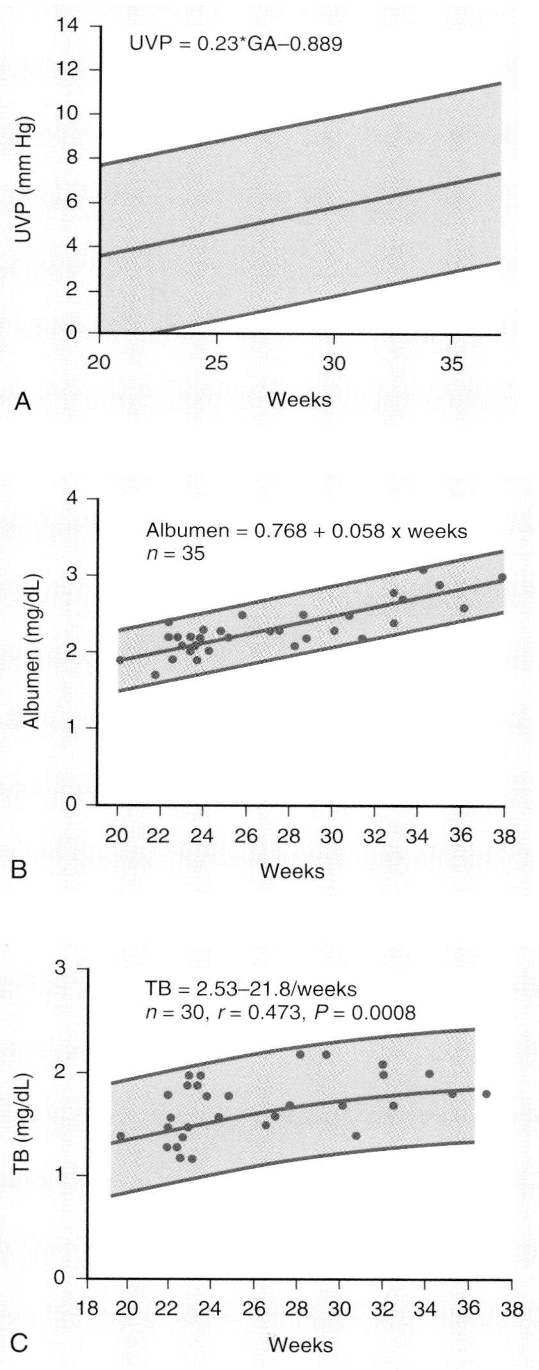

dysfunction, the umbilical venous pressure rises to a greater extent in the hydropic fetus after intravascular transfusion compared with the nonhydropic fetus.[36,37] Within 48 hours of the first RBC transfusion and well before the hydrops resolves, the umbilical venous pressure declines into the normal range. This reversal is too rapid for the occurrence of hydrops to be explained solely by hepatosplenomegaly. Thus, cardiac dysfunction is probably the immediate cause of immune hydrops.

Hyperbilirubinemia secondary to erythrocyte hemolysis is an important part of alloimmune hemolytic disease. Heme pigment is first converted into biliverdin by heme oxygenase and then to a water-insoluble, lipid-soluble bilirubin (the indirect fraction) by biliverdin reductase. Both the fetus and the neonate have reduced levels of glucuronyl transferase, the enzyme necessary for the production of the water-soluble diglucuronide. Indirect bilirubin unbound to albumin penetrates the lipid neuronal membrane, causing cell death. During normal pregnancy, both the fetal serum albumin and bilirubin concentrations rise linearly with advancing gestation (see Fig. 13–1*B* and *C*).[35,38] Most fetal bilirubin under normal and hemolytic conditions is indirect (unconjugated) bilirubin; there is no need routinely to fractionate it. The normal fetal total bilirubin is 5 to 10 times above normal adult levels, suggesting placental bilirubin transport is limited. Bilirubin rises progressively as the severity of hemolysis increases. The total bilirubin concentration in fetuses with hemolytic disease often exceeds 3 mg/dL before the development of anemia.[31]

The neonate with severe hyperbilirubinemia is at risk to develop an encephalopathy (kernicterus). The concentration of bilirubin necessary to cause kernicterus also rises with advancing gestational age. Thus, whereas a term neonate can tolerate a total bilirubin of 25 mg/dL, the extremely preterm neonate is at risk for kernicterus when the total bilirubin level exceeds 12 mg/dL. Affected neonates are initially lethargic and then become hypertonic, lying with their neck hyperextended, their back arched, and their knees, wrists, and elbows flexed. They suck poorly and ultimately develop apneic episodes. Fortunately, bilirubin toxicity is rarely observed with current monitoring protocols and treatment. Neural tissue in the auditory center is particularly sensitive to indirect bilirubin. Survivors often have profound neurosensory deafness and choreoathetoid spastic cerebral palsy. When severe signs of toxicity are present, the mortality rate approximates 90%

MANAGEMENT OPTIONS FOR THE DETECTION OF ALLOIMMUNIZATION

The identification and management of potential fetal hemolytic disease employs several methods for the detection of antibodies either in the maternal serum or bound to the fetal RBC. The tests used vary among countries and not all are covered.

Agglutination Tests

Saline

Rh-negative RBCs suspended in saline agglutinate when serum added to the slide contains IgM but not IgG. IgM does not cross the placenta.

Colloid

Rh-positive RBCs suspended in a colloid medium such as bovine albumin agglutinate if serum containing either IgM or IgG is added to the slide. Thus, if both saline and colloid tests are positive, the antibody may be either an IgM or an IgG. Pretreating the serum with dithiothreitol disrupts the sulfhydryl bonds of IgM and prevents its binding to the RBC. IgG is unaffected by dithiothreitol.

Antiglobulin or Coombs Tests

INDIRECT

RBCs of specific or mixed antigen type are incubated with the patient's serum. The addition of antihuman antiglobulin causes agglutination if the RBCs adsorb antibody from the patient's serum. The reciprocal of the highest dilution that causes agglutination is the titer. Indirect antiglobulin titers are one to three times more sensitive for the detection of RBC alloimmunization than colloid agglutination. In Europe and the United Kingdom, the amount of circulating anti-D is compared with an international standard and reported in International Units per milliliter with a threshold of 15 IU/mL recommended for invasive testing because only mild hemolytic disease of the fetus/newborn is usually noted with anti-D levels below this level.

DIRECT

Antihuman antiglobulin is added directly to the RBCs from the patient. Agglutination indicates antibody is bound to the RBC. It may be eluted off and identified by performing an indirect test using type-specific antigen type cells.

ENZYME PRETREATMENT

RBCs are incubated with either a proteinase (e.g., trypsin) or bromelin to reduce the negative electric potential between cells. Treated cells lie closer together in saline and more readily agglutinate by the IgG bound to them. These are the most sensitive manual methods for the detection of RBC alloimmunization. The technique can be automated, permitting detection of microgram quantities of antibody. Unfortunately, the automated techniques also produce false-positive tests, which limit their application.

Other Serum Tests

Two other tests have been suggested—the Marsh Score and the Monocyte Monolayer assay. Neither in comparative study performs significantly better than Coombs titers.[39,40] One study using monocyte-mediated chemiluminescence suggested it has advantages for antibody quantification,[41] but the technique has not been pursued further.

MANAGEMENT OPTIONS FOR THE Rh-NEGATIVE PATIENT IN PREGNANCY

All women, regardless of past medical and obstetric history, should have on record at least two blood type determinations that are in agreement. Typically, blood is drawn from nulliparous women for ABO and Rh blood type during the first prenatal visit and again after delivery. All pregnant women should have an RBC antibody screen (both indirect and direct Coombs tests) performed at booking. This includes women previously typed as Rh-negative or found to have a negative antibody screen. Laboratory errors remain a significant contributing cause of anti-D prophylaxis failure. In addition, almost of the women who require a fetal transfusion have an RBC antibody directed against an antigen other than D.[30] Although there is controversy on how Rh-positive women can be cost-effectively managed after an initial negative screen, the most complete approach is to repeat the antibody screen at 32 weeks in search of newly developed non–anti-D antibodies.

Nonsensitized Rh-Negative Women

The indirect Coombs test is repeated monthly beginning at 18 to 20 weeks in at-risk Rh-negative women without evidence of sensitization. Many units screen for new alloimmunization far less frequently for financial and practical reasons. In some societies, it may be reasonable to test the father, and if he is Rh-negative, repeat the screen only once between 32 and 34 weeks' gestation. However, paternity is on occasion other than claimed or simply unknown. If the father is tested, the patient should be informed in private of the potential risk for management error should paternity be other than that stated. The decision how to approach paternity is best left to the physician's discretion.

Maternal-fetal ABO incompatibility reduces the risk of D alloimmunization.[14] If the father is heterozygous Rh-positive, there is a 50% chance the fetus will be Rh-negative. If the father is also ABO incompatible with the mother, there is a 60% chance that the fetus will be ABO incompatible. If the fetus is both R-positive and ABO incompatible with the mother (0.5 × 0.6 = 0.3% probability), then the risk of maternal Rh alloimmunization is reduced from approximately 16% to 2%.

Successful passive immunization for Rh factor isoimmunization with anti-D immunoglobulin was first achieved in 1964. The U.S. Food and Drug Administration approved its use in 1968 after confirming efficacy in male prisoners. Anti-D immunoglobulin is extracted by cold alcohol fractionation from the sera of individuals with high titers. This extraction process removes viral pathogens such as HIV and hepatitis B, and an infectious risk from anti-D immunoglobulin has not been substantiated. Anti-D immunoglobulin binds D antigen sites on fetal erythrocytes present in the maternal circulation. Presumably, blockade of these sites prevents immune recognition by B lymphocytes, and the transformation of activated B lymphocytes to IgG-producing plasma cells never occurs. Anti-D immunoglobulin has a half-life of 24 days, and a standard 300-μg dose provides 12 weeks of protection against exposure to up to 30 mL of blood, or 15 mL of erythrocytes. Before the introduction of anti-D immunoglobulin, 10% of susceptible pregnancies developed hemolytic disease of the fetus and newborn. Approximately 90% of these were due to fetomaternal hemorrhage at term. Administration of anti-D immunoglobulin within 72 hours of delivery reduces this incidence by 90%. The administration of an additional dose at 28 weeks produces a further decline in incidence from 2% to 0.1%. Lower doses may be effective but have a higher failure rate. Although the 72-hour limit is based on the original study protocol evaluating the efficacy of anti-D immunoglobulin, beneficial effects may still be present with administration up to 28 days after delivery.

Current guidelines for management of Rh-negative women with uncomplicated pregnancy are focused on the prevention of isoimmunization from physiologic fetomaternal hemorrhage (Table 13–3). If a patient is Rh-negative and the antibody screen is negative on the first prenatal visit, the screen is repeated at 28 weeks and anti-D immunoglobulin administered if negative. Another antibody screen is repeated in labor. If the father is Rh-negative and there is no question on paternity, the prophylactic doses of anti-D immunoglobulin can be omitted.

Women with vaginal bleeding of unknown origin should receive anti-D immunoglobulin prophylaxis (see Table 13–3). Routine antenatal anti-D immunoglobulin therapy is

TABLE 13–3

Preventive Guidelines for Rh-Negative Women in Pregnancy

TIME	TEST	ANTI-D-IG DOSE
First prenatal visit	ABO and Rh blood typing, direct and indirect Coombs test	None
28–29 wk	Direct and indirect Coombs test for newly developed antibodies	300 μg*
32 wk	Direct and indirect Coombs test for newly developed antibodies	None
At birth	Neonatal cord blood for ABO and Rh type as well as direct Coombs test for red blood cell–bound antibodies	
Within 72 hr of delivery	Rosette test, Kleihauer-Betke estimate of fetoplacental hemorrhage	300 μg (individualize for Kleihauer-Betke result)
First-trimester spontaneous miscarriage		50–200 μg
First-trimester therapeutic abortion		300 μg
Following prenatal diagnosis by chorionic villous sampling of amniocentesis		300 μg
Other high risk situations—abdominal trauma, placental abruption, antepartum hemorrhage	Rosette test, Kleihauer-Betke estimate of fetoplacental hemorrhage	300 μg (individualize for Kleihauer-Betke result)

* Some protocols recommend the use of a lower dose of anti-D Ig at 28 wk followed by a further dose at 34 wk in nonimmunized Rh-negative women.
Anti-D Ig, anti-D immunoglobulin.

cost-effective and should be administered to all nonsensitized Rh-negative women with an Rh-positive fetus or a fetus whose status is unknown at 28 weeks' gestation.[42,43] Anti-D immunoglobulin is also administered after amniocentesis if the fetal Rh genotype is unknown, because it carries a 2% risk of maternal sensitization even when performed under ultrasound guidance.[44] Umbilical cord blood is obtained at delivery from Rh-negative women to determine the neonatal ABO and Rh blood type and to seek RBC-bound antibodies. Anti-D immunoglobulin (300 mg) prevents maternal sensitization secondary to fetal-maternal hemorrhage when the volume is less than 30 mL of Rh-positive blood.[45,46] Maternal blood is screened by Kleihauer testing for evidence of a fetal-maternal hemorrhage in excess of 30 mL. This test exploits the relative resistance of fetal hemoglobin to acid denaturation. Acid citrate buffer is used to remove adult hemoglobin, leaving RBC ghosts. The maternal blood is examined on a counting chamber after fixation with 80% ethanol and hematoxylin-eosin staining. The amount of fetal blood in the maternal circulation can be approximated from the number of fetal RBCs per grid using this formula:

Fetal cells/Number of maternal cells = Estimated blood loss/Estimated maternal blood volume in milliliters (85 mL/kg).

About 1 in 400 women suffer a larger bleed and require more anti-D immunoglobulin.[45] Cesarean section and manual removal of the placenta each increase the risk and magnitude of fetal-maternal hemorrhage. In situations in which the estimated bleed exceeds 30 mL, 150% to 200% of the estimated anti-D immunoglobulin requirement is given.

Postpartum, anti-D immunoglobulin may be withheld if the last administration was less than 21 days previously and passively acquired antibodies are still demonstrable on the antibody screen. The rosette test may also be performed in maternal blood to assess the need for further administration of anti-D immunoglobulin. Rosette formation indicates the presence of fetal RBCs, and dosage of anti-D immunoglobulin may have to be adjusted, guided by the Kleihauer-Betke test.

Sensitized Rh-Negative Women

Figures 13–2 and 13–3 illustrate two useful paradigms. Rh immune globulin has decreased the prevalence of RhD alloimmunization in pregnancy so that only approximately 6 cases occur in every 1000 live births. Its rarity means that most obstetricians are inexperienced and thus warrants consideration of consultation with, or referral to a maternal-fetal medicine specialist with experience in the monitoring and treating sensitized pregnancies.

Noninvasive Evaluation

Once an alloimmunized woman is identified, the medical professional caring for the mother must make some estimate of the risk of fetal disease. The prediction of fetal risk by combining the maternal obstetric history and serologic examination is an imprecise art. The magnitude of fetal and neonatal disease typically progresses from one pregnancy to another. The risk of hydrops in the undiagnosed and untested pregnancy approximates 10% in the first sensitized pregnancy.[26]

If maternal indirect Coombs antibody titers are performed in the same hospital using constant techniques, the results are typically reproducible and of clinical value in predicting the presence or absence of fetal disease. The practitioner must be familiar with the laboratory's threshold to avoid clinical error. When the maternal titer is below that threshold, it should be repeated at monthly intervals. In the absence of a relevant clinical history, the fetus may be followed noninvasively by the measurement of the peak middle cerebral artery velocities once that critical titer is exceeded. The utility of antibody titers above the threshold in predicting fetal risk is greatest during the first sensitized pregnancy. In subsequent pregnancies, titer and history are inadequate measures upon which to base management. Bowman and Pollack reported in 1965[47] that a lethal management error would occur in a third of severely sensitized fetuses if only maternal obstetric history and antibody titer were relied upon.

One of the most important advances in the management of fetal hemolytic anemia since the late 1990s is the development and application of molecular tools to determine the fetal genotype for most of the offending RBC antigens. It is possible using PCR to rapidly and accurately determine the fetal antigen status from either maternal blood, amniocytes, or a placental biopsy specimen.[48–54] It is time that Rh-negative women were routinely tested for the fetal genotype in the early second trimester using a peripheral blood sample. This practice would reduce the use of Rh immunoglobulin by over 40% with proportional decreases in serial laboratory samples and ultrasound examinations. At the very least, determination of the fetal Rh genotype should be standard after any second-trimester amniocentesis or chorionic villus sampling (CVS) in an at-risk woman.

Ultrasound evidence of fetal anemia determines the timing of invasive fetal testing. Brass and coworkers[55] were the first to observe in adults a relationship between the systolic flow velocity in the middle cerebral artery and hematocrit. Subsequently, several investigators demonstrated that the development of fetal anemia is associated with increased middle cerebral artery peak systolic velocities (Fig. 13–4).[56–58] Though at least half of anemic fetuses have normal peak velocities,[59] high peaks corrected for gestational age typically indicate moderate to severe anemia.

Other sonographic findings have been claimed to either precede the development of hydrops or predict fetal anemia, including amniotic fluid volume, liver and spleen length or thickness, placental thickness, increased bowel echogenicity, and the cardiac biventricular diameter.[32,60,61] Unfortunately, none of these sonographic markers is reliable. Further, the fetal hematocrit may change rapidly from one week to another. We have observed several fetuses with a normal hematocrit become hydropic over a 7-day period without a change in the maternal antibody titer. Each had a completely normal two-dimensional ultrasonographic examination 7 days before the detection of hydrops.

In summary, the measurement of middle cerebral artery peak velocities is an excellent noninvasive tool for the monitoring of fetal anemia. It is the standard of care for the pretherapeutic management of fetal hemolytic disease. Other than that, ultrasonography is an adjunct to, not a replacement for, invasive fetal studies.

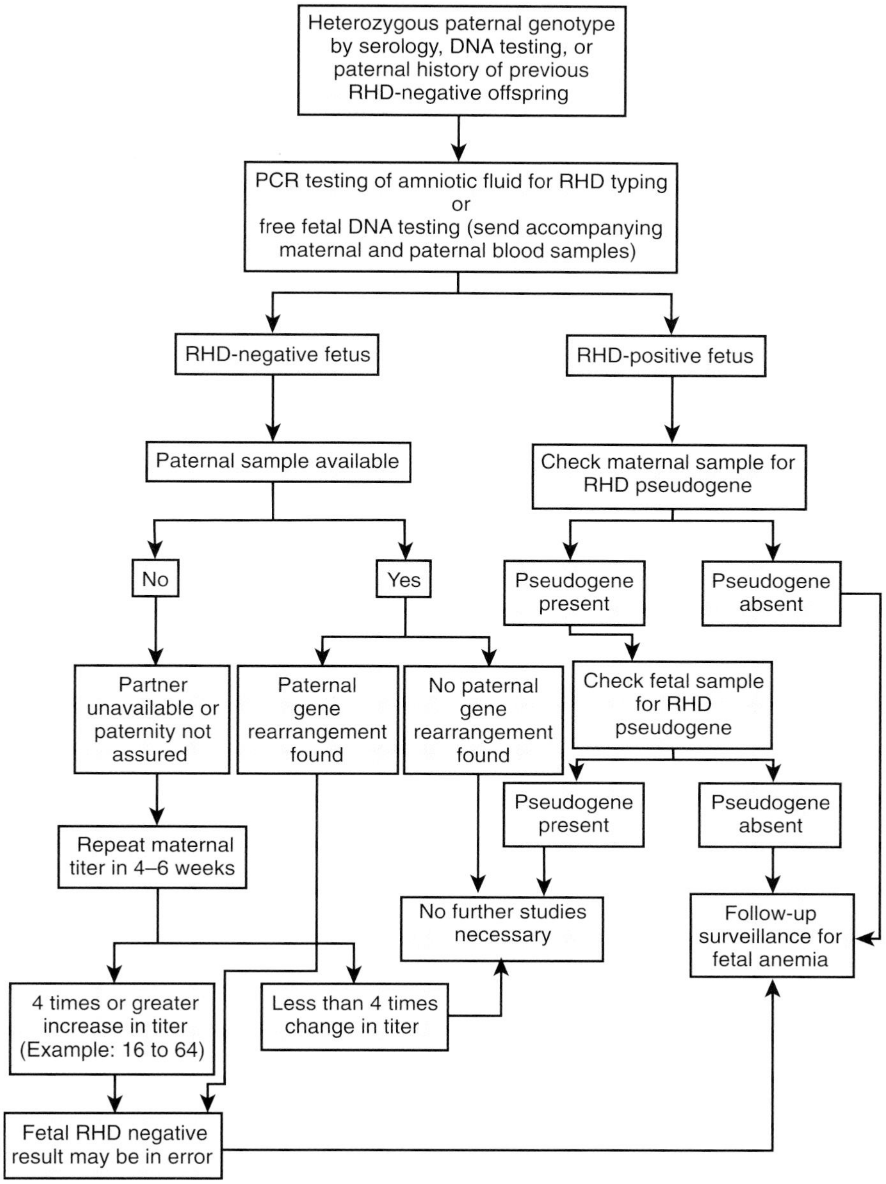

FIGURE 13–2
Sample algorithm for determining the fetal RhD status in the case of a maternal rhesus D antibodies and a heterozygous paternal genotype. PCR, polymerase chain reaction; RHD, rhesus D. (Modified from Moise KJ: Management of rhesus alloimmunization in pregnancy. Obstet Gynecol 2008;112:164-176.)

Invasive Evaluation

Two invasive methods have historically been used to search for fetal anemia secondary to hemolytic disease:

- Indirect: spectrophotometry (the ΔOD450) using a specimen of amniotic fluid obtained by ultrasound-guided amniocentesis.
- Direct: fetal blood studies using a sample obtained by fetal blood sampling.

The argument over which technique to use ended with the development of peak middle cerebral artery flow velocity. If the patient is not already being followed in a center with expertise in the management and treatment of fetal hemolytic disease, she should be referred to one immediately upon discovery of an elevated peak middle cerebral artery flow velocity. There, a fetal blood sample should be obtained and, if fetal anemia is confirmed, treatment initiated. If the fetus is not anemic, the interval until the next sample is determined by the hematologic profile described subsequently. The following information on amniotic fluid spectrophotometry is provided for practitioners who practice in areas with no other options.

AMNIOTIC FLUID SPECTROPHOTOMETRY

The fetus with hemolytic anemia frequently has an elevated serum bilirubin (Fig. 13–5).[31] By the middle of the second trimester, the amniotic fluid consists predominantly of fetal urine and tracheopulmonary effluent; thus, the amniotic fluid

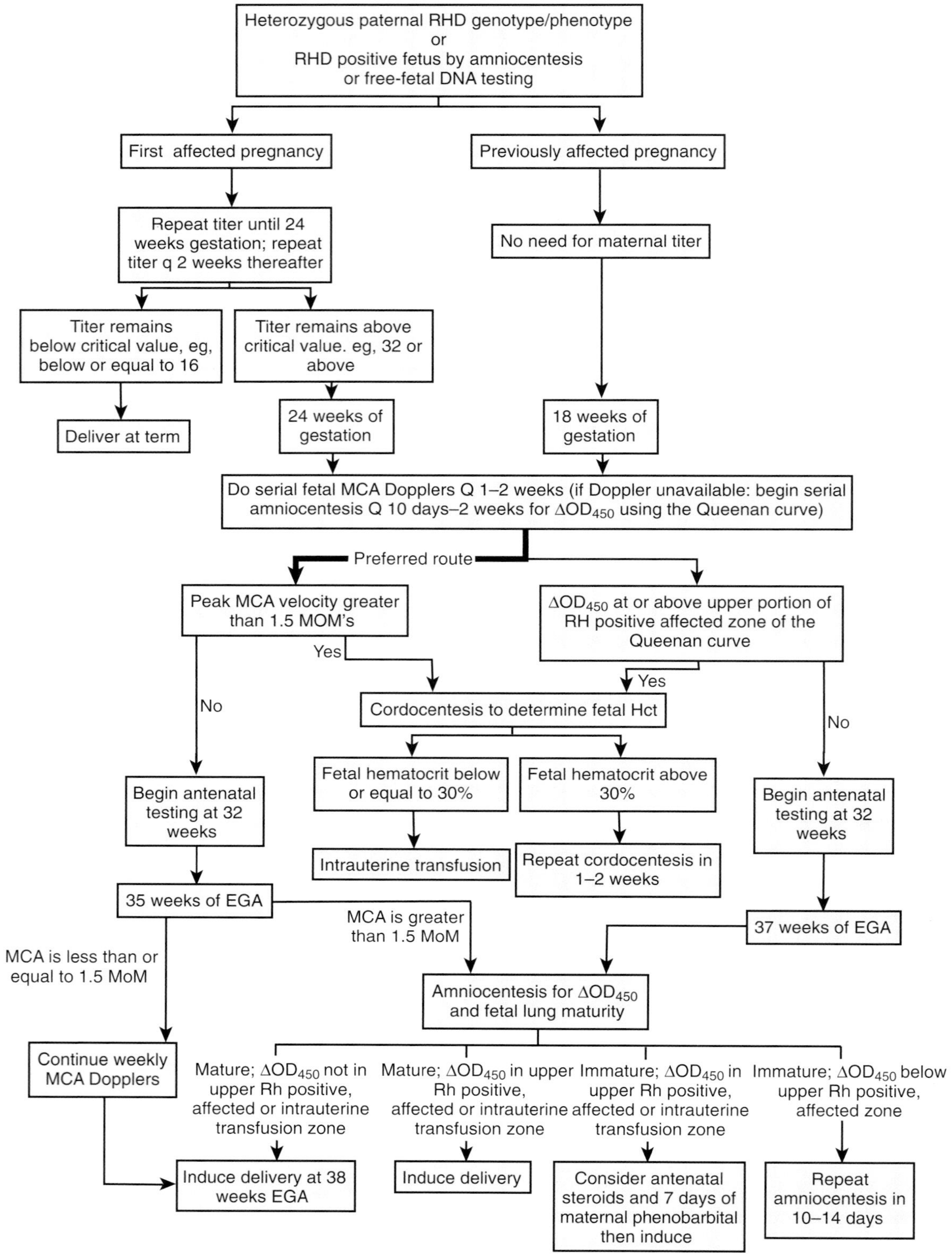

FIGURE 13–3

Algorithm for the overall management of the pregnant patient with RhD alloimmunization. EGA, estimated gestational age; Hct, hematocrit; MCA, middle cerebral artery; MoM, multiple of the median; Rh, rhesus.

(Modified from Moise KJ: Management of rhesus alloimmunization in pregnancy. Obstet Gynecol 2008;112:164-176.)

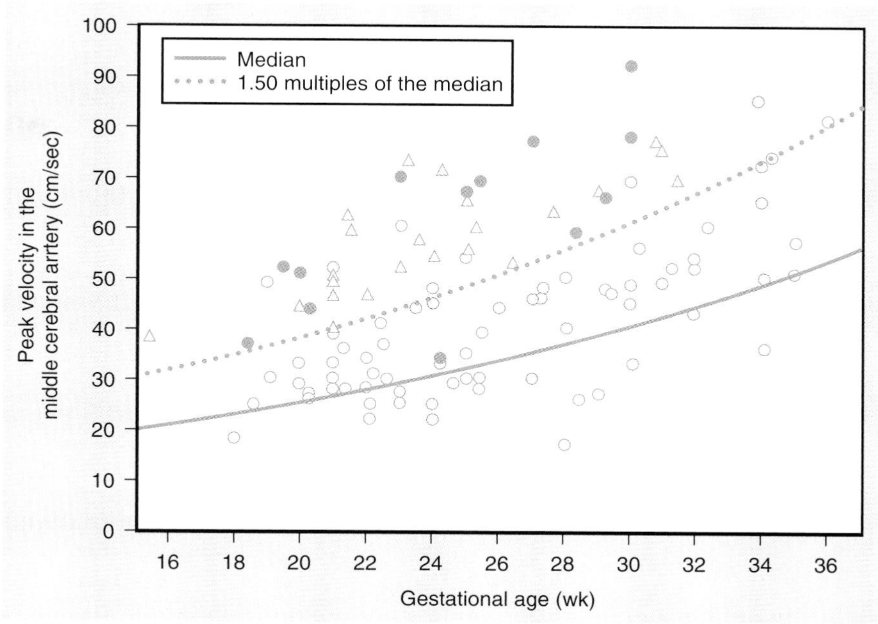

FIGURE 13–4
Peak velocity of systolic blood flow in the middle cerebral artery in 111 fetuses at risk for anemia due to maternal red cell alloimmunization. *Open circles* indicate fetuses with either no anemia or mild anemia (≥0.65 MoM hemoglobin concentration). *Triangles* indicate fetuses with moderate or severe anemia (<0.65 MoM hemoglobin concentration). *Solid circles* indicate the fetuses with hydrops. The *Solid curve* indicates the median peak systolic velocity in the middle cerebral artery, and the *dotted curve* indicates 1.5 MoM.
(From Mari G, Deter RL, Carpenter RL, et al: Noninvasive diagnosis by Doppler ultrasonography of fetal anemia due to maternal red cell alloimmunization. Collaborative Group for Doppler Assessment of the Blood Velocity in Anemic Fetuses. N Engl J Med 2000;342:9–14.)

bilirubin is also elevated. Although William Liley[4] was not the first to use amniotic fluid spectrophotometry for the management of rhesus disease, he standardized an approach that has remained essentially unchanged since first reported in 1961. Although the ΔOD450 satisfactorily predicts the relative fetal hematocrit when used appropriately, it is best at predicting hydrops.

Amniotic fluid is obtained by ultrasound-guided amniocentesis (see Chapter 9), transported to the laboratory in a light-resistant container to prevent degradation of bilirubin, centrifuged, and filtered. If the fetal blood type is unknown, an aliquot of the sample should be subjected to PCR to confirm the fetal genotype is antigen positive.

The optical density (OD) is measured between 700 and 350 nm and plotted on semilogarithmic graph paper with the wavelength on the x-axis. A line parallel to the y-axis is drawn through 450 nm, and the deviation from linearity of the absorption trace measured at that point. The result is plotted on semilogarithmic paper with gestational age on the x-axis and ΔOD450 on the y-axis (Fig. 13–6). Based on the study of 101 amniotic fluid specimens from sensitized pregnancies obtained between 28 and 35 weeks' gestation, Liley[4] observed that the ΔOD450 normally declined with advancing gestation (the opposite direction of the fetal serum bilirubin concentration) (Fig. 13–7). The graph is divided into three ascending zones. Zone 1 represents mild or no fetal disease. Zone 3 indicates severe disease with the possibility of hydrops developing within 7 days. Zone 2 is intermediate, with the disease severity increasing as zone 3 is approached. Amniocentesis is repeated at 1- to 2-week intervals, depending on the gestational age, the zone of the ΔOD450, and the change from the preceding sample. Management is dictated by the trend revealed by serial values. A fetal blood sample is performed when either the ΔOD450 is in zone 3 or serial amniotic fluid specimens reveal a progressive and rapid rise of the ΔOD450 into the upper 80% of zone 2.

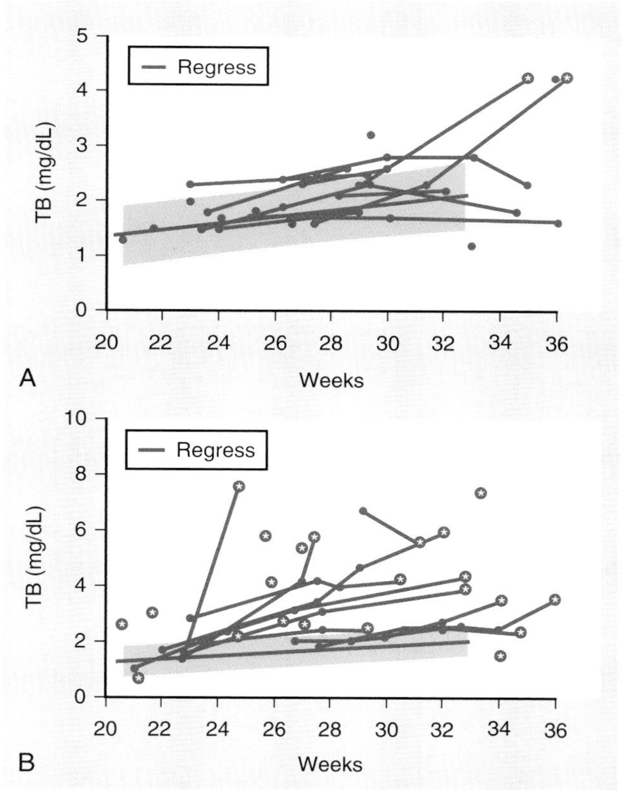

FIGURE 13–5
Effect of hemolytic disease on the fetal total bilirubin (TB) concentration comparing fetuses who do not (*A*) to those who do (*B*) develop anemia. * indicates at which point a hematocrit < 30% was first discovered.
(From Weiner CP, Williamson RA, Wenstrom KD, et al: Management of fetal hemolytic disease by cordocentesis: I. Prediction of fetal anemia. Am J Obstet Gynecol 1991;165:546–553.)

The determination of hemolytic disease severity by amniotic fluid spectrophotometry has several important disadvantages. First, its application requires serial invasive procedures over the space of several weeks. In a 20-year experience that included 1027 women, Bowman[26] performed a mean of 3.1 procedures per patient. Each procedure carries a risk of enhanced maternal sensitization as well as a loss from either amnionitis or premature rupture of the membranes. Though there are no large series reported of women undergoing amniocentesis after 22 weeks' gestation to document the frequency of such complications, some conclusions may be drawn from studies of second-trimester genetic amniocenteses. Amniocentesis performed under ultrasound guidance is clearly associated with sensitization, amnionitis, and rupture of membranes (~1 in 300–400). Simplicity does not mean safe.

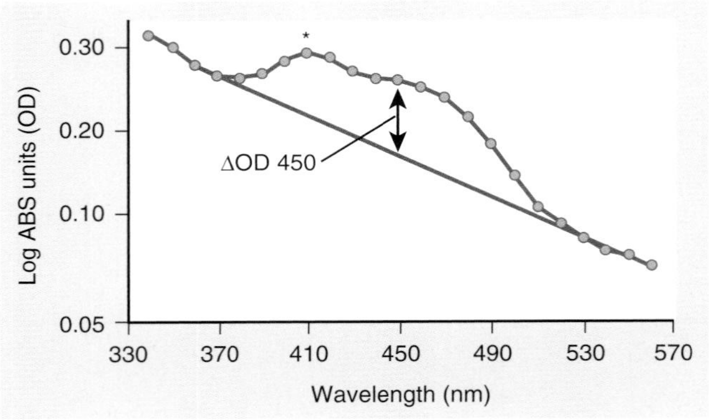

FIGURE 13–6
Semilogarithmic plot of an amniotic fluid ΔOD450. * illustrates a spike in the absorption of light produced by contaminating blood.
(Courtesy of G. Snyder, University of Iowa.)

Second, amniotic fluid spectrophotometry is an indirect test for fetal anemia. The natural history studies by Liley[4,5] revealed a wide range of disease severity for a given ΔOD450 at any gestational age between 28 and 34 weeks (see Fig. 13–7). Liley's postnatal observation is confirmed antenatally using fetal blood sampling. Though most obvious for zone 2, it is also true for zone 3 measurements. In a series of 11 fetuses with a ΔOD450 in zone 3 followed for several weeks, 30% had a clinically acceptable hematocrit at birth.[62] Gottval and Hilden[63] concluded that the maternal indirect Coombs titer was actually superior to the ΔOD450 for the prediction of fetal anemia, and yet the titers were useful only when less than 32 or more than 1000.

The third disadvantage of amniocentesis and the ΔOD450 is that the system was modeled on anti-D alloimmunization. This author and others have shown that Kell

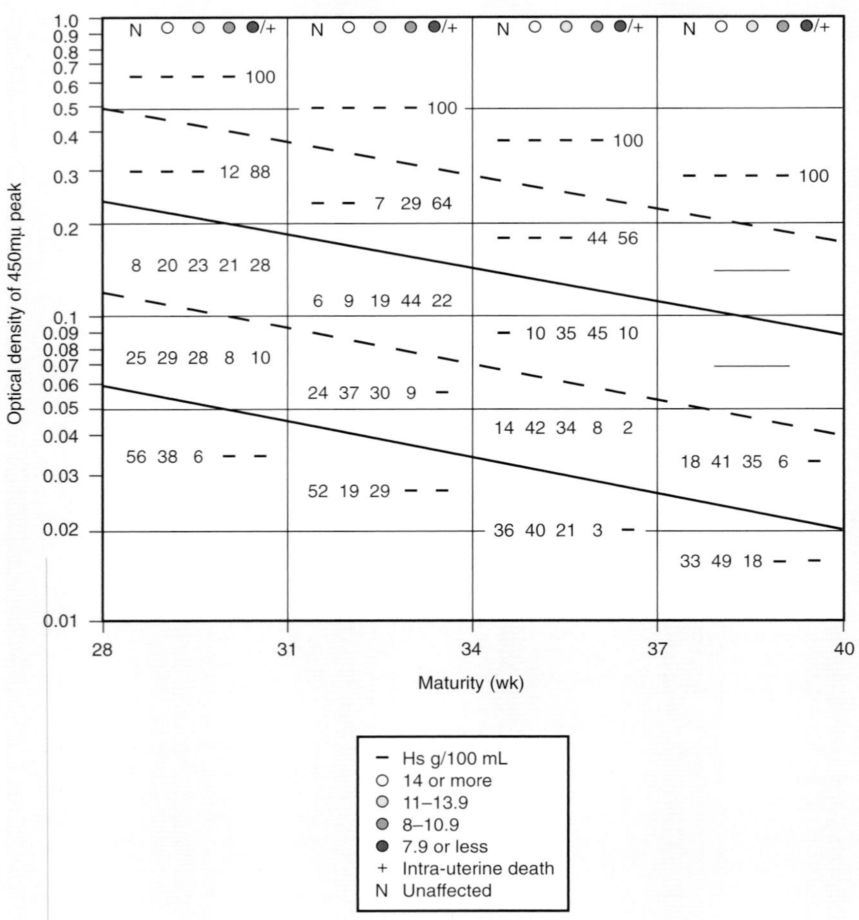

FIGURE 13–7
Relationship between the ΔOD450, hemoglobin, and gestational age. Note, for example, that of fetuses between 28 and 31 weeks and a ΔOD450 in low zone 2, 25% are unaffected, whereas 18% are either profoundly anemic or dead.
(From Liley AW: Liquor amnii analysis and management of pregnancy complicated by rhesus immunization. Am J Obstet Gynecol 1961;82:1359-1368.)

alloimmunization has salient pathophysiologic differences that account for the very poor performance of the ΔOD450 reported in the past.[64,65] Fetuses with Kell alloimmunization have lower serum bilirubin concentrations and lower reticulocyte levels for their degree of anemia compared with D-alloimmunized fetuses. Vaughan and colleagues[66,67] found that monoclonal IgG and IgM anti-Kell antibodies inhibit the growth of Kell-positive erythroid burst-forming units and colony-forming units in a dose-dependent fashion. This suggests that the fetal anemia secondary to Kell reflects erythroid suppression at the progenitor cell level.

The fourth disadvantage of amniocentesis is that the normal ΔOD450 in the second trimester is mid zone 2 of the Liley curve. Some have concluded that there is no clinically useful correlation between the ΔOD450 reading and the fetal hemoglobin before 28 weeks.[68] Yet, amniocentesis is often initiated weeks earlier.

The fifth disadvantage of the ΔOD450 measurement is that it is subject to a variety of extrinsic errors that can interfere with its laboratory measurement, for example, maternal hyperbilirubinemia and specimen contamination with blood or meconium.

In summary, the ΔOD450 is an outdated tool and should be performed only when there is no other option because it is inferior in accuracy and arguably more dangerous for mother and child.

FETAL BLOOD SAMPLING

The safety of fetal blood sampling is detailed in Chapter 9. The loss rate reflects the indication for the procedure, the presence of hypoxemia, the vessel actually punctured, and the technique used (needle guide vs. freehand).[69,70] It has been estimated that technique accounts for at least 30% of losses. Using a needle guide, the loss rate for alloimmunization is less than 0.3%, a rate similar to that of amniocentesis. Further, the size of the fetal-maternal bleed after fetal blood sampling when a needle guide is used and the placenta is not punctured is similar to that after amniocentesis.[71] It has been suggested that the magnitude of the bleed is much greater when the freehand technique is used.

The first fetal blood sample is taken when the peak middle cerebral artery velocity becomes elevated. Laboratory tests performed on the first and subsequent fetal blood samples are listed in Table 13–4. Either a strongly positive direct Coombs test or a manual reticulocyte count outside the 95% confidence interval (Fig. 13–8) is a high risk factor for the development of antenatal anemia if the fetus is not anemic when sampled.[72]

A sensitive and specific assessment of the risk for developing anemia in the 30% to 50% of nonanemic fetuses can be made using direct fetal hematologic and serologic tests (Fig. 13–9). A prospectively validated protocol for risk assessment and the timing of any repeat fetal blood sampling are shown in Table 13–5. There is a direct correlation between the reticulocyte count, the strength of the direct Coombs test, the risk of fetal anemia, and the trimester in which it occurs.[17] Untreated neonates remain at significant risk for postnatal complications (Table 13–6).[72]

Delivery of the nontransfused affected fetus is planned between 37 and 38 weeks' gestation in a medical center capable of caring for a neonate with potentially severe hyperbilirubinemia.

TABLE 13–4

Fetal Hematologic and Serologic Testing for the Prediction of Anemia

First Specimen
ABO and Rh type
Direct Coombs test
CBC
Manual reticulocyte count (%RBCs)
Total bilirubin
Subsequent Specimens
CBC
Manual reticulocyte count (%RBCs)
Total bilirubin

CBC, complete blood count; RBCs, red blood cells.

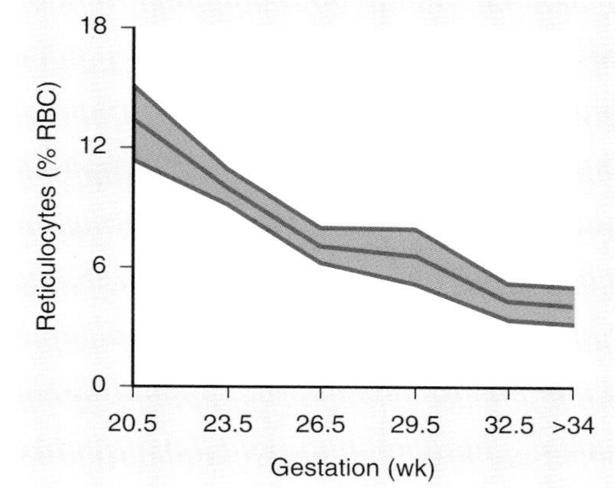

FIGURE 13–8
Normal fetal reticulocyte count across gestation illustrated as the 95% prediction interval.
(From Weiner CP, Williamson RA, Wenstrom KD, et al: Management of fetal hemolytic disease by cordocentesis: I. Prediction of fetal anemia. Am J Obstet Gynecol 1991;165:546–553.)

Treatment Options

SUPPRESSION OF MATERNAL ANTI-ERYTHROCYTE ANTIBODIES

Several methods are used in severely sensitized women to suppress or ameliorate either the maternal antibody concentration or its effect on the fetus. None are of proven efficacy.

Plasmapheresis

Although plasmapheresis reduces antibody concentration by as much as 80%,[73] the decline is transient. Plasmapheresis may delay the need for fetal transfusion by a few weeks. This costly procedure is indicated only when there is a history of hydrops prior to 20 to 22 weeks and the father is homozygous for the offending antigen. Plasmapheresis is begun at 12 weeks, removing 15 to 20 L/wk. It entails a risk of hepatitis and should not be undertaken lightly.

Immunoglobulin

The maternal intravenous infusion of immunoglobulin (400–500 mg/kg maternal weight every 4 wk) reportedly reduces

FIGURE 13–9
Likelihood of a fetus requiring transfusion based on its hematologic pattern.
(From Weiner CP, Williamson RA, Wenstrom KD, et al: Management of fetal hemolytic disease by cordocentesis: I. Prediction of fetal anemia. Am J Obstet Gynecol 1991;165:546-553.)

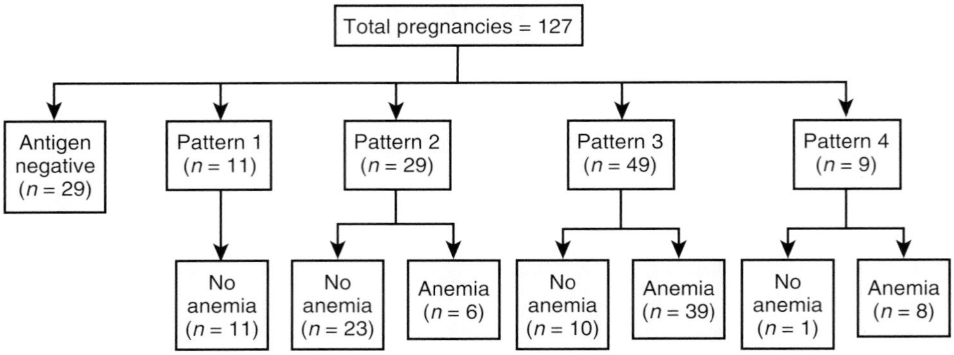

TABLE 13–5

Criteria for Repeat Fetal Blood Sampling with an Affected Fetus

PATTERN	HEMATOCRIT	RETICULOCYTES	AND/OR DC	FBS INTERVAL	SCAN	COMMENTS
1	Normal	Normal	-/tr	–	4-wk interval	Repeat if initial maternal indirect Coombs <128 and twofold increase documented.
2	Normal	Normal or < 2.5th percentile	J+/2+	5-6 wk	2-wk interval	Do not repeat after 32 wk if studies unchanged. Delivery at term.
3	Normal	>97.5th percentile	3+/4+	2 wk	1-wk interval	Continue through 34 wk if hematocrit stable. Deliver at 37-38 wk if not transfused.
4	<2.5th percentile but >30%	Any	Any	1-2 wk	1-wk interval	Repeat as long as hematocrit criteria fulfilled. Deliver with pulmonary maturity if not transfused.

DC, direct Coombs; FBS, fetal blood sampling.
Modified from Weiner CP, Heilskov J, Pelzer G, et al: Normal values for human umbilical venous amniotic fluid pressures and their alteration by fetal disease. Am J Obstet Gynecol 1989;161:714–717.

TABLE 13–6

Neonatal Complications in Affected, Untreated, Pregnancies

	N	%	MEAN	SD	RANGE
Gestation (wk)	48	100	38	2	34-41
Birth weight (g)	48	100	3176	552	2010-4171
Hematocrit (%)	23	47	47	9	24-59
Reticulocytes	10	21	9.2	7	2.8-28
Maximum total bilirubin (mg/dL)	28	58	14.9	5	5-23
Phototherapy (hr)					
No	17	36	–	–	–
Yes	31	64	110	60	23-240
DVET	8	17	–	–	–
Late transfusion*	6	13			

* Late transfusion, performed in the first 3 wk of life for anemia not present.
DVET, double-volume exchange transfusion; SD, standard deviation.
Modified from Weiner CP, Grant SS, Hudson J, et al: Effect of diagnostic and therapeutic cordocentesis upon maternal serum alpha fetoprotein concentration. Am J Obstet Gynecol 1989;161:706–708.

the severity of fetal hemolytic disease.[74] There are no prospective randomized trials. Rarely indicated alone in light of the currently available therapies, intravenous immunoglobulin may be effective as an adjunct to plasmapheresis.[75] Another option is to administer the immunoglobulin directly to the infused fetus. Several abstracts suggest that such fetal therapy has the potential to reduce the frequency of transfusion therapy.[76–80] Yet, the usual interval between transfusions at those institutions was shorter than recommended here.

FETAL TRANSFUSION

Fetal transfusion therapy should not be undertaken in the absence of hydrops without first confirming that the fetus has significant anemia. The author has recommended a hematocrit below 30% because it is below the 2.5th percentile for all gestational ages older than 20 weeks.[72] These procedures should be performed only by individuals with considerable and regular experience whenever possible.

Intraperitoneal Injection

The original, but least preferred, method for fetal transfusion is the intraperitoneal injection of packed RBCs that are

TABLE 13–7
Protocol for Fetal Intraperitoneal Transfusion

Preparation	
Confirm fetal hematocrit <30%	
Prepare donor blood as fresh as possible and compatible with both mother and fetus	
Buffy coat poor, washed in saline ×3, and irradiated	
Final hematocrit 90% ideal	
Prepare two sets of tubing with three-way valves for transfusion; filters are mandatory	
Diazepam, 5–10 mg slow IV for maternal comfort	
Lateral displacement of the uterus, support lower back	
Acetone wipe to remove ultrasound contact gel from the skin	
Povidone-iodine or alcohol surgical preparation of the skin	
Drape as desired and prepare surgical tray	
20-g Tuohy needle 25 cm long	
20-mL syringe	
5-mL normal saline	
Pancuronium, 0.3 mg/kg estimated fetal weight	
Sterile prepare ultrasound transducer	
Transfusion	
Target fetal abdomen between umbilicus and bladder; avoid liver	
Administer pancuronium intramuscularly targeting the fetal buttock	
Insert Tuohy needle into selected site	
Confirm intra-abdominal, extravascular location by injecting saline	
Infuse donor blood in 1-mL aliquots over 10 min checking the fetal heart rate after each aliquot	
Continue transfusion until planned volume infused calculated by volume = (wk gestation − 20) × 10 mL	
Follow-up	
Continuous heart rate monitoring until fetal movement resumes	
Document complete absorption of donor blood by serial ultrasonography	
Examinations every 2–3 days	
Second transfusion after complete absorption; thereafter, repeat at 4-wk intervals	

absorbed via the lymphatic vessels with fetal respiration for absorption. It is rarely indicated in modern fetal medicine, typically with severe disease prior to 18 weeks' gestation. The protocol used in our unit is shown in Table 13–7. Approximately 10% of the transfused cells are absorbed daily by the nonhydropic fetus; absorption is greatly decreased in hydrops. The volume infused is a compromise between the amount necessary to correct the estimated hemoglobin deficit and the amount that will safely fill the intra-abdominal cavity. The formula of Bowman is practical:

$$\text{Volume} = (\text{weeks' gestation} - 20) \times 10\ \text{mL}$$

Once absorption is complete, the residual hemoglobin concentration may be estimated by the following equation:

$$\text{Residual hemoglobin concentration} = ((0.8x)/(125y)) \times ((120 - z\ \text{days})/120\ \text{days})$$

where x is the amount of donor blood in grams transfused, y is the estimated fetal weight, z is the interval in days since the last transfusion, and 120 is the estimated life (in days) of the transfused blood.

The second transfusion is performed after the first has been completely absorbed and subsequently at 3- to 4-week intervals. If the fetus is hydropic and survives the first intraperitoneal transfusion, the fetal abdomen is drained at the time of second transfusion to minimize pressure and maximize the volume of fresh cells infused. The last transfusion is performed no later than 32 weeks' gestation.

Intraperitoneal transfusion has many drawbacks. In addition to a slow correction of the hemoglobin deficit, there is a higher risk of trauma and the unique risk of obstructing cardiac return should intra-abdominal pressure rise too high. Intraperitoneal transfusion should be performed only when percutaneous access to the fetal vasculature is problematic (e.g., <18 wk). Nor is there any advantage to combining intravascular and intraperitoneal transfusions. The combined intraperitoneal/intravascular procedure does not reduce the actual number of required needle punctures. The highest reported survival rates with intraperitoneal transfusion are well below those for intravascular transfusion.[81–83] The risk of fetal death per transfusion was six times that of intravascular transfusion in a comparison of historical data from an experienced team in Winnipeg, Canada.[83]

In summary, intraperitoneal transfusion is rarely indicated in the modern practice of fetal medicine.

Intravascular Transfusion

In contrast to intraperitoneal transfusion, the goal of intravascular transfusion therapy is the delivery of a healthy, nonanemic neonate at term when it can better transition to ex utero life and withstand the associated hyperbilirubinemia. Transfusions are begun when the fetal hematocrit declines below 30%.[35] Though most fetuses tolerate a hematocrit of 25% or lower without clinically significant sequelae, this cutoff point has proved a pragmatic threshold for the following reasons:

- Hematocrit of 30% is below the 2.5th percentile after 20 weeks' gestation (Fig. 13–10).
- Women referred often travel great distances and cannot come either semiweekly or even weekly without great hardship.
- It is difficult to predict with certainty how fast the fetal hematocrit will decline.
- Treatment of anemia prevents the development of hydrops that would greatly increase the chance of an adverse outcome.

The protocol used in our unit for intravascular transfusion is shown in Table 13–8. Blood for the transfusion should be fresh when available, and compatible with both mother and fetus. Infectious agents routinely tested for include cytomegalovirus (CMV), hepatitis A through C, and HIV. Some blood banks use a lymphocyte filter in lieu of serologic testing for CMV. This procedure has the added benefit of reducing the risk of graft-versus-host disease without irradiating the blood. The blood is prepared on the day of transfusion, rendered leukocyte poor, and washed several times in saline to remove particles associated with viral transmission infection. It is then resuspended in saline to a hematocrit between 70% and 80%. Blood with a higher hematocrit mixes poorly; that with a lower hematocrit unnecessarily increases the volume required.

The patient is made comfortable with pillows under her knees to take pressure off the lower back. The uterus is

FIGURE 13–10
Normal fetal hematocrit across gestation illustrated as the 95% prediction interval.
(From Weiner CP, Williamson RA, Wenstrom KD, et al: Management of fetal hemolytic disease by cordocentesis: I. Prediction of fetal anemia. Am J Obstet Gynecol 1991;165:546–553.)

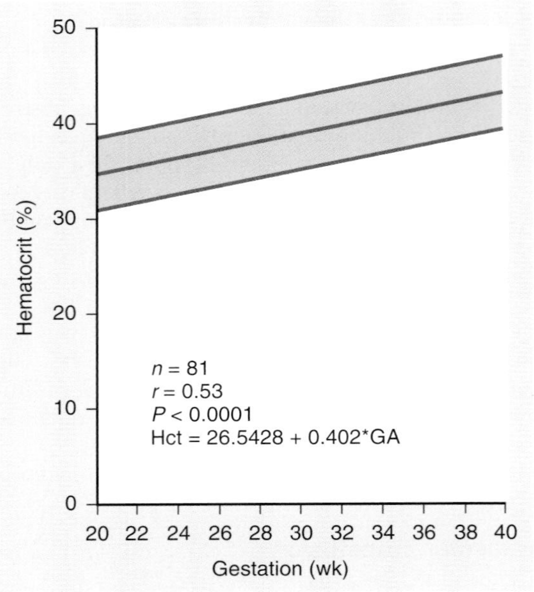

TABLE 13–8

Protocol for Fetal Intravascular Transfusion

Preparation

Confirm fetal hematocrit <30%
Preparation of donor blood as fresh as possible and compatible with both mother and fetus
Buffy coat poor, washed in saline ×3, irradiated
Final hematocrit 70%–80%
Preparation two sets of tubing for transfusion and measurement of UVP
Filters are mandatory
Diazepam, 5–10 mg slow IV for maternal comfort
Lateral displacement of the uterus, support lower back
Acetone wipe to remove ultrasound contact gel from the skin
Povidone-iodine or alcohol surgical preparation of the skin
Drape as desired and prepare surgical tray
- Eight 1-mL tuberculin syringes
- Flush three with heparin (100 U/mL); fill one with lidocaine (1%), and fill one with desired dose of pancuronium (0.3 mg/kg sonographically estimated fetal weight)
- Three 3-way valves
- One 5 inch (12 cm) 22-gauge needle
- Three 4 × 4 gauze sponges

Prepare transducer

Transfusion

Puncture vein at most accessible site
Immediately administer pancuronium—paralysis will be rapid
Aspirate 1 mL for complete blood count, Kleihauer stain, and reticulocyte count; check hematocrit immediately
Aspirate 1 mL for venous blood gases
Measure pressure and confirm puncture is of umbilical vein
Begin infusion of packed red blood cells after double-checking that there is no air in the system
Infuse half the estimated requirement (see Table 13-9)
Repeat blood sampling and pressure measurement
Halt transfusion if the rise in the UVP has exceeded 10 mm Hg; check heart rate to rule out bradycardia as an explanation
If UVP is acceptable, calculate remaining volume necessary to achieve a hematocrit of 50%; infuse that volume
Repeat blood sampling and pressure measurement; remove needle if UVP is at acceptable level
Monitor fetus until spontaneous movement resumes

UVP, umbilical venous pressure.

displaced laterally to avoid supine hypotension during the transfusion. Because the transfusion takes on average 25 to 30 minutes for completion, diazepam 5 to 10 mg intravenously is given to enhance maternal comfort and cooperation. The abdomen is surgically prepared and draped, and the operator's hands are gloved. Neither a surgical mask nor a cap is necessary. Nor is there evidence that prophylactic antibiotic administration is either effective or cost-efficient. The skin is the main source of bacterial contamination. The operator must never touch the shaft of the needle. A new needle is used if one must be removed after insertion into the skin. With this protocol, the incidence of amnionitis is less than 0.5%. The skin is infiltrated with 1% lidocaine in light of the duration of time the needle is in situ.

The easiest approach to the umbilical vein is selected and punctured with a 22-gauge needle. Forty percent of the author's transfusions are performed in a free loop of cord. The intrahepatic portion of the umbilical vein is preferred by some operators. A larger-gauge needle unnecessarily increases the risk of premature rupture of the membranes. Immediately following the free return of blood, the fetus is paralyzed with pancuronium (~0.3 mg/kg of the estimated fetal weight [EFW], range 0.2–0.6 mg/kg), regardless of the puncture location, because any fetal movement may lacerate the vessel or dislodge the needle. Should the latter occur during transfusion, a catastrophic Wharton jelly hematoma with concomitant decrease in umbilical blood flow can sult. Pancuronium, as opposed to other agents used for uromuscular blockade, has the advantage of increasing rt rate secondary to catecholamine release. There is no advantage to not paralyzing the fetus. Without pancuronium, intravascular transfusion decreases both the fetal heart rate and cardiac output, prolonging the time required for the fetus to clear the acid contained in the preserved banked donor blood. With pancuronium, the fetal heart rate remains at or above the pretransfusion rate. The injection of the pancuronium, followed by the measurement of the umbilical venous pressure, allows for the definitive identification of the vessel punctured. The needle is removed if the artery is inadvertently entered because the risk of fetal bradycardia is fivefold greater than that for the vein. Though furosemide is used (3 mg/kg EFW) by some, including the author, clinical and laboratory investigations have failed to show measurable benefit.[84]

The equipment for an intravascular transfusion is illustrated in Figure 13–11. The blood must be filtered immediately prior to transfusion to remove aggregates that could occlude the microvasculature. Careful attention is paid so as to purge the system of all air. Using a series of three-way valves, an assistant injects the donor blood while the operator is free to concentrate on the fetus and needle placement.

FIGURE 13–11
Setup for an intravascular transfusion.

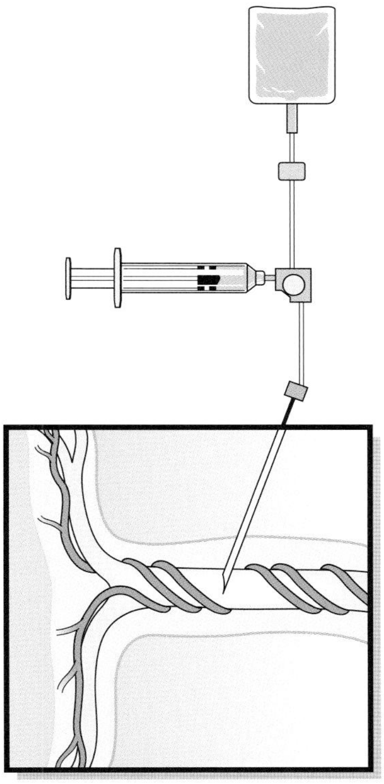

TABLE 13–9

Approximate Volumes of 72% Hematocrit Blood Required for Intravascular Transfusion after the First Transfusion

GESTATION (WK)	VOLUME (ML)
≤22.5	25-40
22.5-27.49	45-65
27.5-32.49	75-90
≥32.5	100-120

The assistant must remain poised to halt the infusion if there is any abrupt change in flow resistance. To minimize the time the needle is in place, the blood is infused with haste (5–10 mL/min).

Except for the first transfusion of a hydropic fetus described later, the post-transfusion target for the fetal hematocrit is 48% to 55%. The volume required depends on gestational age and the initial hematocrit. Assuming similar opening and closing hematocrit measurements at each transfusion, the volume infused is dependent on the gestational age (Table 13–9).

HYDROPS

Because hydropic fetuses have myocardial dysfunction that prevents them from tolerating the required infusion volume,[37] the target hematocrit after their first transfusion is only 25%. Twenty-four hours later, the hematocrit can be safely brought to 50% during a second transfusion. The decline in umbilical vein pH (UVpH) that normally occurs during transfusion is especially important to the severely anemic fetus. The RBC is the principal fetal buffer, and the pH of the citrated banked blood is 6.98 to 7.01. Our losses of hydropic fetuses after transfusion occurred even though the increase in their umbilical venous pressure during the procedure was acceptable and there was no acute bradycardia. All losses, however, were associated with a profound acidemia, and the deaths occurred hours after transfusion. It is suggested the acidemia aggravates myocardial failure. We now infuse bicarbonate in 1-mEq increments to maintain the UVpH above 7.30. There have been no further losses since that practice was initiated in 1988, and the overall survival rate for hydropic fetuses using this protocol now exceeds 95% in our center.

Several formulas have been proposed to calculate the volume of blood necessary to correct the hemoglobin deficit. Though reasonably accurate, none is reliable enough to remove the needle without first checking the hematocrit. Further, there is a possibility of overtransfusion when any formula is relied upon blindly. The author prefers to transfuse half the estimated total volume and then check the hematocrit. Based on the increase in hematocrit achieved following the first aliquot, the remaining volume necessary is rapidly and accurately calculated. Contrary to the adult or child, donor blood with a hematocrit below 80% equilibrates rapidly, perhaps because of the rapid fluid exchange across the placenta. On multiple occasions, the author has found that the hematocrit 24 hours after the transfusion to be within a few percentage points of the closing hematocrit. However, transfused blood with a hematocrit higher than 80% is more viscous and does not equilibrate as rapidly.

The decline in hematocrit after transfusion is more rapid and variable between the first and second transfusions compared with subsequent procedures. This variability results from the differing rates of destruction of disparate amounts of fetal antigen-positive and banked antigen-negative RBCs. Except for the hydropic fetus, the second transfusion is performed 2 weeks after the first. Subsequently, the decline in hematocrit per week is predictable for any given fetus (Fig. 13–12). The rate at which the hematocrit declines between transfusions with advancing gestation is such that by 34 to 35 weeks, delivery may be safely delayed 4 to 5 weeks until term without another transfusion. These findings have been confirmed.[85]

The fetus is monitored during transfusion. Many prefer to image the fetal heart at periodic intervals to rule out bradycardia; although important, it is of limited value. A second option is umbilical venous pressure measurement, which has several advantages. First, an occasional nonhydropic fetus (~5% in the author's experience) with a low hematocrit does not tolerate the transfusion volume necessary to correct the hemoglobin deficit. An increase in the umbilical venous pressure of more than 10 mm Hg is associated with an increased perinatal mortality rate. Either the transfusion should be halted or an appropriate volume of blood removed to reduce preload if the pressure rises more than 10 mm Hg.

FIGURE 13–12
The rate at which the hematocrit (HCT) declines per week after a transfusion. *Open triangles* reflect the interval decline between the first and the second transfusion. *Solid triangles* and the regression line reflect the decline in hematocrit per week between subsequent transfusions. Thus, if the fetus was transfused to 50% hematocrit at 22 weeks, we would expect it to decline approximately 9%/wk. Based on this estimate, the transfusion would be repeated in 2.5 weeks.

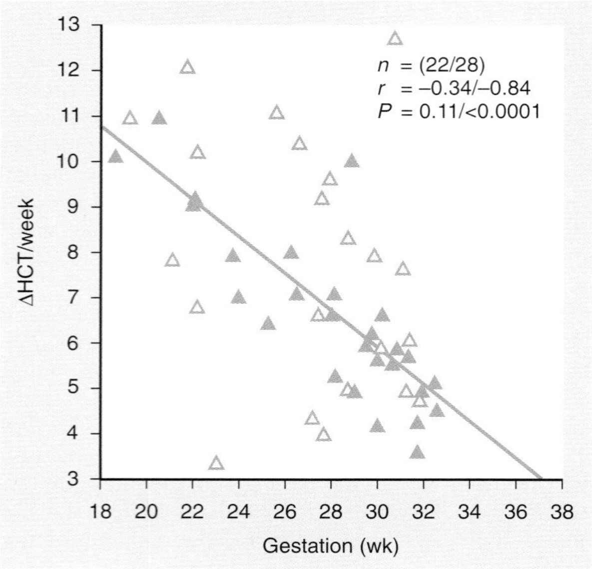

TABLE 13–10

Acute Nonhematologic Effects of Intravascular Transfusion

Cardiovascular
Increased intravascular volume
Decreased heart rate (without pancuronium)
Decreased cardiac output (without pancuronium)
Increased umbilical venous pressure
Increased renal blood flow
Decreased placental resistance measured by Doppler
Decreased aortic resistance measured by Doppler
Biochemical
Acidemia (blood preservative, inadequate fetal buffer capacity)
Increased oxygen-carrying capacity
Increased viscosity
Increased atrial natriuretic peptide
Increased prostacyclin
Increased prostaglandin E_2
Increased iron stores (chronic)

Second, fetal bradycardia increases the umbilical venous pressure. The third option is pulsed Doppler, which can also help differentiate the two causes of an elevated umbilical venous pressure by dropping a Doppler gate on the umbilical artery. Whichever technique is selected, it is important to keep the needle in place because any resuscitative efforts necessitated by a fetal bradycardia are facilitated by access to the fetal circulation.

Intravascular transfusion has many effects on the fetus (Table 13–10) other than raising the hematocrit.[86–88] Some, such as the increases in atrial natriuretic peptide and prostacyclin, help the fetus tolerate a volume load that postnatally would be lethal. Prostaglandin synthetase inhibitors are contraindicated for two reasons: (1) an increase in fetal prostacyclin and prostaglandin E_2 (PGE_2) is part of the normal adaptive response to the abrupt increase in intravascular volume[88] and (2) there is no evidence they are of any utility.

Adequate transfusion therapy rapidly suppresses fetal erythropoiesis. The fetal erythropoietin level declines and the average reticulocyte count is less than 1% by the third transfusion. It is advantageous to perform at least two transfusions 3 weeks apart prior to delivery because postnatal complications of hyperbilirubinemia are significantly less likely to occur after two or more antenatal transfusions.[36] In experienced hands, losses are uncommon and confined to e previable fetus. In the author's view, there is no justifican for routine preterm delivery. The last transfusion can ›erformed at 34 to 35 weeks' gestation and labor induced 7 to 38 weeks.

DELIVERY

The obstetric philosophy need not be altered for the nonanemic, transfused fetus. Antenatal transfusion is not a reason to deny a vaginal birth after cesarean section. If the final hematocrit at the end of the last transfusion was 50%, it will be in the mid-30s in the umbilical cord at delivery. Typically, the neonatal hematocrit increases approximately 15% within 8 hours of delivery, reflecting a massive shift of extracellular and intravascular fluid. The hematocrit then declines to or below the delivery level over the next few days to weeks.

POSTNATAL CARE

Postnatally, infants who received in utero transfusion therapy do remarkably well with an average hospitalization stay of less than 7 days (unpublished data). Because they are delivered at term, a higher peak neonatal bilirubin concentration is tolerated and is normally manageable with just phototherapy. Double-volume exchange transfusion is rarely needed when two or more antenatal transfusions are performed. Small, simple ("top-up") transfusions are frequently necessary, beginning at a few weeks of age, because fetal erythropoiesis has been suppressed by the regular transfusions (see later) and the banked blood transfused 5 weeks earlier is at the end of its life span. This anemia is typified by a low reticulocyte count. The neonatal hematocrit and reticulocyte count should be monitored weekly. If not, a severe anemia may escape detection with resulting high output cardiac failure and failure to thrive. The pediatric goal is to keep the neonate asymptomatic but with a modest anemia so as to drive erythropoiesis. Newborns may be 16 weeks old before reticulocytes reappear on the peripheral smear. Once a reticulocytosis is noted, further transfusion therapy is generally not needed. The need for neonatal transfusion can be decreased significantly by the administration of recombinant human erythropoietin.[89]

Effect of Anemia and Treatment on the Fetus

It is remarkable how well the fetus tolerates all but the most severe anemia. Fetuses who have a mild, chronic anemia are neither growth deficient nor acidemic. Though mild to moderate anemia is not associated with dramatic antenatal sequelae, severe anemia clearly is. As dramatic as hydrops fetalis may be, it is for the most part preventable and completely reversible. Hydropic fetuses not yet severely acidemic recover quickly with appropriate transfusion therapy and on long-term follow-up appear without specific sequelae.[90,91]

Transfusion therapy has a predictable and desirable effect on fetal erythropoiesis. With adequate RBC replacement, the reticulocyte count and percentage of circulating RBCs of fetal origin drops rapidly (Fig. 13–13). Part of this decline is due to consumption of newly formed fetal RBCs as they emerge from the fetal bone marrow and liver. However, after two transfusions correcting the hematocrit to 50%, smears of neonatal bone marrow reveal decreased erythrogenic precursors.[82] The greater the number of antenatal transfusions (i.e., the longer the period of fetal erythrocytic suppression) performed, the less severe the hyperbilirubinemia postnatally and the longer the suppression of erythropoiesis postnatally.[25] These findings coupled with the decrease in fetal plasma erythropoietin concentrations after several transfusions are indicative of marrow and liver suppression.

The long-term outcomes of the most severely affected fetuses have until recently been the subject of scant study. We conducted a case-control study of all 16 consecutive children born at the University of Iowa between July 1985 and August 1990 who as fetuses had intrauterine intravascular transfusion therapy for alloimmune hydrops fetalis.[87] Eight nonhydropic older siblings were control subjects. Hospital records were reviewed and parents completed behavioral questionnaires and were interviewed. Affected children and their sibling controls received comprehensive neuropsychological evaluations, hearing tests, and neurologic examinations. The hydrops children had cranial computed tomography (CT) scans for the measurement of brain and ventricular volumes. No significant differences were noted between the hydrops group and the sibling control group on neuropsychological measures (Table 13–11). Modest but statistically significant correlations were noted between the severity of anemia at the time of hydrops and composite standardized testing of nonverbal and computational skills at follow-up. The first child treated was electively delivered at 35 weeks. He suffered complications of kernicterus associated with a maximum bilirubin of 28 mg/dL. A second child who at 25 weeks' gestation experienced a prolonged fetal bradycardia (heart rate of 40 beats/min for 5 min) due to technical difficulties during an intra-arterial transfusion followed by delivery had cerebral palsy. The remaining 13 children had physical, neurologic, and neuropsychological findings within the normal range. Of the 16 CT scans, 14 were normal, and 2 revealed minor structural abnormalities. Mean total intracranial volume was 1477 mL. All intracranial volumes were within published normative values.

ABO INCOMPATIBILITY AND MINOR BLOOD GROUP ANTIGENS

ABO incompatibility rarely causes fetal disease because the antibodies are often IgM and because these antigens are not

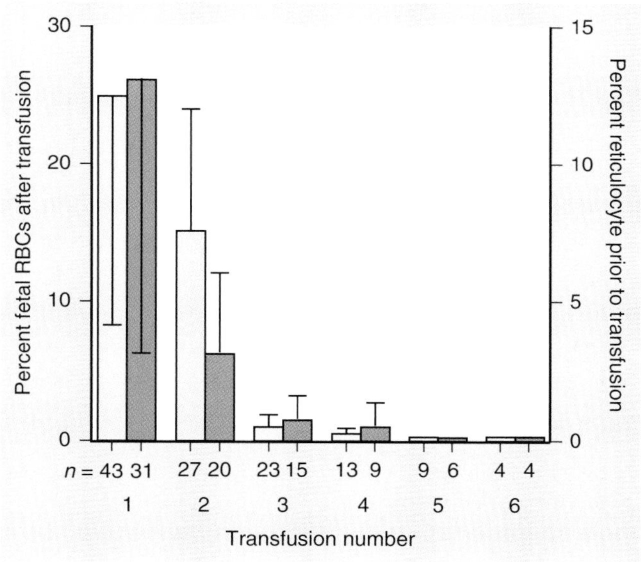

FIGURE 13–13
Effect of simple intravascular transfusion on the circulating fetal red blood cell (RBC) percentage (*M* left x-axis) and the percentage of RBCs that are reticulocytes (*M* right x-axis).

TABLE 13–11
Long-Term Outcome of Consecutive Hydropic Fetuses Treated in Utero

GROUP	HEMOGLOBIN AT g/100 mL	AGE F/U (yr)	COGNITIVE ACHIEVEMENT	VISUAL/ MOTORSPATIAL	ATTENTIONAL PROBLEMS (%)	MEMORY
Hydrops (*n* = 16)	3.5 ± 1.5	9.43	99.33	100.25	40	9.16
Sibcontrol (*n* = 8)	NA	11.93	107.50	107.37	25	10.58

F/U, follow-up; NA, not available.
From Swingle HM, Harper DC, Bonthius D, et al: Long-term Neurodevelopmental Follow-up and Brain Volumes of Children Following Severe Fetal Anemia with Hydrops. American Academy of Cerebral Palsy and Developmental Medicine, Sept. 29 to Oct. 1, Los Angeles, 2004.

SUMMARY OF MANAGEMENT OPTIONS

Fetal Hemolytic Disease

Management Options	Evidence Quality and Recommendation	References
Prevention of Rh Hemolytic Disease in Nonimmunized Women		
Routine screening in Rh-negative women at booking and regularly through pregnancy	III/B	30
Antenatal prophylaxis at delivery	Ib/A	46
Antenatal prophylaxis at 28–34 wk and at delivery	IIb/B	42
Prophylaxis after potential sensitizing events	III/B	44
Prediction of Disease Severity in Immunized Women		
Refer to experienced center when critical antibody titer reached	—/GPP	—
Noninvasive determination of fetal RhD status	III/B	48–54
Measure maternal serum anti-D antibody concentration serially	III/B	40
Sonographic imaging to predict severity of disease—poor without evidence of frank hydrops	III/B	61
Middle cerebral Doppler is reliable for noninvasive screening for the presence of fetal anemia	III/B	57
Amniocentesis bilirubin/ΔOD450 from 27–41 wk—three zones helpful in managing patients (true level of anemia not known)	III/B	4
Liley curves of amniotic fluid bilirubin/ΔOD450 between 18 and 25 wk detected only 32% of fetuses with an Hb <6 g/dL (appropriate management and survival may not be directly correlated with Hb <6 g/dL)	III/B	68
Fetal blood sampling is to be performed whenever the peak middle cerebral artery velocity is elevated to confirm the presence of anemia	III/B	57
Treatment		
Fetal blood transfusion is treatment of choice; intravascular (see Table 13–8) is preferable to intraperitoneal (see Table 13–7)	IIa/B	83
Intravascular transfusion is associated with a >90% survival rate	III,IIa/B,B	36,83
Decline in donor red blood cells is ~2%/day	III/B	85
The efficacy of IVIG as a treatment for severe fetal hemolytic disease has not been established; the same is true for plasmapheresis; many reserve these for women with a history of early-onset hydrops (presenting before 22 wk)	IIb/B	74
Long-term neurodevelopmental outcome after intravascular transfusion is normal in most cases	III/B	92
Kell sensitization does not behave like Rh disease	IV/C	65
Kell sensitization is due to inhibition of erythroid progenitor cells by anti-Kell antibodies	III/B	67
Delivery Options		
In Nontransfused Fetus	—/GPP	—
At 37–38 wk		
In Transfused Fetus	—/GPP	—
Last intravascular transfusion at 34 wk (unless dangerous or difficult) and deliver at 37–38 wk		
32–34 wk (with prior maternal steroid therapy) for intraperitoneal transfusion		
Neonatal Care		
Pediatric surveillance from birth	—/GPP	—
Phototherapy		
Exchange transfusions if severe		
Top-up transfusions and long-term hematinic supplementation may be necessary		

GPP, good practice point; Hb, hemoglobin; IVIG, intravenous immunoglobulin; RhD, rhesus D.

strongly expressed on the fetal erythrocyte. Alloimmunization to minor blood group antigens is usually due to blood transfusion. Although Lewis antibodies are most common, they are almost always IgM and do not pose a risk for fetal disease. Further, the antigen is poorly expressed on the fetal erythrocyte. Therefore, the risk for hemolysis is low.

Kidd, Kell, and Duffy are the most common minor blood group antigens that cause perinatal hemolytic disease. Kell alloimmunization is of particular interest because the pathophysiology differs from the others. The clinical course is particularly unpredictable by indirect fetal assessment because the anti-Kell IgG antibodies damage or inhibit erythrocyte progenitors. Severe anemia and hydrops may develop rapidly with low antibody titers and ΔOD450 values. Management is similar to Rh isoimmunization with monitoring and intervention tailored to the individual circumstances.

OTHER CAUSES OF HEMOLYTIC DISEASE

Rare causes of fetal and neonatal hemolytic disease include hemoglobinopathies, RBC membrane defects, and RBC enzyme deficiencies. Because thallassemia can affect the α and β hemoglobin chains, it may result in disease in utero. Bart's hemoglobin (deletion of all four α chain genes) is the most severe form and causes hydrops fetalis. Hemoglobin H disease (deletion of three α chain genes) is less severe, but the affected patient requires lifelong transfusion treatment. In contrast, sickle cell disease (defective β chain) does not manifest in utero owing to the protective effect of fetal hemoglobin.

FUTURE PREGNANCIES, PREPREGNANCY CONSULTATION

Modern approaches to fetal hemolytic disease have drastically reduced the impact of this disease on the family. Though we may be cognizant that it may occur, we do not expect to lose a fetus to hemolytic disease. Several women under our care have, after presenting with a hydropic fetus in the first treated pregnancy, gone on to a second and a third treated pregnancy. Though not unreasonable to suggest, there is no reason to badger these women toward either an undesired surgical sterilization or a pregnancy by artificial insemination with an Rh-negative donor to avoid a recurrence. It is, however, essential they understand the time demands required of them, along with the costs and risks involved. This information is best supplied prior to conception.

SUGGESTED READINGS

Bennet PR, LeVanKim C, Colin Y, et al: Prenatal determination of fetal RhD type by DNA amplification. N Engl J Med 1993;329:607–610.

Chown B, Duff AM, James J, et al: Prevention of primary Rh immunization: First report of the Western Canadian Trial. Can Med J 1969;100:1021–1047.

Harper DC, Swingle HM, Weiner CP, et al: Long-term neurodevelopmental outcome and brain volume after treatment for hydrops fetalis by in utero intravascular transfusion. Am J Obstet Gynecol 2006;195:192–200.

Liley AW: Errors in the assessment of hemolytic disease from amniotic fluid. Am J Obstet Gynecol 1963;86:485–494.

Mari G, Deter RL, Carpenter RL, et al: Noninvasive diagnosis by Doppler ultrasonography of fetal anemia due to maternal red cell alloimmunization. Collaborative Group for Doppler Assessment of the Blood Velocity in Anemic Fetuses. N Engl J Med 2000;342:9–14.

Nicolaides KH, Rodeck CH, Mibashan RS, Kemp JR: Have Liley charts outlived their usefulness? Am J Obstet Gynecol 1986;155:90–94.

Weiner CP, Pelzer GD, Heilskov J, et al: The effect of intravascular transfusion on umbilical venous pressure in anemic fetuses with and without hydrops. Am J Obstet Gynecol 1989;161:149E.

Weiner CP, Williamson RA, Wenstrom KD, et al: Management of fetal hemolytic disease by cordocentesis: I. Prediction of fetal anemia. Am J Obstet Gynecol 1991;165:546–553.

Weiner CP, Williamson RA, Wenstrom KD, et al: Management of fetal hemolytic disease by cordocentesis: ii. Outcome of treatment. Am J Obstet Gynecol 1991;165:1302–1307.

Yankowitz J, Li S, Weiner CP: Polymerase chain reaction determination of RhC, Rhc, and RhE blood types: An evaluation of accuracy and clinical utility. Am J Obstet Gynecol 1997;176:1107–1111.

REFERENCES

For a complete list of references, log onto www.expertconsult.com.

CHAPTER 14

Fetal Thrombocytopenia

FRANK P. H. A. VANDENBUSSCHE, ANNEKE BRAND, and HUMPHREY H. H. KANHAI

INTRODUCTION

Platelets are first seen in the embryonic circulation at 5 to 6 weeks' postconceptual age.[1] Normal fetal mean (standard deviation) values are 159 (34) × 10^9/L in the first trimester,[2] 245 (65) × 10^9/L in the second and third trimesters,[3] and 308 (69) × 10^9/L at term birth.[4]

Fetal and neonatal thrombocytopenias are defined as a platelet count below 150 × 10^9/L and can be further classified according to the severity:

- Mild thrombocytopenia (100–149 × 10^9/L) does not require treatment.
- Moderate thrombocytopenia (50–99 × 10^9/L) also does not require treatment, but both mild and moderate thrombocytopenias may trigger additional diagnostic tests.
- Severe thrombocytopenia (20–49 × 10^9/L) requires diagnostic evaluation and treatment.
- Very severe thrombocytopenia (<20 × 10^9/L) is associated with a high risk of spontaneous intracranial hemorrhage (ICH) and requires urgent diagnostic evaluation and treatment.

At birth, only 1% to 2% of term infants are thrombocytopenic, but the incidence of thrombocytopenia during the neonatal period then rises to 3% to 5%[5] and may even reach 35% to 72% in preterm infants undergoing intensive care.[5,6]

The focus of this chapter is the immune-mediated thrombocytopenias. Thrombocytopenia secondary to either platelet allo- or isoimmunization is found in 0.3% of newborns.[7] Fetal/neonatal alloimmune thrombocytopenia (FNAIT) is the most frequent cause of severe and very severe fetal thrombocytopenia, and it is amenable to prevention and treatment.

ALLOIMMUNE THROMBOCYTOPENIA

Incidence

Alloimmune thrombocytopenia results from maternal antibodies directed against an antigen on the fetal platelet membrane, localized on glycoprotein (GP) IIIa (CD61) of the GP IIb/IIIa complex. The preferred terminology for these alloantigens is at present human platelet antigen (HPA). The first discovered antigen system was named Zw (Zw^a and Zw^b) after the first two letters of the patient's family name.[8] A few years later, the PL^A system, which appeared to be identical to Zw, was described.[9] The International Platelet Antigen Working Party suggests the name *human platelet antigen* (HPA).[10] The nomenclature is based on the chronologic numbering of alloantibodies in the order of their discovery. The letter "a" or "b" is assigned to the high- and low-frequency alleles, respectively. "W" marks an HPA system antigen of which only one allele is identified so far.

The incidence of a particular HPA varies by race.[11] In whites, 2% are negative for HPA-1a, which accounts for about 85% of FNAIT. Anti-HPA-1a antibodies are produced in approximately 11% of the HPA-1a–negative mothers.[12,13] The other antigens most commonly involved in FNAIT among whites are HPA-5b and HPA-3a.[11]

The development of anti-HPA-1a antibodies is strongly associated with the presence of the HLA class type II DRB3*0101. The absence of DRB3*0101 in an HPA-1a–negative woman virtually precludes the development of antibodies. About one third of HPA-1a–negative women who are DRB3*0101-positive develop antibodies.[12,14,15] The incidence of severe thrombocytopenia caused by anti HPA-1a antibodies approximates 1 in 1100 pregnancies.[12]

Risks

In contrast to red blood cell immunization, platelet alloimmunization affects the first pregnancy in half of the cases.[16] Most infants with FNAIT are born either without symptoms or with petechiae or bleeding from puncture sites. The most serious complication of FNAIT is internal hemorrhage, such as gastrointestinal, lung, and intracranial bleeding (ICH), occurring in either the fetus or the newborn. ICH is the most frequently occurring internal hemorrhage in FNAIT and causes serious perinatal morbidity and even death.[17] The risk of perinatal ICH as a result of HPA-1a–induced fetal thrombocytopenia approximates 11% excluding fetal deaths and 15% including fetal deaths.[18] Prospective studies with HPA-1a antibody screening programs document in aggregate an incidence of severe FNAIT of 0.04%, of intrauterine death of 0.002%, and of ICH of 0.006%.[19] Most cases of FNAIT are identified after the birth of an affected child. The degree of fetal thrombocytopenia reportedly remains similar or increases in 80% of subsequent pregnancies when the father is homozygous for the offending antigen.[20,21] HPA antibody detection is possible using the monoclonal antibody-specific immobilization of platelet antigens assay (MAIPA) (both sensitivity and specificity >90%), but MAIPA is rather complex and time-consuming and should be used only by experienced laboratories. Simpler techniques based on the MAIPA have been developed, but unfortunately, some have lower sensitivity (70%–75%) and specificity (85%).[22] Several prospective studies have shown a correlation between anti-HPA-1a antibody level and severity of thrombocytopenia in the newborn.[12,13,23,24] A correlation was also found in two retrospective studies,[25,26] whereas one other retrospective study did not find such a relationship.[27] One study on antenatal HPA-1a antibody screening and intervention with cesarean section and neonatal platelet transfusion has been published.[19] Antenatal screening, however, is not routine practice, given the low prevalence of ICH in an unselected population, the low sensitivity of screening tests, and uncertainty about the most appropriate prophylactic interventions.

The risk for ICH in a subsequent pregnancy of HPA-1a–alloimmunized women depends on the obstetric history. In the large majority of FNAIT cases, the risk of an ICH in a subsequent pregnancy with an HPA-1a–positive fetus, after the birth of a thrombocytopenic sibling without ICH, approximates 7%.[18] In contrast, the recurrence rate of ICH in subsequent offspring of women with a history of FNAIT approximates 75%.[18] Most cases of ICH in utero occur in the third trimester, though ICH has also been documented before 20 weeks.[28] ICH in utero may cause either fetal death or, if the fetus survives, fetal hydrops or hydrocephalus.

It is not known why one fetus with FNAIT may experience antenatal ICH whereas another fetus with a comparable degree of thrombocytopenia does not. In addition, fetuses and neonates with comparable degrees of thrombocytopenia caused by isoimmune thrombocytopenia (ITP) are not at risk for ICH or other life-threatening internal bleeding. The GP IIb/IIIa complex on the platelet membrane carries not only the HPA-1a or HPA-1b antigen but also most of the autoantigens involved with ITP antibodies. The IIb/IIIa complex is also expressed on vascular endothelium. Although no data are available, one may postulate that the density of antigenic molecules of HPA-1a and the autoantigens on IIb/IIIa may be different.

FIGURE 14–1
Management of platelet immunization.

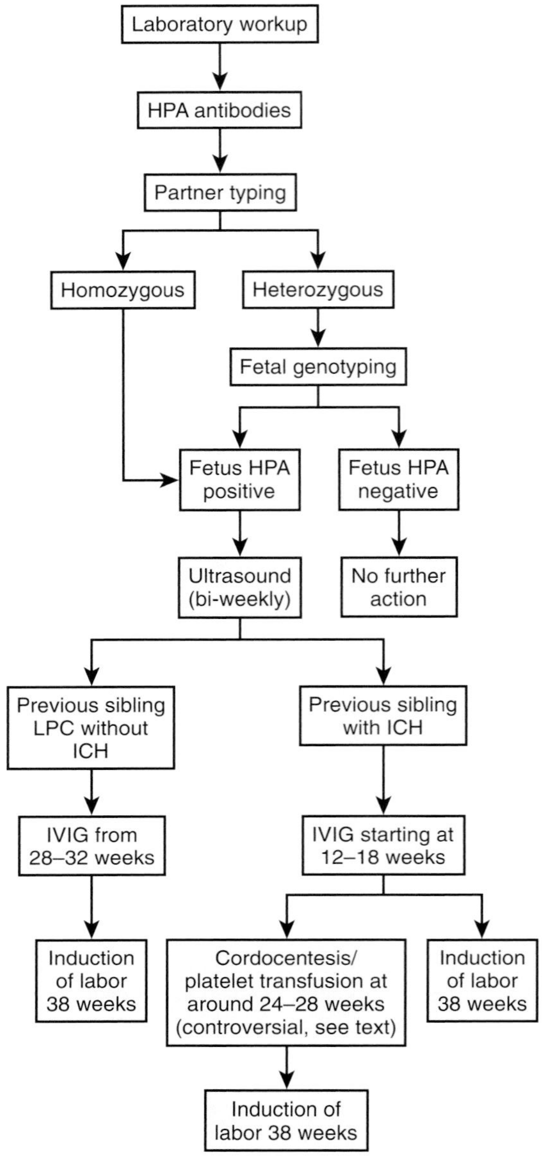

HPA: human platelet antigen; LPC: low platelet count; ICH: intracranial hemorrhage;
IVIG intravenous immunoglobulins to the mother (1g/kg/week; dose finding studies are underway, see for example www.noich.org)

Management Options (Fig. 14–1)

Prepregnancy

Prepregnancy management begins with an accurate diagnosis of FNAIT in the previous pregnancy. Platelet alloimmunization should be part of the differential diagnosis in all cases of neonatal thrombocytopenia (platelet count $< 100 \times 10^9$/L in term infants). The laboratory evaluation includes

- Confirming the presence of anti-HPA antibodies in maternal serum.
- Cross-matching of the maternal serum with paternal platelets, both untreated and chloroquine-treated (to remove HLA antigens that may cause a "false-positive" test).
- HPA pheno- or genotyping of mother and father.
- Exclusion of maternal thrombocytopenia.

When the diagnosis of FNAIT is established, and the couple is considering another pregnancy, prepregnancy counseling in a specialized center is advised. Counseling should include documentation of disease severity in the index case, the antibody specificity, and the hetero-/homozygosity of the father. In very severe instances, donor insemination or preimplantation diagnosis using a single cell of the blastomere can be considered.[29]

Prenatal

When the father is heterozygous for the offending antigen, fetal HPA-typing is advised. Genotyping for all important HPAs is possible using polymerase chain reaction (PCR). Fetal genotyping using cell-free fetal DNA in maternal plasma is now reliable from the early second trimester onward (de Haas M, personal communication). When the fetus is positive for the offending antigen, and thus at risk for severe thrombocytopenia, the pregnancy should be managed in collaboration with a specialized fetal medicine center.

Several strategies can be used for the monitoring and treatment of pregnancies at risk for FNAIT,[20,30–32] including fetal blood sampling (FBS) with platelet transfusion when indicated, and maternal treatment with intravenous immunoglobulin (IVIG) and corticosteroids. In one review of the literature, 26 different combinations of treatment were reported.[17] Unfortunately, there are no reports of controlled trials that compare intervention to nonintervention, and all recommendations are based on historical control subjects and natural history surveys. With these limitations, the current treatment of choice is a weekly maternal infusion of immunoglobulin at a dose of 1 g/kg of maternal weight. Several case series, published since the initial report of Bussel and associates in 1988,[33] confirm that weekly IVIG increases the fetal platelet count to a variable degree.[20,34,35] The result of a multicenter, prospective, randomized trial comparing IVIG with or without dexamethasone revealed a 70% response rate with IVIG alone.[36] Dexamethasone did not improve the effect when used routinely.[36] Significantly, in this study and in others, there were no instances of ICH in IVIG-treated perinates, even if they failed to respond with an increased platelet count.[35,37–39] Further trials are needed to determine the optimal dose of IVIG.[30] Recently, the NOICH study group (www.noich.org) conducted a multicenter study comparing the standard dose of 1 g/kg/wk with a lower dose of 0.5 g/kg/wk. This study was stopped after 2 years of recruitment because only 23 patients of the calculated sample size of 106 patients had been randomized. The outcome in this underpowered trial showed no difference between the standard and the lower doses. None of the neonates had an ICH.

Although FBS is the only tool available to directly monitor the severity of fetal thrombocytopenia, its routine use is not advised. FBS has caused fatal hemorrhage from the umbilical cord puncture site in fetuses with a low platelet count. Special precautions may lower the risk of complications in these patients (Table 14–1). The published literature reports a mean fetal loss rate of FBS in FNAIT pregnancies of 1.6% per procedure. In addition, there is a risk of procedure-related complications such as emergency cesarean section for fetal bleeding and bradycardia of 2.4% per procedure.[18,35,37,39] The reported complications might be method-related, because no increased risk was seen when a needle guide was used.[40] Platelet transfusion is problematic because the half-life of transfused platelets is only 4 to 5 days. Thus, FBS and platelet transfusions are required frequently throughout pregnancy once initiated, introducing a cumulative risk for complications. Transfused platelets may degranulate and release serotonin, compounding the risk of a bradycardia. The cumulative risk of fetal loss with transfusion therapy approximates 6% per pregnancy.[40,41] Given the 70% likelihood that the initial fetal platelet count between 20 and 28 weeks in FNAIT pregnancies with affected siblings is 50 × 10^9/L or less,[20] we suggest IVIG be started as a precaution after the fetal genotype results confirm an affected fetus.

TABLE 14–1

Extra Safety Precautions for Fetal Blood Sampling in Pregnancies at Risk for Severe Thrombocytopenia

The procedure should be performed by the most experienced members of a fetal medicine unit.
Sample in the umbilical vein and thus avoid puncturing the artery.
Use a hematologic cell counter in order to obtain the platelet count within 2 min.
If the fetal platelet count <50 × 10^9/L, compatible platelets may be infused before withdrawal of the needle.

The antenatal management protocols in FNAIT should be based on the following principles. First, the primary goal is the prevention of ICH and not just fetal thrombocytopenia per se. Second, the protocol should reflect the obstetric history. Given the fact that the large majority of patients have a sibling with a history of more or less severe thrombocytopenia, but without ICH, and that the risk of ICH approximates the procedure-related complication rate of invasive therapy, it is best to avoid FBS. Considering that the majority of in utero ICH occurs later in pregnancy and the cost of IVIG, treatment of pregnancies with no ICH history may be delayed to 28 to 32 weeks (see Fig. 14–1). We have seen no ICH or other serious morbidity applying this approach to 48 women in Leiden since the mid 2000s.[38] In fetuses whose siblings experienced an ICH, IVIG should be initiated at 12 to 18 weeks. FBS at 24 to 28 weeks to evaluate the response might be considered. When the anticipated risk of complication from FBS is higher (e.g., less experienced operators), the IVIG can be continued until delivery without periodic sampling (see Fig. 14–1). In recent years, we have treated seven pregnancies in five women with an older sibling with ICH, according to this less invasive protocol.[37] Each received 1 g IVIG/kg/wk (median 16 wk; range 16–29 wk) without initial or follow-up FBS. None of the neonates showed any signs of internal or external bleeding.

Labor and Delivery

Labor should be planned by the obstetrician in close consultation with the fetal medicine and pediatric teams and the blood bank to ensure that compatible platelets are available shortly after birth. A term delivery can be achieved in almost all pregnancies treated with IVIG. If serial fetal platelet transfusions are necessary, we suggest elective delivery after 32 weeks because of the risks of continued cordocentesis and platelet transfusions.

There is no consensus about the safety of vaginal birth in FNAIT infants. However, there is no evidence that a vaginal birth increases the risk of ICH in a treated term infant with FNAIT. The preponderance of perinatal ICH in FNAIT occurs before the start of labor.[17,18] More recently, we showed that in pregnancies with FNAIT and a thrombocytopenic sibling without ICH, vaginal delivery was not associated with neonatal ICH.[42] Similar to ITP, we suggest that an instrumented vaginal delivery be avoided if the fetal platelet count is unknown. In Leiden, in women with FNAIT, whose prior child did not suffer ICH and who have received IVIG, we perform cesarean delivery for obstetric indications only. Lastly, cesarean delivery does not guarantee protection against ICH in a severely thrombocytopenic infant.

Postnatal

In platelet alloimmunized pregnancies, the newborn's platelets count should be tested daily for the first 5 to 7 days. Thrombocytopenia in the neonate may respond to IVIG.[43] In severe cases and in infants treated prenatally with at least four infusions of IVIG, transfusion with compatible platelets is the first-line treatment to obtain immediate correction of thrombocytopenia.[44] However, if immediate correction of the platelet count is warranted, and HPA-compatible platelets are not available, random platelet transfusions can give transient improvement without causing side effects.[45] Breastfeeding is not contraindicated in FNAIT newborns. In cases of severe fetal thrombocytopenia, brain imaging should be performed.

Summary

Severe platelet alloimmunization leading to perinatal ICH is a rare but potentially disastrous condition. Management strategies should focus on the prevention of ICH and not thrombocytopenia per se. There is a lack of adequately sized, well-designed studies regarding management.[30] The index pregnancy is the most important factor for risk estimation of ICH. The majority of ICH cases occur during fetal life. Maternally administered IVIG is the first-line therapy in pregnancies at risk of severe disease and appears to reduce the risk of ICH even when the fetal platelet count has shown no response.

SUMMARY OF MANAGEMENT OPTIONS

Alloimmune Thrombocytopenia

Management Options (see Fig. 14–1)	**Evidence Quality and Recommendation**	**References**
Prepregnancy		
Review history of index case, including severity.	—/GPP	—
Investigate: • Confirm HPA antibodies in mother. • HPA genotyping of both parents. • Exclude maternal thrombocytopenia. • Cross-match maternal serum with paternal platelets.	—/GPP	—
Provide counseling of parents about risks (principally ICH) and potential management.	—/GPP	—
Sister(s) should be typed to establish whether they are at risk during pregnancy.	—/GPP	—
Prenatal		
Management should be in a specialist center.	—/GPP	—
With a heterozygous father, perform fetal genotyping early in second trimester, preferably from ffDNA in maternal plasma.	—/GPP	—
No further action if the fetus is HPA-negative.	—/GPP	—
Maternal anti-HPA antibody titer has limited value in the prediction of severity.	III/B	12,13,22–27
Treatment regimen varies and is controversial:	IV/C	17,31,38
• Maternal IVIG weekly (0.5–2 g/kg) is the main approach; timing may be determined by severity in previous baby.	III/B	20,34,35,38
• FBS for fetal platelet count might be reserved only for those with previous ICH; advisable to defer sampling until after IVIG started.	III/B	39
• Oral corticosteroids do not improve platelet response to IVIG alone.	Ib/A	30
• Reserve corticosteroids for IVIG-resistant cases.	III/B	33
• Limit repeated FBS and intravascular transfusions of fresh platelets to cases that fail to respond to maternal therapy.	III/B	20,34,35
Regular ultrasound of the fetal brain.	—/GPP	—

Management Options (see Fig. 14–1)	Evidence Quality and Recommendation	References
Labor and Delivery		
Close liaison with pediatric staff.	—/GPP	—
Fetal platelet transfusion just before delivery may be considered even if a cesarean section is contemplated; there is no evidence that abdominal delivery reduces risk of ICH.	III/B	38
Postnatal		
Monitor neonatal platelet count daily for the first 7 days; platelet transfusion and IVIG for 4 wk if platelets <50 × 10^9/L.	—/GPP	—
In cases with a low platelet count managed with IVIG during fetal life, consider platelet transfusion only.	—/GPP	—
Breastfeeding is not contraindicated.	—/GPP	—

FBS, fetal blood sampling; ffDNA, cell-free fetal DNA; GPP, good practice point; HPA, human platelet antigen; ICH, intracranial hemorrhage; IVIG, intravenous immunoglobulin.

ISOIMMUNE THROMBOCYTOPENIC PURPURA

Incidence

Adult ITP has an annual incidence of 6 per 100,000 population and most often affects young women.[46] Consequently, a past or present history of ITP complicates 1 to 5 per 10,000 pregnancies.[47] Typically, the woman has a history of ITP and presents with or without thrombocytopenia in pregnancy. However, a first presentation of ITP in pregnancy is not rare. The general issues relating to ITP are covered in Chapter 40.

Risks

Maternal

Platelet counts in pregnant women with ITP tend to decrease, reaching their nadir during the third trimester.[48] Unless the counts are very low, the patient either is asymptomatic or experiences easy bruising. However, some patients do bleed despite platelet counts above 20 × 10^9/L ("wet" thrombocytopenia). In these instances, it is assumed that the autoantibodies interact with functional receptors on the platelet surface.[49] Women who do not respond to treatment are at risk of bleeding during pregnancy and delivery. The lowest maternal platelet count during the prior pregnancy is fairly predictive of the extent of thrombocytopenia in successive pregnancies. One third of pregnant ITP patients need treatment to increase the platelet count. Moderate to severe bleeding occurs in only about 5% of the cases.[50]

Fetus and Newborn

The perinatal mortality rate is around 0.6% with virtually all losses secondary to related medical illnesses, rather than fetal thrombocytopenia.[51] Severe in utero bleeding is not documented in ITP. The risk of severe neonatal thrombocytopenia needing treatment ranges from 9% to 15%.[51–53] In large series, neonatal ICH is reported in 0% to 1.5%.[50,54,55] The nadir neonatal platelet count with inherent major risk for hemorrhage occurs 1 to 4 days after birth.[48,56]

Because the majority of cases with ITP during pregnancy have a benign course, several investigators have sought to predict the risk of fetal thrombocytopenia. Such information could be of practical importance because it would dictate the center selected for delivery. In most studies, however, there was only a weak correlation between newborn platelet counts and maternal platelet counts or the presence of antibodies in the maternal serum.[46,51,55,57] Several studies have reported a better correlation between the newborn platelet count and a maternal history of splenectomy.[53,58] Perhaps the strongest predictive factor for neonatal thrombocytopenia is an older sibling with a platelet count below 50 × 10^9/L.[59] A report that HLA (DRB3*) type in the mother is protective against neonatal thrombocytopenia requires confirmation.[60] Even though each of these factors in isolation is a weak predictor, we think that the combination of a prior sibling with severe thrombocytopenia, together with a mother with a history of splenectomy and severe maternal thrombocytopenia during the current pregnancy, indicates a high probability of severe neonatal thrombocytopenia and indicates the need for delivery in a tertiary hospital.[61]

Management Options (Fig. 14–2)

None of the published guidelines for the management of ITP in pregnancy and during the neonatal period are based on a high level of evidence, and most are based on cohort studies.[46,55,63,64]

Prepregnancy

ITP is not a reason to advise against pregnancy, except perhaps for those women refractory to corticosteroids and splenectomy and who cannot maintain a platelet count above 30 × 10^9/L despite immunosuppressive drugs.[55,63] The risk of fetal morbidity and mortality are never a reason to advise against pregnancy, given the virtual absence of severe fetal bleeding and low risk of severe neonatal bleeding complications.[56] A history of a thrombocytopenic older sibling, together with maternal thrombocytopenia and need of maternal treatment to increase the platelet count, may be indications for pregnancy care in a hospital with multidisciplinary experience with these patients.[59,60]

FIGURE 14–2
Management of maternal thrombocytopenia (<100 × 10^9/L) in pregnancy and before birth.

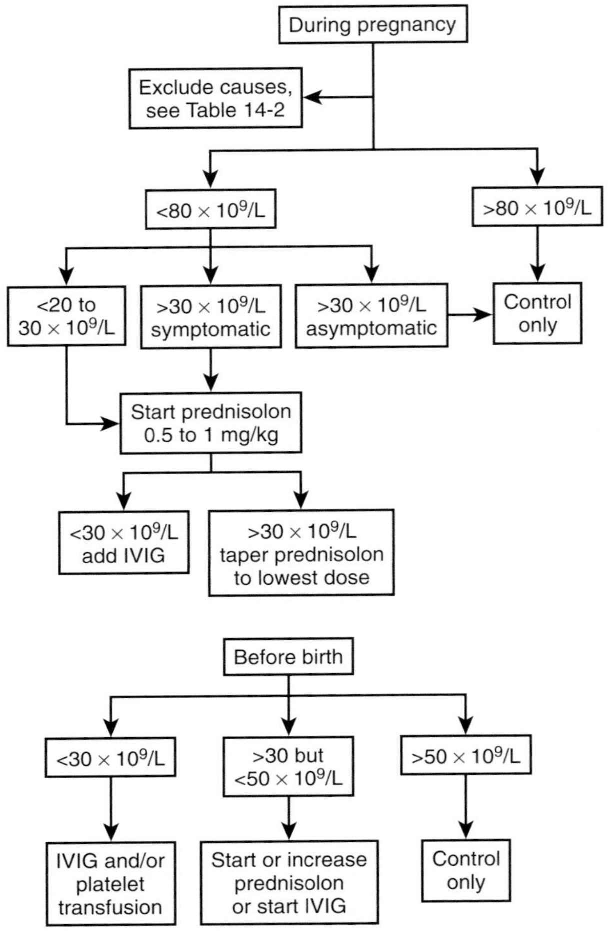

IVIG: intravenous immunoglobulin, suggested dose is 1g per kg body weight weekly

TABLE 14–2

Laboratory Investigations in a Pregnant Woman with Thrombocytopenia

TEST	AIM
Blood film	Exclude spurious thrombocytopenia, HELLP, TTP, other hematologic diseases
Liver function	
Proteinuria	
Coagulation tests–aPTT, lupus anticoagulant	Exclude rare causes of thrombocytopenia
SLE serology	Consider when indicated
HIV	
Thyroid function tests	
Heparin-dependent antibodies	Exclude HIT

aPTT, activated partial thromboplastin time; HELLP, hemolysis, elevated liver enzymes, liver function disturbances, low platelet count; HIT, heparin-induced thrombocytopenia; SLE, systemic lupus erythematosus; TTP, thrombotic thrombocytopenic purpura.

PRENATAL MANAGEMENT IN THROMBOCYTOPENIC WOMEN WITHOUT A HISTORY OF ISOIMMUNE THROMBOCYTIC PURPURA

The most common cause of a maternal platelet count of 100 to 150 × 10^9/L, occurring in 6% to 7% of pregnancies, are incidental thrombocytopenia of pregnancy or gestational thrombocytopenia (GT). GT accounts for more than 70% of cases of maternal thrombocytopenia and has no detrimental effect on mother and child. Hypertensive disorders and some very rare causes, such as HIV, von Willebrand's disease type IIB, and underlying systemic diseases such as systemic lupus erythematosus (SLE), antiphospholipid syndrome, thyroid dysfunction, and hematologic diseases must be excluded (Table 14–2). No further analysis is indicated to distinguish GT from ITP once these conditions are excluded. Bone marrow aspiration is reserved for suspected hematologic malignancy. Thrombocytopenia below 100 × 10^9/L occurs in 1% to 2% of pregnant women.[48] Even then, guidelines do not recommend testing for maternal platelet-associated immunoglobulin G (IgG) antibodies because the rates of false-positive and false-negative results are high.[46,53,57,63] However, the platelet count should be monitored every 2 weeks and, if it falls below 50 × 10^9/L, the patient should be managed based on the assumption she has ITP, although rare cases of severe GT, refractory to corticosteroids and IVIG, have been described.[64]

WOMEN WITH A HISTORY OF ISOIMMUNE THROMBOCYTIC PURPURA

Treatment indications for ITP during pregnancy are similar to those for ITP in nonpregnant individuals. Platelet count should be monitored at an interval dependent on the initial platelet count and every 2 weeks if it is below 50 × 10^9/L. The need for prenatal therapy is based exclusively on maternal indications, with the goal of maintaining the count above 20 × 10^9/L (or higher in case of bleeding symptoms).[46,55] First-line therapy is the lowest effective dose of corticosteroids (see Fig. 14–2). In case of corticosteroid refractoriness or side effects, IVIG is the second-line treatment. The effect of IVIG lasts only 2 to 3 weeks and sometimes decreases with repetitive dosing. Therefore, IVIG is best reserved for use late in pregnancy or immediately prior to delivery. Immunosuppressive drugs (such as azathioprine, rituximab, or vincristine) are best avoided in the first trimester. Splenectomy is rarely needed during pregnancy. There has been no demonstrable effect of maternal treatment such as corticosteroids or IVIG on the fetal platelet count.[65,66]

The association of ITP with other autoimmune diseases is well known. In SLE, patients may present with immune thrombocytopenia and have clinical features and therapeutic responses similar to those with ITP. However, thrombocytopenia in SLE associated with antiphospholipid antibodies (aPLs) may overlap with syndromes associated with small vessel occlusions such as thrombotic thrombocytopenic purpura (TTP), HELLP (hemolysis, elevated liver enzymes, and low platelets) syndrome, and even catastrophic antiphospholipid syndrome.[67,68]

Labor and Delivery

A history of splenectomy, current maternal thrombocytopenia, or treatment for ITP or thrombocytopenia in a sibling at birth dictates delivery at a center with expertise in maternal-fetal medicine. A maternal platelet count above $50 \times 10^9/L$ is generally considered safe for either vaginal or cesarean delivery, though the factual basis for this recommendation is weak. The majority of members of a consensus panel considered a platelet count higher than $30 \times 10^9/L$, without bleeding symptoms, safe for vaginal delivery.[55] A low platelet count may even be an argument against cesarean delivery. Should the count be below $50 \times 10^9/L$, IVIG, platelet transfusions, or both may be given to raise the count by the time of delivery. American and Dutch guidelines consider $50 \times 10^9/L$ as a safe level for epidural anesthesia.[46,69]

There is convincing evidence that the route of delivery does not alter the risk of severe fetal or neonatal internal hemorrhage,[46,51,55,63] and cesarean delivery is undertaken for standard obstetric indications. However, it is prudent to avoid manipulations such as fetal scalp blood sampling, vacuum extraction, or rotational or mid-forceps delivery.[46,55,69] Several investigators have suggested either FBS or scalp blood sampling to estimate the fetal platelet count. However, this practice cannot be condoned because altering the route of delivery based on the fetal platelet count does not change the outcome. Further, scalp blood samples do not provide reproducible platelet counts,[53] and the fetal risks of FBS exceed the risk of fetal hemorrhage from ITP.[70]

Routine thrombosis prophylaxis in cases of surgical delivery, immobilization, or individual risk factors should be undertaken unless there is either bleeding or severe thrombocytopenia ($<50 \times 10^9/L$). When the platelet count is between 50 and $100 \times 10^9/L$, the risks of thrombosis and bleeding should be carefully weighed against each other.[46] One third of ITP patients have antiphospholipid syndrome and these patients have a higher risk of thrombosis.[71]

Postnatal

Maternal platelet counts often improve over the first 6 weeks. Tranexamic acid (1 g given three times daily) may reduce excessive vaginal bleeding. Breastfeeding is not contraindicated.[55,65] The newborn's platelet count, even if normal at birth, should be tested for at least the first 5 days, because one third develop a delayed thrombocytopenia.[51] Neonates with counts below $50 \times 10^9/L$ may bleed and the risk for ICH is 0% to 1.5%.[50,51,54] It is estimated that 15% of neonates require treatment.[72] IVIG and corticosteroids are both recommended as first-line treatment and are combined with platelet transfusion if counts are below $20 \times 10^9/L$ or if there is bleeding.[46,51,63,73] Ultrasound brain imaging is recommended in these cases.

Summary

The management of ITP during pregnancy is based on several large and well-designed clinical cohort studies demonstrating that ITP runs a benign course in pregnancy for both mother and child. Severe fetal bleeding and in utero ICH remain unreported. If confronted with such a case, other bleeding disorders and alloimmune antibodies must be sought before assuming the explanation is ITP.

SUMMARY OF MANAGEMENT OPTIONS

Isoimmune Thrombocytopenia

Management Options	Evidence Quality and Recommendation	References
Prepregnancy		
Risk of neonatal thrombocytopenia is increased if there was a previously affected pregnancy.	III/B	59,61
Avoidance of pregnancy may be an issue in women refractory to splenectomy, steroids, and immunosuppression.	III/B	62
Prenatal		
Laboratory investigations:		
• Exclude other causes (see Table 14–2).	II/B	48,51
• Monitor maternal platelet count every 2 wk during pregnancy in cases with a history of ITP or platelet count $<50 \times 10^9/L$.	IV/C	46,55
Maternal treatment:		
• Threshold count varies between 30 and $50 \times 10^9/L$.	III/B	46,63
• Corticosteroids are first-line therapy; taper to lowest dose.	IV/C	46,55
• IVIG is best reserved for administration between 36 and 37 weeks (predelivery).	IV/C	46,55
• Consider splenectomy with severe ITP in early pregnancy with no response to steroids or IVIG; immunosuppressives (vincristine and azathiaprine) are options for refractory disease in late pregnancy.	—/GPP	—

SUMMARY OF MANAGEMENT OPTIONS

Isoimmune Thrombocytopenia—cont'd

Management Options	Evidence Quality and Recommendation	References
Labor and Delivery		
Plan delivery in a center with appropriate multidisciplinary expertise.	—/GPP	—
Aim for platelet count >50 × 10^9/L before delivery.	III/B	46,63,66
Maternal platelet transfusion is needed to cover delivery if platelet count <50 × 10^9/L.	—/GPP	—
Epidural anesthesia is considered safe if platelet count >50 × 10^9/L.	III/B	69
FBS at 38–39 weeks and fetal scalp blood sampling in labor are not justified.	III/B	46,48,55,63
Cesarean section is performed for obstetric indications; no evidence shows that the risk of fetal/neonatal hemorrhage is lessened by elective cesarean section.	III/B	46,48,53,55,63
Minimize (some advocate avoidance of) fetal scalp sampling and assisted vaginal delivery, especially by vacuum extraction.	III/B	46,55,63
Episiotomy should be avoided if possible with low maternal platelet counts.	—/GPP	—
Postnatal		
Monitor neonatal platelet counts for 5 days:	III/B	46,51,63
• IVIG if <50 × 10^9/L.	IV/C	73
• Platelet transfusion if <20 × 10^9/L or if clinically indicated.	—/GPP	—
Breastfeeding is not contraindicated.	III/B	55,65

FBS, fetal blood sampling; GPP, good practice point; ITP, isoimmune thrombocytopenic purpura; IVIG, intravenous immunoglobulin.

OTHER CAUSES OF FETAL THROMBOCYTOPENIA

Fetal Infections

Petechiae at birth were reported in 14 % of neonates born after maternal cytomegalovirus (CMV) infection in the first trimester of pregnancy.[74] Neonates with symptomatic CMV infection have petechiae in 75% of cases,[75] and ICH has been reported with fetal CMV infection.[3,76] Other fetal infections have also been associated with thrombocytopenia: toxoplasmosis, rubella, syphilis, HIV and Epstein-Barr virus.[3,77,78] Maternal infection with parvovirus B19 may be followed in 5% to 10% of cases by inhibition of fetal erythropoiesis, severe anemia, and hydrops. Fetal thrombocytopenia in parvovirus infection is most probably caused by bone marrow suppression.[78] In a series of 30 severe cases of parvovirus infection, treated with fetal erythrocyte transfusions because of hydrops, de Haan and coworkers[79] found severe thrombocytopenia in 46%. Although in their series no fetal ICH or procedure-related bleeding occurred, Segata and colleagues[78] reported two procedure-related fetal deaths in a series of 11 fetuses in which the FBS was performed at the placental insertion or in a free loop.

Aneuploidy

Fetal triploidy is the aneuploidy most frequently associated with severe thrombocytopenia.[80] There is also an association between fetal trisomies and thrombocytopenia; 6% of newborns with Down syndrome are diagnosed with severe thrombocytopenia,[81] and more than half of newborns with trisomy 18 and 13 present with thrombocytopenia, but this is rarely severe.[82]

Genetic Syndromes

Severe thrombocytopenia is a hallmark of fetuses or newborns with a variety of rare autosomal recessive or X-linked genetic syndromes:

- Thrombocytopenia with absent radius (TAR) syndrome associated with skeletal and nonskeletal abnormalities. The pathogenesis of thrombocytopenia is unknown, but it is thought that there is a decreased response to thrombopoietin.[83] Platelet counts generally improve over the first year of life and may later approach normal adult levels.
- Congenital amegakaryocytic thrombocytopenia (CAMT) often presents with bleeding symptoms within the first week after birth with no other abnormalities but

thrombocytopenia. It is caused by mutations in the c-Mpl gene, leading to an absent or defective thrombopoietin receptor, a severe reduction or absence of megakaryocytes in bone marrow, and up to 10-fold increased serum levels of thrombopoietin. Patients with CAMT finally develop bone marrow failure.[83]

- Bernard-Soulier syndrome (BSS) is due to quantitative or qualitative abnormalities in the GP Ib/IX complex, a platelet von Willebrand factor adhesion receptor. Severe thrombocytopenia in homozygous newborns has been reported.[84] During pregnancy, females with BBS lacking GP Ib/IX, can produce antibodies to the GP Ib/IX complex on fetal platelets. The offspring may consequently develop severe thrombocytopenia and fetal ICH similar to FNAIT.[85]
- Gray platelet syndrome is associated with lifelong bleeding disorders and may present with fetal or neonatal thrombocytopenia.[86]
- Neonatal hemochromatosis is characterized by hepatocellular failure and is often associated with severe thrombocytopenia. It has been considered as a gestational alloimmune disorder that may be responsive to maternal high-dose IVIG.[87]
- Wiskott-Aldrich syndrome (WAS) has an X-linked inheritance and is due to abnormalities in platelet and lymphocyte cytoskeleton and signaling. It presents with severe thrombocytopenia, very small platelets, and associated features of eczema and recurrent infections.[88]

Thrombocytopenia may also be found in fetuses or newborns with other genetic syndromes:

- Amegakaryocytic thrombocytopenia with radioulnar synostosis (ATRUS) has been associated with mutations in HoxA11 and with high levels of thrombopoietin.[83]
- Paris-Trousseau thrombocytopenia is an autosomal dominant macrothrombocytopenia with deletion of the q23-24 region on chromosome 11, a region also deleted in Jacobsen's syndrome.[89]
- Kasabach-Merritt sequence, also called hemangioma-thrombopenia syndrome, may present with severe fetal thrombocytopenia.[90]
- X-linked thrombocytopenia (XLT), like WAS, is associated with an abnormality in the WAS protein, but these abnormalities give rise to a milder phenotype.
- MYH9-related thrombocytopenia syndromes include May-Hegglin anomaly, Fechtner's syndrome, Sebastian's syndrome, and Epstein's syndrome. These are autosomal dominant mutations, leading to a defective cytoskeletal contractile protein in hematopoietic cells. In general, affected individuals do not have life-threatening bleeding events.[91]
- Niemann-Pick is a lysosomal storage disease that is often associated with in utero thrombocytopenia.
- Osteopetrosis is a heterogeneous disorder characterized by osteoclast failure that may present with severe anemia, thrombocytopenia, infections, progressive deafness, and blindness.
- Hemophagocytic lymphohistiocytosis, an immune dysregulation of the monocyte-macrophage lineage, typically represents with pancytopenia.
- Bone marrow involvement is the cause of thrombocytopenia in metastatic neuroblastoma, glycogen storage diseases, organic acidemias, and aminoacidemias.

Severe Rhesus D Hemolytic Disease

In a large cohort of symptomatic rhesus D alloimmunized pregnancies, severe thrombocytopenia was found in 3% of cases prior to the first fetal red cell transfusion.[92] There was an association between the presence of severe hydrops and severe thrombocytopenia. Perinatal mortality in the severely thrombocytopenic group was 36%, compared with only 5% in the nonthrombocytopenic group. Furthermore, 2 of 14 survivors in the thrombocytopenic group had an ICH in the neonatal period. In contrast, fetuses with severe anemia due to Kell immunization are generally not at risk of severe thrombocytopenia.[93] Severe thrombocytopenia probably carries an increased risk of bleeding from the puncture site in the umbilical cord.[94]

Drug Exposure

Drug-induced thrombocytopenia has been described after administration of antibiotics, antiepileptics, and antidepressants, but case reports mostly concern adults. Theoretically, these effects could also occur in fetuses and neonates.

Management Options

Both in rhesus D disease and in fetal infections, a low platelet count seems to be a marker for poor outcome rather than a cause of bleeding, and evidence is lacking that platelet transfusion prevents hemorrhagic complications in fetuses with severe thrombocytopenia. Bleeding after cordocentesis, despite immediate platelet transfusion, has been reported in red cell and platelet alloimmunization.[94,95] Moreover, a platelet transfusion may be associated with complications, such as volume overload, cardiac arrest, or thromboembolic events, supposedly because of release of vasoactive substances.

Summary

Most instances of spontaneous fetal ICH due to severe thrombocytopenia are caused by FNAIT or CMV infection. However, a fetal medicine specialist may be confronted, unexpectedly, with a low platelet count while performing an intrauterine transfusion or a diagnostic FBS. The risk of procedure-related complications may then be increased. It is unclear whether platelet transfusions are beneficial in these circumstances.

SUGGESTED READINGS

All R, Ozkalemkas F, Ozcelik T, et al: Idiopathic thrombocytopenic purpura in pregnancy: A single institutional experience with maternal and neonatal outcome. Ann Hematol 2003;82:348–352.

Birchall JE, Murphy MF, Kaplan C, Kroll H: European Collaborative Study of the Antenatal Management of Feto-maternal Alloimmune Thrombocytopenia. Br J Hematol 2003;122:275–288.

Gernsheimer T, McGrae KR: Immune thrombocytopenic purpura in pregnancy. Curr Opin Hematol 2007;14:574–580.

Kanhai HH, Porcelijn L, Engelfriet CP, et al: Management of alloimmune thrombocytopenia. Vox Sang 2007;93:370–385.

Porcelijn L, van den Akker ES, Oepkes D: Fetal thrombocytopenia. Semin Fetal Neonatal Med 2008;13:223–230.

Rayment R, Brunskill SJ, Stanworth S, et al: Antenatal interventions for fetomaternal alloimmune thrombocytopenia. Cochrane Database Syst Rev 2005;25:CD004226.

Suri V, Aggarwal N, Saxena S, et al: Maternal and perinatal outcome in idiopathic thrombocytopenic purpura (ITP) with pregnancy. Acta Obstet Gynecol Scand 2006;85:1430–1435.

van den Akker ES, Oepkes D, Lopriore E, et al: Noninvasive antenatal management of fetal and neonatal alloimmune thrombocytopenia: Safe and effective. BJOG 2007;114:469–473.

Webert KE, Mittal R, Sigouin C, et al: A retrospective 11-year analysis of obstetric patients with idiopathic thrombocytopenic purpura. Blood 2003;102:4306–4311.

REFERENCES

For a complete list of references, log onto www.expertconsult.com.

CHAPTER 15

Fetal Cardiac Arrhythmias: Diagnosis and Therapy

MERT O. BAHTIYAR, BEVIN WEEKS, and JOSHUA A. COPEL

Videos corresponding to this chapter are available online at www.expertconsult.com.

INTRODUCTION

Clinical Significance

Fetal cardiac arrhythmias are common in clinical practice and may be associated with significant morbidity and mortality. Most reflect transient, isolated ectopic beats with less than 2% of fetal rhythm disturbances resulting in a sustained and clinically significant arrhythmia. However, sustained episodes can occur and, if not treated appropriately, lead to congestive heart failure, nonimmune hydrops, and even fetal or neonatal demise. In this chapter, we define fetal arrhythmias and review their frequency, the methods of detection, and their basic mechanisms, as well as their management. We illustrate the importance of a team approach to fetal arrhythmia management, involving physicians from each subspecialty needed to care for mother, fetus, and newborn.

History

Cremer[1] first described fetal electrocardiography in 1906. Fetal electrocardiography proved reliable for identifying tachycardias but was limited in its ability to determine the etiology. In the 1950s, Smyth[2] described invasive electrocardiographic monitoring with an intra-amniotic electrode. Despite this technologic advance, its use remained limited because it required ruptured membranes for access.

Fetal rhythm assessment became practical with the advent of echocardiography, specifically M-mode. Robinson and Shaw-Dunn[3] detailed the use of M-mode in the evaluation of fetal arrhythmias during the early 1970s. As ultrasound technology expanded to include two-dimensional and both spectral and color Doppler modes, numerous authors described additional echocardiographic techniques for the identification and differentiation of fetal arrhythmias. More recently, fetal magenetocardiography has been shown to be able to detect fetal arrhythmias.[4]

Definition

A *fetal dysrhythmia* is best defined as an irregularity in the fetal cardiac rhythm or a regular rhythm that remains outside the normal range. The currently accepted normal range in clinical practice is between 110 and 160 beats/min, although somewhat higher rates may be seen during labor, especially with maternal fever or dehydration. The American College of Obstetrics and Gynecology (ACOG)[5] and 2008 National Institute of Child Health and Human Development Workshop Report on Electronic Fetal Monitoring[6] established the normal range of fetal heart rate between 110 and 160 beats/min. This range does not exclude hypoxic fetuses. Davignon and coworkers[7] found the heart rate for infants younger than 1 day of age was between 88 and 168 beats/min with mean of 123 beats/min. Any of these ranges may serve as a guide, and the identification of heart rate may be based on data collected for an extended period to ensure that any deviations are not associated with uterine contractions, decelerations, maternal fever, or physiologic fetal activity such as hiccupping.

Frequency

Fetal arrhythmias are relatively common at routine obstetric visits, with a frequency ranging from 1% to 3% of all pregnancies.[8,9] In our experience, they account for approximately 10% to 20% of referrals for fetal echocardiography.[10] Few of these referrals to fetal cardiologists are for dysrhythmias determined to be of clinical significance.[11] In newborns, the most common causes of irregularities are either extrasystoles or respiratory sinus arrhythmia, the variation in the heart rate related to respiration, increasing with inspiration and decreasing with expiration, which is a normal finding and requires no further evaluation. Extrasystoles occur in upward of 14% of term, healthy newborns[12] and account for 43% to 98% of fetal arrhythmia referrals.[13,14] The vast majority of the extrasystoles are atrial in origin, with premature ventricular contractions accounting for less than 4%.[13–15]

The fetal arrhythmias diagnosed in 1384 patients evaluated at our institution over 20 years are listed in Table 15–1. The experience reflects the general findings of others: that extrasystoles are the most common cause of fetal arrhythmias and that tachycardias are more than twice as common as bradycardias.[9,14] The most common causes of fetal tachycardias are atrioventricular (AV) reentry supraventricular tachycardia (SVT), atrial flutter, and sinus tachycardia. Rare causes of SVT include chaotic atrial or atrial ectopic tachycardia, atrial fibrillation, junctional tachycardia, and ventricular tachycardia, each constituting less than 1% of fetal

TABLE 15-1

Incidence of Fetal Cardiac Arrhythmias—Department of Maternal-Fetal Medicine, Yale University School of Medicine

ARRHYTHMIA	NUMBER
Isolated extrasystoles	1213
Tachycardias	114
Supraventricular tachycardia	69
Atrial flutter	21
Sinus tachycardia	7
Ventricular tachycardia	7
Atrial fibrillation	4
Atrial ectopic tachycardia	4
Junctional tachycardia	2
Bradycardias	51
Complete AV block	39
Second-degree AV block	10
Sinus bradycardia	2

AV, atrioventricular.

arrhythmias.[13,14,16] The most common cause of fetal bradycardia is complete atrioventricular block (CAVB), which accounts for more than three quarters of cases. Other, less frequent causes of bradycardia include isolated sinus bradycardia, advanced second-degree AV block, prolonged QT interval syndrome, and fetal toxicity.[17,18]

ASSESSMENT OF A FETAL ARRHYTHMIA

A variety of methods are available for the evaluation of fetal cardiac arrhythmias. The majority of techniques are noninvasive, though invasive techniques, such as scalp electrodes, are used occasionally. We focus on commonly used noninvasive techniques, their advantages and disadvantages, and the future of fetal arrhythmia detection and differentiation.

When a fetal dysrhythmia is detected, the first step is to determine the etiology of the abnormal rhythm. Multiple factors must be considered, because fetal dysrhythmias can result from maternal connective tissue disorders, drugs, hyperthyroidism, or infection or can be a sign of fetal compromise or an intrinsic fetal rhythm disturbance. A complete maternal assessment should be made, including inquiries regarding recent illnesses, medicinal and recreational drug use, caffeine intake, and signs of hyperthyroidism. A complete family history is essential with an emphasis on the presence of inherited causes of arrhythmia, such as prolonged QT interval syndrome, congenital deafness (associated with prolonged QT interval syndrome), previous fetal demise, sudden unexplained death in family members younger than 50 years of age, and tuberous sclerosis. In addition, the fetus must be thoroughly evaluated for signs of hydrops, compromise, or structural cardiac disease.

Auscultation

The simplest method to detect a dysrhythmia is by auscultation with a stethoscope. The technique is a quick, easy, and readily reproducible tool. It was also the most common method of fetal heart rate assessment prior to electronic fetal monitoring (EFM).[19] Since the advent of EFM in the 1960s, the use of fetoscopic auscultation has dwindled. If a brady- or tachyarrhythmia is detected during auscultation, further investigation into the cause of the dysrhythmia is indicated.

Doppler

Doppler ultrasound is the most commonly used screening tool for fetal dysrhythmia. A beam of sound is directed toward fetal cardiac structures such as valves, walls, or aortic pulsations, which is reflected back to the transducer at a slightly different frequency due to tissue or blood movement. Doppler principles are employed in two readily available methods: the handheld Doppler device, which is frequently used for routine office assessment of the fetal heart rate, and as part of cardiotocography. Both devices have proved to be highly effective tools for the detection of fetal dysrhythmias. The handheld devices can be used from the 12th week of gestation, whereas cardiotocography is not usually used before 24 weeks.

Fetal Electrocardiography

Fetal electrocardiography (FECG) is another method for the detection of fetal dysrhythmia. It is similar in principle to standard electrocardiography, with the placement of electrodes on the maternal abdomen to record the differences in electrical potential arising from the fetal cardiac electrical activity. Most fetal QRS complexes are easily identified from the raw signal with FECG, and with signal averaging, the P-waves can be located occasionally. T-waves are rarely seen on these recordings. However, because it requires signal averaging over time to assess P-wave morphology, it is not useful in real-time examinations (e.g., for occasional extrasystoles or intermittent tachycardias). Despite some limitations of use later in pregnancy owing to the electrical insulating nature of vernix caseosa, serial noninvasive FECG of normal fetuses from 18 to 41 weeks' gestation has been shown to achieve good success in FECG detection.[20]

Intrapartum ST segment analysis forms the basis of the STAN ECG system.[21] However, this requires direct application of a scalp electrode, which can be done only if the amniotic membranes are ruptured. In addition, the STAN ECG waveform is achieved by signal averaging, so this technique cannot be used for fetal rhythm anomalies.

Magnetocardiography

Described by Kariniemi in 1974,[22] fetal magnetocardiography (FMCG) has potential utility in the evaluation of ventricular arrhythmias. FMCG noninvasively records the magnetic activity of the fetal heart generated by electrical excitation after maternal signals are filtered out. With specialized offline analysis of the magnetic activity, an equivalent of the surface electrocardiogram (ECG) is created. Its use and reliability are documented from 20 weeks to birth.[23] Numerous studies demonstrate the accuracy of FMCG for the diagnosis of fetal arrhythmias such as atrial and ventricular ectopy, SVT, atrial flutter, CAVB, torsades de points, and ventricular tachycardia (VT).[24–26]

The advantages to FMCG over FECG include the following: it takes less time (seconds vs. minutes), it overcomes the assumption that mechanical activity correlates with electrical activity, and it has greater reliability. FMCG is currently the only antenatal method of measuring cardiac repolarization, which can identify long QT syndrome (LQTS). The disadvantages of FMCG include its size, high cost, and severely limited availability of the equipment, resulting in restricted use in current clinical practice.

Echocardiography

Fetal echocardiography is the current gold standard for the diagnosis and monitoring of fetal arrhythmias and relies on the extrapolation of mechanical events back to presumed antecedent electrical events and the assessment of their temporal relationship. Its status is due, in part, to its widespread availability and relative ease of use. Ongoing improvements in ultrasound technology make this diagnostic modality an increasingly effective means of defining fetal arrhythmias. A significant advantage of fetal echocardiography is its safety throughout pregnancy, starting as early as 11 weeks[27] with a transvaginal probe and 14 weeks transabdominally. Both fetal atrial and ventricular rates along with the AV activation sequence are readily seen. Knowledge of the activation sequence facilitates differentiation of the arrhythmia into ventricular or supraventricular and long or short ventriculoatrial (VA) time interval tachycardia. Limitations associated with the use of fetal echocardiography for arrhythmia assessment are primarily due to fetal lie and difficulty in accurately interrogating structures that represent atrial and ventricular electrical activity. In addition, fetal well-being, cardiac structure, and hemodynamics can be evaluated concurrently with the arrhythmia assessment.

In addition to a careful examination of the fetal heart and circulation, assessment of a fetal arrhythmia should include a detailed, full sonographic examination of the fetus, looking for syndromic features, especially those associated with chromosomal abnormalities. Fetal echocardiography is also crucial in the chronic follow-up of fetuses with clinically significant arrhythmias to assess hemodynamic consequences and overall fetal well-being.

The two most common echocardiographic methods of arrhythmia analysis are M-mode and spectral Doppler. Although either method alone is reliable in the majority of fetuses, comfort in performing and interpreting both techniques is essential in the event that fetal position or a restricted ultrasound window limits the use of one or the other method.

M-Mode

In M-mode echocardiography, the M-mode line is positioned by two-dimensional (2D) image guidance to transect one structure that represents atrial contraction (atrial wall or AV valve) and one that represents ventricular contraction (ventricular wall or aortic or pulmonary valve). Atrial systole is represented by the onset of atrial wall movement or the A-wave of the mitral or tricuspid valve inflow, and ventricular systole is represented by the onset of ventricular wall movement or the opening of either the aortic or the pulmonary valve. The fetal cardiac mechanical movements are then plotted against time. From a hard copy of the M-mode tracing, a "ladder diagram" of atrial and ventricular activity can be constructed[28] (Fig. 15–1). Cardiac time intervals are then measured from the M-mode tracing along with the sequence of atrial and ventricular events and intervals (VA and AV).

The main limitations of M-mode echocardiography are technical (obtaining properly positioned and interpretable tracings) and the assumption that mechanical cardiac events reflect electrical events. The latter can lead to an errant diagnosis with junctional ectopic tachycardia, which occurs when the electrical focus originates in the AV node. In this case, by M-mode echocardiography, the mechanical activity of the ventricle precedes the atrium, thus mimicking VT. Atrial wall motion may be minimal in atrial fibrillation or in the setting of a dilated, poorly contractile atrium. Lastly, discerning the A-waves of the mitral or tricuspid valve can be quite challenging.

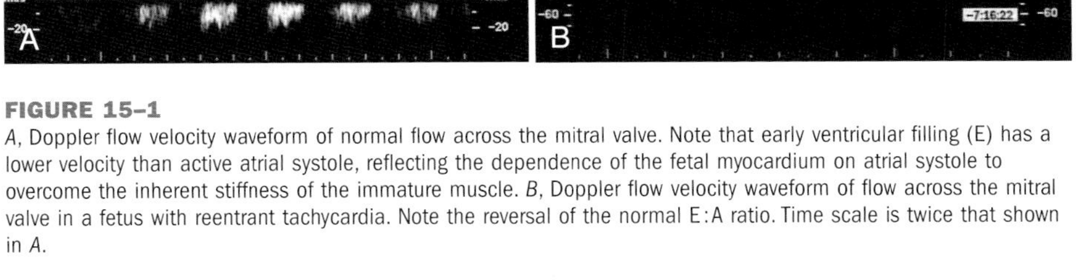

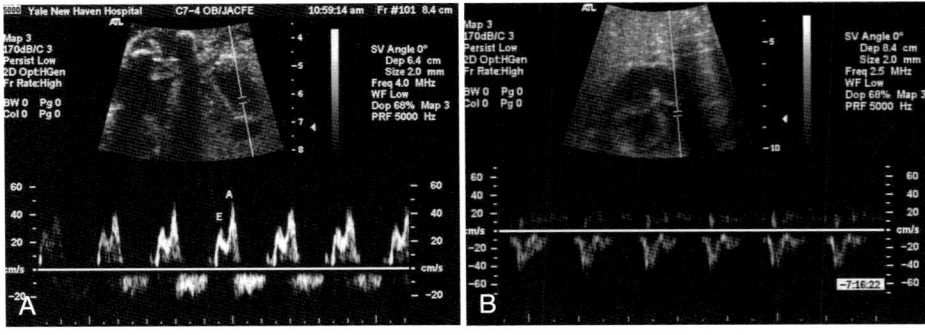

FIGURE 15–1
A, Doppler flow velocity waveform of normal flow across the mitral valve. Note that early ventricular filling (E) has a lower velocity than active atrial systole, reflecting the dependence of the fetal myocardium on atrial systole to overcome the inherent stiffness of the immature muscle. *B*, Doppler flow velocity waveform of flow across the mitral valve in a fetus with reentrant tachycardia. Note the reversal of the normal E:A ratio. Time scale is twice that shown in *A*.

Spectral Doppler

Spectral Doppler is the second echocardiographic method of fetal arrhythmia assessment. Similar to M-mode, under 2D image guidance, the sample volume is placed in a location that allows for the simultaneous recording of flow representing atrial and ventricular systole. The sample volume can be placed in a number of locations, such as the left ventricular outflow tract, which will record mitral valve inflow and ventricular outflow, the pulmonary vein and pulmonary artery, the inferior vena cava and the aorta, or the superior vena cava and aorta.[29–33] We find that the simplest to obtain is left ventricular inflow and outflow from an apical four-chamber view (see Fig. 15–1). After the appropriate sample volume position has been attained, a tracing of the flow velocity is recorded, a ladder diagram is constructed, and the sequence of atrial and ventricular events and intervals is deduced similar to M-mode. The main limitation is that this requires proper fetal positioning and the need to place the Doppler sample volume from an apical four-chamber view so as to maximize both inflow and outflow velocities.

Tissue Doppler Analysis

Tissue Doppler analysis, using myocardial depolarization signals of simultaneous sampling sites in the atrium and ventricular myocardium to assess temporal events in the fetal heart, has been shown to correlate well with intervals obtained on electrocardiography.[10] This technique eliminates some of the limitations that arise in more conventional methods including those that are positional and gestational age–related. Rein and colleagues described a method of independently obtaining timing data from the wall velocities of all four cardiac chambers that was used to construct a "fetal kinetocardiogram," which permitted precise calculation of timing intervals even when atrial and ventricular activity occurred simultaneously or when early atrial activity was weak and, thus, accurate analysis of the mechanism of fetal arrhythmias.[34]

MECHANISMS OF TACHYARRHYTHMIAS

Fetal arrhythmias are generally first detected during routine prenatal visits or ultrasound examinations. Transient fetal rhythm disturbances represent up to 10% to 20% of all indications for fetal cardiac evaluations at tertiary centers.[13] The cause of these transient arrhythmias is usually extrasystoles, typically atrial in origin. The incidence of malignant fetal arrhythmias, ventricular and supraventricular, is unknown but is believed to be rare. The most common causes of fetal tachycardias are AV reentry SVTs, atrial flutter, and sinus tachycardia. Rare causes of fetal tachycardia include atrial ectopy, atrial fibrillation, and junctional and ventricular tachycardia, which constitute less than 1% of fetal arrhythmias. Knowledge of the incidence, mechanism, and associated morbidity and mortality rates of the different arrhythmias is critical in determining the appropriate treatment for the fetus.

IRREGULAR HEART RATE

Premature Atrial Contractions

Premature atrial contractions (PACs) are the result of nonsinus atrial depolarization that occurs earlier than the expected sinus beat. PACs are the most common fetal dysrhythmia, with a prevalence of 1% to 3% of all pregnancies.[35] They may originate from either the right or the left atrium and may be conducted through the AV node either in the normal fashion or aberrantly or they may block at the level of the AV node. PACs are associated with illicit drug use, trisomy 18, and hyperthyroidism[36] and occur more commonly later in gestation. It is also hypothesized that some fetal PACs are caused by an aneurysm of the flap valve of the foramen ovale.[37] Rarely, isolated PACs are reported to trigger episodes of sustained SVT. Fetal PACs are easily recognized either by their characteristic early atrial wall movement (M-mode), mitral inflow (Doppler) pattern, or inferior vena cava flow (Doppler) pattern.

Management Options

Isolated PACs require no treatment, but because of their association with SVT, recurrent auscultation of the fetal heart rate is prudent until the ectopic beats resolve. This management strategy also permits recognition of the infrequent cases of isolated extrasystoles that may go on to develop a clinically significant arrhythmia. There is no increase in the incidence of structural heart disease in affected fetuses[13]; however, fetuses with congenital heart disease as well as those with normal hearts may not tolerate even the minor hemodynamic changes that can be associated with extrasystoles. Frequent, blocked PACs (e.g., fetal bigeminy) may appear to be a fetal bradycardia. Patients are advised to avoid caffeine and medications that may increase ectopy, such as β-adrenergic drugs (e.g., terbutaline). Persistent postnatal ectopy warrants only a neonatal ECG and consideration for a 24-hour Holter monitor.

Premature Ventricular Contractions

Premature ventricular contractions (PVCs) are caused by early, nonsinus depolarization of the ventricles. A compensatory pause may be observed if the PVC is conducted in retrograde fashion through the AV node to the atrium. PVCs produce a characteristic Doppler flow pattern with absence of diastolic flow across the AV (mitral) valve prior to the initiation of ventricular systole (aortic outflow). They account for approximately 2% to 4% of all fetal ectopy.

Management Options

PVCs are usually benign and generally warrant simple maternal avoidance of cardiac stimulants such as caffeine. Under rare circumstances, PVCs may be a harbinger of cardiomyopathy, myocarditis, structural cardiac malformations, or LQTS.[38] Postnatal ventricular ectopy requires an ECG to evaluate the corrected QT interval as well as consideration of placement of a 24-hour Holter monitor in order to quantify the frequency of the ectopy. An echocardiogram may also be recommended to assess the neonatal cardiac structure and function as well as for the presence of intracardiac tumors.

TACHYCARDIA

Sinus Tachycardia

Sinus tachycardia in a fetus is defined as a sustained heart rate between 160 and 210 beats/min with 1 : 1 AV concordance. If the rate is greater than 210 beats/min and nonvariable, SVT should be considered. Persistent fetal sinus tachycardia may be secondary to acidosis, hypoxic ischemic encephalopathy, anemia, myocarditis, infection, maternal fever, and maternal drug ingestion or use of stimulants.[39] Although maternal thyroid hormone does not cross the placenta, prenatal thyrotoxicosis secondary to transplacental passage of thyroid-stimulating immunoglobulin (TSIG) with maternal Graves' disease has also been associated with fetal sinus tachycardia.[40] Management of persistent sinus tachycardia involves recognition and treatment of the underlying cause. Sinus tachycardia should be differentiated from ventricular tachycardia (see later discussion). In sinus tachycardia, atrial systole precedes ventricular contraction, whereas in ventricular tachycardia, ventricular contraction precedes the atrial systole. This can be difficult to distinguish in utero. Sinus tachycardia may be suspected if there are gradual accelerations or decelerations in fetal heart rate rather than abrupt changes as well as preserved heart rate variability.[10]

Supraventricular Tachycardia

Fetal SVT may present at any time after 15 weeks. SVT is a general term used to describe an arrhythmia of nonsinus origin at or above the bundle of His, and thus characterized by a narrow QRS complex (Fig. 15–2) with 1 : 1 AV conduction. The causes of SVT are categorized by their dependence on the AV node for propagation of the arrhythmia. Those that require the AV node to maintain the tachycardia (Wolff-Parkinson-White [WPW] syndrome, atrioventricular node reentry tachycardia [AVNRT], permanent junctional reciprocating tachycardia [PJRT], concealed accessory pathway [CAP], and Mahaim pathways) are referred to as *AV node–dependent*. In these cases, the presence of an accessory pathway in conjunction with the normal AV node allows formation of a circuit through which electrical activity can be propagated both anterograde and retrograde between the atria and the ventricles. Those forms of SVT that do not require the AV node to be maintained (atrial fibrillation, atrial flutter, atrial and junctional ectopic tachycardia) are referred to as *AV node–independent tachycardias*. Reentrant tachycardias are the most common mechanism of fetal tachycardia, accounting for 70% to 80% of fetal SVT.[41]

Based upon their mechanism of propagation, the AV node–dependent SVTs are further divided into the short and long VA tachycardias. This distinction is important in determining the correct medication to control fetal tachycardia. The VA time in tachycardia is determined by simultaneous Doppler interrogation of either the SVC (A) or the ascending aorta (V) or by measuring mitral (A) and aortic (V) flow in the left ventricular outflow. The VA time is considered long if it is greater than one half of the V-V interval. The use of fetal echocardiography and Doppler interrogation is particularly useful in distinguishing between these types of SVT because it allows easy measurement of time intervals.[10]

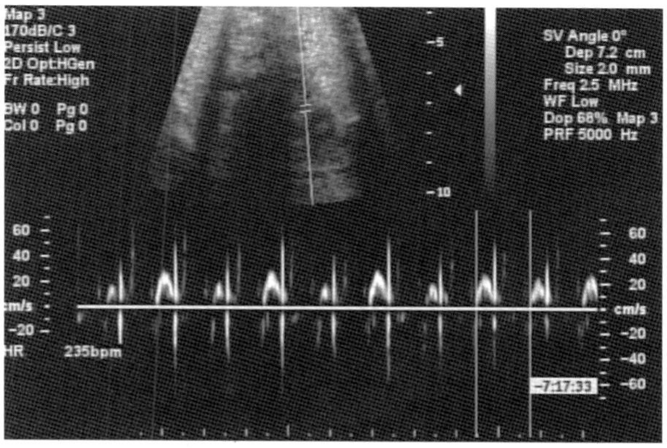

FIGURE 15–2
Doppler flow velocity waveform of flow into pulmonary artery in a fetus with reentrant supraventricular tachycardia. Typical rate of 235 beats/min is shown.

Atrioventricular Node–Dependent Supraventricular Tachycardia

SHORT VENTRICULOATRIAL TACHYCARDIA

The most common form of SVT is the short VA, AV node–dependent SVT. This category includes concealed accessory pathways, WPW syndrome, and typical AVNRT. Characteristics unique to these tachycardias include rates of 220 to 300 beats/min (typically close to 240 beats/min), little rate variability, and 1 : 1 VA concordance. In these forms of tachycardia, the VA interval is less than half the duration of the R-R interval. Atrial and ventricular ectopic beats typically trigger abrupt initiation and cessation of the tachycardia, which may be intermittent or sustained. These arrhythmias generally cannot be differentiated in utero. On rare occasions, a short VA SVT occurs in conjunction with structural cardiac disease (e.g., rhabdomyoma, ventricular inversion, or Ebstein's anomaly of the tricuspid valve). In this instance, WPW syndrome should be suspected because of its known association with these lesions.

Management Options

In general, these arrhythmias respond to transplacental digoxin or β-blocker therapy unless hydrops is already present. Occasionally, when digoxin or β-blockers fail or when there is already hydrops, second-tier antiarrhythmic agents such as flecainide, sotalol, or amiodarone become necessary and are usually effective. Preterm delivery is rarely, if ever, indicated in nonhydropic fetuses with this form of SVT. Close to term or with documented fetal lung maturity, delivery is preferable to continued unsuccessful attempts at in utero treatment. At a minimum, all patients should have a postnatal ECG to determine the etiology of the tachycardia, which will help guide further medication. If structural cardiac disease is suspected, a transthoracic echocardiogram should be performed. Usually, the antiarrhythmic medication(s) are continued up to a year postnatally to avoid recurrence.

LONG VENTRICULOATRIAL TACHYCARDIA

Incessant slow fetal SVT may be due to a slowly conducting accessory pathway found in PJRT. The incidence of this fetal tachycardia is extremely rare. It is characterized by long VA times, an incessant nature, and slower rates (180–220 beats/min) and can readily be misdiagnosed as sinus tachycardia. Owing in part to its incessant nature, it is a relatively dangerous arrhythmia, capable of causing severe cardiac dysfunction and hydrops fetalis.

Management Options

PJRT rarely responds to digoxin or β-blockade, so flecainide or sotalol would be the appropriate choices.

Atrioventricular Node–Independent Supraventricular Tachycardia

ATRIAL FLUTTER

Atrial flutter accounts for approximately one third of fetal tachycardias.[36] This rapid, regular atrial rhythm is propagated by reentrant pathways contained within the atrium itself and is characterized by atrial rates of 400 to 550 beats/min typically with a slower ventricular response. Because the reentry cycle occurs within the atrium, propagation through the AV node is not necessary to maintain the tachycardia. The ventricular rates vary, depending on whether there is uniform conduction of atrial beats. The most common form of AV conduction in fetal atrial flutter is 2 : 1 AV block. The diagnosis of atrial flutter can be made by fetal echocardiogram showing a fast atrial rate with variable AV conduction, or the typical sawtooth appearance on a fetal magnetocardiogram (Fig. 15–3). Atrial flutter is often an isolated finding but may be associated with structural cardiac defects that dilate the atrium, such as Ebstein's malformation, atrial septal defects, hypoplastic left heart syndrome, and cardiomyopathy as well as with WPW syndrome[35] and associated AV node–dependent reentry tachycardia. Hydrops occurs in upward of 35% of the fetuses with incessant atrial flutter.

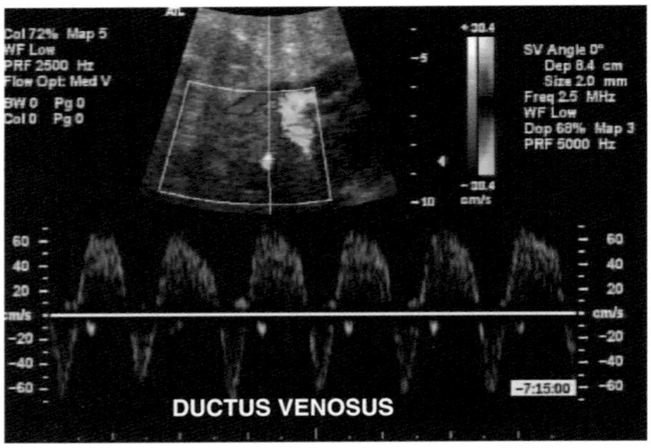

FIGURE 15–3
Flow in ductus venosus of a fetus with reentrant supraventricular tachycardia. Normal flow is unidirectional in contrast with bidirectional flow shown here.

Management Options

The management of atrial flutter is based on either termination of the intra-atrial reentry or by ventricular rate control. Ventricular rate control can be accomplished with the maternal administration of digoxin in the absence of hydrops fetalis. Sotalol has shown to be effective for arrhythmia termination in 80%.

It is prudent to continue transplacental treatment throughout pregnancy once the fetal rate is successfully converted, with careful attention to maternal drug levels, ECG, and symptoms to avoid adverse treatment effects. The prognosis for fetal atrial flutter is excellent if delivery is at term and there is no associated structural cardiac disease. After successful conversion to sinus rhythm, the majority of pediatric patients do not experience recurrence and require no treatment. Early delivery is indicated only if the fetus fails to respond to medications or has hydrops fetalis.

ATRIAL FIBRILLATION

Atrial fibrillation is a rare fetal arrhythmia with a reported incidence of 0.2%.[36] It is characterized by an extremely rapid, chaotic atrial rate of greater than 500 beats/min with variable ventricular conduction due to blocking at the level of the AV node. In cases of fine atrial fibrillation, the atria may appear to actually stand still during fetal echocardiography. Atrial fibrillation can occur in association with Ebstein's malformation of the tricuspid valve, thyrotoxicosis, and cardiac tumors.

Management Options

No antiarrhythmic agent has to date been used to convert fetal atrial fibrillation to sinus rhythm. Ventricular rate control can usually be achieved with transplacental digoxin administration. The prognosis for atrial fibrillation is unknown, owing in part to its relative rarity and the fact that the majority of cases are associated with structural and other conduction abnormalities. Postnatally, newborns are converted to a sinus rhythm through direct current cardioversion. Atrial fibrillation is not an indication for early delivery unless hydrops fetalis develops or fetal compromise is suspected based on biophysical testing.

ATRIAL TACHYCARDIA

Ectopic or *chaotic atrial tachycardias* are rare but are occasionally seen in the later stages of pregnancy. This arrhythmia is characterized by regular or irregular atrial and ventricular Doppler flow patterns, depending on the atrial rate and AV conduction. Gradual speeding and slowing of the heart rate may be identified. Atrial tachycardia is typically well tolerated and hydrops fetalis is rare.

Management Options

Once the diagnosis is established, medical management should be initiated, but the arrhythmia is frequently resistant to basic drug therapies such as digoxin and β-blockers.[42] Flecainide is the drug of choice for fetal atrial ectopic tachycardia. Postnatal recognition and treatment might be needed if the tachycardia is persistent.

JUNCTIONAL ECTOPIC TACHYCARDIA

Congenital *junctional ectopic tachycardia (JET)* is an extremely rare, incessant form of ectopic focus SVT. The focus is located within the AV node, resulting in near-simultaneous electrical activation of the atria and ventricles and superimposition of the A-wave on the V-wave, though more pronounced dissociation of the ventricles from the atria can occur, mimicking VT. This arrhythmia is unique in its inheritance pattern; approximately 50% have a close family member affected. JET is very difficult to diagnose in utero without FMCG and is frequently resistant to conventional therapy. The mortality rate approaches 35% in infancy.[43]

Management Options

Fetuses with JET may respond to either amiodarone or sotalol.

VENTRICULAR TACHYCARDIA

VT is another relatively rare form of tachycardia with the focus originating in the ventricle(s). It may be associated with fetal myocarditis, myocardial dysfunction of any cause including hypertrophic cardiomyopathy, tuberous sclerosis, or LQTS. The most common form of VT is called *slow ventricular tachycardia* or *accelerated idioventricular rhythm*. The rate is between 160 and 200 beats/min and does not warrant any intervention. VT is diagnosed when faster heart rates, greater than 200 beats/min, are observed. In addition, AV dissociation is frequently seen, with the ventricular rate being faster than the atrial rate, although 1 : 1 AV rates can be seen in the setting of retrograde VA conduction.

Management Options

Sustained fast fetal VT with or without hydrops fetalis is often refractory to treatment, which requires agents such as amiodarone, lidocaine, or sotalol. β-Blockers should be considered in suspected LQTS in an effort to minimize fetal sympathetic stimulation and reduce the incidence of fetal VT.

BRADYCARDIAS

Fetal bradycardia is defined as a persistent heart rate below 100 beats/min not associated with uterine contractions or periodic decelerations. A thorough investigation into fetal well-being and cause of the dysrhythmia is warranted when fetal bradycardia is detected. First, extrinsic, noncardiac causes of fetal bradycardia such as drugs, maternal hypothermia, and mechanical compression of the umbilical cord must be excluded.[18,44] If the bradycardia persists and no obvious extrinsic causes are evident, the next step is to determine the exact rhythm (e.g., sinus bradycardia, partial or CAVB, or atrial bigeminy with blocked premature beats) to facilitate appropriate management. As previously noted, a maternal history or screening for connective tissue disorders or drug use, along with a complete family history, probing for arrhythmias, pacemakers, and structural heart disease or congenital deafness in close family members, is warranted.

Sinus Bradycardia

Sinus bradycardia can be differentiated from other causes of fetal bradycardia by Doppler or M-mode echocardiography. The hallmark of sinus bradycardia is the presence of a normal AV activation sequence with 1 : 1 conduction. Confirmation that any slow heart rate is due to sinus bradycardia is mandatory to rule out advanced AV block or CAVB or blocked premature atrial ectopic beats. In addition to rhythm confirmation, a thorough fetal assessment is necessary to seek signs of fetal compromise, hydrops fetalis, or structural cardiac disease. Well-known causes of fetal sinus bradycardia include fetal hypoxia, sinus node dysfunction, LQTS, and heterotaxy syndrome with left atrial isomerism, in which the fetus has two left atria and thus lacks a true sinus node, which is a right atrial structure.

Management Options

The management of a fetal sinus bradycardia depends on the cause as well as the clinical status of the fetus. Close observation generally is all that is necessary if the fetus is not compromised, and all extrinsic causes of sinus bradycardia are removed. A postnatal ECG should be performed to rule out or confirm the presence of a prolonged QT interval.[45]

Atrioventricular Block

The designation *AV block* describes an abnormality in the conduction of atrial impulses through the AV node to the ventricles. This abnormality can range from a simple delay in impulse transmission, as in first-degree AV block, to a complete interruption of signal transmission with failure of AV communication, classified as CAVB or third-degree AV block. Each form of AV block has a distinct anatomic or physiologic cause for the electrical abnormality, and some can be either transient or permanent in nature. In utero, these abnormalities are diagnosed using either fetal echocardiography or FMCG with postnatal confirmation by electrocardiography. The following sections focus on the definition, evaluation, and treatment of more advanced forms of fetal AV block.

Second-Degree Atrioventricular Block

Second-degree AV block is defined as the failure of at least one nonpremature atrial impulse to be conducted to the ventricles. A number of different forms of second-degree AV block exist. Mobitz type I, or Wenckebach, is the most common, but least significant. Wenckebach is characterized by a progressive prolongation of the PR or AV interval with an eventual dropped ventricular beat. The delay occurs in the AV node, proximal to the bundle of His.[46] This conduction abnormality is generally transient in nature and is caused by vagal influence. In rare instances, it can be caused by digitalis toxicity or inflammatory disorders that affect the cardiac muscle. No treatment is necessary in asymptomatic fetuses. Mothers should be screened for presence of anti-Ro anti-La antibodies and the fetus observed closely for progression.

The more pathologic forms of second-degree AV block include Mobitz type II and the advanced types. Type II second-degree AV block is characterized by constant P-P and PR intervals followed by a nonconducted atrial impulse, whereas nonconducted atrial bigeminy may have more variability of atrial events resulting in nonconduction of an early atrial impulse through a refractory AV node. The anatomic site of block is at or below the bundle of His.[47] High-grade or advanced second-degree AV block occurs when two or more successive sinus atrial impulses are not propagated through the AV node. If either form of AV block is identified, the presence of prolonged QT interval syndrome or maternal connective tissue disorders must be investigated and the perinate followed closely for progression to CAVB.[48]

Complete Atrioventricular Block

Fetal CAVB or third-degree AV block is the complete failure of sinus or atrial impulse conduction to the ventricles. The atrial rate must be faster than the ventricular rate to ensure that the AV dissociation is not due to accelerated junctional or ventricular rhythm (e.g., sinus bradycardia with appropriate junctional response or an accelerated junctional or ventricular rhythm). The prevalence of CAVB in liveborn infants is 1 in 20,000.[49] The majority of affected fetuses fall into one of two distinct groups: those with structural cardiac disease and those with maternal connective tissue disorders.[50–52]

The association between fetal CAVB and maternal autoimmune disorders is well established.[53–56] It occurs typically after 18 weeks' gestation in fetuses of women with systemic lupus erythematosus (SLE), Sjögren's syndrome, rheumatoid arthritis, scleroderma, and undifferentiated connective tissue disorders[57–59] who have maternal autoantibodies designated anti-SS-A/Ro, anti-SS-B/La, or both.[59,60] Many women carrying a fetus with CAVB do not have symptoms of any connective tissue disorder at the time, with half demonstrating only serologic evidence of disease.[61] In addition, the vast majority of mothers with SLE do not have children with CAVB.[62] The risk of a woman with SS-A/Ro and SS-B/La antibodies and no prior affected infant having a fetus with heart block is 1% to 2%.[63] There are no reliable markers to detect which fetuses of affected women will go on to develop CAVB, and the onset of lower-order AV block and the progression to CAVB might be quite sudden. The risk of recurrence of CAVB in subsequent pregnancies after delivering an affected infant is 10% to 16%.[51,60]

The conduction system is damaged by maternal antibodies that cross the placenta and react with their corresponding antigens expressed on the surface of cells in the fetal cardiac conduction system, resulting in immunoglobulin deposition on the cells and fibrosis of the affected cells. The resulting local inflammatory reaction leads to permanent damage of the fetal cardiac conduction system and developing myocardium due to localized cellular apoptosis.[64–68] It has been proposed that impaired physiologic clearance of those apoptotic cells results in their accumulation and that in turn leads to inflammation and cellular injury.[69]

The second group of fetuses with CAVB have structural cardiac disorders. The etiology of nonimmune complete AV block was postulated by Lev[70] to be a developmental abnormality of the AV node. This abnormality results from either complete absence of the AV node, lack of union between the AV node and the distal conduction system, or the presence of an aberrant, non- or poorly functioning system.[70] The most common structural cardiac abnormalities associated with CAVB are AV septal defects, both with and without associated left atrial isomerism, and AV-VA discordance (corrected transposition of the great arteries).[50,52] Additional cardiovascular malformations (tetralogy of Fallot, atrial septal defects, transposition of the great vessels, and tricuspid atresia) are described in conjunction with conduction disorders, without any clear association between the structural abnormality and the conduction defect.[50,52]

In addition to those with well-known immunologic and structural causes, a small group of patients has been identified with a genetic mutation that results in CAVB. An autosomal dominant mutation in the cardiac transcription factor Nkx2.5 can result in familial atrial septal defects and AV node conduction abnormalities including Holt-Oram syndrome. There are also fetuses with structurally normal hearts but a mutation in SCN5A, a sodium ion channel, that is responsible for long QT interval and Brugada's syndrome, who can have a range of AV conduction abnormalities including CAVB.[71]

In contrast to the oft-quoted dogma that the majority of fetuses with CAVB without structural cardiac abnormalities have few if any problems with gestation and delivery, several studies document an exceptionally high mortality rate among these fetuses and neonates. The mortality rates range from 7% to 33% in the setting of a structurally normal heart and as high as 86% for those with structural cardiac lesions.[50–52,61,72] Poor outcomes are especially associated with structural cardiac disease, left atrial isomerism, hydrops, ventricular rates below 55 beats/min, atrial rates below 120 beats/min, AV valve regurgitation, dilated cardiomyopathy, endocardial fibroelastosis, prolonged corrected QT interval, or delivery at less than 33 weeks' gestation.[50,73]

Management Options for Heart Block

Second-degree AV block (Mobitz type I/Wenckebach): No treatment is necessary in asymptomatic fetuses. Mothers should be screened for presence of anti-Ro and anti-La antibodies and the fetus observed closely. If the dysrhythmia is transient and there is no evidence of either congenital heart disease or maternal autoimmune disorders, then consideration should be given to the possibility of LQTS, particularly if there is a coexisting history of sinus bradycardia or ventricular arrhythmias or a family history of LQTS.[74,75]

SECOND-DEGREE ATRIOVENTRICULAR BLOCK (MOBITZ TYPE II AND ADVANCED TYPES)

Management of these conduction abnormalities is similar to that of complete AV block (see next item).

THIRD-DEGREE OR COMPLETE ATRIOVENTICULAR BLOCK

The goal of management of a fetus with CAVB is the birth of a healthy, viable infant. This outcome is best achieved through a two-tiered approach. First, early identification of the fetus at risk for developing CAVB is extremely important, allowing for the initiation of therapies in an attempt to prevent the onset or progression of the conduction abnormality or its sequelae. These goals may be accomplished by increasing the fetal heart rate or contractility or by blunting or removing the inflammatory stimulus through immune suppression. Second, early intervention(s) is required at the first sign of fetal compromise including consideration of premature delivery.

Maternal or direct fetal administration of sympathomimetic agents such as terbutaline, isoproterenol, and salbutamol have some efficacy in increasing both fetal heart rate and contractility.[50,76–79] Reported fetal responses to these agents range from no improvement to complete resolution of hydrops and survival.[50,76,77,79,80] The wide applicability of these results is limited by the small number of patients treated, the highly variable clinical situations, and concomitant use of additional therapies. We believe it is unlikely this therapy works in a sustentative fashion, because it does nothing to restore AV concordance. The relative stiffness of the fetal ventricular myocardium, and the consequent reliance of the fetus on atrial systole for normal ventricular filling, makes the fetus exquisitely sensitive to interruption of this relationship.

Another approach to increase the fetal heart rate is through ventricular pacing. Transvenous and epicardial ventricular pacing has been performed in fetal animal models, and transuterine-transthoracic pacing has been reported in a few human fetuses.[81–83] Despite technical successes, all reported treated fetuses have died. With the advent of new, smaller (1.4-Fr), soft-tipped temporary pacing wires, transvenous ventricular pacing mighty become more feasible and less risky to mother and fetus in the future, although placement would require open fetal surgery with the pacemaker generator itself buried under the fetal skin to avoid exposure of the fetus to entanglement with free-floating wires in the amniotic sac.

Reduction of the maternal antibody titer or the fetal inflammatory response to the antibodies is accomplished through either suppression or removal of the offending agents. Removal of the anti-SS-A/Ro and anti-SS-B/La antibodies was reported in a few cases by plasmapheresis with variable results. Intravenous gammaglobulin has also been reported to reduce the maternal anti-Ro antibody titer.[84] Despite their encouraging results, only a limited number of patients have undergone these therapies during pregnancy.

Fluorinated steroids such as dexamethasone and betamethasone have been used for prevention and treatment of CAVB.[65,66,85–87] A retrospective case-control investigation compared pregnancy outcomes of those treated with fluorinated steroids to those untreated.[88] Although steroid use for fetuses with complete AV block failed to resolve the AV conduction defect, it was associated with some improvement in hydrops and other symptoms. Steroids administered shortly after the onset of early AV block (second-degree) may have reversed the block or prevented its advancement in at least some fetuses.[88] Maternal high-dose dexamethasone initiated at the diagnosis of fetal CAVB and continued for the remainder of the pregnancy has also been suggested to improve fetal and neonatal survival.[73] These findings suggest fluorinated steroids are a therapeutic option in fetuses with early forms of AV block to prevent progression and potentially cure the abnormality. However, a recent multicenter prospective study of dexamethasone failed to alter the progression of second- to third-degree block. In rare cases, dexamethasone was successful in reverting first- or second-degree block.[89] Although steroids will not reverse CAVB, they may ameliorate myocardial inflammation and dysfunction and help optimize fetal cardiac output. Steroids can also be considered in fetuses with hydrops, although lack of response should prompt rapid taper of the steroids to avoid complications of long-term steroid use in pregnancy.

In summary, fetal CAVB is a relatively rare condition with rapidly evolving management. We recommend early fetal echocardiography in all mothers with anti-Ro and anti-La antibodies (SS-A and SS-B). Fetuses with structural cardiac disorders associated with CAVB should be closely observed for signs of an arrhythmia. In the fetus of a mother with a connective tissue disorder, early detection of advanced AV conduction abnormalities should at least prompt the consideration of fluorinated steroids with the goal of preventing the progression of the inflammatory process. The presence of hydrops or ventricular rates below 55 beats/min should trigger the reconsideration of therapy with steroids if not previously utilized. Additional studies on the benefits of plasmapheresis and intravenous immunoglobulins are needed. In addition, the patient should be referred to a center with expertise in high risk obstetrics and fetal cardiology as well as pediatric and neonatal pacemaker implantation and management.

Management of Fetal Tachyarrhythmias—General

The management of a fetus with a dysrhythmia should involve a coordinated team approach including experts in obstetric imaging, fetal medicine, electrophysiology, and pediatric cardiology and typically coordinated by the fetal medicine expert. Strasburger and coworkers[29] observed a higher rate of cesarean section (84% vs. 18%) and lower gestational age at delivery (37 wk vs. 39 wk) in infants managed at nontertiary centers without prenatal pediatric cardiology support suggesting a high level of physician discomfort. Medications are often administered to pregnant women with hopes that the beneficial effects of the drug will be transferred to the fetus. For many of these medications, the kinetics of drug transfer is poorly studied. When transplacental antiarrhythmic therapy is to be administered, the authors also work with an adult electrophysiologist to guide dosage selection and assist in monitoring the mother for adverse events and side effects.

Hydrops Fetalis (See also Chapter 24)

Hydrops fetalis is defined as skin edema plus an abnormal collection of fluid in at least two other areas such as ascites, pleural or pericardial effusions, polyhydramnios, or placental edema. Cardiac reasons for the development of hydrops include structural cardiac defects and rhythm disturbances, which are the primary causes of up to 50% of all cases of nonimmunologic hydrops.[90] Rhythm disturbances are thought to lead to fetal heart failure and hydrops secondary to reduced diastolic filling time in conjunction with the normally decreased compliance of the fetal myocardium in comparison with postnatal myocardium and resulting in increased fetal filling pressures. Risk factors for hydrops fetalis and subsequent poor outcome include prematurity, sustained SVT exceeding 12 hours resulting in impaired ventricular filling and/or cardiac dysfunction, and structural cardiac defects. The ventricular rate and the mechanism of tachycardia have not been clearly shown to be risk factors for the development of hydrops.[11] Untreated hydrops fetalis can be associated with decreased fetal movement, fetal metabolic acidemia, myocardial dysfunction, and poor tolerance of labor. In addition, placental edema may contribute to decreased placental drug transfer requiring higher doses, more drugs (two vs. one), or more days (12.5 vs. 3) to control their arrhythmia.[91] Mortality may be as high as 13% at term for fetuses with hydrops and rises as gestational age falls.[92]

Therapeutic Options

One must balance the risks and benefits before initiating medical therapy for fetal tachyarrhythmia. We are currently unsure of the exact pharmacokinetics of many of the medicines used in transplacental treatments. All the drugs we might use have potentially dangerous side effects and might be proarrhythmic for both the mother and the fetus. They might not be effective, and there could be spontaneous resolution of the tachycardia even without treatment. Therefore, the treatment for fetal tachycardia depends on a multitude of factors including the type of arrhythmia, gestational age of the fetus, maternal and fetal health, and the presence of either structural cardiac disease or hydrops.

Therapeutic options for a fetal tachyarrhythmia include monitoring without pharmacologic intervention, transplacental or direct administration of antiarrhythmic medications to the fetus, or delivery of the fetus with postnatal arrhythmia management. Intermittent tachycardia in the near-term fetus is often well tolerated, but the management choice for most fetuses with tachycardia at or very near term (≥34–35 wk) is delivery. The nonhydropic fetus with an intermittent tachyarrhythmia can often be safely and effectively induced with oxytocin for vaginal delivery as long as there are sufficient intervals of normal rhythm present to permit electronic fetal heart rate monitoring. In pregnancies with evidence of fetal compromise or cardiac dysfunction, a complete fetal and maternal assessment must be performed and the pros and cons of all available treatment options weighed by the treatment team and family. Treatment is typically undertaken for fetuses with existing heart failure or those at high risk of developing heart failure, whereas no intervention other than intensive fetal surveillance is a reasonable therapeutic option for fetuses with intermittent tachycardia and the absence of any evidence of hemodynamic compromise.

When the treatment of a fetal arrhythmia is indicated, a number of options are available. Transplacental therapy is preferred for a stable arrhythmia when both the fetus and the mother are in excellent health. If for some reason transplacental therapy is not an option, consideration must be given to direct fetal therapy with drug infusion into the umbilical vein, into the amniotic fluid, or by direct fetal intramuscular injection. The following sections review the advantages as well as the risks of each of these therapeutic options and provide data and clinical scenarios that apply to each therapy.

Signs of fetal compromise must be sought whenever a fetal arrhythmia is detected. Delivery of a hydropic fetus prior to 34 to 35 weeks' gestation is associated with a very high mortality and is indicated only under exceptional circumstances, such as failed transplacental/direct therapy, worsening diastolic dysfunction, or a poor fetal biophysical profile.[79] When iatrogenic premature delivery is desirable rather than mandatory, documentation of fetal lung maturity by amniocentesis may help with the decision. If the pregnancy is at or before 34 weeks, appropriate doses of betamethasone or dexamethasone should be administered to hasten fetal lung maturation.

Pregnancies close to term should be delivered rather than exposing the mother to these potent medications. The aim of transplacental therapy is to use the normal function of the placenta as a fetal drug delivery mechanism. Transplacental therapy is indicated in fetuses with a stable biophysical profile and sustained tachycardia.[93] Those fetuses with tachycardia less than 30% of the time and without hydrops can probably be left untreated and instead followed closely. This decision should be individualized and based on the ability to follow the patient closely. We believe twice-weekly echocardiographic evaluation of nonhydropic infants is warranted. In contrast, many neonates with any episode of nonsinus, AV node–dependent tachycardia will receive antiarrhythmic medications for up to 1 year of age to minimize their risk of developing congestive heart failure.

Antiarrhythmic medicines should be initiated under close supervision. With the exception of β-blockers, most antiarrhythmic drugs require close monitoring of both fetus and mother for side effects as well as successful conversion to sinus rhythm. We believe that when most antiarrhythmic drugs are initiated, the mother should be monitored as an inpatient on cardiac telemetry in consultation with an adult electrophysiologist to monitor the maternal ECG, electrolytes, and vital signs. Conversion can generally be achieved within a few days. Once control or steady state is achieved, the patients may be discharged with close follow-up. Conversion rates of fetal SVT range from 80% to 90% and are lowest when there is already hydrops present.[94] The resolution of hydrops after successful treatment of tachycardia may take several weeks. Acceleration of fetal maturity with corticosteroids should be considered if elective preterm delivery seems likely.[95]

Pharmacokinetics and Choice of Antiarrhythmic Agents

Transfer of any drug across the placental barrier is promoted by low molecular size, low ionization, and high lipid solubility.[96] The rate of diffusion is also dependent on fetal-maternal concentration gradient and the thickness of the placental membrane. Higher doses of drugs are often required to achieve therapeutic levels during pregnancy because of increased blood volume and volume of distribution, increased protein binding of drugs, increased hepatic metabolism, and greatly increased glomerular filtration rate in the mother. The placenta is able to transfer, concentrate, and metabolize drugs to inactive metabolites, although it is worth noting that some antiarrhythmic metabolites are themselves active agents. Fetal metabolism of drugs is primarily renal or placental because hepatic enzymes are immature (only 20%–50% active). The potential myocardial depressant effects of these medications must be considered, especially in the setting of existing or potential myocardial dysfunction in affected fetuses. The transplacental transfer of drugs, particularly digoxin, may be poor in the presence of hydrops fetalis, making management of fetal SVT with associated hydrops more difficult. To circumvent mitigating factors that affect transplacental transfer, direct umbilical or fetal intramuscular administration of drugs has been used successfully to treat the fetus directly after a transplacental approach had failed.[97,98]

The proper diagnosis of the type of tachycardia is required to guide therapy. Based on a 1998 survey of 15 institutions treating fetal arrhythmias, the most commonly used drug was digoxin (78%) followed by flecainide (18%), verapamil (7%), procainamide (6%), quinidine (6%), amiodarone (6%), propranolol (2%), and sotalol (2%).[82] Verapamil and other calcium channel blockers are contraindicated in newborns owing to the risk of profound hypotension and shock and should be used rarely and with extreme caution, if at all, in fetuses. In addition, quinidine has proarrhythmic effects and also should be used rarely. Amiodarone is effective in 90% of reentrant SVTs and 60% of atrial flutter. However, the half-life of amiodarone after prolonged usage is measured in weeks, and the potential for profound fetal hypothyroidism, and consequent goiter and even cretinism, mandates great caution. The maternal ECG and side effects including thyroid, liver, and pulmonary should be monitored along with desired fetal effect, and the dose titrated for optimal response. Standard doses and some common side effects of different drugs are listed in Table 15–2.

Prognosis

The perinatal mortality rate for fetal tachycardia with hydrops ranges from 3.5% to 30% in different studies. The differences may relate to the use of different antiarrhythmic agents, some with proarrhythmic effects, the incidence of premature delivery, and fetal interventions including cordocentesis.[99] Marked acidosis, prematurity, and prolonged tachycardia are also associated with hydrops and long-term postnatal sequelae including neurologic problems.[100]

TABLE 15–2

Pharmacologic Agents Used to Treat Fetal Arrhythmias

DRUG	ADVERSE EFFECT	DOSING RANGE	MECHANISM OF ACTION	THERAPEUTIC LEVEL
Digoxin	Nausea, bradycardia, vision disturbance, first- and second-degree AV block, rhythm disturbances	Loading dose: 1200–1500 μg/24 hr IV Maintenance: 375–875 μg/day PO divided bid	Slows ventricular rate by partially blocking the AV node	0.8–2.5 ng/dL
Propranolol	Low birth weight, hypoglycemia, bradycardia, increased uterine tone	80–320 mg/day PO in three to four divided doses	β-Blocker	25–50 ng/mL
Flecainide	Fetal demise, conduction defects, QT interval prolongation, proarrhythmia	100–400 mg/day PO divided bid-tid	Class Ic; slows conduction velocity in most cardiac pathways by effects on Na channels	0.2–10 μg/mL
Sotalol	Tiredness, dizziness, nausea, QT interval prolongation, torsades de pointes	80–160 mg PO bid-tid	β-Blocker with additional class III antiarrhythmic properties with prolongation of cardiac action potential through blockage of K channels	Not known
Amiodarone	Nausea, thrombocytopenia, visual disturbances, QT interval prolongation, hypothyroidism	Loading dose: 1200 mg PO q6h Maintenance: 600–900 mg/day	Primarily class III antiarrhythmic with prolongation of phase 3 of cardiac action potential through blockage of K channels. Also has β-blocker-like and K channel blocker-like actions as well as Na channel effects	0.7–2.8 μg/mL

AV, atrioventricular.

SUMMARY OF MANAGEMENT OPTIONS

Fetal Cardiac Arrhythmias

Management Options	Evidence Quality and Recommendation	References
Irregular Fetal Heart Rate		
Prenatal Diagnosis		
Careful history and examination to exclude • Familial long QT interval syndrome. • Maternal illicit drug use. • Maternal hyperthyroidism.	IV/C	36
Fetal echocardiography to confirm cardiac normality; detailed fetal sonography to exclude syndromes; consider karyotype if aneuploidy (especially trisomy 18) suspected.	III/B IV/C	13 36

SUMMARY OF MANAGEMENT OPTIONS

Fetal Cardiac Arrhythmias—cont'd

Management Options	Evidence Quality and Recommendation	References
Prenatal Treatment		
No treatment if isolated (as in the majority of cases).	—/GPP	—
Avoid caffeine and drugs that promote ectopy (e.g., β-sympathomimetics).	—/GPP	—
Weekly ausculation to confirm no progression to SVT.	—/GPP	—
Postnatal		
If ectopic beats persist in the neonatal period, perform ECG and consider 24-hr Holter monitor as well as echocardiography.	IV/C	38,45
Tachycardias		
Prepregnancy		
Counseling of those with history of		
• WPW syndrome.	IV/C	36
• Familial long QT interval syndrome.	IV/C	38,45
Prenatal Diagnosis		
Auscultation and fetal echocardiography for sustained fetal rate >180 beats/min.	—/GPP	—
Ultrasound evaluation of cardiac structure, function, presence of hydrops, and mechanism of arrhythmia (including M-mode and spectral Doppler).	III/B	8
Search for other abnormalities with ultrasound; consider karyotype if aneuploidy suspected.	—/GPP	—
Prenatal Treatment		
Depends on • Underlying mechanism/diagnosis. • Persistence of tachyarrhythmia. • Presence of hydrops. • Gestational age.	—/GPP	—
Nonsustained tachycardia requires monitoring but no treatment unless hydrops is present.	—/GPP	—
Medical (Transplacental) control of sustained tachycardia; five drugs are commonly used: Digoxin. β-Blockers. Flecainide. Soltalol. Amiodarone. **Sinus tachycardia**—Treat cause (e.g., maternal thyrotoxicosis). **Short VA SVT**—preceding five drugs have been used. **Long VA SVT**—use flecainide, soltalol. **Atrial flutter**—digoxin, soltalol. **Atrial fibrillation**—no intrauterine drug is effective; DC after birth. **Atrial tachycardia**—flecainide. **Junctional ectopic tachycardia**—soltalol, amiodarone. **Ventricular tachycardia**—soltalol, amiodarone.	III,IV/B,C	44,91,99
Monitor maternal ECG and drug levels with use of these drugs.		
Therapy delivered directly to the fetus has been effective, particularly in the setting of hydrops.	III/B	97,98
Delivery is an option if close to term (34+ wk); short trial of drug therapy before delivery if hydrops even if close to term is a possible option because newborns with hydrops have poor prognosis.	—/GPP	—

Management Options	Evidence Quality and Recommendation	References
Postnatal		
12-lead ECG to confirm WPW or long QT interval syndrome and precise diagnosis.	IV/C	38,45
Take local advice re prophylactic treatment for tachycardia—some will not use this routinely. Some centers will treat asymptomatic neonates for 6–12 mo and review.	—/GPP	—
Treat recurrent tachycardia in infancy (medical therapy or ablation).	III/B	91,93
Bradycardias		
Prepregnancy		
Counseling of women with the following risk factors for CAVB:		
• Previous child with CAVB.	III/B	98
• Maternal anti-SSA (Ro) or SSB (La) antibodies (1%–2% risk).	III/B	59,63
• Maternal heart block.	—/GPP	—
• Previous child with left atrial isomerism.	—/GPP	—
• Familial prolonged QT interval syndrome is a possible risk factor.	IV/C	38,45
Prenatal Diagnosis		
Detailed and serial echocardiography (every 1–2 wk) of antibody-positive mothers and those with a positive family history.	—/GPP	—
Fetal echocardiography for persistent fetal rate <100 beats/min.	—/GPP	—
Serial echocardiography (every 1–2 wk) for emerging block (second- or third-degree heart block).	—/GPP	—
Irregular rhythms • If occasional, clinical follow-up. • If persistent, fetal echocardiography and intensify follow-up.	—/GPP	—
Evaluation of asymptomatic mothers for anti-Ro and anti-La antibodies and autoimmune disease (rheumatoid arthritis, Sjögrens syndrome, systemic lupus erythematosus, or undifferentiated autoimmune syndrome).	III/B	59,63
Prenatal Treatment		
Early steroids (dexamethasone/betamethasone) are common first-line treatment; no evidence of benefit of prophylactic steroids.	III/B	78,84,88
More research is needed into role of plasmapheresis and IVIG.	IV/C	78,84
Inotropic/chronotropic support is of limited benefit.	III/B	72,86
Fetal pacing has been attempted but without success.	IV/C	79,85
Consider early delivery in tertiary center if hydrops is evident, but generally try to avoid preterm delivery.	—/GPP	—
Mode of delivery—intrapartum monitoring of fetal distress may be difficult in CAVB.	—/GPP	—
Postnatal		
Temporary pacing may be necessary.	III/B	51,72
Permanent pacemaker for rate <60 beats/min, symptoms, or structural disease.	III/B	51,72

CAVB, complete atrioventricular block; DC, dilation and curettage; ECG, electrocardiogram; GPP, good practice point; IVIG, intravenous immunoglobulin; SVT, supraventricular tachycardia; VA SVT, ventriculoatrial supraventricular tachycardia; WPW, Wolff-Parkinson-White.

SUGGESTED READINGS

Buyon J, Heibert R, Copel J, et al: Autoimmune-associated congenital heart block: Demographics, mortality, morbidity and recurrence rates obtained from a national neonatal lupus registry. J Am Coll Cardiol 1998;31:1658–1666.

Ferrer PL: Fetal arrhythmias. In Deal BJ, Wolff GS, Gelband H (eds): Current Concepts in Diagnosis and Management of Arrhythmias in Infants and Children. Armonk, NY, Futura, 1998, pp 17–63.

Friedman DM, Kim MY, Copel JA, et al: Prospective evaluation of fetuses with autoimmune-associated congenital heart block followed in the PR Interval and Dexamethasone Evaluation (PRIDE) study. Am J Cardiol 2009;103:1102–1106.

Kaaja R, Julkunen H, Ammala P, et al: Congenital heart block: Successful prophylactic treatment with intravenous gamma globulin and corticosteroid therapy. Am J Obstet Gynecol 1993;82:11–16.

Macones GA, Hankins GDV, Spong CY, et al: The 2008 National Institute of Child Health and Human Development Workshop Report on Electronic Fetal Monitoring: Update on definitions, interpretation, and research guidelines [see comment]. Obstet Gynecol 2008;112: 661–666.

Reed K: Fetal arrhythmias: Etiology, diagnosis, pathophysiology, and treatment. Semin Perinatol 1989;13:294.

Simpson JM, Sharland GK: Fetal tachycardias: Management and outcome of 127 cases. Heart 1998;79:576–581.

Srinivasan S, Strasburger J: Overview of fetal arrhythmias. Curr Opin Pediatr 2008;20:522–531.

Strasburger JF: Fetal arrhythmias. Progr Pediatr Cardiol 2000;11:1–17.

Van Engelen AD, Weitjens O, Brenner JI, et al: Management outcome and follow-up of fetal tachycardia. J Am Coll Cardiol 1994;24: 1371–1375.

REFERENCES

For a complete list of references, log onto www.expertconsult.com.

CHAPTER 16

Fetal Cardiac Anomalies

GIUSEPPE RIZZO and DOMENICO ARDUINI

Videos corresponding to this chapter are available online at www.expertconsult.com.

INTRODUCTION

Examination of the fetal heart is a part of the comprehensive fetal scan, but a complete examination can be a challenge to even an experienced sonographer. Ultrasound techniques used in fetal cardiology have evolved impressively over the years; no other fetal organ is examined with so many modalities as the heart including two-dimensional imaging, M-mode examination, spectral Doppler, color Doppler, power, high-definition digital Doppler as well as tissue Doppler.[1] Very recently, three-dimensional (3D) and four-dimensional (4D) technology were introduced into fetal cardiology and first experiences reported.[1]

Structural and functional abnormalities do affect later cardiac development, and the importance of antenatal diagnosis is well recognized in modern perinatal medicine. Congenital heart disease (CHD) complicates 0.4% to 1.1% of live births[2] and accounts for 35% of infant deaths secondary to congenital disease.[3] Cardiovascular anomalies are frequently associated with other anomalies.[4,5] In this chapter, the indication and the sonographic technique for assessing fetal cardiac status are reviewed, the principal structural cardiac diseases described, and the available management options discussed.

INDICATIONS FOR FETAL ECHOCARDIOGRAPHY

"Routine" Fetal Echocardiography

Despite the high incidence of CHD, "routine" fetal echocardiography (i.e., all pregnancies) remains unavailable in many locations because it requires sophisticated equipment, a skilled operator, and meticulous scanning. It is simply not practical to screen the entire obstetric population at the present. Moreover, the pregnancies at greatest risk of CHD are those in which an abnormality of the fetal heart is suspected during the routine 18- to 23-week anatomic scan. This underscores the importance of a meticulous scanning of the fetal heart in all pregnancies at this gestational age in order to identify those who should be referred for fetal echocardiography.

Selective Fetal Echocardiography

Fetal echocardiography is performed in selected pregnancies at increased risk of carrying a fetus with a CHD. Risk factors can be divided into familial, maternal, and fetal (Table 16–1).

There is an association between increased nuchal translucency (NT) measured between 11 and 13 + 6 weeks of gestation and CHD (see Chapter 7).[6,7] The prevalence of major cardiac defects increases exponentially with NT thickness,[7] from 4.9 per 1000 when the NT thickness is below the median to 8.7 per 1000 when the NT is between the median and the 95th percentile to 18.2 per 1000 when the NT is between the 95th and the 99th percentiles.[7] Further, abnormalities of cardiac function have been demonstrated in fetuses with normal cardiac anatomy but increased NT,[8] suggesting a pivotal role for NT measurement in the screening of fetuses who should undergo fetal echocardiography.

More recently, several new ultrasonographic markers were added to first-trimester screening for fetal aneuploidies including the presence of tricuspid regurgitation (TR) and reverse flow in the ductus venosus (DV). Each is an independent predictor of CHD. In euploid fetuses with an increased NT, TR is present in half of those cases with CHD but in only 5.6% of those without CHD.[9] Likewise, the finding of an absent or reversed A-wave in the DV in euploid fetuses with an increased NT is associated with a threefold increase in the likelihood of CHD, whereas a normal DV halves the risk for such defects.[10] As a consequence, studies of both DV flow and TR at 11 + 0 to 13 + 6 weeks' gestation promise to be good markers for CHD with and without an abnormal NT.

Reports on the efficacy of screening for CHDs vary widely with sensitivities ranging between 10% and 81%.[11–13] These differences may reflect the characteristics of study population (low or high risk), type of study (prospective and retrospective), level of experience of operators, modality of examination (four-chamber view or four-chamber view + outflow tract visualization), and quality of follow-up (postnatal clinical examination or postnatal echocardiography). With the current technology and with a proper training of examiners, demonstration of the four-chamber view allows

TABLE 16–1

Indications for Fetal Echocardiography

Family History

- Previous affected fetus or child
- Maternal or paternal congenital heart disease
- History of a single gene disorder (Di George's, Noonan's, Marfan's, William's, Holt-Oram syndromes)

Maternal History

- Metabolic diseases
  - Insulin-dependent diabetic mother
  - Maternal phenylketonuria
  - Connective tissue disease
- Exposure to teratogens
  - Alcohol
  - Valproic acid
  - Phenytoin
  - Isoretinoin
  - Lithium
  - Hydantoin
- Infections
  - Rubella
  - Parvovirus
  - Coxsackievirus
  - Cytomegalovirus

Fetal

- Arrhythmias
- Extracardiac anomalies
- Hydrops
- Hydramnios
- Growth restriction
- Chromosomal defects
- Increased nuchal translucency thickness at 11 + 0 – 13 + 6 weeks' gestation
- Trucuspid regurgitation at 11 + 0 – 13 + 6 weeks' gestation
- Retrograde flow in the ductus venosus at 11 + 0 – 13 + 6 weeks' gestation
- Abnormal heart at 18–20 weeks routine scan (usually abnormal four-chamber view)

TABLE 16–2

Schematic Approach to Scanning the Fetal Heart

Cardiac Malformations

- **Make diagnosis**—see later for systematic approach
- **Inform the patients** (possibilities and limitations)
- **Fetal position**
- **Fetal situs** (transverse section of the upper abdomen)
- **Real-time view of the fetal heart**
- Apical four-chamber view
  - Size of heart (one third of the thorax)
  - Two atria of approximately equal size
  - Two ventricles of equal size, normally contracting
  - Morphologically right ventricle on right
  - Two opening atrioventricular valve
  - Pulmonary veins
- Lateral four-chamber view
  - Integrity of interventricular septum (muscular portion)
  - Foramen ovale flap
- Left ventricle outflow tract, aortic arch
  - Aorta arise from left ventricle
  - Integrity of interventricular septum (membranous portion)
  - Opening aortic valve
  - Regular size of aortic arch
- Right ventricle outflow tract, ductus arch
  - Pulmonary artery rise from right ventricle
  - Opening of pulmonary valve
  - Regular size of main pulmonary artery
  - Branching of pulmonary artery and continuity with ductus arteriosus
- Three-vessel view
  - Pulmonary artery, aorta, and superior vena cava visualization
  - Identification of trachea and thymus
- Systemic venous return
  - Transverse section of upper abdomen position of aorta (left and posterior) and inferior vena cava (right anterior)
  - Parasagittal view of fetal trunk (inferior and superior vena cava)
- Pulmonary venous return
  - From apical four-chamber view, identify inlet in left atrium

Doppler Echocardiography

Color

- Apical four-chamber view
  - Normal ventricular filling
  - Absence of regurgitation
- Ventricle outflow tracts
  - Normal aortic and pulmonary artery color visualization
  - Absence of flow reversal
- Three-vessel view
  - Same color direction in pulmonary artery and aorta

Pulsed

- Apical four-chamber view
  - Mitral and tricuspid velocity waveforms flow only during diastole (E- and A-waves)
  - Ventricle outflow tract
  - Aortic and pulmonary velocity waveforms flow only during systole (peak velocity, time to peak velocity, cardiac output?)
- Ductus arteriosus flow
  - Flow throughout all cardiac cycle
  - Highest velocities in fetal circulation
  - Exclude ductal constriction (PI < 2)
- Venous flow
  - Inferior vena cava reflects overall cardiac function
  - Poor cardiac function is associated with increased reverse flow during atrial contraction (high preload index)

for the detection of 40% to 50% CHDs in low risk pregnancies. Additional visualization of the outflow tracts increases the detection rate to 65% to 70%. Experience has a significant impact on the examination of the fetal heart and the prenatal detection rate of major CHDs. The learning curve is fairly flat because a sonographer already confident in obtaining the four-chamber view may require another 3 years to properly visualize the outflow tracts.[14]

ULTRASONOGRAPHIC EXAMINATION OF THE FETAL HEART (TABLE 16-2)

Timing of Fetal Echocardiography

Women should be seen within 48 hours of referral when an anomaly is suspected to avoid growing parental anxiety during the interval between detection and consultation. Planned fetal echocardiography is typically performed between 20 and 22 weeks.[15] The maternal abdominal wall thickness, prior abdominal surgery, and the number of fetuses each influence the ideal time for study.

Transvaginal ultrasonography or high-resolution transabdominal probe permits a detailed view of the fetal anatomy early in gestation from 11 weeks onward.[16,17] We currently limit performance of these early scans to woman with an increased NT with or without TR or abnormal DV flow, with a prior affected child, or with insulin-dependent diabetes.[18] At this gestational age, fetal echocardiography is mainly used to confirm or refute normal cardiac anatomy rather than to establish a specific diagnosis, Because the sensitivity of early echocardiography is at a maximum 60%,[16] it should be repeated between 20 and 22 weeks even if the first is normal; an additional 20% of the CHDs will be evident.[17]

General Principles

It is imperative that the mother is informed before the examination in a clear and considerate manner about the reason for the fetal cardiac evaluation and its efficacy and limitations.[19] The findings of the scan should then be explained at the end of the examination. Fetal echocardiography consists of several steps:

1. Determine the fetal cardiac orientation and position.
2. Evaluate the cardiac anatomy.
3. Evaluate the cardiac hemodynamics and function using color and pulsed Doppler.

Fetal Cardiac Orientation and Position

The examination begins with identification of the fetal head and spine so that the fetal right and left sides are known. The fetal visceral orientation, known as *situs*, is easily identified by noting the location of the following landmarks while viewing a transverse section of the upper abdomen (Fig. 16–1).

1. The stomach and spleen are on the left.
2. The abdominal aorta is a circular, pulsating structure on the left, anterolateral to the spine without another vessel posterior.
3. The inferior vena cava (IVC) is an elliptical structure on the right of the spine in a plane anterior to the aorta.
4. The umbilical vein bends to the right, continuing in the portal sinus.

The arrangement described previously constitutes *situs solitus*. An abnormal visceral-vascular arrangement may be either *situs inversus* or *situs ambiguous*. In the former, the visceral-vascular arrangements are the mirror image of *situs solitus*, so that the stomach and aorta are on the right and the IVC and the liver are on the left side. *Situs ambiguous* refers to a condition in which there is an abnormal arrangement of the abdominal and thoracic organs and is usually associated with cardiosplenic syndromes.

Normal Fetal Cardiac Anatomy

A sequential approach is applied to fetal echocardiography based on the pathologic and angiographic examination of the heart.[20] The main steps include identification of the cardiac position within the body, identification of the cardiac chambers, study of atrioventricular (AV) connections, study of ventriculoarterial connections, and study of venous return to the atria. This is accomplished by examining the following standardized, echocardiographic planes.

APICAL FOUR-CHAMBER VIEW

The apical four-chamber view is found in a cross-sectional scan of the fetal thorax just above the level of the diaphragm where the normal heart is almost horizontal, mainly on the left side of the chest with the apex pointing left. The apical four-chamber view is the single most important view of the heart and provides the following anatomic information (Fig. 16–2):

1. The heart is correctly situated in the thorax with the apex on the left, and it occupies about one third of the thorax. The ratio between the cardiac and the thoracic circumferences in this view during end-diastole (i.e., while the AV valves are closed) is constant across gestation with an upper limit of 0.58.[21] Larger values suggest either cardiomegaly or a small chest.
2. There are two atria of equal size. The two ventricles are approximately equal in size and thickness, and in real time, their contractility appears similar.
3. The right ventricle is on the right and near the anterior thoracic wall. It has a septomarginal trabeculum, or moderator band, located near the apex in contiguity with the interventricular septum. The left ventricular cavity is smooth.

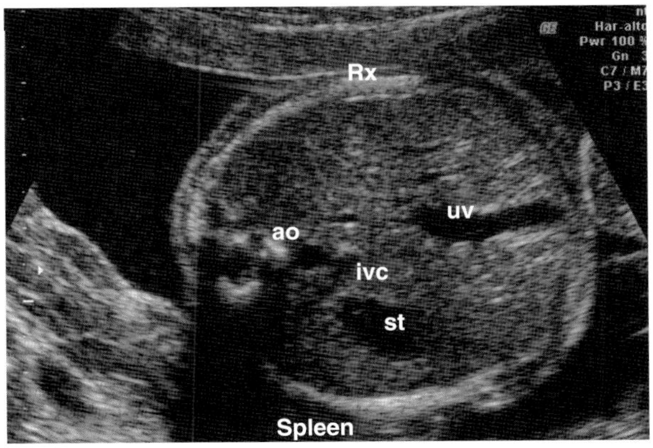

FIGURE 16–1
Transverse section of the upper fetal abdomen shows the spleen, stomach (ST), aorta (AO), inferior vena cava (IVC), and umbilical vein (UV).

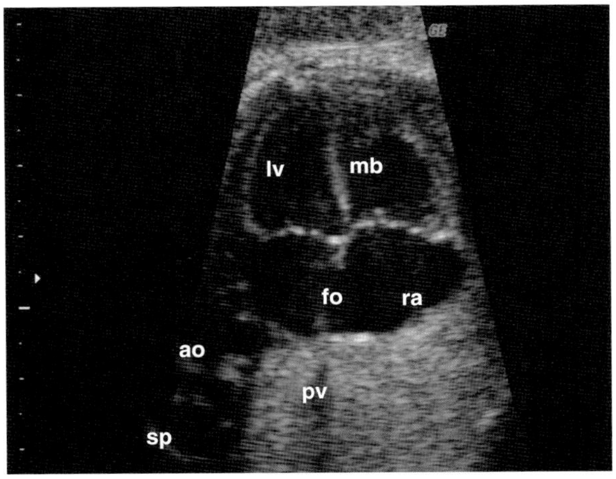

FIGURE 16–2
Apical four-chamber view of the fetal heart. Ao, aorta; Fo, foramen ovale; LV, left ventricle; MB, moderator band; PV, pulmonary vein; RA, right atrium.

4. Two AV valves open in real time, and the insertion of the tricuspid valve is located more toward the apex than the mitral valve.
5. The interatrial septum, the foramen ovale, and the interventricular septum are visualized. The atria and ventricular septa meet at the level of AV valve, generating a crux.
6. The pulmonary veins enter the left atrium.

The four-chamber view is an essential component of any study of the fetal heart, but alone is insufficient, because less than a third of congenital defects are detectable.

LATERAL FOUR-CHAMBER VIEW

This view allows visualization with higher resolution of certain structures lying perpendicular to the line of ultrasound transmission. The artifactual dropout at the level of the high portion of the interventricular septum and of the atrium septum secundum common in the apical four-chamber view is avoided, and the integrity of the interventricular and interatrial septa is optimally demonstrated. This view also allows enhanced imaging of the foramen ovale and the movement of its valve into the left atrium (Fig. 16–3).

LEFT VENTRICLE OUTFLOW TRACT

It is possible to obtain a long-axis view of the fetal heart in an oblique section of the fetal thorax. This section reveals the following landmarks (Fig. 16–4):

1. The mitral valve is seen between the left atrium and the left ventricle, and the posterior leaflet is shorter than the anterior leaflet.
2. The anterior leaflet of the mitral valve is continuous with the posterior wall of the aorta.
3. The anterior wall of the aorta is continuous with the interventricular septum.
4. The aortic valve and its movement are seen at the base of the aorta. By orienting the transducer from the left shoulder to the right hemithorax, the aortic arch and the origin of the brachiocephalic vessels are fully visualized (Fig. 16–5).

RIGHT VENTRICLE OUTFLOW TRACT

This view is a transverse cross-section of the fetal thorax. The pulmonary artery is seen arising from the right ventricle anterior to and left of the ascending aorta (circle and sausage image) (Fig. 16–6). The movement of the pulmonary valve is seen. With slight movement of the transducer, the

FIGURE 16–3
Transverse section of the fetal thorax shows the lateral four-chamber view. The *dotted line* connect the spine(s) with the sternum and allows calculation of the cardiac axis (angle between the *dotted line* and the intraventricular septum). ao, aorta; dx, right side; L, lung; bm, band moderator; pv, pulmonary vein; sx, left side; vs, left ventricle.

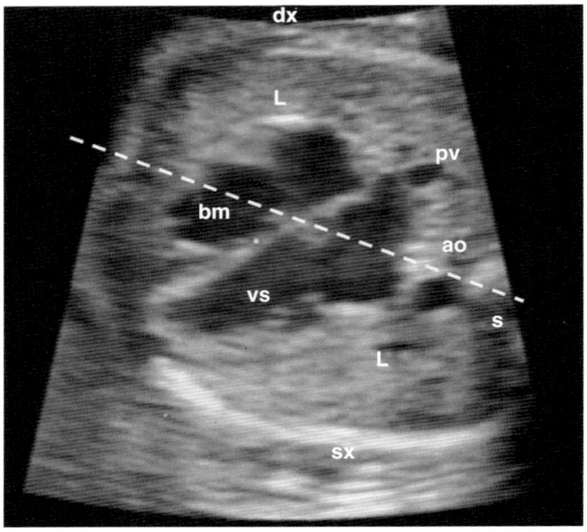

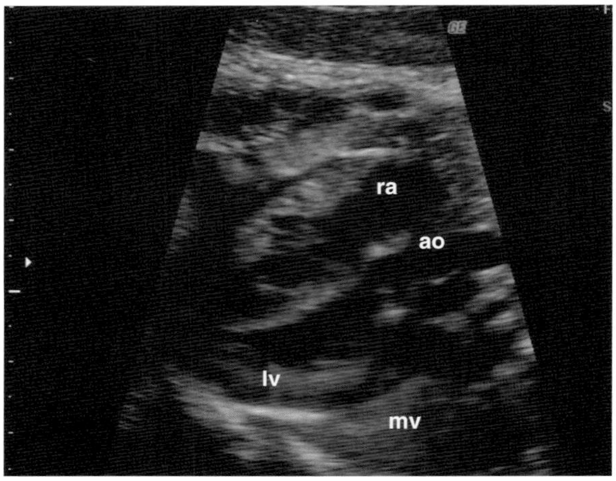

FIGURE 16–4
Long-axis view of the fetal heart shows the continuity between left ventricle (LV) and aorta (ao). mv, mitral valve; ra, right atrium.

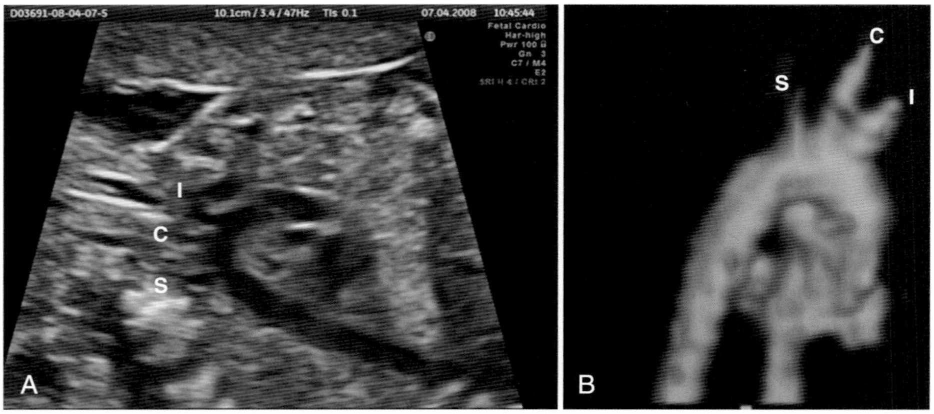

FIGURE 16–5
A, Longitudinal view of the aortic arch and the brachiocephalic vessels. *B*, Same section with flow Doppler superimposed shows the arch with its three branches: innominate artery (I), left carotid artery (c), and subclavian artery (s).

longitudinal view of the ductal arch is obtained. It is also possible to visualize the bifurcation of the main pulmonary artery and the ductus arteriosus connecting to the descending aorta in this section (Fig. 16–7).

THREE-VESSEL VIEW

From the four-chamber view, the transducer is moved parallel in the direction of the upper thorax. In this view, the pulmonary trunk with the ductus arteriosus, the aortic arch with the aortic isthmus, and the superior vena cava are seen (Fig. 16–8). The aorta and pulmonary trunk are seen in a longitudinal view and form a V-shaped area in the posterior thorax on the left side of the spine.[22] In this section, the trachea is a circular structure with an echogenic wall adjacent and to the right of the aorta. In front of the trachea, the superior vena cava can be seen. The landmarks contained in this view include

1. Three vessels seen from left to right: pulmonary artery, aorta, and superior vena cava.
2. In descending order of size: pulmonary artery > aorta > superior vena cava.

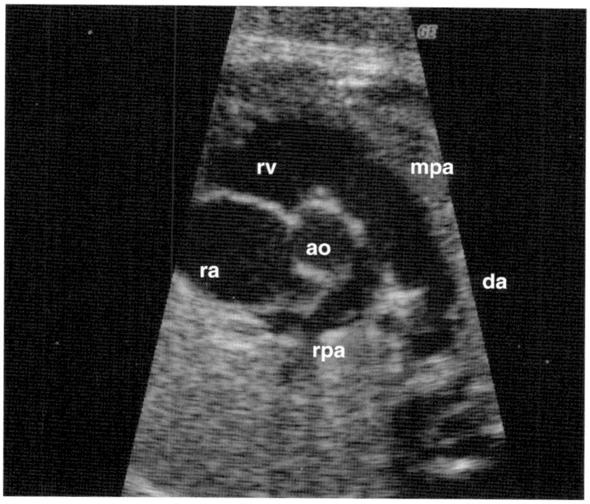

FIGURE 16–6
Short-axis view of the fetal heart shows the outflow tract of the right ventricle (RV). AO, aorta; DA, ductus arteriosus; MPA, main pulmonary artery; RPA, right pulmonary artery; RA, right atrium.

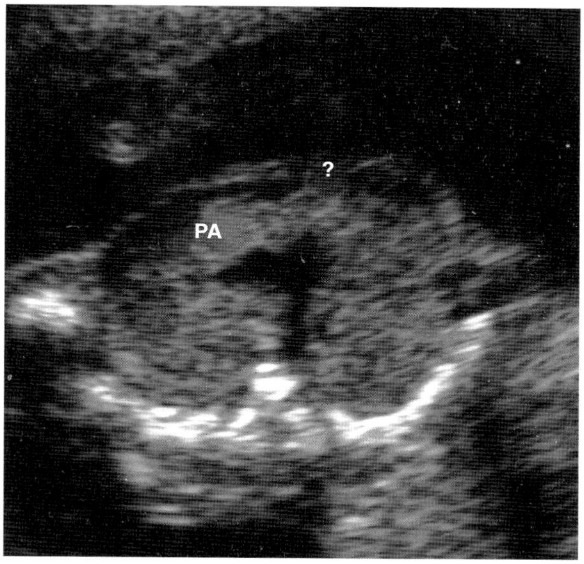

FIGURE 16–8
Three-vessel view in a fetus with a microdeletion of chromosome 22q11 with an absent pulmonary valve resulting in a dilated pulmonary artery (PA) and absent thymus (?).

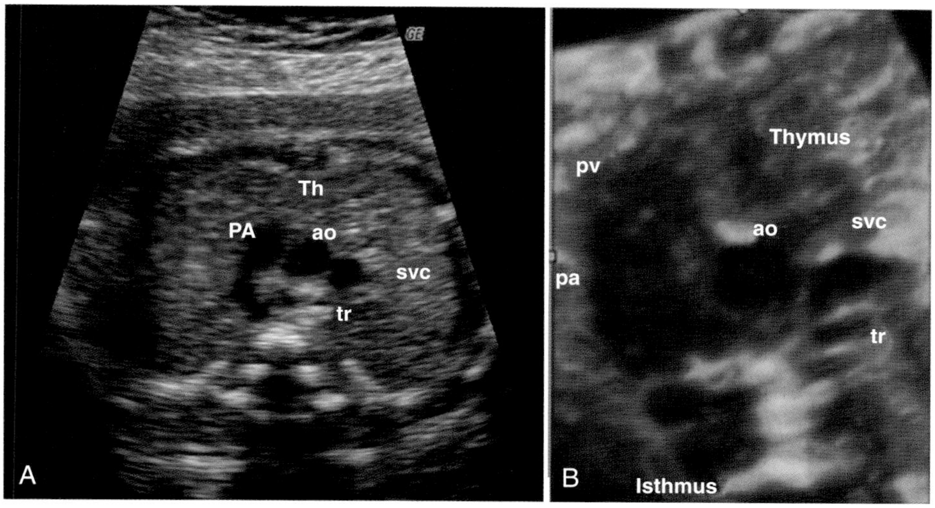

FIGURE 16–7
A, Transverse section of the fetal thorax at the level of the three-vessel view. The pulmonary artery (PA) is the largest of the three vessels; the aorta (AO) is between the PA and the superior vena cava (SVC), which is the smallest and most posterior vessel. The trachea (Tr) is visualized posterior to the aorta, and the thymus (th) is situated anteriorly. *B*, Three-dimensional display of the three-vessel view.

FIGURE 16–9
Three-vessel view of the fetal heart shows the persistence of left superior vena cava (LSVC) lateral to the pulmonary artery (PA). Ao, aorta; svc, superior vena cava.

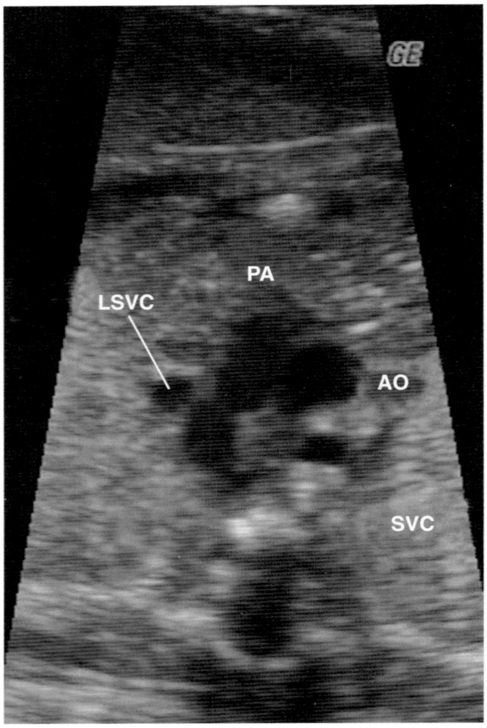

FIGURE 16–10
Parasagittal view of the fetal trunk shows the inlet in the right atrium (RA) of the superior (SVC) and inferior (IVC) venae cavae.

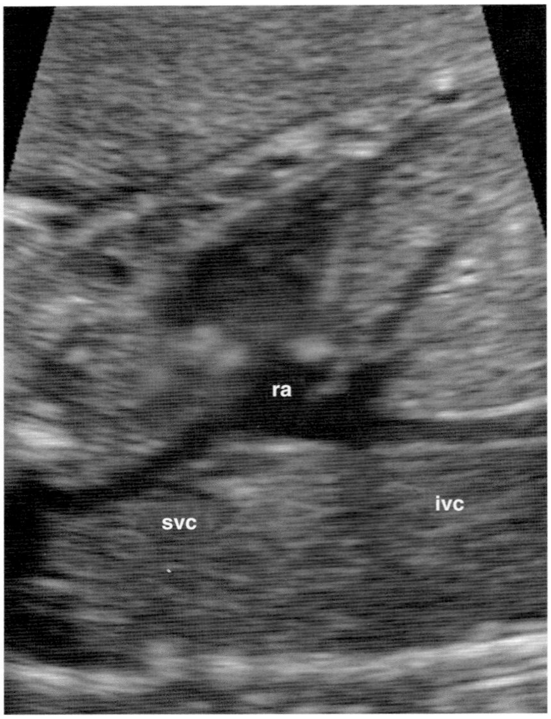

3. Each lies posterior to the other: pulmonary artery anterior to aorta, aorta anterior to superior vena cava.
4. Pulmonary artery arises closest to the anterior chest wall.
5. Trachea and thymus can be visualized.

The position of the trachea in relation to these vessels may be used to differentiate a normal, left-sided aortic arch from an abnormal right-sided aortic arch.[23] Furthermore, the thymus can be seen in front of these vessels (Fig. 16–9), and its absence is a possible marker of CHD associated with a microdeletion of chromosome 22q11.[24]

From this view, a fourth vessel lateral to the pulmonary artery can be seen and represents the persistent left superior vena cava (PLSVC), an anomaly present in about 0.2% of fetuses, and the use of the multiplanar approch of 4D fetal echocardiography facilitates the diagnosis.[25] Isolated PLSVC is a benign vascular anomaly and may not affect the outcome. However, when PLSVC is detected, a meticulous study of the fetal anatomy is necessary because it is frequently associated with heterotaxy syndromes, other cardiac/noncardiac malformations, and aneuploidies.[26]

VENOUS RETURN

The systemic venous return is assessed using a right, parasagittal scan of the fetal thorax to demonstrate the IVC and superior vena cava entering the right atrium (Fig. 16–10). The pulmonary veins are seen entering the left atrium from either the apical or the lateral four-chamber view (Fig. 16–11).

DOPPLER EXAMINATION OF THE FETAL HEART

General Principles

Whereas real-time imaging provides information on the structural integrity of the fetal heart, Doppler ultrasonography provides information that enhances both the definition of the presence and the severity of structural and functional cardiac disease. The parameters used to describe fetal cardiac velocity waveforms differ from those used to describe the peripheral fetal vessels. In the latter, pulsatility, resistance, or systole/diastole indices are used. They are derived from the relative ratios of systolic, diastolic, and mean velocities and are independent of the absolute velocity and the angle of insonation[27] (see also Chapter 10).

In contrast, measurements at the cardiac level are absolute values and require knowledge of the angle of insonation, which might be difficult to obtain accurately. The error in the absolute velocity measurement resulting from angle uncertainty is strongly dependent on the magnitude of the angle itself. For example, the error is insignificant if the angle is less than about 20 degrees. However, when the angle is greater than 20 degrees, the cosine term in the Doppler equation converts the small uncertainty in the measurement to a large error in the velocity equations.[27] Thus, recordings should be obtained with the Doppler beam as parallel to the bloodstream as possible. All recordings with an estimated angle greater than 20 degrees should be rejected.

FIGURE 16–11
Apical four-chamber view of the fetal heart shows the inlet of the pulmonary veins (PV) in the left atrium (LA) in real time (*A*) and with the help of color (*B*) and power (*C*) Doppler.

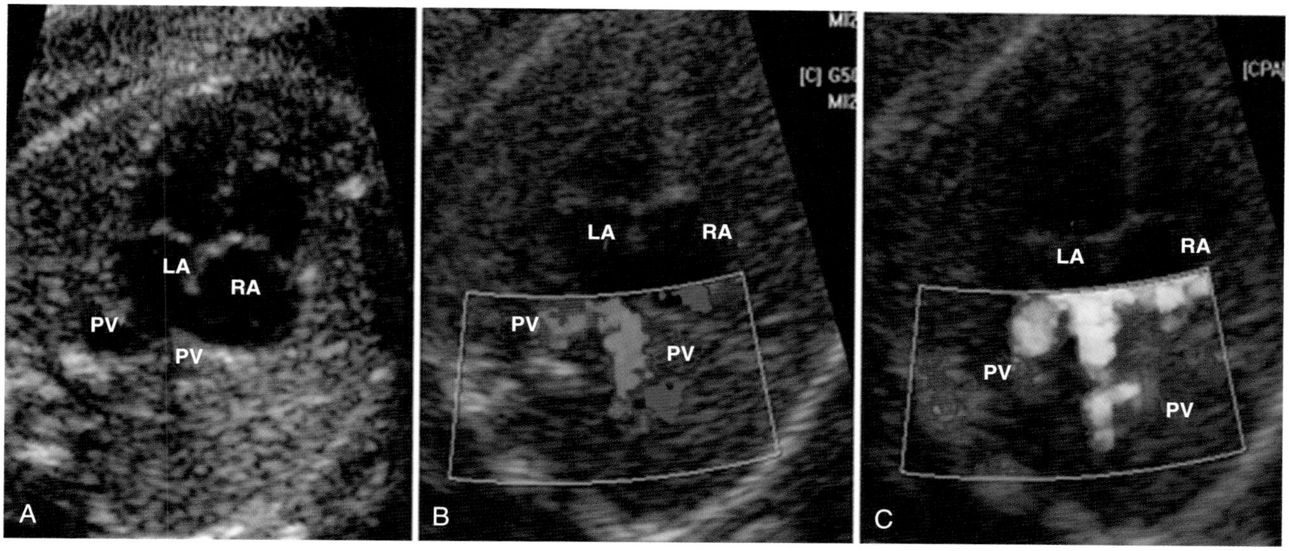

The use of color Doppler velocimetry can help solve many of these problems by revealing in real-time the flow direction so that the beam can be properly aligned. Pulsed Doppler is generally preferred over continuous-wave Doppler because of its superior range of resolution. The sample volume is placed immediately distal to the location to be studied (e.g., distal to the aortic semilunar valves to record the left ventricle outflow). The continuous-wave Doppler may be useful when velocities are particularly high (e.g., in the ductus arteriosus) because it avoids the aliasing effect.

Parameters Measured

The parameters commonly used to describe the cardiac velocity waveforms include

1. The *peak velocity* (PV), which is expressed as the maximum velocity at a given moment (e.g., systole, diastole) on the Doppler spectrum.
2. The *time to peak velocity* (TPV) or acceleration time, which is expressed as the time interval between the onset of the waveform and its peak.
3. The *time velocity integral* (TVI), which is calculated by planimetering the area underneath the Doppler spectrum.

It is possible to calculate absolute cardiac flow from both AV valve and outflow tracts by multiplying:

$$\text{TVI} \times \text{valve area} \times \text{fetal heart rate}$$

The measurement of the valve area is also prone to inaccuracy. It is derived from the measurement of a valve diameter that is near the limit of ultrasonographic resolution. The measurement is then halved and squared in the calculation, amplifying potential errors. Despite these limitations, absolute cardiac flow can be used in longitudinal studies over a short duration during which the valve dimensions are assumed constant. It is also possible to calculate accurately the relative ratio between the right and the left cardiac output (RCO/LCO) and avoid the valve measurement completely because the relative dimensions of the aortic and pulmonary valves remain similar through gestation in the absence of cardiac structural diseases.[1]

Sites of Recordings, Velocity Waveform Characteristics, and Their Significance

Blood flow velocity waveforms can be recorded at all cardiac levels including venous return, foramen ovale, AV valves, outflow tracts, pulmonary arteries, and ductus arteriosus. Factors affecting the morphology of the velocity waveforms include preload, afterload, myocardial contractility, ventricular compliance, and fetal heart rate.[1,27] Because it is impossible to obtain simultaneous recordings of pressure and volume, these factors cannot be fully investigated in the human fetus. However, because each waveform parameter and the site of its recording are specifically affected by one of these factors, it is possible to elucidate indirectly the underlying pathophysiology by performing the measurements at various cardiac levels.

Venous Circulation

Blood flow velocity waveforms can be recorded in the superior and IVC, ductus venosus, and pulmonary, hepatic, and umbilical veins. The vessel most intensively studied to date is the DV.

IVC waveforms recorded just distal to the entrance of the DV[28,29] have a triphasic profile. There is a first forward wave concomitant with ventricular systole, a second forward wave of smaller dimension occurring in early diastole, and a third but reverse wave occurring during atrial contraction (Fig. 16–12). Several indices have been proposed for the analysis of the IVC waveforms. We found that the preload index (PLI) expressed as the ratio between the peak velocities during atrial contraction and systole (PLI = A/S) is the most

FIGURE 16–12
Velocity waveforms from the inferior vena cava. Note the typical triphasic morphology with the reverse flow (*upper channel*) during atrial contraction (A-wave).

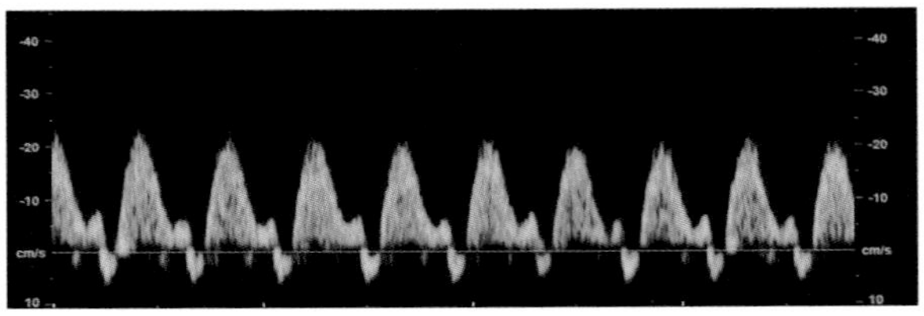

FIGURE 16–14
Velocity waveforms from the pulmonary vein show the presence of forward flow for all the cardiac cycle.

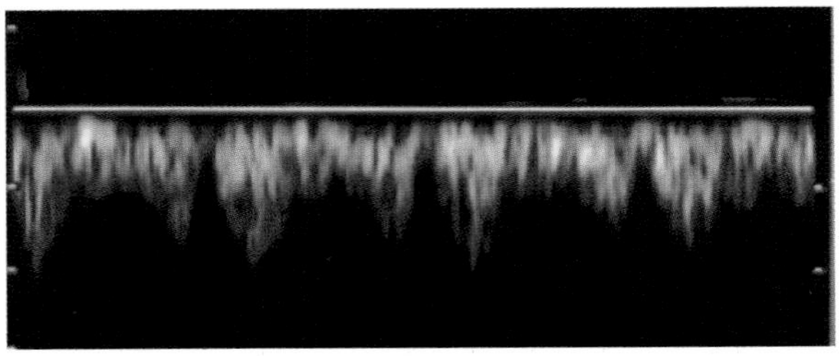

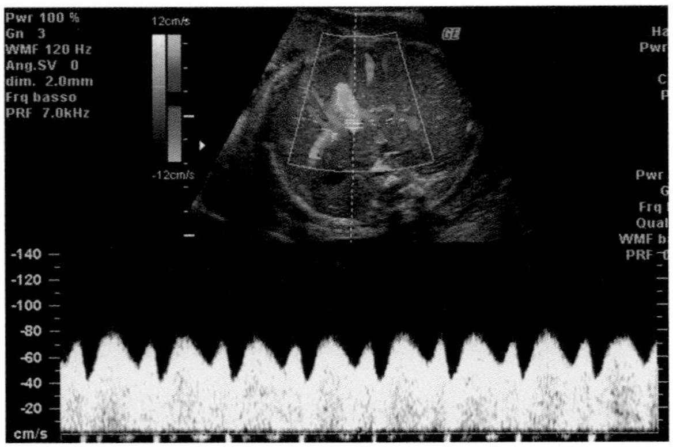

FIGURE 16–13
Transverse section of the upper fetal abdomen with the sample volume placed on the ductus venosus. Note the typical biphasic morphology.

reproducible and efficient index.[29] This index is related to the pressure gradient between the right atrium and the right ventricle during end-diastole, which is a function of both ventricular compliance and ventricular end-diastolic pressure.[30] Decreased cardiac function is associated with an increase in the A-wave, and as a consequence, the PLI increases.

The DV is seen in a transverse section of the upper fetal abdomen at the level of its origin from the umbilical vein. Color Doppler is superimposed and the pulsed Doppler sample volume placed just above its inlet (close to the umbilical vein) at the point of maximum flow velocity as expressed by color brightness. The DV flow velocity waveform has a biphasic pattern with a first peak concomitant with systole (S), a second peak concomitant with diastole (D), and a nadir during atrial contraction (A) (Fig. 16–13). Among the indices suggested to quantify DV velocity waveforms is the ratio of the S peak velocity to the A peak velocity (S/A). This index is angle-independent and describes DV hemodynamics efficiently.[30] The hemodynamic significance of the DV is similar to that of the IVC. In the presence of poor cardiac function, the A-wave is reduced or negative and the S/A ratio increases.

Pulmonary vein velocity waveform is recorded at its entrance into the left atrium. The waveform morphology is similar to that of the DV and characterized by positive velocities during atrial contraction (Fig. 16–14). The striking variation in the velocity waveform morphology between the IVC and the pulmonary vein reflects the different hemodynamic conditions of the fetal systemic and pulmonary venous circulations. Indeed, an abnormal pattern has been described in corrected transposition of the great arteries, a condition in which the afterload of the left ventricle is altered.[31]

Umbilical venous blood flow is usually continuous. However, pulsations in the umbilical venous flow reflecting the heart rate occur in the presence of a relevant amount of reverse flow in the IVC during atrial contraction. In normal pregnancies, these pulsations cease after the 12th week of gestation. Before 12 weeks, they are secondary to ventricular stiffness, which causes a high percentage of reverse flow into the IVC.[1] The presence of pulsations in the umbilical vein after 12 weeks indicates severe cardiac compromise.[1] In clinical practice, the venous circulation is evaluated in sequence moving away from the heart. The further the pulsations are from the heart, the greater the stiffness/cardiac compromise.

Atrioventricular Valves

Flow velocity waveforms at the level of the mitral and tricuspid valves are recorded in the apical four-chamber view of the fetal heart. They are characterized by two diastolic peaks corresponding to early ventricular filling (the E-wave) and active ventricular filling during atrial contraction (the A-wave) (Fig. 16–15). The ratio between the E- and the A-waves (E/A) is a widely accepted index of ventricular diastolic function and an expression of both the cardiac compliance and the preload conditions.[32,33]

Outflow Tracts

Flow velocity waveforms from the aorta and pulmonary artery are recorded respectively from the five-chamber and short-axis views of the fetal heart (Figs. 16–16 and 16–17). PV and TPV are the most commonly used indices. The former is influenced by several factors including valve size, myocardial contractility, and afterload, whereas the latter is believed to reflect the mean arterial pressure.[34]

Pulmonary Vessels

Velocity waveforms may be recorded from the right and left pulmonary arteries or from peripheral vessels within the lung. The morphology of the waveforms varies according to the sample site, and their analysis has been used to study the normal development of the pulmonary circulation.[35]

Three-Vessel View

In this view, the pulmonary artery and ascending aorta have the same flow direction and thus have the same color when imaged with color-flow Doppler (Fig. 16–18). Severe outflow

FIGURE 16–15
A, Apical flow chamber view of the fetal heart shows the normal filling of the two ventricles (*red color*). *B*, Pulsed Doppler tracing from the tricuspid valve. Note the typical morphology (E- and A-waves) and the absence of flow during systole.

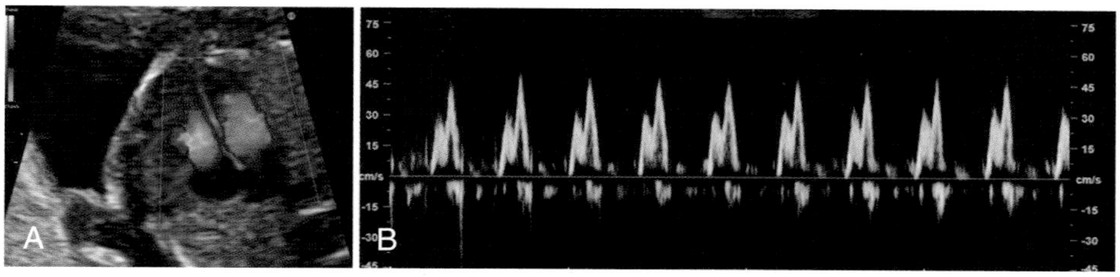

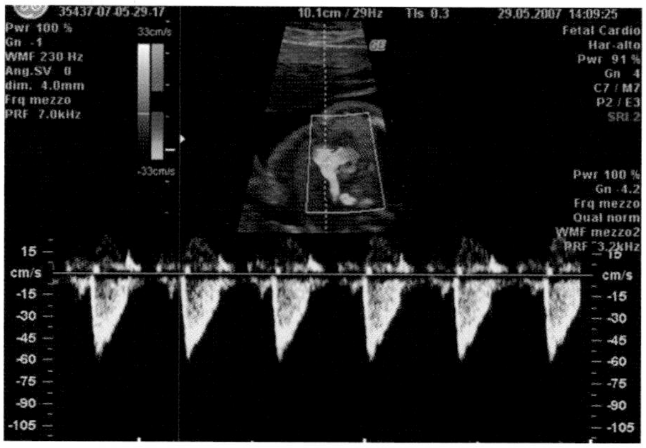

FIGURE 16–16
Short-axis view of the fetal heart with the color Doppler superimposed shows the outflow of the right ventricle (*blue*) and pulsed Doppler tracing at the level of the pulmonary valve and the typical velocity waveform recorded.

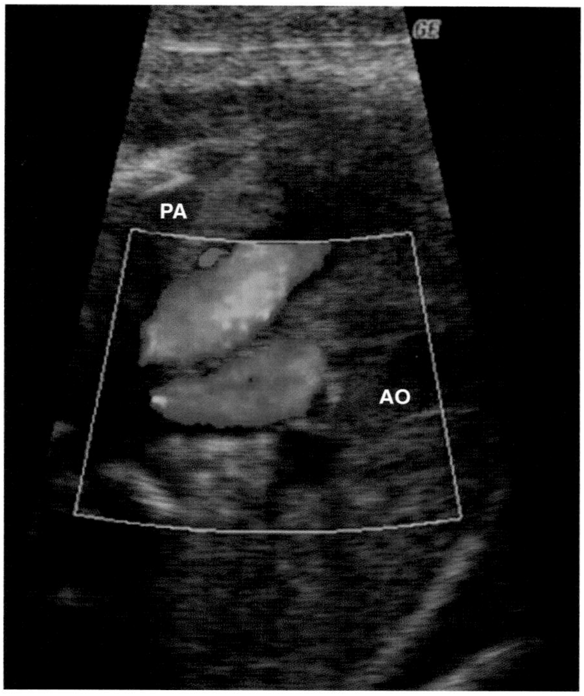

FIGURE 16–18
Three-vessel view with the color Doppler superimposed shows the pulmonary artery (PA) and the ascending aorta (AO) with the same flow direction.

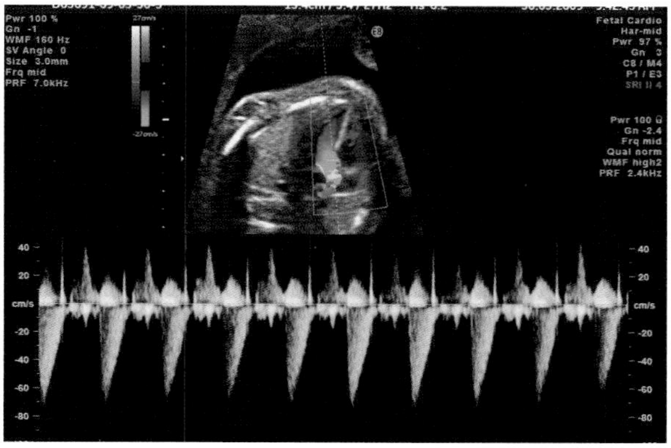

FIGURE 16–17
Long-axis view of the fetal heart with the color Doppler superimposed shows the outflow of the left ventricle (*red*). The sample volume is placed at the level of the aorta and the velocity waveform recorded.

obstruction to one of the ventricles leads to reverse flow in the pulmonary artery (right side obstruction) or in the aorta (left side obstruction) (Fig. 16–19).

Ductus Arteriosus

Ductal velocity waveforms are recorded in a short-axis view showing the ductal arch. They are characterized by continuous forward flow throughout the cardiac cycle.[26] The parameter most commonly analyzed is the PV during systole, or similarly to peripheral vessels, the pulsatility index (PI = [systolic velocity − diastolic velocity]/mean velocity).[36]

Normal Ranges of Cardiac Doppler Indices

The velocity waveforms are recordable from 11 weeks on.[1] The cardiovascular indices change dramatically at all levels up to 20 weeks. The PLI of the IVC decreases significantly,[1,24,26] the E/A ratio at both AV levels increases dramatically,[1,34] and the PV and TVI of the outflow tracts, particularly at the level of pulmonary valve, increase.[34] These changes are consistent with rapid development of ventricular compliance (explaining the decrease in the IVC PLI and

FIGURE 16–19
Three-vessel view in a fetus with pulmonary atresia. The pulmonary artery is evidenced with reversed flow (*red*) indicating retrograde perfusion from the systemic circulation to the pulmonary circulation.

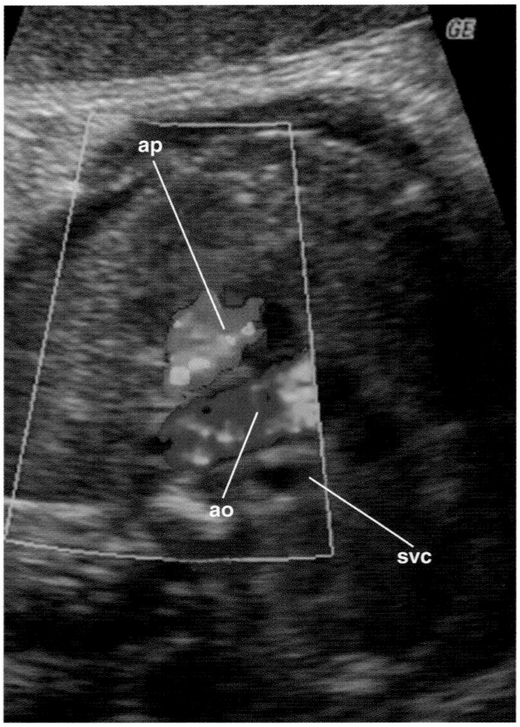

FIGURE 16–20
Multiplanar display of the fetal heart after four-dimensional volume acquisition.

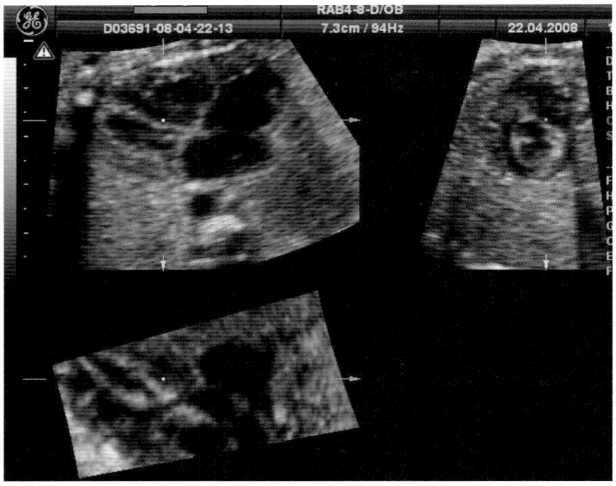

the increase in the E/A) and a shift in the cardiac output toward the right ventricle as placental resistance falls, decreasing right ventricular afterload.

After 20 weeks, the IVC PLI declines less dramatically whereas there is a significant decline in the S/A ratio of the DV.[30] At the level of AV valves, the E/A ratios increase progressively, reaching a value near 1 at term.[34] Similarly, the PV increases linearly at the level of both the pulmonary and the aortic valves.[34] The PV of the aortic valve is usually greater than the pulmonary artery and, under normal conditions, is always below 100 cm/sec. The change in TPV is minimal.[34] TPV measurements at the level of pulmonary valve are lower than at the level of the aortic valve, suggesting the blood pressure in the pulmonary artery is slightly higher than in the ascending aorta.[26] Quantitative measurements reveal the RCO is higher than the LCO and that the RCO/LCO ratio remains constant from 20 weeks onward with a mean value of 1.3.[1,34] This is lower than that reported in fetal sheep (RCO/LCO = 1.8) and may reflect the higher brain weight of humans requiring a higher left cardiac output.[34]

The ductus arteriosus PV increases linearly with advancing gestation, and its values represent the highest velocities in the fetal circulation under normal conditions.[36] Ductal constriction is suggested by a systolic velocity measurement greater than 140 cm/sec in conjunction with a diastolic velocity greater than 35 cm/sec or a pulsatility index value less than 2.[36]

FOUR-DIMENSIONAL STUDY OF THE FETAL HEART

Detection of CHD in the general population, even when the outflow tracts are visualized routinely, depends as previously reported, on the skill of the sonographers and on their ability to interpret the findings.

Spatiotemporal image correlation (STIC) is a technique that allows examination of the fetal heart within a real-time 4D volume, displayed in a cineloop. It has been proposed that fetal echocardiography using STIC has the potential to increase the detection rates for CHD because it decreases the dependency on the sonographer's skill.[37–39] Indeed, it is possible with this technique to acquire a volume starting from the standard four-chamber view and then offline navigating inside the volume in a multiplanar way to obtain all the diagnostic planes (Fig. 16–20). We recently described a technique of analysis known as the "three-steps view" that allows us to obtain in less than 4 minutes the four-chambers-view and the outflow tract[40] (Fig. 16–21).

In order to further facilitate the identification of CHD, computer aid diagnosis software was recently developed (SonoVCAD) that allows a fully automated visualization of the diagnostic plane from volumes acquired from the chamber view.[41] Preliminary applications of this software in fetuses with transposition of the great artery suggest a clinical applicability.[42]

4D echocardiography also can be used to provide enhanced characterization of the CHD either by showing multiple diagnostic planes in a tomographic way or by allowing rendering all the heart or a portion such as a valve in a 3D way (Fig. 16–22). In this manner, it is easier to show the defect to consulting physicians from pediatric cardiology and cardiac surgery.

A further advance of 4D fetal echocardiography is that the acquisition of cardiac volumes can be performed locally at the screening center, but the subsequent analysis of suspect cases can be performed by an expert fetal echocardiographer at a remote site, reducing the number of referrals to tertiary centers of prenatal diagnosis.[43]

CARDIAC STRUCTURAL ANOMALIES

Septal Defects

Septal defects are the most common CHDs with an estimated incidence of about 0.5 per 1000 live births.[2] They are either atrial, ventricular, or AV septal in location.

Isolated atrial septal defects have been diagnosed in utero, but the diagnosis remains difficult because of the foramen ovale. Echocardiographic diagnosis requires demonstration of either the absence or the reduction in the dimension of the foramen ovale valve flap (ostium secundum defect). Dropout of echoes at the level of the outlet of the atrial septum in a perpendicular view suggests the presence of an ostium primum defect or an incomplete form of AV canal.

Atrial septal defects do not impair fetal cardiac function and do so only rarely in the neonate. However, atrial septal defects are associated with other cardiac malformations (coarctation and conotruncal anomalies), an abnormal karyotype (e.g., trisomy 21), and genetic syndromes (e.g., Holt-Oram syndrome).

Ventricular septal defects are classified by their location in the septum: perimembranous, inlet, trabecular, and outlet. Perimembranous defects are most common (80%) and involve the membranous portion of the interventricular septum just below the aortic valve (Fig. 16–23). They can extend a variable degree into the muscular portion. Septal defects are not responsible for fetal compromise. Because the pressure of both ventricular cavities is similar, even large defects cause but small bidirectional shunts that do not affect intracardiac hemodynamics. The great majority of infants

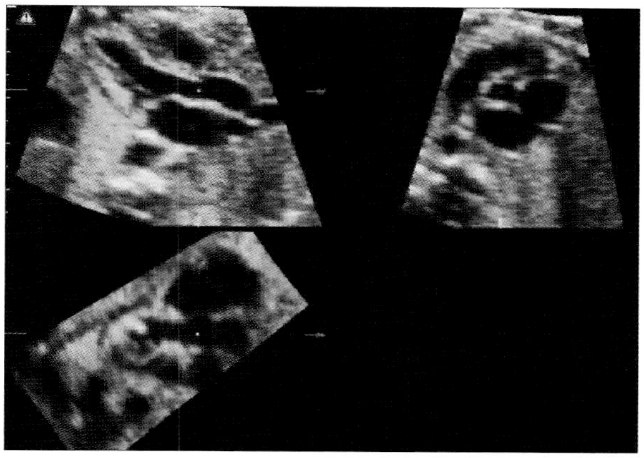

FIGURE 16–21
Simultaneous display of left and right outflow tracts after navigation in the four-dimensional acquired volume following the three-steps technique. (From Rizzo G, Capponi A, Cavicchioni O, et al: Examination of the fetal heart by four-dimensional ultrasound with spatio-temporal image correlation during routine second trimester examination: The "three steps technique." Fetal Diagn Ther 2008;24:126-131.)

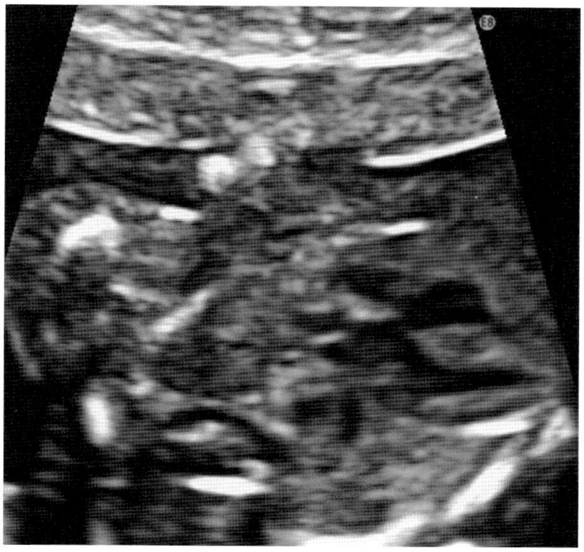

FIGURE 16–23
Lateral four-chamber view shows the interventricular septum with an evident perimembranous defect.

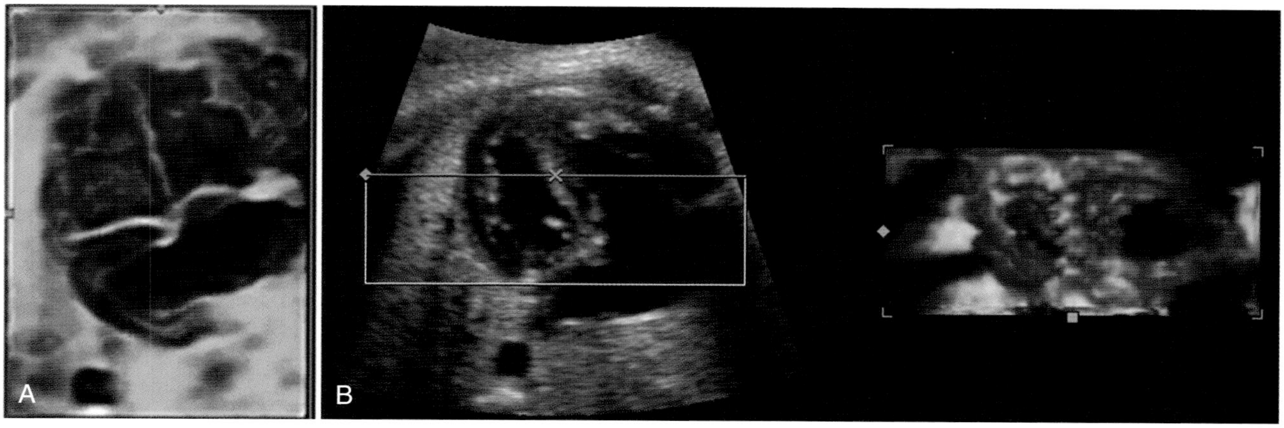

FIGURE 16–22
Three-dimensional rendering of the fetal heart from the four-chamber view (*A*) and of the atrioventricular valves (*B*).

with interventricular septal defects are asymptomatic in the neonatal period. It is calculated that a quarter of the ventricular septal defects close spontaneously during intrauterine life[44] and another third of the remaining ones close during the first year of life.[45]

Echocardiographic diagnosis relies on the demonstration of echo dropout in the interventricular septum (see Fig. 16–23). Care is necessary to avoid artifact due to the inherent limitations in the lateral resolution of ultrasound. The diagnosis is made only when the ultrasound beam is perpendicular to the septum (see Fig. 16–20). Color Doppler is useful for demonstrating the shunt between ventricles (Fig. 16–24). This is particularly clear when the outflow of one ventricle is obstructed (unidirectional shunt) (see Fig. 16–21). The application of new-generation equipment with high-resolution color and power energy Doppler (in which flows are independent of the angle of insonation) are also helpful for detection of isolated ventricular septal defects.[32] Further the use of 4D ultrasonography with tomographic reconstruction seems to improve diagnosis[46] (Fig 16–25). The prognosis for an infant with an isolated interventricular septal defect is good. However, it is essential that other cardiac and extracardiac anomalies be carefully excluded and a normal fetal karyotype documented.[4,5]

Abnormal development of both the atrial and the ventricular septa is described as an AV septal defect—either the endocardial cushion or an AV canal form. The typical appearance is of a single, AV valve opening above and bridging the two ventricles (Fig. 16–26). The common AV valve may be incompetent, with systolic regurgitation leading to fetal heart failure and hydrops. AV septal defects are frequently associated with fetal aneuploidy (50% of the cases, particularly trisomy 21),[5] cardiac isomerism (cardiosplenic syndromes), and other extracardiac anomalies.[4]

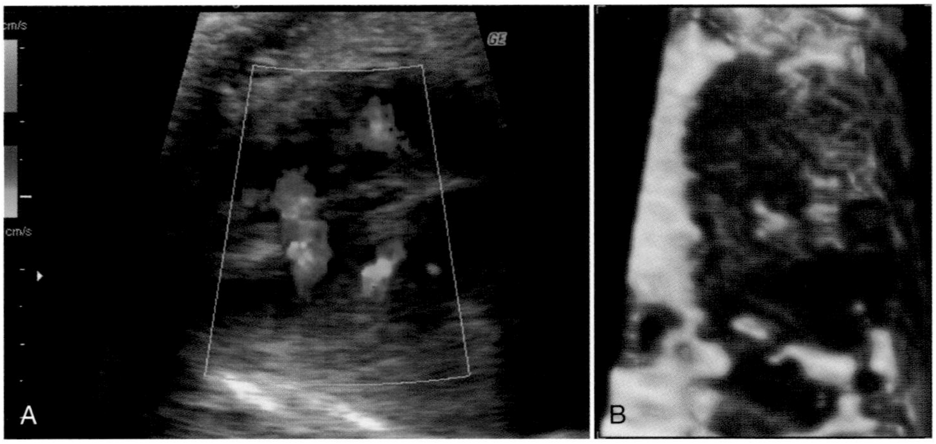

FIGURE 16–24
Example of a muscular septal defect visualized with the help of color Doppler (*A*) and three-dimensional representation of the defect (*B*).

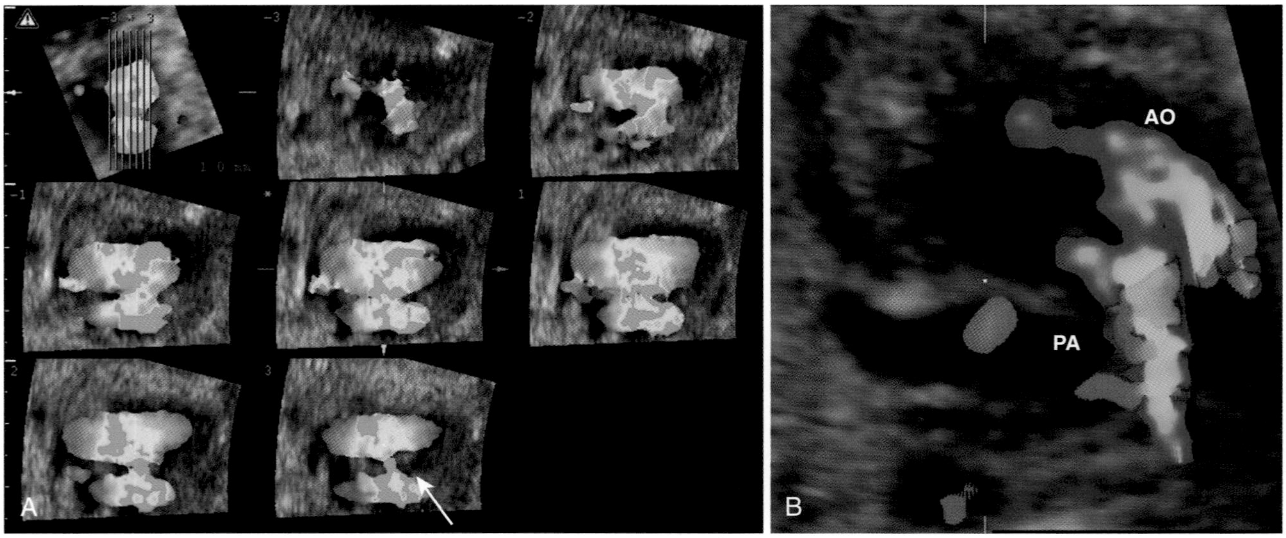

FIGURE 16–25
Tomographic reconstruction of the fetal ventricular septum after four-dimensional acquisition with color Doppler that allows demonstration of a tiny muscular defect (*arrow*).

FIGURE 16–26
A, Apical four-chamber view shows a defect of the atrioventricular septum in a case of atrioventricular canal. *B*, Color Doppler shows the wide connection between left and right heart. *C*, Three-dimensional rendered reconstruction.

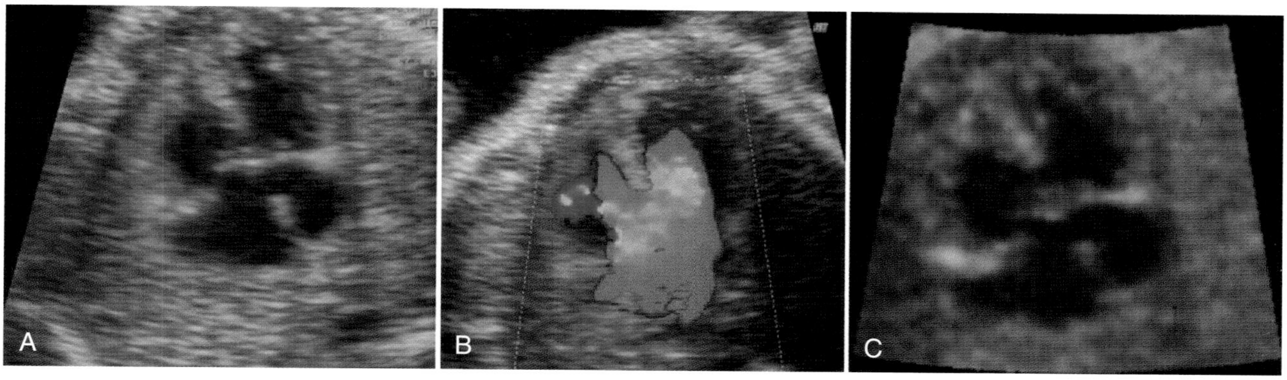

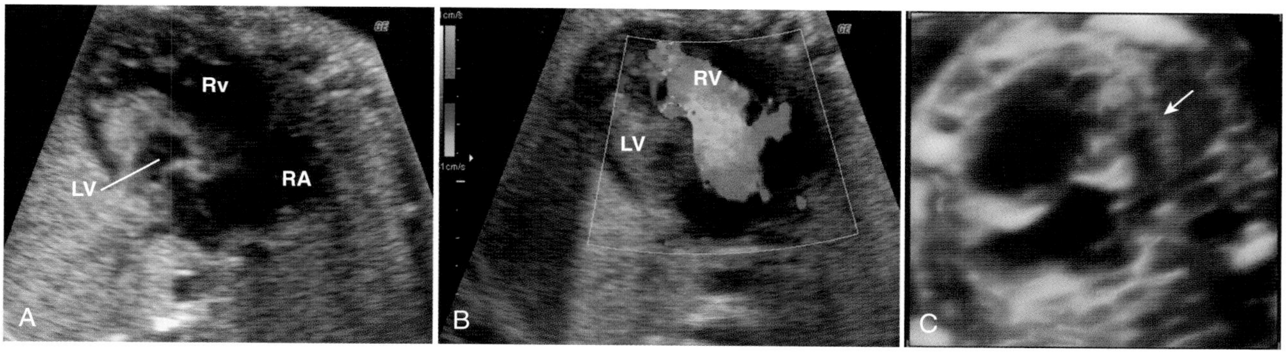

FIGURE 16–27
A, Four-chamber view shows the hypoplasia of the left ventricle. The absent filling during diastole is demonstrated by color Doppler (*B*) and the four-dimensional rendered view (*C*) of the small ventricle (*arrow*). LV, left ventricle; RV, right ventricle.

Hypoplastic Left Heart

A small left ventricle secondary to mitral and/or aortic stenosis/atresia characterizes the hypoplastic left heart syndrome. Blood flow to the head and coronary artery is supplied by retrograde flow through the ductus arteriosus and the aortic arch. The incidence of hypoplastic left heart syndrome approximates 0.16 per 1000 live births and constitutes about 10% of infants with CHDs[47] and up to 20% of those detected in utero.[48]

Echocardiographic diagnosis begins with the demonstration of a small left ventricle (Fig. 16–27). The ascending aorta is severely hypoplastic, and the right atrium, right ventricle, and pulmonary artery are relatively enlarged. Color and pulsed Doppler flow examination may reveal absent flow from the left atrium to the left ventricle (mitral atresia) (see Fig. 16–25) and retrograde flow in the aortic arch.

A hypoplastic left heart is well tolerated in utero, and congestive heart failure is unusual. However, the postnatal prognosis is poor. This lesion is responsible for 25% of cardiac deaths during the first week of life.[49,50] Surgical options are limited. Norwood's three-stage operation was developed to correct this disease, and although the reported survival in selected centers reaches 60%, the long-term prognosis for these children after three procedures remains uncertain.[51,52] Cardiac transplant programs for the neonate have also been developed, but the long-term results of these too are disappointing.[53]

Pulmonary Atresia with Intact Ventricular Septum

Pulmonary atresia with intact ventricular septum makes up 3% to 4% of neonatal and prenatal series.[2,48] Two forms of pulmonary atresia are found in the fetus. In about 75%, the right ventricle is hypoplastic,[48] and in the remaining 25%, the right ventricle is enlarged (Fig. 16–28).[48] In the former instance, the tricuspid valve is atretic (see Fig. 16–26); in the latter, it is typically insufficient (Fig. 16–29). Echocardiographic diagnosis relies on the demonstration of a small pulmonary artery with an atretic pulmonary valve. The four-chamber view is abnormal and shows variable degrees of right ventricular hypoplasia.

Color and pulsed Doppler studies reveal retrograde flow in the pulmonary artery and either absent (atresia) or retrograde flow (insufficiency) across the tricuspid valve (see Figs. 16–28 and 16–29). Heart failure and hydrops often develop with tricuspid regurgitation. Anomalies of the

FIGURE 16–28
Four-chamber view of the fetal heart in the presence of a pulmonary atresia and intact septum. *A*, The right ventricular size is reduced and the tricuspid valve is hyperechogenic. *B*, Color Doppler shows the absent filling of the right ventricle. *C*, The four-dimensional rendered view of the small ventricle). vd, right ventricle; vs, left ventricle.

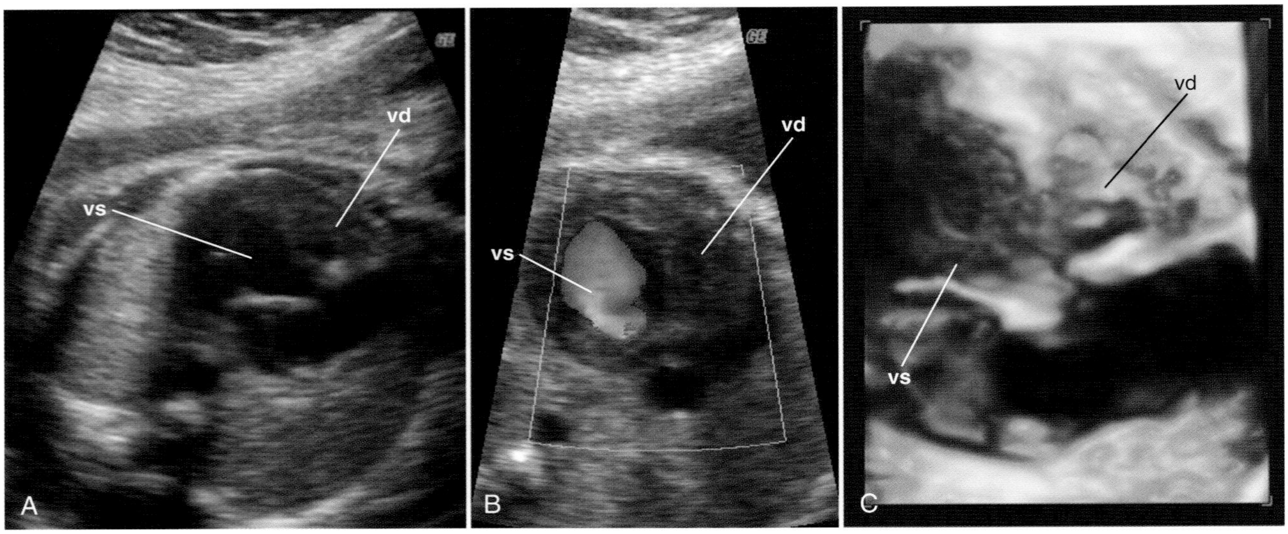

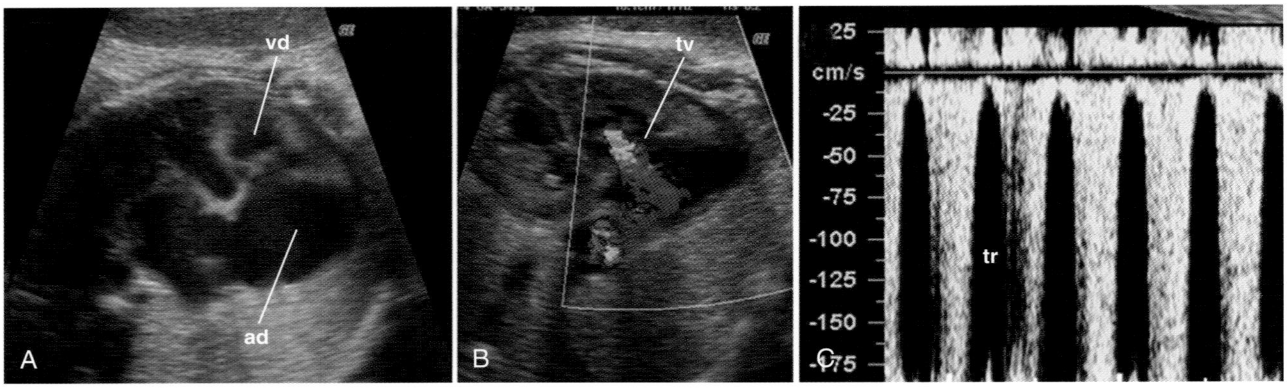

FIGURE 16–29
Apical four-chamber view in the presence of a pulmonary atresia and intact septum. *A*, The echogenicity of the right ventricle is increased and the right atrium is increased. *B*, When the color Doppler is superimposed, a high-velocity retrograde jet is seen (*blue*). *C*, A holosystolic high-velocity (>175 cm/sec) tricuspid regurgitation is measured by pulsed Doppler. ad, right atrium; vd, right ventricle; tv, tricuspid valve; tr, tricuspid regurgitation.

coronary arteries are common and can complicate surgical correction. Extracardiac anomalies are unusual.

Factors that affect prognosis are strictly related to ventricular size and the presence of coronary fistulas.[54] If a postnatal two-ventricular repair can be achieved, the long-term outcome can be good. Conversely, if the right ventricle is severely hypoplastic and addressed therapeutically with a Fontana procedure (placement of a circuit between the right atrium and the main pulmonary artery),[55] the action is considered palliative, associated with several short- and long-term complications.[56]

Outflow Tract Obstructions

Aortic Stenosis and Coarctation of the Aortic Arch

Aortic stenosis is found in 0.04 per 1000 live births[2] and may be supravalvular, valvular, or subvalvular.[57] The pressure in the left ventricle is increased. In severe cases, the left ventricular pressure overload decreases coronary perfusion, leading to subendocardial ischemia, secondary endocardial fibroelastosis, and in utero congestive heart failure. The echocardiographic diagnosis requires demonstration of a small and abnormal aortic valve, usually associated with an enlarged, poststenotic ascending aorta (Fig. 16–30). Doppler examination will show increased flow velocities in the ascending aorta distal to the stenotic site and, in the severe cases, regurgitation across the mitral valve (see Fig. 16–30).

Several fetal medicine specialists have attempted in utero balloon dilation of the stenotic aortic valve by transthoracic puncture of the fetus. In several instances, the procedure was a technical success with a reduction in severity[58,59]; long-term quality survival has been elusive. Although prenatal intervention might be an option, the selection of suitable cases is difficult as is the timing of the procedure.[60]

FIGURE 16–30
A, Four-chamber view shows a reduction of the left ventricle due to aortic stenosis. *B*, Color flow mapping demonstrates turbulent flow on the aortic valve (*arrow*). C, Pulsed Doppler shows high systolic velocity (>200 cm/sec). *D*, Mitral regurgitation (*blue jet*) is also evident by color Doppler. LV, left ventricle; RV, right ventricle.

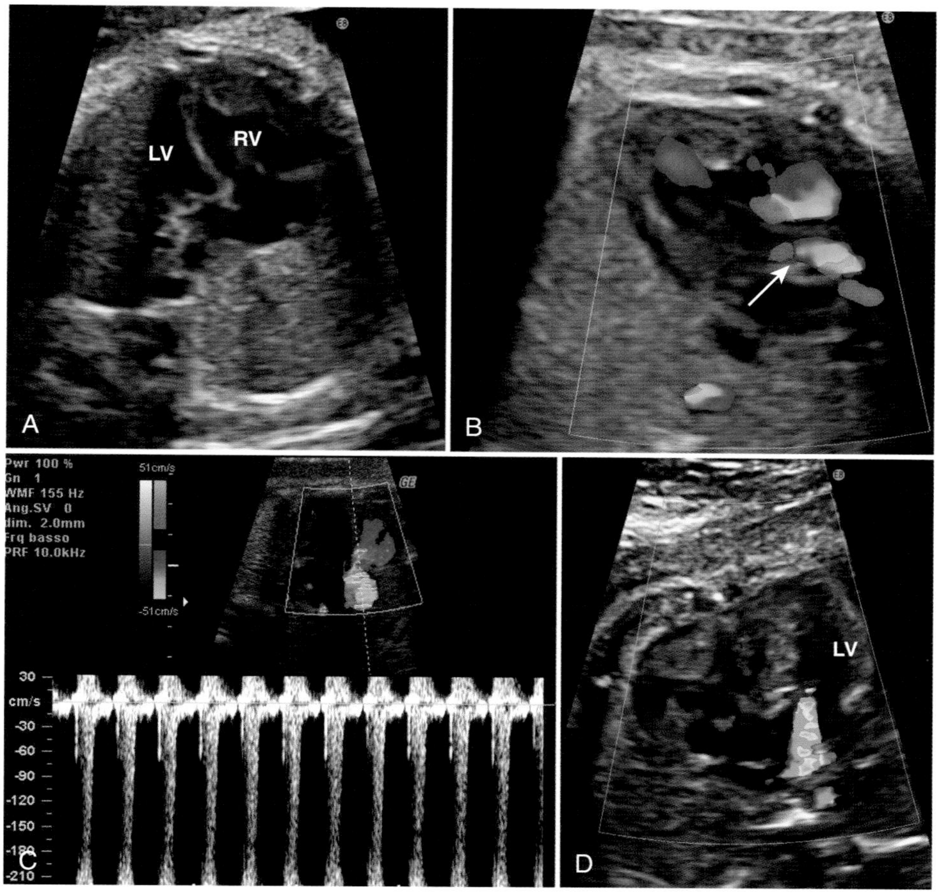

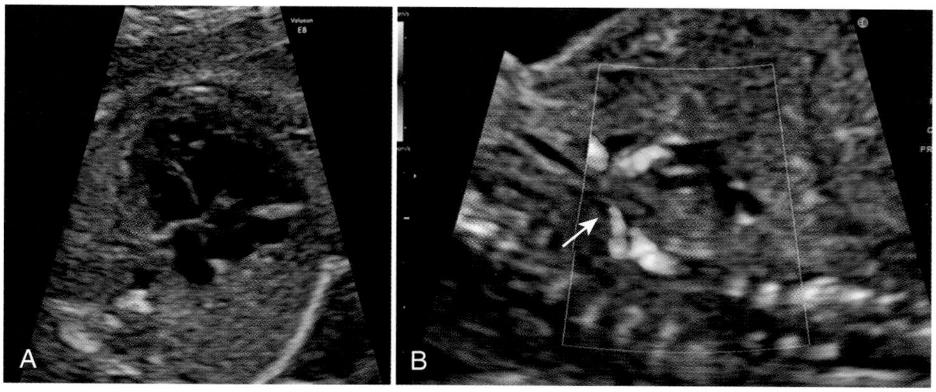

FIGURE 16–31
A, Four-chamber view shows a reduction of the left ventricle due to aortic coarctation. *B*, High definition (HD) color flow demonstrated the small caliper of the aortic arch and the presence of reverse flow (*arrow*), demonstrating retrograde perfusion from the ductus arteriosus.

Coarctation is a narrowing of a portion of aortic arch, usually between the left subclavian artery and the ductus arteriosus. In some cases, the narrowing encompasses the proximal aortic arch and is defined as a hypoplastic aortic arch or, if completely interrupted, an interrupted aortic arch (Fig. 16–31). The incidence approximates 0.18 per 1000 live births and is frequently associated with other cardiac anomalies (≤90%) including ventricular septal defect, aortic stenosis, and transposition of the great arteries.[2,61] Extracardiac anomalies including diaphragmatic hernia, renal agenesis, esophageal atresia, Turner's syndrome, and the chromosome 22q11 deletion syndrome (interruption of the aortic arch) are also frequent.

Coarctation has no significant impact on intrauterine hemodynamics because it is the right ventricle that mainly supplies the descending aorta via the ductus arteriosus. Rather, symptoms develop in the neonatal period. The only in utero echocardiographic evidence of coarctation may be a relatively enlarged right ventricle compared with the left ventricle. Additional signs of coarctation include an echogenic shelf in the aortic lumen at the level of the isthmus, a relative decrease in the diameter of the aorta compared with the pulmonary artery, and a hypoplastic arch (see Fig. 16–31).[61] Hypoplasia of the left ventricle may develop in more severe cases (hypoplastic arch or interruption).[45] The surgical mortality reported for coarctation of the aorta is lower than 10%. However, the surgical mortality may be higher because the surgical approach is similar to that for the hypolastic left heart syndrome, particularly if there is a significant left heart obstruction.[46,62]

Pulmonary Stenosis

Pulmonary stenosis occurs in about 0.9 per 1000 live births and is generally thought to result from fusion of the pulmonary valve leaflets.[2] Associated cardiac and extracardiac anomalies are less common than aortic stenosis but can include atrial septal defects and total anomalous pulmonary venous return. It is typically present in Noonan's syndrome.

The relevant hemodynamic concerns for pulmonary stenosis are the same as those for aortic stenosis. Right ventricular pressure is increased proportional to the degree of stenosis. The resulting ventricular wall hypertrophy can cause tricuspid regurgitation. The echocardiographic diagnosis relies on identification of a small, sometimes thickened, pulmonary valve with a characteristic abnormal movement (doming).[63] Poststenotic enlargement of the pulmonary artery is common. Doppler interrogation reveals increased velocities at the level of the pulmonary valve (Fig. 16–32), frequently associated with tricuspid insufficiency. The progression from stenosis to atresia in utero is well documented.[64] The prognosis is usually good, and postnatal balloon valvuloplasty is the only treatment usually required.

Conotruncal Malformations

Conotruncal malformations are a heterogeneous group of defects affecting the connection between the ventricles and the great arteries. They constitute 20% to 30% of all cardiac anomalies.[2] Conotruncal malformations include transposition of the great arteries, tetralogy of Fallot, double-outlet right ventricle, and truncus arteriosus. Unfortunately, these lesions are frequently missed during the routine obstetric sonographic examination if it is limited to the four-chamber view because the ventricles are usually similar in size. Undiagnosed conotruncal malformations can lead to neonatal emergency with considerable morbidity and mortality. However, the outcome is generally good if promptly recognized and early corrective surgery undertaken.

Transposition of Great Arteries

The prevalence of transposition approximates 0.2 per 1000 live births.[2] The complete form, characterized by AV concordance and ventricle-arterial discordance is most common. The aorta arises from the right ventricle and the pulmonary artery from the left ventricle. Either a ventricular septal defect or pulmonary stenosis is present in about half, though complete transposition is only rarely associated with extracardiac anomalies or an abnormal karyotype. Echocardiographic diagnosis requires demonstration that the left ventricle in the long-axis view connects to a great vessel with a posterior course that bifurcates (pulmonary artery) (Fig. 16–33). In the short-axis view, the vessel originating from the right ventricle has an upward course and gives rise to the brachiocephalic vessels (see Fig. 16–33).

The parallel circulatory model of the fetus allows normal development, and hemodynamic compromise is unusual in utero. However, newborns may be cyanotic and deteriorate rapidly depending on the size of the shunt at the level of the foramen ovale or across any associated ventricular septal defect. Identification of a small foramen ovale prenatally might be an indication for balloon atrial septostomy (Rashkind's procedure) immediately after birth. Cardiac surgery consists of switching the great arteries and is usually performed during the neonatal period. The survival rate is 85% to 90%, particularly when the diagnosis is performed prenatally.[65]

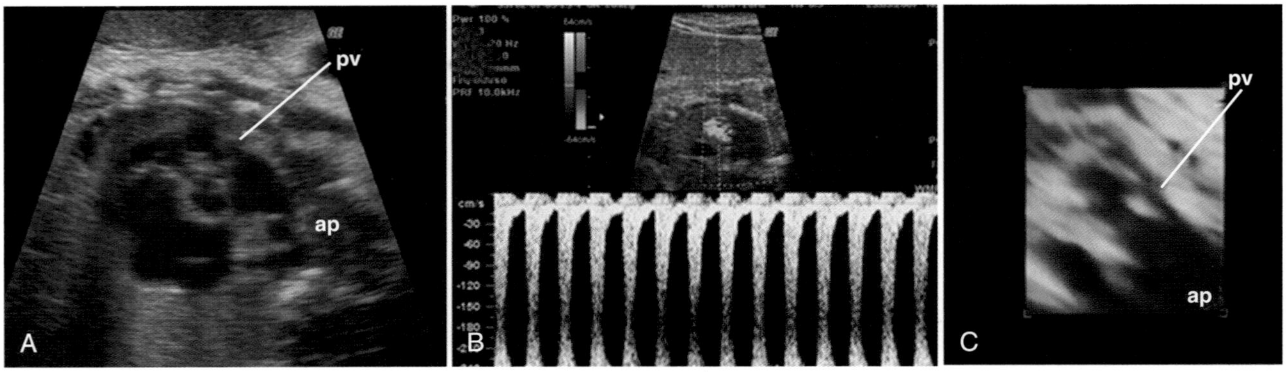

FIGURE 16–32
Short-axis view of the fetal heart in a fetus with pulmonary stenosis. *A*, The narrowing of the valve and the poststenotic dilation. *B*, Color Doppler superimposed on *A* shows high velocities in the pulmonary artery (AP) with pulsed Doppler demonstrating high-velocity waveforms (>160 cm/sec) consistent with pulmonary stenosis. *C*, Resulting in a thickened pulmonary valve (PV) .

FIGURE 16–33
A, Correct transposition of the great artery with intact septum with an apparently normal four-chamber view (*A*). The study of outflow tracts demonstrated the pulmonary artery (PA) (branching vessel) originating from the left ventricle (LV) (*B*) and the aorta (AO) originating from the anterior right ventricle (RV) (*C*).

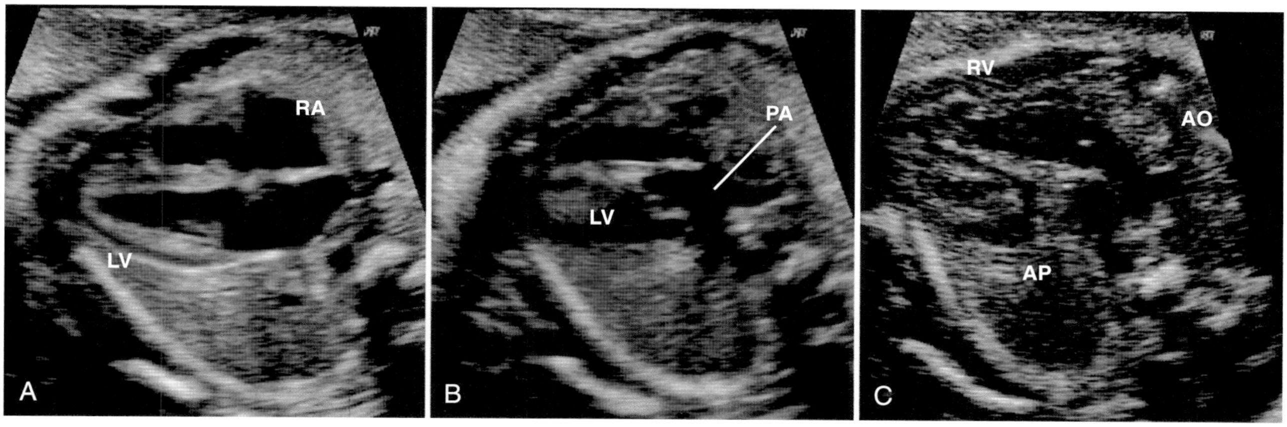

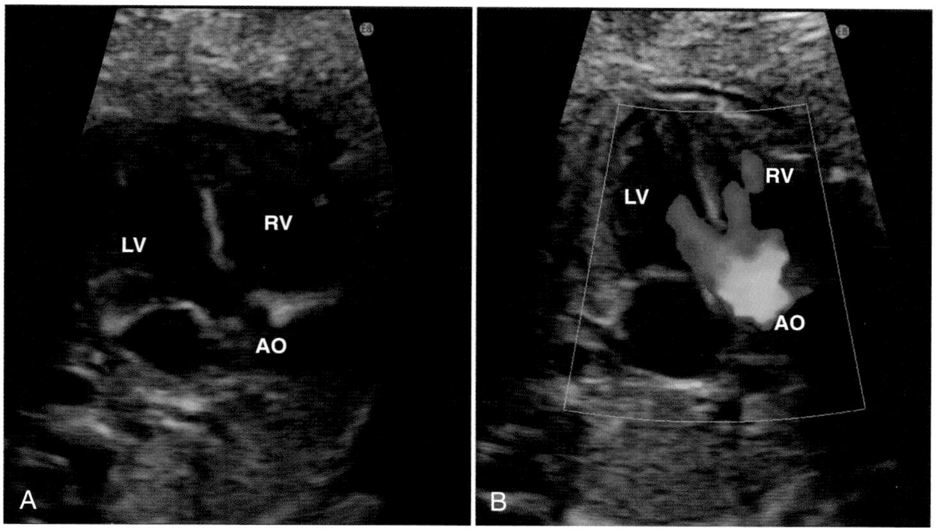

FIGURE 16–34
Tetralogy of Fallot. *A*, Presence of a ventricular septal defect with the aorta (AO) overriding the right (RV) and left (LV) ventricles. *B*, Color Doppler demonstrates the presence of the ventricular septal defect with the Y sign.

Tetralogy of Fallot

Tetralogy of Fallot occurs in 0.4 in 1000 live births[2] and includes stenosis of the infundibulum of the pulmonary artery, a ventricular septal defect, an aortic valve overriding the interventricular septum, and hypertrophy of the right ventricle that usually develops after birth. The pulmonary valve is atretic in about 20%, a condition described as pulmonary atresia with ventricular septal defect. Tetralogy of Fallot is associated with other cardiac defects such as an AV canal (4%) or pulmonary valve absence (1%). Extracardiac anomalies (particularly chromosomal) are frequent.

The echocardiographic diagnosis requires demonstration of an enlarged aortic root overriding the intraventricular septum (Fig. 16–34*A*),[61] an intraventricular septal defect (see Fig. 16–34), and a small pulmonary valve. Color-flow mapping will reveal systolic jets from both the right and the left ventricle into the overriding aorta with a Y shape (Y sign) (see Fig. 16–34*B*). Cardiac failure in utero or during the first days of life is infrequent. In the absence of extracardiac defects, the survival rate after corrective surgery approximates 95%.[66] This percentage is lower when associated with pulmonary atresia[61]; in that instance, the diameter of any available pulmonary artery is crucial.

Double-Outlet Right Ventricle

The prevalence of double-outlet right ventricle approximates 0.32 per 1000 live births.[2] It is characterized by a ventricular septal defect associated with an aorta and a pulmonary artery that originates from the right ventricle anterior to the ventricular septum (Fig. 16–35). The position of the great arteries relative to each other may vary from normal to transposition (see Fig. 16–35). Associated anomalies include mitral valve atresia, AV canal, and pulmonary

FIGURE 16–35
Double-outlet right ventricle. Both great vessels originate from the right ventricle (RV) and a wide septal defect is present (*). However, there is an associated transposition of the great vessels and the aorta (AO) is posterior to pulmonary artery (AP).

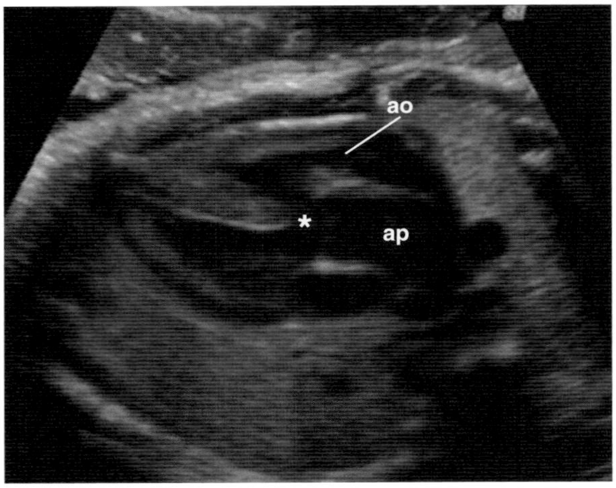

FIGURE 16–36
Truncus arteriosus. A single vessel (T) overrides the two ventricles. LV, left ventricle; RV, right ventricle.

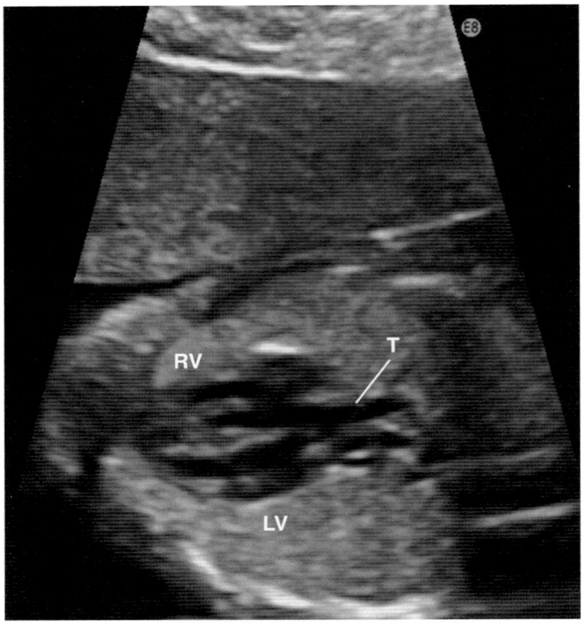

stenosis. Extracardiac and chromosomal anomalies are common. Distinguishing double-outlet right ventricle from tetralogy of Fallot can be difficult when the relationship between the great arteries is normal and pulmonary artery stenosis is present.

The hemodynamic effects of this malformation are similar to those of tetralogy of Fallot. Cardiac decompensation is unusual in utero as well as in the early neonatal period. Long-term survival after corrective surgery is good (70%–80%) in the absence of associated anomalies.[67]

Truncus Arteriosus

Truncus arteriosus complicates approximately 0.01 in 1000 live births.[2] It is characterized by a single great artery, usually larger than the aorta, arising from both ventricles and overriding the ventricular septum. The truncus supplies the systemic, coronary, and pulmonary circulations. A ventricular septal defect may be present (type A) or absent (type B). Type A has four subclasses according to the origin of the pulmonary arteries.[68] Associated intracardiac anomalies are common and include mitral atresia and aortic arch hypoplasia and interruption (type A4). Extracardiac malformations are also common.

The echocardiographic diagnosis is based on the identification of a single great vessel overriding both ventricles whose dimensions are usually larger than the aorta (Fig. 16–36). The diagnosis requires that the pulmonary arteries originate from the truncus. Distinguishing truncus arteriosus from a tetralogy of Fallot with an atretic pulmonary valve may be difficult in utero.

As with other conotruncal malformations, truncus arteriosus is not associated with cardiac decompensation in utero, but it may occur during the first days of life. Surgical correction is often complex, because the dysplastic truncal valve must be transformed into an aortic valve and a circuit created from the right ventricle to the pulmonary arteries. The survival rate at 10 years is less than 80%.[68]

Tumors of the Heart

Congenital tumors of the heart are extremely rare with an incidence estimated at 0.1 per 1000 live births. The most common is rhabdomyoma. These tend to be multiple and involve the septum. Cardiac tumors are usually isolated, but are present in 50% to 86% of fetuses with tuberous sclerosis. Frequently, they are the only detectable sign of tuberous sclerosis in utero.

The echocardiographic diagnosis is based on finding one or more hyperechogenic masses within the heart (Fig. 16–37). They can create mechanical obstruction to ventricular inflow and outflow with the subsequent development of congestive heart failure. Cardiac dysrhythmias are also seen. The postnatal prognosis depends on the presence of tuberous sclerosis. Surgical excision is necessary in selected cases. Intracardiac tumors not associated with tuberous sclerosis may also shrink postnatally and remain asymptomatic.[69]

DOPPLER EXAMINATION OF THE STRUCTURALLY ABNORMAL HEART

Real-time ultrasonography remains the primary tool for the examination of the fetal heart. However, color and pulsed Doppler flow studies are essential for a complete study. The demonstration of normal blood flow direction, a lack of turbulence, and normal velocity waveforms confirms "normal flow" in the cardiac structures and supports the impression of an anatomically and functionally normal heart. Conversely, Doppler studies may reveal abnormal flow patterns in a heart that on real-time ultrasonography appears to be structurally normal, indicating the need for additional study.

FIGURE 16–37
Apical four-chamber view shows a rhabdomyoma (*) in the right atrium (RA).

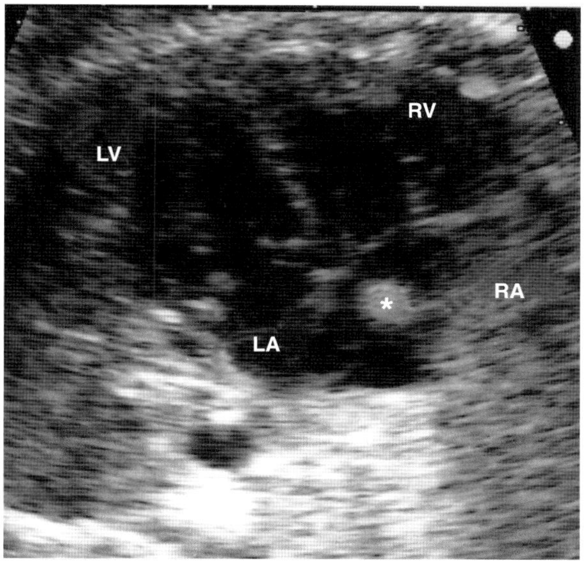

Valve Regurgitation

Valve regurgitation is characterized by bidirectional flow across the valve on Doppler interrogation. There is unidirectional flow from the atrium to the ventricle during diastole with regurgitant flow during systole. Regurgitation is uncommon across the fetal semilunar valves, where if it occurs, the regurgitation occurs during diastole.

Valve regurgitation may be either primary from valve dysplasia (e.g., tricuspid dysplasia,[70] or secondary due to increased ventricular pressure (e.g., pulmonary atresia or stenosis with intact septum) or papillary muscle dysfunction (cardiomyopathy).[71] The diagnosis of AV valve regurgitation requires demonstration of an abnormal color jet from the ventricle into the atrium during systole when imaged in the apical four-chamber view (see Figs. 16–29 and 16–30). The amount of regurgitation is proportional to the peak velocity of the regurgitant jet. High velocities can cause frequency aliasing on pulsed Doppler. As a result, continuous-wave Doppler is preferable when measuring the peak velocities. Although the amplitude of the jet is directly related to the pressure gradient across the valve by the Bernoulli equation ($P = 4V2$), it should not be used to quantify the severity of the disease because the pressure is influenced by both the severity of the obstruction and the ventricular contractility. A severe obstruction can be associated with a low-amplitude jet if ventricular contractility is too impaired to generate an adequate pressure gradient. Likewise, a low-grade stenosis associated with a normally functioning ventricle can generate a high-velocity jet in the absence of hypertension.

The duration of the regurgitant jet is of particular clinical importance.[70] Regurgitation limited to early systole is typically benign, whereas a holosystolic jet suggests severe hemodynamic compromise. Here, venous return is impaired, venous hypertension develops, and heart failure/hydrops may result.

Normal Flow Direction with High Velocities

This pattern of flow may result from hemodynamic adaptation to a hypoplastic or atretic structure in the contralateral side. For example, the flow across the tricuspid and pulmonary valves is increased in the presence of a hypoplastic left ventricle. Likewise, the flow across the mitral and aortic valves is increased in the presence of pulmonary atresia. The diagnosis is made when pulsed Doppler interrogation reveals a normal velocity waveform associated with increased PV and TVI.

Increased velocities can also occur with stenotic lesions such as pulmonary or aortic stenosis. In this setting, the flow is turbulent and the velocities high (see Figs. 16–30 and 16–32). Color Doppler allows for the identification of turbulent flow, and the velocity waveforms obtained with pulsed or continuous-wave Doppler reveal an irregular profile and a high PV. However, the PV is not used clinically to define the severity of stenosis because it also reflects ventricular contractility.

Absent Filling

No flow in a cardiac chamber suggests atresia of either the mitral (left ventricle) (see Fig. 16–27) or the tricuspid (right ventricle) valves (see Fig. 16–28). The equipment must have the correct settings and the angle of insonation must parallel the expected direction of flow (apical four-chamber view). Further, the gain, pulse repetition frequency, and filter must be correctly set to avoid artifact. Flow in the contralateral ventricle (apical four-chamber view) is proof of proper technique.

Abnormal Flow Direction

Because of the parallel nature of the fetal circulation, arterial blood can flow in a reverse direction if the flow from one ventricle is either absent or severely reduced. Examples include hypoplastic left heart or a severe coarctation in which the aortic arch is perfused in a retrograde fashion from the ductus arteriosus (see Fig. 16–31). In this way, the right ventricle can supply the cerebral and coronary circulations. Conversely, both pulmonary atresia and severe ductal stenosis are associated with reversed aortic arch flow because the pulmonary circulation depends on the left ventricle (see Fig. 16–19). Such abnormal hemodynamics are particularly important after birth.

Abnormal flow direction may be detected at the level of the foramen ovale or at the level of a ventricular septal defect, suggesting the presence of a malformation that alters the pressure equilibrium between the right and the left heart chambers. Examples include reverse direction flow (left to right) through the foramen ovale with a hypoplastic left heart or a unidirectional jet across an interventricular septal defect when there is an outflow tract lesion.

Advantages of Doppler for the Evaluation of Fetal Heart Diseases

An investigation of the cardiac flows helps to

1. Define the nature of the cardiac malformation. Copel and coworkers[72] observed retrospectively that color

Doppler was essential for establishing the correct diagnosis in 29%, helpful in 47% and neither helpful nor misleading in the remaining fetuses. We analyzed prospectively 145 fetuses with CHD and found that the combination of color and spectral Doppler was essential for the diagnosis in 34 fetuses (23%, mainly outflow tract stenosis or complex heart diseases [isomerism, double-outlet right ventricle with atresia of one semilunar valve]), useful in 62 fetuses (42%, mainly CHD complicated by valve atresia or outflow tract obstruction causing abnormal flow direction), and not helpful in the remaining 49 fetuses (34%, mainly complete AV canal and ventricular septal defects).[1]

2. Evaluate the hemodynamic consequence of CHD. The consequences of the sonographically same CHD may range in utero from no effect to cardiac failure and hydrops. This wide range of hemodynamic effects reflects the severity of the primary lesion, the presence of associated anomalies, the cardiac rhythm, and any impairment of ventricular function. The detection of regurgitation at the level of the AV valve by Doppler is a particularly useful predictor of hydrops. The presence of holosystolic, tricuspid regurgitation either isolated or associated with mitral regurgitation predicts the development of hydrops fetalis with subsequent poor prognosis. Study of the systemic venous circulation also provides a valuable index of the overall cardiac performance. Although there is no general agreement on the significance of the venous indices and on the vessel of choice, it is our experience that the velocity waveforms from IVC show a higher correlation with cardiac function than either the DV or the umbilical vein.[22] This information is helpful as the health care team formulates a plan, predicts prognosis, and counsels the parents (see also Chapter 11).
3. Monitor the evolution of CHDs. Doppler echocardiography is not only helpful in establishing the correct diagnosis but also valuable longitudinally to follow the natural history and progression of a malformation. One example is the evolution of pulmonary stenosis or atresia in fetuses with primary TR, which is presumably due to the lack of forward flow in the pulmonary artery. This has been described in fetuses with TR due to a dysplastic tricuspid valve and in fetuses with presumed cardiac overload secondary to twin- twin transfusion syndrome.[73] Similarly, a progressive increase in the severity of pulmonary stenosis of tetralogy of Fallot up to atresia is documented.[74,75] Knowledge of the pathologic evolution can be useful for the timing of delivery and/or for developing prenatal treatments such as balloon valvuloplasty in fetuses with deteriorating function.

PLANNING NEONATAL MANAGEMENT

The hemodynamic information gained from antenatal Doppler studies help predict problems after birth. For example, the neonate with a critical stenosis or atresia at the level of the outflow tract (e.g., hypoplastic left heart, pulmonary atresia with intact septum) is ductal-dependent after birth and will require continuous intravenous prostaglandin E_1. Closure of the ductus would have disastrous consequences because either the systemic (left obstruction) or the pulmonary (right obstruction) blood flow depends on ductal patency. Another example is the detection of a small (restrictive) foramen ovale in a fetus with complete transposition of the great arteries and an intact septum. Here, it can be anticipated the shunt between the two circulations will be insufficient after birth, with cyanosis and rapid deterioration expected. A pediatric cardiologist should be present at delivery to promptly perform a balloon septostomy (Rashkind's procedure) if needed. Advanced knowledge of these issues permits a planned delivery at a tertiary center where the facilities exist to optimize outcome.[76]

Management Options for the Fetus with Congenital Heart Disease

Cardiac malformations are the most common birth defects, and experienced fetal diagnosis units can detect a high percentage of major malformations (i.e., lesions typically requiring surgical treatment). Once the diagnosis of a cardiac malformation is made, the following steps are recommended.

Prenatal

CORRECTLY DEFINE THE MALFORMATION

A plan of management should be formulated in concert with a multidisciplinary team that includes a fetal medicine expert and a pediatric cardiologist.

SEARCH FOR ASSOCIATED STRUCTURAL ANOMALIES

Extracardiac anomalies and a normal karyotype are common in fetuses with congenital heart defects (10% in our series). A detailed ultrasonographic evaluation in an experienced fetal medicine center is mandatory. The presence of an associated anomaly may well influence the prognosis and postnatal management.

SEARCH FOR ASSOCIATED CHROMOSOMAL ANOMALIES

A fetal karyotype is mandatory because the result will alter management. The choice of the technique is based on the gestational age of the fetus and the experience of the center (see Chapter 9). Chromosomal abnormalities are present in 10% to 40%.[5] In our prospective series of 489 fetuses with CHDs, autosomal trisomy (trisomy 18, 13, and 21) and Turner's syndrome (45XO) were the most common abnormalities and accounted for 19.4% (see Table 16–2). The incidence of aneuploidy varies with the type of malformation, being extremely high with some (e.g., AV canal) or unusual with others (e.g., transposition of a great artery). This information should be part of the patient counseling.

A detailed study of chromosome 22 is indicated in fetuses with a conotruncal malformation because a microdeletion at the critical region 22q11,2 occurs in a high frequency of fetuses with this anomaly. The 22q11,2 syndrome (also called in the past CATCH 22)[77] consists of several genetic syndromes including velocardiofacial syndrome, Di George's syndrome, Opitz G/BBB syndrome, and conotruncal anomaly face syndrome. Patients with these syndromes have some or all the following features:

Mental retardation, learning disabilities and psychiatric illness.

CHDs: mainly conotruncal defects.

Palatal anomalies: overt and submucous cleft palate, velopharyngeal insufficiency.

Facial anomalies: long face with prominent nose, malar hypoplasia, retrognathia, and minor ear anomalies.

Thymus aplasia or hypoplasia associated with hypocalcemia and immunologic deficiency.

The estimated prevalence of this deletion in the general population is 1 in 4500,[78] which makes the 22q11.2 deletion syndrome the second most common genetic condition after Down syndrome. The prevalence of this syndrome in fetuses with conotruncal anomaly approximates 20%[24] and cannot be detected by routine karyotypic analysis. It is necessary to use either quantitative hybridization or fluorescence in situ hybridization (FISH) techniques that are now standard in most genetic laboratories. It is also important to extend the genetic diagnosis of affected fetuses to the parents, because inherited microdeletions occur in 30% with the remainder being de novo. Because the transmission is autosomal dominant, a parent with the syndrome has a 50% risk of transmitting the deletion to their offspring.[78]

COUNSELING THE PARENTS

The parents are formally counseled by the care team after all useful information is acquired (correct and complete diagnosis of the malformation, presence or absence of associated structural and/or chromosomal abnormalities). It is essential that the care team include, when possible, a fetal medicine physician, a pediatric cardiologist, and a cardiac surgeon. They should describe the malformation, the possibility of surgical correction, the chance of short- and long-term survival, and the quality of life after the correction. Further information on the possible neurologic complications after the surgical procedures should be provided. Indeed, malformations requiring deep hypothermic cardiopulmonary bypass surgery may be associated with neurologic impairment in up to 10% of the cases.[79] After complete information has been provided and all questions asked and answered, the parents should be allowed freedom of choice to continue or end the pregnancy. It is particularly helpful to make an appointment a few days later to discuss their thought process or decision and, when available, to offer psychological support.

PRENATAL MONITORING

The development of the malformation should be followed serially, particularly by using Doppler ultrasonography every 2 to 4 weeks. The interval is based on the likelihood of an in utero complication developing (e.g., 4 wk for a transposition of great artery, 2 wk for a tetralogy of Fallot). Furthermore, it is important in the third trimester to monitor fetal growth, amniotic fluid volume, Doppler velocity waveforms from peripheral fetal vessels, and fetal heart rate patterns, because the prevalence of suboptimal growth and acute fetal distress is increased.

PLACE, TIMING, AND METHOD OF DELIVERY

The need to deliver in a tertiary referral center varies with the diagnosis and upon the local resources and geographic constraints. It is important to predict before birth the type of assistance that may be needed. This may range from simple observation in the nursery (e.g., small ventricular septal defect) to assistance in the neonatal intensive care unit or pediatric cardiology unit (e.g., ductal-dependent CHD, hydrops, immaturity) to immediate postnatal treatment (e.g., balloon septostomy in transposition of a great artery with small foramen ovale).

Most fetuses with CHD tolerate labor well in the absence of uteroplacental dysfunction. There is no a priori indication for cesarean delivery. Furthermore, it is rarely necessary to induce labor early for a cardiac reason, though it may facilitate postnatal management if the delivery is planned between 38 and 40 weeks.

Postnatal

Postnatal management includes further cardiac evaluation by the pediatric cardiologist to confirm the diagnosis and to assess the hemodynamic environment. The neonate is stabilized and the treatment plan activated (interventional catheterization or surgery). Continued communication with the parents during the inevitable additional postnatal diagnostic steps and on the therapeutic strategies is extremely important.

SUMMARY OF MANAGEMENT OPTIONS

Fetal Cardiac Abnormalities

Management Options	Evidence Quality and Recommendation	References
Prepregnancy		
~1% risk of congenital heart defects in pregnancy.	III/B	2,3
Counsel women at risk (see Table 16–1).	III/B	19
Prenatal		
Screening		
Increased nuchal translucency with normal karyotype indicates higher risk of cardiac anomaly and need of careful cardiac scan in second trimester.	III/B	7,8

SUMMARY OF MANAGEMENT OPTIONS
Fetal Cardiac Abnormalities—cont'd

Management Options	Evidence Quality and Recommendation	References
Routine level 2 anomaly scanning at 20 wk should include situs and orientation, apical four-chamber view, lateral four-chamber view, left outflow tract, right outflow tract, three-vessel view, and venous return.	III/B	20–22
General		
Refer all high-risk pregnancies (see Table 16–1) to specialized center for complete fetal echocardiography (see Table 16–2)	GPP	
Meticulous visualization of the fetal heart during routine ultrasound scan at 18–20 wk of gestation, especially looking for the four-chamber view.	III/B	19
After Diagnosis of a Fetal Cardiac Abnormality		
Multidisciplinary team includes specialist obstetrician, pediatric cardiologist, and where appropriate, cardiac surgeon. Establish clear plan of management.	—/GPP	—
Define the defect and the severity of hemodynamic compromise by Doppler ultrasonography.	III/B	19
Search for other cardiac and extracardiac anomalies.	IV/C	4
Offer fetal karyotyping including 22q deletion.	IV/C	4
	III/B	5
Multidisciplinary counseling and psychological support for parents: • Give full explanation of all findings. • Discuss possible treatments (medical and surgical) and their implications and complications, prognosis (short- and long-term), and impact on neurodevelopment. • Offer further meeting/discussions. • In most cases, the only options are to continue with pregnancy or termination.	—/GPP	—
In Continuing Pregnancies		
Serial monitoring of • Fetal cardiac function by real-time and Doppler echocardiography (progression of congenital heart disease). • Fetal growth (IUGR common). • Fetal well-being by NST, biophysical profile, Doppler of peripheral vessels (avoid fetal distress).	—/GPP	—
Labor/Delivery		
Delivery at tertiary center with the appropriate obstetric, pediatric, and cardiologic facilities required by the type of cardiac malformation.	III/B	65
Vaginal delivery usually possible.	—/GPP	—
Close monitoring of fetal condition (continuous fetal heart rate monitoring), though this may not be possible if arrhythmia.	—/GPP	—
Consider planned delivery after 38 weeks for cardiac malformations that may require intensive care after birth.	III/B	76
Postnatal and Neonatal		
Stabilize the neonate, confirm the diagnosis by detailed echocardiography, and plan subsequent management.	—/GPP	—
After termination of pregnancy or perinatal death: • Obtain postmortem examination whenever possible. • Arrange for bereavement counseling.	—/GPP	—
Discuss implications for future pregnancies with parents.	—/GPP	—

GPP, good practice point; IUGR, intrauterine growth restriction; NST, nonstress test.

SUGGESTED READINGS

Achiron R, Glaser J, Gelerenter I, et al: Extended fetal echocardiography examination for detecting cardiac malformations in low risk population. BMJ 1992;404:671–674.

Copel JA, Pilu G, Kleiman GS: Congenital heart disease and extra-cardiac malformations: Associations and indications for fetal echocardiography. Am J Obstet Gynecol 1987;154:1121–1130.

Gardiner HM: In-utero intervention for severe congenital heart disease. Best Pract Res Clin Obstet Gynaecol 2008;22:49–61.

Goncalves LF, Lee W, Chaiworapongsa T, et al: Four-dimensional ultrasonography of the fetal heart with spatiotemporal image correlation. Am J Obstet Gynecol 2003;189:1792–1802.

International Society of Ultrasound in Obstetrics and Gynecology: Cardiac screening examination of the fetuses. Guidelines for performing the "basic" and "extended basic" cardiac scan. Ultrasound Obstet Gynecol 2006;27:107–113.

Miller G, Eggli KD, Contant C, et al: Postoperative neurologic complications after open heart surgery on young infants. Arch Pediatr Adolesc Med 1996;150:560–561.

Randall P, Brealey S, Hahn S, et al: Accuracy of fetal echocardiography in the routine detection of congenital heart disease among unselected and low risk populations: A systematic review. BJOG 2005;112:24–30.

Rizzo G, Arduini D, Romanini C: Doppler echocardiographic assessment of fetal cardiac function. Ultrasound Obstet Gynecol 1992;2:434–445.

Rizzo G, Arduini D (eds): Four Dimensional Fetal Echocardiography. Oak Park, IL, Bentham Science Publishers, 2010. Available at http://www.bentham.org/ebooks/9781608050444/

Roberts D: How best to improve antenatal detection of congenital heart defects. Ultrasound Obstet Gynecol 2008;32:846–848.

Tennstedt C, Chaoui R, Körner H, Dietel M: Spectrum of congenital heart defects and extracardiac malformations associated with chromosomal abnormalities: Results of a seven year necropsy study. Heart 1999;82:34–39.

Westin M, Saltvedt S, Bergman G, et al: Routine ultrasound examination at 12 or 18 gestational weeks for prenatal detection of major congenital heart malformations? A randomised controlled trial comprising 36,299 fetuses. BJOG 2006;113:675–682.

REFERENCES

For a complete list of references, log onto www.expertconsult.com.

CHAPTER 17

Fetal Craniospinal and Facial Abnormalities

ROBIN B. KALISH and FRANK A. CHERVENAK

Videos corresponding to this chapter are available online at www.expertconsult.com.

INTRODUCTION

Craniospinal and facial defects are among the most commonly diagnosed congenital anomalies and have a profound impact on survival, physical appearance, and function. Because the central nervous system (CNS) is the earliest organ system to form and facial development is completed near the end of embryogenesis, teratogenic exposures such as drug ingestion, maternal illness, and infection may cause craniospinal or facial malformations at any time during embryogenesis. Genetic syndromes and chromosomal abnormalities frequently affect the development of the neuraxis and face. Further, the fetal brain continues to develop throughout gestation. Consequently, it is vulnerable to disorders of growth as well as vascular, infectious, and traumatic insults.

OPEN NEURAL TUBE DEFECTS: ANENCEPHALY, CEPHALOCELE, AND SPINA BIFIDA

General

Neural tube closure occurs in the third to fourth weeks after fertilization. Fusion begins in the region of the fourth somite and then extends both rostrally and caudally. Closure in the region of the developing head and sacrum is completed approximately 24 and 26 days after conception, respectively. Neural tube defects most likely result from either a primary overgrowth of neural tube tissue within the line of closure or a failure of induction by adjacent mesodermal tissues that interrupt closure. Depending on the timing and the extent of the interruption, defects may occur at both cranial and caudal ends of the neural tube. Large or small and continuous or noncontinuous regions of the neuroaxis can be affected. Anencephaly is a lethal disorder in which the brain and the overlying calvarium are absent. It is thought to result from failure of the entire rostral portion of the neural tube to close. Less extensive failure of closure in the rostral region results in cephalocele. Failure of neural tube closure in the more caudad regions results in spina bifida.

Open neural tube defects (ONTDs) are multifactorial in origin, arising from a combination of genetic and environmental factors that exhibit a threshold effect. Thus, the incidence of ONTD is highly variable, depending on geographic location, ethnicity, and gender. In particular, the incidence of ONTD is reportedly higher in Hispanic patients,[1,2] in female fetuses,[3] and in areas with low maternal folic acid intake.[4] Additional high risk groups include women with insulin-requiring diabetes,[5] obese women,[6,7] women with a seizure disorder taking anticonvulsants including valproic acid,[8] women consuming high doses of vitamin A,[9] and women with folate or vitamin B_{12} insufficiency.[10] Women who themselves are affected, or who have had an affected infant or sibling, have a higher incidence of ONTD than the general population. ONTDs also may be associated with aneuploidy and other rare genetic syndromes.[11]

Diagnosis

Screening for ONTD may be either biochemical or ultrasonographic. Maternal serum α-fetoprotein (MSAFP) screening does not detect all cases of ONTD, because the MSAFP concentration can be normal if the lesion is predominantly skin-covered. Amniocentesis for the measurement of amniotic fluid α-fetoprotein (AFP) and the detection of acetylcholinesterase (AChE) is usually no longer required but remains an adjunct to ultrasonography when the MSAFP is elevated but no defect is visualized. Most ONTDs can be definitively diagnosed ultrasonographically, even as early as the first trimester,[12] and do not require amniocentesis.[13] The use of three-dimensional (3D) ultrasound and fetal magnetic resonance imaging (MRI) is reputed to assist in the detection and localization of ONTDs in high risk patients.[12,14–16]

Anencephaly

The antenatal ultrasonographic diagnosis of anencephaly is based on the absence of the fetal calvaria, the domelike portion of the cranial vault. A mass of thin-walled channels, known as the *area cerebrovasculosa*, is often seen protruding from the base of the skull above the orbits (Fig. 17–1). Though easily diagnosed during the second and third trimesters, first-trimester diagnosis of anencephaly is sometimes difficult because the normal immature brain may be difficult to differentiate from the area cerebrovasculosa. However, the bony structures of the skull above the orbits should be visualized by 10 weeks' gestation. Other diagnoses

FIGURE 17–1
Coronal sonogram of the fetal head demonstrates anencephaly (note the absent cranium and small neurogenic bundle seen above the orbits).

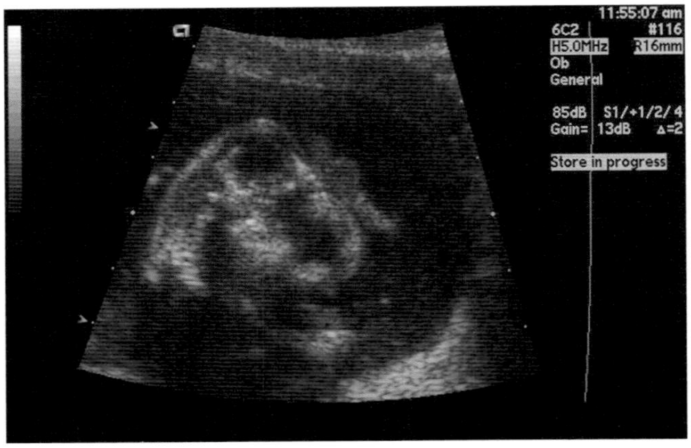

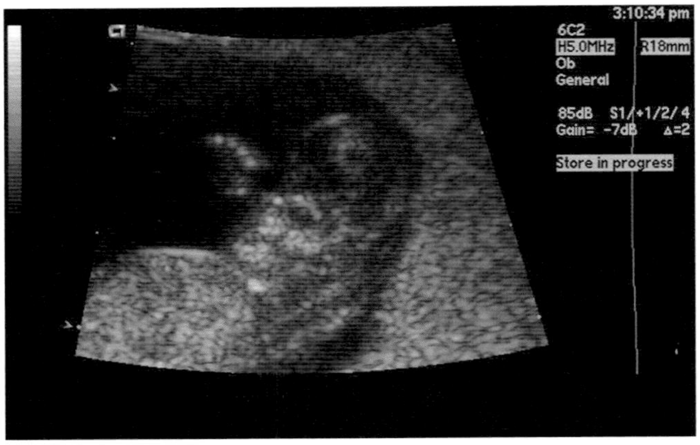

FIGURE 17–2
Sonogram of the first-trimester fetal head demonstrates acrania.

FIGURE 17–3
Encephalocele. *A*, Sagittal sonogram of the fetal head demonstrates posterior encephalocele with herniated brain protruding through the calvarium. *B*, Transverse view of the fetal head demonstrates a small posterior skull defect consistent with cephalocele. *C*, Defect in the posterior skull with herniated brain tissue and membranes.

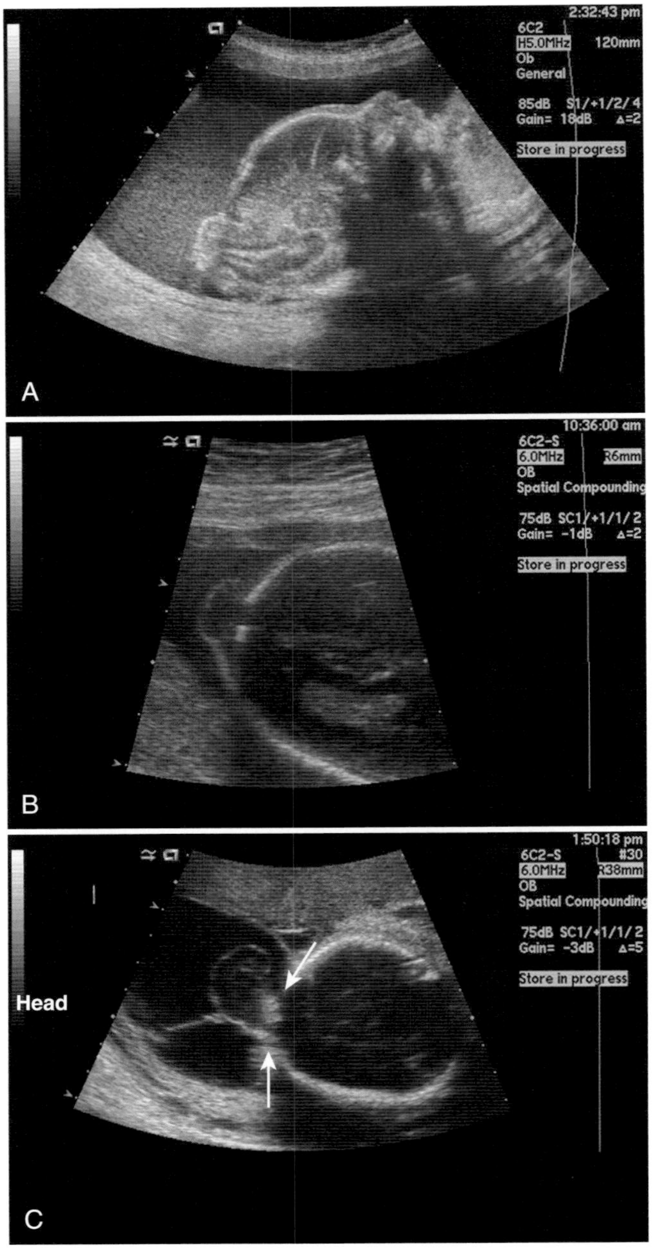

should be excluded; in severe microcephaly, the bones of the skull are present but might be difficult to see ultrasonographically. In the early amnion-rupture sequence, constricting bands may prevent the normal formation of the skull. In this instance, the malformation is usually asymmetrical and brain tissue is present. Amniotic bands may produce a spectrum of abnormalities from anencephaly to asymmetrical defects. Encephalocele may simulate anencephaly until a brain-filled sac is identified. Lastly, acrania, in which there is a normally formed brain with an absent skull, is often difficult to distinguish from anencephaly and, indeed, can be an early phase in the development of anencephaly (Fig. 17–2).

Cephalocele

A cephalocele resembles a saclike protrusion from the head not covered with bone. The malformation is termed an *encephalocele* when the brain has herniated into the sac. In contrast, a *cranial meningocele* does not contain brain substance. Although large amounts of brain tissue are readily seen on ultrasound, the precise diagnosis can be difficult because smaller amounts may be undetectable by ultrasonography (Fig. 17–3).[17] The contents of the herniated sac are typically heterogeneous. The position of the defect can be determined using the bony structures of the face, spine, and when possible, the midline echo of the brain for orientation. Most cephaloceles are occipital, but they may also be parietal, frontal, or nasopharyngeal.[18] The incidence of anterior lesions is considerably higher in Asia.[19,20] Defects away from the midline or in other atypical locations are suggestive of the amnion-rupture sequence. The diagnosis of cephalocele is certain only if the bony defect in the skull is detected. Otherwise, the diagnostic possibilities include cystic hygroma, teratoma, hemangioma, and subcutaneous cyst (Fig. 17–4).

Spina Bifida

Viewed longitudinally on ultrasound, the normal spine narrows caudally. In defective vertebrae, the posterior ossification centers are more widely spaced than those in vertebrae above and below the defect. Whereas an ONTD is detectable on a longitudinal ultrasound image by the loss of skin continuity (Fig. 17–5*A*), meticulous transverse examination of the entire vertebral column is usually necessary to detect smaller defects. In the transverse view, spina bifida appears as a splaying of the posterior ossification centers (see Fig. 17–5*B*). In the second and third trimesters, posterior vertebral elements, including the laminae and spinous processes, are normally visible sonographically. Their absence supports the diagnosis of spina bifida. When the ultrasound examination is not definitive, 3D ultrasound and fetal MRI can be useful, allowing precise localization of the lesion and evaluation of any associated hydrocephalus.[14–16] However, two-dimensional ultrasound remains the diagnostic method of choice for evaluation of fetal anomalies including myelomeningocele.

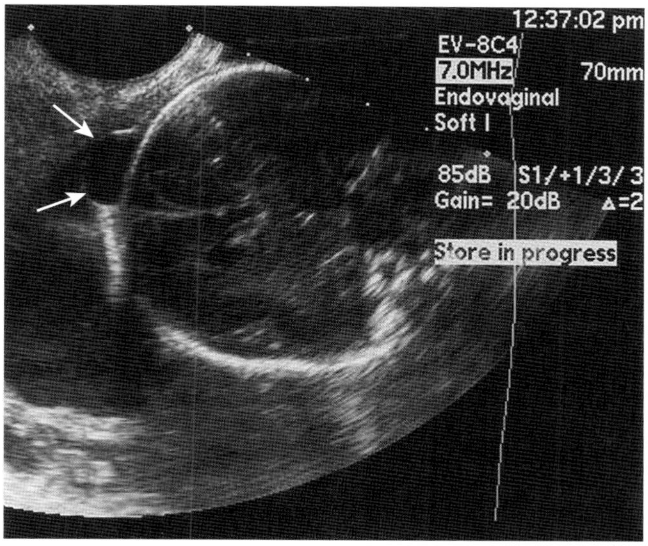

FIGURE 17–4
Coronal view of the fetal skull demonstrates a subcutaneous cystic structure (*arrows*). The skull is intact.

The majority of cases of spina bifida are associated with the Arnold-Chiari malformation in which the cerebellar vermis, fourth ventricle, and medulla are displaced caudally. Nicolaides and coworkers[21] described the now-classic sonographic signs of the Arnold-Chiari malformation: the "lemon" and the "banana" signs (Fig. 17–6*A*).[21] A lemon-like configuration is seen in axial section during the second trimester and is caused by scalloping of the frontal bones owing to caudal displacement of the cranial contents within a pliable skull (see Fig. 17–6*B*). As the cerebellar hemispheres are displaced into the cisterna magna, they are flattened rostrocaudally and the cisterna magna is obliterated, causing a flattened, centrally curved, banana-like sonographic appearance (see Fig. 17–6*C*). These ultrasound markers are present in over 95% of second-trimester fetuses with open spina bifida.[22] Eventually, the flow of cerebrospinal fluid (CSF) becomes obstructed, causing some degree of ventriculomegaly in most cases.

Management Options

Prenatal

The management of pregnancies with ONTD depends on the severity of the lesion and parental wishes. A comprehensive survey of the entire anatomy must be undertaken in all fetuses with an ONTD by an experienced sonographer to exclude other structural anomalies. Ventriculomegaly is present in the majority of cases, and the degree of hydrocephalus and subsequent macrocephaly likely affects the prognosis.[23] ONTDs are also seen in association with a variety of genetic syndromes, features of which may be detectable by ultrasonography. A fetal karyotype is

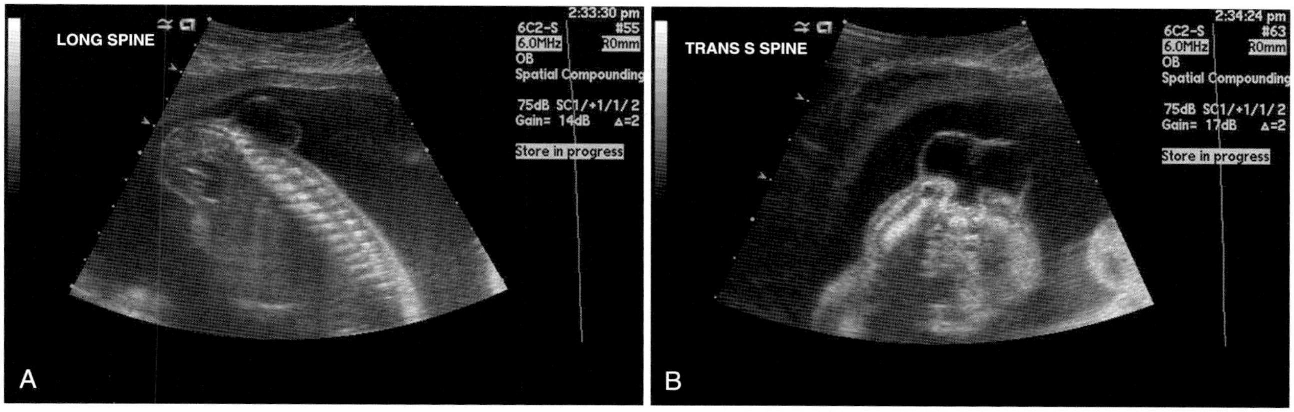

FIGURE 17–5
Spina bifida. *A*, Sagittal view of the fetal spine with sacral spina bifida demonstrated by the loss of skin continuity caudally. *B*, Transverse section of sacral spine demonstrates open spina bifida.

FIGURE 17–6
A, Schematic representation of the "lemon" and "banana" signs described by Nicolaides and coworkers. *B*, Transverse section of fetal head in a fetus with open spina bifida shows the "lemon" sign. *C*, Transverse section of fetal head in a fetus with open spina bifida shows the "banana" sign on the left of the image.
(*A*, From Nicolaides KH, Campbell S, Gabbe SG, Guidetti R: Ultrasound screening for spina bifida. Cranial and cerebellar signs. Lancet 1986;ii:72–74.).

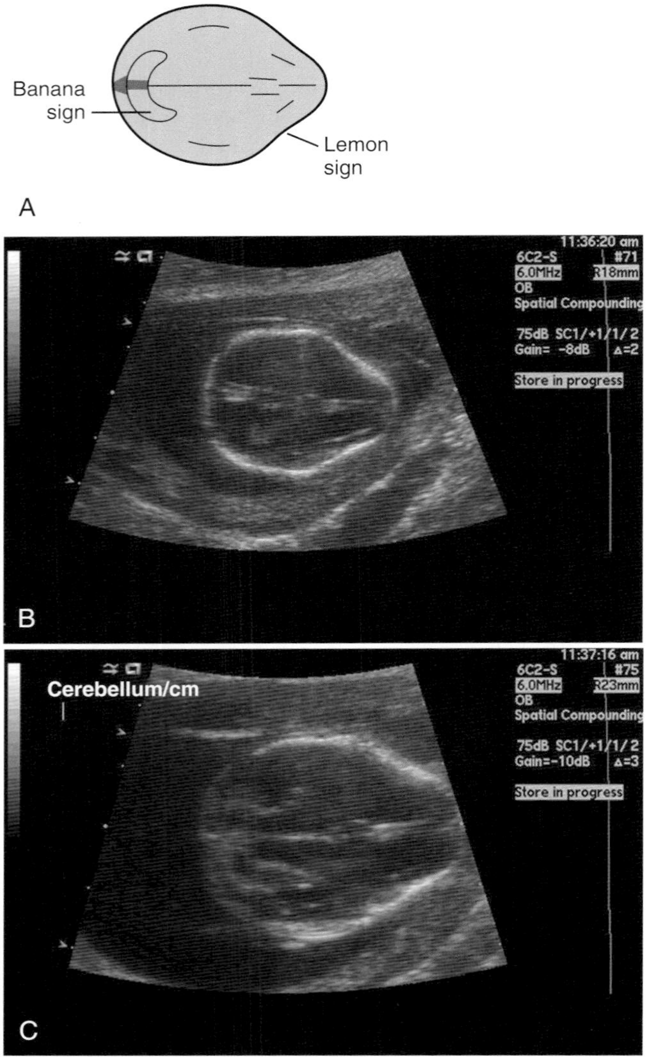

recommended in all instances. The incidence of aneuploidy varies with the type of ONTD, but the lowest reported figure is 2%.

Most fetuses with anencephaly are stillborn or die shortly after birth.[24] Because anencephaly can be diagnosed by antenatal ultrasound with a high degree of accuracy, termination of pregnancy is an ethical option at any time in gestation.[25] If it is diagnosed in the third trimester and the parents elect termination, a number of methods are available.

The most important prognostic indicators for a poor outcome with cephalocele are the presence of brain in the protruding sac and the presence of additional abnormalities.[26–28] A comprehensive fetal ultrasound examination should be performed to exclude genetic syndromes associated with encephalocele. In several series, 50% to 65% of affected fetuses had additional anomalies. Budorick and colleagues[29] observed that only 2 of 8 liveborns survived infancy. Brown and Sheridan-Pereira[30] reviewed 34 cases of neonatal cephalocele and noted an overall mortality rate of 29%. The most optimistic report came from Martinez-Lage and colleagues[31] who reported an overall mortality rate of 36% in 46 newborns with cephalocele, with 20 infants free of neurologic sequelae. In general, about half the infants with an isolated occipital cephalocele develop normally after surgery. The outlook is dismal for children with microcephaly secondary to brain herniation. The impact of concurrent hydrocephalus has been reduced by modern shunt therapy, and thus, hydrocephalus has less impact than the presence and amount of brain herniation. Frontal cephaloceles have a better prognosis than those in other locations because they tend to be smaller with less brain herniation.[32] Further, the loss of frontal cortex may produce fewer or less significant neurologic deficits than other areas of cortical loss.

The prognosis for spina bifida is variable. The extent and severity of the neurologic deficits depend on the presence of neural tissue in the meningeal sac and the spinal level and length of the lesion, because the spinal cord below the lesion is dysplastic.[33,34] Generally, lower extremity paralysis and incontinence of bowel and bladder are common; intelligence may be affected from either the lesion itself or the impact of treatment (e.g., shunt placement). Overall, 75% of infants born with spina bifida survive long term.[35] Twenty- to 25-year outcome was reported in one study of 118 children treated neonatally for the myelomeningocele.[35] Of the 99 patients with follow-up, 28 had died. Of the 71 survivors, 85% reached high school. One quarter suffered seizures. In another study of 117 patients born with open spina bifida, 54% had died within 38 years of closure.[36] The neurologic status of the survivors ranged from normal to severe disability. Thirty-nine of the 54 survivors had an IQ of 80 or higher; 16 could walk without assistance; 22 lived independently in the community; and only 11 were fully continent. Although improvements in the management of patients with open spina bifida have reduced the infant mortality rate, long-term disability is still significant, and late deterioration is common. Dise and Lohr[37] examined the cognitive skills of adolescents born with spina bifida up to 23 years of age. All patients, regardless of IQ, had significant impairments of mental flexibility, efficiency of processing, conceptualization, or problem-solving ability. There was a high degree of variability within profiles, all containing at least one area of dysfunction. These deficits may underlie the "motivational" and academic difficulties commonly observed in these patients.

Still, affected children can grow to be productive adults with normal intelligence. Early closure of the defect, ventriculoperitoneal shunting of any associated hydrocephalus, management of urinary and fecal incontinence by surgery, dietary management and feedback techniques are in part responsible for these improvements. It is unclear whether cesarean delivery improves the prognosis.[38] A selection bias brought about by antenatal diagnosis with termination of the most severely affected fetuses may account, at least in part, for the reportedly improved outcomes. The prognosis for the severely affected newborn remains poor, with gross permanent multisystem defects. It is difficult to accurately predict the prognosis in the first half of pregnancy when the diagnosis is frequently made. The option for pregnancy termination should be included in counseling the patients.

Alternatively, in utero repair of myelomeningocele to stop or slow any progression in damage to the exposed spinal cord reportedly decreases the incidence of hindbrain herniation and shunt-dependent hydrocephalus.[39] The rationale for the procedure is that closure antenatally may decrease spinal cord dysplasia and preserve neurologic function by protecting it from potential insults such as amniotic fluid trauma. Although fetal surgery is promising on a theoretical basis, significant complications are associated with in utero repair, including prematurity and lethal pulmonary hypoplasia secondary to oligohydramnios. In addition, the evidence of long-term benefit, including improved lower limb motor function and bladder and bowel continence, is at this time unclear.[40,41] Danzer and colleagues[42] reviewed 54 children over the age of 3 who underwent fetal myelomeningocele closure. Although the authors observed better lower limb neuromotor function than expected, the toddlers continued to demonstrate significant deficits in motor coordination. In addition, other researchers have found no improvement in bowel or bladder function or ambulatory ability beyond the degree of impairment predicted by the level of the lesion.[43,44] In utero repair of myelomeningocele should be considered experimental until the availability of evidence shows that the benefits outweigh the risks to both mother and fetus. Currently, there is a multicentered randomized clinical trial under way in the United States in order to compare the outcomes of fetal surgery with postnatal management for spina bifida.[34]

When a meningomyelocele is diagnosed and the patient plans to continue the pregnancy, a multidisciplinary team consisting of a pediatric neurologist, neurosurgeon, obstetrician, and neonatologist should discuss the implications with the family. Support is invaluable before and after birth. Fetal surveillance is recommended for all ongoing pregnancies with the exception of anencephaly, including serial ultrasonography to assess fetal growth, head size, and severity of ventriculomegaly. Unless maternal or other obstetric indication take precedence, delivery should occur at term or with documentation of fetal lung maturity.

Labor and Delivery

Postmaturity is common in pregnancies complicated by anencephaly. Cesarean delivery is not indicated for fetal distress, but may be necessary for maternal indications. Humane care is provided to the liveborn anencephalic infant until death. The use of anencephalic newborns as organ donors remains widely debated.[45,46] Pathologic examination of the fetus is important to confirm the diagnosis and to exclude conditions in which anencephaly is part of a genetic syndrome.

The optimal mode of delivery for the fetus with cephalocele is controversial. If a large amount of brain tissue is observed in the sac, and especially if one of the more grave prognostic factors (e.g., microcephaly or associated anomalies) is also present, the parents should be counseled that the chance of a good outcome is remote and cesarean delivery for fetal indications avoided. Decompression of a large sac or associated hydrocephalus might be necessary to allow vaginal delivery. However, cesarean delivery is an option in those rare instances in which a cephalocele is very large and sufficiently solid to cause dystocia. There is no clear objective evidence that cesarean delivery reduces birth trauma and improves neonatal outcome when a cephalocele is present. However, this does not exclude the possibility that trauma during vaginal delivery could, in theory, worsen the prognosis.

Similarly, there is no conclusive information about the optimal route of delivery for the vertex fetus with a meningomyelocele. One retrospective clinical study concluded that elective cesarean delivery prior to the onset of labor improved outcome in terms of the functional level of the spinal defect at age 2 years.[47] However, this study contained numerous sources of bias. Multiple subsequent studies, which have sought to eliminate some of the design flaws of the first study, could identify no benefit from cesarean delivery.[48–51] A randomized trial to study this question has not been done. Until it is clear whether or how the method of delivery affects the neurologic outcome in theses infants, cesarean section remains the delivery method of choice in our institution.

Care must be taken during delivery to minimize traction on the spine regardless of the route of delivery. If there is an indication for cesarean delivery, a low transverse incision is acceptable if the lower uterine segment is well developed. Otherwise, a vertical incision should be performed. After the head is delivered, the bisacromial diameter is positioned horizontally. Both fetal flanks are grasped and gentle traction applied in an outward direction away from the uterine wall near the meningomyelocele. The assistant retracts the edge of the uterine incision as the body of the infant is delivered (Fig. 17–7).

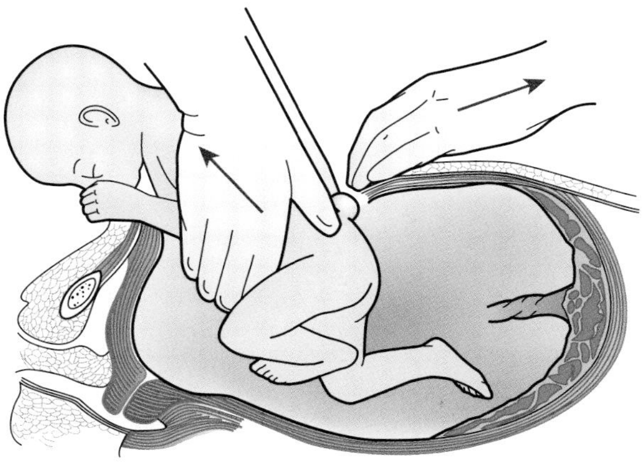

FIGURE 17–7
Fetus with a meningomyelocele is delivered through a low transverse uterine incision. Both fetal flanks are grasped, and gentle traction is applied in an outward direction. Assistant retracts the edge of the uterine incision as the body is delivered.
(From Chervenak FA, Duncan C, Ment LR, et al: Perinatal management of myelomeningocele. Obstet Gynecol 1984;63:376.)

Postnatal and Prepregnancy

In the United States, the recurrence risk for any neural tube defect after one affected child may be as high as 3% to 5%[52,53] and up to 10% after having two affected offspring. The risk is greater in populations in which ONTDs are more common. The recurrence risk is 4% to 5% if one parent is affected, and 25% when the ONTD is part of the Meckel-Gruber syndrome. A cephalocele may also occur as part of other autosomal recessive syndromes.

Randomized, placebo-controlled trials demonstrate that the likelihood of recurrence is reduced by periconceptual administration of folate (4–5 mg orally daily). This treatment should be offered to all women with a prior affected child. Antenatal ultrasonography should be performed in future pregnancies initially at 11 to 14 weeks in search of a recurrent ONTD.

SUMMARY OF MANAGEMENT OPTIONS

Open Neural Tube Defects: Anencephaly, Cephalocele, and Spina Bifida

Management Options	Evidence Quality and Recommendation	References
Prenatal		
Search for skull defect in cephalocele and associated anomalies in all cases of open neural tube defects, including MRI.	III/B	23,90,106
Prognosis for cephalocele depends on amount of herniated brain tissue; prognosis for spina bifida is difficult to predict early and depends on level and extent of lesion.	—/GPP	—
Offer karyotype.	—/GPP	—
Monitor for hydrocephalus.	—/GPP	—
Provide multidisciplinary counseling and care.	—/GPP	—
Offer termination where appropriate.	—/GPP	—
Monitor ongoing pregnancies (growth, umbilical artery Doppler, amniotic fluid volume).	—/GPP	—
Regard fetal surgery for spina bifida as experimental at present.	III/B	39–41
Labor and Delivery		
Deliver by vaginal route for anencephaly and humane neonatal care.	—/GPP	—
Mode of delivery for cephalocele is uncertain; no evidence that cesarean section is beneficial.	—/GPP	—
Where appropriate, offer cephalocentesis	—/GPP	—
Optimal route of delivery is unknown for spina bifida.	III/B	48–51
Great care is needed with delivery of the back, regardless of delivery route.	—/GPP	—
Postnatal and Prepregnancy		
Offer postmortem for abortuses/stillbirths/neonatal deaths.	—/GPP	—
Offer karyotyping if not already done.	—/GPP	—
Assess for diabetes, teratogens (anticonvulsants, vitamin A).	—/GPP	—
Provide counseling.	—/GPP	—
Give periconceptual high-dose folate to women with a history of neural tube defect.	Ia/A	113
Provide pediatric neurosurgical management.	—/GPP	—

GPP, good practice point; MRI, magnetic resonance imaging.

HYDROCEPHALUS

General

Hydrocephalus is defined as ventriculomegaly and macrocephaly associated with increased intracranial pressure. As such, hydrocephalus is a description and not a diagnosis. It results from an abnormal increase in the cerebral ventricular volume compared with brain tissue. There are many causes of hydrocephalus; it may result from abnormal formation of CNS structures, as in hydrocephalus inherited along a mendelian pattern or hydrocephalus associated with a malformation syndrome; it may result from defects acquired in utero, from infection with subsequent scarring, or inflammation and CSF obstruction, from intraventricular hemorrhage, or from intracranial tumors and mass lesions. Many cases of hydrocephalus cannot currently be assigned to any one specific etiologic category.

In general, there are four ways in which the ventricles grow to an abnormal size (Fig. 17–8):

- Obstruction to outflow (noncommunicating hydrocephalus), usually at a point of narrowing in the system (frequently the aqueduct of Sylvius or the foramina of either Luschka or Magendie).
- Impaired resorption of CSF by the arachnoid granulations (communicating hydrocephalus).
- Overproduction of CSF.
- Underdevelopment or destruction of cortical tissue with a relative increase in the size of the ventricles (hydrocephalus ex vacuo).

Obstructive causes are the most common in both fetus and newborn.[54,55] In the United States, the incidence of congenital hydrocephalus unassociated with a neural tube defect is 5.8 per 10,000 total births. This is likely an underestimate of the true incidence because both spontaneous regression and antepartum death occur in some cases.[54]

Diagnosis

A variety of techniques are advocated for the diagnosis of ventriculomegaly. Measurement of the atrium of the lateral ventricles is most common (Fig. 17–9*A*). This method is optimal because the width of the atrium remains constant throughout the second and third trimesters despite the fact

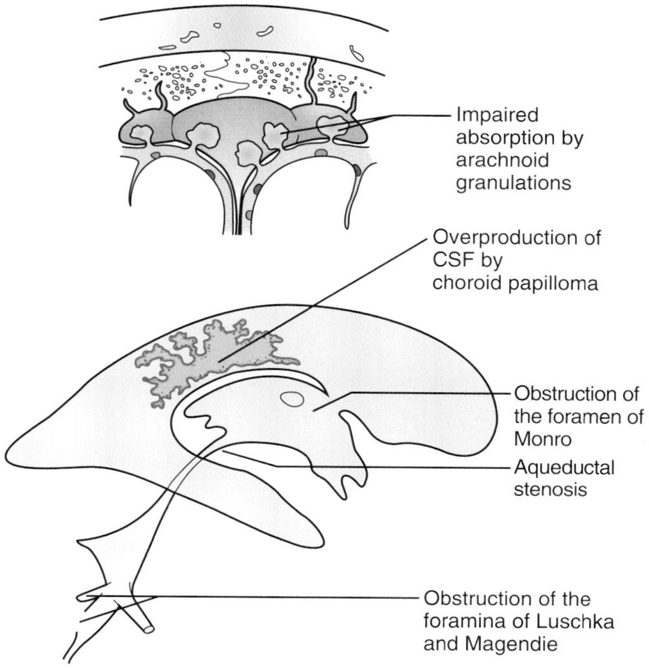

FIGURE 17–8
Diagrammatic representation of the mechanisms of ventriculomegaly.

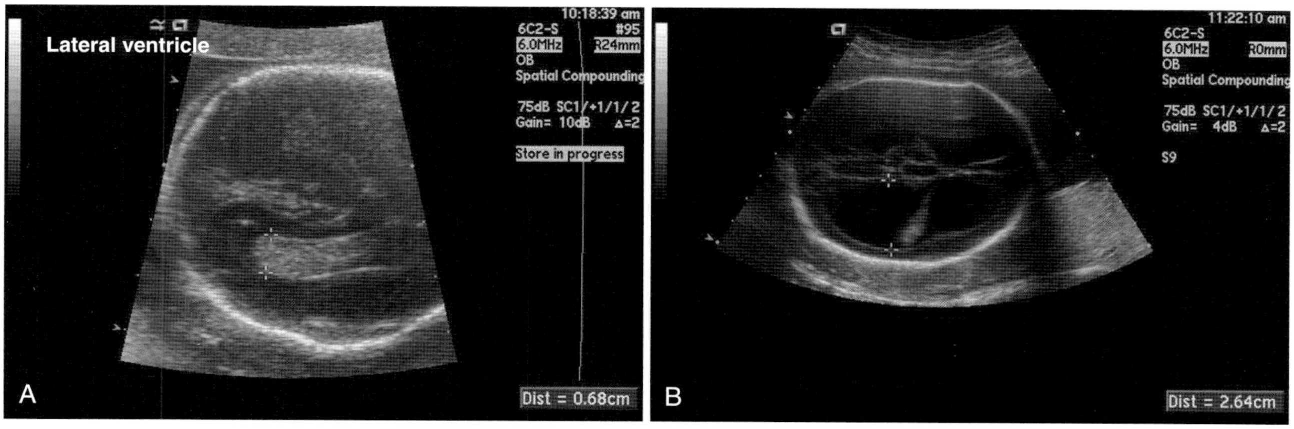

FIGURE 17–9
A, Transverse section demonstrates the distal lateral ventricle with its atrial measurements. *B*, Transverse section of the fetal head demonstrates dangling of the choroid plexus within the dilated lateral and third ventricles, consistent with hydrocephalus.

FIGURE 17–10
Holoprosencephaly. Transverse view of the fetal head demonstrates holoprosencephaly at 13 weeks' gestation. The falx cerebri is noted to be absent anteriorly. The anterior aspect of the fetal brain demonstrates a single ventricle.

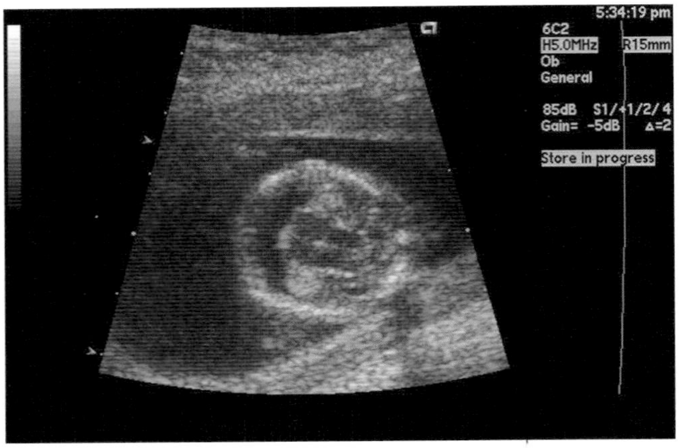

FIGURE 17–11
Arachnoid cyst. *A*, Transverse section through the fetal head demonstrates a midline cyst. *B*, This cystic structure is shown to have no flow on color Doppler and to be separate from the cavum septum pellucidum, consistent with an arachnoid cyst.

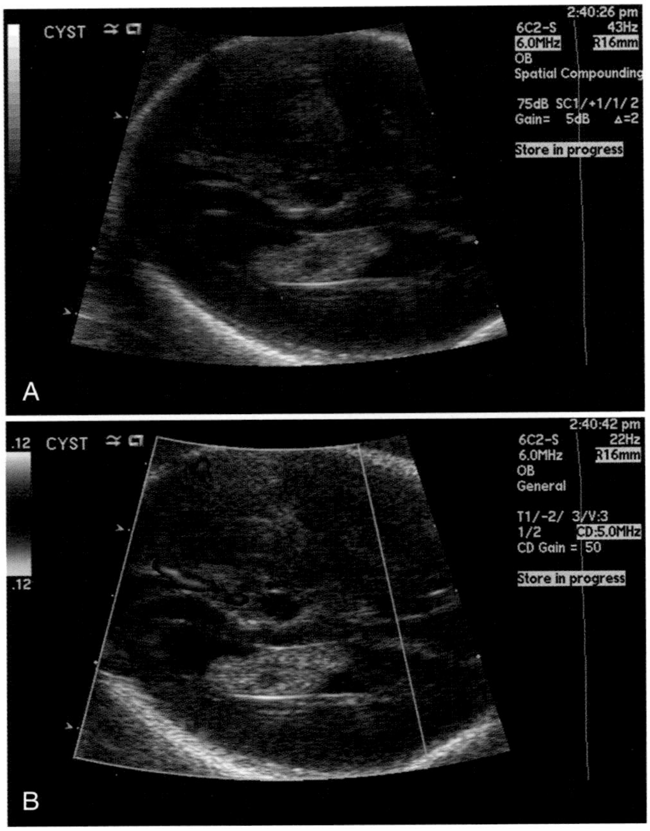

that there is a decrease in the proportion of the cross-section of the brain occupied by the lateral ventricles as pregnancy advances. Cardoza and colleagues[56] presented strong evidence that a single measurement of the lateral ventricle atrium accurately differentiates a normal ventricle system from one that is pathologically enlarged.

Evaluation of the choroid plexus can also be useful when ventriculomegaly is suspected.[57] The choroid plexus usually fills the posterior portion of the lateral ventricles and appears symmetrical bilaterally, regardless of the orientation of the fetal head. In ventriculomegaly, the choroid plexus assumes a dependent position in the enlarged ventricle and appears as a dangling structure (see Fig. 17–9*B*). Serial ultrasound examinations are especially important for at-risk pregnancies. The absence of hydrocephalus early in gestation does not preclude its development later in gestation. Once hydrocephalus is diagnosed as an isolated abnormality, serial scans are important to identify in utero progression. The differential diagnoses for severe hydrocephalus includes alobar holoprosencephaly, hydrancephaly, porencephaly, and arachnoid cyst (Figs. 17–10 and 17–11). Another rare cause of large, intracranial fluid–like collection is an aneurysm of the vein of Galen, characterized by blood flow that can be visualized by color Doppler.

Management Options

Prenatal

Prior to the development of postnatal surgical shunting of the dilated ventricular system, the outlook for the infant with hydrocephalus was generally poor. Although some cases of unoperated obstructive hydrocephalus progressed slowly, or arrested spontaneously, massive head enlargement with blindness and mental retardation were far more common and still occur in underdeveloped parts of the world.[58]

After the development of postnatal shunting, the prognosis of isolated hydrocephalus improved greatly. Most neonatal deaths are attributable to associated anomalies as well as obstetric trauma from cephalocentesis. Intellectual development is related to the etiology, and not necessarily to the severity of the hydrocephalus.[59,60] The association between the age at initial shunt placement and intellectual development is controversial.[61,62] Infants with associated CNS anomalies or hydrocephalus secondary to other defects, such as Dandy-Walker malformation or porencephaly, have significantly lower IQs than infants with isolated hydrocephalus.[63,64] In addition, infants with congenital hydrocephalus have somewhat lower overall survival rates than infants who develop hydrocephalus in the neonatal period.[65] A 10-year follow-up study of 129 consecutive children with non–tumor-related hydrocephalus who underwent their first shunt insertion before age 2 years[66] reported an overall mortality rate below 10%. However, motor deficits were found in 60%, visual or auditory deficits in 25%, and epilepsy in 30%. Intellectual deficits were common and 40% had an IQ below 70. Only 32% of the children had an IQ above 90. Other studies have reported a similar long-term intellectual prognosis.[67,68]

Once fetal hydrocephalus is identified, a careful sonographic search for associated fetal anomalies, including meningomyelocele, is mandatory. Because hydrocephalus is among the extracardiac anomalies associated with congenital heart disease, fetal echocardiography should also be performed. Up to 10% have a chromosomal abnormality.[69,70] The obstetric management of fetal hydrocephalus reflects the gestational age at diagnosis, the presence of other anomalies, the results of the karyotype and infection studies, and the views of the parents. If the diagnosis is made prior to fetal viability, the patient may consider pregnancy termination. If the karyotype is normal, and the parents wish to continue the pregnancy, serial ultrasound examinations are performed to identify progressive ventricular enlargement. In some cases, ventriculomegaly may regress in utero.

Although experimental placement of ventriculoamniotic shunts in fetal rhesus monkeys yielded encouraging results, the experience in human pregnancies has been disappointing. A study of 39 fetal ventriculoamniotic shunt placements reported to the International Fetal Surgery Registry in 1993[71] listed 34 survivors: 14 had apparently normal neurodevelopment, and 18 had severe handicaps. The remaining 2 survivors had varying degrees of neurologic impairment. Children with intact intellectual development were all diagnosed with simple aqueductal stenosis. Of a total of 7 deaths, 4 were directly attributed to the procedure. Many of the fetuses were misdiagnosed, errors that would be less likely to occur using MRI. Although most fetal medicine practitioners are not placing intrauterine ventriculoamniotic shunts, others believe it is time to revisit the issue.[72]

Labor and Delivery

Serial ultrasonography may detect worsening hydrocephalus. In this situation, delivery should be considered as soon as pulmonary maturity is achieved in hopes of minimizing the potential ill effects of progressive ventricular enlargement. There is no clear indication for preterm delivery if the hydrocephalus is rapidly progressive prior to fetal lung maturity because respiratory distress syndrome, which would delay shunt placement, could actually worsen the final outcome. If delivery before fetal lung maturity is elected, maternal corticosteroids should be administered to hasten pulmonary maturity and reduce the risk and severity of respiratory distress syndrome. Fetuses with isolated disease and moderate to severe macrocephaly should be delivered by cesarean section to facilitate the atraumatic delivery of the enlarged fetal head. Attempted vaginal delivery is appropriate when the fetus is in vertex presentation and has only mild macrocephaly.

Fetal cortical mantle thickness correlates poorly with subsequent intelligence. Further, normal intelligence is possible for infants with hydrocephalus who receive optimal neonatal neurosurgical care. In cases of fetal hydrocephalus with associated anomalies that are either incompatible with life or associated with the severest forms of neurologic dysfunction (e.g., alobar holoprosencephaly, hydrancephaly, or thanatophoric dysplasia with cloverleaf skull), cephalocentesis and subsequent vaginal delivery are an acceptable alternative to cesarean delivery. Cephalocentesis is performed by passing a 14- to 18-gauge needle transabdominally or transvaginally under ultrasound guidance (Fig. 17–12). Sufficient CSF is removed to allow overlapping of the cranial sutures. This is a destructive procedure. In a small series reported by Chasen and colleagues,[73] all three fetuses were stillborn with two delivering vaginally and one abdominally through a low transverse uterine incision.

Postnatal and Prepregnancy

Hydrocephalus has diverse etiologies and the identification of the specific cause aids greatly the subsequent genetic counseling. A postmortem examination is essential. Several heritable patterns are recognized. X-Linked recessive aqueductal stenosis carries a 1:4 risk of recurrence in future pregnancies, or 1:2 risk for male fetuses. Cerebellar agenesis with hydrocephalus is extremely rare, but also might be X-linked. Hydrocephalus is also associated with a variety of chromosomal abnormalities including triploidy, trisomies 13, 18, and 21, and certain balanced translocations. The risk of recurrence is relatively low for sporadic chromosomal abnormalities but is much higher for balanced translocations.

In addition, hydrocephalus is associated with several syndromes that manifest dominant inheritance (e.g., achondroplasia and osteogenesis imperfecta).[74] The Dandy-Walker syndrome has been reported in siblings, suggesting the possibility of autosomal recessive inheritance. Several studies suggest an increased risk of uncomplicated hydrocephalus in families with neural tube defects. Lorber and De[75] studied uncomplicated congenital hydrocephalus and found an empirical risk of 4% for a CNS malformation and 2% for spina bifida or hydrocephalus in future pregnancies. Other causes of fetal hydrocephalus include prenatal infection (e.g., toxoplasmosis), intracranial tumors or cysts, and vascular malformations. Such causes are unlikely to result in an increased risk of hydrocephalus in future pregnancies.

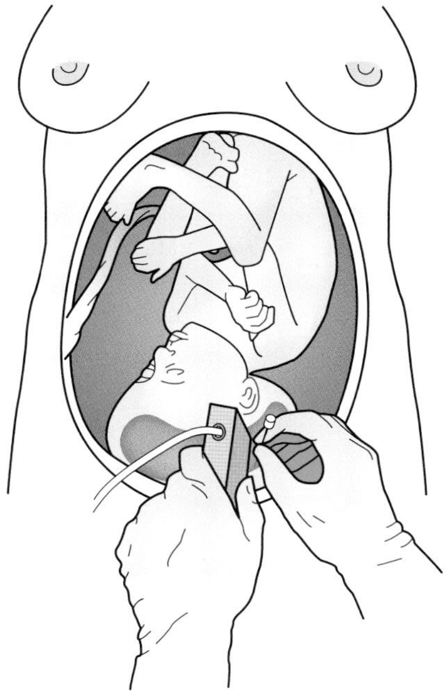

FIGURE 17–12
Sonographic guidance of the needle during cephalocentesis.

SUMMARY OF MANAGEMENT OPTIONS

Hydrocephalus

Management Options	Evidence Quality and Recommendation	References
Prenatal		
Search for other anomalies including karyotype; MRI often helps to clarify diagnosis; full workup is recommended for congenital infection.	III/B	69,70,90,107,108
Provide cautious counseling regarding prognosis if isolated finding.	—/GPP	—
Provide multidisciplinary counseling.	—/GPP	—
Offer termination where appropriate.	—/GPP	—
In continuing pregnancy:		
• Multidisciplinary care	—/GPP	—
• Serial scans to identify progressive dilation of ventricles and head enlargement	—/GPP	—
• No basis for fetal shunt placement	III/B	72
Labor and Delivery		
No evidence supports preterm delivery with worsening ventriculomegaly; deliver fetus when risk of prematurity is low.	—/GPP	—
No evidence supports cesarean delivery a priori, but cesarean section with excessive ventriculomegaly is common.	—/GPP	—
Cephalocentesis is potentially destructive and should not to be used if optimal survival is the aim.	III/B	73
Postnatal and Prepregnancy		
Establish cause and type.	—/GPP	—
Provide counseling.	—/GPP	—
Provide pediatric neurosurgical management.	—/GPP	—
Offer postmortem for abortuses/stillbirths/neonatal deaths.	—/GPP	—

GPP, good practice point.

CRANIOFACIAL DISORDERS OF VENTRAL INDUCTION: THE HOLOPROSENCEPHALY SEQUENCE

General

The prechordal mesoderm, an embryonic connective mass between the undersurface of the neural tube and the oral cavity, is thought to be responsible for both the division of the prosencephalon or forebrain and the production of the nasofrontal process. The term *holoprosencephaly* includes several cerebral abnormalities that share incomplete cleavage of the primitive prosencephalon. Because of the underlying embryologic insult, various midline facial abnormalities are closely associated with holoprosencephaly, although the face can be normal (Fig. 17–13). The incidence of holoprosencephaly approximates 1 in 10,000 live births.[76] Holoprosencephaly is divided into alobar, semilobar, and lobar categories, based on the degree of separation of the cerebral hemispheres (Fig. 17–14). The alobar form is the most severe, with no evidence of cerebral cortical division. The falx cerebri and the interhemispheric fissure are absent. There is a common ventricle with fused thalami. The semilobar and lobar forms represent a higher degree of brain development, with the semilobar having partial separation of the hemispheres. Although there is much variability in the types of defects in the midline cerebral structures (e.g., corpus callosum, septum pellucidum, thalamus), the olfactory tracts and bulbs are usually absent, explaining the older term "arrhinencephaly."

The holoprosencephaly sequence results in the following characteristic facial findings (Fig. 17–15):

- Cyclopia with one median orbit, proboscis from the lower forehead, and absent nose.
- Ethmocephaly with proboscis between two narrowly placed orbits and absent nose.
- Cebocephaly with hypotelorism and rudimentary nose (single nostril).
- Hypotelorism (decreased intraorbital distance), median cleft lip, and flat nose.
- Bilateral cleft lip.

FIGURE 17–13
Embryology of holoprosencephaly and midline facial defects.

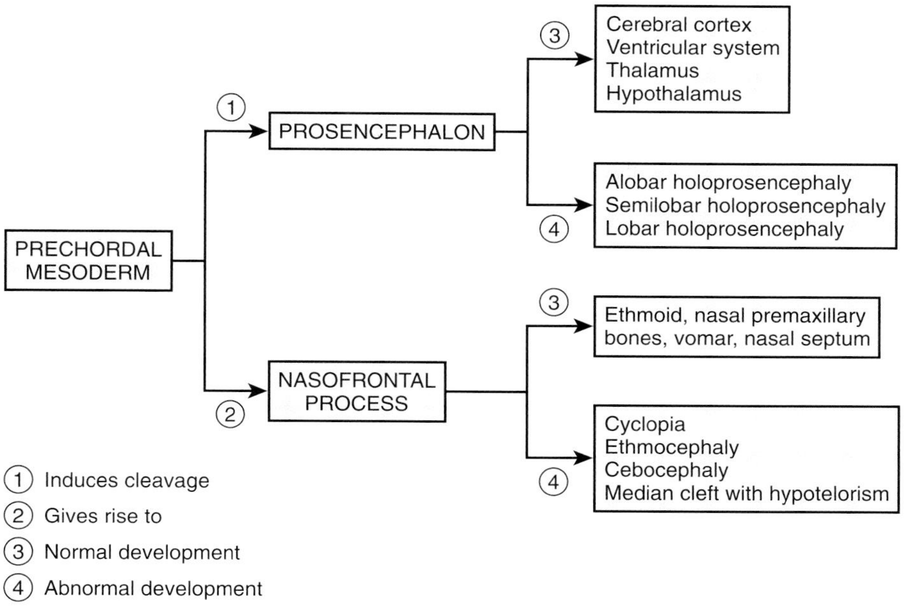

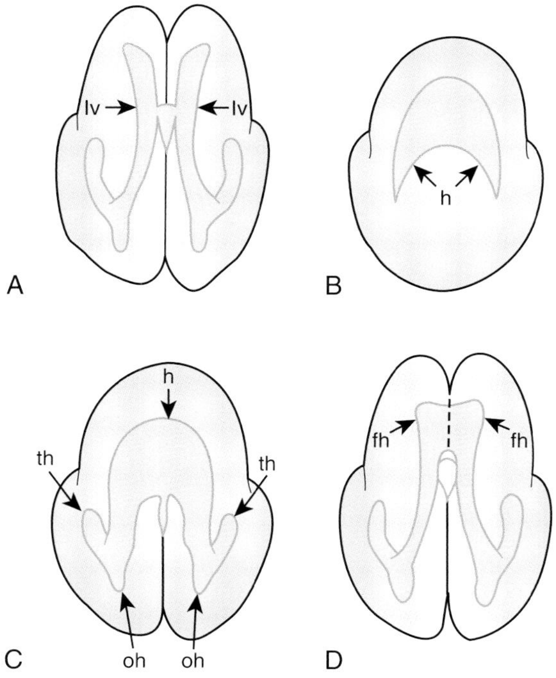

FIGURE 17–14
Holoprosencephaly. *A*, Normal brain. Both the cerebral hemispheres and the lateral ventricles are separated. *B*, Alobar holoprosencephaly. The normal division of the cerebral hemispheres is absent, and there is a single ventricular cavity. *C*, Semilobar holoprosencephaly shows an incomplete separation of the cerebral hemispheres in the occipital area and partial development of the occipital and temporal horns of the lateral ventricles. *D*, Lobar holoprosencephaly. Separation of the cerebral hemispheres and lateral ventricles is nearly complete except for the frontal portions. The frontal horns of the lateral ventricles are usually mildly dilated.
(*A–D*, From Pilu G, Romero R, Rizzo N, et al: Criteria for the prenatal diagnosis of holoprosencephaly. Am J Perinatol 1987;4:41–49.)

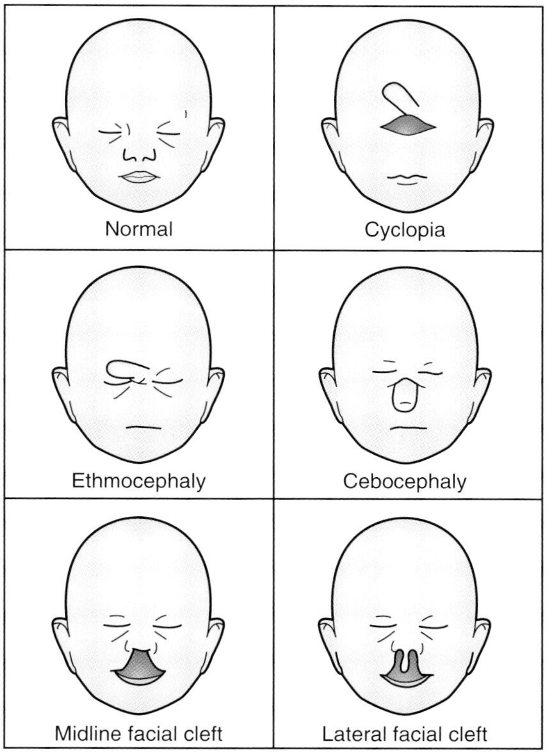

FIGURE 17–15
Holoprosencephaly. Schematic drawings of the facies associated with holoprosencephaly.
(From Mahony BS, Hegge FN: The face and neck. In Nyberg DA, Mahony BS, Pretorius DH [eds]: Diagnostic Ultrasound of Fetal Anomalies: Text and Atlas. Chicago, Year Book, 1990, pp 203–261.)

Diagnosis

The dictum "the face predicts the brain" is often used to describe holoprosencephaly, because cyclopia, ethmocephaly, cebocephaly, and hypotelorism with midline cleft lip are commonly found in association with this CNS anomaly.[77] Ultrasonographic markers include hypotelorism and a single common cerebral ventricle with absent midline echo. The general appearance of the face, the position and configuration of the nose, and the integrity of the upper lip should be observed closely for clues. It may be impossible to differentiate semilobar from lobar holoprosencephaly before birth. Holoprosencephaly can be detected sonographically as early as the first or second trimester (see Fig. 17–10).

It is not sufficient to diagnose holoprosencephaly based solely on a central fluid collection in the brain, because this may also represent hydranencephaly or a midline porencephalic cyst. Other anatomic aberrations associated with holoprosencephaly detectable by ultrasound include hydrocephalus, polydactyly, and hydramnios.

Management Options

Prenatal

The prognosis for alobar holoprosencephaly is uniformly poor. Most infants die shortly after birth, and the survivors have profound mental retardation.[78] Less is known about the prognosis for lobar and semilobar varieties. A normal life span is reported, but many are severely mentally retarded. Subtle forms of lobar holoprosencephaly with little neurologic abnormality may exist. Karyotyping should be offered because of the association with aneuploidy (especially trisomy 13).

Labor and Delivery

The obstetric management of holoprosencephaly is dependent on gestational age at the time of diagnosis. Many patients opt for pregnancy termination when the diagnosis is made in the first or second trimester. Macrocephaly in the third trimester may obstruct labor and cephalocentesis should be considered to avoid cesarean delivery. The destructive nature of this procedure must be explained to the parents.

Postnatal and Prepregnancy

The diagnosis of holoprosencephaly signals the need for a careful postmortem examination and a fetal karyotype to guide the management of future pregnancies. A chromosomal anomaly may predict either a recurrence risk less than 1% (as when a trisomy is demonstrated) or a much higher risk if there is a translocation in one of the parents.

In the absence of a chromosomal abnormality, the reported empirical risk for recurrence ranges from 6% to 14%,[79,80] although some families have a 25% risk associated with autosomal recessive inheritance. Rarely, autosomal dominant inheritance is present, predicting a 50% recurrence rate. A close examination of both parents for minor signs of midline facial abnormalities (e.g., hypotelorism) is essential to rule out this possibility. Maternal diabetes should also be excluded because it significantly increases the risk of holoprosencephaly.[81]

SUMMARY OF MANAGEMENT OPTIONS

Disorders of Ventral Induction: The Holoprosencephaly Sequence

Management Options	Evidence Quality and Recommendation	References
Prenatal		
Scan and MRI are used to clarify the extent of abnormalities.	III/B	90,107
Offer karyotyping	III/B	78
Provide counseling.	III/B	78
Multidisciplinary approach.	—/GPP	—
Offer pregnancy termination where appropriate or induction of labor.	—/GPP	—
Labor and Delivery		
Aim for vaginal delivery; cephalocentesis is ethically justified in cases of severe macrocephaly to avoid cesarean section, but warn parents that this is a destructive procedure.	III/B	73
Postnatal		
Offer postmortem for abortus/stillbirth/neonatal death.	—/GPP	—
Offer karyotyping if not already done.	III/B	78
Check family history.	—/GPP	—
Screen for diabetes.	III/B	81
Provide counseling.	—/GPP	—

GPP, good practice point; MRI, magnetic resonance imaging.

FACIAL CLEFTS

General

Cleft lip or palate is the most common congenital facial deformity.[82] It results from failure of the nasofrontal prominence to fuse with the maxillary process. Clefts may be complete, incomplete, unilateral or bilateral, or symmetrical or asymmetrical. Although more than 100 syndromes are associated with cleft lip or palate, these syndromes probably account for fewer than 10% of cases, because the majority are isolated. A multifactorial etiology is reflected in the varied incidences depending on race, sex, and geographic location. Similar to other lesions with a multifactorial etiology, the empirical recurrence risk increases with the number of previously affected siblings.

Diagnosis

The lower portion of the face must be anterior and clearly visualized in order to demonstrate a facial cleft on antenatal ultrasound (Fig. 17–16). The coronal, sagittal, and transverse planes are used to assess the features of the lower face. Facial clefts may be suspected when either undulating tongue movements, hypertrophied tissue at the edge of the cleft, or hypertelorism is seen on ultrasound. An intact lip does not mean the palate is intact. Transverse sections may reveal a break in the maxillary ridge. Caution is necessary to avoid a false-positive diagnosis from a shadowing artifact produced by the maxillary bones. The availability of 3D ultrasound may facilitate visualization of the precise location and extent of facial clefting.[83,84]

Management Options

It is important to search carefully for other anomalies after a facial cleft is identified. Fetal karyotyping should be offered. The prognosis and management depend on the presence of associated abnormalities and the severity of the defect. If the cleft appears isolated, then the prognosis is excellent. Staged plastic surgical correction is typically offered early in infancy, though the timing of the repairs remains controversial. Prior to surgery, the newborn may experience some difficulty feeding, but this is usually remedied with a specially designed artificial palate. Antenatal diagnosis of a cleft may help the parents prepare for a visually disturbing deformity that is typically correctable and allows the birth to occur with a treatment plan in place.

DANDY-WALKER MALFORMATION

General

The Dandy-Walker malformation is characterized by the complete or partial absence of the cerebellar vermis and an enlarged posterior fossa cyst continuous with the fourth ventricle (Fig. 17–17). Hydrocephalus with ventriculomegaly is often present. Theories on pathogenesis include atresia

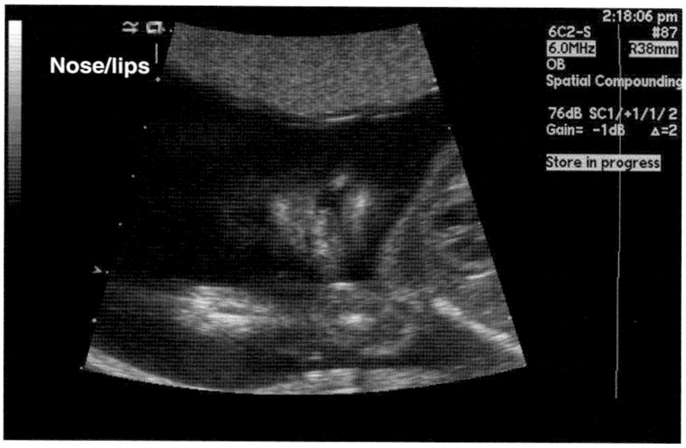

FIGURE 17–16
Coronal section through the lower face demonstrates a unilateral cleft lip.

SUMMARY OF MANAGEMENT OPTIONS

Facial Clefts

Management Options	Evidence Quality and Recommendation	References
Prenatal		
Carefully search for other anomalies.	—/GPP	—
Offer karyotyping.	—/GPP	—
Prognosis depends on cause and severity (good if isolated).	—/GPP	—
Provide counseling with multidisciplinary approach.	—/GPP	—
Postnatal		
Provide counseling.	—/GPP	—
Special measures are needed for infant feeding.	—/GPP	—
Early pediatric surgery is indicated.	—/GPP	—

GPP, good practice point.

of the foramina of Lushka and Magendie and hypoplasia or gross alteration of the cerebellum. In addition to the classic Dandy-Walker malformation, a Dandy-Walker variant indicates a spectrum of anomalies classified by variable hypoplasia of the cerebellar vermis with or without enlargement of the posterior fossa. The Dandy-Walker malformation occurs in approximately 1 in 30,000 births and is diagnosed in 4% to 12% of all cases of infantile hydrocephalus.[85] There is an increased risk of chromosomal anomalies and mendelian syndromes.

Diagnosis

Dandy-Walker cyst appears on ultrasound as an echolucent area in the posterior fossa. The cerebellar vermis, a bright echogenic midline structure caudal to the fourth ventricle, is absent or defective. As a result, the Dandy-Walker cyst is seen communicating with the fourth ventricle. Hydrocephalus usually involves all four ventricles.

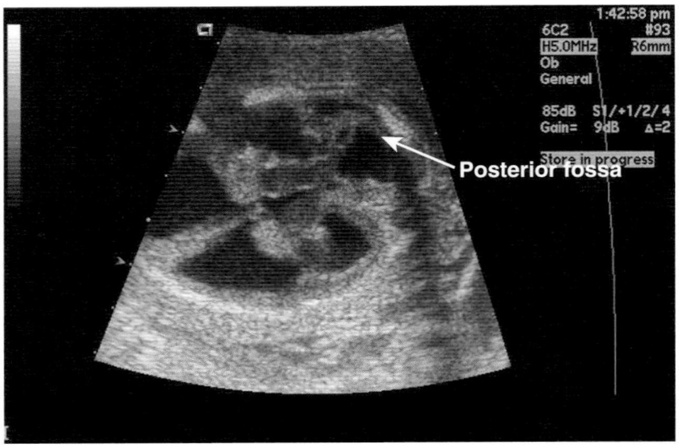

FIGURE 17–17
Dandy-Walker cyst. Transverse view of fetal head demonstrates a Dandy-Walker cyst with a defect in the cerebellar vermis. In addition, the lateral and third ventricles are dilated.

Management Options

The prognosis for infants with a Dandy-Walker malformation is quite variable. A review of 50 cases of Dandy-Walker malformation and 49 cases of Dandy-Walker variant diagnosed by antenatal ultrasound[86] noted a frequent occurrence of associated anomalies and aneploidy. Of fetuses with a classic Dandy-Walker malformation, 85% had other anomalies (32% ventriculomegaly and 38% cardiac defects) and 46% were aneuploid. Of the fetuses with Dandy-Walker variant, 85% had other anomalies (27% ventriculomegaly and 41% cardiac defects) with a 36% aneuploidy rate. Fifty of the 99 women elected pregnancy termination. Of the remaining 49 fetuses, 16 survived the neonatal period with only 8 having a normal pediatric examination at 6 weeks, including 6 with an isolated finding of Dandy-Walker variant. The overall prognosis is therefore poor and the presence of other anomalies is associated with the worst prognosis.

Hydrocephalus and associated anomalies are more common in cases diagnosed in utero and the prognosis is less favorable. The option of pregnancy termination should be discussed with the parents. There is an increased risk of chromosomal anomalies and mendelian syndromes. The Dandy-Walker malformation occurs with increased frequency in families with a history of polycystic kidney disease and after the birth of a child with Dandy-Walker malformation or another CNS abnormality. Autosomal recessive inheritance is documented in some families. In the absence of a clear genetic syndrome, the recurrence risk is between 1% and 5%.[87]

SUMMARY OF MANAGEMENT OPTIONS

Dandy-Walker Malformation

Management Options	Evidence Quality and Recommendation	References
Prenatal		
Careful detailed scan and MRI are needed.	III/B	87,90,107
Multidisciplinary approach includes cautious counseling; prognosis is difficult to predict and largely influenced by other abnormalities.	III/B	10–12
Genetic counseling is needed if there is a family history.	III/B	85
Offer termination where appropriate	—/GPP	—
Labor and Delivery		
Aim for vaginal delivery.	—/GPP	—
Postnatal and Neonatal		
Provide careful neonatal review and follow-up.	—/GPP	—

GPP, good practice point; MRI, magnetic resonance imaging.

ANEURYSM OF THE VEIN OF GALEN

The cerebral veins may enlarge as a direct result of arterial fistula or adjacent arteriovenous malformation. Aneurysmal dilation of the great vein of Galen from an arteriovenous malformation is well documented. The dilated vein appears on ultrasound as a nonpulsatile, midcerebral tubular structure often seen behind the third ventricle.[88,89] MRI and 3D ultrasonography can be useful adjuncts to definitive diagnosis antenatally.[90,91] The lesion may be isolated or associated with fetal hydrocephalus or other abnormalities. The increased intracranial blood flow to a low-resistance shunt can cause cardiomegaly and hydrops, and serial studies are indicated to monitor for the development of fetal hydrops. Traditionally, the prognosis for neonates with an aneurysm of the vein of Galen was considered poor, because many die from heart failure.[92] However, therapeutic advances may be improving outcome. In one study of 18 cases of antenatally diagnosed vein of Galen aneurysm, the neonatal mortality rate was 25% despite evidence of cardiac deterioration in 94%. All survivors required digoxin therapy. Neurologic development was normal in 67% of the surviving neonates.[93]

HYDRANENCEPHALY

General

Hydranencephaly is characterized by replacement of the cerebral hemispheres with fluid covered by leptomeninges such that no cerebral cortex is present. Only the basal ganglia and remnants of the mesencephalon remain within a normally formed skull above the tentorium cerebelli. The subtentorial structures are usually intact, and the falx cerebri is frequently present. Hydranencephaly is thought to result from a severe destructive insult, most likely bilateral occlusion of the internal carotid arteries.

Diagnosis

Ultrasonographic findings include a normal cranial vault filled with fluid. The cerebral cortex is absent, but a midline echo, the tentorium cerebelli, and cerebellum may be visible. This disorder is differentiated from hydrocephalus, holoprosencephaly, and porencephaly by the absence of cerebral cortex. In severe hydrocephalus, the thin cortical mantle may be hard to detect ultrasonographically and MRI or, less frequently, intrauterine computed tomography scanning may aid diagnosis (Fig. 17–18).

Management Options

Most infants with hydranencephaly die in the first year of life. Survivors are profoundly retarded. Sporadic familial recurrences are reported, but these are the exception. In general, the recurrence risk is negligible. The option for pregnancy termination should be offered to the parents.

SUMMARY OF MANAGEMENT OPTIONS

Aneurysm of the Vein of Galen

Management Options	Evidence Quality and Recommendation	References
Prenatal		
Color-flow Doppler is used to differentiate from hydrocephalus and porencephalic cyst.	III/B	90
Three-dimensional ultrasound and MRI help to elucidate the extent of the lesion.	III/B	90,106,107
Multidisciplinary counseling	—/GPP	—
Prognosis is difficult to predict but is no longer uniformly poor.	III/B	93
Maintain vigilance for the development of hydrops, hydrocephalus, or other abnormalities.	—/GPP	—
Labor and Delivery		
No data guide the mode of delivery; many avoid vaginal delivery empirically to avoid cerebral (and hence aneurysm) trauma.	—/GPP	—
Delivery should take place in a tertiary center with appropriate facilities.	—/GPP	—
Postnatal and Neonatal		
Main significant therapeutic advance is in the use of embolization for occluding the aneurysm.	III/B	93

GPP, good practice point; MRI, magnetic resonance imaging.

FIGURE 17–18
Hydranencepahly. In utero computed tomogram shows widening of the sutures of the fetal calvarium. Skull is filled by homogeneous low-density fluid with no evidence of cortex present. MP, maternal pelvis; SS separated suture.
(From Chervanak FA, Berkowitz RL, Romero R, et al: The diagnosis of fetal hydrocephalus. Am J Obstet Gynecol 1983;147:703–716.)

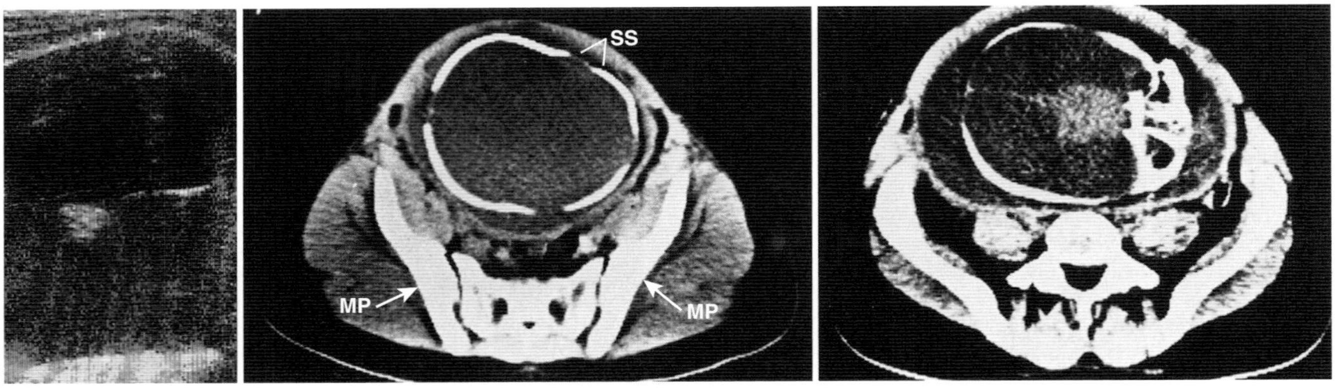

SUMMARY OF MANAGEMENT OPTIONS
Hydranencephaly

Management Options	Evidence Quality and Recommendation	References
Prenatal		
Offer karyotyping.	—/GPP	—
Counsel parents about poor prognosis.	—/GPP	—
Offer termination or induction of labor.	—/GPP	—

GPP, good practice point.

MICROCEPHALY

General

Strictly translated, *microcephaly* means "small head." The clinical importance of the entity is its association with mental retardation. Some authors classify postnatal microcephaly as a head perimeter smaller than 2 standard deviations (SDs) below the mean.[94] Alternatively, a definition of 3 SD below the mean for gender and age may correlate better with mental retardation.[95]

Diagnosis

The postnatal diagnosis of microcephaly is made simply by measuring the neonatal head circumference, but the antenatal diagnosis is more difficult. The head circumference is preferable to the biparietal diameter, which carries a high false-positive rate because of such normal variants as dolichocephaly. Serial ultrasound examinations are important in suspected cases because significant microcephaly may not manifest until the third trimester.

Management Options

Prenatal

Because microcephaly is a part of many different malformation syndromes, a careful search for associated anomalies is mandatory. Cortical mass may be decreased in microcephaly, leading to ventriculomegaly in the absence of an obstructive process. A careful pedigree should be taken and a search made for causes, including possible teratogen exposure, alcohol abuse, and infection. The definitive diagnosis of fetal infection requires an invasive procedure; amniocentesis and even fetal blood sampling are often necessary.

The majority of microcephalic children are mentally retarded, many severely so. As a rule, the smaller the head, the worse the prognosis. If microcephaly occurs as part of a genetic syndrome (e.g., Meckel-Gruber syndrome), the outcome is uniformly poor. However, children born with microcephaly may have normal intelligence despite their very small head size.

SUMMARY OF MANAGEMENT OPTIONS

Microcephaly

Management Options	Evidence Quality and Recommendation	References
Prenatal		
Perform a careful ultrasound search for other anomalies.	—/GPP	—
Use MRI to elucidate the extent of cortical loss.	III/B	90,107
Offer karyotyping and workup for congenital infection.	—/GPP	—
Look for history of teratogens, alcohol use, family history, infection.	—/GPP	—
Exercise caution with counseling because prognosis is difficult to predict.	—/GPP	—
Labor and Delivery		
Aim for vaginal delivery; shoulder dystocia is very rare.	—/GPP	—
Postnatal and Prepregnancy		
Establish cause if not already done (teratogens, alcohol use, family history, karyotype, infection serology, necropsy).	—/GPP	—
Counsel depending on cause.	—/GPP	—

GPP, good practice point; MRI, magnetic resonance imaging.

Labor and Delivery

Vaginal delivery of a microcephalic infant is appropriate. Shoulder dystocia due to incomplete dilation of the cervix by the small fetal head is a rare occurrence.

Postnatal and Prepregnancy

The risk of recurrence for microcephaly depends on the underlying etiology. The search for an etiology should include a physical examination of the infant; a maternal history for teratogenic exposure; a careful family pedigree; chromosomal, microbiologic, and serologic studies; and an autopsy should death occur. Alcohol abuse is a common cause of mental retardation and often associated with microcephaly. Several patterns of inheritance are described within the subgroup of microcephaly without associated anomalies, which is termed "true" microcephaly. These patterns include autosomal recessive, autosomal dominant with incomplete penetrance, and sporadic patterns of inheritance.

AGENESIS OF THE CORPUS CALLOSUM

General

The corpus callosum is the great commissural plate of nerve fibers interconnecting the cortical hemispheres. It lies at the base of the interhemispheric fissure and curves in the midline, forming the roof of the third ventricle. Agenesis of the corpus callosum can occur either as an isolated anomaly or in association with other anomalies, such as hydrocephalus and holoprosencephaly. It is usually a sporadic occurrence, although it has been associated with various genetic syndromes, chromosomal abnormalities, and prenatal exposure to teratogens such as alcohol.

Diagnosis

Agenesis of the corpus callosum is diagnosed in utero on coronal and midline sagittal views of the fetal head, including the routine transverse planes. Transvaginal ultrasonography improves access to these planes by providing an acoustic window through the anterior fontanelle.

On a midsagittal ultrasound examination, the corpus callosum appears as a hypoechoic structure below the pericallosal artery, where it forms the roof of the cavum septum pellucidum and cavum vergae (Fig. 17–19). Failure to image it suggests agenesis of the corpus callosum. However, it is quite difficult antenatally to be definitive. The pathognomonic "sunburst lesion" is seen on midsagittal section and represents the radial orientation of the gyri and sulci of the cerebral cortex to the third ventricle (Fig. 17–20). Normally, the gyri and sulci parallel the corpus callosum.[96] Because the corpus callosum itself cannot be seen on transverse scan, it is necessary to search for the anatomic alterations produced by its absence. These indications include lateral displacement of the bodies of the lateral ventricles, enlargement of the atria and occipital horns producing a characteristic teardrop shape, and enlargement or upward displacement of the third ventricle (Fig. 17–21).

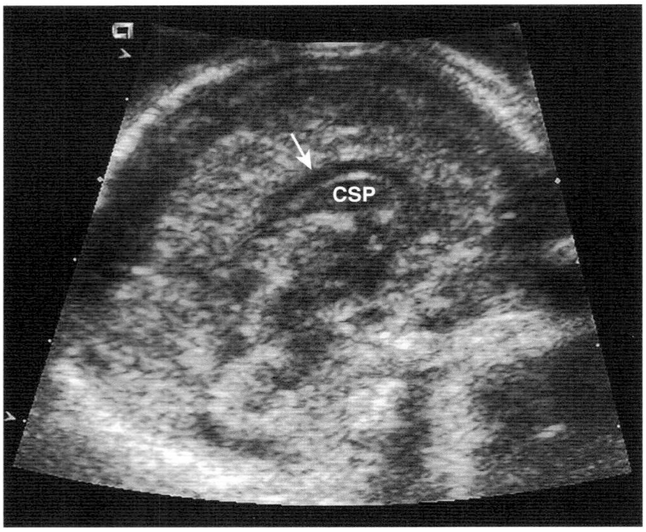

FIGURE 17–19
Corpus callosum. Midsagittal section through normal fetal cranium demonstrates the corpus callosum (*arrow*), the hypoechoic structure superior to the cavum septum pellucidum (CSP).

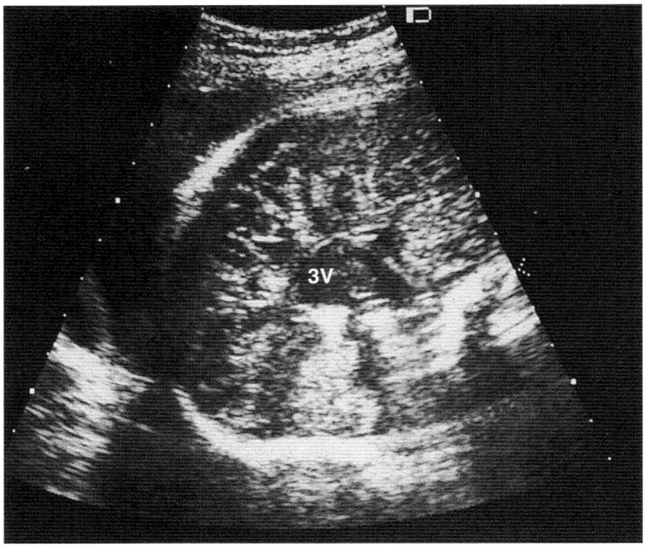

FIGURE 17–20
Agenesis of the corpus callosum. Midsagittal view of the fetal head with agenesis of the corpus callosum demonstrates the pathognomonic "sunburst lesion" representing the radial orientation of the gyri and sulci of the cerebral cortex to the third ventricle (3V).

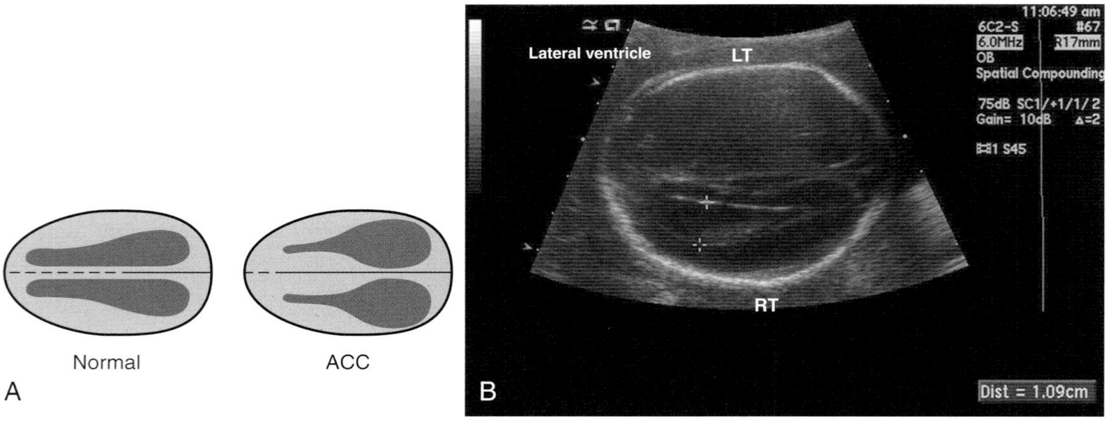

FIGURE 17–21
Agenesis of the corpus callosum. *A*, Schematic representation of agenesis of the corpus callosum in the coronal view. *B*, Transverse section of a fetus with agenesis of the corpus callosum. Note the teardrop shape of the lateral ventricle, with dilation of the posterior portion of the lateral ventricle.

Management Options

The prognosis for a fetus with agenesis of the corpus callosum is highly variable and depends on the presence of associated defects. Management is based on these underlying anomalies. Agenesis of the corpus callosum has been reported as an incidental autopsy finding in intellectually normal adults,[97] and caution should be exercised in counseling patients when isolated agenesis of the corpus callosum is suspected. 3D ultrasonography and MRI may provide additional prognostic information.

INTRACRANIAL HEMORRHAGE AND PORENCEPHALY

General

Intraventricular hemorrhage is well recognized in the newborn and often associated with prematurity. Neonatal intracranial hemorrhage is classified into grade 1 when there is isolated periventricular hemorrhage, grade 2 when there is intraventricular hemorrhage with normal ventricular size, grade 3 when intraventricular hemorrhage is associated with

SUMMARY OF MANAGEMENT OPTIONS

Agenesis of the Corpus Callosum

Management Options	Evidence Quality and Recommendation	References
Prenatal		
Perform a careful search for other anomalies.	—/GPP	—
MRI may be helpful in further evaluation.	III/B	90,103
Counsel depending on other lesions; prognosis for isolated condition is difficult to predict.	—/GPP	—
Offer termination where appropriate.	—/GPP	—

GPP, good practice point.

acute ventricular dilation, and grade 4 when there is intraventricular hemorrhage with parenchymal involvement.[98] When severe, it can produce obstructive hydrocephalus and intraparenchymal hemorrhage. Conversely, the antenatal diagnosis of intracranial hemorrhage is uncommon. In most instances, hydrocephalus is first identified in association with echogenic areas of hemorrhage in the dilated ventricular system.

Porencephaly describes a condition in which a portion of the cerebral cortex is replaced by a cystic cavity and is thought to represent the remains of a severe intrauterine insult. The cavity may communicate with the subarachnoid space or a ventricle. Most cases result from a vascular lesion, either hemorrhagic or embolic. Areas of prior hemorrhage or tissue necrosis resorb, leaving behind porencephalic cysts. In rare cases, an infection or traumatic insult might result in porencephaly.

Diagnosis

Antenatal hemorrhage typically appears as an echogenic mass in the region of the germinal matrix or within the lateral ventricles. MRI of the fetal brain can often assist in making the diagnosis of a brain hemorrhage (Fig. 17–22). Antenatally diagnosed intracranial hemorrhage is predominantly grade 3 or 4. Consequently, these lesions are associated with a high perinatal mortality rate. These cases demonstrate that high-grade intraventricular hemorrhage can occur in the absence of birth trauma.

Porencephalic cysts appear ultrasonographically as solitary or multiple echolucent areas of variable size and location within the brain. The midline echo is present but may be displaced. Some cortical tissue may be preserved in each cerebral hemisphere. These distinctions help differentiate a large porencephalic cyst from unilateral hydrocephalus, holoprosencephaly, and hydranencephaly.

Although the prognostic validity of the grading system for neonatal intracranial hemorrhage is well established, it has not been extensively evaluated in the antenatal period. Ghi and colleagues[99] followed 109 cases of antenatally diagnosed intracranial hemorrhage and concluded that intracranial hemorrhage could be accurately identified and categorized by antenatal sonography.

Management Options

When antenatal intracranial hemorrhage is diagnosed in the absence of an identifiable cause, a search for alloimmune thrombocytopenia is warranted. Serologic studies for intrauterine infection, a fetal karyotype, and screening for maternal infections, including hepatitis and pancreatitis, might also be of value.

The prognosis for porencephaly depends on the underlying etiology, location, and volume of tissue loss. The outcome in the majority of reported cases is poor.[100] Fortunately, there is no increased risk of recurrence unless alloimmune thrombocytopenia is diagnosed. Alloimmune thrombocytopenia carries a greater than 75% recurrence risk.[101]

CHOROID PLEXUS CYST

General

Small areas of cystic dilation are seen in the choroid plexus of the lateral ventricles in 1% to 2% of all fetuses (Fig. 17–23). They typically resolve before the end of the second trimester and lack clinical significance. Choroid plexus cysts may be associated with trisomy 18. However, the great majority of fetuses with trisomy 18 have other structural abnormalities detectable by ultrasonography.

Management Options

A karyotype is recommended for all fetuses with choroid plexus cysts associated with other structural abnormalities. However, the vast majority of isolated choroid plexus cysts are clinically insignificant, and the need for karyotyping is controversial. A meta-analysis reported that the risk of trisomy 18 associated with an isolated choroid plexus cyst in all women was 1 : 374.[102] Another large study concluded that an isolated choroid plexus cyst increased the

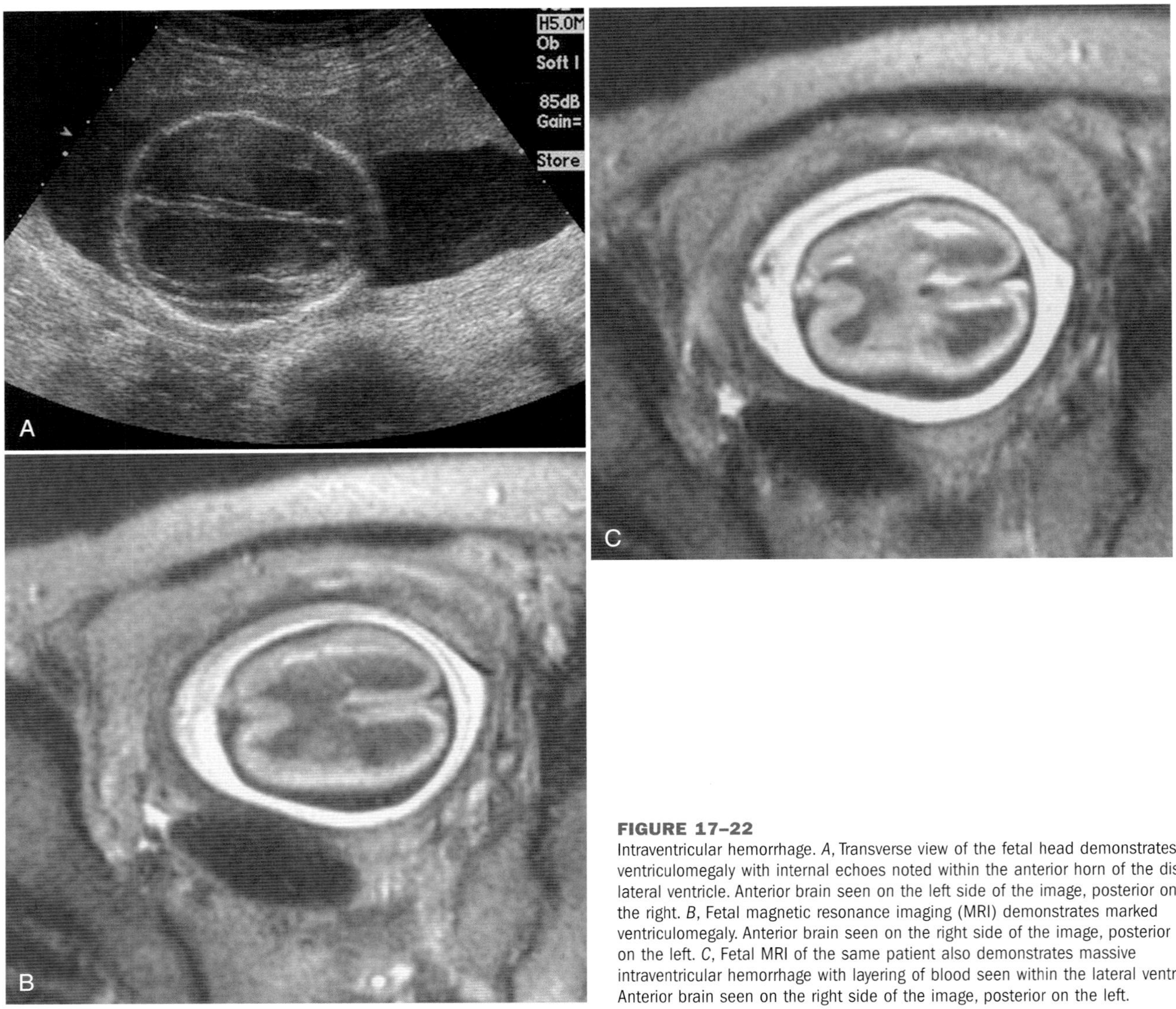

FIGURE 17–22
Intraventricular hemorrhage. *A*, Transverse view of the fetal head demonstrates ventriculomegaly with internal echoes noted within the anterior horn of the distal lateral ventricle. Anterior brain seen on the left side of the image, posterior on the right. *B*, Fetal magnetic resonance imaging (MRI) demonstrates marked ventriculomegaly. Anterior brain seen on the right side of the image, posterior on the left. *C*, Fetal MRI of the same patient also demonstrates massive intraventricular hemorrhage with layering of blood seen within the lateral ventricle. Anterior brain seen on the right side of the image, posterior on the left.

SUMMARY OF MANAGEMENT OPTIONS

Choroid Plexus Cyst

Management Options	Evidence Quality and Recommendation	References
Prenatal		
Perform a careful search for other structural abnormalities.	IIa/B	102
Offer karyotyping if other anomalies found.	IIa/B	102
With isolated cyst, risk of amniocentesis likely exceeds risk of aneuploidy in an otherwise low risk woman.	III/B	103–105
Benign if isolated with normal chromosomes.	IIa/B	103–105

FIGURE 17–23
Choroid plexus cyst. Transverse section demonstrates a choroid plexus cyst in the proximal lateral ventricle.

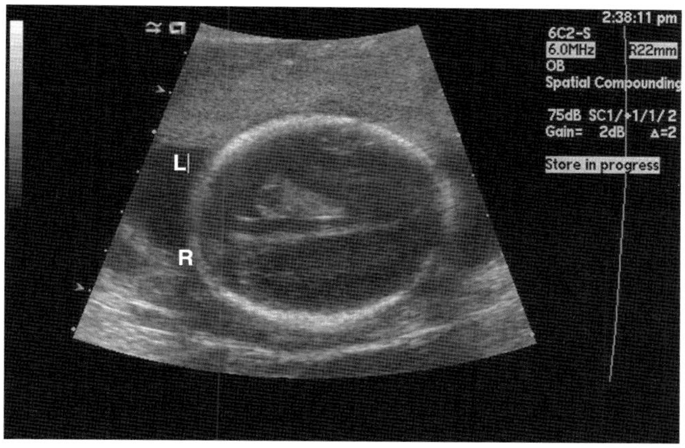

mid-trimester risk of trisomy 18 enough to justify karyotyping only in women older than 35 years.[103] Other large studies have concluded that isolated choroid plexus cysts in women younger than 35 years do not increase the risk of trisomy 18 to a degree that amniocentesis is warranted.[104,105] We believe the presence of a choroid plexus cyst should be disclosed to the patient. However, counseling should take into account the presence of associated anomalies, the age of the patient, and the results of first- and second-trimester screening tests for aneuploidy.

CAUDAL REGRESSION SYNDROME

Caudal regression syndrome describes an embryologic malformation leading to structural defects in the caudal region. The severity is quite variable and may include incomplete development of the sacrum and lumbar vertebrae and disruption of the distal spinal cord, causing neurologic impairment. Caudal regression syndrome is strongly associated with maternal diabetes. Although this disorder was previously considered a severe form of sirenomelia, some evidence suggests the two defects are pathogenetically unrelated.[73] The etiology of caudal regression syndrome is unknown and most likely heterogeneous.

MAGNETIC RESONANCE IMAGING OF FETAL CENTRAL NERVOUS SYSTEM ANOMALIES

Ultrasonography is currently the primary imaging technique used for antenatal evaluation of fetal CNS anomalies. The ability to make a definitive diagnosis by ultrasound alone

SUMMARY OF MANAGEMENT OPTIONS
Intracranial Hemorrhage and Porencephaly

Management Options	Evidence Quality and Recommendation	References
Prenatal		
These anomalies may be associated with severe maternal illness.	—/GPP	—
In absence of identifiable cause, workup for alloimmune thrombocytopenia and congenital infection; offer karyotyping.	—/GPP	—
Prognosis is related to location and degree of tissue loss and is usually poor with larger lesions.	III/B	100
Postnatal and Prepregnancy		
Recurrence risk is relevant only for alloimmune thrombocytopenia.	III/B	101

GPP, good practice point.

SUMMARY OF MANAGEMENT OPTIONS
Caudal Regression Syndrome

Management Options	Evidence Quality and Recommendation	References
Prenatal		
Determine degree of malformation.	—/GPP	—
Offer termination where appropriate	—/GPP	—
Screen for diabetes.	—/GPP	—
Provide multidisciplinary counseling.	—/GPP	—
Postnatal		
Screen for diabetes.	—/GPP	—
Provide counseling.	—/GPP	—

GPP, good practice point.

might be restricted by various factors, including reverberative artifacts from the bony calvarium, fetal position, oligohydramnios, and maternal body habitus. Although transvaginal sonography can sometimes complement or enhance the transabdominal examination,[106] ultrasound often does not have the sensitivity to detect subtle abnormalities of fetal brain development.

MRI can enhance the diagnostic accuracy of ultrasound for the assessment of fetal brain abnormalities (Figs. 17–24 and 17–25).[107,108] MRI permits acquisition of multiplanar views of the fetal brain, allowing for a detailed evaluation of the CNS anatomy that is not possible using ultrasound alone. In addition, MRI is not hindered by the same technical limitations as ultrasound, such as reduced amniotic fluid or fetal position. The use of ultrafast MRI techniques permits good quality brain images, even when there is fetal movement.[109,110] To date, there have been no reports of adverse fetal effects from MRI. Baker and colleagues[111] evaluated children 3 years after prenatal MRI exposure and reported no deleterious effects. The information obtained from MRI may change management by enhancing the diagnostic accuracy. Sharma and colleagues[112] described a series of pregnant patients with fetal brain abnormalities in whom MRI provided valuable additional information in all cases. MRI of the fetal CNS is evolving as a useful adjunct for obtaining additional information in cases in which confirmation of a suspected abnormality or further clarification is sought.

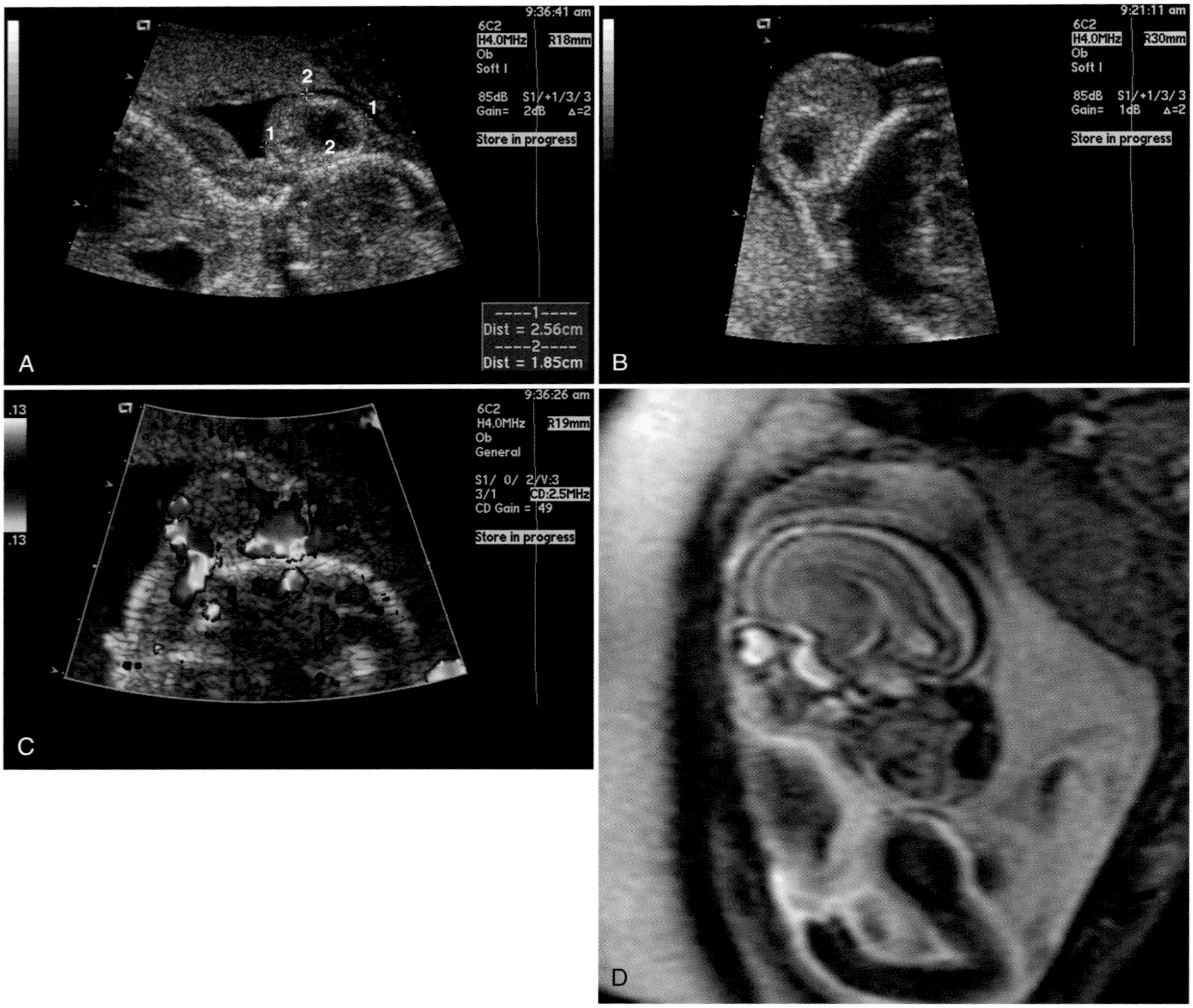

FIGURE 17–24
Hemangioma. *A*, Sagittal view of the fetal head and neck demonstrates a subcutaneous mass. *B*, Transverse view of the fetal head through the occipital bone shows a posterior echogenic mass with a cystic component. The occipital bone appears intact. *C*, Color-flow Doppler demonstrates increased vascularity within the mass. *D*, Subcutaneous midline mass adjacent to the posterior fossa of the brain noted on fetal MRI was diagnosed in the neonate as a hemangioma.

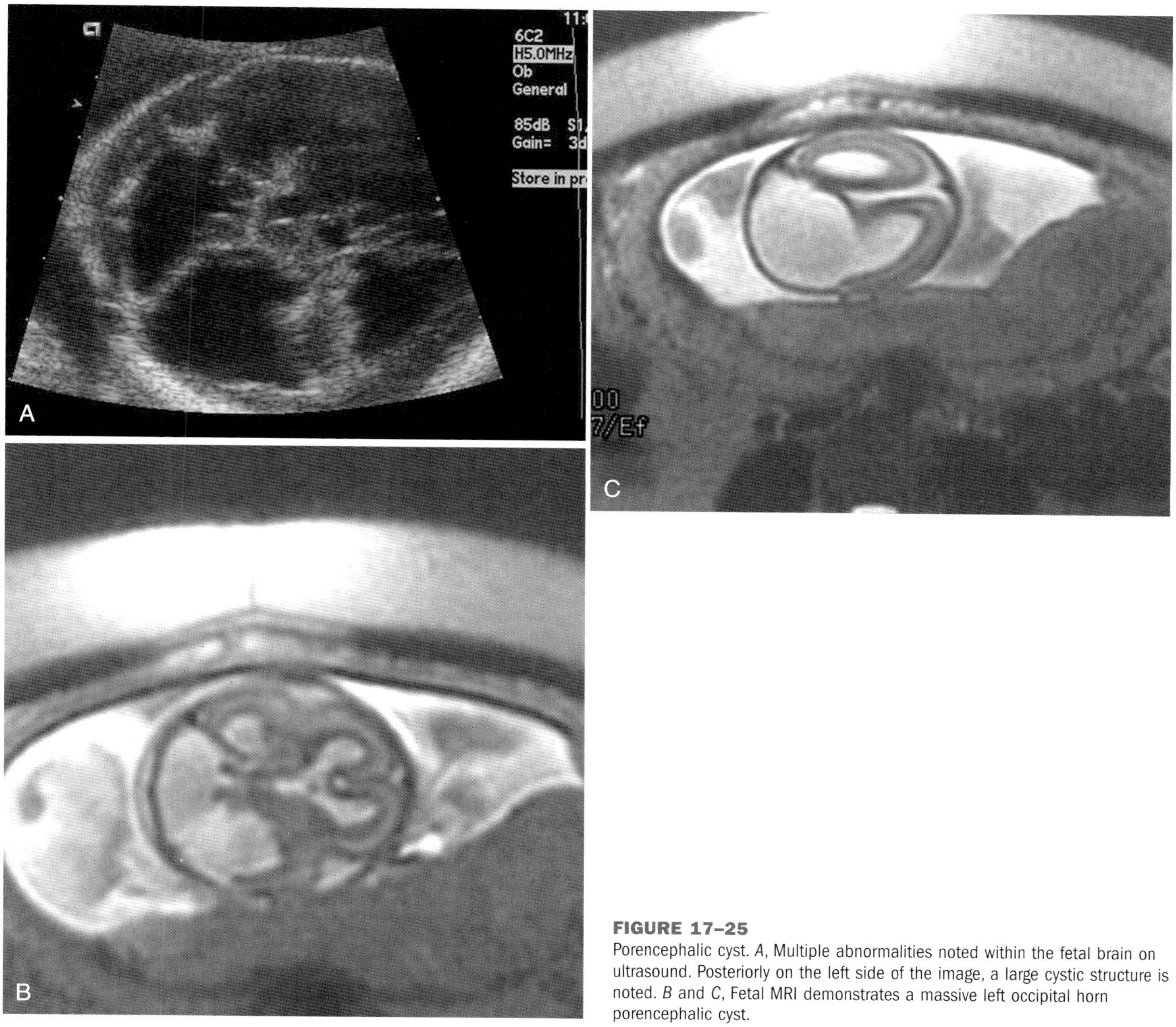

FIGURE 17–25
Porencephalic cyst. *A*, Multiple abnormalities noted within the fetal brain on ultrasound. Posteriorly on the left side of the image, a large cystic structure is noted. *B* and *C*, Fetal MRI demonstrates a massive left occipital horn porencephalic cyst.

SUGGESTED READINGS

Bell WE: Abnormalities in size and shape of the head. In Shaffer AJ, Avery ME (eds): Diseases of the Newborn, 4th ed. Philadelphia, WB Saunders, 1977, pp 717–719.

Chervenak FA, Berkowitz RL, Tortora M, et al: Management of fetal hydrocephalus. Am J Obstet Gynecol 1985;151:933–942.

Chervenak FA, Duncan C, Ment LR, et al: Perinatal management of myelomeningocele. Obstet Gynecol 1984;63:376–380.

Cohen HL, Haller JO: Advances in perinatal neurosonography. AJR Am J Roentgenol 1994;163:801–810.

Ghi T, Simonazzi G, Perolo A, et al: Outcome of antenatally diagnosed intracranial hemorrhage: Case series and review of the literature. Ultrasound Obstet Gynecol 2003;22:121–130.

Gupta JK, Khan KS, Thorton JG, Lilford RJ: Management of fetal choroid plexus cysts. Br J Obstet Gynaecol 1997;104:881–886.

Osenbach RK, Menezes AH: Diagnosis and management of the Dandy-Walker malformation: 30 years of experience. Pediatr Neurosurg 1992;18:179–189.

Pistorius LR, Hellmann PM, Visser GH, et al: Fetal neuroimaging: Ultrasound, MRI, or both? Obstet Gynecol Surv 2008;63:733–745.

Rodesch G, Hui F, Alvarez H, et al: Prognosis of antenatally diagnosed vein of Galen aneurysmal malformations. Childs Nerv Syst 1994;10:79–83.

Stewart RE: Craniofacial malformations. Clinical and genetic considerations. Pediatr Clin North Am 1978;25:485–515.

REFERENCES

For a complete list of references, log onto www.expertconsult.com.

CHAPTER 18

Fetal Genitourinary Abnormalities

MARC DOMMERGUES, RODRIGO RUANO, and MARIE-CÉCILE AUBRY

Videos corresponding to this chapter are available online at www.expertconsult.com.

INTRODUCTION

Genitourinary abnormalities consist of a wide spectrum of heterogeneous malformations. Urinary tract dilations and kidney abnormalities are relatively common with a prevalence ranging from 1 in 250 to 1 in 1000 deliveries.

The majority of genitourinary abnormalities are detected during routine second-trimester screening ultrasound in the absence of any significant clinical or family history. Generally, the sensitivity of antenatal screening depends on the experience of the ultrasonographer and on the timing of the onset of detectable consequences of the abnormality.[1] The diagnosis of a lethal form may become evident with severe oligohydramnios and dilation of the urinary tract. In contrast, some abnormalities, such as urinary reflux, might remain undetectable in utero. Urinary dilation above an incomplete obstruction may occur in the third trimester, when urinary volume exceeds the obstructed capacity. These will be missed unless there is a policy of routine third-trimester ultrasound. Renal abnormalities without urinary tract dilation can be detected if examination of the fetal kidneys is included in the screening ultrasound. Fetal uropathies are rarely diagnosed in the first trimester. An intra-abdominal transonic mass suggests a dilated bladder. However, it may resolve spontaneously, and follow-up is needed to confirm the diagnosis of fetal urinary tract dilation.

In contrast to uronephrologic abnormalities, isolated genital malformations are rare disorders. There is no consensus on whether the structure of the fetal genitalia should be imaged as part of a screening ultrasound examination. Minor abnormalities are virtually impossible to identify, and counseling may be extremely difficult when ambiguous genitalia are identified.

FETAL UROPATHIES

Pathophysiology

Uropathies potentially detectable in utero may be classified according to their pathophysiology:

- Obstruction of the ureteropelvic junction: This is the most common abnormality of the fetal urinary tract. The obstruction may result from compression by an ectopic vessel or may occur in the setting of duplication or ectopy
- Megaureter: True megaureter is the result of ureterovesical junction dysfunction. Megaureter associated with mild hydronephrosis often spontaneously resolves during the first years of life, whereas major hydronephrosis or a retrovesical ureteral diameter greater than 1 cm tends to resolve slowly and might require surgery.[2,3]
- Ureterocele: Cystic dilation of the distal intravesical ureter usually arises from an abnormal location of the ureteral meatus in the bladder. Ureterocele is often associated with double ureter, in which the ureterocele at the lower ureteric orifice drains the upper pole of a duplicated kidney. The lesion is associated with obstruction, accounting for the dilation of the corresponding ureter and renal pelvis. A large ureterocele can even obstruct the bladder neck with features resembling an infravesical obstruction. Antenatal diagnosis is important to plan postnatal management and to avoid future complications.[4]
- Bladder outlet obstruction: This obstruction usually occurs in the urethra, causing bladder dilation with muscle hypertrophy and hydronephrosis. The kidneys may be dysplastic, resulting in a variable degree of renal failure.[5] The most common cause of bladder outlet obstruction is posterior urethral valves. Urethral atresia is less common, causing lethal lesions with fetal anuria in the early second trimester. In spite of advances in antenatal care, posterior urethral valves may still result in postnatal renal failure.[6]
- Reflux: This common disorder is often suspected antenatally but is rarely diagnosed definitively. Occasionally, it may be diagnosed based on dynamic dilation of the upper urinary tract or dynamic imaging of reflux. In severe cases, the bladder and ureters appear dilated owing to a functional increase in urinary outflow. Antenatal diagnosis permits the initiation of prophylactic antibiotic therapy to avoid postnatal urinary infection and subsequent kidney damage. Postnatal surgery may be required for severe forms.[7]
- Prune-belly sequence: This abnormality consists of deficient abdominal wall musculature, bladder distention with renal dysplasia, absence or hypoplasia of the prostate, and cryptorchidism.[8] A patent urachus is common. The uropathy usually consists of urethral obstruction and dysfunction resulting in megacystis and bilateral megaureter. It is rare in females in whom the uropathy and the abdominal wall defect are associated with vaginal atresia, rectovaginal or rectovesical fistula, and bicornuate uterus. The prognosis depends on the amount of functional renal tissue.

FIGURE 18–1
Normal urinary tract at 12 weeks. *A*, Kidneys (frontal view). *B*, Bladder (sagittal view).

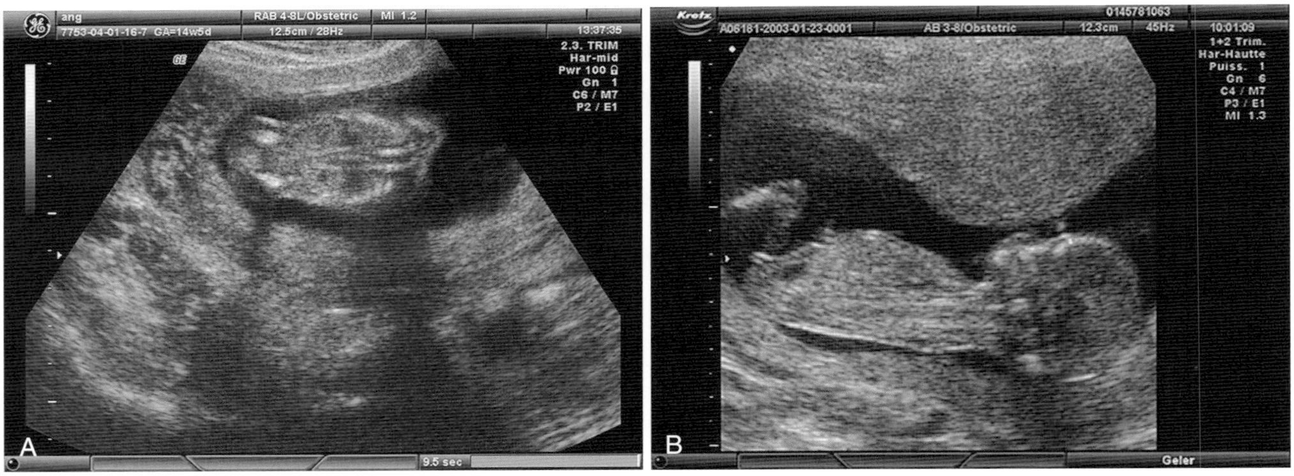

Sonographic Assessment of Normal Development of the Fetal Kidneys, Urinary Tract, and Genitalia

The fetal bladder and kidneys are identifiable by 11 to 12 weeks' gestation (Fig. 18–1) when the kidneys appear as homogeneous echoes on each side of the spine. Between 18 and 24 weeks' gestation, the medulla becomes hypoechogenic and is distinguishable from the echogenic renal cortex (Fig. 18–2). The growth of fetal kidneys parallels the fetus and can be evaluated in a quantitative manner.[9–11]

The image of the genital tubercle should be interpreted carefully during the first trimester,[12,13] although it is possible to identify fetal gender at 12 to 14 weeks in 70% to 90% of cases.[14] In boys, the urethral canal can be seen at 26 to 27 weeks, but it is easier to see in the third trimester (Fig. 18–3). Undescended testes are physiologic until 32 weeks but should be intrascrotal near term. In girls, vulval structures can be identified as early as 15 weeks and seen clearly by 22 weeks. However, a detailed analysis of a vulva anomaly is not usually feasible until 24 weeks (Fig. 18–4). In the third trimester, the external genitalia are large and easier to visualize.

It is not always possible to identify the uterus, even late in gestation. However, using three-dimensional (3D) ultrasound techniques, the uterus can be identified in 50% to 80% of cases depending on the gestational age.[15,16] The fetal sacrum is an indirect but useful marker of the harmonious development of the fetal pelvis. It curves inward progressively during the second trimester (Fig. 18–5). The anal sphincter can also be seen (Fig. 18–6).

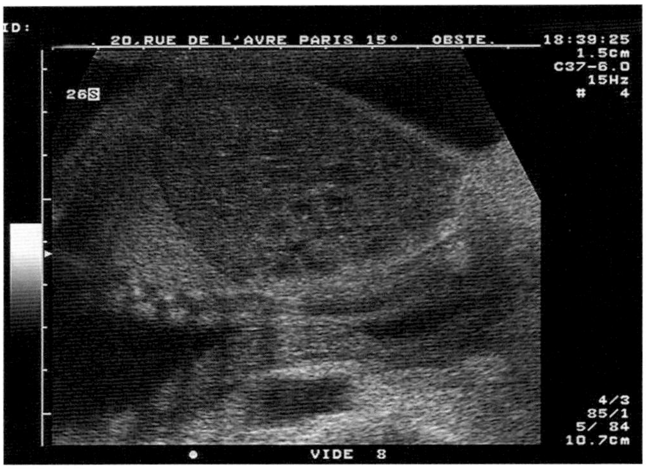

FIGURE 18–2
Normal kidney at 23 weeks shows corticomedullary differentiation of the parenchyma.

Management Options—Overview

Once fetal urinary tract dilation is detected, the following issues should be addressed rapidly:

- The diagnosis should be confirmed.
- Associated abnormalities should be ruled out by an expert in fetal ultrasound.
- The risk of aneuploidy should be evaluated and weighed against the risks of amniocentesis.
- The risk of postnatal respiratory distress (due to severe oligohydramnios leading to pulmonary hypoplasia) should be evaluated.
- The risk of developing postnatal renal failure should be evaluated.
- A perinatal management plan should be established in collaboration with a pediatric urologist/nephrologist. The potential need for emergency neonatal surgery should be evaluated in order to plan the site of delivery.

FIGURE 18–3
Normal male external genitalia at 33 weeks. *A*, Two-dimensional view (note the urethral canal). *B*, Three-dimensional view.

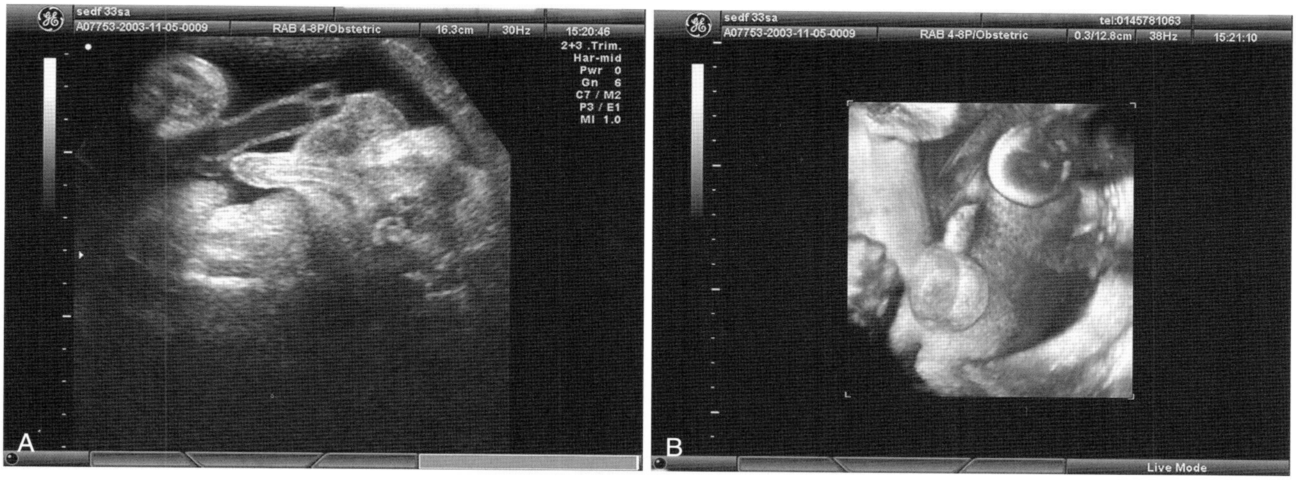

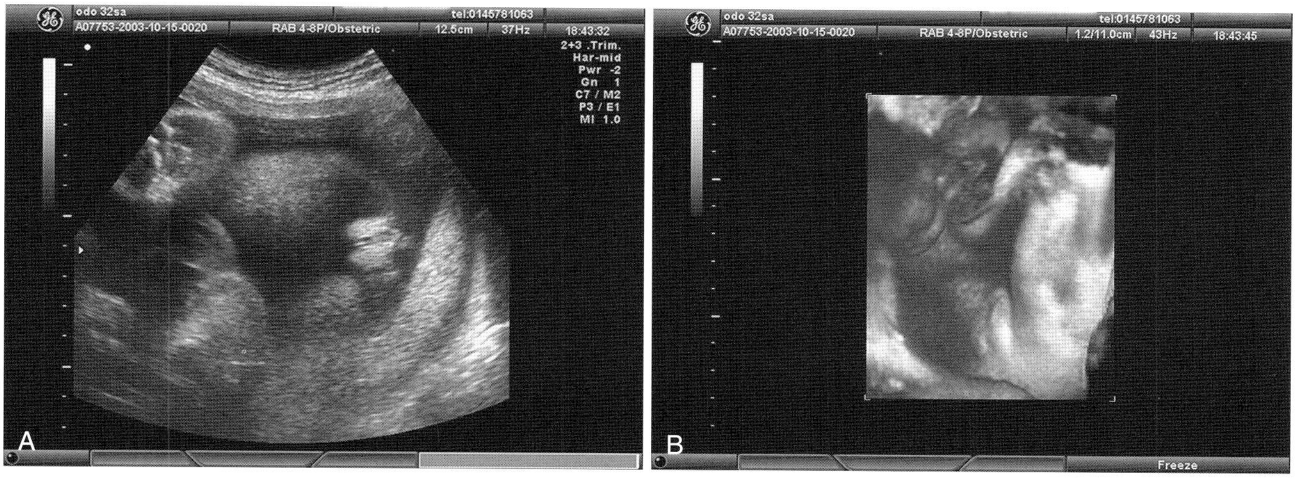

FIGURE 18–4
Normal female external genitalia at 32 weeks. *A*, Two-dimensional view. *B*, Three-dimensional view.

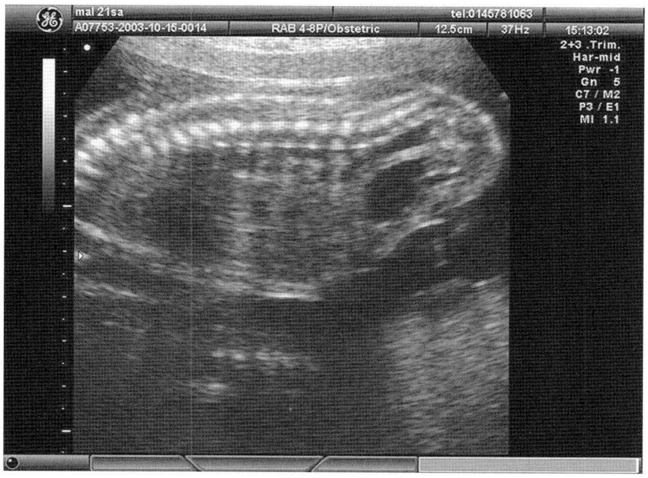

FIGURE 18–5
Normal curvature of the sacrum at 21 weeks (sagittal view).

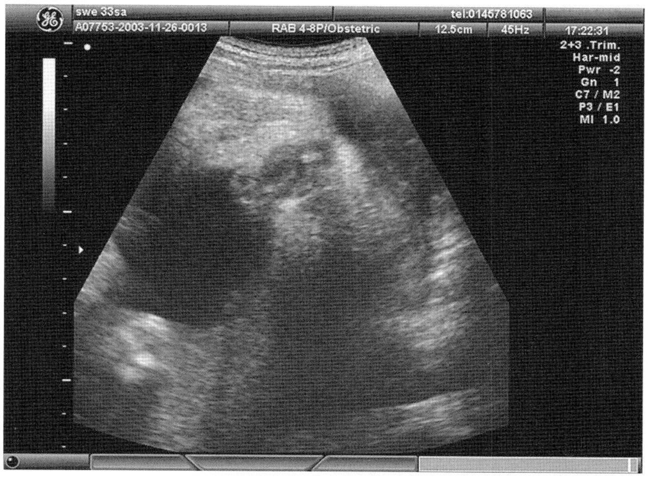

FIGURE 18–6
Normal anal margin at 30 weeks (tangential view).

Sonographic Diagnosis of Fetal Urinary Tract Abnormalities

Antenatal diagnosis of fetal urinary tract anomalies is relatively easy based on the identification of a dilated urinary tract. However, it is not always possible to ascertain the mechanism of the uropathy in utero, because the obstructive lesion cannot be imaged directly and urinary tract dilation resulting from vesicoureteral reflux may mimic the dilation of a true obstruction. Nevertheless, it is rarely important to recognize the exact cause of the dilation before birth. A satisfactory surgical repair can be achieved postnatally in most cases, resulting in a good pediatric outcome provided the renal function is not altered and there is no associated malformation.

Apparent Level of Urinary Dilation

Fetal uropathies can be classified by the level of dilation.[17–21] Only the renal pelves are dilated in upper dilations, whereas the ureters are also involved in midlevel dilations. Upper and midlevel dilations are also categorized as unilateral or bilateral, an important prognostic feature because postnatal renal function should be normal in unilateral cases. Dilation of the upper urinary tract may result from either ureteropelvic junction obstruction or ureteropelvic reflux. Midlevel dilation may be an ultrasonographic feature of vesicoureteral reflux as well as congenital megaureter. The bladder is involved in low-level dilations. Low urinary tract obstruction (LUTO) is mainly the result of posterior urethral valves. However, a dilated bladder may be a feature of major vesicoureteral reflux, which increases urine output through the bladder. More complex urinary defects, for example, cloacal malformations, may appear as a bladder dilation and, occasionally, as a midlevel dilation associated with minor abnormalities of the fetal pelvis. Complex pelvic floor malformations are the most common LUTO diagnosed antenatally in females, and posterior urethral valves are the most frequent cause of LUTO in males.

UPPER URINARY TRACT DILATION

There is no universally accepted definition and grading of fetal upper urinary tract dilation.

Pyelectasis

Pyelectasis is defined by moderate dilation of the renal pelvis without associated dilated calyces. The renal pelvis is measured in the anteroposterior (AP) plane on cross section. However, the upper size limit of a normal fetal renal pelvis remains controversial, partly because there is substantial overlap in renal pelvic size between normal fetuses and those who later prove to have reflux or obstruction. Low thresholds may stimulate unnecessary and potentially dangerous intervention whereas high threshold values will lead to false-negative conclusions.[22] Pyelectasis is variously defined as an AP pelvic diameter exceeding 4 to 7 mm in the second trimester and 8 to 10 mm in the third.[23–30] Depending on the definition, pyelectasis (Fig. 18–7) occurs in 1% to 3% of pregnancies. In most cases, isolated fetal pyelectasis is physiologic. However, it may be secondary to mild reflux or a ureteropelvic junction syndrome. The likelihood of pyelectasis being associated with substantial morbidity requiring postnatal surgery increases with the degree of antenatal pelvic dilation.[7,31,32] Fetuses with pyelectasis should be followed serially to determine whether dilation increases with advancing gestational age.[22,33]

Postnatal evaluation is required but should not be performed immediately after delivery because the false-negative rate is increased. At-risk neonates should have a renal ultrasound between 1 and 3 weeks of age. There is no consensus on whether and when postnatal ultrasound should be repeated and on which patients should be offered a retrograde cystogram and when. Irrespective of the postnatal strategies for the diagnosis of reflux or for the prevention of urinary tract infections, the prenatal history should be kept in mind when unexplained symptoms occur postnatally.[34–36] The sensitivity of antenatal ultrasound for

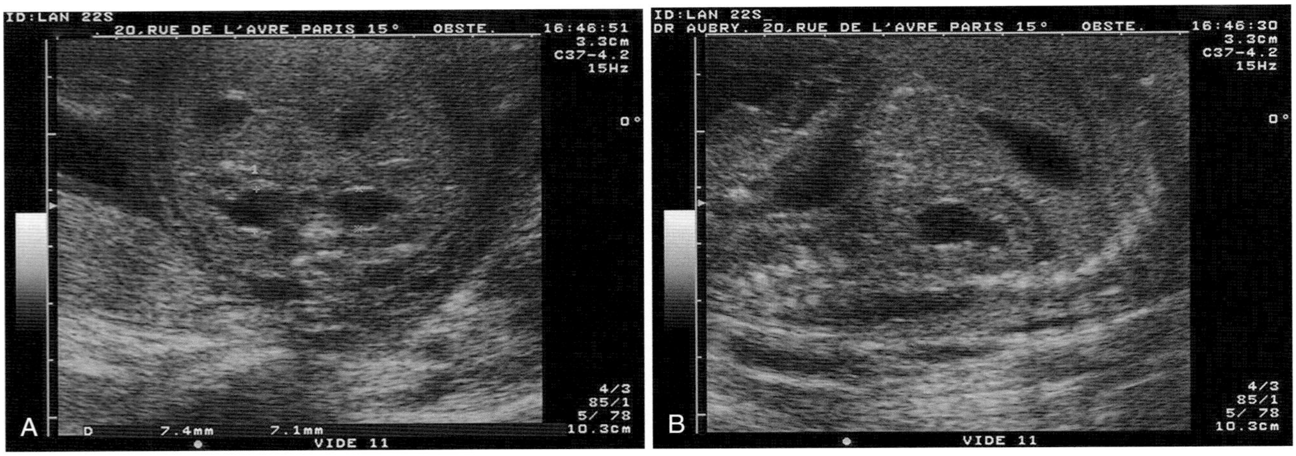

FIGURE 18–7
Mild pyelectasis at 22 weeks. *A*, Transverse view. *B*, Parasagittal view.

the detection of clinically significant reflux remains low,[20,21] and most cases of reflux are discovered after postnatal symptoms.

Hydronephrosis

Hydronephrosis is defined by an AP pelvic size of more than 1.5 cm or calyceal involvement.[37–39] In mild hydronephrosis, the calyces are slightly dilated and retain their shape. With greater upper urinary tract dilation, the calyces become rounded (Fig. 18–8). Dilated calyces are distributed regularly and connect to the renal pelvis, in contrast to the irregular pattern of a multicystic kidney in which the cysts are separate from the pelvis. In severe cases, the calyces are no longer identified separate from the pelvis, appearing instead as a large single transonic image (Fig. 18–9). The renal parenchyma is considered thinned when it is less than 3 mm thick. This finding is not always ominous because large dilations with thin parenchyma can be associated with normal renal function. The presence or absence of corticomedullary differentiation should be noted, as well as the parenchymal echogenicity and the presence of cysts. Although subjective,[40–44] evaluation of the ultrasonographic structure of the renal parenchyma may be a useful predictor of renal function, although it is less sensitive than urinalysis to predict postnatal survival with altered renal function.[45,46]

MIDLEVEL DILATIONS

Hydroureter is a dilated ureter that appears as a convoluted transonic image, located between the kidney and the bladder (Fig. 18–10); normally, the ureter is not seen ultrasonographically. Peristaltic activity suggests a megaureter. A dilated ureter may also result from vesicoureteral reflux.[47] or a ureterocele. A ureterocele appears as a round transonic image located inside the bladder and lined by a thin border (Fig. 18–11).

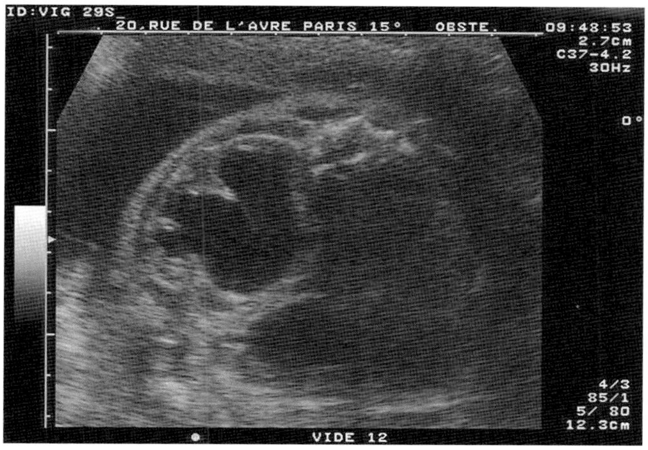

FIGURE 18–8
Unilateral hydronephrosis with rounded calyces at 29 weeks (transverse view).

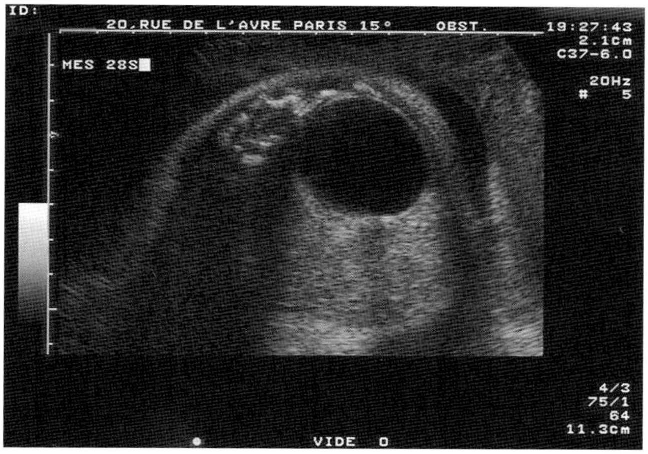

FIGURE 18–9
Large unilateral hydronephrosis at at 28 weeks (transverse view).

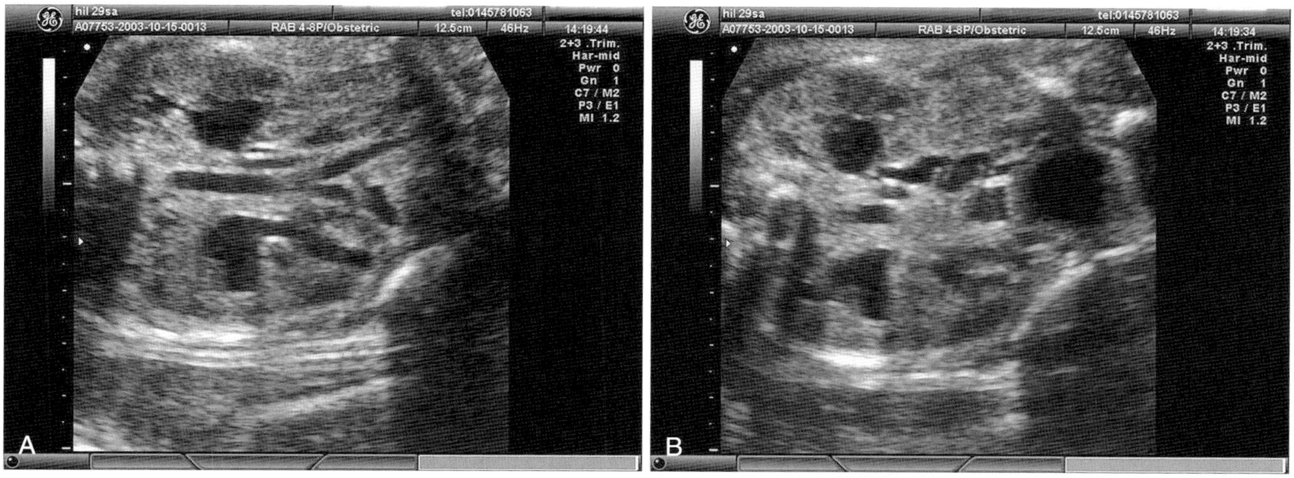

FIGURE 18–10
Dilated ureter at 29 weeks. *A*, Frontal view. *B*, Transverse view.

FIGURE 18–11
Bladder ureterocele. *A*, Frontal view at 25 weeks. *B*, Frontal view at 23 weeks. Note renal duplication.

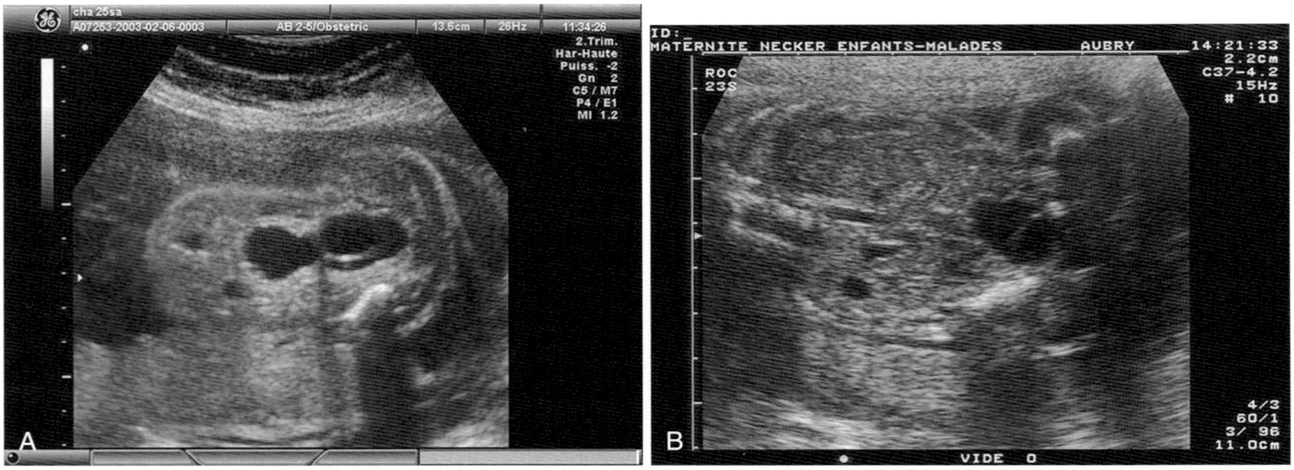

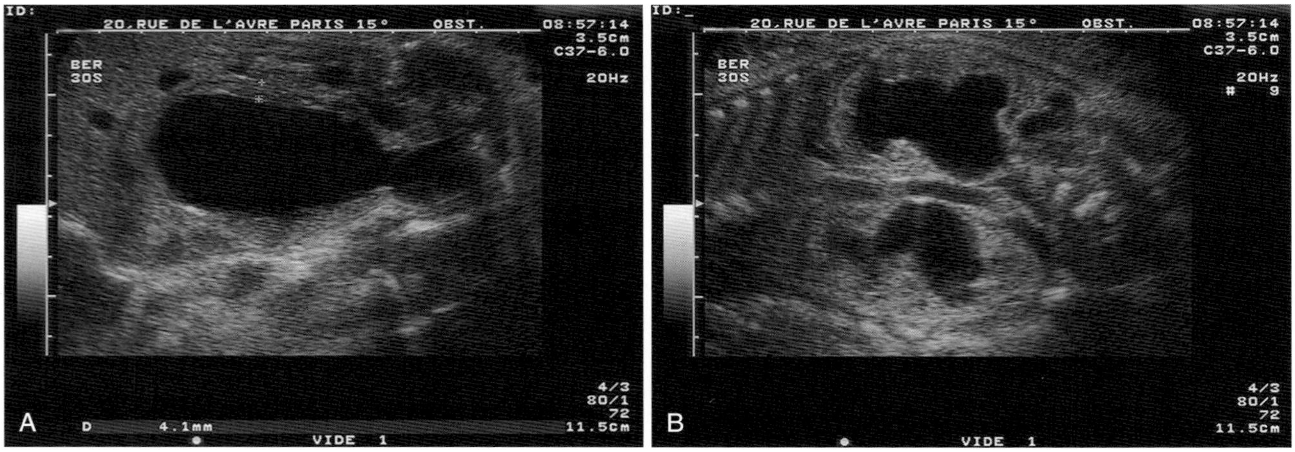

FIGURE 18–12
Posterior urethral valves at 30 weeks. *A*, Enlarged bladder (frontal view). Note the thickened bladder wall and infravesical image of the dilated urethra (posterior urethral valves). *B*, Hydronephrosis with hyperechogenic renal parenchyma (frontal view).

LOW-LEVEL DILATION

A dilated bladder that does not empty over the course of the ultrasound examination suggests an outlet obstruction. The dilated bladder is usually round, but may be larger above the umbilical arteries than below, evoking the shape of a champagne bottle cork. The image of a dilated urethra is specific for posterior urethral valves especially if seen during fetal bladder voiding, but is far from constant. At a later stage, bladder outlet obstruction can result in muscular hypertrophy imaged as a bladder wall thicker than 3 mm (Fig. 18–12). Bladder diverticula may also form. Although posterior urethral valves are the most common cause of bladder dilation in males, other etiologies are possible. Urethral atresia is an almost universally lethal condition. The atresia cannot be directly imaged, and it is usually diagnosed at pathologic postmortem examination (Fig. 18–13). Complex genitourinary anomalies should also be considered. Keep in mind that an LUTO, including posterior urethral valves, can present as a midlevel or even an upper-level obstruction with subsequent evidence of bladder enlargement.

Ascites and Urinoma

Urine may leak into the peritoneal cavity through minor and usually unidentifiable disruptions of the urinary tract wall, causing ascites. Urinary ascites is not specific for a particular uropathy and is not necessarily an ominous finding. The urinary origin of the ascites is usually apparent. Similarly, disruption of the urinary tract in the retroperitoneal space may lead to a urinoma (Fig. 18–14), which appears as a transonic image surrounding the kidney and confined within Gerota's fascia.[48] Urinomas are usually easy to differentiate from renal masses, lymphangioma, neuroblastoma, mesenteric cyst, and enteric duplications.

FIGURE 18–13
Urethral atresia at 15 weeks. Enlarged bladder (sagittal view). Note the infravesical image of the dilated urethra.

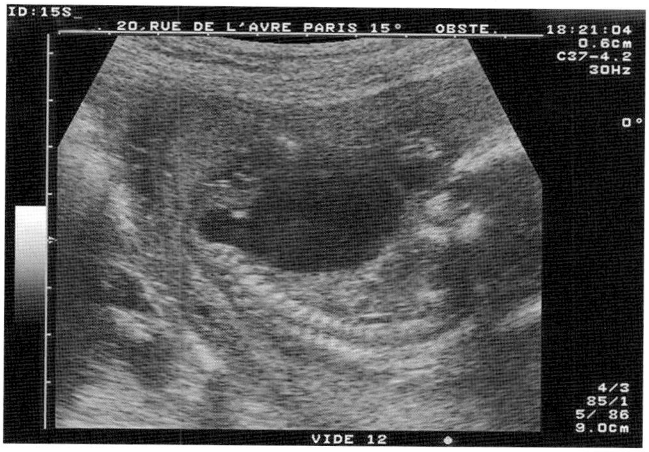

FIGURE 18–15
Bladder exstrophy at 25 weeks. Note the abnormal appearance of the anterior abdominal wall, the absence of vesical image, and the low-lying fetal insertion of the umbilical cord.

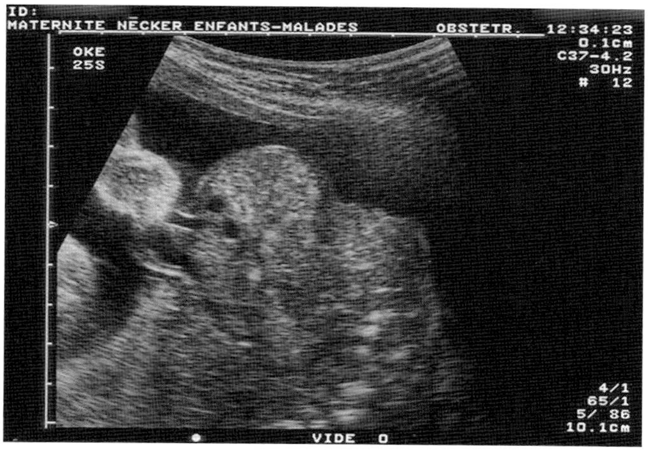

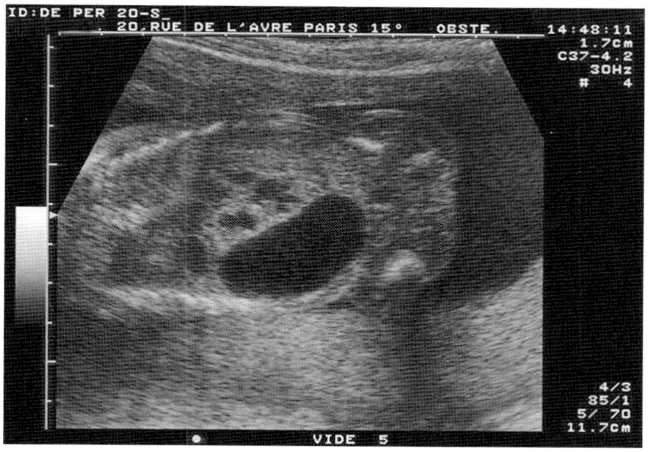

FIGURE 18–14
Urinoma at 20 weeks (frontal view).

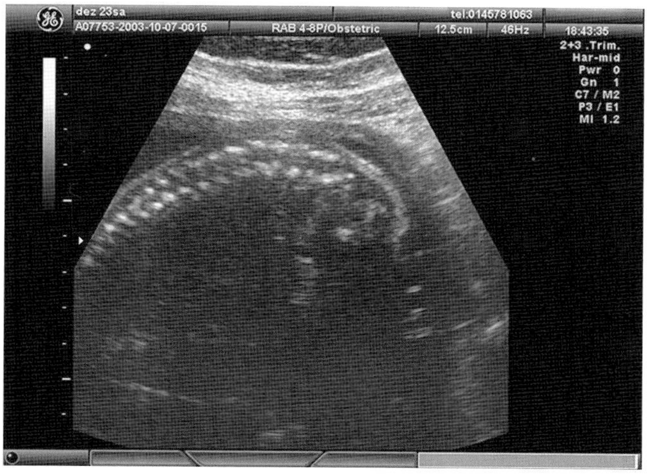

FIGURE 18–16 Cloacal abnormality at 23 weeks (sagittal view). Note the straightened and shortened sacrum.

Exclusion of Associated Anomalies

The first step in the management of a fetus with a urinary tract abnormality is to rule out extraurinary anomalies by a detailed ultrasonographic assessment by an experienced practitioner.[49–51] Soft markers suggestive of a chromosomal abnormality should be sought, as well as complex pelvic malformations.

Bladder exstrophy is characterized by the absence of a vesical image[52,53] and can sometimes be imaged directly (Fig. 18–15). The antenatal diagnosis of cloacal malformations is based on the association of a variety of relatively minor signs that may appear only in the third trimester.[54–58] Rectal atresia is suggested when the sacrum appears too straight (Fig. 18–16). A urodigestive fistula is suspected when the bowel is dilated with hyperechogenic material (Fig. 18–17). The image of an enlarged duplicated vagina is quite specific of a cloacal malformation[59] but might not appear until the third trimester. Visualization of the anal sphincter does not rule out the diagnosis of anal atresia (Fig. 18–18). The external genitalia should also be carefully imaged. Fused labia may appear "floating" in the amniotic fluid. The potential for surgical repair might be difficult to establish when a complex malformation of the pelvic floor is diagnosed in utero, and the management should be discussed with an expert pediatric surgeon. Magnetic resonance imaging may be helpful in some instances. In the VACTERL association, spinal, heart, limbs or the digestive tract anomalies are associated with renal malformation.

The prune-belly sequence is another complex malformation in which the prognosis may be difficult to establish. The diagnosis is suspected antenatally when a large bladder and substantial ureteral dilation are seen with mild hydronephrosis (Fig. 18–19). Undescended testes are common. It is possible to depress the fetal abdomen with a moderate amount of pressure by the ultrasound probe.

Some less common conditions are even more difficult to diagnose than the prune-belly sequence. For example, a microcolon megacystis syndrome[60,61] is suspected when

FIGURE 18–17
Urodigestive fistula with hyperechogenic content of the small bowel at 23 weeks. *A*, Transverse view. *B*, Frontal view.

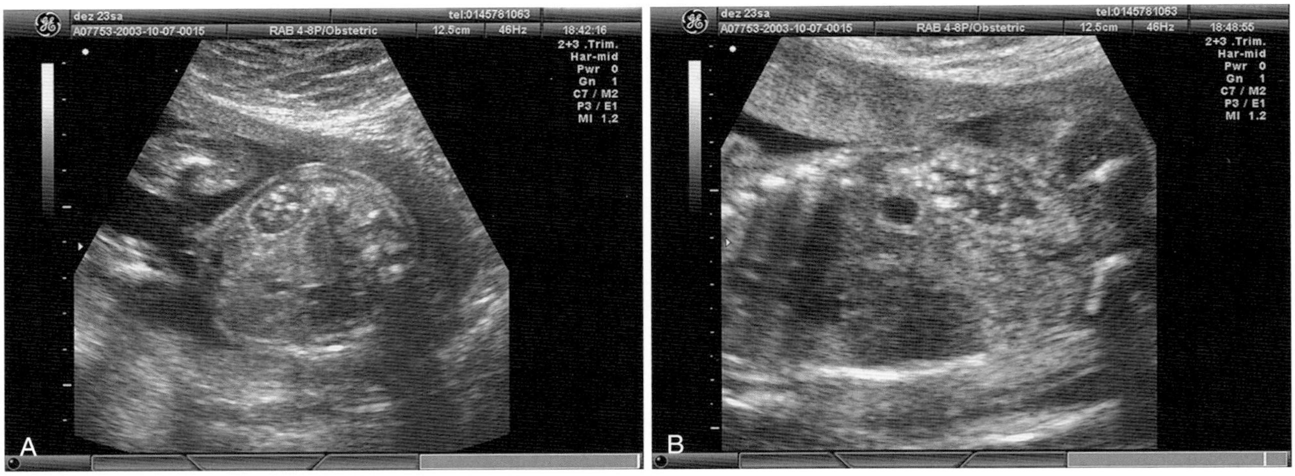

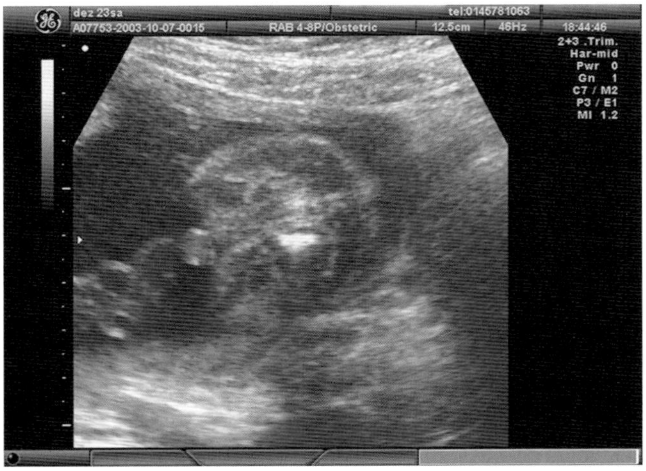

FIGURE 18–18
Absence of image of the anal margin at 23 weeks (tangential view of the perineum).

there is a large bladder and bowel dilation. However, the bowel dilation may occur only late in the third trimester. This syndrome has a poor prognosis owing to associated abnormalities in digestive function.

Karyotyping

The second step in the diagnostic workup is to consider fetal karyotyping. The incidence of chromosomal abnormalities associated with genitourinary defects was initially reported to be 12%.[62] However, in many uropathies secondary to chromosomal abnormalities, additional extrarenal defects are detectable, reducing the prevalence of aneuploidy in truly isolated uropathies such as posterior urethral valves or hydronephrosis. Thus, the risk of aneuploidy should be evaluated and weighed against the risk of an amniocentesis.[63–66] The finding of at least one ultrasound soft marker, such as a short femur or humerus, a minor anomaly of the fingers or toes, or a facial or other structural anomaly, indicates a high risk of aneuploidy. When previous aneuploidy screening such as nuchal translucency measurement or maternal serum markers yield "borderline" risks, one should consider the finding of a fetal uropathy as raising the risk above the "action line." Unfortunately, large studies that would allow calculation of the likelihood ratio of aneuploidy associated with isolated unilateral hydronephrosis or posterior urethral valves are lacking. Regardless of the risk of aneuploidy, some parents may request karyotyping in order to maximize their opportunities of excluding associated abnormalities in a baby for whom neonatal surgery and long-term uronephrologic follow-up are likely.

Whether or not pyelectasis is an indication for karyotyping has been a matter of controversy owing to the high incidence of pyelectasis in normal children. When pyelectasis is associated with another fetal anomaly, even minor, the risk of aneuploidy is increased 10 to 20 times the maternal age–related risk[67,68] and karyotyping is indicated. Early studies suggested isolated pyelectasis to be associated with a substantial risk for Down syndrome. However, more recent studies have shown the risk of aneuploidy is increased by a likelihood ratio of only 1 to 1.5.[64,69] It is likely that in later studies, associated soft markers were diagnosed more frequently than in early reports. Careful ultrasonographic evaluation is therefore necessary to rule out associated minor abnormalities when pylectasis is diagnosed at routine ultrasound. Pylectasis should be considered as a part of the sequential screening process for aneuploidy using multiple parameters including maternal age, nuchal translucency measurement, and maternal serum markers (see Chapters 7 and 8).[25–28,66,70–77] The integrated risk of aneuploidy should then be weighed against the risks of amniocentesis.[64]

FIGURE 18–19
Prune-belly sequence at 34 weeks. *A*, Enlarged bladder with no infravesical urethral dilation and a normal bladder wall. *B*, Bladder, ureter, and kidney (oblique view). *C*, Mild pyelectasis (parasagittal view).

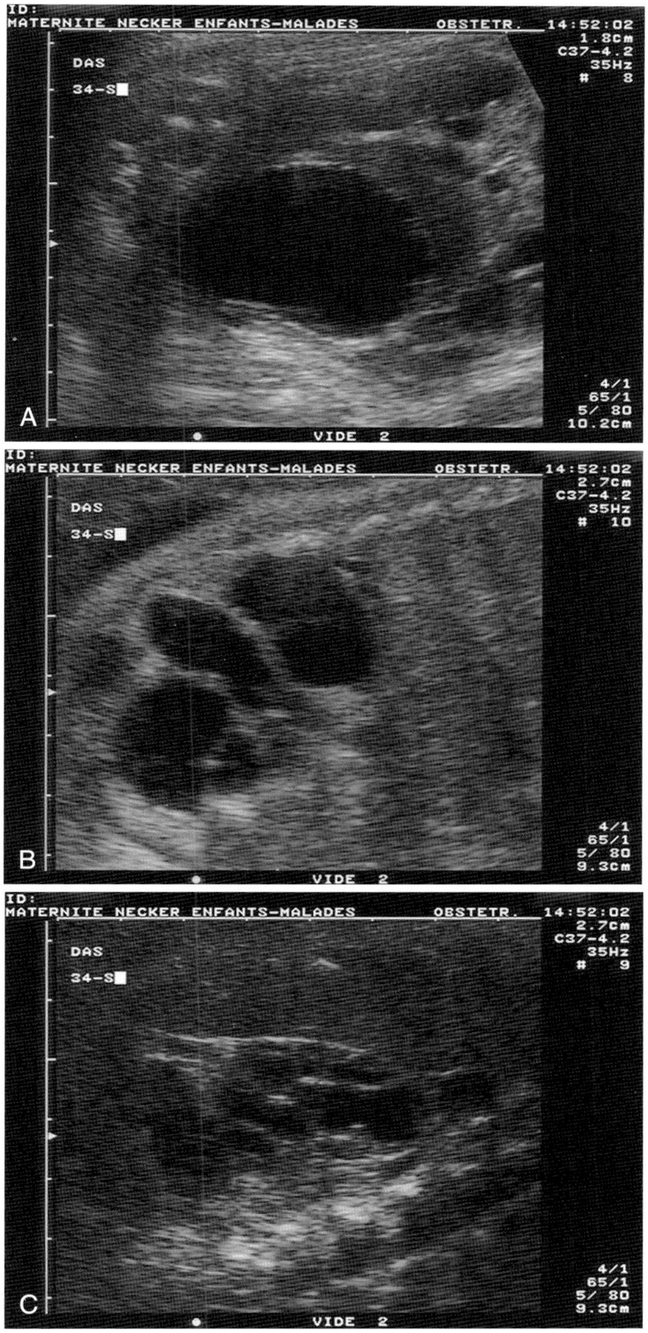

Predicting Postnatal Pulmonary Function

Pulmonary hypoplasia (PH) is a disorder of impaired lung growth characterized by diminished size, generational branching, and vasculature. Severe oligohydramnios from 16 weeks onward appears to preclude further pulmonary development. In contrast, oligohydramnios developing after the second trimester is unlikely to result in PH because the crucial canalicular phase of lung development (occurring between 16 and 25 weeks) has largely been completed by this stage. Predicting the likelihood of PH is difficult. Most studies reporting predictive data have used cases with preterm premature membrane rupture (PPROM),[78–80] and it is not clear how applicable such data are to cases of olgohydramnios secondary to fetal uropathy. In the case of PPROM, additional factors such as preterm delivery and infection contribute to the outcome, and one might speculate that they will worsen the prognosis in contrast to oligohydramnios alone. However, the PPROM data suggest the following:

- If there is a mean vertical pocket of amniotic fluid on ultrasound prior to 26 weeks of greater than 10 mm, PH is very unlikely to occur.[78]
- If the mean vertical pocket of amniotic fluid on ultrasound prior to 26 weeks is less than 10 mm, there is a 90% neonatal mortality rate.[78]
- If the mean vertical pocket of amniotic fluid on ultrasound after 26 weeks is less than 10 mm, PH is very unlikely to occur.[78–80]

Thus, although absence of severe oligohydramnios before 26 weeks probably means that PH is unlikely, predicting which fetus will develop PH after birth is more difficult. New imaging methods such as magnetic resonance imaging and 3D ultrasonography have been used to evaluate fetal lung volumes and might improve the prediction of PH.[81–83]

Predicting Postnatal Renal Function

Unilateral uropathies are associated with a good functional outcome, and it is unnecessary to perform invasive fetal studies to obtain biochemical data from the abnormal kidney, regardless of renal ultrasonographic appearance. Serial examinations are required to ensure that contralateral lesions do not appear later in gestation.

The evaluation of fetal renal function with bilateral renal dilation or LUTO is based mainly on ultrasound and, in selected cases, on fetal urine analysis or fetal blood sampling. Ultrasound permits assessment of the parenchyma and the amniotic fluid volume.[18,40,84] Fetal urine analysis assesses the ability of the renal tubule to reabsorb a variety of compounds, including sodium, β_2-microglobulin, calcium, phosphorus, and glucose.[37,51,85–95] The β_2-microglobulin level in the fetal serum is thought to reflect fetal glomerular function.[96–99] Fetal sonographic features related to terminal renal failure include severe oligohydramnios and abnormal images of the renal parenchyma, such as loss of the normal corticomedullary differentiation, hyperechogenicity, and cortical cysts (see Fig. 18–12*B*). In these instances, fetal urinalysis might confirm renal failure, showing high fetal urinary concentrations of sodium and β_2-microglobulin.[100] Conversely, the functional prognosis is usually good and fetal urine sampling unnecessary in cases of upper obstruction with normal amniotic fluid volume and normal renal parenchyma throughout pregnancy.

In select cases, the functional prognosis cannot be established ultrasonographically. These cases include fetuses with bilateral lesions and moderately decreased amniotic fluid volume and fetuses with mild alterations of the renal parenchyma. Moreover, in cases in which the antenatal diagnosis of posterior urethral valves is almost certain, the relatively high incidence of postnatal renal failure may support fetal urine sampling, even in the absence of any ominous ultrasonographic finding. For such cases, the key issue is to identify, among the children expected to survive, those who are at risk for developing postnatal renal failure from those whose renal function will remain normal after surgical repair. The establishment of prognostic values for any marker is complicated by the fact that renal failure may occur relatively late in life, underscoring the need for long-term follow-up of children in whom fetal urine analysis was performed in utero. Some studies show that fetuses with a normal urinary sodium but a urinary β_2-microglobulin above the 95th percentile are at increased risk of having a serum creatinine greater than 1 standard deviation (SD) above the mean by 1 year of age.[87] When both markers are increased, neonatal renal failure is likely. In contrast, a good postnatal outcome is anticipated when both markers are within the normal range.[87] Others report higher thresholds for fetal urinary β_2-microglobulin to predict a postnatal serum creatinine greater than 2 SD above the mean, thereby increasing specificity.[92] To increase the predictive accuracy of fetal urinalysis, sampling of the apparently less affected kidney[45] or serial vesicocentesis (as long as the values continue to improve or until they normalize) has been advocated.[92,101] In our experience, the results of fetal urinalysis should be interpreted with great care because, in the absence of ominous sonographic findings, only very high levels of urinary β_2-microglobulin (i.e., >10 mg/L) are reliable predictors of renal failure at the age of 10 to 16 years (unpublished data).

Management Options

GENERAL

Once the prognosis is determined, management options, including termination of pregnancy, occasionally fetal therapy, postnatal care, and follow-up, should be discussed with the parents. The option of pregnancy termination should be raised whenever there is terminal renal failure or multiple malformations. Fetal intervention is not indicated when there is unilateral disease or an isolated uropathy with normal renal parenchyma and normal renal function. In these instances, care is focused on postnatal management. It is important to refer the couple antenatally to a pediatric urologist/nephrologist.

IDENTIFICATION OF CONDITIONS REQUIRING EMERGENCY NEONATAL SURGERY

Some isolated uropathies in which postnatal renal function is anticipated to be reasonably good may require emergency postnatal surgery, requiring delivery in a tertiary care center with pediatric surgery facilities. These include posterior urethral valves, obstructive ureterocele, major bilateral hydronephrosis, and more generally, cases with late-onset oligohydramnios leading to the diagnosis of acute obstruction of urinary output.

Fetal Therapy

Fetal therapy for uropathies may be considered because, although obstruction of the urinary tract may be treated by relatively simple postnatal procedures, some abnormalities are associated with severe renal lesions that manifest before birth. These lesions include severe renal dysplasia, severe oligohydramnios, and pulmonary hypoplasia, leading to either perinatal death or end-stage neonatal renal failure. Although intrauterine decompression of experimental urinary tract obstruction in the fetal lamb has been shown to prevent renal dysplasia,[102–105] a positive impact of fetal urinary decompression on chronic renal disease in the human has not been demonstrated.[106–112]

Lower urinary obstruction in the human fetus has been treated by open fetal surgery, endoscopic ablation of posterior urethral valves, percutaneous vesicoamniotic shunting, serial vesicocentesis, or more recently, percutaneous fetal cystoscopy. Some of these techniques can also be applied to upper tract obstruction. Open fetal surgery was abandoned with the development of percutaneous techniques. Serial vesicocentesis has been performed as early as the first trimester,[113] but its efficacy remains unclear. Indeed, resolution of first-trimester urinary dilation following percutaneous needling may reflect the natural history of the condition rather than the intervention.[114]

Percutaneous ultrasound-guided vesicoamniotic shunting was first reported in the 1980s.[115] Briefly, a cannula is inserted through the maternal abdomen under ultrasound guidance and after local analgesia into the dilated fetal bladder or kidney. A double pigtail catheter is introduced through the cannula with the distal end placed into the dilated urinary tract and the proximal end in the amniotic cavity. Complications include chorioamnionitis, premature rupture of membranes, or preterm delivery in around 10% of cases.[116,117] Up to half of the shunts are displaced after a few days or weeks. Migration of the amniotic end into the peritoneal cavity can cause urinary ascites, which can be treated, with modest success, by placing a peritoneoamniotic shunt.[118,119] Other complications include iatrogenic gastroschisis.

Some reviews[120,121] concluded there is a lack of high-quality evidence to guide clinical practice regarding prenatal bladder drainage.[106,109,122–125] In utero drainage may improve survival in severely affected fetuses by improving lung function, but this is achieved at the expense of increasing pediatric morbidity. Long-term follow-up of shunt survivors reveals that some form of chronic renal disease is the rule. Many are ultimately transplanted. A multicenter randomized trial comparing expectant management with percutaneous shunting for lower urinary tract obstruction (PLUTO) is under way with the aim of determining whether or not fetal therapy improves survival and reduces long-term morbidity.[126] Percutaneous fetal cystoscopy has been used to directly visualize the fetal urinary tract.[127–129] This allows differentiation of posterior urethral valves from urethral atresia and fulguration of posterior urethral valves.[130]

SUMMARY OF MANAGEMENT OPTIONS

Fetal Uropathies/Dilation of the Renal Tract

Management Options	Evidence Quality and Recommendation	References
Diagnosis		
Confirm diagnosis with detailed ultrasound by expert.	III/B	42
Search for other abnormalities.	III/B	50
Consider karyotype.	III/B	62
Management		
Assess risk of pulmonary hypoplasia.	IIa/B	80–83
Assess risk of renal failure:		
• Ultrasound	III/B	40
• Urinalysis	IIa/B	87,88,91,93
Interdisciplinary management and planning includes pediatric nephrologist/urologist.	—/GPP	—
Counsel parents.	—/GPP	—
Consider termination of pregnancy in severe cases.	—/GPP	—
Plan for delivery depends on anticipated need for early pediatric surgery.	—/GPP	—
The role of fetal therapy is unclear: decompression probably reduces deaths from pulmonary hypoplasia but at the expense of long-term renal dysfunction in survivors.	Ia/A	120–125
Perform careful examination and assessment of baby after delivery or postmortem examination after perinatal death.	III/B	100

GPP, good practice point.

KIDNEY ABNORMALITIES

General

Fetal renal anomalies include those of number, location, size, and structure. These malformations are primarily renal and usually occur in the absence of a urinary tract defect. Some, such as renal agenesis or multicystic kidney disease, are common and easy to diagnose. The diagnosis and antenatal management can be more difficult when renal structural anomalies present as hyperechogenic or enlarged kidneys. The first step after a renal abnormality has been identified is to exclude associated anomalies and, if necessary, offer fetal karyotyping.

The prognosis of isolated unilateral renal abnormalities is uniformly good, whereas bilateral anomalies associated with severe oligohydramnios are lethal. In bilateral cases with normal amniotic fluid, the long-term postnatal morbidity is difficult to predict. Biochemical markers that have proved predictive of postnatal morbidity in uropathies have not been useful in fetal nephropathies. Our personal experience suggests that neither fetal urinary electrolytes nor serum β_2-microglobulin is a reliable predictor of postnatal renal function in fetuses with bilaterally enlarged and hyperechogenic kidneys and normal amniotic fluid volume (unpublished data).

Anomalies of Number

Renal agenesis can be unilateral or bilateral. It may result from early degeneration of the ureteric bud or from a failed interaction between the ureteric bud and the blastema (Figs. 18–20 and 18-21). The corresponding adrenal gland assumes a globoid shape and should not be mistaken for a hypoplastic kidney.[131] Bilateral agenesis results in the oligohydramnios sequence (pulmonary hypoplasia, dysmorphic face, and limb deformities) and is lethal.[68,132] In contrast, fetuses with unilateral renal agenesis remain symptom-free during postnatal life in the absence of associated anomalies. Minor genital anomalies such as duplicated/hypoplastic uterus, absent fallopian tube, and absent epididymis and vas efferens can be found on the ipsilateral side. They cannot be diagnosed in utero and would not alter the prognosis for survival.[118,119]

Duplication of the kidney is caused by the premature division of the ureteric bud before it connects to the nephrogenic mesoderm (Fig. 18–22). This explains its association with a double or bifid ureter. The upper ureter typically enters the bladder more caudally but might also connect ectopically to the urethra, vagina, seminal vesicle, or rectum. The upper kidney usually shows some degree of outflow obstruction and parenchymal dysplasia. Typical findings include a dilated pelvis in a dysplastic part of the kidney

FIGURE 18–20
Bilateral renal agenesis at 20 weeks. *A*, Transverse view. *B*, Frontal view. Note the bilateral absence of renal vessels.

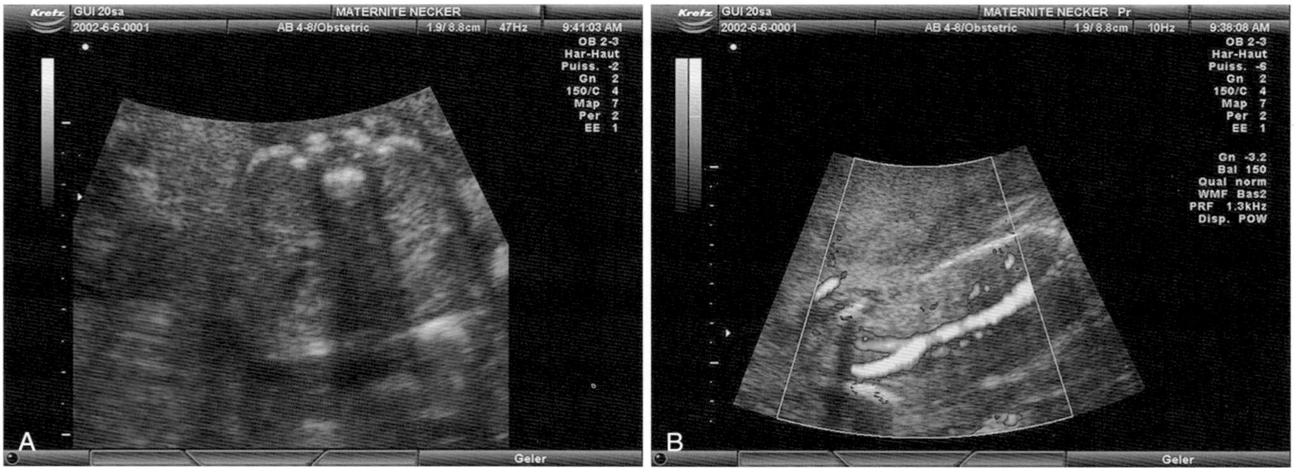

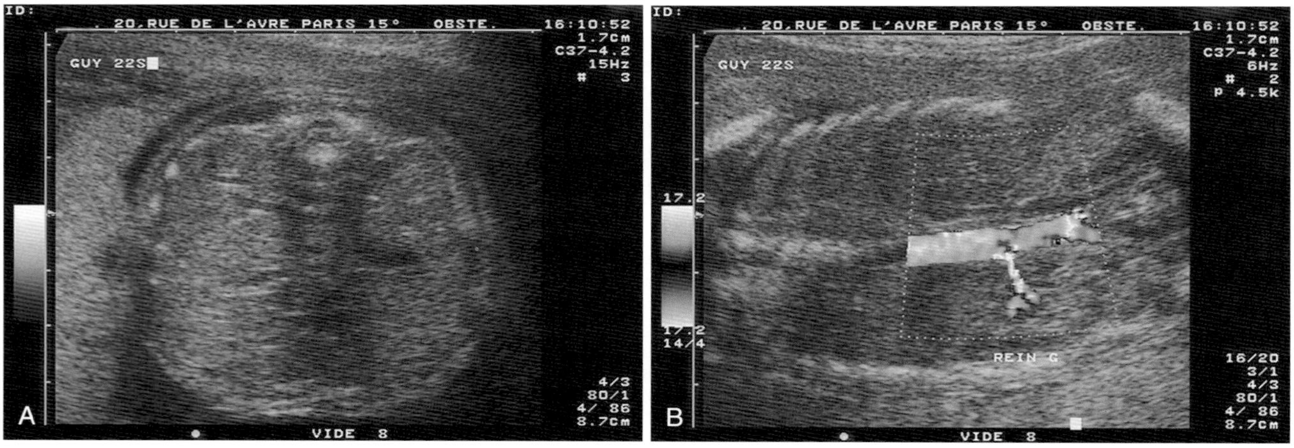

FIGURE 18–21
Unilateral renal agenesis at 22 weeks. *A*, Transverse view. *B*, Frontal view. Note the unilateral absence of renal vessels.

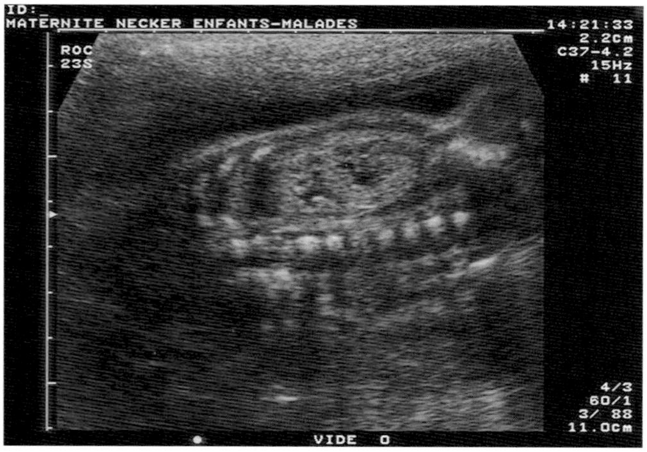

FIGURE 18–22
Renal duplication at 23 weeks (frontal view).

associated with a ureterocele at the connection of the distal ureter to the bladder.[133] The accuracy of antenatal ultrasound for the diagnosis of fetal duplex kidney approximates 75%, based on two main ultrasonographic features: two separate poles in the affected kidney and a ureterocele.

Supernumerary kidney results from premature branching of the ureteric bud. The supernumerary kidney has its own ureter and blood supply and is frequently obstructed or dysplasic.

Abnormalities of Position

Ectopic kidneys are usually displaced caudally One or both kidneys may be involved and the shape is abnormal due to malrotation. Affected individuals are asymptomatic provided the renal parenchyma is well differentiated and free of dysplasia.[134] In crossed renal ectopia, both kidneys are located on the same side of the body and may be fused.

Horseshoe kidney results from the fusion of the kidneys, usually by their lower poles.[135] Fusion of both upper and lower poles produces the ring kidney. When isolated, horseshoe kidneys are usually asymptomatic. However, they are also associated with aneuploidy (trisomy 18, Turner's syndrome, and triploidy).

Isolated Abnormalities of Size and Structure

Renal hypoplasia is defined as kidney mass more than 2 SD below the mean. This condition is diagnosed postnatally except in its most severe form.

Multicystic dysplasia manifests antenatally as kidneys that have lost their normal shape (Fig. 18–23) due to macrocysts of variable diameter (≥0.5–3 cm) that are connected neither to each other nor to the rest of the urinary tract. Some clusters of tubules, rudimentary glomeruli, primitive ducts, and bars of metaplastic cartilage may be irregularly distributed within the loose mesenchyme. Multicystic dysplasia usually occurs in the absence of any obstructive uropathy. Whereas bilateral disease is lethal, unilateral forms have a good prognosis. Spontaneous involution of the multicystic kidney is usual during postnatal life and may on occasion occur in utero. The cyst size is usually constant throughout fetal life, but rarely, extremely large cysts may compress the fetal abdomen or cause dystocia and therefore require intrauterine drainage. These macrocystic lesions are easy to distinguish from polycystic kidney diseases, which present antenatally as enlarged hyperechoic kidneys. The sonographic pattern of the latter conditions is due to the microscopic cysts that fill the renal parenchyma.[136]

Autosomal recessive polycystic kidney disease (ARPKD), also referred to as *infantile polycystic kidney disease*, is an inherited disorder. It is characterized by enlarged kidneys that retain their shape. The cut surface has a spongy appearance due to elongated microcysts that have a radial orientation extending from the medulla to the cortical surface. These cysts correspond to dilated collecting ducts.[118,119] The liver is always involved with portal fibrosis and proliferation of bile ducts.[137,138] Postnatally, the diagnosis is easy to make based on typical anatomic features. Pathologic diagnosis, however, may be more difficult in the second-trimester fetus, underscoring the need for referring abnormal kidneys to pathologists familiar with fetal renal development.

Disease expression in utero is variable.[139–143] In some affected fetuses, the kidneys remain ultrasonographically normal. In this instance, renal enlargement develops during infancy, and renal failure occurs relatively late in the second decade. At the other end of the spectrum, ARPKD manifests in the second trimester as an anuric fetus with absent amniotic fluid and dramatically enlarged, hyperechogenic kidneys with no corticomedullary differentiation (Fig. 18–24). Intermediate forms are the norm, with a variable combination of renal enlargement and late-onset oligohydramnios.[142] The responsible gene has been mapped.[144]

Autosomal dominant polycystic kidney disease is also referred to as adult polycystic kidney disease because its clinical onset usually occurs in adulthood. This term, however, is misleading because autosomal dominant polycystic disease may manifest early and occasionally quite severely, including during fetal life. Autosomal dominant polycystic kidney is a common cause of enlarged hyperechogenic kidneys in the fetus because of the relatively high frequency of the mutation in the general population.[143,145–147] Fetal autosomal dominant polycystic kidney disease often presents as moderately enlarged hyperechogenic kidneys with increased corticomedullary differentiation,[148] with normal amniotic fluid volume and bladder. It may also present as enlarged hyperechogenic kidneys with no specific feature. Fetal terminal renal failure associated with very large kidneys is a rare occurrence in autosomal dominant polycystic kidney disease. The diagnosis is easy when renal cysts are present in one of the parents. However, this hint may be lacking either because of the variability of disease expression or because the fetus has a new mutation.

In the adult, the kidneys are enlarged and their surface distorted by bulging macrocysts. During fetal life, however, the cysts are usually very small, producing a sonographic pattern of enlarged, hyperechogenic kidneys similar in appearance to that of the recessive disease.[143] In the most

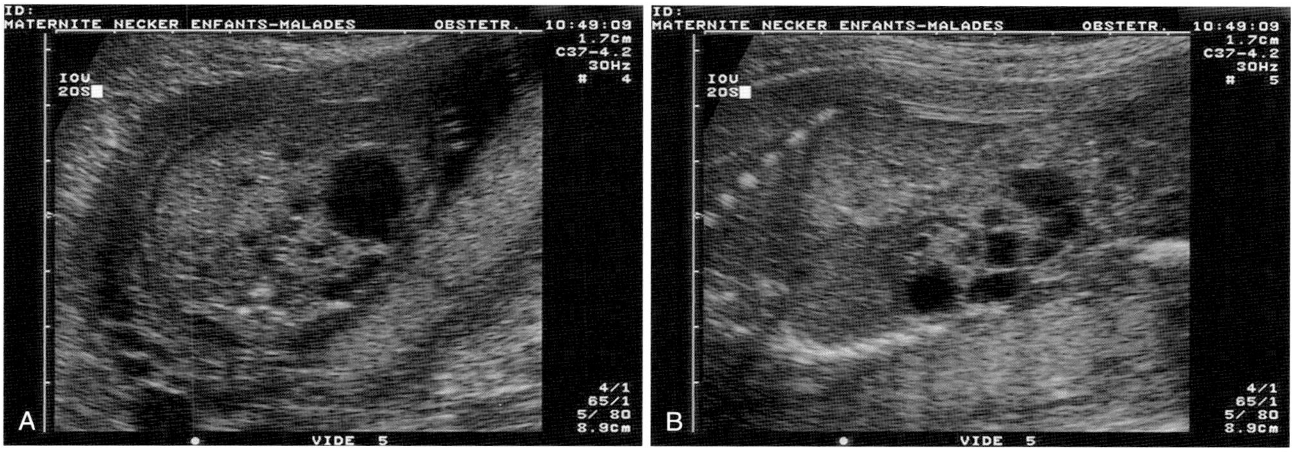

FIGURE 18–23
Unilateral multicystic kidney at 20 weeks. *A*, Transverse view. *B*, Frontal view.

FIGURE 18–24
Enlarged hyperechogenic kidney (autosomal recessive polycystic kidney disease) at 36 weeks. *A*, Transverse view. *B*, Parasagittal view. Note the absence of corticomedullary differentiation of the renal parenchyma.

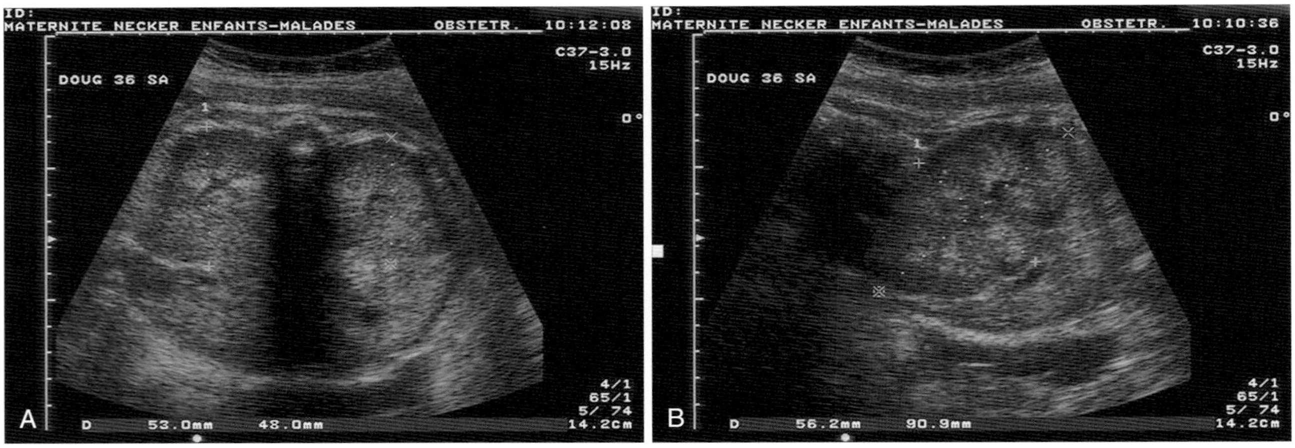

severe cases with terminal renal failure in utero, the diagnosis is made post mortem by showing both collecting tubules and nephrogenic cysts. Several mutations can result in disease. Known sites include chromosome 16 (PKD1 locus) and chromosome 4 (PKD2 locus).[149,150]

Transient nephromegaly is a poorly understood condition and can be defined as renal enlargement without any alteration of renal function. These patients may present as fetuses with moderately enlarged kidneys in which corticomedullary differentiation is usually retained. The kidneys may appear slightly hyperechogenic. The amniotic fluid volume remains normal. The ultrasonographic abnormalities tend to regress during infancy and the children remain symptom-free.[151] The uneventful postnatal course may be the only way to distinguish this condition from a true renal disease, such as polycystic kidney disease, or from less common causes of enlarged fetal kidneys.[143] Renal vein thrombosis may result in unilateral renal enlargement and hyperechogenicity.

Prenatal Management of Isolated Hyperechogenic Kidneys

The counseling of a pregnant woman after a prenatal diagnosis of isolated hyperechogenic fetal kidneys is challenging, because providing patients with overly pessimistic information leads to unnecessary pregnancy termination, whereas unrestricted reassurance may be inappropriate. Fetal ultrasonography usually fails to provide an accurate etiologic diagnosis, and fetal hyperechogenic kidneys can result from a variety of etiologies, including ARPKD, ADPKD, and transient nephromegaly.[152,153] Further, there is a wide range of outcomes within each etiologic group. Postnatal series are likely to overlook the most severe cases leading to perinatal death, as well as the mildest ones, which may remain clinically undetectable over a long period. A TCF2 gene mutation with Mody type diabetes is occasionally associated with moderately enlarged hyperechogenic kidneys.

The outcome can be predicted accurately in the most severe cases, in which terminal renal failure is certain with the discovery of severe oligohydramnios in the second trimester. If the pregnancy is terminated, it is crucial to obtain an accurate etiologic diagnosis and to store fetal DNA, because this information may lead to first-trimester molecular prenatal diagnosis in subsequent pregnancies, should ARPKD or ADPKD be identified. A wrong histopathologic diagnosis might have dramatic consequences in terms of genetic counseling and prenatal diagnosis.

In less severe cases, antenatal counseling should be based on prospective studies with long postnatal follow-up. In our experience of a consecutive series of 45 fetuses with bilateral isolated hyperechogenic kidneys, there were 20 with ARPKD, 8 with ADPKD, 9 with other renal disorders, and 6 symptom-free survivors without an etiologic diagnosis.[143] There were 19 pregnancy terminations, 5 neonatal deaths, and 19 survivors, of whom 14 had normal renal function, 3 had mild renal failure, and 2 had end-stage renal failure. None of those with severe oligohydramnios and fetal kidneys greater than 4 SD survived (n = 14, 10 terminations, 4 neonatal deaths), whereas 13 of 16 with normal amniotic fluid volume and kidneys less than 4 SD survived; 9 were symptom-free with a follow-up of 34 to 132 months.

Rare Etiologies of Fetal Nephropathies

Renal tubular dysgenesis is a rare condition characterized by poorly developed or undeveloped proximal tubules, causing severe oligohydramnios.[154] It is thought to be due to an abnormality of the renin-angiotensin system because similar renal anomalies are reported after prenatal exposure to angiotensin-converting enzyme inhibitors. This lethal condition is probably inherited as an autosomal recessive disorder and should be recognized at fetal autopsy in order to provide appropriate genetic counseling. Prolonged exposition to indomethacin may also induce renal failure, but probably by a different mechanism.[155]

Nephroblastomatosis is characterized by the presence of nephrogenic rests of metanephric blastema in both kidneys.[156] The kidneys may appear hyperechogenic with an unusually disorganized pattern of corticomedullar differentiation and this may be associated with overgrowth syndromes such as Beckwith-Wiedemann syndrome. Affected patients are also at increased risk for developing Wilms' tumor (see Chapter 22).

Renal tumors that present during fetal life are rapidly growing solid heterogeneous masses.[157] They are easy to distinguish from single transonic cysts that can also be recognized in utero but remain asymptomatic postnatally. Mesoblastic nephroma are reported to have a typical "ring" sign on color Doppler examination consisting of an anechoic ring surrounding the tumor signal.[158]

Fetal Nephropathies with Polyhydramnios

The Finnish type of congenital nephrotic syndrome may present antenatally with hydramnios, placentomegaly, and moderate growth restriction. Modest alterations in the renal parenchyma such as hyperechogenicity are inconsistent, making the antenatal diagnosis difficult in the absence of an index case.[159–161] Biochemical analysis of amniotic fluid should be considered in cases of unexplained hydramnios because this may lead to a diagnosis of fetal proteinuria (high concentration of α-fetoprotein and other proteins). Anomalies of electrolyte or aldosterone concentrations in the amniotic fluid may suggest Bartter's syndrome,[162–166] which is characterized by early-onset hydramnios and mild pyelectasis resulting from fetal polyuria.

Cystic Kidneys and Multiple Malformation Syndromes

Cystic kidneys are part of several multiple malformation syndromes.[167] The autosomal recessive Meckel-Gruber syndrome is one of the most common and lethal. It is characterized by severe oligohydramnios during the second trimester with markedly enlarged kidneys containing multiple cysts.[168,169] Encephalocele and postaxial polydactyly are characteristic of the syndrome but can be difficult to see with severe oligohydramnios.[160] Severe oligohydramnios and enlarged dysplastic kidneys can also be sonographic features of chromosomal abnormalities such as trisomy 13. Horseshoe kidney is associated with trisomy 18, Turner's syndrome, or triploidy.

The Laurence-Moon-Bardet-Biedl syndrome presents antenatally as hyperechogenic kidneys with polydactyly. Growth is usually normal during fetal life. In the Beckwith-Wiedemann syndrome, the enlarged kidneys are part of a more generalized visceromegaly, occasionally associated with an omphalocele. DiGeorge's syndrome may manifest as a heart defect associated with renal abnormalities. Zellweger's syndrome appears as renal cortical cysts with cerebral periventricular pseudocysts. Smith-Lemli-Opitz syndrome is suggested by the findings of dysplastic kidneys, fetal growth restriction, abnormal fingers, and ambiguous genitalia.

Dysplastic kidneys are also found in a variety of other syndromes, but usually as a secondary finding (e.g., short rib polydactyly associations). This underscores the need for careful ultrasonographic evaluation when abnormal kidneys are found. Fetal karyotyping should be considered when the structure of the kidneys is abnormal (hyperechogenicity/suspected dysplasia). However, isolated multicystic kidneys, renal agenesis, and ectopic kidneys are not associated with an increased risk of aneuploidy.

SUMMARY OF MANAGEMENT OPTIONS

Kidney Abnormalities

Management Options	Evidence Quality and Recommendation	References
Search for other abnormalities.	III/B	152
Consider karyotype in specific conditions:	—/GPP	—
• Identify inherited disease based on family history, postnatal follow up or postmortem examination.	—/GPP	—
• Store fetal DNA where appropriate.	—/GPP	—
Evaluate fetal renal function based on ultrasound (amniotic fluid volume). Renal function is good in unilateral cases.	III/B	143,152
Arrange prenatal ultrasonographic follow-up.	—/GPP	—
Consider termination of pregnancy in the most severe cases.	III/B	143,152
With ongoing pregnancies, and particularly in bilateral cases, plan perinatal management with pediatric nephrologist/pediatrician.	III/B	143,152
Plan for delivery depends on anticipated need for immediate neonatal care.	—/GPP	—
Perform careful examination and assessment of baby after delivery or postmortem examination after perinatal death.	—/GPP	—

GPP, good practice point.

ABNORMAL GENITALIA

General

Although fetal ultrasound is widely used to determine fetal gender, there is no consensus as to whether the structure of external genitalia should be part of routine ultrasound screening. Genital abnormalities can have a devastating impact on postnatal life and may be the hallmark of a multiple malformation syndrome. Ambiguous genitalia can be a medical emergency in neonates with salt-wasting forms of congenital adrenal hyperplasia. An examination of the fetal genitalia is mandatory whenever a uronephrologic abnormality is found to rule out a complex malformation of the fetal pelvis (Fig. 18–25).

Sonographic Diagnosis

Abnormal fetal genitalia may be identified under different circumstances:

- A specific genetic risk based on family history. This includes 5α-reductase deficiency, androgen insensitivity, and congenital adrenal hyperplasia. However, in an increasing number of cases, the molecular defect responsible for the disease is known, allowing first-trimester genetic diagnosis using chorionic villi.
- A discrepancy between the fetal gender established on routine ultrasound and fetal karyotyping.
- Abnormal or ambiguous genitalia found during routine ultrasound, either isolated or as part of a complex anomaly of the fetal pelvis or of a multiple malformation syndrome.

Undescended testis (Fig. 18–26) can be physiologic in the second trimester. Associated abnormalities, including uropathies and the prune-belly syndrome, should be ruled out. The diagnosis of hypospadias is usually made during the third trimester. Even in experienced hands, antenatal diagnosis of hypospadias may be impossible because of fetal position or technical limitations, including oligohydramnios. Anterior or middle hypospadias is rarely identified antenatally, although it is usually self-evident on examination of the neonate. Occasionally, the fetal penis is suspected to be shorter than usual or to have an abnormal curvature (Fig. 18–27). The tip of the penis may seem blunt. Ventral deflection of urinary stream can occasionally be seen using color Doppler.[170] Posterior hypospadias may be diagnosed antenatally based on the finding of a bifid scrotum, a short, curved penis, and no urethral canal (Fig. 18–28). The angulated penis located between the two scrotal folds is said to resemble a tulip flower.[171] When associated with undescended testis, posterior hypospadias may be difficult to differentiate from masculinized female genitalia with fused labia and an enlarged clitoris.[172] Rare conditions identifiable antenatally by ultrasound include distal obstruction of the fetal urethra (Fig. 18–29), perineal tumors, congenital hernia, and penoscrotal transposition.[173]

Gender discrepancies may be explained by a variety of mechanisms.[174] A discrepancy between the phenotypic fetal gender and the fetal karyotype may result from a labeling error of the amniotic fluid sample, a typing error

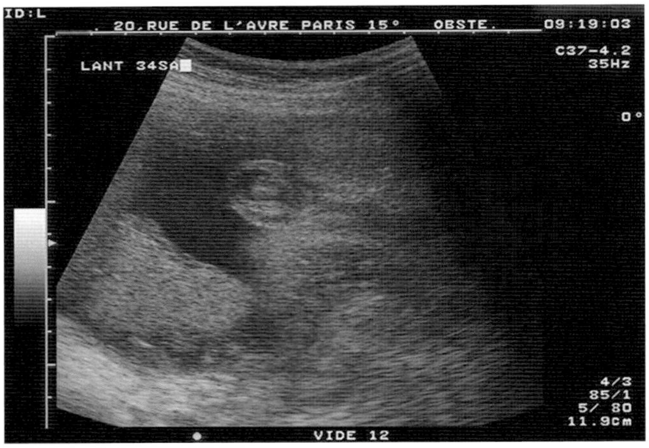

FIGURE 18–26
Unilateral undescended testes at 34 weeks.

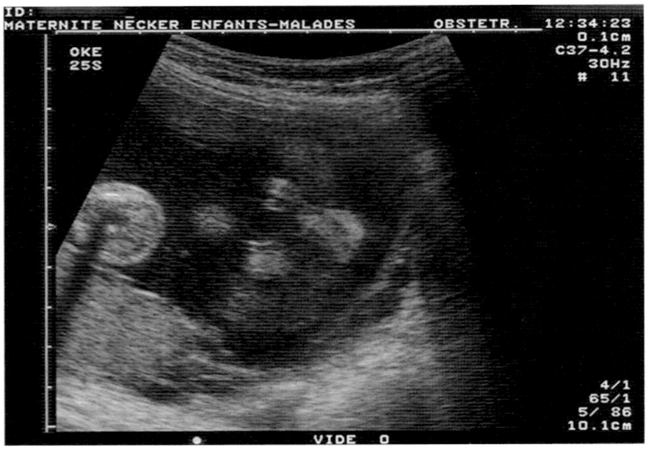

FIGURE 18–25
Bifidity of external genitalia in a girl with bladder exstrophy at 25 weeks (tangential view of the perineum).

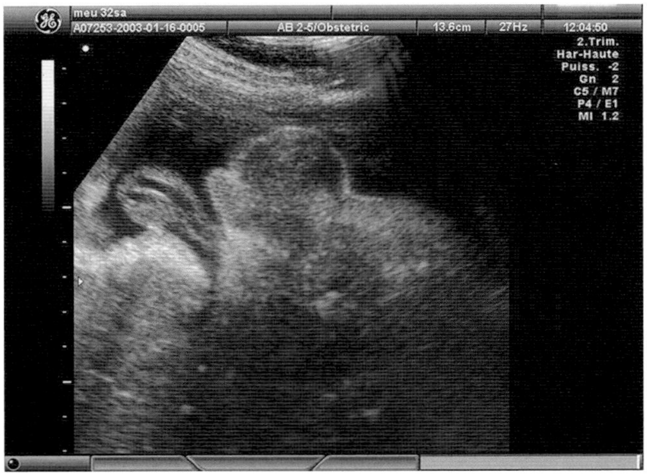

FIGURE 18–27
Short penis at 32 weeks (sagittal view).

FIGURE 18–28
Hypospadias at 32 weeks. Note the short penis with abnormal curvature.

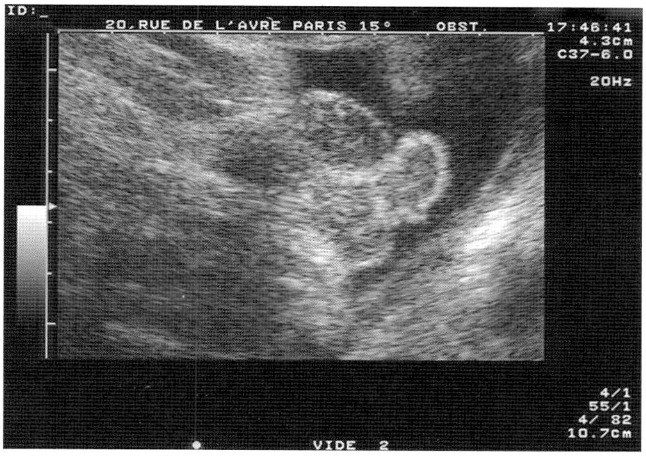

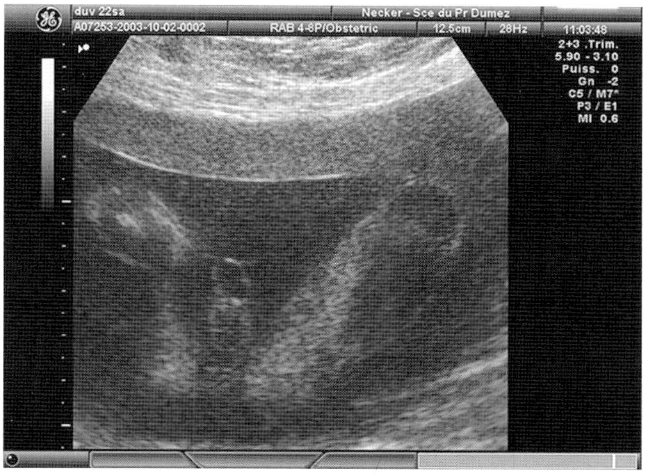

FIGURE 18–29
Distal urethral obstruction with dilated penile urethra at 22 weeks.

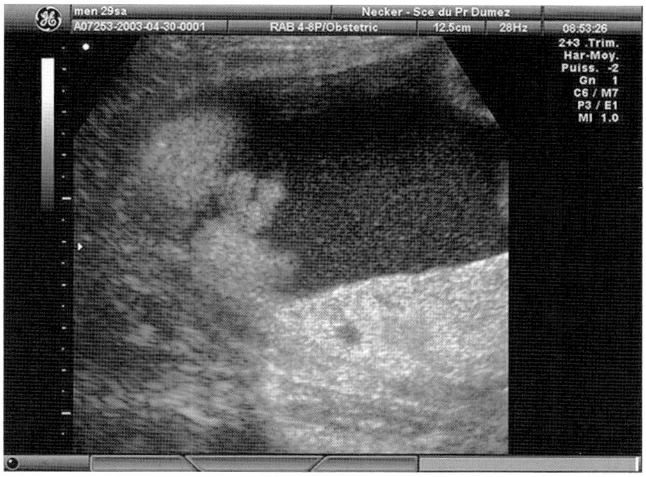

FIGURE 18–30
Ambiguous genitalia at 29 weeks with virilization of an XX fetus (congenital adrenal hyperplasia).

in ultrasonographic or genetic records, or maternal contamination of amniotic fluid cultures. The ultrasound examination should seek to establish whether the external genitalia seem structurally normal or ambiguous. Enlarged adrenal glands in the third trimester are suggestive of adrenal hyperplasia and result more often in ambiguous virilized female genitalia than in a male phenotype with an abnormal scrotum (Fig. 18–30). The presence of a fetal uterus can occasionally be documented sonographically, but its absence can never be ascertained confidently. Conversely, when abnormal genitalia are first identified by ultrasound, fetal genetic sex is the first step toward an antenatal diagnosis. This can be achieved by fetal karyotyping[172] or by analyzing the presence of the *SRY* gene in maternal plasma.[175–177]

Management Options

In addition to establishing the anatomy of the fetal genitalia, associated abnormalities should be sought. A number of multiple malformation syndromes including Smith-Lemli-Opitz, CHARGE (coloboma, heart disease, atresia choanae, retarded growth and retarded development and/or central nervous system anomalies, genital hypoplasia, and ear anomalies and/or deafness), Prader-Willi, and camptomelic dwarfism can be associated with genital abnormalities. Cloacal malformations may be part of a more complex entity, such as the VATER (vertebral defects, imperforate anus, tracheoesophageal fistula, and radial and renal dysplasia) association or a caudal regression syndrome. Fetuses with bladder exstrophy have abnormal genitalia. A bifid genital tubercle with epispadias may be found in males. The diagnosis is based on the absence of a fetal bladder associated with a low-lying fetal umbilical cord insertion and an abnormal bony pelvis. Cloacal exstrophy can produce bowel abnormalities suggestive of gastroschisis associated with vesical exstrophy.

The results of the fetal karyotype should be interpreted with great care, for the "genetic" gender may not be the "true" gender of the infant. For example, XX males bearing the *SRY* gene are unambiguously boys and XY fetuses with complete androgen insensitivity present as females. Adrenal hyperplasia may be suspected by ultrasound and confirmed by measuring the amniotic fluid 17-OH progesterone concentration.

In families with a history of congenital adrenal hyperplasia, management options include first-trimester gender determination by fetal DNA analysis in maternal serum (see Chapter 21). Both male and female fetuses are at risk for adrenal insufficiency. Only female fetuses are at risk for genital anomalies, and therefore, they may benefit from dexamethasone administration via the mother as early as possible during gestation in order to limit virilization.[178,179]

In general, counseling after the antenatal diagnosis of an apparently isolated abnormality of external genitalia is challenging and might be devastating for the family. Identifying the mechanism of the anomaly is helpful. Determining the anatomy of the fetal genitalia is crucial to establish the prognosis in terms of the potential for surgical repair. Counseling by a pediatric surgeon and a pediatric endocrinologist with experience of intersex states is warranted to provide the parents with information on postnatal management and gender assignment.

SUMMARY OF MANAGEMENT OPTIONS

Abnormal Genitalia

Management Options	Evidence Quality and Recommendation	References
Search for other abnormalities.	—/GPP	—
Karyotype for gender and to exclude other chromosomal abnormalities, but exercise care in assigning gender even after birth.	—/GPP	—
Arrange prenatal ultrasonographic follow-up.	—/GPP	—
Interdisciplinary approach: plan perinatal management with pediatric surgeon, pediatric endocrinologist, and geneticist.	—/GPP	—
Delivery is probably best in a center where assessment and plans for management can be made after birth.	—/GPP	—

GPP, good practice point.

SUGGESTED READINGS

Brun M, Maugey-Laulom B, Eurin D, et al: Prenatal sonographic patterns in autosomal dominant polycystic kidney disease: A multicenter study. Ultrasound Obstet Gynecol 2004;24:55–61.

Carr MC, Benacerraf BR, Estroff JA, Mandell J: Prenatally diagnosed bilateral hyperechoic kidneys with normal amniotic fluid: Postnatal outcome. J Urol 1995;153:442–444.

Cheikhelard A, Luton D, Philippe-Chomette P, et al: How accurate is the prenatal diagnosis of abnormal genitalia? J Urol 2000;164:984–987.

Clark TJ, Martin WL, Divakaran TG, et al: Prenatal bladder drainage in the management of fetal lower urinary tract obstruction: A systematic review and meta-analysis. Obstet Gynecol 2003;102:367–382.

Daikha-Dahmane F, Dommergues M, Muller F, et al: Development of human fetal kidney in obstructive uropathy: Correlations with ultrasonography and urine biochemistry. Kidney Int 1997;52:21–32.

Gunn TR, Mora JD, Pease P: Antenatal diagnosis of urinary tract abnormalities by ultrasonography after 28 weeks' gestation: Incidence and outcome. Am J Obstet Gynecol 1995;172:479–486.

Muller F, Dommergues M, Bussieres L, et al: Development of human renal function: Reference intervals for 10 biochemical markers in fetal urine. Clin Chem 1996;42:1855–1860.

Nicolaides KH, Cheng HH, Abbas A, et al: Fetal renal defects: Associated malformations and chromosomal defects. Fetal Diagn Ther 1992;7:1–11.

Sepulveda W, Stagiannis KD, Flack NJ, Fisk NM: Accuracy of prenatal diagnosis of renal agenesis with color flow imaging in severe second-trimester oligohydramnios. Am J Obstet Gynecol 1995;173:1788–1792.

Tsatsaris V, Gagnadoux MF, Aubry MC, et al: Prenatal diagnosis of bilateral isolated hyperechogenic kidneys. Is it possible to predict long term outcome? BJOG 2002;109:1388–1393.

REFERENCES

For a complete list of references, log onto www.expertconsult.com.

CHAPTER 19

Fetal Gastrointestinal Abnormalities

PETER STONE

Videos corresponding to this chapter are available online at www.expertconsult.com.

INTRODUCTION

Fetal gastrointestinal and abdominal wall malformations are easily visualized by ultrasound and may be detected either during a routine second trimester scan or during an examination for a raised maternal serum α-fetoprotein, poor fetal growth, or hydramnios. The most common gastrointestinal abnormalities detected antenatally are omphalocele, gastroschisis, and diaphragmatic hernia. The accuracy of ultrasound in such conditions is high with a very low false-positive rate.[1] Gastrointestinal anomalies should be managed by a fetal medicine specialist in collaboration with a neonatal pediatrician, pediatric surgeon, clinical geneticist, and anesthesiologist. The patient should meet this multidisciplinary team before delivery either on an individual basis or as a group. Parental informational needs vary with the stage in the diagnostic and treatment pathway.[2]

OMPHALOCELE (EXOMPHALOS)

General

This is an extraembryonic hernia due to the arrest of ventral medial migration of the dermatomyotomes. Omphalocele occurs in between 1 in 2500 and 1 in 5000 pregnancies, though this may vary with location and ethnicity.[3] "Physiologic" herniation of abdominal contents into the base of the umbilical cord is normal up until approximately 11 weeks' gestation (Fig. 19–1) and must be distinguished from an omphalocele. Importantly, omphalocele is associated with other malformations 60% to 80% of the time,[4] especially when the omphalocele is superior to the umbilicus. Pentalogy of Cantrell is a particularly severe defect consisting of a supraumbilical omphalocele, a defect in the lower sternum, deficiency of the anterior part of the diaphragm, defects of the diaphragmatic part of the pericardium, and a range of cardiac abnormalities.[5] Survival is poor, particularly with major cardiac abnormalities and aneuploidy.[6] The genomic imprinting disorder Beckwith-Wiedemann syndrome (macroglossia, organomegaly, and hypoglycaemia) is also associated with omphalocele.

Diagnosis

An omphalocele is an extra-abdominal mass enclosed in a membrane. The diagnosis is made after 11 weeks' gestation when an anterior, extra-abdominal mass is detected upon which the umbilical cord inserts rather than into the anterior abdominal wall (Fig. 19–2). Hydramnios may be present. Defect size and type have some prognostic significance. Although the omphalocele contents are usually contained in a membrane, this may rupture spontaneously. A rare variant is the "giant" omphalocele (Fig. 19–3) in which the abdominal defect is massive with a base greater than 6 cm in diameter and most of the liver is extracorporeal. Giant defects and those in which the membrane has ruptured are often associated with a small or defective thoracic cage, pulmonary hypoplasia, and postnatal respiratory complications.[7] There may be difficulty distinguishing gastroschisis from ruptured omphalocele, but the latter is commonly associated with other abnormalities (Table 19–1). Fetal growth restriction is common, and approximately one in six fetuses will be chromosomally abnormal. A small omphalocele may be missed on ultrasonography, especially if the fluid volume is reduced. However, the sensitivity of ultrasound detection exceeds 95% with a specificity of 100%.[6] The presence of a thickened cord insertion without definite signs of an omphalocele should raise the possibility of an occult omphalocele or umbilical hernia. Care should be taken to clamp the umbilical cord at delivery at least 5 cm from the neonate's abdominal wall to avoid inadvertent bowel occlusion.[8] Similarly, the presence of umbilical cord cysts requires careful follow-up.[9]

Both omphalocele and gastroschisis produce a very high maternal serum α-fetoprotein concentration during the second trimester. Amniotic fluid, if sampled, will show a faint acetylcholinesterase band and a dense pseudocholinesterase band. This pattern is opposite that of a neural tube defect.[10]

Risks

There are few obstetric risks to the mother apart from the rare complication of hydramnios. Perinatal risks include those of invasive diagnostic testing, the implications of

FIGURE 19–1
Normal ultrasound appearance of fetus at 11 weeks shows the abdominal contents (*arrow*) outside the body cavity.

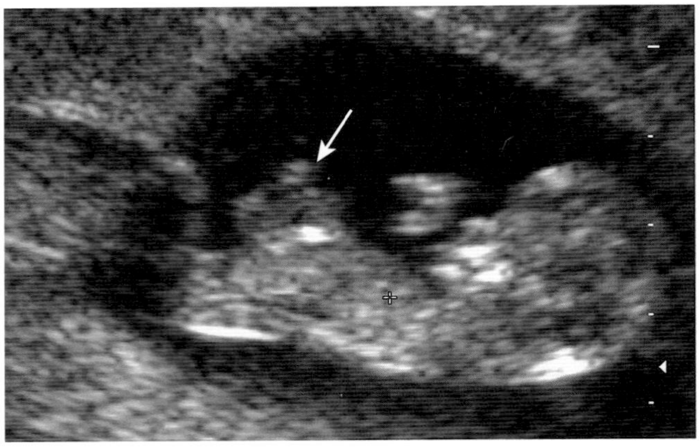

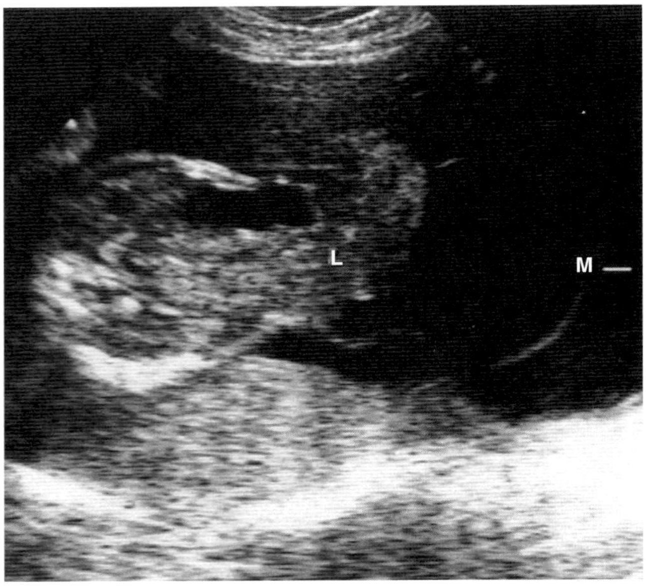

FIGURE 19–2
Omphalocele. Characteristic ultrasound appearance of omphalocele with a membrane (M) surrounding the liver (L) and bowel.

associated abnormalities, and postnatal surgery that may be complicated when the liver is extracorporeal.

Management Options

Prenatal

The first step is to exclude other abnormalities. This mandates a detailed ultrasonographic examination, including a fetal echocardiogram and a fetal karyotype. Abnormal cardiac findings occur in 45% of fetuses with omphalocele.[11] The ultrasonographic differentiation between omphalocele and gastroschisis is important and generally not difficult. The presence of a sac or membrane around the contents with the umbilical cord inserting upon it is pathognomonic. Difficulties arise when the sac has ruptured spontaneously or when the relationship of the herniated tissue to the umbilical cord insertion is unclear. On occasion, thickened loops of bowel in the fetus with gastroschisis may appear as a covering membrane. The peritoneal membrane can also be

FIGURE 19–3
Giant omphalocele. Ultrasound appearance of a giant omphalocele shows a massive amount of extracorporeal tissue and cord insertion.

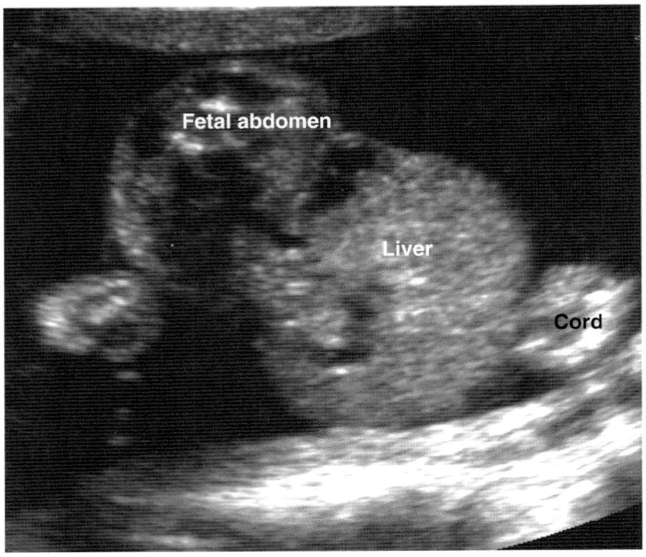

TABLE 19–1
Associated Anomalies in Omphalocele

Pentalogy of Cantrell
Diaphragmatic hernia
Pericardial defect
Distal sternal defect
Omphalocele
Cardiovascular malformations
Cloacal Exstrophy—OEIS
Omphalocele
Bladder or cloacal extrophy
Other caudal abnormalities
Beckwith-Wiedemann Syndrome
Omphalocele
Macroglossia
Generalized organomegaly (autosomal dominant)
Hypoglycemia
Aneuploidy
Trisomies (13, 18, and 21)
Triploidy
Turner's syndrome
Other Abnormalities
Cardiac (atrial septal defect, ventricular septal defect, patent ductus arteriosus, pulmonary stenosis)
Gastrointestinal (atresias, Meckel's diverticulum, imperforate anus)
Renal
Neurologic (meningocele, holoprosencephaly, microphthalmos)

OEIS, omphalocele, exstrophy of the bladder, imperforate anus, and spina bifida.

difficult to visualize when there is oligohydramnios. In contrast to gastroschisis, extracorporeal liver is common (40%). Fetuses with intracorporeal liver are more likely to have chromosomal abnormalities, as are fetuses with other malformations and those with mothers of advanced age. There is probably little prognostic significance of the omphalocele contents if the karyotype is normal, except for a worse prognosis with large defects.

Parental counseling should stress the importance of a fetal karyotype. Studies based on prenatal as opposed to postnatal diagnosis show a generally poor prognosis owing to the large number of associated abnormalities and aneuploidy, especially trisomy 18.[7] Fetuses with isolated omphalocele generally have a good prognosis (although not all abnormalities may be detected before birth). Even with postnatal diagnosis, the survival rate of otherwise normal infants exceeds 75%.[12] Large abdominal wall defects can pose particular problems for both neonatal respiratory management and surgical closure, and these issues should be covered during counseling with the neonatologist and pediatric surgeon. Death of the otherwise normal infant results from prematurity sepsis or problems with short gut syndrome, which is more common with gastroschisis than with omphalocele. Long-term follow-up suggests that the quality of life for adults is similar to that of the general population, although disorders of the abdominal wall scar are reported in 37% of cases and functional gastrointestinal disorders in 51%.[13] Various orthotic interventions are available to assist in the management of giant omphalocele.[14] Parents may benefit from illustrations showing typical defects before (Fig. 19–4) and after surgery. The option of termination of pregnancy should be discussed with parents, especially when other abnormalities are present. Prolonged hospitalization, repeat surgery, and quality of life are all issues that influence parental decision-making.

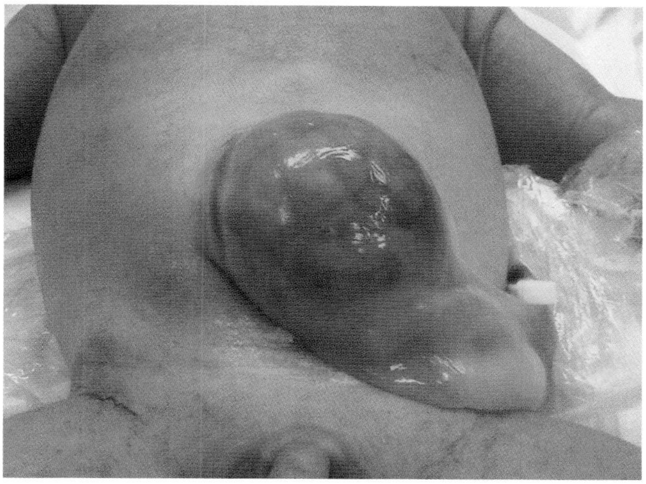

FIGURE 19–4
Omphalocele at delivery. The lesion is epigastric and at the site of the umbilical cord insertion. The contents of the omphalocele may be seen through the membrane.

Labor and Delivery

Delivery should occur in a center with a neonatal medical and surgical team in attendance to optimize the transition to ex utero life and the preoperative care. There is no evidence that elective cesarean delivery a priori confers any benefit to the fetus or neonate with omphalocele with or without a ruptured sac and irrespective of the contents of the sac.[15] Theoretical concerns for vaginal delivery, including visceral trauma, dystocia, and infection, are unsupported. In one series in which the diagnosis was known in only a minority of cases, cesarean delivery made no difference to neonatal outcome.[16] There are untested scenarios in which cesarean delivery might be considered, such as extracorporeal liver when torsion with obstructed cardiac return is a theoretical concern. Neonatal morbidity in all recent series relates to associated anomalies and prematurity. Isolated cases with late morbidity and death relate mostly to complications of bowel obstruction or short bowel syndrome in association with intestinal atresia.[17]

Postnatal

Prevention of heat and fluid loss and infection are the initial goals after delivery while the neonatal evaluation is completed and the surgery planned. These infants are at increased risk of hypothermia owing to the large surface area of exposed viscera. The neonate is immediately lowered into a sterile plastic bag containing warm electrolyte (no warmer than 37.5°C), plasma solution, and antibiotics (e.g., Vi-Drape isolation bag). In emergencies, any sterile bag with warmed normal saline or lactated Ringer's solution and antibiotics will suffice. A suitable solution consists of 1 L lactated Ringer's solution, 0.5 L stable plasma protein or similar solution, and 1 million units of penicillin. The bag is tied at the level of the axillae and care is taken to avoid torsion of viscera. Alternatively, a sterile plastic bag without the fluid may be used. A nasogastric tube is passed to keep the bowel decompressed, and ventilatory support is provided when necessary.

Neonates with associated lethal structural malformations or trisomy 13 or 18 are typically managed nonsurgically. Untreated neonates generally die of dehydration or sepsis. There are two main options for comfort care: either keep the neonate comfortable, providing supportive care only, or paint the unruptured omphalocele sac with 1% mercurochrome solution, although this has been associated with renal failure. Silver sulfadiazine is now the preferred compound when surgical closure is not planned or possible in the short term.

All other infants are managed surgically with operative repair as soon as the general condition is stable. It is difficult to predict antenatally whether a primary surgical closure is possible. Small defects less than 4 cm in diameter and without extracorporeal liver are almost always closed primarily. Large defects, or those containing liver, may not be closable at the first operation. When primary closure is not feasible, the defect and contents are covered with a Silastic silo sutured to the edge of the defect. Over the following days, the contents of the silo gradually enter the abdominal cavity under the influence of gravity coupled with the silo being compressed daily. Care must be taken to avoid respiratory or circulatory compromise during these maneuvers.

Postoperative problems common to all abdominal wall defect repairs include respiratory embarrassment, pulmonary hypertension, small bowel perforation, bowel obstruction, and malrotation. The average neonatal hospital stay after a silo ranges from 3 to 4 weeks. Parenteral nutrition is often necessary for days or weeks postoperatively. In some cases, it may be 3 months before satisfactory bowel function is achieved. Weakness of the anterior abdominal wall or a poor cosmetic result after the initial surgery may be corrected in a subsequent plastic surgical revision. Adhesive small bowel obstruction is not uncommon after surgical correction of congenital abdominal wall defects, particularly in the first year of life, but this together with pain and constipation may be long-term complications.[18]

The long-term prognosis for surviving infants is generally very good, and in the absence of associated structural or chromosomal abnormalities, the risk of recurrence in a subsequent pregnancy is extremely low. The main recurrence risk is that for the associated abnormalities, although case reports of a familial recurrence have been recorded.[19] Evidence from studies of the prevalence of fetal abnormalities after grain fortification with folic acid suggests that folate supplementation reduces the risk of omphalocele but not gastroschisis.[20]

GASTROSCHISIS

General

Gastroschisis is a paraumbilical defect, usually on the right side of the anterior abdominal wall lateral to the umbilical vessels. Left-sided defects are rare but may be associated with increased risks of other abnormalities.[21] The annual prevalence of gastroschisis approximates 1 in 2500 to 1 in 3000 live births with an equal sex ratio. Many studies appear to confirm an increasing incidence of gastroschisis, particularly in young, low-parity women.[22,23] The reason for the increase is not entirely explained by increased recognition of the problem. Gastroschisis has been considered a developmental accident (disruption), but the available genetic and epidemiologic evidence, as well as that from animal models, is more consistent with it being an abnormality during embryogenesis (malformation).[24,25] However, the precise etiology remains controversial.

Recent studies have suggested associations with recreational drug use, vasoactive substances, and aspirin,[26] although not all authors have implicated aspirin.[27] Iatrogenic abdominal wall defects have also resulted from placement of a vesicoamniotic shunt for obstructive uropathy. Large birth

SUMMARY OF MANAGEMENT OPTIONS

Exomphalos/Omphalocele

Management Options	Evidence Quality and Recommendation	References
Prenatal		
Offer karyotyping (aneuploidy more likely if the liver is intra-abdominal).	III/B	4,6,12
Assess for other structural defects (especially cardiac) with ultrasound.	III/B	4,6,7,11
Anticipate risk of prematurity.	III/B	7,19
Offer multidisciplinary counseling.	—/GPP	
Offer termination of pregnancy especially with associated abnormalities.	III/B	4,7
Labor and Delivery		
Mode of delivery does not affect outcome.	III/B	15,16
Delivery is recommended in a tertiary unit with neonatal surgical facilities.	—/GPP	—
Respiratory distress may occur with ruptured or giant omphalocele.	IV/C	7
Neonatal Management		
Necrotizing enterocolitis is associated with increased mortality rate.	III/B	12
Place abdominal contents in a sterile plastic bag with isotonic solutions to prevent heat loss.	GPP	
Assess for associated bowel malformations.	III/B	17
Counsel parents that recurrence risk is low.	III/B	19

GPP, good practice point.

FIGURE 19–5
Gastroschisis. *A*, Transverse section of a 14-week fetus shows the cord insertion adjacent to the abdominal wall defect on two-dimensional scanning and color-flow Doppler. *B*, Sagittal section of a fetus with gastroschisis. Note the absence of a membrane surrounding the bowel. *C*, Gastroschisis at 14 weeks' gestation shown on three-dimensional ultrasound.

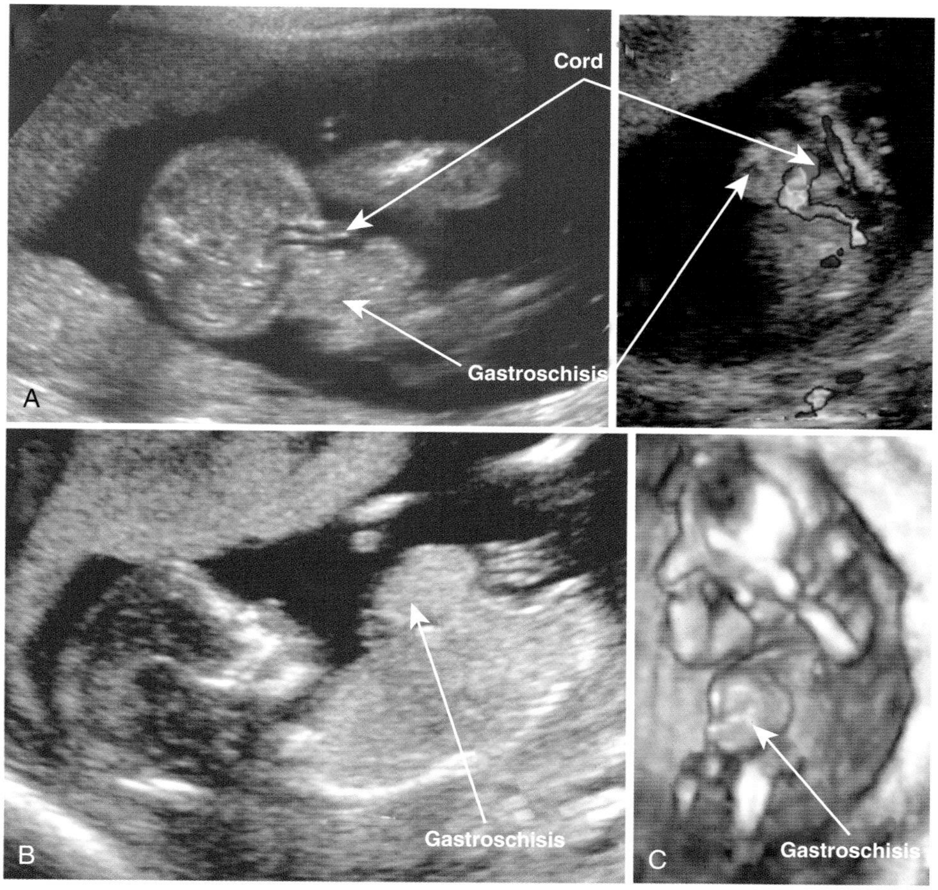

defect registers suggest an incidence of associated defects of around 10%,[28] with cardiac defects being seen in 10% of cases.[29]

Diagnosis

The ultrasonographic image is one of free-floating loops of bowel with no covering membrane, typically appearing like a clump of grapes (Fig. 19–5).

Risks

Maternal risks are similar to those for omphalocele, reflecting complications of the anomaly. Fetal risks are associated with complications of bowel torsion that compromise the vascular supply or obstruction associated with atretic segments of intestine. The mechanism of damage to the extruded bowel serosa in contact with amniotic fluid remains unclear, and there are a number of theories for the formation of the so-called peel or perivisceritis. Matting of the bowel, detected on ultrasound, has been associated with the presence of meconium in the amniotic fluid and peel formation.[30] However, there is little evidence that the presence of peel affects the outcomes after surgical repair. Fetal growth restriction frequently complicates gastroschisis but is not necessarily secondary to uteroplacental vascular dysfunction.

Neonatal complications include not only reduction and closure of the gastroschisis but also atretic segments and critical shortening of the bowel. Other short-term complications relate to the use of total parental nutrition, and some children suffer longer-term bowel dysfunction and neurodevelopmental delay, especially when there has been fetal growth restriction.[31]

Management Options

Prenatal

Although the risk of associated structural abnormalities is lower than that for omphalocele, a detailed ultrasonographic search remains important. The risk of an abnormal karyotype is 1% to 3%,[28] with trisomy 18 being the most common aneuploidy. Many physicians do not consider a karyotype necessary if the gastroschisis is isolated. The most common associated abnormalities are cardiac. Other abnormalities such as bowel stenosis and/or atresia are complications of the gastroschisis itself. Cleft palate and diaphragmatic hernia have also been reported. On rare occasions, other viscera may be present within the gastroschisis including liver, uterus, and testes.

Serial ultrasonographic examination is recommended to assess fetal growth, amniotic fluid volume, and bowel appearance. However, any appraisal of fetal nutrition based on the abdominal circumference measurement is limited because any defect will artifactually reduce the circumference. Oligohydramnios may be associated with fetal growth restriction secondary to uteroplacental dysfunction. Hydramnios is the only antenatal ultrasonographic finding correlated with severe neonatal bowel complications.[32] The appearance of the bowel and the diameter of the bowel loops are not of prognostic significance.[33,34] Increased echogenicity and apparent thickening of the bowel wall after 28 weeks may represent a fibrinous coating or peel covering binding together loops of bowel. The etiology of the peel and interventions to prevent it are debated. There is conflicting evidence for the hypothesis that amniotic fluid components cause a chemical peritonitis. Although there is evidence of intra-amniotic inflammation in human gastroschisis,[35] prolonged intestinal exposure to amniotic fluid does not invariably lead to peel formation.[36] Amnioinfusion or amnioexchange procedures are reported,[37] but there is little evidence of benefit.

An alternative explanation for peel formation is venous and lymphatic obstruction, a hypothesis supported by the observation that the intra-abdominal peritoneum does not always show a peel, although it too is exposed to amniotic fluid. Although the presence of peel can make the surgical closure more difficult, it has little correlation with outcome and resolves quickly after surgical closure. Although increasing dilation of bowel loops might appear worrisome, it is not an indication for delivery (Fig. 19–6).[38] There is no evidence to suggest that early delivery to decrease exposure to amniotic fluid improves outcome. Term delivery at 37 weeks' gestation allows for an earlier, definitive closure of the defect and shorter times to full oral feedings.[39]

Parental counseling should emphasize the high chance of a good outcome with over 90% survival and a primary closure rate over 60%, reaching almost 100% in some units (Vipul Upadhyay, personal communication). Median hospitalization time is 27 days, although prolonged hospitalization up to 444 days has been recorded.[40,41] Repeated admission is often necessary with short bowel syndromes. Long-term follow-up studies suggest some morbidity related to bowel dysfunction and an increased risk of neurodevelopmental delays in fetuses with growth restriction.[31] Uncontrolled psychological studies have suggested that children followed to 10 years of age after surgery for abdominal wall defects may have more behavioral and learning problems than expected.[42]

Epidemiologic studies have shown a relationship between intrauterine death and abnormalities of amniotic fluid volume, especially oligohydramnios, and growth restriction.[22,43] The median gestational age of fetal death in one study was 34 weeks.[22] Close monitoring during the last trimester and especially toward term is therefore recommended. In the absence of abnormalities of growth, amniotic fluid volume, umbilical artery Doppler, or cardiotocography, the pregnancy may continue to term. There is little evidence that delivery before 37 weeks improves outcome.

Labor and Delivery

Fetuses with a gastroschisis should be delivered at a referral center equipped with the appropriate facilities and staff. Cesarean delivery does not improve outcome,[44] and there is some evidence that survival rate is higher in fetuses subjected to labor. Thus, in the absence of other complications, vaginal delivery should be anticipated.

Postnatal

The immediate postnatal management is similar to that for omphalocele, but the preoperative workup and stabilization of the newborn should be expedited, because there is no protecting membrane over the bowel (Fig. 19–7). The neonate is immediately placed into a Lehey bag (or even a sterile plastic oven bag) containing the warmed electrolyte and antibiotic solution, as described under "Omphalocele." The bag is carefully tied at the axillae so not to kink or rotate the bowel, and a nasogastric tube is passed to keep the bowel decompressed.

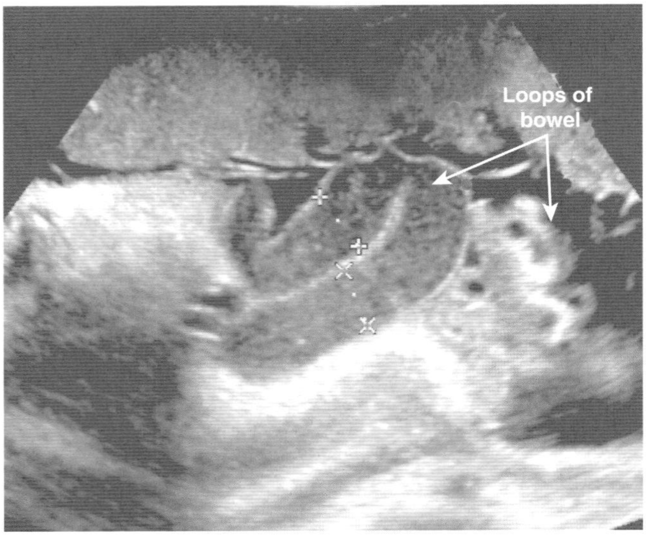

FIGURE 19–6
Gastroschisis. Dilated loops of bowel. This fetus was delivered vaginally at term and primary abdominal wall closure was achieved.

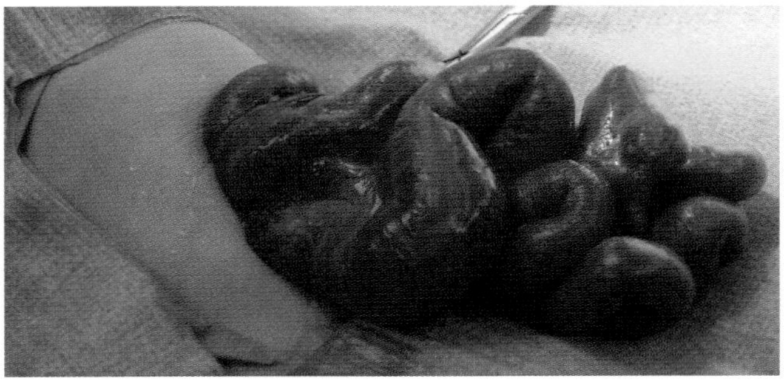

FIGURE 19–7
Gastroschisis at delivery, unusually containing the liver. The baby was delivered by cesarean section, the indications being a footling breech presentation.

Primary closure is achieved in over 80% of cases.[45] Postoperative ventilation is generally required for about 72 hours, and total parenteral nutrition is generally required until oral feeding can commence. The surgical approach is generally a transverse incision at the level of the defect if required. A careful examination of the bowel is made for atretic segments. Any bowel incision made is closed transversely to minimize the risk of a subsequent stricture, and the abdominal wall defect is closed vertically with the umbilical cord left in place to produce a "normal" umbilicus (Fig. 19–8). When primary closure is not possible, a Silastic silo is created as with omphalocele (Fig. 19–9). Failure to pass stool by 28 days mandates a new search for atresia,, which occurs in up to 5%.[46]

The mortality rate is between 3% and 10% and is associated with prematurity, intestinal ischemia or necrosis, late sepsis, or the effects of other abnormalities. Prolonged bowel dysfunction, especially motility disorders or malabsorption, occurs in a small number of cases. Postoperative hospitalization, duration of ventilation, total parenteral nutrition, and establishment of oral feeding are generally longer after repair of gastroschisis than omphalocele.[47] One of the only long-term studies of patients with gastroschisis found that development beyond 5 years of age was normal in fetuses with isolated lesions.[48] Those with bowel atresia or complications requiring bowel resection had a higher frequency of long-term bowel problems or nonspecific abdominal complaints. Rarely, in centers where available, intestinal transplantation may be a therapy for short bowel syndrome.[49]

The risk of recurrence in subsequent pregnancies is very low, though isolated case reports indicate that familial recurrence is possible.[50] Fear of recurrence of an abdominal wall defect may affect the reproductive choices of couples.[51]

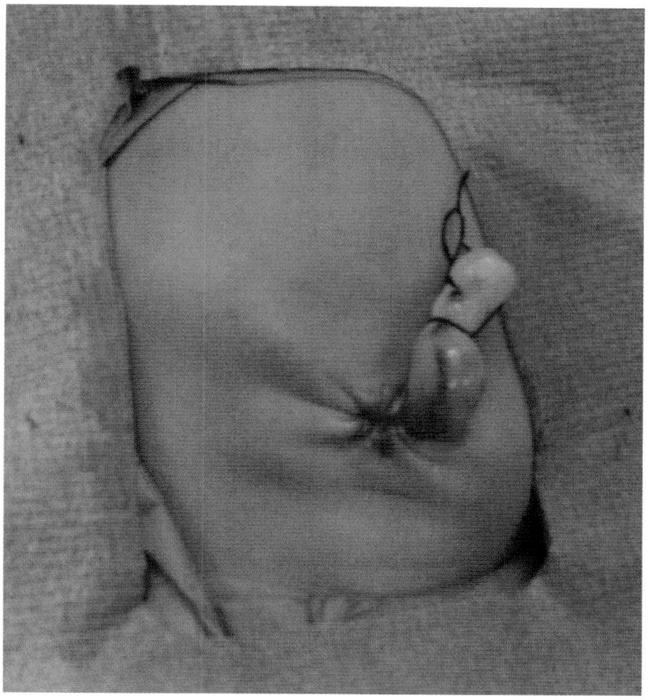

FIGURE 19–8
Abdominal wall closure in gastroschisis. Similar results are usually obtained with or without previous use of a silo.

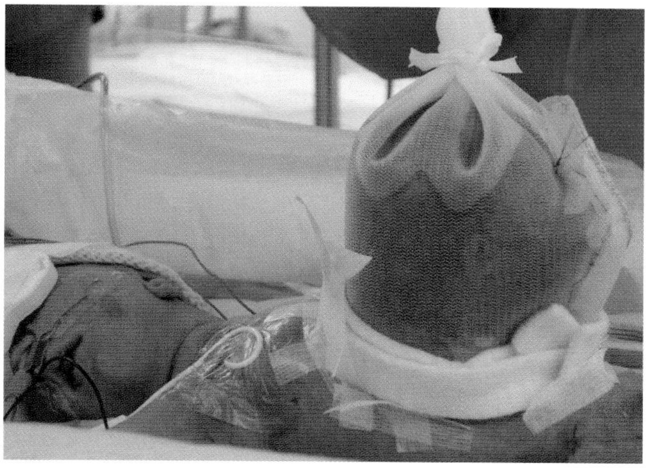

FIGURE 19–9
Silastic silo used to cover the bowel. The silo is reduced in size over 7 days as its contents are returned to the abdomen.

SUMMARY OF MANAGEMENT OPTIONS

Gastroschisis

Management Options	Evidence Quality and Recommendation	References
Prenatal		
Assess for other anomalies (especially cardiac) with ultrasound.	III/B	28,29
Need for karyotyping is unclear.	III/B	11,28
No indication to deliver prematurely.	III/B	38,39
Increased surveillance to assess risk of death, prematurity, and fetal growth restriction.	III/B	43
Provide multidisciplinary counseling.	—/GPP	—

SUMMARY OF MANAGEMENT OPTIONS

Gastroschisis—cont'd

Management Options	Evidence Quality and Recommendation	References
Labor and Delivery		
Mode of delivery does not affect outcome.	III/B	44
Monitor for intrapartum fetal distress.	III/B	43
Deliver a center with neonatal surgical facilities.	—/GPP	—
Handle bowel carefully; place contents in a sterile plastic bag with isotonic solutions.	—/GPP	—
Neonatal Management		
Primary early closure minimizes morbidity.	III/B	34,44
Assess for associated bowel malformations.	III/B	34,40
Prevent heat and fluid loss; plan early surgery.	—/GPP	—
Counsel parents that recurrence risk low.	III/B	50

GPP, good practice point.

CONGENITAL DIAPHRAGMATIC HERNIA

General

Diaphragmatic hernia is a protrusion or herniation of the abdominal contents into the thoracic cavity. Herniation may occur through a posterolateral defect in the pleuroperitoneal canal (the most common is the hernia of the foramen of Bochdalek), a defect in the sternocostal hiatus, the retrosternal or Morgagni hernia, a hiatus hernia, a defect in the central tendon of the diaphragm, and through complete eventration of the diaphragm. The reported annual prevalence is 1 in 3500 live births,[52] but this does not include terminations and stillbirths. Left-sided hernias are more common. Up to 50% of antenatally diagnosed cases have associated abnormalities,[53] and diaphragmatic hernia is associated with a number of syndromes, including Beckwith-Wiedemann, Pierre Robin, Fryns, and chromosomal defects such as trisomy 13, trisomy 18, and deletion 9p. Lung hypoplasia, central to the poor prognosis of diaphragmatic hernia, may originate during embryogenesis and before the visceral herniation into the thoracic cavity.[54] However, a recent study of fetal lung growth in 84 fetuses with congenital diaphragmatic hernia has challenged this view; differences in both alveolar and pulmonary vascular development were evident only in the third trimester compared with gestation-matched controls.[55] Postnatally, both pulmonary hypoplasia and pulmonary hypertension may be lethal.

Diagnosis

The most common postnatal presentation is cyanosis shortly after clamping the umbilical cord. Other signs include a scaphoid abdomen (Fig. 19–10), a barrel-shaped chest, and dextrocardia. Diaphragmatic hernia is the most common cause of dextrocardia diagnosed in the delivery suite.

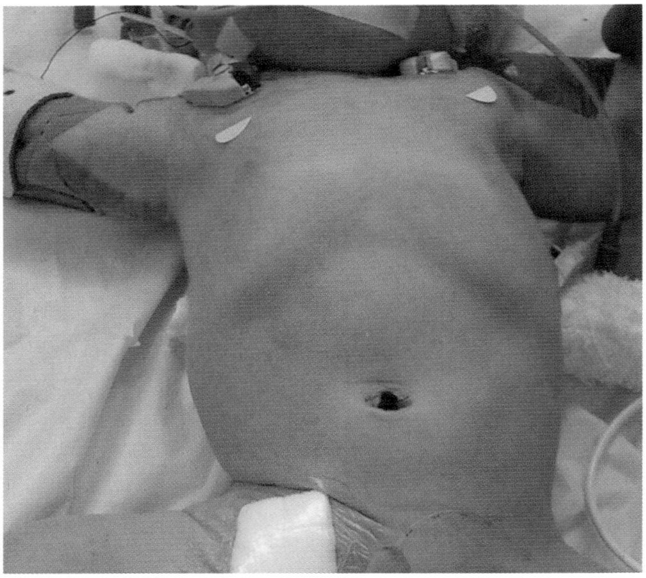

FIGURE 19–10
Neonate with congenital diaphragmatic hernia shows scaphoid abdomen.

The antenatal ultrasonographic diagnosis can be difficult. A multinational study achieved an overall detection rate of 59%. Diaphragmatic hernia was detected in 51% of isolated cases and 72% of cases with additional malformations.[56] Small hernias may be missed by even the most experienced ultrasonographers. A right-sided diaphragmatic hernia is extremely difficult to identify because the liver and lung are of similar echogenicity in early pregnancy. As pregnancy advances, the lungs become more echogenic. The hypoechoic line seen on ultrasonography separating the thoracic from the abdominal cavities is an unreliable sign for the exclusion of diaphragmatic hernia. The most sensitive sign is an abnormal thoracic location of the heart[57] (Fig. 19–11). Other signs, which are not necessarily prognostic, include hydramnios, visualization of the bowel or stomach at the level of the heart, and absence of the stomach in the abdomen. Hydramnios may result from either impaired swallowing (due to mediastinal compression) or obstruction of the upper gastrointestinal tract.

Several techniques can be used to aid diagnosis if there is uncertainty. Color and pulsed Doppler ultrasonography can help delineate the vascular anatomy when there is an echogenic mass in the fetal thorax. Magnetic resonance imaging (MRI) is especially helpful to confirm the presence of the liver in the thorax.

Management Options

Prenatal

The differential diagnosis of an intrathoracic ultrasonographic abnormality includes

- Diaphragmatic hernia.
- Cystic adenomatoid malformation of the lung.
- Extralobar sequestration (may be intra-abdominal).
- Bronchial atresia.
- Other cystic and solid mediastinal masses.

It is important to exclude other structural abnormalities notably in the cardiovascular (e.g., ventricular septal defect, tetralogy of Fallot), gastrointestinal, skeletal, and genitourinary systems because they may profoundly affect the prognosis. A karyotype is indicated. A summary of seven series revealed an overall incidence of aneuploidy of 18%; only 2% when the diaphragmatic hernia was isolated but up to 34% when other abnormalities were present.[58]

One of the challenges of antenatal assessment of congenital diaphragmatic hernia is the prediction of postnatal outcome. The option of pregnancy termination should be discussed with the parents, especially when other abnormalities are present, because the combination is generally fatal. Population-based studies indicate an overall survival rate for isolated diaphragmatic hernia of approximately 65%.[59] Although some units with extracorporeal membrane oxygenation (ECMO) facilities[60] quote survival rates over 90%, others do not.[61] Survival rates depend on a number of prenatal factors. Thus, definitive statements on the optimal management providing the highest survival rates are difficult to make at present.

There is considerable debate on the accuracy of antenatal prediction of postnatal prognosis. Early diagnosis (<25 wk) appears to be associated with poor prognosis (mortality rate ≤58%).[59,62] Hydramnios and the location of the fetal stomach do not appear to be prognostic factors,[62] nor do fetal echocardiographic variables in structurally normal hearts.[63] The presence of liver in the chest is a poor prognostic sign[62] and is associated with the triad of hydramnios, mediastinal shift, and intrathoracic stomach. This is consistent with the finding of right-sided diaphragmatic hernia being an independent risk factor for decreased survival.[59,62] The ratio of the fetal lung diameters to the head circumference (lung-to-head circumference ratio [LHR]) (Fig. 19–12) has been used as a guide to prognosis, but results have been inconsistent, possibly due to differing methods of determining the ratio, correcting for the presence of intrathoracic liver, or the effect of gestation.[64] Most series have reported measurement of LHR between 22 and 28 weeks' gestation; a ratio less than 0.8 has been associated with a 100% mortality whereas values greater than 1.4 have been associated with virtually no mortality.[65] Liver herniation and the LHR

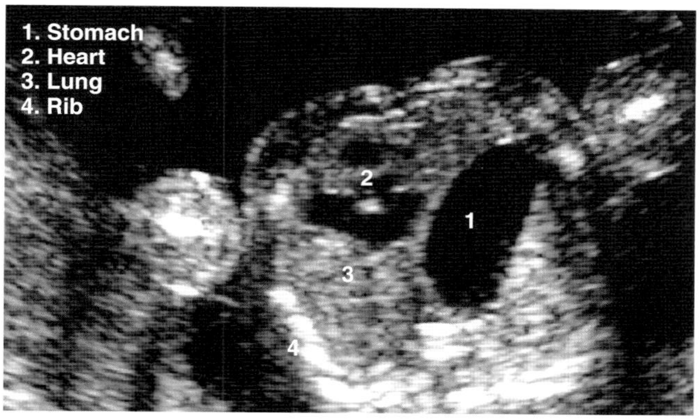

FIGURE 19–11
Ultrasound image of fetal thorax shows the appearances of a diaphragmatic hernia. Note that the heart and stomach are visualized in the same imaging plane.

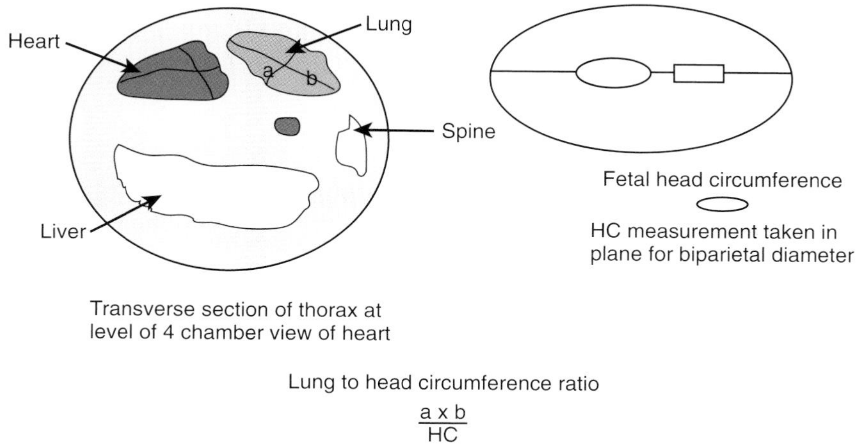

FIGURE 19–12
The lung-to-head circumference ratio. The two diameters of the contralateral lung, "a" and "b," are multiplied together, that is, a × b and divided by the head circumference.

have been found to be independent predictors of survival; in a review of 184 cases of left-sided congenital diaphragmatic hernia with intrathoracic liver, the overall survival was 50% and an LHR less than 1.0 was associated with a very poor prognosis.[66] When there was no liver herniation, the survival was 76.5% after 32 weeks and the LHR did not provide independent prognostic information. It is likely that changes in case selection rather than new postnatal therapies have resulted in the improved survival data. A low lung-to-heart ratio has also been reported to be a poor prognostic sign, but this is not consistent in the literature.[66]

Determination of the fetal lung volumes can be achieved by both three-dimensional (3D) ultrasound and MRI,[67] and there is a high correlation between the two modalities.[68] MRI may provide superior imaging of the ipsilateral lung compared with ultrasound. Total lung volumes, measured by MRI, were compared with LHR in one study of 148 infants born after 30 weeks' gestation. Prediction of postnatal survival was comparable between the two methods.[69] It remains to be shown whether volumetric approaches will improve the prediction of survival or guide management.

A summary of the factors considered influential on outcome is shown in Table 19–2. None are accepted as completely reliable because this condition has a spectrum of fatality or morbidity owing to varied factors, including pulmonary hypoplasia, pulmonary hypertension, morphologic and biochemical abnormalities of the lungs, and the longer-term sequelae of treatment. Consequently, some parents may opt for termination of the pregnancy rather than the uncertainty of continuing with antenatal or postnatal treatments.

Recent experience has clarified the role of fetal surgery. There is no benefit from open fetal surgery for isolated congenital diaphragmatic hernia because the results have been shown to be worse than conventional management after birth.[70] The procedure that appears to be most effective in the prevention of the egress of lung fluid from the trachea, thereby stimulating lung growth and development, is tracheal occlusion with a balloon. The indications for percutaneous fetoscopic endoluminal tracheal occlusion (FETO) have been reported as intrathoracic liver and LHR less than 1.0 at a gestation of 26 to 28 weeks.[71]

Initially, removal of the tracheal occluding balloon was done at delivery and access to facilities to perform ex utero intrapartum treatment (EXIT) were necessary. However, it now appears that endoscopic deflation or removal of the tracheal balloon is associated with high survival. In this poor prognosis group of fetuses, survival rates of 55% are reported.[71] The timing and duration of tracheal occlusion are under investigation.

Obstetrically, the pregnancy is monitored closely for the development of hydramnios. There is limited evidence that the antenatal administration of corticosteroids reduces the severity of lung disease, and pulmonary surfactant deficiency and human trials remain incomplete. When the parents elect to continue with the pregnancy, they should meet with a member of the surgical team before delivery who will explain that a period of preoperative stabilization after birth yields better results than immediate surgical repair. Poor ventilatory parameters that fail to improve with preoperative stabilization generally do not improve postoperatively, and the prognosis is poor.

Labor and Delivery

There is no a priori indication for cesarean delivery. In the absence of massive hydramnios, labor and delivery are generally normal. However, these deliveries should be planned and occur at a referral center equipped for all likely complications.

Postnatal

Immediate intubation, ventilation, and paralysis of the newborn facilitate care, because the maintenance of good oxygenation is a good prognostic sign. Typically, the chest radiograph shows mediastinal shift with abdominal contents in the thorax (Fig. 19–13). A small study reported that maintenance of the mediastinum in a central position by preventing overdistention of the larger lung is associated with improved postoperative survival.[72] This suggests that special care should be taken during the resuscitation to avoid

TABLE 19–2

Factors Reported to Adversely Affect Prognosis in Diaphragmatic Hernia

Additional anomalies
Early diagnosis (<25 wk' gestation)
Liver in the chest
Small lung size–lung head ratio or lung volumes
Bilateral diaphragmatic hernias

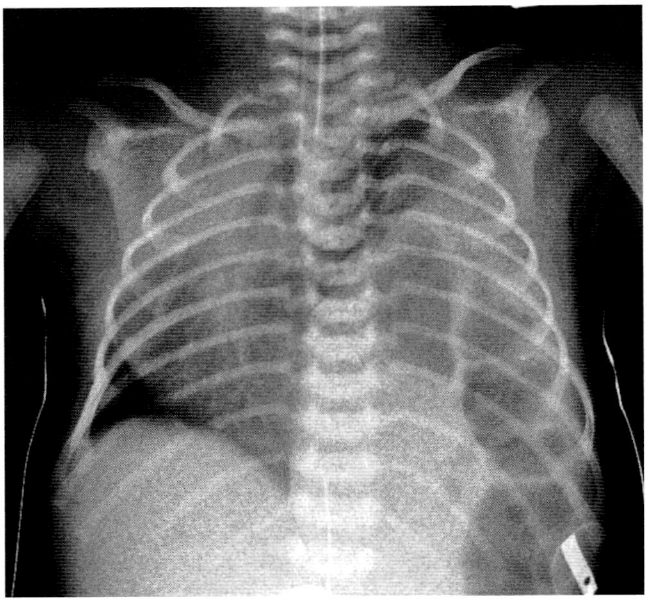

FIGURE 19–13
Diaphragmatic hernia. Neonatal chest radiograph shows the heart displaced to the right and abdominal contents in the left thorax.

FIGURE 19–14
Diaphragmatic hernia. *A*, At surgery, the defect is shown as the contents of the hernia are being removed from the thorax. *B*, A large defect after the contents have been removed. *C*, Closure of the diaphragmatic defect. *D*, Wound closure and chest drain.

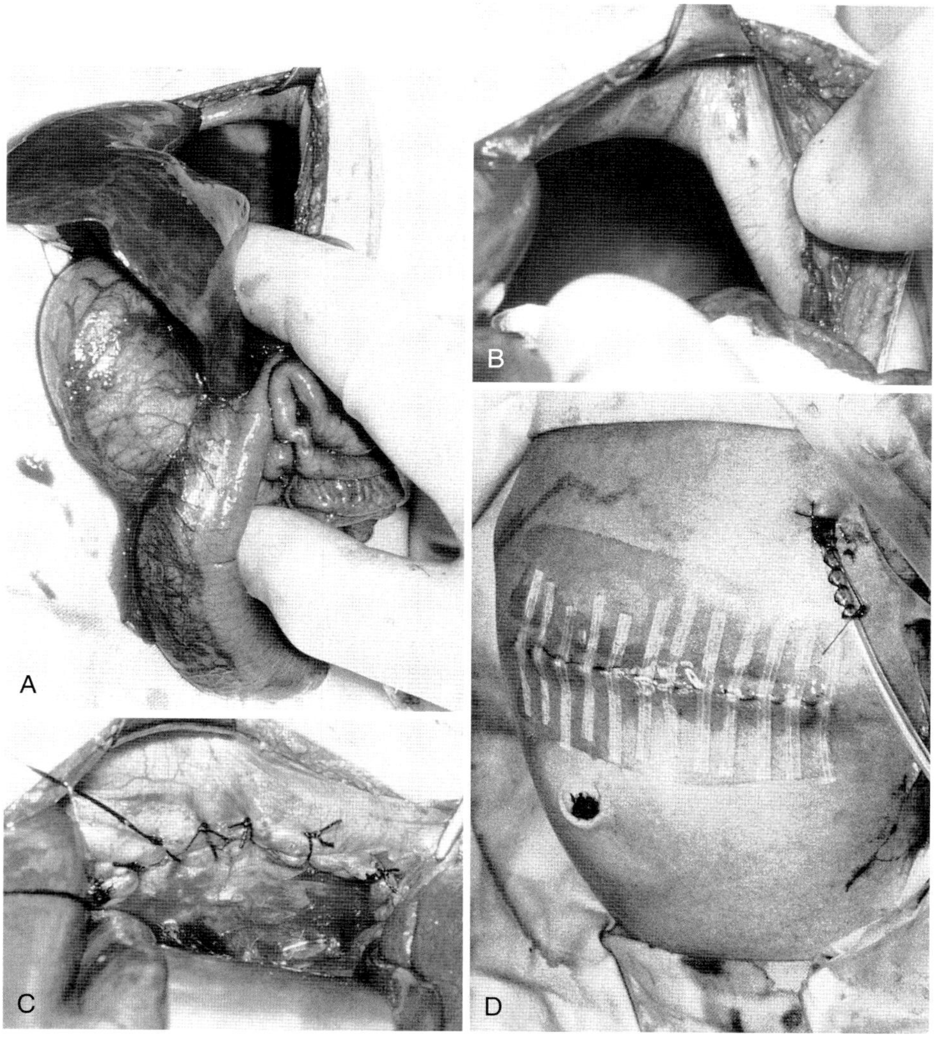

causing excessive mediastinal shift or lung overdistention. There is presently insufficient evidence to support either a policy of early (<24 hr) or late (>24 hr) repair after delivery.[73]

ECMO is available in some centers for those neonates who cannot be adequately oxygenated using conventional ventilatory techniques. The criteria for ECMO vary between centers, as may the criteria for what constitutes good response. The role of ECMO remains controversial,[74] but its main place is probably in the stabilization of the neonate at the time when the fine pulmonary vasculature is very reactive, because the usual run times on ECMO are too short to permit postnatal lung growth. Use of ECMO to treat respiratory failure in congenital diaphragmatic hernia appears to be associated with a consistent 50% mortality.[74] The place of other postnatal treatments, including surfactant, partial liquid ventilation, pulmonary vasodilators, and lung transplantation, remains to be determined. A diaphragmatic hernia and its repair are illustrated in Figure 19–14.

Survivors of postnatal repairs may suffer long-term morbidity secondary to bronchopulmonary dysplasia or other lung degenerative disorders, such as emphysema. As the numbers of survivors increases so to do the neurologic, nutritional, and musculoskeletal morbidities.[75] However, overall these problems occur in the minority of affected children, and in general, the long-term prognosis is good if the neonate survives beyond surgery.

The recurrence risk is low, except where the defect occurs as part of a genetic syndrome such as Fryns syndrome, which is an autosomal recessive trait including diaphragmatic hernia, dysmorphic facies, and distal digital hypoplasia. A number of reports have expanded the phenotype of Fryns syndrome.[76]

SUMMARY OF MANAGEMENT OPTIONS

Congenital Diaphragmatic Hernia

Management Options	Evidence Quality and Recommendation	References
Prenatal		
Offer karyotyping.	III/B	53,58
Assess for other anomalies with ultrasound.	III/B	53,58
Prognosis is difficult to predict.	III/B	59,60,66
Lung size–to–head circumference ratio of prognostic value.	III/B	65
Termination is an option before viability.	—/GPP	—
Provide multidisciplinary counseling.	—/GPP	—
Endoscopic fetal tracheal occlusion of some benefit in poor prognosis groups.	III/B	71
Labor and Delivery		
Normal management but conducted in a tertiary center.	—/GPP	—
Neonatal Management		
Provide immediate pediatric resuscitation and ventilation.	—/GPP	—
Optimal timing for repair unclear.	IIb/B	73
There is limited evidence that ECMO improves survival.	III/B	72,74
Counsel parents that recurrence risk is low.	—/GPP	—

ECMO, extracorporeal membrane oxygenation; GPP, good practice point.

BODY STALK ANOMALY/LIMB BODY WALL COMPLEX

General

These rare abdominal wall defects have an annual prevalence ranging from 1 in 7500 to 1 in 42,000 pregnancies. The defect is now considered to result from early embryonic maldevelopment as a result of abnormal folding of the trilaminar disc, such that the amnion appears to form a continuous sheet between the anterior abdominal wall and the placenta.

Diagnosis

It is essential to differentiate a body stalk anomaly from other abdominal wall defects, because the former is incompatible with extrauterine life. Multiple organ system anomalies are present in most cases. Characteristically, there are neural tube and lower limb defects with scoliosis. The viscera of the fetus may appear either attached to the placenta (Fig. 19–15) or entangled with the fetal membranes. Sometimes, it may be difficult to distinguish from amniotic band sequence, but in that situation, scoliosis is not a major finding. During the first trimester, fetal parts are seen outside the amniotic cavity. The umbilical cord appears absent or abnormal.[77] The karyotype is usually normal, and amniocentesis is not required.

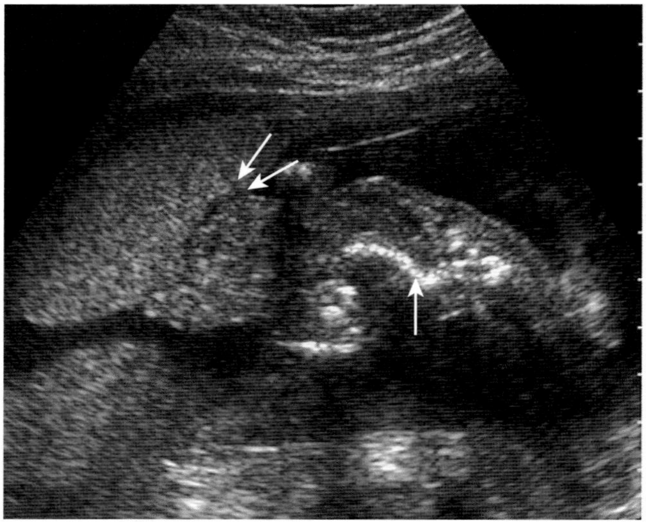

FIGURE 19–15
Body stalk anomaly shows the abnormal fetal spine (*arrow*) and the appearance of the fetus being stuck to the placenta (*double arrows*).

SUMMARY OF MANAGEMENT OPTIONS

Body Stalk Anomaly/Limb Body Wall Complex

Management Options	Evidence Quality and Recommendation	References
Prenatal		
Confirm diagnosis (umbilical cord absence is a clue) and assess for other abnormalities.	IV/C	77
Offer termination of pregnancy.	GPP	
Labor and Delivery		
Aim for vaginal delivery.	—/GPP	—
Neonatal Management		
Provide supportive/palliative care.	—/GPP	—
Recurrence risk is low.	GPP	

GPP, good practice point.

Management Options

Prenatal

The option of pregnancy termination should be offered. Vaginal delivery is the goal. When a body stalk abnormality may affect one fetus in a twin pregnancy, as has been reported after use of artificial reproductive technologies, selective fetal reduction may be offered.[78]

Postnatal

This defect is lethal. It is thought to be sporadic, and thus, the recurrence risk is extremely low.

BLADDER AND CLOACAL EXSTROPHIES, OMPHALOCELE, BLADDER EXTROPHY, IMPERFORATE ANUS

General

Both exstrophies are rare, constituting less than 2% of anorectal malformations.[79] Bladder exstrophy is around four times more frequent than cloacal exstrophy; 1 in 35,500 compared with 1 in 200,000.[80] Bladder exstrophy is distinct from cloacal exstrophy. The group of anomalies termed OEIS[81] (omphalocele, exstrophy of the bladder, imperforate anus, and spina bifida) always includes cloacal exstrophy with imperforate anus. The estimated incidence of OEIS is 1 in 200,000 births. It is unclear whether the two disorders are distinct entities or part of a continuum because some authors have considered OEIS and cloacal exstrophy to be synonymous, though the full OEIS complex includes spinal abnormalities. The primary defect is believed to be a failure of development of the caudal fold of the anterior abdominal wall leading to a defect in forming the urogenital septum. The result of this is a common cloaca with a wide range of urogenital and spinal anomalies. Suspicion of cloacal exstrophy may occur in the presence of an omphalocele associated with an infraumbilical anterior abdominal wall defect and absence of the bladder.[82]

Whatever the cause, the defects produced are severe and lead to lifelong impairments of urinary, gastrointestinal, reproductive, and likely, psychological function.

Diagnosis

Bladder Exstrophy

On ultrasound scanning, typically the fetal bladder is not seen within the abdomen. There is a soft tissue mass on the lower anterior abdominal wall with an abnormally low insertion of the umbilical cord. In severe cases, the pelvic bones will be abnormal with a wide symphysis pubis and genital anomalies. For prognostic reasons, it is important to distinguish this from cloacal exstrophy.

Cloacal Exstrophy

Cloacal exstrophy is a complicated abnormality that should be suspected in the presence of a low anterior abdominal defect and absent fetal bladder on ultrasound scanning. The defect contains an omphalocele, the bladder exstrophy, and the ileum, which herniates between the two halves of the bladder. The exposed ileum has described as looking like an "elephant's trunk." Other findings on ultrasound include multiple abnormalities.

Management Options

Bladder Exstrophy

PRENATAL

When the diagnosis of bladder exstrophy is suspected antenatally, other causes of failure to visualize the bladder should be sought. In bladder exstrophy, the amniotic fluid volume is usually normal. The maternal serum α-fetoprotein may be raised, but chromosomal anomaly is infrequent.

When the diagnosis is made, parental counseling should include the long-term prognosis in terms of urinary continence, renal function, and sexual and reproductive function in both males and females; that is, physiologic function, cosmetic appearance and body image, and psychological well-being. Recent approaches to repair rather than urinary diversion procedures appear to be leading to much improved outcomes,[83] but surgical and functional morbidities remain significant ongoing issues for many children and adults. There appears to be an increase in urinary bladder or colorectal cancer in patients with exstrophies, and therefore, long-term follow-up would seem prudent.[84] Despite advances in surgical management, termination of pregnancy is an option for parents, given the long-term problems associated with bladder exstrophy.

LABOR AND DELIVERY

Labor and delivery are not influenced by the malformation, which would not be expected to increase complications or perinatal mortality. Delivery in a unit equipped with neonatal intensive care and surgical facilities would facilitate planning for surgery, which is now frequently performed early in the neonatal period.

Cloacal Exstrophy

PRENATAL

The antenatal diagnosis of cloacal exstrophy has been reported infrequently. It is typically associated with severe oligohydramnios, probably due to the associated genitourinary abnormalities. The maternal serum α-fetoprotein may be high when associated with either a neural tube defect or an omphalocele. Amniocentesis may be offered to establish the genetic sex of the fetus. The anomalies create difficult management issues, including neonatal gender assignment. As with OEIS, the prognosis in terms of survival depends on the severity of the defects and the associated malformations.

Termination of pregnancy is an option in view of the associated genital abnormalities, the difficult surgical repair, and the long-term problems of achieving continence and sexual and reproductive function. The clinical management of the pregnancy is otherwise unaltered. Should the patient consider continuing the pregnancy, detailed pediatric surgical consultation prior to delivery is recommended to maximize understanding of future medical care.

LABOR AND DELIVERY

There is no a priori reason for cesarean delivery. Standard obstetric management is appropriate with delivery in a unit equipped with neonatal intensive care and surgical facilities.

Omphalocele, Exstrophy of the Bladder, Imperforate Anus, and Spina Bifida Sequence

PRENATAL

Diagnosis by ultrasound is highly accurate (Fig. 19–16). Counseling for parents should include discussion of long-term morbidities and multiple hospitalizations even when neurodevelopmental progress is likely to be normal.[85,86] Some parents may wish karyotyping to determine the genetic sex of the fetus. Because reconstructive surgery would be required, the parents may wish to discuss the prognosis with a multidisciplinary team to maximize the understanding of future medical requirements. Termination of pregnancy may be offered.

LABOR AND DELIVERY

If the parents opt to continue the pregnancy, delivery should be in a tertiary center. Vaginal birth is anticipated.

POSTNATAL

Management will involve reconstructive surgery with multiple hospitalizations. Recurrence risks are difficult to determine, but there are rare cases of familial recurrence.

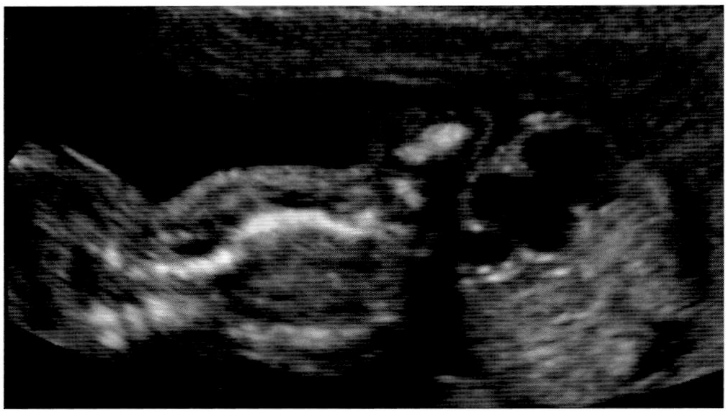

FIGURE 19–16
Omphalocele, exstrophy of the bladder, imperforate anus, and spina bifida (OEIS). Ultrasound image shows abnormal spine and the omphalocele with the bladder in the lower part of the abdominal wall defect.

SUMMARY OF MANAGEMENT OPTIONS

Bladder and Cloacal Extrophies

Management Options	Evidence Quality and Recommendation	References
Prenatal		
Be certain of diagnosis and assess for other abnormalities.	—/GPP	—
Provide multidisciplinary counseling regarding prognosis and management.	—/GPP	—
Offer termination of pregnancy if appropriate, depending on long-term morbidities (physical and psychological).	—/GPP	—

Management Options	Evidence Quality and Recommendation	References
Labor and Delivery		
Normal management.	—/GPP	—
Deliver in a unit with appropriate neonatal medical and surgical facilities.	—/GPP	—
Neonatal Management		
Assessment and planning of surgery (often multiple operations) are a priority after birth.	—/GPP	—
Long-term follow-up of exstrophy repair recommended owing to risks of cancers	IV/C	84

GPP, good practice point.

ESOPHAGEAL ATRESIA

General

The total annual prevalence of esophageal atresia (EA) and tracheoesophageal fistula (TEF) is about 1 in 3500.[87] Half of these anomalies are isolated, with a low recurrence risk, and 50% are associated with syndromes especially the VATER (vertebral defects, imperforate anus, tracheoesophageal fistula, and radial and renal dysplasia) or VACTERL (vertebral abnormalities, anal atresia, cardiac abnormalities, tracheoesophageal fistula and/or esophageal atresia, renal agenesis and dysplasia, and limb defects; see later) groups of abnormalities. Cardiac abnormalities are the most common single anomaly seen with EA or TEF. TEF and EA typically occur together because the esophagus and trachea develop from a common diverticulum of the primitive pharynx. The upper respiratory and gastrointestinal tracts separate at between 3 and 5 weeks' gestation. The most common anomaly is esophageal atresia with a distal TEF (87% of cases). The variants of TEF are illustrated in Figure 19–17. Isolated EA and isolated TEF account for 8% and 4% of the cases, respectively.

Diagnosis

The most common antenatal presentation is hydramnios associated with preterm labor. Fetal swallowing begins around 16 weeks' gestation, and failure to visualize the stomach after this time is unusual. Failure to visualize the fetal stomach on serial scans from 20 weeks should alert the sonographer to the possibility of EA.[88] Other clues to the diagnosis are hydramnios and fetal growth restriction in the late second and third trimesters. However, the prenatal diagnosis of EA or TEF remains limited, ultrasound series reporting no more than a 56% positive predictive value for absent stomach and hydramnios.[89] In addition, nonvisualization of the thoracic esophagus on MRI is not uncommon and cannot be used as an independent reliable marker for esophageal abnormality. The differential diagnosis for the ultrasonographic absence of the stomach includes three possibilities:

- Esophageal atresia.
- Congenital diaphragmatic hernia.
- Impaired fetal swallowing from "neurologic" causes or cleft lip and palate.

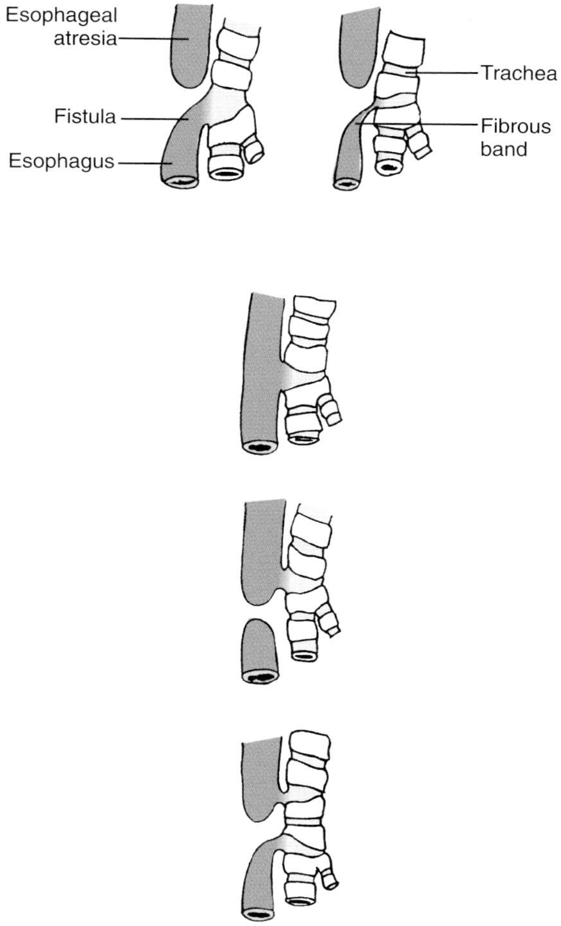

FIGURE 19–17
The main types of tracheoesophageal fistula.

The stomach may simply be empty at the time of the scan, but after 20 weeks. typically it will fill over the course of the examination. In the absence of other abnormalities, a repeat scan within a few days is warranted. The diagnosis should be suspected in all cases of hydramnios (Fig. 19–18). and a targeted ultrasound examination should be part of the management of women with preterm labor. EA with TEF allows for the passage of amniotic fluid into the stomach and is not

FIGURE 19–18
Esophageal atresia. Scan shows hydramnios and absent stomach in the imaging plane for the abdominal circumference measurement.

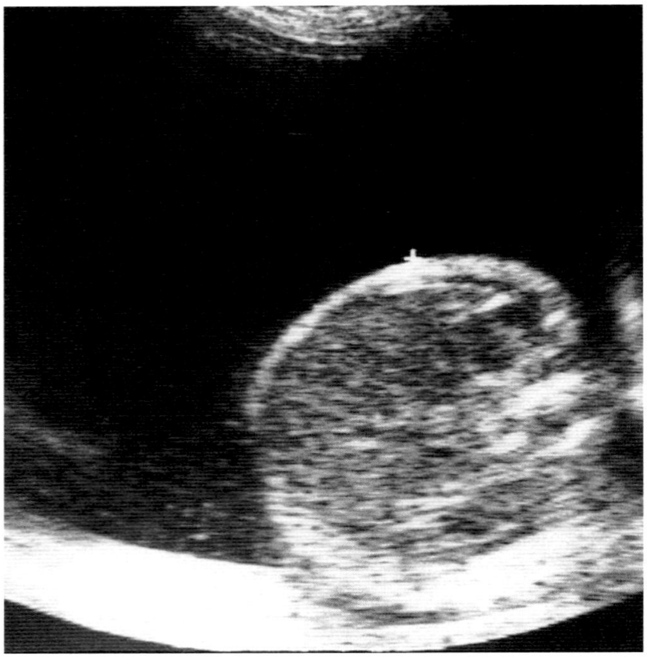

TABLE 19–3
Components of the CHARGE Association Compared with the VATER Complex

Colobomatous malformation
Heart defect
Atresia choanae
Retarded growth and CNS abnormalities
Genital abnormalities and hypogonadism
Ear anomalies and deafness
CHARGE association may also include
Renal anomalies
Tracheoesophageal fistula
Facial palsy
Micrognathia
Cleft lip and palate
Omphalocele
Most have some degree of mental retardation
VATER-VACTERL
Vertebral defects
Anorectal (imperforate anus)
Cardiac
Tracheo
Esophageal fistula or atresia
Radial (and **R**enal) aplasia (may have single umbilical artery)
Limb defects

CNS, central nervous system.

usually associated with either hydramnios or an absent stomach. In many cases, therefore, the diagnosis may not be possible antenatally. A very small stomach in the presence of hydramnios suggests the diagnosis. A high proportion of fetuses have aneuploidy or other malformations. The prognosis for the fetus with EA is worse than for the neonate with EA first suspected postnatally.

Occasionally, the proximal esophageal pouch can be imaged in the fetus with EA when the stomach is absent. This has been referred to as the "pouch" or "upper pouch" sign and can be seen as early as 23 weeks.[90] A blind pouch in the neck appears to have a worse outcome than a mediastinal pouch.[91] MRI has been successfully used to confirm ultrasonically suspected EA.[92] Currently, it is not possible to accurately determine the predictive value of the pouch sign nor its relationship to outcomes.[89] Failure to demonstrate the stomach necessitates a careful search for other abnormalities including the VATER or VACTERL group of abnormalities. Originally, a cluster of abnormalities including *v*ertebral, *a*nal atresia, *t*racheoesophageal atresia, and *r*adial dysplasia was termed VATER.[93] The group was subsequently expanded to *v*ertebral, *a*norectal, *c*ardiac (especially atrial and ventricular septal defects), *t*racheoesophageal atresia, *r*enal and *l*imb defects, or VACTERL.[94] Otocephaly, a major malformation of the mandible and temporal bones associated with abnormally placed ears, may also be present. These anomalies need to be considered in the assessment of the fetus and subsequent counseling.

Management Options

Prenatal

A karyotype should be obtained to rule out aneuploidy (particularly triploidy or trisomy 18), which is present in over 10% of cases.[95] EA may be present in association with a number of complex fetal abnormalities including the DiGeorge sequence identifiable by a characteristic deletion in chromosome 22.[96] More than half of the fetuses with EA in one series had multiple malformations,[96] the VATER complex in either its complete or its incomplete forms being the most common abnormality in another series.[97] The other cluster of abnormalities sufficiently different from the VATER complex to warrant distinction is the CHARGE (coloboma, heart disease, atresia choanae, retarded growth and retarded development and/or central nervous system anomalies, genital hypoplasia, and ear anomalies and/or deafness) association (Table 19–3). These infants usually have some degree of mental retardation. In contrast, the majority of neonates with VATER-VACTERL have normal intelligence (except those associated with either trisomy 18 or 13q deletion syndromes).

When the diagnosis is made before viability, parental counseling should include the influence of any associated abnormalities on neonatal outcome, the possible related problems during pregnancy (e.g., hydramnios), and the short- and long-term prognosis after surgical repair. The latter has improved dramatically since the first recorded survival in 1939,[98] owing to improvements in both surgical technique and neonatal intensive care. Although long-term evaluation after repair suggests that respiratory and gastrointestinal morbidities improve as the individual grows into adulthood, approximately 25% will have significant pulmonary dysfunction, gastroesophageal reflux, or chest wall and spinal deformity.[99,100] The option of pregnancy termination should be offered, especially if there are multiple anomalies.

The most common anomaly is EA with a distal TEF. This is usually managed by thoracotomy with division of the fistula and then end-to-end esophageal anastomosis. In the absence of other abnormalities, survival rates of up to 100% are reported.[98] However, birth weight and the presence of other anomalies, especially cardiac, remain the key prognostic factors; birth weight greater than 1500 g and the absence of major cardiac defects have been associated with greater than 95% survival when lethal anomalies such as trisomy 18 and complex CHARGE syndrome were excluded.[101] Another review of 176 repairs between 1985 and 1997 reported a perinatal and infant mortality rate of 22%, with a further 21% of infants having significant morbidity after 2 years of age.[102] The length of the atresia (gap length) has been also associated with prognosis,[103] but this is virtually impossible to determine on prenatal ultrasound.

Continuing pregnancies are managed along standard obstetric lines. Hydramnios complicating EA may prove difficult to manage and is associated with preterm labor. Medical management of hydramnios using indomethacin may be of value in certain fetal abnormalities, but in the one report with EA, its use was unsuccessful.[104] Other adverse fetal effects of indomethacin or cyclooxygenase inhibitors class II generally preclude their use in the third trimester of pregnancy. Therapeutic amniocentesis is an option after antenatal corticosteroids have been given to enhance pulmonary maturity.

Labor and Delivery

Labor and delivery management are not influenced by the malformation.

Postnatal

Awareness of the possibility of EA in all cases of hydramnios and in any newborn with excessive oral secretions, particularly if there are breathing difficulties or cyanosis, should lead to the same management as planned for the neonate diagnosed or suspected antenatally. Oral feeds are avoided until the diagnosis is clear to reduce the risk of aspiration pneumonia. Definitive surgery is offered once the infant's condition is stable.

The most important single determinant of outcome is the severity of the associated anomalies followed by ventilator dependence.[101] Outcome is usually good if the birth weight is over 1500 g.[104] Immediate surgical complications include anastomotic leaks, tracheal perforation, and chest infection. Late complications are related either to the development of an esophageal stricture, with obstruction to solids at the anastomotic site, or to respiratory complications including pneumonia, tracheomalacia, and tracheal compression by the upper pouch. Only 10% have respiratory complications beyond the first year and 8% an esophageal stricture. Gastroesophageal reflux and its complications remains the biggest single long-term morbidity, affecting 18% to 40% of survivors.[105,106] The less common types of EA with or without fistula (producing an airless abdomen because of either blind upper and lower pouches or an atretic fistula) might require more complex surgery, and the prognosis, especially in terms of morbidity, is worse albeit improving. In this group, gastrostomy feeding, with delay of the repair until the child grows, is more frequently required. Long-term morbidity, both respiratory and gastrointestinal, tends to improve.[105]

Although EA is said to be a sporadic abnormality, a familial form is described and recurrence risk, including that of associated abnormalities, needs to be considered.[87]

ATRESIAS OF THE BOWEL

A wide variety of congenital anomalies can occur in perinates with either gut atresias or stenoses. The specific pattern of anomalies depends on the location of the atresia. For example, cardiac and renal anomalies are associated with EA or duodenal atresia.[107] Other associations are discussed in the sections on the respective abnormality. Overall, although hospitalization may be prolonged, mortality associated with bowel atresias is low and relates primarily to birth weight and the presence of other abnormalities.[108] Pyloric atresia is a rare lesion associated with junctional epidermolysis bullosa.

Duodenal Atresia

General

Atresia of the duodenum occurs around 11 weeks' gestation after an insult to the duodenum, most commonly either just proximal or just distal to the ampulla of Vater, causes failure of canalization. Occasionally, vascular accidents or midgut strangulation associated with omphalocele are implicated. The annual prevalence of duodenal atresia approximates 1 in 6000 live births. Approximately 30% of cases of isolated duodenal atresia are associated with trisomy 21 or other aneuploidies.

Diagnosis

Hydramnios is common with upper intestinal atresias and implies total obstruction. Half the pregnancies complicated by duodenal atresia are associated with hydramnios. The sonographic diagnosis is typically made by the appearance of a "double bubble" (Fig. 19–19*A*) late in the second trimester, but it has been suspected as early as 12 weeks[109] and positively detected at 19 weeks.[110] Like all forms of gastrointestinal obstruction, duodenal atresia may not be diagnosable by ultrasound until the third trimester. It is important that a true transverse section of the abdomen be obtained and that a connection between the two bubbles is seen (see Fig. 19–19*B*). This avoids the potential confusion of an oblique scan of the stomach artificially producing a double bubble or confusing the stomach and a choledochal cyst with a duodenal atresia. Increased peristaltic waves may be seen during real-time imaging.

Management Options

PRENATAL

Associated anomalies are present in over 50%. In addition to trisomy 21 (in 30%), duodenal atresia is associated with abnormalities of chromosome 9. Other gastrointestinal malformations occur in 25% and include malrotation (28%), annular pancreas (33%; especially with duodenal stenosis), EA, imperforate anus, jejunal atresia, duplication of the duodenum, and Meckel's diverticulum.[111] Cardiac, tracheal and esophageal, renal, hepatobiliary, and pancreatic ductal abnormalities have been reported in up to 48%.

FIGURE 19–19
Duodenal atresia. *A*, Oblique longitudinal ultrasound image of fetal abdomen shows the "double bubble." *B*, True transverse section shows communication between the stomach and the duodenum. Increased amniotic fluid is noted.

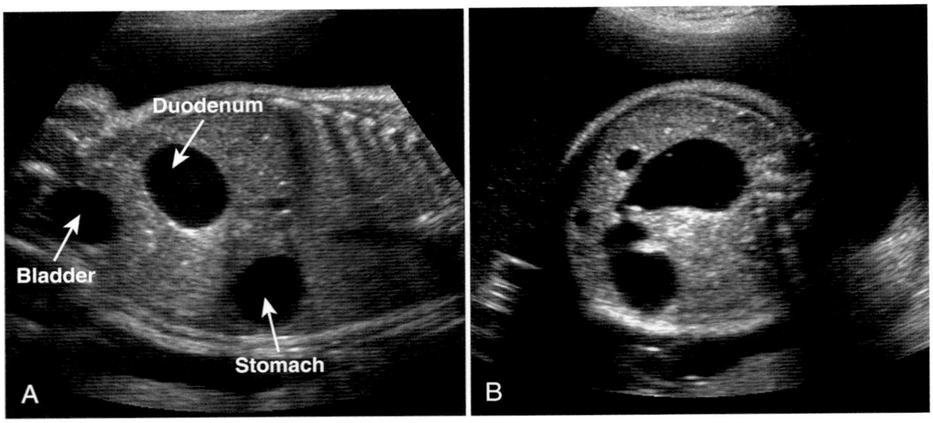

Duodenal atresia may be associated with multiple atresias of the bowel. About half the infants have early-onset growth restriction.

This range of associated anomalies mandates a detailed ultrasonographic examination and the offer of karyotyping. Fetuses with trisomy 21 have a high risk of cardiac abnormalities. They may also have heart rate abnormalities in labor not necessarily indicative of hypoxia. Indomethacin (or similar cyclooxygenase inhibitors) has been given in an attempt to treat the hydramnios.[112] Few clinically adverse effects on the fetus are documented when given for a short time before 32 weeks.

LABOR AND DELIVERY

There is no a priori indication for cesarean delivery because of duodenal atresia. As in any situation with gross hydramnios, delivery in a tertiary center is advised, both to manage the potential complications of the hydramnios and for access to neonatal surgical services. Because a double bubble is not absolutely diagnostic of duodenal atresia, other possibilities must be excluded after delivery. Passage of an orogastric or nasogastric tube after delivery followed by radiographs of the neonate will help confirm the diagnosis. The differential diagnosis includes annular pancreas, peritoneal bands, duodenal stenosis, more distal atresias, and other cystic structures such as choledochal, ovarian, and duplication cysts.

POSTNATAL

After delivery, a tube is passed into the stomach and abdominal radiographs are taken. The diagnosis can be confirmed at this stage by examination of the gas pattern. The atretic area is excised (Fig. 19–20) when the infant is stable. The prognosis for this condition, if recognized and isolated, is good and the recurrence risk is low. Operative mortality rate is up to 4%, with long-term survival rate quoted as 86%. A series of 169 patients with over 30 years follow-up showed a late complication rate of 12% with a 6% mortality.[113] Cardiac lesions or associated abnormalities such as trisomy 21 are the main contributors to long-term morbidity and death.[113]

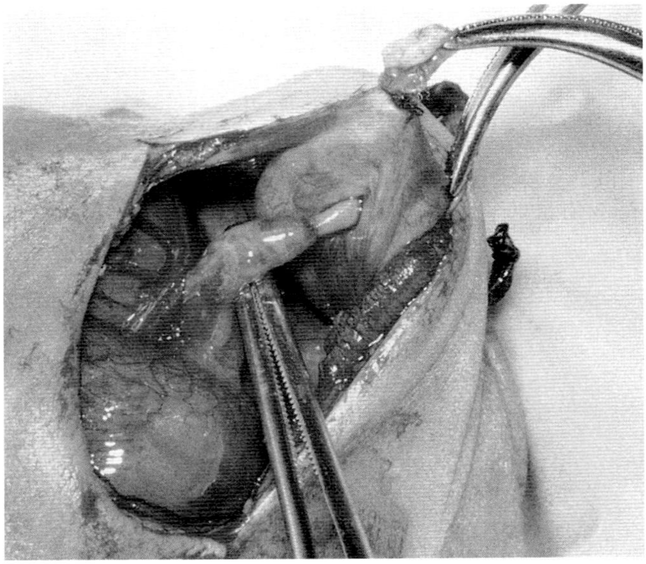

FIGURE 19–20
Duodenal atresia. Atretic segment as seen at neonatal surgery (segment above surgical forceps).

Jejunal and Ileal Atresia

General

Jejunal and ileal atresia have an annual prevalence approximating 1 in 5000 live births. They are the second most common forms of neonatal bowel obstruction.[114] These atresias are thought to result from vascular compromise of a bowel segment after organogenesis is complete. Intestinal atresias are categorized according to the degree of occlusion or separation of the bowel on either side of the atretic segment.

Associated anomalies are less common than with duodenal atresia. Five cases of trisomy 21 were reported in one

FIGURE 19–21
Jejunal atresia. *A*, Bowel dilation at 29 weeks' gestation. *B*, Appearance of bowel at 33 weeks' gestation.

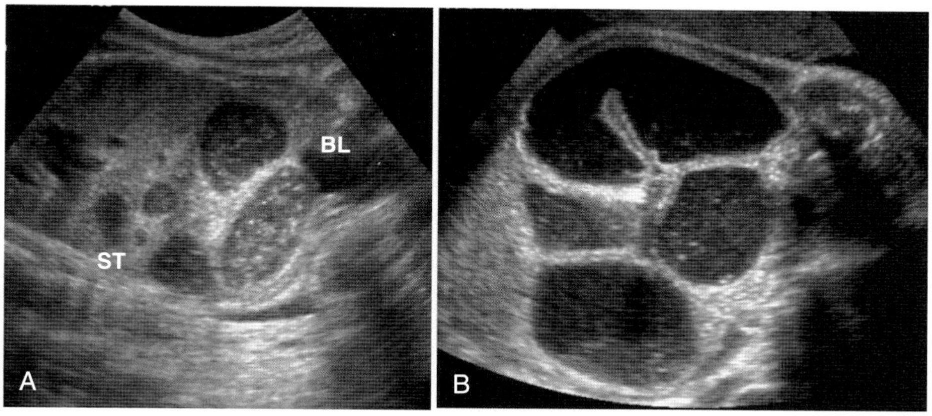

series of 589 perinates with jejunoileal atresia,[115] and none in a more recent series.[108] A special form, the "apple peel" deformity, is an autosomal recessive trait and may have a worse prognosis than the other forms of atresia.[116] Another review noted gastroschisis in 16% of cases, intrauterine volvulus in 27%, and meconium ileus in 11%.[111]

Diagnosis

The ultrasonographic appearance of jejunal atresia is that of multiple distended bowel loops (Fig. 19–21). Hydramnios is more common with upper gastrointestinal obstruction (duodenal and jejunal) than with lower obstructions. The development of ascites or an echogenic mass is a sign of bowel perforation. Detailed examination of the wall of cystic or echogenic intra-abdominal structures for peristalsis is important, because it can be associated with bowel perforation and development of a meconium pseudocyst. Other features useful antenatally for diagnosing bowel obstruction are increased peristalsis, failure to detect a normal colon late in gestation, and a disproportionately large abdominal circumference for dates.

Management Options

PRENATAL

Jejunal and ileal atresias are usually isolated from other gastrointestinal lesions. It is important to exclude other causes of echolucent structures within the abdomen, such as a urinary tract obstruction. It is suggested that serial measurements of the bowel loop diameter are of value, but these measurements correlate with neither the diagnosis of bowel obstruction nor the prognosis. The appearance of the bowel is quite variable, particularly in the third trimester, and in our experience, mild bowel dilation is typically associated with a normal outcome. However, a bowel obstruction should be suspected whenever the internal diameter of the small bowel is greater than 7 mm.[117] There is little evidence to support early delivery based on bowel loop diameter.

LABOR AND DELIVERY

Fetuses with a presumptive bowel obstruction should be delivered in a center with neonatal surgical facilities. Otherwise, obstetric management is unaltered by the presence of the abnormality. Hydramnios is not an indication for a cesarean delivery.

POSTNATAL

After delivery, the neonate is evaluated to determine the site of obstruction and the presence of any associated congenital anomalies or meconium peritonitis. The radiologic features of jejunal atresia are shown in Figure 19–22. The prognosis is very good following repair, with survival in excess of 95%.[108] Even in the group with apple peel deformity, early diagnosis and prolonged parenteral nutrition have resulted in a dramatic improvement in survival.

The risk of recurrence for jejunal and ileal atresia is small except in the group with apple peel syndrome, which would appear to follow autosomal recessive inheritance.[118]

Large Bowel Obstruction, Anal Atresia, and Imperforate Anus

General

Colon atresia is rare and largely confined to the right colon. Anorectal malformation including imperforate anus has an annual prevalence of around 1 in 2500 to 1 in 5000 live births. In the embryo, lumen development begins in the region of the descending colon. Anorectal malformations are complex, and there are several classifications aimed at producing a consistent description of the anomaly to permit comparison and assessment of outcomes with differing surgical treatments. The Krickenbeck simplification of the Wingspread classification is widely used.[119] Constipation, soiling, and complications associated with other abnormalities are all long-term morbidities, which occur in more than 50% cases. Such problems have a major impact on the survivors' lives.[120] Anal anomalies may be part of multiple malformation syndromes, including the VATER-VACTERL and CHARGE complexes and cloacal exstrophy. They are also associated with spinal and genitourinary defects.[121]

Management Options

Large bowel abnormalities are rarely diagnosed antenatally except when part of other multiple malformation syndromes. Apart from mechanical abnormalities such as malrotation or volvulus, other reasons for dilated large bowel or increased echogenicity are meconium ileus, aganglionosis (Hirschsprung's disease), and congenital syphilis. Generally, the ultrasound findings are nonspecific, and the diagnosis is made postnatally. The fetal karyotype is generally normal.

The prenatal diagnosis of imperforate anus is made in less than 20% of cases. Overall, approximately 85% of cases are associated with additional anomalies, including 53% with urogenital abnormalities, and 13% have an abnormal karyotype.[122] Prenatal diagnosis may be made when bowel dilation is seen on ultrasound scanning, but this may be a transient finding.[123] The findings of an abdominopelvic mass or intraluminal calcification might be signs of lower bowel abnormality with communication between the urinary and the gastrointestinal tracts. Because the postnatal consequences of complex anorectal and cloacal anomalies include fecal and urinary continence problems as well as sexual and fertility difficulties, careful investigation and counseling need to be offered to parents.

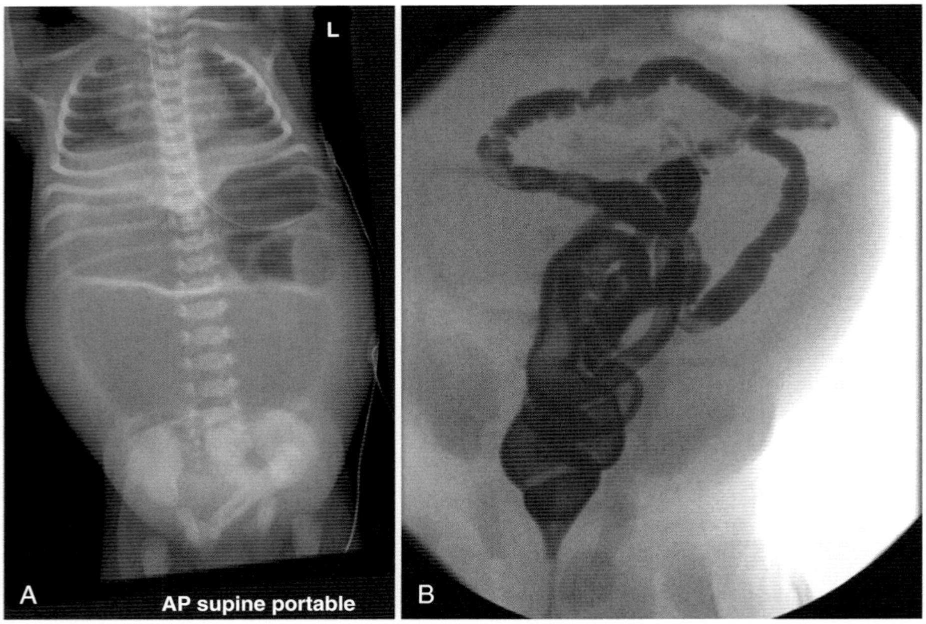

FIGURE 19–22
Neonatal radiology in a case of jejunal atresia. *A*, Plain abdominal x-ray. *B*, Enema shows normal large bowel and ileum.

SUMMARY OF MANAGEMENT OPTIONS

Bowel Atresias

Management Options	Evidence Quality and Recommendation	References
Esophageal Atresia with/without Fistula		
Prenatal		
Diagnosis by ultrasound is uncommon. Raised α-fetoprotein is reported. Suspect diagnosis in all cases of hydramnios.	III/B	88,89
Assess for associated abnormalities with ultrasound and karyotyping.	III/B	89,96,97
Provide multidisciplinary counseling.	—/GPP	—
Offer termination of pregnancy in the presence of associated abnormalities.	IV/C	101

Management Options	Evidence Quality and Recommendation	References
Labor and Delivery		
Normal management in center with facilities for advanced neonatal resuscitation, intensive care, and surgery.	—/GPP	—
Postnatal		
Remove excess secretions at birth; use esophageal tube to maintain low-pressure suction.	—/GPP	—
Early diagnostic imaging should include a chest x-ray.	—/GPP	—
Avoid oral feeding.	—/GPP	—
Assess for other abnormalities	—/GPP	—
The risk of recurrence is small but consider impact of associated anomalies.	—/GPP	87
Duodenal Atresia		
Prenatal		
Diagnosis is made by ultrasound: double bubble.	III/B	109,110
Assess for other structural abnormalities.	III/B	108,111
Offer karyotyping.	III/B	108,111
Provide multidisciplinary counseling.	—/GPP	—
Labor and Delivery		
Normal management in a tertiary center.	—/GPP	—
Vigilance for complications of hydramnios.	—/GPP	—
Postnatal		
Pass nasogastric tube, maintain nil by mouth until bowel atresia excluded.	—/GPP	—
Confirm diagnosis by radiography.	—/GPP	—
Surgical correction is needed; search for other abnormalities at surgery.	—/GPP	—
Recurrence risk is that of associated anomalies.	GPP	
Jejunoileal Atresia		
Prenatal		
Suspect bowel atresia if bowel dilation >7 mm on scan	IV/C	117
Hydramnios may develop.	III/B	111
Assess for other abnormalities.	III/B	108,111
Value of karyotype is uncertain.	GPP	
Serial ultrasound scans to detect perforation (ascites, echogenic mass).	—/GPP	—
Provide multidisciplinary counseling.	—/GPP	—
Labor and Delivery		
Normal management in a tertiary center.	—/GPP	—
Exercise vigilance for complications of hydramnios.	—/GPP	—
Postnatal		
Pass nasogastric tube.	—/GPP	—
Maintain neonate nil by mouth until bowel atresia excluded.	GPP	
Confirm diagnosis by radiography.	—/GPP	—
Surgical correction is needed; search for other abnormalities at surgery.	—/GPP	—
Recurrence risk is low (except for apple peel deformity where risk is 1:4).	—/GPP	118

SUMMARY OF MANAGEMENT OPTIONS
Bowel Atresias—cont'd

Management Options	Evidence Quality and Recommendation	References
Large Bowel Obstruction, Anal Atresia and Imperforate Anus		
Prenatal		
Where diagnosis suspected offer karyotyping.	GPP	122
Assess for hydramnios (rare).	—/GPP	—
Provide multidisciplinary counseling.	—/GPP	—
Assess for other abnormalities.	—/GPP	123
Labor and Delivery		
Normal management in a tertiary center.	—/GPP	—
Postnatal		
Maintain nil by mouth until diagnosis is made.	—/GPP	—
Pediatric assessment and management.	—/GPP	—
Recurrence risk low.	GPP	

GPP, good practice point.

MECONIUM ILEUS AND MECONIUM PERITONITIS, HYPERECHOGENIC BOWEL

General

Hyperechogenic bowel, defined sonographically as echogenicity at least equal to the surrounding bone, occurs in 0.1% to 1.8% of pregnancies in the second or third trimesters.[124] It may be transient. Meconium ileus is an obstruction of the lower ileum by thick meconium. Perforation can occur after bowel obstruction secondary to any cause, including meconium ileus, producing meconium peritonitis, intestinal atresia, volvulus, and malrotation. These conditions are rare. Meconium ileus is most commonly associated with cystic fibrosis. In contrast, most cases of meconium peritonitis are not (though cystic fibrosis should be considered). Bayesian analysis of the risk of prevalence of cystic fibrosis in a fetus with echogenic bowel yields a range of 3.3% to 13% in a mixed North American population.[125] In addition to cystic fibrosis, hyperechogenic bowel is associated with bowel obstruction, viral infection, aneuploidy, and fetal growth restriction. Intraluminal calcification may result from the mixing of meconium and fetal urine, and such findings should suggest the possibility of communication between the urogenital tract and the bowel as may occur in anorectal and cloacal anomalies. An echogenic mass in the stomach may be swallowed blood, for example, after an abruption or invasive procedure.

Diagnosis

Both meconium ileus and peritonitis have been diagnosed in the second trimester. Meconium ileus presents as either a cluster of bright echoes or the bowel appearing dilated and echogenic. Hyperechogenic bowel is present when the echogenicity is at least as bright as adjacent bone (Fig. 19–23). This definition overcomes variation in description owing to ultrasound machine settings. Distinguishing it from normal, especially late in the third trimester, may be difficult. Fetal ascites and hydramnios are signs of perforation. A hyperechoic mass or diffuse hyperechoic deposits in the fetal abdomen suggest meconium peritonitis (Fig. 19–24). The thorax may be compressed if there is a volvulus or massive bowel distention.

Management Options

Prenatal

Screening for cystic fibrosis should be offered when meconium ileus is suspected. The parents should be tested, and if at least one is a carrier (not all mutations are known), testing the fetus by either chorionic villus sampling or amniocentesis should be offered. Meconium ileus affects 15% of neonates with cystic fibrosis,[126] although a recent review of 77 cases of meconium plug syndrome showed 13% with Hirschsprung's disease but none with cystic fibrosis.[127] Meconium peritonitis is a serious condition, and the guidelines for management may be determined by the ultrasonographic appearance. For example, a discrete lesion within the fetal abdomen that appears unchanging and free of ascites or hydramnios does not warrant intervention. However, the presence of ascites, increasing abdominal distention, and hydramnios may warrant preterm delivery if the estimated risks of prematurity do not exceed the potential benefit of early intervention. There are no data to allow clear

FIGURE 19–23
Ultrasound scan shows echogenic bowel (*arrow*) in the third trimester. This fetus had a normal outcome.

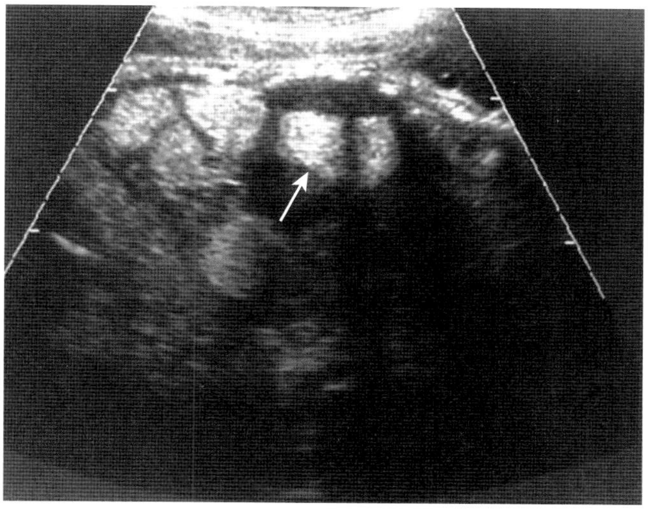

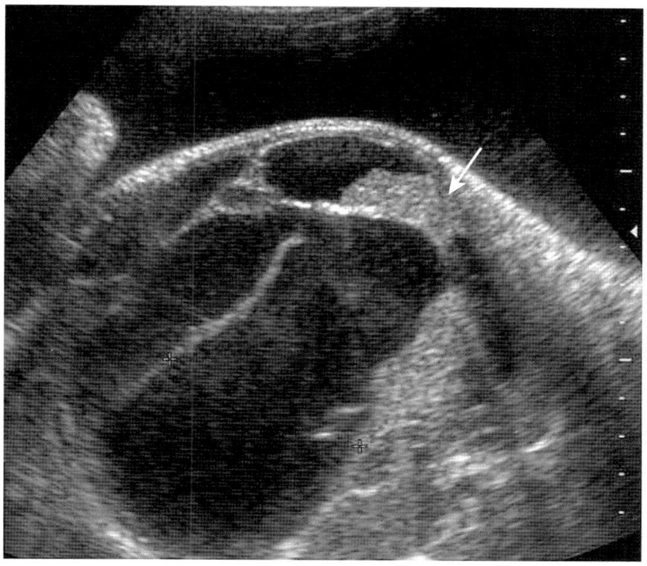

FIGURE 19–24
Longitudinal section of fetal abdomen shows massive bowel dilation. The bowel is surrounded by meconium (*arrow*), indicating the development of peritonitis in a fetus with cystic fibrosis. There is gross hydramnios.

guidance. In this situation, antepartum corticosteroid administration should be considered to hasten pulmonary maturation. Drainage of the ascites, especially if there is lung compression, has been associated with a good outcome, possibly by facilitating the transition to ex utero life. Therapeutic amniocentesis is also an option for pronounced hydramnios. Unexplained death is reported in up to 5% of fetuses with echogenic bowel presenting in the second trimester in the absence of cystic fibrosis, aneuploidy, or infection.[128] Death was associated with fetal growth restriction and oligohydramnios.[128]

FIGURE 19–25
Longitudinal scan of a fetus shows hyperechoic liver (*crosses*). This fetus had a normal outcome.

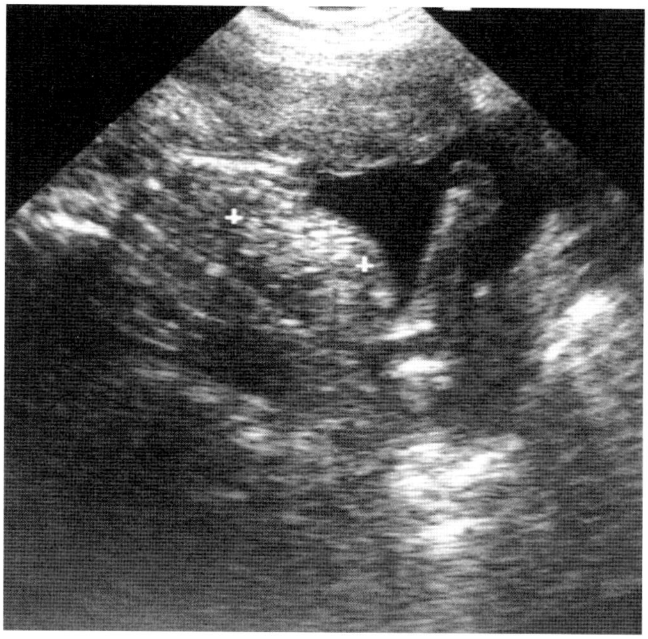

Labor and Delivery

Expectant management is standard in the absence of perforation, though the neonatal intensive care team should be informed of the possible diagnosis. The management of meconium peritonitis in labor is determined by obstetric factors (e.g., the gestation and the ease with which labor can be induced). There is no information to suggest that cesarean delivery benefits the fetus with meconium peritonitis.

Postnatal

Infants with meconium ileus typically become symptomatic within the first 24 to 48 hours of life. Abdominal distention and delayed passage of the meconium plug are characteristic. Vomiting is a relatively late sign. The overall prognosis is determined in part by the success of either a Gastrografin enema or surgery in relieving the obstruction, but mainly by the severity of underlying conditions such as cystic fibrosis. The prognosis for meconium peritonitis is not good, in part due to prematurity. The recurrence rate is low except when the condition is secondary to cystic fibrosis.

ECHOGENIC ("BRIGHT") LIVER AND HEPATIC CALCIFICATIONS

General

Echogenic ("bright") liver (Fig. 19–25) is an uncommon finding with a number of causes or associations, including liver tumors, congenital viral infection, and vascular congestion. Hepatomegaly may occur in hemolytic disease or as part of a visceromegaly syndrome (e.g., Beckwith-Wiedemann syndrome). Splenomegaly in association with hepatomegaly may suggest the occurrence of fetal anemia, extramedullary hematopoiesis, or infection.

SUMMARY OF MANAGEMENT OPTIONS

Meconium Ileus/Peritonitis/Echogenic Bowel

Management Options	Evidence Quality and Recommendation	References
Prenatal		
Diagnosis is made by ultrasound (strict criteria for echogenic bowel/liver [bone-white]).	III/B	124,126
For all, consider diagnosis of cystic fibrosis.	III/B	125,126
For echogenic bowel, consider diagnosis of cytomegalovirus or parvovirus, aneuploidy, intestinal obstruction, intra-amniotic/placental bleed, fetal growth restriction, risk of late fetal death.	III/B	126,128
Maintain vigilance for hydramnios and/or ascites.	—/GPP	128
No data support drainage or delivery if ascites or hydramnios develops.	—/GPP	—
Provide multidisciplinary counseling.	—/GPP	—
Labor and Delivery		
Timing depends on obstetric factors and/or presence of ascites/hydramnios.	—/GPP	—
Delivery in a tertiary center with full pediatric resources but otherwise normal management.	—/GPP	—
Postnatal		
For meconium ileus and peritonitis, outcome depends upon surgical feasibility of repair, associated abnormalities, perforation, and gestation.	III/B	127,128
Consider possibility of Hirschsprung's disease where cystic fibrosis excluded.	GPP	
For echogenic bowel/liver, implement pediatric assessment and management.	—/GPP	—
Recurrence risks are associated with diagnosis.	GPP	

GPP, good practice point.

Hepatic echogenic areas ("calcifications") may be on the surface or within the parenchyma (Fig. 19–26) or be associated with the vasculature.[129] The cause is not always known, and postnatal scanning does not invariably confirm their presence. Subcapsular calcifications may be seen with meconium peritonitis. Intrahepatic calcification may be associated with fetal infection or thromboses.

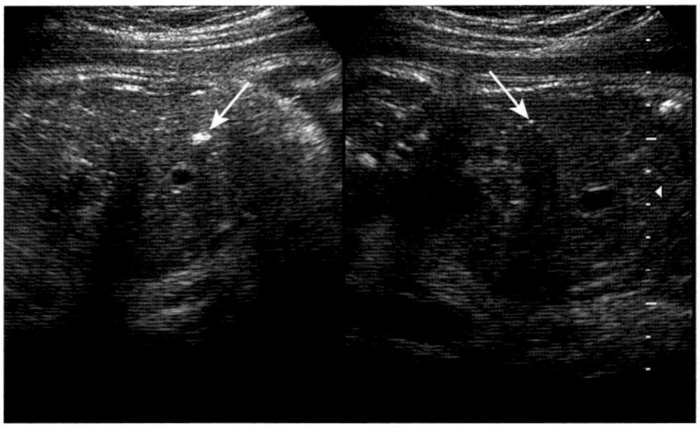

FIGURE 19–26
Hepatic calcifications in the fetal liver (*arrows*). Note the shadowing.

Management Options

Prenatal

Management is directed toward making a diagnosis. The etiology depends on the pathology. Malformations and abnormal karyotypes are seen in association with hepatic calcifications. Single or isolated liver calcification is usually of little consequence.[129] The association of hepatic calcification with congenital toxoplasmosis or viral infection is well documented. Serologic screening is commonly employed but assumes one knows which infectious agent to screen for and that a maternal response has occurred. The risks of infection and effects of toxoplasmosis on the fetus relate to gestation. Toxoplasmosis immunoglobulin G (IgG) avidity testing provides guidance as to the duration of infection in the mother; a low-avidity result would be consistent with maternal infection of less than 12 weeks' duration.

Herpesvirus, echovirus, varicella, coxsackievirus, and adenovirus all have similar hepatic manifestations of infection. Hepatitis leading to ascites is not rare. The ultrasonographic appearances are nonspecific, and invasive tests are usually necessary for a definitive diagnosis.

In addition to infection, hepatomegaly may be associated with Beckwith-Wiedeman syndrome, inborn errors of metabolism, such as glycogen storage diseases, hydrops, and neoplasms. Hepatic tumors are rare. A review of fetal and neonatal liver tumors has shown that hemangiomas account for 60%.[130] A well-defined right upper quadrant mass is suggestive. Hydramnios and hydrops might be present. Management involves observation until delivery, though the fetus may develop congestive heart failure. A search for markers of aneuploidy is indicated when hepatic calcifications are seen because there is an increased risk, but typically aneuploidy is associated with other findings.[131]

Labor and Delivery

Standard obstetric management is generally appropriate, though there is an undefined risk of hepatic bleeding in labor with very large tumors.

Postnatal

Care is determined by the likely diagnosis. Delivery in a center with pediatric surgical facilities as well as neonatal intensive care is advisable.

MEGACYSTIS MICROCOLON INTESTINAL HYPOPERISTALSIS SYNDROME

General

This is a rare autosomal recessive condition manifest in utero by the findings of a dilated urinary bladder with bilateral hydronephrosis, normal amniotic fluid, and abnormal appearance of the bowel. Bowel dilation might not be apparent unless vesicocentesis has been performed.[131] The condition is more common in females. Although the etiology is unknown, histology of the bowel wall shows vacuolated smooth muscle,[132] suggesting abnormality of development and function. The prognosis is grave, but as in other fetal-neonatal dysfunctional bowel lesions resulting in short bowel syndromes and malnutrition, bowel or liver/bowel transplantation has been reported.[133]

Management Options

Prenatal

When the diagnosis has been made, termination of pregnancy may be offered. Counseling may include discussion with neonatologists, pediatric surgeons, and clinical geneticists.

Labor and Delivery

Standard obstetric management is appropriate for those opting to continue the pregnancy. Should dystocia due to fetal bladder dilation be considered likely, vesicocentesis may be offered.

SUMMARY OF MANAGEMENT OPTIONS

Echogenic Liver, Hepatic Calcifications, Hepatomegaly

Management Options	Evidence Quality and Recommendation	References
Prenatal		
Diagnosis is made by ultrasound.	III/B	129,130
Consider infection, fetal thrombosis; where there is hepatomegaly consider infection, Beckwith-Wiedemann syndrome, inborn errors of metabolism, and neoplasms.	III/B	129,130
Consider karyotyping.	III/B	130
Monitor for ascites, hydrops, and hydramnios.	III/B	129
Labor and Delivery		
Timing depends on obstetric factors and/or presence of ascites/hydramnios.	—/GPP	—
Delivery in a tertiary center with full pediatric resources but otherwise normal management.	—/GPP	—
Postnatal		
Implement neonatal pediatric assessment and management directed toward diagnosis.	—/GPP	—
Recurrence risks are rare.	GPP	

GPP, good practice point.

SUMMARY OF MANAGEMENT OPTIONS

Megacystis–Microcolon–Intestinal Hypoperistalsis Syndrome

Management Options	Evidence Quality and Recommendation	References
Prenatal		
Diagnosis is made by ultrasound.	III/B	131
Provide multidisciplinary counseling and offer termination of pregnancy.	III/B	133
Labor and Delivery		
Normal management at a tertiary center.	—/GPP	—
Postnatal		
Recurrence risk consistent with autosomal recessive inheritance.	GPP	

GPP, good practice point.

SUMMARY OF MANAGEMENT OPTIONS

Intra-abdominal Echolucent (Cystic) Structures

Management Options	Evidence Quality and Recommendation	References
Prenatal		
Determine the organ of origin and diagnosis.	—/GPP	
Assess for other abnormalities.	III/B	137
Continue surveillance by ultrasound during pregnancy.	III/B	134–136
Labor and Delivery		
Normal management but in a center with pediatric assessment available.	GPP	
Postnatal		
Implement pediatric assessment and management, including early neonatal ultrasonography.	—/GPP	—
Maintain neonate nil per mouth where bowel duplication or other cysts likely to require early surgical management are present.	GPP	

GPP, good practice point.

Postnatal

Delivery in a center with pediatric surgical and neonatal intensive care facilities is advisable.

ECHOLUCENT STRUCTURES WITHIN THE FETAL ABDOMEN

General

Echolucent or "cystic" structures separate from normal bowel or the urinary tract may be identified on ultrasonography, even as early as the first trimester. The differential diagnosis includes omental cysts, mesenteric cysts, ovarian cysts, urachal cysts, hepatic cysts, choledochal cysts, duplication cysts of the bowel, and retroperitoneal cysts.

Management Options

Prenatal

Intra-abdominal cysts are usually a chance finding on ultrasound. The sonographer should attempt to determine the origin of the structure and exclude other fetal abnormalities. Massive intra-abdominal cysts, especially those detected early in pregnancy, seem to have a poor prognosis, but in many cases, they remain unchanged or resolve.[134] In a recent small series of five cases of fetal abdominal cysts detected in the first trimester, three resolved but one had neonatal bowel abnormalities. In the two that did not resolve, one fetus required prenatal aspiration and the other was found to have a choledochal cyst necessitating postnatal surgery. These cases suggest the need for follow-up even if the cyst appears to resolve on ultrasound.[135]

Hepatic cysts may be isolated or associated with adult type polycystic renal disease. Isolated liver cysts are rare, but usually remain stable during pregnancy and regress postnatally without treatment.[136] Choledochal cysts (single or multiple) occur in the right upper quadrant, below the liver, and are intraperitoneal. Similar to most cystic lesions, their significance relates to postnatal management. Untreated, choledochal cysts can lead to biliary cirrhosis and portal hypertension.

Labor and Delivery

Obstetric care is unaltered by these abnormalities.

Postnatal

Knowledge of the differential diagnosis is important. The neonate should undergo an ultrasound examination as soon after delivery as feasible. Duplications of the small and large bowel may rarely communicate with normal bowel lumen. In this instance, the neonate will present with signs of bowel obstruction. Intestinal duplications in association with spinal cord and vertebral body anomalies are reported.[137]

Acknowledgments

I would like to acknowledge the assistance of Mr. Vipul Upadhyay and Prof. Kevin Pringle (pediatric surgeons), Ms. Louise Goossens (medical photographer), and Ms. Jennie Flower and Mrs. Jenny Mitchell (ultrasonographers) with illustrations.

SUGGESTED READINGS

Abdel-Latif ME, Bolisetty S, Abeywardana S, Lui K, and the Australian and New Zealand Neonatal Network: Mode of delivery and neonatal survival of infants with gastroschisis in Australia and New Zealand. J Pediatr Surg 2008;43:1685–1690.

Deprest J, Jani J, Van Schoubroeck D, et al: Current consequences of prenatal diagnosis of congenital diaphragmatic hernia. J Pediatr Surg 2006;41:423–430.

Gargollo PC, Borer JG: Contemporary outcomes in bladder exstrophy. Curr Opin Urol 2007;17:272–280.

Houben CH, Curry JI: Current status of prenatal diagnosis operative management and outcome of esophageal atresia/tracheoesophageal fistula. Prenat Diag 2008;28:667–675.

Mann S, Blinman TA, Wilson D: Prenatal and postnatal management of omphalocele. Prenat Diagn 2008;28:626–632.

Piper HG, Alesbury J, Waterford SD, et al: Intestinal atresias: Factors affecting clinical outcomes. J Pediatr Surg 2008;43:1244–1248.

Puri P, Shinkai M: Megacystis, microcolon intestinal hypoperistalsis syndrome. Semin Pediatr Surg 2005;4:58–67.

Simchen MJ, Toi A, Bona M, et al: Fetal hepatic calcifications: Prenatal diagnosis and outcome. Am J Obstet Gynecol 2002;187:1617–1622.

Simon-Bouy B, Satre V, Ferec C, et al, and the French Collaborative Group: Hyperechogenic fetal bowel: A large French collaborative study of 682 Cases. Am J Med Genet 2003;121A:209–213.

Smrcek JM, Germer U, Krokowski M, et al: Prenatal ultrasound diagnosis and management of body stalk anomaly: Analysis of nine singleton and two multiple pregnancies. Ultrasound Obstet Gynecol 2003;21:322–328.

REFERENCES

For a complete list of references, log onto www.expertconsult.com.

CHAPTER 20

Fetal Skeletal Abnormalities

DAVID R. GRIFFIN and LYN S. CHITTY

Videos corresponding to this chapter are available online at www.expertconsult.com.

INTRODUCTION

The sonographic detection of a fetus with a skeletal disorder presents the clinician with challenging diagnostic dilemmas and management options. In some instances, the lethality of the disorder is apparent and a discussion of pregnancy termination is appropriate. The estimated prevalence of skeletal dysplasias varies from 2 to 7 in 10,000,[1] and diagnosis might require biochemical, cytogenetic, molecular genetic, or hematologic investigation. Clinical genetic input is often required because the family history or parental examination may yield valuable clues to the diagnosis. Furthermore, a geneticist may be best placed to offer advice with regard to further investigations because the genetics of these conditions is a rapidly changing field. Consultation with a geneticist specializing in dysmorphology may be invaluable. Table 20–1 lists some of the commoner terminology used in describing skeletal anomalies.

Women typically present for the prenatal diagnosis of a skeletal abnormality in one of three ways: with a relevant family history, with an abnormality found during routine ultrasound, or because of a maternal condition. Inheritable skeletal disorders may be autosomal dominant, autosomal recessive, or sex-linked. The gene locations for an increasing number of conditions are now known, making antenatal diagnosis possible early in gestation in families at increased risk, often before any skeletal manifestation is evident ultrasonographically. In many disorders and in new presentations, ultrasound is the prime method for diagnosis. Carriers of dominant disorders have a 50% offspring risk and are expressed in the heterozygous form. Some show variable expression which may be barely noticeable in a mildly affected individual (e.g., ectrodactyly, Holt-Oram syndrome). Many dominant conditions are new mutations and thus appear sporadically. In these cases, the risk of recurrence to unaffected parents is low (~1%). If recurrence does occur, it is generally attributed to gonadal mosaicism in which some of the germ-line cells (but not the somatic cells) of one parent carry the mutation. Recessive disorders are manifest in the homozygous form and occur in the offspring of unaffected heterozygous carriers. There are also a few X-linked disorders in this group (e.g., X-linked chondrodysplasia punctata).

Several ultrasonographic abnormalities may lead to the detection of conditions with limb defects, most commonly the identification of a short femur. Sometimes, close questioning or maternal examination may reveal maternal factors relevant to the etiology, for example, insulin-dependent diabetes mellitus or drugs (Table 20–2).

ULTRASOUND SCANNING FOR FETAL LIMB ABNORMALITIES

A full examination of a fetus at risk for a skeletal abnormality requires a detailed study of the general fetal anatomy, which can provide important clues to the diagnosis. Indeed, detailed examination can help classify the underlying pathology by considering the pattern of anomalies and may indicate other aids to diagnosis (Table 20–3). In early human pregnancy, the upper limbs develop a few days in advance of the lower limbs, with the arm buds appearing at about 5½ postmenstrual weeks followed by the leg buds a few days later. Fetal ossification begins in the clavicle at around 8 weeks' gestation, followed by the mandible, vertebral bodies, and neural arches around 9 weeks, the frontal bones at 10 to 11 weeks and the long bones at approximately 11 weeks.[2] Most skeletal structures can be identified ultrasonographically by 14 to 15 weeks,[3] but the earliest clue to musculoskeletal problems is often an increased nuchal translucency.[4] Later in pregnancy, this is reflected by an increased nuchal fold and generalized skin thickening. In some conditions, frank hydrops can also occur.

If limb shortening appears to be isolated, then fetal growth retardation (FGR) must be considered as a possible etiology.[5] In these circumstances, review of maternal serum screening results for levels of pregnancy-associated plasma protein-A (PAPP-A), β-human chorionic gonadotropin (β-hCG), and maternal serum α-fetoprotein (MSAFP) and assessment of fetal and maternal Doppler results can be useful diagnostic aids (see Table 20–3). Of 130 fetuses referred to the author's unit with abnormal femora (short, bowed, hypoplastic), 42 were thought to have short straight femurs with no other abnormalities. Only 2 of these had a skeletal dysplasia. Many were normal and had had either an incorrect assignment of gestational age or familial short stature, but 31% had FGR.[6]

TABLE 20–1

Terminology Used in Describing Skeletal Abnormalities

Achiria	Absent hand(s)
Achiropodia	Absent hand(s) and foot (feet)
Acromelia	Shortening of distal segments of limbs, hands, and feet
Adactyly	Absent fingers and/or toes
Amelia	Complete absence of one or more limbs from shoulder or pelvic girdle
Apodia	Absent foot (feet)
Arthrogryposis	Congenital restriction of joint movement
Brachydactyly	Short fingers
Camptomelia	Bent limb or bent fingers
Clinodactyly	Incurved fifth finger
Diaphysis	Central shaft of long bone
Ectrodactyly	Split hand(s) or foot (feet; lobster claw deformity)
Epiphysis	End growing plate of bones
Hemimelia	Absence of distal arm or leg below elbow or knee
Kyphosis	Dorsal convex curvature of the spine
Kyphoscoliosis	Combination of lateral and anteroposterior curvature of spine
Lordosis	Dorsal convex curvature of the lumbar spine
Mesomelia	Shortening of middle segment of limb (radius/ulna and tibia/fibula)
Micrognathia	Small jaw or mandible
Micromelia	Shortening of all long bones
Oligodactyly	Absent or partially absent finger(s) and toe(s)
Phocomelia	Absence or hypoplasia of long bones, may have hands or feet attached
Platyspondyly	Flattening of the vertebral bodies
Preaxial polydactyly	Extra fingers or toes on radial or tibial side
Postaxial polydactyly	Extra fingers or toes on ulna or fibular side
Rhizomelia	Shortening of proximal long bones (femur and humerus)
Syndactyly	Fused fingers ± toes (skin or bone)
Scoliosis	Lateral curvature of spine
Talipes equinovalgus	Clubfoot—foot twisted outward
Talipes equinovarus	Clubfoot—foot twisted inward

TABLE 20–2

Skeletal Anomalies Associated with Maternal Disease or Maternal Drug Ingestion

UNDERLYING ETIOLOGY	SONOGRAPHIC FINDINGS	OTHER DIAGNOSTIC AIDS
Warfarin	Rhizomelic shortening of limbs. Stippled epiphyses, kyphoscoliosis, flat face, depressed nasal bridge, renal, cardiac, and CNS anomalies.	Maternal drug history
Sodium valproate	Reduction deformity of arms, polydactyly, oligodactyly, talipes, cardiac and CNS anomalies.	Maternal drug and medical history
Methotrexate	Mesomelic shortening of long bones, hypomineralized skull, syndactyly, oligodactyly, talipes, CNS anomalies including neural tube defects, micrognathia.	Maternal drug history
Vitamin A	Hypoplasia or aplasia of arm bones, CNS and cardiac anomalies, spina bifida, cleft lip and palate, diaphragmatic hernia, exomphalos.	Maternal drug history
Phenytoin	Stippled epiphyses, micrognathia, cleft lip, cardiac anomalies.	Maternal drug and medical history
Alcohol	Short long bones, reduction deformity of arm bones, preaxial polydactyly of hands, oligodactyly, stippled epiphyses, FGR, cardiac anomalies.	Maternal history
Cocaine	Reduction deformities of arms ± legs, ectrodactyly, hemivertebrae, absent ribs, CNS, cardiac, renal anomalies, anterior abdominal wall defects, bowel atresias.	Maternal history
Diabetes	Caudal regression, femoral hypoplasia.	Maternal medical history, glucose tolerance test
Myasthenia gravis	Multiple joint contractures, arthrogryposis.	Measurement of maternal anticholinesterase antibodies
Myotonic dystrophy	Talipes and polyhydramnios.	Examination of mother for signs of myotonia, facial appearance; genetic referral
Systemic lupus erythematosus	Short limbs, Stippled epiphyses, depressed nasal bridge.	Maternal medical and obstetric history, autoimmune screen

CNS, central nervous system; FGR, fetal growth retardation.

Long Bones

The long bones are measured in a plane as near to the horizontal as possible to avoid shadowing artifact (Fig. 20–1). As a result, the longest measurement is the true measurement. Each bone should be measured independently. The pattern of shortening is a useful diagnostic aid and the length of all long bones should be checked against appropriate charts to compare both limb length and measurements of head and abdominal circumference.[7–10] Long bone shortening may be generalized (micromelia), more marked in the proximal long bones (rhizomelia) or the forearms and lower

TABLE 20–3

Sonographic Features to Be Examined When Suspecting a Skeletal Abnormality with the Major Associations and Other Diagnostic Aids

SONOGRAPHIC FINDING	CONDITION	OTHER INVESTIGATIONS TO BE CONSIDERED
Skull—Shape, Mineralization (Acoustic Shadow)		
Hypomineralized	Osteogenesis imperfecta IIA and IIC Achondrogenesis type I Hypophosphatasia (severe neonatal form)	(Phosphoethanolamine in parental urine) Parental serum alkaline phosphatase levels
Mild hypomineralization	Achondrogenesis type 2 Cleidocranial dysostosis Osteogenesis imperfecta IIB	Examine parents
Cloverleaf	Thanatophoric dysplasia type II Occasionally in short-ribbed polydactyly syndromes Antley-Bixler Craniosynostosis syndromes (Pfeiffer/Crouzon/ Saethre-Chotzen)	Screen for mutations in FGFR3 and 2 genes
Spine—Length, Mineralization, Alignment (Hemivertebrae), Organization (Stippling)		
Hypomineralized	Achondrogenesis type I	
Disorganized	Jarcho-Levin Spondylocostal dysplasia Dyssegmental dysplasia Some chondrodysplasia punctatas VATER/VACTERL	
Face—Profile (Frontal Bossing, Depressed Nasal Bridge, Micrognathia), Cleft Lip and/or Palate, Orbital Diameters for Hypo- or Hypertelorism		
Frontal bossing	Thanatophoric dysplasia Achondroplasia Acromesomelic dysplasia	Screen for mutations in FGFR3 gene
Depressed nasal bridge	Chondrodysplasia punctatas Warfarin embryopathy	Drug history, mutations in ARSE gene, metabolic investigations—very long chain fatty acids and sterol profile, maternal history of autoimmune disease
Micrognathia	SEDC Stickler's syndrome Campomelic dysplasia	Examine parents
Cleft lip	Majewski's syndrome	
Long Bones—Length, Pattern of Shortening, Which Bones Are Affected, Symmetrical or Asymmetrical, Bowing/Evidence of Fractures, Ossification, Epiphyses for Stippling		
Isolated, straight short long bones	Fetal growth retardation Constitutional short stature	Fetal and maternal Dopplers Family history Parental stature
Femoral bowing	Campomelic dysplasia Osteogenesis imperfecta Hypophosphatasia	
Talipes	Campomelic dysplasia Diastrophic dysplasia	
Stippled epiphyses	Rhizomelic chondrodysplasia punctata Conradi Hunerman X-linked recessive chondrodysplasia punctata Warfarin embryopathy	Drug history, mutations in ARSE gene, metabolic investigations—very long chain fatty acids and sterol profile, maternal history of autoimmune disease
Limb Girdles—Appearance of Clavicles and Scapulae		
Short clavicles	Campomelic dysplasia Cleidocranial dysostosis	Examine parents
Small scapula	Campomelic dysplasia	
Hands and Feet—Short Fingers (Trident Hand), Short Feet, Camptodactyly, Ectrodactyly, Polydactyly, Oligodactyly		
Polydactyly	Jeune's asphyxiating thoracic dystrophy Ellis-van Creveld syndrome Short-ribbed polydactyly syndromes	
Short fingers/trident hand	Achondroplasia Acromesomelic dysplasia Thanatophoric dysplasia	Screen for mutations in FGFR3 gene
Oligodactyly	Brachmann de Lange Idiopathic limb reduction defects	
Short feet	Brachmann de Lange	

TABLE 20–3

Sonographic Features to Be Examined When Suspecting a Skeletal Abnormality with the Major Associations and Other Diagnostic Aids—cont'd

SONOGRAPHIC FINDING	CONDITION	OTHER INVESTIGATIONS TO BE CONSIDERED
Joints—Contractures, Pterygia, Talipes, Radial Club Hand		
Contractures		
Pterygia		
Talipes	Diastrophic dysplasia Campomelic dysplasia	
Radial club hand	VATER/VACTERL	
Thorax—Size, Length, Rib Length, Shape, Beading (Fractures)		
Narrow with short ribs	Short-ribbed polydactyly syndromes Jeune's asphyxiating thoracic dystrophy Thanatophoric dysplasia Osteogenesis imperfecta types IIA, C and B Campomelic dysplasia Achondrogenesis Hypochondrogenesis Paternal UPD14	
Beaded ribs	Osteogenesis imperfecta type IIA and C	
Associated Abnormalities—Cardiac, Renal, Intracranial, Genital		
Cardiac	Campomelic dysplasia Ellis-van Creveld Short-ribbed polydactyly syndromes VATER/ VACTERL	
Renal	Jeune's asphyxiating thoracic dystrophy Short-ribbed polydactyly syndromes	
Intracranial	Majewski, Beemer Langer Thanatophoric dysplasia type II.	
Genital	Campomelic dysplasia Short-ribbed polydactyly syndromes	Karyotyping to confirm genetic sex
Liquor Volume—Polyhydramnios, Oligohydramnios		
Polyhydramnios	Achondroplasia Thanatophoric dysplasia Paternal UPD14 VATER/VACTERL	
Oligohydramios	Short-ribbed polydactyly syndromes with severe renal anomalies	
Maternal and Fetal Dopplers		
Abnormal Dopplers	Fetal growth retardation	Past obstetric history, maternal autoantibodies, maternal serum PAPP-A, β-HCG, and AFP levels

AFP, α-fetoprotein; ARSE, arylsulphatase E; β-hCG, β-human chorionic gonadotropin; FGFR3, fibroblast growth factor receptor 3; PAPP-A, pregnancy-associated plasma protein-A; SEDC, spondyloepiphyseal dysplasia congenita; UPD14, uniparental disomy 14; VATER/VACTERL, vertebral defects, anal atresia or stenosis, tracheoesophageal fistula, radial defects and renal anomalies.

legs (mesomelia) (Fig. 20–2). In some conditions, the changes may be confined to the legs (e.g., campomelic dysplasia) or arms (e.g., Holt-Oram). Hypomineralized long bones reflect less ultrasound at the proximal interface. Thus, they appear less echo-dense across the diaphysis and have a reduced acoustic shadow. Minor degrees of hypomineralization are likely to go undetected. Hypomineralization may result in fracturing, and the position and degree of bowing or fracturing should be noted. Bones may appear short, thick, and crumpled, indicating severe degrees of fracturing and undermodeling as found in osteogenesis imperfecta (OI) types IIa and IIc. It is important to note which bones are affected and where because this can help with the diagnosis. The ends of the bones should be carefully examined to exclude ephyphyseal stippling which might indicate a chondrodysplasia punctata as in rhizomelic chondrodysplasia punctata. If stippling is identified, various metabolic and cytogenetic investigations can be done in order to try and define the underlying etiology (see Table 20–3). Examination of the joints may be useful because talipes can be a feature of several dysplasias (see Table 20–3).

Skull

Skull hypomineralization reduces both the echogenicity of the skull and the acoustic shadowing beyond it. The cranial contents are seen more clearly than normal. In severe cases of hypomineralization, such as OI types IIA and IIC and achondrogenesis type 1, the cerebral hemispheres are almost anechoic, giving the appearance of ventriculomegaly. This is excluded by showing that the choroid plexus and the walls of the lateral ventricle antrum are normally situated within the hemisphere. The skull bones are soft and can deform when subjected to pressure from the transducer.

FIGURE 20–1
A–E, Normal long bones. The bones are measured as near as possible to horizontal in the scanning plane. The limb segment soft tissue extremity is clearly visible beyond the end of the metaphyses. *A*, T, tibia; F, fibula; K, knee. *B*, F, femur; H, hip. *C*, H, humerus; E, elbow; S, scapula. *D*, R, radius; E, elbow; H, hand. *E*, U, ulna; E, elbow; H, hand.

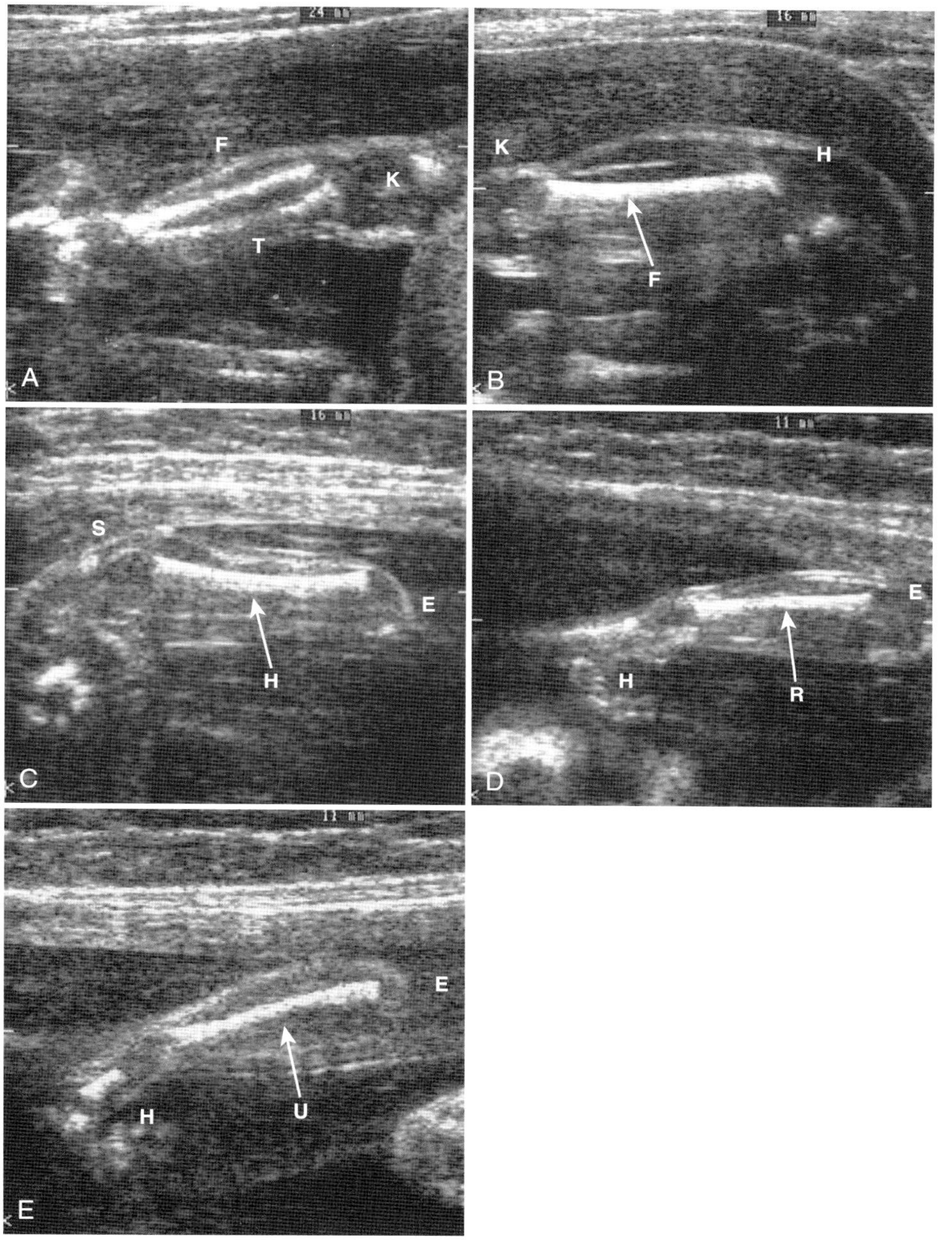

Hypomineralization may be less obvious in disorders such as hypophosphatasia or OI types IIB and III. Variation in skull shape can also be seen in some craniosynostosis syndromes. The cloverleaf skull is seen in thanatophoric dysplasia type II.

Spine

The spine should be examined carefully in all three planes. Absent or decreased mineralization is a feature of some dysplasias (see Table 20–3). Ossification of the cervical and sacral vertebral bodies is a late event; the sacral vertebral bodies are not ossified until 27 weeks' gestation. Diagnosis of pathologic hypomineralization must be made with care. Vertebral anomalies (e.g., hemivertebrae) can occur with or without associated rib anomalies. The appearance of general disorganization may indicate ectopic calcification seen in some chondrodysplasia punctatas or bony abnormalities as in Jarcho-Levin syndrome.[11]

Face

Cleft lip or palate is a feature of many skeletal dysplasias (see Table 20–3) and may on occasions be very subtle, for example, the small midline cleft seen in Majewski's short-ribbed polydactyly syndrome (SRPS) type 2. Measurement

FIGURE 20–2
Femur length measurements in skeletal dysplasias.
(Modified from Griffin DR: Detection of congenital abnormalities of the limbs and face by ultrasound. In Chamberlain G [ed]: Modern Antenatal Care of the Fetus. Oxford, UK, Blackwell Scientific, 1990, pp 389-427; and Griffin DR: Skeletal dysplasias. In Brock DJH, Rodeck CH, Ferguson-Smith MA [eds]: Prenatal Diagnosis and Screening. Edinburgh: Churchill Livingstone, 1992, pp 257-313.)

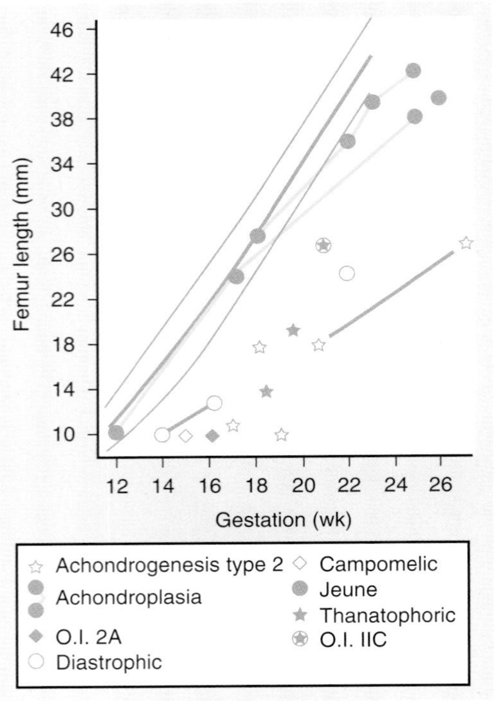

of the intraorbital diameter may reveal hyper- or hypotelorism in some syndromes. Micrognathia is also associated with a number of conditions (see Table 20–3) and the mandible can be measured in the axial plane from the temporomandibular joint to the mental eminence.[12] Measurement of the mandible and orbital diameters might be more difficult in later pregnancy with increasing acoustic shadowing from surrounding bony structures.[12] A facial profile in the sagittal plane may show frontal bossing (achondroplasia, thanatophoric dysplasia), a depressed nasal bridge (chondrodysplasia punctata), or micrognathia (campomelic dysplasia) (see Table 20–3).

Thorax

Examination of the fetal thorax should include an estimation of thoracic size and examination of the ribs and length of the thoracic cavity. Many dysplasias are lethal because of associated pulmonary hypoplasia. Nomograms of thoracic circumference are available,[13] but a small chest can often be inferred by observation alone. In normal circumstances, the thorax and abdomen should be approximately the same size when viewed in the axial plane. The thorax may be normal, constricted, short, or long. Normal liver size and abdominal circumference cause the abdominal wall to protrude, giving a "champagne cork" appearance when viewed in the sagittal plane. When constricted, the ratio of heart circumference to thoracic circumference (normally ~1 : 3)[14] is increased and the heart may appear to lie outside the chest in extreme cases. The chest can also be small secondary to a short spine, as in some of the spondylodysplasias. In these situations, the chest may appear small in a sagittal plane, but when viewed in the axial plane, the ribs appear of normal length and the heart occupies the appropriate proportion of the thoracic cavity. The ribs may be short, thick, thin, beaded (i.e., fractured), flared, or irregular in shape, arrangement, or number. Examination in the axial plane may reveal short ribs, but the longitudinal plane is more likely to reveal the beading indicative of fracturing seen in OI IIA and IIC. Disorganiszation of the ribs (and spine) may be features of conditions such as Jarcho-Levin syndrome. The heart should be carefully examined because several skeletal dysplasias are associated with cardiac anomalies, for example, Ellis–van Creveld (EVC) syndrome (50%) and campomelic dysplasia (see Table 20–3).

Other Anomalies

A detailed fetal anomaly scan is recommended because there are a number of other anomalies that may give a clue to the underlying diagnosis and help target investigations. In most cases, referral to a clinical geneticist is advisable to identify further investigations and to examine the parents (see Tables 20–2 and 20–3).

CLASSIFICATION OF SKELETAL DYSPLASIAS

The genetic and pathologic etiology of skeletal anomalies is wide. Classifications can be on clinical and/or radiologic grounds,[15] by molecular/genetic etiology, or by structure and function of responsible genes and proteins (e.g., defects in structural proteins, metabolic pathways, transcription factors),[16] or a hybrid.[17] For the prenatal diagnostician, a classification based on sonographic findings is the most useful (see Table 20–3), but there can be considerable overlap in conditions and so a table listing the common diagnoses with gene location, where known, inheritance, and main sonographic findings can also be very helpful.[18] In this chapter, the gene, if known, is placed in parentheses at the heading for the appropriate syndrome.

EARLY-ONSET SEVERE SYMMETRICAL SHORT STRAIGHT LONG BONES

Achondrogenesis

Diagnosis

TYPE 1 (PARENTI-FRACCARO SYNDROME) (5q31-5q34) DTDST

The long bones show extreme micromelia with very poor modeling (e.g., femur length of 10 mm at 19 wk).[19] The calvarium and vertebral column are severely hypomineralized (see Fig. 20–2).

TYPE 2 (LANGER-SALDINO SYNDROME) (12q13-12q14; *COL2AI*)

The long bones are better modeled than in type 1 but are still extremely short, thick, and straight (Fig. 20–3*A*; see also

FIGURE 20–3
Achondrogenesis. *A*, Short (13-mm) humerus of a fetus with achondrogenesis type II at 18 weeks. *B*, Ultrasound scan of the trunk and head (H) of the same fetus shown in *A*. The spinal column is shown (*arrow*) as an anechoic cartilaginous column. The skull shows some mineralization. *C*, Radiograph of the fetus in *A* shows total absence of ossification in all elements of the spinal column. The ribs are short and the thorax small. There is little mineralization of the skull. *D*, Postnatal radiograph of a different fetus with achondrogenesis type 2 at a similar gestation to that in *C*. In this case, only the vertebral bodies show lack of calcification. Other features are similar to those in *C* with short, straight, reasonably modeled long bones showing flared, cupped metaphyses. The ischial bones are unossified and the ilia small and halberd shaped.
(*A* and *B*, From Griffin DR: Skeletal dysplasias. In Brock DJH, Rodeck CH, Ferguson-Smith MA [eds]: Prenatal Diagnosis and Screening. Edinburgh: Churchill Livingstone, 1992, pp 257–313.)

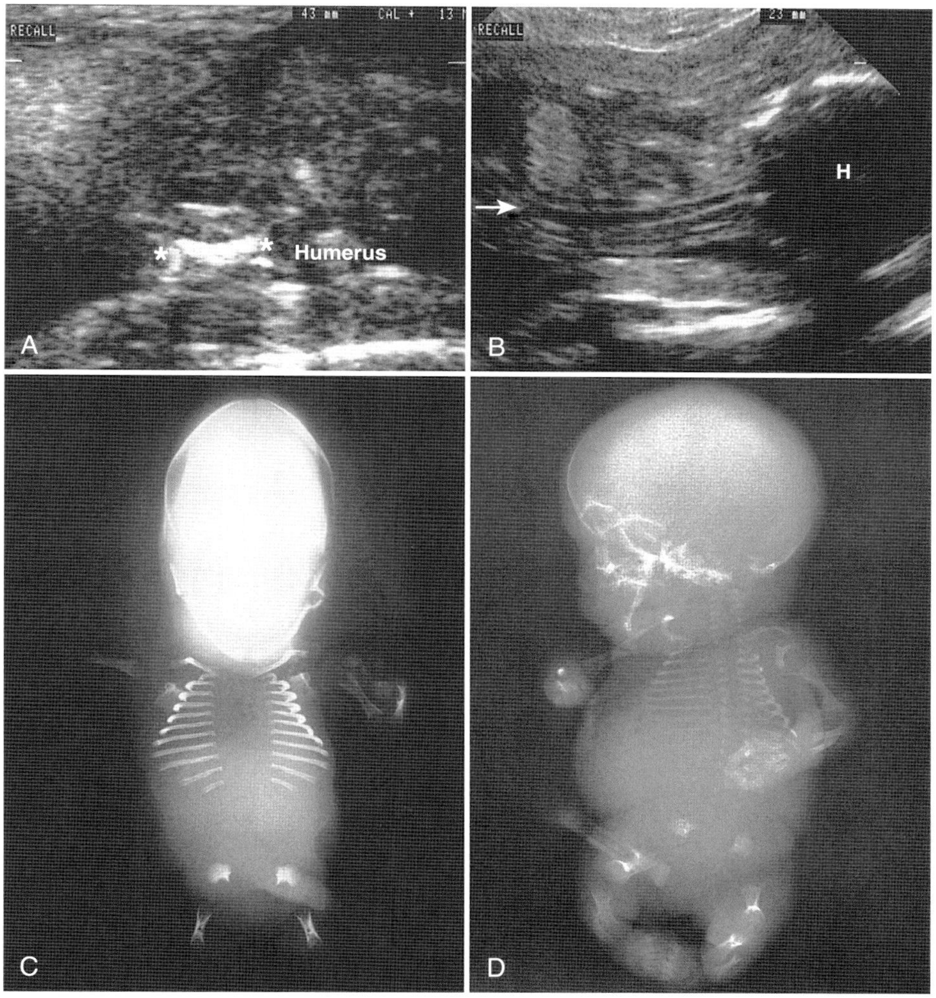

Fig. 20–2). The calvarium is normally ossified, and although hypomineralization of the spine is variable, it can be striking (see Fig. 20–3*B*–*D*).

Risks and Management Options

Achondrogenesis types 1 and 2 are lethal conditions at or before birth. Termination of pregnancy should be included as an option during counseling. The diagnosis is supported by postnatal radiography and expert pathology. Where possible, it should be confirmed by DNA analysis. The recurrence risk is 1 : 4 for achondrogenesis type 1. Achondrogenesis is usually a new dominant mutation.

Thanatophoric Dysplasia (4p16; *FGFR3*)

Diagnosis

Thanatophoric dysplasia is the most common lethal skeletal dysplasia. A definitive diagnosis is possible by 12 to 14 weeks,[20] but is more commonly made at 18 to 20 weeks.[21,22] The femur and other limb-length measurements are well below the 3rd percentile (see Fig. 20–2) and display a characteristic thickening of the metaphyses. Measurements from 14 to 21 mm at 18 to 20 weeks to 26 mm at 32 weeks are reported.[23–26] The femurs may appear bowed in some cases and straight in others (Fig. 20–4*B*). The feet and hands are

FIGURE 20–4
Thanatophoric dysplasia. *A*, Skull showing the cloverleaf deformity. *B*, Lower limbs showing the short legs and femurs in the typical frog-like position. *C*, Transverse sections of the trunk of the fetus at the level of the umbilical vein and the heart showing marked reduction of the thoracic circumference and short ribs with the heart appearing to bulge out of the thorax. *D*, Longitudinal anteroposterior sagittal scan of the trunk of the fetus in *B* shows the narrow thorax and abdomen protruding anteriorly: the "champagne cork" appearance. The prominent forehead (frontal bossing) is also seen in this view.

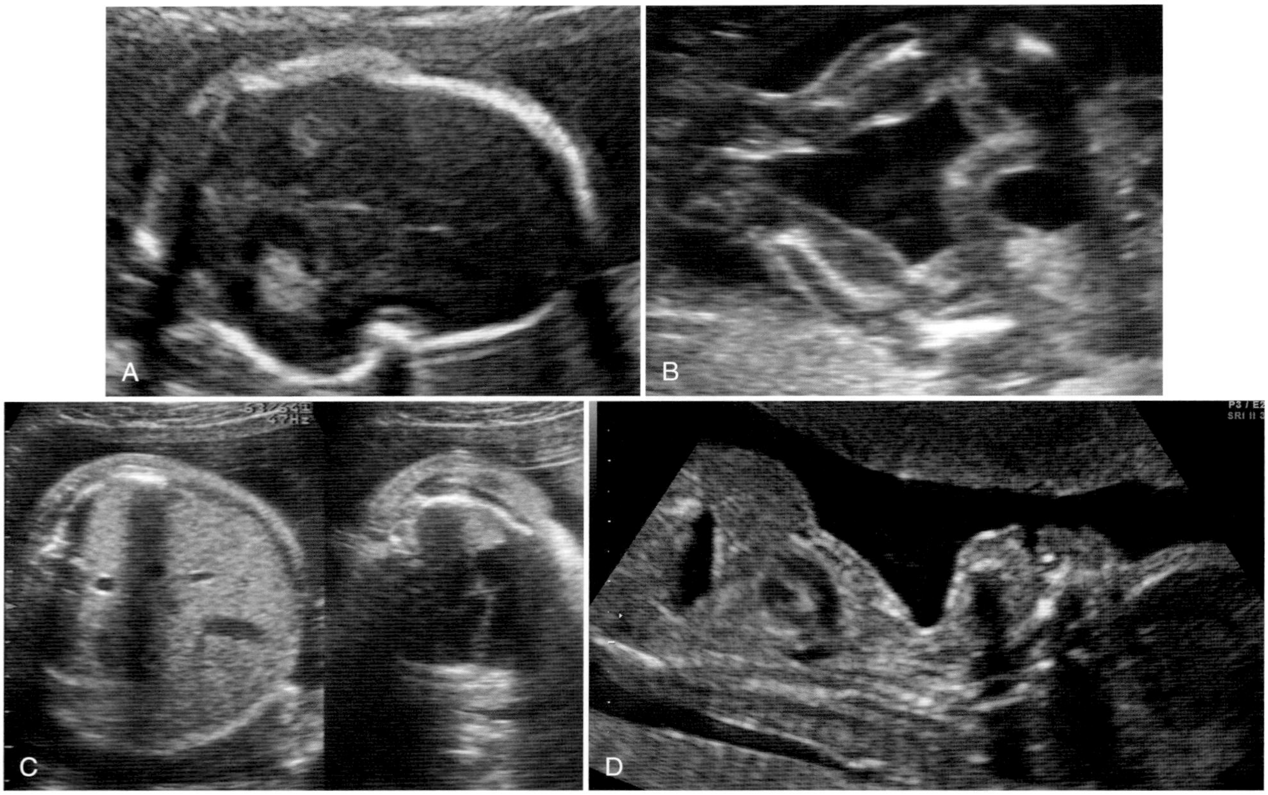

short. The short, splayed fingers are described as a "trident hand." Short stubby ribs produce a markedly small thorax (see Fig. 20–4C). The cardiothoracic ratio is high (see Fig. 20–4C) and the characteristic truncal champagne cork appearance is seen in the sagittal plane (see Fig. 20–4*D*). Some cases show flattening of the vertebral bodies (platyspondyly) and a short spine. The skull is normally ossified and may be macrocephalic or brachycephalic. Some variants with straight, long bones show the cloverleaf deformity (see Fig. 20–4*A*) produced by prominence of the parietal bones.[20,21,23,26] This sign can be recognized in the first trimester[20] but is usually more evident later in pregnancy. Cerebral ventriculomegaly may occur. The facial profile shows a depressed nasal bridge and frontal bossing. Late in pregnancy, soft tissue folds can often be seen on the arms (the "Michelin man" appearance). Hydramnios is also a later feature.

Because the majority of cases result from a mutation in fibroblast growth factor receptor (*FGFR*) 3 gene at 4p16,[27] it can be useful to test the index case. The recurrence risk is small (<1%), but confirmation by DNA analysis will allow early prenatal diagnosis and reassurance in subsequent pregnancies, although a careful scan at 12 to 14 weeks could also exclude a recurrence.

Risks and Management Options

Thanatophoric dysplasia is lethal and pregnancy termination should be included as an option during counseling. Prenatal diagnosis using free fetal DNA extracted from maternal plasma can be used to confirm the diagnosis before delivery.[28] Postnatal confirmation of the diagnosis by radiography or DNA analysis is essential in the absence of a definitive prenatal diagnosis. Parents should be advised that recurrence risks are low because this is a new dominant sporadic condition.

CONDITIONS ASSOCIATED WITH BOWED OR SEVERELY FRACTURED LIMBS

Campomelic Dysplasia (17q24-17q25; *SOX9*)

Diagnosis

Early diagnosis is possible.[29–33] The characteristic midshaft bowing of the femur should be recognized during a routine ultrasound (Fig. 20–5), although there is considerable variation in presentation.[34,35] The tibia is short and bowed and the fibula hypoplastic. Marked talipes may cause the whole lower limb to be grossly bowed inward (campomelia). The ribs may be short and the thorax constricted. Brachycephaly, micrognathia, and short clavicles may be detected. Associated anomalies are found in a third of cases and include atrial/ventricular septal defect, hydronephrosis, and ventriculomegaly. Hydramnios may occur late in pregnancy. Phenotypic sex reversal in males is common; karyotyping to

FIGURE 20–5
Campomelic dysplasia. *A*, Showing bowing of the femur with short lower leg and talipes. *B*, Profile of this fetus demonstrating micrognathia.
(From Griffin DR: Detection of congenital abnormalities of the limbs and face by ultrasound. In Chamberlain G [ed]: Modern Antenatal Care of the Fetus. Oxford, UK, Blackwell Scientific, 1990, pp 389–427.)

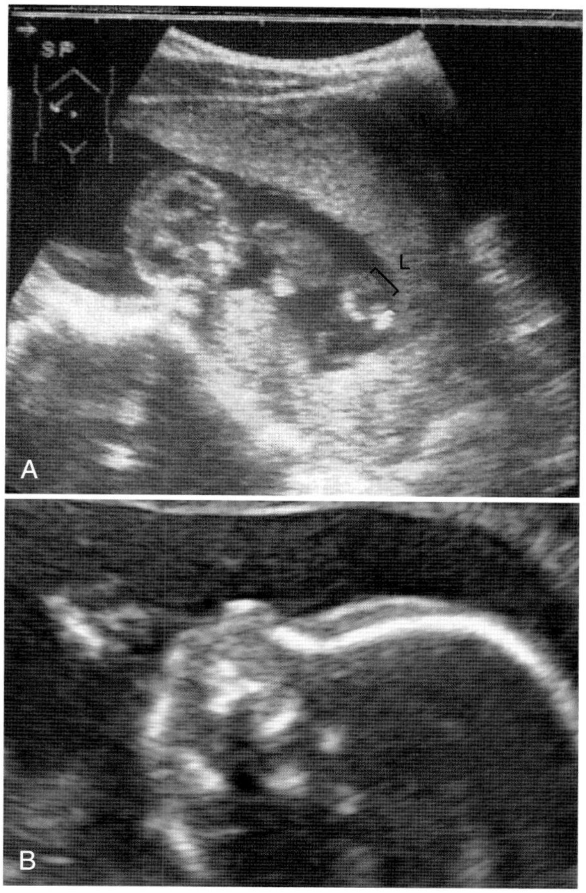

confirm genetic sex in fetuses with bowed lower limbs should therefore be offered. This is now possible by analyzing cell free fetal DNA in the maternal blood, thereby avoiding the risks of invasive testing.[36]

Risks and Management Options

Three quarters of infants die during the neonatal period from pulmonary hypoplasia and 90% die by the age of 2 years. The prognosis depends on the severity of associated malformations. Survivors fail to thrive and can show neurologic impairment. The recurrence risk is around 5%; many cases are thought to be the result of a new dominant mutation.[34] The option of pregnancy termination should be offered. Support for the diagnosis by pathologic examination and radiography is essential before counseling the parents about the recurrence risk. Antenatal ultrasonographic diagnosis should be offered in subsequent pregnancies.

Osteogenesis Imperfecta (*COL1A1, COL1A2*)

OI is characterized by poor bone mineralization. Based on the clinical and radiologic findings, it was originally divided into four types,[37] although further subgroups have since been added[38]; all are due to mutations in the *COL1A1* and *COLIA2* genes[38] (Table 20–4). The overall incidence approximates to 1 in 10,000. Types I and IV are probably not amenable to early ultrasound diagnosis, although diagnosis has been reported in the second trimester for type IV[39] and the third trimester for type I. Types IIA, B, C, and type 3 have all been diagnosed before 22 weeks' gestation.[40–48] Some evidence suggests that recurrences are due to gonadal mosaicism and the recurrence risks should be quoted at 5% to 7%.[49,50] Type I is inherited in an autosomal dominant fashion. In type III, there is genetic heterogeneity and recurrence is reported. There is the possibility of autosomal recessive inheritance and, again, gonadal mosaicism. Recurrence risks after an isolated case are approximately 7%.[51]

Diagnosis

OI type IIA is the most common form. It is recognizable early in pregnancy by hypomineralization of the skull and

TABLE 20–4
Sonographic Features and Prognosis in Different Types of Osteogenesis Imperfecta

TYPE OF OI	GESTATION AT PRESENTATION	PRENATAL FEATURES	PROGNOSIS
Type I	Usually postnatal, occasionally third trimester	Occasional fractures late in third trimester	Variable fracturing
Type IIA	>12 wk	Hypomineralized easily deformable skull; beaded ribs; small chest; very short, crumpled long bones	Lethal
Type IIB	>16 wk	Mild hypomineralized skull, short and bowed long bones, short flared ribs with occasional beading	Usually perinatally lethal
Type IIC	>12 wk	As with IIA, but a greater degree of hypomineralization	Lethal
Type III	~20 wk	Bowed leg bones, occasional bowed radius and ulna; normal skull mineralization, normal chest with very occasional beading; long bones progressively fall below 5th percentile	Early lethality common; fractures, and progressive deformity in survivors
Type IV	≥20 wk	Long bones often within normal range; normal skull and chest; mild bowing of femur and tibia	Variable prognosis; may have rib fractures at birth

OI, osteogenesis imperfecta.

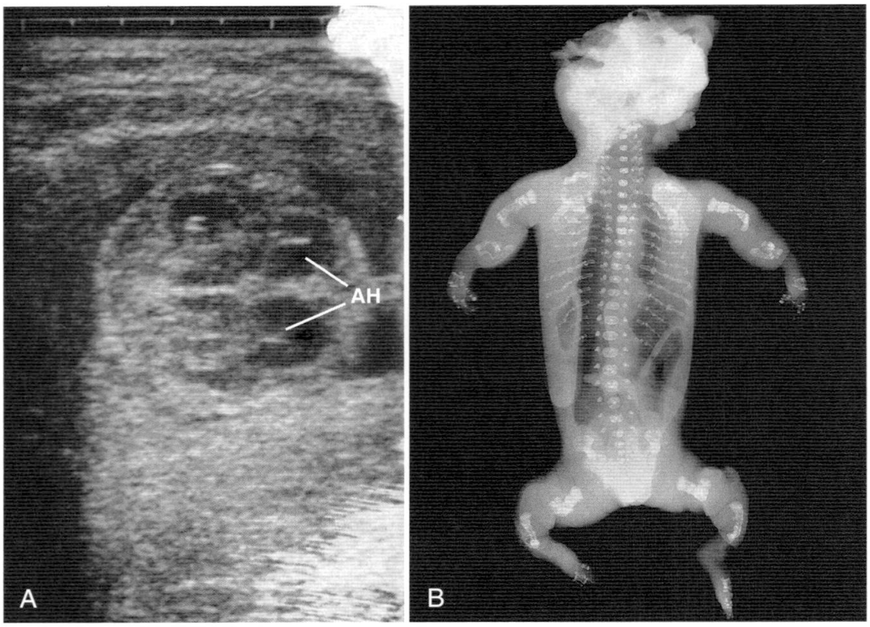

FIGURE 20–6
Osteogenesis imperfecta type IIA. *A*, Skull of a 20-week fetus shows the features of severe hypomineralization. The skull bones are poorly echogenic and cast no acoustic shadow. The cerebral hemispheres are anechoic, giving the appearance of cerebral ventriculomegaly (pseudohydrocephaly). However, the echoes from the anterior horns (AH) are normally placed. *B*, Postnatal radiograph of a fetus shows the short, bowed long bones, crumpled by multiple intrauterine fractures. The lower limbs are held in a camptomelic (bent) posture. The ribs are "beaded" from fractures, and hairline fractures are also evident in the vertebral bodies (the skull was lost in delivery).
(*A* and *B*, From Griffin DR: Detection of congenital abnormalities of the limbs and face by ultrasound. In Chamberlain G [ed]: Modern Antenatal Care of the Fetus. Oxford, UK, Blackwell Scientific, 1990, pp 389–427.)

long bones with severe micromelia.[40–47] The usual bright echo of the skull bones is lost and there is no acoustic shadow (Fig. 20–6*A*). The orbits may be unusually prominent. The cerebral hemispheres take on a transsonic character. There may appear to be ventriculomegaly, though it can be excluded by identifying the choroid plexus within normal ventricular walls and a normal posterior horn measurement. The head is brachycephalic and easily deformed by pressure from the ultrasound transducer even late in pregnancy. The long bones are hypoechoic, irregularly bowed, and crumpled as a result of multiple fractures and callus formation (see Fig. 20–6*B*). The limbs show marked, fixed campomelia and talipes. Other features, such as beading of the ribs and a small thorax, may be recognized. Amniotic fluid abnormalities can occur later in pregnancy. Type IIC has skeletal features similar to those of type IIA.

Fetuses with type IIB or III rarely have a poorly calcified skull. The femurs may show bowing (Fig. 20–7) or fracture with mild to moderate shortening, but are generally well modeled. Lower legs may be bowed and measure below the 5th percentile.[39,48] Other long bones tend to be at or just below the 5th percentile at 20 weeks, with measurements decreasing with gestation. Type I cannot reliably be excluded before viability. The clinical presentation and prognosis of types I and IV are quite variable and can show considerable overlap. Expert advice is recommended before counseling. The antenatal diagnosis of type IV has also been reported. The features are usually mild, with minimal bowing of the femurs and preservation of long bone growth.[39]

Risks and Management Options

Types IIA and C are lethal. Although type IIB is often lethal, a child may survive to infancy.[49–51] Children with type III can survive but with significant physical handicap owing to multiple deforming fractures.[52] Early postnatal treatment with bisphoshanates may improve prognosis in cases that survive.[53] Pregnancy termination is an option that should be discussed following the diagnosis of OI types II or III in view of the severity of the condition. Abdominal delivery might reduce the risk of either trauma or intracranial hemorrhage.

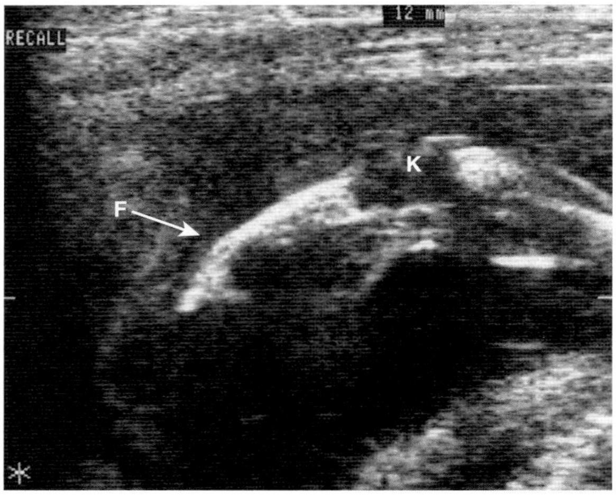

FIGURE 20–7
Osteogenesis imperfecta type III. Femur (F) with midshaft bowing and poor mineralization. The cartilagenous epiphyses are evident at the knee (K).

Hypophosphatasia (1p34-1p36)

Bone hypomineralization results from a deficiency of alkaline phosphatase. This heterogeneous group of disorders varies from a lethal condition to milder forms, which become apparent only in childhood. The appearance of the lethal form is similar to that of OI type II. Although the bones are generally less crumpled, they may show marked angulation.

Diagnosis

The diagnosis may be based on biochemical, ultrasonographic, or molecular methods, or a combination. There are very few reports of the antenatal diagnosis of hypophosphatasia.[54,55] If cranial hypomineralization is marked, the skull appears similar to that in OI type II with anechoic calvarium, prominent intracranial structures, and an easily deformed skull. The femurs and humeri are short and may be so bowed at the midshaft with osseous spurs that measurement is difficult.[56] The ribs are thin and may show fractures. The spine may be markedly demineralized, particularly in the area of the neural arch. In a case report of the milder form, the femoral bowing appeared to resolve during pregnancy.[57] Measurement of alkaline phosphatase (ALP) in amniotic fluid[58] or in cultured amniocytes is unreliable until after 20 weeks. Successful confirmation of diagnosis is possible by measuring cellular ALP in a chorionic villus sample.[59,60]

Risks and Management Options

The severe recessive form is lethal, and the option of pregnancy termination should be included in the counseling session. The osseous maldevelopment in the milder, autosomal dominant forms tends to improve with advancing age. The diagnosis must be confirmed by expert radiography and also by biochemical or genetic investigation of the parents. It is unclear whether milder forms should be delivered abdominally to avoid trauma.

SHORT LONG BONES: MILD TO MODERATE SYMMETRICAL

Fetal Growth Restriction

One of the first conditions to be considered when finding isolated mild to moderate shortening of long bones is FGR.[5,6] In this condition long bones will be normally modeled and there will be no associated visceral anomalies.

Diagnosis

The following investigations should be considered to define the etiology, which includes constitutional short stature, aneuploidy, placental insufficiency, or early signs of a late-onset skeletal dysplasia such as achondroplasia (Table 20–5):

- Detailed anomaly scan.
- Fetal and maternal Doppler scans.
- Family history.
- Amniotic fluid index.
- Down syndrome screening results.
- Karyotyping.
- Maternal blood for *FGFR3* mutation analysis.

Jeune's Thoracic Dystrophy (Asphyxiating Thoracic Dystrophy) (15q13)

Diagnosis

The severity of this condition and the degree of limb shortening are variable. The reports of prenatal diagnosis of Jeune's syndrome are based on the finding of a small thorax in high risk families.[61] The chest is reduced in the anteroposterior diameter with consequent protrusion of the anterior abdominal wall. Limb shortening is variable and can be present from early gestation (~15 wk) but, in some cases, might not be apparent until later in pregnancy (Fig. 20–8). Hydramnios may occur in late pregnancy. Associated features include renal, hepatic, pancreatic, and pulmonary dysplasia, and occasionally, postaxial polydactyly.

Risks and Management Options

Approximately 70% of liveborn children die from respiratory failure during the neonatal period. Survivors are small in stature and often succumb to respiratory, renal, hepatic, or pancreatic complications in childhood. Intelligence is normal. The option of pregnancy termination should be included in counseling if the diagnosis is made in a timely fashion, because the mortality and morbidity rates are high. This autosomal recessive disorder has a 25% recurrence risk.

Short-Ribbed Polydactyly Syndromes

There is some overlap between the main subdivisions of SRPSs[62]:

- I (Saldino-Noonan type) is associated with micromelia characterized by distinct, pointed ends to long bones and associated urogenital and anorectal anomalies.
- II (Majewski type)[63] is characterized by median cleft lip/palate and disproportionately short, ovoid tibiae. The differential diagnosis prenatally includes the orofacial digital (OFD) syndrome type 4.

TABLE 20–5

Etiology and Aids to the Differential Diagnosis of Isolated Long Bone Shortening

CONSTITUTIONAL SHORT STATURE	PLACENTAL INSUFFICIENCY	LATE-ONSET SKELETAL DYSPLASIA
Parental short stature	Past history of FGR	Long bones may show bowing
Normally modeled long bones	Maternal autoimmune disease	Decline in long bone growth
Normal growth velocity of long bones	Generalized slowing of long bone growth	
Normal HC and AC	Decrease in AC	Normal AC; may have relative macrocephaly
Normal amniotic fluid volume	Reduced amniotic fluid volume	±Increased amniotic fluid
Normal fetal Dopplers	±Abnormal fetal Dopplers	Normal fetal Dopplers
Normal uterine artery Doppler	Abnormal uterine artery Doppler	Normal maternal Doppler
Normal anomaly scan	Normal anomaly scan	Other anomalies may be present (see Table 20-3)
Normal karyotype	±Normal karyotype	Normal karyotype

AC, abdominal circumference; FGR, fetal growth retardation; HC, head circumference.

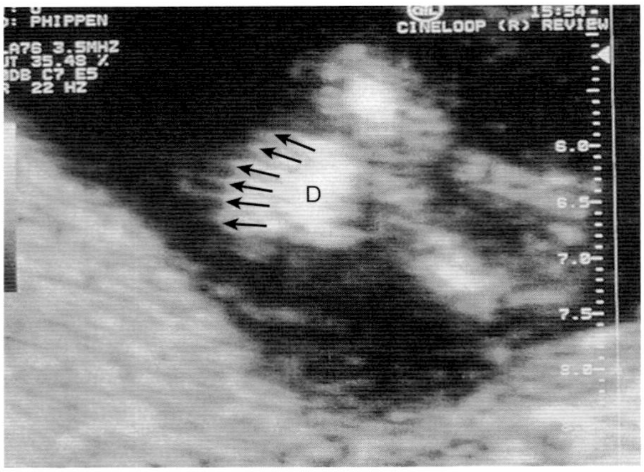

FIGURE 20–8
Short-rib polydactyly syndrome. Scan of the foot shows six digits (*arrow*, D). (With thanks to Mr. P. Smith.)

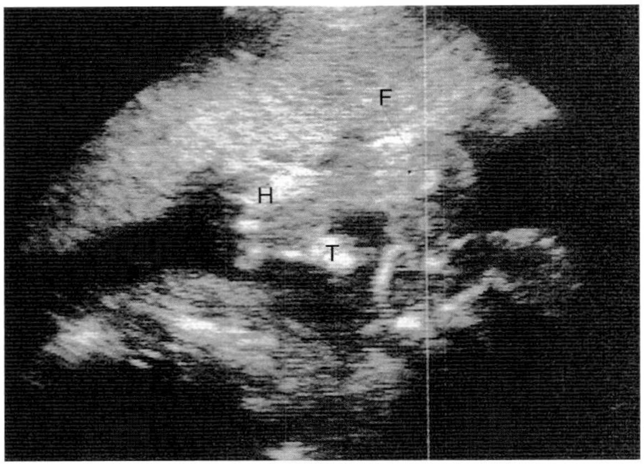

FIGURE 20–9
Diastrophic dysplasia. Scan of the hand (H) shows proximal displacement and abduction of the thumb (T) (the "hitchhiker" thumb). Femur length measurement from this fetus at 22 weeks is shown in Figure 20–2. F, forearm.

- III (Verma-Naumoff type) is associated with short, straight long bones, a midline cleft lip, and other visceral anomalies.
- IV (Beemer-Langer type) is characterized by median cleft lip/palate, bowed forearms, and talipes and may also have a cloverleaf skull and exomphalos.

All types have a small chest secondary to short ribs and can be associated with multiple abnormalities of other organ systems. Fetal hydrops is common. Ambiguous genitalia is a common finding and requires a karyotype for confirmation of genetic sex.

Diagnosis

Prenatal diagnosis is based on the identification of a small, narrow thorax with short ribs, short limbs, and polydactyly (see Fig. 20–8). Other distinguishing features may occasionally help. A number of other uncommon SRPSs have been described.

Risks and Management Options

SRPSs are lethal owing to pulmonary hypoplasia. The option of termination of pregnancy should be included in counseling. These are autosomal recessive disorders with a 25% recurrence risk.

Ellis–van Creveld Syndrome (Chondroectodermal Dysplasia) (4p16)

Diagnosis

Limb shortening is more pronounced in the forearm and lower leg (mesomelic). Polydactyly (hands more commonly than feet) is common.[64] The diagnosis should be considered when these findings are present in association with a small thorax. A fetal echocardiogram is indicated, as more than half of these fetuses have congenital heart disease, typically an atrial septal defect.

Risks and Management Options

One third of affected children die during infancy. Survivors have normal intelligence but a final height of 105 to 150 cm. The inheritance is autosomal recessive with a 25% chance of recurrence. The gene is known,[65] and DNA should be stored so that early antenatal diagnosis can be offered in subsequent pregnancies. The option of pregnancy termination should be discussed. Obstetric management of a continuing pregnancy is unaltered. Neonatal echocardiography is advisable.

Diastrophic Dysplasia (5q21-5q34) DTDST

Diagnosis

This condition has a variable presentation. Antenatal diagnosis is possible in severe cases based on the combination of rhizomelic limb shortening and bowing in association with the hitchhiker thumb and talipes. Diagnosis is possible in early pregnancy using transvaginal ultrasound (Fig. 20–9).[66,67] Other features may include micrognathia and cleft palate. It may be difficult to exclude the diagnosis before viability in milder cases of high risk families because the degree of limb shortening can be minimal. Identification of normal thumbs is helpful in excluding the diagnosis.

Risks and Management Options

Diastrophic dysplasia is an autosomal recessive disorder with a 25% risk of recurrence. DNA should be stored so that early antenatal diagnosis can be offered in subsequent pregnancies. A significant number of newborns die from respiratory failure and pneumonia. No specific measures are needed before birth in continuing pregnancies. Survivors have normal intellect but suffer significant and progressive physical handicap coupled with limited mobility secondary to the kyphoscoliosis and arthropathy. They require considerable mobility and physiotherapy support. Surgical release of contractures is possible but of limited value. In light of the disease severity, the option of pregnancy termination should be discussed when the diagnosis is made.

Chondrodysplasia Punctatas

For this heterogeneous group of conditions, definitive diagnosis can be difficult before birth and indeed frequently after birth as well.[68] Among the many forms, the three most common are X-linked dominant (Conradi-Hunermann disease), X-linked recessive, and rhizomelic.

Diagnosis

X-LINKED DOMINANT CHONDRODYSPLASIA PUNCTATA (XP11) EBP

This mildest form is seen only in females because the heterozygous male form is lethal. The condition is associated with asymmetrical shortening of bones; icthyosis and other patchy skin changes; areas of alopecia and sparse, coarse hair; and occasional cataracts. Intelligence is usually normal. Prenatal ultrasonographic detection has been reported in high risk cases[69] based on epiphyseal stippling and mild limb shortening.

X-LINKED RECESSIVE FORM (Xp22.22) ARYLSULPHATASE

Affected males have generalized but moderate shortening of the long bones with epiphyseal echogenicities, particularly in the femurs. There may be extensive, paravertebral epiphyseal stippling, giving the impression of a disorganized spine, and a flat face with nasal depression. Echogeniciy may be seen in the larynx. This disorder also may be seen in association with visible cytogenetic deletions of the X chromosome when it may also be associated with intellectual impairment.[70] Heterozygous female carriers are clinically normal but tend to be slightly shorter than noncarrier relatives.

RHIZOMELIC CHONDRODYSPLASIA PUNCTATA (*RCDP*)

RCDP1 (6q22-q24) *PEX7* gene encoding the peroxisomal type 2 targeting signal (PTS2) receptor
RCDP2 (1q42) *acyl-CoA:dihydroxyacetone phosphate acyltransferase (DHAPAT)* gene
RCDP3 (2q31) *alkyldihydroxyacetonephosphate synthase (alkyl-DHAP synthase)* gene

Individuals with RCDP have rhizomelic shortening that is more pronounced in the humerus than in other long bones. The characteristic feature on an ultrasound examination is stippled epiphyses.[71–73] There may also be stippling around the pelvic bones, trachea, and larynx. Fixed flexion deformities of the limbs can be seen, more pronounced in the arm than the leg (Fig. 20–10). Cataracts may be detected later in pregnancy.[72] Cultured amniocytes and fibroblasts have low *DHAPAT* activity.[74]

Risks and Management Options

Many newborns with RCDP die from respiratory failure. Survivors fail to thrive and develop microcephaly associated with severely retarded neurologic development. Survival beyond the first year is unusual; the longest reported survival is 5 years. Measurements of *DHAPAT* activity in amniocytes or chromosome/molecular analysis are helpful adjuncts to the ultrasonographic diagnosis.[74] The option of pregnancy termination should be discussed.

FIGURE 20–10
Rhizomelic chondrodysplasia punctata. Scan of the arm and shoulder of a 21-week fetus; the humerus (H) is short (25 mm) and bowed. At both the upper (UHE) and lower (LHE) humeral epiphyses, there are echogenic accumulations representing disorganized calcification. Movement of the upper limb was limited during examination.

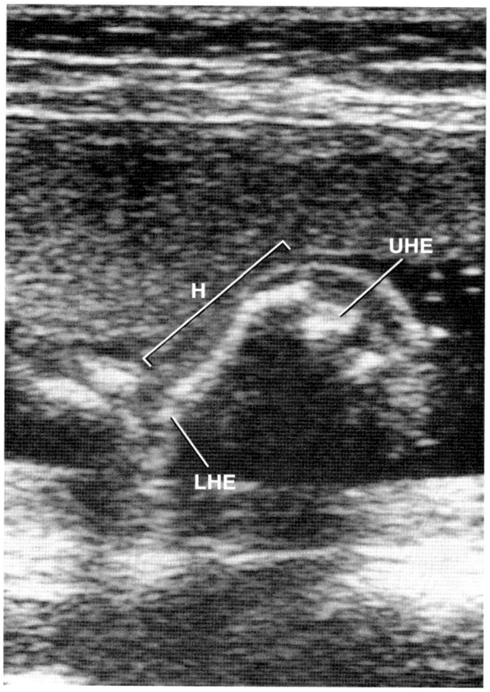

Kniest's Dysplasia (12q13-12q14; *COL2AI*)

Diagnosis

Kniest's dysplasia is characterized by moderately short, dumbbell-shaped long bones with metaphyseal flaring, restricted joint mobility, platyspondyly with vertebral clefts, and a flat face with depressed nasal bridge. Although the limbs are noticeably short at birth, antenatal diagnosis has been reported only once.[75] In this instance, the features were not evident at 16 weeks but were apparent at 31 weeks. In the author's experience of three cases, limb length was around the 5th percentile for most of pregnancy. Other features that were detected included mild micrognathia, talipes, and a short thorax.

Risks and Management Options

Affected children may survive with normal intelligence but are short (106–145 cm) and have limited mobility and severe orthopedic disabilities. Ophthalmic complications and deafness may occur in childhood.

Spondyloepiphyseal Dysplasia Congenita (12q13-12q14; *COL2AI*)

Diagnosis

This condition is associated with short limbs and a short spine, with final stature being approximately 120 cm. The antenatal sonographic findings have been reported.[76,77] In one case, there was moderate shortening of the femur at 16 weeks followed by more marked rhizomelic shortening at 27 weeks.[76] No other distinguishing features were evident and a definitive diagnosis was not made. In the author's experience of one case, the chest did appear small in the parasagittal plane, but when viewed in transverse section, the ribs were of normal length and the heart occupied one third of the chest. In this condition, the chest appears small secondary to the short spine.[77] The disorder is characterized by deficient ossification of the spine, pubis, talus, and calcaneum and delayed appearance of the lower femoral and upper tibial epiphyses. Vertebrae show marked platyspondyly with ovoid vertebral bodies. The thorax is narrow and bell-shaped and the long bones are moderately short. Cleft palate might also occur.

Risks and Management Options

The disorder is compatible with prolonged survival. Myopia and retinal detachment occur in about half the survivors. Hypotonic muscle weakness and restricted joint mobility reduce overall mobility, and the spinal deformities cause progressive kyphoscoliosis.

ACHONDROPLASIA (4p16; *FGFR3*)

Achondroplasia is the most common nonlethal skeletal dysplasia with an incidence of around 5 to 15 in 100,000 births. It results from a mutation in the *FGFR3* gene located on 4p16.3.[78,79] The majority of cases are sporadic and result from a de novo paternal mutation.[80] The diagnosis is not usually evident ultrasonographically until after 24 weeks' gestation when the long bone shortening manifests (see Fig. 20–2). Achondroplasia is characterized by predominantly acromesomelic limb shortening with short fingers (trident hand). Typical facial features include a wide, prominent forehead (frontal bossing) and a depressed nasal bridge. Thoracic dimensions may be reduced and can occasionally cause transitory respiratory at birth. Relative macrocephaly is usual and ventriculomegaly can occur. The diagnosis can be confirmed prenatally by analysis of cell free fetal DNA in the maternal blood to look for one of the common mutations in the *FGFR3* gene.[81,82]

Risks and Management Options

Life expectancy and intellectual performance are good. Hydrocephaly secondary to partial obstruction of the restricted foramen magnum is usually mild and nonprogressive. Progressive neurologic problems can result from spinal cord compression secondary to progressive narrowing of the interpedicular distance, particularly in the lumbar spine as the degree of lordosis increases.[83] Corrective orthopedic surgery may be required to correct the spinal deformities and bowed legs.

Affected women often require cesarean section because of a contracted pelvis. Cephalopelvic disproportion may also occur during the delivery of an affected fetus to a normal woman if the macrocephaly is marked. The recurrence risk for two unaffected parents is low, because in these circumstances, achondroplasia usually results from a new mutation.

SHORT LONG BONES: ASYMMETRICAL

Isolated Limb Reductions

Risks and Management Options

The majority of isolated limb reductions are nongenetic, but some may occur as part of a genetic syndrome or chromosomal abnormality when there are usually other anomalies.[84] A detailed ultrasonographic examination is therefore essential. Karyotyping is recommended if associated with other nonskeletal anomalies, particularly when involving the forearms or if there are other risk factors. The prognosis for unilateral, isolated arm or leg reduction is generally good, depending on the degree of reduction, in the absence of other visceral or chromosomal abnormalities. Advances in prosthetics and orthopedics are such that much can be done to restore function and appearance of the reduced limbs. Parents should be encouraged to discuss these possibilities with appropriate professionals. There are, however, some specific syndromes associated with asymmetrical limb reduction deformities (Table 20–6).

Robert's Syndrome (Pseudothalidomide Syndrome) (8p21.1; *ESCO2*)

Diagnosis

Typically all four limbs (tetraphocomelia) are affected, similar to the teratogenic effects of thalidomide. Median facial clefting, microcephaly, joint flexion deformities, talipes, syndactyly, and extremely short or missing fingers and toes are accompanying features. Other associated anomalies include hydrocephaly, encephalocele, and renal abnormalities such as cystic or horseshoe kidneys.[85] First-trimester diagnosis has been reported using cytogenetic studies to demonstrate the premature separation of the centromeres, which produces a characteristic phenomenon of chromosome "puffing."[86]

Risks and Management Options

Affected individuals have a high perinatal mortality rate (70%–80%) and severe FGR. Survivors are often profoundly developmentally delayed. The option of pregnancy termination should be discussed. Survivors with hypoglossia-hypodactyly syndrome generally have satisfactory intellectual development, and the level of handicap depends on the severity of limb anomalies.

Femoral Hypoplasia: Unusual Faces Syndrome

This condition appears more common in the progeny of diabetic women. Cleft palate and micrognathia are associated with varying degrees of hypoplasia/aplasia of the femur. The tibia and fibula may be hypoplastic. Humeral reduction with a flexion deformity at the elbow can also be seen. Other associated abnormalities include vertebral anomalies of the lower spine, pelvic anomalies, and urogenital anomalies. The main differential diagnosis is caudal regression syndrome,

TABLE 20–6

Selected Genetic Syndromes and Chromosomal Anomalies Associated with Limb Reduction Defects

	FOREARMS	LOWER LIMBS	CARDIAC ANOMALY	GROWTH	OTHER USS FINDINGS	FH	OTHER DIAGNOSTIC AIDS
BDLS	Asymmetrical and variable forearm reduction, oligodactyly, syndactyly	Small feet	±	FGR, microcephaly	Diaphragmatic hernia		Low PAPP-A
TAR	Bilateral radial aplasia, thumbs always present and normal; ulna hypoplasia.	Absent/abnormal tibia, fibula, femur, talipes	±	Usually normal	Absent/abnormal humeri, flexion deformities	AR	Platelet count DNA analysis
Trisomy 18 Trisomy 13	Radial club hand, flexed fingers, polydactyly, absent thumbs	Talipes, rocker-bottom feet, polydactyly	+	FGR	Multiple		Karyotype
Holt-Oram	Bilateral radial abnormalities of variable severity, absent digits (especially thumb)	Normal	+	Normal		AD	Examine parents X-ray parents echocardiography
Fanconi	Hypoplastic thumbs, radial anomalies, polydactyly	Normal	±	FGR	Cryptorchidism, renal anomalies	AR	Chromosome breakage studies
Nager	Bilateral radial defects, absent/hypoplastic thumbs, preaxial polydactyly	Normal, occasional syndactyly of toes	±	Microcephaly	Micrognathia, cleft lip, absent/ abnormal fibula, renal anomalies	AD	Genetic consultation
Robert's	Bilateral radial and ulna hypo/aplasia	Hypoplastic or absent lower limb bones	±	Normal	Cleft lip, cystic kidneys	AR	Karyotype: chromosome puffing
VATER/ VACTERL	Asymmetrical radial defects	Normal	±	Normal	Hemivertebrae, renal anomalies	–	±Hydramnios, genetics
FFU	Variable hypoplasia of forearms	Asymmetrical bowing/ hypoplasia of lower limbs	–	Normal	Ectrodactyly	–	

AD, autosomal dominant; AR, autosomal recessive; BDLS, Brachmann de Lange syndrome; FFU, femur-fibula-ulna complex; FGR, fetal growth restriction; FH, family history; PAPP-A, pregnancy-associated plasma protein-A; TAR, thrombocytopenia with absent radius syndrome; VATER/VACTERL, vertebral defects, anal atresia or stenosis, tracheoesophageal fistula, radial defects and renal anomalies.

but this syndrome is not associated with the facial dysmorphisms or humeral reduction. Most individuals have normal intelligence and are ambulatory.[87]

Femur-Fibula-Ulna Syndrome

This syndrome is characterized by femoral and fibula hypoplasia/aplasia and varying degrees of ulna hemimelia.[88] It has been diagnosed antenatally.[89]

Holt-Oram Syndrome (12q21) *TXB5*

Diagnosis

The cardinal features of Holt-Oram syndrome are congenital heart disease (usually atrial or ventricular septal defect) associated with anomalies of the upper limb shoulder girdle. Abnormalities in the hand and forearm include aplastic, hypoplastic, or triphalangeal (finger-like) thumb and syndactyly and hypoplasia of the radius, ulna, humerus, clavicles, scapula, or sternum.[90,91] Ultrasonographic diagnosis has been reported.[92] This is a dominant condition, and affected individuals have a 50% offspring risk. There is no consistent pattern, and expression is very variable.[90]

Risks and Management Options

Management options depend on the severity of the cardiac malformation and the skeletal deformities. Parents should be examined because the condition is extremely variable and gene carriers may have minimal manifestations.

Thrombocytopenia with Absent Radius Syndrome (1q2.1)

The skeletal manifestations of thrombocytopenia with absent radius (TAR) syndrome are variable; bilateral radial aplasia/hypoplasia is sometimes associated with humeral or ulnar reduction or bowing. The pathognomic feature is that the thumbs are always present regardless of the degree of radial hypoplasia. The femurs can be affected, and cardiac anomalies are relatively common.[93] Thrombocytopenia is a marker of an underlying hematologic abnormality. Antenatal diagnosis is based on both the ultrasonographic findings and the documentation of fetal thrombocytopenia.[94] TAR is associated with a microdeletion at 1q21.1. In a large clinical study, the deletion occurred de novo in 25% of cases and was inherited equally from the mother or the father in the other cases.[95] The inheritance pattern resembles an autosomal recessive pattern, and it is hypothesized that an additional modifier is required.

Cleidocranial Dysostosis (6p21; *CBFA1, RUNX2*)

Diagnosis

The characteristic findings are mild femoral shortening with hypoplastic clavicles (Fig. 20–11). Although the clavicle is not generally included in routine ultrasound examinations of the fetus, nomograms of clavicular length are published.[96] Examination of the clavicle may be helpful in defining the underlying pathology in the presence of short limbs. A hypomineralized cranium with wide fontanelles might also be evident.[97]

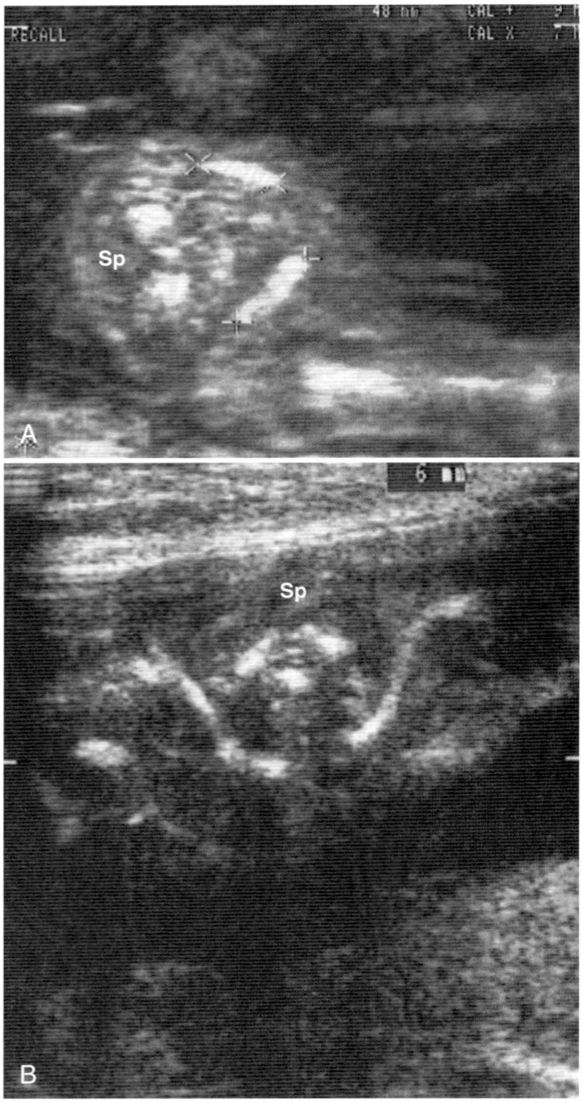

FIGURE 20–11
Cleidocranial dysostosis. *A*, Transverse scan of the clavicles of the fetus of a mother with cleidocranial dysostosis. The clavicles are short, thick, and straight. *B*, Similar posteroanterior scan of the clavicles of a normal 22-week fetus. Note the sigmoid form of the clavicle. Sp, spine.

Risks and Management Options

Individuals with cleidocranial dysostosis are generally short. They may have respiratory difficulties in infancy if the thorax is restricted. Dental and hearing problems can present in later childhood. However, the absent or hypoplastic clavicles do not cause significant handicap, and intelligence is unimpaired. Poor skull ossification tends to improve with age. Affected mothers may require cesarean section because of a small pelvis. The condition is very variable, and parents should be examined for minor manifestions.[97]

Polydactyly/Syndactyly

These conditions frequently coexist. The polydactyly can be either preaxial (on the radial side of the hand or medial side of the foot, including bifid thumb or great toe) or postaxial (on the ulnar side of the hand or lateral side of the foot). Polydactyly is associated with numerous genetic and chromosomal syndromes (see Tables 20–3 and 20–6). Isolated polydactyly can be inherited as an autosomal dominant trait with variable penetrance, particularly in some ethnic groups (e.g., Afro-Caribbean).

Ectrodactyly

Ectrodactyly (split hand) is a variant of syndactyly in which the hands resemble a "lobster claw" (Fig. 20–12). It may occur either as an isolated phenomenon or as part of several syndromes,[80] the most common of which is the ectrodactyly ectodermal dysplasia clefting (EEC) syndrome. Isolated ectrodactyly and EEC syndrome are both inherited as autosomal dominant traits with a 50% risk of recurrence.

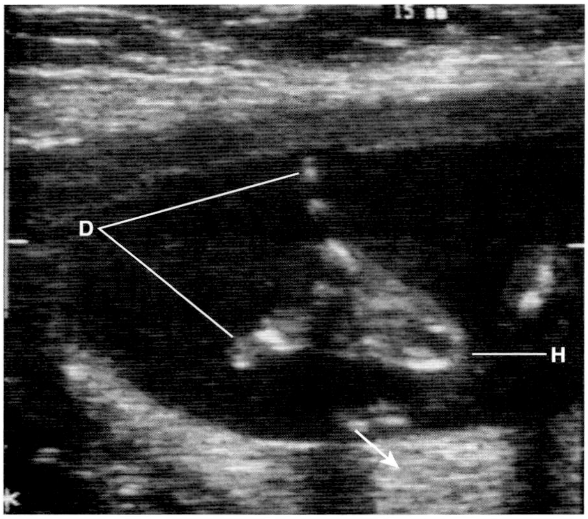

FIGURE 20–12
Ectrodactyly. Scan of a fetal foot showing ectrodactyly. H, heel; D, digits.
(From Griffin DR: Skeletal dysplasias. In Brock DJH, Rodeck CH, Ferguson-Smith MA [eds]: Prenatal Diagnosis and Screening. Edinburgh: Churchill Livingstone, 1992, pp 257-313.)

Diagnosis

Isolated ectrodactyly may affect one or more limbs and has extremely variable penetrance. At the worse end of spectrum, it can be associated with limb reduction defects. Parents of an affected child may show only minimal changes.[98] Antenatal diagnosis is possible in more severe cases. In the EEC syndrome, ectrodactyly is associated with cleft lip or palate and skin, hair, and teeth dysplasia. Renal defects may also be present.

Risks and Management Options

Prognosis depends on the underlying etiology, and when detected antenatally, parents should be referred to a clinical geneticist for careful examination and discussion of possible underlying conditions.

JOINT DEFORMITIES

Detailed discussion of joint deformities is beyond the scope of this review. They can occur as part of a skeletal dysplasia (see Table 20–3), in chromosomal disorders or other genetic conditions (see Table 20–6), as part of a generalized contractural or neurologic syndrome, or from a deformity as a result of intrauterine pressure secondary to oligohydramnios or uterine anomalies.

Talipes

The most common positional deformity is talipes equinovarus, in which the foot is adducted and plantar inverted so that the sole points medially. In the equinovalgus (calcaneovalgus) deformity, the heel is elevated and the foot is plantar everted. Talipes occurs as an isolated phenomenon in approximately 1 in 1200 births with varying degrees of severity, as a marker for chromosomal abnormalities, or as part of many genetic syndromes.[80,99]

Diagnosis

Positional deformities of the feet are best sought in the sagittal and coronal scanning planes (Fig. 20–13). When severe talipes equinovarus is present, the plantar view of the foot is seen in continuity with the leg in sagittal section (Fig. 20–14). Because of the many associated syndromes, a careful search for other abnormalities is mandatory before counseling. The combination of talipes and hydramnios raises the suspicion of congenital myotonic dystrophy[100] or distal dominant arthrogryposis.[101] Thus, parental examination may be helpful, particularly to look for evidence of early signs of myotonic dystrophy in the mother.[100]

Risks and Management Options

Isolated talipes is usually amenable to orthopedic correction. Karyotyping is recommended if other markers of aneuploidy or risk factors are present. Management depends on the severity of any associated structural defects and the karyotype. In the presence of a normal karyotype and other ultrasonographic anomalies, including hydramnios, genetic referral should be considered.

Rocker-Bottom Feet

The typical appearance of rocker-bottom feet, usually caused by a vertical talus, is a posteriorly prominent heel and convexity of the normally concave contour of the plantar arch (Fig. 20–15). Rocker-bottom feet are associated with trisomy

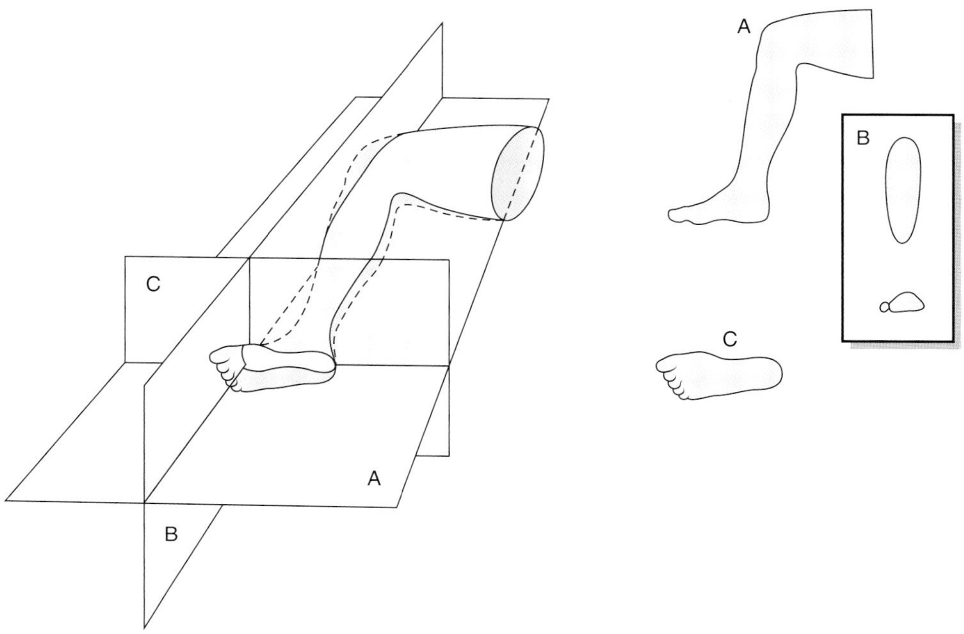

FIGURE 20–13
Diagram represents the scanning planes employed to visualize the foot. Plane A will show rocker-bottom feet; planes A and B will show talipes; planes B and C reveal polysyndactyly.
(From Griffin DR: Skeletal dysplasias. In Brock DJH, Rodeck CH, Ferguson-Smith MA [eds]: Prenatal Diagnosis and Screening. Edinburgh: Churchill Livingstone, 1992, pp 257-313.)

FIGURE 20–14
Positional deformities. Longitudinal view of the leg shows the lower end of the femur, knee (K), tibia/fibula, and foot with talipes. The plantar view of the foot would not normally be seen in this plane.

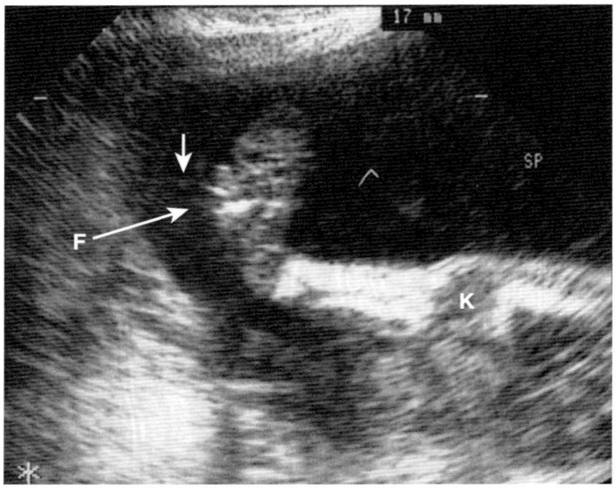

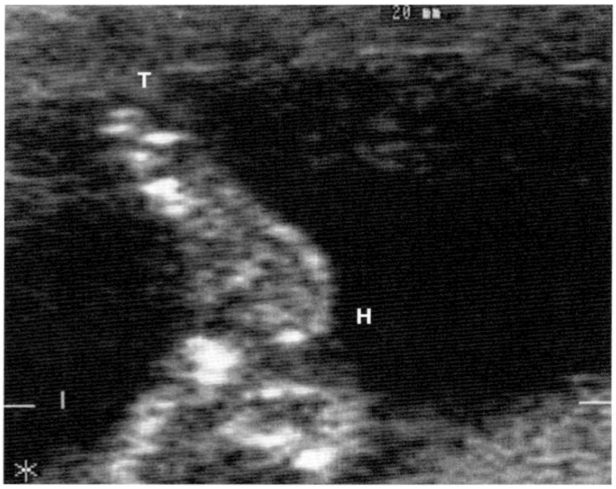

FIGURE 20–15
Rocker-bottom foot. Sagittal scan of the foot of a fetus with confirmed trisomy 18 shows prominent heel (H) and loss of the plantar arch. T, toe.

18, 18q syndrome, trisomy 13, Pena-Shokeir sequence, and other syndromes. The finding requires a diligent search for other abnormalities. Karyotyping is indicated if other abnormalities are present.

MULTIPLE JOINT CONTRACTURES

This heterogeneous group of disorders is characterized by multiple flexion deformities of the limbs, hands, and feet, resulting in fixed immobile limbs, sometimes with cutaneous webbing (pterygia) at joint flexures. The causes include[102]

- Central nervous system disease (55%).
- Peripheral neuromuscular disorder (8%).
- Connective tissue disease (11%).
- Miscellaneous skeletal or other abnormality (19%).

Oligohydramnios is present in 7%.[66] Increased first-trimester nuchal translucency and fetal hydrops in the second trimester are reported.[103] Deficient swallowing and fetal breathing may result in hydramnios and pulmonary hypoplasia. The etiology is broad and includes specific central nervous system abnormalities, primary myopathy, congenital muscular dystrophy, lethal multiple pterygium syndrome, and the Pena-Shokeir spectrum.[104]

Risks and Management Options

Definitive diagnosis is rarely made antenatally. At the severe end of the spectrum, these conditions are perinatally lethal. Detailed postmortem examination is advised with subsequent referral to a clinical geneticist for further investigations (see Tables 20–2 and 20–3) and counseling with regard to recurrence risks, which can be high.

SPINAL DEFORMITIES

These deformities can occur as a consequence of neural tube defects, hemivertebrae, dysplasia or agenesis of the vertebrae, or asymmetrical muscle action (severe abdominal wall defects). Neural tube defects and abdominal wall defects are reviewed in Chapters 17 and 19.

Hemivertebrae

Hemivertebrae occur when one of the pair of chondrification centers that normally combine to form the vertebral body fails to appear. Only half of the vertebral body develops and the result is lateral angulation of the spine (scoliosis). Hemivertebrae may be isolated or associated with cardiac, renal, radial, or digital anomalies, tracheoesophageal fistula, and anal atresia in the VACTERL (vertebral abnormalities, anal atresia, cardiac abnormalities, tracheoesophageal fistula and/or esophageal atresia, renal agenesis and dysplasia, and limb defects) association, or as a part of numerous other genetic syndromes.

Diagnosis

Hemivertebrae are recognized ultrasonographically by spinal scoliosis and asymmetry in the vertebral echoes (Fig. 20–16). A careful search for associated abnormalities is essential. Hydramnios may be the only clue to tracheoesophageal atresia. A karyotype is indicated if other anomalies are seen, because similar abnormalities may be found in trisomy 18 and 13q syndromes.

Risks and Management Options

These options depend on the presence and severity of associated anomalies. The parents should meet with an orthopedic specialist to discuss the postnatal management including surgical correction of the spinal deformity. Individuals with VACTERL association generally have normal intellectual potential.

Jarcho-Levin Syndrome (Spondylothoracic Dysplasia)

Diagnosis

The Jarcho-Levin syndrome is an autosomal recessive disorder characterized by a grossly disorganized axial skeleton and thorax (Fig. 20–17). Vertebral bodies may be missing or fused and the hemivertebrae and ribs are frequently reduced in number with posterior fusion and anterior flaring (the "crab chest" deformity). Visceral and urogenital anomalies along with diaphragmatic hernia are also reported.[11,80]

Risks and Management Options

The majority of individuals with this condition die in the neonatal period or during early infancy as a result of respiratory insufficiency. The option of pregnancy termination should be discussed.

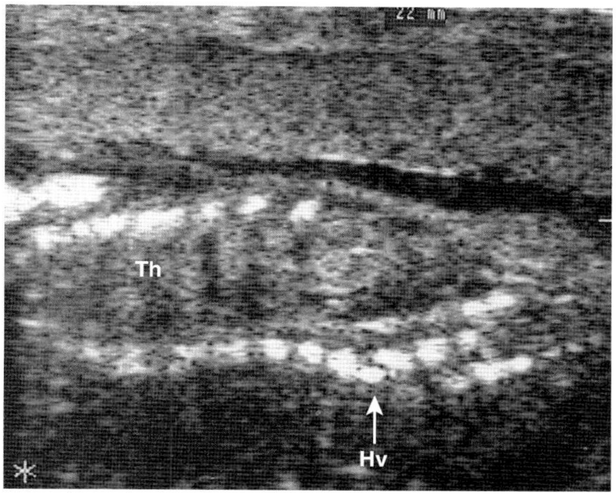

FIGURE 20–16
Hemivertebra. Longitudinal scan of the vertebral bodies of one of twin fetuses shows a midlumbar hemivertebra (HV). The spinal canal showed no evidence of narrowing on scan. Spinal deformity was minimal at birth. Th, thorax.

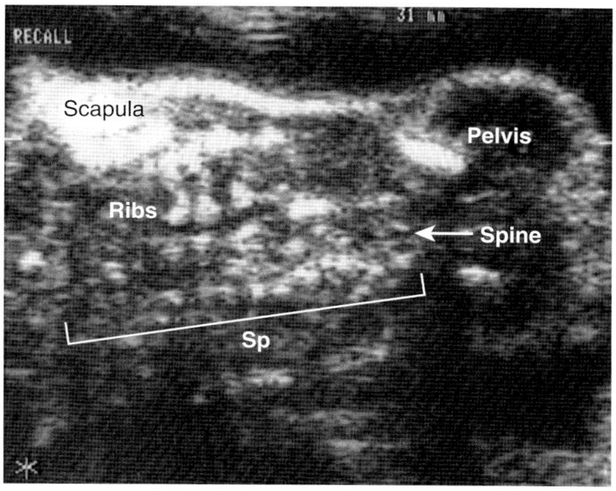

FIGURE 20–17
Jarcho-Levin syndrome. Longitudinal coronal scan of the trunk. The ribs are thick and irregular and the spinal components (Sp) grossly disorganized.
(From Griffin DR: Skeletal dysplasias. In Brock DJH, Rodeck CH, Ferguson-Smith MA [eds]: Prenatal Diagnosis and Screening. Edinburgh: Churchill Livingstone, 1992, pp 257–313.)

SUMMARY OF MANAGEMENT OPTIONS
Skeletal Abnormalities

Management Options	Evidence Quality and Recommendation	References
Prepregnancy		
Ensure accuracy of diagnosis before counseling (review radiographs, postmortem, genetic referral).	—/GPP	—
Genetic counseling about recurrence risks and prenatal diagnostic options.	—/GPP	—
Prenatal		
Careful ultrasonography by experienced sonographer, including examination of fetus for other anomalies.	—/GPP	—
Consider a karyotype or other additional tests if other anomalies or suspicion of genetic condition.	—/GPP	—
Refer for genetic counseling and/or orthopedic discussion before counseling parents (differential diagnosis rather than definitive diagnosis might be all that is possible).	—/GPP	—
Ongoing review of ultrasonographic findings if pregnancy continues (further features may develop, allowing definitive diagnosis).	—/GPP	—
Offer pregnancy termination with severe and/or lethal anomalies.	—/GPP	—
Psychological support of parents.	—/GPP	—

SUMMARY OF MANAGEMENT OPTIONS
Skeletal Abnormalities—cont'd

Management Options	Evidence Quality and Recommendation	References
Labor and Delivery		
Cesarean section for normal obstetric indications, although conditions associated with hypomineralization may be delivered by cesarean section.	—/GPP	—
Postnatal		
If lethal, encourage postmortem by experienced perinatal pathologist including radiography and CT scanning.	—/GPP	—
Tissue for karyotyping and other tests if not performed prenatally.	—/GPP	—
Refer for expert genetic counseling about recurrence risks and future prenatal diagnostic options.	—/GPP	

CT, computed tomography; GPP, good practice point.

SUGGESTED READINGS

Brown N, Lumley J, Tickle C, Keene J: Congenital Limb Reduction Defects. Clues from Developmental Biology, Teratology and Epidemiology. London, HMSO Stationary Office, 1996.

Chitty LS, Altman DG: Charts of fetal size: Limb bones. BJOG 2002;109:919–929.

Chitty LS, Campbell S, Altman DG: Measurement of the fetal mandible—Feasibility and construction of a centile chart. Prenat Diagn 1993;13:749–756.

Chitty LS, Griffin DR: Prenatal diagnosis of fetal skeletal anomalies. Fetal Mat Med Rev 2008;19:135–164.

Hall CM: International nosology and classification of constitutional disorders of bone (2001). Am J Med Genet 2002;113:65–77.

Hyett JA, Griffin DR. Chitty LS: Short femora—Achondroplasia or IUGR: Use of growth patterns as an aid to diagnosis. J Obstet Gynaecol 2002;22(Suppl 1):S32.

Irving M, Chitty LS, Mansour S, Hall CM: Chondrodysplasia punctata: A clinical diagnostic and radiological review. Clin Dysmorphol 2008;17:229–241.

Orioli IM, Castilla EE, Barbosa-Netos JG: The birth prevalence rates for the skeletal dysplasias. J Med Genet 1986;23:328–332.

Sherer DM, Sokolovski M, Dalloul M, et al: Fetal clavicle length throughout gestation: A nomogram. Ultrasound Obstet Gynecol 2006;27:306–310.

Winter RM, Baraitser M: Winter-Baraitser London Medical Databases. Version 1.0, 2006.

REFERENCES

For a complete list of references, log onto www.expertconsult.com.

CHAPTER 21

Fetal Thyroid and Adrenal Disease

STEPHEN C. ROBSON

Videos corresponding to this chapter are available online at www.expertconsult.com.

FETAL THYROID DISEASE

Introduction

Thyroxine (T_4) is synthesised and secreted by the thyroid gland. The active hormone triiodothyronine (T_3) is predominantly produced by deiodination of T_4 in peripheral tissues by the action of deiodinases. Thyroid hormone receptors (TR-α and TR-β) bind T_3 with high affinity and function as ligand-inducible transcription factors that regulate expression of T_3-responsive target genes.

The embryonic thyroid is derived from the endoderm of the buccal cavity. The gland enlarges and migrates to the lower neck by the seventh week of development. Thyroid hormone synthesis begins at 10 to 12 weeks, but appreciable amounts are released only from 14 to 16 weeks onward.[1,2] Thus, the availability of free T_4 (FT_4) to early fetal tissues is dependent on maternal T_4 levels. Whereas levels of total T_4 are very low in the fetus, FT_4 levels are actually comparable with maternal levels because of differences in T_4-binding proteins. Once fetal thyroid hormone production begins, total and FT_4 concentrations increase, reaching adult levels by the third trimester (total T_4 100–150 nmol/L, FT_4 15–25 pmol/L), while levels of total and free T_3 (FT_3) remain very low.[2] Maternal thyroid hormones continue to contribute to fetal T_4 levels until birth, as demonstrated in neonates with complete thyroid agenesis. Thyroid-stimulating hormone (TSH) remains low until 15 to 18 weeks, then increases to around 8 mU/L at term.[2] The fetal pituitary is capable of responding to thyrotropin-releasing hormone (TRH) from 20 weeks but is relatively insensitive to negative feedback from thyroid hormones until late in the second trimester.

The placenta is freely permeable to iodide substrates, TRH, thionanides. and thyroid-stimulating hormone receptor antibodies (TRAbs) but is impermeable to TSH. Transfer of T_3 and T_4 is controlled through the action of placental deiodinase enzymes. During pregnancy, differential expression of deiodinases maintains a suitable maternal-fetal gradient.[2,3] The placenta produces several peptides, including human chorionic gonadotropin (hCG), capable of stimulating the maternal thyroid. As a result, maternal FT_4 concentrations increase in early pregnancy.

Thyroid hormones are essential for optimal growth and development of the central nervous system (CNS), lung, gut, and liver and the regulation of carbohydrate, lipid, and protein metabolism. Three stages of thyroid hormone–dependent neurologic development are recognized.[3] The first occurs before the onset of fetal thyroid hormone synthesis and influences neurogenesis and neuronal migration in the cerebral cortex, hippocampus, and medial ganglionic eminence. The second occurs during the remainder of pregnancy when additional thyroid hormone–dependent processes include axon and dendrite migration, synapse formation, glial cell proliferation, and myelination. During the third (postnatal) stage, specific cell types in the cerebellum, hippocampus, and cortex (Purkinje cells) are sensitive to thyroid hormones and thyroid hormone–dependent gliogenesis and myelination continue.[3] Thus, the specific types of deficit appear to reflect the timing and duration of thyroid hormone insufficiency.[3]

Fetal Hyperthyroidism

Fetal or neonatal hyperthyroidism is a rare condition affecting fewer than 1 in 5000 pregnancies.[4] The disorder is almost invariably secondary to maternal autoimmune thyroid disorders, principally Graves' disease (GD) (Table 21–1). GD is responsible for 85% to 90% of cases of maternal hyperthyroidism, which complicates 1 in 500 to 1000 pregnancies.[5,6] The disease is caused by TRAbs that usually stimulate the receptor but occasionally block the normal effect of TSH. Fetal hyperthyroidism is caused by transplacental passage of stimulating TRAbs. This can occur in euthyroid-treated mothers, although the risk is dependent on the method and time of treatment; both medical therapy and surgery are followed by a decline in TRAbs with disappearance of TRAbs in 70% to 80% after 18 months.[7] Remission of TRAb autoimmunity is less common after radioiodine therapy.[7] Hyperthyroidism occurs in 1% to 5% of infants born to women with a history of GD,[4,8] although only half require antithyroid therapy because of symptomatic disease.[4,8] Thyroid hormone concentrations are also increased in fetuses with anemia secondary to red cell alloimmunization.[9]

TABLE 21–1

Causes of Fetal Thyroid Dysfunction

Hyperthyroidism

- Maternal autoimmune disease
  - Graves' disease (TSH receptor stimulating antibodies)
  - Chronic autoimmune (Hashimoto's) thyroiditis
- Anemia (secondary to alloimmunization)

Hypothyroidism

- Dysgenesis
  - Athyreosis
  - Hypoplasia
  - Ectopic thyroid
- Graves' disease (TSH receptor blocking antibodies)
- Defects in thyroid hormone synthesis and metabolism
- TSH receptor mutations
- Thyroid hormone resistance
- Hypothalamic-pituitary dysfunction
- Iatrogenic
  - Inadvertent use of radioiodine in pregnancy
  - Excessive iodine/iodide
  - Antithyroid drugs
- Iodine deficiency
- Sick preterm infants
- Hypoxic fetal growth restriction

TSH, thyroid-stimulating hormone.

TABLE 21–2

Guidelines for Measurement of Thyroid-Stimulating Hormone Receptor Antibodies in Pregnancy

1. A euthyroid pregnant woman without medication but who has previously received antithyroid drugs for Graves' disease: the risk for fetal and neonatal hyperthyroidism is negligible. Measurements of TRAbs are not necessary.
2. A euthyroid pregnant women (with or without thyroid hormone substitution therapy) who has previously received radioiodine therapy or undergone thyroid surgery for Graves' disease: the risk of fetal and neonatal hyperthyroidism depends on the level of TRAbs in the mother. TRAbs* should be measured early in pregnancy;
   - If absent or low, no further evaluation is recommended.
   - If high,† the fetus should be followed carefully for signs of hyperthyroidism. TRAbs should be measured again in the last trimester to evaluate the risk of neonatal hyperthyroidism.
3. A pregnant women who takes antithyroid drugs for Graves' disease to keep thyroid function normal: TRAbs should be measured in the last trimester;
   - If absent or low, neonatal hyperthyroidism is unlikely.
   - If high,† evaluation for neonatal hyperthyroidism is needed (clinical evaluation and thyroid function tests on cord blood and again after 4–7 days).

* The generally available and technically simple assays measuring TRAbs by competitive inhibition (not indicating whether the immunoglobulins are stimulating the thyroid) predict nearly all cases of neonatal hyperthyroidism.

† In Europe, a widely used method is TRAK (Brahms, Berlin, Germany). With this method, levels > 40 U/L are considered high enough to indicate risk of neonatal hyperthyroidism.

TRAbs, thyroid-stimulating hormone receptor antibodies.

From Abalovich M, Amino N, Barbour LA, et al: Management of thyroid dysfunction during pregnancy and postpartum. An Endocrine Society Clinical Practice Guideline. J Clin Endocrinol Metab 2007;92:S1–S47.

Diagnosis

Fetal hyperthyroidism should be suspected in any woman with a history of active or treated GD or clinical features suggestive of hyperthyroidism.

MATERNAL THYROID FUNCTION AND ANTIBODY TESTS

Decreased TSH and increased FT_4 concentrations are diagnostic of maternal hyperthyroidism. However, maternal thyroid function does not predict fetal thyroid function. The value of measuring TRAbs is controversial and a variety of assays exist. All antibodies that can compete with TSH for binding to the TSH receptor (TSH-R) are identified as thyroid-stimulating hormone–binding inhibitory immunoglobulins (TBII). A range of commercial kits are available that record the percentage of inhibition of TSH binding to a membrane preparation of TSH-Rs (elevated levels >15%).[10] TBII is often used as a surrogate for an assay of thyroid-stimulating hormone receptor–stimulating antibodies (TSAbs), because binding and stimulation frequently go in parallel.[11] Assays are also available for both TSAbs and thyroid-stimulating hormone-receptor–blocking antibodies (TBAbs). TSAbs can be measured by immunoassay or more commonly by biologic assay involving release of cyclic adenosine monophosphate (cAMP) from thyroid cell cultures by purified immunoglobulin G (IgG; elevated values >130% or >1.3 index units [IU]).[12] Approximatey 20% of women with GD have TRAbs. Improvement of Graves' hyperthyroidism is often associated with a reduction in TSAb levels and a shift from stimulatory to blocking antibodies; Kung and Jones[12] reported that median levels of TSAb fell from 280% in the first trimester to 130% at term whereas TBAb increased from 16% to 43%.

The risk of fetal hyperthyroidism correlates with maternal TBII and TSAb.[5,8,13] The incidence of neonatal thyroid dysfunction (including overt and chemical thyrotoxicosis) was 67% if TRAbs were greater than 130% and 83% if greater than 150% compared with 11% with less than 130% antibody response.[8] Peleg and coworkers[13] reported that a TSAb of 5 IU or greater predicted neonatal hyperthyroidism with a sensitivity of 100%, specificity of 76%, positive predictive value of 40%, and negative predictive value of 100%. The risk of fetal/neonatal hyperthyroidism is very small if TRAbs are negative; of 72 women with GD and at least one prior positive test for TRAb (measured by radioreceptor TRAK assay) prospectively followed throughout pregnancy, 31 women had persistently negative TRAbs and all infants were euthyroid at birth.[14] In contrast, fetal hyperthyroidism was detected in 4 of 33 cases in which the woman had at least one positive TRAb test during pregnancy.[14] Guidelines for the measurement of TRAb in pregnancy have been produced by the European Thyroid Association[15] (Table 21–2).

FETAL IMAGING

Fetal hyperthyroidism can be associated with fetal goiter, tachycardia, fetal growth restriction (FGR), hydrops, and fetal death.[13,14,16,17] The fetal thyroid is visible in a transverse section of the neck, lying between and immediately in front of the carotid arteries, which are easily visualized with color Doppler, and in front of the trachea, which appears as a central echo-free disk[14] (Fig. 21–1). Fetal goiter is defined as a thyroid circumference greater than the 95th percentile for gestational age[18] (Fig. 21–2). Luton and colleagues[14] reported fetal goiters in 2.6% of pregnancies in women with a history of thyroid disease and in 19% of mothers with GD. In

FIGURE 21–1
Transverse section of fetal neck at 24 weeks' gestation indicates normal appearance of the thyroid. The thyroid (highlighted with calipers) lies between and anterior to the carotid arteries (*open arrows*) and immediately anterior to the trachea (*solid arrow*). Note that there is also a nuchal cord.

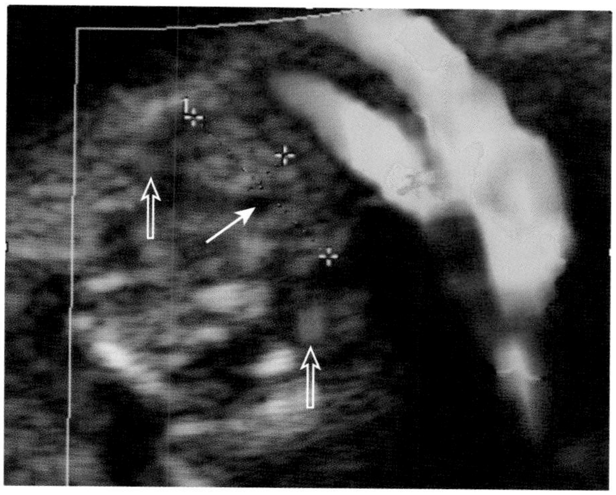

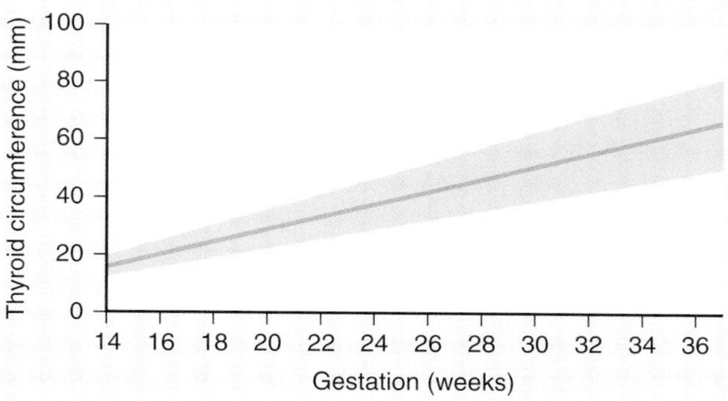

FIGURE 21–2
Ultrasound measurements of fetal thyroid circumference. Data are mean and 95% confidence limits based on 193 normal fetuses.
(Reproduced from Achiron R, Rotstein Z, Lipitz S, et al: The development of the foetal thyroid: In utero ultrasonographic measurements. Clin Endocrinol 1998;48:259–264, with permission.)

another series of 39 cases of fetal goiter (7 of which were related to fetal hyperthyroidism), Huel and colleagues reported that the diagnosis was made at an average of 29 (range 22–38) weeks' gestation.[16] Large goiters (Fig. 21–3) may be associated with esophageal/tracheal compression and hydramnios and have been reported to cause malpresentation in labor owing to hyperextension of the neck and mechanical obstruction.[19] The differential diagnosis of an anterior neck mass on ultrasonography includes a hygroma, teratoma, hemartoma, or hemangioma. Magnetic resonance imaging (MRI) has also been used to assess fetal thyroid size with a diffuse goiter showing homogeneously elevated signal on T1-weighted images.[20] However, it remains to be determined whether MRI is more sensitive than ultrasound. A goiter may also be evident on three-dimensional ultrasound.[21]

FIGURE 21–3
Sagittal section of fetal neck at 26 weeks' gestation in a woman with Graves' disease illustrates a large goiter (*arrow*).
(Image courtesy of Dr. Melissa Manusco and Dr. Joseph Biggio.)

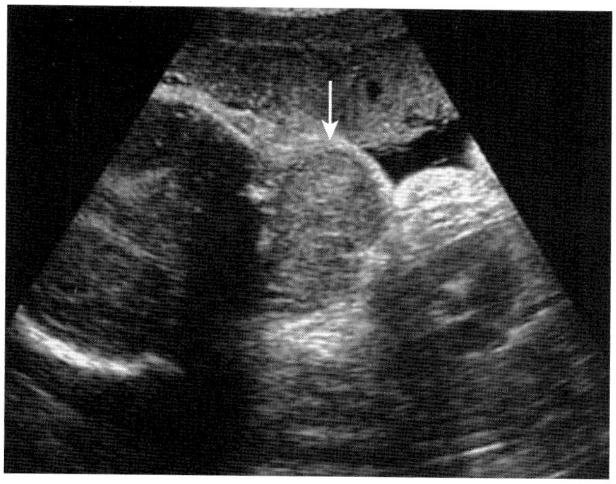

TABLE 21–3
Ultrasound Score to Distinguish Hyperthyroidism from Hypothyroidism in Fetuses with Goiter

		SCORE
Fetal heart rate	Normal	0
	Tachycardia*	1
Vascularization of goiter on color Doppler†	Peripheral or absent	0
	Central	1
Bone maturation‡	Delayed	−1
	Normal	0
	Accelerated	1
Fetal movements	Normal	1
	Increased¶	0

An overall score ≥ 2 is suggestive of hyperthyroidism and a score < 2 is suggestive of hypothyroidism.

* Heart rate > 160 beats/min.
† Color Doppler interrogation of gland performed with the velocity scale adjusted to 13 cm/sec.
‡ Bone maturation was evaluated at 32 wk' gestation. Normally, the distal femoral ossification center is undetectable before 28 wk' gestation, is dotlike around 32 weeks, < 3 mm before 33 wk, and is consistently visible after 35 wk' gestation. Delayed bone maturation was defined as the absence of the femoral ossification center after 33 wk' gestation. Accelerated bone maturation was defined as the presence of the femoral ossification center before 31 wk' gestation.[14]
¶ Broad movements of the limbs and trunk throughout the examination.
From Huel C, Guibourdenche J, Vuillard E, et al: Use of ultrasound to distinguish between fetal hyperthyroidism and hypothyroidism on discovery of a goiter. Ultrasound Obstet Gynecol 2009;33:412–420.

Huel and colleagues[16] have proposed several ultrasound parameters (and a score based on these parameters) to distinguish goitrous hyperthyroidism from hypothyroidism (Table 21–3; Fig. 21–4). In their study of 39 cases of fetal goiter, four out of seven (57%) with hyperthyroidism had tachycardia, six of seven (86%) had accelerated bone growth,

FIGURE 21-4
Color Doppler examination of a transverse section of fetal neck (velocity scale adjusted to 13 cm/sec). *A*, Peripheral vascularization of a goiter. *B*, Central vascularization of a goiter.
(*A* and *B*, Reproduced from Huel C, Guibourdenche J, Vuillard E, et al: Use of ultrasound to distinguish between fetal hyperthyroidism and hypothyroidism on discovery of a goiter. Ultrasound Obstet Gynecol 2009;33:412-420, with permission.)

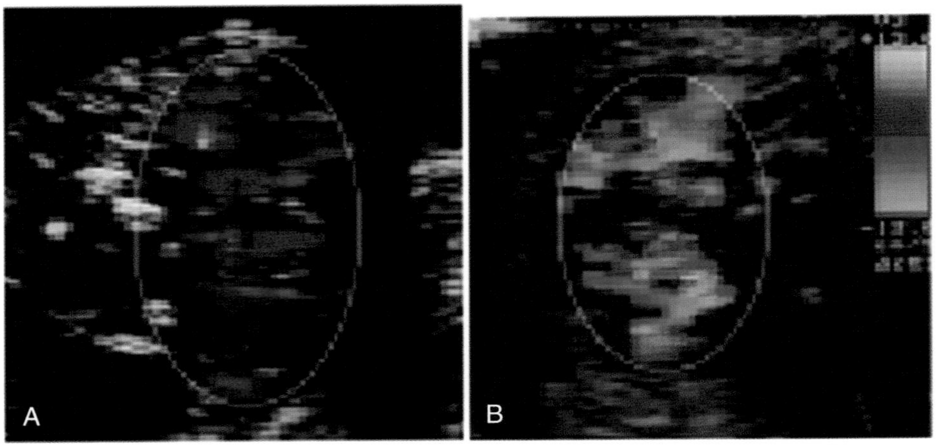

three of five fetuses who had color Doppler assessment of the goiter had central vascularization, and none had increased fetal movements. In all five hyperthyroid cases in which all four parameters were recorded, the overall score (see Table 21–3) was 2 or greater.[16] One case also had tracheal compression and another had cardiomegaly. Peleg and coworkers[13] reported that five of six cases with neonatal thyrotoxicosis manifested fetal tachycardia, one had FGR, and another had hydrops.

Serial fetal ultrasonography is generally recommended in women with hyperthyroidism.[18] Assessment of fetal heart rate, growth, and thyroid size every 4 to 6 weeks from 22 weeks' gestation is reasonable, although more frequent scans may be prudent in women with high TRAbs.[14,22]

FETAL THYROID FUNCTION TESTS

Amniotic fluid thyroid hormone concentrations do not reliably predict fetal thyroid status.[23] Fetal blood sampling (FBS) is therefore the only method of directly assessing thyroid function. Normograms for fetal thyroid hormone and TSH levels are available.[2] In fetal hyperthyroidism, TSH concentrations are low.[19] However, FBS is associated with a small risk of pregnancy loss. This risk is justified in cases of maternal GD in which there is ultrasound evidence of a fetal goiter in order to distinguish hyper- from hypothyroidism. FBS should also be offered to women with GD with isolated sustained fetal tachycardia.[13] There is controversy regarding the role of FBS in women with GD and no ultrasound evidence of fetal involvement. Accumulating evidence suggests that invasive testing is not justified in women with negative or low TRAbs,[14] whereas there is a case for offering FBS in those with high TRAbs[24]; of 14 cases undergoing FBS because of high TRAbs (defined as TSAb levels >160% on bioassay or >10 U/L on immunoassay) or ultrasound evidence of fetal involvement, one of the two cases of fetal hyperthyroidism (with TSAb of 259%) had neither fetal goiter nor tachycardia.[5] Further studies are needed to determine whether the ultrasound score recently reported by Huel and colleagues[16] can replace invasive assessment of fetal thyroid status.

Risks

Perinatal risks of fetal hyperthyroidism include FGR, hydrops, and hydramnios with the associated risks of preterm delivery and malpresentation. Early studies reported a perinatal mortality from fetal hyperthyroidism of up to 50%,[23] but more recent studies, incorporating maternal and fetal surveillance, indicate the risks are much lower than this.[25]

Overt neonatal thyrotoxicosis is associated with tachycardia, tachypnea, flushing, difficulty in feeding, hyperirritability, and poor weight gain. There may be associated jaundice, hepatosplenomegaly, and a bleeding tendancy due to thrombocytopenia and low prothrombin levels.[25] In severely affected babies, mortality may be as high as 25% owing to cardiac arrhythmias or high output failure.[25] Long-term sequelae include craniosynostosis and neurodevelopmental impairment.[26] The half-life of antithyroid drugs in the neonate is shorter than the maternal TRAbs, and therefore, symptoms of neonatal thyrotoxicosis might not present until 5 to 10 days of age.[26] Further, TRAbs are excreted in breast milk, and there is some evidence that neonatal thyroid disease may be worse and more prolonged in TRAb-positive women who breast-feed.[27]

FETAL RISKS OF MATERNAL HYPERTHYROIDISM

In women who become pregnant while their thyrotoxicosis is under control and in those in whom the condition is diagnosed and treated early, the prognosis for mother and fetus is excellent. However, untreated or poorly controlled maternal hyperthyroidism is associated with early pregnancy loss, stillbirth, FGR, and preterm birth.[28,29] These adverse fetal effects are due to direct toxic effects of high levels of thyroid hormone because they occur in fetuses of euthyroid mothers with resistance to thyroid hormone secondary to mutations in the TR-β gene.[30] In one large retrospective review of 249 cases of GD published in 1992, the fetal death/stillbirth rate was 5.6%.[31] Millar and coworkers[32] reported preterm delivery in 33% of hyperthyroid mothers (odds ratio [OR] 16.5, 95% confidence interval [CI] 2.1–130), and 12% gave birth to a small-for-gestational age (SGA) infant (OR 2.2, CI 0.4–11.5). Thyrotoxicosis for 30 weeks or more during pregnancy, GD for 10 years or longer, onset of GD before 20 years of age, and high TBII at delivery (>30%) are each associated with an increased risk of delivering an SGA infant.[8] Pregnancy outcome is closely associated with maternal thyroid status, with poorer outcomes in uncontrolled women at delivery.[29,32]

Management Options

THERAPY FOR MATERNAL HYPERTHYROIDISM (See Also Chapter 45)

Effective treatment of maternal hyperthyroidism is associated with improved maternal and fetal outcome.[8,29,32] Ideally, this should be undertaken prior to pregnancy. Mothers who remain euthyroid throughout pregnancy do not appear to be at increased risk of preeclampsia, preterm delivery, or delivery of an SGA infant.[28]

Antithyroid Drugs

Thionamides inhibit the synthesis of thyroid hormone by preventing iodination of the tyrosine molecule. Early evidence suggested that propylthiouracil (PTU) crossed the placenta more slowly than methimazole and carbimazole (which is metabolized to methimazole),[33] but this has not been confirmed in subsequent studies.[34] Case reports have linked methimazole with fetal scalp defects (aplasia cutis) and choanal or esophageal atresia.[35] However, the overall incidence of major malformations is comparable in women taking PTU and methimazole (2%–3%),[34,36] and in a prospective cohort study comparing methimazole exposed infants with controls, there was no difference in the incidence of major malformations.[37] Further, there is no evidence that the use of PTU is associated with a reduced incidence of neonatal thyroid dysfunction.[34,38] PTU, however, remains the initial preferred drug for maternal hyperthyroidism according to an expert consensus recommendation of the Endocrine Society.[35] In utero exposure to antithyroid drugs has not been associated with long-term differences in IQ scores or psychomotor development compared with unexposed siblings.[39,40]

Methimazole and, to a lesser extent, PTU are excreted in breast milk. However, studies have reported no alteration in thyroid function in infants breast-fed by mothers treated with daily doses of PTU (50–300 mg), methimazole (5–20 mg), or carbimazole (5–15 mg) for up to 8 months.[35] Mothers should be advised to take their antithyroid medication just after a feed and wait 3 to 4 hours before feeding again.

In newly diagnosed cases of maternal hyperthyroidism, the initial dose of PTU is usually 150 mg every 8 hours. The equivalent dose of carbimazole is 20 mg twice daily. Clinical and biochemical improvement is usually evident after 2 to 4 weeks, although the fetal response may take longer. Once maternal symptoms have improved and thyroid function is within the normal range, the dose should be halved. Further reductions may be possible owing to the tendency for GD to ameliorate during the last trimester, and it is usually possible to reach a maintenance dose of 150 mg/day or less of PTU (or ≤15 mg/day of carbimazole). Side effects include nausea, arthralgia, skin rash, metallic taste, and fever. Leucopenia, agranulocytosis, and hepatitis can also occur.

The aim of therapy is to keep the mother euthyroid using the minimum amount of thionamide. Maternal thyroid function should be monitored every 4 to 6 weeks, aiming to keep the FT_4 at the upper third of the normal nonpregnant range.[6,35] With this management, serum FT_4 levels are normal in more than 90% of neonates.[37] In contrast, FT_4 levels are low in 36% of neonates when the maternal FT_4 is in the lower two thirds of the nonpregnant range.[37] If the mother remains euthyroid with a small dose of PTU (50–100 mg) or methimazole (5–10 mg), therapy should be discontinued. This may be possible in up to 30% of patients after 32 weeks.[28]

Reliable differentiation of thionamide-induced hypothyroidism (see later) from TRAb-induced hyperthyroidism in GD requires measurement of fetal FT_4 and TSH. Although fetal heart rate alone is unreliable in detecting thyroid dysfunction,[5] serial measurement of fetal thyroid size may allow early noninvasive detection of thyroid dysfunction.[14,22] Cohen and colleagues[22] measured thyroid size in 20 consecutive women with GD on PTU (1050–1150 mg/wk); thyroid width and circumference were above the 95% percentiles in 5 fetuses; in 3, thyroid size decreased concurrently with a decrease in maternal PTU dosage and all were born euthyroid. In 2 fetuses, thyroid size was unaffected by a decrement in maternal PTU dose and both were hyperthyroid at birth. Luton and colleagues[14] measured fetal thyroid size monthly from 22 weeks' gestation in 72 mothers with past or present GD; fetal thyroid circumference was normal in all 31 fetuses whose mothers were TRAb-negative and took no antithyroid drugs during late pregnancy. Thirty of the 41 other fetuses (of which 16 were exposed to maternal PTU) had normal fetal thyroid circumference; 29 were euthyroid and one hypothyroid at birth. Eleven fetuses developed a goiter; based on associated ultrasound features (see Table 21–3) and/or FBS (performed in 6 cases), 7 fetuses were diagnosed as hypothyroid and 4 as hyperthyroid. Overall, the sensitivity and specificity of fetal thyroid circumference at 32 weeks' gestation for clinically relevant thyroid dysfunction were 92% and 100%, respectively.[14] Thus, accumulating evidence suggests that serial measurement of fetal thyroid size is extremely valuable in monitoring thionamide dosage, although it remains to be determined whether, with the addition of other ultrasound parameters (see Table 21–3), ultrasound can replace FBS in the initial assessment of fetal goiter.

Surgery

Subtotal thyroidectomy can be performed successfully during pregnancy but is usually considered only for those women who develop a serious adverse reaction to thionamides or who require persistently high doses to control hyperthyroidism.[35] Maternal thyrotoxicosis must be adequately controlled preoperatively. This is most rapidly achieved with β-blocking agents and iodide. Surgical thyroidectomy of women with GD does not lead to immediate remission of the autoimmune abnormality and there is a risk, with withdrawal of antithyroid therapy and T_4

(see Table 21–3).[14,16] Hydramnios, fetal tachycardia, and FGR may also be present.[5,16] In the presence of a goiter, a color flow Doppler signal confined to the periphery of the gland is considered suggestive of fetal hypothyroidism (see Fig. 21–4); of the 32 fetuses with a hypothyroid goiter reported by Huel and colleagues,[16] 22 (69%) had peripheral vascularization of the thyroid and none had central vascularization. Fifteen (47%) also showed delayed bone maturation, 14 (44%) had increased fetal movements, and 2 (6%) had tachycardia. Using their ultrasound score (see Table 21–3), all the fetuses with a hypothyroid goiter had a score lower than 2.[16]

The majority of cases of fetal hypothyroidism occur as a consequence of sporadic, embryologic malformations and are not detected on routine ultrasound screening at 18 to 20 weeks' gestation. Occasionally, a goiter may be detected later in pregnancy at an ultrasound examination performed for other reasons.[60] When there is family history of congenital hypothyroidism due to defects in thyroid hormone synthesis or metabolism, serial ultrasound screening may detect a large goiter.

FETAL THYROID FUNCTION TESTS

The development of a goiter and/or polyhydramnios does not correlate closely with the degree of fetal hypothyroidism.[5,61] Definitive antenatal diagnosis, therefore, requires FBS and confirmation of an elevated TSH and low FT_4. Reported values of TSH in fetuses with goiter have ranged from 25 to 1640 mU/L.[60–62] If the ultrasound score reported by Huel and colleagues[16] is confirmed to reliably differentiate hypo- from hyperthyroidism goiter in prospective series, it may be possible to avoid FBS in the future. Although elevated amniotic fluid TSH levels have been reported in fetal hypothyroidism, the sensitivity of this method is unclear.[63] In many countries, all newborns are screened for congenital hypothyroidism by the measurement of TSH on a blood spot.

Risks

CONGENITAL HYPOTHYROIDISM

In congenital hypothyroidism (in which maternal thyroid function is normal), the fetal thyroidal supply is deficient to varying degrees in utero and during early infancy. Transplacental passage of maternal thyroid hormones, along with compensatory deiodinase activity, ensures thyroid hormone sufficiency during the first half of pregnancy. However, the fetal contribution is reduced or totally lacking in the second half of gestation and hypothyroxinemia persists until the diagnosis is made and treatment takes effect. As a result, children with congenital hypothyroidism manifest motor and cognitive defects, with a mean IQ significantly lower than controls. Infants with severe congenital hypothyroidism, particularly those with absent thyroid glands or who show ultrasonographic and/or serum evidence of hypothyroidism in utero, have lower IQ scores than those with less severe hypothyroidism.[64,65] Perinatal hypothyroidism appears to contribute particularly to visuospatial and fine motor deficits.[1] Although neonatal screening programs enable early T_4 supplementation, subtle deficits in cognitive and motor skills are reported even into adolescence.[66,67]

MATERNAL HYPOTHYROIDISM

In iodine-sufficient areas, overt maternal hypothyroidism occurs in 0.3% to 0.5% of pregnancies, whereas subclinical hypothyroidism (normal FT_4 but elevated TSH) has been reported in 2% to 3% of pregnancies.[68,69] In areas of endemic iodine deficiency, the incidence is even higher. Autoimmune thyroiditis is present in 15% to 55% of women with subclinical hypothyroidism and in more than 80% of women with overt hypothyroidism.[69,70]

The rate of miscarriage is increased approximately twofold in women with overt hypothyroidism. This risk appears to be related more to the presence of circulating thyroid antibodies than thyroid function.[71] Pregnancy-induced hypertension, preeclampsia, and placental abruption are purported to be more common, leading to an increased rate of preterm delivery and stillbirth.[70,72,73] Severe maternal hypothyroidism in early pregnancy has also been associated with a 56% rate of intrapartum cesarean section for fetal distress.[74] Complications are more common with overt than subclinical hypothyroidism. However, one recent study found no adverse outcomes in women with subclinical hypothyroidism (TSH levels > 97.5th percentile and FT_4 between the 2.5th and the 97.5th percentiles).[69] In contrast, women with first-trimester hypothyroxinemia (TSH levels between the 2.5th and the 97.5th percentiles and FT_4 < 2.5th percentile) had an increased risk of preterm labor (adjusted OR 1.62, 95% CI 1.00–2.62) and macrosomia (adjusted OR 1.97, 95% CI 1.37–2.83). Adequate T_4 treatment greatly reduces the risk[75,76]; in a recent randomized trial in thyroid antibody–positive women, the rate of miscarriage was reduced by 75% and preterm delivery by 69% in those given T_4 (started at 5–10 wk) throughout gestation compared with antibody-positive women who did not receive T_4 and in whom TSH levels gradually rose during gestation.[77]

Infants born to hypothyroid women are at increased risk of impairment in neuropsychological development, IQ scores, and school learning abilities. The degree of impairment is dependent on the severity, duration, and timing of the maternal thyroid insufficiency.[35] Man and Serunian[78] initially reported that mean IQ at 7 years of age was 13 points lower in children born to women who were hypothyroid during pregnancy than in those born to women who were euthyroid on T_4 replacement. Klein and associates[79] measured maternal TSH levels in 25,216 pregnant women at 15 to 18 weeks' gestation (from frozen samples obtained for Down syndrome screening) and found 2.5% had elevated TSH levels (≥6 mU/L), of which 12% (6/49) also had low FT_4 levels. Children of mothers with high TSH levels scored lower than controls on all 15 of the neuropsychological tests and attained an average IQ that was 4 points below controls.[80] Of the 62 women with thyroid deficiency, 48 were not treated during pregnancy and the IQ of their children averaged 7 points lower than children born to euthyroid and T_4-treated women.[80] Further, there were three times as many children with IQs more than 2 SDs below the mean IQ of controls (i.e., <85) in the children born to untreated hypothyroid women. Further, preschool children born to hypothyroid women with suboptimal replacement (mean TSH 5–7 mU/L) have also been shown to have a mild decrease in IQ, although no deficits in language, visuospatial ability, or fine-motor performance.[81] Even isolated first-trimester hypothyroxinemia (FT_4 < 10.4 pmol/L at 12 weeks' gestation, i.e., in the lowest 10th decile and a normal TSH) that persists until 24 weeks or later has been shown to be associated with delayed mental and motor function (mean deficit of 8–10 points on Bayley Scales of Infant Development) at 2 years of age compared with controls (FT_4 between the 50th and the 90th percentiles).[82] However, when FT_4 recovered spontaneously to normal later in pregnancy, outcome was normal.

IODINE DEFICIENCY

In iodine deficiency, both maternal and fetal thyroid glands are affected early in pregnancy. In a meta-analysis of 19 studies, infants were found to have an overall reduction in cognitive function of 13.5 IQ points.[83] Even when limited to mild to moderate iodine deficiency, there is clear evidence of retarded psychomotor development with low motor and attentive functions.[35]

As more information becomes available concerning the detrimental and long-term effects of maternal hypothyroidism on the fetus, many authorities have advocated screening all women as early as possible in pregnancy.[84] However, it is not certain whether FT_4 or TSH should be used, what cutoff to adopt, or what treatment should be instituted for screen-positive women. Ultimately,the value of screening and treating mildly hypothyroid women in nonendemic areas can be addressed only in large trials with adequate follow-up.

Management Options

FETAL THERAPY

Fetal therapy is indicated in cases with confirmed fetal hypothyroidism because of the risk of neurologic damage. Relatively little T_4 crosses the placenta and the amount of T_4 that would be needed to treat the fetus adequately would result in the development of maternal hyperthyroidism. Direct fetal therapy is therefore necessary. Weiner and colleagues[85] reported the first use of intra-amniotic T_4 in the treatment of fetal goiter. Subsequent reports have confirmed that effectiveness of this mode of administration with reduction in goiter size, resolution of hydramnios, and improvement in fetal thyroid function.[5,60,62] A weekly dose of 250 μg appears to be effective. This is consistent with the neonatal T_4 requirement of 10 μg/day and animal data that suggest that 90% of T_4 administered intra-amniotically is absorbed within 24 hours.[86] Whether this is the optimum dose and frequency is unclear, and larger doses (500–600 μg) given every 14 days may be as effective.[5,61] Fetal therapy should be started as early as possible once the diagnosis of fetal hypothyroidism has been made. Intra-amniotic injections of T_3 (60–120 μg) have also been used.[87] Although uptake of T_3 may be faster (with effects evident within 4–8 hr), it has a shorter half-life than T_4 (1–2 days vs. 6–7 days), and therefore, more frequent intra-amniotic injections are required.

A possible noninvasive alternative to treat fetal hypothyroidism is maternal administration of 3′-tryiodothyroacetic acid (Triac), a T_3-derived analogue that binds to thyroid hormone receptors with higher affinity than T_3. Triac crosses the placenta[88] and has been used successfully to reduce TSH concentrations and goiter size in fetal hypothyroidism secondary to PTU therapy[61,88] and to reduce TSH concentrations in a fetus affected by a mutation in the TR-β gene leading to resistance to thyroid hormones.[89] In both case reports, Triac was increased from a starting dose of 2.1 mg/day to 2.8 mg/day[61] and 3.5 mg/day,[89] respectively, in an attempt to normalize fetal TSH levels. Further experience is needed with this therapy before it can be recommended as a safe alternative to invasive therapy.

Repeat FBS 1 to 2 weeks after starting therapy appears justified to confirm that TSH and FT_4 have returned to normal. Repeat sampling is particularly important if there is a worsening in the fetal condition, failure of the goiter to resolve, or the development of polyhydramnios.[90] Worsening fetal hypothyroidism, despite repeated intra-amniotic injections of T_4, may be an indication for injection of levothyroxine into the umbilical vein.[91] In women with GD with fetal hypothyroidism, assessing the fetal response to reduction in maternal antithyroid therapy may be appropriate before considering direct fetal therapy.[5]

MATERNAL THERAPY (See Also Chapter 45)

Most women with hypothyroidism are already taking T_4 prior to pregnancy. The dose of T_4 should be adjusted preconception to ensure serum TSH is not higher than 2.5 mU/L.[35] Adequate T_4 replacement eliminates or reduces the risks of adverse pregnancy outcome. The serum FT_4 levels should be kept in the upper normal range, necessitating increased T_4 in up to 75% of patients during the first trimester.[92,93] A further 35% of women who maintain a normal serum TSH until the second trimester without increasing their T_4 replacement will require an increment during late pregnancy to maintain a euthyroid state.[92,93] Average T_4 requirements are increased by 25 to 100 μg/day during pregnancy, although this depends on the etiology of the hypothyroidism; women without residual thyroid tissue require a greater increment than women with autoimmune thyroiditis.[93] The increase in T_4 dose can be based on the initial serum TSH: 25 to 50 μg if TSH is 5 to 10 mU/L, 50 to 75 μg if TSH is 10 to 20 mU/L, and 100 μg if TSH is greater than 20 mU/L.[68] However, the maternal dose should not be increased without objective proof of the need.

Maternal TSH and FT_4 should be measured at booking, at 16 to 20 weeks, and at 28 to 32 weeks, although it has been suggested that repeat testing is not necessary unless clinically indicated.[94] Ferrous sulfate reduces the absorption of T_4, and ingestion of these drugs should be separated by at least 2 hours. After pregnancy, T_4 is reduced to the pre-pregnancy dose over a period of 2 to 4 weeks.[68] It is safe for women taking T_4 to breast-feed.

In severe iodine deficiency, iodine supplementation during pregnancy prevents the occurrence of hypothyroid cretinism and neonatal hypothyroidism, increases birth weight, reduces neonatal mortality, and improves developmental quotients.[95] The recommended nutrient intake for iodine during pregnancy was reevaluated in 2005 with a recommendation of between 200 to 300 μg/day, with an average of 250 μg/day.[35] Iodine can be given in the form of iodized salt, potassium iodide drips, or iodized oil.

NEONATAL THERAPY

Infants confirmed to be hypothyroid after screening should be started on replacement T_4 (15 μg/kg orally once daily) immediately. The dose is adjusted according to the TSH and FT_4.[1] Recent data confirm that it is better to suppress TSH levels as quickly as possible rather than simply normalize FT_4 levels.[96] Marginal overreplacement can usually be compensated for by endogenous deiodination.[96] After infancy, the required dose is approximately 100 μg/m^2/day and FT_4 should be rechecked at 3 months, 6 months, and annually thereafter. Response to treatment appears to vary with the etiology of hypothyroidism; athyrotic infants take longer to normalize their thyroid function and probably justify more frequent monitoring in early life.[97]

FETAL ADRENAL DISEASE

Introduction

The adrenal cortex arises from the mesoderm of the mesonephros during the fifth week of embryonic development. The cells that form the medulla are derived from adjacent neural crest cells and come to be encapsulated by the fetal cortex, which rapidly increases in size from the end of the second trimester to occupy 80% of the adrenal cortex by term. The adult (or definitive) cortex, also derived from mesenchymal cells, forms a thin outer layer.

All adrenal steroids are formed from cholesterol (Fig. 21–5). In the zona fasciculata of the definitive cortex, steroid precursors are used to synthesize cortisol under the influence

SUMMARY OF MANAGEMENT OPTIONS

Fetal Hypothyroidism

Management Options	Evidence Quality and Recommendation	References
Prepregnancy		
Offer genetic counseling if previous inherited defect of thyroid hormone synthesis.	III/B	45
Iodine supplementation (250 μg/day) in areas of iodine deficiency.	Ia/A	83,95
Check maternal TSH and FT_4 and adjust thyroxine dose (aim for TSH ≤ 2.5 mU/L) (see Chapter 45).	III/B	35
Prenatal		
In fetus at risk, sonographic surveillance for reduced fetal movements, cardiomegaly, bradycardia/heart block, FGR, goiter.	III/B	5,14,16
Measure maternal TSH and FT_4 at first antenatal visit and adjust thyroxine dose accordingly (see Chapter 45).	III/B	35,68
Measure TSH and FT_4 at 16–20 and 28–32 wk and adjust thyroxine dose accordingly.	III/B	35,68
When goiter detected during a routine or indicated ultrasound examination (e.g., women with Graves' disease on antithyroid therapy) assess thyroid vascularization (by color Doppler) and bone maturation.	III/B	14–16
Measure fetal TSH and FT_4 in fetuses with goiter or delayed bone maturation.	III/B	5,16
If fetal hypothyroidism confirmed, administer intra-amniotic thyroxine and monitor response with repeat fetal blood sampling. In women with Graves' disease on antithyroid therapy, reduce dose initially and monitor response.	IIb/B	5,60–62
Postnatal		
Measure TSH and FT_4 in cord blood in at-risk fetuses.	—/GPP	—
Replace thyroxine in infants confirmed to be hypothyroid on screening/testing.	III/B	35,78,80,82
When necessary, reduce maternal thyroxine dose to prepregnancy levels.	—/GPP	—

FT_4, free thyroxine; GPP, good practice point; TSH, thyroid-stimulating hormone.

FIGURE 21–5
Pathways of adrenal hormone synthesis. Major pathways are indicated by *thick arrows*, minor ones by *thin arrows*. Extra-adrenal conversion of sex steroids is denoted by *double arrows*. Numbers indicate enzymatic steps as follows: 1, cholestrol side chain cleaving system; 2, 3β-hydroxysteroid dehydrogenase; 3, 21-hydroxylase; 4, 11β hydroxylase; 5, 18-hydroxylase; 6, 18-dehydrogenase; 7, 17α-hydroxylase; 8, 17,20-lyase; 9, 17β-hydroxy-steroid dehydrogenase.

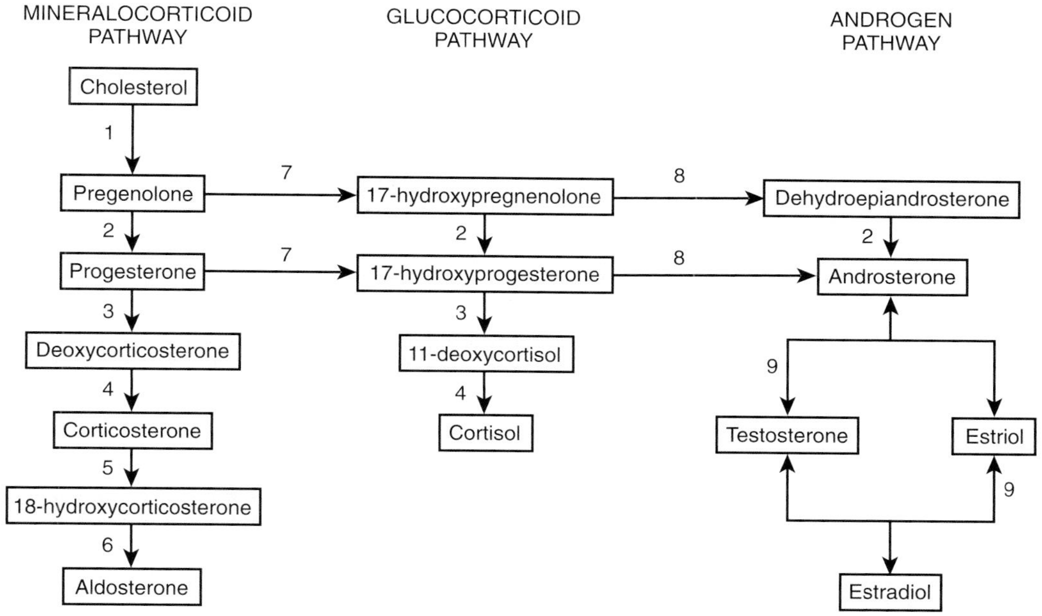

of 17α-hydroxylase. Fetal cortisol concentrations rise, particularly toward term, stimulating the maturation of several enzyme systems in the lungs and gastrointestinal tract. Glucocorticoid synthesis is under the control of pituitary adrenocorticotropic hormone (ACTH). Both hypothalamic corticotropin-releasing hormone (CRH) and arginine vasopressin (AVP) stimulate the release of ACTH, which is cleaved from a large prohormone pro-opiomelanocortin (POMC) containing the sequences of several other peptide hormones. 17α-Hydroxylase is inactive in the zona glomerulosa and precursors are used to synthesize aldosterone under the control of the renin-angiotensin system. Adrenal androgen production is insignificant during fetal life.

The fetal adrenal gland provides precursors for maternal estrogen production. The cortex contains inactivated 3β-hydroxysteroid dehydrogenase. Therefore, pregnenolone is converted primarily into dehydroepiandrosterone sulfate (DHAS), which appears in the fetal circulation from 8 weeks. DHAS is hydroxylated in other fetal tissues, particularly the liver, to 16-hydroxy DHAS, which then passes to the placenta, where it is converted into androstenedione and subsequently to estrogens.

Congenital Adrenal Hyperplasia

Congenital adrenal hyperplasia (CAH) refers to a group of autosomal recessive disorders of adrenal steroidogenesis. The disorder may result from a defect in any of the five enzymes required to synthesize cortisol from cholesterol.

21-HYDROXYLASE ($P450_C21$) DEFICIENCY

In 90% to 95% of cases, CAH is due to 21-hydroxylase deficiency (21-OHD) resulting in a blockade of the conversion of 17-hydroxyprogesterone into 11-deoxycortisol (see Fig. 21–5). Reduced synthesis of cortisol leads to increased ACTH and shunting of precursors into the pathways of androgen synthesis. Steroid 21-OHD occurs in two forms: a severe ("classic") form and a mild ("nonclassic") form. Among severe 21-OHD patients, three quarters have the salt-wasting (SW) type, with a concurrent defect in aldosterone synthesis, and the remainder have the simple virilizing (SV) form with preserved ability to retain salt. The incidence of severe CAH is approximately 1 in 13,000 live births, but there are marked ethnic differences.[98,99]

21-OHD results from mutations in the *CYP21A2* gene, located with its pseudogene (CYP21A1P) in the polymorphic human leukocyte antigen (HLA) histocompatability complex on chromosome 6p21.3. The nucleotide sequences of these two genes are 98% identical in exons and 96% identical in introns, permitting two types of recombination events: (1) unequal crossing-over during meiosis, which results in complete deletions/duplications of CYP21A2 and (2) gene conversion events that transfer deleterious mutations present in the pseudogene to CYP21A2. More than 100 mutations have been described in 21-OHD, the two most common being a 30-kb deletion or genomic rearrangement/conversion fusing CYP21A2 with CYP21A1P (30%) and IVS2-13 A/C → G (28%).[98,100] More than 90% of these deletions are derived from 10 mutations within the CYP21A pseudogene with the remainder caused by rare sporadic mutations.[100] Correlations exist between the genotype and the phenotype; 21-OHD mutations that totally ablate enzyme activity are associated with the SW form whereas those that produce enzymes with 1% to 2% normal activity, permitting adequate aldosterone synthesis, lead to SV disease. A third group of mutations produce enzymes retaining 20% to 60% normal activity and are responsible for the nonclassic form.[99]

OTHER FORMS

11β-Hydroxylase (P450$_c$11) deficiency accounts for approximately 5% of CAH. 11-Deoxycortisol is not converted into cortisol, leading to a shunting of precursors into the pathway for androgen synthesis. The enzymatic defect also leads to an accumulation of deoxycorticosterone, which has significant salt-retaining properties. Two copies of the 11β-hydroxylase gene are present on chromosome 11q, and several mutations have been identified. Deficiencies of 3β-hydroxysteroid dehydrogenase, 17α-hydroxylase, and cholesterol side chain cleavage enzyme account for fewer than 1% of CAH cases. Mild or partial defects may occur more frequently.

Diagnosis

Patients with the classic SW form may present with hyponatremic dehydration, vomiting, and shock in the early neonatal period.[96,99] Female fetuses with classic 21-OHD are exposed to excess androgens from the seventh week of gestation. This leads to virilization of the external genitalia, which can vary from clitoral hypertrophy to complete formation of a phallus and fusion of the labia (Fig. 21–6), causing erroneous assignment of gender. Affected males have normal external genitalia. In the nonclassic form, virilizing symptoms appear postnatally. Females affected with 11β-hydroxylase deficiency also have ambiguous genitalia at birth. The excess deoxycorticosterone generally leads to hypertension and hypokalemia. Virilization of female fetuses is much less marked in 3β-hydroxysteroid dehydrogenase deficiency, and in the other two forms, the male is incompletely masculinized.[96,99]

The diagnosis of 21-OHD is confirmed by measurement of neonatal plasma 17α-hydroxyprogesterone (17-OHP), which typically exceeds 300 nmol/L. Classic 21-OHD deficiency is more common than phenylketonuria, and neonatal screening of blood spots to measure 17-OHP has been introduced in many countries in view of the risks from SW and late diagnosis.[96] In the United Kingdom, however, screening as part of the "Guthrie test" is not supported by the National Screening Committee.[101] This decision, made in 2006, is to be reviewed in 2010/2011. Whereas advocates of screening feel that there is insufficient acknowledgment of the considerable morbidity of CAH, there are little published data on improvements in morbidity resulting from early detection and treatment.[96] In 11β-hydroxylase deficiency, plasma deoxycorticosterone is elevated. The profile of urinary steroids by gas chromatography and mass spectrometry provides a definitive diagnosis.

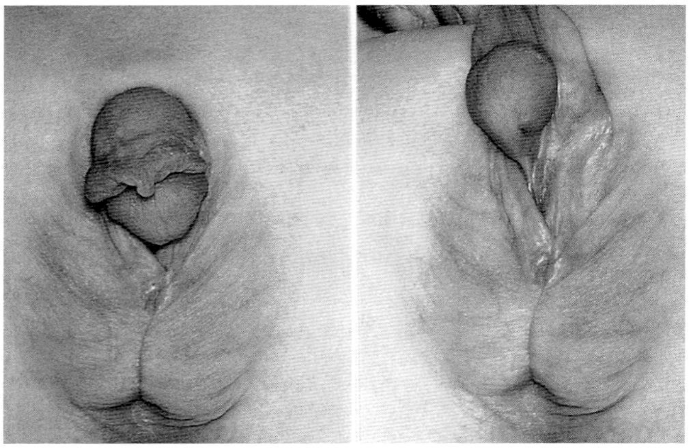

FIGURE 21–6
Severe virilization in two untreated female infants with 21-hydroxylase deficiency. There is almost complete formation of a phallus and scrotum.

Risks

Emergency treatment with sodium replacement and intravenous normal or even hypertonic saline is necessary to prevent death. Once sodium balance is restored, mineralocorticoid replacement is started with 9α-fluorcortisol (fludrocortisone) 0.1 to 0.15 mg/m^2/day. Appropriate glucocorticoid replacement therapy will suppress androgen levels and allow normal growth, skeletal maturation, and puberty.[96] Hydrocortisone 12 to 15 mg/m^2/day is usually given in two or three divided doses.

Postnatally untreated androgen excess may manifest as progressive virilizing changes and accelerated growth and development. The majority of female infants born with virilized genitalia require corrective surgery. More than one operation is required in 50%. Clitoral reduction is best undertaken before 6 months of age, but the timing of vaginal reconstructive surgery is controversial; previously, this was delayed until after puberty, but more recently, single-stage surgery at 2 to 6 months has been advocated.[102] In addition to progressive virilization, the high androgens affect the hypothalamic-pituitary-gonadal axis in both sexes, leading to subfertility. Follow-up studies of adult females with CAH diagnosed in infancy or early childhood suggest that one third are hirsute and their ovulation rate is less than 50%.[103] After reconstructive surgery, about 75% have an adequate vaginal introitus; in this group, pregnancy rates are approximately 60%.[103] Early treatment with glucocorticoids improves fertility. It has also been suggested that prenatal exposure to excess androgens affects subsequent sexual behavior in adolescent and adult females.[104]

Management Options

PRENATAL DIAGNOSIS

All affected families should be offered genetic counseling. Ideally, this should be performed prior to conception. Subsequent offspring have a 1 in 4 chance of being affected, with a 1 in 8 chance of a virilized female. Prenatal diagnosis was initially accomplished by measuring 17-OHP in amniotic fluid, but direct DNA analysis of the *CYP21A2* gene on chorionic villus samples obtained at 10 to 11 weeks' gestation is now standard. Between 95% and 98% of causative mutations can be identified using a combination of molecular genetic techniques (e.g., locus-specific polymerase chain reaction [PCR] and minisequencing-based arrays).[98,100] In some families, prenatal diagnosis is not possible because of either undetectable mutations, drop-out alleles, or maternal DNA contamination. Determination of satellite markers may increase the accuracy of molecular genetic analysis.[98] Molecular diagnosis is possible in some families with other forms of CAH. Otherwise, antenatal diagnosis is dependent on the measurement of steroids in the amniotic fluid.

MATERNAL DEXAMETHASONE THERAPY

The fetal adrenal gland can be pharmacologically suppressed by maternal administration of dexamethasone. Synthetic fluorinated steroids bind minimally to cortisol-binding globulin and are poor substrates for placental 11β-hydroxysteroid dehydrogenase. Thus, dexamthasone readily crosses the placenta and suppresses fetal ACTH. Because differentiation of the external genitalia begins at approximately 7 weeks of pregnancy, dexamethasone (20 μg/kg prepregnancy weight/day given in two or three divided doses) should begin before this time. Compared with previously affected sisters, treated females have reduced virilization; 25% to 50% require no genital surgery, and the extent of genital surgery is reduced in those who do require it.[105–107] However, therapeutic failures occur[108] (Fig. 21–7), and although some cases have been attributed to late initiation or early cessation of therapy, non-compliance, or suboptimal dosing, there is no obvious explanation in others. The extent of virilization can vary among affected females in the same family even without treatment.[109]

Dexamethasone can be discontinued if the fetus is male or an unaffected female (i.e., in seven of eight pregnancies initially treated). Therapy can be monitored by measurement of maternal urine estriol after 15 to 20 weeks of pregnancy. Excessive weight gain, cutaneous striae, edema, hirsutism, and mood fluctuations are the most common problems in women treated throughout pregnancy.[105,106] Hypertension and gestational diabetes do not seem to be increased.[110] Overall side effects necessitate reducing the dexamethasone dose in up to a quarter of women.[107] Reduction of the dose of dexamethasone later in pregnancy (≤5 μg/kg/day) has been reported to maintain fetal and maternal adrenal suppression, as evidenced by urinary estriol and cortisol metabolites, but the efficacy of this regime in preventing virilization remains to be determined.[111]

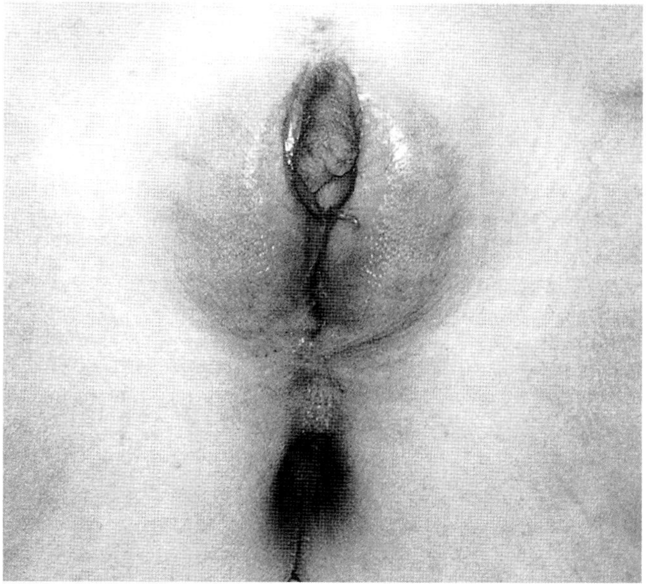

FIGURE 21–7
Partial virilization in a female infant with 21-hydroxylase deficiency treated prenatally with dexamethasone from 8 weeks' gestation. There is clitoromegaly with posterior labial fusion.

No teratogenic effects have been reported in fetuses treated to term with dexamethasone; specifically, the incidence of facial clefting does not appear to be increased.[105,112] The long-term safety of prenatal treatment remains uncertain. Administration of low doses of glucocorticoids to children has been reported to produce retarded growth, diabetes, and hypertension.[113] Follow-up studies of prenatally treated CAH children suggest that birth weight, length, and head circumference are normal, as are subsequent growth and development.[105,113] However, numbers and duration of follow-up remain limited. Concerns remain about the long-term implications of antenatal therapy with respect to metabolic and cardiovascular disease as well as psychosexual/behavioral development. No negative effects on developmental milestones or cognitive development have been found in small studies,[105,114] although Trautman and colleagues[114] did find increased internalizing behavioral traits in prenatally treated children at 2 to 3 years of age. Another group reported adverse effects of prenatal dexamethasone on verbal working memory, but again the numbers studied were small.[115] Although antenatal dexamethasone appears justified, it is important to inform parents that the long-term safety and outcome of this therapy are not established.

DETERMINATION OF FETAL SEX

Fetal sex can be determined by ultrasound from 11 weeks of pregnancy, but reliable assignment is not possible until 12 to 13 weeks' gestation,[116] and a phenotypic male fetus can be a virilized female. Thus, ultrasound is of limited value in the management of an at-risk fetus, other than possibly monitoring the success of prenatal therapy.[117]

Of far greater value is the determination of fetal sex from cell-free DNA in maternal blood. Using real-time PCR, Y chromosome–specific sequences can be amplified from the plasma of women carrying a male fetus.[118] Targetting the multicopy sequence DYS14 appears more sensitive than the single copy SRY sequence (98.8% vs. 65.8% at 11–12 weeks' gestation).[119] Both SRY[120] and DYS14[121] have been detected in maternal plasma as early as 5 weeks' gestation, and recently, Martinhago and associates[121] reported accurate prediction of fetal sex in 25 of 27 cases (92.6%) at 5 weeks using DYS14. Using a protocol of duplicate DNA isolation from 2 mL of maternal plasma, Rijnders and coworkers[118] reported a negative PCR result in all 29 female fetuses. In 35 of 36 male fetuses, SRY was amplified in both DNA isolations (positive predictive value 100%), and in 1 case, only one SRY amplification was positive (negative predictive value 96.7%). Early fetal sexing allows avoidance of unnecessary dexamethasone treatment and invasive prenatal diagnosis in male fetuses.[122] When possible, dexamethasone and weekly plasma DYS14 testing should be started from 5 weeks' gestation. Dexamethasone can be stopped if DYS14 PCR is positive in two separate samples. Male sex should be subsequently confirmed as early as possible with ultrasound. When the DYS14 PCR is negative, testing should be repeated weekly until 10 weeks with a diagnostic chorionic villus sampling at 11 weeks. Dexamethasone can then be discontinued in unaffected females.

SUMMARY OF MANAGEMENT OPTIONS

Congenital Adrenal Hyperplasia

Management Options	Evidence Quality and Recommendation	References
Prepregnancy		
Identify genetic mutation and feasibility of prenatal diagnosis by direct mutation detection.	III/B	98,99
Counsel families regarding risks and options for prenatal diagnosis and treatment.	—/GPP	—
Prenatal		
Start dexamethasone (20 µg/kg/dy) once pregnancy is confirmed.	III/B	105–107
Weekly maternal blood sampling for fetal sexing by PCR amplification of Y-specific DYS14 sequences.	IIa/B	120,121
If male fetus is confirmed, stop dexamethasone and confirm sex as early as possible with ultrasound.	IIb/B	105,107,121,122
If female fetus is confirmed, perform CVS at 10–11 wk' gestation—if affected, continue dexamethasone.	IIb/B	105,107,121,122
In women who continue dexamathasone:		
• Measure maternal serum estriol every 6–8 wk to confirm compliance and adrenal suppression.	III/C	105
• Ultrasound assessment of external genitalia; if there is evidence of virilization, measure amniotic fluid 17-OHP and androstenedione and, if elevated, increase dose of dexamethasone.	III/C	105,122
• Monitor for maternal side effects and if necessary reduce dose of dexamethasone.	III/C	105,107,111
Postnatal		
Examine child carefully for evidence of virilization and salt wasting.	III/C	96,99
Corticosteroid ± mineralocorticoid replacement in affected infants.	III/C	96,99
Long-term developmental follow-up of affected infants.	—/GPP	—

CVS, chorionic villus sampling; GPP, good practice point; 17-OHP, 17-hydroxyprogesterone; PCR, polymerase chain reaction.

SUGGESTED READINGS

Abalovich M, Amino N, Barbour L, et al: Management of thyroid dysfunction during pregnancy and postpartum: An Endocrine Society Clinical Practice Guideline. J Clin Endocrinol Metab 2007;92(Suppl):s1–s47.

Chan S, Rovet J: Thyroid hormones in fetal central nervous system development. Fet Mat Med Rev 2003;14:1–32.

Glinoer D, Abalovich M: Unresolved questions in managing hypothyroidism during pregnancy. BMJ 2007;335:300–335.

Haddow JE, Palomaki GE, Allan WC, et al: Maternal thyroid deficiency during pregnancy and subsequent neuropsychological development of the child. N Engl J Med 1999;341:549–555.

Huel C, Guibourdenche J, Vuillard E, et al: Use of ultrasound to distinguish between fetal hyperthyroidism and hypothyroidism on discovery of a goitre. Ultrasound Obstet Gynecol 2009;33:412–420.

Marx H, Amin P, Lazarus JH: Hyperthyroidism and pregnancy. BMJ 2008;336:663–667.

Nachum Z, Rakover Y, Weiner E, Shalev E: Graves' disease in pregnancy: Prospective evaluation of a selective invasive treatment protocol. Am J Obstet Gynecol 2003;189:159–165.

New MI, Carlson A, Obeid J, et al: Prenatal diagnosis for congenital adrenal hyperplasia in 532 pregnancies. J Clin Endocrinol Metab 2001;86:5651–5657.

Nimkarn S, New MI: Prenatal diagnosis and treatment of congenital adrenal hyperplasia due to 21-hydroxylase deficiency. Mol Cell Endocrinol 2009;300:192–196.

REFERENCES

For a complete list of references, log onto www.expertconsult.com.

CHAPTER 22

Fetal Tumors

MELISSA S. MANCUSO and JOSEPH BIGGIO

Videos corresponding to this chapter are available online at www.expertconsult.com.

INTRODUCTION AND GENERAL APPROACH

Fetal tumors are rare, but can be associated with serious fetal morbidity and mortality. Recent technologic advances in ultrasound imaging have made antenatal detection possible. Early detection has significant implications for maternal and fetal well-being.[1] Once a fetal neoplasm is identified or suspected, a management strategy should be formulated based on the presumptive diagnosis and the prognosis for the specific lesion. An understanding of the ultrasonographic appearance of specific lesions, the differential diagnosis, available treatment modalities, and overall prognosis is critical in providing families with accurate information. A multidisciplinary team, with representatives from maternal-fetal medicine, neonatology, pediatric hematology-oncology, and pediatric surgery, provides an excellent source of information for the parents and allows for an integrated approach.

The prevalence of fetal tumors is difficult to estimate because of variations in the definition of congenital tumors prior to the near-universal application of ultrasonography. Historically, studies included only those tumors apparent at birth or diagnosed within the first 2 to 3 months of life.[2–4] Furthermore, tumors found in stillbirths and nonmalignant tumors may not have been reported to cancer registries. A 30-year population study in the United Kingdom from 1960 to 1989 reported an incidence of 7.2 congenital tumors, both benign and malignant, per 100,000 live births. The incidence of malignancy in neonates is estimated at 36.5 per million live births.[5] In a more recent U.S. survey of infant cancer, the average annual incidence rate for all histologies combined was 223 per million infants in the first year of life. Extracranial neuroblastoma accounted for the largest percentage of neoplasms (26%), followed by leukemias (17%), central nervous system (CNS) tumors (15%), and retinoblastoma (12%).[6]

Although the histology of congenital tumors is similar to that in older children, the incidence, presentation, degree of differentiation, and biologic behavior frequently differ.[7] Teratomas and neuroblastomas are the most common solid tumors reported, but the behavior of these lesions in fetuses and neonates is markedly different from that observed in older children.[2,7,8] The prevalences of these and other neoplasms are listed in Table 22–1.

Prior to antenatal ultrasound, the first sign of a fetal tumor was often hydramnios, which resulted from either neurologic or mechanical interference with fetal swallowing. Frequently, the diagnosis was made in the perinatal period after dystocia, fetal hemorrhage, tumor rupture, or fetal hydrops was diagnosed. Ultrasonography and magnetic resonance imaging (MRI) now allow for a thorough antenatal investigation of suspected fetal masses. Harrison and Adzick[9] observed the natural history of several tumor types and found that some fetuses were able to tolerate the mass, whereas others developed hydrops. Imaging does not provide a histologic diagnosis, but even if a biopsy were taken antenatally, the prognosis might still be obscure because the histologic appearance of malignancy in the fetus or neonate often reflects the immaturity of the patient and not tumor biology.[8] Moreover, even histologically benign lesions can cause fetal or neonatal death if the tumor mass disrupts other vital structures.[10] The location of the mass and the ability to predict the potential for impingement on vital structures are critical in assessing prognosis.

INTRACRANIAL TUMORS

Congenital brain tumors develop rarely during fetal life, with an estimated prevalence of 14 per million live births.[5] Approximately 10% of all tumors diagnosed in the perinatal period arise in the brain.[11,12] Although congenital tumors account for only 0.5% to 1% of all brain tumors diagnosed during childhood, they cause 5% to 20% of perinatal deaths due to neoplasms.[2,5,8,11–13] Fetal intracranial tumors are usually first identified during the third trimester and generally carry a poor prognosis with a global postnatal survival of only 28%. The definite diagnosis usually requires postnatal histology; however, a tentative prenatal diagnosis made via ultrasonography or MRI affords an opportunity to provide the parents with management options and prognosis.[14]

There are several differences between perinatal brain tumors and those occurring in older children. First, primary intracranial tumors in older children are mainly infratentorial (located in the cerebellum and brainstem), whereas the majority of those in the fetus and neonate are supratentorial.[8,11,12,15–17] Second, the initial presenting sign is macrocephaly due to the tumor mass, hydrocephaly, or hemorrhage, with resulting dystocia and stillbirth. The lack of fusion of the calvaria and the patent fontanelles permit expansion of the skull without increased intracranial pressure.[12,15] In contrast, older children develop signs of increased intracranial pressure, such as vomiting and focal neurologic deficits. Third, intracranial teratomas are the most frequent

SUMMARY OF MANAGEMENT OPTIONS

Fetal Tumors—General

Management Options	Evidence Quality and Recommendation	References
Uterine size greater than dates, hydramnios, and fetal hydrops are common presenting signs.	III/B	5–9
Diagnosis usually made by ultrasonography, although MRI may be helpful in some cases.	IIb/B	2–9,39,106,197,198
Consider genetic syndromes and associated malformations/deformations.	III/B	2–9
Multidisciplinary counseling and coordination of care with a team of specialty consultants.	—/GPP	—
The development of hydrops is a poor prognostic sign.	III/B	2–9

GPP, good practice point; MRI, magnetic resonance imaging.

TABLE 22–1

Most Common Perinatal Tumors*

TUMOR TYPE	NUMBER	PERCENTAGE OF TOTAL
Teratoma	113	37
Neuroblastoma	51	17
Soft tissue	52	17
Brain	20	6.6
Renal	16	5.3
Hepatic	13	4.3

* Compiled from three large series of 302 tumors (Isaacs, 1985[8]; Werb et al, 1992[7]; Parkes et al, 1994[2]).

intracranial neoplasms, but they are unusual in older children. Finally, some tumor types behave differently. For example, medulloblastoma is more aggressive in the perinatal period, and choroid plexus papilloma is more benign.[12] Discovery of a brain tumor in the perinatal period requires a careful search for additional defects, because 12% of congenital brain tumors result from a familial cancer syndrome.[12,18]

Teratomas

Teratomas account for 26% to 50% of intracranial masses.[12,15] They are thought to arise from midline locations within the CNS, including the pineal gland, the hypothalamus, the suprasellar area, and the cerebral hemispheres. Intracranial teratomas occur supratentorially in at least two thirds of cases.[19] However, teratomas often become so large as to preclude determination of the exact site of origin.[12] Rapidly growing tumors have been reported to erode through the orbit, oral cavity, and skull, resulting in spontaneous rupture of the scalp and skull during delivery.[20,21]

Prenatal diagnosis with ultrasonography is possible when intracranial complex masses disrupt the underlying brain architecture. Teratomas tend to appear as large cystic areas with solid components. Histologically, mature elements from all three germ layers are usually identified along with immature neuroglial components.[12]

Diagnosis

Intracranial teratomas may present in the second trimester with elevated maternal serum α-fetoprotein (AFP)[22] or an abnormal scan. However, these investigations have been reported to be normal in a fetus later found to have a massive teratoma.[23] The most common presentation is rapid uterine growth. Macrocephaly, hydrocephaly, and an intracranial mass of mixed echogenicity with solid and cystic components are identifiable ultrasonographically.[12,21,23] There may be areas of calcification. The tumor mass can cause distortion or destruction of the normal intracranial architecture. Hydramnios occurs in 15% to 20% of cases.[12]

The differential diagnosis includes other intracranial neoplasms, intraparenchymal hemorrhage, arachnoid or porencephalic cysts, hydrocephaly, hydranencephaly, holoprosencephaly, and encephalocele. Ultrasonographic detection of a complex intracranial mass with the loss of normal intracranial architecture is highly suggestive of teratoma. In cases in which the diagnosis is uncertain, MRI can be helpful (Fig. 22–1).

Risks

Uterine enlargement and hydramnios increase the risk of preterm labor. In rare cases, the fetus may develop hydrops due to high-output cardiac failure secondary to arteriovenous shunting within the tumor,[24] which increases the risk of preeclampsia (the "mirror syndrome"). Perhaps the most significant maternal risk is dystocia due to macrocrania, and in most cases, cesarean section is required (often with a vertical incision) or cephalocentesis is necessary for vaginal delivery.[21,23,25] The massive uterine distention increases the risk of postpartum hemorrhage.

Management Options

The prognosis for a fetus with an intracranial teratoma is dismal. Most infants diagnosed antenatally are stillborn or

FIGURE 22–1
Intracranial teratoma. *A*, A large intracranial mass with solid and cystic components, as well as calcification, was noted in this fetus at 28 weeks' gestation. The mass measured approximately 5 × 3 × 7 cm and caused compression of the ventricular system and development of ventriculomegaly. *B*, A fetal magnetic resonance imaging (MRI) scan was obtained to better define the extent of the lesion. The mass appeared to be arising from the base of the brain and was associated with disruption of normal architecture.

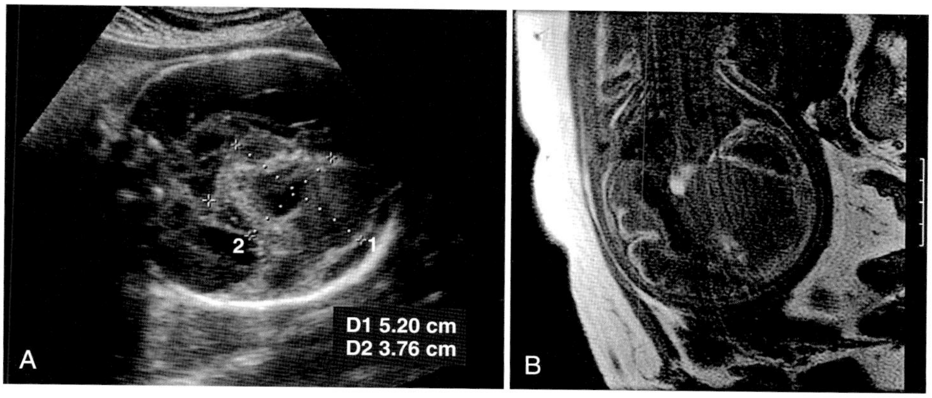

die in the immediate perinatal period.[12] Although one case report described prolonged survival following tumor resection on the first day of life, that infant had severe motor and mental retardation.[23] In spite of the advances in neonatal surgery, intracranial teratomas are still considered a fatal condition. Given the bleak prognosis and the maternal risks, termination of pregnancy should be offered. In ongoing pregnancies, the primary goal is to minimize maternal morbidity. Women who present in preterm labor should not be treated with tocolytic agents. Every effort should be made to avoid cesarean delivery. Cephalocentesis may be required to facilitate decompression of an enlarged fetal head and allow vaginal delivery.[21]

Other Intracranial Tumors

This group predominantly comprises neuroepithelial tumors of which the common types are astrocytomas, medulloblastomas, choroid plexus papillomas, and gliomas. Mesenchymal tumors such as meningioma and craniopharyngioma are also reported in the perinatal period.

Primitive neuroectodermal tumors (PNETs) are highly malignant, small, blue-cell tumors, which are characterized by early recurrence, metastasis, and high mortality rate. They account for 13% of all fetal and neonatal brain tumors. In the three reported cases of prenatal diagnosis, PNETs were associated with progressive hydrocephalus and enlarged biparietal diameter.[26]

Some intracranial masses are associated with genetic syndromes such as tuberous sclerosis or neurofibromatosis.[27–29] Tuberous sclerosis is associated with multiple discrete echodense nodules in the cerebral cortex or ventricles. This finding or a family history of the disorder requires a careful search for other lesions, especially in the heart. Although typically not associated with antenatal cortical findings, rare patients with severe neurofibromatosis have diffuse tumor nodules throughout the entire CNS.[30]

Both neurofibromatosis and tuberous sclerosis can also be the result of a new mutation, especially in cases of advanced paternal age. Hypothalamic hamartomas are rare solid, echogenic tumors associated with Pallister-Hall syndrome.

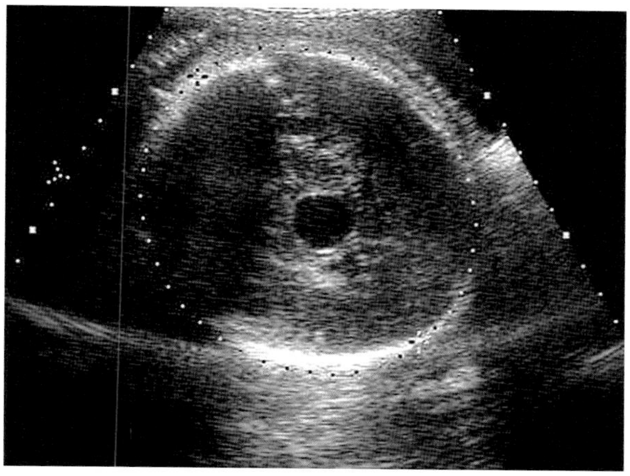

FIGURE 22–2
Vein of Galen aneurysm. A cystic, anechoic mass in the area of the brainstem was identified at 22 weeks in this fetus. Using Doppler interrogation, the lesion was identified as a vein of Galen aneurysm.

Other anomalies associated with this syndrome include holoprosencephaly, hydrocephaly, polydactyly, palatal abnormalities, renal and cardiac malformations, and imperforate anus. Identification of a tumor in the hypothalamic area mandates a search for these other defects.[31,32]

Hyperechoic areas with marked vascularity on Doppler interrogation suggest an arteriovenous malformation. Although the leptomeningeal angiomatosis associated with Sturge-Weber syndrome may appear hyperechoic, other vascular malformations,[33] such as a vein of Galen aneurysm, may appear as a hypoechoic, cystic structures until Doppler mapping is performed[34] (Fig. 22–2).

Diagnosis

Several of the more frequent intracranial neoplasms have a characteristic appearance that aids identification. The differential diagnosis for an intracranial mass includes neoplastic lesions, vascular malformations, parenchymal or intraventricular bleeding, and infarction.[35] Astrocytomas typically present as an intracranial mass associated with macrocrania. These tumors display a wide spectrum of cellular differentiation. The most poorly differentiated tumors (glioblastoma multiforme) generally appear as unilateral, echogenic, rapidly growing solid masses that cause either a shift or destruction of the normal intracranial architecture and contralateral hydrocephalus.[12,13,36] Enlargement of the tumor over a short interval suggests hemorrhage, which occurs more frequently in the perinatal period than in childhood.[15] Medulloblastomas originate from the cerebellar vermis and grow into the fourth ventricle and cerebellar hemispheres, giving rise to the typical ultrasound findings of an echogenic cerebellar mass, hydrocephaly, and macrocrania.[12,26] Metastasis via the cerebrospinal fluid or vascular route occurs in up to 18%.

Choroid plexus papillomas are histologically benign tumors composed of mature epithelial cells. They account for 5% of perinatal brain tumors[11] and typically appear ultrasonographically as a nodular space-occupying lesion arising from the lateral ventricle, although third and fourth ventricle lesions are reported.[11,37,38] Tumor growth results in massive production of cerebrospinal fluid and severe dilation of the ventricular system.[11] These tumors have a more favorable prognosis than other intracranial neoplasms.

Although craniopharyngiomas are a relatively common tumor of childhood, they are rarely discovered perinatally. The most frequent ultrasound findings are hydramnios, a large, cystic, calcified mass in the suprasellar region, and macrocephaly. Craniopharyngiomas may grow quite large, replacing much of the normal brain tissue. The prognosis is poor.[11]

Neoplasms involving nearly all other intracranial tissues (e.g., meningiomas and ependymomas) are reported in the perinatal period, but their occurrence is less frequent.[11]

Risks

The maternal risks are similar to those of a fetal intracranial teratoma. The propensity for the development of hydrocephaly and macrocrania predisposes to dystocia. The identification of an intracranial mass associated with a familial tumor syndrome (e.g., medulloblastoma and Gorlin's syndrome or cerebellar hemangioblastoma and von Hippel–Lindau syndrome) suggests an increased risk of malignancy in family members.

Management Options

Because teratomas tend to destroy normal intracranial architecture, the prognosis is universally poor. The prediction of prognosis is more difficult with other intracranial neoplasms. Choroid plexus papillomas have a more favorable prognosis, with a survival rate of 73%.[11] The prognosis for astrocytomas is dependent on the degree of cellular differentiation, but overall is poor, with only 37% survival rate. Neonates with glioblastomas or anaplastic astrocytomas have a survival rate of only 14%.[11] Medulloblastomas have a propensity to spread throughout the CNS and bloodstream and, therefore, have an extremely poor prognosis, with a less than 10% survival rate.[11] Intracranial lesions characteristic of phakomatoses, neurofibromatosis, or tuberous sclerosis are in general not predictive of the severity of disease.

Parents should be counseled on the differential diagnosis of the intracranial mass and the likely prognosis. Because ultrasound may not completely define the extent of the lesion, MRI can provide additional information.[39] In general, large or rapidly growing tumors that result in distortion of normal anatomy or massive hydrocephaly with macrocrania are likely to be lethal. In these cases, the option of pregnancy termination should be offered and cesarean section avoided wherever feasible.

FACIAL TUMORS

Facial tumors most commonly involve the orbits, the paranasal sinuses, the tongue, the nasopharynx, and the oropharynx. Teratomas are the most frequent tumor type, but mesenchymal tumors are also encountered.

SUMMARY OF MANAGEMENT OPTIONS

Intracranial Tumors

Management Options	Evidence Quality and Recommendation	References
Teratomas and Other Tumors		
Supratentorial location and macrocephaly are common. Teratomas cause destruction of normal brain tissue and have a dismal prognosis. Prognosis is variable for other tumor types: large tumors associated with hydrocephalus or hemorrhage are likely to be lethal.	III/B	8,10–12,15
Assess for maternal respiratory compromise, preterm labor, and abruption in the presence of hydramnios, preeclampsia, or hydrops.	—/GPP	—
Counsel about poor prognosis. Most reported cases have been lethal. Consider termination.	III/B	11,12,21,23,25
Cesarean delivery or cephalocentesis may be required if macrocephaly develops.	III/B	11,12,21,23,25

GPP, good practice point.

Orbital Tumors

The antenatal diagnosis of an orbital tumor is infrequent. The differential diagnosis includes a number of nonneoplastic entities such as encephalocele, vascular malformation, orbital cyst, and lesions of the conjunctiva, eyelid, and lacrimal apparatus. In addition, conditions that cause structurally shallow orbits, such as craniosynostosis, can cause proptosis and give the ultrasound appearance of an orbital mass.

Diagnosis

An orbital teratoma presents as a unilateral mass arising within the orbit that both displaces the globe and enlarges the bony orbit. The globe may have degenerative changes and appear small because of compression. As with other teratomas, both solid and cystic components are present, but there is no evidence of communication between the cystic areas and the intracranial cavity.[40] These tumors occur twice as often in females and are more common on the left side.[41]

Retinoblastomas are the most frequent intraorbital tumors of childhood. Only rarely are these tumors large enough to visualize on antenatal ultrasound. However, giant congenital retinoblastomas protruding from the orbit are reported and can present as an exophytic, solid mass that may compress and destroy the normal ocular structures.[42]

Tumors may also arise within the ocular apparatus. Medulloepithelioma, a malignant tumor arising from the ciliary body, has an exophytic appearance and mixed cystic-solid composition that may mimic the appearance of a teratoma.[43] Massive retrobulbar orbital cysts have also been diagnosed antenatally.[44] Epibulbar tumors can also present as orbital masses. Epibulbar dermoids are cystic lesions that contain pilosebaceous epithelial elements. They are associated with Goldenhar's syndrome.[45] Dacryocystocele, secondary to obstruction of the lacrimal duct, has a characteristic cystic appearance and is located along the inferomedial border of the fetal orbit[46] (Fig. 22–3).

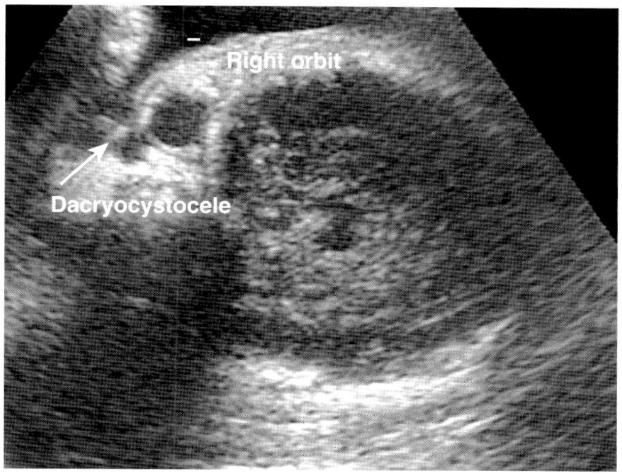

FIGURE 22–3
Dacrocystocele. A cystic area between the nasal bone and the right orbit was identified on ultrasound in the mid trimester. The differential diagnosis included encephalocele, epibulbar dermoid, and dacryocystocele. At birth, the overlying skin had a bluish tinge characteristic of a dacryocystocele.

Risks

Orbital tumors are unlikely to result in pregnancy complications. The degree of fetal risk depends on the nature of the lesion, because even some benign lesions can compromise future vision. Retinoblastomas diagnosed during the perinatal period are commonly due to a hereditary germ-line mutation in the retinoblastoma gene or a deletion of chromosome 13q; these mutations predispose to the development of other malignancies.[47]

Management Options

The tumor type and degree of impingement on surrounding structures determine the prognosis. In general, orbital teratomas have a favorable prognosis; even large lesions that require enucleation of the ipsilateral eye tend to have mature elements and an exceedingly low recurrence rate.[41,42] The prognosis for malignant orbital tumors such as retinoblastoma depends on the degree of spread outside the globe and the presence of any associated anomalies. A karyotype is indicated once the diagnosis of retinoblastoma is suspected. Parents should be counseled regarding the potential for postnatal treatment. Epibulbar tumors and abnormalities of the lacrimal apparatus have a favorable prognosis for survival and normal vision.[45,46] Cesarean delivery is occasionally necessary for large, exophytic tumors when there is a risk of dystocia or hemorrhage.

Nasal and Oral Tumors

Congenital vascular lesions, neoplasms, hamartomas, dental anomalies, and salivary gland lesions can occur in the oral cavity. Tumors of these cavities are rare and are most often teratomas, but granular cell tumors also occur.[48]

Diagnosis

Teratomas of the nasopharynx and oropharynx originate from the sphenoid bone, the hard or soft palate, the jaw, or the tongue. Ultrasonographically, they appear as complex heterogeneous masses that protrude from the mouth.[49–54] A subset of oropharyngeal teratomas are highly organized with recognizable organs suggestive of a parasitic twin; these tumors carry the special appellation of "epignathus."[50,55] Their location can prevent fusion of the palatal shelves, resulting in a cleft palate. Up to 9% of cases are associated with other organ system anomalies.[49] These tumors may cause hydramnios by occluding the pharynx or impeding fetal swallowing.[49,50,52,53] The maternal serum AFP was elevated in several cases.[49–52,54] Three-dimensional ultrasonography has been used to provide detailed visualization of the mass.[56]

Other rare facial tumors are reported including nasal hemangiopericytoma,[57] nasal glioma,[58] mesenchymal tumors of the paranasal sinuses, granular cell tumors of the gingiva,[59,60] and leiomyoma of the tongue.[61]

Risks

The majority of nasopharyngeal and oropharyngeal teratomas interfere with fetal swallowing and cause hydramnios.[49,50,52] For fetuses with large teratomas, there is a significant risk of malposition of the fetal head and dystocia leading to cesarean section.[52]

Although these tumors may be massive in size at birth, most are benign and have a low risk of recurrence after appropriate surgical resection.[49,52] The greatest risk to the fetus is respiratory distress resulting from an inability to establish a patent airway. Arteriovenous shunting has been reported with pharyngeal teratomas leading to placentomegaly, high-output cardiac failure, and fetal hydrops with a maternal risk of mirror syndrome.[52]

Management Options

A large tumor mass within the nasopharynx or oropharynx can impede normal gas exchange. In some cases, tumor may extend into the trachea so that even if an oral airway is attainable, respiration is still impaired. With large pharyngeal masses, delivery coordination with a team including an anesthesiologist, neonatologist, and pediatric surgeon may prove lifes-aving. The ex utero intrapartum treatment (EXIT) procedure allows either endotracheal intubation or tracheostomy to be performed while the placental circulation is maintained.[50,55,62–66] General anesthesia is used to maximize uterine relaxation and fetal anesthesia, a hysterotomy is performed, and the fetus is partially delivered to the level of the shoulders. Endotracheal intubation can then be attempted, with either a laryngoscope or a fiberoptic endoscope; if unsuccessful, tracheostomy can be performed. Some advocate having extracorporeal membrane oxygenation equipment in the operating suite.[67] Fetoplacental circulation has been maintained for more than 50 minutes, during which time fetal oxygen saturation can be easily monitored with reflectance pulse oximetry.[62,63,68]

A substantial number of women will present in preterm labor associated with hydramnios. The presence of these tumors is not a contraindication to either therapeutic amniocentesis or tocolysis, because most of these infants have a favorable long-term prognosis if they survive the perinatal period and initial surgical resection. Prematurity is not a contraindication to the EXIT procedure.[62,63]

NECK TUMORS

Masses in the fetal neck can be divided into those occurring anteriorly or posteriorly. The differential diagnosis depends on the location of the mass. Anteriorly, the most common diagnoses are goiter, thyroid/thyroglossal duct cyst, teratoma, nonseptated cystic hygroma, and branchial cleft cyst.[69] Posteriorly, the differential diagnosis includes nuchal edema, cystic hygroma, meningomyelocele, and rarely, teratoma.[70] The fetal neck is usually in a neutral position; any deviation, such as hyperextension, should prompt an investigation of possible etiologies because of the propensity for airway obstruction.[69]

Teratoma

Although cervical teratomas are the most common fetal neck tumor, only about 5% of all teratomas are located in the neck.[71,72] Extragonadal teratomas are believed to develop during early gestation when all three germ layers are in close approximation.[73] Historically, a distinction has been made between cervical and thyroid teratomas.[74] These tumors can

SUMMARY OF MANAGEMENT OPTIONS

Facial Tumors

Management Options	Evidence Quality and Recommendation	References
Orbital Tumors		
Counseling depends on prognosis; teratomas are most common; although the ipsilateral eye may be lost, overall prognosis is favorable but depends on tumor type, size, and local pressure effects.	IV/C	40,41
Prognosis for orbital retinoblastoma depends on tumor stage, which cannot be determined antenatally. Parents should be counseled that neonatal management of retinoblastoma includes enucleation as well as radiotherapy and chemotherapy.	IV/C	42
Cesarean delivery may be necessary for large tumors likely to cause dystocia.	—/GPP	—
DNA-based prenatal diagnosis is available for hereditary retinoblastoma.	IV/C	47
Nasal and Oral Tumors		
Assess for hydramnios and its complications.	—/GPP	—
Greatest risk to the fetus is severe respiratory compromise at delivery. If tracheal occlusion is anticipated, delivery should be by cesarean section in cooperation with pediatric and surgical consultants to ensure prompt intubation, tracheostomy, or tracheoplasty. In some babies, an EXIT procedure may be required.	III/B	50,55,62,63

EXIT, ex utero intrapartum treatment; GPP, good practice point.

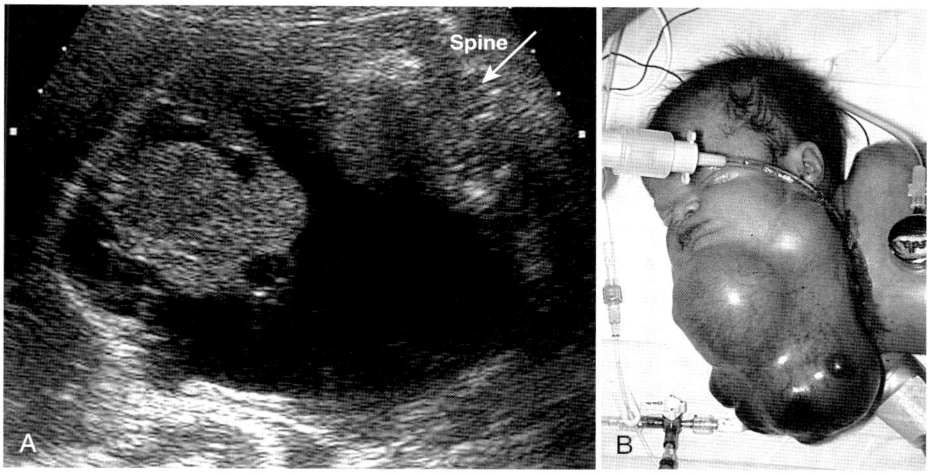

FIGURE 22–4
Cervical teratoma. *A*, A large cervical teratoma was identified in this fetus at 22 weeks. Hydramnios developed and preterm labor ensued at 32 weeks. The fetus was delivered via the EXIT (ex utero intrapartum treatment) procedure. *B*, A postnatal image of the infant with an endotracheal tube in the left aspect of the neck demonstrates the distorted position of the trachea.
(*A and B*, Courtesy of J. C. Hauth.)

achieve a massive size prior to birth and distort the anatomy in the neck, face, and even thorax, but only rarely have malignant components or metastatic foci been reported.[75–78]

Diagnosis

On antenatal ultrasound, the lesion has a characteristic appearance with large solid and cystic areas extending from the anterior surface of the neck (Fig. 22–4). Calcification within the mass occurs in 40% to 50%.[69,76,78] Although maternal serum AFP is not routinely helpful in diagnosis, those with endodermal sinus derivatives may produce AFP. Hydramnios complicates 25% to 55% of cases, especially those with large tumors causing esophageal and tracheal occlusion, and may provide a clue to the extent of the lesion.[69,75,78] Fetal MRI is a useful adjunct to antenatal ultrasound, often providing clearer details of the extent of the lesion to aid in postnatal surgical planning.[78–80]

Risks

Hydramnios increases the maternal risk of preterm labor, respiratory compromise, and postpartum hemorrhage. The most substantial neonatal risk is respiratory distress due to airway obstruction leading to hypoxia and resultant neurologic injury.[77] The overall survival rate with modern surgical care is 85% to 95%, even with large tumors. The most important prognostic factor is the ability to achieve complete surgical resection of the tumor.[77,78]

Management Options

The size of the tumor and the resulting hyperextension of the fetal neck frequently cause dystocia and necessitate cesarean delivery. Because of the potential for airway complications, an EXIT procedure should be anticipated. Surgical resection is usually performed as soon after birth as possible to avoid loss of a previously secure airway. Although an operative mortality rate of 15% was reported in the past, more recent series report exceedingly low mortality rates.[78,79] The risk of morbidity due to operative injury to the thyroid and parathyroid glands, the neck vessels, and the recurrent laryngeal nerve remains significant, but an excellent functional and cosmetic result can be expected in 70% of cases.[79]

Cystic Hygroma

Cystic hygromas are malformations of the lymphatic system that appear as fluid-filled, membranous cysts, lined by true epithelium in the anterolateral or occipitocervical area. The hygroma may be small, simple, and transient or large, multiseptated, and persistent. These lesions result from the jugular lymphatic obstruction sequence, in which either the normal communication between the jugular lymphatic sacs and the jugular veins fails to form by 40 days' gestation or there is an overall lymphatic hypoplasia (Fig. 22–5).[81,82] If the lymph sacs eventually connect with the venous system or an alternative route of lymphatic drainage develops, the cystic hygroma can spontaneously resolve. However, stigmata, such as low posterior hairline and neck-webbing, may persist.[81]

Diagnosis

Ultrasound allows ready diagnosis of cystic hygroma. Their location in the posterolateral portion of the neck and their cystic multiseptated appearance are characteristic (Fig. 22–6). Large hygromas are frequently divided by incomplete septa and often have a dense midline septum extending across the full width of the hygroma. The differential diagnosis includes encephalocele, meningomyelocele, nuchal edema, and the rare posterior teratoma.[70,81,83] Differentiating features include an intact skull and spinal column, lack of a solid component, a constant position of the mass relative to the fetal head, and the separation of cysts by septa. Nuchal translucency or edema may represent the most mildly affected end of the spectrum of the lymphatic obstruction sequence. In contract to cystic hygroma, the subcutaneous fluid is more subtle (usually < 10 mm in thickness) and continuous.[70] Cystic hygroma is associated with either an

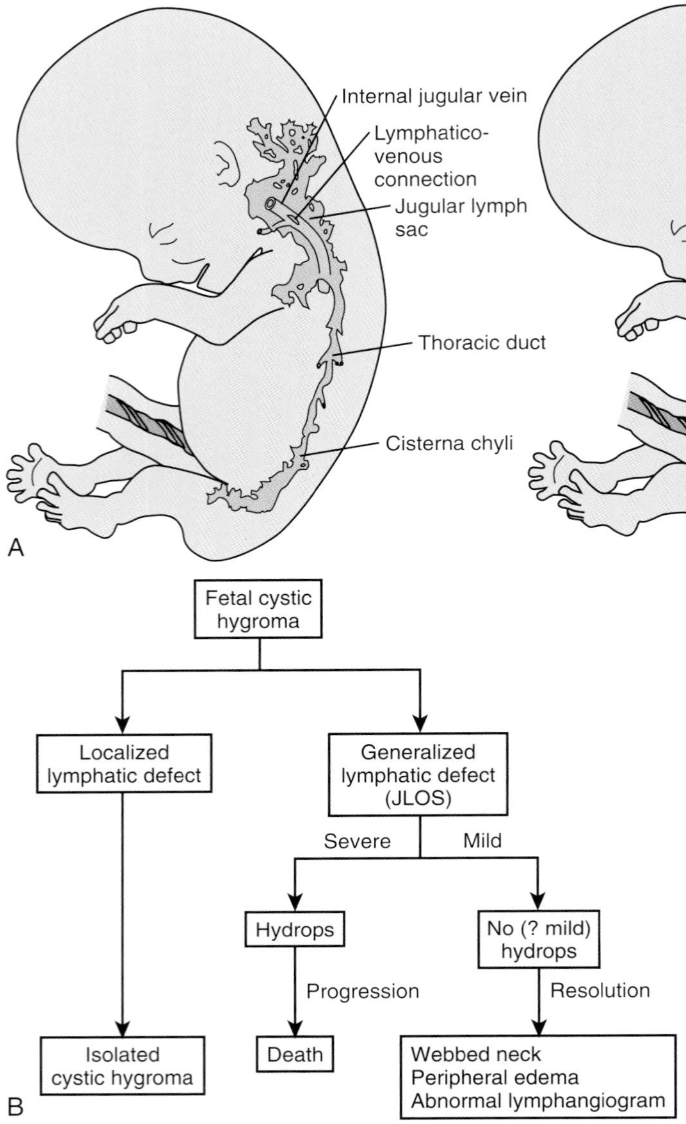

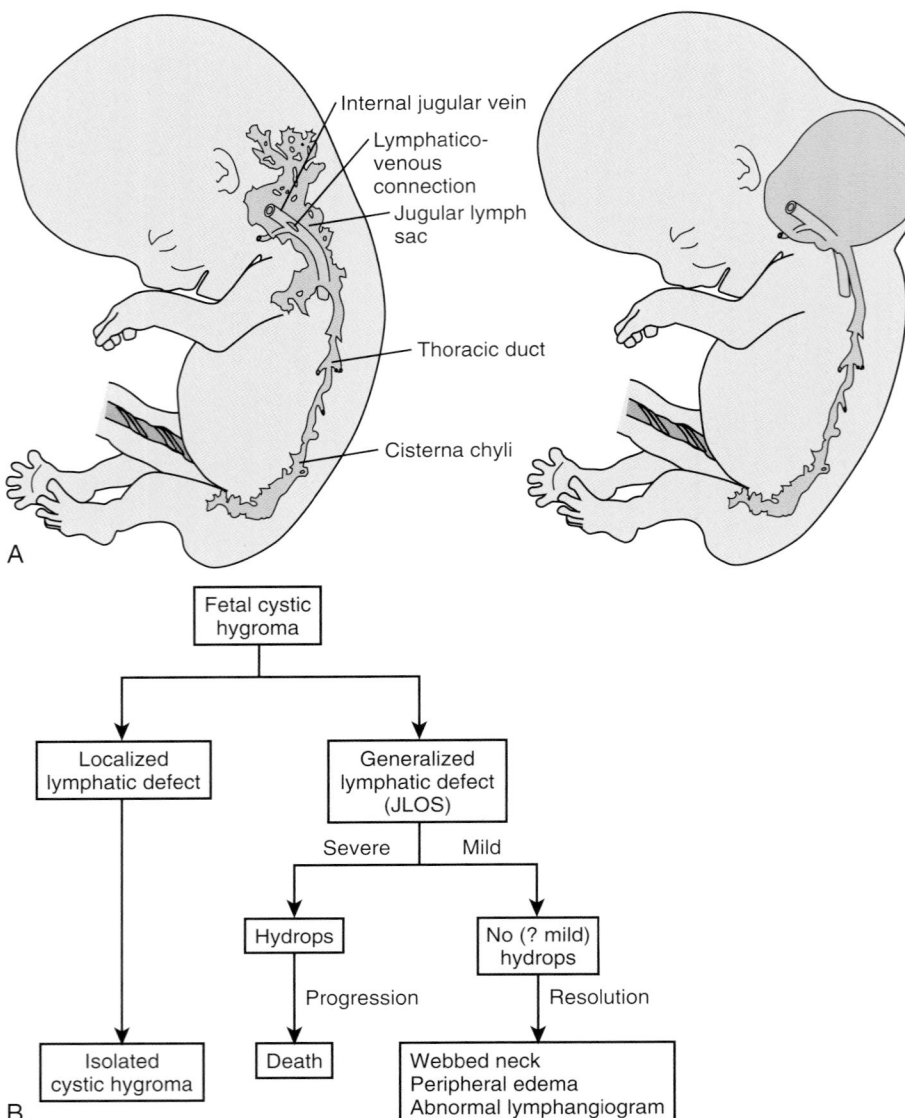

FIGURE 22–5
Cystic hygroma. *A*, Lymphatic system in a normal fetus (*left*) with a patent connection between the jugular lymph sac and the internal jugular vein and a cystic hygroma and hydrops from a failed lymphaticovenous connection (*right*). *B*, Natural history of fetal cystic hygroma. Generalized edema results from jugular lymphatic obstruction sequence (JLOS).
(*A* and *B*, Modified from Chervenak FA, Isaacson G, Blakemore KJ, et al: Fetal cystic hygroma. Cause and natural history. N Engl J Med 1983;309:822–825.)

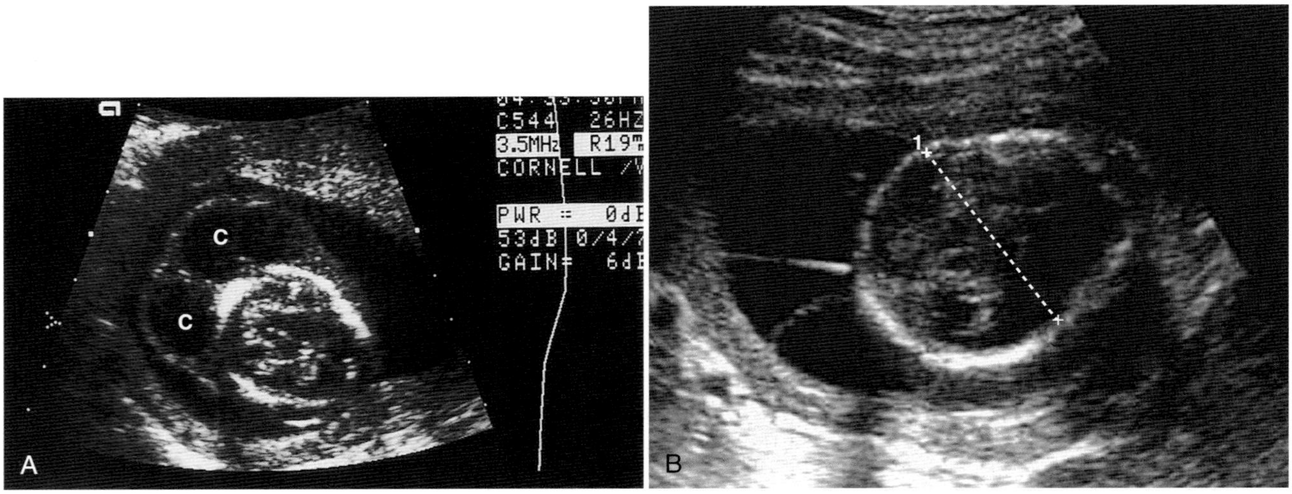

FIGURE 22–6
Cystic hygroma. *A*, First-trimester fetal head demonstrates scalp edema with septations. *B*, Multiseptated cystic hygroma identified at 17 weeks' gestation. The hygroma extended from the occiput to the level of the thoracic spine.
(*A*, Courtesy of R. B. Kalish and F. A. Chervenak.)

elevated maternal serum AFP or human chorionic gonadotropin (hCG).[84,85] Other anomalies may be detected in part because of the association with fetal aneuploidy. Hydrops is often associated with cystic hygroma, because both result from a defect in lymphatic formation. Associated cardiac anomalies, particularly aortic coarctation and hypoplastic left ventricle, may occur as the enlarged thoracic duct impinges on the developing heart.[86] The development of hydramnios or hydrops may reflect fetal cardiac decompensation, which reduces the chances of resolution or survival.[81]

Risks

Between 50% and 75% of fetuses with cystic hygromas are aneuploid; Turner's syndrome (45,X and variants) accounts for 75% of the aneuploidies,[81,87] with the remainder being autosomal trisomies, especially chromosomes 13, 18, and 21.[88] There is controversy as to whether anterloateral hygromas are associated with other anomalies and aneuploidy.[69] One report, however, documents an increased risk of aneuploidy and cardiovascular anomalies with both anterior and posterior hygromas.[89] Noonan's syndrome, multiple pterygium syndrome, and the Klippel-Feil sequence are each associated with cystic hygroma, as are abnormalities related to environmental exposures such as fetal alcohol syndrome.[81,88] Associated congenital heart defects are relatively common.[88,90] Hydrops occurs in 50% to 90% of fetuses with cystic hygroma because both result from a defect in lymphatic formation. Hydrops is associated with an exceedingly low survival rate.[88,91,92] Dilated lymph sacs cause elevation, protrusion, and angulation of the ear, redundant skin in the nuchal region, and altered patterns of hair growth. Dilated lymphatic channels near the heart increase the resistance to blood flow through the ascending aorta, leading to left-sided hypoplastic cardiac lesions.[86,88,90]

Management Options

Once a cystic hygroma is identified, a careful search for skin edema, ascites, pleural and pericardial effusions, and cardiac and renal anomalies is indicated. Karyotyping should be offered. When there is little fluid and the hygromas are large, the cyst can be aspirated and the karyotype obtained from the contained lymphocytes. Counseling and pregnancy management are guided by the presence of other malformations and the fetal karyotype. Because the prognosis for a fetus with a large, persistent cystic hygroma and hydrops is dismal, pregnancy termination should be offered. If the hygroma decreases in size or resolves, the overall prognosis is more favorable. Nonseptated cystic hygromas are more likely to resolve than septated lesions (98% vs. 44%) and have a higher survival rate (94% vs. 12%).[92] Fetuses with persistent cystic hygromas should be scanned periodically for hydrops.

There is no evidence that cesarean delivery improves outcome and should be avoided once a fetus with a cystic hygroma develops hydrops because of the poor prognosis. Ogita and coworkers[93] reported their experience with in utero sclerotherapy and noted the most favorable response in those fetuses without hydrops fetalis, chromosomal abnormalities, or structural abnormalities. This treatment, however, remains investigational. Isolated cystic hygromas may be surgically corrected postnatally and the prognosis for survival is then good.

When the parents opt for termination of pregnancy or when fetal death occurs, a postmortem examination should be recommended. Karyotyping should also be recommended if this has not been performed antenatally. In live births, tissue samples may be taken from fetal membranes or from the newborn itself. Because these fetuses may have chromosomal mosaicism, several tissues should be studied before concluding they are euploid. The content of postpartum counseling depends on the underlying cause.

THORACIC TUMORS

Primary tumors of the fetal lung (blastoma, fibrosarcoma, myofibromatosis, and hemangiomas) are rare, and most diagnoses are made during the neonatal period.[94] Metastatic lesions, especially from hepatoblastoma, neuroblastoma, or Wilms' tumor, are more frequent. Other mass lesions detected within the lung include vascular malformations, congenital lobar emphysema, and bronchogenic cysts.

Mediastinal and thoracic wall masses are also reported. The differential diagnosis of a mediastinal mass includes bronchogenic cyst, neurenteric cyst, esophageal duplication cyst, diaphragmatic hernia, pericardial cyst, lymphangioma, teratoma, and neuroblastoma.[95] Chest wall masses include hemangiomas, lymphangiomas, and mesenchymal tumors.

Diagnosis

Bronchogenic cysts result from abnormal budding of the bronchial tree between 4 and 8 weeks' gestation and usually lack a normal connection to the tracheobronchial tree.[96] They typically appear ultrasonographically as fluid-filled cystic areas located within either the lung or the mediastinum, most commonly in the subcarinal area. The antenatal detection of a chest wall mesenchymal hamartoma is reported.[97] With metastatic lesions, the primary tumor is often identifiable in another organ system. Approximately 15% of neuroblastomas are located in either the thoracic cavity or the mediastinum. On ultrasound, the lesions can appear either solid with calcification or cystic, which is more common.[98–100] Thoracic neuroblastomas tend to be diagnosed earlier than their intra-abdominal counterparts, and therefore, have a better prognosis. Chylothorax attributed to compression of pulmonary lymphatics by a mediastinal tumor has also been reported.[98] Lymphangiomas can occur in either the anterior or the posterior mediastinum. Vascular malformations in the pulmonary tree may be part of a genetic syndrome that is associated with multiple hemangiomas such as Osler-Weber-Rendu syndrome.

Risks

Any lesion that creates a mass effect within the fetal thorax has the potential to alter pulmonary development and cause hydrops by obstructing cardiac return. A large intrathoracic mass may compress the contralateral lung.[101] Compression of the trachea and esophagus can cause hydramnios independent of cardiac function.[102] The ultimate prognosis depends on the nature of the tumor, its resectability, the degree of lung involvement, and the extent to which pulmonary development is impeded by the mass effect. Hydramnios and mediastinal shift are poor prognostic indicators.[103]

SUMMARY OF MANAGEMENT OPTIONS

Neck Tumors

Management Options	Evidence Quality and Recommendation	References
Teratomas		
Assess for hydramnios and its complications.	—/GPP	—
Cesarean section may be necessary in cases of extreme dorsiflexion of fetal head or dystocia caused by large tumor.	—/GPP	—
EXIT procedure may provide up to 1 hr of uteroplacental support to allow time to secure an airway.	III/B	50,55,62,63
Plans for intrapartum intubation, ex utero tracheoplasty or ECMO should be coordinated with pediatric and surgical specialists. Surgical resection is usually performed as soon as possible after stabilization to avoid loss of secure airway.	III/B	50,55,62,63
Prompt surgery for appropriate cases after delivery has reduced the mortality rate to 15%.	III/B	76,77
Cystic Hygroma		
Search for hydrops and associated abnormalities. Offer karyotyping.	GPP	
Prognosis and management depend on cause, other anomalies, and whether the hygroma resolves.	GPP	
Offer termination of pregnancy when appropriate	GPP	
If pregnancy continues and cyst is massive, transabdominal aspiration may allow vaginal delivery; cesarean delivery is rarely justified.	GPP	
Establish cause including postmortem for abortus/stillbirth/neonatal death.	GPP	
"Cosmetic surgery" may be necessary if baby survives with a "web neck."	GPP	
Counseling depends on cause	GPP	

ECMO, extracorporeal membrane oxygenation; EXIT, ex utero intrapartum treatment; GPP, good practice point.

Management Options

The progressive growth of a bronchogenic cyst can lead to hydrops as well as bronchial abnormalities.[96] Percutaneous drainage via repeated thoracentesis or thoracoamniotic shunt placement has been reported.[104,105] The shunt will relieve hydrops only if secondary to mediastinal shift. It is unclear whether a shunt improves outcome in the absence of hydrops. MRI may assist the evaluation of large or atypical chest masses.[106] Because of the potential for respiratory compromise, fetuses with thoracic lesions should be delivered at a center prepared for appropriate fetal resuscitation and support.

TUMOR-LIKE CONDITIONS OF THE LUNG

Congenital Cystic Adenomatoid Malformation

Congenital cystic adenomatoid malformation (CCAM) is a developmental anomaly of the lung consisting of abnormal tertiary bronchioles. Most lesions are unilateral, but up to 15% have bilateral components.[107] Bronchioles display either hamartomatous changes or an arrest in embryologic development with the formation of cystic lesions of various sizes.[102,107] They usually communicate with the bronchial tree. The blood supply derives from the pulmonary circulation.

Diagnosis

CCAM lesions are classified by their histologic appearance: type I lesions account for more than 50% and are composed of large cysts; type 2 lesions make up 40% and are composed of multiple small cysts; type 3 lesions are microcystic, homogeneous, solid-appearing masses[108,109] (Fig. 22–7). Adzick and colleagues[101,110] proposed a simplified approach based on the antenatal sonographic findings; macrocystic lesions contain single or multiple cysts at least 5 mm in diameter, whereas microcystic lesions have cysts less than 5 mm in diameter and appear more echodense. For cystic lesions, the differential diagnosis includes diaphragmatic hernia, bronchogenic or enteric cysts, bronchial atresia, neuroblastoma, anterior meningomyelocele, and teratoma. For solid lesions, the main differential diagnosis is bronchopulmonary sequestration. Demonstration that the blood supply comes from

FIGURE 22-7
A type 2 congenital cystic adenomatoid malformation (CCAM) was identified in this fetus. Although there was evidence of mediastinal shift and mild cardiac deviation, the CCAM decreased in size during gestation, and the fetus was asymptomatic at birth.

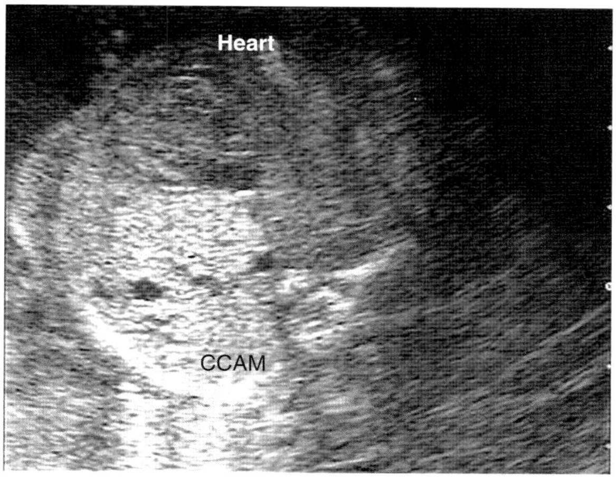

the aorta excludes a diagnosis of CCAM.[88,101] Fetal MRI can provide additional anatomic detail and is helpful in distinguishing CCAM from diaphragmatic hernia.[111,112]

Risks

The antenatal natural history of CCAM is variable, and the prognosis is guided by the size and type of the mass, the progression or regression of the mass, and the presence of cardiac axis deviation, hydrops, and associated anomalies. Although initial reports suggested that solid lesions had a worse prognosis, more recent evidence suggests the overall size of the mass is more important.[88] Large lesions that cause cardiac deviation and compression of the great vessels, esophagus, or trachea, leading to hydrops and hydramnios, have a worse prognosis. Without antenatal intervention, the development of hydrops is a harbinger of fetal demise.[101,113,114] In addition, large lesions may cause compression of normal lung tissue leading to pulmonary hypoplasia. Between 10% and 20% of fetuses develop hydrops, and up to 70% develop hydramnios. Crombleholme and colleagues[113] described a technique for measuring the size of the CCAM that generates a volume ratio and then applied the ratio to predict the likelihood of hydrops developing. Approximately 15% of CCAM lesions shrink in utero with resolution of any mediastinal shift. Although many of these lesions appear ultrasonographically to involute or "disappear," this may be due in part to changes in tissue echo texture, because postnatal radiographic or antenatal MRI studies confirm the persistence of at least some lesions.[101,106,112] In the absence of hydrops, more than 90% survive with most lesions resectable postnatally.[101,107]

Although 26% of fetuses had associated anomalies in Stocker and colleagues' original report,[108] a more recent series observed that only 2% of fetuses with CCAM had associated anomalies.[101,115] Development of hydrops or hydramnios is associated with increased risks.

Management Options

A complete anatomic survey is required to rule out associated malformations, determine the size and type of lesion, and detect any cardiac deviation or evidence of hydrops. Karyotype determination should be offered if there are associated malformations. If multiple anomalies or hydrops are identified, the parents should be counseled regarding the poor prognosis and pregnancy termination offered. In ongoing pregnancies, serial ultrasound scans are indicated to identify hydramnios or hydrops. Corticosteroids for pulmonary maturation followed by delivery are options after consultation with neonatal and pediatric surgical specialists should hydrops develop at a gestation when survival is possible. The delivery of any viable fetus with a persistent thoracic mass should occur at a center prepared for potential neonatal respiratory compromise.

The management of fetuses that develop hydrops prior to viability is more problematic. In such cases, the mortality rate is 100% with expectant management. In a number of reports, decompression of a large dominant cyst by thoracentesis or thoracoamniotic shunt placement successfully reversed the mediastinal shift, pulmonary compression, and hydrops, and survival rates of up to 80% to 90% have been reported.[101,104,113] The initial procedure should be thoracentesis with cyst drainage, because in some cases this can result in complete resolution of the cyst.[113] If the fluid rapidly reaccumulates, shunt placement can be considered. The utility of shunts is limited by occlusion or dislodgment, which occurs in up to 29% of cases.[116]

Thoracoamniotic shunting is ineffective for the treatment of multicystic and solid lesions. When these lesions are large and associated with hydrops, antenatal fetal surgery is an option. Adzick and colleagues[101] described the outcomes of 13 hydropic fetuses with CCAM who underwent antenatal resection of an abnormal pulmonary lobe at 21 to 29 weeks' gestation. Eight (62%) survived. Crombleholme and colleagues[113] reported only 2 of 7 (29%) similar fetuses surviving antenatal surgery. Fetal surgery is limited to a few centers worldwide and is associated with considerable risks including chorioamnionitis, preterm premature rupture of the membranes, preterm labor, postoperative infection, pulmonary edema, and anesthetic complications, as well as an upper segment uterine scar. Percutaneous fetal sclerotherapy has also been used to successfully treat a type 3 CCAM.[117]

Bronchopulmonary Sequestration

Bronchopulmonary sequestration is an isolated mass of lung tissue that does not communicate with the tracheobronchial tree and derives its blood supply from the systemic circulation, usually from the aorta or a major branch. The lesion is thought to result from a supernumerary lung bud that arose caudal to the normal lung bud and migrated with the esophagus.[102,118] Intralobar sequestrations develop early in embryogenesis, are surrounded by lung tissue, and are covered by the same pleura. Extralobar sequestrations develop later, grow separately from the lung, and become covered by their own pleura. The lesions are typically unilateral; left-sided lesions being twice as common. Although intralobar lesions typically involve the lower lobe of the lung, extralobar regions may be found between the lower lobe and the diaphragm, within the diaphragm, in the mediastinum, or below the diaphragm. Extralobar lesions predominate in the fetus and neonate.[119,120]

Diagnosis

Bronchopulmonary sequestration appears ultrasonographically as a solid, highly echogenic, homogeneous mass. Confirmation of a systemic vascular supply using color-flow Doppler is diagnostic.[121,122] It can be very difficult to distinguish a sequestration from a microcystic CCAM if the vascular supply cannot be identified. It is usually not possible to determine ultrasonographically whether an intrathoracic sequestration is intralobar or extralobar. The differential diagnosis includes microcystic CCAM, diaphragmatic hernia, teratoma, and neuroblastoma. For extralobar lesions, the differential diagnosis includes neuroblastoma and renal tumors. Although it is usually possible to demonstrate the well-demarcated boundaries of sequestrations by ultrasound, an MRI scan can help to identify other conditions that can present with a solid echogenic mass in the lower thorax, such as diaphragmatic hernia with liver herniation.[106]

Risks

The prognosis is variable, although large sequestrations can cause pulmonary compression, mediastinal shift, and hydrops. The presence of hydrops is the most important prognostic sign. In one early series, only 36% of fetuses survived, and all fetuses with hydrops (35% of all cases) died.[126] The incidence of hydramnios was 80% and isolated pleural effusion 70%. A more recent experience of 39 continuing pregnancies reported 100% survival of nonhydropic fetuses.[101] Only 4 fetuses developed hydrops, and the only death occurred in the 1 fetus not treated antenatally.[101] Significantly, 72% of sequestrations regressed or resolved spontaneously and were asymptomatic at birth.[101] Postnatal imaging revealed residual evidence of the lesions. Regression appears more common with extralobar sequestration, possibly because the separate pleural investment allows torsion on its vascular pedicle.[123,124] Intra-abdominal extralobar bronchopulmonary sequestration is rarely associated with hydrops and has a better prognosis than intrathoracic lesions.

Even in the absence of a significant mediastinal shift, fetuses with bronchopulmonary sequestration may develop hydrothorax. This phenomenon is more common with extralobar lesions, possibly as the result of lymphatic and venous obstruction due to torsion.[119] The pressure gradient between the systemic artery and the pulmonary vein and the resultant left-to-left shunting has been postulated as an explanation with intralobar lesions.[125]

Associated foregut anomalies include tracheoesophageal fistula, esophageal duplication, diaphragmatic hernia, funnel chest, and cardiac defects. Additional malformations occur more commonly with extralobar lesions (58%) than with intralobar lesions (14%).[126,127]

Management Options

Once the diagnosis of bronchopulmonary sequestration is suspected, a complete anatomic survey is required. Although the majority of intrathoracic lesions will regress to some degree, the possibility of hydrops justifies serial ultrasound examinations. If the lesion is large and associated with either hydrothorax or hydrops, antenatal therapy may be considered, given the dismal prognosis. Weekly thoracentesis and thoracoamniotic shunt placement are reported to effectively treat hydrops and pleural effusion when there is a mediastinal shift, but do not address the underlying lesion. Any fetus that fails to respond to these therapies or has hydrops due to a large lesion without a significant pleural effusion can be considered a candidate for in utero resection of the lesion. The maternal risks of such intervention should be carefully weighed against the potential fetal benefit.[101,102,118,128–130] Isolated intra-abdominal bronchopulmonary sequestrations have a better prognosis than intrathoracic masses because these lesions do not cause pulmonary compression and hypoplasia. Like those above the diaphragm, regression occurs. Hydramnios may occur secondary to esophageal or gastric compression preventing fetal swallowing. All fetuses with bronchopulmonary sequestration should be delivered at a tertiary center equipped for appropriate resuscitative and treatment measures.

CARDIAC TUMORS

Primary cardiac tumors are rare with a reported frequency of 2.7 per 10,000 infants and young children; the prevalence in utero is unknown.[131,132] Cardiac rhabdomyoma is the most common cardiac tumor detected in infancy, accounting for 62% of cases, followed by teratoma in 21%, fibroma in 13%, and only rarely, hemangioma, myxoma, or sarcoma.[133–135]

Diagnosis

Rhabdomyoma is thought to be a hamartoma and not a true neoplasm. It can be solitary or multiple and located within any of the cardiac chambers (Fig. 22–8). The ultrasonographic appearance of rhabdomyoma is of a discrete echogenic mass, but whether the mass is mobile or fixed depends on the location.[136] Rhabdomyomas can be isolated, but they are more frequently found in association with tuberous sclerosis. Between 51% and 86% of neonates born with cardiac rhabdomyomas will subsequently be diagnosed with tuberous sclerosis. Conversely, these lesions may be found in 50% to 60% of patients with tuberous sclerosis.[136–138] The tumors associated with tuberous sclerosis are typically multiple and range in size from 3 to 25 mm. The differential diagnosis

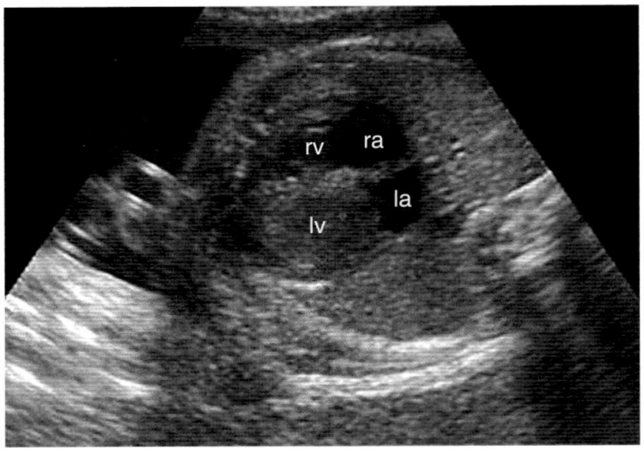

FIGURE 22–8
Prenatal ultrasound demonstrates a mass within the left ventricle (lv) with a small pericardial effusion. la, left atrium, ra, right atrium; rv, right ventricle.

SUMMARY OF MANAGEMENT OPTIONS

Intrathoracic Tumors

Management Options	Evidence Quality and Recommendation	References
Lung Tumors		
Exclude other malformations.	—/GPP	—
Assess for hydramnios and hydrops.	III/B	103
Multidisciplinary care is indicated. Deliver in tertiary center with appropriate specialists.	—/GPP	—
Cystic Adenomatous Malformation		
Exclude other malformations.	—/GPP	—
Assess for hydramnios and hydrops.	III/B	103
Multidisciplinary care is indicated.	—/GPP	—
Cyst aspiration or placement of a cystoamniotic shunt in the setting of hydrops may relieve intrathoracic pressure and reverse hydropic changes.	III/B	104,105
The place of antenatal fetal surgery is not clear.	III/B	101
Deliver in center with appropriate specialists.	—/GPP	—
Pulmonary Sequestration		
Exclude other malformations.	—/GPP	—
Assess for hydramnios and hydrops.	III/B	103
Multidisciplinary care is indicated.	—/GPP	—
Placement of thoracoamniotic shunt may relieve pleural effusion and correct hydrops.	III/B	104,105
The place of antenatal fetal surgery is not clear.	III/B	101
Deliver in center with appropriate specialists.	—/GPP	—

GPP, good practice point.

includes fibroma, myxoma, and sarcoma, although these lesions are less common in the fetus.

Pericardial teratomas appear ultrasonographically similar to teratomas in other locations—a complex echogenic mass with cystic and solid components and occasional calcifications.[139] These tumors are located outside the heart, attach to the base of the heart and great vessels via a broad stalk, and are usually on the right. In nearly all cases, a pericardial effusion is present that assists in narrowing a differential diagnosis that includes mediastinal teratoma, extralobar bronchopulmonary sequestration, and CCAM in which pericardial involvement is rare.

Risks

All cardiac tumors have the potential to cause hemodynamic compromise and hydrops due to obstruction of normal blood flow through either the cardiac chambers or the great vessels. This risk depends on the number, size, and location of the tumors.[134] The prognosis for fetuses with a cardiac tumor and hydrops is dismal. Pediatric patients with intramural tumors are at increased risk for cardiac arrhythmias such as ventricular tachycardia and Wolff-Parkinson-White syndrome. The tumor (especially rhabdomyomas, which have conductive capability) is believed to act as an accessory conduction pathway.[136,140,141] Whether fetuses have a similar risk is unknown. Cardiac tumors are also associated with several genetic syndromes including Beckwith-Wiedemann syndrome, tuberous sclerosis, Gorlin's (basal cell nevus) syndrome, and neurofibromatosis. A detailed ultrasonographic anatomic survey should be performed to search for these stigmata.

Tuberous sclerosis is an autosomal dominant disorder, though approximately two thirds result from new mutations. Most mutations are in the *tuberin* or *hamartin* genes on chromosomes 16 or 9, respectively. Consultation with a geneticist is recommended because a mutation can be identified in some families. Although the disorder has 95% penetrance, there is markedly variable expressivity, and evaluation of the parents and the fetus' siblings by a geneticist can help confirm or refute the diagnosis. Children diagnosed with tuberous sclerosis are at risk for mental retardation and seizures, but it is not possible to predict mental function based on either the antenatal findings or the family history. It is suggested that children with cortical tubers or subependymal nodules are more likely to have unremitting seizures and severe mental retardation. Fetal MRI has been used to identify these cortical abnormalities, which may not be visible on ultrasound.[142,143]

Management Options

The fetus with a cardiac mass should undergo serial ultrasonographic examinations to search for hydrops or an arrhythmia. If hydrops develops at a gestational age when survival is expected, the administration of antenatal corticosteroids followed by delivery should be considered. Should hydrops develop prior to viability, pregnancy termination may be offered. In the absence of hydrops, the prognosis for the fetus with a cardiac mass is favorable. Delivery should be planned at a tertiary center capable of providing pediatric cardiac surgical intervention. Intrauterine pericardiocentesis is reported to relieve cardiac tamponade with a successful outcome of pregnancy in a fetus with pericardial teratoma and a pericardial effusion.[144,145] The majority of cardiac rhabdomyomas spontaneously regress after birth.[136,141] For this reason, intervention is considered only in the presence of hemodynamic compromise. All true cardiac tumors should be evaluated postnatally and surgical resection planned. Although malignant components have only rarely been identified in pericardial teratomas, all become symptomatic eventually, thus justifying surgical therapy.[139,146]

ADRENAL TUMORS: NEUROBLASTOMA

Neuroblastoma is the most common malignant congenital tumor, with a prevalence of 0.6 to 2.0 per 100,000 live births. It originates from the neural crest cells that migrate along each side of the spine and give rise to the adrenal medulla and the sympathetic ganglia. Although tumor can arise anywhere along this path, the most common location is intra-abdominal, involving the adrenal gland. Other locations include the neck, thorax, and pelvis.[147] More than 90% of antenatally diagnosed neuroblastomas are adrenal in origin.[148]

Normal fetal adrenal development can be difficult to distinguish from neuroblastoma. Neuroblasts normally mature to form ganglion cells referred to as "neuroblastoma in situ," with a prevalence of 1 in 250 at term. The development of a clinical neuroblastoma represents a defect in the cellular maturation and differentiation. This defect may be temporary in some cases, accounting for the 15% to 20% rate of spontaneous regression.[149]

Diagnosis

The ultrasonographic appearance of adrenal neuroblastoma is variable, ranging from cystic with a thick-walled complex to solid with hyperechogenicity and foci of calcification.[99,148,149] Approximately 40% to 50% of antenatally diagnosed neuroblastomas have a cystic appearance, which may represent a stage of involution.[148] Doppler flow mapping may aid the diagnosis, because the nest of tumor cells is highly vascular, and the pulsatile flow observed in such tumors is suggestive of neovascularization.[150] The differential diagnosis includes adrenal hemorrhage, renal mass, and intra-abdominal extralobar pulmonary sequestration. Neo-

SUMMARY OF MANAGEMENT OPTIONS

Cardiac Tumors

Management Options	Evidence Quality and Recommendation	References
Determine the tumor type and likely diagnosis; search for ultrasound markers of syndromes.	—/GPP	—
Rhabdomyoma is the most common tumor; consider the diagnosis of tuberous sclerosis. Linkage studies may confirm a familial case, but no genetic test is available to diagnose new mutations. Counseling is difficult. Fetal MRI may detect brain abnormalities that are not visible by ultrasound. Referral to a geneticist for counseling is suggested.	III/B	142,143
Assessment for hydrops and arrhythmias is needed; in the absence of hydrops, prognosis is favorable, often with spontaneous regression.	III/B	134
If hydrops develops, timing affects response:		
• Previability—offer termination.	—/GPP	—
• If pericardial effusion with tamponade develops, pericardiocentesis is necessary.	III/B	144,145
• Preterm delivery after maternal steroids is indicated if there are early signs of hydrops and gestational age is acceptable.	—/GPP	—
Tumors can resolve after birth; surgery is indicated for those that persist with hemodynamic compromise.	III/B	136

GPP, good practice point; MRI, magnetic resonance imaging.

natal diagnosis is frequently prompted by hemorrhage into nests of tumor cells.[99,149] Antenatal adrenal hemorrhage is rare but reported with Beckwith-Wiedemann syndrome.

Metastases occur frequently in utero and can be visualized with ultrasound. Hepatic metastases are seen in up to 25% of fetuses with near-total replacement of the hepatic parenchyma reported.[148,149] Other sites of metastasis include the retroperitoneal lymph nodes, bone marrow, umbilical cord, and skin. Although nearly 90% of children with neuroblastoma have elevated urinary levels of vanillylmandelic acid (VMA) or homovanillic acid (HVA), only 30% to 35% of prenatally diagnosed cases have elevated levels postnatally. Although the measurement of maternal urinary VMA or HVA has prompted diagnosis, the yield is relatively low.[148]

Hydramnios or hydrops is reported in association with neuroblastoma, and may prompt the initial ultrasound examination. The mechanism is unknown, but possibilities include fetal anemia due to bone marrow infiltration, fetal arrhythmia due to catecholamine excess, placental vascular obstruction due to tumor metastases, and vena caval obstruction due to tumor compression.[147–149] In rare cases, the presenting complaints are maternal signs of catecholamine excess such as hypertension, coagulopathy, or renal abnormality.[151] Several genetic disorders associated with abnormalities of neural crest derivatives (Beckwith-Wiedemann syndrome, DiGeorge's syndrome, and CHARGE [coloboma, heart disease, atresia choanae, retarded growth and retarded development and/or central nervous system anomalies, genital hypoplasia, and ear anomalies and/or deafness] association) are associated with neuroblastoma. In addition, a familial form of neuroblastoma is described. Thus, a prior affected child should prompt antenatal screening of subsequent pregnancies.[152]

Risks

The prognosis for the fetus depends on tumor stage and the clinical manifestations of the disease. Although the survival rate in children older than 1 year at diagnosis is only 10% to 20%, the survival rate in neonates is greater than 90%.[99,147–149] Fetal hydrops is strongly correlated with advanced disease and increases the risk of the mother developing preeclampsia. In a review of 21 fetuses with an antenatal diagnosis of neuroblastoma, 3 fetuses developed hydrops. All had advanced stage disease, and all 3 mothers had preeclampsia.[149] Two of the 3 fetuses died antenatally.

The prognosis for a fetus with either stage I or stage IV tumors (metastases involving liver, skin, or bone marrow) is excellent, with survival rates of 90% or better after resection of the primary lesion. The high survival rate reflects the tendency for these tumors to undergo spontaneous regression.[99,148] The prognosis for stages II and III disease is poor, but fortunately, they are rare. Tumor hemorrhage and rupture during labor are reported, but their occurrence is rare.

Management Options

Most women whose fetus has neuroblastoma are asymptomatic. Serial ultrasound examinations are indicated to assess tumor size, amniotic fluid volume, and fetal growth and to detect hydrops. Because dystocia can develop when the fetus has massive hepatomegaly, the abdominal circumference should be regularly monitored in fetuses with metastatic disease; cesarean section is an option should the abdominal circumference be markedly enlarged.[147,153–155] Surveillance for maternal hypertension is critical. In the setting of hydrops, the decision to deliver is based on the gestation and the potential for survival. In fetuses less than 32 weeks' gestation, antenatal corticosteroids may be administered to enhance pulmonary maturity prior to delivery. If maternal symptoms of preeclampsia develop, delivery should be considered regardless of gestation. Any fetus suspected of having a neuroblastoma should be delivered at a tertiary center where the appropriate support staff are available.

RENAL TUMORS

Although renal tumors account for only 5% of all perinatal tumors, renal masses account for 70% of all abdominal masses in the perinatal period. The majority of these masses are hydronephrotic or multicystic dysplastic kidneys.[8,156] Despite their low frequency, renal tumors are often identified antenatally because of the relative ease with which the kidneys are visualized ultrasonographically.

SUMMARY OF MANAGEMENT OPTIONS

Adrenal Tumors: Neuroblastoma

Management Options	Evidence Quality and Recommendation	References
Assess for hydramnios, hydrops and maternal hypertension/ preeclampsia; measurement of maternal urinary catecholamines may help confirm diagnosis.	III/B	149
Delivery may be the only effective treatment, but consider gestational age, the likelihood of fetal viability, and the maternal condition; use steroids if preterm.	—/GPP	—
Serial measurement of fetal abdominal circumference: a very large renal mass may cause dystocia, necessitating cesarean delivery.	IV/C	147

GPP, good practice point.

Diagnosis

Congenital mesoblastic nephroma is a benign renal tumor composed of spindle cell mesenchymal elements that grow between intact nephrons and replace normal renal parenchyma.[157] It is the most common renal tumor in neonates and is distinguished from Wilms' tumor by its benign clinical behavior.[8,158] Ultrasonographically, these lesions usually appear as an isolated solid mass without a distinct capsule. However, occasional cystic changes, nodular densities, or diffuse enlargement of one kidney are reported.[147] The majority of the antenatal cases reported have been associated with hydramnios.[7,8,157] The mechanism of the hydramnios is unclear, but increased renal blood flow, impaired renal concentrating ability, and impaired gastrointestinal motility due to a mass effect are all implicated.[147] The differential diagnosis includes hydronephrosis and multicystic dysplastic kidney (which can usually be excluded because of their predominantly cystic nature), Wilms' tumor, and metastasis from hepatic and adrenal gland malignancies.

Wilms' tumor appears ultrasonographically very similar to congenital mesoblastic nephroma, except a distinct capsule may be identifiable.[8,147,159] This tumor is believed to be derived from the metanephric blastema, which is the embryonic precursor of nephrons and the renal interstitium.[8] It is typically unilateral (95%) and does not cross the midline. Associated congenital anomalies are common, and Wilms' tumor is described as a component of several genetic syndromes or associations, including WAGR (Wilms' tumor, aniridia, genitourinary malformations, and mental retardation) syndrome due to an 11p13 deletion and VATER (vertebral malformations, imperforate anus, tracheoesophageal fistula, limb abnormalities, and renal abnormalities) association.[160] It is also associated with several overgrowth syndromes including Beckwith-Wiedemann syndrome, Sotos' syndrome (cerebral gigantism), Perlman's syndrome (nephromegaly, hydramnios, macrosomia, cardiac defects, and diaphragmatic hernia), and Simpson-Golabi-Behmel syndrome (coarse facies, cardiac defects, islet cell hyperplasia, vertebral abnormalities, and vestigial tail).[161] Suspicion of nephromegaly or a family history of these disorders requires a detailed ultrasound examination and careful postnatal surveillance for the development of a tumor mass. Fewer than 1% of Wilms' tumor cases are familial with autosomal dominant inheritance. However, 20% of familial cases are bilateral, compared with only 3% of sporadic cases, thus warranting a thorough postnatal evaluation of both kidneys.[162]

Risks

Congenital mesoblastic nephroma is commonly associated with hydramnios. High renin levels are reported, and hyperreninism may precipitate fetal hypertension and rarely hydrops. Other potential causes of hydrops include obstruction of the portacaval circulation, arteriovenous shunting through the tumor, and hemorrhage into the tumor.[7,147,157] The prognosis for an affected fetus depends on the identity of the mass and the presence of hydrops or associated anomalies. Simple nephrectomy is usually curative. The prognosis for Wilms' tumor depends on the stage of disease at diagnosis. Survival after surgery and adjuvant therapy is greater than 90% when disease is confined to the area of the kidney, as is usual for prenatally diagnosed tumors. The prognosis for the hydropic fetus is more guarded. Fetuses with associated anomalies should be carefully evaluated to determine whether the constellation of findings represents a defined genetic syndrome.

Management Options

Because the majority of solid renal tumors are congenital mesoblastic nephromas with a benign clinical course, pregnancy should be allowed to go to term. Periodic ultrasound examinations are indicated to monitor fetal growth and amniotic fluid volume and to exclude hydrops. Delivery should be contemplated if hydrops develops at a gestation when survival is expected. Before 32 weeks, antenatal corticosteroids should be considered prior to delivery.[147] Dystocia is reported in cases with large renal masses. Cesarean section may be considered if the abdominal circumference is markedly enlarged.

HEPATIC TUMORS

Hepatic tumors account for 5% of the total neoplasms in the fetus and neonate.[163] Embryologically, the liver is derived from endoderm and mesoderm and is the potential site for

SUMMARY OF MANAGEMENT OPTIONS

Renal Tumors

Management Options	Evidence Quality and Recommendation	References
Assess for hydramnios and hydrops.	—/GPP	—
Majority are mesoblastic nephromas; prognosis overall is favorable.	Ib/A	157,161
Preterm delivery with maternal steroid therapy may be necessary if hydrops develops.	IV/C	147
If the abdominal circumference is enlarged, cesarean delivery may be required.	—/GPP	—

GPP, good practice point.

a wide spectrum of neoplasms.[164] The most frequently identified lesions in the perinatal period are hemangioendothelioma, hemangioma, mesenchymal hamartoma, and hepatoblastoma.

Diagnosis

Hemangioendothelioma and hemangioma are vascular tumors derived from endothelial cells forming vascular channels. A hemangioendothelioma has focal or diffuse hypercellular areas, whereas a hemangioma contains flat, inconspicuous endothelium with dilated vascular spaces.[164] Hemangioendothelioma is the most common hepatic vascular lesion in the perinate, but hemangioma is the most common vascular lesion in all age groups. Ultrasonographically, these lesions may appear hypoechogenic, hyperechogenic, or mixed, depending on the degree of fibrosis, hypercellularity, and extent of involution.[147] Hepatomegaly and multifocal lesions are seen. Doppler interrogation of the lesion confirms its vascular nature. Large vascular spaces within the mass are frequently seen with hemangioendotheliomas, and dominant feeding or draining vessels may also be identifiable.[165] Hydramnios is reported and may be due to either arteriovenous shunting or gastrointestinal tract compression. Mid-trimester maternal serum AFP levels are frequently elevated.[165]

Mesenchymal hamartomas are composed of connective tissue stroma, serous cysts, bile ducts, hepatocytes, and angiomatous components.[8,166] These lesions typically have a complex sonographic appearance with irregular solid and cystic components that can become enlarged and calcified.[167] Hepatoblastoma is the most common hepatic malignancy in the first year of life when 50% to 60% of all hepatoblastomas present. Although hepatoblastoma is believed to develop in utero, fewer than 10% of tumors are detectable antenatally.[8] Ultrasonographically, these lesions appear solid with occasional calcifications. Two thirds involve only one liver lobe, although occasionally, only diffuse hepatic enlargement causing abdominal distention may be seen.[168] Although 80% to 90% of childhood or adult patients with hepatoblastoma have an elevated AFP level, the maternal serum AFP levels are not useful for a fetal diagnosis.[8,168]

Risks

Although hemangioendothelioma and hemangioma are benign tumors, they are associated with life-threatening perinatal complications: hydrops secondary to high-output congestive heart failure and arteriovenous shunting, consumptive coagulopathy due to platelet sequestration (Kasabach-Merritt syndrome), and hemoperitoneum from intrapartum hepatic rupture. Cutaneous hemangiomas and hemangiomas in other sites, such as the eye, are reported in 40% to 45% of children with hemangioendothelioma.[164,165] There also appears to be an association between hemangioendothelioma and placental chorioangioma.[169] Although the majority of lesions regress and involute during early infancy, the size of the lesion and the degree of arteriovenous shunting will determine the antenatal risk of complications such as hydramnios, hydrops, and preterm delivery. The prognosis for the fetus that remains free of hemodynamic compromise is excellent; the prognosis is poor if hydrops develops.[170]

Rapid growth of mesenchymal hamartomas characterized by enlargement of the cystic components is common and increases the risk of hydrops. Of 13 antenatally diagnosed cases, 5 were complicated by hydrops or maternal pre-eclampsia, necessitating delivery; the perinatal mortality rate was 25%. Intrauterine drainage of the cystic lesions has not proved beneficial; drainage does not decrease fluid production and may precipitate hemodynamic compromise. Further, most cysts are multiloculated and not amenable to a single drainage procedure. In the asymptomatic fetus delivered near term, the prognosis is favorable after surgical resection. Owing to a propensity for spontaneous regression, some pediatric surgeons recommend a conservative strategy.[167]

Hepatoblastoma is a locally invasive tumor that can, on occasion, metastasize to the lung, brain, adrenal gland, and placenta. Large tumors are associated with hydramnios and hydrops due to a combination of factors including gastrointestinal obstruction, anemia from tumor hemorrhage, vascular compression, and possibly decreased colloid oncotic pressure secondary to altered hepatic synthesis.[168] Hepatoblastoma, as well as adrenocortical and Wilms' tumors, can occur in association with Beckwith-Wiedemann syndrome; 1% of patients with this syndrome develop hepatoblastoma. Other anomalies associated with hepatoblastoma include hemihypertrophy in 2% to 3%,[164] trisomy 18, Schinzel-Giedion syndrome (congenital heart defects, midface retraction, hypertrichosis, and embryonal malignancies), trisomy 21, and genitourinary abnormalities.[147] There are few reports of antenatally diagnosed hepatoblastoma. The prognosis for these lesions is uncertain but appears dismal in the setting of hydrops.[168,171] Complete surgical resection is possible in 40% to 75% of patients, and the survival rate in this group is 60%. The prognosis is poor if complete resection is not possible owing to infiltrative or metastatic disease.[8,172]

Management Options

Once a hepatic mass is identified, serial ultrasonographic studies are indicated to monitor fetal status, tumor size, and amniotic fluid volume. The ideal mode of delivery is unclear; intrapartum rupture of large hepatic masses with fetal death is reported.[147] Therefore, cesarean delivery should be considered in cases with marked hepatic enlargement. However, the risks of operative delivery need to be carefully considered in the context of the fetal prognosis. If the fetus has no signs of decompensation, delivery occurs at term. The role of intratumor injection of corticosteroids is uncertain.[173]

INTRA-ABDOMINAL CYSTS

Although not strictly tumors, a wide variety of cystic masses are detectable in the fetal abdomen including ovarian, mesenteric, urachal, choledochal, renal, hepatic, and splenic cysts. Enteric duplication, bowel obstruction, and meconium pseudocyst may also present as cystic lesions.[174] The location, size, and appearance of the cyst usually suggest the diagnosis.[175]

Ovarian cysts are common. Approximately 95% are unilateral and the majority are benign, functional cysts that occur in response to maternal hormones and resolve spon-

SUMMARY OF MANAGEMENT OPTIONS

Hepatic Tumors

Management Options	Evidence Quality and Recommendation	References
Assess for hydramnios and hydrops.	—/GPP	—
Cesarean section may be necessary for large tumors with possibility of dystocia or tumor rupture (vascular tumors are most common).	IV/C	147
Role of intratumor injections of corticosteroids with tumor enlargement and hydramnios is uncertain.	IV/C	173

GPP, good practice point.

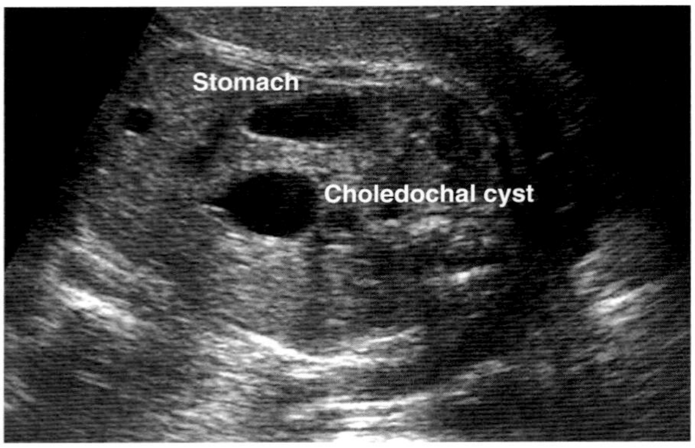

FIGURE 22–9
A choledochal cyst was identified in this fetus at 20 weeks' gestation. The cyst was located in the common bile duct.

taneously after delivery. Ultrasonographically, an ovarian cyst appears as a regular, hypoechoic structure in the lower abdomen. Septations or solid components may be seen if torsion or hemorrhage has occurred. Rarely, a cyst may become so large as to impinge on other organs, cause ovarian torsion and subsequent infarction, or result in dystocia. Ultrasound-guided in utero aspiration of large cysts is reported and may reduce these risks.[176]

Choledochal cysts represent a dilation of the common bile duct arising from either a weakness in the wall of the bile duct or a developmental anomaly and distal obstruction elsewhere in the biliary tree. These cysts have a prevalence of 1 in 2 million live births and occur more frequently in females and Asians.[177,178] Ultrasonographically, they appear as simple, anechoic cysts in the upper abdomen, usually medial to the gallbladder. Occasionally, a tubular structure is seen at the junction of the right and left hepatic ducts or the cystic and common bile ducts (Fig. 22–9). Choledochal cysts are not associated with an increased rate of fetal or maternal complications.[179] However, the patency of the biliary tree must be evaluated in the neonate because it is impossible to distinguish biliary atresia from a choledochal cyst on ultrasound.[177,180,181] All infants with these lesions require surgical treatment and reconstructive surgery of the biliary connections. However, the long-term prognosis with appropriate surgical treatment is excellent.

Solitary cysts are occasionally identified in the hepatic parenchyma. These lesions are usually small and unilocular. Embryologically, they are thought to reflect interruptions in the development of the intrahepatic biliary tree and frequently resolve spontaneously.[174]

Bowel atresia or stenosis may produce cystic dilation of bowel segments proximal to the obstruction. Megacystis–microcolon–intestinal hypoperistalsis syndrome, an autosomal recessive disorder associated with vacuolation and degeneration of the smooth muscle in the bowel and bladder walls, may present as multiple cystic structures in the abdomen that represent dilated segments of proximal small intestine and bladder. No specific antenatal intervention is required. A pediatric surgical evaluation should be obtained after birth prior to the initiation of enteral feeding should bowel atresia be suspected.

Mesenteric and omental cysts represent the benign proliferation of ectopic lymphatic ducts that lack communication with normal lymphatic channels. They occur most commonly in the small bowel mesentery. Most are asymptomatic antenatally and do not require intervention, although there is one report of an enteric cyst associated with hydrops (cause and effect unlikely).[182] Postnatally enlarging lesions may cause partial bowel obstruction, but the prognosis following surgical resection is excellent.[183] Enteric duplication cysts have a similar sonographic appearance and can be distinguished only postnatally.

SACROCOCCYGEAL TERATOMA

Sacrococcygeal teratoma (SCT) is one of the most common tumors of the perinatal period, with a prevalence of 1 in 35,000 to 40,000 live births. It is four to nine times more common in females than in males.[72,147,184–186] Like other teratomas, these tumors contain elements derived from all three germ cell layers. Sacrococcygeal tumors are believed to arise from either Hansen's node or ectopic primordial germ cells.[185,186] The majority of SCTs diagnosed perinatally are benign, but malignant degeneration complicates up to 10%, especially when there is a delay in resection or when the tumor is not entirely resected.[185,186] Lesions with foci of immature cells are described in 10% to 15% of cases.[187,188] The American Academy of Pediatrics (AAP) has adopted a staging system for SCTs that grades the involvement of intrapelvic structures and, hence, the complications associated with surgical resection. Type I tumors, the most common type, are predominantly external and protrude from the perineal region with minimal, if any, presacral component. Type

SUMMARY OF MANAGEMENT OPTIONS

Intra-abdominal Cysts

Management Options	Evidence Quality and Recommendation	References
Assess for cyst enlargement and pressure effects, hydramnios, and hydrops.	—/GPP	—
Rarely, an ovarian cyst impinges on other organs, causes an ovarian torsion, or results in dystocia. Transabdominal aspiration and decompression of the cyst may be preferable to cesarean delivery.	III/B	176
Delivery in center with appropriate specialists as neonatal surgery may be required.	—/GPP	—

GPP, good practice point.

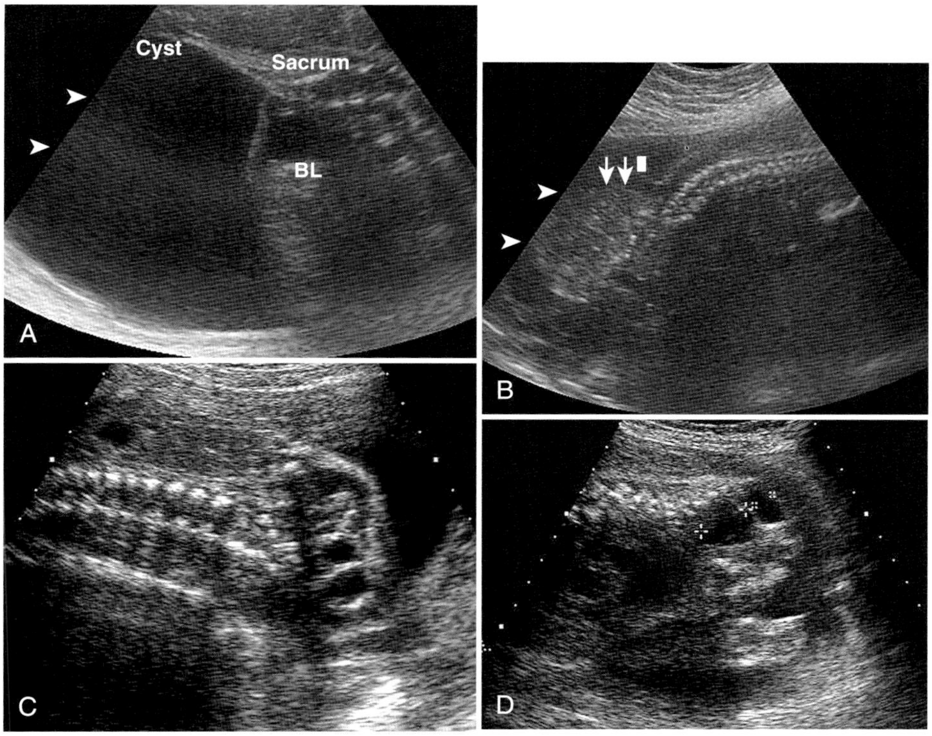

FIGURE 22–10
Sacrococcygeal teratomas. *A*, Type 1 lesion—the tumor is entirely extrapelvic and predominantly cystic. *B*, Type 1 lesion—although the tumor is entirely extrapelvic, it is more solid appearing. *C*, Type 2 lesion—the predominant portion of the tumor is extrapelvic, but intrapelvic portions are visible. *D*, Type 4 lesion—the tumor appears to be located entirely within the fetal pelvis with no external component evident.

II lesions are primarily external but have a significant intrapelvic portion. Type III lesions are primarily intrapelvic with a small external component. Type IV tumors are completely presacral with no external component.

Diagnosis

Teratomas are generally well circumscribed without direct invasion of adjacent tissues. The most common appearance is that of a complex mass, although predominantly solid or cystic masses are also described. The most common location is caudal and dorsal in close proximity to the coccyx[186] (Fig. 22–10). Teratomas with a significant intrapelvic component can compress the urinary and gastrointestinal tracts. Fluid-filled anechoic areas may be visualized proximal to the obstruction. Immature teratomas tend to have a more solid than cystic appearance.[72] Doppler interrogation of the tumor confirms the highly vascular nature. The feeding vessels have blood flow velocities similar to the descending aorta and may have a diameter similar to the external iliac arteries.[189,190] The middle sacral artery and branches of the internal iliac artery are usually the main sources of blood.[191,192] The differential diagnosis includes meningomyelocele, hemangioma, lipoma, and other rare soft tissue tumors. A lumbosacral meningomyelocele is differentiated from teratoma based on the presence of spinal dysraphism and intracranial changes. Hydramnios, placentomegaly, and fetal hydrops are associated with SCTs containing arteriovenous malformations.[185,190]

The incidence of associated anomalies ranges from 0% to 35%.[7,184,189,193] A detailed anatomic survey focusing on skeletal/vertebral anomalies is obligatory. Defects in the area of the tumor, such as distal sacral agenesis, rectovaginal fistula, and imperforate anus, are reported and likely related to tumor growth during gestation. Aneuploidy has not been reported with SCT.[147] Maternal serum AFP levels may be elevated, especially in those tumors with foci of endodermal sinus tumor. The amniotic fluid AFP and acetylcholinesterase levels may also be elevated.[194,195] MRI can aid in ascertaining intrapelvic involvement. This information is useful in both counseling the parents and planning surgical resection.[196–198]

Risks

The prognosis for antenatally diagnosed SCT differs from that of postnatally diagnosed lesions, with estimates of mortality rate ranging from 12% to 68%.[184,190,199,200] The main causes of perinatal death are hydrops, intrapartum trauma, and postnatally either difficulties with resection or hemorrhage secondary to tumor vascularity.[185] An arterial steal syndrome often develops if the tumor contains arteriovenous malformations. The fetus may develop high-output failure due to limited cardiac pumping ability and anemia secondary to sequestration of blood in the tumor.[187–190] Because larger tumors require greater blood flow, fetuses with large, vascular, and especially solid tumors are more likely to develop hydrops.[186–188,190] The mortality rate is greater than 90% if hydrops develops.[184,185,190,200,201]

Other predictors of poor outcome include a second-trimester diagnosis and delivery before 34 weeks' gestation.[185] The risk of preterm delivery correlates with the size of the tumor and the presence of hydramnios.[187] Survival has been reported to increase from 25% for fetuses delivered before 34 weeks' gestation to 88% for those born after 34 weeks' gestation.[185] Survival was halved when the diagnosis was made prior to 30 weeks' gestation (41% vs. 84%).[185] In cases of large teratomas, defined as diameters greater than 10 cm, there was no relationship between survival and gestational age, suggesting that the risks of prematurity must be weighed against complications from further enlargement of the SCT.[202] Not only are large tumors associated with an increased risk of hydramnios, hydrops, and prematurity, they are also associated with an increased risk of dystocia, intrapartum injury, hemorrhage, or rupture, regardless of the mode of delivery.[184–186,188]

The most important variable affecting long-term outcome is the adequacy of tumor removal.[72] The presence of a substantial presacral component is associated with a worse prognosis because of the complexity involved with resection. Optimal treatment consists of an en bloc removal of the tumor and coccyx. However, with extensive presacral involvement, this cannot always be accomplished. Although both mature and immature teratomas are equally resectable, there is a greater risk of intraoperative hemorrhage with an immature teratoma, reflecting its increased vascularity. The identification of frankly malignant elements, especially endodermal sinus or embryonal cell tissue, markedly worsens the prognosis. If the primary tumor is not completely resected, there is an increased risk for recurrence, often with malignant components.[72]

Management Options

Counseling should be provided when the evaluation, including MRI, is complete. If the tumor is identified at an early gestational age or is associated with hydrops, termination of pregnancy should be offered. Serial antenatal ultrasound examinations are indicated to assess fetal well-being and to evaluate tumor growth. If hydramnios develops, amnioreduction may improve maternal symptoms and delay the onset of preterm delivery. If preterm labor develops, tocolysis can be attempted. In the fetus without evidence of cardiac decompensation, delivery is planned at or near term in a tertiary center. If signs of fetal cardiac decompensation develop after 30 weeks, corticosteroids should be administered to improve postnatal pulmonary function and delivery expedited. The optimal management for the fetus with hydrops at earlier gestational ages is unclear, but the prognosis for these fetuses is dismal.

Operative intervention to interrupt the vascular shunt in preterminal fetuses with hydrops has been attempted. Open fetal surgery with in utero debulking or complete resection of the tumor was reported in eight cases, with three long-term survivors.[203,204] Radiofrequency ablation via a percutaneous electrode has been reported in four fetuses; two died after the procedure owing to intratumor hemorrhage. The hydrops reversed in the two surviving fetuses, but both were found at birth to have large areas of soft tissue necrosis requiring reconstructive surgery.[191] Further refinement is needed.

Because of the risk of intrapartum traumatic injury, rupture, and hemorrhage, cesarean delivery prior to the onset of active labor is recommended for fetuses with an SCT greater than 5 to 10 cm in diameter.[184–188] A large vertical uterine incision is required to minimize delivery trauma, which may trigger massive hemorrhage. Type O-negative blood should be available for the neonate. Vaginal delivery may be considered if the tumor is smaller than 5 cm, with an emergency cesarean delivery should any evidence of fetal hemodynamic compromise develop.[186,192] Percutaneous aspiration of a large, predominantly cystic teratoma to facilitate vaginal delivery has been reported.[205] Regardless of the mode of delivery, successful management requires the multidisciplinary efforts of maternal-fetal medicine specialists, neonatologists, anesthesiologists, and pediatric surgeons.

Neonates who are stable and have no complications of prematurity will typically undergo surgical resection within the first few days of life. Although, in some, surgical trauma to the sacral and pelvic nerves results in urologic or bowel dysfunction, most neonates have excellent functional and cosmetic outcomes.[187,188] The long-term prognosis is determined by the extent of intrapelvic involvement and the ability to completely resect the tumor mass.

SUMMARY OF MANAGEMENT OPTIONS

Sacrococcygeal Teratoma

Management Options	Evidence Quality and Recommendation	References
Search for other abnormalities.	III/B	184,189
Cystic lesions have better prognosis.	III/B	179,185,190
Early diagnosis, especially with development of hydrops, allows termination of pregnancy to be considered.	—/GPP	—
Assess for hydramnios and hydrops.	III/B	185,190
Amnioreduction with hydramnios may be indicated.	—/GPP	—
Deliver in center with appropriate specialists	—/GPP	—
Preterm delivery with maternal corticosteroid administration is an option if hydrops develops (prognosis poor).	—/GPP	—
In utero surgery experimental.	IV/C	203,204
Classical cesarean section may be required to facilitate atraumatic delivery.	IV/C	186,192
Have O-negative blood available at delivery.	—/GPP	—
Neonatal stabilization and surgery may be indicated.	III/B	187,188

GPP, good practice point.

LIMB TUMORS

Limb masses are usually either soft tissue tumors (such as fibrous connective tissue tumors, lipomas), skeletal muscle tumors, or tumor-like conditions such as vascular or lymphatic anomalies or hamartomas.

Diagnosis

Soft tissue tumors are usually identified at birth or during neonatal life. In the neonate, most soft tissue limb tumors present as a palpable mass in fascia, muscle, or subcutaneous tissue or a smooth, solid, asymmetrical enlargement of a digit or extremity.[8] Hemangiomas are the most common tumors diagnosed in the neonate, but they are rarely identified before birth.[206]

Infantile fibromatosis is a benign neoplasm of fibrous tissue that occurs in fascia, muscle, or periosteum. This lesion is a type of proliferative fibroblastic disorder difficult to distinguish from low-grade fibrosarcoma and, although locally aggressive and subject to recurrence, is not associated with metastases.[8] Digital fibromas are among the most common of these lesions.[206]

Fibrosarcoma and rhabdomyosarcoma are the two most common malignant soft tissue tumors. Fibrosarcoma is usually cured by local resection, but rhabdomyosarcoma has a propensity for early metastasis and has, therefore, a less favorable prognosis.[207,208]

Congenital lymphangiomas appear ultrasonographically as multicystic masses with anechoic cyst cavities and often result in hypertrophy of the affected extremity. Because of an association with fetal aneuploidy, especially Turner's syndrome, fetal karyotyping should be offered.

Klippel-Trenaunay syndrome is a rare congenital syndrome with generalized mesodermal abnormalities including macular vascular nevus, skeletal and soft tissue hypertrophy, and venous varicosities due to abnormal small vessels.[209,210] Unilateral leg hypertrophy is the most frequent finding on ultrasound, but any extremity may be involved, as may an entire half of the body including the head and brain.[210] The finding of a complex mass in the subcutaneous tissue in the presence of hypertrophy of a limb or other body part is highly suggestive.[210] Proteus syndrome shares several features with Klippel-Trenaunay syndrome, including asymmetrical focal overgrowth, hemihypertrophy, and subcutaneous vascular abnormalities but is distinguished by the presence of warty pigmented nevi and lipoid visceral tumors.[211] This distinction may not be possible antenatally. Both syndromes have a variable prognosis.[211,212]

Risks

Vascular tumors are associated with an increased risk of fetal cardiac decompensation. Kasabach-Merritt syndrome, a consumptive coagulopathy due to intralesional clotting and platelet sequestration, occurs in superficial vascular malformations and can be life-threatening. It is reported in the neonatal period.[209]

Management Options

Close antenatal ultrasonographic monitoring is warranted once a lesion is suspected, not only to identify early signs of fetal compromise but also to monitor the size of the affected area. A markedly enlarged extremity or body wall can lead to dystocia; cesarean delivery may be necessary.

SUMMARY OF MANAGEMENT OPTIONS

Limb Tumors

Management Options	Evidence Quality and Recommendation	References
Assess for tumor growth, hydramnios, and hydrops.	—/GPP	—
Cesarean section may occasionally be necessary to avoid dystocia.	—/GPP	—

GPP, good practice point.

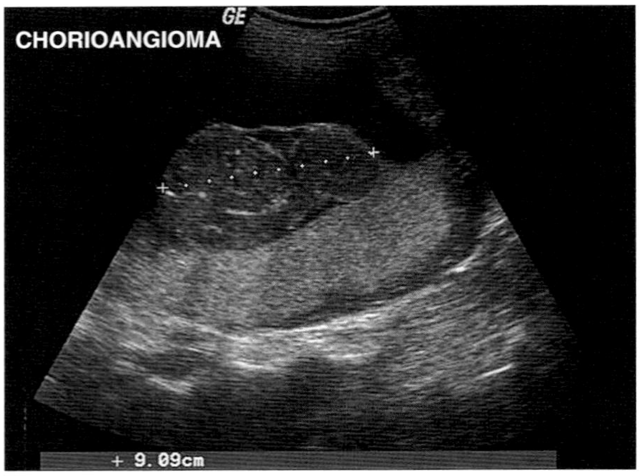

FIGURE 22–11
A large chorioangioma was diagnosed at 22 weeks' gestation. The tumor continued to grow over the subsequent weeks and the fetus developed severe hydramnios. Intractable preterm labor occurred at 29 weeks.

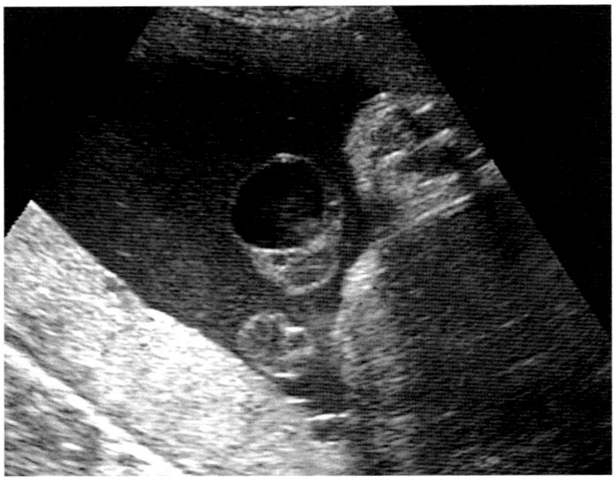

FIGURE 22–12
An isolated umbilical cord cyst was identified near the fetal end of the umbilical cord in this fetus. Doppler studies confirmed normal blood flow in the umbilical vessels.

PLACENTAL AND UMBILICAL CORD TUMORS

Tumors of the umbilical cord and placenta are rare. Most masses identified in these structures are vascular malformations or hematomas.

Diagnosis

Chorioangioma is the most common benign tumor of the placenta and is thought to be either an angioma or a hamartoma derived from primitive chorionic mesenchyme.[213] Small lesions are found in up to 1% of placentas. Tumors ranging in size from a few millimeters to more than 10 cm have been reported.[214]

The ultrasonographic appearance of a chorioangioma is that of a solid or complex mass on the fetal surface of the placenta (Fig. 22–11). Doppler interrogation will confirm the highly vascular nature of the mass and is required to distinguish these lesions from a placental or subchorionic hematoma.[214–216] The maternal serum AFP levels may also be elevated.[214]

Although exceedingly rare, placental teratomas are reported.[217,218] As with other teratomas, these tumors appear ultrasonographically as a complex mass.

Other solid masses identified in placental tissue include metastases from fetal and maternal primary tumors, especially melanoma.[219] Although antenatal identification of such lesions has yet to be described, they should be considered in the differential diagnosis of solid placental masses when the clinical scenario warrants.

The most commonly identified umbilical cord masses are hematomas, true cysts, and pseudocysts. An umbilical cord hematoma appears ultrasonographically as a cylindrical solid mass occluding the umbilical vein. Doppler studies may reveal turbulent flow in the area of the hematoma. True cysts in the umbilical cord are remnants of the omphalomesenteric duct or allantois and are usually located near the fetal end (Fig. 22–12). Pseudocysts are more common and represent localized degeneration and edema of Wharton's jelly, usually near the fetal end of the cord.[220,221] The differentiation between pseudocysts and true cysts cannot be made on ultrasound. Hemangiomas of the umbilical cord and varicosities of the umbilical vein are also seen antenatally, as are teratomas. Masses located at the fetal cord insertion site must be distinguished from omphalocele.[222–224]

Risks

If a chorioangioma is 4 cm or larger, the risk of hydramnios, and its attendant risks of preterm delivery and maternal morbidity, is at least 30%.[214] Large chorioangiomas contain significant arteriovenous shunts and are associated with an increased risk of high-output fetal cardiac failure due to sequestration of blood within the tumor. The prognosis is

SUMMARY OF MANAGEMENT OPTIONS

Placental and Umbilical Cord Tumors

Management Options	Evidence Quality and Recommendation	References
Carefully search for other abnormalities with umbilical cord cysts.	IIb/B	219
Assess for hydramnios and hydrops.	IV/C	212
Role of transfusion or sclerosing/occlusive therapies when hydrops develops is uncertain.	IV/C	224,227

poor if the fetus develops hydrops.[214,215] The development of fetal hydrops increases the risk of the mother developing mirror syndrome.[204] Chorioangioma of the placenta is often associated with cutaneous and visceral hemangiomas in the fetus.

Any umbilical cord mass that obstructs blood flow to the fetus can lead to heart failure and hydrops. Large umbilical cord hemangiomas may be associated with sequestration or shunting leading to hydrops. True cysts of the umbilical cord are associated with other anomalies including omphalocele, patent urachus, hydronephrosis, and mesenteric duct cysts.[221] Pseudocysts of the umbilical cord are also associated with omphalocele, hemangioma, and chromosome abnormalities, especially trisomy 18 (identified in two of seven fetuses with umbilical cord cysts in one study).[221] These conditions are thought to impair local fluid transport in the umbilical cord leading to edema and myxoid degeneration of Wharton's jelly.[221]

Management Options

Once a placental lesion is identified, close antenatal surveillance is essential to follow fetal well-being and observe for cardiac decompensation. Delivery should be considered if fetal hydrops occurs after 32 weeks. At earlier gestational ages, antenatal corticosteroids should be administered and further management individualized. Fetal intrauterine transfusion has been performed in cases of fetal cardiac decompensation as a temporizing measure.[225–227] Large chorioangiomas are associated with a perinatal mortality rate of 40%. Interventions to try to decrease the arteriovenous shunting include fetoscopic coagulation, alcohol injection, and microcoil embolization of feeding vessels.[227–229] Only alcohol injection met with reported success.[228,229]

If an umbilical vein hematoma is identified, antenatal surveillance is required to demonstrate regression of the lesion. If the hematoma appears to be growing, delivery may be required to prevent complete occlusion of venous flow. The identification of a cystic structure in the umbilical cord should prompt a detailed anatomic survey. Although the true incidence of chromosome abnormalities in the presence of a cystic cord lesion is unknown, karyotype analysis should be offered, especially if other anomalies are present.

SUGGESTED READINGS

Brace V, Grant SR, Brackley KJ, et al: Prenatal diagnosis and outcome in sacrococcygeal teratomas: A review of cases between 1992 and 1998. Prenat Diagn 2000;20:51–55.

Bromley B, Benacerraf BR: Solid masses on the fetal surface of the placenta: Differential diagnosis and clinical outcome. J Ultrasound Med 1994;13:883–886.

Chiu HH, Hsu WC, Shih JC, et al: The EXIT (ex utero intrapartum treatment) procedure. J Formos Med Assoc 2008;107:745–748.

Geipel A, Krapp U, Germer R, et al: Perinatal diagnosis of cardiac tumors. Ultrasound Obstet Gynecol 2001;17:17–21.

Hubbard AM, Adzick NS, Crombleholme TM, et al: Congenital chest lesions: Diagnosis and characterization with prenatal MR imaging. Radiology 1999;212:43–48.

Hyett J: Intra-abdominal masses: Prenatal differential diagnosis and management. Prenat Diagn 2008;28:645–655.

Isaacs H Jr: II. Perinatal brain tumors: A review of 250 cases. Pediatr Neurol 2002;27:333–342.

Kamil D, Tepelmann J, Berg C, et al: Spectrum and outcome of prenatally diagnosed fetal tumors. Ultrasound Obstet Gynecol 2008;31:296–302.

Koken G, Yilmazer M, Kir Sahin F, et al: Prenatal diagnosis of a fetal intracranial immature teratoma. Fetal Diagn Ther 2008;24:368–371.

McVicar M, Margouleff D, Chandra M: Diagnosis and imaging of the fetal and neonatal abdominal mass: An integrated approach. Adv Pediatr 1991;38:135–149.

Wenstrom KD, Williamson RA, Weiner CP, et al: Magnetic resonance imaging of fetuses with intracranial defects. Obstet Gynecol 1991;77:529–532.

REFERENCES

For a complete list of references, log onto www.expertconsult.com.

CHAPTER 23

Fetal Problems in Multiple Pregnancy

LIESBETH LEWI and JAN DEPREST

Videos corresponding to this chapter are available online at www.expertconsult.com.

INTRODUCTION

The incidence of multiple births in the developed world has increased dramatically over the past few decades from 1 in 100 to about 1 in 60 to 1 in 70 deliveries, with a 40% increase in twinning rates and a three- to fourfold rise in higher-order multiple births. This rise in multiple births is largely attributable to the increased application of assisted reproductive techniques (ARTs), although advanced maternal age accounts for a slight increase in spontaneous conceived multiplets.[1] At present, a policy of single-embryo transfer is encouraged in an attempt to contain this multiple birth pandemic.[2,3]

In twins, about 30% are monozygotic and 70% are dizygotic (Fig. 23–1). Although mechanisms of twinning are incompletely understood, it is commonly assumed that monozygotic twins result from the fertilization of a single egg followed by early cleavage into two halves, which develop further separately. Monozygotic twins may be dichorionic, monochorionic diamniotic, monochorionic monoamniotic, and even conjoined, depending on the time between fertilization and cleavage. The longer the time span, the more structures the fetuses will share. In terms of the presence of separate placentas for each twin, the time period around the 3rd day may be important, though this theory is not based on any firm knowledge. Further, embryo cleavage has never been observed in ART laboratories before blastocyst hatching. Nevertheless, in about 30% of monochorionic twins, cleavage is thought to occur shortly after fertilization, leading to a separate placenta for each twin (dichorionic); twins that have their own placentas are always in separate amniotic sacs and, by definition, diamniotic. However, in 70% of monozygotic twins, cleavage occurs later on, resulting in a single placenta for two fetuses (monochorionic). Rarely, cleavage takes place after the 9th day, resulting in monoamniotic monochorionic twins. Finally, cleavage after the 12th day is thought to result in conjoined twins.

It is generally accepted that dizygotic twins result from the fertilization of two different eggs, and therefore, each twin has its own placenta and amniotic sac (dichorionic diamniotic). However, some experts recently questioned this assumption of double ovulation and suggest that naturally conceived dizygotic twins also result from a single ovulation and fertilization by two sperms.[4,5] The increasing number of reports on dizygotic monochorionic twins also supports the concept that dizygotic twins may arise from within the same zona pellucida.[6,7] Nevertheless, the incidence of dizygotic twins has a hereditary component and also varies with ethnic group (up to five times higher in certain parts of Africa and half as high in some parts of Asia), advanced maternal age (2% at 35 yr), increasing parity (2% after four pregnancies), and method of conception. In contrast, the incidence of monozygotic twins is fairly constant throughout the world at 4 per 1000 births.[8] After ART, the overall majority of twins are dizygotic (95%), yet 5% are monozygotic.[9] Actually, ART may increase the risk of monozygotic twinning 5- to 10-fold, with about 1 in 20 to 1 in 50 of all iatrogenic conceptions being monozygotic compared with 1 in 250 of natural conceptions.[9] Ovulation induction rather than in vitro fertilization (IVF) seems to carry the highest risk of monozygotic cleavage: 1 in 20 versus 1 in 50.[9] Several mechanisms have been put forward to explain why ART would predispose to embryo cleavage, such as hardening of the zona pellucida with ovulation induction, extended culture, and blastocyst transfer with IVF, micromanipulations of the zona pellucida with intracytoplasmic sperm injection as well as assisted hatching.[10] As for triplets and higher-order multiplets, the overall majority now result from ART and are usually polyzygotic and therefore polychorionic/polyamniotic. Nevertheless, 5% to 10% of multiple pregnancies after ART[11] and up to 50% of naturally conceived higher-order multiplets contain a monochorionic pair.[12]

CHORIONICITY

Multiplets have a more complicated in utero stay than that of singletons, with higher incidences of growth restriction, congenital anomalies, and intrauterine demise. Monozygotic twins are at higher risk for complications than their dizygotic counterparts.[13] However, at closer look, it is chorionicity rather than zygosity that determines outcome.[14] The increased morbidity and mortality rates in monochorionic twins are primarily related to the angioarchitecture of the monochorionic placenta with its almost ever-present (96%) vascular anastomoses (Fig. 23–2),[15,16] which are virtually absent in dichorionic twin pregnancies. These vascular

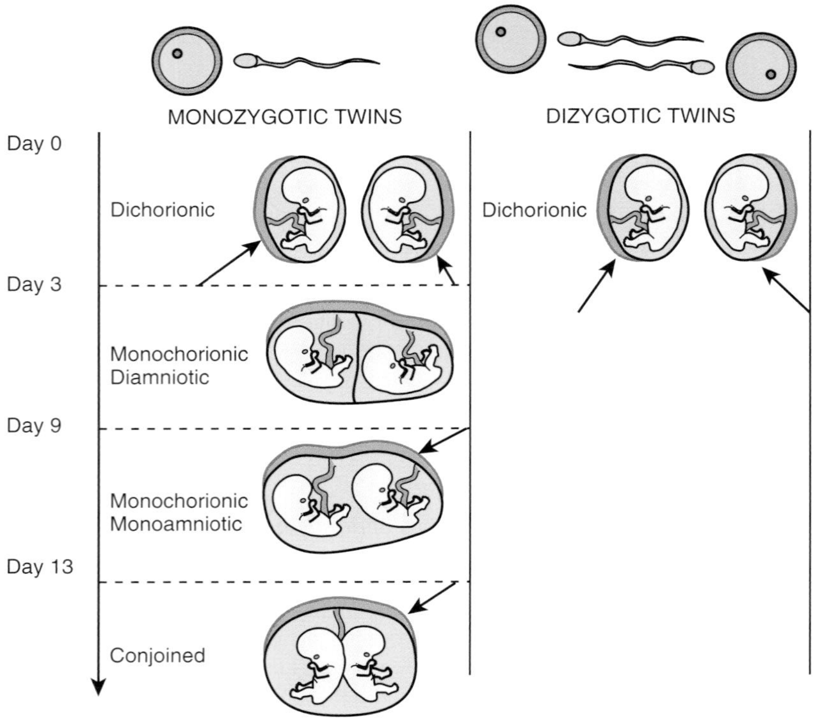

FIGURE 23–1
Zygocity and chorionicity in twin pregnancies.
(Courtesy of T. Van den Bosch, H. Hart Hospital, Tienen, Belgium.)

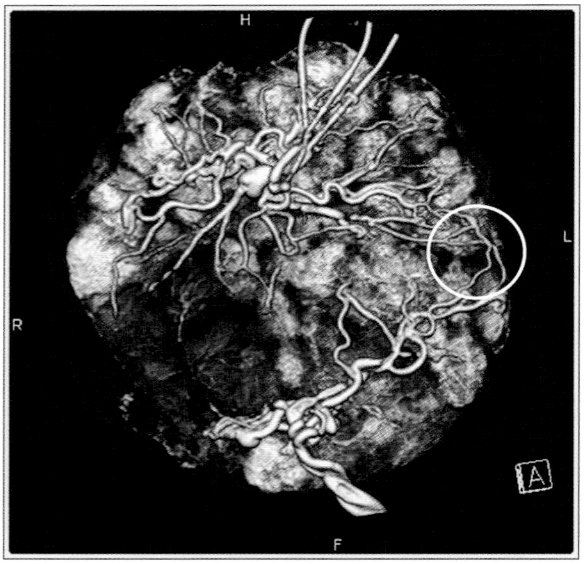

FIGURE 23–2
Three-dimensional reconstruction of a computed tomography (CT) angiogram of a monochorionic placenta at term shows an equal distribution of the placental mass and a large arterioarterial and venovenous superficial anastomosis (*circled*).
(In collaboration with M. Cannie, UZ Leuven, Belgium.)

anastomoses are randomly distributed and can cause significant blood volume shifts between the fetuses, leading to unique complications such as twin-twin transfusion syndrome (TTTS), twin reversed arterial perfusion (TRAP), and acute fetofetal transfusion after single intrauterine fetal demise (sIUFD).[17]

Important to some selected situations, the shared circulation precludes the injection of potassium chloride for selective feticide into the target fetus' circulation. Furthermore, this single placenta, originally designed to support one fetus, has to care for two or more fetuses and is often not equally divided, explaining the increased incidence of poor growth in monochorionic compared with dichorionic multiplets.[16,18] Consequently, perinatal mortality of monochorionic twins is nearly twice as high as dichorionic twins (2.8% vs. 1.6%) and four times as high as singletons (2.8% vs. 0.7%). However, perinatal statistics underestimate the problem, because the highest fetal loss rate occurs prior to viability. As such, monochorionic twins have a sixfold higher fetal loss rate (12%) between 10 and 24 weeks than that of dichorionic twins and singletons (2%), which is largely attributable to complications of the TTTS.[19] Also, there is a direct relationship between the timing of embryo cleavage and the risk of adverse outcome, with monoamniotic and conjoined twins having the highest complication rate. For these reasons and until a proper regimen has been established, we currently perform an ultrasound scan every 2 weeks in all monochorionic twins, whereas dichorionic twins are seen on a monthly basis.

Management issues are also complicated by the fact that two or more fetuses have to be taken into account. This especially applies to monochorionic multiplets, in whom the well-being of one fetus critically depends on that of the other, because their fates are invariably linked by the vascular anastomoses in the shared placenta.

Correct determination of chorionicity is, therefore, of utmost importance to identify this high risk group, for which increased monitoring may improve outcome. Moreover, it is essential for genetic counseling and for the management of

FIGURE 23–3
Chorionicity determination on the first-trimester ultrasound scan. *A*, Monochorionic diamniotic twins: only two thin amniotic membranes (*arrows*) separate the two fetuses. *B*, Both yolk sacs are in a common coelomic cavity. *C*, The insertion of intertwin membrane on the chorionic surface is T-shaped; dichorionic diamniotic twins. *D*, The fetuses are separated by three layers (amnion, chorion-chorion, amnion), and the yolk sacs are in separate coelomic cavities. *E*, Where the placentas fuse, a wedge-shaped junction (Y sign) is seen.

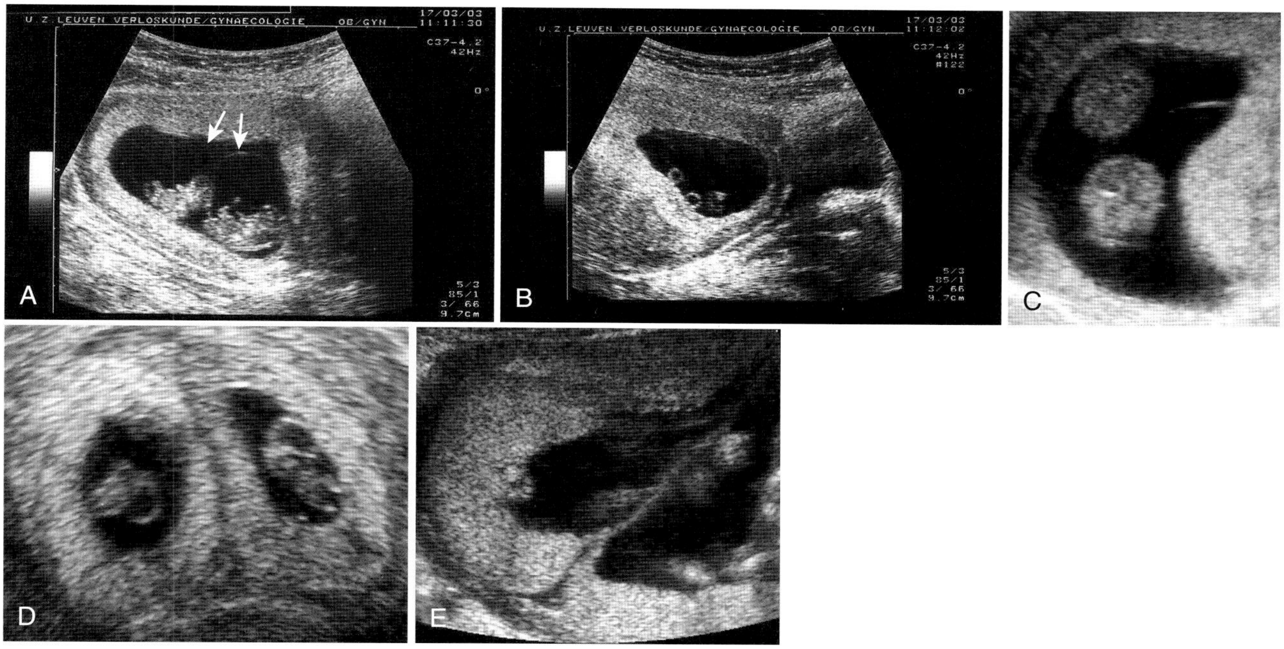

discordant anomalies, discordant growth, and in utero demise of one twin.

Determination of chorionicity is highly accurate when performed prior to 14 weeks' gestation (100% sensitivity and 99% specificity).[20,21] At these early stages in pregnancy, the amniotic membrane is still separated from the chorion. Chorionicity determination is, therefore, simply a matter of counting the layers that separate the twins (Fig. 23–3). If there are two thin layers (two amniotic sacs) and two thick separate chorionic plates or one fused chorion (beyond 9 wk) that forms a lambda at insertion on the placenta, then they are dichorionic diamniotic. However, if there are only two thin layers (two amniotic sacs) separating the two twins, then they are monochorionic diamniotic twins. Later on in pregnancy, because of close apposition of the amnion and chorion and regression of the chorion laeve, it becomes far more difficult and often not possible at all to determine whether same-sex twins do or do not share a common placenta. Only examination of the placenta after birth will give a definite answer. Therefore, failure to determine chorionicity in multiple pregnancies undergoing first-trimester scanning is now considered substandard care. In contrast to chorionicity, it is not possible to determine zygosity of dichorionic same-sex twins on ultrasound scan: approximately 8 out of 10 will be dizygotic, but still 2 out of 10 will be monozygotic. Only genetic examination (DNA fingerprinting) can then determine zygosity, which prenatally would require an amniocentesis of both sacs. After birth, zygosity of same-sex dichorionic twins is best determined on buccal smears from both twins.[22]

Fetal Risks

Poor Growth

Multiplets are particularly prone to poor intrauterine growth, because the human uterus appears less capable of adequately nurturing more than one fetus to term.[23] Consequently, the percentage of small–for–gestational age (SGA) babies (birth weight < the 10th percentile of singleton nomograms) is about 27% in twins[24] and 46% in triplets.[25] Growth curves for twins and triplets are similar to those of singletons up to 28 weeks' gestation, when the growth velocity of multiplets begins to fall. In twins and triplets, the average birth weight crosses the 10th percentile for singletons after 38 and 35 weeks' gestation, respectively,[23] when the majority of twins and triplets actually have already been born.[26] Some authors consider this growth restriction physiologic and therefore advocate for the use of twin-[24] or triplet-[25] specific nomograms. However, twins who are SGA according to singleton standards are at equal risk of perinatal mortality compared with SGA singletons.[27] Thus, the concept that being small is "normal" for twins creates a false sense of security, with possible deleterious consequences in this high risk population. Because the similar impact of size on outcome for singletons and multiplets, singleton growth charts should be used for the clinical management of twin pregnancies.

Accurate pregnancy dating and knowledge of the chorionicity are essential, and both are most reliably determined in the first trimester.[20,21] Two methods are used to describe growth in multiplets: the growth of each individual fetus and the difference (Δ) in sonographic estimated fetal weight (EFW) between the individual fetuses (discordant growth).

A fetus is considered SGA when both the abdominal circumference and the EFW are below the 10th percentile. The EFW prediction in twins is reliable and as accurate as it is in singletons.[28] The chance of both fetuses being SGA is twice as high in monochorionic (17%) as in dichorionic (8%) twins,[19] revealing that a single placenta is less efficient for two fetuses.

The degree of discordant growth, expressed in percentages, is determined as (A – B) × 100/A, where A is the weight of the heavier fetus and B is the weight of the lighter fetus. Severe growth discordancy is usually defined as a weight difference of 25% or more. It occurs in about 12% of twins[19] and 34% of triplets[29] and more commonly affects primiparous women.[30] The most accurate parameter to detect growth discordance is to compare the abdominal circumferences: a difference of more than 20 mm after 24 weeks has a positive predictive value of 83% for a birth weight difference of greater than 20% (Fig. 23–4).[31] Nevertheless, even ΔEFW may accurately predict the actual discordance at the time of birth.[32] In each pair of discordant twins, the heavier twin is usually appropriate for gestational age (AGA), whereas the lighter twin eventually becomes growth-restricted.[33]

Although severe growth discordancy complicates monochorionic (11%) as often as dichorionic (12%) twins,[19] the growth pattern and underlying pathophysiology are probably different. The onset of discordant growth in monochorionic twins is unpredictable and might present early as well as late in pregnancy,[34] whereas in dichorionic twins, the discordancy usually becomes apparent only later in pregnancy.[33] Monochorionic twins are, by definition, monozygotic and thus have the same genetic growth potential. Occasionally, unequal allocation of blastomeres may alter the growth potential of some monochorionic twins and account for very early discordant growth.[35]

Three factors seem to influence growth in monochorionic twins: the division of the single placenta between the fetuses,[17,18] the vascular anastomoses,[17,36] and the effectiveness of invasion of each placental portion into the spiral arteries.[37] These factors determine the magnitude of venous return upon which the fetus depends for its oxygen and nutritional supply. Unequal placental sharing is probably the most important determinant for discordant growth in monochorionic twin pregnancies.[16,18] Although it remains impossible to adequately assess the venous return and functional placental territory for each individual twin antenatally, the umbilical cord insertion site provides a good estimate.[18,38] Placental studies reveal that the combination of a velamentous and eccentric cord insertion is three times more common in monochorionic than in dichorionic twins (18% and 6%, respectively). In addition, nearly half of these monochorionic twins have a birth weight discordancy of 20% or more.[39] The site of the umbilical cord insertion can be accurately determined sonographically between 18 and 20 weeks' gestation (Fig. 23–5)[40] and identifies a group of monochorionic twins at high risk for discordant growth. Vascular anastomoses also influence fetal growth in monochorionic twins. Unequally shared placentas usually have larger anastomoses and thus a more elaborate intertwin transfusion, which may decrease the birth weight discordancy by increasing the oxygen and nutrient supply to the twin on the smaller placental share.[17] In scenarios with an unbalanced intertwin transfusion as in TTTS, the net flow will reduce and increase the birth weight of the donor and recipient, respectively. When the unbalanced flow is toward the twin with the smaller placental share, this may be advantageous. This so-called rescue transfusion could explain concordant growth in some monochorionic pairs with gross unequal placental sharing.[15] Conversely, an unbalanced flow may also lead to severe discordant growth in pairs with an equally shared placenta, especially if the flow is toward the twin with the larger placenta part.[41] Finally, growth in monochorionic twins may be determined by suboptimal implantation of the placental portion of the smaller twin, as suggested by the increased resistance of the blood flow in the spiral arteries of the smaller twin's portion of the placenta.[37]

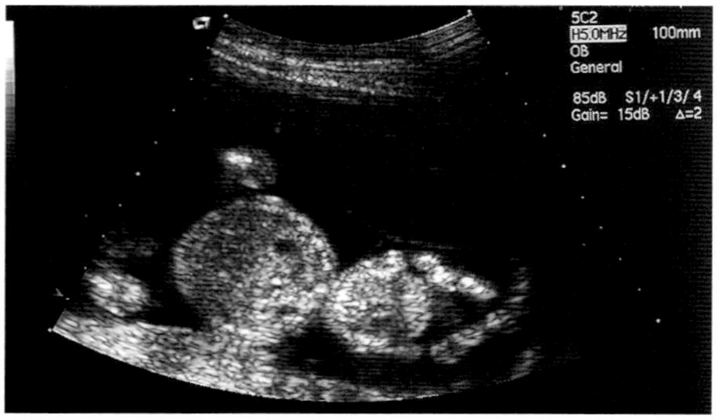

FIGURE 23–4
Ultrasound image illustrates the difference in abdominal circumference in a monochorionic twin pair with discordant growth at mid gestation.

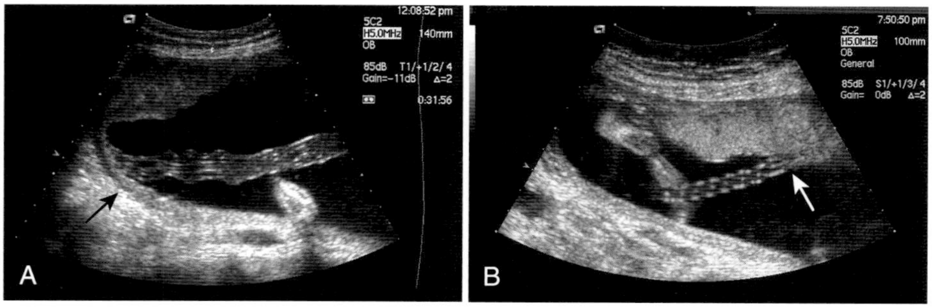

FIGURE 23–5
Ultrasound image of umbilical cord insertion at midgestation. *A*, Velamentous cord. *B*, Nonvelamentous cord inserting in the placenta.

DIFFERENCE BETWEEN TTTS AND DISCORDANT GROWTH

TTTS	Discordant growth
• Hydramnios (DVP > 8 cm) in sac recipient	• Normal amniotic fluid (DVP < 8 cm) in appropriately grown fetus
• "Stuck twin" = donor	• "Stuck twin" = growth restricted fetus

FIGURE 23–6
Differential diagnosis of twin-twin transfusion syndrome and discordant growth. DVP, deepest vertical pocket.

Dichorionic twins are dizygotic in about 90% of cases, and therefore, a different genetic growth potential might account for discordant growth; one twin may be "normal" SGA whereas the other may be "normal" AGA. In addition, each twin has its own placenta without vascular anastomoses connecting the separate fetoplacental circulations. Suboptimal trophoblastic invasion of placenta of the smaller twin may also account for growth restriction via similar mechanisms as in singletons.[42] Furthermore, growth discordance in dichorionic twins has been found to be greater in fused placentas than in separate placentas.[43]

Several investigators have addressed the use of uterine artery Doppler velocimetry at 18 to 24 weeks' gestation to predict growth restriction in twin pregnancies,[44,45] demonstrating a disappointing sensitivity of 10%. Mean uterine artery resistance is lower in twin than in singleton pregnancies, probably because of a larger placental implantation area. In addition, the normally implanted portion of the placenta supplying the AGA twin may attenuate the hemodynamic effects of suboptimal implantation of the portion of the placenta supplying the SGA twin.[46]

Other Fetal Risks

Fetal risks associated with growth restriction for multiplets are similar to singletons (see Chapter 11) and include intrauterine fetal demise and neurologic morbidity due to chronic oxygen and nutrient deprivation. Erythropoietin levels are elevated in SGA compared with AGA twins, and in twins with discordant growth, in the lighter of twins compared with the heavier.[47] Likewise, nucleated red blood cells tend to be higher in the lighter twin than in the larger; the difference increasing with greater discordancy.[48] These findings further support the concept that poor growth in twins is not "physiologic" but rather indicative of chronic hypoxia. SGA dichorionic twins have similar risks of perinatal mortality compared with singletons, whereas the perinatal mortality for SGA monochorionic twins is twice as high.[27]

Growth discordancy (birth weight difference ≥ 25%) as well as being SGA confers an increased risk for adverse perinatal outcome. Although most discordant pairs contain one or two SGA infants,[49] discordant pairs in which both are AGA still face elevated risks compared with nondiscordant pairs[50]; twins who are both SGA and discordant have the highest risks.[51] The same applies for triplets with higher degrees of discordancy associated with increasing rates of in utero demise in the smaller and middle-sized fetuses.[52]

As mentioned previously, growth-discordant monochorionic twins are at higher risk of adverse outcome than discordant dichorionic twins.[53] Unfortunately, most of the earlier data was a mixture of pregnancies with TTTS and discordant growth. Although TTTS is frequently associated with discordant growth, its distinction from isolated discordant growth is essential and based on the sonographic absence of hydramnios (deepest vertical pocket ≥ 8 cm prior to 20 wk, ≥10 cm after 20 wk) in the AGA twin in cases with discordant growth (Fig. 23–6).

Recently, several studies have addressed the pregnancy outcome of isolated discordant growth in monochorionic pairs. It complicates about 10% to 15% of all monochorionic twin pregnancies and carries an overall mortality rate of about 10%.[54,55] In about half of these, the discordancy presents at or prior to 20 weeks (early-onset), whereas in the other half, it appears only later on (late-onset). Pairs with early-onset discordant growth usually have an unequally shared placenta with large intertwin anastomoses. Also, most have abnormal umbilical artery Doppler measurements from 16 weeks onward, and consequently, the mortality is highest in this group with early-onset discordant growth (17%). Conversely, pairs with late-onset discordant growth usually have equally shared placentas with smaller anastomoses. Also, umbilical artery Doppler measurements are usually normal throughout pregnancy and their mortality rate is much lower (4%) than those with early-onset discordant growth. In a third of the pairs with late-onset discordant growth, severe hemoglobin differences are present at the time of birth. This complication is referred to as TAPS (twin anemia polycythemia sequence). This late intertwin transfusion imbalance may account for the growth discordancy and measurement of the peak systolic velocity (PSV) of the middle cerebral artery (MCA) plays an important role in the follow-up of these cases.[34]

Classification of growth restriction or discordance can also be based on the Doppler characteristics of the umbilical artery in addition to the gestational age at first presentation.[56] If a large arterioarterial (AA) anastomosis is present, such as is typically seen in cases with early-onset discordant growth, this may result in a cyclic variation in the diastolic flow component of the umbilical artery Doppler image and, thus, an intermittent absent or reversed end-diastolic flow pattern in the umbilical artery of the smaller twin that shows cyclic variations. Growth-discordant monochorionic pairs may thus have either a normal umbilical artery flow pattern (type I), a persistent absent or reversed end-diastolic flow (type II) or an intermittent absent or reversed end-diastolic flow (type III). Each of these types has distinct placental features and a different clinical outcome. Large AA anastomoses (>2 mm) are present in 70%, 18%, and 98% of type I, type II, and type III, respectively. Pregnancies with normal umbilical artery Doppler measurements (type I) have the most favorable outcome with a low risk of deterioration or unexpected demise, whereas a persistent absent end-diastolic flow (type II) carries the worst prognosis because 90% eventually show signs of deterioration and imminent demise. In fact, type II cases behave quite similar to severely growth-restricted singletons with an abnormal umbilical artery Doppler pattern. Finally, pregnancies with an intermittent absent end-diastolic flow pattern (type III) have an intermediate prognosis, but are the most unpredictable. Because of the presence of large AA anastomoses, unexpected demise without any signs of deterioration occurs in about 15% of fetuses and half of these are double demises.[57] As mentioned previously, abnormal umbilical artery Doppler patterns are largely restricted to the group with early-onset discordant growth and most have an intermittent absent end-diastolic flow pattern (type III).[34] Better criteria are urgently needed to distinguish the discordant-growth pairs with favorable outcome from those with high risk of an adverse pregnancy and long-term neurodevelopmental outcome. A subclassification based on uterine artery Doppler may help refine the prognosis. However, a large prospective series of monochorionic pairs is first necessary to document the prognosis according to the different Doppler patterns and to refine the current classification system.

In dichorionic twins with discordant growth, the pattern of deterioration of the growth-restricted twin follows that of a growth-restricted singleton. In a series of growth-discordant dichorionic twins managed expectantly until 32 weeks, the mortality was 24% with the larger twins surviving in all cases.[58]

Twins with growth restriction and discordant growth also face increased risks of neonatal morbidity and mortality.[59,60] In discordant pairs, the lighter twin more frequently has a low 5-minute Apgar score and is at higher risk of neonatal demise, whereas the heavier twin has more respiratory difficulties when delivered between 33 and 36 weeks.[50] The fear of an intrauterine demise may prompt obstetric intervention, adding complications of iatrogenic preterm birth to the inherent complications of multiple gestations.[61] Clearly, any decision for iatrogenic preterm delivery to prevent intrauterine demise must be weighed against the risks of demise and handicap for each twin as determined by gestational age and EFW.

Finally, growth restriction is associated with increased risks of neurodevelopmental delay[62] and cerebral palsy.[63] Likewise, twins with discordant growth are at increased risk of neurodevelopmental morbidity and cerebral palsy compared with nondiscordant twins, and monochorionic pairs probably have the highest risk. Nevertheless, the magnitude of this risk for monochorionic twins is unclear and the reports conflicting. In one series of preterm twin pregnancies born between 24 and 34 weeks, the rate of impairment and cerebral palsy in growth discordant monochorionic twins was 42% and 19%, respectively, compared with 13% and 1% in growth-discordant dichorionic twins.[64] Other reports also suggest a high risk of parenchymal brain damage (12%–20%), particularly in the larger twin of a monochorionic twin pair with intermittent absent end-diastolic flow in the umbilical artery (type III).[57,65,66] Yet, all of these studies include referral cases, which likely creates a bias toward worse outcome. Other studies failed to find that either discordant growth or a birth weight less than the 10th percentile are significant risk factors for impairment.[67,68] As such, only large prospective follow-up studies of pairs with follow-up from the first trimester until infancy will establish the true morbidity of discordant growth in monochorionic twin pregnancies and can identify risk factors for adverse outcome.

Management Options

Similar to singletons, the goals of management are to prevent intrauterine demise and long-term neurologic damage due to poor oxygenation and nutritional supply. Though this discussion is restricted to twins, because twins are far more common than triplets, growth problems are more frequent and occur earlier in higher-order multiplets, and the management issues are comparable. Because of the different pathophysiology and prognosis, the managements of monochorionic and dichorionic twin gestations are discussed separately.

Dichorionic Twins

Dichorionic twins are conceptually singletons who happen to occupy the same womb at the same time. Thus, the diagnostic workup and follow-up are comparable with those of a growth-restricted singleton (see Chapter 11).

Prenatal Diagnosis

In instances of severe early-onset growth restriction, it is important to look for signs of aneuploidy and rule out structural anomalies and congenital infection because these fetuses will not, for the most part, benefit from intense antenatal surveillance and iatrogenic early birth. Study of Doppler flow profiles in multiple vessels can help to differentiate the hypoxic, growth-restricted fetus from the constitutionally or abnormal SGA but normoxic fetus.

Fetal Surveillance

Methods of fetal surveillance for growth restriction in dichorionic twins include a combination of fetal growth and amniotic fluid assessment, nonstress test, biophysical profile score, and Doppler velocimetry. Similar to singletons, uteroplacental dysfunction is associated with a sequence of Doppler and fetal biophysical profile changes, suggesting progressive deterioration and hypoxia.

Treatment

The risk of intrauterine demise with expectant management must be balanced against the risks of iatrogenic preterm birth. When both twins are growth-restricted to a similar degree (which is rare), the risks are similar for both. However, the most common scenario is discordant growth with one growth-restricted twin. The Doppler changes that allow the reliable identification of fetal hypoxemia are discussed in Chapter 11. Early delivery to rescue the hypoxemic twin may expose the AGA twin to the risks of prematurity. Therefore, it may be preferable in dichorionic twins with severe early-onset discordant growth to delay delivery until the risk of demise and handicap due to prematurity are minimal for the AGA twin, irrespective of the condition of the SGA twin. In one series, such an expectant management until 32 weeks or when EFW of the AGA twin was more than 1500 g resulted in intrauterine demise of the SGA twin in 35% of pregnancies, but no death or handicap in the AGA co-twins.[58] The initiation of intensive fetal surveillance must be planned accordingly. The timing of any intervention depends on the clarity of the diagnosis in the SGA twin and the chances of survival with and without handicap for each fetus. Though the efficacy of antenatal corticosteroid therapy to enhance maturation has not been sufficiently studied in twins, the available information suggests it is reasonable to use with discordant twins whenever an early delivery is contemplated. One can also test for fetal lung maturity if there is an option to delay delivery; it is generally recommended to sample both sacs, especially before 32 weeks.[69]

Monochorionic Twins

Monochorionic twins have an identical genetic constitution (though they will differ epigenetically) and share a single placenta with their circulations connected through vascular communications in the placenta. As such, the management of growth restriction in monochorionic twin pregnancies poses some unique challenges.

Prenatal Diagnosis

The need to search for signs of aneuploidy and exclude discordant structural anomalies and congenital infection also applies to monochorionic twins. Monochorionic twins can be discordant for most common human aneuploidies.[35,70–72] Both amniotic sacs must be sampled in order to diagnose these rare heterokaryotypic monochorionic twins. In addition, structural anomalies are more common in monochorionic twins[73] and usually affect only one fetus.[55,74] Conversely, congenital infection typically affects both twins, although the severity may vary. It is equally important to distinguish discordant growth from TTTS by the absence of hydramnios in the sac of the AGA twin.

Fetal Surveillance

It is unclear what the best method is to monitor fetal well-being in growth-restricted monochorionic twins. Doppler velocimetry of the umbilical artery may not have the same prognostic value that it has in singletons and dichorionic twin gestations. Umbilical artery waveforms reflect downstream vascular resistance, which in monochorionic twins is determined not only by the adequacy of spiral artery invasion but also by the direction and shunting across the vascular anastomoses. Large AA anastomoses can, therefore, influence umbilical artery waveforms, leading to intermittent absent end-diastolic or even reversed flow.[75] This phenomenon occurs typically in the SGA twin of a monochorionic pair with severe early-onset growth discordance (Fig. 23–7).[56,76,77] Intrauterine demise may occur unexpectedly in these fetuses, without additional signs of deterioration of either the Doppler flow profile or the biophysical profile score, because these large AA anastomoses may facilitate acute exsanguination or other hemodynamic aberrations. Conversely, the SGA twin in some cases of discordant growth may have absent end-diastolic flow from early on in pregnancy for up to 15 weeks, without any adverse effect on fetal survival.[78] Prior to 28 weeks, we usually review growth-discordant monochorionic pairs with abnormal umbilical artery Doppler patterns and/or discordant amniotic fluid on a weekly basis for Doppler studies and assessment of amniotic fluid volumes. From 28 weeks onward, we admit those with abnormal umbilical artery Doppler patterns for twice-daily cardiotocography (CTG) and twice-weekly Doppler and biophysical profile scores and administer corticosteroid agents. Those with normal umbilical artery Doppler patterns are further followed on a weekly basis. In cases in which the discordant growth presents for the first time in the latter half of pregnancy, measurement of the PSV of the MCA may play an important role to detect the occurrence of TAPS as a cause of the late-onset discordant growth.[34]

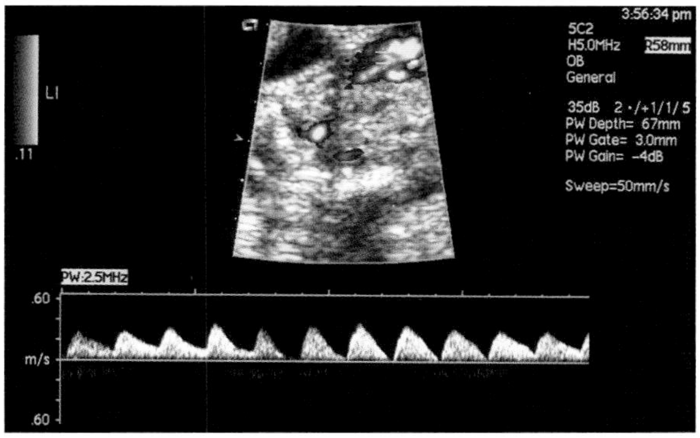

FIGURE 23–7
Doppler pattern of intermittent absent end-diastolic flow as typically seen in the smaller twin of a monochorionic pair with discordant growth.

Treatment

In monochorionic twins, the management is complicated by the almost obligatory presence of a shared circulation. In dichorionic twins, sIUFD is associated with demise or handicap of the surviving twin in 4% and 1% and is largely attributable to extreme preterm birth. In contrast, sIUFD in monochorionic twins leads to double intrauterine fetal demise (dIUFD) in about 12% and neurologic impairment in 18% of surviving co-twins.[79] This extra morbidity and mortality is due to a combination of pressure instability as the first twin dies and acute exsanguination in the fetoplacental unit of the demised twin, all in addition to the effects of extreme preterm birth. Expectant management irrespective of the condition of the SGA until 32 weeks is, therefore, not appropriate in monochorionic twins. Possible management options for severe early-onset discordant growth in monochorionic twins are expectant management with timely birth, selective feticide by umbilical cord occlusion, or selective coagulation of the vascular communications. The problems with expectant management are that intrauterine demise may occur before viability, is difficult to predict, and might have major consequences. Demise is especially dramatic once a viable stage of gestation has been reached. As a result, some advocate elective preterm birth of all monochorionic twins with a growth discordance of more than 25% at 32 weeks after the administration of maternal corticosteroids or, at the latest, after confirmation of fetal lung maturity.

Umbilical cord occlusion may be considered prior to viability when there are signs of imminent fetal demise. The rationale for cord occlusion is that it may better protect the surviving twin against the adverse effects of spontaneous demise. However, a major drawback is that the maximum survival rate is 50%. Further, it is not always clear which signs predict impending demise in monochorionic twins. We usually offer cord coagulation when the smaller twin develops anhydramnios, persistent absent or reversed flow in the ductus venosus, or an arrest of growth over a 3-week observation period prior to viability.

Selective photocoagulation of the vascular anastomoses as it is currently performed in the treatment for TTTS also seeks to protect the AGA twin against the adverse effect of sIUFD of the SGA twin by "unlinking" the two fetal circulations. However, a small case series comparing treated and expectantly managed cases series did not show any significant difference in survival or short-term neurologic morbidity.[80,81] Several explanations for this apparent lack of benefit are possible. First, selective coagulation is technically more challenging for discordant growth than for TTTS owing to the absence of hydramnios. Second, unequal sharing is frequently the reason for discordant growth, and coagulation of the vascular anastomoses might further diminish the already critical placental reserve of the SGA twin. Third, the elaborate intertwin transfusion in these unequally shared placentas may benefit the SGA twin by increasing its oxygen and nutrient supply. And finally, the survival rate of early-onset discordant growth is about 85%,[34,57] in contrast to a nearly 100% mortality of untreated mid-trimester TTTS. Also, long-term neurologic outcome of discordant growth appears to be much better than that of TTTS.[68] As such, a recent series on laser coagulation of the vascular anastomoses as a treatment for discordant growth with intermittent absent or reversed end-diastolic flow (type III) showed a survival of only 64% in contrast to the 85% survival rate in conservatively managed cases.[57] An overactive management might risk the loss of pregnancies that would have reached viability without demise of the SGA fetus. The potential role of laser coagulation of the vascular anastomoses in the management of discordant growth is currently the subject of a randomized controlled trial.[82]

Twins of Unknown Chorionicity

Determining chorionicity in same-sex twins with discordant growth in the second trimester can be challenging. Oligohydramnios with the intertwin membrane plastered around the SGA twin makes assessment of membrane thickness or the presence or absence of a lambda sign especially unreliable. It is estimated that just 3 out of 10 same-sex twins have monochorionic placentation. In these instances, the detection of an AA anastomosis with its characteristic bidirectional waveform (Fig. 23–8) confirms monochorionicity with 100% reliability.[83] Also, DNA determination of zygosity by amniocentesis generally rules out monochorionicity if dizygosity is confirmed.[84] In cases of persistent doubt, it is prudent to manage the pregnancy as a monochorionic twin gestation.

FIGURE 23–8
Characteristic bidirectional Doppler pattern in an arterioarterial anastomosis, which confirms monochorionicity.

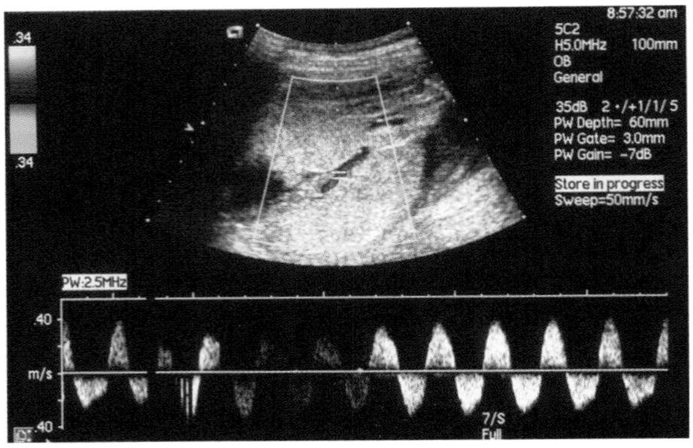

SUMMARY OF MANAGEMENT OPTIONS
Poor Fetal Growth in Twin Pregnancies

Management Options	Evidence Quality and Recommendation	References
Dichorionic Twins		
Exclude aneuploidy, structural anomalies, and congenital infection.	—/GPP	—
Determine when to intervene upon signs of fetal distress of the SGA twin and plan fetal surveillance accordingly.	See Chapters 10, 11 and 12	
In severe early discordant growth, it may be preferable not to intervene to maximize the chances of the AGA twin at the expense of spontaneous demise of the SGA twin.	III/B	58
Fetal surveillance is usually done by a combination of fetal growth assessment, biophysical profile scoring, and Doppler velocimetry.	See Chapter 10	
Consider administration of corticosteroids and fetal lung maturity testing whenever early delivery is contemplated.	Ia/A	299
Monochorionic Twins		
Exclude aneuploidy, structural anomalies, congenital infection, and TTTS.	IIa/B	70,71,73
Consider referral to a tertiary care center.	—/GPP	—
If spontaneous demise is presumed imminent and in the previable period, selective feticide by cord occlusion may protect the AGA twin better against the side effects of spontaneous demise.	IV/C	81
Consider elective preterm delivery at 32 wk for cases with a growth difference of ≥ 25% and abnormal umbilical artery Doppler pattern after administration of corticosteriods or at the latest when lung maturity has been established.	—/GPP	—
Fetal surveillance is usually done by a combination of fetal growth assessment, biophysical profile scoring, and Doppler velocimetry.	See Chapter 10	

Management Options	Evidence Quality and Recommendation	References
Nonstress testing and biophysical profile score are currently the best methods to ascertain acute fetal well-being, although IUFD can occur unexpectedly, despite normal biophysical profile scoring.	III/B	75–77
Assess for TTTS.	—/GPP	—
Twins of Unknown Chorionicity		
Consider DNA fingerprinting to exclude monochorionicity.	III/B	84
Check for arterioarterial anastomoses to confirm monochorionicity.	III/B	83
If chorionicity remains unconfirmed, manage as monochorionic twins.	—/GPP	—

AGA, appropriate for gestational age; GPP, good practice point; IUFD, intrauterine fetal demise; SGA, small for gestational age.

MONOAMNIOTIC TWINS

General

Cleavage of the inner cell mass day 9 to day 12 after fertilization is thought to result in monochorionic monoamniotic twins. These twins share not only their placenta but also their amniotic sac. Monoamniotic twins are rare, occurring in about 1 in 10,000 pregnancies and, as such, constitute 5% of monochorionic twins.[85] The umbilical cords insert usually close to each other mid placenta with multiple deep and superficial large-caliber (8–12 mm) anastomoses connecting the placental stem vessels of the twins (Fig. 23–9).[86,87]

The diagnosis of monoamniotic twin gestation is reliably made in the early first trimester by the presence one amniotic cavity containing two fetal poles and a single placenta. In contrast to what was previously suggested,[88] the presence of a single yolk does not necessarily prove monoamnionicity, as is the case in up to 15% of diamniotic twins.[89] Cord entanglement is diagnostic of monoamniotic twins and often already demonstrable in the first trimester by imaging two heart rates on pulsed Doppler in an entangled mass of umbilical cord vessels (Fig. 23–10).[90,91] Current ultrasound technology with sharper resolution usually permits the distinction between diamniotic and monoamniotic monochorionic twins. On occasion, transvaginal scanning at high frequencies will help confirm or refute any dividing membrane. The "stuck twin phenomenon" is regularly mistaken for a monoamniotic twin pregnancy because of the difficulty of seeing the dividing membrane. However, the fixed position of the stuck twin rules it out because in a monoamniotic gestation both fetuses move freely about.

Fetal Risks

Monoamniotic twins are at increased risk of congenital malformation and IUFD. Although rare, conjoined twins must be excluded. Conjoined twins are thought to arise when the embryonic disk incompletely divides beyond the 12th day of fertilization and has an estimated incidence of 1 in 50,000 pregnancies. The diagnosis is possible as early as the first trimester by the close and fixed apposition of the fetal bodies with fusion of the skin lines at some point (Fig. 23–11).[92] Intrauterine demise occurs in 60% of conjoined twins, and of those that are liveborn; the majority die owing to severe anomalies or as a consequence of surgery.[93] Except for conjoined twinning, congenital malformations occur in 38% to 50% of monoamniotic twins, usually affecting only one twin.[66,94] Up to a third of the perinatal mortality in monoamniotic twins is caused by congenital malformations.[95] Late embryonic cleavage and hemodynamic imbalances due to the large and multiple anastomoses may account for the extremely high prevalence.

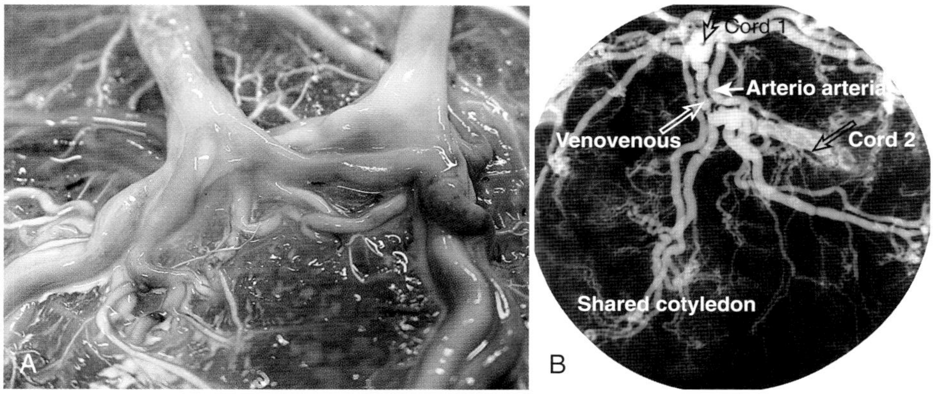

FIGURE 23–9
A, Macroscopic image of large diameter anastomoses and side-to-side insertion of the umbilical cords as typically seen in a monoamniotic twin pregnancy. *B*, Diagnostic angiography in which injection of the umbilical vessels of one twin was sufficient to visualize the placental vascularization of both twins owing to the presence of a large arterioarterial and venovenous anastomosis. Furthermore, about half of the placenta consisted of shared cotyledons.

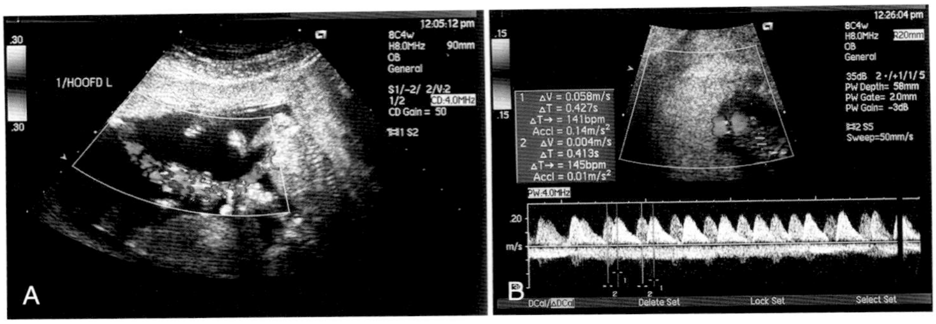

FIGURE 23–10
Ultrasound image of cord entanglement at 14 weeks' gestational age in monoamniotic twins. *A*, Doppler demonstrates cord entanglement. *B*, Pulsed Doppler of the entangled mass shows two different heart rates.
(*A* and *B*, Courtesy of D. Van Schoubroeck, UZ Leuven, Belgium.)

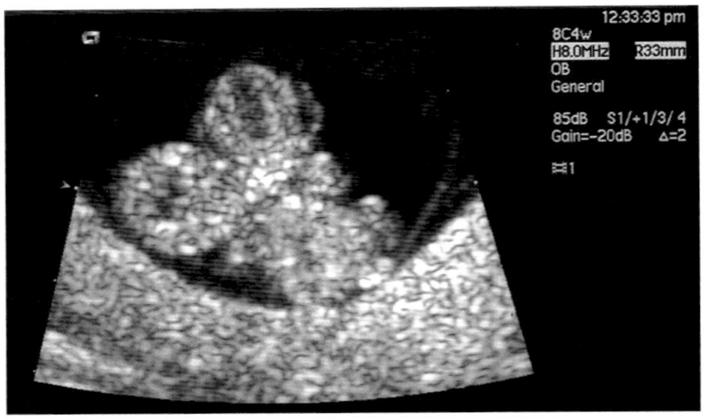

FIGURE 23–11
Ultrasound image of conjoined twins at 9 weeks' gestational age.
(Courtesy of I. Witters, UZ Leuven, Belgium.)

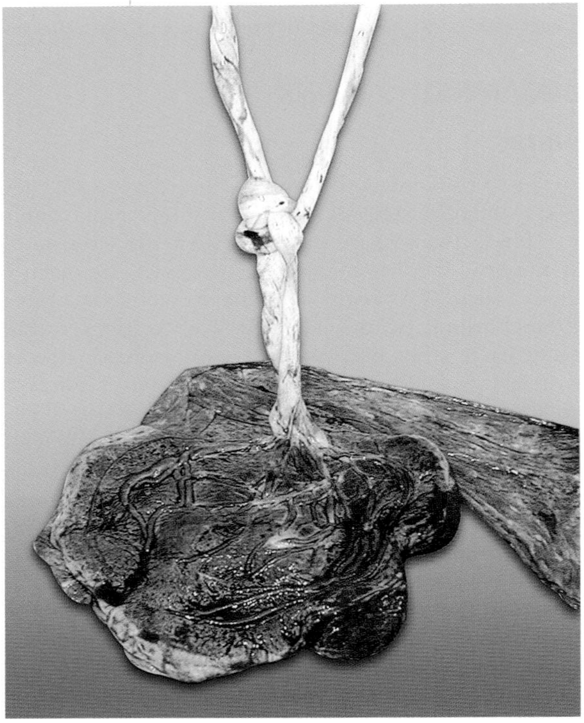

FIGURE 23–12
Cord entanglement and knotting at birth in a monoamniotic twin pregnancy.
(Courtesy of S. Dobbelaere, H. Hart Hospital, Lier, Belgium.)

In structurally normal monoamniotic twins, IUFD is the most important cause of mortality. More recent series report mortality rates of 0%[96,97] to 17%[95,98] with careful fetal surveillance and elective preterm birth compared with previously quoted risks of 30% to 70%.[99,100] However, most pregnancies included in these series were diagnosed in the second trimester, and the mortality would likely be higher should first-trimester diagnoses be included.[85] Umbilical cord entanglement was long considered the only reason for the high mortality rate, but almost all monoamniotic twins have entangled cords at birth (Fig. 23–12) and usually from early in gestation. "Acute" TTTS may be an important contributing factor, perhaps triggered by cord compression. Acute hemodynamic imbalances across the large-caliber anastomoses may also explain the 70% rate of dIUFD in monoamniotic twins compared with 25% in diamniotic twins.[86] Indeed, chronic TTTS is only rarely reported in monoamniotic twins,[98] probably because volume shifts through the large-caliber anastomoses are not tolerated for long periods and are more likely to lead to sudden death typically of both twins within a short time of each other. However, cord entanglement may still cause in utero demise[101] or asphyxia later in gestation if the co-twin survives.[102]

Management Options

The cornerstone of management is a targeted anomaly scan at 18 to 22 weeks to rule out associated anomalies, followed by scans every 2 weeks for growth and amniotic fluid volume, intense antenatal surveillance from 26 to 28 weeks onward, and timely delivery. It is the author's opinion that birth should be planned around 32 weeks, or at the latest when lung maturity is established, because unexpected intrauterine demise may occur even after 32 weeks.[95,98] However, others have suggested the loss rates are extremely low after 32 weeks, possibly because there is less room for fetal movement.[103] Selective feticide for discordant anomalies in monoamniotic twins can be accomplished by fetoscopic/ultrasound-guided coagulation and laser transsection of the umbilical cord (Fig. 23–13).[104,105] The procedure is technically more challenging than in diamniotic twins owing to cord entanglement. An accessory port for fetoscopy may facilitate cord transsection and, to a lesser degree, help identify the correct cord, albeit with an unknown additional risk of preterm premature rupture of the membranes (PPROM) when compared with single-port procedures.

Although intrauterine demise in monoamniotic twins may be sudden and unpredictable, as mentioned previously, the best way to manage these cases is simply not known. Careful antenatal surveillance and elective preterm birth appear to improve perinatal survival to about 90%. Generally, it is

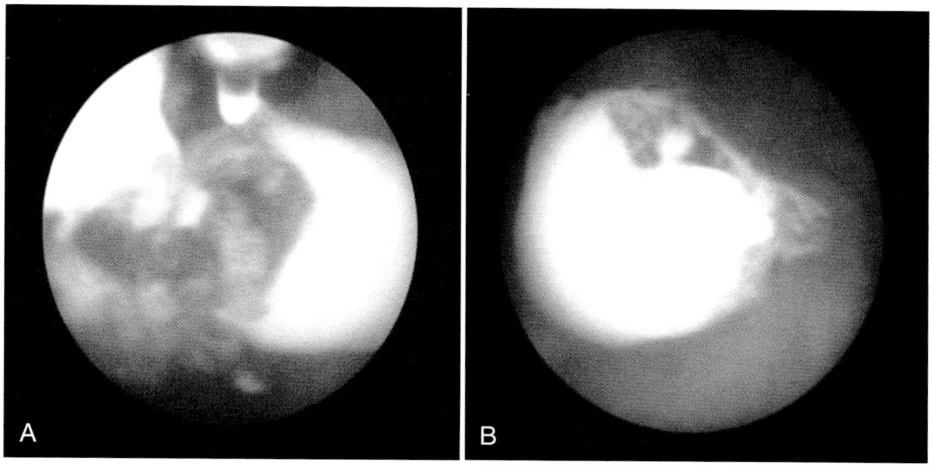

FIGURE 23–13
Fetoscopic image during (*A*) and after (*B*) umbilical cord transsection by laser in a monoamniotic twin pregnancy with a severe discordant anomaly.

agreed that intense fetal surveillance should be started from 26 to 28 weeks onward, with regular nonstress testing to identify symptomatic cord compression and ultrasound scans for a biophysical profile score, Doppler, and growth checks. The recommended frequency is disputed, and in the literature, nonstress testing varies from twice weekly to several times a day. The high frequency of nonstress testing is justified by the suddenness of the events, but fetal demise in between remains possible. Some advocate weekly ultrasound examinations with a biophysical profile score, yet these fetuses are lost because of acute events and not because of chronic hypoxemia. Abnormal umbilical artery Doppler flow waveforms such as diastolic notch[106] or absent/reversed end-diastolic flow may indicate cord compression. But similar to monochorionic twins in general, the predictive value of an abnormal umbilical artery Doppler waveform may be different than in singletons and, like biophysical profile scoring, requires additional validation.[107] The need for hospitalization is likewise controversial and should be individualized based on the results of the ultrasound scan and antenatal testing,[108,109] although surveillance as an inpatient may improve survival rates.[110] The administration of sulindac was suggested as a means of medical amniodrainage to reduce fetal mobility in monoamniotic twins and thereby cord entanglement.[97,111] Yet, because acute transfusion seems to be an important cofactor, intrauterine demise can still occur after 32 weeks[95,98] despite sulindac.[85] For all of these reasons, we advocate birth at 32 weeks when feasible. Even though cases of successful vaginal birth are reported, cesarean delivery is preferred to avoid cord entanglement and inadvertent clamping of the cord of the second twin, which may be tightly around the neck of the first.[112]

SUMMARY OF MANAGEMENT OPTIONS
Monoamniotic Twins

Management Options	Evidence Quality and Recommendation	References
Exclude structural anomalies.	—/GPP	—
Consider referral to tertiary care center.	—/GPP	—
Determine when to intervene upon signs of fetal distress and plan fetal surveillance accordingly.	III/B	95,96
Fetal surveillance is usually done by a combination of fetal growth assessment, biophysical profile scoring, and Doppler velocimetry.	See Chapter 10	
Acute fetal surveillance consists of daily to twice-weekly nonstress testing and biophysical profile scoring.	III/B	95,96
Value of hospitalization is uncertain.	III/B	108
Risk of fetal death does not decline after 32 wk; thus, some advocate delivery at 32 wk after maternal steroids are given.	IIa/B	108,111
Others advocate delivery at term, or sooner if evidence of fetal compromise, but consider steroid administration.	III/B	69
Most advocate cesarean section; vaginal delivery requires continuous fetal heart rate monitoring of both twins and facilities for immediate cesarean section.	IIa/B	103,112

GPP, good practice point.

IN UTERO DEMISE OF ONE FETUS

General

Fetuses of multifetal pregnancies are more likely to die in utero than singletons.[113] Not unexpectedly, the risk grows with an increasing number of fetuses.[114] The rate of sIUFD in twins or higher-order multiplets is difficult to ascertain during the first trimester, because the loss might occur before the diagnosis of either a multifetal pregnancy or an sIUFD. Also, the "vanishing embryo syndrome" might go unrecognized or be wrongly diagnosed as a retromembranous blood collection (Fig. 23–14). The diagnosis of sIUFD should be made when fetal remnants are clearly identified or when a later ultrasound scan demonstrates the demise or disappearance of a previously known fetus. The risk of sIUFD in twin pregnancies resulting from IVF, which are regularly followed throughout the first trimester, is maternal age–dependent and ranges from 10% to 20%, with most cases occurring prior to 12 weeks.[115] These figures are currently the best estimates available for first-trimester sIUFD in dichorionic twins, because about 90% of IVF pregnancies are dichorionic.[116] In one general population scanned between 10 and 14 weeks' gestation, the prevalence of sIUFD was 4% in dichorionic and less than 1% in monochorionic twin pregnancies (compared with 2% in singletons), with dIUFD in 1.6% of dichorionic and 2% of monochorionic twin pregnancies.[117] Thus, dIUFD appears more common than sIUFD in monochorionic twins. Gross unequal placental sharing or hemodynamic imbalances in monochorionic twins may cause sIUFD, with the connected fetal circulations leading to dIUFD. Also, chromosomal abnormalities or an adverse maternal factor (infection, teratogens) will affect both fetuses similarly. In contrast, sIUFD in dichorionic twins is twice as common as dIUFD and may be explained by either a discordant chromosomal or structural anomaly or suboptimal placentation. Because each fetus has a separate fetoplacental circulation, sIUFD will not cause co-twin demise per se, though whatever killed one may harm or ultimately kill the other. About 10% of dichorionic twins are monozygotic and, therefore, concordant for chromosomal anomalies.

From 10 to 14 weeks onward, sIUFD occurs in about 2% of dichorionic but 4% of monochorionic twin pregnancies, and dIUFD occurs in 0.2% of dichorionic and in at least 6% of monochorionic twins. This extra fetal loss of monochorionic twins occurs before 24 weeks and is largely attributable to complications of the connected fetoplacental circulations.[19,55]

Toward the end of gestation, the risk of in utero demise in twins increases from 1 in 3333 at 33 weeks to 1 in 313 at 36 weeks and 1 in 69 beyond 39 weeks. The intrauterine mortality of twins at 37 to 38 weeks is equal that of postterm singleton pregnancies, and elective birth at 37 to 38 completed weeks may be justified when uncomplicated twin pregnancies reach that milestone.[118]

Recently, several studies have addressed the risk of unexpected late intrauterine demise in monochorionic twin pregnancies. Barigye and associates reported that after 32 weeks unexpected stillbirth occurred in 4% of otherwise uncomplicated pairs, supporting a policy of elective preterm birth of all monochorionic twins at 32 weeks.[119] This figure was contradicted by other retrospective analyses[120–122] and one prospective series[55] that all report lower rates (1.2% and 2.1%) in complicated and uncomplicated monochorionic pairs. After 37 weeks, up to 2% of monochorionic twin pregnancies may be complicated by unexpected intrauterine demise.[123] Based on these figures, we now see all monochorionic twin pregnancies on a weekly basis for Doppler velocimetry, biophysical profile score, and nonstress testing from 32 weeks onward; for uncomplicated cases, we plan an elective birth around 37 weeks.

Fetal Risks

The prognosis of sIUFD for the surviving fetus depends first and foremost on chorionicity. To a lesser degree, outcome is determined by the gestational age of sIUFD. There is little evidence regarding the implications of sIUFD in the first trimester. Nonetheless, it seems most likely that sIUFD in a monochorionic twin pregnancy leads to either dIUFD or miscarriage. Rarely, the surviving co-twin may prevent the "vanishing" of the dead twin by reversed perfusion along the vascular anastomoses—a TRAP sequence.[124] Color Doppler should be used to exclude TRAP whenever sIUFD occurs in a monochorionic twin pregnancy, and if there is any doubt, follow-up scans should be arranged. It is also hypothesized that unrecognized early sIUFD in a monochorionic twin pregnancy may explain some cases of cerebral palsy and certain congenital anomalies such as renal agenesis and intestinal atresia in birth singletons, attributable to the

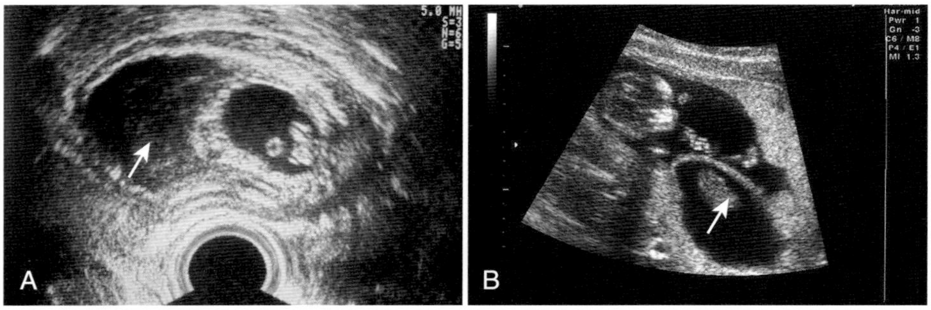

FIGURE 23–14
Ultrasound image of a retromembranous blood collection (*arrow*) in a singleton pregnancy (*A*), which must be differentiated from "vanishing twin syndrome" (*B*) in which felt remnants (*arrow*) can be clearly identified.

agonal hemodynamic events.[125] The outcome of sIUFD in the first trimester in dichorionic twins is usually favorable, although the rate of preterm birth and subsequent miscarriage may be increased especially if the sIUFD occurs toward the end of the first trimester. In the case series of sIUFD diagnosed between 10 to 14 weeks, 18% (3/16) of dichorionic twins subsequently miscarried.[91] This contrasts with the low rate of loss following selective embryo reduction.

A recent meta-analysis showed that sIUFD in dichorionic twins during the second and third trimester leads to co-twin demise or neurologic abnormality in 4% and 1%, respectively,[79] presumably in great part secondary to the conditions that lead to extreme preterm birth. Conversely, the same meta-analysis showed that in monochorionic twins, sIUFD results in dIUFD in 12%, and cerebral damage in 18% owing in part to acute intertwin transfusion plus the risks of extreme preterm birth.[79] Yet, this meta-analysis most likely underestimates co-twin mortality rate, because it covers survival only after sIUFD whereas a significant proportion of monochorionic twins present as dIUFD at first diagnosis. Also, immediate delivery after the diagnosis of sIUFD will reduce the rate of co-twin intrauterine demise, while increasing the neonatal death rate.[126] In a prospective series from Sebire and associates[19] that was not included in the meta-analysis, 10 monochorionic twin pregnancies were complicated by intrauterine demise, 6 were dIUFD from the start and only 4 presented as a sIUFD.

In dichorionic twins, survival seems inversely related to the gestational age at which the sIUFD occurred, with infant survival rates improving from 71% when the sIUFD occurs between 20 and 24 weeks to 98% for sIUFD occurring beyond 37 weeks.[114] In monochorionic twins, the influence of gestational age of sIUFD on outcome is less clear. It seems that early sIUFD is more often associated with death of the co-twin. However, if the co-twin survives, severe morbidity is less common. In contrast, a late sIUFD more frequently results in the birth of a liveborn infant who is neurologically damaged.[127,128]

The reported rate of cerebral palsy after sIUFD in dichorionic twins is 30 per 1000 infant survivors, with preterm birth the greatest association with this excess risk, compared with 1 per 1000 in singletons.[129,130] Specific cerebral palsy rates are not available for sIUFD in monochorionic twins. However, the cerebral palsy rate in same-sex twins (30% monochorionic and 70% dichorionic) after sIUFD is 106 per 1000 survivors, which is about three times higher than that of different-sex twins (100% dichorionic).[129] In addition, most of the twins in the same-sex group with cerebral palsy had monochorionic placentation.[130] Cerebral damage is often detectable sonographically but does not usually become apparent until weeks after the insult. Prenatal magnetic resonance imaging (MRI) may detect brain lesions earlier and with better definition.[131,132] Sonographic evidence of brain injury includes porencephaly, multicystic periventricular leukoencephalomalacia, ventriculomegaly, cerebral atrophy, and cerebellar or cerebral infarcts. Less frequently reported complications include renal cortical necrosis, small bowel atresia, aplasia cutis, and limb infarction. Originally, thromboembolic phenomena with passage of thromboplastin from the dead to the living twin were thought to be responsible for these lesions.[133] There is no evidence to support this line of reasoning, though circulatory instability and acute exsanguination are well documented.[134] Reversed perfusion of the dead twin has been demonstrated by Doppler interrogation of the chorionic plate vessels,[135] and fetal blood sampling within 24 hours of sIUFD has consistently revealed a decreased hematocrit in the survivors with normal coagulation profiles.[136] Further, fetoscopy within 3 hours of the donor twin dying has documented reversal of transfusion with a plethoric donor and anemic recipient.[137] The outcome of the survivor may depend not only on the gestational age at sIUFD but also on the type and direction of vascular anastomoses and the fetoplacental mass of the dead twin. The presence of superficial AA anastomoses is associated with higher rates of death and neurologic damage.[126] However, significant anemia and co-twin demise may occur, even in the absence of AA anastomoses.[127] The outcome of sIUFD associated with TTTS treated by amniodrainage does not differ from sIUFD in untreated cases, and the risk of sIUFD is similar for donors and recipients. It has been suggested that the risk of co-twin death and neurologic damage is lower with sIUFD of the donor compared with sIUFD of the recipient, because transfusion is more likely to be directed toward the recipient.[126] However, small series show similar prevalences of anemia and adverse outcome in surviving recipients and donors.[127,138] Even though treatment by laser coagulation of the vascular anastomoses more frequently results in sIUFD than amniodrainage, it consistently leads less often to a dIUFD.[139,140] Significantly, anemia in the survivor is rare in the event of sIUFD after laser,[141] and the neurologic morbidity is lower than after amniodrainage.[142,143] These findings provide further support for the concept that the vascular anastomoses are responsible for most of the adverse outcomes associated with sIUFD in monochorionic twins.

Management Options

Knowledge of chorionicity is fundamental to the management of sIUFD in multiple pregnancies because the pathophysiology and prognosis varies, though not to complicate matters unnecessarily, our discussion is restricted to twins. Although sIUFD is more common in higher-order multiplets and management issues are more complex, they are based largely on the same principles as in twins. A small paragraph is dedicated to issues that are relevant to both groups of twins.

Dichorionic Twins

The main risks of sIUFD in dichorionic twins are miscarriage and severe preterm birth. Conservative management is advocated with regular ultrasound scans to check the growth and well-being of the survivor. Admittedly, parental anxiety may be an important factor in persuading the obstetrician to intervene, and these complex emotional responses should be adequately addressed by education rather than a precocious response.[144]

Monochorionic Twins

The main risks of sIUFD in monochorionic twins are co-twin demise and ischemic brain lesions secondary to acute exsanguination. Depending upon gestational age, there are additional risks of either miscarriage or severe preterm birth. It is presumed that death and especially ischemic brain damage

FIGURE 23–15
Doppler examination of the middle cerebral artery of the surviving twin of a monochorionic pair at 20 weeks' gestation, within 4 days after single intrauterine fetal demise (sIUFD) of the growth-retarded co-twin.

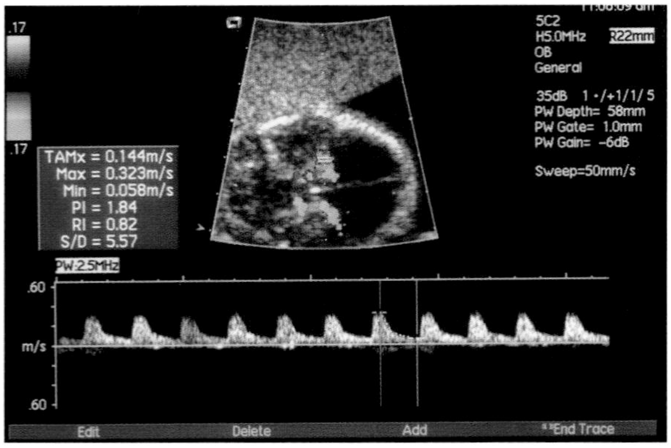

in the survivor occurs during or soon after the death of the co-twin. Therefore, a preemptive preterm birth is inappropriate once an sIUFD has been diagnosed, because this would only worsen the outcome of the surviving twin by adding the complications of preterm birth. Moreover, a long demise-to-birth interval is associated with a better outcome than a short demise-to-birth interval, supporting the premise of conservative management.[128] Monochorionic twin pregnancies with an sIUFD should be managed in a tertiary referral center with sufficient neonatal support. Also, regular detailed (transvaginal if vertex) ultrasound examinations of the fetal brain are indicated to detect brain injury. Unlike hemorrhage, ischemic brain injury is difficult to visualize in the early phase, and MRI scan may aid early detection.[131,132] MRI is also more sensitive than ultrasound scan to detect more subtle brain lesions.[145] It is recommended that an MRI be performed at least 2 weeks after sIUFD to optimize the detection of any injury. Fetal blood sampling shortly after sIUFD may have prognostic value because all nonanemic fetuses in one study had a good outcome and did not develop any brain injury.[127] MCA Doppler velocimetry effectively predicts fetal anemia after sIUFD in cases associated with TTTS and obviates the need of cordocentesis (Fig. 23–15). There is currently insufficient evidence that a rescue intrauterine transfusion improves outcome, though it may prevent co-twin demise probably too late to prevent brain injury.[127,138,146] Intrauterine transfusion may thus increase survival of severely handicapped infants. Additional multicenter studies are necessary to determine the benefit of rescue transfusion. In the meantime, it is best performed only in settings in which a late termination is an option if cerebral lesions are detected later in pregnancy.[146]

After birth, a thorough neonatal evaluation should be performed to detect any neurologic, renal, circulatory, and cutaneous defects. All survivors should undergo an early neonatal brain scan and ideally be enrolled for long-term neurodevelopmental follow-up.

Issues Applicable to Dichorionic and Monochorionic Twins

It seems justified to administer rhesus (Rh) prophylaxis whenever an sIUFD is diagnosed in a Rh-negative woman. Maternal disseminated intravascular coagulation does occur in singletons after intrauterine demise and retention of the fetus for more than 5 weeks. However, in twins, its incidence with conservative management appears extremely low, and it can be treated with heparin should it occur.[147,148] Vaginal birth is not contraindicated after sIUFD, but labor may be obstructed, especially if the sIUFD occurs late and the dead twin is presenting. A postmortem examination of the dead twin is advisable, especially if the cause is unknown, and the placenta should be sent for histologic examination to confirm chorionicity.

The family will require psychological support and counseling prior to, during, and after birth. The grief experienced after an sIUFD equals that for a singleton loss, and yet the parents rarely receive equal sympathy.[149] The death is invisible for the parents and their immediate associates, which hampers the grieving process. Many parents worry the dead twin will have an adverse effect on the remaining fetus and need reassurance that no additional harm is expected except for the possibility of an earlier birth. The delay between diagnosis and birth permits some grieving, but sorrow resurfaces at birth.[150] It is important not to ignore the deceased twin; the parents may wish to see it during ultrasound examination and after birth. Death after 12 to 15 weeks should end with an identifiable fetus at birth, though compressed and mummified, and parents should be prepared and told what to expect.[151]

SUMMARY OF MANAGEMENT OPTIONS

Single Fetal Death in Twins

Management Options	Evidence Quality and Recommendation	References
Issues Applicable to All Twins		
Offer counseling and psychological support to patient and family.	III/B	149,150
Administer rhesus prophylaxis if Rh-negative.	—/GPP	—
Give steroids if preterm delivery is contemplated.	Ia/A	299
Dichorionic Twins		
Check for signs of threatening miscarriage and severe preterm delivery.	III/B	144
If dichorionic pregnancy, continue fetal surveillance in survivor.	III/B	144

Management Options	Evidence Quality and Recommendation	References
Monochorionic Twins		
Check for signs of threatening miscarriage and severe preterm delivery.	III/B	144
Continue fetal surveillance in surviving twin with a combination of fetal growth assessment, biophysical profile scoring, and Doppler velocimetry (see Chapter 10).	III/B	144
Consider Doppler of the middle cerebral artery to detect anemia, which may predict the risk of brain damage.	III/B	127,138
Check for brain injury by (transvaginal) ultrasound scan or MRI.	III/B	131,132
Preemptive preterm delivery is no longer advocated.	III/B	128
Perform pediatric assessment and neurodevelopmental follow-up.	III/B	144

GPP, good practice point; MRI, magnetic resonance imaging.

TWIN REVERSED ARTERIAL PERFUSION

General

The TRAP sequence, also known as "acardiac twinning," is an anomaly unique to monochorionic multiple pregnancies that affects approximately 1 of 35,000 pregnancies and 1% of monochorionic twins.[152] In TRAP, blood flows from an umbilical artery of the pump twin in a reverse direction into the umbilical artery of the perfused twin via an AA anastomosis. The perfused (or acardiac) twin is a true parasite. Its blood is poorly oxygenated, and the hypoxemia contributes to variable degrees of deficient development of the head, heart, and upper limb structures. The lower half of the body is usually better developed, which may be explained by the mechanism of perfusion. Blood enters the acardiac twin via the umbilical artery and flows through the common iliac artery and aorta. What little oxygen is present is extracted in the lower part of the body, allowing at least partial development of the lower limbs and abdomen. By the time the blood reaches the upper body, most of the oxygen will already have been extracted, leading to poor development of upper body structures (Fig. 23–16).[148]

Two criteria must be fulfilled for the development of a TRAP sequence. The first is an AA anastomosis and the second discordant development[153] or in utero demise[101] of one of monochorionic twins, allowing for the blood flow reversal. Not infrequently, chromosomal abnormalities are identified in the acardiac twin, whereas the pump twin has a normal karyotype.[154,155] Embryos/fetuses with chromosomal abnormalities have a high risk for spontaneous intrauterine demise, which in dichorionic twins would lead to a "vanishing" twin. However, in monochorionic twins, the "vanishing" can be prevented by the occurrence of persistent, yet reversed, flow to the chromosomally abnormal twin via the vascular anastomoses. Therefore, whenever sIUFD is suspected in monochorionic twins on a first-trimester scan, the differential diagnosis or development of TRAP should be kept in mind and follow-up scans arranged.[124]

The diagnosis can be reliably made on ultrasound scan in the first trimester.[156] TRAP sequence is characterized by a grossly abnormal fetus that grows, may even show movements, but has no functional cardiac activity of its own. Rarely, a rudimentary heart may show pulsatility (Fig. 23–17). Marked hydrops and cystic hygroma are frequently

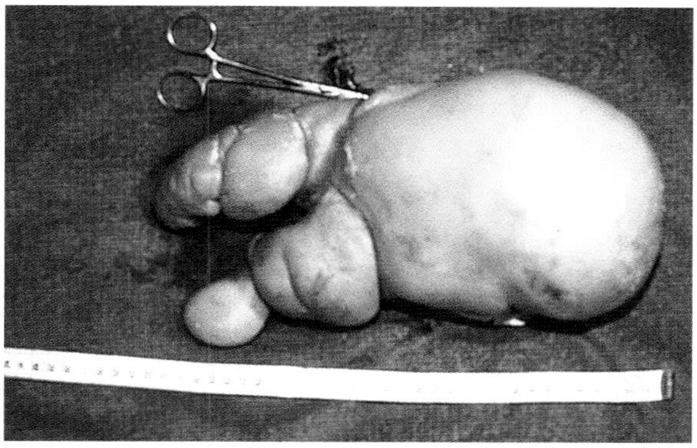

FIGURE 23–16
Macroscopic image of an acardiac twin with absent head and partial development of lower limbs and abdomen. This acardiac mass weighed about 4 kg and was not diagnosed until the third trimester. The patient delivered at 37 weeks, and the pump twin survived.

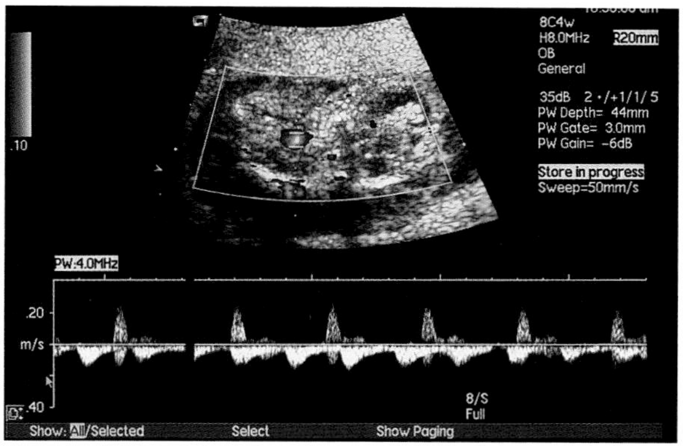

FIGURE 23–17
Doppler examination demonstrates cardiac activity in the rudimentary heart (70 beats/min) of the acardiac twin, with flow in the opposite direction in the aorta (140 beats/min).

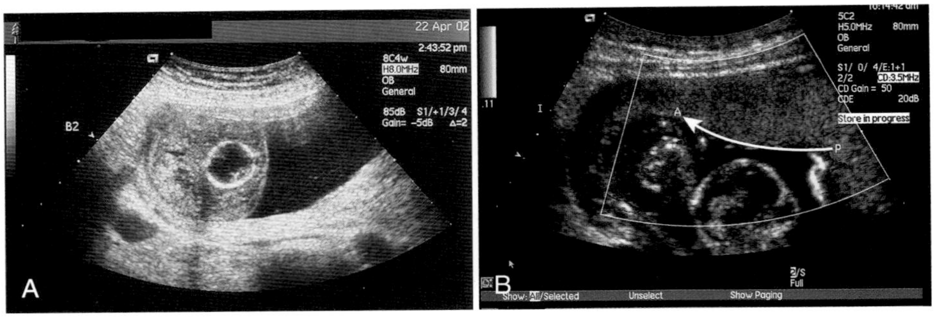

FIGURE 23–18
A, Ultrasound image of an acardiac twin at the level of the rudimentary head with typical, severe subcutaneous edema. *B*, Doppler examination at 15 weeks' gestation demonstrates the typical retrograde flow from the pump twin toward the acardiac twin over an arterioarterial anastomosis (*arrow*).

present, especially toward the end of pregnancy. Doppler studies reveal pathognomonic features of reversed arterial perfusion through an AA anastomosis (Fig. 23–18). TRAP can easily be distinguished from sIUFD by the presence of fetal movements and the typical retrograde perfusion.

Fetal Risks

The pump twin is at risk for high-output cardiac failure secondary to the strain of perfusing the acardiac twin and extreme preterm birth associated with hydramnios.[154,157] The pump twin may be chronically hypoxemic if the deoxygenated blood from the acardiac returns by a vein-to-vein anastomosis.

The natural history of TRAP is poorly documented owing to the rarity of the disorder. Reported perinatal mortality rates for the pump twin vary between 35% to 50%[154,157] of cases diagnosed at birth, whereas some series of antenatally diagnosed cases report better,[158] similar,[159,160] and worse[161] outcomes. One explanation for a better outcome in antenatally diagnosed cases may be spontaneous resolution of the TRAP sequence following complete cessation of flow to the acardiac twin.[158,160,162] Conversely, outcome may be worse due to spontaneous demise of the pump twin leading to an early second-trimester loss not otherwise identified as a TRAP.[158] Long-term outcome data are not available for pump twins, although it is reasonable to speculate the risk of long-term cardiac and neurodevelopmental sequelae is high[163,164] owing to vascular imbalances in utero.

The prediction of outcome for antenatally diagnosed TRAP is challenging. An acardiac–to–pump weight ratio above 70% at birth was associated with increased rates of high-output cardiac failure, hydramnios, and preterm birth, suggesting that a relatively small acardiac mass is a good sign. Certainly, a larger acardiac mass will put a greater hemodynamic strain on the pump twin. However, antenatal weight estimation of the acardiac mass is hampered by the absence of normal biometric structures, and the errors are likely large. Others suggest a rapid increase in the acardiac mass to be indicative of poor prognosis.[159] Doppler velocimetry is probably the best tool to predict outcome. Large differences in the umbilical artery Doppler values suggest relatively little flow to the acardiac twin, thereby predicting a more favorable outcome.[159–161,165] In contrast, small differences in the umbilical artery Doppler values would signify similar flows, the presence of large anastomoses placing a greater hemodynamic strain on the pump twin. Additional factors thought predictive of poor outcome are high-output cardiac failure with hydrops, hydramnios,[154] and certain morphologic characteristics of the acardiac twin such as the presence of a head and upper limbs.[157] It is unknown to what degree these parameters apply in the early second trimester, and spontaneous resolution as well as sudden demise of the pump twin remains largely unpredictable.

Management Options

As the natural history of antenatally diagnosed TRAP remains poorly documented, its treatment is equally controversial, ranging from conservative to palliative to causative. Conservative management consists of close antenatal surveillance and timed birth for signs of cardiac failure, whereas palliative treatment involves prolongation of pregnancy by serial amniodrainage and maternal administration of indomethacin for preterm labor and digoxin for cardiac failure. Reported perinatal mortality rates from conservative and palliative treatment vary widely between 10%[158] and 50%.[154] This is not surprising considering how poor the placental transport of digoxin is normally, much less when the fetus is hydropic. Also, little or no data are available on the long-term outcome of surviving pump twins, but as stated previously, there is concern about long-term neurologic and cardiac sequelae.

Causative treatment seeks to arrest the flow of blood to the acardiac twin. Several methods are proposed, ranging from hysterotomy and birth of the acardiac twin[166] to embolization of the acardiac twin's circulation[167] to fetoscopic cord ligation[168] to ultrasound-guided or fetoscopic coagulation of the umbilical cord[169,170] or intrafetal vessels.[171] Clearly, hysterotomy with selective birth of the acardiac twin is unacceptable because of the high maternal morbidity. Also, embolization by the injection of thrombogenic substances into the acardiac twin's circulation (e.g., absolute alcohol, coils, and enbucrilate gel) is also unacceptable as a first-line treatment, because dIUFD due to incomplete vascular

FIGURE 23–19
A, This 1.0-mm fetoscope is used for fetoscopic interventions early in the second trimester (Karl Storz). *B*, Doppler examination confirms arrest of flow after laser cord coagulation at 16 weeks' gestation.

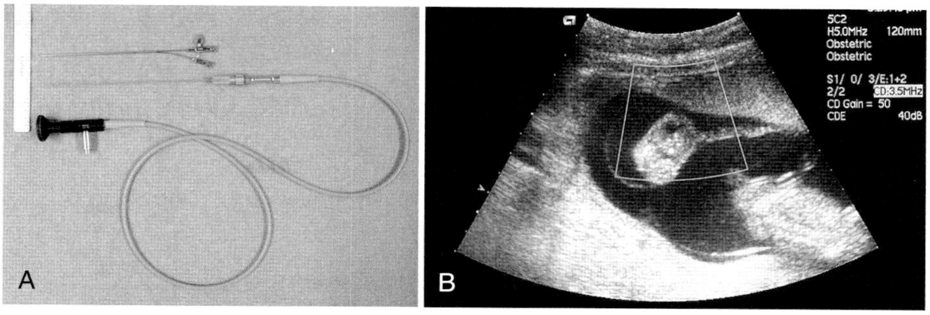

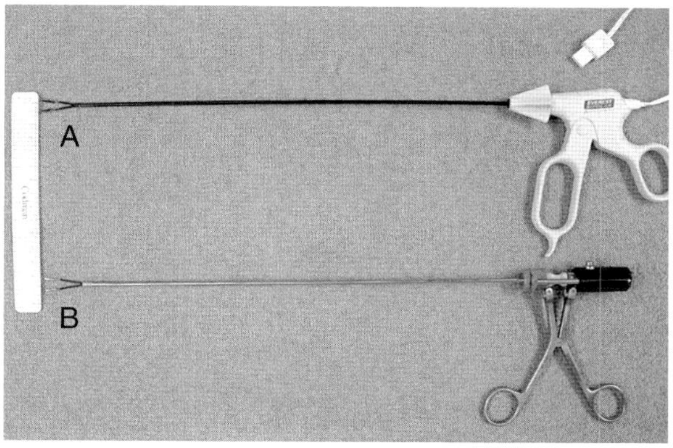

FIGURE 23–20
A, Disposable 3-mm bipolar forceps (Everest Medical). *B*, Reusable 2.4-mm bipolar forceps (Karl Storz).

occlusion or embolization of the product to pump twin is not uncommon.[172,173]

A number of minimally invasive techniques are now available to produce complete circulatory confinement of the acardiac twin. Fetoscopic cord ligation causes immediate and complete interruption of both arterial and venous flow, irrespective of umbilical cord size, but is cumbersome and has a high risk of PPROM. At present, ultrasound- or fetoscopic-guided cord coagulation together with needle-based intrafetal coagulation appear to yield the most consistent results. The method of cord coagulation by laser is derived from that used for the coagulation of vascular anastomoses in TTTS.[170] It can be performed as early as 16 weeks using a double needle loaded with a 1.0-mm fetoscope and a 400-μm laser fiber (Fig. 23–19).[174] Fetoscopic laser coagulation is performed percutaneously under local or regional anesthesia using a single 1.3-mm operating sheath or 10-Fr (3.3-mm) trocar depending on the gestation. Fetoscopically guided laser offers good visual control of the coagulation site, but may fail if the umbilical cord diameter is large or, more rarely, if the amniotic fluid is stained. In these instances, bipolar cord coagulation with purpose-designed 2.4- to 3-mm bipolar forceps under ultrasound guidance is a secondary technique (Fig. 23–20). A recent series reported on the outcome of 60 pregnancies complicated by TRAP and treated with laser coagulation of the anastomoses or the umbilical cord.[175] The survival rate was 80%, and 67% gave birth after 36 weeks. In 15%, additional bipolar coagulation was necessary to achieve arrest of flow.

Needle-based coagulation techniques using laser,[176] monopolar technique,[171] or radiofrequency[177] each involve the insertion of a 14- to 18-gauge needle into the fetal abdomen under ultrasound aiming for the intra-abdominal rather than the umbilical vessels. This technique is attractive for its simplicity, the smaller membrane defect produced, and the seemingly lower risks of PPROM. It may be the preferred technique when the acardiac twin has a short umbilical cord and/or oligohydramnios. Two small recent series reporting on 13[178] and 29 cases[179] with TRAP treated with intrafetal radiofrequency ablation report survival rates for the pump twin of more than 90%. However, in monoamniotic pregnancies, the umbilical cord cannot be transected and thus late dIUFD remains a risk owing to cord entanglement.

Currently, it is not possible to conclude what the best management is for TRAP. Most cases of TRAP are diagnosed early in the second trimester when it is impossible to predict outcome. The outcome may be good without treatment if spontaneous arrest of flow occurs. Conversely, the pump twin may die unexpectedly or sustain sequelae from very preterm birth, cardiac failure, and chronic hypoxia. Early intervention may preclude the difficulties of arresting blood flow in larger, often hydropic acardiac masses, and it seems preferable not to await signs of decompensation. We believe it is justifiable to offer prophylactic, minimally invasive intervention if no spontaneous arrest of flow has occurred by 16 weeks, recognizing the pump twin may survive without any intervention in at least half of cases. The choice of technique will reflect gestational age and access to and the size of the acardiac twin. These procedures should be performed in specialized units by fetal medicine specialists familiar with different techniques in order to tailor therapy to the needs of each individual case.

SUMMARY OF MANAGEMENT OPTIONS

Twin Reversed Arterial Perfusion Sequence

Management Options	Evidence Quality and Recommendation	References
Conservative with no hydramnios or hydrops—maintain surveillance in "pump twin" for the development of hydramnios and/or hydrops and timely delivery.	III/B	154
Palliative with hydramnios or cardiac failure (variable prognosis)—serial amniodrainage and tocolysis for hydramnios and digoxin for the cardiac failure. This is a backup option if intervention is not possible.	III/B	154,158
Intervention with hydramnios or cardiac failure (hydrops)—arrest of flow toward the cardiac twin by a number of possible methods:		
• Coagulation of cord to acardiac twin.	III/B	169,170
• Ligation of cord to acardiac twin.	III/B	168
• Intrafetal (in acardiac twin) coagulation of fetal vessels.	III/B	171
For invasive treatment before 21 wk, intrafetal coagulation and cord coagulation (laser and bipolar) are effective methods to arrest flow.	III/B	169,170,172
Beyond 21 wk and in cases with hydropic cord, bipolar cord coagulation may be more effective.	III/B	169
It is justifiable to offer invasive treatment if no spontaneous arrest has occurred by 16 wk.	—/GPP	—
Mode of delivery depends on factors such as presentation and fetal health,	III/B	154

GPP, good practice point.

TWIN-TO-TWIN TRANSFUSION SYNDROME

General

TTTS is another complication unique to monochorionic multiple pregnancies. In most monochorionic twin gestations, interfetal transfusion across the anastomoses is a constant, but balanced, phenomenon. However, in 10% of monochorionic twins, a chronic imbalance in net flow develops, resulting in TTTS.[54,55] Hypovolemia, oliguria, and oligohydramnios develop in the donor twin, producing the stuck twin phenomenon. Hypervolemia, polyuria, and hydramnios evolve in the recipient twin, who can develop circulatory overload and hydrops (Fig. 23–21). TTTS usually occurs between 15 and 26 weeks and is a sonographic diagnosis based on the following criteria: hydramnios in the sac of the recipient twin (defined as deepest vertical pocket of ≥ 8 cm prior to 20 wk and ≥ 10 cm after 20 wk) secondary to polyuria, combined with oligohydramnios in the donor's sac (deepest vertical pocket ≤2 cm) secondary to oliguria. Quintero and coworkers[180] suggested a cancer-like staging system, which despite its several limitations, is still widely used. Stage I cases include those with hydramnios in the recipient sac but the bladder of the donor twin still visible. In stage II, the bladder of the donor twin remains empty (stuck twin). Stage III is characterized by severely abnormal Doppler studies: absent or reversed end-diastolic flow in the umbilical artery of the donor or abnormal venous Doppler pattern in the recipient, such as reverse flow in the ductus venosus or pulsatile umbilical venous flow. Fetal hydrops means stage IV, and the end-stage V corresponds to fetal demise of one or both twins. The purpose of any classification system in medicine is to assess disease severity, to

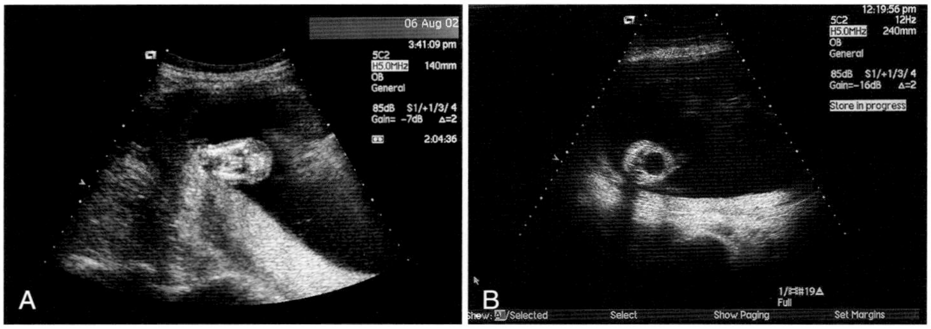

FIGURE 23–21
Ultrasound image of twin-twin transfusion syndrome. *A*, The donor is stuck to the uterine wall without bladder filling. *B*, There is hydramnios in the sac of the recipient, who has a distended bladder.

stratify therapy, and to predict the response to a given therapy. The Quintero staging system only weakly correlates with outcome[181] and the treatment is the same for stage I to stage IV. Further, the Quintero staging system does not reflect a timescale of progressive deterioration. As such, TTTS can present as stage III from the start. Also, stage I disease can progress to stage V directly, without passing through stages II, III, and IV. At best, the Quintero staging system reflects the different possible clinical manifestations that may result from a variable contribution of intertwin transfusion imbalance, hormonal factors, and the degree of placental sharing.

As discussed previously, the differential diagnosis includes discordant growth in which the growth-restricted twin can appear "stuck" owing to oligohydramnios, but in which hydramnios is absent in the larger twin. Likewise, the isolated presence of hydramnios in one sac with normal amniotic fluid in the other precludes the diagnosis of TTTS, and in that case, other causes for hydramnios must be sought.

Many questions remain concerning the exact pathophysiology of TTTS. Nevertheless, TTTS remains best explained by the angioarchitecture. Placental anastomoses can be AA, arteriovenous (AV or VA), and venovenous (VV).[182] AA and VV anastomoses are typically superficial, bidirectional anastomoses on the surface of the chorionic plate, forming direct communications between the arteries and the veins of the two fetal circulations. The direction of flow depends on the relative interfetal vascular pressure gradients. AV anastomoses are usually referred to as "deep" anastomoses. They occur at the capillary level deep within the depth of the placenta, receiving arterial supply from one twin and providing venous (well-oxygenated) drainage to the other. The supplying artery and draining vein of the AV anastomosis can be visualized on the placental surface as an unpaired artery and vein that pierce the chorionic plate at close proximity to each other (Fig. 23–22). The AV anastomoses allow flow in one direction only and, hence, may create an imbalance in the interfetal transfusion leading to TTTS, unless balanced by an oppositely directed transfusion through other superficial or deep anastomoses.

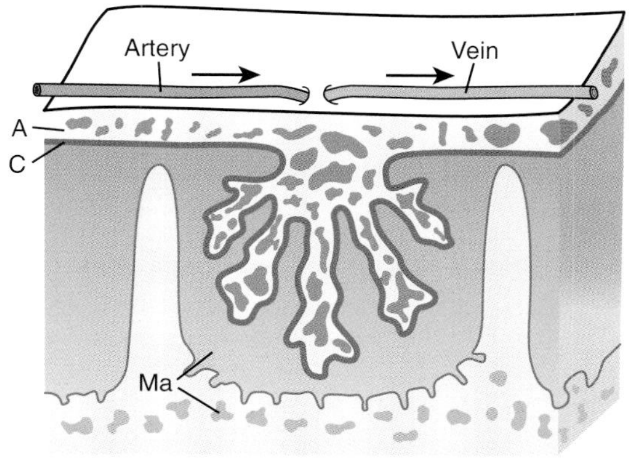

FIGURE 23–22
Schematic three-dimensional drawing of the human "shared" cotyledon. Artery and vein enter the chorionic plate very close to each other. A, amnion; C, chorion; Ma, maternal circulation; depicted as *solid shading*.
(Drawing by Luc Brullemans.)

Both postnatal injection studies[15] and in vivo fetoscopic observations[183,184] indicate the presence of at least one unidirectional AV anastomosis as an anatomic prerequisite for the development of TTTS. Although a TTTS case was reported with only superficial anastomoses (one AA and one VV),[184] this seems the exception confirming the rule. The presence of bidirectional AA anastomoses is believed to protect against the development of TTTS because most non-TTTS monochorionic placentas have AA anastomoses (84%) in contrast to TTTS placentas (20%–30%).[15,184]

Although vascular anastomoses are an anatomic prerequisite for the development of TTTS, other pathophysiologic mechanisms are likely involved. Because 75% of sonographically defined TTTS has an intertwin hemoglobin difference of less than 15%,[185] this syndrome cannot be explained by the simple transfer of blood from one twin to the other. Further, there is no increased erythropoietin production in the donor[186] and no evidence of iron depletion/overload in the donor/recipient.[187] It is suggested that discordant placental function may offset TTTS, because placental dysfunction is associated with an increased fetoplacental resistance, which may promote transfusion from the growth-restricted donor twin to the recipient twin. Reduced insulin growth factor-II[188] and decreased leptin levels[189] in donors compared with recipients may indicate discordant placental development rather than transfusion as a cause of the growth restriction. Other hormonal changes occur in donors and recipients. Raised endothelin-1 levels were observed in recipients, potentially causing increased peripheral vasoconstriction and hypertension. Recipients have increased levels of atrial natriuretic peptide,[190] and those with severe cardiac dysfunction have higher levels of brain natriuretic peptide, suggestive of cardiac remodeling. Increased renin gene and protein expression are found in donor kidneys, but the expression is virtually absent in the recipient kidneys,[191,192] implicating a role of the renin-angiotensin system in TTTS. Thus, the pathophysiology of sonographically defined TTTS is most likely multifactorial with vascular anastomoses providing the anatomic basis, whereas hemodynamic and hormonal factors contribute in varying degrees to its clinical development.

Early identification of the monochorionic twin pregnancies at increased risk of TTTS would assist patient counseling and planning of follow-up. As such, pregnancies at increased risk may be followed in a fetal medicine center, which is especially relevant in geographic settings in which access is problematic. Further, for dichorionic triplets, an increased risk in the first trimester might be an argument in favor of reduction of the monochorionic pair. Finally, timely treatment of TTTS might improve outcome by preventing PPROM and/or cervical shortening, which is an important risk factor for preterm birth.[193,194]

An increased nuchal translucency (NT) (>95th percentile) in at least one fetus during the 11 to 14 weeks' examination occurs in 13% of monochorionic twins and is a marker for chromosomal anomalies, cardiac defects, and a wide range of genetic syndromes. In monochorionic twins, an increased NT may reflect early cardiac dysfunction due to hypervolemic congestion in the recipient and, thus, herald the subsequent development of TTTS. Indeed, fetuses of monochorionic twin pregnancies with increased NT have a higher likelihood for the subsequent development of TTTS (likelihood ratio 3.5; 95% confidence interval [CI]

FIGURE 23–23
Ultrasound image of membrane folding in a monochorionic twin pregnancy, which reflects discordant amniotic fluid in a monochorionic twin pregnancy.

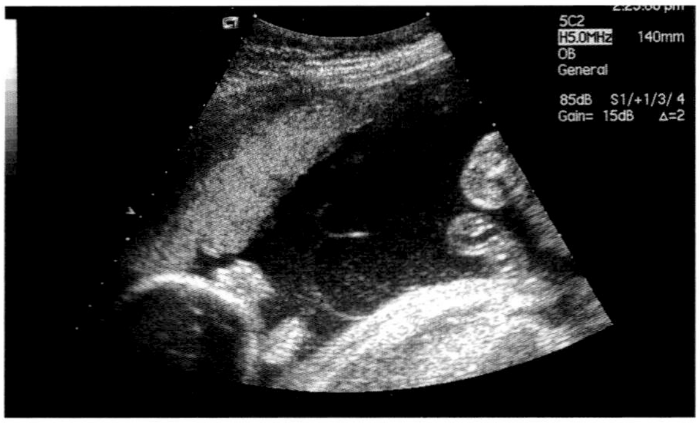

1.9–6.2).[195] However, the sensitivity of the NT measurement for TTTS is only 28%, with a positive predictive value of 33%. These figures were somewhat improved in a more recent study by the same group, in which an NT discordance of 20% or more detected 52% of cases with TTTS with a positive predictive value of 24%.[196] In the same series, the difference in crown-rump length (CRL) had a similar predictive value as NT discordance. However, two other studies did not confirm NT discordance to be a significant risk factor for the subsequent development of TTTS,[197,198] although both demonstrated the difference in CRL to be predictive. As such, difference in CRL of 6 mm or more detected 52% of cases TTTS with a positive predictive value of 19%. It seems unlikely that all TTTS cases will be predictable in the first trimester. The intertwin transfusion equilibrium is probably fragile and might become unbalanced at any stage in pregnancy without any warning. Further, TTTS may result from a random and asymmetrical reduction in vascular anastomoses with placental expansion later on in pregnancy.[199]

Folding of the intertwin membrane (Fig. 23–23) at 15 to 17 weeks may be a more promising sign for the prediction of TTTS. It is present in 32% of monochorionic twin pregnancies and believed to reflect oliguria and a reduced amniotic fluid in the sac of the donor. It is associated with an increased likelihood for the development of TTTS (likelihood ratio 4.2; 95% CI 3.0–6.0). Early mid-trimester membrane folding identifies 91% of TTTS with a positive predictive value of 43%.[195]

Another proposed marker for the prediction of TTTS is the absence of AA anastomoses. These anastomoses can be detected by color-flow mapping and pulsed Doppler[83] as early as 12 weeks, though the majority become detectable after 18 weeks.[200] The difficulty with using the absence of AA anastomoses as a prognostic sign is that it is impossible in early pregnancy to ascertain whether they are truly absent or just undetected. However, when an AA anastomosis is identified, 15% of monochorionic twin pregnancies develop TTTS compared with 61% when no AA anastomosis can be detected.

Finally, a velamentous cord insertion was suggested to increase the risk for TTTS, and cord insertions can be reliably determined at 16 weeks. Fries and colleagues[201] demonstrated a higher prevalence of velamentous cord insertion in TTTS placentas than in non-TTTS placentas, 32% and 9%, respectively. In another series, the combination of an eccentric cord insertion in one twin and a marginal or velamentous cord insertion in the other was more frequently seen in TTTS,[18] though several other studies failed to identify an association.[202,203] Discordant cord insertions reflect unequal placental sharing and, therefore, seem to increase the risk of discordant growth, but not the risk of TTTS.

Within the Eurofoetus consortium,[204] we developed a two-step sonographic scoring system in the first trimester and at 16 weeks to predict a complicated outcome, defined as the occurrence of TTTS, discordant growth, or intrauterine demise.[197] If the CRL difference is 12 mm or more or if there is discordant amniotic fluid in the first trimester, then the probability of a complicated fetal outcome is about 80% and the survival rate only 50%, as compared with an 80% uncomplicated outcome and a survival rate of 93% in the screen-negative group. At 16 weeks, significant predictors for a complicated fetal outcome were difference in abdominal circumference, discordant amniotic fluid, and discordant cord insertions. This two-step risk assessment in the first trimester and at 16 weeks identified a high risk group with a more than 70% risk of complicated outcome, in contrast to an 86% uncomplicated outcome in the group predicted to be at low risk. This information is useful for patient counseling and to identify patients who may benefit from follow-up in a dedicated fetal medicine center, especially in areas where access is limited.

Fetal Risks

Untreated, TTTS has been quoted to have a mortality of nearly 100%, although advances in neonatal care mortality rates may have decreased that rate to 63%.[205] Spontaneous abortion and extreme preterm birth are associated with hydramnios, and fetal demise may result from cardiac failure in the recipient or poor perfusion in the donor. Substantial cerebral and cardiac sequelae may occur in survivors owing to the chronic hemodynamic imbalances. Both the donor and the recipient are at risk of antenatally acquired cerebral lesions with, depending on the therapy used, reported incidences of 10%[206] to 50%.[207] In donor twins, hypovolemia, hypotension, and anemia may induce cerebral hypoxia and brain damage, whereas in the recipient, hyperviscosity and cardiac failure may impair cerebral perfusion. Again depending on the therapy used, the reported incidences of cerebral palsy and major neurologic deficiencies range from 6%[208] to 26%.[143]

The risks of neurologic damage are dramatically increased after an sIUFD when the vascular anastomoses remain patent, presumably due to acute exsanguination of the survivor into the fetoplacental unit of the deceased co-twin. MCA PSV measurement seems a reliable noninvasive method to detect anemia after sIUFD in TTTS.[138] Though it is tempting to intervene based on this finding, it remains to be demonstrated whether a rescue transfusion decreases risks of neurologic sequelae.[146]

Monochorionic twins with TTTS have a reported 8% prevalence of pulmonary valve stenosis in recipients, regardless of whether these pregnancies were treated primarily by amniodrainage or laser.[209,210] Further, up to 48% of survivors have signs of transient oliguric renal failure affecting the donor as well as the recipient, although long-term renal impairment does not appear to be a problem.[211] Also, limb,[212] gastrointestinal,[213] and cerebral infarctions[214] that preferentially affect the recipient are described and may originate from hyperviscosity or hypoperfusion.

Management Options

Laser Coagulation versus Amniodrainage

In view of the poor survival rates with conservative management, there is no disagreement that therapy should be offered. The two most commonly used therapies for midtrimester TTTS are amniodrainage and fetoscopic laser coagulation of the vascular anastomoses. However, since the Eurofetus randomized, controlled trial comparing laser treatment with amniodrainage, there is general consensus that the best treatment option for all stages of TTTS is currently laser coagulation of the vascular anastomoses.[140,215] Women with suspected TTS should be informed that amniodrainage should be reserved only for regions in which laser coagulation is not available and otherwise referred to a fetal medicine center that performs laser coagulation.

Before the advent of fetoscopic surgery, amniodrainage was the most commonly used treatment for TTTS. It controls the amniotic fluid volume, is relatively simple to perform, and is widely available. It was suggested the fetal condition might be improved by reducing the amniotic fluid pressure and perhaps enhancing uteroplacental perfusion.[216,217] The evidence for such benefit is scant. Decompression does appear to prolong pregnancy. However, amniodrainage does not address the vascular basis of TTTS and usually needs to be repeated several times to control the amniotic fluid volume. In addition, because it does not cure the disease, amniodrainage often leads to the preterm birth of two sick neonates, which increases their risk of neonatal mortality and morbidity.[218] Also, in the event of an sIUFD, the surviving twin is at high risk for anemia and neurologic sequelae.[138,214] Available data suggest that amniodrainage is "effective" only in mild cases of TTTS (stages I–II) and outright fails in a third. Such a high failure rate may indicate that its purported efficacy is a reflection of the disease's natural history. The overall perinatal survival rate with amniodrainage in uncontrolled series with cases diagnosed prior to 26 weeks was 57%.[205] This rate was confirmed in a literature review by Skupsi and associates[219] (double survival 50%; single survival rate 20%; total survival rate 61%). Worse yet, amniodrainage is associated with a 16% to 26% risk of severe sequelae in survivors.[143,205]

Whereas amniodrainage is a palliative and repetitive measure, fetoscopic laser coagulation of the vascular anastomoses seeks to address the underlying cause of the disease through a single intervention. Complete coagulation of all visible anastomotic occlusion results in the resolution of TTTS.[220] Most fetoscopic laser centers agree that coagulation of nonanastomosing vessels should be avoided whenever possible, because this increases the area of nonfunctional placental territory and, therefore, the risk of intrauterine demise.[221,222] Most centers have abandoned the nonselective technique of simply coagulating all vessels crossing the intertwin septum.[223] The vascular equator does usually not coincide with the membranous equator, and coagulation along the intertwin septum will, therefore, lead to unnecessary placental loss. In some monochorionic pregnancies with unequal placental sharing or a large shared part of the placenta, coagulation of all anastomoses may leave too little unshared placenta for one or both fetuses, leading to sIUFD or even dIUFD. As a result, most centers now are selective, coagulating all visibly communicating vessels between the two fetuses as well as the ones from which it could not be excluded that they are anastomosing (Fig. 23–24). A "hyperselective" approach, as discussed by Feldstein and coworkers,[224] coagulating only the causative AV anastomosis is interesting from a theoretical point of view because it is simply not possible to identify this anastomosis in the presence of others. Also, leaving certain anastomoses open places the remaining fetus at risk for hypovolemic events in case of sIUFD and might lead even to a reversal of transfusion.

FIGURE 23–24
Macroscopic image of a placenta at birth demonstrates "bichorionization" and laser impact (*arrows*) on the monochorionic placenta after laser coagulation for twin-twin transfusion syndrome.

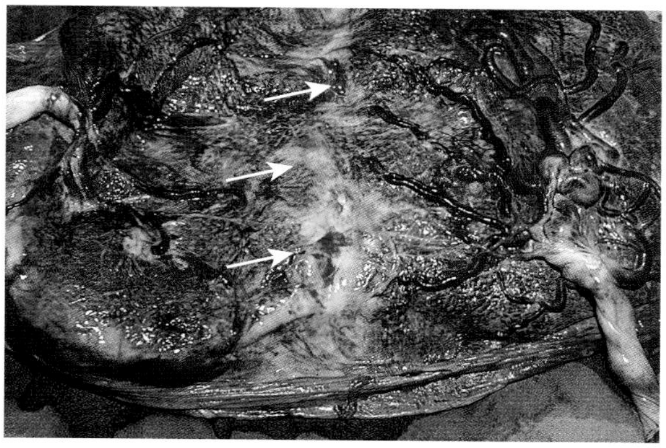

Two adaptations of the currently practiced technique have been suggested to improve survival rates. One is to draw a complete line of coagulation between the two vascular territories to avoid small and potentially invisible anastomoses (unpublished). Another is a sequential technique in which all AV anastomoses from the donor to the recipient are coagulated first in an attempt to minimize blood loss from the already hypovolemic donor and increase its survival rate.[225]

Laser coagulation is performed percutaneously (Fig. 23–25) under local or locoregional anesthesia. A cannula or fetoscopic sheath is inserted into the hydramniotic sac and the placenta inspected. For coagulation, the laser tip is directed toward the target vessels at as close to a 90-degree angle as possible, and with a nontouch technique, a 1- to 2-cm section of the selected vessel is photocoagulated (Fig. 23–26). At the conclusion, amniodrainage is performed until the amniotic fluid pockets on ultrasound are normal. With an anterior placenta, the amniotic sac as well as the vessels on the placenta might be more difficult to access. Some instruments have been purposely developed, but it is yet unclear whether they improve performance.[226] Placental localization does not appear to influence outcome.[227]

Few laser procedures have been reported before 16 weeks and after 26 weeks. Similar to amniocentesis, the minimum requirement for intervention should be chorioamniotic membrane fusion. Therefore, the lower limit for safe laser coagulation seems to be 15 weeks, when the use of a 1.2-mm scope is recommended to reduce membrane trauma. After 26 weeks, the procedure is more challenging because the amniotic fluid is often turbid and the anastomotic vessel much larger. Nevertheless, laser separation seems preferable to serial amniodrainage or elective preterm birth. Curing the disease prior to birth may indeed reduce the incidence of cerebral lesions.[228]

In uncontrolled series, the overall fetal survival has consistently been between 62% and 77%,[140,221] with a risk for long-term neurologic morbidity in survivors of 13% to 18%.[208,229] The Eurofetus research consortium granted by the European Commission was the first to conduct a randomized trial comparing serial amniodrainage withlaser coagulation as a primary therapy for TTTS prior to 26 weeks. The primary outcome measure was survival of at least one twin at 6 months of age, and the secondary outcome measure was intact neurologic survival (Table 23–1).[140] Compared with the amniodrainage group, the laser group had a higher likelihood of survival of at least one twin to 28 days of age (76.4% vs. 51.4%). Infants in the laser group also had a lower incidence of cystic periventricular leukomalacia (laser 6% vs. drainage 14%) and were more likely to be free of neurologic complications at 6 months of age (52% vs. 31%). A recent long-term follow-up study conducted in three European centers showed an incidence of neurodevelopmental impairment of 18% at the age of 2 years.[229] Cerebral palsy was diagnosed in 6%. Donors were similarly affected as recipients. Only a low gestational age at birth was independently associated with the risk of neurodevelopmental impairment.

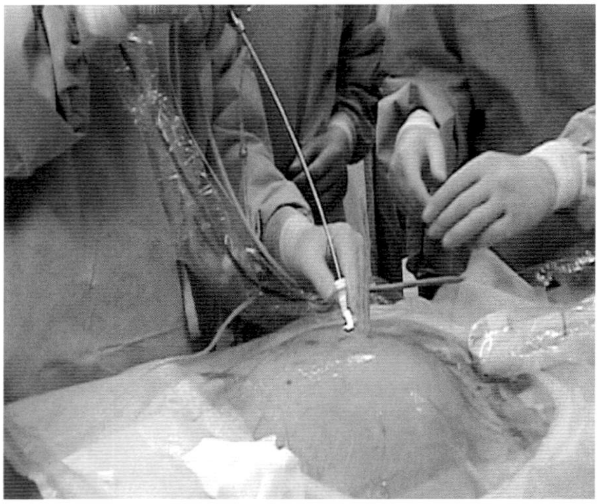

FIGURE 23–25
Image of the operative setup and percutaneous access used for fetoscopic interventions.

Another randomized controlled trial comparing laser with amniodrainage sponsored by the National Institutes of Health was stopped at 40 patients because of poor recruitment and was inconclusive.[230] Surprisingly, they reported a 70% intrauterine demise rate for the recipient and an overall survival rate of only 45% after laser treatment. A major difference with the European trial was that all patients underwent a test amniodrainage, and only patients who failed to respond were randomized. It is well established that an amniodrainage may hamper later laser treatment because of septostomy, intra-amniotic bleeding, or membrane detachment. The high mortality of the recipient might be due to the detrimental effect of the failed amniodrainage on recipient cardiac function. A recent meta-analysis that covered the Eurofetus trial as well as nine other observational cohorts concluded that laser as compared with amniodrainage was associated with an odds ratio of 2.0 for perinatal survival and 0.24 for short-term neurologic morbidity.[231] Recipients appear more likely to survive than donors. At present, laser coagulation is therefore the best available treatment and amniodrainage should be performed as an obstetric emergency in places in which there is no access to fetoscopic laser surgery or when

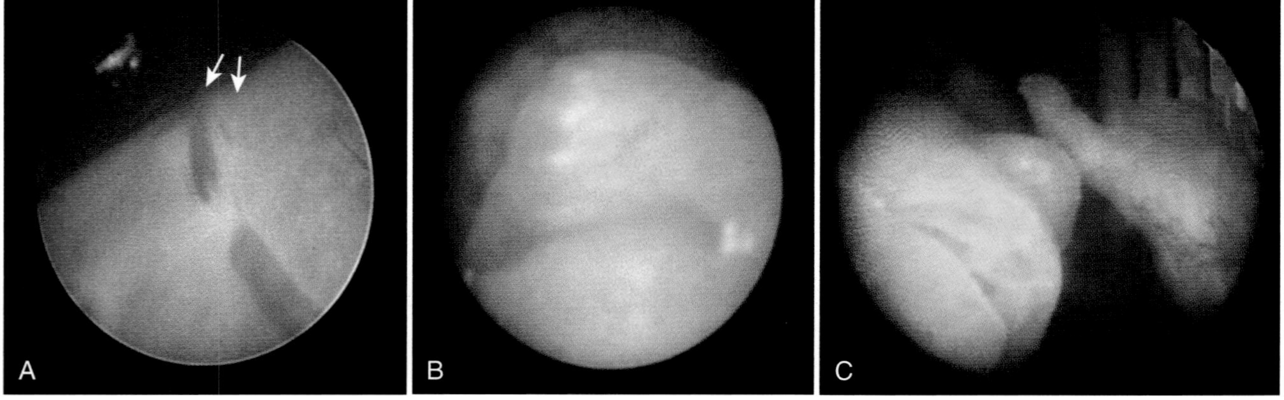

FIGURE 23–26
A, Fetoscopic image of laser coagulation of an arteriovenous anastomosis for twin-twin transfusion syndrome. *B*, Fetoscopic image of the hands of the donor twin, who is stuck behind the intertwin septum. *C*, Fetoscopic image of the face of the recipient, who moves freely in the hydramniotic sac.

TABLE 23-1

Randomized Controlled Trial of Fetoscopic Laser Surgery versus Serial Amniodrainage*

	LASER (*N* = 72)	AMNIOREDUCTION (*N* = 70)	*P* VALUE
Gestational age at randomization (wk)	20.6 (±2.4)	20.9 (±2.5)	ns
Quintero stage at randomization			
Stage 1	6 (8%)	5 (7%)	ns
Stage 2	31 (43%)	31 (44%)	ns
Stage 3	34 (47%)	33 (47%)	ns
Stage 4	1 (1%)	1 (1%)	ns
Number of procedures	1†	2.6 (±1.9)	–
Volume of amniotic fluid drained per procedure–mL‡			–
Median	1725	2000	
Range	500-5500	243-4000	
Total volume of amniotic fluid drained–mL‡			<.001
Median	1725	3800	
Range	500-5500	600-18,000	
Pregnancy loss at or within 7 days of the initial procedure	8 (12%)	2 (3%)	.10
Premature rupture of membranes at or within 7 days of the first procedure	4 (6%)	1 (1%)	.37
Premature rupture of membranes at or within 28 days of the first procedure	6 (9%)	6 (9%)	.98
Intrauterine death within 7 days of the first procedure§	16/138 (12%)	9/136 (7%)	.23
At least one survivor at 6 mo of life	55 (76%)	36 (51%)	.002
No survivors	17 (24%)	34 (49%)	
One survivor	29 (40%)	18 (26%)	
Two survivors	26 (36%)	18 (26%)	
At least one survivor at 6 mo stratified by stage			
Quintero stages I and II	32/37 (86%)	21/36 (58%)	.007
Quintero stages III and IV	23/35 (66%)	15/34 (44%)	.07
Gestational age at delivery–median (interquartile range)	33.3 (26.1-35.6)	29.0 (25.6-33.3)	.004
Neonatal and infant death	12 (8%)	41 (29%)	
Intraventricular hemorrhage (grades III-IV)‖	2 (1%)	8 (6%)	.10
Donor	2 (3%)	2 (3%)	1.0
Recipient	0 (0%)	6 (9%)	.02
Cystic periventricular leukomalacia¶	8 (6%)	20 (14%)	.02†
Donor	2/72 (3%)	5/70 (7%)	.27
Recipient	6/72 (8%)	15/70 (21%)	.03

* Baseline characteristics according to group, results reported as number of pregnancies (*n*), percentage, means (standard deviation [SD]).
† Two patients had two laser procedures.
‡ The median in the laser group is the median volume drained at the end of a single procedure.
§ With number of fetuses as denominator (*P* value adjusted for clustering).
‖ Severe intraventricular hemorrhage was defined as ventricular bleeding with dilation of the cerebral ventricles (grade III) or parenchymal hemorrhage (grade IV).
¶ Cystic periventricular leukomalacia was defined as periventricular densities evolving into extensive cystic lesions (grade III) or extending into the deep white matter evolving into cystic lesions (grade IV).
ns, not significant.
From Senat MV, Deprest J, Boulvain M, et al: Endoscopic laser surgery versus serial amnioreduction for severe twin-to-twin transfusion syndrome. N Engl J Med 2004;351:136–144.

elective preterm birth after lung maturation is an option.[232] Future randomized trial(s) probably will address the need to perform laser in stage I disease. Because of the low number of stage I cases in the Eurofetus randomized trial, expectant management might result in better survival rates by obviating the fetal loss associated with laser coagulation.[233] Nevertheless, these trial(s) will need to address the long-term neurodevelopmental outcome, because expectant management of stage I TTTS may result in better survival rates, but not necessarily in a better long-term neurodevelopmental outcome.

Potential Complications and Follow-up after Laser Treatment

PPROM remains the most important complication of any invasive antenatal procedure. After fetoscopic laser coagulation, the incidence of PPROM prior to 34 weeks is estimated to be 28%.[234] In 12%, PPROM occurred within 3 weeks after the procedure. At present, there is no validated method to prevent PPROM. First, there is the iatrogenic membrane defect that does not seem to close spontaneously. Perhaps because of its avascular nature and detachment from the decidua on the uterine wall, the amnion shows no sign of wound healing.[235] Second, there is probably an inflammatory response in the fetal membranes due to hydramnios (stretching) and the iatrogenic membrane defect. This may activate an enzymatic cascade that degrades the membranes and eventually leads to PPROM.[236] Although prophylactic patching of the membrane defect with collagen plugs seems promising in vitro[237] and in animal models,[238] its true role in clinical practice still needs to be established. The intra-amniotic injection of platelets may occasionally be successful to stop postoperative leakage, but it carries a risk of intrauterine demise or antenatal brain damage, probably due to the platelet release of vasoactive substances or to the formation of fibrinous bands that may constrict the umbilical cord.[239]

Preterm birth is, next to PPROM, a common cause for adverse outcome. In the Eurofetus randomized trial, one in five patients gave birth between 24 and 32 weeks' gestation. A short cervical length at the time of laser increases the likelihood of severe preterm birth.[194] An emergency cerclage immediately after laser in those patients with a cervical length of less than 15 mm may prolong the pregnancy and allow for a better outcome.[240]

In contrast to amniodrainage in which the demise of one or both fetuses often occurs remotely from the procedure, 60% of intrauterine deaths with laser are diagnosed within 48 hours and 75% within 1 week.[241] However, the surviving twin is far less likely to be anemic after laser[138] or to sustain neurologic sequelae[142] compared with survivors after amniodrainage[143] in which the anastomoses remain patent.

About 1 in 10 pregnancies of which both fetuses survive are complicated by persistent TTTS or develop TAPS.[242] These complications are most likely related to missed anastomoses,[220] which may occur in up to one third of placentas after laser treatment[243] and are usually situated near the edge of the placenta.[220,244] Missed large anastomoses may result in dIUFD or persistent TTTS, whereas missed small anastomoses may lead to iatrogenic TAPS.[220] The technique of drawing a complete coagulation line that separates the two vascular territories may reduce the number of missed anastomoses and will be tested in a randomized controlled trial.

Other fetal complications are uncommon but include limb reduction deformities,[212,245] cerebral anomalies,[214] intestinal atresia,[213] and congenital skin loss.[246,247] Each of these anomalies has been described in TTTS not treated by laser[212,248,249] and are probably related more to the disease process than the treatment.

Maternal safety should remain a priority, and serious maternal complications should be registered carefully in a registry, such as the one set up by Eurofetus.[250] Transient maternal mirror or Ballantyne's syndrome with pulmonary edema, placental abruption, chorioamnionitis, and bleeding requiring transfusion are reported, but none yet leading to maternal demise. Hecher and colleagues[251] demonstrated a learning curve and argue against scattering the experience over too many centers.

Intensive surveillance remains indicated for treated pregnancies because of the frequent occurrence of postoperative complications. We recommend weekly sonographic evaluation for the first month and then every 2 weeks thereafter. It is important that the PSV of the MCA be measured at each visit to detect postoperative TAPS, which typically occurs within the first 5 postoperative weeks. The demonstration of bladder filling and increasing amniotic fluid of the donor is a sign of TTTS resolution. Fluid usually takes a week to normalize in the donor twin, so equal fluid levels shortly after the procedure indicates that an accidental septostomy occurred during the procedure. It is important to look for possible cord entanglement thereafter and to check the limbs for any evidence of reduction deformities due to amniotic bands or to vascular insults, especially in the recipient. We also recommend detailed surveillance of the fetal brain. MRI appears more sensitive in detecting more subtle brain lesions, especially in the third trimester, and we therefore recommend a routine MRI to assess the fetal brain around 30 weeks' gestation. In cases in which severe antenatal brain damage is diagnosed, parents can be offered a late (selective) termination where jurisdiction permits. Cardiac assessment is important as well, because laser coagulation does not seem to prevent the occurrence of right ventricular outflow tract obstruction. In terms of monitoring fetal growth, there is usually a decrease in discordancy in successful procedures and more than half of the donors with growth restriction at the time of laser show catch-up growth, ultimately resulting in a normal birth weight.[252]

Alternative Management Options

Termination of the entire pregnancy may be justified based on the risk for adverse outcome and, although it is rarely pursued by parents, this option should be part of counseling. Selective feticide was suggested in 1993 as a way to try to salvage at least one twin in complicated cases of TTTS.[253] Selective feticide by bipolar cord occlusion has also been suggested for the treatment of stage III/IV TTTS.[254] This approach is certainly open for debate and the associated decisions difficult. It is not necessarily easy to determine which fetus will have the worst outcome, a major drawback because the maximum survival rate of selective feticide is 50%. At present, selective feticide should be reserved for instances of severe discordant anomalies, when imminent demise of one twin is anticipated, or in cases in which full visualization of the vascular equator is likely to be technically impossible. If in the future we are able to predict postoperative demise more accurately, then selective feticide might be a valid alternative to laser treatment in those cases with a high likelihood of recipient or donor demise.

Finally, it was suggested that intentional puncturing of the intertwin septum ("septostomy") with or without amniodrainage was beneficial by equilibrating the amniotic fluid volume. The technique is based on the observation that TTTS is rare in monoamniotic twins. It definitely increases the amniotic fluid volume in the donor's sac, but also creates an iatrogenic monoamniotic state with possibility of cord entanglement and might hamper subsequent laser therapy. Not surprisingly, a randomized controlled trial comparing amniodrainage to septostomy ($N = 14$) failed to identify any survival benefit with septostomy.[255] Therefore, septostomy is no longer recommended as treatment for TTTS.

SUMMARY OF MANAGEMENT OPTIONS

Twin-Twin Transfusion Syndrome (TTTS)

Management Options	Evidence Quality and Recommendation	References
Serial amniodrainage does prolong pregnancy and improves fetal condition by reduced intrauterine pressure, although it does not protect the surviving twin in the event of sIUFD and is only effective in mild cases of TTTS.	IIb/B	141
Laser coagulation, as compared with amniodrainage, has been shown to have better survival rates and neurologic outcome, and is therefore considered to be the best first-line treatment for TTTS in centers experienced in this technique.	Ib/A	140
Septostomy does not seem to have a survival benefit as compared with amniodrainage.	IIb/B	253
Selective feticide by cord occlusion does arrest the transfusion process and is indicated for TTTS with associated discordant anomalies or in rare cases of imminent fetal death, or when laser coagulation with full inspection of the vascular equator is technically not feasible.	III/B	254

sIUFD, single intrauterine fetal demise.

TWIN ANEMIA POLYCYTHEMIA SEQUENCE

General

TAPS refers to the occurrence of a chronic and severe hemoglobin discordancy in a monochorionic pair (hemoglobin ≤ 11 g/dL with reticulocytosis in the donor and hemoglobin ≥ 20 g/dL in the recipient), in the absence of the severe amniotic fluid discordance that fulfills the criteria for TTTS. It also results from an intertwin transfusion imbalance, but rather than discordant amniotic fluid, TAPS presents as chronic and severe intertwin hemoglobin discordance. Indeed, TAPS represents the "TTTS of the neonatologist," because it usually presents late in pregnancy and results in the birth of a large plethoric twin and usually small anemic twin that does not show signs of hypovolemic shock. Signs of chronic anemia in the donor and the absence of hypovolemic shock differentiate TAPS from acute intrapartum transfusion.[256] TTTS as it is known to the fetal medicine specialist with the predefined amniotic fluid discordances usually occurs in mid trimester and either is treated or leads to miscarriage and is therefore unknown to the neonatologist. TAPS can occur spontaneously in previously uncomplicated monochorionic twin pregnancies[41] or, as mentioned previously, after incomplete laser surgery as a treatment for TTTS[242] with small missed AV anastomoses.[220]

Iatrogenic TAPS is diagnosed antenatally by an elevated PSV of the MCA above 1.5 multiple of the median (MoM) in one twin (usually in the previous recipient) suggesting anemia and below 0.8 MoM in the other (usually in the previous donor) suggesting polycythemia.[242] Spontaneous TAPS occurs in about 5% of monochorionic twin pregnancies, usually after 30 weeks,[55] especially in pairs with progressive discordant growth after 26 weeks.[34] Also, TAPS may account for some late and previously unexplained intrauterine deaths.[55] It remains to be demonstrated whether measurement of the MCA PSV also identifies TAPS in these previously uncomplicated pregnancies. Nevertheless, MCA PSV measurements are an integral part of our routine follow-up of monochorionic twins.

The placentas of spontaneous TAPS pregnancies show a striking similarity to those of iatrogenic TAPS after incomplete laser surgery. Most spontaneous TAPS placentas have a few small (≤1 mm) unidirectional AV anastomoses without a compensating AA anastomosis,[41,220] suggesting that TAPS results from a slow net transfusion of blood across the tiny anastomoses that are typically present in these cases. Similar to TTTS, the donor may be relatively small compared with its placental territory, whereas the recipient twin may be relatively large, suggesting the intertwin transfusion imbalance in TAPS also reduces and increases the birth weight of the donor and recipient, respectively.[41]

Fetal Risks

TAPS may be involved in the etiology of previously unexplained late intrauterine demise.[55,119] Severe anemia may result in hydrops and intrauterine death of the donor, whereas at least theoretically, severe polycythemia may cause cardiac failure or vascular accidents and death in the recipient. In contrast to TTTS, fetal loss due to miscarriage prior to 20 weeks is less common because TAPS usually occurs in the third trimester and severe hydramnios is unusual.

Management Options

The optimal management of iatrogenic as well as spontaneous TAPS is unknown. Depending on the characteristics of each individual case, such as gestational age, recurrence after intrauterine transfusion, fetal hemodynamic condition, and placental localization, definitive management may consist of elective birth, cord occlusion, or fetoscopic laser coagulation.[242] For fetoscopic laser, the surgeon should be aware that visibility may be impaired by the lack of severe hydramnios and the advanced gestational age at which TAPS usually presents. Conversely, usually only few and tiny anastomoses will need to be coagulated.

CONGENITAL ANOMALIES IN TWINS

General

Structural Anomalies

Structural anomalies are 1.2 to 2 times more common in twins than in singletons. Unfortunately, most studies do not subgroup incidence by either zygosity or placentation. Nevertheless, probably the rate per fetus in dizygotic twins is the same as that in singletons, whereas it is two to three times higher in monozygotic twins.[73] Abnormalities associated with twins include neural tube defects, brain lesions, facial clefts, gastrointestinal defects, anterior abdominal wall defects, and cardiac anomalies.[257] Even in monozygotic twins, concordance (both fetuses similarly affected) for a structural anomaly is rare (<20%).[74] Further, discordance for genetic diseases is frequently reported in monozygotic twins and may reflect variations in gene expression secondary to postzygotic mutation, parental imprinting effects, asymmetrical X inactivation,[35] and differential DNA methylation.[258] The exact mechanism of the increased prevalence of structural anomalies in monozygotic twins remains largely unknown, although several mechanisms are proposed. It is possible the twinning process itself is teratogenic owing to an unequal distribution of the inner cell mass or to cleavage after laterality gradients have already been determined, resulting in such abnormalities as midline defects.[35] Vascular events in early embryogenesis and later fetal life might account for part of the observed discordant brain and heart anomalies. In our prospective series of 202 monochorionic twin pairs, major discordant congenital anomalies occurred in 6% and always affected only one twin.[55] The prevalence of cardiac anomalies in monochorionic twins is reported to be 2.3% in those without TTTS, and 7% in those with TTTS, compared with 0.6% in the general population. Pulmonary valve stenosis in recipients accounts for all the additional congenital heart defects found in TTTS cases, suggesting a causative role for the hemodynamic imbalance. The global prevalence of congenital heart defects in monochorionic twins (3.9%) is thus comparable with that in a family with a history of congenital heart disease (2.5%). Therefore, detailed echocardiography is indicated in both the second and the third trimesters, because pulmonary artery stenosis is a dynamic process that may evolve until birth.[209] Anomalies unique to monochorionic twins are the TAPS sequence and conjoined twinning as discussed previously.

Chromosomal Anomalies

RISKS OF CHROMOSOMAL ABNORMALITIES

In dizygotic twins, the age-related risk of Down syndrome for one twin is independent of the risk for the other and should be the same as in singletons. Therefore, the risk of at least one fetus having Down syndrome should theoretically be double that in singletons. Whereas chorionicity can be accurately determined during the first trimester, there are no noninvasive means to establish zygosity antenatally. Nonetheless, dichorionic twins are dizygotic in about 90% of cases, and all dichorionic twins are, for risk assessment, considered to be dizygotic. In a dichorionic twin pregnancy, the age-related risk of at least one twin having Down syndrome can then be calculated by adding the age-related risks together (e.g., for a 40-year-old woman: $1/100 + 1/100 = 1/50$), whereas the risk of both fetuses being affected is obtained by multiplying the age-related risks ($1/100 \times 1/100 = 1/10{,}000$).

In a monochorionic (and, by definition, monozygotic) twin pregnancy, the age-related risk is the same for both twins and similar to that in singletons with usually both twins affected, although discordances in the phenotypic expression of the aneuploidy are frequently observed.[259,260] It is important to note that, though rare, even monochorionic twins may be discordant for chromosomal anomalies and discordancy for nearly all common human aneuploidies (trisomy 13,[70] trisomy 21,[71] monosomy 45, X[261]) is reported. Most involve one twin with Turner's syndrome and the other twin with either a female or a male phenotype but a mosaic karyotype. This rare phenomenon is called "heterokaryotypic monozygotism," and it reflects either a postzygotic mitotic event (nondisjunction or anaphase lag) or prezygotic meiotic errors. Several mechanisms may be involved. The zygote may initially have been karyotypically normal (46), but a trisomic (47) and monosomic cell line (45) develop due to a mitotic nondisjunction or anaphase lag. Conversely, the zygote may initially have been trisomic (47), but a diploid cell line (46) may be established due to a mitotic disjunction or anaphase lag, a phenomenon known as "trisomic rescue." At the blastocyst stage, the embryo proper originates from only three to five progenitor cells, and cleavage at this stage will give rise to monochorionic twinning. If a mitotic error takes place in any of these cells, it may actually trigger the twinning process with the proliferative advantaged diploid cell line separating out the aneuploid progenitors (Fig. 23–27). If the aneuploidy is nonviable, then this aneuploid "twin" will vanish without leaving any detectable remnants.[262] However, if the aneuploidy is viable, it may give rise to hetorokaryotypic monozygotic twins.

SCREENING FOR ANEUPLOIDIES IN TWINS

Screening for aneuploidy is more complex in multiple pregnancies than in singletons because, although selective

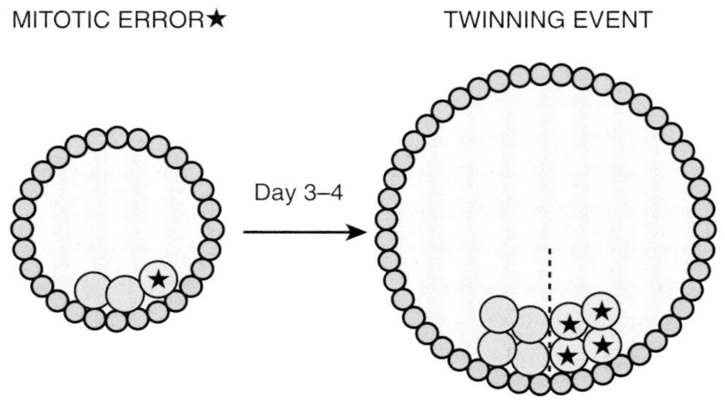

FIGURE 23–27
Illustration of mitotic error in an initially euploid zygote leading to a twinning event.
(Courtesy of T. Van den Bosch.)

feticide is an option if only one fetus is affected, the procedures can cause the loss of the unaffected co-twin. It is essential the parents are adequately counseled on the pros and cons of screening in multiple pregnancy. The screening tests should have good detection rates and an acceptably low false-positive rate, because invasive testing carries a higher risk and is technically more challenging in multiple pregnancy.

Second-trimester serum screening for aneuploidy has disappointingly low detection rates in twins (45% for a 5% screen-positive rate), presumably because the altered biochemical markers of the aneuploid fetoplacental unit are masked by the presence of an euploid co-twin. Also, serum screening provides only the risk of at least one affected fetus being affected (pregnancy-specific risk) and cannot identify which fetus is at increased risk (fetus-specific risk). In contrast, first-trimester nuchal translucency measurement has higher detection rates, identifies the fetus at increased risk, and allows for a selective feticide in the first trimester. It is, therefore, the preferred screening method in twins. The combination of NT with first-trimester serum biochemistry further increases the detection rate. In a 3-year review of combined NT and serum screening in the first trimester on 230 twin pregnancies, detection rates of Down syndrome were 75%, with 7% of fetuses and 9% of pregnancies (with at least one fetus) having a risk above 1 in 300.[263]

Although combined NT and biochemistry screening allows a fetus-specific risk, it seems logical to quote only one risk for monochorionic fetuses (pregnancy-specific risk), because both will be affected or both will be unaffected in nearly all cases. Quoting the risk of the fetus with the largest NT may overestimate the true risk, especially because an increased NT in one twin of a monochorionic pair may be an early sign of unbalanced intertwin transfusion.[195] Screening for Down syndrome in a monochorionic pair is best achieved by quoting the average of the two NT measurements.[264] Conversely, for dichorionic twins, it makes sense to quote the fetus-specific risk, although it is probably more relevant to the parents to hear what the risk is that at least one fetus will be affected (pregnancy-specific), which is obtained by adding the two fetus-specific risks. The risk that both are affected is extremely rare and, as mentioned previously, is obtained by multiplying the two fetus-specific risks.

INVASIVE PRENATAL TESTING IN TWINS

Fetal karyotyping requires invasive testing by either amniocentesis or chorionic villus sampling (CVS). Because these procedures are technically more demanding in multiple pregnancies, they should be performed in tertiary referral centers. The choice of technique depends on the procedure-related risk, the accuracy of obtaining a result from both fetuses, and technical circumstances. Although genetic amniocentesis is a well-accepted procedure, it remains unclear whether the postprocedural loss is higher in twins than in singletons, and whether the risk increases with increasing number of fetuses. Historically, amniocentesis in twin pregnancies was considered to have higher procedure-related loss rates (2.7%–8.1%).[265] However, this may be largely attributable to the higher background risk of fetal loss in twins (6%)[266] rather than to the procedure. As such, Ghidini and associates[267] observed that amniocentesis in experienced hands did not increase loss rates significantly. Conversely, Yukobowitz and coworkers[268] reported loss rates within 4 weeks after the procedure using a double uterine puncture that were five times higher in twins (2.6%) than in singletons (0.6%) and unexposed twins (0.6%).

Several methods can be used to ensure that all fetuses are correctly sampled. No method is demonstrably superior, and the choice reflects operator preference. In any event, great care must be taken to note distinguishing features, such as gender, placental localization, umbilical cord insertion, and fetal positions. A diagram should be made to prevent the potentially disastrous consequence of incorrect sampling. Samples should also be meticulously labeled. Amniocentesis in twins can be done through a single or double uterine entry. With the double-needling technique, each sac is sampled separately and consecutively. The injection of dyes after sampling of the first sac to ensure it is sampled only once is no longer recommended. Methylene blue is contraindicated because of its well-documented fetal risks, such as intestinal atresia, hemolytic anemia, and fetal demise.[269] Methylene is a classic, nonselective pharmacologic inhibitor of soluable guanylate cyclase, and the resulting vasospasm may explain the adverse events. Although no similar fetal risks are reported with indigo carmine, it has serotonergic properties[270] that in theory may lead to hypertension and bradycardia and is thus best avoided. A less commonly used technique is the double-needle simultaneous visualization technique.[271] An amniocentesis needle is advanced into the first cavity while a second needle is introduced into the other amniotic cavity without altering the position of the transducer. This technique permits visualization of both needles simultaneously on either site of the septum, but necessitates the presence of two operators. Finally, a single uterine entry technique is described in which the needle is first advanced into the proximal sac and fluid aspirated.[272] The stylet is replaced, and under direct visualization, the needle is advanced through the septum into the second sac. After discarding the first 1 mL of fluid to avoid contamination, a sample is aspirated from the second sac. This technique has the advantage of creating only one membrane defect and, to date, no cytogenetic errors have been reported, although there is the theoretical concern of contamination and the creation of an iatrogenic monoamniotic pregnancy.

CVS in multiple pregnancy can be performed using either the transabdominal approach, the transcervical approach, or a combination of the two. In the hands of an experienced operator, the loss rate attributable to CVS in twins may be comparable with that after amniocentesis. However, cytogenetic results are incorrect in 1.5% to 2% of cases because of contamination of one sample with villi from the other, placental mosaicism, culture failure, or sampling the same fetus twice. As a result, the resampling rate approximates 2%. To reduce the rate of incorrect sampling, it is imperative that placental localizations are accurately mapped and the extreme ends of each placenta preferentially sampled. For example, in those cases with a lower and an upper placenta, a combined technique with a transcervical approach for the lower placenta and a transabdominal approach of the upper placenta may be used.

Which technique (amniocentesis or CVS) should be used and should both be sampled? The answer largely depends on chorionicity and the risk of one or both being affected. For dichorionic twins, both CVS and amniocentesis are valuable options. Because CVS can be performed in the first trimester, selective feticide in the event of discordant chromosomal anomaly can be done at an earlier stage with the potential for a reduced risk for the healthy co-twin. Conversely, it may be preferable to restrict CVS to fetuses at especially high risk because the higher rates of contamination (e.g., first-trimester screening risk > 1/50), and defer invasive testing to 15 weeks for amniocentesis in lower risk cases. It is generally recommended both fetuses be sampled. Even though only one has an increased NT or anomaly, 10% of dichorionic twins are monozygotic. Amniocentesis is preferred to CVS in monochorionic twins, because rare heterokaryotypic monozygotic twins can be diagnosed only by sampling both sacs. Only if monochorionicity is accurately documented in the first trimester and none of the twins shows any discordant features is it possibly justifiable to sample only one fetus (by CVS or amniocentesis). In heterokaryotypic monozygotic twins, CVS of the common placenta may show mosaicism, a normal or abnormal karyotype, depending on the type and timing of postzygotic event.[70,72] If trisomic rescue is the mechanism involved, then the diploid fetus will have a one in three risk of uniparental disomy (UPD) for the specific chromosomal pair that is trisomic in its co-twin. UPD, om which both chromosomes in a pair are inherited from the same parent, will produce an abnormal phenotype if the involved chromosomal pair carries an imprinted region/gene or homozygous recessive mutation.[273] The presence of UPD should be excluded in heterokaryotic monozygotic twins. Counseling may be very difficult in heterokaryotypic twins because it is not possible to exclude the presence of hidden, but phenotypically important, mosaicism in the twin with normal karyotype on amniotic fluid cells. Cordocentesis is of little help in monochorionic twins because blood chimerism is invariably present, making genotyping of lymphocytes unreliable.

Fetal Risks

In dichorionic twins, the presence of a discordant anomaly usually does not affect the well-being of the other twin unless associated with hydramnios (such as anencephaly, duodenal atresia) or spontaneous demise, which increases the risk of preterm birth for the healthy co-twin. An ethical dilemma arises when elective preterm birth for ex utero treatment or antenatal invasive procedures with risk of iatrogenic PPROM (such as shunt placement) to ameliorate the outcome for the affected twin places the normal co-twin at risk of iatrogenic preterm birth. In contrast to dichorionic twins, the spontaneous demise of the anomalous twin may have disastrous consequences in a monochorionic twin pregnancy, because in addition to the consequences of severe preterm birth, it may lead to acute exsanguination of the healthy co-twin with dIUFD in about 12% and cerebral damage in 18%.[79]

Management Options

There are essentially three management options for discordant structural and chromosomal anomalies:

- Conservative management.
- Selective feticide.
- Termination of the whole pregnancy..

Paramount to safe management is an accurate determination of chorionicity in the first trimester because the methods for selective feticide differ between mono- and dichorionic twins.

Management in Dichorionic Twins

In cases in which the abnormality is nonlethal but might well result in serious handicap, parents must decide whether the burden of a handicapped child is enough to risk the loss of the healthy twin from feticide-related complications. In cases in which the abnormality is lethal, it may be best to avoid such risk and conservative management is preferable, unless the condition threatens the well-being of the healthy twin. Such a dilemma is illustrated by dichorionic twins discordant for anencephaly, which is always lethal but the associated hydramnios places the healthy co-twin at risk of severe preterm birth. However, expectant management in such cases is shown to have a favorable outcome for the unaffected fetus in dichorionic twins, with about half developing hydramnios and none delivering before 28 weeks (mean 36 wk).[274,275] Nevertheless, selective feticide appears associated with a higher gestational age at birth for similar perinatal survival rates.[276]

Selective feticide in dichorionic twins is performed by intracardiac or intrafunicular injection of potassium chloride/lidocaine under continuous ultrasound guidance. It is of utmost importance to ascertain that the correct fetus is terminated by identification of gender differences, obvious structural anomalies, placental localizations, and umbilical cord insertions. The risks of selective termination are loss of the entire pregnancy and preterm birth. The overall loss rate reported by the International Selective Feticide Registry of 402 multiple pregnancies including some higher-order multiple pregnancies is 7.5%. A breakdown by gestation (5.4% at 9–12 wk; 8.7% at 13–18 wk; and 6.8% at 19–24 wk) reveals no significant differences, but a suggestion of an increase after 13 weeks. Preterm birth before 33 weeks occurred in 22%, with 6% delivering between 25 and 28 weeks.[277] One center with 200 selective feticides reported an overall loss rate of only 4%, with significantly higher loss rates in triplets or higher-order multiplets (11%) than those in twins (2.4%), with 16% of patients delivering before 32 weeks.[278] This underlines the importance of referring to experienced centers. Some have suggested deferring selective feticide to 28 to 32 weeks in order to reduce loss rates, but this is an option only in countries in which late termination is legal and this is emotionally more difficult for both parents and doctors to accept. In one series of 23 dichorionic twins with a discordant nonlethal anomaly, there were no fetal losses and all patients delivered beyond 35 weeks.[279]

Selective Feticide in Monochorionic Twins

For selective feticide in monochorionic twins, the conventional techniques of potassium chloride/lidocaine injection used in multichorionic pregnancies cannot be used because the agent can reach the other fetus by the obligatory anastomoses.[280] In addition, patent intertwin vessels may lead to acute fetofetal hemorrhage into the terminated twin's fetoplacental unit, placing the surviving twin at risk for central nervous system damage or co-twin demise.[128] Therefore, the appropriate techniques arrest and isolate the target twin's circulation completely and permanently,[281] although all have considerably higher risks for fetal loss and very early PPROM compared with systemic injection of an agent. Further, while expectant management may be preferable in dichorionic twins with an expected spontaneous demise of the anomalous twin, monochorionic gestations specifically warrant a preventive selective feticide. This is particularly relevant for discordant chromosomal anomalies in which aneuploidy has a high spontaneous intrauterine demise rate.[282,283]

As discussed in the section on the management of TRAP, the preferred method for selective feticide is cord occlusion by either laser or bipolar coagulation. The initially reported method of umbilical cord embolization using a variety of agents, including absolute alcohol, coils, and enbucrilate gel, is no longer recommended in light of failure rates exceeding 60%.[173,284] Anecdotal successes are reported, but dIFD is unfortunately common, probably owing to incomplete vascular obliteration or migration of the sclerosants or thrombogenic products to the co-twin.

Fetoscopic cord ligation is already a historical technique, although it does cause immediate, complete, and permanent interruption of both arterial and venous flow in the umbilical cord. Though co-twin survival rates are over 70% when done fetoscopically,[285] these procedures are quite cumbersome with a high risk for PPROM. In comparison, laser cord coagulation (Fig. 23–28) is a relatively simple and straightforward procedure and uses similar instruments and setup as for coagulation of the vascular anastomoses in TTTS. It is the preferred method, especially before 21 weeks. It can be performed as early as 16 weeks, using a double needle loaded with a 1.0-mm fetoscope and a 400-μm laser fiber.[286] However, it may be difficult to coagulate the umbilical cord at later gestational ages.

For this reason, bipolar energy was explored. Initially, a large-diameter forceps was used, but now purpose-designed devices of 3.0 mm or less are on the market as well as adapted cannulas and trocars. Most procedures can be done with a single port under ultrasound guidance (Fig. 23–29), but rarely an ancillary port is used for the fetoscope to identify the correct umbilical cord (e.g., monoamniotic twins). Under ultrasound guidance, a portion of the umbilical cord is grasped at the abdominal wall, at its placental insertion, or at any other appropriate place in order to ensure correct identification and enhance stability. We try to work completely within the sac of the target fetus and use amnioinfusion only where needed. Direct contact with the placenta, fetus, or membranes is avoided. Coagulation starts at power settings of 15 W applied for approximately 15 seconds with progressive increments of 5 W until the appearance of turbulence and steam bubbles indicative of local heat production and, hence, eventual tissue coagulation between the forceps' blades (usually between 30 and 45 W). Higher initial energy settings are avoided to prevent tissue carbonization, which may lead to the cord becoming stuck to the forceps' blades and eventual cord perforation. Confirmation of arrest of flow distal to the occlusion is performed by color Doppler after the forceps is freed from the umbilical cord by gentle manipulation. Even if there is no longer any visible

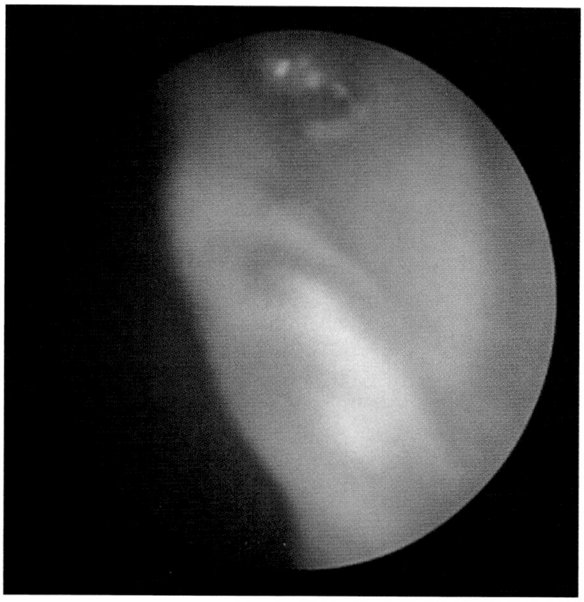

FIGURE 23–28
Fetoscopic image of laser cord coagulation.

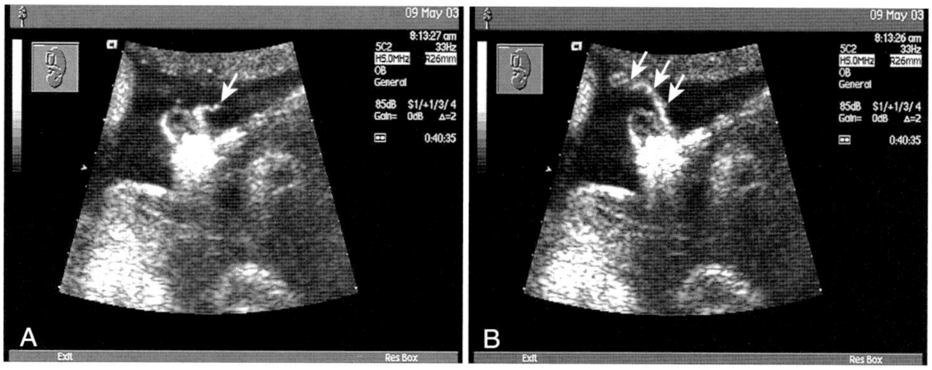

FIGURE 23–29
A, Ultrasound image of a bipolar cord coagulation in a monochorionic twin pregnancy. *B*, Ascending steam bubbles (*arrows*) confirm adequate coagulation impact.

flow, two additional cord segments (preferentially at a site more proximal toward the target fetus) are coagulated. This is an additional safety precaution, because absence of Doppler flow may be caused by temporary vasospasm or asystole rather than by true vascular obliteration. We now fetoscopically inspect all coagulation sites for completeness. In monoamniotic twins or after septostomy, the cord is first coagulated and then transected with laser in contact mode to avoid later cord entanglement. After completion of the procedure, amniodrainage of excessive fluid is carried out before removal of the cannula. PSV of the MCA is measured postoperatively to detect any fetal anemia.

In our initial series of 10 affected pregnancies, 2 patients had PPROM and underwent termination. The other 8 patients delivered at a mean gestational age of 35 weeks (>15 wk after the procedure).[169] Nicolini and colleagues[287] reported their experience with 17 cases. The survival rate was 81% (13/16 survivors; 1 patient had a termination of pregnancy because of an abnormality diagnosed later in gestation). There was 1 fetal hemorrhage caused by cord perforation, which is a complication of too much energy. We reported the outcome of 80 consecutive cord coagulations in complicated monochorionic multiplets (including 7 triplets) by laser and/or bipolar coagulation performed between 16 and 28 weeks (mean 21 wk).[288] Indications were TRAP (27.5%), discordant anomaly (35%), severe TTTS (30%), and selective growth restriction (7.5%). In 70%, the laser was used as the primary technique; additional bipolar was necessary in about half of cases. Overall survival was 83% with normal neurodevelopmental outcome in 92% of infants. Persistent PPROM occurred in 38%, and if prior to 25 weeks, this was associated with a mortality of 80%. There were no serious maternal complications, except for one mild transient mirror or Ballantyne's syndrome. Five cases involved heterokaryotypic monochorionic twins (46, XY/47,XY,+21; 46, XX/47,XX,+13; 46,XY/45,X; 2 46,XX/45,X), and umbilical cord occlusion resulted in a successful outcome in all 5 cases. All 5 surviving children were phenotypically normal at birth (range 34–40 wk) and are developing normally.[72] Robyr and associates[289] reported their experience with umbilical cord coagulation in 46 consecutive cases. They reported a 72% survival rate. In their series, there was a higher incidence of intrauterine demise in procedures performed prior to 18 weeks.

Putting all the previously mentioned series together, the overall survival of umbilical cord coagulation is about 80%. About half of the losses are attributable to intrauterine demise of the healthy co-twin and about half to postnatal losses due to very preterm birth, mostly related to PPROM. Again, about half of the intrauterine deaths occur within 24 hours of surgery, and may reflect either intraoperative vessel perforation, incomplete cord coagulation by laser coagulation, or exsanguination of the surviving twin into the placenta of the dead twin, which may be especially relevant prior to 18 weeks when the placental mass is still relatively large compared with the fetal mass. Late intrauterine death has been diagnosed up to 10 weeks after the procedure and was commonly related to cord entanglement after septostomy. This finding supports the use of cord transection after septostomy or in monoamniotic gestations. Postoperative anemia diagnosed by MCA PSV measurements within 24 hours and requiring an intrauterine transfusion occurred in 2% to 3% of cases and resulted in a normal outcome in all instances.

Similar to the treatment for TTTS, PPROM is an important complication of umbilical cord coagulation, accounting for miscarriage, severe preterm birth, neonatal death, and developmental delay. We demonstrated a significant decrease from 42% to 6% in PPROM prior to 31 weeks with increasing experience, which again underscores the need to restrict this procedure to a limited number of hands.[290] To avoid the risks of early PPROM for the healthy co-twin, it may be preferable to defer selective feticide until after 24 weeks in highly selected cases of discordant anomaly in which the risk of spontaneous intrauterine demise is small (such as in severe discordant central nervous system, genitourinary, skeletal anomaly). Bipolar coagulation can then be performed using the 3.0-mm forceps by overstretching the blades, whereupon the forceps opens more widely to accommodate for the larger cord diameter. We reported on a consecutive series of five cases in which selective feticide was performed between 26 to 30 weeks' gestation. All deliveries occurred beyond 31 weeks (range 31–37 wk). All infants survived, except for one unrelated neonatal demise of a child born at 36 weeks due to a complication of failed therapy for pulmonary stenosis.[290]

It remains to be demonstrated whether needle-based intrafetal coagulation techniques[291,292] are as effective to achieve selective feticide for discordant monochorionic twins as for TRAP. As such, radiofrequency ablation for non-TRAP indications resulted in an overall survival rate of only 60% (9/15 fetuses intended to continue).[293–295] Similar survival rates were reported after intrafetal laser coagulation.[296] Although these techniques perform well in the low-flow conditions of acardiac twins in TRAP, they may fail in the normal flow conditions of a monochorionic twin with a discordant anomaly. Accordingly, larger series with long-term neurodevelopmental follow-up are necessary to establish the efficacy of intrafetal coagulation for non-TRAP monochorionic pathologies.

Currently, it is not possible to state the single best method for selective feticide in monochorionic pregnancies. The surgeon should be familiar with several techniques in order to tailor therapy to the individual requirements of each case. Generally, we recommend laser fetoscopic cord coagulation as a primary technique before 21 weeks, whereas beyond 21 weeks, laser or bipolar coagulation can be used depending on cord diameter.[297] Cord ligation should be available as back up should all other methods fail. These procedures should be performed in experienced tertiary referral centers to ensure a large enough caseload. Also, the surviving twin should be followed carefully throughout pregnancy and after birth with the minimum of an early neonatal brain scan and developmental assessment at 1 year of age.

Issues Applicable to Monochorionic and Dichorionic Twins

As for singletons, Rh prophylaxis should be given in all instances of invasive antenatal procedures in Rh-negative women in which the fetal genotype is unknown. As with the intrauterine death of one twin, the incidence of maternal disseminated intravascular coagulation appears rare and routine checks of coagulation parameters may therefore be unnecessary. From 20 weeks onward, the use of fetal analgesia or anesthesia by administration of fentanyl or other opioid alternative should be considered prior to feticide to reduce fetal awareness and pain sensation.[298] To many people, any deliberate termination of a fetus is controversial and the decision to proceed to selective feticide may be difficult. Therefore, psychological support and counseling for the family is strongly recommended before and after the selective feticide.

Acknowledgment

Dr. L. Lewi is beneficent from a grant of the European Commission in its 5th Framework Programme (#QLG1-CT-2002-01632 EuroTwin2Twin). The other members of the EuroTwin2Twin Consortium are thanked for setting up the group: Y. Ville (Poissy), K. Hecher (Hamburg), E. Gratacos (Barcelona), R. Vlietinck (Leuven), M. van Gemert (Amsterdam), G. Barki (Tuttlingen), K. Nicolaides (London), R. Denk (Munchen), and C. Jackson (London).

SUMMARY OF MANAGEMENT OPTIONS

Congenital Abnomalies in Twins

Management Options	Evidence Quality and Recommendation	References
Issues Applicable to All Twins		
Options	—/GPP	—
Conservative management.		
Selective feticide of the abnormal fetus.		
Termination of the pregnancy.		
Offer counseling and psychological support.	—/GPP	—
Accurate chorionicity determination is essential.	IIb/B	20,21
Anti-D prophylaxis for procedures.	—/GPP	—
Dichorionic Twins		
Conservative management is usually preferred if the condition is lethal to avoid intervention loss rates.	III/B	279
Selective feticide is performed by intracardiac or intrafunicular injection of KCl.	III/B	279
Loss of the healthy fetus occurs in about 7.5% with delivery before 33 wk in 22%.	III/B	277,279
Monochorionic Twins		
Conditions with a high risk of IUFD may indicate selective feticide.	—/GPP	—
Selective feticide is performed by cord occlusion (to avoid the loss of normal co-twin if KCl used).	III/B	281,290
After cord occlusion, the healthy fetus survives in about 80%, with 80% delivering after 32 wk.	III/B	290
Careful follow-up of surviving normal twin.	—/GPP	—

GPP, good practice point; IUFD, intrauterine fetal demise.

SUGGESTED READINGS

Allen VM, Windrim R, Barrett J, Ohlsson A: Management of monoamniotic twin pregnancies: A case series and systemic review of the literature. BJOG 2001;108:931–936.

Denbow ML, Cox P, Taylor M, et al: Placental angioarchitecture in monochorionic twin pregnancies: Relationship to fetal growth, fetofetal transfusion syndrome, and pregnancy outcome. Am J Obstet Gynecol 2000;182:417–426.

Eddleman KA, Stone JL, Lynch L, Berkowitz RL: Selective termination of anomalous fetuses in multifetal pregnancies: Two hundred cases at a single center. Am J Obstet Gynecol 2002;187:1168–1172.

Gratacós E, Lewi L, Muñoz B, et al: A classification system for selective intrauterine growth restriction in monochorionic pregnancies according to umbilical artery Doppler flow in the smaller twin. Ultrasound Obstet Gynecol 2007;30:28–34.

Lenclen R, Paupe A, Ciarlo G, et al: Neonatal outcome in preterm monochorionic twins with twin-to-twin transfusion syndrome after intrauterine treatment with amnioreduction or fetoscopic laser surgery: Comparison with dichorionic twins. Am J Obstet Gynecol 2007;196:450.e1–450.e7.

Lewi L, Blickstein I, Van Schoubroeck D, et al: Diagnosis and management of heterokaryotypic monochorionic twins. Am J Med Genet A 2006;140:272–275.

Lewi L, Gucciardo L, Huber A, et al: Clinical outcome and placental characteristics of monochorionic diamniotic twin pairs with early- and late-onset discordant growth. Am J Obstet Gynecol 2008;199:511.e1–511.e7.

Lopriore E, Ortibus E, Acosta-Rojas R, et al: Risk factors for neurodevelopment impairment in twin-twin transfusion syndrome treated with fetoscopic laser surgery. Obstet Gynecol 2009;113:361–366.

Senat MV, Deprest J, Boulvain M, et al: Endoscopic laser surgery versus serial amnioreduction for severe twin-to-twin transfusion syndrome. N Engl J Med 2004;351:136–144.

Tan TY, Sepulveda W: Acardiac twin: A systematic review of minimally invasive treatment modalities. Ultrasound Obstet Gynecol 2003;22:409–419.

REFERENCES

For a complete list of references, log onto www.expertconsult.com.

CHAPTER 24

Fetal Hydrops

JOHN S. SMOLENIEC

Videos corresponding to this chapter are available online at www.expertconsult.com.

INTRODUCTION

Fetal hydrops is associated with high perinatal morbidity and mortality rates at all gestational ages. However, outcome statistics are greatly influenced by such factors as the etiology (immune vs. nonimmune), gestation at diagnosis, timely referral, prenatal compared with neonatal study groups, and the available health resources in the particular population and their use in the implementation of preconception and antenatal screening programs[1–3] (see Chapters 4 and 7–9). These factors are reflected in the range of reported incidences from 1 : 424[2] to approximately 1 : 1700[4] to 1 : 2000[3] neonatal admissions for hydropic fetuses born alive in developed countries. Traditionally, fetal hydrops is categorized into immune (IH) and nonimmune (NIH) disease. Although rhesus (RhD) hemolytic disease was the most common cause of hydrops in the past (see Chapter 13), the widespread implementation of anti-D immunoglobulin prophylaxis and the improved antenatal management of at-risk fetuses have led to a significant decrease in its incidence and associated morbidity and mortality (e.g., perinatal mortality decreased from 50% to 2% in Canada[5]; see Chapter 13). In contrast, the survival rates for NIH remain less than 10%[4] and as low as 1.5% (2/138).[1] At present, NIH is more prevalent than IH (4 : 1)[3] in most countries with adequate anti-D immunoglobulin prophylaxis supplies and fetomaternal expertise.

Human fetal hydrops is the endpoint of a multitude of pathophysiologic pathways, a number of which have not been elucidated. Advances in ultrasound make fetal hydrops easy to diagnose. The "causes" or rather associations with NIH are many[1–4,6] (Table 24–1). Research using animal models[7–9] provides some understanding of the complexity of fluid dynamics within the uterus (fetal, fetoplacental, fetoamniotic fluid, and between the uterine decidua and the placenta and membranes).

INCIDENCE

The incidence is regionally dependent[1,3,4] (e.g., alpha-thalassemia) and subject to seasonal variation (e.g., parvovirus B19 epidemics.[10,11] Alpha-thalassemia is the most common cause of fetal hydrops in Southeast Asia,[2,12] where the carrier frequency ranges from 4.14%[2] for alpha-thalassemia caused by the Southeast Asian deletion in southern China to 14% in northern Thailand,[13] accounting for between 28%[13] and 55%[2] of cases in these regions. Considering the population density in this region, alpha-thalassemia is probably the leading cause of NIH in the world. Population screening can reduce the incidence of thalassemia,[1,12,13] as it has in Cyprus, providing the resources are available. Similarly, the incidence of NIH associated with aneuploidy and congenital heart disease[14,15] is likely to decrease with the implementation of first-trimester screening (see Chapter 7).

DEFINITION

Hydrops is defined as the excessive extravascular accumulation of fluid in the interstitial compartment secondary to the disruption of the normal intravascular interstitial fluid homeostatic mechanisms. The excessive accumulation of interstitial fluid, particularly in serous cavities (peritoneal, pleural, pericardial), placenta, and amniotic fluid, facilitates the sonographic diagnosis of fetal hydrops (Figs. 24–1 to 24–3). Classically, the sonographic diagnosis of hydrops requires the presence of generalized edema plus the accumulation of fluid within two or more serous cavities. However, many of the pathophysiologic pathways leading to such a diagnosis go through progressive phases in which initially fluid may be recognized sonographically in only one site.

PATHOPHYSIOLOGY

Hydrops occurs when the microvascular fluid exchange regulatory system is disturbed. Microvascular fluid exchange mechanisms in the human fetus are complex, gestational age–dependent, and poorly understood. The number of fluid exchange pathways in the fetus is greater than in either the infant or the adult. They include transplacental, transmembrane, and transcutaneous pathways. Transplacental fluid exchange has a large influence on blood volume, because the placental blood volume accounts for approximately 40% of the total fetal circulation.[16] Fetal development is associated with a continual change in the different fluid exchange pathways and forces. These routes of fetal fluid exchange may be important compensatory mechanisms when fluid homeostasis is disturbed, as shown by the common clinical

TABLE 24–1
Abnormalities Associated with Hydrops*

- Immune (see Chapter 13)
  - Anti-D and other Rh antibodies
  - Antibodies to K in Kell system
  - Antibodies to Fya in Duffy system
- Nonimmune
- Idiopathic/unknown
- Anemia (other than alloimmunization)
  - Alpha-thalassemia major 1 (see Chapter 38)
  - Parvovirus B19 congenital infection (see Chapter 29)
  - Fetomaternal transfusion
  - TTTS and variants (see Chapter 23)
  - Erythroleukemia
  - Congenital erythropoietic porphyria[35] (Gunther's disease)
- Cardiovascular (see Chapters 15 and 16)
  - Severe congenital heart disease[43] (atrial septal defect, ventriculoseptal defect, hypoplastic left heart, pulmonary valve insufficiency, Ebstein's anomaly, subaortic stenosis, atrioventricular canal defect, tetralogy of Fallot, heterotaxy; premature closure of foramen ovale)
  - High-output cardiac failure: associated with large arteriovenous malformation within the fetal vasculature or tumors
  - Premature closure of ductus (? indomethacin therapy)
  - Myocarditis (coxsackievirus, cytomegalovirus, parvovirus B19, adenovirus infections)
  - Tachyarrhythmias (supraventricular tachycardia, atrial flutter)[88]
  - Bradyarrhythmias (heart block)
  - Wolff-Parkinson-White syndrome
  - Intracardiac tumors (teratoma, rhabdomyoma[84]) (see Chapter 22)
  - Cardiomyopathy (e.g., fibroelastosis)
  - Myocardial infarction
  - Arterial calcification (e.g., idiopathic infantile arterial calcification[85])
- Chromosomal (see Chapter 4)
  - Trisomies
  - Turner's syndrome (45 XO)
  - Triploidy
- Pulmonary
  - Congenital hydro-/chylothorax
  - Pulmonary lymphangiectasia
  - Congenital pulmonary tumors/anomalies[46,47,48]
    - CCAM (see Chapter 23)
    - Pulmonary sequestration
    - Bronchogenic cysts and other tumors (see Chapter 23)
  - Diaphragmatic hernia (see Chapter 19)
  - Chondrodysplasia
  - Pulmonary hypoplasia
- Renal (see Chapter 18)
  - Congenital nephrosis (Finnish type)
  - Renal vein thrombosis
  - Urethral obstruction (atresia, posterior valves)
  - Spontaneous bladder perforation
  - Cloacal malformation
  - Prune-belly syndrome
- Infection (intrauterine) (see Chapters 29–32)
  - Parvovirus B19[36,69] (either by anemia, myocarditis, or hepatitis)
  - Syphilis[1]
  - Cytomegalovirus (primary & secodary[34]; adenovirus; coxsackievirus)
  - Toxoplasmosis
  - Herpes simplex
  - Leptospirosis
  - Chagas' disease
- Liver
  - Hepatic calcifications
  - Hepatic fibrosis
  - Congenital hepatitis (see Chapter 47)
  - Cholestasis
  - Polycystic disease
  - Biliary atresia
  - Familial cirrhosis
- Inborn errors of metabolism[74,75]
  - Congenital disorder of glycosylation[74]
- Lysosomal storage diseases (>20) include[75]:
  - Gaucher's disease
  - GM_1 gangliosidosis
  - MPS types VIa and VII
  - Iron-storage disease
- Anomalies (many associated with fetal immobility) (see Chapter 20)
  - Achondroplasia
  - Achondrogenesis type 2
  - Thanatophoric dwarfism
  - Arthrogryphosis
- Multiple pterygium syndrome
  - Neu-Laxova syndrome[76]
  - Pena-Shokeir type 1 syndrome
  - COFS syndrome
  - Noonan's syndrome[83]
  - Myotonic dystrophy
- Neuronal degeneration
- Tumors[63]
- Sacrococcygeal teratoma (see Chapter 22)
- Tuberous sclerosis (see Chapter 22)
- Miscellaneous
  - Nonaneuploid cystic hygroma (see Chapter 22)
  - Meconium peritonitis
  - Fetal neuroblastosis
  - Small bowel volvulus (see Chapter 19)
  - Amniotic band syndrome
  - Torsion of ovarian cyst
  - Polysplenia syndrome
- Lymphatic: intestinal lymphatic hypoplasia[26]
- Placental
  - Monochorionic twins–TTTS (see Chapter 23)
  - Chorioangioma[67] (see Chapter 22)
  - Umbilical cord anomalies[86]
    - Umbilical vein thrombosis
    - True cord knots
    - Umbilical cord cysts
  - Hemagioma
- Maternal
  - Diabetes mellitus (see Chapter 44)
  - Thyroid disease (see Chapter 45)
  - Preeclampsia (see Chapter 35)[27,28]
  - Severe anemia (see Chapter 38)
  - Hypoalbuminemia

* Chapter numbers in text refer the reader to detailed discussion of management options for specific conditions within a given group.

CCAM, congenital cystic adenomatoid malformation; COFS, cerebro-oculofacial-skeletal; Rh, rhesus; MPS, mucopolysaccharidosis; TTTS, twin-twin transfusion syndrome.

FIGURE 24–1
Ascites and cardiomegaly associated with alpha-thalassemia major (Bart's hemoglobin) at 29 weeks' gestation.

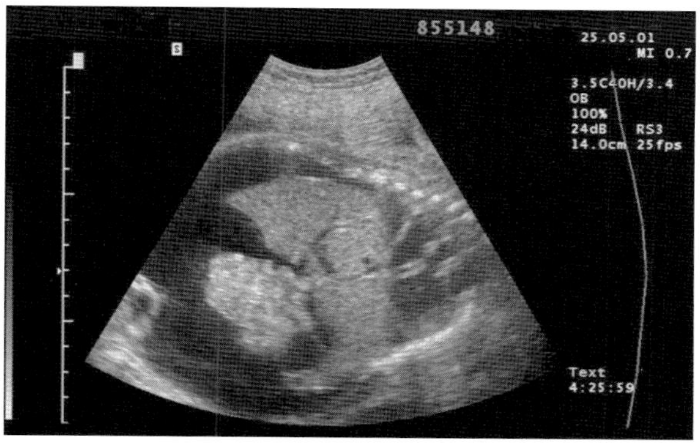

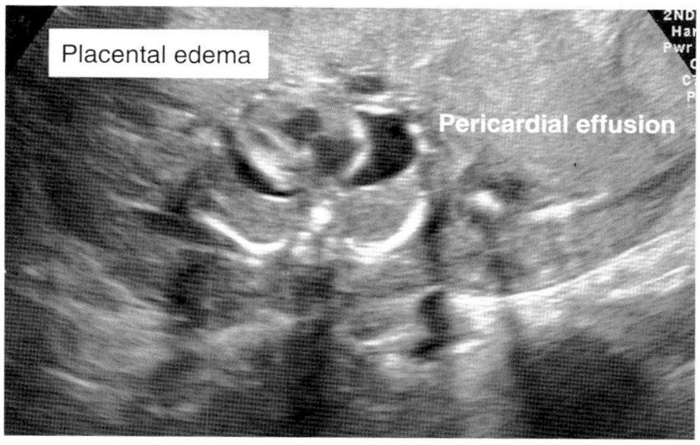

FIGURE 24–2
Pericardial effusion, cardiomegaly and placental edema associated with parvovirus B19 infection at 19 weeks' gestation.

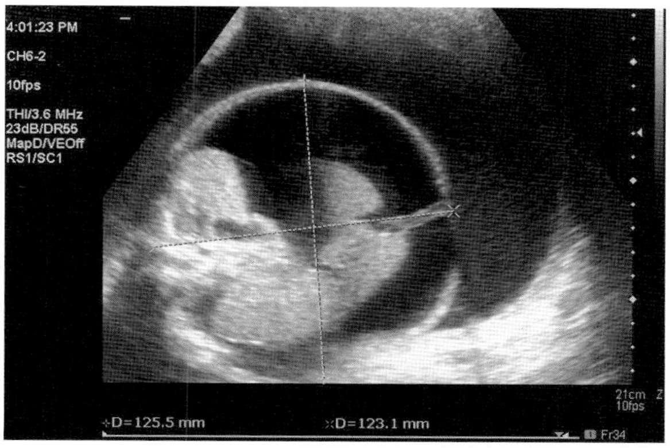

FIGURE 24–3
Polyhydramnios and massive ascites associated with Niemann-Pick type C inborn errors of metabolism.

association of hydramnios and placental edema with fetal hydrops regardless of the underlying cause. The fetal extracellular fluid volume (ECF) exceeds the intracellular fluid volume (ICF), though the ECF:ICF ratio declines progressively with gestation, becoming less than 1 after birth.[17] The interstitial–to–plasma volume ratio is therefore greatest in the fetus and then declines into adulthood. Control of this relatively large interstitial fluid compartment is fundamental to the understanding of fetal hydrops. Unfortunately, interstitial fluid control mechanisms are poorly understood because of the difficulty of measuring plasma and interstitial volumes.[18] The many influences on fetal fluid homeostasis make it unlikely there is a single or simple pathophysiologic explanation for all cases of fetal hydrops. The "Starling equation" does not provide pathophysiologic explanations in the fetus.[19] The fluid-dominated milieu of the fetus and the specific physiologic characteristics of the fetal heart and the lymphatic system make it particularly susceptible to hydrops. Animal research[7,8,20,21] coupled with clinical studies[19,22,23] suggest that raised central venous pressure (CVP) is a critical step in the pathophysiology of hydrops, at least with a cause associated with poor heart function (e.g., myocardopathy, obstructed cardiac return or outflow, profound anemia). The clinical use of umbilical venous pressure (UVP) in the investigation and management of some cases of fetal hydrops is a vindication of the physiologic research findings on the importance of the CVP and the lymphatic system.[22,23] At the same time, some of the traditional pathophysiologic forces such as colloid oncotic pressure are being relegated to a lower tier of importance.

RISKS

Fetal Risks

The fetal risks from hydrops are mainly fetal death with infant morbidity, an important risk in the few survivors. The commonly reported conditions associated with fetal hydrops are

- Alpha-thalassemia; aneuploidy; congenital malformations, infection, and the idiopathic (unknown) group.
- *Fetal death* is mostly influenced by the associated condition, gestation at diagnosis, gestation at delivery, and management. The reported mortality rate ranges between 45%[2] and greater than 90%.[1,3] Management options include elective abortion, various invasive diagnostic and fewer therapeutic procedures, which are in themselves associated with a risk of pregnancy loss, preterm delivery, intrauterine fetal death, and fetal trauma (see Chapters 9 and 25).
- *Infant mortality* is influenced by the etiology, severity, and duration of the hydrops, prenatal procedures performed, gestational age at delivery, and neonatal management. Congenital anomalies are consistently reported with a 57% mortality.[2] In contrast, mortality associated with primary chylothorax, an uncommon association with NIH, may be as low as 6%[2] after admission to a neonatal unit in a developed country.
- *Infant morbidity*. The short- and long-term prognosis depends on many of the factors associated with mortality. The range of more severe morbidity includes terminal cardiac failure and heart transplantation,[24] fetal cerebellar

hemorrhage associated with parvovirus B19 infection,[25] cardiac anomaly needing surgical correction, chromosomal abnormality, persistent generalized edema as a result of protein-losing enteropathy associated with congenital intestinal lymphatic hypoplasia,[26] and cerebral palsy.

Maternal Risks

- Antenatal consequences of fetal hydrops may be classified as direct or indirect:
  - *Direct consequences* include associated hyperplacentosis and hydramnios. Hyperplacentosis is a large placental mass with associated dysfunction such as villus edema, impaired oxygen exchange–hypoxia–increased angiogenic factors (i.e., soluble fms-like tyrosine kinase 1 [sFlt-1]).[27,28] This pathophysiologic process is associated with maternal dilutional anemia, edema, proteinuria, and gestational hypertension (i.e., preeclampsia or "mirror syndrome").[27,28] Hydramnios is associated with malpresentation, preterm labor, and preterm rupture of membranes (PROM) with the associated risk of placental abruption and chorioamnionitis.
  - *Indirect consequences* include the complications of intrauterine investigations and therapy, namely, PROM, chorioamnionitis, abruption (associated with amniodrainage), anemia, and maternal red blood cell alloimmunization. In the event of fetal surgery, the maternal risks include anesthetic risks, fluid overload and electrolyte imbalance, uterine hemorrhage (during entry for fetal shunting and intrauterine laser procedures[29,30]), psychological stress and associated mental illness, and even maternal death.[30] In patients undergoing open fetal surgery, the risks include adverse reproductive outcomes in 35% of future pregnancies, including uterine rupture or dehiscence, antepartum hemorrhage, and cesarean hysterectomy.[31]
- *During labor and delivery*: Hydrops may be associated with preterm labor, the side effects of tocolysis, dystocia (e.g., large tumors), cesarean delivery (e.g., associated with malpresentation, cord prolapse), abruption associated with membrane rupture in cases with hydramnios, postpartum hemorrhage (primary and secondary), and retained placenta.

MANAGEMENT OPTIONS

Prepregnancy

Prevention initiatives are based on the prevalence of conditions associated with fetal hydrops ideally identified by an audit in the region.

Prevention initiatives may include

- Prenatal screening for preventable conditions such as
  - Alpha-thalassaemia.[1,12,13]
  - Inborn errors of metabolism.
- Assessing immunity:
  - Of at-risk women of exposure to parvovirus B19 infection in densely populated areas[10] during an outbreak.
  - Possibly cytomegalovirus (CMV).
  - Syphilis.[1]

Prenatally

Once fetal hydrops is identified, the mother should be counseled regarding the following:

- Diagnosis: based on maternal and fetal investigations (Tables 24–2 and 24–3) and associated fetal risks from invasive procedures.
- Prognosis: fetal risks, both short and long term, which are influenced by the diagnosis and may remain unknown.
- Treatment: if available and feasible in the circumstances.

DIAGNOSIS

Presentation

Fetal hydrops clinically presents in one of several ways (Table 24–4). The fetal sites of fluid collection and the amount of fluid (severity) may be helpful in the management of the hydrops once the cause is ascertained. In general, oligohydramnios is a poor prognostic sign.

Investigations

A comprehensive search in the mother and fetus for the "cause" usually involves antenatal invasive procedures (see

TABLE 24–2

Maternal Investigations for Fetal Hydrops

Maternal History
Parvovirus B19 epidemic and close proximity to children, immunity[10]
Previous fetal hydrops or diagnosis associated with hydrops[74,75]
Previous baby with jaundice
Ethnic origin[1,12,13]
Hemoglobinopathy trait (e.g., alpha-thalassemia[1,12,13,38])
Consanguinity[75]
Congenital heart disease
Family history of hydrops (inborn errors of metabolism)[74,75]
Endocrine disorder
Symptoms of "mirror syndrome"[27,28] (i.e., preeclampsia; see Chapter 35)
Maternal Blood
Complete blood count (e.g., microcytosis–alpha-thalassemia trait)
Electrophoresis (depending upon blood count result and ethnic background)
Blood group and antibody screen (titer if antibodies present)[37]
Glucose-6-phosphate dehydrogenase and pyruvate kinase carrier status
α-Fetoprotein
Serologic tests (of limited value; see Chapters 29–32)
Syphilis[1]
Parvovirus B19[36,69]
Toxoplasmosis
Cytomegalovirus (primary and also secondary)[34]
Herpes simplex virus
Adenovirus
Coxsackievirus
Uric acid, urea, and electrolytes
Liver function including albumin
Kleihauer (-Betke) test[42]
Test of glucose tolerance
SLE, especially anti-Ro/SSA or anti-La/SSB antigens, if bradycardia/heart block
Thyroid function tests including antibodies: TSH and TSH-binding inhibitor IgG (see Chapter 21)

IgG, immunoglobulin G; SLE, systemic lupus erythematosus; TSH, thyroid-stimulating hormone.

TABLE 24-3
Fetal Prenatal Investigations for Fetal Hydrops

Ultrasound

Sites and severity of hydrops (see Figs. 24-1 to 24-5)
Detailed real-time ultrasound for congenital abnormality[14] and abnormality of placenta (chorioangioma[63,67]) and cord (cysts[86])
Fetal echocardiography,[44] pulsed[43] and color Doppler studies and M-mode
Amniotic fluid volume
Biophysical assessment (nonstress testing or biophysical profile score).

Invasive (Mainly Fetal Blood)

Hematologic tests: full blood count, hemoglobin electrophoresis (depending on ethnic background); group and Coombs'
Infection: polymerase chain reaction, serologic tests for acute phase-specific IgM antibodies for infection; culture
Blood gas analysis and pH estimation to provide an indication of the immediate well-being of the fetus
Karyotype (blood, placenta, amniotic fluid, ascitic or pleural fluids are suitable sources)
Intrathoracic pressure[58]/UVP[23]
Liver function tests (albumin)
Cultured amniotic fluid cells enzyme testing for lysosomal storage diseases (e.g., Gaucher's mucopolysaccharidoses[75])

IgM, immunoglobulin M; UVP, umbilical venous pressure.

TABLE 24-4
Presentation of Fetal Hydrops

By chance:
Ultrasound examination
Fetal heart rate recording
Ultrasound surveillance of pregnancies at risk of fetal hydrops (i.e., TTTS in monochorionic twin pregnancy; alpha-thalassemia trait parents[1]; large fetomaternal hemorrhage following trauma; fetal arrhythmia; fetal anomaly [e.g., congenital heart defect[44]]; fetal tumor,[63] cystic hygroma, large nuchal translucency)
Large-for-dates/hydramnios
Reduced fetal movements
Placental abruption (e.g., associated with "mirror syndrome"[28] or chorioangioma[67])
Maternal diabetes
Maternal SLE/anti-Ro antibodies
Maternal preeclampsia/mirror syndrome[27,28]
Maternal parvovirus B19 primary infection or contact/at risk for infection[10,28,31,69]

SLE, systemic lupus erythematosus; TTTS, twin-twin transfusion syndrome.

Tables 24–2 and 24–3). The hydrops severity, gestational age, ultrasound identified anomalies, ultrasound Doppler assessment, and the parents' consent will influence the decision to perform these procedures. The ultrasound scan (Figs. 24–4 and 24–5; see also Fig. 24–1) may in the majority of cases assist in the diagnosis. The diagnosis may escape antenatal detection in 10%[1] to 33%.[32] Real-time gray scale and pulsed Doppler ultrasound assessment of the hydropic fetus are assuming an ever-increasing important role in the noninvasive assessment of associated causes such as structural cardiac anomalies or cardiac dysfunction secondary to hyperdynamic flow (i.e., anemia or associated with tumors or twin-twin transfusion syndrome [TTTS]). On completion of both the noninvasive fetal assessment and, ideally, the

FIGURE 24–4
Twin-twin transfusion syndrome. Recipient hydropic at 20 weeks' gestational age.

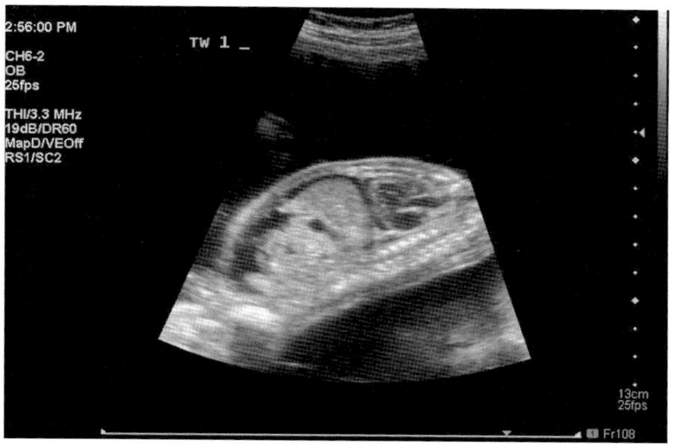

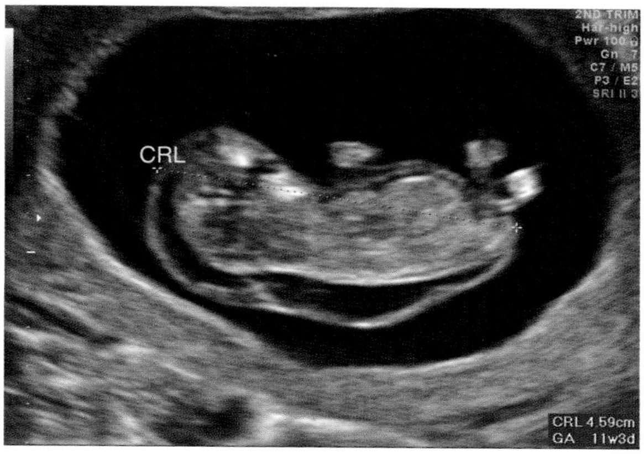

FIGURE 24–5
First-trimester large nuchal translucency and hydrops associated with aneuploidy.

maternal investigations, the most common invasive procedures will be fetal blood sampling (FBS) and/or amniocentesis. FBS is preferred (Table 24–5), but the associated mortality rates higher than for nonhydropic indications,[33] especially if the fetus is thrombocytopenic (e.g., parvovirus B19 infection) and when it is technically more difficult (e.g., maternal obesity, <20 wk' gestational age).

It is important to optimize the information available when planning intrauterine procedures (amniocentesis or FBS). For example, in the case of severe lung compression with heart axis deviation associated with large pleural effusions, a pleural tap may be combined with either procedure to determine the effect of decompression on the lungs and the restoration of the heart to its normal midline position. Pleural fluid can be used for investigations (karyotype, infection screen, cell type and count). Intrathoracic pressure and UVP measurements before and after the drainage may be used prognostically. The UVP is used as a surrogate for fetal CVP, and an elevated UVP for gestational age suggests cardiac dysfunction is involved. Limited human study notes a good correlation between the fetal UVP and CVP, but this relationship did not hold true in the anemic fetal sheep.[9]

TABLE 24–5

Comparative Diagnostic Value of Amniocentesis and Fetal Blood Sampling

Amniocentesis	
Karyotyping (FISH for chromosomes 13, 18, 21, sex chromosomes, and culture may take up to 2 wk for a result)	
Infection screen–PCR	
CEP—amniotic fluid is dark brown, which fluoresces red under Wood's light; increase in type 1 uro- and coproporphyrin isomers[35]	
Inborn errors of metabolism screen[74] (i.e., lysosomal storage diseases[75])	
Fetal Blood Sampling	
Karyotyping (48–72 hr for a result in many centers)	
Hematologic causes (anemia; hemoglobinopathies)	
Infection screen	
UVP	

CEP, congenital erythropoietic porphyria; FISH, fluorescence in situ hybridization; PCR, polymerase chain reaction; UVP, umbilical vein pressure.

Role of Umbilical Vein Pressure Measurement in the Treatment of Nonimmune Hydrops

The measurement of UVP is a helpful guide in the management of fetal hydrops. There are no reports of reproducibly effective therapy or NIH associated with a normal UVP.[19] This suggests that such fetuses should not be subjected to additional invasive procedures in hopes of therapy. Normalization of an elevated UVP after treatment suggests that the therapy will be successful and the hydrops will resolve. Hydrops characterized by an elevated UVP not remedied by either surgical or medical therapy is usually progressive, and the fetus either dies in utero or requires preterm delivery for postnatal therapy.[23] It seems, therefore, that measurement of the fetal UVP should be viewed as a guide to therapy when FBS is planned but is not, in and of itself, an indication for the sampling.

Amniotic fluid may be used to karyotype and to screen for infections associated with hydrops, such as parvovirus B19, CMV primary and secondary maternal infection,[34] syphilis,[1] toxoplasmosis, and herpes simplex virus (HSV), inherited disorders of metabolism (e.g., lysosomal storage diseases; see Chapters 29–32). It is also useful in the diagnosis of the rare condition of congenital erythropoietic porphyria.[35] However, FBS provides more information (e.g., anemia, Coombs' test, UVP) along with quicker karyotyping of all 23 pairs of chromosomes than amniocentesis. Furthermore, treatment can be administered at the time of the procedure in cases of anemia, especially when suspected on the basis of an elevated middle cerebral artery peak systolic velocity (MCAPV).[36] It is important to screen for rare antibodies (Coombs' test), which can be comprehensively done only in regional blood transfusion laboratories, before making the diagnosis of NIH.[37]

Polymerase chain reaction investigation has revolutionized the diagnosis of fetal infection. A maternal infection screen should be performed before the fetal screen in order to optimize the use of the relatively small fetal sample. An extra 2-mL aliquot should be stored at −20°C in case the need for additional tests becomes apparent after the preliminary laboratory results have been completed (e.g., to screen for secondary CMV infection).[34]

The optimal time for prognostic counseling is after the results of the maternal and fetal investigations are available. After multidisciplinary counseling, the patient may elect to undergo a termination of pregnancy, should this be an acceptable option.

The study of fetal nucleic acids in maternal plasma is opening up the possibility of the diagnosis of fetal chromosomal aberrations without the risk of intrauterine invasive procedures.[38] This methodology is already in clinical use in RhD typing of the fetus (see Chapter 13).

Postmortem Examination (See Chapter 25)

When antenatal treatment has not been either possible or successful (e.g., stillbirth or termination of pregnancy), a postmortem examination of the fetus and placenta is potentially important to reduce the percentage assigned to the idiopathic category and to facilitate risk recurrence counseling.

TREATMENT

General

The overall number of NIH cases amenable to antenatal therapy is small, the exception being during parvovirus B19 outbreaks. To date, fetal hydrops has proved amenable to fetal therapy only when associated with the following:

- Anemia.
- Arrhythmia.
- Hydrothoraces.
- TTTS.
- Some tumors (case reports).

Infection, arrhythmia, and TTTS are conditions in which spontaneously reversible hydrops has been reported. The management of TTTS is detailed in Chapter 23.

Anemia

Fetal blood transfusion is the treatment of choice for hydrops secondary to anemia. The prognosis, however, may be poor in some cases of anemia (i.e., when associated with homozygous alpha-thalassemia, CMV infection, trisomy 21, or Gunther's disease).[24,25] It is important, therefore, to determine the cause of the anemia before offering intrauterine transfusion. This may mean not transfusing the fetus (with the patient's agreement) before all investigations (especially on the parents for alpha-thalassemia trait) and fetal karyotype are available. This point should be discussed during the initial counseling session; otherwise, ill-advised transfusions of the fetus with homozygous alpha-thalassemia may result in lifelong transfusions or bone marrow transplantation, iron chelation, and the associated serious neonatal complications.[38]

In Southeast Asia, alpha-thalassemia is the predominant cause of fetal hydrops.[1,12,13,39] Alpha-thalassemia major (no functional α genes) is incompatible with life. Most fetuses develop hydrops by the early third trimester (see Fig. 24–1) and, if born alive, die within hours. This is in contrast with other common causes of fetal anemia for which the prognosis is generally good. Antenatal diagnosis using noninvasive means (ultrasound diagnosis of placental thickness and cardiothoracic ratio before 20 wk or MCAPV thereafter) or invasive methods to obtain fetal tissue samples (amniocentesis, CVS or FBS) is an option for those pregnancies at risk. Preconceptual education, screening, and counseling are to be encouraged (see Chapter 38). The prognosis may improve with advances in intrauterine therapy.[40,41]

Fetomaternal hemorrhage associated with hydrops is rare and is diagnosed based on a strongly positive Kleihauer-Betke test in the mother, an ultrasound showing hydrops, and an elevated MCAPV. It is treated by a fetal intravascular transfusion(s). Presenting symptoms are nonspecific, with the most common being decreased fetal movements. Fetomaternal hemorrhage has been associated with a number of placental disorders (e.g., chorioangioma, abruption) and external forces acting on the mother or uterus (e.g., trauma, external cephalic version, invasive procedures). Regular surveillance of the fetus using ultrasound measurement of the MCAPV for anemia for further episodes[42] is recommended, because they may be fatal. Under these conditions, delivery should be considered once the pregnancy has reached an appropriate gestation.

Glucose-6-phosphate dehydrogenase (G-6-PD) deficiency is, although a common enzyme deficiency, an extremely rare cause with NIH with anemia being more common after birth. There are no effective antenatal treatments at present. However, gene therapy may prove possible in the future, and interdisciplinary counseling including pediatric colleagues and clinical geneticists is advisable.

Monochorionic Multiple Pregnancy Conditions Associated with Hydrops (See Chapter 23)

TTTS is the most common cause of NIH in monochorionic multiple pregnancy (see Fig. 24–4). It may also occur as a complication of laser treatment (i.e., reverse TTTS; see Chapter 23). The optimal management of hydrops associated with TTTS is intrauterine laser ablation of placental anastomoses.[29,30] Other proposed treatments such as amniodrainage, umbilical cord occlusion, delivery, intrauterine fetal transfusion (following failed laser), and termination are clearly less desirable. Another complication of monochorionic multiple pregnancy associated with NIH is twin reversed arterial perfusion, the management of which is based on the same principle as that for TTTS (i.e., interrupt the blood flow between the twins; see Chapter 23).

Cardiovascular Defects (See also Chapters 15 and 16)

Cardiac anomalies are the most common anatomic anomaly associated with fetal hydrops.[1,2] However, many of these anomalies do not affect function to the extent that they can explain the hydrops. There is a strong association with aneuploidy (10%–40%). The implementation of first-trimester screening should reduce the prevalence of hydrops (see Chapter 7).

Cardiac dysfunction leading to hydrops may be caused by structural anomalies, arrhythmias, or both (e.g., heterotaxy). In general, hydrops associated with a structurally abnormal heart carries a poor prognosis, with a survival rate of 0%[43] to 17%.[44] In contrast, the prognosis is good for the majority of hydrops cases associated with a tachyarrhythmia and a structurally normal heart. The response for supraventricular tachycardia is good in the majority of cases whether the approach is transplacental or direct. In a minority of cases, the arrhythmia may be secondary to thyroid-stimulating antibodies, viral infections (myocarditis, e.g., parvovirus/coxsackie/adenovirus) or maternal autoantibodies (e.g., SSA/Ro and SSB/La antibodies), which would influence management. One mechanism by which congenital infection might cause fetal hydrops is a fetal myocarditis that in turn generates either ventricular dysfunction or tachyarrhythmia resulting in hydrops. Fetal myocarditis has even required perinatal heart transplantation.[24] Pediatric follow-up is recommended because there may be neurologic morbidity associated with a long duration of hydrops.[45]

Involvement of a pediatric cardiologist in the antenatal management (especially diagnosis and prognostic counseling[44]) is advisable. The management options for these conditions are discussed in Chapter 16.

Pulmonary Defects

The prognosis for thoracic conditions associated with hydrops is generally poor.[46,47] These conditions include congenital cystic adenomatoid malformation (CCAM), bronchopulmonary sequestration (BPS), tracheal laryngeal atresia or congenital high-airway obstruction (CHAOS), teratomas (see Chapter 22), and primary hydrothorax. The prognosis is better for conditions predominantly associated with collections of fluid such as CCAM Stoker types I and II, with the greatest therapeutic success achieved treating primary hydrothorax.[48,49] In contrast, fetal hydrops associated with solid lung masses has been more difficult to treat (e.g., CCAM type III, some type II; pulmonary sequestration; see Chapter 22). The survival of newborns with solid CCAM masses and hydrops ranges from 0% to 34%.[46,47]

The low survival has led some to offer open fetal surgery to a few highly selected cases. It is associated with an estimated 60% survival but with significant fetal morbidity and maternal morbidity that affects future pregnancies.[48] Moreover, there are an increasing number of successful therapeutic options for solid lung lesions using ultrasound-guided percutaneous injection of a sclerosant or laser vaporization.[50–52] There are also reports of spontaneous resolution of the hydrops[53] associated with regression of the lesion. Even maternal betamethasone has been reported to slow or decrease large CCAM growth.[54] In cases of hydrops associated with large pulmonary masses in which delivery is the chosen treatment option (usually when a late diagnosis is made ~ 35 wk), an EXIT (ex utero intrapartum treatment) procedure is indicated for delivery (see Chapter 22).

Fetal hydrops associated with isolated primary or congenital hydrothorax has a much improved prognosis in contrast to the poor prognosis with solid thoracic lesions. The survival rate of untreated hydrops and pleural effusions approximates 35%, but increases to 62%[49] to 67%[55]

after placement of a pleuroamniotic shunt (unscreened by UVP).

The diagnosis of congenital hydrothorax is a diagnosis of exclusion—excess pleural fluid in the absence of another detectable cause. The hydrothorax typically presents after 24 weeks when human lung development has entered the canalicular phase. The pathogenesis is unknown but is often attributed to abnormalities of the lymphatic system of the lung and/or thoracic duct.[56] The lymphocyte content of the fluid is irrelevant to either the prognosis or the diagnosis.[57] Although it has been known since the mid-1980s that placement of a thoracoamniotic shunt could reverse the hydrops, reported success rates are quite variable.[49,55] This suggests that more than one mechanism underlies the hydrops, and shunting is targeted.[49,56] Although shunting is the most common treatment, other, less frequently reported treatment options question whether it is the best treatment.[55] The therapeutic mechanism of pleuroamniotic shunting is thought by some to be related to the decrease in intrathoracic pressure allowing improved cardiovascular function.[49,58] Others suggest the improved cardiac function reflects the correction of a mechanical obstruction to cardiac return. An initially elevated UVP associated with elevated intrathoracic pressure, both of which normalize after the effusion(s) has been, drained is consistent with the latter.[58] If the effusion recurs, placement of a thoracoamniotic shunt should be curative (Fig. 24–6). Conversely, if the UVP is normal prior to decompression of the chest, or remains elevated after the chest has been drained and the heart has returned to its normal midline position, the placement of a thoracoamniotic shunt is unlikely to be beneficial. It is also believed, based on animal models, that relief of lung compression decreases the risk of pulmonary hypoplasia.

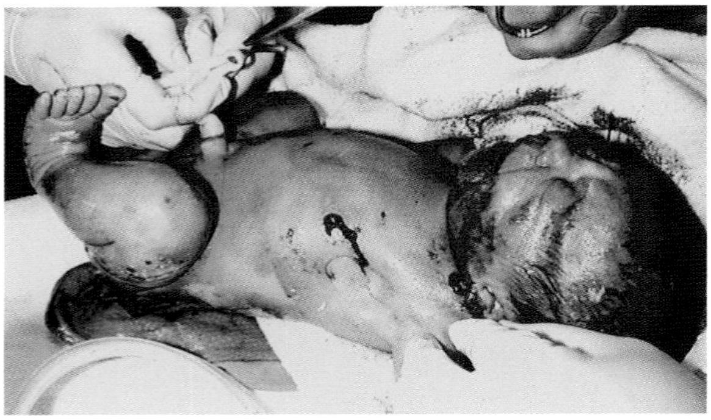

FIGURE 24–6
Infant at birth with pleuroamniotic shunt in situ immediately before removal; no need for respiratory support.

PROCEDURE: INSERTION OF FETAL THORACOAMNIOTIC SHUNT (FIG. 24–7)

Intrauterine shunts available include the larger Rocket Medical (2.1-mm diameter shunt) and Karl Storz introducers (3-mm cannula size) and the smaller Harrison shunt (Fetal Bladder Stent Set, Cook Medical, Inc.) (1.67-mm shunt diameter) introduced via a smaller 13-gauge needle (used in early gestations[59]).

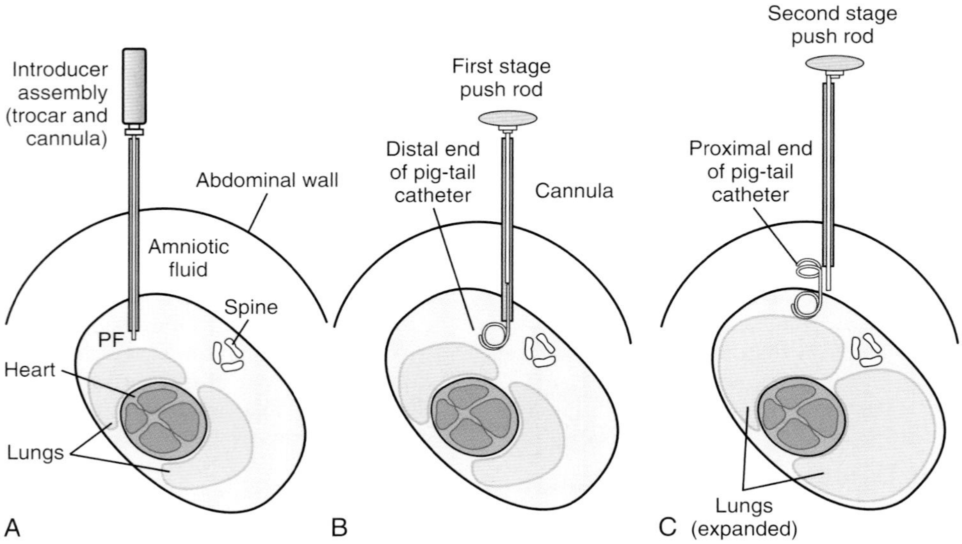

FIGURE 24–7
Procedure for the insertion of a pleuroamniotic shunt. *A*, The introducer (trocar and cannula) are sited under ultrasound guidance in the left side of the fetal chest. *B*, The trocar has been removed, the pigtail catheter sited into the cannula, and the "first-stage push rod" (*shorter rod*) used to push the distal end of the pigtail catheter in the fetal chest. *C*, The tip of the cannula is withdrawn from the chest into the amniotic space and the "second-stage punch rod" (*longer rod*) is inserted into the cannula and displaces the proximal/maternal end of the pigtail out of the end of the cannula into the amniotic space, resulting in a pleural amniotic pigtail shunt.

METHOD (USING A ROCKET SHUNT SET) (SEE VIDEO)

Hydramnios and iatrogenic oligohydramnios complicate the procedure. The usual preparations for a major invasive procedure (such as fetal blood transfusion) should be followed (see Chapter 13). The majority of procedures are performed under local anesthesia with the option of premedication. The practice of using fetal paralysis varies. Fetal analgesia may also be considered.[60]

In preparation, the ultrasound transducer is positioned to provide a transverse view of the fetal chest at the level of the maximal fluid collection. The optimal line of approach is chosen to avoid (if possible) the placenta and the broad ligament vessels (identified with color Doppler interrogation). The goal is puncture of the anterolateral aspect of the fetal thorax (as the space between ribs laterally is wider, though the arms may need to be displaced and can become entangled if lateral). Once the line of approach is determined, the maternal abdomen is cleaned, draped, and a local anesthetic instilled down to the uterine visceral peritoneum.

In order to overcome the problems with insertion of the pigtail catheter into the cannula, a guidewire and pusher are now available from the supplier. The double-pigtailed catheter with its forming wire in place is gently straightened just before inserting the introducer into the fetal chest to avoid delay. A stab incision (5 mm) is made with a blade into the maternal abdomen to minimize the resistance of insertion. The introducer (trocar and cannula) is inserted along the optimal line of approach into the amniotic cavity, taking care to minimize amnion separation and to avoid contact with the fetus. The line of entry into the fetal chest is then reviewed and adjusted as necessary. Once this secondary adjustment is made, the introducer is inserted into the pleural cavity with a sharp, stabbing motion, taking care not to traumatize intrathoracic organs and vessels. The trocar is removed, and the elongated double-pigtailed catheter with introducing guidewire carefully slid down into the cannula by an assistant, taking care not to remove the guidewire before the proximal end of the pigtail is sited within the shaft of the cannula using the guidewire pusher (to prevent jamming). Once the guidewire is removed, pleural fluid will escape the cannula. After checking that the end of the cannula is still within the fetal chest, the shorter of the two push rods (i.e., the "first-stage" pusher rod) is used to advance the distal part of the catheter (fetal component) into the fetal chest, where it should be seen to adopt its natural coiled shape. The introducing cannula is withdrawn from the fetal chest, into the amniotic cavity, taking care (while observing under ultrasound) not to withdraw the cannula too far away from the fetal chest wall lest the distant end of the catheter be pulled out of the chest. The maternal component of the double-pigtailed catheter is now pushed out of the cannula into the amniotic cavity using the longer "second-stage" push rod. The correct position of the pigtail catheter is confirmed ultrasonically. The cannula can now be removed from the uterus and the wound sutured and dressed. If there are bilateral large effusions, a second shunt will be required because decompressing only one side actually worsens cardiac displacement.

A sonographic examination is performed 8 to 24 hours postoperatively to assess shunt function. Resolution of the majority of the effusion is expected if the shunt is working well. The hydrops itself (and the hydramnios if initially present) may take an additional 10 to 14 days to resolve. The shunt will continue to function for a variable time interval.[49] If the pleural fluid reaccumulates, it is due to either blockage or displacement. At this juncture, the decision is made whether to replace the shunt or to deliver the fetus after thoracocentesis to facilitate resuscitation at delivery. The decision will reflect the severity of any residual hydrops, the duration of the functional shunt, and the current gestational age. At delivery, the pigtail drain must be immediately occluded and removed to prevent a pneumothorax (see Fig. 24–6).

COMPLICATIONS

Insertion of a pleuroamniotic shunt is not without complications, and the patient must be carefully counseled. Maternal complications include those associated with maternal analgesia, anesthesia (with or without epidural), hemorrhage, broad ligament hematoma, abortion, PROM, preterm labor and delivery, maternal trauma, and red blood cell alloimmunization. Fetal complications include death, prematurity, fetal injury to thoracic organs and vessels, severe hypoproteinemia, shunt obstruction or actual migration into the fetal chest, and even limb entanglement with the development of circulatory compromise.[61]

Other Treatments

Single or serial thoracocentesis has been successful (54%),[55] though the success rate is as low as 10%.[49]

Percutaneous ultrasound-guided pleurodesis using OK-432 is an option. OK-432 is a preparation of *Streptococcus pyogenes*, which induces a strong inflammatory response and causes pleurodesis. The technique involves percutaneous aspiration followed by injection of OK-432. It has been used with varying success in only a few cases of fetal hydrops associated with hydrothorax. It may be more successful if used in primary hydrothorax before the development of hydrops.[62] The number of cases with fetal hydrops is small and long-term follow-up lacking. The potential systemic long-term effects of this inflammatory agent are unknown. Termination of pregnancy is also an option if there is no improvement in the hydrops after treatment especially at previable gestations.[62]

Diaphragmatic hernia is discussed in Chapter 19.

Tumors (See Chapter 22)

The prognosis for hydrops associated with tumor is poor (19%).[63] Cardiac tumors are most common in cases of hydrops. In selected cases with a poor prognosis, open fetal surgery[48] has been used for a small number of surgically correctable conditions, in particular, solid pulmonary and sacrococcygeal tumors. Only a few centers in the world are willing to attempt such therapy. Other, less invasive (percutaneous) therapeutic options for the treatment of tumors are being tried to circumvent many of the problems of open fetal surgery with varying success. These include percutaneous laser,[52] sclerotherapy alcohol,[50,51,64] radiofrequency ablation,[65] thermocoagulation,[66] and percutaneous ultrasound-guided injection of alcohol for the treatment of sacrococcygeal teratoma; even coils have been tried (Dr. Suresh, Chennai, India, personal communication) in placental chorioangioma, the most common placental tumor.[67]

Chromosomal Abnormalities

The most common aneuploidies associated with fetal hydrops are 45XO and trisomy 21. The proportion of cases of fetal hydrops associated with chromosomal anomalies (4.3%[2]–44.8%[4]) is influenced by the availability of prenatal screening programs, especially those in the first trimester (see Fig. 24–5). It is important to exclude aneuploidy by karyotyping in all cases of fetal hydrops (see Table 24–3) before offering therapy. Aneuploidy with hydrops has a dismal prognosis, and the option of pregnancy termination is often exercised by parents (see also Chapter 4).

Infection (See also Chapters 29–32)

Fetal infection may be the primary etiology in a number of fetuses with NIH, with the reported prevalence (6.9%[4]–15%[1]) being influenced by the types of testing employed and the availability and implementation of prenatal screening (e.g., syphilis[2] was found to be the most common cause in a region where it was not routinely screened for). The application of polymerase chain reaction technologies has revealed a number of previously unsuspected fetal infections. Viral hepatitis is the most common cause of noncardiac hydrops in some populations (see Table 24–1). Hydrops of noncardiac origin does not generally progress, and preterm delivery is not usually required.

The common infectious causes of hydrops include parvovirus B19 (see Fig. 24–2), CMV, syphilis,[1] and toxoplasmosis. Less common viruses associated with hydrops include coxsackievirus and adenovirus. Apart from parvovirus-induced fetal anemia, very little can currently be done antenatally to treat these conditions once they produce hydrops.

Parvovirus B19 infection is a common cause of human fetal hydrops, and during epidemics, it may be the leading cause of hydrops fetalis in the region.[10,11] Hydrops is mainly due to profound hypoplastic anemia, but can also be associated with myocarditis[24] and hepatitis.[36] Susceptibility to infection varies up to 50%.[68] The risk of fetal hydrops is greatest during the first half of pregnancy (i.e., ~3% <20 wk compared with ~1% > 20 wk).[69] The risk of fetal hydrops may be higher in mothers with asymptomatic infection.[10] The management reflects the mechanism. Cordocentesis is the first step. A profoundly anemic fetus with no circulating reticulocytes will continue to deteriorate and should be transfused immediately. Like with rhesus disease, parvovirus

TABLE 24–6

Approximate Survival Rates for Major Treatable Causes of Fetal Hydrops

CAUSE	SURVIVAL RATES (%)
Anemia–parvovirus B19 infection	62.5[36] to 77[71]
Cardiovascular–supraventricular tachyarrhythmia	60[87] to >95[88]
Pulmonary–primary hydrothorax	62[49] to 67[55]

B19 hydrops secondary to anemia is associated with an elevated UVP. Anemic fetuses with reticulocytes present are likely on their way to recovery and may or may not benefit from a "top-off" transfusion. Serial ultrasound examinations have been used to assess severity, but are of little practical use in isolation.[11,36,70] The risk of FBS and therapy may be increased specifically in parvovirus infection because of the associated risk of thrombocytopenia.[71] However, a successful outcome may be expected in the majority of cases (77%[71]) but is influenced by fetal vascular access (i.e., method of puncture), maternal obesity, and fetal gestational age younger than 20 weeks (Table 24–6). Myocarditis secondary to parvovirus is characterized by hydrops, a normal or near-normal hemoglobin, but an elevated UVP. Hydrops secondary to B19 myocarditis has been treated with fetal digitalization. Lastly, hydrops secondary to hepatitis/peritonitis is characterized by ascites, little truncal edema, normal UVP and hemogrobin by grossly elevated hepatic transaminases. Infant follow-up is mandatory in view of the rare complications (e.g., risk of congenital red blood cell aplasia)[72] or even the need for perinatal heart transplantation.[24]

Other Causes

Generalized lymphatic dysfunction (e.g., primary hydrothorax is believed to be a variant) can be associated with abnormal vascular development. The prognosis is guarded and may include significant infant morbidity[25] and recurrence with autosomal recessive inheritance.[73]

Forms of recurrent NIH associated with inborn errors of metabolism (see Fig. 24–3) and autosomal recessive inheritance are being increasingly recognized (1%–2% of NIH cases[74,75]). Once recognized, there is the potential for prenatal diagnosis in subsequent pregnancies.

Fetal akinesia (arthrogryphosis) is another collection of conditions with numerous causes (cerebro-oculofacial-skeletal syndrome, Pena-Shokeir, multiple pterygium syndrome, Neu-Laxova syndrome) associated with fetal hydrops each of which carries a poor prognosis. The risk of recurrence is generally low, but certainly influenced by the cause (e.g., Neu-Laxova syndrome has autosomal recessive inheritance[76]).

Renal associations with hydrops are discussed in detail in Chapter 18.

Fetal Albumin "Therapy"

Pathophysiologic research suggests that fetal hypoproteinemia or hypoalbuminemia may occur as a secondary effect[9,19]

in approximately a third of nonimmune hydrops fetuses, but is distributed with equal frequency in groups with a high and low UVP (the exception being TTTS, which is discussed in Chapter 23). Clearly, the practice of giving the fetus albumin[77] in the absence of a clear understanding of the pathophysiology cannot be recommended (e.g., albumin would aggravate hydrops associated with increased capillary permeability). A more productive approach would be to conduct a comprehensive investigation to reduce this "idiopathic" group.

Outcomes

Long-term follow-up data are sadly lacking, being sporadic and by nature condition-specific.[45,78–81] The challenge aside, such follow-up is particularly important with the emergence and rapid increase in research into the developmental origins of health and disease.[82] One may speculate that fetal hydrops puts survivors at increased risk for a wide range of adult diseases via environmental and/or epigenetic mechanisms.[82] Such knowledge would be indispensable for families attempting to make an informed decision.

SUMMARY OF MANAGEMENT OPTIONS

Fetal Hydrops (See also Chapter 13)

Management Options	Evidence Quality and Recommendation	References
Prevention		
Preconceptual and prenatal screening for		
• Alpha-thalassemia.	III/B	38
• Fetal aneuploidy.	IIb/B	15
• Fetal anomalies, especially severe cardiac disease.	III/B	14
• Monochorionicity screening for TTTS.	III/B	89
Diagnosis—Investigations		
Maternal (see Table 24–2).	III/B	1,3,4,6
Fetal (see Table 24–3).	III/B	
Diagnosis will be made in 75%–90% of cases.	III/B	1,3,4,6,32
Risks of fetal invasive procedures are increased in presence of hydrops.	III/B	33
Counseling and Prognosis		
Counseling is given before and after investigations.	—/GPP	—
Prognosis is determined by the underlying etiology.	III/B	1,3,4,6,32
The earlier it is detected, the worse the prognosis.	III/B	15,69
Earlier detection is more likely to be associated with chromosomal abnormality.	III/B	1,3,4,6,15
Presence of a congenital anomaly worsens the prognosis.	III/B	43,44
Prognosis for isolated hydrothorax with hydrops is fairly good.	III/B	49,55
Generally, prognosis is good for psychomotor development in survivors.	III/B	79–81
Management—Treatment		
In utero, therapy can be effective in selected cases:		
• Intrauterine transfusions for fetal anemia (hemolytic disease [see Chapter 13], fetomaternal bleed, parvovirus)	III/B	36,70,77,79
• Antiarrhythmic medication	III/B	88
• Laser for TTTS stages 2–4 (see Chapter 23)	Ib/A	29,30
• Pleuroamniotic shunts for primary hydrothorax, cystic adenomatous malformation.	III/B	49,55
• Open surgery for chest lesions should be regarded as exceptional.	IV/C	48

SUMMARY OF MANAGEMENT OPTIONS

Fetal Hydrops (See also Chapter 13)**—cont'd**

Management Options	Evidence Quality and Recommendation	References
Management—General		
Interdisciplinary approach is used for ongoing pregnancies.	III/B	2,36,43–45,48
Consider termination in those with severe hydrops at a previable gestation with a condition for which there is no effective treatment.	III/B	1,38
Postnatal		
Perform postmortem examination in cases of fetal/neonatal death.	III/B	90–92
Pediatric follow-up and counseling are needed in survivors.	III/B	78–82

GPP, good practice point; TTTS, twin-twin transfusion syndnrome.

SUGGESTED READINGS

Fairley CK, Smoleniec JS, Caul OE, Miller E: Observational study of effect of intrauterine transfusions on outcome of fetal hydrops after parvovirus B19 infection. Lancet 1995;346:1335–1337.

Haverkamp F, Noeker M, Gerresheim G, Fahnenstich H: Good prognosis for psychomotor development in survivors with non-immune hydrops fetalis. BJOG 2000;107:282–284.

Isaacs H Jr: Fetal hydrops associated with tumors. Am J Perinatol 2008;25:43–68.

Kooper A, Janssens P, de Groot A, et al: Lysosomal storage diseases in non-immune hydrops fetalis pregnancies. Clin Chim Acta 2006;371:176–182.

Leung WC, Leung KY, Lau ET, et al: Alpha-thalassemia (review). Semin Fetal Neonat Med 2008;13:215–222.

Liao C, Wei J, Qiuming L, et al: Nonimmune hydrops fetalis diagnosed during the second half of pregnancy in southern China. Fetal Diagn Ther 2007;22:302–305.

Roberts D, Neilson J, Kilby M, Gates S: Interventions for the treatment of twin-twin transfusion syndrome. Cochrane Database Syst Rev 2008;1:CD002073.

Rustico MA, Lanna M, Coviello D, et al: Fetal pleural effusion (review). Prenat Diagn 2007;27:793–799.

Smoleniec JS, Pillai M: Fetal hydrops associated with parvovirus B19 infection: Management. Br J Obstet Gynaecol 1994;101:1079–1081.

Wald NJ, Morris JK, Walker K, Simpson JM: Prenatal screening for serious congenital heart defects using nuchal translucency: a meta-analysis (review). Prenat Diagn 2008;28:1094–1104.

REFERENCES

For a complete list of references, log onto www.expertconsult.com.

CHAPTER 25

Fetal Death

CARL P. WEINER

INTRODUCTION

Though 80% of pregnancies are unplanned, a fetal death is virtually always viewed as a tragedy. The known threat of an embryonic loss has passed, and both patient and caregiver are optimistic about the future. Whether the death occurs in a single or multiple gestations, it spurs the search for an explanation and changes both pregnancy management and the patient's psychosocial needs. The resulting grief may begin prior to fetal death when associated with the antenatal diagnosis of a lethal abnormality. The successful identification of the etiology may be crucial for the management of any subsequent pregnancy and have a profound impact on the woman's long-term health.

MANAGEMENT OPTIONS

Giving Bad News

Providing a patient bad news is one of the most difficult tasks a physician faces on a regular basis. The problem now is not whether it is necessary to tell the patient, but how to deliver it. There is no room for physician paternalism. Unfortunately, the act of teaching techniques for the breaking of bad news may seem as awkward as the teaching of contraception must have been in the Victorian era. Yet, these techniques can be learned and used in a busy clinical practice.

There are a number of plausible explanations as to why is it difficult to give bad news including the fear of causing emotional pain, sympathetic pain, fear of being blamed for the poor outcome, fear of a therapeutic failure and all that it entails, fear of the medical-legal consequences, fear of eliciting a loud or threatening reaction, fear of saying "I don't know," and fear of expressing emotion to a patient.

Why are patients unhappy with the way they are told bad news? The most common complaints are that the physician is not listening, is using jargon, or is "talking down" to them. The process of informing a patient about bad news should follow the basic steps of the traditional medical interview:

- Prepare for listening.
- Question.
- Listen actively.
- Show verbally that you have heard.
- Respond.

The necessary modifications and additions to the basic interview as they relate to fetal medicine include first finding out how much the patient knows or understands of the events and identifying the misinformation that must be corrected and how much the patient wants to know before beginning to share the information in an unambiguous, plain-spoken fashion that minimizes the chance of denial; responding to the patient's feelings; and then presenting an appropriate action plan.

Perhaps the most difficult component of the interview arises when the patient starts reacting to the news. People perceive bad news in a myriad of ways, some of which may not be clear to the health care provider. A mentally competent and informed patient has the right to accept or reject any treatment offered and to react to the news or express their feelings in any (legal) way they choose. Unexpected reactions often reflect a misunderstanding of the information presented. It is important to reinforce those parts of what the patient has said that are correct and then continue on from there. Avoid jargon, use diagrams and written messages, and then look for evidence of understanding. Listen for and try to address the patient's concerns; do not dismiss them as irrelevant. Common reactions run the gamut and include disbelief, anger, blame, shock, guilt, denial, hope, despair, depression, displacement, fear and anxiety, crying, bargaining, awkward questions, relief, threats, and humor. There is no question that giving parents bad news tests the entire range of one's professional skills and abilities. But if it is done poorly, the family will never forgive and their anger will grow. But if the interview is done well, they will never forget their physician's kindness.

Evaluation

The investigation of a fetal death involves both fetus and mother. It is essential that the cause of death be determined whenever possible. Only then can the likelihood of a recurrence and the possibility of prevention be ascertained. An understanding of the actual cause aids the grieving process by eliminating the natural tendency for self-recrimination. A thorough maternal past and current medical history should again be obtained and the physical examination repeated in search of an unsuspected preexisting or acquired systemic illness. If the fetus is still in utero, a targeted ultrasound examination of the uterus and contents is performed in search of fetal or placental malformations and evidence of fetal growth restriction.

The more common, known causes of fetal death are listed in Table 25–1. The fetal death rate has declined since the late 1960s and the "causes" changed.[1] For example, fetal death due to intrapartum asphyxia and Rh disease has

TABLE 25–1

Causes of Fetal Death

Maternal Systemic Illness

Diabetes mellitus
Hypertension—includes prepregnancy and pregnancy-associated connective tissue disorders
Any disorder causing septicemia with associated hypoperfusion—fetal malformations, structural and chromosomal

Fetal

Infection—bacterial, viral
Fetal immune hemolytic disease
Cord accident—includes prolapse, thrombosis, strangulation
Bands or knots and torsion (likely to be greatly overdiagnosed)
Metabolic disorders
Placental dysfunction includes those associated with fetal growth restriction, postmaturity, and abruption causing hypoxemia, placenta previa, or infarction, twin-twin transfusion, fetal-maternal hemorrhage
Inherited disorders: thombophilias

TABLE 25–2

Routine Laboratory Evaluation and Follow-up of Fetal Death

Maternal (On Detection)

Fasting blood glucose
Platelet count, fibrinogen
Indirect Coombs' test
Stain of a peripheral smear for fetal red blood cells (Kleihauer-Betke test)
Anticardiolipins, antinuclear antibodies, lupus anticoagulant
Fetal karyotype
Thrombophilia workup
Polymerase chain reaction studies of fetal products for evidence of viral infection
Amniotic fluid culture for cytomegalovirus, anaerobic and aerobic bacteria
Subsequent maternal weekly fibrinogen measurements and platelet counts if fetal death is of 4 wk' duration or more

Fetal (At Delivery)

Repeat infection workup (see Chapter 26)
Karyotype (if not done antenatally)
Postmortem examination
Fetogram (total body radiograph) if dysmorphic stigmata at postmortem examination

declined dramatically in the industrialized world, as has the death rate from unexplained growth restriction also declined. Adolescents too are at increased risk of having a fetal demise.[2] Unless the history and physical examination pinpoint the cause, a basic group of laboratory tests (Table 25–2) should be performed. A chromosome abnormality underlies about 15% of second-trimester stillbirths. An amniocentesis to both search for fetal infection (see Chapter 9) and obtain a karyotype is recommended in all cases of fetal death,[3] even in the apparent absence of extrinsic structural malformations, because the usual dysmorphic features of aneuploidy may be obscured by postmortem changes. Amniocytes can be cultured successfully weeks after the death in contrast to fetal fascia, muscle, or subcutaneous tissue, which commonly fail to provide viable cells for culture. Another advantage of amniotic fluid is that it can be used to conduct viral polymerase chain reaction (PCR) studies. Placental tissue is also a viable source for karyotyping.

After delivery, photographs of the child are made for both the medical record and the parents. If the parents decline the photographs (a common grief/fear response), the pictures are stored with the medical record in case the parents change their minds subsequently. A checklist describing the gross presentation is a useful document, a fetogram made (xerography is an excellent modality), and permission for an autopsy sought. The performance of an autopsy significantly increases the likelihood of discovering a presumed cause.[4] Ideally, an individual with both an interest and experience in perinatal pathology should perform the autopsy. The placenta is an important component of that examination. The fetal organ cavities are cultured for both bacteria and viruses, even if an infection workup was initiated antenatally. If amniotic fluid was obtained prior to delivery, an aliquot is sent for viral PCR. There is a growing body of evidence that viral infection can have a role in poor fetal outcome. Maternal serology is, however, rarely useful.[5]

Many stillborn fetuses are small for gestational age. Customized fetal growth charts may required to demonstrate this because the use of preterm neonatal birth weight charts, derived from preterm newborns who are commonly growth-restricted, might obscure this finding.[6,7] In the absence of another explanation, growth restriction increases the likelihood that severe placental dysfunction of some etiology is the explanation.[3]

Pregnancy Management

The approach to the pregnancy after a fetal loss depends on whether it is a single or a multiple gestation, the gestational age at death, and the parents' wishes.

Singleton Gestation

At least 90% of women with an intrauterine demise labor spontaneously within 3 weeks of its detection.[8,9] About a quarter of women who retain their dead fetus for 4 or more weeks after 20 weeks' gestation develop a chronic, consumptive coagulopathy. It is a true disseminated intravascular coagulopathy (DIC) characterized by degrees of decreased fibrinogen, plasminogen, antithrombin III, and platelets and increased fibrin degradation products.[10–14] The etiology of the coagulopathy has never been conclusively determined. Using sensitive coagulation tests, pathologic activation of the clotting cascade is demonstrable within 48 hours of the demise. The incidence of the coagulopathy increases with the duration of the delay, but fewer than 2% of these women experience a hemorrhagic complication. Traditionally, labor was induced after treatment of the coagulopathy even if the cervix was unfavorable and the coagulopathy resolved within 48 hours of the delivery. Fortunately, this coagulopathy can be reversed by the administration of low-dose heparin.[15–17] However, delay decreases any hope of an informative autopsy.

A dilation and evacuation can be performed prior to 15 weeks' gestation. It remains an option until 24 weeks if the practitioner is so skilled, but the risk of maternal hemorrhage may be increased after fetal death.[18] Caution is advised. The second and more common alternative after 15 weeks' gestation is an induction of labor. This has the advantage of leaving the fetus intact for autopsy. The method of termination has no significant impact on the rate of grief resolution.[19]

Oxytocin is not the agent of choice because it is frequently ineffective early in gestation. And although instillation of intra-amniotic hypertonic saline or glucose may shorten the time interval, it has been associated with several maternal deaths.

The development of the stable prostaglandin E and F analogues for the induction of labor has simplified induction because the efficacy of these agents exceeds 90%.[20–23] Delivery shortly after detection of the demise has several advantages. First, it brings an end to an emotionally painful event and allows the psychological healing process to begin. Second, any postmortem examination is more likely to yield useful information if done before the development of severe autolysis.

The various prostaglandin preparations may be administered via oral, vaginal, intracervical, extraovular, or intramuscular routes, depending on regional availability. Misoprostol (either per vaginam or by mouth) has a favorable cost profile and is at least as effective as other forms of prostaglandin. When used specifically for pregnancy termination in the second trimester, misoprostol administered orally is less effective (i.e., more failures) than the vaginal route (relative risk [RR] 3.00, 95% confidence interval [CI] 1.44–6.24) and side effects are more common.[24] Misoprostol regimens used for the induction of labor with fetal death during the second and third trimester range from 50 to 400 μg every 3 to 12 hours; all are clinically effective.[25] The current scientific evidence supports vaginal misoprostol dosages that are adjusted to gestational age: between 13 and 17 weeks, 200 μg q6h; between 18 and 26 weeks, 100 μg q6h; and after 27 weeks, 25 to 50 μg q4h. Caution is advised in women with a previous cesarean and lower doses should be used. In all instances, the patient should be monitored after delivery because of the risk of postpartum atony and/or placenta retention. Common complications of misoprostol include nausea and vomiting, fever, and tachycardia. Their prevalence is generally dependent on route of administration and dose and is greatly reduced by premedication.[17] Their use is discussed further in Chapter 66.

Multiple Gestation (See also Chapters 23 and 59)

The optimal management of the multiple gestation with a singleton demise reflects chorionicity. The incidence of this complication is low (<1% of all twin gestations), but the risk of prematurity, morbidity (especially neurologic), and neonatal death is high among antenatal survivors, especially in monochorionic diamniotic twins (see Chapters 23 and 59).[26,27] There are several potential explanations. First is the cause of death. Could the same stimulus, such as congenital infection or a maternal systemic illness, have caused a sublethal insult yielding a damaged survivor? If so, will continuation of the pregnancy worsen the outcome by prolonging the exposure? An informed decision requires knowledge of the cause and is a matter for individualization.

The second item to consider is whether the dead twin's continued presence poses a risk to the surviving twin. In monochorionic twin gestations, approximately half of the co-twins in an affected pregnancy will either die or experience serious morbidity[28] (see Chapters 23 and 59). Sequelae in survivors of monochorionic gestations with a single demise include bilateral renal cortical necrosis, multicystic encephalomalacia, gastrointestinal structural malformations, and even a DIC.[29–34] It was previously thought the sequelae result from the fetus-to-fetus transfer of necrotic, thromboplastic emboli through placental anastomoses. If this were true, delivery of the surviving twin as soon as possible would be prudent. However, this long-stated explanation has never been supported by a shred of evidence and can now be definitively categorized as a myth. The explanation is one or more hypotensive events occurring either during the co-twin's death associated with extensive vascular anastomosis or after the death as the surviving twin acutely hemorrhages into the dead twin's placenta.[35] As a result, preterm delivery is too late to prevent the sequelae and can only add complications of prematurity. Thus, it is prudent to observe the surviving co-twin very closely, if not continuously for the first 7 days, should the gestation appear monochorionic. It is unclear whether "prophylactic" laser photocoagulation of anastomotic placental vessels will prevent damage once the death has occurred. Survivors should be watched serially for evidence of multicystic leukoencephalomalacia.

If the pregnancy is dizygotic, the risk of death for the surviving co-twin is less than 5%.[26] There is no reason for an iatrogenic delivery prior to 36 weeks solely for the indication of a dead co-twin.

The third and final concern after the death of a co-twin is that the mother will develop coagulopathy should the pregnancy continue. This is an uncommon but treatable event. Laboratory testing for hypofibrinogenemia and thrombocytopenia should be done biweekly after the first 4 weeks. Low-dose heparin, between 10,000 and 30,000 units given subcutaneously in divided doses, is usually adequate to reverse the hypofibrinogenemia.[36,37] There is no need to prolong the partial thromboplastin time. The amount of heparin necessary may seem quite high, and is likely explained by the DIC-mediated decrease in antithrombin. Heparin can usually be discontinued 6 to 8 weeks later without recurrence of the hypofibrinogenemia.

Parental Psychosocial Care

Grief is a normal part of the process. Many hospitals have a counselor or psychologist on the perinatal team to facilitate the grieving process. There may also be local support groups consisting of women who have experienced an intrauterine demise. When appropriate, pastoral care may also be helpful. The woman's partner is encouraged to remain and provide support during labor and after delivery when the couple should be encouraged to view and hold the newborn. Too often, patients incorrectly assume they have conceived a monster. They should also be informed that any bruising and facial marks are normal. Neonatal footprints and handprints are made, and the parents should be encouraged to name the child. Photographs are taken, and if the patient does not want to keep any of these remembrance items, they should be stored. Many women change their mind and later write to request them.

The grieving process may begin prior to the fetus' actual death when associated with the antenatal diagnosis of a lethal congenital or acquired abnormality. Whereas termination shortens the pregnancy, it does not necessarily hasten the resolution of grief.[38] Many couples electively or are required by misguided local laws to continue a pregnancy that has no hope of a living offspring. In this instance, a palliative perinatal care program might prove beneficial.[39,40]

Upon discharge from the hospital, the patient is given an appointment to return after an interval, which should be individualized to her needs. The results of all studies performed are reviewed and the parents given an opportunity to voice any questions they may have about their care.

Evaluation prior to Next Pregnancy

If the cause of death was ascertained, its implications (if any) to subsequent pregnancies should be discussed at their initial postpartum meeting, and again prior to conception if desired. The actions needed should be cause-specific. For example, the discovery of a maternal thrombophilia or connective tissue disorder coupled with the history of a prior stillbirth warrants either medical therapy, prophylactic anticoagulation, or both (see Chapters 42 and 43). The practice of ordering a barrage of antenatal surveillance tests when the cause of death was not hypoxemia due to placental dysfunction is a waste of resources if the subsequent pregnancy is characterized by normal placentation. When the cause of death has escaped detection, it is important to again reinforce to both parents that these events are usually not under their control and that they bear no guilt for its occurrence.

SUMMARY OF MANAGEMENT OPTIONS

Fetal Death

Management Options—For Singleton Pregnancy Unless Stated Otherwise	Evidence Quality and Recommendation	References
Singleton Fetal Death		
Psychosocial Support	III/B	38,40,41
Investigate for a Cause (see Tables 25–1 and 25–2):	III,IV/B,C	41–46
Maternal.		
Fetal.		
Screen for Maternal Coagulopathy		
If death of 4 wk' duration or more.	III/B	10–13
Empty Uterus (See also Chapter 66)		
Many options:		
• **<13–15 Wk**		
Vacuum evacuation/curettage.	III/B	51
Oral mifepristone followed by oral or vaginal prostaglandin 48 h later.	Ia,Ib/A	24,49,50
• **13/15–22 Wk**		
Ripen cervix with laminaria and:	—/GPP	—
Dilation and evacuation (has not been formally compared with contemporary medical methods but safer in comparison to older methods).	III/B	52
Or		
High-dose oxytocin induction.	III/B	47,53
Prostaglandin E_2 vaginal pessaries.	III/B	21,23,47
Misoprostol is very effective (usually oral mifepristone followed by oral or vaginal prostaglandin 48 h later).	Ib/A	22
• **22–28 Wk**		
Ripen cervix with laminaria and oxytocin induction.	—/GPP	—
	III/B	47
Prostaglandin E_2 vaginal pessaries with oxytocin augmentation.	III/B	21,23,48

Management Options—For Singleton Pregnancy Unless Stated Otherwise	Evidence Quality and Recommendation	References
Oral mifepristone followed by oral or vaginal prostaglandin 48 h later. This regimen may need to be supplemented by oxytocin infusion.	III/B	49,50,53
Misoprostol is very effective.	Ib/A	21
• **>28 Wk**		
Cervix favorable:		
Oxytocin induction.	IV/C	47,52
Misoprostol.	Ib/A	53
Cervix unfavorable:		
Ripen cervix with low-dose prostaglandin E_2 vaginal suppositories or misoprostol *without* concurrent oxytocin.		
Overall, vaginal prostaglandin E_2 is superior to oxytocin at inducing labor.	Ia/A	21,23,47, 53
Single Fetal Death in Twin Pregnancy	See Chapters 23 and 59	
Prior to next pregnancy: Review causation and plan appropriate management for pregnancy.	GPP	

GPP, good practice point.

SUGGESTED READINGS

Burgoine GA, Van Kirk SD, Romm J, et al: Comparison of perinatal grief after dilation and evacuation or labor induction in second trimester terminations for fetal anomalies. Am J Obstet Gynecol 2005;192:1928–1932.

de Vienne CM, Creveuil C, Dreyfus M: Does young maternal age increase the risk of adverse obstetric, fetal and neonatal outcomes: A cohort study. Eur J Obstet Gynecol Reprod Biol 2009;147:151–156.

Fretts RC, Boyd ME, Usher RH, Usher HA: The changing pattern of fetal death, 1961–1988. Obstet Gynecol 1992;79:35–39.

Fusi L, McParland P, Fisk N, et al: Acute twin-twin transfusion: A possible mechanism for brain-damaged survivors after intrauterine death of a monochorionic twin. Obstet Gynecol 1991;78:517.

Incerpi MH, Miller DA, Samadi R, et al: Stillbirth evaluation: What tests are needed? Am J Obstet Gynecol 1998;178:1121–1125.

Kulier R, Gulmezoglu A, Hofmeyr G, et al: Medical methods for first trimester abortion. Cochrane Database Syst Rev 2004;1:CD002855.

Lerner R, Margolin M, Slate WG, et al: Heparin in the treatment of hypofibrinogenemia complicating fetal death in utero. Am J Obstet Gynecol 1967;97:373–381.

Silver RM: Fetal death (review). Obstet Gynecol 2007;109:153–167. Erratum appears in Obstet Gynecol 2007;110:191.

REFERENCES

For a complete list of references, log onto www.expertconsult.com.

SECTION FOUR

Infection

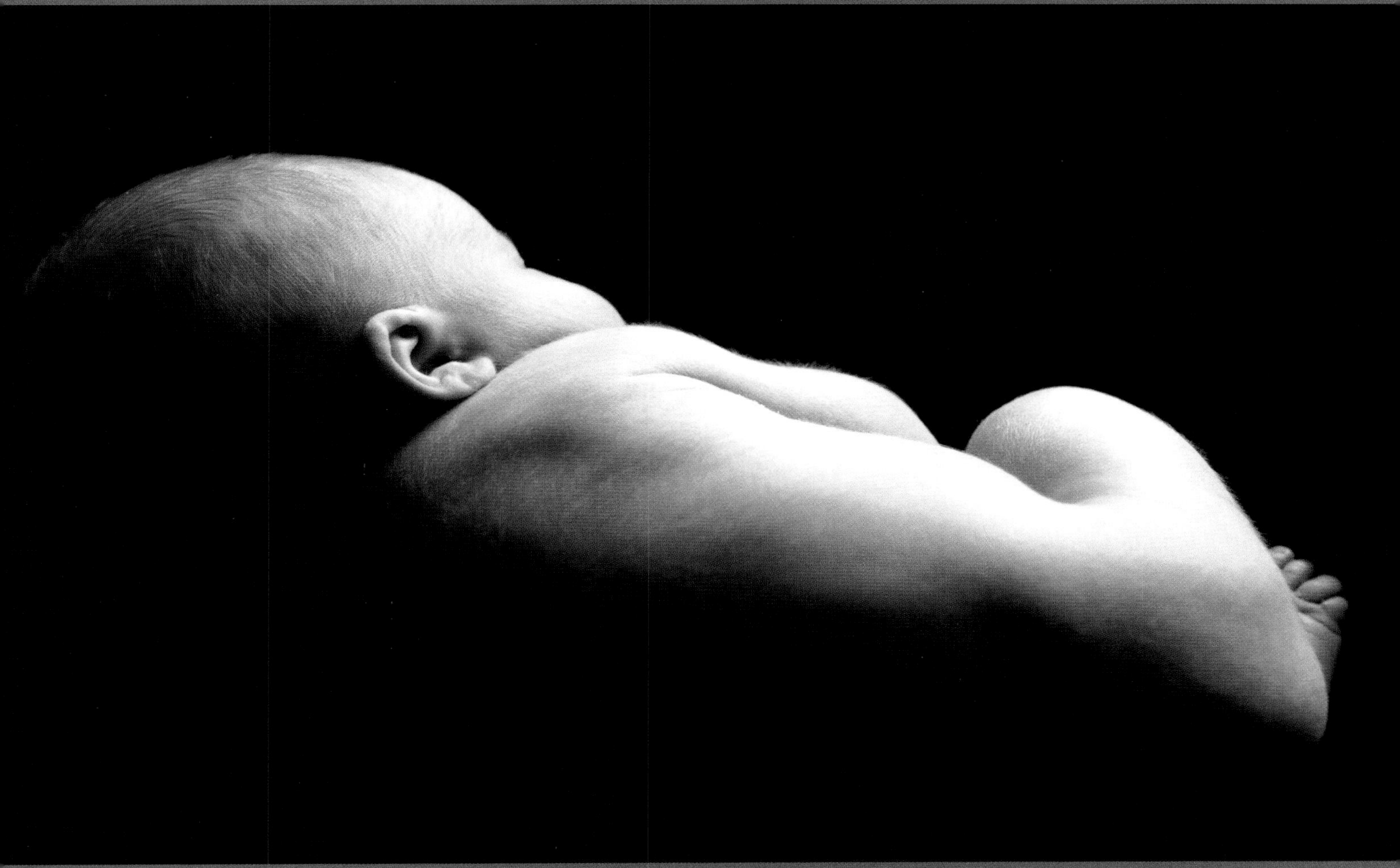

CHAPTER 26

Intrauterine Infection, Preterm Parturition, and the Fetal Inflammatory Response Syndrome

FRANCESCA GOTSCH, ROBERTO ROMERO, and JUAN PEDRO KUSANOVIC

INTRODUCTION

Infection is a frequent and important cause of preterm parturition.[1–8] Indeed, it is the only pathologic process for which both a firm causal link with spontaneous preterm birth has been established and a precise molecular pathophysiology defined.[9,10] Fetal infection/inflammation has been implicated in the genesis of fetal and neonatal injury[11,12] leading to cerebral palsy (CP)[13] and chronic lung disease.[14]

PATHWAYS OF INTRAUTERINE INFECTION

Microorganisms may gain access to the amniotic cavity and the fetus through the following pathways: (1) ascending from the vagina and the cervix; (2) hematogenous dissemination through the placenta; (3) retrograde seeding from the peritoneal cavity through the fallopian tubes; and (4) accidental introduction at the time of invasive procedures.[15–18] The most common pathway for intrauterine infection is the ascending route.[9,15–17] Evidence in support of this includes (1) histologic chorioamnionitis is more common and severe at the site of membrane rupture[5]; (2) in virtually all cases of congenital pneumonia (stillbirths or neonatal), inflammation of the chorioamniotic membranes is present[15,17,19]; (3) bacteria identified in cases of congenital infections are similar to those found in the lower genital tract[16]; and (4) in twin gestations, histologic chorioamnionitis is more common in the first-born twin and has not been demonstrated only in the second twin. This suggests ascending infection, because the membranes of the first twin are apposed to the cervix.[16] This observation is consistent with microbiologic studies of the amniotic fluid (AF) in twin gestations. When AF infection is present, the presenting sac is always involved.[20]

STAGES OF ASCENDING INTRAUTERINE INFECTION

Ascending intrauterine infection has four stages (Fig. 26–1).[3] Stage I consists of a change in the vaginal/cervical microbial flora or the presence of pathologic organisms in the cervix. Some forms of aerobic vaginitis may be an early manifestation of this stage. Once microorganisms traverse the endocervical canal, they reside in the lower pole of the amniotic cavity (stage II). A localized inflammatory reaction causes local chorioamnionitis. The microorganisms may then traverse intact membranes and invade the amniotic cavity (stage III).[21] The last stage of ascending intrauterine infection is fetal infection (stage IV). Once in the amniotic cavity, the bacteria may gain access to the fetus by several ports of entry. Aspiration of the infected fluid by the fetus may cause congenital pneumonia. Otitis, conjunctivitis, and omphalitis are localized infections that occur by direct seeding of the microorganisms from infected AF. Seeding from any of these sites to the fetal circulation results in bacteremia and sepsis.

The fetus is exposed to microorganisms and their products (i.e., bacterial endotoxin)[22] in the amniotic cavity and responds by mounting a cellular and humoral immunoresponse.[23] The overall mortality rate of neonates with congenital neonatal sepsis ranges from 25% to 90%. This wide range may reflect the effect of gestational age on survival; the mortality of infants born before 33 weeks' gestation has been reported to be 33% for infected and 17% for noninfected fetuses.[24] Carroll and coworkers[25] reported fetal bacteremia in 33% of fetuses with positive AF culture and in 4% of those with negative AF culture. Goldenberg and colleagues[26] reported that 23% of neonates born at 23 to 32 weeks' gestation have positive umbilical blood cultures for *Ureaplasma urealyticum* and *Mycoplasma hominis*. Newborns with positive blood cultures had a higher frequency of a neonatal

FIGURE 26–1
The stages of ascending infection. *Stage I*: Consists of an overgrowth of facultative organisms or the presence of the pathologic organisms in the vagina, cervix, or both. *Stage II*: Once microorganisms traverse the endocervical canal, they reside in the lower pole of the amniotic cavity. A localized inflammatory reaction causes local chorioamnionitis. *Stage III*: The microorganisms may then traverse intact membranes, leading to microbial invasion of the amniotic cavity. *Stage IV*: Once in the amniotic cavity, the bacteria may gain access to the fetus by different ports of entry.
(Modified from Romero R, Mazor M: Infection and preterm labor. Clin Obstet Gynecol 1988;31:553–584.)

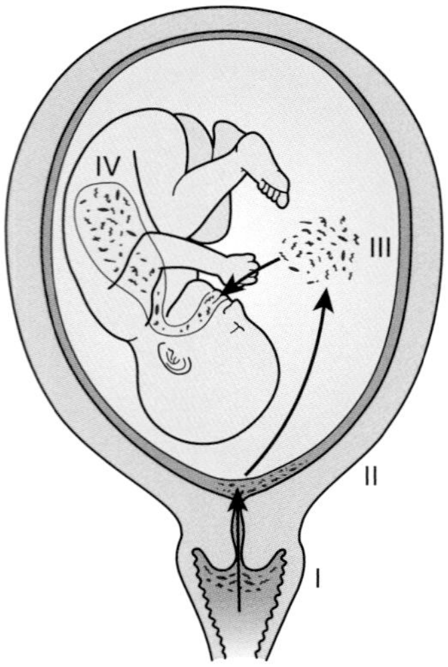

systemic inflammatory response syndrome, higher umbilical cord serum concentrations of interleukin (IL)-6, and more frequent histologic evidence of placental inflammation than those with negative cultures.

MICROBIOLOGY OF INTRAUTERINE INFECTION

The most common microbial isolates from the amniotic cavity of women with preterm labor (PTL) with intact membranes are *U. urealyticum*, *Fusobacterium* spp., and *M. hominis*.[3,8,27] In patients with preterm premature rupture of membranes (PPROM), microbial invasion of the amniotic cavity (MIAC) by *U. urealyticum* is associated with a robust inflammatory response in the fetal, amniotic, and maternal compartments.[28] *U. urealyticum* is implicated in the genesis of clinical chorioamnionitis, puerperal endometritis, postoperative wound infections, neonatal sepsis, meningitis, and bronchopulmonary dysplasia. Other microorganisms found in the AF include *Streptococcus agalactiae*, *Peptostreptococcus* spp., *Staphylococcus aureus*, *Gardnerella vaginalis*, *Streptococcus viridans*, and *Bacteroides* spp. Occasionally, *Lactobacillus* spp., *Escherichia coli*, *Enterococcus faecalis*, *Neisseria gonorrhoeae*, and *Peptostreptococcus* spp. are encountered. *Haemophilus influenzae*, *Capnocytophaga* spp., *Stomatococcus* spp., and *Clostridium* spp. are rarely identified.[29,30] Among patients with PTL, 50% of those with MIAC have more than one microorganism isolated from the amniotic cavity. The inoculum size varies considerably, and in 71% of the cases, more than 10^5 colony-forming units per milliliter (CFU/mL) are found.[5]

FREQUENCY OF INTRA-AMNIOTIC INFECTION IN PRETERM GESTATION

One third of all patients with preterm delivery present with PTL and intact membranes and one third with PPROM. The remaining third are the result of delivery for maternal or fetal indications (e.g., preeclampsia, fetal growth restriction [IUGR]). Microbiologic investigations suggest that intrauterine infection is present in 25% to 40% of spontaneous preterm births.[7] However, this is probably an underestimate because some pathogens are difficult to identify by conventional cultivation techniques. Indeed, using molecular microbiologic techniques, additional bacterial rDNAs have been identified in culture-negative AF from women in PTL.[29,31,32] Further, microbial colonization of the chorioamnion was shown to be twice that of the amniotic cavity.[33,34]

Microbial Invasion of the Amniotic Cavity

In patients with PTL and intact membranes, the mean rate of positive AF cultures for microorganisms is 12.8% (379/2963), based on a review of 33 studies.[8] Women with positive AF cultures generally do not have clinical evidence of infection at presentation, but are more likely to develop clinical chorioamnionitis (37.5% vs. 9%), be refractory to tocolysis (85.6% vs. 16.3%), and rupture their membranes spontaneously (40% vs. 3.8%) than women with negative AF cultures.[8] Neonates born to women with MIAC have more complications than those born to women without infection.[27] Moreover, the earlier the gestational age at birth, the more likely MIAC is present.[35]

In patients with PPROM, the rate of positive AF cultures for microorganisms is 32.4% (47/142).[8] Clinical chorioamnionitis is present in only 29.7% of those with proven MIAC.[8,9] The rate of MIAC in PPROM is probably an underestimate. In addition to the reasons cited with PTL, women with oligohydramnios and those with PPROM admitted in labor are less likely to have an amniocentesis. Yet, women with PPROM and severe oligohydramnios have a higher incidence of intra-amniotic infection/inflammation (IAI)[36] than those without oligohydramnios and those admitted in labor have a higher rate of MIAC than those admitted without labor (39% vs. 25%; $P < .05$).[37] Finally, 75% of women who are not in labor on admission have a positive AF culture at the time of the onset of labor.[37] This means that patients with PPROM acquire MIAC and that they often go into labor when IAI is present. Antibiotic administration to patients with PPROM does not always eradicate IAI, and MIAC may be acquired while receiving antibiotics.[38]

Women presenting with a dilated cervix, intact membranes, and few, if any, contractions before 24 weeks' gestation are considered to have clinical cervical insufficiency. In one study, 51.1% of these patients had a positive AF culture for microorganisms.[39] The outcome of patients with MIAC was uniformly poor because these individuals developed subsequent complications (rupture of membranes, clinical chorioamnionitis, or pregnancy loss). Therefore, infection is frequently associated with dysfunctional cervical ripening. The contribution of subclinical inflammation to dysfunctional cervical ripening has been investigated.[40] In women with dysfunctional cervical ripening undergoing rescue cerclage between 15 and 27 weeks' gestation, the median AF IL-6 concentration (prior the cerclage placement) was higher than in controls (women undergoing amniocentesis for karyotyping at 16–27 weeks' gestation). Moreover, an inverse relationship was found between the AF IL-6 concentration and the latency interval from cerclage to delivery.[40] Among patients with dysfunctional cervical ripening between 17 and 29 weeks' gestation, the prevalence of IAI was reported to be 81%.[41] Among those with dysfunctional cervical ripening and IAI, in the absence of infection, preterm delivery within 7 days occurred in 50% of cases, 84% of patients delived at less than 34 weeks' gestation, and 55% of newborns died immediately after birth (<1 day). It is possible that clinically silent cervical dilation with protrusion of the membranes into the vagina leads to a secondary intrauterine infection.

A sonographic short cervix is considered a powerful predictor of spontaneous preterm delivery.[42–45] The shorter the sonographic cervical length (CL) in the mid trimester of pregnancy, the higher the likelihood of spontaneous preterm delivery.[42–45] Hassan and associates[46] conducted a retrospective study of 57 patients with a CL less than 25 mm at 14 to 24 weeks' gestation. The prevalence of IAI was 9% (5/57). Among these patients, the rate of preterm delivery less than 32 weeks was 40% (2/5), suggesting that a short cervix may be the only manifestation of subclinical MIAC. A CL of 5 mm or less at 16 to 24 weeks' gestation is associated with higher AF concentrations of inflammatory cytokines, even in the absence of proven infection or labor.[47] An inverse correlation was found between AF concentrations of proinflammatory cytokines and sonographic CL. Of 25 cytokines assayed, monocyte chemotactic protein (MCP)-1 was the most differentially regulated.[47]

Microbial invasion of the amniotic cavity occurs in 11.9% to 13% of twin gestations presenting with PTL and delivery[20,48] compared with a 21.6% culture-positive rate in singleton gestations with PTL and delivery.[5] Microorganisms are more frequently isolated from the presenting sac (55.6%) or both sacs (33.3%) rather than from the upper sac alone (11.1%).[48] These data suggest that IAI is a possible cause of PTL and delivery in twin gestation, but does not support the hypothesis that IAI is responsible for a large part of the excessive rate of preterm delivery observed.

CHORIOAMNIOTIC INFECTION, HISTOLOGIC CHORIOAMNIONITIS, AND PRETERM BIRTH

Inflammation of the placenta and chorioamniotic membranes is a nonspecific host response to a variety of stimuli, including infection. Acute inflammation of the chorioamniotic membranes has traditionally been considered an indicator of AF infection.[15–17,19,49,50] Indeed, several studies demonstrated an association between acute inflammatory lesions of the placenta and the recovery of microorganisms from the subchorionic plate and chorioamniotic space. Furthermore, there is a strong correlation between positive AF cultures for microorganisms and histologic chorioamnionitis.[49,50] Cassell and coworkers[33] reported an association between positive microbial cultures obtained from the chorioamniotic interface and histologic chorioamnionitis. The presence of inflammation in the umbilical cord (funisitis) represents evidence of a fetal inflammatory response.[51] Collectively, the evidence indicates an association between preterm birth and the occurrence of acute chorioamnionitis; it also indicates that the lower the gestational age at birth, the higher the frequency of histologic chorioamnionitis and funisitis.[52]

The rate of microbial colonization in the chorioamniotic space is higher than that observed in the amniotic cavity. If the infection is localized to the decidua or the space between the amnion and the chorion, microorganisms may not be detected in the amniotic cavity. Thus, intrauterine infection can be present without a positive AF culture for microorganisms or a positive polymerase chain reaction (PCR).[53] Patients with positive membrane cultures, but negative AF cultures, often have elevated AF concentrations of inflammation indicators, such as IL-6.[53] Therefore, some patients with IAI but negative cultures in the AF may have intrauterine infection in the extra-amniotic space. Fluorescence in situ hybridization (FISH) with a DNA probe specific for conserved regions of bacterial DNA (the 16S ribosomal RNA) has detected bacteria in the fetal membranes of up to 70% of women undergoing elective cesarean section at term.[54] Organisms were also detected in fetal membranes after preterm delivery without labor.[54] Inflammatory cells were found frequently in the amnion or chorion of preterm fetal membranes but not in term tissues. These findings suggest that the presence of bacteria alone is not sufficient to cause PTL and delivery and that microbial colonization of the chorioamniotic membranes may not always elicit a fetal or maternal inflammatory response. In recent studies, we were unable to identify bacteria in the fetal membranes of normal patients at term using FISH for the 16S ribosomal DNA. Moreover, even in the cases of IAI, most of the organisms were in the amnion rather than in the chorion. These observations challenge the conventional view of ascending intrauterine infection.[55]

INTRAUTERINE INFECTION/INFLAMMATION AS A CHRONIC PROCESS

Microbial invasion of the amniotic cavity has been reported at the time of genetic amniocentesis. Cassel and colleagues[56] recovered genital mycoplasmas from 6.6% (4/61) of AF samples collected by amniocentesis between 16 and 21 weeks. Two patients with *M. hominis* delivered at 34 and 40 weeks without neonatal complications, whereas two with *U. urealyticum* had premature delivery, sepsis, and neonatal death at 24 and 29 weeks. Subsequently, Gray and associates[57] reported a 0.37% prevalence (9/2461) of positive cultures for *M. hominis* or *U. urealyticum* in AF samples. Except for 1 woman who had a therapeutic abortion, all patients with a positive AF culture had either a fetal loss within 4 weeks of the amniocentesis ($n = 6$) or preterm delivery ($n = 2$). Horowitz and coworkers[58] detected *U. urealyticum* in 2.8% (6/214) of AF samples obtained between 16 and 20 weeks' gestation. The rate of adverse pregnancy outcome was higher in patients with a positive AF culture than in those with a negative culture (50% vs. 12%; $P = .04$).[58] In a retrospective study, Berg and colleagues[59] found 1.8% (49/2718) positive cultures for *Ureaplasma/Mycoplasma*, and 34 patients were treated with oral erythromycin. Mid-trimester pregnancy loss was lower in the 34 patients treated with erythromycin than in the untreated group (11.4% vs. 44.4%; $P = .04$). However, no differences were observed in the rates of preterm delivery (19.4% vs. 20%) and adverse pregnancy outcome (28.6% vs. 55.6%).[59] In summary, these observations suggest that MIAC may be clinically silent in the mid trimester of pregnancy and that pregnancy loss/preterm delivery can take weeks to occur.

AF IL-6 concentration is a marker of IAI and is frequently associated with microbiologic infection in either the AF or the chorioamniotic space.[60,61] Romero and associates[62] conducted a case-control study in which IL-6 was measured in the stored AF of women who had a pregnancy loss after a mid-trimester amniocentesis and compared them with a control group who delivered at term. Patients who lost their pregnancies had a higher median AF IL-6 concentration. Similar findings were reported by Wenstrom and coworkers.[63] In contrast, maternal plasma IL-6 concentration is not associated with adverse pregnancy outcome. Chaiworapongsa and colleagues[64] measured AF MCP-1 at the time of genetic amniocentesis and reported higher concentrations in 10 patients who had a pregnancy loss after the procedure compared with 84 patients with a normal pregnancy outcome. An MCP-1 concentration greater than 765 pg/mL was strongly associated with pregnancy loss (odds ratio [OR] 7.35; 95% confidence interval [CI] 1.7–31.0).

An association can also be demonstrated between markers of inflammation (matrix metalloproteinase [MMP]-8,[65] IL-6,[66] tumor necrosis factor-α [TNF-α],[67] angiogenin,[68] and C-reactive protein[69]) in mid-trimester AF samples and preterm delivery. Goldenberg and associates[70] demonstrated that the maternal plasma concentration of granulocyte colony-stimulating factor (G-CSF) at 24 and 28 weeks' gestation was associated with early preterm birth, suggesting that a chronic inflammatory process, identifiable in the maternal compartment, is associated with early preterm birth. Collectively, the evidence suggests that a chronic IAI process is associated with both spontaneous abortion and spontaneous preterm delivery.

IS THE RELATIONSHIP BETWEEN INTRAUTERINE INFECTION AND SPONTANEOUS PRETERM BIRTH CAUSAL?

An association of intrauterine infection with spontaneous preterm delivery does not mean that infection *causes* preterm delivery. Indeed, it has been argued that MIAC is merely a consequence of labor.[71,72] The evidence supporting a causal role for infection in preterm parturition includes (1) biologic plausibility, (2) temporal relationship, (3) consistency and strength of association, (4) dose-response gradient, (5) specificity, and (6) animal experimentation. Administration of bacterial products or microorganisms to pregnant animals can lead to premature labor and delivery. Three sets of observations suggest that infection precedes the spontaneous onset of PTL and delivery: (1) subclinical MIAC or intrauterine inflammation in the mid trimester of pregnancy leads to either spontaneous abortion or premature delivery, (2) patients with PPROM who had a positive AF culture for genital mycoplasmas on admission have a shorter amniocentesis-to-delivery interval than those with sterile AF,[73] and (3) abnormal colonization of the lower genitourinary tract with microorganisms is a risk factor for preterm delivery. These conditions include asymptomatic bacteriuria, bacterial vaginosis, and infection with *N. gonorrhoeae*. The consistency and strength of association between infection and preterm delivery is demonstrated by the many studies in which AF was cultured in women with PPROM and PTL; the relative risk for preterm delivery in patients with PTL and MIAC is high (>2) and the hazard ratio for the duration of pregnancy after PPROM is also high.

The likelihood of a causal relationship is increased if a dose-response gradient can be demonstrated. Evidence supporting the existence of this includes (1) the median concentration of bacterial endotoxin is higher in patients in PTL than in patients not in labor,[74] (2) a microbial inoculum greater than 10^5 CFU/mL is more common in women with PPROM admitted with PTL than in those admitted without labor (41.6% vs. 15%; $P = .03$),[37] and (3) the rate of abortion/preterm delivery after administration of *E. coli* bacterial endotoxin to pregnant mice exhibits a clear dose-response gradient.

One criterion for causality that is not met is specificity. Although intrauterine infection appears sufficient to induce PTL and delivery, it is not specific because many patients have a preterm delivery in the absence of evidence of IAI. However, the formulation of "the necessary and sufficient cause" can inappropriately restrict the conceptualization of cause. Although the causal relationship between smoking and lung cancer is accepted, it is also nonspecific; lung cancer occurs in nonsmokers and smoking causes other diseases. Microbiologic, cytologic, biochemical, immunologic, and pathologic data indicate that PTL is a syndrome and infection is but one of its causes.[9]

An important criterion for causation is whether eradication of the agent decreases the frequency of outcome or illness. There is evidence that treatment of patients with asymptomatic bacteriuria reduces the rate of prematurity/low birth weight[75] and that antibiotic treatment of patients with PPROM prolongs the latency period and reduces the rate of maternal and neonatal infection.[76] However, antibiotic treatment in patients with PTL has not yielded positive results in most trials.[77–80] The reasons for this are complex and are probably related to the syndromic and chronic nature of preterm parturition and the inclusion of many patients who do not have intrauterine infection and, thus, cannot benefit from antimicrobial treatment.

DETECTION OF MICROBIAL FOOTPRINTS IN THE AMNIOTIC FLUID WITH SEQUENCE-BASED TECHNIQUES

Estimates of the frequency and type of microorganisms participating in intrautering infections are based on standard microbiologic techniques (e.g., culture). Surveys of terrestrial and aquatic ecosystems indicate that more than 99%[81] of existing microorganisms may not be cultivated using standard microbiologic techniques (e.g., culture) and that only molecular diagnosis can provide identification of these microorganisms.[82] Sequenced-based methodologies are likely to demonstrate how insensitive conventional microbiology methods are for the detection of already known and potentially "new" microorganisms in perinatal medicine. However, application of these techniques to clinical practice poses clinical, technological, and conceptual questions and challenges.

Two strategies have been used to detect microorganisms in the AF with PCR. The broad-range PCR uses primer pairs designed to anneal with highly conserved DNA regions of all bacteria, such as the 16S ribosomal DNA. A positive result indicates the presence of bacteria, but identification of the specific organism requires subsequent sequencing of the PCR products. The second approach is to use specific primers for a particular microorganism. Four studies used primers for the conserved sequence,[29,31,83,84] five used specific primers to recover bacterial DNA from AF,[85–89] while one applied both approaches.[90] Blanchard and coworkers[87] were the first to report the recovery of *U. urealyticum* from AF using specific primers for the urease structural genes. Ten of 293 AF samples collected at cesarean section were PCR-positive but only 4 were also culture-positive. Others have applied broad-spectrum bacterial 16S rDNA PCR for the detection of bacteria in AF.[31,29,83] Hitti and colleagues[29] studied 69 women in PTL with intact membranes. PCR was positive in 94% of the culture-positive AF samples (15/16) and in 36% of the patients with a negative culture. Five of the 14 women with an elevated IL-6 concentration had bacteria detected by PCR. In Markenson and associates' study,[83] 55.5% of the 54 women with PTL but without clinical evidence of infection were PCR-positive, whereas only 9.2% of the cultures recovered a microorganism ($P < .05$). Two thirds (6/9) of the AF samples with an elevated IL-6 were also PCR-positive.

Oyarzun and coworkers[85] described a PCR amplification technique aimed at detecting the 16 microorganisms most commonly cultured from the AF of patients in PTL. AF samples were examined with bacterial culture and PCR in 50 patients with PTL and 23 patients not in labor. All control samples were both culture- and PCR-negative. A higher proportion of samples were positive by PCR than by culture (46% vs. 12%; $P < .05$). The sensitivity of PCR for the prediction of PTL before 34 weeks was better than culture (64% vs. 18%; $P < .05$). However, there were patients with positive PCR who delivered at term without maternal or neonatal complications.

The clinical implications of detecting *U. urealyticum* in AF by PCR in patients with PPROM[86] or PTL[88] were evaluated by Yoon and colleagues. Patients with a positive PCR assay, but a negative culture, had a stronger AF inflammatory reaction (higher AF white blood cell [WBC] count and IL-6 concentration), a shorter interval to delivery, as well as a higher rate of histologic chorioamnionitis, funisitis, and neonatal morbidity than those with a negative AF culture and negative AF PCR assay. These studies reveal that patients with PPROM or PTL and a positive PCR assay for *U. urealyticum* (but a negative culture) have worse pregnancy outcomes than those with a sterile AF culture and negative PCR.

Gerber and associates[89] used PCR to detect *U. urealyticum* DNA in the AF of asymptomatic patients undergoing genetic amniocentesis. Test results were positive in 11.4% (29/294) of the pregnancies and, among these, 58.6% delivered preterm. In contrast, only 4.4% of the PCR-negative patients delivered prematurely ($P < .0001$). This study is consistent with the premise of chronic *U. urealyticum* infection because women with a positive *U. urealyticum* DNA in the AF had a higher frequency of preterm birth in previous pregnancies than women with PCR-negative AF (20.7% vs. 2.7%; $P = .0008$). In a smaller study of women undergoing genetic amniocentesis, bacterial 16S ribosomal DNA was detected in 18% (14/78) of AF samples.[90] No samples tested positive for *Mycoplasma* spp. DNA using a PCR/enzyme-linked immunosorbent assay. No association was found between the recovery of bacteria at the time of amniocentesis and either increased IL-6 concentration in the AF or preterm delivery. Nguyen and coworkers[91] identified *M. hominis* in 6.4% (29/456) of AF samples obtained at 15 to 17 weeks' gestation. The rate of PTL and delivery less than 37 weeks' gestation was higher in women with a positive PCR for *M. hominis* than in those with negative PCR (14.3% vs. 3.3%; $P = .01$; and 10.7% vs. 1.9%; $P = .02$, respectively). Perni and colleagues[92] detected *M. hominis* and *U. urealyticum* by PCR in 6.1% (11/179) and 12.8% (22/172) of asymptomatic women at 15 to 19 weeks' gestation, respectively. PPROM occurred in 2.8% (5/179) of women, and the same proportion of patients had a spontaneous preterm birth with intact membranes. All women with PPROM were positive for either *M. hominis* or *U. urealyticum*, whereas none of those with spontaneous preterm birth. Finally, Wenstrom and associates[93] compared AF samples from a group of 62 pregnancy losses following mid-trimester amniocentesis with 60 controls. PCR was performed for the presence of adenovirus, parvovirus, cytomegalovirus (CMV), Epstein-Barr virus (EBV), herpes simplex virus (HSV), β-actin DNA, enterovirus, and influenza A. No difference in the prevalence of viruses was observed between cases and controls (8% vs. 15%). Adenovirus was identified in 6% of cases but also in 8% of controls.

We have recently compared the results of culture and molecular techniques[84] and demonstrated that the AF of women in PTL and intact membranes harbors DNA from a greater diversity of microbes than previously suspected. This includes uncultivated, previously uncharacterized taxa (bacteria, fungi, and archea). The combined use of molecular and culture methods revealed a greater prevalence (15%) and diversity (18 taxa) of microbes in AF than did the culture alone (9.6%, 11 taxa). A positive PCR was associated with histologic chorioamnionitis (adjusted OR 20; 95% CI 2.4–172), and funisitis (adjusted OR 18; 95% CI 3.1–99). Moreover, the positive predictive value of PCR for preterm delivery was 100%.[84]

MOLECULAR MECHANISMS FOR PRETERM PARTURITION IN THE SETTING OF INTRAUTERINE INFECTION

A considerable body of evidence supports a role for inflammatory mediators in the mechanisms of preterm parturition associated with infection.

Prostaglandins and Lipoxygenase Products

Intrauterine prostaglandins (PGs) are considered by many to be the key mediators of the biochemical mechanisms regulating the onset of labor. They can induce myometrial contractility[94,95] as well as changes in the extracellular matrix metabolism associated with cervical ripening[96] and are thought to participate in decidual/fetal membrane activation.[9] The evidence invoked in support of a role for PGs in the initiation of labor includes (1) administration of PGs induces early and late termination of pregnancy (abortion or labor),[97,98] (2) treatment with indomethacin or aspirin delays the spontaneous onset of parturition in animals,[99,100] (3) PG concentrations in plasma and AF increase during labor,[101,102] and (4) intra-amniotic injection of arachidonic acid can induce abortion.[103]

Infection can increase PG production by amnion, chorion, or decidua through the activity of bacterial products, pro-inflammatory cytokines, growth factors, and other inflammatory mediators. Indeed, AF concentrations of PGE_2 and PGF_2 and their stable metabolites, PGEM and PGFM, are higher in women with PTL and MIAC than in women with PTL without infection.[104] Similar observations have been made in patients with labor and high AF concentrations of IL-1β, TNF, and IL-6. Moreover, amnion obtained from women with histologic chorioamnionitis produces higher amounts of PGs. More recent evidence also suggests that PGD_2 and its active metabolites are involved in the mechanism leading to term and preterm parturition.[105,106]

Metabolites of arachidonic acid derived through the lipoxygenase pathway, including leukotrienes (LTs) and hydroxyeicosatetraenoic acids (HETEs), are also implicated in the mechanisms of spontaneous preterm and term parturition. Concentrations of 5-HETE, LTB_4, and 15-HETE are increased in the AF of women with PTL and MIAC.[107,108] Similarly, amnion from patients with histologic chorioamnionitis releases more LTB_4 in vitro than amnion from women delivering preterm without inflammation.[109] 5-HETE and LTB_4 can also stimulate uterine contractility, and LTB_4 is thought to play a role in the recruitment of neutrophils to the site of infection.[110]

Inflammatory Cytokines

Strong evidence suggests that pro-inflammatory cytokines (IL-1, TNF, IL-18) and chemokines (IL-8, MCP-1, macrophage inflammatory protein [MIP]-1α, requested on activation, normal T cell expressed and secreted [RANTES], and epithelial cell-derived neutrophil-activating peptide-78) are involved in the mechanisms responsible for PTL associated with infection. IL-1β and TNF-α are the most extensively investigated pro-inflammatory cytokines in the context of PTL: (1) IL-1β and TNF-α stimulate PG production by amnion, decidua, and myometrium[111–114]; (2) human decidua produces IL-1β and TNF-α in response to bacterial products[112,114]; (3) AF IL-1β and TNF-α bioactivity and concentrations are elevated in women with PTL and IAI[113,114]; (4) in women with PPROM and IAI, IL-1β and TNF-α concentrations are higher in the presence of labor[116,117]; (5) IL-1β and TNF-α induce preterm parturition when administered systemically to pregnant animals[118,119]; (6) pretreatment with the natural IL-1 receptor antagonist prior to the administration of IL-1 to pregnant animals prevents preterm parturition[120]; and (7) fetal plasma IL-1β is elevated in the context of PTL with intrauterine infection.[121] However, there is considerable redundancy in the cytokine network, and it remains unclear whether a particular cytokine signals the onset of labor.

Adipocytokines

Adipose tissue is a highly active endocrine organ[122,123] that can orchestrate a metabolic response to insults and mount an inflammatory response via the production of soluble adipocytokines (cytokines that are produced mainly, but not exclusively, by adipose tissue). Adipocytokines such as resistin[124] and visfatin[125] participate in the modulation of the innate immune responses, whereas leptin and adiponectin regulate the innate[126] and adaptive[127] immune responses.

Adiponectin, the most abundant gene (*AMP1*) product of adipose tissue, has profound insulin-sensitizing and anti-inflammatory properties. Our group[128] has recently reported that PTL is characterized by a change in the maternal serum profile of adiponectin multimer concentrations that favors insulin resistance and a pro-inflammatory state. These changes were more pronounced in the presence of IAI.[128] Consistent with these observations, preterm parturition and IAI were associated with alterations of AF concentrations of adiponectin.[129] Visfatin is produced preferentially by visceral adipose tissue and exerts insulin-mimicking and pro-inflammatory and immunomodulating effects. PTL and MIAC[130] were both associated with alterations in maternal plasma[131] and AF[130] concentrations of visfatin. Resistin is mainly produced by circulating monocytes and macrophages. AF concentrations of resistin are higher in patients with PTL and in those with PPROM with IAI than in those without IAI.[132] This evidence suggests that adipocytokines may play a role in maternal metabolic adaptations to PTL in the presence of IAI as well as in the regulation of the host response against infection.

Anti-inflammatory Cytokines and Preterm Labor

The resolution of the inflammatory response is an active process that encompasses the removal of the inflammatory stimulus, a decrease in bioavailability of pro-inflammatory mediators with a switch to an anti-inflammatory milieu, followed by tissue repair. Several cytokines have anti-inflammatory properties, including IL-4, IL-10, and IL-27.[133,134]

IL-10 is a cytokine highly expressed in the uterus and placenta and is implicated in pregnancy maintainence.[135] Down-regulation of placental IL-10 has been implicated in the onset of spontaneous labor at term.[133] In addition, IL-10 plays an important role in controlling inflammation-induced pathologies of pregnancy,[136] and it has been implicated in the preterm parturition associated with inflammation.[135] Women with PTL and IAI have higher median AF IL-10 concentrations than those without IAI, suggesting that IL-10 is present to dampen the inflammatory response associated with severe infection.[137] The abundance of endogenous IL-10 in gestational tissues has been identified as a determinant of resistance to PTL, because IL-10 is thought to modulate resistance to inflammatory stimuli by down-regulating pro-inflammatory cytokines.[136] Evidence that IL-10 confers resistance to PTL includes (1) IL-10 knock-out mice experience pregnancy loss in response to very low doses of lipopolysaccharide (LPS)[138]; (2) the IL-10 -1082A/-819T/-592A (IL-10 ATA)-haplotype, associated with low IL-10 production, was found to be independently associated with early preterm birth[139]; (3) administration of IL-10 to pregnant rhesus monkeys results in a reduction of IL-1β–induced uterine contractility as well as the TNF-α and WBC count in the AF[140]; and (4) the administration of IL-10 in animal models of infection has been associated with improved pregnancy outcome.[141]

Pattern Recognition Receptors Identify Microorganisms

The first line of defense against infection is provided by the innate immune system. One of the mechanisms by which the innate immune system recognizes microorganisms is by using pattern recognition receptors (PRRs), which bind to patterns of molecular structures present on the surfaces of microorganisms.[142] Toll-like receptors (TLRs) are a group of transmembrane PRRs.[143] Ten different TLRs have been identified in humans. TLR-2 recognizes peptidoglycans, lipoproteins, and zymosan (gram-positive bacteria, mycoplasmas, and fungi); TLR-4 recognizes LPS (produced by gram-negative bacteria); and TLR-3 recognizes double-stranded RNA (viruses).[143,144] Ligation of TLRs results in activation of nuclear factor κB (NF-κB), which, in turn, leads to the production of cytokines, chemokines, and antimicrobial peptides. Moreover, activation of the Toll pathway also induces surface expression of costimulatory molecules required for the induction of adaptive costimulatory immune responses, such as CD80 and CD86. In combination with antigenic microbial peptides, these molecules presented by major histocompatability complex class II proteins in dendritic cells and macrophages can activate naïve CD4 T cells that initiate an adaptive immune response.[142]

Expression of TLRs has been reported in the fetal membranes,[145] placenta,[146,147] and placental bed.[148] Expression of TLRs within the placenta is not restricted to the infiltrating immune cells and Hoffbauer cells,[147] but it is a feature of human trophoblasts as well.[146,147,149] This suggests a participation of the placenta itself in the induction of immune responses against pathogens.[149] Expression of TLR-2,[149] TLR-4,[149] and TLR-3[150] has been demonstrated by immunohistochemistry in first-trimester trophoblasts. Abrahams and coworkers[149,150] observed that cytotrophoblast and extravillous trophoblast, but not syncytiotrophoblasts, expressed TLR-2 and TLR-4 during the first trimester, suggesting that the placenta is able to respond only to those pathogens that breached the syncytiotrophoblast layer and entered either the placental villous or the decidual compartments.[151] Ligation of TLR-2 in first-trimester trophoblast cells by bacterial product results in the activation of the apoptotic pathway.[149] In contrast, ligation of TLR-4 by LPS results in the production of both pro- and anti-inflammatory cytokines.[150] TLR-3 mediates responses to viral dsRNA.[152] Ligation of TLR-3 in first-trimester trophoblasts is followed by up-regulation of a cytokine profile that is distinct from that induced following bacterial stimulation.[153]

Accumulating evidence suggests that TLRs participate in the onset and/or maintenance of infection-induced PTL[154] and that the innate immune system plays a role in parturition. Because TLRs are crucial for the recognition of microorganisms, it could be anticipated that defective signaling through this PRR would impair bacteria-induced PTL. Indeed, mice that have a spontaneous mutation for TLR-4 are less likely to deliver preterm after intrauterine inoculation of heat-killed bacteria or LPS administration than wild-type mice.[155,156] More recently, it was been demonstrated that preterm delivery in the mouse can be induced by TLR-2 stimulation with peptidoglycans and TLR-3 stimulation with polyinosinic acid.[157] In humans, spontaneous labor at term or preterm with histologic chorioamnionitis is associated with an increased mRNA and protein expression of TLR-2 and TLR-4 in the chorioamniotic membranes.[145] Further evidence for the role of TLRs in the infection-associated PTL comes from genetic studies; a polymorphism, which is known to confer impaired TLR-4 function and higher likelihood of gram-negative sepsis, is carried more often by preterm infants than by term infants and by mothers delivering preterm than at term.[158]

Matrix-Degrading Enzymes

The mechanisms responsible for PPROM are only partially understood. The tensile strength and elasticity of the chorioamniotic membranes are attributed to extracellular matrix proteins. Matrix-degrading enzymes have therefore been implicated in PPROM and there is now compelling evidence of increased availability of MMP-1, MMP-8, MMP-9, and neutrophil elastase, but not MMP-2, MMP-3, MMP-7, and MMP-13, in PPROM. Proposed mechanisms to regulate the expression and activity of matrix-degrading enzymes in fetal membranes include apoptosis[159] and increased availability of superoxide anions,[160] respectively.

Fetal carriage of functional polymorphisms that lead to overproduction of MMP-1, MMP-9, and MMP-8 in response to microorganisms have been associated with PPROM.[161–163] In addition to genetic variation, epigenetic mechanisms (DNA methylation) play a role in controlling MMP-1 expression in the human amnion and the risk of obstetric adverse outcome.[164]

Our group has proposed that the management of patients with PTL[165] or PPROM[166] should be based on the diagnosis of intra-amniotic inflammation rather than the diagnosis of IAI, because (1) the outcome of patients with MIAC is similar to that of patients with intra-amniotic inflammation and a negative AF culture and (2) results of AF culture are not available for 48 hours. MMP-8 is an excellent marker of intra-amniotic inflammation[167] and a bedside test is now available to detect elevated concentrations of MMP-8 in AF. The MMP-8 PTD (preterm delivery) Check test (SK Pharma Co, Ltd, Kyunggi-do, Korea) requires only 20 μL of AF and no laboratory equipment. The results are available within 15 minutes. Nien and colleagues[168] performed the MMP-8 rapid test in 331 patients admitted with increased preterm uterine contractions and intact membranes; the positive predictive values for spontaneous delivery within 48 hours and 7 days were 70% and 94%, respectively. Kim and associates[169] retrieved AF from 141 women with PPROM. Patients with a positive MMP-8 rapid test had a higher rate of IAI, proven AF infection, and adverse outcome than those with negative test results. A positive MMP-8 rapid test had a sensitivity of 90%, a specificity of 80%, a positive predictive value of 77%, and a negative predictive value of 92% in the identification of IAI.[168] In another study of 139 patients who delivered at less than 35 weeks, Park and coworkers[170] reported a positive MMP-8 rapid test that had a sensitivity of 97%, a specificity of 63%, a positive predictive value of 50%, and a negative predictive value of 99% in the identification of funisitis. Further clinical trials are needed to determine whether treatment with antibiotics and/or anti-inflammatory agents based on the MMP-8 rapid test results improves pregnancy outcome.

FIGURE 26–2
Analysis of cordocentesis-to-delivery interval according to fetal plasma interleukin-6 (IL-6) concentrations. Fetuses with fetal plasma IL-6 concentrations greater than 11 pg/mL have a shorter cordocentesis-to-delivery interval than those with plasma IL-6 concentrations of 11 pg/mL or less (median 0.8 days [range 0.1–5 days] vs. median 6 days [range 0.2–33.6 days]; respectively; $P < .05$).
(Modified from Romero R, Gomez R, Ghezzi F, et al: A fetal systemic inflammatory response is followed by the spontaneous onset of preterm parturition. Am J Obstet Gynecol 1998;179:186-193.)

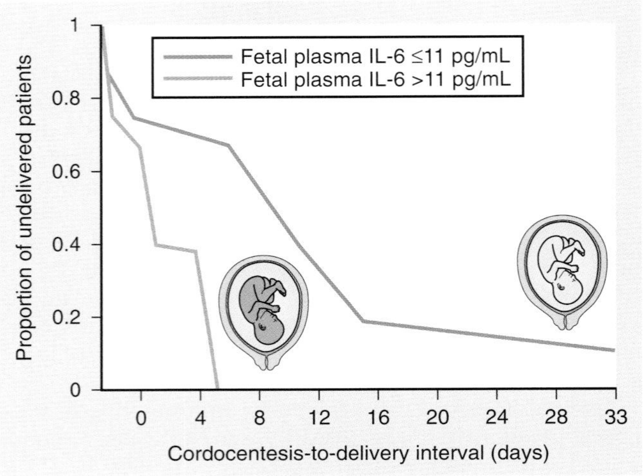

THE FETAL INFLAMMATORY RESPONSE SYNDROME

The term *fetal inflammatory response syndrome* (*FIRS*) was coined to define a subclinical condition originally described in fetuses of women presenting with PTL as well as those presenting with PPROM.[11,12] The definition was an elevation of fetal plasma IL-6 above 11 pg/mL.[11] The original work was based on fetal blood samples, but the association with elevated pro-inflammatory cytokines and sepsis has since been confirmed in umbilical cord blood at the time of birth.[14] Pathologic examination of the umbilical cord is an easy approach to determine whether fetal inflammation was present before birth. Funisitis and chorionic vasculitis are the histopathologic hallmark of FIRS.[51] Neonates with funisitis are at increased risk for neonatal sepsis[171] as well as long-term handicap such as bronchopulmonary dysplasia (BPD)[14] and CP.[13] Among women with PPROM, FIRS is associated with the impending onset of PTL, regardless of the inflammatory state of the AF (Fig. 26–2).[12] This suggests that the human fetus plays a role in initiating the onset of labor. However, maternal cooperation must be present for parturition to occur.

Fetal Target Organs during Fetal Inflammatory Response Syndrome

Fetuses with FIRS are frequently born to mothers with subclinical MIAC.[12] Affected fetuses have evidence of multiorgan involvement with a higher rate of severe neonatal morbidity after adjustment for gestational age[12] and cases of PPROM had a shorter cordocentesis-to-delivery interval.[11] Fetal microbial invasion results in a systemic fetal inflammatory response that can progress toward multiple organ dysfunction, septic shock, and death in the absence of timely delivery.

Hematopoietic System

Neutrophilia is present in two thirds of fetuses with FIRS, whereas neutropenia is observed in 7%.[172] FIRS has also been associated with changes in the immunophenotype of monocyte and granulocytes consistent with activation.[173] Numbers of circulating nucleated red blood cells are also increased. IL-6 has been proposed to have a role in elevating the fetal nucleated red blood cell count.[174]

Lung

FIRS is associated with BPD.[175] Amniotic fluid and its contents can be inhaled by the fetus and reach the distal parts of the airways and the alveoli. Ghezzi and colleagues[176] reported that fetuses who subsequently developed BPD had a higher AF IL-8 concentration than those who did not. These observations were confirmed in another study that reported higher AF concentrations of IL-6, TNF-α, and IL-8 in fetuses who eventually developed BPD,[177] suggesting that antenatal exposure to pro-inflammatory cytokines is also a risk factor for the development of BPD. As for whether fetal systemic inflammation is a risk factor for chronic lung disease, neonates who develop BPD have a higher IL-6 concentration in umbilical cord plasma at birth than those who do not (68.3 pg/mL vs. 6.9 pg/mL; $P < .001$).[14] The same group[175] has also found FIRS in 76% on infants with atypical chronic lung disease (defined as chronic lung disease in the absence of respiratory distress syndrome).

Kidneys

Yoon and associates[36] reported an association between oligohydramnios and fetal infection/inflammation in patients with PPROM. In view of the antimicrobial properties of the AF, oligohydramnios may reduce the protective effect of this component of innate immunity. Alternatively, oligohydramnios may be the result of a redistribution of blood flow away from the kidneys occurring during the host response to microbial products.[36]

Heart

In the presence of IAI, fetuses show changes in cardiac function consistent with a high left ventricular compliance.[178] In cases of overwhelming fetal sepsis, myocardial depression may lead to fetal death. In the context of FIRS, bacterial products and cytokines may contribute to the myocardial depression. Fetuses that are unable to modify their cardiac compliance or maintain ventricular cardiac output may suffer an inadequate brain perfusion, predisposing to hypotension and brain ischemia in utero.[179] This could create conditions for the development of periventricular leukomalacia (PVL) and brain injury.

Adrenal Glands

FIRS is associated with endocrine evidence of "stress," which is expressed by an elevated cortisol–to–dehydroepiandrosterone sulfate (DHEA-S) ratio.[180] These endocrine changes may contribute to the onset of spontaneous PTL. Indeed, Yoon and coworkers[180] reported that in patients with PPROM, there is an association between the fetal plasma cortisol-to-DHEA-S ratio and a shorter interval from cordocentesis to delivery (hazards ratio 2.9; 95% CI 1–8.4). Patients with PPROM who went into spontaneous labor and delivered within 7 days of cordocentesis had a higher fetal plasma cortisol than those delivered after 7 days ($P < .0001$). Fetal plasma cortisol, but not maternal cortisol, was an independent predictor of the duration of pregnancy. These endocrine changes may have short- and long-term implications given the recent observations about the effect of glucocorticoids in fetal programming of several metabolic functions.[181,182]

Skin

Fetal dermatitis is a new entity described in FIRS. Skin samples from fetuses delivered between 21 and 24 weeks' gestation had histologic evidence of dermatitis.[183] TLR-2 expression in the skin was dramatically increased in fetuses born from mothers with histologic chorioamnionitis. Moreover, TLR-2 and TLR-4 were also expressed in the mononuclear inflammatory infiltrate of the dermal-epidermal junction, suggesting that microorganisms are recognized by the fetal skin through PRRs and, thus, participate in the fetal inflammatory response to microbial products.[183]

Thymus

Subclinical chorioamnionitis has been associated with a small thymus,[184] and thymus involution has been demonstrated antenatally with ultrasound in fetuses exposed to IAI in patients with PTL[185] and in those with PPROM.[186] In another study, infants born at less than 28 weeks' gestation and with ultrasonographic signs of cerebral white matter damage (WMD) were more likely to have undergone thymic involution.[187]

CONTRIBUTION OF FETAL INFECTION/ INFLAMMATION TO LONG-TERM HANDICAP

Cerebral Palsy

CP is a symptom complex characterized by aberrant control of movement or posture that appears in early life and can lead to costly lifelong disability. The estimated annual prevalence of CP ranges from 1.5 to 2.5 per 1000 live births, depending on the cohort studied.[188,189] Prematurity has a strong association with CP[190]; one third of all neonates who later have signs of CP weigh less than 2500 g.[191] Newborns with birth weights less than 1500 g have a rate of CP 25 to 31 times higher than those with a normal birth weight.[191] The most common form of CP affecting preterm babies is spastic diplegia.[191] In turn, preterm babies that subsequently develop spastic diplegia have a high rate of PVL.[190,192,193] Strong evidence links brain injury and infant exposure to perinatal infection and inflammation.[194–196] In 1955, Eastman and Deleon[197] observed that intrapartum maternal fever was associated with a sevenfold increase in the risk of CP. In 1978, Nelson and Ellenberg[198] showed, using data from the Collaborative Perinatal Project, that among low–birth weight infants, chorioamnionitis increased the risk of CP from 12 in 1000 to 39 in 1000 live births. The general view is that an initiator event (either systemic or intrauterine infection) leads to maternal and fetal inflammatory responses that, in turn, contribute to adverse outcomes such as preterm delivery, IVH, WMD, and neurodevelopmental disability (mainly CP).

PVL describes foci of coagulation necrosis of the white matter near the lateral ventricles. This condition is frequently associated with the subsequent development of CP,[199,200] is more common in infants born between 28 and 31 weeks, and is nine times more common among those with documented bacteremia.[190] Among preterm neonates, the frequency of IVH and PVL is higher for those born after spontaneous PTL or PPROM than for infants delivered for fetal or maternal indications.[201,202]

Experimental Evidence Linking Infection with White Matter Damage

WMD is more common among children of pregnancies complicated by chorioamnionitis[202] and purulent AF[192] as well as among neonates with bacteremia.[190] Experimental evidence indicates that intrauterine infection results in WMD and neuronal lesions.[203–205] Yoon and coworkers[203] experimentally induced ascending intrauterine infection with *E. coli* rabbits. Histologic evidence of WMD was identified in 12 fetuses born to 10 *E. coli*–inoculated rabbits compared with none in the control group ($P < .05$). All cases with WMD had evidence of intrauterine inflammation. Similar findings were reported by Debillon and colleagues.[204]

Fetal Cytokinemia Is Associated with Intraventricular Hemorrhage, White Matter Damage, and Long-Term Disability

Leviton[206] proposed that inflammatory cytokines (TNF-α) released during the course of intrauterine infection could play a central role in the pathophysiology of WMD. TNF could participate in the pathogenesis of PVL by four different mechanisms: (1) induction of fetal hypotension and brain ischemia[207]; (2) stimulation of tissue factor production and release, which activates the hemostatic system and contributes to coagulation necrosis of white matter[208]; (3) release of platelet-activating factor, which could act as a membrane detergent causing direct brain damage[209]; and (4) a direct cytotoxic effect on oligodendrocytes and myelin.[210]

The hypothesis that fetal inflammation is linked to brain injury is supported by studies documenting higher concentrations of IL-6 in the umbilical cord plasma[201] and AF[195] of fetuses who subsequently develop WMD. Moreover, increased expression of TNF-α and IL-6 is observed in hypertrophic astrocytes and microglia cells obtained from subjects with PVL.[211] Yoon and associates[195] advanced one mechanism to explain how inflammatory cytokines might lead to WMD and CP. According to their theory, MIAC (which occurs in 25% of preterm births) results in congenital fetal infection/inflammation that stimulates fetal mononuclear cells to produce IL-1β and TNF-α. These cytokines increase the permeability of the blood-brain barrier, facilitating the passage of microbial products and cytokines into the brain.[212] Microbial products then stimulate the human fetal microglia to produce IL-1 and TNF-α with subsequent activation of astrocyte proliferation and production of TNF-α. Oligodendrocytes, the cells responsible for the deposition of myelin, are damaged by TNF-α.

Fetal Vasculitis, Intraventricular Hemorrhage, White Matter Damage, and Cerebral Palsy

Yoon and coworkers[13] observed in a study of 123 preterm infants followed to age 3 years that the odds of developing CP were higher in the presence of funisitis (OR 5.5; 95% CI 1.2–24.5), increased AF IL-6 concentrations (OR 6.4; 95% CI 1.3–33.0), and increased AF IL-8 concentrations (OR 5.9; 95% CI 1.1–30.7). All 14 children who developed CP had evidence of WMD and 11 had evidence of intrauterine inflammation. Fifty percent of the children had positive AF cultures. Histologic chorioamnionitis was not associated with subsequent development of CP after adjusting for gestational age at birth, suggesting that it is the fetal, rather than the maternal, inflammatory response that predisposes to CP. Nonetheless, neither infection nor inflammation was considered a sufficient causal factor for WMD or CP, because the latter did not develop in 82% of fetuses with documented MIAC and in 76% of those with evidence of intrauterine inflammation. Factors implicated in the genesis of brain injury include (1) gestational age, (2) virulence of the microorganisms, (3) fetal attack rate, (4) the nature of the fetal immunoresponse, and (5) vulnerability of the central nervous system.

APPROACHES TO FETAL IINFLAMMATORY RESPONSE SYNDROME

Three approaches can be used to interrupt the course of FIRS: (1) delivery, (2) antimicrobial treatment of women in whom the FIRS is due to microbial invasion of susceptible bacteria, and (3) administration of agents that down-regulate the inflammatory response. Preterm delivery places the unborn child at risk for complications of prematurity. Therefore, the risks of prematurity and intrauterine infection must be balanced.

The administration of antimicrobial agents may eradicate MIAC in cases of PPROM. The results of the ORACLE I trial suggest that antibiotic administration may not only delay the onset of labor but also improve neonatal outcome.[76] These findings are supported by experimental evidence in pregnant rabbits inoculated with *E. coli*. Antibiotic administration within 12 hours of microbial inoculation (but not after 18 hours) effectively prevented maternal fever, reduced the rate of preterm delivery, and improved neonatal survival.[213] It is tempting to postulate that this was accomplished by improving or preventing a fetal inflammatory response. It is important to note that the 7-year follow-up of infants in ORACLE trial I did not demonstrate any reduction in the rate of CP in infants given antibiotics.[214]

Agents that down-regulate the inflammatory response, such as anti-inflammatory cytokines, antibodies to macrophage migration inhibitory factor, and antioxidants, may also play a role in preventing preterm delivery, neonatal injury, and long-term perinatal morbidity. A combination of antibiotics and immunomodulators (dexamethasone and indomethacin) given to nonhuman pregnant primates was effective in eradicating infection, suppressing the inflammatory response, and prolonging gestation in experimental premature labor induced by intra-amniotic inoculation with group B streptococci.[215] The administration of magnesium sulfate as a neuroprotective agent has also been found to be beneficial for fetuses of less than 34 weeks' gestation.[216–221]

Acknowledgment

This research was supported by the Perinatology Research Branch, Division of Intramural Research, Eunice Kennedy Shriver National Institute of Child Health and Human Development, NIH, DHHS. The authors wish to acknowledge the contribution of authors of chapters published in previous editions of this book. The current authors also gratefully acknowledge the intellectual contributions of Luís F. Gonçalves and Tinnakorn Chaiworapongsa.

SUMMARY OF MANAGEMENT OPTIONS

Intrauterine Infection, Preterm Parturition, and the Fetal Inflammatory Response Syndrome

Management Options	Evidence Quality and Recommendation	References
Diagnosis of Intra-amniotic Infection/Inflammation (IAI)		
Perform amniocentesis to retrieve AF	III/B	222
• **Rapid tests**: Gram stain, WBC count, glucose, and IL-6 concentration.		
• **Culture**: Aerobic, anaerobic bacteria, and genital mycoplasmas.		
• **PCR** with specific primers for the detection of organisms in patients with IAI and negative culture.		

Management Options	Evidence Quality and Recommendation	References
Diagnosis of a Fetal Inflammatory Response Syndrome (FIRS)		
General:		
• The diagnosis of FIRS suggests antenatal exposure to an agent that promoted inflammation.	—/GPP	—
• It may have medicolegal value because there is no current evidence that treatment can modify the natural history and the risk for adverse outcome conferred by fetal systemic inflammation.	—/GPP	—
Collect umbilical cord blood at delivery:	III/B	51,171,201,223–226
• CBC and differential, platelet count.		
• C-Reactive protein; elevated levels associated with		
• Histologic chorioamnionitis.		
• Funisitis.		
• Neonatal sepsis.		
• IL-6 concentration; elevated levels associated with		51,224,225,227
• Positive AF cultures (MIAC).		
• Histologic chorioamnionitis.		
• Funisitis.		
• Neonatal sepsis.		
• Congenital pneumonia.		
• Necrotizing enterocolitis.		
• Intracranial hemorrhage.		
• White matter damage.		
• Impaired neurologic outcome (lower Bayley psychomotor developmental index scores).		
Examine the placenta:	III/B	51,52,171,228
• Histologic chorioamnionitis.		
• Funisitis is a marker for fetal inflammation.		
For Premature Neonates		
Perform pathologic examination of the placenta.	III/B	13,192,229,230
• Histologic chorioamnionitis associated with		
• Intracranial hemorrhage.		
• Funisitis associated with		
• Neonatal sepsis.		
• White matter damage.		
• Cerebral palsy.		

AF, amniotic fluid; CBC, complete blood count; IL-6, interleukin-6; MIAC, microbial invasion of the amniotic cavity; PCR, polymerase chain reaction; WBC, white blood cell.

SUGGESTED READINGS

Conde-Agudelo A, Romero R: Antenatal magnesium sulfate for the prevention of cerebral palsy in preterm infants less than 34 weeks' gestation: A systematic review and meta-analysis. Am J Obstet Gynecol 2009;200:595–609.

DiGiulio DB, Romero R, Amogan HP, et al: Microbial prevalence, diversity and abundance in amniotic fluid during preterm labor: A molecular and culture-based investigation. PLoS ONE 2008;3:e3056.

Gomez R, Romero R, Ghezzi F, et al: The fetal inflammatory response syndrome. Am J Obstet Gynecol 1998;179:194–202.

Gomez R, Romero R, Nien JK, et al: Antibiotic administration to patients with preterm premature rupture of membranes does not eradicate intra-amniotic infection. J Matern Fetal Neonatal Med 2007;20:167–173.

Gonçalves LF, Chaiworapongsa T, Romero R: Intrauterine infection and prematurity. Ment Retard Dev Disabil Res Rev 2002;8:3–13.

Kenyon SL, Taylor DJ, Tarnow-Mordi W: Broad-spectrum antibiotics for preterm, prelabour rupture of fetal membranes: The ORACLE I ran-

domised trial. ORACLE Collaborative Group. Lancet 2001;357:979–988.
Kenyon S, Pike K, Jones DR, et al: Childhood outcomes after prescription of antibiotics to pregnant women with preterm rupture of the membranes: 7-year follow-up of the ORACLE I trial. Lancet 2008;372:1310–1318.
Leviton A, Paneth N: White matter damage in preterm newborns—An epidemiologic perspective. Early Hum Dev 1990;24:1–22.
Nien JK, Yoon BH, Espinoza J, et al: A rapid MMP-8 bedside test for the detection of intra-amniotic inflammation identifies patients at risk for imminent preterm delivery. Am J Obstet Gynecol 2006;195:1025–1030.
Romero R, Brody DT, Oyarzun E, et al: Infection and labor. III. Interleukin-1: A signal for the onset of parturition. Am J Obstet Gynecol 1989;160:1117–1123.

REFERENCES

For a complete list of references, log onto www.expertconsult.com.

CHAPTER 27

Hepatitis Virus Infections

JANET I. ANDREWS

INTRODUCTION

Viral hepatitis is one of the more commonly diagnosed viral infections in pregnancy. Six subtypes of the hepatitis virus have been identified (A, B, C, D, E, and G). These viral subtypes differ according to structure, routes of transmission, and implications for management during pregnancy and the neonatal period (Table 27–1). In general, diagnosis of viral hepatitis is based on specific clinical symptoms (malaise, fever, abdominal pain, and/or jaundice) and virus-specific laboratory criteria including serology. The purpose of this chapter is to describe each of the viral hepatitis subtypes and their maternal and perinatal implications as they relate to prevention and treatment.

HEPATITIS A

General

Although person-to-person contact resulting in "infectious jaundice" was described in a review of hepatitis epidemics published by Blumer in 1923,[1] the hepatitis A virus (HAV) was not identified until 1973, when Feinstone and colleagues,[2] using immunofluorescent electron microscopy, described virus-like particles in filtered stool samples that stained positively when mixed with HAV convalescent serum. Subsequent work by this group then demonstrated a temporal link between detectable shedding of the HAV antigen in feces and symptomatic illness in experimentally infected subjects.[3]

As a member of the Picornaviridae family, HAV is nonenveloped and resistant to organic solvent dissolution owing to its lipid-poor coating. Compared with other picornaviruses such as poliovirus, HAV is relatively stable in the environment. The virus is resistant to heat and inactivation by drying for up to 1 month.[4] Autoclaving, heating food to above 185°F for 1 minute, or disinfecting surfaces with dilute chlorine bleach will inactivate the virus.[5] This latter effect helps explain the propagation of HAV in areas of poor sanitation.

The distribution of HAV is global, though outbreaks are typically seen in areas with crowded conditions, inadequate water supplies, or poor hygiene and sanitation. The virus is highly contagious and can be isolated from the feces of all infected persons, which facilitates the fecal-oral route of person-to-person transmission. Outbreaks and sporadic cases also can occur from exposure to contaminated food and water. Contaminated food needs to be cooked to the appropriate temperature to kill the virus. Parenteral transmission is rare, because the virus is present only transiently in serum.

Prior to the introduction of the HAV vaccine in 1995, HAV accounted for approximately one third of cases of hepatitis in the United States. Since 1995, HAV rates in the United States have declined by 89%. In 2006, 3579 acute symptomatic cases of HAV were reported, the lowest rate recorded. After adjusting for underreporting bias and asymptomatic cases, the estimated number of cases in 2006 was 32,000.[6] The rate of HAV infection during pregnancy is unknown, but retrospective reviews estimate that HAV is a rare cause of acute hepatitis in pregnancy. In large retrospective case series from Ireland and Isreal, the incidence of HAV infection during pregnancy was extremely low with reported rates of 1/13,181 and 13/79,458 pregnant women, respectively.[7,8]

Major risk factors for HAV infection in pregnant women in developed countries include (1) travel to developing countries (especially Southeast Asia, Africa, central America, Mexico, and the Middle East), (2) household or sexual contact with infected individuals, and (3) contact with contaminated food or water. In the United States, person-to-person transmission is the primary means of HAV transmission via a close personal contact with a household member or sex partner. Because most HAV-infected children are asymptomatic, they serve a key role in the transmission of the virus.[9,10]

Bivalve mollusks such as clams and oysters can act also as reservoirs for HAV within contaminated waters; crustaceans such as shrimp do not seem to carry the same infectious risk. Infected food handlers have also been implicated in HAV outbreaks, especially when they are from global areas with endemic HAV infection rates.[11]

Although HAV infection tends to be clinically less severe than infection with other viral hepatitides, and serious complications are uncommon, distinction between infection with HAV and other viruses can only be made serologically. Conversely, not all HAV infections are symptomatic. Before immune globulin was available for preventive passive immunization, 80% to 95% of infected adults in HAV epidemics were symptomatic, two thirds of whom were icteric.[12]

TABLE 27–1
Comparison of Hepatitis Virus Subtypes

	HEPATITIS A	HEPATITIS B	HEPATITIS C	HEPATITIS D	HEPATITIS E
Virus family	Picornaviridae	Hepadnaviridae	Flaviviridae	Deltavirus genus	Similar to Calciviridae
Diagnosis	Anti-HAV	HBsAg, anti-HBs, anti-HBc, HBeAg	Anti-HCV by ELISA (see text for confirmatory testing)	Anti-HDV and D antigen	Anti-HEV
Primary route of transmission	Fecal-oral	Blood/body fluids	Blood/body fluids	Blood/body fluids (requires HBV for replication)	Fecal-oral
Average incubation period in days (range)	28 (15-50)	90 (60-150)	28-84 (14-168)	21-49	40 (21-56)
Incidence rate* (United States)	1.2/100,000	1.6/100,000	0.3/100,000	N/A	N/A
Rate of vertical transmission risk	Rare	10%-20% if no immunoprophylaxis	2%-7% (unless high HCV-RNA and/or HIV-positive)	Rare	Rare
Vaccine available?	Yes	Yes	No	No	No
Breast-feeding contraindicated?	No	No (risk unknown if HBeAg-positive mom)	No (unless nipples cracked or bleeding)	No	No

* Centers for Disease Control and Prevention: Surveillance for Acute Viral Hepatitis—United States, 2006. MMWR Surveill Summ March 21, 2008. MMWR 2008;57/No. SS-2.
ELISA, enzyme-linked immunosorbent assay; HAV, hepatitis A virus; HBeAg, hepatitis Be antigen; HBsAg, hepatitis B surface antigen; HCV, hepatitis C virus; HDV, hepatitis D virus; HEV, hepatitis E virus; N/A, not applicable.

Severity of illness with HAV infection appears to be directly related to the patient's age (older patients are more severely ill) as well as to the size of the viral inoculum. Virus transmissibility is of greatest concern during the incubation period, which has a mean of 28 days and range of 15 to 50 days.

Diagnosis

The initial clinical symptoms of acute HAV infection are nonspecific, consisting of fatigue, malaise, fever, nausea, and anorexia. Significant weight loss may be a presenting complaint in pregnant women. The classic picture of icteric illness becomes apparent within 10 days of the generalized symptoms and is usually preceded by palpable hepatosplenomegaly. Liver function abnormalities, typically characterized by elevations in serum alanine aminotransferase (ALT) higher than aspartate aminotransferase (AST), peak prior to the appearance of jaundice. They may remain elevated for over a month in adults. Prolonged illness, with elevations in liver functions tests (LFTs) lasting over 12 months, has been reported in 8% to 10% of older patients, and jaundice and pruritus may persist despite an overall improving trend in symptoms and LFTs. Fulminant hepatitis, resulting in death, occurs in fewer than 1% of cases.[13]

HAV-specific immunoglobulin M (IgM) is the serologic marker for acute infection and can be reliably identified with an automated enzyme-linked immunosorbent assay (ELISA).[14,15]

By the time a patient is symptomatic, she will almost uniformly be seropositive for IgM anti-HAV. IgM levels drop below the detectable range within 4 to 6 months in most patients and parallel a concomitant normalization of LFTs in 80% to 85% of cases.[16] HAV-specific IgG, however, will remain positive for years after acute infection.

Maternal and Fetal Risks

As an almost entirely self-limited illness, acute HAV infection usually does not confer an increased risk of adverse outcome to a pregnant woman. Supportive care for the woman is essential, and in areas where the virus may be endemic as the result of sanitation or housing issues, the availability of such care might not exist. Nutritional needs should be addressed, and infected pregnant women may require hospitalization with strict contact isolation precautions. A chronic carrier state for HAV does not exist. Perinatal transmission of HAV is rare.[17–19]

Administration of immune globulin is recommended for neonates born within 2 weeks of acute maternal illness with HAV conferring protection for up to 3 months at 80% to 90% efficacy level.[20]

Management Options

No specific antiviral treatment of HAV is currently available. However, both preventive vaccination and postexposure prophylaxis with immunoglobulin are available. The current HAV vaccine is available either as a single-agent vaccine (Havrix and Vaqta) or as one combined with hepatitis B virus (HBV) vaccine (Twinrix). Single-agent HAV vaccine is given as two doses, 6 to 12 months apart. Currently, the Advisory Committee on Immunization Practices (ACIP) recommends a single-antigen vaccine series for all children at age 12 to 23 months, catch-up vaccination of older children in selected areas, and vaccination of persons at increased risk for HAV (e.g., travelers to endemic areas, users of illicit drugs, or men who have sex with men).[21] As an inactivated-virus vaccine, there is no contraindication to the use of HAV vaccine during pregnancy.

Individuals who have close personal or sexual contact with an HAV-infected person should receive postexposure prophylaxis unless they have been immunized. Until recently, immune globulin was the recommended choice for postexposure prophylaxis. The 2007 ACIP guidelines were revised to recommend the HAV vaccine be given following exposure, based on the data indicating that immune globulin and vaccine have similar postexposure efficacy among healthy persons younger than 40 years of age.[22] The current recommendations state that for healthy persons aged 1 to 40 years, single-antigen HAV vaccine at the age-appropriate dose is preferred to immune globulin for postexposure prophylaxis because of vaccine advantages that include long-term protection and ease of administration. For persons older than 40 years, immune globulin is preferred because of the absence of information regarding vaccine performance and the more severe manifestations of HAV in this age group. A single intramuscular dose of 0.02 mL/kg should be given as soon as possible after contact with the infected individual, within 2 weeks of exposure. The efficacy of immune globulin after 2 weeks from exposure is unknown.[21] Administration of immune globulin is still recommended for neonates born to mothers with recent HAV infection.[23]

HEPATITIS B

General

According to the World Health Organization (WHO), approximately 2 billion people have been infected with worldwide and 350 million are chronically infected.[24] HBV infection is a major global health problem with 600,000 annual deaths attributable to the consequences of HBV infection.[24] In areas of Asia, 8% to 10% of the adult population is chronically infected with HBV, and liver cancer attributable to HBV is a major cause of cancer in women. High rates of chronic infections are also found in the Middle East and the Indian subcontinent, with an estimated 2% to 5% of the adult population infected.[24] In many of these endemic areas, perinatal and childhood infections exist as a primary route for perpetuating the reservoir of carriers. The likelihood that a person infected with HBV will develop a chronic infection depends upon the age at which the person is infected. The earlier in life that a person is infected, the higher the risk of being a chronic carrier. This finding is especially significant because the risk of chronic HBV infection for a child infected in the newborn period, in the absence of prophylactic therapy, is 70% to 90%.[25,26]

In areas of low endemicity for HBV carriage, such as the United States, screening programs for the general population have been targeted to decrease household, transfusion, sexual, and perinatal transmission risks among contacts of hepatitis B surface antigen (HBsAg)–positive individuals. Population subsets have been identified that are at increased risk for HBV acquisition, and HBV vaccination is recommended for individuals within those groups who are serologically negative for HBsAg and hepatitis B surface antibody (HBsAb). The efficacy of a serum-derived HBV vaccine was demonstrated initially on a large scale in a cohort of more than 1000 homosexual men in the United States; this trial showed an antibody (HBsAb) response in 96% of those vaccinated, with an overall protective efficacy of 88% against all HBsAg-positive events for vaccine compared with placebo.[27]

More recently, two single-antigen and three combination vaccines were developed and licensed in the United States. These vaccines are prepared from yeast culture and utilize a recombinant HBsAg protein dose.

In 2006, an estimated 46,000 persons in the United States were newly infected with HBV after taking into account asymptomatic infections and underreporting. This estimate represents a decline by approximately 81% since 1991.[6] Among pregnant women, Asian American women from urban areas have the highest HBsAg prevalence rate of 6%, followed by blacks (1%), whites (0.6%), and Latinos (0.14%).[28] Blood and blood products are the most thoroughly established sources of HBV infection, although HBsAg has been demonstrated in a variety of body fluids. Of those, however, only serum, saliva, and semen have been associated consistently with transmission in experimental models.[29] Percutaneous transfer of the virus is the most obvious route of transmission in the medical setting, through either blood products or needle-stick accidents. Contact of infectious material with broken skin or mucous membranes also can result in effective transmission.

Compared with other transmissible viruses, such as HIV, HBV is a fairly stable virus and remains infectious on household surfaces up to 7 days. Although transmission in households is more common through sexual contact than through fomite contact,[30] nonsexual household transmission has been established as a route for HBV infection.[31] Therefore, any surfaces potentially contaminated with infectious blood should be cleaned with 1 : 10 dilution of bleach solution. In areas of the world with higher HBV carrier rates than the United States, nonparenteral transmission would be expected to constitute the major route of person-to-person HBV infection. Vertical transmission is a major source; investigators in Taiwan estimated that 40% to 50% of HBsAg carriers became infected in the perinatal period.[25,32]

Children born to carrier mothers who escape the neonatal period without evidence of infection are still at risk for childhood acquisition of HBV. One of the early vaccine trials conducted in Senegal showed that among children seronegative at the beginning of a randomized HBV vaccination trial, almost 10% acquired HBV infection in the absence of vaccination by the end of a 12-month follow-up period.[33]

Diagnosis

HBV is distinguished from the other viral hepatitides by its long incubation period (1–6 mo), by the presence of extrahepatic symptoms in up to 20% of patients (arthralgia, rash, and myalgia thought to be a result of antigen-antibody complex deposition),[34] and by the detection of HBV-specific serum markers (Table 27–2).

HBV consists of three structural antigens: surface, core, and e antigen. The appearance of surface antigen (HBsAg) in the serum usually predates any clinical symptoms by 4 weeks on average and remains detectable for 1 to 6 weeks in most patients.[35] In the 90% to 95% of patients in whom chronic infection does not develop, HBsAg titers decrease as symptoms diminish. The appearance of HBsAb defines the absence of the carrier state; titers increase slowly during the clinical recovery period and may continue to increase up to 10 to 12 months after HBsAg is no longer detectable. In most patients with self-limited, acute HBV, HBsAb is

TABLE 27–2
Interpretation of Hepatitis B Panel

TESTS	RESULTS	INTERPRETATION
HBsAg Anti-HBc Anti-HBs	Negative Negative Negative	Susceptible
HBsAg Anti-HBc Anti-HBs	Negative Positive Positive	Immune due to natural infection
HBsAg Anti-HBc Anti-HBs	Negative Negative Positive	Immune due to hepatitis B vaccination
HBsAg Anti-HBc IgM anti-HBc Anti-HBs	Positive Positive Positive Negative	Acutely infected
HBsAg Anti-HBc IgM anti-HBc Anti-HBs	Positive Positive Negative Negative	Chronically infected
HBsAg Anti-HBc Anti-HBs	Negative Positive Negative	Interpretation unclear; four possibilities: 1. Resolved infection (most common) 2. False-positive anti-HBc, thus susceptible 3. "Low level": chronic infection 4. Resolving acute infection

HBc, hepatitis B core antigen; HBs, hepatitis Bs; HBsAg; hepatitis B surface antigen; IgM, immunoglobulin M.
Adapted from A comprehensive immunization strategy to eliminate transmission of hepatitis B virus infection in the United States: Recommendations of the Advisory Committee on Immunization Practices (ACIP) part 1: Immunization of infants, children, and adolescents. MMWR Recomm Rep 2005;54(RR-16):1–31.

detectable only after HBsAg titers in serum disappear.[36] A "window" of time has been described in which a patient still with clinical hepatitis is negative for both HBsAg and HBsAb. During this time, HBV infection still can be diagnosed by the detection of hepatitis B core antibody (HBcAb), which begins to appear 3 to 5 weeks after HBsAg does. HBcAb titers may drop off in the first 1 to 2 years after infection, although the antibody is still detectable years after acute disease in most patients.[36] The appearance of hepatitis Be antigen (HBeAg) parallels that of HBsAg; in self-limited infections, HBeAb is detectable shortly after the time that HBeAg disappears. The chronic HBV carrier state usually can be predicted by HBsAg seropositivity for 20 weeks or longer. HBcAb is detectable in the serum of carriers at levels higher than those seen in either acute or recovering self-limited infections, and e antigen markers are variable. The presence of HBsAb in the absence of HBsAg and HBcAb differentiates vaccine-mediated immunity from natural-infection–mediated immunity.

Maternal and Fetal Risks

Risks during Pregnancy

Acute HBV infection during pregnancy is usually a mild illness with only up to 30% of patients reporting icterus, nausea, vomiting, and right upper quadrant discomfort.[37] Treatment during pregnancy is mainly supportive, as in the nonpregnant state. Symptoms generally resolve within several weeks; however, 0.5% to 1.5% of infective individuals will develop fulminant liver failure.[38] Hospitalization should be considered for pregnant women with acute HBV infection if they have encephalopathy, coagulopathy, or severe fluid and nutritional imbalances. The diagnosis of acute HBV during the later stages of pregnancy can be differentiated from preeclampsia or HELLP (hemolysis, elevated liver enzymes, and low platelets) syndrome using normal blood pressure criteria and presence of jaundice. Encouragement is necessary to maintain adequate nutrition during the early symptomatic phase, and liver-metabolized drugs, if not avoidable, need to be monitored carefully through blood levels. In addition, household and sexual contacts of patients should be offered appropriate immunoprophylaxis. No teratogenic association has been established for maternal HBV infections,[39,40] despite evidence of viral infection within the placenta.[41,42]

The rate of vertical transmission during acute maternal HBV infection depends on the gestational age of the fetus. When maternal infection occurs during the first trimester, up to 10% of neonates will be infected. In contrast, 80% to 90% of neonates are HBsAg-positive when maternal infection occurs during the third trimester.[20,43] Although evidence is limited, there is an association between prematurity and acute HBV infection (32% vs. 11% in controls).[39]

Chronic HBV is endemic in certain areas of Asia where the estimated prevalence among women of reproductive age is 10% to 20%. Studies from these areas indicate that the presence of HBsAg does not appear to increase the risk of adverse pregnancy outcomes.[44] In addition, pregnancy does not exacerbate chronic HBV infection or alter HBV viral levels.[45]

Hepatitis B Screening in Pregnancy

The opportunity to provide almost complete protection against perinatally acquired HBV infection makes antenatal identification of HBV carriers critical so that combined neonatal prophylaxis can be administered in a timely fashion. Previously, in nonendemic areas such as the United States, risk factor–based prenatal screening protocols were implemented, but these protocols detected only up to 60% of HBV carriers. Therefore, the American College of Obstetricians and Gynecologists and the Centers for Disease Control and Prevention (CDC) recommended routine prenatal screening with HBsAg for all pregnant women regardless of risk factors.[20,43] Furthermore, the CDC recommends that pregnant women who are HBsAg-negative and at high risk for HBV infection (including >1 sex partner in past 6 mo, evaluation or treatment for sexually transmitted infection, recent or current injection drug use, or HBsAg-positive sex partner) should be retested upon admission to labor and delivery.

Management Options

Prevention of Hepatitis B Virus Infection

Immunoprophylaxis regimens to prevent HBV transmission in the perinatal period were a direct extension of the success of these therapies in high risk adult populations. Postexposure immunization was first demonstrated through the use of immunoglobulin preparations with high titers of HBsAb, when given within 4 hours of experimental infection with HBV.[46] Before the development of an effective HBV-specific vaccine, transient preexposure prophylaxis was demonstrated using hepatitis B immunoglobulin (HBIG),[47] although such use of HBIG is now of purely historical interest in terms of understanding the evolution of therapeutic standards. Currently, postexposure treatment consists of a single dose of HBIG administered as temporally as possible to the exposure. Immediate therapy is optimal for maximal protection, although 75% efficacy has been shown when HBIG is given within 7 days of exposure.[48]

Although it does not increase the efficacy of HBIG therapy, a series of HBV vaccinations also should be initiated if the exposure was within a setting of ongoing risk, such as a health care or institutional setting. This regimen consists of injections at 0, 1, and 6 months and results in high antibody titers in more than 90% of those younger than 60 years of age. Administration of HBV vaccine simultaneously with HBIG does not diminish the immunologic response to the vaccine.[49] Still, the currently available HBV vaccine's efficacy is conferred by stimulating production of HBsAb by exposure to HBsAg; vaccine-related immunity can be distinguished from natural immunity in most cases by the absence of HBcAb in the serum of successfully vaccinated patients.

Prevention of Hepatitis B Virus in Utero Infection

In utero HBV infection is determined by multiple potential factors including HBV DNA level, gestational age, placenta integrity, and possibly genetic susceptibility of fetus.[50] Several prophylactic therapies (including hyperimmunoglobulin, HBV vaccine, and lamivudine) have been proposed to possibly reduce the risk of in utero transmission. Lamivudine is approved for treatment and can achieve suppression of HBV replication and remission.[20,51–53] Although well-controlled, large studies are needed, several reports have shown potential benefit from maternal lamivudine therapy to reduce the risk of in utero infection.[52,53] However, there is currently no effective, well-studied prophylactic treatment aimed at prevention in utero transmission.[54–57]

Preventing Perinatal Hepatitis B Virus Transmission

Although there may be a theoretical risk of HBV transmission, a lack of data exists regarding risk of transmission with fetal scalp monitoring and operative vaginal delivery. The route of delivery has not demonstrated to influence of the risk of perinatal HBV transmission.[20] According to the CDC, an HBsAg-positive mother can breast-feed even prior to the infant receiving the HBV vaccine and HBIG. The potential for vertical transmission of HBV at birth is significant. Most infants born to carrier mothers are HBsAg-negative at birth but seroconvert in the first 3 months after delivery, suggesting acquisition of the virus at birth.[58] Early attempts at interrupting the perinatal transmission cycle employed HBIG alone, administered in the neonatal period. Globulin alone had a protective efficacy against the carrier state of 70% to 75%, although the protection was not permanent, and many children eventually became infected after the passively acquired antibody was cleared, undoubtedly through household contact.[59,60]

With the advent of the HBV vaccine, trials were established to test its efficacy when administered in the newborn period, both alone and in conjunction with HBIG. A combination of HBIG and vaccine in the newborn period conferred significantly greater protection against perinatally transmitted HBV than even the vaccine alone, increasing efficacy from a range of 75% to 85% up to 90% to 95%.[59] The small but identifiable percentage of infants who become infected, despite even combined HBV therapy at birth, is believed to represent in utero infection.[61,62]

Combination HBV-specific immunotherapy provides the best opportunity to prevent the chronic carrier state in the offspring of HBsAg-positive mothers. CDC guidelines have been changed recently to reflect timing of the vaccine based on infant birth weight. Infants born to HBsAg-*positive* women should receive HBIG (0.5 mL) intramuscularly (IM) and HBV vaccine concurrently at a different site (0.5 mL, IM) within 12 hours of birth. For infants weighing less than 2000 g, the vaccine dose does not count as the first dose in the vaccine series and the full vaccine series should be initiated at 1 to 2 months. Infants (>2000 g) born to women of HBsAg-*negative* status receive the HBV vaccine prior to discharge. Infants (<2000 g) receive the first dose of vaccine 1 month after birth or at hospital discharge. If the mother's HBV status is unknown, the infant will receive HBIG and HBV vaccine within 12 hours of birth. The timing of HBIG appears to be more critical than that of vaccine in achieving maximal effectiveness of passive-active therapy. Subsequent vaccination is performed, also 0.5 mL IM, at 1 month and 6 months of age. Follow-up for these infants is crucial, because one study confirmed the concern that in the United States, groups at highest risk for HBV infection are also least likely to be compliant with follow-up care.[63]

Impact of Perinatal Hepatitis B Virus Vaccination Programs

The efficacy of perinatal HBV vaccination programs in preventing infection in children born to carrier mothers has led to the inclusion of the HBV vaccine series in the American Academy of Pediatrics' current recommendations for childhood vaccines for the general population.[64] Since 1982, over 1 billion doses of HBV vaccine have been administered worldwide. At the end of 2006, 164 countries had instituted HBV vaccination programs for infants in comparison with 31 countries in 1992 according WHO.

The beneficial impact of adequate childhood vaccination for HBV has been demonstrated dramatically in reports from Taiwan, where large-scale mass vaccination programs were begun in 1984. Researchers there have conclusively proven a link between HBV and hepatocellular carcinoma (HCC) by showing a significant decrease in the average annual incidence of HCC since the institution of the program.[65,66] The decline in the rate of HCC was also paralleled by a drop in the rate of HBsAg carriage among children born before the vaccination program was started, suggesting a herd immunity effect from the mass inoculation of children in the much more infectious younger birth cohorts, and resulting in a lower rate of horizontal HBV infection among the older unvaccinated children.[65] These results even further bolster the need to identify HBsAg carrier mothers and provide timely and complete HBV vaccination to their children.

HEPATITIS C VIRUS

General

Hepatitis C virus (HCV) is the most common bloodborne infection in the United States, although the incidence of acute infection has been decreasing steadily since 1992.[67] In 2006, an estimated 3.2 million persons were chronically infected with HCV, largely due to infection during the 1970s and 1980s when the rates were highest.[43] Since 2003, HCV rates in the United States have remained stable with intravenous drug (IV) use being the most commonly identified risk factor.[6] The prevalence of HCV infection in pregnant women with IV drug use approaches 70% to 95%[68] As the risk of HCV infection resulting from blood transfusions has diminished, a result of the mass screening of blood products since 1992, the proportion of HCV infections attributable to drug use has markedly increased.[67] Transfusion-associated HCV infection is now extremely rare, with an estimated risk of less than 1 in 2 million units transfused.[69]

The significance of sexual transmission of HCV is controversial, though the overall rate of infection between HCV-discordant sexual partners appears to be rare.[70] It is likely that the observed association of HCV with high risk sexual practices is a result of the confounding effect of injection drug use associated with high risk sexual practices.[71] In addition, an interaction increasing the risk of concomitant transmission of HCV and HIV has been described. Heterosexual men with HCV and HIV infection were five times more likely to transmit both viruses to a female partner than would have been expected by chance.[72] This potential interaction of HIV and HCV to increase transmissibility of either or both agents also has become important in describing issues surrounding maternal-fetal HCV transmission.

Another important risk factor for HCV infection is transmission in the health care setting. With the introduction of standard precautions, nosocomial transmission has decreased dramatically with three exceptions: sharp injuries, hemodialysis, and iatrogenic therapeutic practices.[73] Needle-stick or sharp injuries from an HCV-positive source confer an estimated risk of HCV seroconversion of 1.8%.[73] Effective October 2008, all dialysis facilities are directed to follow CDC guidelines[74] for prevention of iatrogenic infection in hemodialysis patients as a condition for receiving Medicare payment for services.[75] Overall, prevention of nosocomial HCV transmission is targeted at minimizing the use of multiple-use vials, bottles, and/or IVs fluids where contaminated therapeutic injections can occur.

Acute HCV infection occurs after an incubation period of 30 to 60 days. Asymptomatic infection occurs in 75% of patients; the remaining 25% of infected individuals present with fatigue, abdominal pain, anorexia, or jaundice. Fulminant hepatitis and hepatic failure attributable to HCV are uncommon.

Chronic liver disease (defined as persistent infection for >3 mo) occurs in 75% to 85% of acutely infected individuals. Chronic HCV infection is the leading cause of liver transplantation in the United States.[69]

Diagnosis

Laboratory tests for diagnostic confirmation of acute HCV include at least a sevenfold increase in serum ALT levels, IgM anti-HAV–negative, IgM anti-HBc– or HBsAg–negative, and either a positive anti-HCV screening test with a cut-off predictive of a true positive OR anti-HCV–positive screening test verified with a more specific assay.[6] In a patient at high risk for HCV infection with a positive anti-HCV test result, the chance of a false-positive ELISA is exceedingly low. However, recognizing that most clnical laboratories report positive anti-HCV results using screening assays alone despite previous recommendations, the CDC expanded its HCV testing algorithm to include an option for supplemental testing based on "signal-to-cut-off (s/co)" ratios of positive commercial assay results.[76] The s/co of anti-HCV screening test positive results can be used minimize the number of specimens that require supplemental testing while providing results that have high probability of reflecting the person's true antibody status. Because pregnant women without risk factors do not constitute a high risk group requiring HCV screening by CDC guidelines, it is critical for clinicians to understand the limitations and interpretations of the currently available HCV screening assays.

At least six HCV genotypes and 50 subtypes have been identified. Viral genotyping is valuable to help guide therapy.[77] Genotype 1 is the most common HCV genotype found in the United States and is less responsive to treatment than genotypes 2 and 3. Genotypes 2 and 3 are almost threefold more likely than genotype 1 to respond to therapy with interferon-α (IFN-α) or IFN-α and ribavirin.[77] This variation may limit the reproducibility of results in clinical trials, and therefore, genotyping information should be included for subjects enrolled in these trials. HCV genotype has not been determined to be an independent risk factor for perinatal HCV transmission, although data are very limited.[78,79]

Maternal and Fetal Risks

The prevalence of HCV infection among pregnant women ranges from approximately 0.3% to 2% in the United States and Europe, with higher rates in urban settings.[64,80,81] Routine prenatal screening for HCV is not recommended because of the lack of proven cost-effectiveness and available safe treatment.[82] However, screening is recommended for the subset of women with known risk factors for HCV infection as listed in Table 27–3.[20] Identifying HCV-seropositive pregnant women is important to guide postnatal follow-up and potential therapy for both women and neonates.

Overall, pregnancy does not significantly affect the clinical course of acute or chronic HCV infection. Studies have demonstrated decreases in transaminase levels as pregnancy progresses in HCV-infected women, although there are conflicting results regarding whether pregnancy alters viral load.[83–85] It is postulated that immunomodulatory factors play a role in these findings. Conversely, HCV infection may lead to adverse maternal or neonatal outcomes. Several studies have suggested that maternal HCV reactivity is associated with an increase risk of cholestasis of pregnancy and increased neonatal methadone withdrawal in those infants born to women taking methadone.[86,87] Therefore, clinicians should be aware of the increased risk of cholestasis and its associated morbidity.

Vertical HCV transmission rates range between 2% and 7%.[77,78,80,88,89] Although reported rates of transmission have been variable, overall it is encouraging that most series show the risk to be generally less than 5%. Maternal viremia (HCV RNA detected in maternal blood) near the time of delivery is a key determinant for vertical HCV transmission, regardless of maternal HIV status.[90–92] If an HCV-infected pregnant woman has no detectable HCV RNA, the risk of

TABLE 27–3

Risk Factors Warranting Hepatitis C Screening: Centers for Disease Control and Prevention Guidelines

Individuals Who Should Be Screened Routinely?

- Persons who ever injected illegal drugs (even once)
- Persons notified that they received blood/blood products from a donor who later tested positive for HCV
- Recipients of transfusions or organ transplants, particularly if received before July 1992
- Persons ever on long-term hemodialysis
- Persons with persistently elevated alanine aminotransferase (ALT) levels or other evidence of liver disease
- Persons seeking evaluation or care for a sexually transmitted infection, including HIV

Individuals for Whom Routine Testing Is of Uncertain Need

- Recipients of tissue transplants (e.g., corneal, skin, sperm, ova)
- Users of intranasal cocaine or other illegal noninjected drugs
- Persons with a history of tattooing or body piercing
- Persons with a history of sexually transmitted diseases or multiple sexual partners
- Long-term steady sex partner of an HCV-infected individual

HCV, hepatitis C virus.
From Centers for Disease Control and Prevention (CDC): Recommendations for prevention and control of hepatitis C virus (HCV) infection and HCV-related chronic disease. MMWR 1998;47(RR-19):1–33; and CDC: Sexually transmitted diseases treatment guidelines, 2006. MMWR 2006;55(RR-11):1–94.

transmission is approximately 0% to 3%.[80,93] In a recent study of over 500 HCV-infected women, the vertical transmission rate was 7.1% (95% confidence interval [CI] 6.3%–7.9%) in those women with detectable HCV RNA and 0% in those women who were HCV RNA–negative.[80] In contrast to HIV, the critical titer predictive of perinatal transmission remains unknown.

Women coinfected with HCV and HIV have consistently higher rates of perinatal transmission than women infected with HCV alone. Recent series have demonstrated that the risk may be lower that previously reported, ranging from 5.4% to 13.6% [80,88,94] The interaction between maternal and fetal humoral and immunologic factors is thought to be a critical contributor to both the occurrence and the persistence of perinatally acquired neonatal HCV infection. The fact that maternal or neonatal co-infection with HIV increases the risk of vertical HCV infection suggests that HIV-infected infants, who are known to have early deficits in cell-mediated and humoral immunity, may be less able to clear small amounts of perinatally presented HCV than HIV-uninfected infants.[95,96] Although no large-scale longitudinal follow-up studies exist into the natural history of perinatal HCV infection through childhood, at least one published case report has documented clearance of neonatally documented HCV RNA by 24 months of age in a child born to an HIV-negative, HCV RNA–positive mother.[72] Therefore, an intact neonatal immune system may allow for HCV clearance in early infancy, as can occur in HIV-uninfected adults.

Management Options

Similar to HBV, invasive monitoring during labor should be avoided if possible in HCV-infected women. Internal fetal heart rate monitoring is associated with a 6.7-fold (95% CI 1.1–35.9) increased risk of transmission.[79] Optimal route of delivery, in the context of maternal HCV infection, has been an area of controversy. This debate, to some degree, parallels the one that evolved regarding maternal HIV infection. However, unlike with HCV infection, maternal HIV viral load was a clearly established independent predictor of vertical transmission[97] and had a direct bearing on the current guidelines regarding route of delivery and maternal HIV infection, specifically when maternal HIV viral load is durably suppressed to greater than 1000 RNA copies/mL.[98] Several studies indicate that route of delivery is much less clearly associated with an increased risk of HCV transmission.[68,80,89] Current consensus opinions, therefore, recommend cesarean delivery in HCV-infected women only for usual obstetric indications.[20,80]

The experience with antiretroviral treatment in decreasing both maternal viral load and the risk of neonatal HIV infections raises the question of potential comparable treatment options in the context of maternal HCV infection. Currently, there is no safe treatment for chronic HCV infection during pregnancy. The standard combination therapy for nonpregnant adults consists of weekly injections with pegylated IFN-α and daily ribavirin.[99] Ribavirin is contraindicated during pregnancy and in male partners of pregnant women due to potential teratogenic effects.[73,100,101]

Finally, questions surrounding the safety of breast-feeding frequently arise from HCV-infected women. Many of these women have other risk factors, such as ongoing substance addiction or coexisting HIV infection, which preclude breast-feeding in general and override concerns about transmission of HCV through breast milk. For those women who have no other obstetric or medical issues that prevent nursing, data have failed to demonstrate breast milk as an effective route for HCV transmission. Although most of these studies were not designed to specifically address this topic, the authors' evaluation of mother-infant pairs enrolled in some of the published vertical HCV transmission studies failed to document any neonatal HCV infection in breast-fed infants, even when the mother was HCV RNA–positive. One study from China that did look at breast milk specifically found a correlation between maternal HCV serum titer and detection of HCV by means of polymerase chain reaction (PCR) in breast milk; however, no infants in this small series (n = 15) became infected with HCV.[102] Additional studies from Australia,[103] United Arab Emirates,[104] and Switzerland[105] examined 100 pregnancies in HCV-infected women who breast-fed (up to two thirds of whom were HCV RNA–positive in sera), with no detectable impact of breast-feeding on the risk of neonatal infection. As a result of the available supporting data, consensus opinions do not view maternal HCV infection as a contraindication to breast-feeding except, perhaps, in cases in which a mother experiences cracked or bleeding nipples.[20,77,106]

A survey study, in fact, did demonstrate that that the majority of community-based obstetricians are questioning patients about issues that could relate to HCV infection risk. However, the authors showed that HCV screening practices and counseling provided were discrepant with CDC recommendations up to 53% of the time, particularly in the area of counseling against breast-feeding in the face of maternal HCV infection.[107]

SUMMARY OF MANAGEMENT OPTIONS

Hepatitis Virus Infections

Management Options	Evidence Quality and Recommendation	References
Hepatitis A		
Prenatal		
• Women traveling to endemic areas during pregnancy should be vaccinated.	III/C	23
• Vaccine is recommended for postexposure prophylaxis for women aged up to 40 yr.	Ia/B	23
• Hepatitis A vaccine not contraindicated during pregnancy.	IV/C	20
• Supportive care for acute infection.	GPP	—
Labor and Delivery		
• Supportive care for acute infection.	GPP	—
Postnatal		
• Newborn immune globulin if acute maternal infection occurs proximate to delivery.	IV/C	23
• Hepatitis A vaccine recommended for all children aged 12–23 mo.	Ib/A	21
Hepatitis B		
Prenatal		
• Supportive care.	GPP	—
• Universal HBsAg screening of all pregnant women.	Ib/A	20,43
• No contraindications to HBV vaccine during pregnancy.	IV/C	49
Labor and Delivery		
• Route of delivery does not influence vertical transmission.	III/B	20
Postnatal		
• Newborns of chronic carrier mothers should all receive HBIG within 12 hr of birth and HBV vaccine within 12 hr of birth.	Ib/A	20,60
• Encourage breast-feeding.	IIa/B	20,43
Hepatitis C		
Prenatal		
• Screen pregnant women in high risk groups.	IV/C	20,77
• Most cases asymptomatic; supportive care for clinical illness.	GPP	—
• Counsel regarding increased risk of cholestasis.	III/B	87,88
Labor and Delivery		
• Route of delivery does not influence risk of vertical transmission.	III/B	79,80,83,89
• Avoid invasive monitoring during labor if possible.	III/B	79
Postnatal		
• Encourage breast-feeding.	II/B	102,104,105
• Referral to specialist for potential combination therapy (interferon and ribavirin).	IV/C	73,86

GPP, good practice point; HBIG, hepatitis B virus immunoglobulin; HBsAg, hepatitis B surface antigen; HBV, hepatitis B virus.

SUGGESTED READINGS

Advisory Committee on Immunization Practices (ACIP), Fiore AE, Wasley A, Bell BP: Prevention of hepatitis A through active or passive immunization: Recommendations of the Advisory Committee on Immunization Practices (ACIP). MMWR Recomm Rep 2006;55:1–23.

American College of Obstetricians and Gynecologists (ACOG): Viral hepatitis in pregnancy (ACOG Practice Bulletin No. 86). Obstet Gynecol 2007;110:941–956.

Berkley EM, Leslie KK, Arora S, et al: Chronic hepatitis C in pregnancy. Obstet Gynecol 2008;112:304–310.

Gambarin-Gelwan M: Hepatitis B in pregnancy. Clin Liver Dis 2007;11:945–963,x.

Gonik B: The role of obstetrician/gynecologists in the management of hepatitis C virus infection. Infect Dis Obstet Gynecol 2008;2008:374517.

Mast EE, Weinbaum CM, Fiore AE, et al: A comprehensive immunization strategy to eliminate transmission of hepatitis B virus infection in the United States: Recommendations of the Advisory Committee on Immunization Practices (ACIP) part II: Immunization of adults. MMWR Recomm Rep 2006;55:1–33; quiz CE1–4.

McMenamin MB, Jackson AD, Lambert J, et al: Obstetric management of hepatitis C–positive mothers: Analysis of vertical transmission in 559 mother-infant pairs. Am J Obstet Gynecol 2008;199:315.e1–315.e5.

Victor JC, Monto AS, Surdina TY, et al: Hepatitis A vaccine versus immune globulin for postexposure prophylaxis. N Engl J Med 2007;357:1685–1694.

Wasley A, Grytdal S, Gallagher K, Centers for Disease Control and Prevention (CDC): Surveillance for acute viral hepatitis—United States, 2006. MMWR Surveill Summ 2008;57:1–24.

REFERENCES

For a complete list of references, log onto www.expertconsult.com.

CHAPTER 28

Human Immunodeficiency Virus*

D. HEATHER WATTS

INTRODUCTION

The management of HIV infection continues to evolve rapidly. Amazing advances have been made in therapy of primary infection, prevention of opportunistic infections, and prevention of perinatal transmission since the first cases of AIDS were described in 1981. Perinatal transmission rates have decreased from 20% to 30% early in the epidemic to 1% to 2% in developed countries with the use of antiretroviral therapy and scheduled cesarean delivery. While reducing transmission, these interventions have increased the complexity of prenatal care for HIV-infected women. As standards of care evolve rapidly, providers are urged to access resources available on the Internet such as www.aidsinfo.nih.gov or www.WHO.int/hiv/topics/arv/ for the most recent update.

Women represent the fastest growing group of persons with new HIV infections. In the United States, over 130,000 women are estimated to be infected, and worldwide, the number is over 15 million.[1,2] Approximately 6000 HIV-infected women deliver annually in the United States, with approximately 144 to 236 infants acquiring HIV infection compared with 2 million deliveries to HIV-infected women worldwide resulting in over 600,000 HIV-infected infants.[2,3] Improvements in availability of prenatal care, HIV counseling and testing, antiretroviral therapy, and strategies to reduce HIV transmission through breast-feeding are vitally needed in areas of the world most affected by HIV to improve maternal health and survival and reduce perinatal transmission.[4] This chapter focuses on interventions currently available to maximize maternal health and minimize perinatal transmission in resource-rich countries.

DIAGNOSIS

All pregnant women should be tested for HIV infection to allow optimal care for maternal health and prevention of perinatal transmission. A policy of universal HIV testing, with patient notification and right of refusal, is recommended.[5] All pregnant women should be encouraged to be tested regardless of perceived risk factors or local seroprevalence, because many HIV-infected women were infected heterosexually and are unaware of their risk. If women decline testing, the reasons for declining should be explored and further education provided regarding the benefits and risks of testing. Federal policy recommends universal HIV testing along with other prenatal laboratory studies unless the woman refuses testing, but state laws may require detailed pretest counseling and written informed consent. Providers should be aware of their own local and state requirements while striving for universal testing for pregnant women.

HIV testing should be repeated in the third trimester for all women in high-prevalence areas (HIV incidence >17/100,000[5]) and for those with ongoing risk factors in pregnancy including injection drug use, an HIV-infected partner, or new or multiple partners during pregnancy.[5] In addition, pregnant women with symptoms suggestive of acute HIV infection, such as fever, rash, sore throat, and myalgias, should undergo both antibody testing and HIV RNA testing to diagnose infection as early as possible.

The recommended algorithm for HIV testing consists of initial screening with a U.S. Food and Drug Administration (FDA)–licensed enzyme immunoassay (EIA) or rapid test followed by confirmatory testing with an FDA-licensed supplemental test, usually a Western blot (WB), if the initial test is repeatedly reactive.[6] If the EIA is repeatedly reactive and the WB is positive, HIV infection is confirmed, because false-positive WB results are rare.[7] However, given the implications of a positive HIV test result, repeat testing on a separate blood sample is recommended to rule out any possibility of mislabeling or other clerical error. A more common, though still infrequent, event is an indeterminate WB. Indeterminate WB results can be caused by incomplete antibody response seen with recent HIV infection or late-stage disease or by nonspecific reactions in uninfected persons, possibly related to recent immunizations or current or previous pregnancy. Although indeterminate results are more common among pregnant or parous women, they are estimated to occur during pregnancy at a rate of fewer than 1 per 4000 samples based on a study of over 1 million specimens.[8,9] Pregnant women with indeterminate WB results should be queried regarding potential recent exposures to HIV through occupational, sexual, or needle-sharing activity; have repeat testing to evaluate for evolving infection versus resolution of nonspecific reactivity; and consider testing of sexual partners to clarify risk. For women with repeatedly indeterminate testing, alternate testing for HIV itself using an approved HIV RNA test may be helpful,

*This chapter is in the public domain.

although these tests are not approved for diagnosis of HIV infection. If no recent high-risk exposures are identified, women with repeatedly indeterminate WB results should be reassured that HIV infection is unlikely.

Women delivering with no prenatal care represent a group at high risk for perinatal HIV transmission. During the period 1993 to 1996, approximately 15% of HIV-infected pregnant women in the United States received no prenatal care, compared with 2% in the general population.[10] Given the reduction in transmission achieved with several different intrapartum/neonatal prophylaxis regimens[11–14] and the increased risk of HIV infection among women presenting without prenatal care, rapid HIV testing should be offered to all pregnant women presenting in labor without prenatal care or documentation of previous testing during pregnancy.[5] Testing should be done only after pretest counseling, including discussion of the need for confirmatory testing if rapid assays are positive, and informed consent. Rapid testing may be done using approved rapid tests or EIA testing.[15] Because of the relatively low prevalence of HIV even in this setting, the negative predictive value of a single negative rapid test is high, so no further testing is required to confirm a negative rapid test.[15] All positive rapid tests should be confirmed by supplemental testing with either a WB or an immunofluorescence assay but decisions regarding use of antiretrovirals for prevention of perinatal transmission may need to be made pending confirmatory test results because initiation of therapy during labor or shortly after birth is required to reduce risk of transmission.[15]

MATERNAL AND FETAL RISKS

Disease Progression

Studies in the United States and Europe have been consistent in not demonstrating an effect of pregnancy on HIV disease progression.[16–18] More recently, a report from the Women and Infants Transmission Study (WITS) did not show a difference in CD4+ lymphocyte count or HIV RNA trajectory or clinical AIDS rate between women with one or multiple pregnancies after HIV diagnosis.[19] Studies in developing countries suggest that pregnancy may enhance disease progression, but they included small numbers and might have had selection bias in HIV testing.[20,21]

Increased Toxicity of Antiretroviral Therapy

The hormonal effects of pregnancy may increase the risk of toxicity of antiretroviral therapy, especially the nucleoside reverse transcriptase inhibitors. Several cases of lactic acidosis and hepatic failure, some resulting in maternal deaths, have been reported among women on long-term nucleoside therapy during pregnancy, most frequently stavudine and didanosine in combination.[22,23] Clinical findings were similar to those seen in acute fatty liver of pregnancy, which occurs more frequently among women with heterozygous defects of mitochondrial fatty acid metabolism carrying fetuses homozygous for the defect.[24] Similar enhancement of mitochondrial toxicity due to reduced fatty acid oxidation has been shown in pregnant mice and in mice treated with high doses of estrogen and progesterone to simulate pregnancy.[25,26] The potential for lactic acidosis and hepatic failure is present with the use of any nucleoside agent, with the binding affinity for mitochondrial polymerase gamma, the key enzyme, highest for zalcitabine, then decreasing for didanosine, stavudine, lamivudine, zidovudine, and abacavir.[27] Thus, all pregnant women on nucleoside antiretroviral therapy should be educated regarding the signs and symptoms of lactic acidosis and hepatic dysfunction including nausea, vomiting, fatigue, tachycardia, dyspnea or hyperventilation, and abdominal pain, and clinicians should be vigilant for these signs and symptoms that might be difficult to distinguish from normal pregnancy symptoms.

Impact on Future Therapy

Current indications for initiation of antiretroviral therapy in nonpregnant adults are a CD4+ lymphocyte count below 500 cells/μL or opportunistic infections.[28] Many pregnant women do not meet these criteria for therapy but will take antiretrovirals to reduce the risk of perinatal transmission and stop therapy after delivery. As discussed in more detail later, these women should receive highly active therapy with a combination of three or more drugs to minimize HIV RNA levels and risk of transmission.[29] Although aggressive combination therapy with suppression of HIV RNA to undetectable levels during pregnancy should minimize the risk of resistance, the impact of short-term highly active antiretroviral therapy on future response to therapy and maternal health has not been well studied. Although studies following women postpartum after zidovudine monotherapy and dual nucleoside therapy in pregnancy have not suggested an increased risk of disease progression with stopping therapy,[30,31] studies of structured treatment interruption have raised concern about stopping highly active antiretroviral therapy (HAART) once initiated.[32] However, most subjects in treatment interruption studies had lower nadir CD4+ cell counts, longer duration of antiretroviral therapy, and older age than the pregnant women using HAART during pregnancy for interruption of transmission, making extrapolation of results difficult. More research is needed on the risks of stopping or continuing HAART after use in pregnancy among women with higher CD4+ lymphocyte counts.

Pregnancy Complications

The effect of HIV infection and antiretroviral therapy on pregnancy outcome is another issue for consideration. The majority of studies in developed countries done before the availability of antiretroviral therapy did not demonstrate an increased rate of adverse pregnancy outcomes such as preterm birth and stillbirth among HIV-infected women compared with uninfected women with similar risk profiles.[33–35] Conversely, most studies in developing countries have suggested an increased risk of preterm birth, low birth weight, intrauterine growth restriction, stillbirth, and infant death among infants born to HIV-infected women, with increasing risk with more advanced HIV infection.[33,36] Factors associated with an increased risk of preterm birth and low birth weight among HIV-infected women included previous adverse pregnancy outcome, hypertension, multiple gestation, smoking, bleeding, alcohol use, low maternal weight, *Trichomonas vaginalis* infection, and other sexually transmitted infections, similar to risk factors in

HIV-uninfected women.[35,37,38] Low CD4+ percentage was an additional risk factor for adverse outcome among women not receiving antiretroviral therapy,[37] but neither CD4+ lymphocyte count nor HIV RNA levels were associated with adverse outcomes among women receiving zidovudine therapy.[38]

Zidovudine monotherapy has not been associated with an increased risk of preterm birth or low birth weight in any study to date, but the potential impact of combination antiretroviral therapy on pregnancy outcome is less clear.[39,40] In the early HAART era, a small study from Europe[41] and an analysis of the European Collaborative Study[42] found an increased risk of preterm birth with increasing numbers of drugs, with the highest rate occurring among women receiving protease inhibitor (PI) therapy. A combined analysis of several cohorts in the United States did not find an increased risk of preterm delivery among women on dual therapy or regimens including PIs, although there was a slight increase in risk of very low–birth weight infants born to women receiving PI therapy compared with those on no therapy or zidovudine.[43] A meta-analysis published in 2007 incorporating 14 studies found no increase in risk of preterm birth with antiretroviral therapy compared with no therapy.[44] HAART regimens including PIs did not increase the risk of preterm birth compared with the no therapy group, but were associated with an increased risk compared with combination regimens without PIs (odds ratio [OR] 1.35; 95% confidence interval [CI] 1.08–1.70).[44] Among the subset starting any HAART before pregnancy or in the first trimester, the risk of preterm birth was increased compared with those starting HAART later in pregnancy (OR 1.71; 95% CI 1.09–2.67).[44] Subsequent studies have found an increased risk of preterm birth with HAART, in some cases specifically with PI therapy. A large, population-based study from the United Kingdom and Ireland found an adjusted odds ration (AOR) of 1.51 (95% CI 1.19–1.93) for preterm birth with HAART compared with mono- or dual therapy, regardless of whether a PI was included in the HAART.[45] A Brazilian study found in increased rate of preterm birth (AOR 5.0; 95% CI 1.5–17.0) with HAART started preconception compared with therapy started later in pregnancy.[46] Recent studies from the United States, Germany/Austria, and Italy have found increased risks of preterm delivery with PI-based HAART in pregnancy, with AORs ranging from 1.21 to 3.40.[47–49] Clinicians should be aware of a possible increased risk of preterm birth with PI use, but given the clear benefits for maternal health and reduction in perinatal transmission, these agents should not be withheld because of these concerns.

Perinatal Transmission

A major concern with HIV infection in pregnancy is the risk of perinatal transmission of HIV to the infant. Among untreated women who do not breast-feed, transmission will occur in 20% to 30%.[50] Estimates are that about two thirds of transmissions from untreated women occur at delivery and one third occur in utero, many late in pregnancy.[51] An additional transmission risk of 15% to 20% occurs during breast-feeding.[52] Maternal HIV RNA levels appear to be the factor most predictive of transmission.[53,54] Antiretroviral therapy during pregnancy and in the neonatal period clearly reduces the risk of perinatal transmission of HIV. The first study demonstrating this benefit was the Pediatric AIDS Clinical Trials Group (PACTG) 076 study[39] with a transmission rate of 8.3% among those receiving oral antepartum, intravenous intrapartum, and oral neonatal zidovudine for 6 weeks compared with 25.5% among those receiving placebo. The PACTG 185 trial[55] found no benefit from addition of HIV immunoglobulin to the PACTG 076 regimen but demonstrated benefit of zidovudine among women with CD4+ lymphocyte counts under 500 cells/μL at enrollment, with a transmission rate of 4.6%. Subsequent trials have demonstrated benefit from shorter courses of antepartum/intrapartum or antepartum/intrapartum/neonatal zidovudine or zidovudine/lamivudine compared with placebo, but no benefit was seen from intrapartum zidovudine/lamivudine alone.[14,56–61] In addition, the HIVNET 012 trial[11] demonstrated the benefit of a two-dose nevirapine regimen (one dose intrapartum to the mother and one dose to the infant at 48 hr of age) compared with oral intrapartum and 1 week of neonatal zidovudine. A subsequent trial demonstrated that intrapartum and 1 week of neonatal zidovudine/lamivudine therapy was similar in efficacy to the HIVNET 012 nevirapine regimen.[14] These trials provide data for implementation of shorter, less complex regimens for reduction of transmission of HIV in resource-limited settings or for women diagnosed in the peripartum period as being HIV-infected.

A trial in the United States, Europe, and Latin America (PACTG 316) evaluating addition of the HIVNET 012 nevirapine regimen to established antiretroviral therapy demonstrated no benefit of adding nevirapine to ongoing therapy.[62] However, this trial provides updated data regarding transmission of HIV with the use of combination antiretroviral therapy. The transmission rate overall was 1.5%, with rates of 2.1% for women on zidovudine alone, 1.1% with combination nucleoside therapy, and 1.6% with combination with PI.[62] Similarly, an analysis from WITS, including women enrolled from 1990 through 2000, observed transmission rates of 20.0% for women not receiving antiretroviral agents, 10.4% for women receiving zidovudine monotherapy (not necessarily the complete 076 regimen), 3.8% for those receiving dual nucleoside therapy, and 1.2% for those receiving highly active antiretroviral regimens.[50] These low rates of transmission with highly active regimens occurred despite potential confounding by indication in which women with the highest HIV RNA levels and lowest CD4+ lymphocyte counts were most likely to be treated with highly active regimens, especially early in the period of availability. More recent data from a study of HIV transmission among women delivering in the United Kingdom and Ireland from 2000 to 2006, transmission occurred in 0.7% of 2845 women on HAART, regardless of mode of delivery.[63] Thus, current data demonstrate significant fetal benefit from combination antiretroviral regimens, which would require significant evidence of harm to negate.

Antiretroviral Therapy

Teratogenesis

Another concern with the use of antiretroviral drugs in pregnancy is the potential for birth defects, especially with first-trimester exposure. Limited data from animal studies are available for most of the drugs (Table 28–1). Of concern,

TABLE 28–1

Preclinical and Clinical Data Relevant to the Use of Antiretrovirals in Pregnancy

DRUG	FDA PREG CAT	NEWBORN:MATERNAL DRUG RATIO	ANIMAL STUDIES	MAJOR TOXICITIES	HUMAN STUDIES; CONCERNS SPECIFIC TO PREGNANCY
Nucleoside/Nucleotide Reverse Transcriptase Inhibitors				**Class effect: Rare, but potentially fatal, lactic acidosis with hepatic steatosis.**	
Zidovudine (Retrovir, AZT, ZVD)	C	~0.8 human	No effect on rodent fertility, but cytotoxic to mouse embryos. Positive teratogenicity in rodents only at near-lethal doses.	Bone marrow suppression, myopathy	ARV agent most used in pregnancy, safe in short term. See discussion of rodent tumors, mitochondrial toxicity in text.
Emtricitabine (Emtriva, FTC)	B	0.4–0.5 mice, rabbits	Negative teratogenicity studies in mice and rabbits.	Hyperpigmentation of palms/soles. Possible hepatitis B flare when stopping.	Pk study shows slightly lower levels in third trimester compared with postpartum but no clear need to increase dose. Alternate NRTI for use in pregnancy.
Didanosine (Videx, ddI)	B	0.5 human	No effect on rodent fertility or mouse embryos. No teratogenicity in mice, rats, rabbits.	Pancreatitis, peripheral neuropathy, nausea, diarrhea	Pk study (n = 14) shows no need for dose modification, well-tolerated. Alternate NRTI for use in pregnancy. Do not use with d4T in pregnancy because of enhanced toxicity.
Stavudine (Zerit, d4T)	C	0.76 rhesus monkey	No effect on rodent fertility, but cytotoxic to mouse embryos. No evidence of teratogenicity. Ossification delay at high doses in rats.	Peripheral neuropathy	Phase I/II study indicated no change in pk in pregnancy; well-tolerated. Do not use with ddI in pregnancy because of enhanced toxicity. Antagonizes ZDV, do not use together.
Lamivudine (Epivir, 3TC)	C	~1.0 human	No effect on rodent fertility or mouse embryos. No teratogenicity.	Pancreatitis increased in children. Possible hepatitis B flare when stopping.	Pk study (n = 20) shows no need for dose modification, well-tolerated. Preferred NRTI in pregnancy based on experience with use.
Abacavir (Ziagen, ABC)	C	Passage in rats	No effect on fertility in rodents. Anasarca, skeletal abnormalities at 35 times human dose in rodents, not seen in rabbits.	Potentially fatal hypersensitivity reactions, symptoms: fever, rash, fatigue, nausea, vomiting, diarrhea, abdominal pain in 2%–9%.	No change in pk in pregnancy. Alternate NRTI for use in pregnancy. Screen for HLA-B*5701 before use to reduce risk of hypersensitivity reaction.
Tenofovir (Viread)	B	0.6–1.0 human	No effect on fertility. No birth defects, but growth restriction, reversible bone changes with chronic use in monkeys.	Asthenia, nausea, vomiting, diarrhea, headache, flatulence. Possible hepatitis B flare when stopping.	Limited data in human pregnancy thus far. Use only after careful consideration of alternatives.
Non-nucleoside Reverse Transcriptase Inhibitors				**Class effects: rash with rare cases of Stevens-Johnson syndrome; increased transaminase levels.**	
Nevirapine (Viramune)	C	~0.9 human	Impaired fertility in female rats. Not teratogenic in rats, rabbits.	Rash, drug interactions, potential for fulminant hepatitis and hepatic failure, especially among women with CD4 counts >250 cells/mL at initiation.	No change in pk in pregnancy. Not recommended for women initiating therapy with CD4 count >250 cells/mL due to increased risk of potentially fatal liver toxicity. Single dose at delivery not associated with increased risk. See text for use of NRTI "tail" after single dose in labor.
Delavirdine (Rescriptor)	C	Unknown	No effect on fertility in rodents. Embryotoxic in rabbits. VSD in rats, maternal toxicity, developmental delay, decreased pup survival.	Rash, drug interactions.	No studies. Not recommended for use in pregnancy.
Efavirenz (Sustiva)	D	0.13 human	Increased fetal resorptions in rats. Defects (anencephaly, anophthalmia, cleft palate) in 3/20 monkeys treated with human doses.	Rash, drug interactions, CNS symptoms such as dizziness, insomnia, confusion.	Avoid use in first trimester. May be considered for use later in pregnancy. Ensure adequate contraception postpartum.
Etrvirine (Intelence)	B	Unknown	Negative in rats, rabbits.	Rash, rare hypersensitivity reactions; drug interactions	No data on use in human pregnancy so not currently recommended.
Protease Inhibitors				**Class effects: Hyperglycemia, possible fat redistribution and lipid abnormalities, increased bleeding episodes in hemophiliacs.**	
Indinavir (Crixivan)	C	Minimal	No effect on fertility in rodents. No teratogenicity in rats, rabbits or dogs. Extra ribs in rats.	Kidney stones, hyperbilirubinemia, drug interactions, nausea.	Use with low-dose ritonavir boosting to assure adequate dosing in pregnancy. Alternate PI for use in pregnancy.

TABLE 28-1

Preclinical and Clinical Data Relevant to the Use of Antiretrovirals in Pregnancy—cont'd

DRUG	FDA PREG CAT	NEWBORN:MATERNAL DRUG RATIO	ANIMAL STUDIES	MAJOR TOXICITIES	HUMAN STUDIES; CONCERNS SPECIFIC TO PREGNANCY
Ritonavir (Norvir)	B	Minimal	No effect on fertility in rodents at half the human dose. Hepatotoxicity at higher doses. Developmental toxicity at toxic doses but no teratogenicity in rats, rabbits.	Nausea, vomiting, diarrhea; increased triglycerides, transaminases; drug interactions, paresthesias.	Use only at low doses to boost levels of other PIs in pregnancy.
Saquinavir hard gel capsules (Invirase)	B	Minimal	No effect on fertility in rodents. Negative teratogenicity.	Nausea, diarrhea, elevated transaminases.	Use with low-dose ritonavir boosting to ensure adequate dosing in pregnancy. Alternate PI for use in pregnancy.
Nelfinavir (Viracept)	B	Minimal	No effect on fertility in rodents. Studies negative in rats, rabbits.	Diarrhea, drug interactions	Extensive experience in pregnancy but not recommended for treatment in nonpregnant adults. May be used as part of triple-agent regimen for pregnant women receiving HAART for prophylaxis rather than therapy.
Fosamprenavir (Lexiava)	C	Unknown	No effect on fertility in rodents. Negative teratogenicity studies.	Nausea, vomiting, diarrhea, rash, oral paresthesias, increased liver function tests. Drug interactions.	No studies in human pregnancy, not recommended.
Lopinavir/ritonavir (Kaletra)	C	0.20 human	No effects on fertility. No teratogenicity in rats, rabbits.	Nausea, vomiting, diarrhea, asthenia, elevated transaminase levels.	Preferred PI in pregnancy based on experience. Pk studies of new tablet under way; increased dosing in third trimester required with capsule. Monitor virologic response in third trimester with standard dosing. Once-daily dosing not recommended in pregnancy.
Atazanavir (Reyataz®-)	B	Minimal (<10%)/ variable in humans.	No effect on fertility. No teratogenicity in rats, rabbits.	Drug interactions, prolonged PR interval, hyperbilirubinemia, rash.	Limited experience in human pregnancy. Theoretical concern of hyperbilirubinemia in neonate from maternal exposure. May be considered as alternate PI.
Darunavir	C	Unknown	Negative teratogenicity studies; decreased pup weight after prenatal exposure.	Headache, nausea, diarrhea, hypertriglyceridemia, nasopharyngitis, drug interactions.	No studies in human pregnancy, not recommended.
Entry Inhibitors					
Enfurvirtide (Fuzeon, T-20)	B	None based on limited human data	No effect on fertility. No teratogenicity in rats, rabbits.	Injection site reactions, eosinophilia, rare systemic hypersensitivity	No studies in human pregnancy. Consider use only as salvage therapy.
Maraviroc (Selzentry)	B	Unknown	Negative teratogenicity studies in rats, rabbits.	Hepatoxicity, allergic rash, increased upper respiratory infections, possibly other infections, dizziness, drug interactions.	No experience in human pregnancy, not recommended.
Integrase Inhibitors					
Raltegravir (Isentress)	C	2.0 in rats, 0.02 in rabbits	Negative in rabbits, supernumerary ribs in rats.	Creatine kinase elevations, possible myopathy.	No experience in human pregnancy. Consider use only as salvage therapy.

FDA preg cat, U.S. Food and Drug Administration pregnancy category: A, adequate and well-controlled studies of pregnant women fail to demonstrate a risk to the fetus during the first trimester of pregnancy (and there is no evidence of risk during the later trimesters); B, animal reproduction studies fail to demonstrate a risk to the fetus, and adequate and well-controlled studies of pregnant women have not been conducted; C, safety in human pregnancy has not been determined, animal studies are either positive for fetal risk or have not been conducted, and the drug should not be used unless the potential benefit outweighs the potential risk to the fetus; D, positive evidence of human fetal risk based on adverse reaction data from investigational or marketing experiences, but the potential benefits from the use of the drug in pregnant women may be acceptable despite its potential risks; X, studies in animals or reports of adverse reactions have indicated that the risk associated with the use of the drug for pregnant women clearly outweighs any possible benefit.

ABC, abacavir; ARV, antiretroviral; AZT, azidothymidine; CNS, central nervous system; ddI, dideoxyinosine; d4T, stavudine; FTC, emtricitabine; HAART, highly active antiretroviral therapy; HLA, human leukocyte antigen; NRTI, nucleoside/nucleotide reverse transcriptase inhibitor; PI, protease inhibitor; pk, pharmacokinetic; 3TC, lamivudine; VSD, ventricular septal defect; ZVD, zidovudine.

From Panel on Antiretroviral Guidelines for Adults and Adolescents: Guidelines for the Use of Antiretroviral Agents in HIV-1-infected Adults and Adolescents. Washington, DC, Department of Health and Human Services. December 1, 2009, pp 1–144. Available at http://www.aidsinfo.nih.gov/ContentFiles/AdultandAdolescentGL.pdf (accessed March 25, 2010); and Public Health Service Task Force Recommendations for Use of Antiretroviral Drugs in Pregnant HIV-1–infected Women for Maternal Health and Interventions to Reduce Perinatal HIV-1–Transmission in the United States. April 29, 2009. Available at http://aidsinfo.nih.gov/guidelines/ (accessed March 25, 2010).

birth defects, including anencephaly, anophthalmia, microophthalmia, and cleft palate, were seen in 3 (20%) of 15 monkeys exposed to efavirenz in the first trimester.[29] Several cases of meningomyelocele after first-trimester efavirenz exposure have been reported retrospectively to the Antiretroviral Pregnancy Registry (APR), an important source for data on birth defects among infants born to antiretroviral-exposed pregnant women.[64] Among prospective cases with first-trimester efavirenz exposure reported to the APR, defects have occurred among 13 (3.2%) of 407 live births, not different from the overall rate of 2.7% among all prospective cases reported to APR or the rate of 2.9% among all prospective cases with first-trimester exposure to antiretroviral agents.[64] Of note, however, the defects after first-trimester efavirenz exposure include one case of sacral meningomyelocele with hydrocephalus and one case of bilateral facial clefts, anophthalmia, and amniotic band, indicating that further surveillance is required. Based on animal data and concerning case reports, favirenz use should be avoided during the first trimester of pregnancy, and women of reproductive potential on efavirenz should be counseled regarding potential risks and provided with effective contraception. No increase in birth defects associated with first-trimester antiretroviral therapy has been noted among prospective cases reported to the APR, with adequate numbers to rule out a twofold or greater increased risk of overall birth defects reported for the following drugs: zidovudine, lamivudine, stavudine, nelfinavir, nevirapine, abacavir, efavirenz, didanosine, ritonavir, lopinavir, tenofovir, indinavir, emtricitabine, and atzanavir.[64] Providers caring for pregnant women receiving antiretroviral drugs are urged to report cases as early in pregnancy as possible to the Registry (1–800–258–4263 or http://www.apregistry.com) to allow better assessment of risks.

Additional data are available from prospective cohorts, some of which overlap with cases reported to the APR. A report from the WITS found no increase in birth defects after first-trimester exposure to antiretrovirals compared with later exposure or no exposure, but did find a marginally significant increase in risk of hypospadias in male infants after first-trimester zidovudine exposure.[65] An analysis of data from the European Collaborative Study,[66] including women and infants enrolled between 1986 and 2003, did not find an increase in birth defects with first-trimester antiretroviral exposure compared with later or no exposure, and there was no discernible pattern of defects related to type or timing of therapy. Likewise, an analysis of births in the United Kingdom and Ireland to HIV-infected women between 1990 and 2007 did not find an increased risk of birth defects related to timing or class of antiretroviral exposure in pregnancy.[67] Thus, with the exception of animal data and case reports for efavirenz, data are reassuring so far that use of antiretrovirals in pregnancy does not increase the risk of birth defects overall. Continued vigilance is indicated, though, as new drugs become available and expanded access leads to treatment of more pregnant women.

Mitochondrial Toxicity in Offspring

Another concern, potential mitochondrial toxicity in the children of women treated with antiretrovirals, was first raised by French researchers. Eight children with clinical or laboratory abnormalities, including two who died, were reported from a cohort of 1754 HIV-uninfected children exposed to zidovudine or zidovudine/lamivudine during pregnancy and the neonatal period.[68,69] Findings were consistent with mitochondrial pathology seen in HIV-infected adults on nucleoside analogue therapy and in animal studies and have since been confirmed in other cohorts.[70,71] Two different syndromes of mitochondrial dysfunction have been described in infants after perinatal antiretroviral exposure.[72] The first is hyperlactatemia, usually asymptomatic, occurring in up to one third of antiretroviral-exposed newborns and reversible with cessation of therapy. The long-term impact of this transient hyperlactatemia is unknown. The second includes severe neurologic symptoms manifesting in the first 2 years of life and associated with biochemical and ultrastructural changes characteristic of mitochondrial dysfunction. This severe manifestation has been seen at a rate of 0.3% or less, depending on the cohort and the intensity of surveillance.[72] The risk of clinically apparent mitochondrial toxicity related to antiretroviral therapy is low and must be balanced against the known benefits in reduction of perinatal transmission. However, long-term follow-up of children exposed to antiretrovirals is required to assess for toxicity.

Transplacental Carcinogenesis

Another concern requiring long-term surveillance of children exposed to antiretrovirals is transplacental carcinogenesis. One study in rats treated with zidovudine in utero at about 30 times the human dose found an increase in liver, lung, and reproductive system tumors, yet a similar study using lower doses did not find an increased rate[73,74] No cancers were seen in a follow-up study of PACTG 076 and WITS, including 727 children or among 1859 antiretroviral-exposed but uninfected children in PACTG 219/219C.[75,76] A study of HIV-infected children with malignancies did not identify zidovudine exposure, either in utero or after birth, as a risk factor for developing cancer.[77] A study linking HIV, cancer, and death registries in England and Wales found no cases of cancer among 2612 HIV-exposed children born between 2001 and 2004.[78] Therefore, human data thus far do not support zidovudine use as a risk factor for carcinogenesis, but long-term follow-up of exposed children is required.

MANAGEMENT OPTIONS

Prepregnancy

Ideally, all HIV-infected women would have a preconceptional visit to optimize their status before pregnancy.[29] Issues to be discussed include current maternal status and indications for antiretroviral therapy and opportunistic infection prophylaxis, choice of antiretroviral drugs to minimize risk of birth defects and toxicity, risk of perinatal transmission and strategies to reduce transmission, immunization status, optimal nutritional status and use of folate supplements, and assessment of other preconceptional issues such as family history pertinent to genetic screening, screening for other infectious diseases, and assessment for other medical or psychological conditions. The risk of perinatal transmission is most strongly related to HIV RNA levels, with the lowest transmission risk associated with undetectable HIV RNA.[53,54]

For women planning pregnancy or currently on antiretroviral therapy or with indications for antiretrovirals based on current guidelines (CD4+ lymphocyte count <500 cells/μL), a highly active regimen that does not include efavirenz should be used. Pregnancy should be delayed until HIV RNA levels are undetectable, if possible. For women not meeting criteria for therapy for their own health, initiation of therapy to prevent transmission after the first trimester should be discussed. Need for opportunistic infection prophylaxis should be assessed.[79] Ideally, if CD4+ lymphocyte counts are in the range at which opportunistic infection prophylaxis is indicated, highly active antiretroviral therapy should be initiated to enhance immunity and obviate the need for prophylaxis during pregnancy. Pregnancy should be delayed until sustained CD4+ lymphocyte counts over 200 cells/μL are achieved to minimize the number of drugs needed during pregnancy. Any indicated immunizations should be provided before pregnancy to avoid the theoretical risk of increased transmission risk related to HIV RNA rebound after immunization. If the HIV-infected woman has not previously been tested for antibodies to *Toxoplasma gondii*, hepatitis C virus, or cytomegalovirus, antibody status should be documented at the preconceptional visit to establish risk for seroconversion or reactivation. Tuberculin skin testing should be done if not done within the past year. The range of transmission risks based on maternal HIV RNA levels and antiretroviral therapy should be discussed, and the woman must understand that, although the risk is now low, there is no guarantee that transmission will not occur. If the HIV-infected woman's sexual partner is HIV-uninfected, there should be discussion of methods to avoid unprotected intercourse including the use of male condoms and alternate methods for conception, such as artificial insemination.

Prenatal

The same principles as outlined for preconceptional care should be followed for HIV-infected women presenting already pregnant. Women newly diagnosed with HIV infection during pregnancy should be assessed for any signs or symptoms suggestive of acute HIV infection or opportunistic infection and undergo laboratory testing (HIV RNA and CD4+ lymphocyte testing) to establish the stage of HIV infection. HIV infection should be confirmed by repeat testing if not previously done. In general, highly active combination antiretroviral therapy is indicated during pregnancy to prevent perinatal transmission and may also be indicated for maternal health.[29] A regimen recommended as first-line or alternate therapy for nonpregnant adults, generally including two nucleoside reverse transcriptase inhibitors with either one or more PIs or a non-nucleoside reverse transcriptase inhibitor, should be chosen.[28] However, nevirapine should not be initiated in women with CD4+ lymphocyte counts over 250 cells/μL because the risk of potentially fatal hepatotoxicity is greatly increased in this group compared with women with lower CD4+ lymphocyte counts.[29] Highly active antiretroviral therapy is indicated to lower HIV RNA levels to undetectable levels to minimize transmission risk and also to minimize the risk of development of resistant virus. Extensive discussions with the woman should emphasize the importance of complete adherence to the regimen to prevent development of resistance. Unless contraindicated or not tolerated, the regimen should include zidovudine, which has the most data on efficacy in reducing transmission. Intravenous zidovudine should be given during labor, and the infant should receive zidovudine for 6 weeks after birth. For women with HIV RNA levels below 1000 copies/mL off antiretroviral therapy who want to minimize their exposure to antiretrovirals, monotherapy with the PACTG 076 zidovudine regimen can be offered. In an analysis of data from several studies, transmission among women with HIV RNA levels below 1000 copies/mL during pregnancy was 9.8% among 368 untreated women and 1% among 834 women receiving zidovudine.[80] Zidovudine monotherapy during pregnancy was not associated with a difference in disease progression postpartum among women in several studies.[30,31,81] The risk of developing resistance to zidovudine among women with HIV RNA below 1000 copies/mL is expected to be low given limited viral replication. The option of stopping therapy after delivery should be discussed with women who initiate therapy solely for prevention of perinatal transmission.

Indications for resistance testing during pregnancy should be the same as for nonpregnant adults.[29] Technical aspects of resistance testing have been reviewed elsewhere.[82] The use of resistance testing to optimize therapy during pregnancy and to reduce the rate of perinatal transmission has not been studied specifically, but resistance testing in adults has been shown to be cost-effective in both treatment-naïve patients and those on failing antiretroviral regimens.[82] Pregnant women not on antiretroviral therapy should have genotypic resistance testing obtained before initiation of therapy unless results from previous testing with no intervening therapy are available.[82] Therapy may be started pending receipt of test results and modified if indicated. If the expected response of at least a one log drop in HIV RNA in the first 8 weeks is not obtained, specimens for resistance testing should be obtained while the woman is on therapy before switching to an alternate regimen. For women entering pregnancy already on therapy, resistance testing is indicated if persistently detectable HIV RNA levels are present despite adequate adherence to the regimen and adequate dosing or if HIV RNA levels become persistently detectable after a period of undetectable levels. The specimen for resistance testing should be drawn while still on the failing regimen to maximize detection of resistance. An HIV RNA level above 500 copies/mL is required for resistance testing. Pregnant women with virologic failure after multiple treatment regimens should have both genotypic and phenotypic resistance testing obtained and should be managed in consultation with an HIV expert.[82]

The majority of studies evaluating the impact of resistance on risk of perinatal transmission have not found the presence of zidovudine, lamivudine, or nevirapine resistance to increase the risk of transmission.[83] Given the currently observed rates of transmission of under 2% among women on highly active antiretroviral therapy during pregnancy, antiretroviral resistance does not appear to be a major issue in perinatal transmission. However, as the prevalence of resistant HIV increases among those with recent infection[82] and as women have repeat pregnancies, the chance of coexistent resistant HIV and pregnancy will increase and might become a larger problem. Resistance patterns among pregnant women and among infected infants must be monitored to allow adaptation of treatment guidelines.

For women presenting during pregnancy already taking antiretroviral therapy, management will depend on gestational age, regimen, HIV levels before starting therapy and time to response, and current symptoms such as nausea that may interfere with adherence during pregnancy. Women presenting after the first trimester should continue on their current regimen as long as HIV RNA levels are below the level of detection. Women presenting early in the first trimester should be counseled regarding the potential teratogenic risks of antiretroviral exposure in the first trimester versus the competing risk of rebound in HIV RNA levels if therapy is stopped, with potential risk for perinatal transmission. Women on efavirenz-containing regimens should be switched to alternate regimens if they choose to continue therapy in the first trimester. In general, women on other regimens should be encouraged to continue therapy. If a woman chooses to discontinue therapy during the first trimester, she should stop and restart all agents concurrently to minimize the risk of development of resistance, unless a drug with a long half-life, such as nevirapine or efavirenz, is included in the regimen. These drugs should be stopped first and the additional drugs stopped in 7 to 10 days to minimize the potential for resistance.[29]

If not previously documented, antibody status for *T. gondii*, hepatitis C, and cytomegalovirus should be obtained. Tuberculin skin testing should be performed if not done within the past year. Prophylaxis and treatment of opportunistic infection in pregnant women is generally the same as for nonpregnant women.[79] Ideally, use of highly active antiretroviral therapy should optimize the immune status so that prophylaxis is not indicated. For more detailed information regarding prophylaxis of opportunistic infections in pregnancy, providers should consult current guidelines at http://aidsinfo.nih.gov/guidelines

HIV-infected pregnant women should receive counseling regarding issues of HIV and pregnancy and should be provided with psychosocial support during pregnancy and the postpartum period. Women can be reassured that pregnancy per se does not appear to have an impact on the progression of HIV infection. Women should be educated regarding signs and symptoms such as rash, nausea, vomiting, extreme fatigue, and muscle aches that may indicate toxicity related to antiretroviral drugs. The risks of perinatal transmission of HIV and the evaluation of the infant for infection should be discussed. The need for careful adherence to therapy to maximize response and minimize the development of resistance should be emphasized.

In addition to use of antiretroviral therapy to lower HIV RNA levels and reduce transmission, performance of cesarean delivery before the onset of labor and membrane rupture has been shown to reduce transmission among women on no antiretrovirals or on zidovudine.[84,85] In a meta-analysis of data from 15 cohorts, the AOR for transmission was 0.43 (95% CI 0.33–0.56) for those with cesarean delivery before labor or membrane rupture compared with those with other modes of delivery.[84] A similar benefit was seen among the subset receiving zidovudine. In a randomized trial of planned cesarean section compared with vaginal delivery, transmission occurred in 1.8% of infants assigned to planned cesarean group and 10.5% of 200 who delivered vaginally ($P <$ .001).[85] A similar magnitude in reduction of transmission was seen among the subset receiving zidovudine, although small numbers did not reach statistical significance. Given transmission rates of less than 2% among women receiving highly active antiretroviral therapy or with HIV RNA below 1000 copies/mL receiving zidovudine, it is difficult to assess for any additional benefit of planned cesarean delivery. In the most recent data, the rate of transmission among women on HAART was 0.7% among 2286 women with planned cesarean delivery and 0.7% among 559 women with planned vaginal delivery.[63] Currently, cesarean delivery before labor or membrane rupture is recommended for women with HIV RNA levels above 1000 copies/mL in the third trimester.[86] Women with HIV RNA levels below 1000 copies/mL should have the option of planned cesarean delivery discussed with them, along with the lack of clear data regarding benefit in this setting. All HIV-infected pregnant women should be informed of the increased risks, primarily infectious, associated with cesarean compared with vaginal delivery. Despite early case-control studies suggesting increased rates of morbidity among HIV-infected compared with uninfected women undergoing cesarean delivery, more recent cohort studies suggest that the increased risk is similar in magnitude to that observed in similar HIV-uninfected women.[29,87] Cesarean delivery may be scheduled at 38 weeks' gestation without amniocentesis, rather than the usually recommended 39 weeks, to minimize the risk of labor or membrane rupture, although this increases the risk of respiratory distress in the newborn.[88] To minimize risks of perioperative infection, genital infections such as bacterial vaginosis should be treated, and the use of antibiotic prophylaxis should be considered, although these interventions have not been specifically evaluated in HIV-infected women. Scheduled cesarean delivery also appears to confer a reduced risk of hepatitis C transmission to the infant among HIV-infected women with detectable hepatitis C viremia.[89]

HIV-infected women should undergo baseline testing of renal and hepatic function. The schedule of testing for drug toxicity will vary with drugs chosen. In general, visits for assessment for any new symptoms and laboratory testing should occur about every 2 to 4 weeks during the first 1 to 2 months of therapy. An optimal schedule of testing for early diagnosis of such complications as hepatic toxicity or lactic acidosis has not been established, but clinicians should consider evaluating hepatic function and electrolytes monthly in the third trimester and certainly in the presence of any new symptoms. Accurate blood lactate levels are difficult to obtain, and normal values in pregnancy have not been established. Routine testing of lactate levels is not recommended, but may be helpful during pregnancy if values are elevated above nonpregnant adult levels in the presence of suggestive symptoms. CD4+ lymphocyte counts should be done every 3 months during pregnancy. HIV RNA levels should be monitored as per guidelines in nonpregnant adults (i.e., every 4 wk after initiating or changing therapy until undetectable, then every 3 mo on stable therapy).[28] A drop of at least one log on HIV RNA levels should be seen after 4 to 8 weeks of therapy.

PI therapy has been associated with an increased risk of glucose intolerance and diabetes in nonpregnant adults.[90] Most studies in pregnancy have not found differences in gestational diabetes, glucose intolerance, and insulin resistance among HIV-infected women on PIs compared with other regimens, although rates of glucose intolerance were high in both groups related to other risk factors such as obesity and ethnicity.[91,92] Clinicians may consider early 50-g glucose load testing in pregnant women on PI therapy with repeat testing at 24 to 28 weeks of gestation if earlier testing is normal.

Clinicians caring for HIV-infected pregnant women on methadone should be aware of potential drug interactions when initiating or changing therapy. Nevirapine, efavirenz, and PIs other than indinavir may decrease methadone levels and precipitate drug withdrawal so pregnant women should be monitored for symptoms in this setting.[28]

Counseling regarding options for prenatal diagnosis is complicated by HIV infection. Amniocentesis and other invasive procedures such as scalp electrode placement increased the risk of transmission by two- to fourfold in early studies among women not receiving antiretrovirals.[93,94] In more recent cohort studies among women receiving antiretroviral therapy, invasive testing has not been identified as a risk factor for transmission, but amniocentesis is uncommon and chorionic villus sampling is rare among HIV-infected women. Thus, specific risk figures are not available to use in counseling. Further complicating the discussion is the recent suggestion that median serum human chorionic gonadotropin and α-fetoprotein values may be higher among HIV-infected women and elevations may correlate with increasing disease severity, although more recent, larger studies have not found clinically relevant differences in levels.[95–97] If an invasive prenatal diagnostic procedure is planned for an HIV-infected woman, she should be on optimal antiretroviral therapy with an undetectable HIV RNA level beforehand to minimize the risk of transmission.

Labor and Delivery

Ideally, the decision regarding mode of delivery should be made after discussions throughout pregnancy, based on HIV RNA results obtained at 34 to 36 weeks' gestation. If the decision is made to attempt vaginal delivery, zidovudine infusion at a dose of 2 mg/kg of body weight over 1 hour, followed by a continuous infusion of 1 mg/kg/hr should be given until delivery.[39] Other antiretroviral drugs should be continued as scheduled during labor, except stavudine, which may antagonize zidovudine and should be discontinued when zidovudine infusion is begun. If the woman is unable to tolerate zidovudine, then stavudine may be continued during labor. During labor, artificial rupture of membranes should be avoided if possible, and labor should be augmented as needed to minimize the duration of ruptured membranes. Fetal scalp electrodes, scalp blood sampling, and instrumented delivery should be avoided to limit fetal exposure to maternal blood. Infants should be washed before undergoing blood draws, injections, or other procedures.

If cesarean delivery is planned, it should be scheduled at or after 38 weeks' gestation.[86] Infusion of intravenous zidovudine as described earlier should be begun at least 3 hours before surgery and continued until cord clamping. Other medications should be continued as scheduled. For women who had planned on a scheduled cesarean delivery presenting with ruptured membranes, management must be individualized based on HIV RNA levels, time since rupture, stage of labor, and patient preference. The benefit of cesarean delivery shortly after rupture of membranes or onset of labor is unclear. Among women not receiving antiretrovirals or receiving zidovudine monotherapy, transmission rates increase with increasing duration of rupture before delivery.[98,99] However, in most studies, transmission rates were similar among women delivering vaginally and those delivering by cesarean after labor or rupture. Women with a short duration of ruptured membranes and an unripe cervix in whom a prolonged labor is anticipated may benefit from urgent cesarean delivery, and those progressing rapidly in labor may be less likely to benefit. In the setting of ruptured membranes without labor before 34 weeks' gestation, expectant management with continuing antiretroviral therapy, potentially including intravenous zidovudine, should be offered to attempt to prolong gestation and reduce complications of prematurity.[100] HIV-infected women with preterm labor should be treated the same as HIV-negative women, with a decision regarding delivery mode based on obstetric considerations and recent HIV RNA levels once delivery is deemed to be inevitable.

For HIV-infected women presenting or diagnosed in labor or postpartum without antiretroviral therapy during pregnancy, several options are available. Observational data from Wade and associates[12] demonstrated transmission rates of 6.1% with zidovudine begun prenatally and continued intrapartum and to the neonate for 6 weeks, 10.0% given intrapartum and to the neonate for 6 weeks, 9.3% when started within 48 hours of birth and continued for 6 weeks, 18.4% when started after 48 hours, and 26.6% with no zidovudine for mother or infant. Subsequent studies have demonstrated transmission rates at 14 to 16 weeks of 13.1% with a single dose of 200 mg nevirapine to mother and 2 mg/kg to the infant compared with 25.1% with oral zidovudine during labor and for 1 week for the infant,[11] a rate at 6 weeks of 10.8% with oral zidovudine/lamivudine in labor and for 1 week in mother and infant compared with 17.2% for placebo,[13] and a rate at 8 weeks of 13.3% with the maternal/infant nevirapine regimen compared with 10.9% for zidovudine/lamivudine orally in labor and for 1 week in the infant.[14] The latter three trials were done in predominantly breastfeeding populations. Thus, any of these three regimens (intravenous zidovudine in labor and oral for the infant for 6 wk; the maternal/infant nevirapine dosing; or oral zidovudine/lamivudine in labor and for 1 wk in the infant) could be used for women presenting in labor without therapy during pregnancy. Some clinicians would choose to use a combination of zidovudine and nevirapine in this setting, although a trial comparing this regimen has not been studied specifically. If single-dose nevirapine is used in the mother, 1 week of dual nucleoside therapy, usually zidovudine/lamivudine, should be provided for the mother to minimize the risk of nevirapine resistance mutations developing with the prolonged nevirapine levels occurring after dosing.[101,102] One trial has compared neonatal therapy–only regimens, finding that single-dose nevirapine compared with oral zidovudine for 6 weeks in the infant had similar transmission rates overall and in formula-feeding infants, but nevirapine had a significantly lower transmission rate among breastfeeding infants.[103] Some clinicians might choose to add additional drugs to the 6 weeks of infant zidovudine to mimic postexposure prophylaxis recommendations, although formulations and dosing recommendations for neonates are limited.

Postnatal

The postpartum period is a very demanding period for all women, but HIV-infected women have the added stresses of administering medication to the infant and waiting to discern the infant's infection status. Additional psychosocial support is needed during this period. If the woman plans to continue antiretroviral therapy after delivery, measures to enhance adherence are indicated.[28] For women stopping antiretroviral therapy, all drugs should be stopped simultaneously to minimize the development of resistance unless nevirapine or efavirenz are included, in which case the nucleoside agents should be continued for 7 to 10 days after stopping the non-nucleoside reverse transcriptase inhibitor to decrease the risk of resistance development.[29] HIV-infected women should be counseled against breast-feeding because it increases the risk of transmission by 15% to 20%, based on studies of women not receiving antiretrovirals.[52]

Follow-up care for the woman, both reproductive and HIV-specific, and her infant should be ensured before hospital discharge. During prenatal care, women should be counseled regarding contraceptive options. Condom use should be reinforced. Hormonal contraceptives may be used by HIV-infected women, although estradiol levels are reduced by nevirapine, ritonavir, nelfinavir, rifampin, rifabutin, and possibly amprenavir.[27] The impact on contraceptive efficacy of these interactions is unknown, although these changes may increase the risk of irregular bleeding. No significant interactions were found between depomedroxyprogesterone acetate (DMPA) and nucleosides, nevirapine, efavirenz, or nelfinavir, suggesting that DMPA can be used safely among HIV-infected women on antiretroviral therapy.[104] Studies in HIV-infected women suggest that intrauterine contraceptive devices may be used safely by HIV-infected women at low risk of sexually transmitted infections without severe immune compromise.[105]

Infants born to HIV-infected women require HIV-specific as well as routine pediatric care. Infants should receive zidovudine syrup 2 mg/kg of body weight every 6 hours, or equivalent dosing schedule, for 6 weeks after birth.[29] A complete blood count should be obtained from the neonate before starting zidovudine because anemia is the primary side effect of the zidovudine. Use of additional antiretrovirals in the infant may be considered in some situations, such as for an infant born to women not receiving antiretrovirals during pregnancy.[29] Observational data suggest that transmission is reduced with 6 weeks of oral zidovudine in the infant if started within 24 hours of birth, even in the absence of antepartum and intrapartum use.[12] Testing of the infant should be done at 14 to 21 days of age, 1 to 2 months, and 4 to 6 months of age or as soon as any positive result is obtained. Some providers also perform at test shortly after birth.[106] HIV DNA or RNA polymerase chain reaction (PCR) are the preferred methods for infant diagnosis. Infants with two positive HIV virologic tests on separate samples are considered to be HIV-infected. Infants with two or more negative virologic tests, wtih one sample drawn at or after age 14 days and at least one sample at or after 1 month, can be considered to be HIV-uninfected if not exposed through ongoing breast-feeding. Many experts also perform an HIV antibody test at 12 to 18 months to confirm seroreversion among infants with negative PCR testing. Infants should be started on prophylaxis for *Pneumocystis carinii* pneumonia at 4 to 6 weeks of age unless infection has been presumptively excluded with two negative tests by then, with prophylaxis continued until the infant is confirmed to be HIV-uninfected.[106] HIV-infected children should be managed by or in consultation with a specialist in pediatric HIV infection.

The Summary of Management Options Box contains recommendations for appropriate care for HIV-infected pregnant women to maximize maternal health and minimize the risk of perinatal transmission. Although huge advances have been made in management of HIV infection and prevention of transmission in developed countries, the greater challenge is to translate these interventions into practical and sustainable interventions throughout the world. Ultimately, the goal must be to prevent transmission of HIV to avoid the coexistence of HIV infection in pregnancy.

SUMMARY OF MANAGEMENT OPTIONS
Human Immunodeficiency Virus

Management Options	Evidence Quality and Recommendation	References
Prepregnancy		
Counsel regarding HIV prevention and offer testing for HIV to all reproductive-age women.	Ia/A	29
Assess indications for antiretroviral therapy and opportunistic infection prophylaxis with HIV RNA, and CD4+ cell counts. Initiate highly active antiretroviral therapy if CD4+ cell count <500/μL. Avoid regimens containing efavirenz because of teratogenicity concerns.	Ia/A	28,29,79

Management Options	Evidence Quality and Recommendation	References
Recommend against conception until HIV RNA level undetectable and no indication for opportunistic infection prophylaxis (CD4+ cell count >200/mm^3 for >6 mo).	IIa/B	29,79
Complete other routine preconception assessments such as genetic screening, evaluation for other medical conditions.	IIa/B	29
If partner is HIV-negative, discuss methods to avoid unprotected intercourse: male condoms for all intercourse and artificial insemination for conception.	GPP	
Recommend folate supplementation.	Ia/A	29
Prenatal Screening Policy		
Offer opt-out testing for HIV to all pregnant women, rescreen in third trimester in high-prevalence areas and in women with ongoing risk.	—/GPP	—
Prenatal HIV-positive Patients		
Assess immunization status and update as needed for pneumococcus, influenza, hepatitis A and B, tetanus.	Ia/A	79
Assess antibody status to hepatitis C, *Toxoplasma gondii*, and CMV if not previously documented.	IIa/B	79
Perform tuberculin skin test if not done in past year.	Ia/A	79
Counsel regarding risk of transmission, methods to minimize risk (antiretroviral therapy with scheduled cesarean delivery if HIV RNA >1000 copies/mL after 34 wk), lack of impact of pregnancy on maternal disease progression, symptoms of drug toxicity, possible effects of therapy on infant, evaluation of infant after birth for HIV status.	Ia/A	29
Assess indications for antiretroviral therapy and opportunistic infection prophylaxis with HIV RNA level, CD4+ lymphocyte count. For women already on therapy, discuss risks/benefits of continuing or stopping. Modify regimen if first trimester and on efavirenz. If not on therapy, recommend highly active antiretroviral regimen including zidovudine for all women starting after first trimester, regardless of HIV RNA and CD4+ cell count. Provide opportunistic infection prophylaxis according to adult guidelines.	Ia/A	29,79
Monitor HIV RNA levels monthly after changing or initiating therapy. Level should drop by ≥1 log in first 4–8 wk.	II/B	28
Monitor CD4+ lymphocyte counts each trimester.	Ia/B	29
Perform complete blood count, liver enzymes, renal function frequently (every 2–4 wk) on new regimen, monthly in third trimester.	Ia/A	29
Perform HIV resistance testing for women with detectable HIV RNA levels before initiating therapy or if not responding appropriately to therapy or if rebound from undetectable.	II/B	28,82
Perform ultrasound at 18–20 wk' gestation to rule out anomalies and confirm dates	—/GPP	—
Discuss risks versus benefits of scheduled cesarean delivery. Recommend for HIV RNA levels >1000 copies/mL after 34 wk. Schedule at or after 38 wk' gestation if dating criteria adequate. Perform vaginal delivery only if on antiretroviral therapy with undetectable HIV RNA.	Ia/A	29,86

SUMMARY OF MANAGEMENT OPTIONS

Human Immunodeficiency Virus—cont'd

Management Options	Evidence Quality and Recommendation	References
Routine prenatal care. If indicated, discuss unknown risk of transmission with amniocentesis or chorionic villus sampling.	III/B	29
Labor and Delivery		
Start intravenous zidovudine infusion: a. For those choosing vaginal delivery 2 mg/kg over 1 hr followed by 1 mg/kg/hr until delivery with onset of labor. b. Same regimen at least 3 hr before scheduled cesarean delivery.	Ia/A	29,39
Continue other medications orally except stavudine, which may antagonize zidovudine.		
If vaginal delivery, minimize duration of ruptured membranes as much as possible.	II/B	29,98,99
Avoid scalp electrodes, scalp sampling, instrumented delivery.	II/B	93,94
Wash infant before blood draws, injections.		
Postnatal		
Discuss option of stopping or continuing antiretroviral therapy if initiated solely for transmission prophylaxis. Reinforce adherence if continuing therapy.	Ia/A	29
Counsel against breast-feeding.	Ia/A	29
Provide contraception and ensure continued HIV and reproductive health care. If partner is HIV-negative, advise male condom to avoid unprotected intercourse.	Ia/A	29
Provide psychosocial support as infant infection status assessed.	Ia/A	29
Ensure routine and HIV-specific care for infant including zidovudine 2 mg/kg every 6 hr or equivalent until 6 wk of age, HIV DNA PCR testing, initiation of prophylaxis against *Pneumocystis carinii* pneumonia beginning at 4–6 wk of age unless infant presumptively HIV-infected based on serial testing.	Ia/A	106

CMV, cytomegalovirus; GPP, good practice point; PCR, polymerase chain reaction.

SUGGESTED READINGS

The Antiretroviral Pregnancy Registry: Interim Report. 1/1/89–7/31/08; issued December 2008. Available at www.APRegistry.com

Centers for Disease Control and Prevention: Achievements in public health: Reduction in perinatal transmission of HIV infection, United States, 1985–2005. MMWR Morb Mortal Wkly Rep 2006;55:592–597.

Centers for Disease Control and Prevention: Rapid HIV antibody testing during labor and delivery for women of unknown HIV status: A practical guide and model protocol. January 30, 2004. Available at http://www.cdc.gov/hiv/topics/testing/resources/guidelines/pdf/Labor&DeliveryRapidTesting.pdf

Centers for Disease Control and Prevention: Revised recommendations for HIV testing of adults, adolescents, and pregnant women in health care settings. MMWR Morb Mortal Wkly Rep 2006;55(RR-14):1–17.

Kourtis AP, Schmid CH, Jamieson DJ, Lau J: Use of antiretroviral therapy in pregnant HIV-infected women and the risk of premature delivery: A meta-analysis. AIDS 2007;21:607–615.

Panel on Antiretroviral Guidelines for Adults and Adolescents: Guidelines for the Use of Antiretroviral agents in HIV-1–infected Adults and

Adolescents. Washington, DC, Department of Health and Human Services. November 3, 2008, pp 1–139. Available at http://www.aidsinfo.nih.gov/ContentFiles/AdultandAdolescentGL.pdf (accessed February 19, 2009).

Public Health Service Task Force Recommendations for Use of Antiretroviral Drugs in Pregnant HIV-1–infected Women for Maternal Health and Interventions to Reduce Perinatal HIV-1–Transmission in the United States. July 8, 2008. Available at http://aidsinfo.nih.gov/guidelines/ (accessed February 19, 2008).

Townsend CL, Cortina-Borja M, Peckham CS, et al: Low rates of mother-to-child transmission of HIV following effective pregnancy interventions in the United Kingdom and Ireland, 2000–2006. AIDS 2008;22:973–981.

USPHS/IDSA Guidelines for the Prevention and Treatment of Opportunistic Infection in HIV-infected Adults and Adolescents. June 18, 2008. Available at http://aidsinfo.nih.gov/guidelines/

Working Group on Antiretroviral Therapy and Medical Management of HIV-infected Children: Guidelines for the Use of Antiretroviral Agents in Pediatric HIV Infection. February 23, 2009, pp 1–139. Available at http://aidsinfo.nih.gov/ContentFiles/PediatricGuidelines.pdf

REFERENCES

For a complete list of references, log onto www.expertconsult.com.

CHAPTER 29

Rubella, Measles, Mumps, Varicella, and Parvovirus

LAURA E. RILEY

Videos corresponding to this chapter are available online at www.expertconsult.com.

RUBELLA

Maternal and Fetal Risks

Rubella (German measles or third disease) is an exanthematous disease caused by a single-stranded RNA virus of the togavirus family.[1] Like rubeola, rubella is acquired via respiratory droplet exposure. After a 2- to 3-week incubation period, symptomatic patients develop a rash that spreads from the face to the trunk and extremities, lasting about 3 days. Fever, arthralgias, and postauricular, posterior cervical, and suboccipital lymphadenopathy are characteristic. Severe complications such as encephalitis, bleeding diathesis, and arthritis are rare. Overt clinical symptoms occur in only 50% to 75% of rubella-infected patients, and thus, clinical history is not a useful marker of prior illness.[2]

Rubella infection is usually a mild illness in both adults and children. However, fetal infection may be devastating. Congenital rubella syndrome (CRS) may produce transient abnormalities, including purpura, splenomegaly, jaundice, meningoencephalitis, and thrombocytopenia, or permanent anomalies such as cataracts, glaucoma, heart disease, deafness, microcephaly, and mental retardation. Long-term sequelae might include diabetes, thyroid abnormalities, precocious puberty, and progressive rubella panencephalitis.[2,3] Defects involving virtually every organ have been reported (Table 29–1).[4] A 50-year follow-up of 40 survivors of CRS born between 1939 and 1943 revealed that all had hearing impairment; 23 had eye defects related to the rubella.[5]

The results of one large survey of maternal rubella infection in pregnancy are summarized in Table 29–2.[6] The rate of fetal infection is highest at 11 weeks and greater than 36 weeks. However, the overall rate of congenital defects is greatest in the first trimester (90%) and declines steadily in the second and third trimesters.

Rubella vaccine became available in the United States in 1969. Vaccination given as a trivalent preparation of measles, mumps, and rubella (MMR) vaccine produces long-term immunity in 95% of vaccinees. The rates of rubella dropped precipitously after introduction of the vaccine. Ten years later, the annual incidence of rubella infections, including CRS, had decreased by 99.6%.[7] However, in the 1990s, there were several outbreaks in groups of adults with unknown vaccination status living in close quarters.[8] The largest outbreak in the United States occurred in Nebraska in 1999 and involved 125 cases; 87% of these patients were born in Latin America.[9] In this outbreak, 7 pregnant women were infected and 1 child was born with CRS. Almost half of these women had prior births in the United States and had missed prior vaccination opportunities. Since then, the number of CRS cases has steadily declined in part due to rubella immunization campaigns in Latin America and Mexico.[10,11]

Diagnosis

The clinical diagnosis of rubella infection is difficult. Most infections are subclinical, and the rash is nonspecific. Serologic testing is the primary mode of diagnosis using enzyme-linked immunoassay (ELISA). In a woman with exposure or suspected illness, seroconversion demonstrated by paired acute and convalescent specimens is indicative of acute infection. Acute infection may also be diagnosed by isolation of virus from the blood, nasopharynx, urine, or cerebrospinal fluid. Serologic testing for immunity is based on the assumption that rubella-specific antibodies of the immunoglobulin G (IgG) class are present for life after natural infection or vaccination.

Management Options

Prepregnancy

Vaccination of all children and susceptible adults will help prevent outbreaks of rubella. All children should receive a single dose of live attenuated rubella vaccine at 12 to 15 months of age in a trivalent preparation of MMR strains. The second dose of MMR may be administered at least 1 month after the first dose but before 6 years of age. Susceptible young women should be vaccinated and refrain from pregnancy for 1 month following vaccination.[12] Evidence of immunity is required of health care workers and women of childbearing age.[13] Studies on a MMR-vaccinated cohort followed for 20 years shows that rubella antibodies remain elevated for at least that long in many individuals.[14] However, individuals with low levels of antibody after vaccination may be susceptible to viremia and clinical infection.[15] CRS after previous maternal rubella vaccination has been rarely reported.[16]

The rubella vaccine is a live virus preparation, which may cross the placenta; thus, it should not be administered to

TABLE 29–1

Abnormalities in Congenital Rubella: Triad of Gregg

ABNORMALITY	DESCRIPTION
Eye	
Cataract	Usually bilateral and present at birth.
Retinopathy	"Salt and pepper" appearance, may have a delayed onset, frequently bilateral, visual acuity is not affected.
Microphthalmia	Often associated with cataract.
Glaucoma	Rare but leads to blindness if not recognized.
Heart	
Patent ductus arteriosus	Common, often associated with persistence of the foramen ovale.
Pulmonary valvular stenosis	Common, due to intimal proliferation and arterial elastic hypertrophy.
Pulmonary artery stenosis	
Coarctation of the aorta	Infrequent.
Ventricular septal defects	Rare.
Atrial septal defects	Rare.
Ear	
Commonly damaged	Injury of cells of the middle ear leading to sensorineural deafness may also have a central origin.
Bilateral and progressive	May be present at birth or develop later in childhood. Severe enough for the child to need education at a special school; rare when maternal rubella occurs after the fourth mo of pregnancy.

Adapted from Freij BJ, South MA, Sever JL, et al: Maternal rubella and the congenital rubella syndrome. Clin Perinatol 1988;15:247–257.

pregnant women. However, the Centers for Disease Control and Prevention (CDC) have monitored inadvertent rubella vaccination during pregnancy, collecting over 500 cases. No case of CRS due to vaccination was documented, although virus was isolated from the conceptus in several cases.[17] Thus, patients inadvertently vaccinated during pregnancy, or becoming pregnant shortly after vaccination, should be reassured and counseled that the risk of fetal infection is negligible.[18,19] Furthermore, follow-up studies on fetuses inadvertently exposed to rubella vaccine RA27/3 in pregnancy in Costa Rica did not have increased rates of miscarriage or stillbirth.[20]

Prenatal

A pregnant woman infected with rubella is at little risk. However, depending on the gestational age at infection, the fetus may be at great risk for congenital anomalies. Methods for in utero diagnosis include fetal blood sampling measurement of rubella-specific IgM,[21] rubella-specific reverse transcriptase polymerase chain reaction (RT-PCR), and virus isolation from amniotic fluid or products of conception.[22,23] RT-PCR can detect the presence of viral RNA even when the fetal rubella virus–specific IgM obtained by fetal blood sampling is negative.[24] Although these tests may indicate fetal infection, the counseling is largely based on the gestational age–related risk of congenital abnormalities due to CRS. No treatment other than pregnancy termination is available.

Treatment for acute maternal rubella is generally symptomatic. Rarely, patients who develop thrombocytopenia or encephalitis may benefit from glucocorticoids or platelet transfusion. Immunoglobulin for pregnant women with acute infection is controversial. Furthermore, no data suggest that immunoglobulin will prevent fetal anomalies.

Labor, Delivery, and Postnatal

Acute infection during these time periods is unlikely. If suspected, appropriate infection control measures should be instituted. The neonate should be evaluated for infection following birth.

TABLE 29–2

Fetal Consequences of Symptomatic Maternal Rubella during Pregnancy

	INFECTION		DEFECTS		
STAGE OF PREGNANCY (WK)	NO. TESTED	NO. POSITIVE	NO. FOLLOWED	RATE (%)	OVERALL RISK OF DEFECT (RATE OF INFECTION × RATE OF DEFECTS) (%)
<11	10	9 (90%)	9	100	90
11-12	6	4 (67%)	4	50	33
13-14	18	12 (67%)	12	17	11
15-16	36	17 (47%)	14	50	24
17-18	33	13 (39%)	10	0	0
19-22	59	20 (34%)			
23-26	32	8 (25%)			
27-30	31	11 (35%)			
31-36	25	15 (60%)	53	0	0
>36	8	8 (100%)			
Total	258	117 (45%)	102	20	9

From Miller E, Cradock-Watson JE, Pollock TM: Consequences of confirmed maternal rubella at successive stages of pregnancy. Lancet 1982;2:781–784.

SUMMARY OF MANAGEMENT OPTIONS
Rubella

Management Options	Evidence Quality and Recommendation	References
Prepregnancy		
Prevent by childhood vaccination.	III/B	13
Vaccination programs for girls in their early teens contribute to prevention.	III/B	13
Serologic evaluation and, if negative, vaccination of woman inquiring about status.	III/B	13
Prenatal		
Routine check of rubella immunity status at first visit for all women is standard practice in many centers.	III/B	13,19
Accidental vaccination in early pregnancy is not an indication for termination.	IIa/B	13,16–20
If suspected exposure in woman with immunity:	—/GPP	—
• Confirm presence of rubella-specific IgG (if immediately after exposure).		
• Confirm failure of appearance of IgM (acute phase) antibodies with two serum samples 2–3 wk apart.		
• Reassure patient.		
If suspected exposure in susceptible woman:		
• Establish validity of diagnosis serologically in index case if possible.	III/B	13
• Check for appearance of IgM (acute-phase) antibodies.	III/B	13
• If there is no serologic evidence of infection, reassure patient.	—/GPP	—
If maternal infection is confirmed serologically, options will depend on gestation at time of infection:		
• In early pregnancy, termination should be discussed; it may be performed immediately or only after confirmation by invasive procedure.	IIb/B	5,6
• In late pregnancy, confirmation of fetal infection by invasive procedure can be considered; fetal growth and health should be monitored if infection is suspected or confirmed.	—/GPP	—
Labor, Delivery, and Postnatal		
If fetal infection is suspected, cord blood should be sent for serologic confirmation.	III/C	13
If fetal infection is confirmed, careful pediatric assessment and follow-up are needed.	—/GPP	—

GPP, good practice point; Ig, immunoglobulin.

RUBEOLA

Maternal and Fetal Risks

Rubeola (red measles or first disease), caused by a paramyxovirus, is highly infectious and commonly attacks children. The illness is spread by respiratory droplet and may include high fever, rash, cough and rhinorrhea, conjunctivitis, and the pathognomonic Koplik spots on the oral buccal epithelium. The incubation period is generally 10 to 14 days. The infection is usually self-limited in children.[25] Rarely, the disease might be severe and might be complicated by bronchopneumonia, hepatitis, otitis media, diarrhea, or death.[13,26] Encephalitis occurs in 1 of every 1000 reported cases and may lead to permanent brain damage and mental retardation. Death, usually due to pneumonia or encephalitis, is reported to occur in 1 to 2 per 1000 cases in the United States. The fatality rate is greater in infants, young children, and adults. In addition, subacute sclerosing panencephalitis, an extremely rare degenerative disease of the central nervous system, is caused by this virus presenting years after the initial measles infection.

The number of cases of measles in the United States and other industrialized countries has decreased markedly since the introduction of an effective vaccine in 1963.[13,27] Still, in 1990, there were 55,000 cases and 120 measles-related deaths. This resurgence was largely due to an increase in unvaccinated preschool children, particularly in urban areas.[27,28] Although data from the National Health and Nutrition Examination Survey show that the overall seroprevalence of measles IgG antibody was 95.9% between 1999 and 2004, outbreaks continue to occur.[29,30]

Some report that measles during pregnancy is not associated with increased maternal or fetal death rates.[31] Others find higher rates of measles-related hospitalization, pneumonia, and death for infected pregnant women.[32] Placental damage from the infection has been implicated in stillbirths.[33] Furthermore, measles infection of mothers in developing countries is associated with an increase in the perinatal mortality rate.[34] As with any febrile illness, measles infection may precipitate premature uterine activity and lead to premature delivery.[35]

No specific syndrome is attributed to intrauterine measles infection. However, the newborn delivered to a woman with active disease is at high risk for severe neonatal measles. Pneumonia is the primary cause of death and is more common in the premature newborn. Some reports suggest an association between in utero measles infection and postnatal development of Crohn's disease.[36] This potential relationship has yet to be confirmed and does not warrant prenatal diagnosis in the fetus.

Diagnosis

The clinical diagnosis of rubeola is based on the presence of a maculopapular rash occurring 1 to 2 days after a specific exanthematous rash (Koplik's spots), photophobia, and upper respiratory symptoms. Serologic tests can provide a definitive diagnosis. In addition, a diagnosis can also be confirmed by isolating the virus or using RT-PCR from serum or throat swabs.[37]

Management Options

Prepregnancy

Prevention is the best available mechanism to protect against measles. All children should receive one dose of the live measles virus vaccine as part of MMR between 12 and 15 months of age, followed by a second dose at age 6. Vaccination results in long-lasting immunity in over 95% of recipients.

Likewise, immunity to natural infection is lifelong, and the high infectivity of the virus during childhood leaves few susceptible adults. Women contemplating pregnancy with a negative or questionable history of measles illness or vaccination or laboratory evidence of susceptibility should receive the live attenuated virus vaccine followed by a second dose not less than 1 month later. Women vaccinated before 1967 (and likely to have received a heat-killed viral vaccine), or who were vaccinated before 1 year of age, or those with equivocal serology should also receive two doses of vaccine.[13] Pregnancy should be delayed 1 month after receiving MMR vaccine.

Prenatal

The upper respiratory symptoms of acute measles can be ameliorated with cough suppressants. Fever, especially if high, should be treated aggressively with antipyretics. Measles pneumonia may require respiratory support, and if superimposed bacterial pneumonia develops, antibiotic therapy is required. Even when there is no life-threatening disease, pregnant women should be closely monitored during the acute illness for evidence of uterine activity.

Although pregnant women are not candidates for vaccination with any live virus vaccine, accidental vaccination with rubeola vaccine is not a cause for alarm or an indication for pregnancy termination. Immune serum globulin (ISG) may be given to susceptible pregnant women exposed to rubeola in an attempt to prevent or modify the clinical expression of the disease. The intramuscular preparation (0.25 mL/kg, maximum 15 mL) should be given within 6 days of exposure.[13]

Labor, Delivery, and Postnatal

There are no specific management recommendations for these intervals because acute disease is unlikely. Clinicians, however, should be aware of appropriate isolation precautions instituted for rubeola in the hospital. Observation of the neonate for infection is mandatory.

SUMMARY OF MANAGEMENT OPTIONS

Measles (Rubeola)

Management Options	Evidence Quality and Recommendation	References
Prepregnancy		
Prevent by childhood vaccination.	III/B	13
Serologic evaluation and, if negative, vaccination of woman inquiring about status.	III/B	13

Management Options	Evidence Quality and Recommendation	References
Prenatal		
Treat acute infection symptomatically.	—/GPP	—
Antibiotics are given if secondary bacterial infection is suspected.	—/GPP	—
Immunoglobulin should be considered for the susceptible woman exposed to the infection.	III/B	13
Inadvertent vaccination is not an indication for termination.	III/B	13
Labor, Delivery, and Postnatal		
Appropriate isolation precautions must be taken when in hospital.	—/GPP	—

GPP, good practice point.

MUMPS

Maternal and Fetal Risks

Mumps is a contagious acute viral illness caused by a paramyxovirus, primarily infecting children and young adults. Human beings are the only recognized natural host for this pathogen. The classic presenting symptom for mumps is either unilateral or bilateral parotitis, which usually develops 14 to 18 days after exposure. Respiratory droplets typically transmit the virus. Prodromal symptoms include fever, chills, malaise, and myalgias. The disease can also remain asymptomatic in 20% of cases. Persons are considered infectious from 2 days before the onset of symptoms to approximately 9 days after the parotitis is noted.

Although generally a self-limited disease with symptoms resolving within 5 to 7 days, mumps can result in significant complications, particularly in the adult population. Orchitis occurs in up to 38% of cases in postpuberal males and may lead to infertility.[13] Conversely, mastitis and oophoritis have been reported in women, but infertility is rare.[38] Other complications include aseptic meningitis, pancreatitis, and thyroiditis. Mumps meningoencephalitis can cause permanent sequelae such as sensorineural hearing loss, seizures, nerve palsies, and hydrocephalus.[13]

There are limited data on mumps in pregnancy. In a cohort study of measles, mumps, and rubella, Siegel[39] reported an increased incidence of first-trimester pregnancy loss with acute mumps infection. No data suggest mumps specifically increases the incidence of stillbirths or preterm deliveries. Early studies suggested an association between endocardial fibroelastosis and mumps virus antigen; however, a clear relationship of mumps to this or other congenital malformations has not been confirmed.[40]

The number of reported cases of mumps in the United States has decreased dramatically since the broad institution of effective vaccination. In 1968, over 180,000 cases of mumps were reported in the United States compared with 266 cases reported in 2001.[41] Most cases occurred in persons younger than 20 years. Although the presumption was that these outbreaks were due to failure to vaccinate, surveillance data suggested that there may be a waning of vaccine-induced immunity over time, allowing for susceptibility to wild virus infection.[42] Hence, current recommendations, which were enacted in 1989, include a second dose of MMR vaccine given at age 6 years. This practice has resulted in a further decline in mumps infection.[43] A remaining concern is that only 38% of countries worldwide use routine mumps vaccination. Still, outbreaks occur intermittently such as the outbreak in Iowa among 605 18- to 25-year-olds in which the source is unknown but the G genotype of mumps was isolated. The latter is the same strain found in a large outbreak (>70,000 cases over 3 yr) in the United Kingdom.[44] The importation of mumps into previously protected communities has become increasingly recognized.

Diagnosis

The diagnosis of mumps is usually suspected based on presenting features of the disease in the appropriate clinical setting. Although the virus can be isolated in culture or by RT-PCR detection from a clinical specimen (saliva, cerebrospinal fluid, urine, or other infected organ system), the diagnosis is more typically established by serologic techniques. Enzyme immunoassay (EIA) is the most widely used methodology and is more sensitive than complement fixation or hemagglutination inhibition. Both IgM and IgG antibody testing is available. A positive mumps-specific IgM result from a reliable laboratory or a significant rise between acute and convalescent titers of IgG antibody helps establish the diagnosis of acute infection. After acute infection, it is presumed that one has lifelong immunity and persistent IgG titers.

Management Options

Prepregnancy

Two doses of mumps vaccine in combination with measles and rubella (MMR) are routinely recommended for children in the United States. Therefore, adequate protection against infection should be established prior to a woman reaching her reproductive years. There are no current routine recommendations to test for mumps immunity prior to conception. However, if there is reasonable concern that prior vaccination is not adequate, IgG testing can be obtained. If susceptible, a dose of MMR vaccine should be administered at least 1 month prior to attempting pregnancy.[45]

Prenatal

Because the mumps component in MMR is a live attenuated virus, the vaccine is contraindicated in pregnancy. Because no data indicate that mumps vaccination is associated with congenital malformations or other specific adverse outcomes, the inadvertent administration of the vaccine during pregnancy is not an indication for pregnancy termination.

During pregnancy, if exposure to an infected individual is reported, immediate testing for IgG antibody will in most cases confirm immunity and can be used to reassure the patient. In those individuals who lack proven immunity, postexposure immunoglobulin has not been shown to be beneficial as a prophylactic agent. Careful surveillance and symptomatic care should be instituted. Appropriate infection control procedures should be undertaken. These procedures can be rapidly procured from hospital infection control authorities and via the CDC website.

Labor, Delivery, and Postpartum

There are no specific recommendations for these periods of time because an acute outbreak is unlikely to occur. However, in suspected cases in the laboring gravida, the previously mentioned infection control measures should be started as the diagnostic workup is begun. The neonate should be carefully observed for early signs of infection manifested by parotitis or aseptic meningitis. Pediatric infectious disease consultation should be sought.

SUMMARY OF MANAGEMENT OPTIONS

Mumps

Management Options	Evidence Quality and Recommendation	References
Prepregnancy		
Prevent by childhood vaccination.	III/B	13
Prenatal		
Accidental vaccination is not an indication for termination.	III/B	13
If suspected exposure in woman with "immunity," confirm presence of mumps-specific IgG.	III/B	13
Labor, Delivery, and Postnatal		
Observe neonate for parotitis or aseptic meningitis.	—/GPP	—

GPP, good practice point; IgG, immunoglobulin G.

VARICELLA

Maternal and Fetal Risks

Varicella-zoster virus (VZV) is a member of the herpesvirus family and is the causative agent of varicella (chickenpox) and herpes zoster (shingles). Varicella is generally a mild, self-limited illness in healthy children. It is transmitted by infected secretions from the nasopharynx, by direct contact with vesicular fluids, or by airborne spread of the virus. This is followed by viral replication in regional lymph nodes and the tonsils. Viral replication continues for approximately 4 to 6 days. Primary viremia develops and virus spreads to internal organs. When the virus replicates again and is released into the bloodstream, it invades the skin, resulting in the classic viral exanthem by 14 days. Therefore, patients are infectious 1 to 2 days prior to developing this rash.

The incubation period of chickenpox is 10 to 12 days. Many patients have a prodrome of fever, malaise, or myalgia a few days prior to the rash, which is vesicular and erupts in crops over the trunk, face, oropharynx, and scalp. Several crops erupt every 2 to 3 days and last 6 to 10 days. Complications are rare but may include bacterial superinfection of vesicles, pneumonia, arthritis, glomerulonephritis, myocarditis, ocular disease, adrenal insufficiency, and central nervous system abnormalities.[46]

Retrospective studies suggest that varicella pneumonia in pregnant women is more severe than in nonpregnant adults.[47] In a case-control study, smoking and the occurrence of 100 or more skin lesions were risk factors for developing pneumonia.[48] A pregnant woman with varicella and cough, dyspnea, fever, or tachypnea warrants immediate attention. Pneumonia generally develops within a week of the rash and may rapidly progress to hypoxia and respiratory failure. The mortality rate in untreated varicella pneumonia in pregnancy exceeds 40%.[49] If treated aggressively with intravenous acyclovir and supportive measures, reported mortality rates are less than 15%, but patients may still require intubation and ventilatory support.[50]

Congenital varicella syndrome (CVS) is characterized by dermatomal scarring; ocular abnormalities such as cataracts, chorioretinitis, and microphthalmia; low birth weight; cortical atrophy; and mental retardation (Table 29–3). Most cases occur in infants whose mothers were infected between 8 and 20 weeks' gestation. However, the number of cases is low. Data compiled from multiple retrospective cohort studies have determined the rate of embryopathy is approximately 2%.[51–54] In fact, in a prospective study of 347 varicella-infected mothers, the incidence of CVS was 3 per 231 births (1.3%; 95% confidence interval [CI] 0.3–0.7) where follow-up was complete.[55] In a study of babies who were

TABLE 29–3

Fetal Abnormalities Associated with Congenital (Intrauterine) Varicella Infection

Cutaneous scarring
Limb hypoplasia
Missing/hypoplastic digits
Limb paralysis/muscle atrophy
Psychomotor retardation
Convulsions
Microcephaly
Cerebral cortical atrophy
Chorioretinitis
Cataracts
Chorioretinal scarring
Optic disk hypoplasia
Horner syndrome
Early childhood zoster

exposed in utero to primary varicella and did not develop CVS, there appeared to be no differences in neurobehavioral outcomes when compared with uninfected controls.[56]

Neonatal varicella generally occurs in neonates born to mothers who are infected with varicella within 2 weeks of delivery.[57] It is a serious illness characterized by fever and vesicular rash, which resolves, but in some cases, disseminated disease or visceral involvement may ensue. In the latter, the mortality rate may be as high as 25%.

Herpes zoster or shingles, which arises from reactivated VZV, which had been dormant in the dorsal root ganglia, does not lead to CVS.

Diagnosis

Varicella is usually diagnosed clinically based on the characteristic exanthem. Culture of the vesicular fluid is a lengthy process. Serologic tests are useful to document immunity (when IgG is present) in a patient immediately following exposure. IgM antibody specific to VZV may be identified as soon as 3 days after the onset of symptoms in an acutely infected gravida. IgG seroconversion can be seen by 7 days after VZV symptom onset. Paired sample analysis for IgG may be useful to establish the diagnosis of primary infection.

Prenatal diagnosis of varicella is possible. Ultrasonography may detect limb abnormalities, and fetal blood or amniotic fluid may be tested for VZV antibody or DNA.[58,59] However, despite detection of virus, the presence of embryopathy cannot be predicted.

Management Options

Prepregnancy

Varivax, a live attenuated varicella vaccine, is recommended for susceptible children under age 13 and susceptible adults.[60] The vaccine is given in two doses 4 to 8 weeks apart, and approximately 82% of adults will seroconvert. Women should avoid pregnancy for at least 1 month after vaccination. Results from a voluntary registry of Varivax administered in early pregnancy gathered between 1995 and 2005 revealed no cases of CVS among 131 live births.[61] Thus, inadvertent Varivax exposure should not prompt medical recommendations for pregnancy termination.

Pregnancy

Varicella zoster immunoglobulin should be administered to pregnant women who are susceptible to VZV and are exposed to varicella or herpes zoster. The only product currently available is VariZIG, an investigational varicella immune globulin product that may be obtained under expanded access following patient consent.[62] VariZIG should be administered with 48 hours of exposure but may be effective up to 96 hours. Although it diminishes the severity of maternal disease, there is no evidence that VariZIG prevents congenital varicella.

If a pregnant woman becomes infected with chickenpox, she may be offered oral acyclovir to decrease the number of febrile days and shorten the duration of active lesions.[63] As previously noted, parenteral antiviral therapy is indicated in cases of varicella complicated by pneumonia or central nervous system involvement.

Labor, Delivery, and Postnatal

There are no specific management recommendations for labor. Infected pregnant women should be placed in a negative-pressure room for labor, delivery, and the postpartum period in accordance with infection control protocols. Neonates should be given VariZIG after birth and monitored closely because the neonate at greatest risk for chickenpox is born within 4 days prior to or 2 days after maternal chickenpox.[62] A small study of 24 prenatally infected newborns suggests that VariZIG in conjunction with intravenous acyclovir is a more effective prevention strategy than VariZIG alone.[64]

SUMMARY OF MANAGEMENT OPTIONS

Varicella-Zoster Virus Infection

Management Options	Evidence Quality and Recommendation	References
Prepregnancy		
Prevent by childhood vaccination.	III/B	60
Vaccinate susceptible adults.	IV/C	60
Prenatal		
If mother exposed to VZV, check immunity status.	—/GPP	—

SUMMARY OF MANAGEMENT OPTIONS

Varicella-Zoster Virus Infection—cont'd

Management Options	Evidence Quality and Recommendation	References
If mother is IgG-negative (susceptible), give VariZIG within 96 hr of exposure.	IV/C	60,62
If mother develops chickenpox:		
• Counsel about minimal fetal risks.	IIa/B	51–57
• Offer acyclovir to decrease lesions.	IIa/B	63
• Monitor for signs of pneumonia or disseminated infection.	III/C	47–50
Labor, Delivery, and Postnatal		
Take appropriate infection control measures.	—/GPP	—
Evaluate newborn clinically and serologically.	—/GPP	—
Administer active or passive immunization to neonate if not infected.	IV/C	60,62

GPP, good practice point; IgG, immunoglobulin G; VZV, varicella-zoster virus.

PARVOVIRUS B19

Maternal and Fetal Risks

Human parvovirus B19 (erythema infectiosum, fifth disease) is an infectious exanthematous childhood illness transmitted by droplet. Parvovirus B19 viremia occurs 6 to 8 days after exposure and may persist for up to a week. An infected individual is contagious before the onset of symptoms, and the virus can be detected in the blood or secretions as early as 5 to 10 days after exposure. Parvovirus B19 infection is characterized by fever, rash, and arthropathy. The rash has a "slapped cheek" appearance on the face and a "lacelike" appearance on the trunk and extremities. The arthropathy may affect the joints of the hands, wrist, knees, and ankles. In addition, the virus may cause aplastic crisis in patients with sickle cell disease[65] and other hemolytic states,[66] chronic bone marrow failure in patients with immunodeficiency,[67] a chronic arthropathy,[68] and the childhood illness fifth disease (erythema infectiosum).[69]

Parvovirus B19 infection preferentially infects rapidly dividing cells and is cytotoxic for erythroid progenitor cells.[70,71] As a result, B19 virus also may stimulate a cellular process involving programmed cell death.[72] Parvovirus B19 infections during pregnancy might rarely be associated with fetal loss or hydrops fetalis. The risk of fetal loss appears highest in the first 20 weeks of pregnancy. In a prospective study of 186 pregnancies with confirmed parvovirus B19 infection, there were 27 first-trimester spontaneous abortions versus 7 abortions or fetal deaths in the second trimester and only 1 death in the third trimester.[73] Several additional series of parvovirus infection in pregnancy have been reported. When these series are summarized, the risk of fetal loss among pregnancies infected prior to 20 weeks' gestation is approximately 10%.[74–76] The risk of loss after 20 weeks' gestation is less than 1% and the risk of hydrops is 0.3%.[77] A prospective study of 618 exposed pregnancies showed no hydrops or fetal death attributable to B19 in 52 babies born to infected mothers.[78] The hydrops may develop rapidly within 7 to 14 days and can either lead to fetal death or resolve spontaneously.[79] In the largest prospective study of 1018 women with acute parvovirus infection, 6.3% of pregnancies ended with fetal death, and all were infected prior to 20 weeks' gestation.[80] The rate of death in the first trimester was 13% (34/256 < 12 weeks' gestation); 9% (30/222 13–20 weeks' gestation); and 0/439 after 20 weeks' gestation. There were a total of 6 stillbirths, 4 prior to 24 weeks' gestation and 2 at term. These term deaths were not attributed to B19.

Although B19 infection appears to be teratogenic in fetal animals (cerebellar hypoplasia and ataxia in cats and anencephaly, microcephaly, facial defects, and ectopic hearts in hamsters have been described), epidemiologic studies do not suggest that B19 infection is teratogenic in human fetuses.[81] Furthermore, long-term follow-up of offspring of women with B19 infections suggests the children are normal.[82,83]

Parvovirus B19 infection is distributed worldwide. Antibody to B19 virus occurs in 30% to 60% of adults.[84,85] Secondary attack rates for household contacts may be as high as 50% but as low as 20% to 30% for classroom contacts.[86] Serologic surveys of pregnant women revealed that 35% to 65% are B19-seropositive.[75,78] In one large study during an epidemic, the risk of seroconversion for pregnant women was highest in those with the greatest exposure to young children.[87]

Diagnosis

B19 virus is difficult to culture, and clinical manifestations are often lacking. Serology is the easiest method to detect infection using either IgM antibody capture radioimmunoassay or ELISA. These tests will detect between 80% and 90% of B19 seropositive individuals.[88] IgM, indicating acute infection, can be detected approximately 10 days after exposure and can last for 3 months or longer.[89,90] IgG antibodies may be detected several days after IgM and can persist for years as markers of past infection. Polymerase chain reaction

(PCR) to detect small amounts of B19 virus is useful to diagnose in utero infection from amniotic fluid.[91–93] In cases of unexplained hydrops, the presence of B19 DNA in maternal blood is useful for diagnosis, although avidity testing and EIA for specific parvovirus IgG epitope might be more useful for timing of infection.[94] Additional methods such as electron microscopy, detection of viral DNA, and hybridization assays for nucleic acids may be useful for pathologic specimens in the evaluation of stillbirths.

Management Options

Prepregnancy

Immunocompetent adults rarely need treatment; however, patients at risk for hemolysis may need multiple transfusions.

Prenatal

Pregnant women following exposure to B19 virus should have immediate serologic testing. Presence of IgG and absence of IgM suggests prior exposure to B19 virus and that the fetus is protected from infection. If the IgG is negative or positive and the IgM is positive, this finding is consistent with acute infection. Women should be counseled about the low risk of fetal loss in the first trimester and low risks of hydrops or stillbirth in the second and third trimesters. Prior to 20 weeks' gestation, no further action is required. However, after 20 weeks' gestation, periodic ultrasound examinations may be useful to identify hydrops. In addition, Doppler studies of the fetal middle cerebral artery peak velocity may yield an accurate reflection of fetal anemia.[95] In some reported cases, hydrops did not appear until 8 weeks following maternal infection; hence, the recommendation to continue monitoring for 8 to 12 weeks after infection.[96] If hydrops is noted, percutaneous umbilical blood sampling may be warranted to determine fetal hematocrit and provide transfusion.[97,98] Although some small series show improvement following transfusion, other reports note spontaneous resolution in the absence of intervention.[99,100] Further discussion of fetal hydrops can be found in Chapter 24.

The pregnant woman who is IgG-negative and IgM-negative is susceptible to infection. She should be counseled that repeat testing may be required if her serologic results were obtained within 2 weeks of her exposure. Preventive measures include minimizing contact with known parvovirus infection and good contact precautions. According to the CDC, there is no proven benefit to removing seronegative women from high risk employment for the duration of the pregnancy.

Labor, Delivery, and Postpartum

Onset of signs and symptoms suggesting acute infection during these time periods requires appropriate infection control measures. The neonate should be carefully observed for vertical transmission of the infection. Neonatal IgG levels immediately after birth reflect transplacentally passed maternal immunoglobulin.

SUMMARY OF MANAGEMENT OPTIONS

Parvovirus B19 Infection

Management Options	Evidence Quality and Recommendation	References
Prepregnancy		
If the diagnosis is confirmed before pregnancy, avoid contraception until clinical cure and antibody response.	—/GPP	—
Prenatal		
If mother is exposed to B19 parvovirus or symptoms are noted, check immunity status.	—/GPP	—
If mother is IgG-negative/IgM-negative (susceptible), repeat testing in 3–4 wk.	—/GPP	—
If mother is IgG-negative/IgM-positive:		
• Counsel that risks are small.	IIb/B	73–78,80
• If greater than 20 wk, screen with serial ultrasound for hydrops.	III/B	73–77
• If hydrops is detected, consider intrauterine fetal transfusion.	III/B	97,98
Labor, Delivery, and Postnatal		
Take appropriate infection control measures.	—/GPP	—
Evaluate newborn clinically and serologically.	—/GPP	—

GPP, good practice point; Ig, immunoglobulin.

SUGGESTED READINGS

American College of Obstetricians and Gynecologists: Immunization during pregnancy (ACOG Committee Opinion No. 282). Obstet Gynecol 2003;101:207–212.

Centers for Disease Control and Prevention: A new product (VariZIG(tm)) for postexposure prophylaxis of Varicella available under an investigational new drug application expanded access protocol. MMWR Morb Mortal Wkly Rep 2006;55:209–210.

Centers for Disease Control and Prevention: Rubella and congenital rubella syndrome—United States, 1994–1997. MMWR Morb Mortal Wkly Rep 1997;46:350–353.

Davidkin I: Persistence of measles, mumps, and rubella antibodies in an MMR-vaccinated cohort: A 20 year follow-up. J Infect Dis 2008;197:950–956.

Enders G, Miller E, Cradock-Watson J, et al: Consequences of varicella and herpes zoster in pregnancy: Prospective study of 1739 cases. Lancet 1994;343:1547–1550.

Enders M, Weidner A, Rosental T, et al: Improved diagnosis of gestational parvovirus B19 infection at the time of nonimmune fetal hydrops. J Infect Dis 2008;197:58–62.

Enders M, Weidner A, Zoellner I, et al: Fetal morbidity and mortality after acute human parvovirus B19 infection in pregnancy: prospective evaluation of 1018 cases. Prenat Diagn 2004;24:513.

McQuillan GM, Kruszon-Moran D, Hyde TB, et al: Seroprevalence of measles antibody in the US population, 1999–2004. J Infect Dis 2007;196:1459–1464.

Siegel M: Congenital malformations following chickenpox, measles, mumps, and hepatitis: Results of a cohort study. JAMA 1993;226:1521–1524.

Wilson E, Goss MA, Marin M, et al: Varicella vaccine exposure during pregnancy: data from 10 years of the Pregnancy Registry. J Infect Dis 2008;197(Suppl 2):S178–S184.

REFERENCES

For a complete list of references, log onto www.expertconsult.com.

CHAPTER 30

Cytomegalovirus, Herpes Simplex Virus, Adenovirus, Coxsackievirus, and Human Papillomavirus

THOMAS ROOS and DAVID ALLAN BAKER

INTRODUCTION

Viral infections can pose a serious threat to the fetus and the newborn. In the healthy adult, infections might be asymptomatic or cause only mild unspecific symptoms. Some viruses may reside dormant for prolonged periods, and asymptomatic virus shedding may occur unnoticed. Viruses can be transmitted by trivial interpersonal contacts such as occurs when handling a baby (cytomegalovirus [CMV], herpes simplex virus [HSV], adenovirus, coxsackievirus) or in a swimming pool (adenovirus). Sexual activities with multiple partners confer a high risk for infection with some viruses associated with severe disease in the adult and in the infant. Pregnancy is associated with decreased maternal cell-mediated immunity to viral infections; thus, the pregnant woman and her fetus are theoretically at increased risk for serious illness. Depending on gestational age, transplacental viral infection may range from asymptomatic to severe, causing fetal or neonatal death or long-term sequelae in the survivors. Intrauterine growth restriction (IUGR), nonimmune hydrops, isolated ascites, intracranial calcifications, microcephaly, and hydrocephaly are common ultrasound findings associated with some in utero viral infections. The possible severe impact of viral infections and the lack of specific antiviral treatment options in the fetus and newborn available to date imply that prevention is the most important approach to disease containment. The development of antiviral drugs and vaccines in progress holds the promise of a reduced incidence of fetal viral infections and of their sequelae in the future.

CYTOMEGALOVIRUS

General

CMV, a DNA virus, is a member of the herpes family of viruses, which causes a number of infectious syndromes in humans. However, because CMV is highly efficient in remaining dormant or silent in the host, the most common manifestation of CMV infection in humans is the lack of demonstrable disease. Three disease states are particularly important: intrauterine and neonatal infection, heterophil-negative mononucleosis, and infection in the immunocompromised patient.

Diagnosis

Human CMV is readily grown in cell lines of human fibroblasts. In patients with symptoms suggestive of acute CMV infection, viral culture from urine, nasopharynx, or blood may document the presence of the organism. Direct immunofluorescence tests in combination with a limited culture can detect the virus more rapidly. More recently, nucleic acid amplification systems using polymerase chain reaction (PCR) techniques have been used to identify the virus in amniotic and other fluid samples and in dried newborn blood.[1–4] High numbers of virus copies in the amniotic fluid can possibly signal a fetus at risk for severe CMV disease; however, this relationship remains controversial.[5–7] Viral load detected in newborn dried blood spot test might indicate children at increased risk of sensoneurinal hearing loss.[8] Tissue specimens (biopsy, necropsy) may also be evaluated for virus by immunofluorescence, in situ hybridization, or PCR techniques,[9] thus, providing a better understanding of fetal CMV infection mechanisms.[10,11]

Because many previously infected patients excrete CMV intermittently throughout their lives depending on certain circumstances (e.g., pregnancy, immunosuppression), the presence of CMV in a specimen does not automatically confirm that the illness in question is caused by this particular virus. The physician must be extremely careful with the interpretation of these results.

Approximately 50% of reproductive age women have antibody to CMV. Thus, paired specimens are necessary if seroconversion from negative to positive has not been documented. A significant rise in titer is usually consistent with a primary infection. Immunoglobulin M (IgM)–specific antibody is usually present 4 to 8 weeks after a primary infection but can increase periodically or persist at a low titer for years. IgM and, less frequently, IgA are of use in distinguishing transplacental transfer of maternal antibodies in the diagnosis of congenital infection.[12]

Serologic testing consists of the older complement fixation test or the more current indirect fluorescent antibody (FA) and anticomplement immunofluorescent tests. In a primary infection, these tests become positive sooner than the complement fixation test.[13] Enzyme immunoassay (EIA) methods also have been used to detect CMV-specific IgG, IgM, IgA, and IgE antibodies.[14] This is important because reactivation of latent CMV during pregnancy may be accompanied by either an increase or a reappearance of IgM antibodies (depending on the methodology used), which theoretically would help differentiate it from new infection.[15] More recently, more labor-intensive EIA assays have been used to detect low-avidity IgG antibodies that are produced early in infection.[16–18] In one study, CMV immediate-early messenger RNA in maternal blood was detected only in cases of primary CMV infection and not in immune subjects; thus, this later EIA test has been suggested to be helpful in differentiating primary from recurrent infection.[19]

Isolation of the virus or DNA from amniotic fluid and demonstration of viral DNA, immunologic response, or nonspecific markers in fetal blood collected by cordocentesis have all been used to supplement antenatal diagnosis.[20–23] A prospective evaluation of 1771 pregnant Belgian women by serial serology and culture of urine, saliva, and cervical secretions at each prenatal visit revealed a seronegative rate of 49%.[24] Of this group, seroconversion occurred in 20 susceptible women (2.3%). Five of the 7 who agreed to cordocentesis and amniocentesis had positive amniotic fluid cultures for CMV; 3 had a positive fetal IgM for CMV. The presence of CMV in fetal tissue was confirmed after termination, supporting the authors' contention that amniotic fluid culture is superior to fetal IgM in diagnosing fetal infection.[24] Others have reported either a lack of fetal CMV seropositivity for IgM in culture-positive fetuses or the failure of the fetus to sustain the IgM response. Thus, amniotic fluid culture or PCR analysis of amniotic fluid is superior to fetal CMV-specific IgM.[25,26] There have been a few reports of false-negative amniotic fluid cultures, as ascertained by neonatal shedding, but the relationship of these apparently negative results to the timing of infection and to long-term sequelae is unclear. Culture failure may be related to performance of amniocentesis too close to the time of initial maternal infection or too early in gestation, that is, before the fetal kidneys produce sufficient amounts of urine containing shedded virus.[27,28] The best results for detecting congenital CMV infection by testing amniotic fluid samples occur when amniocentesis is performed after 21 weeks' gestation and after an interval of at least 6 weeks from the first diagnosis of maternal infection.[29,30] Sensitivity to CMV can be enhanced using PCR or nested PCR assays.[16,31] Nested PCR technique has effectively been applied in a dried blood spot test of newborn Guthrie card in a trial evaluating newborn CMV screening.[4] Because all of these techniques can produce false-negative results, a negative diagnostic workup does not guarantee absence of infection.

Detection of specific IgM in fetal blood has been found to be associated with severe CMV disease.[29] Some, but not all, infected fetuses have sonographic abnormalities (e.g., intracranial calcifications, growth restriction), anemia, thrombocytopenia, and elevated liver function test results.[20,32] The natural history of the disease was followed antenatally by serial ultrasound and cordocentesis in at least one reported case.[33] Hyperechoic bowel may precede development of ventriculomegaly, IUGR, nonimmune hydrops, and fetal death in infected fetuses.[34] In a group of 50 pregnant women (51 fetuses) with primary CMV infection and confirmed in utero transmission, abnormal fetal ultrasound findings could be demonstrated in 22% (11 of 51 fetuses). In the same study, 3 out of 16 newborns (19%) with normal ultrasound findings had neurologic abnormalities.[35] Thus, normal mid-trimester ultrasound findings in infected fetuses can exclude neither an abnormal ultrasound later in pregnancy or the birth of a severely affected child. Recently, in addition to ultrasonography, magnetic resonance imaging (MRI) in proven CMV-infected fetuses has demonstrated to be helpful in providing additional information on gyration, cerebellar hypoplasia, and changes in the white matter of the fetal brain. However, MRI may not detect brain anomalies in cases of normal ultrasound findings; thus, MRI is not recommended as a first-line diagnostic procedure in evaluating CMV-infected fetuses.[36,37]

Maternal and Fetal Risks

Approximately 10% of healthy adults infected with CMV for the first time may develop a syndrome of fever, atypical lymphocytosis, malaise, and mild lymphadenopathy, which generally follows a benign course. This illness is clinically indistinguishable from Epstein-Barr virus (EBV) mononucleosis, save that the heterophil-antibody test is negative in patients with CMV infection. Patients with CMV mononucleosis tend to be slightly older than patients with EBV infection. This syndrome is generally self-limiting, although the fever may last for over a month. Serious complications of the acute infection rarely occur, including interstitial pneumonitis, hepatitis, Guillain-Barré syndrome, meningoencephalitis, myocarditis, thrombocytopenia, and hemolytic anemia.[38] The virus may be excreted in tears, saliva, breast milk, cervical secretions, and urine for weeks, months, or years after a primary infection. A latency period eventually occurs, but reinfection and reactivation are common.[39]

CMV infection in the immunosuppressed patient can be serious, depending on the type and degree of immunosuppression.[40] Patients on immunosuppressive drugs because of organ transplantation or patients with AIDS most commonly exhibit the mononucleosis syndrome. The next most frequent manifestation is interstitial pneumonia, which may progress rapidly from asymptomatic to fatal disease (often in association with *Pneumocystis* infection in AIDS patients). A large percentage of persons suffering primary CMV infection exhibit hepatitis; severely immunosuppressed patients may develop clinical symptoms, including malaise, nausea, and vomiting. Gastrointestinal disease, including ulceration leading to hemorrhage and perforation, is another effect of CMV in the immunocompromised patient. The AIDS patient may suffer coexistent CMV infection with other infections such as cryptosporidiosis and *Mycobacterium avium-intracellulare*. In fact, endoscopic examination of the AIDS patient with colitis due to CMV may demonstrate lesions that resemble Kaposi's sarcoma. Finally, in the AIDS patient specifically, CMV infection of the eye may produce retinitis, typically noted in neonates with the disease, and miscellaneous effects on endocrine organs, including adrenals, pancreas, parathyroids, pituitary, and ovaries.

Venereal spread of CMV is conceptually attributed to the presence of virus in the semen and to cervical shedding. CMV has been isolated from semen of both homosexual and heterosexual men.[41] Heterosexual transmission has been demonstrated by outbreaks of CMV mononucleosis among populations of sexual partners.[42] Aside from the fact that differences in rates of cervical shedding are noted in different patient groups throughout the world, it is fairly clear that sexual activity, in particular higher numbers of sexual partners and earlier age at onset of sexual activity, is positively correlated with CMV isolation from the cervix.[43]

Whereas CMV is transmitted by such routes as transfused blood[44] and bone marrow,[45] a common route of acquisition is through perinatal transmission. The fetus may be infected either transplacentally or by exposure to the virus from the cervix and birth canal. The neonate may also be infected by virus excreted in breast milk[46]; however, the risk appears to be low.[47,48] Another source of childhood infection is exposure to other babies in nurseries and daycare centers,[49–51] because infected children tend to shed virus from the urine and respiratory tract for a prolonged time (unlike infected but otherwise healthy adults).

The rate of seropositivity varies by age and multiple demographic factors. The rate increases steadily after the first year or two of life. The prevalence is higher in underdeveloped countries[52] and in lower socioeconomic patient populations.[53] One study of over 21,000 women attending a prenatal clinic in London revealed marked variation by race (white, 46%; Asian, 88%; black, 77%), parity (increasing seropositivity with increasing parity), and socioeconomic status.[54,55] Among most middle-income women in Alabama, 54% were seropositive, with whites having a lower rate than blacks.[53] The incidence of seroconversion in women of childbearing age approximates 2% in high socioeconomic groups and up to 6% in lower socioeconomic groups. The higher infection rate in young adults (hence mothers) does not necessarily lead to higher congenital infection rates.[56]

Primary infection occurs in 1% to 3% during pregnancy, with approximately 40% to 50% of women of childbearing age being serologically determined to be susceptible to such primary infection.[53,57] Estimates are that each year in the United States, approximately 340,000 non-Hispanic white persons, 130,000 non-Hispanic black persons, and 50,000 Mexican American women of childbearing age experience a primary CMV infection.[58] Serologic or culture evidence of in utero CMV infection is present in 0.2% to 2.2% of all liveborns. Thus, congenital CMV infection is a major health problem; CMV is still thought to be the most common congenital infection in the United States based on serologic study.[39,59,60]

Unlike other viral infections, CMV, on the basis of its latency and intermittent shedding from the female genital tract, may infect a fetus or neonate despite the presence of maternal antibody. Virus is shed from the cervix more readily as gestation progresses and occurs in approximately 0% to 2% of women in the first, 6% to 10% in the second, and 11% to 28% in the third trimester.[13] The infection rates at birth are higher in newborns whose mothers excrete virus. The most severe neonatal disease usually occurs in children born to women who experience primary infection during pregnancy. Vertical transmission of CMV occurs in 21% to 50% of fetuses following primary maternal infection.[29,30,61] A study of preconceptional and periconceptional primary CMV infection in 25 women identified a 9% risk for congenital fetal infection in the preconceptional group (1 of 12 newborns) and a 31% risk in the periconceptional group (4 of 13 newborns).[62]

Naturally acquired immunity results in a 69% reduction in the risk of congenital CMV infection in future pregnancies.[63] In addition, severe transplacental infection is not usually seen in children of women with preexisting antibody.[64] However, maternal preconceptional immunity to CMV does not provide complete fetal protection, and secondary CMV infection might cause severe sequelae in the fetus.[65–67] Thus, sonographic findings suggestive of CMV infection should prompt further investigation even if maternal serology does not support recent maternal infection.

CMV infection occurs in approximately 1 of 150 newborn infants. In the United States, this results in an estimated 33,000 infected newborns annually[68–70]; in the United Kingdom, CMV causes much more neonatal disease than rubella.[59] Approximately 5% to 10% of infected newborns are clinically symptomatic at birth. This is one of the classic TORCH (toxoplasmosis, other infections, rubella, CMV infection, and HSV) syndromes, consisting of hepatosplenomegaly, hyperbilirubinemia, petechiae, thrombocytopenia, intracranial calcifications, microcephaly, and often growth restriction. In primary infection, mortality may be as high as 20% to 30%, with 90% of survivors suffering late complications (Fig. 30–1) using "averaged" published data.[71] Of the asymptomatic infected neonates, 5% to 15% develop some abnormality attributable to CMV before their second birthday, primarily sensorineural hearing loss.[60,72] Vertical transmission may also occur in recurrent CMV infection[73]; however, the percentage of symptomatic children at birth or of those developing sequelae is much lower (Table 30–1).[74]

CMV is the most common cause of congenital sensorineural hearing loss, developing in 30% of neonates symptomatic at birth.[75] Hepatosplenomegaly is the most common clinical finding. Microcephaly, frequently associated with paraventricular cerebral calcifications, is also common.[76] Chorioretinitis, optic atrophy, mental and psychomotor delay, learning disabilities, and dental abnormalities are reported. Overall, congenital CMV infection leads to severe sequelae in 1 of 750 newborn infants, affecting close to 8000 children annually. Thus, congenital CMV infection is the most common cause of birth defects and childhood disabilities. Better-known childhood disabilities such as Down syndrome affect approximately 4000 children per year, fetal alcohol syndrome approximately 5000 infants per year, and spina bifida approximately 3500 newborns annually. Public and physicians awareness of these conditions are high compared with congenital CMV disease.[68–70] In a recent survey, 44% of obstetrician-gynecologists counseled their patients on preventing CMV infection, emphasizing the need for

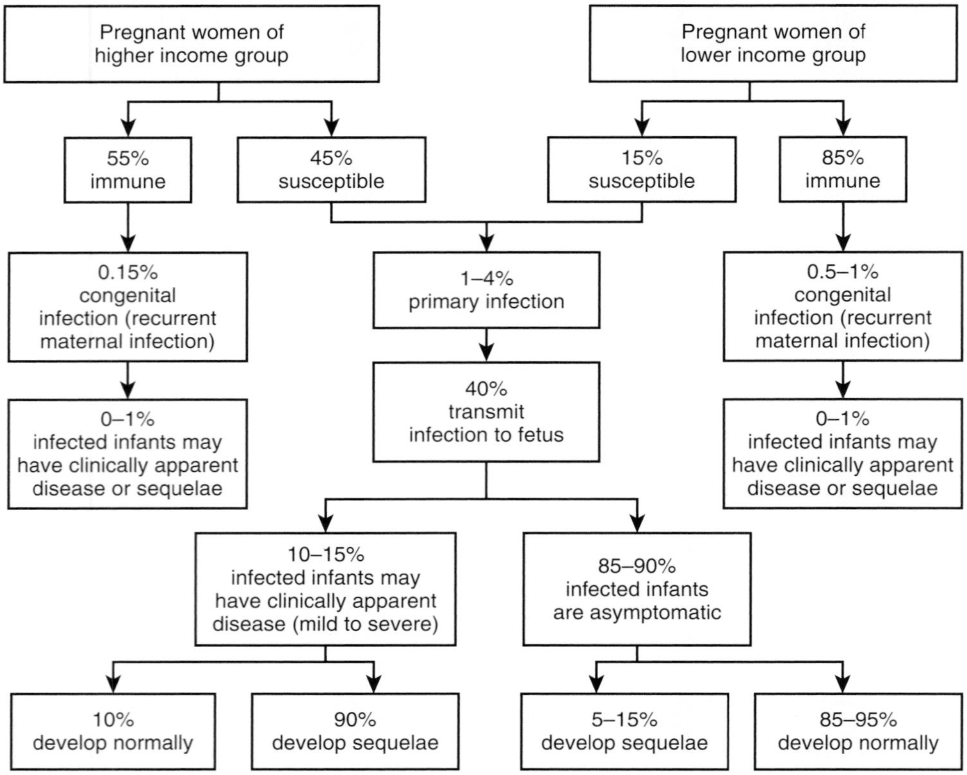

FIGURE 30–1
Infant outcome following cytomegalovirus (CMV) maternal infection in pregnancy. (Adapted from Stagno S: Cytomegalovirus. In Remington JS, Klein JO (eds): Infectious Diseases of the Fetus and Newborn Infant, 4th ed. Philadelphia, Saunders, 1995, p 322.)

TABLE 30–1

Sequelae in Children with Congenital Cytomegalovirus Infection According to Type of Maternal Infection

	PRIMARY	RECURRENT
Symptomatic disease at birth	24/132 (18%)	0/65 (0%)
Any sequelae	31/125 (25%)	5/64 (8%)
More than one sequela	7/125 (6%)	0/64 (0%)
Sensorineural hearing loss	18/120 (15%)	3/56 (5%)
Bilateral hearing loss	10/120 (8%)	0/56 (0%)
Microcephaly	6/125 (5%)	1/64 (2%)
Seizures	6/125 (5%)	0/64 (0%)
IQ < 70	9/68 (13%)	0/32 (0%)
Death	3/125 (2%)	0/64 (0%)

From Fowler KB, Stagno S, Pass RF, et al: The outcome of congenital cytomegalovirus infection in relation to maternal antibody status. N Engl J Med 1992;326:663–667.

additional training.[68] In a different study, only 14% of women had heard of CMV, indicating the potential of preventional behavior education.[77]

Management Options

Treatment of acute, symptomatic CMV infection in the immunocompetent normal individual is palliative. The vast majority of infections are asymptomatic; the remainder are mild. Currently, eradication of the virus is beyond the capacity of modern medicine. In the patient with compromised immunity, such as the transplant patient or the patient with AIDS, the antiviral drug ganciclovir provides temporary relief from such severe effects as retinitis.[13] To date, there is no accepted therapy for acute maternal or neonatal infection.[78]

There is progress in the development of a specific CMV vaccine,[79] although a number of real and theoretical obstacles remain.[80] Even though complete eradication of the virus may appear unlikely, antibody presence similar to that after primary human infection could reduce the rate of congenital fetal infection and its sequelae. Thus, an effective CMV vaccine will be a significant step forward. Passive immunization with specific anti-CMV immunoglobulins appears to be useful as prophylaxis in cases of renal and marrow transplantation.[81] Thus, prevention of maternal infection is clearly the strategy to avert intrauterine infection. Three different areas offer potential to reduce the likelihood of maternal CMV infection in pregnancy: patient education, physician education, and vaccine development. CMV is typically spread by interpersonal contact with transmission of infected secretions from person to person, so, in particular, pregnant women working in high risk situations (e.g., daycare centers) should be counseled to wash their hands carefully after changing diapers and after any contact with children's secretions (e.g., saliva).[78,82] Mouth-to-mouth kissing with children should be discouraged. Physicians need to be aware of the risk of transfusion-related CMV transmission.[83] Thus, when transfusing women of childbearing age who could potentially be or soon become pregnant, CMV-negative blood products should be used whenever possible. Any fetal transfusion in utero must use CMV-negative washed packed cells to avoid fetal CMV contamination. It is not appropriate, however, to screen all pregnant women for either anti-CMV IgG or viral excretion with the aim of isolating them for the duration of the pregnancy. The most reasonable course is to serologically screen all women in high risk areas (e.g., daycare workers) and recommend to susceptible individuals that they pay attention to hygiene measures. For prevention of CMV as well as other sexually transmitted diseases (STDs), all women with nonmonogamous relationships should be strongly encouraged to use condoms during sexual contact.[78]

No effective fetal therapy is yet available. Ganciclovir has been administered into the umbilical vein of a fetus at about 27 weeks. The dosage was 10 mg/day for 5 days, 15 mg/day for 3 days, and 20 mg/day for 4 days. Several episodes of bradycardia were noted after administration. Although the viral load in amniotic fluid decreased dramatically over the time of treatment and liver function tests improved, a fetal demise was noted at 32 weeks.[84] Antiviral treatments in pregnant women have been performed only on a small scale and with moderate effect.[85,86] Toxicity and cost-effectiveness are the main concerns. CMV hyperimmunoglobulin therapy in women with primary CMV infection during pregnancy appears to be promising in reducing CMV disease in the infants; however, the effectiveness and safety of this treatment await results of an international trial under way.[87–89]

Therapy of severely infected newborns with antiviral drugs had only a moderate effect.[90] In the absence of safe and effective treatment of fetal CMV infection, prevention through education of patients and physicians remains the most effective means to reduce the incidence of congenital CMV disease to date.

Assessment of effective newborn screening is the next step in order to early identify infants at risk for CMV disease and to reduce sequelae. Advances in the development of vaccines are promising; however, a licensed CMV vaccine appears to be years away.

SUMMARY OF MANAGEMENT OPTIONS

Cytomegalovirus

Management Options	Evidence Quality and Recommendation	References
Prepregnancy		
Advise women working in high risk environment (e.g., child care) about risks.	III/B	50,78,82
Counsel pregnancy planning in women with history of proven CMV infection	—/GPP	—
• Establishing their "shedding status" may help.	—/GPP	—
Encourage use of condoms in nonmonogamous relationships.	IV/C	78
Use CMV-negative blood products in transfusions.	IV/C	83
Prenatal		
Advise women working in high risk environment (e.g., child care) about risks.	III/B	50,78,82
Use CMV-negative blood products in transfusions.	IV/C	83
If patient is diagnosed to have CMV infection in pregnancy:	—/GPP	—
• Offer careful counseling about fetal risks.		
• Consider invasive procedure to establish fetal risk.		
• Check fetal growth and health.		
• Consider pregnancy termination (if early gestational age).		
• No effective treatment, although acyclovir, ganciclovir, valaciclovir, CMV-specific hyperimmunoglobulin have been used.	IV/C	13,84,85, 88,89
Labor, Delivery, and Postnatal		
If patient is diagnosed to have CMV infection in pregnancy:	—/GPP	—
• Put infection control measures in place.		
• Conduct clinical and serologic evaluation of the newborn with pediatric follow-up if infection confirmed.		

CMV, cytomegalovirus; GPP, good practice point.

HERPES SIMPLEX VIRUS

General

HSV is a DNA virus of the herpes family. HSV-1 has classically been considered the cause of orolabial herpes, referred to commonly as *fever blisters*; HSV-2 has been considered the cause of genital herpes infection, a well-known STD. Although these two types of HSV are generally thought to be segregated in this way, there is a great deal of overlap, that is, of HSV-2 causing oral disease and HSV-1 causing genital infection. In fact, up to a third of genital infections may be due to HSV-1. However, HSV-1 is somewhat less prone to produce recurrent infection than HSV-2. Generally, the two viruses may be considered identical in the clinical circumstance of a patient with characteristic ulcerative lesions.[91]

Diagnosis

HSV is relatively easy to culture; viral culture is the preferred test of genital HSV infection in patients who present with genital ulcers. The sensitivity of culture declines rapidly as lesions begin to heal, usually within a few days of onset. When more rapid diagnosis is desirable, FA staining performed on short-incubation tissue culture slides allows identification within 48 hours, especially when the original specimen contains large numbers of virus. In high-inocula situations, direct FA staining of the original specimen may give the diagnosis, though it is neither as sensitive nor as specific as tissue culture.[92,93] PCR assays for HSV DNA are highly sensitive and can be used to rapidly detect HSV DNA in pregnant women.[94]

Type-specific antibodies to HSV develop during the first 6 to 8 weeks after infection and persist indefinitely. Accurate type-specific assays must be based on the HSV-1–specific glycoprotein G1 for diagnosis of infection with HSV-1 and on the HSV-2–specific glycoprotein G2 for diagnosis of infection with HSV-2.[95,96] Sensitivity of serology tests vary between 80% and 90%, and false-negative results may occur, especially at early stages of infection. Specificity is greater than 96%, and false-positive results can occur. Thus, repeat testing may be indicated in some settings. Type-specific serology in combination with HSV culture and DNA testing by PCR might prove helpful in confirming a clinical diagnosis of genital herpes, especially in patients with healing sores or recurrent episodes of genital herpes when HSV culture provides false-negative results.[97] Clinical examination is likely to miss many cases of genital herpes,[98] and antepartum cultures do not predict viral shedding at the time of delivery.[99]

The Centers for Disease Control and Prevention (CDC)[95] provides guidelines on the use of type-specific serologic tests. The CDC recognize the significance of using serologic testing: (1) to confirm clinical diagnoses, (2) to diagnose people with unrecognized infection, and (3) to manage sex partners of persons with genital herpes. Because cultures are frequently false-negative, serologic tests can be useful in confirming a clinical diagnosis. The guidelines note that some specialists believe that type-specific serologic tests are useful to identify pregnant women at risk for HSV infection and to help them with counseling regarding the risk of acquiring genital herpes during pregnancy. There is no place for using IgM antibody testing to determine primary versus recurrent HSV infection.

There are three stages of HSV infection based on clinical presentation and serology.

Primary Infection

Primary HSV infection is confirmed when no HSV-1 or HSV-2 IgG antibodies are present. Primary genital infection, due to HSV-2 or HSV 1, when symptomatic, presents with mild to severe symptoms and numerous genital lesions. Genital lesions occur on the vulva, vagina, and cervix, between 2 and 14 days, and are multiple and more numerous than those observed in recurrent disease. Vaginal discharge, dysuria, and vaginal burning can be presenting symptoms. Regional lymphadenopathy is caused by virus replication in the sites of lymphatic drainage. Systemic symptoms (malaise, myalgia, and fever) are found during primary herpetic infection. It is important to appreciate that primary infection may be asymptomatic.

Nonprimary First-episode Disease

In nonprimary first-episode disease, HSV-1 antibodies are present in the woman who acquires genital HSV-2 infection for the first time. If the infected person possesses preexisting anti-HSV 1 antibody, there are fewer constitutional symptoms, lesions, and complications, and the duration of the lesions and the time of viral shedding are reduced.[91]

Recurrent Infections

In recurrent infections, homologous antibodies are present.[100] Routine screening in the general population appears not to be cost-effective[101] and is not recommended.[95] However, identification of seronegative women provides the opportunity to properly address the risk of primary transmission during pregnancy and counsel serologically discordant couples, in particular.[102]

In recurrent genital herpes, lesions tend to be limited in size and number. They recur usually on one area of the external vulva, and no more than three lesions are found with clinical examination. A diffuse cervicitis or a single large ulcer may demonstrate cervical involvement. Local irritation or pain is the presenting complaint, and there may be an increase in vaginal discharge or dysuria. The external genital tract is the site of intermittent virus replication. Virus shedding without a lesion (asymptomatic shedding) can occur from the vulva and cervix intermittently in subsequent years after primary infection. Asymptomatic shedding of virus lasts an average of 1.5 days.

Epidemiology and Transmission of Herpes Simplex Virus-1 and Herpes Simplex Virus-2

A susceptible partner can acquire this virus during times of asymptomatic shedding.[103] Shedding of virus without any symptoms or signs of clinical lesions (asymptomatic shedding) makes this viral STD difficult to control and prevent. Patients will experience recurrent disease after clinical or asymptomatic primary HSV genital infection. Recurrences of genital HSV infection can be symptomatic or asymptomatic, and there is significant variation from patient to patient in the frequency, severity, and duration of symptoms and viral shedding. Young adult women typically acquire the first episode of genital herpes between the ages of 20 and 24 years.

Primary orolabial herpes is mainly a disease of childhood, children acquiring the infection from family members through close contact. Although 90% to 95% of primary oral infections are asymptomatic, a few may consist of a rather florid vesiculoulcerative outbreak in the oropharynx and lips about a week after exposure. Adenopathy and viremia, along with fever and malaise, may persist for a week or two, with viral shedding for up to 6 weeks. Thereafter, antibody production limits the virus such that it remains dormant, occasionally flaring up as localized blisters on the lips in times of stress, sunburn, or febrile systemic illness (hence the term *fever blisters*). During recurrent disease, viral shedding lasts up to a week.[104]

Genital herpes may occur after sexual contact, either genital-genital or orogenital, with an infected person. The incubation period is 2 to 14 days. Persons transmitting the virus may be asymptomatic themselves,[105] confusing identification of the origin of the infection. In one study, 10% of pregnant women were at risk for contracting primary HSV-2 infection from their HSV-2–seropositive husbands.[102] Asymptomatic cervical and vulvar shedding following a primary HSV infection occurs in 2.3% of women with HSV-2 infection and 0.65% with HSV-1 infection.[106] In the absence of circulating antibody, primary HSV genital infection can be severe, with symptoms of fever, malaise, myalgias, and aseptic meningitis. HSV encephalitis[107] and hepatitis[108] have proved fatal. Lower motor neuron and autonomic dysfunction may lead to bladder atony and urine retention. Increased viral shedding occurs for nearly 3 weeks in severe cases if untreated. Local disease may recur weeks or months later if the offending virus is HSV-2, in particular, which recurs much more frequently than does HSV-1, especially in the genital area.[109]

Genital herpes infection is common in the United States, with 45 million people ages 12 and older, or one out of five of the total adolescent and adult population, infected with HSV-2.[110] Since the late 1970s, the number of people in the United States with genital herpes infection has increased by 30%. HSV-2 infection is more common in women (~1 of 4) than in men (~1 of 5), and more in blacks (45.9%) than in whites (17.6%). The largest increase is now occurring in young white teens. HSV-2 infection is now five times more common in 12- to 19-year-old whites, and it is twice as common in young adults ages 20 to 29 than it was in the late 1980s.[110] Among sexual partners discordant for HSV infection, the annual risk of acquisition of genital HSV infection was 31.9% among women who were both HSV-1– and HSV-2–negative versus 9.1% among women who were HSV-1–positive.[111] Approximately 1.6 million new HSV-2 infections are acquired yearly, and approximately 2% of women seroconvert to HSV-2 during pregnancy.[112,113]

Maternal and Fetal Risks

Because of the relative immunosuppression during pregnancy,[114] dissemination of HSV may lead to death from hepatitis, encephalitis, and general viral dissemination.[115] Primary infection early in pregnancy, perhaps due to a viral endometritis ascending from cervical infection, may end in spontaneous abortion. However, there are no consistent reports of a congenital syndrome due to intrauterine infection with HSV. The spectrum of fetal/neonatal infection includes abortion, prematurity, and intrapartum infection with resultant disseminated HSV infection.[116]

Primary HSV infection in the second or third trimester increases the risk for preterm delivery as well as the risk of virus transmission to the newborn.[117] The fetus acquiring HSV, especially if the mother suffers an acute, primary infection, may sustain severe neonatal morbidity, including chorioretinitis, meningitis, encephalitis, mental retardation, seizures, and death.[118]

Since the late 1980s or 1990s, industrialized countries have reported a decrease in seropositivity rates of HSV-1, due perhaps to increasing sanitation measures, and increasing rates of HSV-2, due to increasingly permissive sexual behavior.[119] The rates of clinical genital HSV infection have risen dramatically since the 1960s in the United States,[120] United Kingdom, and other parts of Europe.[119]

The incidence of a positive culture in laboring women is 0.5% in the general population.[121] Rates of 0.96%[99] to 2.4%[122] have been reported in asymptomatic women with known histories of genital HSV infection. The rate of neonatal disease is in the range of 0.01% to 0.05%. The variability is due to differences in maternal antibody (and thus passively acquired fetal antibody) levels and the size of the viral inoculum (i.e., primary, severe infection versus mild, recurrent infection in the mother). The majority of infants developing neonatal HSV infection are born to mothers without symptoms or even a history of genital herpes infection and who test seronegative for specific HSV antibodies.[99,121,123] In Seattle, a prospective study was conducted in a cohort of 58,362 pregnant women, of whom 40,023 had genital HSV cultures at the time of labor and 31,663 had HSV specific serology; 202 women (0.5%) had a positive HSV culture, of whom 10 (5%) had neonates with HSV infection.[121] Women without a history of genital herpes were more likely to shed HSV asymptomatically than women with such a history. However, women with a history of genital herpes were more likely to have cesarean deliveries. The rate of vertical HSV transmission was 31.3% (5/16) in HSV-1–culture-positive mothers, and 2.7% (5/186) in HSV-2–positive mothers. Neonatal HSV infection rates per 100,000 live births were 54 among HSV-seronegative women, 26 among women who were HSV-1–seropositive only, and 22 among all HSV-2–seropositive women. Thus, the highest rate of neonatal HSV infection occurred in women who were seronegative and had no specific HSV antibodies. Heterologous antibody in this study did not seem to protect against transmission for primary versus nonprimary first-episode as, in contrast, did homologous antibody. The results emphasize the need for counseling seronegative women, in particular, to reduce the risk of neonatal HSV infection.

Most neonatal HSV infection is the consequence of delivery of a neonate through an infected birth canal. Most infants have localized skin, eye, and mouth disease, which usually is a mild illness. However, localized disease may progress to encephalitis or disseminated disease. Disseminated disease is associated with a 57% mortality rate; central nervous system (CNS) disease has 15% mortality; and localized disease shows no mortality.[124] In a group of 202 women from whom HSV was isolated, HSV transmission occurred in 9 of 117 (7.7%) infants after vaginal delivery, and in 1 of 85 (1.2%) newborns delivered by cesarean section.[121] Thus, cesarean section could reduce the rate of HSV transmission from mother to infant, but cannot completely prevent HSV infection in the newborn.

Management Options

Prepregnancy

The consistent, correct use of latex condoms can help protect against infection, particularly in women.[125] However, condoms do not provide complete protection because the condom may not cover the herpes sore(s) and viral shedding may nevertheless occur, which makes this STD difficult to prevent. In case of symptomatic genital herpes, it is best to abstain from sex and to use latex condoms between outbreaks. More recently, daily valacyclovir (500 mg) suppressed overt acquisition of HSV-2 in susceptible sexual partners. Overall acquisition, symptomatic and asymptomatic, was reduced by 48% in the valacyclovir group compared with the placebo group. Treatment with valacyclovir 500 mg daily decreases the rate of HSV-2 transmission in discordant, heterosexual couples in which the source partner has a history of genital HSV-2 infection. Such couples should be encouraged to consider suppressive antiviral therapy as part of a strategy to prevent transmission, in addition to consistent condom use and avoidance of sexual activity during recurrences.[95,103]

Prenatal

It is important that women avoid contracting herpes during pregnancy because a primary infection during pregnancy causes a greater risk of transmission to the newborn. All pregnant women should be asked whether they have a history of genital herpes. However, history is an unreliable method for identifying women at risk of acquiring genital herpes or those who are already infected.[110] Women without known genital herpes should be counseled to avoid intercourse during the third trimester, in particular, with partners known or suspected of having genital herpes. In addition, women with no history of orolabial herpes should be advised to avoid cunnilingus during the third trimester with partners known or suspected to have orolabial herpes.[95] When a woman's sex partner has a history of HSV infection, serologic testing for HSV-1 and HSV-2 antibodies might prove to be helpful to identify and consequently counsel seronegative women at risk for primary HSV infection during pregnancy. Pregnant women with a significant primary HSV infection may need to be hospitalized and monitored closely for evidence of sequelae. Premature labor should be appropriately treated when identified. Evidence of severe, disseminated disease such as hepatitis (elevated hepatic transaminase levels) and encephalitis (abnormal neurologic testing) should trigger the administration of intravenous acyclovir to prevent serious morbidity.[115] Treatment of primary genital herpes with oral antiherpetic agents is indicated to reduce viral shedding, reduce pain, and heal lesions faster.[126] Different studies have demonstrated that the use of acyclovir and valacyclovir is safe during pregnancy and does not impose an increased risk to the developing fetus even during the first trimester.[126–128] Dosing schedules are presented in Table 30–2. No induction of acyclovir-resistant HSV strains was noted in immunocompetent patients.[129] However, the extent to which suppressive therapy prevents HSV transmission to the infant is unknown.[95] In severe HSV disease, intravenous acyclovir is given at 5 to 10 mg/kg body weight every 8 hours for 2 to 7 days or until clinical improvement is observed. Oral antiviral therapy should follow to complete at least 10 days total therapy.[95] Oral acyclovir or valacyclovir and intravenously administered acyclovir reached therapeutic concentrations in the breast milk, the amniotic fluid, and the fetus.[130] Topical treatment with acyclovir offers no clinical benefit and should not be used to treat genital herpes.[95] Newer antiherpetic drugs, valacyclovir and famciclovir, demonstrate increased bioavailability over acyclovir and thus require less frequent dosing.

Antiviral prophylaxis of the mother to prevent maternal symptomatic and asymptomatic viral shedding during the intrapartum period is now recommended by the American College of Obstetricians and Gynecologists.[131–134] Acyclovir, valacyclovir, and famciclovir are class B medications as categorized by the U.S. Food and Drug Administration. Starting in 1984, an acyclovir pregnancy registry has been compiled. The CDC published data in 1993 showing there was no increase in fetal problems in women who received acyclovir in the first trimester of their pregnancy.[135] Ongoing studies examining newer recommendations to reduce the number of newborns infected with HSV are focused on identifying pregnant women susceptible to HSV infection.[135] The strategy is to test all pregnant women for antibodies to HSV-1 and HSV-2 (using a type-specific glycoprotein G-based testing) and to initiate the antiviral prophylaxis starting at 36 weeks' gestation in selected cases. Intervention is aimed at preventing primary infection in those at risk.

TABLE 30–2

Treatment Recommendations for Genital Herpes in the Nonpregnant Patient

CLINICAL SETTING	RECOMMENDED REGIMEN
First clinical episode of genital herpes	Acyclovir 400 mg orally three times a day for 7–10 days* OR Acyclovir 200 mg orally five times a day for 7–10 days OR Famciclovir 250 mg orally three times a day for 7–10 days OR Valacyclovir 1 g orally twice a day for 7–10 days
Suppressive therapy for recurrent genital herpes	Acyclovir 400 mg orally twice a day OR Famciclovir 250 mg orally twice a day OR Valacyclovir 500 mg orally once a day OR Valacyclovir 1.0 g orally once a day
Episodic therapy for recurrent genital herpes	Acyclovir 400 mg orally three times a day for 5 days OR Acyclovir 800 mg orally twice a day for 5 days OR Acyclovir 800 mg orally three times a day for 2 days OR Famciclovir 125 mg orally twice daily for 5 days OR Famciclovir 1000 mg orally twice daily for 1 day OR Valacyclovir 500 mg orally twice a day for 3 days OR Valacyclovir 1.0 g orally once a day for 5 days

* Treatment might be extended if healing is incomplete after 10 days of therapy.

From Centers for Disease Control and Prevention, Workowski KA, Berman SM: Sexually transmitted diseases treatment guidelines, 2006. MMWR Recomm Rep 2006;55(RR-11):1–91.

Labor and Delivery

On admission to the delivery suite, all women should be questioned carefully about symptoms of genital herpes, and all women should be examined carefully for herpetic lesions.[95] In the absence of visible lesions in the genital area at the onset of labor, vaginal delivery is permitted. If active genital lesions or prodromal symptoms of vulvar pain or burning (which may indicate an impending outbreak) are present, cesarean delivery is indicated. The incidence of infection in newborns whose mothers have recurrent infection is low, but cesarean delivery is warranted because of the serious nature of the disease.

The extent to which maternal antibodies will protect a neonate from an infection during a recurrence has not been determined with certainty. Cesarean delivery is not recommended in women with a history of HSV infection but no active disease during labor.[95,136]

In women with premature rupture of membranes (PROM) near term and active HSV infection, cesarean delivery should be performed as soon as possible. It should not, however, be assumed the fetus is infected just because of prolonged rupture of membranes. Women with preterm PROM and active lesions are considered individually, taking into account gestational age and other relevant factors. Remote from term, expectant management and use of glucocorticoids are increasingly supported, and antiviral therapy is indicated because premature neonates are at greatest risk of infection.[136]

Fetal HSV infection has been attributed to the use of fetal scalp electrodes even in the absence of active lesions.[121,137] Thus, fetal scalp monitoring should be used cautiously even in women with a history of recurrent HSV and no active lesions.

Postnatal

Postpartum, endometritis due to HSV infection has been reported[138] and is responsive to acyclovir. Postnatally acquired HSV infections in the newborn can be severe, and mothers with skin or oropharyngeal lesions should use caution when handling their babies. HSV-1 is more likely to cause nosocomial infections in the infant than is HSV-2. Breast-feeding is unlikely to cause infection in the infant; only in the case of an obvious lesion on the breast is breast-feeding contraindicated.[130]

SUMMARY OF MANAGEMENT OPTIONS
Herpes Simplex Virus

Management Options	Evidence Quality and Recommendation	References
Prepregnancy and Prenatal		
Inform about nature of the disease and that sexual transmission can occur during asymptomatic periods; counsel about condom protection during asymptomatic intervals and sexual abstinence during active disease.	IV/C	95,125
Perform HSV type-specific serology testing; allows more specific advice by identifying seronegative women at risk for HSV acquisition.	IV/C	95
• Advise HSV-2–negative women to abstain from intercourse during third trimester with men who have genital herpes.		
• Advise HSV-1–negative women to avoid intercourse with a partner who has genital HSV-1 infection; no cunnilingus with a partner who has orolabial herpes.		
Provide symptomatic treatment of infections (primary and recurrent); hospitalize for severe cases.	—/GPP	—
Give acyclovir for active disease:		
• Oral (7–14 days) for primary local infection.	Ib/A	126
• IV (for 2–7 days then oral) for primary systemic disease.	IV/C	115
• Oral (5 days) for recurrent disease.	III/B	136
Provide prophylactic acyclovir (400 mg bid) for last trimester in patients with previous HSV to reduce recurrence risk (no known effect on fetal/neonatal transmission).	Ib/A	131,132
No information about newer anti-HSV drugs; not recommended for pregnancy.	—/GPP	—
Remain vigilant for dissemination.	—/GPP	—
Remain vigilant for preterm uterine activity.	—/GPP	—
Serial viral cultures are no longer recommended in the last trimester for patients who are asymptomatic; culture only to document a new case.	IV/C	95
Consider delivery with septicemic cases.	—/GPP	—

SUMMARY OF MANAGEMENT OPTIONS

Herpes Simplex Virus—cont'd

Management Options	Evidence Quality and Recommendation	References
Labor and Delivery		
Inquire and inspect perineum, vagina, and cervix for HSV in all women at onset of labor (especially those with history of HSV).	IV/C	95
Allow vaginal delivery if no active lesions and no prodromal symptoms at time of labor.	—/GPP	—
Active lesions at time of labor is considered an indication for cesarean section by most obstetricians, though the risk of fetal infection is less with recurrent disease.	—/GPP	—
Counseling about the benefits of cesarean section in preventing fetal infection with membrane rupture is controversial, although most would still advise cesarean section. Expectant approach with suspected preterm labor and PROM is reasonable.	—/GPP	—
Avoid fetal electrodes and fetal scalp sampling.	Ib/A	121,137
Postnatal		
Maintain infection control measures if mother has active lesions.	—/GPP	—
Treat maternal infection; reduces dissemination and morbidity.	III/B	136
Perform clinical, microbiologic, and serologic evaluation of the newborn if active maternal lesions are present.	—/GPP	—
Give IV acyclovir to HSV-infected newborns.	III/B	136

GPP, good practice point; HSV, herpes simplex virus; PROM, premature rupture of the membranes.

ADENOVIRUS

General

Adenoviruses are medium-sized (90- to 100-nm) double-stranded DNA viruses. There are 6 subgenera (A through F) with 49 immunologically distinct types that can cause infection in the human. Most commonly, in the healthy adult, adenovirus infection causes gastrointestinal and respiratory tract illness with a wide range of symptoms.

There has been considerable interest in developing adenoviruses as defective vectors to deliver and express foreign genes for therapeutic purposes.[139–141] Furthermore, adenovirus vectors have been used to better understand mechanisms of intrauterine inflammation and fetal programming.[142,143] Adenovirus is relatively easy to manipulate in vitro, and the coupled genes are effectively expressed in large amounts. Direct administration of adenovirus gene vectors to the fetus can be achieved by fetoscopy or ultrasonographic guidance.[144,145] However, repeated prenatal exposure to an adenovirus vector was associated with pulmonary inflammation as reported in newborn sheep.[146] Alternatively, selective placental and maternal intravenous adenovirus vector application has demonstrated only low numbers of adenovirus replication in the fetus, thus reducing the risk of fetal exposure to the virus.[147] In addition, intraplacental adenovirus-mediated gene delivery showed only low numbers of virus in the mother, thus possibly providing a suitable strategy for basic studies of placental function or even a method of correcting placental dysfunction in the future.[148] Amniotic fluid–derived stem cells have been effectively transduced by adenovirus vectors, thus possibly providing pluripotent stem cells for use in gene therapy treatment.[149]

Diagnosis

Conventional virus culture, electronmicroscopy and serology tests,[150,151] and modern laboratory techniques such as antigen detection by immunofluorescence tests[152] and PCR assay[23] are all suitable means to identify adenovirus disease. Adenovirus typing requires the use of type-specific antisera in hemagglutination-inhibition and/or neutralization tests.[150,151] Adenovirus infection in tissues or cell smears can be identified using in situ hybridization technique.[153] The presence of adenovirus does not necessarily mean disease because viruses can be shed for a prolonged time. Adenovirus genome could be identified in amniotic fluid of 30 of 91 (33%) fetuses with ultrasound evidence of nonimmune hydrops. However, concomitant infection with parvovirus, CMV, enterovirus, HSV, and respiratory syncytial virus was found in the majority of cases by PCR technique.[23]

Maternal and Fetal Risks

In healthy adults, adenoviruses commonly cause respiratory illness with symptoms that range from the common cold to pneumonia, croup, and bronchitis. However, depending on the serotype or route of infection (inhalation or ingestion), adenoviruses might cause febrile disease and keratoconjunctivitis, rash illness, gastroenteritis, or cystitis. Immunocompromised patients are susceptible to severe complications of adenovirus infections.

Transmission is by direct contact and the fecal-oral route. Adenoviruses are unusually stable in adverse conditions. Occasionally, waterborne transmission occurs, often centering around swimming pools and small lakes. Infection is usually acquired during childhood and at a higher incidence in late winter, spring, and early summer. Depending on the serotype, adenovirus infection can persist in either the tonsils, the adenoids, or the intestines of infected patients. Virus shedding can continue for years. Adenovirus types 40 and 41 are known to cause gastroenteritis, primarily in children. Inhalation of adenovirus type 7 is known to cause severe lower respiratory tract infection, and acute respiratory disease is most often associated with types 4 and 7.[150,151]

Adenovirus infection of the infant might occur transplacentally or at delivery via birth canal or contact with feces. Amniotic fluid obtained from 303 pregnancies with abnormal ultrasound findings tested positive for adenovirus infection in 124 cases (41%). PCR technique could demonstrate adenovirus to be the only viral genome present in the amniotic fluid of oligohydramnios in 18% (2/11; 2 additional patients positive for CMV), hydrothorax/pleural effusion in 22% (4/18; 2 additional patients positive for enterovirus and CMV), ventriculomegaly in 23% (6/26; 1 additional patient positive for CMV), microcephaly in 20% (1/5), and echogenic bowel in 5% (1/22; 5 additional patients positive for CMV and HSV). In the control group of 154 structurally normal fetuses, viral infection of the amniotic fluid was detected in 4 cases (3%), and adenovirus was the only microorganism in 2% (3/154; 1 additional patient positive for CMV). Intrauterine adenovirus infection might cause fetal myocarditis with tachyarrhythmia, dilated cardiac chambers, poor ventricular function, and subsequent hydrops fetalis.[154,155]

Severe neonatal adenovirus illness is rare, but is most often manifested as necrotizing pneumonitis.[152,153,156,157] Within 10 days of birth, infected infants demonstrate rapidly progressing pneumonia, thrombocytopenia, disseminated intravascular coagulopathy, hepatomegaly, and hepatitis. Respiratory failure might require extracorporeal membrane oxygenation in the newborn.[158] Case fatality might be as high as 84% and death often occurs around day 16.[156,159,160] Neonatal infection may also be seen in epidemic proportions in neonatal nurseries.[161] Severity of the disease in newborns seems to be less pronounced in the presence of maternal antibodies.

Management Options

Prepregnancy and Prenatal

To date, no specific therapy is available for adenovirus infections in pregnancy or for the infected newborn, although new antiviral drugs (cidofovir, ribavirin) show promising results in pediatric patients.[162,163] Thus, the best treatment of adenovirus infection is prevention. Women should be counseled on proper hygiene measures to avoid fecal-oral transmission. Also, inadequately chlorinated swimming pools should be avoided. Most infections are mild and require no therapy.

Severe adenovirus infection can be managed only by treatment of symptoms and complications. Fetal tachyarrythmia and associated fetal hydrops may be treated by maternal oral digoxin and other agents (see Chapter 15). Maternal therapy with oral digoxin at 0.5 mg loading, and 0.125 to 0.25 mg/day maintenance dose has shown to convert fetal tachyarrhythmia to normal sinus rhythm and to produce spontaneous resolution of hydrops. Transplacental transfer of digoxin is at an estimated rate of 60% to 100%. Maternal digoxin levels or persistent fetal tachyarrhythmia might require adjustment of the daily administered digoxin dosage. Vaccines for adenovirus types 4 and 7 were developed for military use only. Risk to the general population is so low that vaccination is not a viable proposition.

Labor, Delivery, and Postnatal

Strict attention to good infection control practices is effective in stopping nosocomial outbreaks of adenovirus disease such as epidemic keratoconjunctivitis.

SUMMARY OF MANAGEMENT OPTIONS

Adenovirus

Management Options	Evidence Quality and Recommendation	References
Prepregnancy and Prenatal		
Route of transmission is fecal-oral and waterborne; thus, transmission can be prevented by	—/GPP	—
• Personal hygiene.		
• Public hygiene (chlorinated swimming pools).		
Treat adenovirus infections symptomatically because there is no proven therapy for maternal infection.	—/GPP	—
If hydrops develops due to fetal tachyarrhythmia, see Chapters 15 and 24.	—/—	—
Labor, Delivery, and Postnatal		
Strictly implement infection control policies.	—/GPP	—
No neonatal therapy other than symptomatic and supportive.	—/GPP	—
Severe pneumonitis in the newborn might require extracorporeal oxygenation.	—/GPP	—

GPP, good practice point.

COXSACKIEVIRUS

General

Coxsackievirus is a single-strand RNA virus, a member of the picornaviridae, which includes human enteroviruses and rhinoviruses. The enterovirus serotypes are determined by type-specific antisera and are traditionally grouped into four classes: poliovirus, group A coxsackievirus, group B coxsackievirus, and echovirus. Newly discovered serotypes are assigned enteroviral numbers (e.g., hepatitis A virus: enterovirus 72).

In northern latitudes, enterovirus infections are more firmly associated with a seasonal periodicity (pronounced in summer and fall) than can be observed in more tropical climates. However, infections may occur at any time of the year. Group B coxsackievirus serotypes 2 to 5 are isolated more frequently, whereas other serotypes are rarely reported. Group A coxsackievirus infections have been identified less frequently, possibly owing to poor growth in routine cell culture.

Enteroviruses are transmitted by direct contact with nose and throat discharge or feces of infected humans. Because many infections are clinically not apparent, spread of coxsackievirus infection may occur accidentally; the incubation period is 3 to 5 days (range 2–15 days).[164]

In healthy, nonpregnant adults, enterovirus infections either are asymptomatic or cause simple febrile illness with or without signs of upper respiratory tract infection or rash. However, some clinical syndromes are characteristically associated with enterovirus infection, including aseptic meningitis, pleurodynia, and the hand-foot-and-mouth disease. The rate of infection is higher in young children than among older children and adults.

Diagnosis

Coxsackievirus infection can be identified by virus culture from the oropharynx, stool, blood, urine, cerebrospinal fluid, and amniotic fluid. After virus isolation by culture, virus typing is performed by conventional neutralization tests. More rapid specific virus identification techniques using immunofluorescence assay (IFA) or enzyme-linked immunosorbent assay (ELISA) have not proved to be useful because of the large number of different serotypes.[165] However, development of monoclonal group-specific antibodies that can be used for rapid identification of enterovirus groups by IFA and ELISA is in progress.[166–168] Modern laboratory methods provide accurate and fast diagnosis of coxsackievirus infection by PCR technique.[23,169] In addition, PCR seems to be more suitable for detection of group A coxsackievirus that grows poorly in culture, which has led to a possible clinical underrecognition of this virus as a cause of disease.

Serology using hemagglutination-inhibition, complement fixation, and ELISA tests can readily identify IgG, IgM, IgA, and IgE classes of specific antibodies; however, the large number of different enterovirus type-specific antigens requires the performance of large numbers of serologic tests. Gene-sequencing technology has identified a common epitope in a number of enteroviruses, which might prove to be helpful for serology tests in the future.[168] When case serology is performed, paired specimens should be obtained to ensure proper diagnosis.

Tissue samples can be examined for specific enteroviral antigens by immunofluorescence or PCR technique.[170]

Maternal and Fetal Risks

The prevalence of enterovirus infection is inversely related to socioeconomic status and age, whereas individual factors, including age, sex, immune status, and pregnancy, are important determinants of the severity of infection.[171]

In pregnancy, most maternal coxsackievirus infections either are not apparent or cause only minimal symptoms similar to a viral upper respiratory tract infection or viral gastroenteritis[172]; however, hepatic failure has been reported.[173] The exact incidence of coxsackievirus infections in pregnancy is not known. There is no direct virologic evidence available that suggests that coxsackievirus infections in pregnancy may result in miscarriage.[165] However, an increased frequency of coxsackievirus IgM in women with spontaneous abortion has been reported.[174] In a collaborative study, serologic evidence of coxsackievirus B (types 1–6) infection during pregnancy was demonstrated in 9% of 198 women[175]; during peak enterovirus season, a seroconversion rate of 25% was noted during the last 2 to 6 weeks of pregnancy among 55 women.[176] Most women either were asymptomatic or had only mild symptoms, and no newborn had signs of severe enterovirus infection. The incidence of neonatal coxsackievirus B infection, based on laboratory records, was estimated at a minimum of 50 per 100,000 liveborn children.[177] Thus, enterovirus infection during late pregnancy might be a rather common event; however, most infections did not produce a significant maternal or neonatal morbidity. Alternatively, in women delivering newborns with evidence of group B coxsackievirus infection, 59% to 65% had symptomatic illness during the perinatal period with febrile disease and upper respiratory symptoms, pleurodynia, myocarditis, and aseptic meningitis.[171,177]

In animal studies, pregnant mice experimentally infected with different strains of enterovirus have a shorter incubation period, develop higher titers in blood and various organs, and remain viremic longer. Susceptibility increases with advancing gestation and rapidly reverts to that of nonpregnant animals within days of delivery. In nonpregnant female mice, administration of corticosterone or estrogen reduced the resistance to encephalomyocarditis virus infection, but this resistance was not altered by exogenous progesterone. Group B coxsackievirus infection of the pregnant mouse may also result in infection of the fetus before delivery or in infection of the mouse intrapartum.[171]

In humans, in vitro experiments demonstrated that vertical infection from mother to fetus rarely happens through transplacental passage.[178] However, 22% to 25% of neonatal group B coxsackievirus infections have been attributed to antepartal transmission.[172,177] The mechanisms of intrauterine coxsackievirus infection are poorly understood. Evidence of congenital disease is inconsistently related to recovery of virus from the placenta and the respective fetus,[165,176,179] and it is assumed that besides hematogeneous transmission involving the placenta, a number of fetuses might be infected by ingesting coxsackievirus contained in the amniotic fluid.[180] Transplacental infection of the fetus occurs in the absence of maternal immunity and is unrelated to the clinical severity of the disease in the mother. Viral shedding from the cervix has been reported; however, ascending viral infection seems to be a rare event.[181] At the time of delivery, infection of the infant might occur by cervical or fecal contamination. Fecal carriage rates of coxsackievirus was reported to range from 0% to more than 6% in different population groups.[165,166]

In a study of 630 infants with 778 anomalies of different organ systems, intrauterine infection with coxsackievirus B2 and B4 was associated with urogenital anomalies and coxsackievirus B3 and B4 with cardiovascular anomalies. The likelihood of congenital heart disease was increased by maternal infection with two or more coxsackievirus B serotypes rather than one. Also, first-trimester infection with coxsackievirus B4 occurred more frequently in mothers of infants with any anomaly than in the control group.[182] In 28 newborns with severe congenital defects of the CNS, neutralizing antibody to coxsackievirus B6 was demonstrated in 4 cases (14%); 2 had hydranencephaly, 1 had occipital meningocele, and 1 had aqueductal stenosis.[183] In a stillborn infant with calcific pancarditis and hydrops fetalis, coxsackievirus B3 antigen could be demonstrated.[179]

Newborns who acquire coxsackievirus infection in the immediate peripartum period are more likely to experience severe disease in the absence of protecting maternal antibodies. Neonatal infection might range from asymptomatic viral shedding to severe and rapidly fatal illness. Infection that occurs more than 5 days before delivery is likely to induce production of maternal IgG that can cross the placenta and protect the newborn from severe disease, but not necessarily from infection. In the newborn, coxsackievirus infection may cause benign neonatal arrhythmias[184]; fever[177]; oral vesicular lesions[185]; vesiculopapular rash[186]; severe respiratory failure[187]; pneumonitis[172]; fatal pulmonary hemorrhage[177,188]; hepatitis, hepatomegaly, jaundice, bleeding diatheses, hepatic failure, and necrosis[165,177]; aseptic meningitis[177]; meningoencephalitis, fatal encephalomyocarditis, and encephalohepatomyocarditis[172,189]; acute aseptic and interstitial myocarditis[190]; and result in heart disease.[191] A study of 16 neonates with enterovirus hepatitis and coagulopathy demonstrated hemorrhagic complications in 10 of 16 cases (63%); 5 infants had intracranial bleeding.[192] The overall fatality rate was 31% (5/16). In the group of 5 neonates with intracranial bleeding, 4 (80%) died. Overall, mortality rates are highest in children with myocarditis, encephalitis, or sepsis-like illness with liver involvement. In addition, prognosis seems to be related to the infecting viral strain. In general, infection with coxsackievirus B1 to B4 seems to carry the most ominous prognoses. Long-term sequelae are mostly reported with regard to heart and CNS-related impairment. Animal studies of coxsackievirus myocarditis demonstrated a T-cell–mediated immunopathic process and a virus-induced autoimmunity. In a study of 7 newborn infants with neurodevelopmental delays, coxsackievirus was retrieved from the respective placenta in 6 of the 7 cases (86%).[187] A 28-year follow-up study of 145 patients, particularly those with coxsackievirus B5 CNS infection during childhood, demonstrated an increased risk for adult onset of schizophrenia or other psychoses.[193] In a group of 15 children who had meningoencephalitis due to coxsackievirus B5, 2 were reported to have developed spasticity, and their intelligence was low.[194] Epidemiologic and serologic studies suggest a role for intrauterine coxsackievirus infection for the onset of insulin-dependent diabetes mellitus (IDDM) in childhood.[195–197] However, conflicting serologic data exist that do not indicate an association of coxsackievirus infections during pregnancy with the development of islet autoantibodies; these results do not support a major role of fetal coxsackievirus infection in the development of IDDM.[198,199]

Infection with coxsackievirus A in neonates has been reported less frequently than with coxsackievirus B. Coxsackievirus A infection has been associated with small–for–gestational-age newborns,[172] sudden infant death,[200–202] anorexia, fever, bronchopneumonia, pericarditis, and meningitis.[165]

A number of reports have confirmed that coxsackieviruses may be responsible for outbreaks of apparent infections with fatalities among neonates in obstetric wards and maternity homes.[203–205] Most commonly, mild nonspecific febrile illness is observed in full-term infants. A careful history frequently reveals a trivial illness in a family member. Feeding difficulties are frequently observed, and short periods of vomiting and diarrhea may occur. The most consistent source of original nursery infection is coxsackievirus transmission from mother to her child, but introduction of the virus into the nursery by personnel also occurs. After infection of the pharynx and lower alimentary tract, minor viremia with spread to regional lymph nodes and secondary infection sites (CNS, heart, liver, pancreas, respiratory tract, skin) occurs on the third day. Major viremia ceases with the appearance of antibodies on day 7. Infection can continue in the lower intestinal tract for prolonged periods, and isolation measures are warranted.[165]

Management Options

Prenatal, Labor, and Delivery

Coxsackievirus infections during late pregnancy seem to be a common event, in particular during late summer and early autumn in temperate climates. Epidemics in the region may be signaled by the occurrence of aseptic meningitis, pleurodynia, or Bornholm's disease (myalgia epidemica). Unseasonal respiratory tract infection or symptoms of fever, muscle pain, neck stiffness, skin rashes, and vesicular lesions (mouth, hand, foot) are suggestive of an enteroviral infection. Ultrasound examination in some cases may reveal an enlarged fetal heart with dilated chambers and unusually thick myocardium. Fetal arrythmias and congestive heart failure in combination with nonimmune hydrops may be treated by maternal digoxin or other agents (see Chapter 15) (oral digoxin at 0.5 mg loading, and 0.125–0.25 mg/day maintenance dose). Conversion of fetal arrhythmia to normal sinus rhythm and, consequently, spontaneous resolution of hydrops may be observed. If a woman is suspected of having an acute coxsackievirus infection, she is a potential risk for transmitting coxsackievirus in the obstetric wards. Isolation measures for delivery, newborn care, and postpartum care are warranted.[165] Coxsackievirus infection in the adult usually takes a benign course. If delivery occurs within 4 days of maternal infection, the newborn is at risk for severe disease.

Postnatal

No specific therapy is available to treat coxsackievirus infection in the newborn. Commercially available immune serum globulin contains titers of antibodies to coxsackievirus; however, no beneficial clinical effect has been observed when administered to an infected infant.[206,207] However, viremia and viruria ceased earlier in treated infants than in the control group. Some studies with new antiviral drugs (e.g., pleconaril) seem promising.[208]

In most cases, transmission of coxsackievirus occurs by direct contact from mother or staff members to the newborn or by mouth and gavage feeding. Coxsackievirus B and echoviruses have been recovered from specimens obtained from nurses and physicians caring for infected patients.[205] Rigorous attention to hygienic measures and handwashing after handling each baby are imperative to avoid the transmission of enteroviruses. Infected newborns should be isolated, and closure on the neonatal unit to new admissions has been advocated.[165]

In sudden and virulent nursery outbreaks passive immunization by intramuscular or intravenous immunoglobulin can be useful in preventing disease.[206,209]

A vaccine to prevent coxsackievirus infection is not available. However, an experimental attenuated vaccine has been developed.[210] Because of the considerable morbidity and mortality associated with coxsackievirus B infection in neonates (and in older persons as well), these agents should be candidates for vaccine development.

SUMMARY OF MANAGEMENT OPTIONS

Coxsackievirus

Management Options	Evidence Quality and Recommendation	References
Prenatal, Labor, and Delivery		
Suspect coxsackievirus infection if unseasonal respiratory tract infection and/or clinical signs of meningitis.	—/GPP	—
Treat infections symptomatically (hospitalize severe cases).	—/GPP	—
Evaluate hydropic fetuses for tachyarrhythmia, congestive heart failure; see Chapters 15, 16, and 24 for management options.	—/GPP	—
Deliver women suspected for acute coxsackievirus infection in an isolated unit.	IV/C	165
Postnatal		
Isolate women known to have coxsackievirus infection during postpartum care.	IV/C	165
Maintain strict attention to infection control measures.	IV/C	165
Provide clinical, microbiologic, and serologic evaluation of the newborn if acute maternal infection is present within the peripartum period.		
Isolate newborns of mothers suspected of having coxsackievirus infection.	IV/C	165
Consider passive immunization of newborns in case of sudden virulent coxsackievirus infection outbreak.	III/B	206,209

GPP, good practice point.

HUMAN PAPILLOMAVIRUS

General

Human papillomavirus (HPV) is a double-stranded DNA virus that can persist as a latent provirus in epithelial cells after infection. Nucleotide sequencing of the DNA has identified more than 100 genotypes of HPV associated with epithelial neoplasias of the skin and mucosa. More than 30 different HPV types can infect the genital tract, and 8 HPV types are predominantly identified in the most common HPV-associated genital diseases.

HPV types 6 and 11 are detected in more than 90% of condylomata acuminata (genital warts), and also in laryngeal papillomatosis, and conjunctival, oral, and nasal warts. HPV types 16, 18, 31, 33, 51, and 54 have been designated high risk HPV types because they have been strongly associated with cervical intraepithelial neoplasia (CIN) and cervical cancer.[211] Genital warts are contagious and are spread during oral, genital, or anal sex. About two thirds of people who have sex with a partner with genital warts will develop warts, usually within 3 months after contact.

Diagnosis

The diagnosis of condylomata acuminata can be made visually by the appearance of white or pink verrucous friable growths. However, most cases of HPV infection are subclinical. Cytologic evaluation of the Pap smear may reveal evidence of infection in 31% to 71% of cases, depending on age.[212] If koilocytosis is noted on the Pap smear, liberal use of colposcopy is warranted, given the association of HPV infection and CIN. Colposcopy may identify up to 70% of infected cases; however, colposcopy during pregnancy is challenging. Directed biopsies can support diagnostic evaluation in certain cases (e.g., unresponsiveness to therapy, uncertain clinical diagnosis). During pregnancy, limiting biopsy to lesions suspicious for CIN 2 or 3 or cancer is preferred, but biopsy of any lesion is acceptable. Biopsy during pregnancy has not been linked to fetal loss or preterm delivery, whereas failure to perform biopsy during pregnancy has been linked to missed invasive cancer.[95,212] The goal of cytology and colposcopy during pregnancy is to identify invasive cancer that requires treatment before or at the time of delivery. However, unless cancer is identified or suspected, treatment of CIN is contraindicated during pregnancy.[212] HPV isolation in culture is difficult to accomplish. Highly specific and sensitive DNA methods utilizing type-specific HPV gene probes can identify HPV infection in vaginal washings, Pap smears, and amniotic fluid. In situ hybridization technique is useful to demonstrate type-specific HPV infection in tissues and cervical cell scrapings. PCR methods can identify even the lowest levels of HPV infection in blood and other kinds of fluids or in tissue samples. Identification of high risk HPV types might prove helpful for follow-up strategies of women in whom cervical cytology has demonstrated atypical squamous cells of undetermined significance (ASCUS).[212] The usefulness of DNA technology in the clinical diagnosis of genital warts is not supported by any data.[95] Routine screening for subclinical HPV infection by DNA tests should be reserved for women aged 30 years and older.[95,212]

Maternal and Fetal Risks

Epidemiologic data suggest that HPV infection is the most prevalent STD. Although the occurrence of grossly visible genital warts is infrequent, sensitive detection tests utilizing dot blot DNA analysis or PCR for detection of HPV DNA indicate that as many as 30% of sexually active adults in the United States may be infected,[213] with a similar rate seen in pregnancy.[214] The highest rates of genital HPV infection (71%) are detected in adults aged 18 to 28. Many adolescents experience multiple sequential HPV infections; thus, repetitively positive HPV DNA tests in this group may represent consecutive incident infections rather than a single persistent infection. Consequently, routine subclinical HPV screening should not be used in this age group, and if inadvertently performed, a positive result should not influence management.[212] Major risk factors to acquiring genital HPV infection include multiple sex partners, younger age at first intercourse and first pregnancy, oral contraceptive use, pregnancy, and impairment of cell-mediated immunity.[213,215,216] Estimates indicate that approximately 1% of the sexually active population have clinically apparent genital warts.[213] Controversial data exist on a possible increase in the prevalence of HPV infections during pregnancy. A threefold increase in HPV DNA–positive women during the third trimester compared with nonpregnant controls has been reported.[217,218] Possible underlying reasons to facilitate HPV infection during late pregnancy could involve hormonal changes inducing virus transcription and the transient immunosuppression experienced by pregnant women.

Genital HPV infections in pregnant women have long been suspected to cause genital warts or laryngeal papillomatosis in the respective infants.[219] Juvenile laryngeal papillomatosis represents the most common neoplasm of the larynx in infants and young children and usually occurs by age 5.[220] The symptoms range from hoarseness to complete upper airway obstruction. A history of genital warts can be obtained from over 50% of women whose infants subsequently develop laryngeal papillomatosis.[221] However, the absolute risk of laryngeal papillomatosis following exposure to maternal infection is extremely low. Conservative estimates suggest the risk of papillomatosis developing in an offspring of a mother with HPV genital infection is approximately 1 in 400.[220] Surgical excision is the mainstream therapy, and most afflicted patients experience spontaneous remission. However, some endure several hundred surgical procedures. Further development of new antiviral drugs (e.g., cidofovir) and preventive and therapeutic vaccines hold promise for reducing the incidence of recurrent respiratory papillomatosis and, at best, eliminating the virus.[222,223] Genital warts in children show spontaneous resolution in up to 75% of cases. In a cohort of 41 children, overall resolution of condylomata was noted in 31 infants (76%), with spontaneous resolution in 22 of 41 (54%); girls were affected three times more often than boys.[224] HPV vaccination should reduce the incidence of vertical HPV transmission.[225]

Vertical transmission and persistence of high risk cancer-associated HPV in the infant is of great concern.[226] Amniotic fluid samples of 37 women with cervical lesions tested positive for HPV in 24 cases (65%) using PCR technique.[227] HPV type 16 amniotic fluid infection was present in 54% (13/24), and HPV type 18 was detected in 21% (5/24). A correlation was noted between viral DNA amplification and grade of the cervical lesions. In a group of 11 women carrying HPV type 16, 7 infants of 11 (64%) tested positive for HPV type 16.[228] Viruses were detected in buccal or genital swabs collected 24 hours after delivery, demonstrating infection rather than contamination. Persistence of HPV type 16 infection after a 6-month interval was noted in 83% of infants. In 270 healthy children between the ages of 3 and 11, 131 (49%) buccal swabs tested positive for HPV type 16. Serologic study performed on 229 children demonstrated IgM seropositivity rates indicative of acute infection that peaked between ages 2 and 5, and again between ages 13 and 16.[228] Thus, given the lack of demonstrable disease in children, consequences of perinatal high risk HPV transmission need to be clarified in long-term studies to establish whether perinatal acquisition of high risk HPV types predisposes for an increased risk of cervical neoplasia later in life.

The frequency of perinatal HPV transmission is a controversial subject. Transmission rates may be as low as 2.8%–12.2%,[228–230] whereas other studies demonstrate vertical transmission in up to 73% of newborns.[231] Discrepancies in infection rates of the newborn may be due to different PCR techniques, with up to a 100-fold difference in sensitivity, differences in study population (e.g., concomitant STDs), sampling technique (nasopharyngeal, buccal, genital), and timing (immediately after birth, contamination versus infection). HPV is thought to cause infection in the infant by direct contact during the passage through the birth canal. However, several studies have shown infants being infected with different strains of HPV despite being delivered by cesarean section.[232,233] In a study of 68 HPV-positive women, 35 delivered vaginally and 33 by cesarean section,[234] at 3 to 4 days of age, buccal and genital swabs were collected. In the group of vaginally born infants, 18 of 35 (51%) had a positive HPV test, whereas in 9 of 33 (27%) infants delivered by cesarean section, HPV was detected. Although the study did show a lower incidence of HPV infection in infants delivered by cesarean section, the study also demonstrated that cesarean section did not consistently protect from vertical HPV transmission. In addition, the presence of HPV has been demonstrated in amniotic fluid, placenta, and cord blood; thus, the fetus is at risk for exposure to the virus prior to delivery.[227,230,231,233,235]

Management Options

Prepregnancy

Parents and women should be advised on HPV vaccination. Two vaccines, a bivalent (HPV 16, 18) and a quadrivalent (HPV 6, 11, 16, 18) are available. Vaccine efficacy for the prevention of the primary composite endpoint (CIN grades 2–3, adenocarcinoma in situ, or cervical cancer related to HPV-16 or HPV-18) was greater than 90%. The quadrivalent vaccine also demonstrated high efficacy against HPV-6 and HPV-11 related external genital lesions. Maximum efficacy is suggested in girls receiving the vaccine prior to sexual activity. However, women who were already infected with one or more of the respective HPV types targeted by the vaccine were protected from clinical disease caused by the remaining HPV types in the vaccine.[236] The recommended age for vaccination of girls is 11 to 12 years, with catch-up vaccination for females aged 13 to 26 years who have not been previously vaccinated. Vaccination during pregnancy is not advocated; however, it appears to be safe.[237] Finishing trials on HPV vaccination of women aged 30 to 45 years are under way. Vaccination of males has been approved in 40 countries worldwide, including a recent permissive approval for the quadrivalent vaccine in the United States.

Widely applied HPV vaccination holds the promise of greatly reducing the incidence of genital warts, precancerous lesions, vulvovaginal and cervical cancer, as well as penile and anal cancer. In addition, reduction of severe respiratory problems due to a laryngopapillomtosis in children infected by vertical transmission from their mothers during pregnancy is expected to occur. Vaccination is not a substitute for routine cervical cancer screening, and vaccinated females should have cervical cancer screening as recommended.[225]

Patients should be counseled on the nature of genital warts and advised on using protection (e.g., latex condoms) when having sex with an infected partner.[216] Some genital warts may resolve spontaneously; however, treatment should be considered for expanding genital warts. Treatment for genital warts reduces but does not eradicate infectivity. In nonpregnant women, podophyllum resin 10% to 25% antimitotic solution, podofilox 0.5% solution, and 5-fluorouracil are commonly used for topical treatment. However, they should not be applied during pregnancy because of the potential for fetal toxicity. All treatments show a 10% to 40% probability of recurrence. Intralesional injections of different types of interferon have demonstrated efficacy comparable with other modalities for the treatment of genital warts; however, use of interferons has been frequently associated with systemic adverse effects.[238] Interferons should not be used during pregnancy.[239] Although some HPV types are associated with CIN and cervical cancer, HPV infection does not necessarily progress to cancer. It is important for women with a history of abnormal Pap smears to receive appropriate cytologic testing on a regular basis so that early treatment, if necessary, can be instituted.

Prenatal

There is no single definitive treatment for HPV infection in pregnancy. Treatment is dependent on the size, location, and number of identified lesions and entails the removal or ablation of all visible warts. Owing to the subclinical and multifocal nature of HPV infection, recurrences are common. Certain treatment modalities that are effective in the nonpregnant patient are contraindicated during pregnancy.

In pregnant women, topical application of 80% to 90% trichloroacetic acid (TCA) can be used for small lesions and is the least expensive treatment.[240] TCA is not absorbed systemically and can be used in pregnancy. However, it has a cure rate of only 20% to 30% after a single application; therefore, weekly applications may be required until the lesions are resolved. TCA solutions have a low viscosity and can spread rapidly, thus damaging adjacent tissues. If an excess amount is applied, the treated area should be powdered with talc, sodium bicarbonate, or liquid soap preparations to remove unreacted acid.[95] Cryotherapy with liquid nitrogen has also been successfully used in pregnancy and is a reasonable first-line treatment option. Cryotherapy is not recommended for use in the vagina because of the risk of vaginal perforation and fistula formation.[95,238] Surgical removal by tangential scissor excision, tangential shave excision, curettage, or electrosurgery has the advantage of eliminating warts at a single visit in most cases.[238] Carbon dioxide laser vaporization has been used successfully in pregnancy, although recurrence rates of 10% to 14% have been reported. In particular, laser therapy is recommended for those patients with large or multiple lesions or with lesions refractory to TCA application or cryotherapy.[240] Recurrences usually occur during the first 3 months after treatment, and a follow-up evaluation should be offered.

Imiquimod 5% cream, an immune-response modulator that induces host T helper-1 (Th-1) cytokines, including interferon-γ, has been demonstrated to be effective in eradicating genital warts when applied topically three times weekly in nonpregnant patients. Although not yet recommended in pregnancy, imiquimod may represent an effective alternative to other topical or destructive therapies during pregnancy. New antiviral drugs (e.g., cidofovir) have not been evaluated for safety and efficacy during pregnancy.[241]

Labor and Delivery

Elective debulking of genital warts should not be done at the time of delivery for two reasons: first, these lesions may be very vascular and obstetric hemorrhage may ensue; second, most lesions regress to some extent after delivery.

Because of the lack of substantial evidence for the preventive value of cesarean delivery, cesarean section should not be performed solely to prevent transmission of HPV infection to the newborn.[95] However, cesarean section may be indicated in women with genital warts obstructing the pelvic outlet or when vaginal delivery would result in excessive bleeding.

Postnatal

Large lesions should be observed for secondary infection, if they involve an episiotomy site. Sitz baths may be particularly useful in comforting and cleansing the perineal area with multiple HPV lesions.

Parents should be counseled on HPV vaccination in order to reduce HPV infection and related disease in the future.[225,236]

SUMMARY OF MANAGEMENT OPTIONS
Human Papillomavirus

Management Options	Evidence Quality and Recommendation	References
Prepregnancy		
Counsel about HPV vaccination	IIa/B	225
Identify and treat lesions:	—/GPP	—
• Topical therapy (podophyllum, podofilox, 5-fluorouracil).		
• Ablation (e.g., cryocautery).		
• Removal.		
Counsel about risks (infectious condition) and use of condoms if partner infected.	IIa/B	216,226
Advise that treatment does not eradicate infectivity.	—/GPP	—
Implications from cervical smear screening programs:	—/GPP	—
If Pap smear reports ASCUS but no other types of abnormalities:		
• Consider HPV testing.	Ib/A	212
If Pap smear reports ASCUS, and high risk HPV types are detected:		
• Perform colposcopy, consider biopsy.	Ib/A	212
• Perform pelvic examination, Pap smear on a regular basis.	Ib/A	212
Screening for subclinical HPV infection is not recommended in women aged 29 and younger.	IV/C	212
Prenatal		
Topical 80% TCA.	III/B	240
Cryotherapy.	IV/C	238
Electrodiathermy.	IV/C	238
Laser vaporization (carbon dioxide).	III/B	240
Excision (tangential scissors, excision, curettage).	IV/C	238
Contraindicated preparations:		
• Podophyllum.	IV/C	238
• Podofilox.	—/GPP	—
• 5-Fluorouracil.	—/GPP	—
• Interferon	IV/C	237
Counsel about low newborn risk, and about nature of HPV infection in the infant.	—/GPP	—

SUMMARY OF MANAGEMENT OPTIONS

Human Papillomavirus—cont'd

Management Options	Evidence Quality and Recommendation	References
Labor and Delivery		
Avoid treatment at delivery, especially debulking, because of risk of hemorrhage.	—/GPP	—
Cesarean section may be indicated in women with genital warts obstructing labor or vaginal delivery that would result in excessive bleeding; not recommended solely to prevent HPV transmission to the infant.	III/B	95
Postnatal		
Maintain vigilance for secondary infection, especially in episiotomy site.	—/GPP	—
Offer sitz baths.	—/GPP	—

ASCUS, atypical squamous cells of undetermined significance; GPP, good practice point; HPV, human papilloma virus; TCA, trichloroacetic acid.

SUGGESTED READINGS

Boppana SB, Rivera LB, Fowler KB, et al: Intrauterine transmission of cytomegalovirus to infants of women with preconceptional immunity. N Engl J Med 2001;344:1366–1371.

Brown ZA, Wald A, Morrow A, et al: Effect of serologic status and caesarean delivery on transmission rates of herpes simplex virus from mother to infant. JAMA 2003;289:203–209.

Cheeran MC, Lokensgard JR, Schleiss MR: Neuropathogenesis of congenital cytomegalovirus infection: Disease mechanisms and prospects for intervention. Clin Microbiol Rev 2009;22:99–126.

Corey L, Wald A, Patel R, et al: Once daily valacyclovir reduces transmission of genital herpes. N Engl J Med 2004;343:11–20.

FUTURE II Study Group: Quadrivalent vaccine against human papillomavirus to prevent high-grade cervical lesions. N Engl J Med 2007;356:1915–1927.

Ross DS, Dollard SC, Victor M, et al: The epidemiology and prevention of congenital cytomegalovirus infection and disease: Activities of the Centers for Disease Control and Prevention Workgroup. J Womens Health 2006;15:224–229.

Sheffield JS, Wendel GD, Laibl V, et al: Valacyclovir prophylaxis to prevent recurrent herpes at delivery: A randomized controlled trial. Obstet Gynecol 2006;108:1550–1552.

REFERENCES

For a complete list of references, log onto www.expertconsult.com.

CHAPTER 31

Other Infectious Conditions

MARK H. YUDIN

INTRODUCTION

Infections are an important contributor to maternal and perinatal morbidity and mortality rates. The relative immunosuppression that occurs during pregnancy may alter the natural course of many infectious diseases. Higher attack rates for a variety of bacterial and viral infections are seen in pregnancy. Furthermore, many of these infections may be associated with adverse outcomes, including preterm labor and delivery, low birth weight, and stillbirth. This chapter addresses a large group of infectious diseases and conditions not discussed in other chapters, including streptococcal infections, listeriosis, common sexually transmitted infections (STIs), and vaginitis.

GROUP A STREPTOCOCCUS

Group A streptococcus (GAS; *Streptococcus pyogenes*) has been associated with obstetric and neonatal infections since the 16th century. It is probable that GAS was responsible for much of puerperal sepsis, or "childbed fever," described by Semmelweis in 19th-century Vienna.[1] However, with the advent of the antibiotic era, GAS infections became increasingly infrequent until the 1980s, when GAS infections dramatically increased again for poorly understood reasons.[2] GAS causes a broad spectrum of invasive and noninvasive diseases, including bacterial pharyngitis, impetigo, scarlet fever, necrotizing fasciitis, and the more recently recognized streptococcal toxic shock syndrome (STSS), as outlined in Table 31–1.[2,3]

S. pyogenes, the etiologic agent for GAS infections, was first described by Louis Pasteur in 1879. The *Streptococcus* genus is classified into groups, based upon polysaccharide capsular antigens and the cell wall M protein, as first described by Lancefield.[4] *S. pyogenes* is divided into serotypes according to the M protein, and to date, more than 80 M protein serotypes have been identified. Different serotypes are associated with different forms of infection, and M1 and M3 have been the most common serotypes identified in serious infection in more recent years.[5]

M protein is also important as a virulence factor because of its antiphagocytic properties. Other significant virulence factors are the streptococcal pyrogenic exotoxins (SPE), which act as superantigens. Superantigens are able to bind to T-cell receptors and the class II major histocompatibility complex (MHC) without first undergoing antigen processing and presentation. The cross-linking of a T-cell receptor with a class II MHC molecule by a superantigen stimulates the proliferation and activation of T cells and macrophages, causing them to release large amounts of cytokines, which can cause shock or inflammation and tissue damage.[2,6] A large number of SPE superantigens have been identified, but SPE A, SPE B, SPE C, SPE F, and streptococcal superantigen (SSA) are among the best characterized. By stimulating cytokine production, these streptococcal exotoxins likely play an important role in the pathogenicity of invasive GAS infections by exacerbating the onset of clinical signs and symptoms of infection.

Maternal and Fetal Risks

GAS may be recovered from the skin or mucous membranes of asymptomatic colonized patients. GAS may gain entry to the body via the skin, mucosa, pharynx, and vagina and cause infections with both suppurative and nonsuppurative complications.[2,7] The most notable GAS infections encountered during pregnancy are presented in Table 31–2 and include bacteremia without a focus of infection and endometritis, but invasive infections including STSS and necrotizing fasciitis also occur. The reasons for the increased susceptibility seen during the puerperium include the breach of integrity in the integumentary system associated with either vaginal delivery or cesarean section. Invasive infections are characterized by hypotension and shock, multiple organ failure, systemic toxicity, severe local pain, rapid necrosis of subcutaneous tissues and skin, renal dysfunction, and fever.[2,7] GAS invasive disease is characterized by a rapid, often fatal course and by difficulties in the early diagnosis, when intervention may be more successful.

Postpartum invasive GAS infection occurs in approximately 1 in 11,000 to 1 in 17,000 births, with an average of 220 cases occurring in the United States every year.[8,9] The rate of invasive GAS infection is 1.6- to 2.0-fold greater among black patients than white patients.[8] Maternal case fatality rate ranges from 3.5% to 30% in postpartum invasive GAS. Maternal GAS disease has also been associated with stillbirth.

TABLE 31–1

Classification of Group A Streptococcal Infections

1. Streptococcal toxic shock syndrome (streptococcal TSS)
2. Other invasive infections (isolation of *Streptococcus pyogenes* from a normally sterile site in patients not fulfilling criteria from streptococcal TSS)
   a. Bacteremia with no identifiable focus
   b. Focal infection with or without bacteremia (meningitis, pneumonia, peritonitis, puerperal sepsis, osteomyelitis, septic arthritis, necrotizing fasciitis, surgical wound infections, erysipelas, cellulitis)
3. Scarlet fever
4. Noninvasive infections (recovery of *S. pyogenes* from a nonsterile site)
   a. Mucous membranes (pharyngitis, tonsillitis, otitis media, sinusitis, vaginitis)
   b. Cutaneous (impetigo)
5. Nonsuppurative sequelae (specific clinical findings with evidence of a recent group A streptococcal infection)
   a. Acute rheumatic fever
   b. Acute glomerulonephritis

Adapted from The Working Group on Severe Streptococcal Infections: Defining the group A streptococcal toxic shock syndrome. JAMA 1993;269:390–391.

TABLE 31–2

Diseases Seen among Patients with Postpartum Group A Streptococcus Infection

INFECTION	NUMBER OF PATIENTS (*N* = 87)
Bacteremia without focus	40 (46%)
Endometritis	24 (28%)
Peritonitis	7 (8%)
Septic abortion	6 (7%)
Cellulitis	3 (3%)
Septic arthritis	3 (3%)
Necrotizing fasciitis	3 (3%)
Streptococcal toxic shock syndrome	3 (3%)
Chorioamnionitis	3 (3%)
Pneumonia	1 (1%)
Other	3 (3%)

Adapted from Chuang I, Van Beneden C, Beall B, Schuchat A: Population-based surveillance for postpartum invasive group A streptococcus infections, 1995–2000. Clin Infect Dis 2002;35:665–670.

Neonatal invasive GAS has also been reported and has a case fatality rate of up to 30%.[9–11] Although the neonate may be colonized following horizontal transmission within the nursery, vertical transmission from a colonized mother has also been demonstrated.[10,12] Furthermore, 50% of neonatal cases of invasive GAS disease occur within the first week of life, suggesting that vertical transmission from a colonized parturient may be the most important route of infection. The most frequent manifestation of neonatal GAS disease is omphalitis, but cellulitis, meningitis, sepsis, and fasciitis may also occur. Fortunately, neonatal GAS disease is rare, with an estimated incidence of 1 in 18,000 births.

TABLE 31–3

Diagnostic Criteria for Streptococcal Toxic Shock Syndrome

I. Isolation of *Streptococcus pyogenes*
   A. From a normally sterile site
   B. From a nonsterile site (throat, sputum, vagina, superficial skin lesion)
II. Clinical evidence of severity
   A. Hypotension (systolic blood pressure ≤ 90 mm Hg in adults or ≤ 5th percentile for age in children) and
   B. Two or more of the following:
      1. Renal impairment (serum creatinine ≥ 2.0 mg/dL or a twofold elevation over baseline level in patients with preexisting renal impairment)
      2. Coagulopathy (platelets ≤ 100 × 10^6/L or disseminated intravascular coagulation)
      3. Liver involvement (AST, ALT, or total bilirubin ≥ two times upper limits of normal)
      4. Adult respiratory distress syndrome
      5. Generalized erythematous macular rash
      6. Soft tissue necrosis (necrotizing fasciitis, myositis, or gangrene)

ALT, alanine aminotransferase; AST, aspartate aminotransferase.
Adapted from The Working Group on Severe Streptococcal Infections: Defining the group A streptococcal toxic shock syndrome. JAMA 1993;269:390–391.

Diagnosis

GASs can be readily recovered from most patients with evidence of GAS disease. GASs are catalase-negative gram-positive cocci that are β-hemolytic on blood agar. The colonies may appear as highly mucoid to nonmucoid, and the organisms are usually 1 to 2 mm in diameter. Although cultures may be helpful in confirming the diagnosis of GAS disease, they are seldom available when considering the initial diagnosis. GAS disease may progress rapidly, and therapy must be initiated before cultures are generally available.

Therefore, the diagnosis of GAS disease depends upon a high index of suspicion. Fever is the most common presenting sign, and 20% of patients have a flulike syndrome with fever, chills, myalgia, nausea, vomiting, and diarrhea.[13] Confusion or altered mental status is present in over one half of patients. Renal dysfunction occurs in 80% of patients and may precede hypotension or shock. The presence of hemaglobinuria or an elevated serum creatinine is evidence of renal involvement. Hemoconcentration, as a result of a fluid shift to the extravascular compartment, and leukocytosis (often > 20,000/mm^3), with a predominance of immature neutrophils, are common. Respiratory failure and adult respiratory distress syndrome occur in approximately 50% of patients but usually develop after the onset of clinically recognized shock. Criteria for the diagnosis of STSS are outlined in Table 31–3.

Eighty percent of patients have evidence of soft tissue infection characterized by induration and erythema, which progress to necrotizing fasciitis in 70% of cases.[13] The hallmark of these soft tissue infections is the abrupt onset of severe pain, which usually precedes physical findings or is out of proportion to physical findings. Any patient suspected of having GAS-associated necrotizing fasciitis must have the diagnosis confirmed by immediate wound exploration and débridement. A purulent discharge is usually not present, and a limited wound inspection may fail to confirm the diagnosis. When the wound is opened, a thin, watery, nonmalodorous discharge is frequently present. The diagnosis of necrotizing fasciitis can be easily confirmed by the bloodless blunt dissection of the superficial fascia and by pathologic frozen section.

In summary, the diagnosis of GAS disease should be considered in any patient with the sudden onset of hypotension and shock, the abrupt onset of severe pain in a wound, or systemic signs and symptoms such as confusion, renal impairment, or respiratory distress in a patient with a wound or episiotomy infection. Aggressive intravenous fluid resuscitation, antibiotic therapy, and wound débridement are necessary in these patients.

Management Options

Prepregnancy

No current evidence suggests that the identification of GAS carriers prior to pregnancy is predictive of subsequent pregnancy outcome or effective in reducing puerperal infectious morbidity. Therefore, prepregnancy screening is not recommended.

Prenatal

Women may be identified as being GAS carriers as a result of routine screening for group B streptococcus (GBS) near the end of pregnancy. In one study, 0.03% of women screened at 35 to 37 weeks' gestation were found to have vaginal colonization with GAS.[14] At present, there are not sufficient data to make a recommendation regarding management of asymptomatic carriers. However, there are published case reports of women identified as carriers during pregnancy who then developed GAS sepsis after delivery.[15] A case of puerperal sepsis in a woman with a strain of GAS identical to that identified in her husband's throat swab has also been reported.[16]

A high index of suspicion is necessary for the early diagnosis of GAS infection. Unfortunately, diagnosis may be difficult in the early stages of GAS infection, and delays in therapy may be associated with increased morbidity and mortality rates. Many patients die within 24 to 48 hours of infection.[17] In general, treatment must be directed at hemodynamic stabilization with intravenous fluids and vasopressors, antibiotic therapy, and in the case of soft tissue infections, surgical exploration and aggressive débridement of involved tissues. Massive amounts of intravenous crystalloids, in the range of 10 to 20 L/day, are often necessary to maintain blood pressure and tissue perfusion. Vasopressors such as dopamine are also frequently required. In soft tissue GAS infections such as necrotizing fasciitis, antibiotic therapy alone, without surgical débridement, usually results in maternal death. Intraoperative Gram stain and histologic frozen section may be necessary to fully delineate the extent of involved tissues. Hyperbaric oxygen therapy has no role in the treatment of necrotizing fasciitis but might be a useful adjunct in delineating necrotic tissue that must be surgically débrided.

Broad-spectrum parenteral antibiotics should be administered promptly. Penicillin G (200,000–400,000 U/kg/day) is the drug of choice for GAS invasive infections. However, studies in mice have demonstrated that even a short delay of 2 hours after initiation of infection dramatically reduces the efficacy of penicillin G.[17] Some studies indicate that clindamycin may be more efficacious than penicillin when therapy is delayed. In an experimental model with mice, survival was 70% even when initiated 16 hours after GAS infection.[17] Several potential advantages to clindamycin therapy (900 mg IV q8h) have been identified.[7] First, in contrast to penicillins, clindamycin is not affected by bacterial inoculum size or rate of growth. Second, clindamycin suppresses the synthesis of bacterial toxins. Third, clindamycin facilitates phagocytosis of *S. pyogenes* by inhibition of M protein synthesis. Fourth, clindamycin has a longer postantibiotic effect than penicillin. Last, clindamycin suppresses lipopolysaccharide-induced monocyte synthesis of tumor necrosis factor-alpha (TNF-α), a cytokine that contributes to hypotension and shock. However, a small proportion of GAS infections are resistant to clindamycin, and clindamycin should not be used alone until the organism is demonstrated to be susceptible by susceptibility testing. Therefore, initial therapy usually includes a combination of both penicillin G and clindamycin.

Some data also indicate that intravenous immunoglobulin (IVIG) (1–2 g/kg given once) may be a useful adjunct to antibiotic therapy in the treatment of STSS. Commercial preparations of IVIG have been shown to contain neutralizing antibodies to several streptococcal virulence factors.[18] Recently, investigators reported a significant reduction in mortality rate among patients with GAS disease treated with IVIG when compared with a historical cohort.

Thus, the optimal treatment for invasive GAS disease includes a high index of suspicion, aggressive fluid resuscitation and hemodynamic support, surgical exploration and aggressive débridement, parenteral antibiotics including penicillin G and clindamycin, and possibly IVIG.

Labor and Delivery

GAS may be associated with intra-amniotic infection and with stillbirth. However, most patients with invasive GAS disease usually present in the postpartum period, frequently within the first 24 to 48 hours. Treatment should follow the general guidelines provided earlier.

Postnatal

There are no current recommendations for screening for or treating asymptomatic parturients colonized with GAS. However, careful attention should be given to any parturient with the sudden onset of systemic signs such as hypotension or shock or to parturients with severe pain out of proportion of physical findings or rapidly progressive soft tissue infections, as noted earlier. Although these findings, which are consistent with necrotizing fasciitis, usually suggest a polymicrobial infection, GAS should be considered in the diagnosis, and broad-spectrum antibiotics including penicillin and clindamycin should be utilized in the initial management.

SUMMARY OF MANAGEMENT OPTIONS

Group A Streptococcal Infection

Management Options	Evidence Quality and Recommendation	References
Prepregnancy		
No benefit to screening.	—/GPP	—
Prenatal, Labor, and Delivery		
No benefit to screening.	—/GPP	—
May cause intra-amniotic infection.	—/GPP	—
Diagnosis requires a high index of suspicion: • Severe pain. • Hypotension or shock. • Altered mental status. • Renal or respiratory impairment.	III/B	13
Treatment requires prompt intervention: • IV antibiotics (penicillin G, clindamycin). • IV fluids and circulatory support including vasopressors. • IVIG in nonresponsive cases. • Surgical débridement if appropriate	Ib/A	17,18
Postnatal		
Infection may cause toxic shock syndrome or soft tissue infection.	—/GPP	—
Diagnosis requires a high index of suspicion: • Severe pain. • Hypotension or shock. • Altered mental status. • Renal or respiratory impairment.	III/B	13
Therapy: • Broad-spectrum antibiotics (penicillin and clindamycin). • Surgical wound exploration and débridement.	Ib/A	17,18

GPP, good practice point; IVIG, intravenous immunoglobulin.

GROUP B STREPTOCOCCUS

GBS (*Streptococcus agalactiae*) has become recognized since the 1980s as one of the most important causes of neonatal infection and is currently considered one of the leading infectious causes of neonatal morbidity and death. Although early reports in the 1930s and 1940s linked GBS with postpartum infections and neonatal meningitis, it was not until the early 1960s that the scope of perinatal and neonatal GBS infections became evident.[19] Initial case series reported case fatality rates as high as 50%. In the 1980s, trials of empirical intrapartum antibiotics to women at risk of transmitting infection to their newborns demonstrated a protective benefit against neonatal infection in the first week of life (early-onset disease). In the 1990s, these efforts led to the implementation of guidelines for intrapartum antibiotic prophylaxis of at-risk mothers, endorsed and issued by the American College of Obstetricians and Gynecologists (ACOG),[20] the Centers for Disease Control and Prevention (CDC),[21] and the American Academy of Pediatrics (AAP).[22] This practice has resulted in a significant reduction in early-onset disease, as well as a smaller impact on maternal morbidity. Based upon these results, updated guidelines were issued by the CDC in 2002[23] to recommend optimization of screening and treatment of pregnant women in an attempt to improve upon the success already demonstrated.

GBSs are one of many serologically distinct species within the genus *Streptococcus*. Streptococci are facultatively anaerobic gram-positive cocci, usually arranged in chains on Gram stain. The most important pathogenic streptococcal species for humans include group A (*S. pyogenes*), group B (*S. agalactiae*), group D (enterococci), *Streptococcus pneumoniae*, and *Streptococcus viridans*. Definitive identification is based on the presence of a polysaccharide group-specific antigen common to all group B streptococcal strains as determined by serologic testing. GBSs can be further subdivided into eight distinct serotypes (Ia, Ib, Ia/c, II, III, IV, V, and VI) on the basis of distinctive type-specific polysaccharide antigens. About 99% of strains can be typed into one of these six antigen types. GBSs can be recovered from the vagina or cervix in 10% to 30% of pregnant women at some point during gestation.[24] The colonization may be transient, chronic, or intermittent, and the rate of colonization does not vary with gestational age. Women with GBS colonization in one pregnancy are at increased risk, relative to women who are negative in the initial pregnancy, for colonization in a subsequent pregnancy.[25] There is evidence that the gastrointestinal tract is the major primary reservoir and that vaginal or cervical contamination and colonization occur from a gastrointestinal source. The frequency of GBS isolation increases as one proceeds from the cervix to the introitus, and GBS can be recovered twice as frequently from rectal cultures as from vaginal cultures. GBSs can also be recovered from the urethra of 45% to 63% of the male consorts of female carriers, implying that sexual transmission may also occur.

Neonatal GBS colonization may occur either by vertical transmission from a colonized mother as the neonate passes through the birth canal or by horizontal transmission, including both nosocomial spread in the nursery from colonized personnel or other colonized neonates and acquisition from community sources. Overall, 3% to 12% of all neonates are colonized with GBS in the first week of life. Forty percent to 70% of neonates born to colonized mothers become colonized, usually with the same serotype that is present in the mother. In contrast, only 1% to 12% of neonates born to noncolonized mothers will become culture-positive. Several additional factors may modify or enhance the risk of GBS vertical transmission. Higher neonatal transmission rates occur when women are persistently culture-positive carriers or when women are heavily colonized with GBS as demonstrated by semiquantitative vaginal cultures.[26] The site of maternal carriage is also important; vertical transmission is more likely to occur with cervical GBS carriage than with rectal carriage.

The most important determinant of susceptibility to invasive infection after colonization may be maternal antibodies directed against the capsular polysaccharide antigens of GBS. Immunity to GBS is mediated by antibody-dependent phagocytosis. Mothers of infants with type III GBS invasive disease have lower serum levels of type-specific antibodies than women giving birth to asymptomatically colonized infants. This antibody, which has some broad reactivity to all GBS types, is an immunoglobulin G (IgG) that readily crosses the placenta. When measured in mother-infant pairs, an excellent correlation exists between maternal and cord antibody levels. Baker and associates[27] demonstrated that 73% of 45 GBS-colonized mothers with healthy neonates had high serum levels of type III antibody in contrast to only 19% of 32 GBS-colonized mothers whose neonates developed early-onset septicemia or meningitis ($P < .001$). Strain virulence is also an important determinant of disease. Although type III strains of GBS represent approximately one third of isolates from symptomatically colonized infants, they account for over 85% of the isolates from early-onset meningitis or late-onset disease. Overall, type III strains account for more than 60% of isolates from infants with all varieties of invasive GBS infections.

Maternal and Fetal Risks

Although most research has focused on GBS neonatal infection, GBS is also an important pathogen for maternal intrapartum, postpartum, and occasionally prenatal infections. Data from an early report suggest puerperal septicemia due to GBS occurs with an incidence of approximately 1 to 2 per 1000 deliveries and accounts for up to 15% of positive blood cultures from postpartum patients.[28] Postpartum endometritis is reported to be more frequently observed among GBS-colonized parturients than among noncolonized parturients. GBS is also associated with clinical intra-amniotic infection and is a frequent isolate from amniotic fluid of patients with intra-amniotic infection. Finally, GBS has been isolated from the urine of pregnant women, with or without symptoms of urinary tract infection. Untreated antepartum GBS bacteriuria has been associated with intrapartum chorioamnionitis.[29]

GBS has also been associated with premature rupture of membranes (PROM) and with preterm delivery prior to the 32nd gestational week in some, but not all, studies.[30] Previous studies have indicated that this association may be strongest for patients with GBS bacteriuria.[31] Thomsen and coworkers[32] have demonstrated significant reductions in PROM and preterm labor among patients with asymptomatic GBS bacteriuria who were treated with penicillin. However, antepartum antibiotic treatment to eradicate GBS from patients with asymptomatic vaginal colonization without bacteriuria has not been demonstrated to alter pregnancy outcome. Thus, a causal relationship between GBS colonization and prematurity remains to be established.

Since the 1970s, GBS has become a leading cause of septicemia and meningitis during the first 3 months of life in neonates. Early surveillance data in the 1990s suggested an incidence of 1.8 cases per 1000 live births. Two distinct clinical syndromes occur among neonates with GBS infections. These differ in the age at onset, pathogenesis, and outcome. The first clinical syndrome, early-onset infection, occurs within the first 7 days of life and represents nearly three fourths of all cases in infants younger than 3 months. The mean age at onset is 20 hours of life, and 72% will present within the first 24 hours of life.[33] A significant portion of these infections are apparent at birth or become symptomatic within the first 90 minutes of life, indicating that in utero GBS exposure and infection often occur. Early infection attack rates were estimated at 1.5 per 1000 for all live births prior to widespread use of intrapartum antibiotics. Among offspring of maternal GBS carriers, however, the attack rate is much higher, ranging from 10 to 60 per 1000 live births.

Early neonatal infection is presumed to result from vertical transmission of GBS from a colonized mother. There is a direct relationship between neonatal attack rates and the size of the inoculum and number of colonized neonatal sites. In one epidemiologic review, early-onset infection presented as bacteremia (80%), pneumonia (7%), or meningitis (6%).[33] Eighty-three percent of cases were in term infants (≥37 wk' gestation). The overall case fatality rate was approximately 4% but was significantly higher in preterm infants, approaching 30% in infants of 33 weeks' gestation or less.

The second type of disease (late-onset infection) occurs in infants after the first week of life until 3 months of age, with a typical range of 3 to 4 weeks. The overall attack rate is estimated to be 0.5 cases per 1000 live births, and these cases represent 28% of infections in infants younger than 3 months.[33] In contrast to early-onset infection, nosocomial transmission may be as important as vertical transmission, although it is believed that some infants are colonized at birth, with subsequent development of invasive disease. The serotype distribution of strains recovered from late-onset infection does not reflect the serotypes present in the maternal genital tract; over 90% of late-onset infection is caused by type III GBS. Late-onset disease also presents most commonly as bacteremia (63%), but may appear as meningitis (24%, relative risk [RR] 4.3 vs. early-onset disease; $P < .001$) and may demonstrate other sites of infection, such as septic arthritis or osteomyelitis. The overall case fatality rate for late-onset disease is 2.8%.[33] Approximately 50% of meningitis survivors will have neurologic sequelae, including cortical blindness, diabetes insipidus, deafness or other cranial nerve deficits, and spasticity.

Diagnosis

The recommended technique for collecting specimens for culture of GBS in pregnant women involves obtaining a combined vaginal-rectal swab. Although some studies have shown that the GBS detection rate is not significantly different when comparing vaginal-rectal specimens with vaginal-perianal specimens,[34,35] the current standard of care is still to obtain a combined vaginal-rectal swab. A speculum is not necessary, and there is no difference in detection rates or accuracy if the culture is collected by the patient or the health care provider.[36]

GBS can be easily grown on selective or nonselective media. Most GBS colonies appear on blood plates as small, 1- to 2-mm, gray-white colonies surrounded by a zone of β-hemolysis, although 2% of strains are nonhemolytic. Preliminary identification and distinction of GBS from other streptococci is based on biochemical reactions including resistance to bacitracin, hydrolysis of sodium hippurate, and the production of a soluble hemolysin that acts synergistically with B-lysin of *Staphylococcus aureus* to produce hemolysis (CAMP [Christie-Atkins-Munch-Petersen] test). Although GBS can be recovered after overnight growth on nonselective media, such as blood agar, the use of a selective broth medium such as Todd-Hewitt broth or Lim broth greatly enhances the isolation rate of GBS from any culture site.

A major limitation of cultures is the length of time necessary for growth and identification. Therefore, research has been focused on developing a more rapid screening test that could be used at the time of labor and delivery to identify colonized women. A number of rapid screening tests have been developed to directly detect GBS in either body fluids or cervical-vaginal secretions. These culture-independent tests include Gram stain, latex particle agglutination (LPA), optical immunoassay, enzyme immunoassay, DNA hybridization, and polymerase chain reaction (PCR). A large number of studies have evaluated the ability of these indirect tests to rapidly detect GBS colonization of the maternal lower genital tract. Such identification is important to interrupt maternal-neonatal vertical transmission that leads to early-onset neonatal disease. Initial results were encouraging,[37,38] although subsequent studies have demonstrated that these tests do not always perform well.[39,40] PCR tests appear to have the most promise and the best test performance characteristics relative to culture.[41–43] Recent studies from the United States and Canada have used PCR assays that demonstrate excellent sensitivity and specificity compared with traditional culture methods, but these assays await further testing to determine the feasibility of widespread application.[43–45] A cost-benefit analysis showed that the use of a rapid PCR test resulted in fewer courses of maternal antibiotics, fewer perinatal GBS infections, and fewer infant deaths compared with culture.[46] However, only culture techniques currently allow for antibiotic sensitivity profiling of positive cultures, which is particularly important in cases of maternal penicillin hypersensitivity.

Management Options

Prepregnancy

No current evidence suggests that the identification of GBS carrier status prior to pregnancy is predictive of subsequent pregnancy outcome. Similarly, treatment of asymptomatic women found to be colonized with GBS prior to pregnancy does not impart any recognized benefit, with the possible exception of women with asymptomatic bacteriuria.

Prenatal, Labor, and Delivery

GBS rarely causes maternal symptoms in the prenatal period, but may cause symptoms of urinary tract infection. However, GBS bacteriuria (whether symptomatic or not) provides a significant risk factor for neonatal disease, as previously mentioned. When detected, GBS bacteriuria should be treated according to current standard of care for urinary tract infections during pregnancy. Pregnant women with documented GBS bacteriuria at any time during their prenatal course do not require routine screening cultures and should receive intrapartum antibiotics, which are discussed in further detail later.

Although the attack rate for neonatal GBS infection is low, a variety of prevention strategies have been advocated because of the high mortality and morbidity rates seen in neonatal GBS disease. These strategies have involved chemoprophylaxis, aimed at eradicating the organism from the mother or the neonate, or immunoprophylaxis, aimed at inducing humoral immunity.

Antibiotic chemoprophylaxis has been advocated for the pregnant patient in either the antepartum or the intrapartum period or for the neonate in the immediate neonatal period. Attempts to eradicate GBS colonization with antepartum treatment have been unsuccessful, and early neonatal prophylaxis is also frequently unsuccessful because many neonates are already septic at birth as a result of in utero infection.[47] Initial chemoprophylactic prevention strategies released in the 1990s focused upon selective intrapartum treatment based on either the presence of risk factors associated with neonatal infection, the maternal genital tract colonization, or both.

Major risk factors for neonatal early-onset GBS disease include low birth weight (<2500 g), premature delivery (<37 wk' gestation), prolonged duration of rupture of membranes (≥18 hr), and intrapartum fever (≥38.0°C). Boyer and colleagues[47] have demonstrated that 74% of neonates with early-onset infection and 94% of those infections with a fatal outcome occur among those neonates with one or more of these risk factors. Additional risk factors include having previously had a neonate with invasive GBS disease and maternal GBS bacteriuria during the current pregnancy. A study in 1985 documented that the overall attack rate for early-onset neonatal GBS disease increased from the then-observed 3.0 per 1000 births in the total population to 8.4 per 1000 births among those pregnancies in which risk factors were present.[48] The attack rate rose even more dramatically to 40.8 per 1000 births if risk factors were present and the mother was colonized with GBS.

Several studies utilizing the presence of risk factors, maternal colonization status, or both, as a determinant for prophylaxis have documented the efficacy of intrapartum chemoprophylaxis in reducing neonatal early-onset GBS disease.[49–55] A meta-analysis of these studies demonstrated a 30-fold reduction in early-onset disease with intrapartum chemoprophylaxis.[56] The two alternative approaches to intrapartum chemoprophylaxis were proposed in the United States by the CDC in 1996[21] and have been endorsed by both ACOG[20] and AAP.[22] The first approach is based upon universal screening for maternal GBS colonization at 35 to 37 weeks' gestation. Cultures remote from term might not be accurate and should not be used. Intrapartum chemoprophylaxis is offered to all pregnant women identified as GBS carriers. In addition, intrapartum chemoprophylaxis is offered to women with a previous neonate with GBS infection, GBS bacteriuria during the current pregnancy, or delivering prior to 37 weeks' gestation, regardless of maternal colonization status. Women with an unknown carrier status are offered prophylaxis in the event of an intrapartum fever of 38.0°C or higher or rupture of membranes at 18 hours or before. It was estimated that this screening-based approach would result in intrapartum chemoprophylaxis of 26.7% of all deliveries and prevent 86% of early-onset neonatal GBS disease (Table 31–4).[21]

An alternative prophylactic strategy, also initially endorsed by the CDC, is based upon offering intrapartum chemoprophylaxis only in the presence of risk factors. In this risk-factor approach, antepartum cultures are not obtained, and prophylaxis is offered only to those women with delivery prior to 37 weeks' gestation, rupture of membranes for greater than 18 hours, an intrapartum fever at or above 38.0°C, a previously infected neonate, or with GBS bacteriuria in the current pregnancy. With this approach, 18.3% of pregnancies were estimated to merit chemoprophylaxis and 68.8% of early-onset neonatal disease would be potentially prevented.[21]

The impact of implementing these guidelines has been studied extensively in the period following their initial recommendation. In the surveillance areas studied, the incidence of early-onset disease declined from 1.7 per 1000 in 1993 to 0.6 per 1000 in 1998, a 65% reduction, with the steepest decline occurring in 1996 following the initial release of consensus guidelines from the CDC. Schrag and associates[57] published the first comprehensive study directly comparing the two management strategies and found that the universal screening-based approach was greater than 50% more effective in preventing perinatal GBS disease. This result was felt to stem from two main factors. First, the screening-based approach identified mothers who were GBS-positive but did not exhibit risk factors during pregnancy or labor, a group representing 18% of all parturients during the study period. Second, women identified as being GBS-positive were more likely to receive intrapartum antibiotics than women who qualified on the basis of risk factors (89% vs. 61%, $P < .001$), indicating improved compliance with the guidelines utilizing the screening-based approach. In this study, similar numbers of patients (24%) in each group received intrapartum prophylaxis, negating previous concerns that the screening-based approach would result in a significant increase in the use of antibiotics and potential contribution to antibiotic resistance. Also, other studies have suggested that the increased cost of performing routine cultures on all eligible pregnant women would be offset by the impact of disease prevention. This idea led to the release of new guidelines by the CDC in 2002,[23] recommending a universal screening-based approach (Fig. 31–1). The risk-based approach should be used only for women who arrive in labor with no documented culture results. In addition, a new algorithm was provided for the management of women with preterm delivery, summarized in Figure 31–2. An evaluation of the universal antenatal screening approach for GBS was recently published, highlighting the efficacy achieved and areas in which further improvements in management might result in the additional reductions in neonatal disease.[58]

TABLE 31–4

Intrapartum Chemoprophylaxis Trials for the Prevention of Neonatal Early-onset Group B Streptococcus Disease

STUDY	CASE SELECTION	COMPARISON GROUP	EARLY-ONSET DISEASE: ICP	EARLY-ONSET DISEASE: NO ICP	*P* VALUE
Allardice[49]	I	Nonrandom	0/57	9/136	.06
Boyer[50]	PC	Random	0/85	5/79	.02
Morales[51]	PC	Random	0/135	3/128	.2
Morales[52]	I	Nonrandom	0/36	13/48	.002
Tuppurainen[53]	PC	Random	1/88	10/111	.03
Matorras[54]	I	Random	0/60	3/65	.14
Garland[55]	PC	Nonrandom	16/30,197	27/26,915	.04

I, intrapartum colonization; ICP, intrapartum chemoprophylaxis; PC, prenatal colonization.
Adapted from American Academy of Pediatrics: Revised guidelines for prevention of early-onset group B streptococcus (GBS) infection. Pediatrics 1997; 99:489–496.

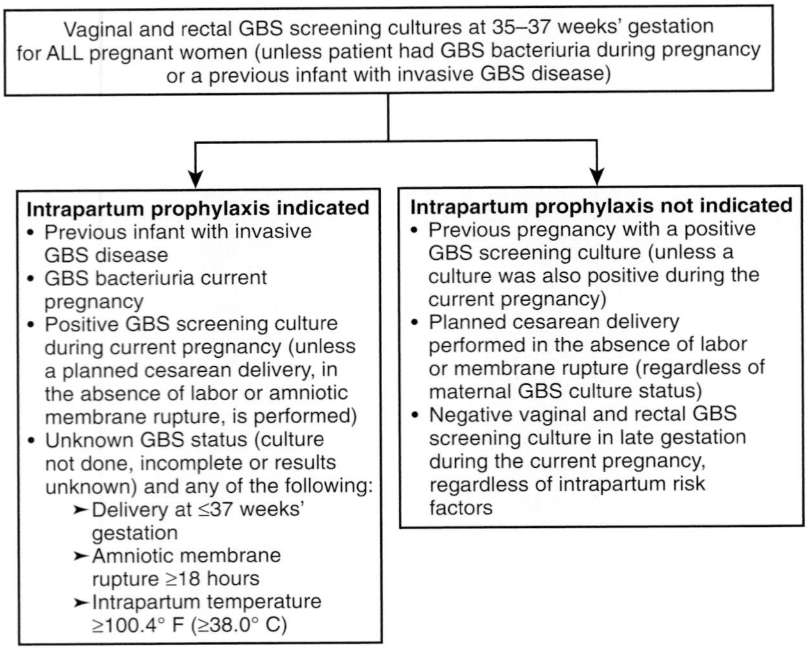

Vaginal and rectal GBS screening cultures at 35–37 weeks' gestation for ALL pregnant women (unless patient had GBS bacteriuria during pregnancy or a previous infant with invasive GBS disease)
Intrapartum prophylaxis indicated
• Previous infant with invasive GBS disease
• GBS bacteriuria current pregnancy
• Positive GBS screening culture during current pregnancy (unless a planned cesarean delivery, in the absence of labor or amniotic membrane rupture, is performed)
• Unknown GBS status (culture not done, incomplete or results unknown) and any of the following:
➢ Delivery at ≤37 weeks' gestation
➢ Amniotic membrane rupture ≥18 hours
➢ Intrapartum temperature ≥100.4° F (≥38.0° C)
Intrapartum prophylaxis not indicated
• Previous pregnancy with a positive GBS screening culture (unless a culture was also positive during the current pregnancy)
• Planned cesarean delivery performed in the absence of labor or membrane rupture (regardless of maternal GBS culture status)
• Negative vaginal and rectal GBS screening culture in late gestation during the current pregnancy, regardless of intrapartum risk factors

FIGURE 31–1
Indications for intrapartum antibiotic prophylaxis to prevent prenatal group B streptococcus (GBS) disease under a universal prenatal screening strategy based on combined vaginal and rectal cultures collected at 35 to 37 weeks' gestation from all pregnant women. (From Centers for Disease Control and Prevention [CDC]: Prevention of perinatal group B streptococcal disease: Revised guidelines from CDC. MMWR Morb Mortal Wkly Rep 2002;51[RR-11]:1–18.)

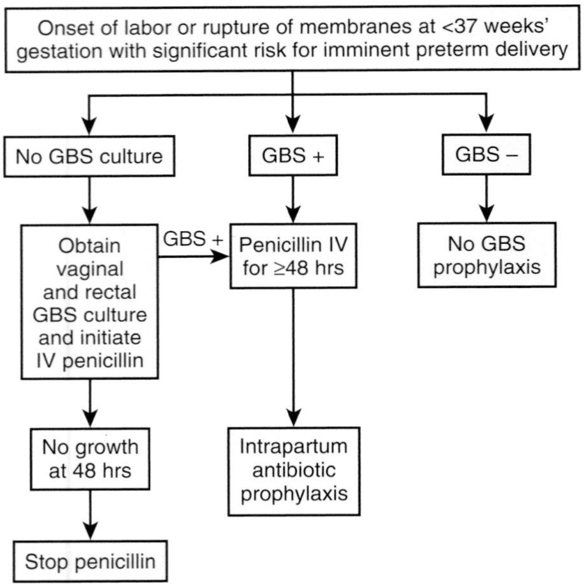

FIGURE 31–2
Sample algorithm for GBS prophylaxis for women with threatened preterm delivery. This algorithm is not an exclusive course of management. Variations that incorporate individual circumstances or institutional preferences may be appropriate. (From Centers for Disease Control and Prevention [CDC]: Prevention of perinatal group B streptococcal disease: Revised guidelines from CDC. MMWR Morb Mortal Wkly Rep 2002;51[RR-11]:1–18.)

Intravenous penicillin G (5 million units IV initially, then 2.5 million units q4h until delivery) is preferred for intrapartum chemoprophylaxis. Ampicillin (2 g IV initial dose, then 1 g q4h until delivery) is an acceptable alternative, but penicillin G is preferable because its narrower spectrum of activity may be less likely to select for antibiotic-resistant microorganisms. Previous debate had centered on the minimum duration of therapy for effective prophylaxis, in terms of length of therapy versus number of doses of antibiotics administered prior to delivery. Vaginal GBS colony counts fall rapidly after intrapartum penicillin administration.[59] Some evidence has confirmed that an initial dose of antibiotics at least 4 hours prior to delivery is as effective as two or more doses of antibiotics in preventing GBS transmission[60] and early-onset disease,[61] and this emphasis is maintained in the current guidelines.

If penicillin resistance is documented but the risk of anaphylaxis is judged to be low, cefazolin (2 g IV initial dose, then 1 g q8h) may be used. Clindamycin (900 mg IV q8h) or erythromycin (500 mg IV q6h) may be used in the severely penicillin-allergic patient. However, increasing resistance to both of these agents has led to the recommendation of routine susceptibility testing of positive cultures if penicillin allergy is suspected or documented. In surveillance studies in the United States covering the time period 1999 to 2005, 32% of isolates were resistant to erythromycin and 15% were resistant to clindamycin.[62] In cases of resistant organisms (or unknown susceptibility) and high risk for anaphylaxis to penicillins and cephalosporins, vancomycin (1 g q12h) is the preferred treatment. This underscores the need to accurately determine true β-lactam allergy as well as risk for anaphylaxis.

An alternative approach to intrapartum chemoprophylaxis is to immunize pregnant women. As noted previously, women delivering neonates with invasive early-onset disease usually have very low (<2 μg/mL) serum concentrations of type III GBS antibody.[27] More recent preliminary trials have been conducted among nonpregnant adults utilizing monovalent protein-conjugate vaccines containing capsular polysaccharide antigens against serotypes Ia and Ib,[63] type II,[64] and type III.[65] Further work is needed in this area prior to the implementation of a vaccination strategy toward women of childbearing age and pregnant women.

Postnatal

In the asymptomatic parturient receiving intrapartum chemoprophylaxis, there is no need to continue antibiotics following delivery. Conversely, in the symptomatic patient with intra-amniotic infection, therapy should be continued as described previously. Because GBS may also be associated with postpartum endometritis, known carriers should be observed closely for this and treated accordingly. Of note, Schrag and associates[57] reported a modest but significant reduction in invasive GBS disease, including postpartum endometritis, among pregnant women following implementation of the original guidelines for intrapartum prophylaxis, from 0.29 cases per 1000 live births in 1993, to 0.23 per 1000 in 1998 ($P < .03$). It should be recognized that postpartum endometritis is frequently a polymicrobial infection and broad-spectrum antibiotics should be utilized, even among those patients known to be colonized with GBS.

SUMMARY OF MANAGEMENT OPTIONS
Group B Streptococcal Infection

Management Options	Evidence Quality and Recommendation	References
Prepregnancy		
Treatment of GBS carriers before pregnancy has no benefit.	—/GPP	—
Immunization strategies are being evaluated currently.	—/GPP	—
Prenatal, Labor, and Delivery		
Treat symptomatic bacteriuria during prenatal period.	IIa/B	29
Recommended universal screening–based approach: • Perform combined vaginal and rectal cultures on all pregnant women at 35–37 wk' gestation. (Exception: women with documented GBS bacteriuria during current pregnancy or history of previous GBS-infected infant warrant intrapartum prophylaxis and do not require screening.) • IAP is recommended for all women with positive culture unless delivery by cesarean section prior to rupture of membranes and onset of labor. • If culture status is unknown at time of delivery, administer IAP for gestation < 37 wk, rupture of membranes ≥ 18 hr, or intrapartum temperature ≥ 38.0°C.	IIa/B	23,57
Suggested management of threatened preterm delivery: • No culture done: obtain cultures and initiate IAP for 48 hr until results obtained or delivery occurs. • Culture positive prior to or during labor: IAP for 48 hr or until delivery occurs. • Culture negative prior to labor (or after 48 hr): no IAP (or stop IAP).	III/B	21
Recommended prophylaxis regimens: • Penicillin G 5 million U IV followed by 2.5 mU IV q4h until delivery (ampicillin 2 g IV initially followed by 1 g IV q4h until delivery is acceptable but less preferred owing to broader-spectrum activity). • For penicillin allergic (low anaphylaxis risk), cefazolin 2 g IV initial dose followed by 1 g IV q8h until delivery. • For penicillin allergic (high anaphylaxis risk, documented susceptibility of GBS), clindamycin 900 mg IV q8h, or erythromycin 500 mg IV q6h. • For penicillin allergic (high anaphylaxis risk and resistance to clindamycin and erythromycin or susceptibility unknown), vancomycin 1 g IV q12h.	Ia/A	23,56,60,61
Postnatal		
Antibiotic prophylaxis need not be continued after delivery.	—/GPP	—
Diagnosis of postpartum endometritis in a GBS-positive woman should be treated with broad-spectrum antibiotics.	—/GPP	—

GBS, group B streptococcus; GPP, good practice point; IAP, intrapartum antibiotic prophylaxis.

METHICILLIN RESISTANT STAPHYLOCOCCUS AUREUS

Maternal and Fetal Risks

Staphylococcus aureus is a commonly encountered organism, colonizing the anterior nares, other mucus membranes and skin surfaces. Resistance to penicillin, and later methicillin, has made these bacteria of particular concern as a nosocomial pathogen. Over the last decade, methicillin resistant strains (MRSA) have been increasingly isolated from patients in the community setting, without typical risk factors such as recent antibiotic treatment, ICU admission, known contact with an infected individual or surgical exposure.[66] Community acquired MRSA usually has chromosomal DNA restriction patterns that are different from the hospital-associated strains, commonly contain the Panton Valentine Leukocidin (PVL) virulence toxin, and are generally less resistant to multiple antibiotic classes of drugs.[67] Whereas hospital-acquired strains most commonly present within the bloodstream, urinary tract, or in association with device or surgical site infections, community associated MRSA presents as "spider bite" lesions, localized skin or other soft tissue infections or as necrotizing pneumonia after an influenza episode.[67] Community associated MRSA has now been identified as an emerging concern among pregnant and postpartum women, with infections in the breast, buttocks, vulva and groin reported.[68,69] More invasive disease has also been noted, including nonmenstrual toxic shock syndrome and neonatal sepsis due to this organism.[67] Recent United States national surveillance data have documented an MRSA nasal colonization rate of 1.5%.[66] Prevalence studies specific to pregnancy have reported recto-vaginal colonization rates of 0.5–3.5%.[68,69] Fortunately only a small fraction of those who are colonized go on to develop clinical disease. Vertical transmission to the neonate has been suggested in isolated case reports, although the frequency of this event must be exceedingly low.

Management Options

Prenatal, Labor, and Delivery

Regardless of the source of infection, antibiotic treatment usually begins with systemic vancomycin for invasive disease. Incision and drainage of any localized abscess collection is required. These infections are often slow to respond, and sensitivity testing should be initiated early to assess adequacy of therapy. Alternative or adjunctive agents include daptomycin, linezolid and tigecycline. Few data, and much debate, surround the discussion of the merits of these latter agents; consultation with a health care provider with expertise in this area would likely be beneficial.[67]

Mild to moderate skin and soft tissue infection due to community associated MRSA begins with incision and drain. Again, despite a paucity of data, the CDC has published guidelines for the outpatient antimicrobial theraphy of MRSA (www.cdc.gov/ncidod/dhqp/ar_mrsa_ca_skin.html) not specific to pregnancy.

Whether to perioperatively decolonize the nose, genital tract or skin to prevent MRSA infection before vaginal or cesarean delivery remains controversial.[67] At the present time, the cumulative data do not support routine screening for MRSA carriers or decolonization with mupirocin ointment (for nasal site) or oral or vaginal chlorhexidine (genital site). An exception may be if the patient has a prior history of MRSA infection, or is at particularly high risk for postoperative infection. This latter consideration would also apply to perioperative antimicrobial prophylaxis prior to cesarean delivery, where an agent that is active against MRSA should be considered for those known to carry or be at risk for MRSA.

MRSA carriage or infection is not a contraindication to breast feeding. As with other types of mastitis, breast feeding may be continued as antimicrobial therapy is instituted. Any draining lesion should be covered to limit infant exposure. If a significant breast abscess is identified, temporary cessation of feeding on that side may be needed for a few days after surgical drainage.[67]

SUMMARY OF MANAGEMENT OPTIONS

Methicillin Resistant Staphylococcus Aureus

Management Options	Evidence Quality and Recommendation	References
Prenatal, Labor, and Delivery		
For Severe Invasive Disease		
Systemic vancomycin (alternative or adjunctive agents include daptomycin, linezolid and tigecyline).	IV/C	67
Incision and drainage of abscess.	IV/B	67
For Mild to Moderate Skin and Soft Tissue Infection		
Incision and drain.	IV/C	67
For recommendations pertaining to oral antimicrobial therapy, see www.cdc.gov/ncidod/dhqp/ar_mrsa_ca_skin.html.		

Management Options	Evidence Quality and Recommendation	References
General		
Decolonization of nose (mupirocin), genital tract (oral or genital chlorhexidine) or skin (chlorhexidine) to prevent MRSA infection before vaginal or cesarean delivery is controversial.	IV/C	67
Current cumulative data do not support routine screening for MRSA carriers or decolonization. Exceptions: Prior history of MRSA infection High risk for infection	IV/C	67
MRSA and its associated antimicrobial treatment are not contraindications to breast feeding. Cover any draining lesion to limit infant exposure. Temporary cessation of feeding on relevant side if abscess occurs.	IV/C	67

LISTERIOSIS

Listeriosis is caused by the organism *Listeria monocytogenes*, an aerobic and facultatively anaerobic, non–spore-forming, motile, gram-positive bacillus. This bacterium is widespread in the environment in soil, vegetation, water, and sewage. It is also found in humans and has been isolated in the stool of 1% to 5% of healthy adults. It is a relatively uncommon infection, although there is a predilection for populations with relative immunosuppression, including infants, the elderly, and the pregnant woman, with the latter group demonstrating an incidence of 12 per 100,000 (compared with 0.7 per 100,000 in the general population, a 17-fold increase).[70] Most cases of human listeriosis during pregnancy are sporadic with occasional epidemic common-source outbreaks. It can contaminate a variety of foods including uncooked meat and vegetables, raw milk, and processed foods that become contaminated after processing, such as soft cheeses and cold cuts at the deli counter. In certain ready-to-eat foods such as hot dogs and deli meats, contamination can occur after cooking but before packaging. Contaminated food looks, tastes, and smells normal. Unlike most bacteria, *Listeria* can survive on food stored in the refrigerator. It is killed with proper cooking and pasteurization procedures.

Maternal and Fetal Risks

Listeria exhibits an unusual life cycle, demonstrating obligate intracellular replication and spread, without significant exposure to the extracellular environment and its defense mechanisms. Thus, cell-mediated immunity is the primary host defense, and this may explain the unique susceptibility of humans to this infection during periods of relative suppression of cell-mediated immunity, including pregnancy.[71]

Listeria infection is well established as a cause of pregnancy loss in domestic and wild animals. Subsequently, it was implicated as a possible cause for recurrent spontaneous abortion in pregnant women. An Israeli study reported a significantly increased rate of multiple positive cervical cultures for *Listeria* in women with a history of recurrent losses compared with a control group without such history.[72] However, subsequent studies failed to replicate this association, and at this time, the association is controversial.[73–75] Multiple gestation pregnancies may also be at increased risk for listeriosis, as reported by Mascola and coworkers.[76]

Pregnant women with listeriosis most commonly suffer from a flulike illness, with fever, general malaise, and other nonspecific symptoms. Rarely, it might cause meningoencephalitis or sepsis-like manifestations. In one large series, 65% of patients had fever (defined usually as temperature ≥ 38.2°C), 32% a "flulike" illness, 21.5% abdominal or back pain, and less commonly, headache, myalgia, or sore throat.[77] The average duration of symptoms prior to diagnosis was 6.6 days. Of note, 29% of patients were asymptomatic.

The primary mode of transmission to the fetus or newborn has not been proved, but is suspected to occur either via ascending infection through the vagina or transplacentally secondary to maternal bacteremia.[70] Neonatal listeriosis might present as respiratory distress, fever, neurologic symptoms, or skin rash, or it might be asymptomatic. Rarely, the infant might present with granulomatosis infantisepticum, which classically exhibits disseminated granulomatous reaction in the lung, skin, liver, and other locations. Similar to GBS infection in the neonate, there is a bimodal distribution of disease. Early-onset infection (usually defined as < 5 days of life) is more commonly associated with maternal illness and produces a sepsis-like illness, with onset of disease exhibited within hours of birth. Late-onset disease presents more commonly as meningitis, is less commonly associated with maternal symptoms or positive *Listeria* cultures, and may be associated with nosocomial or environmental acquisition.[78]

Outcomes of pregnancies complicated by listeriosis vary. In the study by Mylonakis and colleagues,[77] one in five pregnancies resulted in spontaneous abortion or stillbirth. In the remainder, 68.3% of the infants demonstrated infection with a positive culture from one or more sites. Of these infants for which follow-up was available, 62.8% recovered completely, 24.5% died, and 12.7% recovered with neurologic sequelae or other long-term complications. The worst prognosis occurred in patients with meningeal involvement. Similar data were reported in a British review of 248 perinatal cases of listeriosis from 1967 to 1985 in which 19% of cases in which the outcome was known resulted in abortion or stillbirth.[78] Of the remaining infants in which gestational age was known, 58% were delivered prematurely (defined as < 38 wk). The overall neonatal mortality rate in known outcome cases was 35%.

Diagnosis

Listeria grows well on most routine media, although the use of selective media may be required when cultures are obtained from sites of heavy bacterial colonization such as the vagina or rectum. Owing to morphologic similarity, it may be confused with nonpathogenic diphtheroids. However, the organism produces a characteristic tumbling motion when viewed on wet preparation, allowing it to be distinguished. Of the four serotypes, subtypes 1/2a, 1/2b, and 4b are responsible for the vast majority of infections, and serotype analysis may be useful in epidemic settings.[70]

The diagnosis depends upon clinical suspicion and isolation of the organism from a culture of appropriate source. In the large series mentioned previously, *Listeria* was most commonly isolated from cultures of the blood (43%), cervix/vagina (34%), and placenta (12%). It may also be cultured from amniotic fluid obtained by amniocentesis performed for suspected intra-amniotic infection. Staining of amniotic fluid by meconium, especially in the preterm infant, may increase clinical suspicion for listeriosis, because this was observed in 12 of 23 infants in a reported series from Australian authors.[79]

TABLE 31–5

Dietary Recommendations for Pregnant Women

Do not eat hot dogs, luncheon meats, or deli meats **unless they are reheated** until steaming hot.

Do not eat soft cheeses such as feta, Brie, Camembert, blue-veined cheeses, and Mexican-style cheeses such as "queso blanco fresco." Hard cheeses, semisoft cheeses such as mozzarella, pasteurized processed cheese slices and spreads, cream cheese, and cottage cheese can be safely consumed.

Do not eat refrigerated pâté or meat spreads. Canned or shelf-stable pâté and meat spreads can be eaten.

Do not eat refrigerated smoked seafood **unless** it is an ingredient in a **cooked** dish such as a casserole. Examples of refrigerated smoked seafood include salmon, trout, whitefish, cod, tuna, and mackerel, which are most often labeled as "nova-style," "lox," "kippered," "smoked," or "jerky." This fish is found in the refrigerated section or sold at deli counters of grocery stores and delicatessens. Canned fish such as salmon and tuna or shelf-stable smoked seafood may be safely eaten.

Do not drink raw (unpasteurized) milk **or eat** foods that contain unpasteurized milk.

Management Options

Prepregnancy

Treatment of listeriosis in the nonpregnant woman is identical to that of other adult patients and dependent on the site of the infection (i.e., bacteremia vs. meningitis or other location). As mentioned, the possibility of *Listeria* colonization or carriage as a risk factor for subsequent pregnancy loss has been previously evaluated with inconclusive results. Thus, the role of *Listeria* as a cause of poor obstetric outcome in asymptomatic patients is questionable, and routine screening is not recommended at this time.[70]

Prenatal, Labor, and Delivery

Prevention of maternal listeriosis has been targeted as a primary objective following epidemiologic data confirming the role of contaminated food products as a major source for listeriosis, in both epidemic and sporadic cases. The first outbreak confirming an indirect transmission from animals to humans was reported in 1983 in Canada's Maritime Provinces.[80] A subsequent large outbreak occurred in 1985 in the Los Angeles area, in which 65.5% of all cases were pregnant women or their offspring.[81] In 2008, a large outbreak occurred in several Canadian provinces resulting in 56 confirmed cases and 20 deaths.[82] A surveillance project followed the Los Angeles outbreak, beginning in 1986, coordinated between the U.S. Food and Drug Administration (FDA) and CDC over multiple diverse demographic areas throughout the United States. This effort led to identification of many at-risk food sources and implementation of more stringent regulations for these food groups over the next several years.[83] In 1992, multiple agencies including the CDC, FDA, and Food Safety and Inspection Service (FSIS) issued dietary recommendations for persons at increased risk, including pregnant women. Results of this project resulted in a decrease of perinatal listeriosis in the surveillance areas from 17.4 per 100,000 (1989) to 8.6 per 100,000 (1993), ($P < .003$).[83] A list of at-risk food substances has been summarized in a handout for pregnant women on the FSIS website and may be viewed in Table 31–5.[84]

For women with suspected or confirmed listeriosis during pregnancy, intravenous antibiotics are indicated. Multiple cases have been reported of successful antepartum treatment of listeriosis with normal neonatal outcome, including cases diagnosed in the first and second trimesters.[84–86] First-line therapy consists of ampicillin 2 g given every 6 hours for 10 to 14 days. The addition of gentamicin for synergistic activity has been recommended in some cases but lacks adequate study to determine a conclusive advantage. Because of its bactericidal activity and excellent intracellular concentration, trimethoprim/sulfamethoxazole (20 mg/kg/day TMP component IV divided into four daily doses) is the recommended second-line therapeutic agent in cases of penicillin-allergic patients.[71] However, because of fetal effects, its utility must be evaluated in each case individually, weighing the potential risks and benefits. This underscores the necessity of accurately determining true penicillin-allergy status and consideration of desensitization therapy. Other second-line considerations include erythromycin, vancomycin, or the carbapenems, but experience is limited. Cephalosporins are not effective against *Listeria*.

Postnatal

For mothers with proven listeriosis, antibiotic therapy should be continued for a total of 10 to 14 days for bacteremia or superficial infections or 14 to 21 days for meningitis. Care of the neonate should involve obtaining blood and cerebrospinal fluid (CSF) cultures to assess potential infection and empirical treatment with ampicillin and gentamicin pending culture results. Antibiotic therapy is recommended for a minimum of 14 days in cases of bacteremia or pneumonia and 21 days in cases involving the central nervous system.

SUMMARY OF MANAGEMENT OPTIONS

Listeriosis Monocytogenes

Management Options	Evidence Quality and Recommendation	References
Prepregnancy		
No benefit to screening.	III/B	70
Treatment of documented infection depending on the site (see later).	IV/C	84–86
Prenatal, Labor, and Delivery		
Avoid unpasteurized dairy products and certain meat products (see Table 31–5)	III/B	83,84
Culture appropriate sites if listeriosis suspected (blood, CSF, cervix, amniotic fluid).	—/GPP	—
Treatment	IV/C	84–86
• **First-line therapy**: IV ampicillin 200 mg/kg/day (divided into four doses), max = 12 g/day.		
• **For penicillin-sensitive patients**: trimethoprim/sulfamethoxazole (20 mg/kg/day in three or four doses).		
• **Other antibiotics**: erythromycin, vancomycin. *Note*: cephalosporins not effective.		
• **Duration of therapy**: 10–14 days for superficial infection/bacteremia; 14–21 days for meningitis.		
Postnatal		
Evaluate neonate with blood and CSF cultures.	—/GPP	—

CSF, cerebrospinal fluid; GPP, good practice point.

SEXUALLY TRANSMITTED INFECTIONS

Gonorrhea

Gonorrhea is the second most commonly reported bacterial STI in the United States. It is caused by *Neisseria gonorrhoeae*, a gram-negative diplococcus. The prevalence of gonococcal infection in pregnancy varies, depending upon the population studied, from 0.5% to 7.4% in the United States.[87,88] Nationally reported gonorrhea rates have been roughly stable since 1996, although the rate increased in 2005 for the first time since 1999 to 115.6 cases per 100,000 population.[89] Risk factors for gonococcal infection include multiple sexual partners, young age, nonwhite race, low socioeconomic status, and being unmarried.

Maternal and Fetal Risks

The most prevalent type of gonococcal infection in pregnancy is asymptomatic infection of the cervix. *N. gonorrhoeae* may also cause acute cervicitis, proctitis, pharyngitis, and disseminated systemic infection. The rate of pharyngeal gonococcal infection increases during pregnancy, possibly as a result of altered sexual practices.[90] Disseminated gonococcal infection (DGI) also occurs more frequently in pregnant than in nonpregnant women.[91] DGI is characterized by a bacteremic phase associated with malaise, fever, and a pustular hemorrhagic rash and a secondary septic arthritis stage usually with asymmetrical involvement of the knees, wrists, or ankles. Acute salpingitis secondary to gonococcal infection may occur during the first trimester but is rare after the 12th week of gestation because obliteration of the endometrial cavity by the pregnancy prevents ascending infection. In pregnancy, gonococcal cervicitis has been associated with PROM, premature delivery, chorioamnionitis, and both postabortion and postpartum endometritis.[92,93] In addition, gonococcal ophthalmia neonatorum may develop in up to 40% of newborns exposed to maternal infection who did not receive ocular prophylaxis.

Diagnosis

It is estimated that up to 80% of women with gonococcal infection of the cervix are asymptomatic; for this reason, prevention of sequelae of gonorrhea depends upon prenatal screening to detect infected parturients. Screening should occur during pregnancy, and late pregnancy rescreening is advised for patients in a high-prevalence population.[94] Diagnosis depends upon the demonstration of gram-negative intracellular diplococci within leukocytes of a smear obtained from an exudate, if present, or upon culture. Cultures should be inoculated immediately after collection onto a selective medium such as Thayer-Martin. Culture-independent identification of *N. gonorrhoeae* by immunoassay or DNA detection assays are also available and have been demonstrated to be highly specific and sensitive for the detection of gonococcal infections.

TABLE 31–6

Treatment of Uncomplicated Gonococcal or Chlamydial Infections in Pregnancy

Gonococcal Infection

Recommended:
- Cefixime 400 mg orally in a single dose or
- Ceftriaxone 125 mg IM in a single dose

Alternative:
- Spectinomycin 2 g IM in a single dose
- All regimens followed by azithromycin 1 g orally in a single dose or amoxicillin 500 mg orally three times daily for 7 days

Chlamydial Infections

Recommended:
- Azithromycin 1 g orally in a single dose or
- Amoxicillin 500 mg orally three times daily for 7 days

Alternative:
- Erythromycin base 500 mg orally four times daily for 7 days
- Erythromycin base 250 mg orally four times daily for 14 days
- Erythromycin ethylsuccinate 800 mg orally four times daily for 7 days
- Erythromycin ethylsuccinate 400 mg orally four times daily for 14 days

From Centers for Disease Control and Prevention (CDC): Sexually transmitted diseases treatment guidelines, 2006. MMWR Morb Mortal Wkly Rep 2006; 55(RR-11):1–94.

Management Options

PREPREGNANCY

The CDC published new guidelines for the treatment of STIs in 2006.[95] Guidelines are similar for most STIs with regard to the identification and treatment of these diseases prior to pregnancy, with partner notification and treatment an important component to prevent reinfection. For nonpregnant women, recommended antibiotics for treatment of gonorrhea include cephalosporins and quinolones.[95]

PRENATAL

Uncomplicated gonorrhea in pregnancy should be treated with cefixime 400 mg orally in a single dose, ceftriaxone 125 mg intramuscularly in single dose, or spectinomycin, 2 g intramuscularly in a single dose (Table 31–6). Because concurrent cervical infection with *Chlamydia trachomatis* occurs frequently,[96,97] azithromycin 1 g orally in a single dose or amoxicillin 500 mg orally three times daily for 7 days should also be administered, unless specific testing for *C. trachomatis* has been done and the results are negative. For DGI, hospitalization and parenteral therapy are recommended for initial therapy. Recommended regimens include ceftriaxone 1 g intramuscularly or intravenously once daily, ceftizoxime 1 g intravenously every 8 hours, or cefotaxime 1 g intravenously every 8 hours. Parenteral therapy should be continued until 24 to 48 hours after symptoms resolve and then converted to oral therapy for a total of 1 week of antibiotics. Identification, screening, and treatment of sexual contacts of patients with gonococcal infection are recommended.

Tetracyclines and the quinolone antibiotics may be used in the nonpregnant population, although they are contraindicated in pregnancy because of potential adverse fetal effects. As well, because of the emergence of quinolone resistance in some areas of the United States, quinolones are not recommended for areas with increased prevalence of quinolone-resistant *N. gonorrhoeae*.

LABOR AND DELIVERY

Rapid diagnostic screening tools such as Gram stain, immune-based assays, and DNA detection assays are available. These tests can be useful in evaluating the intrapartum patient at risk for infection. Intrapartum treatment of the mother may reduce the neonate's risk for infection, although specific treatment and ocular prophylaxis of the infant after delivery are usually done.

POSTNATAL

Treatment guidelines for the postpartum patient are similar to those outlined previously. However, doxycyline or the quinolone antibiotics may be used in nonlactating women.

Chlamydia Trachomatis

C. trachomatis is the cause of one of the most prevalent sexually transmitted bacterial infections in the world and is the most prevalent sexually transmitted bacterial organism in the United States.[75] Chlamydiae are obligate intracellular organisms. *C. trachomatis* may be differentiated into 15 serotypes. Serotypes A, B, and C cause endemic trachoma, a chronic ocular infection considered to be the leading cause of blindness in the world. Serotypes L1, L2, and L3 cause lymphogranuloma venereum, discussed later in this chapter. Serotypes D through K cause genital and ocular infections, discussed in this section. The prevalence of genital infection in pregnant women in the United States has been reported as between 2% and 37%, with an average estimate of 5% to 7%.[98–100] Risk factors for cervical infection include young age, single marital status, multiple sexual partners, and previous history of sexually transmitted disease.[101]

Maternal and Fetal Risks

The majority of infected patients have asymptomatic cervical infection. In the nonpregnant female, chlamydial infections may cause mucopurulent cervicitis, endometritis, acute salpingitis, infertility and ectopic pregnancy, and acute urethral syndrome. The role of maternal chlamydial infection in pregnancy is more controversial. Several studies have found an association between maternal cervical infection and preterm delivery, PROM, low birth weight, perinatal death, and late-onset postpartum endometritis.[102–106] Two prospective studies have found that only those women with recently acquired infection, as detected by the presence of IgM serum antibody to *C. trachomatis*, are at increased risk for PROM, preterm delivery, and low birth weight.[100,107] Treatment and eradication of maternal cervical chlamydial infection reduces the risk of PROM and premature delivery.[108–110] Thus, the available data suggest an association between maternal chlamydial infection and adverse pregnancy outcome and that screening and treatment in pregnancy is warranted.

Maternal chlamydial infection also poses significant risk to the neonate. Approximately 50% to 60% of the neonates delivered vaginally to women with chlamydial cervicitis will be colonized with *C. trachomatis*.[99] The most common manifestations of neonatal infection are inclusion conjunctivitis and pneumonia. Eighteen percent to 50% of exposed infants develop conjunctivitis within the first 2 weeks of life, and 11% to 18% will develop pneumonia in the first 4 months of life.

Diagnosis

The diagnosis of chlamydial infections is based upon isolation of the organism, or culture-independent detection by immunoassay and DNA detection by PCR and serologic testing. Because chlamydiae are obligatory intracellular bacteria, isolation by culture requires inoculation onto a susceptible tissue culture cell line. Cell cultures are both labor-intensive and expensive and are not readily available to most clinicians. Antigen detection kits are widely available to detect chlamydia and represent a less costly alternative to culture. More recently, detection of *C. trachomatis* DNA from the genital tract, or from urine, by PCR or ligase chain reaction (LCR) has been demonstrated to be greater than 90% sensitive and specific for the detection of *C. trachomatis* and has largely replaced cultures and antigen detection assays. A serum microimmunofluorescent antibody test is also available to detect recent or past infection but is more useful as a research tool than for the clinical diagnosis of chlamydial infection.

Management Options

PREPREGNANCY

C. trachomatis is susceptible to a wide range of antibiotics including azithromycin, erythromycin, doxycycline, tetracycline, and ofloxacin. For the nonpregnant patient, azithromycin 1 g orally in a single dose or doxycycline 100 mg orally two times a day for 7 days is the recommended regimen.[95] Alternate regimens include erythromycin base 500 mg orally four times daily for 7 days, erythromycin ethylsuccinate 800 mg orally four times daily for 7 days, ofloxacin 300 mg orally twice a day for 7 days, or levofloxacin 500 mg orally once daily for 7 days. For nonpregnant women, test of cure is not required, but follow-up testing approximately 3 months after treatment is recommended.[95]

PRENATAL

In pregnancy, azithromycin 1 g orally in a single dose or amoxicillin 500 mg orally three times a day for 7 days is recommended. Alternate regimens include erythromycin base 500 mg orally four times a day for 7 days or 250 mg orally four times daily for 14 days, or erythromycin ethylsuccinate 800 mg orally four times a day for 7 days or 400 mg four times daily for 14 days (see Table 32–6).[95] Erythromycin estolate should probably not be used because it may be associated with hepatotoxicity when given during pregnancy. Because erythromycin therapy is frequently associated with gastrointestinal intolerance in pregnancy, regimens avoiding erythromycin might be preferable. Therapy with either amoxicillin, 500 mg orally three times a day for 7 days, or clindamycin, 450 mg orally four times a day for 14 days, results in cure rates (98% and 93%, respectively) comparable with cure rates with erythromycin base therapy and are better tolerated by the patient.[111,112] Sexual contacts should be examined and treated.

LABOR AND DELIVERY

See the section on "Gonorrhea."

POSTNATAL

The incidence of neonatal inclusion conjunctivitis can be reduced by ocular prophylaxis at birth with 0.5% erythromycin ocular ointment or 1% tetracycline ointment, but not as well by 1% silver nitrate drops. Conjunctivitis that does occur, or pneumonia, should be treated with oral erythromycin for 2 weeks.

Genital Mycoplasmas

Maternal and Fetal Risks

Mycoplasmas are a ubiquitous group of microorganisms that inhabit the mucosa of the genital and respiratory tracts. They differ from bacteria in that they lack a cell wall, but they are susceptible to antibiotics that inhibit protein synthesis. The two most common genital mycoplasmas are *Mycoplasma hominis* and *Ureaplasma urealyticum*. The prevalence of these two microorganisms in the lower genital tract in sexually active women has been reported to be 40% to 95% for *U. urealyticum* and 15% to 70% for *M. hominis*. Their high prevalence rates among otherwise healthy women make it difficult to determine their role in adverse pregnancy outcomes. In general, *M. hominis* has been associated in some, but not all, studies with septic abortion, postpartum endometritis, and postpartum fever.[107,108,114] *U. urealyticum* has been associated with histologic chorioamnionitis, low birth weight, and perinatal death.[115–119]

Serologic evidence of infection with *M. hominis* has been found in 50% of febrile abortions versus 17% of afebrile abortions.[113] In one study of early postpartum endometritis among women, genital mycoplasmas, including *M. hominis*, accounted for 30% of the total endometrial isolates and 19% of the total blood isolates, but were usually recovered in association with other pathogenic bacteria, suggesting a mixed infection.[114] *M. hominis* has also been isolated from amniotic fluid of patients with amniotic fluid infection, but almost always in association with other bacteria, again implying a mixed infection.[28] Significantly, infected patients from whom *M. hominis* is recovered almost always respond to therapy with β-lactam antibiotics, which have no activity against genital mycoplasmas.

A number of studies have found an association between *U. urealyticum* and chorioamnionitis[116,117,119] and with perinatal death.[117,120] In one study, *U. urealyticum* was isolated as the sole isolate from fetal lungs in 24 (8%) of 290 perinatal deaths.[120] Twenty-two of these deaths occurred in utero and all but 1 were associated with pneumonia and chorioamnionitis, implying an ascending intrauterine infection. Some studies have also found decreased birth weight among offspring of women colonized with *U. urealyticum*,[115] but this association has not been confirmed by others.[106] Intervention treatment trials have also been inconclusive. McCormack and associates[121] demonstrated an increase in birth weight among the offspring of women colonized with *U. urealyticum* treated with erythromycin in the third trimester compared with colonized women treated with placebo. Because the presence of potential genital pathogens was not ascertained, their potentially confounding influence upon birth weight cannot be excluded. In contrast, Eschenbach and coworkers[122] found no beneficial effect of erythromycin taken for up to 14 weeks by a large cohort of women colonized for *U. ureaplasma* on birth weight, gestational age at delivery, frequency of PROM, or neonatal outcome. In this study, women also colonized with either *C. trachomatis* or GBS were excluded from analysis, eliminating any potential confounding bias from co-infection.

Management Options

Taken collectively, the data linking either *M. hominis* or *U. urealyticum* to adverse pregnancy outcome are inconclusive. At present, antenatal vaginal cultures for either of these mycoplasmas cannot be recommended. Current evidence does not support the treatment of colonized patients for the prevention of adverse pregnancy outcomes. If treatment is deemed necessary, tetracycline is effective against both *M. hominis* and *U. urealyticum* but should not be used in pregnancy. *U. urealyticum* is also sensitive to erythromycin but is resistant to clindamycin; *M. hominis* is resistant to erythromycin but sensitive to clindamycin. Because the mycoplasmas lack a cell wall, they are resistant to β-lactam antibiotics.

Chancroid

Chancroid is an acute ulcerative disease, usually of the genitals, caused by infection with *Haemophilus ducreyi*, a facultative gram-negative bacillus. Although rare in North America and Europe, it remains an important public health concern in developing countries and can potentially be introduced into other geographic areas as a result of travel. Chancroid may occur more frequently in individuals infected with HIV, genital herpes, or syphilis. Chancroid is spread only through sexual contact with individuals with ulcers and is much more prevalent in men than in women. The incubation period after transmission is usually between 4 and 7 days. A painful chancre then develops at the site of entry, beginning as a small papule that over the course of 1 to 2 days, becomes eroded and ulcerated. Multiple ulcers are common, with the majority occurring on the external genitals and only rarely on the cervix or vagina. The classic ulcer of chancroid is shallow with an irregular border surrounded by erythema. The base of the ulcer is frequently covered with a necrotic exudate. Painful inguinal adenopathy develops in about 50% of cases and may lead to suppuration and spontaneous rupture if untreated. These buboes appear 7 to 10 days after the initial ulcer and are unilateral in two thirds of cases.

Maternal and Fetal Risks

H. ducreyi has not been shown to cause systemic infection or spread to distant sites and poses no special risk to pregnancy.

Diagnosis

The diagnosis of chancroid is based upon clinical characteristics (the presence of a painful ulcer and tender adenopathy) and Gram stain and culture of the ulcer or aspirated bubo. The Gram stain may reveal gram-negative rods that form chains but has a sensitivity of only 50%.[123] Cultures should be taken from the base of the ulcer and placed on selective media. Cultures are both sensitive and specific in the diagnosis of *H. ducreyi* infection, but might not be readily available from commercial sources. An enzyme-linked immunosorbent assay has been developed that is both sensitive and specific and may represent a good alternative when culture is not available.

Management Options

H. ducreyi is susceptible to a variety of antibiotics, although resistance to sulfonamides and tetracycline has emerged that precludes their use. Quinolones, which are very active against *H. ducreyi*, are contraindicated during pregnancy. Current recommended regimens that may be given in pregnancy include (1) azithromycin 1 g orally in a single dose; (2) erythromycin base 500 mg three times daily for 7 days; and (3) ceftriaxone 250 mg intramuscularly as a single dose. Azithromycin and ceftriaxone offer the advantage of single-dose therapy. It is recommended that patients are tested for HIV at the time of diagnosis, and retested for syphilis and HIV 3 months after diagnosis, and that sexual partners of patients are examined and treated.[95]

Lymphogranuloma Venereum

Lymphogranuloma venereum (LGV) is a sexually transmitted disease caused by *C. trachomatis* serovars L1, L2, and L3. Transmission occurs through vaginal, anal, or oral sexual contact with mucosal damage. It is characterized by inguinal lymphangitis, anogenital lesions, and fibrosis with gross distortion of the perineal tissues. LGV is endemic in certain parts of the world, including Africa, India, Southeast Asia, and parts of South America.[124] It occurs sporadically in other geographic locations and was very rarely seen in industrialized countries in North America, Europe, or Australia until more recently. Beginning in 2003, clusters of cases have been identified in Europe, Canada, and the United States.[125] LGV is predominantly a disease of lymphatic tissue characterized by thrombolymphangitis and spread of the inflammatory process into the adjacent tissues. Three stages of infection are recognized: primary, secondary, and tertiary. The primary lesion is characterized by a small shallow genital papule or ulcer that appears at the site of infection after an incubation period of 3 to 12 days, heals rapidly, and is often associated with few symptoms. The secondary stage occurs 10 to 30 days later and is characterized by systemic symptoms and painful inguinal lymphadenitis or buboes, loculated abscesses, and anorectal symptoms such as pain and bleeding. The tertiary stage is characterized by a chronic inflammatory response with progressive tissue destruction, ulceration, fistula formation, and lymphatic obstruction. Antibiotic treatment during the secondary stage will prevent these tertiary complications.

Maternal and Fetal Risks

The course of the disease is not dramatically altered by pregnancy, and transmission to the fetus does not occur. However, infection may be acquired during birth and passage through the infected birth canal.

Diagnosis

The diagnosis of LGV is based upon clinical appearance, serologic tests, and recovery of *C. trachomatis* from infected tissue or its identification by the direct immunofluorescent antibody test. Serology showing complement fixation titers greater than 1 : 64 support the diagnosis. Routine testing for *C. trachomatis* is not specific enough, and confirmatory serovar-specific testing using DNA sequencing techniques is necessary to confirm the diagnosis.

Management Options

A variety of antibiotics have been used to treat LGV. First-line treatment for nonpregnant patients and sexual partners of pregnant patients is doxycycline 100 mg orally two times a day for 21 days.[95] An alternative regimen is erythromycin base 500 mg orally four times a day for 21 days. Pregnant women should be treated with erythromycin.[95] Azithromycin may be an alternative, but there are not yet any published studies regarding its efficacy and safety. Late sequelae such as fistulas or strictures may require subsequent surgical repair.

Granuloma Inguinale (Donovanosis)

Granuloma inguinale (GI) is a rare, chronic genital infection characterized by granulomatous ulcers. It is common in tropical climates and developing countries, but extremely rare in temperate climates.[126] GI is caused by infection with *Klebsiella granulomatis*, formerly known as *Calymmatobacterium granulomatis*, a facultative, gram-negative bacillus. Although most infections probably result from sexual transmission, autoinoculation and nonsexual transmission also occur. The infection is only mildly contagious, and repeated close physical contact is necessary for transmission.[127] Following acquisition of infection, the incubation period varies from 8 to 80 days. The disease begins as a subcutaneous nodule that erodes through the skin and slowly enlarges to form an exuberant, granulomatous heaped ulcer, which is usually painless. Redundant, beefy-red granulation tissue may be present, giving an exophytic appearance to the lesion. These lesions are highly vascular and may bleed on contact. In the female, these lesions are found most commonly on the labia.

Maternal and Fetal Risks

Pregnancy may accelerate the growth of these lesions. The effects of GI upon the fetus are not completely understood, but perinatal transmission at the time of birth through an infected birth canal has been reported.[128]

Diagnosis

The diagnosis of GI is based upon the clinical appearance of the disease. The diagnosis is readily confirmed by examination of a smear of a crushed tissue preparation of the lesion. The smear is stained with Wright or Giemsa stain and examined for Donovan bodies. Donovan bodies are the darkly stained organisms within cytoplasmic inclusions contained in infected mononuclear cells. Their presence is diagnostic for GI. Neither cultures nor serologic tests are available.

Management Options

The recommended treatment of GI for nonpregnant patients is doxycycline 100 mg orally twice daily for a minimum of 3 weeks and until all lesions have completely healed.[91] Chloramphenicol and gentamicin have been used successfully for resistant cases. Pregnant women should be treated with erythromycin base 500 mg orally four times a day for at least 3 weeks. Azithromycin may also be effective, but published data are currently lacking. The addition of a parenteral aminoglycoside should be considered if improvement is not evident within the first few days of therapy. Treatment should continue for a minimum of 3 weeks and until lesions are completely healed to prevent recurrence. Treatment of asymptomatic sexual partners is generally not recommended.

SUMMARY OF MANAGEMENT OPTIONS

Sexually Transmitted Diseases

Management Options	Evidence Quality and Recommendation	References
Gonorrhea		
Prepregnancy		
Identify and treat prior to pregnancy.	III/B	92,95
Contact tracing and treatment.	III/B	92,95
Confirm response with follow-up swabs.	III/B	92,95
Prenatal		
Give antibiotics (see Table 31–6).	III/B	92
Contact tracing and treatment.	III/B	92
Exclude chlamydia infection.	III/B	96
Postnatal		
Screen newborn for infection, although most units treat anyway.	—/GPP	—

SUMMARY OF MANAGEMENT OPTIONS

Sexually Transmitted Diseases—cont'd

Management Options	Evidence Quality and Recommendation	References
Chlamydia		
Prepregnancy		
Identify and treat with doxycycline or ofloxacin.	Ia/A	95,109,111,112
Contact tracing and treatment.	Ia/A	95,109,111,112
Prenatal Treatment		
If diagnosed, give antibiotics (see Table 31–6).	Ia/A	95,109,111,112
Contact tracing and treatment.	Ia/A	95,109,111,112
Mycoplasma		
Prenatal		
If treatment necessary, use erythromycin.	Ia/A	122
Chancroid		
Prenatal		
Treatment of patient and partner with either azithromycin, erythromycin, or a cephalosporin.	IV/C	95,124
Lymphogranuloma Venereum		
Prenatal		
Erythromycin if diagnosed in pregnancy. Azithromycin is a possible alternative.	IV/C	95,124
Fistulas or strictures may need repair after pregnancy.	IV/C	95,124
Granuloma Inguinale		
Prenatal		
Erythromycin if diagnosed in pregnancy. Azithromycin is a possible alternative. Treatment should continue for a minimum of 3 wk.	IV/C	95,126,127

GPP, good practice point.

VAGINITIS

Vaginal discharge is one of the most common complaints of pregnant patients. The discharge may be the result of normal physiologic adaptations of pregnancy or may result from infectious vaginitis, with possible increased risk for pregnancy complications. The vagina has both a nutrient-rich biochemical milieu and a complex microbial flora. Normal vaginal discharge consists of water (primarily as a serum transudate), desquamated epithelial cells, microorganisms, electrolytes, and organic compounds including organic acids, fatty acids, proteins, and carbohydrates (primarily glycogen).[129] Normal vaginal fluid contains two to nine species of facultative and anaerobic bacteria in concentrations of 10^9 colony-forming units/mL.[130] Normally, facultative *Lactobacillus* species account for the majority of the total organisms present. These microorganisms utilize the available glycogen, producing lactic acid, which serves to acidify the vaginal pH to less than 4.5, inhibiting the growth of non–acid-tolerant, potentially pathogenic microorganisms. They also produce hydrogen peroxide, a potent antimicrobial toxin to other microorganisms including *Candida albicans*, *Gardnerella vaginalis*, and anaerobic bacteria.[130,131] When this complex relationship is changed, potentially pathogenic microorganisms indigenous to the vagina such as *C. albicans* or *G. vaginalis* and anaerobes may proliferate and cause vaginal discharge. Alternatively, sexually transmitted exogenous microorganisms, such as *Trichomonas vaginalis*, may disrupt the normal vaginal ecosystem and lead to symptomatic vaginitis.

Pregnancy itself may also lead to physiologic changes of the lower genital tract, which may predispose to vaginitis. During pregnancy, the vaginal walls become engorged with blood, leading to increased transudation, and the glycogen content of the vagina increases.[130] Elevated levels of progesterone seen during pregnancy enhance the adherence of *C.*

albicans to vaginal epithelial cells. Finally, cell-mediated immunity is impaired during pregnancy, predisposing to candidal infections.

The three most commonly occurring causes of infectious vaginitis in pregnancy are bacterial vaginosis, candidiasis, and trichomoniasis. Although frequently asymptomatic, these infections have been implicated in a variety of adverse pregnancy outcomes.

Bacterial Vaginosis

Bacterial vaginosis is the most common lower genital tract disorder among women of reproductive age (pregnant and nonpregnant) and the most prevalent cause of vaginal discharge and malodor.[132,133] It is a polymicrobial syndrome resulting in a decreased concentration of lactobacilli and an increase in pathogenic bacteria (mainly anaerobic). Specifically, there is an increased prevalence of *G. vaginalis*, selected anaerobes (*Bacteroides*, *Peptostreptococcus*, and species), and *M. hominis* and a decreased prevalence of hydrogen peroxidase–producing *Lactobacillus*.[131,134] In addition, there is a 100-fold increase in the intravaginal concentration of *G. vaginalis* and a 1000-fold increase in the concentration of anaerobes.[134] Thus, the diagnosis of bacterial vaginosis does not depend upon the recovery or identification of any single microorganism from the vagina, but rather requires the recognition of an altered vaginal microbial milieu.

Maternal and Fetal Risks

The presence of bacterial vaginosis has consistently been shown to be a risk factor for adverse pregnancy outcomes such as preterm labor and delivery, preterm PROM, spontaneous abortion, chorioamnionitis, and postpartum infections such as endometritis and cesarean section wound infections.[118,135–139] Table 31–7 presents a summary of studies demonstrating an association between bacterial vaginosis and preterm birth. Despite this evidence, the strategy of screening for and treatment of bacterial vaginosis in large-scale studies of women at low risk of adverse obstetric outcomes has not resulted in a reduction in the incidence of prematurity. Thus, the U.S. Preventive Services Task Force published a statement in 2001 concluding that the available evidence was insufficient to recommend for or against routinely screening women at high risk preterm birth for bacterial vaginosis and recommending against screening average risk asymptomatic pregnant women.[139]

Little is known about the mechanisms by which bacterial vaginosis may cause prematurity. The increased intravaginal concentrations of bacteria may simply overwhelm the local host defenses, allowing for ascending infection. Alternatively, these bacteria could also produce protease or phospholipases, which weaken the membranes or stimulate prostaglandin production.[140] Although the magnitude of the increased risk for prematurity noted in these studies is modest (approximately a twofold increased risk compared with patients without bacterial vaginosis), the total impact upon prematurity may be much greater given the high prevalence of 20% for bacterial vaginosis in pregnancy. It has been estimated that as many as 6% of preterm deliveries of infants with low birth weight may be attributable to bacterial vaginosis.[135]

TABLE 31–7

Association between Bacterial Vaginosis and Preterm Labor or Preterm Birth

STUDY	RISK RATIO OR ODDS RATIO	95% CONFIDENCE INTERVAL
Case-Control		
Eschenbach, 1984[131]	3.1	1.6-6.0
Gravett, 1986[166]	3.8	1.2-11.6
Martius, 1988[167]	2.3	1.1-5.0
Prospective Cohort		
Minkoff, 1984[136]	2.3	0.96-5.5
Gravett, 1986[103]	2.0	1.1-3.7
McGregor, 1990[168]	2.6	1.1-6.5
McDonald, 1991[169]	1.8	1.01-3.2
Kurki, 1992[170]	6.9	2.5-18.8
Riduan, 1993[171]	2.0	1.0-3.9
McGregor, 1994[146]	3.3	1.2-9.1
Hay, 1994[172]	5.2	2.0-13.5
McGregor, 1995[173]	1.9	1.2-3.0
Meis, 1995[174]	1.8	1.15-2.95
Hillier, 1995[135]	1.4	1.1-1.8

Diagnosis

The most common symptom among women with bacterial vaginosis is a thin, watery, nonpruritic discharge with a fishy odor. However, one half of women with bacterial vaginosis are asymptomatic.

Criteria for the clinical diagnosis of bacterial vaginosis are well established, with the diagnosis confirmed if three of the four following signs are present[141]: (1) an adherent and homogeneous vaginal discharge; (2) a vaginal pH above 4.5; (3) detection of clue cells on saline wet mount; and (4) the release of an amine (fishy) odor after the addition of 10% potassium hydroxide (positive whiff test). The diagnosis of bacterial vaginosis can also be made by direct Gram stain of the vaginal discharge. The Gram stain is the most widely used and evaluated microbiologic diagnostic method for this condition. Most laboratories use an objective diagnostic scheme that quantifies the number of *Lactobacillus* morphotypes and pathogenic bacteria, resulting in a score that is used to determine whether the infection is present. The most commonly used system is the Nugent score.[142] The criterion for bacterial vaginosis is a score of seven or higher. A score of four to six is considered intermediate, and a score of zero to three is considered normal.

Management Options

The treatment of choice for symptomatic bacterial vaginosis in pregnancy is metronidazole given orally in a dose of 500 mg twice daily for 7 days or 250 mg three times daily for 7 days.[95] This results in cure rates of 90%. A single 2-g oral dose of metronidazole is also effective. Oral clindamycin 300 mg twice a day for 7 days may be used as an alternative. Nitroimidazoles cross the placenta and are mutagenic in bacteria and carcinogenic in some animals. However, there is no evidence that metronidazole is teratogenic or mutagenic in human studies, and it is considered safe for use in pregnancy.[143,144] Cure rates utilizing topical therapy are comparable with those of systemic therapy.[145] However, vaginal preparations such as metronidazole vaginal gel 0.75%, given intravaginally once daily for 5 days, or clindamycin cream 2.0%, given intravaginally once daily for 7 days have not been shown to be effective for preterm birth prevention, and therefore, oral agents are preferred. Further studies are necessary to address this important consideration.

The results of trials examining whether the treatment of bacterial vaginosis in pregnancy can affect the frequency of adverse pregnancy outcomes, especially preterm birth, have been inconsistent. In trials enrolling women from the general population who are not at increased risk for preterm birth, there does not appear to be any benefit to screening for and treating bacterial vaginosis. These results have been replicated in many studies from different countries, enrolling women at a range of gestational ages, and using both oral and vaginal medications (metronidazole and clindamycin).[146–151] However, in women at increased risk for premature birth (often defined as having a history of a previous preterm delivery), there have been more promising results. Several studies have shown that women randomized to treatment with oral metronidazole had lower rates of adverse outcomes, including preterm labor and delivery, than women randomized to placebo.[150,152,153] In a Cochrane Collaboration review[154] of 15 treatment trials involving 5888 women, there was a statistically significant decrease in the rate of preterm prelabor rupture of membranes and low birth weight in treated women with a history of previous preterm birth, but no effect on preterm delivery rates. However, in the same review, there was a statistically significant decreased risk of preterm birth in five trials of 2387 women treated before 20 weeks' gestation.[154]

In published studies, vaginal therapy has not been shown to be effective in preventing preterm birth in women with bacterial vaginosis.[146–149] The one exception to this is a trial by Lamont and colleagues[155] that demonstrated a statistically significant reduction in preterm birth (4% vs. 10%) in women randomized to clindamycin vaginal cream at 13 to 20 weeks' gestation compared with placebo. A meta-analysis exploring the issue of oral or vaginal treatment in women at low risk versus those at high risk for preterm birth found no significant reduction in preterm delivery by treatment of all women, women with a previous preterm birth, or women at low risk for preterm birth.[156] However, in the subgroup of women who had a previous preterm delivery and who had received oral treatment for at least 7 days, there was a highly significant decrease in preterm delivery (odds ratio [OR] 0.42; 95% confidence interval [CI] 0.27–0.67). There was no benefit seen in the group of women receiving vaginal treatment.

Candida Vaginitis

Maternal and Fetal Risks

Candida vaginitis may be caused by many species of *Candida*, but the predominant species is *C. albicans*, which is responsible for 80% to 90% of infections. The remainder of cases are caused by *Candida (Torulopsis) glabrata* and other *Candida* species. These organisms are saprophytic fungi, which may be recovered from the vagina in 25% to 40% of asymptomatic women. *Candida* also accounts for approximately 25% of all symptomatic vaginitis among nonpregnant patients and up to 45% of vaginitis in pregnancy. In pregnancy, alterations in the vaginal microflora, glycogen availability, and a depression in maternal cellular immunity may all contribute to increase the risk of *Candida* overgrowth leading to vaginitis. Although rare, *C. albicans* has been reported as a cause of amniotic fluid infection and congenital cutaneous candidiasis of the newborn.[157]

Diagnosis

Women with vaginal candidiasis experience vulvar and vaginal pruritus, external dysuria, and a nonmalodorous flocculent discharge. Examination usually reveals an erythematous vulvar rash and a characteristic white "cottage cheese" discharge that adheres to the vaginal walls. The vaginal pH is usually normal (<4.5) and no odor is present. Microscopic examination of material suspended in 10% potassium hydroxide reveals typical mycelial forms and pseudohyphae in 80% of patients with symptomatic infection. Because *Candida* species may exist in the vaginal flora in low concentrations among normal asymptomatic patients, cultures are usually not indicated. Cultures should be limited to women in whom candidiasis is suspected but cannot be confirmed by microscopic examination.

Management Options

Treatment by local application of antifungals results in relief of symptoms and eradication of yeast in 70% to 90% of patients. The mainstay of treatment has been with imidazoles. These broad-spectrum antifungals include miconazole, clotrimazole, teraconazole, and butaconazole. These agents inhibit fungal ergosterol synthesis, resulting in disruption of the cell membrane. They are available as a one-time intravaginal suppository or as either 3-day or 7-day courses of intravaginal suppositories or creams given once daily at bedtime. These imidazoles are not absorbed systemically and are safe to use in pregnancy. In pregnant women, the 7-day course is recommended.[95] Boric acid powder, in 600 mg vaginal suppositories, placed intravaginally daily for 14 days is also 90% effective in eradicating symptomatic vaginal candidiasis and has the advantage of being very inexpensive.[158] Although borate is poorly absorbed systemically in nonpregnant women, its absorption during pregnancy is uncertain, and therefore, alternative therapies with topical imidazoles are preferable. Two other antifungal agents that are systemically absorbed after oral or intravenous administration are ketoconazole, an imidazole, and fluconazole, a triazole. These both have superb activity against *Candida* species and are useful in the treatment of systemic fungal infections or vaginal candidiasis in nonpregnant women.

Trichomoniasis

Trichomoniasis is caused by *T. vaginalis*, a sexually transmitted anaerobic protozoan. *T. vaginalis* may be recovered from 40% of women screened in sexually transmitted disease clinics and from the prostatic fluid of 70% of the male contacts of the women with symptomatic trichomoniasis.[159,160] The prevalence of trichomoniasis in pregnancy ranges from 6% to 22%. Risk factors associated with *T. vaginalis* colonization include black race, cigarette smoking, greater number of sexual partners, and a history of gonorrhea.[161] It is estimated that approximately 50% of women harboring *T. vaginalis* are asymptomatic.[159]

Maternal and Fetal Risks

Pregnant women with *T. vaginalis* infection may be asymptomatic or may have clinical vaginitis. *T. vaginalis* may also cause other infections of the lower genitourinary tract including bartholinitis, urethritis, periurethral gland infection, and cystitis. Although the risk of infection to the neonate is low (<1%), vaginitis and cystitis may occur as manifestations of neonatal disease. *T. vaginalis* has also been rarely suspected as a cause of neonatal pneumonitis. Although the relationship between vaginal trichomoniasis and adverse pregnancy outcome has not been well studied, two prospective studies have found a decrease in mean gestational age at delivery and an increase in PROM among women infected with *T. vaginalis*.[99,136] Further studies are necessary to confirm these relationships.

Diagnosis

Women with symptomatic trichomoniasis characteristically complain of a profuse and malodorous vaginal discharge. Vulvar pruritus, dysuria, dyspareunia, and lower abdominal tenderness may also be present. On examination, a gray or yellow-green frothy discharge is frequently present. The pH of the discharge is usually higher than 4.5 and may have an amine odor after addition of 10% potassium hydroxide. Small submucosal punctate hemorrhages of the cervix, the so-called strawberry cervix, are sometimes present. Microscopically, motile trichomonads may easily be identified on a saline wet mount by their characteristic pear shape, flagella, and rapid, jerking motility. Polymorphonuclear leukocytes are also present on saline wet mount microscopy and may be so abundant that they obscure the trichomonads. The sensitivity of the saline wet mount, when compared with culture, is 60%, but its specificity is near 100%.[162] *Trichomonas* cultures are easily performed utilizing Diamond's medium and are highly sensitive (92%–95%) and specific. However, cultures have limited practicality in the clinical setting because 3 to 7 days are needed for growth before the diagnosis can be confirmed. Trichomonads can also be seen on a Pap smear with a similar sensitivity to the wet mount, but with a higher rate of false-positive results. Other sensitive and specific rapidly performed diagnostic tests have recently been developed, including direct immunofluorescence assay, enzyme-linked immunoassay, and LPA. These are not, however, in widespread use currently. All women with trichomoniasis, whether symptomatic or not, should have a culture taken for *N. gonorrhoeae* because of the frequency of coinfection.

Management Options

Because *T. vaginalis* resides not only in the vagina but also in the urethra and bladder, systemic therapy is necessary for treatment. The only effective therapy for trichomoniasis are the nitroimidazole antibiotics, including metronidazole, ornidazole, and tinidazole. For pregnant women who are symptomatic, treatment is recommended. However, it is important to note that, although trichomoniasis has been associated with adverse pregnancy outcomes, treatment has not been shown to reduce the incidence of these adverse events,[135] and some studies have even documented an increased risk with treatment. Therefore, treatment is not indicated in asymptomatic *T. vaginalis* infection in pregnancy. In a randomized, controlled trial of pregnant women with asymptomatic trichomoniasis, the preterm birth rate was 19% in those given two 2-g doses of oral metronidazole and 10% in the placebo group (RR 1.8; 95% CI 1.2–2.7; $P = .004$).[163] In another randomized trial, children of women treated with several antibiotics including metronidazole had an increased risk of low birth rate, preterm delivery, and 2-year mortality.[164] Finally, a meta-analysis of 14 studies revealed that metronidazole treatment increased the incidence of preterm birth.[165]

For pregnant women in whom treatment is chosen, the preferred regimen is a single 2-g dose of oral metronidazole. Simultaneous treatment of sexual partners is required to prevent reinfection. As previously mentioned, there is no evidence that metronidazole is teratogenic or mutagenic in human studies, and it is considered safe for use in pregnancy.[143,144]

SUMMARY OF MANAGEMENT OPTIONS
Bacterial Vaginosis, Candidiasis, Trichomonas

Management Options	Evidence Quality and Recommendation	References
Bacterial Vaginosis		
Prepregnancy and Postnatal		
Treat with oral metronidazole.	Ib/A	95
Give intravaginal metronidazole gel or clindamycin cream.	Ib/A	95

SUMMARY OF MANAGEMENT OPTIONS

Bacterial Vaginosis, Candidiasis, Trichomonas—cont'd

Management Options	Evidence Quality and Recommendation	References
Prenatal		
For symptom relief, treat with oral metronidazole or intravaginal metronidazole gel.	Ib/A	145
For preterm birth prevention in women at increased risk, consider screening for and treating with oral metronidazole.	Ia/A	139,146–156
Candidiasis		
Prepregnancy and Postnatal		
Treat topically with an imidazole (miconazole, clotrimazole, teraconazole, butaconazole) or oral fluconazole.	—/GPP	95
Prenatal		
Topical therapy should be administered with a 7-day course.	GPP	95
Ketoconazole and fluconazole are best avoided in pregnancy except for severe systemic infection.	—/GPP	—
Trichomonas		
Prepregnancy and Postnatal		
Treat patient and partner systemically with a nitroimidazole antibiotic (metronidazole, ornidazole, tinidazole).	IV/C	95,162
Prenatal		
For symptom relief, treat with oral metronidazole.	Ib/A	95
If asymptomatic, do not treat because treatment has been associated with an increased risk of preterm birth.	Ib/A	163,164

GPP, good practice point.

SUGGESTED READINGS

Amsel R, Totten PA, Spiegel CA, et al: Nonspecific vaginitis: Diagnostic criteria and microbial and epidemiologic associations. Am J Med 1983;74:14–22.

Centers for Disease Control and Prevention (CDC): Prevention of perinatal group B streptococcal disease. Revised guidelines from CDC. MMWR Morb Mortal Wkly Rep 2002;51(RR-11):1–18.

Centers for Disease Control and Prevention (CDC): Sexually transmitted diseases treatment guidelines, 2006. MMWR Morb Mortal Wkly Rep 2006;55(RR-11):1–94.

Klebanoff MA, Carey JC, Hauth JC, et al: Failure of metronidazole to prevent preterm delivery among pregnant women with asymptomatic trichomonas vaginalis infection. N Engl J Med 2001;345:487–493.

Meis PJ, Goldenberg RL, Mercer B, et al: The Preterm Prediction Study: Significance of vaginal infections. National Institute of Child Health and Human Development Maternal-Fetal Medicine Units Network. Am J Obstet Gynecol 1995;173:1231–1235.

Nugent RP, Krohn MA, Hillier SL: Reliability of diagnosing bacterial vaginosis is improved by a standardized method of Gram stain interpretation. J Clin Microbiol 1991;29:297–301.

Regan JA, Klebanoff MA, Nugent RP, et al: Colonization with group B streptococci in pregnancy and adverse outcome. VIP Study Group. Am J Obstet Gynecol 1996;174:1354–1360.

Schrag SJ, Zell ER, Lynfield R, et al: A population-based comparison of strategies to prevent early-onset group B streptococcal disease in neonates. N Engl J Med 2002;347:233–239.

Schrag SJ, Zywicki S, Farley MM, et al: Group B streptococcal disease in the era of intrapartum antibiotic prophylaxis. N Engl J Med 2000;342:15–20.

Stevens DL: The flesh-eating bacterium: What's new? J Infect Dis 1999;179(Suppl 2):s366–s374.

REFERENCES

For a complete list of references, log onto www.expertconsult.com.

CHAPTER 32

Parasitic Infections

ALBERT FRANCO and JOSEPH M. ERNEST

INTRODUCTION

In the developing world, pregnant women frequently experience a cycle of undernutrition and parasitic infections, resulting in adverse pregnancy outcomes, including abortion, malformation, and neonatal death. Although malnutrition in general and parasitic infections specifically are less common in developed countries, no society is immune from their potential effects during pregnancy. Six parasitic infections that have major health, financial, or combined consequences worldwide are Lyme disease, malaria, tuberculosis (TB), syphilis, toxoplasmosis, and schistosomiasis.

LYME DISEASE

General

In the early 1970s, a mysterious clustering of juvenile rheumatoid arthritis–like cases occurring in children in and around Lyme, Connecticut, was subsequently recognized as a distinct disease and named Lyme disease. Further investigation revealed that tiny deer ticks infected with a spirochetal bacteria, later named *Borrelia burgdorferi*, were responsible for the outbreak.[1] Subsequent research has discovered additional vectors, three distinct stages of the disease, and multiple therapy options.

Ticks are divided into two families of medical importance: the Ixodidae (hard ticks) and Argasidae (soft ticks). Family Ixodidae contains ticks of the genera Ixodes which are responsible for transmitting spirochetal bacteria responsible for Lyme disease.[2] Black-legged ticks (*Ixodes scapularis*) are responsible for transmitting *B. burgdorferi* to humans in the northeastern and north central United States; on the Pacific Coast, the bacteria are transmitted to humans by the western black-legged tick (*Ixodes pacificus*). The life cycle of ticks is 2 years and includes egg, larva, nymph, and adult. *Ixodes scapularis* nymphs appear to be the most important vector for transmission of *B. burgdorferi*. *Ixodes* ticks are much smaller than common dog and cattle ticks and usually feed and mate on deer during the adult part of their life cycle. The larvae (or seed ticks) are six-legged, whereas adult and nymphs are eight-legged. In their larval and nymphal stages, these ticks are no bigger than a pinhead. According to laboratory studies, a minimum of 36 to 48 hours of attachment of the tick is required for transmission,[3] presumably because of the time required for the bacteria to travel from the midgut of the tick to its salivary glands.

In the United States, Lyme disease is mostly localized to states in the northeastern, mid-Atlantic, and upper north central regions and to several counties in northwestern California, although it has been reported in all 50 states. In 2000, 17,730 cases of Lyme disease were reported to the Centers for Disease Control and Prevention (CDC), making it the most common vector-borne illness in the United States.[4] In 2007, 27,444 cases of Lyme disease were reported yielding a national average of 9.1 cases per 100,000 persons. Ninety-two percent of these were from the states of Connecticut, Rhode Island, New York, Pennsylvania, Delaware, New Jersey, Maryland, Massachusetts, and Wisconsin. In these states, the average was 34.7 cases per 100,000 persons. Most cases occur in the United States between May and August, corresponding with increased outdoor human activity and nymphal activity.

Diagnosis

Clinically, Lyme disease has three stages:

- Early-localized.
- Early-disseminated.
- Late-stage disease.

Only the early-localized stage contains a hallmark unique to Lyme disease—the erythema migrans rash—which is present in 60% to 80% of patients at the site of the bite.[5] Adding to this difficulty in diagnosis is the frequent absence of notable tick bites in many individuals who subsequently have symptoms of Lyme disease.

Although the gold standard for diagnosis of an infectious disease is isolation of the causative organism, this confirmation is often difficult in Lyme disease, and the reliability of other methods currently available is questionable.[6] The diagnosis of Lyme disease is, therefore, based on the history of a tick bite in an endemic area and on characteristic clinical findings. Serology using enzyme-linked immunosorbent assay (ELISA) is the most common laboratory test to screen for antibodies to *B. burgdorferi*, but the test is not standardized and results may vary between laboratories, with false-negatives and false-positives commonly seen.[7] Given the high rate of false-positive serology associated with ELISA, a positive or equivocal ELISA should be followed by an immunoblot (Western blot) on the same specimen to detect immunoglobulin M (IgM) and IgG antibodies. If positive, the diagnosis is confirmed.[6] IgM antibodies appear 2 to 4 weeks following onset of rash and decline to low levels at 4 to 6 months. IgG antibodies appear at 6 to 8 weeks, peak at 4 to 6 months, and remain elevated even with treatment. In patients with only cutaneous disease (erythema migrans rash), laboratory testing is neither necessary nor recommended because laboratory studies may be negative at this early stage; in suspected cases of extracutaneous Lyme diseases, laboratory studies are essential.

Diagnosis of Early-Localized Disease

The hallmark of Lyme disease—the erythema migrans rash—typically occurs within 1 week of infection, but can develop as late as 16 weeks after the tick bite. The rash develops centrifugally as an erythematous, annular, round to oval, well-demarcated plaque and can reach a diameter of more than 30 cm. Occasionally, the lesion might be hemorrhagic or nonmigratory. The rash may be accompanied by constitutional symptoms such as myalgia, arthralgia, low-grade fever, and regional lymphadenopathy. Untreated, the lesions usually resolve within 3 to 4 weeks. Within days to a few weeks after the infection, hematogenous and lymphatic dissemination of the organism to distant sites occurs, leading to the early-disseminated stage.

Diagnosis of Early-Disseminated Disease

The most characteristic manifestations of this stage occur in the skin, musculoskeletal system, and neurologic system.[8] Skin manifestations during this stage include the development of other annular plaques resembling erythema migrans, found in up to half of patients. About 6 months after infection, approximately 60% of patients develop musculoskeletal symptoms, including arthralgias and myalgias early in the process, and asymmetrical, oligoarticular arthritis primarily of the large joints (especially the knee) later in the disease. The most common neurologic feature is cranial neuropathy, including unilateral or bilateral facial paralysis. Cardiac involvement, a less common component of this stage, may include atrioventricular block (in ≤ 8% of patients), left ventricular dysfunction, pericarditis, or fatal pancarditis.[9]

Diagnosis of Late-Stage Disease

Manifestations of late-stage disease can occur months to years after the initial infection and most commonly involve the skin, musculoskeletal system, and neurologic system. Localized scleroderma-like lesions may involve the skin, and approximately 10% of patients in the United States with untreated disease will develop chronic Lyme arthritis, an asymmetrical oligoarticular or monoarticular arthritis. Permanent joint disease is unusual. The central and peripheral nervous system can be affected, most commonly with intermittent distal paresthesias or radicular pain.[7]

Maternal and Fetal Risks

Although transplacental transmission of *B. burgdorferi* has been reported, it seems to be infrequent.[10,11] In a report by Markowitz and colleagues,[12] in which 19 cases of Lyme disease were collected retrospectively, 5 had adverse outcomes, including syndactyly, cortical blindness, intrauterine fetal death, prematurity, and rash. Neither trimester of acquisition nor therapy administered seemed to be associated with the outcome. Weber and Pfister[13] collected 58 cases from Slovenia, including 13 in the first trimester, 27 in the second trimester, and 18 in the third trimester, and concluded that the outcomes of 1 missed abortion and 5 preterm infants revealed no causal connection between the organism and adverse fetal effects. Likewise, Williams and Strobino[14] divided a group of 463 infants after birth into those serologically positive and negative to *B. burgdorferi* and found no difference in the incidence of malformations based on the infant's serology or geographic location. Therefore, recommendations for therapy during pregnancy are similar to those for nonpregnant individuals, with the exception of avoidance of tetracyclines and doxycycline in pregnancy.

Management Options

Prepregnancy and Prenatal

With the exception of the avoidance of tetracyclines during pregnancy, management options are similar before and during pregnancy. Four clinical situations can occur during which the practitioner may need to consider Lyme disease and the need for therapy:

- Tick bites without signs of infection.
- Early-localized.
- Early-disseminated.
- Late-stage disease.

TICK BITES WITHOUT SIGNS OF INFECTION

The best method of preventing Lyme disease is to avoid exposure to the vector ticks. If the patient resides in an endemic area, most practitioners recommend the use of DEET (*N,N*-diethyl-3-methylbenxamide). There is no evidence of risk in pregnancy with its use.[15]

The Infectious Disease Society of America recommends antibiotic prophylaxis only in those who meet four specific criteria: (1) attached tick identified as an adult or nymphal *I. scapularis* tick (deer tick), (2) it is estimated that the tick has been attached for 36 hours or longer, (3) prophylaxis is begun within 72 hours, and (4) doxycycline is not contraindicated.[16] As a result, pregnant patients are not candidates for prophylactic antibiotics. However, pregnant patients who remove attached ticks should be monitored closely for signs and symptoms of tick-borne diseases for up to 30 days and should be especially observant for the occurrence of a skin lesion at the site of the tick bite (which might suggest Lyme disease) or a temperature higher than 38°C (which may suggest other tick-related illnesses). Persons who develop a skin lesion or other illness within 1 month after removing an attached tick should promptly seek medical attention. Owing to the early appearance of both IgM and IgG antibodies, there is no utility in these serologic tests at the time of a tick bite.

EARLY-LOCALIZED STAGE

Identification of the bull's-eye rash of erythema migrans should prompt early oral treatment for nonpregnant adults with doxycycline 100 mg PO twice a day for 10 to 21 days. Pregnant women should be given amoxicillin 500 mg PO three times a day for 21 days, or if allergic to penicillin, cefuroxime axetil 500 mg PO twice a day for 14 to 21 days. Macrolides have been shown to be less effective. As a result erythromycin 250 to 500 mg PO four times a day for 21 days may be substituted only if the patient is intolerant to cefuroxime, and these patients should be monitored closely for evidence of treatment failure.[16] More than 90% of infected individuals respond to antibiotic therapy; when prompt and complete response is not seen the practitioner should consider a later or underdiagnosed stage of disease (such as unsuspected neurologic disease) or co-infection with other tick-borne infections, such as ehrlichiosis or babesiosis.

A Jarisch-Herxheimer–type reaction may occur in the first 24 hours of treatment, consisting of fever, chills, myalgia, headache, tachycardia, increased respiratory rate, and mild leukocytosis.[17] Defervescence usually takes place within 12 to 24 hours, and the patient can be managed by bedrest and appropriate antipyretics.

EARLY-DISSEMINATED AND LATE-STAGE DISEASE

In the absence of neurologic involvement or third-degree atrioventricular heart block, oral doxycycline or amoxicillin are recommended for early-disseminated disease. Cefuroxime axetil is an acceptable alternative when the patient is unable to take either doxycycline or amoxicillin. Parenteral antibiotics such as ceftriaxone 2 g IV daily for 14 to 28 days may be used for acute neurologic disease and third-degree atrioventricular heart block.

Labor and Delivery

No specific recommendations apply to the intrapartum period.

Postnatal

Women who develop Lyme disease during pregnancy should be monitored for up to 1 year for symptoms that may represent late-stage disease. These include localized scleroderma-like lesions of the skin, chronic Lyme arthritis involving single large joints such as the knee, and intermittent distal paresthesias or radicular pain.

SUMMARY OF MANAGEMENT OPTIONS

Lyme Disease

Management Options	Evidence Quality and Recommendation	References
Prepregnancy and Prenatal		
Tick bites: Avoid tick-infested areas when possible and carefully remove all ticks as soon as recognized.	IV/C	16
Observe skin after tick bites for up to 30 days for signs of infection.	IIb/B	16
Prophylactic antibiotics are usually not warranted in absence of infection.	Ib/A	15
Early-stage disease: Doxycycline 100 mg PO bid for 10–21 days for nonpregnant or amoxicillin 500 mg PO tid for 21 days for pregnant adults are comparable therapies.	Ib/A	13,16
Late-stage disease: Intravenous therapy should be considered.	III/B	13,16
Postnatal		
Observe the patient for up to 12 mo for signs of chronic Lyme disease.	IV/C	13,16

TUBERCULOSIS

General

TB is a disease with enormous worldwide implications. There were approximately 8.3 million cases of TB and 1.8 million deaths due to TB in 2000. The highest incidence rate exists on the African continent where approximately 290 of 100,000 persons contract TB on a yearly basis.[18–20]

TBs may be caused by any one of three mycobacterial pathogens: *Mycobacterium tuberculosis* (the most common), *Mycobacterium bovis*, and *Mycobacterium africanum*. *Mycobacterium microti*, also a tubercle bacilli, does not cause disease in humans.

TB is spread from person to person through the air by droplet nuclei, particles 1 to 5 μm in diameter, that contain *M. tuberculosis* complex.[21] Droplet nuclei are produced when persons with pulmonary or laryngeal TB cough, sneeze, speak, or sing. Droplet nuclei, containing two to three *M. tuberculosis* organisms, are so small that air currents normally present in any indoor space can keep them airborne for long periods of time.[22] These particles are small enough to reach the alveoli within the lungs, where the organisms replicate.[23] Organisms deposited on intact mucosa or skin do not invade tissue. After inhalation, the droplet nuclei are carried down the bronchial tree, where the tubercle bacilli are ingested by alveolar macrophages. The organisms can multiply there, growing for 2 to 12 weeks until a critical number of 10^3 to 10^4 is reached, which is sufficient to elicit a cellular immune response that can be detected by a reaction to the tuberculin skin test (TST).[24]

Before the infected individual develops cellular immunity, tubercle bacilli spread via the lymphatics to the hilar lymph nodes and through the bloodstream to more distant sites. After cellular immunity develops, granulomas are formed that limit multiplication and further spread.

Diagnosis

In non–HIV-infected patients, the majority of reported TB cases are limited to the lungs. Advanced infection with HIV, however, results in extrapulmonary involvement over 60% of the time.[25]

Systemic effects of TB include fever (present in ≤ 80% of patients),[26] weight loss, increases in peripheral leukocyte count and anemia (present in ~10% of patients),[27] and hyponatremia, occurring in as many as 11% of patients.[28]

Cough is the most common symptom of pulmonary TB, beginning as nonproductive but subsequently becoming sputum-producing. Hemoptysis is uncommon early in the disease process. Physical findings in pulmonary TB are generally unhelpful, although the chest film almost always reveals abnormalities, generally seen as a middle or lower lung zone infiltrate, often associated with ipsilateral hilar adenopathy when the disease is primary and is occurring as a result of a recent infection. TB that develops as a result of endogenous reactivation of latent infection usually causes abnormalities in the upper lobes of one or both lungs and may also involve cavitation.[29]

Pending confirmatory cultures, which may take several weeks, pulmonary TB can be diagnosed with sputum samples that show the presence of acid-fast bacilli (AFB), identified in 50% to 80% of patients with pulmonary TB.[29] A series of at least three single specimens should be collected on different days. Specimens should be transported to the laboratory and processed as soon as possible. If delay is inevitable, the specimen should be refrigerated until prompt delivery can be ensured. No fixative or preservative agents should be used. Direct amplification tests using gene probes or polymerase chain reaction (PCR) testing and high-performance liquid chromatography may also be useful in some circumstances in evaluating the patient. Regardless of the method used to diagnosis TB, cultures of the organism are essential for confirmation and to allow for drug susceptibility testing, a critical component of TB infection management.

Extrapulmonary TB can present as a disseminated form or in the lymph nodes, pleural cavity, genitourinary system, skeleton, central nervous system, abdomen, or pericardium. The ease and accuracy of diagnosis of extrapulmonary TB depend on the system involved.

In addition to symptomatic TB, patients who may have asymptomatic latent infection require careful consideration and thoughtful diagnosis as well. Current recommendations discourage screening of low risk populations because of false-positive results and subsequent inappropriate and potentially hazardous drug administration.

Annual TST administration is recommended in the following asymptomatic individuals:

- Potential close contact with infected individuals (health care workers, prison guards, laboratory personnel).
- Persons who are HIV-infected or who have another medical condition placing them at high risk for infection (chronic illness, immune deficient, homeless, medically underserved).
- Long-term care facility resident.

A one-time TST is indicated in the following situations:

- Single exposure with low risk for repeated exposures (if recent exposure, repeat TST 6–12 wk later).
- Recent visit to an endemic area in which the person was in a health care, relief, or refugee setting.
- Less than 5 years after arrival of a foreign-born individual from an endemic area.
- Incidental finding of a fibrotic lung lesion.

When screening for latent infection is considered, the preferred skin test for *M. tuberculosis* is the intradermal, or Mantoux, method. It is administered by injecting 0.1 mL of 5 tuberculin units (TU) PPD (purified protein derivative) intradermally into the dorsal or volar surface of the forearm. Tests should be read 48 to 72 hours after test administration, and the transverse diameter of induration (not inflammation) should be recorded in millimeters. Multiple puncture tests (Tine and Heaf) and PPD strengths of 1 TU and 250 TU are not sufficiently accurate and should not be used.

Three cutoff levels have been recommended for defining a positive tuberculin reaction: 5 mm or greater, 10 mm or greater, and 15 mm or greater of induration, depending on the risk group in which the patient resides. If there is no underlying disease causing immunosuppression, 75% to 95% of individuals with active TB will have a positive TST (≥10 mm). Specificity is 98% to 99%. For persons who are at highest risk for developing TB disease if they become infected with *M. tuberculosis*, a cutoff level of 5 mm or greater is recommended. This group contains immunosuppressed patients, those with recent close contact with a patient with infectious TB, and individuals with fibrotic changes on chest x-ray consistent with prior TB. A reaction of 10 mm or greater of induration should be considered positive for those persons with an increased probability of recent infection or with other clinical conditions that increase the risk of TB, such as recent immigrants from endemic areas, intravenous drug users, or those with normal or mildly impaired immunity including groups with poor access to health care. This level is reasonable for pregnant patients. A reaction of 15 mm or greater of induration should be used for groups at low risk for latent infection, should that group be tested.[30] In most individuals, PPD skin test sensitivity persists throughout life. Over time, however, the size of the skin test may diminish or disappear. If a PPD test is administered in this situation, the initial test result may be small or nonidentifiable. However, there may be accentuation of response on repeated testing. This is called the *booster effect* and does not represent a skin test conversion. This two-step method is commonly used in health care workers who undergo repeated tests and involves an initial test that, if negative, is followed in 1 to 3 weeks by a second and similar TB skin test, administered at a different site. The second test should be considered the "correct" one and the results from its induration measurement used. Because of the small amount of antigen administered, repeated skin testing with tuberculin will not induce a positive skin test reaction in individuals who have no cellular immunity to the antigens in PPD.[31]

Previous immunization with bacillus Calmette-Guérin (BCG) has been shown to protect against disseminated TB and meningitis in children, but has not been conclusively demonstrated to have protective effects against pulmonary disease in children or adults.[32] Millions of people around the world have been vaccinated with this attenuated strain of *M. bovis*, which frequently causes a false-positive Mantoux skin test. However, to avoid undertreatment of those truly infected, it is considered prudent by many experts to consider induration of more than 5 mm as indicating infection with *M. tuberculosis*, even with a history of BCG immunization.

Maternal and Fetal Risks

TB during pregnancy appears to progress in a similar fashion as in the nonpregnant individual. There appears to be no risk to the fetus with maternal exposure or positive skin testing in the absence of active pulmonary or extrapulmonary disease, although the tubercle bacillus has been reported to cross the placenta and granulomas rarely are found in the placenta.[33–35] Because of these reassuring findings, the risks to the mother are similar to those of the nonpregnant individual, and both mother and fetus share potential medication side effect risks.

Management Options

Prepregnancy and Prenatal

A positive TST in a low risk asymptomatic pregnant patient should prompt a chest radiograph to be performed after the 12th week of pregnancy to exclude asymptomatic pulmonary TB.[36] The main points about prepregnancy and prenatal care in patients with TB are

- Pregnancy does not affect the course of TB.[30,34]
- TB is unlikely to have fetal effects, and maternal effects of latent disease are primarily related to side effects of medications.[34]
- Latent disease should be treated with isoniazid and pyridoxine during pregnancy if risk factors such as HIV infection or known contact with an infected individual are present or immediately postpartum in the absence of risk factors.[30,34]
- If active disease is suspected, a chest radiograph should be performed regardless of gestational age and, if present, TB should be treated aggressively during pregnancy, with a combination of isoniazid, rifampin, and ethambutol for 9 months. Addition of pyrazinamide should be included only if a multiresistant strain is suspected.[34,36]
- Streptomycin should be avoided during pregnancy.[34]

Labor and Delivery

Factors that should be considered when managing an intrapartum patient with TB include

- Masks worn by persons exposed to an infectious source are less effective than are masks worn by patients with TB, because most airborne droplet nuclei are much smaller than their parent droplets.
- Droplet nuclei do not settle but remain suspended in the air for long periods of time.[22]

Asymptomatic patients under appropriate medical therapy do not pose a risk to health care providers. However, patients with untreated or undiagnosed disease may pose a serious threat to the health care team. In labor and delivery, any coughing patient who comes in contact with the health care team should immediately be provided a surgical mask, tissues, and a container to collect tissues. Patients with any of the following symptoms should be evaluated for the presence of TB: persistent cough for 3 weeks or more, bloody sputum, night sweats, weight loss, or fever. If any of these are noted, a chest x-ray should be obtained and sputum sent for AFB. If active TB is suspected, use of an isolation room with airborne transmission precautions should be implemented until further workup is complete. Health care workers should wear respirators capable of filtering particles to 1 μm in diameter with facial leak of 10% or less. Health care workers exposed to patients with active disease should have a PPD administered immediately and again in 12 weeks. Nursery personnel should be alerted when a newborn has an actively infected mother.

Postpartum

Patients with recent skin test conversion who have not been treated during pregnancy should be considered for therapy in the postpartum period. Although anti-TB drugs can be measured in breast milk, breast-feeding is safe during therapy for TB. Some anti-TB drug may reduce the efficacy of the oral contraceptive pill.

SUMMARY OF MANAGEMENT OPTIONS
Tuberculosis

Management Options	Evidence Quality and Recommendation	References
Prepregnancy and Prenatal		
Pregnancy does not affect the course of TB.	III/B	30,34
TB is unlikely to have fetal effects, and maternal effects of latent disease are primarily related to side effects of medications.	III/B	34
Latent disease should be treated with isoniazid and pyridoxine during pregnancy or immediately postpartum.	III/B	30,34
Active disease should be treated aggressively during pregnancy, with a combination of isoniazid, rifampin, and ethambutol.	III/B	34
Streptomycin should be avoided during pregnancy.	III/B	34

SUMMARY OF MANAGEMENT OPTIONS

Tuberculosis—cont'd

Management Options	Evidence Quality and Recommendation	References
Labor and Delivery		
Take special anesthetic precautions if general anesthesia is necessary.	—/GPP	—
Place patients suspected of having active TB on respiratory isolation.	III/B	22
Postnatal		
Continue treatment until course completed.	—/GPP	—
Breast-feeding is not contraindicated.	III/B	34
If mother has been treated, give baby isoniazid-resistant BCG and a course of prophylactic isoniazid.	III/B	34
Treat any untreated patients with recent TB skin test conversions after delivery.	III/B	34
Notify nursery personnel about the neonate exposed to active disease.	III/B	34
Some antituberculous agents may reduce efficacy of oral contraceptives.	—/GPP	—

BCG, bacillus Calmette-Guérin; GPP, good practice point; TB, tuberculosis.

MALARIA

General

Malaria is produced by intraerythrocytic parasites of the genus *Plasmodium* that are transmitted by the bite of the infective female anopheline mosquito. One billion people worldwide are estimated to carry parasites at any one time and approximately 50 million are pregnant.[37,38] It is estimated that between 10,000 to 200,000 newborns die as a result of infection in pregnancy.[38] Its name is derived from the belief of the ancient Romans that *mal-aria* was due to the bad air of the marshes surrounding Rome.

Four plasmodia produce malaria in humans: *Plasmodium falciparum*, *Plasmodium vivax*, *Plasmodium ovale*, and *Plasmodium malariae*. Most deaths are the result of *P. falciparum* and occur in children younger than 5 years, although pregnant women are also at increased risk for severe disease. Early treatment usually results in cure without recurrence, although *P. ovale* and *P. vivax* may remain dormant and recur months or years after the initial infection. Once infected, partial immunity may develop.

Human infection begins when sporozoites in the salivary gland of the female *Anopheles* mosquito are inoculated into the human host as the insect feeds. These parasites infect human hepatocytes within 30 minutes of entering the human body.[39] In the hepatocyte, each sporozoite divides and differentiates to form up to 30,000 merozoites, which rupture the hepatocyte and enter the bloodstream to infect erythrocytes.[40] Sporozoites of *P. vivax* and *P. ovale* may also form hypnozoites, dormant forms that remain in hepatocytes and may lead to recurrent infection months or years later. Merozoites actively enter the host erythrocytes, where they differentiate into ring-shaped trophozoites. These trophozoites develop into a schizont, which fills with merozoites, subsequently rupturing the erythrocyte and infecting other red blood cells (RBCs). Periodically, merozoites differentiate into male or female gametocytes, sexual forms that are ingested by *Anopheles* mosquitoes feeding on the infected human host. In the mosquito midgut, gametocytes merge to form a diploid zygote that differentiates into a motile ookinete that enters the gut wall to form an oocyst. Sporozoites released from the oocyst migrate to the salivary glands of the mosquito to repeat the cycle.[39]

Rupture of erythrocytes by proliferating merozoites occurs with a periodicity related to the species of plasmodia. This cycle repeats every 72 hours for *P. malariae* (*quartan malaria*) and every 48 hours for other malaria species (*tertian malaria*). Fever greater than 40°C is lethal to schizonts; consequently, the life cycle tends to be synchronized over the course of the infection, leading to periodic fever spikes rather than continuous fever.[41] Anemia develops in the infected human as a result of erythrocyte rupture by merozoite proliferation and by sequestration of normal uninfected RBCs by an engorged liver and spleen. Iron stores are depleted as hemoglobin from lysed RBCs is lost in urine.

Renal failure can result from a number of causes, including the rigidity of RBCs filled with merozoites that fail to pass through venules and capillaries, leading to microvascular sludging and ischemia in the kidneys. Cerebral malaria (the most common cause of death in this disease) occurs only with *P. falciparum* infection, because clumps of erythrocytes occlude the cerebral microvasculature, causing diffuse cerebral ischemia.

Acutely ill patients with malaria typically have either *P. falciparum* or *P. vivax* infections.[41] Partial resistance to malaria occurs in the presence of sickle cell trait (owing to decreased intraerythrocytic adenosine triphosphatase [ATPase] activity, which decreases surplus energy available to support parasite proliferation[39]) and in the absence of the Duffy antigen (owing to the propensity of merozoites of *P. vivax* to invade erythrocytes by binding to that antigen).

Diagnosis

Fevers, chills, and headaches are the hallmark of malarial infection. The chills can last for periods of 1 to 2 hours. Concomitant with lysis of RBCs, the febrile stage is characterized by rigors, flushing, headache, and muscle aches with temperatures of 39°C to 42°C. This stage can last for up to 6 hours, followed by profuse sweating and, as these symptoms disappear, excessive fatigue. Although most cases of malaria are classified as mild or uncomplicated, as the degree of parasitemia in patients with *P. falciparum* rises above 2%, the risk of severe malaria grows. Severe malaria is characterized by renal failure (sometimes accompanied by gross hemoglobinuria from lysed RBCs, termed *blackwater fever*), noncardiogenic pulmonary edema, severe anemia, jaundice, seizures, parasitemia of greater than 5%, coma, circulatory collapse, or hypoglycemia, in the presence of either recent exposure to malaria or *P. falciparum* on smear.[42]

For the past 100 years, confirmation of the diagnosis of malaria has been made with the demonstration of intraerythrocytic parasites by Giemsa-stained thick and thin smears of fresh fingerprick blood. All four *Plasmodium* species may be identified in this fashion. Although the thin smear is easier to read, the thick smear is 10 to 40 times more sensitive and can detect as few as 50 parasites/μL.[43] Detectable parasitemia may lag behind aches, fevers, and chills by 2 days. If malaria is suspected, thick and thin smears should be done every 8 to 12 hours on at least three occasions, the collection of which should not be tied to fever spikes. Persistently negative smears after this time period argue against the presence of malaria.[41]

Several alternative laboratory methods have been developed, including the quantitative buffy-coat centrifugal hematology system, immunofluorescence, ELISA tests for the detection of the *P. falciparum* antigen, and the PCR technique. Because of cost and complexity, none of these tests is used routinely.[44] Rapid blood tests using a dipstick or test strip with monoclonal antibodies directed against the target parasite antigen histidine-rich protein 2 (Pf HRP2) or parasite-specific lactate dehydrogenase (pLDH) are currently commercially available. Limitations in these methods include persistent Pf HRP2 antigenemia despite microscopic and clinical cure and positivity of pLDH only when viable parasites are present.[41]

Maternal and Fetal Risks

Pregnant women have an increased risk of malarial infection compared with their nonpregnant adult counterparts,[45] the difference being most marked during the first pregnancy and after the first trimester. In one study in Malawi, the incidence of parasitemia in primigravidas was 66%, falling to 29% in the second and 20.9% in subsequent pregnancies.[46] This increased susceptibility may be due to a number of reasons. Pregnant women seem to be more attractive to the female *Anopheles* mosquito than nonpregnant women and incur a significantly greater number of bites.[47] Sequestration of *P. falciparum* in the placenta may be another; in one case in which a woman's peripheral blood parasitemia was 3% at presentation (and presumably less after treatment), her placenta at delivery showed a local parasitemia of 70%.[48]

Although the major adverse effect of malaria in pregnancy on the mother is anemia, the risk of developing severe and complicated malaria is three times higher in pregnancy[49] and that of developing hypoglycemia is seven times more likely.[50] Malaria presents a significant risk for morbidity and mortality in pregnancy. Intrauterine growth restriction, miscarriage, preterm birth, congenital infection, and perinatal death have been seen in pregnancies infected with malaria. Studies have demonstrated an increased incidence of intrauterine growth restriction when parasitemia is found during the antenatal period and an increased incidence of premature birth when cord blood parasitemia (probably reflecting recent active infection) is seen.[50–53]

Management Options

Prepregnancy

Malaria chemoprophylaxis and therapy before pregnancy is similar to that administered to other adults, and can be reviewed at www.cdc.gov. Management principles are similar to those discussed in the following sections, with the exception that additional drugs are available to the nonpregnant adult that are not appropriate for the pregnant woman.

Prenatal

Management of the pregnant patient involves two components: prevention of infection and treatment of disease. To prevent serious infection in pregnancy, pregnant women should be advised to avoid travel into areas where there is chloroquine-resistant *P. falciparum* malaria. There are an increasing number of chloroquine-resistant strains worldwide. When travel is unavoidable into these regions, use of pyrethroid-containing flying-insect spray in living and sleeping areas during evening and nighttime hours is advisable. Bednets, especially those sprayed with the insecticide permethrin, are effective in limiting mosquito bites, and use of the insecticide DEET is a safe and effective means to minimize bites during pregnancy as well.[54] Recommended chemoprophylaxis in areas *without* chloroquine-resistant *P. falciparum* is chloroquine phosphate (Aralen) 500 mg/wk (300 mg chloroquine base) once weekly beginning 2 weeks before travel and during exposure and for 4 weeks after leaving the endemic area. Recommended chemoprophylaxis in areas *with* chloroquine-resistant *P. falciparum* is mefloquine (Lariam) 250 mg/wk, following the same schedule as chloroquine. It is critical that the patient continue the medication for 4 weeks after leaving the endemic area because infection is not prevented by the chemoprophylaxis, because sporozoites released into the bloodstream by the biting mosquito still reach the liver even in the presence of these medications. As the developing merozoites are released into the bloodstream, the infection succumbs to the drugs at this point.[55]

Before treating a pregnant patient with malaria, one should consider the place where the infection occurred, the trimester of pregnancy, and whether the clinical and parasitologic situation is severe. Consideration of the place where the infection occurred allows the clinician to use drugs that should meet with the least chance of resistance in the parasite. Consideration of the trimester of pregnancy allows the clinician to use drugs with the least chance of fetal toxicity, and consideration of the clinical and parasitologic situation allows the clinician to determine the aggressiveness and length of therapy. The drug or drugs chosen should be effective in the reduction of the asexual forms in the blood and in the placenta in order to prevent or reduce the severe clinical forms. Although the latest recommendations regarding specific treatment from certain regions may be obtained from the CDC, we review concepts of malaria therapy and drugs useful in the pregnant patient. Of note, CDC clinicians are available 24 hours a day to help with questions of diagnosis and treatment of malaria through the Malaria Hotline (770-488-7788 or 770-488-7100 on holidays, weekends, and off-hours).[43]

CHLOROQUINE

Although in many areas of the world, 80% or more of *P. falciparum* infections exhibit a high degree of chloroquine resistance,[56] chloroquine is still considered one of the safest antimalarials. It is not considered to be a cause of spontaneous abortion or teratogenesis when used for chemoprophylaxis or in recommended dosages for treatment,[57] but when given in large doses, it has been reported to cause alterations of the eighth cranial nerve and retinal pigmentation in the fetus.[58]

QUININE AND QUINIDINE

Quinine and quinidine remain effective therapies for malaria, and a quinine-tetracycline combination cures nearly 100% of *P. falciparum* infections no matter in which region of the world the disease is contracted.[41] Unfortunately, although quinine may be used during pregnancy, tetracyclines should be avoided because of adverse fetal effects. Quinine may cause cinchonism (headache, tinnitus, nausea, vision disturbances) and, if glucose-6-phosphate dehydrogenase deficiency is present, hemolysis. Quinidine may be used intravenously with caution because of its cardiosuppressant effects and its tendency to cause severe hypotension when administered rapidly. It can also cause hypoglycemia in the pregnant patient because of its tendency to stimulate the β cells to produce insulin.[42]

Quinine has been shown to be safe in therapeutic doses in the first trimester of pregnancy.[59]

ANTIFOLATE DRUGS

The drug combinations sulfadoxine/pyrimethamine and sulfamethoxazole/trimethoprim work synergistically on two enzymes of the *Plasmodium* organism: dihydropteroate synthase and dihydrofolate reductase. Pyrimethamine has produced a teratogenic effect in laboratory test animals (which can be avoided by the administration of folinic acid), and sulfa administration to the mother near delivery has a theoretical risk to the fetus of kernicterus. Because of these concerns, these combinations should be limited to the second or early third trimester.

MEFLOQUINE

Mefloquine is critical for chemoprophylaxis or therapy in areas of chloroquine-resistant *P. falciparum*. Studies have not shown significant adverse effects on the mother or fetus when mefloquine is administered in the second or third trimester of pregnancy. Observations made on a group of 1627 women who used mefloquine before conceiving or during pregnancy failed to demonstrate an increased risk of toxic or teratogenic effects on the embryo.[60] Side effects in general may include the induction of neuropsychiatric alterations including anxiety, affective disorders, hallucinations, psychosis, and convulsions.[61]

CLINDAMYCIN

Clindamycin is useful in the treatment of resistant *P. falciparum* and is an alternative to tetracycline or doxycycline, because it does not produce important adverse effects in the pregnant patient or fetus. Clindamycin in combination with quinine has been used since 1982 in Brazil and has been found to be an effective therapy for multiresistant strains of malaria, with no observed significant side effects in mother or fetus.[45]

ARTEMISININS

These antimalarials, isolated by Chinese scientists from *Artemisia annua*, currently are the fastest acting of all antimalarial drugs and have not shown significant toxicity.[62]

Resistance is rare, and although experimental studies with laboratory animals showed that doses above 10 mg/kg weight cause fetal resorption,[63] preclinical studies did not show any mutative or teratogenic effects. Increasing evidence of their safety has prompted the WHO to release a statement allowing the use of these compounds in the second and third trimesters of pregnancy. Their use is also allowed in the first trimester in complicated, severe, or recurrent cases in which no other medicines are effective.[64]

Labor and Delivery

No specific recommendations are needed for labor and/or delivery in these patients.

Postpartum

Breast-feeding patients should use the same chemoprophylaxis schedule and medication regimen for therapy as the pregnant patient.

Malaria Vaccines

Owing to the various life cycles of the protozoan and other features of the infection, development of a malaria vaccine remains elusive.[65]

SUMMARY OF MANAGEMENT OPTIONS

Malaria

Management Options	Evidence Quality and Recommendation	References
Prepregnancy		
If possible, women trying to conceive should avoid travel to endemic areas.	IV/C	45
If such travel is unavoidable, prophylaxis should be taken.	Ib/A	54
Consult www.cdc.gov for appropriate chemoprophylaxis and therapy; significant resistance exists in various regions of the world.	—/GPP	—
Advise patient that use of pyrethroid-containing insect spray and permethrin-impregnated bednets with liberal use of DEET insect spray topically will reduce frequency of mosquito bites.	Ib/A	54
Currently, no effective vaccines are available.	IV/C	44,65
Prenatal–General		
If possible, women trying to conceive should avoid travel to endemic areas, especially those with drug-resistant strains.	IV/C	45
If such travel is unavoidable, prophylaxis should be taken and spray and nets used as recommended.	Ib/A	54
Prenatal–Treatment		
Chemoprophylaxis should begin 2 wk *before* travel and continue for 4 wk *after* leaving the endemic area.	III/B	43
Chloroquine is a safe, effective chemoprophylactic drug for susceptible strains of *Plasmodium*.	IIa/B	45,59
Quinine, mefloquine, and clindamycin are also appropriate and safe therapies in pregnancy.	IIa/B	45,59
Monitor electrolytes, renal and liver functions, and hematology during treatment.	—/GPP	—
After therapy, maintain vigilance/surveillance for IUGR and preterm labor.	IIb/B	52
Labor and Delivery		
No specific recommendations are necessary.	—/—	—
Postnatal		
Breast-feeding is not contraindicated, but the same chemotherapeutic regimens should be used as in pregnancy.	III/B	43
Consider malaria for as long as 1 yr after travel to endemic areas when evaluating a patient with fever or other signs that may indicate malaria.	III/B	43

DEET, *N,N*-diethyl-3-methylbenzamide; GPP, good practice point; IUGR, intrauterine growth restriction.

SYPHILIS

General

Syphilis is a complex systemic illness caused by the spirochete *Treponema pallidum*. Debate about the origin of syphilis has continued for nearly 500 years, with 16th-century Europeans blaming each other, referring to it variously as the Venetian, Naples, or French disease. Evaluations of several hundred skeletons from archaeological sites in the United States and Ecuador ranging in age from 400 to 6000 years favor a New World origin.[66] Syphilis currently is a worldwide malady that can lead to serious maternal and fetal complications. The nickname "lues" came from the Latin *lues venereum*, which means "disease," "sickness," or "pestilence," and originally was loosely applied to any venereal disease. It became a synonym for syphilis at the beginning of the 20th century.

Despite continued declines among African Americans and women of all races, overall rates of primary and secondary syphilis have recently increased for the first time in more than a decade. After declines from 1992 to 2003, the rate of primary and secondary syphilis among women increased from 0.8 cases per 100,000 population to 1.1 cases per 100,000 population in 2007.[67]

The causal agent of syphilis is *T. pallidum* spp. *pallidum*, which belongs to the family Spirochaetaceae. Other members of the genus *Treponema* that can infect humans are *Treponema pallidum* spp. *pertenue* (yaws), *Treponema carateum* (pinta), and *Treponema pallidum* spp. *endemicum* (bejel, nonvenereal, or endemic syphilis). A number of nonpathogenic treponemes have also been isolated from humans, particularly from the oral cavity. Other pathogenic organisms of the family Spirochaetaceae belong to the genera *Borrelia* and *Leptospira*.[68]

Syphilis can be acquired by sexual contact, by the fetus during pregnancy or birth, by kissing or other close contact with an active lesion, by transfusion of fresh human blood (banked < 24–48 hr), or by accidental direct inoculation. The overwhelming majority of cases of syphilis are transmitted by sexual intercourse, but for all practical purposes, a patient cannot spread syphilis by sexual contact 4 years or more after acquiring the disease.[68] Clinically, syphilis can be divided into five stages: incubating, primary, secondary, latent, and late syphilis. Diagnosis, therapy, and risk to the fetus vary with the stage of the disease.

Within hours or days after *T. pallidum* penetrates the intact mucous membrane or gains access through abraded skin, it enters the lymphatics or bloodstream and disseminates through the body. Virtually any organ, including the central nervous system, may be invaded. The minimum dose for human infection is not known, but in rabbits, an inoculum containing as few as four spirochetes can establish an infection. The incubation period is directly related to the size of the inoculum.[69] The median incubation period is 21 days, but can range from 3 to 90 days. During this stage, a spirochetemia develops that sets the stage for subsequent multiple organ invasion. The first symptomatology to develop occurs in the primary stage, which can last for 4 to 6 weeks (range 2–8 wk) and which usually includes development of the chancre. This painless ulcer (which may be slightly tender to the touch) occurs at the site of inoculation. A small inoculum produces only a papular lesion; a larger inoculum produces the ulcerative chancre. Persons with a history of previous syphilitic infection fail to develop any lesion or develop only a small, darkfield-negative papule.[69] Multiple chancres may occur.[70] Chancres heal spontaneously in 3 to 6 weeks (range 1–12 wk), leaving no trace or a thin atrophic scar. The manifestations of secondary syphilis often develop while the chancre is still present,[71] especially in HIV-infected patients.

The secondary or disseminated stage becomes evident 2 to 12 weeks (mean 6 wk) after contact. The generalized nature of this stage becomes evident as parenchymal, constitutional, and mucocutaneous manifestations may develop. The greatest number of treponemes is present in the body during this stage, and the classic and most commonly recognized lesions involve the skin. Macular, maculopapular, papular, or pustular lesions, and combinations and variations thereof, all may occur.[71] Vesicular lesions are notably absent. In warm, moist intertriginous areas, the papules enlarge, coalesce, and erode to produce painless, broad, moist, gray-white to erythematous, highly infectious plaques called *condylomata lata*. Constitutional symptomatology is also frequently present during the secondary stage and may include low-grade fever, malaise, pharyngitis, laryngitis, anorexia, weight loss, arthralgias, and generalized painless lymphadenopathy. The central nervous system may be involved in up to 40% of patients—headache and meningismus are common. The differential diagnosis of secondary syphilis is extensive—hence, the name "the great imitator."

Latent syphilis is by definition that stage of the disease during which a specific treponemal antibody test is present but during which there are no clinical manifestations of syphilis. It does not imply a lack of progression of disease. Early latent syphilis distinguishes the first year of that period, and late latent syphilis begins after 1 year. Only during the first 4 years of latent syphilis may a relapse occur; thus, the patient must continue to be considered infectious during those 4 years. After 4 years of late latent syphilis, the patient develops host resistance to reinfection and to infectious relapse. However, a pregnant woman with late latent syphilis can transmit the infection vertically to her fetus.

Late or tertiary syphilis is a slowly progressive, inflammatory disease that may affect any organ system and is usually subdivided into neurosyphilis, cardiovascular syphilis, and gummatous syphilis.

Diagnosis

Unlike many nonpathogenic treponemas, the virulent treponemes, including *T. pallidum*, cannot be cultivated in vitro.

Direct Examination for Spirochetes

In primary, secondary, and early congenital syphilis, the darkfield examination (a wet-preparation method for direct visualization of living *T. pallidum* spirochetes) or immunofluorescence staining of mucocutaneous lesions are the quickest and most direct laboratory methods of establishing the diagnosis.[72] Examination of a serous transudate from moist lesions such as a primary chancre or condyloma latum is productive because these lesions contain the largest number of treponemes. *T. pallidum* may be demonstrated from dry skin lesions or from lymph nodes by saline aspiration, if the saline is free of bactericidal additives. Specimens from mouth lesions are not accurate because *T. pallidum* cannot be distinguished from nonpathogenic treponemes with certainty.

Serologic Tests

Two different types of antibodies are measured in the evaluation of syphilis: the *nonspecific* nontreponemal reaginic antibody and the *specific* antitreponemal antibody.

Syphilis reaginic antibodies are IgG and IgM directed against a lipoidal antigen resulting from the interaction of host tissues with *T. pallidum* or from the organism itself. The earliest antigens used to measure reaginic antibody were phospholipid extracts made from beef livers and subsequently from beef hearts (hence, the name *cardiolipin*). The standard nontreponemal test is the VDRL (Venereal Disease Research Laboratories) slide test, although most laboratories have adopted a modification for routine screening called the rapid plasma reagin (RPR) test or other similar method. The quantitative RPR test should become nonreactive 1 year after successful therapy in primary syphilis and 2 years after successful therapy in secondary syphilis.[73] A patient with late syphilis should have a negative response after 5 years.[74] However, the longer the disease has been present before treatment, the longer the VDRL takes to become nonreactive. In many cases after the secondary stage, it will never become nonreactive, even with adequate treatment (this is called *Wasserman fastness*). A prozone phenomenon occurs in about 2% of infected patients, especially in secondary syphilis and pregnancy, and appropriate dilutions should be performed whenever the index of suspicion is high.[75]

The principal specific antitreponemal antibody tests done today are the fluorescent treponemal antibody absorption test (FTA-abs), the *T. pallidum* particle agglutination (TPPA) test, *T. pallidum* hemagglutination assay (TPHA), and the microhemagglutination assay–*T. pallidum* (MHA-TP) test. The FTA-abs is a standard indirect immunofluorescent antibody test that uses *T. pallidum* harvested from rabbit testes as the antigen. Because of the difficulty with standardization between laboratories and with quantifying results and the meticulousness with which the test must be performed, the TPHA, which uses a sorbent for increased specificity, or the MHA-TP, an adaptation of the TPHA, is commonly used today. Once positive, the patient usually remains positive for life, although patients treated early may revert to a nonreactive state in up to 10% of cases.[68] Acute or transient false-positive nontreponemal reaginic test reactions may occur whenever there is a strong immunologic stimulus, such as with an acute bacterial or viral infection, vaccination, or early HIV infection. Positive reactions that last for months may occur with parenteral drug abuse, in those with autoimmune or connective tissue diseases, and in patients in hypergammaglobulinemic states. Syphilis may be excluded if a biologic false-positive (BFP) test is suspected by obtaining a negative specific treponemal antibody test, such as the FTP-abs or MHA-TP. Other spirochetal illnesses, such as relapsing fever (*Borrelia* spp.), yaws, pinta, leptospirosis, or rat-bite fever (*Spirillum minus*) may also yield a positive nontreponemal test. Infection with *B. burgdorferi* (Lyme disease) results in a positive FTA-abs test but does not cause a positive nontreponemal reaginic reaction with either the VDRL or the RPR.

Because of expense and ease of performance, screening large numbers of patients such as in pregnancy is usually done with reaginic antibody tests (RPR, VDRL), and confirmation is done with the specific treponemal tests (FTA-abs or MHA-TP).

Ultrasound

The prenatal diagnostic test with the greatest potential for identifying the severely infected fetus is ultrasound. Ultrasound findings suggestive of in utero infection include placentomegaly, intrauterine growth restriction, microcephaly, hepatosplenomegaly, anemia, and hydrops.

Maternal and Fetal Risks

Maternal risks of syphilis acquired during pregnancy are similar to those for acquisition in the nonpregnant state. *T. pallidum* readily crosses the placenta and up to 75% of infants born to mothers with active syphilitic infections will become infected in utero.[76] It is critical to identify infections as early in pregnancy as possible to reduce this risk. Although vertical transmission can occur during any stage of infection in the untreated or inadequately treated gravida, infection of the fetus before 16 weeks' gestation is rare; therefore, early abortion is unlikely to be the result of syphilis. Perinatal transmission occurs in approximately 50% of patients with primary or secondary syphilis. This decreases among women with latent infection (40%) or late latent/tertiary disease (10%). Treatment of the mother decreases risk of infection to approximately 1%. Later in pregnancy, depending on the severity of the maternal infection, abortion, stillbirth, neonatal death, neonatal disease, or latent infection may be seen.[72] More recent evidence indicates that these manifestations appear to be caused largely by dysfunction of the maternal-fetal endocrine axis, resulting in decreased levels of dehydroepiandrosterone produced by the fetal adrenal glands.[77] Neonatal manifestations of congenital syphilis include rhinitis (snuffles), which may be followed by a diffuse maculopapular, desquamative rash with extensive sloughing of the epithelium, particularly on the palms, on the soles, and around the mouth and anus. Hepatic involvement with associated splenomegaly, anemia, thrombocytopenia, and jaundice is also common. Neonatal death is usually caused by liver failure, severe pneumonia, or pulmonary hemorrhage. Renal involvement and a generalized osteochondritis and perichondritis may be seen as well.

Management Options

Prepregnancy

Although the efficacy of penicillin in the treatment of syphilis is well established, there remains uncertainty regarding optimal dose and duration of therapy, especially during pregnancy.[78] Therefore, treatment regimens must be viewed with this in mind and with the understanding that treatment failures do occur and must be recognized and retreated. From work with experimental infections, it is known that penicillin concentrations as low as 0.018 μg/mL sustained for 7 days in the nonpregnant adult results in almost 100% treponemicidal activity.[79] It has also been recognized that *T. pallidum* has been isolated from the cerebrospinal fluid (CSF) of patients with only a chancre.[80] Therefore, to adequately treat this infection that may affect the central nervous system, one must treat the parasite in the CSF. However, despite the fact that benzathine penicillin does not reliably achieve treponemicidal levels in the CSF[81] and that retreatment may be required in as many as 1 in 33 cases,[82] clinical experience continues to suggest that benzathine penicillin remains a mainstay of therapy. When an early diagnosis is made, fewer treponemes exist and the likelihood of a complete cure is greatly enhanced. Because of the high risk of infection, treatment should be given to anyone exposed to infectious syphilis within the preceding 3 months. Serologic studies must be done to establish the diagnosis and monitor success of therapy.

Prenatal

Pregnant patients should receive penicillin in the same dosage schedules as nonpregnant adults for comparable stages of the disease. When a well-documented penicillin allergy exists, desensitization (which can be accomplished in as few as 3–4 hr) is recommended.[83,84]

For primary and secondary syphilis and for early latent syphilis, administer benzathine penicillin G 2.4 million units

IM once. For late latent syphilis or for latent syphilis of unknown duration, administer benzathine penicillin G 7.2 million units total, as three doses of 2.4 million units IM each at 1-week intervals. Regimens for syphilis in pregnancy that do not include penicillin have not been documented to be adequate therapy to prevent congenital syphilis. Pregnant patients with concomitant HIV infections should be considered for treatment as if they have neurosyphilis, regardless of their clinical findings. The only effective treatment demonstrated for penicillin-allergic pregnant patients is desensitization followed by penicillin therapy. True penicillin allergy (except in those with history of an anaphylactic reaction) can be demonstrated by skin allergy testing.[85]

All women should be screened serologically for syphilis at the first prenatal visit. In populations in which prenatal care is not optimal, RPR test screening and treatment (if the RPR test is reactive) should be performed at the time a pregnancy is confirmed. For communities and populations in which the prevalence of syphilis is high or for patients at high risk, serologic testing in addition to routine early screening should be performed twice during the third trimester: at 28 weeks' gestation and at delivery.

The fetus with hepatomegaly or ascites is more likely to fail prenatal therapy and may benefit from a more extended course than usual and more intense monitoring throughout the remainder of the pregnancy.[86]

The Jarisch-Herxheimer reaction is a systemic reaction that occurs 1 to 2 hours after the initial treatment of syphilis with effective antibiotics. It consists of the abrupt onset of fever, chills, myalgia, headache, tachycardia, hyperventilation, vasodilation with flushing, and mild hypotension. Additional findings at or beyond 24 weeks' gestation include uterine contractions (42%) and recurrent variable fetal heart rate decelerations (38%).[87] It lasts for 12 to 24 hours and may be treated in pregnancy with antipyretics or prednisone, although no studies have documented a clearly effective prophylaxis.

Labor and Delivery

In the United States, some states mandate screening for syphilis at delivery for all women. Any woman who delivers a stillborn infant after 20 weeks' gestation should be tested for syphilis.

Postpartum

No infant should leave the hospital if maternal serologic status has not been determined at least once during pregnancy and preferably again at delivery. All patients with early or congenital syphilis should have repeat quantitative nontreponemal tests at 3, 6, and 12 months. All patients with secondary syphilis or syphilis of more than 1 year's duration should also have a nontreponemal serologic test 24 months after treatment. Many experts recommend examination of the CSF for those patients treated with benzathine penicillin because of its poor ability to penetrate the CSF. Retreatment should be considered whenever clinical signs and symptoms of syphilis persist or recur, whenever there is a sustained level or an increase in the titer on the nontreponemal test, or whenever a positive RPR reaction persists beyond 12 months in primary syphilis, 24 months in secondary or latent syphilis, or 5 years in late syphilis.[68]

SUMMARY OF MANAGEMENT OPTIONS

Syphilis

Management Options	Evidence Quality and Recommendation	References
Prepregnancy		
Identify and treat with penicillin (provided not allergic) before pregnancy.	IV/C	78
Initiate contact tracing and treatment.	—/GPP	—
Confirm response with serial serology.	—/GPP	—
Prenatal		
Provide routine serologic screening in early pregnancy.	IV/C	78
Treat with penicillin (provided not allergic) all with *Toxoplasma palladum*–positive lesions (rare).	IV/C	78
Treat all women with positive serology with penicillin (provided not allergic) even if history suggests they have been treated in the past	IV/C	78
If significant penicillin allergy is determined, the pregnant patient should be desensitized.	III/B	83,84
Initiate contact tracing and treatment.	—/GPP	—
Confirm response with serial serology.	IV/C	78

Management Options	Evidence Quality and Recommendation	References
Labor and Delivery		
Some states in the United States require testing of all women at delivery.	—/GPP	—
Evaluate all cases of stillbirth > 20 wk for the presence of syphilis.	IV/C	68
Inform pediatricians of prenatal syphilis.	IV/C	86
Postnatal		
Alert pediatricians to the presence of syphilis during pregnancy so that they can properly evaluate the neonate for early (snuffles, rash, hepatosplenomegaly, jaundice) and late (deafness, hydrocephalus, optic nerve atrophy, mental retardation) manifestations of congenital syphilis.	IV/C	86
Follow-up tests should occur up to 2 yr after treatment, with concomitant fall in titers during that period.	III/B	68,76

GPP, good practice point.

TOXOPLASMOSIS

General

Toxoplasmosis is caused by the obligate intracellular parasite *Toxoplasma gondii*. Its name is derived from "toxon" (Greek for *arc*, the shape of the parasite during its acute infectious phase in humans) and "gundi" (the North African rodent from which the parasite was originally identified). Infections in immunocompetent individuals are frequently subclinical and innocuous unless the individual is pregnant, during which time, vertical transmission can occur and lead to significant disease and possibly death in the fetus or neonate. The organism has three distinct forms: the tachyzoite, or arc form, found in the parasitemic or acute phase of infection; the tissue cyst, found in the quiescent or latent phase in many organs of humans and animals; and the oocyst, which originates only in the digestive tract of members of the family Felidae (including domestic and feral cats).

Toxoplasmosis can be transmitted to humans by three principal routes. It is estimated that approximately 50% of the toxoplasmosis cases in the United States are caused by eating inadequately cooked meat[88] (especially pork, mutton, and wild game meat) containing the tissue cyst form of the organism.[89] A second means of acquiring toxoplasmosis is by inadvertently ingesting the oocysts that cats have passed in their feces, either from a cat litter box, from infected soil where a cat has defecated, or from unwashed fruits or vegetables that have contacted infected soil. Under favorable conditions (i.e., in warm, moist soil), oocysts can remain infectious for approximately 1 year. A third means of transmission is transplacentally, when a primary infection occurs during pregnancy. Other than vertical transmission and the rare incidence of blood or organ donation between individuals, it is not possible to acquire toxoplasmosis from either a neonate or another adult. In adults, the incubation period ranges from 10 to 23 days from ingestion of undercooked meat and from 5 to 20 days from ingestion of oocysts from cat feces.[90]

Since the 1960s, rates of infection with *Toxoplasma* in the United States appear to have declined from 14% (in a study of U.S. military recruits at that time)[91] to a seroprevalence of 9.6% in a second study of recruits in 1989.[92] In the Third National Health and Nutrition Examination Survey (NHANES III) conducted in the United States from 1988 to 1994, 17,658 individuals were tested for *Toxoplasma*-specific IgG antibodies; 23% were found to be positive. Of 5988 women of child-bearing age (12–49 yr) in that series, 14% were seropositive.[93]

Determining the number of cases of congenital toxoplasmosis is more difficult than estimating seroprevalence, although prospective studies in the United States from the 1970s[94,95] and from the period 1986 to 1992[96] indicate an infection rate of between 1 in 10,000 to 10 in 10,000 live births. With an estimated 4 million births annually in the United States, 400 to 4000 neonates yearly will be born with congenital toxoplasmosis.

Although some studies identify cleaning the cat litter box[97] or owning a cat[98] as risk factors, the presence of a cat has not been a consistent risk factor for *T. gondii* infection. Owning a cat was not shown to be a risk factor for *T. gondii* infection in two studies of pregnant women[99,100] and in a study of HIV-infected persons.[101] Cats generally only shed oocysts for several weeks during their lives if they become infected with *T. gondii*. Cats kept indoors that do not hunt prey or are not fed raw meat are not likely to acquire *T. gondii* infection and, therefore, pose little risk. Because of their grooming habits, fecal matter has not been found on the fur of clinically normal cats, and adult cats are not diarrheal during the period in which they are shedding oocysts.[88] Therefore, the possibility of transmission to human beings via touching cats is minimal to nonexistent.[88] Because cats may not develop antibodies to *T. gondii* during the oocyst-shedding period, serologic examination of cats does not provide useful information regarding the ability of a particular cat to transmit the infection.[88]

Outbreaks of toxoplasmosis in humans have been attributed to ingestion of raw or undercooked ground beef, lamb, pork, or venison[102–107]; unpasteurized goat's milk[108]; contaminated unfiltered drinking water[109–110]; soil exposure[111]; and aerosolized soil exposure.[112]

Diagnosis

Because most acute *Toxoplasma* infections are relatively asymptomatic, a universal challenge for obstetricians is how to identify acute infections during pregnancy. In France and Austria, where the incidence of toxoplasmosis is much higher than in the United States, universal screening is mandatory.[113] In the United States, although universal screening has frequently been discussed, it is not generally practiced. An article using decision analysis estimated that universal screening with medical treatment would result in 18.5 additional pregnancy losses for each case of toxoplasmosis avoided (12.1 additional pregnancy losses were estimated to occur if infected pregnancies underwent termination rather than treatment).[114]

When screening is performed or when a pregnant woman's clinical presentation leads the practitioner to suspect acute toxoplasmosis, the diagnosis may be established by serologic tests, amplification of specific nucleic acid sequences (using PCR), histologic demonstration of the parasite and/or its antigens (immunoperoxidase stain), or isolation of the organism. Ultrasound also has an important role in the evaluation of this infection.

Serologic Tests

The use of serologic tests for demonstration of specific antibody to *T. gondii* in maternal blood is the initial and primary method of diagnosis. IgG antibodies usually appear within 1 to 2 weeks of acquisition of an infection, peak within 1 to 2 months, decline at various rates, and usually persist for life. The most common methods of measurement of IgG include the Sabin-Feldman dye test, the ELISA, the immunofluorescence assay (IFA), and the modified direct agglutination test.[115] IgM antibodies, conversely, may appear earlier and decline more rapidly than IgG antibodies. They are measured by ELISA, IFA, and the immunosorbent agglutination assay.[115] False-positive results for the presence of IgM may occur when rheumatoid factor or antinuclear antibodies are present. Commercial kits often have low specificity, and positive results must be interpreted with great caution. Although IgM antibodies usually decline rapidly after the onset of infection, they may persist for years in some individuals, further complicating the interpretation of a positive serologic test.

A combination of serologic tests is usually required to establish whether an individual has most likely been infected in the distant past (which should pose minimal to no risk to an ongoing pregnancy) or has been recently infected. The traditional acute and convalescent titers of IgM and IgG are most helpful when either both are negative in two samples 3 or more weeks apart (no acute or chronic infection) or IgG is positive and IgM is negative in both samples (distant infection but no acute infection). When IgM is positive in either (especially when titers are drawn after the first trimester of pregnancy) or when IgG is negative in the first and positive in the second (or with a greater than fourfold rise in IgG antibody titer from the first sample) with or without positive IgM, concern about a recent infection must be raised. Owing to lack of standardization, serologic diagnosis should be confirmed by a reference laboratory such as the Palo Alto Medical Foundation Research Institute's Toxoplasma Serology Laboratory (650-853-4828).[116] Another reported means by which acute and chronic infections may be distinguished is by measuring the binding strength of specific IgG antibodies to multivalent *Toxoplasma* antigen. This binding strength, or IgG avidity, increases as the duration of infection lengthens. Thus, higher IgG avidity indicates a more long-standing infection and may be useful in early pregnancy when other tests are inconclusive.[117]

Polymerase Chain Reaction

PCR amplification for detection of *T. gondii* DNA in amniotic fluid has been used to accurately and rapidly diagnose intrauterine infection with the parasite. The sensitivity is high (81%–88%),[118,119] and the overall accuracy is comparable with or better than fetal blood testing by cordocentesis[118,119] with less risk to the fetus.

Histology

Demonstration of tachyzoites in amniotic fluid or placental tissue establishes the diagnosis of an acute infection. This is best accomplished with the immunoperoxidase technique with antisera to *T. gondii*.[120]

Isolation of Toxoplasma gondii

Isolation of the organism from tissue or fluid establishes the infection as acute. Mouse inoculation coupled with PCR analysis of amniotic fluid has sensitivities of 91% to 94%.[118,121]

Ultrasound

Ultrasound findings of fetal infection with *T. gondii* are generally nonspecific; however, ventricular dilation (the most common finding), intracranial calcifications, increased placental thickness, hepatic enlargement, and ascites may be seen in over one-third of cases of fetal infection and may be useful in evaluation.[122] In highly suspicious cases in which serology or PCR is nonconclusive, follow-up ultrasound has been found to be valuable in confirming a diagnosis of congenital toxoplasmosis.[123]

Maternal and Fetal Risks

Maternal risks of toxoplasmosis in the immunocompetent gravida are minimal, and 90% of infections are asymptomatic and self-limited. Symptoms most commonly resemble infectious mononucleosis with posterior cervical or axillary lymphadenopathy that is discrete, nontender, and nonsuppurative. Other maternal symptoms may include malaise and muscle pain.

Fetal risks, conversely, vary widely, depending on the trimester of acquisition and presence or absence of maternal treatment. In general, the earlier the infection is acquired, the lower the risk of fetal transmission, but the greater the risk of serious sequelae to the fetus when congenital infection does develop.[124] A recent meta-analysis by Thiebaut and coworkers[125] estimated the risk of transmission at 13 weeks, 26 weeks, and 36 weeks to be approximately 15%, 44%, and 71%, respectively. As many as 85% of congenitally infected neonates have subclinical infections that will later surface as chorioretinitis, hearing loss, or developmental delays. Serious sequelae noted at or after birth, including intrauterine death, neurologic abnormalities, hydrocephalus and cerebral calcifications, and chorioretinal scars with or without severe visual impairment, may be reduced by the use of prenatal antibiotic therapy even though the rate of congenital infection may not change.[118,126]

Management Options

Prepregnancy

Preconception infection with toxoplasmosis generally conveys immunity to subsequent pregnancies against congenital toxoplasmosis. Reports exist describing preconception seroconversion and subsequent fetal infection, but these are extremely rare,[127] and gravidas with IgG positivity at the onset of pregnancy should be considered at low risk for subsequent congenital infection.

Prenatal

Prevention of acute infection during pregnancy is much preferred to treatment of toxoplasmosis. Pregnant women, especially those determined to be IgG-negative during pregnancy, should be advised of appropriate preventive measures to use. When acute toxoplasmosis is suspected during pregnancy, appropriate laboratory testing is critical (see "Diagnosis"). If serologic testing confirms acute *maternal* toxoplasmosis, amniocentesis with PCR testing of amniotic fluid should be performed to document presence of *fetal* infection. Cordocentesis is no longer considered an essential component of the evaluation of fetal infection, having been replaced by PCR owing to its simplicity and relative safety. Spiramycin 3 g/day should be administered as soon as maternal infection is documented, adding pyrimethamine/sulfadiazine if fetal infection is confirmed by PCR testing. Doses and dosing schedules and the addition of folinic acid with pyrimethamine vary, taking into consideration the trimester and local preferences. Pyrimethamine is not recommended for use in the first trimester.[128,129] In the United States, spiramycin may be obtained through special permission from the CDC after confirmation of acute maternal infection by a reputable reference laboratory.[130]

Labor and Delivery

Patients with ongoing or recent toxoplasmosis infection pose a transmission risk only to their fetus and do not require isolation for themselves or for their newborn. The pediatrician caring for the neonate should be alerted to the possibility of congenital toxoplasmosis so appropriate follow-up studies can be performed on the infant. Congenital infection can be excluded if IgG does not persist in the infant beyond age 12 months.

Postpartum

After delivery, the parturient may be managed routinely, again emphasizing to the health care team that neither she nor the newborn poses a risk of transmission to others.

SUMMARY OF MANAGEMENT OPTIONS
Toxoplasmosis

Management Options	Evidence Quality and Recommendation	References
Prepregnancy		
Toxoplasmosis infection before conception (documented by the presence of IgG antibodies) conveys a relative immunity to the gravida and makes congenital infection extremely unlikely.	III/B	127
Prenatal–Prevention		
Teach patient to prevent *Toxoplasma* infection: • Cook meat to well done (industrial deep-freezing also seems to destroy parasites efficiently). • When handling raw meat, avoid touching mouth and eyes. • Wash hands thoroughly after handling raw meat or vegetables soiled by earth. • Wash kitchen surfaces that come into contact with raw meat. • Wash fruit and vegetables before consumption. • Avoid contact with items that are potentially contaminated with cat feces. • Wear gloves when gardening or handling cat litter box. • Disinfect cat litter box for 5 min with boiling water.	—/GPP	—
The policy of routine screening for toxoplasmosis varies between countries; it is not practiced universally in the United States.	III/B	114

SUMMARY OF MANAGEMENT OPTIONS

Toxoplasmosis—cont'd

Management Options	Evidence Quality and Recommendation	References
Prenatal–Diagnosis		
Maternal infection should be confirmed by an appropriate laboratory using reliable testing, which may include Sabin-Feldman dye test for IgG and ELISA; testing for IgM, IgA, and IgE along with IgG avidity testing; or differential agglutination test for chronicity of infection.	III/B	116
IgM antibodies for toxoplasmosis are frequently false-positive or may represent chronic infection, and should *always* be confirmed by a reference laboratory.	IIb/B	116
Prenatal–Treatment		
When maternal infection is confirmed, begin spiramycin as soon as possible.	IIa/B	122,129
Fetal infection may be diagnosed by PCR testing of amniotic fluid, obviating the need for cordocentesis (though not possible to determine prognosis).	IIa/B	118,121
Documented fetal infection necessitates addition of pyrimethamine/sulfadiazine.	IIa/B	122,129
Serial ultrasound will give an identification of signs of fetal infection.	IIa/B	121,123
Labor and Delivery, Postpartum		
Neither the mother nor the infant is infectious to the health care team and may be handled normally.	IV/C	120

ELISA, enzyme-linked immunosorbent assay; GPP, good practice point; Ig, immunoglobulin; PCR, polymerase chain reaction.

SCHISTOSOMIASIS

General

Schistosomiasis, also known as bilharziasis, is caused by a parasitic trematode blood fluke[131] first discovered by Theodor Bilharz in 1852. Schistosomiasis is endemic to 74 countries. This disease infects more than 200 million people, of which 40 million are women of childbearing age. At any one time, 120 million have symptoms of the disease and approximately 20 million have severe disease.[132–134] Estimates indicate that global deaths as a result of schistosomiasis may be as high as 200,000 per year and serious disability results in up to 15% of those infected.[135,136]

Five species of schistosomes have been reported to infect the intestines or urinary tract of humans. In Africa, the Eastern Mediterranean, the Caribbean, and South America, intestinal schistosomiasis is caused by *Schistosoma mansoni*. In central Africa, another species, *Schistosoma intercalatum*, has been found to cause intestinal schistosomiasis. In Asia and Western Pacific countries, intestinal schistosomiasis is caused by *S. japonicum* and *S. mekongi*. Urinary schistosomiasis, caused by *S. haematobium* is endemic to Africa and the Eastern Mediterranean region. 85% of persons with the disease are infected by either *S. mansoni* or *S. haematobium* and live in sub-Saharan Africa.[132]

Schistosomes have a complex life cycle and require two hosts in their development. The parasite's eggs are released into fresh water by way of defecation or, in the case of *S. haematobium*, by urination. The hypotonic environment of fresh water triggers the eggs to mature and release a male or female miracidia. The miracidium swims searching for a susceptible, species-specific snail. Miracidia do not feed and if a suitable host is not found, their life span is limited. Once a suitable snail is found, the miracidium enters through the foot process and subsequently transforms into a primary sporocyst and matures in either the foot process or the snail's digestive gland. Within the primary sporocyst, germinal cells replicate, mature, and bud off as many secondary sporocysts, which migrate to the snail liver and mature into cercariae.[131] Most infected snails are not significantly injured by this process and can survive for prolonged periods of time.

Cercariae are fork-tailed, infective larval forms of the schistosoma and are free-swimming. They exit the snail in search of a host and, like the miracidia, do not feed. Once in water, their ability to optimally infect a host diminishes significantly after 4 hours, although they may survive for as long as 48 hours. The cercariae attach to human skin using an oral sucker containing glands that release enzymes allowing migration through the skin epidermis. During migration, the forked tail is discarded and the larva develops a double-lipid bilayer tegument that effectively protects it from the host's immune system by mimicking the host and inhibiting the immune system. At this point, the cercariae has developed into a schistosomula.[137]

Over several days, the schistosomula (parasite stage) uses lytic enzymes to migrate through the dermis and access the venous system. It is then pumped through the right side of the heart and into the lungs where it migrates along pulmonary capillaries and enters the systemic circulation through the left side of the heart. At this point, the schistosomula travels to the mesenteric arteries and splanchnic capillaries and, finally, through the portal veins where it gains access to the liver. In the liver, the organism matures and pairs with a schistosomula of the opposite sex (a trait that is unique among trematodes). The thin female schistosomula resides within the gynecophoric canal of the male. The female is carried by the male, and they migrate against portal blood flow to either the mesenteric or the vesical veins. At this point, the pair migrates along the veins and deposits eggs.[131,137]

Although the average life span of the schistosomula is 3 to 5 years, cases have been reported of adult schistosomula living up to 30 years.[138] The adult causes little direct damage to the host, clinical sequelae being the result of the immune response to the deposited eggs. Whereas the parasite effectively evades the immune system, the eggs lodged in the host tissue elicit an aggressive T helper-2 (Th-2)–mediated immune attack. Despite this robust immune reaction, the eggshell is extremely resistant to proteases. This results in a granulomatous reaction that may be used by the egg to migrate across the intestinal or urinary bladder wall and allow deposition into stool or urine where the life cycle begins again.[131,138–142]

Acute infection is usually asymptomatic and if clinical symptoms do occur, they usually manifest among individuals who are new to an endemic area and who have no prior immunity. The most common clinical symptom is generalized fatigue. Acute infection can also manifest in the form of "swimmer's itch" or Katayama fever. Swimmer's itch is caused by a local dermatologic reaction to the cercariae that starts as local itching at the site of entry and progresses to an intense pruritic papular or urticarial rash within 24 hours of exposure. The pruritus and itching can last for up to a week.[143,144]

Katayama fever is believed to be a result of a hypersensitivity reaction to the migrating parasite. Onset begins approximately 35 to 40 days following contact with infested water. Clinical symptoms include fever, malaise, diarrhea, arthralgia, myalgia, and cough. Eosinophilia is a component of the acute infection. Although transaminases are not elevated, hepatic tenderness and enlargement are commonly present.[131,145,146] Symptoms usually resolve after a few weeks as the infection enters the chronic stage, although there have been cases of coma and even death reported, especially with *S. japonicum*.[144,147]

Chronic schistosomiasis and its clinical sequelae are the result of egg deposition followed by granuloma formation and scarring. The granulomas that form around the schistosomula egg are composed of eosinophils (50%), mast cells, macrophages, lymphocytes, and fibroblasts. Burden of disease is related to the number of eggs deposited in tissue. Symptoms begin slowly but are progressive without treatment. They commonly involve the intestinal, hepatic, and urinary systems, but in some cases, neurologic, pulmonary, and genital involvement may occur.[131,143]

The most common presenting symptom of intestinal schistosomiasis is bloody diarrhea, which can lead to iron deficiency anemia. Patients also may have abdominal tenderness and tenesmus. In some asymptomatic cases, patients may present with guaiac-positive stools. Rarely, intestinal schistosomiasis will present with inflammatory colonic polyps or intestinal obstruction.[148–150]

Hepatic schistosomiasis may have two clinical presentations. In children and adolescents, there may be hepatomegaly and/or splenomegaly due to an inflammatory response to deposited eggs.[151] The more common form occurs years after infection and is defined by portal hypertension as a result of granulomas that have healed and formed fibrotic scars. Before healing and resolution of one fibrotic lesion is completed, another granuloma is formed, initiating a pattern that can lead to Symmer's pipestem fibrosis. Symmer's pipestem fibrosis results from the portal vein and its tributaries becoming fibrotic, causing impediment of portal blood flow, thus producing portal hypertension. Although hepatic function remains largely unaffected, ascites and esophageal varices can form and lead to hemorrhage.[131,151,152]

Urinary schistosomiasis is caused by *S. haematobium*. The pathophysiology involves deposition of eggs in the mucosa of the genitourinary system. Presentation may be asymptomatic or the infection may manifest as hematuria severe enough to cause anemia, dysuria, and frequency. If untreated, the infection may progress to obstruction, hydroureter, and hydronephrosis. As a result, susceptibility to serious bacterial infections can occur leading to kidney damage.[153] Kidney damage may also occur as a result of deposition of immune complexes leading to proteinuria and nephrotic syndrome.[154] *S. haematobium* can also induce squamous cell metaplasia of the urinary bladder and urethral mucosa and may increase the risk of developing squamous cell carcinoma of the bladder.[131,154]

In some cases of schistosomiasis, neurologic sequelae may occur as a result of deposition of eggs in the spinal cord and its resulting granulomatous inflammatory reaction. This can cause a myelopathy. There may also be migration of the parasite to cerebral or cerebellar tissue manifesting in seizures, focal neurologic impairment, or increased intracranial pressure.[155,156]

Pulmonary complications may occur as an extension of hepatic disease and portal hypertension. The portosystemic collaterals that develop in this scenario allow embolization of schistosome eggs into the pulmonary circulation. This can lead to a granulomatous pulmonary endarteritis, which can cause pulmonary hypertension.[157] Clinical signs may include coughing and wheezing, and a chest x-ray may show infiltrates, military nodules, and heart enlargement with dilated pulmonary arteries.[158,159]

Possible gynecologic involvement includes ulcerative and hypertrophic lesions of the cervix, uterus, vagina, and vulva. In rare cases, ectopic pregnancies have been reported, as has infertility.[151,160,161]

Ultrasound imaging in acute schistosomiasis usually demonstrates normal or nonspecific findings such as hepatomegaly, splenomegaly, or periportal adenopathy. In chronic schistosomiasis, periportal fibrosis and signs of portal hypertension such as an increase in caliber of the portal vein and its tributaries may develop. Ultrasound is mainly helpful for tracking long-term changes and directing further therapy.

Diagnosis

Suspicion of a possible acute schistosomal infection in a patient should develop with a history of recent travel to an endemic area and with recent onset of fatigue, fever, bloody diarrhea, hematuria, abdominal pain, arthalgias, or cough. On physical examination, the addition of hepatosplenomagaly should increase suspicion for the infection. Nonspecific laboratory abnormalities commonly seen with schistosomiasis include eosinophilia in approximately 50% of patients[162] and iron deficiency anemia, which may be present owing to chronic blood loss. Thrombocytopenia may also be present owing to splenic sequestration.[131] Seventy-eight percent of those infected with *S. haematobium* in the bladder will have positive hematuria on dipstick.[163]

Diagnosis of schistosomiasis is usually made by parasitologic (microscopic detection of eggs) or antibody and antigen detection. Demonstrating eggs in the feces or urine indicates the presence of the organism. The classic method used for detecting parasite eggs in the stool is the Kato-Katz thick smear preparation, which uses glycerol to allow for visualization of entrapped eggs. This smear is not routinely used by many laboratories as part of their standard ova and parasite evaluation, necessitating the notification of the microbiology laboratory about a specific concern for schistosomiasis when stool is submitted for evaluation.[131] Disadvantages of searching for parasite eggs in the feces or urine directly include the large fluctuations in egg counts resulting in infections during the nadir of egg release being easily missed and the time-consuming nature of these tests.[164]

Immunologic methods such as ELISA measurement of circulating anodic antigen (CAA) or circulating cathodic antigen (CCA) on serum or urine samples have a higher sensitivity and maintain high specificity.[164] In addition, these methods allow for demonstration of active infections and can be used to monitor the effects of treatment. A disadvantage is the need for sophisticated laboratory equipment that is often not available in the field, and attempts are being made to develop a rapid field-applicable test for the detection of these antigens.[164,165]

Maternal and Fetal Risks

There are little data addressing the pregnancy-related burden of schistosomiasis. The morbidity experienced by pregnant mothers and their newborns remains unclear.[134] In Africa, where greater than 85% of people with schistosomiasis live, it is estimated that 10 million women per year have schistosomiasis during pregnancy. However, the number of pregnant women who are infected worldwide is unknown.[136] Many of the morbidities in pregnancy are likely the cause of the profound undernutrition and anemia caused by schistosomiasis.[166–168]

There is also evidence of potential fetal effects of schistosomiasis. A cross-sectional survey of 972 women in Tanzania demonstrated that heavy infection with *S. mansoni* was associated with increased risk of anemia and reduced hemoglobin levels (adjusted odds ratio 1.82; $P = .026$). The effects persisted after controlling for potential confounders.[169] A prospective study in Ghana compared births outcomes of 41 infected pregnant women with a control group of 500 noninfected women. Delivery data were available for 23 of these infected cases. They demonstrated a larger percentage of preterm births (34.8% vs. 23.8%) among infected females and lower birth weight among the preterm infants (1768 g vs. 2457 g).[170] Another study from an endemic region of China compared 244 infected women with 236 healthy controls. They also showed significant differences in weight among infants born to infected women (3229 g vs. 3355 g).[171] Unfortunately, these two studies were not adjusted for potential confounders such as prepregnancy weight, nutritional status, and socioeconomic status, making their results inconclusive. Vertical transmission has been demonstrated in one study in which schistosoma infection was diagnosed in 3 of 22 newborns who were examined for infection.[134,172] Infection and inflammation has been demonstrated in the placenta of women infected with schistosomiasis, demonstrating a potential mechanism for placental insufficiency.[173,174]

Management Options

Prepregnancy

Owing to the importance of prepregnancy nutritional status, all patients with evidence of infection should be treated. The treatment of choice for all schistosoma species is praziquantel. Praziquantel paralyzes the adult schistosome by increasing calcium ion influx across the tegument membrane and also by exposing parasite antigens to the host immune system.[175] For most schistosoma species, a dose of 40 mg/kg in one or two doses is adequate. When treating *S. japonicum or S. mekongi*, a dose of 60 mg/kg divided in two or three doses is recommended.[176] Cure rates approach 85% to 90%[177] and at present, no vaccine is available.

After therapy, monitoring mainly involves examination of the stool or urine, depending on species of schistosmiasis, and monitoring of eosinophil count in cases with eosinophilia.

In endemic areas, follow-up evaluation of specimens is performed approximately 6 weeks after treatment. In nonendemic areas, reexamination is recommended 3 to 6 months after treatment owing to the low risk of reinfection.[143]

Unfortunately, praziquantel is ineffective in early infection or Katayama fever. In these situations, supportive care with the addition of prednisone (40 mg daily for 5 days), if needed, can be used to relieve some of the host symptoms as a result of hypersensitivity. Praziquantel can then be given 6 to 10 weeks later, once adult worms have developed.[178]

Prenatal

If pregnant women plan on visiting an area endemic to schistosomiasis, care should be taken to avoid swimming in fresh water that may not have proper sewage control and to use footwear when coming into contact with water sources. Nutrition status should be assessed with close monitoring of hemoglobin levels.

The World Health Organization in 2003[136] gave an informal recommendation that pregnant and lactating women should not be excluded from treatment. Although the toxicity of praziquantel has not been formally evaluated, more recent reports have supported its safety in pregnancy. In a report of 88 pregnancies with inadvertent exposure to praziquantel in the first trimester that were compared with 549 pregnant controls, there were no differences between the two groups in rates of abortion and preterm deliveries. In addition, no congenital anomalies were observed.[179] In a separate study conducted in the Sudan, 25 pregnant infected women were treated with a single dose of praziquantel during different semesters. There were no differences in the abortion rate when compared with the background rate of the community.[180]

Labor and Delivery

Schistosomiasis cannot be transmitted from human to human. As a result, patients in labor do not need to be isolated. The pediatrician should be notified of the mother's infection status owing to some reports of vertical transmission.

Postpartum

Routine postpartum management can be continued. No adverse effects of the use of praziquantel during lactation have been reported. Lactating women with evidence of infection should not be excluded from treatment, particularly if they are being treated in endemic areas.[136]

SUMMARY OF MANAGEMENT OPTIONS

Schistosomiasis

Management Options	Evidence Quality and Recommendation	References
Prepregnancy		
Owing to importance of prepregnancy nutritional status, all patients with evidence of infection should be treated with praziquantel.	IIa/B	176
Prenatal–Prevention		
Teach patient to prevent *Schistosoma* infection: • Avoid visiting endemic areas during pregnancy if possible. • Avoid swimming in fresh water that may not have proper sewage control. • Use footwear when coming into contact with water sources.	—/GPP	—
Prenatal–Diagnosis		
Maternal infection should be suspected if history of recent travel to an endemic area with recent onset of fatigue, fever, bloody diarrhea, hematuria, abdominal pain, arthralgias or cough.	—/GPP	—
Diagnosis is usually made by detecting parasite eggs in the stool or urine.	IIb/B	131
Immunologic methods using ELISA measurement of CAA or CCA on serum or urine samples demonstrate higher sensitivity but are not yet commercially available.	IIb/B	164,165
Prenatal–Treatment		
The World Health Organization has given an informal recommendation that pregnant and lactating women should not be excluded from treatment.	IV/C	136
Praziquantel is generally considered safe in pregnancy.	IIb/B	179,180
No increased risk for congenital anomalies or abortion rate with the use of praziquantel in pregnancy.	IIb/B	179,180
Labor and Delivery; Postpartum		
Schistosomiasis cannot be transmitted from human to human. As a result, patients in labor do not need to be isolated.	IIb/B	130,136
The pediatrician should be notified of the mother's infection status owing to some reports of vertical transmission.	IV/C	134,172
Lactating women with evidence of infection should not be excluded from treatment, particularly if they are being treated in endemic areas.	IV/C	136

CAA, circulating anodic antigen; CCA, circulating cathodic antigen; ELISA, enzyme-linked immunosorbent assay; GPP, good practice point.

SUGGESTED READINGS

European Multicentre Study on Congenital Toxoplasmosis: Effect of timing and type of treatment on the risk of mother to child transmission of *Toxoplasma gondii*. BJOG 2003;110:112–120.

Friedman JF, Mital P, Kanzaria HK, et al: Schistosomiasis and pregnancy. Trends Parasitol 2007;23:159–164.

Gryseels B, Polman K, Clernix J, et al: Human schistosomiasis. Lancet 2006;368:1106–1118.

Jones JL, Lopez A, Wilson M, et al: Congenital toxoplasmosis: A review. Obstet Gynecol Surv 2001;56:296–305.

Markowitz LE, Steere AC, Benach JL, et al: Lyme disease during pregnancy. JAMA 1987;255:3394–3396.

McGready R, Hamilton KA, Simpson JA, et al: Safety of the insect repellent *N,N*-dimethyl-M-toluamide (DEET) in pregnancy. Am J Trop Med Hyg 2001;65:285–289.

Riley L: Pneumonia and tuberculosis in pregnancy. Infect Dis Clin North Am 1997;11:119.

Thiebaut R, Leproust S, Chene G, et al: Effectiveness of prenatal treatment for congenital toxoplasmosis: A meta-analysis of individual patients' data. Lancet 2007;369:115–122.

Walker GJA: Antibiotics for syphilis diagnosed during pregnancy. Cochrane Pregnancy and Childbirth Group. Cochrane Database Syst Rev 2004;4:CD001143.

Workowski KA, Levine WC: Sexually Transmitted Diseases Treatment Guidelines—2002. MMWR Morb Mortal Wkly Rep 2002; 51(RR-06):1–77.

REFERENCES

For a complete list of references, log onto www.expertconsult.com.

SECTION FIVE

Late Prenatal

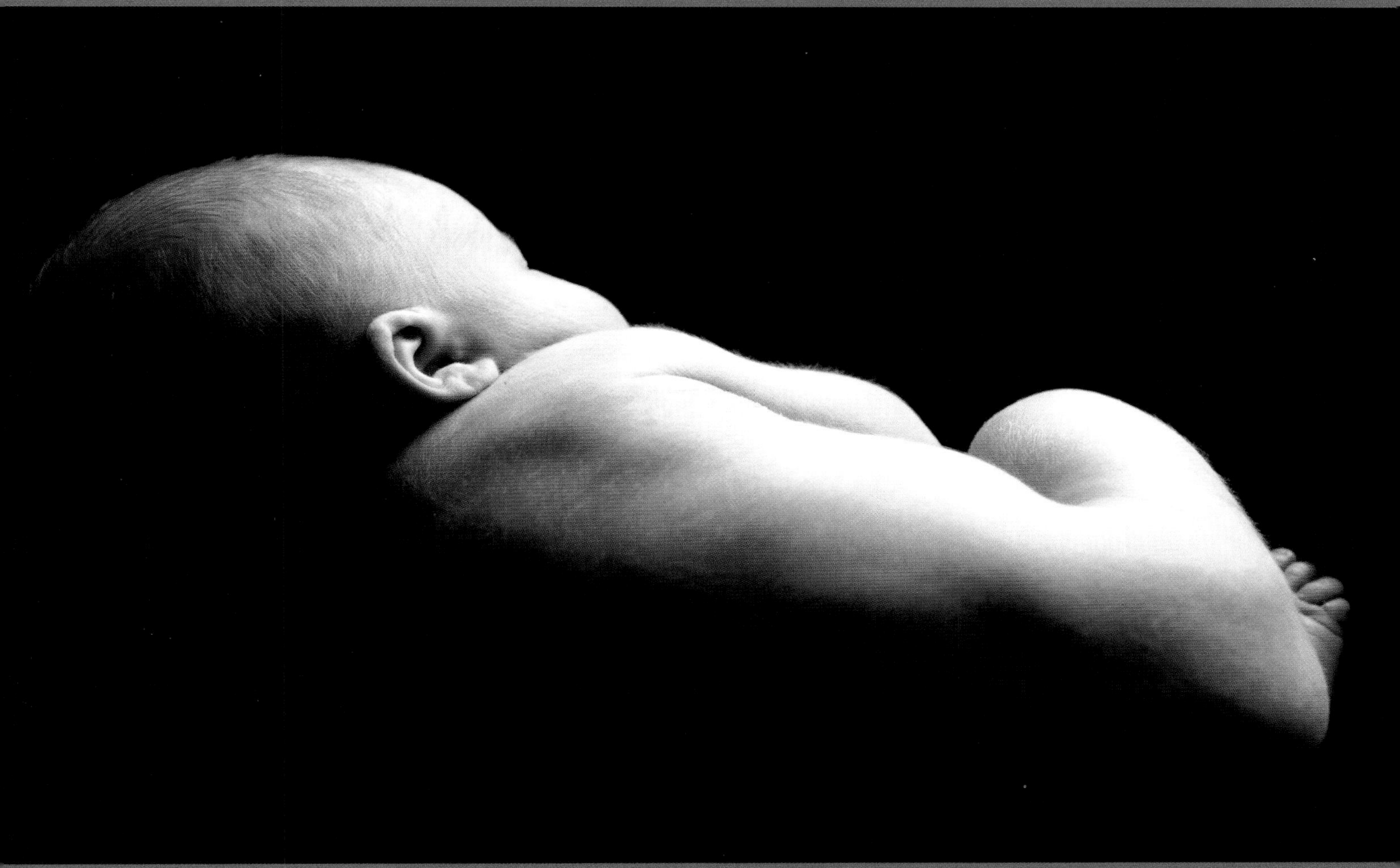

CHAPTER 33

Substance Abuse

JAMES J. WALKER and ANN M. WALKER

INTRODUCTION AND OVERVIEW

Substance abuse is common in our society, including the widespread use of tobacco and alcohol as well as illicit drugs. Substance abuse is increasing in young women,[1] and this produces significant maternal and fetal morbidity during pregnancy. The complication for the clinician is that the mother is complicit with the problem and there are often associated legal, social, and environmental problems[2] that can complicate the provision of care as well as the woman's ability to care for her child after birth. The aim of service provision is to provide an environment that is nonjudgmental and supportive to minimize the risk to the mother and her baby, not only during pregnancy and the neonatal period but also in the long term. Care does not necessarily require abstinence from drug use because the ultimate goal is to keep the mother within the care system and encourage her to take responsibility for herself and her child. To achieve this goal, the caregivers must be multidisciplinary, supportive, and tolerant.[3,4]

Programs of comprehensive antenatal care that provide social and behavioral support along with medical care do not universally improve maternal health and pregnancy outcome.[3,5] The specifics of the care provided are probably less important than the quality of care given and the degree of engagement of the individual.[6,7]

Major life events, such as pregnancy, can be a turning point allowing the women to take control of her life to the benefit of herself and her infant. It is often the first time she has been given any attention or responsibility. She may not be interested in harm reduction for herself, but she is likely to wish to protect her child. Unfortunately, the associated social problems of poor hygiene, nutrition, and social deprivation are responsible for much of the risk, rather than the abuse itself. The use of drugs or alcohol is often a symptom of these problems. Because most users abuse more than one substance and have multiple social complications, it is often difficult to evaluate the risk of any given substance.

TOBACCO SMOKING

Background

Smoking is a legal and socially tolerated form of substance abuse. Although it is accepted that smoking is harmful to general health and to pregnancy in particular, the incidence of smoking in the pregnant population has increased in recent decades to between 16.3% and 52%, depending on the characteristics of the patient group.[8–11] However, there is evidence that it is declining in some populations.[9,11] Smoking is more common in the socially deprived population and varies with race. It is also heavily dependent on family and partner influences.[7,12] Although the incidence of smoking decreases throughout pregnancy, this is largely due to voluntary cessation[8,13] because most intervention programs are only marginally successful.[14,15] As with many addictions, of those who do stop, most relapse in the first year.[14,16]

Maternal and Fetal Risks

Maternal smoking increases almost all placental complications and is dose-related.[14,17] These include placental abruption, placental insufficiency, placenta previa, and low birth weight.[11,14,18,19] Many infants are admitted to the neonatal unit,[11] largely owing to an increase in premature birth.[20] However, the increased risk is eliminated when women with proven placental pathology are excluded, suggesting that smoking produces most of its effects through placental damage.[21] There is also an increased risk of neonatal death and sudden infant death syndrome,[11,14] but this is partly due to secondhand smoke after birth rather than prenatal exposure.[14] Interestingly, smoking in pregnancy is a significant protective factor against preeclampsia, reducing the incidence by up to 50%[22]; however, women with preeclampsia who smoke have a worse outcome, which can be reduced by smoking cessation.[23] Data on miscarriage are contradictory, with some evidence of an increased incidence[14] but large cohort studies found no link.[24,25] However, there is an increased risk of ectopic pregnancy.[14,26] There are also varied data on the role of smoking and cleft lip and palate, but the increase in incidence appears to be small,[14] especially with heavy use.[27] No evidence links maternal smoking to childhood cancer.[14,28]

The risk of growth restriction increases with the number of cigarettes smoked per day. Although the average effect is 200 g,[14] heavy smokers deliver babies up to 458 g lighter than those of nonsmokers.[29] The effect of smoking on birth weight also increases with maternal age. Passive smoking produces risks similar to those seen in women who smoke 1 to 5 cigarettes/day. The effect on growth is largely in the second and third trimesters, so women who stop smoking during pregnancy deliver babies that are, on average, 120 g larger than babies of those who do not stop smoking, although these infants are still 39 g smaller than infants of those who never smoked. Interestingly, the offspring of women who smoke tend to be overweight during infancy. This effect is reduced in those mothers who cease smoking during pregnancy.[30]

Complications do not stop at birth, with neonatal neurobehavioral abnormalities[31] and reduced arousal reflexes seen in infants of mothers who smoke, which may explain the increase in sudden infant death syndrome in these infants. There is evidence that children whose mothers smoked during pregnancy have early neurodevelopmental impairment and behavioral problems,[32] but these effects appear to decrease with age.[33] However, some long-term effects remain, with maternal smoking increasing the risk of conduct disorders and criminal behavior in male offspring.[34] This effect can be alleviated if the mother is responsive to the child in infancy,[35] suggesting that at least some of these changes depend on the social environment and not just the effect of intrauterine exposure to smoking.

There is some evidence that women who smoke breastfeed for less time and produce less milk,[14] although nicotine patches do not produce the same effect.

Management Options

Prepregnancy and Prenatal

Although the strategy appears simple, most smoking cessation programs only have a minimal effect.[14] Most women who stop do so voluntarily, often prior to or early after conception.[14] This is not due to a lack of awareness of the risks to the unborn child as shown by a study which targeted high risk women.[36] After the campaign, more people understood the risks to the unborn child, but there was no significant change in smoking prevalence or consumption. Therefore, information itself does little to change practice, and more active intervention is required. Cessation can be increased by partner's support.[37]

Despite this recognized failure of intervention strategies, smoking cessation is a major drive in most prenatal health care provision. Various studies of the role of a specially designed self-help manual to help stop smoking show that some women had already stopped before recruitment and the effect of the intervention ranges from 10% to 20%.[38,39] Better results (38%) occurred with a more intensive program targeting the specific psychological problems the women have.[40]

Therefore, although smoking cessation is beneficial, intervention programs have limited effect because some women do not comply,[41] partly because of environmental,[42] and psychological[40] factors.

Most studies used patient histories to assess smoking habits. If smoking status in pregnancy is determined by a serum cotinine assay, the rate correlates well with declared smoking.[43] However, in studies in which the percentage of self-reported quitting was higher with intervention programs compared with control groups, cotinine-verified quit rates were not significantly different. These results suggest that as with any addiction program, biochemical verification is essential to evaluate smoking cessation interventions[44] and that previously reported successful intervention programs might have overestimated their success.

Originally, nicotine replacement therapy was not approved for use in pregnancy, but some studies suggest that this therapy may be safe because the amount of nicotine transferred to the baby may be reduced compared with smoking itself[45] and the U.S. Food and Drug Administration (FDA) no longer states pregnancy as a contraindication to its use.[46] However, nicotine is cleared more quickly during pregnancy, and the effects of replacement may be minimal.[14]

Therefore, no particular approach or advice appears to prevent smoking relapse during pregnancy, but repeated support and encouragement provided to women who quit early in pregnancy may be beneficial[47] by encouraging them not to relapse. The effect of family and peer pressure is important, with increasing success occurring when there is family or peer support.[7,48]

In the nonpregnant population, other interventions have been tried including antidepressants. These have mixed results, although bupropion, which is an atypical antidepressant that acts as a norepinephrine and dopamine reuptake inhibitor and nicotinic antagonist, appears to be effective. Initial reports suggest safety in pregnancy, but no trials in smoking cessation in pregnancy have been undertaken.[14]

Therefore, if smoking cessation programs are going to be cost-effective, it is in the high risk group of heavy smokers where most benefits can be achieved but where intervention programs appear to fail. An additional factor is that women find it more difficult to stop smoking compared with men.[14] It may be that greater benefits may be achieved by programs to prevent nicotine addiction among adolescent girls or by encouraging cessation before pregnancy, when cessation may be easier. There is some evidence that this is occurring because the rate of smoking in pregnancy appears to be decreasing in some populations.[49]

Labor and Delivery

Women who smoke are more likely to have preterm prelabor rupture of the membranes and preterm birth, possibly because of increased oxytocin sensitivity,[50] but there is no difference in management. Because the risk of placental insufficiency is increased, the infant may have growth restriction, with an increased possibility of fetal distress. Therefore, close vigilance in labor is recommended, with assessment of the fetal heart rate on admission and again near the end of labor, when the risks to the fetus are greatest. Interestingly, because of the effect on fetal growth, smoking is protective against macrosomia.

If a general anesthetic is required, women who smoke are at increased risk. Normally, smokers are asked to stop at least 24 hours before the anesthetic is administered, but labor is not predictable. Women should be told not to smoke once contractions have started.

Postnatal

Cigarette smoking during pregnancy is a significant health risk to the fetus, but most women continue to smoke during pregnancy, and most who quit relapse postpartum. This can have a significant effect on the future health of the child as well as on subsequent pregnancies.[12] Smoking cessation is easier in the nonpregnant state, but cessation appears to be more closely related to environmental and social factors than to any medical intervention. Failure to stop smoking also has a detrimental effect on long-term maternal health. A 28-year follow-up study of women who smoked during pregnancy in northern Finland showed that the mortality ratio, adjusted for age, place of residence, years of education, and marital status, in women who smoked during pregnancy was more than twice that in nonsmokers.[51] The difference was related to an increase in expected smoking-related diseases.[51]

SUMMARY OF MANAGEMENT OPTIONS

Cigarette Smoking

Management Options	Evidence Quality and Recommendation	References
Train staff to give advice and support.	III/B	179
• Tell women that smoking puts their baby at risk.	III/B	180
• Stopping smoking by midpregnancy will improve the outcome.	III/B	180,181
• Reducing smoking is better than not reducing but not as good as stopping.	III/B	180
• Repeated encouragement and specially designed programs increase the chance of success and reduce relapse.	Ia/A	181
• Low risk, more educated, lighter smokers are more likely to stop.	III/B	181
• Specific targeted intervention programs have benefit for both the mother and the newborn.	Ia/A	181,182
• Women underreport failure to stop smoking and smoking relapse.	Ia/A	183
• Nicotine patches can be beneficial and are safe for use in pregnancy	IIa/B	46

ALCOHOL

Background

The consumption of excessive amounts of alcohol is detrimental to health. After many historical references to the harmful effects of alcohol consumption in pregnancy, Lemoine and colleagues[52] described defects in fetal growth and development associated with maternal alcohol abuse in 1968. Further studies described the range of fetotoxicity attributed to both heavy and social maternal alcohol consumption.[53] Although the risk depends on the level and frequency of alcohol use, therapy is dependent on the degree of maternal dependency. In women who are not dependent, there is a high success rate with simple educational and motivational methods.[54] However, those who are dependent need greater supportive input and often require pharmacologic intervention.[55]

Maternal and Fetal Risks

Excessive Alcohol Consumption

Jones and Smith[56] were the first to coin the phrase "fetal alcohol syndrome" to describe the features associated with heavy maternal alcohol consumption, but the signs had been described before.[57] The main features include

- Growth deficiency, both prenatally and postnatally.
- Central nervous system disturbance that affects intellect and behavior.
- Abnormal facial characteristics, particularly low-set, unparallel ears; a short, flattened philtrum; an elongated midface; a small head; and a short, upturned nose.
- Malformation of major organs, especially the heart, and skeletal deformities.

Newborns with the syndrome may be irritable, with hypotonia, severe tremors, and withdrawal symptoms. The main physical and cerebral signs are usually apparent at birth. Mild mental retardation, the most common and serious deficit, and other anomalies may accompany fetal alcohol syndrome, and the degree of facial abnormality is directly related to the long-term physical and intellectual deficits.[58] Sensory deficits include optic nerve hypoplasia, poor visual acuity, hearing loss, and receptive and expressive language delays. Atrial and ventricular septal defects as well as renal hypoplasia, bladder diverticula, and other genitourinary tract abnormalities may occur. Only complete abstinence during pregnancy is considered safe. Alcohol consumption in each trimester is associated with abnormalities, and the lowest innocuous dose of alcohol is not known.[59] However, abnormal facial features are apparent only at the highest levels of exposure.[59]

Fetal alcohol syndrome is relatively rare, with an incidence of less than 1 in 1000 live births, increasing to 4.3% among "heavy" drinkers. The general incidence is more than 20 times higher in the United States (1.95 in 1000) than in Europe and other countries (0.08 in 1000). Therefore, relatively few women who drink alcohol during pregnancy give birth to children with fetal alcohol syndrome. The problem would appear to be multifactorial including genetic factors, social deprivation, nutritional deficiencies, and tobacco and other drug abuse.[60,61] Intrauterine growth restriction (IUGR) is also more frequent in women who drink alcohol during pregnancy. This effect is aggravated by maternal smoking.[59]

Maternal alcohol intake of more than 20 g/day is associated with an increase in preterm delivery and neonatal jaundice.[62] Therefore, these effects are associated with excessive consumption, poor diet, and smoking.

"Social" Alcohol Consumption

The evidence against more moderate consumption is controversial. Although effects are seen at all intake levels, the results are not conclusive.[63] Approximately 50% of women consume alcohol on a moderate and occasional basis during pregnancy, although more abstain in the first trimester.[64] This behavior is socially acceptable and considered normal. The consequences on pregnancy are difficult to assess because quantification of alcohol consumption is difficult to assess accurately. In addition, there are confounding factors, particularly socioeconomic group and tobacco consumption.

Far more studies have reported no significant effects of mild alcohol intake than have reported problems. The effect of smoking on birth weight is three times greater than the effect of alcohol.[59] When data are stratified by smoking status, moderate maternal alcohol consumption usually has no significant effect on birth weight in nonsmokers, but among smokers, there is a significant linear trend, with a threshold for decreased birth weight at an average of approximately two drinks per day (14 units/wk).[65] Lower consumption levels are associated with an increase in birth weight, suggesting an inverted J-shaped function between drinking during pregnancy and birth weight.[66] On its own, moderate intake of alcohol during pregnancy of less than 12 to 14 units/wk has no apparent detrimental effect on fetal growth.[66]

Although some studies show that children exposed to alcohol prenatally had significantly lower weight, height, head circumference, and palpebral fissure width at 6 years,[67] most show that the effect on growth is transient and the differences are not measurable after 8 months of age.[68]

So low alcohol intake in pregnancy may not have a substantial effect on child development, but there is concern about long-term neurodevelopment. Dose-dependent effects on neurobehavioral function from birth to 14 years have been established and are described as "fetal alcohol effects".[69] Specific problems include attention deficit,[70] slower information processing, and learning problems, especially with arithmetic,[71] as well as slower reaction times, suggesting an alcohol-related deficit in "speed of central processing." Reaction time deficits were dose-dependent,[72] as were attention and memory deficits.[70] The number of drinks per occasion was the strongest predictor of deficits. Fluctuating attention states, problems with response inhibition, and spatial learning also showed a strong association.[71] The higher the average number of drinks per occasion, the poorer the performance of the adolescent offspring on tasks believed to underlie numeric problem-solving and reading proficiency.[73] As with fetal alcohol syndrome, not all exposed offspring studied showed neurodevelopmental deficits. The effects appear to increase with advancing maternal age[74] and associated maternal smoking.[70]

However, because the lower safe limit cannot be determined with any surety, many agencies including the American College of Obstetricians and Gynecologists recommend abstinence for all pregnant women.[75]

Management Options

Prepregnancy and Prenatal

Because most women are not addicted to alcohol, they often take a "better safe than sorry" approach and reduce or stop drinking in pregnancy.[64] A successful previous pregnancy experience or a previous alcohol-related problem can influence this decision.[76] However, it is not the social drinker who concerns the obstetrician because these women are relatively easily educated about risks and tend to reduce their intake.[64] The few heavy drinkers, either dependent or binge drinkers, are more likely to harm their unborn child and are difficult to manage. Smokers and older women are particularly at risk because of the associated additive effects.

Formalized questionnaires on alcohol use can be used to screen either the entire population or targeted at-risk groups. The T-ACE questionnaire has been validated and appears to be accurate in detecting women who drink more than 1 oz of absolute alcohol/day (~25 g, or 2.5 units). Screening is most sensitive during the first 15 weeks of pregnancy.[77] This has been adapted for use in pregnancy.[75]

T-ACE is an acronym for the following:

- T: TOLERANCE
  How many drinks does it take to make you feel "high"?
- A: ANNOYED
  Have people ANNOYED you by criticizing your drinking?
- C: CUT DOWN
  Have you felt you should CUT DOWN on your drinking?
- E: EYE OPENER
  Have you ever had a drink first thing in the morning?

Scoring of the test is straightforward. If the answer to the tolerance question is more than 2, a score of 2 is given. A score of 1 is assigned to a positive answer to all of the other questions. A total score of more than 2 is considered positive for problem drinking, and this score correctly identifies more than 70% of women who drink heavily during pregnancy. Although this questionnaire is better than traditional alcohol questionnaires, its sensitivity can be improved with the use of a further test.[78]

An alternative is the Leeds Dependence Questionnaire, which is a 10-item, self-completion questionnaire designed to measure dependence on a variety of substances. It is understood by users of alcohol and opiates. The questionnaire is sensitive to changes over time from severe to mild dependence. Test-retest reliability is 0.95.[79]

Biochemical markers, such as blood γ-glutamyltransferase, alcohol concentration, thiocyanate, and mean corpuscular volume, can be used as surrogates of excessive alcohol consumption, but they are not accurate and can be used only to identify potential at-risk women. Abnormalities of liver enzymes in women who drink heavily should be taken into account if these tests are used during pregnancy to monitor other diseases, such as preeclampsia.

As with smoking, studies show that approximately one third of women who drink alcohol before pregnancy stop drinking during pregnancy and those who continue to drink tend to reduce their consumption.[64] A few women continue high levels of alcohol intake, and if they can be identified, preventive efforts should be focused on this group.[80] In contrast to smoking, many of these women are in higher socioeconomic groups.[81]

Adults have a significantly higher average daily intake of alcohol than adolescents. However, adults are more likely to reduce their intake in pregnancy and have a reduced incidence of binge drinking during the first trimester, which puts the offspring of adolescents at greater risk.[82]

If intervention programs are established, help from outside agencies, such as the local addiction unit, is invaluable. As with smoking, these programs are more likely to be successful in women who want to stop and when supportive care is provided. Motivational intervention with close monitoring of alcohol consumption with a planned reduction program is of benefit, often with the help of friends, family, and organizations such as Alcoholics Anonymous, with their 12-step program.[83] Because the effects of alcohol are associated with dietary deficiencies, the importance of a good diet and vitamin supplementation should be discussed.[84] Many complications of alcohol abuse may be attenuated by these measures.

If there is continued dependent drinking and the women is motivated to stop, planned detoxification should be considered, possibly with hospitalization or regular daily monitoring of withdrawal symptoms. Sudden withdrawal can lead to acute maternal symptoms, including convulsions, which may be detrimental to the fetus. Detoxification is normally undertaken with benzodiazepines, such as chlordiazepoxide, with the possible addition of phenobarbitone, if required, to manage convulsions.[85] These are given by reducing the regimen over 7 to 10 days. Benzodiazepines given in the first trimester may be associated with cleft palate abnormalities.[86] However, the benefits of stopping alcohol use outweigh this risk because alcohol is by far the greater teratogen. If delivery is likely within the next few days, benzodiazepines should be given with care because neonatal sedation and "floppy baby syndrome" can occur.[87] Disulfiram (Antabuse) should not be used because it is considered a potential teratogen, although the evidence is conflicting.[88] These women should also be given vitamin B supplementation.

Labor and Delivery

There are no problems with labor and delivery, except for the occasional need for higher levels of opiate analgesia or problems with general anesthesia because of induced liver enzymes. Alcohol withdrawal occurs after 48 hours and may be a problem postnatally. Appropriate sedation can be used with vitamin, particularly thiamine, supplementation. Symptoms subside after a few days. Women may appear agitated and have difficulty caring for their infant during this time.

If alcohol abuse continues after delivery, breast-feeding should be discouraged. Alcohol crosses over to the baby, and there may be continued effects of alcohol on the neonate.[59] Alcohol abuse during breast-feeding can cause drowsiness in the baby and may aggravate existing nutritional problems, increasing the need for dietary supplementation. However, alcohol may interfere with milk production, necessitating artificial feeding.

Postnatal

In most follow-up studies, a significant percentage of women relapsed. In one study of adolescents, more than 30% reported using alcohol within 3 months of delivery. These women are more depressed, are under greater stress, and report a greater need for social support. Therefore, the use of alcohol, as with other drugs of abuse, may be a marker for other problems that would benefit from intervention.

There is increasing concern about children of parents who abuse alcohol. These children have a higher risk of psychiatric disorders, cognitive deficits, and substance abuse that may be genetic or a long-term effect of in utero alcohol exposure.[89] Significant alcohol use affects family functioning, and children of alcohol-abusing parents are at risk for abuse and neglect.[90] Family drinking patterns are associated with adolescent alcohol abuse.[89] Children of alcohol-abusing parents have a higher incidence of emotional and behavioral disturbances and are at risk of future adult morbidity other than alcoholism. Therefore, women who abuse alcohol during pregnancy require careful follow-up from the appropriate agencies.

SUMMARY OF MANAGEMENT OPTIONS

Alcohol Abuse

Management Options	Evidence Quality and Recommendation	References
Obstetric risks are related to alcohol exposure itself as well as other associated social factors.	III/B IIa/B	53,184 42,185
A multidisciplinary approach is valuable in the care of these families.	III/B	54
Cessation help should be given to all "at-risk" groups.	III/B	82
	IIa/B	186
Some heavy alcohol users require specific counseling, with support from outside agencies.	IIa/B	186
Some heavy alcohol users require pharmacologic support.	III/B	85
Dietary advice and vitamin supplementation should be given.	III/B	84
Breast-feeding should be discouraged if the woman is still drinking heavily because there can be ongoing neonatal damage.	III/B	58

DRUG ABUSE: GENERAL

Maternal and Fetal Risks

The effects of maternal drug abuse on the mother and infant are difficult to assess because most users are low-income women with multiple drug use along with social and psychological problems.[91–94] When matched for social factors, mothers who use heroin have similar birth outcomes to non–drug-using mothers.[3] Therefore, many effects attributed to maternal drug abuse may be related to socioeconomic deprivation or associated factors, such as smoking, rather than to in utero drug exposure. The only effects that can be definitely blamed on drug abuse are neonatal withdrawal. However, some specific complications are associated with particular substances (discussed later).

Management Options

Prepregnancy and Prenatal

ESTABLISHING A SPECIAL CLINICAL SERVICE FOR THE PREGNANT ADDICT

The social factors are made worse by the fact that the drugs used are illegal. The women often live in a subculture of illegal behavior, including theft and prostitution.[95] Many mothers attempt to hide their lifestyle and claim fictitious support. They are often reluctant to be honest and may fear criticism, legal action, or removal of the child. They may resist antenatal care and must believe that the care is beneficial.[96] The service must be flexible and understanding enough to cope with these problems. In Glasgow, Scotland, a multidisciplinary approach was used to provide economic, social, and antenatal care during pregnancy.[3] This model has been copied elsewhere.[4] However, these approaches may not lead to great improvements in outcome,[5] but do support issues related to social problems and substance misuse that, because they persist after delivery, require close collaboration with local addiction services.[97]

Care programs that have been developed attempt to modify the external influences as much as possible to stabilize the mother's substance misuse.[4] Some women can stabilize their habit, detoxify, leave the drug culture, become healthy and responsible, and keep and care for their infant. However, others struggle to stay within the system, and care should be directed at the best possible outcome for each individual rather than optimal outcome. These care systems may change the pattern of abuse, but not necessarily the neonatal outcome.[5,98]

The systems that work best are multidisciplinary, with input from obstetricians, midwives, pediatricians, community-based health workers, social workers, drug abuse counselors, and others who can offer support.[3,4]

Caregivers should not be judgmental, although they must establish boundaries and maintain discipline. It is important to keep the trust of women and encourage them to obtain care, regardless of whether they still use drugs. A system based on rewards structure is better than one based on punishment. The ultimate reward for the mother is to be able to keep and care for the infant after birth. Care programs are more successful when friends and family are supportive.[99]

It is difficult to believe addicts, and urine screening is beneficial to assess program compliance.[100] Inpatient care can be useful to detoxify the patient; remove her from an unhealthy, stressful street environment; and provide adequate nutrition. However, the patient may be disruptive, cause stress to other women, and continue to abuse substances. In an attempt to overcome these problems, some hospitals have a segregated area for the care of addicts.[101] Our approach in Leeds, has been to treat them as normally as possible and to house them in the regular areas,[4,97] although the need for admission is now rare because the current approach is to reduce narcotic use in a gradual way in their normal environment along with psychosocial support and counseling which helps to maintain success.[97] Protocols must be in place and sympathetic staff available.

In Leeds, a special pregnancy addiction service was set up within an antenatal clinic.[97] This allows women to have all of their needs met at a single site. The clinic is coordinated by a liaison midwife with an obstetrician and an addiction worker. This ensures access to necessary antenatal care and addiction advice. The service provides a regular clinic that is available by appointment as well as on a drop-in basis. Providing care at a single site avoids the potential stigma of a separate clinic as well as possible loss of confidentiality. The availability of the service is promoted in health centers, hospitals, and local relevant organizations.

To achieve this, a close working relationship was developed between the obstetric and the addiction services, with links with community midwives, general practitioners, pediatricians, health visitors, child protection services, social services, and general support services, such as housing, probation, and community care projects. With so many individuals involved, regular meetings are held to exchange information and discuss concerns. Treatment protocols are available for all staff, particularly those who share responsibility with other services.

Regular reviews of the women are important. The Standing Conference on Drug Addiction guidelines are followed.* An initial assessment is performed at presentation, and a full review of progress made and work outstanding is completed at 32 weeks. By that time, a care plan should be in place to deal with outstanding issues. Other professionals, usually social services or housing authorities, can be contacted at that time. This process occurs with the consent of the woman, unless the infant is considered "at risk". In this case, authorities must be involved, even if the woman fails to give consent. When significant concern is present, a full prebirth assessment by social services may be needed. The 32-week meeting generates a report that is circulated to all relevant professionals involved in the care of the mother or child. A postnatal review at 3 months is scheduled to assess the progress of the mother and infant.

Labor and Delivery

The labor and delivery unit must be prepared to provide the care required. As with alcohol, problems include issues of

*Standing Conference on Drug Abuse (SCODA) 1997: Drug using parents: Policy Guidelines for Inter-Agency Working, Local Government Forum and Association, United Kingdom.

drug withdrawal and complications with analgesia, but also include the possibility of HIV and hepatitis infection. Specific problems depend on the drugs used.

Postnatal

The neonatal unit should be ready to care for an infant with withdrawal symptoms. The incidence and severity of these symptoms are related largely to the type and amount of drug used. In the past, babies of drug-using women were usually admitted routinely to the special care nursery and often treated for or in anticipation of withdrawal symptoms. These symptoms are a source of distress to the mother, but separation can cause further distress. In the United Kingdom, most infants do not require admission to a neonatal unit and can be cared for in a transitional care area, where the mother is directly involved.[4] At delivery, a "cause for concern" sheet is made up for the neonatal and other staff involved in the postdelivery care. This lists all relevant details of drug use, infection status, current care plans, and child protection issues.

Drug abuse was formerly considered incompatible with adequate child care, but it is now realized that drug cessation and postnatal abstinence is largely unachievable. An attempt to enforce drug cessation is likely to drive the women away from the supportive environment that was carefully established during pregnancy. However, harm reduction and stabilization should be the goal, and this goal is compatible with maternal and child health. In the United Kingdom, methadone maintenance is the main treatment for opiate addicts who are unable or unwilling to stop using drugs.[97] This approach may allow the women to live a reasonably stable life and care for her children. Many studies show that infants who remain with their biologic parents do better than those who do not.[102] To achieve these outcomes, a good working relationship with the local addiction unit is necessary to ensure that adequate follow-up and support are available.[4,97]

The success of these policies is varied. More than 50% of women who stop abusing drugs resume drug use within 6 months of delivery. Many of their infants are cared for by extended family members on a voluntary basis; others enter foster care or are adopted. This outcome may be upsetting to staff working in this area, but one success can lead to long-term benefit to at least two people (i.e., the mother and her child), and even a temporary success might reduce the long-term effects on the infant.

SUMMARY OF MANAGEMENT OPTIONS

Drug Abuse, General

Management Options	Evidence Quality and Recommendation	References
Provide accurate rather than alarmist information.	IV/C	4
General guidelines include assessing the patient's living environment and whether her partner uses drugs, encouraging the woman to take some responsibility for herself, making sure that she understands what is expected of her, improving her general health, and working toward achievable goals.	III/B	3,4,187
A multidisciplinary approach may be beneficial.	III/B	3,5
Wear gloves to take blood from all patients (not just addicts).	—/GPP	
The increased risk of sexually transmitted disease, including HIV, should be discussed (see also Chapters 27, 28, 30, and 31).	III/B	188
Screen for fetal normality and growth with ultrasonography.	III/B	189
Babies should be assessed for neonatal abstinence syndrome.	III/B	124

GPP, good practice point.

HEROIN ADDICTION: SPECIFIC PROBLEMS

Background

Heroin is processed from morphine, a naturally occurring substance extracted from the seedpod of the Asian poppy plant. Heroin usually appears as a white or brown powder. Street names for heroin include "smack," "H," "skag," and "junk." Other names refer to types of heroin produced in a specific geographic area, such as "Mexican black tar."

Most addiction services see more users of heroin than of any other illicit drug.[103] It is a highly physically addictive substance, and its use is a serious worldwide problem. It can be injected, snorted, or smoked, and like many drugs of abuse, the ritual of preparation is an important part of the attraction. After heroin injection, there is a surge of euphoria ("rush") accompanied by warm flushing of the skin, dry mouth, and a heavy sensation of the extremities. A drowsy state occurs, and mental functioning becomes clouded as a result of central nervous system depression. This leads to a lack of motivation and reduced social interaction.

Maternal and Fetal Risks

The main clinical problems related to heroin use are direct drug effects on the fetus and neonate and the reduced ability of the mother to care for the child.[102] Opiates are not teratogenic.[104] However, their use is associated with IUGR and premature delivery,[102,105] a higher incidence of fetal distress, and a greater need for neonatal care.[106] Although other factors, such as poor antenatal attendance, poor nutrition, mixed drug use, and cigarette smoking, are undoubtedly involved, it is important to realize that these pregnancies are at risk, regardless of whether the drug is primarily responsible.[107] Longitudinal studies found an increased incidence of deficits in cognitive development and more behavioral problems but no differences in motor development. It is difficult to separate the effects of in utero exposure to heroin from the problems of deficient child care.[108] Children who are adopted at an early age into nurturing families develop normally, suggesting that there is no inherent problem in these babies, and if the mother is stabilized and succeeds in changing her lifestyle, the long-term outcome for the infant can be good. However, these mothers have child care problems, and there is an increased risk of sudden infant death syndrome.[5,109] Pregnancy care is only the starting point, and there is a need for ongoing support after delivery, requiring collaboration with addiction services.[97]

Management Options

Prepregnancy and Prenatal

The main aim of care for the pregnant drug-abusing woman is engagement. With this, the rest of the care follows. She should be cared for by a multidisciplinary team (including the addiction service), with the goal of risk reduction and regular follow-up.[4,97,110] The core of risk reduction is the drug substitution program; methadone is the therapy most often used, although there is increasing interest in the use of buprenorphine.[107,111–113]

METHADONE USE IN PREGNANCY

Methadone use in pregnancy varies. In the United States, higher doses are used to block opiate receptors and reduce cravings, whereas in the United Kingdom, the approach is often to find the lowest dose to prevent withdrawal symptoms. Studies show that reducing the dose to a minimum improves birth weight and prolongs gestation.[114] It is difficult to determine whether these benefits result from the use of methadone, the reduction of other drug use, an improved lifestyle, or a combination of these factors.[114] However, the risk and severity of neonatal abstinence syndrome (NAS) appear to be increased by methadone compared with heroin,[115] but methadone stabilization has considerable overall benefits for the mother and infant. The purpose of substitution therapy is to reduce illegal heroin use as well as the crime, disease, and other consequences of street use. Reducing intravenous injection has the added benefit of reducing the risk of HIV infection and hepatitis B and C infection as well as other health risks. Because methadone, at therapeutic levels, does not create euphoria, sedation, or analgesia and has no adverse effects on motor skills, mental capability, or employability, it is compatible with a reasonably normal lifestyle. Therefore, it is suitable for stabilization during pregnancy and for short- to medium-term use after delivery to maintain stability. Although many patients reduce their opiate use, only a few (10%–25%) become drug-free,[104,105] and many of these return to heroin use after delivery. So the aim should be to maintain rather than abstain.[111]

The amount of methadone required should be assessed in the usual way. Women who are not regular (daily) users do not need substitution therapy. Those who are given methadone should have a clear history of daily use, withdrawal symptoms, and positive urine toxicology findings. The amount of methadone required can be assessed by the declared amount of heroin used or the amount of money spent per day. However, because the cost and purity of street heroin vary considerably, this guidance can only be approximate. Dosage is then titrated against withdrawal scores until stabilization is achieved. The aim is to find the lowest dose of methadone that is compatible with an absence of withdrawal symptoms or cravings. The dosage regimens in pregnancy are the same as those used in the nonpregnant user. In Leeds, it is rare to require a dose of methadone above 100 mg/day. If a higher dose is required, an electrocardiogram should be undertaken to exclude cardiac conduction defects.[116] Because the metabolism of methadone is increased in pregnancy, leading to a shorter half-life, the dose may need to be split into a twice-daily dose in later pregnancy to maintain a satisfactory steady state.[117] This dosing can increase compliance without the need to increase the total dose. Methadone maintenance treatment is more successful within a supportive environment and is largely independent of methadone dose or plasma concentration.[100] Therefore, the supportive nature of the service is more important than the drug regimen used.[97]

Once stabilization is achieved and lifestyle issues are addressed, the main aim is to maintain a stable state.[97] However, if the woman is motivated and wishes to, a gradual dose reduction can begin. Because of the danger of miscarriage, this is more safely carried out between 12 and 30 weeks' gestation. After this point, it is better simply to stabilize the patient at the lowest possible dose in preparation for labor and delivery. However, because of the changes in maternal metabolism, the maintenance dose may need to be increased to sustain maternal stability. Reduction should be done slowly, by decreasing the daily dosage by 5 mg, no more often than every 2 weeks, and then, from 20 mg/day, by 2 mg every 2 weeks, to achieve the lowest sustainable dose without the mother resorting to street heroin or suffering withdrawal symptoms.[105] It is important to aim for the lowest maternal dose to reduce the possibility of NAS. Although not strictly dose-related, a dose of less than 20 mg is not usually associated with significant NAS, unless there is concurrent street drug use. Regular urine toxicology testing allows accurate assessment of the success of the treatment program and assists in the planning of dose adjustments.[100]

ALTERNATIVES TO METHADONE

Because of the well-recognized limitations of methadone treatment, alternatives have been sought. Buprenorphine appears to be a potential option,[107,112,113,118–121] and studies showed that stabilization is as good as methadone and the risk of NAS lower. Studies show that NAS still occurs in 40% to 60% of cases, usually within 12 to 48 hours, peaks at approximately 72 to 96 hours, and lasts for 5 to 7 days.[120,122] However, NAS appears to be of less duration and severity than methadone and is related to polydrug use in at least

40% of cases.[109,122] The infants appear to have normal physical and psychological development. Also buprenorphine taken at the time of conception has been reported with no teratogenic effects.[123] It would appear buprenorphine offers a real alternative to methadone, with a reduced risk profile, although good-quality randomized trials are lacking.

Labor and Delivery

The attendant staff must be trained in the care of pregnant drug users and treat them in the same way as other women in labor. On admission, a history of recent drug use (i.e., before admission) must be obtained. Many mothers use heroin before hospital admission to help them tolerate labor.

No specific problems are associated with labor or delivery, except for maternal analgesia. Methadone should be continued, with additional opiate analgesia as required. Because high doses of narcotic analgesia may be necessary because of tolerance, epidural analgesia has advantages. At delivery, the infant should not be given naloxone (Narcan) because it causes a severe withdrawal reaction.

Postnatal

After delivery, normal support should be continued, ideally in a transitional unit. This allows the mother and infant to be together, which is important for bonding and establishment of parenting skills. This is the ideal time for staff to promote support and assess possible risk.

The incidence and severity of NAS are partially related to the type and amount of drug used and the degree of polydrug and street drug use.[124,125] Both benzodiazepines and cocaine delay the onset of NAS, but cocaine also appears to reduce the severity of symptoms.[125] The pediatric unit should be alerted to the potential clinical problems and involved in the case discussion and the development of management protocols.

In Leeds, a modified Finnegan scale is used to monitor the infant for signs of NAS.[126] This is initially carried out every 4 hours, and monitoring is reduced when appropriate. Three scores of 8 or more should be used for the diagnosis. It is useful for the mother to be involved in these assessments because many drug-using mothers have strong feelings of guilt and want to feel that they can make a useful contribution. They can also improve the continuity of assessment. Withdrawal from heroin occurs over 1 to 3 days, whereas methadone has a longer clearance time, and symptoms in the newborn may not occur for up to 7 days after delivery. Buprenorphine would appear to fall in between these lengths. Assessment should last at least 7 days, although some centers advocate earlier discharge if there are no signs by 72 hours.[127] The classic symptoms are restlessness, jitteriness, failure to feed, tremors, a high-pitched cry, arching of the back, yawning, sneezing, and sweating.[126] Convulsions may also occur. Narcotics, either morphine or methadone, are the best drugs for the treatment of NAS, although phenobarbitone may be required if convulsions occur or appear imminent.[127,128] Although most babies show some withdrawal symptoms, fewer than 50% require treatment and most can be safely cared for in a transitional unit.[4,127] Of 200 babies born in Glasgow in the 1980s and early 1990s to mothers using illicit drugs or legal methadone, only 7% required treatment for withdrawal and even fewer required admission to the special care nursery.[101] However, other centers, including more recent figures from Glasgow, quote incidences of 10% to 80% of cases, depending on the amount of antenatal drug used and the success of the clinic maintenance program.[113,124,125,127]

Continuing supportive care, including methadone maintenance, may allow the new mother to live a reasonably stable life and care for her child, which is the best outcome for the child. This requires a continued good working relationship with general practitioners, health visitors, community pediatricians, and the local addiction service. However, many babies are eventually cared for by extended family members, placed in foster care, or released for adoption.[129]

BREAST-FEEDING

If the mother is stable on methadone, is not supplementing with street drugs, and is believed to be HIV-negative, breast-feeding should be encouraged. The secretion of methadone in breast milk is variable,[130] but it may help to reduce withdrawal symptoms.[131] A stable lifestyle helps successful breast-feeding. However, if the mother is still injecting street heroin, is known to be or is at risk for being HIV-positive, or is using other street drugs (e.g., cocaine), breast-feeding is not advisable.

HUMAN IMMUNODEFICIENCY VIRUS AND OTHER INFECTIOUS DISEASES (see also Chapters 27, 28, 30, and 31)

HIV infection is associated with drug abuse because of needle sharing and heterosexual spread from associated prostitution. The danger, particularly in the United Kingdom, has been overstated, although in some areas, the incidence of HIV infection is particularly high. In Edinburgh, in 290 at-risk pregnancies, 93 (32%) of the women were HIV-positive. However, of these 93 pregnancies, only 8 (8.7%) resulted in an HIV-infected child.[132] Since then, the prevalence of HIV has declined from 0.5% of all pregnancies in 1986 to 0.1% in the 1990s.[133] The risk of vertical transmission has been significantly reduced by the use of antiviral drugs and obstetric intervention.[134] Targeting of antiviral treatment is difficult because not all HIV-positive women are known to the medical authorities.[135,136]

Because many HIV-positive patients are not known to the service, single-tier management of all pregnant women is important to minimize the risk of transmission to health care workers. This also helps to reduce discrimination against substance-misusing women. In the United Kingdom, HIV testing is offered to all pregnant women after appropriate counseling. The benefits of testing must be explained to the mother. Current therapy improves maternal health and significantly reduces vertical transmission to the baby with the opportunity for a vaginal delivery.[134]

Intravenous drug users are also at risk for hepatitis B and C infection, and screening is routinely offered. The most common infection found is hepatitis C, which is found in approximately 40% to 60% of women who abuse intravenous drugs.[103] Evidence suggests that hepatitis C does not adversely affect the pregnancy and the pregnancy does not worsen the viral load or prognosis of the disease, although many women have a slight rise in alanine aminotransferase levels postpartum.[137] Vertical transmission of hepatitis C infection occurs in approximately 1% to 6% of cases and is usually in women with detectable hepatitis C virus RNA in the peripheral blood.[138] It is increased by concurrent HIV infection[139,140] and longer labors. Breast-feeding is not a risk because hepatitis C virus RNA is not detected in breast milk. Infants who are hepatitis C virus–positive should be followed up for at least 1 year because some become seronegative over time. No treatment or vaccination is available.

Less frequently, women are hepatitis B–positive.[103] Pregnancy does not appear to affect the course of the disease in the mother, but the rate of vertical transmission without intervention is 80% to 90%. Of these infants, more than 85% become clinical carriers of the virus. Infection in the baby usually occurs at or directly after delivery, so the babies are candidates for post-exposure prophylaxis. An at-risk infant should be given HepB immunoglobulin within 12 hours of delivery while concurrently being given the first dose of HepB vaccination.[141] This should be completed with follow-up vaccinations at 1 month and 6 months. This intervention is safe and provides 90% protection against infection. One study suggested that maternal lamivudine treatment may also help to reduce neonatal infection.[142]

COCAINE ADDICTION: SPECIFIC PROBLEMS

Background

Cocaine is a vasoactive drug and can cause specific problems in the baby as a result of placental damage[143] and direct fetal vascular effects. Unlike alcohol, cocaine has no specific associated syndrome or cluster of signs.[144] Its effects are varied and may be more closely related to other drug use and associated social problems.[143,145]

It comes in the following two forms:

- Pure cocaine, or "coke," which is a white powder that is generally snorted through the nasal mucosa.
- "Crack," which is more addictive and dangerous. Crack is produced by mixing cocaine crystal or powder with water and baking soda or sodium bicarbonate. The mixture is boiled until the water evaporates, leaving brown and white rocks. It is usually smoked with special glass pipes or silver foil, although it can be injected after a solution is made with water.

The use of crack cocaine has been reducing since the late 1980s, but overall cocaine use has increased greatly due to the widespread use of powder cocaine.[146] Many studies, particularly in the United States, found higher rates of cocaine abuse than of heroin abuse, with an incidence of between 0.8% to 31%.[143,146] Radioimmunoassay of hair samples obtained immediately postpartum show much underreporting of cocaine use. Underreporting is more common among women who are unmarried, African American, and multiparous.

Maternal and Fetal Risks

Cocaine is absorbed rapidly into the bloodstream, producing a high in approximately 6 to 8 minutes. Unlike the physical addiction of heroin, cocaine addiction is more psychological. Users often do not eat or sleep while under the influence of the drug and often become dehydrated. Although these effects may not present problems with occasional use, heavy use may be associated with exhaustion, dehydration, and poor nutrition. Some people use heroin to "come down" from cocaine highs, further complicating the medical problems. Because crack can be smoked, it can affect other people nearby; this has implications for children and babies in the room with a user.

Heavy usage of cocaine is associated with an increase in preterm delivery, low birth weight, the need for resuscitation at birth, and prolonged postnatal stay, although significant problems are rare.[147,148] The effect of cocaine on birth weight may be related to shorter gestation and poor maternal nutrition. Women who use cocaine use prenatal care less often, smoke more cigarettes, and drink more alcohol, all of which are associated with poor growth.[72] When these variables are excluded, identifiable differences in birth weight between cocaine-using mothers and control subjects are no longer present.[145] However, peripartum exposure to cocaine is associated with an increased frequency of abruptio placentae; thick, meconium-stained amniotic fluid; and prelabor rupture of the membranes.[143] There is also an association with fetal abnormalities, including genitourinary anomalies and abdominal wall defects.[143]

Cocaine-exposed infants with very low birth weight had an increased incidence of mild intraventricular hemorrhage. The incidence of developmental delay was significantly higher, even after controlling for the effects of intraventricular hemorrhage and gestational age,[149] although there is no place for routine neonatal brain ultrasonography.[150] Cocaine-exposed infants with very low birth weight were also more likely to be living with relatives or in foster homes, which further affects their development.[149] Long-term assessment showed reduced head circumference, low Stanford-Binet Intelligence Scale (SBIS) verbal reasoning, and low SBIS abstract/visual reasoning. These children were also more aggressive.[151] These findings are similar to those associated with alcohol.

Binge cycles are a particular problem and reflect the chaotic lifestyle of many drug abusers. Binges range from 26.4 to 34.4 hours.[152] Bingeing is associated with preterm birth and an increased incidence of acute problems, such as vaginal bleeding (21.8%), abruptio placentae (14.3%), and stillbirth (20.5%). Erratic use of cocaine or crack results in perinatal complications that are as severe as those occurring with daily use.[152]

Like heroin, maternal cocaine exposure during pregnancy is associated with acceleration of amniotic fluid and fetal lung maturity, which may reflect increased fetal stress.[153]

Not all substance-exposed children have the same poor prognosis, suggesting that maternal and environmental factors modify the damage.[151] Surveys show that most cocaine users also use alcohol.[154] Comparison with alcohol shows that alcohol is the more potent teratogen. Those who use both agents are more likely to have troubled backgrounds, indulge in antisocial behavior, and drop out of treatment programs than those who use only alcohol. Good nutrition is very important in preventing congenital anomalies and fetal death, and cocaine use during pregnancy is more dangerous to the street person who uses multiple drugs and alcohol than to the middle-class woman who takes antenatal vitamins.[155]

Management Options

Prepregnancy and Prenatal

Again, the basis of care is trust between the woman and her caregivers. The true nature of cocaine or crack abuse may not be easily divulged, and support may be rejected. The risk to the fetus must be made clear and the particular risk of binge use emphasized. No substitute drug is available to help with stabilization in pregnancy. However, sudden cessation is not associated with adverse fetal effects. Although the desire for a healthy baby may be an incentive to stop using cocaine, success is rare because psychological addiction is usually strong. If a woman wishes to stop using cocaine or crack, hospital admission may be beneficial to remove her from her usual environment. Constant social support and encouragement increases the chance of success. If use is stopped at any time during pregnancy, the outcome is improved.

Labor and Delivery

There is no major problem with labor or delivery other than an increased need for narcotic analgesia. There can be specific problems in anesthetizing a woman who uses cocaine or crack.[156] Drug-related hypertension may mimic preeclampsia. Excessive uterine activity may result in fetal compromise or acute separation of the placenta.

Postnatal

After birth, the symptoms of fetal cocaine withdrawal may not reach a peak until 3 days of life, and they may persist for 2 to 3 weeks. Many babies are discharged home before symptoms occur, so community midwives should be vigilant. Common signs are irritability, tremulousness, mood alterations, and hypertonia; in addition, the infants may be difficult to console.

As with heroin, relapse to drug abuse may occur in the postpartum period. Close community support from the relevant agencies can help women to stay drug-free and develop parenting skills.

CANNABIS: SPECIFIC PROBLEMS

Background

Marijuana is the most prevalent illicit drug used in pregnancy (4%–30%).[94,157–159] Despite this, there are few reports on fetal effects.

Maternal and Fetal Risks

Studies suggest that there is no increase in the rate of morphologic anomalies, low birth weight, preterm delivery, or abruptio placentae.[67,108,160,161]

A study in Jamaica assessed newborns exposed to marijuana antenatally in a blinded fashion and compared them with nonexposed babies from socioeconomically matched mothers. At 1 month, marijuana-exposed infants scored higher on autonomic stability, reflexes, general irritability, and weight. No ill effects from marijuana were found, and there may have been dose-related positive effects. The Jamaican mothers reported that cannabis increased their appetite during pregnancy and relieved pregnancy-related nausea.[161] More recent studies suggest the possibility of more subtle problems.[70]

Therefore, the use of marijuana is not a major problem and may even be beneficial in pregnancy. However, some may see marijuana as a gateway drug that potentially leads to harder drugs because of its association with the drug culture. Users should be warned against progression to drugs that are more harmful. It is also associated with other substances of abuse including alcohol and tobacco that are far more dangerous. There is a recent trend of medicinal use of marijuana for the treatment of nausea in pregnancy. This may increase the exposure of the early fetus to this substance.[162]

Management Options

No management problems are specifically associated with cannabis use, although a careful drug history should be taken and a reduction of use encouraged.

BENZODIAZEPINES: SPECIFIC PROBLEMS

Background

Benzodiazepines are commonly used as anxiolytics and sedatives.[163] Their legitimate use in pregnancy has varied over the years, including the management of preeclampsia.[164] However, because of the fear of harmful effects, many women and their physicians recommend stopping their medication acutely, often with adverse maternal effects.[165] There are no apparent fetal effects, although the fetus may be at risk if the mother has a convulsion. These substances are also taken as part of polydrug abuse,[166] making assessment of their risk difficult.

Maternal and Fetal Risks

Large epidemiologic studies show no teratogenic effects and no obvious problems related to withdrawal from various benzodiazepines. However, some abnormalities, particularly cleft palate,[86] are associated with its use. This finding is not conclusive, and other studies found no link.[167] Further, cleft palate is a common abnormality that occurs with other drug use.[168] However, there is evidence of hypotonia and problems with feeding because of its sedative effect when taken immediately before delivery.[87]

Management Options

No specific management in pregnancy is needed, except to discourage its use or stabilize the patient to the lowest level tolerated. Further reduction and cessation is possible in motivated patients. However, stopping suddenly can produce severe maternal side effects such as convulsion, but it is safe for the baby. Benzodiazepines are excreted in breast milk, but the levels are low and should not cause neonatal problems.[87]

AMPHETAMINES: SPECIFIC PROBLEMS

Amphetamines are synthetic amines that are similar to the body's own adrenaline (epinephrine). They exaggerate the normal reaction to emergency or stress. Common slang terms for amphetamines include "speed," "wizz," "crystal," "meth," "bennies," "dexies," "A," "uppers," "pep pills," "diet pills," "jolly beans," "truck drivers," "co-pilots," "eye openers," "wake-ups," "hearts," and "footballs." The stimulating effects of amphetamines have been widely used to counteract fatigue. These drugs are also used by athletes to increase performance and by others for general stimulation, pleasure, or fun. Their use in pregnancy varies but is usually less than 1%.[169] In the younger age group, approximately 9% describe past use.[158] Overall, its use appears to be decreasing.

The drug is usually taken orally but can be injected or sniffed. It is sometimes used interchangeably with cocaine. Because amphetamine use produces undesirable personality changes, "speed freaks" are highly unpopular with other addicts. They may be aggressive and violent. Most drug users consider amphetamines extremely dangerous and do not use them.

After continued administration of moderate doses, recovery is associated with fatigue, drowsiness, and often depression. The increased energy produced by the drug merely postpones the need for rest. Regular users rely on the drug when fatigued and often do not get proper rest for long periods. Near the end of such a "run" (usually < 1 wk), toxic symptoms dominate and the effects become intolerable. If the drug is discontinued, fatigue sets in and prolonged sleep follows, sometimes lasting days. After wakening, the user feels lethargic, sometimes depressed, and extremely hungry. These effects can be overcome by further drug use, which restarts the cycle. To stop runs, or "downers" opiates are sometimes used. Amphetamines do not produce a physical dependence, and psychological and environmental factors appear to be the motivating factors in the addiction.

Maternal and Fetal Risks

The effect on the baby is not well documented, but it appears to be associated with congenital abnormalities, particularly an increased occurrence of cleft palate.[170] Because amphetamine use is associated with hypertension, the incidence of preeclampsia and convulsions is also increased, with associated IUGR and death. Preterm labor is also more common, but this may be due to associated lifestyle factors. The long-term growth of infants born to mothers who were addicted to amphetamines during pregnancy was found to be impaired.[171] This reduction appeared to be global, suggesting symmetrical growth impairment, which is usually associated with direct injury to the developing fetus rather than placental insufficiency.

Management Options

Amphetamines are dangerous and should be discontinued. There is no drug substitute. Success in stopping the use of this drug is poor, and these addicts are probably the most difficult and problematic to treat. They value their sick appearance and often claim that they will die. Death as a result of amphetamine use is relatively rare. The best approach is to provide close, supportive care and constant encouragement to stop using the drug. The problem is that few engage in care, and if they do, stopping is relatively easy, but so is restarting.

D-LYSERGIC ACID DIETHYLAMIDE-25: SPECIFIC PROBLEMS

Background

D-Lysergic acid diethylamide-25 is an unusual, controversial drug better known as "LSD" or simply "acid." It is usually taken orally but may be sniffed or injected. LSD is one of the most potent biologically active substances known. It is well absorbed from the gastrointestinal tract, is distributed in the blood, easily diffuses into the brain, and crosses the placental barrier.

The psychological effects are not predictable and are affected by the user's personality and current thoughts. However, its use is compatible with a reasonably normal life and is not necessarily associated with the normal drug culture. In the younger age group, approximately 7% describe past use.[158]

Maternal and Fetal Risks and Management Options

High doses of LSD given to pregnant animals produce deformities in the offspring of some species and not others.[172,173] There are little data on LSD use in human pregnancy.[174] Until more information is known, the most sensible approach is to recommend that pregnant women avoid LSD use. No other particular care is required.

BARBITURATES: SPECIFIC PROBLEMS

Background

The incidence of barbiturate use in pregnancy is relatively low and is falling.[175,176] There do not appear to be specific fetal effects, except for fetal dependence. Acute withdrawal during pregnancy can affect the fetus in utero and is not recommended, although the precise risk is unknown. Gradual withdrawal can be achieved with reducing doses of short-acting barbiturates, such as pentobarbitone.

Maternal and Fetal Risks

The main risk to the mother and neonate is associated with withdrawal. This can be alleviated with a gradually reducing regimen that includes supplementary drugs. Acute withdrawal is associated with seizures and mental instability, usually occurring approximately 48 hours after the last dose. The neonate may take longer to show symptoms because the clearance of barbiturates is slower in the newborn.

Management Options

Slow reduction and cessation of drug use is the mainstay of management.

SOLVENT ABUSE: SPECIFIC PROBLEMS

Background

Solvent abuse is extremely common, and up to 19% of schoolchildren in parts of the United States have used them.

Along with alcohol, marijuana, and tobacco, they are considered gateway drugs. There are many types of inhalants, including spray paint, liquid correction fluid, hair spray, nail polish remover, paint thinners, felt-tip markers, air fresheners, octane booster, glues and adhesives, fabric protectors, acetone products, carburetor cleaner, gasoline, propane gas, gas inside Ping-Pong balls, VCR head cleaner, and vegetable cooking sprays. Other examples are butyl nitrates, called "locker room" or "rush," and amyl nitrate capsules, called "snappers" or "poppers."

Maternal and Fetal Risks

Solvent abuse produces clinical signs, such as irritation and sores around the mouth and nose, nausea and headache, coughing, memory loss, lack of concentration and coordination, and odd behavior or irritability.

Sniffing leads to rapid entry of the drugs into the brain and organ systems, producing a high that lasts 15 to 45 minutes. Inhaling from a plastic or paper bag ("bagging") or inhaling from a soaked rag placed in the mouth ("huffing") greatly increases these effects. Damage can occur to the brain, liver, kidneys, blood, and bone marrow, and unconsciousness is common. In a study in pregnant solvent users, renal tubular acidosis was diagnosed in 5.3%, and 3.6% had adverse neurologic sequelae. One patient was diagnosed with brain damage, including expressive aphasia. The incidence of premature delivery was 21.4%. The substances in solvents can cross the placenta and enter the fetal bloodstream. In the same study, 16.1% of infants had major anomalies. Most of these had facial abnormalities similar to those seen in fetal alcohol syndrome, and a further 10.7% had hearing loss.[177]

In another study of infants exposed to toluene, there was a 10% incidence of neonatal death as well as an increased incidence of prematurity (42%), low birth weight (52%), and microcephaly (32%). In addition, some infants had craniofacial features similar to those seen in fetal alcohol syndrome as well as other minor anomalies.[178]

Management Options

Solvent use is associated with erratic behavior, is dangerous for the mother and fetus, and should be strongly discouraged. Close observation and monitoring are required because of the high incidence of premature delivery and IUGR. Because there is evidence of neonatal abnormalities similar to those seen with alcohol and there may be developmental problems, the babies require close long-term follow-up.

SUMMARY OF MANAGEMENT OPTIONS

Specific Drugs of Abuse (e.g., Heroin, Cocaine, Barbiturates)

Management Options	Evidence Quality and Recommendation	References
Use a multidisciplinary approach.	IIb/B	4,187
Explain the risks of low birth weight, intrauterine growth restriction, and preterm delivery and the need for neonatal care, especially if withdrawal symptoms occur.	III/B	106
Explain the risk of developmental abnormality in infants.	III/B	102
In women using heroin, encourage detoxification or substitution with methadone or buprenorphine.	III/B	110
Encourage cessation with cocaine and amphetamines.	IIb/B	190
Solvent abuse produces effects similar to those of alcohol.	III/B	178
Screen for fetal abnormality, growth, and well-being.	III/B	106
The patient may need an increased dose of narcotic analgesia (an epidural is preferable).	IV/C	191
Provide fetal monitoring if intrauterine growth restriction occurs.	—/GPP	—
If the patient is HIV-positive or is still injecting, discourage breast-feeding (see also Chapter 28).	IV/C	134
Watch for symptoms of withdrawal in the infant (starting at 3 days with heroin, cocaine, and solvents; 7 days with methadone, barbiturates, and amphetamines).	IV/C	127,192
Provide follow-up by an addiction team.	IV/C	193,194

GPP, good practice point.

SUGGESTED READINGS

Binder T, Vavrinkova B: Prospective randomised comparative study of the effect of buprenorphine, methadone and heroin on the course of pregnancy, birthweight of newborns, early postpartum adaptation and course of the neonatal abstinence syndrome (NAS) in women followed up in the outpatient department. Neuroendocrinol Lett 2008;29:80–86.

Frank DA, Augustyn M, Knight WG, et al: Growth, development, and behavior in early childhood following prenatal cocaine exposure: A systematic review. JAMA 2001;285:1613–1625.

Hodnett ED, Fredericks S: Support during pregnancy for women at increased risk of low birthweight babies. Cochrane Database Syst Rev 2003;3:CD000198.

Jones KL: From recognition to responsibility: Josef Warkany, David Smith, and the fetal alcohol syndrome in the 21st century. Birth Defects Res Part A Clin Mol Teratol 2003;67:13–20.

Lumley J, Oliver SS, Chamberlain C, Oakley L: Interventions for promoting smoking cessation during pregnancy. Cochrane Database Syst Rev 2004;4:CD001055.

Naughton F, Prevost AT, Sutton S: Self-help smoking cessation interventions in pregnancy: A systematic review and meta-analysis. Addiction 2008;103:566–579.

Schuler ME, Nair P, Kettinger L: Drug-exposed infants and developmental outcome: Effects of a home intervention and ongoing maternal drug use. Arch Pediatr Adolesc Med 2003;157:133–138.

Sokol RJ, Delaney-Black V, Nordstrom B: Fetal alcohol spectrum disorder. JAMA 2003;290:2996–2999.

Testa M, Quigley BM, Eiden RD: The effects of prenatal alcohol exposure on infant mental development: A meta-analytical review. Alcohol Alcohol 2003;38:295–304.

Walker AM, Walker JJ: A methadone programme for substance-misusing pregnant women. In Tober GS (ed): Methadone Matters. London, Martin Dunit, 2003.

REFERENCES

For a complete list of references, log onto www.expertconsult.com.

CHAPTER 34

Medication

CATALIN S. BUHIMSCHI and CARL P. WEINER

INTRODUCTION

Drug use during pregnancy and lactation remains one of the least developed areas of clinical pharmacology and drug research. Pregnancy risk factors together with an increased incidence in chronic diseases and a rise in the average maternal age predict medication use will increase during gestation. Common primary exposure categories include over-the-counter medication, psychiatric agents, gastrointestinal medications, herbals, vitamins, antibiotics, and topical products. Sadly, only a few medications have been tested specifically for safety and efficacy during human gestation. Profound physiologic changes occur during both normal and pathologic pregnancy that may dramatically alter drug clearance, efficacy, and safety. In such an environment, the danger of a drug to mothers, their fetuses, and nursing infants cannot be determined with any confidence until it is widely used. It is important that women with medical disorders such as diabetes, hypertension, epilepsy, and inflammatory bowel disease continue necessary therapy while pregnant. Unfortunately, many physicians stop or delay medically important agents precisely because of the lack of information. Innovative research in genomics and proteomics should facilitate the development of medications exponentially as part of the new scientific field of "theranostics." Theranostics holds great potential for personalized medicine in order to tailor medical treatments for individual patients. Perhaps we should start with a whole class of patients—pregnant women—in desperate need of tailored products.

In this chapter, we seek to provide a general but concise resource of drugs commonly used during pregnancy and lactation. It is critical that clinicians become familiar with all the aspects of the drugs they recommend and consult with a maternal-fetal medicine specialist, when appropriate, so that the best possible evidence-based counseling and treatments are provided.

MATERNAL PHYSIOLOGIC ADAPTATION TO PREGNANCY

Pregnancy is characterized by profound changes in the cardiovascular, respiratory, renal, gastrointestinal, and endocrine systems.[1] These changes begin early and evolve steadily. By 6 to 8 weeks' gestation, the plasma volume begins to rise, reaching 50% above the nonpregnant level by the end of the third trimester.[2,3] Given this increase in the extracellular space and total body water, physiologic dilution occurs and may explain some of the effects of pregnancy on drug efficacy. The efficacy of any medication used is highly dependent on the dose and route of delivery, absorption, plasma level achieved, engagement of the receptors, functionality of the effector mechanisms, and clearance of the drug by liver and kidneys.[4] The physiologic increase in the maternal blood volume provides a rationale for the clinical observation that the doses of many medications must be adjusted during pregnancy to maintain efficacy.

Cardiac output increases during pregnancy by 30% to 50% and begins to do so by 8 weeks' gestation. It is caused by an elevation in both stroke volume and heart rate.[5,6] In addition, there is a significant redistribution of this increased cardiac output.[7] The impact of this on drug clearance might be great because glomerular filtration rate increases while the percentage of the cardiac output delivered to the liver, the organ crucial for drug disposal, declines. Therefore, adaptation to normal pregnancy might increase renal clearance but decrease hepatic clearance. In addition, gastric and intestinal transit is prolonged during pregnancy owing, at least in part, to progesterone-induced inhibition of intracellular calcium movement within smooth muscle cells.[8] This adaptation will alter the bioavailability of oral agents. Further, up to 80% of pregnant women experience nausea and vomiting at least during the first trimester, which can influence compliance with treatment.[9]

Numerous medications are bound by albumin, which declines during pregnancy. Decreased albumin and α_1-acid glycoprotein concentrations increase the free drug concentration of drugs that are normally highly bound, shortening their elimination half-life.[10,11] Pregnancy causes a partially compensated respiratory alkalosis, which also may affect the protein binding of some drugs.

Knowledge of pharmacokinetics and the application of mechanism-based approaches will improve our ability to predict the effects of pregnancy on medications with limited experience.[10] In pharmacology, "bioavailability" describes the fraction of an administered dose of unchanged drug that reaches the systemic circulation. It measures the extent to which a therapeutically active compound reaches the systemic circulation and is present at the site of action. The good news is that despite the many physiologic changes that occur during pregnancy that could affect absorption, drug bioavailability does not appear to be profoundly altered.[10]

GENERAL PRINCIPLES OF TERATOLOGY

Teratology—Definition

Teratology is the study of the biologic mechanisms and causes of abnormal human development coupled with the development of preventive strategies.[12] According to Shepard and Lemire,[12] the following conditions are required to establish proof of teratogenicity:

- Established exposure of the embryo or fetus at a critical time during development.
- Consistent dysmorphic findings recognized in well-conducted epidemiologic studies.
- Specific defects or syndromes consistently associated with a specific teratogen.
- Association of environmental exposure with rare anatomic defects (e.g., carbamazepine with facial dysmorphism and nail hypoplasia).
- Proven teratogenicity in experimental animal models.

Teratogen—Definition

A *teratogen* acts to irreversibly alter growth, structure, or function of the embryo or fetus and refers to any agent that causes an anatomic structural abnormality. This definition can reasonably be expanded to include alterations in function. Although 2% to 3% of all pregnancies are complicated by congenital abnormalities, less than 10% can be associated with a particular drug exposure. Known teratogens include viruses (e.g., rubella, cytomegalovirus, congenital lymphocytic choriomeningitis virus), parasites (toxoplasmosis), spirochetal bacterium (*Treponema pallidum*), environmental factors (e.g., hyperthermia, irradiation), chemicals (e.g., mercury, alcohol), and therapeutic agents (e.g., *lithium*, *methotrexate*, inhibitors of the renin-angiotensin system, *thalidomide*, *streptomycin*, *isotretinoin*, *warfarin*, *valproic acid*, *phenytoin*, *carbamazepine*).[1,13]

Embryonic versus Fetal Exposure to Teratogens

The extent of embryonic and fetal exposure depends on factors such as gestational age, dose, route of administration, absorption of the drug, maternal serum levels, and/or liver or kidney clearance system.[14] Placental passage is also critical for a drug medication to exercise its specific embryonic or fetal teratogenic effect.

Based on the gestation at exposure, a teratogen can induce either an *embryopathy* or a *fetopathy*. From this perspective, several critical periods of embryonic or fetal development are described:

1. "Preimplantation" (fertilization to implantation).
2. "Embryonic" (the second through the ninth week).
3. "Fetal" (the ninth week to term).

The preimplantation period is generally characterized as "all or nothing," meaning that injury to a large number of cells will predictably cause an embryonic loss. In turn, if only a small number of cells are disrupted, the embryo is protected through a phenomenon called "compensation" that facilitates survival without birth defects.[15]

The period of organogenesis (2–8 wk postconception) is the time of maximal vulnerability, and each embryonic system has a period of maximum susceptibility (e.g., the heart is typically affected if the teratogen acts between 6 and 8 wk' gestation). Conversely, the fetus might be affected by alterations in the structure and function of organs that initially develop. For example, a variety of central nervous system (CNS) malformations (e.g., anencephaly, spina bifida, encephalocele, craniorachischisis) arise owing to the failure of closure of the neural tube during the process of neurulation (17th–30th postfertilization days). Other neural tube defects (e.g., encephaloceles) may occur postclosure during the fetal period.[14,16]

Human teratogens may act and induce a different spectrum of malformations during specific stages of fetal developmental. For instance, nonsteroidal anti-inflammatory drugs (NSAIDs; e.g., *indomethacin*, *ibuprofen*) are associated with vascular disruptions (e.g., gastroschisis) if the embryo is exposed early in gestation.[17] In contrast, closure of the ductus and/or kidney failure might occur when the fetus is exposed to an NSAID after 32 weeks.[18] Similarly, *warfarin* is a well-recognized teratogen that carries a 4% to 10% risk of a dose-dependent and specific embryopathy if used during the first trimester.[19,20] Whereas first-trimester exposure to *warfarin* leads to embryopathy, exposure of the fetus during the second and third trimesters causes abnormalities related to hemorrhage, primarily in the CNS and skeleton.[21]

Placenta and Teratogenicity

Placental transfer depends greatly on maternal metabolism, gestational age, protein binding and storage, charge, pH, drug ionization, liposolubility, and molecular size (e.g., most substances <500 daltons diffuse rapidly across the placenta).[22,23] Probably the most eloquent example of this phenomeon may be found in anticoagulation therapy. Whereas the relatively low-molecular-weight *warfarin* is transported across the placenta, the high-molecular-weight *heparin* is not, explaining in part why *warfarin* but not *heparin* is a teratogen agent.[24] The increased circulating sex hormone levels characteristic of pregnancy have a profound impact on at least some placental drug-metabolizing enzymes, drug bioavailability, and receptor coupling. Steroid hormones directly influence the expression and function of placental transporters involved in drug passage to the fetus.[25] Of particular interest in the future is the manipulation of placental transporter activity (either increasing or decreasing) to optimize the fetal therapeutic impact. Lastly, differences in placentation are likely to be a key factor responsible for interspecies variability in response to many agents and might explain why a drug may act as a teratogen in humans but not in animals and vice versa.[22]

Genetic Variation and Teratogenicity

Genetic variation is a relevant determinant of drug clearance in pregnant women. Likewise, the effect of pregnancy on systems subject to genetic variation is likely to affect the efficacy and teratogenic effect of a specific drug. Several drug groups whose metabolic pathways are known to be greatly affected by genetic heterogeneity are widely used during pregnancy, and changes in their clearances are reported.[26–29] For example, developmental effects of certain anticonvulsants (e.g., *phenytoin*) suggest that prenatal exposure may result in gender-determined developmental changes and deficits.[30] Clearly, the fetal genotype determines susceptibility of the fetus to a given agent. Furthermore, all vertebrates carry a group of highly conserved genes—the homeobox genes. These regulatory genes (especially the HOX family) encode for transcriptional factors that control the expression of several other regulatory genes.[31] The HOX genes are essential to establish positional identity of various body structures from the head to the tail. For example, upper arm development is regulated by genes in the 9 to 10 group; the lower arm by the 10, 11, 12 groups; and the digits by the 11, 12, and 13 groups.[32] Several teratogenic agents (e.g., retinoids) activate homeobox genes, causing chaotic gene expression at different times of development. Several patterns of malformations are explained by such pathways, including spina bifida associated with *valproic acid*.[33] The world painfully learned in the 1970s that in utero exposure to diethylstilbestrol (DES) induces various abnormalities in the müllerian duct. Animal studies suggest that organ-specific gene expression patterns in the mouse müllerian duct are altered by in utero DES exposure.[34] DES-induced changes in expression of genes include Dkk2 (Dickkopf gene family), Nkd2 (naked cuticle drosophila), and sFRP1 (secreted frizzled related protein 1) as well as changes in genes of the HOX family that, in the female fetal reproductive tract, could be the basis for various abnormalities.[34]

Drug Risk Classification in Pregnancy

Physicians in the United States rely almost routinely on U.S. Food and Drug Administration (FDA) drug classification (A, B, C, D, or X) (Table 34–1) to ascertain risks and counsel patients regarding the safety of a drug during pregnancy. Other classifications are used worldwide (see Table 34–1). All differ in their conclusions on the safety of numerous agents commonly used during pregnancy.[35] In one comparison, only 61 (26%) of the 236 drugs common to all three systems in Table 34–1 were placed under the same risk factor category. Though these classifications seek simplicity, they are often difficult to interpret and are only rarely updated after a drug is marketed.

Under the FDA taxonomy, less than 1% of drugs are classified as category A (controlled studies in women fail to demonstrate a risk for the fetus and the possibility of fetal harm appears remote).[36] In point, the majority (66%) of all drugs marketed in the United States are classified category C (risks cannot be ruled out in humans, but the benefits of the medication may outweigh the potential risks).[36] Many angiotensin-converting enzyme (ACE) inhibitors are or were initially classified as such. In the same FDA risk classification, some category X drugs (7%; evidence that the medication causes abnormalities in the fetus) are not absolutely contraindicated during pregnancy. One such example is *ribavirin*, which is used in combination with *interferon*, for the treatment of chronic hepatitis C.[37] Although *ribavirin* is considered contraindicated in pregnancy, there is no adequate study demonstrating a teratogenic effect of this drug in human pregnancy.[38]

Given these limitations, the FDA has proposed to revise the content and format of labeling for human prescription drug and biologic products. Detailed information about this proposal can be found at http://www.fda.gov/cber/rules/frpreglac.htm. The new categorization will eliminate the alphabetical (A, B, C, D, and X) category of risk. Two major subsections of the drug labeling are proposed:

- Pregnancy.
- Lactation.

These subsections will replace the existing "Pregnancy," "Labor and Delivery," and "Nursing Mothers" sections of the current drug labeling scheme and include three main components: risk summary, clinical considerations, and data available from animal and human studies. This layout approximates that used by our text *Drugs for Pregnant and Lactating Women*.[36] It is encouraging that under the new rules, postmarketed experience will be provided.

Pregnancy Registries and Case-Control Surveillance Studies as a Resource for Identification of Drug Teratogenicity

Unfortunately, manufacturers, physicians, and patients are often reassured and believe that the most serious short-term adverse effects of a drug were identified in premarketing studies. The reality is that many human teratogenic effects were discovered only after a drug received marketing approval and was used broadly. Although the endorsement of a drug by the FDA requires comprehensive animal and human studies, such surveillance models are limited in their ability to accurately predict whether an agent is a human teratogen. Factors such as dose and route of administration, gestational age at exposure, maturation of the fetus, and its genotype all are important in limiting the identification of drug teratogenicity prior to commercialization. Variations in placentation, species-specific effects, and even between mammalian species are described.[15,22]

Identification of a de novo birth defect is always problematic, given that the caregiver should provide answers to two main questions:

- Was this defect the consequence of a genetic defect?
- Was this defect the result of exposure to a teratogen during gestation?

Most congenital defects associated with prenatal exposure to a drug are identifiable by their pattern of major and minor malformations, rather than a single major malformation. Thus, traditional epidemiologic methods are not always effective in identifying new teratogens.[39] Therefore, two main strategies for the identification of teratogens are proposed:

- Pregnancy registries.
- Case-control surveillance.[40]

The FDA defines a "pregnancy exposure registry" as a prospective observational study that collects information on women who take medicines and receive vaccines during pregnancy. Recruitment of large numbers of exposed pregnancies and successful long-term follow-up of the patients coupled with the complete and accurate ascertainment of pregnancy outcomes are critical attributes of a well-designed

TABLE 34–1

Pregnancy Drug Categories from Different Countries

FDA CATEGORY (USA)	PREGNANCY CATEGORY DEFINITION
A	Adequate, well-controlled studies in pregnant women have not shown any risk to the fetus in the first 3 months of pregnancy, and there is no evidence of later risk either. *Very few medications have been tested to this level.*
B	There have been no adequate, well-controlled studies in women, but studies using animals have not found any risk to the fetus, or animal studies have found risk that was not confirmed by adequate studies in pregnant women. *Not many adequate studies have been performed in pregnant women, so the first situation (not enough information) usually applies if a medication is assigned to this category.*
C	There have been no adequate, well-controlled studies in women, but studies using animals have shown a harmful effect on the fetus, or there have not been any studies in either women or animals. Caution is advised, but the benefits of the medication may outweigh the potential risks.
D	There is clear evidence of risk to the human fetus, but the benefits may outweigh the risk for pregnant women who have a serious condition that cannot be treated effectively with a safer drug.
X	There is clear evidence that the medication causes abnormalities in the fetus. The risks outweigh any potential benefits for women who are (or may become) pregnant.
FASS CATEGORY (SWEDEN)	**PREGNANCY CATEGORY DEFINITION**
A*	Drugs taken by a large number of pregnant women with no proven increase in the frequency of malformations or other observed harmful effects on the fetus
B1*	Limited experience in pregnant women, no increase observed in the frequency of malformations or other observed harmful effects on the fetus. Animal studies reassuring.
B2*	Limited experience in pregnant women, no increase observed in the frequency of malformations or other harmful effects on the fetus. Animal studies inadequate or lacking.
B2*	Limited experience in pregnant women, no increase observed in the frequency of malformations or other harmful effects on the fetus. Animal studies inadequate or lacking.
B3†	Limited experience in pregnant women, no increase observed in the frequency of malformations or other harmful effects on the fetus. Animal studies have shown evidence of an increased occurrence of fetal damage.
C†	May cause pharmacologic adverse effects on the fetus or neonate.
D‡	Suspected or proven to cause malformations or other irreversible damage.
ADEC CATEGORY (AUSTRAILIA)	**PREGNANCY CATEGORY DEFINITION**
A–D	Categories A,a B1,a B2,a B3,b C,b Dc similar to the FASS definitions.
Xc	Limited experience in pregnant women, no increase observed in the frequency of malformations or other observed harmful effects on the fetus. Animal studies reassuring.

* Drugs grouped as probably safe.
† Drugs grouped as potentially harmful.
‡ Drugs grouped as clearly harmful.
ADEC, Australian Drug Evaluation Committee (Australian categorization); FASS, Farmaceutiska Specialiteter i Sverige (Swedish categorization); FDA, U.S. Food and Drug Administration (U.S. categorization).
Adapted from Blackwell Publishing Ltd., Malden, Mass 02148-5020, USA. Buhimschi CS, Weiner CP: Medications in pregnancy and lactation. In Queenan JT, Spong CY, Lockwood CJ (eds): Management of High Risk Pregnancy, 5th ed. An evidence based approach. Malden, Mass: Blackwell Publishing, 2007, pp 38–58.

registry.[41] There is consensus that pregnancy registries are a useful resource of information, and the FDA has required some pharmaceutical manufacturers to maintain a pregnancy exposure registry. The most up-to-date *List of Pregnancy Exposure Registries* is available at the FDA website (http://www.fda.gov/womens/registries/). Recently, the Research Committee for the Organization of Teratology Information Specialists (OTIS) concluded that more specific information on the timing and the dose of drug was necessary in pregnancy birth defect registries sponsored by pharmaceutical companies to improve the accuracy of risk estimates for developmental toxicity.[42] Specifically, the Committee recommended that

- The exposure should be stated in gestational weeks and days rather than simply weeks.
- The exposure dose should be stated in patient-specific terms, such as body weight (milligrams per kilogram) or body surface area (milligrams per square meter), rather than simply the dose strength. OTIS maintains a specialized telephone information service that is a valuable resource available to patients and health care practitioners (http://www.OTISpregnancy.org).

Other online databases about the effect of exposure to a significant number of medications during pregnancy are

- REPROTOX (http://www.reprotox.org).
- TERIS (http://depts.washington.edu/terisweb).

REPROTOX offers information on the effects of medications, chemicals, infections, and physical agents on pregnancy, reproduction, and development. It includes more than 4000 agents along with references. Likewise, TERIS is designed to help physicians assess the risks of possible teratogenic exposures during pregnancy based on a thorough review of published clinical and experimental literature.

Given that randomized studies are in most cases impossible to conduct for detection of teratogenicity, physicians must rely on case-control studies.[43] Even so, case-control studies are used mainly to identify possible associations and their interpretation should be cautious.[44]

Similar to our recent publications,[1,45] the objective of this chapter is to provide a general overview of selected drugs with a large or small potential for teratogenicity. First, we present a list of the most common drugs or drug groups (in alphabetical order) known or strongly suspected to cause developmental defects (Table 34–2). Second, we list and provide information on some of the most common medications or medication groups with minimal or no known human teratogenic effect (Table 34–3). Because information changes rapidly, it is critical that clinicians become familiar with the most up-to-date aspects of the drugs they recommend and consult, when appropriate, with a maternal-fetal medicine specialist so that patient counseling and decisions are based on the best possible evidence. For detailed information regarding all medication drugs, the interested readers should consult a text such as *Drugs for Pregnant and Lactating Women*[36] or a continuously updated database such as REPROTOX, OTIS, or ENTIS.

TABLE 34–2

Drugs or Drug Groups Known or Strongly Suspected to Cause Developmental Defects, and Their Pregnancy Safety Categorization*

DRUG	FDA
Agents acting on renin-angiotensin system (enalapril, captopril, lisinopril)	C (1st trimester) D (2nd and 3rd trimesters)
Antidepressants (paroxetine–only)	D
Antiepileptic drugs (valproic acid, carbamazepine, phenytoin)	D
Anxiolytics (diazepam)	D
Alkylating agents (cyclophosphamide)	D
Hormone androgens (methyltestosterone, medroxyprogesterone acetate, danazol)	X
Antimetabolites (methotrexate)	D, X
Antithyroid (methimazole)	D
Coumarin derivatives (warfarin)	X
Estrogens (diethylstilbestrol)	X
Antifungals (fluconazole)	C
Antipsychotics (lithium)	D
Prostaglandins (misoprostol)	X
Oral contraceptives	X
Penicillamine	D
Retinoids (isotretinoin)	X
Radioactive iodine (sodium iodide-131)	X
Dermatologics; immunomodulators (thalidomide)	X

* See Table 34–1 for an explanation of the safety categories.
FDA, U.S. Food and Drug Administration (FDA). These categories change on occasion. Please review before prescribing any drug you are unfamiliar with.
Modified from Blackwell Lippincott Williams & Wilkins, Baltimore, Md USA. Buhimschi CS, Weiner CP: Medications in pregnancy and lactation: Part 1. Teratology. Obstet Gynecol 2009;113:166–188.

HUMAN TERATOGENS (see Table 34-2)

Angiotensin-converting Enzyme Inhibitors (Enalapril [Vasotec], Captopril [Capoten, Lopurin], Lisinopril [Prinivil; Zestril])

MATERNAL CONSIDERATIONS

There are no adequate reports or well-controlled studies in pregnant women in great part because ACE inhibitors are generally contraindicated throughout pregnancy. This prohibition would include women receiving renoprotective medications.[46] In extremely rare cases, ACE inhibitors may be indicated for the control of severe hypertension in a woman refractory to other medications.[47,48] In this scenario, close consultation with a cardiologist and/or a nephrologist coupled to the serial monitoring of amniotic fluid and fetal well-being is recommended.[49] Should oligohydramnios be detected, the ACE inhibitor must be discontinued immediately unless it is deemed life-saving for the mother.

FETAL CONSIDERATIONS

Both *lisinopril* and *enalapril* cross the human placenta.[50–52] It was long held that exposure of the embryo to ACE inhibitors was safe during the first trimester and that only second- and third-trimester exposure resulted in oligohydramnios,

TABLE 34–3

Drugs or Drug Groups with Minimal or Not Known Human Teratogenic Effect*

DRUG	FDA
Analgesics (aspirin, acetaminophen, ibuprofen)	B-D (see class)
Antibiotics (penicillin G, tetracyclines, ciprofloxacin, metronidazole, tetracycline, nitrofurantoin, azithromycin)	B-D (see class)
Anticholinergics (albuterol, atropine, dimenhydrinate)	B-C (see class)
Antihypertensive agents (methyldopa, hydralazine, labetolol, propranolol)	B-C (see class)
Antihistamines (cetirizine, diphenhydramine)	B
Antivirals (acyclovir)	B
Corticosteroids (prednisone, betamethasone, dexamethasone)	B
Tumor necrosis factor modulators (infliximab)	C

* See Table 34–1 for an explanation of the safety categories.
FDA, U.S. Food and Drug Administration. These categories change on occasion. Please review before prescribing any drug you are unfamiliar with.
Modified from Blackwell Lippincott Williams & Wilkins, Baltimore, Md USA. Buhimschi CS, Weiner CP: Medications in pregnancy and lactation: Part 2. Drugs with minimal or unknown human teratogenic effect. Obstet Gynecol 2009;113:417–432.

hypocalvaria, anuria, renal failure, patent ductus arteriosus, aortic arch obstructive malformations, or death.[53–55] However, one report concluded that infants exposed to ACE inhibitors during the first trimester have an increased risk for cardiovascular (pulmonic stenosis, atrial and ventricular septal defects) and CNS (microcephaly, eye anomaly, spina bifida, coloboma) malformations.[56] Although the strength of this conclusion is limited by the relatively small number of fetuses in the final analysis and its retrospective design, we suggest avoidance of ACE inhibitors in the first trimester until there is evidence of safety. Antenatal surveillance must be initiated should inadvertent exposure occur and the fetus is potentially viable. Oligohydramnios may not appear until after the irreversible renal injury. Fetal exposure to ACE inhibitors is associated with increased neonatal morbidity and mortality. Neonates exposed to ACE inhibitors in utero should be observed closely for hypotension, oliguria, and hyperkalemia. Long-term follow-up after fetal ACE exposure reveals impaired renal function, severe hypertension, and proteinuria.[57]

BREAST-FEEDING CONSIDERATIONS

ACE inhibitors are considered compatible with breast-feeding. Trace quantities of ACE inhibitors (*captopril*, *enalapril*) are excreted into breast milk, though the kinetics remains to be clarified.[58,59] It is unknown whether *lisinopril* enters human breast milk. For this reason, the lowest effective dose should be used, infants should be monitored for possible adverse effects, and breast-feeding should be avoided at times of peak maternal drug levels.

Antidepressant (Fluoxetine [Prozac, Sarafem], Sertraline [Zoloft, Lustral], Paroxetine [Paxil])

MATERNAL CONSIDERATIONS

The use of psychotropic medications during pregancy is increasing and a matter of concern for the physicians and patients. Because depression is common and typically unrecognized, universal screening is recommended at the time of the first prenatal visit, each trimester, and postpartum.[60,61] Pregnancy is not a reason a priori to discontinue psychotropic drugs.[62] Discontinuation of needed antidepressant medication during pregnancy exchanges the risk of embryopathy/fetopathy for debilitating depression. Recently, the manufacturer of *paroxtine* changed its classification from C to D (see Table 34–1). In response, the American College of Obstetricians and Gynecologists (ACOG) issued both a Commitee Opinion and a Practice Bulletin to provide guidelines for the use of selective serotonin-reuptake inhibitor (SSRIs) and psychiatric medications during pregnancy and lactation.[60,61] It recommended that the treatment of depression with SSRIs be in the context of an increased risk of maternal relapse following discontinuation of antidepressive medication. ACOG suggests that a team composed of a psychiatrist and an obstetrician work together to decide on the need for continuing treatment and to discuss the known risks with the mother. *Fluoxetine* is effective treatment for postpartum depression and is as effective as a course of cognitive-behavioral counseling in the short term.[63] There are no adequate reports or well-controlled studies of *sertraline* in pregnant women, though there is growing experience with its use for the treatment of postpartum depression.[63] In general, women taking SSRIs during pregnancy require a higher dose to maintain euthymia.[64] If possible, *paroxetine* should be avoided during gestation and in women planning pregnancy.[61] Other alternatives should be sought in collaboration with the mental health provider.

FETAL CONSIDERATIONS

Most data related to the use of antidepressants in pregnancy are derived from the use of SSRIs (*fluoxetine*, *sertraline*, *paroxetine*). *Fluoxetine*, *sertraline*, and *paroxetine* cross the human placenta and there is evidence of teratogenicity.[65–68] The teratogenic effect of SSRIs has been examined in two other large case-control studies suggesting a 1.5 to 2-fold increased risk of congenital cardiac malformations (atrial and ventricular septal defects) after first-trimester exposure to *paroxetine*.[69,70] In the Slone Epidemiology Center Birth Defects Study, *paroxetine* use was associated with right ventricular outflow defects and *sertraline* use was associated with omphalocele and atrial and ventricular septum defects.[69] Not all studies find the same risks from SSRI use in pregnancy. There was no significant association between SSRIs and congenital heart defects in the National Birth Defects Prevention Study.[70] They did observe an association between *paroxetine* and anencephaly, craniosynostosis, and omphalocele. The small number of exposed infants for each individual malformation and identification of these risks only after performance of more than 40 statistical tests represent the major drawbacks of the studies. An FDA public health advisory note highlighted concerns about a possible association between SSRI use during gestation and newborn persistent pulmonary hypertension.[71]

In summary, exposure to SSRIs, specifically *paroxetine*, during early pregnancy may be associated with an increased risk of cardiac defects. A more recent study did not confirm that *paroxetine* is associated with an increased risk of congenital cardiovascular defects.[72] The absolute risk is small and generally not greater than 2 per 1000 births. Although caution should be exercised (mostly with the use of *paroxetine*), these agents are not considered major teratogens.[73] Late exposure to SSRIs is linked with transient neonatal complications, including jitteriness, mild respiratory distress, transient tachypnea of the newborn, weak cry, poor tone, and neonatal intensive care unit admission.[74–76]

BREAST-FEEDING CONSIDERATIONS

Most psychotropic medications are transferred to breast milk in varying amounts and potentially passed on to the nursing infant. Breast-feeding is not contraindicated in women using either *fluoxetine*, *sertraline*, or *paroxetine*.[77] Maternal serum and peak breast milk concentrations of *fluoxetine* and its active metabolite norfluoxetine predict nursing infant serum norfluoxetine concentrations. Limited data suggest that *paroxetine* is not detectable in the neonates who are exclusively breast-fed.[78] The infant should be monitored for possible adverse effects if breast-fed; the drug should be given at the lowest effective dose; and breast-feeding should be avoided at times of peak drug levels if possible. In theory, discarding breast milk obtained at the time of peak drug concentration could allow the mother to reduce the infant's exposure to her medication.[77]

Anticonvulsants (Valproic acid [Depakene], Carbamazepine [Tegretol, Atretol, Convuline, Epitol], Phenytoin [Dilantin, Aladdin, Dantoin], Lamotrigine [Lamictal])

MATERNAL CONSIDERATIONS

Almost half a million women in the United States have a medical condition that requires psychiatric care, ensuring that the use of such medications during pregnancy would receive much attention.[61] Several anticonvulsants (*valproate, carbamazepine, lamotrigine*) are used for the treatment of epilepsy as well as mood stabilization (bipolar disorders). Many anticonvulsants induce hepatic enzymes that decrease the serum concentrations of estrogen and progesterone, a potential problem for women using oral contraceptives.[79] The risk for contraceptive failure appears greatest with cytochrome P-450 enzyme-inducing agents, such as *carbamazepine* or *phenytoin*. Conversely, the available information suggests that *valproic acid* does alter steroid levels in women taking oral contraceptives.[80] There is no reliable information to assess the relationship between *lamotrigene* and combined hormonal contraceptive failure.[61] Clinicians frequently recommend contraceptives with a higher ethinyl estradiol level (50 μg) to avoid first-trimester exposure, although there is no real experience to support such a practice. Despite the lack of supportive data, ACOG recently suggested that women taking anticonvulsants proven to reduce oral contraceptive steroid levels be switched to a 30- to 35-μg estrogen oral contraceptive.[61] Patients planning pregnancy should be counseled on the risks and the importance of periconceptual folate supplementation (4 mg/day).[81] Some authorities recommend measuring serum concentrations of old- and new-generation antiepileptic drugs.[82]

Valproate is the sodium salt of *valproic acid*. Although there is a long clinical experience with *valproate* and *carbamazepine*, there are no adequate reports or well-controlled studies of these medications in pregnant women. *Phenytoin* is a first-generation, enzyme-inducing anticonvulsant. Stable *phenytoin* serum levels are achievable in most pregnant women, though there is wide variability on equivalent doses.[83] It is unknown whether women with unusually low levels of *phenytoin* are noncompliant subjects or hypermetabolizers. Unusually high levels can result from hepatic disease, congenital enzyme deficiency, or other drugs that interfere with metabolism. To reduce the risk of a seizure, dosage adjustments should be based on clinical symptoms, and not solely on serum drug concentrations. *Phenytoin* may impair the efficacy of corticosteroids, coumadin, digitoxin, doxycycline, estrogens, furosemide, oral contraceptives, quinidine, rifampin, theophylline, and vitamin D.[84]

Lamotrigene is a new-generation antiepileptic drug also useful for the treatment of bipolar depression.[85] It is generally well tolerated, and its reproductive safety profile is superior to that of other antiepileptics. There are no adequate reports or well-controlled studies of *lamotrigene* in pregnant women. *Lamotrigene* levels vary widely during pregnancy, and patients may experience a loss of seizure control without close monitoring.[86–88]

The most common treatment strategy is to use the appropriate antiepileptic drug for the woman's seizure disorder as monotherapy at the lowest effective dosage throughout pregnancy. If necessary, a single medication at a higher dose is preferable to a multidrug regimen.[61] The goal is to use antiepileptic drugs in such a way that generalized tonic-clonic seizures are avoided in hopes of minimizing risk to the fetus.

FETAL CONSIDERATIONS

Valproic acid is a recognized human teratogen.[89,90] The likelihood of an affected offspring is dose-dependent, and the risk is enhanced by a low serum folate level. A recent analysis indicates that the risk of congenital abnormalities in children exposed in utero to anticonvulsant therapy is reduced but not eliminated by folic acid supplementation between 5 and 12 weeks after the last menstrual period.[91] *Valproic acid* is rapidly and actively transported across the human placenta, reaching an fetal-to-maternal ratio exceeding 2.[92] The fetal "*valproate* syndrome"[93] includes a distinct craniofacial appearance, limb abnormalities, and heart defects, coupled with a cluster of minor and major anomalies and CNS dysfunction.[94,95] Affected fetuses may have an increased nuchal translucency measurement between 11 and 13 weeks.[96] After delivery, 10% die in infancy, and 1 of 4 survivors has either developmental deficits or mental retardation.

Carbamazepine crosses the human placenta and is also a teratogen.[97] The fetal "*carbamazepine* syndrome" includes facial dysmorphism, developmental delay, spina bifida, and distal phalanx and finger nail hypoplasia.[98,99]

Phenytoin is also a teratogen specifically associated with congenital heart defects and cleft palate (fetal *hydantoin* syndrome).[100,101] As with most psychotropic drugs, monotherapy and the lowest effective quantity given in divided doses to lower the peak levels can theoretically minimize the risks to the fetus.[102]

Lamotrigene crosses the human placenta.[103] Fetal exposure to *lamotrigene* does not appear to increase the risk of major fetal anomalies.[104] However, because *lamotrigene* crosses the placenta, close monitoring of both mother and newborn is receommended.[105]

BREAST-FEEDING CONSIDERATIONS

Valproic acid enters human breast milk. Fortunately, the peak neonatal serum concentration is less than 10% of the maternal level.[106] *Carbamazepine* is also excreted into human breast milk. Limited study suggests that *carbamazepine* is safe for breast-feeding women, although rare cases of neonatal cholestatic hepatitis have been previously reported.[107] Little *phenytoin* and *lamotrigene* are excreted into human breast milk, and both drugs are considered safe for breast-feeding.[108] Infants of mothers treated with anticonvulsant drugs should be monitored for possible adverse effects; the lowest effective dose should be given; and breast-feeding should be avoided at the time of peak drug levels.

Anxiolytics (Diazepam [Valium], Alprazolam [Xanax], Clonazepam [Klonopin])

MATERNAL CONSIDERATIONS

Anxiety disorders include panic disorders, generalized anxiety disorders, post-traumatic stress disorder, social anxiety, and phobias.[61] Collectively, these disorders are the most common psychiatric conditions, with a prevalence in the United States of approximately 18%.[109] Treatment options include benzodiazepines, antidepressants, and psychotherapy. Currently available information is insufficient to determine whether the potential benefits of benzodiazepines to the mother outweigh the risks to the fetus.[110]

There are no adequate reports or well-controlled studies of *diazepam* use in pregnant women. Although not an integral part of the ACOG protocol for the treatment of nausea and vomiting of pregnancy, *diazepam* may be a beneficial adjunct to intravenous fluids and vitamins for the treatment of hyperemesis gravidarium. *Diazepam* is a useful anxioloytic for women undergoing fetal therapy procedures. It has been used for both prophylaxis and treatment of eclamptic convulsions, but it is clinically inferior to *magnesium sulfate* and is not recommended as first-line therapy.[111–113]

Alprazolam is rarely indicated during pregnancy. There are only few reports of its use during pregnancy.[114,115] Abrupt cessation of therapy is associated with a discontinuation-emergent syndrome that includes neuropsychiatric, gastrointestinal, dermatologic, cardiovascular, and visual symptoms.

Clonazepam is a widely used benzodiazepine for the treatment of seizures and conditions such as panic attack and anxiety disorder. Unfortunately, there is limited study of its safety during pregnancy.[116] Several investigators have used *clonazepam* to treat dystonia gravidarium[117] (muscle contractions, frequently causing twisting and repetitive movements) and seizure prophylaxis in women with severe preeclampsia.

FETAL CONSIDERATIONS

Benzodiazepine use during pregnancy does not appear to carry a significant risk for teratogenesis. *Diazepam* rapidly crosses the human placenta.[118] Though several studies suggested an increased risk of oral clefts if used during the first trimester,[119] these findings were not confirmed in long-term follow-up studies.[115,120] Nor is there convincing evidence of an adverse effect on neurodevelopment. Intravenous *diazepam* may decrease fetal movement; thus, it may be used in select cases as an adjuvant to fetal therapy. Prolonged CNS depression may occur in neonates exposed to *diazepam* in utero. Symptoms vary from mild sedation, hypotonia, reluctance to suck to apneic spells, cyanosis, impaired metabolic responses to stress, floppy infant syndrome, and marked neonatal withdrawal symptoms[121] and may persist for hours to months after birth. Thus, the shortest course and the lowest dose should be used when indicated.

There is no evidence that *alprazolam* is a human teratogen.[122] Neonatal withdrawal syndrome may occur following exposure, and the measurement of *alprazolam's* main metabolite (α-hydroxyalprazolam) may be useful to differentiate between a drug effect and neonatal sepsis.[123]

Clonazepam also crosses the human placenta.[124] Although congenital anomalies are reported in 13% of infants whose mothers took clonazepam during pregnancy in combination with other antiepileptic drugs, there is no pattern of anomalies. Exposure in the late third trimester and during labor seems to carry the greatest risks to the perinate. Although the neonatal withdrawal syndrome is rare, children born to treated women may have symptoms varying from mild sedation, hypotonia, and reluctance to suck to apnea spells, cyanosis, and impaired metabolic responses to cold stress. These symptoms can persist from hours to months after birth.

BREAST-FEEDING CONSIDERATIONS

Benzodiazepines are excreted into human breast milk, but the maximum neonatal exposure is estimated at 3% of the maternal dose.[125] Neonatal lethargy, sedation, and weight loss are each reported and special attention should be paid if the neonate was premature or the maternal dose particularly high.

Alprazolam enters breast milk by passive diffusion.[126] It should be avoided during lactation because of its potential to alter neurodevelopment and because of the documented risks of withdrawal.[110,123]

Clonazepam is excreted into breast milk, but the detected levels in milk are low. The nursing infant is unlikely to ingest significant amounts of the drug. However, special attention should be paid if the infant is premature or has been exposed to high concentrations of drug either during pregnancy or at delivery.[125]

Alkylating Agents (Cyclophosphamide [Cytoxan])

MATERNAL CONSIDERATIONS

Cyclophosphamide is an integral part of numerous multiagent regimens to treat cancer of the ovary, breast, blood, and lymph systems. The most common complications reported following *cyclophosphamide* treatment are transient sterility and secondary malignancy. Several case reports note that *cyclophosphamide* can be used during pregnancy with a good outcome.[127–129]

FETAL CONSIDERATIONS

Cyclophosphamide crosses the human placenta, and neonatal hematologic suppression and secondary malignancies are reported.[130,131] The spectrum of malformations associated with in utero exposure to *cyclophosphamide* is highly variable (high-arched palate, microcephaly, flat nasal bridge, syndactyly, hypoplasia of the fingers). Growth deficiency and anomalies of the craniofacial region and limbs are most common.[132]

BREAST-FEEDING CONSIDERATIONS

Cyclophosphamide is not safe with breast-feeding because it enters human breast milk in high concentration. Neonatal neutropenia is common.[133,134]

Hormones-Androgens (Methyltestosterone [Androral, Testred], Medroxyprogesterone Acetate [Depo-Provera, Med-Pro, Provera], Danazol [Danocrine, Danatrol])

MATERNAL CONSIDERATIONS

Methyltestosterone is used for the treatment of endometriosis and for palliation of advancing inoperable breast cancer.[135] Some recommend *methyltestosterone* with estrogens to enhance libido in women, though its efficacy is unclear.[136] There are no indications for *methyltestosterone* during pregnancy. Inadvertent pregnancy exposures are reported because many pregnancies escape recognition until after the first trimester.[137] Progestational agents such as *medroxyprogesterone* have long been prescribed during early pregnancy to prevent first-trimester spontaneous abortion. This practice continues in some locales despite the failure of well-conducted studies to show effectiveness. Fortunately, epidemiologic studies are reassuring and there is no demonstrable increase in the prevalence of ectopic pregnancy following treatment with *medroxyprogesterone*.

Danazol, a derivative of the synthetic steroid 17-α-ethinyltestosterone is considered one of the most effective treatments for endometriosis.[138] *Danazol* is not an effective contraceptive, and it should be discontinued immediately should the patient become pregnant. There are no indications for *danazol* during pregnancy.

FETAL CONSIDERATIONS

Whether or not *methyltestosterone* crosses the human placenta is unknown. Animal studies reveal pseudohermaphroditism in female fetuses exposed to *methyltestosterone*.[139] Similarly, in utero exposure of male fetuses to *methyltestosterone* increases the risk of hypospadias.[140,141] Although there are insufficient human data to quantify the risk to the female fetus, some synthetic progestins have reportedly caused mild virilization of the external genitalia.[142,143]

It is unknown whether *danazol* crosses the human placenta. In addition, although the FDA classifies *danazol* as category X, there is no a priori reason to terminate an exposed pregnancy. *Danazol* may have an androgenic effect on female fetuses (vaginal atresia, clitoral hypertrophy, labial fusion, ambiguous genitalia).[144,145] First-trimester exposure to androgen-"like" hormones is an indication for a detailed anatomic ultrasound between 18 and 22 weeks' gestation.

BREAST-FEEDING CONSIDERATIONS

It remains unknown whether *methyltestosterone* enters human breast milk. In addition, although small quantities of *medroxyprogesterone* are excreted into human breast milk, it does not suppress lactation or adversely affect the newborn.[146,147] *Medroxyprogesterone* is typically given as a contraceptive 3 days after delivery because progesterone withdrawal may be one stimulus for the initiation of lactogenesis. It is unknown whether *danazol* enters human breast milk, and perhaps as a result, it is generally considered contraindicated during breast-feeding.

Antimetabolites (Methotrexate [Folex, Mexate, Rheumatrex, Tremetex])

MATERNAL CONSIDERATIONS

Methotrexate is an antimetabolite with multiple uses in reproductive-age women, including the treatment of ectopic pregnancy, neoplastic disease, autoimmune disorders, and inflammatory conditions (Crohn's disease, rheumatoid arthritis).[148] It is also considered an efficient medical abortifacient. It is even more efficient when combined with misoprostol (the efficacy ranges from 70% to 97%).[149,150] However, because *methotrexate* is not 100% effective, women must be followed until their serum β-human chorionic gonadotropin (β-hCG) titer returns to normal.[151,152]

FETAL CONSIDERATIONS

First-trimester exposure to *methotrexate* increases the risk of several malformations including craniofacial, axial skeletal, cardiopulmonary, and gastrointestinal abnormalities and developmental delay, though most pregnancies exposed to low doses are unaffected.[153,154] But even a single dose of *methotrexate* and *misoprostol*, used for medical termination of pregnancy, is associated with multiple congenital anomalies.[153] Exposure to *methotrexate* later in pregancy seems to be reasonably safe.[133]

BREAST-FEEDING CONSIDERATIONS

Methotrexate is generally considered contraindicated in nursing mothers,[155] but it is unknown whether *methotrexate* is excreted into human breast milk. Women with rheumatoid arthritis often experience a disease flare within 3 months of delivery, and drug treatment is required. Experts differ regarding the use of *methotrexate* during lactation, in part because of varying views on the potential for short- and long-term adverse effects.[156]

Antithyroid (Propylthiouracil [PTU], Methimazole [Favistan, Mercazole, Tapazole])

MATERNAL CONSIDERATIONS

Graves' disease is the most common cause of hyperthyroidism during pregnancy. Medical treatment involves either *propylthiouracil (PTU)* or *methimazole*.[157,158] Hyperthyroid women should have their thyroid function checked every 3 to 4 weeks throughout pregnancy. There is a general consensus among clinicians that the lowest dose of *PTU* or *methimazole* needed to keep free triiodothyronine (T_3) and free thyroxine (T_4) within the upper normal range for these women should be used.[159,160] Improvements in thyroid-stimulating hormone assay methodology have resulted in accurate identification of high thyroid-stimulating antibodies in pregnancy. Because women previously ablated with either a radioactive iodine (^{131}I) or a thyroidectomy may still be producing thyroid-stimulating antibodies (even though they are themselves euthyroid) the fetus remains at risk. The fetal status, whether the mother is receiving antithyroid medication or previously received definitive treatment, cannot be accurately predicted by ultrasound. The selection of *PTU* versus *methimazole* for the treatment of Graves' disease during pregnancy should not be based solely on the assumptions that *PTU* crosses the placenta less than *methimazole*, or that *PTU* causes less fetal hypothyroidism, or that exposure to *methimazole* leads to decreased intellectual function in the offspring. Rather, *PTU* is preferred because *methimazole* is more likely than *PTU* to be associated with fetal anomalies such as aplasia cutis, esophageal atresia, and choanal atresia.[161] *Methimazole* is a reasonable choice if the patient is allergic to *PTU* or fails to have a therapeutic response to *PTU*.[161] Agranulocytosis remains a major clinical concern when antithyroid drugs are used.[162] In 2009, the FDA issued a warning of increased risk of hepatotoxicity with *PTU* compared with *methimazole* (see http://www.fda.gov/Safety/MedWatch/SafetyInformation/SafetyAlertsforHumanMedicalProducts/ucm164162.htm).

FETAL CONSIDERATIONS

PTU crosses the human placenta, which in the case of Graves' disease, may be desirable. Fetal evaluation is recommended to directly confirm that the fetus is neither severely hyper- or hypothyroid.[163] A hypothyroid fetus can be given T_4 intra-amniotically. If hyperthyroid, the *PTU* can be increased and the mother supplemented with oral thyroxine if necessary. Aplasia cutis is a rare complication of maternal therapy. *Methimazole* also crosses the human placenta and is an alternative to *PTU* for the treatment of fetal hyperthyroidism.[164] The detailed placental kinetics for either agent is unknown. Both *methimazole* and *PTU* can induce fetal goiter and even cretinism in a dose-dependent fashion. Fortunately, long-term follow-up studies of exposed children reveal no deleterious effects on either thyroid function or physical and intellectual development with doses up to 20 mg daily.[165] At least for now, *PTU* remains a first-line treatment for Graves' disease during pregnancy because of the more frequent association of *methimazole* with fetal anomalies such as aplasia cutis, esophageal atresia, and choanal atresia.[161,166,167]

BREAST-FEEDING CONSIDERATIONS

Methimazole and *PTU* are excreted in the human breast milk at low concentrations.[168,169] No deleterious effects on neonatal thyroid function or physical and intellectual development of breast-fed infants have been described when mothers are treated with either *methimazole* or *PTU*.[170,171]

Coumarin Derivatives (Warfarin [Coumadin])

MATERNAL CONSIDERATIONS

Despite significant preventive efforts, thromboembolic disease remains a major cause of maternal morbidity and mortality. *Warfarin* is a teratogen and contraindicated in pregnancy with but a few exceptions, the principal one being a mechanical heart valve in which an International Normalized Ratio (INR) of 2.3 to 3.0 is recommended for either prophylaxis or treatment of venous thromboembolism. The risk of a bleeding complication during pregnancy approximates 18%. It is believed an INR of 2.3 to 3 will minimize the risk of hemorrhage.[172] Women requiring a dose above 5 mg/day have a greater risk of an adverse outcome. Previous studies consistently show that maternal morbidity is higher in women with bioprosthetic valves.[173] One therapeutic approach to minimize risk in a woman receiving therapeutic-dose anticoagulation with *warfarin* before pregnancy owing to a hereditary or acquired condition is to convert her to therapeutic doses of unfractionated *heparin* or low-molecular-weight *heparin* within the first 6 weeks of gestation.[174] When used in this fashion, coumarin derivatives are safe and effective and avoid embryopathy. Therapeutic *heparin* may not be as effective for prophylaxis, though most physicians recommend *heparin* or low-molecular-weight *heparin* for the first 6 to 12 weeks.[175]

If the mother's condition requires anticoagulation with *warfarin*, it should be substituted with *heparin* at 36 weeks to decrease the risk of epidural/spinal anesthesia (subdural hematoma).[176] *Warfarin* treatment should be resumed postpartum.

FETAL CONSIDERATIONS

Warfarin is a recognized teratogen. Exposure from 6 to 10 weeks' gestation is associated with an embryopathy and subsequent exposure with a fetopathy. The fetal "*warfarin* syndrome" consists of a varied spectrum of manifestations that include nasal hypoplasia, microphthalmia, hypoplasia of the extremities, intrauterine growth restriction, heart disease, scoliosis, deafness, and mental retardation.[177,178] In one large series of women treated with *warfarin* throughout pregnancy for a prosthetic valve, the incidence of fetal *warfarin* syndrome was 5.6%, the pregnancy loss rate was 32%, and the stillbirth rate was 10% of pregnancies achieving at least 20 weeks. It is proposed that the embryopathy occurs secondary to vitamin K deficiency and the fetopathy results from microhemorrhages. Agenesis of the corpus callosum, Dandy-Walker malformation, and optic atrophy are the most common CNS malformations. Long-term follow-up studies reported that school-age children exposed in utero have an increased frequency of mild neurologic dysfunction and an IQ less than 80.[179]

BREAST-FEEDING CONSIDERATIONS

Warfarin is not excreted to any degree into breast milk and is compatible with breast-feeding.[180,181]

Antipsychotics (Lithium [Calith, Lithocarb, Lithonate])

MATERNAL CONSIDERATIONS

Lithium is used for the treatment of psychiatric disorders (prevention of recurrent mania and bipolar depression and to reduce the risk of suicidal behavior), but not typically for the rapid control of acute mania.[182] The decision to discontinue *lithium* therapy during pregnancy because of fetal risks must be balanced against the maternal risks of exacerbation.[61] In addition, although pregnancy and especially the puerperium are high risk times for the recurrence of bipolar disease, physicians should be aware that sudden discontinuation of *lithium* is associated with a high rate of disease relapse.[183]

In 2008, ACOG issued a series of recommendations regarding the use of *lithium* during pregnancy or in women who are planning to conceive:

- In women who experience mild and infrequent episodes of illness, *lithium* should be gradually tapered before conception.
- In women who have more severe episodes but are only at moderate risk of relapse, *lithium* should be tapered before conception but restarted after organogenesis.
- In women who have especially severe and frequent episodes of illness, *lithium* should be continued throughout pregnancy and the patient counseled regarding the risks.[61,184]

When *lithium* is indicated, the serum levels should be maintained between 0.5 and 1.2 mEq/L.[185] As delivery approaches, several authorities recommend that the drug be tapered gradually beginning at 36 weeks or decreased by one quarter 2 to 3 days before delivery.[61,102,184,185]

FETAL CONSIDERATIONS

Lithium crosses the placenta. Fetal exposure to *lithium* may be associated with fetal and neonatal cardiac arrhythmias, hypoglycemia, nephrogenic diabetes insipidus, polyhydramnios, changes in thyroid function, premature delivery, large–for–gestational age infant, and floppy infant syndrome.[61,186] There may also be a small increase in congenital cardiac malformations.[187] Several studies have reported an increased prevalence of Ebstein's anomaly, though this was not confirmed in a prospective, multicenter study.[188] The risk ratio for cardiac malformations is approximately 1.2 to 7.7, and the overall risk ratio for congenital malformations 1.5 to 3.[189] Fetal echocardiography is recommended in women exposed to *lithium* during the first trimester.[190]

BREAST-FEEDING CONSIDERATIONS

Lithium is excreted into human milk, and detectable levels can be measured in the nursing newborn.[191] Whether nursing mothers should continue *lithium* therapy while breast-feeding is controversial.[192] The neonatal clearance rate is slower than in the adult, and the circulating level may be higher than expected. If *lithium* must be continued during breast-feeding, neonatal levels should be measured if any apparent adverse effects are noted.[193]

Prostaglandins (Misoprostol [Cytotec])

MATERNAL CONSIDERATIONS

Misoprostol is a prostaglandin E_1 analogue. Though approved by the FDA only for the treatment and prevention of intestinal ulcer disease secondary to NSAID use, there is compelling evidence that *misoprostol* is effective in ripening the cervix and inducing labor during either the second or the third trimester.[194,195] Combined with *mifepristone*, *misoprostol* provides for safe and effective medical termination during early pregnancy.[196] In August 2000, the manufacturer (Pfizer) issued a warning letter to American health care providers on the appropriate use of *misoprostol*. In that letter, the manufacturer cautioned against the use of *misoprostol* during pregnancy because of a perceived lack of safety data for use in obstetric practice. In 2003, the ACOG Committee Opinion on Obstetric Practice[197] concluded that the risk of uterine rupture during vaginal birth after cesarean section is substantially increased by the use of *misoprostol* as well as other prostaglandin cervical-ripening agents. In 2003, ACOG issued specific recommendations in regard to the use of *misoprostol* for labor induction[197]:

- If *misoprostol* is used for cervical ripening or labor induction in the third trimester, 25 μg should be considered for the first dose.
- Higher doses (50 μg q6h) can be used in some situations. Uterine tachysystole and uterine hyperstimulation and meconium staining of amniotic fluid are recognized complications.
- *Misoprostol* should not be given more frequently than every 3 to 6 hours.
- *Oxytocin* should not be administered sooner than 4 hours after the last *misoprostol* dose.
- Fetal heart rate and uterine activity should be monitored when *misoprostol* is used for labor induction in a hospital setting.
- *Misoprostol* is contraindicated in women with prior uterine scar.

FETAL CONSIDERATIONS

Misoprostol is associated with a higher rate of fetal variable decelerations and likely a higher prevalence of meconium.[198] Even though such complications occur more frequently with *misoprostol* than with *oxytocin*, there is no increase in the incidence of cesarean delivery for fetal distress or umbilical artery acidemia. Congenital defects (skull defects, cranial nerve palsies, facial malformations, limb defects) occur following unsuccessful first-trimester medical termination.[153]

BREAST-FEEDING CONSIDERATIONS

Misoprostol is secreted in the breast milk. The levels rise and then decline rapidly, becoming essentially undetectable by 5 hours, significantly lowering infant exposure.[199]

Oral Contraceptives

MATERNAL CONSIDERATIONS

Numerous studies have confirmed the relative safety and effectiveness of hormonal contraceptives in healthy women. The data are far less robust for women with underlying medical problems.[200] Decisions regarding contraception, especially for women with medical problems, may be complicated. Age, tobacco use, hypertension, diabetes, dyslipidemia, and migraine headaches are important risk factors to consider before recommending any form of hormonal contraception. In some cases, medications taken for certain chronic conditions might alter the effectiveness of hormonal contraception, and pregnancy in these cases might pose substantial risks to the mother and her fetus. For details, the reader is referred to the most recent ACOG Practice Bulletin—2006, where this topic is extensively reviewed.[200] Although there are many anecdotal reports of oral contraceptive failure in women taking concomitant antibiotics, pharmacokinetic evidence of lower serum steroid levels exists only for *rifampin*.[201] In addition, although several studies demonstrate reduced serum levels of contraceptive steroids in women treated with anticonvulsants, investigators have not been able to demonstrate an excess of ovulation cycles or accidental pregnancy during anticonvulsant use.[200] However, there is a higher risk of oral contraceptive failure in obese women. This does not preclude their use in overweight women motivated to use these methods in preference to other less effective techniques.[200]

FETAL CONSIDERATIONS

About 1% of pregnant women unknowingly use oral contraceptives during the first part of their pregnancy and expose their fetus to estrogens. However, exposure to specific estrogens or progestogens seems unrelated to the prevalence of malformations. A causal relationship was reported between a syndrome of multiple congenital anomalies (vertebral abnormalities, anal atresia, cardiac abnormalities, tracheo-esophageal fistula and/or esophageal atresia, renal agenesis and dysplasia, and limb defects [VACTERL]) and maternal progesterone/estrogen exposure.[202] However, this link remains weak and may more reflective of other simultaneous exposures. For example, the likelihood of delivering a malformed infant to a woman who used an oral contraceptive at the beginning of pregnancy is increased by concomitant tobacco use.[203] One study concluded that early, high-dose in utero exposure to *medroxyprogesterone* may affect fetal growth.[204] Others notes that *medroxyprogesterone* does not have a measurable teratogenic risk, especially for congenital heart disease and limb reduction defects.[205] Several studies addressed the issue related to fetal exposure to *levonorgestrel* in women who seek emergency contraception. It appears neither the woman nor the fetus will be harmed if hormonal emergency contraception is inadvertently used in early pregnancy.

BREAST-FEEDING CONSIDERATIONS

Women remain in a hypercoagulable state during the puerperium. Product labeling for combination oral contraceptives recommends they not be used until 4 weeks postpartum, and then only in non–breast-feeding women. Because progestin-only oral contraceptives and *depomedroxyprogesterone acetate* do not contain estrogen, these methods may be started safely immediately postpartum.

Retinoids (Isotretinoin [Accutane])

MATERNAL CONSIDERATIONS

Isotretinoin is contraindicated during pregnancy. Before prescribing, physicians must assure themselves that the woman is capable of complying with mandatory contraceptive measures. Two reliable forms of birth control must be used at the same time (unless abstinence is the chosen method) for 1 month before, during, and for at least 1 month after concluding treatment with *isotretinoin*. The most recent, and most stringent, system aimed to avoid exposure to *isotretinoin* is an Internet-based, performance-linked system called iPLEDGE (http://www.fda.gov/cder/drug/infopage/accutane/iPLEDGEupdate).[206] Only manufacturer-approved physicians may prescribe it.[207]

FETAL CONSIDERATIONS

Isotretinoin and its active metabolites cross the human placenta. *Isotretinoin* is one of the strongest human teratogens known today. The prevalence of birth defects after exposure during embryogenesis is estimated to be as high as 30%.[208] Multiple organ systems are affected, including CNS, cardiovascular, and endocrine organs, and the damage can be severe.[209] Mental retardation without malformation has also been reported.

BREAST-FEEDING CONSIDERATIONS

It is unknown whether *isotretinoin* is excreted into human breast milk. Considering its potential adverse impact on the fetus, breast-feeding is contraindicated.

Iodine 131

MATERNAL CONSIDERATIONS

Radioactive iodine (sodium iodide 131) is a cost-effective, safe, and reliable treatment for hyperthyroidism in nonpregnant women.[210] However, radioactive iodine is contraindicated during pregnancy. Although all of the ^{131}I is excreted within 1 month, the current recommendation is that women avoid pregnancy for 4 to 6 months after treatment.[160]

FETAL CONSIDERATIONS

There are no adequate reports or well-controlled studies in human fetuses. Treatment during pregnancy after the first trimester can result in fetal thyroid destruction.[211] Fetal thyroid damage may be ameliorated by treating the mother as soon as the pregnancy is diagnosed with large doses of solution of potassium iodide (SKI) to dilute the effect of the I^{131}.

BREAST-FEEDING CONSIDERATIONS

Breast-feeding should be avoided for at least 120 days after ^{131}I treatment.[212]

Dermatologics; Immunomodulators (Thalidomide [Thalomid])

MATERNAL CONSIDERATIONS

Thalidomide is a known human teratogen and contraindicated during pregnancy.[213] After normal reproductive studies in rodents, *thalidomide* was prescribed to treat morning sickness in Canada and Europe during the early 1960s. Reports of defects followed and *thalidomide* was banned from the market. In 1998, the FDA approved *thalidomide* for use in treating erythema nodosum leprosum. Its potential indications (Behçet's disease, lupus erythematous, Sjögren's syndrome, rheumatoid arthritis, AIDS, inflammatory bowel disease, cancer) are growing, increasing the likelihood of an inadvertent pregnancy.[214–216] *Thalidomide* is excreted in the semen of treated males, necessitating the use of a condom during coitus.[217]

FETAL CONSIDERATIONS

Thalidomide crosses the human placenta and is a potent human teratogen, causing limb abnormalities after first-trimester exposure. A common effect of *thalidomide* is either duplication (preaxial polydactyly of hands and feet) or deficiency (absence of thumbs).[218] No other human teratogen identified to date has this effect on the developing limb. If pregnancy occurs, the drug should be discontinued and the patient referred to a fetal medicine expert for evaluation and counseling. In the United States, any suspected fetal exposure to *thalidomide* must be reported to the FDA, which is controlling *thalidomide's* marketing in the United States via the System for Thalidomide Education and Prescribing Safety (S.T.E.P.S.) Program. This mandatory registry includes authorized patients, prescribers, and pharmacies, offers extensive patient education regarding *thalidomide's* safety, and is designed to prevent fetal exposure (see http://www.fda.gov/cder/Offices/OODP/whatsnew/thalidomide.htm).

BREAST-FEEDING CONSIDERATIONS

There is no published experience with *thalidomide* in breast-feeding women. It is unknown whether *thalidomide* is excreted into human breast milk.

DRUGS WITH MINIMAL OR NO KNOWN HUMAN TERATOGENIC EFFECT (see Table 34-3)

Analgesics (Aspirin, Acetaminophen [Tylenol, Apacet], Ibuprofen [Advil, Alaxan, Brofen, Motrin, Paduden])

MATERNAL CONSIDERATIONS

Our understanding of the action of *aspirin* remains incomplete. Considerable individual variation in the pharmacokinetics of *aspirin* in both nonpregnant and pregnant women increases the task. It is believed that the cyclooxygenase-1 (COX-1) and COX-2 pathways are most frequently involved.[219] Gastrointestinal lesions, renal or hepatic dysfunction, asthma, hypoprothrombinemia, tachypnea, hyperthermia, and lethargy are the most significant risks associated with *aspirin* use.[220] A large cohort study concluded the antenatal use of NSAIDs such as *ibuprofen*, *naproxen*, and *aspirin* but not *acetaminophen* increased the risk of spontaneous abortion.[221] *Aspirin* treatment after the first trimester may provide a small but significant reduction in the rate of preterm birth but not perinatal death.[222]

Aspirin is used to improve pregnancy outcomes in women who have both antiphospholipid antibodies *and* a history of recurrent pregnancy loss. At the base of this practice is an assumption that *aspirin* interferes with the ability of antiphospholipid antibodies to compromise implantation and placental angiogenesis.[223,224] *Aspirin* is also frequently prescribed to reduce the risk of maternal thrombosis. However, *aspirin* alone is not sufficient to prevent thrombosis. Further, this medication is not risk-free. *Aspirin* may increase the risk of fetal malformation and contribute to maternal bleeding due to its effect on platelet COX enzymes. Many clinicians do not recommend its use in the third trimester.

The optimal approach for women with obstetric manifestations of antiphospholipid syndrome is uncertain. *Aspirin* plus *heparin* remains the most effective treatment[225] for women with a history of at least two spontaneous miscarriages or one intrauterine fetal death without apparent cause other than inherited or acquired thrombophilia.[226] Perhaps one explanation for the lack of consensus regarding management reflects the wide range of clinical manifestations. Yet, in a 2002 randomized, controlled trial of *aspirin* alone versus low-dose *aspirin* plus low-molecular-weight *heparin* prophylaxis for the prevention of recurrent pregnancy loss associated with antiphospholipid syndrome and recurrent miscarriage, low-molecular-weight *heparin* did not improve the outcome achieved with low-dose *aspirin* alone.[227]

The benefit of low-dose *aspirin* for the prevention of preeclampsia also remains controversial.[228,229] The most recent meta-analysis available at this writing indicates that antiplatelet agents produce a moderate but consistent reduction in the relative risk of preeclampsia.[230]

Collectively, large trials demonstrate low-dose *aspirin's* relative safety during pregnancy (especially after the first trimester) and generally positive effects on reproductive outcomes.

Acetaminophen is a component of a long list of over-the-counter medications and is one of the most widely used medications during pregnancy. The most common maternal problems relate to overdose and chronic abuse. The tissue damage is thought to be secondary to free radical toxicity with the consumption of glutathione during the *acetaminophen* metabolism. *N-Acetylcysteine* is the treatment of choice for an acute overdose.[231] *Ibuprofen* remains the drug of choice for management of postabortal pain and acute postoperative and postpartum pain.[232,233]

FETAL CONSIDERATIONS

Aspirin crosses the human placenta,[234] and its use is associated with an increased risk of fetal vascular disruptions, particularly gastroschisis, small intestinal atresia, and possibly premature closure of the ductus arteriosus.[17,223,235] It should be avoided in the first trimester.

Use of *acetaminophen* to treat the fever of chorioamnionitis during labor is associated with improved umbilical blood gases (improvements in the umbilical cord bicarbonate concentration and base deficit)[236] apparently by reducing fetal oxygen demand as the maternal core temperature declines. A prior suggestion that first-trimester exposure to *acetaminophen* in combination with *propoxyphene* is associated with clubfoot and digital abnormalities was not sustained by large series.[237] However, there is a link between *acetaminophen*, gastroschisis, and small bowel atresia. One recent study concluded that genetic variation represents a risk factor for the development of gastroschisis in the offspring of mothers exposed to *acetaminophen* early in pregnancy.[238] Unlike *aspirin*, *acetaminophen* has no antiplatelet activity and does not pose a hemorrhagic risk to the fetus.[239]

Ibuprofen crosses the human placenta. Fetal levels are dependent on maternal excretion since NSAIDs are not efficiently metabolized by the fetal kidney. *Ibuprofen* is as effective as *indomethacin* in closing the ductus arteriosus, but may have less impact on fetal renal function.[240] Thus, chronic exposure of the fetus to *ibuprofen* requires fetal surveillance for evidence of fetal right heart decompensation following critical constriction of the ductus arteriosus.

BREAST-FEEDING CONSIDERATIONS

Low-dose *aspirin*, *acetaminophen*, and *ibuprofen* are considered compatible with breast-feeding.[241–243] Patients often question the safety of cough and cold preparations during breast-feeding.[244] Some experts suggest that breast-feeding mothers use the lowest effective dose and for the shortest duration taken after a feeding. Women requiring high doses of *aspirin* such as that used for arthritis or rheumatic fever should avoid breast-feeding because neonatal salicylate levels may reach toxic levels.

Antibiotics (Penicillin G, Tetracycline [Achromycin, Telmycin, Tetocy, Tetracap], Ciprofloxacin [Ciloxan, Cipro], Metronidazole [Flagyl], Nitrofurantoin [Furadantin, Furatoin, Macrodantin, Macrobid], Azithromycin [Aruzilina, Zithromax])

MATERNAL CONSIDERATIONS

Penicillin and its derivatives (ampicillin, cephalosporins) are considered safe during pregnancy.[245–248]

Tetracycline is a broad-spectrum antibiotic avoided during pregnancy for fetal considerations.[249] *Tetracyclines* are alternative treatment for gonorrhea, syphilis, *Listeria monocytogenes*, *Clostridium* species, *Bacillus anthracis*, *Fusobacterium fusiforme* (Vincent's infection), and *Actinomyces* species.

Ciprofloxacin is a bactericidal antibiotic belonging to the fluoroquinolone group. It is recommended when penicillin-class agents have no effect on gram-negative rods (e.g., gonorrhea). It has the best safety profile of any second-line drugs for drug-resistant tuberculosis.[250] *Ciprofloxacin* is the drug of choice for prophylaxis among asymptomatic pregnant women exposed to *B. anthracis* and for the treatment of Q fever during pregnancy.[251,252] Because the prevalence of fluoroquinolone-resistant gonorrhea is growing, the U.S. Centers for Disease Control and Prevention (CDC) no longer recommends fluoroquinolones as first-line therapy (http://www.cdc.gov/std/treatment/2006/updated-regimens.htm). When penicillins and fluoroquinolones are contraindicated, *erythromycin* (a tetracycline-class agent without the fetal sequelae) is an alternative for the treatment of gonorrhea and syphilis.[253,254] A test for cure is indicated in both adolescents and pregnant women.[255]

Metronidazole is widely used during pregnancy for such indications as bacterial vaginosis (BV), trichomoniasis, inflammatory bowel disease, *Clostridium difficile* colitis, and anaerobic and protozoal infections.[256,257] Several large randomized trials to determine whether the treatment of BV reduced the prevalence of adverse outcomes, such as preterm birth,[258–261] had mixed results. Treatment has no effect on the prevalence of preterm birth in women with asymptomatic BV but no prior preterm birth.[262] Women who experienced a prior preterm birth in association with symptomatic BV appear to have a lower risk of recurrent preterm birth if treated with *clindamycin* and *erythromycin*, but not *metronidazole*.[263] Similarly, *metronidazole* failed to prevent preterm birth in women with asymptomatic trichomoniasis.[264] One major concern is the observation that in most randomized trials, *metronidazole* was actually associated with an increased rate of preterm birth.[260,265] The absence of benefit coupled with a potentially serious complication indicates that *metronidazole* should be avoided in preterm women unless there is no option. High risk conditions that require the treatment of BV with oral *clindamycin* and *erythromycin* include women with prior preterm birth associated with symptomatic cervicitis, those with a body mass index (BMI) less than 19.8 kg/m^2, and those with evidence of endometritis before pregnancy. A test of cure is obtained 1 month later.[266]

Nitrofurantoin is safe and effective for the treatment of asymptomatic bacteriuria as well as acute and recurrent urinary tract infections. Resistance rates are less than 10%. Women with recurrent urinary tract infections are candidates for long-term antibiotic prophylaxis. Acute pulmonary reactions to *nitrofurantoin*, presumably immune-mediated, are uncommon but potentially life-threatening. Patients with glucose-6-phosphate dehydrogenase (G-6-PD) deficiency may experience hemolytic reactions. It remains unclear how long a woman with asymptomatic bacteriuria should be treated. Some suggest that short-term administration combined with continued surveillance for recurrent bacteriuria is sufficient. Pyelonephritis occurs in about 7% of women despite adequate treatment.

Azithromycin is probably the treatment of choice for *Chlamydia*. It is also used in combination with *artesunate* for malaria prophylaxis. It is ineffective for delaying preterm birth when given to reduce lower genital tract colonization with *Ureaplasma urealyticum* in women with preterm labor.

FETAL CONSIDERATIONS

Most penicillins cross the human placenta.[267,268] A large clinical experience is reassuring.[269]

Tetracycline crosses the human placenta and may cause a yellow-gray-brown discoloration of the permanent adult tooth.[270] It is unlikely that topically applied *tetracycline*, such as that used to prevent acne, achieves a relevant systemic level. Another tetracycline, *oxytetracycline* (but not *doxycycline*), is associated with an increased risk of neural tube defects, cleft palate, and cardiovascular defects. Treatment with *tetracycline* derivatives such as *doxycycline* has little, if any, teratogenic risk.[271]

Only a small number of fluoroquinolones (*ciprofloxacin*, *ofloxacin*, *levofloxacin*) are known to cross the human placenta.[272] Short-duration treatment with *ciprofloxacin* appears free of adverse fetal effect. As a class, the new quinolones (*irloxacin*, *trovafloxacin*, *sparfloxacin*) are not associated with an increased risk of malformation or musculoskeletal abnormalities in either animals or humans.[272,273] There are no clinically significant musculoskeletal problems reported in children exposed to fluoroquinolones in utero.[273,274] Because these studies include a relatively low number of children exposed during the first trimester, a longer period of follow-up coupled with magnetic resonance imaging of the joints at 1 or 2 years of age may be warranted to exclude subtle cartilage and bone damage.

Metronidazole crosses the human placenta and does not appear to have a teratogenic risk when used at recommended doses.[275]

It is unknown whether *nitrofurantoin* crosses the human placenta, but it is considered compatible with pregnancy. There are no well-documented cases of hemolytic reactions in neonates despite its use either during labor or in the neonate. It is typically avoided for that express reason.

Less than 3% of maternally administered *azithromycin* crosses the placenta. There have been no adverse effects reported in humans.

BREAST-FEEDING CONSIDERATIONS

Trace amounts of *penicillin G* are excreted into human breast milk,[276] and it is believed the infant has little exposure when the mother is treated with a *penicillin*.[277]

Tetracycline is excreted into human breast milk but is considered compatible with breast-feeding.[278]

Ciprofloxacin is concentrated in human breast milk,[279] and neonatal *C. difficile* pseudomembranous colitis is reported in neonates breast-fed by mothers treated with *ciprofloxacin*.[280] There are alternative agents with a superior safety profile.

Metronidazole is excreted into human breast milk but is considered compatible with breast-feeding.[281]

Nitrofurantoin is actively transported into human milk. However, maternal ingestion of *nitrofurantoin* is not associated with adverse neonatal events with the possible exception of a family with a G-6-PD deficiency.

Small amounts of *azithromycin* are excreted in breast milk in a dose-dependent fashion. No neonatal adverse effects have been reported.

Anticholinergics (Albuterol [Proventil, Ventolin], Atropine [Atropen, Atropinol, Atropisol, Borotropin], Dimenhydrinate [Amosyt, Biodramina, Dimetabs, Wehamine])

This class of pharmaceuticals antagonizes the actions of acetylcholine in the central and peripheral nervous systems.

Albuterol

MATERNAL CONSIDERATIONS

Albuterol has been used in the past for the control of asthma during pregnancy. There are superior agents.[282] The mean maternal blood pressures and heart rates are unaffected. In some countries, *albuterol* is used as a tocolytic agent, but there is no evidence to support this practice.

FETAL CONSIDERATIONS

Albuterol crosses the human placenta, though the detailed kinetics of transfer remains to be elucidated. Less than 10% is absorbed when administered by inhalation. There is no convincing evidence of teratogenicity after first-trimester exposure, and long-term follow-up studies of infants exposed to betamimetic tocolytic agents in general are reassuring.

BREAST-FEEDING CONSIDERATIONS

It is unknown whether *albuterol* enters human breast milk, but it is considered compatible with breast-feeding.

Atropine

MATERNAL CONSIDERATIONS

There are no adequate reports or well-controlled studies of *atropine* use in pregnant women. It is used for the treatment of symptomatic bradycardia and organophosphate poisoning or as an adjunct to anesthesia.

FETAL CONSIDERATIONS

Atropine rapidly crosses the human placenta, and the tachycardic fetus will respond to the direct administration of *atropine*.

BREAST-FEEDING CONSIDERATIONS

It is unknown whether *atropine* is excreted into human breast milk.

Dimenhydrinate

MATERNAL CONSIDERATIONS

Dimenhydrinate is a popular agent for the relief of nausea and vomiting during pregnancy. A recent randomized trial concluded that ginger is as effective as *dimenhydrinate* for the treatment of hyperemesis gravidarum and has fewer side effects.[283] Both *dimenhydrinate* and *diphenhydramine* are treatment options for severe migraine headache during pregnancy.[284] Some caution is warranted, however, because several investigators have noted an increase in uterine activity with *dimenhydrinate*.[285]

FETAL CONSIDERATIONS

It is unknown whether *dimenhydrinate* crosses the human placenta. There is no indication that *dimenhydrinate* increases the risk of fetal abnormalities when given at any stage of pregnancy.

BREAST-FEEDING CONSIDERATIONS

Dimenhydrinate is excreted in small quantities into human breast milk. In addition, though the kinetics remains to be elucidated, a long clinical experience is reassuring.

Antihypertensives (Methyldopa [Aldomet, Alfametildopa], Hydralazine [Apresoline], Labetolol [Coreton, Normodyne, Trandate], Propranolol [Inderal])

MATERNAL CONSIDERATIONS

Approximately 3% of the women take an antihypertensive agent during pregnancy.[286] ACOG recommends the treatment of women with a systolic blood pressure higher than 170 mm Hg and/or a diastolic blood pressure above 109 mm Hg. There is no consensus whether lesser degrees of hypertension require treatment during pregnancy because antihypertensive therapy does not improve the fetal outcome in women with mild to moderate chronic hypertension.[287] Not treating requires the assumption that untreated mild to moderate hypertension in the short term has no lasting effect on the mother.

Methyldopa is one of the best-studied antihypertensives during pregnancy and remains a popular agent for the treatment of moderate to mild hypertension despite it being a particularly effective agent.[288,289] *Methyldopa* acts through the sympathetic nervous system (both centrally and peripherally) via an α_2-receptor negative feedback mechanism. Oral *methyldopa* requires 48 to 72 hours to act. *Methyldopa* is less effective than *metoprolol*, but is similar to *nifedipine*, *labetalol*, and *ketanserin* in decreasing both systolic and diastolic blood pressure in women with chronic hypertension in whom speed of control is not critical.[290]

Hydralazine and *labetolol* are the most widely used drugs for the treatment of acute hypertension during pregnancy.[291] The mechanism of action for *hydralazine* is poorly understood. It is thought that *hydralazine* works through a cyclic guanosine monophosphate–mediated mechanism, resulting in smooth muscle relaxation. In two recent randomized trials, *hydralazine* was as safe and as effective as *diazoxide* and *labetalol* for the treatment of hypertensive emergencies during the antenatal and in the postpartum periods.[292,293]

Labetalol combines α- and β-adrenoceptor antagonist properties. Despite its popularity, *labetalol* is associated with a higher risk of hypotension and cesarean section than *diazoxide* when given intravenously.[294]

Propranolol has been used extensively during pregnancy for the treatment of maternal hypertension, arrhythmia, and migraine headache and is generally considered safe unless the dose given decreases maternal cardiac output.[295] It is also used to provide symptomatic relief of symptoms from thyrotoxicosis and pheochromocytoma.[296,297] Although the studies of *propranolol* use for hypertension are small, it appears as effective as *methyldopa* and is often coupled with other hypotensive agents such as *hydralazine* with which its actions are synergistic.[298]

FETAL CONSIDERATIONS

Most antihypertensive agents cross the placenta. *Methyldopa* is considered safe for use during the first trimester.[299] It neither alters fetal cardiac activity nor produces fetal hemodynamic changes as measured by Doppler velocimetry.[300] The effects of various antihypertensive medications on fetoplacental circulation were studied in vitro.[301] *Hydralazine*, *nifedepine*, and *methyldopa* had little or no direct effect on the fetal vasculature in contrast to *labetalol*, which was a vasodilator.

Clinical experience suggests *hydralazine* is safe during the first trimester. Large doses of *labetalol* given intravenously can cause fetal bradycardia, hypoglycemia, bradycardia, hypotension, pericardial effusion, myocardial hypertrophy, and fetal death due to acute hypotension.[302,303] Based on these risks, an initial intravenous dose of 5 to 10 mg is recommended. Similar responses are unlikely with oral therapy. Overall, neonatal outcome is similar to that achieved with *hydralazine*.[304] Simultaneous occurrence of maternal and fetal thyrotoxicosis is not rare, and in this instance, *labetalol* may be useful for symptomatic treatment of the thyrotoxicosis.[305]

BREAST-FEEDING CONSIDERATIONS

Although most antihypertensive medications (*methyldopa*, *hydralazine*, *labetolol*, *propranolol*) are excreted into human breast milk, breast-fed neonates are normotensive.[306] *Labetalol* increases the risk of neonatal hypoglycemia, but this effect is blunted by supplementing with glucose-fortified formula.[307]

Antihistamines (Cetirizine [Zyrtec], Diphenhydramine [Benadryl])

MATERNAL CONSIDERATIONS

Despite a long clinical experience in obstetrics, neither *cetirizine* nor *diphenhydramine* has been adequately studied during human pregnancy. Allergic rhinitis is the most common indication for *cetirizine* during pregnancy. The advantage of *cetirizine* over many other antihistamines is that it does not cause clinically significant cardiac QT interval prolongation.[308] The product label frequently states that medications for allergic rhinitis are to be avoided during pregnancy owing to lack of fetal safety. The human data refute this position.

Diphenhydramine is a useful adjunct for women who have allergic reactions to local anesthetic agents, laminaria, and serum albumin or for the treatment of severe migraine headaches.[309,310]

FETAL CONSIDERATIONS

It is unknown whether *cetirizine* crosses the human placenta. *Cetirizine* is not incriminated as a human teratogen. *Diphenhydramine* crosses the human placenta, but the detailed kinetics remains to be elucidated. There is no evidence of increased fetal risk when administered at any stage of pregnancy. *Diphenhydramine* may cause neonatal depression if administered during labor.[311]

BREAST-FEEDING CONSIDERATIONS

Cetirizine is excreted into human breast milk. It is unknown whether *diphenhydramine* does so. Irritability is the most common adverse reaction reported in the newborns of women using antihistamines while breast-feeding.

Antivirals (Acyclovir)

MATERNAL CONSIDERATIONS

All suspected herpesvirus infections should be confirmed by viral or serologic testing.[312] Treatment of genital herpes with *acyclovir* during pregnancy is not curative but does reduce the duration of symptoms and viral shedding.[313] Extensive clinical experience with *acyclovir* is reassuring. Based on several studies, ACOG recommends prophylactic *acyclovir* from 36 weeks until delivery to reduce the risks of recurrent genital herpes and thus potentially avoid cesarean delivery.[314] Suppression therapy is both effective and cost-effective whether or not the primary infection occurs during the current pregnancy.

FETAL CONSIDERATIONS

Acyclovir crosses the human placenta and is concentrated in the amniotic fluid. However, there is no evidence of preferential drug accumulation in the fetus.[315] Long-term follow-up studies have not revealed any increase or pattern of malformations after first-trimester exposure.[316]

BREAST-FEEDING CONSIDERATIONS

Acyclovir is excreted into human breast milk, reaching a milk concentration higher than maternal serum.[317] It is considered safe with breast-feeding.

Corticosteroids (Prednisone [Cortan, Dacortin], Betamethasone [Celestone], Dexamethasone [Decadron])

MATERNAL CONSIDERATIONS

There are no adequate well-controlled studies of *prednisone* use during pregnancy. The authors of several trials conclude that women with antiphospholipid syndrome treated with *prednisone* and *aspirin* have higher loss rates than women treated with *heparin* and *aspirin*.[318]

Betamethasone and *dexamethasone* are used routinely to accelerate fetal lung maturation. Their administration is standard of care in women with threatened preterm birth.[319,320] A recent multicenter, randomized, double-blind, placebo-controlled trial demonstrated that the administration of a single "rescue course" of corticosteroids before 33 weeks improves neonatal outcome without apparent increased short-term risk.[321]

Corticosteroids may increase the risk of maternal infection in women with preterm premature rupture of the fetal membranes, though most large studies reveal no such increased risk.[322] They can transiently cause an abnormal glucose tolerance test,[323] worsen existing diabetes mellitus, and are associated with pulmonary edema when given with a tocolytic agent in the setting of an underlying infection.[324] Repeat doses of corticosteroids do not reduce the maternal perception of fetal movement.[325,326]

Dexamethasone is an effective postoperative antiemetic following general anesthesia for pregnancy termination.[327] There are reports that intravenous *dexamethasone* modifies the clinical course of the HELLP (hemolysis, elevated liver enzymes, and low platelets) syndrome during both the antenatal and the postpartum periods,[328] though a more recent study contradicts that conclusion.[329]

FETAL CONSIDERATIONS

The human placenta metabolizes *prednisone*, reducing fetal exposure to less than 10% of the maternal level.[330] Evidence that corticosteroids are human teratogens is weak and confined to cleft lip.[331–334] *Betamethasone* and *dexamethasone* cross the human placenta and are two of the few drugs proven to enhance perinatal outcome after preterm birth.[335] An increased risk of neonatal sepsis has been suggested but remains unconfirmed despite large prospective trials with thousands of deliveries. Multiple courses of glucocorticoids for fetal lung maturation are not recommended.[336] Adverse effects noted in animal and/or human studies include profound suppression of fetal breathing and movement (altering the biophysical profile score), impaired myelination, intrauterine growth restriction, and microcephaly.[337,338] The fetal heart rate pattern may also become transiently nonreactive.[339] There is controversy as to the earliest gestational age at which corticosteroids effective.[340] The National Institute of Child Health and Human Development and the Office of Medical Applications of Research of the National Institutes of Health recommend a single course of glucocorticoid to all pregnant women between 24 and 34 weeks' gestation at risk for preterm delivery within 7 days.[341] Repeat corticosteroid courses should not be used routinely. Recently, it was demonstrated that repeat courses of corticosteroid were accompanied by a reduction in birth weight and an increase in the prevalence of small–for–gestational age infants.[326] Some studies suggest that *betamethasone* can alter fetal breathing when administered for the enhancement of lung maturation.[342] Apparently, this does not occur with *dexamethasone*.[325] Complete fetal heart block has been treated successfully with *dexamethasone*.[343] *Dexamethasone* can prevent or diminish virilization due to congenital adrenal hyperplasia if administered early during the first trimester.[344,345]

BREAST-FEEDING CONSIDERATIONS

Although it is unknown whether *prednisone* is excreted into human breast milk, a long clinical experience suggests that this drug is safe during breast-feeding. It is still unclear whether maternal treatment with *betamethasone* or *dexamethasone* increases the concentration of cortisone in breast milk.

Infliximab (Remicade)

MATERNAL CONSIDERATIONS

Infliximab is a monoclonal antibody that specifically binds to tumor necrosis factor-α (TNF-α), blocking its activity. Given the evidence that TNF-α is involved in the pathogenesis of many conditions with an inflammatory component, *infliximab* has been used for treatment of psoriasis, inflammatory bowel disease, spondylarthropathies, rheumatoid arthritis, and juvenile idiopathic arthritis.[346–348] There are only limited data on the use of *infliximab* during pregnancy. Most studies examining the effects of *infliximab* on pregnancy in women with inflammatory bowel disease are confounded by the fact that most of these patients are on multiple medications and have varying levels of disease activity.[349] There is consensus that women on remission therapy can continue their *inflixumab*, given that the disease may flare if the therapy is stopped.

FETAL CONSIDERATIONS

Most of the available data suggest that the benefits of achieving and maintaining remission in mothers with Crohn's disease using *infliximab* outweigh the potential fetal risk.[350] To date, there is no evidence that TNF-α antagonists are associated with embryotoxicity, teratogenicity, or increased pregnancy loss.[351] However, caution continues to be advised because human experience is still extremely limited.

BREAST-FEEDING CONSIDERATIONS

Studies monitoring the level of *infliximab* in human breast milk suggest that targeted monoclonal antibodies and other biologic agents can be used with caution in breast-feeding patients.[352] *Infliximab* is considered compatible with breast-feeding.

CONCLUSIONS

- The decision to prescribe a medication to a pregnant woman must take into consideration many factors such as the risk of teratogenicity, previous experience with that medication, gestational age, route of drug administration, and whether or not the drug crosses the placenta or is excreted into breast milk.
- Comprehensive information on currently prescribed drugs with unknown teratogenicity or classified as nonteratogenic is essential for physicians recommending drug treatment for pregnant and breast-feeding women.
- Up-to-date information about the effect of exposure to a large number of medications during pregnancy can be obtained from textbooks or in electronic format through consultation of pregnancy exposure registries and several databases such as REPROTOX, OTIS, or ENTIS.

SUMMARY OF MANAGEMENT OPTIONS

Medication during Pregnancy

Management Options	Evidence Quality and Recommendation	References
Preconceptual counseling can minimize the risk for the mother and her fetus.	GPP	
During first prenatal visit, obtain a thorough medical, allergy, and drug medication history of the mother.	GPP	
Recommend first-trimester ultrasound surveillance of the fetus for early detection of fetal anomalies.	GPP	
Counseling of the patients should include the background risk for fetal anomalies.	GPP	
Team approach for care of pregnant women with medical conditions is the best strategy.	GPP	
Be aware of known teratogens.	GPP	
Provide the best counseling and treatment recommendations by consulting a text or a continuously updated database such as ReproTOX, OTIS, or ENTIS.	GPP	
Advise that for most drug medications, there are no adequate reports or well-controlled studies in human fetuses.	GPP	
In general, monotherapy with the lowest effective dosage is recommended.	GPP	
Medication should be used during pregnancy and lactation only if the benefit justifies the potential risk.	GPP	
Recommend medications with known safety records rather than new or untested drugs.	GPP	
Human Teratogens (See Table 34–2)		
Agents Acting on the Renin-Angiotensin System		
Enalapril	III/B	56
Antidepressant		
Paroxetine	IV/C	60,62,69–72
Antiepileptic Drugs		
Valproic acid	III/B	89
Carbamazepine	III/B	97
Phenytoin	III/B	100,101
Anxiolytic		
Diazepam	IIa/B	120
Alkylating Agent		
Cyclophosphamide	III/B	127–129
Antimetabolite		
Methotrexate	IV/C	153,154
Antithyroid		
Methimazole	III/B	167
Anticoagulant		
Warfarin	III/B	181
Antipsychotic		
Lithium	IIb/B	190

Management Options	Evidence Quality and Recommendation	References
Retinoid		
Isotretinoin	III/B	210
Dermatologic; Immunomodulator		
Thalidomide	III/B	215
Drugs with Minimal or Not Known Human Teratogenic Effect (See Table 34-3)		
Analgesic		
Aspirin	Ib/A	229
Antibiotics		
Penicillin G	Ib/A	250
Tetracycline	IIa/B	272
Antiviral		
Acyclovir	Ib/A	315
Corticosteroid		
Betamethasone	Ib/A	323
Tumor Necrosis Factor Modulator		
Infliximab	III/B	352

GPP, good practice point.

SUGGESTED READINGS

Bleyer WA, Breckenridge RT: Studies on the detection of adverse drug reactions in the newborn. II. The effects of prenatal aspirin on newborn hemostasis. JAMA 1970;213:2049–2053.

Clayton-Smith J, Donnai D: Human malformations. In Rimoin DL, Connor JM, Pyeritz RE (eds): Emery and Rimoin's Principles and Practice of Medical Genetics, 3rd ed. New York, Churchill Livingstone, 1996, p 383.

Einarson A, Pistelli A, DeSantis M, et al: Evaluation of the risk of congenital cardiovascular defects associated with use of paroxetine during pregnancy. Am J Psychiatry 2008;165:749–752.

Holmes LB: Teratogen-induced limb defects. Am J Med Genet 2002;112:297–303.

Marks PW: Management of thromboembolism in pregnancy. Semin Perinatol 2007;31:227–231.

Matheson I, Samseth M, Sande HA: Ampicillin in breast milk during puerperal infections. Eur J Clin Pharmacol 1988;34:657–659.

Slone D, Shapiro S, Miettinen O: Case-control surveillance of serious illnesses attributable to ambulatory drug use. In Colombo F, Shapiro S, Slone D, Tognoni G (eds): Epidemiological Evaluation of Drugs. Amsterdam, Elsevier-North Holland Biomedical, 1977, pp 59–70.

Spinillo A, Viazzo F, Colleoni R, et al: Two-year infant neurodevelopmental outcome after single or multiple antenatal courses of corticosteroids to prevent complications of prematurity. Am J Obstet Gynecol 2004;191:217–224.

Teixeira NA, Lopes RC, Secoli SR: Developmental toxicity of lithium treatment at prophylactic levels. Braz J Med Biol Res 1995;28:230–239.

REFERENCES

For a complete list of references, log onto www.expertconsult.com.

CHAPTER 35

Hypertension

GUSTAAF DEKKER

Videos corresponding to this chapter are available online at www.expertconsult.com.

INTRODUCTION

Some form of hypertension occurs in approximately 15% to 20% of pregnancies. According to the World Health Organization, hypertensive disease during pregnancy is a major cause of perinatal mortality and morbidity. However, in developed countries, nonproteinuric hypertension arising late in pregnancy is associated neither with any increase in perinatal mortality or morbidity nor with a decreased birth weight. In this chapter, these cases are designated *gestational hypertension*. It appears that an increase in blood pressure (BP) is in some way an adaptive phenomenon of intrinsic survival value that, in some women, breaks down, converting a physiologic process into one of pathology, that is, preeclampsia.[1–3] Preeclampsia, occurring in 3% to 8% of pregnancies, is a major cause (15%–20%) of maternal mortality (in developed countries) and of (often iatrogenic) preterm birth, intrauterine growth restriction (IUGR), and perinatal mortality. The main maternal and fetal risks are listed in Table 35–1.[1]

DEFINITION, CLASSIFICATION, AND RISK

Classification schemes of hypertensive disorders can overemphasize the importance of hypertension in the pathophysiology so that patients with other signs of preeclampsia but without an increase in BP may be mismanaged. Historically, a range of definitions has served to confuse clinicians and researchers as to the most appropriate definition to use.[4] More recent classifications are more closely aligned.

Definition of Hypertension

BP changes throughout normal pregnancy, with a fall in the first and second trimesters and a rise toward term to levels similar to those in the nonpregnant level. The concept of hypertension is artificial, with an arbitrary threshold used to divide a continuously distributed variable into two artifactual categories of "normotension" and "hypertension." The conventional dividing line is 140/90 mm Hg. Any definition of hypertension is inevitably arbitrary, but the use of diastolic BP of 90 mm Hg or greater throughout pregnancy as originally proposed by Nelson[5] has as advantages that (1) readings above this level are beyond 2 standard deviations in normal pregnant women[6] and (2) it corresponds with the point of inflexion of the curve relating diastolic BP to perinatal mortality with a significant increases above a diastolic BP of 85 mm Hg.[7] The criterion of a rise in BP to diagnose pregnancy-induced hypertensive disorders is usually unreliable, because a gradual increase in BP from the second to the third trimester is seen in most normotensive pregnancies.[8] Currently, the following thresholds to define "hypertension" have been accepted by most national bodies and international organizations.[9–11] Thus, ***hypertension in pregnancy*** is defined as

- Systolic BP greater than or equal to 140 mm Hg and/or
- Diastolic BP greater than or equal to 90 mm Hg (Korotkoff 5 [K5]).

These measurements should be confirmed by repeated readings over 4 to 6 hours. Where K5 is absent, K4 (muffling) should be accepted.

Severe hypertension in pregnancy is defined as

- Systolic BP greater than or equal to 170 mm Hg and/or
- Diastolic BP greater than or equal to 110 mm Hg.

This represents a level of BP above which cerebral autoregulation is overcome in normotensive individuals, with the risk of cerebral hemorrhage and hypertensive encephalopathy. It is important to acknowledge that systolic as well as diastolic hypertension increases the risk of cerebral hemorrhage.[9,10]

Classification of Hypertensive Disorders in Pregnancy

The classification adopted by the International Society for the Study of Hypertension in Pregnancy (ISSHP) reflecting both the pathophysiology of the condition and the risks and potential outcomes for both mother and baby is[9–11]

- **Gestational hypertension.**
- **Preeclampsia.**
- **Chronic hypertension**
  - Essential.
  - Secondary.
- **Preeclampsia superimposed on chronic hypertension.**

Gestational hypertension is diagnosed when there is new-onset hypertension after 20 weeks without any systemic

TABLE 35-1

Maternal and Fetal Complications in Severe Preeclampsia

Maternal Complications
Abruptio placentae (1%–4%)
Disseminated coagulopathy/HELLP syndrome (10%–20%)
Pulmonary edema/aspiration (2%–5%)
Acute renal failure (1%–5%)
Eclampsia (<1%)
Liver failure or hemorrhage (<1%)
Stroke (rare)
Death (rare)
Long-term cardiovascular morbidity

Neonatal Complications
Preterm delivery (15%–67%)
Fetal growth restriction (10%–25%)
Hypoxia-neurologic injury (<1%)
Perinatal death (1%–2%)
Long-term cardiovascular morbidity associated with low birth weight (fetal origin of adult disease)

Magnitude of risk depends on gestational age at time of diagnosis, delivery, severity of disease process, and presence of associated medical disorders.
HELLP, hemolysis, elevated liver enzymes, and low platelets.
Modified from Sibai B, Dekker G, Kupferminc M: Preeclampsia. Lancet 2005;365:785–799, with permission.

TABLE 35-2

Society for Obstetric Medicine Australia and New Zealand Definition of Preeclampsia

A clinical diagnosis of preeclampsia can be made when hypertension arises after 20 wk' gestation and is accompanied by one or more of the following:

- Renal involvement:
  - Proteinuria ≥ 300 mg/24 hr or a urine protein/creatinine ratio ≥ 30 mg/mmol
  - Serum/plasma creatinine ≥ 0.09 mmol/L or oliguria (< 500 mL/24 hr)
- Hematologic involvement
  - Thrombocytopenia
  - Disseminated intravascular coagulation
  - Hemolysis
- Liver involvement
  - Abnormal liver function (AST and/or ALT > 50 IU/L, raised bilirubin > 25 IU/L)
  - And/or severe epigastric or right upper quadrant pain.
- Neurologic involvement
  - Convulsions (eclampsia)
  - Hyperreflexia with sustained clonus
  - Severe headache (persisting, atypical)
  - Persistent visual disturbances (photopsia, scotomata, cortical blindness, retinal vasospasm)
  - Stroke
- Pulmonary edema
- IUGR and/or signs of fetal distress
- Placental abruption

ALT, alanine aminotransferase; AST, aspartate aminotransferase; IUGR, intrauterine growth restriction.
From Lowe SA, Brown MA, Dekker G, et al: Guidelines for the management of hypertensive disorders of pregnancy. Aust N Z J Obstet Gynaecol 2009;49:242–246.

features of preeclampsia and BP levels return to normal within 3 months postpartum. This diagnosis will include some women who are in the process of developing preeclampsia but do not yet have proteinuria or other manifestations. Some women initially diagnosed in this category will have BP elevation that persists beyond 12 weeks postpartum and may eventually be classified as having chronic hypertension. Gestational hypertension near term is associated with little increase in the risk of adverse pregnancy outcome. The earlier the gestation at presentation and the more severe the hypertension, the higher the likelihood that the woman with gestational hypertension will progress to develop preeclampsia or have an adverse pregnancy outcome, in particular IUGR, placental abruption, and (often iatrogenic) preterm birth.[12,13]

Preeclampsia is a pregnancy-specific syndrome characterized by variable degrees of placental dysfunction and a maternal response featuring systemic inflammation. Most consider hypertension and proteinuria to be the hallmarks of preeclampsia,[9–11] but the clinical manifestations of this syndrome are very heterogeneous.

Urinary protein excretion increases in normal pregnancy, with the upper 95% confidence limit of total protein excretion being 200 to 260 mg/24 hr and urinary albumin excretion of 29 mg/24 hr.[14,15] The gold standard for determining proteinuria remains the 24-hour urinary protein excretion. Proteinuria, as used in the classification of hypertensive disorders of pregnancy, is defined as excretion of 300 mg/24 hr or a urine protein/creatinine ratio of 30 mg/mmol, or if these methods are not available, as a concentration of 30 mg/dL (≥1+ on dipstick) or more in at least two random urine samples collected at least 4 to 6 hours apart.[1,10,11,14,15] Urinary tract infection should be excluded. Dipstick testing for proteinuria is a screening test with very high false-positive and, more important, false-negative rates.[16–18] The use of automated dipstick readers can improve false-positive and false-negative rates for the detection of proteinuria.[16,17] Dipstick testing should really be used only in scenarios in which access to more reliable methods of establishing the degree of proteinuria is absent. In all women presenting with gestational hypertension, the presence of proteinuria should be confirmed with at least a urine protein-to-creatinine ratio or, preferably, a 24-hour urine collection; for clinical screening purposes, there is a reasonable correlation between these two methods. The protein-to-creatinine ratio has not been found to be an accurate method of quantifying protein excretion and should not be used to track progression of proteinuria in preeclampsia. Centers will need to evaluate local performance of the protein-to-creatinine ratio, because performance may be influenced by the method of measuring protein.[4,16–18]

The traditional criteria to confirm a diagnosis of preeclampsia (new onset of hypertension and new onset of proteinuria after 20 wk' gestation) are appropriate to use in the majority of healthy nulliparous women. However, hypertension and/or proteinuria may be absent in 10% to 15% of women who develop the HELLP (hemolysis, elevated liver enzymes, or low platelets) syndrome[19,20] and in 38% of those who develop eclampsia.[21] In recognition that severe disease may occur in the absence of proteinuria, the Society for Obstetric Medicine Australia and New Zealand (SOMANZ) has widened these criteria to include the presence of other multisystem manifestations, whether or not proteinuria is present[10] (Table 35–2).

The ISSHP[11] has adopted the following research definition of preeclampsia: (1) de novo hypertension after 20 weeks' gestation, (2) properly documented proteinuria of greater than 300 mg/24 hr, and (3) both hypertension and proteinuria disappearing postpartum.

Severe preeclampsia is defined by the presence of

- Severe hypertension in association with proteinuria
  or
- If there is hypertension in association with severe proteinuria (≥5 g/24-hr period)[1,2,10,11]
  or
- If there is multiorgan involvement such as pulmonary edema, seizures, oliguria (<500 mL/24-hr period), thrombocytopenia (platelet count < 100,000/mm^3), abnormal liver enzymes in association with persistent epigastric or right upper quadrant pain, or persistent severe central nervous system symptoms (altered mental status, headaches, blurred vision, or blindness).[1,2,10]

The course of disease in an individual preeclamptic patient is highly unpredictable and a patient's status can evolve from apparently mild preeclampsia to fulminating severe preeclampsia in hours. It should be noted that

- Edema is not included in the diagnostic features of preeclampsia, though rapid development of generalized edema should alert the clinician to screen for preeclampsia.
- Many disorders may present with similar features to preeclampsia, such as acute fatty liver of pregnancy, hemolytic uremic syndrome, thrombotic thrombocytopenic purpura, autoimmune thrombocytopenia, severe folate deficiency, and exacerbation of systemic lupus erythematosis or cholecystitis.[19,20]
- The HELLP syndrome represents a particular presentation of severe preeclampsia.[10,19,20]
- Hyperuricemia is a common feature of preeclampsia. The degree of hyperuricemia may correlate with fetal risk,[22,23] although some studies have questioned its utility.[24,25] A rapidly rising plasma urate in a hypertensive patient can indicate herald progressive preeclampsia.

Chronic hypertension: ***Essential hypertension*** is defined by a BP of 140 mm Hg or greater systolic and/or 90 mm Hg or greater diastolic diagnosed preconception or in the first half of pregnancy without an apparent underlying cause. It may also be diagnosed in women presenting in the pregnancy on antihypertensive medications in whom no secondary cause for hypertension has been determined.[26] ***Secondary hypertension*** may be caused by renal parenchymal disease or scarring, renovascular disease, endocrine disorders, or aortic coarctation. Chronic hypertension is a strong risk factor for the development of preeclampsia.[1,10,26]

Preeclampsia superimposed on chronic hypertension is diagnosed when one or more of the features of preeclampsia develop after 20 weeks' gestation. In women with chronic renal disease, the diagnosis of superimposed preeclampsia is often difficult because preexisting proteinuria normally increases during pregnancy. In such women, sudden dramatic increases in proteinuria and hypertension should raise suspicion of preeclampsia, but the diagnosis is not secure without the development of other systemic features.

PREECLAMPSIA

Epidemiology

The frequency of preeclampsia is between 2% and 7% in healthy nulliparous women.[2,27,28] In these women, the disease is mostly mild, the onset is mostly near term or intrapartum (75% of cases), and it conveys only a negligible increased risk for adverse pregnancy outcome. By contrast, frequency and severity of the disease are substantially higher in women with multifetal gestation,[29,30] chronic hypertension,[26,31] previous preeclampsia,[31,32] pregestational diabetes mellitus,[31] and preexisting thrombophilias.[33-35] Maternal and couple-specific risk factors for preeclampsia are listed in Table 35–3. Preeclampsia is a disease of first pregnancy within a couple (primipaternity). A previous abortion (spontaneous or induced) or healthy pregnancy with the same partner is associated with a reduced risk of preeclampsia, although this protective effect is lost with a change of partner.[36-40] The risk increases in those who have limited sperm exposure with the same partner before conception.[55,56] Also, men who fathered one preeclamptic pregnancy are nearly twice as likely to father a preeclamptic pregnancy in a different woman, irrespective of whether or not she had already had a preeclamptic pregnancy.[41,54] Advances in assisted reproductive technology have also increased the risk of preeclampsia. These include women who are older than 40 years, obese with polycystic ovaries syndrome, and/or pregnant by donated gametes. In addition, many of these women will have multifetal gestations.[39,40,57] Obesity is a definite risk for preeclampsia. The worldwide increase in obesity is probably one of the main reasons for the increased frequency of preeclampsia in many developed countries with a "western" lifestyle.[36,45,46] Factors triggering or augmenting a maternal systemic inflammatory response (e.g., chronic infections and autoimmune disorders) are also known to increase the preeclampsia risk.[43,44,58,59]

TABLE 35–3
Risk Factors for Preeclampsia

Couple-related Risk Factors
Primipaternity[36-38]
Limited sperm exposure[36-39]
Pregnancies after donor insemination; oocyte donation; embryo donation[36,37,40]
Protective effect of "partner change" in case of previous preeclamptic pregnancy[36-38]
"Dangerous male partner" (paternal effects)[41]
Maternal- or Pregnancy-related Risk Factors
Extremes of maternal age[36]
Multifetal gestation[29,30]
Preeclampsia in a previous pregnancy[31,32]
Chronic hypertension and/or renal disease[26,31]
Maternal chronic inflammatory conditions (e.g., rheumatologic disease, systemic lupus erythematosus)[42]
Maternal (chronic) infections[43,44]
Maternal low birth weight[36]
Obesity and insulin resistance (with and without the polycystic ovary syndrome; the risk proportionate to BMI)[45-47]
Pregestational diabetes mellitus[31]
Preexisting thrombophilias[33-35,48-50]
Maternal susceptibility genes[51-53]
Family history of preeclampsia[54]
Smoking (reduced risk)[36]
Hydropic degeneration of the placenta[36]

BMI, body mass index.
Modified from Sibai B, Dekker G, Kupferminc M: Preeclampsia. Lancet 2005;365:785–799, with permission.

Pathogenesis

Shallow, endovascular cytotrophoblast (CTB) invasion in the spiral arteries, inappropriate endothelial cell activation, and an exaggerated inflammatory response are key features in the pathogenesis of preeclampsia.[1,58] The clinical findings of preeclampsia can manifest as a maternal syndrome (hypertension and proteinuria with or without other multisystem abnormalities) and/or as a fetal syndrome (IUGR, reduced amniotic fluid, and abnormal oxygenation).[1,58] The syndrome "preeclampsia" probably encapsulates more than one disease process. Thus, near-term preeclampsia without demonstrable fetal involvement is different from preeclampsia associated with low birth weight and preterm delivery,[28,60] and preeclampsia in nulliparous women may be different from that in women with preexisting vascular disease, multifetal gestation, diabetes mellitus, or previous preeclampsia.[1,2,10,60,61] The main pathogenetic processes demonstrated to be involved in the development of preeclampsia are discussed in the following sections.

Inflammation

Pregnancy imposes a substantial systemic inflammatory stress on all pregnant women in the second half of pregnancy. The inflammatory stimulus may arise from "debris" shed into the maternal circulation from the syncytiotrophoblast (STB), which, if excessive, may signal "danger" to the maternal innate immune system. Preeclampsia occurs when this response is increased to the point of decompensation.[58,62] These features, which are clinically apparent, form the so-called second stage of preeclampsia. The two-stage model of preeclampsia (Fig. 35–1), originally proposed more than a decade ago by Redman and coworkers,[63,64] envisages that preeclampsia arises in various ways including from placental ischemia-reperfusion injury[65] secondary to deficient placentation. Whereas some consider abnormal placentation to be the start and invariable cause of preeclampsia, it is much more likely that it is a completely separate but predisposing condition. Some, but certainly not all, cases of preeclampsia are associated with poor placentation. Poor placentation defines the first stage, which would appear to have a different origin; first-stage decidual immune responses account for the primipaternity and possible partner specificity of preeclampsia.[1,64] Second-stage responses,[58,64] all secondary to the systemic inflammatory response, could also explain why women bearing pregnancies with unusually large placentas are susceptible to preeclampsia. In a completely normal woman, although normal pregnancy stimulates a systemic inflammatory response, it is not intense enough to generate the signs of preeclampsia. To do that requires the abnormal stimulus from an oxidatively stressed placenta ("placental preeclampsia").[66] In a woman with a chronic systemic inflammatory response associated with conditions such as chronic hypertension, diabetes, or obesity, the starting point is abnormal enough that even a normal placenta can stimulate a systemic response of an intensity to give the signs of preeclampsia ("maternal preeclampsia") (Fig. 35–2). In clinical practice, there are many mixed presentations with maternal constitution and placental ischemia-reperfusion contributing to the presentation. Based on the "inflammatory" paradigm,[58,64] preeclampsia is not a separate entity but the extreme end of a range of maternal systemic inflammatory responses engendered by pregnancy itself. The corollary is that any factor enhancing this response would predispose to preeclampsia. Indeed, recent studies have shown that, not only auto-immune disorders, but also certain maternal infections (e.g., urinary tract,[59] periodontal disease,[44] chlamydia,[43] and certain viruses[67]) are associated with preeclampsia.[59] Inflammation is

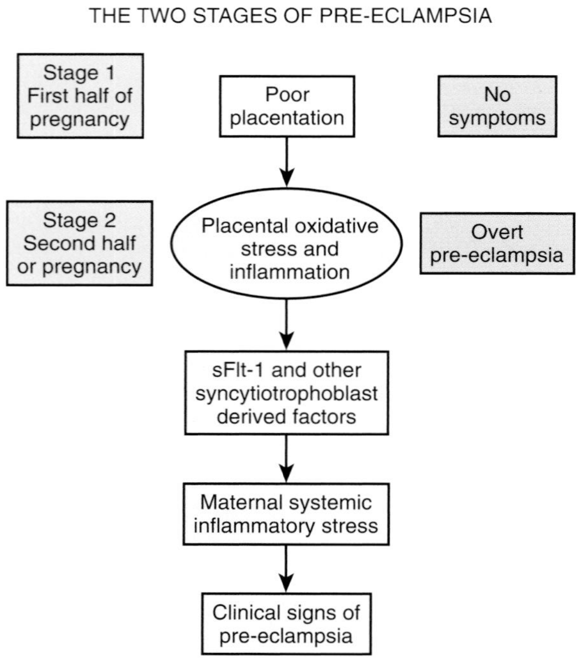

FIGURE 35–1
The two-stage model of preeclampsia. Placental oxidative stress and maternal systemic inflammatory stress are the two central events.
(From Redman and Sargent[64] with permission.)

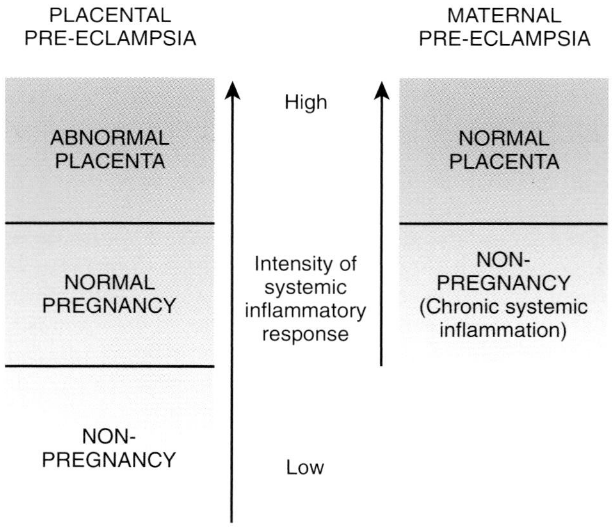

FIGURE 35–2
Placental and maternal preeclampsia. A hypothetical gray scale of increasing systemic inflammation is shown.
(From Redman and Sargent[64] with permission.)

probably also an important part of the causal pathway through which obesity predisposes to preeclampsia.[68]

Endothelial Cell Activation

Endothelial cell activation is part of the generalized inflammatory reaction also involving leucocytes as well as the clotting and complement systems.[58,64] The endothelium is one of the key organs involved in the pathophysiology of preeclampsia, as evidenced by the prostacyclin (PGI_2)/thromboxane A_2 (TXA_2) imbalance, impairment of the nitric oxide–cyclic guanosine monophosphate (NO-cGMP) pathway and a series of markers indicating endothelial activation.[68–76] Glomerular endotheliosis, but also ultrastructural changes in the placental bed and uterine boundary vessels, provides morphologic evidence of endothelial cell "injury" in preeclampsia.[72,73] Absence of normal stimulation of the renin-angiotensin system, despite relative hypovolemia in severe preeclampsia, increased vascular sensitivity to vasoconstrictors, and increased endothelial cell permeability can all be explained on the basis of this endothelial cell activation.[76] Endothelial cell activation fits the selective platelet activation and consumption (sometimes accompanied by microangiopathic hemolysis) and the resulting reduction in uteroplacental blood flow due to spiral artery thrombosis and placental infarction. An inadequate production of either antiaggregatory PGI_2 or NO, or both, increased platelet-derived TxA_2 and serotonin,[76,77] and increased local tissue factor[78,79] provide an attractive explanation for surface-mediated platelet activation occurring on the inner lining of spiral arteries. Platelets adhere to and release α- and dense granule constituents, specifically, TxA_2 and serotonin, contributing to platelet aggregation and inducing fibrin formation in particular in the uteroplacental circulation.[76,77] In preeclampsia, endothelial cell dysfunction and platelet aggregation precede the increase in thrombin and fibrin formation.[80]

Impaired Cytotrophoblast Invasion in Spiral Arteries and Placental Pathology in Preeclampsia

In normal pregnancies, endovascular CTBs replace endothelial cells in the spiral arteries; this invasion results in the destruction of the medial elastic, muscular, and neural tissue. These so-called physiologic changes normally reach the inner third of the myometrium.[81] These physiologic changes create a low-resistance arteriolar system and the absence of maternal vasomotor control, which allows the dramatic increase in blood supply necessary to serve the growing fetus. Fetal and maternal bloods are, at all times, separated by a layer of STB, a variable layer of CTB and mesenchyme, and the walls of the fetal capillaries. Therefore, the fetus can secrete substances directly into the maternal blood, but maternal products must cross trophoblast membranes and cytoplasm before they reach fetal blood.[81] A true intervillous blood flow is established by about 12 weeks' gestation. Initially, CTB plugs in the spiral arteries may act as valves and may protect the early gestation from the forces of arterial blood flow.[82,83] Uterine natural killer (NK) cells produce a series of cytokines involved in angiogenesis and vascular stability, including vascular endothelial growth factor (VEGF), placental growth factor (PLGF) and angiopoietin 2,[84] and play a pivotal role in regulating trophoblast invasion and the maternal placental bed vascular changes.[81,84] The end result is that 100 to 120 spiral arteries are remodeled by the invading "foreign" CTBs into dilated, inelastic tubes without maternal vasomotor control. Only humans have such extensive placental invasion, arguably because of the long intrauterine period required for the development of the fetal brain.[84,85]

In preeclampsia, physiologic changes in many but not all spiral arteries are confined to the decidual portion of the arteries. In these arteries, the myometrial segments remain anatomically intact, do not dilate, and the adrenergic nerve supply to the spiral arteries remains intact. About 30% to 50% of placental bed spiral arteries escape entirely from the endovascular invasion of trophoblast.[81] In addition, many vessels are occluded by fibrinoid material and exhibit adjacent foam cell invasion (atherosis). Acute atherosis is characterized by fibrinoid necrosis of the vessel wall, with an accumulation of lipid-laden macrophages (foam cells) and a perivascular mononuclear cell infiltrate. Acute atherosis and the associated thrombosis are the cause of placental infarctions, which are more common in preeclampsia.[81] Preeclamptic patients are also at higher risk for abruption. Placental abruption in preeclamptic patients probably results from thrombotic lesions in the placental vasculature, leading to decidual necrosis, separation, and hemorrhage. A vicious circle then continues as the decidual hemorrhage results in further separation.[86] Similar pathologic vascular changes exist in a significant proportion of normotensive pregnancies complicated by IUGR and/or preterm labor and are certainly not specific for preeclampsia.[87]

Pro- and Antiangiogenic Proteins in Normal and Preeclamptic Pregnancies

VEGF and PLGF induce vasodilator autocoids including NO and PGI_2 in endothelial cells and play a major role in pregnancy-associated vasodilation and the pregnancy-associated increase in glomerular filtration rate. VEGF-A and PLGF are produced by villous and extravillous CTBs, STBs, and decidual leukocytes. The receptors for VEGF-A, fms-like tyrosine kinase-1 (Flt-1) and kinase-insert domain-containing receptor (KDR),[88] are both expressed on human trophoblasts in addition to endothelial cells. In the placental bed, at time of implantation, VEGF is expressed dominantly in the epithelial cells. Later, expression increases in the decidual leukocytes, which remain a major source of VEGF in placental tissues.[84,88–92] The production of VEGF and PLGF by decidual NK cells and macrophages and the presence of Flt-1 on human intermediate and extravillous trophoblasts are an important part of the complex interplay between the immunologically driven expression of growth factors by decidual leukocytes and trophoblast receptors.[1,84,93] VEGF is up-regulated by hypoxia. The control is homeostatic; neovascularization induced by hypoxia corrects tissue oxygenation and VEGF release is down-regulated. The up-regulation of VEGF by hypoxia may provide an important mechanism through which the placenta develops according to its metabolic requirements. This mechanism may have particular relevance in the first 10 weeks of pregnancy, when oxygen tension of trophoblastic villi is particularly low.[91,94,95] In contrast to VEGF, PLGF is down-regulated by hypoxia in trophoblastic cell cultures grown in vitro.[96,97]

Soluble Flt-1 (sFlt-1), a soluble version of the VEGF receptor generated by alternative splicing of the Flt-1 gene, is a major endogenous angiogenesis inhibitor because it retains the ability to bind to VEGF and PLGF while preventing VEGF and PLGF binding to cell-surface receptors. The subsequent deficiency of free VEGF and PLGF leads to a state of endothelial dysfunction.[93] Early in pregnancy, proangiogenic proteins are overexpressed (placental angiogenesis and increasing placental mass), whereas toward the end of pregnancy, antiangiogenic factors increase in expression, possibly in preparation for delivery[88,93]; as such, sFlt-1 might be involved in the return to booking BP often observed near term. Messenger RNA for sFlt-1 is up-regulated in preeclamptic placentas, leading to increased systemic levels of sFlt-1 falling to baseline 48 hours after delivery.[90,93] These increased sFlt-1 levels result in decreased circulating levels of free VEGF and PLGF in preeclampsia and endothelial cell dysfunction.[88,90,93,98] Excessive levels of sFlt-1 are not the only player causing the antiangiogenic state in preeclampsia.[99] A novel soluble form of endoglin (sEng) of placental origin is present in the sera of pregnant women, is elevated in preeclamptic individuals, and correlates with disease severity.[99] Notably, sEng acts in concert with sFlt-1 to amplify endothelial dysfunction and induce clinical signs of severe preeclampsia, including HELLP syndrome and IUGR. Analogous to sFlt-1, circulating sEng starts rising 6 to 10 weeks before clinical symptoms of preeclampsia.[99] A recent development was the discovery of a human-specific splicing variant of VEGF receptor 1, designated sFlt1-14, qualitatively different from the previously described sFlt-1 and a potent VEGF inhibitor.[100] The fact that preeclampsia is a human-specific disease and that sFlt1-14 is a human-specific protein raises the speculation that a unique aspect in sFlt1-14 regulation or a unique, yet unidentified, biologic property of this protein is responsible for this disease.[100]

Immunology of Preeclampsia

The invasion of trophoblasts into the decidua and myometrium appears to be primarily controlled by immune mechanisms. STBs do not express class human leukocyte antigen (HLA) mRNA. Whereas all of the classic class I HLA antigens are absent, apart from HLA-C, the invading CTBs express the nonclassic HLA-G and HLA-E. Initially, it was thought that the presence of HLA-G, being monomorphic, played an important role in the afferent arm of maternal tolerance to the fetus, through failing to be perceived as "foreign" while still protecting the trophoblast from NK cell–mediated cytotoxicity. Today, we know that HLA-G expressed on the invading CTB plays an even more important role in the required vascular adaptations in the placental bed.[84] Because T cells were believed to be the unique immune cells required for adaptive immune responses, absence of major T-cell interaction in preeclampsia appeared to negate the immune maladaptation hypothesis.[76] This concept was radically changed by the realization of the major role played by the decidual NK cells. The predominant population of lymphoid cells in the decidua consists of NK cells; T and B cells are rare. NK cells express inhibitory and activatory killer cell immunoglobulin-like receptors (KIRs) capable of recognizing HLA-class I molecules. Uterine NK cells influence both trophoblast invasion and the maternal placental bed vascular changes by producing a series of cytokines involved in angiogenesis and vascular stability, in particular VEGF, PLGF, and angiotensin-2.[84,89] Moffett-King and colleagues[84] changed our understanding of the importance of the HLA-C–NK cell receptor interaction. HLA-C loci are dimorphic for residues 77 to 80 and these two HLA-C groups interact with different NK cell receptors. There is great diversity of NK KIR haplotypes in humans with variations in the number of genes as well as polymorphisms at individual loci. All women express KIRs on decidual NK cells for both groups of HLA-C alleles, and because HLA-C is polymorphic, each pregnancy will involve different combinations of paternally derived fetal HLA-C and maternal KIRs. Therefore, each pregnancy is based on a unique couple-specific immune interaction not necessarily involving T cells but NK cells interacting with "paternal" HLA. Mothers lacking most or all activating KIRs (AA genotype) when the fetus had HLA-C, belonging to the HLA-C2 group, are at a substantial risk of preeclampsia.[101] Interestingly, recent studies have also shown that regulatory T cells are involved in specific immune tolerance to fetal alloantigens during pregnancy.[102–104] A major part of the protective effect of previous sperm exposure[55,56] is conveyed by sperm cells.[39] Intercourse provokes a cascade of cellular and molecular events that resemble a classic inflammatory response. The critical seminal factor appears to be seminal vesicle derived transforming growth factor-b1 (TGF-b1). By initiating a postmating inflammatory reaction, TGF-b1 increases the ability to sample and process paternal antigens (HLA-C?) contained within the ejaculate. The processing of paternal antigens by antigen-presenting cells in an environment containing TGF-b1 will initiate a "type 2" immune response. By initiating a type 2 immune response toward paternal ejaculate antigens, seminal TGF-b1 may inhibit the induction of type 1 responses against the semiallogenic conceptus that are thought to be associated with poor placental and fetal development.[40,105,106]

Placental Ischemia/Placental Debris Hypothesis

Circulating placental debris (STB microvillous membrane particles, free fetal DNA, and cytokeratin) is likely to be an important part of the systemic inflammatory stimulus associated with normal and preeclamptic pregnancies. Increased deportation of placental tissue in future preeclamptics is already detectable at 16 to 18 weeks.[107–109] The increased STB deportation in preeclampsia is explained by the presence of syncytial sprouds that may be elongated on long pedicles—interestingly, also the source for sFlt-14.[100] Apoptosis plays a central role in the formation of STB from the underlying villous CTB. Apoptosis, causing controlled cell fragmentation and allowing continuous renewal of the syncytial surface, is increased in preeclampsia.[110–112] In maternal blood, there are more apoptotic microparticles than trophoblastic microparticles, particularly in preeclampsia. The maternal inflammatory response is the likely cause of the increased endothelial cell and leukocyte apoptosis.[113] In the earlier stages of a preeclamptic pregnancy, increased apoptosis could be explained by the maternal-fetal immune maladaptation (tumor necrosis factor [TNF], interferon-γ [IFN-γ], Fas-FAS ligand)[114,115]; later on, placental ischemia-reperfusion probably plays a major role.[113] Not only "placental debris" but many other placental factors are found in the maternal circulation in normal pregnancy, with increased

levels in preeclampsia. These include several inflammatory cytokines, corticotropin-releasing hormone (CRH), and activin A; all could be potential stimulators of the maternal inflammatory response.[113] The maternal inflammatory response syndrome and placental ischemia-reperfusion injury are also responsible for the oxidative stress in preeclampsia.[66,116]

Genetic Conflict Hypothesis

According to Haig's genetic conflict theory,[117] fetal genes will be selected to increase the transfer of nutrients to the fetus, and maternal genes will be selected to limit transfers in excess of some maternal optimum. The phenomenon of genomic imprinting means that within fetal cells, a similar conflict exists between genes that are maternally derived and genes that are paternally derived. The conflict hypothesis predicts that placental factors (fetal genes) will act to increase maternal BP, whereas maternal factors will act to reduce BP. Placental factors have this opportunity to preferentially increase nonplacental resistance because the uteroplacental arteries are highly modified and unresponsive to vasoconstrictors. The intrinsic effects of a high maternal systemic BP are ultimately beneficial to the fetus. Thus, the genetic conflict hypothesis[117] predicts that fetal genes will enhance the flow of maternal blood through the intervillous space by increasing maternal BP (perfusion pressure). The genetic conflict hypothesis predicts that a mother's BP, as a continuum, is determined by the balance between fetal factors increasing BP and maternal factors decreasing BP. Causing maternal endothelial cell activation may have evolved as a high risk fetal strategy to increase nonplacental resistance when the uteroplacental blood supply is inadequate. Small increments in birth weight of semistarved fetuses may often have caused major increases in subsequent survival despite substantial costs to the mother. The balance between angiogenic growth factors and sFlt-1 (and the human-specific sFlt-14) provides a prime example of the molecular pathways predicted by Haig.[117] The magnitude of increase in sFlt-1 levels correlates with disease severity, lending further support that the VEGF–sFlt-1 (sFlt-14) balance represents a major final common pathophysiologic pathway.[118]

Maternal Susceptibility

There is a well-described maternal predisposition to preeclampsia, a clear and important maternal contribution that is of pivotal importance in determining the individual disease phenotype.

Maternal Susceptibility Genes

It is unlikely that there is just one major critical "preeclampsia" gene. Such a gene should have committed "evolutionary" suicide, unless it also carried a major reproductive advantage. More likely, we will see a rapidly growing number of susceptibility genes, many of these interacting with the maternal cardiovascular/hemostatic system and/or regulation of maternal inflammatory responses. Current models suggest a heritability estimate of 30% for preeclampsia.[119]

Thrombophilias

After initial studies[50,120,121] showed a clear association between maternal thrombophilias and early-onset preeclampsia, several studies were unable to reproduce these findings.[122,123] However, systematic reviews[48,49,124,125] have confirmed an overall higher rate of acquired (primarily antiphospholipids) and genetic thrombophilias in women with severe early-onset preeclampsia compared with controls. The apparent controversy probably reflects the heterogeneous nature of preeclampsia and the heterogeneity of the patients being studied.[125] In a "two-hit" type model of preeclampsia in which a triggering event is exacerbated by other factors, thrombophilias clearly function as the exacerbating factor or "second hit." The surface of apoptotic cells is highly procoagulant activity.[126] Apoptotic CTBs in spiral arteries could elicit fibrin deposition as well as platelet activation. Any underlying thrombophilia will greatly augment this pathophysiologic process.[1]

Age

Extremes of age are known risk factors for preeclampsia. A short period of sperm exposure is the most likely explanation for the high risk of preeclampsia among teenagers.[55,56] For the more advanced maternal age categories, the significant positive relation between age (as a continuum) and the incidence of preeclampsia probably reflects a combined effect of "ageing" endothelium and the higher incidence of other adverse factors, in particular increased booking BP and body mass index (BMI).[127]

Chronic Hypertension

Increased booking BP is a major risk factor for preeclampsia.[26,128]

Obesity

Obesity is a definite risk for both gestational hypertension and preeclampsia. The risk of preeclampsia typically doubles with each 5 to 7 kg/m^2 increase in prepregnancy BMI.[45,46] In addition to the increased cytokine-mediated inflammation and oxidative stress,[68] possible explanations[76] include increased shear stress, dyslipidemia,[68] and increased sympathetic activity.[129] Figure 35–3 provides an overview of the major processes involved in the pathogenesis of preeclampsia.

Maternal Changes and Risks

Cardiovascular System

Total body water increases by 6 to 9 L during normal pregnancy, equally divided between the fetus and the mother. Expansion of the plasma volume accounts for 20% to 25% of the increase in extracellular space; the other 75% to 80% are increments in interstitial fluid. The greatest increase in interstitial fluid occurs in the third trimester, contrasting with the increment in plasma volume, taking place primarily in the first and second trimesters. The increase in blood volume is already detectable at 6 weeks. It reaches a level about 40% higher than that in nonpregnant values at 30 weeks and then remains stable until term.[130,131] The increase in plasma volume correlates closely with newborn weight, even if fetal growth is impaired.[130] The average plasma volume in women with established pregnancy-induced hypertensive disease is about 9% below expected values and as much as 30% to 40% below normal in cases of severe preeclampsia. Hypovolemia in pregnancy-induced

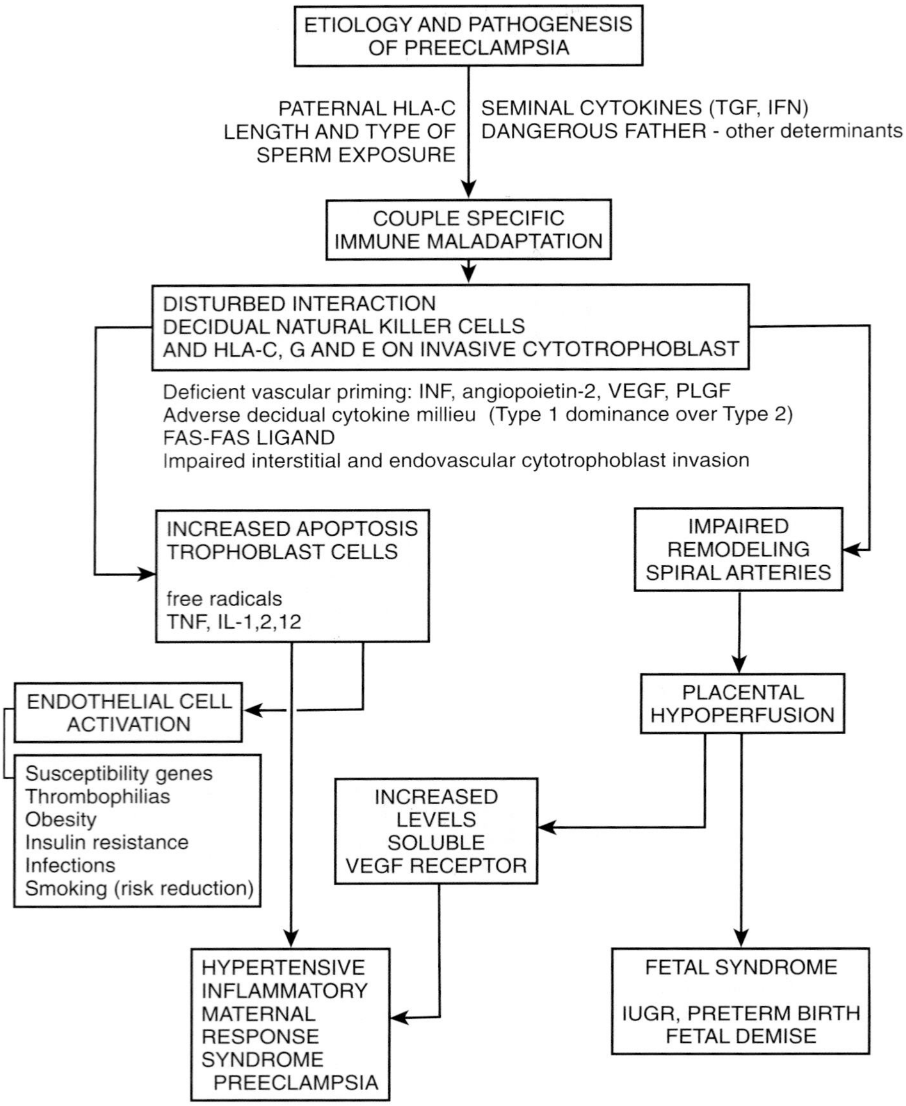

FIGURE 35–3
Etiology and pathogenesis of preeclampsia. HLA, human leukocyte antigen-C; INF, interferon; IL, interleukin; IUGR, intrauterine growth restriction; PLGF, placental growth factor; TGF, transforming growth factor; VEGF, vascular endothelial growth factor.

hypertensive disorders has been identified in particular in cases associated with IUGR, oligohydramnios, and preterm labor.[132–136]

Whereas the mean red cell mass rises during pregnancy, the relatively greater increase in plasma volume results in a gradual fall of the hematocrit until week 30, followed by a gradual rise. The physiologic hemodilution is associated with a decreased viscosity, which may be beneficial for intervillous space perfusion.[130]

Severe preeclampsia is characterized by vasoconstriction and a "leaky" microcirculation, resulting in fluid moving into the extracellular interstitial space and relative hypovolemia. The red cell volume in preeclampsia is no different than in normotensive pregnancy. Thus, the hemoglobin concentration or hematocrit is a reasonable surrogate measure of plasma volume in preeclampsia. Abnormally high hemoglobin levels correlate with adverse perinatal outcome including low birth weight, low placental weight, increased incidence of prematurity and perinatal mortality, and hypertension.[137–142] Hemoglobin concentrations may be elevated in the first and second trimesters in advance of clinical disease.[142–144] Edema and swelling, although not reliable signs of pregnancy-induced hypertensive disorders, are the clinical expression of this shift in the distribution of extracellular fluid. Pathologic edema is not caused by an increased intracapillary hydrostatic pressure, as is the case in normal pregnancy. Because of the increased precapillary resistance in preeclampsia, the intracapillary hydrostatic pressure is actually decreased. Pathologic edema is caused by increased microvascular permeability to plasma proteins, a reduction in plasma colloid osmotic pressure, and an increase in interstitial protein mass.[141] Pathologic edema appears suddenly and is associated with an accelerated rate of weight gain. Chesley[132,133] stated that if pedal edema does not regress overnight, the pregnant woman bears careful watching. Sudden swelling linked with a gain greater than 1 kg/wk over 2 to 3 weeks or greater than 2 kg in 1 week should warn the clinician. A woman with established preeclampsia will often have facial and particularly periorbital edema in contrast to the physiologic pedal edema.

BP falls in the first and second trimesters, followed by a rise to levels similar to the nonpregnant level close to term. By 6 to 8 weeks' gestation, mean arterial blood pressure (MAP) is already decreased relative to the preconceptional reference levels.[145] Cardiac output begins to rise shortly after conception; 50% of the final increase in cardiac output is realized by 8 weeks' gestation. Cardiac output reaches a peak of 35% to 50% higher than resting, nonpregnant levels at the end of the second trimester. The increase in cardiac output is due to an increase in both stroke volume (10%) and pulse rate (5%–15%) and is accompanied by enlargement of the left ventricle. The sequential rise in heart rate before, and in stroke volume after, the fifth week is related to the underfilled state of the vascular bed and is triggered in an attempt to maintain cardiac output in a state of relative underfill. Cardiac output remains elevated until delivery, if not measured in the supine position. In the third trimester, about 65% of the additional cardiac output is distributed to the uteroplacental and renal circulation.[146–149] Because BP falls and cardiac output increases in pregnancy, systemic vascular resistance (SVR) must decrease. In the average woman, SVR falls from 1700 dynes/sec/cm^{-5} before pregnancy to about 900 dynes/sec/cm^{-5} in midpregnancy, rising to 1300 dynes/sec/cm^{-5} toward term. A decrease in SVR is one of the earliest maternal adjustments to pregnancy and is already observed during the luteal phase in women that subsequently become pregnant. The fall in arterial BP and afterload leads to a rise in cardiac output, primarily through an increase in heart rate.[150,151] The fall in arterial BP, together with the concomitant fall in venous tone, activates the volume-retaining mechanisms such as the renin-angiotensin-aldosterone system (RAAS) and the osmoregulatory system. The induced volume retention enhances preload and stroke volume.[150,151]

In preeclampsia, cardiac output, as measured with thermodilution, has been described as decreased, unchanged, and increased, and likewise, there are conflicting data regarding alterations in SVR and pulmonary capillary wedge pressure (PCWP).[152–156] Visser and Wallenburg[154] compared results of pulmonary artery catheter measurements in 87 preeclamptic women who had received no treatment with those obtained in 47 preeclamptic women who had received various drugs and intravenous fluids; 10 normotensive pregnant women served as controls. All measurements were performed between 25 and 34 weeks' gestation. The median (range) cardiac index in the untreated patients of 3.3 (2.0–5.3) L · min^{-1} · min^{-2} was significantly lower than that in the treated patients of 4.3 (2.4–7.6) L · min^{-1} · min^{-2}. The median (range) PCWP in the untreated group was 7 (1–20) mm Hg and did not differ from that of 7 mm Hg (0–25) in the treated group. The variability of all hemodynamic variables was much lower in untreated than in treated patients. Thus, the majority of the extremes in dynamic profiles in severe established preeclampsia, as reported in the literature, are probably related to a combination of iatrogenic artifacts, differences in disease severity, obesity, and the presence of underlying chronic hypertension and/or renal disease. Untreated patients with severe established early-onset preeclampsia, mostly associated with IUGR, show a rather uniform pattern of a low cardiac index, a high SVR index, and low-normal filling pressures.[154] Longitudinal ultrasound studies have demonstrated, however, that preeclampsia is characterized by a high cardiac output before the onset of clinically severe disease; so patients may cross over from a high cardiac output–low SVR state in earlier stages to one of lower output and higher SVR in cases with severe early-onset established disease.[156]

Renal System

Glomerular endotheliosis, swollen intracapillary endothelial cells in the glomeruli, the hallmark renal lesion of preeclampsia, represents the primary renal manifestation of the aforementioned systemic endothelial cell activation. An increase in renal vascular resistance causes a reduction of renal blood flow. The excess sFlt-1 (sFlt-14) probably plays a major role in the causation of glomerular endotheliosis.[93] Glomerular filtration rate, ERPF (effective renal plasma flow), and filtration fraction all decrease in preeclampsia. After delivery, the functional decrements usually reverse quickly but can sometimes progress to acute tubular necrosis (ATN).

In 1983, MacGillivray[157] stated that "oliguria or anuria is a most important sign to look for in preeclampsia, as is an indication that the baby and placenta should be delivered promptly." Although oliguria is indeed a serious sign, it is not, as such, an indication for immediate delivery. Oliguria/anuria may be classified as prerenal, renal, and postrenal. In preeclampsia, hypovolemia, without serious intrarenal vasoconstriction, may cause oliguria. However, in most patients, oliguria/anuria is a consequence of a combination of glomerular endotheliosis, intrarenal vasoconstriction, and hypovolemia. Although acute renal failure (ARF) is a rare complication of preeclampsia (1 in 10,000–15,000),[158] preeclampsia is a major cause of obstetric ARF. ARF in preeclampsia is mostly caused by ATN, but sometimes, it is caused by the more ominous bilateral cortical necrosis variety. Relative oliguria in the early postpartum period is common, but this generally resolves spontaneously and can be treated conservatively, providing that the serum creatinine and urea levels do not increase alarmingly. ARF in a preeclamptic patient who is otherwise well has a good prognosis, with full recovery being the norm. Patients who develop renal complications of preeclampsia superimposed upon preexisting renal disease are at increased risk of bilateral renal cortical necrosis, which is associated with increased maternal mortality and persistent renal compromise. Renal failure due to preeclampsia in antenatal patients will almost always prompt delivery.

Abnormal Hemostasis

Platelet activation, a feature of normal pregnancy, is exaggerated in preeclampsia.[159] Abnormalities of the hemostatic system in preeclampsia are compatible with a local grade of compensated intravascular coagulation, secondary to platelet adherence at sites of endothelial cell damage, instead of the fibrinogen depletion and thrombocytopenia that occur in case of disseminated intravascular coagulation (DIC). Only in certain sites (such as uteroplacental vascular bed, liver, and kidneys) is there a local increase of thrombin formation and fibrin deposition. Vascular damage and platelet aggregation precede an increase in thrombin and fibrin formation.[80,160,161]

TABLE 35–4

Criteria for the Diagnosis of the HELLP Syndrome*

Hemolysis
Abnormal peripheral blood smear (burr cells, schistocytes)
Elevated bilirubin ≥ 1.2 mg/dL
Increased LDH of > twice the upper limit of normal for the laboratory
Elevated liver enzymes
Elevated ALT or AST ≥ twice the upper limit of normal for the laboratory
Increased LDH > twice the upper limit of normal for the laboratory
Low platelet count (<100,000/mm^3)

* Requires at least two of the abnormalities listed.

ALT, alanine aminotransferase; AST, aspartate aminotransferase; HELLP, hemolysis, elevated liver enzymes, and low platelets; LDH, lactate dehydrogenase.

From Sibai BM: Diagnosis, controversies, and management of HELLP syndrome. Obstet Gynecol 2004;103:981–991.

Thrombocytopenia (platelet count < 150,000 μL^{-1}) is common (5%–7%) in late pregnancy.[162] The most common cause of isolated thrombocytopenia in pregnancy is gestational thrombocytopenia. Gestational thrombocytopenia characteristically has its onset earlier in gestation than does preeclampsia, it is commonly detected as part of routine prenatal screening, and platelet counts rarely fall below 70,000 μL^{-1}. Thrombocytopenia is the most frequent hemostatic abnormality in established preeclampsia; 20% of all patients with a pregnancy-induced hypertensive disorder develop mild thrombocytopenia (>50,000 μL^{-1}) varying between 7% in mild disease to 30% to 50% in severe preeclampsia and eclampsia.[132,163–165] Preeclamptic patients, in particular when IUGR is present, may show a marked day-to-day variability in platelet counts as well as in platelet volume distribution.[166] The thrombocytopenia in severe preeclampsia does not commonly fall below 50,000 μL^{-1},[165] and when it does, other diagnoses should be considered (see Chapter 40).

The key features of the HELLP syndrome[167] are shown in Table 35–4.[19] Most patients with HELLP syndrome show decreasing platelet counts until 24 to 48 hours after delivery. Although more than 90% of cases of thrombocytopenia associated with preeclampsia should resolve by postpartum day 4, women with severe thrombocytopenia (platelet count < 50 × 10^9/L) may require more than 10 days to achieve a platelet count greater than 100,000 μL^{-1}. Recovery is typically followed by a marked thrombocytosis. HELLP syndrome is a manifestation of a microangiopathic process and not a form of DIC, although there are often signs of locally increased localized coagulation (uteroplacental vascular bed, kidney, and liver). The localized increase in intravascular coagulation is secondary to endothelial cell injury. The high incidence of DIC reported by some authors is probably caused by the fact that the patients in these studies are already in the (pre) terminal stage of their disease process. In general, only if a patient's platelet count falls consistently lower than 80,000 μL^{-1}, an increasing percentage of patients with HELLP syndrome show evidence of increased intravascular thrombin production and accelerated fibrin consumption that can be documented with more or less sophisticated coagulation studies, such as antithrombin (AT), thrombin-antithrombin (TAT) complexes, fibrininopeptide A, and D-dimer measurements. Only in well-advanced cases of HELLP syndrome with platelets lower than 50.000 μL^{-1} and lactate dehydrogenase (LDH) levels greater than 600 IU/L do routinely available clinical laboratory tests of fibrinogen and fibrinogen degradation products (FDPs) become abnormal, occasionally with some prolongation of the prothrombin time (PT) and activated partial thromboplastin time (aPTT). In case of HELLP syndrome, microangiopathic hemolytic anemia (MAHA) and severe thrombocytopenia precede the appearance of fibrin consumption and DIC and not the reverse, as seen, for instance, in patients with placental abruption.[80] The corollary of all of this is that a HELLP syndrome patient with DIC is really in the very advanced stage of the disease process.

The Liver

Hepatic involvement in the HELLP syndrome is not caused by excessive vasoconstriction of the hepatic arterial circulation,[168] but related to excessive fibrin-fibrinogen deposition in the hepatic sinusoids. In severe preeclampsia, large deposits of fibrin-like material obstruct blood flow in sinusoids and cause hepatic capsular distension, which may cause upper epigastric pain.[1] This is a problem in 90% of HELLP syndrome patients. In addition, 50% have nausea and/or vomiting, and others have nonspecific viral syndrome–like symptoms.[19,169] The majority of patients (90%) will have a history of malaise for a few days prior to presentation. On physical examination, 80% will have right upper quadrant tenderness and 60% significant weight gain with generalized edema. Hypertension may be absent (20%), mild (30%), or severe (50%).[169] Some patients may present with gastrointestinal bleeding, hematuria, flank or shoulder pain, and jaundice. Such patients are often misdiagnosed as having various medical and surgical disorders. Cholelithiasis, cholecystitis, hepatitis, acute fatty liver of pregnancy, pancreatitis, perforated peptic ulcer, severe hiatus hernia, pyelonephritis, and Budd-Chiari syndrome should be included in the differential diagnosis of epigastric or right upper quadrant pain during pregnancy and ,thus, in the differential diagnosis of HELLP syndrome. Subcapsular hematoma and liver rupture are further extensions of the HELLP syndrome with patients presenting with severe epigastric pain, shoulder pain, shock, evidence of massive ascites (hemoperitoneum), respiratory difficulties, or pleural effusions. When the rupture is contained within the capsule, the patient experiences severe pain but is hemodynamically stable. Subcapsular hematomata are clearly visible by ultrasonography and computed tomography (CT) scanning. The CT scan is likely more useful, because it is less operator-dependent and can visualize the entire abdomen. Ultrasonography, however, is more practical to perform, because the equipment is often on hand in an obstetric unit. Most often, the hematoma is on the anterior or inferior surface of the right lobe of the liver. A right pleural effusion may occur in some cases. A peritoneal tap may be used to differentiate between ascites and peritoneal blood.[19,169]

The Brain

Eclampsia is defined as the onset of convulsions and/or coma in women who have either gestational hypertension or preeclampsia. However, a series in the 1990s demonstrated that at the onset of convulsions, 23% had minimal or absent hypertension, 19% did not have proteinuria, and edema was absent in 32%.[170] This said, eclampsia occurs seven to eight times more commonly in the context of proteinuric than in nonproteinuric pregnancy-induced hypertensive disease, and the average BPs of women with eclampsia are higher than those with severe preeclampsia.[171] In general, eclamptic seizures are grand mal in character with tonic/clonic phases; focal seizures have been described occasionally. Cerebral signs and symptoms of preeclampsia-eclampsia are headache, dizziness, tinnitus, hyperreflexia, clonus, drowsiness, mental changes, visual disturbances, paresthesias, and seizures. Headache has long been recognized as a harbinger of eclampsia. The headache is unrelieved by salicylates or phenacetin and is frequently described as "throbbing." The precise mechanism of these headaches is not certain, although hypertensive encephalopathy, cerebral vasospasm, and abnormal cerebral perfusion pressure are intimately involved.[172] To distinguish eclampsia from preeclampsia by the occurrence of at least one convulsion is too restrictive. For instance, cortical blindness is excluded even though the pathology is identical to the lesions causing convulsions. Furthermore, preeclamptic patients can become comatose without convulsing.[173] Hyperreflexia and clonus are hallmarks of severe preeclampsia. However, seizures may occur in the absence of hyperreflexia, and many young subjects have a consistent physiologic hyperreflexia. Clonus is "always" a pathologic sign and must warn the obstetrician of impending eclampsia.[174]

The most frequent symptoms preceding convulsions are headache (82.5%), visual disturbances (44.4%), and upper abdominal pain (19%).[174] Visual symptoms include scintillation (scotomata), chromatopsia, blurring of vision, diplopia, homonymous hemianopsia, and amaurosis. Visual disturbances in severe preeclampsia may be similar to the "aura" preceding migraine attacks, may include flashing or multicolored lights, and may range from blurring to scotomata and temporary blindness. Retinal arteriolar spasm, ischemia, and edema are believed to produce these visual disturbances.[175] Blindness is uncommon (1%–3% incidence in eclampsia). Chesley[132] reported an incidence of amaurosis of 4.3% among 330 eclamptic women. Women with amaurosis usually recover completely within 1 week. Retinal detachment also may cause altered vision, although it is usually one-sided and seldom causes total loss of vision. Without surgical treatment, vision returns to normal within approximately 1 week.[176] Magnesium intravenously is known to cause neuroophthalmic effects, which may thus cause a differential diagnostic problem. However, there are significant differences between preeclamptic visual complaints and those induced by magnesium. Preeclampsia-eclampsia is associated with positive and negative scotomata and/or segmental visual blurring; use of magnesium intravenously is associated with blurred vision and diplopia.[177]

Current data suggest that hypertensive encephalopathy and overperfusion of the brain occur in women with preeclampsia. Middle cerebral artery (MCA) and posterior cerebral artery (PCA) blood flow (as determined by magnetic resonance imaging [MRI]) and MCA velocity and cerebral perfusion pressure are increased in women with severe preeclampsia when compared with normotensive pregnant women.[178] These women are different from normotensive women, who have decreases in the MRI-calculated blood flow in large arteries (MCA and PCA) and Doppler-calculated velocities with increasing gestational age.[179] This overperfusion is coupled with capillary leak and vasogenic edema in most cases of eclampsia and may, in some cases of severe eclampsia, result in local areas of infarction (cytotoxic edema). MRI findings of focal and generalized vasogenic edema are more apparent in eclampsia than in severe preeclampsia, and permanent infarction with the development of cytotoxic edema was demonstrated in about 20% of women with eclampsia in whom MRI of the brain is performed. The role of vasospasm as the primary mechanism of eclampsia in women with severe preeclampsia is challenged by the more recent data that suggest hypertensive encephalopathy as the initiating injury. Secondary vasospasm may well then follow the primary pathophysiology, and the reported vasospasm in cases of eclampsia may be a reflection of the severity of the case, the long interval between the seizure and the imaging, and the development of cytotoxic edema and cerebral infarction. In the future, it may be possible to delineate different groups of patients with predominant vasogenic or cytotoxic edema, and this may significantly influence management.[178–181] Cortical blindness in preeclampsia-eclampsia is caused by multiple microinfarctions and microhemorrhages with edema in the occipital gray matter. Each flash or streak of light experienced in cases of severe preeclampsia could signal the occurrence of another small lesion. In aggregate, these lesions cause cortical blindness, although the syndrome may not be complete because light is perceived. The pupils continue to react to light (midbrain reflex), but the ability to blink in response to a threat is lost. If the lesion is complete, optokinetic nystagmus is absent, and the patient is indifferent to the blindness (Anton's symptom).[173] The so-called posterior reversible encephalopathy syndrome (PRES), with cortical blindness as its cardinal clinical feature, should have the same clinical significance as eclamptic seizures, because the pathology is probably more or less identical.[182] Papilledema in eclampsia signifies cerebral edema.

Fetal/Neonatal Risks and Overall Outcome

Maternal and perinatal outcomes in preeclampsia are dependent on gestational age at time of onset and/or at time of delivery, severity of disease process, quality of management used, and presence or absence of preexisting medical conditions.[1–4,61,183] Maternal and perinatal outcomes are usually favorable in women with mild preeclampsia developing beyond 36 weeks' gestation.[2,9] In contrast, maternal and perinatal morbidities and mortalities are increased in women who develop preeclampsia before 33 weeks' gestation,[2,184] in those with preexisting medical conditions,[19,26,32,34,48–50,183] and in those from the developing countries.[185]

Approximately 1 in 6 babies born to mothers with preeclampsia is very preterm (<32 weeks' gestation), and often severely growth-restricted. In contrast, two thirds are delivered after 37 weeks, most of whom are normally grown, healthy babies.[1,4] The increased risk of prematurity is both iatrogenic and spontaneous. Several studies have shown that term and post-term preeclampsia is associated with an increased mean birth weight.[1] The rate of neonatal complications is markedly increased in those who develop severe preeclampsia in the second trimester, whereas it is minimally increased in those with severe preeclampsia beyond 35 weeks' gestation. Perinatal risks relate largely to the gestational age at delivery, and also to the degree of IUGR.[184] Neonatal complications are also worse if there is associated perinatal hypoxia.

Severe preeclampsia is also associated with an increased risk of maternal mortality (0.2%) and increased rates of maternal morbidity (5%) with conditions such as convulsions, intracranial hemorrhage/infarction, pulmonary edema, acute renal or liver failure, liver hemorrhage, pancreatitis, and DIC. These complications are usually seen in women who develop preeclampsia before 32 weeks' gestation and in those with preexisting medical conditions.[2,169]

Management Options

Prepregnancy

PRIMARY PREVENTION

Several factors known to increase the risk of preeclampsia can be addressed before pregnancy and are, therefore, at least potentially amenable to intervention before attempts at conception.[186] Lengthier sexual relationships preceding the first pregnancy would be expected to translate in a lower risk for preeclampsia,[55,56] but for mostly pragmatic reasons, it will difficult to introduce this as primary preventive strategy. Weight control might offer the potential for affecting gestational outcomes. Women who are overweight or obese should be encouraged to achieve an ideal body weight before conception in an attempt to reduce their risk of preeclampsia. There are no randomized studies, however, to prove this benefit.[187,188] Pre-, periconception, and first-trimester vitamin B supplementation, in particular folate and B_{12}, might reduce the risks not only for neural tube defects, congenital cardiac defects, and cleft palates but also for preeclampsia (risk reduction > 50%).[189,190] Interestingly, this "preventive" effect appears to be limited to lean, multivitamin users.[189] It is not certain whether or this preventive effect operates via lowering maternal homocysteine levels.

Women with Chronic Hypertension and/or Diabetes

Women with chronic hypertension should achieve control of their BP before conception. Again, there are no randomized studies to prove such a benefit. Women with pregestational diabetes mellitus should be encouraged to complete childbearing as early as possible and before vascular complications develop and to aggressively control their diabetes and hypertension (if present) for at least several months before conception and throughout the pregnancy.[191]

Prenatal

PREDICTION

Increased vigilance is advisable in patients a increased risk factors (e.g., chronic hypertension, renal disease, connective tissue disorder, diabetes mellitus, previous preeclampsia).[189,191]

Numerous clinical and biochemical markers have been proposed to predict which women are destined to develop preeclampsia, and a detailed overview of this extensive literature is outside the scope of this chapter. For many of these tests, low predictive values have been established convincingly (e.g., mean BP in second trimester; rollover test; isometric exercise test; platelet count; microalbuminuria, hematocrit; and serum uric acid and magnesium, calcium, and total proteins); others are too invasive as well as costly (e.g., intravenous infusion of angiotensin II).[185] Most biochemical markers were chosen on the basis of specific pathophysiologic abnormalities that have been reported in association with preeclampsia.[185,192] Thus, these markers have included markers of placental dysfunction,[59,193] endothelial and coagulation activation,[70,185,192] renal involvement, and markers of systemic inflammation.[60,64,194] These biomarkers have been reported to be either elevated or reduced in the maternal circulation early in gestation before the onset of preeclampsia. Table 35–5 presents a list of those markers studied intensively since the 1980s.[185] However, the results of various studies evaluating the reliability of these markers in predicting preeclampsia have been inconsistent, and many of these markers suffer from poor specificity and predictive values for routine use in clinical practice.[185,192]

Not surprisingly, there has been a search of interest in circulating antiangiogenic and angiogenic factors before and after the onset of preeclampsia.[193] PLGF is reduced whereas sFLt-1 and endoglin levels are elevated before and after the onset of preeclampsia.[193] Some studies also have found that the magnitude of the imbalance between serum sFLt-1 and serum PLGF (sFLt-1/PLGF ratio) correlates with disease severity as well as early onset of preeclampsia.[90,99,193,195] However, a 2006 systematic review[90] concluded that the evidence is insufficient to recommend these markers for use as screening tests because of differences among the various studies regarding gestational age at time of measurements, methods used for analysis, study population, and reporting of results.[90] More recent studies[196–198] have evaluated first-trimester levels of angiogenic factors as predictors for preeclampsia; only two of these studies found that reduced levels of PLGF are associated with subsequent preeclampsia,[196,197] whereas two found that sFlt-1 levels are not associated with preeclampsia.[197,198] Three other studies evaluated second-trimester levels of angiogenic factors for the prediction of preeclampsia.[199–201] One found that PLGF levels were lower but that sFLt-1 levels were not elevated in women who later developed severe preeclampsia.[199] Another study found serum-soluble endoglin levels were elevated in the second trimester in women who later developed severe, particularly early-onset, preeclampsia.[200] Moore Simas and associates[201] measured serial serum levels of PLGF and sFLt-1 from 22 to 36 weeks in 94 high-risk women and found the sFLt-1/PLGF ratio at 22 to 26 weeks to be highly predictive of early-onset preeclampsia.

Another novel biomarker, placental protein-13, is produced in the placenta and involved in implantation and maternal vascular remodeling. First-trimester placental protein-13 levels are significantly lower in preeclampsia compared with controls; placental protein-13 alone or in combination with the slope between the first and the second trimester may be a promising marker for preeclampsia.[202,203]

Currently, Doppler ultrasound of uterine artery velocity waveforms is the only method used in clinical practice, either as a general screening or in selected patients with a high a priori risk for preeclampsia and/or IUGR.[204,205] An abnormal uterine artery velocity waveform is characterized by a high resistance index and/or by the presence of an early

TABLE 35-5

Screening Tests for Preeclampsia Identified in the Literature

Placental Perfusion and Vascular Resistance Dysfunction–related Tests
Mean blood pressure in second trimester
Rollover test
Isometric exercise test
Intravenous infusion of angiotensin II
Platelet angiotensin II binding
Platelet calcium response to arginine vasopressin
Renin
24-hr ambulatory blood pressure monitoring
Doppler ultrasound
Fetoplacental Unit Endocrinology Dysfunction–related Tests
Human chorionic gonadotropin
α-Fetoprotein
Estriol
Inhibin A
Pregnancy-associated plasma protein-A
Activin A
Corticotropin release hormone
Renal Dysfunction–related Tests
Serum uric acid
Microalbuminuria
Urinary calcium excretion
Urinary kallikrein
Microtransferrinuria
N-Acetyl-β-glucosaminidase
Endothelial and Oxidant Stress Dysfunction-related Tests/Inflammatory Markers
Platelet count
Fibronectin
Platelet activation and endothelial cell adhesion molecules
Endothelin
Prostacyclin
Thromboxane
Cytokines
Homocysteine
Isoprostanes
Asymmetrical dimethylarginine
Serum lipids
Insulin resistance
Antiphospholipid antibodies
Plasminogen activator inhibitor
Placenta growth factor
Leptin
Hematocrit
Total proteins
Antithrombin III
Magnesium
Calcium
Ferritin
Transferrin
Haptoglobin
Atrial natriuretic peptide
β_2-Microglobulin
CRP
Genetic Markers

CRP, C-reactive protein.
Modified from Conde-Agudelo A, Villar J, Lindheimer M: World Health Organization systematic review of screening tests for preeclampsia. Obstet Gynecol 2004;104:1367–1391, with permission.

diastolic notch (unilateral or bilateral). Pregnancies complicated by abnormal uterine artery Doppler findings in the second trimester are associated with more than a three- to sixfold increase in the rate of preeclampsia.[204,205] However, the sensitivity of an abnormal uterine artery Doppler for predicting preeclampsia and/or IUGR, as reported in systematic reviews, ranges from 20% to 60% with a positive predictive value of 6% to 40%.[185,204,205] Current data do not support this test for routine screening of pregnant women for preeclampsia, but uterine artery Doppler could be beneficial as a screening test in women at high risk for preeclampsia if an effective preventive treatment is available. Most authors and researchers agree that uterine artery Doppler has quite a high sensitive for early-onset preeclampsia associated with IUGR.[185,204,205] If overall test performance could be enhanced by the addition of clinical data, biomarkers, or both, 20 weeks would be the best time to perform uterine artery Doppler studies.[206]

SECONDARY PREVENTION

The overall risk for recurrence of preeclampsia is in the range of 14% for preeclampsia and the same for developing gestational hypertension in a next pregnancy,[207] whereas women with prior early-onset preeclampsia and/or significant chronic hypertension have recurrence rates exceeding 50%.[191,208] A number of agents have been studied for their ability to reduce the risk of preeclampsia and improve maternal and fetal outcomes. These include antiplatelet agents, vitamins, calcium, and heparin. Table 35–6 presents an overview of current strategies to prevent preeclampsia with the degree of supportive evidence.[1]

Antiplatelet Agents

The majority of randomized trials for the prevention of preeclampsia have used low-dose aspirin (LDA; 50–150 mg/dL). The rationale for recommending LDA prophylaxis is the theory that LDA in pregnancy inhibits platelet TxA_2 biosynthesis with minimal effects on vascular PGI_2 production, thus altering the balance in favor of PGI_2, and thus preventing the development of preeclampsia.[209] LDA has been the subject of a large number of studies and various statistical reassessments. The Perinatal Antiplatelet Review of International Studies (PARIS) Collaborative Group[209] performed a meta-analysis of the effectiveness and safety of LDA for the prevention of preeclampsia; 31 randomized trials involving 32,217 women are included in this review. For women assigned to LDA, the relative risk (RR) of developing preeclampsia was 0.90 (95% confidence interval [CI] 0.84–0.96). For women with a previous history of hypertension or preeclampsia (n = 6107) who were assigned to LDA, the RR for developing preeclampsia was 0.86 (95% CI 0.77–0.97). The reviewers concluded that LDA has small to moderate benefits when used for prevention of preeclampsia and is also safe. Results from a meta-analysis suggested that LDA improves pregnancy outcome in women with persistent increases in uterine Doppler resistance index at both 18 and 24 weeks' gestation.[210] However, in other studies with abnormal Doppler measurements of uterine arteries at 22 to 24 weeks' gestation, LDA after 23 weeks' gestation did not prevent preeclampsia.[211,212] A large, multicenter study including 2539 high-risk women with pregestational insulin-treated diabetes mellitus, chronic hypertension, multifetal

TABLE 35–6

Prevention of Preeclampsia

	PREGNANCY OUTCOME	RECOMMENDATION
Diet and exercise (I)	No reduction in preeclampsia	Insufficient evidence to recommend.*
Protein or salt (II) restriction	No reduction in preeclampsia	Not recommended.
Magnesium or zinc supplementation (I)	No reduction in preeclampsia	Not recommended.*
Fish-oil supplementation and other sources of fatty acids (I)	No effect in low risk or high risk populations	Insufficient evidence to recommend.*
Calcium supplementation (I)	Reduced preeclampsia in those at high risk and with low baseline dietary calcium intake No effect on perinatal outcome	Recommended for women at high risk of gestational hypertension and in communities with low dietary calcium intake.
Low-dose aspirin (I)	19% reduction in risk of preeclampsia, 16% reduction in fetal or neonatal deaths	Consider in high risk populations.
Heparin or low-molecular-weight heparin (III-3)	Reduced preeclampsia in women with renal disease and in women with thrombophilia	Lack of randomized trials, not recommended.
Antioxidant vitamins (C, E) (I)	No reduction in preeclampsia	Number of adverse effects including increased risk of stillbirth and of birth weight < 2.5 kg. Not recommended.
Antihypertensive medications in women with chronic hypertension (I)	Risk of women developing severe hypertension reduced by half, but not risk of preeclampsia	No evidence to recommend for prevention.

* Insufficient evidence = small trials or inconclusive results.
Modified from Sibai B, Dekker G, Kupferminc M: Preeclampsia. Lancet 2005;365:785–799, with permission.

gestation, or preeclampsia in a previous pregnancy showed no beneficial effects from LDA.[31] However, almost all studies on the prevention of preeclampsia so far focus on poor or inconsistent definitions of the disorder and not on actual perinatal outcome.[213] LDA use should be based on individualized risk assessment for preeclampsia.[36,209,214] In translating these results into clinical practice, the underlying risk of preeclampsia in the population being treated must be taken into consideration. If the baseline risk is 8%, treating 114 women will prevent 1 case of preeclampsia. In a population with a 20% risk of preeclampsia, the number needed to treat to prevent 1 case of preeclampsia is 50. In view of this potential benefit, and the relative absence of maternal or neonatal complications, LDA is indicated for the secondary prevention of preeclampsia in women at increased risk. In most cases, LDA may be ceased at 37 weeks' gestation, although continuation beyond this period is not unsafe.[209]

Calcium Supplements

A possible mode of action for calcium supplementation is that it reduces parathyroid and/or renin release, thereby decreasing intracellular calcium, and as such, reducing smooth muscle contractility. Calcium might also have an indirect effect on smooth muscle function by increasing magnesium levels. A theoretical risk of increased renal tract stone formation with calcium has not been substantiated, and no other adverse effects of calcium supplementation have been documented. Twelve clinical studies compared the use of calcium versus no treatment or a placebo in pregnancy.[215] These trials differ in the populations studied (low risk or high risk for hypertensive disorders of pregnancy), study design (randomization, double-blind, or use of a placebo), gestational age at enrollment (20–32 weeks' gestation), sample size in each group (range 22–4151), dose of elemental calcium used (156–2000 mg/day), and definition of hypertensive disorders of pregnancy used. These 12 trials involving 15,206 women were included in a Cochrane review.[215] For women assigned to calcium, the RR for developing preeclampsia was 0.48 (95% CI 0.33–0.69). This systematic review concluded that calcium supplementation reduces the risk of preeclampsia and hypertensive disorders during pregnancy, particularly in populations that have diets deficient in calcium.[215] In contrast, a recent evidence-based review by the U.S. Food and Drug Administration (FDA)[216] concluded that "the relationship between calcium and risk of hypertension in pregnancy is inconsistent and inconclusive, and the relationship between calcium and the risk of pregnancy induced hypertension and preeclampsia is highly unlikely." None of the published randomized trials with calcium supplementation included women with a history of previous preeclampsia; therefore, the benefit of calcium supplementation for recurrent preeclampsia prevention remains unclear.[191] Calcium supplementation has also not been shown to have a significant beneficial effect on fetal and neonatal outcomes including preterm birth, low birth weight, IUGR, stillbirth or death before discharge from hospital.[191,215] The ideal patient to consider calcium supplementation appears to be the obese patient with a mildly elevated booking BP and a low dietary calcium intake.[215]

Other Therapies

Randomized, placebo-controlled trials of antioxidant vitamins C and E failed to demonstrate any significant effect on the incidence of preeclampsia. Of concern, a number of adverse effects were seen including an increased risk of stillbirth and of birth weight less than 2.5 kg, but there were fewer fetal deaths due to immaturity. Prophylactic antioxidant therapy with vitamins C and E is, therefore, not recommended.[217,218]

To date, there are no large randomized trials assessing the effect of heparin with or without aspirin in prevention of preeclampsia. As discussed previously, women with thrombophilias have an increased incidence of preeclampsia, and there has been enthusiasm for prophylactic treatment with anticoagulants, particularly low-molecular-weight heparin, with or without aspirin. Other than in the specific case of antiphospholipid antibody syndrome (for prevention of recurrent pregnancy loss), there is no randomized study to support this practice.[219]

PRENATAL CARE AND GENERAL MANAGEMENT PRINCIPLES

Most patients with a pregnancy-induced hypertensive disorder have no clinical symptoms. So it can be reliably detected only by screening for the early signs and symptoms in the second half of pregnancy. Adequate and proper prenatal care is the most important part of management of preeclampsia.[2,10,61,205] Maternal prenatal monitoring includes identifying women at increased risk, early detection of preeclampsia by recognizing clinical signs and symptoms, and observing progression to the severe form.[2,10,20,61]

The only effective treatment is to deliver the infant and placenta; ancillary therapy is predominantly symptomatic and not directed at underlying causes. Once the diagnosis of preeclampsia is made, subsequent therapy will depend on the results of initial maternal and fetal evaluation. The primary objective of management of preeclampsia must always be the safety of the mother. Although delivery is always appropriate for the mother, it may not be optimal for the fetus that is extremely premature. The decision between delivery and expectant management depends on fetal gestational age, maternal and fetal status at time of initial evaluation, presence of labor or rupture of fetal membranes (Fig. 35–4), and level of available neonatal and maternal services. The proposed management algorithm[1] and the following recommendations are based on observational studies and expert opinion. The individual components have not been subjected to appropriate large prospective, randomized, controlled clinical trials.

In general, women with mild preeclampsia developing at 38 weeks' gestation or longer have a pregnancy outcome similar to that found in normotensive pregnancy. Those patients should undergo induction of labor for delivery.[1,2,9] Induction of labor and/or delivery is also recommended for those at or beyond 34 weeks' gestation in the presence of severe preeclampsia, labor or rupture of membranes, or non–reassuring tests of fetal well-being (see Fig. 35–4) because the mother is at slightly increased risk for development of placental abruption and progression to eclampsia.[2,61] In women who remain undelivered, close maternal and fetal evaluation is essential. The type of test and frequency of evaluation will depend on fetal gestational age as well as severity of maternal condition and presence or absence of IUGR.[2,9,10,61]

EXPECTANT MANAGEMENT OF SEVERE PREECLAMPSIA

The clinical course of severe preeclampsia may be characterized by progressive deterioration in both maternal and fetal conditions.[220] There is universal agreement that such patients be delivered if the disease develops after 34 weeks' gestation.[1,2,9,10,61,220] Delivery is also indicated when there is imminent (persistent severe symptoms) or actual eclampsia, multiorgan dysfunction, severe IUGR, and/or placental abruption with non-reassuring fetal testing before 34 weeks' gestation.[1,2,61,220] There is disagreement, however, about treatment of patients with severe preeclampsia before 34 weeks' gestation in which the maternal condition is stable and the fetal condition is reassuring.[2,220] The Cochrane review on interventionist versus expectant care[221] states that it is not possible to draw firm conclusions, because there are only two small trials (133 women) that have compared a policy of early elective delivery with a policy of delayed delivery, and the CIs for all outcomes are wide. However, the evidence is promising that short-term morbidity for the baby may be reduced by a policy of expectant care.[221–223] A recent review on expected management of severe preeclampsia remote from term concluded that the results of all these studies suggest that expectant treatment in a select group of women with severe preeclampsia between the beginning of the 24th week and 33 weeks' gestation in a suitable hospital is safe and improves neonatal outcome.[224] Most studies on expectant management report 7 to 10 days of prolongation. For gestational age less than 24 weeks, expectant treatment

FIGURE 35–4
Overall management plan of preeclampsia.
(Adapted from Sibai B, Dekker G, Kupferminc M: Preeclampsia. Lancet 2005;365:785-799, with permission.)

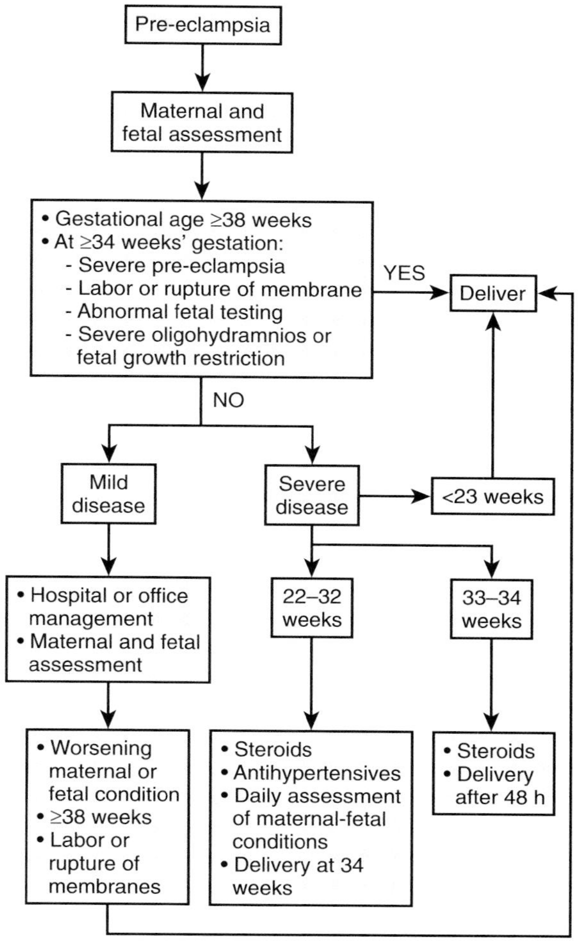

was associated with high maternal morbidity with limited perinatal benefit.[224] Ganzevoort and coworkers[225] studied expectant management in 216 patients presenting with early-onset hypertensive disease (24–34 wk' gestation). In this study, 74% of the women with HELLP syndrome improved after inclusion and had a low risk of major complications, which did not differ from the other inclusion groups. All three inclusion groups (HELLP syndrome, severe preeclampsia, and gestational hypertension combined with IUGR) had a similar rate of major complications, and the median prolongation of pregnancy was of a similar duration. These authors concluded that prolongation of pregnancy in early-onset hypertensive disorders results in the development of further HELLP syndrome episodes and reversible major maternal morbidity but may improve perinatal healthy survival.[225]

If expectant management is undertaken, this should include serial investigation of maternal platelet count, hepatocellular enzymes, and renal function.

ANTIHYPERTENSIVE THERAPY

Although hypertension is only one manifestation of the disease, it is directly related to the cerebral complications.[184,223,226,227] The benefits of acute pharmacologic control of severe hypertension prior to delivery are generally accepted. The more contentious issues are the role of pharmacologic therapy in allowing prolongation of pregnancy and the ability of such therapy to modify the course of the underlying systemic disorder and affect fetal and maternal outcome. Some antihypertensive drugs affect the mother, some the fetus or newborn, some both mother and fetus/neonate.[228] The effects of antihypertensive drugs on the fetus may be indirect, by impairing uteroplacental perfusion, or direct, by influencing the fetal cardiovascular circulation. Although never formerly subjected to randomized, controlled trials, there is consensus that pregnant women with severe hypertension, that is, with diastolic BP values greater than 110 mm Hg, should receive pharmacologic treatment and that the goal in treatment of hypertension in pregnancy is to keep the systolic BP between 140 and 160 mm Hg and the diastolic BP between 90 and 105 mm Hg. Decreasing BP below 130/80 mm Hg is to be avoided. A sudden severe decrease in BP may cause poor uteroplacental perfusion and, therefore, fetal distress.[228,229]

Although the use of antihypertensive agents in women with preeclampsia and severe elevations in BP may prevent cerebrovascular accident, such treatment does not prevent preeclampsia or alter the natural course of the disease in women with mild preeclampsia.[2,230] Use of antihypertensive drugs for mild to moderate hypertension during pregnancy is still controversial. The most recent Cochrane review[231] included 40 studies (3797 women), 24 of which compared an antihypertensive drug with placebo/no antihypertensive drug (2815 women). The risk of developing severe hypertension associated with the use of antihypertensive drugs (17 trials, 2155 women; RR 0.52, 95% CI 0.41–0.64) was halved, but there was no difference in the risk of preeclampsia (19 trials, 2402 women; RR 0.99, 95% CI 0.84–1.18). Similarly, there was no clear effect on the risk of the baby dying (23 trials, 2727 women; RR 0.7, 95% CI 0.46–1.09), preterm birth (12 trials, 1738 women; RR 0.98, 95% CI 0.85–1.13), or small–for–gestational age babies (17 trials, 2159 women; RR 1.13, 95% CI 0.91–1.42). In addition, 17 trials (1182 women) compared one antihypertensive drug with another. There was no clear difference between any of these drugs in the risk of developing severe hypertension and proteinuria/preeclampsia. The reviewers concluded that it remains unclear whether antihypertensive drug therapy for mild to moderate hypertension during pregnancy is worthwhile.[231] A meta-regression of antihypertensive drugs in pregnancy suggested that excessive lowering BP in women with mild disease may increase the risk of a small–for–gestational age baby.[232]

DRUGS FREQUENTLY USED IN THE MANAGEMENT OF PREECLAMPSIA

Methyldopa

Methyldopa lowers BP by reducing overall sympathetic outflow. Methyldopa reduces systemic vascular resistance without causing significant physiologic changes in heart rate or cardiac output.[233] Methyldopa is effective in mild to moderate hypertension, but a fall in arterial BP is achieved only 4 to 8 hrs after an oral dose. As monotherapy, it is not effective in severe hypertension.[233] Although methyldopa when administered to pregnant women with mild or moderate hypertension will reduce the risk of developing severe hypertension, it has no effect on the incidence of proteinuria, IUGR, preterm birth, or cesarean section. Methyldopa is, however, a very well established, useful drug in the management of chronic hypertension in pregnant women.[229–232] The safety of methyldopa during pregnancy in terms of its fetal effects has been followed for longer than 7 years, and no detrimental effects have been observed in exposed offspring.[234]

Hydralazine

During the past decades, intravenous hydralazine has been the drug of choice in the management of severe preeclampsia, given intravenously by continuous infusion or intermittent boluses or by intramuscular or subcutaneous injections. However, up to 50% of patients treated with hydralazine may demonstrate tachycardia, hypotension, palpitations, headache, nausea, vomiting, anxiety, tremors, epigastric pain, and fluid retention,[228] all side effects simulating features of impending eclampsia, and 15% of patients taking high doses of hydralazine daily will develop a lupus-like syndrome after long-lasting administration.[228] More important, hydralazine might cause a too drastic decrease in BP. Such a sudden decrease in BP might adversely affect uteroplacental blood flow and thus cause fetal distress. Fetal distress has been frequently observed with hydralazine infusion. Hydralazine does not inhibit vasoconstrictor responses to noradrenalin, vasopressin, and angiotensin II in human uteroplacental arteries. The uteroplacental vasoconstriction seen with intravenous hydralazine is attributed to increased plasma concentrations of noradrenaline.[228,235,236] The major disadvantages are delayed onset of action, variable peak effect, and fetal distress. Hydralazine is certainly effective, but mainly due to its commonly appearing maternal side effects and the relatively high incidence of overshoot hypotension and subsequent fetal distress, alternate treatments are preferred.[229] Hydralazine is no longer available in many European countries.

Labetalol

Labetalol is a competitive antagonist at β_1- and β_2-adrenoreceptors and has some intrinsic activity at β_2-adrenoreceptors. In addition to its β-blocking action, labetalol has a competitive action at postsynaptic α-adrenoreceptors. It lowers high BP by blocking α_1-adrenoreceptors in peripheral vessels and thereby reducing peripheral resistance, and the heart rate is reduced because of its β-blocking effect. Labetalol has become popular for the treatment of hypertension in pregnancy and preeclampsia. It has been used both intravenously and orally for rapid BP reduction. It effectively decreases maternal BP and, according to some studies, may reduce the occurrence of proteinuria and of fetal or neonatal complications.[237–239] In normotensive pregnancies, a single dose of labetalol does not affect the fetoplacental blood flow.[240]

Diazoxide

Diazoxide, a nondiuretic benzothiadiazine derivative, is a powerful direct vasodilator. Diazoxide also produces a prompt increase in blood glucose. It produces acute BP reduction in patients with severe pregnancy-induced hypertensive disorders. Diazoxide's effects are more rapid and longer lasting than those of hydralazine. Maternal cerebral ischemia, maternal death, and fetal distress following precipitous hypotension have been reported with its use.[241,242] Most units would not use diazoxide for the management of high BP in pregnancy, except in cases of extremely elevated BPs.[228] However, recently, Hennessy and colleagues[243] directly compared the efficacy of mini-bolus diazoxide with intravenous hydralazine; 124 women with severe ante- or postpartum hypertension were randomized to either intravenous hydralazine (5-mg doses) or mini-bolus diazoxide (15-mg doses). Reduction in systolic and diastolic BP was 34 minutes for hydralazine versus 19 minutes for diazoxide ($P < .001$). The mini-bolus doses of 15 mg of diazoxide did not precipitate maternal hypotension as previously described and reduced episodes of persistent severe hypertension compared with results with hydralazine.

Dihydropyridine Derivatives

Calcium antagonists are potent direct vasodilators. Most calcium channel blockers have a rapid onset of action and are effective and safe. Common side effects include severe headache, which can mimic impending eclampsia, hypotension, flushing, and ankle edema. Theoretically, magnesium salts potentiate the hypotensive actions of nifedipine because both drugs have calcium channel functions.[244,245] Indeed, two cases of profound muscle weakness and respiratory arrest have been reportedly associated with the combined use of nifedipine and magnesium.[246,247] However, several leading experts have emphasized that this is a very rare interaction, and this interaction has not been described in any of the randomized trials, including the so-called Magpie trial, in which 29% of patients received this combination.[229,248]

Thus, the five drugs most commonly used for managing severe hypertension in pregnancy all have potentially significant side effects and/or are not always effective in the acute situation or in the management of severe hypertension. In addition, all these drugs are not tailored in any way to the pathophysiology of preeclampsia. According to the Cochrane Database,[249] there is no evidence to justify a strong preference for one of the various drugs discussed so far, although hydralazine is clearly no longer the drug of choice as first-line treatment. Magee and associates[250] reviewed outcomes in randomized, controlled trials comparing hydralazine against other antihypertensives for severe hypertension in pregnancy; 21 trials (893 women), 8 compared hydralazine with nifedipine and 5 with labetalol. Hydralazine was associated with more maternal hypotension (RR 3.29, 95% CI 1.50–7.23), more cesarean sections (RR 1.30, 95% CI 1.08–1.59), more placental abruption (RR 4.17, 95% CI 1.19–14.28), more maternal oliguria (RR 4.00, 95% CI 1.22–12.50), more adverse effects on fetal heart rate (RR 2.04, 95% CI 1.32–3.16), and more low Apgar scores at 1 minute (RR 2.70, 95% CI 1.27–5.88). Hydralazine was also associated with more maternal side effects (RR 1.50, 95% CI 1.16–1.94). The authors concluded that the results are not robust enough to guide clinical practice, but they certainly do not support the use of hydralazine as first-line choice for treatment of severe hypertension in pregnancy.[250]

USE OF CORTICOSTEROIDS TO IMPROVE PREGNANCY OUTCOME IN WOMEN WITH SEVERE PREECLAMPSIA/HELLP SYNDROME

Accelerated fetal lung maturation does not occur in preeclampsia.[220] Infants born to pregnancies complicated by hypertension syndromes treated with corticosteroids have significantly reduced risk of neonatal death, respiratory distress syndrome, and cerebrovascular hemorrhage.[251] There is insufficient evidence to support antenatal corticosteroids for those pregnancies that have reached 34 weeks' gestation.[251] A randomized trial demonstrated a small benefit of antenatal corticosteroids to mothers undergoing a term (37–39 wk' gestation) elective cesarean section.[252]

With the recognition that inflammation plays a key role in the pathophysiology of preeclampsia, it was in itself not surprising to see a series of case-control studies published since the 1990s suggesting that high-dose steroids, mostly dexamethasone, could have a beneficial impact in modulating maternal disease severity, in particular, platelet count and, to a lesser extent, liver transaminases in patients with HELLP syndrome. However, two more recent large studies have demonstrated that the use of high-dose steroids in patients with HELLP syndrome, both antenatally[253] and postpartum,[254] is not associated with a demonstrable improvement in maternal outcome. However, a smaller Dutch trial[255] ($n = 31$) in women at less than 30 weeks' gestation with HELLP syndrome comparing 50 mg of prednisolone with placebo showed contrasting results. Patients in the prednisolone group had a significantly lower risk of a recurrent HELLP exacerbation after the initial crisis had subsided than patients in the placebo group (RR 0.3, 95% CI 0.3–0.9), and platelet counts recovered faster in the prednisolone group than in the placebo group (mean 1.7 days vs. 6.2 days; $P < .01$). The authors concluded that HELLP syndrome remote from term causes a high risk for serious maternal morbidity and mortality (in the placebo group, 1 maternal death occurred as a consequence of liver rupture), but suggested that when expectant management is pursued in selected patients with a HELLP syndrome remote from term, prolonged administration of prednisolone reduces the risk of recurrent HELLP syndrome exacerbations.[255]

PLASMA VOLUME EXPANSION, FLUID BALANCE, AND URINE OUTPUT

The observation that women with severe preeclampsia may have a restricted circulating plasma volume has led to the recommendation that plasma volume should be expanded with either colloid or crystalloid solutions in an effort to improve maternal systemic and uteroplacental circulation.[256] However, intravascular volume expansion carries a risk of volume overload, which might lead to pulmonary or cerebral edema. Also, large volume expansion often requires invasive monitoring of intravascular pressure, procedures carrying risks of their own. A large trial has demonstrated that ongoing plasma volume expansion has no demonstrable maternal and/or perinatal benefits.[257] Administration of fluid at a rate greater than normal requirements should be considered only for (1) women with severe preeclampsia immediately prior to parenteral hydralazine, regional anesthesia, or immediate delivery; or (2) initial management in women with oliguria in whom there is a suspected or confirmed deficit in intravascular volume.[10,258] In established preeclampsia, it is obligatory to monitor daily fluid intake and output. In severe preeclampsia, urine output should be measured on an hourly basis with a urinary catheter. In these patients, kidney function should be assessed at least twice daily. Most patients with acute renal failure (ARF) have a marked decrease in urine flow (<600 mL/24 hr).[258] Total anuria is rare in intrinsic renal failure but, if observed, suggests cortical necrosis as a possible diagnosis, although postrenal (obstructive) failure must always be considered. The initial treatment of ARF in the preeclamptic patient will depend upon the precipitating cause. Restoration of the intravascular volume with appropriate fluids should be carefully monitored to avoid precipitating pulmonary edema. The volume status in such patients can be very difficult to assess, and this is a situation in which central pressure monitoring can be useful. The development of progressive oliguria in preeclampsia despite prudent fluid challenge (≤2000 mL of crystalloid over 2 hr) is an indication for central hemodynamic assessment via a Swan-Ganz catheter.[259] Evidence of hypovolemia in the form of depressed PCWP should be treated with colloid and/or crystalloid infusion to maintain urinary output greater than 30 mL/hr and PCWP below 12 to 16 mm Hg, depending on the colloid osmotic pressure (COP) and clinical situation. Following improvement in urinary output, further fluid management should be directed toward correcting electrolyte and serum osmolarity imbalances. Oliguria in the context of elevated PCWP must be treated only after full assessment of cardiac output and SVR and an evaluation of cardiac function. The latter can be derived by graphing the left ventricular stroke work index versus PCWP. This modified Starling curve can be used to evaluate and subsequently maximize left ventricular function. In the patient with preeclampsia and oliguria with a normal or increased PCWP, increased SVR, and decreased cardiac output, vasodilators might improve renal perfusion. However, if the SVR is normal and the cardiac output is increased, a preload reducer, such as nitroglycerin, may be beneficial.[260]

Meticulous fetal surveillance is required in the context of antepartum preeclampsia-induced oliguria, because uteroplacental blood flow might be compromised. Diuretics are sometimes used to treat the oliguric phase of ATN, but there is no evidence that this will improve the speed of recovery or the eventual outcome.[261,262] Meticulous attention to fluid balance should ensure that urine output is replaced along with insensible losses, blood losses (from delivery), and other losses (diarrhea, vomiting).

PREVENTION OF CONVULSIONS AND CONTROL OF ACUTE CONVULSIONS

The basic principles of management of eclampsia involve (1) maternal support of vital functions; (2) control of convulsions and prevention of recurrent convulsions; (3) correction of maternal hypoxemia and/or acidemia; (4) control of severe hypertension to a safe range; and (5) initiation of the process of delivery. Eclamptic convulsions constitute a life-threatening emergency. During the eclamptic seizure, measures should be taken to prevent maternal injury, such as insertion of a padded tongue blade between the teeth, and to safeguard against potential maternal morbidity after the convulsion. The most urgent parts of the therapy are to assess airway patency, to ensure maternal oxygenation, and to minimize the risk of aspiration. Most eclamptic convulsions resolve in 60 to 90 seconds. Oxygen should be administered during the convulsive episode to improve maternal oxygen concentration and to increase oxygen delivery to the fetus. Eclampsia represents a maternal crisis; a crash cesarean section in an unstable eclamptic patient may result in the birth of a healthy baby but carries tremendous risks for the mother.[226,258] Transient fetal bradycardia lasting at least 3 to 5 minutes is a common finding after an eclamptic seizure and does not necessitate immediate delivery. Resolution of maternal seizure activity is often associated with compensatory fetal tachycardia and even with transient fetal heart rate decelerations that typically resolve within 20 to 30 minutes.[263] Every attempt should be made to stabilize the mother before making a decision about delivery.[226]

Magnesium

A 1995 landmark study compared the efficacy of magnesium sulfate with other anticonvulsants in women with eclampsia. This trial compared magnesium sulfate with diazepam, phenytoin, or a lytic cocktail. This study demonstrated that magnesium sulfate is associated with a significantly lower rate of recurrent seizures and a lower rate of maternal death than that observed with other anticonvulsants.[264] Magnesium is also the drug of choice for seizure prophylaxis in women with preeclampsia. Four large randomized, controlled trials compared the use of magnesium sulfate to prevent convulsions in patients with severe preeclampsia. The overall results of the four trials demonstrate that magnesium sulfate prophylaxis compared with placebo (two trials, 10,795 women), nimodipine (one trial, 1750 women), and no treatment (one trial, 228 women) in severe preeclampsia is associated with a significantly lower rate of eclampsia (RR 0.39, 95% CI 0.28–0.55).[251,265] The largest trial to date, the Magpie trial,[248] enrolled 10,141 women with preeclampsia (largely in the developing countries). Most of the enrolled patients had severe disease, and the rate of eclampsia was significantly lower in those assigned to magnesium sulfate (0.8% vs. 1.9%; RR 0.42, 95% CI 0.29–0.60). However, among the 1560 women enrolled in the western world, the rates of eclampsia were 0.5% in the magnesium group and 0.8% in the placebo, a nonsignificant difference (RR 0.67, 95% CI 1.19–2.37). In addition, two randomized trials compared magnesium sulfate with a placebo in women with mild preeclampsia.[266] The results of these six trials demonstrate no benefit of magnesium sulfate on perinatal outcome and/or serious maternal complications of severe preeclampsia, such as pulmonary edema, stroke, liver, hematoma, or renal failure.[265,266] Available evidence suggests that magnesium sulfate should be given during labor and immediately postpartum in a select group of women with severe preeclampsia because the benefit of magnesium sulfate in women with mild preeclampsia remains unclear. The importance of magnesium sulfate in severe preeclampsia is illustrated by the results of a recent Dutch population-wide study demonstrating that the excess of eclampsia in the Netherlands compared with other Western European countries was found to be related to the fact that patients with classic symptoms of severe preeclampsia did not receive appropriate antihypertensive therapy and magnesium.[267]

Magnesium does not cause any significant maternal-neonatal central nervous system depression when used properly. During its administration, the mother is awake and alert with intact laryngeal reflexes, which helps to protect against aspiration. Fetal magnesium levels tend to equilibrate with maternal levels after prolonged administration; however, neural muscular depression in the newborn is rarely seen with proper use of the drug. In contrast, the use of other anticonvulsants, such as narcotics, sedatives, tranquilizers, and barbiturates, can cause significant maternal-neonatal central nervous system and respiratory depression. The use of these agents may decrease the laryngeal reflexes and allow aspiration.[268,269] As any potent drug, magnesium has significant side effects with the potential for serious magnesium toxicity. Table 35–7 shows the relationship between blood levels of magnesium and symptoms and signs. Magnesium toxicity can be reversed by slow intravenous administration of 10% calcium gluconate and nasal administration of oxygen. If toxicity is not reversed, respirations must be supported until plasma magnesium levels decrease.

FETAL SURVEILLANCE (see also Chapters 10 and 11)

Although fetal surveillance is commonly recommended and performed in women with hypertensive disease in pregnancy,[9,10] there is no consensus on how this should be performed.[2,270] Frequency, intensity, and modality of fetal evaluation will depend on the individual maternal and fetal characteristics. Individual obstetric units should devise their own protocols for monitoring the fetus in pregnancies complicated by hypertension. In compiling such protocols, the following issues should be considered[9,10]:

- Accurate dating of pregnancy is important for women at high risk of preeclampsia.
- Symphysis–to–fundal height measurement is a poor screening tool for detection of IUGR.[271] Therefore, ultrasound should be performed by an experienced operator to assess fetal size, amniotic fluid volume, and umbilical artery Doppler flows in such women. Assessing growth trends by serial ultrasound is recommended if pregnancy continues.
- Umbilical artery Doppler flow is the only fetal surveillance modality that has been shown by systematic review to reduce the need for fetal interventions, improve neonatal outcome, and predict adverse perinatal outcome.[272,273] Severe early-onset IUGR should be monitored at institutions experienced in advanced fetal Doppler waveform analysis. Absent or reversed end-diastolic flow is unlikely to occur within 7 to 10 days after a normal umbilical artery Doppler waveform analysis. Umbilical artery Doppler flow studies have limited value after 36 weeks' gestation.
- Although numerous observational studies have suggested improved outcome in high risk pregnancies monitored using protocols that included biophysical profile, cardiotocography, and combinations of both,[274–276] none of these has shown significant benefit in systematic reviews.[277,278] No fetal testing can predict an acute obstetric event such as placental abruption or cord accident. In practice, many use a comprehensive approach to fetal assessment employing several monitoring modalities.
- Fetal surveillance via a day assessment unit is associated with good perinatal outcome in women with various obstetric complications, including women with well-controlled hypertension.[279]
- An appropriately grown fetus in the third trimester in women with well-controlled chronic hypertension without superimposed preeclampsia is generally associated with a good perinatal outcome. Fetal monitoring using methods other than continued surveillance of fetal growth, umbilical artery blood flow, and amniotic fluid volume in the third trimester is unlikely to be more successful in preventing perinatal mortality/morbidity.

Table 35–8 demonstrates one example of commonly used international and national protocols for fetal surveillance in women with hypertensive disease in pregnancy in whom immediate delivery is deferred. However, none of these protocols has been tested in prospective, randomized trials.[10] Because preeclampsia is an ever-changing and unpredictable disease, for those women in whom expectant management is employed, the frequency and modality of fetal surveillance should be adjusted based on the current maternal and/or fetal condition. Each obstetric unit should develop an agreed institutional approach to fetal surveillance and/or fetal medicine referral.[10]

Early-onset preeclampsia with IUGR still represents a major obstetric dilemma. How IUGR progresses is determined by when it starts and how it starts, that is, gestational age and degree of umbilical artery abnormality at onset. In patients presenting much before 30 weeks, a pattern of worsening umbilical artery Doppler established in the first 7 to 10 days reliably predicts progression to venous Doppler

TABLE 35–7

Magnesium Sulfate Blood Levels

BLOOD LEVELS (MG/DL)	SYMPTOMS AND SIGNS
4–8	Therapeutic
9–12	Nausea, warmth, flushing, somnolence, double vision, slurred speech, weakness, loss of patellar reflexes
15–17	Muscular paralysis and respiratory arrest
30–35	Cardiac arrest

TABLE 35-8

Protocol for Fetal Surveillance in Women with Hypertension in Pregnancy

HYPERTENSION	MODALITY	FREQUENCY
Chronic hypertension	Early dating ultrasound	First trimester
	Ultrasound for fetal growth/AFV/UAD	As per clinical assessment
Gestational hypertension	Ultrasound for fetal growth/AFV/UAD	At time of diagnosis and every 3-4 wk
Preeclampsia	Ultrasound for fetal growth/AFV/UAD	At time of diagnosis and every 2-3 wk
	Cardiotocography	Twice weekly
Preeclampsia with IUGR	Cardiotocography	Twice weekly
	AFV/UAD	On admission and twice weekly
	Ultrasound for fetal growth	Every 2 wk

AFV, amniotic fluid volume; IUGR, intrauterine growth restriction; UAD, umbilical artery Doppler.
From Vatten LJ, Skjaerven R: Is preeclampsia more than one disease? BJOG 2004;111:298–302.

abnormalities and very early intervention (severe early-onset placental dysfunction). In those presenting closer to 30 weeks with decreased (but still present) umbilical artery end-diastolic velocity, Doppler progression is also typically forecast within the first 2 weeks of monitoring and falls into one of two patterns. If initial Doppler abnormalities have not worsened in that first interval, they are unlikely to do so, and abnormalities remain confined to umbilical and mild cerebral changes. These fetuses do not develop venous Doppler abnormalities and are likely to deliver near term (mild placental dysfunction). If the first few weeks of monitoring show progressive elevation of umbilical artery Doppler indices, progression to abnormal venous Doppler findings and preterm delivery become more likely (progressive placental dysfunction).[280] These fetuses require antenatal testing using multiple surveillance modalities to enhance prediction of birth pH. The incorporation of venous Doppler achieves the best prediction of acidemia. Although computerized analysis enhances fetal heart rate assessment, it has limitations as a stand-alone test in IUGR. Computerized cardiotocography performs best when combined with venous Doppler or as a substitute for the traditional nonstress test in the biophysical profile score.[280]

Labor and Delivery

All women with preeclampsia should receive continuous monitoring of fetal heart rate and uterine activity with special attention to avoiding hyperstimulation and development of vaginal bleeding during labor. The presence of uterine irritability and/or recurrent variable or late decelerations may be the first sign of abruptio placentae in these women. All women with severe preeclampsia should have BP recordings at least every hour during labor, and control of BP should be continued. Maternal pain relief during labor and delivery can be provided by either systemic opioids or segmental epidural anesthesia. Epidural anesthesia is safe in women with severe preeclampsia and may assist in BP stabilization. Regional anesthesia is contraindicated in the presence of coagulopathy or severe thrombocytopenia (platelet count < 50,000 μL^{-1}).[61] A plan for vaginal delivery should be considered in all women with severe disease, particularly those beyond 30 weeks' gestation.[1,2,61] The decision to perform cesarean delivery should be based on fetal gestational age, fetal condition, presence of labor, and cervical Bishop score. In general, the presence of severe preeclampsia is not an indication for cesarean delivery. A common policy is to recommend elective cesarean delivery for all women with severe preeclampsia below 30 weeks' gestation who are not in labor in the presence of an unfavorable Bishop score.[281] In the management of the third stage, oxytocin is allowed, whereas ergometrin is contraindicated because of the risk of provoking a hypertensive crisis and cerebral vasospasm.

Postnatal

POSTPARTUM PREECLAMPSIA

In general, preeclampsia is cured by delivery of the placenta; however, it is common for the disease to worsen during the first 48 hours after delivery. Postpartum preeclamptic women are at risk for pulmonary edema, ARF, HELLP syndrome, postpartum eclampsia, and stroke. Therefore, women with diagnosed hypertension and/or preeclampsia require very close monitoring of BP, maternal symptoms, and measurements of fluid intake and urine output as well as laboratory parameters.[1,2,19] Severe hypertension or preeclampsia may develop for the first time in the postpartum period. Hence, postpartum women should be educated about signs and symptoms of preeclampsia. Women who report persistent severe headaches, visual changes, epigastric pain with nausea or vomiting, or respiratory symptoms require immediate evaluation and potential hospitalization.[282,283]

Seizure prophylaxis and antihypertensive medication should continue after delivery, the duration being determined by the clinical and laboratory status. All commonly used antihypertensive drugs, including labetalol, methyldopa, nifedipine, and captopril, are compatible with lactation, based on their pharmacology and low detectable drug levels in breast milk.[229]

Following severe preeclampsia, women will need appropriate counseling and debriefing about their disease and management. In many countries, it is routine practice to test women with early-onset preeclampsia (<32 wk' gestation), in particular those with major placental vasculopathy for underlying disorders such as antiphospholipid syndrome and thrombophilias.

THROMBOPROPHYLAXIS

Preeclampsia is a risk factor for thrombosis, particularly in case of nephritic-range proteinuria or likely inpatient stay more than a few days.[284] When women are admitted for observation in the hospital, they will usually be relatively immobile, and graduated compression stockings should be considered, with or without prophylactic low-molecular-weight heparin. With regard to thromboprophylaxis, the postpartum preeclamptic patient needs to be recognized and treated as a high risk patient; that is, in case of cesarean section, postpartum thromboprophylaxis should be administered to all women with preeclampsia except where there is a surgical contraindication.[285,286] Units should have clear protocols to deal with timing of low-molecular-weight heparin administration in regard to insertion and withdrawal of epidural and spinal cannulae.[285,286]

SUMMARY OF MANAGEMENT OPTIONS
Preeclampsia

Management Options	Evidence Quality and Recommendation	References
Prepregnancy		
Advise early prenatal care.	—/GPP	—
Control diabetes prepregnancy.	IIa/B	191
Control hypertension prepregnancy.	IIa/B	191
Provide advice on good nutrition for those at risk.	—/GPP	—
Advise weight reduction.	—/GPP	—
Supplement B vitamins.	III/B	189,190
Sexual relationship for > 8 mo (not a pragmatic management option).	IIa/B	55,56
Prenatal—Prediction of Preeclampsia		
Counsel on increased risk and vigilance in patients with chronic hypertension, renal disease, connective tissue disorder, diabetes mellitus, previous preeclampsia, positive family history, obesity.	Ia/A	186,191
Abnormal uterine Doppler flow velocity waveforms at 20 wk' gestation are associated with three- to sixfold increase in rate of preeclampsia; poor prediction from clinical and biochemical markers.	Ia/A	185,204,205
Prenatal—Prevention of Preeclampsia		
Calcium supplementation results in a modest reduction in risk and severity in patients with a low dietary calcium intake.	Ia/A	215
Low-dose aspirin reduces risk in women at high risk for preeclampsia.	Ia/A	209,214
Supplementation with vitamin E and C does not reduce the risk for preeclampsia.	Ia/A	217,218
Antihypertensives for mild to moderate hypertension prevent severe hypertension but have no effect on overall maternal and perinatal outcome.	Ia/A	228,229,231
Excessive lowering of blood pressure in women with mild disease may increase the risk of a small–for–gestational age baby.	Ia/A	232
Prenatal—Management		
Mild gestational hypertension without IUGR can be managed expectantly up to 40 wk' gestation.	IV/C	2,9,27
Diagnosis of preeclampsia at term mandates delivery.	IV/C	2,9
Severe preeclampsia at ≥ 34 wk' gestation mandates delivery.	IV/C	1,2,9,10,61
Preeclampsia remote from term (24–33 completed wk) can be managed conservatively with fetal surveillance and monitoring for disease progression.	Ib/A	221,224,225
Management of severe early-onset preeclampsia is best accomplished in a tertiary setting with adult and neonatal intensive care facilities.	—/GPP	—
Principles of Expectant Management		
• Reduce blood pressure (main aim is prevention of cerebral vascular accident).	—/GPP	—
• Prevent convulsions with $MgSO_4$	Ia/A	265,266
• Use IV fluids carefully to avoid fluid overload; there is no maternal and/or perinatal benefit associated with ongoing plasma volume expansion.	Ib/A	257

SUMMARY OF MANAGEMENT OPTIONS
Preeclampsia—cont'd

Management Options	Evidence Quality and Recommendation	References
Laboratory Studies during Expectant Management		
• Platelet count.	—/GPP	—
• AST, ALT, LDH, creatinine.		
• Clotting studies not required in preeclampsia not associated with drop in platelets; D-dimer (not INR and aPTT) useful in detecting early stages DIC.		
• A spot urine protein-to-creatinine ratio is the preferred way to screen for protein when compared with dipstick; 24-hr urine collection for protein and creatinine remains the gold standard.	Ia/A	16–18
Eclampsia Management		
Resuscitate, maintain airway, give oxygen, nurse semiprone.	—/GPP	—
Control and prevent further convulsions with $MgSO_4$; a loading dose of 4 g should be given by infusion pump over 5–10 min, followed by further infusion of 1 g/hr.	Ia/A	264
Recurrent seizures should be treated with either a further bolus of 2 g $MgSO_4$ or an increase in the infusion rate to 2 g/hr	Ia/A	264
Control blood pressure.	III/B	266,267
Check platelet count, renal function, liver enzymes, D-dimer.	—/GPP	—
Deliver when stable.	—/GPP	—
Mode of delivery based on obstetric indications.	—/GPP	—
Maintain high-dependency for 24–48 hr.	—/GPP	—
Maintain $MgSO_4$ for at least 24–48 hr, based on maternal assessment.	—/GPP	—
Fetal Assessment during Expectant Management (See also Chapters 10 and 11)		
Umbilical artery Doppler reduces need for fetal interventions, improves neonatal outcome, and predicts adverse perinatal outcome.	Ia/A	272
• Fetal heart rate monitoring (indicative of more immediate fetal health) is undertaken frequently	—/GPP	—
• US documentation of fetal growth at a minimum interval of every 2 wk.	—/GPP	—
• Growth-restricted fetuses with placental insufficiency require antenatal testing using multiple surveillance modalities to enhance prediction of birth pH.	IIa/B	280
Maternal Steroids		
Steroids for fetal lung maturation if indicated preterm delivery is anticipated.	Ia/A	252
Labor and Delivery		
Cesarean section for obstetric reasons, not for preeclampsia per se.	—/GPP	—
Epidural.	IV/C	296
Intravenous antihypertensive drugs in case of severe hypertension.	—/GPP	—
Select antihypertensive agent on basis of local expertise and drug availability.	Ia/A	250
Hydralazine is no longer first choice.	Ib/A	243
Mini-bolus diazoxide (15 mg) is at least as effective as intravenous hydralazine and blood pressure control is achieved more quickly.		

Management Options	Evidence Quality and Recommendation	References
Postnatal		
Clinicians should be aware that ≤ 44% of eclampsia occurs postpartum, especially at term, so women with signs and symptoms compatible with preeclampsia should be carefully assessed.	—/GPP	—
Continue seizure prophylaxis for 24 hr postpartum.	—/GPP	—
In patients with severe disease, close monitoring (neurologic status, renal and pulmonary function, liver enzymes, and hemostasis) and seizure prophylaxis continue for 2–4 days until disease resolves; close fluid balance with charting of input and output is essential. A catheter with an hourly urometer is advisable in the acute situation.	—/GPP	—
Steroids have no beneficial effects on recovery in case of post-partum HELLP.	Ia/A	253,254
Patients who require antihypertensive medication at discharge should remain under surveillance.	—/GPP	—
Women with persisting hypertension and/or proteinuria at 6 wk may have renal disease and require further investigation.	—/GPP	—
Even those with severe disease whose blood pressure settles are at increased risk for hypertension and other cardiovascular disorders in later life and regular review is prudent.	—/GPP	—
Women whose pregnancies have been complicated by severe disease should be offered a formal postnatal review to discuss the events of the pregnancy.	—/GPP	—
Preconceptional counseling should be offered in which the events that occurred, any risk factors, and any preventive strategies can be discussed.	—/GPP	—
Women with a history of severe early-onset preeclampsia, especially if associated with IUGR or late fetal loss, should be screened for antiphospholid syndrome and may be tested for other thrombophilias, but the implications for future pregnancies have yet to be determined.	IIa/B	33,34,120–125

ALT, alanine aminotransferase; aPTT, activated partial thromboplastin time; AST, aspartate aminotransferase; DIC, disseminated intravascular coagulation; GPP, good practice point; HELLP, hemolysis, elevated liver enzymes, and low platelets; INR, International Normalized Ratio; IUGR, intrauterine growth restriction; LDH, lactate dehydrogenase; US, ultrasound.

CHRONIC HYPERTENSION

Introduction and Maternal and Fetal Risks

Depending on the population studied and the criteria used, the incidence of chronic hypertension in pregnancy is 0.5% to 3%. Essential hypertension is responsible for 90% of cases of chronic hypertension associated with pregnancy. Causes of secondary hypertension include renal disease (glomerulonephritis, nephropathy, renovascular disease), endocrinologic disorders (diabetes with vascular involvement, thyrotoxicosis, pheochromocytoma), and collagen vascular disease (systemic lupus erythematosus, scleroderma).[287,288] Chronic hypertension in pregnancy may be subclassified into mild hypertension (diastolic BP ≥ 90 to < 110 mm Hg or systolic BP ≥ 140 to < 180 mm Hg) or severe hypertension (diastolic BP ≥ 110 mm Hg or systolic BP ≥ 180 mm Hg).[287,288] For the purpose of clinical management, chronic hypertension in pregnancy may also be divided into a low risk group (hypertension with no end-organ damage or associated significant comorbidities) or a high risk group (hypertension with end-organ damage or associated morbidities). Maternal and perinatal morbidity and mortality rates are not generally increased for patients with uncomplicated mild chronic hypertension. However, the risks to mother and fetus increase dramatically when the pregnancy is complicated by severe disease or superimposed preeclampsia. Other risk factors include maternal age older than 40 years, hypertension lasting longer than 15 years, BP greater than 160/110 mm Hg early in pregnancy, diabetes classes B through F, renal disease, cardiomyopathy, connective tissue disease, and coarctation of the aorta.[26] Maternal risks include exacerbation of hypertension, superimposed preeclampsia, congestive heart failure, intracerebral hemorrhage, ARF, placental abruption with DIC, and death as a result of any of these. Superimposed preeclampsia and abruptio placentae are the two most common complications. Superimposed preeclampsia complicates approximately 5% to 50% of pregnancies of women with chronic hypertension, depending on whether the diagnosis of preeclampsia was made simply on the basis of exacerbation of hypertension or whether significant proteinuria was included. In patients with risk factors, the incidence of superimposed preeclampsia is 25% to 50%. The incidence of placental abruption is 0.5% to 2% in patients with mild, uncomplicated hypertension and 3% to 10% in those with severe hypertension. The incidence of superimposed preeclampsia or abruption is not affected by antihypertensives.[26,191] Fetal morbidity and mortality rates are directly related to the severity of hypertension. They are particularly high in patients with superimposed preeclampsia and abruptio placentae. Decreased uteroplacental perfusion (often iatrogenic) can lead to IUGR. Spontaneous or iathrogenic preterm birth adds the compounding complications of prematurity. The risk of mid-trimester death in utero is higher in patients with chronic hypertension, especially those who do not receive prenatal care.[26,191,288]

Management Options

Prepregnancy

Women with chronic hypertension who desire pregnancy should be encouraged to receive prepregnancy care. The cause and severity of chronic hypertension should be established, if possible. Antihypertensives with potential adverse effects on the fetus, such as angiotensin-converting enzyme (ACE) inhibitors and diuretics, should be discontinued and switched to preparations with a strong safety record in pregnancy. These changes should be under physician supervision. Adequate time must be allowed preconceptionally to gauge the patient's response to new medications to control hypertension.[287]

Prenatal

The woman with chronic hypertension should be observed frequently during pregnancy by an obstetrician and/or physician familiar with the management of hypertension in pregnancy. During the initial visits, a detailed evaluation of the etiology and severity of chronic hypertension should be made. Careful attention must be given to a history of cardiac or renal disease, diabetes, or thyroid disease and to the outcome of previous pregnancies. A detailed history, physical examination, and appropriate laboratory and cardiac testing are essential in seeking a possible cause for hypertension and to ascertain end-organ damage if present. A pragmatic baseline evaluation and laboratory studies in pregnant patients with chronic hypertension are presented in Table 35–9.[10]

Because women with chronic hypertension are at high risk of developing preeclampsia, close monitoring for its maternal and fetal manifestations is necessary. In addition to standard prenatal care, the following additional monitoring is indicated: (1) monitoring for signs of superimposed preeclampsia after 20 weeks' gestation; (2) assessment for proteinuria using a spot urine protein-to-creatinine ratio at every visit; (3) laboratory assessment (see Table 35–9) if worsening hypertension or proteinuria; and (4) assessment of fetal growth and well-being (see Table 35–8).

Admission to a hospital or day assessment unit is recommended for women with worsening hypertension or proteinuria at any stage of pregnancy. This enables assessment of maternal and fetal welfare and facilitates discussion among all involved in the woman's care. When necessary, pharmacologic treatment may be commenced or revised under close supervision. Women who are at low risk (those with mild, chronic hypertension and none of the just-discussed risk factors) should be seen every 2 to 4 weeks in the first two trimesters, and then weekly. In pregnant patients with low risk chronic hypertension, Sibai and coworkers[26,191] recommend discontinuation of all antihypertensives at the first prenatal visit. Only half require subsequent medication; treatment of patients who need antihypertensives can be tailored to their individual needs. If there is no superimposed preeclampsia and fetal well-being is well documented, routine induction of labor before 40 weeks' gestation probably is not warranted.

Pregnancy in women with hypertension and additional risk factors should be managed in consultation with appropriate specialists (e.g., maternal-fetal medicine, cardiology, nephrology). Close monitoring is essential, and multiple hospitalizations may be necessary to control maternal hypertension and associated medical complications. Severe hypertension mandates an aggressive pharmacologic approach. Carefully selected antihypertensives may benefit those with mild hypertension who have additional complicating factors, such as diabetes, renal disease, or cardiac dysfunction. Intensive fetal surveillance is critical to optimize fetal outcome. Serial ultrasonography for fetal growth and weekly (or more frequent, depending on the fetal condition) antepartum fetal testing, beginning as early as 26 weeks, should be used.[26,191] The pregnancy may be continued until term, until the onset of superimposed preeclampsia, or until IUGR or other signs of fetal decompensation occur. The development of severe, superimposed preeclampsia places the patient at highest risk for maternal and perinatal complications. This development after 28 weeks is an indication for delivery. Before 28 weeks, the pregnancy may be followed conservatively in a tertiary center with daily evaluation of the maternal and fetal condition, although this approach is controversial.[26]

TABLE 35–9

Investigation of Hypertension Presenting prior to 20 Weeks' Gestation

All Patients

Establish baseline level of proteinuria; a spot urine-to-creatinine ratio is an acceptable screening method, although many clinicians still favor a 24-hr urinary protein collection to get a reliable baseline.

Microscopy of centrifuged urinary sediment for white and red blood cells (including red cell morphology) and for casts.

Midstream urine culture.

Measurement of serum electrolytes, creatinine, uric acid, and blood glucose.

Full blood examination.

Selected Patients

Electrocardiogram.

Renal ultrasound should be considered, particularly if hypertension is severe.

Fasting free plasma metanephrines or 24-hr urine collection for estimation of catecholamine excretion if there is concern regarding a possible pheochromocytoma. At least two consecutive collections are advised.

ANTIHYPERTENSIVE THERAPY

The continued administration or initiation of antihypertensive therapy in women with chronic hypertension in pregnancy (except for the acute treatment of severe hypertension) remains controversial. Most women manifest a physiologic fall in BP in the first half of pregnancy that may allow withdrawal or a reduction of antihypertensive medication.[26,191] Although treatment of chronic hypertension is associated with a significant reduction in severe hypertension, it has not been shown to alter the risk of superimposed preeclampsia, preterm delivery, placental abruption, or perinatal death.[26,191,287,288] There is insufficient evidence upon which to base a definite recommendation for the levels of BP at which antihypertensive drug treatment should commence.

There are no randomized trials of the treatment of severe chronic hypertension during pregnancy. However, the general consensus is that when diastolic BP reaches 110 mm Hg, it clearly requires treatment to prevent cerebrovascular accident, the largest cause of maternal death in patients with hypertension. The current Australian and New Zealand recommendation is that such treatment should definitely be started when the BP consistently reaches or exceeds 160 mm Hg systolic and/or 100 mm Hg diastolic.[10] Treatment at BPs between 140 and 160 mm Hg systolic and/or 90 and 100 mm Hg diastolic is also common practice, with good documented outcomes but certainly not based on randomized, controlled trials.[26] In patients with target organ damage, it has been recommended to keep systolic BP below 140 mm Hg and diastolic BP below 90 mm Hg.

Overzealous treatment of mild hypertension has been found to be associated with a significant increase in small–for–gestational age infants, today, a major concern because of the more recent insights in the fetal origins of adult disease. Large international trials (CHIPS) are currently in progress to finally get an answer on what BPs require treatment and, just as important, what should be the target BP to be achieved.[229,230,289]

In the third trimester of pregnancy, an increase in the requirement for antihypertensive therapy should be anticipated. The drugs used for treatment of chronic hypertension are the same as those recommended for preeclampsia and gestational hypertension. Atenolol and other highly selective β-blocker drugs are not recommended for prolonged use in pregnancy because they have been associated with IUGR.[290–292] The use of ACE inhibitors and angiotensin-receptor blockers is contraindicated in pregnancy. They have been associated with an increased risk of fetal, particularly cardiovascular, malformations in early pregnancy in one study and are known to cause adverse sequelae for the fetus in late pregnancy.[293] Diuretics, although not teratogenic, may restrict the natural plasma volume expansion of pregnancy and are not recommended for the treatment of hypertension. Management of superimposed preeclampsia should be as outlined previously for preeclampsia unless specific diagnostic issues, such as some secondary causes of hypertension, are present.

Labor and Delivery

Intrapartum management of patients with severe chronic hypertension or in patients with superimposed preeclampsia is similar to the intrapartum management of preeclamptic patients, that is, continuous fetal monitoring, appropriate analgesia, and appropriate use of antihypertensive drugs to keep the BP below 160/110 mm Hg.

Postnatal

High risk patients with chronic hypertension should be monitored closely for at least 48 hours after delivery because they are at risk for hypertensive encephalopathy, pulmonary edema, and renal failure. In many women with chronic hypertension or superimposed preeclampsia, BP is unstable for 1 to 2 weeks after delivery and may be difficult to control. It may be particularly high on days 3 to 6 after delivery, and it is often necessary to increase or commence antihypertensive medication at that time. Oral or intravenous labetalol or hydralazine, ACE inhibitors, methyldopa, or calcium channel blockers can be used to control severe hypertension. Diuretic therapy is used in patients with evidence of circulatory congestion or pulmonary edema. These women must be evaluated after the postpartum period to detect deterioration in cardiac or renal function and to adjust antihypertensive medication. Minute amounts of all antihypertensives are found in breast milk. All of the agents mentioned earlier are compatible with breast-feeding, as are the ACE inhibitors enalapril, captopril, and quinapril. However, thiazide diuretics inhibit adequate breast milk production.[229]

SUMMARY OF MANAGEMENT OPTIONS

Chronic Hypertension

Management Options	Evidence Quality and Recommendation	References
Prepregnancy		
Establish the cause and severity of hypertension.	—/GPP	—
Evaluate renal function.	—/GPP	—
In those with mild to moderate hypertension, stop medication or switch to medication with few fetal side effects.	—/GPP	—
In those with severe or difficult-to-control hypertension, medication may be needed despite the potential fetal risks.	—/GPP	—
Encourage early prenatal care in an appropriate setting.	—/GPP	—

SUMMARY OF MANAGEMENT OPTIONS

Chronic Hypertension—cont'd

Management Options	Evidence Quality and Recommendation	References
Prenatal		
Provide early and frequent prenatal care.	IV/C	26,287,288
Discontinue antihypertensive medication unless maternal diastolic pressure > 100–110 mm Hg.	Ia/A	26,231
Use oral medication in severe hypertension (methyldopa, calcium channel blockers, labetalol) and in those with mild hypertension complicated by risk factors.	Ia/A	231,229,287
Laboratory studies:	—/GPP	—
• Establish baseline level of proteinuria.		
• Baseline serum electrolytes, creatinine, urate, and glucose.		
Fetal surveillance with serial ultrasound		
• Obtain early dating scan.	—/GPP	—
• Start with serial ultrasound for fetal growth, amniotic fluid, and umbilical artery Doppler at 26 wk in women with severe hypertension or mild hypertension with risk factors.	IV/C	10,26
Maintain vigilance for superimposed preeclampsia	IV/C	10,26
Labor and Delivery		
Continuous electronic fetal monitoring.	IV/C	10,26
Use antihypertensives to maintain blood pressure < 160/110 mm Hg.	IV/C	26,230
Postnatal		
Monitor closely in the first 48 hr to anticipate hypertensive encephalopathy, pulmonary edema, or renal failure.	IV/C	26,230
Most antihypertensive drugs are safe during lactation; avoid thiazide diuretics.	III/B	229

GPP, good practice point.

ANESTHETIC CONSIDERATIONS IN HYPERTENSIVE DISORDERS OF PREGNANCY

Whenever possible, an anesthetist should be informed about a woman with severe preeclampsia well in advance of labor or operative delivery to plan appropriate anesthetic management. This is associated with a reduction in both fetal and maternal morbidity.[294] Relevant issues include anesthetic risk assessment, BP control, fluid management, eclampsia prophylaxis, and planning of analgesia or anesthesia.[10,268,295–298]

Risk Assessment

Anesthetists/intensivists form an integral part of the team responsible for the critically sick preeclamptic patient. Women who develop organ failure require intensive monitoring and medical management, within either a high dependency or an intensive care setting. Antenatal and (more commonly) postpartum indications for admission of a patient with severe preeclampsia to an intensive therapy unit include pulmonary edema, intractable hypertension, anuria or renal failure, repeated convulsions, DIC, neurologic impairment requiring ventilation (e.g., intracerebral hemorrhage or infarction, cerebral edema), and critical intra-abdominal pathology (e.g., acute fatty liver; subcapsular liver hematoma).[268,295,296]

Fluid Management

Fluid management is a challenging area in preeclampsia, and there is no clear evidence regarding optimal type or volume of fluid.[296,297] Fluid therapy aims to maintain organ perfusion in the setting of vasoconstriction, endothelial dysfunction, and in some parturients, severe left ventricular diastolic dysfunction. Intravenous fluid should be administered incrementally in small volumes (e.g., crystalloid 250 mL) with monitoring of maternal hemodynamics, urine output, and fetal heart rate, because overhydration contributes to maternal mortality from pulmonary edema and adult respiratory distress syndrome.[226] Fluid loading is not mandatory prior to regional analgesia during labor when low-dose local anesthetic and opioid methods are used.[298] Prior to regional anesthesia, intravenous crystalloid loading is ineffective in preventing hypotension but colloid is effective.[299] Treatment or prevention of hypotension with drugs such as phenylephrine or metaraminol is effective and appears safe in preeclamptic women.[300,301]

Anesthetic Technique for Vaginal Delivery

For labor and delivery, epidural analgesia is a useful adjunct to antihypertensive therapy and improves renal and uteroplacental blood flow. When relatively contraindicated (e.g., severe thrombocytopenia, coagulopathy, or sepsis), fentanyl or remifentanil patient-controlled intravenous analgesia is preferred. Although ephedrine usually does not cause rebound hypertension, occasionally vasopressors and epidural adrenaline (epinephrine) cause significant BP elevation. Other drugs that should be avoided in severe preeclampsia include ergometrin,[226] ketamine (hypertension), and the nonsteroidal anti-inflammatory drugs and cyclooxygenase-2–specific inhibitors (impaired renal function and hypertension).[10,268,300,301]

Anesthetic Technique for Cesarean Section

Unhurried preoperative preparation reduces the risk of anesthesia in women with preeclampsia.[226] Regional anesthesia is preferred to general anesthesia for cesarean section, especially because airway problems including laryngeal edema may be increased.[302–304] However, well-conducted general anesthesia is also suitable[305,306] and may be indicated in the presence of severe fetal compromise, pulmonary edema, hemodynamic instability, intraspinal hematoma risk (e.g., placental abruption, severe thrombocytopenia), or after eclampsia in which altered consciousness or neurologic deficit persists. Emergency cesarean section confers increased maternal morbidity, so early anesthetic notification by the obstetrician and in utero resuscitation provide additional time for assessment, planning, and establishment of regional anesthesia. When a well-functioning epidural catheter is in situ, general anesthesia is achieved only marginally more rapidly than conversion to epidural anesthesia.[307,308] Prophylaxis against pulmonary aspiration is recommended using clear antacid and ranitidine, with or without metoclopramide. Skilled anesthetic assistance is mandatory, as is left lateral tilt on a pelvic displacement wedge or table tilt to minimize aortocaval compression.

Attenuation of Pressor Responses at General Anesthesia for Cesarean Section

Laryngoscopy and tracheal intubation present a particularly dangerous time for the preeclamptic woman, especially if the intracranial pressure is elevated or the BP is inadequately controlled.[226] The transient but severe hypertension that usually accompanies intubation can cause myocardial ischemia, cerebral hemorrhage, or pulmonary edema, all important causes of maternal death.[226] Attenuation of this pressor response is best achieved with additional induction drugs such as remifentanil 1 μg/kg,[309,310] or $MgSO_4$ 40 mg/kg or 30 mg/kg with alfentanil 7.5 μg/kg.[311] Neuromuscular block must always be monitored closely after intravenous magnesium administration.[312]

Regional Anesthesia for Cesarean Section and Preeclampsia

All regional anesthetic techniques (spinal, epidural, or combined spinal-epidural) appear safe, provided meticulous attention is paid to fluid management, preventing aortocaval compression, and dealing with hypotension.[268,296,306] Spinal anesthesia with usual doses is now a recommended technique.[313,314] Cardiac output is well maintained and is associated with less hypotension and lower vasopressor requirements than among healthy parturients.[315] Combined spinal-epidural anesthesia appears to offer further advantages in specific cases. Low-dose aspirin therapy is not a contraindication to regional techniques that, in the absence of bleeding, are considered safe when the platelet count is greater than 75000 μL^{-1}. Platelet counts lower than 50.000 μL^{-1} are generally considered a contraindication. Within the range of 50 to 75,000 μL^{-1}, an individual assessment (considering patient risks; coagulation tests and thermoelastography or platelet function if available) and risk reduction strategies (experienced operator; single-shot spinal anesthesia or flexible-tip epidural catheter) is encouraged.[316]

SUMMARY OF MANAGEMENT OPTIONS

Anesthetic Considerations in Hypertensive Disorders of Pregnancy

Management Options	Evidence Quality and Recommendation	References
• Early involvement of the anesthesist in the management of all patients with severe preeclampsia.	—/GPP	—
• Treatment or prevention of regional block induced hypotension with drugs such as phenylephrine or metaraminol is effective and appears safe in preeclamptic women.	III/C	10,268,301
• Drugs to avoid include ergometrin, ketamine, and NSAIDs.	III/C	10,226
• Epidural analgesia is a useful adjunct to antihypertensive therapy.	Ia/A	268,296,298
• Close monitoring of neuromuscular block is required in patient also receiving $MgSO_4$. Prevent convulsions with $MgSO_4$.	—/GPP	
• Low-dose aspirin is not a contraindication to regional techniques.	Ia/A	31,316

GPP, good practice point; NSAIDs, nonsteroidal anti-inflammatory drugs.

LONG-TERM CONSEQUENCES OF HYPERTENSIVE DISORDERS OF PREGNANCY

Women who develop preeclampsia are at increased risk of cardiovascular complications later in life. Many of the risk factors and pathophysiologic abnormalities of preeclampsia are similar to those of coronary artery disease.[317–320] Insulin resistance, with the associated microvascular dysfunction, has been implicated as a major common factor.[317]

Preeclampsia is characterized by an increased systemic inflammatory response, whereas low-grade chronic inflammation is also a risk factor for cardiovascular disease. The mechanism for this susceptibility to inflammation could be attributable to a generalized up-regulation (genetic?) of a number of inflammatory processes or could be a specific overactivity of a particular tissue such as adipose tissue.[317,319] A recent systematic review[321] determined that the RRs for hypertension were 3.70 after 14 years follow-up, for ischemic heart disease 2.16 after 12 years, for stroke 1.81 after 10 years, and for venous thromboembolism 1.87 after 5 years. Overall mortality after preeclampsia was increased 1.5-fold after 14 years. These associations are likely to reflect a common cause for preeclampsia and cardiovascular disease, an effect of preeclampsia on vascular disease development, or both. It is reasonable to counsel patients who develop hypertension in pregnancy that they will benefit from avoiding smoking, maintaining a healthy weight, exercising regularly, and eating a healthy diet.[320,321] It is recommended that all women with previous preeclampsia or hypertension in pregnancy have an annual BP check and regular (every 5 yr or more frequently if indicated) assessment of other cardiovascular risk factors including serum lipids and blood glucose. Having a history of severe early-onset preeclampsia requiring delivery at less than 28 weeks' gestation could be a marker for underlying acquired and genetic thrombophilias. In addition to this risk for the mother, long-term follow-up studies have demonstrated that babies born growth-restricted, and in particular born preterm and growth-restricted, are more likely to develop hypertension, coronary artery disease, dyslipidemia, and diabetes (insulin resistance syndrome), and for growth-restricted female neonates, preeclampsia in adult life.[322,323]

SUGGESTED READINGS

American College of Obstetricians and Gynecologists (ACOG): Diagnosis and Management of Preeclampsia and Eclampsia (Practice Bulletin No. 33). Obstet Gynecol 2002;99:159–167.

Askie LM, Duley L, Henderson-Smart DJ, Stewart LA, PARIS Collaborative Group: Antiplatelet agents for prevention of preeclampsia: A meta-analysis of individual patient data. Lancet 2007;369:1791–1798.

Conde-Agudelo A, Villar J, Lindheimer M: Maternal infection and risk of preeclampsia: Systematic review and meta-analysis. Am J Obstet Gynecol 2008;198:7–22.

Conde-Agudelo A, Villar J, Lindheimer M: World Health Organization systematic review of screening tests for preeclampsia. Obstet Gynecol 2004;104:1367–1391.

Duley L, Galmezoglu AM, Henderson-Smart DJ: Magnesium sulfate and other anticonvulsants for women with preeclampsia. In Cochrane Library. Oxford: Update Software, Issue 2, 2003.

Oudejans CB, van Dijk M, Oosterkamp M, et al: Genetics of preeclampsia: Paradigm shifts. Hum Genet 2007;120:607–612.

Redman CW, Sargent IL: Placental stress and preeclampsia: A revised view. Placenta 2009;30(Suppl A):S38–S42.

Sibai BM, Barton JR: Expectant management of severe preeclampsia remote from term: Patient selection, treatment, and delivery indications. Am J Obstet Gynecol 2007;196:514.e1–e9.

Sibai BM, Dekker G, Kupferminc M: Preeclampsia. Lancet 2005;365:785–799.

von Dadelszen P, Magee LA: Antihypertensive medications in the management of gestational hypertension-preeclampsia. Clin Obstet Gynecol 2005;48:441–458.

REFERENCES

For a complete list of references, log onto www.expertconsult.com.

CHAPTER 36

Cardiac Disease

MARK W. TOMLINSON

INTRODUCTION: GENERAL COMMENTS

Maternal and Fetal Risks

Serious maternal cardiac disease complicating pregnancy is relatively uncommon; however, it can have a significant adverse effect on maternal and fetal outcomes despite modern cardiac care. The overall incidence of serious heart disease complicating pregnancy is approximately 1%.[1] With a decrease in maternal death as a result of the classic causes of hemorrhage, hypertension, and infection, the relative importance of cardiac disease has increased.[1] During the last few decades, the etiology of heart disease in developed countries has changed from primarily rheumatic to predominantly congenital.[1–4] Despite the potential for significant maternal morbidity, most patients with cardiac disease can expect a satisfactory outcome with careful antenatal, intrapartum, and postpartum management.[1–5] Serious complications during pregnancy and the postpartum period such as congestive heart failure, arrhythmias, and stroke are seen in 12% to 20% of patients. Mortality in some conditions can be as high as 30%. The rate of complications is related to several factors, including maternal functional status, myocardial dysfunction, significant aortic or mitral valve stenosis, and history of arrhythmias or a cardiac event.[2,4,5]

Table 36–1[6,7] shows the estimated qualitative risk of maternal complications associated with various cardiac conditions. Maternal mortality secondary to heart disease is generally uncommon today, particularly in developed countries because (1) most congenital lesions are diagnosed early, allowing appropriate surgical repair, (2) the incidence of rheumatic heart disease has significantly decreased, and (3) patients who are at greatest risk for cardiac decompensation are offered sterilization or termination.

Normal physiologic pregnancy-related changes can aggravate underlying cardiac disease, leading to the associated morbidity and mortality. Total body water increases progressively by 6 to 8 L because an additional 500 to 900 mEq of sodium is retained.[8–10] As a result, plasma volume increases steadily throughout the first two trimesters and into the early third trimester, reaching a plateau at approximately 32 weeks.[11] In a singleton pregnancy at term, plasma volume is nearly 50% greater than that seen in nonpregnant women.[12] Maternal cardiac output starts to increase at approximately 10 weeks and reaches a plateau by the early third trimester at levels 30% to 50% above nonpregnant values.[13–16] This increased output results from increases in stroke volume and heart rate. The increase in heart rate peaks in the third trimester at 10 to 15 beats/min over baseline.[15–17] These physiologic changes increase the demand on the heart, which can become critical if function is already compromised.

The pregnancy-related decrease in blood pressure may offset some of the increased work resulting from increased plasma volume. In some cases, however, the significant decrease in peripheral resistance can be deleterious; for example, it may reverse a left-to-right shunt, resulting in cyanosis. Normally, systolic and diastolic pressures fall throughout the first two trimesters, reaching a nadir between 24 and 28 weeks, before increasing to nonpregnant levels at term.[18] Systolic pressure decreases an average of 5 to 10 mm Hg, and diastolic pressure decreases 10 to 15 mm Hg.[19] Blood pressure and cardiac output may be further affected by maternal posture. Late in pregnancy, the gravid uterus may mechanically obstruct the aorta and vena cava in the supine position, leading to hypotension.[20] In addition, changes in cardiac output and blood pressure cause an initial decrease in systemic vascular resistance, followed by an increase toward nonpregnant values near term.[18] During cesarean section, fundal pressure used to facilitate delivery causes vena cava compression, resulting in decreased preload. Heart rate also decreases, possibly due to vagal stimulation. Aortic compression is usually not seen. The net effect of the changes in preload and heart rate is a decrease in cardiac output.[21] There can also be dramatic changes in venous return immediately following birth. If there is more than average blood loss, then venous return can be markedly reduced. Conversely, delivery of the placenta and the rapid contraction of the uterus can result in blood being squeezed out of the uterus and a sudden increase in venous return. This is particularly marked if the placenta is removed manually at cesarean section and oxytocics are given to make the uterus contract. Such manual removal is probably best avoided. Finally, oxytocics commonly used can have major effects on vascular tone (ergometrine producing an increase, and oxytocin producing a decrease). Although not clinically significant in normal pregnant women, the resulting changes in venous

TABLE 36–1

Risk of Maternal and Fetal Morbidity Associated with Pregnancy

Low Risk

Mitral valve prolapse without severe regurgitation
Atrial and ventricular septal defect previously repaired or without pulmonary hypertension
Corrected congenital heart disease without residual cardiac dysfunction
Patent ductus arteriosus
Pulmonary stenosis
Mild mitral or aortic valvular disease (stenosis or regurgitation) with normal left ventricular function: New York Heart Association class I or II

Moderate Risk

Marfan's syndrome with normal aorta
History of peripartum cardiomyopathy with no residual ventricular dysfunction
Previous myocardial infarction

High Risk

Any condition with New York Heart Association class III or IV
Moderate to severe systemic ventricular dysfunction
Pulmonary hypertension from any cause
Tetralogy of Fallot; uncorrected or with residual disease
Coarctation of the aorta
Mitral stenosis with atrial fibrillation
Severe aortic stenosis
Mechanical valve requiring anticoagulation
Marfan's syndrome with aortic involvement
History of peripartum cardiomyopathy with residual ventricular dysfunction

TABLE 36–2

Risk of Congenital Heart Defect in Offspring of Women with Congenital Heart Disease

CONGENITAL HEART DEFECT	NEONATAL RISK (%)
Any defect	5-6
ASD	4-10
VSD	6-10
Tetralogy of Fallot	3-5
Transposition of the great arteries	0
Aortic coarctation	4
Aortic stenosis	4-18
Pulmonary stenosis	3-4
Ebstein's anomaly	4-6

ASD, atrial septal defect; VSD, ventricular septal defect.
Data from references 7, 26, 60, 81, 82, 84, 88, 94.

return may be important in those with limited cardiac reserve.

Colloid oncotic pressure is another important variable affected by pregnancy. Both plasma and interstitial colloid oncotic pressure decrease throughout gestation, with the latter decreasing to a greater extent.[22] There is an accompanying increase in capillary hydrostatic pressure.[23] These changes lead to the normal physiologic edema of pregnancy, most marked in the lower extremities. Any further increase in hydrostatic pressure or a decrease in plasma colloid oncotic pressure will produce increased edema formation, especially in late pregnancy. After delivery, an additional decrease in plasma colloid oncotic pressure occurs, reaching a nadir between 6 and 16 hours, with a return toward intrapartum levels after 24 hours.[24,25] The marked dependent edema commonly seen in normal pregnant patients can complicate the diagnosis of cardiac decompensation.

Fetal complications in pregnancies associated with maternal cardiac disease commonly include growth restriction and preterm delivery. Despite the risk of low birth weight, overall perinatal mortality is not significantly greater than that in the general population. When a pregnant patient has congenital heart disease, the fetus is at increased risk for this disease. The increase in incidence ranges from 0% to 18%, depending on the specific lesion (Table 36–2). When the fetus is affected, approximately 50% have the same anomaly as the mother.[1,26] The risk of a cardiac lesion in the fetus is also increased when other first-degree family members have a congenital heart lesion.[26]

Management Options

Prepregnancy

Ideally in patients with significant heart disease, pregnancy is a planned event. This assumes regular and reliable use of an effective contraceptive method. Before discontinuation of contraception, preconception evaluation and counseling should take place. The patient's cardiologist should be an active participant in this process. Maternal disease status should be determined. An echocardiogram can be used not only to define the cardiac anatomy but also to describe ventricular function and estimate intracardiac pressure gradients.[27] Magnetic resonance imaging can also be useful, for example, in visualizing the descending aorta in cases of coarctation. Nuclear medicine scans, although helpful in the nonpregnant state, should be avoided during pregnancy.

A careful history is obtained to identify previous cardiac complications, including arrhythmias. The patient's functional status should also be established. The New York Heart Association (NYHA) functional classification system[28] (Table 36–3) is commonly used. Ninety percent or more of patients are categorized as having class I or II disease.[1–3,29] Outcomes are favorable in these two groups, but deterioration may occur. The reported frequency of adverse cardiac events varies from 3% to 69% depending on patient risk factors.[2,4,5] Although few patients have class III or IV disease, historically, nearly 85% of maternal deaths occur in these groups.[30]

The risk of maternal cardiac complications during pregnancy was quantified by Siu and colleagues[5] with a combination of five echocardiographic and historical factors that could be obtained and evaluated at the initial encounter. The complications studied include pulmonary edema, symptomatic arrhythmias, and stroke or transient ischemic attack of cardiac origin. The five predictive indicators were NYHA classification greater than grade II or cyanosis, left ventricular obstruction, cardiac dysfunction, previous arrhythmia, and previous cardiac complication. *Left ventricular outflow obstruction* was defined as aortic valve stenosis with a valve area less than 1.5 cm^2, mitral stenosis with a valve area of less than 2.0 cm^2, or a peak left ventricular outflow tract gradient greater than 30 mm Hg. *Myocardial dysfunction* was

TABLE 36–3

New York Heart Association Cardiac Functional Classification

Class I	No limitations of physical activity; ordinary physical activity does not cause undue fatigue, palpitation, dyspnea, or anginal pain.
Class II	Slight limitation of physical activity; ordinary physical activity results in fatigue, palpitation, dyspnea, or anginal pain.
Class III	Marked limitation of physical activity; less than ordinary activity causes fatigue, palpitation, dyspnea, or anginal pain.
Class IV	Inability to perform any physical activity without discomfort; symptoms of cardiac insufficiency or anginal syndrome may be present, even at rest; any physical activity increases discomfort.

TABLE 36–4

Classification System for Fetal Risk Associated with Medications used during Pregnancy

Category A	Controlled studies in women show no risk to the fetus in the first trimester (and no evidence of risk in later trimesters); the possibility of fetal harm appears remote.
Category B	Either animal reproduction studies show no fetal risk but there are no controlled studies in pregnant women or animal reproduction studies show an adverse effect (other than a decrease in fertility) that was not confirmed in controlled studies in women in the first trimester (and there is no evidence of a risk in later trimesters).
Category C	Either studies in animals show adverse fetal effects (teratogenic, embryocidal, or other) and there are no controlled studies in women or studies in women and animals are not available; drugs should be given only if the potential benefit justifies the potential risk to the fetus.
Category D	There is positive evidence of human fetal risk, but the benefits from use in pregnant women may be acceptable despite the risk (e.g., if the drug is needed in a life-threatening situation or for a serious disease for which safer drugs cannot be used or are ineffective).
Category X	Studies in animals or humans show fetal abnormalities or there is evidence of fetal risk based on human experience, or both, and the risk of the use of the drug in pregnant women clearly outweighs any possible benefit; the drug is contraindicated in women who are or may become pregnant.

defined as an ejection fraction less than 40%, restrictive or hypertrophic cardiomyopathy, or complex congenital heart disease. A *significant history of arrhythmia* was defined as symptomatic bradyarrhythmia or tachyarrhythmia requiring therapy. If no predictive factors were present at the beginning of pregnancy, fewer than 5% of patients have a cardiac complication. When one factor was present, 30% of patients have a complication, and when two or more predictors were present, nearly 70% of patients have a complication. This information is useful in counseling patients.[2,4,5]

Medical management of the patient's cardiac condition should be optimized. During maternal drug therapy, potential fetal effects must be considered. Table 36–4 shows a fetal risk factor classification scheme that is helpful when choosing optimal medical therapy.[31] The corresponding risk factor category is listed, with medications discussed in the next sections. Coexisting conditions that may aggravate preexisting heart disease, such as anemia, arrhythmias, and hypertension, should be appropriately treated and controlled. Ideally, necessary cardiac surgery is carried out before conception.

Prenatal

Few patients are seen for prepregnancy evaluation. Therefore, most evaluation and counseling will be initiated at the first prenatal visit. Cardiac surgery, although not contraindicated, is usually not required during pregnancy.[1] If possible, it is best delayed until postpartum. When the maternal mortality rate is excessive, as in Eisenmenger's syndrome, termination of the pregnancy should be discussed.

During prenatal care, the patient should be routinely questioned and examined for signs or symptoms of cardiac failure. Vital signs and weight gain should be closely monitored. When there is an increased risk of intrauterine growth restriction (IUGR), serial ultrasound examinations every 2 to 4 weeks in the third trimester allow assessment of interval fetal growth. Antenatal testing may begin at 32 to 34 weeks unless earlier surveillance is indicated because of compromised maternal or fetal status. Anesthesiology consultation should be obtained prior to delivery. Future fertility desires and contraceptive plans should be addressed in the antepartum period. Topics should include a discussion of sterilization, depending on future fertility desires, the maternal risk due to pregnancy, and the long-term prognosis.

Labor and Delivery

Ideally, women with significant cardiac disease should be delivered in a unit with 24-hour availability of expert obstetric, cardiology, anesthetic, and midwifery/nursing care, because labor can start unpredictably at any time. However, in the most challenging cases, labor induction may be chosen to maximize availability of a skilled multidisciplinary team. The incidence of cesarean section in patients with cardiac conditions is no higher than that occurring in women without cardiac disease induced for other obstetric indications. The key to successful management is to minimize cardiovascular stress, which can be achieved effectively with the use of regional anesthesia. Cesarean section subjects the mother to more stress than a straightforward labor and delivery. Therefore, cesarean section should not be undertaken simply because the mother has cardiac disease. Moreover, induction of labor is not specifically contraindicated. In one study of women with cardiac disease, the complication rate was not higher in those who were induced than in those who were not.[32] If induction with vaginal prostaglandin is used, it is probably wise to start with a low dosage, because an acute uterine hyperstimulation requiring either tocolysis or an urgent delivery is particularly risky in a woman with significant cardiac disease. Labor should proceed with the patient in the lateral position to avoid aortocaval compression and possible hypotension. Intrapartum fluid balance should be followed closely. Continuous maternal electrocardiographic monitoring may be used, as necessary, to detect arrhythmias. Invasive hemodynamic monitoring with an arterial line should be considered in particularly high risk conditions or in patients with deteriorating cardiovascular status, because if the parturient becomes hypotensive, external blood pressure monitoring can be very difficult. A pulmonary artery catheter (PAC) is recommended by some in particularly challenging cases, but its use has not been rigorously evaluated during pregnancy, and some question the safety and utility of the PAC in critically ill and high risk surgical patients.[33–35] Until more information is available on its safety and efficacy, a PAC should be used cautiously during pregnancy. Close fetal surveillance is needed throughout labor. Operative vaginal delivery is indicated in some patients to shorten the second stage of labor and avoid the blood pressure changes associated with pushing. Cesarean delivery can be reserved for obstetric indications.

An understanding of the principles of and indications for bacterial endocarditis antibiotic prophylaxis in pregnant patients is important. In patients with an uncomplicated labor and delivery, bacterial endocarditis is rare. In two series with a total of 906 pregnant women with cardiac disease, routine prophylactic antibiotics were not used and no cases of bacterial endocarditis were identified.[1,36] The incidence of positive blood cultures is low after uncomplicated vaginal delivery, with a reported range of 1% to 5%.[37] Bacteremia is more common with dental procedures, in which positive blood cultures are obtained in 60% to 90% of patients, depending on the procedure.[38] Recent focus has turned to bacteremia resulting from routine daily activities rather than procedure-related exposure. It has been estimated that over the course of a year, "everyday" exposure is six million times greater than that of a single tooth extraction.[37] Genitourinary procedures such as those common in obstetrics are also associated with a very low risk of endocarditis compared with typical daily exposure. The American Heart Association (AHA) suggests that the risk of adverse events related to antibiotic prophylaxis exceeds the benefit. The increased frequency of drug-resistant bacteria and the potential to add to drug resistance raise further doubts about the efficacy and cost-effectiveness of endocarditis prophylaxis. As such, the AHA[39] does not recommend antibiotic use solely for the purpose of endocarditis prophylaxis. Conversely, The Endocarditis Working Party of the British Society for Antimicrobial Chemotherapy[37] recommends antibiotic prophylaxis at cesarean section for patients at high risk for endocarditis. In any case, routine antibiotic prophylaxis for the prevention of postoperative sepsis is now well established as an appropriate measure by many prospective, randomized trials.[40] Individuals considered at high risk include those with a history of previous endocarditis, a prosthetic valve, a surgically conducted shunt or conduit, complex congenital heart disease, aortic stenosis or bicuspid aortic valve, other valve disease, and mitral valve prolapse with significant valve abnormality and regurgitation. A single intravenous dose of ampicillin 1 g plus gentamicin 1.5 mg/kg prior to the procedure has been recommended. The routine practice of prophylactic perioperative antibiotics with a first-generation cephalosporin provides coverage for some of the offending organisms and seems a reasonable compromise between the AHA and the British Society for Antimicrobial Chemotherapy recommendations.

Teicoplanin 400 mg intravenously plus gentamicin is recommended for penicillin-allergic patients. Prophylaxis is not recommended for an uncomplicated vaginal delivery (in this context, an episiotomy or repair of a vaginal tear is not considered to be a complication, unless there is an extension involving the rectal mucosa).[37] Prior to the revision of the AHA recommendations for infective endocarditis prophylaxis, Pocock and Chen[41] evaluated the intrapartum use of endocarditis prophylaxis. Only 12% of those receiving antibiotics had moderate to high risk cardiac conditions that would have potentially warranted therapy by the older recommendations. An appropriate antibiotic regime was given in only half of these cases, pointing out that even older recommendations were not being followed in clinical practice. The inappropriate and overuse of antibiotics for infective endocarditis prophylaxis highlights the broader concerns related to increasing antibiotic resistance and their effect on child development.

Postnatal

In the postpartum period, fluid balance must be monitored carefully. During the first 24 to 72 hours, significant fluid shifts occur and can lead to congestive heart failure in patients with cardiac disease. Careful attention should be paid to patients who do not have a brisk spontaneous diuresis. In these patients, progressive reduction in oxygen saturation monitored by pulse oximetry often heralds the onset of clinical pulmonary edema.

Formulating an effective contraception plan can be challenging but is essential due to the potential maternal and fetal risks associated with an unintended pregnancy. The potential side effects and complications of various contraceptive methods must be considered in relation to the unique problems associated with specific cardiac conditions. The World Health Organization[42] (WHO) provides a framework to aid in choosing an appropriate and effective contraceptive method based on known risks and contraindications. The categories are presented in Table 36–5. In general, progestin-only pills, progestin implants, and emergency contraception are category 1 and can be used in all cardiac patients. Depo-Provera can be used in most, but should be avoided in patients on warfarin. Combined hormonal contraceptive methods and the standard copper-containing intrauterine contraceptive device (IUD) present risks to some cardiac patients and should be avoided.[43] Where the concern with IUD use is related to increased risk of bleeding or infection rather than insertion complications, the levonorgestrel-releasing intrauterine contraceptive system (Mirena) is probably acceptable because its use of slow-release progestogen into the uterine cavity greatly reduces the risk of infection and heavy bleeding. The utility of these methods is reviewed for the individual conditions.

TABLE 36–5

World Health Organization Contraceptive Criteria

CATEGORY	DEFINITION
1	A condition for which there is no restriction for the use of the contraceptive method.
2	A condition where the advantages of using the method generally outweigh the theoretical or proven risks.
3	A condition where the theoretical or proven risks usually outweigh the advantages of using the method.
4	A condition which represents an unacceptable health risk if the contraceptive method is used.

SUMMARY OF MANAGEMENT OPTIONS

Cardiac Disease: General

Management Options	Evidence Quality and Recommendation	References
Prepregnancy		
Obstetrician and cardiologist in collaboration.	—/GPP	—
Discuss maternal and fetal risks.	III/B	3,5,28
Discuss safe and effective contraception.	—/GPP	—
Evaluate current cardiac status.	III/B	5,28
Optimize medical and surgical management.	III/B	1,5,31
Advise against pregnancy with certain conditions.	III/B	3,5,30
Prenatal		
Assess functional class of heart disease (see Table 36–3).	III/B	3,5
Termination is an option with some conditions.	III/B	3,5
Joint management with a cardiologist.	—/GPP	—
Optimize medical management.	III/B	1,5,31
Avoid or minimize aggravating factors.	III/B	3,5
Anesthesiology consultation.	IV/C	30
Prophylactic antibiotics in some situations.	IV/C	37,39
Fetal surveillance		
• Growth and fetal surveillance (especially if left-to-right shunt).	III/B	1,3,5
• Detailed fetal cardiac ultrasonography if the patient has congenital heart disease.	III/B	1,3,5
Labor and Delivery		
Elective induction may be necessary for maternal or fetal indications.	III/B	1,3,5
Prophylactic antibiotics with certain situations.	IV/C	37,39
Avoid mental and physical stress; consider epidural.	III/B	3,5
Labor in the left lateral and upright position.	III/B	1,3,5
Monitor electrocardiogram; more invasive monitoring is needed with certain conditions.	III/B	102
Administer extra oxygen with certain conditions.	—/GPP	—
Full resuscitation facilities should be available.	—/GPP	—
Provide continuous fetal heart rate monitoring.	—/GPP	—
Assisted second stage with certain conditions.	—/GPP	—
Avoid ergotamine for the third stage; boluses of oxytocin are best avoided and it is most safely given as a slow infusion.	—/GPP	—
Postnatal		
Vigilance for cardiac failure.	III/B	1,3,5
Avoid fluid overload.	III/B	1,3,5
Continued intensive care.	—/GPP	—
Discuss safe and effective contraception.	—/GPP	—

GPP, good practice point.

CARDIAC MURMUR

Maternal and Fetal Risks

Cardiac murmurs result from turbulent blood flow that causes vibration of the cardiac structures. Systolic murmurs are very common during pregnancy, with a reported incidence exceeding 90%.[44,45] Typically, the murmur is early to midsystolic and soft (grades I–II). The left sternal border is usually the area of maximal intensity, followed by the aortic and pulmonic areas.[46] These murmurs are rarely associated with cardiac pathology and are likely secondary to the increased intravascular volume and cardiac output.

Echocardiographic studies of pregnant patients who are referred for evaluation of nonspecific systolic murmurs show normal structure and function in more than 90% of examinations. Most patients had the clinical characteristics of a benign flow murmur.[46–50] Most abnormalities were mild and were associated with a history suggesting pathology.[46,48–50] Clinically significant murmurs differ from the typical benign flow murmur. Systolic murmurs that are "loud or long" are suspicious and are more frequently associated with cardiac pathology. Late systolic, pansystolic, and diastolic murmurs are abnormal and also require further evaluation.[6,48]

Management Options

Echocardiography adds little to the clinical evaluation of nonspecific systolic murmurs, because most significant cardiac conditions seen during pregnancy are diagnosed before conception. Unsuspected mild cardiac disease may initially present during pregnancy or the puerperium. A common benign flow murmur must be differentiated from a pathologic condition. Unfortunately, the accuracy of clinical evaluation of systolic murmurs by noncardiologists is unknown.[47] A history that suggests cardiac disease or a pathologic murmur (late systolic, pansystolic, or diastolic) heard on physical examination should prompt evaluation with echocardiography. When a suspicious systolic murmur is noted, either a cardiologist's clinical examination or an echocardiogram can reliably identify significant pathology.[47] The method of choice depends on institutional resources. If a woman gives a history of repeated referrals because of an unusually loud but nonpathologic murmur, it can be helpful to give her a copy of her echocardiogram report, which she can show to future medical attendants, thus avoiding overinvestigation and the development of cardiac neurosis.

MITRAL VALVE PROLAPSE

Maternal and Fetal Risks

Mitral valve prolapse (MVP) represents a range of valvular abnormalities that allow one or both mitral valve leaflets to extend above the plane that separates the atria and ventricle. There is a wide range in the reported prevalence of MVP depending on the method of diagnosis, the diagnostic criteria, and the population studied. The condition is most common in women of reproductive age, with prevalence rates reported as high as 17%. Standardized echocardiographic criteria and a better understanding of the shape of the mitral valve have dramatically decreased prevalence estimates.[51] The condition remains relatively common, with a prevalence of 0.5% to 3% in the general population.[52,53]

Auscultation or echocardiography may be used to diagnose MVP. A midsystolic click, with or without a midsystolic to late systolic murmur, is the clinical hallmark. With two-dimensional echocardiography, the diagnosis is made when the mitral valve is seen prolapsing into the left atrium 2 mm or more on the long-axis view.[6] Postural maneuvers are sometimes used to aid in the auscultatory diagnosis. Activities that decrease left ventricular volume increase the degree of prolapse. Hydration affects the auscultatory findings of MVP.[54] Pregnancy may have similar effects, with changes in the timing of the click and shortening or softening of the murmur. Serial echocardiograms during pregnancy showed disappearance of MVP during pregnancy in a significant number of patients.[55]

Palpitations, arrhythmias, chest pain, syncope, fatigue, and panic attacks are reported in association with MVP. Together, they make up MVP syndrome, although the existence of a distinct syndrome has been questioned. The symptoms associated with MVP syndrome are very common and are seen with near-equal frequency in patients with and without an echocardiographic diagnosis of MVP.[52,56]

Severe mitral regurgitation requiring surgery, infective endocarditis, cerebral ischemia, and sudden death are serious complications associated with MVP. The complications are uncommon in reproductive-age women because they are typically associated with severe mitral regurgitation, older age, and comorbid conditions.[57,58] In an examination of offspring of the Framingham Heart Study participants, with an average age of 54 years, the occurrence of severe complications in association with MVP was only minimally greater than that in those without the diagnosis.[52] The risk of serious complications in women younger than 45 years of age with uncomplicated MVP is estimated to be 0.2%/yr.[57]

Management Options

Prepregnancy

Prepregnancy management should document any associated mitral regurgitation by either echocardiography or evaluation by a cardiologist.

Prenatal

Patients should be observed for cardiac arrhythmias, particularly supraventricular tachycardia. Although these occur very infrequently, the patient should be counseled to avoid caffeine, alcohol, tobacco, and β-mimetic drugs. When necessary, β-blockers (most category C) may be used.[6]

Labor and Delivery and Postnatal

In addition to continued observation for arrhythmias, The Endocarditis Working Party of the British Society for Antimicrobial Chemotherapy[37] recommends endocarditis prophylaxis prior to cesarean section for high risk patients with MVP and in the presence of significant mitral regurgitation, but this has recently been questioned (see earlier).

CONGENITAL HEART DEFECTS

Atrial Septal Defect

Maternal and Fetal Risks

Ostium secundum atrial defect is one of the most common congenital heart defects seen in pregnancy, and women are more commonly affected than men. Pregnancy is generally well tolerated and uncomplicated, especially in patients with normal systolic function shown by echocardiography and NYHA functional class I or II.[59,60] Significant complications can be associated with uncorrected atrial septal defect (ASD), but these are uncommon before 40 years of age. Supraventricular arrhythmias are more frequent with advancing age and may aggravate right-sided heart failure. Paradoxical emboli from the venous to the systemic circulation can occasionally occur. Pulmonary hypertension is uncommonly associated with ASD and is typically found in older patients.[61] In fetuses born to mothers with an ASD, the risk of congenital heart disease is 4% to 10%.[7,26,60]

Management Options

PREPREGNANCY

The ASD should be evaluated for closure prior to conception and any secondary complications, such as supraventricular arrhythmias or pulmonary hypertension, should be identified. In most cases, a newly diagnosed ASD can be closed with a catheter-placed device. Pregnancy should be discouraged and effective contraception initiated when significant pulmonary hypertension is present.[61] In these patients, combination oral contraceptive pills (OCPs) and IUDs are considered class 4 (see Table 36–5) and contraindicated owing to the risk and consequences of pulmonary embolus. The concern with the IUD is related to the risk of cardiovascular instability that can occur with a vasovagal event at IUD insertion (this risk is approximately 1 in 1000), so if the intrauterine contraceptive system is considered, it should be inserted in a hospital setting with appropriate facilities for resuscitation and an anesthetist in attendance. Depo-Provera is considered a category 1 choice and can be safely used.[43] Permanent sterilization is also an option; however, surgical and anesthetic risks must be considered. The new technique of occluding the fallopian tubes with coils inserted at hysteroscopy (Essure) probably poses less of a risk than laparoscopy.

PRENATAL

Prenatal care is routine in the absence of supraventricular arrhythmias, right-sided heart failure, and pulmonary hypertension. A fetal echocardiogram should be recommended owing to the increased incidence of fetal congenital heart disease.

LABOR AND DELIVERY

Labor is generally well tolerated. Patients are monitored for arrhythmias. Blood pressure is carefully monitored, and fluid is restricted. In addition to pain control, epidural anesthesia reduces systemic vascular resistance and may reduce any left-to-right shunt.

POSTNATAL

In patients without secondary complications, postpartum management is routine. Postpartum management encourages ambulation to decrease the risk of deep venous thrombosis and paradoxical embolization.

Ventricular Septal Defect

Maternal and Fetal Risks

Ventricular septal defects (VSDs) are uncommon in adults. Small defects usually either close spontaneously or are corrected in childhood. Maternal morbidity is related to the size of the VSD and the presence of pulmonary hypertension. Small defects and those that are repaired in childhood usually present no problem during pregnancy. Some asymptomatic patients with a repaired VSD have significant, but unrecognized, pulmonary hypertension, which is manifested clinically in association with the hemodynamic stresses of pregnancy.[62,63] Paradoxical systemic emboli can also occur in patients with an uncorrected VSD. As with ASD, however, patients with good functional status and normal systolic ventricular function usually have a normal outcome.[59,60] Infants born to mothers with a VSD have a 6% to 10% risk of congenital heart disease.[7,26,60]

Management Options

PREPREGNANCY

Before pregnancy, patients with a VSD (corrected or uncorrected) should be evaluated for pulmonary hypertension. Pregnancy is discouraged in patients with pulmonary hypertension. In the absence of pulmonary hypertension, repair of uncorrected lesions should be considered. Patients should be counseled about the increased risk of congenital heart disease in their offspring.

PRENATAL

Patients should be evaluated and followed with serial echocardiography. The size of the lesion, the degree of the shunt, and the presence of pulmonary hypertension should be determined. Termination should be offered to patients with pulmonary hypertension. Owing to the increased incidence of fetal congenital heart disease, a fetal echocardiogram should be recommended.

LABOR AND DELIVERY

Hypotension should be avoided to prevent shunt reversal. Endocarditis prophylaxis is recommended by the Endocarditis Working Party of the British Society for Antimicrobial Chemotherapy[37] in patients undergoing cesarean section (but see earlier).

POSTNATAL

Volume status should be monitored during the postpartum period because of fluid shifts and the potential for congestive heart failure. Ambulation is encouraged to avoid the risk of deep venous thrombosis and paradoxical embolization. There are generally no contraceptive restrictions in the absence of pulmonary hypertension.[43]

Pulmonary Hypertension

Maternal and Fetal Risks

Pulmonary hypertension associated with pregnancy is a grave condition, and the maternal mortality rate is as high as 50%, although a recent survey suggests that improved management is reducing mortality, perhaps to as low as 25%.[64,65] Primary pulmonary hypertension is an idiopathic disease of the pulmonary vasculature that is seen primarily in women. Secondary pulmonary hypertension can result from long-standing increases in pulmonary pressure as a result of underlying cardiac disease, such as ASD or VSD, mitral stenosis, or patent ductus arteriosus (PDA).[66] Fortunately, the condition is rare, with a reported incidence of 1.6/100,000 deliveries in the United States.[67]

With primary pulmonary hypertension, the most dangerous times are labor, delivery, and the early postpartum period. Intravascular volume changes are not well tolerated because of the fixed pulmonary vascular resistance. Increases in cardiac output during labor or as a result of postpartum fluid shifts may lead to sudden right-sided heart failure. At delivery, excessive blood loss decreases preload, resulting in an inability to overcome high pulmonary vascular resistance. Both situations lead to a decrease in left ventricular preload and a dramatic decrease in left ventricular output. A direct consequence is myocardial ischemia, leading to arrhythmias, ventricular failure, and sudden death. Pulmonary thromboembolic events are usually fatal. Even small thrombi in the lungs can dramatically aggravate pulmonary hypertension.[66] There is an increased incidence of hypertensive disorders of pregnancy further complicating the condition.[67] In the fetus, chronic maternal hypoxia can lead to IUGR. Despite this, the neonatal survival rate is nearly 90%.[65]

Management Options

PREPREGNANCY

Despite improvements in maternal outcome with a comprehensive team approach,[66] maternal morbidity and mortality are significant risks. As a result, pregnancy should be discouraged and permanent sterilization should be considered.

PRENATAL

Caution should be exercised in diagnosing pulmonary hypertension during pregnancy. Cardiac catheterization is the gold standard for determining pulmonary artery pressures. In the nonpregnant patient, there is good correlation between echocardiographic-derived pressures and those obtained by cardiac catheterization. In the pregnant patient, however, echocardiographic pulmonary artery pressures tend to be overestimated, with nearly one third of those with elevated pressures found to be normal on subsequent cardiac catheterization.[68,69]

If pregnancy occurs in patients with severe pulmonary hypertension, termination should be offered because of maternal risks. If pregnancy is discovered in the second trimester and termination is chosen, dilation and evacuation in experienced hands is preferred over induction. In a continuing pregnancy, the cardiologist, critical care specialist, and obstetrician must work closely together. An obstetric anesthesiologist should be consulted early in the pregnancy. The use of calcium channel blockers has been reported in some patients, with improvement in maternal cardiac output and successful pregnancy outcome. Nifedipine (category C) in doses of 90 to 120 mg daily was used.[70] Heparin (category C) thromboembolism prophylaxis is initiated early, with doses of 5000 to 10,000 units given subcutaneously twice daily. Patients with more severe disease, manifested by chest pain or oxygen saturation of 80% or less, are at higher risk and full heparin anticoagulation has been used. In the early third trimester, in-hospital bedrest with oxygen therapy (up to an FIO_2 [fractional concentration of oxygen in inspired gas] of 0.4) and frequent monitoring with pulse oximetry is advocated. Late diagnosis and late admission to the hospital were associated with an increased risk of maternal mortality.[65] Lack of improvement in arterial oxygen saturation (SaO_2) with oxygen suggests further increased maternal risk.[66] A recent review has suggested that optimal therapy may include the use of drugs such as prostacyclin analogues, phosphodiesterase inhibitors, sildenafil (Viagra), and inhaled nitric oxide. The use of endothelin-receptor antagonists (e.g., bosentan) has also been reported; however, this agent should be used with caution in the antepartum period because animal studies have reported teratogenicity with this agent.[64]

LABOR AND DELIVERY

Because continuing pregnancy represents such a grave risk to the mother and because 25% of babies of such mothers are growth-restricted, the majority of these women will be delivered at preterm gestations. Although spontaneous labor is preferred to prevent the increased risk of cesarean section associated with preterm induction of labor if the cervix is unfavorable, it will often be necessary to deliver the woman by cesarean section to avoid the stress of a prolonged and potentially failed induction. When indicated, however, oxytocin or E series prostaglandins can safely be used for induction, provided great care is exercised to avoid uterine hyperstimulation. Oxygen flow is increased to 5 to 6 L/min. Oxygen saturation is monitored continuously with pulse oximetry. A radial artery line is placed to allow continuous blood pressure monitoring and facilitate frequent blood gas sampling. Maintenance of stable blood pressure is important. Adequate preload is essential to maintain cardiac output. Routine use of a PAC is discouraged.[65] An alternative is to place a central venous pressure (CVP) catheter early in labor. Arguments against the use of a PAC stem from the fact that information from the right side of the heart can be obtained from the CVP line. Left-sided heart pressure may not be accurately reflected owing to elevated pulmonary artery pressures. Potential complications, such as arrhythmias, thrombosis, and pulmonary artery rupture, must be considered when deciding on PAC use. Despite these concerns, in some patients, cardiac output data obtained from a PAC is useful. The decision to use invasive hemodynamic monitoring should be made on an individual basis, after the risks and benefits are considered.

Several case reports described the use of intravenous prostacyclin or inhaled nitric oxide therapy during labor.[71–73] Both drugs cause vascular dilation and inhibit platelet aggregation, leading to improved oxygenation, decreased pulmonary vascular resistance, and a decreased risk of thromboembolism. Improvement in pulmonary hypertension is similar between the two drugs in nonpregnant patients, and there seems to be no added benefit to a combination of the two agents. Inhaled nitric oxide avoids systemic hemodynamic changes, is easy to administer, and may cost less than other agents. Nitric oxide is typically used at a dose of 5 to 20 ppm. Elevated methemoglobin levels are a potential toxicity, but this problem has not been reported at these doses.[74]

An epidural catheter is placed early in labor and carefully activated when contractions become painful, to avoid hypotension. Intrathecal narcotics can be added to decrease the hypotensive effect of local anesthetics. During labor and delivery, the patient is placed in the left lateral position to avoid supine hypotension. Vaginal delivery, with shortening of the second stage using forceps or a vacuum to decrease the need for pushing, is desirable. Blood loss at delivery is carefully monitored. Crystalloid solution can be used to replace volume and maintain preload if blood loss is greater than normal. Older evidence suggests that cesarean delivery is associated with increased maternal morbidity and mortality and should be reserved for obstetric indications, although some studies suggest that the proportion of women being delivered by cesarean section is in fact increasing, probably due to the increasing recognition of the value of preterm delivery to avoid a third-trimester deterioration in maternal condition.[65,66] Despite the concern of increased morbidity and mortality, nearly 60% of 182 women with pulmonary hypertension were delivered by cesarean section between 2002 and 2004.[67] Although the mortality rate was not reported in that study, a more recent small case series including 15 pregnancies in 14 women with pulmonary hypertension of various etiologies evaluating anesthetic management described a cesarean rate of 69%.[75] The maternal mortality was 25% in those delivering vaginal delivery and 22% in those delivered by cesarean section.[75]

POSTNATAL

Antepartum and intrapartum management principles are continued into the postpartum period. Thromboembolism prophylaxis and oxygen therapy are continued. Excessive blood loss or right-sided heart failure as a result of fluid shifts can lead to sudden death. The patient must be monitored closely during the first 48 to 72 hours. During this time, nitric oxide is slowly weaned.[71] If prostacyclin is used, long-term therapy can continue, if necessary, through a central venous catheter.[73] Controlled diuresis is important during postpartum fluid mobilization to control preload and prevent worsening right-sided heart function.[70] Pulmonary edema may develop rapidly in patients who do not have brisk spontaneous diuresis. Permanent sterilization should be considered in patients with severe pulmonary hypertension. Depo-Provera or progesterone implants may be considered to avoid surgical and anesthetic risks. Combined hormonal contraceptives and standard IUDs should be avoided, as noted in the section on ASD.[43]

Eisenmenger's Syndrome

Maternal and Fetal Risks

Eisenmenger's syndrome is defined as pulmonary hypertension resulting from an uncorrected left-to-right shunt of a VSD, ASD, or PDA, with subsequent shunt reversal and cyanosis. *Pulmonary hypertension* is defined as mean pulmonary artery pressure greater than 25 mm Hg. The increase in blood volume and decrease in systemic vascular resistance can lead to right ventricular failure, with a decrease in cardiac output and sudden death. Maternal mortality with Eisenmenger's syndrome is as high as 40% in pregnancies that continue past the first trimester.[65,76] In contrast, the 15-year survival rate is more than 75% in nonpregnant patients.[77] Postoperative fluid shifts associated with cesarean delivery pose an even greater risk, with mortality rates approaching 70%. Although maternal risk remains high, one report emphasizing a team approach, with close follow-up and careful attention to detail, achieved a more optimistic outcome.[66]

IUGR is a common fetal complication. If the maternal SaO_2 is less than 85%, babies usually die in utero before reaching a viable gestation and early miscarriage is very common. Preterm delivery is also frequent, occurring in up to 85% of pregnancies.[60,76] Despite the maternal and fetal complications, the neonatal survival rate of babies alive at birth approaches 90%.[60,65] Congenital heart defects are seen in approximately 5% of offspring.[60]

Management Options

PREPREGNANCY

Pregnancy should be discouraged and reliable contraception, preferably permanent sterilization, advised because of the extreme maternal risk associated with pregnancy. Depo-Provera or progesterone implants are nonsurgical alternatives.[43] Even first-trimester termination is associated with a maternal mortality rate of 5% to 10%.[66]

PRENATAL, LABOR AND DELIVERY, AND POSTNATAL

Echocardiography is helpful in evaluating shunting, right ventricular function, and pulmonary hypertension. Cardiac catheterization may be necessary to quantify pulmonary hypertension. Pregnancy complications and outcome are related to the degree of pulmonary hypertension. Management of pulmonary hypertension associated with Eisenmenger's syndrome follows the same principles discussed in the section on "Pulmonary Hypertension." Nitric oxide use is described in two case reports that showed improvement in pulmonary hypertension and maternal oxygenation during labor and delivery.[78,79] Unfortunately, despite continued use, progressive deterioration occurred postpartum, and neither patient survived. In one case, doses as high as 80 ppm were used, and an elevated methemoglobin level resulted.[78]

Pulmonary Stenosis

Maternal and Fetal Risks

Pulmonary stenosis is one of the more common congenital heart defects seen in adults. It is often asymptomatic even in patients with severe stenosis. Although reports on pregnancy outcome are limited, it appears that isolated pulmonary stenosis is not associated with significant adverse maternal or fetal effects.[6,7,60,80] One report does suggest, however, that there may be an increased incidence of hypertensive disorders of pregnancy and thromboembolic events.[81] In patients entering pregnancy with good functional status, maternal deterioration is uncommon. There is not an increased incidence of spontaneous preterm delivery or

IUGR. Severe stenosis does not increase the risk of adverse obstetric outcome.[60,80] The risk of congenital heart disease in the offspring is approximately 3% to 4%.[60,81]

Management Options

PREPREGNANCY AND PRENATAL

Maternal functional status and the degree of stenosis should be determined by echocardiography. Balloon valvotomy is done in patients with cardiac symptoms including exertional dyspnea, angina, or syncope when the gradient across the valve is greater than 30 mm Hg. It should also be considered in asymptomatic patients when the gradient is greater than 40 mm Hg.[6,7] Because significant problems during pregnancy are rare even with severe stenosis, balloon valvotomy should usually be delayed until after the postpartum period.[80] This will reduce the risk of thromboembolic complications associated with the sixfold increase in coagulability during pregnancy.

LABOR AND DELIVERY AND POSTNATAL

Cesarean section should be reserved for obstetric indications.[80] Patients should be monitored for signs of right heart failure during the postpartum period, although this is uncommon. There are no contraceptive restrictions.[43]

Coarctation of the Aorta

Maternal and Fetal Risks

Untreated coarctation of the aorta carries a poor prognosis and is uncommon today. As a result, pregnancy is seen almost exclusively in patients who have undergone some type of repair. When the lesions are corrected, maternal and fetal outcomes are not significantly different from those in the general obstetric population.[82] Several cardiovascular anomalies are associated with coarctation of the aorta. A bicuspid aortic valve is the most common, found in 20% to 40% of patients. VSDs, anomalies of the intercostal and subclavian arteries, and aneurysms of the circle of Willis may also be present. The benefit of screening for berry aneurysms is uncertain.[83] Hypertensive disorders of pregnancy are common and reported in more than 15% of patients.[60] Although data are limited, the physiologic changes associated with pregnancy may unmask and aggravate postrepair gradients. Aortic rupture or dissection is rare but has been reported.[82,84] Congenital heart disease is seen in approximately 4% of offspring.[60,82,84]

Management Options

PREPREGNANCY AND PRENATAL

Termination may be considered in patients with uncorrected coarctation of the aorta, especially if it is associated with other anomalies, because of the increase in morbidity and mortality seen in adults. The majority of patients will have had a previous repair and require evaluation of the repair as well as screening for associated cardiac abnormalities. The highest risk of rupture or dissection is in patients with a Dacron patch repair (a Dacron replacement of the whole root is now recognized to be safer) or an aneurysm. A fetal echocardiogram should be considered owing to the increased risk of fetal congenital cardiac anomalies.

LABOR AND DELIVERY AND POSTNATAL

Hypertension should be controlled in both the intrapartum and the postpartum periods. Epidural anesthesia is encouraged because it effectively controls pain and decreases systemic vascular resistance. Endocarditis prophylaxis is recommended by the Endocarditis Working Party of the British Society for Antimicrobial Chemotherapy prior to cesarean section in patients with coexisting aortic valvular disease (but see earlier).

Progesterone-only contraceptive methods and IUDs can safely be used for contraception. In patients with repaired coarctation, combined hormonal methods are also considered safe in the absence of an aneurysm or hypertension.[43]

Tetralogy of Fallot

Maternal and Fetal Risks

Tetralogy of Fallot is the most common cyanotic heart disease, consisting of a VSD, overriding aorta, pulmonary stenosis, and right ventricular hypertrophy. In developed countries, nearly all patients undergo surgical repair in infancy. The majority of these patients are now alive during the reproductive years and leading normal lives. Nearly all patients with corrected tetralogy of Fallot enter pregnancy with NYHA class I and tolerate pregnancy well. Maternal complications can occur, however. Pulmonary regurgitation is seen 70% to 85% of patients.[85,86] Severe pulmonary regurgitation is associated with an increased risk of arrhythmias and right heart failure. These complications also appear to be more common in patients with repair later in life.[86]

Although survival to adulthood with uncorrected tetralogy of Fallot is possible, pregnancy is rarely seen in these individuals owing to a shortened life expectancy as well as decreased fertility. When pregnancy does occur in uncorrected tetralogy of Fallot, patients are at risk of serious maternal morbidity and mortality (see Table 36–1). Preexisting pulmonary hypertension is a concern. In addition, increased cardiac output leads to increased venous return to the hypertrophic right ventricle. These changes, together with decreased systemic vascular resistance, increase the right-to-left shunt. Oxygenation decreases, hematocrit increases, and cyanosis worsens, further stressing an already compromised cardiovascular system. Risk factors that worsen the prognosis include prepregnancy hematocrit exceeding 65%, a history of congestive heart failure or syncope, cardiomegaly, right ventricular pressure exceeding 120 mm Hg or strain pattern on electrocardiogram, or oxygen saturation less than 80%.[87]

Miscarriage, preterm delivery, and perinatal mortality do not seem to be increased.[60,85,86] There may be an increased incidence of growth-restricted newborns, however.[85] Congenital heart disease affects 3% to 5% of infants of mothers with tetralogy of Fallot.[26,60]

Management Options

PREPREGNANCY

Surgery is advocated for patients with uncorrected lesions. Patients who underwent previous corrective surgery should be evaluated for residual defects, such as pulmonary stenosis or residual VSD. If defects are found, the need for repair should be evaluated.[86]

PRENATAL

After surgical correction, patients with pulmonary regurgitation should be monitored for arrhythmias and signs of right heart failure. Patients with uncorrected tetralogy of Fallot should be offered termination. In those who continue, the pregnancy hematocrit should be followed. Supplemental oxygen may be of benefit. In all patients, a fetal echocardiogram should be preformed. In addition, serial obstetric ultrasound examinations should be done to monitor for IUGR. Antenatal testing is started during the third trimester, as indicated.

LABOR AND DELIVERY

In patients with uncorrected defects, careful fluid management and maintenance of blood pressure are the main features of intrapartum care. Central hemodynamic monitoring may be used, but there is a risk of exacerbating arrhythmias. Hypotension should be prevented to avoid shunt reversal. Epidural anesthesia can be used if the patient is adequately hydrated and it is carefully administered. To prevent decreases in venous return with bearing down, operative vaginal delivery may be used to shorten the second stage of labor. This strategy is often applied in patients with corrected tetralogy of Fallot, although it probably is not necessary.[85,86]

POSTNATAL

In patients with uncorrected tetralogy of Fallot, volume status should be monitored during the early postpartum period. A reliable contraceptive plan should be made, with permanent sterilization a good alternative. All reversible forms of contraception are considered category 1 or 2 and can be used in patients with corrected and uncomplicated tetralogy of Fallot.[43]

Transposition of the Great Arteries

Maternal and Fetal Risks

Transposition of the great arteries is a congenital heart disease consisting of discordance between the ventricles and the great arteries, in which the aorta arises from the right ventricle and the pulmonary artery originates from the left ventricle. Two types exist, depending on the concordance of the ventricles and the atria. In the first type, complete transposition, there is atrial concordance. After delivery, two parallel circulations exist. The systemic venous return enters the right atrium, proceeds to the right ventricle, and exits through the aorta, bypassing the pulmonary circulation. The pulmonary venous return enters the left atrium, continues into the left ventricle, and returns to the lungs through the pulmonary artery. Thus, no oxygenated blood reaches the systemic circulation. Without an additional congenital shunt such as a PDA or a surgical procedure to redirect blood flow more appropriately, this condition is not compatible with extrauterine life. Although several procedures are used to repair the condition, the Mustard operation, an atrial switch procedure, has been the most commonly used.[88] In this procedure, a baffle is placed between the right and left atria. Systemic venous return is redirected to the left side of the heart and to the lungs, whereas the oxygenated pulmonary venous blood is shunted to the right ventricle and on to the systemic circulation. Surgery allowed these patients to reach adulthood and contemplate pregnancy but left them with a systemic right ventricle that often fails in the sixth decade because it is unable to cope long-term with the demands of supplying the systemic circulation. Today, the arterial switch procedure is more common, because it results in both ventricles performing their correct function. Little information regarding pregnancy is available in these patients, however, because few of them have yet reached childbearing age.[89]

The second type is congenitally corrected transposition. Both arterioventricular and atrioventricular discordance are present. The right atrium empties its systemic venous blood into the morphologic left ventricle. Oxygenated pulmonary venous blood returns to the left atrium and empties into the morphologic right ventricle. Additional cardiac anomalies are often present, including VSD, pulmonary stenosis, and valve abnormalities.[90] The major concern in both types of transposition is the ability of the morphologic right ventricle to continue to support the systemic circulation as well as the increased cardiac output occurring during gestation. Maternal mortality is uncommon but reported. The risk of significant maternal morbidity is increased in both types of transposition. Cardiovascular complications include arrhythmias, congestive heart failure, myocardial infarction (MI), and cerebrovascular accident.[3,60,88,90] There also appears to be an increased incidence of hypertensive disorders of pregnancy reported in approximately 15% of pregnancies.[60,88]

The incidence of miscarriage is high, ranging from 15% to 40%. The increased risk is primarily related to maternal cyanosis.[60,91,92] In patients with surgically ameliorated transposition, the preterm birth rate is 30% to 40%. The incidence of babies small for gestational age is 20% to 30%.[60,88] The risk of congenital heart disease in offspring of these women does not appear to be increased above that in the general population, although the number of patients evaluated was small.[26,60,88]

Management Options

PREPREGNANCY

As with all cardiac conditions in pregnancy, it is important to determine the patient's functional status. Echocardiography to evaluate the function of the systemic right ventricle is necessary. The patient should also be evaluated for arrhythmias. A cardiologist with experience in treating congenital heart disease in adults should be included in the initial evaluation and throughout pregnancy. Often, this role is filled by the patient's pediatric cardiologist because these physicians frequently follow patients into adulthood. Unfortunately, pediatric cardiologists often have a limited medical knowledge regarding pregnancy and contraception, and increasingly, a joint service between an expert in adult congenital heart disease and a high risk obstetrician is becoming available and should be recommended.

PRENATAL

Decreased activity is advised to minimize further stress on the right ventricle. Patients should have serial echocardiography to evaluate cardiac function. Symptoms of congestive heart failure should be evaluated quickly and treated with diuretics and digoxin, as indicated. An anesthesiologist should evaluate the patient before labor.

LABOR AND DELIVERY AND POSTNATAL

Maternal cardiac monitoring is used to detect arrhythmias. Supplemental oxygen is given, as necessary. Volume overload should be avoided during labor and throughout the postpartum period. Adequate analgesia is important and can be provided with an epidural. Shortening of the second stage with forceps or a vacuum should be considered. Cesarean delivery is reserved for the usual obstetric indications.

Combined hormonal contraceptive methods can be used in patients with transposition of the great vessels (category 2), provided there are no arrhythmias or cardiac dysfunction.[43]

Ebstein's Anomaly

Maternal and Fetal Risks

Ebstein's anomaly is a relatively uncommon congenital heart defect characterized by apical displacement of the tricuspid valve leading to tricuspid regurgitation and right heart enlargement. Varying degrees of right and left ventricular dysfunction are also noted. Additional cardiac anomalies are often present, the most common being an ASD. Right-to-left shunting can occur, resulting in cyanosis. There is an increased incidence of arrhythmias, particularly Wolff-Parkinson-White Syndrome (WPW). Ablation of the accessory pathway has a lower success rate and higher recurrence rate in patients with Ebstein's anomaly than in those without structural cardiac abnromalities.[93]

Pregnancy is generally well tolerated in patients with Ebstein's anomaly; however, serious complications can occur. Arrhythmias and heart failure each occur in 3% to 4% of pregnancies.[60] The rate of preterm delivery is increased to approximately 25%.[60,94] The incidence of low birth weight is only slightly elevated and is seen primarily in women with cyanosis.[94] Congenital cardiac abnormalities are seen in 4% to 6% of offspring.[60,94]

Management Options

PREPREGNANCY

Most patients who require correction will have undergone surgery prior to adulthood. Echocardiography should be undertaken to evaluate ventricular function and the degree of tricuspid regurgitation. Those that have not had surgical correction should be evaluated for this, and if indicated, it should be done prior to pregnancy.

PRENATAL

The patient should be observed for arrhythmias. Serial maternal echocardiograms may be done to monitor cardiac function and evaluate for evidence of right heart failure. Decreased activity may be considered to decrease right heart strain. A fetal echocardiogram is indicated at 20 to 22 weeks to evaluate for fetal cardiac abnormalities. The patient should be educated and monitored for evidence of preterm labor. It may also be prudent to obtain serial ultrasounds for fetal growth with antenatal testing if growth restriction is identified.

LABOR AND DELIVERY AND POSTNATAL

Maternal cardiac monitoring should be considered to detect arrhythmias. Supplemental oxygen may be given, as necessary. Fluid balance should be monitored closely to avoid volume overload during labor and throughout the postpartum period. Adequate analgesia should be provided and can be accomplished with an epidural. Shortening of the second stage with forceps or a vacuum may be considered. Cesarean delivery is reserved for the usual obstetric indications.

Patent Ductus Arteriosus

Maternal and Fetal Risks

Surgical correction of PDA is usually accomplished in childhood. Uncorrected lesions have traditionally accounted for fewer than 5% of pregnancies complicated by congenital heart disease.[1] Maternal complications depend on the size of the ductus. Asymptomatic patients with a small PDA generally tolerate pregnancy without difficulty. Left-to-right shunting may decrease during pregnancy as a result of decreased systemic vascular resistance. A large lesion with a long-standing left-to-right shunt can lead to pulmonary hypertension.[95] In this situation, the normal decrease in systemic vascular resistance during pregnancy can cause shunt reversal, with an increase in maternal mortality.

Management Options

PREPREGNANCY

Before pregnancy, evaluation includes echocardiography to determine the size of the PDA and identify pulmonary hypertension.

PRENATAL

Antenatal management consists of echocardiography to detect pulmonary hypertension. If pulmonary hypertension develops, bedrest and supplemental oxygen should be instituted.

LABOR AND DELIVERY AND POSTNATAL

Intrapartum volume status should be monitored with care to avoid hypotension, which can result in shunt reversal. Use of a PAC may be indicated in patients with pulmonary hypertension. Careful attention to volume status should continue through the postpartum period.

RHEUMATIC HEART DISEASE: GENERAL

Maternal and Fetal Risks

Over the last several decades, a significant decline in the incidence and severity of rheumatic heart disease has occurred in developed countries. A similar pattern has been seen with rheumatic heart disease complicating pregnancy,[1] although recent data suggest that it is increasing again because of increases in immigration.[96] In a multicenter report of 562 women with heart disease managed during pregnancy, only 14% had acquired valvular lesions.[3] The changes were attributed in part to improved socioeconomic conditions. In many parts of the world, however, rheumatic heart disease remains a significant public health problem. Asia,

Africa, and South America have high prevalence rates.[97] Despite the dramatic decline in developed countries, rheumatic heart disease will continue to be seen because of immigration from high-prevalence areas.[98]

Rheumatic heart disease is a complication of rheumatic fever. Cardiac valve damage results from an immunologic injury initiated by a group A β-hemolytic streptococcal infection.[99] During pregnancy, the increased maternal blood volume and heart rate can lead to heart failure and pulmonary edema. Arrhythmias also frequently complicate pregnancy. In a series of 64 women followed in Los Angeles, congestive heart failure occurred in 38% and arrhythmias occurred in 15%. Not surprisingly, poor maternal functional class (NYHA class III or IV) was associated with worse maternal and fetal outcomes.[100] Rates of IUGR and prematurity are increased with complicated rheumatic heart disease.[100,101]

Management Options

General management principles for patients with rheumatic heart disease are aimed at preventing cardiac failure and bacterial endocarditis. Volume status is monitored, and activity should be limited. Antibiotics can be given prior to cesarean section as recommended by the Endocarditis Working Party of the British Society for Antimicrobial Chemotherapy.[37] Specific valvular lesions are discussed individually.

Mitral Stenosis

Maternal and Fetal Risks

Mitral stenosis, either alone or in combination with other lesions, is the most common valvular disorder associated with rheumatic heart disease.[1,101] In a 12-year review of 486 pregnant patients in India through 1999, 63% of lesions affected a single valve. Mitral stenosis was the abnormality in 90% of these women.[101] Although in the past, mitral stenosis was the most common rheumatic lesion associated with maternal mortality, death rarely occurs today, even in developing countries.[1,101–104] Hemodynamically, mitral stenosis is a state of fixed cardiac output caused by left atrial outflow obstruction. Pressures in the left atrium and pulmonary vasculature are increased. Long-standing severe disease may be complicated by secondary pulmonary hypertension and atrial fibrillation. In pregnancy, the increased intravascular volume can further elevate pressures and lead to pulmonary edema and arrhythmias, even in previously asymptomatic patients.[103] For this reason, any administration of intravenous fluid should be closely monitored and kept to a minimum. The risk of cardiac compromise is further aggravated by an increased maternal heart rate and decreased left ventricular filling time, which lead to a decrease in cardiac output.[102] The severity of the stenosis is the best predictor of cardiac compromise.[104,105] If maternal decompensation can be avoided, a good fetal outcome can be expected.[1,102,104]

Management Options

PREPREGNANCY

The goal of preconception care is to define the severity of cardiac compromise. Two-dimensional echocardiography and color-flow Doppler are used to determine cardiac function and the degree of stenosis. Together, these modalities allow noninvasive evaluation and decrease the need for cardiac catheterization.[106] Severe stenosis is defined by a valve area of less than 1.0 cm.[6] Valve areas of 1.2 cm or less are associated with an increased risk of complications during pregnancy.[104] In symptomatic patients or those with severely stenotic valves, surgical correction should take place before conception. Surgical commissurotomy is the traditional treatment modality. Percutaneous mitral valve commissurotomy has emerged as an alternative in patients without calcified valves or significant regurgitation. The percutaneous method is safe and as effective as the surgical approach in appropriate patients. In addition, it is less invasive, less expensive, and the preferred therapy in many centers.[6,7,98,107,108] Satisfactory results persisted beyond 5 years in these reports, delaying and potentially avoiding the risks associated with prosthetic valves.[109]

PRENATAL

The goal of prenatal care is to avoid cardiac decompensation. Special attention should be paid to volume status. Weight gain should be closely monitored. Symptoms or physical findings associated with heart failure should be reported and evaluated promptly. Maternal tachycardia should be avoided to prevent a decrease in cardiac output. Restriction of physical activity can aid in this objective. β-Blockade may be used to control heart rate. It is frequently used empirically in mitral stenosis during pregnancy to prevent the development of tachycardia, with good maternal and fetal outcome.[6,104,110] Atrial fibrillation can be managed with digoxin (category C) or cardioversion, as necessary. If the atrial fibrillation is persistent or long-standing, these patients may also require anticoagulation to prevent atrial thrombi.

Serial echocardiography is indicated to follow cardiac function. Percutaneous mitral balloon valvulotomy may be necessary to treat patients with significant functional deterioration or refractory pulmonary edema, despite optimal medical management. Several series have reported symptomatic improvement with good maternal outcomes in women managed with balloon valvulotomy for severe mitral stenosis during pregnancy.[108,111–113] In experienced hands with abdominal shielding, fluoroscopy time and fetal radiation exposure can be minimal.[6,113] Neonatal outcomes are also reported to be better when compared with closed mitral valvotomy or valve replacement.[108,114] Follow-up of 2 to 5 years has not identified any increase in developmental delay or adverse childhood outcomes following percutaneous valvuloplasty.[111,113,115]

LABOR AND DELIVERY

During the intrapartum and postpartum periods, volume status and cardiac output are critical concerns. In patients with NYHA class III or IV disease, central hemodynamic monitoring has been used. Pulmonary pressures and cardiac output can be measured reliably. Although pulmonary capillary wedge pressure (PCWP) can warn of the potential for pulmonary edema, it does not accurately reflect left ventricular preload. The pressure gradient across the stenotic valve may necessitate a high-normal or even elevated PCWP to allow adequate left ventricular filling and maintain cardiac output. To prevent pulmonary edema after delivery as a result of postpartum fluid shifts, PCWP should be maintained as low as possible without compromising cardiac output. Fluid restriction or careful diuresis, with attention to cardiac output, may be used to obtain desirable pressures. Decreased diastolic filling time associated with tachycardia may also decrease cardiac output. Careful intravenous administration of β-blockers (most category C) may be necessary to control heart rate and maintain cardiac output during labor.[102]

Similar considerations accompany analgesia and anesthesia during labor and delivery. Epidural analgesia is both safe and effective. Slow administration of the anesthetic agent is necessary to avoid hypotension. Control of labor pain removes a stimulus for tachycardia. The increased venous capacitance can also moderate postpartum fluid shifts. Drugs such as atropine, pancuronium, and meperidine can cause tachycardia and should be avoided.

Cesarean delivery is typically reserved for obstetric indications. If abdominal delivery is necessary, epidural is the anesthetic method of choice. Although forceps delivery is advocated to shorten the second stage of labor and reduce bearing down, it is not always required.[102] Endocarditis antibiotic prophylaxis should be given prior to cesarean section as recommended by the Working Party of the British Society for Antimicrobial Chemotherapy (but see earlier).[37]

POSTNATAL

Postpartum fluid shifts increase the risk of pulmonary edema. Clark and associates[102] noted a mean increase in PCWP of 10 mm Hg between the second stage of labor and the postpartum period in eight patients with functionally severe mitral stenosis. Because frank pulmonary edema is unlikely at a PCWP of less than 30 mm Hg, maintaining the PCWP at 14 mm Hg or lower if central hemodynamic monitoring is employed should prevent this complication.[102]

Combined hormonal contraceptive methods should be used only in patients with mild stenosis and no atrial fibrillation. Standard IUDs should be used with caution owing to a potential increased risk of endocarditis,[43] the levonorgestrel intrauterine contraceptive system is preferable because it is associated with a very low risk of infection.

Mitral Regurgitation

Maternal and Fetal Risks

Although mitral stenosis is almost exclusively caused by rheumatic heart disease, mitral regurgitation has several causes. In addition to rheumatic disease, floppy mitral valves in association with MVP, papillary muscle dysfunction, and ruptured chordae tendineae can result in mitral regurgitation.[116] In women of reproductive age, however, rheumatic heart disease is the most common cause of hemodynamically significant regurgitation. It is the dominant lesion in approximately one third of patients with rheumatic heart disease, but it is often associated with mitral stenosis.[1,105] In patients without severe mitral regurgitation or ventricular dysfunction, pregnancy is generally well tolerated. The decrease in systemic vascular resistance associated with pregnancy has a beneficial effect. Supraventricular tachycardia or atrial fibrillation may develop as a result of the increased volume, leading to atrial dilation. These arrhythmias may precipitate congestive heart failure.[105]

Management Options

PREPREGNANCY

NYHA functional status should be determined (see Table 36–3). The degree of regurgitation, atrial size, and ventricular function should be established with echocardiography. If required, digoxin (category C) therapy should be optimized. Although uncommon, if valve replacement is necessary, surgery should be performed before pregnancy. Valve replacement is indicated in asymptomatic patients with mild to moderate ventricular dysfunction and in those with atrial fibrillation, pulmonary hypertension, or symptoms such as dyspnea at rest or orthopnea.[117]

PRENATAL

In patients with NYHA class I or II disease, restriction of activity to prevent fatigue should be all that is required. In patients who have symptoms, serial echocardiography is indicated. Digoxin, diuresis, and afterload reduction should be instituted if left ventricular failure develops.

If medical therapy is unsuccessful, cardiac surgery during pregnancy can proceed, if necessary.[6] Although small case series have suggested that maternal mortality is not increased compared with nonpregnant women,[114,118] a review of the literature suggests that surgery for valvular disease during pregnancy and the early postpartum period is associated with a mortality rate of approximately 9%, roughly four times that of the nonpregnant population.[119] The fetal mortality is as high as 30%.[118,119] Factors that affected survival were gestational age at hospital admission and the degree of emergency necessitating the procedure. During cardiac bypass, fetal bradycardia and even cardiac arrest can occur as a result of maternal hypotension.[120] Fetal risks are minimized with high flow to maintain a mean maternal blood pressure greater than 70 mm Hg. Fetal heart rate can be monitored during the procedure and used as a guide to adjust flow rates. Hypothermia is also a concern because it is associated with fetal bradycardia, and therefore, hypothermia should be avoided. Perfusion temperatures greater than 30°C are generally well tolerated.[118] Uterine contractions are common, further complicating fetal heart rate abnormalities. In the larger review, however, neonatal outcome was not related to the evaluated variables associated with cardiac bypass, including duration of bypass, hypothermia versus normal temperature, and lowest temperature, provided the baby was born alive.[119]

LABOR AND DELIVERY AND POSTNATAL

Volume status should be monitored, and increases in blood pressure should be avoided to prevent worsening of regurgitant flow. When the left atrium is enlarged, cardiac monitoring may aid in the early identification of atrial fibrillation. Regional anesthesia is the method of choice for pain control during labor and delivery because of the decrease in systemic vascular resistance. Endocarditis prophylaxis may be utilized for cesarean sections.[37] Monitoring for congestive heart failure and atrial fibrillation should continue into the postpartum period.

Combined OCPs should be avoided in patients with severe regurgitation at risk for atrial fibrillation.[43]

Aortic Stenosis

Maternal and Fetal Risks

Aortic stenosis is the most common cardiac valve lesion in the United States. It can be congenital or rheumatic in origin, or it may be due to an age-related calcification of the aortic valve. All of these causes are uncommon in women of reproductive age, although congenital aortic stenosis is the most frequent etiology seen during pregnancy.[6] Aortic stenosis of rheumatic origin is typically progressive and tends to be less severe in patients of reproductive age.[121] In addition, it accounts for only 5% to 10% of cases of rheumatic heart disease in pregnancy and is usually seen in conjunction with mitral valve disease.[1]

The normal aortic valve area is 3 to 4 cm^2. The pressure gradient across the valve increases rapidly as the valve area is reduced to less than 2 cm^2, and this increase is associated with left ventricular outflow obstruction.[122] Mild to moderate congenital stenosis (valve area > 1 cm^2) is relatively well tolerated in pregnancy, and cardiac complications typically do not occur[103,105,123,124] Even patients with severe aortic stenosis generally do well. Maternal mortality is rare, although cardiac complications occur in approximately 10% of patients.[103,105,123,124] During 2-year follow-up, 36% of patients had progression of the cardiac condition that required surgery.[124] In these patients, cardiac output is fixed. Increased left ventricular pressure leads to hypertrophy and subsequent atrial enlargement. Tachyarrhythmias and atrial fibrillation may further complicate the condition. A decrease in cardiac output may result in inadequate coronary artery and cerebral perfusion, followed by sudden death.

With severe stenosis, the rate of preterm delivery and low birth weight is increased.[123] If maternal disease is congenital, the incidence of congenital heart disease in the fetus has been reported to be as high as 18%.[7]

Management Options

PREPREGNANCY

Before pregnancy, the severity of aortic stenosis should be determined by echocardiography. Severe disease should be corrected surgically before conception.[6,7]

PRENATAL

Physical activity should be limited. Patients should be observed for signs of congestive heart failure or arrhythmias. Serial fetal ultrasounds should be scheduled to detect evidence of growth restriction.

LABOR AND DELIVERY AND POSTNATAL

Fluid management is the critical component of intrapartum care. Volume overload can lead to pulmonary edema. Of greater concern, however, is hypovolemia or hypotension, with decreased venous return and cardiac output. Use of a PAC may aid in monitoring volume status in selected patients. Patients should labor and deliver in the lateral position to avoid aortocaval compression. Regional anesthesia is administered slowly and cautiously, after adequate volume loading, to avoid hypotension. A narcotic epidural can decrease the occurrence of hypotension. Blood loss should be monitored closely and replaced as necessary. If pulmonary edema develops, overaggressive diuresis is avoided to prevent a decrease in preload. Oxygen supplementation, morphine (category B), and inotropic agents, such as dopamine (category C) or dobutamine (category C), may be needed to maintain cardiac output. Bacterial endocarditis prophylaxis is recommended for cesarean delivery.[37] Close monitoring of volume status is essential in the postpartum period.

Continued follow-up after the postpartum period is important because the condition is typically progressive. Many patients require surgical intervention within 2 years of pregnancy.[103]

Combined hormonal methods and standard IUDs need be avoided only in patients with severe stenosis. The risk of thrombosis with atrial fibrillation is a concern with the OCPs, and the potential for a vasovagal event is of concern with IUD insertion. These methods as well as progestin-only contraception can be used in patients with mild stenosis.[43]

Aortic Regurgitation

Maternal and Fetal Risks

Like aortic stenosis, aortic regurgitation is uncommon in women of childbearing age. Although it is most likely of rheumatic origin, aortic regurgitation is an infrequent rheumatic lesion. Less common etiologies include Marfan's syndrome and syphilitic aortitis. Regurgitation in both is a consequence of aortic root dilation.

With progressive aortic insufficiency, cardiac output is usually maintained by left ventricular dilation and hypertrophy as a result of increased preload and stroke volume. Because the condition is progressive, severe disease, with ventricular dilation, hypertrophy, and widened pulse pressure, typically has not yet developed in women of reproductive age and is not likely to be seen in pregnancy.[125] The decreased systemic vascular resistance and increased heart rate associated with pregnancy may improve the hemodynamics of aortic insufficiency because of decreased resistance to forward flow and decreased time for regurgitant flow during diastole. As a result, pregnancy is generally well tolerated.[126] Patients with severe regurgitation and left ventricular hypertrophy can show cardiac decompensation during the later part of pregnancy or postpartum, however.[105]

Management Options

PREPREGNANCY

Preconceptually, the extent of disease should be defined by echocardiogram. In symptomatic patients, cardiac function should be optimized with digoxin (category C) and afterload reduction, as necessary. If indicated, valve replacement should be done before pregnancy.

PRENATAL

Cardiac status should be optimized, as in the nonpregnant state, and patients should be followed for signs of congestive heart failure. If medical management is inadequate, valve replacement can be performed during pregnancy with generally good maternal outcomes but an increased risk of fetal mortality, as previously noted.[114,118]

LABOR AND DELIVERY AND POSTNATAL

Volume status should be followed during labor and delivery and into the postpartum period while the patient is observed for congestive heart failure.[6] Invasive hemodynamic monitoring is usually unnecessary unless other valvular disease is present. Pain control is best achieved with lumbar epidural anesthesia, which decreases regurgitant flow by reducing afterload.

Combined hormonal contraceptive methods can be used as the benefit generally exceeds the risk (WHO category 2).[43]

PROSTHETIC HEART VALVES

Maternal and Fetal Risks

Surgical valve replacement has allowed many patients with severe valvular heart disease to survive and lead near-normal lives. There are two broad categories of replacement valves, each with advantages and disadvantages. Mechanical valves are made of nonbiologic materials. Bioprosthetic valves are either heterografts, made of bovine or porcine valves or pericardium, or homografts, which are human aortic valves.[127] Autografts of the patient's own pulmonary valve may also be used.[128] The different characteristics of these valves make the optimal choice in women of reproductive age difficult and controversial.[6] Mechanical valves have the advantage of durability, but the risk of thrombosis requires long-term anticoagulation. DeSanto and coworkers[129] followed 267 women with mechanical mitral valves for more than 3700 patient-years. Survival, freedom from thrombotic complications, and reoperation were all high. Survival was 90% at 5 years and 72% at 25 years. Only 6% of patients experienced a thrombotic complication by 5 years after surgery, with 25% experiencing it by 25 years. Fourteen percent of patients required reoperation by 25 years of follow-up. Bioprosthetic valves do not require anticoagulation, but valve failure often occurs within 10 to 15 years.[127] Pregnancy has also been reported to increase the rate of spontaneous valve deterioration. This has not been a consistent finding, however, and may simply represent the spontaneous deterioration that occurs when these valves are implanted in a younger population.[130] In order to reduce the need for replacement, mechanical valves are recommended by some authorities for young patients.[127] Conversely, bioprosthetic valves are advocated by others to decrease the risk of thrombosis during pregnancy as well as the risk of bleeding complications due to the need for anticoagulation. Bioprosthetic valves also eliminate the significant fetal risks associated with oral anticoagulants.[131]

The Ross procedure is an alternative for young women requiring aortic valve replacement. The patient's own pulmonary valve is transplanted into the aortic valve position and an aortic or pulmonary homograft is used to replace the transplanted pulmonary valve.[6,128] The advantages of this procedure include the fact that the valve can grow with the patient and anticoagulation is not required. Disadvantages of the operation include its technically difficulty along with the fact that long-term follow-up is limited and there still is concern over the durability of the valve.[6] A small series of five women with 12 pregnancies reported no significant cardiac complications during pregnancy. There was a suggestion of an increased risk of preterm delivery, although the numbers were small. One patient required reoperation for valve complications of both the aortic and the pulmonary valves 9 years after the original operation and 5 years after the last pregnancy.[128]

The incidence of major thromboembolism in nonpregnant patients with mechanical valves averages 8%. Anticoagulation reduces this risk by 75%.[132] Valve thrombosis causes pulmonary congestion, poor perfusion, and systemic embolization. Rapid clinical deterioration often follows. Most embolization involves the cerebral vessels. Patients with atrial fibrillation or left ventricular dysfunction are at increased risk for embolic events.[129] In addition, increased rates of pregnancy loss,[133–136] prematurity, and low birth weight[135] are reported in patients with mechanical valves.

Bioprosthetic valve dysfunction is often related to rupture or tearing of a leaflet. Progressive dyspnea and congestive heart failure suggest bioprosthetic valve deterioration. Failure in these valves is more common with a mitral valve prosthesis and in patients younger than 40 years.[127] Pregnancy has been associated with an accelerated rate of valve deterioration,[134] although this finding was not confirmed by others.[137,138] In a report by Salazar and coworkers,[138] the need for bioprosthetic valve replacement was associated with the patient's age at the time of initial surgery and not with pregnancy. Bioprosthetic valve dysfunction occurred at a rate of 3.5% per patient-year in the pregnancy group compared with 3.4% per patient-year in the nonpregnant control group. Endocarditis complicates both types of prostheses equally. Reported rates vary from 3% to 6%[127] to as high as 10% to 22%.[137]

North and associates[137] reviewed their experience with valve replacement in a population of more than 230 patients 12 to 35 years of age, with nearly 1500 woman-years of follow-up. The report covered a 20-year period beginning in 1972. Of these women, 71 had a total of 132 pregnancies. Patients with bioprosthetic valves had a significantly lower incidence of thrombosis and bleeding complications as well as greater 10-year survival than those with mechanical valves. Not surprisingly, there was an increased need for replacement of the bioprosthetic valve within 10 years (Table 36–6).

In patients with mechanical valves, anticoagulation is required throughout pregnancy, and there is controversy surrounding the optimal choice of therapy. Heparin use, both low-molecular-weight (LMWH) and unfractionated (UFH) formulations (category C), have been associated with an increased incidence of valve thrombosis compared with warfarin.[136] Although the majority of cases are associated with inadequate heparin dosing or lack of adequate monitoring using anti-Factor Xa levels,[139,140] one manufacturer of LMWH recommends against its use in patients with mechanical heart valves.[139] This may, however, have more to do with reducing medicolegal liability than a true assessment of risk. Osteoporosis and fractures are also potential risks of long-term UFH therapy. LMWH has the advantage over UFH of more predictable therapeutic effect and lower risk of bleeding complications as well as lower risks of osteoporosis and thrombocytopenia. Conversely, warfarin (category D) is associated with increased fetal risk in pregnancy, both early and late, compared with heparin.[136] A specific embryopathic

TABLE 36–6

Comparison of Outcomes Associated with Mechanical and Prosthetic Valves in Young Women

OUTCOME	MECHANICAL (*N* = 178)	BIOPROSTHETIC (*N* = 73)	HOMOGRAFT (*N* = 72)	*P*
10-Yr survival (%)	70	84	96	.12
Thrombotic complications (%)	45	13	1	<.01
Bleeding complications (%)	15	4		.05
10-Yr valve replacement (%)	29	82	28	<.01

TABLE 36–7

Anticoagulation Dosing

REGIMEN	DOSING	MONITORING	THERAPEUTIC GOAL
LMWH throughout pregnancy	Begin with 1 mg/kg enoxaparin q12h	Anti-Factor Xa level 4 hr after dose	Manufacturers upper therapeutic range
UFH throughout pregnancy	Begin at 17,500–20,000 U q12h	aPTT or Anti-Factor Xa level 4–6 hr after dose	>2 × control 0.35–0.70 U/mL
LMWH or UFH through 13 wk and after 36 wk; warfarin from 14–36 wk	Heparin q12h Warfarin daily	As above for heparin INR	As above for heparin 2.5–3.5
Aspirin added to all above regimens	75–100 mg daily	None	

aPTT, activated partial thromboplastin time; LMWH, low-molecular-weight heparin; UFH, unfractionated heparin.
From Bates S, Greer I, Pabinger I, et al: Venous thromboembolism, thrombophilia, antithrombotic therapy, and pregnancy: American College of Chest Physicians Evidence-Based Clinical Practice Guidelines. Chest 2008;133:844–886.

pattern is seen when warfarin is used between weeks 6 and 9. Fetal warfarin syndrome is characterized by nasal hypoplasia and stippled epiphyses.[31] The incidence of fetal complications has been reported to be related to the warfarin dose, with a substantially increased risk noted in patients requiring more than 5 mg/day.[129,133,141] Others have reported increased fetal loss rates despite low-dose warfarin therapy.[142] Because it crosses the placenta, warfarin can also cause fetal anticoagulation and bleeding, particularly if taken within 2 weeks of labor.[143] It is associated with an increased risk of neurologic abnormalities in the baby, probably related to intracerebral bleeding.

Despite the potential fetal consequences associated with oral anticoagulation, a task force of the European Society of Cardiology[7] states that oral anticoagulation is the safest approach for the mother. UFH may be considered during the first trimester after a thorough discussion of both the maternal and the fetal risks with the patient. Warfarin is then used with a switch to UFH at 36 weeks to decrease the risk of fetal bleeding complications at delivery.

The American College of Chest Physicians[139] recommends one of three anticoagulant regimens consisting of UFH, LMWH, or warfarin with UFH or LMWH during the first trimester and at the end of pregnancy. The lack of well-designed trials does not allow identification of one approach as clearly superior to the others. The choice is individualized after a thorough discussion of the risks and benefits (Table 36–7). Low-dose aspirin (75–100 mg/day) should be added to these regimens to further decrease the risk of thrombosis.[6,139] In patients at particularly high risk of thrombotic complications, such as those with older more thrombogenic mitral valves or history of thrombosis, warfarin is recommended throughout pregnancy with heparin being used prior to delivery.[139]

Management Options

Prepregnancy

As with other cardiac lesions, NYHA functional status is determined. Baseline echocardiography is indicated. Patients with bioprosthetic valves should be informed of the symptoms of valve deterioration, although the specific relationship with pregnancy is controversial.[134,137,138] Warfarin embryopathy must be discussed with patients who have a mechanical valve. An informed decision should be made about the potential use, timing, and duration of heparin treatment.[7,139]

Prenatal

Patients with bioprosthetic valves should be followed for signs of valve deterioration. Those with mechanical valves must maintain adequate anticoagulation. In patients who continue treatment with warfarin, the International Normalized Ratio (INR) is maintained near 3.0 with a range between 2.5 and 3.5. If UFH is used, it is dosed every 12 hours with the activated partial thromboplastin time (aPTT) maintained at least twice the control value or an anti-Factor Xa level between 0.35 to 0.70 U/mL 4 to 6 hours after the dose. If LMWH is used, the anti-Factor Xa level should be maintained at the upper limits of the manufacturer's suggested range 4 hours after the dose.[139] Although rare in pregnancy, monitoring for heparin-induced thrombocytopenia should be undertaken.[144] At term, if warfarin has been used, it is discontinued and heparin initiated.[7,139]

Labor and Delivery

Clear recommendations for heparin use during labor and delivery are not available. Intravenous heparin at therapeutic doses may be given until 4 to 6 hours before delivery.[139] This approach has the advantage of preventing thrombotic complications. The benefit is small, however, because the risk of valve thrombosis during the relatively short time of subtherapeutic anticoagulation is low.[132] If necessary, protamine can be used to reverse intravenous heparin anticoagulation at a dose of 1 mg/100 Us heparin up to a maximum dose of 50 mg. The dose is decreased as the time since heparin withdrawal increases. Another approach is to give prophylactic doses of heparin (5000–7500 U q12h) subcutaneously.

Endocarditis prophylaxis may be given prior to cesarean section.[37] Patients with bioprosthetic valves may benefit from operative vaginal delivery to shorten the second stage of labor and avoid the additional hemodynamic stresses of pushing.

Postnatal

Warfarin is initiated in the postpartum period in patients with mechanical valves. Prophylactic doses of heparin may be given while awaiting therapeutic levels of warfarin. Full anticoagulation with intravenous heparin is probably not warranted because the risk of bleeding, particularly after cesarean delivery, exceeds the risk of thrombotic complications.[132] Breast-feeding during anticoagulation with warfarin is not contraindicated, because the levels of warfarin in the breast milk are too low to be significant.[145]

Patients with bioprosthetic valves and no other complications generally can use combined hormonal contraceptive methods (WHO category 2) and IUDs. Those with mechanical valves should generally avoid combined hormonal methods, Depo-Provera, and standard IUDs.[43] The levonorgestrel-containing IUD may be acceptable.

MARFAN'S SYNDROME

Maternal and Fetal Risks

Marfan's syndrome is a connective tissue disorder resulting from a mutation in the *FBN1* gene leading to alterations in fibrillin-1, a protein found in the extracellular matrix. The characteristic findings include abnormalities in the skeletal, ocular, and cardiovascular systems. Cardiac manifestations include MVP, mitral regurgitation, and aortic root dilation. Aortic pathology is associated with increased incidence of aortic regurgitation, dissection, and rupture leading to significant morbidity and mortality.[146] In pregnant patients, morbidity and mortality rates increase when the aortic root diameter exceeds 40 mm with dissection rates reported to be 10%, compared with only about 1% if the aortic root is of normal dimensions.[147,148] However, it is most unlikely that there is a sudden increase in risk when the aortic root dimensions exceed 4 cm, and it is more likely that the risk represents a continuum, increasing with increasing evidence of progressive root dilation both before and during pregnancy. If aortic dissection occurs, mortality rates as high as 25% to 50% have been reported. Even with a normal aorta, maternal mortality has been reported. The elevated risk seen in pregnancy may be related to the increased cardiac output, placing additional stress on the relatively stiff aorta. Pregnancy-associated hypertension may further aggravate the condition.[149] Several reports suggested a better prognosis when there is minimal cardiovascular involvement. These patients had no increase in adverse maternal outcome and no accelerated dilation of the aorta compared with similar patients with Marfan's syndrome who did not become pregnant. Patients without aortic root dilation usually tolerate pregnancy well.[147,148,150] Pregnancy does not appear to be associated with an increased rate of progression of aortic root dilation in patients with a prepregnancy diameter of less than 40 mm. Pregnancy is associated with a slightly increased rate of growth in those with an initial diameter greater than 40 mm.[150]

There is an increased incidence of adverse pregnancy outcomes noted in women with Marfan's syndrome. Incompetent cervix and preterm delivery occur in 15% of pregnancies, and perinatal mortality was reported to be 7%.[151] The syndrome is inherited by autosomal dominant transmission, so there is a 50% chance that the fetus will be affected.

Management Options

Prepregnancy

Genetic counseling is an essential part of family planning in Marfan's syndrome because of the autosomal dominant inheritance. In about 80% of women (or affected men), a specific gene abnormality can be identified, allowing the possibility of prenatal diagnosis (either by preimplantation genetic diagnosis or by chorionic villus sampling in the first trimester). Echocardiographic evaluation of the aorta is performed to define maternal risk status. Pregnancy is discouraged in patients with significant aortic root dilation. If pregnancy is desired, prophylactic repair should be undertaken.[7] In nonpregnant adults, 50 mm is the critical aortic root diameter at which prophylactic repair is recommended.[146] Aortic repair is not completely protective against complications, however. Those with previous dissections are at risk for future events.[148,150] Even when the aortic root size is normal, a risk-free pregnancy cannot be guaranteed.[147,152] If cardiac involvement is minimal, however, women often choose to become pregnant. In this group of patients, initiation of β-blockade should be considered if not already utilized.[7] Although information on its use in pregnancy complicated by Marfan's syndrome is limited, studies of long-term use outside of pregnancy show that it slows the progression of aortic dilation.[146]

Prenatal

Serial echocardiography should be performed every 6 to 10 weeks throughout pregnancy to follow the aortic root size.[7,148] If not initiated preconceptually, the addition of β-blocker therapy should be considered. Little information is available to guide management in patients with progressive aortic root dilation during pregnancy. Patients should be kept at rest to minimize hemodynamic stresses. Hypertension should be avoided because of the increased risk of aortic dissection. Although it is best postponed until postpartum, prophylactic aortic root repair may be considered in extreme cases.

Prenatal diagnosis is now available in most families through linkage analysis or mutation detection.[149]

Labor and Delivery and Postnatal

Epidural anesthesia during labor should be recommended. Adequate oxygenation must be maintained, and hypertension should be avoided. Vaginal delivery is desirable, with shortening of the second stage of labor with the use of a vacuum or forceps.[7,148] Elective cesarean delivery has been recommended in patients with significant aortic dilation, but remains controversial.[7,147] Both patient and physician must remain vigilant because the risk of aortic dissection persists for 6 to 8 weeks postpartum.[148] Combined hormonal contraceptives can be used in patients without aortic dilation (WHO category 2), but should be avoided in those with dilation.[43]

DILATED CARDIOMYOPATHY

Maternal and Fetal Risks

Dilated cardiomyopathy is uncommon in women of reproductive age. Peripartum cardiomyopathy is a subset of dilated cardiomyopathy defined by onset of heart failure in the last month of pregnancy or the first 5 months postpartum, with no other etiology of heart failure identified and no history of cardiac disease. In 1997, echocardiographic evidence of left ventricular dysfunction was added to the diagnostic criteria by a National Institutes of Health and the National Heart Lung and Blood Institute work group. The dysfunction is documented by a reduced ejection fraction or decreased fractional shortening.[153] The reported frequency of the condition varies widely. The reasons for such variations are unknown. In Haiti, the incidence is as high as 1 in 300 live births,[154] whereas in the United States, it is between 1 in 3000 to 4000.[155,156] In the United States, the incidence varies by race, being more common in black women in whom the incidence is reported to be approximately 1 in 1400 births.[155,156] Despite the rarity of the condition, it is accounting for an increasing proportion of maternal mortality in the United States.[157]

The etiology of pregnancy-associated heart failure is unknown, although a number of pathologic theories exist. Evidence of varying degrees of inflammation has been found through serum markers and on endomyocardial biopsy.[158–161] The inflammation has been associated with evidence of viral infection in some cases,[158] as well as autoimmune mechanisms.[162] Hypertensive disorders and black African descent are significant risk factors.[153,155,156] A number of other risk factors have been inconsistently reported including older maternal age, multiparity, twins, and tocolytic use,[153,163] hypertensive disorders of pregnancy, and black African descent.[153] The existence of peripartum cardiomyopathy as a distinct pathologic entity is debated. To minimize confounding by exacerbation of unrecognized preexisting heart disease, the National Institutes of Health work group emphasized the importance of limiting the diagnosis to heart failure occurring within the defined 6-month window.[153] A more recent report of pregnancy-associated cardiomyopathy diagnosed more than 1 month before the end of pregnancy found no difference in risk factors, presentation, clinical course, and outcome, suggesting that there may be a continuum of the disease process during pregnancy.[163]

Regardless of the etiology, cardiomyopathy during pregnancy is associated with significant morbidity and mortality. Reported complication rates vary widely and likely reflect different patient populations and variations in diagnostic criteria. Persistent cardiac dysfunction is seen in 50% to 80% of patients.[154,164,165] A number of echocardiographic findings at initial presentation have been reported to predict persistent dysfunction. These include a decreased fractional shortening to less than 20%, a left end-diastolic dimension greater than 6 cm, a left end-systolic dimension greater than 5.5 cm, an ejection fraction less than 27%, and a left ventricular thrombus.[164–166] Maternal mortality reports vary widely with rates up to 15% in Haiti,[154] and 1% to 4% in larger population-based studies in the United States.[155,156] Survivors often require cardiac transplant.[164,167,168] The rate of recurrence in subsequent pregnancies is as high as 85%.[153] Patients with severe left ventricular dysfunction during the index pregnancy or persistent dysfunction are at increased risk of recurrent or progressive heart failure and death in subsequent pregnancies.[167,169,170] Although those with normal cardiac function 6 to 12 months postpartum fare better, they are still at risk for heart failure and a recurrent decrease in ejection fraction that may not recover after another pregnancy.[169,171] Patients whose cardiomyopathy clinically resolved had decreased contractile reserve with provocative testing.[168] This lack of reserve may cause cardiac decompensation as a result of the hemodynamic stress of a subsequent pregnancy and may contribute to the morbidity after a previous return to normal cardiac function.

Management Options

Prepregnancy

Pregnancy is strongly discouraged in patients with a history of peripartum cardiomyopathy, particularly those with residual cardiac dysfunction. In those with normal cardiac function, pregnancy is less contraindicated. The patient should be informed of the potential for worsening cardiac function during pregnancy, which may not completely resolve postpartum.[169] Combined hormonal contraceptives should be avoided in patients with residual ventricular dysfunction. Depo-Provera or IUDs can be safely used.[43] Permanent sterilization may also be considered.

Prenatal

If pregnancy occurs, echocardiography should be performed to document ventricular size and function as well as the presence of mural thrombi. Termination should be offered, especially to patients who have persistent echocardiographic abnormalities, because of the high associated maternal morbidity and mortality. If the pregnancy is continued, a multidisciplinary team, including a cardiologist, a perinatologist, an anesthesiologist, and a neonatologist, should collaborate to optimize outcome. Decreased activity and potentially even bedrest are recommended, along with salt restriction. Diuretics, digoxin (category C), and afterload reduction with hydralazine (category B) should be used, as necessary. Because of the risk of embolic phenomena, prophylactic heparin (category C) should be given.

Labor and Delivery

Patients are watched closely for signs of heart failure and pulmonary edema. Cardiac monitoring is instituted early in labor. Fluids are restricted, and central hemodynamic monitoring may be considered if decompensation occurs. If a flow-directed PAC is necessary, care must be taken during insertion. Positioning may be difficult because of dilated chambers and decreased ejection fraction. Arrhythmias may also be precipitated during insertion. Heparin can be discontinued prior to a planned delivery or during early labor and resumed in the early postpartum period. Adequate pain control is important, and epidural anesthesia works well. Patients with significant cardiac dysfunction may need to labor in a sitting position to reduce or prevent shortness of breath.

Postnatal

Monitoring of volume status must continue through the postpartum period, with fluid restriction as necessary. Diuretics may be used as necessary, and the patient should be given an angiotensin-converting enzyme (ACE) inhibitor (category D) for afterload reduction.[153] Although uncommonly performed, endomyocardial biopsy is recommended to exclude treatable causes of cardiomyopathy. Some patients with myocarditis found on biopsy respond favorably to immunosuppressive therapy.[153] There are no contraceptive restrictions in patients whose cardiac function has completely recovered. Combined hormonal methods should not be given in the early postpartum period or to those with persistent ventricular dysfunction.[43]

CARDIAC ARRHYTHMIAS

Maternal and Fetal Risks

Cardiac arrhythmias are relatively common during pregnancy. Most are benign and include sinus bradycardia, sinus tachycardia, and atrial and ventricular premature contractions. These patients are often asymptomatic, but may have palpitations, although the correlation between symptoms and the actual arrhythmia is poor. Shotan and associates[172] evaluated symptomatic pregnant patients who were referred to a cardiac clinic and compared them with asymptomatic pregnant patients who were referred for evaluation of a cardiac murmur. The incidence of premature atrial and ventricular contractions was 50% to 60% in each group. Although the frequency of arrhythmias was higher in symptomatic patients, only 10% of symptoms occurred in conjunction with the arrhythmia. Healthy, asymptomatic patients without underlying pathology can often be managed with reassurance, observation, and rest.[173,174] Nearly all women in labor will have tachycardia and isolated premature atrial beats at some point.[175] Aside from this, however, normal labor and delivery does not seem to increase the incidence or type of arrhythmias identified when compared with nonpregnant women.[175,176]

Pregnancy may be associated with an increase in the incidence and severity of arrhythmias.[172,177,178] Supraventricular tachycardia is often seen in pregnancy. Ventricular tachycardia and multiform premature ventricular complexes are much less common but may be recognized for the first time during gestation. Atrial fibrillation is usually associated with underlying cardiac disease.[179] With any of these arrhythmias, cardiac decompensation can occur, resulting in pulmonary edema. This is particularly common with underlying structural heart disease in which cardiac reserves may be limited. Sudden death is a concern in the presence of significant preexisting cardiac conditions. Women with a prior history of significant arrhythmias have a high incidence of recurrence during pregnancy. Atrial arrhythmias occur in approximately half of these patients, whereas ventricular arrhythmias recur in a quarter.[179]

Long QT syndrome is a genetic condition associated with a prolongation of the QT interval along with syncope and sudden cardiac death. β-Blockers are the mainstay of therapy. Women who continue therapy during pregnancy are at low risk of complications.[177,180] An increase in cardiac complications as a result of long QT syndrome has been noted during the postpartum period.[177] Some may benefit from the surgical implantation of a pacemaker.

Prematurity is increased in the presence of many arrythmias.[179] In addition, fetal exposure to drugs used for maternal therapy is a potential concern. Symptomatic and sustained arrhythmias often require appropriate antiarrhythmic therapy. Most antiarrhythmic agents are classified as category C, except when otherwise noted. β-Blockers can be used in patients with sinus tachycardia or frequent premature atrial or ventricular contractions when symptoms persist after conservative management.[178] In patients with long QT syndrome, β-blockers are continued to reduce the incidence of cardiac events.[177] Digoxin can be used safely to control the ventricular rate in atrial fibrillation and flutter and some supraventricular tachycardias.[173,174] Adenosine has a rapid onset and very short duration of action. It is used acutely during pregnancy to treat supraventricular tachycardia and is the drug of choice.[173,178,181] Esmolol and verapamil can be used intravenously in the acute management of supraventricular tachycardia. Quinidine is used to treat some atrial and ventricular arrhythmias. Lidocaine (category B) is used acutely to control ventricular arrhythmias. Procainamide is a second-line agent because of maternal side effects, including cardiac rhythm disturbances, lupus-like syndrome, and blood dyscrasia. Amiodarone (category D) is used to treat life-threatening ventricular arrhythmias when first-line agents are unsuccessful. It is associated with neonatal hypothyroidism, hyperthyroidism, and possibly IUGR, fetal bradycardia, and neurologic abnormalities.[173,182]

Management Options

Prepregnancy

All patients with a sustained arrhythmia should undergo a baseline electrocardiogram to determine whether the rhythm abnormality originates from the atrium or the ventricle. This is followed by a search for an underlying etiology. Patients with unexplained sinus tachycardia or premature atrial or ventricular contractions are questioned about tobacco, caffeine, and illicit drug use. They are also evaluated for anemia and hyperthyroidism. If a contributing factor is identified, behavior modification is attempted, as appropriate. Medical conditions should be treated before conception. Ambulatory monitoring is considered when patients have symptoms that suggest a rhythm disturbance but no objective evidence on examination. Patients who may benefit from ablative therapy should be identified and treated before conception.[173]

Prenatal, Labor and Delivery, and Postnatal

Management during pregnancy consists of maintenance therapy to control arrhythmias. Drug levels should be monitored, as indicated, because of pregnancy-associated changes in volume of distribution and protein binding. Vagal maneuvers can be tried initially in tachyarrhythmias with first onset in pregnancy.[173] Cardioversion can be used safely during pregnancy in unstable patients or when medical therapy is unsuccessful.[173,174,183] In patients with atrial fibrillation, ventricular rate should be controlled with digoxin, a β-blocker, or a calcium channel blocker. Prophylactic anticoagulation with either aspirin or heparin (LMWH or UFH) should be added. In the stable patient, medical cardioversion with quinidine or procainamide may be tried. Electrical cardioversion should be done in those who are hemodynamically unstable.[184] Continuous cardiac monitoring may be necessary intrapartum and postpartum for symptomatic or complex arrhythmias. Occasionally, surgical implantation of automatic defibrillators can be life-saving.

MYOCARDIAL INFARCTION

Maternal and Fetal Risks

MI is still uncommon in women of reproductive age with an incidence ranging from 3 to 7 per 100,000 births in the United States; however, with the current epidemic of obesity, it is likely to become increasingly important. In the United Kingdom, the incidence of MI in pregnancy has doubled since the 1990s, and it is now one of the leading causes of maternal death (16 deaths from this cause in the triennium from 2003 to 2005).[96] Approximately 20% of cases occur during labor, with the remainder nearly equally divided between the antepartum and the postpartum periods. Maternal mortality ranges from 5% to 8% and appears to have decreased in recent years.[185–187] Mortality is approximately 20% when the MI occurs in the peripartum period. This is roughly twice the rate during the antepartum period.[186,187] Prematurity is reported to be 43% in patients with an antenatal MI. Fetal outcome is ultimately related to maternal status and outcome.[186]

Risk factors associated with MI in pregnancy include increasing age, chronic hypertension, diabetes, hypertensive disorders of pregnancy, thrombophilia, and postpartum infection. Obesity is associated with an increased incidence of several of these risk factors. Although MI was reported to be more common in black women, race was not an independent risk factor after controlling for other comorbidities.[185,186] Transfusion has also been identified as a risk factor for MI and may represent a surrogate marker for postpartum hemorrhage.[185] Karpati and coworkers[188] demonstrated elevated troponin I levels, electrocardiographic changes, and decreased cardiac contractility compatible with myocardial ischemia in half of the 55 patients they managed with severe postpartum hemorrhage.

Atherosclerosis is the most common lesion seen with MI during pregnancy and is identified in 40% of patients. Coronary artery dissection is seen in 27%, whereas 13% of patients had normal coronary arteries. A coronary artery thrombosis in the absence of atherosclerosis was seen 8% of women.[187]

Criteria for the diagnosis of MI do not change during pregnancy. The diagnosis remains a challenge, in part because the index of suspicion is often low. Physiologic changes of pregnancy may mimic the symptoms of MI and delay the diagnosis. During labor, the diagnosis is further complicated by the fact that creatinine phosphokinase and the cardiac-specific MB fraction may normally be elevated.[189] Troponin I is a specific marker for cardiac injury that does not increase during normal labor and delivery, making it a potentially useful tool in the diagnosis of MI in the pregnant woman.[190] A few case reports have described the utility of troponin I in the diagnosis of MI during pregnancy.[191,192]

Management Options

Prepregnancy

Because the underlying condition is rare, pregnancy after MI is uncommon. Unfortunately, it is even more uncommon for these patients to seek preconception counseling.[193] When possible, cardiac evaluation should be done, including stress testing and echocardiography. Even if the patient has no cardiac dysfunction, pregnancy should be planned cautiously.[193] Medication should be optimized and statins (category X) should ideally be stopped before conception. ACE inhibitors (category C) used in the second or third trimester are associated with oligohydramnios and neonatal renal failure. An alternative drug should be used beginning before conception or in early pregnancy. β-Blockers (most category C) can be used. Atenolol is a cardioselective β-blocker (category D) that has been associated with IUGR and can be used with caution. Low-dose aspirin (category C) is not associated with adverse effects. There is limited information during pregnancy for clopidogrel (category B), an antiplatelet agent. Animal studies suggest low risk. It is believed to cross the placenta and, in theory, could pose a bleeding risk to the fetus.[31] For this reason, it should thus be used with caution near delivery. Because as many as half of women with ischemic heart disease will be obese, dietary advice and support in achieving weight reduction are important.

Prenatal

Patients should rest and avoid strenuous activity. They should also be monitored for evidence of arrhythmias or congestive heart failure. If an MI occurs during pregnancy, management principles are similar to those for nonpregnant patients.[187] Most drugs used in the medical management of acute MI are category C, except where otherwise noted. Nitroglycerin, oxygen supplementation, morphine (category B), heparin, and continuous cardiac monitoring are initiated. Lidocaine (category B), dopamine, calcium channel blockers, and β-blockers can be used, as indicated. Coronary angiography can be utilized as clinically indicated during pregnancy. Percutaneous angioplasty and stent placement are being used more frequently in pregnant patients with favorable outcomes.[185,187] Coronary artery bypass surgery has also been reported in pregnancy; however, the number of cases is small and conclusions regarding outcomes are limited.[187] Pregnancy is considered a relative contraindication to thrombolytic therapy because of the theoretical increased risk of maternal and fetal bleeding; however, safe and effective use during pregnancy has been reported, as well as cases of significant maternal bleeding and abruption.

The increased incidence of coronary artery dissection also urges caution with the use of thrombolytic therapy because bleeding may worsen the dissection.[185,187]

In cases of cardiac arrest, cardiopulmonary resuscitation proceeds with some notable modifications to the procedure used in the nonpregnant patient. These include lateral displacement of the gravid uterus to prevent aortocaval compression and improve venous return. Cricoid pressure is used when ventilation is required, and early intubation is recommended owing to the increased risk of aspiration. Chest compressions are done just above the mid sternum rather than above the xiphoid. There is no change in the recommendations for defibrillation.[194] If initial attempts at resuscitation are unsuccessful, perimortem cesarean section is indicated. Although a final heroic effort, the procedure is potentially life-saving for a viable fetus, and improved effectiveness of the resuscitation may also be life-saving for the mother. Optimal maternal and neonatal outcomes are seen when delivery occurs within 5 minutes of cardiac arrest.[195] Thus, making the decision to proceed and initiating the cesarean section should occur within 4 minutes of the arrest.[194–196]

Labor and Delivery

Vaginal delivery is believed to be relatively safe in patients who have had an MI. Cesarean delivery should be reserved for the usual obstetric indications as well as those who have had a MI in close proximity to labor or are unstable. External cardiac monitoring is necessary. Supplemental oxygen should be given, and epidural anesthesia is used for pain control. Operative vaginal delivery to shorten the second stage of labor is also recommended.[187]

Postnatal

Volume status is monitored in the postpartum period, and the patient should avoid exertion. A reliable plan for contraception should be made. Combination oral contraceptives, patches, rings, or injectables are usually contraindicated (category 4). Continued use of progesterone-only methods including the mini-pill, Depo-Provera, and implants should generally be avoided because they may have adverse effects on lipid profiles (category 3). Although the risk of atherosclerosis is not increased, estrogen increases thrombotic risk, especially when other risk factors are present. If permanent sterilization is not desired, the copper-containing IUD is a reasonable alternative (category 1).[42]

HYPERTROPHIC CARDIOMYOPATHY

Maternal and Fetal Risks

Hypertrophic cardiomyopathy is an autosomal dominant condition characterized by left ventricular hypertrophy without chamber dilation and no other etiology to explain the hypertrophy. It is classically associated with left ventricular outflow obstruction, but this is not found in most patients. As a result, older names for this condition, such as idiopathic hypertrophic subaortic stenosis and hypertrophic obstructive cardiomyopathy, have been generally replaced. In the general population, the frequency of this condition is approximately 1 in 500.[197]

The presentation and prognosis are clinically variable. Most patients have a normal life expectancy without limitations; however, hypertrophic cardiomyopathy is a common cause of sudden cardiac death in young people. The annual mortality rate is estimated at 1%, substantially less than the rate reported in older series, primarily because of the identification and inclusion of patients with more benign forms of the disease.[197,198] Clinical risk factors for sudden death include a family history of sudden cardiac death, previous syncope, and documented ventricular tachycardia. Maki and colleagues[198] identified an inadequate increase in systolic blood pressure associated with exercise, defined as less than 24 mm Hg on treadmill testing, as a risk factor in patients younger than 50 years. Left ventricular wall thickness greater than 30 mm may be a risk factor in young adults.[197] Septal myectomy in nonpregnant individuals has not only improved the outflow obstruction but also resulted in significant regression of the ventricular hypertrophy.[199] Implantable cardiac defibrillators are used successfully in high risk patients and can be used in pregnant patients.[200]

Physiologic changes associated with pregnancy have variable effects on the condition. Adequate preload and systemic vascular resistance are important factors in maintaining end-diastolic volume and cardiac output. A decrease in end-diastolic volume increases outflow obstruction. The increased blood volume associated with pregnancy has a beneficial effect, whereas the decrease in systemic vascular resistance can worsen outflow obstruction. The increased heart rate can also adversely affect maternal condition as a result of decreased diastolic filling time. Despite these concerns, maternal complications are uncommon and are confined primarily to women with specific risk factors.[201,202] The autosomal inheritance pattern gives the fetus a 50% chance of having the condition.

Management Options

Prepregnancy

Genetic counseling is indicated if either parent is affected. A careful history should be taken to identify patients with historical risk factors. An echocardiogram should be done. Patients should also be seen by a cardiologist who has experience with patients who have this condition to determine the need for exercise testing and the role of Holter monitoring. High risk patients may be evaluated for septal myectomy.

Prenatal

Activity is limited to avoid tachycardia. Adequate hydration should be maintained. Although it is not necessary in all patients, β-blockade may be used in symptomatic patients.[197]

Labor and Delivery and Postnatal

Volume status is monitored to avoid dehydration and hypotension during labor. Regional anesthesia may be used, but should be administered with care after adequate volume loading, again, to prevent hypotension. If tachycardia develops and the patient becomes symptomatic, β-blocking agents (mostly category C) may be used to control the heart rate. The patient should be observed for excessive blood loss and tachycardia in the postpartum period. Volume replacement is given, as indicated.

SUMMARY OF MANAGEMENT OPTIONS
Cardiac Disease: Specific

Management Options	Evidence Quality and Recommendation	References
Cardiac Murmur		
Echocardiogram for patients with a significant history or a pathologic murmur (late systolic, pansystolic, diastolic).	III/B	6,48
Mitral Valve Prolapse		
Echocardiogram evaluation prenatally for mitral regurgitation.	IV/C	57,58
Surveillance and treatment of arrhythmias in pregnancy.	IV/C	6
Atrial Septal Defect		
Pregnancy		
Screen for arrhythmias or pulmonary hypertension; manage accordingly both before and during pregnancy (if undertaken).	III/B	59,61
Prenatal		
Routine unless the patient has arrhythmias or pulmonary hypertension.	III/B	59
Screen fetus for congenital heart defect.	IIb/B	7,26,60
Labor and Delivery		
Screen for arrhythmias, monitor blood pressure, and avoid fluid overload.	III/B	59
Postnatal		
Encourage early mobilization.	III/B	59
Screen newborn for congenital heart defect.	IIb/B	7,26,60
Ventricular Septal Defect		
Prepregnancy		
Screen for pulmonary hypertension and manage accordingly; consider repair of uncorrected lesions.	III/B	62,63
Counsel about the risk of congenital heart disease.	IIb/B	7,26,60
Prenatal		
Obtain serial echocardiograms, and manage accordingly.	III/B	62,63
Screen fetus for congenital defect.	IIb/B	7,26,60
Labor and Delivery		
Avoid hypertension; provide antibiotic prophylaxis unless the patient has an uncomplicated vaginal delivery or if the defect has been repaired.	III/B	62,63
Provide antibiotic prophylaxis prior to cesarean section.	IV/C	37
Postnatal		
Provide careful fluid balance and early ambulation.	III/B	62,63
Screen newborn for congenital heart defect.	IIb/B	7,26,60
Pulmonary Hypertension		
Prepregnancy		
Counsel against pregnancy; offer sterilization if requested.	III/B	65,66

SUMMARY OF MANAGEMENT OPTIONS
Cardiac Disease: Specific—cont'd

Management Options	Evidence Quality and Recommendation	References
Prenatal		
Consider termination.	III/B	65,66
Joint obstetric and cardiology care and early anesthesiology consultation.	III/B	66
Thromboembolism prophylaxis.	III/B	65,66
Consider hospital admission and monitor SaO_2.	III/B	65,66
Provide fetal surveillance.	III/B	65,66
Use of calcium channel blocker has been reported.	III/B	70
Prostacyclin analogues, endothelin-receptor antagonists (e.g., bosentan), phosphodiesterase inhibitors, sildenafil (Viagra), and inhaled nitric oxide may be helpful.	III/B	64
Labor and Delivery		
Intensive care setting (degree of invasive monitoring varies); dilemma over induction (to end the pregnancy) vs. spontaneous onset of labor (because of shorter labor); oxytocin or E series prostaglandins are safe; O_2 is given at 5–6 L/min; Sao_2 is monitored continuously; monitor blood pressure and maintain fluid balance; epidural analgesic is preferable (reduce or stop anticoagulation for a few hours for delivery).	III/B	65,66
Intravenous prostacyclin or inhaled nitric oxide.	III/B	71,73
Postnatal		
Maintain intensive care monitoring; give O_2 therapy and thromboembolism prophylaxis; maintain vigilance for fluid retention and consequences; inhaled nitric oxide and intravenous prostacyclin may be continued or initiated; consider sterilization.	III/B	65,66,71–73
Eisenmenger's Complex		
As for Primary Pulmonary Hypertension.	III/B	76–79
Echocardiography may be helpful in evaluation, shunt, right ventricular function, and pulmonary hypertension.	III/B	76–79
Pulmonary Stenosis		
Prepregnancy and Prenatal		
Determine maternal functional status.	III/B	6,7
Echocardiography to determine degree of stenosis.		
Balloon valvotomy as clinically indicated.	III/B	80
Labor and Delivery and Postnatal		
Monitor volume status and for signs of right heart failure.	III/B	80
Coarctation of the Aorta		
Prepregnancy		
Screen for associated cardiac abnormalities and aortic valve disease, and manage appropriately (i.e., repair) before conception.	III/B	83
Prenatal		
Consider termination in patients with severe uncorrected disease.	III/B	84

Management Options	Evidence Quality and Recommendation	References
Labor and Delivery and Postnatal		
Avoid hypertension.	III/B	84
Provide antibiotic prophylaxis prior to cesarean section.	IV/C	37
Screen the newborn for congenital heart disease.	IIb/B	60,82,84
Tetralogy of Fallot		
Prepregnancy		
Surgical correction and evaluation of cardiac status after corrective surgery.	III/B	86
Prenatal		
Consider termination in patients with uncorrected lesions.	III/B	86
Monitor maternal Sao_2 and exercise tolerance; consider rest and supplemental O_2.	III/B	87
Fetal surveillance.	III/B	85
Fetal echocardiography to screen for congenital heart disease.	IIb/B	26,60
Labor and Delivery		
Provide careful fluid management; monitor the patient's blood pressure, Sao_2, and electrocardiogram; epidural use requires careful preloading, the need to shorten the second stage, and fetal monitoring; avoid fluid overload, maintain blood pressure.	III/B	85,86
Postnatal		
Maintain maternal monitoring and discuss effective contraception.	III/B	85,86
Transposition of the Great Arteries		
Prepregnancy		
Consultation with a cardiologist specializing in adults with congenital heart disease; evaluation of cardiac status with attention to the right (systemic) ventricle; monitor for arrhythmias.	III/B	60,88,90
Prenatal		
Decrease activity; monitor for heart failure and arrhythmias; perform serial echocardiography.	III/B	60,88,90
Labor and Delivery		
Provide careful fluid management; give oxygen as necessary; perform an electrocardiogram; use an epidural, shorten the second stage, and provide fetal monitoring.	III/B	60,88,90
Postnatal		
Monitor volume status.	III/B	60,88,90
Discuss effective contraception.	III/B	43
Ebstein's Anomaly		
Prepregnancy		
Echocardiography to evaluate right ventricular function and tricuspid regurgitation.	III/B	93
Surgical correction as indicated.	III/B	93

SUMMARY OF MANAGEMENT OPTIONS
Cardiac Disease: Specific—cont'd

Management Options	Evidence Quality and Recommendation	References
Prenatal		
Serial echocardiograms; monitor for arrhythmia; decrease activity as indicated.	III/B	60
Fetal echocardiogram.	III/B	60,94
Monitor for preterm labor and intrauterine growth restriction.	III/B	94
Labor and Delivery and Postnatal		
Maternal cardiac monitoring, supplemental O_2, monitor fluid balance, epidural for pain control, vacuum or forceps to shorten the second stage.	III/B	60
Patent Ductus Arteriosus		
Prepregnancy		
Screen for pulmonary hypertension, and manage appropriately before and during pregnancy (if undertaken).	III/B	95
Prenatal		
Screen for pulmonary hypertension.	III/B	95
Labor and Delivery and Postnatal		
Monitor blood pressure and fluid balance.	III/B	95
Rheumatic Heart Disease: General		
Principles		
• Prevent heart failure.	III/B	100
• Prevent bacterial endocarditis.	IV/C	37,39
• Use a team approach, including a cardiologist and an anesthesiologist.	—/GPP	—
Mitral Stenosis		
Prepregnancy		
Assess cardiac function, optimize medical therapy, and consider surgical correction.	III/B	6,7,106–109
Prenatal		
Monitor for excess weight gain; prevent and treat tachycardia and other arrhythmias.	III/B	6,104,110
Serial echocardiography; perform percutaneous commissurotomy or surgery for symptomatic severe disease.	III/B	108,111–113
Labor and Delivery		
Intensive care setting; consider central invasive monitoring, epidural analgesia, shorten the second stage of labor.	III/B	102
Antibiotic prophylaxis; cesarean delivery.	IV/C	37
Mitral Regurgitation		
Prepregnancy		
Evaluate functional status, maternal echocardiography to evaluate cardiac function, valve replacement as indicated.	III/B	117

Management Options	Evidence Quality and Recommendation	References
Prenatal		
Restrict activity; perform serial echocardiography; adjust medical control; consider surgery for symptomatic severe disease.	III/B	6,118,119
Perform fetal surveillance.	III/B	118,119
Labor and Delivery and Postnatal		
Avoid fluid overload and hypertension; provide maternal cardiac monitoring.	—/GPP	—
Provide endocarditis prophylaxis for cesarean deliveries.	IV/C	37
Aortic Stenosis		
Prepregnancy		
Determine severity by echocardiography.	III/B	6,7
Correct severe disease surgically before conception.	III/B	6,7
Prenatal		
Limit physical activity; maintain vigilance for heart failure and arrhythmias.	III/B	105,123,124
Fetal echocardiogram.	III/B	7
Fetal surveillance.	III/B	123
Labor and Delivery and Postnatal		
Avoid fluid overload, hypovolemia, and hypertension.	III/B	105,122–124
Some would use pulmonary artery catheter.	—/—	—
Bacterial endocarditis prophylaxis in patients undergoing cesarean section.	IV/C	37
Aortic Regurgitation		
Prepregnancy		
Echocardiography; optimize medical control (Digoxin); value replacement if indicated.	III/B	125
Prenatal		
Surveillance for cardiac failure; surgery for failed medical therapy.	III/B	114,118
Fetal surveillance.	III/B	114,118
Labor and Delivery and Postnatal		
Avoid fluid overload; invasive monitoring is usually unnecessary; epidural is beneficial; provide fetal surveillance.	III/B	125
Prosthetic Valves		
Prepregnancy		
Assess cardiac status; provide counseling about valve function and risks associated with warfarin.	III/B	7,31,134, 137–139
Prenatal		
If the patient has biosynthetic valves, monitor for deterioration; if the patient has mechanical valves, provide adequate anticoagulation; vigilance for thrombocytopenia when using heparin.	III/B	127,134,139
Labor and Delivery		
Adjust anticoagulation.	III/B	132,139
Endocarditis prophylaxis as indicated.	IV/C	37

SUMMARY OF MANAGEMENT OPTIONS
Cardiac Disease: Specific—cont'd

Management Options	Evidence Quality and Recommendation	References
Postnatal		
Readjust anticoagulation.	III/B	132
Marfan's Syndrome		
Prepregnancy		
Genetic counseling.	III/B	149
Echocardiography to assess aortic root diameter; counsel about pregnancy risks.	III/B	147,148,152
Prenatal		
Serial aortic root echocardiography; give β-blockers; avoid hypertension; encourage rest; surgery in extreme cases.	III/B	7,146,148, 149
Monitor for preterm labor.	III/B	151
Labor and Delivery and Postnatal		
Epidural is beneficial; avoid hypertension; ensure adequate oxygenation; shorten the second stage of labor; maintain vigilance for aortic root dissection for at least 8 wk postnatally.	III/B	7,147,148
Dilated Cardiomyopathy		
Prepregnancy		
Echocardiography.	III/B	169
Counsel regarding the risk of pregnancy if the patient has a history of peripartum cardiomyopathy and counsel against pregnancy if there is residual cardiac dysfunction.		
Prenatal		
Echocardiography.	III/B	164–166
Consider termination in patients with an abnormal echocardiogram; if the patient is symptomatic, provide medical therapy and anticoagulation.	III/B	164,167–169,171
Multidiscliplinary team care	—/GPP	—
Labor and Delivery		
Monitor for heart failure; avoid fluid overload; possibly use pulmonary artery catheter, vigilance for arrhythmias; adequate analgesia.	III/B	154,169
Postnatal		
Avoid fluid overload; discuss contraception.	III/B	153,154,169
Cardiac Arrhythmias		
Prepregnancy		
Investigate and treat.	III/B	173,177,178, 180,181,184
Prenatal, Labor and Delivery, and Postnatal		
Maintenance of therapy to control arrhythmia; cardioversion can be used as indicated.	III/B	173,177,178, 180,181,184

Management Options	Evidence Quality and Recommendation	References
Myocardial Infarction		
Prepregnancy		
Assess cardiac function (especially echocardiography and stress testing); counsel on the basis of results.	III/B	193
Optimize medical therapy.	III/B	31
Prenatal		
Avoid strenuous activity; provide surveillance for failure and arrhythmias; management as for a nonpregnant patient; surgery can be performed in pregnancy.	III/B	187
Percutaneous coronary artery interventions can be used as indicated.	III/B	185,187
Thrombolytic therapy may be used with caution when indicated.	III/B	185,187
Labor and Delivery		
Monitor electrocardiogram; provide supplementary oxygen; epidural is beneficial; consider cesarean section if labor occurs within 4 days of an acute myocardial infarction.	III/B	187
Postnatal		
Avoid fluid overload and exertion; discuss contraception (avoid combination oral preparations).	III/B	42
Hypertrophic Cardiomyopathy		
Prepregnancy		
Genetic counseling; evaluate cardiac status with echocardiography; implantable defibrillator may be used as indicated.	III/B	197,198,200
Prenatal		
Limit activity; give β-blockers for symptomatic patients	III/B	197
Labor and Delivery and Postnatal		
Avoid dehydration or hypotension; give β-blockers for tachycardia.	III/B	197

GPP, good practice point; Sao_2, arterial oxygen saturation.

SUGGESTED READINGS

Bates S, Greer I, Pabinger I, et al: Venous thromboembolism, thrombophilia, antithrombotic therapy, and pregnancy: American College of Chest Physicians Evidence-Based Clinical Practice Guidelines. Chest 2008;133:844–886.

Bédard E, Dimopoulos K, Gatzoulis M: Has there been any progress made on pregnancy outcomes among women with pulmonary arterial hypertension? Eur Heart J 2009;30:256–265.

DeSanto L, Romano G, DellaCorte A, et al: Mitral mechanical replacement in young rheumatic women: Analysis of long-term survival, valve-related complications, and pregnancy outcomes over a 3707–patient-year follow-up. J Thorac Cardiovasc Surg 2005;130:13–19.

James A, Jamison M, Biswas M, et al: Acute Myocardial infarction in pregnancy: A United States population-based study. Circulation 2006;113:1564–1571.

Pearson G, Veille J, Rahimtoola S, et al: Peripartum cardiomyopathy. JAMA 2000;283:1183–1188.

Sadler L, McCowan L, White H, et al: Pregnancy outcomes and cardiac complications in women with mechanical, bioprosthetic and homograft valves. BJOG 2000;107:245–253.

Siu S, Sermer M, Harrison D, et al: Risk and predictors for pregnancy-related complications in women with heart disease. Circulation 1997;96:2789–2794.

Skinner J, Hornung T, Rumball E: Transposition of the great arteries: From fetus to adult. Heart 2008;94:1227–1235.

Thorne S, Nelson-Piercy C, MacGregor A, et al: Pregnancy and contraception in heart disease and pulmonary arterial hypertension. J Fam Plann Reprod Health Care 2006;32:75–81.

Wilson W, Taubert KA, Gewitz M, et al: Prevention of infective endocarditis: Guidelines from the American Heart Association: A guideline from the American Heart Association Rheumatic Fever, Endocarditis, and Kawasaki Disease Committee, Council on Cardiovascular Disease in the Young, and the Council on Clinical Cardiology, Council on Cardiovascular Surgery and Anesthesia, and the Quality of Care and Outcomes Research Interdisciplinary Working Group. Circulation 2007;116:1736–1754.

REFERENCES

For a complete list of references, log onto www.expertconsult.com.

CHAPTER 37

Respiratory Disease

PAUL S. GIBSON and RAYMOND O. POWRIE

INTRODUCTION

A variety of physiologic adaptations to the maternal respiratory system occur in normal pregnancy. Minute ventilation increases, attributable mainly to the effect of high progesterone levels on the maternal respiratory center. Oxygen consumption rises and residual lung volume decreases, particularly in the latter half of pregnancy. Generally, these physiologic changes are well tolerated with minimal symptomatology by the pregnant woman. The interaction of these biologic changes with various pulmonary diseases is less well understood, however, despite the relatively common occurrence of some of these conditions during pregnancy. Respiratory physicians should be involved in the management of many of these disorders when they occur in pregnancy. This is particularly important in conditions such as acute severe asthma, the severity of which may be underestimated by both doctor and patient; severe pneumonia; cystic fibrosis (CF); and tuberculosis (TB), considering that the guidelines for therapy change frequently. Acute pulmonary edema is also one of the most common reasons that pregnant or postpartum women are transferred to critical care units, and appropriate understanding and management of these severely ill women is essential.

BREATHLESSNESS OF PREGNANCY

General

Pregnancy is associated with several significant changes in respiratory function. Pregnant women increase their minute ventilation by nearly 50%. This is achieved by increasing the volume of each breath rather than by increasing respiratory rate. This is an effect of progesterone, leading to a decrease in arterial carbon dioxide pressure ($PaCO_2$) to 27 to 32 mm Hg.[1] Arterial oxygen pressure (PaO_2) is increased to 95 to 105 mm Hg at sea level, as per the alveolar gas equation. A compensatory renal excretion of bicarbonate occurs in response to the chronic respiratory alkalosis, and serum bicarbonate levels normally decrease by approximately 4 mEq/L.

Pulmonary function test results, including forced expiratory volume in 1 second (FEV_1), forced vital capacity (FVC), and peak expiratory flow rates (PEFR), remain largely unchanged in pregnancy. The main change seen on pulmonary function tests (PFTs) is an approximately 20% drop in functional residual capacity (FRC; that portion of a breath that can still be exhaled after normal resting exhalation) due to a decrease in both expiratory reserve volume (ERV) and residual volume (RV).[2,3] Although the diaphragm may be elevated to 4 cm above its usual position by term, this does not have a significant effect on respiratory function because diaphragmatic excursion is not altered.[4]

Mild breathlessness is a common symptom in normal pregnancy and, therefore, does not necessarily indicate cardiorespiratory disease. Up to 70% of pregnant women will report some level of dyspnea. The most typical description of this would be "air hunger."[3,5] This symptom may appear during the late first or early second trimester, though the peak period for the onset of breathlessness is 28 to 31 weeks' gestation. Often the breathlessness occurs spontaneously at rest rather than in association with exertion. The trigger of the symptomatology has not been clearly defined, although the hormonal effect of progesterone on ventilation and the associated fall in $PaCO_2$ seem to be central features. Studies have found that the presence of dyspnea during pregnancy correlates with a relatively high baseline nonpregnant $PaCO_2$ and a low $PaCO_2$ during pregnancy.[6,7]

Management Options

It is a clinical challenge to differentiate benign breathlessness of pregnancy from more serious causes of shortness of breath in pregnancy, such as asthma, pulmonary embolism, and cardiomyopathy. Initial evaluation should be based on a careful history and physical examination. Dyspnea attributable to pregnancy physiology alone is generally episodic, insidious in onset, and not associated with any chest discomfort, cough, or sudden exacerbation. A previous history of reactive airways, the presence of cough or wheezing, or an obstructive pattern on PFT may point to asthma as a cause. Pulmonary embolism is usually characterized by the sudden onset of dyspnea or chest pain, often in association with asymmetrical leg symptoms/signs. Cardiac disease in pregnancy may present with dyspnea as an initial or predominant feature. This may reflect a preexisting cardiac condition, unmasked by the increased blood volume and cardiac work of pregnancy, or may point to a new onset of cardiac disease such as peripartum cardiomyopathy. Findings on physical examination of tachypnea, tachycardia, an elevated jugular venous pulse, a concerning murmur, respiratory "crackles" on auscultation, or an abnormal chest x-ray or electrocardiogram (ECG) can point to a cardiac cause of dyspnea. Suspicion of a cardiac cause should lead to prompt evaluation with transthoracic echocardiography.

History and physical examination can be supplemented with investigations including: complete blood count (CBC), oxygen saturation measurement (SaO_2) with exercise, and, if necessary, a chest x-ray. The CBC can be used to identify those cases of dyspnea attributable to severe anemia. Measurement of SaO_2 (by pulse oximeter) with moderate exertion can also help alleviate a patient's anxiety about her symptoms. If the SaO_2 remains normal (>95%) on exercise, the dyspnea does not limit activity at all, and the onset was not sudden, it is unlikely but not impossible that the patient has a pathologic cause for her dyspnea. Measurement of arterial blood gases (ABGs) will be unnecessary in the vast majority of women presenting with dyspnea in pregnancy.

When clinical evaluation leads the clinician to suspect that a patient's dyspnea is due to more than just the normal physiology of pregnancy, the clinician should be confident that all relevant diagnostic imaging procedures for investigating other causes of dyspnea can be safely performed during pregnancy. This includes chest x-rays, computed tomography (CT) scans of the chest, ventilation-perfusion scans, magnetic resonance imaging (MRI), and occasionally, pulmonary angiography.[8] Most often, if other serious causes of dyspnea do not appear to be present, management of breathlessness in pregnancy is limited to educating the patient regarding these physiologic changes and providing reassurance and follow-up.

SUMMARY OF MANAGEMENT OPTIONS

Breathlessness in Pregnancy

Management Options	Evidence Quality and Recommendation	References
Ask about wheezing, nocturnal worsening, and cough to distinguish from asthma.	IV/C	1,4,7
Ask about orthopnea and paroxysmal dyspnea and perform cardiac examination to distinguish from heart failure.	IV/C	1,4,7
Ask about sudden onset of dyspnea, presence of chest pain, personal or family history of thrombosis and look for tachypnea, tachycardia, or signs of DVT to distinguish from PE. Consider objective testing for DVT/PE if any of the above are present.	IV/C	1,4,7
Key investigations:	IV/C	8
When a diagnosis other than "physiologic" breathlessness of pregnancy is suspected, consider the following tests:		
• Oxygen saturation at rest and with ambulation.		
• Hemoglobin.		
• Chest radiograph.		
• Ventilation-perfusion scan or CT angiogram or MRI.		
• Echocardiography.		

CT, computed tomography; DVT, deep vein thrombosis; MRI, magnetic resonance imaging; PE, pulmonary embolism.

ASTHMA

General

Asthma is the most common potentially life-threatening chronic medical disorder to occur in pregnancy. The worldwide prevalence both outside and during pregnancy has been increasing. Among pregnant women, the prevalence of ever having received a diagnosis of asthma increased from 6.6% to 14.7% from 1988 to 2002.[9] According to the most recent U.S. data, about 8% of pregnant women report current active asthma during pregnancy.[9]

Available data do not describe a consistent effect of pregnancy on the frequency of asthma symptoms or the overall severity of the disease. In one prospective study of 330 asthmatic women, asthma was unchanged in 33%, improved in 28%, and worsened in 35%.[10] A systematic review reported that 69% of women have improved methacholine-induced bronchial hyperresponsiveness during pregnancy, but that 31% have a deterioration.[11] More recent data from the northeastern United States, however, state that 88% of pregnant asthmatic women studied report one or more asthmatic symptoms during pregnancy, and that 16% of these women have symptoms almost daily.[9]

It is not clear whether the severity of asthma before pregnancy predicts its course during pregnancy,[12] but up to 75% of women who have no reported asthma symptoms in the year before pregnancy have some symptoms during pregnancy.[9] Overall, about 6.7% of pregnant asthmatic women require emergency treatment for asthma in pregnancy, and 1.6% require hospitalization. Asthma attacks and asthma-related emergency room visits are more common in pregnant American women who are younger, unmarried, of lower family income, and of Puerto Rican or non-Hispanic black background.[9] It does appear that women tend to have similar courses with respect to their asthma in successive pregnancies.[13] Some investigators suggest that asthma tends to be less severe in the last 4 weeks of pregnancy and that if it does worsen, it tends to do so between 29 and 36 weeks.[14] Asthma exacerbations in labor are uncommon.

A common reason for asthmatic patients to deteriorate in pregnancy is the misperception that treatment for asthma is harmful to the fetus, leading to noncompliance with asthma-controlling medications. A National Institutes of Health (NIH) Consensus Conference has concluded that "undertreatment of pregnant asthmatics, particularly because of unfounded fears of adverse pharmacologic effects on the developing fetus, remains the major problem in the management of asthma during pregnancy in the United States."[15] A recent study reported that only 17% of pregnant asthmatic women took any regular controller medication during pregnancy.[9] Only half of women on a controlling medication continued it in pregnancy, and even among women with asthma symptoms in more than 10 of the preceding 12 months prior to pregnancy, use of an asthma-controlling medication during pregnancy occurred in only 42%. Another recent study of prescription claims found a decrease of 23% in inhaled corticosteroid use, of 13% in short-acting β-agonist use, and of 54% in systemic steroid use in the first trimester of pregnancy.[16] Other treatable reasons why asthma may worsen in pregnancy in individual women include pregnancy-related gastroesophageal reflux disease (GERD) and pregnancy rhinitis. These precipitating factors should be considered and treated as possible contributors in pregnant women with difficult-to-control asthma.

Maternal and Fetal Risks

There are conflicting reports concerning the relationship between asthma and maternal and fetal complications. Risks that are established are an increased risk of preterm delivery[17–22] and maternal gestational hypertension/preeclampsia.[23,24] Possible associations between maternal asthma and hyperemesis gravidarum, vaginal hemorrhage, complicated labor, neonatal mortality, and placenta previa have been noted in some studies but not in others. Intrauterine growth restriction (IUGR) and small–for–gestational age infants do not seem to be caused by maternal asthma.[18–21,25] The risk of the reported complications does appear to be greater in women with severe (steroid-dependent) or poorly controlled asthma.[19] One large study also identified a relationship between lower FEV_1 results and both preterm delivery and gestational hypertension.[26] Lastly, a few studies have suggested a small increased risk of congenital malformations in offspring of women with asthma. One recent study identified a small overall increased risk of congenital malformations (odds ratio [OR] 1.1) in offspring of asthmatic women, which was not explained by exposure to asthma medications in pregnancy.[27] Other recent reports have shown an increased risk of gastroschisis (OR 2.06) in offspring of women who used bronchodilators in pregnancy[28] and an overall increased risk of malformations following pregnancies with an asthma exacerbation in the first trimester (OR 1.48).[29] These results require verification and, if real, the increased risk of malformations appears to be small.

It is not clear whether the relationship between asthma and these obstetric complications represents a direct effect of hypoxia and/or hypocapnia on the developing pregnancy, the effects of medication use, or a fundamental abnormality of smooth muscle in asthmatics manifest as increased contractile tone in the uterus, airways, and vasculature.[25,30] In general, asthma should not be considered a contraindication to pregnancy, although good asthma control should be emphasized as a way to minimize the incidence of many of these complications.

The risk of the child developing asthma in later life varies between 6% and 30%, depending on whether or not the mother is atopic and whether or not the father is also atopic and/or has asthma.[31] Younger maternal age at the time of delivery also appears to increase the lifetime risk of asthma in the offspring.[32]

Management Options

Prepregnancy

Preconception counseling should be included as a routine part of regular health maintenance visits in women of childbearing age who have asthma. The counseling should be individualized with regard to the individual's disease severity and current treatment regimen. Overall, it should be communicated that pregnancy is generally well tolerated, but that compliance with asthma monitoring and maintenance treatments is essential. Patient education regarding the use of maintenance and rescue asthma medications, monitoring via PEFR use, proper use of inhalers, avoidance of asthma precipitants, and an asthma management plan (as described in the following section) are important prior to and during pregnancy. Spirometry may be desirable prepregnancy in order to serve as a baseline reference point, particularly if serial monitoring of air flows is planned as part of the asthma follow-up during pregnancy. Patients should be firmly counseled not to stop necessary medications when they find out they are pregnant.

Prenatal

Whereas asthma care should ideally be optimized prior to conception, patients often present with symptomatology during pregnancy that requires assessment and urgent management. Given the described complications of poorly controlled asthma, close monitoring of the patient's status and appropriate adjustment of treatments are essential to ensuring the best outcome for mother and child.

GENERAL PRINCIPLES

The goal of treatment for asthma in pregnancy is to provide optimal therapy to maintain asthma control, defined as minimal or no chronic symptoms, day or night; minimal or no exacerbations; no limitation of activity; maintenance of (near) normal pulmonary function; minimal use of short-acting inhaled β_2-agonists; and minimal or no adverse effects from the treatment provided. The underlying principle for treatment of asthma during pregnancy is that with few exceptions, the same drugs and dosages that would be used outside pregnancy should be used in pregnancy for a given clinical indication.[33] Inadequate control of asthma is a greater risk to the fetus than asthma medications are. Proper control of asthma should enable a woman with asthma to maintain a normal pregnancy with little or no risk to her or her fetus. Whenever possible, treatment should be by the inhalational rather than the oral route, because this reduces maternal systemic effects[34,35] and also reduces the medication exposure of the fetus.

PREVENTION AND EDUCATION

Patient education is vital to the successful management of asthma in pregnancy because it will lead to improved compliance with monitoring and pharmacologic treatments, thereby reducing the risk of severe asthmatic exacerbations. Pregnant women with asthma should be strongly encouraged to avoid exacerbating factors, including allergens/irritants and particularly tobacco smoke. These women should also have proper inhaler use reviewed with them repeatedly. Proper use includes using a spacer to improve delivery of medication to the lungs, avoiding local side effects of inhaled steroids (such as oral thrush), and decreasing unnecessary systemic absorption of medication through the buccal mucosa.

SPECIFIC ASTHMA MEDICATIONS

Asthma medications are classified as either rescue agents or maintenance agents. *Rescue agents* are those medications used to treat acute bronchospasm and provide symptomatic relief but do not treat the underlying inflammation that causes bronchospasm. Rescue agents include all the inhaled β_2-agonists and ipratropium. The data regarding their effectiveness and the safety of rescue asthma medications in pregnancy are reviewed in Table 37–1. *Maintenance agents* are those medications that help to control airway hyperreactivity and generally treat the underlying inflammation of the airway. The inhaled steroids are the keystones of asthma maintenance. Other maintenance agents include systemic steroids, leukotriene antagonists, and cromolyn. The data regarding the effectiveness and safety of maintenance asthma medications in pregnancy are reviewed in Table 37–2.[15,36]

MONITORING AND DAILY ASTHMA MANAGEMENT WITH A STEPWISE PLAN

Women with asthma in pregnancy should be seen regularly and assessed via both history and physical examination as well some objective measure of pulmonary function (spirometry or PEFR monitoring). This objective data can be especially helpful in determining whether dyspnea is due to breathlessness of pregnancy or an asthmatic exacerbation. Serial fetal evaluations may also be indicated in the setting of significant asthma activity to monitor fetal growth and well-being.

Asthma medications are generally prescribed in a "stepwise" manner. All asthmatics should be given a written asthma management plan outlining recommended medication adjustments according to their symptoms (and PEFR if monitored), and guiding them about when to seek medical advice. Action plans are based on the best PEFR that a patient has ever obtained. Table 37–3 outlines the criteria for classification of asthma into four classes and reviews the treatment recommended during pregnancy for each degree of severity. This stepwise approach is recommended in the current guidelines by the U.S. National Asthma Education and Prevention Program[33] and the British Thoracic Society.[37] A typical action plan for a patient would tell her that if she develops symptoms more than 2 days per week or her PEFR drops below 80% of her personal best, her therapy needs "stepping up"; the patient should have instructions at home as to how to do this. The patient should be told that sustained drops in PEFR of more than 20% below her personal best warrant a call to the physician. A PEFR drop greater than 40% from her personal best warrants a trip to the emergency department (ED). When good control has been maintained for several months, the individual may consider stepping down the treatment to a regimen appropriate for the next lower level of asthma severity.

In pregnancy, GERD,[38,39] vasomotor rhinitis of pregnancy, and medication noncompliance should always also be considered as possible treatable causes of difficult-to-control asthma.

TREATMENT OF ACUTE ASTHMA EXACERBATIONS

Patients with worsening asthma, not improving on home management by the stepwise approach, will need to be seen

TABLE 37–1

Summary of Pregnancy Data on Rescue Agents Commonly Used to Treat Asthma[15,202–209]

CLASS	AGENT	EFFECT ON EMBRYO AND FETUS
Short-acting inhaled β_2-adrenergic agonists	Albuterol, isoproterenol, pirbuterol, metaproterenol, terbutaline	Published experience with these drugs in animals and humans suggests that β-sympathomimetics do not increase the risk of congenital anomalies.[15,202,207] Albuterol is the most studied of these agents. Metaproterenol is the second most studied.
Long-acting inhaled β_2-adrenergic agonists	Salmeterol, formoterol	Animal data about intravenously administered salmeterol have not been reassuring, but this agent is still felt to probably be safe in humans when administered by inhalation.[15] Very limited human data have been published regarding salmeterol, and none regarding formoterol at this point; therefore, salmeterol may be preferred[15] and its use should be reserved for patients who have failed low-potency steroids and/or cromolyn alone.
Inhaled anticholinergic agents	Ipratropium	Reassuring animal studies but no published human data. Poorly absorbed by the bronchial mucosa so fetal exposure is likely minimal.[208] Efficacy in acute asthma attack presenting to the emergency department makes its short-term use seem justifiable, however.

Adapted from Powrie RO: Drugs in pregnancy. Respiratory disease. Best Pract Res Clin Obstet Gynaecol 2001;15:913–936.

TABLE 37–2

Summary of Pregnancy Data on Maintenance Medications Commonly Used to Treat Asthma[15,202,209–211]

CLASS	AGENTS	PREGNANCY DATA
Inhaled corticosteroids	Low potency: beclomethasone, dipropionate Medium potency: triamcinolone, acetonide High potency: fluticasone, propionate, budesonide, flunisolide, mometasone furoate	Inhaled corticosteroids are the most important pharmacologic agents in maintaining asthma control in and out of pregnancy. Only 4% of 257 patients taking inhaled glucocorticoids from the start of pregnancy had acute attacks of asthma during pregnancy, in contrast with 17% of 177 patients who were not.[210] Beclomethasone and budesonide are the most widely studied of the inhaled corticosteroids in pregnancy. The most recent data refer to budesonide, which should now be considered the preferred inhaled steroid in pregnancy.[15] Data regarding triamcinolone and fluticasone suggest no adverse pregnancy effects. Relatively little of these agents is absorbed, and human data have not suggested any teratogenic effects of these agents.[15,211-214]
Mast cell stabilizers	Disodium cromoglycate (cromolyn), sodium nedocromil	Human and animal data suggest these agents are nonteratogenic and well tolerated. These agents are virtually not absorbed through mucosal surfaces, and the swallowed portion is largely excreted in the feces. These agents are less effective than inhaled corticosteroids[15] and thus are useful in mild cases of asthma in which the decision not to use inhaled steroids has been made. Cromolyn[202,215] has been better evaluated in human pregnancy than nedocromil and should be considered the preferred agent of this class.
Leukotriene antagonists	Zafirlukast, montelukast, zileuton	Zafirlukast and montelukast both have favorable animal data, but data about their safety in human pregnancy remain limited at this point.[216] Zileuton has concerning animal data and should be avoided in pregnancy.[15] The use of these agents may be considered in pregnancy to those unusual cases in which a woman has previously had a significant improvement in asthma control with these medications before becoming pregnant, control that was not obtainable through other methods.
Sustained-release methylxanthines	Theophylline, aminophylline	Theophylline and its intravenous form aminophylline do not appear to be human teratogens.[202,207,217] The safety of aminophylline therapy in the second and third trimesters has been demonstrated in a large group of 212 gravidas in Finland.[217] The clearance of aminophylline is increased in pregnancy in a rather variable way.[217] Any patient who is taking more than 700 mg of aminophylline per day should have blood measurements made for optimal dosing. Their present role in treating asthma is generally felt to be as second- or third-line agents; they do not appear to be of benefit in an acute exacerbation.[218]
Systemic steroids	Oral: prednisone Intravenous: methylprednisolone hydrocortisone	Most data suggest that systemic steroids do not present a significant teratogenic risk in human pregnancy. Nonfluorinated systemic steroids do not cross the placenta in significant quantities because of placental metabolism[219-221] (the same is not true for betamethasone or dexamethasone). Even in higher doses, the effect of hydrocortisone or prednisone on the fetus in terms of suppression of the hypothalmic-pituitary-adrenal axis is minimal. There is a significant association with first-trimester use and oral clefts (odds ratio 6.55, 95% confidence interval 1.44-29.76).[221,222] In the setting of severe asthma or a severe exacerbation, however, the benefits of controlling a life-threatening disease make systemic steroid use (even in the first trimester) justifiable.[15]
Immunotherapy	Administration of gradually increasing quantities of an allergen extract to an allergic subject to down-regulate response	Human data from small trials suggest safety of continuing immunotherapy in pregnancy, but most physicians avoid initiation in pregnancy because of fear of provoking anaphylaxis.[223-225]

Adapted from Powrie RO: Drugs in pregnancy. Respiratory disease. Best Pract Res Clin Obstet Gynaecol 2001;15:913–936.

in an ED for evaluation. Treatment in the ED is reviewed in Table 37–4. Acute severe asthma (status asthmaticus) is a life-threatening condition that should be managed by a respiratory physician in an intensive care environment. High-dose intravenous steroids are the cornerstone of treatment for asthmatic exacerbations requiring admission to the hospital. Even in the absence of acute severe asthma, there should be a very low threshold for hospital admission of pregnant asthmatic patients because uncontrolled asthma can deteriorate very quickly.[40] General guidelines for admission to hospital include a sustained drop in PEFR to less than 60% of baseline, a PaO_2 less than 70 mm Hg at sea level, a $PaCO_2$ greater than 35 mmHg, a heart rate of greater than 120 bpm, or a respiratory rate greater than 22/min. It is important to remember that a $PaCO_2$ greater than 40 mm Hg in a pregnant women with an asthmatic exacerbation suggests impending respiratory failure, because the normal $PaCO_2$ in pregnancy is 27 to 32 mm Hg.

Labor and Delivery

An asthma exacerbation is not generally an indication for elective delivery, but if there are other maternal or fetal problems, facilitated delivery may be considered. Asthma exacerbations commencing during labor are rare, presumably owing to the natural outpouring of endogenous steroids and epinephrine associated with the stress of delivery. Exacerbations occurring at this time should always be approached with a differential diagnosis that includes pulmonary edema (from cardiac causes or noncardiac ones such as preeclampsia, tocolysis, and sepsis), pulmonary embolism, and aspiration.

TABLE 37–3

Classification of Asthma and Stepwise Management in Pregnancy[15,202]

CATEGORY	CRITERIA	STEP THERAPY
Mild intermittent	• Symptoms up to twice a week *and/or* • Nighttime symptoms *up to* twice a month • PEFR > 80% predicted and day-to-day variability < 20%	• No daily treatment necessary • Inhaled β_2-adrenergic agonists as needed
Mild persistent	• Symptoms more than twice a week but not daily *and/or* • Nighttime symptoms *more than* twice a month • PEFR > 80% predicted *but* day-to-day variability 20%-30%	• Inhaled β_2-adrenergic agonists as needed ***and*** • Daily treatment with inhaled low-dose corticosteroid (preferably budesonide). • Alternatives include daily cromolyn, a leukotriene receptor antagonist, or a theophylline preparation
Moderate persistent	• Daily symptoms *and/or* • Nighttime symptoms more than once a week • PEFR 60%-80% with day-to-day variability > 30%	• Inhaled β_2-adrenergic agonists as needed ***and*** • Daily treatment with inhaled *low-dose* corticosteroid *and* daily treatment with salmeterol *or* • Daily treatment with inhaled *medium-dose* corticosteroid • If needed, combine treatment with daily *medium-dose* inhaled corticosteroid *and* daily salmeterol • Alternative: daily *low-medium* dose inhaled corticosteroid *and* either theophylline or a leukotriene receptor antagonist
Severe persistent	• Continual symptoms that limit activity • Frequent nighttime symptoms and acute exacerbations • PEFR < 60% predicted and day-to-day variability > 30%	• Inhaled β_2-adrenegic agonists as needed ***and*** • Daily treatment with inhaled high-dose corticosteroid ***and*** • Daily treatment with salmeterol *and, if needed* • Daily treatment with systemic corticosteroids

PEFR, peak expiratory flow rate.
Adapted from Powrie RO: Drugs in pregnancy. Respiratory disease. Best Pract Res Clin Obstet Gynaecol 2001;15:913–936.

TABLE 37–4

Management of the Acute Asthma Exacerbation Presenting to the Emergency Department[15,209]

1. Place patient on oxygen to keep $Sao_2 > 95\%$.
2. Administer inhaled β_2-adrenergic agonist until improvement obtained or toxicity is noted; e.g., albuterol MDI with spacer 3 to 4 puffs *or* albuterol nebulizer every 10–20 min.
3. If exacerbation is mild-moderate (i.e., FEV_1 or PEF > 50% predicted) initiate oral corticosteroids (i,e., prednisone ~ 1 mg/kg)
4. If exacerbation is severe (i.e., FEV_1 or PEF < 50% predicted) administer either oral or systemic steroids (e.g., methylprednisolone 125 mg IV acutely and then 40–60 mg IV q6h *or* hydrocortisone 60–80 mg IV q6h. When the patient improves, she can be switched to a tapering oral regimen of prednisone).
5. Consider use of ipratropium MDI (2 puffs of 18 µg/spray q6h) or nebulizer (one 62.5-mL vial by nebulizer q6h) in first 24 hr after presentation.
6. Initiate assessment of fetal well-being if pregnancy has reached fetal viability.
7. Make individualized assessment of need for hospitalization (see text).

FEV_1, forced expiratory volume in 1 sec; MDI, metered-dose inhaler; PEF, peak expiratory flow.
Adapted from Powrie RO: Drugs in pregnancy. Respiratory disease. Best Pract Res Clin Obstet Gynaecol 2001;15:913–936.

Prostaglandin E_2 compounds and oxytocin can be safely used in asthmatics. 15-Methyl prostaglandin F_2 should not be used in asthmatic patients because it can cause bronchoconstriction.[41,42] Ergonovine and other ergot derivatives should also not be used in asthmatics because they too have caused severe bronchospasm in asthmatic patients, particularly in association with general anesthesia. Although morphine and meperidine may theoretically cause bronchoconstriction through histamine release, this is not generally a problem in clinical practice. Nonetheless, some experts prefer to use butorphanol or fentanyl as alternatives in pregnant asthmatics because these agents are less likely to cause histamine release. Regional anesthesia is preferable to general anesthesia because of the lower risks of pulmonary infection and atelectasis. For those women who do require a general anesthetic, bronchodilatory agents such as ketamine and halogenated anesthetics are preferred.

It is known that supraphysiologic daily doses of systemic steroids, given for as little as several weeks, may suppress the hypothalamic-pituitary-adrenal (HPA) axis for up to 1 year. This could blunt the normal physiologic outpouring of adrenal corticosteroids that occurs with stressors such as illness, surgery, and labor, though the prevalence of clinical complications seems to be low. The significance of this theoretical risk in pregnancy remains unstudied. To avoid the risk of precipitating an adrenal insufficiency crisis, however, many experts advise giving an empirical "stress dose" of systemic steroids (e.g., hydrocortisone 50–100 mg IV q8h on the day of delivery followed by 25–50 mg IV q8h on day 1 after delivery and then back to the baseline dose) to any woman in labor who has received systemic steroids in doses greater than 5 mg.day for longer than 2 to 4 weeks in the preceding year. If stress-dose steroids are not given, it is advisable to watch the patient for signs of adrenal insufficiency (anorexia, nausea, vomiting, weakness, hypotension, hyponatremia, and hyperkalemia) in the peripartum interval and postpartum.

Postnatal

Physicians should ensure that asthmatic women have their asthma medications reordered and continued postpartum. These women should also have their PEFR monitored in the days following delivery. Breast-feeding is recommended in women regardless of their asthma treatment. In fact, breast-feeding for between 1 and 6 months reduces the prevalence of atopy by about 30% to 50% in 17-year-olds who were breast-fed.[43]

SUMMARY OF MANAGEMENT OPTIONS

Asthma

Management Options	Evidence Quality and Recommendation	References
Prepregnancy		
Adjust maintenance medication to optimize respiratory function.	IV/C	15,33,37
Educate patient about use of spacers and peak expiratory flow meters.	III/B	15,33,37
Educate patient to continue maintenance medications in pregnancy.	III/B	15,33,37
Provide patient with a stepwise asthma action plan.	III/B	15,33,37
Advise early referral for prenatal care.	III/B	15
Prenatal		
Use same drugs as outside pregnancy—especially steroids and β-agonists.	III/B	15,33,36
If theophylline is used, monitor blood levels, because blood volume expansion in pregnancy may mandate higher doses of the drug.	III/B	15,33,36
Monitor peak flow and adjust asthma medication as needed to control symptomatology and minimize need for "rescue" therapy.	III/B	15,33,36,37
Utilize inhalation rather than oral route.	III/B	34,35
Ensure adequate fetal oxygenation with acute exacerbation by keeping maternal oxygen saturation > 95%.	III/B	15,36
In the woman with active asthma, increase fetal growth monitoring and assessment of immediate fetal health by fetal heart rate monitoring.	III/B	15,36
Seek anesthesiology consultation in preparation for delivery if general anesthesia is anticipated.	III/B	15
Labor and Delivery		
Regional is preferable to general anesthesia.	III/B	15
Ensure adequate fetal oxygenation with acute exacerbation by keeping oxygen saturation > 95%.	III/B	15,36
Avoid prostaglandin F_2 and ergometrine	III/B	41,42
Consider parenteral "stress-dose" steroids for patients on chronic oral therapy or in those who have received more than 3 wk of systemic steroids in the past year.	III/B	15
Postnatal		
Continue maintenance drug therapy.	III/B	15,36
Encourage breast-feeding.	III/B	15,43
Physiotherapy to maintain adequate pulmonary toilet.	III/B	15,36

SARCOIDOSIS

General

Sarcoidosis is a chronic condition most commonly seen in women of reproductive age, and thus, may complicate pregnancy. The prevalence of sarcoidosis in the general population is estimated to be 10 to 20 per 100,000 population, with a lifetime risk of 0.85% among whites and three to four times more common in the black population.[44]

The lung is the organ most likely to be affected in sarcoidosis, and the majority of cases are found incidentally on routine chest x-rays. The differential diagnosis of pulmonary sarcoidosis includes malignancy, TB, HIV infection, collagen vascular disease, and occupational lung disease. Tissue biopsy is required for an accurate diagnosis in all but the most classic presentations.

Pulmonary involvement in sarcoidosis is classified by the radiographic stage of disease. Stage I is defined by the presence of bilateral hilar adenopathy, often accompanied by right paratracheal lymph node enlargement. Stage II involves bilateral hilar adenopathy along with interstitial infiltrates. Stage III disease consists of interstitial lung disease with shrinking hilar nodes, and stage IV disease is defined by advanced pulmonary fibrosis. Most individuals (~75%) with stage I disease will have spontaneous regression in 1 to 3 years, and about two thirds of patients at stage II will undergo spontaneous resolution. Those with stages III and IV disease are likely to progress to serious lung impairment without treatment.

Sarcoidosis may also involve other organ systems including the skin (maculopapular eruptions, skin nodules, and erythema nodosum), the lymphatic system (lymphadenopathy), the eyes (iridocyclitis, chorioretinitis, and keratoconjunctivitis), and the liver. Rarely, sarcoidosis can occur in the spleen (splenomegaly); the neurologic system; the salivary glands; the bone marrow; the ear, nose, and throat; the heart; the kidneys; bones, joints, or muscle.[45,46] Sarcoidosis can also have effects on calcium homeostasis (hypercalciuria and hypercalcemia).

The cornerstone of treatment for sarcoidosis is systemic corticosteroids. In general, steroid treatment is reserved for those with significant symptoms due to pulmonary compromise or major extrapulmonary involvement. Corticosteroid therapy may also be of some benefit in milder cases of pulmonary sarcoid in which there is chest x-ray evidence of parenchymal disease (i.e., stage II or above). Whether the risks of long-term corticosteroids are worth the modest (~10%) benefit seen in asymptomatic patients remains unclear.[47,48] Chloroquine, hydroxychloroquine, methotrexate, azathioprine, pentoxifylline, thalidomide, cyclophosphamide, cyclosporine, and infliximab have all also been tried in the treatment of chronic or steroid-unresponsive sarcoidosis with variable success.[49]

Maternal Risks

Whereas sarcoidosis rarely infiltrates the female reproductive organs, involvement of the endometrium, ovary, and leiomyoma have all been reported.[50,51] In the absence of significant cardiopulmonary compromise, sarcoidosis does not appear to adversely affect fertility and does not increase the incidence of fetal or obstetric complications.[52]

Although some series have described a pregnancy-associated improvement in sarcoidosis,[53] followed by a postpartum exacerbation, the general consensus is that pregnancy does not predictably influence the natural history of sarcoidosis.[54] It has been postulated that improvement during pregnancy might be due to physiologic increases in maternal free cortisol and/or the immune modulation intrinsic to pregnancy.

Among the unfortunate patients in whom sarcoidosis has progressed to the stage of extensive pulmonary fibrosis and hypoxemia, along with cor pulmonale and pulmonary hypertension, the maternal and fetal prognosis is poor.

Fetal Risks

Beyond severe maternal disease from pulmonary or other organ involvement, leading to fetal compromise, there are no specific risks to the fetus from maternal sarcoidosis. The use of systemic steroids in pregnancy for maternal sarcoidosis poses little risk to the developing fetus. Severe maternal sarcoidosis that is unresponsive to steroids, however, might lead physicians to consider other treatments that are less well studied in pregnancy. Untreated severe hypercalcemia in the mother could precipitate neonatal hypocalcemia and tetany, but the hypercalcemia associated with sarcoidosis is usually mild and unlikely to lead to such neonatal problems. Sarcoid granulomas have occasionally been noted in the placenta[55] but not in the fetus.

Management Options

Prepregnancy

Preconception counseling should be undertaken in women with sarcoidosis, incorporating the previous information.[53] Measurement of baseline parameters should include SaO_2 (both resting and with exercise), PFT (including a diffusing capacity for carbon monoxide [DL_{CO}], as a measure of gas exchange that is sensitive to the presence of interstitial lung disease), a chest x-ray, CBC, liver function tests, blood urea nitrogen, creatinine, and serum calcium. In the setting of moderate to severe pulmonary disease, echocardiography should be considered to evaluate for pulmonary hypertension. On the basis of these data, patients with stage I or II disease (and minor extrapulmonary manifestations) may be advised to expect a good pregnancy outcome. Women with more severe and active disease should be counseled that their pregnancy may be complicated by their disease and/or its treatment and that there is the potential for severe maternal illness to have a secondary effect on the well being of the fetus. Severe pulmonary arterial hypertension of any cause poses a very serious maternal mortality risk, and therefore, such women should be discouraged from proceeding with pregnancy (see Chapter 36).

Prenatal

Breathlessness is common in normal pregnancy but can also be seen in stages II to IV sarcoidosis. Women with sarcoidosis who develop complaints of increased dyspnea require reevaluation with SaO_2 (both resting and with exercise), chest x-ray, and PFT. Comparison with the baseline investigations (listed previously) will facilitate the interpretation of this additional testing. In some circumstances, a high-resolution CT scan may be needed to define the extent of disease. This evaluation may be undertaken with an acceptable degree of risk owing to fetal radiation exposure. Serial monitoring of maternal calcium (ionized or total calcium corrected for decreasing albumin in normal pregnancy), liver enzymes, creatinine, and CBC approximately once per trimester is also advisable. This may be helpful in identifying hypercalcemia prior to delivery as well as establishing a baseline that may help prevent the inappropriate attribution of abnormalities in creatinine or liver tests to preeclampsia later in pregnancy.

Painful joints and erythema nodosum are manifestations of sarcoidosis that may also be seen in normal pregnancies but need to be evaluated carefully, because they may be a manifestation of disease progression.

Symptomatic disease attributable to sarcoidosis should generally be treated with systemic steroids, under the supervision of a pulmonologist/internist experienced in treating this disease. As previously stated, the safety of steroids in pregnancy is well established and is discussed in the preceding section on "Asthma." Symptomatic disease unresponsive to steroids may require treatment with other agents that are less well studied in pregnancy and will require careful consideration of both risk and potential benefits of treatment.

Patients with sarcoidosis have a risk of developing hypercalcemia, particularly in the setting of vitamin D supplementation.[56] Even in women with a normal serum calcium level, sarcoidosis-associated hypercalciuria can lead to nephrocalcinosis. Pregnant patients with sarcoidosis should, therefore, avoid both vitamin D and calcium supplementation, and the ingredients of their prenatal vitamins should be reviewed to prevent unintended supplementation.

The level of angiotensin-converting enzyme (ACE) has been advocated by some experts as an index of disease activity in sarcoidosis, but this may be invalid in pregnancy because ACE levels seem to change independently of sarcoid activity in pregnancy.[57]

Labor and Delivery

Among women with parenchymal lung disease due to sarcoidosis, regional techniques are strongly preferred to general anesthesia for cesarean delivery. Women with severe pulmonary involvement will benefit from an early epidural in labor (to reduce oxygen consumption in response to pain), and an assisted second stage of labor (forceps or vacuum suction) to reduce maternal exhaustion should be considered. Women who have been on supraphysiologic systemic steroids for more than 3 weeks in the preceding year should be considered for stress-dose steroids around the time of labor and delivery.

Postnatal

There are no specific recommendations regarding the postpartum management of the parturient with sarcoidosis.

SUMMARY OF MANAGEMENT OPTIONS
Sarcoidosis

Management Options	Evidence Quality and Recommendation	References
Prepregnancy		
Reassure patient of benign nature of sarcoidosis during pregnancy (unless there is preexisting evidence of pulmonary fibrosis, hypoxemia, or pulmonary hypertension).	III/C	53,54
Obtain baseline laboratory and pulmonary function studies.	IV/C	53,54
If lung disease is significant, obtain echocardiogram for assessment of pulmonary hypertension. Discourage pregnancy in presence of severe pulmonary hypertension.	III/B	53,54
Prenatal		
Avoid multivitamins containing vitamin D.	III/B	53,54
Monitor serum calcium once per trimester (because of potential neonatal toxicities with maternal hypercalcemia).	III/B	53,54
Monitor for signs and symptoms of progressive pulmonary disease; institute steroid therapy if evidence of significant disease advancement.	III/B	53,54
Labor and Delivery		
With substantial parenchymal disease, avoid inhalation anesthesia.	IV/C	53,54
Obtain early anesthesiology consultation in patients with severe disease.	IV/C	53,54
Use parenteral "stress-dose" steroids for patients on chronic oral therapy or in those who have received more than 2–4 wk of systemic steroids in the past year.	III/B	53,54
Watch for neonatal tetany if mother has hypercalcemia.	III/B	53,54
Postnatal		
No specific recommendations.		

TUBERCULOSIS

General

Although TB made a significant resurgence in the western world in the early 1990s, the incidence of TB is once again declining in the United States. In 2004, the Centers for Disease Control and Prevention (CDC) reported a rate of new TB infections of 4.9 per 100,000 individuals.[58] There remain, however, a large number of latent (unidentified) and active cases of TB in the western world.[59,60] Most of these cases are occurring among the homeless and inner-city residents, among recent immigrants from countries with a high prevalence of TB, and among drug abusers and individuals with HIV infection.

Worldwide, TB infection remains a much more daunting problem. It is estimated that one third of the world's population has been infected with TB and that there are 8 million new cases of TB and 2 million deaths worldwide caused by TB each year.[59] Medical contact during pregnancy is an opportunity for the identification and treatment of TB among young women. Such therapy will benefit the mother, her child, and the general public.

Maternal and Fetal Risks

Although the incidence and transmission factors for TB are not altered by pregnancy, management requires additional consideration by the clinician. The main concerns are potential fetal infection and drug safety.

Maternal Risks

Pregnancy does not alter the clinical course of TB for the mother, and with modern antituberculous therapy, immunocompetent women should expect to make a complete recovery even if the TB is first diagnosed in pregnancy. It has been reported in some series that hepatotoxicity due to isoniazid (INH)—one of the key agents in antituberculous therapy—may occur with increased frequency in pregnancy.[61–63]

Fetal Risks

Risks to the fetus in the setting of maternal TB relate to (1) risk of fetal infection, (2) risk of fetal harm from antituberculous medications, and (3) fetal risks from severe maternal illness. Overall, TBs that is confined to the thorax or limited to lymphadenitis poses little risk to the fetus. Adverse fetal outcomes may be more frequent with disseminated disease.[64,65]

Mycobacterium tuberculosis rarely crosses the placenta,[65] although granulomata may be found in the placenta in the setting of primary or disseminated or miliary disease. True congenital infection is therefore extremely uncommon. This may relate to the observation that disseminated TB almost invariably involves the genital tract, which is a cause of infertility. Criteria for congenital TB include (1) confirmed diagnosis of TB in the newborn; (2) primary granulomatous complexes identifiable in the neonatal liver; and (3) in the absence of neonatal liver lesions, the diagnosis of TB in the newborn is made within a few days of birth (in order to differentiate congenital TB from neonatal/postpartum infection).[58,66] The neonate is at risk of postnatally acquired infection only if the mother is still infectious with active TB at the time of delivery. In that unusual setting, the risk of transmission to the neonate is high.[67]

Low birth weight, preterm delivery, and increased perinatal mortality rates have been reported in the setting of incomplete treatment and advanced or disseminated TB. One small study that compared pregnancy outcomes in pregnant women with extrapulmonary TB versus healthy controls found a significantly higher frequency of low–birth weight infants and infants with low Apgar scores among mothers with extrapulmonary TB.[58,67]

Given the very low risk of congenital TB infection and the generally good maternal prognosis, the main risk to the developing fetus is the issue of potential teratogenicity/toxicity of the antituberculous medications.

Management Options

Prepregnancy

Preconception counseling should address the possible effects of the antituberculous drugs on the developing fetus. Women undergoing treatment for active TB should be advised to delay pregnancy until their course of treatment course is complete. They should be counseled that in the event of an unplanned pregnancy, they should seek prompt medical attention rather than abruptly stopping their treatment. Women who have previously completed an adequate course of antituberculous therapy have no contraindication to pregnancy. Women with latent TB should be offered appropriate treatment prior to pregnancy, with a review of effective contraception if necessary in order to delay pregnancy until after the completion of the treatment.

Prenatal

Screening for TB with a tuberculin skin test (TST) is not justified for the whole general obstetric population.[68] Pregnant women from high risk populations for TB, however, should undergo a TST unless documentation of recent TST status is available. High risk populations include HIV-infected women; close contacts of persons known or suspected to have TB; immigrants or visitors from areas with a high prevalence of TB; residents and employees of high risk settings (prison, institutions) including health care workers; injection drug users; and medically underserviced, low-income populations (e.g., inner-city minority populations). TST is both safe and reasonably sensitive throughout pregnancy.[69,70]

Women who have a positive skin reaction according to standard criteria[71] and women with symptoms suggestive of active pulmonary TB (regardless of their TST results) should have a chest x-ray performed to look for evidence of active or latent pulmonary TB. If the chest x-ray is suggestive of active TB, sputum specimens must be obtained to evaluate for *Mycobacteria*.

Susceptibility testing for INH, rifampin, and ethambutol should be performed on a positive initial culture. Prior to commencing antituberculous treatment, baseline measurements of liver enzymes, bilirubin, alkaline phosphatase, serum creatinine, and platelet count should be obtained. HIV testing, if not already completed as part of prenatal care, is recommended for all pregnant patients with evidence of active or prior TB. Testing of visual acuity and red-green color discrimination should be obtained when ethambutol is to be used.

If sputum testing is positive (on acid-fast bacillus [AFB] smear, polymerase chain reaction [PCR] testing, or culture), treatment should be promptly initiated. The maternal and fetal benefits of treatment dramatically outweigh any concerns about potential drug toxicity to the fetus. Tuberculous infections in pregnancy should be managed jointly by an obstetrician and a physician experienced in the treatment of TB. Directly observed therapy is recommended because it ensures compliance. Pregnancy data about the commonly used antimycobacterial agents are reviewed in Table 37–5.[72–76] Streptomycin is the only commonly used antituberculous drug that is clearly contraindicated in pregnancy, because it has the potential to cause eighth cranial nerve damage,[77] leading to neonatal deafness. The recommendations by the World Health Organization (WHO) and the International Union Against Tuberculosis and Lung Disease (IUATLD) for uncomplicated TB in a pregnant individual include an initial 2-month course of INH, rifampin, ethambutol, and pyrazinamide. This is followed by a further 4 months of treatment with just INH and rifampin (for a total of 6 mo of treatment).[71] The current guidelines for Americans by the American Thoracic Society, in contrast, suggest that the initial treatment regimen in pregnancy should consist of INH, rifampin, and ethambutol ***without*** pyrazinamide. They comment that pyrazinamide is excluded "because of insufficient data to determine safety." If pyrazinamide is not included in the treatment regimen, the minimum recommended duration of treatment is 9 months.[72]

All women taking INH should also receive pyridoxine 25 to 50 mg daily to minimize the risk of neuropathy.[78] The amount of pyridoxine in multivitamins is variable but generally less than the needed amount. Vitamin K should probably also be given to the mother from 36 weeks' gestation onward in a dose of 10 mg daily to decrease the risk of

TABLE 37–5

Pregnancy Data Regarding Commonly Used Antimycobacterial Agents[72–76,209]

AGENT AND USUAL DOSE	ADVERSE EFFECTS IN GENERAL	PREGNANCY DATA	ADDITIONAL NOTES
Isoniazid (INH)			
• 5 mg/kg, up to a maximum of 300 mg daily • Dispensed in the United States as 50-, 100-, and 300-mg tablets and 50 mg/5 mL syrup	• Hepatitis • Peripheral neuropathy • Drug interaction with many agents, especially anticonvulsants • Cutaneous hypersensitivity	• FDA pregnancy classification C. • High lipid solubility; easily passes into fetal circulation. • Fair data to suggest this agent is safe in human pregnancy and any risk is outweighed by potential benefit. However, concerns about potential increase in INH hepatotoxicity in pregnancy make its routine use for prophylaxis in pregnancy in low risk cases not advisable.	• Always administer with 25–50 mg/day of pyridoxine (vitamin B_6) to decrease the risk of neurotoxicity in the mother. • Give vitamin K to mother near birth (10 mg PO daily from 36 wk on) and infant at birth to decrease risk of postpartum hemorrhage and hemorrhagic disease of the newborn. • Check transaminases monthly while on the medication.
Rifampin			
• 10 mg/kg, up to a maximum of 600 mg daily • Dispensed as 150- and 300-mg scored tablets in the United States	• Fever • Nausea • Hepatitis • Purpura • Flulike symptoms at high doses • Orange secretions • Increased metabolism of many agents	• FDA pregnancy classification C. • Limited data suggest no adverse fetal effects.	• Give vitamin K to mother near birth (10 mg PO daily from 36 wk on) and infant at birth to decrease risk of postpartum hemorrhage and hemorrhagic disease of the newborn. • Limited data suggest no adverse fetal effects.
Ethambutol			
• 15–25 mg/kg, up to a maximum of 2500 mg daily • Dispensed as 100- and 400-mg tablets in the United States	• Retrobulbar neuritis in 1% of patients • Peripheral neuropathy	• FDA pregnancy classification B. • Limited data suggest no adverse fetal effects.	• At each monthly visit, patients taking this agent should be questioned regarding possible visual disturbances, including blurred vision or scotomata; monthly testing of visual acuity and color discrimination is recommended for patients receiving the drug for longer than 2 mo.
Pyrazinamide			
• 15–30 mg/kg PO daily, up to a maximum of 3000 mg daily	• Thrombocytopenia • Hepatotoxicity • Interstitial nephritis • Nephrotoxicity	• FDA pregnancy classification C. • Human data extremely limited.	• Use in pregnancy supported by international recommendations but current ATS guidelines caution against use. Essential for multidrug-resistant TB and HIV-positive patients.
Streptomycin			
• Dose varies	• Ototoxicity	• FDA pregnancy classification D. • Reports of fetal ototoxicity preclude use.	• Avoid use in pregnancy.

ATS, American Thoracic Society; FDA, U.S. Food and Drug Administration; TB, tuberculosis.
Adapted from Powrie RO: Drugs in pregnancy. Respiratory disease. Best Pract Res Clin Obstet Gynaecol 2001;15:913–936.

hemorrhagic disease of the newborn.[79] The most common serious adverse effect of INH is a toxic hepatitis. Symptoms of hepatotoxicity (e.g., nausea, abdominal pain, hepatic tenderness) in association with hepatic transaminase elevations greater than three times the normal range or asymptomatic elevations in transaminases greater than five times the normal range should prompt discontinuation of therapy (and consideration of an alternative regimen). Pregnant women are at a higher risk of developing INH-related hepatotoxicity; therefore, testing of hepatic transaminases at initiation of treatment and at monthly intervals thereafter is advisable.[61–63]

Management of HIV-related TB is complex and requires expertise in the management of both HIV disease and TB. Because HIV-infected patients are often taking numerous medications, some of which interact with antituberculous medications, it is strongly encouraged that experts in the treatment of HIV-related TB be consulted.

Whether a positive TST, in the absence of active pulmonary TB, merits treatment with antituberculous medications during pregnancy depends on several factors: the size of the woman's TST response, her HIV status, and whether or not the woman has had recent contact with someone with an active case of TB. Indications to treat a positive TST in pregnancy, because of a high short-term risk of progression to active disease, include HIV-infected women exposed to an active case of TB; HIV-infected women with a TST result greater than 5 mm; any woman with recent active TB contact and a TST result greater than 5 mm; and women with a recent conversion from a negative to a positive TST. It remains controversial whether other pregnant women with normal immune status and a positive TST (not previously treated) should receive prophylaxis during pregnancy. A decision analysis found that antepartum treatment of a positive TST would result in fewer active TB cases, would be less expensive, and would improve life expectancy of the pregnant women affected.[80] Nonetheless, among asymptomatic immunocompetent pregnant women who are reliable to follow-up, treatment of a positive TST can generally be delayed until the postpartum period.[81,82]

The standard regimen for treatment of a positive TST is INH 5 mg/kg (up to a maximum of 300 mg) daily for 9 months. Twice-weekly doses of 15 mg/kg (up to a maximum of 900 mg) for 9 months may also be used as an alternative as part of directly observed therapy. Pyridoxine 25 to 50 mg daily should also be given, as in treatment of active TB.

Labor and Delivery

There are no specific recommendations regarding the pregnant woman with TB at the time of labor and delivery, except for appropriate infection control issues in the infectious patient. Because transmission of TB infection from mother to infant (neonatal TB) may occur postpartum, medical contact at the time of delivery may be an opportunity to evaluate the symptomatic woman for active and infectious pulmonary TB.[83]

Postnatal

In the rare circumstance of identifying a woman with active and infectious (sputum-positive) TB in late gestation or at the time of delivery, the neonate must unfortunately be separated from the mother until she is no longer infectious. In this circumstance, the neonate should also be given INH to prevent it acquiring neonatal infection. It is also reasonable to consider treating the neonate with INH-resistant bacilli Calmette-Guérin (BCG) vaccine to boost its immunity.[84]

Breast-feeding should not be discouraged for women being treated with INH, pyrazinamide, ethambutol, and/or rifampin. These agents are found in only small concentrations in breast milk and are not known to produce toxicity in the nursing newborn. These concentrations are also not significant enough to provide any protection to the nursing infant from infection with TB.[85]

SUMMARY OF MANAGEMENT OPTIONS
Tuberculosis

Management Options	Evidence Quality and Recommendation	References
Prepregnancy		
Screen at-risk populations for TB with a TST prior to pregnancy.	III/B	68–70
If positive TST, treat as appropriate and delay pregnancy until after completion of antituberculous therapy.	III/B	71,72
Counsel regarding the potential teratogenesis of streptomycin, if being used.	III/B	77
Prenatal		
Perform TST on all women from high risk populations (see text).	III/B	68–72
Arrange HIV testing for all women with a positive TST.	IV/C	71,72
Administer INH prophylaxis during pregnancy to TST-positive women (without active TB) if they are HIV-positive, have a known recent TB exposure, or are new TST-converters.	IV/C	71,72

Management Options	Evidence Quality and Recommendation	References
Send sputum cultures (with antibiotic sensitivity testing) from women with active TB and start a recommended drug regimen: INH, rifampin, ethambutol ± pyrazinamide.	IV/C	71,72
Give pyridoxine 25–50 mg/day when using INH.	III/B	78
Measure hepatic transaminases monthly in pregnant women on INH.	IV/C	71,72
Labor and Delivery		
No specific recommendations except infection precautions needed with active disease.	IV/C	71,72
Postnatal		
Only separate baby from mother at birth if mother has infectious TB, and only until no longer infectious (~10 days into therapy).	IV/C	71,72
Administer INH and BCG vaccine to neonate if mother infectious at birth.	III/B	84
Encourage breast-feeding.	IV/C	85

BCG, bacillus Calmette-Guérin; INH, isoniazid; TB, tuberculosis; TST, tuberculin skin test.

KYPHOSCOLIOSIS

General

Kyphoscoliosis is usually an idiopathic disorder (>80%) involving kyphosis (anteroposterior spinal angulation) and/or scoliosis (lateral spinal curvature) that begins in childhood—and hence, often affects women of reproductive age. Affected individuals may develop functional lung impairment, the degree of which correlates well with the severity of spinal deformity. The pattern of abnormality on PFTs is restrictive, with decreased total lung capacity (TLC) and vital capacity (VC) and preserved RV. Chest wall compliance also typically decreases with age, increasing the work of breathing.

Kyphoscoliosis that is mild has a good prognosis. Conversely, in severe cases, pulmonary hypertension may develop as a result of persistent hypoxemia and result in cor pulmonale. Such individuals have a life expectancy of less than 1 year. Although various surgical and nonsurgical treatments are often undertaken in childhood, surgery has little role in adults with kyphoscoliosis. Medical therapy can include pulmonary rehabilitation, the use of supplemental oxygen, and occasionally, the use of negative- or positive-pressure ventilators.[86]

Mild degrees of kyphoscoliosis are common among pregnant women. More severe deformity resulting in respiratory impairment occurs in less than 0.1% of pregnancies. In some severe cases, it is remarkable that patients can complete a successful pregnancy despite their degree of deformity; the abdominal cavity may appear so contracted that there seems to be insufficient room for a fetus to develop normally. Nonetheless, positive outcomes are usually seen.[87]

Maternal and Fetal Risks

Among women with significant kyphoscoliosis, the maternal risks are mainly cardiac failure and cor pulmonale in the rare patient with significant pulmonary hypertension. To develop pulmonary hypertension, the condition has to be severe enough to produce hypoxemia at rest. The patient is at risk of respiratory failure if the VC is less than 1.5 L, particularly if it is less than 1 L.[88,89] The main risks to the fetus are IUGR and preterm delivery related to maternal hypoxemia.[90] Fetal hypoxic brain damage has been described in a patient with kyphoscoliosis and severe hypoxia (maternal PaO_2 < 59 mm Hg).[91]

Management Options

Prepregnancy

Preconception counseling should be undertaken, incorporating the previous information. PFTs should be obtained. If the VC is greater than 2 L, patients may be advised that they will generally tolerate pregnancy and delivery. If the VC is less than 2 L, the woman should be advised that she will be at increased risk for pulmonary complications with pregnancy. A blood gas analysis should be obtained in all women with a VC less than 2 L and if the resting PaO_2 is decreased, the fetus should be considered at risk of growth restriction. If the resting $PaCO_2$ is increased prepregnancy, the risk of maternal pulmonary complications in pregnancy is high.

In the setting of significant abnormalities on ABGs and PFTs—particularly resting hypoxia or hypercapnia—the woman should be evaluated for pulmonary hypertension. An ECG may be uninformative at evaluating for right ventricular hypertrophy in kyphoscoliosis, owing to the deformity of the chest. The pulmonary artery pressure and right heart function should therefore be assessed by echocardiography. Moderate to severe pulmonary hypertension is a relative contraindication to pregnancy (see Chapter 36). Before such a drastic recommendation is made, however, the physician may want to consider performing a direct measurement of pulmonary vascular indices via a formal right cardiac catheterization.

Prenatal

Women with significant kyphoscoliosis require comprehensive medical care and follow-up regarding diagnosis and treatment of respiratory infections, bronchospasm, and evidence of cardiac failure. Women with hypoxia should be provided with supplementary oxygen therapy to reduce the risk of adverse fetal effects such as growth restriction. Patients identified to have significantly elevated pulmonary artery pressures and vascular resistance should be offered a termination of pregnancy, in view of the markedly increased risk of maternal mortality or severe morbidity.

These women may require hospitalization in later gestation, owing to impending respiratory compromise or for fetal concerns. Respiratory support with nasal positive-pressure ventilation has been used in some patients who have deteriorated in the third trimester.[92,93] Obstetric prenatal care relates mainly to monitoring for IUGR and preterm labor. Elective preterm delivery may be indicated for either maternal (increasing hypoxemia or frank respiratory failure) or fetal (signs of fetal hypoxia ± IUGR) indications.

Labor and Delivery

Women with severe kyphoscoliosis are often delivered by cesarean section because of concerns about concomitant pelvic deformity.[94] Regional anesthesia is much preferred to general anesthesia, and despite the severity of back deformity, a spinal or epidural puncture and catheterization is often possible in these patients—because the defect in kyphoscoliosis is typically in the upper part of the spine.

Postnatal

After delivery, optimal medical care includes early mobilization, physiotherapy, and ongoing monitoring for cardiac complications and respiratory infections.

SUMMARY OF MANAGEMENT OPTIONS
Kyphoscoliosis

Management Options	Evidence Quality and Recommendation	References
Prepregnancy		
Obtain PFTs for assessment of vital capacity; obtain ABGs to assess O_2 and CO_2 levels.	III/B	88–90
If PFTs/ABGs are abnormal, assess for evidence of pulmonary hypertension; if present, advise against pregnancy.	IV/C	88–90
Counsel regarding risk for increase in pulmonary compromise as pregnancy progresses; discuss risk for fetal growth restriction and possible need for preterm delivery.	IV/C	88–90
Prenatal		
Monitor respiratory function: clinically and with periodic oxygen saturation measurement.	IV/C	88–90
Discuss pregnancy termination if pulmonary hypertension is present.	III/B	88–90
If severe cardiorespiratory compromise develops, initiate surveillance for fetal growth restriction and well-being.	III/B	88–91
Administer oxygen if maternal $Sao_2 < 95\%$. Consider use of nasal intermittent positive-pressure ventilation if respiratory status deteriorating.	IV/C	92,93
Consider elective preterm delivery for frank respiratory failure or severe fetal compromise.	III/B	88–90
Labor and Delivery		
Supplementary oxygen if low Sao_2 values.	III/B	88–90
Consider cesarean section if associated pelvic deformities, though vaginal delivery possible in most cases; regional anesthesia for cesarean section is possible in most cases.	IV/C	88–90
Postnatal		
Chest physiotherapy, especially following general anesthesia.	—/GPP	—

ABGs, arterial blood gases; GPP, good practice point; PFTs, pulmonary function tests; Sao_2, arterial oxygen saturation.

CYSTIC FIBROSIS

General

CF is an autosomal recessive multisystem disorder characterized by recurrent pulmonary infections due to unusually thick bronchial secretions. The incidence of CF is about 1 in 2000 live births. Five percent of whites are carriers of the CF gene. Although CF remains a potentially fatal disease associated with a decreased life expectancy, the therapy of CF has undergone rapid evolution in the past few decades with a resulting significant improvement in patient survival. Many more women with CF are now surviving to reproductive age, and so we can expect to see more cases of CF in pregnancy.[95]

The symptoms and signs of CF include recurrent and persistent pulmonary infections, pancreatic exocrine insufficiency, and elevated sweat chloride levels. A functional defect in the complex chloride channel found in all exocrine tissues results in thick, viscous secretions in the lungs, pancreas, liver, intestine, and reproductive tract.[96] The resulting chronic pulmonary disease is the leading cause of morbidity and mortality in patients with CF. Pulmonary involvement is characterized by recurrent pneumonias, chronic bronchitis (with or without bronchiectasis), and an obstructive pattern on PFTs.

The tenacious respiratory secretions facilitate colonization of the airway and sinuses with pathogenic bacteria. *Staphylococcus aureus* and *Haemophilus influenzae* are common pathogens during early childhood, but over 70% of adults with CF are chronically ultimately infected with *Pseudomonas aeruginosa*, a highly pathogenic and resistant bacteria. Persistent infection with the species *Burkholderia cepacia*, notorious for inducing airway injury and exhibiting high-level antibiotic resistance,[97] is associated with an accelerated decline in pulmonary function and shortened survival among CF patients.

Acute or subacute exacerbations in CF patients are characterized by increased cough, sputum production, fever, and/or shortness of breath. Spirometry usually demonstrates a decline in airflow relative to baseline during these episodes, although chest radiographs may not show significant changes over baseline. Antibiotics are routinely prescribed when patients with CF develop an exacerbation.

Most physicians also prescribe aerosolized β-adrenergic agents to CF patients, particularly those who have clinical or spirometric evidence of reactive airways. Ipratropium bromide is also occasionally prescribed. The nebulized endonuclease DNase I is often used in CF patients with persistent productive cough, because it can decrease the viscosity of expectorated sputum by cleaving long strands of DNA into smaller segments. Patients who chronically produce purulent sputum, particularly those with concomitant bronchiectasis, benefit from chest physiotherapy and postural drainage to assist the clearance of secretions. Inhaled corticosteroids and/or daily azithromycin therapy are also sometimes used in the long-term management of this disease.

Pancreatic insufficiency is another common sequela of CF which may lead to malabsorption of fat and protein, an issue that can often be reversed with oral supplementation of pancreatic enzyme extracts. Nonetheless, many CF patients remain significantly underweight. Endocrine pancreatic insufficiency resulting in diabetes mellitus can also be seen, particularly in individuals surviving into adulthood.

Optimal medical therapy of CF lung disease can delay but does not stop disease progression, and premature death from respiratory failure still occurs in the majority of patients. As in other progressive lung diseases, lung transplantation provides an additional, albeit imperfect, management option for end-stage CF. Thirty-three percent of all double-lung transplants in adults are performed in CF patients.[98]

Maternal and Fetal Risks

Maternal Risks

Women with CF often suffer from reduced fertility, owing to both malnutrition-related amenorrhea and the production of an abnormally tenacious cervical mucus.[99] Data from the United States[100] and the United Kingdom[101] report a pregnancy rate for women with CF of 40 per 1000 per year, compared with 80 per 1000 for unaffected women. Of those who successfully conceive, 70% to 80% of pregnancies in patients with CF will result in a live birth. Among women with CF who do not have frank diabetes, glucose tolerance may be more subtly impaired, and as such, the risk of gestational diabetes appears to be increased.[102]

In contrast to early case reports of poor maternal outcome in CF patients, more recent studies have demonstrated the relative safety of pregnancy among women with CF who have good preexisting lung function.[103–108] It is reported that maternal and fetal outcomes are generally favorable if the prepregnancy FEV_1 exceeds 50% to 60% of the predicted value. If the mother has any evidence of pulmonary hypertension, however, her prognosis is much more guarded. Pulmonary hypertension from any cause confers a significant risk of right ventricular decompensation and maternal mortality in pregnancy.

Available data indicate that pregnancy does not appear to affect the rate of decline in FEV_1 or survival compared with those in nonpregnant reproductive-age women.[108,109] Following pregnancy, deaths among new mothers usually occur in those with the most severe lung disease. The absence of *B. cepacia* colonization, pancreatic insufficiency, or a prepregnancy FEV_1 below 50% of predicted were all associated with better maternal survival rates.

Women with CF who become pregnant face an additional nutritional demand as well. Those who achieve pregnancy despite being significantly underweight may become emaciated if they are unable to keep up with the significant nutritional demands of the fetoplacental unit.[110]

Fetal Risks

Well-nourished mothers with reasonably preserved lung function can expect a good pregnancy outcome. Following successful conception, 70% to 80% of pregnancies in women with CF will result in a live birth. In women with greater disability, however, IUGR and premature labor can result from chronic hypoxia and malnutrition, and maternal diabetes is associated with an increased risk of adverse pregnancy outcome in women with CF. Over half of women with severe CF lung disease deliver prematurely,[108] with acute episodes of pneumonia in pregnancy particularly associated with an increased risk of preterm delivery and pregnancy loss. Malnutrition can also lead to fetal growth restriction.

Although most medications used for treatment of CF are safe for use in pregnancy, infection with some multidrug-resistant organisms may require use of antibiotic agents with less extensive fetal safety data.

All offspring of a mother with CF will be at least heterozygous for the condition and, in view of the high prevalence of the CF gene in the community, will have a considerable risk of being phenotypically affected.

Management Options

Prepregnancy

Preconception counseling should be undertaken in women with CF, including detailed genetic counseling. Genetic counseling is useful to explain to the parents the risk of having a child affected with CF, as determined by the partner's carrier status. Identification of the specific gene mutation in the mother will facilitate screening her partner and fetus, because most CF mutations can be identified by screening for the 20 to 30 most prevalent mutations.[109] If a mutation is identified in both mother and father, prenatal diagnosis with chorionic villus sampling or amniocentesis can be undertaken.[111] Prenatal diagnosis should be undertaken with the understanding that if the fetus is found to be affected, it may help the couple emotionally prepare for an affected child or may lead them to consider pregnancy termination.[112]

General medical care and pharmacologic treatment of CF should also be reviewed and optimized prior to conception. Given the complex nature of the disease, this is best accomplished by a multidisciplinary team led by a physician experienced in the care of CF and involving chest therapists, nutritionists, and social workers.

The nutritional status of the woman should be assessed and optimized prior to pregnancy, with a body mass index (BMI) less than 18 kg/m^2 considered a relative contraindication to pregnancy. The presence of pulmonary vascular disease should be sought, with a clear description of the substantial maternal risks communicated if significant pulmonary hypertension is found.[113,114] Pulmonary function tests, ABGs, and echocardiography (with estimation of pulmonary artery pressures) should be obtained or reviewed. Pregnancy should be strongly discouraged if the FEV_1 is less than 50% of predicted.[115] In the setting of severe disease, the issue that offspring may be left without a mother at a relatively young age needs to be tactfully discussed with the woman, because the 10-year mortality rate among pregnant women with CF is approximately 20%. Although heart and lung transplantation may be a future option for some patients with CF, it will not be available for the majority given the shortage of organ donors.

Prenatal

The primary goals of management for women with CF in pregnancy include optimization of her pulmonary and nutritional status. Women with severe lung impairment and/or pulmonary hypertension presenting in early pregnancy should be informed of the substantial personal risk of a pregnancy to their own health and should be offered a termination of pregnancy.

CF patients require ongoing optimal medical care throughout pregnancy. These women are usually utilizing chest physiotherapy and/or postural drainage on a daily basis, and this treatment should be continued. Exacerbations of lung involvement should be managed as they would be outside of pregnancy, recognizing that severe pulmonary exacerbations can lead to hypoxia and increase the risk of preterm delivery and fetal death. These should be a very low threshold for hospital admission in the setting of respiratory infections. The dosing of antibiotic agents may require adjustment owing to the altered pharmacokinetics of pregnancy. The use of penicillins, cephalosporins, trimethoprim/sulfamethoxazole, and/or aminoglycosides is safe in pregnancy.[116,117] Quinolone antibiotics have limited data regarding fetal safety in humans, but should be used when clinically indicated in pregnancy for the management of CF.[118,119] Bronchodilator drugs can be used safely in pregnancy. The use of supplemental oxygen is essential for maternal and fetal well-being in the setting of hypoxia.

Maternal malnutrition may lead to IUGR. Women who enter pregnancy significantly underweight may become emaciated in pregnancy owing to the additional nutritional demands of the fetoplacental unit. Whereas normal pregnancy is associated with an average weight gain of 10 to 12 kg, this can be difficult for the pregnant woman with CF. These women may need to eat 120% to 150% of their recommended daily caloric intake to maintain their body weight even when not pregnant, and to achieve adequate weight gain in pregnancy, they typically need to consume a further 300 kcal/day.[120] Even among CF women with normal prepregnancy weight, pregnancy-related dyspepsia, reflux, nausea and vomiting, and constipation may lead to a decrease in caloric intake. The additional calories needed for a healthy pregnancy may, therefore, be difficult to meet without resorting to enteral feeding. Involvement of a clinical dietician is thus advisable for monitoring and enhancement of the woman's nutritional status.

Because many women with CF will have underlying impaired glucose tolerance, screening for gestational diabetes should occur early in gestation (i.e., initially at ~18 wk' gestation, repeated at 24 to 28 weeks if initially normal). Most CF patients who are identified to have gestational diabetes will require insulin therapy. CF patients with diabetes should achieve the usual tight control of blood glucose to optimize pregnancy outcome.

If women with CF develop IUGR, decreasing maternal weight, or deteriorating respiratory function despite optimal medical treatment, facilitation of preterm delivery might be considered in individual cases—considering both maternal and fetal risks and benefits.

Labor and Delivery

A vaginal delivery is preferable for women with CF to reduce the risk of postoperative pneumonia and other maternal complications associated with an operative delivery. Use of regional anesthesia is ideal, because it will decrease maternal oxygen requirements associated with pain and avoid the need for general anesthesia should an urgent cesarean delivery be needed. In women with moderate to severe lung disease, an assisted second stage of delivery (with forceps or vacuum suction) should be considered to avoid maternal exhaustion.

Postnatal

The vast majority of women with CF should be strongly encouraged to breast-feed their babies, because the common medications for the treatment of CF are safe to take during breast-feeding. Breast-feeding might not advisable, however, in severely ill or malnourished women. If the mother's general health is very poor, bottle feeding may permit alternate caregivers to assist in feeding and thus allow the mother to rest. The breast milk of mothers with CF has a slightly lower fat content than usual (mainly essential fatty acids) but normal electrolyte content and is adequate to nourish the child.[121–123] Infants of mothers with CF are typically screened for CF by their pediatrician.

SUMMARY OF MANAGEMENT OPTIONS

Cystic Fibrosis (Maternal)

Management Options	Evidence Quality and Recommendation	References
Prepregnancy		
Document baseline respiratory function with PFTs, ABGs, echo.	III/B	103–108,110
Counsel regarding maternal risks of respiratory failure, congestive cardiac failure, IUGR, and preterm delivery if FEV_1 < 50% and/or pulmonary hypertension exists	III/B	103–108,110
Counsel regarding fetal risks of developing CF and certainty of being a carrier.	III/B	109,110
Gene test father for CF carrier status—will determine fetal CF risk and inform the potential for informative prenatal diagnosis (genes for CF identifiable in about 99% of cases).		
Assess patient weight and encourage patient to optimize nutritional status.	III/B	110
Optimize medical management of CF	III/B	110
Prenatal		
Care for patient via multidisciplinary team led by individual with expertise in CF management.	—/GPP	—
Counsel regarding fetal risks of developing CF and certainty of being a carrier—if not done prepregnancy (as above).	III/B	109,110
Optimize medical management:	III/B	110
• Chest physiotherapy.		
• Bronchodilators.		
• Treat pulmonary exacerbations as when nonpregnant.		
Increase calorific intake in pregnancy.	III/B	110,120
Monitor for IUGR and preterm delivery.	III/B	108
Labor and Delivery		
Monitor respiratory function (oxygen saturation).	III/B	110
Supplemental oxygen if hypoxic.		
Hemodynamic monitoring of women with pulmonary hypertension.		
Assisted vaginal delivery may be necessary.	III/B	110
Avoid general anesthesia for cesarean section.	III/B	110
Postnatal		
Monitor respiratory function.	III/B	110
Continue regular medications; breast-feeding is not contraindicated.	III/B	121–123

ABGs, arterial blood gases; CF, cystic fibrosis; FEV_1, forced expiratory volume in 1 sec; GPP, good practice point; IUGR, intrauterine growth restriction; PFTs, pulmonary function tests.

PNEUMONIA

General

Pneumonia and influenza are the seventh leading cause of death in the United States, and the leading cause of infectious death.[124] The incidence of pneumonia in pregnancy is between 0.8 and 2.7 cases per 1000 deliveries,[125,126] a rate similar to that in the nonpregnant population. The onset of pneumonia does not seem to occur at any particular point in gestation, with one study noting an average gestational age at diagnosis of 32 weeks.[127] Respiratory failure develops in up to 10% of pregnant women with pneumonia[128] and accounts for 12% of obstetric patients requiring intubation.[129] Overall, pneumonia accounts for 4.2% of antepartum admissions for nonobstetric causes.[130]

Risk factors for the development of pneumonia in pregnancy are maternal disease, including HIV infection, asthma, and CF; smoking; anemia; cocaine use; alcohol abuse; maternal corticosteroid administration for fetal lung maturity; and tocolytic therapy use. Overall, about 24% of women with pneumonia in pregnancy have a predisposing condition.[131]

Perhaps the most important role for physicians in the assessment and management of suspected pneumonia in pregnancy is to carefully review the differential diagnosis. Community-acquired pneumonia in the pregnant patient generally presents with typical features (abrupt onset of fever and rigors, productive cough, tachycardia, tachypnea, fever, and localized inspiratory "crackles"). Pulmonary embolism is the leading cause of maternal mortality in the United States and the United Kingdom, and it can present very similarly with dyspnea, cough, chest pain, fever, and pulmonary infiltrates. Aspiration pneumonitis and pulmonary edema related to sepsis, tocolysis, or preeclampsia can also present with a similar clinical picture.

The maternal physiologic changes to the respiratory system do not significantly alter the susceptibility to pneumonia. An exception to this principle is the pregnancy-associated reduction in cell-mediated immunity, which leaves pregnant women with an increased susceptibility to viral and fungal pneumonias. As such, pregnant women are at an increased risk of severe pneumonia and disseminated disease from atypical pathogens such as herpesvirus, influenza,[132,133] varicella,[134] and coccidioidomycosis.[135]

Maternal and Fetal Risks

Pneumonia in pregnant women may not be more common than in the general population, but it may result in greater morbidity and mortality owing to the physiologic changes of pregnancy and the needs of the fetus. Maternal prognosis from pneumonia is generally good in the antibiotic era, although severe maternal morbidity and significant mortality from primary varicella (maternal mortality ~14%)[136] and influenza pneumonia remain a major concern. Women with immunodeficiency due to HIV are at the additional risk of opportunistic infections (e.g., *Pneumocystis carinii* pneumonia, TB) and require very careful attention.

Because radiographic evidence of a pulmonary infiltrate is considered the gold standard for diagnosing pneumonia, a chest x-ray should be obtained in almost all patients.[137] Given the negligible fetal radiation exposure of a single chest x-ray with abdominal shielding (approximately equal to 1 day's background radiation), there should be no hesitation about performing chest radiology in pregnant patients suspected of having pulmonary disease. Other fetal risks in the setting of maternal pneumonia include an increased risk of miscarriage, preterm labor, prematurity, and low birth weight. Most cases of pneumonia in pregnancy are caused by organisms that do not directly affect the fetus, but occasionally, the organism causing pneumonia may present a specific risk to the fetus (e.g., varicella pneumonia and congenital varicella syndrome).[138]

Management Options

Prepregnancy

Preconception counseling is usually not relevant to bacterial pneumonia in otherwise healthy women. In HIV-infected women with low CD4 cell counts, however, continuation of *Pneumocystis* prophylaxis during pregnancy should be advised because this infection is the leading cause of AIDS-related death of pregnant women in the United States.[139] Given the increased attack rate and morbidity of influenza infection among pregnant women, the CDC and the American College of Obstetricians and Gynecologists (ACOG) have recommended that women currently pregnant or anticipating pregnancy should routinely receive influenza vaccination during the influenza season regardless of gestational age.[140] Pneumococcal vaccine is advised for women with high risk conditions—such as diabetes mellitus, asthma, chronic cardiac or pulmonary disease, or any other disease or treatment affecting immune function—either before or during pregnancy. Pneumococcal vaccine is also mandatory in women with prior splenectomy and in women with functional hyposplenism (e.g., sickle cell disease) and is recommended for women living in long-term care facilities or prisons.[141] Women without demonstrable immunity to the varicella virus should also be offered immunization with the varicella vaccine prior to pregnancy, though this live attenuated virus should not be administered during gestation.

Prenatal and Postnatal

Recommendations regarding empirical therapy for community-acquired pneumonia, per the American Thoracic Society (ATS),[142] are reviewed in Table 37–6. Per these

TABLE 37–6

Empirical Antibiotic Regimens for the Treatment of Community-acquired Pneumonia in Pregnancy[222,228,229]

- For uncomplicated pneumonia in patients who ***do not require hospitalization***:
  Standard: azithromycin 500 mg PO on day 1 followed by 250 mg daily for 4 days
  Alternate: erythromycin 250 mg qid PO for 10–14 days
- For uncomplicated pneumonia in patients ***requiring hospitalization***: ceftriaxone 2 g IV once daily *with* azithromycin 500 mg IV daily (or erythromycin 500 mg IV q6h). Once patient is afebrile and stable, switch to azithromycin 500 mg PO daily × 7–10 days (or erythromycin 250–500 mg PO qid × 10–14 days) with cefuroxime axetil 500 mg PO bid for 10–14 days.

guidelines, treatment varies according to the severity of illness (as reflected by whether the patient qualifies for inpatient versus outpatient care) and also reflects the increasing prevalence of drug-resistant organisms. In pregnancy, the threshold for hospitalization of borderline patients should be low, given the potential maternal and fetal risks of hypoxia from a worsening condition. Routine collection of sputum and blood cultures before initiation of antibiotic therapy is advisable, at least among hospitalized patients, even though an etiologic organism is found in only about half of cases investigated.[142,143] In the hospital, patients initially treated with intravenous antibiotics can be switched to oral agents once the patient is afebrile and improving. With appropriate antibiotic therapy, some improvement in the clinical course is expected within 72 hours. A full adequate course of therapy is 10 to 14 days, except for azithromycin, which can be given for only a shorter course because of its extended tissue half-life.

Although the ATS guidelines apply quite well to pregnant women, the treating physician should bear a few additional points in mind. If parenteral erythromycin is selected, the use of the estolate ester should be avoided owing to a relatively high incidence of subclinical, reversible hepatotoxicity when used during pregnancy.[144] Although clarithromycin and levofloxacin are often recommended for the treatment of possible drug-resistant pneumococci in the nonpregnant population, these drugs should be avoided in pregnancy. Clarithromycin appears to be teratogenic in the animal model and, therefore, should be used in only situations in which it is the drug of choice. The use of fluoroquinolones such as levofloxacin has also been discouraged owing to a described ability (ciprofloxacin and ofloxacin) to cause an irreversible arthropathy in immature experimental animals. Although subsequent human data have been generally reassuring, these agents should still be considered relatively contraindicated in pregnancy.[118,119] Tetracyclines cause staining of fetal bones and teeth and should not be used in pregnancy.

Doses of antibiotics selected should be in the upper recommended range in pregnancy[145] because of increased renal clearance. Patients may use acetaminophen as an antipyretic. Critically ill women with sepsis or refractory hypoxia may require intubation and assisted ventilation. Fairly standard ventilatory settings can be utilized, with adjustment to maintain the acid-base changes typical of pregnancy (i.e., $PaCO_2$ 28–32, normal pH).

Varicella infection in pregnancy confers a risk of transplacental infection and embryopathy, particularly in the first half of pregnancy, with an incidence of 1% to 2%. Varicella of the newborn is a life-threatening illness that may occur when a newborn is delivered within 5 days of the onset of maternal illness or after postdelivery exposure to varicella. Therefore, if exposure to varicella virus occurs in pregnancy in a woman without protective immunity, varicella zoster immune globulin (VZIG) should be administered within 96 hours in an attempt to prevent maternal infection. Because of the high prevalence and morbidity of pneumonia associated with primary varicella infection in pregnancy, parenteral acyclovir should be given to all women who develop varicella infection in pregnancy.[146–150]

SUMMARY OF MANAGEMENT OPTIONS
Pneumonia

Management Options	Evidence Quality and Recommendation	References
Prepregnancy		
Vaccinate for influenza during flu season.	IV/C	140
Pneumococcal vaccination for women with splenectomy or immunodeficiency.	IV/C	141
In patients with HIV and low CD4, counsel to continue PCP prophylaxis in pregnancy.	IV/C	139
Prenatal		
Vaccinate for influenza during flu season (regardless of gestational age) if not done preconception.	IV/C	132,140
Differentiate pneumonia from other conditions, especially pulmonary embolus and ARDS.	IV/C	58
Perform chest radiographs as needed to confirm diagnosis.	III/B	137
Use standard approach with sputum and blood cultures for seriously ill women.	IV/C	58,142
Begin appropriate antimicrobial therapy based on underlying conditions and presentation:	IV/C	58
• Avoid tetracyclines in pregnancy.		
• Avoid fluoroquinolones unless specifically indicated.		
• Continue treatment for 10–14 days		

SUMMARY OF MANAGEMENT OPTIONS

Pneumonia—cont'd

Management Options	Evidence Quality and Recommendation	References
Oxygen therapy to maintain saturation levels > 94%.	IV/C	58
Treat varicella infection in a pregnant woman with acyclovir.	—/GPP	—
Labor and Delivery		
None specific.		
Postnatal		
None specific.		

ARDS, acute respiratory distress syndrome; GPP, good practice point; PCP, *Pneumocystis carinii* pneumonia

PULMONARY EDEMA, ACUTE LUNG INJURY, AND ACUTE RESPIRATORY DISTRESS SYNDROME

General

The physiologic changes of pregnancy predispose pregnant women to the development of pulmonary edema (Table 35–7), and as such, this dangerous condition is not rare in pregnancy and occurs more frequently than in the nonpregnant population. The overall incidence of pulmonary edema in pregnancy is approximately 80 in 100,000 pregnancies.[151]

Pulmonary edema may be classified as cardiogenic or noncardiogenic. Cardiogenic pulmonary edema is the result of elevated pulmonary venous pressure leading to a hydrostatic pressure gradient that causes the movement of fluid into the alveoli,[152] a phenomenon referred to as *congestive heart failure*. Causes specific to pregnancy include peripartum cardiomyopathy and preeclampsia-associated myocardial dysfunction. The causes and treatment of cardiogenic pulmonary edema are discussed in Chapter 36. Noncardiogenic pulmonary edema, in contrast, is the result of fluid leaking into the alveoli across a leaky pulmonary capillary bed despite normal intravascular pressures. This may be caused by a variety of disorders in pregnancy, some pregnancy-specific and others incidental to or exacerbated by pregnancy (Table 37–8). For a diagnosis of noncardiogenic pulmonary edema to be made, the pulmonary capillary wedge pressure (PCWP) should be less than 18 mm Hg and there should be no evidence of a cardiac cause.[153]

Noncardiogenic pulmonary edema may be subclassified as acute lung injury (ALI) and the acute respiratory distress syndrome (ARDS). These two entities represent a spectrum of disease: the syndrome is defined by a scoring system based on the level of positive end-expiratory pressure (PEEP) required, the PaO_2-FIO_2 (fractional concentration of oxygen in inspired gas) ratio, the degree of static lung compliance, the degree of pulmonary infiltrates, and the clinical cause (as defined in Table 37–9).[154] Patients with less severe lung injury are defined as ALI and those more severely affected have ARDS. ARDS has an incidence in the general population of 13.5 in 100,000 per year.[155] It is considered a relatively rare but often lethal condition in pregnancy, contributing significantly to maternal mortality. Precipitants

TABLE 37–7

Normal Physiologic Changes of Pregnancy That Predispose to and May Exacerbate Pulmonary Edema[230]

20% decrease in colloid osmotic pressure
50% increase in blood volume and cardiac output
Decreased FRC in pregnancy means end-expiratory volumes closer to critical closing volumes

FRC, functional residual capacity.

TABLE 37–8

Select Causes of Noncardiogenic Pulmonary Edema in Pregnancy

Incidental to Pregnancy
Sepsis: appendicitis, bacterial pneumonia
Chemical pneumonitis
Inhalational lung injury
Venous air embolism
Cocaine and high-dose opiates in susceptible patients
Exacerbated or Facilitated by Pregnancy
Aspiration (Mendelson's syndrome)
Sepsis: pyelonephritis, viral pneumonia, listeriosis
Severe hemorrhage, especially related to systemic inflammatory response, low PCOP, and rarely leukoagglutination in the lung
Pancreatitis
Unique to Pregnancy
Tocolytic therapy
Preeclampsia/eclampsia/HELLP syndrome
Amniotic fluid embolism
Neurogenic pulmonary edema after eclamptic seizure
Sepsis: chorioamnionitis, endometritis, septic abortion

HELLP, hemolysis, elevated liver enzymes, and low platelets; PCOP, plasma colloid osmotic pressure.

TABLE 37–9

Diagnostic Criteria for Acute Lung Injury and Acute Respiratory Distress Syndrome[153,154,160,230,231]

1. Acute onset.
2. Bilateral chest radiographic infiltrates.
3. A pulmonary artery occlusion pressure <18 mm Hg or no evidence of left atrial hypertension.
4. Impaired oxygenation manifested by a Pao_2/Fio_2 of 200–300 mm Hg for ALI and ≤200 mm Hg for ARDS.

ALI, acute lung injury; ARDS, acute respiratory distress syndrome; Fio_2, fractional concentration of oxygen in inspired gas; Pao_2, arterial oxygen pressure.

of ALI/ARDS in the general population include sepsis, aspiration, pneumonia, severe trauma and burns, sudden relief of upper airway obstruction, lung and bone marrow transplants, medications (especially aspirin, cocaine, narcotics, and nitrofurantoin), leukoagglutination reactions in the lungs after a blood transfusion, venous air embolism with central venous catheter insertion, and neurocardiogenic (associated with a intracerebral bleed or seizure) causes.[153,156] Those commonly encountered in pregnancy are outlined in Table 37–9.

Although some cases of noncardiogenic pulmonary edema seen in pregnancy will meet the strict diagnostic criteria of ARDS (see Table 37–7), the majority of the pregnancy-related cases will not have the protracted course and poor prognosis typically seen with true ARDS. The mechanism in these cases relates more to transient fluid shifts across the alveolar lining due to acute inciting factors in a host predisposed because of the physiology of pregnancy (discussed later). Most of these pregnancy-related cases will improve rapidly with removal of the inciting factor and urgent medical treatment, and most will not require mechanical ventilation. Some experts suggest that these cases could better be termed *permeability pulmonary edema* rather than true ALI/ARDS. The initial clinical presentations are often indistinguishable from true ALI/ARDS, however, and many of the non–pregnancy-specific causes remain the same.[157–163]

The differentiation between cardiogenic and noncardiogenic pulmonary may be difficult clinically, in part because the clinical presentation may represent a combination of several different disorders. It is important to identify which contributor is predominant, because the optimal treatment varies considerably depending on the underlying pathophysiologic mechanisms.

Physiologic Changes in Pregnancy That Predispose Pregnant Women to Pulmonary Edema

Pregnant women have a clear predisposition to noncardiogenic pulmonary edema, which is attributable to a number of normal physiologic changes that occur in pregnancy. These changes can be viewed as "contributing" factors that increase the likelihood that a pregnant woman with a particular insult or condition will develop pulmonary edema. These changes are discussed later and summarized in Table 37–8.

Pregnancy-associated Increase in Blood Volume and Cardiac Output

Normal pregnancy is characterized by an approximately 50% increase in blood volume and a 40% increase in cardiac output, both peaking and plateauing at 26 to 32 weeks' gestation. Fever, pain, preeclampsia, and multiple gestations can further increase cardiac work and lead to a rise in pulmonary artery occlusion pressure (PAOP) that can, despite remaining within the "normal" (<18 mm Hg) range, lead to pulmonary edema in the setting of low plasma colloid osmotic pressure (PCOP) and/or endothelial damage.

Pregnancy-associated Drop in Plasma Colloid Osmotic Pressure

The pregnancy-associated expansion of blood volume occurs via an increase in plasma free water that is greater than the expansion of blood cells and plasma proteins. This leads to a physiologic anemia and a progressive decrease in the concentration of plasma proteins including serum albumin with advancing gestation. Because the plasma protein concentration is the main determinant of PCOP, this decrease increases the propensity for fluid to move into the interstitial and alveolar spaces in pregnant women. PCOP drops further in women with preeclampsia, contributing to the increased risk of pulmonary edema seen with this entity (as discussed further later).[164,165]

Pregnancy-associated Decrease in Functional Residual Capacity

A third factor predisposing pregnant women to pulmonary edema is the elevation of the diaphragm by the gravid uterus in the latter part of gestation, decreasing the FRC in pregnant women by around 18% compared with that in nonpregnant individuals. As such, at end-expiration, the pregnant woman is closer to her *critical closing volume* (the volume at which alveoli collapse upon themselves). It is believed that this increases the likelihood that small airways and alveoli will collapse when small amounts of pulmonary edema are present and may thereby contribute to a worsening hypoxia due to pulmonary edema.

Precipitating Causes of Pulmonary Edema

Although pregnant women are predisposed to pulmonary edema due to the factors listed previously, the occurrence of pulmonary edema still generally requires an inciting event to "tip the balance" and precipitate movement of fluid into the interstitial spaces of the lung. The myriad conditions that may cause ARDS in the general population can also occur in pregnant women. Some of these conditions, such as severe viral pneumonia and aspiration, occur with increased frequency in pregnancy. Some pregnancy-specific conditions can precipitate pulmonary edema. In any pregnancy, the presence of anemia, a multifetal gestation, or the injudicious administration of intravenous fluids will further increase the risk that a particular inciting cause will result in pulmonary edema. The common precipitants of pulmonary edema in pregnancy are outlined in Table 37–9 and discussed in the following paragraphs.

Tocolysis

A pregnancy-specific cause of noncardiogenic pulmonary edema is the use of β-adrenergic agonists (such as terbutaline) and magnesium for the treatment of preterm labor (tocolysis).[166] The incidence of pulmonary edema in this setting is 0.3 to 9.0%[154] and may be seen during the infusion of the tocolytic agent or up to 12 hours after its discontinuation. Although β-adrenergic agonists have been used extensively in the treatment of asthma in nonpregnant patients without this complication, there is a clear association in the obstetric literature between the systemic use of these agents and pulmonary edema. A recent series noted that tocolysis accounted for 25% of pregnancy-associated pulmonary edema.[151] Possible mechanisms include a β-mimetic–induced increase in cardiac work; possible catecholamine-induced myocardial dysfunction; and the frequent coadministration of excess intravenous fluids and high-dose glucocorticoids. Multiple gestation, maternal infection, and corticosteroid therapy are associated with a further increased risk of pulmonary edema in combination with tocolytic therapy.

The use of β-mimetic agents for tocolysis has been called into question because they have been found to be no more effective than nifedipine or magnesium and are associated with excess maternal morbidity.[167] We anticipate that the incidence of tocolytic-induced pulmonary edema will decrease as the sympathomimetic agents are used less frequently.

Preeclampsia

Preeclampsia is an important cause of pulmonary edema in pregnancy owing to its high prevalence. In one series, 2.9% of preeclamptic women developed pulmonary edema.[168] Maternal mortality from preeclampsia-associated pulmonary edema in this setting may be as high as 10%. About 30% of preeclampsia-associated pulmonary edema will occur antepartum, the remainder usually within the first 72 hours after delivery. The majority of women with antenatal pulmonary edema due to preeclampsia have preexisting chronic hypertension.[154] Excessive intravenous fluid administration, often in response to oliguria, is another important contributing factor in many cases. Perinatal mortality in the setting of antenatal preeclampsia-associated pulmonary edema may be as high as 50%, although this is often related to concomitant placental abruption and, therefore, more a result of the severity of the preeclampsia rather than the presence of the pulmonary edema itself.

Preeclampsia may provoke pulmonary edema by several mechanisms. One factor is the additional drop in PCOP, beyond that seen in normal pregnancy. Another is the endothelial damage, characteristic of preeclampsia, disrupting the endothelial barrier in the lungs and facilitating the leakage of fluid into the pulmonary interstitium and alveoli. In women with preexisting hypertension, diastolic dysfunction due to a thickened and noncompliant ventricle may be an important factor contributing to pulmonary edema—particularly in conjunction with a dramatic increase in afterload due to preeclampsia-associated hypertension. Lastly, preeclampsia-associated transient left ventricular systolic dysfunction may occur and contribute to pulmonary edema. The occurrence of left ventricular dysfunction in preeclampsia has been well described but is poorly understood. It is assumed that the intense vasospasm and endothelial damage that characterize preeclampsia have an impact on myocardial oxygen supply leading to impaired myocardial contractility.[168–173]

Sepsis

Infection is also a common and important mechanism leading to noncardiogenic pulmonary edema in pregnancy. Systemic bacterial infection originating from any primary site can precipitate pulmonary edema in pregnant women. Pneumonia can progress to ALI and ARDS and is an important cause of prolonged mechanical ventilation in pregnant women (see the section on "Pneumonia"). Pyelonephritis is another common cause, because pulmonary edema may complicate up to 10% of cases of pyelonephritis during pregnancy.[174,175] The main mechanism of sepsis-related pulmonary edema in pregnancy appears to be an increased sensitivity of pregnant women to bacterial endotoxin, resulting in increased capillary permeability.

Aspiration Syndromes: Mendelson's Syndrome and Bacterial Aspiration Pneumonia

Aspiration of gastric contents is among the leading nonobstetric causes of ARDS among pregnant women. Aspiration syndromes are more common in pregnancy because of increased GERD due to progesterone-mediated relaxation of the lower esophageal sphincter and reduced gastric motility and delayed emptying; and elevated intragastric pressure due to compression by the enlarging uterus. In the setting of altered mental status related to drug or medication use, seizure activity or in association with anesthesia, stomach contents can be aspirated and lead to Mendelson's syndrome and/or bacterial aspiration pneumonia.

Mendelson's syndrome may occur in association with a difficult intubation during general anesthesia or during the postanesthesia period, when the gag reflex may be depressed. It requires a high index of suspicion at times, because it may occur in association with silent GERD. Gastric secretions aspirated into the lungs lead to intense pulmonary inflammation that can rapidly progress to ALI/ARDS. Clinical manifestations may include tachypnea, hypoxia, wheezing, hypotension, and fever. Gastric contents may be noted in the pharynx or mouth during laryngoscopy. Chest x-ray changes classically show diffuse interstitial and alveolar infiltrates. Despite the rapidity and severity of the syndrome, mild cases generally resolve without antibiotics within 2 to 5 days unless bacterial superinfection intervenes.[176] Modern anesthetic management, with a preponderance of regional anesthesia for cesarean sections, has thankfully made this a far less common event than it was in the past.

Bacterial aspiration pneumonia usually has a more gradual onset than Mendelson's syndrome, presenting 48 to 72 hours after aspiration with clinical manifestations including persistent fever, purulent sputum, and leukocytosis. Chest x-ray findings tend to be localized to the areas of the lung that were dependant at the time of aspiration. The bacterial infection is generally polymicrobial, including a preponderance of oral anaerobes, so treatment with penicillin or clindamycin is usually effective.

Massive Transfusion

Massive red cell transfusion for severe antepartum or postpartum hemorrhage can result in cardiogenic or noncardiogenic pulmonary edema. The mechanism is often multifactorial, including volume overload; reduced PCOP (from replacement of whole blood loss with packed red cells and crystalloids); endothelial damage from a systemic inflammatory response to the massive hemorrhage; and occasionally, transfusion-associated acute lung injury (TRALI), an immune-mediated reaction to human leukocyte antigens (HLA).

Amniotic Fluid Embolism (Anaphylactoid Syndrome of Pregnancy)

Amniotic fluid embolism (AFE) is a rare but catastrophic complication of pregnancy that typically presents as the abrupt onset of hypotension, dyspnea, and altered mental status proceeding to full blown disseminated intravascular coagulation (DIC) and ARDS. AFE syndrome accounts for approximately 10% of all maternal deaths in the United States and results in permanent neurologic deficits in up to 85% of survivors.[177] One U.S. study reported an incidence of 1 in 20,646 singleton pregnancies, with a mortality of 26%.[178] Risk factors for the development of AFE include multiparity, increased maternal age, maternal trauma, prolonged labor, meconium staining of the amniotic fluid, use of oxytocin, instrumental delivery, and cesarean delivery.

The AFE syndrome usually occurs in the immediate peripartum interval but has been reported to occur spontaneously antepartum. The diagnosis is clinical and should be strongly considered in any woman near term (especially in labor) who presents with sudden cardiorespiratory failure.

The mechanism of the AFE syndrome involves the entry of amniotic fluid into the maternal circulation through the endocervical veins or uterine tears. In susceptible individuals, this may precipitate a dramatic systemic reaction. Animal data suggest the initial response is acute right heart failure resulting from embolization of amniotic fluid and fetal debris (squamous cells, mucin) causing occlusion and vasospasm of the maternal pulmonary vasculature, with resulting pulmonary hypertension and systemic hypotension. This is followed by a dramatic maternal systemic reaction resulting in ARDS and DIC. Some researchers would prefer that the syndrome be called *anaphylactoid syndrome of pregnancy*, thereby emphasizing the importance of the maternal immunologic response in this syndrome.

Presentation of Pulmonary Edema in Pregnancy

The symptoms and signs of pulmonary edema in pregnancy are similar to those seen in the general medical population. Early signs and symptoms of pulmonary edema are often mild and may be mistaken for findings of normal pregnancy, given that these young women often maintain respiratory and cardiovascular stability longer than the typical medical patient with pulmonary edema.

Tachypnea is an important clinical sign that a woman's dyspnea represents a more serious condition than dyspnea of pregnancy. The lungs may be clear to auscultation early in the course when only interstitial edema has developed. Affected women will usually exhibit some degree of tachycardia along with anxiety related to dyspnea or hypoxia. As the condition progresses, diffuse "crackles," wheezing, and cough will become apparent in association with alveolar edema.

The chest x-ray in early pulmonary edema may be normal. Diffuse interstitial and alveolar infiltrates, and in some cases pleural effusions, will subsequently become manifest. In some women, the infiltrates may be patchy or even unilateral, particularly if the woman has spent prolonged periods in the lateral decubitus position. The patient can be confidently reassured that the fetal radiation exposure from a chest x-ray with abdominal shielding is negligible.

ABGs initially reveal a decrease in both PaO_2 and $PaCO_2$. As the condition progresses, the PaO_2 may decrease further and the $PaCO_2$ begin to rise, reflecting impending respiratory failure. It is essential to recall the normal ABG parameters for pregnancy, recognizing that a $PaCO_2$ of 40 mm Hg is very abnormal and indicates impending ventilatory failure. Additional laboratory investigations that should be obtained in the setting of suspected pulmonary edema include CBC, blood urea nitrogen (BUN) and creatinine, as well as "preeclampsia laboratories" (alanine aminotransferase [ALT], uric acid, lactate dehydrogenase [LDH], CBC, creatinine, and urine protein–to–creatinine ratio).

Differential Diagnosis of Pulmonary Edema in Pregnancy

The differential diagnosis of pulmonary edema in pregnancy is broad. Diagnostic possibilities include cardiac disease, including peripartum cardiomyopathy, ischemic heart disease, and valvular heart disease. Differentiation of noncardiogenic pulmonary edema from peripartum cardiomyopathy, ischemic heart disease, or occult valvular heart disease should begin with a careful history, physical examination, and ECG. When doubt remains, or to follow up on equivocal or positive cardiac findings, echocardiography should be undertaken. A prospective study of 45 pregnant women with pulmonary edema found that echocardiography identified an unsuspected cardiac abnormality in 47% of cases.[170] Pneumonia (bacterial or viral) is discussed in the "Pneumonia" section. Drug-related lung disease (nitrofurantoin hypersensitivity, cocaine-associated pulmonary edema) should also be kept in mind, and a full medication history should be obtained and a drug screen considered in some cases, recognizing that the vast majority of patients with cocaine-associated pulmonary edema will have severe hypertension.

Treatment of Pulmonary Edema in Pregnancy

Pulmonary edema in pregnancy is a medical emergency. Regardless of the etiology, the immediate goal is to maintain adequate maternal oxygenation ($PaO_2 \geq 70$ mm Hg,

$SaO_2 \geq 95\%$) to avoid potential hypoxic injury to the fetus.[179–181] The next step is to promptly identify and initiate treatment of the underlying cause(s) of the condition. Relief of symptoms to improve patient comfort should also be addressed.

Clear, reassuring communication of maternal and fetal status with the patient and her support person will decrease maternal distress. Unless respiratory failure is imminent, small doses of parenteral morphine sulfate may be given as needed to reduce maternal anxiety and decrease pulmonary congestion. Judicious titration of intravenous fluid administration and careful monitoring of fluid balance should be undertaken. Although most pregnant women with pulmonary edema will not be volume-overloaded, gentle diuresis to try to achieve the lowest PCWP that will still support normal blood pressure is advisable. Data regarding the treatment of ARDS in nonpregnant patients show that decreasing the PCWPs by 25% with diuretics and fluid restriction can improve pulmonary function and perhaps outcome.[182–184] Most patients will respond to tiny intravenous doses of furosemide (i.e., 10–20 mg). Starting with these low doses will avoid overdiuresis, which can lead to hypovolemia and hypotension and might impair placental perfusion (and precipitate fetal distress).

Remove or Treat the Underlying Cause

TOCOLYTIC-RELATED PULMONARY EDEMA

Critical to the management of pulmonary edema in pregnancy is identification and treatment or removal of the underlying cause. In the setting of established or suspected tocolytic-induced pulmonary edema, discontinuation of the tocolytic agents is mandatory. This difficult decision is made easier when one recognizes that (1) fetal well-being is dependent on maternal well-being and (2) tocolytics are of minimal proven efficacy for prolongation of gestation beyond 48 hours.

PREECLAMPSIA-RELATED PULMONARY EDEMA

When the clinical spectrum of preeclampsia evolves to include pulmonary edema, prompt maternal stabilization followed by prompt delivery is the treatment of choice. Sometimes a high index of suspicion for preeclampsia is required, if the preeclampsia is otherwise mild. Blood pressure should be brought down quickly below approximately 160/100, because the decrease in afterload and, therefore, intracardiac pressures may help decrease pulmonary edema. A small dose of furosemide may be given, with close monitoring of mother and fetus. If intravenous magnesium sulfate is felt to be required (for seizure prophylaxis in the setting of severe preeclampsia), it should be administered in the smallest volume considered safe with close following of the total fluid balance.

INFECTION-RELATED PULMONARY EDEMA

Noncardiogenic pulmonary edema due to maternal systemic infection should be promptly treated with judiciously selected broad-spectrum antibiotic(s). Empirical antibiotics should be started pending culture results. In the absence of a clear focus of infection, abdominal pain and tenderness indicative of possible appendicitis or chorioamnionitis/endometritis should be sought. Pyelonephritis should be considered in any woman with pulmonary edema associated with fever, and a urinalysis and urine culture should be obtained.

AMNIOTIC FLUID EMBOLISM/ANAPHYLACTOID SYNDROME

Suspected AFE necessitates aggressive supportive management in a critical care setting. DIC is nearly universal in the evolution of AFE and should be anticipated. Treatment should begin with aggressive volume administration with or without vasopressors to maintain adequate blood pressure. Intubation and mechanical ventilation will almost always be required. Coagulopathy and hemorrhage should be managed with aggressive blood product and factor replacement (fresh frozen plasma and cryoprecipitate as needed).

Endotracheal Intubation

The hemoglobin dissociation curve favors transfer of adequate oxygen to fetal hemoglobin as long as the maternal PaO_2 remains at 70 mm Hg or above, but if oxygenation cannot be maintained or the patient shows evidence respiratory fatigue (either clinically or on the basis of a $PaCO_2$ rising even into the normal nonpregnant range), assisted ventilation should be promptly arranged. In cases in which a normal level of consciousness is maintained, and in which a rapid reversal of the hypoxia is anticipated, a trial of spontaneous breathing with supplemental oxygen and PEEP administered through a tight-fitting mask may be considered. Noninvasive positive-pressure ventilation (NIPPV) may also be used, but concerns about its use in the setting of pregnancy-associated upper airway edema and the propensity of pregnant women to aspiration may limit its use.

Intubation is required if the patient does not improve with attempts at noninvasive assisted ventilation and/or the woman has evidence of respiratory failure ($PaO_2 < 70$ mm Hg or $PaCO_2 > 45$ mm Hg on 100% oxygen administered through a snug non-rebreather mask). Given the delays inherent in assembling the equipment for intubation, it is preferable to intubate a pregnant patient electively in controlled conditions rather than delay intubation until it is required emergently. The clinician should bear in mind that the upper airway in pregnant women is often difficult to visualize because of soft tissue swelling related to physiologic hyperemia of mucosal tissues during gestation. Because of this, the rate of failed elective intubation in pregnant patients is eight times greater than that seen in general surgical patients.

Pregnant women are at higher risk for aspiration during intubation because of reduced lower esophageal sphincter tone and delayed gastric emptying. It should also be recalled that because of reduced FRC in the latter part of pregnancy, there is less available oxygen in their lungs to maintain PaO_2 during periods of apnea. Generous preoxygenation with 100% oxygen should, therefore, always be done prior to and between attempts to intubate a pregnant woman. In light of these considerations, it is imperative that the intubation of a pregnant woman be performed by the most experienced individual available and that every effort be made to ensure that all required equipment is readily available and functioning properly before attempting intubation (Table 37–10).

TABLE 37-10

Equipment and Medications Necessary for the Intubation of a Pregnant Woman[226]

Continuous electrocardiographic monitoring
Blood pressure monitor on patient's arm
Pulse oximeter
High-flow oxygen source
Large-bore intravenous access secured in place
Intubation to be performed by most experienced individual available, with assistant at his or her side; the incidence of failed intubation in pregnancy is 1 in 200 to 1 in 300 cases, almost 10 times as high as for nonpregnant patients[226]
Mask (that fits patient securely) and manual bag-valve inflation device
Oropharyngeal suction equipment
Endotracheal tubes (with tested inflatable cuff) for oral intubation (rather than nasal intubation) with smaller endotracheal tube (6-6.5) than would be used with similar nonpregnant patient preferable owing to upper airway narrowing in pregnancy[226]
Laryngoscope with light
Stylet
Medications for sedation and (if necessary) paralysis of patient, usually thiopental 3-5 mg/kg IV for sedation, and succinylcholine 1-1.5 mg/kg, up to 150 mg IV, for paralysis
Etomidate 0.3 mg/kg IV over 60 sec may be needed in certain circumstances for muscle relaxation
Method readily available to assess that endotracheal placement is not esophageal (listener with stethoscope or CO_2 detector)
Self-inflating bulbs or syringes have been found to be unreliable in pregnant women
Chest x-ray to be done shortly after intubation to ensure endotracheal tube is properly placed 4-7 cm above the carina
Gloves, mask, goggles, and gown available to intubator
Plan in place for next step if intubation attempt fails. Use of the laryngeal mask has been described in pregnancy and should be available in this circumstance[227]

Adapted and updated from material used with permission from Powrie RO.[230]

Mechanical Ventilation

In general, mechanical ventilation for the pregnant woman with pulmonary edema should be undertaken in the same manner as for the nonpregnant patient. For patients with ARDS, this generally involves the use of lower tidal volumes with lower pressures (tidal volumes ≤ 8 mL/kg predicted body weight and inspiratory plateau pressures ≤ 30 cm H_2O)[185] to avoid lung overdistention and ventilator-associated lung injury. Although this ventilation strategy has not been formally studied in pregnant women, it is recommended by the ARDS Network.[186] Although this ventilation strategy generally leads to "permissive hypercapnea" in the general medical population, the associated acid-base changes may not provide an optimal environment for the fetus. Therefore, it is recommended that the ventilatory rate be increased to maintain pH and PCO_2 in the appropriate ranges for pregnancy. The FIO_2 should ideally be kept less than 60% if possible. PEEP is also universally recommended, because it facilitates recruitment of collapsed alveoli. Excessive levels of PEEP (>10 cm H_2O) should be avoided, however, because it may reduce cardiac preload and cardiac output, thereby compromising uteroplacental blood flow. Similarly, respiratory alkalosis from overventilation should be avoided, because alkalemia can also adversely effect uterine blood flow.

Role of Pulmonary Artery Catheters in Pregnant Women with Pulmonary Edema

In most cases of pulmonary edema in pregnancy, central hemodynamic monitoring will not be necessary for diagnostic purposes. In the absence of clinical evidence of cardiac disease or preeclampsia, it can generally be assumed that the PCWP is unlikely to be greater than 18 mm Hg in a pregnant woman. Preeclampsia is an exception, because severe preeclampsia may be associated with systolic and/or diastolic cardiac dysfunction. In cases in which cardiac dysfunction is suspected, an ECG may be useful in deciding if central hemodynamic monitoring may be helpful. Such monitoring may also be useful in the setting of presumed cardiogenic pulmonary edema that does not improve quickly in response to supplemental oxygen and diuresis.

The goal of invasive monitoring in the setting of pulmonary edema in pregnancy is to safely reduce the PCWP and improve left ventricular performance. It must be remembered, however, that a PCWP that is normal outside of pregnancy may represent a level that will still lead to pulmonary congestion given the predisposing physiology of pregnancy/preeclampsia. It is most helpful, therefore, to follow trends in the PCWP during treatment than to look at absolute numbers.

Although central hemodynamic monitoring in a critical care setting may be quite helpful in difficult cases of pulmonary edema in pregnancy, it is widely accepted that beyond complex cardiac disease or sepsis, it is not generally necessary.[187–201]

Use of Vasoactive and Inotropic Medications

Use of vasoactive and/or inotropic drugs to maintain blood pressure and cardiac output may be helpful in some cases of pulmonary edema in pregnancy, particularly when sepsis or cardiac dysfunction is present. It is critical not to withhold any potentially beneficial treatment from a critically ill pregnant woman because of concerns about possible fetal effects. The paucity of human data on the effects of most of these medications on placental blood flow, however, should caution against their use to "fine-tune" maternal hemodynamic parameters.[201]

SUMMARY OF MANAGEMENT OPTIONS

Pulmonary Edema, Acute Lung Injury, and Acute Respiratory Distress Syndrome

Management Options	Evidence Quality and Recommendation	References
High or intensive care setting; nurse patient at 45-degree angle if possible.	—/GPP	—
Provide supplemental oxygen to maintain $Pa_{O_2} > 65$ mm Hg and oxygen saturation > 95%.	III/B	179–181
If patient is maintaining blood pressure and placental perfusion is not in question, consider administration of IV furosemide (at a dose of 10 mg if patient has not received furosemide in past).	IV/C	182–184
Consider possibility of cardiogenic cause of pulmonary edema. Obtain echocardiogram in most cases to rule out cardiogenic causes.	III/B	170
Monitor fluid balance and avoid fluid overload; minimize IV fluids	III/B	182–184
Remove or treat underlying causes of pulmonary edema in pregnancy:	—/GPP	—
• Discontinue tocolytics.		
• Evaluate for presence of preeclampsia and begin active efforts toward delivery of fetus if patient has preeclampsia.		
• Evaluate for presence of infection (especially pyelonephritis) and treat if present.		
• Protect airway if aspiration is suspected.		
• Check INR, aPTT, and CBC if AFE suspected.		
If oxygenation cannot be maintained, consider use of intermittent positive-pressure nasal ventilation or semielective intubation.	IV/C	185,186
Consider placement of central hemodynamic monitoring line if:	IV/C	187–192
• Cardiac cause suspected and patient unresponsive to diuretics.		
• Poor urine output despite diuretic administration.		
• If hypotension present.		
Consider use of inotropic and vasoactive agents to maximize cardiac output in the minority of cases. Therapy should be guided in this setting by central hemodynamic monitoring.	IV/C	201

AFE, amniotic fluid embolism; aPTT, activate partial thromboplastin time; CBC, complete blood count; GPP, good practice point; INR, International Normalized Ratio; Pa_{O_2}, arterial oxygen pressure.

SUGGESTED READINGS

American Thoracic Society/Centers for Disease Control and Prevention/Infectious Diseases Society of America: Treatment of tuberculosis. Am J Respir Crit Care Med 2003;167:603–662.

Bandi VD, Mannur U, Matthay MA: Acute lung injury and acute respiratory distress syndrome in pregnancy. Crit Care Clin 2004;20:577–607.

Bartlett JG, Breiman RF, Mandell LA, File TM Jr: Community-acquired pneumonia in adults: Guidelines for management. Guidelines from the Infectious Disease Society of America. Clin Infect Dis 1998;26:811.

Graves CR: Acute pulmonary complications during pregnancy. Clin Obstet Gynecol 2002;45:369–376.

Laibl V, Sheffield J: The Management of respiratory infections during pregnancy. Immunol Allergy Clin North Am 2006;26:155–172.

National Asthma Education Program: Report of the Working Group on Asthma and Pregnancy. Management of Asthma During Pregnancy. Update 2004 (NIH Publication No. 05-5236). Bethesda, Md, National Institutes of Health, March 2005.

Powrie RO: Drugs in pregnancy. Respiratory disease. Best Pract Res Clin Obstet Gynaecol 2001;15:913–936.

Sciscione AC, Ivester T, Largoza M, et al: Acute pulmonary edema in pregnancy. Obstet Gynecol 2003;101:511–515.

Subramanian P, Chinthalapalli H, Krishnan M, et al: Pregnancy and sarcoidosis. Chest 2004;126:995–998.

Tonelli MR, Aitken ML: Pregnancy in cystic fibrosis. Curr Opin Pulm Med 2007;13:537–540.

REFERENCES

For a complete list of references, log onto www.expertconsult.com.

CHAPTER 38

Anemia and White Blood Cell Disorders

JANE STRONG and JANE M. RUTHERFORD

ANEMIA: OVERVIEW

Anemia is defined as a hemoglobin value that is lower than the threshold of 2 standard deviations below the median value for a healthy matched population. The World Health Organization (WHO) defines anemia in pregnancy as a hemoglobin concentration of less than 11 g/dL.[1] The cutoff point suggested by the U.S. Centers for Disease Control and Prevention (CDC) is 10.5 g/dL in the second trimester.[2]

Marked physiologic changes in the composition of the blood occur in healthy pregnancy. Increased total blood volume[3] and hemostatic changes[4] help to combat the hazard of hemorrhage at delivery. Plasma volume increases by 50%, and red cell mass by 18% to 25%, depending on iron status. These changes cause a physiologic dilution in hemoglobin concentration that is greatest at 32 weeks' gestation. In iron-replete women, hemoglobin returns to normal by 1 week postpartum.

Worldwide, pathologic anemia is the most common medical disorder of pregnancy. Deficiency of essential hematinics usually arises from increased requirements and inadequate intake. Iron deficiency is the most common hematinic deficiency in pregnancy, followed by folate deficiency. Vitamin B_{12} deficiency rarely causes anemia in pregnancy.

In nonindustrialized countries, anemia is associated with up to 13% of maternal deaths.[5] The global prevalence of anemia is 42%, but this ranges from 5% in the United States to more than 60% in parts of Central Africa.[1]

ANEMIA: IRON DEFICIENCY

Maternal Risks

To maintain iron balance, women of reproductive age require 2 mg of iron daily. Pregnancy further stresses iron balance. The total iron requirements in normal pregnancy are approximately 1240 mg.[6] The main demands for iron arise from expansion of the red cell mass (~500–600 mg), and the fetus and placenta require approximately 300 mg. The daily iron requirement in pregnancy is approximately 4.4 mg (0.8 mg/day in the first trimester, increasing to 7.5 mg/day in the third trimester).[6,7] These requirements can be achieved only by maximizing dietary iron absorption and mobilizing iron stores.[8,9] If a woman enters pregnancy with depleted iron stores, the effects of iron deficiency develop. Vegetarians are at an additional disadvantage because heme iron (derived from meat) is more readily absorbed than nonheme iron, and heme iron also facilitates the absorption of nonheme iron in a mixed diet. Absorption of iron is less than 10%, so an average of 40 mg of dietary iron is required daily.

As iron deficiency develops, the ferritin level decreases first and then the serum iron level. A decrease in hemoglobin concentration is a late development. Iron-dependent enzymes in every cell are affected, and there is a profound effect on body functions.[10]

Tissue enzyme malfunction occurs, even in the early stages of iron deficiency. This might explain the reported association between anemia during pregnancy and preterm birth and the anecdotal evidence that blood loss at delivery is greater in women with anemia.[11,12]

In normal pregnancy, hypervolemia modifies the response to blood loss.[4] Blood volume decreases after the acute loss at delivery but remains relatively stable as long as the loss does not exceed 25% of predelivery volume. No compensatory increase in blood volume occurs, and plasma volume decreases gradually, primarily because of diuresis. Thus, hematocrit gradually increases and blood volume returns to nonpregnant values.

Fetal Risks

The fetus obtains iron from maternal transferrin, regardless of maternal iron stores. The placenta traps maternal transferrin, removes the iron, and actively transports it to the fetus, mainly in the last 4 weeks of pregnancy.[6] If maternal iron stores are depleted, the fetus obtains iron from erythrocyte breakdown or maternal intestinal absorption. Most fetal iron is found in fetal hemoglobin, but one third is stored in the fetal liver as ferritin.

When maternal iron stores are depleted, there is a decrease in fetal iron stores,[13] and this might have an important bearing on the development of anemia during the first year of life, when oral iron intake is very poor.[14–16]

Studies suggest that behavioral abnormalities occur in children with iron deficiency.[17] Iron deficiency in the absence of anemia is associated with poor performance on the Bayley

Mental Development Index.[18] Development delays in iron-deficient infants can be reversed by treatment with iron.[17] Cognitive function can also be improved with iron supplementation, as was shown in a randomized study in nonanemic, iron-deficient adolescent girls.[19]

Studies suggest that prophylaxis of iron deficiency during pregnancy might have an important role in the prevention of adult hypertension.[20,21] High blood pressure in adults appears to originate in fetal life and is associated with lower birth weight and high ratios of placenta to birth weight. Placental size at term was shown to be inversely proportional to serum ferritin concentrations at initial evaluation.[21]

Diagnosis

Hemoglobin Concentration

Although reduction in hemoglobin concentration is a relatively late development in iron deficiency, measuring hemoglobin concentration is the simplest noninvasive practical test available. Hemoglobin values of less than 10.5 g/dL in the second and third trimesters are probably abnormal and require further investigation.

Red Cell Indices

The increased drive to erythropoiesis, resulting in a higher proportion of young large red cells, appears to mask the effect of iron deficiency on mean corpuscular volume (MCV) in pregnancy, even when anemia is established. Healthy, iron-replete pregnancy is associated with a small physiologic increase in red cell size, on average 4 femtoliters (fL; 10^{-15} L), but in some women, the increase may be as high as 20 fL.[22] MCV is a poor indicator of iron deficiency that develops during pregnancy.[23] Some women enter pregnancy with established iron-deficiency anemia or with grossly depleted iron stores. These do not present diagnostic problems. Those who enter pregnancy with a precarious iron balance and a normal hemoglobin value present the most difficult diagnostic problems.

Serum Iron and Total Iron-Binding Capacity

Serum iron level and total iron-binding capacity (TIBC) provide an estimate of transferrin saturation. Reduced transferrin saturation indicates a deficient iron supply to the tissues and the development of iron deficiency. At this early stage, erythropoiesis is impaired and iron-dependent tissue enzymes are adversely affected.

In health, the serum iron of adult nonpregnant women shows considerable diurnal variation and can fluctuate from hour to hour. TIBC rises in association with iron deficiency and decreases in chronic inflammatory states. It is increased in pregnancy because of the increase in plasma volume. In nonanemic patients, TIBC is approximately one-third saturated with iron.

In pregnancy, most reports describe a decrease in both serum iron and percentage saturation of TIBC, which can be largely prevented by iron supplements. Serum iron, even in combination with TIBC, is not a reliable indicator of iron stores, because it fluctuates widely and is affected by recent ingestion of iron and other factors that are not directly involved in iron metabolism, such as infection.

Zinc Protoporphyrin

Zinc protoporphyrin increases when there is a defective iron supply to the developing red cell. Although zinc protoporphyrin may increase in patients with chronic inflammatory disease, malignancy, or infection, the increase usually is not as marked as the increase in ferritin.

Ferritin

Ferritin is a high-molecular-weight glycoprotein that is stable and is not affected by recent ingestion of iron. It appears to reflect iron stores accurately and quantitatively in the absence of inflammation, particularly in the lower range associated with iron deficiency, which is so important in pregnancy. In the development of iron deficiency, a low serum ferritin level is the first abnormal laboratory test result.

Transferrin Receptor

Serum transferrin receptor (TfR) is a relatively new method for assessing cellular iron status.[24] It is present in all cells as a transmembrane protein that binds transferrin-bound iron and transports it to the cell interior. A reduction in the iron supply increases TfR synthesis. Sensitive immunologic techniques show that TfR, like ferritin, circulates in small amounts in the plasma of all individuals, and the concentration is proportional to the total body mass of TfR. In iron-deficiency anemia, the plasma receptor is elevated threefold and the density of surface TfR in iron-deficient cells increases. Little or no change in the serum TfR concentration occurs during the early stages of storage iron depletion, but as soon as tissue iron deficiency is established, the serum TfR concentration increases in direct proportion to the degree of iron deficiency. This change, which precedes the reduction in MCV and the increase in zinc protoporphyrin, is a valuable measurement of early tissue iron deficiency. This measurement is particularly helpful in identifying iron deficiency in pregnancy.[25] It differentiates truly iron-deficient women from those who have a low serum ferritin level as a result of storage iron mobilization or those who have a low hemoglobin concentration as a result of hemodilution. It also helps to distinguish those with a normal or high serum ferritin level as a result of chronic inflammatory disease from those who have low stores that lead to genuine cellular iron deficiency. TfR accurately reflects tissue iron deficiency, both in pregnancy and in anemia of chronic disease, in which serum ferritin may be inappropriately elevated because of release from cells. In combination with serum ferritin, TfR gives a complete picture of iron status. Serum ferritin reflects iron stores (in the absence of chronic inflammatory disease), and TfR reflects tissue iron status.[24]

Marrow Iron

The most rapid and reliable method of assessing iron stores in pregnancy is to examine an appropriately stained preparation of a bone marrow sample. Without iron supplementation, there is no detectable, stainable iron in more than 80% of women at term.[26] No stainable iron (hemosiderin) may be visible once serum ferritin has decreased to less than 40 mg/L,[27,28] but other signs of iron deficiency in developing erythroblasts, particularly late normoblasts, confirm that anemia is caused by iron deficiency in the absence of stainable iron. The effects of folate deficiency, which often accompanies iron deficiency, are also apparent (discussed later). Iron incorporation into hemoglobin is blocked if there is acute or chronic inflammation, particularly if it is caused by urinary tract infection, even if iron stores are replete. This problem is shown by examination of the marrow aspirate stained for iron and can be predicted by simultaneous assessment of serum ferritin and TfR and an indicator of chronic inflammatory disease, such as C-reactive protein.

With the development of noninvasive tests of iron status (described earlier), bone marrow examination is reserved for the differential diagnosis of severe anemia during pregnancy when the cause cannot be determined by any other means and for the investigation of other hematologic abnormalities that arise de novo during the index pregnancy.

Management Options

Prepregnancy

Iron and folate supplementation should be considered in all women of childbearing age in areas of high prevalence of iron-deficiency anemia.[29,30]

Prenatal

PROPHYLACTIC IRON SUPPLEMENTATION

Iron supplementation is used to prophylactically treat women with low iron stores or those at risk for low iron levels in pregnancy. Women with iron-deficiency anemia are a different group requiring treatment doses of iron (discussed later).

Iron supplementation in pregnancy is controversial. Despite increased iron absorption from the gastrointestinal tract,[31] physiologic iron requirements in pregnancy often are not met by diet alone. In addition, many women enter pregnancy with depleted iron stores. The goal of prophylactic iron administration is to maintain maternal iron stores during the time of increased physiologic iron demand; it may also prevent anemia in infancy.[13] According to the Cochrane Database, routine supplementation with iron or iron and folate does prevent low maternal hemoglobin at delivery, but there is very little information regarding pregnancy outcomes for mother or baby.[32,33] Unfortunately, few good-quality studies of iron and folate supplementation have been carried out in areas where iron and folate deficiency are common and anemia is a significant health problem.

Some studies have suggested that iron supplementation improves maternal iron status and increases neonatal iron reserves, preventing iron deficiency in the first year of life.[34] In pregnant women who did not receive supplementation, iron deficiency persisted many months after delivery.[35,36] Iron supplementation may prevent reduced or absent iron stores after pregnancy and reduce the risk of iron deficiency in subsequent pregnancies.[37]

Iron supplementation has few adverse effects. The dosage is generally low enough to avoid the gastrointestinal side effects seen with treatment doses. Iron supplements may interfere with the absorption of other trace elements, such as zinc.[38] Zinc depletion may be associated with fetal growth restriction.[39] A study of the effects of oral iron supplementation on zinc and magnesium levels during pregnancy concluded that decreases in the concentration of these elements were physiologic and unaffected by iron supplementation.[40]

High maternal hemoglobin concentrations are associated with poor pregnancy outcome.[41,42] This has led to concerns about iron prophylaxis. However, iron supplementation in iron-replete women does not increase the hemoglobin level.[43] In iron-replete pregnancies, the hemoglobin concentration is largely dependent on the increase in plasma volume. Ineffective plasma volume expansion increases the rate of poor pregnancy outcome.

The other concern about iron prophylaxis is that excess iron can result in the production of free radicals and oxidative damage and may be implicated in cardiovascular disease and cancer.[44,45] Concerns about iron overloading in women with hemochromatosis have been raised. Approximately 12% of western white women are heterozygous for the common mutation of the hemochromatosis gene, and 0.5% are homozygous. A study of hemochromatosis and iron stores in pregnancy suggested that heterozygosity for the hemochromatosis mutation did not affect iron storage levels in reproductive-age women. One woman in the study who had markedly reduced iron stores was homozygous for the gene.[46]

Iron supplementation can be given on a selective or routine basis. Selective administration is appropriate for women with low or depleted iron stores, usually based on ferritin levels in early pregnancy. Ferritin cutoff levels for action vary between publications. A serum ferritin level less than 50 μg/L in early pregnancy is an indication for iron supplements. Some groups further stratify the starting time of these supplements, depending on ferritin levels.[47]

This approach avoids unnecessary supplementation in women with adequate iron stores. It identifies those who are at risk for iron depletion and anemia and targets these women with prophylactic or treatment doses of iron. The need for routine iron supplementation is debatable in western countries, but supplementation is recommended in nonindustrialized countries.[48,49] Various official bodies made recommendations for routine iron supplementation. WHO recommends universal oral iron supplementation with 60 mg of elemental iron daily for 6 months in pregnancy in areas where the prevalence of iron deficiency is less than 40%. In areas where the prevalence is greater than 40%, the recommendation is to continue supplementation for 3 months postpartum.[29] The CDC recommends supplementation with 30 mg of elemental iron daily, as does the American College of Obstetricians and Gynecologists.[50,51] Some consider universal supplementation to be a practical and cost-effective approach.[52] The debate is ongoing, and the decision to choose universal or selective prophylaxis depends on the prevalence of iron deficiency in the obstetric population served, along with nutritional, economic, and social factors.

Prevention of iron deficiency also requires education about diet. Dietary iron has two forms, heme and nonheme iron. Heme iron is the most bioavailable form of iron in the diet and comes from food containing heme molecules, essentially animal meat, viscera, and blood. Nonheme iron is obtained from cereals, vegetables, milk, and eggs. Absorption of nonheme iron is enhanced by ascorbic acid, proteins, and heme and inhibited by phytates, tea, coffee, and calcium. Many countries now fortify food products with iron compounds.[53] In nonindustrialized countries, other actions to prevent iron deficiency include iron prophylaxis in nonpregnant women[29] and treatment of hookworm infestation.[54]

Prophylaxis of iron deficiency is generally provided with oral iron. Various iron salts are available in tablet or syrup form (ferrous fumarate, gluconate, sulfate, and succinate). The elemental iron content of the different salts varies slightly. Compound preparations with folic acid are available, as are modified-release preparations, which release iron into the gastrointestinal tract slowly. However, these preparations may carry iron past the first part of the duodenum, where absorption is optimal, to areas of the gut where iron absorption is poor.

The frequency of oral dosing with iron supplementation has been questioned. Intermittent weekly or twice-weekly dosing schedules are as effective as daily dosing schedules.[55–57] In nonindustrialized countries, intermittent intramuscular iron dextran injections are used to ensure compliance and maintenance of adequate iron stores.[58] Compliance is a major problem with iron supplementation and may be as low as 36%.[59] In oral intermittent iron supplementation, compliance may be an even larger issue than with daily dosing schedules.[60] Iron-rich natural mineral water may be an acceptable alternative to oral iron prophylaxis. For example, Spatone Iron-Plus contains ferrous sulfate 0.20 mg/mL, which is highly bioavailable and maintains ferritin levels more effectively than placebo.[61]

MANAGEMENT OF IRON DEFICIENCY

Iron-deficiency anemia is usually treated with oral iron preparations. The oral dose of elemental iron required to treat iron deficiency is 100 to 200 mg daily. Ferrous sulfate 200 mg three times daily is equivalent to 195 mg of elemental iron daily. Many iron preparations are available, and no scientific evidence suggests that one brand is superior. Treatment doses of iron should continue until hemoglobin normalizes and should be followed with prophylactic or maintenance doses until 3 months postpartum to ensure that iron stores are replenished. Side effects with oral iron are common. Iron salts cause gastrointestinal irritation, with dose-related nausea and epigastric discomfort. Altered bowel habits (constipation or diarrhea) and abdominal cramping are common and have a less clear dose relationship. If side effects occur, reducing the dose or taking the tablets before meals (absorption can be reduced up to 50% if the dose is taken with meals) may help. Alternative iron salts can be tried, but tolerance is often related to reducing the dose of elemental iron. The addition of laxatives should overcome problems with constipation. The response to treatment doses of elemental iron is rapid. Reticulocyte counts increase within 5 to 10 days of initiation, and hemoglobin should rise 0.8 g/dL/wk (1.0 g/dL/wk in nonpregnant women). If no clinical or hematologic response is seen after 3 to 4 weeks of oral iron therapy, diagnostic reevaluation is required. Patients who do not respond to oral iron should be evaluated for ongoing blood loss, concomitant infection, additional hematinic deficiency, noncompliance, and other causes of anemia.

Parenteral iron therapy can be administered intravenously as an infusion or injection and also intramuscularly. It has no advantage over oral therapy if oral iron is well tolerated and absorbed. The response rate to parenteral iron is similar to that with oral preparations.[62] The advantage of parenteral therapy over oral therapy is the certainty of its administration.[63] Parenteral iron is given when oral iron therapy is unsuccessful because of patient intolerance, noncompliance, or malabsorption. Parenteral forms of iron include iron dextran, iron sucrose, and ferric carboxymaltose. Iron dextran is a complex of ferric hydroxide that contains 50 mg/mL of iron and can be given intravenously. Dosage is calculated according to body weight and iron deficit. A small test dose is given, and the patient is observed for 1 hour for evidence of anaphylaxis. If the test dose is tolerated, the total dose can be administered in a 0.9% sodium chloride infusion over several hours. The product is licensed in the United Kingdom in the second and third trimesters but contraindicated in patients with a history of allergy. Anaphylactic reactions have been reported, and facilities for cardiopulmonary resuscitation must be available when these drugs are administered. Patients require close monitoring during and after administration, and treatment should be given in a hospital setting.

Iron dextran is available by deep intramuscular injections. Total dosage is calculated according to body weight and iron deficit. It is administered as a series of undiluted injections of up to 100 mg of iron each. As with the intravenous preparation, anaphylactic emergency treatment should be available.

Preparations of iron sucrose complex contain 20 mg/mL of iron and are used in pregnancy as 5- to 10-mL aliquots up to three times per week in the second and third trimesters.[64]

Ferric carboxymaltose is a new compound that is now available, although there are little human data on pregnancy effects. It does not require a test dose to be administered and can be given by bolus intravenous injection or a fast intravenous infusion.[65]

Blood transfusions are rarely indicated in pregnant women with iron-deficiency anemia. With vigilant antenatal care and appropriate iron prophylaxis and treatment, severe anemia should not be detected late in pregnancy. If a woman has severe anemia beyond 36 weeks' gestation and there is not time to achieve a reasonable hemoglobin concentration before delivery, blood transfusion should be considered.

Recombinant human erythropoietin has also been used in difficult cases. Most experience has been with Jehovah's Witnesses. It does not cross the placenta but carries a risk of hypertension and thrombosis. Its role in pregnancy is not well established. Trials have shown that in combination with intravenous iron, hemoglobin rose more quickly than with parenteral iron alone; however, parenteral iron alone should be the first-line treatment in resistant iron-deficiency anemia.[66]

Treatment of iron-deficiency anemia in pregnancy was the subject of a Cochrane review.[67] Only 17 trials met the inclusion criteria. The reviewers concluded that there was a paucity of good trials assessing the maternal and neonatal effects of iron administration in women with anemia and that large-scale, good-quality trials assessing clinical outcomes and adverse effects are required.

Labor and Delivery

There are no specific recommendations for the management of iron-deficient patients during labor. Cross-matching should be carried out for women who are anemic on admission for labor. Blood transfusion may be necessary if significant blood loss occurs, because these women have little reserve to tolerate bleeding.

Postnatal

As the physiologic effects of pregnancy diminish, hemoglobin levels rise during the puerperium. There is no consensus on the management of severe postpartum anemia. Treatment is usually with either oral supplementation or blood transfusion. The Cochrane review of treatments for women with postpartum anemia concludes that there is some limited evidence of favorable outcomes for the treatment of postpartum anemia with erythropoietin.[68] However, most of the data focus on laboratory hematologic indices rather than clinical outcomes, and further trials are required to assess the treatment of postpartum anemia with blood transfusions and both oral and parenteral iron supplementation.[68] Any women who have clear evidence of iron-deficiency anemia should continue oral supplementation for at least 3 months.

ANEMIA: FOLATE DEFICIENCY

Folic acid, together with iron, has assumed a central role in the nutrition of pregnancy. At a cellular level, folic acid is reduced first to dihydrofolate and then to tetrahydrofolate, which is fundamental to cell growth and division.

Maternal Risks

Megaloblastic anemia in pregnancy is nearly always secondary to folate deficiency. Plasma folate levels decrease as pregnancy advances, reaching approximately half of nonpregnant values at term.[22] Explanations for the reduction in folate levels include reduced dietary folate intake because of loss of appetite,[69] increased plasma clearance of folate by the kidneys (believed to play a minor role),[70,71] transfer of folate from the mother to the fetus (~800 μg at term), and uterine hypertrophy and expanded red cell mass. As pregnancy proceeds, increased folate catabolites are excreted in maternal urine.[72]

Worldwide, folic acid deficiency may complicate one third of pregnancies. The incidence is higher in multiple pregnancies and closely spaced successive gestations.[73] Folate is readily available in most diets. Good sources include broccoli, Brussel sprouts, and spinach. Folate is often lost in the cooking process. It is heat-labile and rapidly destroyed by boiling or steaming.

Body stores of folate are found predominantly in the liver and total approximately 10 mg. Folate stores last approximately 4 to 5 months before symptomatic anemia develops. A survey of reports from the United Kingdom suggests that the incidence of folate deficiency is 0.2% to 5.0%, but more women have megaloblastic changes in their bone marrow that are not suspected based on examination of peripheral blood alone.[74] The incidence of megaloblastic anemia in other parts of the world is considerably greater and is believed to reflect the nutritional standards of the population. Current WHO recommendations advise folic acid intake of 400 μg daily with 60 mg of iron for 6 months during pregnancy and continuing for 3 months postpartum in areas of the world with poor nutrition.[29]

The maternal risk of folate deficiency appears to be megaloblastic anemia. This condition usually has an insidious onset, with gradually progressive symptoms and signs of anemia. It can be abolished with routine use of folic acid supplements during pregnancy.[75]

Fetal Risks

The risk of megaloblastic anemia is increased in the neonate of a folate-deficient mother, especially if delivery is preterm. Data also suggest an association between periconceptional folic acid deficiency and cleft lip and palate and, most important, neural tube defects.[76–82] Folate supplementation has been shown to reduce the incidence of neural tube defects.[78] It is not known how folate supplements reduce the incidence of neural tube defects.

Diagnosis

Outside of pregnancy, the hallmark of megaloblastic hemopoiesis is macrocytosis. This can be more difficult to interpret in pregnancy when there is a physiologic increase in red cell size and the possibility of masking iron-deficiency anemia. Examination of the blood film with oval macrocytes and hypersegmented neutrophil nuclei can provide useful diagnostic clues. The reticulocyte count is also low in relation to the hemoglobin. To diagnose folate deficiency, red cell folate assay is performed. Plasma folate levels fluctuate substantially from day to day, and postprandial increases are noted, limiting the use of serum folate as a diagnostic test. Red cell folate is believed to give a better indication of overall body tissue levels. However, the turnover of red blood cells is slow, and there is a delay before significant reductions in the folate concentration of red cells is evident. Patients who have a low red cell folate concentration at the beginning of pregnancy have megaloblastic anemia in the third trimester.[22] Folate deficiency in pregnancy is not always accompanied by significant hematologic changes. In the absence of changes, megaloblastic hemopoiesis is suspected when the expected response to adequate iron therapy is not achieved. Ultimately, the diagnosis of folate deficiency may depend on bone marrow examination and the finding of large erythroblasts and giant, abnormally shaped metamyelocytes. This test is usually reserved for patients with pancytopenia rather than isolated anemia.

Management Options

Prepregnancy

As with other anemias, a careful diagnostic evaluation should be undertaken, followed by prompt therapy before conception. The risks (described in earlier and later sections) should be discussed before pregnancy, and dietary advice about folate-rich foods should be given. Women who are contemplating pregnancy should be advised to take folate supplements of 400 μg daily.[29,83–85] In the United States, the Food and Drug Administration has made folic acid food fortification mandatory since 1998. All enriched flour, pasta, rice, and grain products contain 140 μg of folic acid per 100 g. Targeted fortification of food is under consideration in the United Kingdom.

Prenatal

PROPHYLAXIS

The case for giving prophylactic folate supplementation throughout pregnancy is relatively strong,[86,87] particularly in countries where nutritional and megaloblastic anemia is common. A systematic review of folic acid supplementation showed that hemoglobin levels were improved with supplementation, but there was insufficient evidence to evaluate other clinical outcomes for the mother or baby.[88] Folate should be given in combination with iron supplements. The folic acid content must be approximately 200 to 300 μg daily. The concern about routine folate supplementation is the risk to a woman with undiagnosed vitamin B_{12} deficiency. Folate treatment can worsen neuropathy in patients with vitamin B_{12} deficiency. The risk is low in pregnancy, and patients with severe vitamin B_{12} deficiency are usually infertile. Pernicious anemia is generally a disease of older people. Not one case of subacute combined degeneration of the spinal cord was reported among the thousands of women receiving folate supplements during pregnancy.[22] Folate deficiency is also an independent risk factor for thrombosis.

MANAGEMENT OF ESTABLISHED FOLATE DEFICIENCY

Severe megaloblastic anemia is uncommon in the United Kingdom and the United States, largely as a result of prophylaxis and prompt treatment. Once megaloblastic hematopoiesis is established, treatment of folic acid deficiency is more difficult, presumably as a result of megaloblastic changes in the gastrointestinal tract that impair absorption. If the diagnosis is made prenatally, initial treatment is with folic acid, 5 mg once daily, continued for several weeks postpartum.

ANTICONVULSANTS AND FOLIC ACID

Outside of pregnancy, folate deficiency can develop in patients who take anticonvulsants. Folate status is further compromised in pregnancy.[86] Interference with epilepsy control by folate supplementation may be overestimated.[89] Anticonvulsant therapy is associated with an increased incidence of congenital abnormalities,[90] prematurity, and low birth weight.[91] Hence, folate supplements should be given to all pregnant epileptic women who take anticonvulsants.

DISORDERS THAT MAY AFFECT FOLATE REQUIREMENTS

Women with hemolytic anemia, particularly hereditary hemolytic conditions, such as hemoglobinopathy and red cell membrane and enzyme disorders, require extra folate supplements from early pregnancy. The recommended supplementation is 5 to 10 mg orally daily. Anemia as a result of thalassemia trait is caused by ineffective erythropoiesis. However, the increased abortive marrow turnover results in folate depletion, and these women probably benefit from routine administration of folic acid, 5.0 mg orally daily, from early pregnancy.

Labor and Delivery

There are no specific management recommendations for folate-associated anemia during labor and delivery, as long as the patient is hemodynamically stable and blood replacement therapy is available, if needed.

Postnatal

In the 6 weeks after delivery, indices of folate metabolism return to nonpregnant values. However, if folate deficiency develops and remains untreated in pregnancy, it may be seen clinically for the first time in the puerperium. Lactation provides an added folate stress. A folate content of 5 μg/100 mL in human milk and a yield of 500 mL daily implies a loss of 25 μg of folate daily in breast milk.[92] Red cell folate levels in lactating women are significantly lower than those in infants during the first year of life.

SUMMARY OF MANAGEMENT OPTIONS

Iron and Folate Deficiency Anemia

Management Options	Evidence Quality and Recommendation	References
At Any Time		
Studies if hemoglobin < 10.5 g/dL (opinions vary; range 10.0–11.0 g/dL): • Complete blood count. • Blood film. • Red cell indices. • Reticulocyte count. • Iron status (e.g., ferritin). • Red cell folate. • Serum vitamin B_{12}. • Other studies as indicated by clinical findings and laboratory results.	—/GPP	—

Management Options	Evidence Quality and Recommendation	References
Prepregnancy		
Provide dietary advice and iron therapy to ensure satisfactory hemoglobin status before pregnancy.	—/GPP	—
Institute public health measures to prevent periconceptual folate deficiency.	Ia/A	82
Use of folic acid periconceptually reduces the risk of neural tube defects.	Ia/A	78
Prenatal		
Prophylactic use of iron or folate is controversial in industrialized countries, but important for pregnant women in developing countries to maintain or increase predelivery hemoglobin levels.	Ia/A	32,33
When iron or folate is prescribed, selective use is better than routine use if women can have their hemoglobin status assessed and followed up reliably.	Ia/A	32,33
Oral iron preparations are preferred; different compounds are used to minimize side effects.	—/GPP	—
Side effects related to dose and weekly oral iron administration may be an alternative to improve compliance without losing efficacy.	Ib/A	56,57
Give parenteral iron therapy if oral iron treatment is unsuccessful because of noncompliance, poor follow-up, or poor absorption.	IIa/B	63
Consider blood transfusion in patients with severe symptomatic anemia close to delivery.	—/GPP	—
Provide folate prophylaxis with anticonvulsants.	—/GPP	—
Continue routine oral folate therapy in cases of autoimmune hemolytic anemia.	—/GPP	—
Give parenteral folate therapy if deficiency is severe.	—/GPP	—
Labor and Delivery		
Cross-match blood if anemia is severe.	—/GPP	—
Postnatal		
Continue iron therapy for patients with iron deficiency.	—/GPP	—

GPP, good practice point.

ANEMIA: VITAMIN B_{12} DEFICIENCY

Muscle, red cell, and serum vitamin B_{12} concentrations decrease during pregnancy.[93,94] Women who smoke tend to have lower serum vitamin B_{12} levels, which may account for the positive correlation between birth weight and serum levels in women without deficiency.

Maternal and Fetal Risks

Vitamin B_{12} absorption is unaltered in pregnancy,[95] but tissue uptake is increased under the influence of estrogens. Oral contraceptives also cause a decrease in serum vitamin B_{12} levels. This decrease in pregnancy is related to preferential transfer of absorbed vitamin B_{12} to the fetus at the expense of maintaining maternal serum concentration. The vitamin B_{12}-binding capacity of plasma increases in pregnancy because of the increased levels of transcobalamin II, which is derived from the liver and affects vitamin B_{12} transport. Cord blood serum vitamin B_{12} levels are higher than maternal vitamin B_{12} levels. Pregnancy does not greatly affect maternal vitamin B_{12} stores. Adult stores are 3000 μg or more, and stores in newborns are approximately 50 μg. Minimal amounts of vitamin B_{12} are required for fetal development, which may account for the few fetal problems seen in pregnancies complicated by vitamin B_{12} deficiency. A deficiency syndrome is described in breast-fed neonates of mothers with significant vitamin B_{12} deficiency. It is usually apparent by 6 months of age and is characterized by failure to thrive, developmental regression, and anemia.[96] Addisonian pernicious anemia is unusual during the reproductive years and is usually associated with infertility. Pregnancy is likely only if the deficiency is corrected.

Dietary deficiency of vitamin B_{12} is possible in strict vegans who consume no animal products. Other disorders associated with vitamin B_{12} deficiency include tropical and nontropical sprue, Crohn's disease, and surgical resection of the distal ileum.

Management Options

Prepregnancy

Women with vitamin B_{12} deficiency should have their therapy optimized and their anemia corrected before they become pregnant. This approach may be needed to restore fertility.

Prenatal

The recommended intake of vitamin B_{12} is 2.6 μg daily during pregnancy.[97] This intake is met by almost any diet that contains animal products. Strict vegans, who do not eat any animal-derived substances, may have a deficient intake of vitamin B_{12}, and this type of diet should be supplemented in pregnancy.

Difficulties can arise when interpreting vitamin B_{12} levels measured in pregnancy because many women have lower values than those quoted as the normal range outside of pregnancy.[98] This decline in vitamin B_{12} levels is not believed to represent a true deficiency.[99] Levels return to normal in the puerperium. Care must be taken in the interpretation of vitamin B_{12} levels in pregnancy. If deficiency is suspected, the etiology should be considered. Intrinsic factor antibodies may be useful if the results are positive. Therapy is instituted empirically if there is clinical concern, especially if neurologic findings are consistent with vitamin B_{12} deficiency. The earliest symptoms are numbness and paresthesia of the fingers and toes, followed by weakness, ataxia, and poor concentration. Patients may have changes in mental status. Treatment of vitamin B_{12} deficiency is generally parenteral because patients usually have absorptive problems. Cyanocobalamin or hydroxycobalamin 1 mg is given three times a week for 2 weeks, and then every 3 months. In patients who have neurologic involvement, the dosage is higher. These patients are given 1 mg on alternate days until no further improvement is noted, and then 1 mg every 2 months. Oral vitamin B_{12} can be used in patients with dietary deficiency.

Labor and Delivery and Postnatal

There are no specific measures for patients with genuine vitamin B_{12} deficiency, apart from continuing maintenance therapy.

SUMMARY OF MANAGEMENT OPTIONS

Vitamin B_{12} Deficiency

Management Options	Evidence Quality and Recommendation	References
Prepregnancy		
Deficiency is rare.	—/GPP	—
Prenatal		
Continue treatment if it was instituted before conception.	—/GPP	—
Consider oral supplementation and other components for strict vegans and women with diets deficient in animal protein.	—/GPP	—
Consider checking intrinsic factor antibodies if the diet is adequate.	—/GPP	—
Labor and Delivery		
Continue treatment if already instituted.	—/GPP	—
Postnatal		
Continue treatment if already instituted; if the patient is not receiving treatment, check vitamin B_{12} levels postpartum.	—/GPP	—

GPP, good practice point.

HEMOGLOBINOPATHIES

Hemoglobinopathies are inherited disorders of hemoglobin. Hemoglobin is composed of heme (a combination of iron and porphyrin) and four globin chains. The type of globin chain determines many of the characteristics of the hemoglobin. Several types of globin chains are present at different times in embryonic development, in fetal life, and through to adulthood (Fig. 38–1 and Table 38–1). Abnormalities of the quantity or quality of the globin chains produced result in conditions known as hemoglobinopathies.

Hemoglobinopathies can be divided into two subgroups:

- Sickling disorders, which are qualitative abnormalities—an amino acid substitution in an α globin or β globin chain results in the synthesis of an abnormal hemoglobin. Many types of hemoglobin can sickle.
- Thalassemia syndromes are usually quantitative problems of globin chain synthesis. They result in impaired production and imbalance of globin chains. α-Thalassemia is caused by reduced α-chain production, and β-thalassemia is caused by reduced or abnormal β chain production.

FIGURE 38–1
Production of different globin chains. (From Hoffbrand AV, Pettit J (eds): Genetic defects of haemoglobin. In: Essential Haematology, 3rd ed. Oxford, Blackwell, 1993, p 95.)

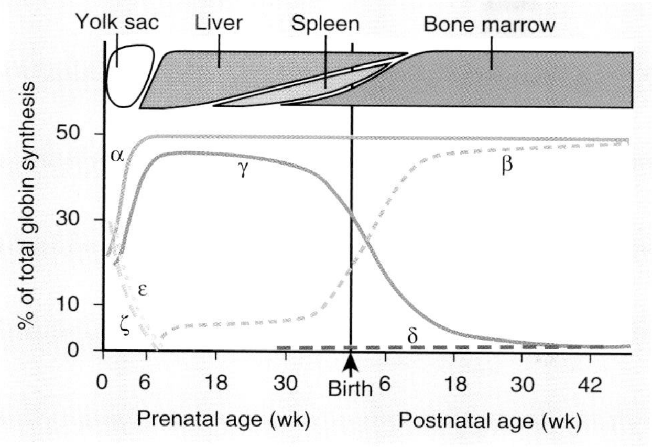

TABLE 38–1
Composition of Adult Hemoglobin

FEATURE	HEMOGLOBIN A	HEMOGLOBIN F	HEMOGLOBIN A_2
Structure	$\alpha_2\beta_2$	$\alpha_2\gamma_2$	$\alpha_2\delta_2$
Normal (%)	97-99	0.5-0.8	1.5-3.7

Women with major sickling and thalassemic conditions require specialized multidisciplinary team management preconception and throughout pregnancy.

Neonates with major sickling and thalassemic conditions require early identification and appropriate referral for specialized management, and this necessitates genetic screening to identify at-risk couples.

Screening for Hemoglobin Disorders[100]

Timely antenatal screening programs identify women and their partners who are carriers of these conditions and couples who are at risk for having an infant affected with a major hemoglobinopathy. This allows informed decisions regarding reproduction and prenatal diagnosis. Detection of major hemoglobinopathies leads to early identification of affected infants with improvements in care and survival.

In sickle cell disease, the first 5 years of life carries a high morbidity and mortality. Protective levels of hemoglobin F have declined by 6 months, and pneumococcal septicemia and acute splenic sequestration pose significant risks. Identification of these infants and targeted antibiotic prophylaxis, pneumococcal vaccination, and education programs have significantly improved survival. Identifying infants at risk of β-thalassemia major ensures timely further investigation and appropriate care for transfusion-dependent anemia.

In the United Kingdom, the National Health Service Sickle and Thalassemia Screening Program is a linked antenatal and neonatal program. Antenatal screening for hemoglobinopathies is universal in high-prevalence areas but selective in low-prevalence areas, depending on ethnicity and red cell indices.

The chance of being a carrier is dependent on ancestry. Tables are available that show the prevalence of traits in different countries and ethnic groups.[101]

Neonatal screening uses blood from the heelprick Guthrie card samples. All births in England are screened. Regional laboratories use high performance liquid chromatography as first-line screening for hemoglobin disorders and isoelectric focusing for confirmation of abnormalities. The Guthrie card hemoglobinopathy results are available to Child Health professionals, allowing appropriate early referrals of children requiring follow-up.

Sickle Cell Syndromes

More than 300 abnormal (variant) hemoglobins are recognized. Sickle cell disease caused by homozygosity of hemoglobin S (i.e., HbSS) is the most common sickling disorder. It is caused by a point mutation in the β globin gene on chromosome 11 that produces an amino acid change at position 6, changing valine to glutamic acid. This enhances the polymerization of hemoglobin S in the deoxygenated state and causes increased red cell rigidity and sickling. Chronic intravascular and extravascular hemolysis is a hallmark of sickle cell disease with significantly reduced red cell survival from 120 days to approximately 20 days. This results in intravascular nitric oxide depletion, endothelial activation, and vasoconstriction. Increased blood viscosity and tissue hypoxia occur as sickled cells occlude the microcirculation. Clinical consequences of sickling include

- Vaso-occlusive crises (micro- and macroinfarcts, leading to a painful crisis and organ damage).
- Anemic crises as a result of severe hemolysis, red cell aplasia, or splenic sequestration.
- Chest and girdle syndrome.
- Neurologic events.

Maternal and Fetal Risks

Sickling occurs in the homozygous condition (HbSS) or in compound heterozygous states (e.g., HbSC or HbS β-thalassemia, HbSD-Punjab, HbSE, HbSLepore, HbSO-Arab). Hemoglobin C, D-Punjab, E, and O-Arab are variant hemoglobins with mutations in the B globin gene. Hemoglobin Lepore is a variant hemoglobin that behaves like β-thalassemia.

The heterozygous state, or sickle cell trait (HbAS), is essentially a benign condition believed to have no particular antenatal sequelae. However, women with sickle cell trait are slightly more prone to renal papillary necrosis and urinary tract infection.[102] Their hemoglobin levels are similar to those of other pregnant women and should be managed similarly. Their sickle cell trait should be noted on their records, and the anesthesiologist should be informed of this condition if a general anesthetic is required. A study showed an increased incidence of preeclampsia in women with sickle cell trait.[103] Women with sickle cell trait should be identified by antenatal hemoglobinopathy screening. If the partner of a woman with sickle cell trait also carries the trait, there is a one in four chance that the offspring will be affected by homozygous sickle cell disease. These couples require counseling and the opportunity for antenatal diagnosis.

Pediatricians must be alerted to the possibility of sickle cell disease in neonates because antipneumococcal vaccines can now be given from 2 months of age and infants with sickle cell disease require long-term prophylactic penicillin treatment and regular evaluation.

People with major sickling disorders start life relatively protected from crises for 3 to 6 months because of the ongoing production of fetal hemoglobin. When hemoglobin A production becomes predominant, chronic hemolytic anemia develops. The severity and complications of the disease vary widely between patients. Many have debilitating chronic disease and frequent crises that require hospital admission. Others appear to be free of complications but have progressive organ damage. The life expectancy of these patients is still 25 to 30 years less than that of the general population, even in the developed world, with access to medical care.[104]

There are increased risks in pregnancy for the mother with sickle cell disease and her fetus.[105] The risks are not so great as to prohibit pregnancy. Maternal mortality is increased but has significantly improved since the early 1980s. Mortality rates of 30% to 40% are reported before the 1970s but have reduced to 1% to 2% in the United States and Europe.[105]

Recognition of this at-risk group along with improvements in medical management, transfusion, and neonatal care has significantly reduced morbidity and mortality.[105] Maternal risks include exacerbated sickle cell disease phenomena,[106] such as anemia, vaso-occlusion, ischemic injury, and organ damage as a result of the physiologic stress of pregnancy. These patients have greater susceptibility to infection (chest and urinary tract), hypertensive disorders of pregnancy, and thromboembolic complications.

Risks to the fetus include increased frequency of miscarriage, intrauterine growth restriction, preterm labor, and preterm birth.[107,108] Perinatal morbidity and mortality rates vary widely in different regions of the world[109–111] but are higher than in the general population. Perinatal mortality rates of 50% to 80% are reported before the 1970s, but more recent studies report rates of 1% to 8% in the United States and Europe.[105]

Diagnosis and Management Options

PREPREGNANCY

Before an affected woman becomes pregnant, a number of issues should be addressed.

Sickle Cell Disease

The frequency and management of crises outside of pregnancy is a useful starting point and may indicate the likelihood of crises throughout pregnancy. The patient's transfusion history and red cell antibody values should be documented. Hydroxyurea should be discontinued 3 months prior to conception in both men and women who are planning to conceive because it is teratogenic in animal models. Although there is little information about its effect on the human fetus, there are case reports in which hydroxyurea was taken throughout pregnancy with no reported adverse fetal effects.[112,113] Hydroxyurea is a disease-modifying drug that increases hemoglobin F, improves red cell hydration, and decreases the rate of polymerization of hemoglobin S. Its use decreases the frequency of crises.[114]

Contraception

Pregnancy planning is useful in women who have a chronic debilitating disease. No contraceptive choices are absolutely contraindicated on the grounds of sickle cell disease. Based on the theoretical risks of thromboembolism, sickle cell disease is listed as a relative contraindication for some combined oral contraceptives. The risks of pregnancy outweigh those of contraception.

Maternal and Fetal Complications

Past obstetric history is important, including a discussion of maternal and fetal risks associated with sickle cell disease. Patients should be told that active prenatal management significantly affects pregnancy outcome, and the importance of attending visits should be emphasized.

Multidisciplinary Team Approach

The community sickle cell service and midwifery team, along with hospital obstetric, hematology, anesthetic, and pediatric teams, plays an important role in the care of the pregnant woman and fetus.

Partner's Hemoglobinopathy Status

It is important to establish the partner's hemoglobinopathy status, ideally, before pregnancy. This information facilitates appropriate, timely, and nondirective counseling about antenatal diagnosis.

PRENATAL

These women should be seen early in pregnancy. Ideally, they should be seen by an obstetrician and hematologist with experience in this area. Partner screening should be carried out if it has not been done. A discussion about prenatal diagnosis should take place, if appropriate, and time should be taken to review the patient's obstetric history and history of sickle cell disease, including a drug history and the typical management of crises.

Laboratory evaluation should include a complete blood count, hemoglobin electrophoresis (if not previously done or available), reticulocyte count, ferritin level, folate level, urea and electrolyte levels, liver function tests, blood typing, and red cell antibody screen. The red cell antibody screen serves two purposes: (1) to identify women whose fetuses and newborns may be at risk of hemolysis because of red cell antibodies and (2) to ensure screening for the most common minor red cell antigens so that phenotypically matched blood will be available for transfusion. This is especially important because the donor population differs in ethnic origin, carries different minor cell antigens, and may sensitize this group of patients. As a result, it may be difficult to obtain suitable blood for transfusion. Blood tests should be performed to determine hepatitis A, B, and C, HIV, and rubella antibody status. Urine dipstick and culture allow identification and treatment of women with asymptomatic bacteruria. This group is more susceptible to urinary tract infections.

People with homozygous sickle cell disease may have a hemoglobin concentration of 5 to 12 g/dL, but concentrations are typically 6 to 10 g/dL. Hemoglobin S has a lower affinity for oxygen. Symptoms of anemia are decreased by the increased delivery of oxygen to the tissues. The reticulocyte count is elevated, reflecting increased red cell turnover. The bilirubin level also indicates the rate of hemolysis. Other abnormal liver function test results may indicate chololithiasis or acute cholecystitis as a result of chronic hemolysis or chronic hepatitis.

Pregnancy outcome appears to be similar in women who undergo prophylactic transfusion compared with those who undergo selective transfusion for clinical reasons.[115] No improvement in obstetric outcome was seen in a retrospective multicenter study in the United Kingdom.[116]

There is debate about the use of blood transfusions throughout pregnancy. Prophylactic versus selective blood transfusions was the subject of a Cochrane review.[117] This review found that there was not enough evidence to reach conclusions about the use of prophylactic blood transfusions. The development of atypical red cell antibodies is a real concern.[118] Transfusion is generally given before anesthesia or as an exchange procedure in severe crises, but no data suggest that transfusions should be given prophylactically.

Red cell indices in patients with sickle cell disease alone should be normal, but low MCV and mean corpuscular hemoglobin (MCH) may indicate iron deficiency or an associated thalassemia trait. The blood film shows variable numbers of sickle cells and features of hyposplenism (Howell-Jolly bodies, target cells, and increased platelet and white cell counts). Hemoglobin electrophoresis and high-performance liquid chromatography can separate out the various hemoglobins and allow detection and characterization of variant hemoglobins. In homozygous sickle cell disease, hemoglobins S, F, and A_2 are seen. Hemoglobin S is usually the predominant hemoglobin, making up 90% to 95% of total hemoglobin. Hemoglobin A is absent. In compound heterozygous states, other hemoglobins are found, except in hemoglobin S β-thalassemia, in which the hemoglobin S level is lower than that in homozygotes.

A sickle solubility test is a quick screening test for sickling hemoglobin, but it does not elucidate the type or quantity of sickling hemoglobin. It does not distinguish between homozygous sickle cell disease and a person with sickle cell trait.

The antenatal care plan should be outlined, with a discussion of the risks for both mother and fetus and strategies to reduce these risks. The patient should be advised to avoid precipitating factors that may cause sickle crises, including education about the signs and symptoms of infection and appropriate analgesics.

Return visits should be scheduled every 2 to 3 weeks to allow early detection of maternal or fetal complications. These visits monitor the course of the pregnancy, with regular monitoring of blood pressure, and assessment of fetal growth and development at appropriate intervals. Patients with sickle cell disease also should be asked about pain and crises and should undergo laboratory assessment, including complete blood counts, reticulocyte counts, and bilirubin measurements.

COMPLICATIONS OF SICKLE CELL DISEASE

Vaso-occlusive or Painful Crisis[119,120]

Crises occur when rigid sickle cells obstruct blood vessels in the microvasculature. This obstruction leads to tissue hypoxia, infarction, and pain. It is the most common type of crisis and the reason for most hospital admissions. Factors that may precipitate or exacerbate a crisis include cold, infection, dehydration, exercise, and stress. The pain is usually bony, although it may occur in the chest or abdomen. Systemic markers include low-grade fever, tachycardia, and mild leukocytosis.

As a result of sickling in the splenic circulation, most patients become hyposplenic at a young age, increasing their susceptibility to encapsulated organisms, such as *Streptococcus pneumoniae* and *Haemophilus influenzae*. This is the rationale for pneumococcal, *H. influenzae* B, and meningococcal vaccination and prophylactic penicillin administration.

Treatment and evaluation are as for nonpregnant women. Most pain occurs in the third trimester and the postpartum period. Underlying precipitants of pain, such as infection and toxemia, should be sought. The management hinges on good rehydration, with careful fluid balance and adequate analgesia. The pain normally requires opioid analgesia as an infusion or patient-controlled analgesia. Nonsteroidal anti-inflammatory drugs are a useful adjunct but should be avoided in the second half of pregnancy because of the risk of patent ductus arteriosus. Oxygen supplementation and intravenous antibiotics covering encapsulated organisms may be required. If intravenous antibiotics are not required, penicillin prophylaxis should be ongoing. Folic acid supplementation (5 mg daily) also should be ongoing. The patient should be kept warm. All of the relevant teams should be involved, including obstetricians, hematologists, and obstetric anesthesiologists. In women who have frequent sickling crises and heavy narcotic use, fetal growth must be monitored carefully because of the risk of intrauterine growth retardation. Pediatricians must be made aware of the risk of opiate dependence in the newborn and the need for opiate tapering. On admission, the patient should have a complete blood count, reticulocyte count, biochemistry testing, blood typing, blood cultures, arterial gases, and/or pulse oximetry. Potential sites of infection require culturing (e.g., throat swab, midstream urine, sputum, blood). Hemoglobin requires regular monitoring. Transfusion is generally given if hemoglobin is less than 5 g/dL. Review is required at regular intervals to assess the response to pain relief and look for evidence of infection, girdle or chest syndrome, splenic or hepatic sequestration, and complications of pregnancy, such as preeclampsia.

Acute Anemia

When a precipitate decrease in hemoglobin occurs, the differential diagnosis includes blood loss, bone marrow suppression secondary to infection, hyperhemolysis, and sequestration. Careful examination and basic blood tests are useful in determining the cause. A reticulocyte count will determine whether the bone marrow is responding appropriately to the anemia. If the count is low or absent, parvovirus B19 infection should be considered. This infection causes red cell aplasia, and transfusion is required. It can also cause miscarriage or hydrops, so careful fetal monitoring is required.

Prompt transfusion in splenic sequestration can be lifesaving when the decrease in hemoglobin is precipitous and hazardous for the mother and fetus. Patients have acute abdominal pain, with rapid enlargement of the spleen. This situation is rare because most patients with homozygous sickle cell disease are hyposplenic. Approximately 5% have splenomegaly, but it is more common in compound heterozygote sickling states, such as HbSC and HbS β^- thalassemia.

Acute Chest Syndrome[121]

Acute chest syndrome is a form of acute lung injury that is distinct from pneumonia. It is believed to be caused by fat emboli from the bone marrow along with red cell sequestration. It does not resolve with antibiotics but may become secondarily infected. It usually causes clinical or radiologic evidence of consolidation, with elevated temperature, cough, and pleuritic chest pain. Hypoxemia, which may be severe, and leukocytosis are also features. Treatment is the same as for a crisis, as discussed earlier, with early recourse to top-up or exchange transfusion, depending on the baseline hemoglobin. Oxygen saturation and blood gas values must be monitored carefully, and antibiotics and bronchodilators are useful. An intensive care setting is often the best place to monitor these patients.

Neurologic Events

Neurologic events are common in patients with sickle cell disease. Thrombotic cerebrovascular accidents and seizures are the main concern. The differential diagnosis (including metabolic disturbances, toxemia, subarachnoid or intracerebral hemorrhage, ischemic stroke, cerebral venous thrombosis, meningitis, cerebral abscess, epilepsy, or tumor) must be considered, and studies may include neuroimaging, examination of the cerebrospinal fluid if fever is present, and assessment for toxemia. Sickle-related central nervous system events should be treated with exchange transfusion to reduce the sickle hemoglobin percentage to less than 30%. This value should be maintained by transfusions to keep hemoglobin levels between 10 and 11 g/dL.

LABOR AND DELIVERY

Close supervision is required during labor. The risk of sickle cell crisis in labor increases if the woman is dehydrated or has hypoxia, acidosis, or infection. Care should be taken to prevent these complications.

Labor is also a time of increased cardiac output, exacerbated by the pain of uterine contractions. Cardiac function may be reduced by chronic hypoxemia and long-standing anemia. Pain relief is important in reducing cardiac work, and epidural is particularly effective.[122] Prolonged labor should be avoided. The woman should be kept warm, well-hydrated, and oxygenated. Continuous intrapartum monitoring should take place. The timing and mode of delivery must be determined by obstetric factors. Transfusion is considered if the hemoglobin is less than 8 g/dL.[123]

Thromboprophylaxis is given to women who are immobilized or experiencing a sickle crisis at the time of delivery. Routine thromboprophylaxis for women with sickle cell disease is controversial. There are no randomized, controlled trials, and efficacy has not been conclusively shown. Patients who have cesarean delivery should have chest physiotherapy, and early mobilization is encouraged.

Cord blood can be sent to the laboratory for hemoglobinopathy screening. Those who interpret the results must be aware of the possibility of maternal contamination. Universal neonatal screening for sickle cell disorders has been introduced in England as part of the newborn blood spot test.

POSTPARTUM

The heightened risks of sickle crisis persist after delivery. Adequate oxygenation and hydration need to be ensured. Patients must be monitored for infection and crises, and thromboprophylaxis may be considered, depending on the degree of mobility and individual risk assessment. Contraception can be discussed at this time (discussed earlier).

The results of neonatal screening and follow-up arrangements with the pediatrician should be confirmed before discharge.

SUMMARY OF MANAGEMENT OPTIONS

Sickle Cell Syndromes

Management Options	Evidence Quality and Recommendation	References
Prepregnancy		
Counsel against conception until disease status is optimized; assess renal and liver function.	—/GPP	—
Counsel about the risks of pregnancy.	—/GPP	—
Screen partner; if the result is positive, counsel about prenatal diagnosis.	Ia/A	100
Review medication—ensure on folic acid supplements, stop hydroxycarbamide 3 mo prior to conception.	—/GPP	—

Management Options	Evidence Quality and Recommendation	References
Prenatal		
Early booking appointment with planned schedule of care between obstetrician and hematologist with expertise and experience in the field of hemoglobinopathies.	—/GPP	—
Hemoglobin electrophoresis screening of the entire population or high risk groups.	Ia/A	100
Screen partner; if the result is positive, consider counseling and prenatal diagnosis.	Ia/A	100
Administer folic acid 5 mg daily.	—/GPP	—
Prompt treatment of crises (adequate hydration, oxygen, screening for infection) may include exchange transfusion.	—/GPP	—
Prenatal fetal surveillance and tests for fetal well-being.	—/GPP	—
Screen for: • Urinary infection. • Hypertension or preeclampsia. • Renal and liver function. • Pathologic fetal growth and umbilical artery blood flow.	—/GPP	—
Labor and Delivery		
Ensure adequate hydration, strict fluid balance.	—/GPP	—
Avoid hypoxia, continuous pulse oximetry.	—/GPP	—
Continuous cardiotocography.	—/GPP	—
Keep warm.	—/GPP	—
Provide thromboprophylaxis.	—/GPP	—
Alert pediatricians.	—/GPP	—
Postnatal		
Use of prophylactic antibiotics is controversial; low threshold for use on clinical grounds especially after an operative delivery.	—/GPP	—
Maintain good hydration and oxygenation, especially for the first 24 hr.	—/GPP	—
Provide contraceptive counseling.	—/GPP	—
Test the neonate for hemoglobinopathies.	—/GPP	—

GPP, good practice point.

Thalassemia Syndromes

Thalassemia syndromes are usually quantitative disorders of globin chain production that affect either the α or the β globin chain.

α-Thalassemia

There are normally two pairs (i.e., four) of functional α globin genes on chromosome 16. If one or two of these genes are missing, the result is an α-thalassemia trait. The type of thalassemia trait is an important factor to consider when offering antenatal counseling and diagnosis. These traits are not detected on hemoglobin electrophoresis because no abnormal hemoglobin is made. In addition, there is neither excess nor lack of any normal hemoglobins.

Deletion of three α globin genes results in hemoglobin H (HbH) disease, a chronic hemolytic anemia, with moderate anemia, hypochromia, and marked microcytosis and normal life expectancy. Nondeletional HbH disease also exists when there is deletion of two α globin genes plus a nondeletional mutation affecting a third α globin gene. The condition can be detected by hemoglobin electrophoresis by an HbH peak on the high-performance liquid chromatography trace and the presence of HbH inclusion bodies in the red cell that appear like "golf ball" cells on supravital staining.

In α-thalassemia major, there is no α chain production and no synthesis of hemoglobin F, A, or A_2. Tetramers of fetal gamma chains (γ_4) form because no α chains are present. This condition is known as hemoglobin Barts. Patients have severe anemia, failure of oxygen delivery to tissues, cardiac failure, and abnormal organogenesis. The condition is incompatible with life and causes intrauterine hydrops. Serious obstetric complications often occur, including preeclampsia and delivery difficulties because of the large fetus and placenta. The nonviability of the fetus and the maternal complications make early termination advisable. Experimental fetal treatment may be available if the condition is detected early in pregnancy. There are ethical issues with this practice, and antenatal screening for α-thalassemia is directed at preventing hemoglobin Barts hydrops. To prevent this condition, women and their partners who have a cis-(2) α gene deletion (i.e., genotype $--/\alpha\alpha$ or $-\alpha_0$-thalassemia trait) must be identified. These couples have a one in four chance of having a fetus with hydrops. In practice, these couples are identified on the basis of otherwise unexplained hypochromic, microcytic red cell indices (iron deficiency and β-thalassemia should be excluded). An MCH of less than 25 pg suggests the genotype $--/\alpha\alpha$ or $-\alpha/-\alpha$. Hemoglobin electrophoresis does not detect α-thalassemia traits, and definitive diagnosis requires DNA analysis to detect thalassemia-causing mutations. This diagnostic procedure is undertaken only if both the woman and her partner have indices and test results that suggest α_0-thalassemia trait or HbH disease or a combination of both within the partnership. Persons particularly at risk for α_0-thalassemia trait are those of Chinese, Southeast Asian, or Mediterranean descent.

DIAGNOSIS AND MANAGEMENT OPTIONS

Prepregnancy

Women who have α_0-thalassemia trait should be identified before pregnancy so that they can be alerted to the one in four chance of having a hydropic fetus if their partner carries the same trait. Early screening of partners is strongly encouraged. If the woman and her partner are at risk, the possibility and techniques of antenatal diagnosis can be discussed. Women with HbH disease should be encouraged to take regular folate supplementation outside of pregnancy to meet the demands of increased bone marrow turnover.

Prenatal

Prenatally, the main issues are antenatal diagnosis (if required) and maintenance of adequate hemoglobin. In women with indices that suggest α_0-thalassemia trait or HbH disease, partner carrier status should be sought early in pregnancy to determine risk, especially in affected racial groups. At-risk couples should be counseled about the risks and offered antenatal diagnosis with chorionic villus sampling or amniocentesis.

Oral iron supplements should not be prescribed on the basis of red cell indices alone (i.e., hypochromia and microcytosis). They are indicated when ferritin levels are reduced.

In HbH disease, folate supplementation (5 mg daily) is recommended, and transfusion may be needed for women with severe symptomatic anemia or early signs of fetal compromise.

Labor and Delivery and Postpartum

There are no specific management recommendations.

β-Thalassemia

MATERNAL AND FETAL RISKS

β-Thalassemia has three phenotypic presentations: the trait, intermedia, and major.

β-Thalassemia trait, or heterozygote state, is important to detect for antenatal screening purposes. It does not affect the mother's health, but causes hypochromic, microcytic red cell indices. Iron therapy must be based on hematinic measurements rather than the complete blood count.

Partner screening should be performed to determine the risk of having a child affected with a major hemoglobinopathy. If the partner carries a sickle cell trait, a β-thalassemia trait, or hemoglobin E, and the mother carries a β-thalassemia trait, there is a one in four risk of having a child with a major hemoglobinopathy. Sickle cell/β-thalassemia is a major sickling disorder, whereas hemoglobin E/β-thalassemia and homozygous β-thalassemia are transfusion-dependent states, with the associated problems of iron overload and iron chelation therapy.

Couples at risk for having a child with a major hemoglobinopathy need timely, nondirective counseling, with education about the possibility and techniques available for antenatal diagnosis.

Partners of women with β-thalassemia or hemoglobin E/β-thalassemia need antenatal screening to determine the risk of major hemoglobinopathy. If the partner has a relevant heterozygous condition, the risk of having an affected fetus increases to one in two. Although fertility is reduced in women with transfusion-dependent thalassemia, pregnancy has been reported.[124–126]

The physiologic stress of pregnancy may exacerbate symptoms of thalassemia. The transfusion regimen needs careful monitoring because blood requirements tend to increase in pregnancy. Iron chelation therapy also needs to be reviewed. Outside of pregnancy, iron chelation is usually performed with desferrioxamine mesylate (Desferal), which is given as a subcutaneous infusion over 12 hours 5 to 7 days per week. Continuing this treatment periconceptually and during pregnancy may put the fetus at risk for skeletal anomalies. This finding was noted in animal studies at doses equivalent to human dosages. The small number of reported cases in pregnant women is not sufficient to establish the safety of desferrioxamine mesylate in this setting. There are case reports of desferrioxamine mesylate use in early pregnancy,[127] but ideally, iron status is optimized prepregnancy and chelation is discontinued periconceptually, at least for the first trimester, but ideally, throughout pregnancy. A risk-benefit assessment of continuing iron chelation in pregnancy is required, and the results will depend on the degree of iron overload at the start of pregnancy. At conception, various organs may already be affected by iron overload, particularly the heart, liver, and endocrine system. These patients require careful evaluation prepregnancy and monitoring throughout gestation.

Patients with β-thalassemia major are often small in stature, and affected women have small pelvic bones. This finding might be the reason for the increased rate of cesarean delivery reported in these women.[126]

The fetus is primarily at risk if the transfusion regimen is inadequate and the mother is anemic. Fetal hypoxia may occur and has been associated with intrauterine growth restriction, pregnancy loss, and preterm labor. These complications do not occur when maternal anemia is managed well. Women with iron overload are at increased risk for maternal diabetes, which can lead to an increased risk of birth defects and prenatal and maternal complications.

DIAGNOSIS AND MANAGEMENT OPTIONS

Prepregnancy and Prenatal

β-Thalassemia trait is indicated by hypochromic, microcytic red cell indices and usually is seen with a finding of increased hemoglobin A_2 on hemoglobin electrophoresis. Complications in diagnosis can arise in patients with iron-deficiency anemia because it can falsely decrease hemoglobin A_2.

Racial groups at greatest risk include those of Mediterranean origin and some Asian populations, but it can occur in any racial group. The overall carrier rate in the United Kingdom is approximately 1 in 10,000 compared with 1 in 7 in Cyprus.

Women who are carriers of β-thalassemia trait need early education about the advisability of partner testing and the availability of antenatal diagnosis.[128,129]

In most cases, women with β-thalassemia intermedia or major are identified well before pregnancy and are receiving regular follow-up. Fertility is often reduced in women with transfusion-dependent thalassemia major owing to iron overload and central hypogonadism, but pregnancy is possible for some. Many require regular transfusion programs and iron chelation therapy. Unnecessary iron loading should be avoided. Oral and intravenous iron supplements are contraindicated. If possible, iron chelation therapy should be optimized prior to pregnancy and then discontinued during pregnancy. Iron chelation can be restarted after delivery. Desferrioxamine is safe to use if breast-feeding. Assessment of the function of organs affected by iron overload (heart, liver, and endocrine system) should be carried out regularly throughout medical follow-up. Assessment includes evaluation of cardiac status, liver function tests, thyroid and parathyroid function tests, and glucose testing.

Baseline cardiac status is important because the demands of a 30% to 50% increase in cardiac output that occurs in pregnancy can lead to cardiac decompensation with serious arrhythmias and heart failure in those with cardiac siderosis. Echocardiography assessment should be carried out, and the magnetic relaxation parameter T2* measured by magnetic reasonance imaging is useful in the quantification of cardiac iron, where available, although its predictive value for heart failure is unknown.[130]

If pregnancy was achieved spontaneously (i.e., without fertility treatment), the pituitary axis is likely to be functioning. Thyroid function and a glucose tolerance test should be carried out. Thyroid dysfunction is present in up to 75% of patients with thalassemia major, and the occurrence of treated hypothyroidism is approximately 9%. There is a high incidence of gestational diabetes among this group of women. If known to be diabetic (incidence of approximately 7% in thalassemia major), the control should be optimized prior to pregnancy.

Bone problems with osteopenia and osteoporosis often occur in transfusion-dependent thalassemics, and these can worsen during pregnancy. Vitamin D and calcium supplements are advisable if bone density is reduced, but bisphosphonates should be discontinued. Transfusion requirements tend to increase in pregnancy, and the transfusion regimen needs monitoring. The fetomaternal medicine team should monitor the health of the mother and the growth and well-being of the fetus. Partner screening should be performed.

Labor and Delivery and Postpartum

There are no specific management recommendations. As discussed earlier, issues relating to pelvis size, diabetes, and cardiac function may require assessment on an individual basis.

SUMMARY OF MANAGEMENT OPTIONS

Thalassemia Syndromes

Management Options	Evidence Quality and Recommendation	References
β-Thalassemia Major		
Prepregnancy and Prenatal		
Pregnancy is rare.	—/GPP	—
Review medication: stop iron chelators, give calcium and vitamin D supplements if bone density is reduced prepregnancy.	—/GPP	—
Avoid iron.	—/GPP	—
Give folate.	—/GPP	—
Give regular transfusions for anemia.	—/GPP	—
Screen partner; if the result is positive, consider counseling and prenatal diagnosis.	Ia/A	100

SUMMARY OF MANAGEMENT OPTIONS
Thalassemia Syndromes—cont'd

Management Options	Evidence Quality and Recommendation	References
Labor and Delivery		
Mode of delivery is dependent on cardiac status and presence of cephalopelvic disproportion.	—/GPP	—
Cord sample.	—/GPP	—
Postnatal		
Neonatal follow-up.	—/GPP	—
β-Thalassemia Minor		
Prepregnancy and Prenatal		
Give folate.	—/GPP	—
Give oral (not parenteral) iron if ferritin level is low.	—/GPP	—
Screen partner; if the result is positive, consider counseling and prenatal diagnosis.	Ia/A	100
Labor and Delivery		
Obtain a cord sample if the patient has an at-risk pregnancy.	—/GPP	—
Postnatal		
Provide neonatal follow-up if the patient has an at-risk pregnancy.	—/GPP	—
α-Thalassemia (Hemglobin-H)		
Prepregnancy and Prenatal		
Give folate.	—/GPP	—
Transfusion for severe anemia.	—/GPP	—
Screen partner; if the result is positive, consider counseling and prenatal diagnosis.	Ia/A	100
Labor and Delivery		
Cross-match blood if the anemia is severe.	—/GPP	—
Postnatal		
Provide hematologic follow-up.	—/GPP	—
α-Thalassemia (Hemoglobin Bart's Hydrops)		
Prenatal		
No treatment for fetal hydrops (incompatible with life).	—/GPP	—
Labor and Delivery		
Problems related to large fetus.	—/GPP	—
Postnatal		
Counsel about events and approaches to future pregnancy.	—/GPP	—
α-Thalassemia Minor/Trait		
Prepregnancy and Prenatal		
Provide iron and folate supplementation.	—/GPP	—
Screen partner; if the result is positive, consider counseling and prenatal diagnosis.	—/GPP	—

GPP, good practice point.

HEMOLYTIC ANEMIAS

Hemolytic anemias are characterized by accelerated red cell destruction, which typically results in an increased unconjugated bilirubin level, increased urobilinogen excretion, and an increased lactate dehydrogenase level. The reticulocyte count increases as the bone marrow responds. If intravascular hemolysis is present, free plasma hemoglobin and absent serum haptoglobins are characteristic findings.

Clinically, patients may have anemia, jaundice, splenomegaly, and pigment gallstones.

Hemolytic anemias are caused by something intrinsic or extrinsic to the red blood cell. Intrinsic causes of hemolysis include abnormalities in hemoglobin structure or function (i.e., hemoglobinopathies), the red cell membrane (e.g., hereditary spherocytosis), or red cell metabolism (e.g., pyruvate kinase, glucose-6-phosphate dehydrogenase [G-6-PD] deficiency). Extrinsic causes may be the result of a red cell–directed antibody (i.e., autoimmune hemolytic anemia), altered intravascular circulation (e.g., disseminated intravascular coagulation, thrombotic thrombocytopenic purpura; see Chapters 78 and 79), or infection.

Red Cell Membrane Disorders

Hereditary spherocytosis occurs in approximately 1 in 2000 individuals of Northern European descent.[131] The inheritance pattern is autosomal dominant. The red cells are spherocytic and osmotically fragile. The condition is caused by a wide range of molecular lesions resulting in defects in red cell membrane proteins. This leads to loss of red cell membrane surface, reduced red cell deformability, and accelerated red cell destruction. It is clinically and genetically heterogeneous. Diagnosis is made by a combination of nonimmune hemolysis and typical blood film findings, with spherocytes and osmotic fragility testing, or flow cytometry using an eosin-5-maleimide probe. This probe is a flow cytometric test that measures the fluorescence intensity of intact red cell membrane labeled with the dye eosin-5-maleimide. This fluorescent label binds to a component of the red cell membrane known as band 3. Binding is significantly reduced in hereditary spherocytosis.[132]

Hemoglobin concentrations are usually between 9 and12 g/dL but may be lower (6–8 g/dL) in up to 10% of patients. A pregnant woman with this condition should be monitored for anemia and should receive folic acid supplementation (≤5 mg daily). Aplastic and hyperhemolytic crises may occur. Aplastic crises are usually caused by parvovirus B19, which switches off erythropoiesis and causes a dramatic decrease in hemoglobin.[133] The virus may also affect fetal erythropoiesis and development. Hyperhemolysis is characterized by increased jaundice and splenic enlargement. In severe anemia, treatment with blood transfusion may be necessary.

Splenectomy ameliorates hemolytic anemia and reduces gallstone formation, but does not alter the underlying red cell defect. After splenectomy, women should ensure that their presplenectomy vaccinations (pneumococcal, *H. influenzae* B, and meningococcal) are current preconception and should take prophylactic penicillin V. Some small case series suggest that maternal morbidity and fetal outcome may be more favorable after splenectomy.[134] Pediatricians should be made aware of infants who are born to these women because there is a 50% chance that these children will be affected with hereditary spherocytosis, which may cause neonatal jaundice. Affected infants require long-term follow-up.

Red Cell Metabolism Disorders

The mature red cell has two principal pathways of glucose metabolism, the glycolytic pathway and the hexose monophosphate shunt. The glycolytic pathway provides the red cell with adenosine triphosphate as an energy source. Other products include the reduced form of nicotinamide adenine dinucleotide to reduce methemoglobin and 2,3-diphosphoglyceric acid to regulate the oxygen affinity of hemoglobin.

Pyruvate kinase deficiency is the most common defect of the glycolytic pathway. It is inherited in an autosomal recessive fashion and is clinically and genetically heterogeneous.[135,136] Varying degrees of nonspherocytic hemolytic anemia are seen. Hemolysis can worsen during pregnancy.[136] The need for transfusion of red cells must be assessed throughout pregnancy. Folic acid supplements are important for these patients, especially during pregnancy. Patients who have had splenectomy should be current with their vaccinations and receiving prophylactic penicillin.

Metabolism of glucose through the hexose monophosphate shunt produces the reduced form of nicotinamide adenine dinucleotide phosphate to maintain the antioxidative activity of the red cell. G-6-PD deficiency is a defect in the hexose monophosphate shunt and is the most common abnormality of red cell metabolism.[137] Worldwide, it affects more than 200 million people and offers a survival advantage in the face of *Plasmodium falciparum* malaria.[138]

G-6-PD deficiency is X-linked. More than 300 genetic variants occur, and they are categorized according to the variant enzyme activity. The severity of this nonspherocytic hemolytic anemia in heterozygous women depends on the degree of lyonization, the type of defect, the level of enzyme activity, and the oxidative challenge (typically, drugs and fava beans). Heinz bodies can be seen on supravital staining of peripheral blood at times of hemolysis, and they indicate the presence of denatured hemoglobin within the red cell.

The G-6-PD A variant is an unstable enzyme, with a half-life of 13 days (normal half-life 62 days) and the enzyme activity decreases as the red cells age. This variant is found in approximately 10% to 15% of African American men. Women with this condition usually are only mildly anemic. Enzyme levels are between 10% and 60% of normal and hemolysis is intermittent and usually secondary to drugs or infection. The G-6-PD B variant (also known as G-6-PD Mediterranean) is found in up to 5% of people with Mediterranean or Asian ancestry and is clinically more severe. The unstable enzyme has a half-life measured in hours. Men and heterozygous women may have severe enzyme deficiency, but the hemolysis is usually only intermittent. The responsible agent must be removed because even the reticulocytes have low enzyme levels and are prone to hemolysis. Some variants cause congenital hemolytic anemia with persistent splenomegaly.

G-6-PD deficiency screening tests are available in most hematology laboratories. Direct quantification of G-6-PD is available at more specialist red cell laboratories and is applicable when screening tests are positive.

In more severe variants, women must be monitored for anemia throughout pregnancy, should avoid oxidant stresses, should take folic acid, and might need transfusion. Women heterozygous for G-6-PD deficiency should avoid oxidant drugs in pregnancy and when breast-feeding because hemolysis may occur in the fetus or neonate if the drugs cross into the fetal circulation or breast milk. The pediatrician must be alerted to the risk of hemolysis and neonatal jaundice because affected patients need careful monitoring and early therapy with phototherapy or exchange transfusion with G-6-PD–screened blood if indicated by the bilirubin levels.

Autoimmune Hemolytic Anemia

Autoimmune hemolytic anemia may be primary or secondary to drugs, infection, autoimmune disease (typically systemic lupus erythematosus), neoplasia, or other hematologic disorders.

Usually, the antibodies are of the immunoglobulin G class, and antibody-coated red cells are cleared by the spleen. Symptoms of autoimmune hemolytic anemia are indistinguishable from those of other causes of hemolysis. The positive direct antiglobulin test (Coombs' test) is the mainstay of diagnosis.

Treatment is usually with glucocorticoids, but some patients have undergone splenectomy or are taking other immunosuppressive agents, such as cyclophosphamide, azathioprine, and cyclosporine. Transfusion may be required in patients who do not respond to treatment, but the autoantibodies may cause difficulties with cross-matching and close liaison with the blood bank is advisable.

Women who have autoimmune hemolytic anemia should have prepregnancy counseling, and treatment should be optimized. Careful antenatal supervision to assess maternal hemoglobin and markers of hemolysis, with adjustment of steroid therapy, is required.[139] Transplacental antibody transfer may occur, and hemoglobin levels in the newborn should be evaluated. Some infants require exchange transfusion,[140] but usually no treatment is necessary.[141]

Autoimmune hemolytic anemia has been reported specifically associated with pregnancy, with remission occurring after delivery. This condition tends to recur in subsequent pregnancies. The anemia responds to steroids, and most infants are not affected.[142]

SUMMARY OF MANAGEMENT OPTIONS

Hemolytic Anemias

Management Options	Evidence Quality and Recommendation	References
Red Cell Membrane Disorders (Hereditary Sperocytosis)		
Prepregnancy and Prenatal		
Consider splenectomy prepregnancy (with appropriate up-to-date vaccination and penicillin V cover for pregnancy).	III/B	134
Monitor hemoglobin, folate supplementation during pregnancy.	III/B	133
Blood transfusion if anemia is severe.	GPP	
Consult with pediatricians to arrange screening of infant.	GPP	
Red Cell Metabolism Disorders		
Prepregnancy and Prenatal		
Consider splenectomy prepregnancy (with appropriate up-to-date vaccination and penicillin V cover for pregnancy).	III/B	136
Monitor hemoglobin, folate supplementation during pregnancy.	III/B	136
Blood transfusion if anemia is severe.	GPP	
G-6-PD patients should avoid antioxidants during pregnancy.	GPP	
Autoimmune		
Prepregnancy and Prenatal		
Prepregnancy counseling and optimization of drug treatment and continue with "pregnancy-safe" drugs during pregnancy.	III/B	139
Blood transfusion if medical treatment not successful.	GPP	

G-6-PD, glucose-6-phosphate dehydrogenase; GPP, good practice point.

ANEMIA: BONE MARROW APLASIA

Aplastic Anemia

Aplastic anemia is a syndrome of bone marrow failure defined by pancytopenia and bone marrow hypocellularity. Normal hematopoietic tissue in the marrow is replaced by fat. Causative agents include infection, medications, and toxins, but most cases are idiopathic. Patients have pallor and fatigue as a result of anemia and bruising and bleeding as a result of thrombocytopenia. Infection is a risk because of neutropenia. Musculoskeletal abnormalities may indicate an inherited syndrome of bone marrow failure. The patient should be examined carefully for organomegaly and lymphadenopathy. These findings suggest viral infection or another underlying disease.

In patients with pancytopenia, testing should be directed by a hematologist and will include bone marrow aspirate and trephine with cytogenetic analysis and chromosome fragility tests.

Treatment of aplastic anemia is initially supportive, with blood products and growth factors. For younger patients with matched sibling donors, bone marrow transplantation is the treatment of choice. Immunosuppressive therapy with antilymphocyte globulin in combination with cyclosporin is also effective.

There are sporadic case reports of aplastic anemia in pregnancy[143–146] and reports of pregnancy occurring in women with underlying aplastic anemia.[147–152] However, overall, aplastic anemia in pregnancy is rare. The relationship between aplastic anemia and pregnancy is uncertain, but the literature suggests that there is not a strong association in most cases.[153] In a few women, however, pregnancy may play an etiologic role. There are case reports of aplastic anemia that are diagnosed for the first time in pregnancy, with spontaneous remission occurring after cessation of pregnancy.[154]

Pregnancy may exacerbate bone marrow depression and cause clinical deterioration.[155]

If severe aplastic anemia occurs in the first trimester, early termination should be considered. If spontaneous recovery does not occur after termination, bone marrow transplantation is performed as soon as possible in women who have a histocompatible sibling donor. In women with severe aplastic anemia later in pregnancy and those who refuse termination, intensive hematologic support with red cells and platelet transfusions is required until delivery. After delivery, bone marrow transplantation should be considered if spontaneous recovery does not occur. There are case reports of the use of antilymphocyte globulin in pregnancy,[154] but each case requires individual assessment and close liaison between obstetricians and hematologists.

SUMMARY OF MANAGEMENT OPTIONS

Aplastic Anemia

Management Options	Evidence Quality and Recommendation	References
Prepregnancy and Prenatal		
Optimize medical treatment prepregnancy.	GPP	
Consider termination of pregnancy if in first trimester.	GPP	
Provide supportive treatment.	GPP	
Provide multidisciplinary approach.	GPP	

GPP, good practice point.

WHITE BLOOD CELL DISORDERS

Neutrophilia

The neutrophil count increases throughout pregnancy. The increase is more marked during labor and immediately postpartum. Occasional band forms and myelocytes in the peripheral blood may be a normal finding during pregnancy. Neutrophilia may be associated with

- Bacterial infection.
- Acute or chronic inflammatory disorders.
- Tissue damage or infarction.
- Preeclampsia.
- Hemorrhage.
- Malignant disease, either hematologic (e.g., chronic myeloid leukemia) or nonhematologic.

Neutropenia

The finding of neutropenia on an automated complete blood count should be verified by examination of the peripheral blood film. Aged samples may show spurious neutropenia or neutrophil clumping. A repeat count should be obtained to ensure that the findings are reproducible. Ethnic origin affects the neutrophil count; persons of African and Caribbean descent tend to have a lower peripheral blood neutrophil count because of an increase in the marginating pool. Neutropenia may be acute or chronic and isolated or part of generalized pancytopenia. It may be caused by peripheral destruction or underlying bone marrow disease. A summary of the causes of nonmalignant neutropenia is shown in Table 38–2. The investigation of neutropenia in the pregnant woman is identical to that outside pregnancy. Drugs that

TABLE 38–2

Nonmalignant Neutropenia

TYPE	CAUSES
Acute	Drug-induced bone marrow suppression
	Agranulocytosis
	Viral infection
	Vitamin B_{12} or folate deficiency
Chronic	Race
	Immune neutropenia
	Primary
	Associated with connective tissue disorder or autoimmune disease
	Felty's syndrome
	Congenital neutropenia
	Kostmann's neutropenia
	Associated with other congenital disorders
	Chronic idiopathic neutropenia
	Cyclic neutropenia
	Aplastic anemia

may be implicated should be discontinued immediately, especially if neutropenia is severe. There are case reports of ritodrine-induced neutropenia.[156] If clinical assessment and examination of the blood film do not show the cause of neutropenia, bone marrow examination is indicated.

Maternal and Fetal Risks

In severe neutropenia, the principal maternal risk is sepsis. A patient with moderate or severe neutropenia (neutrophil count $< 1.0 \times 10^9$/L) and fever should have prompt cultures of blood, urine, and sputum, if available, followed immediately by empirical treatment with broad-spectrum intravenous antibiotics, according to local policy. Antifungal therapy is considered if the fever does not resolve after 48 to 72 hours, especially when neutropenia is prolonged.

There are many case reports of pregnancy in patients with cyclic neutropenia.[157,158] This disorder is characterized by cyclic fluctuations of the neutrophil count, with a periodicity of approximately 21 days. At its nadir, neutropenia is usually severe and is often associated with clinical infection. The onset is usually in childhood, but adult-onset cyclic neutropenia is also described. Pregnancy in cyclic neutropenia is associated with preterm labor and stillbirth, possibly because of chorioamnionitis associated with the neutropenia. There are also reports of improvements in symptoms and neutrophil counts during pregnancy in patients with cyclic neutropenia, possibly because of the production of neutrophil growth factors, such as granulocyte-macrophage colony-stimulating factor, by the placenta.[159] In approximately one third of cases, cyclic neutropenia appears to be inherited in an autosomal dominant fashion; therefore, the fetus may be affected.

Management Options

Recombinant granulocyte colony-stimulating factor is successfully used to treat patients with severe chronic neutropenia of differing etiologies, including cyclic and congenital types.[160] A few pregnancies have occurred in patients treated with granulocyte colony-stimulating factor for severe chronic or cyclic neutropenia.[161] Pregnancy outcome was normal in some, but fetal abnormality, including bilateral hydronephrosis, occurred in others. Data on the safety of the use of granulocyte colony-stimulating factor during pregnancy are inconclusive. Risks and benefits should be evaluated individually.

For a patient with severe neutropenia, prophylactic antibiotics should be considered to cover invasive procedures for labor and delivery.

Some viral infections that cause neutropenia have implications for fetal development and congenital infection (e.g., rubella, parvovirus, cytomegalovirus) or hepatitis. Maternal autoimmune neutropenia may lead to transfer of antineutrophil antibodies across the placenta, resulting in fetal neutropenia.[162,163]

SUMMARY OF MANAGEMENT OPTIONS

White Cell Disorders

Management Options	Evidence Quality and Recommendation	References
Neutrophilia		
Prenatal		
Increase in values for pregnancy.	—/GPP	—
Search for pathology and treat if the count is above normal.	—/GPP	—
Neutropenia		
Prepregnancy and Prenatal		
Give antibiotics for fever (and antifungals if fever persists).	—/GPP	—
For severe cases, consider recombinant granulocyte colony-stimulating factor; experience in pregnancy is limited to case reports.	Ib/A	160
Labor and Delivery		
Consider prophylactic antibiotics.	IV/C	157

GPP, good practice point.

SUGGESTED READINGS

Dodd J, Dare MR, Middleton P: Treatment for women with postpartum iron deficiency anaemia. Cochrane Database Syst Rev 2004;3:CD004222.

Howard RJ, Tuck SM, Pearson TC: Pregnancy in sickle cell disease in the UK: Results of a multicentre survey on the effect of prophylactic blood transfusion on maternal and fetal outcome. Br J Obstet Gynaecol 1995;102:947–951.

Jenson CE, Tuck SM, Wonke B: Fertility in β thalassaemia major: A report of 16 pregnancies, preconceptual evaluation and review of the literature. Br J Obstet Gynaecol 1995;102:625–629.

Mahomed K: Iron and folate supplementation in pregnancy. Cochrane Database Syst Rev 2006;3;CD001135.

Mahomed K: Iron supplementation in pregnancy. Cochrane Database Syst Rev 2006;3:CD000117.

Milman N: Prepartum anaemia: prevention and treatment. Ann Hematol 2008;87:949–959.

Model B, Harris R, Lane B, et al: Informed choice in genetic screening for thalassaemia during pregnancy: Audit from a national confidential inquiry. BMJ 2000;320:337–341.

Singh K, Fon YF, Kuperan P: A comparison between intravenous iron polymaltose complex (Ferram Hausmann) and oral ferrous fumarate in the treatment of iron deficiency anemia in pregnancy. Eur J Hematol 1998;60:119–124.

Smith JA, Espeland M, Bellevue R, et al: Pregnancy in sickle cell disease: Experience of the co-operative study of sickle cell disease. Obstet Gynecol 1996;87:199–203.

Zanella A, Fermo E, Bianchi P, Valentini G: Red cell pyruvate kinase deficiency: Molecular and clinical aspects. Br J Haematol 2005;130:11.

REFERENCES

For a complete list of references, log onto www.expertconsult.com.

CHAPTER 39

Malignancies of the Hematologic and Immunologic Systems

JOHN MAELOR DAVIES and LUCY H. KEAN

INTRODUCTION

Malignancy complicating pregnancy is uncommon; however, hematologic disorders account for most malignancies in women of reproductive age. Acute leukemia complicates approximately 1 in 75,000 pregnancies, and lymphoma complicates 1 in 5000 pregnancies.[1,2] Hematologic malignancies are an important consideration in pregnancy because, although they may threaten life, many are potentially curable. It is also important that the clinician has an understanding of the impact on reproduction of previously treated disease, because many women who have undergone successful treatment will later become pregnant.

The classification of tumors of the hemopoietic and lymphoid tissues is complex and subject to change. The World Health Organization classification[3] provides the major framework for categorizing these disorders. Much of the literature on these conditions in pregnancy predates the introduction of effective modern management. In some areas, data are necessarily limited, but as far as possible, the management principles discussed are evidence-based.

ACUTE LEUKEMIA

Acute leukemia results from malignant change in hemopoietic precursor cells at various stages of differentiation. Acute leukemia is traditionally subdivided into acute myeloblastic leukemia (AML) and acute lymphoblastic leukemia (ALL), depending on the major cell lineage involved. Further subdivision of AML and ALL provides additional prognostic and therapeutic information. Both AML and ALL are usually rapidly progressive and lead to bone marrow failure, with symptoms and signs of anemia, neutropenia, and thrombocytopenia. More unusually acute leukemias may present with extramedullary involvement. The myelodysplastic syndromes (MDSs) represent a heterogenous group of clonal disorders characterized by peripheral blood cytopenias and abnormal marrow morphology often with cytogenetic abnormalities. MDS may behave indolently, in which case outcome for pregnancy is excellent, whereas more aggressive forms of MDS resemble and overlap with AML in their prognosis and management.[4]

Maternal Risks

Pregnancy does not appear to affect either the development or the course of acute leukemia. Patients who have symptoms or signs with abnormalities in the complete blood count suggesting bone marrow failure or infiltration should undergo appropriate investigation. The diagnostic workup in pregnant patients with suspected acute leukemia should not differ from that in nonpregnant patients. This includes bone marrow aspiration, trephine biopsy, and examination of the cerebrospinal fluid, as appropriate. Cytogenetic and molecular diagnostic techniques are now routine and provide rapid additional prognostic information.[3] Blood chemistry including renal and hepatic function and urate should be monitored. Infection and bleeding are major risks in uncontrolled acute leukemia, particularly in some subtypes, such as acute promyelocytic leukemia. Laboratory assessment of the degree of thrombocytopenia is essential, and evidence of coagulation factor depletion and disseminated intravascular coagulation should be sought.

Supportive care, with blood and platelet transfusions and antibiotic administration, should be instituted early. However, chemotherapy offers the only prospect for long-term maternal survival. If delivery is contemplated before complete remission is achieved, then infection and bleeding pose a major risk to maternal survival. Patients may require intensive supportive care including antibiotic administration and appropriate blood, coagulation factor, and platelet replacement.

The outcome in both AML and ALL depends on a number of pretreatment prognostic factors. The prognosis is also determined by the response to treatment and the type of treatment offered. Recent population-based data from the United States show that for AML, approximately 50% of patients in the 15- to 35-year-old age group will be alive at 10 years. Similar Scandinavian data for ALL give a 60% event-free survival in patients aged 17 to 25 years. The acute leukemias are, however, a very heterogeneous group of disorders with widely varying outcomes. For example, patients with acute promyelocytic leukemia treated with modern protocols have an approximately 70% long-term survival,[3] whereas patients with Philadelphia chromosome–positive

ALL continue to present significant management problems. Despite the introduction of tyrosine kinase inhibitors, this disease remains essentially incurable with current chemotherapy regimens alone.[5] Discussion of prognosis should be highly individualized and undertaken only when all necessary information is available. Fertility is likely to be maintained in many patients with AML and ALL treated with conventional chemotherapy, and future pregnancy outcome in survivors of AML and ALL is also likely to be favorable. Counseling and contraceptive advice should include these considerations. Increasing numbers of patients have been treated with high-dose therapy including both autologous and allogeneic hemopoietic stem cell transplantation for acute leukemia. Although successful pregnancy has been reported, in most patients, these procedures significantly impair subsequent fertility.[6,7]

Fetal Risks

The main risks to the fetus are growth restriction, which occurs in both treated and untreated pregnancies, and chemotherapy-induced effects, both reversible and irreversible. Historically, fetal growth restriction and spontaneous preterm delivery occurred in approximately 40% to 50% of cases, and causation appeared to be multifactorial.[8] With modern chemotherapy and the attainment of remission in the majority of patients within 4 to 6 weeks, the fetal survival rate improves significantly.[9] Congenital leukemia is rare and essentially can be discounted. The fetal risks associated with chemotherapy depend, in part, on the timing of the treatment in terms of gestational age and also on the agents used. Although data are limited, general conclusions can be drawn about the fetal risks of chemotherapy.

First, adverse fetal events may occur at any point in gestation, although congenital malformation is more likely to occur with first-trimester exposure to chemotherapy. The literature suggests that the risk of major fetal abnormality with first-trimester exposure is 10% to 30%, depending on the degree of exposure and the agents used.[10] When a patient has known first-trimester exposure to cytotoxic agents, a careful fetal ultrasound should be performed at 18 to 22 weeks. However, not all teratogenic effects are detectable by ultrasound examination, and parents should be carefully counseled. Serial scans may improve the detection of some abnormalities, especially central nervous system (CNS), cardiac, and growth abnormalities.

Second, some chemotherapeutic agents are more likely than others to produce adverse fetal effects. For example, first-trimester use of high-dose methotrexate produces an approximately 25% risk of significant adverse fetal effects, with CNS, skeletal, and facial abnormalities being most common. Data on other agents used to treat acute leukemia are limited, and the degree of fetal risk is not known. However, successful fetal outcomes have been described following fetal exposure to many commonly used classes of cytotoxics particularly in the second and third trimesters. This includes vinca alkaloids, corticosteroids, anthracyclines, and cytarabine.[11–14] The situation is further complicated by an apparent "weakening" of predicted class effects with some agents, in that agents structurally closely linked to known human teratogens may produce less fetal abnormality than expected. All-*trans*-retinoic acid, which is used extensively to treat acute promyelocytic leukemia, is related to other retinoids that are potent human teratogens. These agents are contraindicated in women of childbearing age. There are, however, increasing case reports of the successful use of all-*trans*-retinoic acid in pregnancy, and these data emphasize that maternal versus fetal risk must be balanced at all stages in patient management.[15]

Finally, exposure to many chemotherapeutic agents is associated with the development of markers of chromosomal damage. The significance of this observation is not clear, and data on long-term effects in surviving infants exposed to chemotherapeutic agents in utero are encouraging.[16–18] However, this observation may reflect a lack of good information rather than a true lack of adverse events, with late chemotherapy-induced malignancies representing the major potential concern.[19]

Management Options

Prepregnancy

Women who undergo chemotherapy for acute leukemia should be counseled and advised against conception until remission is achieved and chemotherapy is discontinued. Oral contraceptives are not contraindicated. Methotrexate has a long "wash-out" period and can remain in tissues for periods of at least 3 months. It is, therefore, recommended that women wait at least 6 months before conceiving after receiving the drug. The risk of teratogenesis does not seem to be increased, but spontaneous miscarriage rates are higher.

For women in sustained complete remission, which is now a more common scenario, prepregnancy counseling should include a discussion of the prognosis in terms of the disease and the effect of the disease and its treatment on pregnancy. As a result of the 1994 European Registration of Congenital Anomalies (EUROCAT) study of policies for karyotyping in pregnancy, patients began to seek invasive prenatal testing because of maternal anxiety about exposure to chemotherapy or radiation therapy.[20] As discussed, although chemotherapy may cause chromosome breaks, there does not appear to be a documented increase in the risk of chromosomal or genetic problems in offspring of successfully treated patients. Importantly, previous chemotherapy exposure does not appear to increase the risk of miscarriage, growth restriction, or stillbirth.[21,22] It has not been possible to perform large studies to determine whether the incidence of childhood cancer is increased in the offspring of patients who have undergone chemotherapy. However, smaller studies suggest that there is no increased risk. Given the lack of evidence suggesting an increase in the risk of chromosomal abnormalities in the fetus, invasive prenatal diagnosis should be based on normal criteria in relation to age and screening test results. Women who have undergone pelvic radiation therapy, however, have a significantly increased risk of growth restriction in the fetus and should be counseled that increased surveillance is needed in pregnancy.

Prenatal

A pregnant woman with acute leukemia should be treated aggressively, with full supportive care and combination chemotherapy. A broad-based multidisciplinary team approach is required to manage the hematologic and obstetric aspects of care. Untreated acute leukemia is fatal to both mother and fetus. Standard treatment should be given, when possible, with appropriate counseling about fetal risk. No robust data are available on the need for dosage modifications of chemotherapeutic drugs in pregnancy. In some cases, agents that are less likely to cause fetal abnormalities can be used (e.g., intrathecal cytarabine rather than intrathecal methotrexate for central nervous system prophylaxis in ALL). However, nonstandard regimens of unproven efficacy should not be substituted on the basis of fetal risk without full and informed discussion of maternal risks.

Counseling about the teratogenic risks of treatment should be provided, and fetal and maternal well-being should be monitored throughout pregnancy by a hemato-oncologist and an obstetrician. Regular monitoring of fetal growth is indicated for patients who have received pelvic radiotherapy in the past. Whether more intensive surveillance in all patients previously treated for hematologic malignancy is necessary is unclear. However, it would seem sensible to provide an enhanced level of fetal monitoring when this provides additional reassurance to the mother and the attending physician that the pregnancy is progressing normally.

Labor and Delivery

Delivery should be expedited for normal obstetric indications. The goal of management is to deliver a viable infant while the mother is in hematologic remission. This approach offers the best prospect for uncomplicated delivery and infant survival. There is no contraindication to the use of steroids before delivery to enhance fetal surfactant production. Early assessment of the infant should be undertaken to detect complications from in utero exposure to chemotherapy. This evaluation includes assessment of potential congenital abnormalities and hematologic testing to exclude short-term effects (e.g., neutropenia as a result of recent in utero exposure to cytotoxic agents administered to the mother). When indicated, a cord blood sample should be sent for a complete blood count.

Postnatal

If delivery is inevitable in a patient who is not in remission, vigorous supportive care should be continued peri- and postnatally. If the disease is in remission at the time of delivery, counseling and appropriate contraceptive advice should be given after delivery.

Data on the excretion of cytotoxic drugs in breast milk are variable. Methotrexate is excreted into breast milk in small amounts with a measured milk-to-plasma ratio of 0.08. However, there is a risk for tissue accumulation in the neonate, which may lead to potential problems including myelosuppression. Results of excretion studies for cisplatin are mixed. The maximum reported excretion showed that milk-to-plasma ratios may reach 1, with consequent neonatal concerns regarding breast-feeding. A small number of reports of mothers breast-feeding while taking cyclophosphamide have shown significant neonatal myelosuppression. The data on anthracycline excretion are so limited that no assessment of safety is possible. This is also the case for newer classes of drugs. The absence of good data for most cytotoxics and evidence of potential harm for some lead to the general recommendation of avoidance of breast-feeding while taking cytotoxic drugs.

SUMMARY OF MANAGEMENT OPTIONS

Hematologic Malignancies: Acute Leukemia

Management Options	Evidence Quality and Recommendation	References
Prepregnancy		
Counsel about the prognosis.	—/GPP	—
Advise against conception until the patient is in remission and not on chemotherapy.	IV/C	10,11
Prenatal		
Provide an interdisciplinary approach.	—/GPP	—
Start chemotherapy as for a nonpregnant patient if the disease is diagnosed in pregnancy.	III/B	9,12–14
Provide supportive therapy (e.g., blood, platelets, antibiotics).	—/GPP	—
Counsel carefully, especially if treatment is commenced in the first trimester.	IV/C	10,11
Monitor fetal growth and health.	IV/C	12,13
Labor and Delivery		
Expedite for normal obstetric indications (ideally when the patient is in remission and the fetus is mature).	—/GPP	—
Give steroids if preterm delivery is contemplated.	—/GPP	—

SUMMARY OF MANAGEMENT OPTIONS

Hematologic Malignancies: Acute Leukemia—cont'd

Management Options	Evidence Quality and Recommendation	References
Postnatal		
Provide contraceptive advice.	—/GPP	—
Counsel about the long-term prognosis.	—/GPP	—
Avoid breast-feeding if the patient is receiving cytotoxic treatment.	III/B	48
Examine and follow-up of the newborn.	—/GPP	—

GPP, good practice point.

CHRONIC LEUKEMIA

Chronic Myeloid Leukemia

Chronic myeloid leukemia (CML) is traditionally considered a triphasic disease (chronic phase, accelerated phase, and blast crisis) that is usually diagnosed in the chronic (early) phase. It accounts for 15% to 20% of cases of leukemia, and the median age at diagnosis is in the fifth and sixth decades. CML arises from a cytogenetic abnormality that results in production of the Philadelphia chromosome. As a result, the *BCR/ABL* fusion gene is produced that encodes for a protein with tyrosine kinase activity. CML causes systemic symptoms, such as weight loss, fatigue, and often significant splenomegaly. Laboratory findings include marked leukocytosis, and as discussed earlier, a specific marker chromosome that is detectable in blood and bone marrow. Hyperleukocytosis with ocular and other CNS effects may occur.

Management Options outside Pregnancy

The management of CML has been revolutionized by the introduction of specific tyrosine kinase inhibitors, the first of which was imatinib mesylate.[23] A recent update of one of the major comparative studies with imatinib has demonstrated an estimated event-free survival at 6-year follow-up of 83% with an overall survival of 95% when only deaths from CML are included in analysis. Tyrosine kinase inhibitors have accordingly replaced the now-historic treatment options of hydroxyurea and interferon-alfa as first-line therapy. Related or unrelated allogeneic hemopoietic stem cell transplantation, which traditionally has been used to treat this condition, is now reserved for those failing or intolerant of tyrosine kinase inhibitors.[24] The practical management of patients with CML in the imatinib era including the role of molecular monitoring and approach to imatinib resistance or intolerance has recently been reviewed.[25]

Maternal and Fetal Risks

There is no evidence that the behavior of CML is altered in pregnancy. Control of the maternal white count may be achieved in a number of ways. The risk to the fetus is probably secondary to exposure to maternal therapy, and control of the maternal white count with physical means, such as leukapheresis, should be considered. Patients on treatment with imatinib or other tyrosine kinase inhibitors should currently be counseled against becoming pregnant because good data on their use in pregnancy are insufficient.

Management Options

PREPREGNANCY

The implications and risks of pregnancy should be fully explained, and appropriate contraceptive advice should be given.

PRENATAL

Regular hematologic review is required to determine the need for active treatment. Leukapheresis may be an effective method to control the white cell count, particularly in the first trimester. This approach may be continued throughout pregnancy. Successful pregnancies are described in patients treated with hydroxyurea and interferon-alfa,[26,27] though cumulative data are insufficient to allow an estimate of the real risk of fetal abnormality. Measurement of interferon-alfa in fetuses following administration of high doses has shown that it does not appear to readily cross the placenta. This also appears to be the case for excretion into breast milk, with levels no higher than controls found following high-dose administration. Patients who become pregnant while taking imatinib should be counseled about the uncertainty regarding the risk of fetal abnormality. The degree of risk and the type of potential fetal abnormality are unknown, but this advice is based on lack of extensive evidence that imatinib is safe rather than positive evidence of high risk of harm. However, the safe option for patients in the chronic phase who become pregnant while taking imatinib is to discontinue use of the agent and to institute other methods to control the white cell count. There are, however, several case reports of successful pregnancy outcome in patients treated with imatinib at all stages of gestation.[28,29] Imatinib does not appear to cross the placenta in the third trimester, but data regarding transplacental passage at earlier gestations are not available. Therefore, careful ultrasonographic examination of the fetus should be performed in women who wish to continue the pregnancy after first-trimester exposure. Imatinib is excreted into breast milk with a milk-to-plasma ratio of 0.5 for imatinib and 0.9 for its main metabolite. This could potentially lead to levels in a term infant of 10% of the therapeutic level. The effects of even low-dose exposure to the baby are unknown, and full discussion with the pediatric team should be considered in women who want to breast-feed.

Hematologic abnormalities that suggest disease progression, such as signs of the accelerated phase or blast crisis, should lead to management review. In the accelerated phase, expediting delivery should be considered. Maternal options include reintroduction of imatinib, use of an alternative tyrosine kinase inhibitor, and referral for hemopoietic stem cell transplantation, which is the only likely curative option. Blast crisis in pregnancy may be treated with tyrosine kinase inhibitors, if the patient is not already receiving these agents, or with combination chemotherapy, as for other forms of acute leukemia. However, the maternal outlook long-term is poor, and urgent consideration should be given to early delivery and referral of the mother, if appropriate, for hemopoietic stem cell transplantation, particularly if a second chronic phase can be obtained.[30]

Chronic Lymphocytic Leukemia

Chronic lymphocytic leukemia (CLL) is a disease of older populations[3] and rarely occurs in pregnancy. A "wait-and-watch" approach is often appropriate, and the patient may need treatment only if symptoms occur. When treatment is required, standard first-line therapies include corticosteroids, alkylating agents, fludarabine, and rituximab.[31] Given the usual indolent course of CLL, most pregnancies will be managed without fetal exposure to potentially teratogenic agents and with no detriment to maternal outcome.

Myeloma

Myeloma is also a disease of older age groups and is rare in pregnancy. It presents a unique set of management problems and may cause significant skeletal damage, bone marrow failure, extended risk of infection, and renal failure. Radiologic assessment of potential skeletal damage should be undertaken in a manner that limits fetal exposure to radiation. Magnetic resonance imaging (MRI) may be useful in this regard.[32] A number of chemotherapeutic agents are active in the treatment of myeloma. If treatment is required in pregnancy, then high-dose corticosteroids either alone or in combination with older agents such alkylators and anthracyclines may be preferred to newer agents such as bortezomib in which data on fetal outcome are very limited.[33] Thalidomide and its structural analogue lenalidomide, now commonly incorporated into front-line and salvage regimes, are absolutely contraindicated in pregnancy.[34] Radiotherapy has a significant role in the management of myeloma, particularly in the context of cord compression. The management of maternal spinal cord compression in pregnancy is challenging, and treatment needs to be highly individualized following full interdisciplinary discussion, which includes neurosurgical opinion.

SUMMARY OF MANAGEMENT OPTIONS

Hematologic Malignancies: Chronic Myeloid Leukemia

Management Options	Evidence Quality and Recommendation	References
Prepregnancy		
Counsel about the prognosis for pregnancy and in the long term.	IV/C	26
Give contraceptive advice.	—/GPP	—
Prenatal		
Provide an interdisciplinary approach.	—/GPP	—
Provide regular hematologic monitoring.	—/GPP	—
Consider leukapheresis	—/GPP	—
Control with hydroxyurea or interferon-alfa (avoid cytotoxics in the first trimester); data on imatinib are limited–current recommendation is not to use in pregnancy.	IV/C	27–29
Manage accelerated phase and blast crisis as for nonpregnant patients, and expedite delivery if possible (to allow for the possibility of bone marrow transplantation).	IV/C	30
Postnatal		
Provide contraceptive advice.	—/GPP	—
Counsel about the long-term prognosis.	—/GPP	—
Avoid breast-feeding if the patient is receiving cytotoxic treatment.	III/B	48
Examine and follow-up of the newborn.	—/GPP	—

GPP, good practice point.

LYMPHOMA

The lymphomas are a heterogeneous group of malignant disorders that arise in lymphoid tissue. The major histologic subdivision of lymphoma is into the following categories:

- Hodgkin's disease.
- Non-Hodgkin lymphoma.

Hodgkin's Disease

Hodgkin's disease is an uncommon lymphoid malignancy.[35] However, because of the age distribution of patients with Hodgkin's disease, it is the most common type of lymphoma seen in pregnancy. Hodgkin's disease causes nodal enlargement, classically in the neck, and diagnosis requires biopsy of the affected tissue. Further management depends on the stage of disease. Early-stage or localized Hodgkin's disease may be cured with either radiation therapy alone or a combination of chemotherapy and radiation therapy in modified dosage. More extensive stage disease requires combination chemotherapy for cure. The Ann Arbor system is still the most commonly used staging system, but staging may be refined anatomically with the Cotswolds revision.[36] In addition, information available from laboratory tests (e.g., lymphocyte count, erythrocyte sedimentation rate, serum albumin level) may be used to produce a prognostic index that may affect management. However, none of the commonly used prognostic scoring systems have been validated in pregnancy.

Maternal Risks

Hodgkin's disease in pregnancy does not appear to differ from that in nonpregnant patients, although Hodgkin's disease is less common in multiparous women. Diagnosis is made by biopsy. Further studies in the pregnant patient are associated with specific problems, particularly with regard to computed tomography (CT); however, MRI, which is considered safe in pregnancy, may be used.[37] Staging laparotomy has essentially been abandoned.[38] The outlook for cure in patients with early-stage disease treated with radiation therapy, with or without a short course of chemotherapy, is excellent.[39] The greater than 5-year disease-free survival rate in patients with advanced disease treated with combination chemotherapy is 70% to 80%.[39] After relapse, high-dose therapy may produce additional long-term survivors.[40]

Most patients who are successfully treated for Hodgkin's disease return to a normal or very near normal quality of life on cessation of treatment. Many women who receive combination chemotherapy for Hodgkin's disease remain fertile, although there is a risk of premature menopause.[41] No apparent increase in the complications of pregnancy or fetal abnormality in subsequent pregnancy is seen after combination chemotherapy for Hodgkin's disease.[42]

Fetal Risks

The risks to the fetus stem chiefly from the effects of either radiation therapy or chemotherapy. The risks to the fetus of diagnostic radiation have been reviewed.[43,44] Both CT and positron-emission tomography (PET) scanning are now routinely used in the evaluation of lymphoma including Hodgkin's disease. Exposure of pregnant women to the radiation doses used in standard abdominal and pelvic CT appears to have no substantial effect on the risk of fetal death or malformation. The risk of childhood cancer is more than doubled after fetal irradiation. Where possible, irradiation of the fetus in utero should be avoided, but staging should be sufficient to determine the correct modality of treatment. MRI is an adequate tool for staging evaluation in most circumstances and avoids exposure to ionizing radiation.[37]

The risk to the fetus of therapeutic irradiation depends on whether early-stage Hodgkin's disease involves the abdomen or pelvis. Supradiaphragmatic irradiation with heavy lead shielding of the uterus resulted in no congenital abnormalities in one series.[45] When high-dose irradiation cannot be avoided by field manipulation, infradiaphragmatic radiation therapy even with appropriate shielding carries a substantial risk of spontaneous miscarriage and fetal abnormality throughout pregnancy. Under these circumstances, chemotherapy alone rather than radiation therapy should be considered, with delivery before therapeutic irradiation. The fetal effects of combination chemotherapy used to treat Hodgkin's disease are unlikely to be substantially different from those seen in acute leukemia. The teratogenic risk is potentially greatest with first-trimester exposure. However, one series found no apparent adverse fetal effects even with first-trimester exposure to the current gold standard treatment of doxorubicin (Adriamycin), bleomycin, vinblastine, and dacarbazine (ABVD).[46]

Management Options

PREPREGNANCY

Women with active Hodgkin's disease should be counseled about the risks of pregnancy and should take appropriate contraceptive measures. Pregnancy outcome is good in patients who have been successfully treated for Hodgkin's disease, and routine amniocentesis is not recommended.

PRENATAL

The outlook for patients treated for Hodgkin's disease is good to excellent. Diagnosis and investigation are discussed previously. Patients diagnosed in the first trimester should be counseled about the risks of continuing with the pregnancy.

In highly selected cases, early-stage supradiaphragmatic disease can be successfully treated with radiation therapy alone, with little fetal risk. Historically, early-stage intra-abdominal disease presented a management problem. The options were therapeutic abortion or early delivery, followed by local radiation therapy.

Conventional management of early-stage Hodgkin's disease now uses combined modality treatment; thus, both supradiaphragmatic and infradiaphragmatic disease may be treated with a short course of combination chemotherapy until delivery, with radiation therapy given after delivery. Management decisions are, however, complex and discussion should include the patient, hemato-oncologist, obstetrician, and radiation oncologist.

Patients with more extensive disease should be counseled about the risks of proceeding with pregnancy. Some women may wish to continue with the pregnancy and opt for combination chemotherapy on evidence of disease progression. The optimum management in this context is not clear, but early in pregnancy, patients with symptomatic or progressive disease could reasonably receive standard chemotherapy, currently ABVD or an equivalent. Beyond the first trimester, treatment options include ABVD, corticosteroids, alone or single-agent vinblastine, which is not associated with a teratogenic risk at this point in gestation.[47] After delivery, patients may be treated with more aggressive combination chemotherapy, such as ABVD, as appropriate. There appears to be no detriment to outcome if ABVD is used after corticosteroids or vinblastine in this situation.

POSTNATAL

Careful counseling about the prognosis for both long-term disease-free survival and preservation of fertility should be given. Patients who are undergoing active treatment for Hodgkin's disease with combination chemotherapy should be advised not to breast-feed.[48]

SUMMARY OF MANAGEMENT OPTIONS

Hematologic Malignancies: Hodgkin's Disease

Management Options	Evidence Quality and Recommendation	References
Prepregnancy		
Counsel about risks and prognosis.	IIa/B	42
Give contraceptive advice.	III/B	47
Prenatal		
Provide an interdisciplinary approach.	—/GPP	—
Diagnose by lymph node biopsy.	—/GPP	—
Stage by clinical assessment and magnetic resonance imaging; counsel about the prognosis and risks to the fetus.	IV/C	37,43
Treatment		
Stage IIa/IIa nonbulky (localized disease):		
Extra-abdominal:		
• Radiation therapy with shielding with or without abbreviated chemotherapy.	Ib/A	63
Intra-abdominal (depends on gestation and the patient's wishes):		
• Delivery and radiation therapy with or without abbreviated chemotherapy.	Ib/A	63
• Continue pregnancy with chemotherapy only.	III/B	47
Other stages (extensive-stage disease):		
• Chemotherapy with supportive care.	IIa/B	47
Postnatal		
Provide contraceptive advice	III/C	2
Counsel about the long-term prognosis.		
Avoid breast-feeding if the patient is receiving cytotoxic treatment.		
Examine and follow-up of the newborn.		

GPP, good practice point.

Non-Hodgkin Lymphomas

Non-Hodgkin lymphomas comprise a heterogeneous group of malignancies. Unlike in Hodgkin disease, extranodal presentation of non-Hodgkin lymphoma is not uncommon. The increase in the incidence of non-Hodgkin lymphomas is partly attributable to an aging population and risk factors such as HIV infection, but an unexplained real increase in incidence has been noted. Non-Hodgkin lymphomas are uncommon in the reproductive years. The subclassification of non-Hodgkin lymphomas is complex and changing. However, in general, three types of biologic behavior are seen.[3]

Low-grade, or indolent, lymphomas that are slow-growing do not immediately threaten life and may be treated either on a wait-and-watch basis, with single-agent or combination chemoimmunotherapy or local radiation therapy.[49] More aggressive lymphomas, such as diffuse large B cell lymphoma, have a much shorter clinical history and may cause early life-threatening complications. These are treated with combination chemoimmunotherapy.[50,51] Some lymphomas, such as lymphoblastic lymphoma or Burkitt's lymphoma behave biologically like subtypes of ALL. These are treated with aggressive combination chemotherapy, the nature of which depends on the histologic subtype.

Maternal Risks

Diagnosis is made on biopsy, and testing and staging are as for Hodgkin's disease, although advanced disease is more common in non-Hodgkin lymphomas. Treatment must be highly individualized and may, as discussed earlier, vary from a wait-and-watch policy to administration of intermediate- or high-dose combination chemotherapy.

Fetal Risks

Non-Hodgkin lymphoma does not appear to affect the outcome of pregnancy. The risks to the fetus are those of treatment. In terms of exposure to cytotoxic agents, fetal risk should not be substantially different from that seen in acute leukemia and Hodgkin's disease. The potential long-term effects on the fetus due to the recent introduction of chemoimmunotherapy into the management of many B cell lymphomas are unknown. Insufficient data are available on the effects of rituximab on pregnancy to allow formal risk stratification, and the conventional wisdom is that rituximab is contraindicated in pregnancy.[53] The introduction of an agent such as rituximab, which clearly improves outcome but has limited data in pregnancy, illustrates the dilemma that many physicians face.

Management Options

PREPREGNANCY

Women who have active non-Hodgkin lymphoma should be counseled about the outlook for the particular subtype of disease and receive appropriate contraceptive advice. Patients who are receiving active treatment for non-Hodgkin lymphoma should be advised against becoming pregnant.

PRENATAL

Management depends on the histologic subtype and extent of disease (discussed previously).

POSTNATAL

Although data are limited, patients undergoing active treatment for non-Hodgkin lymphoma should be advised against breast-feeding.

SUMMARY OF MANAGEMENT OPTIONS

Hematologic Malignancies: Non-Hodgkin Lymphoma

Management Options	Evidence Quality and Recommendation	References
Prepregnancy		
As for Hodgkin's disease.	—/GPP	—
Prenatal		
Provide an interdisciplinary approach.	—/GPP	—
See comments about staging and diagnosis as for Hodgkin's disease.	—/GPP	—
Treat as for a nonpregnant patient; options vary from "wait and watch" to aggressive combination chemotherapy with supportive care; termination and preterm delivery before chemotherapy are options.	Ib/A III/C	51,52 49
Counsel about the prognosis and risk to the fetus.	III/C	64
Postnatal		
Provide contraceptive advice.	III/C	2
Counsel about the long-term prognosis.		
Avoid breast-feeding if the patient is receiving cytotoxic treatment.		
Examine and follow-up of the newborn.		

GPP, good practice point.

MYELOPROLIFERATIVE DISORDERS

Essential Thrombocythemia

Diagnosis, Assessment, and Risks

Essential thrombocythemia is a myeloproliferative disorder that usually occurs in older age groups. Occasional cases complicating pregnancy are reported in the literature. Causes of reactive thrombocytosis are much more common and should be carefully excluded. Common causes of reactive thrombocytosis include iron deficiency, hemorrhage, infection, and inflammatory conditions. In essential thrombocythemia, the platelet count is consistently elevated in the absence of an apparent underlying cause. Approximately 50% of patients will have evidence of the JAK 2 mutation, and this may provide the diagnosis.[54] Bone marrow biopsy may have a characteristic appearance and cytogenetic studies should be performed to exclude CML. Essential thrombocythemia may be complicated by abnormal bleeding as a result of defective platelet function or by both arterial and venous thrombosis. The incidence of these complications in younger patients is unknown, and thrombosis in particular may be less common than in older age groups. The literature on pregnancy includes small series and case reports. Spontaneous abortion, intrauterine death, and intrauterine growth restriction are possible risks, due primarily to placental infarction.[38,39] However, other small series have reported good pregnancy outcomes in asymptomatic women.[40,41]

Management Options

If the patient is asymptomatic and the platelet count is only moderately increased, in the range of 400 to 600 × 10^9/L, an expectant approach is reasonable.[38] If thrombosis or hemorrhage occurs, however, treatment is necessary. Because of a reluctance to use cytotoxic agents in pregnancy, plateletpheresis has been used.[38] However, each pheresis is a short-term measure, and it may be practically difficult to achieve good long-term platelet control. If plateletpheresis is used, response may be assessed over a number of days initially and the intervals between phereses extended if possible. Subsequent management decisions should balance the pheresis interval against the degree of platelet control, and alternative treatment should be introduced if necessary. Aspirin may be used to treat thrombotic complications,[39] but may aggravate an underlying platelet function defect. Aspirin may have a role in patients with essential thrombocythemia and a history of previous pregnancy failure or growth restriction, but few data are available.[40] There are anecdotal reports of the use of hydroxyurea in essential thrombocythemia in pregnancy.[39] Most experience with this agent in pregnancy is with CML, when hydroxyurea has been used for prolonged periods. However, because teratogenicity is reported in animals, first-trimester use of hydroxyurea should ideally be avoided. The safety profile is good in the second and third trimesters. Interferon-alfa has been used successfully throughout pregnancy in patients with essential thrombocythemia, without adverse effects.[42,43] More data are needed on the safety of interferon-alfa in pregnancy, but reported experience is encouraging.[42,43] It may emerge as the agent of choice if treatment of essential thrombocythemia is necessary in a pregnant woman.

Similarly, data on the safety of anagrelide, a new agent used to treat essential thrombocythemia, are limited. This agent should currently be avoided in pregnancy, and alternative methods should be used to control the platelet count, when necessary.

Because data are inconsistent, increased fetal surveillance during pregnancy is appropriate, particularly if assessment of growth and umbilical artery Doppler recordings show intrauterine growth restriction and placental dysfunction.

Platelet dysfunction may lead to an increased risk of primary and secondary postpartum hemorrhage. Secondary hemorrhage is exacerbated by the risk of retained placental fragments from an infarcted placenta. Thrombosis prophylaxis in the puerperium should include compression stockings and early mobilization. Patients with uncontrolled platelet count or a previous history of thrombosis should be treated with low-molecular-weight heparin or equivalent according to unit protocol.

Polycythemia

Polycythemia occurs when hemoglobin, hematocrit, and the red cell mass are increased above the upper limit of normal for the patient's age and sex. Polycythemia may be relative or true. Relative, or stress, polycythemia occurs when plasma volume is reduced with no increase in the red cell mass. In true polycythemia, the red cell mass is greater than 32 mL/kg for women and 36 mL/kg for men. True polycythemia may be primary or secondary. Secondary polycythemia occurs in conditions associated with either chronic hypoxia or inappropriate erythropoietin production (e.g., renal cysts or tumors). Primary proliferative polycythemia, or polycythemia vera (PV), is characterized by proliferation of erythroid precursors in the bone marrow arising as a result of a clonal stem cell defect. Understanding of the pathogenesis of PV has been revolutionized by the demonstration of the JAK 2 mutation in approximately 95% of cases. PV is usually seen in older patients, but rare cases are described in women of childbearing age.[44]

The diagnosis of polycythemia is difficult during pregnancy because physiologic changes in plasma volume may decrease hemoglobin and hematocrit.[62] Further, isotopic techniques used to determine the red cell mass are contraindicated in pregnancy. However JAK 2 testing by molecular methods may now be used to diagnose PV with features such as splenomegaly, increased white cell, and platelet counts supporting the diagnosis. However, definitive testing and diagnosis may need to be postponed until after delivery. In women who have a high hematocrit in pregnancy, secondary causes should be excluded, particularly pulmonary disease leading to chronic hypoxia. Other causes such as renal tumor are much less likely to present in this way. If erythropoietin levels are available, a low level suggests primary rather than secondary polycythemia. However, erythropoietin levels increase physiologically during pregnancy,[45] and a normal or high level is difficult to interpret.

Preeclampsia and intrauterine growth restriction can be the result of failure of normal plasma volume expansion. In these conditions, the hematocrit may be relatively increased compared with levels in normal pregnancy, but an increase above the normal range in nonpregnant women usually does not occur.

Maternal and Fetal Risks

In a series of 13 pregnancies in 8 women with PV maternal outcome was good, but fetal outcome was adversely affected. Miscarriage, intra-uterine growth restriction, preterm delivery, and stillbirth were more common than expected.[44] The risk of pre-eclampsia may also be increased. A relationship between pregnancy outcome and maternal red cell count was suggested, but the numbers in this study were too small to allow firm conclusions to be drawn. In some patients, hematocrit values decreased significantly during pregnancy.

Management Options

Venesection may be performed to maintain the hematocrit below 0.45. Myelosuppressive therapy should be avoided but may be necessary in patients with associated marked thrombocytosis. Management principles are similar to those outlined for essential thrombocythemia. Thrombosis prophylaxis in the puerperium should include compression stockings and early mobilization. Peripartum treatment with subcutaneous low-molecular-weight heparin should be considered even in the absence of a previous history of thrombosis, although there are no data specific to this patient group.

SUMMARY OF MANAGEMENT OPTIONS

Myeloproliferative Disorders

Management Options	Evidence Quality and Recommendation	References
Essential Thrombocythemia		
Prenatal		
Provide expectant approach in asymptomatic patients with moderate elevation of platelets.	III/B	56–58
If the patient is symptomatic (thrombosis or bleeding), consider plateletpheresis.	III/B	55
Give low-dose aspirin if the patient has thrombosis; no evidence supports use in all cases.	III/B	56,57
Hydroxyurea has been used, but most experience is with chronic myeloid leukemia.	III/B	56
Limited experience with interferon-alfa.	III/B	59,60
Limited experience with anagrelide thus avoid.	—/GPP	—
Obtain serial fetal growth and umbilical artery Doppler recordings.	—/GPP	—
Labor and Delivery and Postnatal		
Maintain vigilance for PPH. Consider prophylactic low-molecular-weight heparin.	—/GPP	—
Polycythemia		
Prenatal		
Maintain vigilance for hypertensive disease.	III/B	61
Obtain serial fetal growth and umbilical artery Doppler recordings.	III/B	61
Some advocate regular venesection to keep hematocrit < 0.45.	IV/C	61
Labor and Delivery and Postnatal		
Maintain vigilance for PPH. Consider prophylactic low-molecular-weight heparin.	—/GPP	—

GPP, good practice point; PPH, primary postpartum hemorrhage.

SUGGESTED READINGS

Ali R, Ozkalemkas F, Kimya Y, et al: Imatinib use during pregnancy and breast feeding: A case report and review of the literature. Arch Gynecol Obstet 2009;280:169–175.

Aviles A, Diaz-Maqueo JC, Talavera A, et al: Growth and development of children of mothers treated with chemotherapy during pregnancy: Current status of 43 children. Am J Hematol 1991;6:234–248.

Aviles A, Neri N: Haematological malignancies and pregnancy: A final report of 84 children who received chemotherapy in utero. Clin Lymphoma 2001;2:173–177.

Beressi AH, Tefferi A, Silverstein MN, et al: Outcome analysis of 34 pregnancies in women with essential thrombocythemia. Arch Intern Med 1995;155:1217–1222.

Byrne J, Rasmussen SA, Steinhorn SC, et al: Genetic disease in offspring of long-term survivors of childhood and adolescent cancer. Am J Hum Genet 1998;62:45–52.

Chelqhoum Y, Vey N, Raffoux E, et al: Acute leukemia in pregnancy. A report of 37 patients and review of the literature. Cancer 2005;104:110–117.

Friedrichs B, Tiemann M, Salwender H, et al: The effects of rituximab treatment during pregnancy on a neonate. Haematologica 2006;91:1426–1427.

Green DM, Whitton JA, Stovall M, et al: Pregnancy outcome of female survivors of childhood cancer: A report from the Childhood Cancer Survivor Study. Am J Obstet Gynecol 2002;187:1070–1080.

Nicklas AH, Baker ME: Imaging strategies in the pregnant cancer patient. Semin Oncol 2000;27:623–632.

REFERENCES

For a complete list of references, log onto www.expertconsult.com.

CHAPTER 40

Thrombocytopenia and Bleeding Disorders

ELIZABETH HELEN HORN and LUCY H. KEAN

THROMBOCYTOPENIA

Introduction

The normal range for peripheral blood platelet count in nonpregnant individuals is generally reported as 150 to 400 $\times 10^9$/L. If a low platelet count is seen on an automated complete blood count, spurious thrombocytopenia should be excluded. This phenomenon may occur because of a small clot in the blood sample or because of platelet clumping caused by the addition of the anticoagulant ethylenediaminetetraacetic acid (EDTA) to the sample. A repeat count for confirmation and examination of the peripheral blood film can ascertain whether the thrombocytopenia is genuine. If the blood film shows platelet clumps, a repeat complete blood count in a sample anticoagulated with citrate may resolve the problem.

Studies of platelet counts during normal pregnancy differed in their conclusions, with some suggesting no overall effect of pregnancy on platelet count[1–3] and others showing a modest reduction in late pregnancy.[4–6] One study of platelet counts in 6715 consecutive patients delivering in a single Canadian center showed that thrombocytopenia (platelet count < 150 $\times 10^9$/L) occurred in 7.6% of women, and most (65.1%) had no associated pathology.[7] From a practical point of view, any pregnant woman with a platelet count of less than 100 $\times 10^9$/L in pregnancy should undergo further clinical and laboratory assessment. All pregnant women with a platelet count less than 150 $\times 10^9$/L after 20 weeks' gestation should have blood pressure and urinalysis checked. In the absence of hypertension or proteinuria, no pathology is found in most women with mild thrombocytopenia at this stage of pregnancy.[8]

Causes of Thrombocytopenia in Pregnancy

Causes of thrombocytopenia in pregnancy are summarized in Table 40–1. They can be broadly divided into the following categories:

- Platelet destruction or consumption.
- Splenic sequestration of platelets.
- Failure of platelet production in the bone marrow.

Platelet destruction or consumption is much more common than bone marrow failure in obstetric practice. Causes with management implications in pregnancy are discussed in detail.

Investigation of Thrombocytopenia in Pregnancy

As discussed earlier, spurious thrombocytopenia should first be excluded. In assessing pregnant women with genuine thrombocytopenia, close liaison is required between the obstetrician and the hematologist. Clinical assessment and examination of the blood film are the starting points in making a diagnosis. Documentation of previous platelet counts and the timing of development of thrombocytopenia are helpful.

For patients developing thrombocytopenia after 20 weeks' gestation, particular attention should be paid to blood pressure and urinalysis for protein. Renal and liver function should be assessed and the presence of any major obstetric complications such as HELLP (hemolysis, elevated liver enzymes, and low platelets) syndrome or acute fatty liver of pregnancy should be rapidly excluded. The peripheral blood film should be examined for red cell fragmentation, the presence of which suggests HELLP syndrome or another thrombotic microangiopathy. For the remainder of those patients who have developed mild thrombocytopenia after 20 weeks' gestation and who are clinically well and without abnormalities in the peripheral blood film, gestational thrombocytopenia is the likely diagnosis.[9]

More detailed clinical and laboratory assessment are required if the platelet count is less than 70 $\times 10^9$/L, if the blood film is abnormal, if thrombocytopenia occurs before 20 weeks' gestation, or if there is a previous history of thrombocytopenia or bleeding. In such patients who have a normal blood film, autoimmune thrombocytopenia (AITP) is the most likely diagnosis and is a diagnosis of exclusion[9]

In the history, the presence of current or previous bleeding problems should be noted. The clinical severity of any hemorrhagic problems should be assessed. Other medical or obstetric problems, a drug and alcohol history, and a recent transfusion history should be noted. For example, a history of recurrent miscarriage may suggest antiphospholipid syndrome. Risk factors for HIV and hepatitis B or C virus

TABLE 40–1

Causes of Thrombocytopenia in Pregnancy

Platelet Consumption or Destruction
Gestational thrombocytopenia
Autoimmune thrombocytopenia
Primary
Secondary
Antiphospholipid syndrome
Systemic lupus erythematosus and connective tissue disorders
Drug-induced
HIV-associated
Other viral infection (e.g., Epstein-Barr virus)
Lymphoproliferative disorder
Nonimmune
Disseminated intravascular coagulation
Preeclampsia or HELLP syndrome
Thrombotic thrombocytopenia purpura or hemolytic uremic syndrome
Acute fatty liver of pregnancy
Large vascular malformations
Heparin-induced thrombocytopenia (rare in pregnancy)
Splenic Sequestration
Splenomegaly
Portal hypertension
Liver disease
Portal or hepatic vein thrombosis
Myeloproliferative disorders
Lymphoproliferative disorders
Storage disease (e.g., Gaucher's disease)
Infection (e.g., tropical splenomegaly or malaria)
Failure of Platelet Production
Bone marrow suppression
Drug-induced
Aplastic anemia
Paroxysmal nocturnal hemoglobinuria
Infection (e.g., parvovirus B19)
Bone marrow infiltration
Hematologic malignancy
Nonhematologic malignancy
Severe vitamin B_{12} or folate deficiency

HELLP, hemolysis, elevated liver enzymes, and low platelets.

(HCV) should be assessed. Enquiry should be made regarding a family history of hemorrhagic problems.

On examination, important features include petechiae and signs of mucosal bleeding. The clinician should look for clinical features that suggest underlying autoimmune disease or chronic liver disease and should exclude splenomegaly.

Careful examination of the blood film is mandatory because it may give important clues to the diagnosis. For example, red cell fragmentation narrows the differential diagnosis to thrombotic microangiopathies (discussed later) (Table 40–2). Hypersegmented neutrophils and oval macrocytes suggest folate deficiency, and other red and white cell abnormalities may suggest underlying bone marrow disease. In gestational thrombocytopenia and AITP, the blood film is normal except for the apparent reduction in platelet count. Renal and liver function should be routinely checked.

After initial assessment, further tests may be indicated, including antinuclear factor, specific tests for lupus anticoagulant and anticardiolipin antibodies, or tests for the diagnosis and typing of von Willebrand's disease (vWD). The lactate dehydrogenase level is usually elevated in microangiopathic hemolysis. The results of coagulation screening tests and D-dimer may be abnormal in thrombocytopenia associated with consumptive coagulopathy. The serum urate level may be increased in preeclampsia, HELLP syndrome, or acute fatty liver of pregnancy. Bone marrow examination is necessary only when features suggest underlying bone marrow disease. However, bone marrow examination should be carried out in AITP if the patient fails to respond to first-line therapy.[8]

Platelet antibody testing is of little value both diagnostically and prognostically in suspected cases of AITP.[8,10–12] In cases of suspected thrombotic thrombocytopenic purpura (TTP), some specialized laboratories carry out assays of ADAMTS 13 activity. ADAMTS 13 (discussed later) is a plasma von Willebrand's factor (vWf)–cleaving protease whose activity is reduced in most cases of primary idiopathic TTP.[13]

Gestational Thrombocytopenia

Gestational thrombocytopenia, or incidental thrombocytopenia of pregnancy, accounts for approximately 70% of cases of maternal thrombocytopenia at delivery.[7,14] The cause is unknown. There is evidence of a degree of physiologic platelet activation in vivo during pregnancy; platelet life span is reduced, and the site of platelet activation is believed to be the placental circulation.[15,16] These mechanisms and hemodilution may contribute to gestational thrombocytopenia.[9]

Gestational thrombocytopenia usually develops in the third trimester and is usually mild to moderate. Results of other studies are normal. The platelet count is usually greater than 80×10^9/L, but counts of 40 to 50×10^9/L can occasionally occur due to gestational thrombocytopenia.[7,17,18] The platelet count rapidly returns to normal after delivery, usually within 7 days.[7,17] Gestational thrombocytopenia is a diagnosis of exclusion. Antenatally, it can be difficult to distinguish from mild AITP. The diagnosis is suggested by a late decrease in platelet count in a patient with no history of previous thrombocytopenia outside of pregnancy. One group of investigators attempted to define predictors of AITP versus gestational thrombocytopenia in pregnancy. They reported that the detection of thrombocytopenia before 28 weeks' gestation and a platelet count less than 50×10^9/L were independently predictive of AITP.[19] Certainty often rests on observations of platelet counts in the puerperium.

Maternal and Fetal Risks

Gestational thrombocytopenia has no pathologic significance for the mother or fetus.[7,8,14,17,18,20] If AITP cannot be excluded, a potential concern is the transfer of antiplatelet antibodies across the placenta, leading to fetal and neonatal thrombocytopenia. However, neonatal thrombocytopenia is uncommon in women in whom thrombocytopenia is

TABLE 40–2

Variation in the Features and Management of Thrombotic Microangiopathic Hemolytic Anemia

DIAGNOSIS	TTP	POSTPARTUM HEMOLYTIC UREMIC SYNDROME	HELLP SYNDROME	PREECLAMPSIA OR ECLAMPSIA
Time of onset	Usually < 24 wk	Postpartum	After 20 wk, most > 34 wk	After 20 wk, most > 34 wk
Hemolysis	+++	++	++	+
Thrombocytopenia	+++	++	++	++
Coagulopathy	-	-	±	±
CNS symptoms	+++	±	±	±
Liver disease	±	±	+++	±
Renal disease	±	+++	+	+
Hypertension	Rare	±	±	+++
Effect on fetus	Placental infarct can lead to IUGR and mortality	None, if maternal disease is controlled	Placental ischemia/increased neonatal mortality	IUGR; occasional mortality
Effect of delivery	None	None	Recovery	Recovery
Management	PEX	Supportive (±PEX)	Supportive/steroids (±PEX)	Supportive

CNS, central nervous system; HELLP, hemolysis, elevated liver enzymes, and low platelets; IUGR, intrauterine growth restriction; PEX, plasma exchange; TTP, thrombotic thrombocytopenic purpura.

incidentally detected in pregnancy and in whom there is no history of AITP. The incidence of neonatal thrombocytopenia in these patients is approximately 4%,[18,21] which is not statistically different from the incidence of thrombocytopenia in infants of nonthrombocytopenic mothers. Further, no infants in these studies had cord platelet counts less than 50 $\times$ 10^9/L, and none had clinical hemostatic impairment.[18,21]

Management Options

PREPREGNANCY AND PRENATAL

If a woman with previous gestational thrombocytopenia seeks prepregnancy counseling, the most important issue is the exclusion of alternative diagnoses. This is also the case when thrombocytopenia is detected incidentally in the antenatal period. The maternal platelet count should be monitored at a frequency determined by the platelet count, rate of decline, and expected date of delivery.[8] No treatment is necessary for gestational thrombocytopenia. Invasive approaches to fetal monitoring, such as fetal blood sampling to determine the fetal platelet count, are not indicated because the risks are not justifiable (discussed later).[8,20]

LABOR AND DELIVERY

Because the fetus is not at risk for hemorrhage, the mode of delivery is determined by obstetric considerations, and invasive fetal blood sampling to determine the fetal platelet count is not indicated. Although there is no evidence that gestational thrombocytopenia is associated with a risk of maternal bleeding, most anesthetists would not contemplate the use of regional analgesia if the platelet count was below 80 $\times$ 10^9/L.[8] If AITP has not been excluded, management options for labor and delivery are the same as those for AITP.[8]

POSTNATAL

If it is difficult to distinguish between gestational thrombocytopenia and AITP, management of the infant should be the same as in maternal AITP (discussed later). Maternal platelet counts should also be followed postnatally. A rapid return to normal confirms the diagnosis of gestational thrombocytopenia, whereas continued thrombocytopenia after pregnancy should prompt reassessment of the patient.

Autoimmune Thrombocytopenia

AITP is relatively common in women of childbearing age. AITP occurs in approximately 0.14% of pregnant women at delivery and accounts for 3% of cases of thrombocytopenia at that time.[17] AITP is the most common cause of thrombocytopenia in the first trimester of pregnancy.[9]

AITP is caused by autoantibodies, which are usually directed against platelet surface glycoproteins, particularly glycoprotein IIb/IIIa and glycoprotein Ib/IX.[22,23] These antibodies adhere to the platelet membrane, causing platelet destruction through Fc receptors in the reticuloendothelial system. The major site of platelet destruction is usually the spleen. AITP may cause purpura and self-limiting mucosal bleeding. This pattern of acute AITP, often after a viral infection, is most commonly seen in children. Conversely, AITP in adults is usually chronic. The symptoms are variable and often insidious. Although fluctuations in the platelet count may occur, the condition is not self-limiting, and continuing thrombocytopenia is the usual course. Chronic AITP may be asymptomatic and may be found by routine testing, such as the testing that is performed during pregnancy.

AITP may be primary or idiopathic or may be secondary to another disorder (see Table 40–1). In primary AITP, if the thrombocytopenia is severe, the clinical examination may show purpura, bruising, or signs of mucosal bleeding, but findings are otherwise normal. Other than a reduced platelet count, findings on the blood film are normal, and the bone marrow is normal, with normal or increased numbers of megakaryocytes. As noted previously, bone marrow examination is no longer routinely recommended in AITP. In primary or idiopathic AITP, all other test results are normal. Secondary causes of AITP may be associated with antinuclear antibodies or increased levels of antiphospholipid antibodies. HIV and HCV testing should be offered in all cases.

Neither assays of platelet-associated immunoglobulin G (IgG) nor assays of glycoprotein-specific antibodies are reliable as diagnostic tools in suspected AITP.[23] Further, no assay of platelet antibodies has predictive value for maternal or fetal outcome.[8,10–12]

Maternal Risks

The risk of maternal bleeding has generally been thought to relate to the severity of thrombocytopenia. In AITP, clinical bleeding is often less severe for a given platelet count than in conditions in which thrombocytopenia is caused by an underlying bone marrow disorder.

Women with severe thrombocytopenia (platelet count $< 20 \times 10^9/L$) are at risk for spontaneous bleeding antenatally as well as at delivery, and they generally require treatment. Women with platelet counts less than $50 \times 10^9/L$ may be at risk for increased bleeding at delivery[8,24,25]; therefore, treatment may be required in late pregnancy to ensure a safe platelet count for delivery in asymptomatic women. Both British[8] and American[24] guidelines suggest that a platelet count greater than $50 \times 10^9/L$ is safe for a vaginal delivery. British guidelines suggest aiming for a platelet count above $80 \times 10^9/L$ for cesarean section,[8] whereas American guidelines considered a platelet count greater than $50 \times 10^9/L$ was suitable for all modes of delivery.[24] A platelet count of greater than $80 \times 10^9/L$ is recommended for epidural anesthesia by the British Committee for Standards in Haematology (BCSH).[8] These figures are generally accepted by clinicians but are somewhat arbitrary.

A retrospective series of 119 pregnancies in 92 women with AITP reported a 21% incidence of bleeding in pregnancy. Bleeding was uncommon at delivery and was not correlated with the platelet count, even although 15% of women had a platelet count less than $50 \times 10^9/L$.[26] Another observational series showed that bleeding at delivery was increased in women with platelet counts less than $50 \times 10^9/L$ who underwent cesarean section but not vaginal delivery.[25,27] There is no evidence that bleeding time is helpful in predicting hemorrhagic problems in AITP.

Fetal Risks

In mothers with AITP, IgG antiplatelet antibodies may cross the placenta and cause fetal thrombocytopenia, resulting in fetal or neonatal bleeding. Maternal findings, such as platelet count and platelet-associated IgG level, are of no value in predicting fetal thrombocytopenia.[11,28,29] It has been suggested that the only clear predictor of neonatal thrombocytopenia in pregnant women with thrombocytopenia is a history of AITP, and even then, the incidence of neonatal bleeding is low (<2%).[18] Limited data suggest that in women with AITP, the outcome of a previous pregnancy with respect to neonatal thrombocytopenia is a reasonable guide to the likely outcome of a current pregnancy, if there have been no significant changes in the course or management of AITP in the mother.[10,30]

In the early 1990s, large prospective studies helped to clarify that in maternal AITP, the risk to the fetus and neonate of bleeding as a result of thrombocytopenia is extremely low. In these and subsequent studies, the overall incidence of fetal or neonatal thrombocytopenia was 10% to 30%, but severe thrombocytopenia was less common and intracranial hemorrhage was rare.[10,14,18,29] The largest study,[14] which was conducted over 7 years and included more than 15,000 mothers and infants, showed that among 46 mothers with AITP, 4 (8.7%) neonates had cord platelet counts of 20 to $50 \times 10^9/L$. No infant whose mother had AITP had a platelet count of less than $20 \times 10^9/L$, and none had an adverse outcome. In 3 of the 4 cases, delivery was vaginal.[14] In this study, all of the neonates with clinically severe bleeding had alloimmune thrombocytopenia (see Chapter 15). Another study showed that 18 of 88 neonates (20%) born to women with AITP before the index pregnancy had platelet counts of less than $50 \times 10^9/L$. Five had clinically important bleeding, and 2 of these had intracranial hemorrhage.[18] Other studies confirm an approximate 20% incidence of neonatal thrombocytopenia in infants of mothers with AITP,[26,27] and that major neonatal bleeding, including intracranial hemorrhage is uncommon.

Another salient point is the time course of thrombocytopenia and bleeding complications in the fetus and neonate in a pregnancy affected by AITP. Bleeding in utero in maternal AITP is rare.[31] Other studies concluded that after birth, the platelet count continues to decrease in affected neonates, reaching a nadir 2 to 5 days after delivery.[11]

Management Options

PREPREGNANCY

In general, pregnancy does not affect the clinical course of AITP; however, there is anecdotal evidence of worsening of AITP during pregnancy, with improvement after delivery.[32]

In women known to have AITP before pregnancy, therapy should be optimized before pregnancy is planned. The advent of several new treatments for AITP has opened up more management options, but management for most patients continues to be with well-established treatments. Most treatment in AITP is aimed at reducing immune destruction of platelets. Steroids or intravenous immunoglobulin (IVIG) is the usual initial treatment, but neither is curative.[33,34] Splenectomy is the most commonly used second-line treatment in patients who continue to have clinical symptoms following treatment with steroids. Sixty-six percent of patients have a complete remission following splenectomy,[34] which is durable in the majority. A proportion of others have a very useful partial response.[33] In patients with chronic AITP, decisions about splenectomy are best made before the patient becomes pregnant.

More recently, anti-D immunoglobulin has been used as first- or second-line treatment (as an alternative to IVIG) in patients who are RhD-positive. Its efficacy is limited to patients who have not been splenectomized.[33] The mechanism of action is thought to be via preferential removal of antibody-coated red cells via the reticuloendothelial system. Patients who respond to anti-D may be given maintenance treatment, which may be limited by anemia. Treatment with anti-D may postpone the need for splenectomy, but this treatment is unlikely to lead to long-term remission.[34]

A small number of women of childbearing age have refractory AITP. A wide range of treatments have been used in refractory AITP, most of which act as immunosuppressants.[33,34] These include azathioprine, cyclosporine, mycophenolate mofetil, danazol, cyclophosphamide, vinca alkaloids, and more recently, an anti-CD20 monoclonal antibody (rituximab).[35,36]

There are no randomized, controlled trials of any of these agents in refractory AITP. The evidence for their use comes from case series. Many patients with refractory AITP have been treated with the anti-CD20 monoclonal antibody, and it is generally well tolerated. Case series data suggest rates of response of 40% to 50%.[35,36] Sustained responses have been reported, and treatment may be successfully repeated if relapse occurs in previous responders.[37,38] Adverse effects include anaphylactoid reactions, serum sickness, infections and rarely, progressive multifocal leucoencephalopathy.[36,39] There has been debate about whether this treatment may be used as second-line therapy as an alternative to splenectomy.[38] It is not yet recommended that this should be routine practice, but second-line use of anti-CD20 antibodies is acceptable in patients who decline splenectomy or who are unfit for surgery. A further important advance in the treatment of AITP has been made. Thrombopoietin receptor agonists have been shown in randomized, controlled trials to be effective in increasing the platelet count in patients with refractory AITP.[40] One of these agents (eltrombopag) has been granted a limited license for treatment of AITP by the U.S. Food and Drug Administration (FDA). The platelet count falls when the drug is stopped. The future use of these agents is, therefore, likely to be confined to situations in which the platelet count needs to be temporarily increased (e.g., for surgery) or for symptomatic patients refractory to other treatments.

Many third-line agents used for the treatment of AITP should be avoided in pregnancy, and women of childbearing age requiring such treatment should generally be advised to use effective contraception. Until recently, azathioprine was the most commonly used third-line agent for women with AITP who wished to become pregnant. There is considerable experience of the safe use of azathioprine in pregnancy in clinical settings other than AITP.[41,42] In more recent years, many clinicians prefer to attempt to induce a response in AITP with the anti-CD20 monoclonal antibody rituximab, given as a course of four treatments at weekly intervals.[34,36] There are reports of successful outcome of pregnancy following antenatal administration of this treatment.[43,44] It would be preferable, however, to use this agent in advance of pregnancy, to advise contraception at the time of use, and also to allow time to assess the response. There are as yet no safety data for thrombopoietin (TPO) agonists in pregnancy; these agents should, therefore, be avoided in women planning pregnancy.

In summary, the aim of prepregnancy management of symptomatic AITP is to achieve a sustained improvement in platelet count in order to reduce hemorrhagic risk, using the least-toxic therapies.

The potential hazards of AITP and its treatment in pregnancy must be individually assessed, and patients should be counseled carefully. Prepregnancy counseling should cover the risk of bleeding for the mother and fetus and the risks of various treatment options in pregnancy. For very few women with severe refractory AITP, pregnancy may be hazardous and should be avoided.

PRENATAL

In the prenatal period, the aims of management are

- To treat maternal symptoms of hemorrhage at any stage of pregnancy.
- To achieve a safe platelet count for delivery.

There is no evidence that any available modalities of treatment administered to the mother affect the platelet count in the fetus or neonate.[25] The frequency of monitoring of platelet counts should be based on the initial count and the rate of any decline. Closer surveillance is required in the last trimester to ensure a safe count for delivery. Treatment is generally required in symptomatic patients if the maternal platelet count is less than $20 \times 10^9/L$.[8,25] Treatment is also often given in late pregnancy, in the absence of symptoms, to raise the platelet count to $50 \times 10^9/L$ or more for delivery.[8,24,25]

Principal options for the treatment of AITP in pregnancy include corticosteroids and high-dose IVIG. Conventionally, steroids are used by many as the first-line treatment. When steroid therapy is chosen, prednisolone is usually given initially at a dose of 1 mg/kg daily (based on nonpregnant body weight). A response is obtained in most patients, allowing the dose to be tapered gradually to achieve the minimum dose at which a safe platelet count is achieved. Potential disadvantages of steroid therapy during pregnancy are the precipitation or exacerbation of hypertension, excessive weight gain, gestational diabetes, osteoporosis, and psychiatric disorders.[8,24,25] These considerations are particularly relevant when prolonged therapy is required and when high doses are needed to control symptoms. From the fetal point of view, corticosteroids are not teratogenic. Fetal adrenal suppression is unlikely because prednisolone is extensively metabolized in the placenta.[45]

Concerns about potential adverse maternal effects of steroids have led some to use IVIG as first-line therapy in pregnancy.[17,24,25] Others reserve this treatment for patients who do not respond to steroids and for those in whom the maintenance dose of steroids is unacceptably high. IVIG is usually given in doses of 1 g/kg daily for 1 or 2 days.

This regimen increases the platelet count in most cases, but the response to immunoglobulin is temporary in adult AITP. On average, responses are seen by the fifth day of infusion, with a peak response occurring approximately 4 to 5 days after the end of the infusion.[46] Responses tend to be sustained for only 2 to 4 weeks,[24] but the duration of response is extremely variable.[46] When IVIG is used to increase the platelet count before delivery, treatment is initiated approximately 7 to 10 days before delivery is planned. In mothers who need treatment for symptomatic AITP, courses of IVIG may be repeated at intervals to prevent symptoms and ensure a safe platelet count for delivery. One study outside the context of pregnancy showed that approximately one third of patients who require repeated infusions eventually stop responding to immunoglobulin.[47]

IVIG is a pooled blood product. IVIG preparations that have been virally inactivated have an excellent safety record, but the risk of transfusion-transmitted infection cannot be completely excluded.[8,48]

Other adverse effects include allergic reactions, and occasional cases of anaphylaxis have occurred in IgA-deficient patients. Aseptic meningitis is well documented, and there are a few reports of thrombotic complications, mainly in elderly patients.[48] Renal failure may be precipitated by IVIG preparations with a high sucrose content.[49] IVIG is well tolerated in most patients. Other adverse effects tend to be mild.[48]

The placenta contains Fc receptors; therefore, immunoglobulins can cross the placenta. This finding led to hopes that maternal treatment with high-dose IVIG would improve the fetal platelet count.[50,51] There are no controlled studies, but fetal and neonatal thrombocytopenia have been reported following maternal use of IVIG.[48] Evidence does not show a substantial effect of IVIG on fetal platelet counts in maternal AITP, in contrast to fetal alloimmune thrombocytopenia, in which treatment with IVIG is now the first-line management for maintenance of fetal platelet counts.

Patients with severe hemorrhage associated with profound thrombocytopenia require aggressive management. Although platelet transfusion has little efficacy prophylactically in AITP, platelets should be administered in large doses to patients with life-threatening bleeding.[8] Options for further management in severely hemorrhagic patients include intravenous methylprednisolone and IVIG.[8,24] IVIG was shown in one study to be more effective than methylprednisolone in leading to a rapid increase in platelet count in recently diagnosed AITP.[52]

If a pregnant woman with AITP does not respond to standard treatment with steroids and IVIG, decisions about further therapy must be considered. Factors such as gestation and hemorrhagic symptoms should be taken into account. If the woman is not hemorrhagic, an observant approach is the best option. Platelet transfusion may be required at delivery, even if the patient is asymptomatic prenatally. If the patient is hemorrhagic antenatally, several options are available, but supporting evidence is anecdotal. Splenectomy may be carried out in pregnancy, preferably in the second trimester.[53] Splenectomy is commonly performed laparoscopically in nonpregnant patients. In pregnancy, the laparoscopic approach is also preferable and is technically feasible up to 20 weeks.[54] The enlarging uterus, however, may cause difficulties with laparoscopic splenectomy after 20 weeks' gestation. Conventional splenectomy in the third trimester may precipitate premature labor, but in some cases, when the fetus is mature, splenectomy may be combined with cesarean delivery in late pregnancy.[53] Approximately two thirds of patients have a useful response to splenectomy. Prophylaxis against infections with organisms such as pneumococci, *Haemophilus*, and *Neisseria meningitidis* is necessary. When splenectomy is performed during pregnancy, penicillin V prophylaxis should be given in the prenatal period, and vaccination against these organisms should be performed postnatally.

Many of the other therapies discussed in the "Prepregnancy" section ealier are contraindicated in pregnancy. Azathioprine is probably the treatment with most experience in pregnancy. Use in renal transplant recipients suggests that teratogenicity is rare in humans, but intrauterine growth restriction may occur.[41,42]

Anecdotal reports exist of successful use of anti-D[55] and of rituximab in pregnancy.[43,44,56,57] Anti-D was associated with a positive direct antiglobulin test in some neonates, none of whom was anemic or jaundiced.[55] Rituximab crossed the placenta and was associated with a temporary reduction in numbers of B cells in the neonate, but no clinical consequences apparently resulted.[43] Until further studies are available, use of these agents in pregnancy should be restricted to refractory cases in which alternatives are unsuitable or have failed.

Collaboration with an obstetric anesthetist in the third trimester is necessary for all women with platelet counts low enough to affect management of delivery. Regional analgesia is usually ruled out for women with a platelet count below 80×10^9/L.[8,24,25] Alternatives to regional analgesia, such as patient-controlled analgesia, can be offered when epidural analgesia is considered unsafe.

LABOR AND DELIVERY

From the maternal point of view, when possible, vaginal delivery is preferred in mothers affected by AITP.[8,25] If the maternal platelet count remains low at the time of delivery, despite optimal antenatal treatment, and hemorrhagic complications result, platelet transfusion may be required to treat maternal bleeding. Platelets should be available for women who have a platelet count less than 50×10^9/L at delivery, but platelet transfusion given for purely prophylactic reasons is unnecessary and ineffective. For women who have experienced hemorrhage around the time of delivery, the administration of IVIG should be considered with the aim of rapidly improving the platelet count over the next few days to minimize risk of primary postpartum hemorrhage (PPH).

Epidural anesthesia should be avoided if the platelet count is less than 80×10^9/L,[8] although there is little concrete supporting evidence.

Thrombocytopenic women are at risk of bleeding from surgical incisions. Judicious administration of platelets during operative procedures is reasonable in women with severe thrombocytopenia.[24] As discussed earlier, large, well-conducted studies show that the risk to the fetus and neonate of bleeding as a result of thrombocytopenia is low in maternal AITP.[14,18] No maternal findings are of value in predicting fetal thrombocytopenia. There is no role for measuring fetal platelet count in late pregnancy or during labor. Fetal scalp sampling is often inaccurate and can cause significant scalp bleeding or hematoma formation in thrombocytopenic fetuses. Intrauterine fetal blood sampling cannot be justified as a routine practice in maternal AITP because the associated risks outweigh the risk of serious fetal hemorrhage.[8,10]

In AITP, it was previously assumed that cesarean section may protect the fetus from bleeding as a result of head trauma. However, no difference was seen between vaginal delivery and cesarean section in bleeding complications in 474 infants born to mothers with AITP.[58] Because the nadir of the platelet count often occurs several days after delivery, peripartum events may not have a major effect on neonatal bleeding complications.[59]

The low incidence of neonatal bleeding in modern studies and the data on the mode of delivery and time course of thrombocytopenia support a conservative approach to the management of the fetus in pregnancies complicated by AITP, both antenatally and during labor and delivery. Traumatic delivery, delivery by Ventouse extraction, and the use of midcavity rotational forceps should be avoided. Decisions about cesarean section should be made on obstetric grounds, without determining the fetal platelet count. Most authors recommend avoiding the use of fetal scalp electrodes and scalp blood sampling to determine acid-base status.[8]

POSTNATAL

Mothers with thrombocytopenia are unlikely to bleed from the uterine cavity after the third stage of labor, provided that there are no retained products of conception. However, bleeding may occur from surgical wounds, episiotomies, or perineal tears. Prompt suturing and close observation of these sites are required. Immediately after delivery, a cord blood sample should be taken. If the infant is thrombocytopenic but not hemorrhagic, a complete blood count should be repeated over the next few days because the platelet count often continues to decrease, reaching a nadir between days 2 and 5.[8] If the infant has signs of skin or mucosal bleeding or has severe thrombocytopenia (platelet count $< 20 \times 10^9$/L, or $< 50 \times 10^9$/L in a premature sick neonate), cranial ultrasound should be considered and treatment instituted. IVIG 1 g/kg is the preferred treatment in neonates[8,10] and increases the platelet count in most infants affected by maternal AITP. Platelet transfusion is rarely necessary, but is indicated if bleeding is life-threatening (e.g., intracranial hemorrhage). Products that are known to be cytomegalovirus-negative should be used.[60] Preterm infants with very low birth weight (<1.5 kg) are at greater risk for transfusion-transmitted cytomegalovirus infection than are healthy term infants.

AITP should not exclude women from consideration for peripartum thrombosis prophylaxis. Risk assessment should be carried out and consideration given to constitutional and acquired thrombotic risk factors as well as the risk of bleeding. Prophylactic doses of low-molecular-weight heparin (LMWH) are generally safe if the platelet count is greater than 50×10^9/L.[8] Graduated compression stockings may be used for women who require specific thrombosis prophylaxis if the platelet count is less than 50×10^9/L. Nonsteroidal anti-inflammatory drugs should be avoided for maternal postpartum analgesia.

SUMMARY OF MANAGEMENT OPTIONS
Autoimmune Thrombocytopenia

Management Options	Evidence Quality and Recommendation	References
Prepregnancy		
Optimize management and consider splenectomy.	—/GPP	—
Discuss risks in pregnancy if the patient is refractory to treatment.	—/GPP	—
Prenatal		
Monitor platelet count (frequency determined by initial values).	IV/C	8,24,25
Treat if symptoms occur or platelet count $<20 \times 10^9$/L at any stage in pregnancy.	IV/C	8,24,25
Treat if $<50 \times 10^9$/L in late pregnancy even if the patient is asymptomatic:	IV/C	8,24,25
• Treatment option 1: Prednisolone. Debate whether to use as first-line therapy vs. IVIG.	IV/C (Ib for nonpregnant adults)	8,24,25 34*
• Treatment option 2: High-dose IVIG.	IV/C (Ib for nonpregnant adults)	8,24,25 34*
• Treatment option 3: Splenectomy may be performed in refractory cases in the second trimester or occasionally in the third trimester at the time of cesarean section.	IV/C (III for nonpregnant adults)	54
• Treatment option 4: Rituximab or anti-D. For severe cases unresponsive to steroids/IVIG as an alternative to splenectomy.	IV/C (III for nonpregnant adults)	34–38*, 43,44,55
• Treatment option 5: Azathioprine (slow onset of action) may be used in nonresponsive cases. It is safe in pregnancy but beware of IUGR.	IV/C (III for nonpregnant adults)	34*,41,42
Inform anesthetists and pediatricians of impending delivery.	—/GPP	—

SUMMARY OF MANAGEMENT OPTIONS

Autoimmune Thrombocytopenia—cont'd

Management Options	Evidence Quality and Recommendation	References
Labor and Delivery		
Platelets should be available if count <50 × 10^9/L, but use only if the patient is bleeding.	IV/C	8,24
Avoid epidural if platelet count <80 × 10^9/L.	IV/C	8
Avoid traumatic delivery, fetal scalp electrodes, and fetal blood sampling.	IV/C	8,10
Cesarean delivery has no benefit over vaginal delivery.	IV/C	8,25
Postnatal		
Because of the risk of bleeding, repair perineal trauma promptly.	—/GPP	—
Obtain a cord blood platelet count.	IV/C	8,24,25
Obtain a platelet count daily for a few days if count is initially low (nadir = days 2–5).	IV/C	8,24,25
If neonatal count <20 × 10^9/L or symptoms occur, perform ultrasound scan of brain and treat with IVIG.	IV/C	8,24,25
Administer platelets if bleeding is life-threatening.	IV/C	8,24,25

* Refers to evidence in nonpregnant adults.
GPP, good practice point; IUGR, intrauterine growth restriction; IVIG, intravenous immune globulin.

Special Considerations in Secondary Autoimmune Thrombocytopenia: Risks and Management Options

Antiphospholipid Syndrome (See Chapter 43)

Primary antiphospholipid syndrome (APL) includes the reproducible presence of antiphospholipid antibodies (either lupus anticoagulant or anticardiolipin antibody) and one of the following clinical features: venous thrombosis, arterial thrombosis, and fetal loss (recurrent if <10 weeks' gestation).[61]

Thrombocytopenia is not a diagnosis-defining criterion for antiphospholipid syndrome.[61] However, antiphospholipid antibodies are frequently found in patients with AITP,[62] and 20% to 40% of patients with primary antiphospholipid syndrome are thrombocytopenic.[63] In these cases, thrombocytopenia is autoimmune.[63] Antiphospholipid antibodies are probably not the cause of the immune platelet destruction. In some cases, platelet consumption mediated by antiphospholipid antibody–induced platelet activation may contribute.[62]

Outside the context of pregnancy, responses to the treatment of immune thrombocytopenia are similar in patients with and without antiphospholipid antibodies.[64] There is debate about whether the incidental finding of positive antiphospholipid antibodies in a patient with thrombocytopenia leads to an increased risk of thrombosis.[65,66] A panel of experts in antiphospholipid syndrome have suggested that patients with AITP and antiphospholipid antibodies require closer follow-up, because they may be at risk of future thrombotic events, and that these patients should be regarded as having "associated thrombocytopenia."[61]

Management options during pregnancy are similar to those for primary AITP. However, if the patient meets criteria for a diagnosis of primary antiphospholipid syndrome, there are other implications for pregnancy. In addition to recurrent spontaneous abortion, women with antiphospholipid syndrome are at risk for other complications, such as intrauterine fetal death, intrauterine fetal growth restriction, preeclampsia, and maternal thrombosis.[67–70] The mechanism of fetal loss is complex. Thrombosis in the placental vasculature is a contributory factor, but there is also evidence of inadequate trophoblastic invasion, induced by antiphospholipid antibodies.[71,72]

A combination of low-dose aspirin and prophylactic heparin is helpful in preventing recurrent spontaneous abortions in antiphospholipid syndrome.[73] Moderate thrombocytopenia should not alter decisions about antiplatelet or antithrombotic therapy in antiphospholipid syndrome.[63] In patients who have more marked thrombocytopenia, decisions should be made on an individual basis, taking account of the risks and potential benefits of various management options.

Close maternal supervision and fetal monitoring are required antenatally. Antenatal and postnatal thromboprophylaxis is indicated in women with antiphospholipid syndrome and a history of thrombosis.[74,75] As discussed previously, thrombocytopenia should not necessarily preclude this, and the balance of risks should be assessed individually (see Chapter 43).

Systemic Lupus Erythematosus (See Chapter 43)

Immune platelet destruction may occur in systemic lupus erythematosus (SLE) because of antiplatelet antibodies or immune complexes. Thrombocytopenia is not usually severe, but if treatment is required, patients may respond to immunosuppression used for other manifestations of SLE. Otherwise, management is governed by the principles outlined for primary AITP. Thrombocytopenia has been shown to be associated with an increased likelihood of end-organ damage in SLE.[76] Women with SLE are also at risk for preeclampsia, which may be complicated by thrombocytopenia. Other management issues are discussed in Chapter 43.

HIV-Associated Thrombocytopenia (See Chapter 28)

Thrombocytopenia may be associated with HIV infection. A survey of HIV-positive pregnant women showed that 3.2% were thrombocytopenic, and in most cases, thrombocytopenia was believed to be directly related to HIV infection. Slightly fewer than half of the thrombocytopenic women in this series had platelet counts less than 50×10^9/L, and 20% had hemorrhagic complications. Of 28 infants, only 1 had thrombocytopenia.[77]

Thrombocytopenia associated with HIV is multifactorial. In advanced disease, drugs and infection may lead to marrow dysfunction that results in thrombocytopenia. However, thrombocytopenia is relatively common in otherwise-asymptomatic HIV-positive individuals. Immune platelet destruction by antiplatelet antibodies or immune complexes and the formation of antibodies that cross-react with the HIV virus and platelets are likely mechanisms of thrombocytopenia in these patients.[62,78] Thrombotic thrombocytopenic purpura (TTP; discussed later) may also be associated with HIV.[79]

Suppression of viral replication by antiretroviral therapy increases the platelet count in HIV-positive patients with thrombocytopenia. Combinations of antiretroviral drugs are much more effective at suppressing HIV viral load than is monotherapy, and treatment is usually unaltered in pregnancy.[80] All patients with HIV-associated thrombocytopenia should receive treatment with highly active antiretroviral therapy (HAART).[62,81]

Careful evaluation of trends in platelet counts that correspond to changes in therapy and viral load is helpful in assessing thrombocytopenia in HIV-infected patients. Blood film examination (for red cell fragmentation associated with TTP and other cytopenias that may be associated with disease, infection, or therapy) and bone marrow examination to assess whether thrombocytopenia is caused by peripheral consumption may be useful in selected cases, especially if the platelet count does not improve with HAART.

When immune destruction is believed to be a significant component of thrombocytopenia, and the thrombocytopenia does not respond to HAART, IVIG may be required to treat hemorrhagic symptoms or to increase the platelet count before delivery in thrombocytopenic HIV-positive women.[77] Corticosteroids are also effective in HIV-associated immune thrombocytopenia, but prednisolone is associated with oral candidiasis and reactivation of herpes simplex.[78] Many physicians avoid the use of steroids because of the risk of further immunosuppression and infection. Issues related to the management of labor and delivery in HIV-positive women are covered in Chapter 28.

Thrombocytopenia Associated with Hepatitis C Infection

HCV infection has been reported in 10% to 30% of patients diagnosed clinically as AITP.[62,82] HCV testing should be considered in all patients with apparent AITP, and testing is definitely indicated in those with risk factors for HCV. Immune mechanisms may contribute to the etiology. Thrombocytopenia may respond to steroids in such patients, but steroids have been associated with an increase in transaminases and viral load.[62] Treatment should primarily be directed at the HCV. The thrombocytopenia is likely to respond to anti-HCV treatment. In women of childbearing age, this should be carried out prior to pregnancy and women should be advised to use contraception. IVIG or anti-D may also be helpful if thrombocytopenia remains problematic.[62] Recognition is important because of these differences in management. Furthermore, the knowledge that a woman is HCV polymerase chain reaction (PCR)–positive may influence management options around the time of delivery (see Chapter 27).

Drug-Induced Thrombocytopenia

Drugs may cause thrombocytopenia through immune destruction or through suppression of platelet production in the bone marrow. Both are uncommon in pregnancy, but drug-induced causes should be considered and excluded.

One type of drug-induced thrombocytopenia merits further discussion. Heparin-induced thrombocytopenia (HIT) occurs in 1% to 5% of patients receiving unfractionated heparin (UFH). HIT is caused by an antibody directed against the heparin-platelet factor 4 complex, which can induce platelet activation and aggregation in vivo.[83] The mechanism of thrombocytopenia, therefore, differs from classic immune destruction in the reticuloendothelial system. HIT also differs from many other drug-induced thrombocytopenias because the platelet activation induced in HIT is associated with thrombosis and not with bleeding. Thrombosis in HIT may be venous or arterial and may be life-threatening.[83]

The incidence of HIT in patients treated with LMWH is considerably lower than that in patients treated with UFH.[84] Cross-reactivity of antibodies is common, and low-molecular-weight agents are not suitable once HIT has occurred.[85] HIT has been reported in pregnancy,[86,87] although it is considerably less common in pregnant than in nonpregnant individuals.[88] Fetal thrombocytopenia does not occur because heparin does not cross the placenta.

Heparin should be withdrawn immediately on clinical suspicion of HIT. Laboratory tests are available to confirm the diagnosis. The heparinoid danaparoid may be used as an alternative anticoagulant when HIT is diagnosed.[89] Danaparoid has been used successfully to treat HIT in pregnancy.[87] Hirudin is an alternative in nonpregnant patients, but experience is limited in pregnancy and its use is not recommended unless there is no suitable alternative.[90,91] Ancrod has been used in HIT,[90] but great caution should be used in pregnancy. Platelet transfusion should be avoided in patients with HIT.

Routine monitoring of platelet counts in pregnant women on prophylactic LMWH is no longer required because of the very low incidence of HIT in this situation,[92,93] but regular monitoring of the platelet count is still required in pregnant women receiving UFH.[92,93] BCSH guidelines advise that the platelet count should be monitored in women receiving treatment doses of LMWH, on the grounds that most studies on the incidence of HIT with use of LMWH have included very few pregnant patients on treatment doses.[92] The Royal College of Obstetricians and Gynaecologists venous thromboembolism guidelines recommend that monitoring is not necessary unless a woman has received UFH.[93] Recognition of HIT also remains important, and clinicians should consider HIT as a possible diagnosis in any patient who develops thrombocytopenia, skin reactions around injection sites, or new thrombosis in the first 21 days of therapy with heparin.[92]

Thrombocytopenia with Microangiopathy

Several syndromes are associated with thrombocytopenia as a result of platelet activation, red cell fragmentation, and a variable degree of hemolysis (microangiopathic hemolytic anemia). Some syndromes are unique to obstetric practice. The differential diagnosis is particularly pertinent for obstetricians and is important because management options differ.[94]

The differential diagnosis is summarized in Table 40–2.

DISSEMINATED INTRAVASCULAR COAGULATION RISKS AND MANAGEMENT OPTIONS (See later under "Acquired Coagulation Disorders" and Chapter 77)

Platelet consumption and consequent thrombocytopenia occur as part of the process of disseminated intravascular coagulation (DIC). DIC, particularly if chronic, may also occasionally be associated with microangiopathic features on the blood film. DIC is discussed briefly in the section on "Acquired Coagulation Disorders."

PREECLAMPSIA AND HELLP SYNDROME (See Chapters 35 and 78)

Risks and Management Options

Preeclampsia is a multisystem disorder unique to pregnancy. Its pathophysiologic basis lies in widespread damage to the vascular endothelium.[7] The platelet count decreases as a result of platelet activation.[15] A decrease in the platelet count often precedes clinical signs of disease,[95] but thrombocytopenia is rarely severe, and although there may be evidence of consumptive coagulopathy, severe DIC is unusual.[96] The extent and rate of the decrease in the platelet count indicate the severity of preeclampsia,[97] and together with other aspects of clinical and laboratory assessment, these findings may be used to guide the timing of delivery. HELLP syndrome is thought to be a variant of preeclampsia characterized by microangiopathic hemolysis, elevated liver enzyme levels, and a low platelet count.[98] Work on gene expression in the placenta has shown that there are substantial differences in gene transcripts between placentas from women with preeclampsia and HELLP, suggesting that these may be separate disease entities.[99] Hypertension may be minimal. HELLP syndrome carries a particularly bad prognosis for pregnancy outcome if delivery is postponed, so recognition is important. Platelet transfusion is infrequently required in preeclampsia or HELLP[100] but may be needed if bleeding occurs or if thrombocytopenia is severe and cesarean delivery is planned.[101] In both preeclampsia and HELLP, delivery of the fetus and placenta is the only effective treatment, and delivery results in resolution of hematologic and other features of the condition. Regional analgesia is an option if the maternal platelet count is greater than 80×10^9/L and the results of coagulation screening tests are normal. If severe thrombocytopenia, hemolysis, or organ dysfunction persist after delivery, plasma exchange may be considered,[102] but the diagnosis should also be reviewed. A role for postnatal treatment with steroids in HELLP syndrome has been postulated because initial reports suggested a more rapid resolution in platelet counts.[103] However, this initial enthusiasm has not been confirmed in randomized trials, which have shown no benefit.[104]

THROMBOTIC THROMBOCYTOPENIC PURPURA (See Chapters 41 and 78)

TTP is a rare disorder associated with platelet activation that leads to thrombocytopenia and the formation of platelet thrombi in the microcirculation. The clinical features of TTP consist of a classic pentad of thrombocytopenia, microangiopathic hemolysis, renal impairment, neurologic features, and fever.[105] Many patients do not have all of the features. Results of coagulation screening tests are normal, and D-dimer levels are normal or minimally elevated.[105] TTP may be primary with no clear precipitating factors, secondary to infection (including HIV), drugs, underlying malignancy, or occur after transplant procedures. The pathophysiology of primary idiopathic TTP and secondary TTP are different.[13] TTP is more common in women and can occur in association with pregnancy. A large review of the literature reported that 13% of female patients with TTP were pregnant.[106] The pathophysiology of pregnancy-associated TTP is similar to that of primary idiopathic TTP.[13,106] Chronic relapsing TTP may be congenital.[107]

Severe deficiency of a vWf-cleaving metalloproteinase was recognized in patients with both congenital and primary idiopathic TTP.[108,109] This metalloproteinase is a member of the ADAMTS family (ADAMTS 13)[110] and can cleave ultralarge vWf multimers. The presence of ultralarge vWF multimers, not normally present in plasma, is the likely mechanism promoting formation of platelet microthrombi.[111]

ADAMTS 13 deficiency may be heritable, leading to congenital TTP, or may be caused by an inhibitory autoantibody, leading to primary idiopathic TTP.[13,107,109] Most cases of TTP occurring in pregnancy are due to autoimmune severe ADAMTS 13 deficiency, but congenital TTP may present for the first time or relapse during pregnancy.[106] Severe ADAMTS 13 deficiency is not seen in most cases of secondary TTP.[13,112] Levels of ADAMTS 13 decrease in the second and third trimesters of pregnancy, but do not reach the very low levels seen in severe ADAMTS 13 deficiency associated with TTP.[106,113] Variable reductions in ADAMTS 13 are also seen in hepatic failure and sepsis-induced DIC.[13] Preeclampsia and HELLP syndrome are not associated with ADAMTS 13 deficiency.

The diagnostic role of ADAMTS 13 deficiency in microangiopathic syndromes has been debated, and assays to measure ADAMTS 13 levels are available only in laboratories with a research interest in ADAMTS 13. The diagnosis of TTP does not require the demonstration of ADAMTS 13 deficiency,[107] but these assays may be helpful in cases of diagnostic difficulty, particularly in differentiating other microangiopathies in pregnancy.[114] Plasma exchange therapy (see later) should not be delayed until results of these assays are available.

Studies vary in the reported timing of TTP associated with pregnancy, with some reporting the most common occurrence in the second trimester[114,115] and others report the most common occurrence in late pregnancy or the postpartum period.[106] Preeclampsia/HELLP syndrome usually occurs after 20 weeks in pregnancy, and hemolytic-uremic syndrome (HUS) mainly occurs postnatally.[116]

Maternal and Fetal Risks

Untreated TTP is almost uniformly fatal for the mother and fetus. However, treatment with plasma exchange with fresh frozen plasma (FFP) markedly improves the outlook.[116,117] When treated with plasma exchange, the outlook for patients with TTP in pregnancy is similar to that in nonpregnant individuals.[118]

High recurrence rates have previously been reported in subsequent pregnancies, although a large cohort study showed a lower rate of recurrence in subsequent pregnancy if the TTP had originally presented in pregnancy compared with other cases of primary TTP.[119] TTP in pregnancy may be associated with superimposed preeclampsia.[114]

Fetal risks include intrauterine growth restriction and intrauterine fetal death,[114] but comparison of modern and historical data predating widespread use of plasma exchange suggests that fetal risks may be reduced if the condition is quickly recognized and treated with plasma exchange.[114]

Management Options

Plasma exchange with FFP has been shown in randomized, controlled trials to be an extremely effective treatment for idiopathic TTP (including those associated with pregnancy) and is superior to plasma infusion.[116,117] In the United Kingdom, it has been recommended that the replacement fluid of choice for plasma exchange is FFP that has been subjected to pathogen reduction procedures (e.g., solvent detergent–treated) and sourced from donors outside of the United Kingdom.[120] Plasma exchange should be instituted as soon as possible after the diagnosis of TTP (within 24 hr). Daily plasma exchange should continue until at least 48 hours after complete remission is obtained.[116] Exchange is often tapered (e.g., to alternate-day treatments). In pregnancy, repeated maintenance plasma exchange cycles or plasma infusion therapy is often used until delivery, although data to support this approach are lacking. It is possible that measurement of ADAMTS 13 levels could help to guide ongoing therapy in pregnancy after an initial complete response has been obtained.[121,122]

Cryosupernatant was advocated as superior to standard FFP as an exchange replacement fluid,[123] but a subsequent randomized trial did not confirm this.[124] In practice, the use of cryosupernatant is usually reserved for patients with a poor response to exchange with FFP. Furthermore, any advantage is unlikely to apply to solvent detergent–treated FFP as both cryosupernatant and solvent detergent–treated FFP are lacking in very large von Willebrand multimers.[116] There is a rationale for use of immunosuppressive therapy in those patients with inhibitors of ADAMTS 13. Steroids are often given concomitantly with plasma exchange in TTP, but there is no firm evidence of their benefit.[107] Guidelines in the United Kingdom recommended the use of adjuvant steroids in idiopathic TTP.[116] Additional immunosuppression with the anti-CD20 monoclonal antibody, rituximab has been used with success in primary TTP that has relapsed following standard treatment.[36,107] Rituximab has been used for TTP in pregnancy,[121] but experience is limited.

The use of low-dose aspirin has been advocated when the platelet count increases to more than $50 \times 10^9/L$.[116] In pregnancy, LMWH has been administered, in part to reduce the risk of placental failure syndromes.

Platelet transfusion is contraindicated and may lead to rapid worsening of the condition.[125] Red cell transfusion should be given as required, and folic acid is administered as requirements are increased in hemolytic states.

Unlike in preeclampsia/HELLP syndrome, delivery does not necessarily cause rapid resolution, but delivery should be considered in pregnant women with TTP who are unresponsive to standard therapy.[116]

The correct management of subsequent pregnancies in women with previous TTP is unclear. High rates of recurrence have been reported by some investigators. An aggressive approach with the use of prophylactic plasma exchange together with aspirin and LMWH has been reported in one observational case series with an excellent outcome.[121] The authors advocated the measurement of ADAMTS 13 in early pregnancy in women with a previous history of TTP as a guide to selecting patients for prophylactic plasma exchange therapy.[121]

HEMOLYTIC-UREMIC SYNDROME (See Chapter 78)

HUS is characterized by microangiopathic hemolytic anemia, renal impairment, and a variable degree of thrombocytopenia. In most childhood cases and some adult cases, HUS occurs after infection with Shiga toxin–producing organisms such as some types of *Escherichia coli*. In adults, many cases are atypical and are difficult to distinguish from TTP. Fifty percent of cases of atypical HUS are associated with abnormalities of complement regulatory proteins (e.g., mutations in Factor H or CD46).[126]

Pregnancy-associated HUS usually occurs postpartum with acute renal failure.[115,116] Subsequent chronic renal failure is common.

Initial management of atypical HUS including those cases associated with pregnancy should be with plasma exchange, although this is less well proved than in TTP.

The rationale is, first, the difficulty in distinguishing such cases from TTP, and second, anecdotal data suggesting some benefit of plasma therapy in those patients with defects of complement regulatory pathways.[127] Otherwise, management is supportive and includes renal dialysis and red cell transfusion.

SUMMARY OF MANAGEMENT OPTIONS

Secondary Autoimmune Thrombocytopenia

Management Options	Evidence Quality and Recommendation	References
Antiphospholipid Syndrome and Systemic Lupus Erythematosus (See also Chapter 43)		
Manage thrombocytopenia as for autoimmune idiopathic thrombocytopenic purpura.	III/B	62,63,64
Thromboprophylaxis	IV/C	61,66
HIV Thrombocytopenia (See also Chapter 28)		
Platelet count may be improved by the use of HAART, IVIG, or steroids	III/B (nonpregnant adults)	62*
For cesarean section, consider platelet cover, as with autoimmune idiopathic thrombocytopenic purpura, if platelet count is low.	—/GPP	—
Thrombotic Microangiopathy		
Disseminated intravascular coagulation.	See below and Chapter 78	
Preeclampsia or HELLP syndrome.	See Chapters 35 and 79	
Thrombotic thrombocytopenic purpura (see also Chapters 41 and 78)		
• Plasma exchange with fresh frozen plasma is the first-line treatment.	Ib/A	117*
• Steroids may have a role.	III/B	116*
• Consider aspirin when platelet count > 50 $\times 10^9$/L.	IV/C	116*
• Avoid platelet transfusion.	IV/C	116*
Hemolytic Uremic Syndrome (See also Chapter 79)		
Supportive care.	IV/C	115,116
Renal dialysis.	IV/C	115,116
Red cell transfusion.	IV/C	115,116
Plasma exchange has a role in selected cases.	IV/C	127

* Refers to evidence in nonpregnant adults.

GPP, good practice point; HAART, highly active antiretroviral therapy; HELLP, hemolysis, elevated liver enzymes, and low platelets; IVIG, intravenous immune globulin.

COAGULATION DISORDERS

Heritable Coagulation Disorders

Von Willebrand Disease

The primary function of vWf, which is a large, multimeric protein, is to promote platelet adhesion to the subendothelium. It also binds to and stabilizes plasma Factor VIII. vWD is a common bleeding disorder that arises as a result of heritable mutations that result in quantitative or qualitative defects in vWf.

vWD is divided into several types and subtypes.[128] Identification of the type of vWD has implications for management. Type 1 vWD is due to quantitative deficiency of vWF, and type 2 vWD results from qualitative defects in vWf. Some patients have little or no vWf in terms of measurable antigen and function, and these patients have associated marked reductions in Factor VIII activity (type 3 vWD).

Most types of vWD are inherited in an autosomal dominant fashion, but the pattern of inheritance in type 3 disease is autosomal recessive.

Patients with type 1 or 2 vWD usually have a mild to moderate bleeding disorder characterized by skin and mucosal bleeding and bleeding after surgery or trauma. Patients with type 3 disease have a severe bleeding diathesis and may have deep joint and intramuscular bleeding resembling the pattern seen in hemophilia, in addition to skin and mucosal bleeding.

Coagulation screening tests in patients with vWD may show a prolonged activated partial thromboplastin time (aPTT). More definitive diagnostic tests depend on the finding of reduced plasma vWf activity measured by ristocetin cofactor activity (vWf:RCo) or collagen-binding assay (vWf:CB), accompanied by variable reductions (depending on the type) in vWf antigen and Factor VIII (FVIII:C).[129,130]

Several further tests that aid in classification include analysis of ristocetin-induced platelet aggregation, vWf multimer analysis, and assay of Factor VIII binding to vWf.[129,130] Stress, inflammation, physical exercise, recent surgery, and pregnancy increase plasma vWf and Factor VIII levels, and diagnosis may be difficult in these circumstances. A subtype of type 2 vWD, type 2BvWD, is associated with thrombocytopenia.[129,130]

Molecular genetic analysis may be useful as an aid to diagnosis in type 2 or 3 vWD. Knowledge of the mutation may also aid genetic counseling and allow the option of prenatal diagnosis to be offered to women at risk of having a child with severe type 3 vWD.[131]

MATERNAL RISKS

Levels of vWf and Factor VIII tend to increase during pregnancy. This increase results in improvement in the bleeding tendency in most patients with type 1 vWD.[132] In type 2 vWD, vWf antigen and Factor VIII levels may increase, but this increase is not accompanied by clinical improvement.[133,134] The platelet count may decrease further in patients with type 2B vWD during pregnancy, causing diagnostic problems.[135,136] In type 3 vWD, no improvement occurs in either laboratory parameters or clinical severity.[137]

The risk of bleeding in patients with vWD is usually greatest postpartum.[134,137,138] Levels of Factor VIII and vWf may decrease rapidly after delivery.[139] One series showed an 18.5% incidence of PPH and a 20% incidence of secondary PPH in vWD.[140] In type 1 vWD, Factor VIII levels are a good predictor of the risk of bleeding at delivery (minimal if the Factor VIII level > 0.5 IU/mL).[141] Invasive procedures during the first trimester (e.g., chorionic villus sampling [CVS]) may also carry a risk of bleeding in all types of vWD because vWf and Factor VIII levels do not start to increase until late in the first trimester.[142]

FETAL RISKS

There is very little literature on fetal risk in vWD. Two case series suggest a possible increased rate of spontaneous miscarriage,[143,144] but others disagree.[138,140] A survey of risk factors for antenatal fetal intracranial hemorrhage listed maternal vWD as a predisposing factor.[145] General experience, however, is that fetal or neonatal hemorrhage is rarely encountered in infants with vWD. This observation is supported by a retrospective case series that showed no neonatal hemorrhagic complications after pregnancies affected by maternal vWD.[140] Newborns with type 2 and particularly type 3 vWD may be at increased risk of bleeding including intracranial bleeding following trauma during delivery.[146] Identification of infants affected with type 3 vWD before birth is difficult other than in families in which there are consanguineous relationships.

MANAGEMENT OPTIONS

Prepregnancy

One important aspect of pregnancy management in patients with vWD is its recognition. Patients with vWD may have menorrhagia. Recognition and treatment of vWD may allow avoidance of hysterectomy and a more conservative approach to management.[143,147]

In women diagnosed with vWD, counseling should be given about its inheritance, which is autosomal dominant in most cases. Vaccination against hepatitis A and B should be carried out before pregnancy. The type of vWD should be characterized to plan optimal management of pregnancy and delivery.[142]

In patients with type 1 vWD, it is often useful to carry out a trial of therapy with intravenous desmopressin (DDAVP) to determine the patient's response.[142] This agent may help to prevent or control mild to moderate bleeding. A synthetic analogue of vasopressin, DDAVP increases Factor VIII and vWf levels in plasma.[148] Its major advantage is the avoidance of exposure to pooled blood products.

If menorrhagia has been problematic, iron-deficiency anemia should be corrected before pregnancy. For women with vWD who stopped using a combined oral contraceptive to become pregnant, alternative therapies to control menorrhagia may be required (e.g., tranexamic acid)[142] if pregnancy can be excluded at the time of use.

For women at risk of having a child with severe type 3 vWD (most of whom are asymptomatic carriers, recognized in families with consanguineous relationships), the option of prenatal diagnosis should be discussed at prepregnancy counseling. The causative mutation in the family should be identified, where possible, before pregnancy.[131]

Prenatal

Close liaison between the obstetrician and the hematologist is necessary. Factor VIII, vWf antigen, and vWf activity levels should be monitored.[142,146] U.K. guidelines recommend monitoring at booking, 28 weeks', and 34 weeks' gestation and prior to invasive procedures.[146] Management plans should be determined individually, depending on the patient's hemostatic response to pregnancy. As discussed earlier, in patients with type 1 vWD, hemostatic values are more likely to normalize as pregnancy progresses. If hemostatic parameters have not improved, treatment may be required to cover invasive procedures (particularly in the first trimester) or episodes of antenatal bleeding.

Options for the treatment or prevention of bleeding in vWD include DDAVP (in responsive patients, mainly those with vWD type 1) and Factor VIII concentrates that contain sufficient quantities of vWf.[99,142,149] The use of DDAVP has been controversial in pregnancy. Theoretical concerns have existed about possible oxytocic effects and maternal vasoconstriction. However, there are now several published reports of successful use of DDAVP in pregnancy without adverse effects.[148,150–152] Hyponatremia can occur, particularly after repeated dosing or if copious intravenous fluids are given concomitantly.[149] DDAVP should be avoided in women with preeclampsia.[146]

DDAVP is contraindicated in type 2B vWD because it may worsen thrombocytopenia.[148] Patients with type 2A vWD have a variable response to DDAVP, and patients with type 3 vWD are unresponsive.[149]

When DDAVP is considered unsuitable, patients are treated with a Factor VIII concentrate that contains sufficient vWf. Recombinant factor VIII concentrates do not contain vWf; therefore, suitable products are plasma-derived Factor VIII concentrates that have undergone viral inactivation.[148,149] A high-purity, plasma-derived vWf concentrate is also available, but it must be administered initially with Factor VIII.[153]

Public health considerations for management of invasive procedures are covered in the section on "Labor and Delivery."

Labor and Delivery

For all women with vWD, delivery plans should be agreed among the obstetrician, the hematologist, the obstetric anesthetist, and the patient in advance of labor. This is best done with knowledge of the laboratory vW profile in the third trimester.

For women with type 3 vWD, type 2 vWD, and women with more severe forms of type 1 vWD whose hemostatic profile has not corrected in pregnancy, it is preferable for delivery to take place in a major obstetric unit that has close geographic and professional links with a hemophilia center and where appropriate laboratory facilities for monitoring exist.[146] This is also the case if the fetus is at risk for severe vWD. For patients whose von Willebrand's profile has normalized in pregnancy, no specific hemostatic support is required. For patients whose vWf activity has not normalized, hemostatic supportive therapy is necessary to cover either vaginal delivery or cesarean section. Treatment is indicated to raise vWF activity and Factor VIII levels above 0.5 IU/mL.[142,146,148] Patients with type 1 vWD may receive DDAVP if they are responsive and there are no current contraindications; patients with type 2 or 3 vWD will usually require a suitable coagulation factor concentrate. vWF activity and Factor VIII levels should be maintained at greater than 0.5 IU/mL for 3 days following vaginal delivery and for at least 5 days following cesarean section.[146]

Ventouse delivery, rotational forceps, fetal blood sampling, and scalp electrodes should be avoided if the fetus is at risk for type 2 or 3 vWD or more severe forms of type 1 vWD.[146] The third stage of labor should be managed to ensure adequate uterine contractions. Effort should be made to ensure the placenta is complete. Careful and prompt repair of episiotomies or perineal tears should be undertaken. A low threshold for antibiotics should be adopted if the uterine cavity is opened or explored.

Risks of regional analgesia should be considered on an individual basis.[154] Close collaboration between the hematologist and the anesthetist is required. In type 1 vWD when vWf activity and Factor VIII levels have spontaneously corrected, epidural anesthesia is likely to be safe for the majority. Alternatives should be used for patients with type 2 or 3 vWD and in type 1 vWD where vWf activity has remained low.[146] Bleeding in such cases does not always correlate with laboratory parameters after corrective treatment and so caution should be exerted even after treatment has been given. Patient-controlled analgesia with short-acting opioids can be useful when regional analgesia is contraindicated.

For patients previously treated in the United Kingdom, the patient's "at-risk status" for public health purposes with respect to new-variant Creutzfeldt-Jakob disease (nvCJD) should be documented prior to labor and delivery. All recipients of pooled plasma products manufactured from U.K. plasma between 1980 and 2001 are considered "at risk of nvCJD for public health purposes."[155] This is particularly relevant if instrumental or operative delivery is required. The reproductive tissues and the placenta are considered low risk for contamination with prion proteins,[156] but advice should be sought from an expert in infection control in cases deemed "at risk."

Postnatal

All patients should be observed closely for PPH. Uncorrected hemostatic defects should be treated after delivery. In suitable responsive patients, DDAVP is the treatment of choice to prevent and treat mild to moderate postpartum bleeding.[157] Factor VIII and vWf:RCo levels should be checked a few days after delivery because they may fall rapidly after delivery.[139] FVIII:C and vWf:RCo levels should be maintained in the normal range for at least 3 days following vaginal delivery and 5 to 7 days after cesarean section.[137,146,148,157]

It is difficult and unnecessary to diagnose type 1 vWD in the neonate. If type 2 or 3 vWD is suspected, a cord blood sample should be sent for assay of Factor VIII and vWF activity. Affected infants who have clinical signs of significant bleeding should be treated with a coagulation factor concentrate that contains vWf, and infants with severe vWD may require treatment if delivery has been traumatic.[149] Intramuscular injections should be avoided for both mother and newborn. Vitamin K may be given orally.

Nonsteroidal anti-inflammatory drugs should be avoided for maternal analgesia. Tranexamic acid may be used as an adjunct in the management of postpartum bleeding.[146] Women taking tranexamic acid may breast-feed. Individual decisions should be made about thromboprophylaxis in order to balance the thrombotic with the hemorrhagic risk. Mechanical methods are the first-line approach in patients with bleeding disorders.

Carriers of Hemophilia A and B

Hemophilia A (deficiency of Factor VIII) is the most common severe heritable bleeding disorder, with a prevalence of approximately 1 in 5000 in the population. Hemophilia B (deficiency of Factor IX) is approximately five times less prevalent. The conditions are inherited in an X-linked fashion and are clinically identical. Affected males have a bleeding disorder that correlates in severity with the reduction in the level of Factor VIII or IX. Severely affected males have spontaneous bleeding into muscles and joints; mildly affected patients may bleed only after surgery or trauma.

Females in families with a history of hemophilia may be obligate, potential, or sporadic carriers, depending on the details of the pedigree.[158] An obligate carrier is a woman

whose father has hemophilia, a woman who has a family history of hemophilia and who has given birth to a hemophiliac son, or a woman who has more than one child with hemophilia. A potential carrier of hemophilia is a woman who has a maternal relative with the disorder. A woman with one affected child and no family history may be a sporadic carrier.[158] Carriers of hemophilia usually have Factor VIII or IX levels that are approximately 50% of normal, because of lyonization. Abnormal bleeding does not occur at this level of Factor VIII activity. Some carriers have lower Factor VIII or IX levels, and these individuals have a bleeding disorder that varies according to the coagulation factor level.[159]

MATERNAL RISKS

As discussed earlier, Factor VIII levels tend to increase during pregnancy.[160] This increase usually, but not invariably, occurs in carriers of hemophilia A. The risk of bleeding in carriers of hemophilia A is greatest in the postpartum period because Factor VIII levels may decrease rapidly after delivery.[134,137,161] Invasive procedures during the first trimester, such as CVS, also carry a risk of bleeding. No substantial increase in Factor VIII occurs at this early stage in pregnancy.[137] The risk of antepartum hemorrhage is not increased.[161]

There is usually no substantial increase in Factor IX levels during pregnancy.[137,161,162] Consequently, compared with carriers of hemophilia A, carriers of hemophilia B who have low Factor IX levels are more likely to require treatment to prevent bleeding complications during delivery.

The possible need for treatment with coagulation factor concentrate should be pointed out when counseling women who are carriers of hemophilia. The risks of pregnancy and the safety and potential risks of available treatments should be discussed. This is best carried out by medical and nursing staff with expertise in the management of bleeding disorders.

FETAL RISKS

If the mother is a definite carrier of hemophilia A or B, a male fetus has a 50% chance of being affected. The family history predicts the severity of the hemophilia for the affected fetus.[162] Spontaneous fetal or neonatal bleeding is unusual, even in severe hemophilia, but there are well-documented cases after traumatic delivery.[161,163]

The most serious risk is that of intracranial hemorrhage. Cephalohematoma may also lead to serious bleeding. One retrospective series reported a combined incidence of 3.58% for intracranial hemorrhage and cephalohematoma in newborns with hemophilia A and B.[164,165] Other reported areas of bleeding in hemophilic neonates are at puncture sites, the umbilical stump, and during circumcision.[165]

If the parents seek prenatal diagnosis of hemophilia, counseling should cover the fetal risks associated with CVS. This procedure carries a 1% to 2% risk of miscarriage.[166]

MANAGEMENT OPTIONS

Prepregnancy

All women who are potential, obligate, or sporadic carriers of hemophilia require prepregnancy counseling, including genetic counseling. Arrangements for genetic counseling vary from one area to another, but there is general agreement that a genetic counselor and a physician who is responsible for the management of patients with hemophilia should be involved.[167] It should be established that there is truly a history of hemophilia in the family (not, e.g., another bleeding disorder). The pedigree should be established and the possibility of hemophilia carriership confirmed or refuted. Counseling of obligate and potential carriers should include a discussion of the nature and management of hemophilia.[167]

Carrier identification studies with molecular genetic techniques should be offered to all potential carriers of hemophilia A and B. Written informed consent is recommended before blood samples are collected for molecular analysis.[167] Advances in molecular genetics have made accurate diagnosis of carriership possible in most cases.[167–170] Molecular genetic studies should be carried out in laboratories experienced in molecular analysis of the Factor VIII and IX genes.[169,170] Hemophilia A and B are genetically heterogeneous. The starting point is identification of the mutation responsible for hemophilia in an affected male member of the family (direct mutation detection).[169–171] Potential carriers may be screened for this mutation. The availability of a molecular marker in the family is necessary if prenatal diagnosis is required later.

Approximately 20% of cases of hemophilia A (45% of severe hemophilia A) are caused by an inversion in intron 22 of the Factor VIII gene.[169,171,172] An inversion in intron 1 is the molecular basis of 1% to 2% of cases of severe hemophilia A.[169] If an affected male is not available and there is a family history of severe hemophilia A, a potential carrier should be screened for these common molecular defects. Direct mutation detection is difficult if there is no available affected male but may be attempted in specialized laboratories.

Linkage analysis is now rarely used, but may occasionally be useful if the mutation responsible for hemophilia cannot be identified.[169,171] Intragenic polymorphic markers should be used.[169] Blood from an affected male family member is required, and more extensive family testing is needed for successful linkage analysis. Linkage analysis will be unsuccessful if the potential carrier is homozygous (un-informative) for common intragenic polymorphisms.[171] In families in which there is a single affected male (sporadic hemophilia), female family members may be excluded from carriership by linkage analysis, but carriership cannot be positively diagnosed by this method.[169]

Coagulation studies should also be carried out to identify carriers with low Factor VIII or IX levels. Normal levels of Factor VIII or IX do not exclude carriership. Women with low levels of Factor VIII or IX should be offered vaccination against hepatitis A and B. The immunity status should be checked if the patient has been vaccinated. Women who have low levels of Factor VIII may have a useful hemostatic response to DDAVP.[173] To establish whether this response is occurring, a trial of intravenous DDAVP can be attempted, with measurement of the response in Factor VIII levels over the next 24 hours. DDAVP is not useful for women with low Factor IX levels.[174]

Once carriership has been established, careful planning of pregnancies should be encouraged. Partners of hemophilia carriers should be encouraged to attend prepregnancy counseling sessions.[158,162] Couples should be informed that hemophilia "breeds true" in families. In other words, its severity is predictable by the family history.[162] Approximately 25% of patients with hemophilia A will develop an inhibitor to Factor VIII in their lifetime.[175] Inhibitors are less common in hemophilia B. The development of an inhibitor renders usual treatment with Factor VIII concentrate ineffective or less effective and is a serious complication. There is a genetic component to the risk of inhibitor development.[175,176] Some molecular genetic defects are associated with an increased risk of inhibitor formation (e.g., large deletions).[176] This should be addressed during counseling. Couples should be counseled in a nondirective manner about all reproductive options, including the availability of prenatal diagnosis. They should be encouraged to consider the matter in advance of pregnancy,[158,167] although circumstances may change and final decisions must be made given the circumstances in each pregnancy. Prepregnancy counseling may need to be repeated in subsequent pregnancies. Discussion of the techniques and risks associated with prenatal diagnosis is appropriate during preconception counseling sessions.[158] Carriers should be encouraged to seek care early in pregnancy, especially if prenatal diagnosis is being considered or has not been excluded.

Preimplantation genetic diagnosis may be made available by referral to specialized centers for carriers of hemophilia who, after counseling, do not wish to contemplate bringing up a hemophilic child, but would not consider termination.[146] Preimplantation diagnosis is possible only with in vitro fertilization and is available only in a few specialized centers. In the United Kingdom, each new test requires a license from the Human Fertilisation and Embryology Authority. Couples contemplating this procedure require complex counseling with the involvement of an expert in in vitro fertilization and the opportunity to discuss possible pitfalls with the relevant specialist center in advance of the procedure.

Prenatal

Identification and counseling of carriers should be carried out before pregnancy, but may be necessary in early pregnancy if a woman with a family history of hemophilia does not seek care until pregnancy is diagnosed. General practitioners, midwives, and obstetricians should refer these patients for specialized counseling as early as possible.[167]

Pregnancies in patients who are carriers of congenital bleeding disorders should be managed in a hospital with hemophilia expertise.[137,146,161] Close liaison between the obstetrician and the hemophilia team is necessary. Factor VIII or IX levels should be monitored regularly throughout pregnancy. U.K. guidelines recommend measurement of coagulation factor levels at booking, at 28 weeks, and at 34 weeks.[146] Knowledge of coagulation factor levels toward the end of the third trimester (34–36 wk) is necessary to plan management of delivery.[161,162]

If prenatal diagnosis is requested and a suitable molecular marker exists, testing is usually carried out by CVS at 11 to 14 weeks. Amniocentesis from 15 weeks onward is an alternative. CVS is generally considered the method of choice for prenatal diagnosis because it offers early diagnosis.[146] Fetal blood sampling by cordocentesis is now rarely carried out because of hazards. Risks associated with these procedures should be fully discussed with the patient. CVS and amniocentesis carry a 1% risk of miscarriage. Fetal bleeding sufficient to result in death is a recognized risk of cordocentesis.[146]

The use of prenatal diagnosis is decreasing in developed countries. As hemophilia care improves, more couples are willing to contemplate bringing up a child with hemophilia.[162]

If prenatal diagnosis is requested, treatment may be necessary to increase maternal Factor VIII or IX levels if they are less than 0.5 IU/mL. Laboratory measurement of coagulation factor levels should be used to monitor treatment. DDAVP may be used for women with reduced Factor VIII levels for patients demonstrated to be responsive.[148,150,161,162] DDAVP is ineffective in increasing Factor IX levels. Readers are referred to the section on "von Willebrand's Disease" for further discussion on the use of DDAVP in pregnancy. If coagulation factor concentrates are used, a recombinant Factor VIII or IX concentrate should be chosen.[174] Many patients are previously untreated, and even a minimal risk of transmission of infection from plasma-derived products is unacceptable. Further, parvovirus B19, which can cause fetal hydrops, may be transmitted by plasma-derived concentrate, and no method of viral inactivation seems to be effective in eradicating this virus.[177] Women previously treated with plasma-derived factor concentrates manufactured from U.K. plasma between 1980 and 2001 are considered "at risk of nvCJD for public health purposes."[155] When invasive procedures are required in such cases, advice should be taken from an expert in infection control. Reproductive tissues have been considered low risk for transmission of prions by the Health Protection Agency in the United Kingdom.[156]

Fetal sex should be determined in all pregnancies in which the fetus is at risk for hemophilia.[146] Ultrasonography at 20 weeks has been the standard approach.[137,161,162] This information is necessary for the obstetrician and hematologist to plan delivery, even if the parents do not wish to know the sex of the infant. Research into fetal sexing earlier in pregnancy has given rise to two techniques that have been successfully applied in small numbers of pregnancies. The first is detection of free fetal DNA in maternal plasma. This depends on quantitative PCR for Y chromosomal DNA sequence.[178,179] A second technique is that of gender determination by ultrasound at 11 to 14 weeks' gestation.[178] These techniques are, at present, limited to centers with research expertise, and it has been recommended that if used, both techniques should be used to check that the results are in agreement. Fetal sexing by free fetal DNA in the late first trimester has now, however, been shown to have a high rate of accuracy.[180,181] In cases in which fetal sex can be determined by these methods in the first trimester, this may aid decisions regarding CVS for some women.

A delivery plan taking account of the patient's coagulation factor level, the sex of the fetus, and obstetric considerations should be made in the third trimester of pregnancy. This should be agreed among the obstetrician, the hemophilia specialist, the obstetric anesthetist, and the patient. The use of third-trimester amniocentesis to aid delivery planning if the fetus is male has been advocated by some obstetricians (T Overton, personal communication). The rationale is that definite molecular diagnosis may exclude a fetus from having hemophilia and open up more options for management of delivery. There is a small risk of premature labor,[182] which in turn, may increase risk of bleeding for a hemophilic infant (because the coagulation system is less mature). Risks must, therefore, be balanced carefully if this is considered, but this approach may be useful in individual cases. If the fetus is male and hemophilia has not been excluded or if ***baseline*** maternal coagulation factor levels have been low, delivery should be planned in a center where hemophilia expertise, including laboratory monitoring, is readily available.[146]

Labor and Delivery

If maternal Factor VIII or IX levels remain low at 34 to 36 weeks in hemophilia carriers, treatment to correct maternal hemostasis is necessary for delivery.[137,161,162] Factor VIII or IX levels should be maintained at greater than 0.5 IU/mL for all modes of delivery.[146] Considerations similar to those discussed earlier govern the choice of treatment. Recombinant Factor VIII or IX or DDAVP (for carriers of hemophilia A only) should be used.[174] Full laboratory monitoring of hemostatic replacement therapy is necessary. Epidural anesthesia may be used if coagulation defects have been corrected.[161]

As discussed previously, the maternal "at-risk" status for nvCJD should be noted and infection control advice sought when appropriate.[155]

If the fetus is a known hemophiliac, is male and of unknown hemophilia status, or is of unknown sex, care should be taken to avoid traumatic vaginal delivery.[161–163,165] When possible, obstetric problems should be identified before the expected date of delivery, and the mode of delivery should be planned. Routine cesarean delivery is unnecessary,[162,163,165] but cesarean delivery should be carried out if obstetric complications are anticipated.

Fetal scalp sampling and scalp electrodes should not be used if the fetus may have hemophilia.[146,161,162] Similarly, in such cases, ventouse delivery is absolutely contraindicated because major cephalohematoma and intracranial bleeding have been documented after this procedure.[146,162,163,165] Mid-cavity rotational forceps delivery should be avoided, but simple lift-out forceps delivery may be preferable to a difficult cesarean section if the fetal head is low in the pelvis.[162]

Active management of the third stage of labor is recommended.[146] Maternal perineal trauma should be minimized, with suturing performed promptly after delivery.

Postnatal

Most bleeding problems in carriers of hemophilia occur postpartum. There is a 22% risk of primary post partum bleeding and an 11% risk of secondary PPH.[161]

As discussed earlier, replacement therapy should be given immediately after delivery to mothers with an uncorrected hemostatic defect. Coagulation factor levels should be rechecked urgently if postpartum bleeding occurs. Options at this stage include DDAVP for mothers who are carriers of hemophilia A and recombinant coagulation factor concentrates for carriers of hemophilia A or B. Supportive therapy to maintain hemostasis should be continued for 3 to 4 days after vaginal delivery and for 5 to 7 days after cesarean section.[137,146] All hemostatic parameters must be normal before epidural catheters are removed. Nonsteroidal anti-inflammatory analgesics should be avoided. All mothers who are carriers, regardless of whether they need peripartum hemostatic support, should be observed for signs of PPH. Coagulation factor levels should be checked daily after delivery because they may decrease quickly.[146,162]

Women who are carriers of hemophilia should not be excluded from considerations regarding thromboprophylaxis. In general, mechanical methods should be the method of first choice but risks and benefits should be assessed individually. Women with risk factors for thrombosis may merit prophylaxis with LMWH if coagulation factor levels have been corrected. Close clinical monitoring for signs of bleeding and laboratory monitoring to ensure adequate coagulation factor levels is advisable under such circumstances.

In the infant, intramuscular injections (including vitamin K) should be avoided until hemophilia has been excluded.[162] Vitamin K may be given orally.[165] Cord blood should be obtained for appropriate factor assays.[162,165] Except for very mild cases, hemophilia A can be diagnosed easily in the neonatal period. Difficulties may arise with mild or moderate hemophilia B because of the physiologic reduction in Factor IX levels that occurs in the newborn.[165,183] However, severe hemophilia B is usually easily identified.

There has been debate about the routine administration of coagulation factor concentrates to neonates with hemophilia.[184] There is some evidence that the administration of factor concentrate in very early life might increase the risk of inhibitor development.[185] Factor concentrate should not, therefore, be administered routinely. Treatment with recombinant factor concentrate should be considered if there has been trauma at delivery or if the neonate has significant hemorrhagic signs.[146,184] Prompt coagulation factor support is clearly needed if there is clinical evidence of intracranial hemorrhage or significant bleeding from other sites.[165] Cranial ultrasound or computed tomography scanning should be carried out in infants with hemophilia if delivery has been traumatic or if there is clinical suspicion of intracranial bleeding.[146,165]

The hemophilia team should be involved from the outset in counseling parents of infants with newly diagnosed congenital bleeding disorders. A clear follow-up plan should be discussed with the parents at discharge.[165] The community midwife and family physician should be informed if the infant is hemophilic.

Other Heritable Bleeding Disorders

Some women have rare deficiencies of coagulation factors or congenital platelet function disorders.[186] Detailed description is beyond the scope of this chapter. As with all bleeding disorders, close liaison between the obstetrician and the hematologist is required. The principles of management revolve around assessment of the risk of bleeding for the mother and infant. The risks of hemostatic supportive therapy must be taken into account. Many (but not all) disorders are inherited in a recessive manner; therefore, the risk of fetal or neonatal bleeding is often negligible unless there is a consanguineous partnership. For rarer congenital coagulation factor deficiencies, clinical bleeding does not always correlate with coagulation factor levels. This is particularly the case for Factor XI deficiency.[186] Women with deficiency of fibrinogen or Factor XIII may have recurrent fetal loss.[187,188] Placental abruption is reported in congenital afibrinogenemia.[187] Appropriate replacement therapy can help to maintain pregnancy.[187,188]

SUMMARY OF MANAGEMENT OPTIONS

Coagulation Disorders—Inherited

Management Options	Evidence Quality and Recommendation	References
Von Willebrand's Disease		
Prepregnancy		
Establish type of von Willebrand's disease.	IV/C	149
Provide genetic counseling (usually dominant except type 3).	IV/C	131,146
Give hepatitis A and B immunization.	IIa/B	174*
For type 1 von Willebrand's disease, perform a DDAVP trial to establish efficacy (contraindicated in type 2B von Willebrand's disease).	IV (for trial)/C III (for efficacy)/B	149 173*
Prenatal		
Combined or interdisciplinary team approach (obstetric and hemophilia team).	IV/C	146
Monitor vWf:Ag, vWf:RCo, FVIII:C, platelet count (in many cases, parameters improve).	IV/C	146
Treatment is unlikely to be required unless invasive procedures are performed or an episode of antenatal bleeding.	IV/C	146
Labor and Delivery		
Deliver in center with readily available expert hematologic support if severe type 1, 2 or 3.	IV/C	146
Maternal hemostatic support is needed if FVIII:C <0.5 IU/mL or if vWf:RCo significantly reduced.	IV/C	146
DDAVP may be used in responsive patient (except in type 2B von Willebrand's disease), or a plasma-derived concentrate containing vWf may be used.	IV/C	146,149
Aim for atraumatic delivery (vaginal delivery if uncomplicated delivery is anticipated, but avoid fetal scalp electrodes and fetal scalp sampling if risk of severe type 1, 2 or 3).	IV/C	146
Active management of the third stage.	IV/C	146
Prompt repair of perineal trauma.	—/GPP	—
Postnatal		
Vigilance for postpartum hemorrhage.	IV/C	140,146
Cord samples are not indicated unless type 2 or 3 von Willebrand's disease is suspected in the newborn.	IV/C	146
Avoid neonatal intramuscular injections until status is known.	IV/C	146
Recheck maternal FVIII:C, vWf:Ag, and vWf:RCo for a few days after delivery. If parameters fall or if the patient is bleeding, give hemostatic supportive therapy. Maintain support based on laboratory parameters for 3–5 days.	IV/C	140,146
Carriers of Hemophilia A or B		
Prepregnancy		
Provide genetic evaluation and counseling.	IV/C	146,167
Establish mutation, if possible; if not, define whether linkage analysis is of use.	IV/C	167,169,170
If maternal Factor VIII or IX is reduced, obtain baseline virology (including hepatitis B and C, HIV, and immunity vs. hepatitis A and parvovirus).	—/GPP	—

Management Options	Evidence Quality and Recommendation	References
Give hepatitis A and B immunization if the patient is not immune.	IIa/B	174*
For carriers of hemophilia A with low Factor VIII levels, perform a trial of DDAVP to establish efficacy.	III (for efficacy of DDAVP)/B	173*
Prenatal		
Provide combined or interdisciplinary team approach (obstetric and hemophilia team).	IV/C	146
Offer prenatal diagnosis (chorionic villus sampling) at 11–14 wk (cover with factor concentrate if level of Factor VIII or IX < 0.5 IU/mL); use recombinant products, or DDAVP.	IV/C	146
Obtain maternal serial clotting factor levels.	IV/C	146
Fetal sexing either by free fetal DNA with confirmation by ultrasonography at 16–20 wk if invasive prenatal diagnosis is not requested or by ultrasound alone.	IV/C	146,180
Labor and Delivery		
Consider factor concentrate cover for labor and delivery if Factor VIII or IX level <0.5 IU/mL	IV/C	146
For hemophilia A carriers, consider DDAVP alone if the patient is known to be responsive, if normal vaginal delivery is anticipated, and if the coagulation defect is mild.	IV/C	146
If high risk fetus, aim for atraumatic unassisted (no ventouse or forceps) delivery (vaginal delivery if uncomplicated delivery is anticipated, but avoid fetal scalp electrodes and fetal scalp sampling).	IV/C	146
Postnatal		
Obtain cord blood for neonatal evaluation if risk of hemophilia A or B.	IV/C	146,165
Avoid neonatal intramuscular injections until status is known.	IV/C	146,165
Give vitamin K orally if neonate has hemophilia or if hemophilia not excluded.	IV/C	146,165
Consider cranial ultrasound/CT if neonate has severe hemophilia and traumatic delivery.	IV/C	146,165
A clear follow-up plan is needed for the parents and child.	IV/C	146
Vigilance for postpartum hemorrhage.	—/GPP	—
Provide maternal hemostatic support for 3 days if vaginal delivery and for 5 days if cesarean delivery.	IV/C	146

* Refers to evidence in nonpregnant adults.
CT, computed tomography; DDAVP, desmopressin; GPP, good practice point; vWf, von Willebrand factor; vWf:Ag, von Willebrand factor antigen; vWf:RCo, vWf activity measured by ristocetin cofactor activity.

Acquired Coagulation Disorders

Disseminated Intravascular Coagulation (See Chapter 77)

DIC occurs in a wide variety of obstetric complications. It is triggered by vascular endothelial damage, release of procoagulant substances as a result of tissue damage or liquor entering the circulation, or cytokine-mediated up-regulation of tissue factor expression on monocytes and endothelial cells.[189,190] These triggers lead to the generation of thrombin, cause defects in inhibitors of coagulation, and suppress fibrinolysis. These hemostatic changes result in deposition of fibrin in the microcirculation and consumption of coagulation factors and platelets, leading to a bleeding tendency.

In obstetrics, DIC often develops acutely, for example, in placental abruption, and results in rapid defibrination with hemostatic failure. Very long clotting times and marked thrombocytopenia usually occur. At the other end of the spectrum, chronic DIC may cause minimal or no abnormality on standard coagulation screening tests.

No single test is diagnostic of DIC; the diagnosis depends on a combination of clinical findings and laboratory test results.[190,191]

Thrombocytopenia or a decreasing platelet count is a sensitive indicator.[191] In most cases of DIC, whether acute or chronic, the plasma D-dimer level is elevated.[191] In interpreting the results of coagulation screening tests in suspected DIC in pregnant women, it is prudent to note that normal baseline values are altered by physiologic changes. The plasma fibrinogen level is elevated and Factor VIII levels increase in pregnancy, leading to an acceleration of aPTT.[160,192] Fibrinogen levels and aPTT in the normal nonpregnant range in late pregnancy should be regarded suspiciously. Fibrinogen should be assayed by the Clauss method.

The use of a scoring system for diagnosis of DIC has been advocated.[193] This has been evaluated in a wide range of critical care patients but not specifically in obstetric patients.

Because rapid changes in parameters may occur in DIC, repeat testing and ongoing monitoring until resolution are always necessary.[191]

MATERNAL RISKS

Maternal risks arise as a result of the underlying disorder, but there are also risks of bleeding and small vessel occlusion as a direct result of DIC.

FETAL RISKS

Fetal risks in DIC are associated with the underlying cause.

MANAGEMENT OPTIONS

Management of DIC includes treatment of the underlying cause and appropriate resuscitative measures to maintain tissue perfusion. Hemostatic replacement therapy is indicated if there is significant hemorrhage or if invasive procedures are required.[191] When clinically indicated, replacement therapy with FFP, platelet transfusions, and in some cases, a source of fibrinogen (such as cryoprecipitate or fibrinogen concentrate) is based on the results of laboratory tests and clinical findings.[120] Prothrombin time and aPTT provide a guide for FFP usage, and the fibrinogen level can be used to guide the use of both FFP and cryoprecipitate.[191] The goal is to increase the fibrinogen level to 1 g/L. Platelet transfusion is required if bleeding occurs in a patient with a platelet count less than 50 × 10^9/L.[191] However, the goal is not simply to correct laboratory defects, and clinical features are paramount in guiding treatment.[189] Treatment of the underlying cause is the most important consideration.[189,191]

The use of heparin is controversial, and it should be reserved for cases in which microvascular occlusion rather than hemorrhage is the predominant clinical problem. The cautious use of heparin may also have a place alongside replacement therapy in the management of amniotic fluid embolism. The rationale is that the underlying cause cannot be removed, and because of the rate of consumption, it is difficult to keep pace with replacement therapy unless thrombin generation is inhibited concomitantly.[189,190]

For patients who are not bleeding with DIC, prophylactic doses of UFH or LMWH are recommended for prevention of venous thromboembolism.[191]

Concentrates of the anticoagulant protein activated protein C have been used in patients with severe sepsis including those with DIC caused by severe sepsis. Reduction in mortality and improvement in hemostatic parameters have been observed in patients with severe sepsis.[194–196]

Activated protein C increases the risk of major bleeding and should be avoided in patients at particular risk of bleeding or if platelets are less 30 × 10^9/L.[191]

Massive Blood Loss (See Chapters 58 and 78)

Causes of massive obstetric hemorrhage are discussed elsewhere (see Chapters 58 and 78). Massive bleeding in obstetric practice (e.g., as a result of placental abruption) is often accompanied by DIC. Bleeding as a result of placenta previa may be massive but is not necessarily associated with DIC. Resuscitative measures and red cell transfusion are the first considerations. However, dilutional effects on coagulation factors and platelets occur, and bank blood does not provide platelets and labile clotting factors.

MANAGEMENT OPTIONS

The underlying cause should be treated. Resuscitative measures and red cell transfusion are paramount concerns. Blood should be warmed when rapid transfusion is required because cold injury can exacerbate end-organ damage and DIC.[197]

Coagulation defects should be corrected with FFP, and thrombocytopenia is treated with platelet transfusion. Treatment should be guided by the findings on complete blood count, coagulation screening tests, and fibrinogen measurements. Reasonable aims are to keep the platelet count above 50 × 10^9/L and to keep the fibrinogen level above 1.0 g/L[197] and the hemoglobin above 80 g/L (or 8 g/dL). A trigger platelet count of 75 × 10^9/L has been recommended in British transfusion guidelines to ensure that the platelet count is always kept above 50 × 10^9/L.[197] In some cases, cryoprecipitate or fibrinogen concentrate may be required as a source of fibrinogen if the fibrinogen remains below 1 g/L despite transfusion of FFP.[197]

In intractable major hemorrhage, recombinant Factor VIIa may be used to stem bleeding when all other measures have failed. This treatment, which was originally developed for the management of bleeding in hemophilic patients with inhibitors, has been used successfully in a variety of clinical situations associated with major bleeding and is becoming viewed as a "universal" hemostatic agent.[198] Recombinant Factor VIIa is not licensed for control of massive bleeding in such circumstances. DIC is not a contraindication to the use of recombinant Factor VIIa if massive bleeding is occurring. However, caution should be exercised in patients with major DIC because there are occasional reports of thrombosis and DIC after the use of recombinant Factor VIIa.[199] Recombinant Factor VIIa should not be viewed as a replacement for conventional approaches to control bleeding. It is important to correct acidosis and hypothermia and to optimize the platelet count as far as possible in order to maximize the chance of efficacy of recombinant Factor VIIa.[200]

There are several reports of the successful use of recombinant Factor VIIa to control massive hemorrhage in obstetric patients.[201–203]

There are no clinical trials in obstetric practice of the use of Factor VIIa in massive hemorrhage. Nevertheless, a recent European consensus statement included massive PPH as a suitable clinical condition in which to consider use of Factor VIIa (grade E recommendation).[200] Use in this situation may avoid the need for hysterectomy.[203]

Liver Disease (See Chapter 47)

MATERNAL RISKS AND MANAGEMENT OPTIONS

Patients with liver disease, especially if it is advanced, often have significant hemostatic impairment. Several mechanisms contribute to this impairment, including thrombocytopenia as a result of splenic enlargement or alcohol use, impaired production of coagulation factors in the liver, impaired polymerization of fibrin, platelet dysfunction, and hyperfibrinolysis.[204] In pregnant women with liver disease, a complete blood count should be obtained and coagulation parameters monitored. Coagulation screening tests and measurement of fibrinogen levels are indicated. In some cases, screening for DIC or coagulation factor assays is helpful. The risk of bleeding is greatest during and after surgery or invasive procedures. Hemostatic supportive therapy may be required in these situations or if bleeding occurs during labor or delivery. Standard therapy is with FFP and platelets. Efficacy may be limited in patients with liver disease, and large volumes of FFP may be required. In cases of severe bleeding in liver disease that are unresponsive to conventional component therapy, the use of modern prothrombin complex concentrates (PCCs) may be considered. In the past, liver disease has been considered a relative contraindication to the use of PCCs. However, modern PCCs contain less activated coagulation factors and a better balance of procoagulant and anticoagulant proteins.[205] Successful use of such concentrates in patients with liver disease has been reported.[206]

Acquired Inhibitors of Coagulation (Acquired Factor VIII Inhibitor)

MATERNAL RISKS

Rarely, pregnancy is associated with the development of an antibody that inhibits Factor VIII activity. Most reported cases occur postpartum.[207–209] This antibody may lead to postpartum hemorrhage or postsurgical bleeding. Bleeding may be severe and life-threatening; therefore, recognition is important. The pattern of spontaneous bleeding differs in acquired hemophilia compared with that in heritable Factor VIII deficiency. Classically, in acquired hemophilia, subcutaneous bleeding and bleeding from mucous membranes occur. Inhibitors that develop early in the postpartum period are associated with PPH, whereas skin and soft tissue bleeding is a more common presenting manifestation if inhibitors develop later in the postpartum period.[209] The severity of bleeding correlates less well with the Factor VIII level than in males with heritable Factor VIII deficiency.[210]

The timing of the development of these postpartum inhibitors is highly variable. One series reported identification of acquired hemophilia between 3 and 150 days postpartum.[207] Postpartum Factor VIII inhibitors may disappear spontaneously, but the usual pattern is persistent for months or even years.[207,208] The more common pattern seems to be that inhibitors do not recur in subsequent pregnancies.[207]

In the laboratory, a Factor VIII inhibitor is associated with a prolonged aPTT, with normal prothrombin time and fibrinogen levels. The addition of normal plasma in vitro does not correct the aPTT. Specialized tests are necessary to confirm the presence of a Factor VIII inhibitor, and it is important to differentiate a Factor VIII inhibitor from a lupus inhibitor because the clinical implications are profoundly different.[211,212]

FETAL RISKS

Most inhibitors occur postpartum, so there are generally no fetal risks. However, inhibitors that arise antenatally have been reported. These antibodies may cross the placenta and persist for up to 3 months in the neonate. Bleeding complications have not usually occurred, but intracranial hemorrhage has been reported.[208] The management of these pregnancies should be based on the assumption that the fetus potentially is phenotypically hemophilic, regardless of the sex. Delivery plans and immediate neonatal management are as described earlier. The management of a neonate with bleeding complications as a result of a maternal Factor VIII inhibitor requires the expert input of a pediatric hemophilia specialist. Conventional Factor VIII concentrates are likely to be ineffective.

MANAGEMENT OPTIONS

Patients with acquired hemophilia should be managed in a hospital where hemophilia expertise exists.

Conventional Factor VIII concentrates may be ineffective in controlling bleeding. Various coagulation factor concentrates are available for immediate control of bleeding in patients with Factor VIII inhibitors. Detailed discussion is outside the scope of this chapter. In a young woman with bleeding as a result of acquired hemophilia, options include recombinant Factor VIIa[212,213] or larger doses of a recombinant Factor VIII concentrate, if a useful Factor VIII recovery and half-life can be achieved.

It is important to attempt to eradicate the inhibitor because the risk of severe bleeding otherwise persists.[214] Steroids and immunosuppressive therapy have been used.[212,214] Successful use of the anti-CD20 monoclonal antibody rituximab has been reported.[212,214,215]

Combination therapy with steroids and immunosuppressive therapy may be more efficacious in reducing the time to disappearance of inhibitors,[207] but cyclophosphamide should be avoided if possible in women of childbearing age.[214] It has been suggested that postpartum Factor VIII inhibitors may take longer to eradicate than similar autoantibodies occurring in different clinical circumstances.[216] Women should be advised to use effective contraception until the inhibitor has been eradicated. Prepregnancy counseling should be offered prior to the next pregnancy. Although most inhibitors do not recur in subsequent pregnancies, recurrence has been reported and women should be informed about this possibility.[209,216]

SUMMARY OF MANAGEMENT OPTIONS

Acquired Coagulation Disorders

Management Options	Evidence Quality and Recommendation	References
Disseminated Intravascular Coagulation (See also Chapter 77)		
Provide interdisciplinary approach (obstetric and hematology).	IV/C	191*
Treat the cause.	IV/C	191*
Serial monitoring is important because rapid changes may occur.	III/B	191*
Replace fresh frozen plasma, cryoprecipitate, and platelets on the basis of clinical condition and laboratory results.	IV/C	191*
Consider heparin in DIC due to amniotic fluid embolism.	IV/C	189,190
Consider thromboprophylaxis with LMWH or UFH if patient is not bleeding.	Ib/A	191*
Concentrates of activated protein C are useful in DIC due to severe sepsis.	Ib (nonpregnant)/A	194,195*
Massive Hemorrhage (See also Chapters 58 and 77)		
Treat the cause.	IV/C	197*
Resuscitation with volume replacement to maintain tissue perfusion.	Ib/A	197*
Replace red cells, fresh frozen plasma, cryoprecipitate, and platelets on the basis of laboratory results and clinical condition	IV/C	197*
Consider recombinant Factor VIIa if massive bleeding continues despite correction of surgical hemostasis and adequate conventional product replacement; most experience is outside pregnancy, although it is increasing in pregnancy.	IV/C	200
Acquired Factor VIII Inhibitor		
Provide interdisciplinary approach with involvement of experts in hemophilia.	IV/C	214*
Recombinant Factor VIIa if severe acute bleeding is nonresponsive to other therapy.	IIb/B	214*
Provide immunosuppressive therapy (see text).	IIb/B	214*

* Refers to evidence in nonpregnant adults.
DIC, disseminated intravascular coagulation; LMWH, low-molecular-weight heparin; UFH, unfractionated heparin.

SUGGESTED READINGS

Alstead ME, Ritchie JK, Lennard-Jones JE, et al: Safety of azathioprine in pregnancy in inflammatory bowel disease. Gastroenterology 1990;99:443–446.

British Committee for Standards in Haematology Haemostasis and Thrombosis Task Force: Guidelines on the diagnosis and management of the thrombotic microangiopathic haemolytic anaemias. Br J Haematol 2003;120:556–573.

Cooper N, Avangalista ML, Amadori S, Stasi R: Should rituximab be used before or after splenectomy in patients with immune thrombocytopenic purpura? Curr Opin Haematol 2007;14:642–646.

Duguid J, O'Shaughnessy DS, Aterbury C, et al: Guidelines for the use of fresh frozen plasma, cryoprecipitate and cryosupernatant. Br J Haematol 2004;126:11–28.

Galli M, Finazzi G, Barrbui T: Thrombocytopenia in the antiphospholipid syndrome. Br J Haematol 1996;93:1–5.

George JN: The association of pregnancy with thrombotic thrombocytopenic purpura-hemolytic uremic syndrome. Curr Opin Hematol 2003;10:339–344.

Kulkarni R, Lusher JM: Intracranial and extracranial haemorrhages in newborns with haemophilia: A review of the literature. J Paediatr Haematol Oncol 1999;21:289–295.

Laffan M, Brown SA, Collins PW, et al: The diagnosis of von Willebrand disease: A guideline from the UK Haemophilia Centre Doctors Organisation. Haemophilia 2004;10:199–217.

Matthay MD: Severe sepsis: A new treatment with both anticoagulant and anti-inflammatory properties. N Engl J Med 2001;344:759–762.

Morgenstern GR, Measday B, Hegde UM: Autoimmune thrombocytopenia in pregnancy: New approach to management. Br Med J 1983;287:584.

REFERENCES

For a complete list of references, log onto www.expertconsult.com.

CHAPTER 41

Clotting Disorders

CHRISTINA S. HAN, MICHAEL J. PAIDAS, and CHARLES J. LOCKWOOD

INTRODUCTION

Disorders of coagulation can lead to significant maternal and fetal compromise during pregnancy and the puerperium. In 2006, the World Health Organization reported the contrasting disorders of embolism and hemorrhage as the second and third leading causes of maternal mortality in the developed world, contributing to 14.9% and 13.4% of maternal deaths, respectively. Hypertensive disorders, the leading cause, accounted for 16.1% of deaths.[1]

Maintenance of an intact vascular compartment in the face of vessel damage requires meticulous coordination of platelet function, coagulation products, fibrinolytic factors, and the vascular endothelium. Physiologic changes during pregnancy and the puerperium pose a significant challenge to the hemostatic system, evolving from a hypocoagulable state that allows for uterine perfusion to a hypercoagulable state that prevents maternal hemorrhage.

HEMOSTATIC SYSTEM

Coagulation is mediated by a cascade of extracellular clotting factors and cellular components that seal breached endothelium with fibrin-platelet plugs. This procoagulant activity is dampened by endogenous anticoagulants and fibrinolysis.

Platelet Plug Formation

Damage to the endothelial surface exposes collagen in the subendothelial layer to the coagulation factors trafficking within the bloodstream. One factor that is both produced constitutively within the endothelium and freely flowing in the plasma is von Willebrand's factor (vWF), a large multimeric glycoprotein (GP) that binds to the uncovered subendothelial collagen. The A1 domain of vWF binds to the GP1b/IX/V receptor on platelets, recruiting platelets to sites of endothelial disruption.[2] Platelets can also adhere directly to subendothelial collagen via their GP1a/IIa ($\alpha_2\beta_1$ integrin) and GP VI receptors.

Recruited platelets are activated by collagen following binding to the GP VI receptor, which triggers calcium flux and activates protein kinase C. Activated protein kinase C, in turn, triggers platelet secretory activity and activates various signaling pathways. Activated platelets degranulate to release various compounds that biochemically enhance the plug formation.[3] These compounds include thromboxane A2 (TXA_2), dense granules of adenosine diphosphate (ADP), serotonin, vWF, vitronectin, fibronectin, thrombospondin, partially activated Factor V, fibrinogen, β-thromboglobulin, and platelet-derived growth factors. Activation causes the platelet GPIIb/IIIa receptor ($\alpha_{IIb}\beta_3$ integrin) to undergo a conformational change that promotes binding to fibrinogen molecules, which serves as a glue to bind other platelets, causing platelet aggregation.[4] Multiple disorders of the coagulation cascade can occur at this level and result in bleeding diatheses (Table 41–1).

Fibrin Plug Formation

The platelet plug is further enhanced by fibrin formation, thereby creating a synergistic partnership that allows for controlled propagation of the coagulation cascade. The initiation of clotting is triggered by exposure of tissue factor (TF), present on the membranes of subendothelial cells (e.g., fibroblasts, vascular smooth muscle cells, and parenchymal cells), to circulating Factor VII. Factor VII autoactivates upon binding to TF to trigger a greater than 100-fold increase in catalytic activity.[5] The TF/VIIa complex then activates Factors IX and X. Activated Factor Xa binds to its co-factor Va to convert prothrombin (Factor II) to thrombin (Factor IIa). Of note, the co-factor Va is generated from Factor V by either Factor Xa or thrombin. Partially activated Factor Va can also be directly delivered to the damaged site by the platelet α-granule.[6]

Locally generated Factor IXa diffuses to adjacent activated platelet membranes and binds to Factor VIIIa. Factor VIII is activated by thrombin and released from its vWF carrier molecule to form active Factor VIIIa. The Factor IXa/VIIIa complex is able to alternatively generate Factor Xa to further drive production of thrombin. In addition, thrombin on activated platelet surfaces activates Factor XI to XIa, which alternatively activates Factor IX. These redundant pathways all lead to thrombin generation, which converts fibrinogen to fibrin. The final hemostatic plug is formed when fibrin monomers self-polymerize and are cross-linked by thrombin-activated Factor XIIIa (Fig. 41–1). The most well-known bleeding diathesis involving fibrin plug formation is hemophilia, or Factor VIII deficiency (see Table 41–1).

Endogenous Anticoagulants

A system of mechanical and biochemical barriers evolved to confine the extent of coagulation activity. The adherence and activation of platelets diminish over time as a firm network of platelets settles into the breach, concealing the subendothelial collagen. This mechanical blockade of platelet aggregation and platelet-associated clotting is complemented by the action of endogenous anticoagulants, such as tissue factor pathway inhibitor (TFPI), activated protein C (APC), protein Z–dependent protease inhibitor (ZPI), and antithrombin (AT). TFPI rapidly deactivates circulating Xa, which may have diffused away from the TF/VIIa prothrombinase complex. APC, with its co-factor protein S (PS), inactivates Factors VIIIa and Va. ZPI inhibits Factor XIa, and with its co-factor protein Z (PZ), also efficiently inhibits Factor Xa. Lastly, AT, the most potent inhibitor of both Factor Xa and thrombin, binds to endothelial surface heparanoids to enable a greater than 1000-fold inactivation of thrombin.[7] Disorders involving endogenous anticoagulants result in thrombophilias (see Table 41–1).

TABLE 41–1

Disorders of Coagulation Cascade

Disorders of Platelet Plug Formation
- Mutations in vWF receptors (von Willebrand's disease)
- Mutations in platelets receptors (Bernard-Soulier or Glanzmann thrombasthenia)
- Mutations in platelet α-granule proteins (gray platelet syndrome)
- Mutations in dense-granule proteins (Wiskott-Aldrich, Chediak-Higashi, Hermansky-Pudlak, and thrombocytopenia-absent radius syndromes)
- COX-1–mediated inhibition of TXA_2 (nonsteroidal anti-inflammatory drugs)

Disorders of Fibrin Plug Formation
- Factor VIII deficiency (hemophilia)

Disorders of Endogenous Anticoagulant
- APC resistance/Factor V Leiden
- Protein Z deficiency
- AT deficiency

Disorders of Fibrinolysis
- PAI-1 overexpression

APC, activated protein C; AT, antithrombin; COX-1, cyclooxygenase-1; PAI-1, plasminogen activator inhibitor-1; TXA_2, thromboxane A_2; vWF, von Willebrand's factor.

Fibrinolysis

Restoration of the vasculature to its normal state is enabled by fibrinolysis. Fibrinolysis occurs when plasmin degrades cross-linked fibrin polymers to form fibrin degradation products (FDPs).[8] Plasmin is derived from plasminogen via proteolysis by tissue-type plasminogen activator (tPA) and is embedded within the fibrin clot.

As with all systems of checks and balances in the hemostatic system, fibrinolysis is further regulated by a series of inhibitors, including α_2-plasmin inhibitor, plasminogen activator inhibitor-1 (PAI-1), and thrombin-activatable fibrinolysis inhibitor (TAFI). PAI-1 is an inhibitor of tPA and released by platelets and endothelial cells in response to thrombin binding to protease-activated receptors.[9] PAI-1 bound to vitronectin and heparin inhibits thrombin and Factor Xa activity.[10] Overexpression of PAI-1 results in hypercoagulability (see Table 41–1).

EFFECTS OF PREGNANCY ON HEMOSTASIS

Virchow's classic triad of stasis, vascular trauma, and hypercoagulability all occur naturally in pregnancy. Estrogen augments G-protein receptor coupling and drives endothelium-derived nitric oxide production, resulting in vessel dilation and increasing deep vascular capacitance. Venous stasis is further exacerbated by positional obstruction of the lower

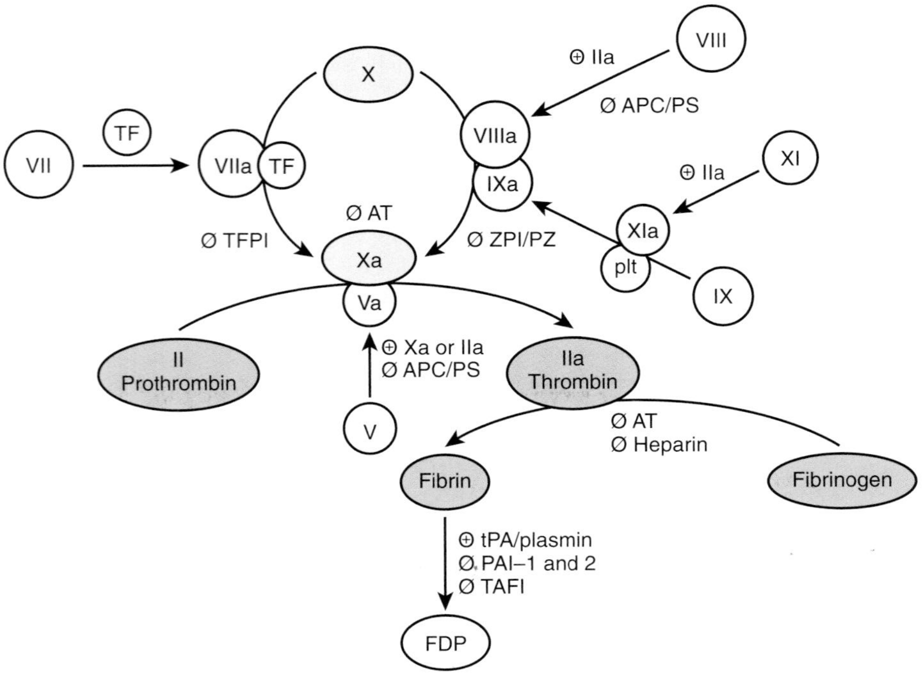

FIGURE 41–1
Hemostatic, thrombotic, and fibrinolytic pathways. Ø, inhibitory effect; ⊕, stimulatory effect.
(From Gabbe SG, Niebyl JR, Simpson JL, et al [eds]: Obstetrics: Normal and Problem Pregnancies, 5th ed. Philadelphia, Churchill Livingstone, 2007.)

extremity vasculature by the enlarging uterus.[11,12] Endothelial damage frequently occurs peripartum, especially when associated with cesarean delivery, hypertension, tobacco use, and infections.

The hypercoagulable state results from changes in the coagulation cascade including

- Increases by 20% to 1000% in fibrinogen, vWF, Factors II, VII, VIII, IX, and X levels.[13]
- Decreases by 60% to 70% in level of PS. Levels nadir at delivery due to hormonally induced increases in levels of the PS carrier protein, complement 4B-binding protein.[14–17]
- Progressive increases in resistance to APC.[18]
- Increases in the levels of antifibrinolytic PAI-1 and PAI-2.[19,20]
- Progressive platelet activation.

HYPERCOAGULABLE DISORDERS

Acquired Thrombophilia

Antiphospholipid antibody syndrome (APAS) is an autoimmune disorder of coagulation that predisposes to clot formation. Anionic phospholipids, such as cardiolipin and phosphatidylserine, are major components of the inner layer of cell membranes, which are exteriorized following endothelial cell perturbations. Proteins binding negatively charged phospholipids such as β_2-glycoprotein-I (β_2GPI) alter their tertiary shape and become neoantigens that are then targeted by the immune system. More than half of the patients with antiphospholipid antibodies have secondary APAS, which is defined by the presence of an underlying disorder, such as systemic lupus erythematosus (SLE).

The multiple pathways by which antiphospholipid antibodies induce a thrombophilia include

- Direct inhibition of the anticoagulant effects of anionic phospholipids-binding proteins such as β_2GPI and annexin V.[21,22]
- Inhibition of thrombomodulin, APC, and AT activity.
- Induction of tissue factor, PAI-1, and vWF expression in endothelial cells.
- Augmentation of platelet activation.
- Induction of complement activation.[23]

Diagnosis

The diagnostic criteria for APAS have evolved through debate in the expert community. The original Sapporo classification from 1999[24] was revised during a recent international consensus conference in 2006.[25] The requirement for one clinical criterion and one laboratory criterion has allowed for uniformity in diagnosis.

CLINICAL CRITERIA

The diagnosis of APAS requires one clinical criterion, which may be either related to an adverse pregnancy outcome (APO) or a nonobstetric thrombotic event.

Obstetric Outcomes

1. History of *three* unexplained consecutive spontaneous abortions at 10 weeks' or less gestational age (GA), or
2. History of unexplained fetal death of 10 weeks' or later GA (morphologically and karyotypically normal), or
3. History of preterm delivery at less than 34 weeks' GA, as a sequelae of preeclampsia or uteroplacental dysfunction, including the following:
   - Non-reassuring fetal testing indicative of fetal hypoxemia (e.g., abnormal Doppler flow velocimetry waveform).
   - Oligohydramnios (amniotic fluid index ≤5 cm).
   - Intrauterine growth restriction (IUGR) below the 10th percentile.
   - Placental abruption.

Nonobstetric Outcomes

Thrombosis in any tissue, diagnosed by objective, validated criteria, such as diagnostic imaging or histopathologic diagnosis.

1. Arterial thrombosis including cerebrovascular accidents, transient ischemic attacks, myocardial infarction, amaurosis fugax.
2. Venous thromboembolism (VTE) including deep venous thrombosis (DVT), pulmonary emboli (PE), or small vessel thrombosis.

LABORATORY CRITERIA

Positive testing for antiphospholipid antibodies is required on two occasions, at least 12 weeks apart, and no more than 5 years prior to clinical manifestations. Any of the three following tests can be utilized to fulfill the criteria:

1. **Anticardiolipin antibody** (ACA) immunoglobulin G (IgG) or IgM isotype, present in medium or high titers (i.e., >40 GPL or MPL, or >99th percentile), or
2. **Anti-β_2GPI antibody** IgG or IgM isotype (>99th percentile), or
3. Presence of **lupus anticoagulant** (LA) in plasma. It is important to recognize that LA is a misnomer that arises from its in vitro ability to prolong phospholipid-dependent coagulation tests, despite its in vivo thrombogenic properties. One common test used is the dilute Russell viper venom time (dRVVT), which utilizes the coagulant properties of the snake venom to activate Factor X and promote thrombin production. The presence of LA will prolong the clotting time.

Maternal and Fetal Risks

THROMBOSIS

Thrombotic outcomes vary depending on the qualifying criteria used to verify the diagnosis of APAS. The presence of ACAs alone entails a lower risk than positive LA, which signifies the presence of downstream effects of these antibodies on prothrombin activation. In a meta-analysis of more than 7000 patients, LA yields an odds ratio (OR) for arterial thrombosis of 8.6 to 10.8 and 4.1 to 16.2 for venous thrombosis.[26] The presence of ACA yields an OR for arterial thrombosis of 1 to 18 and a lower OR for venous thrombosis of 1 to 2.5.

In patients with APAS secondary to SLE, the risk of VTE has been similarly computed from a meta-analysis of 18 studies. ACA carrier status is associated with ORs of 2.50 (95% confidence interval [CI] 1.51–4.14) for acute VTE and 3.91 (95% CI 1.14–13.38) for recurrent VTE, whereas LA-positive status again carries higher ORs of 6.32 (95% CI

3.71–10.78) for VTE and 11.6 (95% CI 3.65–36.91) for recurrent VTE.[27]

ADVERSE PREGNANCY OUTCOMES

The diagnostic criteria for APAS include pregnancy complications that occur from conception through the third trimester. Here, we review the effects of APAS on subsequent pregnancies in a similar, chronologic fashion.

Despite its inclusion as a diagnostic criterion, there is much debate regarding the association of APAS with recurrent pregnancy loss (RPL) prior to 10 weeks' GA. The effect of APAS on pregnancy loss is clearer after the establishment of embryonic cardiac activity. More than 50% of pregnancy losses in patients with APAS occur after 10 weeks' GA.[28] Fetal heart activity was seen prior to fetal death in 86% of women with APAS, compared with only 43% of women without APAS ($P < .01$).[29] Furthermore, there was no significant association between APAS and clinical pregnancy rates (OR 0.99; 95% CI 0.64–1.53) or live birth (OR 1.07; 95% CI 0.66–1.75) in a meta-analysis of seven studies of women undergoing in vitro fertilization (IVF).[30] Finally, treatment of APAS patients does not appear to improve IVF outcomes.[31]

The data on fetal loss after the first trimester are more convincing. In a meta-analysis of 25 studies, LA was associated with late fetal loss with a pooled OR of 7.79 (95% CI 2.30–26.45), whereas moderate to high titers of LA yielded an OR of 4.68 (95% CI 2.96–7.40).[32]

In the second and third trimesters, APAS may manifest as IUGR and/or preeclampsia. The reported frequency of IUGR in APAS ranges from 11.7% to 31%.[33,34] A systematic review of APAS and preeclampsia revealed an OR of 2.73 (95% CI 1.65–4.51) for ACL, and 1.45 (95% CI 0.70–4.61) for LA. The association appears stronger for early-onset, recurrent severe preeclampsia compared with mild, near-term preeclampsia.[35]

The concern for thrombosis in APAS patients is heightened in the setting of pregnancy, given its inherent hypercoagulable state. In one report, more than half of the thrombotic episodes in patients with APS occurred in relation to pregnancy or the use of the combined oral contraceptive pill.[36] Some studies report a significant proportion of patients still have thrombotic episodes, even with medical and mechanical thromboprophylaxis.[34]

A rare but life-threatening variant of APAS with thrombosis is the catastrophic antiphospholipid syndrome (CAPS), characterized by multiple thromboses that lead to multiorgan failure. CAPS can be triggered by infection, trauma, surgery, anticoagulation withdrawal, or flares of underlying autoimmune processes. In a registry-based case series, 43% of CAPS in pregnancy occurred during the puerperium and 46% resulted in maternal mortality.[37]

APAS may affect a pregnancy beyond parturition secondary to the transplacental passage of antibodies. Neonatal antiphospholipid syndrome is a rare clinical condition that can cause neonatal thrombocytopenia, livedo reticularis, effusions, and thrombosis. Only a few cases have been described in the literature.[38]

Management Options

Management of APAS in pregnancy is directed at prevention of maternal and fetal adverse outcomes. Chapter 43 contains a detailed description of the treatment options for APAS.

Inheritable Thrombophilia

Background

Inherited thrombophilias predispose pregnant patients to various morbidities, including VTE, fetal loss, and placental abruption.[39–41] The following mutations are most common: APC resistance (most commonly caused by the Factor V Leiden [FVL] mutation), prothrombin G20210A mutation heterozygosity, hyperhomocysteinemia (most commonly associated with homozygosity for the methylenetetrahydrofolate reductase [MTHFR] mutation), and PAI gene 4G/4G polymorphism homozygosity. Rarer causes of inherited thrombophilias include AT deficiency, PS deficiency, protein C (PC) deficiency, and PZ deficiency (Table 41–2).

Factor V Leiden and Activated Protein C Resistance

MUTATION

FVL refers to a guanine to adenine point mutation at nucleotide 1691 on chromosome 1q23, resulting in the replacement of arginine by glutamine at position 506. The mutated Factor V is resistant to APC cleavage at position 506 and, therefore, retains its procoagulant activities while concealing the anticoagulant function.[42] The mutation is inherited in an autosomal dominant fashion.[43] Screening is done by assessing APC resistance, followed by genotyping for the FVL mutation if APC resistance is found.

FREQUENCY OF MUTATION

Homozygosity is present in 5% to 9% of the European population, 3% of African Americans, and 2.1% of Native American, but is virtually absent in African blacks and Asian populations. FVL is the most common heritable thrombophilia, accounting for 40% to 50% of cases of VTE in pregnancy.[44,45]

MATERNAL AND FETAL RISKS

Thrombotic Effects of Mutation

FVL heterozygosity confers a 5- to 10-fold increased risk of VTE, whereas homozygosity confers a greater than 25-fold increased risk of VTE.[46] Although FVL is present in 40% of pregnant patients with VTE, the estimated risk of VTE among heterozygous pregnant women without a personal or family history of thrombosis is only 1.5%, given the overall incidence of thrombosis in pregnancy (1 in 1400) and the high incidence of the mutation in the European-derived population.[41] The risk may be as high as 17% among pregnant women with a personal or strong family VTE history.[47] However, the applicability of such studies remains unclear because there were no differences in adverse outcomes between FVL carriers and noncarriers in a multicenter, prospective observational study of 134 FVL mutation carriers among 4885 gravidas.[48] Universal screening for FVL is not recommended at this time.

Fetal Loss

Several studies report strong associations between FVL and second- and/or third-trimester fetal loss, but not with early first-trimester losses.

TABLE 41-2

Inherited Thrombophilias and Their Association with Venous Thromboembolism in Pregnancy

TYPE	PREVALENCE IN EUROPEAN POPULATION (%)	PREVALENCE IN PATIENTS WITH VTE IN PREGNANCY	RR/OR OF VTE IN PREGNANCY (95% CI)	PROBABILITY OF VTE IN PREGNANCY WITH HISTORY (%)*	PROBABILITY OF VTE IN PREGNANCY WITHOUT HISTORY (%)*	REFERENCES
High Risk						41,47,69,97, 103,181-188
FVL homozygous	0.07	<1	25.4 (8.8-66)	>10	1.5	
PGM homozygous	0.02	<1	N/A	>10	2.8	
AT III deficiency	0.02-1.1	1-8	119	11-40	3.0-7.2	
FVL/PGM compound heterozygous	0.17	<1	84 (19-369)	4.7 (COMBINED RISK)		
Low Risk						
FVL heterozygous	5.3	44	6.9 (3.3-15.2)	>10	0.26	
PGM heterozygous	2.9	17	9.5 (2.1-66.7)	>10	0.37-0.5	
PC deficiency	0.2-0.3	<14	13.0 (1.1-123)		0.8-1.7	
PS deficiency	0.03-0.13	12.4			<1-6.6	
Hyperhomocysteinemia	<5		6.1 (1.3-28.4)			

* History of personal history of VTE or first degree relative with history of VTE.
AT III, antithrombin III; CI, confidence interval; FVL, Factor V Leiden; N/A, not available; OR, odds ratio; PC, protein C; PGM, prothrombin G mutation; PS, protein S; RR, risk ratio; VTE, venous thromboembolism.

- Roque and coworkers[49] evaluated 491 patients in a retrospective cohort study with a history of various APO and concluded that FVL carrier status was paradoxically protective against losses at less than 10 weeks with an OR of 0.23 (95% CI 0.07–0.77), but significantly associated with losses at greater than 14 weeks with an OR of 3.71 (95% CI 1.68–8.23).
- This protective effect of FVL on early pregnancy is also seen within the IVF population, where implantation rates were substantially higher among FVL carriers than among noncarriers (90% vs. 49%; *P* = .02).[50]
- In a meta-analysis of 31 studies in 2003, FVL was associated with early (<13 wk) pregnancy loss with an OR of 2.01 (95% CI 1.13–3.58), but was more strongly associated with late (>19 wk) fetal loss with an OR of 3.26 (95% CI 1.82–5.83).[51]
- In another meta-analysis of 54 case-control or cohort studies in 2004, pooled OR for association with first-trimester fetal loss with FVL was heterogeneous (*P* = .06) and no dose-response curve could be found. For second- and third-trimester fetal loss, there was a consistent and graded increase in risk, with isolated third-trimester fetal loss having an OR of 2.4 (95% CI 1.1–5.2), and recurrent second- and/or third-trimester fetal loss having an increased OR of 10.7 (95% CI 4.0–28.5).[52]
- In a French study, using a nested case-control group of 4396 pairs from a large cohort of 32,700 patients, multivariate analysis revealed an association between FVL and pregnancy loss after 10 weeks with an OR of 3.46 (95% CI 2.53–4.72), but not for losses occurring between 3 and 9 weeks.[53]
- A large European retrospective cohort involving 1524 pregnancies from 571 women with thrombophilia, compared with 1019 pregnancies from 395 controls, found a trend toward stillbirth for patients with FVL (OR 2.0; 95% CI 0.5–7.7), but no association with spontaneous abortion (OR 0.9; 95% CI 0.5–1.5).[54]

Preeclampsia

The link between FVL and preeclampsia is even more controversial. Overall, there is not sufficient evidence to conclude that FVL is associated with an increased occurrence of preeclampsia, though there is inadequate power to rule out an association between this thrombophilia and severe, early-onset preeclampsia.

- A prospective observational study in 1999 noted a link between FVL and severe preeclampsia in 110 women with APO (OR 5.3; 95% CI 1.8–15.6).[55] However, multiple subsequent case-control studies have failed to find a link between FVL and moderate to severe preeclampsia.[56–58]
- Dudding and Attia's meta-analysis[52] estimated a 2.9-fold (95% CI 2.0–4.3) increased risk of severe preeclampsia among FVL carriers.
- Lin and August[59] conducted a meta-analysis including 31 studies with 7522 patients. FVL associated with any preeclampsia had an OR of 1.81 (95% CI 1.14–2.87) and with severe preeclampsia with an OR of 2.24 (95% CI 1.28–3.94).
- Kosmas and colleagues[60] observed that studies performed before 2000 reported a modest association between FVL and preeclampsia (OR 3.16; 95% CI 2.04–4.92), whereas those published after 2000 did not (OR 0.97; 95% CI 0.61–1.54). A reporting bias appears to be present after the discovery of the mutation in the early 1990s, which may have since dissipated.
- A more recent meta-analysis in 2008 again revealed a significant but weak association with preeclampsia (pooled OR 1.49; 95% CI 1.13-1.96).[61]
- In 2009, the Montreal Preeclampsia Study[62] reviewed 113 preeclamptic patients from a cohort of 5162 patients, compared with 443 control subjects. This case-control study did not find an increased risk of preeclampsia, including early-onset or severe preeclampsia, in association with maternal FVL mutation.

- A risk of recurrent preeclampsia was found in 59% of patients with FVL mutation versus 25.9% of patients without thrombophilia in an Italian prospective cohort study published in 2009 involving 172 patients with a prior history of preeclampsia.[63]

Abruption

There may be an association between FVL and placental abruption.

- Kupferminc and associates[55] reported a modest association between FVL and abruption with an OR of 4.9 (95% CI 1.4–17.4).
- Procházka and coworkers[64] conducted a retrospective case-control study among 102 women with placental abruption and 2371 controls. The increase in FVL carriers among affected patients compared with controls, with an OR of 1.5 (95% CI 0.9–2.7), did not reach significance. However, in 2007, the same group[65] retrospectively reviewed 180 women with placental abruption and 196 controls, and this time noted a significantly increased carrier rate for FVL compared with controls, with an OR of 3.0 (95% CI 1.4–6.7).
- Alfirevic and colleagues[66] conducted a systematic review and reported a strong association between placental abruption and homozygosity for FVL, with an OR of 16.9 (95% CI 2.0–141.9). A milder, but statistically significant, association was also seen for FVL heterozygosity, with an OR of 6.7 (95% CI 2.0–21.6).
- The prospective, observational, nested carrier-control analysis from the National Institute of Child Health and Human Development (NICHHD) in 2005[48] revealed no difference between FVL carriers and noncarriers in development of abruption, but the study was underpowered for this observation.

Intrauterine Growth Restriction

There is no consistent evidence for an association between FVL and IUGR.

- Martinelli and associates[67] noted an association between FVL and IUGR, with an OR of 6.9 (95% CI 1.4–33.5).
- However, multiple large case-control and cohort studies have reported no statistically significant association between FVL and IUGR less than the 10th and less than the 5th percentiles.[55,58,68]
- A systematic review by Howley and coworkers[69] analyzed 10 case-control studies and 5 cohort studies. The case-control studies showed a significant association between FVL and IUGR, with a pooled OR of 2.7 (95% CI 1.3–5.5), whereas the cohort studies (2 prospective and 3 retrospective) showed no association (summative relative risk [RR] 0.99; 95% CI 0.5–1.9). This discrepancy highlights differences in studies based on design may account for many of the conflicts in the field. As a rule, the better the study, the weaker the association.
- The recent meta-analysis in 2008 by Dudding and colleagues[61] failed to identify an association with IUGR, yielding a pooled OR of 1.15 (95% CI 0.95–1.39).

Conclusions Based on Current Literature

Because it is the most common inheritable thrombophilia, there has been debate regarding the effect of FVL on various APOs. There is a positive association between FVL and fetal loss after 10 weeks, with a particularly strong association after 22 weeks. There is also probably an association with abruption. There is no association between FVL and early first-trimester embryonic loss, preeclampsia, or IUGR. Given its prevalence, we do not recommend routine FVL testing as a part of work-up for APO without a history of maternal VTE.

Prothrombin Gene Mutation

MUTATION

The G20210A polymorphism for prothrombin is a point mutation causing a guanine to adenine switch at nucleotide position 20210 in the 3′-untranslated region of the gene at chromosome 11p11-q12.[70] The switch results in increased translation and circulating levels of prothrombin. Other prothrombin gene mutations (PGMs) have been described (e.g., C20209T and A19911G), but literature is sparse regarding their effects.

FREQUENCY OF MUTATION

PGM is less prevalent than FVL and is present in only 2% to 3% of the European population, with the preponderance in southern Europeans.[41] The mutation is exceedingly rare in the black or Asian populations.[71]

MATERNAL AND FETAL RISKS

Thrombotic Effects of Mutation

PGM accounts for 13% to 17% of women with an initial VTE. However, because of the overall low incidence of VTE in pregnancy, the actual risk of clotting in a PGM mutation carrier is 0.5%. Homozygous patients without a personal or strong family history of a VTE have a 2.8% risk for VTE in pregnancy, whereas a positive history confers around a 20% risk in pregnancy. Compound heterozygosity for FVL and PGM results in a 4.6% risk of VTE, even in the absence of a strong family history.[41,72]

Fetal Loss

Analogous to FVL, the association between PGM and pregnancy loss may increase with increasing GA.

- One case-control study reported the presence of the PGM in 9% of recurrent miscarriage patients versus 2% of controls, yielding an OR of 4.7 (95% CI 0.9–23).[73] Finan and associates[74] also noted an association between PGM and recurrent abortion, OR of 5.05 (95% CI 1.14–23.2).
- Other studies failed to identify a link. Carp and coworkers[75] could detect no statistically significant association between PGM and pregnancy loss in a case-control study. Jivraj and colleagues[76] reached similar conclusions in a European white cohort.
- A 2003 meta-analysis of PGM reported an increased risk of recurrent first-trimester loss (OR 2.3; 95% CI 1.1–4.8), fetal loss prior to 28 weeks (OR 2.6; 95% CI 1.0–6.3), and late nonrecurrent fetal loss (OR 2.3; 95% CI 1.1–4.9).[51]
- A 2004 meta-analysis of seven studies evaluating the link between PGM and RPL, defined as 2 or more pregnancy losses in the first or second trimester, found a combined OR of 2.0 (95% CI 1.0–4.0).[77]

- Silver and coworkers, representing the NICHD MFM Unit network, performed a secondary analysis of the FVL study,[78] in patients who were also tested for the PGM polymorphism. They found no association between PGM and any APO in low-risk women without a history of VTE.

Preeclampsia

Multiple studies have failed to establish a link between PGM and either preeclampsia or severe preeclampsia.

- A small case-control study revealed a 5.2% carrier rate for PGM in women with preeclampsia, compared with 4.1% (P = .76) in controls.[58]
- A meta-analysis including 31 studies with 7522 patients by Lin and August[59] observed a pooled OR for PGM and all preeclampsia was 1.37 (95% CI 0.72–2.57) and 1.98 (95% CI 0.94–4.17) for severe preeclampsia.
- Morrison and associates[79] compared 404 women with preeclampsia to gestational hypertensive and healthy controls and found no association between preeclampsia and PGM. Livingston and coworkers[80] performed a prospective cross-sectional study and found no differences of PGM carrier rate between patients with severe preeclampsia and controls (0% vs. 1.1%, P = .92). Similarly, in a 2007 case-control study by Larciprete and colleagues,[81] there was no association between PGM and preeclampsia.
- The Montreal Preeclampsia Study[62] reviewed 113 preeclamptic patients from a cohort of 5162 patients, compared with 443 control subjects in 2009. This case-control study did not find an increased risk of preeclampsia, including early-onset or severe preeclampsia, in association with maternal PGM.

Abruption

There is likely no association between PGM and abruption.

- The case-control study of Kupferminc and associates[55] observed an association between PGM and abruption (OR 8.9; 95% CI 1.8–43.6).
- Procházka and associates noted in the 2003 retrospective case-control study[64] an association between PGM and abruption, OR of 8.9 (95% CI 1.8–43.6).
- The systematic review by Alfirevic and colleagues in 2002[66] also suggests a link between PGM heterozygosity and placental abruption, with an OR of 28.9 (95% CI 3.5–236.7).

Intrauterine Growth Restriction

There is also likely no association between PGM and IUGR.

- Kupferminc and associates[55] found an association between PGM and IUGR (<5th percentile), OR 4.6 (95% CI 1–20). Martinelli and colleagues[66] also noted an association, OR 5.9 (95% CI 1.2–29.4).
- In contrast, the large case-control study of Infante-Rivard and coworkers[68] could identify no link between heterozygotes for PGM and IUGR (OR 0.92; 95% CI 0.36–2.35). Franchi and colleagues[82] and Verspych and associates[83] concluded similarly.
- Facco and coworkers reported in a 2009 meta-analysis[84] that the association between PGM and IUGR was not significant (OR 1.52; 95% CI 0.98–2.35).

Conclusion Based on Current Literature

Uncertainty exists regarding the putative role of PGM in the genesis of APO. We do not recommend PGM testing as a routine part of work-up for APO without a history of maternal VTE.

Hyperhomocysteinemia

MUTATION

Homozygosity for mutations in the MTHFR gene on chromosome 1p36.3, such as C677T and A1298C polymorphisms, is the most common cause of hyperhomocysteinemia. C677T is a thermolabile variant that causes mild enzymatic dysfunction and mild hyperhomocysteinemia in folate-deficient patients. The A1298C mutation alone does not cause hyperhomocysteinemia, but compound heterzogysity of A1298C/C677T may induce a biochemical profile similar to C677T homozygosity.[85]

FREQUENCY OF MUTATION

Homozygosity for the MTHFR C677T and A1298C polymorphisms is present in 10% to 16% and 4% to 6% of all Europeans, respectively.[86] Allele frequency is 7% in sub-Saharan African and 34% in Japanese populations. Little data are available for other populations.[84] Clinical sequelae are rare in the United States because of folate fortification of grains, which has resulted in decreased national homocysteine levels, which are then further decreased by physiologic changes of pregnancy. It is not appropriate to screen by testing for the presence of an MTHFR mutation, which is the second step after first identifying hyperhomocysteinemia. Screening for this disorder in pregnancy should use a cutoff of greater than 12 µmol/L.

MATERNAL AND FETAL RISKS

Thrombotic Effects of Mutation

Hyperhomocysteinemia is a risk factor for VTE with an OR of 2.5 (95% CI 1.8–3.5).[87] Isolated MTHFR mutations without hyperhomocysteinemia do not convey an increased risk for VTE in either nonpregnant[88] or pregnant women.[89] This finding was confirmed in 2008 in a large population-based study of 66,140 individuals from Norway in whom there was no association between VTE and isolated MTHFR mutation in women.

Fetal Loss

As with thrombotic risk, elevated fasting homocysteinemia is associated with RPL rather than isolated MTHFR mutation.

- A meta-analysis by Nelen and colleagues in 2000[90] calculated pooled risk estimates for fetal loss at less than 16 weeks of 2.7 (95% CI 1.4–5.2) for hyperhomocysteinemia and 1.4 (95% CI 1.0–2.0) for isolated MTHFR mutation.
- In a review of 14,492 pregnancy outcomes, the Hordaland Homocysteine Study[91,92] concluded there was an association of elevated homocysteine with stillbirth (OR 2.03; 95% CI 0.98–4.21), though this did not reach statistical significance.

Preeclampsia

There is no clear association between hyperhomocysteinemia or isolated MTHFR mutation and preeclampsia.

- In a case-control study of various polymorphisms of MTHFR, there was no association identified between MTHFR mutation and preeclampsia.[93] The Hordaland Homocysteine Study[91,92] reached a similar conclusion (OR 1.32; 95% CI 0.98–1.77).
- Induced hyperhomocysteinemia is not sufficient to induce a preeclamptic state in the mouse.[94]

Abruption

There is an association between hyperhomocysteinemia and placental abruption, but not with isolated MTHFR mutation.

- In a 2007 case-control study from the New Jersey-Placental Abruption group,[95] neither homozygosity for C677CT (OR 0.60; 95% CI 0.33–1.18) nor A1298C (OR 2.28; 95% CI 0.82–6.35) was associated with placental abruption.
- The Hordaland Study[91,92] observed a clear association between abruption and homocysteine greater than 15 μmol/L (OR 3.13; 95% CI 1.63–6.03); a weaker but significant association was observed between C677T homozygosity and abruption (OR 1.6, 95% CI 1.4–4.8).
- A meta-analysis confirmed the previous finding, with hyperhomocysteinemia yielding a stronger pooled OR for abruption of 5.3 (95% CI 1.8–15.9) than MTHFR mutation homozygosity (OR 2.3; 95% CI 1.1–4.9).[96]

Intrauterine Growth Restriction

A weak association may be present between hyperhomocysteinemia and IUGR, but this may reflect publication bias.

- The Hordaland Study[91,92] showed an association between elevated homocysteine and very low birth weight (OR 2.01; 95% CI 1.23–3.27).
- In a 2009 meta-analysis of case-control studies, Facco and coworkers[84] reported that the association between MTHFR mutation and IUGR was not significant (OR 1.01, 95% CI 0.88–1.17), but was significant for the case-control studies (OR 1.35, 95% CI 1.04–1.75). A funnel-plot analysis of the case-control studies suggests publication bias.

Conclusion Based on Current Literature

Studies strongly suggest that hyperhomocysteinemia, not isolated MTHFR mutations, is linked to VTE and APO. There is a positive association between hyperhomocysteinemia and abruption. There may be a weak association with IUGR and fetal loss. There is no association between hyperhomocysteinemia and preeclampsia. Additional risks include fetal neural tube defects, with C677T heterozygosity yielding an OR of 1.52 (95% CI 1.16–2.00) and homozygosity yielding an OR of 2.56 (95% CI 1.75–3.74).[97]

Protein C Deficiency

MUTATION

Deficiencies of PC result from over 160 distinct autosomal dominant mutations, producing a highly variable phenotype. Two primary types are recognized: (1) type I, with reduced antigen and activity levels and (2) type II, with normal levels but reduced activity. Most laboratories use activity levels below 50% to 60% as abnormal.

FREQUENCY OF MUTATION

PC deficiencies occur with a frequency of 0.2% to 0.5% in the general population.[98]

MATERNAL AND FETAL RISKS

Thrombotic Effects of Mutation

PC deficiency carries a less than 2% to 8% risk of VTE during the antepartum period, a 10% to 20% risk in the puerperium, and accounts for 10% to 25% of all VTEs in pregnancy.[99] RR for VTE is reported as 6.5 to 12.5.[69]

Fetal Loss

There is no clear association between PC deficiency and miscarriage, but there may be an association with stillbirth.

- In a 1996 study, loss rates were 28% for PC deficiency, compared with the control group, which had a loss rate of 11%.[54]
- Preston and associates[54] reported the risk of miscarriage does not appear increased with PC deficiency (OR 1.4; 95% CI 0.9–2.2), and although the risk of stillbirth seemed modestly increased, it did not reach statistical significance (adjusted OR 2.3; 95% CI 0.6–8.3).
- In contrast, Alfirevic and colleagues[66] found no association of PC deficiency with stillbirth in a meta-analysis. Saade and McLintock[101] also failed to find an association between PC deficiency and late fetal loss, with adjusted an OR of 1.22 (95% CI 0.09–15).

Preeclampsia

A limited number of studies note a strong association between PC deficiency and preeclampsia.

- Roque and coworkers[49] reported a strong association between PC deficiency and preeclampsia in a retrospective cohort study (OR 6.85; 95% CI 1.09–43.2). A meta-analysis also concluded there was a strong association (OR 21.5; 95% CI 1.1–414.4).[65]

Abruption

There is a paucity of literature on the potential relationship between PC deficiency and abruption.

- Roque and coworkers[49] observed a strong association between PC deficiency and abruption (OR 13.9; 95% CI 2.21–86.9).

Intrauterine Growth Restriction

There are no reports on the association of PC deficiency with IUGR.

Conclusion Based on Current Literature

There is a positive association between PC deficiency and preeclampsia, and perhaps a weaker association with IUGR (very limited data). There is no clear association between PC deficiency and early miscarriage. There are insufficient data to evaluate the relationship between PC deficiency and abruption or IUGR. It is worth noting that neonatal purpura fulminans may occur with PC deficiency.[102,103]

Protein S Deficiency

MUTATION

Over 130 mutations have been linked to PS deficiency.[69] Two major phenotypes of PS deficiency exist: (1) type I, with low total and free PS antigen levels, and (2) type IIb, with low free PS levels due to enhanced binding to the complement 4B–binding protein. Type IIb phenotype is frequently caused by a serine to proline mutation (PS Heerlen), which is also associated with either FVL or PC mutation in about half the patients, suggesting a synergistic effect.[104]

PS activity assay is associated with substantial inter-assay and intra-assay variability, due in part to frequently changing physiologic levels of complement 4B–binding protein.[105] Paidas and coworkers[106] noted far lower levels in normal pregnancy, suggesting the cutoffs for free PS levels in the second and third trimester of 38.9% ± 10.3% and 31.2% ± 7.4%, respectively.

FREQUENCY OF MUTATION

The prevalence of true PS deficiency is low (0.03%–0.13%).[69,104]

MATERNAL AND FETAL RISKS

Thrombotic Effects of Mutation

The degree of thrombogenicity is modest (OR 2.4; CI 0.8–7.9). Among those with a strong family history, the risk of VTE in pregnancy is 6.6%.[98]

Fetal Loss

There appears to be an association between PS deficiency and fetal loss.

- One meta-analysis observed an association between PS deficiency and recurrent late fetal loss (OR 14.7; 95% CI 1.0–2181), as well as nonrecurrent fetal losses at greater than 22 weeks (OR 7.4; 95% CI 1.3–43).[51]
- A second meta-analysis suggested an even stronger link between PS deficiency and stillbirth (OR 16.2; 95% CI 5.0–52.3).[65]
- Saade and McLintock[101] also noted an association between PS deficiency and late fetal loss, with an adjusted OR of 41 (95% CI 4.8–359).
- In a 2006 systematic review, PS deficiency was associated with late pregnancy loss with an OR of 20.1 (95% CI 3.7–109).[107]

Other Adverse Pregnancy Outcomes

Alfirevic and colleagues[66] concluded after a meta-analysis that there was a link between PS deficiency and preeclampsia-eclampsia (OR 12.7; 95% CI 4–39.7) and IUGR (OR 10.2; 95% CI 1.1–91.0), but not between PS deficiency and abruption.

Conclusion Based on Current Literature

There is a positive association between PS deficiency and fetal loss. There may well be an association with preeclampsia and IUGR, but the data are too limited. There is no association was between PS deficiency and abruption. Note, neonatal purpura fulminans may occur with PS deficiency.

Antithrombin Deficiency

MUTATION

AT deficiency is an autosomal dominant condition. Over 250 mutations of the AT gene contribute to a highly variable phenotype, with three main variants.[69,108] Type I involves reductions in both antigen and activity; type II has normal antigen levels but decreased activity; and type III is a very rare homozygous deficiency associated with little or no activity. Acquired AT deficiency may result from decreased production (hepatic dysfunction), consumptive coagulopathy (disseminated intravascular coagulation [DIC]), or increased excretion (nephrotic syndrome). The laboratory cutoff of 50% function is used.

FREQUENCY OF MUTATION

AT deficiency is the rarest of the heritable thrombophilias, with prevalence from 0.02% to 1.1%.[108]

MATERNAL AND FETAL RISKS

Thrombotic Effects of Mutation

AT deficiency confers the highest thrombogenic risk of the heritable thrombophilias, with a 25-fold increase in the nonpregnant state.[108] However, only 1% to 8% of VTE is due to AT deficiency owing to its low prevalence.[69] Thromboembolism during the antepartum period occurs at a range of 12% to 60%, and in the puerperium of 11% to 33%.[109] Risk can be further stratified based on personal or family history of thromboembolic events, with VTE developing in 3% to 7% without a history and up to 40% with a history.[71]

Obstetric Effects of Mutation

In a large retrospective cohort study, AT deficiency was associated with an increased risk of stillbirth at greater than 28 weeks (OR 5.2; 95% CI 1.5–18.1), but a far more modest association with miscarriage at less than 28 weeks (1.7; 95% CI 1.0–2.8).[54] Given its very low prevalence, there are little data linking it to other APOs. Roque and coworkers[49] observed an increased risk of IUGR (OR 12.93; 95% CI 2.72–61.45) and abruption (OR 60.01; 95% CI 12.02–300.46).

Conclusion Based on Current Literature

There is a positive association was found between AT deficiency and stillbirth after 28 weeks' GA. Possible associations exist with early stillbirth, IUGR, and abruption.

Protein Z Deficiency

MUTATION

Two nonsense mutations in the coding region of the PZ gene account for most cases of PZ deficiency. Normal PZ levels in the second trimester are 2.0 ± 0.5 μg/mL, and in the third trimester, levels are 1.9 ± 0.5 μg/mL, with a statistically significant decrease in patients with adverse outcomes.[105]

FREQUENCY OF MUTATION

Unknown.

MATERNAL AND FETAL RISKS

Thrombotic Effects of Mutation

In one study, PZ deficiency was identified in 4.4% of patients with VTE, compared with 0.8% of controls (OR 5.7; 95% CI 1.25–26.0).[110] In another study, PZ deficiency (activity < 5th percentile) was associated with strokes, but not VTE.[111] Other studies have shown that PZ deficiency influences the prothrombotic phenotype in patients with the FVL mutation.[112]

Obstetric Effects of Mutation

PZ deficiency has been linked to late fetal loss (10–16 wk' gestation) in one study (OR 6.7; 95% CI 3.1–14.8),[132] but not others.[113,114] In the presence of other thrombophilic mutations in patients with prior fetal loss, PZ deficiency may confer resistance to heparin therapy.[111]

Plasminogen Activator Inhibitor-1 Overexpression

MUTATION

Two polymorphisms, A844G and –675 4G/5G, are described in the promoter region of the PAI-1 gene on chromosome 7q21.3-22.[115] In patients homozygous for the 4G/4G allele, the presence of four instead of five consecutive guanine nucleotides in the PAI-1 promoter produces a site that is too small to allow repressors to bind. As a result, circulating PAI-1 levels are modestly increased.[116] Conversely, the A844G polymorphism affects a consensus sequence binding site for the regulatory protein Ets, thereby enhancing PAI-1 transcription. Whereas laboratory testing for the PAI-1 antigen is reliable via immunoassay, PAI-1 activity assay is best performed in a reference laboratory because variable results for PAI-1 activity are common.

FREQUENCY OF MUTATION

The prevalence of the 4G/4G genotype in the general population is high, ranging from 23.5% to 32.3%.[117,118]

MATERNAL AND FETAL RISKS

Thrombotic Effects of Mutation

Most studies have not found an association between the –675 4G/5G polymorphism and VTE.[119–121] However, the 4G/4G genotype, in conjunction with FVL or PS deficiency, has been linked to an increased risk for VTE, suggesting an additive role despite lack of independent thrombogenic activity.[122] No relationship has been identified between the A844G and VTE.[118]

Fetal Loss

There was no association between isolated homozygosity for 4G/4G and recurrent abortion in several small studies.[123,124] Glueck and colleagues[125] conducted a case-control study and observed that compared with patients with 5G/5G or 4G/5G, patients homozygous for 4G/4G had more second- and third-trimester fetal deaths (9% vs. 2%; $P = .004$). However, a larger multicenter study did not find a relationship between fetal loss and 4G/4G, though it had less than 30% power to detect a difference.[126]

Preeclampsia

Yamada and associates[127] described a modest association between 4G/4G homozygosity and severe preeclampsia (OR 1.62; 95% CI 1.02–2.57).

Intrauterine Growth Restriction

Glueck and colleagues's case-control study[125] noted that homozygous 4G/4G allele had higher rates of IUGR (4% vs. 0.4%; $P = .012$). However, caution must be exercised in the interpretation because 30% of patients homozygous for the 4G/4G mutation also had coexisting thrombophilias. In addition, affected patients generally exhibit elevated PAI-1 levels only in the presence of metabolic syndrome, which is itself a major risk factor for preeclampsia.

Conclusion Based on the Literature

The significance of derangements in PAI-1 activity, antigen, or the presence of the 4G/4G mutation remains uncertain with respect to VTE and APOs owing to limited data. Based upon available evidence, screening for PAI-1 activity, antigen, and the genetic 4G/5G mutation should be strongly discouraged in the investigation of APOs.

Management Options for Inheritable Thrombophilias

SCREENING

Patients with a personal history of VTE, a strong family history of VTE, or a history of APO may be candidates for evaluation of inheritable thrombophilias. Screening of an unselected population is not recommended.[128]

DIAGNOSIS

Laboratory testing for thrombophilia should ideally be done in the nonpregnant patient who is not receiving hormonal or anticoagulation therapy and is remote (>6 mo) from a history of VTE.[129] Testing can include APC resistance (with FVL polymerase chain reaction [PCR] for confirmation), PGM G20210A PCR, fasting homocysteine levels, AT activity, PC activity, PS activity (with consideration for normally reduced PS levels in pregnancy), and PAI-1 protein assay. Genotyping for PAI-1 4G/4G mutation and MTHFR mutation are not recommended.

TREATMENT

Prevention of Adverse Pregnancy Outcomes

Several small observational studies suggest a benefit of anticoagulation to prevent APOs in patients with various thrombophilias.[130,131] Gris and coworkers[132] randomized 160 patients with FVL, prothrombin 20210A, or PS deficiency and a history of one unexplained loss after 10 weeks to either low-dose aspirin or enoxaparin (40 mg subcutaneously daily). They observed a significant increase in liveborn rates in the enoxaparin group (86.2% vs. 28.8%; OR 1515; 95% CI 7–34). However, given the lack of consistent evidence of an association between maternal thrombophilia and recurrent early first-trimester loss (<10 wk), anticoagulant therapy does not at present appear justified.[49] Definitive recommendations await further clinical trials of anticoagulation in this population. Vitamin B_{12} and folic acid should be supplemented if hyperhomocysteinemia is diagnosed.

Prevention of Venous Thromboembolism

Women with high risk (more thrombogenic) thrombophilias (AT deficiency, FVL homozygosity, and PGM homozygosity and FVL/PGM compound heterozygosity) should be treated with full therapeutic anticoagulation during pregnancy, and for at least 6 weeks postpartum, regardless of the history. Pregnant women who have low risk (less thrombogenic) thrombophilias (FVL heterozygosity, PGM heterozygosity, PC or PS deficiency, hyperhomocysteinemia [unresponsive to folate therapy]) do not need antepartum anticoagulation if there is no personal history of VTE or affected first-degree relative.[133] However, they should receive postpartum prophylaxis if they require a cesarean delivery because most fatal pulmonary emboli occur during this period.[134] Some experts also recommend postpartum prophylaxis in the setting of vaginal delivery, and especially if the patient has an affected first-degree relative or another thrombotic risk factor (e.g., obesity or immobilization).

Prevention of Recurrent Venous Thromboembolism

Women with VTE during a current pregnancy should receive therapeutic anticoagulation for at least 4 months during the pregnancy, followed by prophylactic therapy for at least 6 weeks postpartum. Women with a history of VTE associated with nonrecurrent risk factors (e.g., surgery, orthopedic immobilization), but without acquired or inherited thrombophilia, appear to be at very low risk for a repeat event. Although anticoagulation during the antepartum period appears unnecessary in these patients, prophylaxis should be used during the higher risk postpartum period.[135]

SUMMARY OF MANAGEMENT OPTIONS

Inherited Thrombophilias

Management Options	Evidence Quality and Recommendation	References
Screening		
Screening should be considered in patients with personal history of VTE or a strong family history of VTE.	III/B	169
Population screening is not recommended.	III/B	128
Screening for inheritable thrombophilia is not recommended in patients with history of APOs.	III/B	128
Laboratory testing should include APC resistance (with FVL PCR for confirmation), PGM G20210A PCR, fasting homocysteine levels, AT activity, PC activity, PS activity, and PAI-1 protein assay.	IV/C	129
Prenatal		
Unclear benefit of treatment for a history of APO with anticoagulation.	IIa/B	172,189
Provide therapeutic heparin or low-molecular-weight heparin with VTE during pregnancy.	IV/C	134
Provide prophylactic or therapeutic heparin or low-molecular-weight heparin for a history of VTE, depending on the level of risk and recurrent features.	IV/C	133
Provide folate and vitamin B12 supplementation for hyperhomocysteinemia.	III/B	133
Intrapartum		
Reduce or stop heparin for labor and delivery; restart after 6 hr.	III/B	173
Postnatal		
Switching to warfarin postpartum is an option.	III/B	174

Essential Thrombocythemia

Essential thrombocythemia is a nonreactive chronic myeloproliferative disorder with sustained elevation of the platelet count.[136] A slight female preponderance is reported, with a overall prevalence of 2.38 patients per 100,000.[137] Proposed etiologies include increased sensitivity to cytokines and decreased inhibition of platelet inhibitory factors.

Diagnosis

Typical criteria used in the diagnosis of essential thrombocythemia include platelet count greater than 600,000/μL, megakaryocyte hyperplasia, splenomegaly, and hemorrhagic or thrombotic complications. Weight loss, sweating, low-grade fever, and pruritus may occur in up to 20% of patients. Although 40% to 50% of patients have splenomegaly and 20% have hepatomegaly, most are undetectable by physical examination and seen only on ultrasound or computed tomography. Typically, prothrombin time and activated partial thromboplastin time (aPTT) are unaffected. One fourth of patients have elevated uric acid and vitamin B_{12} levels. Levels of potassium, phosphorus, and acid phosphatase may be falsely elevated. Elevated levels of acute-phase reactant C-reactive protein, fibrinogen, and interleukin-6 suggest secondary thrombocytosis.[138]

Maternal and Fetal Risks

THROMBOSIS

Essential thrombocythemia may cause arterial or venous occlusive disease. Microvascular disease may involve transient ischemic attacks, migraine, visual dysfunction, digital ischemia, and erythromelalgia.[139,140] Arterial thrombosis may include occlusion of the lower extremity, pulmonary, coronary, or renal arteries. Venous thrombosis of the splenic, hepatic, or pelvic veins may occur.[73,141]

HEMORRHAGE

Hemorrhagic complications are seen in patients with very high platelet counts (>1,000,000/μL) and may include bruising of the skin and bleeding of the mucous membranes or digestive tract. This paradoxical effect occurs via a functional deficiency of von Willebrand's multimers.[142,143]

LEUKEMIA

The evolution of essential thrombocythemia into leukemia is rare, but the incidence may be increased by some chemotherapeutic agents.[144]

ADVERSE PREGNANCY OUTCOMES

Essential thrombocythemia in pregnancy is associated with a 50% risk of obstetric complications, including recurrent abortion, premature delivery, IUGR, and placental abruption. The proposed mechanism of pathogenesis is placental infarction.

Management Options

Some authors recommend treatment during pregnancy with aspirin or subcutaneous heparin.[145,146] Current recommendations for treatment have yet to be defined, as illustrated by a Mayo Clinic study that showed no therapeutic benefit of treatment in 18 women (34 pregnancies) with essential thrombocythemia.[147] In this study, 45% of pregnancies ended in spontaneous abortion, with no specific factors predisposing to miscarriage. Because outcomes were similar in treated versus untreated patients, anticoagulation is not recommended in asymptomatic low risk patients.

Interferon-alfa (pregnancy category C) is a cytoreductive agent that antagonizes platelet-derived growth factor and is associated with a dose-dependent reduction in platelet count. A 90% reduction in the platelet count (<600,000/μL) has been obtained after 3 months of therapy, with an average dose of 3 million IU daily. It has been used in some pregnant patients without apparent harm[148,149] and has been used successfully in those candidates who are at increased risk for thrombosis.[150]

Two pregnancy category D medications used efficaciously outside of pregnancy are hydroxyurea and busulfan.[151] Lastly, anagrelide (pregnancy category C) is a newer imidazoquinolin that causes the suppression of megakaryocytes and thus decreases platelet counts without affecting other hematopoietic cell lines. Significant complications include palpitations, tachycardia, cardiac arrhythmias, and congestive heart failure. Little is known about its use in pregnancy.[148]

SUMMARY OF MANAGEMENT OPTIONS

Essential Thrombocythemia

Management Options	Evidence Quality and Recommendation	References
Prenatal		
Provide interdisciplinary approach.	III/B	176
Use expectant approach in symptomatic patients with only moderate elevation of platelets.	III/B	176
In symptomatic patients (thrombosis or bleeding), consider plasmapheresis in first instance.	III/B	176
Provide low-dose aspirin and heparin if thrombosis occurs; evidence does not support use in all cases.	III/B	176

Management Options	Evidence Quality and Recommendation	References
Hydroxyurea has been used, but most experience is with chronic myelogenous leukemia.	III/B	151
Limited experience with interferon-alfa.	III/B	148,150
No experience with anagrelide; avoid.	III/B	149
Obtain serial fetal growth and umbilical artery Doppler velocimetry.	III/B	147,150
Labor and Delivery		
Maintain vigilance for postpartum hemorrhage.	III/B	142,143

Thrombotic Thrombocytopenic Purpura–Hemolytic-Uremic Syndrome

The classic pentad of thrombotic thrombocytopenic purpura–hemolytic uremic syndrome (TTP-HUS) consists of thrombocytopenia (<30,000/μL), microangiopathic hemolytic anemia (MAHA), fever, and neurologic and renal abnormalities, but the complete complement of findings is seen in only a minority of patients. TTP-HUS may be triggered by pregnancy, pathogenic bacterial diarrhea, autoimmune processes, drugs, HIV, malignancy, or malignant hypertension.

Most patients with TTP-HUS are women (69%), and a significant number are pregnant (25%).[152] Puerperium is the most likely period for TTP-HUS to develop. The clinical picture is often ambiguous in pregnancy, and differential diagnoses may include lupus flare, severe preeclampsia, and HELLP (hemolysis, elevated liver enzymes, and low platelets) syndrome.

Damage to the microvascular endothelial cells, leading to release of usually large von Willebrand's multimers, is the current hypothesis to explain the pathogenesis of TTP-HUS.[153,154] Typically, these large multimers are cleaved to a normal size by a plasma protease specific to vWF.[155] Accumulation of these multimers is associated with the promotion of platelet aggregation,[156] but is not specific for TTP-HUS.[157]

ADAMST13 Deficiency

Patients with TTP-HUS may have an inherited or acquired deficiency of the vWF-cleaving protease, named a disintegrin and metalloproteinase with thrombospondin type 1 (ADAMST13). Deficiencies of ADAMST13 lead to disseminated formation of platelet-rich thrombi in the microcirculation, mechanical hemolytic anemia, consumptive thrombocytopenia, and multivisceral ischemia.[158] Severe ADAMST13 deficiency is associated with TTP-HUS relapses in 37%, compared with 6% of those without severe ADAMST13 deficiency. During remission, persistently undetectable levels of ADAMST13 in patients with severe ADAMST13 deficiency have been associated with a 38% risk of relapse, compared with a 5% risk with detectable levels.

False positives, with less pronounced reductions in ADAMST13 levels, can be seen in patients with DIC, isoimmune thrombocytic purpura, severe sepsis, SLE, cirrhosis, and heparin-induced thrombocytopenia, and even in patients without disease. In pregnancy, these protease levels decline with advancing gestation. Thus, an asymptomatic pregnant patient with decreased baseline levels of cleaving protease may not manifest with TTP-HUS until late gestation.[159]

Diagnosis and Maternal and Fetal Risks

Classically, the diagnosis of TTP-HUS was made only if the patient had the classic pentad of signs and symptoms as described previously. Because of the ability of plasma exchange to improve the survival rate from less than 10% to approximately 80%, the diagnostic criteria have been eased.[160,161] Thrombocytopenia coupled with MAHA without an alternative diagnosis is sufficient to define TTP-HUS and possibly begin plasma exchange. Abdominal pain is another common symptom, including pain, nausea, diarrhea, and vomiting. In contrast, seizures, fever with chills, and extensive purpura suggest an alternative diagnosis.[162] Recently, a characteristic placental feature, called the "snowman sign" has been described in placentas of patients with TTP, referring to alternating zones of vascular dilation and constriction.[163]

Preeclampsia/HELLP syndrome may make the diagnosis of TTP-HUS difficult because both conditions are associated with thrombocytopenia, MAHA, and neurologic symptoms (visual changes or seizures). In preeclampsia/HELLP syndrome, thrombocytopenia typically reaches a nadir soon after delivery, and spontaneously recovers. Hemolytic anemia is much less common in patients with preeclampsia (2%).[164] Patients with HELLP syndrome may have hemolytic anemia that is significantly slower to recover than thrombocytopenia.[165] The changes in mental status that are typical in TTP-HUS are rarely seen in patients with preeclampsia or HELLP syndrome. In these patients, neurologic symptoms usually include blurred vision, headache, visual scotomata, and rarely, eclamptic seizures. Although proteinuria is a diagnostic hallmark of preeclampsia, renal failure is rare in preeclampsia unless the process is complicated by severe hypertension, DIC, hypotension, or sepsis.[166]

Management Options

Plasma exchange is an empirical and effective treatment for TTP-HUS. Mental status changes may be the first to resolve, with slower recovery of more severe neurologic symptoms, thrombocytopenia, MAHA, and renal failure. Days or months of treatment may be required to achieve a lasting remission. Increasing the frequency of plasma exchange may be required in patients who show a poor response. Plasma exchange is usually tapered to reduce the risk of relapse. Complications include those related to central venous catheter placement and the administration of large volumes of plasma.

If plasma exchange is not available, the inferior therapies of plasma infusion and platelet transfusion have been advocated.[167] Although controversial, occasional supplemental treatment with glucocorticoids, vincristine, splenectomy, intravenous immune globulin, immunosuppressive agents, and antiplatelet drugs has been anecdotally recommended.[168]

Observation may be appropriate in a clinically stable patient who is remote from term and has an uncertain diagnosis. Deterioration of clinical status should prompt treatment with plasma exchange or delivery. If the patient's symptoms do not resolve after delivery, the clinician must consider the diagnosis of TTP-HUS, especially if symptoms persist beyond the third postpartum day. TTP-HUS may recur in subsequent pregnancies; however, at least 50% have an uncomplicated pregnancy.[169]

SUMMARY OF MANAGEMENT OPTIONS

Thrombocytopenic Purpura and Hemolytic Uremic Syndrome

Management Options	Evidence Quality and Recommendation	References
Plasmapheresis is the treatment of choice.	IV/C	167
Fresh frozen plasma and platelet transfusions are secondary approaches.	IV/C	167
Use high-dose steroids.	III/B	154
Provide appropriate supportive therapy for renal failure and neurologic features.	III/B	161,164
Use critical care setting and interdisciplinary approach.	III/B	160

SUGGESTED READINGS

Bremme KA: Haemostatic changes in pregnancy. Best Pract Res Clin Haematol 2003;16:153–168.

Dudding T, Heron J, Thakkinstian A, et al: Factor V Leiden is associated with pre-eclampsia but not with fetal growth restriction: A genetic association study and meta-analysis. J Thromb Haemost 2008;6:1869–1875.

Facco F, You W, Grobman W: Genetic thrombophilias and intrauterine growth restriction: A meta-analysis. Obstet Gynecol 2009;113:1206–1216.

Kahn SR, Platt R, McNamara H, et al: Inherited thrombophilia and preeclampsia within a multicenter cohort: The Montreal Preeclampsia Study. Am J Obstet Gynecol 2009;200:151.e1–e9.

Kupferminc MJ, Eldor A, Steinman N, et al: Increased frequency of genetic thrombophilia in women with complications of pregnancy. N Engl J Med 1999;340:9–13.

Lockwood CJ: Inherited thrombophilias in pregnant patients: Detection and treatment paradigm. Obstet Gynecol 2002;99:333

Lockwood CJ, Bauer KA: Inherited thrombophilias in pregnancy. In Barss VA (ed): UpToDate. Waltham, MA, UpToDate, Jan 2009.

Lockwood CJ, Silver RM: Coagulation disorders in pregnancy. In Creasy RK, Resnik R, Iams J (eds): Maternal Fetal Medicine: Principles and Practice, 6th ed. Philadelphia, Saunders, 2008, pp 825–854.

Miyakis S, Lockshin MD, Atsumi T, et al: International consensus statement on an update of the classification criteria for definite antiphospholipid syndrome (APS). J Thromb Haemost 2006;4:295–306.

Rey E, Kahn SR, David M, Shrier I: Thrombophilic disorders and fetal loss: A meta-analysis. Lancet 2003;361:901–908.

REFERENCES

For a complete list of references, log onto www.expertconsult.com.

CHAPTER 42

Thromboembolic Disease

ROY G. FARQUHARSON and MICHAEL GREAVES

INTRODUCTION

Venous thromboembolism (VTE) is one of the most common causes of maternal death. For example, 33 women died during pregnancy or soon after delivery in the United Kingdom between 2003 and 2005,[1] which equates to a rate of 1.56 deaths per 100,000 pregnancies. Despite publicity and the propagation of practice standards, pulmonary embolism remains the leading direct cause of maternal mortality, and the total number is disappointingly similar to that reported in previous 3-year periods with the exception of 1994 to 1996 when the total peaked at 46 deaths. There is room for encouragement, at least in the United Kingdom, after news that the number of fatal VTE events after cesarean delivery continues to decline from the reported peak of 15 to 7 following the introduction of the Royal College of Obstetricians and Gynaecologists (RCOG) guidelines on thromboprophylaxis in 1995.[2] Even early pregnancy is a significant risk period for VTE; 10 cases (30%) occurred before 12 weeks' gestation. Fatal VTE may occur before the first prenatal visit. As such, it would not be possible to prevent all fatalities caused by pulmonary embolism in pregnancy even if the risk of VTE could be predicted accurately.

An accurate measure of the total incidence of pregnancy-related VTE in the United Kingdom is difficult to determine because there is no national registry. The Swedish national register suggests an overall incidence of 1.3 events per 1000 deliveries[3] for all types of VTE, including deep vein thrombosis (DVT) and fatal and nonfatal pulmonary embolism. This rate corresponds closely to the prevalence reported in a large, unselected cohort of pregnant women in Glasgow, Scotland.[4]

MATERNAL RISKS

Pregnancy significantly increases the risk of VTE. Many substantial changes in the coagulation and vascular systems occur during pregnancy, and these changes support the accepted orthodoxy that pregnancy is a state of hypercoagulability. There is a progressive increase in the plasma concentration of several coagulation factors, including Factor VIII, and some reduction in the coagulation inhibitor protein S. As a result, there is increased thrombin generation such that the consumption of antithrombin in normal pregnancy is similar to that seen in nonpregnant subjects with septic shock.[5] In addition, systemic fibrinolysis suppressed and there is altered venous flow in the lower limbs. Table 42–1 summarizes additional features in pregnancy that contribute to VTE, based on individual case analysis.[1]

Inherited thrombophilia, for example, due to factor V Leiden or deficiency of a physiologic coagulation inhibitor, increases the risk of VTE throughout life, and this risk is increased further in pregnancy and during the puerperium (Table 42–2). Screening for thrombophilia has been suggested as part of the first prenatal visit. Yet this approach identifies relatively few women who will go on to develop VTE,[6] and there is a very real risk of exposing large numbers of healthy women to anticoagulant prophylaxis without benefit. Further, screening for the most common heritable thrombophilia, heterozygosity for Factor V Leiden is not cost-effective for the prevention of pregnancy-related VTE.[7] Indeed, the clinical value of testing for heritable thrombophilia is questioned in most clinical situations.[8] Most commonly, inherited thrombophilia represents a nonfatal, late-onset clinical disorder of low penetrance. Testing may lead to inappropriate anxiety and false reassurance. It should be undertaken by specialists, and pretest counseling is mandatory. Non–evidence-based interventions determined by the results of testing must be avoided.[9] We recommend women be assessed for thrombosis risk primarily in relation to clinical risk factors. If an asymptomatic woman has a strong family history of unprovoked or pregnancy-related VTE, testing for heritable thrombophilia can be considered.

The consequences of VTE are clinically important. Untreated pulmonary embolism has a significant mortality. Although recovery from a nonfatal pulmonary embolism may seem to be complete, pulmonary hypertension develops in a proportion of cases. DVT results in damage to venous valves and incompetence. Postphlebitic syndrome is a long-term consequence. Fortunately, symptoms are usually mild, with residual swelling and some skin pigmentation. However, severe postphlebitic syndrome, with skin ulceration, is associated with significant impairment of quality of life.

FETAL RISKS

Most fetal risk is secondary to the maternal consequences of VTE and therapeutic interventions. For example, hypoxia

TABLE 42-1

Risk Factors Identified from Individual Case Analysis of 33 Maternal Deaths from Venous Thromboembolism (2003–2005)

RISK FACTOR	NUMBER OF CASES	COMMENT
Older age	31	The rate of death is doubled in women older than 30 yr.
Obesity	16	Body mass index >30. All patients affected in the third trimester were overweight. Higher doses of low-molecular-weight heparin may be necessary for the treatment of VTE in the obese.
Immobility	1	Prolonged bedrest.
Family history of VTE	2	Strong history of VTE. All deaths occurred in the antenatal period.
Cesarean delivery	7	The number of events decreased dramatically from the previous report after the 1995 Royal College of Obstetricians and Gynaecologists guideline.
History of VTE	2	Both patients were obese.
Air travel	2	Both cases occurred before 24 wk' gestation.

VTE, venous thromboembolism.
From Lewis G (ed): The Confidential Enquiry into Maternal and Child Health (CEMACH). Saving Mother's Lives: Reviewing Maternal Deaths to Make Motherhood Safer—2003–2005. The Seventh Report on Confidential Enquiries into Maternal Deaths in the UK. London, CEMACH, 2007.

TABLE 42-2

Prevalence of Inherited Thrombophilia with the Relative Risk of Venous Thromboembolic Disease

	PREVALENCE (NORTHERN EUROPE) (%)	ESTIMATED LIFELONG RELATIVE RISK OF VTE
Homozygous factor V Leiden	0.1	×80
Heterozygous factor V Leiden	4	×5
Heterozygous prothrombin G20210A	2	×4
Protein C deficiency	0.2	×12
Protein S deficiency	?	?
Antithrombin deficiency	0.02	×30

Note: All values are estimates. Prevalence varies between populations. VTE risk varies between molecular subtypes, for example, in antithrombin deficiency. Reliable data for protein S deficiency and homozygous prothrombin G20210A are not available. Combinations of thrombophilias generally lead to higher risk of VTE.
VTE, venous thromboembolism.

and circulatory failure are consequences of major pulmonary embolism with a high likelihood of an adverse effect on placental and fetal homeostasis. Furthermore, VTE occurring close to term may affect the management of delivery.

Although heparin does not cross the placenta, it may lead to or worsen maternal hemorrhage, with all of its consequences for both mother and fetus. Warfarin and other coumarins do cross the placenta, are teratogenic, and impair fetal hemostasis. Warfarin is seldom used in pregnancy, perhaps the most common indication being a maternal mechanical heart valve.

Whether inherited thrombophilias are associated with poor pregnancy outcomes, including miscarriage and fetal death, remains the subject of investigation.[10] Current data suggest a weak association with pregnancy failure. The role of these, and acquired thrombophilias,[11] is discussed in the chapters on clotting disorders and autoimmune disease in pregnancy (see Chapters 41 and 43).

THROMBOEMBOLISM IN PREGNANCY

General

The key elements of the management of VTE in pregnancy include a high index of clinical suspicion for the diagnosis, objective confirmation by imaging, and the administration of heparin for the rest of the pregnancy followed by heparin or warfarin for at least 6 weeks postpartum, for a minimum of 3 months total.

Clinical Diagnosis

The typical clinical features of DVT in pregnancy differ somewhat from those in the nonpregnant patient in relation to lateralization and extent. In up to 90% of cases, thrombosis affects the left leg, and in most patients, the proximal veins are affected. In contrast to the nonpregnant state, DVT confined to the calf veins is uncommon during pregnancy, although it may occur in the postpartum period.

The differential diagnosis of a painful, swollen lower limb in pregnancy is narrow. Alternative causes, such as ruptured Baker's cyst and hematoma, are rare in this age group, and cellulitis is uncommon and generally easily distinguished from VTE by the history and clinical signs. Superficial thrombophlebitis results in more localized pain, swelling, erythema, and tenderness and may progress to DVT. Although symptoms of DVT may be subtle and mistaken for common benign changes in pregnancy, such as lower extremity edema or muscle cramping, DVT is almost always unilateral. In addition to swelling, there may be pain on compression of the calf or on deep palpation in the femoral triangle. Dorsiflexion of the foot sometimes causes pain (Homan's sign), but this feature is neither reliable nor discriminatory. In the experience of the authors, in an occasional case, the more usual symptoms and signs of lower limb DVT in pregnancy are preceded by severe low back pain. DVT affecting other sites during pregnancy may occur, such as the upper limb or splanchnic veins, but is exceedingly rare compared with lower limb thrombosis.

The clinical features of pulmonary embolism are no different from those in the nonpregnant patient, but may be masked by the perception of dyspnea which is commonly associated with pregnancy. Delayed diagnosis is common because both patient and physician fail to appreciate the significance of the symptoms. In most cases, the common features are those of pulmonary infarction, with pleuritic chest pain of acute or subacute onset, with or without dyspnea. There may be hemoptysis and low-grade fever. The differential diagnosis includes chest infection with pleurisy and pneumothorax, but as a rule, pulmonary infarction should be considered most likely until it has been excluded or an alternative diagnosis identified. In some women, there may be increasing dyspnea only, presenting a diagnostic challenge. A larger embolus may cause severe dyspnea, often of sudden onset, with evidence of arterial oxygen desaturation. There may be visibly increased jugular venous pressure and other evidence of right heart strain. In massive pulmonary embolism, there is hypotension, usually with severe dyspnea, cyanosis, and collapse, or sudden death. There may be no chest pain, or central chest pain as a result of myocardial ischemia from increased right ventricular work in the face of low arterial oxygen tension. Clinical and electrocardiographic evidence of increased right heart pressure and right ventricular strain are evident. In the absence of a high index of suspicion, much valuable time may be lost running through the differential of less dangerous disorders.

Clinical risk factors to consider in addition to pregnancy include family history, high parity, age older than 30 years, obesity, recent immobilization, and operative delivery.[4] About two thirds of patients have an obvious risk factor.

Confirmation of the Diagnosis

A diagnosis of VTE in pregnancy requires full anticoagulant therapy for several months, with its attendant risks of iatrogenic injury and its effect on the management of delivery. A diagnosis of VTE also affects the management of future pregnancies, contraceptive choices, and the use of hormone replacement therapy as well as the perceived level of risk of VTE in first-degree relatives. Objective confirmation is essential because of these considerations and the inaccuracy of clinical diagnosis.

In lower limb DVT, compression ultrasonography is preferred because it is noninvasive and sensitive to thrombi in the proximal veins. The typical criteria for diagnosis are lack of vessel compressibility, absence of blood flow, and vessel dilation or visualization of the thrombus. The principal limitation is reduced sensitivity for thrombi confined to the distal calf veins, although such a distribution of thrombus is rare in pregnancy and thrombi that remain localized to calf veins have a low risk of embolization. Other sources of diagnostic error relate to diminished flow in a patent femoral or iliac vein because of extrinsic compression from the gravid uterus (may occur as early as 18 weeks' gestation), and persistent flow in the face of a nonocclusive thrombus in the iliac vein. For these reasons, many practitioners prefer an imaging test initially whereby the actual clot in the proximal system is demonstrated. When the diagnosis is in doubt, repeat ultrasound examination after a few days or an alternative imaging modality is needed. X-Ray contrast venography with shielding of the uterus is a rarely required option. It is invasive, causes some discomfort, and inevitably involves radiation exposure, but the diagnostic sensitivity is high. An alternative and attractive technique is magnetic resonance imaging (MRI), which may be sensitive to the presence of DVT.[12] However, its role remains uncertain and contraindications to use of some contrast media require consideration.

When there is suspicion of a venous thrombosis restricted to a minor calf vein, one strategy is to withhold anticoagulant therapy after a first ultrasound examination and to repeat the study in 3 to 5 days to exclude progression to the popliteal vein. Anticoagulant therapy is introduced only if progression is seen. This approach is based on observations of nonpregnant subjects that progression occurs in only some cases and that pulmonary embolism is uncommon when the DVT is restricted to an intramuscular calf vein and may not be applicable to the pregnancy situation.

When pulmonary embolism is suspected based on the clinical features, imaging is essential to confirm the diagnosis or establish an alternative one. Although electrocardiography is usually performed as part of the bedside assessment, it is insensitive and insufficiently specific. Arterial blood gas analysis is used to indicate the degree of hypoxia, but may be normal in pulmonary infarction. In several studies of young patients with pulmonary embolus, the average arterial oxygen level exceeded 90 mm Hg. Ultrasonography examination of the lower extremities is sometimes recommended in suspected pulmonary embolism in pregnancy because it is accessible, is noninvasive, and carries no risk from radiation exposure. However, a negative finding on ultrasound study of the legs does not exclude pulmonary embolism because the clot may have embolized in its entirety or there is an alternative source of thrombus (e.g., pelvic veins). A chest x-ray should be obtained with lead apron shielding of the fetus. The most common finding on chest x-ray is a "normal" result. Although not diagnostic in isolation, the chest x-ray may reveal an alternative cause of the symptoms such as pneumothorax or pneumonia. A chest x-ray is also required for interpretation of the results of a ventilation-perfusion scan should one be performed. The unavoidable radiation exposure has been judged acceptable in pregnancy and can be minimized by performing the perfusion scan first, and then proceeding to the ventilation scan only if perfusion is abnormal. The principal limitation of this technique is a lack of specificity. Although a normal scan excludes pulmonary embolism with an acceptable sensitivity, and a scan showing unmatched perfusion defects at the segmental level or greater can be considered diagnostic, many scans are interpreted as intermediate probability. At present, a computed tomography (CT) scan of the chest is thought to have the greatest sensitivity for pulmonary embolus among noninvasive tests. CT angiography may be a preferred approach, although technical limitations in pregnancy have been identified.[13] Radiation scatter to the abdomen is sufficiently low to be considered safe for use in pregnancy. MRI techniques are also being developed for use in diagnosis of pulmonary embolism.

There has been increasing interest in the use of D-dimer assay alongside a clinical algorithm to assess patients with suspected DVT. D-Dimer is a product of the plasmin digestion of cross-linked fibrin. An increased concentration in plasma is a marker for thrombus formation. Although this test is sensitive, it is not specific for VTE and is insufficient to confirm the diagnosis. Further, diagnostic algorithms that use a D-dimer assay were validated only in previously healthy, nonpregnant, nonhospitalized subjects.[14] Products of fibrin digestion increase in concentration in plasma from approximately 10 weeks' gestation in healthy pregnancy and increase further and abruptly immediately postpartum. Therefore, the use of D-dimer in the diagnosis of VTE in pregnancy would require the establishment of

TABLE 42–3

Pharmacologic and Nonpharmacologic Interventions for Prevention and Treatment of Venous Thromboembolism

ANTITHROMBOTIC AND THROMBOLYTIC AGENTS	MECHANICAL MEASURES
Heparins	Graduated compression stockings
Unfractionated heparin	Mechanical calf compression
Low-molecular-weight heparin	
Synthetic pentasaccharide	
Oral anticoagulants	Filters
Vitamin K antagonists	
Direct thrombin and factor Xa inhibitors	
Aspirin	
Thrombolytics	
Streptokinase	
Urokinase	
Recombinant tissue plasminogen activator	

gestation-specific laboratory ranges and local validation. It is not recommended.

Prevention and Treatment

Interventions to prevent and treat VTE include pharmacologic and mechanical measures (Table 42–3). Among the pharmacologic agents, heparins and warfarin are the principal drugs; they are effective in the prevention of VTE in a range of settings as well as in treatment. Aspirin has been promoted for the prevention of postoperative VTE, but its efficacy is debated. There may be some evidence for its efficacy in lower limb orthopedic surgery,[15,16] but the use of aspirin for thromboprophylaxis in pregnancy is not evidence-based. Novel oral anticoagulants are under development, including direct inhibitors of thrombin and Factor Xa, which are active by the oral route. Although promising, their role is not established, and there are no data on their use in pregnancy. In the context of VTE in general, use of thrombolytic drugs such as streptokinase and recombinant tissue plasminogen activator is generally restricted to the emergency management of massive pulmonary embolism or limb salvage in rare cases of massive lower limb DVT with a threat of venous gangrene. The bleeding risk from their use is substantial, although it may be reduced by a catheter-directed approach to drug delivery. Although there are reports of their use in life-threatening pulmonary embolism, thrombolytic therapy is associated with pregnancy loss (miscarriage or fetal death) and maternal bleeding and is relatively contraindicated during pregnancy. Similarly, thrombolytics may induce massive uterine hemorrhage during the puerperium. Under these circumstances, massive pulmonary embolism has been treated with heparin anticoagulation and emergency embolectomy. Despite the previously discussed concerns regarding thrombolytic drugs, one review of anecdotal reports of thrombolytic therapy in pregnancy implied the risks to the mother and fetus may be lower than suggested.[17]

Heparins

Unfractionated heparin (UFH) is manufactured from mammalian intestine or lung. It consists of a heterogeneous mixture of highly sulfated polysaccharide chains with a molecular weight ranging from 5000 to 35,000 daltons. Its anticoagulant action is principally the result of binding through a specific pentasaccharide sequence to antithrombin III, with a resultant profound acceleration in the rate of inhibition of coagulation enzymes, particularly thrombin and Factor Xa. Available formulations must be administered by either a subcutaneous or an intravenous route.

Although UFH is an effective antithrombotic agent, laboratory monitoring of the anticoagulant effect is necessary when it is used to treat established thrombosis. The activated partial thromboplastin time (aPTT) is typically used, but there is marked variation in reagent sensitivity to heparin, and laboratory standardization of heparin dosage control has not been achieved.

Low-molecular-weight heparins (LMWHs) are manufactured from UFH. With an average molecular weight of approximately 5000 daltons, they include a high concentration of molecules with fewer than 18 saccharides. These molecules cannot bind to antithrombin III and thrombin simultaneously, a feature necessary for thrombin inhibition. However, the anti-Xa effect is preserved because there is no requirement for direct binding to Factor Xa for the acceleration of inhibition by the heparin–antithrombin III complex. Consequently, the anti-Xa activity of LMWH is greater than that of UFH, relative to the antithrombin activity. The aPTT is relatively insensitive to LMWH; assay of anti-Xa activity is the method of choice. Like UFH, parenteral administration of LMWH is necessary, but the bioavailability from subcutaneous tissues is greater and the plasma half-life is longer than that of UFH, permitting effective anticoagulation by once- or twice-daily subcutaneous administration without laboratory monitoring in nonpregnant subjects. These attributes of LMWH have led to the replacement of UFH for many clinical indications. This development is supported by clinical trials in nonpregnant subjects that show at least equivalence to UFH in safety and efficacy in the prevention and treatment of VTE. Indeed, DVT can be treated safely with LMWH in the community setting,[18] although data on pregnant patients are limited. Although the available LMWH preparations differ somewhat in their composition and metabolism, there is little to suggest clinically important differences in clinical efficacy in routine use.

The efficacy, ease of administration, and possible greater safety of LMWH suggest that these agents are preferable to UFH in pregnancy. However, the pharmacokinetics of LMWH are altered in pregnancy. This fact is important because the dosing of LMWH has been extrapolated from data in nonpregnant subjects and increased renal clearance during pregnancy has not been considered. Some early observational studies of LMWH in pregnancy had design flaws, including nonstandardized gestation intervals, a nonhomogenous case mix, and small numbers of patients with few serial observation points.[19] One systematic review reported 40 citations of LMWH involving 728 pregnant and postpartum women. However, only 2 articles were categorized at the highest level with regard to the quality of evidence,[20] and 19 of the articles were considered to be of limited quality. Variations in dosage regimens were marked and ranged from 2500 to 22,000 units daily, which included fixed dosages, increasing dosages as pregnancy progressed, dosages based on body weight, and dosages titrated according to anti-Xa levels. The wide variation in dosage regimens highlights the uncertainty about the pharmacokinetics in pregnancy. Some useful data have emerged. In a longitudinal study of LMWH prophylaxis during pregnancy, the mean peak anti-Xa level occurred later, at 4 hours, compared with 2 hours in the nonpregnant state.[19] Mean peak values were significantly different at the 2-hour time point at 12 and 36 weeks' gestation compared with the nonpregnant state (Fig. 42–1).[21] A previous study in a smaller cohort with nonstandardized gestation intervals supports this trend.[22] Compared with the nonpregnant state, the area under the anti-Xa curve (AUC) is lower in pregnancy, with the nadir occurring at 36 weeks' gestation (Fig. 42–2).[21] The AUC reflects anti-Xa activity and, therefore, reduced plasma activity with advancing gestation. Renal excretion is the principal route of clearance of LMWH. In contrast, UFH is also cleared in part by the reticuloendothelial system. Pregnancy-related physiologic adaptations in renal function probably account for the lower AUC of anti-Xa in pregnancy. This observation is supported by higher AUC values in 12 healthy, nonpregnant volunteers given LMWH.[23] Conversely, the biologic half-life of LMWH is increased in renal failure.[24] These issues highlight the unresolved question as to whether dosing regimens based on trials in nonpregnant individuals can be used in pregnancy. Hunt and coworkers[25] recommended dose escalation after 20 weeks' gestation to overcome these altered heparin pharmacokinetics in pregnancy. We suggest that rather than guessing, measurement of the peak anti-Xa level each trimester may give some reassurance that the target degree of anticoagulation has been achieved.

The principal side effect of heparin is bleeding. Spontaneous hemorrhage is uncommon, even when treatment doses are administered, but increased bleeding from surgical incisions is inevitable. Nevertheless, LMWH has proved to be highly effective and safe, with generally acceptable levels of increased bleeding when used as prophylaxis against postoperative VTE.

Heparin-induced thrombocytopenia with paradoxical thrombosis is an uncommon but potentially lethal side effect of heparin exposure (UFH and LMWH). It is caused by a heparin-induced antibody leading to platelet activation and consumption in a new thrombus. Typically, the platelet count begins to decrease 5 to 10 days after first exposure to heparin, even at a low dose, and in many cases, new or worsening thrombosis is noted. It is imperative to discontinue heparin immediately and to substitute an alternative anticoagulant, because the induced prothrombotic state persists for some time. This complication is around 10-fold more likely with UFH than with LMWH,[26] and fortunately, it appears extremely uncommon with LMWH in prophylactic doses during pregnancy.

Clinically significant osteoporosis is a rare consequence of pregnancy and also of long-term (>3 mo) exposure to heparin. It is less likely to occur with LMWH than with UFH. The potential for osteoporosis has been addressed by several prospective studies that concluded the physiologic effect of pregnancy-induced bone loss is probably greater than that seen with long-term heparin use (Table 42–4).[27–30]

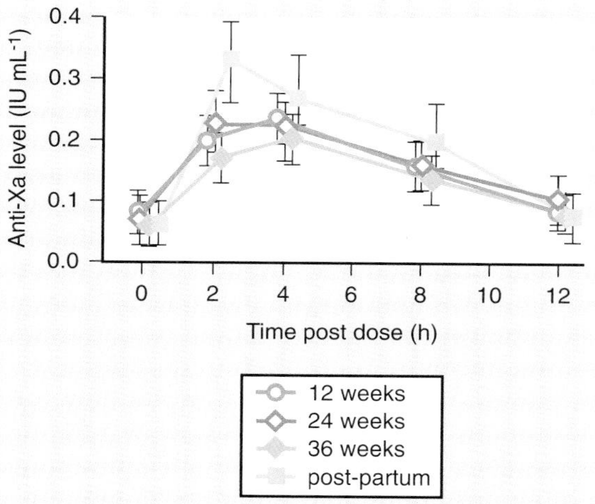

FIGURE 42–1
Anti-Xa levels in the first 12 hours after dalteparin administration, expressed as mean and 95% confidence intervals (12 wk, *n* = 29; 24 wk, *n* = 26; 36 wk, *n* = 24; postpartum, *n* = 24).

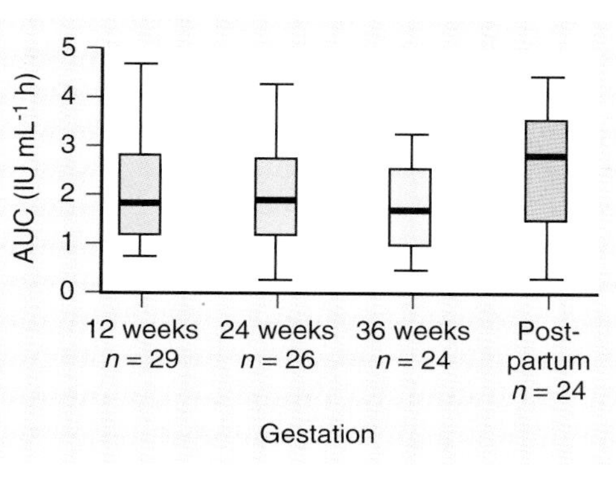

FIGURE 42–2
Area under the curve (AUC) of anti-Xa activity, subclassified by gestational age. *Central bar*, median; *box area*, interquartile range; *whiskers*, range.

TABLE 42–4
Effect of Pregnancy on Bone Mineral Density in the Lumbar Spine (L1–4) Expressed as Percentage Loss (Number of Patients)

STUDY	CONTROL (%)	LOW-MOLECULAR-WEIGHT HEPARIN (%)	UNFRACTIONATED HEPARIN (%)
Shefras and Farquharson, 1996[28]	3.13 (8)	5.1 (17)	
Backos et al, 1999[29]		3.7 (77)	3.7 (46)
Black et al, 2000[27]	3.5 (10)		
Carlin et al, 2004[30]	3.56 (20)	4.17 (55)	

Bone remodeling is uncoupled during pregnancy, with a marked increase in early bone resorption subsequently followed by late bone formation[27] and alteration of bone architecture.[31] Though osteoporotic fracture in pregnancy is an alarming condition, it is rare and sporadic.

Fondaparinux is a synthetic pentasaccharide Factor Xa inhibitor.[32] Like UFH and LMWH, it must be administered parenterally, but it has no antithrombin activity. It is used for prophylaxis and treatment of VTE and to prevent infarct in cardiac ischemia. There are reports of its successful use in the management of VTE in pregnancy.[33]

Coumarins

Coumarins are vitamin K antagonists. They are active orally and inhibit the synthesis of the vitamin K–dependent procoagulants (prothrombin, Factors VII, IX, and X) as well as the anticoagulant proteins C and S. Ingestion of coumarins produces a dose-dependent prolongation of clotting times, especially the prothrombin time, and an anticoagulant effect in vivo. Warfarin is the most commonly used coumarin in clinical practice. There is considerable interindividual variation in the dose-response to warfarin owing in great part to genetic heterogeneity in the genes encoding the cytochromes responsible for coumarin metabolism and those coding for the target enzyme influencing coagulation factor synthesis.[34] The dose-response is also influenced by diet and drug interactions. Close laboratory monitoring is critical. The adoption of the Iinternational Normalized Ratio (INR) system to express prothrombin time ensured uniformity between laboratories. Prospective trials established that the appropriate target INR in a variety of clinical situations is 2.5, range 2.0 to 3.0. Although the risk of bleeding increases markedly with INR greater than 3.0, there is a significant risk even in the target therapeutic range (~25% of bleeds occur when the INR < 3.0), which increases markedly should the INR climb above 5.0. In an unselected series, the prevalence of life-threatening bleeding in subjects treated with warfarin was approximately 1 to 2 events per 100 treatment-years.[35] The greatest risk is to subjects with peripheral or cerebrovascular disease and older patients. It may be lower in women of childbearing age. There have been case reports of intra-abdominal hemorrhage from the site of ovulation, leading to the suggestion that women taking warfarin should use contraceptive methods that suppress ovulation. Bleeding complications are most likely to occur during the first weeks of warfarin therapy. The identification of the genetic influences on individual sensitivity to coumarin has led to the possibility of a pharmacogenomic approach to dosage prediction,[34] but this has not been adopted widely in most countries to date.

Warfarin is a teratogen causing both an embryopathy and a fetopathy (see Chapter 34). Up to 30% of fetuses exposed between 6 and 10 weeks' gestation have been estimated to be affected to some degree, although recent data suggested congenital anomalies in a smaller number of exposed pregnancies—around 6%. The developing skeleton is the principal target, with abnormalities ranging from subclinical stippling of the epiphyses on x-ray, to nasal deformity, and to severe phocomelia. Heparin is a safer alternative, and warfarin is never used to manage VTE during the first trimester. Further, it is rarely the anticoagulant of choice to treat or prevent VTE at any stage of gestation because of reports of intracranial abnormalities and developmental problems attributed to fetal hemorrhage. Commonly, heparin anticoagulation during pregnancy is switched to warfarin postpartum because of the ease of administration.

Mechanical Measures

Well-fitted graduated compression hosiery is widely used to prevent VTE. Although there are few studies of pregnant women, there is evidence of efficacy perioperatively in nonpregnant patients. There is also evidence that symptoms of postphlebitic syndrome are less likely to develop if compression stockings of appropriate class are worn regularly for 2 years after an episode of lower limb DVT.[36] Whether below-the-knee stockings are as effective as full-length hosiery is the subject of debate, although there are some data supporting this practice in the postoperative state,[37] and compliance tends to be better with below-the-knee stockings.

Mechanical devices that stimulate calf muscle contraction or compress the calf intermittently have been used to prevent DVT perioperatively, and may be useful in women who are not candidates for pharmacologic thromboprophylaxis because of a high risk of bleeding.

Filter devices that can be placed in the inferior vena cava either temporarily or permanently have been used in subjects with lower limb proximal DVT considered high risk for pulmonary embolism. The frequency of their use varies among nations. Risks include inferior vena cava thrombosis, vessel perforation, and migration of the filter. They are mostly used in patients in whom either anticoagulant therapy is contraindicated (e.g., those with a recent cerebral hemorrhage) or when a pulmonary embolism has occurred despite therapeutic levels of anticoagulation. Successful use has been reported,[17] but pregnancy poses additional challenges including the need to use radiologic screening to ensure safe placement and the possibility that vena caval compression by the gravid uterus will hinder placement. These devices may be helpful when VTE presents at term, for example.

Management Options: Established Venous Thromboembolism in Pregnancy

Treatment protocols with heparin have been based largely on those used in nonpregnant patients and seem safe and effective. Heparin should be initiated when there is strong clinical suspicion of DVT and continued after the diagnosis is confirmed. Because of the advantages of LMWH, (low injection volume, occasional vs. frequent testing), most clinicians consider LMWH the anticoagulant of choice. LMWH is administered by subcutaneous injection at the recommended dose for the particular product based on early pregnancy body weight. Once-daily administration may be preferred for convenience and is reasonable as long as therapeutic levels can be maintained. Coagulation times, such as aPTT, are not appropriate for this purpose because the aPTT may remain short, even in patients who are given therapeutic doses of LMWH. The anti-Xa assay gives an indication of the pharmacologic response but is a poor predictor of antithrombotic efficacy and provides limited information on bleeding risk in nonpregnant subjects.[38] A peak (4 hr after injection) plasma anti-Xa concentration of around 0.5 to 1.0 anti-Xa international units appears to be acceptable for a 12-hourly regimen, with slightly higher peak levels sought for a 24-hourly regimen. More intensive monitoring by anti-Xa assay has been recommended when the dose-response is likely to be less predictable, for example, in the very over- or underweight patient and when renal function is impaired. UFH may be preferred in renal failure.

If preferred, treatment with UFH can be initiated by intravenous bolus, followed by continuous intravenous infusion, with adjustment to maintain the aPTT ratio to control of 1.5 to 2.5. This value is often difficult to achieve, especially in late pregnancy, because the starting aPTT is short owing to the physiologic increased concentration of several clotting factors, including Factor VIII. There are few indications for use of UFH rather than LMWH in the context of VTE. It may, however, be justified if there is concern that rapid reversal of the anticoagulant effect may be unpredictably and urgently required, in renal failure, and in the initial management of unstable pulmonary embolism.

Whether UFH or LMWH is administered in treatment doses, the platelet count should be monitored from day 5 until around day 20. A progressive, unexplained decrease in the platelet count suggests heparin-induced thrombocytopenia. In the event of this rare complication, heparin should be discontinued. The condition is caused by the development of platelet-activating antibody, and there is a high risk of further thrombosis if the heparin is continued. Warfarin does not appear to be effective for the prevention of thrombosis in this situation. Lepirudin, a direct inhibitor of thrombin, is the alternative anticoagulant of choice in nonpregnant patients with heparin-induced thrombocytopenia, and there are occasional reports of its use in pregnancy.[39] Another alternative is the heparin-like danaparoid, but cross-reactivity may be a problem and there have been problems with availability. It has been used in pregnancy.[40] Fondaparinux can be considered as an alternative. As in all cases of thrombosis in pregnancy, optimal treatment should be determined individually, with consideration for the relative lack of pregnancy-specific evidence on which to base decisions.

The initial management of most cases of pulmonary embolism is comparable with that of DVT. The exception is life-threatening massive pulmonary embolism, in which the relative risks of surgical embolectomy and thrombolytic therapy must be considered urgently.

There are a few additional management issues to consider in VTE. Elevating the affected limb helps relieve symptoms in DVT, and analgesia is frequently necessary because of the considerable swelling and discomfort caused by either proximal venous occlusion or the pain associated with pulmonary infarction. Confinement to bed is not mandatory. Fitted (vs. one size fits all) graduation compression stockings should be used as soon as resolution of swelling allows them to be worn without discomfort.

Full-dose heparin treatment should be maintained to delivery. The patient should be advised to withhold the next due dose of heparin once labor has begun or the morning of a planned induction. There has been some concern about the safety of spinal or epidural anesthesia in laboring women who are receiving anticoagulants.[41] In general, insertion and withdrawal of a spinal catheter should be avoided within 12 hours of a subcutaneous dose of LMWH, and preferably for 24 hours after a treatment dose. Whether the risk is increased after this period is unclear, but the potential risk must be balanced against the needs for analgesia and anesthesia during labor.

If no abnormal bleeding occurs during delivery, heparin can be reintroduced 12 to 24 hours postpartum. Alternatively, warfarin may be initiated along with heparin (until the INR is in the therapeutic range, when heparin can be discontinued) and continued postpartum. Anticoagulation is typically continued 6 to 12 weeks postpartum or a total of 3 months from the initial diagnosis of VTE, whichever is longer. Although warfarin is secreted in breast milk, the breast-fed neonate of a treated mother is not adversely affected. However, warfarin is best avoided when the mother is expressing milk to feed to a severely premature neonate.

SUMMARY OF MANAGEMENT OPTIONS

Established Thromboembolism in Pregnancy

Management Options	Evidence Quality and Recommendation	References
Clinical Diagnosis	III/B	14
DVT: Can be difficult; sometimes different clinical presentation to nonpregnant state.		
PE: Similar presentation to nonpregnant state.		
Key: "High index of suspicion."		
Confirmation of Diagnosis	III/B	14
DVT: Compression ultrasound, venogram.		
PE: Perfusion scan, CT angiogram (ECG insensitive and nonspecific; chest x-ray excludes other pathology; Pao_2 indicates degree of hypoxia).		
D-Dimer is not specific for VTE.		

SUMMARY OF MANAGEMENT OPTIONS

Established Thromboembolism in Pregnancy—cont'd

Management Options	Evidence Quality and Recommendation	References
Initial Management	Ia/Ib/A	18
Heparin: Give UFH IV bolus loading dose then continuous IV, e.g., 1000–2000 U/hr or LMWH in therapeutic doses. LMWH is preferred.	III/B	44
Monitor aPTT (with UFH) or peak anti-Xa level (with LMWH); monitor serial platelet counts.		
Additional measures: Analgesia; elevation and compression stockings with DVT; with severe PE, consider surgical embolectomy and intensive care (see Chapter 78).		
Maintenance	Ia/A	19
Heparin: Give UFH (e.g., 10,000 units SC twice daily) or therapeutic dose LMWH. LMWH is preferred.	III/B	44
Monitor aPTT (1.5–2.5 times control) (UFH) or peak anti-Xa (LMWH); monitor platelet counts.		
Intrapartum	IIa/B	44
Temporarily discontinue heparin therapy with onset of labor.		
The timing of heparin administration should be considered in relation to catheter placement for regional analgesia, and catheter withdrawal.		
Reinitiate treatment with UFH or LMWH approximately 12 hr after delivery if no active bleeding occurs.		
Postpartum	IIa/B	43
Continue LMWH, UFH, or warfarin (with monitoring) for 6 wk or at least 3 mo after an acute event.		
Graduated elastic compression stockings should be worn for 2 yr.	Ia/A	37
Breast-feeding is not contraindicated.		

aPTT, activated partial thromboplastin time; CT, computed tomography; DVT, deep vein thrombosis; ECG, electrocardiogram; LMWH, low-molecular-weight heparin; Pao_2, arterial oxygen pressure; PE, pulmonary embolism; UFH, unfractionated heparin; VTE, venous thromboembolism.

Management Options: Thromboprophylaxis in Pregnancy

Thromboprophylaxis should be offered selectively. All pregnant women should undergo clinical assessment for risk of VTE. Population screening for hereditary thrombophilias is not performed as a routine and should be based on the clinical circumstances and the family history. When a heritable thrombophilia is detected in an asymptomatic subject as part of a family study, this information can be used for an informed risk assessment. Acquired factors are at least as important as genetic predisposition in assessing thrombotic risk. A personal history of VTE is an important consideration for thromboprophylaxis in pregnancy. In addition, patient age, parity, and weight can be considered. Limited mobility and some chronic medical conditions such as systemic lupus erythematosus may be relevant. The risk of venous thrombosis is greatest in the puerperium and higher yet in women who have had cesarean delivery, especially as an emergency procedure, or in preeclampsia.

The risk of VTE in women with a personal history of thrombosis may be lower than previously considered. In a persuasive prospective study of 125 women who had a history of venous thrombosis and in whom antenatal thromboprophylaxis was withheld, the overall rate of recurrence in a subsequent pregnancy was only 2.4%. No recurrence was reported in the subgroup of women who had a temporary risk factor at the time of the first event.[42] This study also suggested that the recurrence rate may be higher in heritable thrombophilia, but was too small to allow firm conclusions to be drawn. The risk of pregnancy-associated first occurrence of VTE in women with heritable thrombophilia may be overstated. Although data from a large cohort study suggest a substantial risk, possibly as high as 1 in 3 in some kindreds with antithrombin deficiency, the risk is much lower, perhaps around 1 in 100 in asymptomatic

TABLE 42–5
Sample Recommendations for Thromboprophylaxis in Pregnancy

RISK CATEGORY	MANAGEMENT
Low	
Women who have no personal history of venous thrombosis, but a positive family history and who are heterozygous for protein S deficiency, heterozygous for factor V Leiden, or heterozygous for prothrombin G20210A. Women with a history of venous thrombosis in association with a temporary risk factor that is no longer present.	In general, pharmacologic thromboprophylaxis is not required antenatally in the absence of additional risk factors, but anticoagulant prophylaxis may be considered after delivery. In reaching a decision, the early pregnancy or antenatal risk assessment at booking should clearly identify the presence of additional risk factors such as advanced maternal age (>35 yr), high BMI (>30 kg/m^2) and smoking. For example, the presence of three risk factors should trigger expert assessment.
Intermediate	
Women who have a personal history of apparently spontaneous VTE and who have a thrombophilic mutation who are no longer receiving anticoagulant prophylaxis. Women who have no personal history of venous thrombosis, but a positive family history of venous thrombosis and who are heterozygous for protein C deficiency, are homozygous for factor V Leiden or the prothrombin G20210A mutation, or have combinations of defects.	Postpartum thromboprophylaxis with heparin or warfarin should be given. Expert review of risk factor assessment is strongly recommended. Antenatal thromboprophylaxis with LMWH or UFH should be considered.
High	
Women who are receiving long-term anticoagulant therapy for VTE. Women who have type I antithrombin deficiency or a type II reactive site antithrombin defect (regardless of whether they have had a thrombotic episode).	Prophylaxis should be strongly considered throughout pregnancy and postpartum. Adjusted doses of LMWH or UFH, higher than those usually used to prevent venous thrombosis, can be considered.

Note: Clinical assessment of risk factors is paramount. The individual patient history and clinical assessment must be considered in each case, especially the presence of combinations of heritable and acquired risk factors, as well as patient preference.
BMI, body mass index; LMWH, low-molecular-weight heparin; UFH, unfractionated heparin; VTE, venous thromboembolism.
From Walker ID, Greaves M, Preston FE: Investigation and management of inherited thrombophilia. Br J Haematol 2001;114:512–528.

subjects with protein C deficiency, and perhaps lower still in asymptomatic women heterozygous for Factor V Leiden.[4] Based on these observations, an attempt to stratify risk has been made with recommendations for thromboprophylaxis of graded intensity depending on these factors.[9] The RCOG in the United Kingdom has recommended an algorithm, based on an assessment of personal and family history, heritable thrombophilia, and acquired risk factors.[44] Table 42–5 is modified from the recommendations of the British Committee for Standards in Haematology.[9] National bodies in other countries have recommended guidelines also. The aim should be to achieve a balance between efficient prevention of VTE and avoidance of exposure of a large number of healthy women to unnecessary pharmacologic thromboprophylaxis throughout their pregnancies. It has to be accepted that it will not be possible to prevent all VTE.

The ideal stage of pregnancy to introduce LMWH prophylaxis is debated. Some clinicians introduce treatment in the second trimester to minimize the duration of exposure. In doing so, it should be remembered that VTE, including fatal pulmonary embolism, may occur during the first trimester.

The use of compression stockings antenatally and postpartum is a reasonable precaution in any woman deemed to be at increased risk of VTE. In general, for the reasons discussed earlier, LMWH is preferable to UFH for pharmacologic thromboprophylaxis. The use of preloaded syringes is convenient and increases safety. Most women can safely self-medicate after instruction. Heparin-induced thrombocytopenia is vanishingly rare in healthy pregnant women receiving LMWH, and the monitoring of the platelet count is not mandatory in women using prophylactic doses only. Warfarin can be used for postpartum prophylaxis with a target INR of 2.5. Updated thromboprophylaxis recommendations have been published by the RCOG,[43] and in addition, acute management recommendations for thromboembolic disease in pregnancy and the puerperium were published in 2007.[44]

SUGGESTED READINGS

Black AJ, Topping J, Durham B, et al: A detailed assessment of alterations in bone turnover, calcium homeostasis, and bone density in normal pregnancy. J Bone Miner Res 2000;15:557–563.

Brill-Edwards P, Ginsberg JS: Safety of withholding antepartum heparin in women with a previous episode of venous thromboembolism. N Engl J Med 2000;343:1439–1444.

Carlin A, Farquharson RG, Quenby S, et al: Prospective observational study of bone mineral density during pregnancy: Low molecular weight heparin versus control. Hum Reprod 2004;19:1211–1214.

Lewis G (ed): The Confidential Enquiry into Maternal and Child Health (CEMACH). Saving Mother's Lives: Reviewing Maternal Deaths to Make Motherhood Safer—2003–2005. The Seventh Report on Confidential Enquiries into Maternal Deaths in the UK. London, CEMACH, 2007.

McColl MD, Ramsay JE, Tait RC, et al: Risk factors for pregnancy associated venous thromboembolism. Thromb Haemost 1997;78:1183–1188.

Royal College of Obstetricians and Gynaecologists: Report of a Working Party on Prophylaxis against Thromboembolism in Gynaecology and Obstetrics. London, RCOG Press, 1995.

Royal College of Obstetricians and Gynaecologists: Thromboembolic Disease in Pregnancy and Puerperium: Acute Management (Greentop Guideline 28). London, RCOG Press, 2007. Available at rcog.org.uk

Royal College of Obstetricians and Gynaecologists: Thrombosis and Embolism during Pregnancy and the Puerperium, Reducing the Risk (Green-top Guideline 37). London, RCOG Press, 2009. Available at www.rcog.org.uk

Sajid MS, Tai NR, Goli G, et al: Knee versus thigh length graduated compression stockings for prevention of deep venous thrombosis: A systematic review. Eur J Vasc Endovasc Surg 2006;32:730–736.

Sephton V, Farquharson RG, Topping J, et al: A longitudinal study of maternal dose response to low molecular weight heparin in pregnancy. Obstet Gynecol 2003;101:1307–1311.

REFERENCES

For a complete list of references, log onto www.expertconsult.com.

CHAPTER 43

Autoimmune Diseases

JEFF M. DENNEY, TROY FLINT PORTER, and D. WARE BRANCH

INTRODUCTION

The immune system's remarkable ability to protect the body from invasion by foreign pathogens stems from its capacity to distinguish biologic "self" from "nonself." An aberration in this normally well-regulated process leads to a state of so-called *autoimmunity*, in which immune effector cells are directed against "self" tissues. Persistent immunologic activation results in an *autoimmune disease*, characterized by a typical pattern of clinical signs and symptoms of disease and confirmed by the serologic presence of immune effector cells, usually autoantibodies. For many autoimmune conditions, serologically detected autoantibodies play an active role in tissue damage. In others, their presence may serve only to confirm the existence of an autoimmune process.

The pathophysiologic mechanisms that lead to autoimmune diseases have been studied extensively. The earliest theory held that autoimmunity resulted from a failure in the normal deletion of lymphocytes that recognized self-antigens. More recently, investigators have suggested that autoimmunity results from a failure of the normal regulation of the immune system (which contains many immune cells that recognize self-antigens but are normally suppressed). Regardless of what fundamental immunologic disturbance allows autoimmunity, it appears that a combination of environmental, genetic, and host factors must be present for the full expression of an autoimmune disease.

Autoimmune diseases have a predilection for reproductive-age women and are frequently encountered during pregnancy. Indeed, more than 70% of patients with autoimmune disease are women of reproductive age.[1] Studies in both animal models and humans support the role that sex hormones play in the development of autoimmunity; estrogens accelerate disease and androgens are protective.[2–6] It should come as no surprise that pregnancy-associated fluctuations in sex hormones may influence disease severity. Interestingly, the effect of pregnancy depends on whether the autoimmune disease is innate (cellular) or adaptive (humoral) in nature. Diseases with strong cellular pathophysiology, such as rheumatoid arthritis (RA) and multiple sclerosis, are associated with remission during pregnancy, whereas diseases characterized by autoantibody production, such as systemic lupus erythematosus (SLE) and Graves' disease, tend toward increased severity in pregnancy. Still others are unique to pregnancy or have unique features associated with pregnancy. Thus, the obstetrician should be familiar with the more common autoimmune diseases, how they influence and are influenced by pregnancy, and what special medical risks may be in store for mother or the conceptus.

SYSTEMIC LUPUS ERYTHEMATOSUS

General

SLE is an idiopathic chronic inflammatory disease that affects skin, joints, kidneys, lungs, serous membranes, nervous system, liver, and other organs of the body. Like other autoimmune diseases, its course is characterized by periods of remission and relapse. The most common complaint among patients with SLE is extreme fatigue (Table 43–1). Fever, weight loss, myalgia, and arthralgia are also particularly common symptoms.

The prevalence of SLE is 5 to 100 per 100,000 individuals, depending on the population studied. The disease is at least 5, and probably closer to 10 times, more common among adult women than adult men.[1] The lifetime risk of developing SLE for a white woman is 1 in 700,[7] with an overall incidence of 1 in 2000 in the United States. The incidence varies among populations and is approximately two to four times higher in African Americans and Hispanic Americans.[7] A genetic predisposition to SLE is likely, given that approximately 10% of patients with SLE also have an affected relative[8]; concordance between twins is reportedly greater than 50%.[9] Several alterations in the human leukocyte antigen (HLA) system have been linked to the development of SLE, and homozygous carriers of mutations responsible for complement deficiency disorders also appear to be predisposed to development of the disease.

Diagnosis

Serologic Markers

The diagnosis of SLE, suspected by the clinical presentation, is confirmed by demonstrating the presence of circulating autoantibodies. Patients are initially screened for nonspecific antibodies directed against nuclear antigens. Cumbersome biologic assays of antibodies directed against nucleoprotein

TABLE 43–1

Approximate Frequency of Clinical Symptoms in SLE

SYMPTOMS	PATIENTS (%)
Fatigue	80–100
Fever	80–100
Arthralgia, arthritis	95
Myalgia	70
Weight loss	>60
Skin	
Butterfly rash	50
Photosensitivity	60
Mucous membrane lesions	35
Renal involvement	50
Pulmonary	
Pleurisy	50
Effusion	25
Pneumonitis	5–10
Cardiac (pericarditis)	10–50
Lymphadenopathy	50
Central nervous system	
Seizures	15–20
Psychosis	<25

(nucleohistone) commonly referred to as the *LE phenomenon*, have been replaced by immunofluorescent assays for nonspecific antinuclear antibodies (ANAs). Findings are interpreted according to antibody titer and, to some degree, on the pattern of antibody binding. The *homogeneous* pattern is found most commonly in patients with SLE (65%), though its specificity is low. A peripheral pattern is the most specific for SLE, even if it is not very sensitive. The speckled and nucleolar patterns are more specific for other autoimmune diseases.

Immunofluorescent assays that identify specific nuclear antigen-antibody reactions are better for confirming the diagnosis of SLE, monitoring disease activity, and guiding immunotherapy. Particularly useful are anti–double-stranded DNA (anti-dsDNA) antibodies, present in 80% to 90% of patients with newly diagnosed SLE, elevations of which precede symptomatic flare in 80% of SLE patients followed prospectively.[10,11] In pregnancy, anti-dsDNA antibodies correlate with flare and preterm delivery.[11,12]

Antibodies to single-stranded DNA (anti-ssDNA) are also found in a large number of untreated SLE patients, but are less specific for SLE than is anti-dsDNA. Patients with SLE may also have antibodies to RNA-protein conjugates, often referred to as *soluble* or *extractable antigens*, because they can be separated from tissue extracts. These antigens include the Sm antigen, nuclear ribonucleoprotein (nRNP), the Ro/SS-A antigen, and the La/SS-B antigen. The Sm and nRNP antigens are nuclear in origin, and the presence of anti-Sm, found in about 30% to 40% of patients with SLE, is highly specific for the disease. Anti-Ro/SS-A and anti-La/SS-B, found in the sera of both SLE patients and patients with Sjögren's syndrome, are of particular importance to obstetricians because they are associated with neonatal lupus.

In addition, rises in the erythrocyte sedimentation rate (ESR) and C-reactive protein (CRP) levels correlated with disease activity.[13] When serum levels of complement C1q are noted to be persistently low, patients are at higher probability for having not only SLE but also SLE-associated proliferative glomerulonephritis.[14] Notably, not all patients with measurable serologic markers have active disease. Moreover, the presence of serologic markers of lupus neither confirms active disease nor reliably predicts exacerbation.[15]

Diagnostic Criteria

In 1971, the American Rheumatism Association devised criteria for SLE as a framework for comparing studies of patients with SLE. These were revised in 1982[16] and again in 1997[17] (Table 43–2). To be classified as having SLE, an individual must have at least 4 of 11 clinical and laboratory criteria at one time or serially. These criteria are very sensitive and specific for SLE, but were never intended to form the sine qua non for the diagnosis of SLE. Many patients have fewer than four clinical or laboratory features of SLE and do not meet strict diagnostic criteria. Exclusion of patients with an autoimmune diathesis from the diagnosis of SLE by the dogmatic use of strict diagnostic criteria can result in patients being confused and frustrated. Although these patients should not be considered to have SLE, they are often referred to as having lupus-like disease. Such individuals may benefit from therapies for SLE and often require special care during pregnancy. A subset of these patients will ultimately develop the clinical syndrome.

Lupus Nephritis

Clinically obvious renal disease is a relatively common complication of SLE, eventually occurring in as many as two thirds of patients with SLE.[18,19] Lupus nephropathy probably results from anti-DNA antibodies and glomerular immune complex deposition leading to complement activation and inflammatory tissue damage in the kidney.[20] The most common presentation is proteinuria, which occurs at some time in up to 75% of patients. About 40% of patients will have hematuria or pyuria, and about a third will have urinary casts. Note that the presence of hematuria, pyuria, and cellular casts in the urine sediment are important distinctions of lupus nephritis as opposed to preeclampsia.

Renal biopsy is necessary to confirm the diagnosis of lupus nephropathy. Because laboratory and clinical manifestations are poor prognosticators for the progression of disease, obtaining biopsy to determine renal histology is key to understanding the prognosis and providing direction for appropriate treatment.[21] Renal biopsy findings are used to group lupus nephropathy into four basic histologic and clinical categories. Of these, *diffuse proliferative glomerulonephritis* (DPGN) is the most common (40%) and most severe, with 10-year survival around 60%. Patients with DPGN typically present with hypertension, moderate to heavy proteinuria and nephrotic syndrome, hematuria, pyuria, casts, hypocomplementemia, and circulating immune complexes. *Focal proliferative glomerulonephritis* is usually associated

TABLE 43-2

Revised American College of Rheumatology Classification Criteria for Systemic Lupus Erythematosus*

CRITERION	DEFINITION
1. Malar rash	Fixed erythema, flat or raised, over the malar eminences, tending to spare the nasolabial folds
2. Discoid rash	Erythematous raised patches with adherent keratotic scaling and follicular plugging; atrophic scarring possible in older lesions
3. Photosensitivity	Skin rash as a result of unusual reaction to sunlight, by patient history or physician observation
4. Oral ulcers	Oral or nasopharyngeal ulceration, usually painless
5. Arthritis	Nonerosive arthritis involving two or more peripheral joints, characterized by tenderness, swelling, or effusion
6. Serositis	a. Pleuritis—convincing history of pleuritic pain or rubbing heard by a physician, or evidence of pleural effusion b. Pericarditis—documented by ECG or rub or evidence of effusion
7. Renal	a. Persistent proteinuria >0.5 g/day or >3+ if quantitation not performed b. Cellular casts—red cell, hemoglobin, granular, tubular, or mixed
8. Neurologic	a. Seizures—in the absence of offending drugs or known metabolic derangements (e.g., uremia, ketoacidosis, or electrolyte imbalance) b. Psychosis—in the absence of drugs or metabolic derangements
9. Hematologic	a. Hemolytic anemia—with reticulocytosis b. Leukopenia—<4,000/μL on two or more occasions c. Lymphopenia—<1500/μL on two or more occasions d. Thrombocytopenia—<100,000/μL in absence of drugs
10. Immunologic	a. Anti-DNA—antibody to native DNA in abnormal titer b. Anti-Sm—presence of antibody to Sm nuclear antigen c. Positive finding of antiphospholipid antibodies based on (1) an abnormal serum level of IgG or IgM anticardiolipin antibodies, (2) a positive test result for lupus anticoagulant using a standard method, or (3) a false-positive serologic test for syphilis for 6 mo
11. ANA	An abnormal ANA titer by immunofluorescence or an equivalent assay at any time and in the absence of drugs known to be associated with "drug-induced lupus" syndrome

* SLE can be said to be present if four or more of the criteria are present simultaneously or serially.
ANA, antinuclear antibody; ECG, electrocardiogram; Ig, immunoglobulin; SLE, systemic lupus erythematosus.
From Tan EM, Cohen AS, Fries JF, et al: The 1982 revised criteria for the classification of systemic lupus erythematosus. Arthritis Rheum 1982;25:1271–1277; and Hochberg MC: Updating the American College of Rheumatology revised criteria for the classification of systemic lupus erythematosus. Arthritis Rheum 1997;40:1725.

with mild hypertension and proteinuria; serious renal insufficiency is uncommon. *Membranous glomerulonephritis* typically presents with moderate to heavy proteinuria but lacks the active urinary sediment and does not cause renal insufficiency. *Mesangial glomerulonephritis* appears to be the least clinically severe lesion and carries the best long-term prognosis.[21]

Notably, both type and severity of disease dictate the protocol for optimal treatment.[22] The first line of therapy in patients with active lupus nephropathy has traditionally been glucocorticoids, usually given as oral prednisone, 40 to 50 mg/day, for several weeks to several months. Thereafter, the dose is tapered while carefully watching the patient for evidence of signs and symptoms of worsening disease. Avoiding conception while on immunosuppressants or glucocorticoids minimizes risk of adverse fetal effects, but the maternal disease may dictate at least a judicious continuation of glucocorticoid therapy of the lowest effective dose.[23] Severe proliferative lesions, such as seen in moderate to severe DPGN, have been shown to respond best to cytotoxic agents. Cyclophosphamide, in a divided monthly dose of 0.5 to 1.0 g/m^2, is now generally used.

Lupus Cerebritis

Ten percent to 35% of patients with SLE develop neurologic and psychiatric manifestations of their disease, also referred to as *lupus cerebritis*.[24–26] Patients most often present with new-onset cognitive dysfunction, seizures, although peripheral neuropathy, headaches, chorea, stroke syndrome (i.e., either transient ischemic attack or ischemic brain infarction), mood disorders, transverse myelitis, and psychosis also are reported. The severity of lupus cerebritis may also be influenced by other problems commonly encountered in patients with SLE, including metabolic abnormalities, infection, and chronic steroid use. Prospective studies suggest that a high percentage—50% to 78%—of neurologic episodes are caused largely by secondary factors: hypertension, corticosteroid toxicity, uremia, and other metabolic complications of other organ system failure.[27,28] An evaluation for lupus cerebritis should include an assessment for the presence of infection, including lumber puncture if necessary, radiologic imaging, and electroencephalogram. Patients with lupus cerebritis who present with chorea, transverse myelitis, or stroke should be tested for antiphospholipid antibodies (aPLs). There is a higher risk for stroke with presence of aPLs in SLE, especially when more than one type is present. These antibodies also correlate with increased incidence of small high-intensity white matter lesions on magnetic resonance imaging (MRI).[29]

Empirical therapy for lupus cerebritis typically includes glucocorticoids (e.g., prednisone 0.5–1.0 mg/kg/day) as a first-line therapy, with cyclophosphamide (0.5–1.0 g/m^2) monthly for 6 months and intravenous immune globulin (IVIG) reserved for refractory cases.[30]

Risks of Systemic Lupus Erythematosus and Pregnancy

The Risk of SLE Exacerbation (Flare)

Whether pregnancy is associated with a higher rate of SLE exacerbation is debated. Early studies on the subject were hampered by poor study design, not to mention the difficulty of differentiating between normal manifestations of pregnancy and the signs and symptoms typically associated with SLE. At the same time, common complications of pregnancy such as preeclampsia may mimic exacerbations of SLE.

Between the early 1950s and the early 1970s, the findings of several small retrospective series suggested that women with SLE were placing themselves at substantial risk for severe morbidity and even mortality during pregnancy.[31] Many also reported relatively high rates of pregnancy wastage among women with SLE.[32] These concerns led many practitioners to the opinion that SLE patients should not become pregnant. However, these early studies were plagued by several problems, and their conclusions should not be the basis of clinical decision-making today. All were retrospective and relatively small and, because of the lack of generally agreed-upon criteria for the classification of SLE, were predisposed to include a disproportionate number of more severe cases. In addition, without standardized diagnostic criteria for SLE exacerbation, early investigators may have incorrectly diagnosed preeclampsia and other obstetric complications as SLE exacerbations.

Studies undertaken since 1980 have done much to clarify the relationship of pregnancy to the rate and nature of SLE exacerbations. Overall, the rate of flare during pregnancy or the postpartum period varies between 15% and 60% of women.[33–45] Several prospective studies deserve special consideration. Lockshin and colleagues[33] matched nonpregnant SLE patients with 28 SLE patients undertaking 33 pregnancies and used a previously published scoring system to define SLE exacerbations. There was no difference in the flare score between the cases and the controls, and a similar number in both groups required a change in their medication. The same investigators have now followed 80 consecutive pregnancies in women with SLE and conclude that exacerbations occur in less than 25% of cases and that most are mild in nature. If only signs or symptoms specific for SLE are included, exacerbations occurred in only 13% of cases.

Mintz and coworkers[35] prospectively studied 92 pregnancies in women with SLE and used a similar group of nonpregnant SLE patients on oral contraceptives derived from a previous study as controls. Exacerbations were defined by criteria different from those used by Lockshin and colleagues. As a matter of policy, all pregnant women were started on 10 mg prednisone daily, even if there was no evidence of SLE activity. The rate of SLE flares per month at risk was similar in both groups. As in Lockshin and colleagues's studies, most of the exacerbations tended to be easily controlled with low to moderate doses of glucocorticoids, but 7 patients (8%) had severe exacerbations requiring more aggressive therapies. Interestingly, the majority (54%) of the exacerbations occurred in the first trimester.

Using criteria for SLE flare that differed from either of the other two studies, Petri and associates[36] found SLE flares (flares/person-years) to be more common among pregnant women than among controls. Fortunately, over three quarters of the flares were mild to moderate in nature.

Urowitz and colleagues[37] reported their experience comparing 79 pregnancies in patients with active SLE with a matched control group of 59 nonpregnant women with active SLE. They also compared these women with 216 women with inactive disease. Using a previously defined SLE exacerbation score, they found no significant differences in disease activity between the three groups. Only inactive patients at the onset of pregnancy showed a significant reduction in SLE activity (41%).

Ruiz-Irastorza and coworkers[38] analyzed the course of SLE in 78 pregnancies in 68 patients and a matched control group of 50 nonpregnant women. Sixty-five percent of the patients experienced an exacerbation of SLE during pregnancy, for a flare rate of 0.082/patient-month. In the control group, 42% of the patients experienced a flare, with a flare rate of 0.039/patient-month, representing a statistically significant difference.

Georgiou and associates[39] prospectively evaluated the frequency of SLE exacerbation during 59 pregnancies in 47 women with SLE and 59 nonpregnant women matched for parameters other than disease activity and duration. Using accepted clinical criteria, they reported SLE exacerbation in 8 (13.5%) pregnant patients compared with 13 (22%) nonpregnant women. More than half of the exacerbations in the pregnant group occurred during the first trimester. As in the previous studies, all exacerbations were mild and easily treated with glucocorticoids.

It follows that whether or not pregnancy predisposes to SLE exacerbation is unsettled. At most, the predisposition to SLE flare during pregnancy is modest. Importantly, in a majority of studies of pregnant women with SLE, flares have been mild to moderate in nature and easily treated with glucocorticoids.[33–45] However, a prospective study of consecutively enrolled pregnant lupus patients in one center found the rate of flare was highest among women who discontinued their prepregnancy hydroxychloroquine compared with those who continued it.[46] The authors concluded that the continuation of prepregnancy hydroxychloroquine during pregnancy promotes the maintenance of "quiet lupus activity."

Preexisting disease activity undoubtedly plays a large role in risk of SLE flare during pregnancy. Derksen and colleagues[42] reported that SLE exacerbation occurred in fewer than 20% of women with sustained remission prior to pregnancy. More recently, Cortez-Hernandez and coworkers[44] studied 60 women with 103 pregnancies and found that SLE exacerbations during pregnancy were more likely in women who discontinued maintenance therapy before pregnancy and/or had a history of more than three severe flares prior to pregnancy. The findings of several other studies support the notion that women with active disease should postpone pregnancy until sustained remission can be achieved.[39,43,45]

Better prognoses are attained for both mother and fetus when the disease and any associated renal dysfunction has been quiescent for 6 months prior to conception. Thus, judicious family planning and contraceptive use are paramount to best outcomes. The mother and fetus face higher risks of adverse outcome with SLE in the presence of comorbidities such as pulmonary hypertension, restrictive lung disease, chronic renal failure, heart failure, history of preeclampsia, history of cerebrovascular accident, and lupus flare within a 6-month period preceding pregnancy.[47]

The Risk of Lupus Nephritis Exacerbation

Women with lupus nephropathy face several challenges during pregnancy.[48–50] Some evidence suggests that pregnancy may worsen renal function. In turn, underlying renal disease presages increased risks of maternal and fetal complications. Those with chronic renal disease are likely to have worsening proteinuria during gestation as renal perfusion increases. In turn, this inevitably poses the question of whether the increased proteinuria represents an exacerbation of underlying renal disease, preeclampsia, or both.

Whether renal flares are more common in pregnancy in all women with SLE remains controversial. Two studies reported high frequencies of renal flares (43%–46%) during pregnancy,[51,52] whereas others have reported lower figures (9%–28%).[35,38,53,54] Three studies describe the patients' status during pregnancy in terms of whether the SLE was active or in remission prior to conception.[55–57] In all three, the rate of SLE exacerbation was lower among pregnancies in which the patient was in remission prior to conception.

Studies of pregnancy outcome in women with past or current SLE nephritis are scarce. This may be explained, in part, by (1) the reduced fertility associated with long-term cyclophosphamide or impaired renal function, or both, and (2) the classic assumption that pregnancy should be discouraged in women with a history of lupus nephritis. The earliest reports suggested that lupus nephropathy was a major contributor to serious maternal morbidity or death.[31,32,58] However, larger, more recent series suggest that the outlook for pregnancy in women with lupus nephropathy is usually favorable if the disease is well-controlled and renal function is preserved.[59] Oviasu and associates[60] reviewed eight studies (151 pregnancies) published between 1973 and 1991 on the effect of completed pregnancy on maternal renal function in established lupus nephritis and reported that transient deterioration of renal function occurred in only 17% of pregnancies and permanent deterioration occurred in 8%.

Even better outcomes were reported in three studies published in the 1990s.[60–62] Of 143 patients with lupus nephropathy, only 1 developed irreversible loss of renal function after pregnancy. Importantly, the majority of women in these studies had normal renal function, mild proteinuria, and well-controlled hypertension *before* conception. Petri and colleagues at the Hopkins Lupus Pregnancy Center reported that only women who began pregnancy with nephrotic syndrome went on to renal failure after delivery.[52] Hayslett and Lynn[55] and Bobrie and coworkers[57] also found that the rate of renal deterioration was somewhat lower among pregnancies in which the patient was in remission prior to conception. Most recently, Moroni and associates[63] reported that renal flare occurred in 5% (1/20) of pregnancies in women with inactive lupus nephropathy prior to conception compared with 39% (12/31) in women with active lupus nephropathy prior to conception ($P < .01$). The sole predictors for renal flare were a plasma creatinine greater than 1.2 mg/dL or proteinuria of 500 mg or greater in the 24-hour collection. Permanent deterioration occurred in 2 women with active lupus nephropathy prior to conception, 1 of whom eventually died.

Based on the published data summarized in Table 43–3, approximately one third of women with lupus nephropathy experience SLE exacerbation during pregnancy and 21%

TABLE 43–3
Renal Deterioration during Pregnancy in Patients with Lupus Nephritis

			EXACERBATIONS		DETERIORATION		
AUTHOR	PATIENTS	PREGNANCIES	NO	YES	NO	YES	PERMANENT
Hayslett[48]							
Inactive PTC	23	31	21/31 (68%)	10/31 (32%)	24/31 (77%)	7/31 (23%)	2/31 (6%)
Active PTC	24	25	13/25 (52%)	12/25 (48%)	16/25 (64%)	9/25 (36%)	5/25 (20%)
Fine et al[66]	13	14	NA	NA	10/14 (71%)	4/14 (29%)	2/14 (14%)
Jungerset al[56]							
Inactive PTC	8	11	9/11 (82%)	2/11 (18%)	9/11 (82%)	2/11 (18%)	1/11 (9%)
Active PTC	8	15	4/15 (27%)	11/15 (73%)	13/15 (87%)	2/15 (13%)	1/15 (7%)
Imbasciati et al[67]	6	18	8/18 (44%)	10/18 (56%)	14/18 (78%)	4/18 (22%)	2/18 (11%)
Devoe and Taylor[68]	14	17	13/17 (76%)	4/17 (24%)	12/17 (71%)	5/17 (29%)	2/17 (12%)
Bobrie et al[57]	35	53	35/53 (66%)	18/53 (34%)	NA	NA	4/53 (8%)
Julkunen et al[61]	16	26	24/26 (92%)	2/26 (8%)	25/26 (96%)	1/26 (4%)	0/26
Packham et al[62]	41	64	NA	NA	52/64 (81%)	12/64 (19%)	1/64 (2%)
Oviasu et al[60]	25	53	NA	NA	22/28 (79%)	6/28 (21%)	0/28
Moroni et al[63]							
Inactive PTC	19	20	19/20 (95%)	1/20 (5%)	NA	NA	0/20
Active PTC	20	31	19/31 (61%)	12/31 (39%)	NA	NA	2/31 (6%)
Total	252	378					
Median rates of exacerbation/ deterioration				**33%**		**21%**	**7%**

PTC, prior to conception.

experience some form of renal deterioration. The median rate for permanent deterioration is 7%. Women with inactive lupus nephropathy prior to conception rarely suffer permanent deterioration during pregnancy.

Medical prudence would strongly suggest that pregnancy is contraindicated in patients with active lupus nephropathy (especially DPGN), nephrotic syndrome, and severe hypertension. Pregnancy should be attempted only if immunosuppressive therapy is effective in reducing disease activity and antihypertensive therapy reduces blood pressure to acceptable levels. Ideally, pregnancy is undertaken without exposure to immunosuppressants or steroids. Hence, azathioprine should be used with caution, and glucocorticoids should be used at the lowest effective dose.[64,65] Moderate renal failure (creatinine 1.5–2.0 mg/dL) is a relative contraindication to pregnancy, and advanced renal failure (creatinine >2.0 mg/dL) should be considered an absolute contraindication to pregnancy.

Problems of Detection of Systemic Lupus Erythematosus Exacerbation (Flare) in Pregnancy

Thorough and frequent clinical assessment remains essential for the timely and accurate detection of SLE exacerbation. However, detection of flare during pregnancy is hampered by the fact that many of the typical signs and symptoms associated with flare are considered normal manifestations of pregnancy.[66–68] In addition, common complications of pregnancy such as preeclampsia may be mistaken for SLE exacerbation. Nevertheless, criteria for measuring SLE flare during pregnancy have been tested and have been found valid.[69] Fever, weight loss, myalgia, and arthralgia are very common.[70] As in all patients with SLE, the most common presenting symptom of flare during pregnancy is extreme fatigue (see Table 43–1). In addition, skin lesions occur in greater than 90% and arthritis/arthralgias in greater than 80% of SLE exacerbations during pregnancy.[39,52]

Serologic evaluation of SLE disease activity may be beneficial in confirming flare in confusing cases. Most specific are elevations in anti-dsDNA titers that precede lupus flare in more than 80% of patients.[10,11] In pregnancy, elevated anti-dsDNA titers have also been shown to correlate with the need for preterm delivery.[12] In combination with anticardiolipin antibodies, elevated levels of anti-dsDNA are associated with an increased risk of fetal loss.

Early reports suggested that serial serologic evaluation of complement components and activation products were beneficial in predicting SLE flare during pregnancy. In two studies, Devoe and colleagues[68,71] found that SLE exacerbation was signaled by a decline of C3 and C4 into the subnormal range. Buyon and coworkers[72] found that SLE exacerbation was associated with an absence of the usual increase in C3 and C4 levels during normal pregnancies. However, the practical utility of serial determinations of complement components or their activation products during pregnancy remains unproved. Lockshin and associates[73] reported that low-grade activation of the classic pathway may be attributed to pregnancy alone. Wong and colleagues[51] prospectively studied 19 continuing SLE pregnancies and found that neither ANA, C3, nor C4 levels predicted which patients were going to have a flare. Nossent and Swaak[74] observed that fewer than half of the pregnancies with decreased serum C3 levels were associated with a clinical SLE flare. Finally, although some have found that hypocomplementemia has been reported to correlate with poor pregnancy outcomes,[75–77] there is also evidence that hypocomplementemia may occur in pregnant patients without SLE and no adverse pregnancy outcomes.[78]

Laboratory confirmation of SLE flare is probably most helpful in women with active lupus nephropathy in whom proteinuria, hypertension, and evidence of multiorgan dysfunction may easily be confused with preeclampsia. Distinguishing between the preeclampsia and the SLE flares is not always possible, and the two conditions may occur concurrently. Nonetheless, both clinical findings and serum markers may be utilized in an effort to differentiate the two.[79] Table 43–4 outlines features that may prove helpful in distinguishing between the two conditions. Preeclampsia is more likely in women with prior history of preeclampsia, diabetes mellitus, aPLs, increased levels of complement, or decreased levels of antithrombin III.[80–82] On the contrary, SLE flares tend to be associated with increased anti-DNA antibody titers, active urine sediment (red and white cells and cellular casts), proteinuria, and hypocomplementemia.[83,84] Complement concentrations are not always helpful because activation may also occur in women with preeclampsia.[85] In the most severe and confusing cases, the correct diagnosis is possible only by renal biopsy. Ultimately, concerns about maternal and fetal well-being often prompt delivery, rendering the distinction between SLE flare and preeclampsia clinically moot.

TABLE 43–4

Distinguishing between Preeclampsia and Systemic Lupus Erythematosus/Lupus Nephropathy Flare

TEST	PREECLAMPSIA	SLE
Serologic		
Decreased complement	++	+++
Elevated Ba or Bb fragments with low CH50	±	++
Elevated anti-dsDNA	-	+++
Antithrombin III deficiency	++	±
Hematologic		
Microangiopathic hemolytic anemia	++	-
Coombs' positive hemolytic anemia	-	++
Thrombocytopenia	+	++
Leukopenia	+	+++
Renal		
Hematuria	- -	+++
Cellular casts	±	++
Elevated serum creatinine	+	++
Elevated ratio of serum blood urea nitrogen/creatinine	±	++
Hypocalciuria	++	±
Liver transaminases	++	+

SLE, systemic lupus erythematosus.

Risks of Immunosuppressive Agents in Pregnancy

GLUCOCORTICOIDS

The group of drugs most commonly given to pregnant women with SLE is the glucocorticoid preparations, both as maintenance therapy and in "bursts" to treat suspected SLE flares. The doses used in pregnancy are the same as those used in nonpregnant patients. Pregnancy per se is not an indication to reduce the dose of glucocorticoids, though a carefully monitored reduction in dosage may be reasonable in appropriately selected women whose disease appears to be in remission.

Some groups have recommended prophylactic glucocorticoid therapy during pregnancy,[35,45,54] but there are no controlled studies to show this practice to be prudent or necessary in the face of inactive SLE. Moreover, good maternal and fetal outcomes are achieved without prophylactic treatment of women with stable disease.[42] In contrast, glucocorticoid treatment of women with active disease and/or elevated anti-dsDNA titers has been shown to result in fewer relapses and better pregnancy outcomes.[11,39]

Although glucocorticoids have a low potential for teratogenesis, they are not without risk during pregnancy. Patients requiring chronic maintenance therapy are best treated with prednisolone or methylprednisolone because of their conversion to relatively inactive forms by the abundance of 11-β-ol dehydrogenase found in the human placenta. Glucocorticoids with fluorine at the 9-α position (dexamethasone, betamethasone) are considerably less well metabolized by the placenta, and chronic use during pregnancy should be avoided. Both have been associated with untoward fetal effects. Maternal side effects of chronic glucocorticoid therapy are the same as in nonpregnant patients and include weight gain, striae, acne, hirsutism, immunosuppression, osteonecrosis, and gastrointestinal ulceration. During pregnancy, chronic glucocorticoid therapy has also been associated with an increased risk of preeclampsia,[86–88] uteroplacental insufficiency, and intrauterine growth restriction (IUGR),[89] and glucose intolerance.[87,88] Women undergoing chronic treatment with glucocorticoids should be screened for gestational diabetes at 22 to 24 weeks', 28 to 30 weeks', and 32 to 34 weeks' gestation.

ANTIMALARIALS

An accumulating body of evidence suggests that antimalarial drugs, such as hydroxychloroquine, may be used safely for the treatment of SLE during pregnancy.[90–94] In the past, many patients and their physicians have discontinued antimalarials during pregnancy because of concerns about teratogenicity, including ototoxicity[95] and eye damage.[96] The latter was of particular concern because of the affinity of antimalarials for melanin-containing tissues found in the eye. However, hydroxychloroquine has been used in women considered at risk for malaria for years without any reported adverse fetal effects. This experience has been confirmed in large series showing hydroxychloroquine to be relatively safe during pregnancy.[90–94] Furthermore, these agents may be more beneficial than glucocorticoids for women who need maintenance therapy during pregnancy. In a randomized controlled trial, women who continued hydroxychloroquine during pregnancy experienced a significant reduction in SLE disease activity compared with women who changed to glucocorticoid therapy.[97] The findings of a case-control trial, which compared the effects of in utero exposure to hydroxychloroquine, were very reassuring.[94] There were no differences between 122 infants with in utero exposure to hydroxychloroquine and 70 control infants in the number and type of defects identified at birth or in the proportion of infants with visual, hearing, growth, or developmental abnormalities at follow-up (median 24 mo).

NONSTEROIDAL ANTI-INFLAMMATORY DRUGS

The most common types of analgesics used in the treatment of SLE outside of pregnancy are nonsteroidal anti-inflammatory drugs (NSAIDs). Unfortunately, they readily cross the placenta and block prostaglandin synthesis in a wide variety of fetal tissues. Maternal ingestion of normal adult doses of aspirin in the week before delivery has been associated with intracranial hemorrhage in preterm neonates.[98] Although short-term tocolytic therapy with indomethacin appears to be safe,[99,100] chronic use has been associated with a number of untoward fetal effects; when used after 32 weeks' gestation, chronic indomethacin therapy may result in constriction or closure of the fetal ductus arteriosus.[101] Long-term use of all NSAIDs has been associated with decreased fetal urine output and oligohydramnios as well as neonatal renal insufficiency.[102] Given these risks, chronic use of adult dosages of aspirin and other NSAIDs should be avoided during pregnancy, especially after the first trimester. Acetaminophen and narcotic-containing preparations are acceptable alternatives if analgesia is needed during pregnancy.

CYTOTOXIC AND IMMUNOSUPPRESSIVE AGENTS

Cytotoxic agents, including azathioprine, methotrexate, and cyclophosphamide, are used to treat only the most severely affected patients with SLE. Limited data suggest that azathioprine, a derivative of 6-mercaptopurine, is not a teratogen in humans, though it has been associated with IUGR[103,104] and evidence of impaired neonatal immunity.[105] Women who require azathioprine to control SLE disease activity should not necessarily be discouraged from becoming pregnant, though potential fetal risks should be carefully weighed against the benefits of the medication.

Cyclophosphamide has been reported to be teratogenic in both animal[106] and human studies[107,108] and should be avoided during the first trimester. Thereafter, cyclophosphamide should be used only in unusual circumstances such as in women with severe, progressive proliferative glomerulonephritis.[109] Methotrexate is known to kill chorionic villi and cause fetal death, and its use should be scrupulously avoided. Cyclosporine, high-dose IVIG, mycophenolate mofetil, and thalidomide have been studied in the treatment of nonpregnant patients with SLE.[109] Cyclosporine is a U.S. Food and Drug Administration (FDA) pregnancy category C agent that should be used in pregnancy only when the benefits clearly outweigh concerns about possible fetal-neonatal effects. Mycophenolate mofetil (CellCept) is associated with an increased risk of first-trimester pregnancy loss and an increased risk of congenital malformations, especially external ear and other facial abnormalities including cleft lip and palate, and anomalies of the distal limbs, heart, esophagus, and kidney. IVIG has been used during pregnancy without reports of adverse fetal effects. Obviously, thalidomide is strictly contraindicated during pregnancy because of

TABLE 43–5
Suggested Methods for Tapering Prednisone

1. Consolidate to a single morning dose of prednisone. Reduce the daily dose by 10%/wk, as tolerated. When a dose of 20–30 mg/day is reached, reduce by 2.5-mg increments/wk. If the patient remains asymptomatic at a dose of 15 mg/day, reduce the dose by 1-mg increments/wk to a dose of 5–10 mg/day.
2. Consolidate to a single morning dose of prednisone. Taper to 50–60 mg/day by reducing the dose 10%/wk. Thereafter, eliminate the alternate-day dose by tapering it 10%/wk, as tolerated. Thereafter, taper the remaining every-other-day dose by 10%/wk, as tolerated.

its known potent teratogenicity. Complete immunoablative therapy followed by bone marrow stem cell transplantation has also been studied in patients with the most severe, unresponsive SLE.[109]

Treatment of Systemic Lupus Erythematosus Exacerbations in Pregnancy

Mild to moderate symptomatic exacerbations of SLE without central nervous system (CNS) or renal involvement may be treated with initiation of glucocorticoids or an increase in the dose of glucocorticoids. Relatively small doses of prednisone (e.g., 15–30 mg/day) will result in improvement in most cases. For severe exacerbations without CNS or renal involvement, doses of 1.0 to 1.5 mg/kg/day of prednisone in divided doses should be used, and a good clinical response can be expected in 5 to 10 days. Thereafter, glucocorticoids may be tapered by several different approaches (Table 43–5).

Severe exacerbations, especially those involving the CNS or kidneys, are treated more aggressively. In recent years, an intravenous pulse glucocorticoid approach has become popular. The initial regimen involves a daily intravenous dose of methylprednisolone at 10 to 30 mg/kg (~500–1000 mg) for 3 to 6 days. Thereafter, the patient is treated with 1.0 to 1.5 mg/kg/day of prednisone in divided doses and rapidly tapered over the course of 1 month. One can expect that 75% of patients will respond favorably to this approach.[110] This regimen may be repeated every 1 to 3 months in severe cases as an alternative to cytotoxic drugs.

In nonpregnant patients, both azathioprine and cyclophosphamide may be used in severe SLE exacerbations to control disease, reduce irreversible tissue damage, and reduce glucocorticoid doses.[111–113] In particular, severe proliferative lupus nephritis may be treated more effectively with cyclophosphamide, usually in combination with glucocorticoids.[113] The drug may be given either orally or intravenously, but the most effective cyclophosphamide regimen is uncertain. Cyclophosphamide appears to be useful in the treatment of severe cerebral lupus as well.

Plasmapheresis and IVIG have been used to treat severe cases of SLE flare unresponsive to standard treatments. Plasmapheresis should be considered in life-threatening disease that is unresponsive to other treatments. A cytotoxic agent should also be administered soon after plasmapheresis is initiated (days 5–10 of therapy) if the patient is no longer pregnant. IVIG has been used for salvage treatment of recalcitrant SLE flare with neuropsychiatric or renal involvement.[114]

Obstetric Complications in Women with Systemic Lupus Erythematosus

GESTATIONAL HYPERTENSION AND PREECLAMPSIA

The exact incidence of pregnancy-related hypertension associated with SLE is difficult to estimate owing to inconsistencies in the definition and classification of these disorders as well as the inclusion of patients with lupus nephropathy in the various studies. Nevertheless, it appears that between 20% and 30% of women with SLE develop either gestational hypertension or preeclampsia (gestational hypertension with proteinuria) sometime during pregnancy.[86,115–117] Women with lupus nephropathy are undoubtedly most vulnerable given the known association between preeclampsia and underlying renal disease of any origin.[118] In one prospective series, preeclampsia occurred in 7 of 19 (37%) women with lupus nephritis, compared with 15 of 106 (14%) without.[86] Other important predisposing factors include chronic hypertension, antiphospholipid syndrome (APS), and chronic steroid use.[60,117,119,120]

PREGNANCY LOSS

Women with SLE are probably more likely to have an unsuccessful pregnancy than women in the general obstetric population. The exact physiologic mechanisms responsible for pregnancy loss in women with SLE and other immunologic diseases remain uncertain, though a clear relationship between pregnancy failure and histologic evidence of inflammation has been well documented. Recent experimental observations suggest that altered complement regulation causes and may perpetuate pregnancy loss.

In most retrospective studies, the rate of pregnancy loss appears to be higher in women with SLE than in the general obstetric population, ranging between 8% and 41%, with a median of 22%.[31,34,55,66,117,121–126] In one case-control trial comparing obstetric outcomes between 481 pregnancies in 203 lupus patients, 566 pregnancies in 177 healthy relatives, and 356 pregnancies in 166 healthy unrelated women, investigators found that pregnancy loss occurred significantly more often in women with SLE (21%) than in either their healthy relatives (8%) or the unrelated healthy controls (14%).[127] In the group of women with SLE and prior pregnancy, those whose diagnosis was made with SLE onset *after* their first pregnancy had a higher rate of loss once the diagnosis was made (27% vs. 19%). The pregnancy loss rates observed in most prospective trials of lupus pregnancies have been better than those found in retrospective trials, possibly because of careful monitoring of SLE activity and routine antenatal surveillance. Still, from the data summarized in Table 43–6, between 11% and 34% of women with SLE experienced pregnancy loss, with a median of 24%. In the well-detailed prospective trials, fetal deaths in the second or third trimester accounted for between 10% and 40% of the total number of losses.[39,43] Though not clearly linked to better management, Clark and coworkers[127] suggested that the incidence of pregnancy loss with SLE has declined over the past several decades from a mean of 43%

TABLE 43–6

Fetal Outcome in Prospective Cohort Studies of Women after the Diagnosis of Systemic Lupus Erythematosus

AUTHOR	PREGNANCIES	LIVE BIRTHS	THERAPEUTIC ABORTIONS*	PREGNANCY LOSSES		TOTAL
				MISCARRIAGE	FETAL DEATHS	
Devoe et al[68]	11	8 (73%)	1 (9%)	2 (18%)	0	3 (27%)
Mintz et al[35]	102	80 (78%)	0	17 (17%)	5 (5%)	22 (22%)
Lockshin et al[33]	80	61 (76%)	NA	NA	NA	19 (24%)
Nossent et al[53]	39	33 (85%)	0	4 (10%)	2 (5%)	6 (15%)
Wong et al[51]	24	17 (71%)	5 (21%)	2 (8%)	0	7 (29%)
Derksen et al[42]	35	25 (71%)	1 (3%)	8 (23%)	1 (3%)	10 (29%)
Huong et al[45]	99	76 (77%)	5 (5%)	13 (13%)	5 (5%)	23 (23%)
Lima et al[129]	108	89 (82%)	2 (2%)	7 (7%)	10 (9%)	19 (18%)
Georgiou et al[39]	59	36 (61%)	3 (5%)	9 (15%)	1 (2%)	13 (22%)
Cortes-Hernandez et al[44]	103	68 (66%)	8 (8%)	15 (15%)	12 (12%)	35 (34%)
Total	**660**					
Median Rates		**75%**	**5%**	**14%**	**5%**	**24%**

* Elective terminations were excluded.
NA, not available.

TABLE 43–7

Pregnancy Outcomes among Women with Systemic Lupus Erythematosus Nephropathy

AUTHOR	PATIENTS	PREGNANCIES	THERAPEUTIC ABORTIONS	PREGNANCY LOSSES		LIVE BIRTHS		TOTAL
				MISCARRIAGES	FETAL DEATHS	PRETERM	TERM	
Hayslett et al[55]								
Remission PTC	23	31	7	1 (4%)	2 (8%)	1 (4%)	20 (84%)	21 (88%)
Active PTC	24	25	3	3 (14%)	5 (23%)	0	14 (64%)	14 (64%)
Jungers et al[56]								
Remission PTC	8	11	0	0	0	1 (9%)	10 (91%)	11 (100%)
Active PTC	8	15	3	3 (25%)	0	2 (17%)	7 (58%)	9 (75%)
Imbasciati et al[67]	6	18	2	0	4 (25%)	10 (62%)	2 (12%)	12 (75%)
Gimovsky et al[124]	19	46	6	16 (40%)	5 (12%)	9 (23%)	10 (25%)	19 (48%)
Devoe and Taylor[68]	14	17	2	2 (13%)	1 (7%)	3 (20%)	9 (60%)	12 (80%)
Bobrie et al[57]	35	53	15	5 (13%)	0	5 (13%)	28 (74%)	33 (87%)
Julkunen et al[61]	16	26	2	1 (4%)	1 (4%)	6 (25%)	16 (67%)	22 (92%)
Packham et al[62]	41	64	5	5 (9%)	10 (17%)	19 (32%)	24 (41%)	43 (73%)
Oviasu et al[60]	25	53	6	8 (17%)	1 (2%)	10 (21%)	28 (60%)	38 (81%)
Huong et al[45]	22	32	0	7 (22%)	2 (6%)	17 (53%)	6 (19%)	23 (72%)
Cortes-Hernandez et al[44]	20	20	1	5 (26%)	6 (32%)	3 (16%)	5 (26%)	8 (42%)
Total	**261**	**411**						
Median Rates				**13%**	**7%**	**19%**	**58%**	**75%**

PTC, prior to conception.

in the 1960s to 17% from 2000 to 2003. The latter figure coincidentally approximates reported pregnancy loss rate of the general American population. In contrast, a 2008 report of a multiethnic, North American cohort with SLE cited an incidence of stillbirths and fetal losses to be 45%.[128] Control of disease activity appears to have a salutary effect on the rate of pregnancy loss,[41] with one early study reporting live births in 64% of women with active disease within 6 months of conception, compared with 88% in women with quiescent disease.[48] In a more recent prospective study of pregnancy in SLE patients, pregnancy loss occurred in 75% of women with active disease compared with 14% of women with inactive disease.[39] Not surprisingly, pregnancy loss is more likely if SLE is diagnosed during the index pregnancy.[56,67,124]

Preexisting renal disease increases the rate of pregnancy loss in women with SLE. Table 43–7 summarizes obstetric outcomes in 411 pregnancies in 261 women with a diagnosis of lupus nephropathy prior to conception. Excluding therapeutic abortions, the median rates of miscarriage, fetal and neonatal death, and live birth were 13%, 7%, and 75%, respectively, figures not remarkably different from those for all patients with SLE shown in Table 43–6. Pregnancy loss rates in individual studies vary widely, probably because of variations in the degree of renal impairment of included patients as well as definitions of pregnancy loss.

The degree of renal impairment no doubt influences the likelihood of pregnancy loss in women with lupus nephropathy. In a study of lupus nephropathy in pregnancy that included only women with inactive disease and normal renal function (serum creatinine <0.8 mg/dL), the overall fetal survival rate was greater than 90%, after exclusion of embryonic losses (losses <10 weeks' gestation).[126] These results contrast markedly to those of another study in which the rate of fetal loss was 50% in pregnant women with lupus nephropathy and moderate to severe renal insufficiency (serum creatinine ≥1.5 mg/dL).[55] In a study comparing obstetric outcomes according to the degree of renal impairment in women with lupus nephropathy, spontaneous abortion occurred in 26% of women with minimally impaired renal function (serum creatinine <1 mg/dL, creatinine clearance >80 mL/min, and proteinuria <1 g/day) and 36% in women with mild impairment (creatinine clearance 50–80 mL/min and proteinuria 1–3 g/day).[66]

Among SLE patients, fetal deaths are associated with the presence of aPLs (see the sections on "Antiphospholipid Syndrome"). In several studies, the presence of aPLs has been the single most sensitive predictor of fetal death.[129] The positive predictive value of aPLs for fetal death is over 50%.[86] For women with SLE and a prior fetal death, the predictive value is over 85%.[130] In a prospective trial, the presence of any aPL was the single strongest predictor of subsequent pregnancy loss, even in women with active disease and underlying renal impairment.[131]

PRETERM BIRTH

Preterm birth has been reported in as few as 3% and as many as 73% of pregnancies complicated by SLE.[35,51,55,56,66,67,125,129,132–134] Not surprisingly, the presence of aPLs, chronic hypertension, and disease activity have all been reported to increase the likelihood of preterm birth in women with SLE.[39,131] Only a handful of studies have compared preterm birth rates in women with SLE with those in healthy controls. In one retrospective case-control study, preterm birth occurred more commonly in a group of women with SLE than in a group of matched controls (12% vs. 4%).[135] This was not the case in a more recent prospective trial, in which the rates of preterm birth in women with SLE and healthy controls were statistically similar (8% vs. 15%).[39] Interestingly, preterm birth was more common among women with active SLE than among those with inactive disease (12.5% vs. 4%).

A substantial proportion of preterm birth associated with SLE is undoubtedly a result of iatrogenic delivery for obstetric and medical indications rather than idiopathic preterm labor. From the few studies that provide sufficient detail, between 28% and 66% of preterm deliveries are indicated because of preeclampsia and another 12% to 33% because of suspected or confirmed fetal compromise.[125,130–132,135] An association between SLE and preterm premature rupture of membranes (PPROM) has also been reported, occurring in 39% of pregnancies delivered at 24 to 36 weeks' gestation.[134]

INTRAUTERINE FETAL GROWTH RESTRICTION

Uteroplacental insufficiency resulting in IUGR or small–for–gestational age neonates has been reported in between 12% and 40% of pregnancies complicated by SLE.[38,41,43,62,116,131] Mintz and coworkers[35] reported higher rates of IUGR in pregnancies complicated by SLE than in pregnancies in normal controls (23% vs. 4%). However, the higher rate of IUGR associated with SLE may have been due to all the women with SLE receiving prophylactic glucocorticoid therapy during pregnancy. In a more recent prospective trial during which glucocorticoids were given only for symptomatic SLE flare, Georgiou and associates[39] reported no significant differences in the rate of IUGR between SLE pregnancies and healthy controls. Factors that have been associated with a higher rate of IUGR in SLE pregnancies include renal insufficiency and/or hypertension.[89,117,131]

NEONATAL LUPUS ERYTHEMATOSUS

Neonatal lupus erythematosus is a rare condition of the fetus and neonate, occurring in 1 in 20,000 of all live births and in fewer than 5% of all women with SLE.[136] Dermatologic manifestations are the most common manifestation of neonatal lupus and are described as "erythematous," "scaling annular," or "elliptical" plaques occurring on the face or scalp, analogous to the subacute cutaneous lesions in adults.[137] Lesions appear in the first weeks of life, probably induced by exposure of the skin to ultraviolet light, and may last for up to 6 months. Hypopigmentation may persist for up to 2 years. A small percentage of affected infants will go on to have other autoimmune diseases later in life.[136] Hematologic neonatal lupus is rare and may be manifest as autoimmune hemolytic anemia, leukopenia, thrombocytopenia, and hepatosplenomegaly.

Cardiac neonatal lupus lesions include congenital complete heart block (CCHB) and the less frequently reported endocardial fibroelastosis. CCHB is due to disruption of the cardiac conduction system, especially in the area of the atrioventricular node. The diagnosis of CCHB is typically made around between 18 to 24 weeks[138] when a fixed bradycardia, in the range of 60 to 80 beats/min, is detected during a routine prenatal visit. The associated mortality approaches 20%, making it a very concerning diagnosis.[139] Sonographic markers in affected fetuses that negatively correlate with survival include ascites, increasing cardiothoracic circumference ratio, and hydrops. In cases of CCHB, fetal echocardiography reveals complete atrioventricular dissociation with a structurally normal heart.[140] Confirmation of neonatal lupus is based on the presence of autoantibodies in maternal circulation. Endomyocardial damage is irreversible; in the most severely affected cases, cardiac failure leads to hydrops fetalis and fetal death. In less severely affected neonates, pacemaker placement is frequently necessary to ensure survival. In the largest series of prenatally diagnosed CCHB, the 3-year survival was only 79%; the majority of deaths occurred before 90 days of life.[138] Cutaneous manifestations of neonatal lupus have also been reported in infants with CCHB.[137]

Not all women who give birth to babies with neonatal lupus have been previously diagnosed with an autoimmune disorder.[137,138,141] However, in one study, 7 of 13 previously asymptomatic mothers who delivered infants with dermatologic neonatal lupus were later diagnosed with one of several autoimmune disorders.[137] Surprisingly, asymptomatic women who deliver infants with CCHB were less likely to develop an autoimmune disorder than those who delivered infants with dermatologic manifestations.[141]

A model of passively acquired autoimmunity, neonatal lupus manifestations are presumed to arise from the transplacental passage of autoantibodies directed against Ro/SS-A ribonucleoprotein antigens.[138,142–145] Anti-Ro/SS-A antibodies are found in 75% to 95% of mothers who deliver babies with neonatal lupus.[138,146,147] A smaller percentage have anti-La/SS-B, and some have both.[147] More than 80% of mothers of infants with CCHB have autoantibodies to the 52-kDa Ro/SS-A protein.[148,149] The finer specificity of this autoantibody has been identified as epitope expressed by amino acids 200-239 of the Ro/SS-A 52-kDa protein.[150] Using sera from a large research registry, other investigators have shown that reactivity to this peptide (aa200-239) is a dominant but not uniform anti-Ro/SS-A 52 response in women whose children have CCHB.[151]

The proposed mechanism of CCHB is that the relevant autoantibodies cross the placenta and damage the myometrium or conduction system of the fetal heart. However, the SS-A antigen containing the SS-A 52 protein is intracellular, and authorities acknowledge that the maternal autoantibody is requisite but not sufficient to cause CCHB. Other factors, including genetic contributions and the fine specificity of the autoantibodies, are likely important. One group has shown that the p200-specific anti-SSA antibodies from humans bind to cultured cardiomyosites, affect cellular calcium homeostasis, and lead to cellular apoptosis.[150] They have further demonstrated that the pups of rats immunized against the p200 amino acid stretch of SS-A 52 develop heart block. The authors suggest that the autoantibodies do not bind to intracellular SS-A, but to a cross-reactive cell surface antigen.

Among all mothers with SLE, the risk of neonatal lupus is less than 5%.[136] Of mothers with SLE who are serologically positive for anti-Ro/SS-A antibodies, 15% will have infants affected with dermatologic neonatal lupus; the proportion that delivers infants with CCHB is much smaller. The latter condition is more prevalent in infants born to women with high anti-Ro/SS-A and anti-La/SS-B titers.[152] Also, once a women with SLE and anti-Ro/SS-A antibodies delivers one infant with CCHB, her risk for recurrence approaches 20%, some three- or fourfold higher than women with anti-Ro/SS-A or anti-La/SS-B antibodies who have never had an affected child.[138,153] Recurrence of dermatologic neonatal lupus is approximately 25%.[153,154]

In women with anti-Ro/SS-A and/or anti-La/SS-B antibodies, the presence of anti-La/SS-B anti-idiotypic antibodies in maternal serum confers lower risk; these anti-idiotypic antibodies may protect the fetus by binding and, in effect, blocking the activity of harmful maternal autoantibodies. Women with neonates with congenital heart block tend not to express these anti-idiotypic antibodies. As such, testing for such "anti-idiotypic" responses has been suggested as being useful for predicting outcomes.[155]

Management Options

Prepregnancy

Women with SLE who are contemplating pregnancy should be counseled before conception about potential obstetric problems, including pregnancy loss, preterm birth, gestational hypertension/preeclampsia, and IUGR. They should also be informed of the risk of SLE flare as well as special concerns related to APS and neonatal lupus. Preconceptional laboratory evaluation should include an assessment for anemia and thrombocytopenia, underlying renal disease (urinalysis, serum creatinine, and 24-hr urine for creatinine clearance and total protein) and aPLs. It is also common practice to obtain anti-Ro/SS-A and anti-La/SS-B antibodies on all patients with SLE, but the cost-effectiveness of these is questionable given the low prevalence of the condition and the lack of proven intervention.

Women with active SLE should be discouraged from embarking on pregnancy until remission can be attained. Cytotoxic drugs and NSAIDs should be stopped before pregnancy. However, maintenance therapy with hydroxychloroquine or glucocorticoids need not be discontinued.

Prenatal

The obstetric management of the patient with SLE is guided by the potential risks to the mother and fetus. Once pregnancy is confirmed in a woman with SLE, the following examinations and tests are recommended: physical examination complete with blood pressure, complete blood count, urinalysis, urine protein–to–urine creatinine ratio, glomerular filtration rate, and aPL antibodies (if not recently performed). Some experts routinely test for anti-Ro/SS-A and anti-La/SS-B antibodies, anti-dsDNA antibodies, and complement (C3 and C4), though the need for these in unselected, and especially in asymptomatic, cases is questionable. Periodic reassessment of platelet count or complete blood count is recommended by some.[156]

As mentioned, prenatal visits should occur every 1 to 2 weeks in the first and second trimesters and every week thereafter. A primary goal of the antenatal visits after 20 weeks' gestation is the detection of hypertension and/or proteinuria. Because of the risk of uteroplacental insufficiency, fetal ultrasonography should be performed every 4 to 6 weeks starting at 18 to 20 weeks' gestation. In the usual case, fetal surveillance (daily fetal movement counts and once- or twice-weekly nonstress tests and amniotic fluid volume measurements) should be instituted at 30 to 32 weeks' gestation. More frequent ultrasonography and fetal testing is indicated in patients with SLE flare, hypertension, proteinuria, clinical evidence of IUGR, or APS. In the patients with APS, fetal surveillance as early as 24 to 25 weeks' gestation may be justified.[157]

In fetuses at risk for CCHB, some experts have used weekly fetal PR interval determinations from 16 to 26 weeks, performed using gated pulsed Doppler techniques, in an effort to detect early evidence of evolving heart block.[158] In the PRIDE (PR Interval and Dexamethasone Evaluation) study,[158] this approach detected a prolonged PR interval (>150 msec) in only a few of nearly 100 fetuses at risk and failed to reliably diagnose impending CCHB. A somewhat similar European study detected a much higher rate of prolonged PR intervals, defined as greater than 135 msec, in an at-risk population.[159] In both studies, though, transiently prolonged PR intervals of uncertain clinical significance were seen, and in neither study was it definitively shown that detection of a prolonged PR interval altered fetal-neonatal outcomes with regard to CCHB. Thus, in a strict sense, PR interval monitoring in fetuses at risk for CCHB remains investigational. Nonetheless, most experts would recommend that at-risk fetuses be monitored frequently from approximately 16 to 26 weeks.

The treatment of fetuses with CCHB is somewhat uncertain. A 2002 report of consecutive cases from a single institution suggested that a combination of dexamethasone, along with a β-mimetic when the fetal heart rate is less than 55 beats/min, results in improved overall survival.[160] These investigators found 1-year neonatal survival rates of in excess of 80% using their management regimen. Less salubrious results come from the recently published PRIDE study.[158] The PRIDE investigators enrolled 40 pregnant women with anti-Ro/SS-A antibodies and a fetus with heart block from 33 centers. Thirty of the mothers elected to take dexamethasone, whereas 10 did not. None of the 22 fetuses with complete (third-degree) heart block recovered any conduction in association with dexamethasone treatment. Of the 6 fetuses with second-degree heart block who were treated with dexamethasone, 3 progressed to third-degree block, whereas 2 stabilized at second-degree and only 1 reverted to normal sinus rhythm. Two fetuses found to have first-degree heart block reverted to normal sinus rhythm with dexamethasone treatment.

Outcomes were fairly similar in the nondexamethasone group, in which 9 of the 10 fetuses presented with third-degree heart block. Though case selection likely played a role, there were no fetal-neonatal deaths in the nondexamethasone group, whereas there were 6 (20%) in the dexamethasone group. The preterm birth rate was higher in the dexamethasone group.

The case of CCHB associated with fetal hydrops may pose a special circumstance. A retrospective analysis of collected cases found that dexamethasone use was associated with improvement in the hydrops, though not the heart block.[161] Based on available evidence, although much of it less than convincing, most experts still recommend a trial of dexamethasone if first- or second-degree heart block is found or in selected cases of CCHB with hydrops (Table 43–8).

Another therapy that has become of interest in the prevention of CCHB is that of IVIG. IVIG has the potential to lower the transplacental passage of autoantibodies against Ro/SS-A-La/SS-B that are responsible for the pathogenesis of CCHB.[162] Favorable outcomes have been reported in case reports.[163] The PITCH (Preventative IVIG Therapy for Congenital Heart Block) study is currently under way to answer the question of whether maternal administration in the context of positive Ro/SS-A and/or La/SS-B titers, maternal rheumatic disease either symptomatic or not, and a previously affected child with CCHB or neonatal lupus.[164] Though the results of two prospective studies (one European and the PITCH study) are as yet unpublished, neither found a decrease in the frequency of CCHB in high risk populations when mothers were treated with periodic infusions of IVIG. These important results strongly suggest that IVIG is not indicated for the prevention of CCHB. Thus, insufficient evidence exists to recommend IVIG therapy except under an approved experimental protocol.

TABLE 43–8

Management Approaches for Anti-Ro/SSA Antibody Associated Risk of Complete Congenital Heart Block or Evidence of Cardiac Conduction Abnormalities

CLINICAL SITUATION	MANAGEMENT
Maternal anti-SSA antibodies; no history of fetus with CCHB	Expectant management. Evaluation of the fetus by serial echosonography is recommended by some experts.
Maternal anti-SSA antibodies; prior fetus with CCHB	Expectant management. Evaluation of the fetus by serial echosonography is recommended by some experts.
Fetal first-degree heart block (prolonged mechanical PR interval)	Repeat echocardiographic assessment within 24 hr. If first-degree heart block persists, treat with maternally administered DEX), 4 mg daily. If first-degree heart block persists or resolves, continue DEX until 24–26 wk, then taper. If there is progression to third-degree heart block, taper DEX to discontinuation.
Fetal second-degree heart block or alternating second-/third-degree heart block	Treat with maternally-administered DEX, 4 mg daily. If second-degree heart block persists or resolves, continue DEX until 24–26 wk, then taper. If there is progression to third-degree heart block, taper DEX to discontinuation.
Fetal third-degree heart block	Expectant management, with monitoring for fetal hydrops. If fetal heart rate <55 beats/min, treat with maternally administered oral terbutaline (2.5–7.5 mg q4–6h) sufficient to result in mild maternal tachycardia.
Fetal third-degree heart block with evidence of myocarditis or fetal hydrops	Treat with maternally administered DEX, 4 mg daily, at least until improvement in fetal sonographic findings.

CCHB, complete congenital heart block; DEX, dexamethasone.

Fetuses with heart rates less than 55 beats/min are more likely to have hydropic changes and demise.[165–168] Because of this, some clinical investigators have used maternally administered β-sympathomimetic agents in a effort to increase the fetal heart rate,[169–171] and reports suggest that the use of these agents may favorably alter signs of cardiac insufficiency and result in higher fetal-neonatal survival rates.[169–171] Jaeggi and associates in 2004[160] analyzed 37 cases of fetal CCHB since 1990. The investigators stratified their data by their institution's initiation of β-sympathomimetic stimulation for fetal heart rates of less than 55 beats/min in 1997 when reports of worse outcomes for this finding surfaced. Significant improvement in neonatal morbidity and 1-year survival rates (80%–95%; $P < .01$) were noted with the addition of β-stimulation to dexamethasone therapy for CCHB when the fetal heart rate was les than 55 beats/min.

Labor and Delivery

The management of the gravida with SLE during labor and delivery represents a continuation of her antenatal care.[172] Exacerbations of SLE can occur during labor and may require the acute administration of steroids. Regardless, stress doses of glucocorticoids should be given during labor or at the time of cesarean delivery to all patients who have been treated with chronic steroids within the previous year. This compensates for the anticipated endogenous adrenal insufficiency in these patients. Intravenous hydrocortisone, given in three doses of 100 mg every 8 hours, is an acceptable regimen. Complications such as preeclampsia and IUGR should be dealt with based on obstetric concerns; their management is not specifically altered by the presence of SLE. Neonatology support may be needed at delivery for problems associated with CCHB and other manifestations of neonatal lupus.

Postnatal

The true predisposition for SLE exacerbation following delivery is uncertain. Regardless, care should be taken to examine for these flares in the symptomatic parturient. If gestational hypertension complicates the intrapartum process, it should be anticipated that the patient will clear these acute effects in a manner similar to otherwise normal women with this condition. Maintenance medications should be restarted immediately after delivery, at similar doses as during the pregnancy. Further dose adjustments can be handled in the outpatient setting.

SUMMARY OF MANAGEMENT OPTIONS

Systemic Lupus Erythematosus

Management Options	Evidence Quality and Recommendation	References
Prepregnancy		
Establish good control of SLE; adjust maintenance medications.	—/GPP	—
Discontinue azathioprine and cyclophosphamide if possible and only under careful supervision; avoid methotrexate.	IIb/B	98,101,103,105, 106,109,110
It is not necessary to discontinue hydroxychloroquine.	IIa/B	88–92
Laboratory assessment for anemia, thrombocytopenia, renal disease, antiphospholipid antibodies (antiphospholipid).	—/GPP	—
Counsel patient regarding risks (exacerbations, preeclampsia, fetal/neonatal).	—/GPP	—
Prenatal		
Provide multidisciplinary care.	—/GPP	—
Encourage early prenatal care.	—/GPP	—
Obtain a dating scan.	—/GPP	—
Obtain frequent antenatal checks: every 2 wk in the first and second trimesters, weekly in third trimester.	—/GPP	—
Maintain vigilance for SLE flare, preeclampsia, IUGR.	—/GPP	—
For SLE patients with renal involvement, perform baseline 24-hr urine collections for creatinine clearance and total protein; repeat as clinically indicated.	—/GPP	—
Drugs		
• Antimalarials.	IIa/B	88–92
• Glucocorticoids.	IIb/B	103
• Azathioprine if steroids are ineffective.	III/B	101
• Cyclophosphamide as third choice.	III/B	103,110
• Avoid full-dose NSAIDs and methotrexate.	III/B	98,105,106,109
Serial biometry (q3–4wk) to assess fetal growth and amniotic fluid from 18-wk anatomic survey to delivery.	—/GPP	—
Begin fetal surveillance at 30–32 wk' gestation (earlier in patients with worsening disease, evidence of fetal compromise, or a history of poor pregnancy outcome).	III/B	157
Consider low-dose aspirin, especially if history of early-onset severe preeclampsia.	Ib/A	57,58

SUMMARY OF MANAGEMENT OPTIONS

Systemic Lupus Erythematosus—cont'd

Management Options	Evidence Quality and Recommendation	References
Labor and Delivery		
Deliver at term; avoid postdates.	—/GPP	—
Continuous fetal heart rate monitoring.	—/GPP	—
Intravenous glucocorticosteroids for delivery in patients who have received maintenance or steroid bursts during pregnancy.	IIb/B	80
Postnatal		
Monitor for SLE exacerbation.	—/GPP	—
Restart maintenance therapy.	—/GPP	—
Check neonate for SLE manifestations.	—/GPP	—

GPP, good practice point; IUGR, intrauterine growth restriction; NSAIDs, nonsteroidal anti-inflammatory drugs; SLE, systemic lupus erythematosus.

ANTIPHOSPHOLIPID SYNDROME

General

APS was first identified as a syndrome of thrombosis or fetal loss in association with circulating lupus anticoagulant (LA) or anticardiolipin antibodies in the mid-1980s.[173,174] Preliminary classification criteria for the syndrome were derived by expert consensus in 1998 and included recurrent preembryonic and embryonic pregnancy loss, fetal death, and severe preeclampsia or placental insufficiency requiring delivery prior to 34 weeks' gestation.[175] This classification was revised in 2004, and both the thrombotic and the obstetric clinical criteria were preserved.[176]

Antiphospholipid Antibodies

Current evidence suggests that the primary clinically relevant epitope for aPLs is on β_2-glycoprotein I. This glycoprotein is a ubiquitous, multifunctional plasma protein with affinity for negatively charged phospholipids and regulatory roles in coagulation, fibrinolysis, and other physiologic systems.[177] Specifically, it appears that autoantibodies that bind a cryptic epitope in domain I of β_2-glycoprotein I correlate best with thrombosis, a primary clinical feature of APS.[178–181] These relevant aPLs can be detected in several different assay systems, including clotting assays that detect LA and enzyme-linked immunosorbent assays (ELISA) for anticardiolipin and anti-β_2-glycoprotein I antibodies (Table 43–9). Importantly, the common feature is a dependency for binding on the presence of β_2-glycoprotein I. aPLs, though, are a heterogeneous, and β_2-glycoprotein I–independent "antiphospholipid" antibodies can be detected in immunoassays. These antibodies appear to play little or no role in APS.

The revised consensus criteria for the diagnosis of definite APS accept one or more of three aPLs as diagnostic. These include LA, anticardiolipin, and anti-β_2-glycoprotein I antibodies. Most experts hold that LA, which is detected via coagulation assays in plasma, is more specific but less

TABLE 43–9

Detection of Antiphospholipid Antibodies

Lupus anticoagulant	1. Screening with two phospholipid-dependent, in vitro clotting assays using patient's platelet-poor plasma. The assays most commonly used in the United States are the aPTT (which tests the intrinsic coagulation pathway) and the dRVVT (which tests the final common pathway). 2. If either of the above is prolonged, the test is repeated with a mix (usually 1:1) of patient and normal platelet-poor plasma. If mixing studies do not "correct" the prolonged clotting time(s), lupus anticoagulant is suspected. 3. Lupus anticoagulant is confirmed by demonstrating marked shortening or correction of the prolonged clotting time after addition of excess phospholipid. This is most commonly done using the platelet neutralization procedure or hexagonal phase phospholipid neutralization. 4. If the confirmatory test is negative or equivocal, additional tests may be done to investigate other possible coagulopathies or specific factor inhibitors.
Anticardiolipin antibodies	ELISA for IgG and IgM antibodies. The assay used should employ available international calibrators, and results should be reported in GPL and MPL units.
Anti-β_2-glycoprotein I antibodies	ELISA for IgG and IgM antibodies. The assay used should employ available international calibrators, and results should be reported in standard units.

aPTT, activated partial thromboplastin time; dRVVT, dilute Russell's viper venom time; ELISA, enzyme-linked immunosorbent assay; GPL, reference reagent for IgG; Ig, immunoglobulin; MPL, reference reagent for IgM.

sensitive than the other two tests.[180] Both anticardiolipin and anti-β_2-glycoprotein I are detected in serum by ELISA. Many patients with APS have all three antibodies detected. However, many also do not, indicating that the three antibodies are not identical. Moreover, LA and anticardiolipin antibodies may be separated in the laboratory.[181] Thus, aPLs are perhaps best viewed as related but distinctly different immunoglobulins.

LA is detected in platelet-poor plasma and is so named because it paradoxically prolongs phospholipid-dependent, in vitro clotting tests such as the activated partial thromboplastin time (aPTT). The presence of LA is detected through a series of tests (see Table 43–9). Screening typically is performed using a sensitive aPTT and the dilute Russell's viper venom time (dRVVT). Prolongation of these tests may be due to plasma factor deficiencies, anticoagulant medications, or factor-specific inhibitors. Thus, if either of the screening tests suggests the presence of LA, subsequent tests are done to exclude other causes of prolonged clotting times and to establish that the prolonged clotting times is caused by a phospholipid-sensitive inhibitor-LA. The latter step usually involves either the platelet or the hexagonal phase phospholipid neutralization procedure. LA is reported as either present or absent. Transient positive tests may occur; the diagnosis of APS requires repeatedly positive aPL tests at least 12 weeks apart.

Anticardiolipin antibodies are most commonly detected using ELISA (see Table 43–9). Experts recommend that immunoglobulin G (IgG) and IgM isotypes be sought. It is widely held that IgG anticardiolipin antibodies are most strongly associated with clinical features of APS.[182] The clinical relevance of IgA anticardiolipin antibodies is poorly characterized and the diagnosis of APS should not be made on the basis of isolated IgA anticardiolipin antibodies. Historically, standardization of anticardiolipin antibody assays has been difficult, resulting in poor concordance between laboratories.[183] More recently, though, interlaboratory agreement, in terms of semiquantitative results, is seemingly improved.[184]

Standard, reference reagents for anticardiolipin antibodies are available, and results are typically reported in arbitrary units, designated "GPL" for IgG and "MPL" for IgM. Because the accuracy and reliability of quantitative anticardiolipin antibody results are somewhat limited, consensus guidelines have emphasized the use of semiquantitative results (e.g., negative, low, medium, or high). Thus, a laboratory might report that a patient's serum is positive at 42 GPL units, a result that is better interpreted as a "medium" positive.

As with anticardiolipin antibodies, anti-β_2-glycoprotein I antibodies are most commonly detected using enzyme-linked immunosorbent assays (see Table 43–9). However, in the case of assays for anti-β_2-glycoprotein I antibodies, high-affinity, hydrophilic, negatively charged immunoassay plates are required.[185] As with anticardiolipin antibodies, experts recommend that IgG and IgM isotypes anti-β_2-glycoprotein I be sought and hold that the IgG isotype is most strongly associated with APS.

Anti-β_2-glycoprotein I antibodies are reported most commonly in standard units known as "SGU" or "SMU" for IgG and IgM, respectively. Optimal interpretation of results is in semiquantitative terms (e.g., negative, low, medium, or high).

Other "Antiphospholipid" Antibodies

The revised criteria for the diagnosis of definite APS include only three aPLs—LA, anticardiolipin, and anti-β_2-glycoprotein I.[176] Some laboratories offer testing for other so-called aPLs, often in a panel of tests. Results from such assays do little to improve the diagnosis of APS and are not recommended.[186]

aPLs represent a special consideration in APS. Some investigators have found the presence of these antibodies to be clinically relevant,[187–189] whereas others have not.[190,191] There is, however, no clear consensus as to how antiprothrombin antibody assays should be performed,[192] and some investigators have found substantial levels of aPLs in the normal population.[179] Thus, aPLs are not recommended for the diagnosis of APS.[176]

The Pathogenesis of Antiphospholipid Syndrome

Whether aPLs per se are the cause of adverse obstetric outcomes remains the subject of some debate. Investigators working with murine models have found that passive transfer of aPLs results in clinical manifestations of APS, including fetal loss and thrombocytopenia.[193,194] One group has used a murine pinch-induced venous thrombosis model to demonstrate that human polyclonal and murine monoclonal aPLs are associated with larger and more persistent thrombi than in mice treated with control antibodies.[195]

In humans, APS-related pregnancy complications are probably related to abnormal placental function. Some authorities have focused on abnormalities in the decidual spiral arteries as the immediate cause of fetal loss in APS pregnancies. Some investigators have found narrowing of the spiral arterioles, intimal thickening, acute athetosis, and fibrinoid necrosis.[196–198] In addition, placental histopathology demonstrates extensive necrosis, infarction, and thrombosis.[196] These abnormalities might result from thrombosis during the development of normal maternoplacental circulation via interference with trophoblastic annexin V[198] or by impairing trophoblastic hormone production or invasion.[199]

aPLs appear to activate endothelial cells, indicated by increased expression of adhesion molecules, secretion of cytokines, and production of arachidonic acid metabolites.[200] The findings that some anticardiolipin antibodies cross-react with oxidized low-density lipoprotein[201] and that human anticardiolipin antibodies bind to oxidized, but not reduced, cardiolipin[202] imply that aPLs may participate in oxidant-mediated injury of the vascular endothelium. However, aPLs do bind perturbed cells, such as activated platelets[203] or apoptotic cells,[204] which typically lose normal membrane symmetry and express anionic phospholipids on their surface.

Some work points to the complement system as having a major role in APS-related pregnancy loss, showing that C3 activation is required for fetal loss in a murine model.[205] Inactivation and inhibition of the complement cascade prevents fetal loss and growth restriction that is associated with addition of aPLs.[206] Tumor necrosis factor-α (TNF-α), a pro-inflammatory cytokine associated with complement activation, has likewise been implicated in the signaling

TABLE 43–10

Revised Sapporo Criteria for the Diagnosis of Definite Antiphospholipid Syndrome

APS is present if at least one of the clinical criteria and one of the laboratory criteria that follow are met.*

Clinical Criteria

1. Vascular thrombosis[†]
   One or more clinical episodes[‡] of arterial, venous, or small vessel thrombosis,[§] in any tissue or organ. Thrombosis must be confirmed by objective validated criteria (i.e., unequivocal findings of appropriate imaging studies or histopathology). For histopathologic confirmation, thrombosis should be present without significant evidence of inflammation in the vessel wall.
2. Pregnancy morbidity
   a. One or more unexplained deaths of a morphologically normal fetus at or beyond the 10th wk of gestation, with normal fetal morphology documented by ultrasound or by direct examination of the fetus, or
   b. One or more premature births of a morphologically normal neonate before the 34th wk of gestation because of (i) eclampsia or severe preeclampsia defined according to standard definitions (ACOG) or (ii) recognized features of placental insufficiency,[¶] or
   c. Three or more unexplained consecutive spontaneous abortions before the 10th wk of gestation, with maternal anatomic or hormonal abnormalities and paternal and maternal chromosomal causes excluded.

In studies of populations of patients who have more than one type of pregnancy morbidity, investigators are strongly encouraged to stratify groups of subjects according to a, b, or c above.

Laboratory Criteria[‖]

1. LAC present in plasma, on two or more occasions at least 12 wk apart, detected according to the guidelines of the International Society on Thrombosis and Haemostasis (Scientific Subcommittee on LAs/phospholipid-dependent antibodies).
2. aCL antibody of IgG and/or IgM isotype in serum or plasma, present in medium or high titer (i.e., >40 GPL or MPL, or >99th percentile), on two or more occasions, at least 12 wk apart, measured by a standardized ELISA.
3. Anti-β_2-glycoprotein-I antibody of IgG and/or IgM isotype in serum or plasma (in titer >99th percentile), present on two or more occasions, at least 12 wk apart, measured by a standardized ELISA, according to recommended procedures.

* Classification of APS should be avoided if <12 wk or >5 yr separate the positive aPL test and the clinical manifestation.

† Coexisting inherited or acquired factors for thrombosis are not reasons for excluding patients from APS trials. However, two subgroups of APS patients should be recognized, according to (a) the presence and (b) the absence of additional risk factors for thrombosis. Indicative (but not exhaustive) such cases include age (>55 in men and >65 in women), and the presence of any of the established risk factors for cardiovascular disease (hypertension, diabetes mellitus, elevated LDL or low HDL cholesterol, cigarette smoking, family history of premature cardiovascular disease, body mass index ≥ 30 kg/m^2, microalbuminuria, estimated GFR <60 mL min^{-1}), inherited thrombophilias, oral contraceptives, nephrotic syndrome, malignancy, immobilization, and surgery. Thus, patients who fulfill criteria should be stratified according to contributing causes of thrombosis.

‡ A thrombotic episode in the past could be considered as a clinical criterion, provided that thrombosis is proved by appropriate diagnostic means and that no alternative diagnosis or cause of thrombosis is found.

§ Superficial venous thrombosis is not included in the clinical criteria.

¶ Generally accepted features of placental insufficiency include (i) abnormal or non-reassuring fetal surveillance test(s), e.g., a nonreactive nonstress test, suggestive of fetal hypoxemia, (ii) abnormal Doppler flow velocimetry waveform analysis suggestive of fetal hypoxemia, e.g., absent end-diastolic flow in the umbilical artery, (iii) oligohydramnios, e.g., an amniotic fluid index ≤5 cm, or (iv) a postnatal birth weight <10th percentile for the gestational age.

‖ Investigators are strongly advised to classify APS patients in studies into one of the following categories: I, more than one laboratory criteria present (any combination); IIa, LAC present alone; IIb, aCL antibody present alone; IIc, anti-β_2-glycoprotein-I antibody present alone.

aCL, anticardiolipin; ACOG, American College of Obstetricians and Gynecologists; APS, antiphospholipid antibody syndrome; ELISA, enzyme-linked immunosorbent assay; GPL, reference reagent for IgG; HDL, high-density lipoprotein; Ig, immunoglobulin; LAC, lupus anticoagulant; LDL, low-density lipoprotein.

Modified from Miyakis S, Lockshin MD, Atsumi T, et al: International consensus statement on an update of the classification criteria for definite antiphospholipid syndrome (APS). J Thromb Haemost 2006;4:295–306.

pathways by T cells that are essential to the pathogenesis of aPL; that is, pregnant TNF-α knock-out murine models do not experience miscarriage when injected with aPLs.[207]

Diagnostic Evaluation of Antiphospholipid Syndrome

Diagnostic Criteria

The 2006 revision of the 1999 International Consensus Statement provides simplified criteria for the diagnosis of APS; such criteria are often referred to as the *Sapporo criteria* (Table 43–10).[176]

For obstetricians, the pertinent differences between the original and the revised criteria are

- The inclusion of anti-β_2-glycoprotein I IgG and IgM antibodies as diagnostic of APS. LA and anticardiolipin antibodies were retained as pertinent aPLs.
- Recognition that the threshold used to distinguish medium levels of anticardiolipin and anti-β_2-glycoprotein I antibodies from low levels has no standard; thus, a positive test for either of these antibodies should be greater than 40 GPL or MPL units or greater than the 99th percentile.
- Repeat testing for an initially positive test for aPLs, which is required for the diagnosis of the syndrome, should be performed 12 weeks or later after the initial clinical manifestation and positive test(s).
- The distinction between "primary" and "secondary" should be abandoned because of the lack of differences in clinical consequences between the two categories.

Essentially, patients with bona fide APS must manifest at least one clinical criterion (vascular thrombosis or pregnancy morbidity) and at least one of three laboratory criteria (positive LA or medium to high titers of β_2-glycoprotein I–dependent IgG or IgM isotype anticardiolipin antibodies or anti-β_2-glycoprotein I antibodies), confirmed on two separate occasions, at least 12 weeks apart. Thrombosis may be either arterial or venous and must be confirmed by an imaging or Doppler study or by histopathology. Pregnancy morbidity is divided into three categories: (1) otherwise unexplained fetal death (10 wk′ gestation), (2) preterm birth (34 wk′ gestation) for severe preeclampsia or placental insufficiency, or (3) otherwise unexplained recurrent preembryonic or embryonic pregnancy loss. Autoimmune thrombocytopenia and amaurosis fugax are often associated with APS but are not considered sufficient diagnostic criteria. APS may exist as an isolated immunologic derangement (primary APS) or in combination with other autoimmune diseases (secondary APS), most commonly SLE.

The assays for anticardiolipin antibodies and anti-β_2-glycoprotein I antibodies are more sensitive tests for detection of APS; the assay for LA is more specific. Low titers of anticardiolipin antibodies and anti-β_2-glycoprotein I antibodies are present in up to 5% of normal individuals and should not be used to make the diagnosis of APS. Women with low levels of IgG anticardiolipin antibodies have been found to have no greater risk for aPL-related events than women who tested negative.[208,209] Medium to high titers of the antibodies are more specific for the diagnosis of APS, as is the specificity of the IgG isotype compared with the IgM isotype. The presence of isolated IgM or IgA aPL levels also is of questionable clinical significance. Women with isolated IgM anticardiolipin antibodies are no more likely to suffer aPL-related morbidity than women who tested negative for all aPLs.[146] Finally, repeatedly positive tests, as required to meet revised Sapporo criteria, are uncommon and thus are more indicative of APS.[208] As a final note, the 2006 International Consensus Statement Criteria[176] were developed primarily for research purposes to ensure more uniform patient characterization as well as disease subcategorization in APS studies. Not unlike the situation with autoimmune conditions such as SLE, some patients will present with one or more clinical or laboratory features suggestive but not diagnostic of APS. In such cases, the decision to proceed with therapies generally reserved for patients with APS should be based on experienced clinical judgment.

Risks of Antiphospholipid Syndrome and Pregnancy

Thrombotic Complications of Antiphospholipid Syndrome in Pregnancy

Venous thrombotic events (VTE) that have been associated with aPLs include that of deep venous thrombosis (DVT) and pulmonary embolus (PE). Transient ischemic attacks (TIA) and cerebral vascular accidents (CVA) are the most common arterial events associated with APS. Numerous retrospective studies confirm a link between aPLs and venous or arterial thrombosis.[173,210] A meta-analysis of studies in the general population found an association of both arterial and venous thromboses in patients with LA antibodies (odds ratio [OR] 8.6–10.8; OR 4.1–16.2, respectively).[211] Approximately 70% of thrombotic events occur in the venous system, although arterial thromboses and CVAs are also common.[211] Transient CNS manifestations of ischemia also are common in APS patients.[212] aPLs are present in approximately 2% of individuals with unexplained thrombosis[213] and are the only identifiable predisposing factor in 4% to 28% of cases of stroke in otherwise healthy patients younger than age 50.[214–217] In the only prospective study of untreated APS patients (who also had SLE), 50% of those with LA had a thrombotic episode during the study period; the annual risk of venous thrombosis and arterial thrombosis was 13.7% and 6.7%, respectively.[218] The lifetime risk of thromboembolism in women with APS is unknown. However, over half occur in relation to pregnancy or the use of combination oral contraceptives.[219] In the two largest series of prospectively followed APS pregnancies, the rates of thrombosis and stroke were 5% and 12%, respectively.[130,220]

Obstetric Complications of Antiphospholipid Syndrome in Pregnancy

GESTATIONAL HYPERTENSION/PREECLAMPSIA

The median rate of gestational hypertension/preeclampsia in pregnancies complicated by APS is 32%, with a range up to 50%.[220,221] Preeclampsia may develop as early as 15 to 17 weeks' gestation.[222] The rate of gestational hypertension/preeclampsia does not appear to be markedly diminished by treatment with either glucocorticoids and low-dose aspirin or heparin and low-dose aspirin.[220,223] In contrast to the high rate of preeclampsia observed in some case series of women previously diagnosed with APS, aPLs are not found in a statistically significant proportion of a general obstetric population presenting with preeclampsia[224,225] or in women at moderate risk to develop preeclampsia because of conditions such as underlying chronic hypertension or preeclampsia in a prior pregnancy.[226] However, two groups of investigators have reported that women with early-onset, severe preeclampsia are more likely to test positive for aPLs compared than are healthy controls.[222,227] Based on these findings, testing for aPLs should be considered only in early-onset, severe preeclampsia.

INTRAUTERINE GROWTH RESTRICTION AND PRETERM BIRTH

Several investigators have found relatively high rates of IUGR in association with aPLs.[139,220,222,228] Even with currently used treatment protocols, the rate of IUGR approaches 30%.[130,220] Pregnancies complicated by APS are also more likely to exhibit non-reassuring fetal heart rate patterns during antenatal tests of fetal well-being and intrapartum monitoring.[129,220] Not surprisingly, the rate of preterm birth in these series ranges from 32% to 65%.[129,220,224]

PREGNANCY LOSS

In the original description of APS, the sole obstetric criterion for diagnosis was fetal loss (>10 menstrual wk' gestation).[173] At least 40% of pregnancy losses reported by women with lupus anticoagulant or medium to high positive IgG anticardiolipin antibodies occur in the fetal period[220,229–232]; this rate is not affected by the administration of prednisone.[233] More recently, APS-related pregnancy loss has been extended to include women with early recurrent pregnancy loss, recurrent pregnancy loss including those occurring in the preembryonic (<6 menstrual wk' gestation) and embryonic periods (6–9 menstrual wk gestation).[175] In serologic evaluation of women with recurrent pregnancy loss, 10% to 20% have detectable aPLs.[232–237]

Fetal death and early recurrent pregnancy loss might be considered two points along the same continuum of APS-related pregnancy loss. However, women with APS identified because of a prior fetal death and/or thromboembolism seem to have more serious complications in subsequent pregnancies than those with early recurrent pregnancy loss.[232] Prospective treatment trials of APS during pregnancy have been composed mainly of women with early recurrent pregnancy loss and no other APS-related medical problems.[234–236,238–240] Accordingly, the rates of obstetric complications were relatively low, with fetal death, preeclampsia, and preterm birth occurring in 4.5% (0%–15%), 10.5% (0%–15%), and 10.5% (5%–40%), respectively. Only 1 of 300 women suffered a thrombotic event, and no neonatal deaths due to complications of prematurity were reported. Thus, women with early recurrent pregnancy loss probably represent a different patient population than those with second- and third-trimester events.[241]

Postpartum and Catastrophic Antiphospholipid Syndrome

Catastrophic APS is a rare but devastating syndrome characterized by multiple simultaneous vascular occlusions throughout the body, often resulting in death.[242] The diagnosis should be suspected if at least three organ systems are affected and confirmed if there is histopathologic evidence of acute thrombotic microangiopathy affecting small vessels. Renal involvement occurs in 78% of patients.[242,243] Most have hypertension; 25% eventually require dialysis. Other common manifestations described by Asherson and colleagues[242] include adult respiratory distress syndrome (66%), cerebral microthrombi and microinfarctions (56%), myocardial microthrombi (50%), dermatologic abnormalities (50%), and disseminated intravascular coagulation (25%). Death from multiorgan failure occurs in 50% of patients.[242] The pathophysiology of catastrophic APS is poorly understood. However, the onset may be presaged by several factors, including infection, surgical procedures, discontinuation of anticoagulant therapy, and the use of drugs such as oral contraceptives.[242–244]

Early and aggressive treatment of catastrophic APS appears prudent.[242] Patients should be transferred to an intensive care unit where supportive care can be provided. Hypertension should be aggressively treated with appropriate antihypertensive medication. Although no treatment has been shown to be superior to another, a combination of anticoagulants (usually heparin) and steroids plus either plasmapheresis or IVIG has been successful in some patients.[242,243,245] Streptokinase and urokinase have also been used to treat acute vascular thrombosis.[242] Women suspected of catastrophic APS during pregnancy should probably be delivered.[242]

Management Options

General Considerations

TREATMENT FOR ANTIPHOSPHOLIPID SYNDROME DURING PREGNANCY

The goals of treatment for APS during pregnancy are

- To improve fetal-neonatal outcome by reducing the risk of pregnancy loss, preeclampsia, placental insufficiency, and preterm birth.
- To reduce or eliminate the maternal thrombotic risk and to appropriately manage the potential impact of gestational hypertensive disease on the mother.

TABLE 43–11

Suggested Subcutaneous Heparin Regimens for the Treatment of Antiphospholipid Syndrome in Pregnancy (See Text for Postpartum Thromboprophylaxis Recommendations)

Antiphospholipid Syndrome without Prior Thrombosis

- Recurrent early (preembryonic or embryonic) miscarriage
  - Unfractionated heparin
    - 5000–7500 U subcutaneously q12h
  - Low-molecular-weight heparin
    - Enoxaparin, 40 mg, or dalteparin, 5000 U, subcutaneously once daily, or
    - Enoxaparin, 30 mg, or dalteparin, 5000 U, subcutaneously q12h
- Fetal death (>10 wk' gestation) or prior early delivery (<34 wk' gestation) due to severe preeclampsia or placental insufficiency
  - Unfractionated heparin
    - 7500–10,000 U SC q12h in the first trimester; 10,000 U SVC q12h in the second and third trimesters, or
    - q8–12h adjusted to maintain the midinterval aPTT* 1.5 times the control mean
  - Low-molecular-weight heparin
    - Enoxaparin, 30 mg, or dalteparin, 5000 U, SC q12h

Antiphospholipid Syndrome with Thrombosis

- Unfractionated heparin
  - q8–12h adjusted to maintain the midinterval aPTT* or heparin level (anti-Xa activity)* in the therapeutic range
- Low-molecular-weight heparin
  - Weight adjusted, e.g., enoxaparin 1 mg or dalteparin 200 U/kg, subcutaneously q12h with monitoring of anti-Xa activity*

* Women without a lupus anticoagulant in whom the aPTT is normal can be monitored using the aPTT. Women with lupus anticoagulant should be monitored using anti-Xa activity.
aPTT, activated partial thromboplastin time.

ANTIPHOSPHOLIPID SYNDROME WITHOUT PRIOR THROMBOSIS

APS patients *without* a prior thrombotic event may be categorized into one of two groups for the purpose of treatment: (1) those with recurrent early (preembryonic or embryonic) miscarriage and no other features of APS and (2) those with one or more prior fetal deaths (>10 wk' gestation) or prior early delivery (<34 wk' gestation) due to severe preeclampsia or placental insufficiency. A third group of patients is composed of those with a history of thrombosis, irrespective of pregnancy history. Table 43–11 summarizes treatments during pregnancy and in the postpartum period for these patients.

RECURRENT EARLY (PREEMBRYONIC OR EMBRYONIC) MISCARRIAGE

Three randomized trials have addressed APS patients with predominantly recurrent early miscarriage. In two trials, unfractionated heparin (UFH) plus low-dose aspirin was compared with low-dose aspirin alone, and in both of these, the proportion of successful pregnancies was significantly improved using heparin.[234,235] A third trial, which proved negative, involved the use of low-molecular-weight heparin (LMWH).[246] A 2005 Cochrane systematic review[247] concluded that women with recurrent miscarriage and APS should be treated with a combination of heparin 5000 U subcutaneously twice-daily and low-dose aspirin. The preponderance of data indicates that good pregnancy outcomes are achieved with heparin initiated in the early first trimester when a live embryo is discernable by ultrasound. Most experts recommend anticoagulant treatment in the postpartum period,[248] though the duration of treatment is debated.

FETAL DEATH (>10 WEEKS' GESTATION) OR PRIOR EARLY DELIVERY (<34 WEEKS' GESTATION) DUE TO SEVERE PREECLAMPSIA OR PLACENTAL INSUFFICIENCY

The optimal treatment for women in this category is not defined by randomized trials. Case series suggest that these women are at risk for thrombosis.[249] Some experts recommend intermediate-dose heparin[248] (see Table 43–11). Others recommend either prophylactic or intermediate-dose UFH or prophylactic LMWH combined with low-dose aspirin. The preponderance of data indicates that good pregnancy outcomes are achieved with heparin initiated in the early first trimester when a live embryo is discernable by ultrasound. Experts recommend a minimum of 6 weeks of postpartum thromboprophylaxis in women with obstetric APS.[248,250] After delivery, this can be safely accomplished with warfarin.

ANTIPHOSPHOLIPID SYNDROME WITH THROMBOSIS

For women with APS who have a thrombotic event, experts recommend full heparin or LMWH anticoagulation[248,250] (see Table 43–11). Patients enrolled in most published series also received low-dose aspirin, but the benefit of adding aspirin is uncertain. Patients should be switched from warfarin to heparin anticoagulation at no later than 6 weeks' gestation. Anticoagulation should be continued for a minimum of 6 weeks postpartum to minimize the risk of maternal thromboembolism.[250] After delivery, this can be safely accomplished with warfarin.

OTHER THERAPIES IN PREGNANCY

Other therapies have been suggested for treatment of pregnancy women with APS including corticosteroids and IVIG. Several case series have reported a 60% to 70% rate of successful pregnancies in women with APS treated with prednisone and low-dose aspirin.[251,252] However, a meta-analysis of therapeutic trials showed no reduction in pregnancy loss in women treated with prednisone and low-dose aspirin.[247] Direct comparison of studies is difficult because subjects had different clinical and laboratory findings and dosing regimens, and many studies were of case series, nonrandomized and poorly controlled.

Treatment with IVIG has been evaluated in the treatment of APS. Randomized trials have demonstrated that either the addition of IVIG to heparin or IVIG alone offers no better outcomes than heparin and low-dose aspirin or prednisone and low-dose aspirin.[253–255] A subsequent Cochrane analysis concluded that IVIG was associated with an increased risk of pregnancy loss or premature birth compared with heparin and low-dose aspirin.[247] Thus, IVIG is not recommended in the treatment of APS in pregnancy.

Prepregnancy

Women with APS will preferably seek preconception counseling. At that time, the presence of clinically significant levels of aPL should be confirmed and potential maternal and obstetric complications discussed, including thrombosis, pregnancy loss, preterm delivery, gestational hypertension/preeclampsia, and uteroplacental insufficiency. APS patients, like patients with SLE, should be assessed for evidence of anemia, thrombocytopenia, and underlying renal disease (urinalysis, serum creatinine, 24-hr urine for creatinine clearance, and total protein).

The various anticoagulation prophylaxis regimens should be discussed, along with their risks and limitations. Patients should also be informed about the risks of heparin-induced osteoporosis and heparin-induced thrombocytopenia (HIT), and recommendations for appropriate protective measures should be provided. Some authorities recommend instituting daily low-dose aspirin (81 mg) prior to conception.

Prenatal

Women with APS who suspect they are pregnant should be evaluated immediately. An early transvaginal ultrasound is useful to confirm an intrauterine pregnancy as well as provide accurate dating of the pregnancy. One of the anticoagulation prophylaxis regimens discussed previously (see Table 43–11) should be instituted, and appropriate precautions against heparin-induced osteoporosis and HIT should be taken. Calcium supplementation is encouraged, as well as the performance of daily weight-bearing exercise.

Prenatal visits should occur every 2 to 4 weeks until 20 to 24 weeks' gestation and every 1 to 2 weeks thereafter. Patient visits should be specifically designed to monitor for the development of preeclampsia and thrombosis and to monitor fetal well-being. Because of the risk of IUGR and oligohydramnios secondary to uteroplacental insufficiency, serial ultrasound examinations should be performed every 3 to 4 weeks after 17 to 18 weeks' gestation. Antenatal surveillance (daily fetal movement counts and at least once-weekly nonstress tests with amniotic fluid volume measurements) should be initiated at 30 to 32 weeks' gestation (or earlier if uteroplacental insufficiency is suspected). More frequent ultrasound examinations and more frequent or earlier fetal testing may be indicated in selected cases.

Labor and Delivery

Labor and delivery in women with APS should be managed in the same way as in any patient who is considered at high risk for preeclampsia and uteroplacental insufficiency. Most authorities recommend continuous electronic fetal monitoring throughout labor, given the increased risk of non-reassuring fetal heart rate tracings noted in women with APS.

The most common management dilemma in women with APS probably involves the need to alter anticoagulation regimens in a way that minimizes the risk of bleeding at the time of delivery without placing the patient at a prohibitively high risk of thromboembolism. Treatment approaches vary, and there is no evidence that one method is better than another. Patients receiving prophylactic anticoagulation with heparin can be instructed to withhold their injections at the onset of labor. Alternatively, injections can be discontinued 12 hours before a planned induction. The most common practice in women with APS on full-dose anticoagulation (UFH or LMWH) is to hold the last injection 24 hours prior to a planned induction of labor or cesarean delivery. As an alternative for women deemed at extremely high risk for thromboembolism, including those with an event within 2 weeks of delivery, intravenous heparin can be started in labor and discontinued 2 to 4 hours prior to anticipated delivery. Intravenous heparin can be resumed 4 to 6 hours after vaginal delivery and 12 hours after cesarean.

Spontaneous labor is problematic for women who are fully anticoagulated, particularly those receiving LMWH preparations. Anti-Factor Xa levels might be helpful but have been found to underestimate the risk of bleeding in some patients. Protamine sulfate may be necessary in the event of surgical intervention. For those on adjusted-dose UFH, careful monitoring of the aPTT (or heparin level) is required. If the aPTT is prolonged near delivery, protamine sulfate may be necessary to reduce the risk of bleeding.

Many anesthesiologists are particularly concerned that anticoagulation in any form increases the risk of spinal hematoma formation in women receiving regional anesthesia in labor or for cesarean delivery. The American Society of Regional Anesthesia (ASRA) recommends that neuraxial blockade should be withheld until 24 hours after the last injection in women on full anticoagulation with LMWH.[256] The same recommendation has been made for women receiving adjusted-dose anticoagulation with UFH. For women receiving low-dose thromboprophylaxis (low-dose twice-daily UFH or once-daily LMWH), ASRA has recommended that needle placement be delayed until 10 to 12 hours after the last dose.[256]

Postpartum

Anticoagulant coverage of the postpartum period in women with APS and prior thrombosis is critical.[257] We prefer initiating warfarin thromboprophylaxis as soon as possible after delivery, with doses adjusted to achieve an International Normalized Ratio of 2.0 to 3.0. There is no consensus regarding the postpartum management of APS patients without prior thrombosis. The recommendation in the United States is to treat with anticoagulant therapy for 6 weeks after delivery. The need for postpartum anticoagulation in women with APS diagnosed solely on the basis of recurrent preembryonic or embryonic losses is uncertain. Both heparin and warfarin are safe for breast-feeding mothers.[257] Finally, oral contraceptives containing estrogen are contraindicated.

SUMMARY OF MANAGEMENT OPTIONS
Antiphospholipid Syndrome

Management Options	Evidence Quality and Recommendation	References
Prepregnancy		
Counsel regarding risks of thromboembolism, pregnancy loss, pregnancy complications.	—/GPP	—
Check for		
• Anemia.	III/B	129
• Thrombocytopenia.	III/B	129
• Renal compromise.	III/B	129
Discuss anticoagulation prophylaxis options and risk of heparin therapy.	III/B	129
Prenatal		
Provide joint obstetrician and physician surveillance.	—/GPP	—
Institute anticoagulation prophylaxis (usually low-dose aspirin and subcutaneous low-molecular-weight heparin) and take the appropriate precautions against heparin-induced osteoporosis and heparin-induced thrombocytopenia (see Table 43-11).	III/B Ib/B	129 146,151,179
Encourage calcium supplementation and weight-bearing exercises.	—/GPP	—
Monitor platelet counts for the first 2–3 wk of heparin therapy.	—/GPP	—
Schedule prenatal visits every 2–4 wk until 20–24 wk' gestation and every 1–2 wk thereafter.	III/B	129
Obtain serial biometry (q3–4wk) following 18–20-wk anatomic survey.	III/B	129
Screen for preeclampsia.	III/B	129
Fetal surveillance should be initiated at 30–32 wk' gestation or earlier if uteroplacental insufficiency is suspected.	—/GPP	—

Management Options	Evidence Quality and Recommendation	References
Labor and Delivery		
Deliver near term. Avoid postdates.	—/GPP	—
Adjust anticoagulation prophylaxis to minimize the risk of thromboembolism (see text).	III/B	129
Consider sequential compression devices.	—/GPP	—
Monitor fetal heart rate continuously through labor.	—/GPP	—
Postpartum		
Resume anticoagulation 4–6 hr after vaginal delivery and 8–12 hr after cesarean delivery.	III/B	129
Warfarin may be substituted.	III/B	129
Continue anticoagulation prophylaxis for at least 6 wk after delivery. Consider consultation with subspecialist in thrombophilic disorders.	III/B	129

GPP, good practice point.

RHEUMATOID ARTHRITIS

General

RA is a debilitating disease, the hallmark feature of which is chronic symmetrical inflammatory arthritis of the synovial joints. RA is more common than SLE, with an incidence of from 2.5 to 7 per 10,000 per year and a prevalence of approximately 1% in the adult U.S. population. Although found in virtually all populations, it is more common in some populations (Native American) and less common in others (Native African). Although it is often said to peak in the 40s or 50s, RA can appear at any age of life (including in children), and the prevalence increases with age into the 60s or 70s in both females and males. As with many autoimmune conditions, RA is more common in women than men, with a ratio of 2 : 1 to 3 : 1 women to men.[258]

Pathogenesis of Rheumatoid Arthritis

Histologic features of RA are described as symmetrical inflammatory synovitis marked by cellular hyperplasia, accumulation of inflammatory leukocytes, and angiogenesis with membrane thickening, edema, and fibrin deposition as common early findings. Inflammatory damage at the synovium eventually leads to typical joint erosion involving a locally invasive synovial tissue called *pannus*.

The characteristic autoantibody in patients with RA is rheumatoid factor (RF), an autoantibody made by oligoclonal activated B cells in the peripheral circulation and synovium of RA patients. This group of autoantibodies, which reacts with antigens on the Fc portion of IgG, is composed of a heterogeneous group of antibodies containing light and heavy chains distributed among all the variable region subgroups. It is unknown whether RF autoantibodies are simply markers for RA or whether they are directly responsible for tissue damage. There is some evidence that RF autoantibodies form IgG aggregates in synovial fluid, resulting in complement activation and local inflammation and eventual joint erosion.

Concordance for RA is found in approximately 15% of monozygotic twins and 5% of dizygotic twins. It is estimated that heritable factors account for approximately 60% of the predisposition to RA.[259] The HLA region (HLA class II gene locus DRB1, encoding HLA-DR), is of primary importance in RA susceptibility. Variant forms of DRB1 have been identified in association with RA, including DRB1*0401, *0404, *0405, *0101, *1402, and *1001. These alleles encode for similar amino acid sequences (*shared epitopes*) that are suspected of bestowing susceptibility to RA. Others suspect HLA complex genes are located on chromosomes 1p and 1q, 9, 12p, 16cen, and 18q.[260,261]

Juvenile rheumatoid arthritis (JRA) is a somewhat different, but related, arthritis. It is probably a heterogeneous group of diseases. By definition, JRA has its onset in individuals younger than 16 years; males and females are equally represented. One prominent subgroup is composed of individuals with Still's disease. This condition is initially systemic in nature and includes fever, skin rash, serositis, and lymphadenopathy. Arthritis occurs late in the course of disease and tends not to be as destructive or chronic as classic RA. Nearly three quarters of children with JRA have spontaneous, permanent remission by the time they reach adulthood.

Diagnostic Evaluation of Rheumatoid Arthritis

Clinical Presentation

The symptoms of RA develop insidiously over several months; the clinical course is variable. Less commonly, disease onset is acute and somewhat rapid.[262] Twice as many patients present during winter months than summer months, and trauma (including surgery) is a frequent precursor. Morning stiffness, pain, and swelling of peripheral joints are the most common initial features. The disease tends to involve primarily the joints of the wrists, knees, shoulders, and metacarpophalangeal joints in an erosive arthritis that typically follows a slowly progressive course marked by exacerbations and remissions. Eventually, joint deformities may occur; these are especially obvious at the metacarpophalangeal joint and proximal and distal interphalangeal joints of the hands.[262] Fatigue, weakness, weight loss, and malaise are also common.

Rheumatoid nodules, present in 20% to 30% of affected patients, are made up of a local proliferation of small vessels, histiocytes, fibroblasts, and other cells and are usually located in the subcutaneous tissues of the extensor surfaces of the forearm. Uncommonly, extra-articular tissues may also be affected, including the lung (pleuritis, pleural effusions, interstitial fibrosis, pulmonary nodules, pneumonitis, and airway disease) and heart (pericarditis, effusion, myocarditis, endocardial inflammation, conduction defects, and arteritis leading to myocardial infarction).

Diagnostic Criteria

The classification criteria published by the American College of Rheumatology are shown in Table 43–12. Physical examination should reveal evidence of joint inflammation, including joint tenderness, synovial thickening, joint effusion, erythema, and decreased range of motion. Symmetrical involvement should be noted. Radiographic evidence of RA includes joint space narrowing and erosion; although too expensive for routine use, MRI may detect synovial hypertrophy, edema, and early erosive changes.

Laboratory Criteria

More than 70% of patients with clinical features of RA are also seropositive for RF. In addition, some of those who are initially seronegative will eventually convert, leaving only 10% of RA patients without a positive RF. Approximately 5% of the general population also test positive for RF, as do many patients with other autoimmune conditions (e.g., SLE, scleroderma, and mixed connective tissue disease), viral infections, parasitic infections, chronic bacterial infections, and after irradiation or chemotherapy.

Rheumatoid Arthritis in Pregnancy

The relationship between RA and pregnancy is fascinating even if the basic scientific understanding of the relationship remains elusive. The observation that in many patients, RA dramatically improves during pregnancy eventually led Philip Hench[263] to discover cortisone. Numerous studies (Table 43–13) show that at least 50% of patients with RA demonstrate improvement in their disease in at least 50% of their pregnancies.[263–269]

For a majority of patients, the improvement in RA starts in the first trimester, heralded by a reduction in joint stiffness and pain.[265,266] The peak improvement in symptoms

TABLE 43–12

Classification Criteria for the Diagnosis of Rheumatoid Arthritis

CRITERIA*	DEFINITION
Morning stiffness	Morning stiffness in and around the joints, lasting at least 1 hr before maximal improvement
Arthritis of ≥ three joint areas	At least three joint areas simultaneously have had soft tissue swelling or fluid (not bony overgrowth alone) observed by a physician. The 14 possible areas are right or left proximal interphalangeal, metacarpophalangeal, wrist, elbow, knee, ankle, and metatarsophalangeal joints
Arthritis of hand joints	At least one area swollen (as defined above) in a wrist, metacarpophalangeal, or proximal interphalangeal joint
Symmetrical arthritis	Simultaneous involvement of the same joint areas (as defined above) on both sides of the body (bilateral involvement of proximal interphalangeals, metacarpophalangeals, and metatarsophalangeals is acceptable without absolute symmetry)
Rheumatoid nodules	Subcutaneous nodules, over bony prominences or extensor surfaces, or in juxta-articular regions, observed by a physician
Serum rheumatoid	Demonstration of abnormal amounts of serum rheumatoid factor by any method for which the result has been positive in <5% of normal control subjects
Radiographic changes	Radiographic changes typical of rheumatoid arthritis on posteroanterior hand and wrist radiographs, which must include erosions or unequivocal bony decalcification localized in or most marked adjacent to the involved joints (osteoarthritis changes alone do not qualify)

* For classification purposes, a patient shall be said to have rheumatoid arthritis if he or she has satisfied at least four of these seven criteria. Criteria 1 through 4 must have been present for at least 6 wk. Patients with two clinical diagnoses are not excluded. Designation as classic, definite, or probable rheumatoid arthritis is *not* to be made.

TABLE 43–13

Improvement of Rheumatoid Arthritis in and outside of Pregnancy

AUTHOR	NONGRAVID PATIENTS WITH RA (*N*)	NONGRAVID PATIENTS WITH IMPROVEMENT IN RA (*N* [%])	GRAVID PATIENTS WITH RA (*N*)	GRAVID PATIENTS WITH IMPROVEMENT IN RA (*N* [%])
Hench[263]	22	20 (91%)	37	33 (89%)
Oka[264]	93	73 (78%)	114	88 (77%)
Betson and Dorn[266]	21	13 (62%)	21	13 (62%)
Ostensen and Husby[267]	10	8 (80%)	10	9 (90%)
Ostensen[271]*	51	NA	76	35 (46%)

* Study of patients with juvenile RA.
RA, rheumatoid arthritis.

generally occurs in the second or third trimester. Other aspects of the disease may also improve during pregnancy, with studies indicating that the subcutaneous nodules associated with RA may disappear during pregnancy.[267] Even with the overall improvement in symptoms, the clinical course of RA during pregnancy is characterized by short-term fluctuations in symptoms, as in the nonpregnant state.[268] Most patients who experience an improvement in RA during pregnancy will have a similar improvement in subsequent pregnancies.[269] In addition, Hazes and coworkers[270] reported a protective effect of pregnancy in development of RA. However, this is not a given, and some patients will have relatively less improvement in a second or third pregnancy. There are no laboratory or clinical features that predict improvement of RA in pregnancy.

A quarter of RA patients have no improvement in their disease during pregnancy, and in a small number of cases, the disease may actually worsen. Unfortunately, nearly three quarters of patients whose disease has improved during pregnancy will suffer a relapse in the first several postnatal months.[265–267] The level of disease during the first postnatal year generally returns to that of a year before conception, but might be worse.[269]

In contrast to SLE, there are no data to suggest that RA in remission is likely to have a better course during pregnancy than active RA. The long-term prognosis for RA patients undertaking pregnancy appears to be similar to those who avoid pregnancy. Oka and Vainio[269] compared 100 consecutive pregnant RA patients with age- and disease-matched controls and found no significant differences between the groups in terms of the severity of their disease. There are few studies of JRA, but Ostensen in 1991[271] found that only 1 case in 20 had a worsening or reactivation of their disease associated with pregnancy.

The mechanism(s) by which pregnancy favorably affects RA has yet to be fully elucidated. Plasma cortisol, which rises during pregnancy to peak at term, was initially thought to be important to the amelioration of RA.[263] However, there is no correlation between cortisol concentrations and disease state.[272] Some studies suggest that estrogens or estrogens and progestagens favorably affect arthritis,[273] but there are conflicting studies,[274] and a double-blind crossover trial found that estrogen did not benefit RA.[275] Sex hormones may interfere with immunoregulation and interactions with the cytokine system.[276] Promising data suggest that certain proteins circulating in higher concentrations during pregnancy or unique to pregnancy are associated with improvement of RA. These include pregnancy-associated α_2-glycoprotein[277] and gamma globulins eluted from the placenta.[278] Other investigators feel that the placenta may modify RA by clearing immune complexes[279] or that modification of immune globulins during pregnancy alters their inflammatory activity.[280] Nelson and associates[281] suggested that amelioration of disease was associated with a disparity in HLA class II antigens between mother and fetus. In fact, these investigators have correlated improvement of RA symptoms of pregnant women with increased HLA mismatch; this mismatch may be mediated by the induction of suppressor mechanisms. Hence, the more "foreign" the fetal HLA type is to the maternal immune system, the more likely the maternal disease is to undergo remission during gestation.[281]

Risks of Rheumatoid Arthritis in Pregnancy

Obstetric Complications and Rheumatoid Arthritis

About 15% to 25% of pregnancies in women with RA end in miscarriage,[282,283] a figure that may or may not be slightly higher than in normal women. One controlled study found that women with RA have a significantly higher frequency of miscarriage than normal women, even before the onset of their disease (25% vs. 17% before disease; 27% vs. 17% after disease).[282] Another controlled study did not find that women with RA have a higher proportion of miscarriage prior to the onset of disease.[268] Interestingly, this same study found that the frequency of fetal death was higher in patients who later develop RA than in nonaffected relatives. There are scant data available, but women with RA do not appear to be at significant risk for preterm birth, preeclampsia, or IUGR.

Management Options

Prepregnancy

The prepregnancy management of RA is similar to that of any of the other autoimmune disorders. This includes stabilization of the underlying disease process, reducing maintenance medications to minimize early fetal risks, and avoidance of known teratogenic agents.

Prenatal

As with SLE, a physician should see a woman with RA every 2 to 4 weeks throughout the pregnancy, especially if the patient is having trouble with her disease. Rest is an important part of the management of RA, and the patient should be counseled to plan adequately for this. Physical therapy can be helpful in patients whose disease does not improve with pregnancy.

It is best to use acetaminophen for simple analgesia. If possible, the patient should avoid NSAIDs and aspirin (see discussion in the "Systemic Lupus Erythematosus" section). Glucocorticoids should be considered for patients whose RA does not improve during pregnancy.[272] Relatively low doses of prednisone are usually adequate for RA during pregnancy and are not often necessary for maintenance therapy. Intra-articular steroids can also be used if necessary in pregnancy. If NSAIDs prove necessary, the minimum dose necessary to control inflammation should be used.[284] Methotrexate is absolutely contraindicated during the first trimester and relatively contraindicated thereafter. The anti-TNF-α agents are of unknown safety in pregnancy and probably should be avoided. Leflunomide (Arava),[285] a pyrimidine synthesis inhibitor, is teratogenic in animals, and is contraindicated not only in pregnant women but also in those of reproductive age who are contemplating pregnancy. In fact, women of reproductive age who wish to become pregnant should not only stop the therapy but also have verification of plasma levels less than 0.02 mg/L.[285]

Labor and Delivery

Because RA has little, if any, adverse effect on pregnancy outcome, there are no special prenatal obstetric concerns. In a rare case, severe deforming RA can pose a problem to the mechanics of vaginal delivery; such cases are obvious and require individualized care.

Postnatal

Postpartum management of the RA parturient is similar to that of patients with other autoimmune disorders (see the section on "Systemic Lupus Erythematosus"). Roughly 90% of women flare within the first 3 months postpartum; this risk may be somewhat more pronounced after a first pregnancy.[286] Lactation has been reported to have a protective effect on the development of RA and decreased mortality of RA, with a direct correlation with total time of lactation.[287]

SUMMARY OF MANAGEMENT OPTIONS

Rheumatoid Arthritis

Management Options	Evidence Quality and Recommendation	References
Prepregnancy		
Counsel regarding risk of exacerbation during pregnancy, risk of medication exposure.	III/B	208–212
Establish good control of RA and adjust maintenance medications.	—/GPP	—
If possible, discontinue cytotoxic medications before conception. This should be done only under careful supervision. Avoid methotrexate.	III/B	208–212
Reduce dosage to lowest levels achieving therapeutic effect.	—/GPP	—
Avoid known teratogens (e.g., leflunomide, methotrexate).	—/GPP	—
Prenatal		
Review regularly (joint obstetrician and physician surveillance).	—/GPP	—
Rest (general and local).	—/GPP	—
Physiotherapy/physical therapy recommended in some patients.	—/GPP	—
Drugs	III/B	208–212
• Avoid full-dose aspirin and NSAIDs if possible (or use minimum doses to control inflammation).		
• Prescribe steroids for worsening disease (RCT not in pregnancy).		
• Avoid methotrexate		
• D-Penicillamine contraindicated		
Use glucocorticoids judiciously for exacerbations of disease. Use lowest dosage possible.	III/B	208–212
Avoid teratogenic medications (consider Embrel as a substitute if indicated).	III/B	208–212
Schedule prenatal visits every 2–4 wk throughout pregnancy.	—/GPP	—
Labor and Delivery		
Individualize care according to physical abilities.	—/GPP	—
Postpartum		
Monitor for RA exacerbations.	—/GPP	—
Consult with rheumatology subspecialist.	—/GPP	—

GPP, good practice point; NSAIDs, nonsteroidal anti-inflammatory drugs; RA, rheumatoid arthritis; RCT, randomized controlled trial.

SYSTEMIC SCLEROSIS

General

The term *scleroderma* is derived from words referring to *hardening* ("scleros") and *skin* ("derma"), the hallmark feature of this disease. *Systemic sclerosis* (SSc) refers to internal organ involvement, characterized histologically by a marked increase in collagen, mostly in the dermis, with hyalinization and often obliteration of small blood vessels.[288] Early in the disease process, the dermis contains mononuclear cell infiltrates and sometimes calcium due to the deposition of calcium hydroxyapatite. Pathologic changes also include thinning of the epidermis and loss of normal dermal appendages. Most patients with SSc report Raynaud's phenomenon, and vascular features are evident in biopsies from SSc patients. Small arteries and arterioles exhibit characteristic endothelial cell proliferation and intimal thickening as well as increased amounts of fibrinogen and fibrin, with lumina often occluded by fibrosis. Remaining vessels become dilated, visible through the skin as telangiectasias.

Internal organs have similar histologic changes. Fibromucoid intimal thickening in the kidney results in narrowing and thinning of the lumen. Cortical glomerular involvement is usually focal and includes endothelial cell proliferation and thickening of the basement membrane. In the lung, the most common finding is interstitial fibrosis with increased numbers of fibroblasts, capillary congestion, and thickening and occlusion of alveolar walls and arteriolar intima. Densely hyalinized fibrosis is found in the gastrointestinal tract and random focal fibrosis in the myocardium.

The disease is uncommon, occurring in no more than 10 to 15 individuals per million per year.[288] The ratio of females to males is 10:1 in the 15- to 44-year-old age group. The mean age of onset is in the early 40s, when many affected women may potentially become pregnant.[289,290]

Pathogenesis of Systemic Sclerosis

The pathophysiologic changes of SSc include vascular abnormalities, immunologic abnormalities, and disordered collagen synthesis. The initial event most likely occurs in small blood vessels with early proliferation of intimal layer endothelial cells that produce cytokines, growth factors, adhesion proteins, vasoactive proteins, coagulation factors, and extracellular matrix.[291] Aberrant production of factors such as von Willebrand's factor also occurs. A hallmark feature of SSc is clearly increased fibroblast activity with an accelerated rate of fibroblast collagen synthesis.

An association between an increase of HLA-DR11 (whites) and HLA-DR15 (Asians) in patients with diffuse SSc has been described. Associations have also been described with the SSc-associated autoantibodies topoisomerase I and anticentromere antibody, although results have varied in different ethnic and racial groups.[292]

A number of different non-HLA genes have most recently been identified in association with SSc. Genes encoding for extracellular matrix proteins have been identified, notably COL1A1 and COL1A2, genes encoding type I collagen. Other interesting studies have identified a candidate gene near the fibrillin 1 gene on chromosome 15q in studies of a Native American population with a particularly high prevalence of SSc. Polymorphisms in transforming growth factor-β1, 2, and 3 genes have also been identified in association with SSc, as have polymorphisms in TNF-α, TNF-β, CXCR2, tissue inhibitor of metalloproteinase-1, and interleukin-4 receptor-α.[292]

Diagnostic Evaluation of Systemic Sclerosis

Clinically, the expression of SSc varies considerably; the morbidity depends on the extent of skin or internal organ involvement. Raynaud's phenomenon is common, especially in patients with CREST syndrome (calcinosis of involved skin, Raynaud's phenomenon, esophageal dysmotility, sclerodactyly, and telangiectasias), a more limited form of scleroderma. Patients who eventually develop diffuse disease involving the internal organs are more likely to present with arthritis, finger and hand swelling, and skin thickening. The skin thickening, which usually starts on the fingers and hands, eventually involves the neck and face. In severe, progressive disease, much of the skin may be involved and marked deformities of the hands and fingers may occur. Raynaud's phenomenon and internal organ damage are attributed to fibrosis of arterioles and small arteries. In these circumstances, the normal vasoconstrictor response to various stimuli, including cold, causes near-complete obliteration of the vessel. As a result, digital ischemia may occur. A similar vasculopathy is probably responsible for internal organ involvement. Lower esophageal dysfunction is most common. Other portions of the gastrointestinal tract may be involved, producing malabsorption, diarrhea, and/or constipation.[288]

A variety of pulmonary lesions may occur, with the most common being progressive interstitial fibrosis. Pulmonary hypertension, a problem of special interest to the obstetrician, may also occur in long-standing disease. Nearly half of the patients with well-established SSc have evidence of myocardial involvement. Arrhythmias are probably the most common sign encountered. Renal disease occurs to some extent in many patients and is a major cause of mortality among patients with SSc. Severely involved cases may present with proteinuria and renal insufficiency, hypertension, or both. Sudden onset of severe hypertension and progressive renal insufficiency with microangiopathic hemolysis is known as *scleroderma renal crisis*. These crises usually occur in cold weather, suggesting that the pathophysiology is similar to that of Raynaud's phenomenon.[288]

ANAs are present in most patients with SSc, but anti-DNA antibodies are not. About half of patients have serum cryoglobulins. Antibodies to centromere detected by indirect immunofluorescence are common among patients with limited scleroderma (CREST syndrome), but not among those with diffuse disease. Up to 40% of patients have antibody to an extractable nuclear antigen designated Scl. The biologic significance of these autoantibodies is unclear.

Risks of Systemic Sclerosis in Pregnancy

Complications of Systemic Sclerosis in Pregnancy

Pregnancy in women with SSc is uncommon, with fewer than 200 reports in the published literature. Early reports suggested that fertility was impaired in women with SSc, although this has not been confirmed in more recent studies.[289,293] Rather, women in the SSc group were older and either had waited to have children or had not desired pregnancy.[289] The effect that pregnancy might have on the course of SSc depends to some extent on the degree of preexisting disease involvement. Published data regarding the risks of pregnancy in women with SSc are scarce, and the findings of case reports and small series that suggest pregnancy should be avoided in women with SSc should be regarded with caution. Historically, the largest and most complete studies suggested that overall maternal outcomes are more salubrious, with worsening of disease in pregnancy in no more than 20% of cases.[289,293,294] Very recent data from an estimated 11.2 million deliveries in the Nationwide Inpatient Sample of the Healthcare Care and Utilization Project included 504 women diagnosed with systemic sclerosis; these women exhibited increased rates of hypertensive disorders like preeclampsia (OR 3.71, 95% confidence interval

[CI] 2.25–6.15), IUGR (OR 3.74, 95% CI 1.51–9.28), and increased length of hospital stay. Such results led Chakravarty and colleagues[295] to recommend extensive preconceptional counseling to women diagnosed with SSc about their risks incurred by conception and subsequent pregnancy. Postpartum, approximately one third of women with SSc have exacerbations of Raynaud's phenomenon, arthritis, and skin thickening.[294]

Pregnancy is probably safest in SSc patients without obvious renal, cardiac, or pulmonary disease. Although data are scant, women with SSc with moderate to severe cardiac or pulmonary involvement likely face increased risks of substantial morbidity or mortality and should not undertake pregnancy. In addition, SSc patients with moderate to severe renal disease and hypertension probably face a substantial risk for preeclampsia and perhaps mortality due to renal crisis. Pregnancy should be discouraged in these women as well. Finally, there may be an increased risk of renal crisis in patients with early diffuse SSc[294]; therefore, some authorities suggest that these patients delay pregnancy.

Obstetric Complications in Women with Systemic Sclerosis

PREGANCY LOSS

Fetal outcomes in SSc pregnancies are mixed, with half or more ending in term live births and another quarter ending in liveborn premature infants.[293,296–302] Preterm birth is particularly prominent in women with early, diffuse disease. Women with late, diffuse SSc may be at increased risk for miscarriage, reported at 65% in one case series. There has been some suggestion that a predisposition to pregnancy loss predates the onset of SSc in some women. Of 154 patients who eventually developed SSc and 115 matched controls, a significantly greater number of women with SSc had a history of miscarriage (29% vs. 17%).[302] However, only 3 met the definition for recurrent miscarriage (three or more consecutive losses). The large case-control trial failed to find any association between a history of pregnancy loss and the subsequent development of SSc.[294]

GESTATIONAL HYPERTENSION, PREECLAMPSIA, AND INTRAUTERINE GROWTH RESTRICITON

Given the microvascular nature of the condition and the relative frequency of renal involvement in SSc, one might speculate that preeclampsia and IUGR would occur significantly more often in SSc pregnancies. This is supported by high rates of preeclampsia in case reports but not by case series. In one case series, 10% of pregnancies were complicated by IUGR.[293] Neonatal involvement with skin sclerosis possibly attributable to SSc has been reported in a few cases. The risks of this condition, as well as its relationship to SSc itself, remain unclear. Among the 29 pregnancies accumulated in case reports, there were 2 miscarriages (7%), 2 fetal deaths (7%), and 1 neonatal death attributable to prematurity. Two other infants died because of multiple anomalies. Among the 103 pregnancies in the small series,[297–300] there were 24 miscarriages (23%), 3 fetal deaths (3%), and 2 neonatal deaths due to prematurity. Thus, noncontrolled reports suggest that 72% to 83% of pregnancies among women with SSc are successful (excluding perinatal deaths due to anomalies). In the case-control study by Giordano and coworkers,[301] 80 SSc patients had 299 pregnancies. Of these, 50 ended in miscarriage (17%), significantly higher than the rate of miscarriage in the matched controls (10%). There was no difference in the miscarriage rate between patients with diffuse versus those with limited SSc. The retrospective study of Steen[294] included 86 pregnancies after the onset of SSc. Of these, 15% ended in miscarriage and 2% ended in mid-trimester fetal deaths. These percentages were not significantly different from those in RA controls or neighborhood controls. The later prospective study by this same group[303] found that 18% of 67 SSc pregnancies ended in miscarriage, compared with 158 control pregnancies. Taken together, the available data suggest that the rate of miscarriages and fetal deaths in patients with SSc might be slightly increased compared with controls.

Management Options

Prepregnancy

Currently, most experts agree that the typical women with mild to moderately severe SSc has a high likelihood for favorable pregnancy outcomes with appropriate preconceptional planning, antepartum management, and close monitoring.[304] However, patients with early diffuse SSc, severe visceral involvement, significant cardiopulmonary involvement (ejection fraction <30%), pulmonary hypertension, severe restrictive lung disease (forced vital capacity <50%), or severe renal insufficiency have significantly increased risk of adverse pregnancy outcomes and, thus, should be counseled against getting pregnant.[303] Patients who have a history of renal crisis but, at present, have disease that has been stable for years may be counseled that their disease does not represent contraindication to future pregnancy.[305] A trial off of angiotensin-converting enzyme (ACE) inhibitors to determine whether blood pressure may be controlled with nonteratogenic antihypertensive medications has been suggested. Naturally, patients who fail the trial should be placed back on the ACE inhibitor.[303] Likewise, women who experience scleroderma renal crisis should be treated aggressively with ACE inhibitors.[303,304]

Prenatal

SSc patients considering pregnancy and any patient with SSc who presents for medical care already pregnant should have her clinical situation thoroughly investigated. Special attention should be given to the evaluation of possible renal or cardiopulmonary involvement. It is prudent to recommend pregnancy termination in patients with diffuse SSc and cardiopulmonary involvement or moderate to severe renal involvement.

Even in the nonpregnant state, there is no satisfactory therapy for SSc. Patients with limited disease are usually managed with vasodilators and anti-inflammatory agents. As discussed previously, NSAIDs should be avoided if at all possible during pregnancy. Oral vasodilators for the prevention and treatment of Raynaud's phenomenon may be continued, although substantial data to prove fetal safety are not available. Patients with diffuse SSc may be taking glucocorticoids (see discussion in the section on "Systemic Lupus Erythematosus"). Nacci and associates[306] recently reported amelioration of joint and skin involvement in SSc during pregnancy. Other immunosuppressive or cytotoxic agents should be avoided. Although sometimes used as therapy in SSc, cyclophosphamide should be avoided in pregnancy because this agent is associated with a 16% to 22% risk of congenital anomalies following exposure during the first trimester.[284] ACE inhibitors appear to be particularly efficacious in treating SSc-related hypertension and renal crises. These drugs have been associated with fetal/neonatal renal insufficiency in a small number of cases. However, in SSc-related hypertension, the benefits of these medications probably outweigh the risks of discontinuing them.[307]

Patients with continuing pregnancies should be seen by a physician every 1 to 2 weeks in the first half of pregnancy and once weekly thereafter. Although serial laboratory testing is not necessary, laboratory assessment of unusual or suspicious symptoms or signs may be helpful. The possible risk of IUGR and fetal death requires serial examination of the fetus by sonography. Fetal surveillance should be instituted by 30 to 32 weeks' gestation, or sooner if the clinical situation demands.

In the event of relapse, risks associated with essential therapies are high in the gravid female. However, low-dosage prednisone has been safely administered without increased risk for development of maternal renal crisis or fetal oral cleft.[308,309]

Labor and Delivery

In patients with mild to moderate disease, few additional precautions are needed during the labor and delivery process. Again, signs of preeclampsia should be sought, because this complication may be more likely with scleroderma. Wound healing may be a problem in patients with advanced disease or those on steroids. Therefore, operative interventions require meticulous attention to this issue. In patients with significant pulmonary, cardiac, or renal impairment, intensive care management may be needed.[303–305]

Postnatal

Postpartum care represents a continuation of the intrapartum management plan. Most often, reinstitution of maintenance medication is all that is required. Complications of scleroderma, as previously outlined, require individualization of care.

SUMMARY OF MANAGEMENT OPTIONS
Systemic Sclerosis

Management Options	Evidence Quality and Recommendation	References
Prepregnancy		
Counsel regarding risk of exacerbation during pregnancy, risk of medication exposure.	IIa/B	231
Establish good control of SSc and adjust maintenance medications.	III/B	232
If possible, discontinue cytotoxic medications before conception. This should be done only under careful supervision.	—/GPP	—
Assess cardiopulmonary and renal function (advise against conception if significantly compromised).	III/B	232
Prenatal		
Provide joint obstetrician and physician surveillance.	III/B	232
Prenatal visits should occur every 2–4 wk until 20–24 wk' gestation and every 1–2 wk thereafter.	III/B IV/C	232 228
Monitor cardiopulmonary and renal function (consider termination of pregnancy if severe compromise).	IV/C	228
Drugs		
• Anti-inflammatory for moderate joint problems.	—/GPP	—
• Vasodilators for pulmonary problems.	—/GPP	—
• Steroids for worsening disease.	—/GPP	—
Maintain vigilance for preeclampsia.	IV/C	228
Use of ACE inhibitors is a dilemma if hypertension is present; avoid if possible.	III/B	232
Check fetal growth (q3-4wk after 18 wk) and health.	IIa/B	231
Fetal surveillance should be initiated at 30–32 wk' gestation or earlier if uteroplacental insufficiency is suspected.	—/GPP	—

SUMMARY OF MANAGEMENT OPTIONS

Systemic Sclerosis—cont'd

Management Options	Evidence Quality and Recommendation	References
Labor and Delivery		
Deliver near term. Avoid postdates.	—/GPP	—
Intensive/high-dependency care may be necessary.	—/GPP	—
Institute special precautions to ensure wound healing if cesarean section delivery.	—/GPP	—
Postnatal		
Provide initial care in intensive/high-dependency care setting.	—/GPP	—
Review dosage of drugs and resume maintenance medications.	—/GPP	—

ACE, angiotensin-converting enzyme; GPP, good practice point.

MYASTHENIA GRAVIS

General

Myasthenia gravis (MG) is an autoimmune disorder affecting neuromuscular transmission, resulting in variable weakness and fatigability of skeletal muscle. Increasing weakness with repetitive use of the muscle(s) is the characteristic feature. Occurring in only 2 to 10 per 100,000 individuals, MG affects twice as many women as men, with an onset usually in the second or third decade in women.[310,311] The immediate cause of the disease is probably an autoimmune attack on the acetylcholine receptor (AChR) complex of the neuromuscular junction. Serum autoantibodies against acetylcholine receptors (anti-AChR) are found in the serum of 85% of patients with MG.[312,313] The disease can be transferred passively to laboratory animals by the injection of IgG from affected individuals.[314] Accordingly, 10% to 20% of infants born to women with MG show signs of neonatal MG, thought to be caused by the transplacental passive transfer of antibodies from mother to child.[315,316]

Ocular muscle weakness resulting in diplopia or eyelid ptosis is the usual presenting problem. Some patients have difficulty with chewing or talking. In a large majority of patients, MG progresses from ocular to generalized skeletal muscle involvement over a 1- to 2-year period. Any trunk or limb muscle may be involved, but the neck flexors, deltoids, and wrist extensors are notable. Death results from severe respiratory muscle fatigue. Muscle weakness varies throughout the day but is usually worse toward the end of the day. The long-term course of disease is likewise variable and is characterized by periodic fluctuations in severity. For unclear reasons, MG tends to be worsened by emotional distress, systemic illness, and increased temperature (fever, hot weather).[311]

Pathogenesis of Myasthenia Gravis

It is apparent that the pathophysiology of disease is not simply the blockade of AChR by antibody. The muscle endplate, wherein the AChR resides, is misshapen and bears a reduced number of AChRs.[317] This is presumed to be due to autoimmune damage, perhaps mediated through complement destruction. The net result is a diminished depolarization response to a normal amount of released acetylcholine at the postsynaptic membrane.

Recent data suggest that a subset of individuals afflicted with MG are seronegative for anti-AChR antibodies. Rather, these individuals test positive for antibodies against the muscle-specific kinase (anti-MuSK–positive).[318] Animal models demonstrate the injection of IgG from anti-MuSK triggers muscle weakness by impairment of the neuromuscular junction, inducing MG.[314]

Abnormalities of the thymus are found in most patients with MG. In total, 75% have lymph follicle hyperplasia and 10% to 15% have lymphoblastic or epithelial thymic tumors. Thymectomy results in remission in 35% and improvement in 50% of patients.[319] These observations suggest that MG may be due to (1) an autoimmune attack on the antigens common to the thymus and motor endplate or (2) abnormal clone(s) of immune cells in the thymus.

Moreover, ectopic germinal centers are found with MG. Meraouna and colleagues[320] used gene chip analysis to identify 88 genes that were both associated with thymic dysregulation and normalized by glucocorticoids. They determined a B-cell chemoattractant (CXCL13) to be overproduced by MG patients and served as a main target of corticotherapy in ex vivo experiments, suggesting that new therapies targeting this chemoattractant might be of interest in the treatment of MG. Autoantibodies to other muscle proteins are suspected. Sera from MG patients induces muscle cell disarray of actin microfilaments, inclusion bodies, intracellular vesicles, and complement-independent induction of cellular death atypical of classic apoptosis. Continuing ex vivo and animal model experimentation is needed to further our knowledge of how this disease manifests through seemingly multiple pathways.[321]

Treatment of Myasthenia Gravis

MG is treatable but not curable. The use of anticholinesterase drugs is reportedly safe during pregnancy. Pyridostigmine, an analogue of neostigmine, is the most commonly used anticholinesterase medication. These medications impede degradation of acetylcholine and bring about improvement in muscle function. Some patients with MG may respond only to immunosuppressive therapy with corticosteroids, azathioprine, and cyclosporine.[319] Remission is often accomplished with high-dose corticosteroids followed by slow tapering to maintain the remission state.[322] In the occasional patient with refractory MG, IVIG and plasmapheresis have been used with some success[310,322,323]; IVIG 2 g/kg appears to be highly effective for MG as measured by The Quantitative Myasthenia Gravis (QMG) Score for Disease Severity.[323]

Diagnostic Evaluation of Myasthenia Gravis

The diagnosis of MG rests on the clinical presentation, physical examination, and confirmatory diagnostic procedures. Repetitive use of the muscle under study results in apparent exhaustion. The muscle vigor can be dramatically restored with short-acting anticholinesterase drugs, such as edrophonium, in doses of 210 mg given by intravenous injection.[322] More sophisticated tests are now available, including single-fiber electromyography and repetitive nerve stimulation studies.

Risks of Myasthenia Gravis in Pregnancy

Complications of Myasthenia Gravis in Pregnancy

Several pregnancy-related physiologic changes may have detrimental effects on MG. Nausea, vomiting, altered gastrointestinal absorption, expanded plasma volume, and increased renal clearance require adjustment of anticholinesterase throughout pregnancy. Elevation of the maternal diaphragm by the gravid uterus causes hypoventilation of the lower portions of the lungs, which exacerbates respiratory compromise in some women with MG. Increased physical exertion in the second and third trimesters and the emotional stress of pregnancy itself may also result in MG exacerbation.[324]

The course of MG during pregnancy is highly variable. Both infection and shorter history of disease increase risk for puerperal flares.[324] Cartlidge[325] recommends postponement of pregnancy in women recently diagnosed with MG because this period represents the time of greatest risk. In an extensive review, approximately 40% of women with MG had exacerbation of their disease during pregnancy; approximately 30% had no change, and 30% had postpartum exacerbations that were frequently sudden and serious in nature.[326] Moreover, of the approximately 30% of MG patients whose disease remained unchanged during pregnancy, several had significant postpartum exacerbations. In a review that included both patients who were in remission prior to pregnancy and patients who were taking therapy, exacerbations occurred in 10 of 54 pregnancies (19%), improvement in 12 (22%), and no change in 32 (59%).[324] Plauche[326] found an overall maternal mortality of 4% (9 of 225 reported cases). The majority of these (7 of 9) were due to refractory MG.

Obstetric Complications in Myasthenia Gravis

The rates of miscarriage and fetal death in pregnancies complicated by MG do not appear to be significantly different from those of the normal population.[310,327] However, early series suggested preterm birth in up to two thirds of patients with MG,[327–330] and anticholinesterase drugs are thought to have an oxytocic action.[310,331] Historically, reports have suggested differences in the prevalence of preterm birth and low birth weight in 54 MG patients compared with the general population.[310] More recently, Hoff and coworkers[331] found that neonatal survival, birth weight, and gestational age at delivery in women with MG were no different than controls.

Mothers with MG are no more likely than controls to require oxytocics in labor. According to the Medical Birth Registry of Norway from 1967 to 2000, cesarean section rates and PPROM were higher in gravidas with MG. Since 1981, assisted vaginal delivery with either forceps or vacuum has been no different from controls.[331] The transplacental passage of anti-AChR antibodies can lead to fetal or neonatal MG. Only about 10% to 15% of infants born to mothers with MG show signs of MG.[332] The relative infrequency of fetal involvement was due to α-fetoprotein, which has been shown to inhibit the binding of anti-AChR to AchR.[333,334] Most infants with neonatal MG have high concentrations of anti-AChR in their circulation.

The diagnosis of neonatal MG is made by observation of poor sucking, feeble cry, and respiratory difficulties that respond to edrophonium. Neonatal MG is transient, usually abating over a period of 1 to 4 weeks. The symptoms usually develop within the first several days of life, but are often absent initially, perhaps because of the presence of α-fetoprotein.[334] When properly recognized, the disease is easily managed with supportive care and anticholinesterase drugs. There does not appear to be any correlation between the risk of neonatal MG and the severity of maternal MG manifestation[331] or the level of maternal anti-AChR antibodies.[335,336] However, there does appear to be a relationship between neonatal levels and the severity of neonatal MG.[315] Arthrogryposis multiplex congenita (AMC), a nonprogressive congenital contraction disorder thought to result from poor fetal movement, has rarely been reported in infants born to women with MG.[332,337,338] There is some evidence that plasmapheresis and immunosuppressive therapy may reduce the recurrence of AMC in MG patients with a prior neonatal death presumably due to AMC.[339]

Management Options

Prepregnancy

Adjustment of medication to establish quiescence/control of the disease process is vital before pregnancy. Patients should be appropriately educated regarding the need for close supervision, the expected increase in fatigue, and the potential for respiratory compromise (especially late in pregnancy). The fetal risks of preterm delivery, the potential for associated anomalies, and the transient nature of neonatal MG should be discussed.[340]

Prenatal

Treatment is frequently necessary before, during, and after pregnancy to ensure maternal and fetal well-being. Pregnancy-related changes in drug absorption, increased renal clearance, and expanded plasma volume may require alterations in medication in order to maintain adequate drug levels. The first line of therapy is quaternary ammonium compounds with anticholinesterase activity. Although neostigmine (Prostigmin) was the first such drug to be used, its short half-life was a major drawback. Pyridostigmine

(Mestinon), which has a longer half-life, is the most popular long-acting medication currently used for maintenance therapy of MG. There is now a sustained-release form of the drug (Mestinon Timespan, 180 mg), but its popularity is limited by concerns about irregular absorption and drug preparation. Oral pyridostigmine is typically given in doses of 240 to 1500 mg/day in divided doses at 3- to 8-hour intervals. When used, the sustained-release preparation is typically given as a single bedtime dose of 180 to 540 mg. If the patient requires more drug, as is often the case with advancing pregnancy, it is best to first shorten the interval between doses. If this fails to control symptoms, the dose of pyridostigmine should be increased by increments of 15 to 30 mg. Such maneuvers usually lead to adequate control of MG during pregnancy. The most common side effects of these medications are due to the accumulation of acetylcholine (muscarinic effects). These include gastrointestinal symptoms (nausea, vomiting, cramping, diarrhea) and increased oral and bronchial secretions. Overdose of anticholinesterase drugs results in the rare so-called cholinergic crisis, which paradoxically includes muscle weakness and respiratory failure.[340]

Glucocorticoids are effective in most patients with MG. Most authorities prefer high doses (prednisone 60–80 mg/day) to start; the dose is tapered over many months after improvement is noted. The disease may transiently worsen soon after the steroids are started; for this reason, patients should be hospitalized for steroid therapy. Unfortunately, remission appears to be maintained only if the patient continues on steroids, and withdrawal of steroids may cause myasthenic exacerbations. For these reasons, pregnant MG patients should maintain glucocorticoid therapy through pregnancy and the postpartum period. Some authors believe that glucocorticoid-induced remission is a particularly good time for pregnancy in patients with MG.[338]

Plasmapheresis has been used with success in severe MG. Most patients were also taking glucocorticoids. There is one case report of using plasmapheresis to successfully treat MG in pregnancy.[339] It may be that maternal plasmapheresis might be the treatment of choice in MG pregnancies in which the fetus has markedly reduced or absent fetal movement predisposing it to AMC.

Thymectomy may result in improvement in many patients with MG by mechanisms that are unknown. However, resorting to thymectomy during pregnancy would seem imprudent because of frequent long delays before improvement and perioperative maternal and fetal concerns. Notably, neonatal myasthenia is less common in neonates born to women who have undergone thymectomy.[336,341] Patients with MG should be seen relatively frequently throughout pregnancy, every 2 weeks in the first and second trimesters, and every week in the third trimester. Undue emotional and physical stress are to be avoided, because they may result in exacerbation of MG. The patient and physician should be alert to the possibility of preterm labor and appropriate preventive steps instituted. Although care must be individualized, limiting exercise and work is probably in order for many patients. Infections may also result in exacerbation of MG. Respiratory and urinary tract infections must be identified and treated promptly.

Fetal involvement with MG is suspected by poor fetal movement and hydramnios. This is not treatable in utero. Differentiating poor fetal movement due to MG from that due to fetal hypoxemia may be difficult, but normal fetal heart rate tests, especially a negative contraction stress test and a normal biophysical profile score, are reassuring.

Labor and Delivery

The management of labor and delivery in patients with MG requires limitation of emotional and physical stress and the appropriate use of parenteral anticholinesterase drugs. Neostigmine can be given subcutaneously, intramuscularly, or intravenously. As a rough guide, 60 mg oral pyridostigmine is equivalent to 0.5 mg intravenous neostigmine and 1.5 mg subcutaneous neostigmine. The usual dose of parenteral neostigmine is 0.5 to 2.5 mg. Maximal effects on skeletal muscle may occur 2 to 30 minutes after intramuscular injection; the effects last for about 2.5 hours. Pyridostigmine can be given intramuscularly or very slowly intravenously. The usual dose is 2 mg (~1/30 of the usual oral dose) every 2 to 3 hours. The course of the first stage of labor in patients with MG is not altered because MG does not affect smooth muscle.[316] The second stage of labor could be affected by the weakened material expulsive efforts, although the average duration of labor in MG patients is normal.

It is important to recognize that certain medications that may be used in the management of obstetric concerns are contraindicated in patients with MG. These are listed in Table 43–14. Magnesium sulfate is absolutely contraindicated because it further interferes with the neuromuscular blockade of MG. Preterm labor can probably be treated with β-sympathomimetics,[331] but the associated hypokalemia should be carefully avoided. A small number of patients with MG have an associated cardiomyopathy, which could increase the risks of β-sympathomimetics.

Because the patient with MG is particularly sensitive to neuromuscular drugs, analgesic and anesthetic considerations are important before the onset of labor. All patients with MG should be seen in consultation with an anesthesiologist early in the course of pregnancy. Epidural anesthesia is probably best because it limits the need for analgesia, may help prevent anxiety and fatigue, and is excellent for forceps procedures. Amide-type local anesthesia agents are used.[337] Some authors recommend general endotracheal anesthesia for cesarean section in patients with respiratory involvement. Myasthenic crises requiring ventilatory support may be precipitated by the stress of labor and delivery,

TABLE 43–14

Medications That May Exacerbate or Cause Muscle Weakness in Patients with Myasthenia Gravis

Magnesium salts	Cholistin
Aminoglycosides	Polymyxin B
Halothane	Quinine
Propranolol	Lincomycin
Tetracycline	Procainamide
Barbiturates	Ether
Lithium salts	Penicillamine
Trichlorethylene	

an inadvertent change in medication, or surgery. Rarely, cholinergic crises may result from overdosage with anticholinesterase drugs. These patients have prominent muscarinic symptoms in addition to respiratory weakness. In all patients with MG, labor and delivery management should include the immediate availability of personnel and equipment for ventilatory support and airway maintenance. Postoperative care may be best accomplished in an intensive care setting.[340]

Postnatal

It would be difficult to find a patient, following delivery, who is not fatigued and weakened. Differentiating this normal state of affairs from exacerbation of MG may be difficult without objective testing. Drug dosages may need to be rapidly adjusted, in particular downward, as the effects of the volume expansion of pregnancy clear.

SUMMARY OF MANAGEMENT OPTIONS
Myasthenia Gravis

Management Options	Evidence Quality and Recommendation	References
Prepregnancy		
Counsel regarding risk of exacerbation during pregnancy, risk of medication exposure	III/B	241
Review therapy; establish good control of SLE; adjust maintenance medications.	III/B	250–256
If possible, discontinue cytotoxic medications before conception. This should be done only under careful supervision.	III/B	250–256
Consider thymectomy in symptomatic women who are refractory to therapy.	III/B	250–256
Prenatal		
Provide joint obstetrician and physician surveillance.	III/B	251
Continue Preexisting Drugs	III/B	241
• Anticholinesterase.		
• Steroids.		
• Azathioprine.		
Consider plasmapheresis and IVIG in refractory cases.	III/B	241
Provide fetal surveillance, especially activity (biophysical profile score).	—/GPP	—
Initiate fetal surveillance at 30–32 wk' gestation.	—/GPP	—
Avoid/minimize physical/emotional stress.	III/B	250–256
Labor and Delivery		
Minimize stress.	III/B	250–256
Continue anticholinesterase drugs (parenteral).	III/B	250–256
Administer intravenous glucocorticosteroids for delivery in patients who have received maintenance or steroid bursts during pregnancy.	—/GPP	—
Regional analgesia is preferable to narcotics for pain relief and general anesthesia.	III/B	250–256
Use experienced anesthetists if general anesthesia (advisable to consult in prenatal period).	III/B	250–256
Assisted second stage is more likely.	III/B	250–256
Avoid magnesium sulfate in patients with preeclampsia (and other contraindicated drugs).	IV/C	255
Postnatal		
Provide special care and surveillance of newborn; may need short-term anticholinesterases.	III/B	241,260
Review dosage of drugs	III/B	241

GPP, good practice point; IVIG, intravenous immune globulin; SLE, systemic lupus erythematosus.

SUGGESTED READINGS

Andrade R, Sanchez ML, Alarcon GS, et al: Adverse pregnancy outcomes in women with systemic lupus erythematosus from a multiethnic US cohort: LUMINA (LVI). Clin Exp Rheumatol 2008;26:2:268–274.

Batocchi AP, Majolini L, Evoli A, et al: Course and treatment of myasthenia gravis during pregnancy. Neurology 1999;52:447–452.

Branch DW, Khamashta MA: Antiphospholipid syndrome. In Queenan JT (ed): High-risk Pregnancy. Washington, DC, American College of Obstetricians and Gynecologists, 2007, pp 60–72.

Empson MB, Lassere M, Craig JC, et al: Prevention of recurrent miscarriage for women with antiphospholipid antibody or lupus anticoagulant. Cochrane Database Syst Rev 2005;(2):CD002859.

Friedman DM, Kim MY, Copel AJ, et al: Prospective evaluation of fetuses with autoimmune-associated congenital heart block followed in the PR Interval and Dexamethasone Evaluation (PRIDE) study. Am J Cardiol 2009;103:1102–1106.

Miniati I, Guiducci S, Mecacci F, et al: Pregnancy in systemic sclerosis. Rheumatology (Oxford) 2008;47(Suppl 3):iii16–iii18.

Ostensen M: Glucocorticosteroids in pregnant patients with rheumatoid arthritis. Z Rheumatol 2000;59(Suppl 2):II70–II74.

Ostensen M, Khamashta M, Lockshin M, et al: Anti-inflammatory and immunosuppressive drugs and reproduction. Arthritis Res Ther 2006;8:3:209.

Preventative IVIG Therapy for Congenital Heart Block (PITCH). Available at http://clinicaltrials.gov/ct2/show/NCT00460928; ClinicalTrials.gov (accessed April 18, 2009).

Ruiz-Irastorza G, Lima F, Alves J, et al: Increased rate of lupus flare during pregnancy and the puerperium: A prospective study of 78 pregnancies. Br J Rheumatol 1996;35:133–138.

REFERENCES

For a complete list of references, log onto www.expertconsult.com.

CHAPTER 44

Diabetes

ROBERT FRASER and TOM FARRELL

INTRODUCTION

Diabetes complicating pregnancy is becoming more common worldwide, but the last 5 years have produced several major advances in the management of the diabetic syndromes from well-designed randomized, controlled trials addressing improvement in outcome. The majority of complications seen in fetal development, growth, and labor and delivery can be ascribed in the broadest context to relative maternal hyperglycemia, and it follows that optimal maternal diabetic control at all stages from pregnancy planning to the postnatal period is critical to the various outcomes. It is important to note, however, that many of the medical complications of diabetes can affect the success or otherwise of pregnancy but also that the pregnancy itself may contribute to a deterioration in the long-term health of the mother. There are short-term risks to the mother as well particularly from hypoglycemia because of the combination of medical and patient attempts to maintain a low blood glucose in preparation for a pregnancy and during the pregnancy. Women with complications such as proliferative retinopathy and large vessel arteriopathy may experience acute deteriorations in their health. Important further considerations include the safety of some drugs used to minimize progression of diabetic complications, such as nephropathy, for use during pregnancy. Obesity is common among women who have type 2 diabetes or gestational diabetes mellitus (GDM). The medical and surgical complications of obesity can be superimposed onto the existing complications associated with hyperglycemia of diabetes in pregnancy.

CLASSIFICATION OF DIABETES

Preexisting Diabetes

This comprises cases of type 1 (insulin-dependent) and type 2 (non–insulin-dependent diabetes). These conditions can have been present for a variable length of time before the onset of a pregnancy, and in particular, type 1 diabetes can have been present from early childhood. Although there is considerable individual variation, as a general guide, the long-term complications of the diabetic state and indeed many of the complications seen in pregnancy become more common when the diabetes has been present for more than 10 years. Type 2 diabetes used to be relatively less common than type 1 in pregnancy, but the ratio is changing because of the increasing proportion of type 2 diabetes now being recognized in women of childbearing age, particularly where childbearing is more common in the late fourth and fifth decades. Taking these two conditions together, approximately 1 pregnancy in 250 will be complicated by preexisting diabetes. A small number of these cases that are starting to become more widely recognized are of monogenic diabetes, also called MODY (mature-onset diabetes of youth), a series of single gene defects that are inherited dominantly and may lead to diabetes complicating pregnancy through several generations of a family.

Gestational Diabetes Mellitus

Although the relative risk of preexisting diabetes remains less than 1% in most populations worldwide, there is a dramatic difference in the number of cases seen with GDM, which is defined as "any degree of glucose intolerance with onset or first recognition during pregnancy."[1] This definition includes women whose glucose tolerance will return to normal after pregnancy and those who will persist with glucose intolerance and type 2 diabetes. The latter group contains individuals who had unrecognized type 2 disease prior to pregnancy. In United Kingdom practice universal screening, where applied, reveals between 3% and 5% of women have biochemically diagnosed GDM. It is felt that the incidence of the condition is increasing in association with increasing obesity in the population at large and the increase in age-specific maximum fertility. In obstetric management terms, GDM probably has most of the risks of preexisting diabetes with regard to the second half of pregnancy but because the majority of women with GDM are normoglycemic at the time of conception, the excess risk of congenital malformation is not seen. It is, however, becoming increasingly recognized that a proportion of women diagnosed as having GDM on provocative screening during pregnancy are in fact previously unrecognized cases of type 2 diabetes,[2] and there is a suggestion from various national and international audits that this proportion, which might be as high as 20%, is increasing. In some populations in which obesity is particularly common or in which the population is dominated by ethnic groups at high risk for diabetes, GDM complicating pregnancy may be seen in up to 40% of women.

Apart from recognizing the adverse effects of GDM on the outcome of pregnancy, it is also of value to make this diagnosis because, after the delivery, interventions such as pharmacologic drugs, dietary modification, and lifestyle modification may reduce the risk of subsequent pregnancies being complicated by diabetes. It may also improve the long-term health of the woman potentially by reducing her risk of developing chronic type 2 diabetes.

PREEXISTING DIABETES

Maternal Risks

The recent national enquiry in the United Kingdom performed by CEMACH (Confidential Enquiry into Maternal and Child Health)[3,4] in women with preexisting diabetes identified the risks for the mother in an intensively studied subset. Recurrent hypoglycemia occurred in 51% of women, and in 20% of women, there was at least one episode of hypoglycemia requiring "third-party assistance," meaning another person was required to assist in the reversal of insulin-induced hypoglycemia and implying a more serious condition. Most severe hypoglycemic episodes occur between 8 and 16 weeks' gestation, probably associated with nausea and anorexia at this stage of pregnancy. Twenty-three percent of women entered pregnancy with some degree of retinopathy and a further 9% were recognized as having retinopathy for the first time during the pregnancy. Pregnancy is associated with an independent risk of progression of retinopathy. Twelve percent of pregnancies of women with preexisting diabetes were complicated by nephropathy. Preeclampsia is more common by a factor of two to four times in women with preexisting diabetes than in women free of diabetes. In a large case series from the United States, there was a stepwise increase in preeclampsia frequency with the duration and complication rate in preexisting diabetes, from 10.8% in those with the disease for less than 10 years to 22.0% in those with a longer duration but no vascular complications to 36.2% in those with proliferative retinopathy, nephropathy, or both.[5]

Fetal and Neonatal Risks

Congenital Abnormality

Congenital anomalies are now the leading single cause of perinatal death among infants of diabetic mothers, accounting for 40% to 50% of all perinatal deaths.[6–8] The nature of the congenital abnormalities are blastogenetic in origin,[9] and as a result, the insult responsible for the congenital malformations must impact on the developing organ systems before the seventh week of pregnancy.[10,11] Maternal hyperglycemia is considered to be the primary factor responsible for increased congenital abnormalities in pregnancy in diabetes. The proportion of pregnancies complicated by congenital malformation in which the periconceptional hemoglobin A_{1c} (HbA_{1c}) is less than 7% is not significantly greater than the rate seen in the nondiabetic population however. Above this percentage, there is a progressive rise with rates of congenital malformation exceeding 8% where the HbA_{1c} level is above 10%[12,13] (Fig. 44–1).

FIGURE 44–1
The risk of major or minor congenital anomaly according to periconceptional hemoglobin A_{1c} (HbA_{1c}; absolute risk ± 95% confidence interval [CI]).
(From Guerin A, Nisenbaum R, Ray JG: Use of maternal GHb concentration to estimate the risk of congenital anomalies in the offspring of women with prepregnancy diabetes. Diabetes Care 2007;30:1920-1925.)

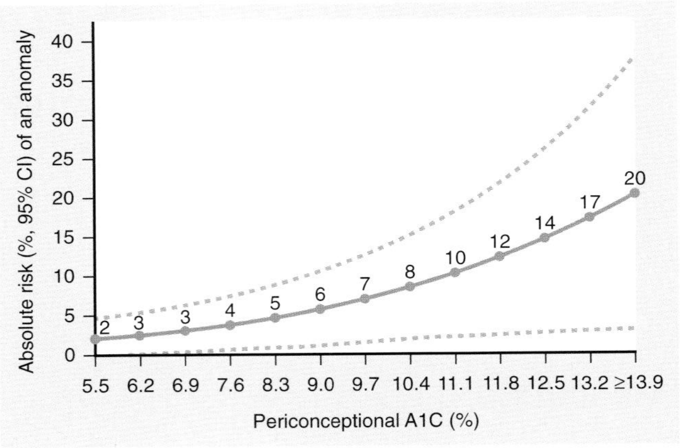

Shields and coworkers[14] in a cohort of women with preexisting diabetes found no cardiac abnormalities in women with an early pregnancy HbA_{1c} level under 6.1%. Similarly, Wong and colleagues[15] demonstrated that no congenital abnormalities were found in a cohort of women when the HbA_{1c} was under 9%.

There do not appear to be specific abnormalities associated with increasing levels of maternal hyperglycemia during embryogenesis. Abnormalities of all organ systems are seen. What is apparent is that the degree of maternal hyperglycemia appears to have a greater influence on the number of organ systems that are adversely affected rather than on which organ system is specifically involved. This is reflected in increased risk of multiple congenital abnormalities with increasing levels of maternal hyperglycemia.[16]

The usually quoted frequency of major congenital abnormalities in pregnancy in diabetes is 6% to 10%.[15–18] More recent data from the CEMACH enquiry found the prevalence of major congenital anomalies to be 46 per 1000 births in women with diabetes (48/1000 births for type 1 diabetes, 43/1000 births for type 2 diabetes), more than twice the population rate.[19] The increase in congenital abnormality rates was mainly due to a 4.2-fold increase in neural tube defects (NTDs) and a 3.4-fold increase in congenital heart disease. Although the spectrum of type of congenital anomalies is varied, it does appear that both neural tube and cardiovascular defects predominate.

There is little difference between preexisting type 1 and type 2 diabetes with regards to both the rate and nature of congenital abnormalities seen.[2,19,20] Women with GDM, conversely, are a heterogeneous group of women containing women with previously undiagnosed preexisting diabetes and glucose intolerance of pregnancy (see earlier).

Farrell and associates[2] reported on major anomalies in a New Zealand population of women with type 1, type 2, and GDM. The incidence of major abnormalities was 5.9% in women with type 1 diabetes, 4.4% with type 2 diabetes, and 1.4% in women with GDM. Women with GDM were then reclassified once the results of the postnatal glucose tolerance test were known. The congenital abnormality rate for those women later reclassified as having unrecognized type 2 diabetes was 4.6%, whereas in the remaining women with GDM, the rate had fallen to 0.9%.

Martinez Frias and coworkers[21] found GDM was associated with an increased of risk of congenital abnormalities (odds ratio [OR] 2.8) in obese women. A strong association between GDM and major congenital anomalies was confirmed when the initial fasting glucose at diagnosis was greater than 6.7 mmol/L. There is an association between maternal obesity and relatively high fasting glucose levels.[22]

Pathologic Fetal Growth

Disordered fetal growth is well recognized as a problem in pregnancy complicated by all types of maternal diabetes, with intrauterine growth retardation being common in those with long-standing diabetes with macrovascular disease, but much more common in all the diabetic syndromes is fetal overgrowth (macrosomia) associated with excess glucose transfer across the placenta and secondary fetal hyperinsulinemia. In the newborn period, complications including hypoglycemia, respiratory distress syndrome (RDS), hyperbilirubinemia, hypocalcemia, and polycythemia may occur. Feeding difficulty associated with delayed gastric emptying secondary to raised serum amylin levels is more common in overgrown newborns.[23]

Fetal Well-being

Despite good glycemic control in pregnancy, there is a persisting increased risk of stillbirth in pregnancy complicated by maternal diabetes in the United Kingdom.[3] This increased risk of stillbirth has led to a generally accepted policy of induction of labor at around 38 weeks to avoid late fetal loss, which has invariably contributed to the higher cesarean section rate experienced by women with diabetes.

The cause of late stillbirth is likely to be multifactorial. Fetal hypoxia and acidosis have been implicated, as has hypokalemia leading to fetal cardiac dysrhythmias, as well as placental dysfunction. The increased risk of late stillbirth was shown many years ago to correlate with poor glycemic control during late pregnancy.[24] Histologic examination of the placenta from women with diabetes demonstrates characteristic changes often described as "immature villi." Blood glucose levels appear to be the metabolic driver responsible for these placental changes that result in milder degrees of uteroplacental compromise being less well tolerated than in pregnancy in women free of diabetes. Identifying the fetus at risk of late intrauterine death remains a challenge.

Stillbirth, perinatal death, and neonatal mortality rates per 1000 births compared with the general population were 26.8, 31.8, and 9.3 versus 5.7, 8.5, and 3.6, respectively, in the U.K. national dataset.

There is agreement in the literature about the late pregnancy risks of women with frank GDM with a fasting plasma glucose above 6.9 mmol/L or a 2-hour plasma glucose above 11.0 mmol/L. Collected series confirm that the adverse outcomes of late pregnancy in such women left untreated are as common as in women with preexisting diabetes and poor control in late pregnancy. There has been, however, lack of agreement over the clinical significance of mild GDM (sometimes called impaired glucose tolerance [IGT]) that comprises a group of women with fasting plasma glucose levels below 7 mmol/L but 2-hour levels above 7.8 mmol/L but below 11.1 mmol/L. This group corresponds to some extent with those diagnosed as GDM by having two abnormal values on a 3-hour glucose tolerance test using the American Diabetes Association (ADA) criteria for diagnosis (Table 44–1). The recent publication of two double-blind studies, the Australian Carbohydrate Intolerance Study in Pregnant Women (ACHOIS) study[25] and the Maternal-Fetal Medicine Units Network (M-FMUN)[26] study, appears to have addressed this question in that both studies demonstrated that significant reductions in pregnancy complications such as preeclampsia and adverse perinatal outcomes were achieved by referral to a joint diabetes antenatal clinic after randomization compared with untreated groups (Table 44–2). The untreated women were blinded, as were their medical attendants, to the presence of GDM and, therefore, attended the routine antenatal clinics. With the evidence from these two studies, most authorities would accept that the diagnosis is worth making because treatment is likely to be effective, and therefore, some form of screening approach is appropriate.

The classical Pedersen hypothesis was that excessive glucose transfer across the placenta stimulated excessive fetal insulin production and that this relative fetal

TABLE 44–1

Diagnostic Criteria for Gestational Diabetes

WHO Criteria[53]	**FASTING**		**2 Hr**	
Plasma glucose after 75-g glucose load	Either > 6.9 mmol/L		Or > 7.7 mmol/L	
ADA Criteria[1]	**FASTING***	**1 Hr**	**2 Hr**	**3 Hr**
Plasma glucose after 100-g glucose load	5.3 mmol/L	10 mmol/L	8.6 mmol/L	7.8 mmol/L
HAPO Consensus Criteria[55]	**FASTING†**	**1 Hr**	**2 Hr**	
Plasma glucose after 75-g glucose load	5.1 mmol/L	10.0 mmol/L	8.5 mmol/L	

* Two or more values are to be met or exceeded for diagnosis.
† One or more values above the threshold for diagnosis.
ADA, American Diabetes Association; HAPO, Hyperglycemia and Adverse Pregnancy Outcomes; WHO, World Health Organization.

TABLE 44–2

Summary Outcomes of ACHOIS and M-FMUN Double-Blind Trials of Treatment of Gestational Diabetes

	ACHOIS[25]				M-FMUN[26]			
OUTCOME	TREATED	CONTROLS	RR	*P*	TREATED	CONTROLS	RR	*P*
Preeclampsia	58 (12%)	93 (18%)	0.70 (0.51-0.95)	.02	12 (2.5%)	25 (5.5%)	0.46 (0.22-0.97)	.02
Cesarean section	152 (31%)	162 (32%)		NS	128 (27%)	154 (34%)	0.79 (0.6-0.97)	.021
Composite							0.87 (0.73-1.05)	
Adverse perinatal outcome	7 (1%)	23 (4%)	0.33 (0.14-0.75)		149 (32%)	163 (37%)		.143
Perinatal loss	0 (0%)	5 (1%)		NS	0 (0%)	0 (0%)		
Shoulder dystocia	7 (1%)	16 (3%)	0.45 (0.19-1.09)	NS	7 (1.5%)	18 (4.0%)	0.37 (0.16-0.88)	.019
Bony injury/birth trauma	0	1 (<1%)	–	–	3 (0.6%)	6 (1.3%)	0.48 (0.12-1.90)	.332
NNU admission	357 (71%)	321 (61%)	1.15 (1.05-1.26)	.02				
LGA	68 (13%)	115 (22%)	0.62 (0.47-0.81)	<.001	34 (7.1%)	66 (14.5%)	0.49 (0.33-0.73)	.0003

ACHOIS, Australian Carbohydrate Intolerance Study in Pregnant Women; LGA, large for gestational age; M-FMUN, Materal-Fetal Medicine Units Network; NNU, neonatal unit; NS, not significant; RR, risk ratio.

hyperinsulinemia in the second half of pregnancy was the driver to hypertrophy of the insulin-sensitive tissues in the fetus leading to the common diagnosis of fetal macrosomia.[27] The Pedersen hypothesis was elaborated by Freinkel and Metzger[28] with the recognition that other nutrient substrates, particularly certain amino acids, were also fetal insulin secretagogues and probably contributed to the development of fetal hyperinsulinemia. In normal pregnancy, glucose becomes a fetal insulin secretagogue only around 26 weeks' gestation. In maternal diabetes with maternal hyperglycemia however, early maturation of the mechanism by which glucose causes secretion of fetal insulin is obtained, and in approximately half of cases of fetal macrosomia, the pattern of excessive growth can be recognized on late midtrimester ultrasound scanning. In the remainder of cases in which macrosomia is developing, it is recognized only in the third trimester.

Figure 44–2 shows the relative incidence of fetal hyperinsulinemia from studies performed in our unit and reveals that despite modern target-oriented hypoglycemic therapy in women with both GDM and preexisting diabetes, a significant number of fetuses are hyperinsulinemic.[29]

Fetal insulin secretion rates play a major role in fetal growth.[27] Increases in fetal plasma insulin levels are directly correlated with increased maternal glucose levels because of the process of facilitated diffusion of glucose across the placenta. This increase in fetal insulin leads to accelerated growth of insulin-sensitive tissues in the fetus such as bone, muscle, and adipose tissue.[30] As a result, macrosomia associated with maternal diabetes results in larger shoulder diameters, increased skinfold thicknesses, and lower head–to–abdominal circumference ratios[31] than "constitutional" macrosomia seen in pregnancies free of maternal diabetes. The increase in biacromial distance may explain why the incidence of shoulder dystocia reported by birth weight in the CEMACH Enquiry rose from 0.9% in infants of birth weight below 2.5 kg to 4.7% between 2.5 and 3.9 kg, 23.0% between 4.0 and 4.5 kg, and 42.9% over 4.5 kg.[3]

The reported incidence of macrosomia in pregnancies in diabetes ranges between 8% and 43%.[32] This variation may simply reflect differing populations, different targets for maternal glucose control in pregnancy, or the influence of other factors predisposing to fetal macrosomia such as maternal weight, weight gain during pregnancy, parity, and genetic factors.[33]

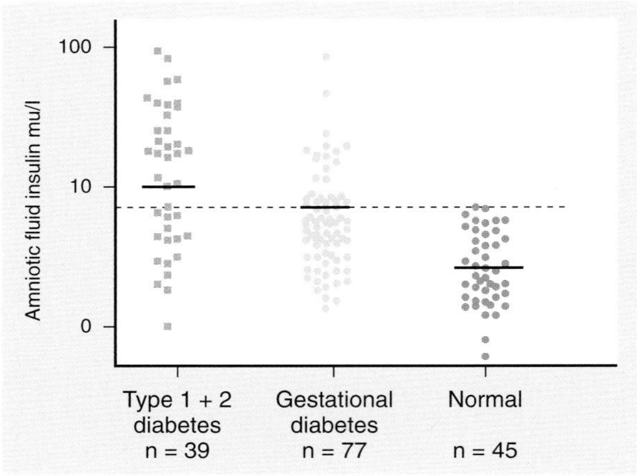

FIGURE 44–2

Amniotic fluid insulin levels and type of diabetes. Amniotic fluid insulin levels (mU/L) at delivery in women with type 1 or 2 diabetes and gestational diabetes mellitus (GDM) compared with a nondiabetic group. *Bars* represent geometric means of each distribution, and the *dotted line* is the upper limit of liquor insulin levels measured in nondiabetic women.

(From Fraser R, Bruce C, further data collected since the authors' publication: Fraser RB, Bruce C: Amniotic fluid insulin levels identify the fetus at risk of neonatal hypoglycemia. Diabet Med 1999;16:568–572.)

Traditionally, fetal macrosomia was considered to be driven by maternal glucose control in the third trimester with the 1-hour postprandial blood glucose level strongly associated with fetal birth weight.[34] There is now evidence to suggest that diabetic control in the first and early second trimesters is also important in the development of a macrosomic infant.[35–37] Increased maternal glucose levels in early pregnancy may result in the fetal pancreas being "reprogrammed" in terms of insulin secretion and additionally result in hyperplasia of fetal adipose cells that become hypertrophied in response to third-trimester glucose transfer to contribute to fetal macrosomia.

Neonatal Complications

From a combination of spontaneous and elective delivery, the preterm birth rate in preexisting diabetes is 4.9% at less than 32 weeks' gestation and 32% between 32 and 36 completed weeks.[3] RDS is more common at all gestational ages in infants of women with diabetes.[38] Other causes of respiratory distress such as transient tachypnea of the newborn (TTN) are also more common. Intrapartum difficulties with delivery, particularly shoulder dystocia, are responsible for neonatal complications such as bony injuries, particularly fractures to the humerus or clavicle, and brachial plexus trauma resulting typically in Erb's palsy. This was reported in 0.45% of births in the CEMACH audit.[3] This complication is more common in fetal macrosomia driven by fetal hyperinsulinism. Neonatal hypoglycemia resulting from autonomous insulin secretion and delayed gastric emptying induced by high levels of amylin is more likely in these overgrown infants.[23] Chronic intrauterine hypoxia is thought to be the mechanism underlying excessive erythropoietin production and polycythemia, which leads to increased blood viscosity and secondarily to hyperbilirubinemia in the newborn. Hypocalcemia is also more common in the newborn of the diabetic mother and enters into the differential diagnosis with hypoglycemia of the infant with symptoms such as jitteryness and convulsions.

Management Options

Prepregnancy

All women of reproductive age with preexisting diabetes should be advised about the potential benefits of prepregnancy planning at their regular contacts with medical services in which their diabetes is reviewed. Women with diabetes should also be aware of the options with regard to effective contraception in an attempt to reduce the number of unplanned pregnancies, particularly when adequate preparation for pregnancy with regard to diabetes control has not been undertaken.

From adolescence onward, women with diabetes and, if possible, their partners should be offered education on the role of diet, body weight, and exercise as well as the importance of planning any pregnancy. They should be made aware that the risks of pregnancy are associated with both the quality of diabetes control and the presence and duration of any complications of their diabetes. The value of measurement of glycated HbA_{1c} in preparation for pregnancy is well established from observational studies if not from any randomized, controlled trials.[39,40] The nomenclature for laboratory-based measurements of HbA_{1c} is about to change, as detailed in Table 44–3.[41] A reasonable target for HbA_{1c} in prepregnancy counseling is to aim for 6%, and when such a target has been chosen, outside pregnancy, in randomized, controlled trials of intensified insulin treatment, it has been associated with successful achievement of levels of approximately 7% to 7.4% compared with mean levels of HbA_{1c} of 9% when conventional insulin regimes are followed. In women participating in the Diabetes Control and Complications Trial who became pregnant, there were 8 congenital malformations among 86 women randomized to conventional treatment but only 1 in 94 in those randomized to intensive insulin treatment.[42]

TABLE 44–3

New Reporting Standards for Glycated Hemoglobin (International Federation of Clinical Chemistry and Laboratory Medicine) Compared with Percentage Glycation Using Diabetes Control and Complications Trial–Aligned Criteria

HbA_{1C} (DCCT) (%)	HBA_{1C} (IFCC) (%)	eAG (mmol/L)
6.0	42	7.0
6.5	48	7.8
7.0	53	8.6
7.5	59	9.4
8.0	64	10.1
9.0	75	11.8
9.5	80	12.6
10.0	86	13.4

DCCT, Diabetes Control and Complications Trial aligned laboratory method; eAG, estimated average blood glucose; HbA_{1c}, hemoglobin A_{1c}; IFCC, International Federation of Clinical Chemistry and Laboratory Medicine.
From Kahn R, Fonseca V: Translating the A1C assay. Diabetes Care 2008;31:1–4.

An improvement in HbA_{1c} levels can also be achieved by switching to short-acting modern analogue insulins and by enrolling the prepregnant subject into education programs that teach enhanced carbohydrate counting. Examples include the Dose Adjustment for Normal Eating (DAFNE)[43] for women with type 1 diabetes. Similar structured education programs exist for type 2 diabetes, such as Diabetes Education and Self-Management for Ongoing and Newly Diagnosed (DESMOND).[44] Switching someone who has established diabetes with which they are able to cope and lead a normal lifestyle into an enhanced program of tight diabetic control is not without its risks from the point of view of hypoglycemia.[45,46] There are important social considerations if hypoglycemia becomes more common including the threat of loss of the driving license and problems with maintaining employment and normal lifestyle if hypoglycemic episodes become frequent. At the time of submitting women to enhanced prepregnancy glycemic control regimes, education should be provided on recognition and management of hypoglycemia for both the patient and her partner. Third-party administered glucose supplements such as buccal glucose gel and intramuscular glucagon must be made available. These regimes are intensive and demanding, and once an acceptable target range for HbA_{1c} has been achieved, contraception can be safely discontinued. The situation should be closely monitored, and an early resort to referral to the infertility service should be considered, perhaps as early as 6 months after trying has failed to achieve a pregnancy. When women, despite their best efforts, do not achieve an optimal percentage of HbA_{1c}, more detailed investigation into the pattern of diabetes control such as that obtained by continuous glucose monitoring (CGMS) should be considered. When conventional insulin regimes do not appear to be effective, some women would benefit from continuous subcutaneous insulin infusion (CSII) using an insulin pump.

As a counseling guide, women with HbA_{1c} above 10% might reasonably be recommended to continue contraception and avoid pregnancy until there has been a significant improvement. Data from a recent large case series suggest that the relative risk for perinatal mortality is also correlated with levels of periconceptional HbA_{1c}.[12] It is important during prepregnancy counseling to discuss the still relatively high rate of congenital malformations that can complicate pregnancy in women with diabetes even if they achieve HbA_{1c} targets (see Fig. 44–1).[13] In practice, however, the uptake of prepregnancy counseling remains poor in proportionate terms, and many pregnancies are unplanned or occur with a relatively high HbA_{1c} value.

Attitudes to antenatal diagnosis and termination of pregnancy should be explored. Women who have obesity with preexisting diabetes, commonly type 2 diabetes, should have expert dietetic advice in the prepregnancy period. In gross obesity, it may be considered that preconceptional bariatric surgery has a place for a small number of women. As a guide, to reduce the superimposed complications of obesity on type 2 diabetes in pregnancy, a target body mass index (BMI) of 27 might be considered, although there will be large individual variation of what can be achieved by dietary advice, lifestyle modification, and perhaps, the use of biguanide drugs such as Metformin rather than sulfonylureas or insulin. Both of the latter can be associated with increased fat deposition.[47]

In prepregnancy counseling, the current drug regime should also be reviewed. Some hypoglycemic drugs have not been evaluated for safety in pregnancy, including some of the newer long-acting insulin analogues. Antihypertensives, particularly angiotensin-converting enzyme (ACE) inhibitors[48] and angiotensin II receptor antagonists,[49] should be discontinued prior to pregnancy or as soon as pregnancy is recognized. The former are teratogenic and the latter can cause fetal anuria, though this risk to the fetal kidney does not appear to be related to first-trimester drug exposure. Medication with statins would generally be discontinued, although there is no consistent evidence of a teratogenic effect,[50] but stopping them during pregnancy should have no detrimental effect on long-term therapy of hyperlipidemia.

All women with preexisting diabetes should have been subject to regular digital imaging of the retina, preferably with mydriasis using tropicamide or with dilated retinoscopy when digital photography is not available. Women with any degree of previously unrecognized retinopathy should have a referral to an ophthalmic surgeon prior to discontinuing contraception. It should also be pointed out to them that rapid optimization of glycemic control can be associated with a deterioration in retinopathy. One cohort study of 171 pregnant diabetic women reported a more rapid rate of progression of retinopathy with an OR of 1.8 (95% confidence interval [CI] 1.1–2.8) compared with 298 nonpregnant women with type 1 diabetes over a comparable period of time independent of HbA_{1c}, blood pressure, number of previous pregnancies, and duration of diabetes.[51] Continued monitoring of the retina during any pregnancy and during periods of enhanced prepregnancy diabetic control is essential. Those at greatest risk appear to be those entering pregnancy with established retinopathy, but in one cohort study in 154 women, there was progression in 23% of women with no retinopathy in the first trimester, 41% with nonproliferative retinopathy deteriorated, and 63% of those with established proliferative disease experienced progression.[52]

When pregnancy occurs without any prepregnancy counseling, then an urgent assessment of all the previous factors should be undertaken as soon as possible at the antenatal clinic.

Prenatal

GESTATIONAL DIABETES: DIAGNOSIS, AND SCREENING

The diagnosis of GDM is based on World Health Organization (WHO) criteria with a 75-g oral glucose load with fasting and 2-hour glucose levels[53] or the ADA criteria using a 100-g load[1] (see Table 44–1). Many national bodies, including National Institute for Clinical Excellence (NICE),[54] have recommended screening for GDM in pregnancy either in the whole population or in identified high risk groups. A new diagnostic criterion, also included in Table 44–1, is based on fasting, 1-hour, or 2-hour levels has been suggested by a consensus group reviewing the Hyperglycaemia and Adverse Pregnancy Outcomes (HAPO) study.[55]

As a rough guide to the various approaches to screening (which are summarized in Appendix B of the NICE guideline *Diabetes in Pregnancy*[56]), screening can be selective or universal. Individual units may choose their own approach, but one consideration is the likely prevalence of GDM in any particular country or, indeed, individual obstetric unit within any country. Where the disorder has an expected prevalence of less than 3%, screening based on historic risk factors might be considered an acceptable approach, but where prevalence is expected to be above 3%, provocative testing by either one- or two-step glucose loading with a 50-g glucose challenge test (GCT) or diagnostic screening with a 75-g oral glucose tolerance test (OGTT) might be considered. Rationalization could be applied by offering universal screening, but with the exclusion of women recognized as being at "low risk" on the grounds of age and/or ethnicity. The ADA defines these women as age younger than 25 years, normal BMI, and not from a high-prevalence ethnic minority group.[1]

When a selective approach to screening is to be applied, then the recommended screening historic risk factors are as follows[54]:

- BMI of 30 or above.
- Previous macrosomic infant.
- Previous pregnancy complicated by GDM.
- Family history of diabetes in first-degree relatives.
- Ethnic origin with known high prevalence of diabetes including subcontinental Asia, black Caribbean, and Arabic, particularly of Middle Eastern origin.

It is acknowledged that a selective screening approach will miss a proportion of women with GDM, perhaps up to 30%.

When a case of GDM is recognized by a screening program, the woman should be referred to a joint antenatal/diabetes clinic where she can be instructed in self-monitoring of blood glucose levels. Having made the diagnosis of GDM, usually in the last trimester, and enrolled the

TABLE 44–4

Summary Outcomes of Postprandial Monitoring versus Preprandial Monitoring of Blood Glucose in Insulin-Dependent, and Gestational Diabetes

	TYPE 1 DIABETES			GESTATIONAL DIABETES MELLITUS		
OUTCOME	PREPRANDIAL	POSTPRANDIAL	*P*	PREPRANDIAL	POSTPRANDIAL	*P*
N	31	30		33	33	
Success in meeting targets (%)	30.3	55.5	<.001	86	88	
Insulin dose (U/day)	103.0 ± 51.3	120.4 ± 52.37	NS	76.8 ± 21.4	100.4 ± 29.5	<.003
Final HbA_{1c} (%)	6.3 ± 0.7%	6.0 ± 0.8%	NS	8.1 ± 2.2%	6.5 ± 1.4%	.006
Preeclampsia	6 (21%)	1 (3%)	.048	–	–	
Cesarean section (%)	68	47	NS	39%	24%	NS
Birth weight (g)	3509 ± 684	3270 ± 565	NS	3848 ± 434	3469 ± 668	.01
LGA	18 (58%)	15 (50%)	NS	14 (42%)	4 (12%)	.01
Shoulder dystocia/birth trauma	1 (3%)	2 (7%)	NS	6 (18%)	1 (3%)	NS
Neonatal hypoglycemia	9 (29%)	8 (26.7%)	NS	7 (21%)	1 (3%)	.05
Mean cord insulin (mU/L) (range)	34.4 (7.8-95.8)	11.4 (5.8-41.4)	NS	–	–	

HbA_{1c}, hemoglobin A_{1c}; LGA, large for gestational age.
From Manderson JG, Patterson CC, Hadden DR, et al: Preprandial versus postprandial blood glucose monitoring in type 1 diabetic pregnancy: A randomized controlled clinical trial. Am J Obstet Gynecol 2003;189:507–512; and De Veciana M, Major CA, Morgan MA, et al: Postprandial versus preprandial blood glucose monitoring in women with gestational diabetes mellitus requiring insulin therapy. N Engl J Med 1995;333:1237–1241.

patients into a program of self-monitoring and diet with or without hypoglycemic agents, the antenatal care and targets for glycemic control should be the same as those described in the next section for women with preexisting diabetes.

GLYCEMIC TARGETS

The evidence suggests that therapeutic approaches that succeed in reducing the rate of fetal hyperinsulinemia will also be associated with improved obstetric outcomes and a reduction in the typical neonatal morbidity of the macrosomic newborn. Two small, but well-conducted, randomized, controlled trials, one in women with type 1 diabetes[57] and one in women with GDM,[58] confirm that postprandial, compared with preprandial, glucose monitoring with a target in both studies of a 1-hour blood glucose level lower than 7.8 mmol/L is associated with important reductions in birth weight and in typical neonatal morbidity (Table 44–4).

A likely cause of fetal hyperinsulinemia despite apparently well-controlled maternal glycemia based on the previous target is that in many women with type 1 diabetes experience high postprandial peaks of glucose or high fasting levels of glucose on some days but not others.[59] This phenomenon has been well described in observational studies using continuous glucose monitoring systems (CGMS), and a new randomized, controlled trial by Murphy and colleagues[60] from the United Kingdom randomizing women to intermittent use of adjunctive CGMS or conventional intermittent self-monitoring also reveals a major stepwise improvement in reduced birth weight and perinatal morbidity. A small randomized, controlled trial of the use of CGMS in GDM reported an increase in the use of hypoglycemic therapy (31% vs. 8%) in the self-monitored group. There were no differences in pregnancy outcomes; however, the study was underpowered to assess these.[61] CGMS technology is expected to become more widely available for use in pregnancy with the hope of improving pregnancy outcomes and in particular in those with ultrasound evidence of incipient macrosomia.

Conventionally, intermittent sampling is used in all types of diabetes, and it is recommended that the target for glucose levels after an overnight fast should be maintained between 3.3 and 5.9 mmol/L of glucose and the 1-hour postprandial glucose level should be maintained at less than 7.8 mmol/L, except in cases in which this regime provokes frequent severe maternal hypoglycemia.[57,58]

HYPOGLYCEMIA

Both hypoglycemia and hyperglycemia can complicate diabetes control in pregnancy, particularly in women with type 1 diabetes. The greatest frequency of hypoglycemia occurs between weeks 8 and 16, corresponding with the time at which most women who are susceptible will experience nausea and vomiting and anorexia. Although some authors have suggested this is a likely etiologic factor,[62] others have reported no difference in the self-reported incidence of nausea and/or vomiting in the previous week between those with and those without episodes of severe hypoglycemia.[63] A further complicating factor that women should be made aware of in prepregnancy counseling or in early pregnancy is that their usual subjective experience of hypoglycemia awareness may be obtunded in pregnancy and this is an independent risk factor for requiring third-party assistance because of hypoglycemic coma in the first half of pregnancy.[63] Vulnerable women should be instructed in the more frequent use of self-monitoring of blood glucose sampling and to particularly increase the frequency of sampling before planned activities such as driving. Obviously, they will be familiar with the requirement to carry readily available calories with them, but also their partners and close relatives, friends, or work colleagues might be advised about the use of preparations such as buccal glucose gel and indeed intramuscular glucagon, as stated in the "Prepregnancy" section earlier.

HYPERGLYCEMIA

Hyperglycemia with the risk of diabetic ketoacidosis (DKA) in type 1 diabetes is fortunately less common in pregnant than in nonpregnant women. It is potentially a very serious problem because untreated mild or moderate DKA can be associated with intrauterine fetal death. Women with type 1 diabetes in pregnancy should be offered or advised to use a blood glucose monitoring system that can also measure ketones and to test themselves when they become unexpectedly hyperglycemic or otherwise feel unwell. Early admission to the hospital is appropriate when DKA is suspected, and rapid correction of the acid-base balance is essential if fetal viability is to be preserved. Accident and emergency units, acute medical admission units, and/or obstetric units should have written protocols for the management of DKA in pregnancy, and if the diagnosis is confirmed, it is recommended that treatment is offered on a suitable high-dependency unit. An assumption of incipient or actual DKA should be made if an urgent serum bicarbonate level on admission is less than 20 mmol/L or if an arterial blood gas analysis confirms maternal acidosis (Table 44–5).

Iatrogenic DKA and on some occasions fetal death have been provoked in the past by treatment of suspected preterm labor with β-sympathomimetic drugs and/or maternal steroids, both of which have insulin counterregulatory actions (see the section on "Preterm Labor," later). In addition to the urgent treatment of DKA, underlying causes such as maternal urinary infection or respiratory infection should be sought and treated as appropriate. The recognition of fetal distress in association with DKA in late pregnancy will generally provoke urgent delivery, but here close cooperation with an experienced obstetric anesthetist is essential because there are maternal risks of induction of anesthesia in someone who may have a deteriorating pattern of metabolic acidosis.

TABLE 44–5

Recognition and Management of Diabetic Ketoacidosis in Pregnancy

Clinical Suspicion

- All pregnant women with Type 1 diabetes should be provided with Optimum Xceed Meter (or equivalent) and B-ketone test strips.
- If feeling unwell for any reason, or any vomiting, or blood sugars above target having been within normal range before test blood for ketones: if <0.6 mmol/L, repeat in 2 hrs if symptoms persist or if blood sugar rising despite normal insulin doses; if ≥0.6 mmol/L, arrange self-referral/urgent professional review.

Biochemical Confirmation

- Urgent FBC/U & E venous bicarbonate, or arterial blood gases.

Urgent Management

- Venous bicarbonate:
  - If <20 mmol/L, commence DKA regime.
  - If <16 mmol/L, commence DKA regime and seek urgent assistance from diabetes physician.
- DKA regime:
  - Admit HDU: Commence IV normal saline and administer 1000 mL in first hr. Give second 1000 mL over 2 hr.
  - K^+ replacement in normal saline, based on serum potassium measurement:
    - >5.5 mmol/L no KCl supplement, repeat U & E in 2 hr.
    - 4–5.5 mmol/L 20 mmol KCl/1000 mL saline.
    - <4.0 mmol/L 40 mmol KCl/1000 mL saline.
- Insulin
  - 50 U Actrapid in 49.5 mL normal saline by pump/syringe driver 6 U/hr; if blood glucose not falling after 2 hr, increase to 12 U/hr.
- Fetal monitoring
  - CTG if fetal viability established.
- Maternal investigations (for C & S in microbiology)
  - Throat swab
  - MSU
  - Vaginal swab
  - Blood culture

C & S, culture and sensitivity; CTG, cardiotocogram; DKA, diabetic ketoacidosis; FBC, full blood count; HDU, high-dependency unit; MSU, midstream urine; U & E, urea and electrolytes.

DIETARY MANAGEMENT

In modern obstetric practice, diabetes management is offered by a multidisciplinary team, usually working in a joint antenatal clinic. Women with all types of diabetes will generally benefit from either a prepregnancy or an early pregnancy review of their "normal" diet. Where available, women who have not had the benefit of attending DAFNE[43] or similar courses when not pregnant (see earlier) should be offered a place in such a course as early as possible during the pregnancy. The importance of adopting appropriate dietary patterns should be emphasized so that the doses of insulin or oral hypoglycemic drugs can be minimized. For many women with GDM, oral hypoglycemic or insulin therapy may be avoided altogether with no increase in adverse perinatal outcomes. In women with GDM, observational studies have shown an inverse relationship between birth weight and proportion of dietary energy obtained from carbohydrate.[64] Low–glycemic index (GI) carbohydrate sources are associated with enhanced maternal sensitivity to endogenous insulin,[65] a mechanism that should contribute to several benefits such as reduced likelihood of requiring hypoglycemic therapy, lower rates of fetal macrosomia, and lower maternal net body weight gains after the completion of the pregnancy. One recent randomized, controlled trial of low GI versus a conventional high dietary fiber diet resulted in insulin being required in 29% of low GI but 59% of high dietary fiber. There were no differences in obstetric or fetal outcomes.[66] Prepregnancy dietary advice is adaptable to use in pregnancy with all types of diabetes.

The first approach to glycemic control should be dietary advice based on Diabetes UK[67] or ADA[1] criteria (Table 44–6). These recommend a diet relatively high in carbohydrate sources of known low GI, lean proteins including oily fish, and a balance of polyunsaturated and monounsaturated fats. Women with a high BMI might be advised to restrict calorie intake with expert dietetic advice and consider suitable enhanced mild or moderate exercise during the pregnancy.

INSULIN THERAPY

If insulin therapy is required or has been chosen in type 2 or GDM, intermittent bolus doses of insulin to cover each main meal will usually be prescribed with the pregnant woman given telephone access to a diabetes specialist nurse or diabetes specialist midwife for advice on dose adjustment. More severe type 2 diabetes and type 1 diabetes are generally treated by a combination of long-acting basal insulins with three or four times daily short-acting insulins. Modern short-acting analogue insulins are known to be safe for use

TABLE 44-6

Dietary Advice for Pregnant Women with Diabetes

COMPOSITION OF THE DIET	NUTRITIONAL ADVICE FOR PEOPLE WITH DIABETES
Protein	Not > 1 g/kg body weight
Total fat	<35% of energy intake.
Saturated + transunsaturated fat	<10% of energy intake.
ω-6 polyunsaturated fat	<10% of energy intake
ω-3 polyunsaturated fat	Eat fish, especially oily fish, once or twice weekly. Fish oil supplements not recommended.
cis-monounsaturated fat	10%–20% } 60%–70% of energy intake
Total carbohydrate	45%–60% } 60%–70% of energy intake
Sucrose	≤10% of daily energy.
Fiber	No quantitative recommendation. *Soluble fiber*—has beneficial effects on glycemic and lipid metabolism. *"Insoluble" fiber*—has no direct effects on glycemic and lipid metabolism, but its high satiety content may benefit those trying to lose weight and is advantageous to gastrointestinal health.
Vitamins and antioxidants	Encourage foods naturally rich in vitamins and antioxidants.
Salt	≤6 g sodium chloride/day.

Modified from Nutrition Subcommittee of the Diabetes Care Advisory Committee of Diabetes UK: The implementation of nutritional advice for people with diabetes. Diabet Med 2003;20:786–807.

in pregnancy and probably have advantages in their speed of action helping to reduce postprandial peaks.[68,69] There is some theoretical risk associated with the use of longer-acting insulin analogues, but small observational studies have reported no adverse outcomes.[70] Larger-scale randomized, controlled trials addressed to the safety and effectiveness of these drugs are currently in progress. Many women entering pregnancy on a combination of short- and long-acting analogue insulins will wish to continue using these drugs. If they do so, they should be aware of the uncertainty of the risks of the long-acting analogue preparations, pending the performance and publication of suitable randomized, controlled trials. If commencing long-acting insulins for the first time in pregnancy or in women who are not taking long-acting analogue insulins, the more traditional human isophane (NPH) insulin should be prescribed.

Some women are using continuous subcutaneous insulin infusion (CSII), the "insulin pump," when they enter pregnancy and there is no reason to discontinue these devices. A systematic review of randomized, controlled trials comparing CSII with intensified conventional insulin regimens has revealed no advantage or disadvantage to either regime.[71] It is also likely that a small number of women who find that their control, in terms of both hypoglycemia and/or hyperglycemia, has been disturbed by the adjustments they need to make for pregnancy will benefit from either a short-term or a long-term switch to CSII. In the future, it is likely that women who have difficulty with glycemic control will be helped by feedback devices combining CGMS with automatic insulin infusion by a CSII regime.

ORAL HYPOGLYCEMIC DRUGS

The conventional recommendation for women with type 2 diabetes has been to discontinue oral hypoglycemic drugs when planning a pregnancy or as early as possible in any unplanned pregnancy because of concerns about teratogenesis. However, systematic reviews and meta-analyses have failed to demonstrate any increase in structural congenital malformations associated with use of these drugs in pregnancy and suggest that when a woman with type 2 diabetes has satisfactory control maintained on an oral hypoglycemic agent, she should continue it during pregnancy unless she chooses to switch to insulin.[72,73]

The other concern about the continuation of oral hypoglycemics during pregnancy is the greater likelihood of poor glucose control compared with insulin. One retrospective cohort study from South Africa reported a higher perinatal mortality rate in women on oral hypoglycemics compared with those switched to insulin during the pregnancy.[74] In GDM, new-generation short-acting sulfonylureas were the subject of one large-scale randomized trial by Langer and associates.[75] Four hundred four women with GDM were randomized between 11 and 33 weeks' gestation to receive glibenclamide (glyburide) or insulin with a primary endpoint of maternal glycemic control with targets of 5.3 mmol/L fasting and 6.7 mmol/L 2 hours postprandial. Four percent of women in the glibenclamide group could not maintain these levels of control without supplementary insulin. The dose of glibenclamide was started at 2.5 mg daily in the morning and then increased on a weekly basis by 2.5 or 5 mg/day up to a maximum of 20 mg. No significant differences emerged between the groups: the rate of birth weight above the 90th percentile was 12% on glibenclamide and 13% on insulin. Neonatal respiratory distress was seen in 8% versus 6%, neonatal hypoglycemia 9% versus 6%, and cord serum insulin concentrations were identical, suggesting a similar quality of maternal glycemic control. No glibenclamide was detected in the in cord serum, suggesting that this short-acting sulfonylurea does not cross the placenta in significant amounts.

A more recent study randomizing women similarly to insulin or metformin for the treatment of GDM has been reported by Rowan and coworkers.[76] There were 363 women randomized to metformin and 370 randomized to insulin. In that study, the dosage of metformin was started at 500 mg once or twice daily and increased every first or second week toward glycemic targets up to a maximum daily dose of 2500 mg. Seven women randomized to metformin had to discontinue the drug because of gastrointestinal side effects. The outcomes of the pregnancy for mothers and infants were not significantly different, apart from an excess of preterm birth, 12% versus 7.6% in the metformin group. There was, however, only 1 birth before 32 weeks' gestation in each group, and 9 infants in each group required transient treatment with continuous positive airway pressure. Forty percent of women in this study required supplementary insulin, however.

Perhaps more important in terms of long-term maternal prognosis, particularly in this group of women who are often obese, there was a net increase in weight loss from enrollment to the postpartum visit of 8.1 kg in the metformin group versus 6.9 kg in the insulin group.

In conclusion, modern short-acting sulfonylurea drugs and metformin are likely to have an increasing place in the management of GDM. Metformin may become the drug of choice for those entering pregnancy who are overweight or obese.

RETINAL ASSESSMENT

During pregnancy, digital retinal imaging should be performed with mydriasis at or as soon as practicable after the first antenatal clinic appointment. The Diabetic Retinopathy Study Research Group[77] reported that the presence of any of the following high risk characteristics at any stage of life is associated with a 2-year risk of developing severe visual loss:

- Presence of vitreous or preretinal hemorrhage.
- Presence of new vessels.
- Location of new vessels on or near the optic disk.
- Severity of new vessels.

In randomized studies, photocoagulation in the presence of these abnormalities reduced the risk of severe visual loss by 50% or more. Background or mild nonproliferative retinopathy should be followed by a further digital retinal imaging at 16 to 20 weeks. With a normal retina in early pregnancy, the second assessment can be deferred to 28 weeks' gestation.[78]

There is a particular concern about the risk of visual loss if diabetic macular edema is detected, and in nonpregnant randomized, controlled studies, photocoagulation is associated with a reduced risk of visual loss from 24% to 12% at 3-year follow-up. No such study has been reported in pregnancy, but it seems likely that the ophthalmologist would wish to consider urgent treatment of macular edema, should it be detected.

DIABETIC NEPHROPATHY

Renal function should be assessed not only prepregnancy but also as early as possible during pregnancy. Diabetic nephropathy is classified as

- Stage 1: microalbuminuria (albumin-to-creatinine ratio ≥3.5 mg/mmol).
- Stage 2: macroalbuminuria (albumin-to-creatinine ratio ≥ 30 mg/mmol) or urinary albumin concentration of 200 mg/L or more.
- Stage 3: end-stage renal disease.

Early consultation with a nephrologist is indicated if the serum creatinine is above 120 μmol/L or urinary protein excretion exceeds 2g/day.

A systematic review of progression and development of nephropathy showed that for most women, pregnancy was not associated with either an increased incidence or a deterioration in mild nephropathy, but some women with moderate or advanced nephropathy may progress to end-stage renal disease during the pregnancy.[79] When nephropathy is present throughout pregnancy, intrauterine growth retardation, chronic hypertension, preeclampsia, and preterm birth are all more common and appropriate maternal and fetal surveillance should be undertaken during the pregnancy. Pharmacologic treatment of nephropathy with ACE inhibitors is generally contraindicated in pregnancy (see earlier) but should be recommenced after the completion of the pregnancy.

SCREENING FOR CONGENITAL MALFORMATIONS

The NICE Antenatal Guideline[54] currently recommends that all women should be offered first-trimester screening for Down syndrome. The combined nuchal translucency test (nuchal translucency, free β-human chorionic gonadotrophin [β-hCG], and pregnancy-associated plasma protein A [PAPP-A] is the test of choice). Levels of free β-hCG and PAPP-A have been found to be unaffected by diabetes in pregnancy.[80] As a result, the detection rate and screen-positive rates remain 80% and 5% for the combined nuchal translucency test for pregnancy with diabetes.

Increased nuchal translucency thickness (>3.5 mm) is associated with an increased risk of cardiac anomalies in chromosomally normal fetuses. A first-trimester nuchal translucency thickness of greater than 4.5 mm has been reported to be associated with a 15-fold increased risk of congenital cardiac disease. These findings may prove selective fetal echocardiography for women with diabetes and increased nuchal translucency thickness to be a more cost-effective approach.

Diabetes in pregnancy is associated with an increased risk of NTDs.[3] There is an association between maternal serum α-fetoprotein (AFP) and NTD, however, the weighted-corrected median multiple-of the mean value is lower in pregnancies affected with preexisting diabetes than in pregnancy not complicated by diabetes.[81] In practice, many consider that there is no benefit from maternal AFP screening in women with diabetes if routine 20-week anomaly screening is in place.[17,82]

Ultrasound screening for fetal anomaly should be routinely offered between 18 and 21 weeks' gestation.[56] A comprehensive ultrasound examination is of paramount importance given the increased risk of congenital anomaly. A cohort study compared 130 women with diabetes (85 type 1 diabetes, 45 type 2 diabetes) with 12,169 low risk pregnant women over the same period.[15] All women had a routine ultrasound scan at 16 to 24 weeks' gestation. Ten major anomalies (7.7%) were present in fetuses of women with diabetes compared with 1.4% in nondiabetic women. Ultrasound antenatal detection of the fetal abnormality was significantly lower in women with diabetes compared with the low risk group (42% vs. 86%). An increased BMI was responsible for 35% of the ultrasound scans performed in women with diabetes being considered suboptimal. Of the 7 major congenital anomalies missed by antenatal ultrasound, 3 were abnormalities of the cardiovascular system. This does raise the question of whether routine fetal echocardiography is warranted in the diabetic population. Most of the common cardiac defects seen in diabetic pregnancy are of conotruncal or septal origin.[83–85] As such, a standard four-chamber view including the two ventricular outflow tracks should detect the majority of cardiac abnormalities. Smith and colleagues[86] reported a detection rate of major congenital cardiac abnormalities of 82% using the four-chamber view and outflow track ultrasound views. They concluded there was no benefit in universal fetal echocardiography in women with diabetes if a comprehensive anatomic ultrasound survey, which included four-chamber and outflow tracks, was reported as normal.

A cost-effectiveness analysis of fetal echocardiography screening of pregnant diabetic women demonstrated an increased detection rate of cardiac abnormalities using fetal echocardiography compared with standard comprehensive ultrasound. Selective fetal echocardiography after an abnormal detailed comprehensive anatomic survey was more cost-effective than a policy of universal fetal echocardiography screening of women with diabetes of pregnancy. Fetal echocardiography should be restricted to those women with diabetes who had increased nuchal translucency in the first trimester or either have a cardiac anomaly suspected at routine fetal anatomic survey ultrasound scan or when cardiac views are restricted by increased body fat and confirmation of normal cardiac structure cannot be made.

MONITORING FETAL GROWTH AND WELL-BEING (See Also Chapters 10 and 11)

Excessive birth weight is defined as either large for gestational age (LGA) or fetal macrosomia. Large for gestational age relates to a birth weight equal to or greater than the 90th percentile for gestational age. A macrosomic fetus is, however, variously defined as a birth weight greater than either 4 kg or 4.5 kg regardless of gestational age. This is recognized clinically by a disproportionate increase in abdominal circumference on ultrasound (see later). Excessive fetal growth is associated with increased maternal and infant morbidity. Shoulder dystocia rates and subsequent brachial plexus injuries are increased as are fetal asphyxia, operative deliveries, and the incidence of postpartum hemorrhage.

Ultrasound prediction of fetal weight in pregnancy in diabetes is inaccurate and sometimes technically difficult. Accuracy of fetal weight estimation decreases with increasing birth weight, a fact compounded in women with both obesity and diabetes.[87,88] A comparison was made between a single biometric measurement, abdominal circumference greater than 36 cm, and fetal weight estimation using multiple standard ultrasound biometry measurements in predicting birth weight greater than 4 kg (estimated fetal weight [EFW]).[89] There was no difference in accuracy between EFW and abdominal circumference in the prediction of macrosomia at birth likelihood ration (LR) 5.7 (95% CI 4.3–7.6) and LR 6.9 (95% CI 5.2–9.0), respectively. This demonstrates that both a single abdominal circumference measurement and an EFW are only moderately predictive of birth weight.

Examination of neonates of women with diabetes clearly shows that these infants have different anthropometric features than macrosomic babies of nondiabetic women. The phenotypic features are a result of excess growth in the insulin-sensitive tissues such as liver, bone, and abdominal and subcutaneous fat. Perhaps because of the distortion of normal body composition parameters, prediction of fetal weight by ultrasound in pregnancies in diabetes underestimates fetal weight by more than 15% of true birth weight in a quarter of cases compared with only 5.4% in nondiabetic women.[87] The measured parameters in standard formulas for EFW are less accurate in pregnancy in diabetes often underestimating but sometimes overestimating true fetal weight.[87,90]

Fetal subcutaneous fat layers, three-dimensional upper arm volumes, fetal liver volumes, and cheek-to-cheek measurements have all been compared with standard ultrasound biometry in the prediction of macrosomia in diabetes and have, in small studies, been found to be perform well when compared with abdominal circumference or EFW.

It is important to note that infants of mothers with diabetes have an accelerated growth pattern unless coexisting vasculopathy complicates the pregnancy.[91] Management of such a pregnancy would deviate from standard protocols for diabetic pregnancy and involve fetal heart rate monitoring, umbilical and middle cerebral Doppler velocimetry, and biophysical profile (BPP) testing owing to the increased fetal risk.

The NICE Guideline on Diabetes in Pregnancy[56] recommends that fetal growth is assessed on a 4-weekly basis from 28 to 36 weeks' gestation. This would seem a reasonable proposal; however, one would advise that interpretation of any ultrasound scan in a women with diabetes is carefully made. Evidence of disproportion between the measurements may indicate truncal adiposity. The EFW is likely to be underestimated, and the presence of a macrosomic fetus and polyhydramnios may reflect a hyperinsulinemic fetus with the greatest risk of late stillbirth.

Pregnancy in diabetes complicated by vascular disease appears to confer the greatest risk of uteroplacental insufficiency and subsequent fetal intrauterine growth restriction (IUGR) and its sequelae. Antenatal surveillance of fetal well-being in this group of women is likely to have a favorable effect on perinatal outcome, and management of such pregnancies would follow strategies similar to those for fetal IUGR in nondiabetic pregnancies. Those women with preexisting diabetes, no vascular complications, and good maternal glycemic control rarely have fetal compromise and are, therefore, unlikely to benefit from a policy of universal antenatal surveillance using fetal well-being protocols.

Antenatal fetal surveillance of high risk pregnancy is usually performed using a combination of fetal heart rate monitoring, BPP testing, and umbilical artery Doppler velocimetry. Each method has been independently found to be predictive of fetal compromise in high risk pregnancy groups. However, whether the tests are equally predictive in pregnancies with diabetes is questionable.

Umbilical artery Doppler velocimetry is an indirect measure of placental flow resistance. An abnormal umbilical Doppler result is usually associated with chronic placental insufficiency typically associated with preeclampsia and IUGR. The use of umbilical artery Doppler velocimetry in high risk pregnancies has demonstrated a significant reduction in cesarean section for fetal distress and resulted in a nonsignificant trend in reducing perinatal mortality in high risk women.[92] An abnormal umbilical artery Doppler does appear to predict fetal compromise in pregnancy complicated by diabetes if there is coexisting diabetic vasculopathy, hypertension, or IUGR.[93] The absence of these comorbidities does significantly reduce the effectiveness of umbilical artery Doppler in predicting adverse fetal outcome in these women.

The BPP is an ultrasound assessment of fetal well-being that incorporates fetal movements, fetal tone, fetal breathing movements, and liquor volume. It is a time-consuming test but does have a role in the antenatal assessment of high risk pregnancy. The role of the BPP test in antenatal surveillance of pregnancy complicated by diabetes is controversial because the test has been shown to be a poor predictor of adverse pregnancy outcome.[94] A normal test result, however, is usually thought to be reassuring of fetal well-being.[95]

A rise in maternal glucose levels is known to stimulate fetal breathing movements, contributing to a positive score for one of the components of the BPP. In addition, maternal diabetes is often associated with increased amniotic fluid, again a positive score in the BPP. It is, therefore, easy to see why the role of the BPP is controversial because two of the five tests of fetal well-being are influenced positively simply by having diabetes in pregnancy.

Brasero and associates[96] compared the ability of the BPP, the cardiotocogram (CTG), and the assessment of umbilical artery Doppler in pregnancies complicated by diabetes to predict adverse outcome. Adverse outcome was categorized as cesarean section for fetal distress, hypocalcemia, hypoglycemia, hyperbilirubinemia, fetal respiratory distress, and/or preterm delivery under 37 weeks. The relative risk was 1.7 for both the BPP and the fetal heart rate pattern. Umbilical artery Doppler velocimetry had a relative risk of 2.6 in predicting one of the composite outcomes. As is often a problem with such studies, perinatal mortality is low, there were no stillbirths in this series, and therefore, the ability to predict perinatal mortality remains unknown.

Given the paucity of good randomized, controlled studies on assessment of fetal well-being in pregnancies with diabetes, a pragmatic approach to monitoring these fetuses must be taken. The presence of either diabetic vasculopathy, hypertensive disease, or the identification of a growth-restricted fetus should trigger comprehensive fetal surveillance, the frequency of which will be determined by the severity of the underlying comorbidity. In those women with well-controlled diabetes and no additional obstetric risk factors, the value of antenatal fetal well-being testing is questionable because it will not improve the already good outcome in these pregnancies. If delivery beyond 38 weeks is anticipated, however, then despite the absence of good-quality evidence, weekly tests including CTG, umbilical artery Doppler, and possibly BPPs would seem appropriate.

ANTENATAL CARE SCHEDULES IN MATERNAL DIABETES

The pattern of antenatal care offered to women with diabetes in pregnancy should incorporate appointment times and investigations that would be applicable to all pregnant women as stipulated by the recent NICE Diabetes in Pregnancy Guideline.[56] The relevant flowcharts are shown in Table 44–7. The number of additional antenatal units

TABLE 44–7

Specific Antenatal Care for Women with Diabetes

APPOINTMENT	CARE FOR WOMEN WITH DIABETES DURING PREGNANCY*
First appointment (joint diabetes and antenatal clinic)	Offer information, advice, and support in relation to optimizing glycemic control. Take a clinical history to establish the extent of diabetes-related complications. Review medications for diabetes and its complications. Offer retinal and/or renal assessment if these have not been undertaken in the previous 12 mo.
7–9 wk	Confirm viability of pregnancy and gestational age.
Booking appointment (ideally by 10 wk)	Discuss information, education, and advice about how diabetes will affect the pregnancy, birth, and early parenting (such as breast-feeding and initial care of the baby).
16 wk	Offer retinal assessment at 16–20 wk to women with preexisting diabetes who showed signs of diabetic retinopathy at the first antenatal appointment.
20 wk	Offer four-chamber view of the fetal heart and outflow tracts plus scans that would be offered at 18–20 wk as part of routine antenatal care.
28 wk	Offer ultrasound monitoring of fetal growth and amniotic fluid volume. Offer retinal assessment to women with preexisting diabetes who showed no diabetic retinopathy at their first antenatal clinic visit.
32 wk	Offer ultrasound monitoring of fetal growth and amniotic fluid volume.
36 wk	Offer ultrasound monitoring of fetal growth and amniotic fluid volume. Offer information and advice about: • Timing, mode and management of birth. • Analgesia and anesthesia. • Changes to hypoglycemic therapy during and after birth. • Management of the baby after birth. • Initiation of breast-feeding and the effect of breast-feeding on glycemic control. • Contraception and follow-up.
38 wk	Offer induction of labor, or cesarean section if indicated, and start regular tests of fetal well-being for women with diabetes who are awaiting spontaneous labor.
39 wk	Offer tests of fetal well-being.
40 wk	Offer tests of fetal well-being.
41 wk	Offer tests of fetal well-being.

* Women with diabetes should also receive routine care according to the schedule of appointments in reference 54, including appointments at 25 wk (for nulliparous women) and 34 wk, but with the exception of the appointment for nulliparous women at 31 wk.

From National Collaborating Centre for Women's and Children's Health: Diabetes in Pregnancy. London, RCOG Press, 2008.

required would be based on whether the diabetes was preexisting or gestational.

For preexisting diabetes, it would be anticipated that the woman would attend for preconception advice and counseling. Information would be imparted on the type of care she would receive within the joint care diabetes clinic and would be given education and advice in relation to achieving optimal glycemic control. If the woman has not attended for preconception advice, this information should be given at the first hospital visit. Clinical history and investigations would establish the extent of diabetes-related complications such as neuropathy and vascular disease. Retinal assessment would be recommended at this time if this has not been performed in the preceding 12 months. Additional retinal assessment would be required between 16 and 20 weeks if diabetic retinopathy had been present at the time of the booking assessment. In the absence of prepregnancy or booking retinopathy, further assessment is indicated at 28 weeks' gestation.

At 20 weeks' gestation, ultrasound anatomic examination of the fetus should be performed and include a four-chamber view of the heart and outflow tracks. Thereafter, serial assessment of fetal growth and amniotic volume should take place at 28, 32, and 36 weeks' gestation. Following the 36-week ultrasound scan, information and advice with regard to timing and mode of delivery and management of labor and birth should be discussed. At 38 weeks' gestation, delivery, whether by induction of labor or cesarean section if indicated, should be offered to all women with diabetes in pregnancy (see below). If the decision is made to await spontaneous labor, weekly assessment of fetal well-being should be performed. Those women who have been diagnosed with GDM as a result of routine antenatal screening should also be offered serial fetal growth and amniotic fluid volume assessment at 28, 32, and 36 weeks.

PRETERM LABOR MANAGEMENT AND OUTCOMES

The etiology and management of preterm labor is discussed in detail in Chapter 61. There is an increased risk of spontaneous preterm birth in diabetes, however, that may be inversely proportional to the quality of maternal diabetic control and the corresponding frequency of polyhydramnios. There is some evidence in women free of diabetes that the preterm birth rate goes up with mean HbA_{1c}.[97] If tocolytic agents are being considered for use in women with diabetes, β-minetics should be avoided because they have an acute hyperglycemic effect and can provoke DKA in type 1 diabetes. When preterm delivery is anticipated, antenatal steroids, usually in the form of betamethasone injections, 12 mg intramuscularly, repeated after 24 hours, can be administered. Glucocorticoids cause insulin resistance and hyperglycemia, and the inadequately supervised use of these drugs has been associated in some cases with hyperglycemia and even DKA. To avoid this in women with type 1 diabetes, one group recommended that daily insulin doses should be increased by enhancement of their existing regimes as follows[98]:

Day 1 Insulin dose increased by 25%.
Day 2 Insulin dose increased by 40%.
Day 3 Insulin dose increased by 40%.
Day 4 Insulin dose increased by 20%.
Day 5 Insulin dose increased by 10%.
Day 6 Return to previous insulin doses.

Alternative approaches to managing the steroid induced relative hyperglycemia include

- Titration of intermittent subcutaneous short-acting insulin on a sliding scale based on 4-hourly glucose values.
- Titration of an intravenous insulin infusion on a sliding scale based on 4-hourly glucose values. This may be of value particularly in those who may not be eating normally because of abdominal pain or uterine contractions and when delivery may be imminent.

Elective or spontaneous preterm birth of an infant of a mother with diabetes should wherever possible be in a unit with neonatal intensive care facilities. There should be joint consultation with neonatal pediatricians because of the potential neonatal complications.

Labor and Delivery

TIMING AND MODE OF DELIVERY

In pregnancy complicated by diabetes, timing of delivery presents a challenge. Elective delivery by induction of labor or cesarean section after 37 completed weeks has the potential advantage of reducing the risk of shoulder dystocia secondary to macrosomia and the risk of mature stillbirth. Twenty-seven percent of nonmalformed stillbirths in women with preexisting diabetes in the CEMACH data[3] occurred after 37 completed weeks, when it might be assumed that had the baby been born alive, it would have been a healthy survivor. Against the apparent advantages of early elective delivery are the relatively high cesarean section rates that are often associated with a diagnosis of failed induction of labor and the relatively high incidence of respiratory difficulty, including RDS, in the newborn because of pulmonary immaturity that is often associated with fetal hyperinsulinemia.

Only one randomized, controlled trial of expectant management has been performed in 200 women the majority of whom had insulin-treated GDM.[99] They were randomized to active management, which consisted of induction of labor in the 38th week of gestation, or expectant management, which consisted of weekly physical examination, twice-weekly CTG, and weekly ultrasound estimates of amniotic fluid volume. The expectant group had a doubling of the rate of spontaneous labor (44% vs. 22%), but they also had a doubling of babies born above the 90th percentile for gestational age (23% vs. 10%). The expected endpoint of a reduction in cesarean section rate was not obtained (31% vs. 25%). There were three cases of mild shoulder dystocia, all of which occurred in the expectantly managed group.[99]

One further randomized, controlled trial was undertaken in 273 women with an ultrasound estimate of fetal macrosomia (4.0–4.5 kg), but this was performed in nondiabetic women.[100] The rates of mode of birth were almost identical in the induced and the expectant groups, the mean birth weights were 4.06 versus 4.13 kg, and there were 5 cases of shoulder dystocia in the induced group and 6 in the expectant group.[100] The relevance of this study to management of women with diabetes may be questioned because of the increased risk of shoulder dystocia associated with the disproportionate growth seen in macrosomia in the hyperinsulinemic fetus of the mother with diabetes. Many authorities would opt for elective cesarean section when an ultrasound EFW exceeds 4.5 kg, not least because current methods of EFW are likely to overestimate the weight of the hypertrophic fetus (see "Prenatal Care" section, earlier). It is the case, however, that this policy has not been subject to any randomized, controlled trial. A small number of case series and cohort studies would suggest that vaginal birth after cesarean section is often successful in the absence of antenatally diagnosed fetal macrosomia.

ANALGESIA AND ANESTHESIA (See Also Chapter 70)

There are limited data on the risks and benefits of various methods of analgesia and anesthesia available for labor and delivery, but all commonly used modalities appear to be suitable for women with diabetes. Obesity in type 2 diabetes and GDM may introduce its own complications for both the anesthetist and the obstetrician, and joint consultation with the anesthetist in the antenatal period for women with a high BMI above 35 might be considered worthwhile.

GLYCEMIC CONTROL IN LABOR OR FOR CESAREAN SECTION

On the day of labor and/or delivery for most women, their usual approach to glycemic control will have to be replaced to allow flexibility in calorie intake for the demands of labor, to maintain nil by mouth for those going for elective, or potentially for emergency, cesarean section, and finally to maintain glycemia in a range that minimizes neonatal hypoglycemia.

A reasonable approach is to aim to maintain the plasma glucose level in the physiologic range (between 4 and 7 mmol/L), and in particular in women with type 1 diabetes, an adequate insulin regime must accompany oral or intravenous feeding. Common practice would be to secure the maintenance of blood glucose within the physiologic range in spontaneous or induced labor or on the day of elective cesarean section by a balanced regime of intravenous dextrose and insulin such as the one in Table 44–8.[101] There should be a flexible approach to the way euglycemia is achieved in labor, however, and some women will choose to continue CSII throughout labor if they have been used to this technique for insulin replacement; others will be able to maintain their glycemic targets with intermittent subcutaneous injections of short-acting insulin. These latter two approaches may have some advantages for the woman in terms of mobility and the adoption of more comfortable positions in labor. As a general guide, women who have not required insulin during the pregnancy for type 2 or GDM and those women whose insulin dose has totaled less than 20 U/day will often maintain their blood glucose levels within the physiologic range without resorting to an intravenous dextrose and insulin regimen.

TABLE 44–8

Standardized Intravenous Protocol and Insulin and Dextrose Therapy

- Nil by mouth until after the birth of the baby.
- Start intravenous dextrose 10% in 500 mL, 100 mL/hr by electronic pump.
- Hourly blood glucose estimation by glucose meter.
- Insulin infusion by intravenous pump through the same or an alternate intravenous line commencing at 2 U/hr if blood glucose > 7 mmol/L (for most syringe pumps, 50 U of short-acting insulin in 50 mL or 0.9% saline by electronic pump 1 mL is equivalent to 1 U).
- If initial blood glucose is in the physiologic range, 4–7 mmol/L commence infusion at 1 mL (1 U)/hr.
- Adjust insulin infusion rate to maintain blood glucose between 4.0 and 7.0 mmol/L by glucose meter, decreasing insulin rate by 1 U/hr if glucose <4 mmol/L and increasing by 0.5 U/hr when any reading >7 mmol/L.
- After delivery of the placenta, halve the insulin infusion to a minimum of 0.5 U/hr adjust insulin rate to maintain blood glucose at 4.0–7.0 mmol/L. When discontinuing, stop the intravenous fluids and insulin 30 min after self administration after first dose of subcutaneous insulin.

Note: These regimes require constant supervision by midwifery/nursing and medical staff in particular to be sure that both pumps are functioning normally and at the set rate and that no lines to the patient are obstructed.
Based on reference Lean ME, Pearson DW, Sutherland HW: Insulin management during labour and delivery in mothers with diabetes. Diabet Med 1990;7:162–164.

MODE OF DELIVERY

For women in whom the intravenous dextrose insulin regimen is indicated, this can be commenced as soon as the diagnosis of labor is confirmed. For those women in whom induction of labor is planned, a satisfactory regimen on the morning of induction after any treatment required for cervical favorability the previous evening is to allow a light breakfast accompanied by the normal dose of short-acting insulin but to omit any morning dose of intermediate- or long-acting insulin. The intravenous dextrose and insulin regime can be commenced after induced labor has been established.

For those women who are to have an elective cesarean section in type 1 diabetes, it is recommended that the intravenous dextrose and insulin regimen be commenced in the morning of surgery and maintained until the postoperative woman is able to eat and drink normally. At this time, insulin can be recommenced based on either the prepregnancy doses of insulin or the woman's self-direction if she has been trained on a DAFNE course or similar regimen.

For those with type 2 or GDM having elective cesarean section, preoperative blood glucose may be checked and, if it is within the physiologic range, most women will be able to have the surgical procedure without the need for intravenous dextrose or insulin, although obviously it is sensible to retain this as an option and in particular to consider it for women whose return to normal eating and drinking postsurgery is delayed for any reason.

NEONATAL HYPOGLYCEMIA AND MATERNAL GLYCEMIA IN LABOR

The newborn infant of the mother with diabetes complicating pregnancy is at risk of potentially harmful hypoglycemia in the newborn period as a result of three mechanisms, only one of which is modifiable. The two unmodifiable ones are, first, that the newborn who had hyperinsulinemia established in fetal life may in the first 24 or 48 hours of neonatal existence have persisting autonomous increased secretion of insulin unmatched by oral calorie intake. Second, it has now been established that because amylin is cosecreted with insulin and is a potent cause of delay in gastric emptying, the hyperinsulinemic newborn may be unable to maintain its blood glucose despite an apparently adequate calorie intake (often with an increased glucose component).[23] For these reasons, a significant minority of newborn infants will require transfer to a neonatal care unit for intravenous dextrose feeding to bypass the gastrointestinal tract. The third mechanism for neonatal hyperglycemia is in the fetus who is not necessarily severely hyperinsulinemic but who has β cells sensitive to transplacental glucose infusion, and relative maternal hyperglycemia in labor can provoke transient neonatal hypoglycemia that may be severe. Several observational studies have been published typically showing that neonatal hypoglycemia is seen in about 30% to 50% of the infants of mothers whose blood glucose was 7 mmol/L or more in the hours prior to delivery compared with rates between 0% and 20% in those in which maternal blood glucose was maintained between 4 and 7 mmol/L in the hours prior to birth.[102] In addition to this, two uncontrolled prospective studies suggest that fetal distress in labor and perinatal asphyxia are more common with a mean blood glucose in labor above 7 mmol/L.[103,104]

Postnatal

MATERNAL POSTNATAL CARE IN RELATION TO TYPE OF DIABETES

Following delivery, insulin requirements fall immediately in both women with preexisting and those with GDM. Women with insulin-treated preexisting diabetes should reduce their insulin immediately after birth to near prepregnancy levels and monitor their blood glucose levels carefully to establish the appropriate dose. The immediate postnatal period is a time of increased risk of hypoglycemia, especially when breast-feeding, and women with insulin-treated preexisting diabetes should be advised to have a meal or snack available before or during feeds. Those women with preexisting type 2 diabetes should resume or continue with their oral hypoglycemic medication. However, if breast-feeding, only metformin and glibenclamide should be considered suitable.

In those women with GDM, a small subgroup will have persisting hyperglycemia postnatally and be subsequently diagnosed to have type 2 diabetes. In a New Zealand population, 13% of women with GDM was subsequently found to have type 2 diabetes on postnatal glucose tolerance testing.[2] Following delivery in women with GDM, insulin therapy and oral hypoglycemic agents should be discontinued and blood glucose monitoring extended into the immediate postnatal period. Those with persisting hyperglycemia and newly diagnosed diabetes would then be identified and referred to the diabetes team for consideration of subsequent management. For the majority of women whose blood glucose levels are normal, monitoring can discontinue and a fasting plasma glucose measurement offered at a 6-week postnatal check.

All women with diabetes in pregnancy should, prior to discharge, be reminded of the importance of contraception and the need for preconception care when planning future pregnancies.

Women who develop GDM have a lifetime risk of developing type 2 diabetes of approximately 40%.[105] All women should, therefore, be advised of the symptoms of hyperglycemia and offered lifestyle advice that includes weight control, diet, and exercise in order to reduce this risk of developing type 2 diabetes. It is important that an annual fasting glucose test is performed to enable prompt detection of diabetes and early management to reduce longer-term associated morbidity.

Those with GDM should be informed of the risks of GDM in future pregnancies and should be offered a fasting plasma glucose or OGTT to exclude diabetes when planning future pregnancies.

NEONATAL CARE OF THE INFANT OF THE MOTHER WITH DIABETES

The more common neonatal complications are RDS and neonatal hypoglycemia, necessitating careful supervision of the infant of the mother with diabetes. Other complications, particularly in the macroscomic hyperinsulinemic infant, include cardiomyopathy, hypocalcemia, hypomagnesemia, polycythemia, hyperbilirubinemia, and hyperviscosity. Women with diabetes should not be delivered in obstetric units where there are no facilities for neonatal intensive care. Although routine admission to the neonatal unit is not required, these mothers and babies must be admitted to a transitional care unit or similar facility in which monitoring of the newborn is of high quality.

Breast-feeding should be encouraged in women with diabetes, and there is no indication that the quality of milk is significantly different in women with diabetes than in those who do not have this disorder. Because early feeding may be indicated to prevent neonatal hypoglycemia, women with diabetes may consider banking colostrum in the antenatal period, but in many cases, formula feeding may be required to manage hypoglycemia in the short term in the newborn period to avoid the need for neonatal unit admission and intravenous dextrose. Neonatal hypoglycemia should be tested for either in the laboratory, or in a laboratory-certified bedside method that is accurate in the severe hypoglycemia range. Testing should be commenced at approximately 3 hours of age and a level below 2.0 mmol/L should lead to the encouragement of early oral feeding or tube feeding. Intravenous dextrose should be withheld in the absence of clinical signs of hypoglycemia, or a falling level 1 hour after a recording of 2.0 mmol/L or less to 1.4 mmol/L or less.

SUMMARY OF MANAGEMENT OPTIONS

Diabetes

Management Options	Evidence Quality and Recommendation	References
Prepregnancy		
Advise all women with diabetes in the reproductive years about the benefits of prepregnancy planning.	III/B	45,46
Screen for complications of diabetes and review therapeutic options.	IV/C	77
Target prepregnancy HbA_{1C} level at 6.1% to reduce rate of structural malformation.	Ib/A	13,42
Refer for DAFNE or alternative structured education programs.	Ib/A	43,44
Commence folic acid supplements.	IV/C	4,56
Switch to short-acting insulin analogues/consider CSII to improve prepregnancy glycemic control.	Ib/A	68
Continue contraception if HbA_{1C} >10%.	III/B	42
Recognize risks of complications of hypoglycemia from intensified regime and provide appropriate emergency treatments.	III/B	45
Continue oral hypoglycemic regimes with short-acting sulfonylureas/metformin if judged effective.	III/B	72,73
Discontinue potentially teratogenic drugs used for complications of diabetes.	III/B	48,49
Prenatal		
Screen for GDM universally or according to expected prevalence within geographic areas or by ethnic and age groups.	Ia/A	25,26
Enroll cases of GDM in joint diabetes/antenatal clinic, commence fetal growth monitoring.	Ia/A	25,26
Treat GDM unresponsive to diet by glycemic criteria with insulin or glibenclamide.	Ib/A	58,75
Refer women with preexisting diabetes to calorie counting/DAFNE course as early as possible in pregnancy—if not previously attended.	Ib/A	43
Advise target-orientated therapy, based on fasting and 1-hr postprandial levels.	Ib/A	57,58
Use CGMS intermittently if available.	Ib/A	60
Advise about management of hypoglycemia and supply hypostop/glucagon for those at risk.	GPP	—
Advise women how to suspect early DKA and how to self-monitor for ketonemia or ketonuria.	GPP	—
Arrange admission of any pregnant woman suspected of DKA to high dependency unit, and maintain unit protocol for management.	GPP	—
Offer antenatal care through a multidisciplinary clinic.	GPP	—
Arrange dilated retinal photography as soon as referred with pregnancy and preexisting diabetes. Arrange follow-up retinal scans based on initial findings.	—/GPP	—
Measure albuminuria and refer to nephrology if serum creatinine > 120 μmol/L.	III/B	79
Offer first-trimester screening for Down syndrome if requested.	GPP	
Arrange anatomy scan at 18–21 wk.	GPP	
Include cardiac outflow tracts in anatomy scan.	III/B	86
Refer for fetal echocardiography selectively.	III/B	86
Scan for fetal growth and amniotic fluid index at 4-wk intervals from 26 wk' gestation.	GPP	

Management Options	Evidence Quality and Recommendation	References
Review and intensify hypoglycemic (insulin) regime if incipient macrosomia.	GPP	
Initiate tests of fetal well-being if IUGR is diagnosed.	GPP	
Offer induction of labor/elective CS if indicated after 37 completed wk' gestation.	Ib/A	99
Monitor fetal well-being weekly in women who wish to continue their pregnancy beyond 38 wk.	Ib/A	99
Avoid β-sympathomimetics in preterm labor	GPP	
Establish in-house protocols for insulin dose increases when administering maternal steroids.	GPP	
Elective preterm birth in maternal diabetes should be in a unit with neonatal ICU facilities.	GPP	
Labor and Delivery		
Maintain plasma glucose levels between 4.0 and 7.0 mmol/L in labor and during elective or emergency CS.	III/B	102
Monitor newborn infant for evidence of respiratory distress and/or clinical or biochemical hypoglycemia.	GPP	
Postnatal		
Return women with preexisting diabetes to their prepregnancy insulin/hypoglycemic therapy.	GPP	
Discontinue hypoglycemic therapy in women with GDM, and monitor blood glucose levels for evidence of newly diagnosed type 2 diabetes.	GPP	
Offer contraceptive advice.	GPP	
Check fasting plasma glucose at 6 wk postdelivery and annually to exclude a new diagnosis of type 2 diabetes.	III/B	105

CS, cesarean section; CSII, continuous subcutaneous insulin infusion; CGMS, continuous glucose monitoring system; DAFNE, dose adjustment for normal eating; DKA, diabetic ketoacidosis; GDM, gestational diabetes mellitus; GPP, good practice point; HbA_{1c}, hemoglobin A_{1c}; IUGR, intrauterine growth restriction.

SUGGESTED READINGS

Confidential Enquiry into Maternal and Child Health (CEMACH): Diabetes in Pregnancy: Are We Providing the Best Care? Findings of a National Enquiry: England, Wales, and Northern Ireland. London, CEMACH, 2007.

Confidential Enquiry into Maternal and Child Health (CEMACH): Pregnancy in Women with Type 1 and Type 2 Diabetes in 2002–2003. England, Wales, and Northern Ireland. London, CEMACH, 2005.

Crowther CA, Hiller JE, Moss JR, et al: Effect of treatment of gestational diabetes mellitus on pregnancy outcomes. N Engl J Med 2005; 352:2477–2486.

The HAPO Study Cooperative Research Group: Hyperglycemia and adverse pregnancy outcomes. N Engl J Med 2008;358:1991–2002.

National Collaborating Centre for Women's and Children's Health: Diabetes in Pregnancy. London, RCOG Press, 2008.

Rowan JA, Hague W, Gao W, et al: Metformin versus insulin for the treatment of gestational diabetes. N Engl J Med 2008;358:2003–2015.

REFERENCES

For a complete list of references, log onto www.expertconsult.com.

CHAPTER 45

Thyroid Disease

ANNA P. KENYON and CATHERINE NELSON-PIERCY

Thyroid disease is the second most common cause of endocrine dysfunction in women of childbearing age (diabetes is the first). It can often be challenging to diagnose and manage because many of the symptoms of the disease are common symptoms in pregnancy. Physiologic changes in the serum levels of pituitary and thyroid hormones may hamper diagnosis, and a clear understanding of these changes is needed when managing those women with suspected or known thyroid disease.

The thyroid gland is a bilobed gland composed of spherical follicles. A follicle comprises a colloid center surrounded by a single layer of follicle cells. Intimately involved with follicle cells are parafollicular C cells, lymphatic drainage channels, and capillary networks.

Iodide ions are actively transported from the blood into the apical surface of follicle cells and, via the action of thyroid peroxidase (TPO), are oxidized to iodine. The thyroid regulates the amount of iodide it actively traps and is able to withstand fluctuations in dietary supply. In the lumen, (colloid) iodide is incorporated into the tyrosine residues of thyroglobulin (also made in the follicle cells) to produce inactive monoiodotyrosine and diiodotyrosine. This process is termed the *organification* of iodide. Combinations of these products result in formation of the active thyroid compounds thyroxine (T_4) and triiodothyronine (T_3), which are released into the capillary network at the apical surface of follicle cells after reentering from the colloid at their basal surface (endocytosis).

Production is controlled by the hypothalamus-pituitary-thyroid axis. Thyroid-releasing hormone (TRH) is released from the hypothalamus, and thyroid-stimulating hormone (TSH) from the anterior pituitary. TSH is a glycoprotein with α- and β-subunits. Many anterior pituitary hormones share the α-subunits, but the β-subunit is unique. TSH has many actions, one of which is to increase release of T_4 and T_3 via increased iodide transport into follicular cells, organification and release of thyroglobulin into the follicular lumen, and endocytosis of colloid.

More T_4 than T_3 is produced by the thyroid gland, but T_4 is converted in some peripheral tissues (liver, kidney, and muscle) to the more potent T_3.

In the plasma, more than 99% of all T_3 and T_4 is carrier protein–bound to thyroid-binding globulin (TBG), albumen, and transthyretin (previously known as thyroid-binding prealbumen). TBG has the highest affinity for T_3 and T_4, so although it is present in the lowest concentration, 75% of all thyroid hormones are bound to it. Only the free hormones (free T_4 and free T_3) are biologically active (0.04% of total T_4 and 0.5% total T_3). Pregnancy results in a rise in TBG (and transthyretin) via the effects of estrogen favoring increased synthesis but also decreased clearance. The elevation is present at 2 weeks' gestation and peaks at 20 weeks' gestation.[1] Because only the free hormone is biologically active, only free hormone measurements should be used in pregnancy.

Pregnancy is a state of relative iodine deficiency secondary to an increase in renal loss (increased glomerular filtration rate in the early first trimester) and transfer of iodine to the developing fetus. In order to compensate, the thyroid gland increases its uptake of iodine from the blood, and if this is lacking, cellular hyperplasia and goiter will result. It is suggested that, although a physiologic goiter may be seen on ultrasound examination by a change in gland size of up to 10% to 20%, this is not clinically detectable. If apparent clinically, it suggests iodine deficiency or pathology.[1]

Fetal thyroid disorders are discussed in Chapter 21.

THYROID-STIMULATING HORMONE CHANGES IN PREGNANCY

Human chorionic gonadotrophin (hCG) and TSH share a common α-subunit and their β-subunits share some similarities, as do their receptors. The rise in hCG of early pregnancy is thought to "spill over" and stimulate the TSH receptor, causing a suppression of TSH (and a rise in T_4). The longitudinal study by De Geyter and coworkers[2] of 18 women attending for infertility investigations preconception suggested that in very early pregnancy, TSH was present in rising concentrations peaking at week 6 with levels declining thereafter. In contrast, serum hCG levels increased progressively to weeks 9 to 12[2,3] with stable levels thereafter[2]; however, free T_4 and T_3 remained unchanged during the whole sampling period.[2]

A large American study of 9562 women attending antenatal screening for aneuploidy with paired samples in the first and second trimesters confirmed TSH levels to be lower and to show greater variability in the first trimester than in the second. The median first-trimester TSH (1.05 mIU/L) was lower than in the second trimester (1.23 mIU/L) and the

98th percentile was higher (4.15 mIU/L vs. 3.77 mIU/L). The variance (spread) of TSH values was greater at 10 to 13 weeks than at 15 to 18 weeks at both the lower and the upper extremes of the distribution. Of those with TSH above the 98th percentile in the first trimester, 68% had second-trimester values over the 95th percentile,[3] suggesting that in some, the relative rise was sustained. In 2004, Haddow and colleagues[4] studied 1126 pregnant women and confirmed lower median TSH in the first trimester (1.00 mIU/L vs. 1.29 mIU/L) but a higher 98th percentile (5.20 mIU/L vs. 4.18 mIU/L). A Scandinavian longitudinal study of 52 normal pregnancies confirmed that in weeks 7 to 17, the lower limit of normal (2.5th percentile; and 95% confidence interval [CI]) for TSH was 0.09 (0.00–0.26) rising to 0.78 (0.52–1.04) and the upper limit (97.5th percentile; and 95th CI) was 3.39 (3.02–3.76).[5]

A recent longitudinal study of a U.K. general antenatal population (307 women) demonstrated that for TSH, the range is broader and higher than outside pregnancy. In addition, the median expected value rises throughout pregnancy.[6] Thus, it seems that after an initial rise in TSH, concentrations fall to a nadir at week 12 and thereafter rise with advancing gestation; however, the normal range in the first trimester remains wide (Table 45–1).

THYROXINE LEVELS IN PREGNANCY

The elevated concentrations of hCG of early pregnancy "spill over" and stimulate the TSH receptor resulting in a rise in T_4 in early pregnancy. This may have the advantage of providing the fetus with T_4 before it becomes autonomous. The rise in TBG necessitates a small rise in production of T_4 (1%–3%) and T_3 until a plateau level is reached when hCG levels are maximal. In addition, there is enhanced peripheral conversion of free T_4 to free T_3, and it has been suggested that this increased efficiency may be in preparation for the exertions of labor and delivery.[7] Lambert-Messerlian and associates[8] confirmed that free T_4 concentrations are higher in the first trimester than in the second at all percentiles ($P < .001$). In contrast to TSH, however, the within-person correlation of T_4 between trimesters is weak. The previously cited study in the U.K. general antenatal population (307 women) reported that compared with levels outside pregnancy, free T_4 has a narrower and lower range and falls throughout pregnancy and free T_3 has a broader and higher range, falling through most of gestation to a nadir at 30 weeks and 5 days; then the upper end of the range increases and the lower end of the range reduces to term.[6] Thus, T_4 concentrations appear to be highest in the first trimester (but still lower than nonpregnant values) and fall with rising gestational age.

Table 45–1 shows normal values for thyroid function tests throughout pregnancy. Whereas the literature is useful in identifying trends, the reference ranges cited are not easily translated into meaningful values to guide clinical practice. Older free hormone[6] or TSH assays may be less accurate and values may vary between laboratories.[3] The studies use differing sample sizes, populations of different ethnicities and fertility and study women from geographically discrete areas with different iodine intakes. The studies may restrict investigation to one trimester, use different gestational age

TABLE 45–1

Reference Ranges for Thyroid Function Tests in Pregnancy (See also Appendix of Normal Values)

		TSH (MU/L)	THYROXINE (PMOL/L UNLESS OTHERWISE STATED)	TRIIODOTHYRONINE (PMOL/L)
Nonpregnant	Guys & St. Thomas' NHS Foundation Trust, United Kingdom, 2009	0.27-4.2	12-22	3.1-6.8
First trimester	Cotzias[6]	0-5.5	10-16	3-7
	Shan[9]	0.09-4.38	11.41-23.76	
	Marwaha[10]	0.6-5	12-19.45	1.92-5.86
	Larsson[5]	0.09-3.39		
	Lambert-Messerlian[8]	0.12-2.68	0.87-1.38 ng/dL	
Second trimester	Cotzias[6]	0.5-3.5	9-15.5	3-5.5
	Marwaha[10]	0.435-5.78	9.48-19.58	3.2-5.7
	Larsson[5]	0.37-3.88		
	Lambert-Messerlian[8]	0.35-2.77	0.72-1.26 ng/dl	
Third trimester	Cotzias[6]	0.5-4	8-14.5	2.5-5.5
	Marwaha[10]	0.74-5.7	11.3-17.71	3.3-5.18
	Larsson[5]	0.23-2.83		

Key:
Cotzias[6]: Cross-sectional analysis of 307 women. Median trimester thyroid hormone intervals rounded to nearest 0.5.
Shan[9]: 4800 women, cross-sectional study. Samples drawn at 4, 8, 12, 16, and 20 wk. Antibody-positive women excluded. Only those <12 wk shown here. 5th and 95th percentiles.
Marwaha[10]: 331 Indian women. Singleton pregnancies. Antibody-positive women excluded. Cross-sectional study. 107, 137, and 87 women recruited in first, second, and third trimester, respectively. 5th and 95th percentiles.
Larsson[5]: 52 normal pregnancies. Longitudinal study. Samples drawn at 12 and 20 wk and at 4-weekly intervals thereafter. "Upper" and "lower" limit of the calculated reference range.
Lambert-Messerlian[8]: 8531 and 8415 singleton antibody-negative women in first and second trimesters, respectively. 5th and 95th percentiles. Paired first- and second-trimester samples.
NHS, National Health System; TSH, thyroid-stimulating hormone.

ranges, and use different statistical methods to define "normal" ranges.[4–6,9,10] This can make clinical decisions regarding dosage adjustments in pregnancy problematic. Target ranges are not clear.

HYPOTHYROIDISM

General

Hypothyroidism affects 1% of pregnant women, and as with hyperthyroidism, many of the symptoms are encountered in normal pregnancy. Discriminatory symptoms are cold intolerance, slow pulse rate, and delayed relaxation of deep tendon reflexes, particularly those of the ankle.

The most common cause of hypothyroidism is autoimmune in origin associated with TPO autoantibodies leading to destruction of the gland, lymphoid infiltration, and eventual atrophy and fibrosis. This is termed *atrophic (autoimmune) hypothyroidism*. In some cases, antibodies blocking the TSH receptor have been implicated. Hashimoto's thyroiditis is a different form of autoimmune thyroiditis also with TPO (microsomal) autoantibodies, often in high titers. However, in this condition, there are atrophic changes with regeneration resulting in goiter formation. Where the origin is autoimmune, there are associations with other autoimmune disease (e.g., pernicious anemia, insulin-dependent [type 1] diabetes mellitus, and vitiligo).

Hypothyroidism may be iatrogenic following lithium, amiodarone, or antithyroid medication. Alternatively, it may be transient, occurring as part of the disease course in subacute de Quervain's thyroiditis or postpartum thyroiditis.

Any woman on T_4 for iatrogenic hypothyroidism should have a careful history taken to determine the original cause of her disease. This is particularly true in those women on T_4 following thyroidectomy or radioiodine therapy in which the original indication for the surgery may have been hyperthyroidism. Thyrotoxic symptoms in such women should not be attributed to treatment excess until a flare of residual disease has been excluded.[11]

Diagnosis

Hypothyroidism may be diagnosed in those with a reduced free T_4 concentration in association with an elevated TSH, which outside pregnancy, is a sensitive indicator of the degree of thyroid hormone deficiency. However, pregnancy represents a challenge for establishing reliable reference ranges and cutoffs.[8] Identifying TPO autoantibodies can confirm the diagnosis, but these are nonspecific, being present in 20% to 30% of the normal population.[12]

Maternal and Fetal Risks

The most serious consequence of hypothyroidism is myxedema coma. This is extremely rare in pregnancy, but it represents a true medical emergency with a 20% mortality rate. The clinical picture of myxedema coma includes hypothermia, bradycardia, decreased deep tendon reflexes, and altered consciousness. Hyponatremia, hypoglycemia, hypoxia, and hypercapnia may also be present. Once the diagnosis is made, therapy should begin immediately with supportive care and thyroid hormone replacement. Improvement in symptoms usually occurs after 12 to 24 hours of therapy.[13]

One study addressing outcome in hypothyroidism demonstrated that gestational hypertension, (eclampsia, preeclampsia, and pregnancy-induced hypertension) occurred more commonly in the overt and subclinical hypothyroid patients than in the general population, with rates of 22%, 15%, and 7.6%, respectively. In addition, 36% of the overt and 25% of the subclinical hypothyroid subjects who remained hypothyroid at delivery developed gestational hypertension. Low birth weight in both overt and subclinical hypothyroid patients was secondary to premature delivery for gestational hypertension. Older studies have suggested a link with congenital malformations, but more recently, no such association has been reported.[14]

Little T_4 crosses the placenta after the first trimester, and the placenta is relatively impermeable to TSH and T_3. The fetal thyroid gland begins to form at 5 weeks' gestation and has some function at 10 weeks but is only autonomous at 12 weeks when T_4, T_3, and TSH can all be measured in fetal serum.[15] Levels continue to rise until 35 to 37 weeks' gestation when they reach adult levels. The gland, however, is relatively immature with high TSH levels relative to the amount of T_4 produced.

T_4 is important in early development of the fetal brain. Haddow and coworkers[16] have suggested impaired neuropsychiatric development in the offspring of hypothyroid mothers. Pop and colleagues[17] demonstrated that children of women who had hypothyroxinemia (free T_4 levels below the 10th percentile and TSH levels within the reference range) during the first trimester of pregnancy are at risk of having a baby with delay in both mental and motor development at 1 and 2 years, with the effect being most pronounced in those whose levels remained low throughout gestation. Those children born to mothers in whom T_4 was maintained between the 50th and the 90th percentile during early pregnancy showed normal neurodevelopment.[17] A study examining IQ scores in offspring born to mothers who were hypothyroid in early pregnancy who were subsequently treated failed to show any adverse effect on mental development when compared with their siblings born when the same mothers' were euthyroid.[18] Haddow and coworkers[16] studied 25216 women and found 62 had TSH above the 98th percentile in conjunction with a low T_4 at the time of screening for prenatal diagnosis in the second trimester. These women were then matched to 124 control women. The children born to mothers with high TSH performed less well on IQ tests. Forty-eight of the women were not treated and these had the lowest scores.[16] The fetus is thus reliant on maternal T_4 prior to 12 weeks' gestation, and correction of maternal hypothyroxinemia in the first 12 weeks of pregnancy might, therefore, be expected to improve neurodevelopmental outcome.[16]

Cretinism (deaf mutism, spastic motor disorder, and hypothyroidism) is a distinct and severe form of brain damage caused by severe maternal iodine deficiency.

Neonatal or fetal hypothyroidism secondary to transplacental transfer of maternal autoantibodies is extremely rare (1 in 180,000 neonates or ~2% of babies with congenital hypothyroidism)[19] if it occurs at all.[20]

Congenital absence of the thyroid gland is also exceptionally rare, and in these cases, the fetus is reliant on transfer of maternal T_3 and T_4 across the placenta[21] throughout gestation.

All infants are screened for hypothyroidism via the blood spot Guthrie card collected via a heelprick on day 6 of life. Those with an abnormality are recalled for further testing (0.2%–0.3% of the general population).

The fetus is not thought to be at risk of hyperthyroidism from maternal T_4 therapy because placental transfer is so poor.

Management Options

Prepregnancy

In hypothyroidism, the frequency of menstrual irregularities has been variously reported as between 56% and 80% of patients. Oligomenorrhea, amenorrhea, polymenorrhea, and menorrhagia have all been reported. Most are likely to be attributed to anovulatory cycles. However, a recent study reported far fewer menstrual irregularities; 23.4% among 171 hypothyroid patients studied (three times more frequent than in 124 controls).[22] The most common manifestation in this group was oligomenorrhea (42.5%) followed by menorrhagia in 30%. Reduced libido may be an associated feature.

Ovulation and conception can occur in mild hypothyroidism.[23] It is likely, however, that severe hypothyroidism is associated with failure of ovulation, and therefore, tests of thyroid function are appropriate in the investigation of an infertile couple. The guidelines issued by the National Collaborating Center for Women's Health in 2004 suggest that testing should be done only when the woman reports menstrual irregularities or other symptoms consistent with thyroid disease.

Given the association of hypothyroidism and other autoimmune diseases, performing thyroid function tests in women with insulin-dependent (type 1) diabetes mellitus prior to pregnancy may be a useful screening tool.

Patients with hypothyroidism should be counseled to delay pregnancy until maintenance T_4 levels have been achieved. Reassurances should be given for the safety of T_4 during pregnancy. It is useful to perform a baseline TSH and free T_4 measurement in those contemplating a pregnancy in the near future or as early as possible postconception. Recent guidelines produced by the Endocrine Society[24] have advised that in those known to be hypothyroid prior to pregnancy, adjustment of the preconception T_4 dose to reach TSH less than 2.5 μIU/L before pregnancy is advisable.

Prenatal

A new diagnosis of hypothyroidism in pregnancy is uncommon, given its association with infertility. A more common problem is someone who is inadequately replaced embarking on a pregnancy or in those labeled with hypothyroidism following an episode of postpartum thyroiditis that resolved but the diagnosis was never reviewed.

Those who enter pregnancy euthyroid can expect a good outcome. Hypothyroidism requires treatment with T_4. If there is no coexisting heart disease, an initial dose of 100 μg of T_4 is usually required. In women who are stable on treatment, checking thyroid function in each trimester will suffice. However, if dosage changes are implemented, thyroid function tests (TSH and free T_4) should be measured after 4 to 6 weeks. More frequent testing (every 2 wk) may be needed in those with very poor control in early pregnancy. When making dosage adjustment, the free T_4 should be used rather than TSH, which can take time to fall. However, poor compliance may also result in a raised TSH with a normal free T_4. Several investigators have variously advocated increasing doses of T_4 with advancing gestation.[25–27] Alexander and associates[3] prospectively studied 20 women who were hypothyroid and planning a pregnancy. Samples were taken preconception, every 2 weeks during the first trimester, and then monthly thereafter. The T_4 dose was increased in order to keep the TSH concentration at prepregnancy values or increased if TSH was greater than 5 mIU/L The serum TSH level increased during the first 10 weeks of gestation, prompting an increase in the levothyroxine dose in 85% of the group. A mean increase in dose by 47% was required in these women to keep TSH at prepregnancy concentrations. The increased doses were required during the first 16 to 20 weeks. In the hypothyroid women studied, the peak in TSH at 8 to 10 weeks was accompanied by a downward trend in free T_4, as is observed in normal subjects. The authors concluded that women on treatment for hypothyroidism should be advised to increase their current dose of levothyroxine by taking two extra daily doses during each week (i.e., to increase the dose by 29%) beginning the week pregnancy is confirmed and to continue doing so until they are able to undergo thyroid function testing; thus, additional T_4 is provided during this time of increased demand.[3] The small Abalovich and coworkers' study[28] suggested that in hypothyroid women attending their clinic, 69.5% required a dose increase to achieve a target of TSH 0.5 to 2.0 mIU/L (but considered a TSH to be adequate if < 4 mIU/L), and of their population, 69% needed a reduction in dose postnatally. Suggested mechanisms for this increased requirement were of an elevated extrathyroidal pool of T_4, the need to saturate large quantities of TBG, increased degradation of T_4, reduced absorption of T_4, and increased transfer of T_4 from mother to fetus.[29] However, Girling[7] and Chopra and Baber[30] suggest that there is no need to adjust doses of T_4 replacement provided replacement was adequate before the pregnancy. The Chopra and Baber study[30] also stresses the point that taking T_4 at the same time as iron supplements may reduce its absorption and, therefore, its effectiveness. It is not currently routine UK practice to routinely increase thyroxine dose on diagnosing pregnancy though some guidelines do advocate this.[31] Instead dosage adjustments may be made when necessary with reference to thyroid function tests early in pregnancy. A reasonable approach is to measure thyroid function tests as soon as pregnancy is confirmed, and adjust the dose if necessary, aiming for a free T_4 at the upper end of the normal range and TSH in the lower half of the normal range. Thyroid function tests should then be repeated once each trimester, or every 4 to 6 weeks if there has been a dose adjustment.

Labor and Delivery

In the patient who is adequately controlled, no specific measures are needed for labor or delivery. However, when a large goiter causes respiratory compromise, anesthetic and/or surgical advice may be required.

Postnatal

The presence of TPO autoantibodies is significantly associated with not only postpartum thyroiditis (see later) but also postpartum depression.[32]

Clinically Euthyroid—Subclinical Hypothyroidism

Subclinical hypothyroidism (SCH) describes those patients with a high TSH and normal thyroxine concentration with no specific symptoms or signs of thyroid dysfunction. Outside pregnancy, there is not considered to be an absolute threshold between hypothyroidism and euthyroidism, but it is suggested that a normal TSH is likely to be below 5 to 6 mU/L.[33] SCH affects 5% of the general population[2] and is more common in women, particularly those who have antithyroid antibodies.[33] There is an association with hypothyroidism, but outside pregnancy in those with TSH lower than 10 mU/L without thyroid antibodies, the conversion rate is less than 3%/yr.[33] In 1999, Haddow and coworkers[16] reported that when noted in pregnant women (unrecognized TSH > the 99.7th percentile), 58% (26/45) progressed to a clinical diagnosis of hypothyroidism in 5 years. Diagnosing SCH in pregnancy is usually an incidental finding, and screening for the condition has not been recommended. The prevalence with which SCH is observed will vary depending on the reference range (and gestation) used for diagnosis and whether antibody-positive women are included or not. Lambert-Messerlian and associates[8] noted 0.16% (16/9562) of women had a TSH greater than 10 mIU/L, and Allan and colleagues[34] systematically screened an antenatal population (9403 unselected women) in the second trimester and reported a TSH greater than 6 mU/L in 2.2%. Casey and associates[35] noted that among 25,756 women with singleton pregnancies of whom 67% were enrolled at 20 weeks' gestation, SCH (TSH > 97.5th percentile for gestational age) was noted in 2.3%. Marwaha and coworkers[10] reported SCH in 14.2% (78/541) of normal pregnant women across all gestations. The higher prevalence may be explained by their definition of SCH (TSH > 4.2 μIU/L) and the inclusion of antibody-positive women. However, the authors did determine pregnancy-specific ranges for thyroid function (see Table 45–1) but did not reevaluate the SCH population. The importance of pregnancy-specific ranges was highlighted in a Chinese cross-sectional study of 480 women at less than 20 weeks (excluding those with antithyroid antibodies) when up to 4% of women were reclassified with SCH using pregnancy-specific ranges who would have been "normal" if nonpregnant reference ranges were used.[9] On screening 10,990 pregnant women, Cleary-Goldman and colleagues[36] noted SCH (TSH > 97.5th percentile and normal free T_4 of 2.5 in the 97.5th percentile) in 2.2% of women in the first and 2.2% of women in the second trimester. SCH in pregnancy is appearing increasingly in the literature because of a suggested association with adverse obstetric outcome. Indeed much of the drive for determining a "normal" range for thyroid function in pregnancy has been fueled by emerging evidence of adverse obstetric outcome in those with SCH or poorly controlled thyroid function. Allan and colleagues[34] reported a significantly higher rate of fetal death (3.8%) in those women with TSH greater than 6 mU/L (2.2%) compared with those with TSH lower than 6 mU/L (0.9%) (odds ratio [OR] 4.4, 95% CI 1.9–9.5). The other complications of pregnancy occurred at rates similar to the rest of the population, and gestational ages and delivery and birth weights were similar.[34] Casey and associates[35] noted that placental abruption and preterm birth (<34 wk) were both observed more frequently in the SCH group than in the controls (relative risk [RR] 3.0, 95% CI 1.1–8.2, and RR 1.8, 95% CI 1.1–2.9, respectively). Stagnaro-Green and associates[37] compared 124 women delivering at less than 37 weeks to 124 controls. Elevated TSH (≥3 mIU/L as measured at "entry to care," ~16 wk' gestation) was associated with an increased risk of very preterm (<32 wk) delivery (adjusted odds ratio [AOR] 3.13, 95% CI 1.02–9.63) after control for the mother's history of prior preterm delivery and parity. However, in the Cleary-Goldman and colleagues study,[36] SCH in either the first or the second trimester was not associated with an adverse obstetric outcome.

In order to justify seeking a diagnosis of SCH and then managing women with SCH in pregnancy in light of this evidence, one would need to be convinced of evidence that intervention improved outcome. Data from randomized controlled trials are lacking. However, Negro and coworkers[38] randomized 115 TPO antibody (TPO-Ab)–positive women to receive T_4 or no treatment and compared outcomes with those of the antibody-negative women. The given dose of T_4 was maintained throughout gestation. Women were recruited at their first prenatal visit (~10 wk) and blood was sampled again at 20 and 30 weeks and 3 days after delivery. TSH concentrations were initially higher in the antibody-positive women and remained high in those not receiving treatment. Those antibody-positive women not on treatment had a higher percentage (13.8%) of pregnancy loss than those on treatment (3.5%, $P < .05$, RR 1.72, 95% CI 1.13–2.25) or antibody-negative women (2.4%, $P < .01$, RR 4.95, CI 2.59–9.48). Preterm deliveries also occurred more frequently (22.4%) in the group not on treatment than in those on treatment (7%, $P < .05$, RR 1.66, 95% CI 1.18–2.34) or antibody negative women (8.2%, $P < .01$, RR 12.18, CI 7.93–18.7). Other complications of pregnancy (hypertension, preeclampsia, placental abruption) did not vary between the groups. Because the pregnancy losses all occurred early, the authors concluded that T_4 supplementation should occur early.[38] After parturition, half of the patients studied had a free T_4 lower than the normal range.[38] A further study, though not randomized and looking at both SCH and overt hypothyroidism, by Ablovich and coworkers[28] retrospectively examined hypothyroid women delivering their unit. Thirty-five of 150 women were diagnosed with SCH (TSH 12.87 ± 8.43 mIU/L, T_4 6.93 ± 1.88 μg/dL) as defined at conception and were given T_4 to achieve TSH between 0.5 and 2.0 mIU/L. Blood was then tested each trimester. Those with overt hypothyroidism were similarly managed. In those who were euthyroid at conception, the miscarriage rate was 4%, and in those hypothyroid at conception, it was 31.5%. Gestations at delivery were similar. In those with SCH who were inadequately treated, the miscarriage rate was 71.4%. There were no miscarriages in the adequately treated group ($P < .006$). The term delivery rate was 21.4% in the inadequately treated SCH group (20.8% total for the hypothyroid group) and 90.5% in those on adequate treatment ($P < .006$).[28] It has been suggested that those with a reduced functional thyroid reserve (hypothyroid, raised TSH, thyroid antibodies) cannot compensate for the increased hormone requirement of early pregnancy (described earlier) caused by higher thyroid-binding globulin, increased volume distribution of thyroid hormones, and increased placental transport and degradation.[38] Negro and coworkers[38] suggested a potential benefit of treatment. On examining the effects of treatment on TSH profiles in early pregnancy, they found that T_4 does not appear to completely correct these values. De Geyter and coworkers[2] recruited 16 women attending for infertility investigation preconception. Eight were defined as SCH (TSH > 4.5 mU/L) and 8 were euthyroid controls. Blood was sampled weekly. Those with SCH were all given 50 μg T_4 until 12 weeks' pregnancy. TSH levels remained higher in the SCH group than in the controls, and for both groups, TSH was present in rising concentrations peaking at week 6. Thereafter, levels declined. Serum hCG levels increased progressively to week 9 with stable levels thereafter. Free T_4 and T_3 remained unchanged during the whole sampling period. Of note is that a proportion of these pregnancies received exogenous gonadotrophins[2] when elevations in TSH are of greater magnitude and occur earlier.[3]

Several authors suggest that SCH may have a better prognosis than overt hypothyroidism because of normal concentrations of T_4, but a worse outcome when compared with the general antenatal population,[28] and thus represent a continuum of reducing thyroid reserve.

Screening of the general population at booking for raised TSH has not yet been recommended.[39] One study has suggested that screening using TSH or TSH and antibody positivity are both cost-effective strategies.[39] Outside pregnancy, treatment of SCH is advised only insofar as it is better to treat SCH before overt hypothyroidism develops.[33] The Endocrine Society Clinical Practice Guideline[24] advocated that in patients previously known to be antibody-positive or in those who have been screened with TSH (e.g., as part of subfertility investigations), in those with a previous history of miscarriage or preterm delivery, aggressive case finding using TSH should be carried out. However, what concentration of TSH to use for diagnosis, what dose of T_4 to commence, what target TSH to aim for, and what is the important gestation to diagnose and commence treatment to improve outcome has not been agreed on.

Clinically Euthyroid—Thyroid Antibody–Positive

Higher TSH levels are consistently seen in those who are TPO-Ab or TBG antibody–positive, and a high prevalence of SCH is noted in these women.[24] A prospective study by Glinoer and coworkers[40] was undertaken in 87 healthy pregnant women with thyroid antibodies (TPO or TG) and normal thyroid function (T_3 and T_4 within normal reference ranges adjusted for gestational time and TSH 0.20–4 mU/L) at initial presentation. Antibody-positive women had a basal TSH value significantly higher, though normal, in the first trimester (1.6 vs. 0.9 mU/L, $P < .001$) than controls, as previously reported elsewhere. At delivery, 40% of the cases had serum TSH levels above 3 mU/L, and 16% had serum TSH levels above 4 mU/L. Furthermore, free T_4 concentrations were in the range of hypothyroid values in 42% of the women.[40] Among the 87 women in the Glinoer and coworkers study,[40] 7% (75 women) miscarried compared with 3.3% in 606 pregnant women, and the rate of premature delivery doubled (16% vs. 8%). A higher rate of miscarriage was confirmed by Stagnaro-Green and colleagues[41] who reported that among 552 women screened in the first trimester, 17% of antibody-positive women miscarried compared with 8.4% of antibody-negative women.[24] Cleary-Goldman and colleagues[36] screened 10,990 women and found 15% were antibody (TPO and TG) positive in the first and second trimesters. All had higher TSH concentrations than antibody-negative women and, when antibodies were positive in both the first and the second trimesters, preterm premature rupture of membranes (PPROM) was significantly increased compared with antibody-negative women. No other associations were reported.[36] It has been suggested that TPO-Ab and TG-Ab are found more commonly in those women with recurrent (≥3) miscarriages,[42] the risk of which may be associated with antibody titer and avidity.[26,42,43] These studies tested women because of their history of recurrent miscarriage (and were, therefore, at risk of miscarrying again anyway) rather than any clinical or biochemical features of hypothyroidism. Cleary-Goldman and colleagues[36] discuss whether their observed association of antibody-positivity and PROM might just be a marker of an inflammatory process placing women at risk of PPROM. Of note is that thyroid antibody-positivity is seen more frequently with advancing age (also a risk factor for miscarriage) and is a risk factor for subfertility.[38]

Glinoer and coworkers[40] systematically screened 234 women attending for assisted reproductive technology (ART) for TPO antibodies (TPO-Ab), serum TSH, and free T_4 before the first ART cycle. Women with overt thyroid dysfunction were excluded. Fourteen percent of the cohort had positive TPO-Ab. Concentrations of TSH (1.6 [0.02–4.1] mU/L) and T_4 (12.2 [9.1–18] ng/L) were comparable with those of the 86% of women without antibodies (TSH, 1.3 [0.05–3.6] mU/L) and free T_4 (11.7 [9.5–16.5] ng/L). In the antibody-positive group, the pregnancy rate was 53% versus 43% in the antibody-negative group, with an OR of 0.67 (95% CI 0.32–1.41, P = not significant); however, within the group that was pregnant, the miscarriage rate was 53% and 23%, respectively, with an OR of 3.77 (95% CI 1.29–11.05, $P = .016$). The age of the women was also an independent risk factor for miscarriage (OR 1.08, 95% CI 1.03–1.15, $P = .005$).[44] Several other papers have reported increased rates of miscarriages among antibody-positive women.[45] It has thus been suggested that antibody positivity reflects or is a cause of reduced or imminent reduction in thyroid reserve (discussed earlier). What is not clear is whether this increased risk of adverse pregnancy outcome (e.g. miscarriage) is a manifestation of an altered humoral response to pregnancy, or whether the thyroid autoantibodies themselves are implicated in the pathophysiology. It has been suggested that those who are known to be antibody positive but euthyroid should have their TSH monitored serially[24] because they are at risk of developing hypothyroidism. In those who are antibody-positive and have SCH, whether treatment with T_4 may improve outcome, as suggested by the Negro study,[38] needs to be subjected to further randomized, controlled trials. There is currently insufficient evidence to support T_4 treatment for pregnant women who are antibody-positive with normal thyroid function.[24]

SUMMARY OF MANAGEMENT OPTIONS

Hypothyroidism

Management Options	Evidence Quality and Recommendation	References
Prepregnancy		
Consider diagnosis in those with subfertility/menstrual disorders.	IIa/B	23
Optimize medical therapy; delay pregnancy until good control.	IIa/B	16,17
Prenatal		
Obtain baseline thyroid function tests as soon as possible.	—/GPP	—
Use pregnancy-specific reference ranges when interpreting thyroid function tests.	III/B	3,5,6,9,10
Obtain thyroid function tests every 3 mo. More frequently if dosage adjustments are made.	—/GPP	—
Routine increases in thyroxine doses are not required. Make dosage adjustments based on results of thyroid function tests.	III/B	4,30
Avoid taking iron supplements at the same time as oral thyroxine therapy.	III/B	30
Check compliance in those with vomiting.	—/GPP	—
Clinically Euthyroid with Subclinical Hypothyroidism		
Early thyroxine treatment appears to reduce the miscarriage rate.	Ib/A	38
Clinically Euthyroid and Thyroid Antibody–Positive		
Monitor TSH levels and give thyroxine only if patient becomes hypothyroid.	III/B	24
Labor and Delivery		
Large maternal goiter may cause anesthetic complications.	—/GPP	—
Postnatal		
Observe for signs of postpartum thyroiditis.	—/GPP	—
Screen for postpartum depression.	III/B	32

GPP, good practice point; TSH, thyroid-stimulating hormone.

HYPERTHYROIDISM

General

Hyperthyroidism affects 0.2% of pregnant women,[46,47] and 95% of these will have a diagnosis of Graves' disease, an autoimmune disorder associated with circulating immunoglobulin G (IgG) antibodies to the thyroid TSH receptor, which stimulate thyroid hormone production.

Possible causes of hyperthyroidism are

- Graves' disease.
- Toxic multinodular goiter.
- Toxic nodule/adenoma.
- Subacute thyroiditis.
- Acute thyroiditis (De Quervain's [viral] or postpartum).
- Iodine treatment.
- Amiodarone therapy.
- Lithium therapy.
- Hyperfunctioning ovarian teratoma (Struma ovarii)
- TSH-producing adenoma.
- hCG-producing tumor.
- Thyroid carcinoma.

Diagnosis

Thyrotoxicosis usually presents in the late first or early second trimester. Symptoms are as for thyrotoxicosis outside pregnancy, but these may be unhelpful and commonly reported by many euthyroid pregnant women (e.g., palmar erythema, emotional lability, vomiting, goiter. and heat intolerance). Discriminatory symptoms may be weight loss, tremor, lid lag, lid retraction. and a persistent tachycardia greater than 100 beats/min.

Diagnosing hyperthyroidism in early pregnancy may be difficult.

Careful consideration of normal ranges must be made when contemplating a diagnosis of hyperthyroidism in early pregnancy. This is especially so in the context of hyperemesis gravidarum, in which hCG secretion may be exaggerated, or in trophoblastic disease, in which it is grossly elevated. Two thirds of women with hyperemesis will have abnormal thyroid function tests in the absence of thyroid disease with 30% having undetectable TSH, 60% suppressed TSH, and 59% an elevated free T_4.[48]

Symptoms that persist beyond 10 to 20 weeks' gestation that antedate the pregnancy and the presence of thyroid-stimulating antibodies suggest true hyperthyroidism. The diagnosis of hyperthyroidism is confirmed by an elevated free T_4 and/or free T_3 with suppressed TSH levels.

Carbimazole, methimazole (a metabolite of carbimazole), and propylthiouracil are all used to treat hyperthyroidism in and out of pregnancy. All are of the thionamide class and act by competitively inhibiting the peroxidase-catalyzed reactions necessary for iodine organification. They also block the coupling of iodotyrosine, especially diiodothyronine formation. Their onset of action is delayed until the preformed hormones are depleted, a process that can take 3 to 4 weeks.

Maternal and Fetal Risks

Important maternal side effects of thionamides are agranulocytosis and hepatitis that is idiosyncratic with propylthiouracil but dose-related with carbimazole. Monitoring of liver function tests may be necessary. It is essential that in those women with sore throat or a fever, a white blood cell count be performed to exclude agranulocytosis. A neutropenia should prompt discontinuation of therapy, and thionamides should not be given again. A drug rash or urticaria is reported in 1% to 5% and would necessitate a switch to an alternative preparation. Additional symptoms sometimes reported are nausea, vomiting, and diarrhea.

The two most serious maternal complications of untreated hyperthyroidism are heart failure and thyroid storm, a medical emergency associated with a maternal mortality rate of 25% even with appropriate management.[49] Heart failure is the more common of the two serious maternal complications. It is caused by the long-term myocardial effects of T_4 and is intensified by other pregnancy conditions such as preeclampsia, infection, or anemia.[50]

When diagnosed in pregnancy, thyrotoxicosis is associated with adverse outcomes including miscarriage, growth restriction, preterm labor, placental abruption, pregnancy-induced hypertension, preeclampsia, infection, and increased perinatal mortality. One study has suggested an increased risk of chromosomal abnormalities.[51] The relative risk for low birth weight is reported as 0.74 in one euthyroid (controlled hyperthyroidism) population, 2.36 in the same population with uncontrolled hyperthyroidism in the first half of pregnancy, and 9.24 in those hyperthyroid throughout pregnancy.[52] The same study showed an OR for developing preeclampsia of 4.74 in those with uncontrolled hyperthyroidism at term.[52] This study suggests that treatment improves outcome and is supported by another study[16] showing stillbirth in 24% of those untreated hyperthyroid pregnancies, falling to 5% to 7% in those on treatment. The incidence of prematurity was 53%, falling to 9% to 11% with treatment.

There is a risk of fetal and/or neonatal thyrotoxicosis due to the passive transplacental passage of immunoglobulins associated with Graves' disease. Such antibodies are able to exert an effect on the fetal thyroid at 20 weeks' gestation.[53] Infants born to mothers with high titers of antibodies or poorly controlled disease[46,53] are particularly at risk. Studies report varying prevalences between 1% and 17%,[53,54] with fewer cases being diagnosed in utero than in the neonatal period.

Fetal thyrotoxicosis may be suspected in a fetus with a persistent tachycardia (>160 beats/min), a goiter, or growth restriction,[53] and as such, may be diagnosed with antenatal ultrasound screening.[55,56]

Fetal thyrotoxicosis may result in preterm delivery[53] and the development of fetal craniosynostosis, exophthalmos, heart failure (hydrops fetalis), hepatosplenomegaly, thrombocytopenia, exophthalmos, goiter (with neck obstruction and polyhydramnios), and growth restriction. Additional neonatal features include jaundice, poor feeding, poor weight gain, and irritability.[53] The mortality of the condition may be as high as 25%.[47]

Thyrotoxicosis presenting in the neonatal period is usually transient, lasting only 2 to 3 months after delivery. Presentation may be delayed up to 2 weeks postnatally if the mother was on medication at the time of delivery. The effects of maternal antithyroid medication are eventually cleared from the neonates' circulation but the thyroid-stimulating antibodies are cleared at a slower rate.

In order to predict fetal thyrotoxicosis, maternal TSH receptor autoantibodies should be tested in early pregnancy; to predict neonatal disease, they should be tested again in late pregnancy.[57] One suggested protocol is to test in the first trimester and again at 6 months' gestation.[26] If high titers of antibodies are detected in early pregnancy or if levels have not fallen with advancing gestation, fetal thyrotoxicosis should be anticipated and obstetric ultrasound scans may be recommended to assess fetal growth, heart rate, and the presence of goiter. If antibodies are detected in late pregnancy, then cord blood and neonatal (days 3–4 and 7–10)[47,58] thyroid function tests (TSH and free T_4) should be performed.[57] It is important to recognize the risk of neonatal/fetal thyrotoxicosis in women who appear at first glance to have hypothyroidism because they are on T_4 replacement for previous thyroidectomy or radioiodine treatment but, in fact, may have high titers of TSH receptor autoantibodies.

Treatment for fetal thyrotoxicosis is possible in utero by giving the mother increased doses of antithyroid medication. Any subsequent maternal hypothyroidism can be treated with T_4, which will not cross the placenta in significant amounts. Percutaneous fetal blood sampling to measure thyroid function (for which normal ranges exist) is technically possible and may play a role in management.[15]

Fetal effects of maternal antithyroid medication have been reported, particularly the association of carbimazole or methimazole with aplasia cutis.[59] This condition results in patches of absent skin at birth, 70% to 85% of which occur on the scalp. However, the condition is rare. The natural incidence of the condition is 0.03%,[60] but in this study in a population of 49,000 babies, none of the mothers[58] on antithyroid medication had affected babies, and in 643 women with Graves' disease, there were no cases.[29]

High doses of antithyroid medication may cause fetal hypothyroidism but only rarely goiter. In one study, 43 women treated with thionamides until delivery were compared with 27 women in whom treatment was discontinued in the pregnancy. Free T_4 levels were slightly lower in fetuses compared with mothers in the first group and higher in the second group in which some maternal and cord T_4 levels were in the thyrotoxic range at delivery.[61] This suggests that if maternal disease is controlled too tightly, some infants may become hypothyroid. Neonatal hypothyroidism usually spontaneously resolves by day 5 of life[62] and is said to occur in 10% to 20% of patients treated with thionamides.[63]

Management Options

Prepregnancy

Menstrual abnormalities are less common now than in previous series. The most common manifestations are hypomenorrhea and oligomenorrhea. However, most thyrotoxic women are thought to remain ovulatory.[23]

Therapy for hyperthyroidism is best begun prior to pregnancy. This will allow for the use of radioactive iodine studies for diagnosis, higher initial doses of pharmacologic agents without fetal concern, and surgery when needed for unresponsive cases. Those having had radioiodine are advised not to conceive until 4 months after their last treatment.[64] Some would argue for establishing a euthyroid state 3 months prior to conception. Counseling should be supportive and reassuring, because treated thyrotoxicosis has a low risk of adverse obstetric outcome. Women should be counseled against discontinuing medication either prepregnancy or antenatally.

Prenatal

The aim of treatment is to maintain the euthyroid clinical state and maintain a level of free T_4 at the upper limit of normal (with reference to pregnancy-specific ranges). This allows the lowest possible dose of medication and minimizes the risks of fetal hypothyroidism. Women should be seen and have thyroid function tests monthly in newly diagnosed cases, but less frequent testing is required in those with stable disease.

In Graves' disease, there is often a temporary worsening of control in early pregnancy due to rising hCG levels and perhaps reduced absorption of medication secondary to vomiting. There is then an improvement with women often requiring less medication because the relative immune suppression of pregnancy results in a fall in antibody levels. Thirty percent can stop all medication in the last weeks of pregnancy.[65]

Block and replace regimes sometimes used outside pregnancy are not suitable for pregnant women. Antithyroid medications cross the placenta freely, whereas T_4 does not. Such a regime would, therefore, place the fetus at risk of hypothyroidism. Fetal abnormalities are seen more commonly in the offspring of women receiving T_4 and carbimazole (9.5%) than in those on carbimazole alone (4.1%).[29,55] Such regimens may be of some use in the treatment of fetal thyrotoxicosis.

Therapeutic modalities for hyperthyroidism can be divided into five categories:

- Thionamides (propylthiouracil, carbimazole, methimazole).
- β-Blockers.
- Iodides.
- Radioactive iodine.
- Surgery.

Propylthiouracil, methimazole, and carbimazole are the mainstays of treatment for hyperthyroidism in pregnancy. Carbimazole is a pro-drug as it converts to methimazole after absorption. Propylthiouracil is more highly protein bound than the other two agents and thus crosses the placenta less readily. A disadvantage with propylthiouracil is that more frequent dosing is often necessary than with carbimazole. Newly diagnosed cases should be aggressively treated initially with high doses for 4 to 6 weeks, which can then gradually be reduced by up to a quarter.

In the United States, propylthiouracil had been considered the drug of choice in pregnancy for the treatment of hyperthyroidism until recently. This related to concerns regarding possible teratogenic effects of methimazole. However, reports of severe propylthiouracil-related liver failure in adults, including during pregnancy, have raised concerns about its routine use.[68] The incidence of this adverse occurrence is approximately 1 in 10,000 adults. Teratogenic concerns of prenatally administered methimazole include choanal atresia and aplasia cutis (approximate risk 0.03%). The American Thyroid Association and the U.S. Food and Drug Administration now suggest that propylthiouracil use be limited to the first trimester only, and that patients be switched to methimazole in the second trimester.[66] Methimazole is approximately 20–30 times as potent as propylthiouracil. Therefore a propylthiouracil dose of 300 mg would be roughly equivalent to 10–15 mg of methimazole. Thyroid function testing should be performed within a few weeks of switching drugs to confirm maintenance of a euthyroid state. Propylthiouracil is still recommended in preference to methimazole in the setting of life-threatening thyrotoxicosis to take advantage of its ability to inhibit peripheral conversion of T4 to T3. In the United Kingdom it is common practice to continue a patient already on carbimazole throughout the pregnancy.

In those with troublesome autonomic (sympathetic) symptoms of palpitations, tachycardia, and tremor, propranolol may be used for up to a month until longer-term treatment with thionamides becomes effective. Longer treatment courses should be avoided because of the risk of growth restriction.[67] β-Blockers have the additional beneficial action of reducing peripheral conversion of T_4 into T_3.

Iodide treatment is an older mode of therapy and essentially now limited to preoperative use. Otherwise, this therapy results in a high incidence of fetal goiter and hypothyroidism when used long-term and does not result in adequate control of thyrotoxicosis.[68]

The fetal thyroid concentrates iodine at a significantly higher rate than the maternal thyroid. Therefore, the use of radioactive iodine (131-I) or any radioactive tracers such as iodine-131 or technetium-99, although widely used outside pregnancy for treatment of Graves' disease and in high doses for carcinoma, are absolutely contraindicated in pregnancy, because they ablate the fetal thyroid gland causing fetal and neonatal hypothyroidism.[3] There is some additional concern about possible effects on the parental gonads, and it is usually advised that pregnancy be delayed following treatment. Radioactive iodine also frequently results in maternal hypothyroidism.[16,29]

Surgery is reserved for patients who do not respond to medication, who develop intolerance to the medication, or those with compressive symptoms from a large goiter. Thyroid surgery is associated with a high incidence of hypothyroidism postoperatively. Other postoperative complications include hypoparathyroidism (1%–2%) causing hypocalcemia, and recurrent laryngeal nerve palsy

(1%–2%). Surgical and anesthetic morbidity and mortality are also increased in pregnancy. The reported pregnancy loss associated with general anesthesia and surgery of all types in the first trimester is approximately 8%, and decreases to 6.5% in the second trimester. Prior to surgery, patients should be prepared medically with 7 to 10 days of iodide to decrease gland vascularity and prevent thyroid storm. Overall, surgery is reserved for failures of the standard medical management and/or in those women with a significant goiter causing stridor, respiratory distress, dysphagia, or carcinoma.

Labor and Delivery

In women with adequately treated thyrotoxicosis, labor and delivery are not associated with increased risks. However, labor and delivery are events that may precipitate thyroid storm in pregnant women with poorly controlled or untreated thyrotoxicosis. The patient may present with extreme symptoms of hyperthyroidism particularly cardiovascular symptoms (palpitations, tachycardia, and atrial fibrillation with rapid ventricular response), and if severe, high-output cardiac failure. Blood pressure is usually normal, though there may be an increased pulse pressure. With prolonged duration of symptoms, shock may ensue.[69]

Fever is invariably present, is progressive, begins a few hours after a stressful event, and may exceed 40°C. Mental status is commonly altered, ranging from restlessness and confusion to psychosis, seizures, and coma. Severe diarrhea, nausea, vomiting, and nonspecific abdominal pain may also be present.[70] If the patient has a large goiter, exophthalmos, or a known history of hyperthyroidism, the diagnosis of thyroid storm is usually not difficult to establish. However, without the obvious findings or history, it may be difficult to make the diagnosis because biochemical tests may not differ from those with thyrotoxicosis without thyroid storm. Treatment should not be delayed if the condition is suspected.

The aims of treatment in thyroid storm are (1) to decrease thyroid hormone production, (2) to decrease the effect of circulating hormone, (3) to provide supportive therapy, and (4) to treat the underlying cause. Methimazole/carbimazole may be used, although propylthiouracil (300–400 mg q8h orally, nasogastrically, or rectally) is preferred because it decreases peripheral conversion of T_4 to T_3 as well as decreasing thyroid hormone production. Potassium iodide (2–5 drops orally) or sodium iodide (0.5–1.0 g intravenously) every 8 hours should be commenced approximately 1 to 2 hours after the initiation of therapy with thionamides. This is done in an attempt to block preformed thyroid hormone release from the colloid space.

Supportive therapy involves maintenance of blood volume, glycemic control, temperature control, and restoring electrolyte balance. Propranolol (40–80 mg orally or 1 mg/min intravenously) should be given to reduce adrenergic overactivity.

Postnatal

To exclude hyperthyroidism secondary to passive antibody transfer and hypothyroidism secondary to transfer of antithyroid medications, perform thyroid function tests on umbilical cord blood and in the neonate in women who are breast-feeding. For propylthiouracil, only 0.07% of the maternal dose is excreted in breast milk, with a slightly higher dose (0.5%) excreted for carbimazole and for methimazole (10%).[55] Breast-feeding is, however, generally thought to be safe in those on less than 150 mg/day of propylthiouracil and less than 15 mg/day carbimazole.[55,71]

Graves' disease can flare postnatally as maternal antibody levels rise postpartum. In those having stopped medication, it is often necessary to re introduce it at 2 to 3 months postpartum. It is important to distinguish such changes from a true postpartum thyroiditis.

SUMMARY OF MANAGEMENT OPTIONS
Hyperthyroidism

Management Options	Evidence Quality and Recommendation	References
Prepregnancy		
Establish the diagnosis of hyperthyroidism (elevated free T_4 and/or free T_3 with suppressed TSH levels) prior to pregnancy so that a complete diagnostic workup (including radioiodine studies) can be performed and therapy instituted.	—/GPP	—
Avoid conception until 4 mo after radioiodine therapy. Advise euthyroid state for 3 mo prior to conception.	IV/C	64
Prenatal		
Use pregnancy-specific reference ranges when interpreting thyroid function test results.	III/B	3,5,6,9,10
Caution interpreting thyroid function tests in early pregnancy: TSH levels fall as result of rising hCG.	IIa/B	48
If autoimmune etiology, disease may improve as pregnancy advances and antibody levels fall.	—/GPP	—

Management Options	Evidence Quality and Recommendation	References
Continue therapy; keep T_4 at upper limit of normal.	—/GPP	—
Test thyroid function every 3 mo, more frequently if dose adjustments are made.	—/GPP	—
Screen for agranulocytosis and hepatitis in those on thionamides.	—/GPP	—
Measure TSH receptor antibody titer early pregnancy (1 mo); if high, there is a risk of fetal thyrotoxicosis.	III/B	26,57
Perform fetal USS for fetal growth, tachycardia, or goiter.	III/B	47,58
Measure TSH receptor antibody titer in late pregnancy (6 mo); if high, there is a risk of neonatal thyrotoxicosis.	III/B	26,57
Labor and Delivery		
May precipitate thyroid storm.	—/GPP	—
Large maternal goiter may cause anesthetic complications.	—/GPP	—
Postnatal		
Observe for worsening symptoms in postpartum period, especially in those whose medications were reduced. If medications were stopped, these may need to be reintroduced at 2–3 mo postpartum.	—/GPP	—
If high TSH receptor antibody titer in late pregnancy, screen for neonatal thyrotoxicosis by testing infant on days 3–4 and 7–10 of life.	III/B	26,57
Observe neonate for signs of hypothyroidism if born to mothers on high doses of antithyroid medication. Test cord blood and neonatal blood if breast-feeding.	III/B	47,57,58
Perform complete diagnostic evaluation.	—/GPP	—

GPP, good practice point; hCG, human chorionic gonadotropin; T_3, triiodothyronine; T_4, thyroxine; TSH, thyroid-stimulating hormone; USS, ultrasound screening.

THYROID NODULES AND THYROID CANCER

General

Thyroid nodules or solitary toxic nodules or adenomas are found in 2% of pregnant women[72] and usually present with hyperthyroidism. An important consideration is that, although rare overall,[50] 90% of thyroid cancers present as thyroid nodules. Carcinomas derived from thyroid epithelium may be papillary, follicular (differentiated), or undifferentiated. They are only rarely active hormonally, but 90% secrete thyroglobulin, which is used outside pregnancy as a tumor marker. It has been suggested that there is an increased incidence of malignancy in pregnancy (40%).[55] Indeed, an association between enlargement of the thyroid gland in pregnancy[73] or a recent pregnancy (within 5 yr) has been linked with the development of thyroid cancer.[74,75] However, because these malignancies are most commonly seen in women of childbearing age, any additional risk in pregnancy may be difficult to determine. Only those nodules thought to be malignant need further investigation or treatment, which is usually by surgery with or without radioiodine. Following such treatment, T_4 may be used to suppress production of TSH and so prevent any stimulation of residual thyroid tissue or tumor. One study has suggested a target TSH of 0.5 to 5.0 μU/mL[3] in those with previous thyroid cancer.

Diagnosis

Outside pregnancy, radioiodine is used to distinguish "cold" (more likely to be malignant) from "hot" (functioning) nodules. However, such studies are avoided in pregnancy. Ultrasound, therefore, forms the main investigative tool. Fine-needle aspiration should be reserved for rapidly enlarging nodules, cystic nodules larger than 4 cm or solid nodules larger than 2 cm.[55] Cystic nodules are usually benign (multinodular goiter or solitary toxic adenoma). Those with retrosternal extension or tracheal deviation and respiratory compromise may necessitate further imaging. Biopsy results are usually of four types: insufficient sample (in < 5%), biopsy in these women should be repeated; definitely benign (75%), these women should be reassured; definitely malignant (5%), these women should undergo surgery; and indeterminate (20%), this is usually because follicular cells have been seen and often require surgery. Prognoses are similar for those cases diagnosed in or out of pregnancy.[72]

Management Options

Prepregnancy

Thyroid nodules should be investigated and treated prior to embarking on a pregnancy. Pregnancy should be delayed for 1 year after thyroid cancer has been treated with high-dose radioactive iodine because congenital abnormalities have been reported.[64]

Prenatal

Because of the risk of malignancy, investigation should proceed as outlined previously and not be delayed because of pregnancy. Antithyroid drugs should be used as described earlier to treat any hyperthyroidism, but nodules do not usually remit after such treatment. Only if a nodule is found at greater than 20 weeks' gestation should aspiration wait until the postnatal period. Those in which biopsy confirms malignancy should undergo surgery in pregnancy unless only a few weeks from term. In those in which the histology is not clear, benign, low-grade malignant, or slowly growing lesions, surgery may be deferred until after delivery. Surgery is safest when carried out in the second trimester and, with the previous exceptions, should not be delayed because of pregnancy.[76,77] Radioactive iodine should not be used in pregnancy. Suppressive doses of T_4 should be safe in pregnancy, taking care to avoid maternal thyrotoxicosis

Labor and Delivery

When a large goiter with retrosternal extension is present, careful consideration must be given to possible respiratory compromise and complications of intubation in the event of a general anesthetic. Retrosternal extension should be suspected in those with respiratory symptoms, dysphagia, and rarely with vocal cord paralysis, Horner's syndrome, and vascular or lymphatic compromise.

Postnatal

Radioactive iodine may be administered after delivery but not while breast-feeding. Contact with the baby may also need to be temporarily limited to reduce exposure risk.[78]

SUMMARY OF MANAGEMENT OPTIONS

Thyroid Nodules and Cancer

Management Options	Evidence Quality and Recommendation	References
Prepregnancy		
Delay pregnancy for 1 yr after thyroid cancer has been treated with high-dose radioactive iodine	IV/C	35
Prenatal		
Nodule identified at > 20 wk should be biopsied after delivery.	—/GPP	—
If biopsy confirms malignancy, proceed to surgery.	III/B	76,77
Surgery is safest after second trimester.	III/B	76,77
If biopsy shows intermediate pathology, delay surgery until after delivery.	III/B	76,77
Labor and Delivery		
Watch for anesthetic complications in those with large goiter/retrosternal extension.	—/GPP	—
Postnatal		
Radioactive iodine may be used, but not while breast-feeding, and contact with the infant may need to be temporarily limited.	IV/C	78

GPP, good practice point.

POSTPARTUM THYROIDITIS

General

Postpartum thyroiditis is thought to occur in 5% to 10% of pregnancies,[79] and the frequency with which it is diagnosed largely depends on the extent to which it is sought. Women may not report symptoms, instead attributing them to normal postpartum physiology. The condition occurs 3 to 4 months postpartum but has been reported up to 6 months after delivery.[80] It is an autoimmune disorder, and thyroid antibody–positive women in the first trimester have a 33% to 50% chance of developing thyroiditis in the postpartum period.[79] The disease is seen more commonly (threefold higher) in those with insulin-dependant (type 1) diabetes mellitus,[81] with a family history of the disease, or with TPO-Ab (present in 75% of affected individuals).

Differential diagnosis of hyperthyroidism in the postpartum period includes

- Postpartum painless thyroiditis.
- Postpartum Graves' disease.
- Postpartum Hashimoto's thyroiditis.
- Postpartum toxic multinodular goiter.

The most common is postpartum painless thyroiditis, which is characterized by an initial destructive phase in the first 2 months, with release of preformed thyroid hormone, resulting in hyperthyroidism. This is followed about 3 months later by hypothyroidism as stores of preformed thyroid hormone are depleted and the gland itself is destroyed. However, any combination of clinical states is possible at any time. Most resolve spontaneously.

Diagnosis

Radioiodine uptake studies can be used in those women who choose not to breast-feed. Low uptake is seen in postpartum painless thyroiditis in which T_4 release is all preformed, as distinct from Graves' disease in which new T_4 is generated. In women who are breast-feeding, repeat thyroid function tests 1 month later may reveal a transition from hyperthyroid to hypothyroid, so confirming the diagnosis.

Management Options

Most cases resolve spontaneously. However, a study of 86 women showed only 51% of those not treated were biochemically euthyroid at 9 months, and the authors advocate early institution of permanent T_4 replacement in women with postpartum thyroid dysfunction, elevated TSH, and positive thyroid antibodies.[82] Later hypothyroidism (in 23%–39%) may occur in those who recover, particularly when antibodies are found. For this reason, some would advocate yearly thyroid function tests. T_4 may be discontinued in some. Close observation in the puerperium of any future pregnancies should be undertaken because the risk of recurrence is high.

SUGGESTED READINGS

Abalovich M, Amino N, Barbour LA, et al: Management of thyroid dysfunction during pregnancy and postpartum: An endocrine society clinical practice guideline. J Clin Endocrinol Metab 2007;92:S1–S7.

Alexander EK, Marqusee E, Lawrence J, et al: Timing and magnitude of increases in levothyroxine requirements during pregnancy in women with hypothyroidism. N Engl J Med 2004;351:241–249.

Burrow GN: Current concepts—The management of thyrotoxicosis in pregnancy. N Engl J Med 1985;313:562–565.

Cleary-Goldman J, Malone FD, Lambert-Messerlian G, et al: Maternal thyroid hypofunction and pregnancy outcome. Obstet Gynecol 2008;112:85–92.

Fisher DA: Fetal thyroid function: Diagnosis and management of fetal thyroid disorders. Clin Obstet Gynecol 1997;40:16–31.

Girling J: Thyroid disorders in pregnancy. Curr Opin Obstet Gynecol 2006;16:7.

Kuijpens JL, Vader HL, Drexhage HA, et al: Thyroid peroxidase antibodies during gestation are a marker for subsequent depression postpartum. Eur J Endocrinol 2001;145:579–584.

Poppe K, Glinoer D: Thyroid autoimmunity and hypothyroidism before and during pregnancy. Hum Reprod Update 2003;9:149–161.

Stagnaro-Green A: Recognizing, understanding, and treating postpartum thyroiditis. Endocrinol Metab Clin North Am 2000;29:417–430, ix.

REFERENCES

For a complete list of references, log onto www.expertconsult.com.

CHAPTER 46

Pituitary and Adrenal Disease

MARK B. LANDON

PITUITARY DISEASE

Normal Changes in Pregnancy

The anterior lobe of the pituitary gland may enlarge significantly during pregnancy as a result of lactotroph proliferation. Magnetic resonance imaging (MRI) scans confirm that the gland more than doubles in size by the end of gestation.[1] Accordingly, prolactin levels increase approximately 10-fold in preparation for lactation.[2]

Pregnancy also affects the levels of other pituitary hormones. Gonadotropin concentrations decrease and show a diminished response to gonadotropin-releasing hormone. The response of growth hormone (GH) to insulin or arginine stimulation is similarly blunted. Pituitary GH levels decline and are accompanied by a progressive increase in the placental variant of GH. Plasma levels of adrenocorticotropic hormone (ACTH) increase throughout pregnancy, but absolute levels remain lower in the pregnant than in the nonpregnant state.[3] Curiously, the increase in ACTH levels occurs despite an increase in free and bound cortisol. The placenta produces ACTH, which may explain this phenomenon. The diurnal variation of cortisol, although blunted, is maintained during pregnancy. Thyrotropin levels are unaffected by pregnancy. Free levels of thyroxine and triiodothyronine are unchanged, whereas total levels increase as a result of estrogen-induced synthesis of thyroxine-binding globulin.

Posterior pituitary function is also altered during normal pregnancy. A significant preterm increase in oxytocin is observed, whereas plasma levels of vasopressin remain similar to those obtained in the nonpregnant state. However, plasma osmolality decreases 5 to 10 mOsm/kg in pregnant women, indicating a decreased threshold for vasopressin secretion in pregnancy. During gestation, patients also experience thirst at a lower plasma osmolality.[4]

Prolactin-Producing Adenomas

Maternal and Fetal Risks

Widely available radioimmunoassays for serum prolactin and improved techniques for radiologic diagnosis have led to the detection of an increasing number of prolactin-secreting pituitary adenomas in women. Prolactin-producing tumors represent the most common pituritary neoplasm encountered during pregnancy. Spontaneous ovulation is uncommon in patients with a pituitary tumor. Therefore, most patients with this disorder have amenorrhea-galactorrhea or anovulatory cycles and infertility. With ovulation induction and suppression of prolactin synthesis by dopaminergic agents, such as bromocriptine, pregnancy can often be achieved in patients with prolactinomas.

Much of the normal pituitary gland enlargement that occurs in pregnancy is secondary to hyperplasia of the anterior pituitary lactotrophic cells, which are stimulated by estrogen. Although this stimulus may cause enlargement of adenomas during pregnancy,[5] most patients with a microadenoma, a pituitary tumor of less than 1 cm, have an uneventful pregnancy.[6–8] In the few patients who have symptoms, regression usually occurs after delivery.

Management Options

PREPREGNANCY

Most women with prolactin-secreting adenomas require ovulation induction to conceive. Nonpregnant patients who have amenorrhea-galactorrhea and hyperprolactinemia (prolactin level > 20 ng/mL) should be evaluated for pituitary adenoma. Although serum prolactin levels are correlated with pituitary adenomas, when a patient with hyperprolactinemia is considering pregnancy, a thorough radiologic examination is warranted. MRI has replaced both computed axial tomography and coned-down sella turcica radiographs as the procedure of choice to evaluate the size of the pituitary gland.

Once a pituitary tumor is diagnosed, it may be prudent to reevaluate the gland for growth after several months before attempting ovulation induction. Bromocriptine therapy is often all that is required for patients with microadenomas. Macroadenomas, which are tumors that measure 1 cm or more, should be treated definitively with surgery. These patients are more likely to have symptoms during pregnancy when treated with medical therapy alone.[5,8] Continued bromocriptine therapy after surgery is indicated if symptomatic residual tumor enlargement occurs.

PRENATAL

Evaluation for possible prolactin-secreting tumors is difficult during pregnancy because of the physiologic increase in serum prolactin that occurs in normal gestation. At term,

FIGURE 46–1
Maternal serum prolactin concentration in patients with microadenoma (*shaded bars*, $n = 237$) and control subjects (*open bars*, $n = 215$) in the nonpregnant state (NP) and during each trimester.
(From Divers W, Yen SSC: Prolactin producing microadenomas in pregnancy. Obstet Gynecol 1983;62:425.)

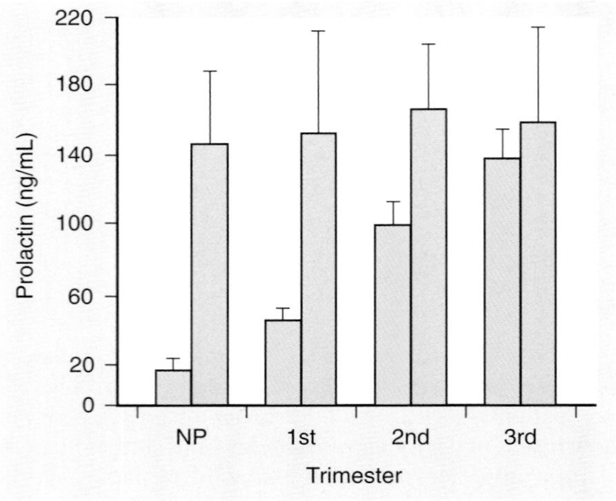

FIGURE 46–2
Time from the beginning of pregnancy to the onset of symptoms (headache or visual disturbances) in 91 pregnancies in women with previously untreated pituitary tumors.
(From Maygar DM, Marshall JR: Pituitary tumors and pregnancy. Am J Obstet Gynecol 1978;132:739.)

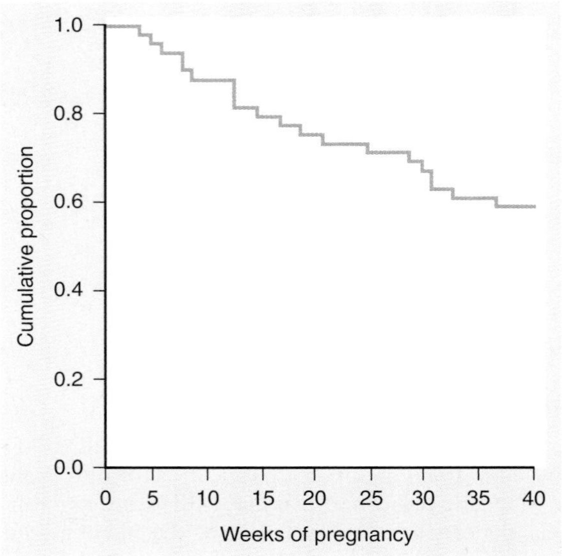

serum prolactin levels may reach values that are 20 times normal. Further, prolactin levels do not always increase during pregnancy in women with prolactinomas, nor do they always increase with pregnancy-induced tumor enlargement (Fig. 46–1).[9] Enlargement usually produces a headache as the first clinical feature, before visual disturbance. Therefore, radiologic diagnosis is necessary for the pregnant patient who has severe headaches or a visual field defect.

Management of the pregnant patient with a previously diagnosed prolactinoma requires careful attention by a team of physicians, including an obstetrician, an endocrinologist, and an ophthalmologist. Women with asymptomatic microadenomas may discontinue bromocriptine and receive routine obstetric care with prompt evaluation for any symptoms of tumor expansion. In contrast, women with asymptomatic macroadenomas should be evaluated with visual field testing at least every 3 months. Women with symptomatic macroadenomas should be seen monthly. Prompt self-referral in patients with headache or visual symptoms should be encouraged. Visual field testing should be performed monthly in women with macroadenomas. Headaches may reflect tumor enlargement and impingement on the diaphragmatic sella or adjacent dura. Visual disturbances are caused by compression of the optic nerve. If the optic chiasm is compressed by superior extension, bitemporal hemianopsia may develop. Although the limitations of serum prolactin levels have been discussed, marked elevations outside the normal range for pregnancy at a given gestational age may signal rapid tumor enlargement.

Gemzell and Wang[5] reviewed the course of 85 women during 91 pregnancies affected by previously untreated microadenomas. Only 5% had complications. Four of the 5 patients with headache and visual disturbances showed resolution after delivery. One patient who had a visual field defect noted early in pregnancy subsequently underwent transsphenoidal hypophysectomy after cesarean delivery for a triplet gestation at 36 weeks. Similarly, Albrecht and Betz[10] reported a low rate of complications in women with untreated

TABLE 46–1
Effect of Pregnancy on Prolactinomas

TUMOR TYPE	PREVIOUS THERAPY?	PATIENTS (*N*)	SYMPTOMATIC ENLARGEMENT
Microadenoma	No	246	4
Macroadenoma	No	45	7
Macroadenoma	Yes	46	2

microadenomas during gestation. Of 352 patients, 8 (2.3%) had visual disturbances and 17 (4.8%) had headaches.

Maygar and Marshall[6] reported that symptoms are more common in the first trimester than in the second or third, with a median time at onset of 10 weeks' gestation. However, the likelihood of visual symptoms did not differ among trimesters (Fig. 46–2). In this series, symptoms requiring therapy occurred in more than 20% of the 91 patients with untreated tumors, but in only 1% of women with previously treated adenomas.

Molitch[8] reviewed 16 series that included 246 cases of prolactin-secreting pituitary microadenomas in pregnancy. Only 4 of the 246 women (1.6%) had symptoms of tumor enlargement, and 11 (4.5%) had asymptomatic enlargement on radiologic examination (Table 46–1). In no case was surgical intervention necessary. Molitch[8] also reviewed 45 patients with macroadenomas, 7 of whom (15.5%) had symptomatic tumor enlargement. Four of these women required surgery during pregnancy. Cabergoline, a dopamine agonist, has been used to treat refractory cases of tumor enlargement during pregnancy.[11] Although data on cabergoline are less extensive, preliminary evidence does not suggest an increase in adverse perinatal outcomes.[12] The risk of symptoms is probably related to the size of the tumor at the onset of pregnancy. Further data are needed to define which group of patients with a microadenoma should be treated with bromocriptine for a prolonged period before conception.

Treatment of complications during pregnancy is influenced by both gestational age and the severity of symptoms. If the fetus is mature, induction of labor or cesarean delivery should be accomplished. Cesarean section is generally performed for obstetric indications. Earlier in gestation, therapy should not be delayed if radiologic evidence suggests tumor enlargement. Medical treatment with bromocriptine or cabergoline is successful in most symptomatic patients and has become the preferred primary approach during pregnancy.[9] Bromocriptine has an established safety profile in early pregnancy, as evidenced by its use to induce ovulation in large groups of women with hyperprolactinemia without an increased incidence of congenital malformations.[13,14] Other treatment modalities used during pregnancy include transsphenoidal surgery,[6–8] and in one case, hydrocortisone therapy.[14] Complications of transsphenoidal surgery include infection, hypopituitarism, hemorrhage, and transient diabetes insipidus. The risk of these complications is probably not increased during pregnancy. However, the risk of preterm delivery is increased in those women requiring surgical intervention.[6]

LABOR AND DELIVERY

Intrapartum care of the patient with a prolactin-producing adenoma does not differ from that of the general obstetric population. Some undiagnosed patients may have sudden visual impairment, and prolactinoma must be differentiated from more common conditions, such as preeclampsia and migraine, which may cause the same symptoms.

POSTNATAL

After delivery, radiologic assessment of tumor size and a serum prolactin assay should be performed at the first postpartum visit. Breast-feeding is not contraindicated in patients with a prolactin-secreting microadenoma.[7] Because serum prolactin levels may remain elevated during breast-feeding, caution must be used in interpreting these results. However, serum prolactin levels do not appear to be significantly higher than prepregnancy levels in women with microadenomas who choose to breast-feed.[15] Counseling patients about future pregnancies requires establishing that progression of tumor growth has not occurred. Some suggest continuing bromocriptine therapy for 12 months before conception to reduce the risk of tumor enlargement during gestation.[12] Gemzell and Wang[5] concluded that in 16 patients with untreated pituitary adenomas, symptoms did not seem to occur with increasing frequency in subsequent pregnancies.

SUMMARY OF MANAGEMENT OPTIONS
Prolactin-Producing Adenomas

Management Options	Evidence Quality and Recommendation	References
Prepregnancy		
Treatment (bromocriptine, cabergoline, surgery, or radiation therapy, depending on tumor size).	III/B	15,55
Advise against pregnancy until cure is achieved.	III/B	7
Prenatal		
Bromocriptine is safe for the fetus.	III/B	7,13,15
Cabergoline is probably also safe, but there is less experience in pregnancy.	III/B	11,12
Screening or monitoring for recurrence or exacerbation is best undertaken by vigilance for clinical features (headaches, visual disturbance) and prompt testing. Some recommend visual field testing every month for women with macroadenomas.	III/B	7,15
Interdisciplinary management.	III/B	7,9,15,53
If enlargement or recurrence is seen:		
• Bromocriptine if the fetus is not mature; delivery and definitive management if the fetus is mature.	III/B	13–15
• Cabergoline for resistant cases (less experience).	III/B	11,12
• Limited experience with hydrocortisone.	IV/C	14
• Surgery in extreme cases that do not respond to medical measures.	III/B	7,8
Postnatal		
Can breast-feed.	III/B	7,15
Monitor symptoms, the prolactin level (may be difficult to interpret in breastfeeding mothers), and tumor size by imaging.	III/B	15

Acromegaly

Maternal and Fetal Risks

Acromegaly is caused by excessive secretion of GH, most often because of an acidophilic or chromophobic pituitary adenoma. Most patients have tumors greater than 1 cm in size. Although amenorrhea is common in women with acromegaly, pregnancy occasionally occurs.[16] Pregnancy may be accompanied by tumor expansion that necessitates medical treatment and surgical resection.[17] Patients with acromegaly are at increased risk for diabetes, hypertension, and cardiomyopathy.

Management Options

Documenting elevation of GH levels during pregnancy may be difficult because of placental expression of a GH variant.[18] Few laboratories offer specific radioimmunoassays to differentiate GH from the placental variant. Lack of suppression of GH levels below 2 mg/mL during a glucose tolerance test can help to establish the diagnosis. Measurement of the level of somatomedin C, which mediates the effects of GH, is more useful in establishing the diagnosis of acromegaly in nonpregnant women. However, levels of this insulin-like growth factor may increase in normal pregnancy. Definitive surgical treatment or radiation therapy is often undertaken before conception. Tumor expansion necessitating hyperphysectomy during pregnancy can be expected to occur in 10% of untreated cases.[19] Dopaminergic agents may paradoxically decrease GH levels in patients with acromegaly. Case reports confirm the lack of tumor expansion during pregnancy in women receiving bromocriptine therapy.[20] More recently, octreotide (Sandostatin) was used to reduce GH levels in women with acromegaly who were pregnant or were attempting pregnancy.[21] Maternal-fetal transfer of octreotide has been shown to occur without side effects. However, few cases have been reported, and the potential benefits of octreotide treatment should be weighed carefully against the potential risks.[21,22]

SUMMARY OF MANAGEMENT OPTIONS

Acromegaly

Management Options	Evidence Quality and Recommendation	References
Prepregnancy		
Definitive surgical management before conception.	—	—
Prenatal		
Normal elevation of growth hormone levels in pregnancy makes the diagnosis difficult. Lack of suppression of growth hormone levels during a glucose tolerance test is suggestive of the diagnosis. Elevation of somatomedin C levels is a more precise indicator of the diagnosis.	III/B	18
Screen for diabetes, hypertension, and cardiomyopathy.	—	—
Vigilance for tumor expansion (headaches, visual disturbance).	—	—
Bromocriptine is an effective and safe treatment in pregnancy.	IV/C	20
Octreotide has been used in pregnancy, but only in a small number of cases, so probably is best avoided.	IV/C	21,22

Diabetes Insipidus

Maternal and Fetal Risks

Diabetes insipidus is rare, with fewer than 100 cases complicating pregnancy reported in the literature. The disease results from inadequate or absent antidiuretic hormone (vasopressin) production by the posterior pituitary gland. The etiology of diabetes insipidus is often unknown, although in most cases, it follows pituitary surgery or destruction of the normal pituitary architecture by tumor. It is a primary idiopathic disorder in up to 50% of cases. Many cases are likely autoimmune, with lymphocytic infiltration of the posterior pituitary gland. Massive polyuria, caused by failure of the renal tubular concentrating mechanism, and dilute urine, with a specific gravity less than 1.005, are characteristic of diabetes insipidus. To combat dehydration and the intense thirst produced by this syndrome, affected individuals consume large quantities of fluid. The diagnosis of diabetes insipidus relies on the finding of continued polyuria and relative urinary hyposmolarity when water is restricted. Administration of intramuscular vasopressin causes water retention and an appropriate increase in urine osmolality. This response is not seen in patients with nephrogenic diabetes insipidus, in which free water clearance is increased because of insensitivity of the renal tubules to antidiuretic hormone. In patients with primary polydipsia or psychogenic diabetes insipidus, urine osmolality increases in response to vasopressin or desmopressin (DDAVP).

However, the increase is not as marked as in individuals with central diabetes insipidus. Other conditions that cause polyuria, such as diabetes mellitus, hyperparathyroidism with hypercalcemia, and chronic renal tubular disease, must be considered in the differential diagnosis. However, these conditions usually can be distinguished from central diabetes insipidus by appropriate laboratory testing.

Hime and Richardson[23] reviewed 67 cases of diabetes insipidus complicating pregnancy and noted that 58% of patients showed deterioration during gestation, whereas 20% of patients showed improvement. To explain this phenomenon, it has been suggested that the increased glomerular filtration rate seen in pregnancy may increase the requirement for antidiuretic hormone.[24] Mild disease may worsen during pregnancy because antidiuretic hormone clearance is increased by increased placental vasopressinase activity.[25] Impaired liver function, including fatty liver of pregnancy, is seen with arginine vasopressin (AVP)–resistant but DDAVP-responsive diabetes insipidus during pregnancy, suggesting that several factors may explain the observed worsening of this condition.

Transient diabetes insipidus of pregnancy has been reported during the last trimester in women with presumed limited vasopressin secretion capacity.[26] Transient diabetes insipidus is associated with acute fatty liver and HELLP (hemolysis, elevated liver enzymes, and low platelets) syndrome as well as twin gestation. Increased placental vasopressinase activity, along with insufficient liver degradation in HELLP syndrome and acute fatty liver, may unmask this condition. Finally, diabetes insipidus can accompany Sheehan's syndrome.

Management Options

Synthetic vasopressin, in the form of 1-deamino-8-D-arginine vasopressin (DDAVP), is the treatment of choice. This drug is given intranasally in doses of approximately 0.1 to 0.25 mg twice daily. Plasma electrolytes and fluid status should be monitored carefully with initiation of therapy. A stable dose is usually easy to achieve. Oxytocic activity is rarely observed. The successful use of DDAVP in pregnancy and the puerperium suggests that this drug is safe for both mother and fetus as well as during lactation.[27]

Spontaneous labor and lactation seem to occur in most patients with diabetes insipidus. Although older reports suggest an increased incidence of dysfunctional labor in affected patients, oxytocin release appears to be independent of vasopressin secretion.[28]

SUMMARY OF MANAGEMENT OPTIONS

Diabetes Insipidus

Management Options	Evidence Quality and Recommendation	References
Prepregnancy		
Vigilance for tumor expansion (headaches, visual disturbance).	—	—
Prenatal		
Continue supplementation with synthetic DDAVP, which is effective and safe in pregnancy. The dose may need to be increased during pregnancy.	IV/C	26,27
Monitor disease control with clinical features and the specific gravity or osmolarity of urine.	IV/C	27
Labor and Delivery		
Vigilance for dysfunctional labor (seen in only a few cases)	IV/C	27,28
Postnatal		
Vigilance for poor lactation (seen in only a few cases)	IV/C	27

DDAVP, desmopressin.

Pituitary Insufficiency

Maternal and Fetal Risks

Approximately 70 years ago, Sheehan[29] described postpartum ischemic necrosis of the anterior pituitary. This form of hypopituitarism is usually observed in patients with severe postpartum hemorrhage and hypotensive shock. Because pituitary necrosis is uncommon in patients with other conditions associated with hypovolemic shock, the hyperplastic pituitary gland of pregnancy may be more susceptible to hypoperfusion. It has been suggested that small sella size may be a risk factor.[30] Lymphocytic hypophysitis, an autoimmune form of hypopituitarism, is also more common in pregnant women and during the puerperium. It should be considered when hypopituitarism is suspected in patients without preceding postpartum hemorrhage. Slow clinical progression suggests that factors other than ischemia may be involved in the pathogenesis of pituitary insufficiency after pregnancy. Tissue necrosis may release sequestered antigens, triggering autoimmunity of the pituitary and delayed hypopituitarism in Sheehan's syndrome.[31] Destruction of the gland as a result of tumor invasion, surgery, or radiation therapy may accompany pregnancy, although fertility is often compromised. Antepartum pituitary infarction is a rare complication of insulin-dependent diabetes mellitus.[32] In these cases, insulin requirements may decrease dramatically.

Patients with Sheehan's syndrome may have varying degrees of hypopituitarism, and specific assays of tropic hormones as well as stimulation and suppression tests may be necessary to establish the diagnosis. During pregnancy, because of normal physiologic changes, adjustments must be made in interpreting both hormone levels and responses to various stimuli. An average delay of 7 years is observed between onset and diagnosis. Hypovolemic shock from postpartum hemorrhage is a precipitating event in up to 79% of cases.[32] There is no apparent correlation between the degree of hemorrhage and the occurrence of Sheehan's syndrome. The characteristic clinical picture begins with failure to lactate. However, this does not occur in all cases. Some patients have late-onset disease and progress to loss of maxillary and pubic hair, oligomenorrhea, or amenorrhea with senile vaginal atrophic changes as well as signs and symptoms of hypothyroidism. Patients with these findings are usually infertile, although the frequency of pregnancy is difficult to ascertain. In a review of 19 patients with Sheehan's syndrome documented by endocrinology studies or postmortem examination, 39 pregnancies occurred after the onset of hypopituitarism.[32] Eleven of these women required hormonal therapy to establish a pregnancy, and replacement therapy was used during 15 (38%) of the 39 pregnancies. The treated group had a live birth rate of 87%, compared with 54% in untreated patients, suggesting that early diagnosis and proper therapy improve outcome.

Because pregnancy may occur in women with Sheehan's syndrome,[33] this diagnosis should be considered in all patients with a history of postpartum hemorrhage. Measuring gonadotropin levels is of little value because levels decrease with normal pregnancy. However, the finding of a low or low-normal level of thyroid-stimulating hormone in conjunction with a low serum thyroxine level is consistent with secondary hypothyroidism. Similarly, low cortisol levels that do not increase with stress and decreased ACTH levels support the diagnosis.

Management Options

The treatment of pituitary insufficiency involves replacement of hormones that are necessary to maintain normal metabolism and respond to stress. Thyroid hormone may be provided as L-thyroxine in doses of 0.1 to 0.2 mg daily. Target free thyroxine levels should be in the mid-normal range. Corticosteroids are essential for patients who have adrenal insufficiency. Maintenance dosage is cortisone acetate 25 mg every morning and 12.5 mg every evening or prednisone 5 mg every morning and 2.5 mg every evening. Mineralocorticoid replacement is rarely necessary because adrenal production of aldosterone is not solely dependent on ACTH stimulation. The dose of glucocorticoids should be increased during the stress of labor and delivery.

SUMMARY OF MANAGEMENT OPTIONS

Pituitary Insufficiency

Management Options	Evidence Quality and Recommendation	References
Prepregnancy and Prenatal		
Give appropriate replacement hormones (usually thyroxine and corticosteroids).	—	—
Monitor clinical features and thyroid-stimulating hormone levels.	—	—
Labor and Delivery		
Increase the dose of glucocorticoids.	—	—
Postnatal		
Readjust glucocorticoid and thyroxine dosage if necessary.	—	—

ADRENAL DISEASE

Normal Changes in Pregnancy

A two- to threefold increase in cortisol levels is observed by the end of normal pregnancy.[34] Most of this increase is caused by an estrogen-induced increase in cortisol-binding globulin levels; however, biologically active free cortisol levels are also elevated.[35] An increase in free, or unbound, cortisol is apparent by the end of the first trimester. The urinary free cortisol concentration is also elevated during gestation.

Increased cortisol-binding globulin levels prolong the half-life of cortisol in plasma, and cortisol production is also increased. Urinary 17-hydroxycorticosteroid levels are actually lower in pregnancy because excretion of cortisol tetrahedron metabolites is decreased.[36] ACTH levels increase throughout pregnancy, but absolute levels remain lower in the pregnant than in the nonpregnant state.[37] Both ACTH and cortisol surge during labor. Unlike cortisol, ACTH does not cross the placenta. ACTH is manufactured by the placenta, as is corticotropin-releasing hormone. The relationship between these placental hormones and maternal adrenal function is unknown. Aldosterone secretion, which is controlled by the renin-angiotensin system, increases in early pregnancy. Finally, the production of dehydroepiandrosterone in the adrenal cortex is elevated in normal pregnancy. This hormone is aromatized to estradiol and estrone by the placenta.

Cushing's Syndrome

Maternal and Fetal Risks

Cushing's syndrome, which is characterized by excess glucocorticoid production, arises from ACTH-dependent or -independent inappropriate hypersecretion of ACTH by a pituitary adenoma (Cushing's disease) or from ectopic production of ACTH.[38] Cushing's syndrome as a result of primary adrenal disease, usually an adrenal adenoma, is more common during pregnancy than in the nonpregnant state. It accounts for approximately 50% of Cushing's syndrome cases during pregnancy.[39] Patients with pituitary disease and secondary adrenal hyperplasia are more likely to have excess androgen secretion, which can inhibit pituitary gonadotropin release. Amenorrhea is common in this setting. In contrast, adrenal adenomas are more likely to be pure cortisol producers and less likely to impair fertility.[34] Other causes of Cushing's syndrome include neoplastic ectopic ACTH production, nodular adrenal hyperplasia, and excessive doses of exogenous corticosteroids.

Because women with Cushing's syndrome are usually infertile, de novo cases are rare in pregnancy. Most cases occur in patients who were previously or partially treated. The clinical features may be difficult to distinguish from many signs and symptoms that accompany normal pregnancy. Weakness, weight gain, edema, striae, hypertension, and impaired glucose tolerance may be observed, both during gestation and in Cushing's syndrome. Early onset of hypertension, with easy bruising and proximal myopathy, strongly suggests the diagnosis and requires further evaluation.

Laboratory diagnosis includes elevated serum cortisol levels without diurnal variation and failure to suppress cortisol secretion with the administration of dexamethasone. Assays for ACTH are of variable accuracy and may confuse the diagnosis. However, an elevated early-morning ACTH value in the presence of high urinary levels of free cortisol suggests ACTH-dependent Cushing's syndrome. During gestation, total and free cortisol levels normally increase. Therefore, laboratory results must be compared with established norms for pregnancy. Diurnal variation in cortisol production is maintained in normal pregnancy, although free plasma cortisol levels at term may be two to three times higher than those in nonpregnant women. Further, even in normal pregnant patients, cortisol secretion may not be suppressed with low doses of dexamethasone (1 mg).[37] The preferred screening test for Cushing's syndrome is a 24-hour urine free cortisol measurement. A mean eightfold increase

FIGURE 46–3
Diagnostic algorithm for the different diagnosis of Cushing's syndrome (CS) in pregnancy.
(From Lindsay JR, Nieman LK: Adrenal disorders in pregnancy. Endocrinol Metab Clin North Am 2006;35:5.)

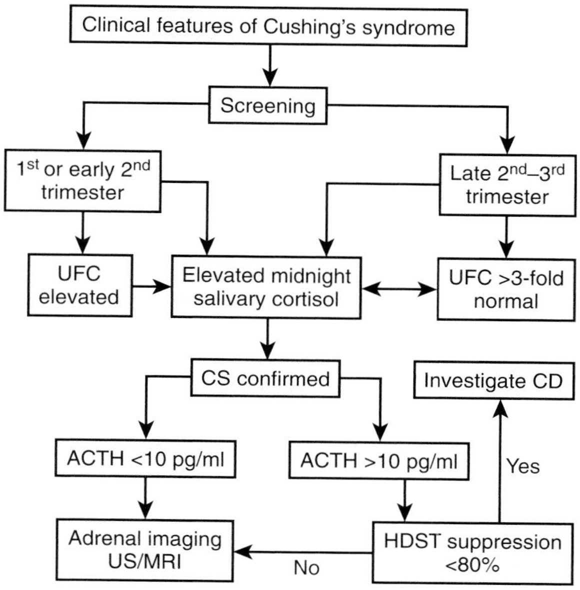

in urinary free cortisol accompanies cases of Cushing syndrome during pregnancy.[38] It has been suggested that if urinary collection shows levels elevated threefold and midnight salivary cortisol is also present, then Cushing's syndrome is diagnosed and the cause of excess cortisol production must be determined[40] (Fig. 46–3). A high-dose dexamethasone test may be helpful in distinguishing the site of excess cortisol production. Most patients with adrenocortical hyperplasia show greater than 50% reduction in plasma and urinary corticosteroid levels with an 8-mg dose (2 mg q6h for 2 days). If suppression is unsuccessful, an adrenal tumor, an autonomous adrenal nodule, or ectopic ACTH production must be considered. After testing, pituitary or adrenal gland imaging should be undertaken. MRI is the optimal imaging modality during pregnancy because no radiation is used.

Several reports suggest that Cushing's syndrome may be exacerbated by pregnancy, with improvement of symptoms after delivery.[34,38,39] In most cases, Cushing's syndrome is associated with an adrenal adenoma.[38] Keegan and colleagues[41] speculated that placental ACTH may stimulate a latent adrenal tumor, with adrenal cortisol secretion decreasing after parturition. The idea that pregnancy may stimulate the development of Cushing's syndrome is supported by the fact that in virtually all reports of Cushing's syndrome in pregnancy, the diagnosis was not established until pregnancy occurred.[34] Several cases of recurrent Cushing's syndrome during pregnancy have been described. These may represent hyperresponsiveness of adrenocortical cells to a non-ACTH or non–corticotropin-releasing hormone substance that is produced during pregnancy.[42]

Pregnancy outcome in Cushing's syndrome is marked by a high rate of preterm delivery (43%) and stillbirth (6%) when elective termination is not performed.[38] Maternal

TABLE 46–2

Cushing's Syndrome and Perinatal Complications in 65 Pregnancies

COMPLICATION	%
Miscarriage	3.1
Perinatal death	
Neonatal death	7.7
Stillbirth	6–7.7
Premature birth	43–64.6
Intrauterine growth retardation	21–26.2

Adapted from Buescher MA, McClamrock HD, Adashi EY: Cushing syndrome in pregnancy. Obstet Gynecol 1992;79:130; and Lindsay JR, Jonklaas J, Oldfield EH, Neiman LK: Cushing's syndrome during pregnancy: Personal experience and review of the literature. J Clin Endocrinol Metab 2005; 90:3077.

hyperglycemia may be a contributing factor to the intrauterine deaths observed (Table 46–2). Hypertension has been reported in 68% of cases, and preeclampsia in 9%.[31,38]

Koerten and coworkers[43] reviewed 33 cases of Cushing's syndrome in pregnancy and concluded that maternal complications are more common with adrenal adenomas than with hyperplasia. In this review, every patient with an adenoma had hypertension if the pregnancy progressed beyond the first trimester. Seven of 16 (47%) patients had pulmonary edema, and 1 died. In contrast, only 1 of the 12 patients with adrenal hyperplasia had hypertensive disease. The overall prematurity rate (delivery after 20 weeks' gestation) was 20 of 33 cases (61%); stillbirth occurred in 4 cases.

Management Options

Management of the pregnant patient with cortisol excess includes identifying the source of hormone production and instituting proper therapy. Surgery is recommended for disease diagnosed during the first trimester.[38] Patients with pituitary disease are most often treated surgically if a tumor can be well defined. Surgical removal of adrenal adenomas can be accomplished through a posterior incision. Bevan and associates[44] examined maternal and fetal outcomes based on the timing of surgery. Fetal loss occurred in 1 of 11 (9%) patients treated during gestation versus 8 of 26 (31%) in whom definitive therapy was delayed. In Buescher and colleagues's review[34] of 105 cases in which 32 women underwent therapy to relieve hypercortisolism, treatment reduced the perinatal mortality rate from 15% to 6.3%. Again, because the incidence of adrenal adenoma and carcinoma appears to be increased in pregnant patients with Cushing's syndrome, prompt evaluation with MRI is warranted, particularly if high levels of dexamethasone do not suppress excess cortisol production. Surgery is indicated if an adrenal tumor is discovered. Treatment may be delayed in the third trimester if an expedited delivery is planned.

SUMMARY OF MANAGEMENT OPTIONS

Cushing's Syndrome

Management Options	Evidence Quality and Recommendation	References
Prepregnancy		
Complete testing and treatment (usually surgical) before conception.	—	—
Prenatal		
If the diagnosis is made during pregnancy, identify and treat the cause or source of hormone production (usually by surgery). The only exception is diagnosis in the third trimester. In this case, delivery and subsequent definitive management may be an option.	III/B	34,39,44
Testing includes magnetic resonance imaging, especially because of the risk of carcinoma.	—	—

Primary Aldosteronism

Maternal and Fetal Risks

Few cases of primary aldosteronism during pregnancy have been reported.[40] The diagnosis is suggested in a patient with hypertension, hypokalemia, and metabolic alkalosis. Adrenal adenoma is the most common etiology, present in nearly 75% of cases. Glucocorticoid-remediable aldosteronism is a hereditary form of primary aldosterone excess that causes hypokalemia and hypertension in childhood. This diagnosis is established before pregnancy and is amenable to medical treatment. The clinical course of these pregnancies has been described, including a high rate of preeclampsia in patients with underlying chronic hypertension.[45] Because aldosterone secretion is increased during pregnancy, the diagnosis of new-onset hyperaldosteronism can be difficult to establish. However, elevated aldosterone levels accompanied by suppressed renin levels support the diagnosis of primary hyperaldosteronism. High levels of urinary potassium with serum hypokalemia also help to establish the diagnosis. Failure to replace serum potassium may also suppress aldosterone secretion, obscuring the diagnosis.[45] Inappropriately high aldosterone levels are present after suppression testing. The potassium level should be normalized before the administration of suppression tests, such as 9-α-fludrocortisone. Amelioration of hypertension and hypokalemia during gestation is attributed to high levels of progesterone, which may block the action of aldosterone. Even so, patients often have severe hypertension and superimposed preeclampsia.

Management Options

The management of patients without toxemia complicating primary aldosteronism is controversial.[46] Although early case reports suggested prompt surgical excision of underlying adrenal adenomas, Lotgerring and associates[47] described successful medical therapy from midgestation with spironolactone, an aldosterone antagonist, and other antihypertensive medications. This therapy should be used cautiously because spironolactone is an antiandrogen that may cause feminization of a male fetus. Laparoscopic adrenalectomy has been used to treat primary hyperaldosteronism during pregnancy.[48]

SUMMARY OF MANAGEMENT OPTIONS

Primary Aldosteronism

Management Options	Evidence Quality and Recommendation	References
Prenatal		
If the diagnosis is made during pregnancy, options are		
• Medical treatment (antihypertensives and spironolactone), although spironolactone is an antiandrogen, with an associated risk of feminization.	IV/C	47
• Laparoscopic adrenalectomy.	IV/C	48
• Open surgery.	IV/C	46

Adrenal Insufficiency

Maternal and Fetal Risks

Adrenal insufficiency is usually primary (Addison's disease) and caused by autoimmune destruction. Granulomatous diseases, such as tuberculosis, bilateral adrenalectomy, fungal infection, and AIDS, are other rare etiologies. Pituitary failure or adrenal suppression as a result of steroid replacement may also lead to adrenal insufficiency. In these cases, mineralocorticoid production is preserved. Adrenal crisis, an acute, life-threatening condition, may accompany stressful conditions, such as labor, the puerperium, or surgery. Unfortunately, the diagnosis of hypoadrenalism is often difficult, particularly in patients who have enough adrenal reserve to sustain normal daily activity. Postpartum adrenal crisis may lead to the diagnosis of adrenal insufficiency for the first time.[49]

The clinical presentation of Addison's disease during gestation is similar to that in the nonpregnant state. Fatigue, weakness, anorexia, nausea, hypotension, nonspecific abdominal pain, hypoglycemia, and increased skin pigmentation are hallmarks of this endocrinopathy. Mineralocorticoid deficiency leads to renal sodium loss, with resultant depletion of intravascular volume. A small cardiac silhouette on chest radiography is often associated with reduced cardiac output and eventual circulatory collapse. Hypoglycemia, which is common in early pregnancy, may be exacerbated by glucocorticoid deficiency.

Management Options

The diagnosis of adrenal insufficiency is based on specific laboratory findings. Plasma cortisol levels are decreased. However, because the level of cortisol-binding globulin is elevated in pregnancy, even low-normal cortisol values may reflect adrenal insufficiency.

Stimulation of the adrenal gland by synthetic ACTH may help to establish a diagnosis.[50] After intravenous administration of 0.25 mg cosyntropin (Cortrosyn), the plasma cortisol level should be increased at least twofold over baseline values. Failure to respond to this stimulus suggests primary adrenal insufficiency. This test may be used in pregnancy because little ACTH crosses the placenta. A longer ACTH stimulation test is used if the short test does not confirm the diagnosis. Measurement of serum ACTH may also help to distinguish primary adrenal insufficiency from hypopituitarism. Low baseline serum cortisol levels, coupled with ACTH levels greater than 250 pg/mL, confirm the diagnosis of primary adrenal insufficiency.

Pregnancy usually proceeds normally in treated patients. Maintenance replacement of adrenocortical hormones is provided by cortisone acetate 25 mg orally each morning and 12.5 mg in the evening. As an alternative, prednisone may be substituted at doses of 5 mg and 2.5 mg, respectively. Mineralocorticoid deficiency is treated with fludrocortisone acetate (Florinef) 0.05 to 0.1 mg daily. Stress doses of glucocorticoids should be administered during labor and delivery. With doses of glucocorticoids exceeding 300 mg in 24 hours, supplemental mineralocorticoid therapy is unnecessary. The use of a mineralocorticoid requires careful observation for symptoms of fluid overload. Patients with edema, excess weight gain, and electrolyte imbalance require dose adjustment.

Adrenal crisis is a rare, life-threatening condition that requires immediate medical attention. Treatment in an intensive care setting is recommended. Women with undiagnosed Addison's disease may have a crisis during the puerperium. Symptoms include nausea, vomiting, and profound epigastric pain accompanied by hypothermia and hypotension. After blood samples are obtained for diagnostic purposes, treatment initially consists of glucocorticoid and fluid replacement. Intravenous hydrocortisone is given at a dose of 100 mg, followed by repeat doses every 6 hours for up to several days. Mineralocorticoid replacement is indicated in cases of refractory hypotension or hyperkalemia.

Patients with adrenal insufficiency should wear an identifying bracelet. Emergency medical kits are available to help these patients when they travel. Women with Addison's disease require an increase in steroid replacement during periods of infection or stress and during labor and delivery. Cortisol is administered at a dose of 100 mg intravenously every 8 hours for the first 24 hours. The dose of steroids is reduced by 50% the next day.

SUMMARY OF MANAGEMENT OPTIONS

Adrenal Insufficiency

Management Options	Evidence Quality and Recommendation	References
Prenatal		
Continue glucocorticoid and mineralocorticoid supplementation.	IV/C	49,50
Vigilance for fluid overload and electrolyte disturbance	IV/C	49,50
Vigilance for adrenal crisis:	IV/C	49,50
• IV hydrocortisone.		
• IV fluids.		
• Supportive medical therapy.		
• Critical care setting.		
Labor and Delivery		
Increase glucocorticoid supplementation.	IV/C	49,50

Pheochromocytoma

Maternal and Fetal Risks

Pheochromocytoma is a rare, catecholamine-producing tumor that is uncommon in pregnancy. Approximately 200 cases have been reported in the literature.[40] The tumors arise from the chromaffin cells of the adrenal medulla or sympathetic nervous tissue, including remnants of the organs of Zuckerkandl, neural crest tissue that lies along the abdominal aorta. In pregnancy, as in the nonpregnant state, the tumor is located in the adrenal gland in 90% of cases.[51] The incidence of malignancy, which can be diagnosed only when metastases are present, is approximately 10%. In patients with a family history of pheochromocytoma, multiple endocrine neoplasia syndrome (MEN types IIa and IIb) should be suspected. Pheochromocytoma is more common in patients with neurofibromatosis. Schenker and colleagues[51,52] reported mortality rates of 55% with postpartum diagnosis versus 11% with diagnosis during pregnancy. Fetal loss rates can exceed 50%.

In pregnancy, pheochromocytoma may cause a hypertensive crisis, with cerebral hemorrhage or severe congestive heart failure. Pheochromocytoma is easily confused with other medical diseases. The signs and symptoms may mimic those of severe pregnancy-induced hypertension (Table 46–3). Hypertension, headache, abdominal pain, and blurring of vision are common to both entities. Although not uniformly present, paroxysmal hypertension (particularly <20 wk' gestation), orthostasis, and absence of significant proteinuria and edema may be helpful in the differential diagnosis. Severe thyrotoxicosis may also resemble this

TABLE 46–3

Symptoms and Signs in 89 Cases of Pheochromocytoma in Pregnancy

SYMPTOM OR SIGN	%
Paroxysmal or sustained hypertension	82
Headaches	66
Palpitation	36
Sweating	30
Blurred vision	17
Anxiety	15
Convulsion and dyspnea	10

Adapted from Schenker JG, Chowers I: Pheochromocytoma and pregnancy: Review of 89 cases. Obstet Gynecol Surv 1971;26:739.

disease. However, significant diastolic hypertension is rarely seen with hyperthyroidism. Aggravation of hypertension with administration of β-blockers suggests pheochromocytoma. An unexplained hypertensive response to anesthesia or circulatory collapse after delivery should also prompt consideration of this diagnosis.

Management Options

PREPREGNANCY

If this condition is suspected, a complete diagnostic evaluation is indicated before pregnancy is attempted. Definitive therapy should be undertaken (discussed later).

PRENATAL

The diagnosis depends on laboratory measurement of catecholamines and their metabolites in a 24-hour urine collection. Elevated metanephrine excretion appears to be the most sensitive and specific finding, although isolated elevated vanillylmandelic acid excretion may be present.[50] Because episodic secretion of catecholamines occurs with some tumors, plasma assay of epinephrine or norepinephrine may be helpful during symptomatic episodes.[52] Levels of catecholamines are unaffected by normal pregnancy. Levels may be elevated after eclamptic seizures. Extra-adrenal tumors have characteristic elevations of norepinephrine, but not epinephrine.

Pharmacologic testing may establish the diagnosis in the nonpregnant patient. The phentolamine (Regitine) test is based on the observation that marked α-adrenergic blockade causes a decrease in blood pressure in many patients with pheochromocytoma. This test is not advised during pregnancy because it is associated with maternal and fetal deaths.[52] Nonetheless, it is extremely importance that the diagnosis be established. Approximately 90% of maternal deaths as a result of pheochromocytoma occur in patients who are undiagnosed before delivery.[53] When symptoms suggest pheochromocytoma and laboratory findings support the diagnosis, the tumor should be localized with radiologic techniques. MRI is the procedure of choice in pregnancy. In the nonpregnant state, selective venous catheterization of the adrenals may be performed. The tumor is bilateral in approximately 10% of cases, including those that occur during gestation.

Before surgery, the patient's condition should be stabilized with oral doses of phenoxybenzamine and α-adrenergic receptor blockers.[54] Careful evaluation of fluid status with central monitoring is essential when using these preparations. β-Blockade with propranolol or similar selective agents is reserved for the treatment of tachyarrhythmias and should not be instituted before α-blockade because hypertensive crisis may ensue. Labetalol is not recommended because it is a combined adrenergic-blocking agent. Hypertensive crisis requires intravenous phentolamine administration in an intensive care setting.

Schenker and Granat[52] recommend prompt surgical removal of pheochromocytomas detected before 24 weeks' gestation. Laparoscopic removal has been achieved during pregnancy.[55] When the diagnosis is made during the early third trimester, maternal stabilization with medical therapy has been successful, allowing further fetal maturation.

LABOR AND DELIVERY AND POSTNATAL

Cesarean delivery is preferred because it minimizes the potential catecholamine surges associated with labor and vaginal delivery. Adrenal exploration is performed at the time of cesarean delivery. Careful follow-up is needed because tumors may recur and are potentially malignant.

SUMMARY OF MANAGEMENT OPTIONS

Pheochromocytoma

Management Options	Evidence Quality and Recommendation	References
Prepregnancy		
Avoid pregnancy until definitive treatment is implemented and cure is achieved.	—	—
Prenatal		
If the diagnosis is suspected clinically, establish the diagnosis with 24-hr catecholamine testing. Establish the location of the tumor (10% are bilateral) with magnetic resonance imaging.	III/B	40,51–53
Establish medical stabilization and control of blood pressure before and during surgery.	III/B	40,47–49
Some give medical treatment and defer surgery until after delivery.	IV/C	54
Laparoscopic surgery has been undertaken.	IV/C	55
Labor and Delivery		
Cesarean delivery is preferable once medical stablization is established.	III/B	51–53
Concomitant surgery at the time of cesarean delivery is debatable.	III/B	51–53
Postnatal		
Monitor for recurrence.	III/B	51–53

SUGGESTED READINGS

Durr JA: Diabetes insipidus in pregnancy. Am J Kidney Dis 1978;9:276.

Frankenne F, Closset J, Gomez F, et al: The physiology of growth hormones in pregnant women and partial characterization of the placental GH variant. J Clin Endocrinol Metab 1988;66:1171.

Gonzalez JG, Elizondo G, Saldwar D, et al: Pituitary gland growth during normal pregnancy: An in vivo study using magnetic resonance imaging. Am J Med 1988;85:217.

Hermann-Bonert V, Seliverstov M, Melmed S: Pregnancy in acromegaly: Successful therapeutic outcome. J Clin Endocrinol Metab 1998;83:727.

Kelestimur F: Sheehan's syndrome. Pitutiary 2003;6:181.

Lindsay JR, Jonklass J, Oldfield EH, et al: Cushing's syndrome during pregnancy: Personal experience and review of the literature. J Clin Endocrinol Metab 2005;90:3077.

Lindsay JR, Neiman LK: Adrenal disorders in pregnancy. Endocrinol Metab Clin North Am 2006;35:1–20.

Liu C, Tyrrell JB: Successful treatment of a large macroprolactinoma with cabergoline during pregnancy. Pituitary 2001;4:85.

Maygar DM, Marshall JR: Pituitary tumors and pregnancy. Am J Obstet Gynecol 1978;132:739.

Schenker JG, Granat M: Pheochromocytoma and pregnancy: An update and appraisal. Aust N Z J Obstet Gynaecol 1982;22:1.

REFERENCES

For a complete list of references, log onto www.expertconsult.com.

CHAPTER 47

Hepatic and Gastrointestinal Disease

CATHERINE WILLIAMSON and JOANNA GIRLING

INTRODUCTION

Anatomy and Physiology of the Liver

An understanding of the physiologic changes of normal pregnancy is vital if pathologic conditions are to be correctly defined. False-positive and false-negative interpretations can result if the normal changes due to pregnancy are not fully appreciated.

The liver moves superiorly and posteriorly in pregnancy, such that a palpable liver edge is likely to be pathologic. Absolute blood flow to the liver is unchanged, although the proportion of cardiac output perfusing the liver falls from 35% to 25%. Venous pressure increases in the esophagus due to increased circulating volume, increased portal pressure, and increased pressure from the gravid uterus, thereby diverting a greater proportion of venous return from the inferior vena cava via the azygos system. This results in transient esophageal varices in up to 60% of healthy pregnant women.[1,2] Spider nevi, palmar erythema, and edema are common findings in normal pregnancy, reflecting, in part, peripheral vasodilation. They should not be assumed to be due to chronic liver disease unless they clearly antedate the pregnancy.

The liver has several important functions, including protein synthesis, metabolism, excretion, and inactivation of a number of substances. Changes in each of these should be considered in relation to both the effect of normal pregnancy and the potential overlap with the changes of liver disease outside pregnancy:

- Protein synthesis increases in pregnancy, with rises in coagulation Factors VII, VIII, and X and fibrinogen: The last of which has usually doubled by the end of pregnancy, so an apparently normal result may reflect a significant abnormality in, for example, disseminated intravascular coagulopathy (DIC).[3] This increase is probably the main cause of the increase in erythrocyte sedimentation rate that occurs in pregnancy; the 95th percentile for the second trimester in a nonanemic woman being 70 mm/hr.[4] In acute liver failure, prolongation of the prothrombin time (PT) may be the first sign of coagulopathy, because prothrombin has the shortest half-life of those coagulation factors manufactured in the liver. Production of albumin is not changed during uncomplicated pregnancy, and hemodilution results in a fall in concentration, so that levels of 28 g/L are commonly seen. These do not reflect failure of hepatic synthesis, as might be the case outside pregnancy. The concentration of many hormone-binding proteins is increased, largely due to reduced metabolism rather than increased hepatic synthesis. For example, the higher concentration of estrogen stimulates greater sialylation of the carbohydrate moieties of thyroxine-binding globulin, which extends its half-life from 15 minutes to 3 days[5] and so greatly increases the total throxine (T_4).
- Amino acids undergo oxidative deamination in the liver to produce ammonia, which is converted to urea in the Krebs cycle. Failure of this process in severe liver disease can contribute to hepatic encephalopathy. It may also be associated with low urea concentrations, which must not be confused with the fall in urea that occurs as a consequence of the increased glomerular filtration rate of normal pregnancy.[6]
- Hypercholesterolemia occurs in some forms of chronic liver disease owing to impaired excretion. Hypertriglyceridemia can occur in chronic alcohol abuse. In normal pregnancy, their concentrations increase by 50% and 300%, respectively,[7] and take several months to return to normal after delivery.
- The liver is responsible for postprandial glucose storage and subsequent release during fasting. Hypoglycemia may occur, despite these large glucose reserves, in patients with massive liver necrosis, for example, in acute fatty liver of pregnancy (AFLP), and is an important cause of liver coma. Serial measurements of blood glucose and, subsequently, intravenous infusion of 50% dextrose are important in preventing hypoglycemic coma in patients with severe liver failure.

Anatomy and Physiology of the Gastrointestinal Tract

The gastrointestinal tract also undergoes extensive physiologic changes in pregnancy. These changes contribute to the common findings of nausea and vomiting, gastroesophageal reflux, constipation, and hemorrhoids, although the exact basis for these changes is not clearly understood. Nausea and

TABLE 47–1

Liver Function Tests in Normal Pregnancy

TEST	NONPREGNANT	FIRST TRIMESTER	SECOND TRIMESTER	THIRD TRIMESTER
AST u/L	7-40	10-28	11-29	11-30
ALT u/L	0-40	6-32	6-32	6-32
Bili μmol/L	0-17	4-16	3-13	3-14
GGT u/L	11-50	5-37	5-43	5-41
Alk phos u/L	30-130	32-100	43-135	130-418

Alk phos, alkaline phosphatase; ALT, alanine aminotransaminase; AST, aspartate aminotransaminase; Bili, bilirubin; GGT, γ-glutamyl transferase.
From Girling JC, Dow E, Smith JH: Liver function tests in preeclampsia: Importance of comparison with a reference range derived for normal pregnancy. Br J Obstet Gynaecol 1997;104:246–250.

vomiting seem to be due to the combined actions of estrogen and progesterone, although this is not certain; human chorionic gonadotrophin may also make a contribution (see the section on "Hyperemesis Gravidarum"). Gastroesophageal reflux occurs in up to 80% of pregnancies[8] and is thought to be due to a combination of reduced lower esophageal sphincter pressure, raised intragastric pressure, reduced pyloric sphincter competence with backwash of alkaline bile, and failure of clearance of acid gastric contents. Constipation is traditionally attributed to progesterone-driven smooth muscle relaxation and increasing transit times allowing more fluid to be absorbed. However, in pregnancy, only small bowel transit times have been reported[9]; colonic times have not been studied directly. Iron supplements, dietary changes, and altered exercise levels may also contribute, as may mechanical problems in the lower gastrointestinal tract, especially the anal sphincter.[10]

Liver Function Tests

So-called liver function tests (LFTs) are really nonspecific tests of liver cell damage: In essence, they reflect the extent of hepatocyte damage, although if damage is extensive and sustained, values may plummet. In pregnancy, significant changes occur in the commonly measured tests of liver function, which must be borne in mind when interpreting blood results. Aspartate transaminase (AST), alanine transaminase (ALT), γ-glutamyl transferase (GGT), and total bilirubin each fall during pregnancy, the upper limit of normal being about 25% lower than outside pregnancy. This is mainly as a result of hemodilution[11] (Table 47–1). Alkaline phosphatase rises steadily through pregnancy, reaching a peak in the third trimester up to 300% above the nonpregnant range, owing to the production of a heat stable placental isoenzyme: If there is a clinical indication to differentiate the hepatic from the placental form, the sample can be heat-treated to 60°C for 10 minutes and then reanalyzed, the fall representing the liver isoenzyme.

In the postnatal period, alkaline phosphatase falls steadily, reaching nonpregnant values by day 13 in most women. The transaminases may rise considerably, especially during the first 5 days of the puerperium, and can exceed both the pregnant and the nonpregnant reference ranges[12] (Table 47–2). This is because they are not specific to liver, occurring also in breast, smooth and striated muscle, and red blood cells. The exercise of labor, the trauma of delivery, and breast-feeding may all contribute to this phenomenon.

TABLE 47–2

Liver Function Tests following Delivery in Normal Pregnancy

TEST	POSTPARTUM PEAK (DAYS)	MEAN RISE (%)	RANGE RISE (%)
AST	2-5	88	0-500
ALT	5	147	0-1140
GGT	5-10	62	0-450
Alk phos	Predelivery	–	–

Alk phos, alkaline phosphatase; ALT, alanine aminotransaminase; AST, aspartate aminotransaminase; GGT, γ-glutamyl transferase.
From David AL, Kotecha M, Girling JC: Factors influencing postnatal liver function tests. BJOG 2000;107:1421–1426.

It is essential to bear this in mind when managing liver disease in the puerperium.

The Fetus and Maternal Liver Disease

In many cases, the fetus is only affected by the maternal liver condition if the pregnant woman is systemically unwell, for example, febrile, dehydrated, hypoglycemic, or profoundly malnourished. Specific issues relating to transmission of infection, the genetic input of the fetus to the maternal condition (e.g., AFLP), the role of the placenta (e.g., preeclampsia and HELLP [hemolysis, elevated platelets, and low platelets] syndrome), and fetal "poisoning" (e.g., obstetric cholestasis [OC]) are covered in the relevant sections. It does not seem that fetal exposure to raised bilirubin, even if prolonged, or toxic metabolites of maternal liver failure influence development.[13] Unconjugated bilirubin crosses the placenta bidirectionally, and this is the main route of fetal clearance. There is not a simple link between maternal and fetal levels of bilirubin.

JAUNDICE

Jaundice may be coincidental to the pregnancy or due to a condition that is specific to the pregnancy. Worldwide, the most common cause of jaundice in pregnancy is viral hepatitis, usually hepatitis A. In some parts of the world, hepatitis B, C, or E is most prevalent. Hepatitis secondary to infection with cytomegalovirus (CMV), Epstein-Barr virus (EBV), toxoplasmosis, or herpes simplex should also be considered as causes of jaundice in pregnancy, not least because of the

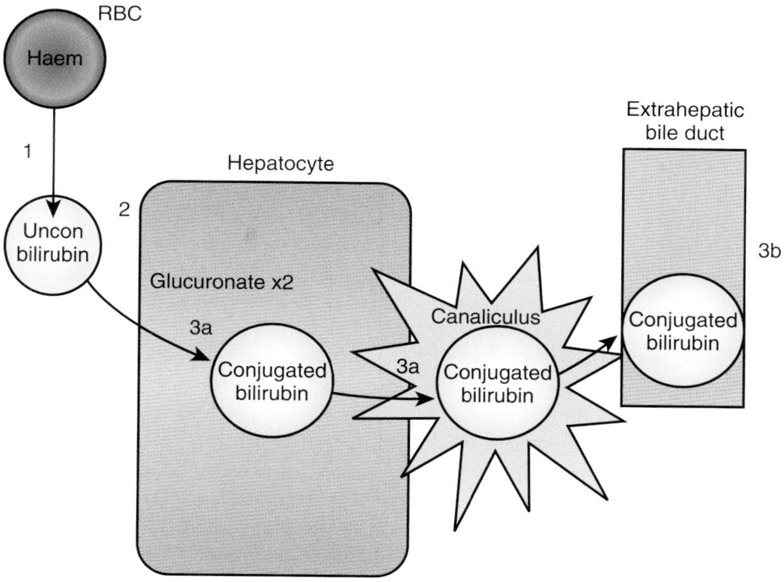

FIGURE 47–1
The potential points for pathologic processes resulting in jaundice.

other important implications that these infections have for the fetus. Other common causes of jaundice not related to the pregnancy are the complications of gallstones, drug reactions (in the United Kingdom co-amoxiclav is the most common prescription-related cause of cholestatic jaundice), and drug abuse, including alcohol.

The pregnancy-specific causes of jaundice are AFLP, HELLP syndrome, OC, and hyperemesis gravidarum. Only in the first of these, which is also the rarest, is jaundice a common feature.

Physiology

When faced with the challenge of a jaundiced pregnant patient, it is easier to reach a diagnosis if a simple logical pathway is followed. Initially, the jaundice should be classified according to its type. Then, its cause can usually be determined. An understanding of the physiology of bilirubin handling makes this much easier.

Following the destruction of a red blood cell, the released hemoglobin is broken down into globin and heme; other heme-containing proteins, such as myoglobin, cytochromes, and catalase, contribute up to 15% of the total heme. The heme is broken down to biliverdin, which is reduced to form bilirubin, usually amounting to 250 to 300 mg daily: This is not changed by pregnancy. This bilirubin is unconjugated and water-insoluble and usually carried to the liver bound to albumin. In this state, it is unable to pass through the kidney or the blood-brain barrier. However, unbound unconjugated bilirubin is lipid-soluble and can cross the blood-brain barrier. This is most likely in neonates with immature conjugating mechanisms or in the presence of either profound hypoalbuminemia or displacement of bilirubin from albumin by, for example, fatty acids, salicylates, or sulfonamides.

At the hepatocyte membrane, unconjugated bilirubin is actively taken up and conjugated to two molecules of glucuronide, by the action of uridine diphosphoglucurosyl (UDP) transferase. This conjugated bilirubin is water-soluble and usually remains in the liver. Hepatocyte (or canalicular) damage allows it to enter the blood, and the part that remains unbound passes into urine and causes the dark urine of cholestatic jaundice; it is always abnormal to find bilirubinuria. The protein-bound conjugated bilirubin contributes to the yellow discoloration of skin and mucus membranes and the hyperbilirubinemia of liver disease.

From the hepatocyte, bilirubin is actively taken up by the bile canaliculus. It is these energy-dependent steps that are most likely to be impaired by either liver damage or increased pressure in the biliary tract. From the canaliculus, conjugated bilirubin drains into the extrahepatic bile ducts, the common bile duct, and finally, the small intestine. The conjugated bilirubin is too large to be absorbed from this location. It passes to the terminal ileum where bacterial action hydrolyzes it to free bilirubin, which is then reduced to urobilinogen. Some of this undergoes further bacterial action in the stool, changing it to stercobilinogen, which contributes to the dark color of feces—reduced entry of bilirubin into the gut accounts for the pale stool of cholestatic jaundice. The rest of the urobilinogen is absorbed and returns to the liver via the enterohepatic circulation; from there it is reexcreted into the bile. This urobilinogen is water-soluble, and in normal circumstances, a small amount passes into the urine. Urinary urobilinogen is increased either if there is an increased load of bilirubin, in which case, the hepatic capacity to reexcrete the urobilinogen may be overwhelmed, or if hepatic damage impairs reexcretion.

Classification and Risks

In Figure 47–1, the potential points for pathologic processes resulting in jaundice are highlighted. Three pathologic processes lead to jaundice:

- Hemolysis
- Congenital hyperbilirubinemia
  - Unconjugated
  - Conjugated
- Cholestasis
  - Intrahepatic
  - Extrahepatic

Hemolytic Jaundice

Hemolytic jaundice occurs when there is excess breakdown of red blood cells and is characterized by increased unconjugated bilirubinemia. There are no abnormalities in AST, ALT, or GGT unless liver disease is present as well. Investigations are centered on causes of hemolytic anemia, including hereditary spherocytosis or elliptocytosis, thalassemia, sickle cell disease, glucose-6-phosphate dehydrogenase, blood group incompatibility, or drug reaction. In HELLP syndrome, the main cause of jaundice may be hemolysis.

Congenital Hyperbilirubinemia

In this group of disorders. raised bilirubin is the only biochemical abnormality. It occurs when there is either defective conjugation or abnormal handling of bilirubin. The most common condition in this category is Gilbert's syndrome. This benign, familial cause of unconjugated hyperbilirubinemia affects up to 7% of the general population. Most patients have a reduced level of UDP transferase, to around 30% of normal. A number of gene mutations have been described, although phenotypic expression of carriers varies widely, with some individuals being asymptomatic and others experiencing intermittent jaundice. Fasting, intercurrent illness, and pregnancy have been reported to increase the level of unconjugated bilirubinemia, with up to half of pregnant women developing worsening of jaundice.[14] Apart from the raised bilirubin, the other LFTs are normal, and there are no stigmata of chronic liver disease. The reticulocyte count is not raised, thus excluding hemolysis.

Crigler-Najjar syndrome is a very rare and much more serious cause of unconjugated hyperbilirubinemia, which is due to either absence of (autosomal recessive) or marked reduction of (autosomal dominant) UDP transferase. This usually presents at birth, with jaundice and sometimes kernicterus.

Conjugated hyperbilirubinemia is due to defective handling of bilirubin within the liver. Dubin-Johnson syndrome is autosomal recessive and results from a mutation in the *MRP2* (multidrug-resistance protein 2) gene, which is responsible for transporting a wide range of compounds out of the hepatocyte across the canalicular border, including bilirubin and bile salts. It is benign, with a good prognosis, with most affected individuals experiencing only mild and fluctuating jaundice. Rotor's syndrome is a similar condition, which is often autosomal dominant. In both conditions, bilirubinuria is present.

Benign recurrent intrahepatic cholestasis (BRIC) and progressive familial intrahepatic cholestasis (PFIC) are rare causes of conjugated congenital hyperbilirubinemia, which in pregnancy may account for a small proportion of cases of OC (see the following sections).

Cholestatic Jaundice

The broad term *cholestasis* refers to failure to excrete bile from the hepatocyte, the canaliculus (intrahepatic), or the common bile duct (extrahepatic) owing to acquired damage or obstruction. Consequently, some or all of the substances usually excreted by this route, including bilirubin, bile salts, cholesterol, and phospholipids, accumulate in the blood. Alkaline phosphatase levels may rise, due to either increased synthesis at the sinusoidal surface of the hepatocyte or reentry from the sinusoids into the systemic circulation in response to raised intraductal pressure. Cholestasis may occur without jaundice if excretion of bilirubin is maintained or only part of the liver is affected. Jaundice occurs when the failure of excretion of bilirubin results in its accumulation in the circulation.

Intrahepatic cholestatic jaundice is due to any of a wide range of abnormalities at a cellular level and has a diverse number of clinical causes. Within this category fall viral hepatitis, drug reactions, alcohol abuse, cirrhosis of any cause, OC, AFLP, and hyperemesis gravidarum. Extrahepatic cholestasis is due to obstruction to the flow of bile at any point beyond the canaliculus; causes include gallstones, biliary stricture, pancreatitis, and malignancy.

In both forms of cholestatic jaundice, there may be pale stool, dark urine, and conjugated bilirubinemia. They must be clearly differentiated from each other by careful history, examination, and investigation because they require different management strategies.

In practical terms, an important step in assessing a patient with jaundice is to establish the type of jaundice (see the section on "Classification" and Table 47–3). This is very simply and quickly done by asking the laboratory to report the bilirubin as both the total amount and divided into conjugated and unconjugated forms (also referred to as "direct" and "indirect" bilirubin). Commercial urine dipsticks should be used to test for bilirubinuria (which is always abnormal) and urinary urobilinogen. Table 47–3 can then be used to establish the most likely type of jaundice.

TABLE 47–3

Serum and Urine Findings in a Jaundiced Patient, Allowing Characterization of the Cause of the Jaundice

	SERUM BILIRUBIN		URINE BILIRUBIN			
CAUSE OF JAUNDICE	UNCONJUGATED	CONJUGATED	BILIRUBIN	UROBILINOGEN	RETICULOCYTE COUNT	ALT
Hemolysis	↑	N	–	↑	↑	N
Gilbert's syndrome	↑↑	N	–	↑	N	N
Crigler-Najjar	↑↑↑	N	–	↑	N	N
Dubin-Johnson	N/↑	↑	✓	↑	N	N
Hepatocellular	N/↑	↑	✓	↑/N	N	↑
Hepatocanalicular	N/↑	↑	✓	↑/N	N	↑
Extrahepatic	N/↑	↑	✓	↑/N	N	↑

✓, present; –, absent; ↑, increased; ↓, decreased; ALT, alanine transaminase; N, normal.

Management Options

Prepregnancy

Some causes of jaundice have long-term implications for maternal health and should be discussed prior to pregnancy.

Prenatal

It is important to determine the type of jaundice and its cause. Management depends on the cause and involves interdisciplinary approaches with health professionals from other specialties according to differential diagnosis.

Labor and Delivery

Planned early delivery may be required as "treatment" for some pregnancy-specific causes of jaundice, but is not inevitable. An epidural should not be sited if a coagulopathy or profound thrombocytopenia is present.

Postnatal

Resolution of jaundice should be confirmed. Care should be taken with the use of the oral contraceptive pill. Implications for future pregnancy depend on the cause and should be discussed with the patient.

SUMMARY OF MANAGEMENT OPTIONS

Jaundice

Management Options	Evidence Quality and Recommendation	References
Prepregnancy		
Jaundice due to conditions with implications for pregnancy should be discussed.	—/GPP	—
Prenatal		
Identify the type of jaundice and its cause.	—/GPP	—
Interdisciplinary management depends on cause.	—/GPP	—
Labor and Delivery		
Plan early delivery if this will improve outcome.	—/GPP	—
Avoid regional analgesia if coagulopathy is present.	—/GPP	—
Postnatal		
Confirm resolution of jaundice	—/GPP	—
Long-term management depends on cause.	—/GPP	—

GPP, good practice point.

OBSTETRIC CHOLESTASIS

General

OC affects 0.7% of pregnancies in whites in the United Kingdom and approximately double this proportion of women of South Asian origin.[15,16] It is associated with maternal hepatic impairment and with fetal morbidity and mortality. OC has a complex etiology, with genetic, environmental, and endocrinologic factors playing a role.[17–22]

Women who develop OC are thought to have an increased sensitivity to the cholestatic effect of raised serum estrogens in pregnancy. The condition occurs most commonly in the third trimester when estrogen levels are highest and some women with a previous history of OC develop similar symptoms when taking the oral contraceptive pill[23] or when challenged with exogenous estrogens.[24] It has also been suggested that progesterone may play a role in the etiology of the condition because 34 of 50 women (68%) in a French prospective series of OC cases had been treated with oral micronized natural progesterone for risk of premature delivery.[25]

Diagnosis

The classic maternal symptom of OC is generalized pruritus without a rash. Dark urine, pale stool, or jaundice may also be present, but these are uncommon. If pruritus is associated with abnormal liver transaminases or raised bile acids, OC should be considered. A U.K. study demonstrated that pruritus without hepatic impairment occurs in approximately 50% of pregnancies.[26] Among women with pruritus, 3% had OC (using a diagnosis of pruritus plus raised serum

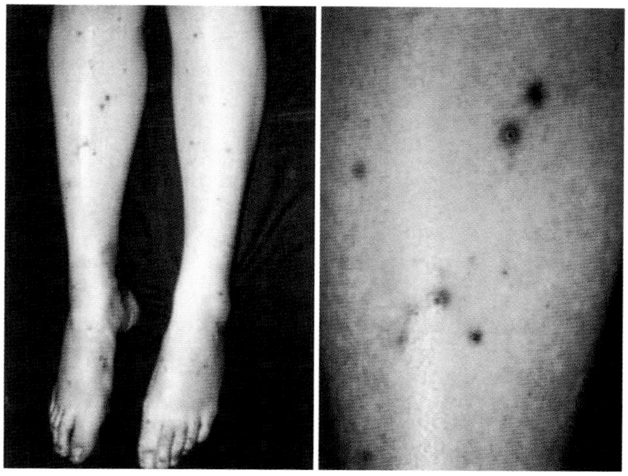

FIGURE 47–2
Dermatologic features observed in obstetric cholestasis cases: Dermatitis artefacta.

transaminases or bile acids), and in this group, the itch was more commonly described as "all over," "on the legs," or "on the palms and soles."

Measurement of bile acids is the most useful test for the diagnosis of OC. In unaffected pregnancies, the levels of serum bile acids change little.[27] The extent of the rise in OC pregnancies is variable and can be marked. A Swedish study of approximately 700 OC pregnancies showed that fetal complications of spontaneous preterm delivery, meconium-stained liquor, and fetal asphyxia occur more commonly in pregnancies in which the fasting serum bile acids are greater than 40 μmol/L[28]; several smaller studies have supported this finding.[29–32] Serum transaminases (ALT and AST) also rise in the majority of cases, but the extent of the rise may not be marked (i.e., two- to threefold). The relative value of serum bile acids, ALT, and AST for the diagnosis of OC is a matter of debate because it is not yet certain which is the best prognostic indicator.[31] In a subgroup of women, the rise in serum bile acids and transaminases can occur up to 15 weeks after the onset of pruritus, so it is advisable to repeat the tests in women with persistent symptoms of OC even if the initial results are normal.[33]

Raised bilirubin can occur in OC, but it is not commonly seen and should not be used alone to make the diagnosis. Alkaline phosphatase rises in the third trimester of normal pregnancies, mainly as a consequence of the placental isoenzyme, and is therefore not of value in the diagnosis of OC. GGT is elevated in approximately 33% of cases.[27]

Women with pruritus and abnormal LFTs should have viral hepatitis (hepatitis A, B, C, CMV, and EBV) and autoimmune hepatitis (antimitochondrial and anti–smooth muscle antibodies) excluded. An ultrasound scan of the liver and biliary tree should be performed to exclude other causes of biliary obstruction. In a study of 227 U.K. cases of OC, gallstones were present in 13%; of these cases, 70% had a history of symptoms of cholelithiasis prior to pregnancy.[34] Asymptomatic gallstones are unlikely to cause OC and are more likely to be present because mutations in at least one gene predispose affected women to both OC and gallstones.[35]

The diagnosis of OC should be one of exclusion and be finally confirmed by resolution of symptoms and biochemical abnormalities postpartum. Antenatally, once the diagnosis of OC has been made, the LFTs, including a PT, should be checked once per week: This will allow monitoring of the decline of serum bile acids or transaminases. It should be borne in mind that some women with other pregnancy disorders (e.g., preeclampsia or AFLP) may present with initial symptoms of pruritus.

It is particularly important to establish whether a woman with OC has hepatitis C, because pregnancies in seropositive women are more likely to be complicated by spontaneous prematurity.[36] In addition, women with hepatitis C infection have a higher prevalence of OC.[36] An additional argument for screening for hepatitis C in women with OC is that treatment with interferon and ribavirin postnatally can be curative.

Maternal and Fetal Risks

Maternal Risks

Pruritus can be a very distressing symptom, and some women may have such marked dermatitis artefacta that they develop permanent scars (see Fig. 47–2). The pruritus and hepatic impairment resolve rapidly after delivery in the majority of cases. If symptoms or biochemical abnormalities persist more than 3 months postpartum, women should be referred to a hepatologist.

There was a 90% risk of recurrence of OC in U.K. cases. Twenty-seven percent of women complained of either cyclical or oral contraceptive-induced pruritus when they were not pregnant.[34] Therefore, women with OC should be advised to avoid estrogen-containing contraceptives. If no alternatives are suitable, the oral contraceptive pill should be introduced only with serial monitoring of LFTs, surveillance for pruritus, and discontinuation if changes develop.

Fetal Risks

OC has been reported to be associated with increased rates of spontaneous prematurity, fetal distress (defined as meconium-stained amniotic fluid or cardiotocography [CTG] abnormalities), and intrauterine death (IUD). However, the rates of these complications vary depending upon the diagnostic criteria used. An increasing number of studies indicate that the level of the serum bile acids is related to the fetal complication rate.[28–30,32] Table 47–4 summarizes the frequency of these complications in each of the studies that have been performed in all successive cases within specific hospitals/regions in which the diagnosis was made using serum bile acids. There is considerable debate about whether the rates of IUD can be decreased with a policy of delivery by 38 weeks' gestation. Some studies revealed that OC-related IUDs cluster at later gestations,[22] and therefore, this policy is relatively prevalent in the United Kingdom. However, there have been no prospective studies to establish whether the policy of early delivery is effective at improving fetal and neonatal outcomes or safety. Some data from in vitro animal studies suggest that ursodeoxycholic acid (UDCA) treatment is safe and may also be protective.[37] Furthermore, UDCA treatment reduced pruritus and maternal serum transaminases, bilirubin, and bile acids in women with serum bile acids greater than 40 μmol/L in a randomized, controlled trial,[38] and the improvement in biochemical abnormalities may further reduce fetal risk.

Iatrogenic prematurity is also more common in OC pregnancies,[34] and it is important not to underestimate the fetal risks of elective delivery at 37 weeks' gestation. A study of neonatal respiratory morbidity following elective cesarean section for all indications reported a higher incidence of respiratory distress syndrome and transient tachypnea of the newborn in those who were delivered during the week 37 + 0 to 37 + 6 compared with 38 + 0 to 38 + 6, and a similar difference was seen when this was compared with deliveries in the following week of gestation.[39]

Management Options

Once the diagnosis of OC has been made, we recommend consideration of delivery between 37 and 38 weeks' gestation in women with raised serum bile acids because this may reduce the risk of IUD. Fetal surveillance can be performed with regular CTG, although there is no evidence that this predicts which pregnancies are at risk of fetal distress or IUD. We recommend that vitamin K, 10 mg orally, should be taken daily to reduce the risk of

TABLE 47-4
Summary of the Major Studies of Fetal Outcome in Obstetric Cholestasis

YEAR	CASES (*N*)	IUD AND/OR NND (%)	MECONIUM STAINING (%)	PRETERM LABOR (%)	PLANNED DELIVERY < 37–38/40 WK*	REFERENCE
1977	55†(m)	0	22	NR	NR	29
	31†(s)	1	43	NR	NR	
1980–1981	96‡(m)	1	8	NR	NR	30
	21‡(s)	0	52	NR	NR	
1989–1997	206	0	16.2	27	Yes	50
1999–2002	409‡(m)	1§	22	2	24%‡	28
	96‡(s)	2	43	16	32%‡	
2000–2007	122	0	13	4	Yes	32
1990–1996	91	0	15	14	Yes	48

* That is, in the majority of cases in the study.
† This study defined mild(m) and severe(s) cholestasis in cases with fasting cholic acid ≤ 15 μmol/L and > 15 μmol/L, respectively.
‡ This study defined mild(m) and severe(s) cholestasis in cases with fasting serum bile acids 10–39 μmol/L and > 40 μmol/L, respectively. The proportions shown indicate the cases in which planned early delivery was reported.
§ There was also a tight knot in the umbilical cord.
IUD, intrauterine death rate as a percentage of all births; NND, neonatal death; NR, not reported.

hemorrhage. UDCA has been shown to improve maternal symptoms and biochemical abnormalities in OC, but there are currently no clinical data on whether it improves fetal outcomes or on safety.

Vitamin K

The active vitamin-K–dependent clotting factors (II, VII, IX, and X) are formed from precursors in the liver, and patients with liver disease are at risk of hemorrhage due to deficiency of these clotting factors. In OC, impaired intestinal absorption secondary to steatorrhea is the most likely cause of vitamin K deficiency, although hepatic impairment may also contribute in some cases. It is possible that the increased prevalence of postpartum hemorrhage in OC is related to vitamin K deficiency, although it is feasible that prematurity, induction of labor, instrumental delivery, or other factors are more relevant.

Ursodeoxycholic Acid

There have been more studies of UDCA than any other drug for the treatment of OC. In the Cochrane Database of Systematic Reviews,[40] three trials totaling 56 women are identified in which UDCA is compared with placebo: In two, there is no difference in relief of symptoms; in one trial, greater reduction in bile salts and liver enzymes was noted with UDCA.[40] When the results of 10 studies with a total of 85 affected women who have been treated with UDCA are combined, 74 (87%) showed clinical or biochemical improvement or both.[41] A more recent study that randomized women with OC to treatment with UDCA, dexamethasone, or placebo only demonstrated benefit in symptoms and biochemical abnormalities in women who received UDCA.[38] In addition, UDCA has been shown to reduce the levels of bile acids in the cord blood and amniotic fluid at the time of delivery.[42] UDCA is commonly started at a dose of 500 mg twice a day, but doses of up to 2000 mg/day were given in several studies, and some women will respond only to higher doses. All babies born to mothers given UDCA were delivered safely, and no problems attributable to treatment have been reported, although there has been no follow-up of these babies.

Dexamethasone

One Finnish case series demonstrated improvement in clinical symptoms and biochemical abnormalities in 10 women with OC who were treated with oral dexamethasone, 12 mg daily, for 7 days, with a gradual reduction in dose over the subsequent 3 days.[43] However, subsequent case reports and case series have not supported this finding.[38,44,45] There have been no long-term studies of the subsequent effects on the child of antenatal exposure to high doses of dexamethasone in the 7- to 10-day regimen used in obstetric cholestasis. However, there are concerns about the potential fetal risks of high doses of antenatal corticosteroids on growth and neuronal development.[46,47]

Other Drugs That Can Be Used to Treat Obstetric Cholestasis

Several other drugs have been used to treat OC, including cholestyramine, *S*-adenosylmethionine, and guar gum (reviewed in Williamson[41]). Although all resulted in clinical improvement in some studies, none of these agents consistently resulted in a biochemical improvement and no studies were powered to show improvement in fetal outcome.[48]

Aqueous cream with menthol often relieves the pruritus for a short time, and some women find this helps them to fall to sleep.

Amniocentesis and Amnioscopy

Meconium staining of the amniotic fluid is reported in almost all cases of IUD that complicate OC in the current literature. Amniocentesis for the presence of meconium has been proposed as the best way to predict the at-risk fetus.[49] No IUDs were reported in a series of 206 women in whom amnioscopy and amniocentesis were used to test for meconium before 37 weeks' gestation as part of a management protocol for OC.[50] However, such an approach may be considered too intrusive to be used routinely by most obstetricians.

SUMMARY OF MANAGEMENT OPTIONS

Obstetric Cholestasis

Management Options	Evidence Quality and Recommendation	References
Prepregnancy		
If previous history of OC, advise of recurrence risk of 90%.	III/B	22,34
Obtain biliary tract ultrasonography to exclude other pathology.	III/B	3
Prenatal		
Confirm the diagnosis with serum bile acid, ALT, or AST measurement.	IIa/B	27–31,33
Monitor serum bile acids in women with a proven diagnosis of OC.	III/B	28–30,32
Exclude viral infection, including hepatitis C, autoimmune hepatitis, and other causes of biliary obstruction.	III/B	34–36
Treat maternal symptoms initially with simple topical measures (e.g., aqueous cream with menthol).	IV/C	22
Consider UDCA 500 mg bid for women with severe symptoms.	Ib/A	38,41
Consider oral vitamin K to reduce risk of PPH.	IV/C	22
Dexamethasone (problem of possible fetal adverse neurologic effects of repeated doses).	IIb/B	41,44,45
Cholestyramine, guar gum.	IV/C	41
Monitor fetal well-being, though it does not predict at-risk fetus.	III/B	16,22
Labor and Delivery		
Consider elective delivery at 37–38 wk.	III/B	16,22
Maintain vigilance for postpartum hemorrhage.	IV/C	22
Postnatal		
Monitor biochemical resolution; generally long-term maternal health and baby health are good.	—/GPP	—
Vitamin K supplement for baby	—/GPP	—
Use oral contraceptives only with close clinical and biochemical monitoring: 27% of cases have cyclical or oral contraceptive-induced pruritus.	III/B	34
Consider referral to hepatologist if symptoms and biochemical abnormalities persist.	—/GPP	—

ALT, alanine aminotransaminase; AST, aspartate aminotransaminase; GPP, good practice point; OC, obstetric cholestasis; UDCA, ursodeoxycholic acid.

ACUTE FATTY LIVER OF PREGNANCY

AFLP is a rare but dangerous disorder. The clinical symptoms and signs are not specific, and because the definition is one of exclusion (rather than inclusion), the diagnosis can be difficult to reach. However, failure to do so may jeopardize the life of the pregnant woman or her fetus.

General

Definition

AFLP may be defined as acute liver failure with reduced hepatic metabolic capacity in the absence of other causes. Histologically, there is panlobular microvesicular steatosis, with sparing of periportal areas and intrahepatic cholestasis: These appearances, which are not unique to AFLP, can be difficult to detect with conventional fixing and staining techniques. The very nature of the illness means that a liver biopsy is often not appropriate. In reviewing the literature, it is clear that subjective diagnoses are often used, and this, in conjunction with the rarity of the condition, makes evidence-based care of women with AFLP challenging. The Swansea criteria (see later) represent a set of standard diagnostic criteria that have recently been validated and, therefore, add some consistency to the diagnosis.[50]

Incidence

The incidence of AFLP has previously been reported to be between 1 in 7000 (diagnosis on clinical criteria alone in 27 of 28 cases)[51] and 1 in 13,000 pregnancies (10 cases, all biopsy-proven).[52] More recently, United Kingdom Obstetric Surveillance System (UKOSS) has reported an incidence of 5 in 100,000 maternities, based on 57 women with AFLP reported during an 18-month period of surveillance of all consultant-led maternity units in the United Kingdom in 2005 and 2006.[53] Approximately three quarters of cases are reported in the third trimester, although it is described as early as 20 weeks, and one quarter in the puerperium. Twin pregnancy is associated with a 14-fold increase in the risk of developing AFLP (odds ratio [OR] 14.3, 95% confidence interval [CI] 6.4–28.6]. AFLP is also more likely in older women and primiparous women.

Diagnosis

The symptoms and signs of AFLP are vague and nonspecific, such that making an early diagnosis is challenging. It is likely that many women experience a prodromal phase in which there is only a gradual deterioration in their condition and when jaundice may not be apparent. In one study, this lasted on average for 9 days (range 1–21 days)[51] prior to the rapid and sometimes catastrophic decline that can occur with AFLP; in the UKOSS study[53] over 80% women experienced a prodromal period. There should be a low threshold for performing LFTs on pregnant women who present in the third trimester with potential prodromal symptoms including new-onset nausea, vomiting, epigastric or right upper quadrant pain, malaise, or polyuria or polydipsia (diabetes insipidus).

The presence of more than 5 Swansea criteria (see later) represents a validated method for supporting the clinical diagnosis of AFLP. Use of these criteria will allow consistency in both clinical management and future research. In the UKOSS study, 55 of the 57 women with AFLP had more than 5 of the 14 criteria present; all 4 women referred to UKOSS, who were deemed on clinical grounds not to have AFLP, had fewer than 5 criteria.

- Vomiting.
- Abdominal pain.
- Polydipsia and polyuria.
- Encephalopathy.
- Elevated transaminases (>42 IU/L; often 3 to 10 times the upper limit of normal; be aware that falling or low levels may be due to very extensive liver damage).
- Elevated bilirubin (>14 μmol/L).
- Hypoglycemia (<4 mmol/L).
- Elevated urate (>340 μmol/L).
- Renal impairment (creatinine > 150 μmol/L).
- Elevated ammonia (>47 μmol/L).
- Leucoytosis (>11 × 10^9/L; often 20–30 × 10^9/L).
- Coagulopathy (PT > 14 sec, activated partial thromboplastin time [aPTT] > 34 sec).
- Ascites or bright liver on ultrasound scan.
- Microvesicular steatosis on liver biopsy.

One of the keys to the diagnosis of AFLP is the rapidity with which LFT can deteriorate in the aggressive phase of the disease. This typically is combined with features of hepatic synthetic failure, including hypoglycemia, deranged clotting, and confusion secondary to hepatic encephalopathy. Other pregnancy-specific liver conditions do not impair liver function in this way. Other causes of fulminating liver failure must be excluded: Paracetamol (acetaminophen) overdose and acute viral hepatitis are the most common causes; rarer causes include Wilson's disease, poisoning with carbon tetrachloride, and drug reactions (e.g., to halothane or isoniazid).

Imaging of the liver has not been successful in accurately detecting fatty infiltration nor, if it is present, in determining its cause. Techniques that have been used include ultrasound, computed tomography (CT), and magnetic resonance imaging (MRI). Apart from ultrasound, it is unlikely that imaging will be either portable or easily accessible to the delivery suite. Abdominal CT is better avoided when possible prior to delivery because of radiation exposure to the fetus, and many pregnant women will be too large to fit inside a standard MRI machine even if they are well enough to be moved there. False-positive and false-negative diagnoses are equally common with all modalities.[54] In the recent UKOSS study,[53] 80% of women had an ultrasound scan, of which only one quarter showed the classic features of bright liver or ascites. If the diagnosis remains in doubt and, in particular, if there is not a rapid improvement after delivery, the place for imaging the liver should be reconsidered.

Liver biopsy is another possibly helpful diagnostic tool. Bearing in mind the histopathologic caveats outlined earlier and the potential complexities of performing a biopsy in the presence of deranged clotting, the need for a tissue diagnosis should be carefully assessed on an individual basis.

Maternal and Fetal Risks

Women experiencing AFLP have increased maternal and fetal mortality and morbidity. However, it is likely that the outcome for mother and baby has improved in recent years. In the 1960s, 16 cases of AFLP associated with the use of tetracycline were reported, with a 70% maternal mortality.[55] Among 33 pregnancies with biopsy-proven AFLP reported in the 1980s, maternal mortality was 21% and fetal mortality was 27%.[56] Castro and associates in the 1990s[51] reported 28 clinically diagnosed cases with no maternal mortality and a 7% neonatal mortality. The UKOSS report,[53] which is the most robust and recent series of cases, gives maternal mortality of 2% (1 death in 57 cases) and 10% fetal mortality. There is an ongoing need for all obstetricians, anesthetists, and midwives to be aware of AFLP, not just those working in large tertiary referral centers.

Etiology

The cause of AFLP is uncertain, but is likely to be multifactorial, with a genetic component in a number of cases. In some women, AFLP may occur because of an autosomal recessive abnormality in fetal long-chain fatty acid beta oxidation. This is an interesting concept, because it demonstrates that the fetus may determine maternal complications of pregnancy. In addition, for these families, the risk of recurrence is significant and in the order of 15% to 20%.

Long-chain hydroxyacyl coenzyme A dehydrogenase (LCHAD) deficiency is a recently described disorder of mitochondrial fatty acid oxidation that is usually asymptomatic in heterozygous carriers. Affected (homozygous) individuals often die in early childhood or sooner from complications of hypoglycemia, cardiomyopathy, or fatty liver failure. Those who live longer develop chorioretinopathy, rhabdomyolysis, and peripheral neuropathy, although these can be ameliorated by a high-carbohydrate and low-fat diet, in which the fat component is medium-chain triglycerides. Several mutations of the α-subunit of the mitochondrial trifunctional protein cause deficiency of LCHAD. In Finland, a guanine cytosine transposition, G1528C, and in America, a glutamic acid to glutamine change, E474Q, have been identified.[57,58] The latter group estimates that 1 in 175 of their population is heterozygous for E474Q and, therefore, that 1 in 62,000 pregnancies results in LCHAD deficiency. Affected fetuses do not metabolize long-chain fatty acids completely, resulting in accumulation of abnormal and highly toxic intermediates in the heterozygous mother's liver, and the acute clinical picture we recognize as AFLP. It is also hypothesized that fat accumulation may occur in the placenta and that this may induce the clinical picture of preeclampsia. Preeclampsia has been described in pregnancies with fetuses affected by homozygous LCHAD deficiency more commonly than would be expected, and more than in pregnancies in the same women with unaffected fetuses.[59]

It is not certain what proportion of cases of AFLP may be due to LCHAD deficiency. It is likely that this will vary between countries, depending in part on the prevalence of the known (and unknown) genetic mutations in the local populations. Mansouri and colleagues[60] reported no carriers of the G1528C mutation in 14 histologically proven cases of AFLP, but Treem and coworkers[61] found that 75% of 12 women with AFLP had LCHAD levels compatible with carrier status. A larger study identified LCHAD mutations in 5 of 27 women with AFLP, all of whom had a fetus with LCHAD deficiency.[62] All 5 affected fetuses had at least one copy of the E474Q mutation, and the authors therefore recommended screening for this mutation in the children of women who have had pregnancies complicated by AFLP. In contrast, the same study demonstrated that only 1 of 81 women with HELLP had an LCHAD mutation, and this was not inherited by the fetus, indicating that it is not justified to screen the offspring from all pregnancies affected by HELLP.

Conversely, not all pregnancies in which the baby has LCHAD deficiency will result in AFLP or other serious maternal liver disease. Ibdah and colleagues[63] found that in 15 of 24 pregnancies in which the baby had LCHAD deficiency, either AFLP (n = 12) or HELLP (n = 3) syndrome developed; in the other 9 pregnancies, there were no complications. These women had 11 other pregnancies with unaffected babies in which maternal liver disease did not occur. Similarly, Tyni and associates[59] found some form of liver disease of pregnancy and/or preeclampsia in 15 of 29 pregnancies in which the fetus was homozygous for LCHAD deficiency and described 7 of the remaining 14 pregnancies as completely normal; none of the other 34 pregnancies from these women (when the fetus did not have homozygous LCHAD deficiency) was complicated by significant liver disease.

Management Options

The ultimate management option is to deliver the baby, because this seems to be the optimal way to improve the maternal condition and to protect the fetus. The decision to deliver brings with it a not uncommon conundrum for obstetricians: A vaginal delivery minimizes the risk of maternal hemorrhage in the face of a coagulopathy but may take several hours or longer to achieve, and this could be significantly detrimental to the mother or fetus; a cesarean section allows delivery to be achieved more quickly but may be complicated by bleeding. An individual decision regarding the severity of the maternal and fetal conditions needs to be made. Often, induction of labor can be started while the maternal condition is stabilized and blood products made available, and then the ongoing management can be reviewed according to the current balance of concerns. A further challenge is the best choice of analgesia and anesthesia, because regional blockade may be contraindicated if coagulopathy ensues, but general anesthesia can worsen hepatic encephalopathy.

From the maternal perspective, she should have one-to-one nursing on the delivery suite, preferably in a high-dependency area. All vital signs should be measured and recorded clearly on a 24-hour spread sheet; it is usually advisable to insert a central line early in the course of the disease before coagulopathy ensues. Glucose assessments should be made at least every 2 hours, and hypoglycemia treated with large doses of high-concentration intravenous glucose via a long line. PT should also be measured every 6 hours along with LFTs, renal function tests and electrolytes, and full blood count. Formal assessment of level of consciousness must be made hourly, because hepatic coma is a potential complication of AFLP.

One of the keys to successful management is a multidisciplinary approach. Senior obstetric, anesthesiology, hematology, and hepatology colleagues should be involved at an early stage. If no hepatologists are in-house, the obstetrician should liaise directly with the nearest liver transplant unit. This serves several purposes: (1) it provides expert advice on both the investigations and the management and (2) it alerts the transplant team who are usually able to accept transfer after delivery if recovery does not commence. Most women will be transferred from the delivery suite to the intensive care unit after delivery.

Follow-up and Recurrence

Once they have recovered, all women affected by AFLP should have the opportunity with their partners to be debriefed about the complications of their pregnancy. In women who survive and do not need a transplant, complete recovery of the liver is expected without long-term sequelae.

Pediatricians should consider screening all babies of women with AFLP for LCHAD deficiency, either by measuring LCHAD activity in cultured skin fibroblasts or liver or by doing DNA studies looking for the common mutations. Affected babies should be placed on the appropriate dietary restrictions. Not only does this screening minimize the complications for the index baby, but also it allows the couple to make an informed choice about the risks to the mother and fetus in a future pregnancy.

The risk of recurrence of AFLP depends largely on whether the baby has LCHAD deficiency. If he or she does, the rate is between 15% and 25% for future pregnancies from the same partnership; if the baby does not, then the recurrence risk is very much lower, although it is difficult to give a precise figure because so many women decide against a further pregnancy.

When a woman has had an affected baby previously, prenatal diagnosis of LCHAD is possible in subsequent pregnancies by enzyme assay in amniocytes[64] or DNA analysis from chorionic villus sampling (CVS).[63]

SUMMARY OF MANAGEMENT OPTIONS

Acute Fatty Liver of Pregnancy

Management Options	Evidence Quality and Recommendation	References
Prepregnancy		
None, unless previous pregnancy is affected, in which case, confirm previous diagnosis, check LFTs, advise risk of recurrence.	IV/C	56
Consider screening for LCHAD deficiency.	III/B	59,63
Prenatal		
If previous AFLP, check baseline LFT; advise to report any new symptoms; start home testing for urinary protein from 24 wk; monitor BP every 2 wk.	—/GPP	—
Establish diagnosis, resuscitate.	—/GPP	—
Intensive care/high dependency setting	—/GPP	—
Provide supportive therapy (see "Labor and Delivery").	—/GPP	—
Plan delivery or end pregnancy.	—/GPP	—
Labor and Delivery		
Maternal resuscitation by correction of • Hypoglycemia. • Fluid balance. • Coagulopathy.	—/GPP	—
Use multidisciplinary approach ideally in liaison with liver unit to manage liver failure.	—/GPP	—
Use intensive fetal monitoring.	—/GPP	—
Perform urgent delivery when maternal condition is stabilized, vaginal delivery preferable for mother.	—/GPP	—
Maintain meticulous hemostasis.	—/GPP	—
Postnatal		
Continue intensive care management	—/GPP	—
Watch for postpartum wound hematoma formation and sepsis, postpartum hemorrhage.	—/GPP	—
Recurrence risk is difficult to estimate, perhaps as high as 10%–20%.	—/GPP	—
Support contraceptive measures.	—/GPP	—
Full hepatic recovery expected without further sequelae; occasionally emergency liver transplant needed.	—/GPP	—
Pediatricians to consider screening baby for LCHAD deficiency.	—/GPP	—
Prenatal diagnosis of LCHAD possible by amniocentesis/CVS if previous baby affected.	III/B	63,64

AFLP, acute fatty liver of pregnancy; BP, blood pressure; CVS, chorionic villus sampling; GPP, good practice point; LCHAD, long-chain hydroxyacyl coenzyme A dehydrogenase; LFT, liver function test.

LIVER HEMATOMA AND NONTRAUMATIC LIVER RUPTURE

General

Liver hematoma is an uncommon and potentially dangerous problem in pregnancy, its most hazardous complication being hepatic rupture. Rupture of the liver capsule occurs in between 1 in 45,000 and 1 in 225,000 deliveries.[65,66]

The vast majority of cases are reported in association with preeclampsia, and a very high proportion are in multiparous women older than 30 years. Only a few cases have been described in the puerperium following a normal pregnancy.[67] In over 85% of cases, the right lobe of the liver is affected. Rinehart and coworkers[68] reviewed the literature and presented figures for the common symptoms and signs of hepatic rupture. Not surprisingly, they found that almost 70% of patients had epigastric pain, 65% had hypertension, and over 50% were shocked. However, there was a wide range of other presentations, including some women with mild symptoms prior to massive circulatory collapse. HELLP syndrome seems to be particularly associated with intrahepatic hemorrhage, subcapsular hematoma, and capsular rupture.

The pathogenesis is debated. One attractive theory suggests that preeclampsia causes hepatic ischemia via intravascular volume depletion, which results in local necrosis and hemorrhage. Subsequently, neovascularization occurs, and these vessels are especially susceptible to rupture and further hemorrhage, particularly during hypertensive episodes. Subcapsular hematoma may then expand sufficiently to result in hepatic rupture.[68]

FIGURE 47–3
Liver hematoma.

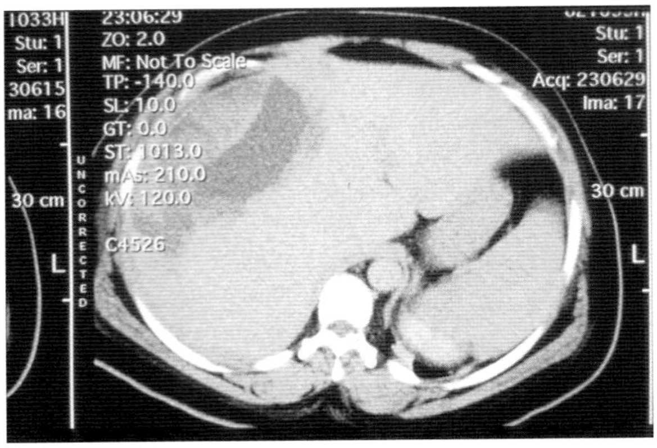

Maternal and Fetal Risks

Hepatic rupture is dangerous for mother and baby. Maternal mortality is between 16% and 60%, and perinatal mortality is between 40% and 60%.[69,70] Current management options have contributed greatly to lowering the mortality rates.

Management Options

The management will obviously be determined by the seriousness of the situation. There should be a low threshold for imaging the liver in older, multiparous women with preeclampsia and epigastric pain. Ultrasound will usually be readily available and is helpful in diagnosing subcapsular hematomas. CT (Fig. 47–3) and MRI hepatic digital subtraction angiography may have greater sensitivity for identifying small amounts of intraperitoneal blood and small hematomas but have the disadvantage of being less readily available and less portable if the patient is unwell.

Treatment of hepatic rupture is based on resuscitating the patient and stopping the hemorrhage. If the diagnosis is suspected, a midline laparotomy with the involvement of an experienced surgeon should be considered: This allows the diagnosis to be confirmed, the baby to be delivered (which will improve the maternal circulation and remove the baby to a place of safety), and treatment to be instituted. If unexplained hemoperitoneum is found at a Pfannenstiel laparotomy for presumed abruption or uterine rupture, careful exploration of the upper abdomen, preferably by an experienced general or hepatic surgeon and possibly with an upper midline incision to improve access, must be strongly considered.

A wide variety of therapeutic maneuvers for liver rupture have been described. Currently, the most successful seem to involve digital compression of the hepatic artery and portal vein to temporarily arrest the hemorrhage (Pringle's maneuver),[69] evacuation of the residual hematoma, and temporary packing with large dry gauze swabs.[71] Packs are removed at a further laparotomy 24 to 36 hours later, once correction of hypovolemia, coagulopathy, acidosis, and hypothermia is complete. Liver resection and transplantation have also been described, but not surprisingly, the mortality rate is very high.

Unruptured small hematomas have been managed conservatively, following delivery of the baby, with serial imaging of their size to exclude expansion.[69] Delayed rupture 6 weeks after initial diagnosis has been reported,[72] so care must be taken if this option is adopted. Tense, large, or expanding hematomas should probably be evacuated surgically to obviate the impending rupture. Hepatic embolization has been described in these circumstances (and in others) but seems to carry a high risk of ischemic necrosis of the liver, liver failure, and sepsis[73] and may not be accessible to many units; others have described this technique as a "gold standard."[67]

SUMMARY OF MANAGEMENT OPTIONS

Liver Hematoma and Rupture

Management Options	Evidence Quality and Recommendation	References
Prepregnancy		
None.	—/GPP	—
Prenatal		
Treat upper abdominal discomfort seriously, especially in parous women with PET or HELLP; consider imaging the liver.	—/GPP	—
Labor and Delivery		
Consider liver rupture in a woman with unexplained shock or if unexpected hemoperitoneum is found at cesarean section.	—/GPP	—

Management Options	Evidence Quality and Recommendation	References
Management:		
• Resuscitation.	—/GPP	—
• Laparotomy and stop hemorrhage (by liver surgeon preferably) with temporary occlusion of portal vein and packing.	IV/C	69,71
• Embolization has varied success.	III/B	67,73
• Manage unruptured hematomas conservatively (though danger of delayed rupture).	IV/C	69
Postnatal		
Patients who survive do not have permanent liver damage.	—/GPP	—
Recurrence has been recorded but very rarely.	—/GPP	—

HELLP, hemolysis, elevated liver enzymes, low platelets; GPP, good practice point; PET, preeclampsia.

HYPEREMESIS GRAVIDARUM

General

Nausea and vomiting affect up to 50% of pregnant women. Most women are able to maintain fluid and nutrient intake by dietary modification, and the symptoms will resolve by the end of the first trimester. Hyperemesis gravidarum affects 0.5% to 1% of pregnancies and causes severe and protracted vomiting that results in ketosis, dehydration, and weight loss. The cause of hyperemesis gravidarum remains unidentified, but it is thought to result from a combination of endocrine, biochemical, and psychological factors. Seropositivity for *Helicobacter pylori* is more common in women with hyperemesis than in controls.[74,75]

Diagnosis

The onset of hyperemesis gravidarum is always in the first trimester. In addition to nausea, vomiting, and weight loss, women often report ptyalism (excessive salivation), and there may be signs of dehydration, including postural hypotension and tachycardia. Hyperemesis gravidarum is a diagnosis of exclusion (Table 47–5), and it is important to make a thorough clinical assessment and to ensure that investigations are performed for common and serious causes of vomiting.

An ultrasound of the uterus should be performed to confirm pregnancy, to establish the number of fetuses, and to exclude hydatidiform mole.

Laboratory investigations commonly reveal hyponatremia, hypokalemia, and raised hematocrit. A biochemical hyperthyroidism and abnormal LFTs may also be present. These are both markers of the severity of the disease and resolve with successful treatment. Women with biochemical hyperthyroidism should be examined for signs of hyperthyroidism, but these are rarely present.

Maternal and Fetal Risks

Maternal Risks

Serious maternal morbidity and mortality may result if hyperemesis gravidarum is not managed correctly. Wernicke's encephalopathy can develop as a result of thiamine (vitamin B_1) deficiency. This is associated with diplopia, sixth nerve palsy, nystagmus, ataxia, and confusion. If untreated, Wernicke's encephalopathy may lead to Korsakoff's psychosis (amnesia, impaired ability to learn) or death. Other vitamin deficiencies may occur, for example, peripheral neuropathy and anemia may result from deficiency of vitamins B_{12} and B_6.

TABLE 47–5

Differential Diagnosis of Hyperemesis Gravidarum

SYSTEM	DIAGNOSIS	INVESTIGATION/INITIAL ASSESSMENT
Genitourinary	Urinary tract infection	Mid-stream urine specimen
	Uremia	Urea and electrolytes
	Molar pregnancy	Ultrasound of the uterus
Gastrointestinal	Gastritis/peptic ulceration	*Helicobacter pylori* antibodies
	Pancreatitis	Amylase, blood glucose, calcium
	Bowel obstruction	Plain supine abdominal radiograph
Endocrine	Addison's disease	Urea and electrolytes, early-morning cortisol, short synacthen test with ACTH
	Hyperthyroidism	Surveillance for symptoms and signs of hyperthyroidism, TFTs, thyroid autoantibodies
	Diabetic ketoacidosis	Blood glucose, urinary dipstick for ketones, glucose tolerance test
CNS	Intracranial tumor	CNS examination, brain imaging
	Vestibular disease	CNS examination
Drug-induced	–	Discontinue agent

ACTH, adrenocorticotrophic hormone; CNS, central nervous system; TFT, thyroid function test.

Hyponatremia (plasma sodium < 120 mmol/L) can cause confusion, seizures, and respiratory arrest. If hyponatremia is severe, or if it is treated too rapidly, women may develop central pontine myelinolysis. This is caused by symmetrical destruction of myelin at the center of the basal pons and can result in pyramidal tract signs, spastic quadraparesis, pseudobulbar palsy, and impaired consciousness.

Other risks include deep venous thrombosis that may result from dehydration and reduced mobility, Mallory-Weiss tear due to prolonged vomiting, and muscle wasting with weakness.

Fetal Risks

The infants of women with hyperemesis gravidarum with low pregnancy weight gain (<7 kg) are more likely to be small for gestational age and to be born before 37 weeks' gestation.[76] These poor outcomes were not seen in the offspring of women with hyperemesis who gained 7 kg or more in pregnancy. If the mother develops Wernicke's encephalopathy, the fetal outcome is worse; of 45 cases in the published literature, only 44% were reported as having been born alive.[77]

Management Options

Rehydration and Vitamin Supplementation

Fluid replacement therapy should be with either normal saline (NaCl 0.9%; 150 mmol/L Na^+) or Hartmann's solution (NaCl 0.6%; 131 mmol/L Na^+). Dextrose-containing fluids should not be used because they do not contain sufficient sodium to correct hyponatremia, and Wernicke's encephalopathy can be precipitated by intravenous dextrose and carbohydrate-rich foods. Double-strength saline should not be used to correct hyponatremia in hyperemesis gravidarum, because central pontine myelinolysis can occur if the serum sodium level is corrected too rapidly. Potassium supplements should be added to the intravenous fluid replacement therapy as required. Thiamine supplements should be given, as a daily dose of either 50 to 150 mg orally or 100 mg diluted in 100 mL normal saline as an intravenous infusion.

Urine output should be monitored and dipsticks used to assess ketonuria. Women should be weighed on admission and regularly thereafter if their symptoms do not resolve. Serial assessments of electrolytes should be carried out.

Antiemetics

There is no evidence for teratogenicity following treatment with dopamine antagonists (metoclopramide, domperidone),[78,79] phenothiazines (chlorpromazine, prochlorperazine),[80,81] anticholinergics (dicyclomine),[82] or antihistamine H_1-receptor antagonists (promethazine, cyclizine). One of these should be tried in the first instance. Women with hyperemesis often find nonoral preparations preferable.

In women with severe hyperemesis who have not responded to these antiemetic therapies, promising results have been reported with both corticosteroids and 5-hydroxytryptamine$_3$ (5-HT_3) receptor antagonists (ondansetron, cisapride).

Corticosteroids

Corticosteroids have been reported to be an effective treatment for hyperemesis gravidarum in several case reports.[83–85] In an American double-blind study of 40 women with hyperemesis who were randomized to receive either oral methylprednisolone 16 mg or oral promethazine 25 mg (three times daily for both), the response to both drugs was similar after 2 days, but no women who received methylprednisolone were readmitted within 1 week of discharge. In contrast, 5 (25%) women who received promethazine were readmitted with hyperemesis.[86] A British double-blind study of 25 women who were randomized to receive either 40 mg prednisolone or placebo daily demonstrated a trend toward improved nausea and vomiting and reduced dependence on intravenous fluids, but this did not reach statistical significance.[87] However, steroid therapy did result in an improved sense of well-being, improved appetite, and weight gain compared with placebo.[87] Overall, the studies of corticosteroid treatment for hyperemesis suggest that the treatment is effective for some patients. We recommend starting intravenous hydrocortisone 100 mg three times a day in women with severe and resistant symptoms who are unable to tolerate fluids, followed by prednisolone 40 mg once daily. This should be reduced by approximately 5 mg every 5 days, provided symptoms are controlled.

5-Hydroxytryptamine Receptor Antagonists

Ondansetron is a 5-HT_3 receptor antagonist and a potent antiemetic drug for the treatment of chemotherapy-associated and postoperative nausea. It has been used to treat hyperemesis successfully in several case reports, in which it was given for between 2 and 19 weeks.[88–90] In all cases, there were no known adverse fetal events. One double-blind, controlled trial in which 30 patients were randomized to receive either 10 mg intravenous ondansetron or 50 mg intravenous promethazine failed to demonstrate any significant difference in the degree of nausea, weight gain, or days of hospitalization between the two groups.[91] However, the entry criteria for this study were less stringent than for the randomized, double-blind studies of corticosteroid treatment for hyperemesis gravidarum.[86,87] Therefore, it remains likely that ondansetron may be an effective treatment for women with more severe disease.

Other Treatment Options

There has been one double-blind, randomized, cross-over trial of the efficacy of powdered root ginger and placebo in which women reported a reduced severity and greater relief of symptoms in the period in which ginger was given and no side effects were observed.[92] Several authors have reported success in managing severe hyperemesis gravidarum using enteral and parenteral nutrition.[93–95] However, because the complications can be serious, such treatment is usually reserved for women whose symptoms are sufficiently severe as to be life-threatening to the mother. In one series of 16 cases with good pregnancy outcomes, there were 3 cases of line sepsis and pneumothorax, thrombosis, and dislodgement of the line.[95]

It is advisable to give thromboembolic deterrent stockings and thromboprophylaxis such as enoxaparine 40 mg daily to women with hyperemesis while they are inpatients.

SUMMARY OF MANAGEMENT OPTIONS

Hyperemesis Gravidarum

Management Options	Evidence Quality and Recommendation	References
Prepregnancy		
Discuss recurrence risk.	—/GPP	—
Give advice on treatment options and provide psychological support at an early stage.	—/GPP	—
Give folate supplements.	—/GPP	—
Prenatal		
Remember alternative diagnoses.	—/GPP	—
Rehydrate with intravenous fluid and electrolyte therapy.	—/GPP	—
Supplement nutrients and vitamins (especially thiamine).	—/GPP	—
Consult dietician, provide parenteral nutrition in extreme cases.	III/B	93–95
Provide psychological and social support.	—/GPP	—
Provide thromboprophylaxis.	—/GPP	—
Treatment:		
• First line = conventional antiemetics.	III/B	77–81
• Alternative agent = corticosteroids.	Ib/A	83–87
• Alternative agent = $5\text{-}HT_3$ antagonist if no response.	Ib/A	88–91
Antigastroesophageal reflux measures may help some.	—/GPP	—
Provide fetal growth surveillance	—/GPP	—
Labor and Delivery		
Women on corticosteroids prenatally should have intravenous hydrocortisone to cover labor/delivery.	—/GPP	—
Postnatal		
Review nutritional status.	—/GPP	—
Wean off steroids; most will not need short synacthen test to exclude adrenal suppression.	—/GPP	—
Discuss contraception.	—/GPP	—

GPP, good practice point; $5\text{-}HT_3$, 5-hydroxytryptamine$_3$.

PEPTIC ULCERATION

General

Dyspepsia is common, affecting up to 50% of pregnant women.[96] It usually worsens as pregnancy progresses, and it is more prevalent in women who are older, multiparous, or carrying multiple pregnancy or have a prepregnancy history of heartburn.[97]

Peptic ulceration, affecting the stomach, duodenum, or lower esophagus is uncommon in pregnancy.[98] In the absence of nonsteroidal anti-inflammatory drug (NSAID) use, nearly all duodenal and most stomach ulceration is caused by *H. pylori*. Eradication of *H. pylori* is very successful in curing peptic ulcer disease and reduces recurrence of ulceration and prevents rebleeding. In pregnancy, some women with established peptic ulcer disease report symptomatic improvement. This is thought to be secondary to reduced gastric acid output and increased protective mucus production associated with raised progesterone levels, in addition to a healthier diet and increased medical supervision.

Diagnosis

It is important to have a high index of suspicion for peptic ulcer disease because the classic symptoms of epigastric pain, nausea, and dyspepsia may be absent or confused with normal features of pregnancy. Also, symptoms may not correlate with severity of disease. Patients who are smokers and have a previous history of peptic ulcer disease or previous NSAID use are at highest risk.

Investigations should include blood tests for hemoglobin, electrolytes, and serum amylase as well as LFTs. An abdominal ultrasound is useful to exclude cholelithiasis and pancreatitis secondary to gallstones. However, if peptic ulcer

TABLE 47–6
Therapeutic Options for *Helicobacter Pylori* in Pregnancy

	ANTIBIOTIC		
ACID SUPPRESSANT	AMOXYCILLIN	CLARITHROMYCIN	METRONIDAZOLE
Omeprazole 20 mg bid	1 g bid	500 mg bid	–
Omeprazole 20 mg bid	500 mg tid	–	400 mg tid
Omeprazole 20 mg bid	–	500 mg bid	400 mg bid

bid, twice a day; tid, three times a day.
Modified from the British National Formulary, No. 59, 2010, www.bnf.org.

disease is suspected from the history and examination, *H. pylori* antibodies should be measured, and if a woman has positive serology, treatment should be considered (Table 47–6). Although endoscopy is the investigation of choice outside pregnancy and is safe in pregnancy,[99] too few cases have been reported for the frequency of complications to be assessed. However, endoscopy does allow direct visualization of upper gastrointestinal tract pathology, permits biopsies to be taken for histopathology, and provides a therapeutic option (e.g., injection of adrenaline for acute bleeding ulcers).

Zollinger-Ellison Syndrome

This syndrome is caused by pancreatic gastrin-secreting tumors that result in a marked increase in gastric acid secretion. If untreated, the condition causes severe gastroesophageal reflux, peptic ulceration, and malabsorption, and therefore, the acid secretion usually requires treatment. There have been reports of the successful management of Zollinger-Ellison syndrome in pregnancy.[100,101]

Maternal and Fetal Risks

Maternal Risks

Complications of peptic ulcer disease in the general, nonpregnant population include bleeding and perforation. These are rarely reported in pregnancy.

Acute gastrointestinal bleeding presents with hematemesis, melena, or the passage of fresh blood from the rectum. It can be associated with hypotension and tachycardia and may result in anemia. It is important to insert a nasogastric tube if gastrointestinal bleeding is suspected. This will allow upper and lower gastrointestinal bleeding to be distinguished and will help to ensure a clear view for endoscopy. When endoscopy is performed, pregnant women should be placed in the left lateral position to reduce inferior vena caval obstruction and reduced venous return. Large-bore cannulae should be sited, the woman should be fasting, and a transfusion should be commenced if acute bleeding is confirmed and the clinical scenario warrants it.

Ulcer perforation is rare in pregnancy. Clinical features include abdominal pain with abdominal guarding and rebound tenderness, nausea, vomiting, pyrexia, dehydration, hypotension, and a leukocytosis. If suspected, an abdominal or chest radiograph should be performed to investigate for the presence of pneumoperitoneum or free gas in the abdomen.

Fetal Risks

The fetus may be compromised if there is major maternal hemorrhage or perforation of a peptic ulcer. Otherwise, few fetal risks arise from the drugs are used to treat peptic ulcer disease, with the exception of sodium bicarbonate–containing preparations and misoprostol (see the subsequent section on "Misoprostol").

Management Options

Antacids, H_2-antagonists, or proton pump inhibitors can be used to treat established peptic ulcer disease in pregnancy, including Zollinger-Ellison syndrome. If gastrointestinal bleeding is present, therapeutic endoscopy or surgery is indicated, and perforation requires surgical management.

Antacids

Aluminum- and magnesium-containing antacids are generally considered to be safe in pregnancy and breastfeeding,[102,103] as are the nonabsorbed alginate-containing drugs such as Gaviscon[104] and the mucosal protective agent sucralfate.[105] Magnesium-based antacids may be preferred to aluminum-based ones, because the latter can be associated with constipation. Sodium bicarbonate–containing antacids should be avoided because they may cause respiratory alkalosis and fluid overload in the mother and fetus.[106]

Acid-Suppressing Drugs

Several studies have indicated that H_2-receptor antagonists[107–110] and proton pump inhibitors[108–111] are safe in pregnancy. Three studies have compared the rate of congenital malformations in pregnancies in which there was first-trimester exposure to either H_2-receptor antagonists or omeprazole. A Swedish cohort study in which H_2-receptor antagonists had been taken in 255 pregnancies, proton pump inhibitors in 275, and both in 20 pregnancies did not demonstrate an increased rate of congenital malformation compared with all births at that time.[108] Similar results were found in a study of 447 British and 108 Italian women with first-trimester exposure to ranitidine, cimetidine, or omeprazole.[110] Similarly, there was no evidence of increased risk of major malformations in a prospective, multicenter, controlled study in which two groups of 113 women were treated with either omeprazole or H_2-receptor antagonists and compared with the same number of controls.[109]

Less is known about lansoprazole than omeprazole, but there has been one reassuring report of good fetal outcomes with lansoprazole treatment in six cases in which there was first-trimester exposure.[112]

One prospective, controlled, multicenter study of the use of cisapride, a 5-HT_3 receptor antagonist for the treatment of gastroesophageal reflux, gastrointestinal pain, and duodenal ulcer in pregnancy, showed no increase in the rate of major or minor malformations nor fetal distress.[113]

Triple Therapy for Helicobacter Pylori

If peptic ulcer disease is suspected, serology should be sent for *H. pylori* antibodies. If a woman has distressing symptoms, appropriate therapy will eradicate the infection and may improve the symptoms. Of the recommended therapeutic regimens at the time of writing, only three include the use of omeprazole (see Table 47–6). The others advise the use of alternative acid-suppressant drugs, about which there is little experience in pregnancy. We therefore recommend that one of the three regimens outlined in Table 47–6 be used for 7 days. The regimens containing amoxycillin are recommended for community-based use. Studies of the incidence of congenital abnormalities and adverse pregnancy outcomes in women who have taken these antibiotics indicate that there is no increased risk for amoxycillin,[114] clarithromycin,[115] or metronidazole.[116,117]

Misoprostol

Misoprostol is a synthetic prostaglandin E_1 analogue that has antisecretory and protective properties believed to promote healing of peptic ulcers. However, its use is contraindicated in pregnancy because it is a potent stimulant of uterine contractions and can induce spontaneous abortion or uterine bleeding. It is also teratogenic.[118–120]

Therapeutic Endoscopy and Surgery

There is very little experience of therapeutic endoscopy in pregnancy. Of four cases in the literature, thermocoagulation was performed in one for bleeding duodenal ulcer,[99] sclerotherapy for bleeding duodenal ulcer was performed in two,[99,121] and sclerotherapy for a bleeding Mallory-Weiss tear in the fourth.[122] The fetal outcome in three cases was good and was not specifically reported in the fourth.[122]

The indications for surgery are the same as in the nonpregnant patient. A perforated ulcer requires emergency surgery, and the patient should receive broad-spectrum antibiotics. Surgery should also be performed in patients with hemorrhage from peptic ulcers if they have not responded to a transfusion of 6 units of blood.

SUMMARY OF MANAGEMENT OPTIONS

Peptic Ulceration

Management Options	Evidence Quality and Recommendation	References
Prepregnancy		
Advise against agents that may exacerbate peptic ulcer disease (e.g., alcohol, smoking).	—/GPP	—
If taking bicarbonate-containing antacids or misoprostol, advise cessation of treatment.	III/B	118–120
Perform investigations to establish the cause of peptic ulceration.	—/GPP	—
Anticipate improvement in clinical symptoms with pregnancy.	—/GPP	—
Aluminum- and magnesium-containing antacids, mucosal protective agents, and histamine receptor blockers are safe in pregnancy.	IIb/B	102–105
Avoid bicarbonate-containing antacids (danger of respiratory alkalosis and fluid overload).	IV/C	105
Consider anti-*Helicobacter* treatment with positive immunologic diagnosis and if other therapy has been ineffective.	—/GPP	—
Endoscopy is also safe with an experienced operator if no response to medical management; surgery is rarely required and mainly needed for those with severe bleeding/perforation.	—/GPP	—
Postnatal		
Symptoms of dyspepsia are likely to improve postnatally.	—/GPP	—
Repeat endoscopy if indicated by initial findings.	—/GPP	—

GPP, good practice point.

CELIAC DISEASE

General

Definition and Incidence

Celiac disease, or gluten-sensitive enteropathy, is a common disorder in which gluten-containing foods trigger inflammation of the jejunal mucosa that improves when a gluten-free diet is taken. In England, it occurs in 1 in 1000, and in Ireland, in 1 in 300 individuals,[123] although more may have silent or undiagnosed celiac disease. It seems to be rare in black Africans, although this may reflect reporting bias. The cause is multifactorial. There is a genetic component, with 10% to 15% of first-degree relatives being affected.[124] However, 30% of identical twins are discordant,[125] suggesting additional factors are involved, such as viral infection.

Etiology

Gluten is present in the cereals wheat, barley, and rye, but not oats. There are four main gluten fractions, but α-gliadin is the most damaging to small intestine mucosa. The enzyme tissue transglutaminase, the main antigen of the endomysial antibody, modifies gliadin and enhances gliadin-specific T-cell responses in genetically predisposed individuals. This is one of several immunologic abnormalities that revert to normal when a gluten-free diet is assumed. Histologically, the small bowel shows partial villus atrophy, with crypt hypertrophy and chronic inflammatory changes, the extent of the damage decreasing toward the ileum as gluten is progressively digested into smaller and less damaging moieties.

Diagnosis

Clinically, celiac disease presents at any age and is more common in females than in males. The symptoms are variable and may include tiredness and malaise (often in conjunction with anemia), diarrhea, steatorrhea, abdominal pain or bloating, weight loss, mouth ulcers, osteoporosis, and neurologic symptoms from folate, B_6, or B_{12} deficiency. In pregnancy, the most common presentation is with nonspecific symptoms without overt malabsorption or with anemia.

A new diagnosis of celiac disease should be considered in pregnant women with iron-deficiency anemia or in the presence of otherwise unexplained folate- or B_{12}-deficiency anemia. There should be a low threshold for investigating unexplained iron-deficiency anemia, diarrhea, or weight loss in pregnancy, especially if the anemia responds poorly to iron supplementation or if folate or B_{12} deficiency is also present. In a study of premenopausal nonpregnant women, 1 in 16 asymptomatic but anemic volunteer blood donors were found to have celiac disease.[126] Among anemic pregnant women, 1 in 43 were found to have antiendomysial antibodies, although apparently none was investigated further for celiac disease.[127] The diagnosis of celiac disease is confirmed by finding endomysial, gliadin, or tissue transglutaminase antibodies, which have high specificity and sensitivity. Outside pregnancy, a jejunal biopsy is usually obtained. Within pregnancy, most experts feel that this is best avoided, although duodenoscopy can be performed if clinically indicated.

It is important not to miss the diagnosis of celiac disease, because left untreated, the condition causes significant morbidity for both the pregnant woman and her fetus and carries with it an increased lifetime increase in mortality, mostly from small bowel carcinomas and lymphomas. All of these risks can be ameliorated by assuming a gluten-free diet.

Maternal and Fetal Risks

Maternal Risks

Untreated celiac disease is associated with later menarche, earlier menopause, and a greater risk of secondary amenorrhea compared with control groups of either unaffected women or women with treated celiac disease.[128] Women with treated celiac disease who adhere to a gluten-free diet have no more gynecologic problems than a group of women without celiac disease. Infertility itself is more common in women with celiac disease than in the general population and has been reported to affect 4% to 8% of cases.[129,130] The pathophysiology of these problems remains uncertain.

Male subfertility is also reported in celiac disease. Abnormal sperm forms, which resolve once dietary gluten is withdrawn, have been observed in nearly half of men with untreated disease. Another group found that male fertility improved after treatment.[131–133]

Anemia is common in women with celiac disease. They should take iron and folate supplements throughout pregnancy; they may also need B_{12} supplementation, and so should be monitored appropriately. Women with celiac disease who are not anemic before pregnancy should be tested for anemia and iron, folate, and B_{12} deficiency regularly throughout the pregnancy. Hypocalcemia is less common but must be considered.

Ideally women with celiac disease should take 5 mg, not 400 μg, of folate preconceptually, in order to optimize their levels of folic acid. There is insufficient evidence to support, or refute, the claim that celiac disease increases the risk of neural tube defect. This may be because most series of women are too small to make meaningful conclusions.

Fetal Risks

Several reports show first-trimester pregnancy loss to be up to nine times more common in women with untreated celiac disease than in those who have received treatment and to be much more common in pregnancies in the same woman before compared with after treatment with a gluten-free diet.[134] Low–birth weight babies are nearly six times more common in women with untreated compared with treated celiac disease, and in a cohort of 12 women, once they assumed a gluten-free diet, the number of low–birth weight babies born fell from nearly 30% to 0%.[140] Similarly, a gluten-free diet increased the duration of breast-feeding more than twofold.

Gasbarrini and colleagues[135] investigated a group of 83 women with either two or more consecutive miscarriages or an unexplained growth-restricted baby (<10th percentile) and 50 controls. In the poor-outcome groups, 8% and 15%, respectively, had immunologic and histologic features of celiac disease, compared with none of 50 controls.[135] They hypothesize that treatment with a gluten-free diet might improve pregnancy outcome. Martinelli and associates[136] found similar results in an Italian population: Among 845 pregnant women screened for celiac disease, 12 cases were discovered and these women had more small–for–gestational-age infants than the other women.

More recently, an intriguing hypothesis suggests that men with celiac disease may father more pregnancies complicated by low birth weight than other men do. In a prospective, population-based cohort of 10,000 pregnancies in Sweden, babies of the 27 fathers with celiac disease were delivered at the same gestational age as the rest of the population, but weighed on average 266 g less and were five times more likely to weigh less than 2.5 kg.[137] Babies of fathers with a wide range of autoimmune conditions were not similarly affected. The babies of the 53 mothers with celiac disease had outcomes similar to those of the babies born to fathers with celiac disease. No difference was noted for babies with siblings or other relatives with celiac disease ($n = 512$). The exact mechanism for this is uncertain but indicates the importance of non-nutritional factors for neonatal outcome in parents with celiac disease. Genetic factors must be implicated.[137]

Management Options

Women with celiac disease should have a strict gluten-free diet prior to conception to minimize the risk of miscarriage. They should persist with this throughout pregnancy to minimize the risks of growth restriction, prematurity, and anemia. In order to achieve this, they should ideally have prepregnancy advice. Once they are pregnant, a management plan should include growth scans, testing for anemia, and iron and possibly folate and B_{12} supplementation. Some women with celiac disease malabsorb calcium: A baseline measurement should be taken, and a calcium-rich diet recommended. Supplementation may be necessary for some women.

SUMMARY OF MANAGEMENT OPTIONS

Celiac Disease

Management Options	Evidence Quality and Recommendation	References
Prepregnancy		
Provide preconception counseling and gluten-free dietary control.	IIa/B	135,144
Supplement folic acid.	—/GPP	—
Prenatal		
Provide careful gluten-free dietary surveillance by dietician.	IIa/B	135,144
Supplement folic acid.	—/GPP	—
Monitor nutritional status.	—/GPP	—
Replace vitamins, minerals as indicated.	—/GPP	—
Give iron; check for anemia.	—/GPP	—
Screen for fetal abnormality, especially neural tube defect.	—/GPP	—
Monitor fetal growth and well-being.	III/B	135,136
Postnatal		
Monitor nutritional and vitamin adequacy, particularly with lactation.	—/GPP	—
Provide contraceptive advice and caution with oral preparations if disease active.	—/GPP	—

GPP, good practice point.

INFLAMMATORY BOWEL DISEASE

General

The term *inflammatory bowel disease* describes Crohn's disease and ulcerative colitis, as well as other less common forms of colitis. Crohn's disease is a chronic, granulomatous inflammatory disease of the intestine in which affected segments of bowel are often separated by normal bowel (skip lesions). It most commonly involves the terminal ileum. Common symptoms are abdominal pain and diarrhea, and there may also be anemia and weight loss, fresh blood or melena per rectum, fistulas, or perianal sepsis. Nonintestinal tract manifestations of the disease include aphthous ulcers, sacroiliitis, sclerosing cholangitis, and uveitis.

Ulcerative colitis is a chronic inflammatory disease of the colon and rectum. It commonly presents with diarrhea and rectal passage of mucus and blood. Typically, the disease starts in the rectum and spreads proximally, without skip lesions. Severe attacks are characterized by passage of a large number of bowel movements a day and can be complicated by fever and abdominal distension (toxic megacolon), which can be fatal. Other complications include anemia, weight loss, hypoalbuminemia, electrolyte imbalances, and carcinoma of the colon (with long-standing disease). Nonintestinal features are similar to those seen in Crohn's.

Although Crohn's disease and ulcerative colitis are both chronic inflammatory disorders of the gastrointestinal tract, the cause of the inflammation does not appear to be the same in each condition. Both are thought to be caused by immune dysregulation in response to constituents of normal gut flora in genetically predisposed individuals. The inflammatory response in Crohn's disease is driven by interleukin-12 (Il-12) and interferon-γ (IFN-γ),[138] whereas in ulcerative colitis it is caused by Il-13 release by natural killer T (NKT) cells in a murine model.[139]

There is evidence for a genetic origin in both Crohn's disease and ulcerative colitis. One study reported that in siblings with similar genetic susceptibility for inflammatory bowel disease, smoking was associated with an increased risk of Crohn's disease and nonsmoking was associated with the development of ulcerative colitis.[140] Laboratory studies have also demonstrated mutations in *NOD2*, a gene that encodes an intracellular receptor for bacterial lipopolysaccharide, in a subgroup of patients with Crohn's ileitis, but not in patients with colitis or anorectal disease.[141]

Diagnosis

If a woman has known inflammatory bowel disease and is complaining of symptoms consistent with an exacerbation, stool culture should be performed to exclude infection. Blood specimens should be taken to establish whether she has anemia, electrolyte imbalance, or hepatic impairment, and inflammatory markers should be checked. The erythrocyte sedimentation rate is raised in normal pregnancy, but the C-reactive protein is not and is of value in the assessment of patients with Crohn's disease and ulcerative colitis. If a flare-up of inflammatory bowel disease is confirmed, care should be shared between obstetricians and gastroenterologists. If there is severe disease or if toxic megacolon is suspected, an abdominal radiograph should be performed, and the woman should be referred for a surgical opinion.

In a woman who does not have a history of inflammatory bowel disease, the diagnosis is based on imaging of the upper and lower gastrointestinal tract, colonoscopy, and biopsy. Most women will have had the diagnosis made before they conceive, but if a new presentation of inflammatory bowel disease occurs in pregnancy, endoscopy and biopsy are preferable to barium studies.

Maternal and Fetal Risks

Maternal Risks

Fertility is reduced in women with active Crohn's disease and possibly in those with ulcerative colitis, but there is no evidence of reduced fertility with quiescent inflammatory bowel disease. The frequency of exacerbations of both Crohn's disease and ulcerative colitis is the same as outside pregnancy (30%–40% women/yr).[142] Flares may occur at any stage of pregnancy, although they occur most commonly in the first trimester.

Women who have had an ileostomy or colostomy usually tolerate pregnancy well, providing at least 50% of the small intestine remains. Complications that can occur in patients who have had gut resection include malabsorption of fat, fat-soluble vitamins, vitamin B_{12}, and water, and electrolyte imbalance. Also, women can have obstruction of ileostomy as pregnancy progresses.

The mode of delivery is not usually influenced by inflammatory bowel disease, even in those with an ileal pouch–anal anastomosis. There are few reports of the management of labor in such cases, but two studies have reported normal vaginal deliveries in the majority of women.[143,144] However, cesarean section should be considered in women with impaired anal continence, in those who have had extensive perineal surgery due to scarring causing skin inelasticity, or in women with active perianal disease, because episiotomy may result in fistula formation. These cesarean procedures may be complicated, and an experienced obstetrician should be present.

Postpartum flare is not a feature of ulcerative colitis but can occur in Crohn's disease.

Fetal Risks

For the majority of cases, if the maternal inflammatory bowel disease is quiescent at the time of conception, the fetal outcome is no different from that in unaffected pregnancies. However, active disease at the time of conception is associated with an increased rate of miscarriage, and flares during pregnancy result in low birth weight and prematurity.[145–147]

Because the etiology of inflammatory bowel disease has both hereditary and immune components, breast-feeding should be encouraged in an effort to reduce the risks to the children of affected women.

Management Options

Acute exacerbations of inflammatory bowel disease can be treated with 5-aminosalicylic acid (5-ASA)–containing compounds and corticosteroids taken rectally, and then orally if local therapy is not sufficient to control symptoms. In severe attacks, intravenous corticosteroids may be required. Loperamide can be used for the treatment of diarrhea. Metronidazole is used to treat anal disease and fistulas, particularly in active Crohn's disease. 5-ASA–containing compounds, corticosteroids, and the immunosuppressives azathioprine and 6-mercaptopurine can be used during remission to prevent relapse rates. Long-term management for recurrent Crohn's disease also includes attention to diet and vitamin supplementation. Pregnant women with inflammatory bowel disease should be advised to take high-dose folate (5 mg daily).

5-Aminosalicylic Acid Derivatives

Many women are now treated with 5-ASA derivatives. Sulfasalazine (Salazopyrin or Azulfidine) is a prodrug that is converted by colonic bacteria into sulfapyridine and 5-ASA. The efficacy of sulfasalazine in the treatment of inflammatory bowel disease resides in the 5-ASA component. Many of the side effects of the drug have been attributed to sulfapyridine, and therefore, newer preparations that do not have this component are now used more commonly than sulfasalazine. These include mesalazine (5-ASA), balsalazine (a prodrug of 5-ASA), and olsalazine (a dimer of 5-ASA that is cleaved in the lower bowel). Both oral and topical preparations of 5-ASA and sulfasalazine are safe in pregnancy. In a U.S. study that included 186 cases in which the mother was treated with sulfasalazine, the fetal complication rate was lower than the reported rates in the general population.[148] A prospective Canadian study of 165 women who were exposed to oral mesalazine in pregnancy, 146 of whom had first-trimester exposure, demonstrated no increase in major congenital malformations when compared with matched controls who had not been exposed to teratogenic drugs.[149] In a French study designed to address whether treatment with high doses of mesalazine in pregnancy were associated with an adverse fetal outcome, 86 women who received less than 3 g mesalazine daily were compared with 37 who received more than 3 g daily. The results revealed no difference in the rates of congenital malformations, prematurity, or fetal death between the groups, and the prevalence of these complications was not different from the quoted rates from the general population.[150] Only very small amounts of 5-ASA pass into breast milk, and the drug is therefore also thought to be safe in lactating women.[151]

Corticosteroids

Corticosteroids taken orally in low doses may reduce recurrence rates, and in higher doses are used for acute intestinal symptoms, orally or intravenously. Distal disease can respond to steroid enemas.

Azathioprine

Azathioprine is an immunosuppressant that is metabolized to 6-mercaptopurine. There are many reports of renal transplant recipients who have conceived while taking azathioprine and who have had normal children. Thus, the drug is thought to not be teratogenic in humans. Azathioprine crosses the placenta, but the fetal liver lacks the enzyme that converts it to its active metabolite; this is thought to explain the fetal protection from teratogenic effects. There is no reason to suspect that the risks in women with inflammatory bowel disease should be different from those who have had renal transplants. One case series reported the outcome of 16 pregnancies in 14 women with inflammatory bowel disease who were treated with azathioprine.[152] There were no congenital abnormalities, and the children's growth and development were normal.

6-Mercaptopurine

There have been very few reports of 6-mercaptopurine use in pregnancy. In one large case series of patients with inflammatory bowel disease treated with the drug, two women had ongoing pregnancies after having stopped the drug at 3 and 4 weeks' gestation, respectively, and no congenital abnormalities were found in their children.[153]

Metronidazole

Because metronidazole is used to treat *Trichomonas vaginalis*, there have been several studies of its use in the first trimester. A Canadian meta-analysis of all studies that contained at least 10 women exposed to metronidazole in the first trimester and untreated controls did not find evidence that the drug is teratogenic.[116] A Spanish meta-analysis that included five cohort and case-control studies reported similar results.[117] This study included three series that were also included in the Canadian study.

Antidiarrheal Agents

Loperamide is a synthetic piperidine derivative that is used for the treatment of diarrhea. In a prospective, controlled, multicenter study of loperamide in pregnancy in which 105 women were studied and 89 were exposed to loperamide in the first trimester, there were no significant differences in the rate of major or minor congenital malformations when compared with matched controls.[154]

Biologic Therapy

The most commonly used biologic agent is infliximab, an immunoglobulin G_1 (IgG_1) antibody. Although infliximab does not cross the placenta in the first trimester, it can cross in the third trimester.[155] It is also detectable in the infant for several months after birth. The data on fetal risk following infliximab treatment in pregnancy are limited. However, there is no evidence of an increased congenital malformation rate in more than 100 pregnancies reported in the two largest registries (the TREAT registry[156] and the Infliximab Safety Database[157]). There is a theoretical concern that treatment with infliximab and other biologic agents could affect the infants' immune system, but there have not been sufficient numbers of cases treated in the third trimester to assess this at present. There are currently very limited data about the effects of other biologic agents in pregnancy.

SUMMARY OF MANAGEMENT OPTIONS

Inflammatory Bowel Disease

Management Options	Evidence Quality and Recommendation	References
Prepregnancy		
Provide preconception counseling and control and encourage conception when disease is quiescent.	IIa/B	145,147
Consider modification of drug therapy to those with a good safety record in pregnancy (see later); steroids do not reduce the risk of relapse.	—/GPP	—
Ensure folate supplementation (5 mg/day).	—/GPP	—

SUMMARY OF MANAGEMENT OPTIONS

Inflammatory Bowel Disease—cont'd

Management Options	Evidence Quality and Recommendation	References
Prenatal		
Continue appropriate drug therapy prenatally:		
• Salicylates.	IIa/B	148–150
• Corticosteroids (oral or rectal).	III/B	148
• Azathioprine.	III/B	152
• 6-Mercaptopurine—limited experience in pregnancy.	III/B	153
• Metronidazole.	III/B	116,117
• Loperamide.	IIa/B	154
Treat flares in the same way as outside pregnancy.	—/GPP	—
Pay attention to nutrition, iron, and folate supplementation	—/GPP	—
Monitor fetal growth.	IIa/B	145–147
Labor and Delivery		
Cesarean section is rarely indicated.	—/GPP	—
Exceptions are women with severe perianal disease, postoperative perineal scarring, or impaired anal continence with an ileal pouch–anal anastomosis.	—/GPP	—
Pay scrupulous attention to wound repair (abdominal and perineal) with Crohn's disease.	—/GPP	—
Postnatal		
If severe diarrhea and malabsorption are present, consider alternatives to oral contraceptives.	—/GPP	—
Breast-feeding is safe for women taking sulfasalazine, mesalazine, corticosteroids, and metronidazole.	IIa/B	116,117, 148–151
Data are currently insufficient about azathioprine and breast-feeding to give evidence-based guidance, although most experts in the field feel that the benefits of maintaining remission and achieving lactation outweigh the risks of discontinuing therapy.	III/B	152
An increased frequency of flares in the postpartum period is reported in Crohn's disease but not in ulcerative colitis.	—/GPP	—

GPP, good practice point.

SUGGESTED READINGS

Avery AJ, Carr S: Treatment of common minor and self-limiting conditions. In Rubin P(ed): Prescribing in Pregnancy, 3rd ed. London, BMJ Publishing Group, 2000, pp 15–28.

Dodds L, Fell DB, Joseph KS, et al: Outcomes of pregnancies complicated by hyperemesis gravidarum. Obstet Gynecol 2006;107:285–292.

Geenes VL, Williamson C: Intrahepatic cholestasis of pregnancy. World J Gastroenterol 2009;15:2049–2066.

Girling JC, Dow E, Smith JH: Liver function tests in pre eclampsia: Importance of comparison with a reference range derived for normal pregnancy. Br J Obstet Gynaecol 1997;104:246–250.

Glantz A, Marschall HU, Mattsson LA: Intrahepatic cholestasis of pregnancy: Relationships between bile acid levels and fetal complication rates. Hepatology 2004;40:467–474.

Knight M, Nelson-Piercy C, Kurinczuk JJ, et al: A prospective national study of acute fatty liver of pregnancy in the UK. Gut 2008;57:951–956.

Martinelli P, Troncone R, Paparo F, et al: Celiac disease and unfavourable outcome of pregnancy. Gut 2000;46:332–335.

Milkovich L, Van Den Berg BJ: An evaluation of the teratogenicity of certain antinauseant drugs. Am J Obstet Gynecol 1975;125:245.

Morales M, Berney T, Jenny A, et al: Crohn's disease as a risk factor for the outcome of pregnancy. Hepatogastroenterology 2000;47:1595–1598.

Yang Z, Yamada J, Zhao Y, et al: Prospective screening for pediatric mitochondrial trifunctional protein defects in pregnancies complicated by liver disease. JAMA 2002;288:2163–2166.

REFERENCES

For a complete list of references, log onto www.expertconsult.com.

CHAPTER 48

Neurologic Complications

J. RICARDO CARHUAPOMA, MARK W. TOMLINSON, and STEVEN R. LEVINE

INTRODUCTION

Neurologic conditions seen in reproductive-age women will be encountered during pregnancy. Table 48–1 shows the incidence of several such neurologic diseases. The relative rarity of many of these conditions limits the actual clinical experience of both the managing obstetrician and the neurologist. In addition, the individual practitioner is further hampered by the limited amount of pregnancy-specific information available. The frequent overlap of symptoms associated with common pregnancy complaints, the sometimes disabling and lethal consequences of the disease, and the fetal effects of maternal treatment make the diagnosis and management of neurologic disease during pregnancy an often-daunting task.

Optimal and effective management commonly requires the expertise of several disciplines. This obviously includes the obstetrician or maternal-fetal medicine specialist and the neurologist in combination. Involvement of an anesthesiologist is essential at the time of labor and delivery to provide appropriate analgesia or anesthesia. Early involvement of the pediatrician or neonatologist is important to anticipate neonatal needs and adequately care for the newborn. Drugs discussed are listed with a risk factor category used by the U.S. Food and Drug Administration (FDA). The categories and definitions are shown in Table 48–2.[1] There are very few randomized clinical trials to guide evidence-based medicine in the field of neurologic complications of pregnancy.

SEIZURES

Neurologic Complications of Preeclampsia/Eclampsia

Maternal and Fetal Risks

Preeclampsia and eclampsia are also discussed in Chapters 35 and 78. The reported incidence of eclampsia in both the United Kingdom and the United States is approximately 0.05% of births. As with preeclampsia, the specific etiology and pathophysiology leading to eclampsia are unknown. Postulated contributing factors include cerebral edema, vasospasm/cerebral vasculopathy, ischemia, hemorrhage, a cerebrovascular dysregulation or central dysautonomia, and hypertensive encephalopathy.[2]

Hypertension is an important factor associated with convulsions. Increasing systolic and diastolic blood pressures in a previously normotensive patient challenge the autoregulatory properties of cerebral blood vessels. In normotensive patients, autoregulation is preserved between mean arterial pressure (MAP) values from 50 to 150 mm Hg. Beyond this range, cerebral blood vessels lose their tone and an angiographic pattern of vasodilation with segments of vasoconstriction develops. The blood-brain barrier and its "tight junctions" are disrupted and vasogenic edema ensues.[3–8] This process occurs preferentially in the occipital lobes and in "watershed" areas of the brain.[9] The neuropathologic changes are widespread throughout the neuraxis.[10] Cerebral edema is evident and the presence of petechial hemorrhages surrounding arterioles is conspicuous, conceivably rendering certain neuronal populations hyperexcitable. Although hypertension through this cascade of events can initiate the pathogenic process of convulsions in many instances, it does not explain all cases. Eclampsia can be seen in patients without significant blood pressure elevations.[2] As many as 38% of all eclamptics have been reported to have no hypertension or proteinuria identified before the initial seizure.[11]

In addition to convulsions, a variety of visual symptoms may be seen. These may be nonspecific, but can include retinal detachments and cortical blindness, secondary to hypertension-induced retinal arteriolar dilation, papilledema,[12] central retinal artery occlusion,[13] and vasospasm.[14] Visual changes generally improve with delivery and hypertension control. Headache (see Table 48–7) is also a common complaint and may involve increased intracranial pressure (ICP) resulting from vasogenic edema.[15] More severe findings such as worsening headache, lethargy, focal neurologic findings, stupor, and coma in a preeclamptic patient should always raise the suspicion of an intracerebral hemorrhage or of worsening brain edema with the subsequent risk of brain herniation.[16]

Although maternal mortality has decreased over the past several decades, eclampsia continues to be a significant contributor, particularly in underdeveloped countries. In a large U.S. hospital system managing nearly 1.5 million births from 2000 to 2006, preeclampsia and its related complications was the leading cause of maternal deaths, accounting for

TABLE 48–1

Incidence of Neurologic Disease in Childbearing Population

DISEASE	INCIDENCE
Migraine	1:5
Epilepsy	1:150
Multiple sclerosis	1:1000
Cerebral venous thrombosis	1:2500–10,000 deliveries
Ruptured cerebral aneurysm	1:10,000 pregnancies
Bleed from cerebral AVM	1:10,000 pregnancies
Myasthenia gravis	1:25,000
Malignant brain tumor	1:50,000
Guillain-Barré syndrome	1.5:100,000

AVM, arteriovenous malformation.

TABLE 48–2

Classification System for Fetal Risk Associated with Medications Used during Pregnancy

Category A	Controlled studies in women fail to demonstrate a risk to the fetus in the first trimester (and there is no evidence of a risk in later trimesters), and the possibility of fetal harm appears remote.
Category B	Either animal reproduction studies have not demonstrated a fetal risk but there are no controlled studies in pregnant women or animal reproduction studies have shown an adverse effect (other than a decrease in fertility) that was not confirmed in controlled studies in women in the first trimester (and there is no evidence of a risk in later trimesters).
Category C	Either studies in animals have revealed adverse effects on the fetus (teratogenic or embryocidal or other) and there are no controlled studies in women or studies in women and animals are not available. Drugs should be given only if the potential benefit justifies the potential risk to the fetus.
Category D	There is positive evidence of human fetal risk, but the benefits from use in pregnant women may be acceptable despite the risk (e.g., if the drug is needed in a life-threatening situation or for a serious disease for which safer drugs cannot be used or are ineffective).
Category X	Studies in animals or human beings have demonstrated fetal abnormalities or there is evidence of fetal risk based on human experience, or both, and the risk of the use of the drug in pregnant women clearly outweighs any possible benefit. The drug is contraindicated in women who are or may become pregnant.

16% of these deaths. The Confidential Inquiry into Maternal Deaths in the United Kingdom from 2003 to 2005, preeclampsia and eclampsia were the second leading cause of direct maternal mortality, accounting for 18% of the deaths.[17] In other series, approximately 1% of pregnancies complicated by eclampsia still resulted in maternal death.[11,18] In developing countries, maternal mortality is reported in 8% to 14% of patients with eclampsia.[19] Fetal and neonatal complication rates also tend to be high and are attributed to prematurity, placental insufficiency, and placental abruption.[20]

Management Options (See also Chapters 35 and 78)

PRENATAL, LABOR AND DELIVERY, AND POSTNATAL

Eclampsia most frequently occurs during the antepartum and intrapartum periods, but approximately one third of cases are seen postpartum.[21] Between 28% and 56% of postpartum convulsions occur more than 48 hours after delivery.[22,23] The diagnosis is clinical, and additional diagnostic evaluation is not always necessary in cases in which typical preeclampsia precedes the seizure. When the presentation is not classic, however, imaging studies such as brain computed tomography (CT) and preferably magnetic resonance imaging (MRI) including diffusion weighted imaging can be helpful in identifying complications or other seizure etiologies such as hemorrhage, cerebral infarction, infection/inflammation, or cerebral venous thrombosis (Fig. 48–1).

Magnesium sulfate continues to be the mainstay of both seizure prophylaxis and abortive therapy in the United States.[24] The precise mechanism of action remains poorly understood. Current hypotheses include reduction in cerebral vasospasm through calcium antagonism and *N*-methyl-D-aspartate (NMDA) receptor channel blockade providing "neuroprotection" from ischemic injury resulting from vasospasm.[25–28] The efficacy of magnesium has been established.[29] Large trials provide compelling evidence that magnesium sulfate is superior to phenytoin and diazepam in both treatment and prophylaxis of eclamptic seizures.[30] A multicenter worldwide trial including more than 1600 eclamptic patients reported that magnesium sulfate was associated with a 52% lower risk of recurrent seizures than diazepam and a 67% lower risk than phenytoin. Furthermore, maternal and neonatal morbidity were lower in the magnesium group than in those receiving phenytoin. Magnesium sulfate has also been shown to be superior to placebo and phenytoin when used prophylactically to prevent seizures. A large North American study comparing the efficacy of magnesium and phenytoin for seizure prophylaxis was stopped early when interim analysis demonstrated that phenytoin provided ineffective seizure prophylaxis.[30] Management differences between eclampsia and epilepsy should not be surprising because the pathophysiology of the two conditions is likely to be different. A Cochrane Review showed that magnesium sulfate more than halves the risk of eclampsia and probably reduces the risk of maternal death (relative risk [RR] 0.41, 95% confidence interval [CI] 0.29–0.58).[29] Magnesium sulfate does not improve outcome of the newborn. The risk of placental abruption was also reduced.[29]

Specific dosing recommendations for magnesium sulfate have varied, but generally consist of a 4- to 6-g intravenous load given over 5 to 30 minutes. This is followed by a maintenance dose of 1 to 3 g/hr intravenously. Therapeutic serum levels are in the range of 4 to 8 mEq/L. The magnesium infusion is usually continued for approximately 24 hours into the postpartum period. The duration of therapy is empirical and based on the distribution of postpartum seizure risk. Complications associated with the use of magnesium center on its calcium antagonism at the neuromuscular junction, which can result in neuromuscular blockade. At levels above 10 mEq/L, deep tendon reflexes are lost. Lethargy and respiratory depression are also seen. Levels of 12 to 15 mEq/L result in respiratory paralysis. Higher levels can result in

FIGURE 48–1

Axial head T_2-weighted magnetic resonance imaging (MRI) scan of a woman with headaches, proteinuria, and postpartum seizures. There are multiple regions of T_2 hyperintensity in the cerebellum, pons, basal ganglia, and the hemispheric white matter consistent with changes seen in eclampsia. These radiologic abnormalities reversed on subsequent MRI evaluation that followed the complete clinical resolution of this patient's initial neurologic presentation.

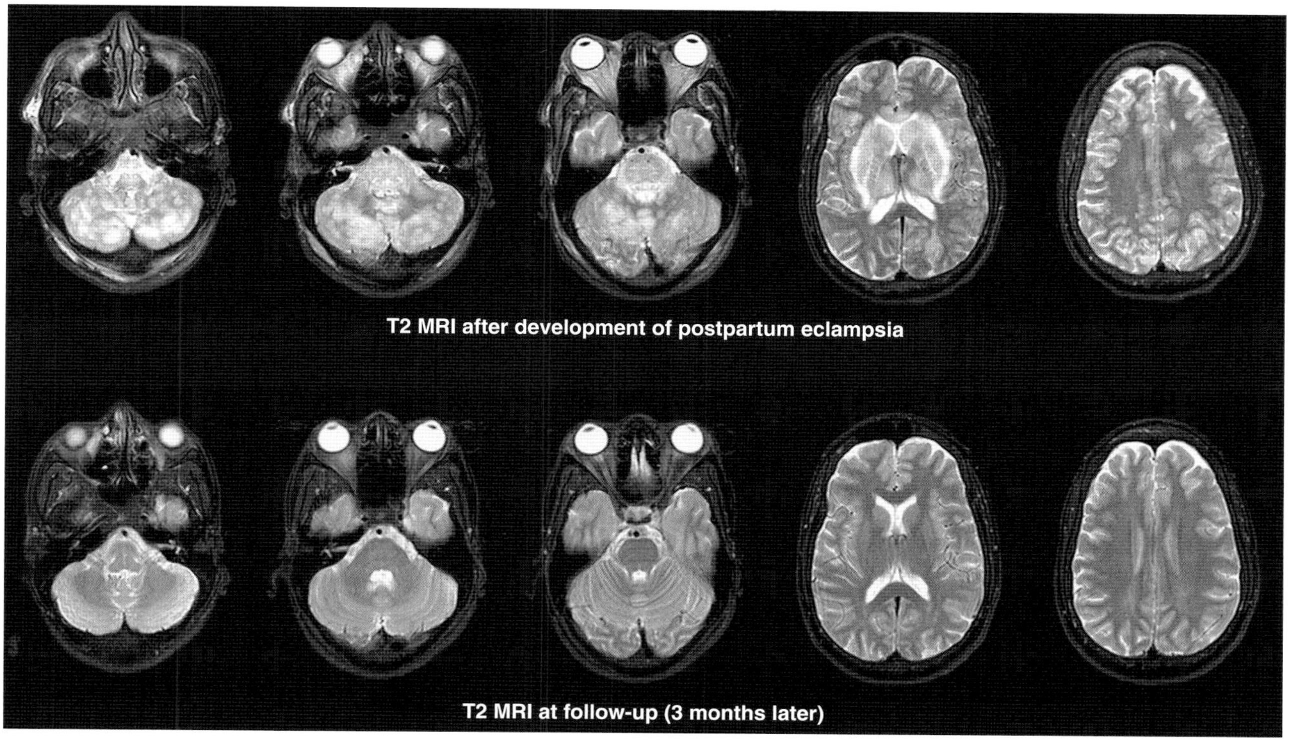

cardiac standstill. Management of overdose includes respiratory support, calcium gluconate (1 g), and cardiac monitoring.

Low-dose aspirin use in preeclampsia was evaluated in a meta-analysis involving over 40 trials and more than 30,000 women.[31] Limited data prevented conclusions regarding the use of aspirin to treat preeclampsia; however, a moderate decrease in the incidence of preeclampsia was found when aspirin was used prophylactically.

Blood pressure control is also important in both preventing and managing neurologic complications associated with preeclampsia/eclampsia.[32] Some investigators have suggested that a greater emphasis should be placed on blood pressure control, with the potential elimination of seizure prophylaxis. Hydralazine and labetalol are frequently used as first-line agents, with continuous intravenous infusions of nicardipine, sodium nitroprusside, and nitroglycerin used in refractory cases.

Simple first-aid measures (avoiding injury, nursing semiprone, maintaining airway, and giving oxygen) should not be forgotten.[32] Maternal renal, liver, and coagulation status should be monitored together with the fetal condition if the eclampsia is prenatal. Fluid overload should be avoided. The majority of obstetricians would deliver the fetus once the mother is stable if the eclampsia occurs during pregnancy (see Chapters 35 and 78 for further discussion).

SUMMARY OF MANAGEMENT OPTIONS

Neurologic Complications of Preeclampsia/Eclampsia

Management Options (See also Chapters 35 and 78)	**Evidence Quality and Recommendation**	**References**
Prenatal, Labor and Delivery, and Postnatal		
First-aid measures • Avoid injury. • Place in semiprone position. • Maintain airway. • Administer oxygen. • Monitor maternal and fetal condition.	Ia/A	32

SUMMARY OF MANAGEMENT OPTIONS

Neurologic Complications of Preeclampsia/Eclampsia—cont'd

Management Options (See also Chapters 35 and 78)	Evidence Quality and Recommendation	References
Control and prevent recurrence of seizures; magnesium sulfate is the drug of choice.	Ia/A	30
Treat hypertension.	Ia/A	32
Avoid fluid overload.	—/GPP	—
Check renal, liver, and coagulation status.	—/GPP	—
Deliver when stable.	—/GPP	—

GPP, good practice point.

Epilepsy

Maternal and Fetal Risks

Epilepsy is probably the most common serious neurologic problem faced by obstetricians. There are approximately 1 million women of childbearing age with epilepsy in America, delivering roughly 20,000 babies annually. Seizures during pregnancy have an incidence of 0.15% to 10%.[33] The interrelationship of maternal epilepsy, antiepileptic drug (AED) metabolism and pharmacodynamics, genetics, drug-induced embryopathies, and maternal behavior is complex and has led to considerable controversy concerning epilepsy in pregnancy.

One area of unresolved controversy involves the effect of pregnancy on seizure frequency.[34–36] Approximately one third of patient's will have an increase in frequency, whereas the remainder will experience no change or a decrease.[35] Some of the change can be attributed to physiologic changes and psychological stress associated with pregnancy.[36] These factors include increased steroid hormone levels, sleep deprivation, and metabolic changes. More commonly, when seizure frequency is increased, deliberate patient noncompliance secondary to fear of fetal drug effects is likely to blame.[37] The effect of pregnancy on epilepsy may be inferred from the women's seizure frequency before pregnancy. As a rule, the fewer the number of seizures occurring in the 9 months before conception, the less the risk of worsening epilepsy during pregnancy.[35,37] If the seizure frequency is at least one seizure monthly before pregnancy, there is a high probability that increased seizure frequency will be seen during pregnancy. This is in contrast to women having only one seizure during the 9 months before pregnancy. These patients have only a 25% risk of seizing during pregnancy.

Decreases in most AED levels occur during pregnancy and can affect seizure frequency.[38] Gastrointestinal absorption decreases, whereas hepatic and renal clearance increase for most AEDs. Albumin levels decrease, leading to lower total drug levels.[39] Pregnancy-associated changes in specific agents are described in Table 48–3. Postpartum, these changes reverse with a resultant increase in drug levels. In reality, the availability of serum drug level testing allows women to maintain prepregnancy therapeutic levels. When this is accomplished, only 10% of patients will experience increased seizure frequency during pregnancy.[35]

The effects of AEDs on the fetus are complex and controversial.[40,41] The four most commonly used agents (carbamazepine, phenobarbital, phenytoin, and valproic acid) are known to cross the placenta and all are believed to have teratogenic effects. The rate of congenital malformations in patients using these drugs is approximately two to three times that of infants of nonepileptic mothers (i.e., 6%–8% in epileptic pregnancies).[37] Thus, more than 90% of mothers taking AEDs during pregnancy will deliver normal children.

Additional factors have been linked to the increased rate of anomalies seen in patients using AEDs. Multiagent therapy appears to enhance malformation rates.[42] In addition, phenytoin,[43] primidone,[44] and carbamazepine[45] have been associated with patterns of malformation that are quite similar. Common anomalies include a mildly dysmorphic face and fingers with stubby distal phalanges and hypoplastic fingernails, suggesting a "fetal antiepileptic drug syndrome."[37] A genetic predisposition might play a role in development of these malformations. Such a link has been reported for the enzyme epoxide hydrolase.[46] A reduction in the enzyme's

TABLE 48–3

Antiepileptic Drug Level Changes in Pregnancy Compared with Nonpregnant Baseline

DRUG	TOTAL DRUG LEVEL (%)	FREE DRUG LEVEL (%)
Phenytoin	−56*	−31
Phenobarbital	−55*	−50*
Carbamazepine	−42*	−28*
Valproic acid	−39*	+25

* Significantly different from baseline ($P < .005$).
Adapted from Yerby MS, Friel PN, McCormick K: Antiepileptic drug disposition during pregnancy. Neurology 1992;42(Suppl 5):12–16.

activity was seen in amniocytes of fetuses who developed findings of fetal hydantoin syndrome, but not in those lacking any findings. Further confusing the issue is evidence that some of the anomalies associated with AEDs are found in mothers with epilepsy but no exposure to these medications.[47]

Despite the etiologic uncertainty, individual drugs have been associated with specific anomalies. Cleft lip and palate, as well as cardiac and urogenital defects, are reported with phenytoin. Spina bifida is found in 1% to 2% of patients taking valproic acid.[48] The malformation pattern associated with phenobarbital is similar to that seen with phenytoin. Carbamazepine was felt to be the safest of the AEDs, but it too has been associated with spina bifida at a rate of approximately 1%.[42] Developmentally, most children have normal motor function but may have some degree of cognitive dysfunction. The latter-observed abnormalities appear more likely to relate to seizures during pregnancy and lower levels of paternal education rather than AEDs. Valproate appears to be an exception, however. It has been associated with increased cognitive impairment in children evaluated at 3 years of age compared with those taking carbamazepine, lamotrigine, or phenytoin.[49]

Coagulopathies have been reported in approximately half of all babies born to mothers taking phenobarbital, primidone, or phenytoin. A deficiency of vitamin K–dependent clotting factors is responsible. Few infants actually develop clinical symptoms.[50]

Levetiracetam (LEV; FDA category C) is an AED approved for use as adjunct agent in partial-onset seizures in adults and children aged 4 years or older. Recently, it has been approved as adjunctive therapy in the treatment of myoclonic seizures in adults and adolescents aged 12 years or older. Although not formally approved by the FDA for its use in primary generalized epileptic syndromes, its use as monotherapy or first-line therapy for generalized seizures is increasing. The mechanism of action of this drug is not well understood. The absence of hepatic clearing and lack of drug interactions make this drug particularly attractive in patients who are on multiple agents. The most common side effects—asthenia, somnolence, and dizziness—are mild to moderate and usually do not require discontinuation of the drug. Few data are available on human teratogenicity of LEV. In 11 pregnancies during treatment with LEV, 1 spontaneous abortion, 1 termination, and 9 live births were noted. None of the live births had evidence of malformations. Two infants were found to have low birth weight. Data from women with epilepsy treated with LEV suggest transfer of the drug from mother to fetus and into breast milk. However, infants had very low LEV levels and did not show signs of adverse effects. In general, women on LEV should be encouraged to breast-feed.[51–54]

Management Options

PREPREGNANCY

Ideally, patients are seen prior to conception to optimize antiepileptic therapy.[55] The patient should be evaluated in conjunction with a neurologist for withdrawal of AEDs. Some patients who have been seizure-free for greater than 2 years are potential candidates. However, other factors must also be considered before a decision is made. Age of onset, seizure type, electroencephalographic findings, and number of seizures occurring before control was achieved all affect the risk of recurrence.[56,57] If complete withdrawal is not possible or practical, monotherapy should be attempted to reduce the risk of fetal malformations. The drug chosen should be that which is most effective for a given seizure type.[37] Vaproate should be avoided in women of reproductive age whenever possible.

Those who will be continuing on AEDs should be counseled about the importance of seizure control and the current understanding of fetal risks for malformations. Such counseling may decrease the number of patients who inappropriately discontinue their medication. Initiation of folic acid supplementation should also be considered preconceptionally. Although there is no direct evidence of benefit in epileptic patients, the recommendation is based on findings demonstrating a decrease in recurrence of neural tube defects in women with a previously affected child. The goal of therapy is to maintain normal serum and red cell folate levels.[37]

PRENATAL

Patients on AEDs should have drug levels monitored.[55] They should be maintained on the lowest effective dose. If valproic acid must be used, multiple doses at intervals during the day are preferred. A fall in drug level is common and does not necessarily require an increase in dose. Decisions to change the drug dose should be based on the clinical status, with drug levels used to guide such changes. Free drug levels change to a lesser degree than the total levels and may be used to serially monitor the patient.[37] A targeted ultrasound examination should be performed in the second trimester to search for fetal anomalies. Maternal serum α-fetoprotein may be considered in addition to ultrasound to screen for neural tube defects in patients taking valproate or carbamazepine. Vitamin K can be given to the mother during the final 4 weeks of gestation to decrease the risk of fetal coagulopathy.[37] Should seizures recur, short-acting benzodiazepines may be used acutely. Free serum levels should be rechecked and drug dosage optimized.

In recent years, the use of new AEDs has become widespread in patients with epilepsy. However, the alterations in the pharmacokinetics of these agents during pregnancy have not been adequately studied. Data are lacking for drugs such as gabapentin, topiramate, tiagabine, oxcarbazepine, LEV, and zonisamide, but no definitive adverse effects have been demonstrated in humans. All these drugs are classified as category C. Their use during pregnancy should be based on an evaluation of the benefits of the drug in a given patient versus the unknown potential for adverse outcome.

The majority of AEDs are characterized by significant increases in clearance during pregnancy.[58] Limited studies of the newer AEDs (lamotrigine, OXC, TPM, and ZNS) indicate similar extensive transplacental transfer. Current recommendations are that ideal AED concentration should be established for each patient before conception and that monitoring of AED levels should be performed during each trimester and the last month of pregnancy.[58]

LABOR AND DELIVERY

Most patients with epilepsy are able to labor normally and achieve a vaginal delivery. Elective cesarean section may be considered in patients refractory to treatment during the third trimester or in those that exhibit status epilepticus (SE) with significant stress. During labor, repeated seizures that cannot be controlled or SE may require an operative delivery. Fetal asphyxia can occur with prolonged or repeated seizures. Cesarean delivery may also be considered when repeated absence or psychomotor seizures limit maternal awareness and ability to cooperate. Tonic-clonic seizures are seen in approximately 1% to 2% of women during labor. Lorazepam, a short-acting benzodiazepine, is the drug of choice for treating seizures acutely.[37] The drug is administered in 2-mg boluses every 5 minutes as necessary. Some use 5- to 10-mg boluses of diazepam as an alternative.

POSTNATAL

AED levels must be monitored after delivery because reversal of the physiologic alterations causing a decline in levels during gestation leads to a rise postpartum. If the medication dose was increased during pregnancy, the regimen should be returned to that used prior to pregnancy to avoid toxicity. During the first postpartum day, an additional 1% to 2% of women will have tonic-clonic convulsions. Again, lorazepam is the agent of choice for acute control. New-onset seizures in the postpartum period require complete evaluation to rule out intracerebral hemorrhage, cortical vein thrombosis, infection, or eclampsia.

Neonates should be given vitamin K 1 mg intramuscularly after birth to prevent a coagulopathy. All AEDs can cross into the breast milk, but breast-feeding is not contraindicated for most agents. The effects of diazepam on nursing infants are unknown and it should be used with caution. Phenobarbital should be used only when no alternatives exist because neonatal sedation can occur along with neonatal withdrawal upon weaning.[59]

Contraception is an important consideration for women with epilepsy. Although the condition itself does not limit the choice of method, anticonvulsant therapy can have a significant impact on contraceptive effectiveness. Many of the drugs increase hepatic enzymes, thus increasing drug metabolism. The World Health Organization (WHO) states that there are no contraindications to intrauterine devices (IUDs) or depomedroxyprogesterone acetate use. The benefit of hormonal implants or other injectable hormones outweighs the risks. Combined oral or progestin-only pills along with the patch and vaginal ring should be avoided, if possible, owing to the increased risk of failure. If oral contraceptives are to be used, low-dose estrogen formulations should be avoided.

Status Epilepticus

Maternal and Fetal Risks

SE is defined as ongoing seizure activity lasting greater than 30 minutes or recurrent seizures without full recovery of consciousness between episodes. The actual incidence during pregnancy is unknown. The important causes are listed in Table 48–4. Predisposing factors include poor compliance with AEDs, central nervous system infections, trauma, and illicit drug use.[35] SE represents a medical emergency. Most seizures are generalized tonic-clonic. During the tonic phase, contractions of the respiratory muscles impair adequate maternal oxygenation, leading to fetal hypoxia and potentially asphyxia. During the convulsive (clonic) phase, metabolic acidosis ensues. Rhabdomyolysis occurs and can lead to acute renal failure. After 30 minutes of continuous brain electrical activity, even in the absence of the metabolic derangements, irreversible neuronal injury can occur. The hippocampus and amygdala of the temporal lobe are particularly sensitive to permanent damage.[60] Trauma from recurrent seizure activity can result in preterm labor, rupture of membranes, abruptio placenta, and fetal death.[35]

TABLE 48–4
Causes of Prolonged Convulsions

Uncontrolled epilepsy
Eclampsia
Encephalitis
Meningitis
Cerebral tumor
Cerebral trauma
Drug withdrawal
Toxicity (e.g., heavy metals)
Metabolic disturbance
Cerebrovascular disease

Management Options

ANTENATAL, LABOR AND DELIVERY, AND POSTNATAL

Diagnostic and therapeutic interventions should be performed simultaneously. A patent airway must be secured and supplemental oxygenation given. Hypotension should be avoided to prevent decreased cerebral perfusion pressure. Complete blood count (CBC) with differential, electrolyte profile, blood urea nitrogen, creatinine, urine toxicology screen, and AED levels should be obtained. Cerebrospinal fluid (CSF) analysis is performed if meningoencephalitis is suspected.

Intravenous benzodiazepines are used acutely. Again, lorazepam is the drug of choice. It is given in 2-mg boluses every 5 minutes. Simultaneously, the patient is loaded with phenytoin, 18 mg/kg, administered at a rate not exceeding 50 mg/min. The administration of intravenous valproic acid (20 mg/kg loading dose) is an alternative if phenytoin is otherwise contraindicated. The combination of phenytoin and benzodiazepines is effective in controlling 75% to 85% of SE patients. In those with persistent seizures, higher levels of phenytoin can be achieved with an additional 5 mg/kg. In refractory cases in which barbiturates or a continuous infusion of benzodiazepines is needed, elective intubation is required to protect the airway. Continuous electroencephalographic monitoring should also be initiated. Once identified, the underlying etiology should be treated.

SUMMARY OF MANAGEMENT OPTIONS

Epilepsy

Management Options	Evidence Quality and Recommendation	References
Prepregnancy		
Check clinical control and serum anticonvulsant levels regularly.	Ia/A	37
Adjust anticonvulsant dose to control seizures with serum levels as a guide; avoid toxic doses.	Ia/A	37
Supplement folate.	Ia/A	55
Status Epilepticus		
First-aid measures (see "Preeclampsia/Eclampsia").	—/GPP	—
Investigate and treat simultaneously.	Ia/A	55
Control convulsions:		
• Anticonvulsant drugs (IV benzodiazepine as boluses plus either IV phenytoin or IV magnesium if eclampsia is the cause).	Ia/A	37
• Ventilate while maintaining anticonvulsants if anticonvulsants alone fail to control seizures.	—/GPP	—
Avoid hypertension.	—/GPP	—
Prenatal		
Check clinical control and serum anticonvulsant levels regularly.	Ia/A	37
Adjust anticonvulsant dose to control seizures with serum levels as a guide; avoid toxic doses.	Ia/A	37
Obtain detailed fetal anomaly scan at 20 wk.	Ia/A	37
Administer short-acting benzodiazepine acutely if seizures recur.	Ia/A	37
Information about safety of more recent anticonvulsants is lacking.	IV/C	58
Labor and Delivery		
Continue anticonvulsant medication.	—/GPP	—
Administer short-acting benzodiazepine acutely if seizures recur.	Ia/A	37
Postnatal		
Examine newborn to confirm normality.	—/GPP	—
Administer vitamin K to newborn.	—/GPP	—
Monitor seizure control and serum levels; dose adjustment may be necessary.	Ia/A	37

GPP, good practice point.

CEREBROVASCULAR DISEASE

Ischemic Stroke and Transient Ischemic Attacks

Maternal and Fetal Risks

For many years, it was believed that the incidence of cerebral ischemia is significantly higher during pregnancy. Currently, controversy exists because the evidence is inconclusive.[61] In a population-based report, the relative risk of stroke during gestation was found to be 0.7.[62] Most of the risk in the population-based report appears to be from increased occurrence of hemorrhagic stroke. The relative risk of stroke increased to 8.7 during the postpartum period. During the years 2000 and 2001, the incidence of pregnancy-associated stroke was found to be 34 cases/100,000 deliveries using the Nationwide Inpatient Sample from the Healthcare Cost and Utilization Project of the Agency for Healthcare Research and Quality.[63] The stroke-related mortality was 1.4 in 100,000 deliveries. For reasons that are unclear, there may be an overrepresentation of middle cerebral artery occlusions during pregnancy and internal carotid artery occlusions during the postpartum period.

Most of the conditions associated with "stroke in the young" are shared by pregnant women suffering cerebral ischemia and, therefore, demand an extensive diagnostic evaluation to identify the cause and provide optimal treatment. The etiologies can be divided into processes that

TABLE 48–5

Causes of Stroke in Pregnancy

Arteriopathies
Atherosclerosis
Arterial dissection
Moyamoya disease
Takayasu's arteritis
Fibromuscular dysplasia
Syphilis
Chronic meningitis
Systemic lupus erythematosus
Pregnancy-related intimal hyperplasia
Hematologic Disorders
Sickle hemoglobinopathies
Antiphospholipid antibody syndrome
Thrombotic thrombocytopenic purpura
Protein C or S or antithrombin III deficiency
Activated protein C resistance
Paroxysmal nocturnal hemoglobinuria
Polycythemia vera
Thrombocytosis
Leukemia
Systemic malignancy
Disseminated intravascular coagulation
Cardioembolism
Valvular disease
Mitral valve prolapse
Atrial septal defect with paradoxical embolism
Atrial fibrillation
Subacute bacterial endocarditis
Nonbacterial thrombotic endocarditis
Peripartum cardiomyopathy

FIGURE 48–2
Conventional cerebral angiography in a young cocaine user shows severe basilar artery irregularities, stenosis, and filling defects (*arrows*).

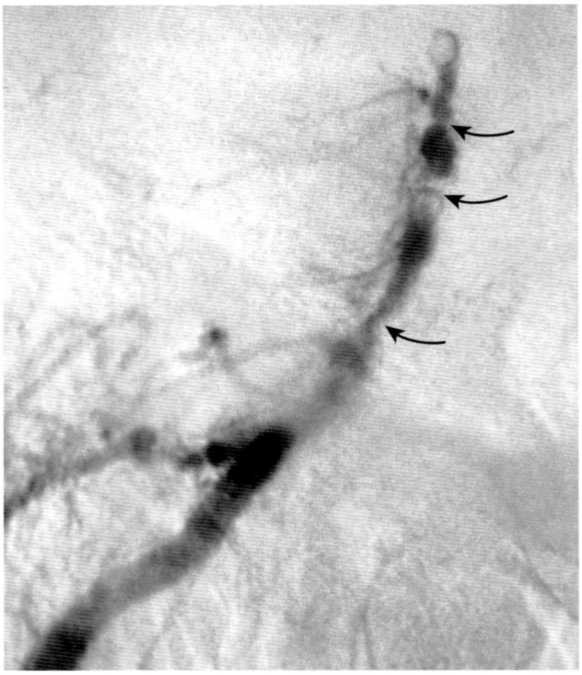

involve the "ABCs" of stroke: arteries, blood components, and cardiac sources of emboli. A detailed list of specific causes is given in Table 48–5. Pregnancy-specific complications that are associated with an increased risk of stroke include preeclampsia and gestational hypertension, postpartum infection, and postpartum hemorrhage, especially when blood transfusion is required.

Premature or accelerated atherosclerosis accounts for almost 25% of ischemic strokes in pregnant women. Women with hypertension, diabetes mellitus, tobacco use, hyperlipidemia, and family history of premature atherosclerotic disease are especially at risk for this stroke mechanism. Less common vascular etiologies include arterial dissection during labor and delivery,[64] inflammatory arteritis such as Takayasu's arteritis,[65] and fibromuscular dysplasia. The latter has been associated with cerebral ischemia as well as intracranial aneurysms, carotid artery dissection, and carotid-cavernous fistula.[64,66,67] Fibromuscular dysplasia appears to occur more commonly in young women and might also affect the renal arteries.[68]

Physiologic alterations seen in pregnancy may theoretically predispose the pregnant woman to develop cerebral ischemia. Increases in clotting factors including fibrinogen, increased platelet aggregability, decreased antithrombin III concentration,[69] and impaired fibrinolytic activity all occur during normal pregnancy.[70,71] These changes persist through the first several postpartum weeks and may be the only identifiable predisposing risk factors during pregnancy. The risk of thrombosis due to congenital deficiencies in antithrombin III, protein C, or protein S is compounded by pregnancy (see also Chapters 41 and 42). Activated protein C resistance is a recently identified cause of thrombosis resulting from a point mutation in Factor V, rendering it resistant to inactivation by activated protein C. The abnormal Factor V (Factor V Leiden) is the most common hereditary cause of thrombosis.[72] The Leiden mutation may be a risk factor for stroke during pregnancy.[72] It has also been identified in neonates with cerebral ischemic or hemorrhagic infarct and placental infarcts.[73] Thrombotic thrombocytopenic purpura may initially present during pregnancy and is often mistaken for eclampsia.[74]

Substance abuse is an underrecognized cause of stroke, especially in poor, urban woman (see also Chapter 33). Cocaine (Fig. 48–2), amphetamines, heroin, and other sympathomimetics are associated with both ischemic and hemorrhagic stroke.[75,76] Mechanisms of injury include vasospasm (Fig. 48–3), vasculitis, endocarditis, drug-induced cardiomyopathy with cerebral embolism, foreign material embolism, rupture of preexisting arteriovenous malformations (AVMs) and aneurysms, and acute hypertensive hemorrhage.

Antiphospholipid antibody syndrome is also associated with cerebral arterial occlusive disease (Fig. 48–4) (see also Chapter 43).[77] The diagnostic criteria require the presence of one clinical and one laboratory criteria to be present. The clinical criteria include arterial or venous thrombosis, recurrent pregnancy loss prior to 10 weeks' gestation, one or more unexplained fetal losses after 10 weeks' gestation, premature birth due to placental insufficiency, and preelampsia. Laboratory criteria consist of a medium or high titer of anticardiolipin immunoglobulin G (IgG) or IgM or positive lupus

FIGURE 48–3
Histopathology of a cerebral vessel shows an excessively corrugated internal elastic lamina (*arrows*) separated from the media seen after presumably prolonged vasospasm in a young mother with a massive stroke from crack cocaine use.

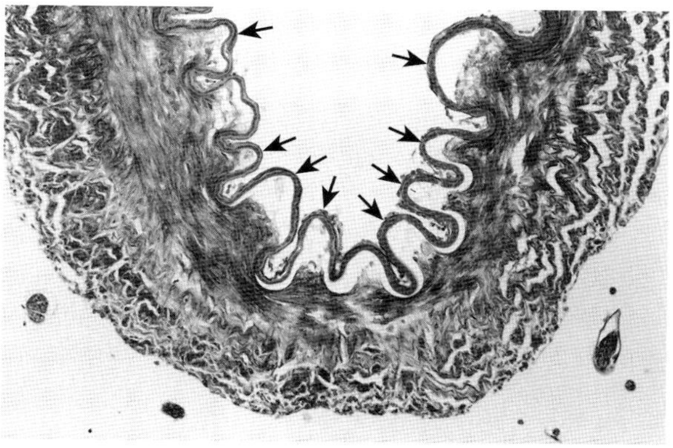

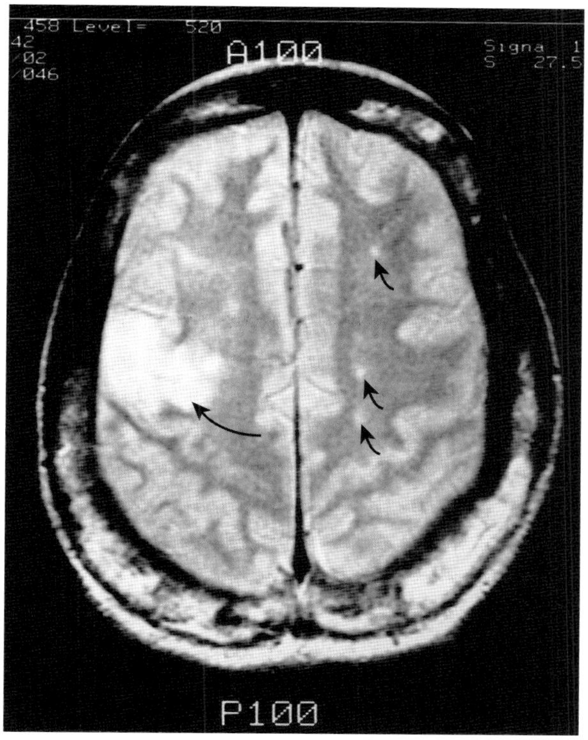

FIGURE 48–4
Axial head MRI (proton-weighted) of a young woman with the antiphospholipid syndrome including recurrent miscarriages. A right middle cerebral artery infarct (*long arrow*) and multiple smaller ischemic lesions in the left cerebral hemisphere (*short arrows*) can be seen.

anticoagulant on two occasions at least 6 weeks apart. Only a portion of these patients has coexistent systemic lupus erythematosus. Patients with higher titers of IgG anticardiolipin antibodies may be at higher risk for recurrent thrombo-occlusive events.[78–84]

Sickle cell disease and sickle cell trait are associated with an increased risk of stroke. Vessel wall injury may occur during periods of crises. The recurrent vascular damage can lead to endothelial proliferation and subsequent vessel occlusion. Frequent blood transfusions can dramatically reduce the vessel damage.[85]

Congestive heart failure during pregnancy or the postpartum period is associated with significant maternal morbidity and mortality (see also Chapter 35). Pulmonary or systemic emboli occur in as many as 50% of these patients. Peripartum cardiomyopathy and rheumatic heart disease are causes of congestive heart failure in pregnancy. Emboli result from ventricular wall thrombosis secondary to a low cardiac output or atrial thrombosis from atrial fibrillation.[86] "Watershed infarction" in the brain has also been reported secondary to low cardiac output.[87]

Cerebral embolism has been associated with mitral valve prolapse (MVP) in case reports.[88] MVP is a common condition with a prevalence of 0.5% to 3% in the general population and as high as 17% in reproductive-age women.[89] The rarity of stroke in pregnancy makes it unlikely to be a significant complication for pregnant women with MVP. Complications associated with atrial septal defects (ASDs) are uncommon in reproductive-age women. However, ASD has been found in up to 50% of young patients with unexplained ischemic stroke.[90] Paradoxical emboli from the venous to the systemic circulation are the cause. Mechanical heart valves may also cause stroke in pregnant women secondary to emboli from valve thrombosis.[91,92] Bacterial endocarditis can also result in ischemic or hemorrhagic stroke.[93] Cardiac disease associated with systemic lupus erythematosus and antiphospholipid syndrome represents another potential etiology.[94]

Management Options

PRENATAL, LABOR AND DELIVERY, AND POSTNATAL

Any focal neurologic deficit in the pregnant woman, transient (<24 hr) or persistent, should raise the suspicion of cerebral ischemia. A careful history and physical examination often give enough information to narrow the diagnostic evaluation. An early imaging study of the brain is essential to exclude hemorrhage or a mass lesion. CT is not contraindicated in pregnancy under these circumstances. Abdominal shielding further limits the minimal fetal radiation exposure. MRI can also be used during pregnancy. Although it is more sensitive than a CT scan, it is tolerated less well by critically ill patients and is often less available.

Initial blood work should include a CBC with differential and platelet count, electrolytes, serum glucose, blood urea nitrogen, creatinine, and prothrombin time (PT)/activated partial thromboplastin time (aPTT). Antinuclear antibody, lupus anticoagulant, and anticardiolipin antibodies, rheumatoid factor, Venereal Disease Research Laboratory (VDRL), and HIV testing should be obtained. Other blood studies include Factor V Leiden, prothrombin gene mutation and with serum protein, and hemoglobin electrophoresis. Protein C and antithrombin III assays may also be done if there is a suggestive family history because these abnormalities are uncommon especially in the absence of such a history. Protein S normally decreases in pregnancy, and testing should be deferred until after pregnancy, if possible, owing to the difficulty in interpreting the results. Blood and urine toxicology evaluation should be obtained. Carotid and transcranial Doppler should be considered. If cardiac etiology is suspected, an electrocardiogram, echocardiogram, Holter monitor, and possibly evaluation for deep venous thrombosis can be performed. A lumbar puncture may also be indicated. In the absence of identified etiology, cerebral angiography is recommended. Despite a thorough evaluation, the etiology of ischemic stroke remains elusive in 20% to 40% of nonpregnant patients. Although no specific data are currently available, this probably holds true for pregnant patients as well.

The use of antithrombotics or anticoagulants for stroke prevention in the first trimester of a pregnancy woman with a history of stroke is controversial and without an evidence base. A recent survey of neurologists through the American Academy of Neurology found that 75% of neurologists would recommend some form of antithrombotic therapy for a history of stroke not related to pregnancy and 88% for women with a history of prior stroke related to pregnancy.[95] Aspirin and low-molecular-weight heparin were chosen by 51% and 7%, respectively, for stroke unrelated to pregnancy and by 41% and 25%, respectively, for stroke related to pregnancy. There remains a significant amount of disagreement over which drugs to use.

When anticoagulation is deemed necessary, heparin is the agent of choice in most instances. Warfarin is an option, but first-trimester embryopathy and the potential for fetal hemorrhage limit its usefulness. Heparin does not cross the placenta and is shorter = acting than warfarin. This decreases fetal risk while making peripartum management easier and more predictable. Complications associated with heparin include thrombocytopenia and osteopenia in addition to bleeding.[96,97]

Prophylactic doses of heparin tend to need to be higher in pregnancy and increase with increasing gestational age.[88] Typical doses are 7500 to 10,000 IU/mL subcutaneously every 12 hours. As in the nonpregnant patient, full anticoagulation aims to maintain the aPTT at 1.5 times control. Therapy is individualized with subcutaneous heparin two to three times daily.

Low-molecular-weight heparin is now commonly used in pregnancy. Advantages over unfractionated heparin include longer duration of action, more reliable antithrombotic effect, and a suggestion of decreased risk of thrombocytopenia and osteopenia.[98,99] Increasing data on use during pregnancy suggest it is safe and effective in preventing noncerebral thrombotic complications.[100,101] Treatment of acute ischemic stroke with low-molecular-weight heparin is of uncertain benefit. Patients with inherited thrombophilias requiring full anticoagulation before pregnancy should be placed on therapeutic doses of heparin preconceptually or once pregnancy is discovered. The optimal therapy for activated protein C resistance during pregnancy is unknown, but likely should at least utilize prophylactic doses of heparin.

Current recommendations for the management of antiphospholipid antibody syndrome in patients with a previous thrombotic episode include therapeutic anticoagulation with unfractionated or low-molecular-weight heparin and low-dose aspirin (60–80 mg/day).[78,79] In those without a prior history of thrombosis, low-dose aspirin should be used. The addition of prophylactic unfractionated or low-molecular-weight heparin is more controversial; however, most authorities would recommend its use. The role of corticosteroids, immunosuppression or plasma exchange, and intravenous gamma globulin is not well defined. In patients with cardiomyopathy or atrial fibrillation, heparin has been used in both prophylactic and therapeutic doses.[102]

Thrombolytic therapy for acute ischemic stroke is indicated in carefully selected patients within a carefully defined time window from symptom onset using a defined protocol. Such time window is currently 180 minutes, but recent evidence strongly suggest that it could be expanded to 4.5 hours.[103] Its use in pregnancy is uncertain, however, because pregnant or lactating women were excluded from the trial that demonstrated efficacy. Case reports have documented the relative safety of intravenous and intra-arterial thrombolysis for neurologic and medical indications throughout pregnancy.[104,105] Nevertheless, the widespread use of thrombolytics during pregnancy cannot be recommended, and they should be used only after a careful discussion of the risks and benefits of this form of treatment with the patient or surrogates and documented in the medical record. Plasmapheresis has been used successfully in some patients with thrombotic thrombocytopenic purpura.[106]

Cerebral Venous Thrombosis

Maternal and Fetal Risks

Cerebral venous thrombosis has been traditionally associated with pregnancy, especially the puerperium. The condition is seen throughout gestation but most commonly is identified during the second to third week postpartum.[107–109] The incidence is highest in developing countries. The original description of severe headache, papilledema, and seizures has evolved through the years. Additional findings at presentation include focal neurologic deficits, bilateral long tract signs, aphasia, visual disturbances, headache, focal seizures, and the syndrome of idiopathic intracranial hypertension. When the deep cerebral venous system is involved, lethargy and coma are common manifestations. The superficial venous sinuses, particularly the superior sagittal sinus, are commonly involved.

Cerebral venous thrombosis has classically been associated with infection and dehydration. Other underlying conditions such as hemoglobinopathies, hyperviscosity syndromes, anemia, leukemia, collagen vascular diseases, malignancy, AVM, and paroxysmal nocturnal hemoglobinuria should be sought.[110] In addition, hypercoagulable states such as protein C and S deficiencies have been implicated.[71,111] More recently, activated protein C resistance,[112,113] lupus anticoagulants, and anticardiolipin antibodies have been identified in patients with cerebral venous thrombosis.[78,114,115]

Management Options

PRENATAL, LABOR AND DELIVERY, AND POSTNATAL

Timely diagnosis of cerebral venous thrombosis requires a high index of suspicion. During pregnancy, the initial evaluation begins with a brain CT without contrast. A partially filled posterior segment of the superior sagittal sinus is seen (empty delta sign) (Fig. 48–5). MRI with magnetic resonance venography can identify the thrombus. It provides greater sensitivity and is currently the test of choice within the limitations previously described.

FIGURE 48–5
Axial head computed tomography (CT) scan demonstrates cerebrovenous thrombosis of the straight sinus (*arrowhead*) and the empty delta sign (*arrow*).

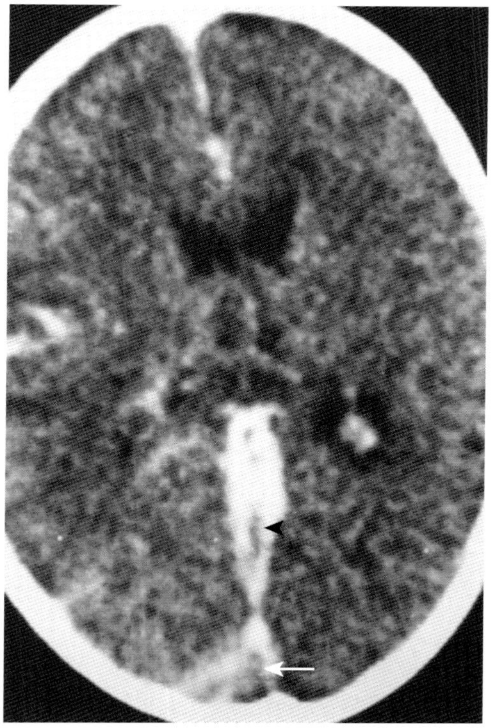

FIGURE 48–6
Conventional cerebral angiography documents large, bilateral cerebral arteriovenous malformations (*arrows*).

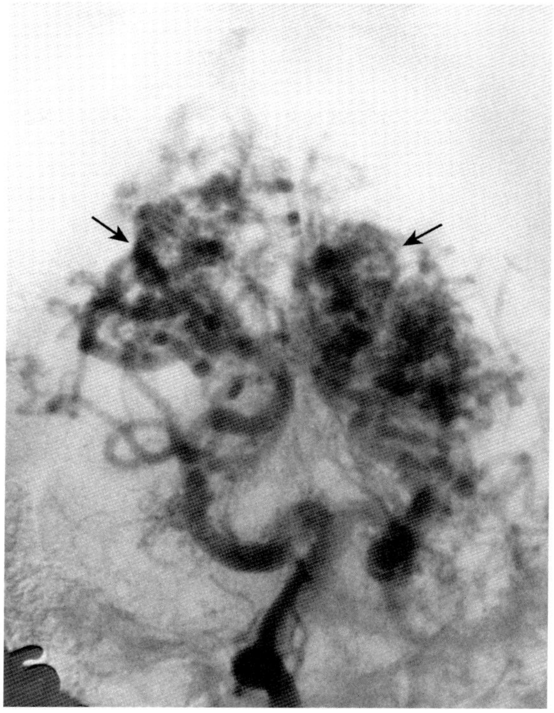

The only prospective, randomized, case-control study evaluating acute treatment found systemic anticoagulation to be the treatment of choice, even in the presence of intracerebral hemorrhage.[116] Thrombolytic therapy is an emergent therapeutic approach; however, owing to the lack of experience in pregnant patients, caution should be exercised.[117] In selected cases of refractory brain edema and ICP elevation, the use of decompressive hemicraniectomy can be entertained.[118] The overall prognosis is generally good in the absence of coma, recurrent seizures, or rapid decline in neurologic function. Long-term outcome is generally better than for arterial stroke. Prolonged anticoagulation with warfarin is required postpartum.

Subarachnoid Hemorrhage

Maternal and Fetal Risks

Subarachnoid hemorrhage (SAH) is a rare but often catastrophic event that can occur during pregnancy. The incidence of SAH is 1 to 5 per 10,000 pregnancies. Maternal mortality is 30% to 40%, but rates as high as 80% have been reported.[119] Fetal outcome parallels that of the mother and reflects the maternal condition as well as gestational age at delivery.[119] The primary etiology during gestation is ruptured cerebral aneurysms or AVMs. Less common causes include Moyamoya disease,[120] dural venous sinus thrombosis, mycotic aneurysm, choriocarcinoma, vasculitides, brain tumors,[121] and coagulopathies. Drugs such as cocaine and phenylpropanolamine have also been linked with SAH in pregnant patients.[122–124]

Aneurysms and AVMs are believed to develop secondary to congenital defects in cerebral vasculature formation. Aneurysms are generally located at an angle of vessel bifurcation in or near the circle of Willis. AVMs, conversely, can be located anywhere between the frontal region and the brainstem, but occur with a higher frequency in the frontoparietal and temporal regions (Fig. 48–6). The anatomic distribution of both lesions is similar to that in the nongravid population.[119] Information describing the natural history of intracranial aneurysms during pregnancy is scarce. In the nonpregnant patient, asymptomatic lesions account for 95% of intracranial aneurysms and are typically identified incidentally. They rupture at a rate of 1% to 2% per year.[125] Activities reported to precede aneurysmal rupture include emotional strain, heavy lifting, coughing, coitus, urination, and defecation. Outcomes of patients with AVMs are influenced by the presenting symptoms and subsequent treatment. Most present with spontaneous bleeding, and these patients have the worst prognosis. Other presenting symptoms in order of frequency include seizures, headache, and neurologic deficit. If left untreated, there is an annual hemorrhage rate of 4%.[125]

Rarely, unruptured aneurysms are first identified during pregnancy. Because SAH is uncommon during gestation, the effect of pregnancy on cerebral aneurysms or AVMs remains controversial. More than 85% of SAH cases occur during the second or third trimester.[126] Several physiologic changes occur during pregnancy, which may theoretically predispose these cerebrovascular abnormalities to bleed. These factors include increases in blood volume, stroke volume, and cardiac output. Estrogen levels are also increased and may result in vasodilation of already abnormal vessels. The many dynamic events occurring during labor and delivery would seem to make this a particularly high-risk time.

Despite the associated physiologic changes, pregnancy does not appear to increase the incidence of SAH, and surprisingly, bleeding during the time of labor and delivery is infrequent.[119,127] Most pregnancies complicated by SAH are preceded by unaffected gestations. In a review of 154 patients prepared by Dias and Sekhar,[119] only 25% were nulliparous, and the mean parity of patients with aneurysmal and AVM ruptures were 2.0 and 1.4, respectively. Barno and Freeman[128] reviewed 24 years of maternal mortality in Minnesota resulting from SAH. The mean parity among the 37 deaths was 2.9. Forster and coworkers[127] reported their experience with AVMs in reproductive-age women. Although the annual hemorrhage rate was higher when these women were pregnant than when not (9.3% vs. 4.5%), it was no different from the 9.6% annual rate in reproductive-age women who never became pregnant. Although Horton and colleagues[129] identified a lower annual rate of hemorrhage in both their pregnant and their nonpregnant patients with AVMs (3.5% vs. 3.1%), they too concluded that pregnancy was not a risk factor for bleeding.

Once bleeding has occurred, the patient's course is significantly modified by the patient's neurologic condition at presentation. The Hunt and Hess classification system has prognostic implications and is shown in Table 48–6. Untreated, half of all nonpregnant patients will die as a result of the initial event, with another 25% to 35% succumbing to a subsequent bleed. Other factors affecting the patient's ultimate outcome are neurologic status, presence of vasospasm, and blood pressure. Maternal mortality associated with aneurysmal bleeding is not increased owing to pregnancy.[119] Conversely, AVM-associated mortality appears to be increased in gravid compared with nongravid patients. This is likely related to the poor neurologic condition of these patients at presentation.[119]

Pregnancy does not significantly alter the clinical presentation of SAH. Signs and symptoms of aneurysmal or AVM bleeding are indistinguishable. A sudden-onset, "bursting" headache is generally the initial symptom. Frequently, other signs and symptoms accompany the headache. These may include nausea and vomiting, meningeal signs, decreased level of consciousness, hypertension, focal neurologic signs, and seizures. Specific findings are dependent on the size, location, and rapidity of the bleed. When the hemorrhage is massive, the patient may be moribund at presentation.

TABLE 48–6

Hunt and Hess Scale for Grading the Clinical Severity of Subarachnoid Hemorrhage

GRADE	EXAMINATION FINDINGS
I	Normal neurologic examination, mild headache, and slightly stiff neck
II	Moderate to severe headache and stiff neck; no confusion or neurologic deficit except for cranial nerve palsy
III	Persistent confusion and/or focal deficit
IV	Persistent stupor; moderate to severe neurologic deficit
V	Coma with moribund appearance

Major complications associated with SAH include vasospasm and recurrent hemorrhage. Vasospasm is a serious problem seen in 30% to 40% of aneurysm patients, but much less commonly in those with AVMs. The resultant ischemia is a major cause of permanent disability and death. Recurrent hemorrhage is a particularly morbid complication. In the untreated nonpregnant, patient the risk of rebleeding is 6% during the first 48 hours. Rebleeding continues to occur at a rate of 1.5% per day for the remainder of the first 2 weeks.[125] Mortality increases with each successive bleed with a rate of 64% and 80% after the first and second rebleed, respectively. Although considerably fewer data are available for the pregnant patient, the risk of recurrent bleeding appears to be similar in this population.[126]

Management Options

PRENATAL

Owing to the rare and life-threatening nature of the condition, it is important to maintain a high index of suspicion. Occasionally, SAH is confused with eclampsia, resulting in diagnostic delays and often a worse outcome. All abnormal neurologic signs and symptoms in the gravida should be thoroughly evaluated. CT scan of the brain, lumbar puncture (if necessary), and cerebral angiography is the common sequence of testing. The CT scan can predict, with a high degree of accuracy, the type of hemorrhage and its site of origin. If the CT scan is normal, the cerebrospinal fluid (CSF) should be examined for blood or xanthochromia. Nonclearing bloody CSF found at lumbar puncture supports the diagnosis of SAH, but it may also be seen with other conditions such as preeclampsia. Cerebral angiography remains the best diagnostic tool for identifying any vascular abnormality. Angiography may fail to visualize the cause of SAH in 20% of patients, however. In these cases, a repeat angiogram may be necessary to rule out false-negative results secondary to vasospasm or clot filling of the aneurysm. MRI scan may also be helpful in situations in which the initial angiogram fails to identify the lesion. Abdominal shielding should be considered during any radiologic examination of the gravid patient.

Management of SAH is based on standard neurosurgical principles with only slight alterations during pregnancy. The clinical goals remain prevention and treatment of neurologic complications. Early aneurysm clipping (<4 days) is now commonly recommended in the post-SAH period for conscious patients. Early operation also allows for therapies such as induced hypertension and volume expansion to be instituted to combat vasospasm without increasing the risk of rebleeding. Improved outcomes for both the mother and the fetus have been realized with early surgical intervention in pregnant patients.[119] Patients with significant neurologic deficits are less likely to undergo early aneurysm clipping owing to an extremely high operative mortality. Advances with endovascular procedures in the treatment of cerebral aneurysms (e.g., guglielmi detachable coils [GDC]) allow the early securing of these vascular lesions in high risk patients.[130] Medical therapy alone and careful monitoring of these high risk patients always remains as an alternative to any intervention if the patient is too unstable to leave the intensive care unit.

The proper timing for resection of AVMs is more controversial owing to the smaller number of cases. No clear benefit to surgery in these patients has been found,[119] with some surgeons advocating operative intervention in AVMs only to remove clinically significant hematomas. One alternative is embolization of the AVM under angiographic control prior to surgical excision.

A complete discussion of the neurosurgical and anesthetic principles of craniotomy for aneurysm clipping is beyond the scope of this chapter. However, there are two intraoperative therapies—hypotension and hypothermia—commonly instituted to reduce complications, which raise special concerns in the pregnant patient. Hypotension is sometimes instituted to reduce the risk of rupture of the aneurysm during surgical dissection. Although maternal hypotension may pose a threat to fetal well-being, it has been successfully induced with sodium nitroprusside or isoflurane in a number of cases.[131,132] Based on experimental evidence, administration of sodium nitroprusside in pregnant patients has raised concerns regarding potential fetal cyanide toxicity. Thus, if surgery is to be preformed during pregnancy, it is recommended that infusion rates not exceed 10 mg/kg/min.[132] The fetal effects of maternal hypotension should be evaluated throughout the perianesthetic period with electronic fetal heart rate monitoring. Adverse changes in fetal cardiac activity suggest the need for elevation in maternal blood pressure if safe and feasible from the maternal standpoint. Many of the drugs used in anesthesia may decrease fetal heart rate variability, thereby complicating fetal heart rate monitor interpretation. Excessive hyperventilation has been shown to further decrease uterine blood flow during sodium nitroprusside administration and should be avoided.[133,134] Because of the potential fetal risks of maternal hypotension, some authors recommend cesarean delivery immediately prior to intracranial surgery if the fetus is mature enough.[135]

Hypothermia is instituted during cerebral aneurysm clipping as a means of cerebral protection from potential ischemia due to aneurysm rupture, retraction injury, or hypotension. Stånge and Halldin[136] have suggested that hypothermia is well tolerated by the mother and fetus, provided that other confounding variables (such as respiratory exchange, acidosis, and electrolyte balance) are controlled. However, the majority of experience with hypothermia and hypotension in pregnancy is anecdotal. Regardless of the neurosurgical technique employed, maternal outcome remains the most important predictor of eventual fetal outcome.

Adjunctive medical therapy for SAH is directed toward reducing the risks of rebleeding and cerebral ischemia due to vasospasm. Patients are generally confined to bedrest in a dark, quiet room. They are administered stool softeners and analgesics. Because of the presumed benefits of volume expansion, colloid solutions are frequently administered. Nimodipine, a dihydropyridine calcium channel blocker, is often given because it has been shown to improve neurologic outcome following SAH. Caution is advised in using this drug in pregnancy because the fetal effects have not been completely defined. In a small number of preeclamptic patients taking nimodipine for seizure prophylaxis, no apparent adverse fetal outcomes were reported.[137] However, in an animal model, nicardipine (another dihydropyridine calcium channel blocker) led to the development of fetal acidosis and hypoxemia.[138]

Epsilon-aminocaproic acid (EACA) and tranexamic acid have been used to block the activation of plasminogen, a precursor of plasmin, a major fibrinolytic protein, and decrease the incidence of rebleeding. Initial clinical trials did find a reduction in the incidence of rebleeding with these agents; however, later work failed to demonstrate significant improvement in outcome.[139] EACA, because of the lack of proven benefit and potential interference with fetal fibrinolysis, which may be linked to the development of hyaline membrane disease, is not used in current clinical practice.[140]

Cerebral edema can result in elevated ICP. Intracranial invasive monitoring may be necessary. If there is ICP elevation secondary to cerebral edema, mannitol, an osmotic diuretic, may be used. Typically, 1 g/kg of mannitol is administered intravenously, as frequently as needed to keep the ICP below 20 mm Hg. The development of hyperosmolality due to dehydration is a potential hazard of mannitol therapy and can be monitored by frequent determinations of the patient's intravascular volume status. Normal values are 280 to 300 mOsm/L; the drug should be withheld when a level of 315 to 320 mOsm/L is reached. Care must be taken to prevent hypovolemia resulting from the accompanying diuresis, which could aggravate both cerebral and placental hypoperfusion. The use of hypertonic saline solutions (2% and 3% sodium chloride/acetate) is becoming a popular alternative to mannitol owing to their efficacy and hemodynamic profile. Nevertheless, their safety during pregnancy is not defined, and the use of these solutions should, therefore, be limited to only extreme cases of refractory ICP elevation.

LABOR AND DELIVERY

After a successful repair of an aneurysm or AVM, the most frequent obstetric concern relates to mode of delivery. Earlier authors routinely recommended elective cesarean section for these patients. This was particularly true along with consideration of sterilization if an AVM was responsible for the SAH.[141] More recent data and reanalysis of some older studies suggest that labor and vaginal delivery pose no additional risk to mother or fetus.[119,127,129,142] These recommendations probably also hold true for the patient who begins labor before surgical correction is attempted or in the case in which the intracranial lesion is inaccessible to surgical intervention, but the data are very limited. Young and associates[143] have suggested that the rise in physiologic blood pressure known to occur in labor are counterbalanced by a parallel increase in CSF pressure, offering a potential explanation for the foregoing clinical observations. Despite the suggested safety of labor, minimizing the hemodynamic stresses of labor is still advocated by using epidural anesthesia and shortening the second stage of labor with outlet forceps. In reality, with cesarean section rates exceeding 30% in the United States, many of these patients will be delivered by elective cesarean section to minimize any perceived risk. Ultimate management decisions should be individualized based primarily on the maternal condition with modifications for fetal intervention based on gestational age.

SUMMARY OF MANAGEMENT OPTIONS

Cerebrovascular Disease

Management Options	Evidence Quality and Recommendation	References
Ischemic Stroke (Arterial) and Transient Ischemic Attacks		
General supportive measures (see Chapter 78)	—/GPP	—
Search for cause/associated factors:	III/B	62,66
• Investigate CBC, clotting and thrombophilia screen, renal and liver function routinely; other investigations determined by possible cause.		
• Treat thrombolic/embolic conditions (see Chapters 41, 42, 43, and 78).		
• Cause is unknown in 20%–40%.		
Consider anticoagulation with heparin if no evidence of hemorrhage on MRI or CT.	III/B	62,66
Indications for surgery are as for nonpregnant patients.	III/B	62,66
Cerebral Venous Thrombosis		
Control seizures.	III/B	107,111
Ensure adequate hydration.	III/B	107
One randomized case-controlled study suggests anticoagulation beneficial.	Ib/A	116
No experience in pregnancy with thrombolytic therapy.	III/B	117
Subarachnoid Hemorrhage		
Diagnosis		
(following high index of clinical suspicion) by, in order:	IV/C	119
• CT scan.		
• Lumbar puncture.		
• Cerebral angiography (or MRI).		
Management—Prenatal		
Arrange for interdisciplinary care with neurosurgeons.	—/GPP	—
In general, normal neurosurgical principles of management apply in pregnancy, though care needed intraoperatively with		
• Hypotension.	IV/C	132
• Hypothermia.	IV/C	136
Anticonvulsants, high-dose steroids, mannitol, and nimodipine (safe in limited pregnancy experience) are used depending on clinical picture/problems.	IIb/B	137
Use caution with EACA.	Ia/A	139
Trend for early surgery.	III/B	119
Embolization prior to or without surgery is a new development.	IV/C	131
Management—Labor and Delivery		
Regional analgesics preferable to narcotics and general anesthetics.	—/GPP	—
No evidence to support blanket policy of elective cesarean section, but most advocate	III/B	40,119, 127,129
• Minimizing pushing in second stage.		
• Cesarean section for normal obstetric reasons.		
• Consider life-support machine and care in patient with brain death to gain fetal maturity.		

CBC, complete blood count; CT computed tomography; EACA, epsilon-aminocaproic acid; GPP, good practice point; MRI, magnetic resonance imaging.

TABLE 48–7
Types and Causes of Postpartum Headache

Primary Headache Disorders
Migraine
Tension-type headache
Causes of Secondary Headaches
Postdural puncture headache
Embolic stroke
Carotid or vertebral artery dissection
Subarachnoid hemorrhage
Parenchymal brain hemorrhage
Cerebral venous sinus thrombosis
Meningitis, encephalitis
Pituitary disorders
Postpartum preeclampsia
Reversible posterior encephalopathy syndrome
Postpartum angiopathy
Coincidental conditions (e.g., cerebral vasculitis or brain tumor)

HEADACHE

Maternal Risks

Headaches during pregnancy and postpartum are extremely common. The most common categories are migraine and tension-type. Although a new-onset headache during pregnancy and in the postpartum period is most likely either a migraine or a tension-type, it may be the first manifestation of an intracranial process that needs immediate attention[144,145] (Table 48–7). Such conditions include aneurysm rupture, AVM, intracranial hypertension, cerebral ischemia, cerebral venous thrombosis, meningitis, sinusitis, and intracranial masses. In addition, benign intracranial hypertension or pseudotumor cerebri may be seen with pregnancy, but it is uncommon. Patients receiving spinal or epidural analgesia or anesthesia may experience a spinal headache during the postpartum period.

Evaluation of the pregnant patient with headache represents a clinical challenge. The ailment's prevalence and typically benign nature make it desirable to minimize costs by limiting diagnostic testing while being certain to promptly diagnose the uncommon but more serious conditions. The medical history is usually very helpful. Migraines are often associated with a history of similar previous episodes. With a past history suggestive of migraine headaches, a normal neurologic examination, and resolution with simple measures, the patient may be followed clinically. A new-onset headache severe enough to justify an emergency room visit or a preexisting condition becoming progressively worse, presence of an "aura," or a new neurologic deficit warrants a diagnostic evaluation.

Migraine

Maternal and Fetal Risk

Migraines can be subdivided into those with and those without an aura. The aura is described as the presence of transient neurologic signs or symptoms before, during, or even after the headache. The pain is often associated with nausea, vomiting, and photophobia. Sleep often provides relief. As with headaches in general during gestation, the course of migraines is variable. A decrease in frequency is seen in 50% to 80% of women, particularly in the third trimester.[144] Those patients experiencing migraines associated with menstruation are especially likely to show improvement. The headaches tend to worsen postpartum with as many as 40% of patients complaining of pain during this time. Migraine recurred during the first week after childbirth in about one third of women.[146] Migraines may present for the first time during the puerperium in 4.5% of patients, however, and an aura may initially appear during this time period. There is no demonstrated adverse fetal outcome associated with migraines.[147]

Management Options

PRENATAL, LABOR AND DELIVERY, AND POSTNATAL

A carefully obtained history and physical examination are essential. With a prior personal or family history of migraine and a typical presentation, no further investigation is needed. New-onset migraines represent a diagnosis of exclusion. In the absence of a past history or with focal neurologic findings, neuroimaging studies such as brain CT or MRI are indicated.[144] It is desirable to minimize x-ray exposure to the abdomen and pelvis and avoid contrast agents if possible. Radiologic studies should not be avoided on the basis of pregnancy alone, however. Prothrombin time, aPTT, fibrinogen, and CBC with platelets should be obtained. Additional investigations should include anticardiolipin antibodies, antithrombin III, and protein C as indicated to exclude thrombophilias. Physiologic decreases in protein S levels make these levels difficult to interpret in pregnancy. Lumbar puncture is indicated once the absence of an intracranial mass effect has been ruled out by imaging studies. A normal opening pressure (range 5–15 mm Hg) excludes pseudotumor cerebri.

Migraine treatment during pregnancy is complicated by the fact that most drugs cross the placenta and many have potential adverse fetal effects. As a result, physicians often avoid indicated drug therapy despite relatively safe and effective options.[144] Therapy can be divided into abortive and prophylactic measures. The latter approach is reserved for patients with debilitating headaches or those with a frequency, for example, exceeding three migraine episodes per month. β-Blockers (categories B and C) are often helpful in this situation. Tricyclic antidepressants (most category D) are a useful second-line approach.

A variety of interventions are available once a headache has begun. In patients in which normal daily function is not significantly compromised, nonpharmacologic measures are advised. Such strategies include coping mechanisms such as ice, massage, sleep, and biofeedback. Reassurance is also of value, because many migraine sufferers experience improvement during gestation. When drug therapy is needed, acetaminophen and low-dose caffeine (both category B) can be used as first-line agents. During the first two trimesters, a short course of nonsteroidal anti-inflammatory drugs (NSAIDs) can be tried (many are category B in early pregnancy). Extended use of NSAIDs should be avoided, however, because of potential constriction of the fetal ductus arteriosus and oligohydramnios particularly in the later part of gestation (category D in the third trimester). Narcotics such as meperidine, morphine, and hydromorphone (category B) can be used if severity warrants.[148] Glucocorticoids (category B) are safe when used for short periods and may help in migraines refractory to standard treatment. Magnesium sulfate can be used for prophylactic or abortive therapy. Benzodiazepines (category D), ergot derivatives (category D), and sumatriptan as well as the newer triptans (category C) should be avoided.[149] Although the association of benzodiazepines with birth defects is not clear, neonatal depression and withdrawal are problems encountered with use during the latter part of pregnancy. Vasoconstriction caused by the ergot derivatives may lead to fetal vascular disruption. In addition, these agents may increase uterine activity by an oxytocin-like action. In the most extreme cases, intravenous hydration, prochlorperazine 10 mg intravenous, and intravenous narcotics or corticosteroids may be necessary.[144]

Nausea is a common accompanying complaint. Mild symptoms can usually be successfully treated with phosphorylated carbohydrate solution (emetrol) or doxylamine succinate (category B) and pyridoxine (vitamin B_6). In more severe cases, trimethobenzamide (category C) and some phenothiazine compounds including chlorpromazine, prochlorperazine, and promethazine (all category C) can be used parenterally or as suppositories. Most of the medications described previously enter the breast milk. Those that can be used in pregnancy can continue to be utilized during breast-feeding. Chlorpromazine is an exception, because it can cause neonatal lethargy.

Tension-type Headaches

Maternal and Fetal Risks

Tension-type headaches are characterized by daily headaches of mild to moderate severity with a global distribution. They typically worsen throughout the day, and nausea and vomiting are seldom reported. Patients may exhibit symptoms such as depressed mood, anorexia, and insomnia. In contrast with migraine, tension-type headache symptoms do not improve during pregnancy, and may actually worsen. The pathogenesis is unclear. Contracture of the neck muscles and stretching of aponeurotic connections may be the result rather than the cause of the headache. Characteristically, the neurologic examination is normal and no neuroimaging studies are required.

Treatment is aimed at behavioral aspects of the condition. Mild analgesics are indicated only in the presence of considerable pain. Acetaminophen is preferable to aspirin. If depression is a cardinal component, antidepressant agents can be used. Despite their classification, the tricyclic antidepressants (most category D) appear to be relatively safe during pregnancy and can be used when clinically indicated. The serotonin uptake inhibitors (most category C) have been associated with a neonatal abstinence syndrome characterized by jitteriness, poor tone, and mild respiratory morbidity. The available information suggests that these agents may also be used relatively safely when indicated.[150,151]

Spinal Headache (See also Chapter 70)

Maternal Risks and Management Options

Spinal headaches are commonly seen after accidental dural puncture during epidural placement. The typical history is that of a moderate to severe headache that is exacerbated with sitting or standing and palliated with lying flat. The frequency of symptoms is related to the large-bore needle used. Such headaches less commonly follow the use of spinal anesthesia. The symptoms are believed to be due to leakage of CSF and subsequent CSF hypotension. Initial management consists of intravenous hydration and bedrest lying flat. If the patient fails to show improvement within 24 hours of conservative management, a blood patch is indicated and brain imaging should be strongly considered. About 2 to 3 mL of autologous blood is injected near the area of the dural puncture. Dramatic resolution of symptoms is typically observed,[152] although it may take 1 to several days for resolution.

Benign Intracranial Hypertension (Pseudotumor Cerebri)

Maternal Risks

Benign intracranial hypertension is characterized by the presence of diffuse global headache, nausea, vomiting, papilledema, and at times, horizontal diplopia. It is typically worse during early morning hours. The cause of increased ICP is due to either increased production or decreased reabsorption of CSF.[153] This condition is seen more frequently in young, obese, reproductive-age women. There is no evidence that the incidence is higher during pregnancy. Although benign intracranial hypertension can develop throughout pregnancy, it is most often seen during the first half of gestation. Other causes of increased ICP are listed in Table 48–8.

TABLE 48–8

Causes of Raised Intracranial Pressure

Benign intracranial hypertension
Cerebral edema
Hypertensive encephalopathy
Lead poisoning
Viral encephalitis
Impaired reabsorption CSF
Venous sinus thrombosis
High CSF protein
Guillain-Barré syndrome
Spinal cord tumor
Postmeningitis
Drugs
Hypervitaminosis A
Tetracycline
Indomethacin
Nitrofurantoin
Space-occupying lesion

CSF, cerebrospinal fluid.

Management Options

PRENATAL AND LABOR AND DELIVERY

The diagnosis is one of exclusion. It is confirmed by demonstrating a high opening pressure at the time of lumbar puncture in the presence of a normal CT scan. Although weight reduction is a part of treatment in nonpregnant individuals, it is not encouraged during pregnancy. Excess weight gain should be avoided. Treatment is aimed at avoiding visual complications.[154] Acetazolamide, a carbonic anhydrase inhibitor (category C), is used along with repeated lumbar puncture and CSF drainage. Refractory cases may be treated with a lumbar subarachnoid-peritoneal shunt. When vision is threatened, optic nerve sheath fenestration can be performed to relieve pressure on the optic nerve.

Cesarean section is reserved for obstetric indications. Because lumbar puncture is a mainstay of treatment, regional anesthesia with either spinal or epidural is not contraindicated.

SUMMARY OF MANAGEMENT OPTIONS
Headache

Management Options	Evidence Quality and Recommendation	References
General		
Indications for Further Investigation	—/GPP	—
• Focal/abnormal neurologic signs.		
• Impaired intellect.		
• Worsening and/or intractable pain.		
• Pain that disturbs sleep.		
Migraine		
Avoid Precipitating Factors; Nonpharmacologic Measures	IV/C	144,148
• Bedrest.		
• Avoidance of light.		
• Coping mechanisms.		
• Ice.		
• Massage.		
• Sleep.		
Analgesics		
Simple agents (e.g., acetaminophen)	IV/C	144,148
Short course of NSAIDs in first two trimesters but not third.	IV/C	144,148
Narcotics (e.g., meperidine, morphine) for severe cases.	IV/C	144
Short course of adjuvant glucocorticoids for refractory cases (**avoid** benzodiazepines, ergot preparations, and sumatriptan).	IV/C	144,149
Prophylaxis	IV/C	144,148
Propranolol (trial excluded pregnant women).		
Tricyclic antidepressants.		
Antiemetics		
Phenothiazines (Trial excluded pregnant women.)	IV/C	144,148
Tension Headaches		
Provide reassurance, bedrest.	—/GPP	—
Use simple analgesia.		
Administer tricyclic antidepressants in extreme cases.		

SUMMARY OF MANAGEMENT OPTIONS

Headache—cont'd

Management Options	Evidence Quality and Recommendation	References
Spinal Headache		
No evidence that injection of physiologic saline at time of dural tap/puncture is of benefit.	—/GPP	—
Analgesia.	—/GPP	—
Lying flat.	Ib/A	7
Autologous blood patch if analgesia and lying flat fail to work after 24 hr.	Ib/A	7
Benign Intracranial Hypertension		
Exclude other causes of raised intracranial pressure.	—/GPP	—
Monitor visual function.	—/GPP	—
Avoid excess weight gain.	III/B	154
If evidence of visual function deterioration, consider		
• Acetazolamide.	III/B	154
• Serial lumbar puncture.	III/B	154
If these conservative measures fail (extrapolated from management in nonpregnant subjects):		
• Shunting.	—/GPP	—
• Optic nerve sheath fenestration if vision is still threatened.	—/GPP	—

GPP, good practice point; NSAIDs, nonsteroidal anti-inflammatory drugs.

VENTRICULOPERITONEAL SHUNTS

Maternal Risks

Advances in extracranial shunt technology during the 1960s have improved the prognosis for patients with hydrocephalus. As a result, an increasing number of women with ventriculoperitoneal shunts in place are reaching reproductive age and becoming pregnant.[155] Pregnancy is associated with signs and symptoms of elevated ICP in as many as 58% of patients with previously well-functioning shunts.[156] Several case reports would suggest that shunt malfunction is more common in the third trimester. The causes of the malfunctions have been postulated to be functional rather than mechanical, due to increased intraperitoneal pressure associated with advancing gestational age.[157]

Management Options

PREPREGNANCY

A baseline CT scan or MRI preconceptually may be of value. Further investigation is indicated if there is any suggestion of shunt malfunction.[156] The baseline study can also be of benefit for comparison purposes in the diagnostic evaluation of symptoms suggestive of increased ICP that may occur later in pregnancy. Patients using AEDs should have their therapy reevaluated. Genetic counseling and preconceptual folic acid should be provided in cases in which a maternal neural tube defect is present.

PRENATAL

Patients should be monitored for evidence of increased ICP including headaches, nausea, vomiting, visual changes, and altered sensorium. In the presence of these symptoms, a CT scan or MRI should be obtained. With radiologic evidence of elevated ICP, conservative management with bedrest, fluid restriction, and corticosteroids may be tried. More rapid relief and direct measurement of the ICP can be obtained during aspiration of the shunt reservoir.[158] Pumping of the shunt may also provide symptomatic relief.[159] This method is less invasive and theoretically can decrease the risk of shunt infection. Shunt replacement should be reserved for those patients who fail conservative treatment.

LABOR AND DELIVERY

Intrapartum management of women with ventriculoperitoneal shunts centers on the optimal mode of delivery and the need for prophylactic antibiotics. The majority of reported cases were allowed to labor and deliver vaginally. No complications were noted.[155] Concern with the potential for intra-abdominal scarring associated with surgery and the favorable outcomes seen with vaginal delivery would suggest that cesarean section should be reserved for routine obstetric indications. Shortening of the second stage with forceps or vacuum can be considered, but it does not appear to be universally necessary.[155] Analgesia and anesthesia choices during labor and delivery are limited. Narcotic use should be minimized because of the potential further increase in ICP and altered sensorium. Epidural anesthesia can be used with caution. In patients with elevated ICP or a neural tube defect, regional anesthesia should be avoided and general anesthesia used.

The use of prophylactic antibiotics during the intrapartum period is controversial, but the presence of a foreign body with a direct connection to the brain makes prophylaxis theoretically sensible.[156] No adverse outcomes have been reported in several patients managed without the routine use of prophylaxis.[157] It should be noted, however, that the number of involved patients was small and increased experience will be required before a true lack of benefit is determined.

SUMMARY OF MANAGEMENT OPTIONS

Ventriculoperitoneal Shunts

Management Options	Evidence Quality and Recommendation	References
Prepregnancy		
Check clinically for symptoms suggestive of shunt malfunction; MRI/CT if suspected (? useful as baseline for pregnancy even if asymptomatic).	Ib/A	156
Review and rationalize anticonvulsant medication (see earlier under "Epilepsy").	—/GPP	—
Administer folate for all and provide specific genetic counseling if neural tube defect.	Ib/A	156
Prenatal		
Maintain vigilance for raised intracranial pressure (and shunt malfunction).	—/GPP	—
MRI/CT if suspected.	—/GPP	—
If confirmed:	IV/C	158,159
• Bedrest.		
• Fluid restriction.		
• Reservoir aspiration or pumping.		
Replace shunt for those who fail conservative measures.	—/GPP	—
Labor and Delivery		
Vaginal delivery is acceptable; assisted procedure only for normal obstetric indications.	III/B	155
Epidural with care; avoid narcotic analgesia (raises intracranial pressure).	GPP	
No evidence of need for prophylactic antibiotics.	III/B	155,156

CT, computed tomography; GPP, good practice point; MRI, magnetic resonance imaging.

SPINAL CORD INJURY

Maternal Risks

Modern rehabilitation practices allow many patients with spinal cord injuries to lead increasingly independent lives. Often included is the desire to develop a family. Many of the medical problems common to patients with spinal cord problems may be exacerbated during pregnancy. Urinary tract infections (UTIs) often with resistant organisms are common in all patients with spinal cord injury owing to incomplete bladder emptying and indwelling or intermittent catheterization. During gestation, 75% or more women will develop a UTI. This increases the risk of pyelonephritis.[160] Anemia is present in 60% to 100% of patients. Chronic constipation, another problem seen in nearly all patients with spinal cord injury, is compounded both by pregnancy itself and by iron supplementation used in anemia treatment.[161] Immobility associated with many spinal lesions places patients at risk for pressure ulceration. One quarter to a half of gravid patients develop pressure sores, with gestational weight gain a potential aggravating factor. Patients with lesions above T10 may not feel contractions, resulting in failure to appreciate the onset of term or preterm labor, increasing the risk of precipitous or preterm delivery.

Autonomic dysreflexia is a potentially life-threatening complication, which can occur in patients with spinal cord lesions at or above T5. The condition results from stimulation of pelvic or abdominal organs with resultant sympathetic activation uncontrolled by higher centers. Clinical manifestations can include headache, flushing, sweating, cardiac arrhythmias, and hypertension. Several activities common to pregnancy may precipitate autonomic dysreflexia, making this a time of particular concern, including bowel or bladder distention, bladder catheterization, labor, and even vaginal examination.

Management Options

PRENATAL

Management is aimed at minimizing the risk of the common complications. Urine should be screened for bacteria with appropriate treatment when significant bacteriuria is identified. Prophylactic antibiotics for suppression may be considered. If bladder catheterization is necessary, intermittent is preferred over an indwelling catheter. Dietary changes, stool softeners, or enemas may be necessary to control constipation, with manual disimpaction in extreme cases. Attention to padding and position changes is important to avoid skin breakdown. Patients should be monitored for preterm labor. Uterine palpation and serial cervical examinations can be utilized.

LABOR AND DELIVERY

Unnecessary stimuli that may lead to autonomic dysreflexia should be avoided. Because uterine contractions are often associated with the condition, epidural anesthesia may be placed early in labor to eliminate sympathetic tone. This should be done even if the patient does not feel the pain of contractions.

SUMMARY OF MANAGEMENT OPTIONS

Spinal Cord Injury

Management Options	Evidence Quality and Recommendation	References
Prenatal		
Administer prophylactic antibiotics.	—/GPP	—
Screen for bacteriuria.	III/B	160
Provide dietary adjustment and bowel softener.	—/GPP	—
Provide nursing care including attention to pressure areas.	—/GPP	—
Maintain vigilance for preterm labor.	—/GPP	—
Labor and Delivery		
Avoid unnecessary stimuli; epidural even if no sensation.	—/GPP	—

GPP, good practice point.

NEUROMUSCULAR DISEASES: MONONEUROPATHIES

Facial Nerve Palsy ("Bell's Palsy")

Maternal Risks

Peripheral facial nerve palsy is characterized by acute onset facial-weakness, occasionally preceded by ipsilateral retroauricular pain. The sense of taste may be diminished over the anterior two thirds of the tongue in lesions proximal to the origin of the corda tympani. Viral infection may play an etiologic role. Bell's palsy appears to be more prevalent during pregnancy, with an increased frequency during the third trimester and postpartum. More than three quarters of the pregnancy-related cases occur during this time period. The reported incidence is approximately 50 per 100 000 pregnancies, but only 17 per 100 000 in nonpregnant women of childbearing age.[162]

Management Options

Although the benefit of prednisone (category B) is uncertain, it is frequently used at a dose of 1 mg/kg daily for 5 to 7 days. Success rates are higher if therapy is started within 7 days of the onset of symptoms. The eye should be protected with drops and glasses or a patch. The outcome is quite favorable, with most women recovering completely within 3 to 6 weeks.

Carpal Tunnel Syndrome

Maternal Risks

Carpal tunnel syndrome results from entrapment of the median nerve in the carpal tunnel of the wrist. It is one of the most common mononeuropathies encountered during pregnancy, with a prevalence of up to 20%.[163] The syndrome is manifested by wrist pain and numbness in the first three digits (and occasionally part of the fourth) of the affected hand. The symptoms may often be severe enough to interfere with the sleep; however, significant weakness and muscle wasting are uncommon. Excessive weight gain and fluid retention are predisposing factors. Symptoms typically begin in the second half of pregnancy; however, carpal tunnel syndrome may initially present in the puerperium.[164,165]

Management Options

The diagnosis is typically made clinically. Electrophysiologic studies may be used if necessary. A decreased conduction velocity in the median nerve across the wrist is seen.

Initial therapy is conservative and consists of rest and wrist splinting. Resolution of symptoms usually occurs within a few weeks after delivery. In those cases that first present postpartum, resolution is seen 2 to 3 weeks after breast-feeding is stopped. Very few patients will require surgical nerve decompression.

Lateral Femoral Cutaneous Neuropathy (Meralgia Paresthetica)

Maternal Risks

Meralgia paresthetica is a minor but bothersome sensory disturbance caused by stretching or compression of the lateral femoral cutaneous nerve under the inguinal ligament.[166] Numbness, tingling, burning, or pain in the lateral aspect of the thigh and no other neurologic deficits characterize it. Standing or walking aggravates the symptoms. Symptoms usually begin during the third trimester and are often associated with obesity and exaggerated lumbar lordosis. Prolonged labor may cause or precipitate this neuropathy due to straining with hips flexed.

Management Options

During pregnancy, pain relief can usually be achieved with sitting. Resolution occurs postpartum without treatment in most instances. Occasionally, AEDs or antidepressant drugs such as carbamazepine or amitriptyline, respectively, may be required. Local steroid or lidocaine injections may be useful.

Lumbar Disk Disease

Maternal Risks and Management Options

Lower back pain is one of the most common complaints during pregnancy, affecting more than 50% of pregnancies from the mid-second trimester onward.[167] Significant lumbar disk disease is relatively uncommon, however. Clear clinicoradiologic evidence of herniated disk was found in only 5 of nearly 49,000 consecutive deliveries.[168] Fifty-six of 6048 (0.92%) interviewed women had a confirmed new nerve injury of the lower extremities.[169] Factors associated with nerve injury were nulliparity and prolonged second stage of labor. Median duration of symptoms was 2 months. Diagnostic studies include nerve conduction velocities and electromyography. MRI studies should be used cautiously because there is a significant prevalence of disk bulges and frank disk herniations in asymptomatic individuals.[170] Patients who are refractory to medical therapy after delivery may benefit from lumbar laminectomy. Intraoperative positioning during cesarean section may cause sciatica neuropathy.[171]

SUMMARY OF MANAGEMENT OPTIONS

Mononeuropathies

Management Options	Evidence Quality and Recommendation	References
Facial Nerve Palsy (Bell's Palsy)		
Administer high-dose steroids, especially if severe and early presentation, though it may not be as effective in pregnancy.	III/B	162
Protect eye on affected side.	—/GPP	—
Carpal Tunnel Syndrome		
Provide explanation and reassurance.	III/B	163,164
Perform wrist exercises during day; use elevation at night.	III/B	163,164
Splint wrist.	III/B	163,164
Diuretics have been used in severe cases.	III/B	165
Administer local steroid injection for relief of symptoms.	III/B	165
Surgical decompression is not usually necessary in pregnancy.	III/B	165
Lateral Femoral Cutaneous Neuropathy (Meralgia Paresthetica)		
Provide explanation and reassurance.	IV/C	166
Relief with certain positions, especially when sitting.	IV/C	166
Rarely are anticonvulsants (carbamazepine) or antidepressants (amitriptyline) required.	—/GPP	—
Lumbar Disk Disease		
Use conservative approach (bedrest, firm supporting mattress).	III/B	167,168
Surgery reserved for cases refractory to conservative measures persisting after pregnancy.	III/B	167

GPP, good practice point.

NEUROMUSCULAR DISEASES: POLYNEUROPATHIES

Acute Inflammatory Demyelinating Polyneuropathy (Guillain-Barré Syndrome)

Maternal Risks

Acute inflammatory demyelinating polyneuropathy is an acquired condition characterized by demyelination of the motor roots and the proximal segments of the peripheral nerves.[172] Pregnancy appears to have no effect on the incidence or course of the disease. Guillain-Barré syndrome also does not adversely affect pregnancy.[173,174] Presentation usually consists of ascending paralysis associated with lower back pain and radicular symptoms. Deep tendon reflexes are typically very depressed or lost. In the most severe cases, respiratory muscle paralysis is seen and mechanical ventilation is required. Viral infections such as cytomegalovirus (CMV), Epstein-Barr virus (EBV), HIV-1, and hepatitis virus may play a causative role. Flulike symptoms often precede the onset of weakness by 2 to 3 weeks. In addition, *Campylobacter jejuni* has been implicated as an etiologic agent.

Management Options

The diagnosis is made based on the history and physical examination. Confirmation is obtained with electrophysiologic studies. Abnormal findings become evident more than 7 days after the onset of symptoms. Plasmapheresis has been used in the treatment during pregnancy since 1980.[175] Volume status and fetal well-being should be monitored during therapy because significant hypovolemia can result from fluid shifts occurring during therapy. Intravenous immunoglobulins have been used as an alternative to plasmapheresis.[176] Intubation and mechanical ventilation along with appropriate supportive care should be utilized as indicated. Spontaneous labor and vaginal delivery can be allowed. There is no contraindication to epidural anesthesia.

Chronic Inflammatory Demyelinating Polyneuropathy

Maternal Risks

Chronic inflammatory demyelinating polyneuropathy is a condition with clinical features similar to those of Guillain-Barré syndrome. A protracted course extending beyond 6 months and a tendency to relapse differentiates the two conditions. During pregnancy, recurrence is seen more often in the last half of gestation.[177] There are no known adverse fetal effects.

Corticosteroids, plasmapheresis, and immunoglobulins have been used therapeutically individually or in combination. Treatment response is variable, and sometimes, poor outcomes result. Data during pregnancy are limited, but labor and delivery are usually uneventful.

Multifocal motor neuropathy has been reported to worsen during pregnancy and to improve with intravenous immunoglobulin (IVIG).[178]

SUMMARY OF MANAGEMENT OPTIONS

Polyneuropathies

Management Options	Evidence Quality and Recommendation	References
Acute Inflammatory Demyelinating Polyneuropathy		
Monitor respiratory function; ventilatory support may be necessary.	—/GPP	—
Provide nursing and physiotherapy care.	—/GPP	—
Administer prophylactic heparin.	—/GPP	—
Therapy options:		
• Plasmapheresis.	IV/C	175
• IVIG.	Ib/A	176
Chronic Inflammatory Demyelinating Polyneuropathy		
Management similar to Guillain-Barré syndrome.	IV/C	177
Treatment with	IV/C	177
• Corticosteroids.		
• Plasmapheresis.		
• IVIG.		
• Interferon.		

GPP, good practice point; IVIG, intravenous immunoglobulin.

NONINFLAMMATORY MYOPATHIES (MYASTHENIA GRAVIS IS DISCUSSED IN CHAPTER 43)

Myotonic Dystrophy

Maternal and Fetal Risks

Myotonic dystrophy is an autosomal dominant genetic condition characterized by a progressive distal muscle weakness and wasting. There is an associated delay in relaxation in affected muscles. The effect of pregnancy on myotonic dystrophy is variable. Symptoms may first present during pregnancy,[179] exacerbations may occur particularly in the third trimester,[180] or the patient may remain asymptomatic.[181] Cardiac disease can occur in association with myotonic dystrophy, presenting as conduction defects, arrhythmias, or congestive heart failure.[182,183]

An elevated risk of poor fetal outcome is associated with myotonic dystrophy. There is an increased incidence of spontaneous abortion, preterm labor and delivery, and neonatal death.[179] Polyhydramnios is frequently present and may be associated with an affected fetus.[184] Preterm labor is likely a result of the increased amniotic fluid volume and myotonic involvement of the uterus.[185] Congenital myotonic dystrophy presents as generalized hypotonia and weakness. The respiratory muscles may be involved, resulting in inadequate ventilation at birth. Neonatal death is frequent, but if the affected infant is able to survive the first few weeks, some improvement may be seen.[186] The overall long-term prognosis remains generally poor, however. Developmental milestones are delayed and the incidence of mental retardation is increased.[187] Congenital myotonic dystrophy is usually found only in neonates born to mothers with the disease and differs from the adult form of the disease.[188]

Management Options

PREPREGNANCY AND PRENATAL

Any maternal cardiac or pulmonary compromise should be determined. A baseline electrocardiogram and pulmonary function tests should be obtained and the patient informed of the signs and symptoms of arrhythmias. Physical activity should be encouraged to slow clinical progression. Genetic counseling and prenatal diagnosis using DNA linkage analysis should be offered. Serial ultrasonography should be used to assess the amniotic fluid volume. In the presence of polyhydramnios, patients need to be followed for evidence of preterm labor. In the third trimester, fetal surveillance may be indicated.

LABOR AND DELIVERY AND POSTNATAL

Despite the risk of preterm labor, myotonic involvement of the uterine smooth muscle can result in dysfunctional labor. Augmentation with oxytocin is often effective.[189] Shortening of the second stage of labor may be helpful in women with significant weakness. Postpartum hemorrhage is a common complication and should be anticipated.

Respiratory muscle weakness may be present and must be considered when offering analgesia and anesthesia. Local or regional anesthesia is preferred. The risk of apnea with narcotics may be increased, and these agents should be used with caution. Nondepolarizing neuromuscular blocking agents should be avoided because of generalized muscle contracture resulting in difficulty with airway management.[190] Prenatal consultation with an anesthesiologist may be prudent.

A pediatrician should be present in the delivery room to aid in neonatal resuscitation and ventilation. There are no newborn tests for myotonic dystrophy. In those cases in which there are no maternal symptoms and neonatal myotonia is suspected, electromyographic studies on the mother can confirm the neonatal diagnosis.

SUMMARY OF MANAGEMENT OPTIONS

Myotonic Dystrophy

Management Options	Evidence Quality and Recommendation	References
Prepregnancy		
Assess cardiorespiratory status; optimize treatment.	III/B	180
Provide genetic counseling.	III/B	180
Prenatal		
Monitor cardiorespiratory status.	III/B	180
Discuss prenatal diagnosis.	III/B	180
Maintain vigilance for hydramnios.	III/B	180
If hydramnios, vigilance for preterm labor.	III/B	180
Inform and arrange consultation with anesthesiologist; inform pediatricians if fetus affected.	—/GPP	—
Labor and Delivery		
Augment with oxytocin if dystocia in first stage.	IV/C	189
May need assisted second stage if significant weakness.	III/B	180
Provide active management of third stage; vigilance for PPH.	—/GPP	—

SUMMARY OF MANAGEMENT OPTIONS

Myotonic Dystrophy—cont'd

Management Options	Evidence Quality and Recommendation	References
Regional analgesic is preferable to narcotics and/or general anesthetic; avoid nondepolarizing neuromuscular blocking drugs.	III/B	180,190
Pediatrician to be present for delivery.	—/GPP	—
Postnatal		
Provide careful neuromuscular examination and follow-up of newborn.	III/B	180

GPP, good practice point; PPH, postpartum hemorrhage.

DEMYELINATING DISEASES

Multiple Sclerosis

Maternal and Fetal Risks

Multiple sclerosis (MS) is a demyelinating disease that affects the central nervous system at different levels and at varying times.[191] It is a relatively common neurologic disease among young adults, peaking at age 30. The prevalence in the United States is 1 per 1000. Women are affected twice as often as men.

Common symptoms include acute onset of diplopia, vertigo, gait instability, bladder incontinence, loss of vision, and fatigue. Any central nervous system symptom can be a manifestation of MS, however. The disease course in an individual patient is unpredictable. Different general disease patterns are recognized. One type is characterized as relapsing and remitting with an identified onset and resolution of symptoms. The chronic progressive pattern follows a protracted course with worsening of symptoms over a prolonged period of time. Finally, a relapsing progressing course displays identifiable exacerbations with no clear return to baseline neurologic function. Poor prognostic factors include prominent weakness, poor response to steroids, and older age at onset. The common pathologic lesion called a plaque demonstrates myelin loss and gliosis associated with inflammatory infiltrates.

Previous research on the effects of pregnancy on MS has generally been flawed, and well-controlled studies are needed.[192] Pregnancy itself may exert a short-term beneficial effect on the course of MS, including fewer, less severe relapses, especially in the third trimester. However, this protection is lost in the postpartum period. The incidence of new cases of MS is decreased during pregnancy, as is the risk of exacerbation and progression of existing disease. Postpartum, the incidence of new-onset disease is not different from that in the nonpregnant population.[193] Exacerbation is reported to increase 20% to 40% during the first 6 months after delivery.[34,194] Despite the increase in disease activity postpartum, there does not appear to be any increase in long-term disability related to pregnancy.[195–197] Objective evidence of decreased MS activity during the latter half of gestation with a return to baseline postpartum has been demonstrated using serial MRI scans in two patients.[198] The relative immunosuppression associated with pregnancy may play a role in pregnancy-related changes seen in MS. Children of MS mothers have a 3% risk of developing MS compared with a 0.1% risk seen in the general population.[199]

Management Options

PREPREGNANCY

The diagnosis of MS is made clinically. Brain imaging and CSF studies are used to support the clinical impression. High-intensity signal lesions are found in the central nervous system white matter on MRI scanning, and oligoclonal banding is seen in the CSF. There are few data available during pregnancy on the three FDA-approved treatments for MS patients with relapsing-remitting disease. The therapies include copolymer 1 or glatiramer acetate (category B), interferon-β1b, and interferon-β1a (both category C). Corticosteroid therapy is also used.

Preconceptual evaluation and counseling is desirable. Disease activity should be assessed. In times of remission, with the lack of information regarding MS therapies during gestation, and the fact that most patients show improvement during pregnancy, consideration should be given to stopping the drugs or minimizing the dose. Patients should also be informed of the increased risk of their offspring developing the disease.

PRENATAL

Patients should be monitored for evidence of increased disease activity and the risks of therapy weighed against the potential concerns associated with lack of information. In those patients with urinary tract involvement, regular screening for asymptomatic bacteriuria should take place. Physical therapy and stretching exercises required prior to conception should be continued.

LABOR AND DELIVERY AND POSTNATAL

Labor and delivery should not be significantly affected in patients with MS. Prolonged antepartum corticosteroid use requires stress dose steroids during labor. Hydrocortisone

25 mg parenterally every 8 hours in addition to the usual daily dose is an acceptable regimen.[200] Maternal exhaustion seen in the second stage can be managed with operative vaginal delivery. The use of spinal anesthesia has traditionally been avoided owing to fear of increasing the risk of exacerbation. There are no data to support this concern, however, and spinal, epidural, and general anesthesia can all be used safely.[201] Breast-feeding may be encouraged, because there does not appear to be an increase in the frequency or severity of postpartum relapse.[202]

SUMMARY OF MANAGEMENT OPTIONS

Multiple Sclerosis

Management Options	Evidence Quality and Recommendation	References
Prepregnancy		
Counsel about risks to mother and baby.	IV/C	192,199
Consider reducing therapy if disease in remission.	—/GPP	—
Prenatal		
Monitor for relapse or worsening of disease activity (including use of MRI).	IV/C	198
If necessary, increase therapy (lack of information on some drugs in pregnancy).	—/GPP	—
Maintain physical exercises and the like.	—/GPP	—
Labor and Delivery		
Administer "stress dose" steroids for labor/delivery if patient on corticosteroids prenatally.	III/B	200
Assisted second stage may be necessary.	—/GPP	—
No data to suggest spinal, epidural, and general anesthetics are contraindicated.	IV/C	201
Postnatal		
Breast-feeding is acceptable.	III/B	202
Maintain vigilance for relapse.	III/B	193,194

GPP, good practice point; MRI, magnetic resonance imaging.

CEREBRAL TUMORS

Primary Brain Tumors

Maternal and Fetal Risks

All types of brain tumors have been described in pregnant women, but the overall incidence of primary brain tumors in pregnancy is small and not different from that seen in nonpregnant women of childbearing age. Nevertheless, normal physiologic changes such as increased fluid volumes and increased sex hormone levels occurring during gestation may have a profound effect on tumor growth and neurologic symptoms. Growth of some tumors with estrogen and progesterone receptors can be altered.[203,204] Although tumor growth may lead to initial diagnosis during pregnancy, signs and symptoms at presentation are the same as those in nongravid individuals.

Presenting symptoms relate to increased ICP or local mass effect. Common complaints or neurologic findings include headache, nausea, vomiting, visual changes, hemiparesis, cranial nerve deficits, and seizures. Most of these findings are nonspecific and commonly associated with normal pregnancy, potentially leading to a delay in diagnosis.

Management Options

PREPREGNANCY AND PRENATAL

Management of primary brain tumors in pregnancy depends on the type of tumor and whether it is benign or malignant. Maternal outcome will be dependent on these factors as well as the histologic grade of malignant lesions.[205] Gestational age will also be an important consideration in determining timing and mode of therapy as well as maternal and fetal risks and benefits.

The diagnosis is made with neuroimaging studies. MRI is preferred because low-grade tumors may present as nonenhancing lesions on brain CT, making their classification difficult. Surgical therapy is the treatment of choice for most lesions. Resection is best performed prior to conception when a diagnosis is made before pregnancy. In benign tumors such as most meningiomas or in low-grade malignant gliomas diagnosed during pregnancy, resection can often be delayed until after delivery, providing the patient is neurologically stable. Malignant tumors should be resected promptly. Adjuvant chemotherapy can be given after the first trimester when maternal benefit outweighs fetal risk.

In tumors in which radiation therapy is indicated as a primary treatment modality or an adjuvant, this should be delayed until after delivery, if possible. Preterm delivery may be undertaken in the presence of fetal pulmonary maturity to expedite therapy. If gestational age prohibits timely delivery, localized brain radiation may be used with careful abdominal shielding to minimize fetal exposure.

Vasogenic cerebral edema is seen with some tumor types and may require glucocorticoid therapy. Dexamethasone is the drug of choice. Because this agent readily crosses the placenta, if prolonged high-dose treatment is required, prednisone may be considered as a substitiute to decrease fetal exposure. Seizure prophylaxis with appropriate AEDs is also indicated where there is a significant risk of convulsions.

LABOR AND DELIVERY

Little information exists to guide labor and delivery management. Vaginal delivery may be allowed with cesarean section reserved for obstetric indications. The second stage may be shortened with forceps or vacuum to avoid increased ICP with pushing.

Metastatic Brain Tumors (See also Chapter 52)

Maternal Risks and Management Options

The brain is a common site of metastatic cancer. Lung, breast, and gastrointestinal tract are the most frequent site of the primary tumors. Rarely do maternal cancers spread to the fetoplacental unit.

Choriocarcinoma is a trophoblastic tumor that is rarely found associated with a normal pregnancy. The tumor spreads rapidly by the hematogenous route with brain metastasis discovered at the time of diagnosis in as many as 20% of patients.[206–208] Brain involvement presenting as an ischemic stroke,[209] intracerebral hemorrhage,[210] or subdural hematoma resulting from metastatic infiltration and proliferation in vascular spaces may actually lead to the diagnosis. Chemotherapy is considered the treatment of choice in choriocarcinoma. Alternatives in special circumstances include surgical resection of single brain metastasis and cranial irradiation. The presence of brain lesions is associated with an overall worse prognosis.

SUMMARY OF MANAGEMENT OPTIONS

Cerebral Tumors

Management Options	Evidence Quality and Recommendation	References
Primary Tumors		
Prepregnancy		
Tumors are best treated before commencing pregnancy.	III/B	205
Prenatal		
Management depends on:	III/B	205
• Tumor type and whether benign or malignant.		
• Its natural history.		
• Gestation.		
• Patient's wishes.		
Most tumors are treated by surgery.	III/B	205
Adjuvant chemotherapy can be given after the first trimester.	III/B	205
Radiation is best delayed until after delivery.	III/B	205
High-dose steroids may be necessary with cerebral edema.	III/B	205
Labor and Delivery		
Insufficient data to determine whether assisted second stage is of benefit.	—/GPP	—
Secondary/Metastatic Tumors		
Management depends on:	III/B	206–208
• Primary.		
• Site.		
• Its effects.		

GPP, good practice point.

Prolactinoma (See also Chapter 46)

Maternal Risks

Prolactinomas are the most common type of pituitary tumor. Most are microadenomas found during an evaluation for amenorrhea, galactorrhea, or infertility. In addition, macroadenomas (>10 mm diameter) may present with headache or bitemporal hemianopia. The use of bromocriptine to treat infertility has allowed women with prolactinomas to become pregnant. Pregnancy can stimulate tumor growth. Although this is rarely a problem with microadenomas, symptomatology may develop or worsen in the presence of a macroadenoma.[211]

Management Options

If adenoma size has not previously been determined, neuroimaging studies are indicated to define the extent of the tumor. MRI is able to identify small adenomas and their relation to the optic nerve, whereas CT scan provides better definition of any bony erosion resulting from the tumor expansion.[212] With microadenomas, bromocriptine can be stopped once pregnancy is diagnosed, with less than a 5% chance of the lesion becoming symptomatic.[213] Visual fields are periodically tested to detect evidence of tumor growth. Headaches are a useful early symptom of tumor enlargement. Bromocriptine may be started during pregnancy if symptoms develop.[214] Macroadenomas have a 15% to 35% chance of enlargement. Bromocriptine may be continued throughout gestation or patients must be followed closely for symptoms. Hypophysectomy or radiotherapy is reserved for cases that fail medical management. Adenomas generally decrease in size after delivery.[215]

SUMMARY OF MANAGEMENT OPTIONS

Prolactinoma

Management Options (See also Chapter 46)	Evidence Quality and Recommendation	References
Prenatal		
Maintain clinical surveillance (headaches and visual disturbance) for recurrence or expansion in pregnancy.	III/B	214
Some screen visual fields through pregnancy.	—/GPP	—
Bromocriptine with tumor enlargement (confirmed with CT or MRI).	III/B	78,212
Bromocriptine appears to be safe during pregnancy.	III/B	78
Hypophysectomy (radiotherapy rarely needed for failed medical management).	III/B	215

CT, computed tomography; GPP, good practice point; MRI, magnetic resonance imaging.

MOVEMENT DISORDERS

Maternal and Fetal Risks

Life-threatening, new-onset movement disorders are extremely rare during pregnancy.[216,217] Movement disorders are classified based on either excessive ("hyperkinetic" or "dyskinetic") or slowed ("hypokinetic") motor activity. The findings can be persistent or intermittent. In reproductive-age women, the hyperkinetic or dyskinetic disorders predominate. Several of the movement disorders are associated with abnormalities of tone, but most are not associated with actual weakness.

Most movement disorders are the result of disease involving the basal ganglion (caudate nucleus, globus pallidus, putamen, substantia nigra) and its connections. However, abnormalities of the thalamus, cerebellum, spinal cord, and peripheral nerves can cause abnormal movements. A wide spectrum of pathologic processes including degenerative conditions, toxins, metabolic aberrations, cerebrovascular disease, neoplasms, autoimmune conditions, infections, and trauma can lead to movement disorders.[217] In addition, dopamine receptor antagonists commonly used to treat nausea and vomiting in early pregnancy may rarely induce new-onset dystonia, chorea, tremors, and parkinsonism.

Chorea Gravidarum

Maternal and Fetal Risks

Chorea gravidarum, a hyperkinetic disorder, is an uncommon condition that encompasses any cause of chorea occurring during pregnancy.[218–220] In the preantibiotic era, it was commonly due to group A streptococcal infection and rheumatic fever. Clinical manifestations of chorea include abrupt, rapid, unsustained, involuntary, purposeless, irregular, and nonrhythmic movement of a limb or axial structure. The movements may be isolated and of brief duration or they may be more flowing and sustained. Patients are often unable to persist with voluntary motor activity. This is illustrated by difficulty in maintaining protrusion of their tongue or closure of their eyes. There are multiple causes of chorea gravidarum. Most cases are due to medications, toxins,

TABLE 48–9
Causes of Chorea Gravidarum

Sydenham's (rheumatic)
Systemic lupus erythematosus
Antiphospholipid syndrome
Wilson's disease
Cerebrovascular disease
Meningovascular syphilis
Hyperthyroidism
Neuroacanthocytosis
Huntington's disease
Adult-onset Tay-Sachs disease
Medications/drugs
Antiepileptic drugs
Neuroleptics
Theophylline derivatives
Lithium
Tricyclic antidepressants
Lead toxicity
Amphetamines
Cocaine
Metaclopramide

infections (such as HIV or cerebral toxoplasmosis), autoimmune disorders, cerebrovascular disorders, or an endocrinopathy. Specific causes are shown in Table 48–9.

Management Options

Management of chorea depends on the underlying etiology and its severity. The diagnostic evaluation is complex and aimed at excluding the conditions listed in Table 48–9. Therapeutic intervention is aimed primarily at the underlying etiology. The actual chorea is usually benign and of secondary concern. Treatments typically offer only symptomatic relief and have the potential for adverse effects. Expectant management is preferred except in situations in which the movements may lead to dehydration, malnutrition, or insomnia or when they are exceedingly violent and pose a risk of maternal injury. Short-term use of low-dose haloperidol (category C) can reduce chorea movements.

Wilson's Disease

Maternal and Fetal Risks

Wilson's disease is an autosomal recessive disorder of copper metabolism associated with a deficiency of the copper-binding and carrier protein ceruloplasmin. Disease manifestations include chorea, tremors, hypersalivation, dystonia, myoclonus, and slurred speech. Copper deposition in the brain is responsible for the clinical findings. Kayser-Fleischer rings describe copper deposition in the cornea and represent one of the classic physical findings. Other organ systems are also affected. The defective gene is located on chromosome 13 (p14).[216,217] The carrier frequency in the population is between 1 in 90 and 1 in 200.

Management Options

Typically, the diagnosis is made when serum ceruloplasmin levels are less than 20 mg/dL. Half of patients with Wilson's disease will have levels less than 5 mg/dL. The diagnosis may be complicated in pregnancy because increased estrogen levels increase ceruloplasmin levels leading to false-negative assays. Prior to penicillamine therapy, pregnancy was uncommon because of the development of infertility, and when conception did occur, the rate of spontaneous abortions was increased.[221,222]

Penicillamine (category D) therapy is the first-line treatment of Wilson's disease.[223] Five consecutive successful pregnancies in the same woman with Wilson's disease have been reported.[224] Therapy has been associated with adverse fetal effects. Fetal connective tissue anomalies secondary to an inhibition of collagen synthesis can result.[223,225] Also, neonatal inguinal hernia, reversible cutis laxa,[216,217] hyperflexible joints, vascular fragility, and poor wound healing have all been reported.[226,227] Many infants born to mothers taking penicillamine during pregnancy are found to be free of defects, however.

With proper therapy, the course of Wilson's disease does not appear to be affected by pregnancy. Penicillamine therapy should be continued during pregnancy. Halting therapy could lead to irreversible damage to the maternal brain, liver, and other organs. To minimize the risk of poor wound healing following delivery, the daily penicillamine dose should be decreased from 1 g to 250 mg during the third trimester. An alternative therapy uses zinc and trientine. Collagen synthesis is not adversely affected, but experience with this regimen in pregnancy is limited.[221]

Restless Leg Syndrome

Maternal Risks

Restless leg syndrome is a common condition with 11% to 19% of pregnant women affected.[228] It consists of an unpleasant sensation of the legs often associated with periodic movements during or just before sleep or in the late evening when fatigue is present. Clinically, there is flexion of the hip and knee with dorsiflexion of the ankle and extension of the great toe. The etiology is unclear; however, in nonpregnant patients, there has been an association with iron deficiency. Treatment aimed at iron replacement has been associated with an improvement in symptoms.[229] Symptoms are also often noted to disappear with walking.

Management Options

Treatment is supportive and includes reassurance, massage, flexion and extension leg exercises, and walking. With the high incidence of iron deficiency in pregnancy, iron supplementation may be a prudent early intervention. Severe cases can be managed with opiates.

Parkinson's Disease

Maternal and Fetal Risks

Parkinson's disease is an idiopathic hypokinetic disorder typically seen after the age of 40, but approximately 5% of cases may present earlier.[216] Thus, Parkinson's disease may be seen in women of childbearing age. The condition is a degenerative disorder of unknown etiology related to a deficiency of dopamine-secreting neurons in the substantia nigra of the brainstem mesencephalon (midbrain). Manifestations include slowed movements (bradykinesia), increased tone (rigidity), resting tremor, loss of postural reflexes, masked facies, and transient akinesia. Patients often have difficulty initiating movements and automatic movements are reduced. This constellation of findings is termed *parkinsonism* and represents a common clinical presentation for a variety of conditions in addition to Parkinson's disease. The differential diagnosis includes intracranial processes such as hydrocephalus, head trauma, subdural hematomas, cerebrovascular disease, and encephalitis. Carbon monoxide poisoning, metabolic abnormalities, and cyanide and manganese toxicity have also been implicated. Also, several medications including α-methyldopa, disulfiram, dopamine receptor antagonists, lithium, methanol, reserpine, and tetrabenazine may lead to parkinsonism. Discontinuation of the offending drug, if clinically feasible, may lead to varying degrees of symptomatic improvement.

Information describing the course of Parkinson's disease in pregnancy is limited. There are reports of worsening during pregnancy with improvement postpartum.[216,217] Symptoms may be exacerbated by several factors including hormonal changes, medications, weight gain, increased fatigue, and dehydration.

Management Options

Initial evaluation of a patient suspected of having Parkinson's disease should exclude other conditions associated with parkinsonism. As with the condition itself, information regarding the safety of antiparkinsonism medications during pregnancy is limited. Use of the combination of levodopa/carbidopa (category C), a mainstay in the treatment of Parkinson's disease, has been associated with malformations in animals, but adequate human data are not available. These medications should be used with caution. Amantidine (category C) has also been associated with malformations in animals. In humans, the overall malformation rate is reported to be higher, but there is no specific pattern. Again, data are limited and caution should precede its use.[1] Bromocriptine (category C) is a second-line agent for the treatment of Parkinson's disease. Although it is not as efficacious as the levodopa/carbidopa combination, there is considerably more experience during pregnancy. The information is based on lower doses used to treat prolactinomas.[230] It is considered safe without excess risk of complications based on 1335 women receiving it during pregnancy for a prolactinoma. Bromocriptine may be added to the levodopa/carbidopa combination when disabling symptomatology appears such as dopa-induced dyskinesias. Selegiline (category C) and pergolide (category B) are newer treatments that also lack adequate pregnancy data.[231]

SUMMARY OF MANAGEMENT OPTIONS

Movement Disorders

Management Options	Evidence Quality and Recommendation	References
Chorea Gravidarum		
Management depends on cause	IV/C	217
Treatment given only if: • Dehydration. • Malnutrition. • Insomnia. • Violence. • Risk of maternal injury.	IV/C	217
Short-term low-dose haloperidol commonly used.	IV/C	217
Wilson's Disease		
Penicillamine is the treatment of choice, but use lowest dose that gives disease control (risk of fetal defects).	III/B	221–223
Restless Leg Syndrome		
Supportive treatment: • Reassurance. • Massage, exercises, and physiotherapy. • Walking.	III/B	228
Supplement iron if deficient.	IV/C	229
Administer opiates for severe cases	III/B	228

SUMMARY OF MANAGEMENT OPTIONS

Movement Disorders—cont'd

Management Options	Evidence Quality and Recommendation	References
Parkinson's Disease		
Levodopa/carbidopa is probably safe for the fetus (limited human data).	—/GPP	—
Bromocriptine is often added to this with severe cases.	III/B	230
Amantadine, selegiline, and pergolide have limited published data.	—/GPP	—

GPP, good practice point.

CEREBRAL ABSCESS

Maternal Risks

Pregnancy and puerperium-associated cerebral abscesses are exceedingly rare with fewer than 15 cases reported.[232] Although the majority of abscesses are supratentorial and solitary (Fig. 48–7), focal neurologic deficits are not always present despite headache, fever, seizures, or depressed level of consciousness. Sources of infection include otitis media, venous sinus thrombosis, and hemorrhage into the basal ganglia. In most cases, a source is not found. Cerebral abscesses have been reported in immunocompetent hosts. Approximately half the cases have been associated with eclampsia. Overall mortality is 35%, and when the abscess is associated with eclampsia, mortality reaches 50%.

Management Options

Although rare, a cerebral abscess should be a part of the differential diagnosis when a mass lesion is seen on brain imaging. As a rule, aggressive medical management of the abscess is often adequate and surgical evacuation may not be necessary. Medical therapy includes the appropriate use of intravenous antibiotic(s) to cover a broad spectrum of potential organisms. A source for the infection should be promptly and thoroughly sought and treated and, when found, might give information about the responsible organism(s). Surgical drainage may be indicated if there is an initial poor response to the antibiotics.

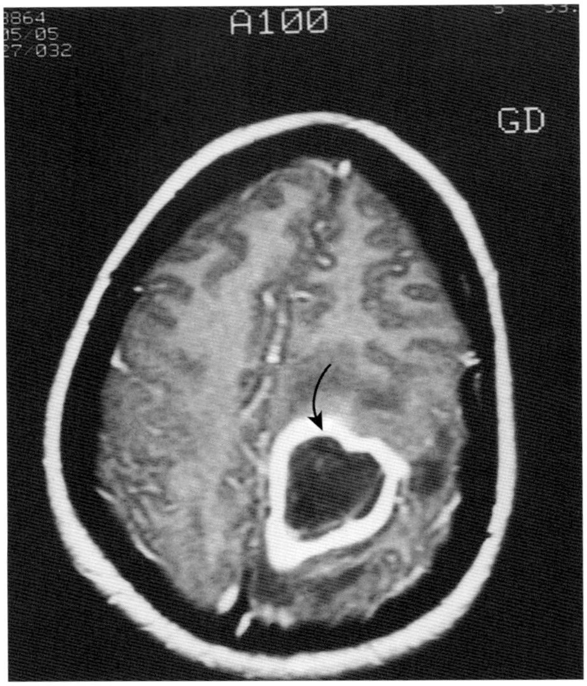

FIGURE 48–7
Axial head MRI reveals a ring-enhancing lesion, proven to be a puerperal cerebral abscess (*curved arrow*) at surgery.

SUMMARY OF MANAGEMENT OPTIONS

Cerebral Abscess

Management Options	Evidence Quality and Recommendation	References
Administer aggressive IV antibiotics (broad spectrum).	III/B	232
Find and treat source of infection.	III/B	232
Provide surgical drainage for the few cases that fail to respond to antibiotics.	III/B	232

SUGGESTED READINGS

Briggs GG, Freeman R, Yaffe SJ (eds): Drugs in Pregnancy and Lactation. Philadelphia, Lippincott Williams & Williams, 2008.

Coutinho JM, Majoie CB, Coert BA, Stam J: Decompressive hemicraniectomy in cerebral sinus thrombosis: Consecutive case series and review of the literature. Stroke 2009;40:2233–2235.

Davis SM, Donnan GA: 4.5 hours: The new time window for tissue plasminogen activator in stroke. Stroke 2009;40:2266–2267.

Helms AK, Drogan O, Kittner SJ: First trimester stroke prophylaxis in pregnant women with a history of stroke. Stroke 2009;40:1158–1161.

Murugappan A, Coplin WM, Al-Sadat AN, et al: Thrombolytic therapy of acute ischemic stroke during pregnancy. Neurology 2006;66:768–770.

Pennell PB: Antiepileptic drug pharmacokinetics during pregnancy and lactation. Neurology 2003;61:S35–S42.

Piotin M, de Souza Filho CB, Kothimbakam R, Moret J: Endovascular treatment of acutely ruptured intracranial aneurysms in pregnancy. Am J Obstet Gynecol 2001;185:1261–1262.

Sances G, Granella F, Nappi RE, et al: Course of migraine during pregnancy and postpartum: A prospective study. Cephalalgia 2003;23:197–205.

Sloan MA, Stern BJ: Cerebrovascular disease in pregnancy. Curr Treat Options Neurol 2003;5:391–407.

Wong CA, Scavone BM, Dugan S, et al: Incidence of postpartum lumbosacral spine and lower extremity nerve injuries. Obstet Gynecol 2003;101:279–288.

REFERENCES

For a complete list of references, log onto www.expertconsult.com.

CHAPTER 49

Renal Disorders

ALEX C. VIDAEFF and SUSAN M. RAMIN

INTRODUCTION

Although renal disorders are relatively uncommon in pregnancy, obstetricians will encounter pregnant women with known underlying renal disease or previously subclinical renal conditions uncovered during pregnancy. In addition, complications of pregnancy such as severe preeclampsia may include acute renal deterioration as part of the clinical spectrum. This chapter discusses the management of acute and chronic renal conditions from an obstetric perspective. Unfortunately, the cumulative knowledge in this field is based almost exclusively on retrospective studies addressing only a small number of cases, underscoring the critical need for large prospective observational studies.

When considering the interaction between renal disease and pregnancy, maternal outcomes are related to the initial level of renal dysfunction more than to the specific underlying disease. With regards to fetal outcomes though, a distinction may exist between renal dysfunction resulting from primary renal disease and that in which renal involvement is part of a systemic condition. Although maternal and fetal outcomes in pregnancies complicated by kidney disease have improved in recent years owing to continuous progress in obstetrics and neonatology, as well as better medical management of hypertension and renal disease, every pregnancy in these women remains a high risk pregnancy.

RENAL CHANGES DURING NORMAL PREGNANCY (Table 49-1)

In normal pregnancy, renal plasma flow (RPF) increases progressively up to a maximum of 80% above nonpregnant levels in the second trimester, before falling to about 50% above nonpregnant levels in the late third trimester.[1] It is presumed that the third trimester decline in RPF is at least in part related to the compression of the intra-abdominal large vessels by the gravid uterus. The increased RPF in pregnancy is the consequence of renal vasodilation. Women with preexisting nephropathy who have further renal deterioration during pregnancy frequently do not manifest the early renal hyperperfusion present in a normal pregnancy because their renal vasodilation is already maximal. Unlike the hyperperfusion that may precede some renal pathologic conditions, gestational hyperperfusion does not lead to increased glomerular capillary pressure as demonstrated by animal studies and indirect evidence from mathematical models of data from fractional dextran sieving in humans.[2]

Renal hyperperfusion is the primary determinant of renal hyperfiltration in pregnancy with resulting increased urinary output and frequency. An increase in glomerular filtration rate (GFR) of approximately 25% is seen as early as 3 to 4 weeks from conception, and by 16 weeks' gestation, GFR is 55% above nonpregnant levels.[3] Consequently, creatinine clearance increases from the nonpregnant normal range of 100 to 180 mL/min to 150 to 200 mL/min, and blood urea nitrogen (BUN) and serum creatinine decline. Thus, values considered normal in the nonpregnant state may be abnormal during pregnancy. A BUN or serum creatinine value greater than 14 mg/dL and 0.9 mg/dL, respectively, may indicate preexisting renal disease or pregnancy-induced complications. In parallel with the decline in effective RPF toward term, the creatinine clearance will decrease by approximately 20% after 36 weeks' gestation and serum creatinine will increase. This should not be interpreted as a decline in renal function. In general, at least a 25% change in creatinine clearance or serum creatinine is required in order to suspect significant alterations in GFR.

The increased RPF in pregnancy is the consequence of renal vasodilation with profound reductions in renal afferent and efferent arteriolar resistances. The mechanism of vasodilation with decrease in vascular resistance in pregnancy is still poorly defined. The ovarian hormone relaxin has been implicated as a mediator.[4] However, relaxin is not the only determinant. Smith and coworkers[5] studied women who conceived with ovum donation, therefore without circulating relaxin, and still demonstrated an increase in creatinine clearance in the first trimester, albeit to a smaller degree than in women with normal ovarian function. A possible role has also been assigned to the natriuretic peptides, a family of peptide hormones shown to be potent natriuretic, diuretic, and vasodilatory agents. It has been posited that natriuretic peptides contribute to the systemic vasodilation of pregnancy, thus increasing RPF, either by a cyclic guanosine monophosphate (cGMP)–mediated vasorelaxant effect or indirectly by antagonizing the activity of the renin-angiotensin system. Sala and colleagues[6] have shown that plasma natriuretic peptides increase in the first trimester and then

TABLE 49–1

Urinary Tract Physiologic Changes during Normal Pregnancy

Renal vasodilation and RPF increase of 50%–80% above nonpregnant level
Renal hyperperfusion and hyperfiltration causing increased urine output, frequency, nocturia
Increased GFR (by 25%–55%) causing increase in proteinuria and creatinine clearance with decline in SCr and BUN
Reduced tubular glucose reabsorption causing glycosuria (in 70% of nondiabetic mothers)
Hypercalciuria
Increased renal size
Pelvicaliceal, ureteral, bladder, and urethral morphologic changes contributing to urinary stasis and VUR
Symptoms mimicking cystitis

BUN, blood urea nitrogen; GFR, glomerular filtration rate; RPF, renal plasma flow; SCr, serum creatinine; VUR, vesicoureteric reflux.

tend to decrease in late pregnancy, a pattern consistent with the reciprocal changes in RPF. Interestingly, the increase in plasma natriuretic peptides is demonstrable only in the supine position, not in the sitting position.[6] This is reflected in the nocturia typically experienced by gravid women, with mobilization of dependent edema and dilution of urine at night.

Urinary excretion of protein is also increased during normal pregnancy secondary to increased GFR, reduced proximal reabsorption, and possibly alterations in the electrostatic charge of the glomerular filter.[4] Proteinuria up to 300 mg/24 hr is considered normal in pregnancy. The specific excretion of albumin in the urine increases three times, contributing to a decline in serum albumin of 0.5 to 1.0 U/L.[7]

The results of a 24-hour urine specimen for proteinuria may be influenced by ambulation, exercise, cold, or heat exposure. Such inaccuracies and practical difficulties associated with the outpatient attempts to collect 24-hour urine specimens have led to an evolving interest in calculating instead the random spot urine protein-to-creatinine ratio or at least obtaining supervised 8- to 12-hour urine collections. A random urine protein (mg)-to-creatinine (mmol) ratio of more than 0.19 predicts significant proteinuria, but is not a substitute for a 24-hour urine collection, owing to the high incidence of both false-negative and false-positive results.[8]

Any gravida with preexisting renal disease or those at risk for renal deterioration during pregnancy should have a baseline determination of serum creatinine, proteinuria, and creatinine clearance early in pregnancy. Ideally, baseline values should be obtained before conception if possible. Baseline creatinine clearance appears to be a more sensitive indicator than a baseline serum creatinine level because the latter can be influenced by muscle mass, physical exercise, racial differences, and dietary intake of meat.[9] After the baseline workup, surveillance with monthly serum creatinine levels is usually sufficient. Although serum creatinine is not linearly correlated with creatinine clearance, a doubling in serum creatinine roughly suggests a 50% reduction in GFR. A 24-hour urine collection may be repeated when indicated.

Another renal tubular change in pregnancy is the reduced tubular glucose reabsorption, which leads to a 10- to 100-fold increase in urine glucose, causing glycosuria in 70% of healthy pregnant women.[10] There is also a threefold increase in urinary calcium excretion during normal pregnancy. However, the additional active vitamin D production by the placenta increases the circulating vitamin D to twice the nongravid levels, resulting in essentially no change in maternal plasma ionized calcium levels.[11]

The gestational rise in RPF causes an increased renal interstitial volume reflected in a 30% increase in overall renal volume and an approximately 1 cm increase in renal bipolar length. Dilation of the urinary tract is another common renal modification in pregnancy. The renal pelvicaliceal system and ureters progressively dilate, particularly on the right side. In 6% of pregnant women, the maximal caliceal diameter may reach 20 mm on the right and 8 mm on the left, as early as 20 weeks' gestation.[12] The pelvicaliceal dilation may persist in the immediate postpartum period. In 90% of pregnant women, the ureters are also dilated, elongated, kinked, and displaced laterally, suggesting obstruction, although in reality, these are normal physiologic changes. In contrast to pathologically dilated ureters, in pregnancy, the physiologically dilated ureter is expected to narrow below the pelvic brim. Physiologic ureteral dilation may begin as early as 6 weeks' gestation and peak at 22 to 24 weeks. At the level of the bladder, pregnancy-related changes include a wider trigon, increased vascular congestion, and increased pressure from approximately 8 to 20 cm H_2O. The urethra is 20% longer and has a higher closure pressure. All these mechanical changes contribute to increased urinary stasis and vesicoureteral reflux (VUR).[13] The changes at the level of the urinary tract may be responsible for an increased risk of urinary tract infection (UTI) in pregnancy. Mechanical effects from the enlarged uterus and the smooth muscle relaxation secondary to changes in the hormonal milieu additionally promote urostasis, incomplete emptying of the bladder, and reflux. Furthermore, glycosuria may encourage bacterial growth, whereas the increases in urinary progesterone and estrogen may lead to decreased ability of the lower urinary tract to repel bacterial attachment to the urothelium.[13]

LOWER URINARY TRACT INFECTION

General

Colonization of the vaginal introitus and periurethral region by *Enterobacteriaceae* and gram-positive organisms from the distal gastrointestinal tract is thought to be the initial step in the bacterial contamination of the lower urinary tract in women. Bacteria ascend into the bladder via the short female urethra, and the incidence of asymptomatic bacteriuria in pregnancy is 2% to 7%, similar to the rate observed in nonpregnant reproductive-age women.[14] Asymptomatic bacteriuria is defined as the growth of 10^5 or more colony-forming units per milliliter of urine (CFU/mL) of a single uropathogen from a first-void midstream clean-catch specimen in a woman with no urinary complaints. If the urine is obtained by urethral catheterization or the specimen is non–first-void, even 10^2 CFU/mL of a single organism may indicate significant bacteriuria. The changes at the level of the urinary tract during pregnancy make it more likely that asymptomatic bacteriuria will progress to a lower UTI (cystitis) that may subsequently ascend to cause acute pyelonephritis. Once infected, the patient becomes symptomatic and the examination of the urine may reveal pyuria, proteinuria, and hematuria in approximately 50% of cases. Acute cystitis affects 1% to 2% of pregnancies.[15]

Diagnosis

Symptoms suggestive of a UTI are dysuria, frequency, nocturia, urge incontinence, voiding difficulty, suprapubic pain, and cloudy, malodorous urine. However, these symptoms are frequently found in healthy pregnant women, and the diagnosis needs to be confirmed by microscopic examination and culture of a freshly voided midstream urine sample. The microscopic examination will visualize the bacteria and allow quantification of leukocytes in the urine. The presence of at least one bacterium per oil-immersion field at gram stain correlates well with a positive urine culture.[16] Pyuria is defined as the presence of more than 10 leukocytes per high-power field in an unspun urine specimen or more than 50 leukocytes per high-power field in a spun urine specimen. Urine yielding more than 10^5 CFU/mL of a single uropathogen in a symptomatic woman is by convention diagnostic of UTI. However, 30% to 50% of women with acute symptoms of lower UTI may have lower counts (10^2–10^4 CFU/mL) that are still significant and may be explained by high fluid intake or a slow-growing organism. According to Tomson,[17] women with "low-count bacteriuria" left untreated will have 10^5 CFU/mL 2 days later.

Positive dipstick testing for nitrites (produced by most uropathogens by conversion of urinary nitrate) or leukocyte esterase (produced by leukocytes) in a symptomatic woman may strongly suggest UTI, allowing the initiation of empirical treatment before the urine culture results are available. The majority of cystitis cases remain uncomplicated and respond readily to empirical treatment with antibiotics, most of which are concentrated in the urine and thus achieve exceedingly high bladder levels. However, for screening of asymptomatic women in early pregnancy, these biochemical urine dipstick tests are not sensitive enough and cannot replace the urine culture. In a prospective international study, the dipstick tests missed 46% of all pregnant women with asymptomatic bacteriuria.[18]

Maternal and Fetal Risks

The major rationale behind screening for asymptomatic bacteriuria in pregnancy is that in the absence of treatment, about 25% to 30% of women with asymptomatic bacteriuria will develop acute pyelonephritis.[19] In a Cochrane review, antibiotic treatment of asymptomatic bacteriuria, compared with placebo or no treatment, significantly reduced the incidence of pyelonephritis (odds ratio [OR] 0.24, 95% confidence interval [CI] 0.19–0.32).[20] Following successful treatment of asymptomatic bacteriuria, rescreening is necessary, because approximately 30% of women will have a relapse of bacteriuria. Women at increased risk of pyelonephritis or renal impairment (previous UTI, diabetes mellitus [DM], hemoglobinopathy, nephropathy, immunodeficiency, neurologic dysfunction such as spinal cord injuries or multiple sclerosis, calculi, anatomic abnormalities of the urinary system, genitourinary instrumentation) should be screened for asymptomatic bacteriuria every 4 to 6 weeks throughout pregnancy.

Asymptomatic bacteriuria has also been associated with an increased risk of preterm delivery and low birth weight.[21] Treatment of asymptomatic bacteriuria has been shown to reduce the incidence of preterm delivery and low–birth weight newborns (OR 0.60, 95% CI 0.45–0.80).[20]

Management Options

The most common uropathogens are gram-negative bacteria such as *Escherichia coli* (about 80% of cases), *Klebsiella*, *Proteus*, *Enterobacter*, *Citrobacter*, and *Pseudomonas* species. Other contributing uropathogens may be gram-positive bacteria including *Staphylococcus saprophyticus* (the most common gram-positive bacteria), *Staphylococcus epidermidis*, enterococci, and group B β-hemolytic streptococci. The increasing resistance rate of gram-negative uropathogens, particularly *E. coli*, to penicillins (28-39%) has disqualified these agents as first-line treatment choices. Even sulfa regimens and first-generation cephalosporins have been reported to be less efficacious (31% resistance rate for trimethoprim-sulfamethoxazole and 9%–19% for cefazolin).[22] For treating asymptomatic bacteriuria or a first episode of cystitis, nitrofurantoin macrocrystals (100 mg twice daily for 7 days) remains an inexpensive and effective oral agent, for which plasmid-mediated resistance is unlikely. In an international double-blind, placebo-controlled, randomized trial conducted by the World Health Organization, the standard 7-day regimen of nitrofurantoin was demonstrated to be significantly more effective than a 1-day nitrofurantoin regimen, reinforcing the current treatment recommendations.[23] Nitrofurantoin should be avoided in patients with glucose-6-phosphate dehydrogenase deficiency owing to the risk of hemolytic anemia. There are a few case reports suggesting a very rare association between the use of nitrofurantoin and pulmonary fibrosis as acute pulmonary toxicity in pregnancy.[24]

A test-of-cure urine culture should be obtained 2 weeks after treatment for cystitis is completed. Women treated for cystitis may have a recurrence in 33% of cases, requiring the use of a second-line antimicrobial agent for prolonged 10-day treatment.[14] The treatment should be based on urine culture with antibiotic sensitivity determination. The recurrence represents either a reinfection or a relapse. Reinfections usually occur more than 2 weeks after cessation of a previous therapy, and are due to a different organism. Reinfections indicate the need for low-dose antibiotic daily suppression guided by the sensitivities of the most recent infective organism until 4 weeks postpartum. Suppressive therapy should not be initiated until a negative test-of-cure confirms eradication of the acute infection. Suitable regimes for long-term antibiotic prophylaxis include nitrofurantoin 100 mg orally at night or cephalexin 250 mg orally at night.[25] Relapse is more rare and usually occurs within 2 weeks of cessation of initial therapy. Relapse or persistence may be associated with calculi or structural abnormalities of the urinary tract and ultrasound evaluation may be necessary.

Quinolone antibiotics should be avoided in pregnancy because of the risk of arthropathy in infants exposed in utero. Single-dose intravenous therapy with gentamicin is not adequately evaluated and should be reserved for those rare cases of allergy to both penicillin and sulfa that markedly limits the options.

Women who remain symptomatic despite treatment and an infecting uropathogen cannot be isolated should be evaluated for other conditions, such as trichomoniasis, herpetic infection, urethritis (possibly with *Chlamydia trachomatis*), or interstitial cystitis. *Lactobacillus* bacteriuria should be treated with erythromycin or clindamycin only if persistent on two consecutive cultures.

SUMMARY OF MANAGEMENT OPTIONS

Lower Urinary Tract Infections

Management Options	Evidence Quality and Recommendation	References
Prenatal Screening		
Screen for asymptomatic bacteriuria early in pregnancy with urine culture.	Ia/A	19–21
Women at increased risk of pyelonephritis or renal impairment should be screened for asymptomatic bacteriuria every 4–6 wk throughout pregnancy.	III/B	19
Dipstick testing for nitrites and leukocyte esterase in asymptomatic women may suggest UTI, allowing the initiation of empirical treatment before the urine culture results are available.	IIb/B	16
Dipstick testing for nitrites and leukocyte esterase is not sensitive enough and cannot replace the urine culture for screening of asymptomatic women in early pregnancy.	IIa/B	16,18
Prenatal Treatment		
For treating asymptomatic bacteriuria or a first episode of cystitis, use nitrofurantoin macrocrystals (100 mg orally twice daily for 7 days) or treat according to antibiotic sensitivities.	Ib/A	22,23
A test-of-cure urine culture should be obtained 2 wk after treatment is completed.	III/B	14
For cystitis recurrence (33% rate), treat with a second-line agent based on urine culture with antibiotic sensitivity for 10 days.	III/B	14
For relapse or persistence, ultrasound evaluation is necessary to exclude calculi or structural abnormalities of the urinary tract.	IV/C	14,25
Reinfections indicate the need for continued low-dose antibiotic suppression guided by the sensitivities of the most recent infective organism until 4 wk postpartum.	IV/C	14,25

UTI, urinary tract infection.

ACUTE PYELONEPHRITIS

Clinical Presentation

Acute pyelonephritis involves the upper urinary tract. Over 80% of women will present with lumbar pain, fever, chills, and costovertebral angle tenderness. Other signs of systemic illness often present include myalgia, headache, malaise, and confusion. Only about half of the cases have associated symptoms of lower urinary tract irritation (urgency, frequency, dysuria) in addition to nausea, vomiting, and anorexia.[26] Costovertebral tenderness is right-sided in 54% of cases, left-sided in 16%, and bilateral in 27%.[26] The right kidney is most commonly affected because of greater obstructive changes owing to the dextrorotated uterus and the course of the right ovarian vessels. Most women (91%) with antepartum pyelonephritis present in the second and third trimester, possibly in relation to increasing urinary obstruction during late pregnancy.[26] In 19% of the peripartum cases, the presentation is in the postpartum period.[26] The same uropathogens that cause asymptomatic bacteriuria and cystitis are responsible for acute pyelonephritis.[26] In a population screened and treated for asymptomatic bacteriuria, the incidence of acute pyelonephritis in pregnancy is less than 1%.[19]

Maternal and Fetal Risks

Unless acute pyelonephritis is treated promptly, there is considerable maternal and fetal morbidity. Treatment itself may be associated with an initial phase of significant side effects secondary to the massive endotoxemia resulting from the lytic action of antibiotics on the cell wall of

TABLE 49–2

Effects of Endotoxemia in Acute Pyelonephritis

Hemolytic anemia
Thrombocytopenia
Decreased GFR
Acute respiratory distress syndrome
Uterine contractions
Shock
Hypothalamic instability

GFR, glomerular filtration rate.

gram-negative bacteria (Table 49–2). Pregnant women are very sensitive to the effects of endotoxins, and it is not uncommon for the patient to appear worse and even more febrile during the first 12 to 24 hours of therapy. Endotoxins increase the release of cytokines and prostaglandins and cause endothelial damage and capillary leak. They may also induce alveolar damage and pulmonary edema. Almost 25% of pregnant women with acute pyelonephritis will manifest mild hemolytic anemia, thrombocytopenia, and transient decrease in GFR with a rise in serum creatinine, and 2% of patients will develop pyelonephritis-associated acute respiratory distress syndrome (ARDS).[27] Pulmonary injury may be further compounded by injudicious fluid replacement or by the use of tocolytic agents (β-adrenergic agents or magnesium sulfate).[28] Increased uterine activity is present in about 20% of gravidas presenting with acute pyelonephritis, and the frequency of contractions increases significantly within the first 2 hours from initiation of antibiotics in response to bacterial endotoxin release.[29] However, uterine activity during treatment for pyelonephritis often occurs in the absence of cervical change.

Approximately 15% of pregnant women with acute pyelonephritis have bacteremia, and a small proportion may develop septic shock.[26] It is important to differentiate on initial presentation cases with impending septic shock from those in which hypotension is secondary to hypovolemia as a result of fever, vomiting, and dehydration. The potent bacterial endotoxins are capable of generating hypothalamic instability and high fever in these patients may be followed by hypothermia during the same day.

Management Options

Women suspected of having acute pyelonephritis should be admitted to the hospital. Laboratory tests should include, but are not limited to, a complete blood count, serum creatinine, BUN, electrolytes, lactate dehydrogenase (LDH), urinalysis, and urine culture. Urinary sediment reveals many leukocytes in clumps and bacteria. Hemolysis is confirmed by a peripheral blood smear and elevation in LDH concentration. Blood culture is indicated if the patient has high fever (>39.4°C), tachycardia (>110), or hypotension. With prior use of antibiotics, the urine culture may be negative while the blood culture will be positive. Another possible cause for a negative urine culture may be the complete obstruction of the unilaterally affected collecting system.

Intravenous antibiotics should be started empirically until sensitivities on blood and urine cultures are known. Intravenous crystalloid solutions are administered along with antibiotics as part of the initial treatment in order to restore the contracted blood volume. In addition to close monitoring of blood pressure, pulse, urinary output, uterine activity, and fetal heart rate patterns, one should promptly investigate any respiratory difficulties by pulmonary auscultation, chest radiography, pulse oximetry, and arterial blood gas analysis. Most respiratory manifestations are transient and respond to increased oxygen delivered by face mask, but the occasional ARDS may require tracheal intubation with mechanical ventilation and positive end-expiratory pressure. Infections caused by *Klebsiella pneumoniae*, second most common after *E. coli*, are more susceptible to pulmonary injury and other organ system derangements. Pregnant women with pyelonephritis and septic shock often require invasive hemodynamic monitoring of fluid balance in order to reduce the risk of pulmonary edema and acute tubular necrosis (ATN).

The outpatient management of pyelonephritis in pregnancy has been evaluated in a randomized clinical trial of 120 women at less than 24 weeks' gestation.[30] Inpatients received intravenous cefazolin until 48 hours afebrile, and the outpatients received ceftriaxone intramuscularly. Both arms completed the antibiotic course with oral cephalexin. Following this regimen, 10% of outpatients required hospital admission owing to sepsis or recurrent pyelonephritis. Based on available data, outpatient management of pyelonephritis in pregnancy cannot be recommended. Women with acute pyelonephritis should always be admitted to the hospital to observe the maternal condition that can deteriorate rapidly and to monitor uterine activity and fetal condition. Acute pyelonephritis increases the risk for preterm birth.[31]

Depending on the severity of the patient's condition, a second- or third-generation cephalosporin (such as cefoxitin sodium 2 g q6–8h or ceftriaxone sodium 1g daily) is an effective (95%) first choice until sensitivities are known. Women allergic to β-lactam antibiotics can be given intravenous gentamicin (100 mg q8h). Gentamicin should be carefully used in cases of renal dysfunction because of possible synergistic nephrotoxicity.[32] Clinically, renal dysfunction is identified by serum creatinine concentrations in excess of 1 mg/dL persisting after adequate hydration. Serum concentrations of gentamicin can be measured and dose adjustments made accordingly. One advantage of gentamicin is that aminoglycosides do not lyse the bacterial cell wall, producing less endotoxemia than other antibiotics.[29] Some practitioners add gentamicin to the initial first-line agent in patients with a poor clinical response.

Intravenous antibiotics should be continued until the patient has been afebrile and asymptomatic for 48 hours. Oral antibiotics should then be given according to bacterial sensitivities to complete a 14-day course.[32] In most women with uncomplicated pyelonephritis, fever abates in 2 to 3 days. Failure of treatment to improve the maternal clinical condition within 96 hours suggests an underlying structural abnormality if microbial resistance to the employed antibiotic has been ruled out. Ultrasonography may be inconclusive in excluding urinary stones. If clinical suspicion is high, a plain abdominal radiograph will identify 90% of renal stones, and an one-shot intravenous pyelography at 20 to 30 minutes after injection of contrast will identify the rest, also excluding other abnormalities of the collecting system.[33]

The risk to the fetus from radiation after one or two radiographs is minimal, especially when compared with the clinical benefit of identifying an obstructed, nonfunctioning kidney. Urinary tract obstruction can also be detected using magnetic resonance urography, especially during the second and third trimesters.[34] Continuing sepsis may also be caused by a renal or perinephric abscess, a rare complication of acute pyelonephritis in pregnancy. Except for obstructive cases requiring the placement of a double-J ureteral stent, instrumentation during pyelonephritis in pregnancy should be avoided because it can precipitate septic shock. If the stent fails, percutaneous nephrostomy should be considered, and ultimately surgical removal of calculi. For pyonephrosis, nephrectomy may be life-saving.

Following one episode of pyelonephritis, pregnant women should have a test-of-cure urine culture 2 weeks after completion of the acute therapy, and the risk of recurrent pyelonephritis can be reduced (from 20% to 8%) with nitrofurantoin 100 mg orally at night continued until 6 weeks postpartum.[33] Alternatively, monthly urine cultures can be obtained to screen for recurrence.[33] Suppressive therapy is always necessary when abnormalities of the urinary tract are present.

SUMMARY OF MANAGEMENT OPTIONS

Acute Pyelonephritis

Management Options	Evidence Quality and Recommendation	References
Prenatal Treatment		
If acute pyelonephritis is suspected, admit to hospital.	Ib/A	30
Investigate: CBC, serum creatinine, BUN, LDH, electrolytes, urinalysis, urine culture, blood culture.	—/GPP	—
IV antibiotic should be started empirically until cultures results are known; cefoxitin 2 g q6–8h, or ceftriaxone 1g daily, or gentamicin 100 mg q8h (95% efficacy).	Ia/A	32,33
IV crystalloid solutions are administered along with antibiotics to restore the contracted blood volume.	—/GPP	—
Promptly investigate any respiratory difficulties by chest radiography and arterial blood gas analysis. Most respiratory manifestations are transient and respond to increased oxygen delivered by face mask. Acute respiratory distress syndrome may require tracheal intubation with mechanical ventilation and positive end-expiratory pressure.	III/B	27,28
Septic shock often requires invasive hemodynamic monitoring.	—/GPP	—
Continue IV antibiotics until the patient has been afebrile and asymptomatic for 48 hr and then switch to oral antibiotics according to bacterial sensitivities to complete a total of 14-day course.	IIb/B	30,32
Failure of treatment to improve clinical condition within 96 hr requires imaging studies to rule out abnormalities of the collecting system. In case of obstruction, placement of a double-J ureteral stent, percutaneous nephrostomy, or surgical removal of calculi may be required.	—/GPP	—
Perform urine culture 2 wk after completion of antibiotic course and then monthly.	IV/C	25,33,34
The risk of recurrent pyelonephritis can be reduced (from 20% to 8%) with nitrofurantoin 100 mg orally at night continued until 6 wk postpartum. Such suppressive therapy is always necessary when abnormalities of the urinary tract are present.	III/B	25,33

BUN, blood urea nitrogen; CBC, complete blood count; GPP, good practice point; LDH, lactate dehydrogenase.

ACUTE RENAL FAILURE IN PREGNANCY

Maternal and Fetal Risks and Management Options

Acute renal failure (ARF) is a rare complication of pregnancy. The causes are listed in Table 49–3. It may be associated with septic shock (endotoxemia or septic abortion), dehydration related to hyperemesis gravidarum, amniotic fluid embolism, severe preeclampsia, obstructive uropathy, or severe hemorrhage. The principles of management are aimed at identification and correction of the precipitating insult and optimal fluid resuscitation. Fluid balance is critical to the management of ARF during pregnancy. Too little intravascular fluid may be especially damaging to chronically

TABLE 49–3

Causes of Acute Renal Failure in Pregnancy

Most Common Causes
Hemorrhage
Severe preeclampsia
Rare Causes
Septic shock
Hyperemesis gravidarum
Nephrotoxic drugs
Amniotic fluid embolism
HUS/TTP
Acute fatty liver of pregnancy
Obstructive uropathy
Postoperative oliguria
Idiopathic postpartum acute renal failure

HUS, hemolytic uremic syndrome; TTP, thrombotic thrombocytopenic purpura.

impaired kidneys, whereas too much fluid risks pulmonary edema and ARDS.

An acute prerenal insult such as hemorrhage, dehydration, or septic shock may lead to transient ATN if inadequately treated. Pregnancy, being associated with heightened inflammation, changes to the vascular endothelium, and a prothrombotic state, is more likely to favor the development of ATN and subsequent progression from temporary ATN to bilateral renal cortical necrosis (BRCN) with permanent renal impairment. This is even more likely to occur if the prerenal insult coexists with preeclampsia, a condition characterized by volemic constriction and endothelial dysfunction. The associated prerenal insult, such as abruption or hemorrhage, will exacerbate the hypovolemic state and precipitate the development and progression of ATN. In a cohort of South African women with severe preeclampsia and renal impairment, 7 of 72 (10%) required temporary dialysis and all had either hemorrhage due to abruptio placentae or HELLP (hemolysis, elevated liver enzymes, and low platelets) syndrome.[35]

With the development of ATN, the amount of sodium in the urine will exceed 25 mEq/L, as opposed to prerenal azotemia without intrinsic renal damage in which the amount of sodium in the urine is expected to be lower than 20 mEq/L. The urine sediment may also help in differentiating uncomplicated prerenal azotemia from renal causes of renal dysfunction. In uncomplicated prerenal azotemia, the urine sediment is negative or has only occasional hyaline and granular casts, whereas with the development of ATN, tubular cell debris and brown granular (pigmented) casts will appear in the sediment. Half of the ATN cases may be nonoliguric.

As a consequence of thrombosis in segments of the renal vascular system, about 20% of ARF cases of obstetric origin progress to BRCN.[36] In early phases, it is not possible to differentiate ATN from BRCN. When anuria persists for longer than a week, BRCN should be suspected. Without dialysis, a patient with BRCN cannot survive more than 3 weeks. Computed tomography with contrast or selective renal angiography may help in confirming the diagnosis, revealing delayed filling and poor arborization of the interlobar arteries, with absent or nonhomogeneous filling at the level of the cortex. Imaging, however, is usually unnecessary and may cause further nephrotoxicity. If oliguria persists longer than 30 days, renal biopsy may be considered, although the patchy nature of cortical necrosis in pregnancy may often preclude the definitive diagnosis. Other forms of BRCN, such as focal, confluent, or gross, are less likely to be encountered in pregnancy. Recovery depends on the extent of cortical necrosis, which is often incomplete (patchy) in pregnancy, and for those women who survive the acute illness, renal function usually returns slowly over the next 6 to 24 months. Long-term renal function remains, however, uncertain because hyperfiltration through remnant glomeruli may lead to subsequent progressive decline in renal function.

Acute Renal Failure Associated with Preeclampsia (See also Chapters 35 and 78)

The histopathologic renal changes classically described in preeclampsia as glomerular endotheliosis consist of swollen, vacuolated endothelial cells with fibrils, swollen mesangial cells (mesangiosis), subendothelial deposits of protein reabsorbed from the glomerular filtrate, and tubular casts. As a consequence of all these changes, glomeruli are enlarged by about 20%. The swollen endothelial cells may block the capillary lumen.

Preeclampsia frequently causes mild transient renal impairment (serum creatinine ≤ 1.4 mg/dL), but with appropriate management, recovery of renal function is usually complete. As in other cases of azotemia of intrinsic renal etiology, urine sodium is increased. Proteinuria in preeclampsia is nonselective as a result of increased tubular permeability to most large-molecular-weight proteins (albumin, globulin, transferrin, and hemoglobin). Urinary calcium declines because of an increased tubular reabsorption of calcium.

The cure for severe preeclampsia with renal failure is delivery of the fetus and placenta. Women with preeclampsia who have a rise in serum creatinine from normal to greater than 1.3 mg/dL should be delivered to prevent ongoing renal impairment. When serum creatinine increases by 1 mg/dL/day, ATN is very probable, but with delivery, the condition is reversible in 80% of cases. Recovery is only 20% in women with preexistent renal pathology. It has been reported that 2% to 5% of women with preeclampsia may have undiagnosed underlying renal disease.[37] Delivery may halt the general progression of preeclampsia, but postpartum maternal renal function usually deteriorates before improving.[35] Doubling of serum creatinine within 48 hours is suggestive of progression to BRCN. BRCN and need for dialysis are rare in preeclampsia, occurring more frequently in association with other obstetric complications.[35]

Oliguria in severe preeclampsia is a consequence of intrarenal vasospasm, with about 25% reduction in GFR. Transient oliguria (<100 mL over 4 hr) is a common observation in labor or the first 24 hours postpartum and a fluid challenge, consisting of 500 mL of an isotonic solution over 20 minutes, may be used to correct the usually inadequate vascular volume, unless signs of pulmonary edema are present (basal crackles and oxygen pressure [PO_2] < 95% on room air). If a preeclamptic woman is not obviously hypovolemic and has a BUN less than 14 mg/dL and serum creatinine less than 1.0 mg/dL, repeated fluid challenges to increase urine output are unnecessary and will only increase the maternal risk of pulmonary edema.

Women with severe preeclampsia and serum creatinine greater than 1.36 mg/dL, refractory hypertension, or multisystem organ failure should have their fluid replacement therapy guided by a pulmonary artery catheter in an intensive care unit.[38] Monitoring only the central venous pressure (CVP) may be inadequate in preeclampsia because in those cases with high systemic vascular resistance (SVR), there is a resultant disparate left and right ventricular function. As a consequence, CVP becomes a poor reflection of the left ventricular tolerance to volume expansion; the increase in CVP may be insignificant despite a markedly increased pulmonary capillary wedge pressure (PCWP). In normal pregnancy, this concern does not exist because SVR is always decreased by 25% compared with the nonpregnant state (600–900 dyne sec cm^{-5} from 800–1200 dyne sec cm^{-5}), and CVP and PCWP are unchanged (1–7 mm Hg and 6–12 mm Hg, respectively).

Once invasive hemodynamic monitoring has been instituted in preeclamptic women based on the previously discussed clinical indications, three different situations may be uncovered:

- Low PCWP and high SVR. The best treatment in this situation is continuation of fluid therapy at 250 mL/hr until the PCWP is 10 to 12 mm Hg. In hypovolemic preeclamptic women, volume expansion will decrease SVR, increase cardiac output, and may even reduce the increased arterial pressure, improving both maternal and fetal well-being.[39] It is important to correct hypovolemia before any attempt to reduce blood pressure in order to avoid abrupt drops in blood pressure. A vasodilator given without such precautions can cause profound hypotension that may threaten maternal renal, cerebral, and uteroplacental blood flow.
- Normal or elevated PCWP and normal SVR. The best treatment in this situation is vasodilator therapy (intravenous hydralazine) or low-dose dopamine. Low-dose "renal" dopamine infusion (2.5 μg/kg/min) will induce vasodilation of the renal vessels, with increased RPF, favoring diuresis and solute excretion.
- Markedly elevated PCWP and high SVR. This situation is rare and requires aggressive afterload reduction with diuretics (furosemide infusion 5 mg/hr) and fluid restriction. Unguided fluid therapy in this group of patients who display poor cardiac function may be detrimental.

Once the patient is euvolemic, the fluid balance has to be rigorously monitored hourly, with a Foley catheter in place. The rate of intravenous fluid replacement should equal the previous hour's urine output plus insensible losses—usually 30 mL/hr, if afebrile. Intravenous fluid regimens administered at a fixed hourly rate can lead to fluid overload in oliguric women or to reduced intravascular volume in those undergoing diuresis. The amount of intravenous fluid replacement can be reduced when the mother can take oral fluids and her renal impairment starts to improve. The invasive central hemodynamic monitoring is continued until the diuretic phase occurs in the postpartum period.

Fluid replacement should include blood to replace blood loses, then isotonic sodium chloride solution or Ringer's lactate solution. Dextrose solutions are hypotonic and lead to maternal hyponatremia (5% dextrose solution contains only 30 mmol/L NaCl, compared with 150 mmol/L NaCl in 0.9% NaCl solution). Colloid solutions (albumin) given to women with severe preeclampsia have the risk of markedly increasing PCWP, even in cases with low serum albumin level, and should be avoided.

TABLE 49–4

Indications for Renal Replacement Therapy (Dialysis)

Electrolyte abnormalities refractory to medical treatment
Volume overload with congestive heart failure and pulmonary edema refractory to standard therapy
Severe metabolic acidosis
Uremia (BUN > 39 mg/dL or SCr > 5.65 mg/dL)

BUN, blood urea nitrogen; SCr, serum creatinine.

TABLE 49–5

Hyperkalemia and Associated Electrocardiographic Changes

SERUM POTASSIUM LEVEL	ECG CHANGES
>5.5 mEq/L	Peaked T waves, atrioventricular block
7.0–7.5 mEq/L	Widening QRS complex
8.0–9.0 mEq/L	Atrial standstill
>9.0 mEq/L	Ventricular fibrillation, asystole

ECG, electrocardiographic.

Persistent oliguria and a rising serum creatinine despite adequate intravascular volume and blood pressure correction would indicate the presence of ATN. Fluid intake should then be restricted to avoid fluid overload. Indications for dialysis are volume overload with congestive heart failure not responding to standard therapy, intractable electrolyte abnormalities, severe metabolic acidosis, or BUN greater than 39.2 mg/dL and serum creatinine greater than 5.65 mg/dL (Tables 49–4 and 49–5). The risk of fetal demise is significantly increased if BUN exceeds 60 to 80 mg/dL. Maternal acidosis will result in progressive fetal acidemia. The goal is to maintain the maternal blood pH greater than 7.2. In a series of 60 postpartum preeclamptic women with oliguric renal failure treated with both furosemide infusion and low-dose dopamine, 13 required at least temporary dialysis.[40] Dialysis in pregnancy should be started before the patient becomes symptomatic secondary to acidosis or electrolyte abnormalities.

Acute Renal Failure Due to Renal Obstruction in Pregnancy

Obstruction of the renal tracts during pregnancy may be due to renal calculi (see later discussion), an overdistended uterus, congenital renal tract abnormalities, or the gestational overdistention syndrome. Women with urinary tract surgery in childhood for congenital obstructive uropathy are at increased risk for urine outflow obstruction in the second half of pregnancy, besides a higher incidence of UTI.[41] Obstruction can cause high back-pressures with damaging effect on the renal medulla, leading to loss of renal concentrating ability and production of dilute urine. Patients may also develop hypertension. With incomplete obstructions, in spite of the renal impairment, the patient may still have an apparently good urine output and the urine sediment is usually negative. The serum and urinary indices are not helpful in differentiating renal from postrenal causes of ARF, and imaging studies must be used to confirm the diagnosis. Urinary outflow obstruction requires ureteric stents that can remain in place for up to 3 months during pregnancy and will be removed 4 to 6 weeks after delivery. A temporary nephrostomy may be necessary if the ureteric stents are ineffective.[42]

During pregnancy, the renal tracts can rarely become grossly overdistended. If untreated, this overdistention can rarely lead to rupture of the kidney or urinary tract.[43] Women with overdistention of the urinary tract present with mild to severe back pain, most commonly on the right side and radiating to the lower abdomen. The pain is characteristically relieved by lying on the opposite side and tucking the knees up to the chest. A palpable, tender flank mass and gross or microscopic hematuria suggest renal tract rupture.[43] Rupture of the kidney usually occurs with preexistent renal conditions, such as hamartomas or chronic infections.[43] Occasionally, a urinoma will be evident around the kidney on ultrasound examination. Rupture of the kidney necessitates immediate surgery and almost invariably an emergency nephrectomy.[43]

Other Causes of Acute Renal Failure during Pregnancy

Nephrotoxic Drugs

Nonsteroidal anti-inflammatory drugs (NSAIDs), when given to the mother peripartum, reduce renal blood flow and can cause acute renal impairment to both mother and fetus.[44] Women with reduced intravascular volume, especially if they have preexisting renal impairment, are particularly vulnerable and should be prescribed NSAIDs with caution. Indomethacin may also precipitate hyperkalemia.

Postoperative Oliguria

Postoperatively, oliguria is usually secondary to hypovolemia from hemorrhage and third-space losses, although renal function may also be depressed by general anesthetics. A decrease in RPF may be seen with regional anesthesia causing sympathetic blockade and cardiac preload reduction. Volume depletion with oliguria may sometimes occur several days after surgery owing to continuous nasogastric suction or third-space sequestration (ileus, ascites, pleural effusion). In the assessment of oliguria after pelvic surgery, exclusion of obstructive uropathy or nephrotoxic agents (drugs or radiologic contrast) should always be considered before proceeding with adequate volume and electrolyte replacement.

Acute Fatty Liver of Pregnancy (See also Chapter 47)

Acute fatty liver of pregnancy (AFLP) is a rare but potentially fatal complication of the third trimester or postpartum period. The typical presentation is with nausea, vomiting, anorexia, malaise, epigastric or right upper quadrant pain, headaches, and jaundice. The laboratory studies usually reveal hemoconcentration, elevated white blood cell count, hypofibrinogenemia, prolonged prothrombin time, low antithrombin, metabolic acidosis, elevated liver enzymes and bilirubin, increased ammonia, and elevated serum creatinine and uric acid. In a series of 28 women with AFLP, mean serum creatinine at the time of delivery was 2.32 mg/dL and mean uric acid 11 mg/dL.[45] Intensive care by a multidisciplinary team is necessary because, in addition to hepatic impairment and coagulopathy, other complications frequently arise. Pulmonary edema and ARDS develop in about 25% of cases, pancreatitis in about 15%, sepsis in 10%, and renal failure in 44% to 50% of cases.[46] The ultimate treatment is maternal stabilization and delivery, with close monitoring before and after delivery of vital signs, intake-output balance, and any hemorrhagic diathesis. It is important to treat maternal hypotension aggressively to avoid further injury to liver, kidneys, and other organs. It may be necessary to use invasive hemodynamic monitoring to adequately correct and maintain the intravascular volume, cardiac output, and renal perfusion. In general, patients with AFLP will start to improve 3 days after delivery and will recover normal renal and liver function. Occasionally, temporary dialysis may be necessary.

THROMBOTIC THROMBOCYTOPENIC PURPURA–HEMOLYTIC UREMIC SYNDROME (See also Chapters 41 and 78)

Maternal and Fetal Risks and Management Options

Thrombotic thrombocytopenic purpura (TTP) and hemolytic uremic syndrome (HUS) are very similar, sometimes even undistinguishable, syndromes characterized by microangiopathic hemolytic anemia and thrombocytopenia (thrombotic microangiopathy). They are extremely rare during pregnancy and postpartum, occurring in less than 1 case in 100,000 pregnancies.[46]

Thrombotic Thrombocytopenic Purpura

The classic pentad of TTP, first described in 1925 by Moschcowitz,[47] consists of thrombocytopenia, hemolytic anemia, neurologic abnormalities, fever, and renal impairment. The complete pentad is present in only 40% of cases, but the first three components are manifested by 50% to 75% of patients.[46] Thrombocytopenia is frequently severe (<25,000 platelets/mm^3), the same as anemia, which often requires transfusion. Although neurologic abnormalities are reported to be present in as many as 90% of patients, they may be nonspecific or difficult to diagnose (headaches, visual changes, confusion, aphasia, weakness, paresis, seizures, and stroke). Fever is usually mild (<38.4°C), being present in 30% to 40% of cases. Renal impairment is manifested as proteinuria, hematuria, increase in serum creatinine, and oliguria. Long-term renal and neurologic impairment is possible. Presenting signs and symptoms may also include abdominal pain, nausea and vomiting, gastrointestinal bleeding, epistaxis, petechiae, purpura, jaundice, and syncope.

There are both congenital (familial) and acquired types of TTP. The familial form is characterized by a chronic relapsing course. The underlying pathologic disturbance involves microthrombi in end-organ microvessels typically resulting in ischemia and multiorgan disorder (kidneys, liver, pancreas, heart, and lungs).[48] ADAMTS13 is a von Willebrand factor–cleaving metalloprotease that normally prevents the persistence in circulation of unusually large von Willebrand's factor multimers. This enzyme produced mainly in the liver is markedly reduced (<5% of normal) in most patients with congenital TTP,[49] and antibodies that neutralize ADAMTS13 have been found in women with acquired TTP.[50] Consequently, large multimers of von Willebrand's factor are in high concentration in the circulation, inducing aberrant platelet aggregation and adhesion with formation of microthrombi, thrombocytopenia, and mechanical injury to erythrocytes with microangiopathic hemolytic anemia. Testing for ADAMTS13 is not readily available in clinical laboratories. On a peripheral blood smear, schizocytosis is noted, and the increased compensatory hematopoiesis is denoted by a high reticulocyte count, many nucleated red blood cells in circulation, and leukocytosis. In the bone marrow, normoblastic erythroid hyperplasia and increase in megakaryocytes may be noted. Hemolysis is responsible for increase in LDH and indirect bilirubin.

During pregnancy, the levels of ADAMTS13 progressively fall.[51] This may explain why TTP is common in association with pregnancy (~13% of all cases).[52] In 89% of cases, the presentation is antepartum with 58% in the second trimester. TTP shares many similarities with preeclampsia, and it is most important to differentiate them, not least because their management is different (Table 49–6). In HUS-TTP, typically there are no coagulation abnormalities, antithrombin III level is unchanged, and liver transaminases may be only modestly elevated, whereas in preeclampsia, anemia is not expected to be so severe. In TTP, maternal condition does not improve with delivery, but pregnancy usually cannot be prolonged for more than 4 weeks from the acute presentation, and given the increased risk of fetal loss, it seems advisable to deliver earlier. Undoubtedly, consideration should also be given to sepsis when the prevailing manifestations are fever, thrombocytopenia, and renal failure.

Without adequate treatment, women with TTP do not survive more than 3 months. With the use of plasmapheresis, first introduced in 1976, 90% maternal survival is expected and the rate of fetal loss is only 20% to 30%.[53] Maternal hypoxia, reduced uteroplacental blood flow, and vascular lesions in the placenta may be contributors to the adverse perinatal outcomes.[54]

Until recently, it was unclear why plasmapheresis worked, but the recent discovery of antibodies to ADAMTS13 (removed with old plasma) and a congenital deficiency of ADAMTS13 (replenished with infusion of fresh plasma) may, at least in part, explain the efficacy of the process. Plasma exchange also helps remove the abnormally large multimers of von Willebrand's factor. Plasma infusion alone has a response rate of 64% and may be employed as the first-line approach in cases with less severe thrombocytopenia. Plasma exchange is effective in approximately 90% of cases and is preferable in cases with severe hematologic manifestations.[46] Plasmapheresis commonly causes mild urticaria or hypotension. Plasma exchanges are performed daily at a rate of 40 mL/kg until a few days after normalization of the platelet count, correction of neurologic symptoms, and elimination of hemolysis as evidenced by decline in LDH and stable hematocrit. If there is a suboptimal response, the rate can be increased to 80 mL/kg, but the risk of hypovolemia should be carefully avoided. When the adequate response is achieved, the frequency of plasma exchanges will be tapered to weekly sessions but never discontinued during pregnancy because relapses are common. Some patients, especially those with high antibody titers against ADAMTS13, may not respond to plasma exchange alone, requiring immunosuppressive therapy (prednisone, cyclophosphamide, vincristine, or rituximab), or splenectomy, or both.[55] Antiaggregant treatment with low-dose aspirin and dipyridamole (225 mg/day) may also be beneficial in conjunction with plasma exchange.[56] Conversely, administration of platelets to thrombocytopenic patients with TTP-HUS can result in a precipitous decline in clinical status due to an increase in microvascular thrombosis. Platelets may still be necessary when there is a potential for life-threatening bleeding.[57] Red cell transfusions are used as needed according to clinical guidelines.

Based on case reports, there may be a risk of recurrence of TTP in subsequent pregnancies, sometimes as early as the first trimester, and also with hormonal contraception.[53] Based on such limited data, the risk magnitude cannot be estimated.

TABLE 49–6
Differential Grid for Imitators of Severe Preeclampsia

	PREECLAMPSIA	AFLP	TTP	HUS
Leukocytosis	-	+	+	-
Anemia	±	-	++	++
Thrombocytopenia	+	-	++	+
Elevated liver transaminases	+	+	±	±
Elevated bilirubin	+	+	+	-
Elevated LDH	+	±	+	+
Elevated ammonia	-	+	-	-
Elevated creatinine	+	++	+	++
Elevated uric acid	+	+	-	+
Coagulopathy	+	+	-	-

AFLP, acute fatty liver of pregnancy; HUS, hemolytic uremic syndrome; LDH, lactate dehydrogenase; TTP, thrombotic thrombocytopenic purpura.

Hemolytic Uremic Syndrome

HUS was first described by Gasser in 1955 in children,[58] in whom it is more frequent and milder than in adults. It is rarely associated with pregnancy, almost universally occurring in the postpartum period (≤10 wk).[54] Clinically, HUS is very similar to TTP, but the microvascular injury mainly affects the kidneys. Thrombi are seen in afferent arterioles and glomerular capillaries, and the renal functional impairment is more severe than in preeclampsia or TTP. Patients present with edema, hypertension, and renal failure. In about 40% of cases, there is a flulike prodromal phase with gastrointestinal symptoms suggesting a possible endotoxin-mediated etiology at least in some cases.[59] The serum creatinine levels increase rapidly, by at least 0.5 mg/dL/day, in addition to proteinuria and microscopic hematuria. Oliguria progresses to anuria, and most patients will need dialysis, with risk for long-term renal deficit.[60] Anemia may be severe, requiring transfusion of red cells, and LDH may be elevated. Thrombocytopenia is less severe than in TTP, there are no coagulation abnormalities, and with the exception of seizures, other neurologic abnormalities are uncommon.

The treatment of HUS is similar to that of TTP. However, the response to plasma infusions alone is not so favorable. A combination of plasma exchange and prednisone at 1 mg/kg/day is frequently used as in nonpregnant protocols. After improvement, the rate of plasma exchange may be reduced and the dose of prednisone tapered down to 5 mg/day and maintained at this dose until 3 weeks postpartum. Thereafter, the prednisone can be completely tapered off.

Until 1996, only nine cases of HUS had been reported during pregnancy.[61] Such cases have been associated with an extremely poor prognosis, including maternal mortality of up to 55% and frequent preterm birth and fetal demise.[62] Because of these major risks, immediate delivery upon diagnosing HUS seems advisable, although in a case report of HUS developing at 18 weeks' gestation, the pregnancy was continued until term.[61]

Another thrombotic microangiopathy with thrombocytopenia and hemolysis similar to TTP/HUS is the *idiopathic postpartum acute renal failure* first described by Robson and associates in 1968.[63] About 100 cases have been reported so far. The diagnosis is made by renal biopsy, which shows thrombosis of the afferent arterioles, necrosis, and glomerular endothelial proliferation. No other organs are affected. The condition is irreversible and may lead to chronic hypertension. Severe forms are complicated by seizures, coma, and cardiac failure. Many treatments have been proposed so far, with different levels of efficacy: plasmapheresis, immunosuppression, heparin, dialysis, dipyridamole, and uterine curettage.

SUMMARY OF MANAGEMENT OPTIONS

Acute Renal Failure

Management Options	Evidence Quality and Recommendation	References
Management is aimed at identification and correction of the precipitating insult and optimal fluid resuscitation.	—/GPP	—
Differentiate uncomplicated prerenal azotemia from renal causes of renal dysfunction.	—/GPP	—
Suspect BRCN when anuria persists longer than a week and consider dialysis.	III/B	36
Severe Preeclampsia (See also Chapters 35 and 78)		
Delivery for oliguria or a rise in serum creatinine from normal to > 1.3 mg/dL	III/B	35
Fluid challenge (500 mL isotonic solution over 20 min) may be considered in cases with suspicion of hypovolemia, serum creatinine 1.0–1.36 mg/dL, and no clinical signs of pulmonary edema.	—/GPP	—
In cases with serum creatinine > 1.36 mg/dL, refractory hypertension, or multisystem organ failure, continuation of fluid therapy should be guided by a pulmonary artery catheter in an intensive care unit. Monitoring only the central venous pressure is inadequate.	IV/C	38
IV hydralazine or low-dose dopamine infusion (2.5 μg/kg/min) if necessary.	Ib/A	35,38,39,40
Furosemide infusion (5 mg/hr) and fluid restriction if necessary.	Ib/A	35,38,39,40
Correct hypovolemia before any attempt to reduce blood pressure to avoid abrupt drops in blood pressure.	IIa/B	39
Once the patient is euvolemic, the rate of IV fluid replacement should equal the previous hour's urine output plus insensible losses. Reduce the amount of IV fluid replacement when the mother can take oral fluids and her renal impairment starts to improve. Continue invasive central hemodynamic monitoring until the diuretic phase in postpartum.	—/GPP	—
Dialysis in rare cases.	IIa/B	40

SUMMARY OF MANAGEMENT OPTIONS
Acute Renal Failure—cont'd

Management Options	Evidence Quality and Recommendation	References
Postoperative Oliguria		
Exclude obstructive uropathy or nephrotoxic agents (drugs or radiologic contrast) before proceeding with adequate volume and electrolyte replacement.	—/GPP	—
Thrombotic Thrombocytopenic Purpura (See also Chapters 41 and 78)		
Differentiate from preeclampsia.	III/B	46
Plasma infusion may be first-line approach in cases with less severe thrombocytopenia (64% response rate).	III/B	46
Plasmapheresis is preferable in cases with severe hematologic manifestations (90% response rate).	Ib/A	46,52,57
Antiplatelet therapy (aspirin, dipyridamole) in conjunction with plasma exchange.	Ib/A	56
Immunosuppressive therapy (prednisone, cyclophosphamide, vincristine, or rituximab), or splenectomy, or both, for non responders to plasma exchange.	III/B	55
Consider delivery at 34 wk.	—/GPP	—
Hemolytic Uremic Syndrome (See also Chapters 41 and 78)		
Dialysis for most cases.	III/B	60
Red cell transfusion for severe anemia.	III/B	62
Plasma exchange and prednisone until 4 wk postpartum.	III/B	57,62
Delivery upon diagnosis.	IV/C	61
Acute Fatty Liver of Pregnancy (See also Chapter 47)		
Admit to intensive care unit. Invasive hemodynamic monitoring may be necessary.	III/B	45,46
Maternal stabilization and delivery.	III/B	45,46
Monitor clotting, hypoglycemia, and fluid balance before and after delivery.	III/B	45,46
Temporary dialysis occasionally.	III/B	45,46
Urinary Tract Obstruction		
Ureteric stents until 4–6 wk postpartum. If ineffective, temporary nephrostomy.	III/B	42
Nephrotoxic Drugs		
Prescribe NSAIDs with caution.	III/B	44

BRCN, bilateral renal cortical necrosis; GPP, good practice point; NSAIDs, non-steroidal anti-inflammatory drugs.

CHRONIC RENAL DISEASE IN PREGNANCY

Maternal and Fetal Risks and Management Options

When considering the interaction between renal disease and pregnancy, two salient questions are frequently asked: what effect will the pregnancy have on the mother's already affected kidneys and what effect will the mother's kidney disease have on the pregnancy? It appears that the major determinant for maternal outcome and for the likelihood of further pregnancy-induced renal damage is the degree of renal function impairment at the beginning of pregnancy. Another overriding prognosticator is the presence of hypertension, which is also associated with increased obstetric risks regardless of the underlying specific renal pathology. Proteinuria, conversely, although predictive for the mother's long-term renal outcome, is poorly correlated with immediate obstetric outcomes.[64] The specific underlying disease becomes relevant when fetal outcomes are considered. A distinction may be drawn from a fetal/neonatal perspective between renal dysfunction resulting from primary renal disease and that in which renal involvement is part of a systemic disease. One has to note, however, that such conclusions are based on studies including only a small number of cases, without an appropriate control group, and virtually all retrospective, underscoring the critical need for large prospective observational studies in this field.

The Influence of Preexisting Renal Impairment

There is a relationship between the degree of renal impairment and the physiologic adaptation to pregnancy. With mild renal impairment (serum creatinine < 1.4 mg/dL), there is normal intravascular volume expansion and only minimal attenuation of the gestational increment in GFR.[65] With moderate impairment (serum creatinine between 1.4 mg/dL and 2.4 mg/dL), in spite of a normal blood volume expansion, only 50% of women will have the expected increase in GFR, whereas with severe impairment (serum creatinine > 2.4 mg/dL), there is a markedly attenuated increase in blood volume and no increase in GFR.[66]

Large multicenter series appear to suggest a linear relationship between the preconception serum creatinine level and the likelihood of further renal damage during pregnancy, although a more reliable interpretation of data should have been based on creatinine clearance rather than conventional serum creatinine levels. Women with mild renal disease who become pregnant have only a slightly increased risk of long-term damage to their kidneys from pregnancy compared with women with mild renal disease who had never become pregnant.[66] Even with moderate renal disease, irreversible deterioration of maternal renal function is uncommon. In an analysis of 82 pregnancies complicated by primary renal disease, Jones and Hayslett[64] reported that pregnancy-related deterioration in renal function occurs in 40% of women with initial serum creatinine level of 1.4 to 2.0 mg/dL. In half of these cases, the deterioration will persist postpartum, but only 2% will rapidly decline to end-stage renal disease (ESRD). When the serum creatinine level is above 2.0 mg/dL at the beginning of pregnancy, 66% of women will have gestational deterioration in renal function, deterioration that nearly always persists in postpartum and progresses to ESRD within 6 months after delivery in 23% of cases.[64] The risk of accelerated progression to ESRD within a few years after pregnancy is 45% when the serum creatinine level is greater than 2.6 mg/dL.

Although termination of pregnancy per se will not result in an improvement in renal function,[67] a rapid and significant decline reflected by changes in serum creatinine or creatinine clearance of at least 25% may justify delivery or termination of pregnancy. However, if the gestational age is between 24 and 31 weeks, with a normally grown fetus and controllable hypertension, expectant management with dialysis as indicated may be considered.

With regard to obstetric outcomes, available data indicate that fetal survival of pregnant women with mild or moderate renal disease is only slightly diminished. In contrast, fetal outcome is particularly reserved with severe disease, when the perinatal mortality rate is approximately four times higher compared with mild or moderate disease (36% vs, 8%).[68] In a Japanese retrospective study of 240 pregnancies in women with underlying renal disease, the rate in perinatal mortality was correlated with the decline in GFR.[69] The rate of perinatal morbidity as a consequence of low birth weight or prematurity doubles from mild to moderate renal insufficiency and again from moderate to severe disease. Reported rates of fetal growth restriction are 24% for pregnancies complicated by mild renal disease, 35% for moderate disease, and approximately 50% for severe disease.[68] Preterm delivery occurs with a frequency of 20%, 48%, and 80%, respectively, for mild, moderate, and severe degrees of renal failure.[68] Furthermore, early pregnancy losses, which are often ignored in analyses of pregnancy outcome, are more common in women with severe renal impairment.[64]

The Influence of Associated Hypertension

The degree of renal function impairment is not the only outcome modifier. Hypertensive renal disease is associated with increased maternal-fetal risk compared with normotensive renal disease, and the presence of hypertension increases the risk of further decline in renal function during pregnancy. Hypertension present at conception or early in pregnancy increases the perinatal mortality rate 6- to 10-fold.[69,70] In a retrospective study of 51 pregnancies from India, all women delivered prematurely when the diastolic blood pressure was greater than 100 mm Hg at initiation of prenatal care.[9] Pregnancy outcome is improved when blood pressure is optimized prior to conception and the control is maintained throughout gestation.[71]

Pregnant women with renal disease have a 50% increased risk of preeclampsia.[72,73] The risk increases to 80% with preexisting hypertension.[66] Such risk levels might have been overestimated as a result of the inherent pitfalls in differentiating an exacerbation of the renal disease with new-onset hypertension from superimposed preeclampsia.

The Influence of Associated Proteinuria

Limited postpartum follow-up of women with proteinuria identified in early pregnancy has shown an increased risk of progressive renal impairment.[74] Approximately 20% of women with nephrotic syndrome (proteinuria > 3 g/day, hypoalbuminemia, and hyperlipidemia) will progress to ESRD within 4 years. It is, therefore, important that women with proteinuria recognized in early pregnancy be investigated for previously occult renal disease and monitored serially throughout pregnancy for changes in renal function, hypertension, and urinary infection. Frequently, in the absence of pregestational information, the diagnosis of preexistent renal disease will be possible only retrospectively, when the manifestations are still present at 6 months postpartum. The only certain way of first making the diagnosis during pregnancy is by renal biopsy, with the theoretical advantage that some primary glomerular diseases that are adversely influenced by pregnancy may be steroid-responsive. However, renal biopsy is considered potentially beneficial only in highly selected women before 28 weeks' gestation who are found to have sudden unexplained deterioration of renal function or new-onset heavy proteinuria (>5 g/24 hr) with no history of renal disease, in the absence of preeclampsia.[68,75] After 28 weeks' gestation, if progressive renal deterioration is noted, early delivery can be considered, with biopsy postpartum if necessary.

There is a poor correlation between the degree of proteinuria and obstetric outcomes. Significant proteinuria may result, however, in a poorer nutritional status and inappropriate maternal weight gain, a known risk factor for both fetal growth restriction and preterm delivery. These women also have an increased risk of preeclampsia (~30%).[74]

Severe proteinuria may contribute to hypoalbuminemia and a diminished capacity to excrete sodium. Retention of salt and water may lead to extensive edema, a situation particularly seen in diabetic nephropathy. In order to reduce the edema, it may be necessary to prescribe a low-sodium diet (1.5 g Na) close to term, bedrest in the lateral decubitus position to increase GFR, and an intermittent, small dose of a loop diuretic.[71] The use of diuretics in these patients should be undertaken very cautiously because they may increase the risk of uteroplacental hypoperfusion and may precipitate circulatory collapse or thromboembolic episodes. Nephrotic syndrome increases the risk of arterial and venous thrombosis, including renal vein thrombosis, but the efficacy of prophylactic anticoagulation has never been proved in pregnancy or outside of pregnancy.

Based on available data, it is difficult to separate the independent contribution to poor fetal outcome of maternal renal impairment, hypertension, and sometimes proteinuria. The evidence suggests that especially the first two parameters are individually and cumulatively detrimental to fetal outcome. For both maternal and fetal monitoring, more frequent prenatal visits are recommended, initially every 2 weeks, and weekly after 32 weeks' gestation. It may be necessary to initiate weekly or twice-weekly biophysical profiles at 28 weeks' gestation depending on the degree of renal insufficiency, hypertension, proteinuria, fetal growth velocity, and past obstetric outcome. In the absence of maternal or fetal deterioration, consideration should be given to delivery at or near term, with cesarean delivery reserved for the usual obstetric indications.

SUMMARY OF MANAGEMENT OPTIONS

Chronic Renal Failure

Management Options	Evidence Quality and Recommendation	References
Any gravida with preexisting renal disease or at risk for renal deterioration during pregnancy needs a baseline determination of proteinuria and creatinine clearance early in pregnancy, then monitoring with monthly serum creatinine levels. Repeat 24-hr urine collections when indicated.	III/B	9
Women with proteinuria recognized in early pregnancy should be investigated for previously occult renal disease. Renal biopsy is potentially beneficial only in highly selected women < 28 wk gestation with sudden unexplained deterioration of renal function or new-onset heavy proteinuria (>5 g/24 hr), with no history of renal disease, in the absence of preeclampsia.	IV/C	68,75
Pregnancy outcome is improved when blood pressure is optimized prior to conception and the control is maintained throughout gestation.	III/B	71
Changes in serum creatinine or creatinine clearance of at least 25% may justify delivery or termination of pregnancy. If the gestational age is between 24 and 31 wk, with a normally grown fetus and controllable hypertension, manage expectantly, with dialysis as indicated.	IV/C	64,67,68
For extensive edema in nephrotic syndrome, prescribe a low-sodium diet (1.5 g Na), bedrest in lateral decubitus to increase GFR, and cautiously, an intermittent, small dose of a loop diuretic.	IV/C	71
Prenatal visits initially every 2 wk, then weekly after 32 wk gestation. Serial measurement of fetal growth and umbilical artery Doppler recordings.	—/GPP	—
Weekly or twice weekly biophysical profiles starting at 28 wk gestation depending on the degree of renal insufficiency, hypertension, proteinuria, fetal growth velocity and umbilical artery Doppler values.	—/GPP	—
In the absence of maternal or fetal deterioration, delivery at or near term, with cesarean delivery reserved for the usual obstetrical indications.	—/GPP	—

GFR, glomerular filtration rate; GPP, good practice point.

SPECIFIC RENAL DISEASES IN PREGNANCY

Maternal and Fetal Risks and Management Options

Primary Glomerulonephritis

Immunoglobulin A (IgA) glomerulonephritis is the most common type of primary nephropathy in young people and the most frequently occurring variety in pregnancy. Information derived from small case series appears to suggest that the histologic type of glomerulonephritis influences the fetal and maternal outcomes, although this conclusion has been challenged in the literature.[76] There is consensus, however, that clinical parameters, such as the presence of impaired renal function, hypertension, and nephrotic range proteinuria in the first trimester, correlate with less favorable fetal and maternal outcomes, regardless of histopathologic diagnosis.[71] No increase in adverse outcomes occurs when nephrotic syndrome develops late in pregnancy.[76] The presence of severe vascular lesions on renal biopsy has also been associated with increased perinatal mortality, but this has no significant effect on maternal complications during pregnancy.[71] Based on more recent data, the overall fetal loss rate in primary glomerular disease is 21%, with the highest fetal loss rate (23%–45%) and low birth weight (32%) being associated with focal glomerulosclerosis.[77]

About 20% of women with chronic primary glomerulonephritis will experience worsening of preexisting hypertension or new-onset hypertension during pregnancy.[78] Changes in the preconceptional immunosuppressive regimen are not advisable during pregnancy.[79] However, chlorambucil is preferably avoided in pregnancy, and cyclophosphamide should not be used in the first trimester. Based on a large cohort study with patient follow-up over an average of 15 years, pregnancy is not an independent contributor to renal function deterioration in patients with chronic primary glomerulonephritis provided that they have normal or near-normal renal function (serum creatinine < 1.4 mg/dL) at conception.[80]

Women who had Henoch-Schönlein purpura (HSP) with primary glomerulonephritis in childhood are at an increased risk of preeclampsia during their pregnancies (70%) according to a small Finnish retrospective study.[81] There are also case reports of pregnancy triggering recurrent HSP.[82] In one such case, early pregnancy was associated with progressive renal failure, purpura, and arthralgia, unresponsive to corticosteroids, requiring treatment with cyclophosphamide.[83]

Autosomal Dominant Polycystic Kidney Disease

Pregnant women with autosomal dominant polycystic kidney disease (ADPKD) frequently manifest hypertension, which may predate the pregnancy or develop during the pregnancy, including superimposed preeclampsia. Increases in serum creatinine and proteinuria may also develop with advancing gestation, but in general, unless renal insufficiency was present before conception, the chance of a successful pregnancy outcome is unaffected.[84]

Extrarenal manifestations are seen in 50% of patients, including cerebral aneurysms (in up to 10%), liver and choledochal cysts, cardiac valvular defects, and aortic aneurysms.[85] The risk of rupture of asymptomatic intracranial aneurysms in pregnant ADPKD women has never been defined, but the event may be devastating, with over 50% mortality or permanent disability.[86] Although the detection of an aneurysm may not lead to immediate treatment, the presence of the aneurysm would influence the mode of delivery. The general consensus is that cesarean delivery is indicated for uncorrected arterial lesions such as arteriovenous malformations and berry aneurysms, because blood pressure elevations with pushing during the second stage can elicit hemorrhage.[87] For these reasons, we feel that screening with magnetic resonance angiography in pregnancy, or ideally in the immediate preconceptional period, is advisable.[88] Genetic counseling should also be considered in pregnancy or preconceptionally because, as with any autosomal dominant condition, the chance for the offspring to be affected is 50%. Genetic linkage analysis is available for in utero molecular diagnosis, but although the results are essentially unequivocal, it is impossible to predict the severity of disease or clinical outcome.

Reflux Nephropathy

Reflux nephropathy is common in women of childbearing age and is characterized by renal scarring and reduced GFR. Women with surgically corrected VUR in childhood remain at increased risk of reflux nephropathy in pregnancy. Pregnancy increases the risk of irreversible renal function deterioration as result of tubulointerstitial disease (in up to 13% of cases) and gestational overdistention (in ~4%).[89] Close monitoring is necessary to detect significant hydroureteronephrosis, particularly if the woman develops flank pain, decreased urinary output, persistent infections, or hypertension. Ultrasonography of the renal pelvis at the end of the first trimester will provide a useful baseline measurement to be compared with subsequent imaging. Worsening proteinuria is rare and more indicative of preeclampsia. Detection of renal deterioration on serial serum creatinine measurements may require temporary urinary drainage. The changes may be reversible, and unnecessary surgical procedures soon after delivery should be avoided.

VUR at the time of conception increases the risk of pyelonephritis. Monitoring for asymptomatic bacteriuria every 4 to 6 weeks throughout pregnancy is essential, and for women with persistent bacteriuria, low-dose prophylactic antibiotics chosen according to the sensitivity of the most recent UTI would prevent symptomatic infection. Women with surgically corrected VUR in childhood also have a high incidence of UTIs in pregnancy (18%–57%), a much higher rate than in women who had correction at adult age or in whom the reflux subsided spontaneously.[89]

The risk of superimposed preeclampsia (≤75%), and the rate of fetal morbidity and mortality are influenced by maternal hypertension and serum creatinine at conception.[89,90] When serum creatinine levels are increased over 1.24 mg/dL, the rate of preterm delivery is as high as 20%, and the fetal loss rate, excluding elective abortions, may reach 37%.[89]

There is increasing evidence that VUR may be a familial disorder affecting 20% of infants who have a parent with a family history of VUR, compared with a 1% to 2% frequency of VUR in the general population.[91] If kidney damage is to be prevented, early diagnosis and treatment of VUR are necessary, before the neonate develops a UTI.[92] It has been suggested that infants of mothers with reflux nephropathy be prescribed prophylactic antibiotics immediately after birth and undergo renal ultrasound and voiding cystourethrogram.[91] Evidence for renal scarring can be sought in those positive for VUR using a 2,3-dimercaptosuccinic acid (DMSA) radioisotope scan at 3 months of age.[91] It seems prudent to also offer screening to infants whose father has VUR.

SUMMARY OF MANAGEMENT OPTIONS

Primary Glomerulonephritis, Autosomal Dominant Polycystic Kidney Disease, and Reflux Nephropathy

Management Options	Evidence Quality and Recommendation	References
Primary Glomerulonephritis		
Changes in the preconceptional immunosuppressive regimen are not advisable.	III/B	79
Autosomal Dominant Polycystic Kidney Disease		
Screen for cerebral aneurysms with magnetic resonance angiography in the immediate preconceptional period or in pregnancy.	IV/C	88
Cesarean delivery for uncorrected cerebral aneurysms.	IV/C	87,88
Hereditary autosomal dominant condition requires preconceptional or prenatal genetic counseling.	—/GPP	—
Reflux Nephropathy		
Baseline renal ultrasound at 12 wk gestation.	III/B	89,90
Repeat renal ultrasound if flank pain, decreased urinary output, hypertension, persistent infections, or increase in serum creatinine.	—/GPP	—
Monitor for asymptomatic bacteriuria with urine cultures every 4–6 wk.	III/B	89
Low-dose prophylactic antibiotics if persistent bacteriuria.	III/B	89
Renal function deterioration may require temporary urinary drainage.	III/B	89
Screen fetus and neonate for VUR and consider neonatal prophylactic antibiotics.	III/B	91

GPP, good practice point; VUR, vesicoureteric reflux.

Urolithiasis

The incidence of urolitiasis during pregnancy is similar to that in the nongravid state.[93] Although gestational hypercalciuria, urinary stasis, and urinary tract dilation may appear as an ideal environment for stone formation, de novo formation of stones during pregnancy is prevented by a concomitant increase in the urinary excretion of crystallization inhibitors, such as magnesium, citrate, and nephrocalcin.[94] Uric acid and cystine stones rarely form in pregnancy owing to the physiologic alkalinization of the urine. The physiologic ureteropelvic dilation in pregnancy favors migration of preexisting stones. Pregnant women in the process of passing a renal calculus usually develop severe colicky lumbar pain associated with fever and hematuria. In the absence of a typical acute renal colic, urolithiasis may be suggested by flank pain or tenderness, hematuria, or persistent bacteriuria.

Symptomatic calculi are more common in white than in African American women and in multigravidas than in primigravidas.[93] Renal colic is also more common in the second and third trimesters.[93] Based on large published series of pregnancies complicated by renal stones, the affected women have an increased frequency of UTI, preterm labor, and preterm rupture of membranes.[95]

The diagnosis may be confirmed by a renal tract ultrasound in about half of the cases.[96] When inconclusive, more definitive information may be obtained with a plain abdominal radiograph or an one-shot intravenous pyelograph.[33] The radiation exposure of the fetus from one or two radiographs is minimal, only 0.4 to 1.0 rads.[96] Alternatively, in an effort to avoid even a small dose of radiation to the fetus, magnetic resonance urography can be used.[34]

Initial conservative management of renal colic during pregnancy is successful in close to 70% of cases.[96] Hydration, bedrest, analgesia with meperidine, and antibiotics will allow the spontaneous passage of the stones in many cases. The passage of the stone may be facilitated by epidural anesthesia, which will relieve the ureteral spasm. Continued symptoms may necessitate cystoscopy for stone removal by ureteroscopy or passage of a double-J stent catheter that will relieve the obstruction and then be maintained in place under antibiotic prophylaxis until delivery. A percutaneous or open nephrostomy is another option, especially for an obstructed single kidney. Nephrostomy is also likely to have to remain in place for the rest of the pregnancy.

Invasive procedures do place the gravida at increased risk of preterm delivery and other complications. They are indicated only in cases of intractable pain, severe infection, or deterioration of renal function. Lithotripsy is generally contraindicated in pregnancy because of fetal safety concerns. An alternative with a 91% success rate for ureteral calculi, as reported in a series of eight pregnant women, is the flexible ureteroscopy with holmium laser lithotripsy.[97] This technique appears to have a good margin of safety because the direct stone-crushing energy is confined to within 0.5 mm of the laser fiber tip. It can be used in all stages of pregnancy.[97]

Women who are recurrent stone formers with persistent gross hypercalciuria, despite increased fluid intake, can use thiazide diuretics in pregnancy to increase distal tubular resorbtion of calcium. For problematic cases of cystinuria or recurrent uric acid calculi, high diuresis should be maintained and the urine should be further alkalinized to a pH greatrer than 6, preferably with potassium citrate.[98] During pregnancy, xanthine oxidase inhibitors for prevention of uric acid stones should be avoided, especially during the first trimester. Although the outcome of most pregnancies is normal under D-penicillamine for the prevention of cystine stones,[99] a teratogenic effect of the drug is suggested by animal studies, and a few cases of children with cutis laxa whose mothers received D-penicillamine during pregnancy are reported in the literature, dictating extreme caution.[100]

SUMMARY OF MANAGEMENT OPTIONS
Urolithiasis

Management Options	Evidence Quality and Recommendation	References
Identify renal calculus with renal tract ultrasound and when inconclusive, KUB, one-shot IV pyelography, or MRU.	III/B	33,34,96
If Renal Colic:		
IV hydration, bedrest, analgesia (meperidine), and antibiotics. Initial conservative management is successful in 70% of cases.	III/B	96
Epidural anesthesia may facilitate the passage of the stone.	—/GPP	—
Continued symptoms, or obstruction, especially in a single kidney, require cystoscopy for stone removal by ureteroscopy or passage of a ureteric stent, or nephrostomy.	III/B	96
Definitive removal of obstructing calculus by ureteroscopic holmium laser lithotripsy.	III/B	97
For Recurrent Stone Formers:		
In case of persistent gross hypercalciuria, increase fluid intake and give thiazide diuretics.	III/B	98,99
In case of cystinuria or recurrent uric acid calculi, maintain high diuresis and alkalinize the urine with potassium citrate.		

GPP, good practice point; KUB, kidneys, ureter, bladder (plain abdominal radiography); MRU, magnetic resonance urography.

Diabetic Nephropathy (See also Chapter 44)

Although only 5% to 10% of pregnant women with pregestational DM have diabetic nephropathy, this is the most common chronic renal disorder in pregnancy. It also represents the highest risk subgroup among pregnant women with DM. When the renal function is only minimally diminished, pregnancy does not have any negative impact on kidney function.[101] Conversely, women with diabetic nephropathy and moderate to severe renal impairment (serum creatinine > 1.4 mg/dL) have a 45% chance of an accelerated decline in renal function, significantly higher than in nonpregnant controls.[102] The prognosis is especially worse if hypertension coexists. The data on the impact of pregnancy on renal function in cases of moderate to severe renal impairment are based almost exclusively on studies conducted on type 1 DM cases, with only limited data from type 2 DM.

Pregnancies in women with diabetic nephropathy are complicated by an overall rate of hypertension of more than 60% and superimposed preeclampsia in 41% of cases.[103] In class F diabetics, the rate of preeclampsia is 50%, and even 60% in association with chronic hypertension. Besides chronic hypertension, other risk factors independently associated with the development of preeclampsia are an elevated glycosylated hemoglobin in the first trimester and the prepregnancy duration of DM.[104] Effective antihypertensive treatment is essential because, even in women with advanced diabetic disease, blood pressure control can considerably slow the deterioration of maternal renal function.[105] The target diastolic blood pressure is 90 mm Hg or less, lower than that usually recommended for nondiabetic pregnant women with chronic hypertension.[106] In all cases of diabetic nephropathy, proteinuria will increase in pregnancy, peaking in the third trimester, and decreasing postpartum.[103] The increase during pregnancy is dramatic in 58% of cases.[107] However, increased protein excretion, in the absence of preeclampsia, does not influence pregnancy outcome or the rate of change in creatinine clearance.[107]

Although pregnancy in women with diabetic nephropathy and moderate renal function impairment appears to accelerate the progression of their disease, fetal prognosis remains generally favorable in the absence of uncontrolled hypertension.[108] With severely impaired renal function, early delivery between 32 and 36 weeks frequently becomes necessary for fetal concerns or superimposed preeclampsia or to prevent further deterioration of maternal renal function. The mainstay of management before conception and during pregnancy is adequate glycemic and blood pressure control. However, even with normoglycemia throughout pregnancy, the risk of preterm delivery remains high (22%–30%). Other pregnancy complications are fetal growth restriction in 16% of cases and more frequent bacteriuria.[103] The willingness to expectantly manage women with increasing proteinuria without other signs of preeclampsia may at least in part explain the current fetal survival rate of 95%.[103]

SUMMARY OF MANAGEMENT OPTIONS

Diabetic Nephropathy (See also Chapter 44)

Management Options	Evidence Quality and Recommendation	References
Adequate glycemic control.	III/B	103
Control hypertension to ≤150/90 mm Hg.	III/B	103,105,106
In cases with severe renal failure, consider early delivery (32–36 wk gestation).	—/GPP	—

GPP, good practice point.

Lupus Nephritis (See also Chapter 43)

Systemic lupus erythematosus (SLE) is a multisystem autoimmune disorder that predominantly affects young women, without impact on their fertility.[109] Renal involvement (lupus nephritis) occurs in 50% of SLE cases and, in pregnancy, is one of the most serious complications of lupus. Possible manifestations include hematuria, proteinuria, elevated serum creatinine, hyperuricemia, thrombocytopenia, and hypertension. Women with active lupus nephritis at conception, especially in association with proteinuria, hypertension, and antiphospholipid antibodies, have an increased risk of fetal loss (≤50%), fetal growth restriction, preterm delivery, preeclampsia, and perinatal and maternal mortality.[110] Severe lupus nephritis with manifestations early in pregnancy may justify termination of pregnancy because this clinical context is not only associated with poor fetal outcome but also life-threatening for the mother. In contrast, women with absent antiphospholipid antibodies, normal or near-normal renal function, proteinuria lower than 500 mg/24 hr, controlled hypertension, and SLE in remission for at least 6 months before conception can expect better fetal and maternal outcomes.[110,111]

The risk of preeclampsia in pregnancies complicated by lupus nephritis is 15%.[111] Differentiating an exacerbation of lupus nephropathy from preeclampsia during the second half of pregnancy is often a diagnostic challenge. Hypocomplementemia (C3 and C4 fractions) and an increase in baseline anti-DNA antibodies favor the diagnosis of lupus flare,[112] although some degree of complement activation may also be present in preeclampsia.[113] Clinical features that may also be discriminatory are the presence of hematuria and red cell casts in the urine sediment in active lupus nephritis, as well as extrarenal manifestations affecting the skin and joints.

Treatment with corticosteroids usually improves the complement level and decreases proteinuria, but the very high doses needed to control the disease activity have been associated with a sharp increase in fetal loss rate. Antepartum fetal surveillance should be utilized. When the response to corticosteroids is suboptimal, it may be necessary to add hydroxychloroquine or even cytotoxic drugs, such as cyclophosphamide, azathioprine, or cyclosporine.[114] Cyclophosphamide should be avoided in the first trimester because of possible teratogenicity.[115] Additional treatment includes antihypertensive medication and, in the presence of antiphospholipid antibodies, prophylaxis with low-dose aspirin and heparin. In a series of 70 pregnancies with lupus, the presence of antiphospholipid antibodies increased the rate of adverse fetal outcome to 76%, compared with13% in antibody-negative pregnancies (OR 17.8).[111] Results of one randomized trial indicated that administration of low-dose aspirin plus heparin in patients with antiphospholipid antibodies improves the rate of live birth in comparison with treatment with low-dose aspirin alone.[116] Lupus nephritis may flare postpartum, especially when the histologic type is active diffuse proliferative glomerulonephritis,[117] but the consensus is not to use prophylactic steroids peripartum unless there are signs of disease activity.[111]

SUMMARY OF MANAGEMENT OPTIONS

Lupus Nephropathy (See also Chapter 43)

Management Options	Evidence Quality and Recommendation	References
Severe lupus nephritis (SCr > 1.4 mg/dL, proteinuria > 500 mg/24 hr, hypertension) with manifestations early in pregnancy may justify termination of pregnancy.	III/B	110,111
Advise increased risk of adverse pregnancy outcome, if active lupus at conception, SCr > 1.36 mg/dL, BP > 140/90 mm Hg, antiphospholipid antibodies.	III/B	110,111
Corticosteroids, hydroxychloroquine, azathioprine, cyclophosphamide (avoid in first trimester), cyclosporine to be used to treat lupus nephritis flare as necessary.	III/B	111,114
Antihypertensive medication as needed.	III/B	110,111
Prophylaxis with heparin and low-dose aspirin if antiphospholipid antibodies are present.	Ib/A	111,116
Advise increased risk of postpartum lupus flare, but no need for prophylactic increase in immunosuppression	III/B	111,117

BP, blood pressure; SCr, serum creatinine.

CHRONIC DIALYSIS AND PREGNANCY

Maternal and Fetal Risks and Management Options

Women with ESRD have reduced fertility, but improvements in renal replacement therapy have increased the likelihood of spontaneous conception, especially with hemodyalisis.[118,119] The available data do not permit comparative statistical interpretations on outcomes between peritoneal dialysis and hemodialysis; however, there does not appear to be any obvious superiority of one modality over the other, and there is no compelling argument for changing dialysis modality in pregnancy.[120] When starting dialysis during pregnancy, the usual criteria for choosing the dialysis modality can be used, with the recommendation of catheter placement higher in the abdomen if the peritoneal modality is elected. Chan and coworkers[121] reported less preeclampsia and higher infant birth weight in pregnancies managed with peritoneal dialysis compared with hemodialysis, but the rate of preterm delivery was higher.

The outcome of pregnancies occurring in women on dialysis has improved in recent years but the prognosis remains limited. The various maternal and fetal complications should temper any optimism and raise questions about the advisability of pregnancy in dialysis patients. Only 60% of pregnancies result in a live infant,[119] with a 85% rate of preterm delivery.[122]

The management of pregnancy for women with ESRD requires knowledge of the pregnancy-related physiologic changes and a willingness to balance maternal benefit and fetal well-being. Gestational reduction in serum sodium concentration necessitates a concomitant reduction in dialysate sodium concentration to around 135 mmol/L, and the gestational reduction in serum bicarbonate concentration should be matched with a low bicarbonate concentration in dialysate.[123] The requirement for calcium and vitamin D supplements is also likely to change as pregnancy progresses, and plasma levels of calcium and phosphate need to be monitored and adjusted accordingly.

Aggressive dialysis can lead to maternal hypovolemia/hypotension and result in fetal hypoxia. Slow rate ultrafiltration, increased frequency of hemodialysis to almost daily sessions, and limitation in the ultrafiltration volume per session limit the risk of hypotension, extracellular volume contraction, and compromised uteroplacental blood flow.[121] Pregnancy outcomes are improved when the sessions are prolonged to 4 hours, occur six times a week, the fluid removal is limited to 400 mL per session, and the predialysis serum creatinine level is maintained at 4.5 mg/dL.[122,124] In those women who had been on dialysis less than 6 years and in those who still produce more than 50 mL of urine daily, fluid balance is easier to manage, and the likelihood of a successful pregnancy increases.[125]

The exchange volumes also have to be decreased in peritoneal dialysis (from 2 L to 1.5 L), and the exchange frequency increased. Because more frequent exchanges increase the risk of peritonitis, it may be necessary to use a combination of daytime with nighttime continuous cycling peritoneal dialysis.

The disadvantages of almost daily hemodialysis may include hypercalcemia, alkalosis, and hypokalemia. If worsening alkalosis is noted, an individually formulated dialysate solution with less bicarbonate may be required, and for hypokalemia, a higher concentration of potassium in the dialysate or potassium supplements. Conversely, an increased dialysis frequency will allow for a more liberal diet and greater protein intake, improving the nutritional status. The protein supply is calculated based on pregravid weight and is recommended to be about 1.8 g/kg/day.[119] Water-soluble vitamins are dialyzed off, and it is important to ensure their supplementation. Vitamin C supplementation is necessary at 170 mg/day and folic acid at 2 mg/day, amounts that may not be present in prenatal vitamin formulations.

Electronic fetal monitoring for viable pregnancies immediately after the dialysis session is important because of the acute fluid shifts that may occur. Increased fetal heart rate after hemodialysis may be an indication of excessive fluid removal with fetal hypovolemia.[126] Uterine contractions frequently occur during and after dialysis but usually resolve and do not require any treatment. Significant changes in amniotic fluid volume have also been reported during hemodialysis.[127]

In ESRD, anemia occurs with almost 100% incidence[128] and the hematocrit will decrease even further when the patient with renal insufficiency conceives.[120] Serum iron, ferritin, and hemoglobin levels need to be monitored monthly, and when the hemoglobin level decreases below 8 g/dL (hematocrit < 25%), erythropoietin (EPO) treatment is indicated to maintain the hemoglobin above 10 g/dL and transferrin saturation above 30%. The dose of EPO needs to be 50% to 100% higher in pregnancy because of relative resistance to EPO. EPO is administered intravenously or subcutaneously and can also be administered at the time of hemodialysis. It does not cross the placenta and there are no reports of teratogenicity or polycythemia in the infant.[122] Rarely, maternal thrombogenic activity may be increased, causing clotting of the dialyzer. Other rare adverse effects may be hyperkalemia, hyperphosphatemia, seizures, and severe hypertension. EPO is contraindicated in women with uncontrolled hypertension. The development of hypertension is more likely when the hematocrit increases rapidly. A rise in hemoglobin of greater than 1 g/dL in 2 weeks requires EPO dose reduction. Adjustments in antihypertensive medication and reduction in EPO dose allowing the hematocrit to decrease slightly will correct the situation.[129] The treatment with EPO frequently has to be supported by 200 mg iron intravenously weekly. With intravenous iron, the rise in hemoglobin concentration is significantly faster than after orally administered iron.[130]

For women on dialysis, pregnancy should not be continued beyond 38 weeks' gestation, and even early delivery at 34 to 36 weeks' gestation with documentation of fetal lung maturity may be advisable.[125] Surveillance of fetal growth and umbilical artery Doppler recordings during pregnancy is common practice. The reported rate of cesarean delivery is about 50%. After cesarean delivery, peritoneal dialysis may be resumed with small 1-L exchange volumes 24 hours after surgery, gradually building back up to 2 L by day 3 after delivery.[131] If there is leakage, hemodialysis may be used instead for 2 weeks. Infants of women on dialysis are born with BUN and creatinine levels equal to the mother's and will experience osmotic diuresis after birth. Without careful monitoring and replacement, they may develop volume contraction and electrolyte abnormalities.[132] Fetuses exposed to hypercalcemia are at risk for hypocalcemia at birth and tetany. Fetal osmotic diuresis caused by high BUN levels is also responsible for the more than 50% rate of polyhydramnios in patients with ESRD.[133]

SUMMARY OF MANAGEMENT OPTIONS

Chronic Dialysis

Management Options	Evidence Quality and Recommendation	References
Advise on increased risk of adverse pregnancy outcome and limited prognosis, raising questions about the advisability of pregnancy.	III/B	119,122
When starting dialysis during pregnancy, the usual criteria for choosing the dialysis modality (peritoneal vs hemodialysis) can be used.	III/B	120
Dialysis regime to mimic physiologic renal changes of pregnancy (lower sodium and bicarbonate concentration in dialysate). Adjust potassium, calcium and phosphate binders according to serum chemistry.	III/B	119,120, 122,123
After first trimester, increase the dialysis regime to almost daily (20–24 hr/wk) to keep predialysis BUN < 50 mg/dL or SCr < 4.5 mg/dL, and limit fluid removal to 400 mL/session.	III/B	119,120, 122,124
Monitor serum iron, ferritin, and Hb monthly, and when Hb decreases below 8 g/dL (hematocrit < 25%), give EPO and iron (may need IV iron) to keep Hb > 10 g/dL. A rise in Hb > 1 g/dL in 2 wk requires EPO dose reduction.	III/B	120,122, 128,129
Fetal surveillance • Fetal monitoring after each dialysis session. • Serial recording of fetal growth and umbilical artery Doppler. • Vigilance for polyhydramnios	—/GPP	—

Management Options	Evidence Quality and Recommendation	References
Consider delivery at 34–36 wk gestation with documentation of fetal lung maturity; pregnancy should not be continued beyond 38 wk gestation.	III/B	125
Infants are born with BUN and creatinine levels equal to the mother's and will experience osmotic diuresis after birth. Careful monitoring and replacement is necessary to avoid volume contraction and electrolyte abnormalities. Fetuses exposed to hypercalcemia are at risk for hypocalcemia at birth and tetany.	III/B	132

BUN, blood urea nitrogen; EPO, erythtropoietin; GPP, good practice point; Hb, hemoglobin; SCr, serum creatinine.

RENAL TRANSPLANT PATIENTS AND PREGNANCY (See Also Chapter 53)

Maternal and Fetal Risks and Management Options

Current consensus opinion is that pregnancy can be relatively safely undertaken by 1 year after transplant if the woman has had no rejections, the immunosuppressive medication dosing is stable, allograft function is adequate (serum creatinine < 1.5 mg/dL and urinary protein excretion < 500 mg/day), and there are no infections that could affect the fetus.[134] About 1 in 20 women of childbearing age who have a functioning kidney transplant will become pregnant, and for those that go beyond the first trimester, fetal survival is 95%.[135]

Pregnancies in renal transplant patients are more likely to be complicated by preterm delivery (55%) and fetal growth restriction (20%).[135] As for all renal disease, obstetric and maternal outcome is worse in the presence of hypertension, recurrent UTIs, proteinuria greater than 500 mg/day, and renal impairment (serum creatinine > 1.5 mg/dL). According to data from the European Dialysis and Transplant Association Registry,[136] if serum creatinine is greater than 1.5 mg/dL, fetal survival is only 75%.

The rate of maternal complications in renal transplant recipients is up to 70%, including worsening of renal function, worsening hypertension, and infectious morbidity.[135] Although the deterioration in renal function cannot be categorically attributed to pregnancy,[137] graft loss can be expected in up to 11% of pregnancies within 2 years of delivery, according to the North American National Transplantation Pregnancy Registry.[138] Long-term maternal renal function correlates with serum creatinine level measured within 3 months before conception. The majority of controlled studies have shown that pregnancy has no influence on renal function if serum creatinine is less than 1.5 mg/dL,[137] but a serum creatinine level in excess of 2.3 mg/dL should be regarded as a contraindication to pregnancy because in the United Kingdom Transplant Pregnancy Registry experience,[139] all transplant recipients with such prepregnancy creatinine levels had progression of renal impairment and required renal replacement therapy within 2 years of delivery.

About one third of pregnancies in renal allograft recipients will develop worsening hypertension, often representing superimposed preeclampsia.[135] The differential diagnosis of preeclampsia from allograft dysfunction or postrenal obstruction may be very challenging because worsening proteinuria, increased uric acid level, and hypertension can occur with many causes of renal deterioration. Biopsy may be necessary to distinguish severe preeclampsia that may require delivery from acute rejection that can be treated with high-dose methylprednisolone as the first-line treatment.

The most frequent intercurrent infections in pregnant renal transplant patients are UTIs (40% risk).[136] Other infections that may be encountered include *Pneumocystis carinii* pneumonia, toxoplasmosis, cytomegalovirus, and herpesvirus infections.[68] Monthly urine cultures are recommended and even asymptomatic bacteriuria should be treated for 2 weeks followed by suppressive therapy.[140] Urethral instrumentation should be minimized during pregnancy and peripartum. Prophylactic antibiotics are indicated before any type of surgery and for vaginal delivery. Live vaccines are contraindicated in immunosuppressed patients, and if necessary, vaccination should ideally be given prior to transplantation.

During pregnancy, the allograft should be followed with monthly ultrasound examinations and a technetium renal scan each trimester, in addition to serum BUN, creatinine, and electrolytes every other week. The pelvic transplant kidney may have some baseline pyelectasis, not necessarily indicative of obstruction. But pelvicaliceal distention is concerning and, if detected preconceptionally, contraindicates pregnancy. Even a small rise in serum creatinine level or oliguria may indicate allograft rejection, the same as renal enlargement, tenderness, and fever. The rate of 2% to 11% allograft rejection episodes in pregnancy[138] would suggest a need for monitoring immunosuppressive levels. In practice, though, prednisone, azathioprine, or tacrolimus dosage alterations are only rarely necessary during pregnancy,[141] and in spite of conflicting opinions, most experts suggest that it is unnecessary to increase the dose of cyclosporine to prevent rejection in pregnancy.[142]

Antepartum exposure to immunosuppressive drugs is frequently associated with low birth weight. The rate of low birth weight may be higher in women requiring cyclosporine

(46%) than in women receiving prednisone and azathioprine (39%), although the two groups are not comparable as clinical condition.[138] Cyclosporine is otherwise well tolerated in pregnancy, and a meta-analysis of 15 studies suggested no increased risk of teratogenesis.[143] Several reports have raised the possibility of autoimmune disorders developing later in life in exposed children, underscoring concerns for still undefined long-term consequences.[144]

Prolonged administration of corticosteroids has been associated with preterm birth, and in utero first-trimester exposure may also increase the risk of facial midline fusion defects by approximately threefold. No definite pattern of teratogenesis has been detected with the use of azathioprine in a prospective, controlled, international study including 189 women who took azathioprine during pregnancy.[145] Although azathioprine crosses the placenta, the immature fetal liver lacks the enzyme inosinate pyrophosphorylase needed for conversion of azathioprine to its active metabolite 6-mercaptopurine, and consequently, the fetus is relatively protected from the effects of the drug. Significant problems attributable to the drug have been reported only rarely, as long as the used dose is low enough to maintain maternal white count greater than 7500/mm^3.[146] Dose reductions in azathioprine may also be necessary to correct maternal liver toxicity when occuring.[147] Cyclosporine has also been associated with maternal liver toxicity, diabetes, tremor, convulsions, and HUS.

A series of 100 pregnancies in which the mother was treated with tacrolimus revealed a side effect profile similar to that of cyclosporine.[148] The incidence of hypertension, including pregnancy-induced hypertension, was lower with tacrolimus- than with cyclosporine-receiving patients (27% vs. 67%), but the incidence of DM was higher (27% vs. 6%).[148]

Because cyclosporine and tacrolimus may be associated with serious adverse effects, particularly nephrotoxicity, new, highly effective immunosuppressive drugs have been introduced, such as mycophenolate mofetil. Mycophenolate mofetil has fewer nephrotoxic effects, but its administration in pregnancy is unadvisable because of documented teratogenicity in animals and humans (18%–26% rate of congenital anomalies based on registry data: www.fda.gov/medwatch/safety/2007/safety07.htm#CellCept2). The reported malformations after first-trimester exposure demonstrate clustering of similar defects and include microtia, micrognathia, cleft lip and palate, hypoplastic nails and shortened fingers, diaphragmatic hernia, and heart defects. If a kidney transplant patient taking mycophenolate mofetil plans a pregnancy, she should consider switching to cyclosporine for a period of time.[149]

The use of sirolimus in pregnancy may be contraindicated because only limited data are available and the animal studies have suggested teratogenicity.[150] There is also very limited experience in human pregnancy with monoclonal antibodies against lymphocytes (OKT3) or antithymocyte globulin (ATG) to recommend their use in pregnancy. Other chemotherapeutics with immunosuppressive activity such as cyclophosphamide, methotrexate, chlorambucil, and leflunomide are better avoided in pregnancy.

Although the available information is often controversial, the Consensus Conference Report published in 2005[144] did not view breast-feeding as absolutely contraindicated in immunosuppressed transplant recipients. Immunosuppressants are excreted in breast milk at drug concentrations similar to maternal blood concentrations, but the dose absorbed by the infant is very small,[79] and the additional exposure for a few weeks postpartum is unlikely to be harmful compared with the in utero exposure over the previous 9 months.

In the absence of complications, pregnancies after transplantation can be delivered at term, with cesarean delivery reserved for usual obstetric indications.[151] The renal allograft is placed extraperitoneally and is not expected to obstruct the birth canal during labor.[136] Cesarean delivery is eventually necessary in 50% of women with renal transplants because of the higher rate of obstetric complications.[137] At cesarean delivery, care should be taken to identify the graft; the ureter may be superior to the uterine artery and may enter the bladder over the lower uterine segment. Cesarean delivery is preferred in combined pancreas-kidney recipients, because the effect of vaginal delivery on a pancreas graft placed in the pelvis is still unknown.

SUMMARY OF MANAGEMENT OPTIONS
Renal Transplant (See also Chapter 53)

Management Options	Evidence Quality and Recommendation	References
Prepregnancy		
Advise that pregnancy can be undertaken 1 yr post-transplantation if the woman had no rejections, the immunosuppressive medication dosing is stable, allograft function is adequate (serum creatinine < 1.5 mg/dL and urinary protein excretion < 500 mg/day), and there are no infections that could affect the fetus.	III/B	134,137
Pelvicaliceal distension detected preconceptionally contraindicates pregnancy.	—/GPP	—
SCr > 2.3 mg/dL contraindicates pregnancy because of universal progression of renal impairment and requirement for renal replacement therapy within 2 yr of delivery.	III/B	139

Management Options	Evidence Quality and Recommendation	References
Prenatal		
Keep maintenance immunosuppression the same as before pregnancy, despite dilutional fall in cyclosporine level	III/B	141,142,148
The use of sirolimus, mycophenolate mofetil, OKT3, ATG, cyclophosphamide, methotrexate, chlorambucil, and leflunomide is better avoided in pregnancy.	III/B	149,150
Monitor BUN, SCr, electrolytes every other wk. Monitor allograft with monthly US and technetium renal scan each trimester.	—/GPP	—
Monthly urine cultures. Treat asymptomatic bacteriuria for 2 wk followed by suppressive therapy.	III/B	140
Screen for and differentiate preeclampsia, allograft dysfunction, or postrenal obstruction. Biopsy may be necessary to distinguish severe preeclampsia from acute rejection	III/B	135
Vigilance for preterm labor.	III/B	135
Fetal assessment		
• Detailed anomaly scan at ~20 wk.	III/B	149
• Serial monitoring of growth and umbilical artery Doppler.	III/B	135
Labor and Delivery		
Prophylactic antibiotics for any type of surgery and vaginal delivery.	—/GPP	—
In the absence of complications, deliver at term, with cesarean delivery reserved for usual obstetric indications.	III/B	151
Temporary stress dose corticosteroids to cover delivery.	—/GPP	—
Cesarean delivery is preferred in combined pancreas-kidney recipients.	—/GPP	—
Postnatal		
No good evidence that limited (≤4 wk) breast-feeding while taking immunosuppressants is harmful.	III/B	79,144

ATG, antithymocyte globulin; BUN, blood urea nitrogen; GPP, good practice point; SCr, serum creatinine; US, ultrasound.

SUGGESTED READINGS

George JN: The association of pregnancy with thrombotic thrombocytopenic purpura–hemolytic uremic syndrome. Curr Opin Hematol 2003;10:339–344.

Gilbert WM, Towner DR, Field NT, Anthony J: The safety and utility of pulmonary artery catheterization in severe preeclampsia and eclampsia. Am J Obstet Gynecol 2000;182:1397–1403.

Gilstrap LC III, Ramin SM: Urinary tract infections during pregnancy. Obstet Gynecol Clin North Am 2001;28:581–591.

Hou SH: Modifications of dialysis regimens for pregnancy. Int J Artif Organs 2002;25:823–826.

Jeyabalan A, Conrad KP: Renal function during normal pregnancy and preeclampsia. Front Biosci 2007;12:2425–2437.

Josephson MA, McKay DB: Considerations in the medical management of pregnancy in transplant recipients. Adv Chronic Kidney Dis 2007;14:156–167.

Moroni G, Quaglini S, Banfi G, et al: Pregnancy in lupus nephritis. Am J Kidney Dis 2002;40:713–720.

Ramin SM, Vidaeff AC, Yeomans ER, et al: Chronic renal disease in pregnancy. Obstet Gynecol 2006;108:1531–1539.

Vidaeff AC, Yeomans ER, Ramin SM: Pregnancy in women with renal disease. Part I: General principles. Am J Perinatol 2008;25:385–397.

Vidaeff AC, Yeomans ER, Ramin SM: Pregnancy in women with renal disease. Part II: Specific underlying renal conditions. Am J Perinatol 2008;25:399–405.

REFERENCES

For a complete list of references, log onto www.expertconsult.com.

CHAPTER 50

Spine and Joint Disorders

DARREN TRAVIS HERZOG and RALPH B. BLASIER

INTRODUCTION

During pregnancy, maternal anatomic changes present mechanical challenges to the musculoskeletal system. Hormonal changes occur that modify the connective tissues and their response to mechanical stress. Complaints of musculoskeletal discomfort during pregnancy are common[1,2] and may be temporarily disabling.[3] These problems usually do resolve spontaneously with completion of pregnancy, but occasionally, they may remain as chronic disorders. Some musculoskeletal conditions that exist prior to pregnancy may affect the course of the pregnancy.

LOW BACK AND PELVIC PAIN

General Considerations

In 2003, Wu and coworkers[3] published a meta-analysis of English-language papers concerning "pregnancy-related pelvic girdle pain (PPP)" and "pregnancy-related low back pain (PLBP)," considered together to be "lumbopelvic pain." They found 761 papers, of which 106 contained sufficient material for analysis. They concluded that about 45% of women have lumbopelvic pain during pregnancy and 25% of women have lumbopelvic pain after pregnancy. They also concluded that about 25% of women have severe lumbopelvic pain during pregnancy, with severe disability in 8%.

The many terms used in the literature such as "sacroiliac joint dysfunction," "pelvic girdle relaxation," "pelvic insufficiency," and even "sacroiliac joint pain" allude to an unjustified knowledge of pain mechanisms and describe a mixed group of patients. Albert and colleagues[4] proposed a more clear delineation between the subtle differences in the types of pregnancy-related pelvic joint pain. In their prospective epidemiologic cohort study of 1460 women, they found a total incidence of 20.1%. This total was subdivided into four groups based on objective findings and symptoms: pelvic girdle syndrome 6%, symphysiolysis 2.3%, one-sided sacroiliac syndrome 5.5%, and double-sided sacroiliac syndrome 6.3%.

Hormonal Considerations

Relaxin is a polypeptide hormone. In the human female, production sites for relaxin are the corpus luteum, the deciduas, and the chorion. The known target organs for relaxin are the uterine cervix, the myometrium, the endometrium, and the decidua. Unproven probable target organs are the pubic symphysis and the sacroiliac joints.[5] It has been taught that relaxin relaxes connective tissue, and a side effect of this instability may be pelvic pain.[6] Mens and associates in a 2009 meta-analysis[7] concluded that in the last months of pregnancy and in the first month after delivery, motion in the pelvic joints (sacroiliac and symphseal areas) is larger in women with pelvic girdle pain and/or low back pain than pelvic joint motion in pain-free controls. Other studies have called into question whether circulating relaxin levels do actually correlate with onset or severity of PPP or PLBP.[5] Björklund and coworkers[8] evaluated symphyseal distention, circulating relaxin levels, and pelvic pain in 68 patients. The patients' pain ranged from little–to–no pain to severe pain. They concluded that severe pelvic pain during pregnancy was strongly associated with an increased symphyseal distention, but relaxin levels were not associated with the degree of symphyseal distention or pelvic pain. The best conclusion is that the relationship between hormone levels and joint pain in pregnancy is unclear.

Mechanical Explanations for Back and Pelvic Pain in Pregnancy

Load on the spine is increased by general weight gain and the weight of the uterus, fetus, and breasts. Theories of increasing lumbar lordosis occurring in response to the more anterior center of mass and increased shear stress across the motion segments of the lumbar spine have long been entertained. The contribution of abdominal musculature to support of the spine may be diminished, and postural adjustments in response to increased loads are required.

Radicular symptoms are commonly noted in pregnancy.[9] This may be caused by direct pressure of the uterus on nerve roots and lumbar and sacral plexi. Bushnell[10] is credited with describing the "parietal neuralgia of pregnancy" as mechanical pressure on nerve roots by ligamentous structures of an increasingly lordotic spine. With descent of the fetus into the pelvis in late pregnancy, radicular symptoms attributed to pressure on the lumbosacral plexus may be experienced.

Ostgaard and colleagues[11] provided a biomechanical analysis, which demonstrates that the flexion moment caused by the more anterior center of increasing mass of the fetus and uterus can be accommodated by large increases in extensor muscle forces and consequential lumbar spine compression forces. Extension of the upper trunk, head, and neck can partially offset the increase in flexion moment by moving the new center of gravity closer to the spine. Ostgaard and colleagues[11] analyzed biomechanical factors and low back pain in 855 pregnant women and found that lumbar lordosis did not increase during gestation. However, a correlation has been identified between back pain and prepartum lumbar lordosis, suggesting that women with increased lumbar lordosis for any reason prior to pregnancy may be at higher risk for back pain while pregnant. However, in two separate prospective studies, no correlation was found between spinal configuration and complaints of back pain.[11,12]

If lordosis does not increase during pregnancy, then hip joint extension, rather than lumbar spine extension, may be a major mechanism used by pregnant women to cope with the increased flexion moment produced by pregnancy. If so, back pain in pregnancy ought to occur more often in women with intrinsic limitation of hip extension, and women with hip flexion contracture ought to have a greater tendency toward back pain with pregnancy. However, these hypotheses are unproved.

Peripheral joint laxity, followed throughout pregnancy in the prospective back pain study by Ostgaard and colleagues[11] of biomechanical factors, was measured by the presence of *striae distensae,* by serial measurement of ulnar deviation angle of the fourth finger to a defined force, and by the Bishop score (a 1–10 scale of cervix "ripeness"). Peripheral laxity was seen to significantly increase from weeks 12 through 20 in primiparous women. Laxity in multiparous women was the same at 12 weeks as that in primigravidas at 36 weeks and did not change during pregnancy. The correlation between increased peripheral laxity and increased abdominal sagittal diameter was strong. These data suggest that an increase in laxity after an initial pregnancy does not return to normal.[11] All persons lose stature (total height) with physical exertion. Control individuals and pregnant women without back pain regain stature after exertion faster than pregnant women with symptoms of back pain.[13]

A presumed common inheritable disorder called *benign joint hypermobility syndrome* has been recognized in the medical literature since 1967. At times linked to entities such as fibromyalgia, osteogenesis imperfecta, and Ehlers-Danlos and Marfan's syndromes, several investigations suggest that the underlying pathophysiology for this ill-defined condition may relate to altered collagen synthesis. Grahame and associates[14] have attempted to establish specific clinical diagnostic criteria for this constellation of joint-related symptoms. Their "revised Brighton criteria" for diagnosis include major and minor articular and extra-articular symptoms or physical examination findings. Relative to spine and joint symptoms in pregnancy, an underlying hypermobility syndrome may add risk to affected individuals.

Lumbar Disk Disease

The association of lumbar disk disease and pregnancy has been suggested by several authors. Relaxin may weaken the annulus of the intervertebral disks.[15] No prospective, controlled studies have related lumbar disk disease to pregnancy, yet the prevalence of symptomatic lumbar disk herniation may be on the rise owing to the increasing age of patients who are becoming pregnant.[16] Thus, the potential for disk herniation and lumbar nerve root compression, with radicular pain and definite neurologic loss, should be considered in the evaluation of the pregnant patient with back pain. Magnetic resonance imaging (MRI), as well as electromyographic studies, may be helpful in diagnosis and management. Initial treatment of the pregnant patient with a documented herniated disk may involve conservative approaches such as bedrest, heat therapy, and lumbrosacral bracing. Progressive paralysis or loss of bowel and bladder control secures the diagnosis of cauda equina syndrome, and this requires urgent imaging studies, usually with MRI, and urgent surgical decompression. Unless decompression of the affected nerve roots is accomplished fairly quickly, the loss of bowel and bladder control becomes permanent. Pregnancy at any stage is not a contraindication to undergoing an MRI, regional or general anesthesia, and surgical diskectomy, if necessary.[17–20]

Vascular Congestion and Night Backache

Back pain in pregnancy is common in the evening. It has been proposed that this pain is due to increased venous flow through lumbar veins, the vertebral venous plexus, paraspinal veins, and azygous veins that occurs at night in response to redistribution of an already large extracellular and venous fluid volume. This may be worsened owinge to mechanical vena caval compression by the gravid uterus in a supine patient. Edema and increased pressure occur, which causes pain.

Sacroiliac Pain and Osteitis Condensans Illii

Inflammatory changes in the sacroiliac joints have been suggested as a cause for sacroiliac pain. "Osteitis condensans illii," as described by Wells,[21] is a "fairly uniform area of increased density in the lower iliac bone, adjacent to the sacroiliac joint, unilateral or bilateral." This finding is most common in women, particularly those who have been pregnant. Of the 67 patients reported by Wells, all were females, 80% had been pregnant, and 30 patients had had low back pain. Shipp and Haggart in 1950[22] suggested that the motion and/or strain associated with pregnancy on the sacroiliac ligaments may explain that osteitis condensans illii is found most often in postpartum women. However, Wells[21] concluded, probably incorrectly, that there is little relationship between back pain and oteitis condensans illii and that the association with pregnancy is due to some unknown mechanism.

Risk Factors

Borg-Stein and coworkers in a 2005 review article[23] summarized risk factors for PLBP. Risk factors for back pain during pregnancy include increasing parity, older maternal age (except one study that said younger maternal age), and back pain during a previous pregnancy.[23] Risk factors for postpartum low back pain include early onset of severe pain during the pregnancy and inability to reduce maternal body weight to prepregnancy levels. Risk factors did not include maternal height, weight, weight gain, or weight of the baby.

Other investigators found that risk factors for pelvic girdle syndrome included history of previous low back pain, history of trauma to the back or pelvis, multiparity, higher maternal body weight, and self-reported on-the-job stress. Risk factors for symphysiolysis included multiparity, higher maternal body weight, and smoking. Risk factors for one-sided sacroiliac syndrome included maternal professional education or vocational training, self-reported stress, history of previous low back pain, history of trauma to the back or pelvis, and history of salpingitis. Risk factors for double-sided sacroiliac syndrome included history of previous low back pain, history of trauma to the back or pelvis, multiparity, poor relationship with the spouse, and low job satisfaction.[24]

General Low Back and Pelvic Pain—Management Options

Evaluation

History and physical examination can give some insight into pain mechanisms and direct the management of back and pelvic pain. Extraskeletal causes for backache must be considered. Obstetric complications and urologic disorders may present with symptoms ranging from vaginal discharge, flank pain, nausea, vomiting, and dysuria. Atypical presentations of refractory pain may indicate more significant and rare pathology such as disk herniation, infection, or tumor. Although complaints of back pain are common, vigilance must be maintained if serious diagnoses are not to be missed.

A history of pain at night, a radicular pain distribution, paresthesias, and bowel or bladder dysfunction may herald radiculopathy from nerve root irritation by lumbar disk disease. Differentiation from similar symptoms related to direct fetal pressure on nerve roots, such as paresthesias, in the distribution of the ilioinguinal and iliofemoral nerves and even of quadriceps weakness and giving-way episodes, is necessary.

A number of physical examination signs may help locate the anatomic site of the pain generator. Straight-leg raise testing (Lasègue's sign) is performed with the patient supine, noting the presence and distribution of pain and the angle of lower limb elevation at which pain occurs as the examiner raises the straight leg from the examining table by flexion at the hip only. In the normal patient, the angle between the leg and the examining table should reach 70 degrees or more without pain, and the maneuver should not cause any pain beyond hamstring discomfort with stretching. A positive test reproduces the patient's radicular pain and suggests nerve root compression.

Posterior superior iliac spine pressure in the standing patient may reproduce sacroiliac pain. Sacrospinous and sacrotuberous ligament tenderness by direct pressure during vaginal examination suggests a pelvic contribution to the patient's pain. Symphyseal pain is reproduced by direct pressure over the pubic symphysis.

The femoral compression test, or "posterior shea," or "thigh thrust" test, is performed with the patient supine and the hip in 90 degrees of flexion. Axial pressure is applied to the femur. The test is positive if pain is produced in the sacral area or ipsilateral buttock. If positive, the test suggests a sacroiliac source of pain on the positive side(s).

The iliac or ventral gapping test involves lateral opening pressure against the medial aspect of the anterosuperior iliac spine, that is, the pelvis of the supine patient is pressed apart. The iliac compression or dorsal gapping test involves compressive or closing pressure against the lateral iliac wings of the patient in a lateral decubitus or supine position. Pain provoked in either right or left sacral area and/or buttock area denotes a positive test. If positive, the test suggests a sacroiliac source of pain on the positive side(s).

The Patrick test is performed on the supine patient by flexing, abducting, externally rotating, then extending the hip, placing the ankle of the side being tested across the thigh of the opposite leg. This is also named the FABERE (flexion, abduction, external rotation, and extension) test. The examiner places one hand on the contralateral pelvis to stabilize it. The test is positive if pain is provoked in the sacroiliac area with the pelvis stabilized. If positive, the test suggests a sacroiliac source of pain on the ipsilateral side(s).

Pain provoked in the groin with rotation of the lower limb suggests the hip joint itself is a source of the pain, whereas posterior pelvic or symphyseal pain indicates sacral or symphyseal causes. Limitation of extension (flexion contracture) may be associated with increased lumbar lordosis, likely of long duration (before pregnancy), and predisposing to low back pain with pregnancy.

Radiographic evaluation, undesirable during pregnancy, may be warranted if pain cannot be explained by the common hormonal, mechanical, and vascular mechanisms, especially if neoplasm or infection is being considered. No harm to the fetus has been demonstrated with fetal exposure of less than 5 rads, a dose greater than that incurred in a routine spine radiography series. MRI may be helpful in diagnosis of tumor and infection or herniated vertebral disk.[20] It is generally agreed now that MRI does not have any deleterious effects on mother or fetus.[17] Mass lesions impinging on nerve roots, such as disk herniations, can be safely evaluated with electromyographic and nerve conduction studies, although these are not highly sensitive and depend strongly upon operator skill and technique.

Treatment

The majority of complaints regarding back and pelvic pain during pregnancy require only symptomatic care. Lumbar disk disease, urologic disorders, venous thrombosis, or other vascular or visceral causes for back pain must be considered in refractory or atypical cases.

The institution of either an individualized physiotherapy or a stretching and/or stabilizing exercise program may be a cost-effective and useful option to alleviate the intensity of pelvic pain in both the pre- and the postpartum periods.[24–26]

In a randomized, controlled trial of 81 postpartum women with pelvic girdle pain, Stuge and colleagues[24] sought to establish whether a program of specific stabilizing exercises would reduce pain, increase functional status, and improve quality of life. The women were assigned randomly to one of two groups for 20 weeks, one received physical therapy with the addition of specific stabilizing exercises and the other received a traditional physical therapy regimen. The study group received specific training, which included stretching and strengthening of the abdominal musculature, the lumbar multifidus, gluteus maximus, latissimus dorsi, erector spinae, quadratus lumborum, hip adductors, and hip abductors. The participants were required to exercise for 30 to 60 minutes a day, three times a week for 18 to 20 weeks. At 1-year follow up, the study group had significant improvements in pain, functional status, and health-related quality of life in comparison with the control group. This study alludes to the probable importance of the musculature surrounding and stabilizing the pelvic girdle, specifically the abdominal musculature, which has been shown in previous studies to play a pivotal role in the stability of the sacroiliac joints.[27,28]

A subsequent study looking at the role of three different regimens of physical therapy instituted during gestation showed no significant difference regarding pain and activity between the groups during pregnancy or at postpartum follow-up.[25] However, in all groups, there was a reduction in pain and an increase in activity ability between gestational week 38 and at 12 months postpartum. The results of this study are obscured by the fact that the home exercise group was not required to record the exercise sessions, which were performed and merely relied on patient compliance. The authors concluded that most pelvic pain will improve with time and recommended patient education and a sacroiliac belt.

Exercise may also play a role in altering the relationship between flexibility of the spine and low back pain during pregnancy. The reason for this may be that as weight gain during pregnancy increases, some instability of the sacroiliac joint must result.[29]

Waller and associates in a 2009 meta-analysis[30] concluded that there is evidence that therapeutic aqua exercise is beneficial to patients with PLBP, but the clinical trials available for inclusion into the meta-analysis were not of good quality. The utility of "water gymnastics" for reduction in PLBP was confirmed in another meta-analysis.[2]

Stuber and Smith,[31] in a 2008 meta-analysis of papers evaluating chiropractic care for PLBP, found that every paper reported positive results. However, they also found that none of the included papers had randomization and a control group and all seemed subject to bias.

Intradermal injection of sterile water has been found to provide analgesia for low back pain in pregnancy.[32–34] However, the pain relief lasts only approximately 2 hours, so this modality is reserved for pain during labor. Acupuncture has been found to decrease pregnancy-related pelvic and low back pain.[2]

SUMMARY OF MANAGEMENT OPTIONS
Back and Pelvic Pain—General

Management Options	Evidence Quality and Recommendation	References
Evaluation		
Consider extraskeletal causes for backache (obstetric complications and urologic disorders).	Ib/A	3
Atypical presentation or pain refractory to the usual care may indicate more significant, rare pathology (disk herniation, infection, tumor).	Ib/A	3
Differentiation from similar symptoms from direct fetal pressure on nerve roots (paresthesias in the distribution of the ilioinguinal and iliofemoral nerves and even of quadriceps weakness) is necessary.	IV/C	9,10
Radiographic evaluation, although undesirable during pregnancy, may be warranted if insidious causes for pain are suspected.	III/B IV/C	17–20
MRI may be particularly helpful in the diagnosis of tumor, infection, or disk herniation.	III/B IV/C	17–20
Mass lesions compressing nerve roots, such as disk herniations, can be initially evaluated with electromyographic and nerve conduction studies without radiation.	GPP	
Treatment		
Physiotherapy for strengthening and/or stretching, aqua therapy, acupuncture, chiropractic manipulation, and subdermal injection of sterile water have all been found to be beneficial in the symptomatic treatment of back and pelvic pain.	Ia/A II/B III/B IV/C	2,24–26, 29–34
For mild to moderate pain, general comfort measures including rest, activity modification, and physical therapy, including massage and pelvic and low back exercises, as well as general back care are helpful.	II/B IV/C	24,26,29
For night pain, the use of a "maternity cushion" may give relief.	Ia/A	2

Management Options	Evidence Quality and Recommendation	References
Elastic compression stockings worn throughout the day may, by limiting lower extremity edema, diminish the fluid shifts and venous engorgement that occur at night.	GPP	
Analgesic options are limited, and NSAIDs should be avoided for potential adverse fetal effects.	GPP	
Persistent pain, including diskogenic pain, not responsive to rest may benefit from lumbar epidural steroids.	GPP	
TENS may be helpful.	GPP	
Acute loss of bowel and bladder function or acute paralysis indicates a need for decompressive surgery during pregnancy.	III/B, IV/C	17–20
Treatment with a trochanteric belt or girdle provides relief, particularly for women with posterior pelvic pain.	Ia/A	2
Sacroiliac injection with corticosteroids and local anesthetic may be indicated in severe cases.	GPP	

GPP, good practice point; MRI, magnetic resonance imaging; NSAIDs, nonsteroidal anti-inflammatory drugs; TENS, transcutaneous electrical nerve stimulation.

SPONDYLOLYSIS AND SPONDYLOLISTHESIS

Spondylolysis is a bony insufficiency at the pars interarticularis of the spine. The condition can cause instability and pain. Spondylolisthesis is the slipping forward of one vertebra on another. This can result from a spondylolytic defect or from degenerative change in the facet joints.[15] Depending on the cause and the nature of the defect, the disorder is classified into five different types. Dysplastic and isthmic spondylolisthesis represent congenital and developmental disorders, which have a high familial incidence. These slips are more common in males than females (2:1), although females have a higher chance of progression. These slips most commonly occur at the L5–S1 level. The condition probably develops or presents in the first 2 decades of life, with the diagnosis most often being made in adolescence.

Risks

Degenerative spondylolisthesis usually occurs at the L4–5 level and presents later in life and more commonly in women than in men (4:1). Sanderson and Fraser[15] found, in a review of radiographs of 949 women, that those who had borne children had a significantly higher incidence of degenerative spondylolisthesis than those who had not. Proposed explanations for their findings include the generalized increase in laxity of pregnancy and residual relative joint relaxation and the effects of relaxin on the collagen of the facet joint capsules and of the annulus of the intervertebral disk. Women have generally greater joint laxity than men. Possibly, compromised abdominal musculature in parous women may allow perpetually increased sheer and rotatory stresses at the L4–5 joints.[15]

Management Options

The management of spondylolysis and spondylolisthesis during pregnancy differs little from that in the nonpregnant patient. Symptomatic relief can be obtained by rest and immobilization. The choice of analgesics is limited in pregnancy and should not include aspirin or nonsteroidal anti-inflammatory agents. In the event that significant neurologic impairment is detected, consultation should be obtained emergently.

SCOLIOSIS

Scoliosis is a three-dimensional deformity of the spine, most prominently manifested by curvature in the coronal plane. The disorder is usually idiopathic, commonly familial, and presents and progresses most dramatically during the adolescent growth spurt. Spinal curvature may also be due to congenital defects in the vertebral bodies, spinal cord disorders, intracranial pathology, or muscle spasm and back pain. Scoliosis is more common in females than in males.

Risks

The influence of pregnancy on preexisting scoliosis, particularly with regard to curve progression, has been controversial. An increase in curve progression during pregnancy has been demonstrated in scoliosis patients in small series. In particular, those treated with bracing who have multiple pregnancies before age 23, those with curves greater than 25 degrees, and patients who already had ongoing curve progression at the time of the pregnancy have been found to have increases in their curves during pregnancy.[35] Subsequent reviews have not found the same associations.[35,36]

Betz and coworkers[36] retrospectively reviewed 355 women with idiopathic scoliosis who had reached skeletal maturity. Two groups, 175 who had had at least one pregnancy and 180 who had never been pregnant, were compared. No effects on curve progression during pregnancy were demonstrated with regard to age of the patient at the time of pregnancy, ongoing progression of the curve at the time of pregnancy, or the number of pregnancies. Those having severe back pain during pregnancy (12%) may be slightly higher in unfused patients with scoliosis than in nonscoliotic patients. In patients who had undergone posterior spinal fusion, no progression of the unfused portion of the curve was demonstrated. In these patients, no problems during the pregnancy were attributed to the scoliosis.

In 159 deliveries of women who had scoliosis without a spinal fusion, spinal anesthesia could not be administered in 2 patients because of the scoliosis and cesarean section was necessary in 12 (7.4%) for reasons unrelated to the scoliosis.[36] In patients who had undergone posterior fusion, 2 patients had minor problems during delivery related to the fusion. In 1, spinal anesthesia could not be administered, and in the other, proper positioning was difficult. The incidence of complications or deformity in the newborn was not increased.

Postpartum back pain in scoliotic women or women with scoliosis who had not been pregnant was no greater than in the general population. As in other series, potential for progression of curves greater than 30 degrees during adulthood at a general rate of 1 degree per year was seen. However, increased progression, especially of the 6 to 8 degrees per pregnancy previously reported, was not found. They recommend that for women of childbearing age with curves greater than 30 degrees, radiographs should be done soon after each delivery to minimize the potential for fetal exposure.[36]

A more recent, long-term, case-control study looked at various outcomes after treatment for adolescent idiopathic scoliosis.[37] In a period between 1968 and 1977, 136 women who were surgically treated with distraction and/or fusion using Harrington rods and 111 who were treated by bracing were followed for 22 years. These women were compared with age-matched controls and displayed no significant difference in regard to the number of children born, rates of low back pain, or necessity to undergo cesarean section during first pregnancy. There was no correlation between progression of spinal curvature and number of pregnancies or between this progression and age at first pregnancy. They did find that the rate of vacuum extractions was greater in the surgically treated group (16%) than in the control group (5%) and the brace-treated group (8%). In addition, there was a significant difference in sexual function between the surgically treated group and the control group, with the surgically treated group reporting more limitation of sexual function owing to back-related issues, 33% versus 15%, respectively. There was no significant difference in sexual function between the surgically treated group and the brace-treated group. The patients reported that pain was not a predominant factor in limiting their sexual activity but was more related to physical difficulty and self-consciousness about appearance.

Management Options

Prepregnancy and Prenatal

The affected patient should be counseled that no significant increase in the rate or incidence of curve progression during pregnancy has been demonstrated in large series of pregnant scoliosis patients compared with nonpregnant ones.[35,36] In patients who had undergone posterior spinal fusion, no progression of the unfused portion of the curve is seen in the majority.

Labor and Delivery

In patients who have undergone posterior fusion, 1.5% have minor problems during delivery related to the fusion.[36] In one report, spinal anesthesia could not be administered, and in another, proper positioning for delivery was difficult.[36] More recent reports have presented successful ultrasound-guided spinal anesthesia after spinal fusion.[38] Overall, fewer than 3% of deliveries in women who had undergone posterior spinal fusion for scoliosis had problems requiring cesarean section. The indications for operative delivery were unrelated to the fusion or the scoliosis. The incidence of complications or deformity in the newborn was not increased in patients who had undergone posterior fusion for scoliosis.

The risk of cardiorespiratory complications during pregnancy should be considered in patients with severe kyphoscoliotic deformity. Involvement of the respiratory team, with possible use of nasal intermittent positive-pressure ventilation, may be of benefit for a successful outcome for both mother and child.

Postpartum

Scoliotic women show no increase in postpartum back pain compared with women with scoliosis who had not been pregnant. Therefore, no specific postpartum recommendations are offered. In general, for women with curves greater than 30 degrees, radiographs should be done every 2 years up to age 25 and every 5 years thereafter. Appropriate radiographic and clinical evaluation by a surgeon who manages scoliosis should be considered in the months following delivery, taking the opportunity to have a radiograph when pregnancy is unlikely.

PELVIC ARTHROPATHY AND RUPTURE OF THE PUBIC SYMPHYSIS

Pelvic arthropathy usually occurs in two recognizable syndromes, though there may be overlap between them:

- Abnormal mobility of the pelvic joints may lead to pain and a waddling gait.
- After a difficult delivery, there may be a rupture of the symphysis.

Pelvic Arthropathy

The weight and position of the developing fetus increases the stress on the lumbosacral junction and the sacroiliac joints. In patients with a more sagittal than oblique orientation of these joints, there is less inherent stability and there may be a predisposition to pelvic laxity. The ligaments of the pubic symphysis and the sacroiliac joints relax during the first half of pregnancy. Excessive relaxation of the ligaments of the pelvis may cause symptoms at about the sixth or seventh month, consisting of pain with walking, turning in bed, or other exertion. There may be a unilateral limp or even a bilateral waddling gait. The pain may rarely be so severe that standing or walking is precluded. Asymmetrical sacroiliac laxity (right different from left) is much more strongly associated with pelvic pain than is the absolute amount of laxity.[28,39,40]

In some cases, symptoms appear only during labor, due to excessive loosening of the symphysis and sacroiliac joints.

Separation of the pubic symphysis during pregnancy is common, varying between 0 and 35 mm (average 7–8 mm). Separation over 8 to 9 mm is considered pathologic. Rupture of the ligaments of the pubic symphysis may occur spontaneously during labor or as a result of forceps delivery. Patients often complain of prelabor pain in the pubis and sacroiliac joints. During and after labor, the patient may complain of pain over the symphysis and sacroiliac joints, radiating down the thighs and often exacerbated by leg movement.

Commonly, there is tenderness over the greater trochanters, and severe pain can be elicited in the pubic symphysis when the greater trochanters are compressed toward the midline. The lower limbs may be externally rotated, and the patient may be unable to walk normally for weeks or months. The diagnosis is made with a history of pregnancy, pain at the pubic symphysis or the sacroiliac joints, tenderness at the pubic symphysis or the sacroiliac joints, and excessive laxity of the ligaments. A gap may be felt at the symphysis externally or by vaginal examination. Relaxation of the symphysis can be ascertained by placing the examiner's fingers on the superior edges of the pubic bones and noting vertical translation during walking. A prevaginal examination of the symphysis can be made while an assistant pulls down on one of the patient's ankles while pushing up on the other.

Ultrasonography has been used to confirm the diagnosis, with symptomatic patients having a symphyseal gap of 20 mm (range 10–35 mm) and asymptomatic controls 4.8 mm (range 4.3–5.1 mm).[41,42] MRI has been used to diagnose postpartum pubic and pelvic pain, but its clinical benefit has not been established.[43,44]

Management Options

Treatment is generally by rest, with or without a pelvic band or girdle. Some investigators report treatment with early injection of steroid or local anesthetic or use of oral anti-inflammatories.[39–41] A limited number of reports mention pelvic arthropathy with onset 1 to 2 days after delivery, characterized by pain and tenderness at the symphysis, but without swelling or bruising and without widening or abnormal mobility of the symphysis.[40] Symptoms abate within a week or 2 with rest and analgesics. It has been speculated that this is caused by swelling and pressure within the fibrous confines of a relatively normal pubic symphysis.

Rupture of the Pubic Symphysis

Separation of the pubic symphysis in association with labor and delivery is rare and is sometimes unrecognized when it does occur. Some widening of the pubic symphysis has been noted as being necessary for normal delivery and some widening normally does occur. Rarely, the separation is greater than 10 mm, and this is usually asymptomatic. The pubic symphysis consists of a thick fibrocartilagenous disk between two thin layers of hyaline cartilage covering the articular surfaces of the bone. It is held together by four ligaments: the anterior pubic (strong), the superior and inferior arcuate, and the posterior pubic (weak).

Occasionally, actual rupture of the pubic symphysis may occur. The onset of pain may be abrupt and may even be accompanied by an audible "crack."[45] Associated factors may include hard labor, precipitous labor, difficult forceps delivery, cephalopelvic disproportion, abnormal presentation, multiparity, forceful abduction of the thighs, or previous pelvic trauma.[46–49] Estimates of incidence range between 1 in 500 and 1 in 30,000.[50,51] The incidence appears to be decreasing over time, because many difficult vaginal deliveries are being replaced by cesarean section.[50] Separations of as much as 120 mm have been reported, and the sacroiliac joints become affected with more than 40 mm of separation.[50]

Management Options

Treatment may begin with tight pelvic binding and/or rest in the lateral decubitus position. Symptoms may last as little as 2 days, typically 8 weeks, or up to 8 months.[50] For inadequate reduction, recurrent diastasis, or persistent symptoms, external skeletal fixation, and open reduction and internal fixation are the treatment options available to maintain stability while the ligaments heal.[45] Pin tract infections in association with external fixation pins are common and are usually readily manageable. Internal fixation by plate and screws or cerclage wire has been reported with good results.[45] In addition, concurrent open reduction and internal fixation at the time of cesarean delivery has been described.[52] Advantages of this option include a definitive treatment that would ensure stability, facilitating pain relief and earlier mobilization. This approach may help avoid rare but potential complications associated with conservative management. Using a pelvic binder or sling may require several weeks of bedrest, thus placing the patient at increased risk of decubitus ulcers, pulmonary and urogenital infections, venous thromboembolism, muscle atrophy, and joint stiffness. There is some concern that if the symphysis has been fixed by a plate and screws, the plate and screws should be removed before the next pregnancy. However, there is a report of two normal vaginal deliveries with symphyseal plate and screws remaining in situ.[53]

Complications of separation of the pubic symphysis include nonunion (failure to heal with reduction), pubic degenerative joint disease, osteitis pubis, and hemorrhage. The separation may occur in association with a connecting vaginal laceration, and there have been reports of these being complicated by suppurative arthritis, abscess of the vulva, and abscess of the space of Retzius.[50] Some investigators report irrigation and immediate closure of such a connecting vaginal laceration, under the belief that lack of a cortical fracture, unexposed bone ends, and coverage of the bone by articular cartilage may decrease the chance of a resulting wound infection.[54]

A previous symphyseal rupture has been found to increase the risk of a recurrence, especially with subsequent vaginal delivery.[49,55] Thus, it may be reasonable to offer cesarean delivery to patients who sustained a severe symphyseal disruption during a prior vaginal delivery.

POSTPARTUM OSTEITIS PUBIS

Osteitis pubis is a self-limited, apparently noninfective, osteonecrosis that begins at the pubic symphysis and extends into the pubic bones. It is rarely associated with pregnancy, either antepartum or postpartum. It is similar to pelvic arthropathy in its presentation, with accompanying pubic tenderness and pain that may prevent ambulation. It is differentiated from pelvic arthropathy and symphyseal disruption by radiographic rarefaction of the pubic bones, without symphyseal widening. It is differentiated from septic symphysitis by its lack of fever, leukocytosis, and radiographic bony sequestrum. Steroids and nonsteroidal anti-inflammatories have been recommended for treatment.[56] Treatment of symptomatic osteitis pubis with intravenous pamidronate has been reported.[57]

SEPTIC PUBIC SYMPHYSITIS AND SACROILITIS

Osteomyelitis in or adjacent to the pubic symphysis has rarely been reported in association with pregnancy. Fever is not universal, though leukocyte count, erythrocyte sedimentation rate, and C-reactive protein levels are usually elevated. Surgical drainage and antibiotics should be curative.[58,59]

STRESS FRACTURES OF THE PUBIC BONE

Stress fracture of the body of the pubic bone has rarely been reported during pregnancy, unrelated to athletics or physical training. In the few cases reported, no underlying pathologic process has been found. The cause is thought to be due to ligament laxity, muscle imbalance, and increased load. Pain is usually insidious in onset. There is tenderness at the fracture. Radiography is diagnostic but not usually until some healing has occurred. MRI has been suggested to diagnose pelvic stress fractures immediately.[60,61] Management is usually directed toward symptomatic relief.

PELVIC TRAUMA AND PREGNANCY

In a study of 34 women who had had a displaced pelvic ring fracture, all of whom had at least one full-term pregnancy after healing, only 2 required elective cesarean section, and the need for the cesarean section was determined at the first presentation by pelvimetry.[62] Of these 34 women, 17 had healed with displacement of the fracture involving the birth canal. Of 8 who had had previous traumatic pubic symphyseal disruption, 2 had recurrence of pain during pregnancy. Recently, orthopedic surgical exposure and fixation techniques have improved to the point at which restoration of the preinjury pelvic size and shape is closely approached, but sometimes that goal is not met. In cases in which the pelvic inlet, the mid pelvis, and/or the outlet measurements are less than 9.5 cm, consideration should be given to cesarean delivery.

TRANSIENT OSTEOPOROSIS OF THE HIP

Transient osteoporosis of the hip is a rare condition. It has been defined by multiple case reports over the last half century.[63] It is characterized by a gradually developing pain in the hip with weight-bearing.[64] Symptoms begin in the third (or late second) trimester. The pain is predominantly in the anterior thigh and groin. The patient often presents with an antalgic gait and functional disability on the affected side. For unknown reasons, the left hip is affected more often than the right, though both may be affected.[63] The pain is relieved by rest. There is no associated history of trauma or illness. Musculoskeletal examination is normal, except for discomfort at the extremes of hip motion and a slight decrease in total range of hip motion.[64] Joints other than the hip may become involved, and the process may regress at one joint and progress at another. Other areas affected may include knee, ankle, foot, ribs, shoulders, and spine.

Radiographic osteopenia can occur, beginning 2 to 4 weeks after onset of symptoms. Radiographically, the joint space is preserved.[63,64] The indistinctness of the subchondral cortical bone on radiographs may be striking. MRI of the involved joint reveals a joint effusion and diffuse signal abnormalities in the marrow, suggestive of marrow edema (decreased signal on T1-weighted images and increased signal on T2-weighted images). This is in contrast to the findings of avascular necrosis, which on MRI, may typically show a focal lesion often in the anterosuperior region of the femoral head and decreased signal intensity on both T1- and T2-weighted images. The differential diagnosis includes joint infection, rheumatoid arthritis, pigmented villinodular synovitis, and osteonecrosis. Radionucleide bone scanning shows an increased uptake in the affected femoral head and often the acetabulum. One report of a case followed by serial dual-energy x-ray absorptiometry (DEXA) over a period of 4 years showed a loss of 20% of bone mineral density (compared with age-matched controls) that resolved rapidly in the first year and returned to the normal range after cessation of lactation.[63]

The cause of transient osteoporosis of the hip is unknown. Some hypothesize that the cause may be neurovascular and perhaps related to reflex sympathetic dystrophy.[64] However, lack of trauma; lack of the characteristic burning, pulsing pain; lack of changes in skin color, temperature, and moisture; and failure to respond to sympathetic blockade all militate against this explanation.[65,66] Some authors have speculated about other causes, including abnormalities in local blood flow, viral infection, rheumatic and other inflammatory conditions, and metabolic abnormalities, but none of these explanations has been convincingly upheld.[67] Other investigators have speculated that mechanical compression of the obturator nerve in pregnancy may be a causative factor, but animal experimentation has failed to produce hip osteoporosis by this mechanism.[68] It appears that by an unknown stimulus, intense bone resorption is initiated in the femoral head.[63,69] Later, during resolution, osteoid is laid down and mineralized. Between resorption and remineralization, the bone is weak and susceptible to microtrauma, thus explaining the pain with weight-bearing. If the microtrauma accumulates faster than it can be repaired, a pathologic fracture may ensue. For this reason, weight-bearing should be limited until resolution of osteopenia.

Management Options

The condition is self-limiting, usually resolving spontaneously in 6 to 8 months. Treatment is conservative, including protection from weight-bearing, maintenance of joint motion, and analgesic medications.[65] Bone and synovial biopsies are not necessary. In cases in which joint aspiration has been performed, the effusion is sterile and the joint fluid is normal. Some cases report associated pathologic fracture of the pubic rami or the femoral neck. In a series by Guerra and Steinberg,[66] the authors report two patients with transient osteoporosis in their third trimester of pregnancy.

They both sustained a subcapital femoral neck fracture after a fall, which was treated with simultaneous pinning and birth by cesarean section. One of these patients went on to have two successful pregnancies with no recurrence of the transient osteoporosis. The authors advised restricted weight-bearing until confirmatory radiographs show the reestablishment of bone mass.

Various treatments have been used, including limitation of weight-bearing by wheelchairs, crutches, or canes. Corticosteroids, phenylbutazone, and calcitonin have been tried without beneficial effect.[65] After delivery, symptoms completely resolve over 3 to 9 months.

AVASCULAR NECROSIS OF THE HIP

Avascular necrosis is not an uncommon disorder. Incidence in the United States has been estimated to be approximately 15,000 new cases annually. However, avascular necrosis during pregnancy has only rarely been reported, and thus, it is difficult to demonstrate a causal relationship between the two.[66,69] Traditionally, the risk factors most commonly associated with nontraumatic avascular necrosis of the hip have included systemic administration of steroids, excessive alcohol consumption, collagen vascular diseases, renal transplantation, and pregnancy, among others. Despite this diverse spectrum of conditions, the most widely accepted precipitating event is a mechanical interruption of the circulation to the femoral head.

It is not entirely clear that there is any difference between pregnancy-related transient osteoporosis of the hip and pregnancy-related avascular necrosis of the hip. Some authors have defined aseptic necrosis of the femoral head during pregnancy as an entity separate from transient osteoporosis of the hip in pregnancy,[66] but the clinical presentation is very similar to transient osteoporosis. Symptoms begin in the third trimester; the hip is painful with weight-bearing; the pain is relieved by rest; there is no associated history of trauma or illness; and the musculoskeletal examination is normal, except for discomfort at the extremes of hip motion and a slight decrease in total range of hip motion. Radiographs show osteoporotic changes, and radionucleide bone scanning shows an increased uptake in the affected femoral head.[66] Unlike nonpregnancy-related aseptic necrosis of the hip, which often mandates operative treatment and often leads to predictable degenerative joint disease, it has been observed that aseptic necrosis of the hip in pregnancy gives good results with conservative treatment, consisting of reduction in weight-bearing. However, the optimum treatment of avascular necrosis in the pregnant patient remains controversial. Accepted surgical treatment options include osteotomy, use of a nonvascularized structural graft, electrical stimulation, core decompression, and use of a vascularized structural graft.[69]

One radiographic finding that may differentiate aseptic necrosis of the femoral head during pregnancy from transient osteoporosis of the hip has been a "crescent sign," with subchondral lucency or subchondral collapse of the weight-bearing dome of the femoral head. Actual bone necrosis, dead osteocytes, or empty osteocyte lacunae have not been well documented. The crescent sign of the femoral head radiographically resembles other proven cases of aseptic necrosis that occur without pregnancy, and this has been the basis for calling the osteoporotic hip with a crescent sign in pregnancy, "aseptic necrosis during pregnancy." However, the crescent sign might as well be a pathologic fracture in osteoporotic bone, making the distinction between these two entities questionable.

With MRI, avascular necrosis typically shows focal lesions in the anterolateral femoral head with decreased signal intensity on both T1- and T2-weighted images. There may frequently be a double-density signal surrounding the lesion. In a series by Montella and colleagues,[69] the authors followed 13 women who developed hip pain during pregnancy and were later diagnosed with avascular necrosis. Eleven of these women were treated with a free vascularized fibular graft. They differentiated necrosis from transient osteoporosis based on the presentation, radiographic characteristics, and natural history. Specifically, the diagnosis was made based on MRI findings of the double-density signal as well as radiographic features, including the crescent sign, progression, and collapse of the femoral head. All 13 of their patients had severe, debilitating symptoms that worsened over 12 months. They also found that there were significant demographic differences in women who have osteonecrosis associated with pregnancy compared with nonpregnant women of childbearing age who have an idiopathic avascular necrosis. The pregnancy-associated form was more likely to be found in older primigravid women with a smaller body frame who gain a relatively larger amount of weight during their pregnancy.

The diagnosis of avascular necrosis is frequently delayed, and thus, the practitioner should have a high clinical suspicion. The use of MRI may be efficacious in earlier diagnosis and a better prognosis. The incidence of this disease in pregnancy may be increasing as more women delay childbearing.

HIP ARTHROPLASTY

Historically, hip joint replacement has not been an option in women of childbearing age, because this operation was typically reserved for patients with limited physical activities and a relatively short expected life span. However, there are a few rare indications for hip joint replacement in the young, such as avascular necrosis of the hip, severe rheumatoid disease, post-traumatic arthritis, or certain aggressive tumorous conditions. With the advent of more durable bearing materials with superior wear characteristics, as well as hip resurfacing designs, younger patients are being more readily considered for hip joint replacement. There have been reports of completely normal impregnation, labor, and delivery in girls who had had a prior total hip replacement.[70] Sierra and associates conducted a survey of 343 women, all of child bearing age with a total of 420 total hip arthroplasties.[70] Of these women, 13.7% had a successful pregnancy after their procedure. The authors concluded that childbirth is not affected by the presence of hip arthroplasty implants, nor is a pregnancy after hip arthroplasty associated with decreased survival of the prosthesis. Previous smaller studies corroborate these findings in the use of both total hip prostheses and bipolar designs.[71,72]

Women who have had a previous total hip replacement may have increased pain during their pregnancy in the respective hip with an increased risk of continued pain postpartum. Persistence of pain in the groin and joint should be investigated to determine whether it is related to implant loosening, wear, or osteolysis, which may necessitate revision. Although the need for revision may increase in these situations, it is not likely attributed to the evolution and completion of pregnancy, but more likely directly related to the age at which the primary arthroplasty was done.

A prosthetic hip does not have as much inherent joint stability as a biologic hip. Dislocation during positioning is a theoretical concern. However, hip flexion as long as it is accompanied by abduction ought to be relatively safe. The dangerous positions are hip flexion with internal rotation and/or adduction and, to a lesser extent, hip extension with external rotation and/or adduction. Neither of these positions would be likely to occur during delivery, with or without stirrups, or squatting with a birthing chair.

Other preexisting hip conditions, such as severe slipped capital femoral epiphysis, especially bilateral or hip fusion, may make positioning for delivery challenging. They do not otherwise preclude vaginal delivery.

SUMMARY OF MANAGEMENT OPTIONS

Back and Pelvic Pain—Specific Conditions

Management Options	Evidence Quality and Recommendation	References
Scoliosis		
Prepregnancy and Prenatal		
Curvature does not usually worsen.	III/B	35,36
Compromise of respiratory function may occur in some (see Chapter 37).		
Labor and Delivery		
Regional analgesia may not be possible.	IV/C	36
Positioning for delivery may have to be individualized.	IV/C	36
For respiratory compromise, see Chapter 37.		
Pelvic Arthropathy		
Rest, with or without a pelvic band or girdle.	GPP	
Analgesia and anti-inflammatory drugs.	III/B	48
If this fails, consider injection of steroids and local anesthetic.	III/B	48
Rupture of the Pubic Symphysis		
Treatment is generally nonsurgical, and complete recovery is to be expected.	GPP	
Steroids and anti-inflammatory drugs.	IV/C	56
Treatment may begin with tight pelvic binding and rest in the lateral decubitus position.	IV/C	50
Symptoms may last as little as 2 days, typically 8 wk, or reportedly up to 8 mo.	IV/C	50
For inadequate reduction, recurrent diastasis, or persistent symptoms, external skeletal fixation is the treatment of choice to maintain stability while the ligaments heal.	IV/C	45,52
Internal fixation by plate and screws or metallic cerclage wire is considered in extreme cases.	IV/C	52,53
Pelvic Problems		
Postpartum Osteitis Pubis		
Needs to be differentiated	GPP	
• From pelvic arthropathy and symphyseal disruption by w-ray.		
• From septic symphysitis by lack of fever, leukocytosis, and radiographic bony sequestrum.		

Management Options	Evidence Quality and Recommendation	References
Steroids and NSAIDs recommended for treatment.	IV/C	56
Treatment with intravenous pamidronate has been reported.	III/B	57
Septic Pubic Symphysitis and Sacroilitis		
A rare condition in pregnancy; surgical drainage and antibiotics should be curative.	III/B	58,59
Stress Fractures of the Pubic Bone		
Radiography is diagnostic, but often after some healing; MRI may give earlier diagnosis. Management is symptomatic relief.	III/B	60,61
Pelvic Trauma and Pregnancy		
Manage as for nonpregnancy. Critical issue is the degree to which pelvic anatomy is distorted and cesarean delivery indicated.	III/B	62
Maternal Pelvic Osteotomy		
If this has been performed before skeletal maturity, there is greater risk of smaller pelvis and greater need for cesarean delivery.	III/B	73
Acetabular rotational osteotomy after skeletal maturation appears to have no effect on pelvic dimensions and need for cesarean delivery.	III/B	74
Hip Problems		
Transient Osteoporosis—Conservative Approach		
Limit weight-bearing.	IV/C	65,66
Encourage movement.	IV/C	65
Analgesia.	IV/C	65
Avascular Necrosis		
Manage as for transient osteoporosis.	GPP	
Hip Arthroplasty		
Usually no significant problem encountered nor special management required.	IV/C	70
Normal birthing position can be used.	GPP	
Avoid flexion to more than 90 degrees and internal rotation or adduction of the hips, which can provoke dislocation.	GPP	

GPP, good practice point; MRI, magnetic resonance imaging; NSAIDs, nonsteroidal anti-inflammatory drugs.

MATERNAL PELVIC OSTEOTOMY

Historically, pelvic osteotomy was reserved for young patients, predominantly female, for the treatment of developmental dysplasia of the hip. When the osteotomies were done at a young age, the pelvis would remodel during growth to a normal size and shape. When the osteotomies were done at an older age, the pelvis might not remodel to a normal size and shape. Loder[73] compiled a series of 40 pelvic osteotomies in 37 patients done for developmental dysplasia of the hips. He was able to follow 30 patients to skeletal maturity. At skeletal maturity, the mid-pelvis and/or outlet measurements were less than 9.5 cm in 6 of the 30 cases, and these tended to be those in whom the osteotomy had been done at an older age.

Recently, the use of pelvic osteotomies has been expanded to patients after skeletal maturity, typically in the childbearing years. Such osteotomies are for the purpose of delaying or avoiding the need for a hip replacement later in life. These osteotomies are typically rotational osteotomies at the acetabulum for the purpose of correcting slight residual hip dysplasia or redirecting a slightly arthritic joint. Masui and colleagues[74] studied 21 patients who had had successful pregnancy and childbirth after rotational acetabular osteotomy. They concuded that rotational acetabular osteotomy caused no substantial difference in the bony birth canal before or after surgery. Fortunately, in case of osteotomy, the treating orthopedic surgeon would most likely have large numbers of the patient's radiographs, so new radiation exposure for pelvimetry might not be needed.

SUGGESTED READINGS

Betz RR, Bunnell WP, Lombrecht-Mulier E, et al: Scoliosis and pregnancy. J Bone Joint Surg Am 1987;69:90–96.

Borg-Stein J, Dugan SA, Gruber J: Musculoskeletal aspects of pregnancy: Am J Phys Med Rehabil 2005;84:180–192.

Danielsson AJ, Nachemson AL: Childbearing, curve progression, and sexual function in women 22 years after treatment for adolescent idiopathic scoliosis: A case-control study. Spine 2001;26:1449–1456.

Goldsmith LT, Weiss G, Steinetz BG: Relaxin and its role in pregnancy. Endocrinol Metab Clin North Am 1995;24:171–186.

Grahame R, Bird HA, Child A: The revised (Brighton 1998) criteria for the diagnosis of benign joint hypermobility syndrome (BJHS). J Rhematol 2000;27:1777–1779.

Mens JM, Pool-Goudzwaard A, Stam HJ: Mobility of the pelvic joints in pregnancy-related lumbopelvic pain: A systematic review. Obstet Gynecol Surv 2009;64:200–208.

Sierra RJ, Trousdale RT, Cabanela ME: Pregnancy and childbirth after otal hip arthroplasty. J Bone Joint Surg Br 2005;87:21–24.

Smith MW, Marcus PS, Wurtz LD: Orthopedic issues in pregnancy. Obstet Gynecol Surv 2008;63:103–111.

Wu WH, Meijer OG, Uegaki K, et al: Pregnancy-related pelvic girdle pain (PPP), I: Terminology, clinical presentation, and prevalence. Eur Spine J 2004;13:575–589.

Wurdinger S, Humbsch K, Reichenbach JR, et al: MRI of the pelvic ring joints postpartum: Normal and pathologic findings. J Magn Reson Imaging 2002;15:324–329.

REFERENCES

For a complete list of references, log onto www.expertconsult.com.

CHAPTER 51

Skin Disease

GEORGE KROUMPOUZOS

INTRODUCTION

Skin problems in pregnancy can be categorized as follows[1]:

- Physiologic skin changes of pregnancy.
- Preexisting skin diseases and tumors affected by pregnancy.
- Pruritus in pregnancy.
- Specific dermatoses of pregnancy.

Prompt recognition and correct classification of the skin problem are essential for treatment, when necessary. The pregnant woman should be counseled about the nature of her skin condition, possible maternal or fetal risks associated with it, and management options.

PHYSIOLOGIC SKIN CHANGES OF PREGNANCY

The skin undergoes changes during pregnancy that are caused by the profound endocrine and metabolic alterations during the gestational period. The physiologic skin changes of pregnancy include pigmentary changes such as hyperpigmentation and melasma, vascular changes such as spider angiomas (Fig. 51–1), palmar erythema, nonpitting edema, and varicosities, stretch marks (*striae gravidarum*) (Fig. 51–2), as well as mucosal, hair (Fig. 51–3), nail, and glandular changes.[1–3] These changes are not associated with any risks for the mother or fetus and are expected to resolve postpartum.

The types of pigmentation seen in pregnancy are summarized in Table 51–1. The most common pigmentary changes of pregnancy are hyperpigmentation and melasma (Fig. 51–4). Uncommon pigmentary patterns, such as pseudoacanthosis nigricans (Fig. 51–5) and dermal melanocytosis (Fig. 51–6), can also be seen.[4–8] Furthermore, postinflammatory hyperpigmentation secondary to specific dermatoses of pregnancy (Fig. 51–7) is particularly common in skin of color. A mild form of localized or generalized hyperpigmentation occurs to some extent in up to 90% of pregnant women[1,3] and shows accentuation of the areolae, nipples, genital skin, axillae, and inner thighs. The most familiar examples are darkening of the *linea alba* (*linea nigra*) (see Fig. 51–2) and periareolar skin (*secondary areolae*).

Melasma (*chloasma* or *mask of pregnancy*) is a type of facial melanosis reported in up to 70% of pregnant women[2] and one third of nonpregnant women taking an oral contraceptive.[9] Although the malar pattern is common, the entire central face is affected in most patients (*centrofacial pattern*) (see Fig. 51–4) and, less often, the ramus of the mandible (*mandibular pattern*).[10] Melasma results from melanin deposition in the epidermis (70%, accentuated by Wood's lamp examination), dermal macrophages (10%–15%), or both (20%). This type of melanosis is thought to be associated with the hormonal changes of gestation and worsens with exposure to ultraviolet and visible light.[10,11] Melasma usually resolves postpartum but may recur in subsequent pregnancies or with the use of oral contraceptives. The dermal type of melasma is less responsive to treatment than the epidermal. Mild gestational melasma can be treated with azelaic acid, which is safe during pregnancy. Persistent melasma can be treated postpartum with topical hydroquinone 2% to 4% and a broad-spectrum sunscreen, with[12] or without a topical retinoid and mild topical steroid. Melasma, whether caused by pregnancy or oral contraceptives,[3] is resistant to treatment in 30% of patients. Combination therapies, including laser treatment[13,14] and chemical peels,[15] may be effective to some extent in resistant cases.

The physiologic vascular, connective tissue, mucosal, glandular, hair, and nail changes of pregnancy are summarized in the Summary of Management Options box. The oral pyogenic granuloma of pregnancy (*granuloma gravidarum* or *pregnancy epulis*) is discussed under "Skin Tumors."

FIGURE 51–1
Spider angioma (telangiectasia) on the arm.

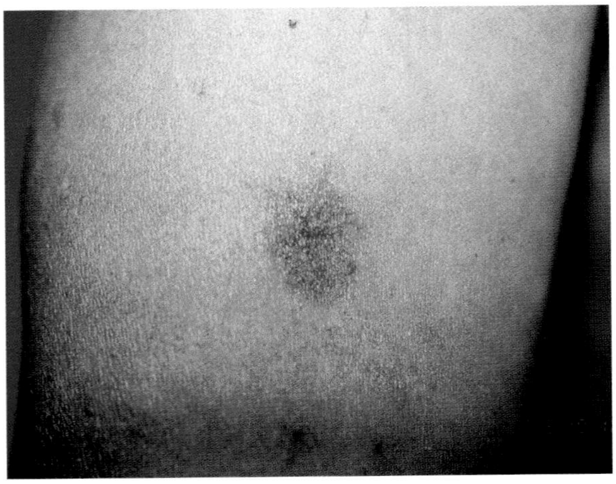

FIGURE 51–2
Stretchmarks (striae gravidarum) on the lateral aspects of the abdomen and hyperpigmentation of the linea alba, causing development of the linea nigra.

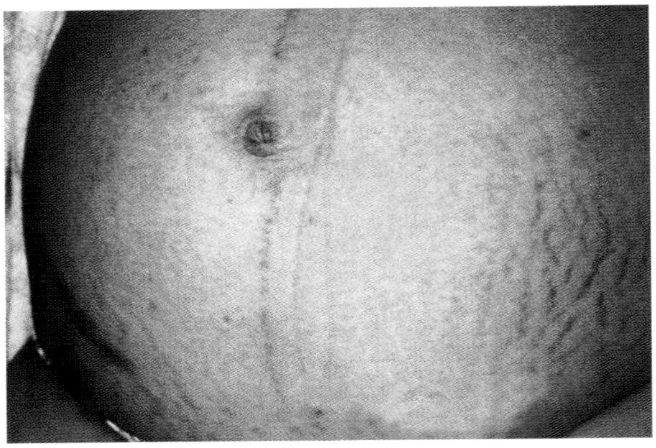

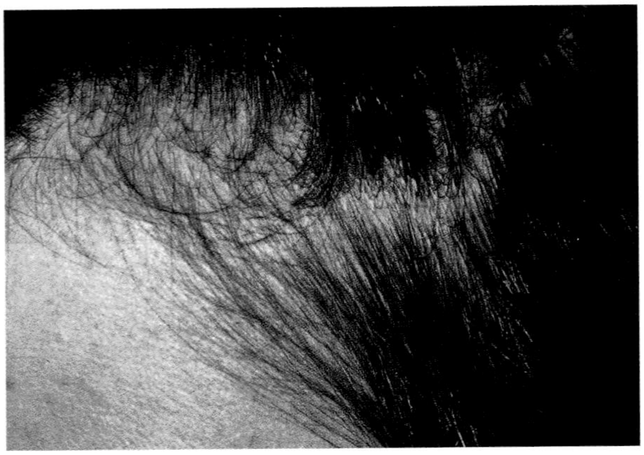

FIGURE 51–3
Telogen effluvium, which developed in the immediate postpartum period, with typical temporal recession and thinning.

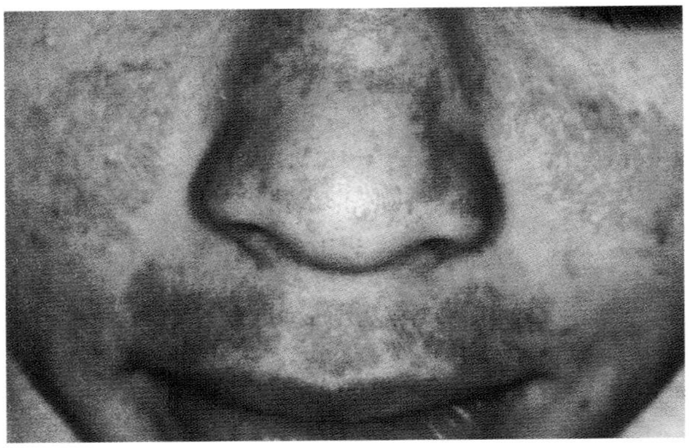

FIGURE 51–4
Melasma of the entire central face.

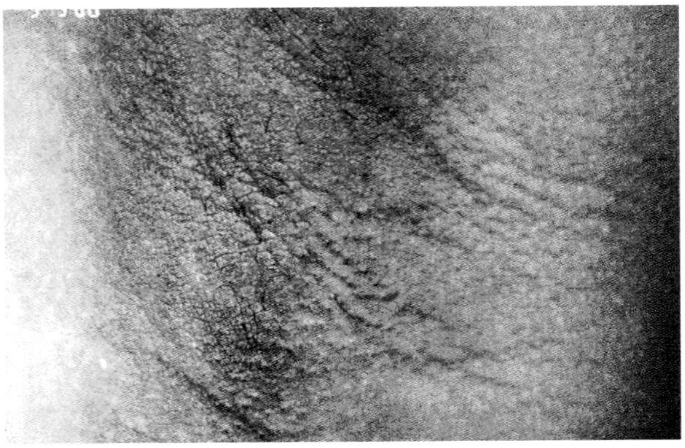

FIGURE 51–5
Pseudoacanthosis nigricans may develop in skin of color during pregnancy and manifests itself as hyperpigmented velvety plaques on the axillae (as shown) and neck.

TABLE 51–1

Patterns of Pigmentation in Pregnancy

Common Hypermelanoses
Hyperpigmentation
Melasma
Uncommon Hypermelanoses
Pseudoacanthosis nigricans
Dermal melanocytosis
Vulvar melanosis
Verrucous areolar pigmentation
Localized reticulate pigmentation
Darkening of Preexisting Pigmentation
Acanthosis nigricans
Pigmentary demarcation lines
Darkening of Benign Skin Lesions
Scars
Melanocytic nevi
Skin tags, seborrheic keratoses
Postinflammatory Hyperpigmentation
Secondary to specific dermatoses of pregnancy (see specific section in text)
Jaundice (see specific section in text)

FIGURE 51–6
Grayish-brown ill-defined patches of dermal melanocytosis may develop in pregnancy and persist in the postpartum period.

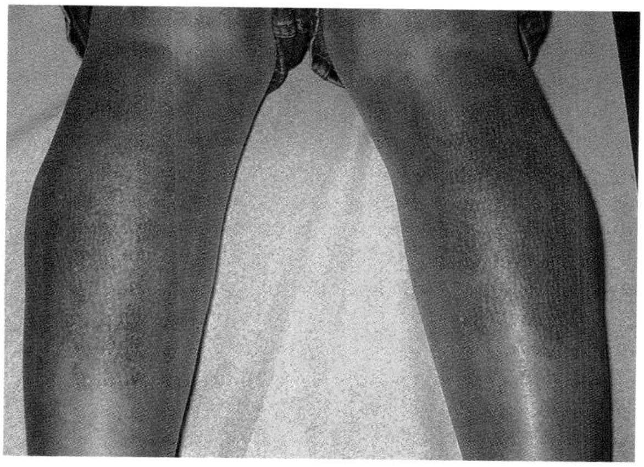

FIGURE 51–7
Extensive postinflammatory hyperpigmentation secondary to pruritic urticarial papules and plaques of pregnancy in an Asian female.

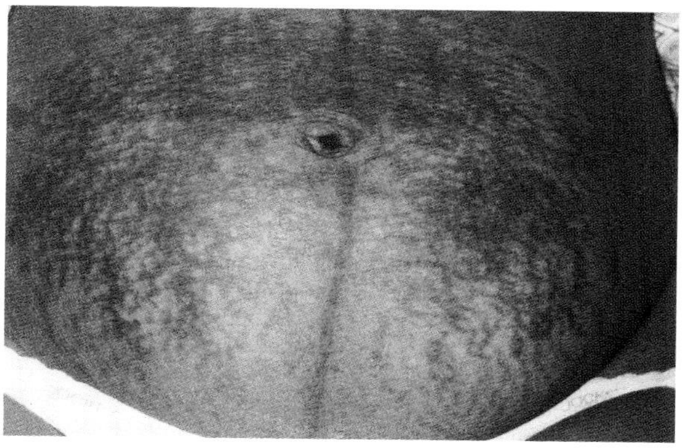

SUMMARY OF MANAGEMENT OPTIONS

Physiologic Skin Changes of Pregnancy

Management Options	Evidence Quality and Recommendation	References
Pigmentation		
Follow-up for spontaneous resolution in postpartum period.	—/GPP	—
Sun protection is mandatory in all cases.	—/GPP	—
For persistent cases postpartum, consider:		
• Hydroquinone 2%–4% cream with or without tretinoin and mild topical steroids.	IV/C	12
• Combination therapies including laser treatment (Er:YAG, Q-switched ruby, or Q-switched Nd:YAG).	IIa/B	13,14
• Combination therapies, including chemical peels (glycolic acid and Jessner's solution).	IIb/B	15
Spider Nervus (see Fig. 51-1)		
Reassure (occurs in 67% of white women, in the second to fifth mo; resolves within 3 mo postpartum); persistent lesions can be treated with fine-needle electrocautery, cryotherapy, or laser.	—/GPP	—
Palmar Erythema		
Reassure (occurs in 70% of white and 30% of African American women).	—/GPP	—
Varicosities		
Explain (occurs in 40% of women; thrombosis in < 10%); recommend leg elevation, compression stockings.	—/GPP	—
To treat symptomatic hemorrhoids, recommend stool softeners, hot sitz baths, topical anesthetics, suppositories, laxatives.		
Nonpitting Edema		
Reassure; exclude preeclampsia. Recommend leg elevation; compression stockings, diuretics if severe.	—/GPP	—

SUMMARY OF MANAGEMENT OPTIONS

Physiologic Skin Changes of Pregnancy—cont'd

Management Options	Evidence Quality and Recommendation	References
Striae Gravidarum (see Fig. 51–2)		
Reassure (occurs in 90% of white women; less common in other groups; less apparent postpartum but may never disappear); prescribe antipruritics, topical steroids if itchy; laser can improve the color changes.	—/GPP	—
Pyogenic Granuloma (*Granuloma Gravidarum*)		
Reassure (occurs in 2% of pregnant women at second to fifth mo; typically on the gingivae; postpartum shrinkage).	—/GPP	—
Recommend good dental hygiene; excision if excessive discomfort or bleeding		
Gum Hyperemia/Gingivitis		
Seen in most pregnant women in the third trimester; resolves postpartum.	—/GPP	—
Reassure; recommend good dental hygiene.		
Hair Changes (see Fig. 51–3)		
Mild hursutism regresses within 6 mo postpartum.	—/GPP	—
Postpartum hair shedding (telogen effluvium) lasts 1–5 mo.		
Frontoparietal hair recession and diffuse thinning also reported.		
Exclude pathologic androgen production if hirsutism.		
Follow-up postpartum hair changes.		
Glandular Changes		
Reassure (enlargement of sebaceous glands of the areolae); axillary sweating can be controlled with aluminum chloride solution (20%).	—/GPP	—
Nail Changes		
Reassure (start in the first trimester; onycholysis, subungual hyperkeratosis, transverse grooving, brittleness).	—/GPP	—

Er:YAG, erbium:yttrium-aluminum-garnet; GPP, good practice point; Nd:YAG, neodymium:yttrium-aluminum-garnet.

PREEXISTING SKIN DISEASES AND TUMORS AFFECTED BY PREGNANCY

The pregnant woman is susceptible to aggravation or, less often, to improvement of skin diseases and tumors.[16] The conditions that may improve during pregnancy are listed in Table 51–2.

TABLE 51–2

Preexisting Disorders That May Improve in Pregnancy

Acne
Atopic dermatitis
Autoimmune progesterone dermatitis
Chronic plaque psoriasis
Fox-Fordyce disease
Hidradenitis suppurativa
Linear IgA disease
Rheumatoid arthritis
Sarcoidosis

IgA, immunoglobulin A.

Inflammatory Skin Diseases

ATOPIC DERMATITIS (ECZEMA)

Eczema is the most common pregnancy dermatosis, accounting for 36% of total cases.[17] Atopic dermatitis is more likely to worsen than remit in pregnancy, although remission has been reported in up to 24% of cases.[17] There is a personal history of atopy in 27% of pregnant females with atopic dermatitis, a family history of atopy in 50% of cases, and infantile eczema in 19% of the offspring.[17] Some studies indicate that atopic dermatitis may start before the third trimester in up to 75% cases.[17] There have been no adverse effects on the fetal outcome. Maternal smoking may be implicated in the development of atopic eczema during pregnancy and lactation.[18] The effect of breast-feeding on atopic eczema has been debated. Gestational atopic eczema is treated with moisturizers and low- to mid-potency topical steroids. A short course of oral steroid may be required for severe eczema. Systemic antibiotics, such as erythromycin base or penicillin, are necessary in superinfected eczema. Systemic antihistamines, such as diphenhydramine, are often required for severe pruritus. Ultraviolet B (UVB) light is a safe adjunct in treating chronic eczema. Irritant hand dermatitis and nipple eczema are often seen postpartum.[1] Nipple eczema can show painful fissures and be complicated with bacterial infection, most commonly from *Staphylococcus aureus*.

ACNE VULGARIS

The effect of pregnancy on acne vulgaris is unpredictable. Some patients may develop acne for the first time during pregnancy, and acne conglobata may worsen during pregnancy. In one study, pregnancy affected acne in approximately 70% of women, with 41% reporting improvement and 29% worsening in pregnancy.[19] Comedonal acne can be treated with topical keratolytic agents, such as benzoyl peroxide, whereas inflammatory acne can be treated with azelaic acid, topical erythromycin, topical clindamycin phosphate, or oral erythromycin base. All these medications are safe to use during gestation.[19]

Urticaria may worsen in pregnancy, whereas **hidradenitis suppurativa** and **Fox-Fordyce disease** may remit during gestation as a result of reduced apocrine gland activity (see Table 51–2).[1]

CHRONIC PLAQUE PSORIASIS

Chronic plaque psoriasis is the most common type of psoriasis to develop or exacerbate during pregnancy.[20] It is more likely to improve (40%–63%) than worsen (14%) during gestation; it commonly flares, however, within 4 months of delivery. Psoriatic arthritis may develop or worsen during pregnancy and often starts postpartum or perimenopausally (30%–45%).[21] Topical steroids and topical calcipotriene as well as topical anthralin and topical tacrolimus appear to be safe treatment options for localized psoriasis in pregnancy.[22] UVB is the safest treatment for severe psoriasis that has not responded to topical medications. A short course of cyclosporine can be administered for psoriasis that has not responded to UVB.

GENERALIZED PUSTULAR PSORIASIS/ IMPETIGO HERPETIFORMIS

A very rare variant of generalized pustular psoriasis develops in pregnancy, often associated with hypocalcemia[23] or low serum levels of vitamin D.[24] When compared with nonpregnant women with various forms of psoriasis, pregnant women with impetigo herpetiformis rarely have a personal or family history of psoriasis, develop the eruption strictly during pregnancy, and improve postpartum. The eruption usually starts in the third trimester. It often persists until delivery and occasionally runs a protracted course postpartum. It can exacerbate with the use of oral contraceptives.[25] Impetigo herpetiformis is manifested as grouped discrete sterile pustules at the periphery of erythematous patches (Fig. 51–8*A*). The lesions start in the major flexures and extend centrifugally onto the trunk and around the umbilicus, usually sparing the face, hands, and feet. The lesions may become crusted (see Fig. 51–8*B*) or vegetative, and the mucous membranes may show erosive or circinate lesions. Postinflammatory hyperpigmentation commonly develops; nail changes secondary to subungual pustules are exceptionally seen.

Skin histopathology shows features of pustular psoriasis, and direct immunofluorescence is negative. The laboratory workup reveals leukocytosis, elevated erythrocyte sedimentation rate, and occasionally, hypocalcemia or decreased serum vitamin D levels. Impetigo herpetiformis is thought to be an outbreak of psoriasis probably triggered by a metabolic milieu, such as pregnancy or hypocalcemia.[1] The latter is known to exacerbate generalized pustular psoriasis and can develop secondary to hypoalbuminemia in pregnancy. A report that showed reduced levels of an inhibitor of skin elastase in a patient with impetigo herpetiformis warrants further investigation.[26] Furthermore, one report raised speculation that infections during pregnancy may trigger a flare

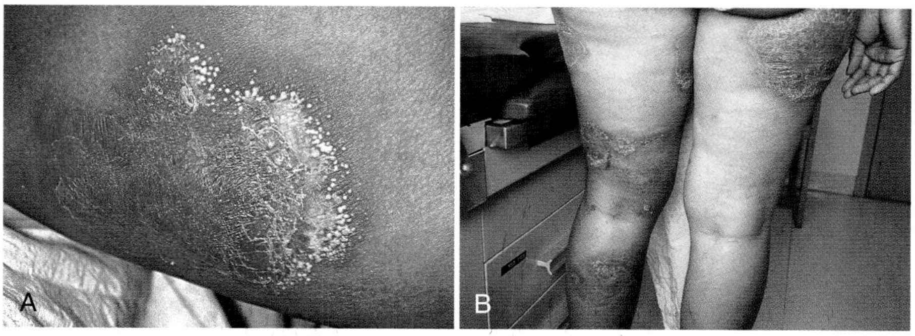

FIGURE 51–8
A, Early impetigo herpetiformis: discrete group sterile papules at the periphery of erythematous patch. *B*, Generalized advanced lesions of impetigo herpetiformis show crusting or vegetations. (*A* and *B*, Photographs courtesy of Aleksandr Itkin, MD.)

of pustular psoriasis in an individual with psoriatic tendency.[27]

Impetigo herpetiformis can be treated with systemic steroids at daily doses up to 60 mg/day of prednisone. Calcium and vitamin D replacement therapy should be undertaken if necessary and can lead to remission of the eruption.[23] A severe case was treated with cyclosporine.[28] Impetigo herpetiformis has been treated postpartum with oral retinoids[29] or PUVA[30] (psoralens with ultraviolet A light). Systemic antibiotics should be administered in superinfected cases. The eruption commonly resolves postpartum but recurs in each successive pregnancy with earlier onset and increased morbidity.[25,31] There are serious risks for the mother and fetus. Maternal risks include tetany, seizures, delirium, and exceptionally, death from cardiac or renal failure. Fetal risks[25] such as stillbirth, neonatal birth, and fetal abnormalities may result from placental insufficiency, which often complicates impetigo herpetiformis, and have been reported even when the skin disease was well controlled.[31] Maternal and fetal monitoring is of utmost importance. In severe cases, termination of pregnancy is warranted, the timing of which depends on the maternal and fetal status. The eruption resolves promptly afterward.

Infections

Pregnancy can affect the vast majority of common infections, causing an increase in the prevalence or exacerbation of candida vaginitis, *Trichomonas*, *Pityrosporum* folliculitis, and papillomavirus infections.[1,16] Other infections, such as recurrent genital herpes simplex virus infection, are not exacerbated in pregnancy but are of critical interest because they significantly increase fetal morbidity and mortality[32] (see Chapter 30). Disseminated infections are more likely to occur during gestation and may have devastating effects for the fetus. Viral exanthems can have significant maternal and/or fetal risks for complications; their management options are summarized in Chapters 29 and 32.

The prevalence of candida vaginitis increases during pregnancy. The infection has been reported in 17% to 50% of pregnant women[33]; of those, 10% to 40% are asymptomatic.[34] *Candida albicans* has been associated with intra-amniotic infection.[35] The organism can be cultured from up to 50% of neonates born to infected mothers.[16] Neonatal candidiasis can result from passage of the infant through an infected birth canal and congenital candidiasis from an ascending infection in utero. The latter is characterized by generalized skin lesions that appear within 12 hours of delivery.[16] *Trichomonas* infection is seen in 12% to 27% of pregnant women.[36] An association with preterm delivery and low birth weight[37] has been debated.[38] *Pityrosporum* folliculitis and tinea versicolor (Fig. 51–9), both caused by yeasts of the *Malassezia* species, occur with greater frequency in pregnant women.[39] Papillomavirus infections may worsen during gestation, and condylomata acuminata can show accelerated growth, blocking the birth canal.[16]

Early studies showed exacerbation of leprosy during pregnancy or within the first 6 months of lactation,[40] a finding that was debated by one study.[41] Leprosy reactions are triggered by pregnancy: type 1 (reversal) reaction occurs maximally postpartum,[42] when the cell-mediated immunity returns to prepregnancy levels, and type 2 reaction (*erythema nodosum leprosum*) throughout pregnancy and lactation.[43] The increased incidence of erythema nodosum leprosum in pregnant women has been associated with early loss of nerve function secondary to "silent neuritis."[44] Multidrug therapy of rifampin, dapsone, and clofazimine is the treatment of choice during pregnancy. Leprosy reactions should be treated with oral steroids and not thalidomide, which is contraindicated in pregnancy. Patients with leprosy should be counseled about the effects of pregnancy on the disease before they become pregnant, and pregnancies should be planned when the disease is well controlled. Leprosy has been associated with increased fetal mortality and low birth weight.[40] Approximately 20% of children born to mothers with leprosy will develop the disease by puberty.

FIGURE 51–9
Hyperpigmented minimally scaly patches on the chest in a pregnant female with tinea versicolor.

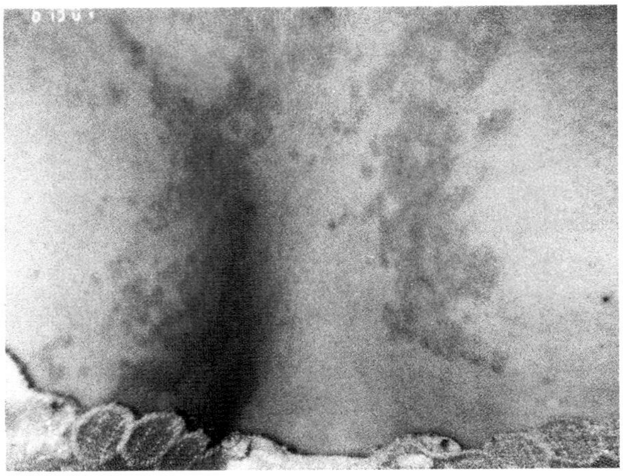

Autoimmune Disorders

SYSTEMIC LUPUS ERYTHEMATOSUS (See also Chapter 43)

Chronic discoid lupus is not affected by pregnancy. The data as to whether flares of systemic lupus erythematosus (SLE) are more common during pregnancy are conflicting.[45–47] The discrepancy among previous studies is due to methodologic differences,[48] including the definition of lupus flare, and the fact that several typical manifestations of active SLE, such as facial erythema (Fig. 51–10), alopecia, fatigue, edema, anemia, musculoskeletal pain, mild proteinuria, and elevated erythrocyte sedimentation rate, are common findings in pregnancy. In most studies, the frequency of flare during pregnancy was higher than 57%.[48] Pregnancy is well tolerated by mothers in remission for at least 3 months before conception, but if conception occurs during the active stage of disease, 50% of gravidas will worsen during pregnancy and might experience life-threatening progression of the renal disease.[45] When SLE first appears during pregnancy, it may show severe manifestations but usually remits postpartum. Cutaneous flares and arthralgias are the

FIGURE 51–10
Malar erythema in a butterfly distribution in a pregnant woman with systemic lupus erythematosus. (Photograph courtesy of Cameron Thomas, Campbell Kennedy, and Phillipa Kyle.)

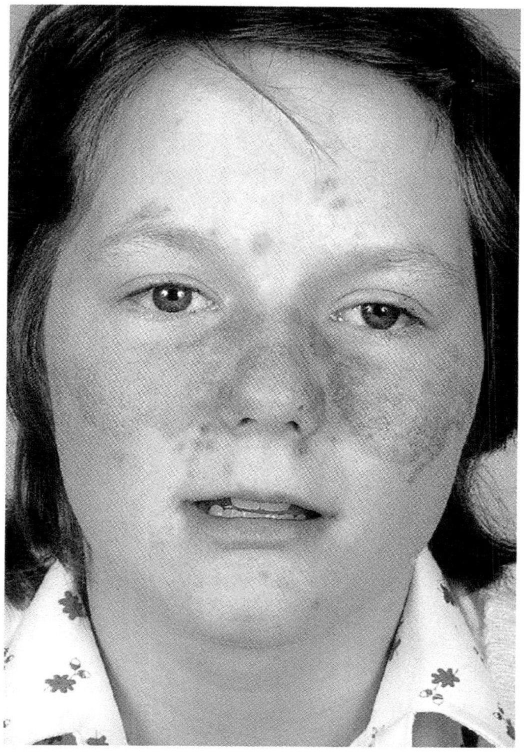

most common manifestations of SLE in pregnancy. Flares are not more severe during than outside of pregnancy and can be treated with oral steroids. Yet, steroids do not prevent flares and should not be prescribed prophylactically.

The effects of lupus on fetal outcome correlate with the severity of maternal lupus, active disease at the time of conception or first presentation of SLE during pregnancy, and presence of anticardiolipin antibody or lupus anticoagulant. Preterm delivery occurs in 16% to 37% of pregnancies, and spontaneous abortion rates are two to four times normal. Other risks include fetal death, intrauterine growth restriction (IUGR), and preeclampsia.[48] These obstetric complications have been associated with uteroplacental hypoperfusion, defective placentation, and chronic inflammation. The antiphospholipid syndrome[49] may complicate SLE, but many patients have primary antiphospholipid syndrome without lupus. It presents with manifestations that can worsen or lead to its initial diagnosis during gestation, such as recurrent miscarriage, thrombosis, livedo reticularis, migraine, stroke, and thrombocytopenia. Treatment with low-molecular-weight heparin or aspirin and close antenatal surveillance for maternal and fetal complications is warranted.

NEONATAL LUPUS (See also Chapter 43)

Neonatal lupus[50] can develop owing to transplacental passage of maternal anti-Ro (SS-A) and, less commonly, anti-La (SS-B) or anti-U1-RNP antibody. The risk is 5% if anti-Ro–positive, and the incidence is 1.6% of all lupus pregnancies. An association with human leukocyte antigen (HLA) DR2 and DR3 positivity in the mother has been reported.[50] The female-to-male ratio is 3 : 1.[50] Neonatal lupus is characterized by a transient skin eruption and systemic manifestations, including congenital heart block (15%–30%), cytopenias, hepatosplenomegaly, and pericarditis/myocarditis. The eruption becomes manifest several weeks into postnatal life and resolves by 6 to 8 months of age, coincident with the clearance of maternal autoantibody from the infant's circulation. The skin lesions frequently affect the face and scalp, with a predilection for the eyelids. Other sun-exposed areas may be also affected; occasionally, the eruption becomes generalized. The lesions are papulosquamous or annular/polycyclic, indistinguishable from subacute cutaneous lupus of the adult. Skin histopathology shows interface dermatitis and superficial dermal mononuclear cell infiltrate. Immunofluorescence shows a particulate pattern of immunoglobulin G (IgG) in the epidermis.

Congenital heart block carries a substantial neonatal morbidity and mortality and can be detected in utero at 18 to 20 weeks' gestation.[50] Twenty-two percent of affected infants die in the perinatal period, and 62% of the infants require a pacemaker.[50] The risk of bearing a second child with heart block is 25%, rising to 50% after two or more affected infants. The maternal and fetal anti-Ro, anti-La, and anti-U1-RNP status should be determined, and the newborn should be screened for heart block. Survivors of neonatal lupus may be at increased risk of developing connective tissue disease in adulthood.

DERMATOMYOSITIS/POLYMYOSITIS

Dermatomyositis/polymyositis may show a flare of the heliotrope rash, worsening of proximal muscle weakness, or subcutaneous calcification in approximately half of the affected individuals.[51] When the disease is in remission during pregnancy, there are no maternal or fetal risks involved. Nevertheless, when the disease starts or relapses during gestation, it can be detrimental to the mother and/or fetus. High doses of oral steroids may be required to control the disease. Fetal demise owing to abortion, stillbirth, or neonatal death has been reported in over half of the cases of active disease, and prenatal surveillance is crucial. An assisted vaginal delivery may be required in case of active myositis during labor. If the disease is diagnosed in the first trimester, the option of therapeutic abortion should be offered to the mother because of the high risk of maternal and/or fetal complications.

SYSTEMIC SCLEROSIS (See also Chapter 43)

The course of scleroderma is not significantly altered by pregnancy. Gravidas with limited scleroderma without systemic disease do better than those with diffuse scleroderma.[52] Women with early (<4 yr) diffuse scleroderma are at high risk for hypertension, renal failure, premature delivery, and small full-term infants. The risk of hypertension and renal failure is greatest during the third trimester and postpartum period. Nevertheless, renal crisis during gestation is less common than previously thought. Successful pregnancy is now reported in 70% to 80% of patients.[52] The skin disease usually does not progress during pregnancy, whereas reflux esophagitis and articular disease worsen. Raynaud's phenomenon usually improves secondary to gestational vasodilation and increased blood flow.

BULLOUS DISORDERS

Pemphigus vulgaris, vegetans, or foliaceus may present or worsen during gestation.[53] Linear IgA disease may improve in pregnancy and relapse postpartum.[54] Pemphigus vulgaris is rare during pregnancy; it usually worsens in the first or second trimester. Skin immunofluorescence studies are required to differentiate pemphigus from herpes gestationis (see "Herpes Gestationis," later). Neonatal pemphigus can develop from transplacental transfer of IgG antibodies. Most neonates require no therapy because the blisters heal spontaneously within 2 to 3 weeks. A recent review of 49 pregnancies complicated by pemphigus vulgaris showed 5 stillbirths and 1 death in the early neonatal period (perinatal mortality 12%).[55] Of the 44 live births, 20 (45%) of neonates had pemphigus lesions of birth.[55] Stillborn infants have been found to have skin lesions and immunofluorescence findings consistent with pemphigus. Pemphigus during pregnancy can be controlled with high doses of oral steroids.

Metabolic Disorders

PORPHYRIA

Porphyria cutanea tarda, acute intermittent porphyria, and variegate porphyria can present problems in pregnancy because they are adversely affected by estrogen. Patients with porphyria cutanea tarda demonstrate bullous lesions, skin fragility, and milia on sun-exposed areas, such as the dorsa of the hands and forearms. Other skin changes include facial hypertrichosis, periorbital hyperpigmentation, scarring alopecia, and dystrophic calcification with ulceration. Reports of porphyria cutanea tarda and pregnancy have been scarce in the literature; these reports have provided conflicting results.[56] Symptomatic exacerbation of the disease has been often reported during the first trimester followed by improvement later in pregnancy. These changes parallel a rise in serum estrogen and porphyrin excretion in the first trimester and a fall in serum iron levels and urinary porphyrins later in gestation. Nevertheless, some authors reported exacerbation of the disease with oral contraceptives and not in pregnancy. The fetal prognosis is not usually affected by this disorder. Lists of drugs that are safe and unsafe for porphyria patients have been published.[57] Management of porphyria cutanea tarda during pregnancy includes sun protection, avoidance of alcohol and iron, and repeated phlebotomies in retractable cases. Chloroquine is contraindicated in pregnancy because of its teratogenicity. The newborn should be assessed and screened for porphyria cutanea tarda in the immediate postpartum period, both for genetic counseling and to avoid inducing factors in the child.

ACRODERMATITIS ENTEROPATHICA

Acrodermatitis enteropathica is a rare autosomal disorder of zinc deficiency characterized by dermatitis, diarrhea, and alopecia. The skin lesions are vesiculobullous and eczematous and are distributed on the extremities and periorificial sites, such as the mouth, anus, and genital areas. The disease usually flares during gestation, because serum levels decrease early in pregnancy.[58] This decline is not attributed to fetal demands only, because acrodermatitis enteropathica can also flare with oral contraceptive use. The skin lesions in pregnancy need to be differentiated from pemphigoid gestationis and impetigo herpetiformis. Most often, having first appeared in childhood, the skin disease reappears during pregnancy, worsens until delivery, and clears postpartum.[57] The disorder usually has no effect on fetal outcome. Fetal malformations and neonatal death have been reported in a few cases of untreated maternal disease.

Connective Tissue Disorders

EHLERS-DANLOS SYNDROMES I TO X

Ehlers-Danlos syndromes I to X are a group of inherited disorders of collagen metabolism that manifest with skin fragility, easy bruising, joint hypermobility, and skin hyperelasticity. Women with Ehlers-Danlos syndromes type I (classic or gravis) and IV (ecchymotic or arterial) are particularly likely to develop complications during pregnancy. The risks include premature rupture of the membranes; postpartum bleeding; rupture of major vessels (especially in type IV), including the aorta and pulmonary artery; poor wound healing and dehiscence; uterine lacerations; bladder and uterine prolapse; and abdominal hernias.[59] The reported maternal mortality in type IV disease is 20% to 25%. The risks are such that women with Ehlers-Danlos syndromes types I or IV should be counseled against pregnancy. A favorable outcome of pregnancy, however, has been reported for types II (mitis) and X (fibronectin abnormality).[2]

PSEUDOXANTHOMA ELASTICUM

Gestation may worsen the vascular complications of pseudoxanthoma elasticum. The main complication is massive hematemesis from gastrointestinal (particularly gastric) bleeding, but repeated epistaxis and congestive heart failure with ventricular arrhythmia have been also reported.[60] Hypertension is frequent and should be treated aggressively. An increased risk of first-trimester miscarriage and IUGR secondary to placental insufficiency has been reported.

Skin Tumors

MISCELLANEOUS LESIONS

Most benign skin tumors can appear for the first time, increase in number, or enlarge during gestation as a result of the effects of high estrogen levels on vascular and soft tissues. The most common lesions that change during pregnancy are melanocytic nevi, seborrheic keratoses, and skin tags. Melanocytic nevi may develop, enlarge, or darken during pregnancy (Fig. 51–11). The pigmentary changes observed in melanocytic nevi during pregnancy are thought to be due to the melanogenic effects of high estrogen levels and increased levels of melanocyte-stimulating hormone. An increase in estrogen and progesterone receptors in melanocytic nevi in pregnancy has been demonstrated. A mild degree of histopathologic atypia has been reported in a few studies. The pregnant woman should be advised that there is no evidence that pregnancy induces malignant transformation of preexisting nevi. Studies that used dermoscopic analysis of nevi showed that the pigment network becomes thicker and more prominent and the globules darker during

FIGURE 51–11
Melanocytic nevus that became darker and developed a mild border irregularity during gestation.

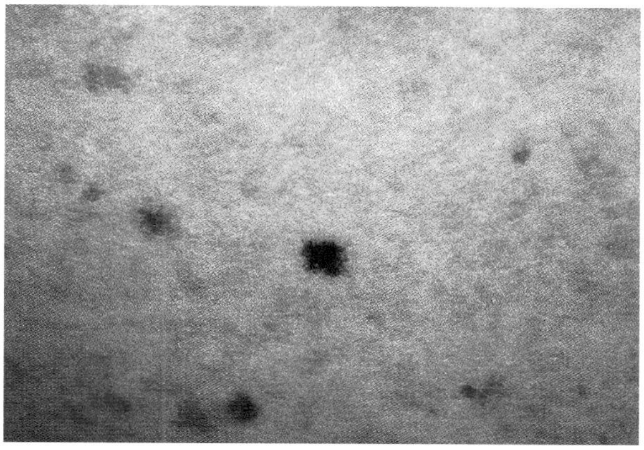

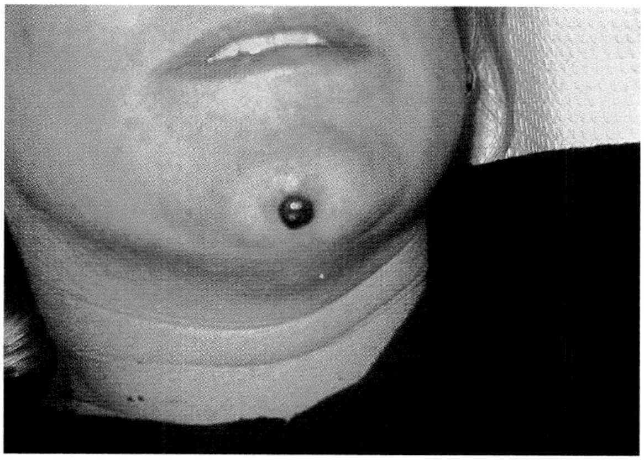

FIGURE 51–12
Pyogenic granuloma of pregnancy (granuloma gravidarum), typically seen on the gingivae, can also develop on extramucosal sites.

pregnancy.[61] These features, however, return to their original condition within 1 year after delivery. Seborrheic keratoses may also enlarge or darken during gestation. Skin tags (*molluscum fibrosum gravidarum*) usually appear during the later months of pregnancy and may partially or completely disappear postpartum. In all these cases, the pregnant woman needs to be reassured that these skin lesions are common during pregnancy and may improve postpartum.

Vascular tumors may also be affected or present during pregnancy. The pyogenic granuloma of pregnancy (*granuloma gravidarum*, *pregnancy tumor*, or *pregnancy epulis*) is a benign proliferation of capillaries within the gingivae that appears between the second and the fifth months of pregnancy. The prevalence of granuloma gravidarum is estimated to approach 2% of all pregnancies. It may be caused by trauma to inflamed mucosa and presents as a vascular deep-red or purple nodule between the teeth or on the buccal or lingual surface of the marginal gingiva. Occasionally, pyogenic granulomas can develop on the lip or extramucosal sites (Fig. 51–12). Typical histopathologic features of a pyogenic granuloma are seen in all cases. Spontaneous shrinkage of the tumor usually occurs postpartum, and most cases do not require treatment. Surgical excision, however, is necessary in cases of excessive

FIGURE 51–13
Keloid that developed during pregnancy without previous trauma.

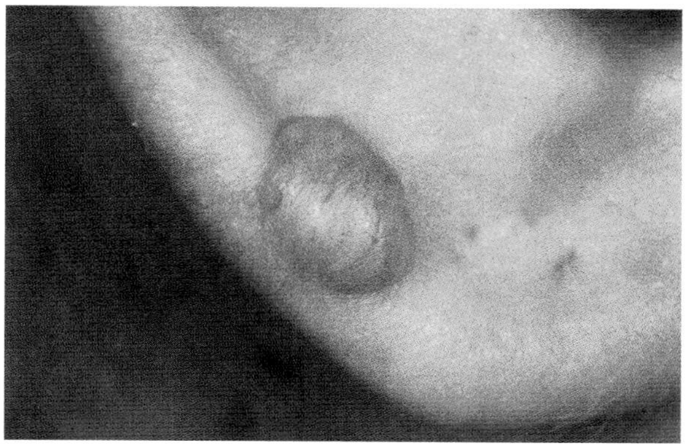

bleeding. An increased frequency of other vascular tumors, such as hemangioma, hemangioendothelioma, glomus tumor, and glomangioma, has been reported in pregnancy. Large hemangiomas that exceptionally cause arteriovenous shunt and high-output cardiac failure in pregnancy partially regress postpartum, tending to enlarge again in subsequent pregnancies.

Dermatofibromata, dermatofibrosarcomata protuberans, leiomyomata, and keloids may develop or enlarge during pregnancy (Fig. 51–13). Desmoid tumors often develop in the rectus abdominis muscle. Neurofibromas may enlarge or arise de novo during gestation, often complicated with massive hemorrhage within the tumor. These lesions may partially resolve postpartum.

NEUROFIBROMATOSIS

Women with neurofibromatosis are at high risk for vascular complications during pregnancy such as hypertension and renal artery rupture.[62] A higher prevalence of maternal and fetal risks, such as first-trimester spontaneous abortion, stillbirth, IUGR, and perinatal complications, has been reported in neurofibromatosis.[63]

MALIGNANT MELANOMA

Malignant melanoma has an incidence of 2.8 cases per 1000 births and accounts for 8% of malignant neoplasms during pregnancy. Several studies have shown that melanomas that develop during pregnancy are thicker than melanomas in nonpregnant women.[64,65] This finding may be due to a delay in the diagnosis of melanoma during gestation, possibly because of a shared misconception by the patient and/or her physician that darkening and changing of a nevus is normal in pregnancy. Despite initial concerns, several epidemiologic studies evaluating the effect of pregnancy status at diagnosis have showed that the 5-year survival rate is not affected after controlling for other factors.[66–68] The protective effect of female gender on prognosis of melanoma has been attributed to the inhibitory effect of estrogens on melanoma cell lines through type II estrogen receptors and the fact that melanoma cells lack type I estrogen receptors. In the largest study to date, the major prognostic determinants of survival in pregnant women with localized melanoma were tumor thickness (Breslow scale) and ulceration status.[68]

Surgery is the treatment of choice in patients with early melanoma. Correct staging is crucial, and sentinel lymph node biopsy using preoperative intradermal injection of technetium-99m-sulfur colloid is considered safe during pregnancy[69] and should be performed as indicated. For pregnant women with advanced melanoma, the prognosis, risks, and benefits from systemic therapy should be discussed, and a special consideration should be given to gestational age at presentation and consequences of delayed treatment on overall survival. Systemic chemotherapy during the second and third trimesters does not usually cause fetal abnormalities, except in the case of alkylating agents.[70] Nevertheless, given that the effectiveness of chemotherapy in advanced melanoma is at present limited, systemic chemotherapy should not be given in pregnancy in other than exceptional circumstances. In some cases, termination of pregnancy in early gestation may be the least damaging course of action to allow systemic therapy to be offered.

Although placental and/or fetal metastasis is extraordinarily rare (19 cases),[69] melanoma is the most common type of malignancy to metastasize to the placenta and fetus, representing 30% of placental metastases and 58% of fetal metastases. Maternal and fetal death invariably occurs; 80% of maternal deaths occur within 3 months of delivery. When a gravida is diagnosed with melanoma, the placenta should be sent for histologic examination. Some authors suggested that blood from both the mother and the umbilical cord be examined cytologically. The effectiveness of systemic treatment in preventing metastases to the placenta and fetus has not been adequately studied.[70]

There are currently no standard guidelines for patients who desire a pregnancy after the diagnosis and treatment of melanoma. Based on the fact that 50% of recurrences develop by 3 years in patients with thick lesions, Mackie[70] suggested that women who have melanoma should not become pregnant nor should they take oral contraceptive or postmenopausal hormonal replacement therapy for 2 years after initial treatment unless there are exceptional circumstances. Nevertheless, pregnancy subsequent to a diagnosis of melanoma was associated with a nonsignificant decrease in mortality,[68] and there is no evidence to support an increased risk of melanoma recurrence with oral contraceptive use. The recommendation of other authors about how long to wait before becoming pregnant after a diagnosis of melanoma is on case-by-case basis, depending on tumor thickness and stage, age of the patient, and desire to become pregnant.[69]

FIGURE 51–14 Minimal residual skin lesions of sarcoidosis on the knee in a pregnant female who showed severe generalized skin sarcoidosis before gestation.

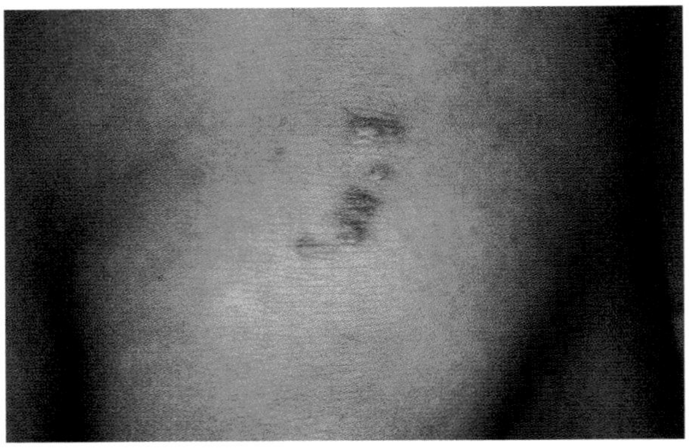

Miscellaneous Skin Disorders

A variety of skin disorders have been reported to start or flare during pregnancy, but large series are missing for most of them. Autoimmune progesterone dermatitis, a condition caused by hypersensitivity to progesterone and characterized by recurrent cyclic skin lesions that appear during the luteal phase of the menstrual cycle, has been reported to improve or flare during pregnancy. The improvement may be due to increased cortisol levels and/or the gradual increase in sex hormone levels during gestation with subsequent hormonal desensitization in some patients. Sarcoidosis of the skin is one of the most studied and has been shown to improve in pregnancy. Figure 51–14 demonstrates minimal residual skin lesions of sarcoidosis in a pregnant female who demonstrated generalized skin sarcoidosis before gestation. Exacerbation or new onset of erythema nodosum (adversely affected by estrogen), keratosis pilaris, erythema multiforme, bowenoid papulosis, mycosis fungoides, Langerhans cell histiocytosis, mastocytosis, erythrokeratodermia variabilis, hereditary angioedema, tuberous sclerosis, Marfan's syndrome, and hereditary hemorrhagic telangiectasia during pregnancy have been reported. The serious maternal risks related to vascular complications of tuberous sclerosis, Marfan's syndrome, and hereditary hemorrhagic telangiectasia should be promptly assessed. The management of the rest of the aforementioned conditions should be individualized.

SUMMARY OF MANAGEMENT OPTIONS

Preexisting Skin Disorders

Management Options	Evidence Quality and Recommendation	References
Atopic Dermatitis (Eczema)	IV/C	19
Emollients.		
Low- or mid-potency topical steroids.		
Oral antihistamines.		
UVB.		
Short-course oral steroid for severe disease.		

Management Options	Evidence Quality and Recommendation	References
Acne Vulgaris		
Comedonal Acne	IV/C	19
May treat with benzoyl peroxide.		
Inflammatory Acne	IV/C	19
Treat with:		
• Azelaic acid.		
• Topical erythromycin or clindamycin.		
• Oral erythromycin base.		
Psoriasis		
Chronic Plaque Psoriasis		
Treat with:		
• Topical steroids, calcipotriene, anthralin, tacrolimus.	IV/C	22
• UVB.	—/GPP	—
• Short-course cyclosporine.	—/GPP	—
Generalized Postular Psoriasis		
Monitor maternal BP, cardiac and renal function.	—/GPP	—
Institute fetal monitoring, vigilance for IUGR.	IV/C	25
Prescribe high-dose oral steroids as first-line therapy.	—/GPP	—
UVB and cyclosporine are second-line therapies.	IV/C	28
Give calcium and vitamin D if necessary.	IV/C	23
Prescribe systemic antibiotics if superinfection.	—/GPP	—
Infections (See Chapters 30–32 and Table 51–3)		
Autoimmune Disorders		
Systemic Lupus Erythematosus		
Give oral steroids for skin and joint exacerbation.	IV/C	48
Neonatal Lupus		
Perform skin biopsy if diagnosis uncertain.		
Screen fetus/newborn for heart block.		
Assess maternal/fetal anti-Ro, anti-La, anti-RNP.		
Test ECG, liver function, platelets in newborn.		
Give topical steroids, UV protection for skin rash.		
See Chapter 37 for discussion congenital heart block.		
Dermatomyositis/Polymyositis	III/B	51
Prescribe oral steroids; second line: methotrexate.		
Be vigilant for IUGR and preterm labor.		
Consider assisted vaginal delivery.		
Systemic Sclerosis		
Monitor for hypertension and renal failure.		
Be vigilant for preterm delivery and small-for-dates infants.		
Bullous Disorders—Pemphigus	III/B	53,54
Prescribe oral steroids.		
Institute vigilance for miscarriage/fetal death.		55
Institute vigilance for neonatal lesions.		55

SUMMARY OF MANAGEMENT OPTIONS
Preexisting Skin Disorders—cont'd

Management Options	Evidence Quality and Recommendation	References
Metabolic and Connective Tissue Disorders		
Porphyria Cutanea Tarda		
Be vigilant for exacerbation. Avoid sun, iron, and alcohol. Consider venesection.	IV/C	56
Avoid chloroquine in first trimester. Avoid drugs that cause exacerbation.	IV/C	57
Acrodermatitis Enteropathica		
Offer zinc supplementation.		
Screen carefully for fetal malformations.		
Ehlers-Danlos Syndromes I and IV	III/B	59
Counsel against conception prepregnancy.		
Maintain vigilance for rupture of major vessels, postpartum hemorrhage, wound dehiscence.		
Maintain vigilance for uterine or bladder prolapse.		
Be vigilant for preterm delivery.		
Provide IV access and cross-match blood for delivery.		
Avoid excessive trauma at operative delivery.		
Use nonabsorbable sutures for cesarean section.		
Consider termination of pregnancy if no response to therapy.		
Pseudoxanthoma Elasticum	IV/C	60
Institute vigilance for GI bleeding, hypertension.		
Institute vigilance for first-trimester miscarriage, IUGR.		
Skin Tumors		
Malignant Melanoma		
Make decisions about conception subsequent to a melanoma diagnosis on a case-by-case basis.	IIa/B	68
Perform prompt excision and staging for definitive management.	IIa/B	68
Chemotherapy may be used after first trimester with low risk of fetal anomaly.	IV/C	70
Perform biopsy of placenta for metastasis (very rare).	IV/C	69,70
Neurofibromatosis		
Monitor for hypertension and vascular complications.	IV/C	62
Monitor fetal growth and health.	IV/C	63

BP, blood pressure; ECG, electrocardiogram; GI, gastrointestinal; GPP, good practice point; IUGR, intrauterine growth restriction; UV, ultraviolet; UVB, ultraviolet light B.

PRURITUS IN PREGNANCY

Pruritus has been reported in up to 17% of pregnancies. As shown in Table 51–3, a broad differential diagnosis needs to be considered, and the constellation of clinical and laboratory findings is the most helpful approach to establishing a diagnosis and reaching management decisions. In summary, a patient with pruritus in pregnancy should be evaluated as follows:

- A detailed history, past medical history, obstetric history, and physical examination are imperative for determining the cause of pruritus. The laboratory workup should be directed by the clinical findings. The constellation of

TABLE 51–3
Etiology of Pruritus in Pregnancy

Common Causes
Intrahepatic cholestasis of pregnancy
Preexisting skin diseases
Specific dermatoses of pregnancy
Systemic diseases with skin involvement
Allergic reactions
Drug eruptions
Pruritus associated with striae gravidarum
Uncommon Causes
Systemic causes of pruritus (lymphoma; liver, thyroid, or renal disease)
Viral hepatitis
Hyperbilirubinemic states
Hyperemesis gravidarum

clinical and laboratory data will help identify pruritic skin diseases that are not specifically related to pregnancy, such as scabies, or systemic disorders with skin manifestations (see the previous section).

- In the patient with pruritus and no eruption, one should consider systemic causes of pruritus such as lymphoma and liver, renal, and thyroid disease.
- In the patient with pruritus, jaundice, and no eruption, one should consider hepatitides, obstetric cholestasis, hyperbilirubinemic states, and other liver diseases.
- In the patient with pruritus and eruption, one should consider specific dermatoses of pregnancy (see the following section), allergic reactions, drug eruptions, and urticarial lesions of hepatitis B.
- In the patient with pruritus, no jaundice, no eruption, no systemic disease, and no specific pregnancy dermatosis, one should consider intrahepatic cholestasis of pregnancy, pruritus associated with striae gravidarum, and hyperemesis gravidarum complicated with cholestasis.

Obstetric Cholestasis (Intrahepatic Cholestasis of Pregnancy) (See also Chapter 47)

Generalized pruritus without a skin rash often results from obstetric cholestasis, the most common pregnancy-induced liver disorder. The condition manifests itself with jaundice (*intrahepatic jaundice of pregnancy*) or without (*pruritus gravidarum*). Viral hepatitis is the most common cause of jaundice in pregnancy, with obstetric cholestasis second. Obstetric cholestasis is very common in South Asia (0.8%–1.46%), South America (9.2%–15.6%), especially Chile and Bolivia, and Scandinavia (1.5% in Sweden).[71] The incidence of obstetric cholestasis is lower in the rest of Europe (0.1%–1.5%), the United States, Canada, and Australia. This geographic variation is thought to be due to environmental and/or dietary factors. Obstetric cholestasis recurs in 60% to 70% of subsequent pregnancies.[72] Oral contraceptives can cause a recurrence of pruritus and cholestasis. In half of the cases, there is a family history of this condition or an association with multiple-gestation pregnancy.[71] Obstetric cholestasis may occur more frequently and at an earlier gestational age in pregnant women who are positive for hepatitis C virus.

Obstetric cholestasis manifests itself in 80% of cases after the 30th week of pregnancy,[71] although initial presentation as early as 6 weeks' gestation has been reported. The pruritus, which may precede the liver function abnormalities of the condition, affects the palms and soles and extends to the legs and abdomen. Excoriations due to scratching are invariably seen. Obstetric cholestasis is occasionally preceded by a urinary tract infection. Mild nausea and discomfort in the upper right quadrant may accompany the pruritus. Mild jaundice (20%) usually develops 2 to 4 weeks after the onset of itching and may be associated with subclinical steatorrhea and increased risk of hemorrhage.[72] Up to 50% of patients develop darker urine and light-colored stools. The symptoms and biochemical abnormalities of obstetric cholestasis usually resolve within 2 to 4 weeks postpartum. An increased risk of cholelithiasis has been debated.

Elevated serum bile acids, especially postprandial elevations, are the most sensitive marker of obstetric cholestasis[71] and correlate with the severity of the pruritus. The serum bile acid profile shows characteristically an increased cholic-to-chenodeoxycholic ratio and a decreased glycine-to-taurine ratio. Mild abnormalities on liver function tests are commonly found, namely elevated cholesterol, transaminases, alkaline phosphatase, γ-glutamyltranspeptidase, and lipids. The conjugated bilirubin is mildly to moderately elevated (2–5 mg/dL) in jaundiced patients. Other authors showed an increase in low-density lipoprotein (LDL) levels as early as the 16th week of gestation and increased glutathione *S*-transferase. Malabsorption of fat may cause vitamin K deficiency, resulting in a prolonged prothrombin time. Skin biopsy is unnecessary because there are no primary skin lesions. Liver biopsy is not indicated, but if performed, shows centrilobular cholestasis, bile thrombi within dilated canaliculi, and minimal inflammatory changes.

Hormonal, immunologic, genetic, environmental, and probably alimentary factors may play a role in the etiology of obstetric cholestasis.[71] It has been suggested that the relative decrease in hepatic blood flow during gestation causes decreased elimination of toxins and estrogens. Some D-ring estrogens, in particular glucuronides like estradiol-17β-D-glucuronide, interfere with bile acid secretion and increase biliary cholesterol secretion. Progestins inhibit hepatic glucuronyltransferase, thus reducing the clearance of estrogens and amplifying their effects.[73] Monosulfated or disulfated progesterone metabolites, in particular the 3α-, 5α-isomers, are substantially increased in obstetric cholestasis secondary to decreased biliary and fecal excretion. The increased serum levels of sulfated progesterone metabolites may saturate the maximal transport capacity of membrane transport proteins of the hepatocyte. The interaction between the high levels of sex steroids produced in pregnancy and the genetically determined dysfunction of biliary canalicular ABC transporters can contribute to the development of cholestasis. An immunologic study showed a predominance of T helper-1 (Th-1) cytokines (cell-mediated immunity) and decreased maternal-fetal lymphocyte reaction in obstetric cholestasis. Another study showed increased natural killer cells and decreased T cells in the decidual parietalis and oversecretion of interferon-γ.

Genetic factors have been suggested by experimental data, the existence of familial cases, and geographic variation of obstetric cholestasis. Mutations in the canalicular transporters ABCB4 (multidrug resistance 3 gene [MDR3]) and MDR-associated protein 2 (MRP2) have been found in several families with intrahepatic cholestasis of pregnancy, and associations with these genes' polymorphisms have been reported.[73] A high prevalence of the HLA haplotype Aw31B8 has been reported. A higher incidence of obstetric cholestasis has been observed in mothers of patients with progressive familial intrahepatic cholestasis (PFIC) or benign recurrent intrahepatic cholestasis. Patients with PFIC type 3 show mutations of the MDR3 gene, which encodes the canalicular phosphatidylcholine translocase, a biliary transport protein. In a family of PFIC type 3 patients, six women with a history of obstetric cholestasis were heterozygous for the familial mutation in the MDR3 gene.[74] Environmental factors, as indicated by the geographic variation of obstetric cholestasis and its higher incidence during the winter, and alimentary factors have been implicated in the pathogenesis of obstetric cholestasis.[71] The importance of these factors, however, has been debated.

Fetal risks in obstetric cholestasis include fetal distress (22%–33%), stillbirth (0.4%–4.1%), preterm delivery (44%), and meconium staining (25%–45%).[73] Acute onset of fetal compromise (22%) and intrauterine demise (2%) have been well-documented complications.[75] Untreated intrahepatic cholestasis is assocated with increased perinatal mortality (11%–20%).[75] A twofold increase in neonatal respiratory distress syndrome has been reported.[75] Malabsorption of vitamin K increases the risk of intracranial hemorrhage. Early onset of pruritus and high levels of serum bile acids have been associated with preterm delivery and define a subgroup of patients at risk for poor neonatal outcome.[76] The pathogenesis of fetal complications is associated with decreased fetal elimination of toxic bile acids, which can cause vasoconstriction of human placental chorionic veins. Furthermore, a higher incidence of meconium passage has been reported in stillbirths in obstetric cholestasis. Meconium can cause acute umbilical vein obstruction. The incidence of meconium passage was increased with the infusion of cholic acid in animal studies.[77] Experimental data indicate that raised levels of bile acid taurocholate in the fetal serum in cholestasis of pregnancy may cause fetal dysrhythmia and sudden intrauterine fetal death.[77]

The risk of serious fetal complications in obstetric cholestasis makes intensive fetal surveillance mandatory.[78–80] Some obstetricians recommend nonstress tests or biophysical assessment, although no test reliably predicts the risk of fetal demise. Obstetric management should weigh the risk of preterm delivery against the risk of sudden death in utero and should be individualized. Glantz and coworkers[81] showed no increase in fetal risk with bile acid levels less than 40 μmol/L and suggested that these patients be managed expectantly. Because the majority of intrauterine fetal deaths in singleton pregnancies complicated by cholestasis occur after 37 weeks' gestation, delivery has been recommended no later than 37 to 38 weeks' gestation.[80,82,83] Delivery around 36 weeks or earlier, if lung maturity is achieved and cervix favorable, should be considered for severe cases with jaundice, progressive elevations in serum bile acids, and suspected fetal distress.[84] Most authors advocate starting treatment with ursodeoxycholic acid (UDCA), which has been shown to decrease fetal risks, in all patients with intrahepatic cholestasis as soon as the diagnosis is established.

Mild cholestasis can be treated symptomatically with topical antipruritics and emollients; oral antihistamines are rarely effective. Epomediol and silymarin have been helpful in mild cases.[71] Treatment with activated charcoal or benzodiazepines has met limited success. Phenobarbital has shown minimal effect on the pruritus of obstetric cholestasis and variable effects on the biochemical abnormalities of the condition.[83] UVB has been variably effective in controlling the pruritus.[68,75] The glutathione precursor *S*-adenosylmethionine has shown some relief of pruritus but does not effectively correct the biochemical abnormalities of cholestasis. Two controlled trials showed that UDCA was superior to *S*-adenosylmethionine in correcting the biochemical abnormalities of the disease[85,86]; relief of pruritus was more effectively achieved with UDCA in one of these trials.[85] Dexamethasone (12 mg/day) suppression of fetoplacental estrogen production was effective in improving the symptoms and biochemical abnormalities of cholestasis in an uncontrolled trial,[72] but a randomized, controlled trial showed that dexamethasone produced no alleviation of pruritus or reduction of alanine aminotransferase and was less effective than UDCA in reducing bile acids and bilirubin.[87]

Cholestyramine decreases the enterohepatic circulation of bile acids. It needs to be administered (≤18 g/day) for several days before a clear benefit for pruritus can be obtained and does not improve the biochemical abnormalities of obstetric cholestasis.[88] Furthermore, it has the disadvantage of precipitating vitamin K and should be administered in conjunction with weekly vitamin K supplementation.[71] A case of severe fetal intracranial hemorrhage during treatment with cholestyramine for obstetric cholestasis has been reported. Vitamin K and cholestyramine should be given at different times of the day so that cholestyramine does not interfere with vitamin K absorption. A decrease in pruritus has been reported in approximately half of the patients studied (uncontrolled), but recurrence of itching was common after the first week of treatment. Patients with high serum bile acids may not respond to cholestyramine,[88] and several patients who did not respond to cholestyramine subsequently responded to other agents, such as UDCA and dexamethasone. It may be concluded that cholestyramine can be effective only in mild to moderate obstetric cholestasis.

UDCA, a naturally occurring hydrophilic bile acid, protects against injury to bile ducts by hydrophobic bile acids and stimulates the excretion of these and other hepatotoxic compounds as well as sulfated progesterone metabolites. The medication restores the ability of the placenta to carry out bile acid transfer and reduces bile acid levels in colostrum, cord blood, and amniotic fluid.[73] It also normalizes the cholic-to-chenodeoxycholic and glycine-to-taurine ratios of the serum bile acid pool. Experimental evidence indicates that UDCA improves impaired hepatocellular secretion by mainly posttranscriptional stimulation of canalicular expression of transporters like the MRP or the bile salt export pump (ABCB11). A meta-analysis of four randomized, controlled trials indicated that UDCA, when administered in doses between 450 and 1200 mg daily, was highly effective in controlling the pruritus and liver dysfunction associated with obstetric cholestasis.[72] A dose of 12 to 15 mg/kg/day has been used in most trials,[72] although some authors reported administration of high-dose (1.5–2 g/day) UDCA with no adverse reactions. The results of this meta-analysis[72] were confirmed by a subsequent retrospective, nonrandomized study[89] over a 12-year observation period, which also showed a greated proportion of deliveries at term in patients treated with UDCA. All children whose mothers were treated with UDCA were healthy in a 12-year follow-up period. A randomized, placebo-controlled trial showed that UDCA has shown a synergistic effect with *S*-adenosylmethionine in reducing the biochemical abnormalities of cholestasis.[90] A synergistic effect on improving pruritus and biochemical abnormalities was also shown in a randomized, prospective trial that compared UDCA with intravenous *S*-adenosylmethionine. The trial, however, showed that the combined therapy had no additive effect on pruritus compared with UDCA monotherapy.[91] Compared with cholestyramine, UDCA is safer, works faster, has a more sustained and profound effect on pruritus, and shows higher efficacy in improving the biochemical abnormalities of obstetric cholestasis.[92] Babies were delivered significantly closer to term by patients treated with UDCA than by those treated with cholestyramine. UDCA has been safe for both mother and fetus and may decrease the fetal mortality associated with obstetric cholestasis.[93] Some authors suggested that it has a cardioprotective effect on the fetus against the possible toxic effect of bile acid. Data that are available support the use of UDCA as a first-line agent and cholestyramine as a second-line agent in the treatment of moderate to severe obstetric cholestasis.

SUMMARY OF MANAGEMENT OPTIONS
Pruritus in Pregnancy

Management Options	Evidence Quality and Recommendation	References
Establish the Diagnosis		
Consider: • **Specific systemic diseases** with skin involvement (see previous sections). • **No eruption**: other systemic diseases with pruritus (lymphoma; liver, renal, thyroid disease). • **No eruption and jaundice**: hepatitides, obstetric cholestasis, hyperbilirubinemic states, and other liver diseases. • **Eruption**: specific dermatoses of pregnancy (see following section), allergic reactions, drug eruptions, and urticarial lesions of hepatitis B. • **No eruption/jaundice/systemic disease or dermatosis**: obstetric cholestasis, pruritus associated with striae gravidarum, and hyperemesis gravidarum complicated with cholestasis.	—/GPP	—
Management depends on cause—see "Obstetric Cholestasis," later.		
Obstetric Cholestasis		
Maternal Treatment		
Symptomatic in mild cases (antihistamines, topical medications, UVB).	—/GPP	—
First line: ursodeoxycholic acid.	Ia/A	72
Second line: cholestyramine plus vitamin K.	Ib/A	92
Consider ursodeoxycholic acid plus *S*-adenosylmethionine (synergistic effect) in severe cases.	Ib/A	90,91
Oral contraceptives with low-estrogen or progesterone-only products can be started postpartum once LFTs normalize.	—/GPP	—
Management of Fetal Risks		
Initiate fetal surveillance as soon as diagnosis of cholestasis is established (typically not before the 30th wk).	IIa/B	78–80
Initiate maternal treatment with ursodeoxycholic acid.	Ib/A	92,93

SUMMARY OF MANAGEMENT OPTIONS

Pruritus in Pregnancy—cont'd

Management Options	Evidence Quality and Recommendation	References
Monitor LFTs and bile acids every 2–4 wk.	III/B	80
Perform elective delivery at 37–38 wk.	III/B	82,83
Perform elective delivery at 36–37 wk if fetal lung maturity and favorable cervix.	IIb/B	84

GPP, good practice point; LFTs, liver function tests; UVB, ultraviolet light B.

SPECIFIC DERMATOSES OF PREGNANCY

Specific dermatoses of pregnancy are encountered predominantly during gestation or in the puerperium and include only those skin diseases that result directly from the state of gestation or the products of conception. The classification of specific dermatoses of pregnancy into herpes gestationis, pruritic urticarial papules and plaques of pregnancy (PUPPP), prurigo gestationis, and pruritic folliculitis of pregnancy that was proposed by Holmes and Black[94] was accepted by most authors. A reclassification[95] that included prurigo gestationis and pruritic folliculitis of pregnancy under the proposed "atopic eruption of pregnancy" was debated.[96]

Pemphigoid (Herpes) Gestationis

Pemphigoid (herpes) gestationis is a rare autoimmune bullous disease of pregnancy and the puerperium. It has been rarely associated with choriocarcinoma and molar pregnancy.[97] The disease is more prevalent in white females and occurs in approximately 1 in 50,000 pregnancies.[98] Pemphigoid (herpes) gestationis usually starts in the second or third trimester, with an average onset at 21 weeks' gestation, although initial onset in the immediate postpartum period occurs in about 20% of cases.[98,99] Pemphigoid (herpes) gestationis starts with severely pruritic urticarial abdominal lesions in half of the cases (Fig. 51–15*A*). The lesions do not spare the umbilicus. A generalized bullous eruption rapidly ensues (see Fig. 51–15*B*), which may affect the palms and soles; facial and mucosal involvement is rare. Bullous lesions arise in both inflamed and clinically normal skin and, unless superinfected, heal without scarring. Annular patterns of new vesicles tend to develop at the periphery of the polycyclic lesions.

A flare at the time of delivery, preceded by a period of quiescence in late pregnancy, is typically seen (75%).[97] The disease spontaneously resolves in the postpartum period, although a protracted course and "conversion" to bullous pemphigoid have been reported. Cases with overlapping features of pemphigoid (herpes) gestationis and bullous pemphigoid have been described. Herpes gestationis often recurs in subsequent pregnancies, usually appearing at an earlier gestational age and more severely. Nevertheless, skip pregnancies occur (8%).[98,99] The postpartum duration of herpes gestationis may increase with the number of involved pregnancies. Recurrence with menses or ovulation or subsequent use of oral contraceptives has been reported.[99] The effects of breast-feeding and prolactin on prolonging the duration of pemphigoid gestationis deserve further clarification. The data previously discussed underscore the importance of hormonal factors in the pathogenesis of the disease.

Histopathology of early urticarial lesions shows a spongiotic epidermis, marked papillary dermal edema, and a mild perivascular infiltrate of lymphocytes, histiocytes, and characteristically, many eosinophils. Focal necrosis of the basal keratinocytes leads to subepidermal blister formation. Direct

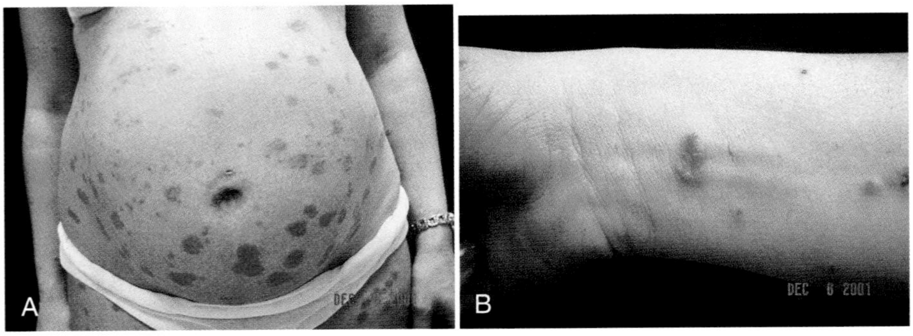

FIGURE 51–15
A, Pruritic abdominal urticarial lesions usually develop in the early phase of herpes gestationis. *B*, Characteristic tense vesicles on an erythematous base on the forearm in a patient with herpes gestationis. (*A* and *B*, Photographs courtesy of Jeffrey Callen, MD.)

immunofluorescence of perilesional skin shows linear C3 along the basement membrane zone.[1] In salt-split skin specimens, the antibody binds to the roof of the vesicle. Concomitant IgG deposition is detected in about 25% to 30% of patients. However, IgG is always positive when indirect complement-added immunofluorescence is used.[1] Deposition of IgG1 has been found in virtually all patients studied with monoclonal antibodies. Linear deposition of C3 and IgG1 has also been seen in the skin of neonates of affected mothers and in the basement membrane zone of amniotic epithelium.[91]

The antibody in pemphigoid gestationis belongs to the IgG1 subclass and is believed to activate complement through the classical pathway. Other studies, however, showed predominance of non–complement-fixing IgG4 subclass.[100] The major pathogenic antigen is the bullous pemphigoid 180-kd hemidesmosomal glycoprotein.[101] Reactivity against both the 180-kd and the 240-kd bullous pemphigoid antigens is detected in 10% of cases—the reactivity against the 240-kd antigen is thought to develop later during the disease process as a secondary response to basal keratinocyte injury[97] (*epitope spreading*). Serum antibody levels and eosinophilia do not correlate with the severity of disease. Antibody titers and immunofluorescence for C3 may remain positive even after clearance of the skin lesions or in subsequent disease-free pregnancies. The available enzyme-linked immunosorbent assays (ELISAs) have greater specificity and specificity for pemphigoid gestationis than indirect immunofluorescence. The major antigenic epitopes (A1, A2, A.25, and A3) are located in the noncollagenous domain (NC16A) of the transmembrane 180-kd antigen[102]; epitopes outside the NC16A domain have been also reported. Autoantibodies and autoimmune T lymphocytes from herpes gestationis patients recognize the NC16A2 (MCW-1) epitope[102]; these T cells express a Th-1 cytokine profile. Several authors postulate that an immunologic insult occurs against class II placental antigens of paternal haplotype, and the antibody then cross-reacts with a maternal skin basement membrane epitope.[103] This hypothesis is strengthened by a recent study that showed that the pemphigoid gestationis autoantigen is localized to the hemidesmosomes of amniotic epithelium, cultured extravillous trophoblast cells, and cells in the amniotic fluid, and its ectodomain in the amniotic fluid is structurally similar to the ectodomain produced by cultured keratinocytes.[104]

The association of pemphigoid gestationis with alleles of HLA-DR3 (61%–80%), HLA-DR4 (52%), or both (43%–50%)[105] and with the C4 null allele indicates that genetic factors may play an important role in the pathogenesis of the disease. Nonetheless, the finding of anti-HLA antibodies in all patients with herpes gestationis is considered an epiphenomenon in the disease process.[97] A change in partner has been occasionally associated with the onset of the disease,[99] and an increased prevalence of HLA-DR2 among husbands has been associated with herpes gestationis among their wives, particularly females positive for HLA-DR3/DR4. Yet, an association between change in consort and development of pemphigoid gestationis has not been consistently found,[98] and skip pregnancies despite having the same partner[98,99] would argue against this association. The role of paternal factors is intriguing but not yet entirely understood.

The differential diagnosis of pemphigoid gestationis includes drug eruptions, erythema multiforme, allergic contact dermatitis, PUPPP, and preexisting bullous disease with exacerbation during gestation, such as bullous pemphigoid. A careful history and clinical examination are usually sufficient to rule out allergic contact dermatitis, drug eruptions, and preexisting bullous disease with flare during pregnancy. Of note, bullous pemphigoid has not been reported during gestation, usually affects the elderly, and is equally common among males and females. The lesions in bullous pemphigoid are more prominent on the lower abdomen and thighs and do not cluster around the umbilicus. Erythema multiforme can be differentiated by histopathologic and immunofluorescence studies. PUPPP is the most common specific dermatosis of pregnancy that needs to be differentiated from herpes gestationis. Interestingly, PUPPP can manifest with urticarial and/or vesicular lesions almost indistinguishable from those of herpes gestationis. The two diseases, however, can be distinguished by direct immunofluorescence, which is negative in PUPPP.

Pemphigoid gestationis is associated with no maternal risks other than an increased risk of Graves' disease. Neonatal vesiculobullous lesions occur in 10% of cases[106] secondary to passive transplacental transfer of herpes gestationis antibody. The eruption is usually mild and resolves spontaneously in a few weeks as the maternal antibodies disappear from the infant's blood. The clinical course of neonatal pemphigoid gestationis is explained by the fact that the plasma elimination half-life of anti-BP 180 antibody has been shown by ELISA to be approximately 15 days. Lesions in the neonate resolve without treatment before antibody titers normalize, which indicates that factors other than the pathogenic antibody may be involved in the pathogenesis of the eruption in the nonate. Superinfection of bullous lesions warrants prompt treatment with systemic antibiotics. Monitoring for evidence of adrenal insufficiency is necessary for infants of mothers treated with oral steroids. Although an association with small–for–gestational age infants and preterm delivery has been reported,[107] no increase in fetal morbidity or mortality has been documented, with the exception of one case of fetal cerebral hemorrhage and one case of convulsions in the neonate. The fetal complications may not be altered by the use of systemic steroids[72] and are thought to be due to low-grade placental insufficiency.[103] A recent retrospective study showed that onset of pemphigoid gestationis in the first or second trimester and presence of blisters may be associated with adverse pregnancy outcomes, including prematurity and low birth weight, whereas systemic steroid treatment and autoantibody titers do not affect pregnancy outcomes.[108]

Early urticarial lesions may respond to topical steroids with or without an oral antihistamine, but most cases require oral steroids. Even though doses of prednisone up to 180 mg daily have been reported, most patients respond to lower doses (20–40 mg daily). The dose should be tapered 7 to 10 days after control is achieved. Most patients can be maintained on 5 to 10 mg of prednisone daily. The dosage should be increased at the time of delivery to control postpartum exacerbation. Plasmapheresis or chemical oophorectomy with goserelin have been used in recalcitrant herpes gestationis with some success.[97] Plasmapheresis can be considered for patients who do not respond to high doses of oral steroids or when oral steroids are contraindicated. High-dose intravenous immune globulin, alone or combined with cyclosporine, has been used to treat herpes gestationis with some success.[109] Early delivery may be warranted in refractory cases. Intractable cases may respond to postpartum administration of cyclophosphamide, pyridoxine, gold, methotrexate, dapsone, rituximab or combination of minocycline with nicotinamide.[1,97] Nevertheless, these agents have not been consistently effective, and their use is limited to patients who are not breast-feeding.

Pruritic Urticarial Papules and Plaques of Pregnancy (Polymorphic Eruption of Pregnancy)

PUPPP is the most common specific dermatosis of pregnancy, affecting approximately 1 in 240 pregnancies.[94] The term *PUPPP* was coined by Lawley and colleagues,[110] who reported a specific self-limited pruritic urticarial eruption in seven pregnant women. PUPPP occurs predominantly in primigravidas in the third trimester, with a mean onset at 35 weeks' gestation, and occasionally postpartum.[94,111] Persistence of PUPPP months to years postpartum has been reported. PUPPP has been associated with predominance of male fetuses (55%) in recent studies.[112] Familial occurrence and recurrence in subsequent pregnancies, with menses, or with oral contraceptive use are uncommon. The lesions start in the abdominal striae in two thirds of the cases, and characteristically show periumbilical sparing (Fig. 51–16*A* and *B*).[1] The eruption is polymorphous, showing urticarial and at times vesicular, purpuric, polycyclic, or targetoid lesions[111] (see Fig. 51–16*C*). Lesions can spread over the trunk and extremities, usually sparing the palms and soles. Involvement of the face and dyshidrosis-like lesions on the extremities are unusual. When generalized, PUPPP may resemble a toxic erythema (see Fig. 51–16*D*) or resolving atopic eczema. On resolution of PUPPP, extensive postinflammatory hyperpigmentation can be seen, especially in skin of color (see Fig. 51–7).

PUPPP is a clinical diagnosis because it lacks pathognomonic histopathologic features and laboratory abnormalities. The histopathology shows spongiotic dermatitis, a perivascular or upper dermal inflammatory cell infiltrate with variable numbers of eosinophils, and occasionally, mild epidermal changes such as parakeratosis, acanthosis, and exocytosis.[1] Results from immunofluorescence and serology studies are negative. Differentiation from the urticarial prebullous phase of herpes gestationis requires immunofluorescence studies (positive in herpes gestationis). Mild PUPPP requires symptomatic treatment with antipruritic topical medications, topical steroids, and oral antihistamines. Rarely, a short course of oral prednisone may be necessary. UVB can be effective (anecdotal).[1]

The pathogenesis of PUPPP has not been fully elucidated. The clinical presentation and immunohistologic profile suggest a delayed hypersensitivity reaction. No immunologic or hormonal abnormalities have been found, with the exception of a decrease in serum cortisol in one study.[17] It has been postulated that rapid abdominal wall distention in primigravidas may trigger an inflammatory process. This hypothesis was proposed by Cohen and associates,[113] who first reported an association with twin pregnancy and excessive maternal and fetal weight gains. The author's meta-analysis[72] of 282 PUPPP cases revealed 29 multiple gestation pregnancies (11.7%). This prevalence is at least 10-fold

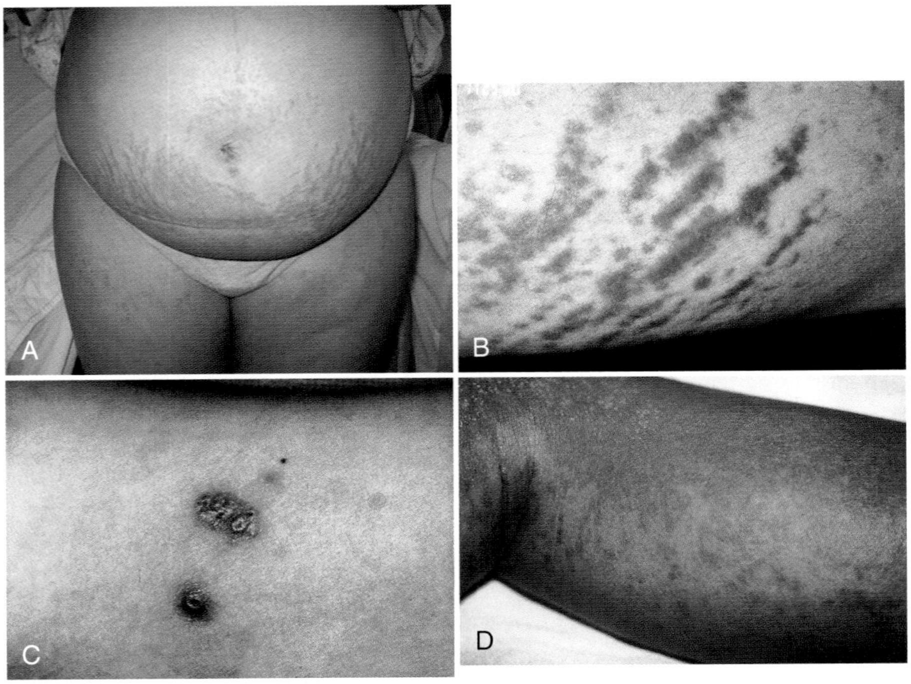

FIGURE 51–16
A, Pruritic urticarial papules and plaques of pregnancy (PUPPP): typical periumbilical sparing and distribution of the lesions along the abdominal striae. *B*, Early PUPPP shows urticarial lesions in the abdominal striae. *C*, Lesions with microvesiculated appearance on the forearm in PUPPP. *D*, Widespread PUPPP may resemble a toxic erythema. (*A–D*, Photographs courtesy of Helen Raynham, MD.)

higher than the prevalence of multiple gestation in the United States (1%).[72] The association of PUPPP with multiple-gestation pregnancy is also supported by other studies.[114,115] Furthermore, multiple gestation is characterized by higher estrogen and progesterone levels, and progesterone has been shown to aggravate the inflammatory process at the tissue level. Interestingly, increased progesterone receptor immunoreactivity has been detected in skin lesions of PUPPP.[116]

Immunohistochemical studies showed an infiltrate composed predominantly of T-helper lymphocytes.[117] Activated T cells (HLA-DR+, CD25+, LFA-1+) were found in the dermis associated with increased numbers of CD1a+, CD54+ ([intercellular adhesion molecule-1 [ICAM]+-1+) dendritic cells, and CD1a+ epidermal Langerhans cells in skin lesions, compared with unaffected skin. This immunohistologic profile may imply a delayed hypersensitivity reaction to an unknown antigen. Fetal DNA was detected in skin lesions of PUPPP by Aractingi and coworkers.[118] The authors suggested that fetal cells can migrate to maternal skin and cause PUPPP because pregnancy is associated with peripheral blood chimerism, particularly during the third trimester. The importance of microchimerism in the pathogenesis of PUPPP awaits further clarification.

PUPPP has not been traditionally associated with any maternal or fetal risks.[119] Two recent studies showed an association with cesarean section, which should be discussed with the pregnant female.[112,115] Early delivery in refractory cases is not indicated because there are no maternal or fetal risks.

FIGURE 51–17
Prurigo gestationis: excoriated papules and nodules on the extensor surfaces of the extremities. (Photograph courtesy of Cameron Thomas, Campbell Kennedy, and Phillipa Kyle.)

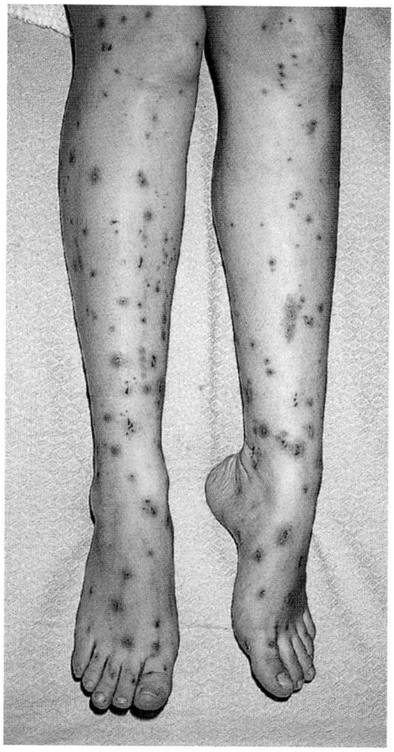

Prurigo of Pregnancy

Prurigo of pregnancy affects between 1 in 300 and 1 in 450 pregnant females.[94] The condition usually begins at about 25 to 30 weeks' gestation and manifests itself with grouped excoriated or crusted pruritic papules over the extensor surfaces of the extremities (Fig. 51–17) and occasionally on the abdomen and elsewhere.[1] The lesions may be nodular, reminiscent of prurigo nodularis. Prurigo of pregnancy commonly resolves in the immediate postpartum period but may occasionally persist for up to 3 months. On resolution of the lesions, postinflammatory hyperpigmentation develops. Recurrence in subsequent pregnancies is variable. Serology may show an elevated IgE.[17] Results of immunofluorescence studies are negative and the histopathology nonspecific. Although Spangler and colleagues[120] reported a dismal fetal outcome in their series, fetal or maternal risks have not been confirmed by any other studies. The differential diagnosis includes other specific dermatoses of pregnancy, pruritic dermatoses unrelated to pregnancy, drug eruptions, arthropod bites, and infestations such as scabies. The treatment is symptomatic with moderately potent topical steroids, if necessary intralesional or under occlusion, and oral antihistamines.[1]

The pathogenesis of prurigo of pregnancy has not been adequately studied. Although its clinical presentation is indistinguishable from that of prurigo nodularis in nonpregnant women, a flare of prurigo nodularis during pregnancy has not been reported. Prurigo of pregnancy has been associated with a family history of obstetric cholestasis. Vaughan Jones and associates[17] postulated that prurigo of pregnancy and obstetric cholestasis are closely related conditions, being distinguished only by the absence of primary lesions in obstetric cholestasis. The authors reported an association with personal or family history of atopic dermatitis and elevation of serum IgE and suggested that prurigo of pregnancy may be the result of obstetric cholestasis in women with an atopic predisposition. Furthermore, they more recently suggested that prurigo of pregnancy be classified under "atopic eruption of pregnancy."[95] Nevertheless, many patients with prurigo of pregnancy fulfilled only minor criteria of atopy in the study,[95] and IgE was not measured by the authors in a control group of pregnant women without the eruption. The regulation of IgE in pregnancy is complex and warrants further investigation. The classification of prurigo of pregnancy under "atopic eruption of pregnancy" has been debated.[96]

Pruritic Folliculitis of Pregnancy

Pruritic folliculitis of pregnancy is a rare specific dermatosis of pregnancy first described by Zoberman and Farmer.[121] In two of the original six cases, pruritic folliculitis of pregnancy had occurred in previous pregnancies. Since the original description, 26 cases have been reported.[122] Decreased awareness of the condition and the fact that many cases may be misdiagnosed as infectious folliculitis[123] or PUPPP may have contributed to an underestimate of its true prevalence. The lesions are pruritic follicular erythematous papules and

FIGURE 51–18

A, Pruritic folliculitis of pregnancy: typical follicular erythematous or pigmented papules on the abdomen. *B*, Follicular acneform pustules and papules on the upper back in pruritic folliculitis of pregnancy. *C*, Follicular erythematous papules on the lower extremities are seen less often in pruritic folliculitis of pregnancy.

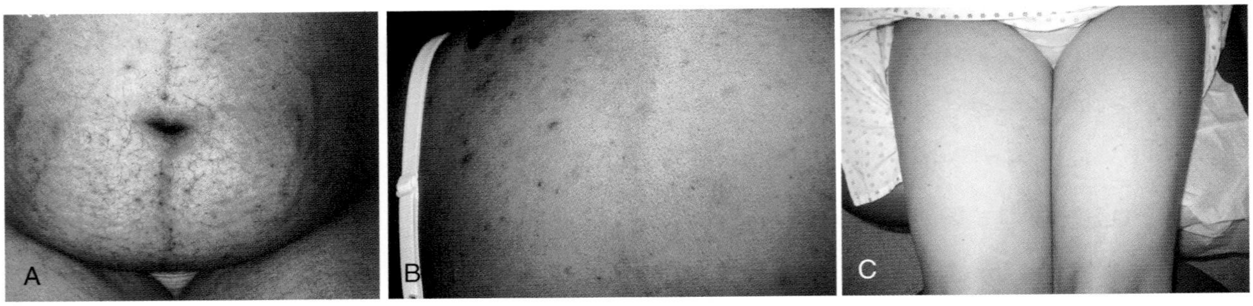

pustules that predominate on the trunk (Fig. 51–18*A* and *B*).[124] Lesions on the extremities are seen less often (see Fig. 51–18C). The eruption develops during the second or third trimester and clears spontaneously at delivery or in the postpartum period. The histopathology is that of a sterile folliculitis. Results of immunofluorescence and serology tests are negative. The differential diagnosis includes infectious folliculitis and specific dermatoses of pregnancy. An infectious folliculitis can be ruled out with special stains and cultures from the pustules. The largest series of pruritic folliculitis of pregnancy patients showed a decreased birth weight and a male-to-female ratio of 2 : 1.[17] Preterm delivery was reported in one case. No other maternal or fetal risks have been documented.

The patient should be reassured that the eruption resolves after delivery and has not been associated with substantial fetal risks. Symptomatic pruritic folliculitis of pregnancy can be treated with low- or mid-potency topical steroids, benzoyl peroxide, and UVB therapy.[1] The pathogenesis of pruritic folliculitis of pregnancy remains elusive. No immunologic or hormonal abnormalities have been found, and associations with increased serum levels of androgens or obstetric cholestasis seem to have veen coincidental. It has been suggested that pruritic folliculitis of pregnancy may be a form of hormonally induced acne, similar to the monomorphic type of acne that develops after the administration of systemic steroids or progestogens.[94] This intriguing hypothesis has not been supported by any data. Other authors have considered pruritic folliculitis of pregnancy to be a variant of PUPPP.[125] Although follicular lesions have been reported in PUPPP, the clinical presentation and histopathology of pruritic folliculitis of pregnancy differ from those of PUPPP. A more recent study classified pruritic folliculitis of pregnancy under "atopic eruption of pregnancy," but this was based on only one case (patient with family history of atopy).[95] For the time being, pruritic folliculitis of pregnancy can be considered a specific dermatosis of pregnancy.[96,126]

SUMMARY OF MANAGEMENT OPTIONS

Rashes in Pregnancy

Management Options	Evidence Quality and Recommendation	References
Establish the Cause—Two Possibilities:		
Preexisting skin conditions.	—/GPP	—
Dermatoses of pregnancy.	—/GPP	—
Pemphigoid (Herpes) Gestationis		
Perform skin immunofluorescence to confirm the diagnosis.	III/B	17
Give topical steroids with or without an oral antihistamine (e.g., diphenhydramine) for early urticarial lesions.	IV/C	97
Give oral steroids in most cases.	III/B	17
Perform plasmapheresis if oral steroids fail.	IV/C	97
Cyclosporine with IVIG may be beneficial.	IV/C	109
Immunosuppressants postpartum in non–breast-feeding mothers can be considered.	IV/C	97

Management Options	Evidence Quality and Recommendation	References
Maintain fetal surveillance (growth and health).	III/B	107,108
Maintain vigilance for neonatal herpes gestations.	IV/C	106
Polymorphic Eruption of Pregnancy		
Perform skin biopsy if herpes gestation is a consideration.	III/B	17
Reassure that there are no fetal risks.	IIb/B	119
Discuss possible association with cesarean section.	IIa/B	112,115
Prescribe topical steroids and/or antipruritic medications with or without an oral antihistamine.	III/B	17
Give oral steroids in severe cases.	III/B	17
UVB can be tried.	IV/C	1
Prurigo of Pregnancy		
Reassure that there are no fetal risks.	III/B	17
Give topical steroids with or without an oral antihistamine.	III/B	17
Give oral steroids in severe cases.	III/B	17
Pruritic Folliculitis of Pregnancy		
Perform cultures and special stains to rule out infectious folliculitides.	III/B	17
Reassure that there are no fetal risks.	III/B	17
Topical benzoyl peroxide, low- or mid-potency topical steroids, and UVB can be tried.	III/B	17

GPP, good practice point; IVIG, intravenous immunoglobulin; UVB, ultraviolet light B.

SUGGESTED READINGS

Ambros-Rundolph CM, Mullegger RR, Vaughan Jones SA, et al: The specific dermatoses of pregnancy revisited and reclassified: Results of a retrospective two-center study on 505 pregnant patients. J Am Acad Dermatol 2006;54:395–404.

Glantz A, Marschall HU, Lammert F, et al: Intrahepatic cholestasis of pregnancy: A randomized controlled trial comparing dexamethasone and ursodeoxycholic acid. Hepatology 2005;42:1399–1405.

Hale EK, Pomeranz MK: Dermatologic agents during pregnancy and lactation: An update and clinical review. Int J Dermatol 2002;41:197–203

Kenyon AP, Nelson-Piercy C, Girling J, et al: Obstetric cholestasis, outcome with active management: A series of 70 cases. BJOG 2002;109:282–288.

Kondrackiene J, Kupcinskas L: Intrahepatic cholestasis of pregnancy-current achievements and unsolved problems. World J Gastroenterol 2008;14:5781–5788.

Kroumpouzos G, Cohen LM: Dermatoses of pregnancy. J Am Acad Dermatol 2001;45:1–19.

Kroumpouzos G, Cohen LM: Specific dermatoses of pregnancy: An evidence-based systematic review. Am J Obstet Gynecol 2003;188:1083–1092.

Ohel I, Levy A, Silberstein T, et al: Pregnancy outcome of patients with pruritic urticarial papules and plaques of pregnancy. J Matern Fetal Neonat Med 2006;19:305–308.

Roger D, Vaillant L, Fignon A, et al: Specific pruritic dermatoses of pregnancy. A prospective study of 3192 women. Arch Dermatol 1994;130:734–739.

Rudolph CM, Al-Fares S, Vaughan Jones SA, et al: Polymorphic eruption of pregnancy: clinicopathology and potential trigger factors in 181 patients. Br J Dermatol 2006;154:54–60.

REFERENCES

For a complete list of references, log onto www.expertconsult.com.

CHAPTER 52

Malignant Disease

ADNAN R. MUNKARAH, CHRISTOPHER S. BRYANT, and VERONICA L. SCHIMP

INTRODUCTION

Cancer is the second leading cause of death in women of reproductive age, and fortunately, a rare cause of maternal mortality.[1,2] Between birth and 39 years of age, 1 in 52 females has invasive cancer, and approximately 3500 women between the ages of 15 and 34 years die annually of cancer in the United States.[1] It is estimated between 1 in 1000 and 1 in 1500 women will be affected by cancer while pregnant each year. The predominant malignancies associated with pregnancy are cervical cancer, breast cancer, melanoma, hematologic cancer, thyroid cancer, and colorectal cancer (Table 52–1).[3] It should be noted that preinvasive cervical cancer is often included in these numbers and that the incidence of invasive cervical cancer is likely lower than estimated.[4] No convincing data show that pregnancy adversely influences the biology, natural history, prognosis, or treatment of maternal cancer.[5]

The evaluation and treatment of pregnant women with cancer are similar to those in nonpregnant women. Both maternal and fetal outcomes should be considered when planning therapy during pregnancy. One major dilemma encountered in the treatment of pregnant women with cancer is the timing of therapeutic intervention with regard to fetal growth, development, and viability. For most malignancies, the presence of the cancer does not adversely affect the fetus. The major risk to fetal survival and normal development is the toxic effect of the various treatment modalities. Conversely, continuation of pregnancy has not been associated with accelerated tumor growth for most malignancies; therefore, elective abortion often appears to have no therapeutic advantage to the mother. Intuitively, however, any cancer left untreated has an opportunity to grow and metastasize. The therapeutic challenge for the medical team is to weigh the need to immediately intervene owing to maternal indications against the need to delay therapy for fetal well-being.

RADIATION

Radiation therapy is an effective treatment modality for a variety of cancers encountered during pregnancy. In addition, many diagnostic procedures, such as regular x-rays, radioisotope scans, and computed tomography, used in the pretreatment evaluation of malignancies are associated with radiation exposure to the mother and, potentially, to the fetus.[6] The effects of radiation on tissues are the result of multiple cellular events that include mitotic delay, cytogenetic abnormalities, mutagenesis, and apoptotic cell death.

The effects of radiation on the fetus depend on the dose of radiation delivered (total dose, field size, and distance) as well as the stage of gestation during which exposure occurred. The dose to the embryo or fetus depends on several factors. These include the teletherapy machine used and its leakage, the target dose, the size of the radiation fields, the distance from the edge of the field to the embryo or fetus, and the use of wedges, lead blocks, compensators, and other scattering objects. Factors that decrease the radiation dose to the embryo or fetus include less leakage, a lower target dose, smaller irradiation fields, greater distance between the edges of the radiation fields and the embryo or fetus, and avoidance of wedges and other scattering objects. Advances in the field of radiation oncology and new technologies have focused on optimizing the dose to the target tissue and minimizing the leakage of radiation to the surrounding organs. A distance of more than 30 cm between the edges of the radiation fields and the embryo or fetus yields a fetal exposure of only 4 to 20 cGy. Lead shielding can further reduce exposure.[7]

Before and during implantation, the embryo is a multicellular organism that is mostly sensitive to the lethal effects of radiation.[8,9] Exposure to high-energy radiation at that stage may induce cytogenetic abnormalities that will result in an abortion.[10–12] An all-or-nothing phenomenon occurs during the first 10 days after conception.

The teratogenic effects of radiation are a significant risk if the fetus is exposed during organogenesis, which usually lasts for 10 days to 7 weeks after conception. The congenital malformations that are most frequently described with exposure to high-dose radiation involve the central nervous system, skeleton, and genitals. Microcephaly is the most common malformation reported.[13] Other malformations

TABLE 52-1
Incidence of Cancer in Pregnancy

SITE OR TYPE	ESTIMATED INCIDENCE PER 1000 PREGNANCIES
Cervix	
Noninvasive	1.3
Invasive	1.0
Breast cancer	0.33
Melanoma	0.14
Ovary	0.10
Thyroid	Unknown
Leukemia	0.01
Lymphoma	0.01
Colorectal	0.02

From Allen H, Nisker J (eds): Cancer in pregnancy: An overview. In Cancer in Pregnancy: Therapeutic Guidelines. New York, Futura, 1986, pp 3–8.

include eye abnormalities, such as microphthalmia, retinal changes, and cataracts. Growth retardation and abortion can also occur during this period.

Later in gestation, the fetal organs, except for the central nervous system, become more resistant to the teratogenic effects of radiation. Exposure to high-dose radiation at that stage mainly results in growth retardation and neurophysiologic and behavioral changes that may become obvious in infancy or childhood. Data show that central nervous system malformations and growth retardation have occurred after acute exposure to more than 50 rad and until 25 weeks after conception.[13] Fetal exposure to less than 5 rad has not been associated with such effects. In utero exposure to radiation may result in an increased risk of leukemia in childhood.[13–16] This effect, however, is a subject of debate among investigators. Although some have suggested that radiation therapy may be compatible with pregnancy under strict conditions,[17] ample evidence exists that radiation therapy delivered to the abdomen and pelvis results in fetal exposure to dangerous radiation doses.

CHEMOTHERAPY

Chemotherapy is an essential part of the treatment of many malignancies, such as breast and ovarian cancers, lymphomas, and leukemias, that can occur during pregnancy.[18–23] Before the initiation of treatment with an antineoplastic agent in a pregnant woman, the potential benefits to the mother should be weighed against the potential risks to the mother and fetus. When cure is a realistic goal, appropriate treatment should be initiated as needed, without modifications that may adversely affect maternal outcome.

The physiologic changes that accompany pregnancy may alter the pharmacokinetics of various drugs, including many chemotherapeutic agents. For water-soluble drugs, the increase in plasma volume and decrease in albumin concentration may lead to a decreased concentration of the drug after bolus administration; however, its half-life will be longer. Conversely, an increase in the activity of the hepatic oxidases and an increase in glomerular filtration may lead to an increase in the hepatic or renal clearance of some agents. As with other substances, the transfer of antineoplastic agents to the fetus through the placenta is controlled by the molecular weight, lipid solubility, and protein binding of the agents. For example, the highly protein-bound nature of vinca alkaloids makes transplacental passage to the fetus inefficient.

The timing of fetal exposure to the chemotherapeutic agents is one of the most important determinants of pregnancy outcome. In the first trimester, exposure to chemotherapy can result in congenital malformations or abortion.[18,24,25] The risk of congenital malformations has been reported to be as high as 17%. The folic acid antagonists aminopterin and methotrexate, when used in the first trimester, seem to be more teratogenic than other antineoplastic agents. Taking into account a background risk of 3% for congenital malformations, the use of cytotoxic drugs during organogenesis is associated with a risk as high as 17%. Excluding folate antagonists, the risk is estimated at 6%.[26] Syndromes of congenital anomalies that include cranial anomalies, cleft palate, anencephaly, and micrognathia have been associated with the use of aminopterin. Similarly, the use of alkylating agents and procarbazine has led to skull abnormalities known as "cloverleaf skull," or oxycephaly.[27–32] First-trimester use of alkylating agents and procarbazine is also associated with an increased risk of fetal malformations.[33] Second- and third-trimester exposure to chemotherapy does not seem to result in an increased risk of congenital malformations except for microcephaly. However, chemotherapy given at those stages has been associated with other complications including spontaneous abortion, low birth weight, intrauterine growth retardation, premature birth, mental retardation, and impaired learning behavior. The alkylating agents cyclophosphamide, cisplatin, and carboplatin seem to be relatively safe to be administered at that stage. Some authors have suggested that cisplatin may be preferable in pregnancy to carboplatin, because carboplatin is more myelosuppressive and less protein-bound and thus possibly more prone to transplacental transfer.[26] However, there are a number of reports regarding the use of carboplatin with normal neonatal outcome; in some of these, it was used in combination with paclitaxel, another commonly used chemotherapy drug.[34] No fetal problems were reported in at least 11 case reports using taxanes alone or in combination regimens for lung, ovarian, and breast cancer.[35]

Myelosuppression is a side effect common to many chemotherapeutic agents. Maternal thrombocytopenia or leukopenia at the time of delivery can result in significant complications including massive hemorrhage and serious infections. Therefore, the timing of delivery should be well planned in a woman who is receiving chemotherapy. Unwanted toxicities to the mother and fetus at the time of delivery commonly result in the discontinuation of chemotherapy administration 3 to 4 weeks preceding delivery.[36] Rarely is chemotherapy indicated after 35 weeks' gestation.

SUMMARY OF MANAGEMENT OPTIONS

Cancer Treatment

Management Options	Evidence Quality and Recommendation	References
Radiation		
Fetal exposure from imaging doses are given in Table 52–2.	III/B	6
Lead screening reduces embryo/fetal exposure and risk.	III/B	7
Main risk to early embryo is miscarriage.	III/B	10–12
Main risks between 10 days and 7 wk is teratogenesis (if >50 rads).	III/B	13
After embryogenesis, the main risks are growth restriction and impaired neurobehavioral development (if >50 rads).	III/B	13–16
Chemotherapy		
Physiologic changes of pregnancy may alter the pharmacokinetics of chemotherapeutic agents.	III/B	25
In first trimester, the main risks are miscarriage and fetal abnormality (17%), especially with the folate antagonists.	III/B	24–32
In second and third trimester, the main risks are growth restriction, preterm delivery, and impaired neurobehavioral development.	III/B	29

TABLE 52–2

Estimated Average Fetal Dose

ROENTGENOGRAM OF MOTHER	DOSE TO FETUS (RAD)
Barium enema	0.800
Upper gastrointestinal series	0.560
Intravenous pyelogram	0.400
Hip	0.300
Abdomen	0.290
Lumbar spine	0.275
Cholecystography	0.200
Pelvis	0.040
Chest	0.008
Skull	0.004
Cervical spine	0.002
Shoulder	0.001
Extremity (upper or lower)	0.001
Computed tomography scan of abdomen and pelvis	3.00

From Deppe G, Munkarah A, Malone JM Jr: Neoplasia. In Gleicher N, Buttino L (eds): Principles and Practice of Medical Therapy in Pregnancy, 2nd ed. Norwalk, CT, Appleton & Lange, 1988, pp 1231–1234.

CERVICAL CANCER

Cervical cancer is diagnosed in pregnancy with a frequency of 10 to 1000 cases per 100,000 pregnancies.[37] The wide variability in the incidence reported in the literature seems to be caused by the inclusion of patients with postpartum cancer, carcinoma in situ, and preinvasive disease. A recent cancer registry study[5] reported cervical cancer as the most common gynecologic malignancy to occur during pregnancy and represented 15% of all cancers during pregnancy. It is estimated that between 1% and 3% of patients with cervical cancer are pregnant at the time of diagnosis.[38] The mean age of pregnant patients at the time of diagnosis of cervical cancer is 31.6 years (range 31–36.5 yr).[39] As in nonpregnant patients, the most common histologic type is squamous cell carcinoma, which accounts for more than 80% of all cervical cancers.[40] More than 70% of patients have early-stage disease, which includes FIGO (International Federation of Gynecology and Obstetrics) stages I to IIA lesions.[40–43] Diagnosis may be made at an earlier stage in pregnancy because pregnant women are seen frequently by health care providers and undergo routine examinations and Pap smears. One third of pregnant patients who are diagnosed with cervical cancer are asymptomatic, with diagnosis made at the time of an abnormal Pap smear result. The interpretation of Pap smears obtained during pregnancy can be problematic, because several common physiologic changes associated with the gravid state can lead to false-positive results.[44–46] For example, eversion of the transformation zone and exposure of columnar cells to the acid pH of the vagina cause squamous metaplasia that may be falsely interpreted as dysplasia. The changes seen with Arias-Stella reaction can resemble those of endocervical adenocarcinoma.[47,48] In one study of gravid hysterectomy specimens, Arias-Stella reaction was reported in 9% of specimens examined.[49] Another cause of false-positive Pap smear is related to the presence of trophoblastic cells that may be misinterpreted as dysplastic cells in the cytologic specimen. It is essential to inform the cytopathologist interpreting the Pap smear that the patient is pregnant.

Historically, it was believed that pregnancy had an adverse effect on the natural history of cervical cancer. Multiple studies have shown that there is no difference in survival between pregnant and nonpregnant cervical cancer patients when matched by age, stage, and year of diagnosis.[5,38–40,43,48,50–52] In addition, the decision for a vaginal delivery versus a cesarean delivery depends on the stage of disease at the time of diagnosis.[44] Microinvasive or early invasion is not a contraindication to vaginal delivery.[44,53] However, gross tumor present at the time of delivery may have a higher likelihood of peripartum complications and potentially higher risk of locoregional recurrence and death.[54,55]

Management Options

Colposcopy is a safe and reliable method for evaluation pregnant patients with abnormal cervical cytologic findings.[56–60] The interpretation of colposcopy during pregnancy is more difficult owing to increased cervical volume, stromal edema, glandular hyperplasia, and increased vascularization.[4] Colposcopy-direct biopsy may be performed during any trimester, although most colposcopists suggest delaying biopsy until the second trimester. The main complication associated with cervical biopsy during pregnancy is bleeding; however, this usually can be controlled with the application of Monsel's solution and pressure. Endocervical biopsy must be avoided during pregnancy because of the risk of premature rupture of the membranes, preterm labor, and uncontrollable bleeding.[55] Many investigators estimate that without colposcopic findings suggestive of cancer, the likelihood of invasive cancer or progression to invasive cancer is low and that carcinoma in situ lesions may be treated conservatively until the postpartum period with periodic control colposcopy antenatally.[61] During pregnancy, diagnostic cervical conization is reserved for selected indications including (1) the diagnosis of minimal stromal invasion on a colposcopically directed biopsy and (2) persistent cytologic abnormalities suspicious of invasive cancer on Pap smear.[44] Fortunately, eversion of the squamocolumnar junction during pregnancy improves access to the endocervix and decreases the necessary volume of tissue to be removed if conization is performed. The risks of immediate and delayed bleeding after conization are 8.9% and 3.7%, respectively.[51] An estimated blood loss of 500 mL has been reported to occur during conization procedures performed during pregnancy.[44] Other infrequent complications include premature labor, chorioamnionitis, and fetal loss.[62]

Pregnant women who are diagnosed with invasive cervical cancer should be counseled extensively about treatment options as well as the effect of the treatment on the mother and fetus. Many factors should be considered in treatment planning, including gestational age, tumor size and stage, and the patient's desire to preserve the pregnancy. Few studies have evaluated the effect of delaying definitive therapy until fetal maturity is reached.[63–70] In these reports, treatment delays ranging from 21 to 212 days to allow for fetal maturity did not result in decreased maternal survival. At last follow-up, 96% of the patients were alive without disease. However, the numbers of patients in these series are small and definitive conclusions should be drawn cautiously. Two intervention options have been described in case reports for patients diagnosed with cervical cancer greater than FIGO stage IA and who desire pregnancy preservation. One is a surgical excision option, which involves an abdominal radical trachelectomy during pregnancy; it is hazardous and associated with significant risk of surgical complication and pregnancy loss.[71] Alternatively, neoadjuvant chemotherapy during pregnancy has been used with the intent to stabilize or reduce the cervical tumor.[67] Cesarean delivery followed by definitive treatment would be performed after fetal maturity. For patients with more advanced disease and at less than 20 weeks' gestation, termination of pregnancy is an option so that definitive management is not delayed.[38,44,72] The choice of treatment modality for pregnant patients with invasive cervical cancer is based on the same principles that are used in the nonpregnant state. Patients with early-stage disease can be treated surgically with radical hysterectomy and bilateral pelvic lymphadenectomy.[63,64,73,74] Depending on the time of diagnosis, surgery can be done early in gestation with termination of the pregnancy or at cesarean delivery. Except for increased blood loss, there is no significant increase in other perioperative complications compared with nonpregnant patients, and the cure rates are comparable.[64] Radiation therapy with chemosensitization is used to treat advanced disease that is not amenable to surgical management. When radiation is administered in the first trimester, spontaneous abortion usually occurs at a cumulative dose of 30 to 50 Gy. Treatment in the second trimester results in abortion at a higher cumulative radiation dose and less reliably. If spontaneous abortion did not occur by the end of the external radiation therapy, surgical evacuation should be performed before brachytherapy.[75] For patients who are treated after delivery, most radiotherapists wait a few weeks for uterine involution before starting treatment. Tumor stage is an important predictor of survival in cervical cancer. The outcome of patients with early-stage disease is excellent, with 5-year survival rates exceeding 90%.[40] In one report, the survival rate was worse and risk of recurrence was higher in women who were diagnosed postpartum than in those diagnosed during pregnancy.[65] One uncommon site of tumor recurrence when cervical cancer occurs in pregnancy is the episiotomy incision line.[76–78] It is believed that tumor cells can implant at the site of the episiotomy incision after vaginal delivery.

SUMMARY OF MANAGEMENT OPTIONS

Cervical Cancer

Management Options	Evidence Quality and Recommendation	References
Diagnosis		
Physical examination and cervical smear at first prenatal visit in high risk and those without smear in previous 3 yr.	III/B	56–61
Colposcopy and directed biopsies for suspicious lesions, though measures are needed to deal with increased bleeding risk.	III/B	51,55–61

Management Options	Evidence Quality and Recommendation	References
Cone biopsy when microinvasion suspected on directed biopsies; loop excision may be associated with increased preterm births.	III/B	55,62
Treatment		
Cervical Intraepithelial Neoplasia		
Follow-up with colposcopy during pregnancy.	III/B	59,61
Microinvasive Cancer		
After careful maternal counseling, consider delaying definitive therapy until fetal maturity is reached (enhance with steroids) and delivery is completed.	III/B	51–53, 63–70,74
Invasive Cancer		
Use same therapy guidelines as for nonpregnant patient:		
• Before 20 wk: consider termination and immediate therapy.	III/B	38,44,63, 64,71–74
• After 20 wk: consider awaiting fetal maturity (enhance with steroids), then deliver and implement therapy postnatally.	III/B	63,64,73, 74,78
Elective cesarean hysterectomy can be considered with early-stage disease.	III/B	53
Careful patient counseling required with either presentation.	III/B	63,64,73, 74,78
Prognosis		
Impact of cervical cancer during pregnancy does not appear to influence outcomes. However, some studies suggest a worse prognosis when diagnosed after pregnancy.	III/B	65,68
Reports of recurrences in episiotomy sites after vaginal birth.	III/B	63,78

OVARIAN CANCER

Ovarian cancer occurs in between 10 and 40 per 100,000 pregnancies and is the fifth most common malignancy diagnosed during pregnancy.[37,79] Most ovarian masses are diagnosed incidentally at the time of obstetric ultrasound. They are frequently nonmalignant and are found on histologic examination to be functional ovarian cysts (41%), endometriomas (24%), dermoid (18%), serous cystadenoma (6%), mucinous cystadenoma (3%), paraovarian cyst (3%), and borderline serous tumor (5%).[80] The risk of malignant or borderline ovarian neoplasm discovered during pregnancy ranges from 2% to 5% compared with 20% outside of pregnancy.[81–83] The histologic distribution of ovarian cancers diagnosed in pregnancy is different from that seen in the general population, partly because pregnant women are relatively young and have a higher incidence of germ cell tumors. Germ cell tumors account for 6% to 40% of malignant neoplasm complicating pregnancy; conversely, epithelial malignancies account for 49% to 75% and gonadal stromal tumors for 9% to 16%.[84–89] The distribution of subtypes of germ cell tumors diagnosed during pregnancy has varied among published series. Whereas some indicate that dysgerminomas are the most common subtype,[82,86,87] others indicate that malignant teratomas[84,85] and endodermal sinus tumors[90] are more common. Most ovarian malignancies diagnosed in pregnancy are stage I, as would be expected with germ cell tumors.

Management Options

Management of an adnexal mass during pregnancy depends on the ultrasonographic characteristics of the mass and the gestational age. Some authors recommend to proceed with surgical exploration early in the second trimester for lesions that are larger than 6 cm, have a significant solid component, are bilateral, or persist after 14 weeks' gestation.[91,92] However, others encourage conservative management secondary to the low risk of malignancy and acute complications.[93] The serum cancer antigen 125 (CA-125) level can be elevated in normal pregnancies, especially in the first trimester, and low-level elevations are typically not associated with pregnancy.[93,94] Ovarian neoplasms, even when benign, are associated with increased risk of complications during pregnancy. Adnexal torsion is reported in up to 25% of patients.[95–97] Other complications include rupture and hemorrhage.[93,98] The risk of pregnancy loss or preterm labor is increased if surgery is performed for one of these acute complications.

Unilateral salpingo-oophorectomy with staging biopsy is the recommended surgery for stage I germ cell tumors.

Patients with stage IA dysgerminomas and stage IA grade 1 immature teratomas do not require further adjuvant therapy. The remaining germ cell tumors behave more aggressively and usually require adjuvant chemotherapy even in early stages. Treatment of advanced germ cell tumors of any histologic subtype includes surgery and chemotherapy. In anecdotal reports of pregnant patients with malignant ovarian germ cell tumors treated with combination chemotherapy (bleomycin, etoposide, cisplatin and vinblastine), good maternal and fetal outcomes were achieved.[99–101] Patients with early-stage epithelial ovarian carcinomas can be treated successfully with conservative surgery, including salpingo-oophorectomy and staging biopsy. Advanced-stage disease presents a management problem. Tumor debulking surgery is often extensive and may result in adverse pregnancy outcome. This surgery may be performed after vaginal delivery or at the same time as the cesarean section. Platinum-based chemotherapy is usually used postoperatively. Few case reports describe successful treatment of advanced ovarian cancer in pregnancy with surgery and chemotherapy.[16,21,26,34–36,92] Gonadal stromal tumors are uncommon in pregnancy. They are often confined to the ovary and have an indolent course. Treatment involves unilateral salpingo-oophorectomy.

SUMMARY OF MANAGEMENT OPTIONS

Ovarian Cancer

Management Options	Evidence Quality and Recommendation	References
Diagnosis		
Often diagnosed as a chance finding during an obstetric ultrasound examination.	III/B	80,91,92
CA-125 levels are unhelpful because they can be raised in normal pregnancy.	III/B	93,94
MRI helpful.	IV/C	89
Treatment		
Surgical exploration ideally performed in second trimester.	III/B	84–86
Pregnancy preservation and conservative surgery with unilateral salpingo-oophorectomy and staging biopsies are possible in most early-stage ovarian cancers (uncommon).	III/B	84–86
Chemotherapy, if needed, has risks (see earlier and Chapter 39).	III/B	16,21,24–32
Salvage of the pregnancy may not be possible with advanced disease.	III/B	16,21,26,34–36, 84–86,92

MRI, magnetic resonance imaging.

OTHER GYNECOLOGIC MALIGNANCIES

Vulvar carcinoma in pregnancy is extremely rare. The most common histologic varieties are invasive squamous cell carcinoma and melanoma.[102] Radical excision of the primary lesion with inguinofemoral node dissection is the treatment of choice for stage I and II tumors.[103] The timing of treatment and mode of delivery are usually dependent on the time of diagnosis during pregnancy. The current recommendation is to proceed with definitive surgical treatment before 36 weeks' gestation.[102,104,105] If wounds have healed, then cesarean is indicated only for obstetric indications. Human papillomavirus–related intraepithelial neoplasia might be treated with laser vaporization, surgical excision, or observation. Although the use of imiquimod has been described during pregnancy,[106] the application of podophylline or imiquimod is contraindicated.

Few cases of endometrial carcinoma have been reported during pregnancy.[107–109] Surprisingly, some were associated with a viable fetus.[84,85] The remaining cases were diagnosed at the time of dilation and curettage performed for miscarriage or postpartum bleeding. This highlights the importance of evaluation of abnormal postpartum bleeding despite the protective effects of pregnancy.[110]

SUMMARY OF MANAGEMENT OPTIONS

Other Gynecologic Malignant Disease in Pregnancy

Management Options	Evidence Quality and Recommendation	References
Vulval Carcinoma		
Histologic varieties most commonly encountered are invasive squamous cell carcinomas and melanomas.	III/B	102–105
Radical excision of the primary lesion and inguinal femoral node dissection is the treatment of choice for stages I and II squamous cell cancer.	III/B	102–105
Timing of treatment and mode of delivery are usually dependent on the time of diagnosis during pregnancy. It has been recommended to proceed with definitive surgical treatment at any time during pregnancy up to 36 wk' gestation. Patients can be allowed to deliver vaginally, provided the wounds have healed.	III/B	102–105
Endometrial Carcinoma		
Endometrial cancers rarely occur during pregnancy. Surprisingly, 30% were associated with a viable fetus. The remaining cases were diagnosed at the time of dilation and curettage performed for irregular bleeding.	III/B	107–110

BREAST CANCER

Pregnancy-associated breast cancer is usually defined as carcinoma that is diagnosed during pregnancy or within 1 year postpartum.[111,112] It is second only to cervical cancer as one of the most common types of pregnancy-associated cancers.[37] Approximately 15% of breast cancers occur in women of childbearing age and 3% of breast cancers occur in pregnancy. The incidence is approximately 10 to 40 per 100,000 pregnancies.[37,113] Pregnancy-associated breast cancer usually presents as advanced disease; the largest proportion of stages II to IV breast cancers are reported among women diagnosed during pregnancy or less than 2 years postpartum.[114] Between 53% and 74% of pregnant women who are diagnosed with breast cancer have evidence of lymph node metastases. A delay in diagnosis has been reported as a potential cause for the advance stage at diagnosis. The estimated delay in the diagnosis of breast during pregnancy is between 1 and 6 months or more.[111] Physiologic changes that affect the breast during gestation make clinical examination difficult and inaccurate. In addition, physicians may be reluctant to perform breast biopsy during pregnancy and lactation because of the increased risk of bleeding, infection, and milk fistulas. Traditionally, it was believed that pregnancy adversely affected the outcome of patients with breast cancer. Earlier reports had shown poor survival in women with pregnancy-associated breast cancer.[115–118] In at least one series, pregnancy was found to be an independent adverse prognostic factor in multivariate analysis; however, it is unclear whether delay in treatment may have contributed to the poorer survival.[115] In contrast, there are data that show identical survival rates in pregnant women and nonpregnant cohorts when matched for disease stage.[5,72,119–121] The 5-year survival rate for pregnant women with stage I disease have been reported to be 90%.[122] In an analysis of selected studies, an expert panel concluded that the worse prognosis in pregnant women with breast cancer is probably caused by the advanced stages of the cancer at diagnosis or a less standardized therapy.[123]

Management Options

Pregnant women should have a baseline breast examination at the first prenatal visit. Diagnostic mammography can be performed safely during pregnancy when clinically indicated; however, it should not be done routinely because of concern about fetal irradiation. A bilateral mammogram performed with modern equipment yields less than 500 μGy to the human embryo, which is well below the 100-mGy toxic level.[7] The mammogram may have limited diagnostic utility because of the hyperemia and edema that affect the mammary tissues and contribute to the generalized radiographic density of the breasts. Mammography is one of the most intensely studied imaging procedures during pregnancy and the only imaging procedure to rule out microcalcifications and should be used if it is necessary.[123] Ultrasound is accurate in differentiating between cystic and solid masses. The detection of a mass necessitates prompt evaluation with fine-needle aspiration or surgical biopsy. An experienced cytologist should evaluate the cells obtained from aspirates because hyperproliferative physiologic changes in the mammary tissue may be mistaken for malignancy. Because atypical cytomorphologic findings are encountered during gestation and lactation, some authors describe a core biopsy as a more sensitive and specific method for evaluating a suspicious, palpable mass.[124] The increased risk of complications associated with breast biopsy during pregnancy should not deter the surgeon from performing these procedures when clinically indicated.[111]

As in the nonpregnant patient, staging of breast cancer during pregnancy involves a complete physical examination, blood testing, and chest x-ray with abdominal shielding. Evaluation of the liver can be safely performed using ultrasound.[125] A radionuclide bone scan can cause significant fetal exposure to radiation. Because of lower yield in early-stage disease, bone scans should be limited to patients with more advanced disease. Magnetic resonance imaging (MRI) during pregnancy is generally considered safe for the mother and fetus; it is being used with increasing frequency to diagnose bone, liver, and brain metastases. MRI has been used to evaluate many obstetric and fetal conditions without any evidence of harmful effects.[126] One advantage of this imaging modality is its avoidance of exposure of the fetus to ionizing radiation. However, gadolinium is known to cross the placenta and was associated with fetal abnormalities in animal models, especially during the first trimester.[127]

Mastectomy with axillary lymph node dissection has been the most common breast surgery for stages I, II and some stage III breast cancers when the patient wants to continue the pregnancy.[128,129] A major advantage of mastectomy is the elimination of the need for breast radiation therapy. The indications for axillary lymph node dissection are similar in the pregnant and the nonpregnant patients with breast cancer. Lumpectomy with axillary lymph node dissection is feasible and safe in pregnant woman with breast cancer[130,131] and is reported to have no adverse impact on locoregional recurrence rates.[132] Owing to the reduction in short- as well as long-term morbidity, there has an increasing interest in sentinel node biopsy. The use of radiocolloid injections during sentinel node localization procedures does not appear to significantly increase the risk of prenatal death, fetal malformation, or mental impairment.[133] A recent review of a prospectively collected database revealed that sentinel lymph node biopsy could be performed safely during pregnancy.[113] Sixty percent of the population had combined sentinel node localization procedures (technetium-99m and blue dye) with 90% achieving successful pregnancy and delivery. The most common reported reason for unsuccessful pregnancy was first-trimester voluntary termination of pregnancy.[113] Alternatively, blue-staining alone can be used and appears to be of little risk to the fetus. More data are needed regarding the use of sentinel node biopsy as a standard in pregnant women with localized disease.[134]

The standard breast radiation therapy course of approximately 5000 cGy exposes the fetus to a radiation dose that varies according to gestational age and the associated anatomic changes. Early in pregnancy, when the uterus is still in the pelvis, fetal exposure may be as low as 10 cGy. However, in late pregnancy, when the fetus moves up into the mother's abdomen, fetal exposure can reach 200 cGy. Conversely, for some women diagnosed with early breast cancer in the third trimester, delaying treatment until after parturition is an acceptable option with minimal maternal risks and obvious fetal benefit.[135,136]

Adjuvant chemotherapy is indicated in patients with specific high risk factors including those with lymph node metastases. During organogenesis in the first trimester, the risks of teratogenicity and fetal malformation should be weighed carefully against the potential benefits. Chemotherapy administration during the second and third trimesters appears to be feasible. Many agents with known activity in breast cancer have been safely administered during pregnancy for the treatment of other cancers.[137–140] However, some agents may offer a potentially excessive risk of fetal toxicity.[141,142] Antimicrotubule agents paclitaxel, docetaxel, and vinorelbine display a high activity against breast cancer and have a favorable toxicity profile when administered during pregnancy.[36] The transplacental transfer of chemotherapy agents varies greatly, and it is commonly recommended that chemotherapy administration be discontinued 3 weeks preceding delivery.[36] Chemotherapy during pregnancy may also result in maternal complications, including sepsis and hemorrhage, with unplanned labor and delivery.

Breast cancer in young patients (≤35 yr) overexpress HER-2 in up to 35% of cases.[143] The HER-2 targeting agent trastuzumab has been used for the treatment of advanced breast cancer in pregnant patients. Although assigned a category B pregnancy risk on the basis of trials in monkeys, fetal effects vary based on gestational age and length of exposure. Its use has been associated with uteroplacental complications.[144] Lapatinib, a tyrosine kinase inhibitor, has been reported in only one patient who unexpectedly became pregnant during a phase I trial. There were no reported adverse events during the pregnancy or delivery.[145] Hormonal therapy with tamoxifen is contraindicated during pregnancy because of its teratogenic effect and the risk of severe fetal malformations.[146] There are no published reports of the use of aromatase inhibitors for the treatment of breast cancer during pregnancy. Animal studies have reported that aromatase is needed during embryo and fetal development. The inhibition of aromatase during the prenatal period may interfere with the development of fetal gonadocytes and sexual differentiation of the brain and significantly impair the pregnancy outcome.[147,148] Advanced-stage disease requires both chemotherapy and radiation therapy. The prognosis is poor, and maternal survival is limited. Management of these patients during pregnancy presents ethical and medical dilemmas and should be planned on an individual basis.

Published literature does not support the routine recommendation of therapeutic abortion in pregnant patients with breast cancer.[111,149] Many authors showed that survival is not improved by pregnancy termination for maternal indications.[150–152] In some cases, therapeutic abortion may be strongly recommended because of potential fetal damage from the proposed chemotherapy or radiation treatments. In early pregnancy, treatment is greatly simplified with therapeutic abortion.[111] Subsequent pregnancy in women who have been treated for breast cancer does not seem to confer a worse prognosis than that in patients who did not become pregnant. Interestingly, few population-based studies have shown that a subsequent pregnancy results in an improvement in survival, with favorable relative risks of 0.2 (range 0.1–0.5)[112] to 0.8 (range 0.3–2.3).[135,136] However, it is difficult to draw definite conclusions from available studies because of the small number of patients reported and the associated selection bias. Because recurrence is most likely to occur in the first 2 years, most investigators recommend delaying conception for 2 to 3 years after treatment. A recent publication has even suggested that premenopausal women with localized disease and good prognosis are unlikely to have a reduced survival if conception is delayed only 6 months after treatment.[153]

SUMMARY OF MANAGEMENT OPTIONS

Breast Cancer and Pregnancy

Management Options	Evidence Quality and Recommendation	References
Diagnosis		
Physiologic changes of pregnancy reduce the sensitivity of physical examination and mammography.	IV/C	111,123
Fine-needle aspiration of any suspicious lesion.	IV/C	111,124
Open biopsy if the results of needle biopsy are equivocal.	IV/C	111,124
Treatment		
Mastectomy with lymph node dissection is the preferred treatment for early cancers. Indications for lymph node dissection are similar in the pregnant and the nonpregnant patients.	III/B	129
Sentinal node localization procedures appear safe during pregnancy.	III/B	113,133,134
Adjuvant chemotherapy may be indicated for some patients with high risk cancers. Both maternal benefits and potential risks to the fetus should be weighed carefully.	III,IV/B,C	111,129
If diagnosis is made late in pregnancy and chemotherapy or radiation treatment is indicated, consider delaying therapy until after delivery.	IIb/B	128,135,136
Routine therapeutic abortions are not indicated.	III/B	111,122,149
Termination of pregnancy may be considered in patients with advanced disease if chemotherapy and/or radiation treatment is indicated in early pregnancy.	IIa/B	136
Recommend delaying conception for 2–3 yr after treatment.	IIa/B	111,136,153

PLACENTAL METASTASES

Metastasis of maternal malignancy into the placenta is rare and poorly understood. Malignant melanoma is the most common maternal malignancy associated with placental metastasis; it accounts for nearly one third of reported cases.[151,154] Next in frequency are hematopoietic malignancies and breast carcinoma.[151,155,156] Fetal metastasis is extremely rare, even when the maternal surface of the placenta contains evidence of metastatic tumor. The low incidence of fetal metastasis has been attributed to two factors: inherent resistance of the trophoblast to tumor invasion and possible immune rejection by the fetal immune system.[155] Interestingly, after delivery, some infants with metastatic melanoma have complete tumor regression and long-term survival. Comprehensive understanding of maternal cancers with metastasis to the placenta or fetus would benefit from a registry of malignancies associated with pregnancy.[156,157]

SUGGESTED READINGS

Amant F, Van Calstseren K, Vergote I, Ottevanger N: Gynecologic oncology in pregnancy. Crit Rev Oncol Hematol 2007;67:187–195.

Behtash N, Zarchi MK, Gilani MM, et al: Ovarian carcinoma associated with pregnancy: A clinicopathologic analysis of 23 cases and review of the literature. BMC Pregnancy Childbirth 2008;8:3.

Cradonick E, Iacobuxxi A: Use of chemotherapy during human pregnancy. Lancet Oncol 2004;5:283–291.

Kal HB, Struikmans H: Radiotherapy during pregnancy: Fact and fiction. Lancet Oncol 2005;6:328–333.

Lee JM, Lee KB, Kim YT, et al: Cervical cancer associated with pregnancy: Results of a multicenter retrospective Korean study (KGOG-1006). Am J Obstet Gynecol 2008;1981:92.e1–92.e6.

Loibl S, von Minckwitz G, Gwyn K, et al: Breast carcinoma during pregnancy. International recommendations from an expert meeting. Cancer 2006:106:237–246.

McIntyre-Seltman K, Lesnock JL: Cervical cancer screening in pregnancy. Obstet Gynecol Clin North Am 2008;35:645–658.

Mir O, Berveiller P, Ropert S, et al: Emerging therapeutic options for breast cancer chemotherapy during pregnancy. Ann Oncol 2008;19:607–613.

Patel SJ, Reede DL, Katz DS, et al: Imaging the pregnant patient for nonobstetric conditions: Algorithms and radiation dose considerations. Radiographics 2007;27:1705–1722.

Stensheim H, Moller B, van Dijk T, Fossa SD: Cause-specific survival for women diagnosed with cancer during pregnancy or lactation: A registry-based cohort study. J Clin Oncol 2009;27:45–51.

REFERENCES

For a complete list of references, log onto www.expertconsult.com.

CHAPTER 53

Pregnancy after Transplantation

VINCENT T. ARMENTI, MICHAEL J. MORITZ, and JOHN M. DAVISON

INTRODUCTION

Transplantation is now an accepted therapeutic option for patients with end-stage organ failure. The first successful human kidney transplant took place in 1954.[1] However, it was not until the 1960s that immunosuppression became available and not until the 1980s, with the introduction of cyclosporine, that consistently acceptable graft and patient survival was achieved. With the restoration of organ function, patients experience an overall improvement in their health, increased libido, and return of fertility.

The first post-transplant pregnancy occurred in March 1958 and was reported in 1963.[2] It occurred in a patient who had received a kidney from her identical twin.[2] This pregnancy resulted in cesarean delivery of a healthy boy. As transplantation has progressed, with improvements in surgical techniques and medical therapy and advances in immunosuppression, pregnancies have been reported in recipients of each organ type. Most outcomes reported are in kidney transplant recipients. Issues that must be considered include maternal graft function and maternal health, the effect of pregnancy on graft function, and the effect of the medications and graft function on the developing fetus. There is also concern about the long-term effects of pregnancy on graft function. Finally, there is the question of whether more subtle and long-term effects, although not apparent at birth, might affect the growth and development of the offspring of these recipients or future generations.

ORGAN TRANSPLANTATION

Patients with end-stage renal disease who are receiving or will soon need dialysis are candidates for renal transplantation. Common indications for renal transplantation are glomerulonephritis, diabetes, polycystic kidney disease, and hypertension. In 2008, in the United States, 16,514 kidney transplants were performed.[3] The 1-year graft survival rate was 90% for deceased donor kidneys and 98% for living donor kidneys.[4] Recent technical advances that allow laparoscopic removal of living donor kidneys have helped to make living donation more acceptable, removing disincentives.[5] Standard requirements for donor-recipient pairs for kidney transplantation are ABO compatibility and a negative pretransplant cross-match (i.e., absence of preformed antidonor antibodies). Efforts to increase the number of kidney transplants include the use of methods to use ABO-incompatible donor treatment protocols to alter antidonor antibodies and exchange programs.

Patients with type 1 diabetes and concomitant end-stage renal disease are candidates for simultaneous kidney-pancreas transplantation. These patients may opt for a kidney transplant first, especially if they have a living donor, and later undergo a pancreas transplant. In 2008, there were 836 pancreas-kidney transplants performed in the United States,[3] with a 1-year graft survival rate of 95% for simultaneous pancreas-kidney allografts.[4]

Patients with end-stage liver disease are candidates for liver transplantation. The first successful human liver transplant was performed in 1967.[1] Of candidates for liver transplantation, 95% have chronic liver disease (i.e., cirrhosis) and 5% have fulminant hepatic failure, a disorder that progresses rapidly. Chronic diseases that require transplantation include cirrhosis as a result of hepatitis C, hepatitis B, alcohol use, biliary cirrhosis, and primary sclerosing cholangitis. In children, the most common cause of liver failure is biliary atresia. Complications of end-stage liver disease that suggest the need for transplantation include ascites, encephalopathy, and bleeding as a result of esophageal varices. In 2008, in the United States,[3] 6318 liver transplants were performed, with a 1-year graft survival rate of 88% for deceased donor liver transplantation.[4] Living donation, in which part of an adult liver is donated, is now an option for both adult and pediatric recipients; 249 living related liver transplants were performed in the United States in 2008.[3]

Cardiomyopathy and coronary artery disease are the most common indications for heart transplantation. Peripartum cardiomyopathy is a rare indication for heart transplantation. On average, these adults are older than patients in other organ groups, which is likely part of the reason why fewer pregnancies have been reported. In the United States, 2163 heart transplants were performed in 2008,[3] with a 1-year graft survival rate of 85%.[4] Fewer heart-lung and liver-kidney transplants are performed, and few pregnancies have been reported in these recipients.

Patients with end-stage lung disease and an anticipated survival of less than 2 years without transplantation are candidates for lung transplantation. Three common indications are emphysema or chronic obstructive pulmonary disease, including α_1-antitrypsin deficiency, primary pulmonary hypertension, and cystic fibrosis. The 1-year graft survival rate is lower than the groups discussed, at 76%,[4] with 1478 transplants performed in the United States in 2008.[3] Living donation has been an option, although none were performed in the United States in 2008 and the number has declined over the last several years.

The majority of patients who receive an intestinal transplant (70%) have had the diagnosis of short gut syndrome. This type of transplant may be performed in conjunction with a liver in up to 71% of the cases.[4] In 2008, 185 transplants were performed with a 1-year graft survival rate of 73%.[3,4]

SUCCESS OF TRANSPLANTATION

Medication regimens to maintain graft survival and prevent rejection have been evolving since the 1960s. In general, these can be divided into the following three categories:

- Induction regimens are used in the first week after transplantation. These include agents such as antilymphocyte sera and interleukin-2–receptor blockade antibodies.
- Antirejection regimens are used to treat episodes of rejection. They typically include high-dose, short-term treatments with either corticosteroids or antilymphocyte sera.
- Maintenance regimens are initiated soon after transplantation to prevent acute rejection episodes and provide long-term immunosuppression. The goal of this treatment is to minimize acute rejection episodes and toxicity. Combination therapies are used to balance benefits against side effects and toxicities.

A major goal of therapy is to avoid acute rejection episodes, which affect graft survival. Different organs show different effects of acute rejection, but the result can be chronic rejection, which has no effective treatment and ultimately leads to graft loss.

Maintenance regimens in the early 1960s included azathioprine and prednisone. In the 1980s, the mainstay of immunosuppression was cyclosporine, either in combination with azathioprine and prednisone or with prednisone alone. Tacrolimus (Prograf), introduced in the 1990s, has a mechanism very similar to that of cyclosporine, but is more potent and with different side effects. Mycophenolate mofetil (CellCept, MMF) was introduced in the mid-1990s. A few years later, mycophenolic acid (Myfortic, MPA), an enteric-coated capsule with less gastrointestinal side effects than MMF, was introduced. These agents have essentially replaced azathioprine and, in most cases, are used as an adjunct. Sirolimus was introduced in 2000 and has a different mechanism of action and the added advantage of not being nephrotoxic. In standard combination regimens, two drugs of the same class are not used together (e.g., cyclosporine and tacrolimus). Table 53–1 summarizes the current agents and their mechanisms of action and side effects, including agents used for induction and rejection.[6] The U.S. Food and Drug Administration (FDA) categories for these drugs are shown in Table 53–2, including information on published reproductive or clinical outcome data.[7]

RISKS OF TRANSPLANTATION

Immunosuppressive Agents and Teratology

Corticosteroids

In animal studies, corticosteroids have caused cleft palate, although this has not been seen in humans.[8] Clinically, these agents are associated with an increased risk of premature rupture of the membranes and adrenal insufficiency in newborns.[9] Prednisone has been used for more than 45 years for maintenance therapy, and intravenous methylprednisolone is used for induction and treatment of rejection. At current doses, it is considered an adjunctive drug. More recently, given the many side effects, steroid withdrawal and steroid avoidance regimens have become common.

Azathioprine

Azathioprine (1.5–3 mg/kg/day), a primary drug used for immunosuppression before the introduction of cyclosporine, is now an adjunctive agent at doses of 0.5 to 1.5 mg/kg/day. Clinical data do not support early concerns about teratogenicity in animal studies, nor has a predominant structural malformation pattern been identified. It is listed as a category D agent, and reviews show occasional attributable newborn problems, including thymic atrophy, leukopenia, anemia, thrombocytopenia, chromosomal aberrations, sepsis, and reduced immunoglobulin levels.[10,11]

Cyclosporine

As the first calcineurin inhibitor, cyclosporine became the mainstay of immunosuppression and remains a commonly used agent. Cyclosporine was originally available as Sandimmune, which was later reformulated as Neoral. The two formulations are not bioequivalent and should not be interchanged. Generic versions are available. It is usually used with one or two adjunctive agents. Maternal problems include hypertension and nephrotoxicity. Although fetal toxicity and abnormality were reported in animal studies, these occurred at dosages higher than those used clinically.[12,13] Some early clinical reports suggested a greater risk of fetal growth restriction, not borne out by later studies.[14] The magnitude of teratogenic risk appears minimal, and no predominant pattern of newborn malformations is evident.

Tacrolimus (Prograf)

Tacrolimus, approved for use in the United States in 1995, is more potent than cyclosporine. In animal studies, fetal resorption occurred at doses higher than those used clinically.[15] Transient neonatal hyperkalemia has been reported,[16] as has a higher incidence of maternal diabetes. Tacrolimus is usually used with an adjunctive agent.

Mycophenolate Mofetil/Mycophenolic Acid

The mycophenolate drugs, first approved for use in 1995, are typically used in combination with a calcineurin inhibitor. In contrast to the calcineurin inhibitors, there is greater concern about the potential risk of teratogenicity with MMF/MPA, based on reproductive toxicity studies in animals. Developmental toxicity in rats and rabbits included malformations and intrauterine growth restriction. Death occurred at dosages that appeared to be within the recommended clinical dosages based on body surface area.[17,18]

TABLE 53–1
Immunosuppressive Drugs

DRUG	USES	EFFECTS	SIDE EFFECTS	COMMENTS
Cyclosporine (Sandimmune, others), cyclosporine modified, USP (Neoral, Gengraf)	Maintenance	Inhibitor of helper T-cell function	Nephrotoxicity, hypertension, tremor, hirsutism	Relatively selective for alloimmune responses; synergistic nephrotoxicity with tacrolimus
Tacrolimus (Prograf)	Maintenance	Inhibitor of helper T-cell function	Nephrotoxicity, neurotoxicity, diabetes	
Corticosteroids (oral prednisone, IV methylprednisolone)	Maintenance, antirejection, induction	Inhibits all leukocytes; high doses cause lymphocytolysis	Cushingoid facies, diabetes, excessive weight gain, aseptic necrosis of joints	Many troublesome side effects; nonspecific immunosuppressant
Azathioprine	Maintenance	Inhibits clonal proliferation of T cells	Leukopenia	Nonspecific
Antithymocyte globulin, antilymphocyte globulin	Antirejection, induction	Depletes T cells	Fevers, chills	Polyclonal serum made in rabbits, horses; Maximum duration of therapy 2 wk
Mycophenolate mofetil (CellCept)	Maintenance	Inhibits lymphocyte proliferation	Diarrhea, leukopenia	More lymphocyte-selective than azathioprine
Mycophenolic acid (Myfortic)	Maintenance	Inhibits lymphocyte proliferation	Leukopenia	More lymphocyte-selective than azathioprine
Sirolimus (Rapamune)	Maintenance	Inhibits helper T cells	Anemia, thrombocytopenia, hyperlipidemia	Site of action distinct from other drugs
Basiliximab (Simulect)	Induction	Inhibits interleukin-2-mediated activation of lymphocytes	Possible anaphylactoid reaction	Immunosuppressive chimeric monoclonal antibody
Daclizumab (Zenapax)	Induction	Inhibits interleukin-2-mediated activation of lymphocytes		Chimeric humanized monoclonal antibody
Muromonab-CD3 (OKT3)	Antirejection, induction	Disables or depletes all T cells	First dose can cause fever, chills, or bronchospasm as a result of cytokine release	Murine monoclonal, maximum duration of therapy 2 wk

USP, U.S. Pharmacopeia.
Adapted from Moritz MJ, Armenti VT: Organ transplantation. In Jarrell BE, Carabasi RA (eds): National Medical Series for Independent Study: Surgery. Philadelphia, Lippincott Williams & Wilkins, 2000, pp 461–477.

TABLE 53–2
Immunosuppressive Drugs Commonly Used in Transplantation

DRUG	USUAL ORAL DOSAGE	ANIMAL REPRODUCTIVE DATA	PUBLISHED PREGNANCY CLINICAL OUTCOMES?	FDA PREGNANCY CATEGORY
Corticosteroids (prednisone, prednisolone, methylprednisolone)	5–20 mg/day	Yes	Yes*	B
	500–1000 mg/day IV (antirejection)	Yes	Yes*	B
Azathioprine	0.5–1.5 mg/kg/day	Yes	Yes*	D
Cyclosporine	3–10 mg/kg/day	Yes	Yes*	C
Cyclosporine modified, USP	3–10 mg/kg/day	Yes	Yes*	C
Tacrolimus	0.05–0.2 mg/kg/day	Yes	Yes*	C
Mycophenolate mofetil	2–3 g/day	Yes	Yes*†	D
Mycophenolic acid	1440 mg/day	No	No	D
Antithymocyte globulin (Atgam, ATG)	15–30 mg/kg/day IV	No	Yes*†	C
Antithymocyte globulin (Thymoglobulin)	1.0–1.5 mg/kg/day IV	No	No*	C
Sirolimus	2–5 mg/day	Yes	Yes*	C
Basiliximab	20 mg/day IV	Yes	No	B
Daclizumab	1 mg/kg/day IV	No	No	C
Muromonab-CD3 (OKT3)	0.5–10 mg/day IV	No	Yes*†	C

* Registry data.
† Case reports only.
B, no evidence of risk in humans; C, risk cannot be excluded; D, positive evidence of risk; FDA, U.S. Food and Drug Administration; USP, U.S. Pharmacopeia.
Adapted from Armenti VT, Moritz MJ, Davison JM: Drug safety issues in pregnancy following transplantation and immunosuppression. Drug Saf 1998;19:219–232.

TABLE 53–3

Structural Birth Defects in Transplant Recipient Offspring with Exposure to Mycophenolate Mofetil during Pregnancy Reported to the National Transplantation Pregnancy Registry

	KIDNEY	LIVER	PANCREAS-KIDNEY	HEART
Recipients (*N*)	34	7	3	7
Pregnancies (*N*)	44	10	6	11
Live births (*N*)	27	5	1	5
Liveborn with birth defects (*N*)	5*	1*	0	2
Incidence of birth defects (%)	19	20	0	40

* Includes one neonatal death.

From Coscia LA, Constantinescu S, Moritz MJ, et al: Report from the National Transplantation Pregnancy Registry (NTPR): Outcomes of pregnancy after transplantation. In Cecka JM, Terasaki PI (eds): Clinical Transplants 2008. Los Angeles, UCLA Terasaki Foundation Laboratory, 2009, pp 89–105.

Clinical data have demonstrated a particular pattern of malformation noted in the National Transplantation Pregnancy Registry (NTPR) database, with additional reports of problems in newborns with exposure to MMF.[19–31] In 2007, the package inserts of MMF and MPA included a change from pregnancy category C to category D.[17,18] These package inserts state that females of childbearing potential must use contraception while taking MMF or MPA, because use during pregnancy is associated with increased rates of pregnancy loss and congenital malformations. This is also the recommendation of the European Best Practice Guidelines.[32] In addition to the NTPR data, in postmarketing data collected by Roche Laboratories, Inc., between 1995 and 2007, among the 77 women exposed to systemic MMF during pregnancy, 25 had spontaneous abortions and 14 had a malformed infant or fetus. Six of these 14 had ear abnormalities. Table 53–3 lists the structural birth defects in transplant recipient offspring with exposure to MMF during pregnancy.[33] Women using MMF or MPA at any time during pregnancy are encouraged to enroll in the NTPR.

Sirolimus

Sirolimus, approved for use in the United States in 1999, is an antiproliferative agent of its own class. It is used in combination with cyclosporine or tacrolimus or with prednisone alone (European and U.S. labeling). There are concerns about its use in pregnancy. Teratogenicity has not been noted in animal studies, although decreased fetal weight and delayed ossification have been reported.[34] When it was used with cyclosporine in pregnant animals, resorption and fetal mortality rates were increased, suggesting increased toxicity; however, there are insufficient data on clinical outcome.[19,35–37] Data remain limited with regard to sirolimus exposure during pregnancy.

Other agents used for short-term induction or rejection have a minor role in pregnancy. In a small series of patients, muromonab-CD3 (OKT3)[7] and corticosteroids were used for rejection in pregnancy (discussed later).

Maternal Risks

Transplant recipients have varying degrees of post-transplant recovery. One difficulty in assessing pregnancy risk in this population overall is that many of the conclusions have been derived only from experience in kidney transplant recipients. In 1976, a management plan was suggested in a detailed case report of a renal transplant recipient during pregnancy.[38] Based on this information and a survey of literature at the time, the following criteria were derived for counseling renal recipients who are contemplating pregnancy:

- Good general health for at least 2 years after the transplant.
- Stature compatible with good obstetric outcome.
- No proteinuria.
- No significant hypertension.
- No evidence of renal rejection.
- No evidence of renal obstruction on excretory urogram or ultrasound.
- Stable renal function.
- Stable immunosuppressive therapy.

Most of these guidelines still apply, although recipients can safely become pregnant sooner than 2 years post-transplant.[39] Drug-treated hypertension is now much more prevalent.[40] It has been more difficult to identify criteria for recipients of other organs, but good, stable graft function would seem to be essential for pregnancy to be well tolerated. The appropriate interval after transplant and the features of good, stable graft function for each group of organ recipients are harder to define. For renal recipients, graft function can be assessed by measuring the serum creatinine level or creatinine clearance. Studies in both clinical and animal models in the nontransplant population have assessed the effect of pregnancy on renal function. Renal function is unaffected if the kidney is stable.[41] In the transplant population, this finding is supported by well-designed case-control studies showing that pregnancy does not cause deterioration of graft function when prepregnancy graft function is stable.[42–46] Factors that must be considered in nonrenal recipients are the nephrotoxic effect of calcineurin inhibitors on native kidney function and the increased likelihood of hypertension. Thus, nonrenal recipients who receive calcineurin inhibitor therapy often have baseline renal impairment.

These guidelines have been revised and published as Consensus Guidelines through the American Society of Transplantation (AST).[39] The European Best Practice Guidelines[32] are also available for clinicians.

Literature surveys from the azathioprine era of the 1970s and 1980s attest to thousands of successful post-transplant pregnancies in renal transplant recipients. The spontaneous abortion rate was approximately 14%, and the therapeutic abortion rate was approximately 20%. Of pregnancies that continued beyond the first trimester, more than 90% were successful. Renal impairment occurred in approximately 15% of women, and hypertension complicated approximately 30% of pregnancies. Preterm delivery was common, affecting 45% to 60% of pregnancies, with fetal growth restriction occurring in approximately 20%.[47,48]

Initial reports of cyclosporine exposure during pregnancy raised concern because a higher rate of fetal growth restriction, which may have been related to higher doses, was

TABLE 53–4

Prepregnancy Renal Function in Renal Transplant Recipients with Estimates for Pregnancy Outcome (>24 weeks) and Impact on Maternal Renal Function

					LOSS OF >25% RENAL FUNCTION		
SCR μMOL/L (MG/DL)	FETAL GROWTH RESTRICTION (%)	PRETERM DELIVERY (%)	PREECLAMPSIA (%)	PERINATAL DEATHS (%)	PREGNANCY (%)	PERSISTS POSTPARTUM (%)	ESRF IN 1 YR (%)
<125 (<1.4)	30	35	24	3	15	4	–
125–160 (1.4–1.85)	50	70	45	7	20	7	10
>160 (>1.85)	60	90	60	12	45	35	70

ESRF, end-stage renal failure; SCr, serum creatinine.
Estimates based on literature from 1991 to 2007, with all pregnancies attaining at least 24 wk' gestation (unpublished data from Dr. John Davison).

noted.[14] Also apparent was a higher incidence of hypertension than was previously noted in the azathioprine era.[40] With the advent of cyclosporine, it was suggested that this drug might not be optimal for use in pregnancy and that patients should be switched back to azathioprine-based regimens because of the longer experience with these drugs. Given the need to provide more consistent and effective surveillance for the transplant community, the NTPR was established in 1991 with the goal of maintaining an ongoing database to assess the safety of pregnancy in female transplant recipients as well as pregnancies fathered by male transplant recipients.[33,49] A pregnancy registry was established in the United Kingdom in 1997[50] but discontinued in 2002, although there has been an updated publication reporting the pregnancy outcomes in the United Kingdom.[51] This report depicts outcomes similar to those of the NTPR.

After the introduction of cyclosporine, case and individual transplant center reports and registry data reported successful pregnancies in female transplant recipients while highlighting potential risks to mothers and newborns. Most conclusions came from data on renal recipients, but information is accruing from other organ recipients, with differences evident among the groups.

Overall, compared with the general population, female transplant recipients are at greater risk for preeclampsia and hypertension during pregnancy. A higher percentage of cesarean deliveries are reported as well. The balance between graft function and management of immunosuppression during pregnancy is crucial. Fortunately, in organ recipients, the incidence of rejection during pregnancy does not appear to be higher than that in the nonpregnant population, and similarly, graft loss within 2 years of delivery does not appear to be affected by pregnancy. When irreversible and unpredictable graft events occur, they more often happen in patients with impaired prepregnancy graft function. Many recipients have had successful successive pregnancies, and some have had successful outcomes with multiple gestations and in vitro fertilization.[52–55] An overview of the literature in renal transplant recipients is summarized in Table 53–4.

Current data for each organ recipient group reported to the NTPR are summarized in Tables 53–5 to 53–9.[33] High incidences of preterm delivery and low birth weight are reported and are more apparent among pancreas-kidney recipients and less apparent in liver and heart recipients. Pancreas-kidney recipients usually tolerate pregnancy without gestational diabetes. Most infectious complications

TABLE 53–5

Pregnancies in Female Transplant Recipients Reported to the National Transplantation Pregnancy Registry as of January 2009

ORGAN	RECIPIENTS	PREGNANCIES	OUTCOMES*
Kidney	834	1301	1339
Liver	143	247	251
Liver-kidney	4	6	7
Pancreas-kidney	43	76	78
Pancreas alone	1	4	5
Heart	48	82	83
Heart-lung	4	4	4
Lung	17	23	25
Totals	**1094**	**1743**	**1792**

* Includes twins and triplets.

involve the urinary tract. Rejection during pregnancy is associated with poorer outcomes for the newborn and for graft survival (Tables 53–10 and 53–11). Rejection should be biopsy-proven, if possible; treatment is with steroids, antilymphocyte sera, or adjustment of baseline immunosuppression.

Fetal Risks

Two large reports on the two primary calcineurin inhibitors, cyclosporine and tacrolimus, examined the overall prevalence of malformations in newborns. In the offspring of cyclosporine-treated recipients, the malformation rate was 4.1% (14 of 339 births), based on a meta-analysis.[56] NTPR data on the offspring of cyclosporine-treated liver or kidney recipients showed malformations in 3% to 5% of a total of 425 liveborn infants.[57] The types of malformations varied among different systems, with no predominant type noted. In a report of patients treated with tacrolimus during pregnancy (84 women, 100 pregnancies), 4 of 71 liveborn infants analyzed (5.6%) had evidence of structural malformations, but no specific pattern was evident.[58] Transplant recipients, on average, delivered 1 month early, with birth weights of 2160 to 2600 g reported. Differences were seen among organ recipient groups. Genetic considerations must be taken into account. They may contribute to organ failure in

TABLE 53–6

National Transplantation Pregnancy Registry: Pregnancy Outcomes in Female Kidney Transplant Recipients with Cyclosporine, Neoral, and Prograf Exposure during Pregnancy

	CSA	NEORAL	PROGRAF
Maternal Factors (*N* = pregnancies)	**(512)**	**(190)**	**(152)**
Transplant to conception interval (yr; mean)	3.5 ± 2.8	5.8 ± 3.9	4.0 ± 2.6
Hypertension during pregnancy (%)	62	66	54
Diabetes during pregnancy (%)	12	2	10
Infection during pregnancy (%)	23	20	24
Rejection episode during pregnancy (%)*	1	2	2
Preeclampsia (%)	29	28	31
Mean serum creatinine (mg/dL)			
Before pregnancy	1.4 ± 0.5	1.3 ± 0.4	1.2 ± 0.4
During pregnancy	1.4 ± 0.7	1.4 ± 0.5	1.3 ± 1.0
After pregnancy	1.6 ± 0.97	1.4 ± 0.6	1.4 ± 0.9
Graft loss within 2 yr of delivery (%)	11	7	9
Outcomes (*N*)†	**(524)**	**(199)**	**(155)**
Therapeutic abortions (%)	8	1	0.7
Spontaneous abortions (%)	12	18	21
Ectopic (%)	0.6	0.5	0.7
Stillborn (%)	3	1.5	2
Live births (%)	76	79	75
Live Births (*N*)	**(400)**	**(158)**	**(117)**
Mean gestational age (wk)	36 ± 3.4	36 ± 2.9	35 ± 3.8
Premature (<37 wk; %)	52	48	54
Mean birth weight (g)	2489 ± 757	2541 ± 703	2437 ± 876
Low birth weight (<2500 g; %)	46	43	58
Cesarean section (%)	52	42	62
Newborn complications (%)	41	42	52
Neonatal deaths (*N* [%]) (within 30 days of birth)	4 (1%)	0	3 (3%)

* Biopsy-proven acute rejection only.
† Includes twins, triplets.
CsA, cyclosporine, Sandimmune brand cyclosporine (336 recipients, 512 pregnancies); Neoral brand cyclosporine (129 recipients, 190 pregnancies); Prograf (107 recipients, 152 pregnancies).
From Coscia LA, Constantinescu S, Moritz MJ, et al: Report from the National Transplantation Pregnancy Registry (NTPR): Outcomes of pregnancy after transplantation. In Cecka JM, Terasaki PI (eds): Clinical Transplants 2008. Los Angeles, UCLA Terasaki Foundation Laboratory, 2009, pp 89–105.

TABLE 53–7

National Transplantation Pregnancy Registry: Pregnancy Outcomes in 138 Liver Transplant Recipients with 241 Pregnancies and 245 Outcomes

Maternal Factors (*N* = pregnancies)	**(241)**
Transplant to conception interval (yr; mean)	5.2 ± 4.4
Hypertension during pregnancy (%)	33.9
Diabetes during pregnancy (%)	6.7
Infection during pregnancy (%)	26.5
Rejection episode during pregnancy (%)	8.4
Preeclampsia (%)	21.5
Graft loss within 2 yr of delivery (%)	8
Outcomes (*N*)*	**(245)**
Therapeutic abortions (%)	4.5
Spontaneous abortions (%)	19.2
Ectopic (%)	0.4
Stillborn (%)	2.1
Live births (%)	73.8
Live Births (*N*)	**(180)**
Mean gestational age (wk)	36.5 ± 3.5
Premature (<37 wk; %)	39.6
Mean birth weight (g)	2645 ± 777
Low birth weight (<2500 g; %)	35.4
Cesarean section (%)	38.9
Newborn complications (%)	35.6
Neonatal deaths (*N*; within 30 days of birth)	1

* Includes twins.
From Coscia LA, Constantinescu S, Moritz MJ, et al: Report from the National Transplantation Pregnancy Registry (NTPR): Outcomes of pregnancy after transplantation. In Cecka JM, Terasaki PI (eds): Clinical Transplants 2008. Los Angeles, UCLA Terasaki Foundation Laboratory, 2009, pp 89–105.

the mother and must be considered in the assessment of risk to the newborn. Table 53–12 summarizes the incidence of malformations reported to the NTPR in transplant recipients receiving the newer immunosuppressants, but prior to reports of additional birth defects with MMF.[59] Of additional concern is the potential for more subtle effects that may not be apparent at birth, but may affect long-term growth and development as well as in the next generation.[60] Clinical reports noted that children of recipients are developing well, although there is concern that alterations in T-cell subpopulations may affect vaccinations or long-term immunity.[61,62] A large series of 175 newborns of cyclosporine-treated kidney recipients reported to the NTPR showed no evidence of an increased incidence of developmental delays over that expected, given the high percentage of premature offspring in this group.[63]

Childhood transplant recipients who subsequently become pregnant in adulthood are of increasing relevance (Table 53–13).[64] The risk of malformations in newborns of these patients is not increased, but a small percentage of recipients have graft rejection, dysfunction, or even loss within 2 years of delivery. Consistent features of obstetric outcomes are higher incidences of prematurity and low birth weight, depending on the type of organ transplant.

TABLE 53-8

Pregnancy Outcomes in 43 Female Pancreas-Kidney Recipients with 76 Pregnancies and 78 Pregnancy Outcomes Reported to the National Transplantation Pregnancy Registry

Maternal Factors	
Transplant to conception interval (yr; mean)	4.1
Hypertension during pregnancy (%)	65
Diabetes during pregnancy (%)	4
Infection during pregnancy (%)	48
Rejection episode during pregnancy (%)	6
Preeclampsia (%)	33
Graft loss within 2 yr of delivery (%)	23
Outcomes (*N*)*	**(78)**
Therapeutic abortions (%)	4
Spontaneous abortions (%)	23
Ectopic (%)	3
Stillbirth (%)	0
Live births (%)	71
Live Births (*N*)	**(55)**
Mean gestational age (wk)	34
Premature (<37 wk; %)	76
Mean birth weight (g)	2112
Low birth weight (<2500 g)	62
Cesarean section (%)	62
Newborn complications (%)	56
Neonatal deaths† (*N* [%]) (within 30 days of birth)	1 (2%)

* Includes twins.
† One neonatal death due to sepsis (26 wk, 624 g).
Adapted from Coscia LA, Constantinescu S, Moritz MJ, et al: Report from the National Transplantation Pregnancy Registry (NTPR): Outcomes of pregnancy after transplantation. In Cecka JM, Terasaki PI (eds): Clinical Transplants 2008. Los Angeles, UCLA Terasaki Foundation Laboratory, 2009, pp 89–105.

These rates are always higher than in the general population.

MANAGEMENT OPTIONS

Prepregnancy and Prenatal

Recommendations for the management of pregnancy after transplantation have been published.[65–83] Transplantation restores fertility, and patients must be advised about appropriate birth control. For all organ recipients, an interval from transplant to conception is advisable to allow establishment of stable graft function and reduction of immunosuppression to maintenance levels, with concomitant reduction of the risk of more serious post-transplant infections. NTPR data showed a higher incidence of pregnancy termination and peripartum rejection with transplant-to-conception intervals of less than 6 months compared with longer intervals in cyclosporine-treated kidney recipients. Waiting at least 6 months, and preferably 1 year, from transplant seems advisable.[39,82,83] It is important to note whether the recipient has been rejection-free (and for how long) as well as the level and stability of graft function.

TABLE 53-9

Pregnancy Outcomes in 48 Female Heart, 4 Heart-Lung Recipients, and 17 Lung Transplant Recipients

ORGAN	HEART	HEART-LUNG	LUNG
Maternal Factors (*N* = pregnancies)	**(81)**	**(4)**	**(23)**
Mean transplant-to-conception interval (yr)	6.2 ± 4.7	4.8 ± 2.4	4.0 ± 3.1
Hypertension during pregnancy (%)	42	25	48
Diabetes during pregnancy (%)	3	0	16
Infection during pregnancy (%)	13	50	22
Rejection episode during pregnancy (%)	14	0	17
Preeclampsia	17	50	7
Graft loss within 2 yr of delivery (%)	2	25	18
Outcomes (*N*)	**(82)***	**(4)**	**(25)†**
Therapeutic abortions (%)	6	0	20
Spontaneous abortions (%)	23	0	24
Ectopic (%)	2	0	0
Stillbirths (%)	1	0	0
Live births (%)	67	100	56
Live Births (*N*)	**(55)**	**(4)**	**(14)**
Mean gestational age (wk)	37 ± 2.7	36.8	33.4 ± 5.7
Premature (<37 wk)	33	75	50
Mean birth weight	2609 ± 548	2537 ± 261	2160 ± 1030
Low birth weight (<2500 g)	40	75	64
Newborn complications	28	50	64
Neonatal deaths (*N*; within 30 days of birth)	0	0	2†

* Includes twins.
† Triplet pregnancy: one spontaneous abortion at 10 wk and two born at 22 wk died within 24 hr of birth.
From Coscia LA, Constantinescu S, Moritz MJ, et al: Report from the National Transplantation Pregnancy Registry (NTPR): Outcomes of pregnancy after transplantation. In Cecka JM, Terasaki PI (eds): Clinical Transplants 2008. Los Angeles, UCLA Terasaki Foundation Laboratory, 2009, pp 89–105.

The potential teratogenicity of MMF/MPA amplifies the dilemma between protecting the transplanted organ from rejection versus fetal risk. The risk to the fetus of a kidney recipient from MMF/MPA of a significant malformation is based on a small experience with varying other immunosuppressants and comorbidities. It is not currently known to what degree this risk is generalizable to other organ

TABLE 53–10

Outcomes of Cyclosporine (Neoral) or Tacrolimus Treatment in Female Kidney Recipients with Biopsy-Proven Acute Rejection Episodes during Pregnancy

CASE	REGIMEN	PREPREGNANCY LEVEL CREATININE (MG/DL)	REJECTION TREATMENT	GRAFT LOSS < 2 YR POSTPARTUM	OUTCOME	GESTATIONAL AGE (WK)	BIRTH WEIGHT (G)
1	Cyclosporine (Neoral) switched to tacrolimus during pregnancy*	1.3	OKT3 and radiation	Yes	Spontaneous abortion	6	N/A
2	Tacrolimus	2.8	Muromonab-CD3 (OKT3) and methylprednisolone	No	Spontaneous abortion	7	N/A
3	Neoral	1.2	Methylprednisolone	No	Live birth	32	1378
4	Neoral	3.0	Methylprednisolone	No	Live birth	29	1247
5	Neoral	2.6	Reinitiate immunosuppression†	No	Live birth	32	1417
6	Tacrolimus	1.0	Antithymocyte globulin (Thymoglobulin) and sirolimus	Yes	Live birth	32	1531

* Both recipients stopped taking their medications during pregnancy.
† The recipient was being treated for cancer.
From Armenti VT, Radomski JS, Moritz MJ, et al: Report from the National Transplantation Pregnancy Registry (NTPR): Outcomes of pregnancy after transplantation. In Cecka JM, Terasaki PI (eds): Clinical Transplants 2002. Los Angeles, UCLA Immunogenetics Center, 2003, pp 121–130.

TABLE 53–11

National Transplantation Pregnancy Registry: Live Birth Outcomes of Liver Recipients with Biopsy-Proven Acute Rejection during Pregnancy

CASE	MATERNAL IMMUNOSUPPRESSION	GESTATIONAL AGE (WK)	BIRTH WEIGHT (G)	NEWBORN COMPLICATIONS
1	Cyclosporine	35	1673	Jaundice
2	Cyclosporine	34	1474	
3	Cyclosporine	37	2693	
4	Cyclosporine	39	2920	
5	Cyclosporine	27	964	Bronchopulmonary dysplasia requiring oxygen for 3 yr and pyloric stenosis repair at 3 mo
6	Tacrolimus	38	2892	
7	Tacrolimus	34	2268	
8	Cyclosporine	27	680	Death at 3.5 mo as a result of complications of prematurity
Mean		33.8	1946	

From Armenti VT, Herrine SK, Radomski JS, et al: Pregnancy after liver transplantation. Liver Transplant 2000;6:671–685.

TABLE 53–12

Reported Birth Defects in Offspring of Female Kidney Recipients Taking Cyclosporine (Neoral) or Tacrolimus during Pregnancy

DEFECT	*N*	REGIMEN
Cleft lip and palate and ear deformity	1	Tacrolimus, mycophenolate mofetil, then sirolimus and prednisone
Hypoplastic nails and shortened fifth fingers	1	Tacrolimus, mycophenolate mofetil, and prednisone
Renal cystic dysplasia	1	Tacrolimus, alone
Submucosal cleft palate	1	Neoral, azathioprine, and prednisone
Tongue-tied	1	Neoral, azathioprine, and prednisone
Pyloric stenosis	1	Neoral, azathioprine, and prednisone
Imperforate anus, clubbed feet, hypospadias	1	Neoral, azathioprine, and prednisone
Total number of liveborn infants with birth defects (*N* [%])	7/140 (5%)	

From Armenti VT, Radomski JS, Moritz MJ, et al: Report from the National Transplantation Pregnancy Registry (NTPR): Outcomes of pregnancy after transplantation. In Cecka JM, Terasaki PI (eds): Clinical Transplants 2002. Los Angeles, UCLA Immunogenetics Center, 2003, pp 121–130.

TABLE 53-13

National Transplantation Pregnancy Registry: Outcomes in Pediatric Female Kidney Recipients (<21 Years at Transplant)

	CYCLOSPORINE (SANDIMMUNE) (86 RECIPIENTS, 142 PREGNANCIES; 1 OUTCOME UNKNOWN)	CYCLOSPORINE (NEORAL) (25 RECIPIENTS, 31 PREGNANCIES)	TACROLIMUS (PROGRAF) (11 RECIPIENTS, 13 PREGNANCIES)
Maternal Factors			
Transplant-to-conception interval (yr)*	3.9	7.2	3.3
Hypertension during pregnancy (%)	56	68	54
Diabetes during pregnancy (%)	2	3	0
Infection during pregnancy (%)	26	26	67
Rejection episode during pregnancy (%)	1	0	15
Preeclampsia (%)	26	45	8
Mean serum creatinine level (mg/dL)			
Before pregnancy	1.4	1.3	1.2
During pregnancy	1.4	1.3	2.9
After pregnancy	1.7	1.4	1.9
Graft loss within 2 yr of delivery (%)	12	0	36
Outcome (*N*)†	145	33	13
Therapeutic abortion (%)	9	0	0
Spontaneous abortion (%)	10	9	15
Ectopic pregnancy (%)	0	0	0
Stillbirth (%)	5	3	15
Live birth (%)	76	88	69
Live Births (*n*)	110	29	9
Mean gestational age (wk)	36	37	35
Mean birth weight (g)	2512 g	2547 g	2422 g
Premature birth (<37 wk; %)	49	52	44
Low birth weight (<2500 g; %)	46	48	56
Cesarean delivery (%)	52	46	67
Newborn complications (%)	38	24	56
Neonatal death (*N* [%]) within 30 days of birth	1 (1)	0	0

* Calculated from the most recent transplant before the estimated date of conception.
† Includes twins and triplets.
From Armenti VT, Moritz MJ, Davison JM: Pregnancy in female pediatric solid organ transplant recipients. Pediatr Clin North Am 2003;50:1543–1560.

recipients. Conversely, the benefit of a lower risk of rejection to the recipient of a regimen including MMF/MPA varies by organ, other immunosuppressants in the regimen, recipient factors, and so on. Further, there are no data available on the risks of switching patients to alternative regimens that have a presumed lower risk of malformations of the newborn. Currently, the most popular regimens at the time of hospital discharge for kidney recipients are cyclosporine or tacrolimus plus MMF/MPA, with or without prednisone. Thus, for each recipient contemplating pregnancy, an individual decision must be made. One must weigh the risks to the transplanted organ of switching immunosuppressants, because organ function directly affects fertility and the ability to safely carry a pregnancy. This must be weighed against the risk of continuing the prepregnancy immunosuppressive regimen, which could harm the fetus. At this time, such decisions are best made preconception with the involvement of the patient, her partner, and the transplant team.

A significant percentage of recipients have hypertension and may be receiving a combination of antihypertensive medications. Angiotensin-converting enzyme inhibitors and angiotensin II receptor antagonists are contraindicated during pregnancy, although some controversy exists with regard to the timing of greatest exposure risk.[39,84] If dosage adjustments or changes to hypertensive agents are needed, these changes can be made in anticipation of pregnancy. In addition to hypertension and preeclampsia, attention should be focused on other comorbid conditions that are likely to occur, including infections and gestational diabetes.

Rejection, although not common, must be considered in the face of graft dysfunction. The etiology of graft dysfunction in any solid organ recipient must be investigated. There are special clinical considerations for each organ group. In the renal transplant group, the group with the most data, the usual pattern for the serum creatinine level is a slight decrease in early pregnancy, with a return to baseline postpartum. Increases during pregnancy and postpartum should be evaluated. Pancreas-kidney recipients usually can tolerate pregnancy without problems with glucose control, but additional comorbid conditions caused by cardiovascular disease must be considered. Lung recipients appear to have a higher incidence of peripartum problems in terms of both graft function and patient survival.

Infectious complications during pregnancy are most often urinary tract infections; therefore, monthly urine culture should be performed. Occasionally, more serious yeast infections, pneumonia, sepsis, or unspecified viral infections complicate pregnancy. Cytomegalovirus is usually asymptomatic and is detected by serologic, antigen, or viral monitoring. If a primary infection occurs during pregnancy, there is a risk of transmission with fetal sequelae, but the effectiveness of treating the mother's infection in preventing or ameliorating fetal sequelae is uncertain.

The rate of hepatitis C transmission from mother to child in the nontransplant population is 5%.[85] Recipients with acute hepatitis B infection may transmit it to their offspring. Administration of hepatitis B immune globulin and hepatitis B virus vaccine to the newborn within a few hours of birth usually prevents transmission. Estimates of the incidence of acute infection with toxoplasmosis are 0.2% to 1%, with most cases undiagnosed and asymptomatic. Congenital toxoplasmosis can have severe consequences, and the diagnosis is dependent on culture, direct antigen detection, or serologic tests.[86]

Scrutiny for hypertensive changes and preeclampsia is essential, although the diagnosis of preeclampsia may be difficult because serum uric acid levels and urinary protein excretion may be well above expected normal ranges without preeclampsia, as a result of drug nephrotoxicity or the renal allograft. Other complications include HELLP (hemolysis, elevated liver enzymes, and low platelets) syndrome, ureteral obstruction, and complications of cesarean delivery. Peripartum ultrasound assessment to exclude urinary obstruction is warranted if the serum creatinine level increases.

Unless obvious immunosuppressive toxicity or rejection occurs, it is best to maintain baseline immunosuppressive dosing. Blood concentrations are likely to decrease during pregnancy, given the increased maternal volume of distribution as well as fetal metabolism of drugs. Some recipients are noncompliant, choosing to stop taking medications during pregnancy for fear that the medication will harm the fetus. Reports to the registry show that, in most pregnancies, immunosuppressive doses have been kept the same or increased during pregnancy. Regardless of dosing during pregnancy, many changes that occur peripartum mandate that postpartum immunosuppressive dosing should be directed by blood level, when possible.

Significant unexplained deterioration in graft function should be assessed with biopsy. For heart recipients to avoid x-ray exposure, biopsy can be done with echocardiographic guidance.[73] If the diagnosis of acute rejection is made, appropriate antirejection treatment is necessary. Given the risk of rejection and preeclampsia, more frequent monitoring is warranted from midpregnancy onward, including blood pressure measurements, assessment of graft function, and measurement of immunosuppressive drug levels.

In liver recipients, worsening liver function with chronic rejection or hepatitis C has been noted, with further deterioration in subsequent pregnancies.[87] Whether such deterioration is time-linked or pregnancy-induced requires further study. Recipients with stable graft function have tolerated subsequent pregnancies. Data to support this observation have been noted in each recipient group but are more easily quantified among kidney recipients.

Labor and Delivery

A high incidence of cesarean section is reported in all organ recipient groups. Cesarean delivery should be performed for obstetric indications only. Immunosuppression must not be interrupted during labor and delivery.

Postnatal

Most oral maintenance agents are easily absorbed, and treatment can usually be resumed shortly after cesarean delivery. When oral treatment cannot be resumed, intravenous formulations are available for most, but not all, agents. Immunosuppressive drug levels should be monitored and dosage adjusted appropriately, which may affect blood pressure, renal function, and other toxicities. One must be aware of postpartum depression among transplant recipients, because medications may be missed or not taken; therefore, close monitoring is required for several months postpartum.

Breast-feeding is controversial. Although exposure of the newborn to an immunosuppressive drug may be detrimental, a newly emerging view is that the benefits of breast-feeding outweigh the minimal risk. Further study of potential long-term effects is needed.

SUMMARY OF MANAGEMENT OPTIONS

Pregnancy after Transplantation

Management Options	Evidence Quality and Recommendation	References
Prepregnancy		
Patients should defer conception for at least 1 yr after transplantation, with adequate contraception.	IIb/B	39,47,79, 82,83,92
Assessment of graft function:	III/B	47,70,92
• Recent biopsy.	III/B	93
• Proteinuria.	III/B	93
• Hepatitis B and C status.	IV/C	69
• Cytomegalovirus, toxoplasmosis, and herpes simplex status.	IV/C	69,70

Management Options	Evidence Quality and Recommendation	References
Maintenance immunosuppression options: • Azathioprine. • Cyclosporine. • Tacrolimus. • Corticosteroids. • Mycophenolate mofetil. • Mycophenolic acid. • Sirolimus.	IV/C	7,19,33,40, 56,58,65,67, 69,73,94,95, 99
The effect of comorbid conditions (e.g., diabetes, hypertension) should be considered and their management optimized; nonrenal recipients should have their baseline kidney function assessed.	III/B	39,41,47,96
Vaccinations should be given, if needed (e.g., rubella).	IV/C	47,69
Explore the etiology of the original disease; discuss genetic issues, if relevant.	IV/C	47,97
Discuss the effect of pregnancy on renal allograft function.	IIa/B	42–47
Discuss the risks of intrauterine growth restriction, prematurity, and low birth weight.	III/B	33,40,47, 48,80
Prenatal		
Accurate early diagnosis and dating of pregnancy.	IV/C	47
Clinical and laboratory monitoring of the functional status of transplanted organs and immunosuppressive drug levels: • Every 4 wk until 32 wk. • Every 2 wk until 36 wk. • Then weekly, until delivery.	III/B	47,69,70, 73,98,100
Monthly urine culture.	IV/C	47,69,71
Surveillance for rejection, with biopsy considered if it is suspected.	III/B	47,60,69,87
Surveillance for bacterial or viral infection (e.g., cytomegalovirus, toxoplasmosis, hepatitis).	IV/C	47,69,70
Fetal surveillance.	IV/C	47,70,79
Monitoring for hypertension and nephropathy.	IV/C	40,47,69,72, 96
Surveillance for preeclampsia.	IV/C	47,70
Screening for gestational diabetes.	IV/C	47
Labor and Delivery		
Vaginal delivery is optimal; cesarean delivery is used for obstetric reasons.	IV/C	47,71
For kidney recipients, episiotomy is performed on the side opposite the allograft.	GPP	
For heart, lung, or heart-lung recipients: • Vigilance for poor or absent cough reflex and the need for airway protection. • Unpredictable response to vasoactive medications. • Judicious use of intravenous fluids.	GPP	
Postnatal		
Monitor immunosuppressive drug levels for at least 1 mo postpartum, especially if dosages were adjusted during pregnancy.	III/B	69,73,94,98

SUMMARY OF MANAGEMENT OPTIONS

Pregnancy after Transplantation—cont'd

Management Options	Evidence Quality and Recommendation	References
Surveillance for rejection, with biopsy considered if it is suspected	III/B	47,60,87
Breast-feeding.	III/B	88–91
Contraception counseling.	IV/C	47

GPP, good practice point.

SUGGESTED READINGS

Armenti VT, Ahlswede KM, Ahlswede BA, et al: National Transplantation Pregnancy Registry: Outcomes of 154 pregnancies in cyclosporine-treated female kidney transplant recipients. Transplantation 1994;57:502–506.

Armenti VT, Constantinescu S, Moritz MJ, Davison JM: Pregnancy after transplantation. Transplant Rev 2008;22:223–240.

Armenti VT, Moritz MJ, Davison JM: Pregnancy in female pediatric solid organ transplant recipients. Pediatr Clin North Am 2003;50:1543–1560.

Christopher V, Al-Chalabi T, Richardson PD, et al: Pregnancy outcome after liver transplantation: A single-center experience of 71 pregnancies in 45 recipients. Liver Transplant 2006;12:1138–1143.

Coscia LA, Constantinescu S, Moritz MJ, et al: Report from the National Transplantation Pregnancy Registry (NTPR): Outcomes of pregnancy after transplantation. In Cecka JM, Terasaki PI (eds): Clinical Transplants 2008. Los Angeles, UCLA Terasaki Foundation Laboratory, 2009, pp 89–105.

Kallen B, Westgren M, Aberg A, Olausson PO: Pregnancy outcome after maternal organ transplantation in Sweden. BJOG 2005;112:904.

McKay DB, Josephson MA, Armenti VT, et al, Women's Health Committee of the American Society of Transplantation: Reproduction and transplantation: Report on the AST Consensus Conference on Reproductive Issues and Transplantation. Am J Transplant 2005;5:1592–1599.

Rahamimov R, Ben-Haroush A, Wittenberg C, et al: Pregnancy in renal transplant recipients: Long-term effect on patient and graft survival. A single-center experience. Transplantation 2006;81:660–664.

Sibanda N, Briggs JD, Davison JM, et al: Pregnancy after organ transplantation: A report from the UK Transplant Pregnancy Registry. Transplantation 2007;83:1301–1307.

Sifontis NM, Coscia LA, Constantinescu S, et al: Pregnancy outcomes in solid organ transplant recipients with exposure to mycophenolate mofetil or sirolimus. Transplantation 2006;82:1698–1702.

REFERENCES

For a complete list of references, log onto www.expertconsult.com.

CHAPTER 54

Trauma

RENEE A. BOBROWSKI

INCIDENCE AND RISKS

General

Trauma occurs in 6% to 7% of all pregnancies and is the leading cause of nonobstetric maternal death.[1,2] Nationwide in 2002, almost 17,000 pregnant women sustained an injury requiring hospitalization, with nearly half the women younger than age 25.[3] For trauma admissions not resulting in delivery, motor vehicle accidents (MVAs) were most common, followed by falls; the reverse is seen with patients requiring delivery at the time of trauma admission. Poisoning, overexertion injuries, assault, and penetrating trauma were next most frequent. MVAs occur with equal frequency across trimesters, whereas falls are most frequent between 20 and 30 weeks, and trauma secondary to abuse and interpersonal violence increases with advancing gestation.[4]

Most injuries during pregnancy are minor, but 2% to 8% of victims have a life-threatening injury and require admission to an intensive care unit.[5] Maternal mortality from trauma approximates 10%, but it is the same as nonpregnant patients when matched for injury severity.[6] Trauma places the mother and fetus at increased risk, and fetal loss occurs in at least 40% of critically injured gravidas. High injury severity and Glascow Coma scores, increasing fluid requirement during resuscitation, and maternal acidosis and hypoxia appear to predict an increase in fetal loss.[5–9] The rate of adverse pregnancy outcome, however, is approximately 4%, even when maternal injuries are minor.[10] Because 90% of all trauma in pregnant women is minor, more fetuses die as a result of lesser injuries than as a result of catastrophic trauma.

Women injured during pregnancy but not requiring delivery at the time of their injury nevertheless appear to be at increased risk for adverse outcome. An increased risk for preterm delivery, low birth weight, and abruption has been reported when injured pregnant women are followed for the duration of their pregnancy.[11–13] Several mechanisms have been proposed. Trauma may be a marker for lifestyle risks that adversely affect pregnancy outcomes. The traumatic event may also result in uteroplacental injury causing uteroplacental insufficiency and/or chronic abruption.[11,12] Thus, ongoing surveillance for the remainder of the pregnancy has been suggested by several authors.[11,12]

The obstetrician must be prepared to work in concert with the trauma team to evaluate and treat an injured pregnant woman (Fig. 54–1). The presence of a fetus may be extremely unnerving to even the most experienced emergency team, and obstetric consultation can be invaluable. Simulation training is ideal for low-frequency, high-acuity events occurring in medicine. Simulated scenarios provide a great opportunity for obstetric and trauma personnel to develop protocols for obstetric trauma and improve communication and teamwork under noncritical circumstances. Simulation as a training tool in medicine provides many opportunities to improve provider knowledge and skills, refine clinical protocols, educate staff and students, and ultimately, improve patient care. The most important component of simulation training, however, is postscenario debriefing to allow participants discuss, analyze, and synthesize their actions.

The basic principles of trauma management apply to injured pregnant women, and maternal resuscitation is the first priority under all circumstances. It is imperative to understand the physiologic changes of pregnancy and the implications for managing gravid trauma patients. Among the many physiologic changes that occur during pregnancy, some assume greater importance in trauma. Understanding a pregnant woman's response to injury will facilitate her care from the moment of arrival in the emergency department. Table 54–1 outlines changes pertinent to the care of gravid trauma victims and their clinical implications. Once the maternal condition is stable, diagnostic evaluation, fetal assessment, and treatment can proceed.

MANAGEMENT OPTIONS—GENERAL

Prehospital Care

Most emergency medical services (EMS) personnel find their anxiety increases upon arrival at the scene of an injured pregnant woman. Thus, familiarity with prehospital procedures is beneficial for hospital staff in providing guidance to those at the scene. EMS should follow standard Advance Trauma Life Support (ATLS) protocols for extrication and spinal immobilization.

A left lateral tilt of 15 degrees should be performed for all women greater than 20 weeks' gestation. If a spine injury is suspected or documented, a rolled towel or blanket can be placed beneath the spine board at the level of the hips without risking neurologic compromise. If a patient in the

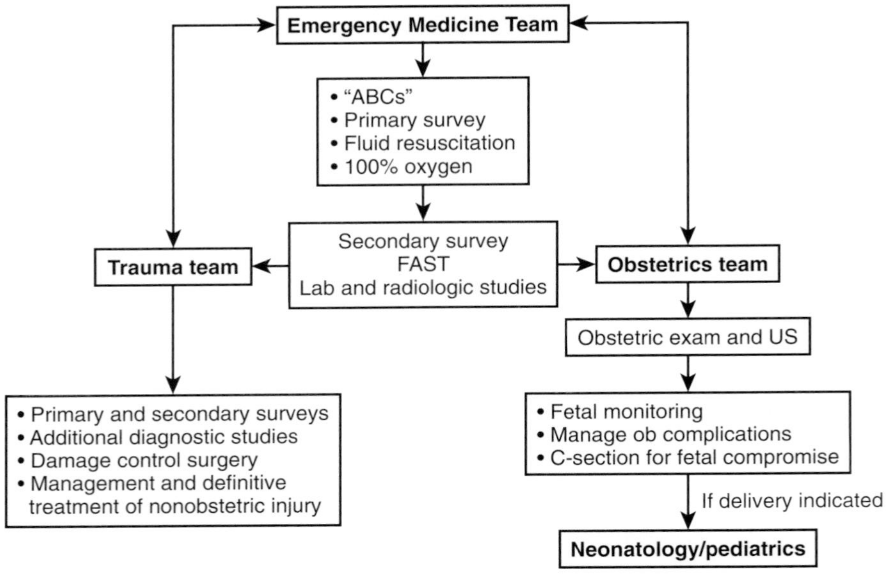

FIGURE 54–1
Interdisciplinary management of the pregnant trauma patient.

TABLE 54–1
Clinical Implications of the Physiologic Changes of Pregnancy in the Patient with Traumatic Injury

PHYSIOLOGIC CHANGE	CLINICAL IMPLICATION
Blood volume increases 50%.	Clinical signs of hypovolemia may not occur until 1500–2000 mL blood loss. Aggressive volume replacement is needed.
Systemic vascular resistance decreases.	Misinterpreted as hemodynamic instability.
Heart rate increases 15–20 beats/min.	Misinterpreted as early decompensation.
Respiratory rate and tidal volume increase.	Normal P_{CO_2} = 27–32 mm Hg.
Minute ventilation and oxygen consumption increase.	More susceptible to hypoxemia with apnea.
Diaphragm is elevated 4 cm cephalad.	Perform thoracostomy one to two interspaces higher than normal.
Gastrointestinal motility decreases.	Aspiration risk increases.
Distended abdomen occurs with advancing gestation.	Sensitivity of peritoneal signs decreases.
Uterine enlargement occurs.	Protects bowel with lower abdominal penetrating trauma.
Uterine blood flow increases to 600 mL/min	Risk of hemorrhage and retroperitoneal bleeding increases
Bladder becomes intra-abdominal after 12 wk.	More susceptible to injury.
Renal blood flow increases 50%.	Serum blood urea nitrogen and creatinine levels = 4 and 0.6–8 mg/dL, respectively.
Hypomotility of the renal collecting system occurs.	Ureteral dilation and mild hydronephrosis (right > left).
White blood cell count may increase.	Nonspecific for injury.
Levels of fibrinogen and Factors VII, VIII, IX, and X increase.	Hypercoaguable state; risk of thrombosis increases.

P_{CO_2}, carbon dioxide pressure.

third trimester is having difficulty lying flat with a left lateral tilt, 30 degrees of reverse Trendelenberg and the tilt may provide some comfort.

Early establishment of an airway in the field is the best option if there is any concern for airway stablility or patency. Practice management guidelines for prehospital fluid resuscitation in the general population have been established by the Eastern Association for the Surgery of Trauma (EAST) Workgroup and can be summarized as follows[14]: The benefit of venous access and fluid resuscitation in the field is not supported in the literature and may be harmful to some critically injured patients. Attempting access at the scene also delays transport and attempts en route are equally successful if indicated. Fluids should be administered to patients with penetrating trauma and altered mental status or lack of a radial pulse and patients with traumatic brain injury to maintain systolic blood pressure greater than 90mm Hg. Small boluses (250 mL) of hypertonic saline are equivalent to large boluses (1000 mL) of standard solutions.[14] Guidelines for transfer of an injured pregnant patient to a level I trauma center (in addition to accepted guidelines for nonpregnant patients) include maternal heart rate greater than 110, chest pain, loss of consciousness, and third-trimester gestation.[15]

Basic Management Principles for Minor Injury during Pregnancy

Patients with minor injuries should receive routine medical treatment and obstetric assessment based upon gestational age and clinical findings. A recent prospective study of a standardized protocol for minor trauma patients demonstrated that extensive evaluation does not appear to be required.[16] Over 300 pregnant women with minor trauma (Index-Injury Severity Score [ISS] = 0) at 23 + 6 weeks or more were prospectively evaluated. Falls were the most common mechanism of injury (48%). All patients had reassuring fetal testing prior to discharge. Pregnancy outcome data was available for 80% of women in the study. Nineteen percent had a low–birth weight infant or preterm delivery.

One patient had an abruption but it occurred 5 weeks after her injury, which is lower than the rate previously reported with minor trauma. No single clinical or laboratory risk factor predicted an adverse outcome.The authors recommend that Kleihauer-Betke (KB), fibrinogen, and coagulation studies not be performed for minor trauma and that a thorough but brief clinical examination is adequate. This study also raises the issue of an increased risk for long-term adverse outcomes as previously discussed,[11–13] even though this is a lower risk group of patients.[16]

Basic Principles of Trauma Resuscitation for Moderate to Severe Injury during Pregnancy

Emergency department evaluation and treatment of the injured gravida should proceed in a timely and organized fashion. Each member of the trauma team is assigned specific tasks to avoid confusion and duplication of services. The management of gravidas with moderate to severe injuries can be divided into steps, some that are performed simultaneously:

- Primary survey.
- Resuscitation.
- Secondary survey.
- Laboratory and diagnostic studies.
- Definitive treatment.

The management scheme is summarized in Figure 54–2.

Primary Survey

The standard ATLS protocol for the primary survey focuses on identifying life-threatening injuries and initiating resuscitative measures. Details of the event, the mechanism of injury, resuscitation attempts in the field, and the patient's medical history should be obtained from the transporting paramedics. The components of the primary survey include the ABCs of resuscitation (airway, breathing, and circulation), an initial physical examination with adequate exposure to identify injuries, and a brief neurologic assessment.

The highest priority is to establish that the patient has an adequate airway. This can be accomplished in many cases by talking to the patient. A patient who can speak in complete sentences, in a normal voice, and can respond appropriately has a patent airway as well as adequate oxygenation and brain perfusion. If there is evidence of airway compromise, endotracheal intubation should be performed without delay.

Once the airway is deemed adequate, breathing is assessed. The chest should be examined for expansion, breath sounds, crepitus, subcutaneous emphysema, and open wounds. Supplemental oxygen, 100% by mask, is administered to all patients until respiratory assessment is completed. Pulse oximetry objectively confirms normal oxygen saturation unless the patient has hypotension, peripheral vasoconstriction, or severe anemia. If there is evidence of maternal hypoxia, arterial blood gas analysis should be obtained while the patient breathes room air if possible. A maternal arterial oxygen pressure (PaO_2) of 60mm Hg or greater is needed to ensure adequate fetal oxygenation. Oxygen can be weaned based on the clinical assessment and the patient's condition. When a nasogastric tube is required for gastric decompression, it should be placed after adequate ventilation is established.

Endotracheal intubation and mechanical ventilation are indicated for a patient who cannot maintain adequate ventilation and/or oxygenation. Indications for intubation and mechanical ventilation include airway obstruction, inability

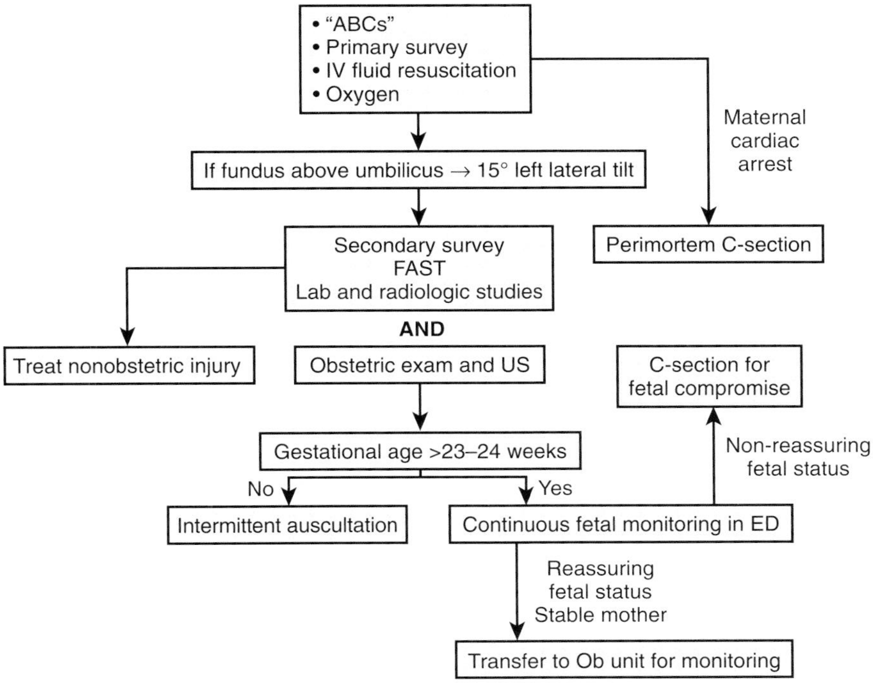

FIGURE 54–2
Initial resuscitation of the pregnant trauma patient.

to protect the airway, hypoxia, coma, shock, flail chest, open chest wounds, and ineffective ventilation. Intubation should not be delayed with the expectation that a patient's respiratory status will quickly and spontaneously improve. Oxygen consumption increases by 20% and functional residual capacity decreases in pregnancy, resulting in rapid development of maternal hypoxia during respiratory compromise. The failed intubation rate during pregnancy is 1 : 300, or sevenfold higher than for the nonpregnant patient.[17] Thus, early intubation under controlled conditions is preferable to an emergent procedure in a profoundly hypoxic gravida. Blood gas analysis can be helpful in the decision-making process, but clinical judgment is equally important. There are several important modifications for intubation of the pregnant patient. Adequate preoxygenation and prompt reoxygenation afterward are important, given the respiratory changes of pregnancy. Lower esophageal sphincter tone is decreased during pregnancy, and rapid-sequence induction with cricoid pressure should be performed. Postintubation chest radiography is mandatory to confirm proper tube placement.

Circulation is the third component of the ABCs that requires immediate assessment. The hemodynamic changes of pregnancy can result in a misleading impression of maternal stability. Blood volume increases 50% during pregnancy, and gravid women tolerate a greater degree of acute blood loss before hemodynamic compromise occurs. Pulse rate and blood pressure may not change until 30% to 35% of blood volume has been lost.[18] Tachycardia and hypotension are absent in a pregnant woman during the early phase of shock, and hemodynamic instability does not occur until 1500 to 2000 mL of blood loss.[19] A gravida with tachycardia and hypotension will need aggressive resuscitation with fluids and blood products. Any pregnant patient beyond 20 weeks' gestation lying supine should have a 15-degree left lateral tilt. This positioning maximizes cardiac output by reducing uterine pressure on the inferior vena cava and allowing adequate venous return. Failure to tilt the patient results in a 30% decrease in maternal cardiac output.

The physical examination during the primary survey should be thorough and efficient. In patients with moderate to severe injuries, all clothing must be removed to allow adequate visualization and assessment of injuries. Obvious hemorrhage should be controlled with direct pressure to the wound. A rapid neurologic assessment is included, and the initial examination includes determination of orientation and responsiveness, pupillary reaction, motor response, and the Glasgow Coma Scale.

Concurrent with the initial evaluation of a moderately to severely injured patient, intravenous access must be established. A large-bore (14–16-gauge) peripheral catheter is preferred because it allows the quickest infusion of fluids and blood products. The number of peripheral catheters placed should increase as injury severity increases; patients with moderate injuries should have two secure catheters in place. Central venous access is required when peripheral access cannot be established because of absent veins, hypotension, or large surface area burns. Subclavian line placement in hypotensive trauma patients, however, carries a 12% complication rate, including pneumothorax, hemothorax, thrombosis, and infection.[20] In addition, the infusion ports of a double- or triple-lumen central venous catheter are generally 18 gauge, and the maximum flow rate is slower than with a large-bore peripheral intravenous line. Another option for central access is placement of a large-bore (8.5-Fr) central catheter; if needed, this line can be converted over a guidewire to a triple-lumen catheter after resuscitation.

Crystalloid (lactated Ringer's solution) is the fluid of choice for initial resuscitation for many physicians. Replacement should be at a rate of 3 : 1 crystalloid to blood lost. Others use colloid or plasma expanders. If the patient remains hypotensive despite infusion of 2 to 3 L of crystalloid, transfusion of packed red blood cells should begin. In the emergency setting, type O-negative blood is administered until blood type and cross-match are obtained. A warming device helps to prevent hypothermia as a result of rapid infusion of crystalloid and blood products. Coagulation products should be administered based on abnormal laboratory parameters.

Military antishock trousers are controversial in the management of traumatic shock. They have not been well studied nor widely used in pregnant women. In the injured gravida, the lower extremity compartments can be inflated, but this may increase bleeding from injured pelvic structures. Generally, the abdominal compartment should not be inflated in the second and third trimesters, because it can compromise venous return and precipitate or exacerbate respiratory compromise from increased intra-abdominal pressure. Military antishock trousers are recommended for an injured pregnant woman only when major pelvic fractures are accompanied by uncontrollable hemorrhage.[21,22]

Resuscitation

The goal of the resuscitation phase is to monitor the patient's response to initial treatment and optimize intravascular volume and oxygen delivery. Adequate maternal resuscitation is of paramount importance to fetal survival. Blood pressure and pulse rate are assessed frequently, although these parameters are not reliable in detecting early shock in the gravida.[6] Measurement of central venous pressure has been used in the acute setting, but absolute values should be viewed with great caution because central venous pressure is lowered by pregnancy. A pulmonary artery catheter is rarely indicated during initial resuscitation attempts. Vasopressors are contraindicated in hemorrhagic shock unless the patient has cardiogenic shock from cardiac contusion or spinal cord injury with neurogenic shock.[22]

A urinary catheter is diagnostic and therapeutic; it allows accurate measurement of urine output, assessment for hematuria, and complete bladder drainage. The kidney is sensitive to the effects of hypotension, and urine output decreases as the kidney attempts to conserve fluid and maintain intravascular volume. An output of 30 mL/hr or more indicates adequate renal perfusion. Evidence of blood at the urethral meatus or difficulty in passing a catheter suggests bladder or urethral injury. If no urine is obtained through the catheter, bladder rupture must be considered. This condition is most commonly associated with a pelvic fracture. Gross or microscopic hematuria mandates evaluation to exclude urinary tract injury.

If an injured patient in shock is unresponsive to aggressive resuscitative measures, immediate operative intervention must be considered. A number of causes of refractory shock in the seriously injured pregnant woman should be eliminated, however, before proceeding to the operating room. Volume replacement may be inadequate, particularly in the third trimester, when blood volume is at its peak. Concealed hemorrhage associated with abruptio placentae can result in maternal shock, and amniotic fluid embolism is a rare but potential cause of cardiovascular collapse. Additional causes of persistent shock include tension pneumothorax, cardiac tamponade, neurogenic shock, uncorrected hypothermia, significant electrolyte and acid-base disturbances, and hypoxia.[18]

Secondary Survey

The secondary survey is performed once there is evidence of response to resuscitation efforts and the maternal condition is stabilized. Ongoing assessment of vital signs and a complete physical examination should be conducted in an ordered fashion. Particular attention must be given to sites of bleeding, injured limbs, and entrance and exit wounds in cases of penetrating trauma. Head injuries account for nearly 50% of deaths in trauma patients, and a complete neurologic assessment should be performed and compared with the initial examination.[23] The most common underlying etiologies of central nervous system impairment in a trauma patient include alcohol intoxication, diabetic ketoacidosis, narcotic and barbiturate overdose, hypovolemic shock, and cerebrovascular accidents. All neck injuries should be presumed to be life-threatening until excluded by appropriate evaluation. Tension and open pneumothorax, flail chest, and massive hemothorax are thoracic injuries that require rapid diagnosis and treatment. A chest tube should be placed one to two interspaces higher in pregnant patients because the diaphragm is elevated.[4] Abdominal injury may also occur with penetrating thoracic trauma secondary to the high diaphragm. An abdominal examination should be conducted, although the absence of findings does not exclude an acute intra-abdominal process. A rectal examination performed in patients with moderate to severe injuries evaluates for gastrointestinal bleeding and documents sphincter tone.

A complete obstetric examination is included in the secondary survey. Fundal height should be measured and fetal heart tones auscultated. A mark can be placed at the level of the fundus to provide a baseline in the case of increasing fundal height due to a concealed abruption. Uterine tone and the presence of contractions and tenderness are assessed. Pelvic examination should be performed on all gravidas unless contraindicated by their injuries. A sterile speculum examination assists in identifying membrane rupture or genitourinary bleeding. Contraindications to the pelvic examination include unstable spine, pelvic, and femur fractures because positioning may risk additional injury. Examination may be possible after orthopedic consultation. AmniSure (AmniSure International LLC) can accurately diagnose rupture of membranes, and speculum examination is not required. Digital examination can be performed if there is no vaginal bleeding or, in the presence of bleeding, once placenta previa has been excluded by ultrasonographic examination.

Fetal assessment begins with estimating gestational age by last menstrual period, fundal height, and ultrasonography. If the gestational age is uncertain, ultrasonographic measurements can quickly approximate dating of the pregnancy. When the potential for fetal survival must be determined urgently, a biparietal diameter of 54 mm or greater measured by ultrasonography has been suggested as more predictive than estimated fetal weight.[24] Fetal heart tones can be auscultated intermittently by Doppler in a previable fetus.

Continuous fetal heart rate monitoring of a viable fetus should be instituted in the emergency room as soon as possible, once initial resuscitation of the mother has begun. Fetal well-being is an excellent indicator of adequate maternal resuscitation. Changes in the fetal heart rate pattern may be the first sign of maternal compromise and generally occur before changes in maternal vital signs. Fetal tachycardia, bradycardia, late decelerations, and decreased beat-to-beat variability can indicate deterioration in fetal status. The tocodynameter is helpful in detecting contractions that an injured patient may not perceive. Obstetric staff must be immediately available to interpret the fetal heart rate tracing while the patient is in the emergency department or other nonobstetric unit.

A variety of laboratory studies and diagnostic modalities are available to assist in evaluating and managing an injured gravida. The study or combination of studies performed should be tailored to the clinical situation as discussed in the following sections.

Laboratory Studies in the Gravid Trauma Victim

Complete laboratory evaluation must be initiated quickly for patients with moderate to severe injuries. Suggested studies are listed in Table 54–2. Additional tests should be ordered as dictated by the patient's condition and the clinical situation.

Pregnant women have a physiologic anemia because plasma volume increases to a greater degree than red cell volume. Nevertheless, the hemoglobin level during pregnancy is normally 10 g/dL or higher. An initial hemoglobin level less than 8 g/dL has been associated with ongoing hemorrhage and an increased mortality rate in nonpregnant trauma patients.[25] A normal hemoglobin level, however, does not exclude excessive bleeding because several hours may be required for equilibration to occur. Activated partial thromboplastin time (aPTT) and prothrombin time (PT) are unaffected by pregnancy. Fibrinogen increases during pregnancy, and a low-normal fibrinogen level (200–250 mg/dL) suggests a consumptive coagulopathy.[26]

TABLE 54–2

Suggested Laboratory Studies for Patients with Moderate to Severe Traumatic Injury

Complete blood count and platelet count
Coagulation profile
Type and cross-match
Serum electrolytes, blood urea nitrogen, and creatinine
Serum glucose
Aspartate aminotransferase and alanine aminotransferase
Amylase
Lipase
Arterial blood gas analysis
Urinalysis
Urine and blood toxicology screens
Kleihauer-Betke stain

Serum chemistry values provide additional information. Although electrolyte levels are usually normal in healthy gravidas, a decreased bicarbonate level is correlated with fetal demise in pregnant trauma patients. Determining a baseline creatinine level is helpful in case renal complications develop. Elevation of the aspartate aminotransferase (AST) or alanine aminotransferase (ALT) level above 130 IU/L is associated with a sixfold increase in the risk of intra-abdominal injury and is an indication to pursue diagnostic imaging in the stable nonpregnant patient.[27] Lactate may have decreased sensitivity due to increased renal clearance in the pregnant patient.

The KB stain determines the presence of fetal blood cells in the maternal circulation as well as the degree of fetomaternal hemorrhage (FMH). Fetal cells and ghost maternal cells are counted after acid elution and staining of the maternal blood sample. A normal maternal blood volume of 5000 mL is commonly assumed. The laboratory reports the ratio of fetal to maternal cells, and the volume of FMH is calculated:

$$\frac{\text{Fetal cells}}{\text{Maternal cells}} \times \text{Maternal blood volume}$$

Alcohol and illicit substance use is common in trauma patients, and urine and blood toxicology screens should be performed. The results of testing provide information that is important for both medical and legal reasons. The physiologic effects of illicit substances can alter a patient's response to the stress of trauma. Alcohol lowers sympathetic response, whereas cocaine can cause sympathetic stimulation or paradoxical depression. Cocaine use has been associated with placental abruption and should be considered in the gravid trauma patient with an adverse fetal outcome. Organic pathology should be excluded in patients with neurologic compromise, but their condition may reflect the effects of an illicit substance.

Diagnostic Studies in the Gravid Trauma Victim

Diagnostic studies are pursued once initial resuscitation is complete and the mother and fetus are stable. Radiographic screening of patients with moderate to severe injuries consists of cervical spine, chest, and pelvis films. Cervical spine films exclude C-spine injury in most patients with blunt trauma. Chest x-ray can detect hemothorax, pneumothorax, or ruptured diaphragm, but there are several limitations in pregnant trauma patients that should be kept in mind. A small pneumothorax may not be evident on initial chest film owing to the reduced inspiratory effort and decreased lung volume. The sensitivity of a chest x-ray in diagnosis of aortic injury is also decreased and transesophageal echocardiography or computed tomography (CT) scan of the chest is the modality of choice to exclude thoracic aortic injury or pericardial tamponade.[4] A plain film of the abdomen should be obtained if abdominal injury or a foreign body is suspected.

Radiation exposure is always a consideration when caring for the pregnant patient, but necessary tests should not be omitted because the patient is pregnant. Fetal risk is negligible if maternal exposure is limited to less than 5 rad (5000 mrad).[28] Abdominal shielding and avoiding duplication of studies minimizes fetal exposure. A review of a large group of pregnant trauma patients found all patients had less than 5 rads of exposure with their trauma evaluation.[29] Radiation exposure to the fetus from specific radiologic studies is outlined elsewhere in this text.

Intra-abdominal injury must be excluded, as in the nonpregnant patient. Clinical examination of the abdomen in nonpregnant patients with blunt trauma detects only 60% of intra-abdominal injuries. During pregnancy, signs and symptoms of an acute intra-abdominal process are often further obscured as the uterus stretches the peritoneum, decreasing the afferent sensory fibers of the peritoneum per square centimeter. Pain may also be referred to an atypical location owing to displacement of organs.[4] The diagnostic modalities available to exclude abdominal injury when the patient does not require emergent laparotomy include diagnostic peritoneal lavage (DPL), CT scan, and focused abdominal sonography in trauma (FAST). Although not established in the trauma literature, magnetic resonance imaging (MRI) may be useful in evaluation of the pregnant trauma patient. Each examination has its advantages, disadvantages, and limitations, as detailed below.

DPL is highly sensitive and accurately detects 94% to 98% of intra-abdominal injuries.[30,31] Traditional indications for DPL include equivocal findings on physical examination, unexplained hypotension, an unresponsive patient, and spinal cord injury. DPL can be performed in a pregnant patient without compromising safety and accuracy.[32,33] Although FAST and CT scan have become the more commonly used modalities, DPL is still useful for evaluation of unstable blunt trauma or an indeterminate FAST study. DPL is more accurate than CT for early diagnosis of hollow visceral and mesenteric injury, but does not reliably exclude retroperitoneal injury. DPL also cannot assess the specific site of bleeding or the extent of injury. Previous laparotomy, massive obesity, and advanced third-trimester pregnancy are relative contraindications to DPL, although no gestational age cutoff has been defined.[34] The complication rate for DPL is 1% in nonpregnant patients and does not appear to be increased during pregnancy.[32–34]

The standard technique for DPL is modified somewhat for the pregnant patient. Location of the incision is dependent on the stage of gestation. During the first trimester, a standard infraumbilical incision may be used. As pregnancy advances, however, the incision must be supraumbilical and above the uterine fundus, and an open technique is employed. A positive DPL is an indication for exploratory laparotomy.[31]

CT scanning is recommended when a patient with blunt trauma is hemodynamically stable but has unreliable or equivocal findings on physical examination or multiple injuries. It is the diagnostic modality of choice for nonoperative management of solid viscus injuries and has the advantage of detecting clinically unsuspected injuries. Its negative predictive value is excellent. Disadvantages of CT include a lower sensitivity for hollow viscus injury, possible dye reactions, and lack of portability, which requires patients to be moved from the resuscitation area of the emergency department.

MRI has not been described for the pregnant trauma patient but might be an option in a stable mother requiring further evaluation. The CT is typically a faster study to perform and more accessible in many emergency departments, and thus, remains the standard. Discussion among the radiologist, trauma surgeon, and obstetrician regarding the utility of MRI for specific trauma patients may be considered.

FAST has become the diagnostic study of choice in many centers for hemodynamically stable patients.[35,36] It is noninvasive, can be performed at the bedside in the emergency room, and can be repeated easily if the results are equivocal. The examination focuses on identifying fluid in the pericardium, pleural cavity, pararenal retroperitoneum, and peritoneal cavity. The sensitivity of FAST to detect intraperitoneal fluid is 73% to 88%, and its accuracy is 96% to 99%.[31] FAST appears to decrease the need for both DPL and CT scan, allowing more selective and cost-effective use of these modalities.[35] The sensitivity and specificity of FAST in pregnant blunt trauma victims is similar to those in nonpregnant patients (80%–83% sensitivity), making it a safe and effective screening examination.[37,38]

An evidence-based algorithm incorporating hemodynamic status and the findings on physical examination was developed by the EAST Practice Management Guidelines Work Group.[31] FAST is considered the diagnostic examination of choice for patients who are hemodynamically unstable, with DPL as an alternative to exclude hemoperitoneum. Patients who are hemodynamically stable, with a reliable physical examination, undergo serial examinations or diagnostic testing, depending on the findings on initial clinical examination. Patients with an unreliable physical examination should undergo FAST or CT scan, depending on institution and physician preference, with subsequent management determined by results.

Definitive Treatment

Definitive treatment is instituted according to the type and severity of injuries as well as the clinical condition. A patient with hemorrhagic shock and obvious intra-abdominal injury is unlikely to remain in the emergency department longer than necessary and will have undergone minimal diagnostic evaluation before operative intervention. In a patient who is hemodynamically stable, adequate time is available to assess the full extent of injuries. Once diagnostic studies have been completed and interpreted, a treatment plan can be devised in consultation with appropriate specialty services.

Trauma victims are frequently transported to the nearest hospital. However, not all institutions are equipped to care for a patient with major injuries, and transfer to a tertiary care center may be necessary for definitive therapy. Maternal stability and fetal well-being must be ensured before land or air transport. A patient should not be transferred if there is any sign of hemodynamic compromise, ongoing hemorrhage, severe uncorrected anemia, non-reassuring fetal status, or danger of delivery en route. Personnel equipped to handle obstetric emergencies should always accompany a pregnant patient during transport.

Tetanus immunization is the first of several general treatment issues. Tetanus occurs almost exclusively in patients who have been inadequately immunized. Preventing tetanus after injury entails ensuring adequate immunity and local wound care, with elimination of necrotic tissue and foreign bodies. Tetanus toxoid (0.5 mL intramuscularly) is administered when a patient has been appropriately immunized but the most recent booster was longer than 5 years ago. Previously unimmunized patients require both tetanus immune globulin (500 U intramuscularly) and the first of three doses of tetanus toxoid. The immune globulin and toxoid must be injected into different sites to ensure adequate protection.

The second issue is the extremely high risk of deep venous thrombosis (DVT) in patients with moderate to severe injuries. Blood transfusion, surgery, femur or tibia fracture, and spinal cord injury are associated with an increased risk of DVT.[39] Young patients with injuries are at high risk, and DVT has been reported to occur in 46% of trauma victims younger than 30 years of age.[39] Pregnant women who suffer a fracture injury have been noted to be at a ninefold increased risk for thrombosis.[40] The American College of Chest Physicians[41] recommends DVT prophylaxis for trauma patients with an identifiable risk factor of which the hypercoaguable state of pregnancy is included. Low-molecular-weight heparin (LMWH) prophylaxis should be administered if the patient has no contraindications to heparin therapy. If LMWH is contraindicated, mechanical prophylaxis (graduated compression stockings, intermittent pneumatic compression devices, or the venous foot pump) should be instituted. An inferior vena caval filter is not recommended for prophylaxis.[41]

Guidelines for stress ulcer prophylaxis have been developed by The EAST Practice Committee.[42] Level 1 recommendations for prophylaxis include all patients with mechanical ventilation, coagulopathy, traumatic brain injury, and a major burn. Prophylaxis is also recommended for all intensive care unit patients with multitrauma, sepsis, or acute renal failure (level 2) as well as an ISS greater than 15 or high-dose steroid administration (level 3). No difference is noted in effectiveness of H_2 antagonists, proton pump inhibitors (PPIs), and cytoprotective agents (level 1). Tolerance has been noted to develop in H_2 antagonists but has not been observed with PPIs. The duration of prophylaxis is less clear but it may be continued throughout the time of mechanical ventilation or intensive care unit stay or until enteral feeding is tolerated.[42]

Damage Control Surgery for the Critically Injured Patient

Damage control surgery is defined as rapid termination of an operation after control of life-threatening hemorrhage and intestinal spillage. It creates a stable anatomic environment to prevent progression to an unsalvageable metabolic state. It is a staged approach to the patient with multiple injuries. If the patient declines owing to hypothermia, acidosis, hypotension, or coagulopathy, only problems that require immediate intervention are addressed in the operating room, with return to the intensive care unit for ongoing resuscitation and stabilization. Pregnancy does not influence the decision for damage control surgery, and there are limited data with regard to its use in the pregnant trauma patient. Nevertheless, delivery of the term or near-term fetus should be considered part of the approach in a woman in extremis.[4]

SUMMARY OF MANAGEMENT OPTIONS

Trauma in Pregnancy—General Management

Management Options	Evidence Quality and Recommendation	References
Overall Primary Survey: Identify and Treat Life-Threatening Injury		
Use a multidisciplinary team approach.	—/GPP	—
Assess airway.	IV/C	18
Assess breathing.	IV/C	18
Assess circulation:	IV/C	18
• Venous access.	Ia/A	20
• IV fluid and blood products.		
• 15-Degree left lateral tilt.	III/B	4,23,61
Perform initial neurologic assessment.	IV/C	22
Perform initial physical examination.	IV/C	22
Resuscitation		
Assess response to initial treatment:	IV/C	6,18
• Pulse and blood pressure.		
• Urine output.		
• Continued resuscitation.		
Secondary Survey		
Initiate after stabilization.	IV/C	18,34
Perform complete physical examination.	III/B	33
Perform obstetric assessment:		
• Fundal height with mark on abdomen.		
• Uterine tone, contractions, tenderness.		
• Fetal assessment: FHR, nonstress test if >23–24 wk, ultrasound examination.		
• Pelvic examination.		
Obtain laboratory investigations (see Table 54–2)		
Obtain diagnostic studies:		
• FAST, CT, and DPL.		
Definitive Treatment		
Assess need for transfer to tertiary center.	—/GPP	—
Thromboprophylaxis.	IV/C	28,41
	III/B	39
Administer tetanus immunization if needed.	—/GPP	—
Administer Rh-immunoglobulin if Rh-negative.	IIa/B	10
Administer stress ulcer prophylaxis.	IIa/B	42

CT, computed tomography; DPL, diagnostic peritoneal lavage; FAST, focused abdominal sonograpy in trauma; FHR, fetal heart rate; GPP, good practice point.

BLUNT TRAUMA

Incidence

MVAs are responsible for 60% to 75% of cases of blunt trauma, making it the most common mechanism of injury and the leading cause of fetal death related to maternal trauma.[6,43] Higher crash severity, severe maternal injury, and lack of restraints are associated with a higher risk of adverse fetal outcome.[44] Although most injuries are minor, each year in the United States, an estimated 1300 to 3900 women experience a fetal loss as a result of an MVA.[45] Obstetric complications associated with blunt trauma include abruptio placentae, preterm labor, uterine rupture, FMH, direct fetal injury, and fetal demise. The incidence of abruptio placentae, direct fetal injury, and fetal death in non–life-threatening blunt abdominal trauma is fortunately low (1.6%, 0.8%, and 1.6%, respectively), but the fetus is nevertheless at risk, even when maternal injuries are minor.[46] The incidence of preterm delivery associated with noncatastrophic blunt trauma is also infrequent, at 0.86%.[47]

Falls are the second most common form of blunt trauma, but direct abdominal assault is occurring with increasing frequency in pregnant women. The prevalence of physical abuse of pregnant women is 6% to 31%. Morbidity and adverse outcomes of pregnancy appear to be more common with direct assaults than with MVAs, including a high risk of uterine rupture.[15,48,49] Women sustaining an assault during pregnancy are also at increased risk for long-term sequelae of abruption, preterm delivery, and low birth weight.[49] Physical abuse is often a repetitive event that may prompt multiple emergency room visits. It is important to ask specific questions about abusive relationships because women frequently do not volunteer such information. As the only health care provider many patients sees regularly during pregnancy, the obstetrician has the best opportunity to offer assistance to victims of abuse.

General Management

The trauma team may have performed a primary survey and begun resuscitation efforts of a woman with blunt trauma before an obstetrician arrives. This approach is appropriate because maternal stabilization is always the priority. The obstetric consultant should assume co-management responsibilities for the mother and fetus once notified of the patient's admission to the emergency department.

Injury patterns associated with MVAs vary depending on whether the victim was restrained, the type of safety belt system in use, and the patient's place in the vehicle. On average, 30% of pregnant women involved in an MVA are unrestrained.[27,28,50] Unbelted individuals usually sustain injuries to the head, face, chest, abdomen, and pelvis when they hit the interior of the car or are ejected. An unbelted pregnant woman is nearly three times more likely to suffer a fetal death compared with a belted gravida.[51] A lap belt prevents ejection from the vehicle, but hollow viscus and lumbar spine injuries are common. Those wearing a shoulder harness without the lap component often have cervical spine, clavicular, chest, liver, and spleen injuries. A three-point lap-shoulder system offers optimal protection, but injuries do occur and include rib, sternum, and clavicular fractures. Air bag deployment may cause face, arm, and chest abrasions, and chemical keratitis has been reported.

Fractures, dislocations, and sprains have been reported to be the most common type of injury in women hospitalized for traumatic injury, with falls being the leading mechanism of injury.[40] Pelvic fractures are the least common type of injury but are associated with the worst outcomes.[40] Detailed information on pelvic fracture during pregnancy is found in a review of 101 cases.[52] Mechanisms of injury included automobile-pedestrian accidents, MVAs, and falls. Overall maternal mortality was 9%, and fetal mortality was 35%. Pelvic fractures in the third trimester were associated with an 18% incidence of fetal skull fracture. As reported by other authors, increasing severity of maternal injury increases both maternal and fetal mortality rates. The trimester of pregnancy during which the injury occurred did not influence fetal death. Repair of the pelvic fracture usually is not performed during pregnancy, and 75% of women deliver vaginally. Mode of delivery should be individualized with consideration for cesarean delivery for pubi rami fractures adjacent to urethra/bladder, severe lateral compression fractures, and acute pelvic fractures with marked displacement.[52]

Abdominal injuries are common in victims of blunt trauma. Specific injuries sustained during pregnancy change with advancing gestation. By 12 weeks, the bladder has become an intra-abdominal organ and thus is more susceptible to injury. As the uterus enlarges and rises out of the pelvis, risk of direct injury to the uterus increases. Life-threatening retroperitoneal hemorrhage occurs more frequently during pregnancy, when pelvic blood flow is markedly increased.[53] Bowel injuries, however, tend to occur less often because the small intestine is compressed into the upper abdomen.

Accurate and timely diagnosis of intra-abdominal injury requiring surgical intervention is one of the challenges in blunt trauma. Findings on initial physical examination of the abdomen may be normal despite visceral injury. Serial examinations are, therefore, important to detect deterioration in the patient's condition. Splenic injury and retroperitoneal bleeds are the most common injuries from blunt abdominal trauma in pregnancy and occur more frequently than in nonpregnant patients.[10] Rib fractures are frequently associated with liver and spleen injuries, and pelvic fractures are associated with genitourinary injuries and retroperitoneal hemorrhage. The choice of diagnostic studies is best made in concert with the trauma team.

Abruptio Placentae

Abruptio placentae occurs in 1% to 5% of gravidas with minor injuries and 6% to 37% of those with major injuries.[19,46,47,53–55] The largest prospective study of minor trauma in pregnancy, however, noted a much lower rate of abruption than prior studies and the single case was remote from the time of injury.[16] It is the most common cause of fetal death when the mother survives blunt trauma. Placental abruption cannot be predicted based on placental location, severity of maternal injury, or vehicle damage (in the case of an MVA), and it can occur without obvious injury to the mother.[8,10,56,57] A small series reported an increased incidence of abruption in patients involved in MVAs at speeds of 30 mph and greater and those with a higher ISS.[9]

When a gravida is involved in an MVA, intrauterine pressure at the time of impact is estimated to be 10 times greater than the forces generated with labor.[58] Although the uterus is considered more elastic than the placenta, recent models indicate that their mechanical properties are similar and there is overlap. The uteroplacental interface appears to fail at a lower strain than either the uterus or the placenta.[45] Increased intrauterine pressure generated on impact may propagate placental separation, with subsequent formation of a retroplacental hematoma.[58]

Placental abruption usually occurs soon after the traumatic event. Classic signs and symptoms include vaginal bleeding, abdominal pain, and fundal tenderness as well as uterine irritability, high-frequency contractions, and increased tone. Back pain and vaginal bleeding may be the most prominent symptoms in women with separation of a posterior placenta.[59] The absence of vaginal bleeding, however, does not exclude the diagnosis. Bleeding can be concealed within the uterus and may be detected only by increasing fundal height, fetal heart rate abnormalities, or maternal hypovolemia. A hypertonic uterus and evidence of fetal compromise are highly suggestive of abruptio placentae. Cardiotocographic monitoring is the most sensitive method of surveillance after a traumatic event and is discussed later in this section.[10,15,47]

Management of a patient with abruptio placentae after traumatic injury is similar to that of an uninjured gravida with this complication. As soon as abruption is suspected, intravenous access must be established. A urinary catheter allows accurate measurement of output. Complete blood and platelet counts, fibrinogen level, aPTT, and PT should be obtained and repeated every 4 to 6 hours to detect disseminated intravascular coagulation. D-Dimer and fibrin split products are often elevated in placental abruption but have not been shown to be a useful screen.[47] A minimum of 2 units of packed red blood cells must be immediately available in the blood bank. Fresh frozen plasma and packed red blood cells should be administered based on abnormal laboratory findings and estimates of ongoing hemorrhage. Obstetric management depends on the maternal condition, fetal status, and severity of abruption. If there are signs of maternal hypovolemia or shock, fluid resuscitation and administration of blood products should begin promptly. Disseminated intravascular coagulation is not an indication to proceed with cesarean section, and abdominal delivery only increases the risk of bleeding complications.

Fetal status and the severity of abruption direct the clinical course once the mother is stable. When the fetus is alive, gestational age and plans for intervention must be established quickly. Hysterotomy offers no benefit to either mother or fetus if a previable fetus shows signs of compromise. Continuous fetal monitoring and close observation are reasonable approaches for a preterm gestation when the heart rate pattern is reassuring. Corticosteroids should be administered to minimize the complications of prematurity if the gestational age is 24 to 34 weeks. As always, the risks of prematurity must be weighed against the risks of continuing the pregnancy. Delivery is generally indicated in a term pregnancy with abruptio placentae, but cesarean delivery is unnecessary if the fetal and maternal status are reassuring. If the fetus has died, induction of labor and vaginal delivery are the safest method of delivery for the mother.

Preterm Labor

Preterm labor requiring tocolysis has been reported in 11% to 28% of gravidas who have blunt trauma.[47,48,60] Delivery before 34 weeks' gestation, however, is uncommon and experienced by only 0.86% of gravidas with blunt trauma.[47] Extravasation of blood into the myometrium is a stimulus for uterine contractions associated with traumatic events. Uterine muscle injury can also cause release of lysosomal enzymes, generation of prostaglandins, and subsequent uterine activity.

When uterine contractions occur after blunt trauma, it may be difficult to determine whether they represent placental abruption or isolated preterm labor. Tocolysis is discouraged by those who believe that uterine activity is an indication of the former. Uterine contractions developing after blunt trauma abate without treatment in 90% of gravidas.[19] Successful tocolysis has been reported after blunt trauma,[60] but close observation is prudent in many cases, given the high rate of spontaneous resolution of contractions. Regardless of whether pharmacologic inhibition of labor is used, fetal heart rate and uterine contractions should be monitored continuously during observation of the patient.

If a tocolytic is administered, the agent should be selected with an awareness of its potential complications. β-Mimetics (ritodrine, terbutaline) are relatively contraindicated in patients at risk for hemorrhage because drug-induced tachycardia may mask early signs of hypovolemia. Magnesium sulfate has fewer cardiac side effects than the β-mimetics. However, patients with renal dysfunction are at increased risk for toxicity because magnesium is excreted through the kidneys. Indomethacin may be used to inhibit preterm labor, although nonsteroidal anti-inflammatory agents, such as indomethacin, may be contraindicated in severely injured patients because the drug can adversely affect platelet and renal function. In addition, it can cause transient premature closure of the fetal ductus arteriosus and oligohydramnios. Calcium channel blockers (e.g., nifedipine) have also been used successfully as an oral tocolytic. This class of drugs may cause maternal hypotension, however, and may imitate early shock in a gravid trauma patient.

Uterine Rupture

Uterine rupture usually occurs as a result of direct abdominal trauma during the late second and third trimesters. It occurs in 0.6% to 1% of gravidas who have blunt trauma and is most frequently associated with maternal pelvic fracture.[61–63] When the uterus ruptures, the site is often fundal.[64] A scarred uterus has a greater propensity to rupture than an unscarred uterus. It is much more devastating for the fetus than for the mother, with a 10% maternal mortality rate but a fetal mortality rate of nearly 100%.[60]

The diagnosis of uterine rupture can be difficult. Signs and symptoms may be limited to vague abdominal pain. Uterine tenderness, a non-reassuring fetal heart rate pattern, absence of the presenting part, palpable fetal parts outside the uterus, fetal demise, and maternal shock are more dramatic presentations. When fetal death occurs after a serious accident, uterine rupture must be considered. Rupture of the uterus may first be suspected when induction of labor is unsuccessful. DPL results are generally positive when the uterus has ruptured and major vessels have been damaged.

If uterine rupture is suspected, exploratory laparotomy should be performed to control maternal hemorrhage. Ideally, a trauma surgeon will be in attendance to explore the abdomen for additional injuries. A vertical abdominal incision allows maximum exposure, particularly if surgical repair of intra-abdominal injuries is required. Conservation of fertility is always a consideration because a patient's wishes may be unknown or uncertain at the time of the accident. However, uterine repair should be undertaken only if the patient is hemodynamically stable and hemorrhage can be controlled. When the uterus is extensively damaged and repair is impossible or the patient is in hemorrhagic shock, hysterectomy is indicated.

If the uterus is to be repaired, the site of rupture should be assessed after delivery of the fetus and once hemostasis is achieved. Necrotic tissue along the rupture site may be excised to allow reapproximation of well-vascularized tissue. The uterine defect can then be repaired in layers. The risk of uterine rupture in future pregnancies is certainly present, but not prohibitive. It would seem prudent to offer elective cesarean delivery in subsequent pregnancies, especially if the rupture site was fundal or the damage was extensive.

Fetal Injury

The exact incidence of fetal injury as a result of maternal trauma is unknown. An incidence of 0.49% has been noted in gravidas with noncatastrophic trauma.[47] Fetal skull fractures, long bone fractures, intracranial hemorrhage, and soft tissue injury have been reported. Skull fracture or head injury is most commonly described and is associated with maternal pelvic fracture late in gestation, when the fetal head is engaged.[52]

The management of fetal injuries must be individualized, and experience is limited. Delivery may be delayed in a very premature gestation if the fetus is alive and without signs of distress. Serial ultrasonography and frequent assessment of fetal well-being may be beneficial until maturity is reached. If pregnancy is advanced or delivery is indicated for fetal compromise, a pediatrician, or neonatologist if available, should be in attendance for delivery. Accurate and unbiased documentation is always important, given the medicolegal ramifications of fetal injury.

Fetal Assessment

The prediction of adverse fetal outcome after a traumatic event has been a controversial subject. Cardiotocographic monitoring is currently the most sensitive method of immediate fetal surveillance and is more sensitive than ultrasound in detecting abruption.[19,61,65] Risk factors for fetal death include ISS, severe abdominal injury, hypotension, hemorrhagic shock, disseminated intravascular coagulation (DIC) with or without abruption, and gestational age less than 23 weeks.[66–70] Because almost all patients who have placental abruption after trauma manifest signs soon after the event, it is important to institute fetal heart rate and uterine activity monitoring in the emergency department as soon as the mother is stable. Delayed abruption several days after an accident is described, but the few patients reported were not monitored immediately after the event and early signs may have been overlooked.[71,72]

Uterine activity appears to be the most sensitive indicator for the risk of abruption after blunt trauma.[15,23,47,73] The presence of six to eight or more contractions per hour identifies a patient who is at risk for adverse pregnancy outcome.[10,15,47] Approximately 14% of women who had contractions every 2 to 5 minutes immediately after blunt trauma subsequently had abruption. No patient with fewer than eight contractions per hour had abruption.[10] Similarly, a second study showed that when uterine contractions, tenderness, or vaginal bleeding were present, 19% of patients had obstetric complications compared with 0.9% who did not have these symptoms.[15]

FIGURE 54–3
Fetal monitoring recommendations for the pregnant trauma patient.

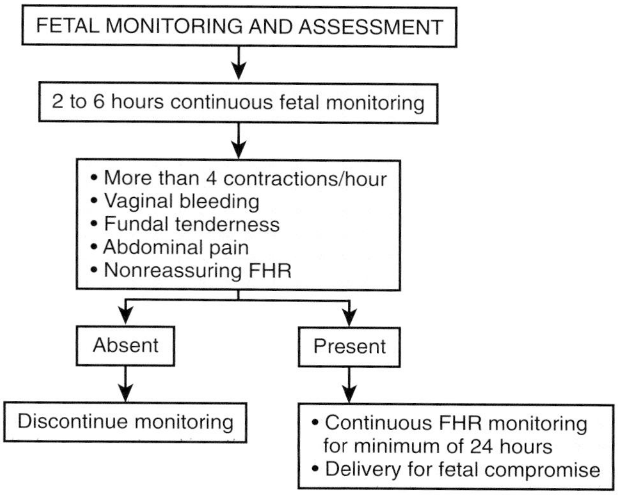

Although obstetric ultrasonographic examination can be helpful in fetal assessment, normal findings do not exclude or reduce the risk of abruption. The sensitivity of ultrasonography in predicting abruption in blunt trauma patients is only 40%.[10,19] Findings suggestive of an abruption include retro- or preplacental hematoma, increased placental thickness and echogenicity, and subchorionic or marginal fluid collection. Ultrasonography is useful to exclude placenta previa, document fetal viability, establish gestational age, estimate fetal weight, measure amniotic fluid volume, and assess fetal well-being.

Guidelines for monitoring pregnant trauma victims have been suggested and are outlined in Figure 54–3. If a patient does not have uterine tenderness, contractions, or vaginal bleeding on presentation, 2 to 6 hours of cardiotocographic monitoring is sufficient.[15,47,48,60,61] Patients may be released home if they do not have symptoms, the fetal heart rate pattern is reassuring, and maternal injuries have been appropriately evaluated and treated. These patients are not at increased risk for adverse pregnancy outcome compared with uninjured control subjects.[10] They should be instructed about the symptoms and signs of preterm labor and abruption as well as indications to return to the hospital.

Approximately 52% of gravidas have uterine tenderness, irritability, or contractions or vaginal bleeding after blunt trauma.[48] These patients require additional observation and continuous fetal monitoring; a minimum of 24 hours has been recommended, even if symptoms resolve.[47] A more recent study also recommends at least 24 hours of fetal monitoring if the maternal heart rate is greater than 110 beats/min, the ISS is greater than 9, the fetal heart rate is less than 120 beats/min or greater than 160 beats/min, or there is evidence of placental abruption, and for victims of ejections or motorcycle or pedestrian collisions.[74] The hospital stay should be extended as maternal and fetal conditions dictate. Seriously injured patients who require surgery or transfer to the intensive care unit present a challenge to the obstetrician. If the fetus is viable, continuous monitoring should be used; obstetrics personnel must be readily available to evaluate the fetal heart rate tracing.

Fetomaternal Hemorrhage

The KB remains controversial and no study has clearly demonstrated usefulness in predicting adverse maternal or fetal outcome in pregnant trauma victims. Although routine testing of all gravid blunt trauma victims has been suggested, the clinical utility of this approach is uncertain.[48] Earlier studies reported that FMH occurs in a significant number of gravidas who are victims of blunt trauma, with an incidence of 8.7% to 30% in gravid trauma patients versus 1.8% to 8% of pregnant controls.[10,15,48,73,75] Another study, however, found no difference in the incidence of a positive KB in pregnant trauma patients (2.6%) versus low risk gravidas undergoing a diabetes screen (5.1%).[76] Patients evaluated in the study of minor trauma had a similar low incidence of a positive KB (2.8%).[16] The KB does not correlate with the occurrence of placental abruption or fetal distress,[16,47,73] but a positive KB has been suggested to predict preterm labor.[77] The KB predicted obstetric complications in only 27% of pregnant trauma patients in one study,[73] and the sensitivity for adverse outcome was only 4% to 18% in another series.[16] Although no clinical signs reliably predict FMH, an increased incidence has been noted in women who have an anterior placenta or uterine tenderness.[10,15]

Most fetuses with FMH have a normal outcome, but anemia, supraventricular tachycardia, and fetal demise are recognized complications.[10,75] No classification for degree of FMH has been established, but a number of studies have attempted to clarify the amount of FMH that predicts adverse fetal outcome. A transfused volume of greater than 20 mL/kg fetal weight has been suggested as the threshold at which adverse perinatal outome is observed.[78] Most recently, the transfused blood volume corrected for fetoplacental weight was shown to best correlate with fetal hemoglobin levels. A KB greater than 2.5% or transfused volume corrected for fetoplacental weight greater than 43 mL/kg was associated with adverse fetal outcome.[79] Middle cerebral artery (MCA) blood flow velocity reliably predicts fetal anemia in isoimmunized pregnancies, but its accuracy in the acute anemia of FMH is less certain. Too few data exist to use the MCA in isolation because severe acute anemia may not be detected.[79] Nevertheless, an elevated peak systolic velocity of the MCA would be very suggestive of fetal anemia.

The importance of KB testing in the pregnant trauma patient remains identification of a large volume of fetomaternal transfusion in the Rh-negative woman. Massive FMH occasionally occurs, so all Rh-negative gravidas should undergo KB testing after any trauma to ensure an adequate dosage of Rhogam is administered. Repeat testing 24 to 48 hours after the initial positive result may be considered to evaluate for ongoing FMH and ensure adequate Rhogam coverage.

Isoimmunization can occur very early in pregnancy because the Rh antigen is present on fetal red blood cells 34 days after conception. The amount of fetal blood required to stimulate maternal antibody formation may be as little as 0.01 mL. The KB test, however, is not sensitive enough to detect such a small amount of fetal blood in the maternal circulation. Because an undetectable amount of fetal blood can lead to sensitization in early pregnancy, all unsensitized Rh-negative women who suffer trauma should receive Rh immune globulin.[47,61]

The amount of immune globulin administered depends on the volume of FMH as calculated from the KB stain results. Anti-D immunoglobulin (300 μg or 1500 IU) administered within 72 hours of the event protects against maternal antibody formation for transfusion of up to 15 mL fetal red blood cells (30 mL whole blood). If KB testing is unavailable, 300 μg is adequate in most women and can be administered empirically.[15,19]

SUMMARY OF MANAGEMENT OPTIONS

Blunt Trauma

Management Options	Evidence Quality and Recommendation	References
General Management		
Perform general trauma resuscitation.	—/GPP	—
Obtain FHR monitoring and fetal ultrasound.	III/B	47
Abruptio Placentae		
Assess maternal condition.	III/B	59
Assess fetal condition with FHR.	IIa/B	10,15
	III/B	47
See Chapter 58 for detailed discussion.	—/—	—
Preterm Labor		
Be alert for evolving abruption.	—/GPP	—
Consider tocolysis.	III/B	47,48
See Chapters 61 and 62 for detailed discussion.	—/—	—

Management Options	Evidence Quality and Recommendation	References
Uterine Rupture		
Exploratory laparotomy when suspected.	III/B	33
Use a midline incision for adequate exposure.		
Perform uterine repair if the patient is hemodynamically stable.		
Perform cesarean hysterectomy if the patient has uncontrollable hemorrhage or excessive uterine damage.		
Fetal Injury		
Individualize management, because experience is limited; gestation and fetal condition will influence the management; ultrasound evaluation may help.	—/GPP	—
Fetomaternal Hemorrhage		
Perform KB test: if positive, confirms significant fetomaternal hemorrhage; if negative, does not exclude a small bleed.	III/B	47
Give Rh immune globulin to all Rh-negative women in accordance with local guidelines; increased doses required with positive KB test.	III/B IV/C	47 61
Fetal Assessment		
FHR monitoring is the most sensitive assessment of immediate fetal condition.	III/B IV/C	19 61
Normal obstetric ultrasound does not exclude fetal risk (e.g., abruption); confirms viability, approximate weight, and presentation; excludes placenta previa.	IIa/B III/B	10 66,67
Clinical risk factors for adverse fetal outcome are severity of injury, shock, disseminated intravascular coagulation, and gestation <23 wk.	III/B	15,47,48
Guidelines for fetal monitoring:	III/B	15,47,48
• No uterine tenderness, contractions or bleeding.	III/B	15,47,48
• 2–6-Hr continuous FHR monitoring.	IV/C	61
• Uterine tenderness, contractions or bleeding: minimum of 24-hr continuous FHR monitoring.		

FHR, fetal heart rate; GPP, good practice point; KB, Kleihauer-Betke.

Seat Belts and Airbags

Passenger restraint systems have saved thousands of lives. The use of lap-shoulder belts reduces the likelihood of fatal injury by 45% and the likelihood of moderate to critical injury by 50%.[80] Safety belts minimize injuries by limiting passenger contact with the interior of the vehicle, preventing ejection, and spreading the force of deceleration over a larger area.

The leading cause of fetal death in MVAs is maternal death, and the most common cause of maternal death is ejection from the vehicle.[81] Maternal mortality rate is 33% when the woman is ejected from the vehicle versus only 5% when she is not. When the mother is ejected, the fetal mortality rate is 47% compared with 11% when the mother remains in the vehicle. The rate of fetal death is decreased by seat belt use because seat belts prevent ejection, thereby decreasing maternal mortality.[81]

The shoulder harness reduces the risk of maternal head injury by preventing jackknifing of the mother's torso over the lap belt and increasing the area over which deceleration forces dissipate. Decreasing force over the abdomen reduced the fetal mortality rate in animal studies from 50% with a lap belt alone to 12% with the three-point restraint system.[82] Crash simulation with a pregnant crash dummy also provides evidence that the three-point restraint system decreases the likelihood of injury.[83]

Although air bags have augmented the reduction in rates of injury and death, they do not offer protection in lateral collisions and do not prevent ejection. Combined lap-shoulder restraint systems must continue to be worn for optimal crash protection. Air bags should not be disconnected during pregnancy and do not appear to worsen fetal outcomes.[44] Peak uterine strain has been shown to be reduced by half in computer simulations of air bag deployment.[84]

Despite the benefits of safety belts, pregnant women often hesitate to use them; 30% of gravidas either do not wear a safety belt or wear it incorrectly.[44,50,85] The perception of increased risk of fetal injury with seat belt use is a major factor contributing to the reluctance of pregnant women to use restraint systems. Unfortunately, only 42% to 55% of gravidas receive information on the use of restraint systems during pregnancy.[50,86,87] Women should be instructed to place the lap portion of the belt under the abdomen and across both the anterior and the superior iliac spines. The belt should be snug, but comfortable. The shoulder restraint should cross the shoulder without rubbing the neck and should be positioned between the breasts. It is helpful to remind pregnant women that women wearing seatbelts at the time of an MVA are not at significantly greater risk for adverse fetal outcomes than pregnant women not in an MVA.[51]

PENETRATING TRAUMA

Incidence

Pregnant women are the victims of penetrating trauma with increasing frequency, particularly in inner-city areas. Gunshot and stab wounds are the most common, but injury occurs by other mechanisms as well and may be self-inflicted.[88] Pregnant women have also been victims in terror-related multiple-casualty incidents and frequently sustain significant injuries.[89]

Mortality in nonpregnant victims with penetrating injury increases with the number of organs injured, but visceral injury and mortality are lower during pregnancy. The mother usually fares much better than the fetus when the injury is caused by a gunshot or stab wound.[22,90] Maternal mortality is 0% to 9% for gunshot wounds during pregnancy, whereas perinatal mortality is 41% to 71%.[90] When the mother is stabbed, fetal injury and fetal death occur in 93% and 50% of cases, respectively.[91]

Fetal survival is affected by several factors, including the severity of fetal and maternal injury, the presence and extent of placental hemorrhage, and gestational age at delivery. Although direct fetal injury is responsible for most perinatal deaths, some deaths results from premature delivery, with its attendant complications.[92] Women in terror-related incidents have a high likelihood of requiring emergent delivery for fetal compromise with bradycardia, uterine rupture, and placental abruption cited in a recent review.[89]

General Management

Maternal injury patterns change with advancing gestation. Penetrating trauma in the first trimester causes wounds similar to those in nonpregnant victims. As the uterus enlarges and occupies more space in the abdominal cavity, it is more likely to be injured than any other intra-abdominal organ. The uterus offers relative protection to other abdominal organs by the third trimester. Hence, bowel injury is less common when a pregnant woman has a penetrating injury to the lower abdomen, but the small bowel is at high risk for injury when entry is in the upper abdomen. Multiple bowel wounds are more common in pregnant victims than in their nonpregnant counterparts because the intestine is compressed in the upper abdomen with advancing gestation.

As with other forms of trauma, the emergency team, trauma surgeon, and obstetrician must coordinate the care of a pregnant woman. Maternal resuscitation and hemodynamic stability are a priority, and the leading cause of early death from gunshot wounds is hypovolemia as a result of major vessel injury. The injured woman must be thoroughly examined and each entrance and exit wound noted. If exploratory laparotomy is indicated, a midline vertical incision offers optimal exposure to the abdomen.

DPL may be used to identify intra-abdominal injury requiring laparotomy, but it has several limitations in patients with penetrating injuries.[6] First, the findings may be negative in nonpregnant victims, despite hollow viscus injury, because bleeding is usually minimal. Second, the leukocyte response to bowel injury may be delayed, causing a false-negative finding. Finally, the accuracy of DPL in pregnant women with stab wounds is unknown. Although a positive finding would be expected when uterine vessels are injured, the size of a uterine wound and the depth of penetration cannot be ascertained.

FAST was prospectively evaluated in 75 patients with penetrating abdominal trauma and was shown to be useful as the initial diagnostic test.[93] It is not, however, as reliable as in blunt trauma, and a negative result requires additional testing. In addition, it has not been studied in pregnant victims of penetrating trauma, and its accuracy is unknown in this setting.

An indication for exploratory laparotomy, however, is not an indication to empty the uterus. Abdominal delivery concurrent with exploratory laparotomy increases operative time and blood loss. A patient may undergo induction of labor and vaginal delivery postoperatively without increased risk of morbidity.[94] The only indication for hysterotomy is to provide adequate surgical exposure for repair of maternal injuries. Cesarean hysterectomy is indicated when damage to the uterus is extensive or uterine injury is associated with uncontrollable hemorrhage. Specific guidelines for treating pregnant women with gunshot and stab wounds are discussed later, but these guidelines should be individualized based on obstetric and surgical needs.

Gunshot Wounds

The size of the entrance wound does not predict the internal damage caused by a bullet. If no exit wound is found, radiographic studies are performed to localize the bullet. A flat plate and lateral film usually suffice. A number of management options exist for intra-abdominal bullet wounds and include exploratory laparotomy with or without cesarean delivery, DPL, laparoscopy, contrast CT, wound exploration, and observation.

Surgical exploration has been considered standard practice for managing bullet wounds of the abdomen and flank. However, careful observation of a wounded gravida has been suggested as an alternative in the following situation[95]:

- The mother is hemodynamically stable.
- The bullet has entered below the uterine fundus.
- The bullet can be localized to within the uterus.
- No maternal genitourinary or gastrointestinal injury has occurred.

The fetus should be free of injury or compromise, or dead, if the mother is managed conservatively.[96,97] Broad-spectrum antibiotic coverage is prudent, at least initially. This conservative approach should be considered only in trauma centers in which experienced surgeons manage trauma care. With this approach, it has been suggested that fewer than 20% of gravidas require surgical intervention for visceral wounds.[95]

Although nonoperative management has been reported, this approach has not been prospectively tested in gravidas with penetrating injuries. Radiologic studies may give a false impression of the location of the bullet in the uterus when significant maternal injury has occurred.[98] DPL can be performed to exclude intra-abdominal hemorrhage. Exploratory laparotomy, however, is the most reliable means for detecting intra-abdominal injury should doubt exist. The ultimate decision about the need for operative intervention rests with the surgical team.

The decision to deliver the fetus is based on gestational age, fetal status, and exposure required for surgical exploration and repair of maternal injuries. If a near-term fetus is alive and the uterus injured, cesarean delivery with uterine repair is reasonable. When a viable fetus is alive but remote from term, suggested indications for delivery include evidence of fetal hemorrhage, uteroplacental insufficiency, and infection.[90]

Although fetal injury can occur when a bullet enters the mother's lower abdomen, the risks of prematurity may outweigh the risk of delaying repair of fetal injuries. Although obstetric ultrasonography and radiography may be helpful, the diagnosis of in utero injuries can be difficult. Neonatal and pediatric surgical consultation is invaluable in planning care.

If the fetus has died, vaginal delivery is preferred if there is no evidence of uterine hemorrhage. Options include awaiting spontaneous labor and induction of labor with prostaglandins or oxytocin once maternal injuries have been addressed. If laparotomy is required and the uterus prevents exposure for repair of maternal injuries, evacuation of the dead fetus is indicated.

Stab Wounds

When a patient has a stab wound, attempts should be made to determine the object used and its length. The longer the object, the more likely it is that the peritoneum was penetrated when the abdomen was wounded. The risk of intestinal injury in nonpregnant stabbing victims is less than that with gunshot injuries because bowel tends to move away from a penetrating object (sliding effect). This effect explains, in part, the lower mortality rate with stab wounds than with gunshot wounds. The sliding effect may be less during pregnancy because bowel is compressed into the upper abdomen with advancing gestation.

Traditionally, all abdominal stab wounds have been regarded as an indication for exploratory laparotomy, but nonoperative management has been considered for some patients.[88] Two of the most important factors in assessing the need for laparotomy in injured gravidas are peritoneal penetration and location of the entrance wound. A wound can be probed, and a fistulogram may assist in determining whether the peritoneal cavity has been entered. If a conservative approach is chosen, the patient must be closely monitored and exploration undertaken without delay if the mother has signs of hemorrhage or evidence of sepsis. Contraindications to observation include

- Penetration of the peritoneal cavity.
- Entry above the fundus.
- Hemodynamic instability of the mother.
- Fetal compromise at a viable gestational age.

The final decision for operative intervention should, as with gunshot wounds, be made by the surgical consultant.

A lower abdominal stab wound with adequate force is likely to damage the uterus as well as the fetus. Management options include observation or laparotomy/uterine repair with or without delivery of the fetus.[99] No outcome data are available comparing repair of a uterine wound with no repair. The risks of infection and uterine rupture associated with each approach are unknown, given the limited number of patients with these injuries. Indications for delivery are the same as those for gravidas with a gunshot wound.

Based on reported cases of stab wounds to the pregnant uterus, Sakala and Kort[91] proposed the following management plan: A nonperforating injury of the uterus may be repaired without disturbing the pregnancy. Perforating injuries, however, carry a much higher rate of fetal injury. A fetus at or near term should be considered for cesarean delivery and uterine repair. If the fetus is premature, alive, and not compromised, the uterus may be repaired, with vaginal delivery anticipated. When the fetus has died, both perforating and nonperforating injuries should be repaired and the fetus delivered vaginally. The injured uterus maintains its ability to labor and deliver an infant.[100] Antibiotic prophylaxis seems reasonable in these cases, although no data are available to support this recommendation.

Stab wounds to the upper abdomen are three times more frequent than lower abdominal wounds. Upper abdominal wounds that penetrate the peritoneum require surgical exploration because of the high likelihood of small bowel injury. If doubt exists, exploratory laparotomy is the safest approach to exclude intra-abdominal injury. When the peritoneum of the upper abdomen has been penetrated, laceration of the diaphragm must be excluded because it can result in bowel herniation, strangulation, and sepsis. After diaphragm repair, labor and second-stage Valsalva efforts should be avoided and cesarean delivery should be performed, presumably to avoid increasing intra-abdominal pressure.[91]

SUMMARY OF MANAGEMENT OPTIONS

Penetrating Trauma

Management Options	Evidence Quality and Recommendation	References
General Management		
See earlier box on "Blunt Trauma."	—/—	—
Examine patient for entrance and exit wounds.	IV/C	22
	III/B	90
Exploratory Laparotomy		
Use a midline vertical incision.	IV/C	22
	III/B	90
Uterine evacuation is not mandatory.	IV/C	22
	III/B	90
Cesarean hysterectomy may be necessary if the patient has uncontrollable hemorrhage or excessive uterine damage.	IV/C	22
	III/B	90
Gunshot Wounds		
Obtain flat plate and lateral radiographs if no exit wound is visible.	IV/C	96
Perform surgical exploration if:		
• Signs of intra-abdominal injury.	III/B	94
• Positive peritoneal lavage.	III/B	6
• Persistent unexplained shock.	—/GPP	—
Consider conservative management if:		
• The mother is hemodynamically stable.	IV/C	95,96
• The bullet entered below the uterine fundus.	III/B	94
• The bullet can be localized to the uterus.	III/B	94
• The fetus is without injury or dead.	III/B	94
• The mother has no genitourinary or gastrointestinal injury.	III/B	94
Deliver fetus if:		
• Evidence of fetal hemorrhage.	IV/C	95
• Uteroplacental insufficiency.	IV/C	95
• Infection.	—/GPP	—
Stab Wounds		
Determine peritoneal penetration; options:		
• Probe wound.	—/GPP	—
• Fistulogram.	IV/C	91
• Diagnostic peritoneal lavage.	III/B	6
Perform surgical exploration if:		
• Peritoneal penetration.	IV/C	91
• Entry above the uterine fundus.	—/GPP	—
• Hemodynamically unstable mother.	IV/C	99
• Fetal compromise at viable gestation.	IV/C	91
Consider conservative management if:		
• No peritoneal penetration.	IV/C	91
• Entry below the uterine fundus.	IV/C	91
• Guidelines for delivery of the fetus are the same as for gunshot wounds (see "Gunshot Wounds," earlier).	IV/C	91

Management Options	Evidence Quality and Recommendation	References
Assess uterine injury with lower abdominal stab wound; options:		
• Observation.	IV/C	91
• Uterine repair with delivery.	IV/C	91
• Uterine repair and fetus remains in utero.	IV/C	91

GPP, good practice point.

ACUTE SPINAL CORD INJURY

The initial management of a pregnant patient with a spinal cord injury includes general resuscitation measures, stabilization of the neck, and airway maintenance. Initiation of high-dose methylprednisolone (30 mg/kg) within 8 hours of the injury followed by 5.4 mg/kg for 23 hours improves motor and sensory function at 6 months.[101] Evaluation for additional injuries should be performed and fetal monitoring instituted as soon as possible given the potential hemodynamic sequelae of cord injury. Neurogenic shock, cardiovascular instability, and autonomic hyperreflexia can develop following complete cord transection. Long-term issues of the patient with a spinal cord injury are beyond the scope of this chapter.

Neurogenic shock develops due to the blockade of sympathetic function associated with the cord injury. Parasympathetic symptoms dominate and include hypotension, bradycardia, decreased cardiac output, and hypothermia, all of which can lead to fetal distress. Fluid replacement and inotropic agents such as dobutamine may be required to maintain hemodynamic stability. This therapy should be guided by central vascular monitoring. Neurogenic shock lasts from 1 to 3 weeks, and its resolution may be signaled by the onset of autonomic hyperreflexia.

Autonomic hyperreflexia develops in 85% of patients with a cord injury above T5-6. It is due to unregulated sympathetic discharge and is triggered by a stimulus below the level of the lesion (full bladder or rectum, labor). Paroxysmal release of catecholamines causes tachycardia, hypertension, flushing, headache, sweating, and feelings of anxiety. Treatment in the laboring patient includes regional anesthesia; labetolol or hydralazine may also be used but with caution to avoid hypotension.

BURNS

Incidence

Fortunately, most burns sustained during pregnancy are minor, and more severe burns are uncommon. Most burns occur in the home and result from a house fire, hot water, flammable liquids, or gases. Pregnant women account for 0.4% to 7% of all patients who are hospitalized with major burns.[102–106]

Maternal survival is dependent on the percentage of total body surface area (TBSA) burned.[105,107,108] When 20% to 39% of TBSA has been burned, 97% to 100% of gravidas survive. The mortality rate for 40% to 59% TBSA burns ranges from 27% to 50%. Burns exceeding 60% TBSA are associated with very high death rates.[104,105,108–111] Survival in pregnant women with burn injuries is comparable with that in their nonpregnant counterparts, when matched for burn severity.[107] Concurrent inhalation injury is associated with increased maternal and fetal mortality.[112]

Fetal survival is also affected by the percentage of maternal TBSA involved. The fetal mortality rate is negligible when the burn affects less than 20% of maternal TBSA. When 20% to 39% of the mother's TBSA is involved, the fetal loss rate ranges from 11% to 27%. The fetal mortality rate increases to 45% to 53% with burns that affect 40% to 59% of maternal TBSA. When a pregnant woman has a burn that involves greater than 60% of TBSA, fetal loss approaches 100%.[104,105,108–111]

Classification of Burns

The depth of a burn is classified by a system that characterizes the need for surgical treatment. A *superficial burn* is confined to the epidermis with pink or red painful skin. *Superficial partial-thickness burns* involve the epidermis and superficial dermis. Adequate epithelial cells remain and allow skin to regenerate. Clinically, blistering, erythema, and pain characterize superficial partial-thickness burns. *Deep partial-thickness lesions* are characterized by blisters, pale white appearance, and no pain. *Full-thickness burns* destroy all dermal elements and regeneration is not possible without grafting. The burned area appears charred and leathery, without blisters; thrombosed superficial vessels may be visible and pain is absent.

Burn size, or the percentage of TBSA, can be estimated by the "rule of nines" and refined with a Lund-Browder or Berkow chart. This system was devised for nonpregnant patients, however, and does not account for the presumed increase in abdominal surface area with advancing gestation.

Burn severity is defined as minor, moderate, or major. A minor burn is a superficial burn, a partial-thickness burn that covers less than 10% of TBSA, or a full-thickness burn that covers less than 2% of TBSA. Moderate burns are those of 10% to 20% TBSA, 2% to 5% full-thickness burn, high-voltage injury, suspected inhalation injury, circumferential burn, and coexisting medical problems that predispose to infection. Moderate burns require hospital admission for management. Major burns include any burn covering more than 20% TBSA; full-thickness burns covering more than 5% of TBSA; burns of the face, eyes, ears, hands, feet, genitalia, or skin over major joints; high-voltage burn, including lightning strike; inhalation injury; patients with other significant injury; and patients requiring special social, emotional, or long-term rehabilitation. Major burns mandate referral to a burn center.[113]

Management of Minor Burns

Minor burns may be treated on an outpatient basis if the burn does not affect an area of critical function (e.g., hand, across a joint) or an area in which cosmesis is a concern (e.g., face). Superficial burns do not require specific treatment beyond keeping the area clean and protected. A mild analgesic may be prescribed. A narcotic, such as oxycodone, may be required for pain control in patients with partial-thickness burns. The burned area should be cleansed with sterile saline and devitalized tissue removed. Large blisters may be incised and débrided. Blisters should not be aspirated because bacteria can be introduced into a closed space. A number of biosynthetic dressings are commercially available and can be used to protect the burned area. Patients with partial-thickness burns should be reevaluated in 24 hours. At this time, the wound is evaluated and the dressing changed. Complete healing can be expected in 2 to 3 weeks, with no adverse effects on the pregnancy.

Management of Major Burns

The basic principles of resuscitation also apply to the patient with a major burn injury. Fluid resuscitation is the most important initial treatment and is commonly required for burns covering greater than 20% TBSA. Venous access should be established with a 14- to 16-gauge catheter placed through unburned skin, when possible. Immediate removal of clothing prevents continued burning by smoldering synthetic fabric. All skin surfaces must be examined, burned areas assessed for depth and surface area involved, and additional injuries excluded. Diligent wound care is critical to preventing infectious complications. Inhalation injury should be suspected and 100% oxygen given by face mask. Arterial blood gas analysis and carbon monoxide level measurements are standard. An intravenous narcotic should be administered, as needed, for pain control.

The systemic response to a major burn is a massive release of vasoactive mediators that cause a decrease in plasma and blood volumes, shifting intravascular fluid to intracellular and interstitial compartments. Thus, the goal of fluid resuscitation is to correct hypovolemia during the initial 24 to 48 hours. Hypovolemic shock develops in a patient with burns covering more than 15% to 20% of TBSA if fluid resuscitation is not instituted promptly.[114] Hypovolemia in the pregnant patient can also lead to decreased placental perfusion and fetal compromise. Therefore, proper resuscitation is critical for both mother and fetus.

The essential component of fluid resuscitation is crystalloid (normal saline or lactated Ringer's solution). Edema formation at the burn site is most rapid during the initial 6 to 8 hours after a burn, and fluid is administered at a rate to compensate for the intravascular loss. The amount of fluid that a patient requires during the first 24 hours after a burn injury can be estimated with one of several formulas. The Parkland formula estimates fluid requirements during the first 24 hours as 4 mL/kg/% TBSA burned. One half of the total fluid required is administered during the first 8 hours after the burn (not after admission), and the remaining half is administered over the next 16 hours. The Brooke and Evans formulas are also used to estimate fluid requirements, but differ in their administration of colloid and free water in addition to crystalloid. Inhalation injury also increases the amount of fluid required during initial resuscitation. A new multifactorial formula has been recently published that may offer a better guide to initial fluid resuscitation.[115]

The standard formulas, however, may not be as accurate for a major burn in pregnancy because they appear to underestimate the amount of fluid required for adequate resuscitation. A case report of a gravida with 38% TBSA burn and inhalation injury required twice the amount of fluid estimated by the Parkland formula.[116] Fluid administration is adjusted to maintain urinary output of 0.5 mL/kg/hr or 30 to 50 mL/hr. Over-resuscitation must be avoided because compartment syndromes can develop as edema accumulates beneath the inelastic burned skin of deep burns (eschar). Most patients remain tachycardic despite adequate fluid resuscitation, and because pregnant women have a mild baseline increase in heart rate, this may not be a reliable clinical measure. Serum electrolytes must be closely monitored during and after resuscitation, with imbalances corrected on an ongoing basis.

Carbon Monoxide Poisoning

Carbon monoxide (CO) poisoning can occur whenever carbonaceous material is released as a result of incomplete combustion. The affinity of CO for hemoglobin is more than 200 times that of oxygen, and it readily displaces oxygen from hemoglobin.[117] CO causes a left shift of the oxyhemoglobin dissociation curve and increases the affinity of hemoglobin for the remaining bound oxygen. Tissue oxygenation decreases as less oxygen is released from hemoglobin in the periphery. Signs and symptoms of CO poisoning correlate with the blood level. A CO level of less than 10% is unlikely to cause symptoms, whereas levels of 10% to 20% cause a mild headache and palpitations. Once the level reaches 20% to 40%, dizziness, agitation, confusion, and incoordination become apparent. Patients with a CO level of greater than 40% are at risk for progressive dyspnea, lethargy, coma, and death.

CO readily crosses the placenta and may cause fetal malformations, hypoxia, neurologic dysfunction, low birth weight, and death in utero. CO levels rise more slowly in the fetus than in the mother and continue to increase for up to 24 hours after the maternal level has reached a steady state. Once fetal CO reaches a steady state, the concentration is 10% to 15% higher than the mother's concentration. Likewise, the fetus requires a much longer time for elimination than the mother does. The maternal half-life of CO in a sheep model was 2.5 hours compared with 7 hours in the fetus.[117]

The blood level determines the urgency of treatment for CO poisoning. Observation is sufficient if the CO level is less than 10%. When the level is 10% to 20%, treatment with 100% inspired oxygen is indicated. High-concentration oxygen administered with a tight-fitting face mask decreases the half-life of carboxyhemoglobin in adults from 2 to 3 hours in room air to 45 minutes.[117] Similarly, 100% oxygen decreases the half-life of carboxyhemoglobin in the fetus from 7 hours to 2 to 3 hours, but it is still longer than that in the mother. Based on mathematical calculations, a pregnant woman with CO poisoning should receive 100% oxygen for up to five times longer than needed to reduce her own level to normal (<5%).[117,118] This extended period of treatment allows for the longer elimination time required by the fetus.

Hyperbaric oxygen therapy is used for nonpregnant patients with a CO level greater than 25% or with neurologic changes, regardless of the blood level. It has been used to treat pregnant women with CO poisoning, with no adverse fetal effect. Therapy has been recommended for pregnant women with a maternal CO level of more than 20%; neurologic changes, regardless of the CO level; or signs of fetal compromise.[119] However, hyperbaric oxygen therapy in patients with a major burn presents a number of logistic problems, and care must be individualized.

Inhalation Injury

Inhalation injury occurs as a result of exposure to smoke particles and chemicals. Patients who are burned in a closed space are at increased risk, and the incidence increases with burn severity. Two thirds of patients with burns affecting more than 70% of TBSA have concurrent inhalation injury.[114] Singed nasal hair, facial burns, inflamed oropharyngeal mucosa, carbonaceous sputum, and a CO level greater than 15% suggest injury. Laryngeal edema should be suspected in a patient with hoarseness, stridor, or cough. Intubation may be required to maintain a patent airway. The initial chest radiograph, however, may not show the severity of injury. If the diagnosis of inhalation injury is in doubt, laryngobronchoscopy can be performed. Treatment includes warm humidified oxygen, bronchodilators, pulmonary toilet, nebulized heparin, and therapeutic bronchoscopy. Mechanical ventilation is required if respiratory failure occurs.

Additional Complications of Burns

Patients with major burns are at risk for many complications, including pulmonary edema, pneumonia, septic shock, electrolyte disturbances, ileus, nutritional deficiencies, and scar formation. Sepsis is the major cause of death in patients with burns, emphasizing the importance of sterile technique.[108] Topical antimicrobial agents delay bacterial colonization of the wounded area. Three have established efficacy in the treatment of major burns: 11.1% mafenide acetate, 1% silver sulfadiazine, and 0.5% silver nitrate. Silver sulfadiazine must be used with caution, and long-term use is relatively contraindicated in pregnant women because of the theoretical risk of kernicterus in the newborn. Iodine-containing solutions are frequently used for wound care, but their use must be limited during pregnancy because of the absorption of the iodine and the risk of fetal thyroid dysfunction.[108] All patients with a burn affecting greater than 10% of TBSA should receive tetanus toxoid with immunoglobulin if their previous immunization status is uncertain

Circumferential burns of the thorax or abdomen may cause respiratory compromise or vena caval compression in pregnant victims. Early escharotomy improves respiratory excursion and relieves increased intra-abdominal pressure. Scar formation can be physically limiting, but successful pregnancies have been reported in patients with significant abdominal scarring after burn injuries. Surgical release and grafting can be performed in a scar that becomes restrictive with advancing pregnancy, and uninvolved expanded abdominal skin has been used as a flap to reconstruct a scar after delivery.[120,121]

Clinically significant thromboembolism is an infrequent complication in patients with a major burn. Nevertheless, prophylaxis has been suggested for patients with additional risk factors, including lower extremity trauma, extensive burns, morbid obesity, prolonged bed rest, and central venous lines.[41] Although data on thromboembolism in pregnant burn victims are not available, the hypercoaguable state of pregnancy is a risk factor for which heparin prophylaxis seems reasonable, providing no contraindications.[112,116]

Obstetric Complications of Burns

Obstetric complications associated with major burns include spontaneous abortion, premature labor, and fetal death in utero. The first week after injury seems to be the period of highest risk, and medical complications often precede obstetric complications. The physiologic response to burns includes hypovolemia, hypoxia, acidosis, electrolyte imbalance, and sepsis. Each of these, alone or in combination, can lead to uterine activity or fetal compromise.[122] Septicemia is the most common cause of spontaneous abortion in women with burns.[102]

An increased incidence of premature labor has been associated with burns affecting more than 30% to 35% of TBSA.[122] Prostaglandins and leukotrienes are released from macrophages, neutrophils, and platelets at the burn site. Prostaglandin F_2, a uterine stimulant, is produced by scalded skin. Because prostaglandins are associated with uterine activity, pregnant women who have a burn injury should be monitored for uterine contractions. Tocolytic agents, particularly β-mimetics, must be used very cautiously, and only after the mother is clinically stable and the fetal heart rate tracing is reassuring.

Intervention on behalf of a viable fetus may be required in a gravida with a major burn. The following recommendations are based on combined experiences of various authors caring for pregnant burn victims: Delivery is suggested when a significant medical complication develops in a woman with moderate burns, because fetal survival in this group appears to be influenced by maternal complications. Likewise, early obstetric intervention has been advocated for a gravely ill woman who has complications that jeopardize the fetus and any woman with extensive burns who is beyond 32 weeks' gestation.[103,107] Fetal death occurs most commonly during the first week after a major burn and is a likely event when a gravida has severe to critical burns.[122,123] Delivery after maternal stabilization is recommended for women at 26 weeks' gestation and beyond with burns affecting greater than 40% to 50% of TBSA.[105,110,111,123] This recommendation is based on older literature, and the gestational age for intervention should be adjusted based on institutional neonatal survival at the limits of viability and on patient and family wishes. Cesarean delivery is reserved for obstetric indications, and vaginal delivery has been accomplished, even in women with perineal burns. If abdominal delivery is indicated, the incision may be performed through burned skin without increasing morbidity.

SUMMARY OF MANAGEMENT OPTIONS
Burns

Management Options	Evidence Quality and Recommendation	References
Minor Burns		
Treat as outpatient if burn does not cover area of critical function or cosmetic importance.	—/GPP	—
Superficial burn:		
• Analgesia.	—/GPP	—
• Keep burned area clean and protected.	—/GPP	—
Partial full-thickness burn:		
• Clean, débride and irrigate.	—/GPP	—
• Bacitracin ointment.	—/GPP	—
• Nonadherent dressing.	—/GPP	—
• Adequate analgesia.	—/GPP	—
• Reevaluate in 24 hr.	—/GPP	—
Major Burns		
Perform resuscitation.		
See "General Management" (earlier)	—/—	—
Manage fluid balance:	IV/C	114,115
• Adequate fluid administration (Parkland, Brooke, or Evans formula).		
• Monitor urinary output to maintain 0.5 mL/kg/hr.		
Examine entire body surface: assess depth of burn and surface area involved.	IIa/B	105,109
Obtain arterial blood gas analysis and carbon monoxide level.	IV/C	117
Wound care:		
• Sterile technique.	—/GPP	—
• Topical antimicrobial agent.	—/GPP	—
• Silver sulfadiazine relatively contraindicated in late pregnancy.	—/GPP	—
• Surgery for débridement, prevention of cicatrization.	—/GPP	—
• Cicatrized abdominal wounds may require release in pregnancy.	IV/C	120
• Minimal use of iodine-containing topical cleansing solutions.	IV/C	108
Carbon monoxide poisoning:		
• 100% inspired oxygen by face mask if CO level ≥10%.	IV/C	117
• Treat five times longer than required to lower maternal level <5%.	IV/C	117
• Hyperbaric oxygen therapy if:	IV/C	119
◦ Maternal CO level >20%.		
◦ Neurologic changes occur (regardless of CO level).		
◦ Signs of fetal compromise are noted.		
Inhalation injury:	IV/C	114
• Intubation if laryngeal edema develops.		
• Warm humidified oxygen.		
• Pulmonary toilet.		
• Mechanical ventilation as indicated.		
• Therapeutic bronchoscopy.		

Management Options	Evidence Quality and Recommendation	References
Preterm labor: • Cautious use of tocolysis if preterm labor. • Steroids if preterm delivery likely.	III/B	122
Consider delivery of the fetus if: • Significant medical complications in a gravida with a moderate to severe burn injury. • Complications occur in a gravely ill woman. • Extensive burns at > 32 wk' gestation. • >40%–50% of the total body surface area is burned.	IIa/B	105,109

CO, carbon dioxide; GPP, good practice point.

ELECTRICAL INJURY

Incidence

Reports of electrical injuries in pregnant women are exceedingly uncommon. A total of 21 pregnant women with electrical injury and 13 gravidas struck by lightning have been reported.[124,125] Although one study reported no maternal deaths from conductive and lightning injuries, the fetal mortality rate was 73%[124] and 50% in a second series,[126] respectively. The fetal death rate was only 6%, however, in 31 women who were followed prospectively after predominantly household electrical injuries.[125] Minor injuries are less likely to be reported than catastrophic events, however, and the true incidence of electrical injury in pregnancy is probably underestimated. Most victims of electrical injury have multisystem trauma and should be transferred to an experienced center for optimal care.

Management Options

The direct effects of the current and the heat it generates cause physical damage, as does trauma as a result of electrical injury. Electrical injury can be thermal, conductive, or caused by lightning; conductive injuries are the most common. The type of current, its path through the body, and its voltage also affect the type of injury. Cardiac and respiratory arrest are the main causes of death after injury from domestic alternating current and lightning. The current passing through the body can cause cardiac dysrhythmia, asystole, respiratory arrest, muscle contraction, tetany, skeletal fractures, and neurologic injury. Continuous cardiac monitoring is recommended for patients who have loss of consciousness, cardiac dysrhythmia, abnormal findings on 12-lead electrocardiogram, abnormal mental status or physical examination findings, or burns or tissue damage expected to cause hemodynamic instability or electrolyte abnormalities.[127] Fractures may be caused by a fall occurring with the shock, and cervical spine injury as a result of muscular contraction must be excluded. Rhabdomyolysis can cause renal failure if adequate intravenous hydration is not maintained until myoglobinuria resolves. Tissue necrosis may be extensive, and antibiotic prophylaxis with penicillin decreases the risk of muscle and fascial infection. Surgical consultation may be required for wound care, débridement, and fasciotomy. Most victims of electrical injury have multisystem trauma and require transfer to an experienced center for optimal care.

Resistance to current varies among tissues of the body. Amniotic fluid, the uteroplacental circulation, fetal skin, nerves, and blood offer low resistance to electrical current flow; much higher resistance is found in tendon, fat, and bone.[124,128] As a result, the fetus is very vulnerable to electrical injury. When the current takes a hand-to-foot path through the mother, it presumably passes through the uterus.[125,128] The current path may, therefore, be an important factor in fetal outcome and may account for the difference in mortality rates among reported cases.[124,125]

The severity of maternal injury is not predictive of fetal outcome, and minor exposure can have a profound fetal effect. Significantly less current is required to produce injury in the fetus than in the mother.[124] In cases of fetal demise, cardiac arrest appears to have been the cause of death. This observation is consistent with maternal reports of sudden cessation of fetal movement after the injury. Intrauterine growth restriction and oligohydramnios have been reported in fetuses surviving maternal electrical injury.[124,128] An animal model also showed growth restriction in 71% of rabbit fetuses subjected to electrically induced thermal injury of the placenta.[129]

The paucity of data makes it difficult to offer management recommendations for a gravida who has an electrical injury. Care of the mother should follow established guidelines. Fetal cardiac activity should be confirmed after electrical injury. If the fetus is alive and viable, continuous cardiotocographic monitoring should be started at the time of initial maternal evaluation. Monitoring for 4 hours is suggested when minor mechanical trauma (e.g., fall to the floor) is associated with electrical injury. Twenty-four hours of maternal and fetal monitoring has been recommended if the results of maternal electrocardiogram are abnormal, maternal loss of consciousness occurred, or there is a history of maternal cardiovascular disease.[127] Monitoring for oligohydramnios and fetal growth restriction throughout the rest of the pregnancy is also recommended for the surviving fetus.[128]

SUMMARY OF MANAGEMENT OPTIONS

Electrical Injury

Management Options	Evidence Quality and Recommendation	References
Maternal Resuscitation		
Manage multisystem trauma in cooperation with subspecialists (see earlier).	—/—	—
Obtain continuous cardiac monitoring with:	III/B	127
• Loss of consciousness.		
• Cardiac dysrhythmia.		
• Abnormal 12-lead electrocardiogram reading.		
• Abnormal mental status or physical examination findings.		
• Burn or tissue damage is expected to cause hemodynamic instability or electrolyte abnormalities.		
Provide adequate intravenous hydration if rhabdomyolysis develops.	III/B	124,125
Provide antibiotic prophylaxis.	III/B	124,125
Provide wound and burn care.	III/B	124,125
Obstetric Management		
Confirm the presence of FHR.	—/GPP	—
Maternal injury does not correlate with fetal injury.	III/B	124
Obtain continuous cardiotocographic monitoring for 4 hr:	III/B	128
• Minor mechanical trauma.		
Obtain continuous cardiotocographic monitoring for 24 hr:	III/B	128
• Abnormal maternal electrocardiogram reading.		
• Maternal loss of consciousness.		
• History of maternal cardiac disease.		
Consider surveillance for oligohydramnios and fetal growth restriction if the fetus survives the event.	III/B	124,128

FHR, fetal heart rate; GPP, good practice point.

PERIMORTEM CESAREAN SECTION

Incidence

The concept of perimortem and postmortem cesarean delivery dates back thousands of years. Fortunately, it is an uncommon occurrence, and the exact incidence is difficult to calculate. It is important to distinguish emergency cesarean section in the emergency department from perimortem cesarean section. Emergency cesarean section is performed for maternal or fetal distress but maternal vitals are present. Perimortem cesarean section is performed concurrent to the mother's cardiopulmonary arrest.

Management Options

The decision to perform perimortem cesarean delivery in an attempt to save the fetus is based on gestational age and the duration of cardiac arrest. The operation is not performed in anticipation of cardiopulmonary arrest, but only once cardiovascular collapse has occurred.

One of the most important questions is the effect of cesarean delivery on the efficiency of cardiopulmonary resuscitation (CPR). Even under optimal conditions, CPR generates a cardiac output that is only 30% of normal.[130] Ten percent of maternal cardiac output is shunted to the uterus, and left lateral tilt as recommended to decrease vena caval compression further reduces the effectiveness of chest compressions. Oxygen consumption increases during pregnancy and predisposes pregnant women to rapid desaturation with hypoventilation. It is presumed that delivery of the fetus allows more efficient CPR by relieving vena caval obstruction and increasing blood volume by autotransfusion.

The sooner the infant is delivered after a maternal arrest, the better the chance of intact neurologic survival. Optimal neonatal outcome is achieved when delivery occurs less than 5 minutes from the arrest. There are no documented cases of intact fetal survival beyond 35 minutes from the onset of cardiac arrest in the mother.[130] Therefore, it seems reasonable to proceed with delivery up to 35 minutes after maternal collapse, although the risk for neonatal compromise is high. If more than 4 minutes have passed, but signs of fetal life are present, proceed with delivery. If the duration of arrest is unknown, proceeding with delivery is also reasonable, although fetal survival becomes unlikely beyond 20 minutes, particularly with catastrophic maternal trauma.

Once maternal cardiopulmonary arrest has occurred and the decision is made to intervene on behalf of the fetus, the following steps are suggested: Initiate delivery 4 minutes after maternal arrest if resuscitation is unsuccessful, with the intention to deliver the fetus 5 minutes after the arrest.[130] Intervention at a gestational age of 24 weeks or more is recommended by the EAST Practice Group.[131] CPR is continued throughout the procedure to offer every chance for maternal survival. Do not waste precious time preparing a sterile field or instrument tray or attempting to perform an ultrasound examination. Each surgeon should approach the abdominal incision in their most efficient fashion. A low transverse uterine incision offers the advantages of less blood loss and quicker closure than with a classic incision.

SUMMARY OF MANAGEMENT OPTIONS

Perimortem Cesarean Section

Management Options	Evidence Quality and Recommendation	References
Perform when maternal cardiopulmonary arrest occurs, not in anticipation of it.	IV/C	130
Initiate delivery 4 min after arrest if maternal resuscitation is unsuccessful: the goal is delivery 5 min after arrest.	IV/C	130
Continue cardiopulmonary resuscitation during delivery.	IV/C	130
Use time efficiently: • Do not prepare a sterile field or a full instrument table. • Use the quickest incision possible. • Consider a low transverse uterine incision.	IV/C	130
Proceed with delivery if >4 min have passed since maternal arrest but signs of fetal life are still present.	IV/C	130

SUGGESTED READINGS

American College of Chest Physicians: Antithrombotic and thrombolytic therapy: Prevention of venous thromboembolism. Evidence-Based Clinical Practice Guidelines. Chest 2008;133:381S–453S.

American College of Obstetricians and Gynecologists: Obstetric Aspects of Trauma Management (ACOG Educational Bulletin No. 251). Washington, DC, September, 1998.

Brown MA, Sirlin CB, Farahmand N, et al: Screening sonography in pregnant patients with blunt abdominal trauma. J Ultrasound Med 2005;24:175–181.

Cahill AG, Bastek JA, Stamilio DM: Minor trauma in pregnancy—Is the evaluation unwarranted? Am J Obstet Gynecol 2008;198:208.e1–208.e5.

Cusick SS, Tibbles CD: Trauma in pregnancy. Emerg Med Clin North Am 2007;25:861–872.

Hoff WS, Holevar M, Nagy KK, et al: Practice management guidelines for the evaluation of blunt abdominal trauma: The EAST Practice Management Guidelines Work Group. J Trauma 2002;53:602–615. Available at www.east.org

Huissoud C, Divry V, Dupont C, et al: Large fetomaternal hemorrhage: Prenatal predictive factors for perinatal outcome. Am J Perinatol 2009;26:227–233.

Muench MV, Canterino JC: Trauma in pregnancy. Obstet Gynecol Clin North Am 2007;34:555–583.

Pacheco LD, Gei AF, VanHook JW, et al: Burns in pregnancy. Obstet Gynecol 2005;106:1210–1212.

Whitty JE: Maternal cardiac arrest in pregnancy. Clin Obstet Gynecol 2002;45:379–392.

REFERENCES

For a complete list of references, log onto www.expertconsult.com.

CHAPTER 55

Psychiatric Illness

ROGER F. HASKETT

INTRODUCTION

Recognition of psychiatric illness during pregnancy and the postnatal period is vitally important for the health of the mother and infant. Psychiatric disorders, such as depression, are commonly associated with impaired functioning that can significantly interfere with a pregnant woman's ability to care for herself, including participating in optimal prenatal care and maintaining an appropriate diet, as well as increasing the risk of using substances such as tobacco and alcohol. Women with psychiatric and substance use disorders during pregnancy are reported to have at least twice the risk of inadequate prenatal care compared with women without these diagnoses.[1] This association with inadequate prenatal care persists after controlling for other known risk factors and is associated with more adverse pregnancy outcomes and decreased use of pediatric care after birth. These findings are consistent with studies of patients in other primary care settings, noting that depressed individuals are much less likely to comply with treatment recommendations. In addition, the presence of mood or anxiety disorders during pregnancy is a strong predictor of psychiatric illness and disability in the postpartum period.

In obstetrics and gynecology practices, the prevalence of psychiatric disorders, including substance abuse disorders, is reported to range from 20% to 48%; this number is even higher in clinics serving low-income women.[2] In particular, the prevalence of major depression in these settings is reported to be as high as 22%.[2] This high prevalence should not be unexpected, considering that adult women suffer from depression and anxiety disorders at rates two to three times higher than men and that the increased prevalence tends to be most prominent following puberty and throughout the reproductive years.[2] When detected, it will be noted that the onset of these psychiatric disorders may predate pregnancy, occur during pregnancy, or most commonly, appear during the postpartum period.

In addition to appropriately administering specific treatments,[3] successful management of psychiatric illness in pregnancy and the postpartum period requires effective collaboration between the obstetrician, the pediatrician, the psychiatrist, and other mental health professionals as well as the participation of relatives and other key social supports.

PREVALENCE OF PSYCHIATRIC ILLNESSES IN PREGNANCY

Recognition of the high frequency of psychiatric symptoms in obstetric and gynecology practices has followed the recent development of screening tools for use in these settings. One study in a university-based obstetric clinic providing prenatal care for low-income minority women reported that 38% of women screened positive for psychiatric disorders including substance abuse.[4] One in five pregnant women screened positive for alcohol or other substance abuse, and more than half of the women who screened positive for a psychiatric disorder (21%) met criteria for a depressive disorder, including 4%, with major depression. Other identified diagnoses were anxiety disorder (5%) and eating disorder (5%). Women with psychiatric disorders were more likely to have public insurance, an unexpected pregnancy, and a previous history of psychiatric treatment. More significantly, they tended to be more likely to have received inadequate prenatal care and to be referred to child protective services. Another study of 766 women attending gynecologic practices in Sweden[5] found that 30% met criteria for a psychiatric disorder, although these investigators deleted the screening questions for alcohol abuse. Overall, 27% of women screened positive for a depressive disorder, including 10% for major depression, and 12% were positive for an anxiety disorder. Of more concern was the finding that only one out of five women with a psychiatric diagnosis was receiving any treatment, either medication or psychotherapy.

The PRIME-MD Patient Health Questionnaire (PHQ) was the screening instrument used in these studies to assess current psychiatric disorders. The PHQ is a four-page self-report measure that assesses eight common psychiatric diagnoses, including mood, anxiety, eating, alcohol, and somatoform disorders. Although developed in other primary care settings,[6] the validity and utility of the PHQ has been assessed in a multisite sample of 3000 patients attending obstetric/gynecology outpatient clinics or office practices.[7] In addition to assessing the eight psychiatric diagnoses, the PHQ screens for disorders that are more common among or restricted to women, such as premenstrual syndrome, postpartum and menopausal mood disorders, and posttraumatic stress disorder. Information about reproductive history, psychosocial stressors, and severity of impairment is also included. In the validation study, 20% of women met criteria for a psychiatric diagnosis; the majority were unrecognized prior to reviewing the questionnaire. Most physicians and nurse practitioners (89%) reported that the diagnostic information provided by the PHQ was "very" or "somewhat" useful in management or treatment planning.[8]

MAJOR DEPRESSION

General

In 2008, the Global Burden of Disease study, 2004 update,[9] again reported that unipolar major depression was the most common cause of disease burden in women aged 15 to 44. This heavy burden of depression-related disability in women results not only from the high prevalence of depression but also from a clinical course that is characterized by early onset, recurrence, chronicity, and co-morbidity.[9] Typically, major depression is found to be 1.5 to 3 times more prevalent in women than in men. This higher prevalence of depression among women has been detected throughout the world using a variety of epidemiologic study designs.[2] Similar gender differences have been found for chronic minor depression or dysthymia and recurrent minor depression. The gender difference in prevalence appears at age 11 to 14 and is consistently found through midlife.[10,11] There does not appear to be a gender difference in the course of depression. The higher prevalence of depression among women is due to a higher risk of first onset, not to a differential risk of recurrence or chronicity of depression.[12] In addition, although limited, research has not found an effect of pregnancy on the onset or recurrence of major depression.[13] Pregnancy does not protect against depression, as was once believed, nor does it appear to increase the risk of depression compared with that in nonpregnant controls. In a review of depression in pregnancy, the prevalence rates were reported as 7.4%, 12.8%, and 12.0% for each trimester of pregnancy.[13] An emerging consensus holds that significant distress and impairment are also associated with the presence of "minor depression," or depressive symptoms that do not reach a level of severity to meet criteria for major depression. When depressive symptoms were monitored through pregnancy, the prevalence of major depression was 12.3% and minor depression was 18.1%, with major depression having a later onset and longer duration than minor depression.[14]

Diagnosis

Depression during pregnancy may be difficult to detect because many symptoms characteristic of depression, such as sleep and appetite disturbance, low energy, and diminished libido, are common in pregnant women who are not depressed. Although five of nine symptoms (Table 55–1) must be present over the same 2-week period to meet criteria for major depression, one of the symptoms must be either (1) depressed mood most of the day and nearly every day or (2) markedly diminished interest or pleasure in activities, often referred to as *anhedonia*. Using these symptoms in a two-question case-finding instrument is an effective means for identifying major depression. A positive response to either of the questions (1) "During the past month, have you often been bothered by feeling down, depressed, or hopeless?" or (2) "During the past month, have you often been bothered by little interest or pleasure in doing things?" had a sensitivity of 96% and a specificity of 57%; a negative response made a diagnosis of major depression very unlikely.[15] In women who give a positive response to either question, additional inquiry should be made about the presence of the other seven features of depression—such as change in sleep or appetite, physical agitation, fatigue, worthlessness or guilt, poor concentration, and suicidal thinking. In pregnant women, the most useful confirming symptoms are anhedonia, guilt, hopelessness, and suicidal thinking.

Many pregnant women do not seek treatment; identification of their depression is dependent on adequate screening by their obstetrician during antenatal visits. Risk factors for depression in pregnancy include a personal and family history of mood disorder, marital conflict, younger age, and limited social support with greater numbers of children. In a study of 3472 women at 10 obstetric clinics who were screened for depression during a prenatal visit,[16] 20% were found to have elevated depressive symptom scores (Center for Epidemiologic Studies—Depression [CES-D] ≥ 16), but fewer than 1 in 7 of these women was receiving treatment for depression. Among the 28% of women who were positive on the lifetime depression screen items ("You had 2 weeks or more when nearly every day you felt sad, blue, or depressed or in which you lost interest in things like work"), nearly one half (42.6%) reported increased depressive symptoms during pregnancy. Women having a prior history of depression were nearly five times more likely to have elevated depressive symptoms during pregnancy than women without this history. Other factors predicting elevated depression scores were a self-rating of poor overall health, greater alcohol use problems, smoking, being unmarried, being unemployed, and lower educational attainment. Other studies have reported low levels of spousal support and conflicts with spouse/partner as predicting depression during pregnancy.[14,17]

TABLE 55–1
Diagnostic Criteria for Major Depression

1. Depressed mood most of the day, nearly every day*
2. Markedly diminished interest or pleasure in activities*
3. Major change in appetite or weight
4. Decrease or increase in sleep
5. Psychomotor agitation or retardation
6. Fatigue or loss of energy
7. Feelings of worthlessness or excessive or inappropriate guilt
8. Diminished ability to think or concentrate; indecisiveness
9. Recurrent thoughts of death or suicide

* Must be present to establish diagnosis.
From American Psychiatric Association: Diagnostic and Statistical Manual of Mental Disorders, Fourth Edition, Text Revision. Washington, DC, American Psychiatric Association, 2000.

Maternal and Fetal Risks

Several literature reviews and cohort studies note the association between depressive symptoms during pregnancy and poor neonatal outcomes, such as low birth weight, increased risk of premature delivery, and maternal preeclampsia.[18–21] In a study of African American women, who have twice the risk of spontaneous preterm birth relative to white women, an association was found between elevated maternal depressive symptoms and spontaneous preterm birth.[22] In addition, there have been reports linking developmental delays, antisocial behavior, and criminality in individuals whose mothers were depressed during pregnancy.[23,24] Pregnant women with depression may have decreased appetite and inadequate weight gain during pregnancy and are more likely to use tobacco, alcohol, or illicit drugs.[25] In addition, depression during pregnancy is a strong predictor of postpartum depression.

Management Options

Screening for depression is feasible, and when using self-report instruments, does not require clinical staff. In the Marcus and coworkers study,[16] 90% of women approached were willing to be screened; in the study by Scholle and colleagues,[26] 82% of screened women agreed to a clinical research review of their results. Identification of risk factors for depression in pregnancy can increase the efficiency of screening; for example, women with a past history of depressive illness should be specifically targeted for appropriate screening.

Standard treatments for depression with demonstrated efficacy include psychotherapy, antidepressant medications, and electroconvulsive therapy (ECT).[27] Selection of a specific intervention will be influenced by the severity of depression and level of impairment, specific information related to use of the intervention in pregnancy, and the woman's preferences.[28–30] Nonpharmacologic treatments such as interpersonal psychotherapy have been adapted successfully for use during pregnancy[31] and are sometimes preferred by women concerned about exposing the fetus to antidepressant medications.

When considering pharmacologic treatments for depression in pregnancy, the risks to the developing fetus can be divided into risks of physical malformations (*teratogenesis*), risks of neonatal toxicity or withdrawal syndromes following delivery, and risks of long-term behavioral effects (*behavioral teratogenesis*). Although the U.S. Food and Drug Administration established a system to advise physicians about the safety of medications in pregnancy, these categories should be used with caution. The majority of psychotropic medications are categorized as category C, which indicates "human studies are lacking … risk cannot be ruled out." No psychotropic medications are in category A, indicating that they are safe for use in pregnancy, because ethical concerns do not permit the randomized studies needed to generate the data for this classification. Clinicians should note that medications in category B should not be assumed to be safer than those in category C because, although the former indicates that there is no evidence of risk in humans, this may be the result of an absence of human studies.

On review of the literature, there is no evidence that tricyclic or selective serotonin-reuptake inhibitor/serotonin and norepinephrine-reuptake inhibitor (SSRI/SNRI) antidepressants are associated with an increased risk of major malformations.[32] Maternal use of antidepressants during early pregnancy was not associated with increased risks of most categories of birth defects, and when associations have been observed, the specific defects are rare and absolute risks are small.[33] Although reports have been inconsistent and generated from small numbers of women, fluoxetine, paroxetine, and sertraline have been linked to transient neonatal difficulties for some women taking these medications in late pregnancy.[33] There are limited data assessing behavioral teratogenesis or neurologic and behavioral developmental outcomes following prenatal exposure of the developing brain to tricyclic and SSRI antidepressants.[34,35] Fortunately, the studies that have been published were unable to detect any differences between children exposed to antidepressants in utero and unexposed children at ages varying from 4 months to 7 years.[36]

The treatment of depression during pregnancy raises the following issues, which must be addressed by the treating physician and the patient:

- Risk of exposing the fetus to antidepressant medication.
- Risk of untreated depression in the mother.
- Risk of relapse of depression in the mother following antidepressant withdrawal.[37]

Obstetricians may encounter these issues in two possible circumstances: a pregnant woman who is recently diagnosed with depression or a woman who is not currently depressed or pregnant and who seeks consultation before conception. In women who present with a new onset or recurrence of depression during pregnancy, the choice of antidepressant treatment will be influenced by the severity of the current episode and any prior episodes of depression. In milder forms of depression, interpersonal or cognitive behavioral psychotherapy alone may be an appropriate treatment. Alternatively, in women who have failed psychotherapy alone or who have severe symptoms, such as weight loss or suicidality, or marked functional impairment, antidepressant medication is likely to be strongly recommended. In these latter women, the risks to the pregnancy associated with their depressive illness will usually exceed the known risks of exposure to an antidepressant medication.[38] Many of the women who seek consultation about antidepressant treatment prior to conception will have suffered prior episodes of depression and may be taking maintenance treatment. In these circumstances, the decision to continue or withdraw antidepressant medications prior to conception will be influenced by the risk for relapse of depression, including the severity and frequency of prior episodes of depression. Up to 68% of women who discontinue an antidepressant during pregnancy will suffer a depressive relapse,[37] although assessing a specific woman's prognosis should focus on the number of prior episodes and the time to relapse after previous attempts at antidepressant discontinuation. Women with a history of rapid and severe relapses following antidepressant discontinuation are likely to be most appropriately treated by continuing medication throughout pregnancy. These risk-benefit discussions with the mother should be documented in the medical record and, if possible, should occur with the father present.

SUMMARY OF MANAGEMENT OPTIONS
Major Depression

Management Options	Evidence Quality and Recommendation	References
Prepregnancy/Prenatal		
Women with previous depressive illness are at risk of relapse during or after pregnancy.	—/GPP	—
Institute specialist team management with access to mother and baby units if available.	—/GPP	—
Psychotherapy (interpersonal and/or cognitive behavioral) has been effective for milder disease.	IV/C	31
Tricyclics and SSRIs have been effective in pregnancy.	Ib/A	32
	IIb/B	33,36
Counsel about fetal risks from medication; withdrawal syndrome reported but no evidence of teratogenic or long-term risks. See also Chapter 34.	Ib/A	32
	IIb/B	33,36
Counsel about danger of relapse with reduction in medication.	IIb/B	37,38
Check for drug/alcohol abuse.	IIb/B	24
Institute surveillance for fetal growth, preeclampsia, and preterm labor.	III/B	18,19
	IV/C	20
Postnatal		
Be vigilant for maternal relapse in postnatal period.	—/GPP	—
Be vigilant for neonatal withdrawal.	IIb/B	33,34

GPP, good practice point; SSRIs, selective serotonin-reuptake inhibitors.

ANXIETY DISORDERS

General

Studies of women in the general population have reported that the 12-month prevalence of anxiety disorders is 4.3% for generalized anxiety disorder (GAD), 3.2% for panic disorder, and 1.8% for obsessive-compulsive disorder (OCD).[39] The prevalence of post-traumatic stress disorder (PTSD) in a cohort of economically disadvantaged pregnant women was 7.7%, with these women being five times more likely to have a major depressive disorder and three times more likely to have a GAD.[40] Unfortunately, in contrast to depression, the systematic data on the frequency and course of anxiety disorders during pregnancy are limited. Some of the difficulty in characterizing anxiety disorders in pregnancy results from the frequent overlap of depressive and anxiety symptoms and from the past convention of subsuming all combined presentations under a depressive diagnosis. Surveys that distinguish between anxiety and depressive disorders, however, find a prevalence of anxiety disorders in obstetrics and gynecology practices that ranges from 5% to 12%.[41] Little is known about the influence of pregnancy on the course of anxiety disorders, although a small number of retrospective accounts and case reports have suggested that symptoms of anxiety and panic disorder decrease and symptoms of OCD increase during pregnancy.[42]

Diagnosis

Anxiety is frequently free-floating, although it may focus on specific pregnancy fears, and is accompanied by symptoms of autonomic arousal. In women with panic disorder, chronic feelings of elevated anxiety are interspersed by the abrupt onset of episodes of pronounced fear, sometimes described as a fear of dying, going crazy, or losing control, which is associated with prominent physical symptoms of distress. These include shortness of breath, dizziness, unsteady feelings or faintness, palpitations or tachycardia, chest pain or discomfort, trembling or shaking, sweating, hot flashes or chills, choking, nausea or abdominal distress, numbness or paresthesias, as well as depersonalization (feeling separated from their body) or derealization (familiar surroundings feel unfamiliar). Episodes of panic usually begin to ease within 30 minutes but may be followed by a lingering period of increased anxiety and impaired function. Women with OCD describe recurrent thoughts that are unpleasant and out of character, often involving personally unacceptable aspects of aggression or sexuality, or repetitive compulsive behavioral rituals that are experienced as unreasonable; attempts to resist are followed by increased and incapacitating anxiety.

Maternal and Fetal Risks

There is some evidence for a deleterious effect of increased maternal stress and anxiety on birth weight and preterm birth.[43,44] Other obstetric complications associated with increased maternal anxiety include preeclampsia, increased analgesic use,[45] and increased rate of cesarean section.[46] Adverse effects on the fetus include increased uterine artery resistance, as well as changes in fetal hemodynamics and autonomic reactivity.[47,48]

Management Options

Nonpharmacologic treatments are often effective in decreasing anxiety symptoms and include cognitive behavioral therapy and relaxation techniques. Pharmacologic treatment of anxiety disorders during pregnancy is indicated in women who have severe symptoms and are unresponsive to psychotherapy. Use of SSRI antidepressants is favored, owing to their demonstrated effectiveness in anxiety disorders and accumulating evidence for their safety in pregnancy. Epidemiologic studies in the 1970s and 1980s suggested an increased frequency of oral clefts as well as signs of toxicity in neonates born to women taking high doses of benzodiazepines in late pregnancy. More recent meta-analyses and case-control studies have concluded that first-trimester exposure to benzodiazepines is associated with minimal risk, although these medications should be used cautiously and at the lowest effective dose.[49] Abrupt withdrawal of benzodiazepines during pregnancy is not recommended. There are insufficient data to determine the safety of buspirone during pregnancy.

SUMMARY OF MANAGEMENT OPTIONS

Anxiety Disorders

Management Options	Evidence Quality and Recommendation	References
Prepregnancy and Prenatal		
Recommend psychotherapy (cognitive behavioral or relaxation techniques).	—/GPP	—
Prescribe SSRIs if medication is required.	—/GPP	—
Avoid benzodiazepines.	—/GPP	—
Institute surveillance for fetal growth, preeclampsia, and preterm labor.	III/B	44–46

GPP, good practice point; SSRIs, selective serotonin-reuptake inhibitors.

BIPOLAR DISORDER

General

The prevalence of mania and bipolar disorder is about 1% and, in contrast to depression, there is no significant gender difference. Despite this, there appears to be a relationship between childbirth and the first episode of mania in women with bipolar illness, as noted by reports that childbirth predated the first episode of mania in 1 of 4 women with this illness.[50,51] A population-based cohort study found that women with a history of bipolar disorder are at particular risk of postpartum psychiatric readmissions.[52] Epidemiologic studies also note a marked excess of postpartum psychosis after the first child compared with subsequent pregnancies, suggesting that there is a particular change occurring at the first delivery that is less evident at other births.[52] Overall, the risk of relapse of mania after delivery is estimated to be between 1 in 3 and 1 in 4. Diagnostic and management issues associated with depressive episodes occurring during the course of a bipolar disorder are similar to those for unipolar depressive episodes, described previously.

Diagnosis

The essential criterion for the diagnosis of mania is the presence of abnormally and persistently elevated, expansive, or irritable mood for at least 1 week. This must be accompanied by at least three of the following clinical features: inflated self-esteem or grandiosity, decreased need for sleep, increased talkativeness or pressure to keep talking, flight of ideas or subjective experience of racing thoughts, distractibility, increase in goal-directed activity (socially, at work or school, or sexually) or psychomotor agitation, disinhibited behavior, and excessive involvement in pleasurable activities with high potential for painful consequences (engaging in unrestrained buying sprees, sexual indiscretions, or foolish business investments). The overall severity must lead to marked functional impairment or need for hospitalization. Women with bipolar illness may also present with less severe forms of mania, diagnosed as *hypomania*, which are of shorter duration and usually associated with less functional impairment. Although the euphoric or irritable mood changes are usually evident in a patient being followed longitudinally, the most informative diagnostic feature of mania, especially during the assessment of current and past episodes in a new patient, is persistently decreased need for sleep without daytime fatigue or lowered energy.

Maternal and Fetal Risks

Risks to the mother and fetus result from the impulsive, disinhibited, or high risk behavior that is seen in mania, as well as from the commonly associated substance abuse and dependence. In addition, women with untreated mania or hypomania are unlikely to participate in appropriate prenatal care or maintain an adequate diet.

Management Options

Treatment considerations should address two separate groups of women:

- Those presenting with mania during pregnancy.
- Women with an established diagnosis of bipolar disorder requesting advice about a planned or recently confirmed pregnancy.

In the former, the risks to the mother and fetus from untreated mania are prominent, and the risks of failure to treat must be balanced against the risks of effective pharmacologic treatment.[53] Admission to a psychiatric facility is necessary if there is a high risk of imminent harm to the mother or fetus and the woman has reduced insight and is unwilling to cooperate with appropriate outpatient treatment. Medication choices for mania in pregnancy should include lithium carbonate, despite early reports about the risk of Ebstein's anomaly and other cardiovascular abnormalities in infants exposed to lithium during the first trimester.[54] Subsequent studies of lithium in pregnancy suggest a more modest teratogenic relationship, with a risk of cardiovascular abnormalities that is 10 to 20 times higher in exposed children than the normal population, but with an actual occurrence rate that is low (0.05%–0.1%).[55,56] It is recommended that fetuses who have first-trimester exposure to lithium should be screened for cardiovascular abnormalities by ultrasound in the mid trimester. Despite these concerns, the risk of lithium for mania must be balanced against the increased teratogenic potential of the anticonvulsants that are the other established pharmacologic treatment for this disorder.[57] Valproate and carbamazepine have been linked to neural tube defects in 2% to 5% of exposed babies; there are insufficient data to assess the risks with the newer, more novel anticonvulsants. It does appear, however, that teratogenic risk is increased by the use of combinations of anticonvulsants and high plasma levels. In addition, a third class of medications is now under consideration for the treatment of mania, the atypical antipsychotics. Olanzapine was the first approved for this indication and has been followed by others in the class. Although, currently, there are limited safety data available, which limits use of these drugs in pregnancy, studies of small numbers of women taking olanzapine during pregnancy have not revealed any teratogenicity. Finally, ECT should also be considered as an alternative to psychotropic medication exposure. It has demonstrated effectiveness for treatment of mania and depression, and reviews support the relative safety of ECT during pregnancy, provided that specific modifications are made to the anesthetic procedure.[58]

Ideally, a woman with well-controlled bipolar illness will address the specific management of pregnancy prior to conception.[59] Unfortunately, the rate of unplanned pregnancy in women with bipolar illness is even higher than the 50% seen in the general population. In these women, pregnancy will commonly be at an advanced gestational age when diagnosed. As neural tube closure usually occurs by the end of the fourth week and development of the heart by the end of the eighth week, the period of risk for major organ malformation may have passed by the time many women taking maintenance psychotropic medication have confirmed pregnancy. This is particularly important information for women considering a rapid discontinuation of medications once pregnancy is detected. Studies have shown a 50% recurrence rate within 2 to 10 weeks of discontinuation of lithium in patients with bipolar illness, and this is increased if medication is discontinued abruptly.[60] Considering the lack of data of a clear safety advantage for a specific mood stabilizer and the risks of relapse following a change in treatment, there is little support for switching a woman from one mood stabilizer to another once pregnancy is detected.[60] If the decision is made to continue medication during pregnancy, the minimum effective dose should be used. In women who are planning pregnancy and report only occasional episodes of moderately severe mania or hypomania, medication discontinuation before conception may be a supportable option, provided that the taper occurs over 2 to 4 weeks minimum and there is close collaboration between the obstetrician and the psychiatrist.

SUMMARY OF MANAGEMENT OPTIONS
Bipolar Disorder

Management Options	Evidence Quality and Recommendation	References
Prepregnancy and Prenatal		
Lithium is effective; increased risk of fetal cardiovascular abnormalities, though low prevalence. See also Chapter 34.	Ia/A	55
	IV/C	56
	III/B	57
Anticonvulsants are effective; increased risk of fetal neural tube defects. See also Chapter 34.	IV/C	57
Atypical antipsychotics (e.g., olanzapine) have no reported risks in pregnancy. See also Chapter 34.	—/GPP	—

Management Options	Evidence Quality and Recommendation	References
For severe episodes, ECT has been used effectively in pregnancy (with appropriate anesthetic precautions).	III/B	58
Perform careful detailed fetal anomaly scan at 20 wk, especially if on medication.	Ia/A	55
	IV/C	56,57
	III/B	57
Hospitalize in a psychiatric facility if safety concerns present (mother and baby unit if postnatal).	—/GPP	—
Screen for substance abuse.	—/GPP	—
Postnatal		
Be vigilant for recurrence after delivery.	III/B	52
Perform careful neonatal examination to exclude abnormality.	Ia/A	55
	IV/C	56,58
	III/B	57

ECT, electroconvulsive therapy; GPP, good practice point.

SCHIZOPHRENIA

General

Pregnancy in women with schizophrenia occurs under very different circumstances today compared with a few decades ago.[61] The first and most influential change resulted from the release of patients to the community instead of confining them to institutions, providing them with increased opportunities to meet partners. Despite this, although the fertility rates for women with schizophrenia have increased, its occurrence remains between 30% and 80% of the general population.[62] Because effective utilization of birth control practices is limited in women with schizophrenia, one important contributing factor for this decrease in fertility is the high prevalence of hyperprolactinemia in patients taking the older class of antipsychotic medications. More recently, the treatment of schizophrenia has seen an increased utilization of a new generation of atypical antipsychotics that are much less likely to produce elevated prolactin levels. As a result, it is very likely that the frequency of pregnancy in women with schizophrenia will increase.

Diagnosis

The diagnostic criteria for schizophrenia require the presence of at least two of the following over a 1-month period: delusions, hallucinations, disorganized speech, grossly disorganized or catatonic behavior, and affective flattening or markedly decreased volition. These features should be associated with prominent social and occupational dysfunction of at least 6 months' duration. The diagnostic evaluation should focus on the chronic and persistent features of the illness because the clinician may have difficulty during a cross-sectional assessment in differentiating psychosis in schizophrenia from psychotic symptoms in a patient with mood disorder. Particular presentations that may have diagnostic challenges are the delusional denial of the pregnancy or the incorporation of the pregnancy into established delusional systems.

Maternal and Fetal Risks

Prenatal care might not be appropriately sought or maintained by these women, especially in cases in which the pregnancy was not planned and in women with prominent volitional deficits. Individuals with this illness are also noted to have great difficulty maintaining healthy lifestyle choices for diet, exercise, and avoidance of alcohol and tobacco. All of these factors are associated with worse outcomes from pregnancy. The use of older antipsychotic medications conveys some increased risk of teratogenicity, although further examination of these data linked the low-potency phenothiazines, such as chlorpromazine, with an increased risk of malformations. The depot antipsychotics are not recommended during pregnancy because they have been associated with an increased risk of extrapyramidal side effects in the neonate (see Chapter 34).

Management Options

Although it may be desired by the patient, discontinuation of psychotropic medication during pregnancy in women with schizophrenia is associated with a markedly increased risk of relapse. Considering that treatment of relapse is likely to require higher doses of medication than maintenance treatment, one alternative is to attempt reduction to the lowest effective dosage of medication, especially during the first trimester. Although low doses of the more potent older antipsychotics, such as haloperidol, are preferred for the treatment of schizophrenia in pregnancy, the new atypical antipsychotics are commonly being continued in pregnancy, despite the limited amount of safety data currently available. Any indication of psychotic relapse should be managed by prompt admission to a psychiatric facility for restabilization. A key aspect of management during pregnancy is to evaluate the options for the mother and child after delivery. Assessment of the woman's capacity to provide appropriate care for the infant should begin during the pregnancy; this should include review of the stability of the illness, the woman's adherence to outpatient care, and the quality of psychosocial supports.

SUMMARY OF MANAGEMENT OPTIONS
Schizophrenia

Management Options	Evidence Quality and Recommendation	References
Prepregnancy, Prenatal, and Postnatal		
Decrease oral medication to lowest level consistent with a therapeutic effect.	—/GPP	—
Avoid depot preparations.	—/GPP	—
Check for substance abuse.	—/GPP	—
Offer psychosocial support and encouragement to take up prenatal care.	—/GPP	—
Hospitalization in a psychiatric facility may be necessary with acute relapses (mother and baby unit preferable).	—/GPP	—
Assess ability of patient to care for baby and need for additional psychosocial support.	—/GPP	—

GPP, good practice point.

SUBSTANCE ABUSE AND DEPENDENCY (see also Chapter 33)

General

Considering that substance abuse and dependence are chronic relapsing disorders, women with these diagnoses are at particular risk when they become pregnant. Identification of prenatal substance use, including alcohol and nicotine, is a critical public health issue in the care of pregnant women.[63] In 1992, the National Pregnancy and Health Survey reported an estimated prevalence among U.S. women during pregnancy of alcohol (18.8%) and illicit drug use (5.5%). Another report of prospectively screened newborns in an urban population noted that 44% of infants tested positive for opiates, cocaine, or cannabis. Although many women report spontaneously quitting substance use on learning of the pregnancy, maintenance of abstinence is problematic without participation in treatment programs.[64] A key strategy in the accurate identification of affected women is the use of self-report screening instruments. These tend to identify much higher rates of substance use than those detected by maternal interview alone. For example, one report contrasted the 65% to 70% correct identification of prenatal drinkers using a questionnaire with the 20% having documentation of alcohol use in the obstetric record.

Diagnosis

One of the strongest risk factors for substance abuse is the presence of other psychiatric disorders. Depression, mania, and schizophrenia are all associated with an increased prevalence of substance use and abuse. Other risk factors identified for frequent drinking in pregnancy were being unmarried, smoking, age 25 years or older, and having a college education, although the applicability of these findings to other populations requires further study.[65] Interviewing individuals who are aware of the mother's behavior, such as the spouse/partner and other relatives, can be informative, although the presence of substance abuse in these individuals may decrease the reliability of their responses. Urine screening of the mother has been controversial, although with the mother's consent, it may be a useful strategy for identifying mothers who should be referred for treatment.

Maternal and Fetal Risks

The legality of substances does not lessen their serious implications for the health of the fetus; legal substances are probably associated with more widespread use.[66] The fetal consequences of maternal smoking are well established. These include intrauterine growth restriction, low birth weight, and developmental delays. Fetal alcohol syndrome (FAS) is associated with alcohol consumption during pregnancy. The three critical features are growth deficiency, facial phenotype, and brain damage dysfunction. A preclinical study showed that alcohol blocked *N*-methyl-D-aspartate receptors and excessively activated γ-aminobutyric acid (GABA) receptors, leading to extensive neuron degeneration. The damage was dependent on the rapidity of dose administration and the duration of blood alcohol level elevation.[67] This suggests that peak levels during a drinking episode are most critical to developing FAS. Maternal use of benzodiazepines and barbiturates is known to be associated with neonatal withdrawal syndromes, but of more concern is the recent report suggesting that these substances may delete neurons from the developing brain through a mechanism similar to that proposed for alcohol. Considering their relatively common use in pregnant women and infants, there is an urgent need for more systematic examination of these risks.

Maternal use of illicit substances is associated with significant risk of adverse effects on the fetus.[68] Cannabis use during pregnancy has been associated with effects on the exposed infant's cognitive development and behavior, with at least one report linking hyperactivity, inattentiveness, and impulsivity at age 10 with first- and third-trimester exposure to cannabis.[69] Prenatal cocaine use is reported to be associated with a dose-dependent decrease in head circumference and head weight.[70] There has been a report of increased frequency of cardiovascular and musculoskeletal anomalies in infants exposed to methyl-enedioxymethamphetamine (Ecstasy) during pregnancy,[71] but further study is needed. Opiate withdrawal is the primary risk for infants born to opiate-dependent mothers and is characterized by autonomic dysfunction as well as gastrointestinal and respiratory symptoms.

Management Options

The key to management of substance abuse is detection. The use of screening instruments is valuable; questionnaires such as CAGE (cut down, annoyed by criticism, guilty about drinking, eye opener) or T-ACE (tolerance, annoyed, cut down, eye opener; Table 55–2) are commonly used for the detection of alcohol misuse.[72] Although the literature suggests that six drinks daily can cause overt FAS, the safe level has not been identified and the comparative risks for binge drinking and daily drinking are not clear. Risk-drinking (enough to *potentially* damage the offspring) has been defined as an average of more than one drink (0.5 oz) per day, or less if massed (binges of > five drinks per episode).[73] In the United States, a conservative position has been adopted that essentially recommends total abstinence during pregnancy.

Unfortunately, there are few screening tools for detection of the use of other substances. When diagnosed, a comprehensive treatment program is indicated, with individual and group therapy, behavioral incentives, and in some situations, pharmacologic agents such as methadone. These interventions have demonstrated positive effects on both maternal and neonatal outcomes.

The Summary of Management Options for this section is found in Chapter 33.

TABLE 55–2

T-ACE Screening Tool for Pregnancy Risk-Drinking*

Tolerance

"How many drinks can you hold?"

(A positive answer, scored a 2, is at least a six-pack of beer, a bottle of wine, or six mixed drinks. This suggests tolerance of alcohol and very likely a history of at least moderate to heavy alcohol intake.)

Annoyed

"Have people annoyed you by criticizing your drinking?"

Cut Down

"Have you felt you ought to cut down on your drinking?"

Eye Opener

"Have you ever had a drink first thing in the morning to steady your nerves or get rid of a hangover?"

* The first question is scored 0 or 2 points. The last 3 questions are scored 1 point if answered affirmatively. A total score of 2 or more is considered positive for risk-drinking.

From Sokol RJ, Delaney-Black V, Nordstrom B: Fetal alcohol spectrum disorder. JAMA 2003;290:2996–2999.

POSTPARTUM DEPRESSION CONDITIONS

General

The psychiatric diagnostic system (i.e., *Diagnostic and Statistical Manual for Mental Disorders*, 4th ed. [DSM-IV]) does not recognize postpartum disorders as discrete diagnoses but permits "postpartum onset" to be used as a specifier for episodes of illness appearing within 4 weeks of childbirth. There is continued debate about this relatively brief interval for the definition of postpartum illness. Most epidemiologic studies use a 3-month period, which captures the peak prevalence of psychiatric illness and hospitalization after childbirth, and other researchers and clinicians are extending their focus to the events occurring during the first postnatal year.[74] Postpartum mood changes include three distinct clinical syndromes: postpartum blues, postpartum depression, and postpartum psychosis, although a single cross-sectional evaluation of all three may be indistinguishable. Fortunately, the prevalence of these three disorders varies inversely to their severity.

Postpartum "Blues"

General

Although not actually listed in *DSM-IV* as a psychiatric disorder, this well-recognized, common disorder occurs in 25% to 80% of women following delivery. Sadness may be prominent, but the syndrome is commonly characterized by emotional lability, bursting into tears without apparent cause; increased anxiety; insomnia; and negative thinking. Symptoms usually appear within the first postpartum week and, in the majority of women, peak around day 5 postpartum and resolve within 2 weeks. Given the timing and self-limiting nature of this syndrome, there have been many reports and hypotheses linking its pathophysiology to the rapid and profound changes occurring at parturition, but so far none has achieved wide support.

Diagnosis

The key to the diagnosis of this state is its time course.[75] Distinguishing between postpartum blues and postpartum depression has great clinical significance. Persistence of depressive symptoms past the second week postpartum should result in a careful reassessment of the original diagnosis. In addition, prominent insomnia and mood lability in a woman with risk factors for postpartum psychosis, even if it occurs in the first 2 weeks after childbirth, should prompt an urgent psychiatric consultation.

Maternal and Fetal Risks

Generally, this syndrome is not associated with significant functional impairment of the mother and does not significantly increase risks to the infant.

Management Options

Provide support and education about the typically self-limiting nature of this condition, but monitor for progression and development of postpartum depression.

SUMMARY OF MANAGEMENT OPTIONS

Postpartum "Blues"

Management Options	Evidence Quality and Recommendation	References
Postnatal		
Confirm that this is not postnatal depression and that it resolves within 2 wk.	—/GPP	—
Offer explanation and support.	—/GPP	—

GPP, good practice point.

Postpartum Depression

General

The prevalence of postpartum depression is 10% to 15%; it occurs in 1 of every 7 to 10 women after delivery, making it the most common complication of childbirth.[76] Women with a past history of depression have an elevated risk of postpartum depression, estimated to range from 25% to 50%.[76] Although the psychiatric diagnostic system focuses on depression appearing up to 4 weeks after delivery, a significant body of data emphasizes the importance of depression having an onset up to 1 year after childbirth. Owing to its temporal association, the cause of postpartum depression is commonly attributed to the rapid and profound hormonal changes occurring after delivery. Other factors that increase the risk of postpartum depression are also seen in women suffering from depression unrelated to childbirth, such as past and family history of depressive episodes, poor marital relationship, low social support, stressful life events, and low socioeconomic status.[17,76]

Diagnosis

The clinical features and diagnostic process for postpartum depression are similar to those for women suffering from depression at other times. The first step is to identify a period of persistent depressed mood or anhedonia lasting at least 2 weeks. Several screening instruments have been utilized for this purpose. The most commonly reported instrument in the literature is the Edinburgh Postnatal Depression Scale (EPDS), a 10-item self-report instrument designed to assess the presence of depressive symptoms in women after childbirth.[77] Each symptom item is scored from 0 to 3 according to severity. A score greater than 9 on the EPDS should be followed by a brief focused interview to determine the presence of a depressive diagnosis. Other instruments include a 2-question case-finding instrument assessing the presence of depressed mood or anhedonia.[15] A positive response to either of the two items suggests that a diagnosis of depression should be explored.

In women who were screened during the second trimester of pregnancy and again during the postpartum year, the two independently predictive risk factors for postpartum depression were high depressive symptoms during pregnancy and a past personal history of depressive disorder.[78] Another study of first-time, otherwise-healthy mothers found that women reporting high levels of depressive symptomatology at 2 months' postpartum had an increased risk of high levels of depressive symptoms continuing through the first year postpartum.[79] This emphasizes the persistence of depressive symptoms with associated impairment of function and reinforces the importance of identifying depressed mothers soon after childbirth, preferably with routine use of screening instruments, and referring for appropriate interventions.[80]

Considering that bipolar illness can present with an episode of depression, it is essential to ask the depressed woman about the features of past hypomania or mania, particularly when psychotic features are present. This can be done by asking about the past occurrence of at least 3 to 4 days of a markedly decreased need for sleep (i.e., feeling rested after 3 to 4 hours sleep per night, without daytime fatigue or decreased energy). A positive response to this question or one about periods of persistently elevated or irritable mood that others thought were abnormal indicates that further evaluation for possible bipolar disorder is indicated and psychiatric referral is recommended.

Maternal and Fetal Risks

Although the overall risk of suicide in postpartum women is low, those who develop a severe psychiatric illness in the first year after childbirth are at a significantly increased risk. In one study, the long-term risk of suicide in women admitted to a psychiatric hospital in the first year after childbirth was increased 17 times.[81] In these women, the risk of completed suicide during the first postpartum year was markedly increased to 70 times greater than the age-specific mortality rate. A report from the United Kingdom noted that suicide was the leading cause of maternal death during the first year after childbirth.[82]

Adverse effects of maternal depression on infant development have been widely reported,[83–85] including reports of an association between maternal depression and an increased risk of sudden infant death syndrome.[86] Children of depressed parents are at high risk for anxiety and depressive disorder in childhood, depression in adolescence, and alcohol dependence as adults.[87] Children of depressed mothers are also less likely to benefit from appropriate parental prevention practices.[88] Depressed mothers reported a three times greater risk of serious emotional problems in their children and more functional disability.[89]

Homicide is the leading cause of infant deaths due to injury, 9 per 100,000 live births from 1988 to 1991.[90] This study revealed that children born to young unmarried and poorly educated mothers were several times more likely to be killed. In this group of mothers, the most important risk factors were maternal age younger than 17 years and birth of the second or subsequent child before age 19; these accounted for 17% of the infant deaths. Five percent of homicides occurred on the first day of the infant's life; 95% of these infants were not born in a hospital compared with 8% of all infants killed during the first year of life who were not born in a hospital. Infants killed immediately after birth appeared to be the result of unwanted or disguised pregnancies. Identification of adolescents who have hidden their pregnancies and provision of appropriate prenatal care are particularly important. Maternal depression may play a role in the deaths occurring after the first day of life. The combination of depressed mood, low self-esteem, pessimism, and hopelessness may reach delusional levels in some mothers, leading them to believe that their babies and themselves are better off dead.[91] In addition, reports suggest that infants of depressed mothers are more irritable, are less easily consoled, and have disrupted sleep and wake cycles, all increasing their risks of being abused.

Management Options

Women receiving a diagnosis of depression after childbirth are commonly treated with antidepressant medication.[92] Uncontrolled studies have reported improvement in postpartum depression after treatment with antidepressants such as sertraline, fluvoxamine, and venlafaxine. Unfortunately, only one placebo-controlled trial of antidepressants in postpartum depression has been published.[93] This study compared antidepressant medication (fluoxetine) with psychotherapy (cognitive-behavioral therapy [CBT]). Results indicated that fluoxetine was more effective than placebo. With regard to the role of psychotherapy, six sessions of CBT were more effective than one session, but the addition of multiple CBT sessions to fluoxetine did not provide any additional benefit.[93] As concluded in the Cochrane Review on the use of antidepressants for postnatal depression,[94] more trials are needed to determine the role of antidepressants in treating women with postnatal depression.

Women with postpartum depression appear abnormally sensitive to the withdrawal of high levels of gonadal steroids following parturition. A preliminary placebo-controlled study showed that transdermal estrogen was an effective treatment for women with severe postpartum depression,[95] although more research is needed to assess the safety of estrogen in the postpartum period.

Owing to the reluctance of some postpartum women to take medication, psychotherapy has been studied as an alternative to antidepressant medication as well as an adjunct to medication. In addition to the study noted previously, several randomized, controlled trials have shown that individual psychotherapy is an effective treatment for postpartum depression.[96] There was greater improvement of maternal mood and social functioning in women receiving interpersonal psychotherapy than in women in the waiting-list control group.[97] Other studies have shown the benefit of including the partner in the psychotherapy sessions, although the results from group therapy are mixed.[98]

The Cochrane Review by Dennis and Hodnett[99] on "psychosocial and psychological interventions for treating postpartum depression" included nine trials and 956 women. Both psychosocial (e.g., peer support, nondirective counseling) and psychological (e.g., CBT and interpersonal psychotherapy) interventions appeared to reduce the symptoms of postpartum depression.

Many women who express reluctance to take medication after childbirth identify concern about the possible adverse effects on breast-feeding infants. Because all antidepressants are excreted in breast milk, many studies have evaluated the serum levels of antidepressants in breast-feeding infants. With few exceptions, these reports have found that the serum levels of antidepressants in infants were either very low or undetectable.[100,101] Reports of adverse effects in breast-fed infants of mothers taking antidepressants have included increased crying, colic, and decreased sleep in three infants whose mothers were taking fluoxetine and who were found to have serum levels of fluoxetine and its metabolite that were in the adult therapeutic range.[100,101] Citalopram, sertraline, and doxepin have been identified in case reports with either adverse effects or elevated serum levels.[100,101] It should be noted that most reports were of one or two cases, methodologies varied, and with the exception of one study, the follow-up was brief.

SUMMARY OF MANAGEMENT OPTIONS

Postpartum Depression

Management Options	Evidence Quality and Recommendation	References
Postnatal		
Maintain vigilance for the condition by all health providers in the puerperium.	—/GPP	—
Antidepressants (SSRIs are first choice) are effective.	III/B	92

SUMMARY OF MANAGEMENT OPTIONS

Postpartum Depression—cont'd

Management Options	Evidence Quality and Recommendation	References
More information is required about estrogen as a therapy.	Ib/A	95
Interpersonal psychotherapy is an effective alternative.	Ib/A	96,99
Cognitive behavioral psychotherapy does not give additional benefit when used with antidepressants.	Ib/A	96,99
Suggest mother and baby unit admission in extreme cases.	—/GPP	—
Breast-feeding is safe with antidepressants.	—/GPP	—

GPP, good practice point; SSRIs, selective serotonin-reuptake inhibitors.

Postpartum Psychosis

General

Postpartum psychosis is the most severe postpartum mood disorder; fortunately, it is rare, affecting 1 to 2 women per 1000 births. Current literature generally reflects the view that postpartum psychosis, in the majority of cases, is a presentation of bipolar disorder following childbirth.[102] Women with a history of bipolar disorder have a 100-fold higher risk of developing postpartum psychosis than women without bipolar disorder.[103] In addition, women with bipolar disorder and a family history of postpartum psychosis have a rate of postpartum episodes twice that seen in women with bipolar disorder and no family history.[104]

Diagnosis

Symptoms of insomnia, prominent mood lability, restlessness, sadness, and irritability appear within 2 weeks of childbirth, followed by the development of psychotic features, such as delusions, hallucinations, and thought disorder. Insomnia is an early and common symptom and is found in 42% to 100% of women with psychosis.[105] The presence of perplexity and confusion are also noted to be common, unlike in nonpuerperal manic episodes. Some researchers have commented on the role of sleep loss in the precipitation of mania generally[106]; this may be of particular importance following childbirth.[107] Studies of sleep in the later stages of pregnancy show prominent sleep disruption, with prolonged sleep latency, more awakenings, decreased total sleep time, and suppression of stage 4 sleep; recovery of stage 4 sleep and reduction in REM sleep occur in the early postpartum period.[108,109] More important, a prospective study of sleep in pregnancy revealed a differential effect depending on the presence of a past history of mood disorders. In addition, sleep disruption during late pregnancy and the early postpartum period appears to be more pronounced in first-time mothers than in multiparous women. This may be relevant for the observed increase in the risk of postpartum psychosis after the first child compared with after later births.

Maternal and Fetal Risks

In almost all instances, women with postpartum psychosis are unable to provide adequate care for themselves or their child and require additional support and supervision. Thoughts of harming the infant are common in women with postpartum psychosis; sometimes, they act on their thoughts. Postpartum women who commit infanticide or suicide more commonly present with depressed mood than with mania.

Management Options

Early identification of sleep impairment is important in the management of women with a history of bipolar disorder or postpartum psychosis. Prevention of sleep loss in vulnerable women by daytime delivery and reduction of nocturnal stimulation may be appropriate. Prompt treatment of decreased sleep in these women, with a high-potency benzodiazepine such as clonazepam or a sedating antipsychotic, is essential. Owing to the high risk of recurrence, prophylactic treatment of women with a history of postpartum psychosis or bipolar disorder is often considered, although there is no consensus about the optimal time to begin prophylaxis. Many patients prefer to defer starting prophylactic medication until immediately after delivery.

Established postpartum psychosis requires admission to a psychiatric hospital. Mother and baby units are optimal but are relatively uncommon in the United States. Because there are no adequately controlled studies of psychopharmacologic treatment of postpartum psychosis, the standard treatments for a psychotic manic or depressed episode are used, including new-generation antipsychotics, lithium, valproate, and antidepressants. If an antidepressant is used, a mood stabilizer such as lithium or valproate should be given in combination. There are numerous reports that ECT is effective in the treatment of postpartum psychosis, but there are no controlled studies of this strategy. A small open-label pilot study of 17β-estradiol in the treatment of postpartum psychosis found encouraging results but requires further investigation.[110]

SUMMARY OF MANAGEMENT OPTIONS
Postpartum Psychosis

Management Options	Evidence Quality and Recommendation	References
Postnatal		
All health providers in the puerperium must maintain vigilance for the condition.	—/GPP	—
Psychiatric admission usually mandatory to protect baby; mother and baby unit preferred if available.	—/GPP	—
Medication may include a combination of lithium, valproate, antidepressants; use benzodiazepines for sleep problems.	—/GPP	—
Role of ECT and estrogen therapy uncertain.	—/GPP	—

ECT, electroconvulsive therapy; GPP, good practice point.

SUGGESTED READINGS

Alder J, Fink N, Bitzer J, et al: Depression and anxiety during pregnancy: A risk factor for obstetric, fetal and neonatal outcome? A critical review of the literature. J Matern Fetal Neonatal Med 2007;20:189–209.

Brockington I: Postpartum psychiatric disorders. Lancet 2004;363: 303–310.

Dennis CL, Hodnett ED: Psychosocial and psychological interventions for treating postpartum depression. Cochrane Database Syst Rev 2007;4: CD006116.

Empfield MD: Pregnancy and schizophrenia. Psychiatr Ann 2000;30: 61–66.

Freeman MP: Bipolar disorder and pregnancy: Risks revealed. Am J Psychiatr 2007;164:1771–1773.

Hendrick V: Treatment of postnatal depression. BMJ 2003;327: 1003–1004.

Hoffbrand SE, Howard L, Crawley H: Antidepressant treatment for postnatal depression. Cochrane Database Syst Rev 2001;2:CD002018.

Johnson K, Gerada C, Greenough A: Substance misuse during pregnancy. Br J Psychiatr 2003;183:187–189.

Marchesi C, Bertoni S, Maggini C: Major and minor depression in pregnancy. Obstet Gynecol 2009;113:1292–1298.

Sit D, Rothschild AJ, Wisner KL: A review of postpartum psychosis. J Womens Health 2006;15:352–368.

REFERENCES

For a complete list of references, log onto www.expertconsult.com.

SECTION SIX

Prenatal—General

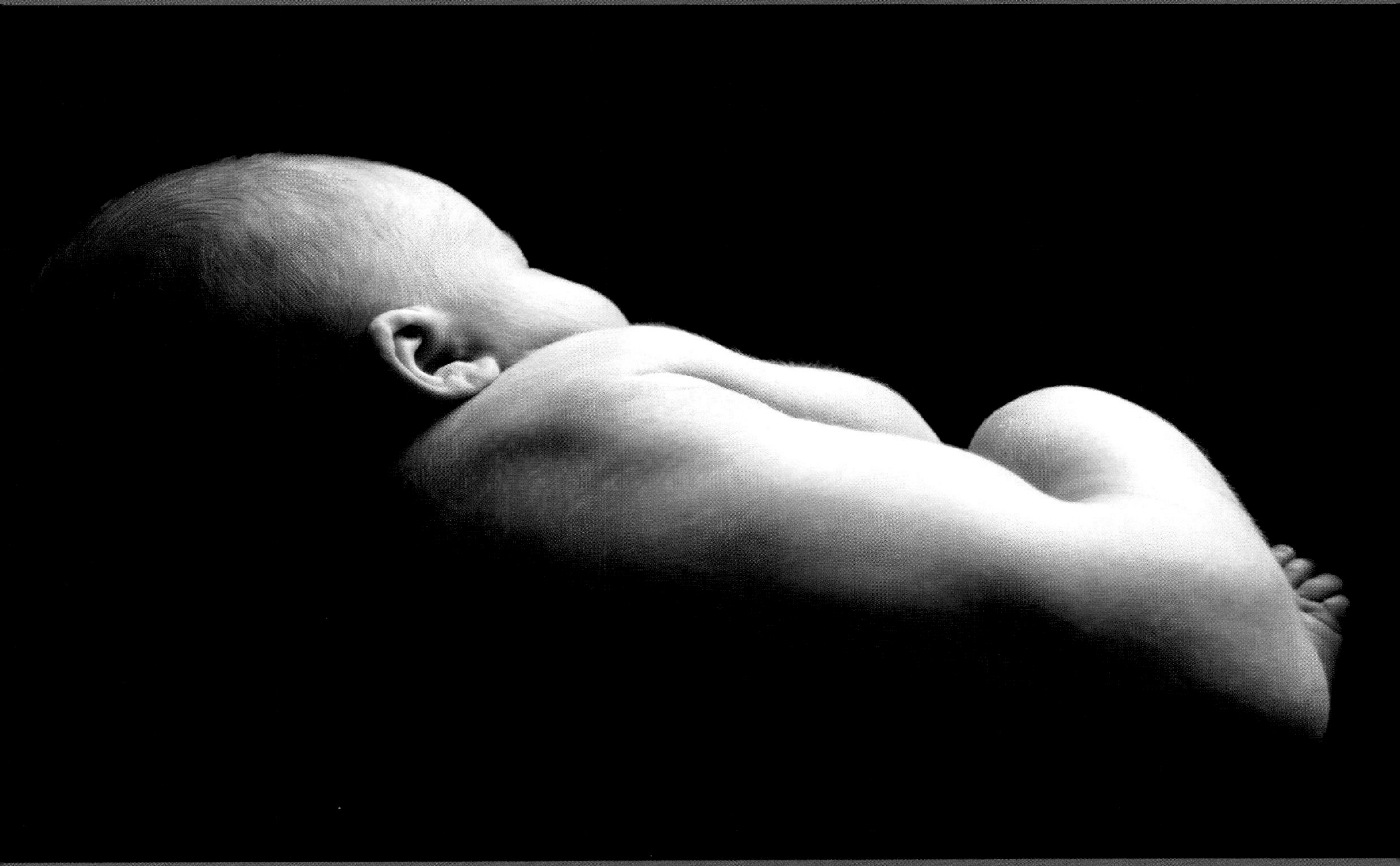

CHAPTER 56

Abdominal Pain

KASSAM MAHOMED

INTRODUCTION AND OVERVIEW

Abdominal pain during pregnancy presents unique clinical challenges; the differential diagnosis during pregnancy is extensive. The pain may result from three sources:

- Physiologic effects of pregnancy.
- Pathologic conditions related to pregnancy.
- Pathologic conditions unrelated to pregnancy.

The clinical presentation and natural history of many abdominal disorders are altered during pregnancy; the diagnostic evaluation is altered and constrained by pregnancy; and finally, the interests of both the mother and the fetus must be considered in pain management.

The initial step in management of abdominal pain is to establish a diagnosis by a detailed history, a thorough physical examination, and specific investigations as summarized in Tables 56–1 to 56–5.

Abdominal assessment during pregnancy is modified by displacement of abdominal viscera by the enlarging gravid uterus, because of which, abdominal masses may also be missed on physical examination.

Physiologic changes in laboratory values during pregnancy that are relevant to interpreting laboratory results include mild leukocytosis, dilutional anemia, increased alkaline phosphatase levels, hyponatremia, hypercoagulability, and fasting hypoglycemia with postprandial hyperglycemia.

DIAGNOSTIC IMAGING IN PREGNANCY

Fetal safety during diagnostic imaging is a concern in pregnancy. Ultrasonography in pregnancy is not associated with adverse maternal or perinatal outcome, impaired physical or neurologic development or an increase in childhood malignancy.[1] Guidelines for computed tomography (CT) and magnetic resonance imaging (MRI) during pregnancy and lactation have recently been published.[2] Radiation dosage is the most important risk factor and is worse in earlier gestation. Exposure of more than 15 rads during the second and third trimester, or more than 5 rads in the first trimester, should be of concern because of the associated increased risk of miscarriage, chromosomal and fetal abnormalities, as well as the increased likelihood of malignancies in childhood.[3] Diagnostic studies with the most radiation exposure, such as intravenous pyelogram (IVP) and barium enema, typically expose the fetus to less than 1 rad.[4]

Sigmoidoscopy, especially flexible sigmoidoscopy, seems to be relatively safe in pregnancy; it does not induce labor and should be considered in medically stable patients with important indications, as opposed to routine screening.[5] Informed consent, however, should be routine in all cases.

PHYSIOLOGIC CONDITIONS IN PREGNANCY (Table 56-1)

Round Ligament Pain

Round ligament pain occurs in 10% to 30% of pregnancies and most commonly occurs toward the end of the first trimester and in the second trimester. It is more common in multigravidae than primigravidae and is said to be due to stretching of the round ligaments, but there is no documented evidence for this. The pain, which is usually described as "cramplike" or "stabbing" and is made worse by movement, is in the lower quadrant and can radiate to the groin. It is often associated with some tenderness over the area of the round ligaments.

Risks

The main risk is failure or delay in diagnosis of a significant pathologic condition (see later discussion).

Management Options

Management is conservative and includes reassurance, reducing physical activity, avoiding movements or postures that exacerbate the symptoms, and in some cases, administering analgesics. Failure to respond to conservative measures or worsening of symptoms is an indication for further investigation.

Severe Uterine Torsion

Mild asymptomatic axial rotation of the uterus (<40 degrees), usually to the right, is observed in the majority of pregnancies.[6] Torsion of the gravid uterus is a rare obstetric complication in humans, but has been reported in association with malpresentation and with uterine leiomyomata; it has also

TABLE 56-1

Physiologic Conditions in Pregnancy

	ROUND LIGAMENT PAIN	UTERINE TORSION	BRAXTON HICKS CONTRACTIONS	MISCELLANEOUS MILD DISCOMFORT
History				
Pain	Cramplike/stabbing, aggravated by movement	Recurrent attacks, pain can be severe	Irregular tightenings	Mild/varied
Urine	–	± Urinary retention		–
Trimester	Late 1st/2nd	3rd	Late	3rd
Previous disease	–	Uterine anomaly, pelvic mass, previous surgery	2nd/3rd	Fibroids
Examination				
Shock	–	+	–	–
Uterus	Soft	Very tender	Irregular contractions	–
Tenderness	Over area of round ligament insertion	Very tender over adnexa	–	–
Others	–	Vagina distorted/changed	No show, no cervical change	–
Investigations				
All	Negative or normal	Negative or normal	Negative or normal	Negative or normal

+, present; –, absent; ±, may be present.

been reported following an external cephalic version.[7] The features of pain, shock, intestinal complaints, urinary symptoms, bleeding, and obstructed labor are related to the degree of torsion and can be acute, subacute, chronic, or intermittent.[8]

Risks

Maternal vasovagal shock and possible fetal asphyxia (both acute and chronic) are the main risks of severe uterine torsion.

Management Options

Conservative measures such as bedrest, analgesia, and altering the position of the mother can be used to try to produce a spontaneous correction of the torsion. Often laparotomy is performed for detorsion of the uterus, hoping the pregnancy will continue. If the fetus is viable, cesarean section is performed following detorsion of the uterus.[7,8]

Braxton Hicks Contractions

Many women experience Braxton Hicks contractions in the latter half of pregnancy.[9] They are irregular in frequency and inconsistent in intensity. Although in the majority of women these contractions are painless, some women find them painful.

Risks

The main danger is to mistake the uterine activity of true preterm labor for Braxton Hicks contractions.

Management Options (See also Chapters 60 and 61)

A careful history and examination should be performed to exclude genuine labor. Absence of a "show" or membrane rupture together with a high presenting part would be reassuring. Cervical ultrasound and fetal fibronectin testing ideally in combination have a very high negative predictive value and would rule out the possibility of threatened preterm labor.[10] In the presence of a positive test, however, a vaginal examination, perhaps repeated in 4 hours, may be the only satisfactory way to assess the significance of these uterine contractions. Once the diagnosis is made, reassurance is all that is necessary.

Miscellaneous Nonpathologic Causes of Discomfort

Heartburn, excessive vomiting, and constipation are common causes of mild discomfort or pain, especially during early pregnancy. A full discussion of the risks and management of hyperemesis gravidarum is given in Chapter 47.

During the third trimester, heartburn may affect up to 80% of women. The reasons for the increase in symptoms in pregnancy are not well understood, but may be due to the effect of pregnancy hormones on the lower esophageal sphincter and gastric clearance.

Risks

The main risk is to miss a pathologic cause for the pain.

Management Options

Heartburn may be helped by reassurance, avoidance of bending, and lying flat in bed. Numerous interventions have been used to relieve these symptoms including advice on diet and lifestyle, antacids, antihistamines, and proton pump inhibitors. The use of these in pregnancy appears to be safe.[11,12] If vomiting is excessive and not relieved by reassurance and dietary adjustments, hospital admission may be required, especially if there is dehydration.

Constipation may be relieved by increasing dietary fiber and avoiding iron unless absolutely necessary. In severe cases, laxatives may be tried.[13]

SUMMARY OF MANAGEMENT OPTIONS

Physiologic Conditions in Pregnancy

Management Options	Evidence Quality and Recommendation	References
Round Ligament Pain		
Exclude pathologic causes of pain.	—/GPP	—
Reassure.	—/GPP	—
Reduce physical activity.	—/GPP	—
Provide local heat.	—/GPP	—
Severe Uterine Torsion		
Exclude pathologic cause of pain.	—/GPP	—
Conservative measures:	—/GPP	—
• Bedrest.		
• Provide analgesia.		
• Alter maternal position.		
• Screen for acute and chronic fetal hypoxia.		
Surgical measures (diagnosed at laparotomy):	IV/C	7,8
• Correct the torsion.		
• Deliver by cesarean section during laparotomy or later (either vaginal or by cesarean) if preterm.		
Braxton Hicks Contractions		
Use cervical ultrasound and biochemical screening methods to exclude preterm labor. See Chapters 60 and 61.	II/B	10
Heartburn, Excess Vomiting, and Constipation		
Heartburn		
Reassure.	—/GPP	—
Avoid bending.	—/GPP	—
Avoid lying flat in bed (more pillows/raise head of bed).	—/GPP	—
Use antacids.	Ib/A	11,12
Use H_2 antagonists if severe.	Ia/A	11,12
Excess Vomiting		
Exclude pathologic cause.	—/GPP	—
Reassure.	—/GPP	—
Provide dietary adjustment.	—/GPP	—
Provide oral antiemetics	—/GPP	—
Consider hospital admission (especially if dehydration/ketosis):	—/GPP	—
• Nothing else as first measure.		
• Consider IV fluids and IV antiemetics if continued problem.		
• See Chapter 47 for discussion of hyperemesis gravidarum.		
Consider steroids in extreme cases.		
Constipation		
Provide dietary adjustment, increase fiber.	III/B	13
Stop iron therapy unless absolutely indicated.	—/GPP	—
Consider laxatives.	III/B	13
Consider suppositories/enema only if severe.	—/GPP	—

GPP, good practice point.

PATHOLOGIC CONDITIONS RELATED TO PREGNANCY (Tables 56-2 and 56-3)

Spontaneous Miscarriage

Chapter 5 provides a detailed discussion of risks and management options.

Uterine Leiomyoma

Chapter 57 provides a detailed discussion of risks and management options.

Placental Abruption

Chapter 58 provides a detailed discussion of risks and management options.

Chorioamnionitis

Chapters 26, 61, and 62 provide detailed discussions of risks and management options.

Preterm Labor

Chapter 61 provides a detailed discussion of risks and management options.

Uterine Rupture

Chapter 75 provides a detailed discussion of risks and management options. Chapters 66, 67, and 73 contain discussions of specific issues.

Ectopic Pregnancy

Chapter 5 provides a detailed discussion of risks and management options.

Ovarian Pathology

Chapter 57 provides a detailed discussion of risks and management options.

TABLE 56-2

Pathologic Conditions Related to Pregnancy: Uterine

	ABORTION/ MISCARRIAGE	FIBROIDS	PLACENTAL ABRUPTION	CHORIOAMNIONITIS	PRETERM LABOR	UTERINE RUPTURE
History						
Pain	+	Localized ± severe	Mild to very ± severe	±	+	+
Vaginal bleeding	++	±	Mild to severe	–	± Show	+
Urinary	–	–	–	–	–	± Hematuria
Alimentary	–	± Vomiting	–	–	–	–
Trimester	1st/early 2nd	Late 2nd/3rd	Late 2nd/early 3rd	3rd	Late 2nd/3rd	3rd
Previous disease	±	+	Hypertension, fibroids	Draining liquor	–	Uterine scar
Others	–	–	Multiple pregnancy	–	Multiple pregnancy, PROM, ± polyhydramnios	Oxytocin
Examination						
Shock	±	–	±	–	–	±
Pyrexia	±	Low-grade	–	±	±	–
Hypertension	±	–	±	–	±	–
Uterus	± Tender	Tender fibroid	± Tender	± Tender	Contractions	++ Tender
Fetal heart	–	–	±	Fetal tachycardia	–	FHR abnormality/ fetal death
Proteinuria	–	–	±	–	±	±
Others	Open cervical os	–	± Oliguria ± Coagulopathy	–	Cervical dilation	±
Investigations						
Hemoglobin	± Low	± Low	± Low	± Low	–	± Low
Leukocytes	± Raised	± Raised	± Low	Raised	± Raised	–
Platelet	–	–	± Low	–	–	–
Ultrasound scan	+	+	± Retroplacental clot	–	Absent fetal breathing movement	–
Others	–	Low-grade fever Malpresentation	± Positive Kleihauer's sign	–	–	–

+, present; –, absent; ±, may be present.
FHR, fetal heart rate; PROM, prelabor rupture of membranes.

TABLE 56-3

Pathologic Conditions Related to Pregnancy: Extrauterine

	ECTOPIC PREGNANCY	CORPUS LUTEUM CYST	HEMORRHAGE INTO CYST/TORSION
History			
Pain	± Severe ± Shoulder tip	+ Aching unilateral	Intermittent lower quadrant
Vaginal bleeding	+	±	±
Trimester	1st	1st	1st/2nd
Previous disease	±	–	±
Others	±	–	Nausea/vomiting
Examination			
Shock	±	–	±
Pyrexia	±	–	± Low grade
Extrauterine	Tenderness ± Mass	Mild tenderness ± Mass	± Tenderness + Mass
Others	Cervical excitation tenderness Os closed		
Investigations			
Hemoglobin	± Low	–	–
White blood cell count	–	–	± Raised
Ultrasound scan	+	+	
Others	β-hCG positive	–	–

+, present; –, absent; ±, may be present.
β-hCG, β-human chorionic gonadotropin.

SUMMARY OF MANAGEMENT OPTIONS COVERED IN OTHER CHAPTERS

Pathologic Conditions Related to Pregnancy

Topics	Summary of Management Options Is Found in Chapter
Spontaneous miscarriage	5
Uterine leiomyoma	57
Placental abruption	58
Chorioamnionitis	26, 61, and 62
Preterm labor	61
Uterine rupture	66, 67, 73, and 75
Ectopic pregnancy	5
Ovarian pathology	57

Abdominal Pregnancy

General

Advanced abdominal pregnancy is a rare event. In the United States, it has been estimated that there are 10.9 abdominal pregnancies per 100,000 births and 9.2 abdominal pregnancies per 1000 ectopic gestations.[14]

It is more commonly seen in patients of low socioeconomic status, in developing countries, and in those patients with a history of infertility or a previous history of pelvic infection.

Advanced abdominal pregnancy has been divided into

- Primary abdominal pregnancy, in which the tubes and ovaries are normal, and there is no evidence of uteroplacental fistula. The pregnancy is related exclusively to the peritoneal surface very early in pregnancy.
- Secondary abdominal pregnancy occurs after tubal abortion or rupture, with subsequent implantation of the conceptus on a nearby peritoneal surface.

Diagnosis

Advanced abdominal pregnancy can have dramatic and catastrophic consequences for the fetus and the mother. Difficult to diagnose preoperatively, it presents special challenges to the physician. Preoperative diagnosis allows time for thoughtful preparation of the patient, family, and medical team; diagnosis requires a high index of suspicion. Abdominal pain is present in 80% of cases, often noticed in early pregnancy, and varies from mild discomfort to severe and unbearable pain. Fetal movements may be painful or absent with fetal death. In 30% of cases, vaginal bleeding is reported in early pregnancy. Examination reveals abdominal tenderness, with easily palpable fetal parts.

Abnormal lie occurs in 15% to 20% of cases. Vaginal examination often reveals a closed, uneffaced cervix occasionally displaced anteriorly. Absence of palpable uterine contractions to oxytocin stimulation or to induction of labor by prostaglandins is one of the most helpful clinical clues to the diagnosis.[15] Even with a high index of suspicion, confirmation of the diagnosis is not always easy.

Ultrasound scan may reveal one or more of the following features: the fetal head is located outside the uterus; the fetal body is outside the uterus, as is the ectopic placenta; failure to demonstrate a uterine wall between the fetus and the urinary bladder; and recognition of a close approximation of fetal parts and the maternal abdominal wall. An unusual echographic appearance of the placenta should prompt a more thorough investigation to confirm the diagnosis.[16]

MRI can safely produce images in different planes without the use of ionizing radiation. This method seems to be a very sensitive diagnostic tool where facilities exist.

Risks

Perinatal mortality rate is reported to be greater than 50%. If there is reduced liquor volume, there is an increased incidence of fetal malformation, pressure deformities, and pulmonary hypoplasia. Maternal mortality rate depends on availability and accessibility of services but has been reported as 5 per 1000 cases.[14]

Management Options

Management is based on an empirical approach derived from a review of cases[15–17] rather than evidence from controlled trials.

Timing and the nature of the intervention will depend on the gestation and viability of the fetus at the time of diagnosis. If the fetus is dead, surgery is indicated. Waiting for a few weeks to allow atrophy of the placental vessels will possibly decrease intraoperative complications. If the fetus is alive but nonviable (before 24 wk), immediate surgery is thought to be indicated. If the pregnancy is 24 or more weeks, a conservative approach may be contemplated to allow time for further development of the fetus. This approach requires thorough and careful counseling of the parents. There are no data that define the risks for the conservative versus surgical options at either gestation.

NATURE OF THE INTERVENTION

Preoperative preparations should include having several units of blood available and, if possible, carrying out the delivery with a general, vascular, or genitourinary surgeon. A midline vertical incision is always advisable to improve access. The amniotic sac should be carefully incised in an avascular area free of placenta. Removal of the fetus should be done in a way to minimize manipulation of the placenta and surrounding membranes and the likelihood of bleeding.

MANAGEMENT OF THE PLACENTA

If the blood supply to the placenta can be safely secured, complete removal of the placenta usually results in an uncomplicated postoperative recovery, and if removal of the placenta is straightforward, this should be the optimal approach.

If the placenta cannot be removed safely, other options include ligating the cord close to the placenta and leaving it in situ or ligating the placental blood supply and removing the pelvic organ upon which implantation has occurred (e.g., hysterectomy or salpingo-oophorectomy).

Partial removal of the placenta when its whole blood supply cannot be ligated may result in massive hemorrhage, shock, and death. This is not recommended. In such situations, it is best that the placenta be left in situ. However, this option is often accompanied by ileus, peritonitis, abscess formation, and prolonged hospital stay.

One possible option would also be to leave the placenta in situ with later use of methotrexate to increase the rate of absorption/destruction of the retained placental tissue. However, this leads to rapid destruction of the placenta with accelerated accumulation of necrotic placental tissue, which often becomes infected. This is, therefore, not a recommended method of treatment.[15,17]

SUMMARY OF MANAGEMENT OPTIONS

Abdominal Pregnancy

Management Options	Evidence Quality and Recommendation	References
Dead Fetus		
Delivery by laparotomy, possibly with a delay to reduce complication rates.	IV/C	15–17
Live Fetus before 24 Weeks		
Deliver by laparotomy.	—/GPP	—

Management Options	Evidence Quality and Recommendation	References
Live Fetus after 24 Weeks	IV/C	15–17
Consider a conservative approach after careful counseling. Possibly undertaken as inpatient.	—/GPP	—
Perform laparotomy and deliver if oligohydramnios and/or compressional deformities.	—/GPP	—
Guidelines for laparotomy and delivery: • Ideally perform jointly with general/vascular surgeon. • Have several units of blood available. • Make midline vertical incision in abdomen. • Incise sac away from placenta. • Avoid placental manipulation during delivery. • If blood supply to placenta can be secured, remove placenta completely. • If blood supply to placenta cannot be secured, ligate cord only (greater postoperative morbidity).	IV/C	15–17

GPP, good practice point.

PATHOLOGIC CONDITIONS UNRELATED TO PREGNANCY (Table 56-4)

Gastrointestinal Tract

Acute Appendicitis

GENERAL

Acute appendicitis is the most common nonobstetric cause of an acute abdomen during pregnancy complicating about 1 in 1000 pregnancies,[18] the same frequency as in nonpregnant women.[19] The incidences are approximately 30%, 45%, and 25% in the first, second, and third trimesters, respectively.[20] An infected appendix appears to be more likely to rupture during pregnancy, especially in the third trimester, possibly because of delay in diagnosis and intervention. The incidence among teenagers is higher than in older age groups.[21]

DIAGNOSIS

The diagnosis is challenging because the typical symptoms—anorexia, nausea, and vomiting—mimic normal pregnancy, and the anatomic location of the appendix during pregnancy can be different from that in the nonpregnant patient. Conventional teaching maintains that appendicitis pain "migrates" upward with the growing uterus. However, ine review of cases over a 10-year period showed that pain in the right lower quadrant of the abdomen is the most common presenting symptom in pregnancy, regardless of gestational age.[18] Appendicitis should always be considered when a pregnant woman presents with persistent abdominal pain and tenderness, nausea, vomiting, and fever. Rebound tenderness and muscle guarding are valuable signs in the diagnosis of appendicitis, but because of the laxity of the abdominal wall, these signs are found less frequently in pregnant women.[21] In several publications, features significantly associated with the diagnosis of acute appendicitis included nausea, vomiting, and peritonism.[22,23]

Normal pregnant women may have mild leukocytosis, but serial white blood cell counts can prove helpful when evaluating patients over several hours.[19] Pyelonephritis is the most common differential diagnosis of abdominal pain that mimics acute appendicitis in pregnancy.[20] Ultrasound, CT scan, and MR imaging have all been used to assist in the diagnosis of acute appendicitis.[22,24,25] A systematic review of studies in individuals 14 years of age and older compared the reported overall accuracy for the diagnosis of appendicitis using CT scan with ultrasound. CT had an overall sensitivity of 0.94 (95% confidence interval [CI] 0.91–0.95), a specificity of 0.95 (95% CI 0.93–0.96), a positive likelihood ratio of 13.3 (95% CI 9.9–17.9), and a negative likelihood ratio of 0.09 (95% CI 0.07–0.12). Ultrasonography had an overall sensitivity of 0.86 (95% CI 0.83–0.88), a specificity of 0.81 (95% CI 0.78–0.84), a positive likelihood ratio of 5.8 (95% CI 3.5–9.5), and a negative likelihood ratio of 0.19 (95% CI 0.13–0.27).[26] In one review of cases over 5-year period, ultrasound was positive in over a third whereas MRI was positive in all cases of acute appendicitis.[24] In patients without appendicitis, a normal appendix was visualized in fewer than 2% with ultrasound but in 87% of cases with MRI. In another review, in 5 out of 19 (25%) patients who had confirmed acute appendicitis the ultrasound was normal.[27]

RISKS

Similarity with normal symptoms in pregnancy can lead to a delay in the diagnosis. Maternal morbidity following appendectomy is low, except when perforation has occurred. Pregnancy complications are frequent, especially when surgery is delayed or performed in the first or second trimester. In one review of 56 women who underwent

TABLE 56-4

Pathologic Conditions Unrelated to Pregnancy

	ACUTE APPENDICITIS	INTESTINAL OBSTRUCTION	CHOLECYSTITIS	INFLAMMATORY BOWEL DISEASE	PEPTIC ULCER	ACUTE PANCREATITIS
History						
Pain	Right lower quadrant, lumbar, loin	Colicky	Right upper quadrant, epigastric colicky/stabbing	+	Epigastric pain	Central upper abdomen, radiating into back
Urinary	± Frequency	–	–	–	–	–
Alimentary	Nausea/vomiting	Nausea/vomiting, constipation	Nausea/vomiting	Diarrhea	Nausea/vomiting	
Trimester	–	Late 2nd/3rd postnatal	–	–	–	3rd/postnatal
Previous disease	–	±	–	+	+	Alcohol gallstones
Others	–	–	Jaundice Weight loss	–	–	
Examination						
Shock	±	±	±	–	If perforation	±
Pyrexia	+	±	±	–	–	–
Extrauterine	Tender	Distention/tenderness	Tenderness	±	Tender epigastrium	Tender
Others	–	Bowel sounds high-pitched	–	–	–	–
Investigations						
Leukocytes	Raised	Raised	Raised	Raised	–	± Raised
Urine	± Pyuria	–	–	–	–	–
Ultrasound scan	–	–	Gallstones	–	–	–
Radiographic abnormality	–	+	–	–	If perforation	–
Others	–	–	–	Endoscopy/biopsy	Endoscopy	Amylase +

+, present; –, absent; ±, may be present.

appendectomy in various trimesters, spontaneous miscarriage occurred in 33% if in the first trimester, and preterm labor in 14% patients operated on in the second trimester.[28] No pregnancy complications were observed in women who underwent appendectomy in the third trimester.

Reluctance to operate in a pregnant woman causes further delay and thus increases the risk of perforation, peritonitis, and septicemia as well as a substantial risk of miscarriage, preterm labor, and fetal demise. The interval between onset of symptoms and surgery has been reported to be the only predictive variable, with a longer interval being associated with appendix perforation. In one study, there was a significant difference in the rate of preterm labor (5.1% vs, 1.3%) and the rate of fetal mortality (25% vs, 1.7%) between patients with and without perforation of the appendix.[29]

MANAGEMENT OPTIONS

Despite the difficulty in making the diagnosis, surgery should not be delayed when the clinical suspicion is high. Laparoscopy appears to be well tolerated in pregnancy,[22,25,27,30] but larger multicenter prospective trials are required to make firm recommendations concerning its use in pregnancy. Use of ultrasound to guide first trocar insertion to prevent injury to the uterus may be a useful adjunct to improve safety.[31] The decision to proceed with a laparoscopic approach or to perform a laparotomy will depend on the skill and experience of the surgeon as well as clinical factors such as the size of the gravid uterus.

If laparotomy is being performed, the incision site needs to be individualized. In the first trimester, because the appendix remains in its usual location and the uterus does not obstruct access to it, a low transverse or McBurney incision can be used. In the second and third trimesters, a right paramedian incision over the area of maximal tenderness allows better access to the appendix and the option of extending the incision if needed. It is thought preferable to extend the incision to gain adequate exposure rather than to extensively compress or manipulate the pregnant uterus. There are, however, no studies that address this issue.

Postoperatively, vigilance should be maintained for signs of preterm labor, monitoring for contractions and cervical dilation. The value of perioperative use of tocolysis is uncertain. The main concern with using tocolysis is the risk of potential fluid overload and adult respiratory distress syndrome.[32] However, many have used prophylactic tocolysis successfully.[33] There are no reported trials to resolve this issue.[33,34]

SUMMARY OF MANAGEMENT OPTIONS

Appendicitis

Management Options	Evidence Quality and Recommendation	References
Diagnosis is not easy; risks to mother and fetus greatly increased with perforation.	III/B	29
Laparoscopy can be performed safely especially before 20 wk.	IV/C	22,25,27,30
Use of ultrasound scan to guide trocar is a useful adjunct for safety.	III/B	31
Laparotomy performed with right paramedian incision at site of maximal tenderness.	—/GPP	—
There is conflicting evidence for the use of prophylactic tocolysis postoperatively for 2–3 days.	III/B	32–34
Administer postoperative antibiotics.	—/GPP	—

GPP, good practice point.

Intestinal Obstruction

Acute intestinal obstruction is the second most common nonobstetric abdominal emergency complicating pregnancy. It occurs in 1 in 1500 pregnancies. Its incidence as a cause of acute abdominal pain requiring surgery in pregnancy is increasing.[35] This trend is attributed to a number of factors, including a rising number of surgical procedures performed in young women[36] and an increased number of pregnancies occurring in older women.[37,38] Obstruction most likely occurs in the third trimester because of the added mechanical effects of the enlarged gravid uterus.[39]

Clinical presentation is similar to that in the nonpregnant state, with colicky abdominal pain, vomiting, and constipation. Abdominal distention and high-pitched bowel sounds are found. If the diagnosis is suspected, there should be no delay in requesting an erect abdominal x-ray to demonstrate dilated loops of bowel with fluid levels.

RISKS

Like appendicitis, delay in diagnosis is common and is often the explanation for the morbidity and fatality that accompany intestinal obstruction in pregnancy. High maternal and fetal mortality rates of 10% to 20% and 30% to 50%, respectively, are reported, especially if the obstruction is complicated by strangulation or perforation or by fluid and electrolyte imbalance.[35,37]

MANAGEMENT OPTIONS

If there are no signs of strangulation, conservative management with intravenous fluids and nasogastric aspiration may be tried for a few hours.[35–37] However, where there is any doubt, early surgery after correcting fluid and electrolyte imbalance would be the safest option in view of the high complication rate. A vertical midline incision is usually necessary, and occasionally, the definitive surgical procedure may have to be preceded by cesarean section if access becomes a problem and fetal maturity is assured. Use of perioperative tocolysis to prevent preterm labor is of uncertain benefit.[31–33]

SUMMARY OF MANAGEMENT OPTIONS

Intestinal Obstruction

Management Options	Evidence Quality and Recommendation	References
Once diagnosis is made, conservative vs. surgical approach are the options: • ***Conservative*** (nasogastric suction and IV fluids) may be considered for a few hours if no strangulation/perforation is present. • ***Surgical*** approach (laparotomy and surgical correction of obstruction) always indicated if strangulation/perforation, though some would advocate early surgery for all cases.	IV/C	35,37

SUMMARY OF MANAGEMENT OPTIONS

Intestinal Obstruction—cont'd

Management Options	Evidence Quality and Recommendation	References
If surgical option chosen: • Obstetrician and surgeon should operate together. • Make adequate vertical incision. • Cesarean section may be necessary for adequate surgical field in late pregnancy.	IV/C	35,37
Give careful attention to fluid and electrolyte balance.	—/GPP	—
Use of tocolysis for 2–3 days after surgery is controversial.	III/B	32–34

GPP, good practice point.

Acute Cholecystitis and Cholelithiasis

Physiologic changes of the biliary system in pregnancy including decreased gallbladder motility and delayed emptying results in an increase in gallbladder disease in pregnancy. In a prospective study of 3254 women having serial ultrasound examination during pregnancy, stones or sludge were present in 5% and 8% of women by the second and third trimesters, respectively, and 10% of women by 4 to 6 weeks postpartum.[40] Spontaneous regression of sludge and stones was common in the postpartum period. Twenty-eight women (0.8%) underwent cholecystectomy within the first year postpartum. The paper also reported that higher body mass index and serum leptin levels were independent predictors of the risk of gallbladder disease.

In another large ultrasound study in Chile, 12% of pregnant women versus 1.3% of nonpregnant control subjects had gallstones.[41] Most gallstones are asymptomatic in pregnancy, but when symptoms occur, they are the same as in nonpregnant women. The obstruction may result in gallbladder distention and acute cholecystitis. When inflammation occurs, it may be aseptic or bacterial. In a audit of over 6500 cases of biliary disease during pregnancy and in the first year postpartum, in the United States, 76% had uncomplicated cholelithiasis, 16% had pancreatitis, 9% had acute cholecystitis, and 8% had cholangitis.[42]

DIAGNOSIS

Pain is located in the epigastrium and right upper quadrant and can vary in severity. It may be sudden in onset and become intermittent. Colicky pain is often a result of a stone obstructing the common bile duct. There may be nausea, vomiting, pyrexia, tachycardia, and right subcostal tenderness. The tenderness on deep palpation under the right costal margin on deep exhalation is known as positive Murphy's sign. Leukocytosis is common. Serum liver function tests and amylase may be mildly abnormal. The differential diagnosis includes viral hepatitis, pneumonia, appendicitis, acute fatty liver of pregnancy, and shingles. Ultrasound scan of the gallbladder and the common bile duct will demonstrate gallstones in more than 90% of cases.[43] Cholangiography is contraindicated in pregnancy.

It is important to differentiate cholecystitis from the hemolysis, elevated liver enzymes, and low platelets (HELLP) syndrome and severe preeclampsia, which are associated with great risk to the mother and fetus (see Chapter 35). Abnormal renal function, raised serum uric acid levels, and low platelet counts will help to make the correct diagnosis of HELLP syndrome.

RISKS

Spontaneous rupture of the gallbladder may occur. There is a possible risk of miscarriage and preterm delivery when surgery is required during pregnancy.

MANAGEMENT OPTIONS

Management is similar to that in the nonpregnant woman. Cholecystectomy is not indicated when asymptomatic gallstones are present. Initially, and particularly in the first and third trimesters, conservative treatment should be advocated.[44–46] This approach includes analgesia (avoid morphine), intravenous fluids, and nasogastric suction. Antibiotics may be used.

Recurrent attacks, failure to respond to conservative treatment, suspected perforation, empyema of the gallbladder, peritonitis, and doubt about the diagnosis are indications for surgery.

If symptomatic, it is safer to operate in the second trimester when the risk of preterm labor is lowest, although more aggressive surgical options have now become more acceptable during all trimesters because of advances in maternal and fetal monitoring and advances in laparoscopic surgery.[47,48] Laparoscopic cholecystectomy has been performed during pregnancy and is thought to be safe if performed by a skilled laparoscopic surgeon and has not been associated with fetal mortality.[49,50]

Use of perioperative tocolysis to prevent preterm labor in a continuing pregnancy is debatable, as has been noted previously.[31–33]

SUMMARY OF MANAGEMENT OPTIONS

Cholecystitis

Management Options	Evidence Quality and Recommendation	References
Prepregnancy		
Consider cholecystectomy prior to conception with symptomatic gallstones.	—/GPP	—
Prenatal		
Conservative approach first: • Bedrest. • Analgesia/sedation. • IV fluids • Nasogastric suction. • Antibiotics (e.g., amoxicillin, cephalosporine, or co-amoxiclav). • Dietary adjustment after attack has subsided (e.g., avoiding fatty foods).	III/B	44–46
Cholecystectomy can be performed in pregnancy if required and can be performed laparoscopically.	III/B	47–50

GPP, good practice point.

Inflammatory Bowel Disease

Chapter 47 provides a detailed discussion of risks and management options.

Gastroesophageal Reflux and Peptic Ulcer Disease

Chapter 47 provides a detailed discussion of risks and management options.

Acute Pancreatitis

Acute pancreatitis is an uncommon complication of pregnancy, and its incidence has been reported to range from 1 in 1000[51] to 1 in 3333 in a recent 10-year audit in the United States.[52] Most cases tend to be associated with gallbladder disease, and more than half (56%) occur in the second trimester.[53] Cases that are biliary in origin have a better outcome than nonbiliary cases.[52] Gallstones probably cause obstruction of the sphincter of Oddi. Preexisting genetic abnormalities in lipid metabolism may be worsened during pregnancy and may also cause gestational hyperlipidemic pancreatitis.[51] In these, a third are reported to develop pancreatitis in their first pregnancy and are associated with a worse outcome. Management may include expectant or surgical. In the 10-year audit, it was noted that patients with gallbladder disease who received surgical or endoscopic treatment during pregnancy had lower preterm delivery rates and recurrences than those that were managed expectantly.[52]

Typical symptoms include fever and often sudden mid-epigastric pain, which may localize to the left upper quadrant and often radiates into the left flank. Anorexia, nausea, and vomiting are common. There may be mild pyrexia with varying degree of abdominal tenderness. Ultrasonography will demonstrate gallstones in more than 70% of cases. Raised serum amylase and lipase concentrations will confirm the diagnosis.[54] False-negative results may occasionally occur with hemorrhagic pancreatitis with massive necrosis or when the blood is taken 24 to 72 hours after the attack. A CT scan may be used for severe cases to delineate areas of pancreatic necrosis.[54] Endoscopic retrograde cholangiopancreatography (ERCP) may be used as a diagnostic tool and has been safely performed during pregnancy,[55] but needs further evaluation.

RISKS

There is increased perinatal mortality and morbidity. An acute episode may be associated with preterm labor and its associated risks.[54] This is especially so with hyperlipidemic pancreatitis.[51]

MANAGEMENT OPTIONS

The recommended treatment is similar to that for the nonpregnant patient and includes intravenous fluids, nil orally, gastric acid suppression, analgesia, and possibly nasogastric suction.[52] Because conservative treatment is associated with a high recurrence rate,[52] especially if associated with gallbladder disease, early surgical intervention is appropriate as soon as inflammation has subsided. This may be cholecystectomy or endoscopic sphincterotomy. Some have, however, recommended early aggressive surgical intervention.[54,56]

SUMMARY OF MANAGEMENT OPTIONS

Acute Pancreatitis

Management Options	Evidence Quality and Recommendation	References
Prepregnancy		
Discuss specific measures in women with risk factors:	—/GPP	—
• Cholecystectomy in women with known gallstones and previous attacks of cholecystitis or pancreatitis. Various strategies in women with alcohol abuse (see Chapter 33). Change treatment in women taking thiazide diuretics		
Prenatal		
Prevent and treat shock with IV fluids and monitoring of electrolyte, calcium, and glucose concentrations.	IV/C	52
Provide analgesia.	—/GPP	—
Administer prophylactic antibiotics	IV/C	52
Suppression of pancreatic activity (no randomized, controlled trials).	—/GPP	—
Prompt recognition and treatment of surgical complications:	—/GPP	—
• Laparotomy usually performed with cholecystectomy if conservative measures fail.	IV/C	52,54,56
• Cholecystectomy can be an early option when pancreatitis occurs with gallstones in first or second trimester.	IV/C	52,54,56
Postnatal		
Cholecystectomy possible if pancreatitis with gallstones successfully treated conservatively in pregnancy.	IV/C	54,56

GPP, good practice point.

Urinary Tract Pathology

Chapter 49 provides detailed discussions of risks and management options.

Liver Disease

Acute Fatty Liver of Pregnancy

Chapter 47 provides a detailed discussion of risks and management options.

Severe Preeclampsia and Eclampsia

Chapters 35 and 78 provide detailed discussions of risks and management options.

MISCELLANEOUS CAUSES (Table 56–5)

Rectus Hematoma

Bleeding into the rectus muscle and subsequent hematoma formation following rupture of a branch of the inferior epigastric vessels may occur following a bout of coughing or direct trauma, usually in late pregnancy. A large unilateral painful swelling may be confused with an ovarian cyst, degenerating fibroid, uterine rupture, or placental abruption. However, its superficial location in the abdominal wall should enable accurate diagnosis.

Management Options

If diagnosed early, treatment consists of analgesia and bedrest. If, however, diagnosis is made only at the time of surgery, the hematoma can be evacuated and hemostasis secured.

Sickle Cell Crisis

Chapter 38 provides a detailed discussion of risks and management options.

Porphyria

Chapter 51 provides a detailed discussion of risks and management options

Malaria

Chapter 32 provides a detailed discussion of risks and management options

Arteriovenous Hemorrhage

Miscellaneous, very rare conditions resulting in intraabdominal hemorrhage can cause abdominal pain in pregnancy. These conditions include rupture of the utero-ovarian veins, rupture of aneurysms (splenic, hepatic, renal, aortic), and spontaneous rupture of the uterine vein.[57] In addition

TABLE 56-5
Miscellaneous Conditions

	RECTUS HEMATOMA	SICKLE CRISIS	PORPHYRIA	MALARIA	ARTERIOVENOUS HEMORRHAGE
History					
Pain	+	+	+	+	+
Alimentary	–	±	±	±	±
Urinary	–	–	±	±	–
Previous disease	–	+	Precipitating factor	–	±
Others	Trauma/cough	Precipitating factor	Psychological, autonomic	Travel to malaria area	–
Examination					
Shock	±	+	–	±	±
Pyrexia	±	±	–	+	–
Uterine	–	–	–	–	Tender if uterine vein rupture
Extrauterine	Tender	–	–	–	–
Others	± Mass	–	–	Spleen enlarged	–
Investigations					
Hemoglobin	–	Low	–	Low	Low
Ultrasound scan	± Mass				±
Radiologically abnormal	–	±	–	–	–
Others	–	HbS, sickling	Urinary porphyrins	Positive malaria slide	–

+, present; –, absent; ±, may be present.
HbS, hemoglobin S.

to the abdominal pain, rapidly progressing shock is a feature.

Risks

The main risks of these conditions are maternal and fetal demise.

Management Options

Speed of action is imperative in these cases, and even then, death may not be avoided. In all conditions, the principles of management are the same: namely, surgical control of the hemorrhage, correction of shock, and specific measures for specific problems (such as splenectomy with splenic rupture or insertion of a graft with aortic rupture). If the patient survives long enough for such definitive measures to be considered, practical assistance from a general or vascular surgeon is mandatory.

Tuberculosis

Chapter 32 provides a detailed discussion of risks and management options.

Psychological Causes

About 1% of laparoscopies performed for abdominal pain in pregnancy reveal no cause for the pain.[58] Many of these patients have psychological stress that affects the irritable bowel syndrome. Pregnant women with idiopathic abdominal pain are often single, are smokers, and have financial problems.[58] This diagnosis should, however, be made only after exclusion of all possible organic causes and requires comprehensive diagnostic evaluation. This would possibly avoid unnecessary surgical intervention. Reporting a high number of ailments during antenatal care may be an indication for psychosocial support.[59] Domestic violence should also be considered in these cases (see Chapter 3).

PROCEDURE

LAPAROSCOPY IN PREGNANCY

Indications

Laparoscopy has become an increasingly popular option for many conditions. The common indications in pregnancy have been acute appendicitis and cholecystectomy, which though initially reserved for the second trimester, are now being more widely and safely being performed in any of the three trimesters as surgeons become more aggressive in their management approach. Other indication includes ovarian cyst complications in early pregnancy.

Procedure

In pregnancy, patients should be counseled adequately regarding the risks from the procedure. In late pregnancy, ultrasound-guided Vers needle insertion has been shown to reduce injury to the uterus.[31] An experienced anesthetist would be recommended to ensure that respiration is not compromised by the pneumoperitoneum.

Complications

Lachman and associates[60] reviewed the literature on the subject and cautioned on the lack of adequate data on the possible harmful effect of intra-abdominal pressure as a result of the pneumoperitoneum as well as any possible effect of carbon dioxide absorption on the fetus. The long-term consequences have also been questioned in another review article.[61] In terms of short-term risks of miscarriage and preterm labor, the numbers studied to date are too small to be reassured and caution would still need to be exercised.

PROCEDURE

LAPAROTOMY IN PREGNANCY

Indications

The indications for laparotomy in pregnancy are discussed in the different sections of this chapter. In general, they are the same as in the nonpregnant patient. Obstetricians arguably are more comfortable with the idea of operating on a pregnant woman than are general surgeons. They are also often more familiar with the alterations in disease presentation and differential diagnosis in pregnancy than are general surgeons. For these reasons, it is advisable that obstetricians do not simply turn the care of their patients over to surgical specialists for diagnosis and treatment, but rather, remain actively involved in their patients' management throughout the period of evaluation, treatment, and postoperative care.[62]

Procedure

Anesthetic Considerations

The choice of the anesthesia for surgery during pregnancy depends on the operation proposed, the skill of the anesthesiologist, and the preference of the surgeon and the patient, Although it has been suggested that chronic exposure of operating room personnel to anesthetic agents leads to an increased rate of miscarriage, the hazard associated with acute general anesthetic administration to the patient is not well characterized. It seems that the risk is very small. It is probably more important that meticulous attention is paid to maintenance of maternal homeostasis. The fetus is totally dependent on adequate maternal oxygenation and uterine perfusion. Any compromise of maternal oxygenation will potentially affect the fetus. Both conduction or regional anesthesia and general anesthesia can be used in pregnancy with safety for both the mother and the fetus.

Operation

Abdominal incisions in pregnancy are the same as those used in nonpregnant patients. McBurney and low transverse incisions are best limited to the first trimester. Later in pregnancy, the enlarged uterus so completely fills the lower abdomen that access to organs other than the anterior, lower uterine segment (as for cesarean section) is extremely difficult. It is generally advisable to make an incision that can be extended if necessary, rather than attempting to use a small and poorly placed incision and being forced to manipulate the uterus in an attempt to accomplish the operation. Midline or paramedian incisions work well. Healing in pregnancy is generally without complications, though there may be some skin scar spreading as the abdomen enlarges through pregnancy and keloid formation in some women. If labor occurs shortly after surgery, the fresh incision may inhibit maternal expulsive efforts during the second stage, necessitating an assisted delivery.

Complications

There is an increased risk of miscarriage in association with laparotomy performed during early pregnancy.[64] This risk exists especially in the first trimester and is considerably reduced on planned procedures carried out in the second trimester. Preterm delivery and technical difficulty are problems encountered when laparotomy is carried out during the third trimester. However, although the risks of laparotomy in pregnancy should not be underestimated, the risks to the mother and baby of the condition for which the surgery is required are usually greater than the risks of the operation itself, and if surgery is indicated, it should not be unduly delayed.

SUGGESTED READINGS

Andersen B, Nielsen TF: Appendicitis in pregnancy: Diagnosis, management and complications. Acta Obstet Gynecol Scand 1999;78:758–762.

Brown JJ, Wilson C, Coleman S, Joypaul BV: Appendicitis in pregnancy: An ongoing diagnostic dilemma. Colorectal Dis 2009;11:116–122.

Eddy JJ, Gideonsen MD, Song JY, et al: Pancreatitis in pregnancy. Obstet Gynecol 2008;112:1075–1081

Kilpatrick CC, Orejuela FJ: Management of the acute abdomen in pregnancy: A review. Curr Opin Obstet Gynecol 2008;20:534–539.

Kirshtein B, Perry ZH, Avinoach E, et al: Safety of laparoscopic appendicectomy during pregnancy. World J Surg 2009;33:475–480.

Ko CW: Risk factors for gall stone–related hospitalization during pregnancy and the post partum. Am J Gastroenterol 2006;101:2263–2268.

Mahajan NN: Advanced extrauterine pregnancy: Diagnostic and therapeutic challenges. Am J Obstet Gynecol 2008;199:11–15.

Pedrosa I, Lafornara M, Pandharipande PV, et al: Pregnant patients suspected of having acute appendicitis: Effect of MR imaging on negative laparotomy rate and appendiceal perforation rate. Radiology 2009;250:749–757.

Torloni MR, Vadmedorska N, Merialdi M, et al: Safety of ultrasonography in pregnancy: WHO systematic review of the literature and meta-analysis. Ultrasound Obstet Gynecol 2009;33:599–608.

Yoneyama K, Kimura A, Kogo, M, et al: Clinical predictive factors for preterm birth in women with threatened preterm labour or preterm premature ruptured membranes. Aust N Z J Obstet Gynaecol 2009;49:16–21

REFERENCES

For a complete list of references, log onto www.expertconsult.com.

CHAPTER 57

Nonmalignant Gynecology

KASSAM MAHOMED

INTRODUCTION

This chapter discusses the significance of a number of gynecologic problems in association with pregnancy that are not covered elsewhere in the book. For malignant gynecologic problems, see Chapter 52. Nonmalignant topics discussed elsewhere include infection (see Chapter 31), female circumcision (see Chapter 71), previous pelvic floor surgery, and previous third-degree tear (see Chapter 71).

OVARIAN CYSTS IN PREGNANCY (See Chapters 52 and 56)

Introduction

With wider routine ultrasound scanning during the first trimester, the discovery of an ovarian cyst has become relatively common. In a retrospective audit, 4.8% of women having a scan before 10 weeks had an ovarian cyst of 3 cm or more.[1] Larger ovarian cysts that are 6 cm or more are estimated to occur in 0.5 to 2 per 1000 pregnancies.[2] Most unilocular and anechoic ovarian cysts with thin borders that are seen during the first trimester are corpus luteum cysts. These cysts are not usually present after the end of the first trimester. The majority are asymptomatic, and most resolve spontaneously.[3] Thus, further evaluation and management of cysts in early pregnancy are usually left until the second trimester.[4]

If cysts are noted after 16 weeks' gestation, pathology needs to be excluded. They may present with torsion or pain or on routine ultrasound scanning. In a recent review of such cases, 20% were functional cysts, 50% were serous cysts, 10% were mucinous cysts, and 35% were dermoid cysts.[5]

Risks

The major risk of ovarian cysts in pregnancy is to the mother, namely pain from torsion, rupture, or hemorrhage into cyst. If the cyst is large enough in the third trimester, it may predispose to malpresentation or obstructed labor.[6] Fetal risks include miscarriage and preterm delivery.[7]

Management Options

Prepregnancy

Surgical treatment is indicated for cysts that are detected before pregnancy, if they are larger than 5 cm, contain echogenic material, or are symtomatic.[8] Aspiration of cysts, either laparoscopically or ultrasonically, with cytologic examination of the fluid, is not favored because cystadenomas or cystadenocarcinomas may be misdiagnosed.[9] However, in one long-term follow-up of patients who had aspiration of simple cysts because they were not suitable for surgery, the main risk was recurrence (75%).[10] No patient developed ovarian malignancy.

Prenatal

Familiarity with the natural history and ultrasound scan features of common adnexal lesions, such as simple cysts, hemorrhagic cysts, endometriomas, mature cystic teratomas, and ovarian conditions specific to pregnancy, may permit stratification of patients into management protocols. More than 90% of cysts that occur in pregnancy are non-neoplastic.[5] Corpus luteum cysts usually begin to regress after 12 weeks.[11] Ultrasound scanning may help to identify those patients in whom conservative management is appropriate. Asymptomatic ovarian cysts with benign sonographic features may be followed closely by serial scanning into the second trimester, when surgery can be planned, if necessary.[12,13] However, if the cyst is not enlarging, conservative management may be preferred. Surgery, even in the second trimester, may result in preterm delivery.[7]

If ultrasound examination of an ovarian cyst larger than 5 cm shows echogenic features, surgery may be indicated.[12] The risk of surgical interventions needs to be balanced against the potential risks of nonintervention, which may include torsion, rupture, and hemorrhage. Laparoscopic management is now the preferred management option if the cyst is not too large.[14,15]

Torsion of ovarian cysts is treated by surgery.[16] If intervention is necessary, laparoscopy is the preferred method.

The use of tocolysis to reduce the risk of preterm delivery is controversial, and there are no reported trials to help to resolve this issue.[17] Aspiration of the cyst is not well evaluated and is not generally recommended.[9] The role of progesterone in women considered to be at risk of preterm birth for "other reasons" is uncertain. Two randomized trials to date indicate no benefit in terms of preterm birth less than 37 weeks' gestation.[18] However, the combined sample size of these two trials is significantly underpowered to detect all but large differences in these outcomes.

Labor and Delivery

If an ovarian cyst causes obstruction in labor, delivery is by cesarean section. The ovarian mass is managed in the usual manner at the same time.[19] Aspiration is generally not recommended.[9]

FIGURE 57–1
Ovarian cystectomy.

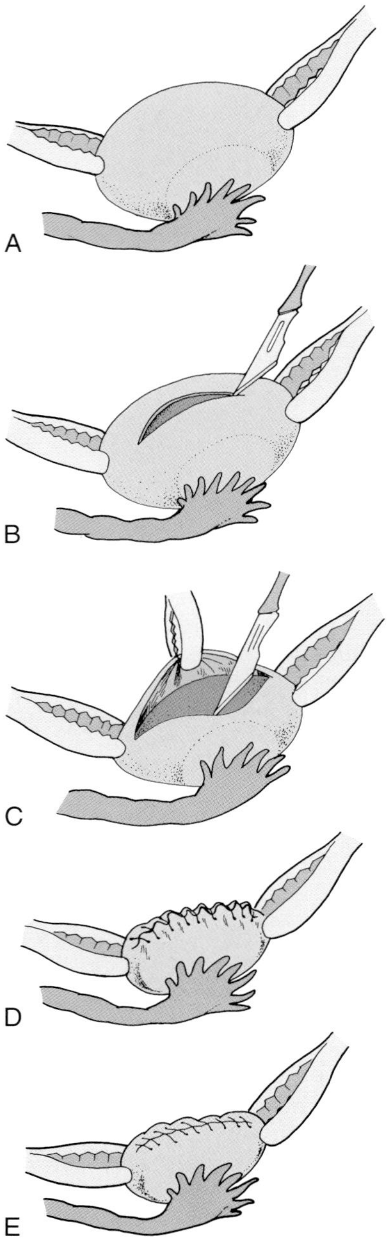

PROCEDURE

OVARIAN CYSTECTOMY IN PREGNANCY

Indications

Cystectomy is performed in patients with a symptomatic cyst (e.g., torsion, hemorrhage, rupture) and in those with an asymptomatic cyst that is recognized ultrasonically but does not regress by 16 weeks. Other indications include echogenic material that suggests a dermoid or has a septate or multilocular appearance.

Gestation

The procedure should be performed ideally at 18 to 20 weeks' gestation. A cyst noted earlier in gestation may be corpus luteum.

Description

Preoperative and perioperative measures include the use of appropriate antithromboprophylaxis.

Anesthesia

A general anesthetic agent is traditionally used, though regional anesthesia is an alternative.

Incision

If laparotomy is being performed, the type of skin incision will depend on the size of the cyst, although in the majority, a lower transverse skin incision would be adequate.

Method

The ovary with the cyst is usually very mobile, unless the cyst is associated with infection, endometriosis, or malignancy. The principles are the same whether performed via laparotomy or laparoscopy. The ovary and cyst are gently grasped at the antimesenteric border near each pole of the ovary (Fig. 57–1*A*).

The ovarian capsule only (not the cyst) is incised along the antimesenteric border, between the two forceps (taking care not to puncture the cysts; see Fig. 57–1*B*).

The handle of the scalpel or dissecting scissor blades are used to bluntly dissect the capsule away from the cyst, using grasping forceps on the margin of the capsule as counteraction (see Fig. 57–1*C*). The blunt dissection is continued close to the cyst, including along the mesenteric aspect. The cyst can then be removed and sent for histologic evaluation.

Hemostasis

Spot diathermy is applied to bleeding points arising from the mesenteric aspect of the ovary.

Repair of the Ovary

Usually, the cut edges of the ovary are everted and repaired with either polyglactic (Vicryl) or polyglycolic

(Dexon) (2/0 or 3/0) (see Fig. 57–1*D*). If hemostasis is satisfactory, and especially with laparoscopy, the ovarian base may be left open unsutured. Careful tissue handling is required, and microsurgical technique (i.e., forceps) is preferred to gross handling (see Fig. 57–1*E*).

Postoperative Management

Narcotic analgesia is used. The use of prophylactic tocolysis is debatable.[17] The histology report should be followed up.

Complications

Complications are miscarriage, preterm labor, and tubal adhesions of the fimbria to the incision in the ovarian capsule, which may impair future fertility. If the lesion appears benign, ovarian cystectomy rather than oophorectomy is probably the treatment of choice, because malignancy is rare. In young women, it is probably better to repeat the laparotomy to remove the ovary later rather than remove an ovary for what may be a benign condition.

SUMMARY OF MANAGEMENT OPTIONS

Ovarian Cysts

Management Options	Evidence Quality and Recommendation	References
Prepregnancy		
Treat symptomatic cysts, sonolucent cysts, and echogenic cysts ≥8 cm in diameter.	III/B	8
Prenatal		
Aspiration of cysts is not recommended.	IV/C	9
Corpus luteum cysts regress by 12 wk.	IV/C	11
Remove cysts that are symptomatic.	—/GPP	8
Laparoscopy is the preferred method of surgical management whenever possible.	III/B	9,14,15
Surgery is best performed in the second trimester.	III/B	12,13
If cysts are asymptomatic with benign features, conservative management is acceptable.	III/B	12,13
Use of tocolysis to prevent miscarriage or preterm labor is debatable.	III/B	17
There is no evidence that progesterone is of benefit to prevent preterm labor.	Ib/A	18
Labor and Delivery		
For cysts impacted in the pouch of Douglas, perform LSCS and ovarian cystectomy rather than cyst aspiration.	IV/C	19

GPP, good practice point.

FIBROIDS (See also Chapter 56)

Introduction

In a review of over 15,000 women with singleton pregnancies undergoing routine second-trimester ultrasound scan, fibroids of 1 cm or more were found in 2.7% of cases.[20] Others have noted 4% of pregnant women having uterine fibroids on routine scanning,[21] and the proportion of women with fibroids increases with age, especially in African American women compared with white women.[22]

Risks

It is widely believed that fibroids increase in size during pregnancy; however, only about 25% of fibroids enlarge during pregnancy.[23,24] In those that enlarge, most of the growth occurs in the first trimester, with little if any further increase in size during the second and third trimesters.[23,24] Larger fibroids (>5 cm in diameter) are more likely to grow, whereas smaller fibroids are more likely to remain stable in size.[25] The mean increase in fibroid volume during pregnancy is 12%, and very few fibroids increase by more than 25%.[23,24] Larger fibroids may undergo hemorrhagic infarction and can cause varying severity of pain, which is often localized to the region of the fibroid. There may be associated nausea, vomiting, and mild pyrexia and mild leucocytosis.[25] Classically, this complication occurs at approximately 20 to 22 weeks' gestation.

There are no well-designed studies that provide adequate data on fibroids and pregnancy outcome. Risks of fibroids in pregnancy probably relate to their number, size, and position. Large submucosal and intramural fibroids that distort the uterine cavity are associated with miscarriage.[26] Antepartum hemorrhage and placental abruption are reported to occur, especially with retroplacental fibroids.[26,27] Other complications include preterm labor and preterm birth,[26] malpresentation (mainly breech presentation),[26,28] and dysfunctional and obstructed labor.[28] Studies have also reported that uterine fibroids are associated with an increased risk of cesarean delivery,[21,26–28] especially when the fibroids are located in the lower uterine segment. This is probably related to the increased risk of malpresentation, dysfunctional and obstructed labor, and placental abruption. Some have reported an increased risk of postpartum hemorrhage, especially if the fibroids are large and retroplacental.[26,29]

Management Options

Prepregnancy

Prepregnancy myomectomy may improve the chances of a successful pregnancy in women with recurrent miscarriages, particularly those in whom no other cause has been found apart from the presence of fibroids.[30] Because most complications of pregnancy are associated with larger submucosal fibroids, removal before pregnancy should be considered in these cases also,[31] usually hysteroscopically, with or without the use of gonadotropin-releasing hormone analogue.[32]

Intramural or subserosal fibroids should be removed only if they are large, distorting the uterine cavity, or are symptomatic and are better performed laparoscopically rather than by open myomectomy.[33] Careful patient counseling[34] is important because hysterectomy may become necessary if excessive bleeding occurs. Preoperative gonadotropin-releasing hormone analogue therapy may reduce the risk of hemorrhage.[32] The appropriate interval from surgery to conception is not known.

Prenatal

Most fibroids are asymptomatic during pregnancy and are diagnosed on routine ultrasound examination. If degeneration occurs and causes pain, analgesia is necessary. Application of local heat or ice packs to the abdomen may provide relief.[35]

Myomectomy has generally been contraindicated during pregnancy.[36] However, several case series have been reported of myomectomy being performed in the first and second trimesters.[37–40] The most common indication would be intractable pain. In a series of 106 pregnant women with uterine fibroids, surgical intervention for recurrent pain, or for rapidly growing fibroid (defined as doubling in size over 8 wk), or if a fibroid larger than 5 cm was located in the lower uterine segment, prenatal surgery was not associated with any increased risk of miscarriage or preterm birth.[41] Despite this reassuring publication, antepartum myomectomy should be avoided if possible until further data are available. A subserosal fibroid that becomes impacted in the pouch of Douglas and interferes with micturition may be managed conservatively by catheterization. The patient should be encouraged to spend time resting prone in the head-down position.[42]

If a fibroid (usually a lower segment fibroid) causes an abnormal lie of the fetus after 36 weeks' gestation, elective cesarean section at 38 to 39 weeks' gestation is advised.[28]

Labor and Delivery

Management during labor of a patient with a fibroid depends on whether the fibroid is obstructing delivery. Cesarean delivery is indicated when a lower segment fibroid causes an abnormal lie at 38 weeks' gestation or is larger than 6 cm at 38 weeks' gestation and is palpable below the fetal head, either abdominally or vaginally.[34] Fibroids are usually soft and "drawn" or "pressed" out of the way during labor. Specific management points for the operation include

- Cross-matched blood should be available.
- Thromboprophylaxis should be undertaken.
- Regional anesthesia is normally used.
- A midline subumbilical incision is advisable if the fibroid is large or if a classic cesarean section is anticipated. However, if the fibroid is small or posterior, a routine lower transverse incision may be performed.
- The type of incision used depends on the observed site of the fibroid. If the lower segment is well formed around the fibroid and a transverse lower segment incision can be made, allowing a 2- to 3-cm margin with the fibroid, a lower segment approach is used. If access through the lower segment with a 2- to 3-cm margin is not possible, a classic cesarean section should be performed, again ensuring a 2- to 3-cm safety margin with the fibroid.

Myomectomy at the time of cesarean delivery may be required if the fibroid makes it impossible to satisfactorily close the uterine incision. Performing an elective myomectomy at the time of cesarean delivery is associated with high risk for postpartum hemorrhage and hysterectomy[42] and should be strongly discouraged, even though this has been reported to have been performed safely.[43] Following delivery, even without any intraoperative problems, postpartum hemorrhage due to poor uterine contractility should be anticipated. Adequate oxytocic therapy should be prescribed and blood transfusion anticipated.[29,31,44]

Pregnancy after Previous Myomectomy

The increased risk of uterine rupture during labor in patients with prior myomectomy is well described.[45] An incidence of zero to 1 in 40 has been reported, mainly from early descriptive studies, and appears to depend on whether the endometrial cavity had been opened.[46,47] The risk of rupture may be higher with laparoscopic myomectomy, which may be related to the efficacy of laparoscopic suturing.[48,49] However, a literature review of pregnancy outcome following laparoscopic myomectomy noted a rupture rate of only 1 in 211 cases.[50]

Until more reassuring data become available, standard advice would be to perform elective cesarean section if the endometrial cavity had been entered during the myomectomy or a large number of fibroids had been removed. However, if the myomectomy was performed for subserosal fibroids only, there is less risk of uterine rupture during labor. In this case, conservative management is usually advised, although labor should be managed as in a patient with a previous cesarean delivery.

Another concern for women who have had a myomectomy is the association with placenta accrete, and a careful search for invasive placentation is warranted.[51]

SUMMARY OF MANAGEMENT OPTIONS

Fibroids

Management Options	Evidence Quality and Recommendation	References
Prepregnancy		
Remove endometrial or submucosal fibroids hysteroscopically, with or without the use of a gonadotropin-releasing hormone analogue, if the patient has a history of subfertility.	III/B	30–32
Most women with fibroids have no problem conceiving and the pregnancy is usually uneventful.	Ia/A	33
Consider myomectomy for other fibroids if they are symptomatic, and only after careful counseling.	Ia/A	33,34
Prenatal		
Red degeneration is treated with bedrest, analgesics, local heat, and ice.	IV/C	35
Need to remove a pedunculated serosal fibroid for severe symptoms is rare. Avoid surgery if possible.	IV/C	36
Consider elective LSCS if: • Lower segment or cervical fibroids cause unstable lie or failure of engagement of the fetal head. • The patient had a previous myomectomy for intramural fibroids.	IV/C	28
Labor and Delivery		
Perform an LSCS if a fibroid leads to obstructed labor or if endometrial cavity opened during previous myomectomy.	IV/C	34,48,49
Be vigilant for postpartum hemorrhage.	IV/C	29,31,44
Avoid myomectomy at LSCS.	IV/C	42
For cesarean delivery, consider a classic or upper segment approach if access through the lower segment with 2 to 3 cm normal tissue is not possible.	IV/C	28
Beware of invasive placentation if previous myomectomy.	IV/C	51

SUBFERTILITY

Introduction

One in six couples of reproductive age needs specialist help because of inability to conceive (primary infertility) or inability to conceive the number of children they wanted (secondary infertility).[52] This figure is increasing because both women and men are delaying having children until after the age of 35 years.[53] In one study, the probability of pregnancy was twice as high for women aged 19 to 26 years compared with women aged 35 to 39 years. Controlling for age of the woman, fertility was significantly reduced for men older than 35 years.[54] The number of couples seeking assisted reproductive technology (ART) has tripled between 1992 and 2004.[55]

A male factor is the dominant cause of subfertility in 20% to 25% of couples.[56,57] Female causes of subfertility include problems with ovulation, defects in sperm-mucus interaction, and tuboperitoneal disorders. In 25% to 30% of couples who undergo evaluation, inability to conceive is unexplained.[56] Endometriosis causes subfertility in approximately 5% of women through any of these mechanisms.

. Whereas tubal causes of subfertilty have decreased, others female factor, male factors, and multiple causes have become more common.[55] In couples without a clear indication for in vitro fertilization (IVF), one study has also shown that, although the cumulative probability of pregnancy was highest for early treatment with IVF, over time, conservative treatment or frequent intercourse approached the same cumulative probability; thus, emphasizing that benefit must be weighed against cost and potential harm and that couples should continue to be encouraged to maintain regular intercourse.[58]

Treatments to assist conception include use of ovulation-inducing agents, tubal or ovarian microsurgery, and various forms of ART.

Risks Associated with Pregnancies Conceived Using Fertility Treatments

Ovarian Hyperstimulation

Ovarian stimulation is associated with a risk of theca-lutein cysts in the ovary; these cysts are more common with gonadotropin (6%) than with clomiphene therapy (3%).[59] Ovarian hyperstimulation syndrome (OHSS) is a potentially life-threatening complication of ovulation induction. Its most severe form is associated with massive ovarian enlargement and multiple cysts, ascites, pleural effusions, hemoconcentration, and hypoalbuminemia. It may result in oliguria and renal failure, hypovolemic shock, thromboembolic episodes, adult respiratory distress syndrome, and rarely, death.[60] Mild OHSS occurs in about 25% of cases, and the severe form occurs in 0.5% to 5% of cases.[61]

Miscarriage

In a large U.S. database, it was noted that the spontaneous miscarriage rate among ART pregnancies was 14.7%, similar to that after normally conceived pregnancies. The increased rate is related to oocyte or embryo quality. Pregnancies conceived with frozen and thawed embryos have a higher miscarriage rate than fresh embryos.[62]

Chromosomal Abnormality

There does not appear to be an increase in the prevalence of karyotype abnormalities in offspring of IVF-conceived pregnancies. However, this may be so with the use of sperm from subfertile men, and the intracytoplasmic sperm injection (ICSI) procedure itself may increase the risk of chromosomal and gene abnormalities in children conceived by ART.[63]

Ectopic Pregnancy

In a large review of 94,118 ART pregnancies, 2.1% were ectopic. The figures were 2% among pregnancies conceived with IVF and 3.6% with zygote intrafallopian transfer (ZIFT).[64]

Multiple Pregnancy

A world collaborative report on IVF pregnancies cites a twin pregnancy rate of 27% and a triplet pregnancy rate of 3%. ART is estimated to account for just over 1% of all births and 18% of all multiple births.[65]

Preterm Birth and Small for Gestational Age and Perinatal Mortality

The 2006 result of the Canadian ART Register[66] have confirmed that clinical pregnancy and live birth rates continue to increase, but multiple birth rates have only slightly decreased despite the recommendation of only one embryo transfer.[67] Although multiple pregnancy remains the principal cause of adverse outcome after ART,[68] a meta-analysis of 15 studies comprising 12,283 IVF and 1.9 million spontaneously conceived singletons, IVF singleton pregnancies were also associated with significantly higher odds of each of the perinatal outcomes examined: perinatal mortality (odds ratio [OR] 2.2; 95% confidence interval [CI] 1.6–3.0), preterm delivery (OR 2.0; 95% CI 1.7–2.2), low birth weight (OR 1.8; 95% CI 1.4–2.2), and small for gestational age (OR 1.6; 95% CI 1.3–2.0).[69] These poor outcomes have also been confirmed in a large case-controlled study.[70] It is possible that these adverse outcomes could be attributable to the factors leading to infertility, rather than to factors related to the reproductive technology.

Cerebral Palsy

An increased risk of cerebral palsy has been reported (OR 2.2; 95% CI 1.7–2.8), but most of the increase may be related to the high risk of multiple pregnancy and of preterm birth.[71]

Intraventricular Hemorrhage

There was a significantly increased risk of grade III/IV intraventricular hemorrhage in infants of IVF pregnancies from a single study,[72] and more information is needed on this issue.

Long-Term Health Implications

There do not appear to be any long-term health implications for children conceived by IVF or ICSI. However, more long-term follow-up is required to fully establish the truth of this statement.[73]

Placenta Previa

There was a sixfold higher risk of placenta previa in singleton pregnancies conceived by assisted fertilization compared with naturally conceived pregnancies. The authors of that report suggest that the increased risk may be caused by factors related to the reproductive technology.[74]

Other Obstetric Complications

Other obstetric complications include gestational diabetes and preeclampsia. In a case-control study, pregnant women with polycystic ovary syndrome (PCOS) had a much higher incidence of pregnancy-induced hypertension (31.8%) than women without PCOS (3.7%).[75] However, confounding factors such as the cause of infertility were not consistently ascertained and adjusted for when interpreting pregnancy outcome data. For example, PCOS is a common cause of infertility and is associated with insulin resistance, which plays a major role in development of gestational diabetes.[76]

Effect of Medical Adjuncts in Assisted Reproductive Technologies on the Fetus

One important outcome of the increase in pregnancies conceived by ART is the number of women who are taking medical adjuvant treatment in the early stages of pregnancy. Table 57–1 reviews the present state of knowledge of such adjuncts in assisting conception.[77] In summary, very few have any evidence to support their use in clinical practice other than as part of a randomized trial. Furthermore, and of greater concern, the impact of most of these treatments on the first-trimester fetus is not known.

Management Options

Prepregnancy

When a couple seeks treatment for infertility, the woman must undergo an assessment that includes a thorough history and examination to ensure that she does not have a medical problem that must be treated or controlled before conception to minimize subsequent risks during pregnancy. All women with infertility should be tested for rubella. Those who are not immune should be vaccinated at least 3 months before pregnancy.[78] Couples considering IVF should be

TABLE 57–1

Medical Interventions in In Vitro Fertilization

INTERVENTION	COMMENT ON EVIDENCE	EVIDENCE GRADE
Investigations		
Measuring uterine natural killer cells	There is no robust evidence that this is clinically useful in predicting the outcome of IVF treatment.	B
Routine testing for antiphospholipid antibodies	There is no evidence that this is of benefit.	A
Testing for thrombophilias	This is justified in patients with a history of repeated implantation failure.	C
Testing for thyroid and ovarian autoantibodies	There is no evidence that this is of benefit.	B
Alloimmune testing	There is no evidence that this is of benefit.	C
Treatments		
IVIG for recurrent failed IVF cycles	There is no evidence for the use of IVIG as adjunctive therapy for recurrent failed IVF cycles	A
TNF-α immune therapy in women undergoing IVF	There are a lack of studies investigating the role and the safety of TNF-α immune therapy in women undergoing IVF; thus, there is no indication for its use.	C
Peri-implantation steroids in ART cycles	There is no evidence to support the use of this treatment.	A
Peri-implantation steroid administration in women undergoing IVF alone	There is limited evidence that peri-implantation steroid administration may improve pregnancy rates in women undergoing IVF alone. These results need to be confirmed in a suitably powered, RCT designed specifically to address this issue.	GPP
NTG or sildenafil citrate	Neither NTG nor sildenafil citrate has beneficial effects on IVF outcome and should not be used.	A
Uterine relaxants (β_2-adrenergic antagonists, progesterone)	These should not be used because their effect is unknown.	GPP
Aspirin	There is no evidence that this is of benefit and should not be prescribed.	A
LMWH alone and in combination with LDA	There is no evidence that this is of benefit.	C
Pragmatic treatment with LMWH and LDA	This should be used only in women with antiphospholipid syndrome and in those with antiphospholipid antibodies and repeated implantation failure.	C
Growth hormone adjuvant therapy	There is no evidence that this is of benefit.	A
Luteal phase estradiol supplementation	There is no evidence that this is of benefit in all patients.	A
	Estradiol supplementation should be used only in recipients of donated oocytes and in patients with hypogonadotrophic hypogonadism.	C

ART, assisted reproductive technology; GPP, good practice point; IVF, in vitro fertilization; IVIG, intravenous immunoglobulin; LDA, low-dose aspirin; LMWH, low-molecular-weight heparin; NTG, nitroglycerin; RCT, randomized, controlled trial; TNF-α, tumor necrosis factor-α.
From Nando LG, Granne I, Stewart J: Medical adjuncts in IVF: Evidence for clinical practice. Hum Fertil 2009;12:1–13.

informed of the increased risks of complications discussed previously and should include provision of genetic counseling.[79]

For all women contemplating pregnancy, folic acid supplementation should be initiated.[80]

Preventive strategies for OHSS attempt to identify women who are at increased risk (using ultrasound and serum estradiol measurements). The lowest possible dose of gonadotropin is used to reduce the granulosa and luteal mass. In patients with a large number of follicles (>20) and an increasing serum estradiol level, the most widely used and most cost-effective approach is to withhold gonadotropin stimulation (coasting) while continuing down-regulation.[81] Other methods include early unilateral ovarian follicular aspiration; administration of glucocorticoids, macromolecules, and progesterone; cryopreservation of all embryos; and electrocautery or laser vaporization of one or both ovaries.[82] Surgical resection of the ovary causes regression of symptoms much faster than pharmacotherapy and should be considered in severe cases that do not respond well to initial management.[83]

Prenatal

The first, and probably most important, management step is to confirm that the missed period is associated with at least one viable intrauterine pregnancy and to identify whether there is a multiple pregnancy, and if present, to determine the chorionicity (see Chapter 59). The prenatal management of multiple pregnancy is discussed in Chapter 59.

All caregivers should recognize the likelihood of anxiety and the need for supportive counseling in patients who conceive after IVF.[84] Ideally, the number of people caring for these patients should be restricted, especially so that consistent information and advice can be given to the couple, who may be anxious. The couple may believe that their only difficulty was in conceiving and that once this goal has been achieved, the pregnancy is not at additional risk.[84]

Vigilance for ectopic pregnancy should be maintained in women with a history of tubal disease.[85]

If pregnancy is associated with the use of hyperstimulatory drugs, corpus luteum cysts are commonly seen until 12 weeks.[86] Surgical therapy or aspiration should be avoided. Sometimes, the need for stimulation of ovulation is associated with an endocrine dysfunction, such as a progesterone defect, in early pregnancy. Use of progesterone has become widely prescribed based on biologic plausibility and reports of successful treatment,[84] though not on any controlled trials.[87]

First-trimester screening (nuchal translucency and biochemistry) should be offered to all women; few patients will need second-trimester screening and invasive testing.[88]

Women with PCOS should be screened for gestational diabetes during pregnancy, with frequent surveillance of blood pressure.[76]

Ultrasound is frequently performed to evaluate fetal growth and well-being, especially to allay the anxiety of the couple.[84]

Labor and Delivery

These pregnancies have an increased rate of operative deliveries, especially cesarean section. Continuous fetal heart monitoring is advisable and may be demanded by the patient. Use of fetal blood sampling for any non-reassuring fetal heart rate pattern may avoid unnecessary cesarean section.

Postnatal

Contraception is not usually an issue in these couples, but it must be discussed. The usual contraindications to the use of intrauterine devices in women with a recent history of tubal disease apply. Contraceptives that may delay the return of ovulation (such as progesterone-only preparations) should be avoided in couples who may want another pregnancy soon.

SUMMARY OF MANAGEMENT OPTIONS

Subfertility

Management Options	Evidence Quality and Recommendation	References
Prepregnancy		
Check for underlying medical disease (e.g., hypertension, diabetes, renal disease, *Chlamydia* infection).	—/GPP	—
Counsel women undergoing assisted reproduction about the rates of multiple pregnancy and other specific risks.	III/B	65
Use pre- and postconceptual folate supplementation.	Ia/A	78
Ensure that the patient is immune to rubella.	III/B	76
Follow protocols to avoid hyperstimulation and multiple pregnancy.	III/B	66,67,79
If the male partner has obstructive azoospermia, the couple should be screened for cystic fibrosis carrier status. Males should also be screened for Y chromosome deletions.	IV/C	62
Prenatal		
Check the viability and number of intrauterine pregnancies and chorionicity if multiple.	III/B	65,66
Diagnose ectopic pregnancy early.	IV/C	83
First-trimester screening should be offered to all women.	IIa/B	86
Screen for hypertension and gestational diabetes in women with polycystic ovary syndrome.	IV/C	75
Check fetal growth and development in pregnancies achieved through an ART.	III/B	70,82
Provide reassurance and counseling.	IIb/B	82
Labor and Delivery		
Provide continuous fetal heart rate monitoring for psychological reasons.	IIb/B	82
Postnatal		
Contraception is not usually an issue.	—/GPP	—
Avoid IUCD use in patients with a history of tubal disease.	—/GPP	—
Avoid progestogens in patients with a history of ovulatory disorders.	—/GPP	—

GPP, good practice point.

OTHER GYNECOLOGIC DISEASES AND PROBLEMS

Congenital Disorders

Some women have congenital abnormalities of the genital tract that affect pregnancy or labor and delivery. Most uterine abnormalities are diagnosed by ultrasound scan and/or hysterosalpingogram. Bicornuate uterus, uterus didelphys, and septate uterus constitute 80% of cases.[89] These conditions are associated with preterm delivery (29%), spontaneous first-trimester miscarriage (24%), ectopic pregnancy (3%), fetal malpresentation (23%), and a high cesarean delivery rate (28%).[89]

Whereas there is overall evidence of benefit from cerclage with short cervix in women at risk of preterm delivery, there are insufficient data for the subgroup of women with congenital abnormality.[90] Progesterone therapy may have a role, but its use to prevent preterm labor awaits evaluation.[18] In women with repeated miscarriages, hysteroscopic metroplasty in the treatment of septate uterus has improved fetal survival rates.[91]

The other disorder of the lower tract is a vaginal septum. A septum that is fenestrated superiorly may obstruct labor. This complication can usually be managed acutely simply by dividing the septum in the second stage under epidural or pudendal anesthesia. Hemostatic measures are not usually required.

Cervical Stenosis or Incompetence as a Result of Previous Cone Biopsy

Cone biopsy may affect conception because the destruction of mucus-producing glands might cause cervical stenosis or incompetence. The overall rate of normal-term vaginal delivery is reported as 46.6% and is inversely proportional to the cone size. The incidence of both spontaneous mid-trimester miscarriage and preterm birth is increased in direct proportion to cone size. Cervical stenosis necessitating cesarean delivery is associated with small rather than large cones.[92] The role of cervical cerclage is uncertain.[90]

Pregnancy after Previous Endometrial Ablative Therapy

Endometrial ablation by numerous methods is used in women with dysfunctional menstrual bleeding and usually is performed only in women who do not wish to retain reproductive capacity. A few women may become pregnant after endometrial ablation (0.7% in one series[93]), and 45 pregnancies have now been reported in the English literature. A large number ended with an ectopic pregnancy or a miscarriage or were terminated (62%). Nine of the 17 that continued beyond 20 weeks' gestation reached 38 weeks with good outcome. Only 1 term pregnancy was complicated by placenta increta and resulted in cesarean hysterectomy.

Vulval Varicosity

Vulval varicosities are common during pregnancy, especially in multipara. This familial condition may be noted in the first pregnancy, but varicosities develop earlier and are larger as the number of pregnancies increases. They cause discomfort, heaviness in the pubic region, and sometimes pruritus or even pain, which is most often relieved by lying flat. They usually disappear completely postpartum. Bedrest and support may provide symptomatic relief. They are also significantly relieved by sclerosing agents.[94]

SUMMARY OF MANAGEMENT OPTIONS

Other Gynecologic Diseases and Problems

Management Options	Evidence Quality and Recommendation	References
Congenital Anatomic Defects		
Evaluate and treat prepregnancy.	IV/C	87
Evaluate prenatally and plan delivery.	IV/C	87
Divide vaginal septa.	IV/C	89
Cervical Stenosis or Incompetence		
Evaluate prenatally and plan delivery.	IV/C	90
Cervical suture may be of benefit	Ia/A	88
Be vigilant for dystocia in labor and the need for LSCS.	—/GPP	—
Endometrial Resection		
Counsel risk of ectopic pregnancy, miscarriage, preterm delivery, and intrauterine growth restriction.	III/B	91
Vulval Varicosity		
Provide symptomatic treatment prenatally (bedrest, support).	—/GPP	—
Sclerosing therapy may be used.	IV/C	92
Avoid trauma during delivery.	—/GPP	—

GPP, good practice point.

SUGGESTED READINGS

Al-Shawaf T, Grudzinskas JG: Prevention and treatment of ovarian hyperstimulation syndrome. Best Pract Res Clin Obstet Gynaecol 2003;17:249–261.

Allen C, Bowdin S, Harrison RF, et al: Pregnancy and perinatal outcome after assisted reproduction: A comparative study. Ir J Med Sci 2008;11:233–241.

Balci O, Gezginc K, Karatayli R, et al: Management and outcomes of ovarian masses during pregnancy: A 6-year experience. J Obstet Gynaecol Res 2008;34:524–528.

Coronado GD, Marshall LM, Schwartz SM: Complications in pregnancy, labor, and delivery with uterine leiomyomas: A population-based study. Obstet Gynecol 2000;95:764–769.

Dupas C, Christin-Maitre S: What are the factors affecting fertility in 2008? Ann Endocrinol (Paris) 2008;69(Suppl):S57–S61.

Glanc P, Brofman N, Salem S, et al: The prevalence of incidental simple ovarian cysts ≥3 cm detected by transvaginal sonography in early pregnancy. J Obstet Gynaecol Can 2007;29:502–506.

Hill LM, Conners-Beauty DJ, Nowak A, et al: The role of ultrasonography in the detection and management of adnexal masses during the second and third trimesters of pregnancy. Am J Obstet Gynecol 1998;179:703–707.

Jackson RA, Gibson KA, Wu YW, Croughan MS: Perinatal outcomes in singletons following in vitro fertilization: A meta-analysis. Obstet Gynecol 2004;103:551–563.

Klatsky PC, Tran ND, Caughey AB, Fujimoto VY: Fibroids and reproductive outcomes: A systematic literature review from conception to delivery. Am J Obstet Gynecol 2008;198:357–562.

Terava AN, Gissier M, Hemminki E, Luoto R: Infertility and the use of infertility treatments in Finland: Prevalence and socio-demographic determinants 1992–2004. Eur J Obstet Gynecol Reprod Biol 2008;136:61–66.

REFERENCES

For a complete list of references, log onto www.expertconsult.com.

CHAPTER 58

Bleeding in Late Pregnancy

OSRIC B. NAVTI and JUSTIN C. KONJE

INTRODUCTION

Vaginal bleeding in late pregnancy, or antepartum hemorrhage (APH), is defined as bleeding from the genital tract after 20 weeks' gestation. This type of bleeding complicates 2% to 5% of all pregnancies[1] and has various causes (Table 58–1). There is no identifiable cause in almost half of cases. Bleeding from the placental bed is the most common identifiable cause.

MANAGEMENT OF BLEEDING IN LATE PREGNANCY

APH is often unpredictable, and the patient's condition may deteriorate rapidly before, during, or after presentation. The initial management is the same regardless of etiology and starts with general measures to treat or prevent deterioration, followed by specific treatment measures. The general measures discussed in this chapter apply to all cases of APH, but they may be modified depending on the severity of bleeding. The specific measures depend on the diagnosis and are discussed under the various causes of bleeding.

INITIAL ASSESSMENT AND MANAGEMENT (Fig. 58–1)

Management of the patient with APH must be in a hospital with adequate facilities for transfusion, cesarean delivery, neonatal resuscitation, and intensive care. In the patient with significant vaginal bleeding, immediate transfer to a hospital by ambulance is recommended. Initial management includes a history, evaluation of the patient's general condition, and initiation of testing and treatment.

History

The history must include the amount, character, and duration of bleeding. It is also important to ascertain whether there is any associated pain or regular uterine contractions. The history should identify initiating factors, such as trauma or coitus, a history of ruptured membranes, or previous vaginal bleeding. The gestational age as determined ideally by early ultrasound scan should be documented and note taken of fetal movements and the placental site recorded in previous scans. Additional information includes details of previous bleeding episodes, past obstetric history, and cervical smear histories.

Physical Examination

Physical examination should assess both the maternal and the fetal condition, including

- Maternal pulse, blood pressure, and respiratory rate.
- Clinical evidence of shock (restlessness; cold, clammy extremities; poor skin perfusion; piloerection response).
- Abdominal examination to determine whether the uterine fundus is compatible with the estimated gestational age and to assess the presence of tenderness, the number and viability of fetuses, the presence of uterine contractions, and the lie and presentation of the fetus or fetuses.
- Vaginal examination. Traditionally, digital and speculum examinations are considered inadvisable unless placenta previa has been excluded. However, despite this conventional guidance, in practice, experienced clinicians can undertake careful vaginal examinations when they are certain that the fetal head is engaged, making the diagnosis of placenta previa unlikely. However, in most cases, only an inspection of the vulva to quickly assess the amount of blood loss and to determine whether bleeding has stopped or is continuing is necessary. When placenta previa has been excluded, a speculum examination can then be performed.

Testing and Immediate Management

Initial management comprises

- Insertion of an intravenous line with a wide-bore cannula (preferably 14–16 Fr). A second line may be needed in cases in which bleeding is severe.
- Obtaining blood for immediate hemoglobin or hematocrit estimation, complete blood count and typing, and holding of serum for potential cross-matching. If bleeding is continuing or is heavy, then at least 4 units of blood must be cross-matched. When placental abruption is suspected, a coagulation profile and measurement of urea and electrolytes should be performed. Another test that may be performed is the Kleihauer-Betke test on maternal blood.

- Administration of intravenous fluids if bleeding is continuing or severe while waiting for cross-matched blood. Colloids are the most suitable fluids. Consideration should be given to transfusing O-negative blood or type-specific blood if cross-matching is delayed.

TABLE 58–1

Causes of Bleeding in Late Pregnancy

CAUSE	INCIDENCE (%)
Placental	
Placenta previa	31.0
Abruptio placentae	22.0
Vasa previa	0.5
Unclassified	
Marginal	60.0
Show	20.0
Genital Tract	
Cervicitis	8.0
Trauma	5.0
Vulvovaginal varicosity	2.0
Genital tumor	0.5
Genital infection	0.5
Hematuria	0.5
Others	0.5

- Performing an ultrasound scan to exclude placenta previa if a scan has not been done previously or to exclude a major abruption with placental separation. However, a scan should be performed only if maternal and fetal conditions are stable.

Subsequent management is determined by the fetal and maternal condition, the severity of the bleeding, and the gestational age of the fetus. Options include immediate delivery versus expectant management. These are discussed under the various types of APH. The flow charts in Figures 58–1 and 58–2 outline the steps in management.

PLACENTA PREVIA

In placenta previa, the placenta is inserted partially or entirely into the lower uterine segment. Although clinical acumen remains vitally important in suspecting and managing placenta previa, the definitive diagnosis of most low-lying placentas is now achieved with ultrasound imaging. Clinical suspicion should always be raised in women with painless vaginal bleeding with a high presenting part or abnormal lie irrespective of previous ultrasound imaging. Four grades have traditionally been defined (Fig. 58–3). Figures 58–4 and 58–5 show two of these grades. If the placenta overlies the cervical os, it is considered as major previa.

Several publications have described the diagnosis and outcome of placenta previa on the basis of localization using

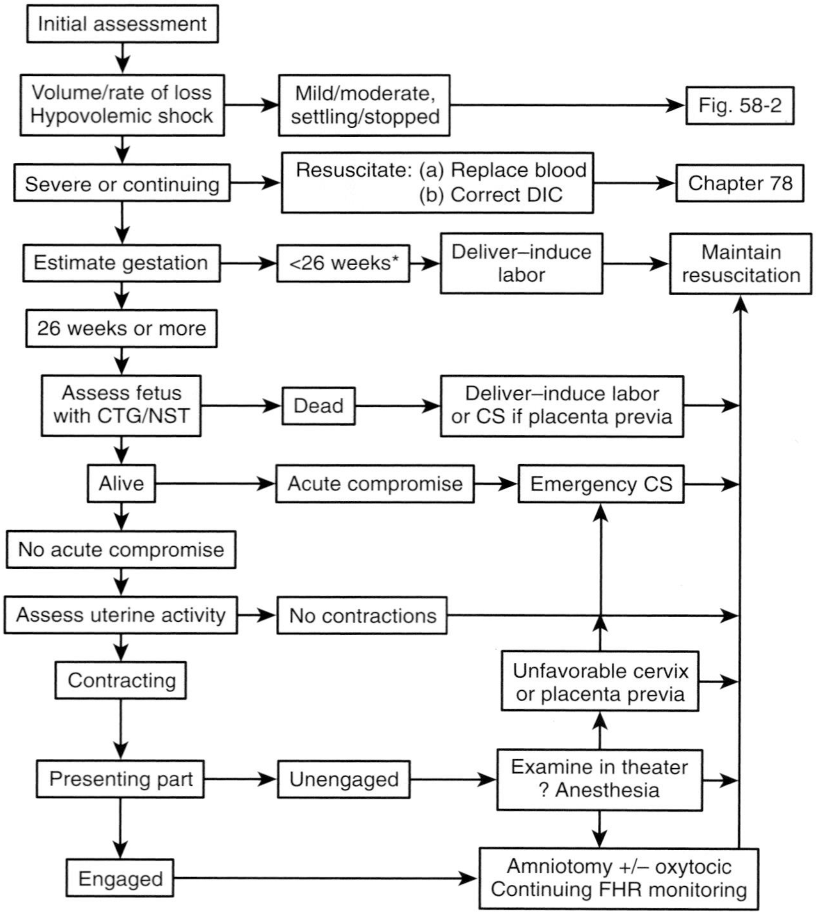

FIGURE 58–1
Management of bleeding in late pregnancy. Initial assessment and management of severe bleeding. *The gestation after which survival rates are considered high enough to influence the mode of deliver of the preterm fetus varies in different centers from 24–28 wk. CS, cesarean section; CTG, cardiotocography; DIC, disseminated intravascular coagulation; FHR, fetal heart rate; NST, nonstress test.

FIGURE 58–2
Management of bleeding in late pregnancy. Subsequent assessment and specific management of mild bleeding. CS, cesarean section; EUA, EWA, examination in the theater with and without anesthesia, respectively; FBC, full blood count; FHR, fetal heart rate.

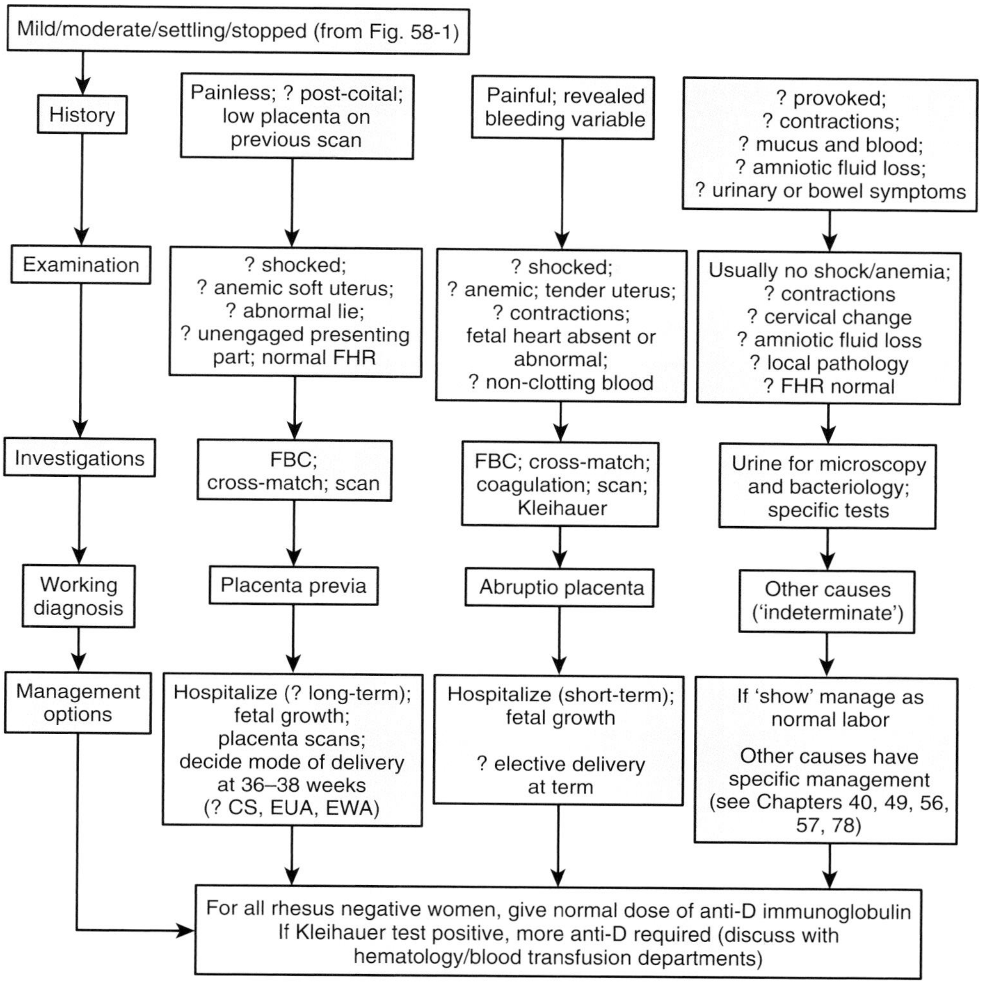

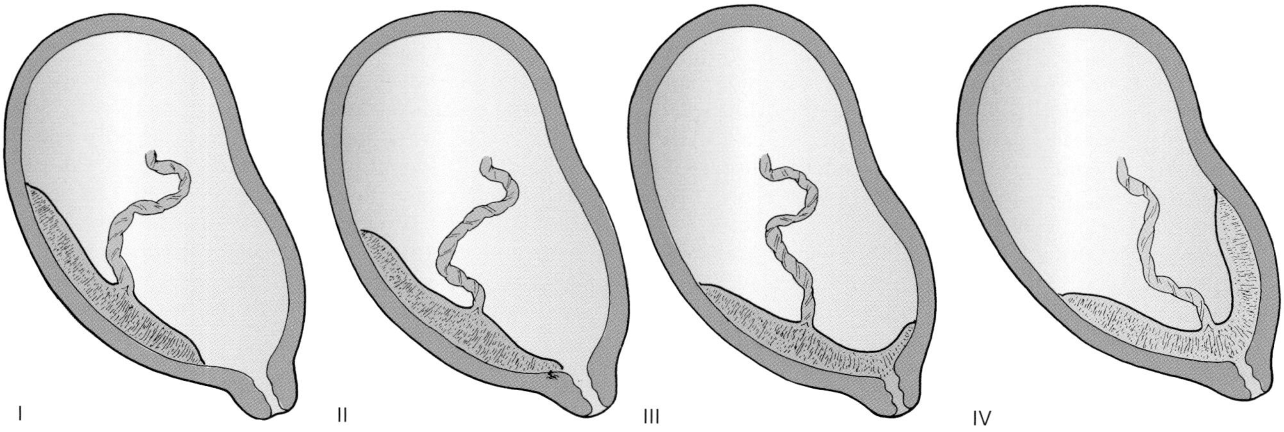

FIGURE 58–3
Grades of placenta previa: I. The placenta is in the lower segment, but the lower edge does not reach the internal os. II. The lower edge of the low-lying placenta reaches, but does not cover, the internal os. III. The placenta covers the internal os asymmetrically. IV. The placenta covers the internal os symmetrically.

FIGURE 58–4
Grade II posterior placenta previa. The placenta extends to the cervical os, but does not cover it.

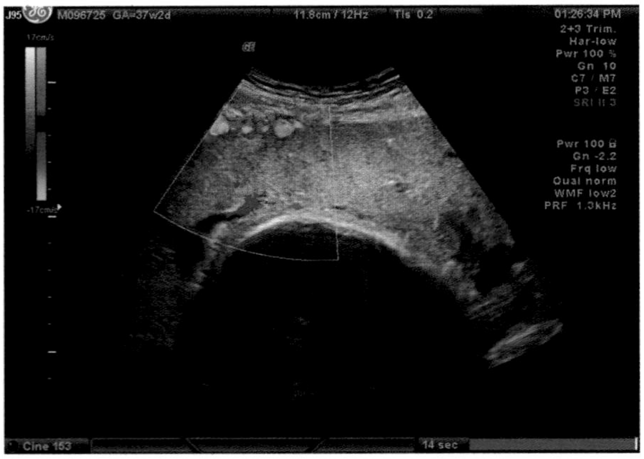

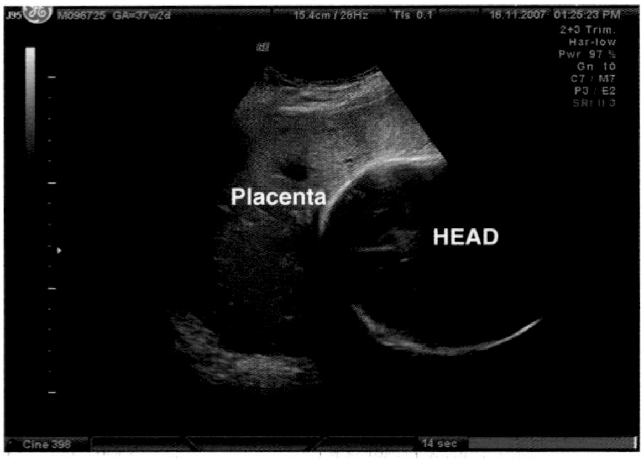

FIGURE 58–5
Grade IV placenta previa. The placenta covers the os symmetrically.

transvaginal ultrasound (TVUS) recording of the exact relationship of the placental edge to the internal cervical os. The increased prognostic value of TVUS diagnosis has rendered the imprecise terminology of the previous classifications obsolete.[2] TVUS is the gold standard in the localization of a low-lying placenta. It is significantly more accurate than transabdominal scanning and its safety is well established.[3] A reasonable antenatal imaging policy is to perform a TVUS on all women in whom a low-lying placenta is suspected from their transabdominal scan (at ~20–24 wk) in order to reduce the number of women requiring follow-up scans.[4]

Placenta previa occurs in 2.8 of 1000 singleton pregnancies and 3.9 of 1000 twin pregnancies[5] and presents a significant clinical problem because patients are at risk for significant hemorrhage needing blood transfusions and preterm delivery. They may need to be admitted to the hospital for long periods of observation with significant impact on family life. Cesarean hysterectomies may be required in cases of intractable postpartum hemorrhage with an incidence of 5.3%[6] with a three- to fourfold increase in perinatal mortality compared with normal pregnancies.[7,8]

The etiology of placenta previa is unknown, but various associations have been identified. These include older age, multiparity, multiple gestation, previous cesarean delivery, previous uterine curettage, and chronic hypertension.[9] Other risk factors include cigarette smoking, drug abuse (especially cocaine), a history of abortion, previous placenta previa, and assisted conception.[10]

A single cesarean delivery increases the risk by 0.65%, two increase the risk by 1.5%, three increase the risk by 2.2%, and four or more increase the risk by 10%.[11] A recurrence risk of 4% to 8% after one pregnancy affected by placenta previa has been reported.[12] The association with abortion (spontaneous or induced) is greater with an increasing number of previous abortions.[13,14]

Placenta accreta and placenta percreta are discussed in Chapter 75.

Maternal Risks

- **Maternal mortality**: The U.K. CEMACH (Confidential Enquiry into Maternal and Child Health) reports have demonstrated an impressive decline in deaths from obstetric hemorrhage over the last 50 years. Maternal mortality as a result of hemorrhage decreased from 29 cases in 1952–1954 to 3 in 2003–2005.[15] Possible reasons for this are
- **Postpartum hemorrhage** is believed to be caused by inadequate occlusion of the sinuses in the lower segment after delivery.
- **Anesthetic and surgical complications** may occur, especially in women with major placenta previa who have emergency cesarean delivery with suboptimal preparation for surgery.
- **Air embolism** occurs when the sinuses in the placental bed are torn.
- **Ascending infection** of the raw placental bed causes postpartum sepsis.
- **Placenta accreta** occurs in up to 15% of women with placenta previa.
- **The risk of recurrence** is approximately 4% to 8% after one previous placenta previa.

Fetal Risks

The fetal risks of placenta previa include

- **Perinatal mortality**: Cotton and colleagues[16] reported a perinatal mortality rate of 100% at less than 27 weeks, 19.7% at 27 to 32 weeks, 6.4% at 33 to 36 weeks, and 2.6% after 36 weeks in 1980. In recent years, the overall perinatal mortality rate has dropped from 126 per 1000 to 42 to 81 per 1000[17] as a result of conservative management and improved neonatal care. In women with placenta previa the odds ratio for having a preterm delivery, need for neonatal intensive care and low birth weight are 27.7, 3.4, and 7.4 respectively.[18]
- **Fetal growth restriction** may occur in up to 16% of cases. The incidence is higher in patients with multiple episodes of APH.[19]
- **Major congenital malformations** are twice as common in women with placenta previa. The most common malformations are those of the central nervous system, cardiovascular, respiratory, and gastrointestinal systems.[20]

- **Unexpected fetal death** can occur secondary to vasa previa (VP) or severe maternal hemorrhage.
- **Other risks** include fetal malpresentation, fetal anemia, umbilical cord prolapse, and compression.[13]

Presentation

Placenta previa characteristically causes unprovoked painless vaginal bleeding. Occasionally, it is caused by sexual intercourse. Threatened second-trimester miscarriage may precede placenta previa,[21] although bleeding may be minor—and in some cases unreported. The initial episode of bleeding has a modal incidence at approximately 34 weeks and occurs before 36 weeks in more than 50% of cases. It occurs after 40 weeks in only 2% of cases.[17]

The absence of pain is often considered a significant distinguishing factor between placenta previa and placental abruption, but 10% of women with placenta previa have coexisting abruption.[13] These patients and those who seek care for the first time while in labor and are therefore experiencing painful uterine contractions (25% of women with placenta previa[22]) may present a diagnostic problem.

Because ultrasound scanning is performed in early pregnancy in most centers, some patients with a low-lying placenta may be identified before 20 weeks' gestation, but the diagnosis of placenta previa cannot be made because the lower segment has not formed at this time.

Abdominal findings in placenta previa include malpresentation, which is either breech or transverse in 35% of cases[16]; slight, but consistent, deviation of the presenting part from the midline; and difficulty with palpating the presenting part.

Diagnosis

Various approaches have been used to diagnose placenta previa.

Vaginal Examination

Digital vaginal examination may cause hemorrhage. Because local causes are likely to be benign, speculum examination is probably best deferred until ultrasonography has excluded the diagnosis. If digital vaginal examination is necessary because of excessive bleeding, it should be performed only in an operating room, with full preparation for cesarean delivery (see later).

Placental Localization

Diagnostic ultrasound scanning is safe, accurate, and noninvasive and is the diagnostic method of choice. Routine placental localization is considered part of the anomaly scan at 20 to 22 weeks' gestation in many centers. Unfortunately, the earlier the scan is performed, the more likely the placenta is to be found in the lower pole of the uterus. For example, approximately 28% of placentas in women who undergo transabdominal scanning before 24 weeks are "low," but by 24 weeks, this number drops to 18%, and only 3% are low-lying by term.[23] Conversely, a false-negative scan for a low placenta is found in as many as 7% of patients at 20 weeks.[24] These results are more common when the placenta is posterior, the bladder is overfilled, the fetal head obscures the margin of the placenta, or the operator does not scan the lateral uterine wall.[25] A low-lying placenta is more common in early pregnancy because the lower segment does not exist. The apparent placental migration is caused by enlargement of the upper segment and formation of the lower segment. Many apparently low placentas are found above the lower segment. Comeau and associates[26] and Ruparelia and Chapman[27] showed that the more advanced the pregnancy, the more accurate the diagnosis of placenta previa based on scanning findings.

TVUS is now well recognized as the preferred method for accurately localizing the placenta. Sixty percent of women may have a reclassification of placental localization following transvaginal scans. Sonographers are encouraged to report the actual distance from the placental edge to the internal os at TVUS, using millimeters away from the os or millimeters of overlap. A placental edge exactly reaching the os is described as 0 mm. When the placental edge reaches or overlaps the internal os on TVUS between 18 and 24 weeks' gestation (incidence 1%–2%), a follow-up scan for placental localization in the third trimester is recommended. Overlap of more than 15 mm is associated with an increased likelihood of placenta previa at term. When the placental edge lies between 20 mm away from the internal os and 20 mm overlap after 26 weeks' gestation, ultrasound repeats should be guided by clinical features such as bleeding, gestational age, and actual distance from the internal os because continued change in placental location is likely. Overlap of more than 20 mm at any time is highly predictive of the need for cesarean section.[28] Although no randomized, controlled trials have been conducted exploring whether this is of benefit, case studies advocate localization of the placenta at the routine anomaly scan. Practitioners must recognize the limitations of this practice, and whenever possible, TVUS should be used to investigate placental localization when the placenta is thought to be low lying.

Because there are no randomized, controlled trials of the maternal and fetal effects of routine localization versus no localization, current practice must be governed by large cohort case studies. It is assumed that when there is a low-lying placenta, education of patients and carers enhances the chance of better maternal and fetal outcome, but this is not always the case. Whether these patients should be admitted routinely at a later gestation is debatable. Most units do not routinely admit these patients, but repeat the scans at 32 to 34 weeks' gestation. Dashe and coworkers[29] observed that in 34% of cases, placenta previa that was diagnosed at 20 to 23 weeks was still present at delivery, whereas 73% of those present at 32 to 35 weeks persisted at delivery. A policy of routine scanning will reduce the false-positive rate, but at the expense of increasing workload and patient anxiety. Unfortunately, none of the studies reported the proportion of patients with low-lying placenta diagnosed at 32 to 34 weeks who had bleeding later in gestation. For units that do not routinely scan for placental site at 20 weeks, this 32- to 34-week scanning is indicated only in patients with an indication such as abnormal presentation, vaginal bleeding, or a chance finding when ultrasound was undertaken in late pregnancy for other reasons. In these cases, a transvaginal approach is recommended because it has a better diagnostic accuracy, especially with posterior placenta previa.[30,31] This approach is safe and well tolerated. Placenta previa is diagnosed on TVUS when the placental edge is less than 20 mm from the internal os.

The findings on placenta previa can be summarized as follows:

- Routine location of the placental site at the 20-week transabdominal ultrasound has a low positive predictive value for placenta previa later in pregnancy.
- TVUS is more accurate than transabdominal in diagnosing placenta previa.
- Transperineal or translabial ultrasound (using a transabdominal probe) can also improve upon the diagnostic accuracy of transabdominal ultrasound and may be a useful alternative when TVUS is not available.[32]
- Recent guidance from the Royal College of Obstetricians and Gynaecologists (RCOG) recommends that patients with a previous cesarean section and an anterior placenta previa should have color-flow Doppler as the investigation of choice pending further evidence about magnetic resonance imaging (MRI) between 32 and 36 weeks.[33] MRI may also be beneficial in defining the degree of myometrial invasion, if any. It has the advantage of being a more objective test.
- There is no evidence that either of these interventions or rescanning "at-risk" patients in the third trimester reduces adverse maternal or fetal outcomes from placenta previa, and randomized trials addressing these issues are needed.

Management Options (See Fig. 58–2)

General management options were discussed earlier (see Fig. 58–1). Specific measures include immediate delivery and expectant management.

Immediate Delivery

If bleeding continues, but is neither profuse nor life-threatening and the gestation is more than 34 weeks, delivery is preferred after resuscitation is initiated. The mode of delivery depends on the grade of placenta previa and the state of the cervix. Occasionally, placental localization leads to inaccurate grading of placenta previa. In addition, some units do not have facilities for emergency placental localization. Options include immediate cesarean section and examination in an operating room, with or without anesthesia ("double setup"). Cesarean section is the only option in patients with profuse, life-threatening bleeding.

PROCEDURE

EXAMINATION IN AN OPERATING ROOM (DOUBLE SETUP)

This procedure is fast becoming obsolete with the advent of all the ancillary diagnostic tools for placenta previa. It is, however, considered important to continue to describe this setting because these tools are not universally available. Examination in an operating room provides the most accurate assessment of the relationship between the lower edge of the placenta and the cervical os. It should be done only when delivery will be undertaken. This approach is contraindicated by active, profuse hemorrhage mandating immediate delivery; fetal malposition or malpresentation precluding vaginal delivery; and fetal heart rate abnormality.

Preparation

Before this procedure is undertaken, cross-matched blood must be available. An anesthetist must be present, a midwife or operating room nurse must be scrubbed and gowned, and a cesarean section tray prepared. A second obstetrician should be scrubbed and ready to operate. The procedure must be performed by an experienced obstetrician, and a pediatrician must be present. Opinions vary as to whether the procedure should be carried out under general anesthesia. A survey of anesthetic management of cesarean section for placenta previa in the United Kingdom showed that 86% of anesthetists were willing to use regional anesthesia for a minor degree of placenta previa, but only 15% were prepared to offer these techniques for all degrees of placenta previa.[34] One advantage of general anesthesia is proper relaxation of the patient, which makes examination easier and allows rapid progression to cesarean section, if necessary. The main disadvantage is the need to wake the patient from anesthesia before inducing labor if vaginal delivery is possible. In addition, if cesarean section becomes necessary, a second anesthetic increases the risks. Performing the procedure under epidural anesthesia is an alternative, but this approach causes peripheral vasodilation and may worsen the effects of hypovolemia if hemorrhage is severe. A compromise appears to be drawing the drugs for induction of general anesthesia and preparing the anesthetic machine and instruments before the procedure. With such precautions, and in experienced hands, the interval between examination and delivery can be short.

Procedure

The patient is placed in the lithotomy position and draped with sterile towels after the vulva, but not the vagina, is cleaned. The bladder is catheterized, and two fingers are gently introduced into the vagina, with care taken to avoid the cervical os. Each vaginal fornix is palpated in turn to feel whether there is placenta between the presenting part and the finger. If placental tissue is present, a sensation of "bogginess" is felt. If the four fornices are empty, the index finger is gently introduced into the cervical os and the surroundings felt for the placental edge. If the cervix is closed, it should not be forced open and cesarean section should be performed. If the cervix admits a finger and no placental tissue is felt, the fetal membranes should be ruptured. An organized blood clot in the cervix may be mistaken for placental tissue. Persistent bright red bleeding after membrane rupture is an indication for cesarean delivery. If the placental edge is felt anteriorly but does not extend to the os and no bleeding is provoked, the decision may be made to rupture the membranes in preparation for vaginal delivery. If brisk vaginal bleeding occurs at any stage during the procedure, the procedure should be abandoned immediately and cesarean section performed.

Expectant Management

The major concern in caring for asymptomatic women with placenta previa is the possibility that the women may bleed suddenly and heavily, requiring speedy delivery. For that reason, the traditional management has involved admitting women with placenta previa even if asymptomatic from about 34 weeks' gestation until delivery. Attempts have been made to predict which women are more likely to bleed. Observational studies so far suggest that women with raised α-fetoprotein levels at 15 to 20 weeks and placentas that encroach on the cervical os, are thick inferiorly, or show turbulent flow at their lower margin on ultrasound are most associated with APH.[35] A review of the evidence from the Cochrane Database[36] to assess the impact of any clinical intervention applied specifically because of a perceived likelihood that a pregnant woman might have placenta previa found three randomized, controlled trials. These included 114 women in total. Both tested interventions (home vs. hospitalization and cervical cerclage vs. no cerclage) were associated with reduced lengths of stay in hospital antenatally: weighted mean difference (WMD) respectively −18.50 days (95% confidence interval [CI] −26.83 to −10.17), −4.80 days (95% CI −6.37 to −3.23). Otherwise, there was little evidence of any clear advantage or disadvantage to a policy of home versus hospital care. The 1 woman who had a hemorrhage severe enough to require immediate transfusion and delivery was in the home care group. Cervical cerclage may reduce the risk of delivery before 34 weeks (relative risk [RR] 0.45; 95% CI 0.23–0.87), the birth of a baby weighing less than 2 kg (RR 0.34; 95% CI 0.14–0.83), or having a low 5-minute Apgar score (RR 0.19; 95% CI 0.04–1.00). In general, these possible benefits were more evident in the trial of lower methodologic quality. The authors of the review concluded that there are insufficient data from trials to recommend any change in clinical practice. Available data should, however, encourage further work to address the safety of more conservative policies of hospitalization for women with suspected placenta previa and the possible value of insertion of a cervical suture.[36]

Severe hemorrhage (causing maternal hypovolemia) was originally considered a contraindication to expectant management.[37] However, in one study in which approximately 20% of the women lost more than 500 mL blood, half were managed expectantly, with a mean gain in gestation of 16.8 days.[38] Crenshaw and colleagues[39] managed only 43% to 46% of patients successfully with an aggressive expectant approach, whereas Cotton and associates[16] successfully managed 66% of women expectantly with an aggressive approach.

During expectant management, preterm labor is a problem. Brenner and colleagues[40] found that 40% of women with placenta previa had rupture of the membranes, spontaneous labor, or other problems that resulted in delivery before 37 weeks' gestation. Inhibiting contractions in those with preterm labor seems logical, but some consider APH a contraindication to the use of tocolytics.[41] When vaginal bleeding and uterine contractions occur, placental abruption, which is widely considered a contraindication to tocolysis, cannot be excluded. In addition, placental abruption may coexist with placenta previa in 10% of cases. Further, tocolytics cause maternal tachycardia and palpitations, features that may be confused with hypovolemia. Sampson and coworkers[42] advocate the use of tocolytics in cases of placenta previa and uterine contractions after 21 weeks and reported a reduction in the perinatal mortality rate from 126 to 41 per 1000. Besinger and colleagues[43] conducted a prospective trial on 112 women with acute vaginal bleeding and known placenta previa and gave tocolysis to the 72 women with significant uterine activity. This resulted in a prolongation of pregnancy (39.2 days vs. 26.9 days; $P < .02$) and an increase in birth weight (2.52 kg vs. 2.124 kg; $P < .03$) compared with the 40 women who were not given tocolysis. A retrospective review by Towers and associates[44] on the use of tocolysis for third-trimester bleeding including 76 of 105 women with placenta previa suggested no increased mortality or morbidity associated with tocolytic use in a tertiary setting. Prophylactic terbutaline to prevent bleeding has, however, not been found to be of benefit in women with placenta previa.

The perinatal mortality rate is also directly related to the total amount of blood lost antepartum. Liberal use of blood transfusions may nullify this effect.[16] There is no limit to the number of blood transfusions a patient can have. To optimize the oxygen supply to the fetus and protect the mother against anticipated blood loss, the aim of transfusion is to maintain hemoglobin of at least 10 g/dL or hematocrit of 30%.

Despite expectant management, 20% of women with placenta previa are delivered earlier than 32 weeks. These cases account for 73% of perinatal deaths.[16] These premature deliveries are a major problem, and although cervical cerclage has been advocated, it is not normally used. Neonatal mortality and morbidity rates are reduced in this group by maternal corticosteroid administration.

The main disadvantages of continuous hospitalization are the cost and the psychological effect of separation on families. For many families, hospitalization means prolonged separation, and in some extreme cases, the break up of marriages. Advantages include easy access to resuscitation and prompt delivery and ensuring bedrest (which may decrease the occurrence of hemorrhage) and limitation of activities. Outpatient management of placenta previa may be appropriate for stable women with home support, close proximity to hospital, and easy access to transportation and telephone. For women who are managed as inpatients, 2 units of cross-matched blood should be readily available, especially if they have had bleeds.

Method of Delivery

The need for cesarean delivery is dictated by the ultrasound findings as well as clinical judgment. Five studies have examined the likelihood of cesarean section for placenta previa based on placental edge–to–os distance on the last scan prior to delivery. The scans were performed between 35 and 36 weeks' gestation, and a distance of more than 20 mm away from the os was associated with a high likelihood of vaginal delivery (range 63%–90%). When the fetal head is engaged, the pregnancy may be allowed to continue beyond 37 to 38 weeks and vaginal delivery anticipated. In these patients, amniotomy followed by oxytocin (Syntocinon) administration can be considered. Where the placental edge is between 0 and 20 mm from the os, the rates of cesarean delivery was 40% to 90%. A placental edge less than 20 mm from the internal os, especially with a posterior or thick (>1 cm), is likely to need delivery by cesarean section. Where the placenta overlaps the cervical os on a third-trimester scan, a cesarean section is invariably required.

In those with major placenta previa, emergency or elective cesarean delivery is commonly used. Elective delivery is ideal because emergency delivery has a negative effect on perinatal mortality and morbidity rates, independent of gestational age. Cotton and colleagues[16] found that 27.7% of infants delivered emergently had anemia compared with 2.9% delivered electively. Cesarean section for placenta previa poses several problems. It should never be left to an inexperienced obstetrician. The RCOG in the United Kingdom recommends that such cesarean sections be performed by senior obstetricians ("consultants" in the United Kingdom). Anesthetists are divided in their opinions regarding the safest method of anesthesia for cesarean section in placenta previa.[34] There is increasing evidence of the safety of regional anesthesia, especially with regards to maternal hemodynamics.[45] However, when prolonged surgery is anticipated, as in women with prenatal diagnosis suggestive of placenta accreta, general anesthesia may be preferable. Regional anesthesia may also be converted to general anesthesia when the clinical situation dictates. Ideally, cross-matched blood should be available on the delivery suite prior to cesarean sections for placenta previa. Cell salvage may be considered in cases at high risk of massive hemorrhage.

Yamada and coworkers[46] suggested some benefit from autologous transfusion of placenta previa women, but further studies are required to establish its benefit.

PROCEDURE

There is increasing evidence to support the safety of regional anesthesia in cesarean sections for placenta previa. The choice of anesthetic technique is usually made by the anesthetist in consultation with the obstetrician and the mother. An experienced obstetrician and anesthetist must be present at the delivery. Because patients and their partners may experience severe anxiety in the presence of profuse bleeding during cesarean delivery, careful consideration should be given to the decision to allow partners in the operating room.

A transverse incision of the lower segment of the uterus is commonly used, provided there is a lower segment. When the lower segment is nonexistent or is very vascular, some obstetricians advocate a classic or De Lee's incision. Scott,[47] however, believes that such incisions are rarely justified because of their consequences and long-term disadvantages. When difficulties occur with transverse incisions of the lower segment, the incision may be converted to an inverted T-, J-, or U-shaped incision.

If the incision in the uterus is transverse and the placenta is anterior, two approaches are available: going through the placenta or defining its edge and going through the membranes above or below the placenta. The former approach requires speed and may cause significant fetal blood loss.[48] The latter approach, however, may be associated with undue delay in the delivery of the fetus, more troublesome bleeding from a partially separated placenta, and resultant fetal blood loss and anoxia. Myerscough[48] advises against cutting or tearing through the placenta because of the inevitable fetal blood loss that occurs as fetal vessels are torn. Because the lower segment is less muscular, contraction and retraction cause inadequate occlusion of the sinuses of the placental bed, and intraoperative hemorrhage is not uncommon.[49] When hemostasis is difficult, bleeding sinuses can be oversewn with atraumatic sutures.[47] If this approach is unsuccessful, uterine balloon tamponade or uterine packing may be considered. However, if the pack is left in situ during closure of the uterus, bleeding may continue but remain concealed for some time. Intramyometrial injection of prostaglandin $F_{2\alpha}$ is useful in these cases.[48] When bleeding is uncontrollable, ligation of the internal iliac artery or even hysterectomy may be necessary as a last resort.

Placenta Previa and Placenta Accreta

There is a well-recognized association between previous cesarean section, placenta previa, and placenta accreta. The increasing incidence of cesarean section deliveries and advanced maternal age has led to a rise in the incidence of placenta accreta, which is 1 in 2500.[50] The risk of placenta accreta increases dramatically in the presence of placenta previa and previous cesarean section, with a risk of 25% for one prior cesarean section and 40% for two previous cesarean sections.[51,52] Placenta accreta is associated with significant risk of massive obstetric hemorrhage, sometimes necessitating hysterectomy. Antenatal diagnosis by ultrasound may be beneficial in allowing preparation for delivery by a multidisciplinary team of obstetricians, anesthetists, radiologists, and surgeons in an appropriate setting. Color-flow Doppler studies on ultrasound[53] and MRI[54] are helpful in making an antenatal diagnosis. In all cases of placenta accreta, increta, or percreta, the risk of hemorrhage, transfusion, and hysterectomy should be discussed with the patient as part of the consent procedure. There are numerous case reports of placenta accreta and its management. Options have included clamping and leaving the placenta in situ at the end of cesarean section in association with prophylactic or therapeutic uterine artery ligation or internal iliac artery ligation at time of initial surgery. Others have been treated with methotrexate following the cesarean section with successful pregnancies being reported subsequently.[55]

PLACENTAL ABRUPTION

Placental abruption is defined as premature separation of a normally situated placenta. The reported incidence varies from 0.49% to 1.8%.[56] The wide variation in reported incidence is believed to be caused by variations in diagnosis. Fox[57] found evidence of abruption in 4.5% of placentas examined routinely, suggesting that small episodes of placental abruption are more common than those diagnosed clinically. Placental abruption is concealed in 20% to 35% of cases and revealed in 65% to 80% of cases.[31,58] The concealed type is more dangerous, with more severe

TABLE 58–2
Grading of Placental Abruption

GRADE	DESCRIPTION
0	Asymptomatic patient with a small retroplacental clot.
1	Vaginal bleeding; uterine tetany and tenderness may be present; no signs of maternal shock or fetal distress.
2	External vaginal bleeding possible; no signs of maternal shock; signs of fetal distress.
3	External bleeding possible; marked uterine tetany, yielding a boardlike consistency on palpation; persistent abdominal pain, with maternal shock and fetal demise; coagulopathy may be evident in 30% of cases.

From Sher G, Statland BE: Abruptio placentae with coagulopathy. A rational basis for management. Clin Obstet Gynecol 1985;28:15–23.

complications. Four grades of placental abruption have been described (Table 58–2). The most severe type (grade 3) occurs in approximately 0.2% of pregnancies.[31]

The etiology of placental abruption is unknown in most cases. In a few, however, the cause is obvious, such as in direct trauma to the uterus. Various risk factors are associated with placental abruption. The risk of recurrence in subsequent pregnancies is significant, varying from 6%[56] to 16.7%.[59,60] It is more common in older women, but this increase has been attributed to parity and is independent of age.[61] Cigarette smoking increases the incidence of placental abruption.[62] Naeye[63] reported an incidence of 1.69% in nonsmokers, 2.46% in smokers, and 1.87% in smokers who had quit. In the smokers, evidence of decidual necrosis at the edge of the placenta was found. This finding may represent the effect of smoking on uteroplacental blood flow[64,65] and decidual integrity.

Other etiologic factors include sudden decompression of the uterus after membrane rupture in patients with polyhydramnios and multiple pregnancy, external cephalic version,[65] placental abnormalities (especially circumvallate placenta),[66,67] abdominal trauma,[68] and increased levels of α-fetoprotein.[69,70] Although maternal hypertension is considered a risk factor, there is no consensus on whether hypertension precedes abruption or vice versa. Naeye[63] found no evidence of placental abruption in patients with hypertension, but Abdella and associates[71] observed that the incidence of placental abruption in patients with preeclampsia was twice that in those without preeclampsia. In a meta-analysis, Ananth and colleagues[72] concluded that chronic hypertension was associated with a threefold increased risk of abruption compared with normotensive patients, whereas the odds ratio for patients with preeclampsia was 1.73. The suggestion that folic acid deficiency may have an etiologic role in placental abruption has not been confirmed. Large prospective studies have not shown an association between placental abruption and folate supplementation.[73,74] More recently, hyperhomocysteinemia and protein C deficiency[75] and other thrombophilias were reported to be more common in women with placental abruption.[76]

There has recently been some evidence suggestive of a genetic influence in the pathogenesis of placental abruption. A review and meta-analysis by Zdoukopoulos and coworkers[77] found a positive association for the F5 Arg506Gln and F2 G20210A polymorphisms. However, considering the multifactorial etiology of abruption and the relatively small numbers of studies and participants, this review provided only the first clues of possible genetic causes, and larger case-control studies that include gene-gene and gene-environment interactions may help to further elucidate the genetics of placental abruption.

Maternal Risks

- The maternal mortality rate is approximately 1%. In the last CEMACH study in the United Kingdom (2003–2005),[15] two maternal deaths were caused by placental abruption. The maternal mortality rate decreased from 8% in 1919 to less than 1% in 1995.[69] Although severe hemorrhage is usually the major cause of other complications that lead to mortality, disseminated intravascular coagulation may cause severe hemorrhage, renal failure, and death.
- The recurrence rate is generally reported as 6% to 17% after one episode and increases to 25% after two episodes. Approximately 7% of women with abruption severe enough to kill the fetus have the same outcome in subsequent pregnancies, and 30% of all future pregnancies of women who have a placental abruption do not produce a living child.[1]
- Hypovolemic shock. Blood loss may be underestimated in placental abruption because concealed bleeding into the myometrium may be difficult to quantify.
- Acute renal failure can result from hypovolemia or disseminated intravascular coagulation.
- Disseminated intravascular coagulation.
- Postpartum hemorrhage can result from coagulation failure or from a couvelaire uterus, in which severe bleeding occurs into the myometrium and impairs the ability to contract.
- Fetomaternal hemorrhage can lead to severe Rh sensitization in Rh-negative patients. All Rh-negative patients must undergo a Kleihauer-Betke test and have anti-D immunoglobulin administered to prevent immunization.

Fetal Risks

Fetal risks include

- In a review of 7,508,655 singleton births delivered in 1995 and 1996 in the United States,[78] placental abruption was recorded in 6.5 per 1000 births. The perinatal mortality was 119 per 1000 births to mothers with abruption compared with 8.2 per 1000 among all other births. The high mortality to mothers with abruption was due, in part, to its strong association with preterm delivery. Babies in the lowest percentile of weight (<1% adjusted for gestational age) were almost nine times as likely to be born to mothers with abruption than those in the heaviest (≥90%) birth weight percentiles. The risk of abruption declined with increasing weight percentiles. Fifty-five percent of the excess perinatal deaths in deliveries linked with placental abruption were due to early gestational age alone. In contrast, the fetal size at delivery contributed only 9% to the perinatal mortality associated with abruption despite the strong predictive value of poor fetal growth as a risk factor for abruption.[78] The fact that babies born to mothers with placental abruption are smaller at most gestational ages than those born without suggests that factors other than prematurity contribute to the increase in perinatal mortality. The association with fetal growth restriction is so strong that growth restriction in itself can serve as a marker for abruption risk. The chronic processes underlying abruption may also contribute to the risk of preterm delivery. More than 50% of the perinatal deaths are stillbirths.[12] Of the infants delivered alive, Abdella and associates[71] reported a 16% mortality rate within 4 weeks, with most infants weighing less than 2500 g. Paterson[61] reported survival rates varying from 23% at 28 to 32 weeks to 87.6% at 37 to 40 weeks. However, survival rates today are probably higher than these figures suggest because they were reported before the advances that have occurred in modern neonatal care. For example, in Norway, the rate decreased from 2.5 per 1000 to 0.9 per 1000 between 1967 and 1991.[60] The higher incidence of fetal malformations[69] and intrauterine growth restriction[1] also contribute to the high perinatal mortality rate. For babies weighing more than 2500 g, the reported survival rate is 98%.[79] In the presence of associated complications, such as hypertension, the fetal mortality rate increases threefold.[71]

- Fetal growth restriction is reported in up to 80% of infants born before 36 weeks' gestation.
- The rate of congenital malformations may be as high as 4.4% (twice that in the general population[80]). The rate of major malformations is increased threefold. Most involve the central nervous system, and these can occur at five times the normal incidence.[69]
- The neonatal hematologic findings may be abnormal. Anemia results from significant fetal bleeding.

Diagnosis

The diagnosis is usually made on clinical grounds, but ultrasonography is helpful in some cases (e.g., when there is a large retroplacental hematoma, although this is uncommon, even in severe cases). The symptoms and signs are diagnostic in moderate to severe cases. In mild forms, the diagnosis may not be obvious until after delivery, when a retroplacental clot is identified.

Placental abruption causes vaginal bleeding, abdominal pain, uterine contractions, and tenderness. Vaginal bleeding occurs in no more than 70% to 80% of cases.[31] This bleeding is characteristically dark and nonclotting. It occurs after 36 weeks' gestation in approximately 50% of cases.[81] In a study of 193 cases, Paterson[61] found that 18% occurred before 32 weeks, 40% occurred between 34 and 37 weeks, and 42% occurred after 37 weeks. Because labor is the most common factor precipitating placental separation,[12] nearly 50% of patients with placental abruption are in established labor. Uterine contractions may be difficult to distinguish from the abdominal pain of abruption. When this distinction is possible, the contractions are characteristically very frequent, often with more than five occurring in 10 minutes.[82]

Although abdominal pain is common, it is not invariable and is less common in posteriorly sited placentas. This is evidenced by unsuspected, or silent, abruption described by Notelovitz and colleagues[83] and the higher pathologic incidence of placental abruption reported by Fox.[57] Pain probably indicates extravasation of blood into the myometrium. In severe cases (grade 3), the pain is sharp, severe, and sudden in onset. In addition, some patients may have nausea, anxiety, thirst, restlessness, and a feeling of faintness, whereas others report absent or reduced fetal movements.

If blood loss is significant, the patient may have signs of shock (tachycardia predominates and blood pressure is poorly correlated with blood volume). Hypertension may mask true hypovolemia, but increasing abdominal girth or fundal height suggests significant concealed hemorrhage. The uterus is typically described as "woody hard" in severe placental abruption. In such cases, the fetus is difficult to palpate, and a continuous fetal heart rate monitor or real-time ultrasonography must be used to identify the fetal heart beat. The fetus may be "distressed," with fetal heart rate abnormalities, or may be dead. Fetal distress occurs in grade 1 to 2 abruption, but in grade 3 abruption, fetal death is inevitable, by definition.[84] In severe cases complicated by disseminated intravascular coagulation, there may be no clotting in the vaginal blood, which is dark. The incidence of coagulopathy is 35% to 38%,[59,85] and it occurs mainly in the severe forms.

Typically, blood clots are found in the vagina, except if the blood is nonclotting. Serous fluid from a retroplacental clot may be confused with liquor. The cervix may be dilating because 50% of patients are in labor. If the membranes are ruptured, blood-stained liquor is seen.

Ultrasonography is not a sensitive method of diagnosing placental abruption, but it is useful in excluding coincident placenta previa, which is present in 10% of cases. When the retroplacental clot is large, ultrasonography identifies it as hyperechogenic or isoechogenic compared with the placenta. This echogenicity may be misinterpreted as a thick placenta.[86] Resolving retroplacental clots appear hyperechogenic within 1 week and sonolucent within 2 weeks. Although ultrasonography is not an accurate diagnostic tool, it is useful in monitoring cases managed expectantly, and Rivera-Alxima and associates[87] used it to determine the time of delivery. The size of the hematoma, its location, change in size over time, and fetal growth are monitored by ultrasound scan. The Kleihauer-Betke test may be useful in making the diagnosis when a patient has abdominal pain without vaginal bleeding and in cases of unsuspected (silent) abruption.

The differential diagnosis of placental abruption includes conditions that can be broadly classified into two groups. These are other causes of vaginal bleeding and causes of abdominal pain. The former groups are discussed elsewhere in this chapter.

Management Options (See Fig. 58–2)

Once the diagnosis of placental abruption has been made, management depends on its severity, associated complications, the condition of the mother and the fetus, and gestational age. Management is divided into general and specific measures. For management, Sher and Statland[88] divided placental abruption into three degrees of severity. These are summarized in Table 58–2.

The general management options were discussed earlier (see Fig. 58–1). Specific measures to be considered are

- Immediate delivery.
- Expectant management.
- Management of complications.

Immediate Delivery

The need for immediate delivery depends on the severity of abruption and whether the fetus is alive or dead. If the fetus is dead, vaginal delivery is the goal. Maternal resuscitation is emphasized because fetal death is common in severe placental abruption, often with coagulopathy. Once resuscitation has been initiated, the fetal membranes should be ruptured to hasten the onset of labor. This approach is effective in most cases, but in a few, augmentation with oxytocin is needed. This drug must be administered cautiously because uterine rupture may be caused by an overstimulated uterus. Barron[89] reported that membrane rupture should be reserved for dead fetuses and patients who are in advanced labor.

If the fetus is alive, the decision as to how best to achieve delivery is not always easy. In addition, the outlook for the fetus is poor not only in terms of immediate survival but also because studies show that as many as 15.4% of liveborn infants do not survive.[71] However, when the mortality rate associated with vaginal delivery is compared with that of cesarean section in nonrandomized, controlled trials (52% vs. 16%, Okonofua and Olatubosun[90]; 20% vs. 15%, Hurd and coworkers[82]), cesarean delivery has advantages. Hibbard[12] stated that many of the poor results associated with cesarean section are largely the result of indecision and delay in the last quarter of pregnancy. He stated that cesarean delivery must be considered when the fetus is alive, particularly if there is evidence of fetal distress. However, coagulopathy adds considerable maternal risk, and the likelihood of injury or death may be increased by surgery.

If the decision is made to deliver and the fetus is alive, the degree of abruption and the state of the fetus are important determining factors. When abruption is severe, cesarean section must be performed once resuscitation has started. Delivery should be performed promptly, especially because most postadmission fetal deaths occur in fetuses delivered more than 2 hours after admission.

In mild to moderate cases of abruption, the mode of delivery is determined by the condition of the fetus, its presentation, and the state of the cervix. Abnormal fetal heart rate patterns are an indication for immediate cesarean delivery. However, if the decision is made to deliver vaginally, continuous fetal monitoring must be available to identify early abnormal fetal heart rate patterns. Golditch and Boyce,[73] Lunan,[79] and Okonofua and Olatubosun[90] showed that the perinatal mortality rate is higher with vaginal delivery in the absence of electronic fetal monitoring. Prostaglandins are used to ripen the cervix in women with mild abruption, but the danger of inducing tetanic contractions must be remembered. When feasible, amniotomy often hastens delivery, but when it is not possible, oxytocin can be used. However, vigilance must be maintained for the development of hyperstimulation.

Expectant Management

The goal of expectant management is to prolong pregnancy, with the hope of improving fetal maturity and survival. Expectant management is usually considered in cases of mild placental abruption occurring before 37 weeks' gestation. Vaginal bleeding is slight, abdominal pain is mild and usually localized, and the patient is cardiovascularly stable. Once conservative management has been chosen, the fetal condition must be monitored closely. No evidence supports the routine admission of patients who are being managed expectantly, especially when there is no evidence of maternal or fetal compromise or uterine contractions. Fetal growth restriction is a common finding in association with placental abruption. The timing of delivery depends on the finding of further vaginal bleeding, the fetal condition, gestational age, and the availability of neonatal care facilities. If bleeding episodes are recurrent, induction at 37 to 38 weeks is usually undertaken if fetal indices of health (e.g., biophysical parameters and growth) are satisfactory. When the initial episode is small and self-limiting and there is no acute (abnormal cardiotocographic findings or biophysical profile score) or chronic (growth restriction, oligohydramnios, or abnormal umbilical artery Doppler recording) fetal compromise, no evidence supports the induction of labor. Despite this lack of evidence, induction of labor at term is often advocated in such patients using the speculative argument that undetected damage might have occurred to the integrity and function of the placenta, and in the face of uncertainty, delivery at term confers more advantages.

If the initial ultrasound scan showed a retroplacental clot, the clot may be monitored by serial ultrasound scans. If the fetal condition deteriorates, delivery is expedited, with the speed and urgency determined by whether fetal compromise is acute or chronic.

Some cases of mild abruption may be complicated by labor. In such cases, it is difficult to establish which came first. Many consider tocolytics contraindicated in the presence of placental abruption because they may worsen abruption.[41] Tocolytics are controversial in the management of abruption and are considered only in patients who are hemodynamically stable with no evidence of fetal compromise and who might benefit from corticosteroids or prolongation of pregnancy. Towers and associates[44] conducted a review on the use of tocolytics in patients with placental abruption and first bleeding at mean of 28.9 weeks. They showed that this resulted in a mean increase in time from bleeding until delivery of 18.9 days. The neonatal mortality rate was 51 deaths per 1000 live births and all the deaths were related to complications of prematurity. An ongoing randomized, double-blind trial of magnesium sulfate tocolysis versus intravenous saline for suspected placental abruption by Stanford University investigators may provide further evidence.[91]

Management of Complications

The major complications of placental abruption are hemorrhagic shock, disseminated intravascular coagulation, ischemic necrosis of the distal organs (especially the kidneys and brain), and postpartum hemorrhage (see Chapter 78).

Rh Isoimmunization

Fetomaternal hemorrhage is a risk in association with all forms of placental bleeding but the risk is arguably higher during abruption.[59] All Rh-negative women with abruption must undergo a Kleihauer-Betke test and receive an appropriate dose of anti-D immunoglobulin to prevent immunization. Repeated doses depend on the amount of fetomaternal

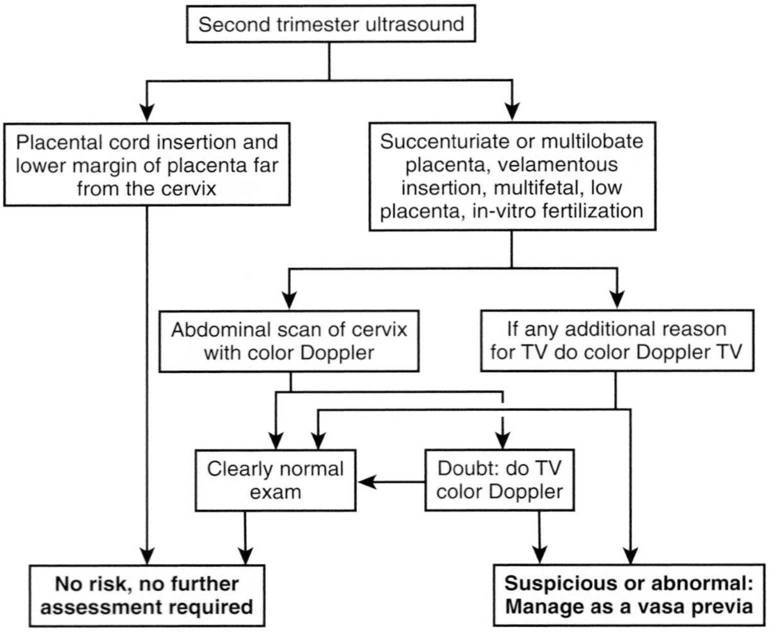

FIGURE 58–6
Proposed diagnostic algorithm for second trimester detection of vasa previa.
(From Derbala Y, Grochal F, Jeanty P: Vasa previa. J Prenat Med 2007;1:2-13.)

hemorrhage as determined by the Kleihauer-Betke test. This treatment must be given within 72 hours of the onset of abruption. When management is expectant in a patient with intermittent recurrent bleeding, regular Kleihauer-Betke testing and assays of anti-D immunoglobulin levels can be performed to guide further anti-D administration. Collaboration with the hematologist and blood bank is advisable to determine the correct dose when the Kleihauer-Betke test result is positive.

VASA PREVIA

VP is a characterized by fetal or placental vessels coursing over the cervix beneath the presenting part. These vessels are vulnerable to laceration and compression during pregnancy because they are unprotected by Wharton's jelly or placental tissue. The reported incidence is 1 per 2500 deliveries.[92] The incidence is reported to be 1 in 300 in vitro fertilization (IVF) pregnancies,[93,94] and this has been attributed to the increased proportion of placental morphologic alterations seen in assisted conceptions.[95,96] The patients usually present in labor, classically with bleeding at the time of artificial rupture of membranes; however, presentation after spontaneous rupture of membranes has been reported in several cases reports.[92] Type 1 VP occurs with a single-lobed placenta with velamentous insertion of the cord (VCI) whereas type 2 VP occurs when vessels join the placenta to an accessory lobe.

Risks

Fetal exsanguination after rupture may cause fetal death with fetal and neonatal mortality rates of up to 75% being reported in the past.[97] The presenting fetal pole may also exert direct pressure on the exposed blood vessels causing death by asphyxiation. The main risk to the mother is bleeding, but often maternal blood loss is mild and therefore not life-threatening.

Management Options

VP typically presents with painless vaginal bleeding at the time of spontaneous or artificial rupture of membranes. Fetal heart rate abnormalities quickly follow, leading to emergency cesarean section delivery for fetal distress. The neonate is usually severely anemic and hypovolemic requiring rapid life-saving blood transfusion and fluid replacement.[98]

Ultrasound scan is the mainstay of antenatal diagnosis of VP. Figure 58–6 shows an algorithm for the antenatal diagnosis of VP. The first reported diagnosis of VP on ultrasound was by Gianopolous and colleagues in 1987.[99] It was, however, only in 1996 that the first case of VP was diagnosed at the time of routine second-trimester anomaly scan.[98] The chances of VP being present are minimal when the umbilical cord inserts into the placental mass or in the absence of a succenturate or bilobed placenta.[100] Determining placental cord insertion during the anomaly scan is reported to take less than a minute and can be easily incorporated into the allocated scanning time with no additional skills required.[101] The ultrasound technique for ruling out VP is based on

- Assessment of placental cord insertion.
- Assessment of placental appearance and location.
- Consideration of other risk factors.

The umbilical cord inserts into the placental mass centrally or paracentrally in 90% of pregnancies. In 10%, the insertion is marginal with 1% being VCI. When the site of cord insertion into the placental mass is clearly identified, the possibility of VP type 1 is extremely low and no further action is required.[100] In contrast, when the insertion site cannot be identified, efforts should be made to exclude VCI because this group has a higher risk of having VP (6%). It is imperative to scan the area above the internal os using a transvaginal approach with color Doppler when a VCI cannot clearly be demonstrated in the upper uterine segment. Some authors have proposed a transperineal approach, but the use of color Doppler is critical.[102]

Placenta previa and marginal placenta are risk factors for VP, and when present, it is important to check for vessels near the cervix. Other risk factors for VP pregnancies include IVF, multiple pregnancies (10% of VP occur in twins), and patients presenting with APH.

When the presentation is with vaginal bleeding or bleeding during labor and VP is suspected, direct visualization of the vessels with an amnioscope may be possible, or alternatively, a blood test is performed to determine the presence of fetal hemoglobin in the vaginal loss.[97] The use of amnioscopes in modern obstetrics practice is, however, not common.

When the diagnosis is made antenatally and cesarean section delivery appropriately scheduled, infant survival rates of up to 97% have been reported compared with 44% survival when the condition was undiagnosed.[103] Even when the infant survives an undiagnosed VP, the study demonstrated an often complicated postnatal course with over 50% requiring a blood transfusion and registering poor Apgar scores. Reported methods for the diagnosis in symptomatic cases include the palpation of velamentous vessels through the dilated cervix.

UNCLASSIFIED BLEEDING

The exact cause of APH is unknown in approximately 47% of patients. The reported incidence varies from 38% to 74%.[102,104] The cause of bleeding may become apparent later, but in most cases, no cause is identified.[58] When causes are identified, they include marginal sinus rupture (60%), "show" (20%), cervicitis (18%), trauma (5%), vulvovaricosities (2%), genital tumors, hematuria, genital infections, and VP (0.5% each). Although this group of causes is referred to as "unclassified bleeding," it invariably includes unrecognized cases of minor abruption or placenta previa. Marginal sinus rupture is the most common source of bleeding in APH of unknown cause.[66]

Risks

The risks of unclassified bleeding depend on the cause. More serious causes are discussed in the relevant sections earlier and in Chapters 40, 49, 56, 57, and 78. This type of bleeding is associated with a higher perinatal mortality rate (3.5%–15.7%).[104–106] This rate is higher than that associated with placenta previa (4.2%–8.1%), suggesting some degree of placental dysfunction. Preterm labor is more common in these patients and is a contributor to the higher perinatal mortality rate.

Diagnosis

There are usually no signs and symptoms diagnostic of either placenta previa or placental abruption. In most cases, bleeding is mild and resolves spontaneously. Approximately 60% of cases occur after 37 weeks, and of these, 15% of patients are delivered within 10 days of the initial hemorrhage.[104] When marginal bleeding occurs with clot formation, serum separated from the clot may be confused with liquor after spontaneous rupture of fetal membranes.[107]

The diagnosis of unclassified bleeding is often made after placental abruption and placenta previa are excluded. An ultrasound scan is necessary to exclude placenta previa because minor grades may present in a similar manner.

Speculum examination should be performed in patients with unclassified bleeding, although opinions differ about the timing of this examination. Some argue that it should be delayed until bleeding has stopped, whereas others advocate immediate examination once placenta previa has been excluded. Those advocating immediate examination do so because they want to exclude advanced labor and local causes of bleeding. Those advocating delayed examination do so because of the belief that a delay does not affect management and that other local causes of bleeding are usually benign and need no immediate action. No controlled trials have compared these different types of management.

Management Options

If placenta previa and abruption have been excluded, further management depends on gestational age, the nature of the bleeding (severity and persistence or recurrence), the state of the fetus (abnormal fetal heart rate patterns), and the presumed cause of bleeding.

Options for further management include delivery and an expectant approach. At or beyond 37 weeks' gestation, when bleeding is recurrent or significant or associated fetal factors (e.g., growth restriction, abnormal heart rate patterns) are present, delivery is the management option of choice. Vaginal delivery is not contraindicated if there is no fetal compromise. Before 37 weeks' gestation, if bleeding is recurrent and significant, delivery may be justified. The mode of delivery is determined by the state of the fetus, its lie, and other associated factors, such as the state of the cervix.

If expectant management is chosen, the patient may be monitored at home or in the hospital. Most units monitor patients in the hospital until bleeding has stopped for at least 24 hours. Watson,[104] in a retrospective review, showed no significant advantage in admitting patients to the hospital. A randomized, controlled trial comparing inpatient versus outpatient care in these cases is needed, especially with the current emphasis on community-based care for pregnancy. Regardless of where the patient is managed, fetal surveillance should be implemented because of the increased risk of perinatal death (discussed earlier). When awaiting the spontaneous onset of labor is the practice,[106] the perinatal mortality rate is not increased. Some advocate elective delivery usually by labor induction at 38 weeks[106] because any bleeding carries a theoretical risk of causing placental separation.[108] However, there is no evidence to support this theoretical risk. Thus, the authors recommend awaiting the spontaneous onset of labor if fetal growth and welfare are satisfactory and use induction only when there is evidence of fetal compromise.

SUMMARY OF MANAGEMENT OPTIONS

Bleeding in Late Pregnancy

Management Options	Evidence Quality and Recommendation	References
Prenatal		
Identification of at-risk women, with delivery in units with facilities for blood transfusion and cesarean delivery:	III/B	94,95
• Previous cesarean delivery (risk of placenta previa).	IIb/B	96
• Proven placenta previa (on ultrasound).	III/B	17
• Clinical diagnosis of abruption.	IV/C	52
• Clinical diagnosis of unclassified bleeding.	IV/C	88
Initial Assessment of Severity of Bleeding		
Severe and continuing bleeding (see also Chapter 78):	III/B	97,98
• Resuscitate (IV access, blood and clotting factors) and correct coagulopathy (if possible).	III/B	97,99
• A major obstetric hemorrhage protocol should be available.	IV/C	12
• Deliver the infant or empty the uterus (the route depends on gestation, fetal condition, maternal condition, amount of blood loss, fetal presentation, and whether the patient is in labor).	GPP	—
• In most cases of placenta previa, cesarean delivery is used.	IV/C	46
Mild to moderate bleeding or bleeding that is resolving:		
Establish the cause and manage bleeding appropriately:		
Placenta previa:		
• Expectant management:	III/B	36,39
• Controversy about whether to admit an asymptomatic patient to the hospital.		
• Hospital admission (and readiness for blood transfusion and cesarean delivery) if the patient is symptomatic (considerable variation in practice).		
• Elective or planned delivery:	IV/C	13
• Anesthesia for cesarean delivery in patients with placenta previa:		
• Emergency delivery: Regional or general anesthesia.	III/B	82
• Elective delivery: Regional anesthesia.	III/B	42,82
Placental abruption or unclassified bleeding:	III/B	100–103
• Serial fetal assessment.		
• Elective delivery at term.		
Anti-D for Rh-negative women.	IV/C	104
Labor and Delivery		
Cross-match in patients with severe or active bleeding or placenta previa.	III/B	97,99
Postnatal		
Vigilance for postpartum hemorrhage.	IV/C	105
Anti-D for Rh-negative women (if not already given).	IV/C	104
Treatment of anemia.	GPP	—

GPP, good practice point.

SUGGESTED READINGS

Cotton DB, Read JA, Paul RH, Quilligan EJ: The conservative aggressive management of placenta previa. Am J Obstet Gynecol 1980;137:687–695.

Crenshaw C, Jones DED, Parker RT: Placenta previa: A survey of 20 years' experience with improved perinatal survival by expectant therapy and cesarean delivery. Obstet Gynecol Surv 1973;28:461–470.

Daly-Jones E, John A, Leahy A, et al: Vasa previa: A preventable tragedy. Ultrasound 2008:16:8–14.

Derbala Y, Grochal F, Jeanty P: Vasa previa. J Prenat Med 2007;1:2–13.

Liston W: Haemorrhage. In Lewis G (ed): Saving mother's lives: Reviewing maternal deaths to make motherhood safer–2003–2005. The Confidential Enquiry into Maternal and Child Health (CEMACH). The seventh report on Confidential Enquiry into Maternal Deaths in the United Kingdom. London, CEMACH, 2007, pp 78–85.

Neilson JP: Interventions for suspected placenta previa. Cochrane Database Syst Rev 2003;2:CD001998.

Oyelese KO, Turner M, Lees C, Campbell S: Vasa previa: An avoidable obstetric tragedy. Obstet Gynecol 2000;18:109–115.

Royal College of Obstetricians and Gynaecologists: Guidelines No. 27. Revised October 2005. Available at http://www.rcog.org.uk/womens-health/clinical-guidance/placenta-praevia-and-placenta-praevia-accreta-diagnosis-and-management

Silver RM, Landon MB, Rouse DJ, et al, National Institute of Child Health and Human Development Maternal-Fetal Medicine Units Network: Maternal morbidity associated with multiple repeat cesarean deliveries. Obstet Gynecol 2006;107:1226–1232.

Zdoukopoulos N, Zintzaras E: Genetic risk factors for placental abruption: A HuGE review and meta-analysis. Epidemiology 2008;19:309–323.

REFERENCES

For a complete list of references, log onto www.expertconsult.com.

CHAPTER 59

Multiple Pregnancy

JODIE M. DODD, ROSALIE M. GRIVELL, and CAROLINE A. CROWTHER

Videos corresponding to this chapter are available online at www.expertconsult.com.

INTRODUCTION

Multiple pregnancy rates vary worldwide, from a low of 6.7 per 1000 births in Japan to 40 per 1000 births in Nigeria. The frequency of twin births in tertiary centers ranges from 1 in 25 to 1 in 100, reflecting the hospital referral population rather than the true population rate. The incidence of monozygous twinning is relatively constant at 3.5 per 1000 births.[1] Dizygous twinning rates and higher-order birth rates vary widely and are affected by age, parity, racial background, and the use of assisted reproductive techniques. This chapter discusses the general and obstetric risks associated with multiple pregnancy. Problems specific to multiple pregnancy are discussed in Chapter 23.

RISKS

Multiple pregnancy is associated with more maternal and fetal risks than singleton pregnancy.

Maternal Risks (Table 59–1)

Increased Symptoms of Early Pregnancy

Nausea and vomiting are three times more common in multiple than in singleton pregnancies,[2,3] with higher levels of pregnancy hormones implicated.[4]

Increased Risk of Miscarriage

Both threatened and actual miscarriage are more common in multiple pregnancy,[2] with the rate of missed abortion approximately twice as high as the 2% rate seen in singletons at 10 to 14 weeks' gestation.[5]

Vanishing Twin Syndrome

Twins and higher-order multiple gestations are more often conceived than born. During the first trimester, arrest of development and subsequent reabsorption of one or more of the fetuses may occur. This event can be seen ultrasonographically and is known as the "vanishing twin" phenomenon.[6] First-trimester vaginal bleeding may be related to this syndrome. Whereas the prognosis for the remaining fetus after loss of a co-twin at this early stage of pregnancy is generally considered to be good,[6] more recent reports suggest an increase in the risk of low birth weight in the surviving twin.[7–9]

Minor Disorders of Pregnancy

The extra weight carried with a multiple pregnancy exaggerates the minor symptoms of pregnancy. Backache, breathlessness, difficulty walking (especially toward the end of pregnancy), and pressure problems (e.g., varicose veins) are more common in multiple pregnancy.

Anemia

Anemia is thought to be more frequent in multiple than in singleton pregnancy. However, the greater increase in blood volume compared with the red cell mass decreases the hemoglobin concentration, producing a more pronounced decrease in hemoglobin than in seen in singleton pregnancy.[10] Mean corpuscular hemoglobin concentration, used as a measure of anemia, does not differ in multiple versus singleton pregnancy. In a retrospective case-control study comparing hemoglobin concentration in twin and singleton gestations matched for parity, no statistically significant differences in third-trimester hemoglobin levels were identified between the two groups.[11] The lower levels identified in the first and second trimesters of pregnancy in twins compared with singletons reflected lower values in multiparous women with a twin pregnancy. Fetal demands in a multiple pregnancy are greater, particularly for folate, and megaloblastic anemia has been reported.

Preterm Labor and Delivery

Preterm birth (birth <37 wk) occurs in over 50% of all twin pregnancies,[12–15] with approximately 10% of these births occurring prior to 32 weeks' gestation.[12,14] The mean duration of pregnancy decreases as the number of fetuses in utero increases. The risks to the mother of a preterm birth relate to the need for hospitalization and the possible use of tocolytic therapy, with potential side effects. Preterm prelabor rupture of the membranes occurs more frequently in multiple gestations and is often followed by preterm labor and birth.

Hypertension

The incidences of pregnancy-induced hypertension, preeclampsia, and eclampsia are all increased in multiple

TABLE 59–1

Maternal Risks Associated with Multiple Pregnancy

Increased symptoms of early pregnancy
Increased risk of miscarriage
Vanishing twin syndrome
Minor disorders of pregnancy
Anemia
Preterm labor and delivery
Hypertension
Antepartum hemorrhage
Hydramnios
Possible need for prenatal hospitalization
Single fetal death in twins
Increased risk of an operative vaginal birth
Increased likelihood of cesarean birth
Postpartum hemorrhage
Postnatal problems
Maternal mortality

TABLE 59–2

Fetal Risks Associated with Multiple Pregnancy

Stillbirth or neonatal death
Single fetal death in twins
Preterm labor and delivery
Intrauterine growth restriction
Congenital anomalies
Congenital anomaly in one twin
Twin reversed arterial perfusion sequence
Conjoined twins
Cord accident
Zygosity
Monoamniotic twins
Hydramnios
Twin-twin transfusion syndrome
Risk of asphyxia
Operative vaginal birth, especially for the second twin
Twin entrapment
Cerebral palsy

pregnancy.[2,16,17] A primigravid woman with a twin pregnancy has a 5 times greater risk of severe preeclampsia than one with a singleton pregnancy, and for a multigravid woman, the risk is 10 times greater.[18] Some report a higher risk of hypertension with monozygotic twins,[19] but others do not.[20,21]

Antepartum Hemorrhage

Antepartum hemorrhage as a result of either placenta previa[22] or placental abruption[23–25] is increased in multiple gestations.

Hydramnios

Hydramnios is suspected clinically in up to 12% of multiple pregnancies[26] and is associated with an increased risk of preterm labor.[27] Acute polyhydramnios may occur, particularly with monochorionic twins, often with significant abdominal discomfort for the mother. This is often associated with twin-twin transfusion syndrome (TTTS) (see Chapter 23).

Possible Need for Prenatal Hospitalization

With the increased risk of threatened preterm labor, hypertension, fetal growth restriction, and minor disorders of pregnancy, women with a multiple pregnancy often require hospital admission, sometimes for prolonged periods, during the prenatal period. For the mother, prolonged separation from her family is often a disruptive and stressful experience. Specific complications of twinning, such as TTTS or single fetal death, may require hospitalization.

Single Fetal Death in Twins

The risk of single fetal death in a multiple pregnancy is 2% to 6%. Psychological trauma may be considerable and is enhanced by concerns about the health of the surviving fetus or fetuses. The mother who experiences fetal death of one twin during the antepartum period must adjust to a future without one of the twins while developing a bond with the surviving twin. The mother also must adjust to the additional risk of death and morbidity from cerebral and renal lesions for the surviving twin (see Chapter 23).

Risk of Operative Vaginal Birth

Compared with a vaginal singleton birth, there is an increased likelihood of operative delivery for one or both twins, with the associated maternal risks of trauma, infection, and hemorrhage.

Increased Likelihood of Cesarean Birth

Twins are more frequently born by cesarean section than are singletons, either as an elective procedure or as an emergency procedure before or after the birth of the first twin. Presentation and gestational age influence this likelihood.[28]

Postpartum Hemorrhage

The risk of postpartum hemorrhage is greater in multiple pregnancy because of the increased placental site, uterine overdistention, and a greater tendency to uterine atony.[29,30]

Postnatal Problems

Learning to cope with the demands of two or more infants can be stressful. A higher percentage of depression is reported in mothers of twins.[31] Given the increased perinatal mortality rate among higher-order multiple pregnancies, the problems of coping with the loss of one or more infants may be an added burden in the postnatal period.

Maternal Mortality

Women with a multiple pregnancy have a twofold increase in the risk of death compared with women with a singleton gestation.[32]

Fetal Risks (Table 59–2)

Stillbirth and Neonatal Death

Multiple pregnancy contributes approximately 10% of total perinatal mortality,[14,33] being up to 10 times greater than in singletons.[26,34,35] If late abortion, late neonatal death, and infant death are included the mortality, the risk is further doubled. Cause-specific perinatal mortality in twins is higher for every major cause of death, and at all weeks of gestation, compared with singletons.[36]

Higher mortality rates are reported for monochorionic compared with dichorionic twins,[37–39] although not in all studies.[40] For dichorionic twins, the risk of death increased throughout gestation, whereas the risk for monochorionic twins reached a maximum at 28 weeks' gestation and then remained constant.[40] In a review of 1051 twin pairs, factors associated with one or both twins dying in utero related to monochorionicity (odds ratio [OR] 2.0; 95% confidence interval [CI] 1.2–3.4) and discordant birth weight (OR 4.3; 95% CI 2.5–7.3), after correcting for gestational age at birth.[41]

Single Fetal Death in Twins

See Chapter 23.

Preterm Labor and Birth

Preterm birth (<37 completed wk) is the major contributor to the poor perinatal outcomes observed in multiple pregnancy. The preterm birth rate in twin pregnancy is consistently reported to be above 50%,[13–15,33] the risk increasing to in excess of 80% among triplet pregnancies.[14,42,43]

The median gestational age at birth for monochorionic twins is 36 weeks compared with 37 weeks for dichorionic twins. However, 9.2% of monochorionic twins are born before 32 weeks' gestation compared with 5.5% of dichorionic twins (Fig. 59–1).[5]

Intrauterine Growth Restriction

The incidence of small–for–gestational age infants (birth weight < 10th percentile for gestational age standards in pregnancy) is common in multiple pregnancy, with up to 50% of infants having birth weight below 2500 g.[14] These infants are at increased risk for perinatal mortality and morbidity.[44–47]

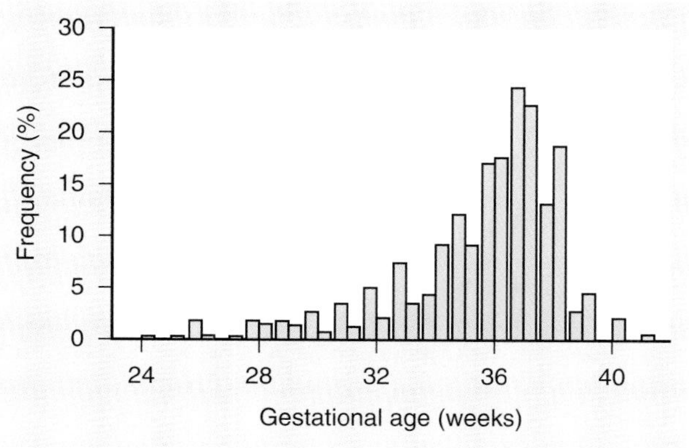

FIGURE 59–1
Gestational age at birth for monochorionic and dichorionic twin pregnancies.
(From Sebire N, Thornton S, Hughes K, et al: The prevalence and consequence of missed abortion in twin pregnancies at 10–14 weeks of gestation. Br J Obstet Gynaecol 1997;104:847–848.)

Fetal Problems Specific to Multiple Pregnancy

Major congenital abnormalities are more common in multiple pregnancies than in singletons, with rates reported as 4.9%.[48] Several fetal problems are specific to multiple pregnancy, including conjoined twins (discussed later), twin reversed arterial perfusion sequence, monoamniotic twins, and TTTS (see Chapter 23).

Conjoined Twins

Conjoined twins is a congenital abnormality that occurs only in multiple pregnancy and affects 1 in 200 monozygotic twins.[49]

Cord Accident

Preterm birth, preterm prelabor rupture of the membranes, hydramnios, malposition, and malpresentation are more likely to increase the risk of a cord accident in multiple pregnancies than in singleton pregnancies.

Chorionicity

Chorionicity has an important effect on pregnancy outcome. Two thirds of monozygous twins are monochorionic and are at increased risk for mortality and morbidity compared with dichorionic twins. Risk factors include increased risk of TTTS, congenital anomalies, single fetal death in utero, and acute hydramnios (see Chapter 23).

Hydramnios

Hydramnios may occur in one gestational sac in both TTTS and the "stuck twin" phenomenon (see Chapter 23). It may be caused by fetal anomalies such as upper gastrointestinal tract atresias, congenital heart anomalies. or hydrops fetalis. In some cases of gross hydramnios in both sacs, no causal factor is evident. Hydramnios is a major cause of preterm birth and the associated perinatal mortality rate is high.[27]

Risk of Asphyxia

The risk of mortality as a result of asphyxia in a twin is four to five times than in a singleton.[50] Important risk factors include the increased occurrence of intrauterine growth restriction, cord prolapse, and hydramnios.

Operative Vaginal Birth, Especially for the Second Twin

The likelihood of operative birth is increased, especially for the second twin, who may require internal podalic version. Operative birth is associated with an increased risk of birth trauma, low Apgar scores, and hyperbilirubinemia compared with a normal vaginal birth.

Twin Entrapment

Twin entrapment is rare and reported to occur in 1 in 817 twin pregnancies.[51] The risk of fetal death of the first twin is high, as is the risk of fetal hypoxia in both twins. Twin entrapment is associated with monoamniotic twins.

Cerebral Palsy

The prevalence of cerebral palsy in triplets is 47 times greater and in twins 8 times greater than in singletons.[52] Lower gestational age at birth is associated with a greater risk of cerebral palsy.[53]

MANAGEMENT OPTIONS

Prepregnancy

The rate of multiple pregnancy for women undergoing ovulation induction is increased to 20 to 40%. For clomiphene, the twinning rate is 9% to 14%.[54] Appropriate counseling about this increased risk should be provided to women who are offered this treatment. The risk of multiple pregnancy from assisted reproductive techniques correlates with the number of embryos or zygotes transferred, increasing from 1.4% with single embryo transfer to 17.9% with two embryos, and 24.1% after transfer of four embryos.[55] Similarly, after gamete intrafallopian transfer, the rate of multiple pregnancy is 18.7% after transfer of two oocytes and 25.8% after transfer of three oocytes.[55] The rate of multiple pregnancy at 20 weeks' gestation after zygote intrafallopian transfer with three zygotes is 27%.[56]

The best way to reduce the risk of multiple pregnancy is to reduce the number of embryos, zygotes, or oocytes transferred after full discussion of the risks (of multiple pregnancy) and benefits (of high successful pregnancy rates) with the couple. Three randomized, controlled trials compared single versus double embryo transfer,[57–59] and another compared double embryo transfer with transfer of four embryos.[60] When single embryo transfer was compared with double embryo transfer, fewer women became pregnant (relative risk [RR] 0.69; 95% CI 0.51–0.93), but the risks of twin pregnancy (RR 0.12; 95% CI 0.03–0.48) and low birth weight (RR 0.17; 95% CI 0.04–0.79) were markedly reduced.[61] No statistically significant differences were identified for outcomes relating to singleton pregnancy, pregnancy loss at less than 20 weeks' gestation, extrauterine pregnancy, or preterm birth at less than 37 weeks.[61] When the transfer of two embryos was compared with the transfer of four embryos, no statistically significant differences were seen in the number of women who became pregnant with a multiple or singleton pregnancy or the risk of pregnancy loss.[60] In view of the risks associated with multiple pregnancy, the Royal College of Obstetricians and Gynaecologists (RCOG) has issued guidelines indicating that consideration should be given to transferring only a single embryo.[62]

Periconceptual folate supplementation is recommended as a general measure for all women to reduce the risk of neural tube defects.[63]

Prenatal

Overall Care

Regular prenatal attendance for pregnancy care is accepted practice. The variation in visit frequency, the health care provider, and screening program seen in practice are of unproven value. Specialized multidisciplinary twin clinics have been advocated, and some nonrandomized cohort data suggest that perinatal outcome can be improved by intensive preterm birth education, continuity of care providers, and individualized care.[64–66] Prospective randomized data are lacking.

Frequent prenatal visits permit extra vigilance in the early detection of pregnancy-induced hypertension.[67] Routine screening for gestational diabetes is often performed, with some reports suggesting an increased risk in twins[68] and others suggesting no increased risk.[69] Antepartum hemorrhage can be neither predicted nor prevented by additional prenatal visits or any other strategy. In addition, iron and folate supplementation is frequently advised from the beginning of the second trimester for women with multiple pregnancy, although the evidence to support this practice is limited.[10,11]

Diagnosis of Chorionicity by Early Ultrasound

Amnionicity and chorionicity can be determined by ultrasound.[70] This knowledge may be useful in predicting which pregnancies are at greater risk for TTTS, and for monoamniotic twins, cord entanglement, or to differentiate TTTS from a twin pregnancy complicated by growth restriction. Similarly, this knowledge may be useful in the management of twin pregnancy when one twin has a major congenital malformation and selective termination is considered or in the management of pregnancy after a single fetal death.[71] Screening for amnionicity and chorionicity is best performed in the first trimester, although it is not always easy, even for a skilled ultrasonographer.[72]

Monochorionic twins are the same sex and have one placental mass, with a thin dividing membrane (two amnions, no chorions) and a T insertion.[41,73] Because the dividing membrane is so thin, it is often difficult to identify, and the pregnancy may be misidentified as monoamniotic. Visualization of the dividing membrane is facilitated by searching over the fetal chin or away from the fetal body and around the limbs. A dichorionic placenta essentially eliminates the diagnosis of TTTS.

The dividing membrane is thicker in dichorionic twins (containing two layers of amnion and two layers of chorion). Measuring the membrane thickness by ultrasound, using a cutoff of 2 mm to characterize a dichorionic or monochorionic placenta,[74] has been described as a good, but suboptimal, test for determining chorionicity.[72] High interobserver and intraobserver variation, together with differences related to gestational age and sampling site, lead to suboptimal accuracy of the determination of chorionicity.[73] Ultrasonic detection of the lambda sign[69] (an echogenic V-shaped chorionic projection of tissue between the dividing membranes in dichorionic placentation) is reported as more reliable, especially if the scan is performed at 10 to 14 weeks' gestation (Fig. 59–2).[75] As gestational age increases, the lambda sign is more difficult to see, and after 20 weeks, it may disappear. The lambda sign is also known as the "twin peak" sign.[76] Given the prognostic value for later risks of pregnancy, attempting to establish the chorionicity of the placenta between 10 and 14 weeks' gestation may be appropriate.

Accuracy rates for determining chorionicity with first-trimester ultrasound, determined by subsequent pathologic examination, are reported as up to 96% with transabdominal sonography[77] and up to 100% with transvaginal sonography.[32]

No prospective clinical studies show that knowledge of chorionicity should alter subsequent clinical management or whether pregnancy outcome can be improved by changes in clinical care. Despite this, many practitioners increase antenatal surveillance in women with a monochorionic pregnancy.

TABLE 59–3

Pregnancy Outcomes in Multifetal Pregnancy Reduction

OUTCOME (% OF PREGNANCIES)	TRIPLETS UNREDUCED (%)	TRIPLETS REDUCED TO TWINS (%)	TWINS UNREDUCED (%)	TWINS REDUCED TO SINGLETONS (%)
Miscarriage rate	20.2	8.6	7.8	5.6
Very preterm birth	22.1*	9.3*	13.8†	13.3†

* <32 wk.
† <34 wk.
From Dodd J, Crowther C: Reduction of the number of fetuses for women with triplet and higher order multiple pregnancies (Cochrane Review). In Cochrane Library. Chichester, UK, John Wiley & Sons, Issue 4, 2003.

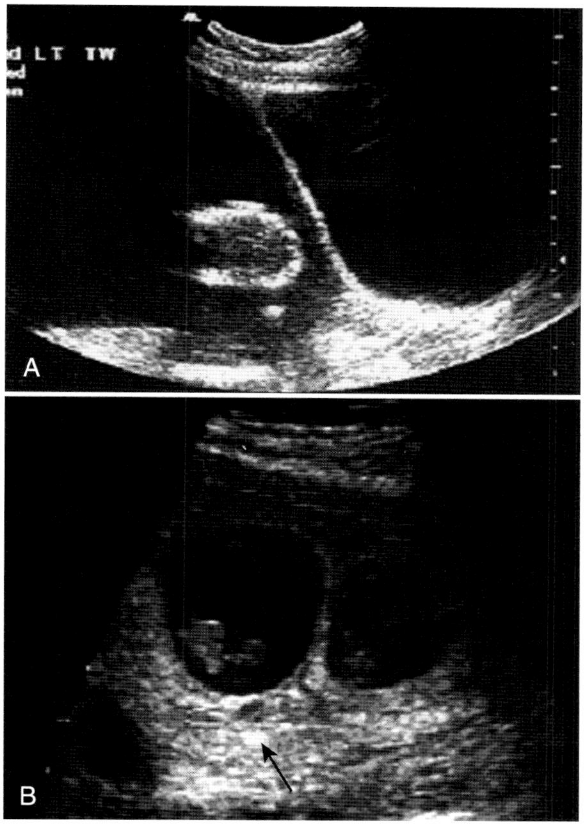

FIGURE 59–2
Ultrasonography to establish chorionicity. *A*, Monochorionic twin pregnancy. B, Dichorionic twin pregnancy showing the lambda sign (*arrow*).

Nuchal Translucency Screening

The use of nuchal translucency screening for aneuploidy in singleton gestation is widespread, and it has been used to screen women with twin pregnancy. In a study of 448 women with twin pregnancy, nuchal translucency was measured for each fetus and combined with maternal age to derive a risk estimate.[78] The detected nuchal translucency was greater than the 95th percentile for gestational age (using crown-rump length derived from singletons) in 7.3% of fetuses, including 88% of those with trisomy 21. These findings suggest that in dichorionic twin pregnancies, the sensitivity and false-positive rate of fetal nuchal translucency as a screening tool for trisomy 21 are similar to those reported for singleton pregnancies.[78] In monochorionic twin pregnancies, the false-positive rate of screening is higher than that reported in singleton pregnancies, and discordance in nuchal translucency measurements raise the possibility of early-onset TTTS.[79] The incorporation of nasal bone assessment has more limited sensitivity in screening for chromosomal anomalies and is technically more difficult to achieve in multiple pregnancies.[80]

Pregnancy Reduction

Couples who are faced with the dilemma of a triplet or higher-order multiple pregnancy have several options. Termination of the entire pregnancy generally is not acceptable to women, particularly those with a history of infertility. Attempting to continue the pregnancy with all of the fetuses is associated with inherent problems related to preterm birth, survival, and long-term morbidity. Reduction in the number of fetuses by selective termination has been advocated in an attempt to reduce the risk of adverse obstetric and perinatal outcomes.[81] The procedure is described in Chapter 23. Many prospective, nonrandomized studies have compared pregnancy outcome after multifetal pregnancy reduction in twins conceived spontaneously or after assisted reproduction[82–84] with multifetal pregnancy reduction in expectantly managed triplet pregnancies.[84–87] A systematic review assessed the effects of multifetal pregnancy reduction on fetal loss, preterm birth, and perinatal and infant mortality and morbidity rates in women with triplet and higher-order multiple pregnancies.[88,89] When pregnancy was reduced to twins, the reported outcomes appeared comparable with those in twins conceived spontaneously or those conceived with assisted reproductive techniques (Table 59–3).[88,89] Counseling these women is further complicated by the varying preterm delivery rates and their consequences (Table 59–4). No randomized, controlled trials have assessed multifetal reduction. The available nonrandomized studies provide limited insight into the benefits and risks associated with fetal reduction procedures.[88,89] Although a randomized, controlled trial would provide the most reliable evidence, selective termination may not be acceptable to couples, particularly those with a history of infertility, and consequently, recruitment to such a trial may be exceptionally difficult.

Fetal Anomaly Scanning

Given the increased risk of congenital abnormalities, an anomaly scan of each fetus by an ultrasonographer with appropriate expertise is suggested, usually between 18 and

TABLE 59–4

Likelihood of Preterm Delivery and Subsequent Preterm Mortality and Neurodevelopmental Morbidity Rates in Unreduced Triplets and Triplets Reduced to Twins

	24 WK		26 WK		28 WK		30 WK		32 WK		
OUTCOME	URT	TWN	URT	TWN	URT	TWN	URT	TWN	URT	TWN	REFERENCE
Percentage of pregnancies undelivered at a given gestation	80	90	75	87	70	87	65	87	55	82	86
Percentage survival if delivered at a given gestation (95% CI)	21 (16-25)		62 (58-65)		88 (68-90)		96 (95-97)		99 (97-99)		167
Percentage with no NDM ("no disability") if delivered at a given gestation (95% CI)	30* (8-58)		55* (35-75)		70* (62-88)		Proportion of survivors with "no disability" continues to rise with gestation at delivery, but no accurate current data are available for each gestational period > 28 wk.*				168,169

* Mortality and neurodevelopment morbidity assessed at 4 yr in survivors.
CI, confidence interval; NDM, neurodevelopmental morbidity; TWN, triplets reduced to twins; URT, unreduced triplets.

20 weeks' gestation. In centers offering routine ultrasound scanning at this stage of pregnancy, undetected multiple pregnancy should be diagnosed. Early diagnosis allows appropriate counseling and planning for future care and has been reported to reduce perinatal loss related to twin pregnancy.[90] Conjoined twins can be diagnosed if an ultrasound scan is performed at this stage.

In one series, prenatal ultrasonography, including cardiac screening limited to the four-chamber view, resulted in the detection of up to 39% of all major congenital anomalies in twins.[91] However, none of the cardiac lesions was detected. Of major noncardiac anomalies, 55% were detected, as were 69% of major anomalies that could alter prenatal management.[91] In a retrospective study of 245 women with twin pregnancy, ultrasound screening for fetal anomalies identified a 4.9% prevalence of congenital malformations.[48] For the detection of each individual anomaly, sensitivity was 82%, specificity was 100%, positive predictive value was 100%, and negative predictive value was 98%.[48]

Conjoined Twins

Conjoined twins are usually diagnosed antenatally.[92] Determination of the conjoined site permits multidisciplinary discussion before birth as to the prognosis and the possibility of surgical correction and allows full involvement of the parents. Unless birth is necessary for other reasons, preterm cesarean section is recommended. The use of one course of steroids to stimulate fetal lung maturity is advisable. Some test for fetal lung maturity before birth. Many obstetricians recommend elective cesarean delivery at 38 weeks; however, this procedure can be difficult technically. Some recommend a classic incision, although this increases the maternal risks, particularly of uterine scar rupture in subsequent pregnancy. At delivery, two neonatal teams should be available, with the neonatal surgical team and operating room on standby.

Preterm Labor

Preterm labor and subsequent birth presents the greatest risk for fetal morbidity and mortality. Maternal counseling as to the signs and symptoms of preterm labor may be of value. If uterine activity is noted, the woman should go to the hospital promptly.

It is difficult to predict which patients will have preterm labor. Cervical assessment by either digital[93–95] or ultrasound examination[96–99] has been suggested as a useful way to evaluate the risk of preterm delivery. How frequently such an assessment should be made (e.g., weekly, every 2 weeks, monthly) is uncertain, and whether such assessment is more beneficial than harmful is not known. Cervical assessment allows calculation of the cervical score (cervical length [in centimeters] – cervical dilation [in centimeters]). A cervical score of 2 or less at or before 34 weeks' gestation has a positive predictive value of 75% for preterm birth,[94] with other authors reporting that a cervical score of 0 or less has a positive predictive value of 75% for preterm birth.[95] As part of a study of the prediction of preterm delivery, cervical length was prospectively assessed by ultrasound in 147 women with a twin pregnancy.[96] A short cervix (<25 mm) was consistently associated with spontaneous preterm birth at less than 32 weeks' gestation (OR 6.9; 95% CI 2.0–24.2), less than 35 weeks' gestation (OR 3.2; 95% CI 2.3–7.9), and less than 37 weeks' gestation (OR 2.8; 95% CI 1.1–7.7).[96]

The presence of fetal fibronectin in cervical secretions has been used to predict preterm birth.[96,99] In multiple pregnancy, a positive fetal fibronectin test result at 28 to 30 weeks was associated with preterm birth before 32 weeks' gestation.[96] A positive fetal fibronectin test result at 28 weeks' gestation predicted birth before 35 weeks, with sensitivity, specificity, positive predictive value, and negative predictive value of 50.0%, 92.0%, 62.5%, and 87.3%, respectively.[99] The ability of fetal fibronectin to predict very preterm birth requires ongoing prospective evaluation to determine whether such prediction can lead to effective interventions that would reduce the risk of preterm birth.

If cervical change is noted, hospital admission is the most generally accepted management. Routine hospital admission and subsequent rest, however, seem to offer little benefit in delaying labor.[100,101] It is unknown whether prophylactic tocolysis is of value in this identifiable group at high risk for preterm birth.

Several prenatal interventions have been tried to reduce the risk of preterm birth in multiple pregnancies and have been evaluated by randomized clinical trials. These include prophylactic cervical cerclage,[102,103] prophylactic β-mimetic agents,[104–106] prophylactic progesterone therapy,[107–109] bedrest in the hospital,[100,110] and home uterine activity monitoring.[111,112] However, none of these haa proved to be of value in reducing the incidence of preterm birth and the associated high perinatal mortality rate in multiple pregnancy.

Prophylactic cervical cerclage in twin pregnancy does not show benefit when the results of randomized trials are reviewed.[113] It seems prudent to reserve the insertion of a cervical suture for women with evidence of cervical incompetence. Prophylactic tocolytic agents are occasionally used in multiple pregnancy. Systematic review of randomized trials of prophylactic β-mimetics does not show a benefit in the incidence of preterm labor,[114] and their use cannot be recommended.

Prophylactic progesterone has been advocated as a treatment for women at risk for preterm birth from multiple pregnancy. Two randomized trials have been identified evaluating the use of 17α-hydroxyprogesterone caproate in women with a twin pregnancy,[108,109] and a single trial involving women with a triplet pregnancy.[107] To date, there is little evidence to support its use, with no demonstrated benefit in either the risk of preterm birth or the neonatal health outcomes.[115,116]

Admission of women with an uncomplicated twin pregnancy to the hospital for rest does not reduce the risk of preterm birth. The Cochrane Systematic Review of randomized trials of routine hospitalization for rest shows an increased likelihood of preterm birth in women who were admitted compared with control subjects who continued normal activity at home.[100] Hospital admission for rest in an uncomplicated twin pregnancy should be considered only if the woman requests admission. Women may request hospital admission for several reasons, including discomfort, difficulty coping at home, or living a significant distance from the hospital.

The value of hospital admission for rest in triplet or higher-order multiple pregnancy is uncertain. Only two small randomized studies have been conducted, with no demonstrable benefit.[110,117]

Home uterine activity monitoring (HUAM) has been suggested to permit the diagnosis of preterm labor at an early stage, allowing successful tocolysis and fewer preterm births. A small randomized trial of 45 women reported these benefits.[112] However, in subgroup analysis of the 844 twin gestations in a multicenter trial comparing HUAM with weekly or daily nursing contact, HUAM did not reduce the risk of preterm birth.[111] HUAM, when combined with daily nursing contact, did result in more unscheduled visits and increased use of tocolytics.

A course of prenatal corticosteroids should be given to improve fetal outcome in women with multiple pregnancy who are considered at increased risk for preterm birth at less than 34 weeks, if birth is planned, or if there is a high risk of birth within the next 48 hours.[118] Whether a larger dose of corticosteroids than that given in singleton pregnancies would be more beneficial in twin gestations has been suggested but not adequately assessed.[118] For women who remain undelivered after 7 days following corticosteroids, repeat doses may be recommended, because they have been shown to reduce the occurrence and severity of neonatal lung disease and other serious health problems in the early neonatal period.[119] However, these benefits are associated with a reduction in some measures of weight and head circumference at birth, and there is still insufficient evidence on the longer-term benefits and risks.[119,120]

Fetal Assessment

Fetal assessment during pregnancy includes regular ultrasound to determine fetal growth and well-being. The recommended frequency of scanning varies (e.g., from every 2 wk from 24 wk' gestation to every 3–4 wk from 20 wk' gestation). Umbilical artery Doppler improves pregnancy outcome in high risk pregnancy and is often included as part of routine fetal assessment.[121] Some centers suggest obtaining biophysical profiles from 30 weeks' gestation, although the evidence to support this strategy is not strong.

The use of umbilical artery Doppler studies in the assessment of twin pregnancy was evaluated in three randomized, controlled trials.[122–124] Giles and colleagues[122] randomly allocated 526 women with a twin pregnancy at 25 weeks' gestation to biometry only or to biometry and umbilical artery Doppler waveform at 25, 30, and 35 weeks' gestation. This study of close antenatal surveillance identified a lower than expected fetal mortality rate from 25 weeks' gestation in both the biometry alone and the combined biometry and Doppler groups.

Maternal Education and Support

During the prenatal period, the couple will need specific information and support to help prepare for the birth and care of their infants.[125] The most likely mode of birth, care in labor, and the use of analgesia, especially epidural, should be discussed.[126] Many countries have multiple pregnancy support groups. The opportunity to contact a local group during the prenatal period, attend meetings, and make personal contact with other families who have had a multiple birth is recommended.

Labor and Delivery

Birth in a hospital is accepted practice,[127] with many advising birth in a tertiary unit, when possible. Induction of labor may be indicated for complications such as preeclampsia or growth restriction. The benefit of elective birth at 37 weeks' gestation to reduce the risk of antepartum stillbirth as a result of intrauterine growth restriction is controversial.

Retrospective data suggest that the lowest rate of perinatal mortality and morbidity in twin pregnancies occurs at 36 to 38 weeks' gestation, with the risk of adverse outcome increasing as gestation advances.[36,128–131] The recent Cochrane Systematic Review of the role of elective birth in twin pregnancy from 37 weeks' gestation[132] identified a single small randomized, controlled trial from Japan assessing elective birth with continued expectant management.[133] This study identified no statistically significant differences. However, the sample size was underpowered to detect meaningful differences, and insufficient data are available to support the practice of elective birth from 37 weeks' gestation in women with an otherwise uncomplicated twin pregnancy. A multicenter randomized, controlled trial is in progress, coordinated by the Maternal Perinatal Clinical Trials Unit at the University of Adelaide, to assess the optimal timing of birth in women with twin pregnancy at term.[134]

Intrapartum blood loss is greater in multiple pregnancy, as is the risk of postpartum hemorrhage. An intravenous access line should be inserted early in labor and blood obtained to estimate maternal hemoglobin or hematocrit and to hold serum for cross-matching, if needed later.

For a vaginal birth, both twins should be monitored continuously.[127] Initially, only external fetal monitoring will be possible. When feasible, a scalp electrode should be placed on the first twin, with continuation of external monitoring of the second twin. The use of a twin fetal heart rate monitor allows simultaneous recording of the two fetal heart rate tracings. If continuous monitoring of the second twin is impossible, some recommend cesarean section because of the higher risk of fetal asphyxia in twins, which may go undetected without adequate monitoring.

Epidural analgesia is widely used, providing the mother with adequate pain relief, and minimizes the risk that she will push before full dilation occurs.[127] In addition, adequate analgesia is provided in the event that operative birth, internal podalic version of the second twin, or cesarean delivery is needed. The widespread use of epidural anesthesia often negates the need for emergency general anesthesia with the complications discussed earlier, although it may still be needed for emergency cesarean section for fetal distress.

The optimal mode of birth in multiple pregnancy is controversial.[135] For triplets and higher-order multiple gestations, the most frequent mode of delivery is cesarean section,[136–138] although no randomized studies are available to support this mode of birth over vaginal birth. Reports suggest that the risk of lower Apgar scores in higher-order multiple gestations is reduced with cesarean delivery[42,139]; in addition, there are fewer perinatal deaths.[42]

Neonatal respiratory disease was more common in twins born by cesarean section at 36 to 38 weeks than in those born vaginally at 38 to 40 weeks.[140] Another report suggested higher perinatal mortality rates with cesarean delivery, primarily as a result of respiratory distress syndrome.[141] This has led to the suggested role of prophylactic corticosteroid administration prior to elective cesarean section.[142]

The Cochrane Systematic Review of the mode of birth for the second twin[143] identified a single randomized trial[144] comparing planned vaginal birth with planned cesarean birth for the second, nonvertex twin. This study highlighted the need for further evidence from randomized, controlled trials to inform practice. To provide more reliable information about the optimal mode of birth for women with twin pregnancy, a randomized, controlled trial (Twin Birth Study) is in progress, coordinated by the University of Toronto's Centre for Mother, Infant, and Child Research.[145]

Based on the literature on twin pregnancy, some recommendations can be made. The mode of birth is often affected by the presentation of the twins, which may be divided into the following three groups:

- First twin vertex, second twin vertex.
- First twin vertex, second twin nonvertex.
- First twin nonvertex.

First Twin Vertex, Second Twin Vertex

The most common presentation of twins is vertex-vertex. In this case, most obstetricians recommend vaginal birth,[146–149] and the literature supports vaginal birth, even of very low–birth weight infants (<1500 g).[147,150,151]

First Twin Vertex, Second Twin Nonvertex

For twins presenting as first twin vertex, second twin nonvertex, opinion is divided as to the optimal mode of birth. Some recommend elective cesarean delivery, reporting reduced neonatal mortality and morbidity rates for the second twin.[146,152] Others suggest that there is no increase in neonatal risk associated with vaginal birth of the second twin weighing 1500 g or more, either as breech presentation after internal podalic version if the fetus does not have a longitudinal lie or as cephalic presentation after external cephalic version.[153–158] The only randomized study found no difference in neonatal outcome in 60 nonvertex second twins at 35 weeks' gestation or more. Study subjects were randomly allocated to either vaginal delivery or cesarean section.[144,159] Assessment of whether vaginal breech delivery is appropriate is necessary using the standard criteria for singleton birth. These include exclusion of cephalopelvic disproportion, estimated fetal weight of less than approximately 3500 g, and the finding of a flexed fetal head on ultrasound.

For a nonvertex second twin of very low birth weight (<1500 g), the mode of birth is controversial. Some reports recommend cesarean delivery to minimize birth trauma to the preterm infant,[147,153,155,158,160] whereas others show no neonatal benefit and emphasize that vaginal delivery has reduced risks for the mother.[151] No randomized studies have compared vaginal and cesarean birth in these infants.

First Twin Nonvertex

When the first twin is nonvertex, cesarean delivery is often preferred[135,148] and advised,[147] although no series suggests that vaginal birth is inappropriate. It is likely that this approach is influenced by the data on the optimum mode of delivery in singleton breech presentations (see Chapter 63). By following such a policy, the risk of twin entrapment by interlocking chins or heads can be avoided.

PROCEDURE

TWIN BIRTH

For a vaginal twin birth, at least one experienced obstetrician, anesthetist, pediatrician, and neonatal nurse should be in attendance. Depending on gestational age (e.g., if preterm) and circumstances (e.g., operative birth, abnormal cardiotocographic findings), a double pediatric team (two pediatricians and two neonatal nurses) may be appropriate. For higher-order multiple births, one pediatric team should be present for each infant. Some recommend having a nurse scrubbed and the operating room prepared for emergency cesarean section.

For a vaginal birth, delivery of the first twin should be as for a singleton. After the birth of the first twin, an experienced obstetrician assesses the lie and presentation of the second twin. This assessment can be

FIGURE 59–3
Modified external version for delivery of the second twin.

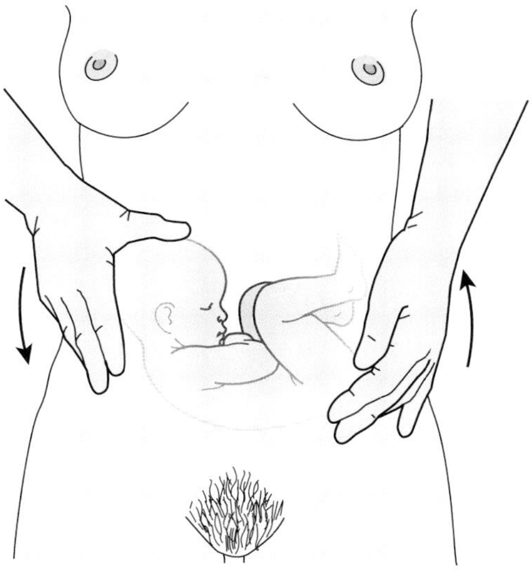

FIGURE 59–4
Internal podalic version.

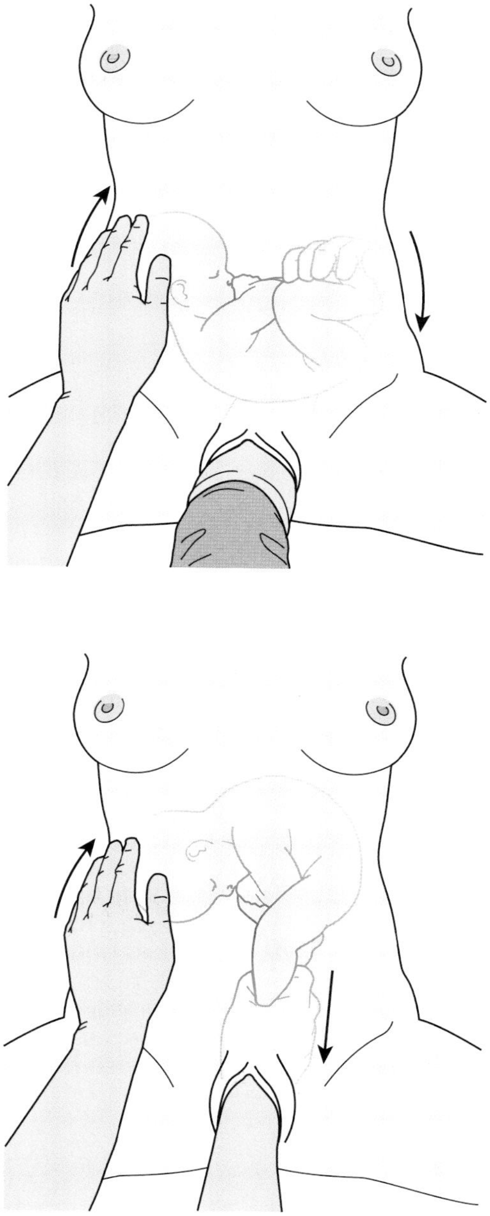

done by vaginal examination, abdominal palpation, or transabdominal ultrasound examination. The lie should be corrected to longitudinal by external version or internal podalic version.[161] External version (Fig. 59–3) gently turns the fetus so that the vertex lies above the pelvic brim. Amniotomy can be performed if there are uterine contractions (discussed later), and then delivery is completed. Version is more likely to be successful with epidural anesthesia and when the twins are of similar weight (difference of <500 g).[156]

In two series, external version was less likely than breech extraction to result in a vaginal birth.[158,162] Emergency cesarean section and complications such as cord prolapse and fetal distress were more frequent in the external version group. Although these were not randomized studies, in view of these findings, internal podalic version, if necessary, and breech delivery are recommended by some obstetricians if the lie is nonlongitudinal or the breech is presenting. However, others prefer to use external cephalic version and perform amniotomy once the lie is longitudinal and there are regular uterine contractions. They advocate cesarean delivery if the lie remains nonlongitudinal. Oxytocin (Syntocinon) infusion is mandatory if there is uterine inertia, and it is normal practice in many units to have an infusion ready at the onset of the second stage of labor. Once there are contractions and the lie is longitudinal, amniotomy is performed and birth proceeds with maternal effort during contractions. A scalp electrode can be applied after amniotomy to permit continuous fetal heart rate monitoring, or an external monitor can be used. Most authors advise continuous monitoring of the second twin throughout the second stage of labor, given the increased risk of intrapartum asphyxia. The risk of fetal distress and acidosis is increased if the twin-twin delivery interval exceeds 30 minutes.[163] If fetal distress develops and birth cannot be achieved safely, or if the second twin does not descend into the pelvis, emergency cesarean delivery is necessary.

After birth of the second infant, active management of the third stage of labor is recommended with an oxytocic agent.[164] To prevent uterine atony, in many units, an oxytocin infusion is continued for 3 to 4 hours.

Internal podalic version with vaginal breech delivery remains an option for birth of the second twin when a nonlongitudinal lie persists and the membranes are intact (Fig. 59–4). This approach involves the following steps:

- Use adequate analgesia, usually epidural, but possibly a general anesthetic.
- Place the patient in the lithotomy position.
- Provide continuous fetal heart rate monitoring.

- Use aseptic technique, and catheterize the patient.
- Ensure that a pediatrician is present.
- Determine the lie of the second twin by abdominal palpation, internal examination, or transabdominal ultrasound examination.
- Locate a fetal foot. Confirm that the structure is a foot rather than a wrist by palpating the heel.
- Perform an amniotomy.
- Grasp the foot, and pull down into the vagina. Grasp both feet, if possible.
- With maternal effort during contractions, deliver the fetus as an assisted breech.

Complications

Complications include
- Fetal anoxia.
- Difficulty with delivery of the head with breech presentation.
- Fetal trauma as a result of breech delivery (e.g., dislocated hips).
- Inadvertent delivery of a hand with shoulder presentation.
- Placental abruption.
- Cord accident.
- Endometritis.
- Maternal trauma (e.g., ruptured uterus).

Twin Entrapment

Twin entrapment may occur if the first twin is delivered as a breech and the second twin is cephalic and the head of the second twin enters the pelvis before the head of the leading twin. Some maintain that the risk of twin entrapment can be avoided by performing elective cesarean section if the first twin is breech and the second twin is cephalic. In an emergency, an attempt may be made to separate the locked twins by passing a hand vaginally between the chins of the fetuses and pushing the second twin upward. If this attempt fails, emergency cesarean section is necessary. Alternatively, an attempt may be made to push back the first twin, presenting as a breech, and allow the "second" twin, presenting cephalically, to deliver first. Again, if this attempt fails, emergency cesarean delivery is necessary.

During cesarean section, the head of the first twin is maneuvered upward, enabling birth of the second twin's head and body. The "first" twin may then be delivered. Some recommend having a second obstetrician available to manipulate the infants vaginally, if necessary.

If the first twin is already dead, rather than cesarean birth, there is the option of decapitation of the first twin, vaginal delivery of the second twin, and delivery of the head of the first twin. Such a destructive procedure should be performed under general anesthesia to protect the mother from seeing it. Many believe that this option should not be used in modern obstetrics, and some would argue that abdominal delivery may be associated with a lower incidence of perinatal asphyxia for the second twin.

Complications

In twin entrapment, the risk of fetal death of the first twin is high, as is the risk of fetal hypoxia for both twins. Maternal risks relate to the need for emergency cesarean section, endometritis, and the possible need for general anesthesia.

Postnatal

After the birth of twins, the mother may require a prolonged hospital stay. Breast-feeding should be encouraged, and additional support is important. The provision of adequate contraception is necessary and should be discussed. Coordinated support to help the parents care for their infants should be available.[125]

Before discharge, if extra help is not available at home, additional community support may need to be arranged. Maintaining contact with the local multiple birth support group during the puerperium is important.

SUMMARY OF MANAGEMENT OPTIONS

Multiple Pregnancy

Management Options	Evidence Quality and Recommendation	References
Prepregnancy		
Counsel women who are undergoing assisted conception techniques about the risks of multiple pregnancy.	III/B	56
No data are available to indicate the "ideal" number of embryos or oocytes to replace. But, there is guidance encouraging the consideration of single embryo replacement.	Ia/A	61
Supplement folate pre- and periconception.	Ia/A	63
Prenatal		
Specialized twin clinics may lessen adverse outcomes. Little evidence supports other forms of prenatal care.	III/B	64–66
Document zygosity or chorionicity at 10–14 wk. But no prospective data are available on whether this documentation improves outcome.	III/B	75

Management Options	Evidence Quality and Recommendation	References
Maintain increased surveillance if twins are monozygous or monochorionic.	IIb/B	165
Monochorionic twins are at increased risk for adverse outcome. But no prospective data are available on whether increased surveillance improves outcome.		
Supplement iron and folate from the second trimester.	IIb/B	11
Screen for hypertension.	IIa/B	67
There is conflicting evidence of the value of screening for gestational diabetes.	IIa/B	68,69
Nuchal translucency measurement of each fetus identifies fetuses at risk for trisomy 21, cardiothoracic abnormalities, and twin-twin transfusion syndrome.	III/B	78
Obtain routine anomaly ultrasound scan at 18–20 wk.	III/B	48
Conjoined twins: • Obtain careful ultrasonographic evaluation of anatomy. • Provide interdisciplinary discussion of therapeutic options.	III/B	92
Be vigilant for early symptoms of preterm labor; prompt self-referral if suspected.	Ib/A	112
Obtain possible ultrasound assessment of cervical changes and fetal fibronectin as part of preterm delivery screening.	IIa/B	96
Provide prenatal corticosteroids if preterm birth before 34 wk is possible.	Ia/A	118
There is no evidence that hospitalization prevents preterm labor and delivery.	Ia/A	100
There is no evidence that prophylactic cervical cerclage prevents preterm labor and delivery.	Ia/A	113
Obtain regular fetal ultrasound assessment of growth and umbilical artery Doppler.	Ib/A	122
Hospitalize at the woman's request or if complications are detected.	Ia/A	100
Consider therapeutic amniocentesis (repeated if necessary) for extreme hydramnios and maternal distress.	IIb/B	166
Provide prenatal education about the possible modes of delivery, analgesia, and care in labor.	IV/C	126
Labor and Delivery		
Arrange for hospital delivery.	III/B	127
Have experienced obstetrician and other health professionals on stand by.	III/B	127
Await spontaneous labor if no complications occur.	Ia/A	132
Have pediatrician, neonatal nurse, and anesthetist available at delivery, with one pediatrician per infant present if preterm or operative delivery or fetal problems are anticipated.	GPP	—
Maintain continuous monitoring of all fetuses during labor.	III/B	127
Provide IV access.	GPP	—
Epidural analgesia recommended.	III/B	127
Aim for vaginal delivery unless the leading twin has a nonlongitudinal lie.	III/B	140,151
Some advocate elective cesarean delivery if the first twin is not cephalic.	III/B	140,151
Arrange for vaginal delivery of the first twin, if appropriate.	III/B	151
Consider synthetic oxytocin infusion for uterine inertia, especially after the first twin is delivered.	GPP	—
If the second twin has a longitudinal lie, perform amniotomy and deliver.	III/B	161

SUMMARY OF MANAGEMENT OPTIONS

Multiple Pregnancy—cont'd

Management Options	Evidence Quality and Recommendation	References
If an infant has a nonlongitudinal lie, convert to a longitudinal lie by external version or internal podalic version.	III/B	161
Infuse oxytocin prophylactically after delivery to reduce the risk of postpartum hemorrhage.	Ia/A	163
Some advocate elective cesarean delivery for triplets and higher-order births.	IIb/B	141
Postnatal		
Provide extra support while in the hospital to assist with infant care.	GPP	—
Offer longer in-patient stay.	GPP	—
Arrange support at home.	GPP	—
Provide adequate contraceptive advice.	GPP	—

GPP, good practice point.

SUGGESTED READINGS

Crowther C: Caesarean delivery for the second twin (Cochrane Review). In Cochrane Library. Oxford, Update Software, Issue 1, 2004.

Crowther C: Hospitalisation for bed rest in multiple pregnancy (Cochrane Review). In Cochrane Library. Oxford, Update Software, Issue 1, 2004.

Crowther CA, Harding JE: Repeat doses of prenatal corticosteroids for women at risk of preterm birth for preventing neonatal respiratory disease. Cochrane Database Syst Rev 2007;3:CD003935.

Dodd J, Crowther C: Elective delivery from 37 weeks gestation in women with a twin pregnancy (Cochrane Review). In Cochrane Library. Oxford, Update Software, Issue 1, 2005.

Dodd J, Crowther C: Reduction of the number of fetuses for women with triplet and higher order multiple pregnancies (Cochrane Review). In Cochrane Library. Oxford, Update Software, Issue 1, 2005.

Dodd JM, Flenady VJ, Cincotta R, Crowther CA: Prenatal progesterone for prevention of preterm birth. Cochrane Database Syst Rev 2006;1:CD004947.

Hofmeyr G, Drakely A: Delivery of twins. Ballieres Clin Obstet Gynaecol 1998;12:91–108.

Keirse M, Grant A, King J: Preterm labour. In Chalmers I, Enkin M, Keirse M (eds): Effective Care in Pregnancy and Childbirth. Oxford, Oxford University Press, 1989, pp 694–749.

Neilson J, Alfirevic Z: Doppler ultrasound for fetal assessment in high risk pregnancies (Cochrane Review). In Cochrane Library. Oxford, Update Software, Issue 1, 2004.

Royal College of Obstetricians and Gynaecologists (RCOG): Consensus views arising from the 50th study group: Multiple pregnancy. London, RCOG, 2006. Available at http://www.rcog.org.uk/files/rcog-corp/uploaded-files/StudyGroupConsensusViewsMultiplePregnancy.pdf

REFERENCES

For a complete list of references, log onto www.expertconsult.com.

CHAPTER 60

Screening for Spontaneous Preterm Labor and Delivery

ROBERT OGLE, JONATHON HYETT, and ANTHONY J. MARREN

Videos corresponding to this chapter are available online at www.expertconsult.com.

INTRODUCTION

Preterm birth is associated with significant perinatal morbidity and mortality rates. Adverse outcomes from preterm birth include cerebral palsy, developmental delay, chronic lung disease, and visual and hearing loss. About 40% of preterm births follow idiopathic preterm labor, 35% follow preterm prelabor rupture of membranes, and the remainder are iatrogenic because of obstetric or medical indications.[1] The early detection of preterm labor or preterm rupture of membranes in traditional antenatal care is often problematic because symptoms or signs may vary only a little from the normal physiologic symptoms and signs of pregnancy. The criteria for diagnosis of preterm labor, defined by the onset of increasingly frequent and painful uterine contractions with progressive effacement and dilation of the cervix, can be assessed most accurately once contractions occur at least once every 10 minutes, there is 80% cervical effacement, and the cervix is at least 3 cm dilated.[2,3] However, the patient may frequently present with relatively mild symptoms and signs suggestive of labor, which may be features of normal pregnancy.[4] Using lower thresholds for contraction frequency and cervical change will, therefore, affect the sensitivity and positive predictive value of clinical assessment for detection of preterm labor.

Prediction of preterm birth would ideally involve a screening test with high sensitivity and high negative predictive value. It should also enable effective intervention if the test gives a positive result. Until recently, the screening tools and interventions that were available did not enable obstetricians to decrease the incidence of preterm birth and, therefore, did not satisfy the requirements of an optimal screening test. However, in 2007, Fonseca and associates[5] published a randomized, controlled trial suggesting that effective screening by measuring cervical length at 23 weeks' gestation and therapeutic intervention with progestins to 34 weeks could reduce the risk of preterm delivery by 42%, which may translate into improved neonatal outcomes. A wide variety of screening tools have been evaluated in research, and those most extensively evaluated fall into four groups:

- Monitoring of uterine activity.
- Assessment of cervical length.
- Measurement of cervical fetal fibronectin.
- Presence of bacterial vaginosis in early pregnancy.

Other forms of screening have been looked at in small series and include estimation of estriol, interleukins, ferritin, and corticotropin-releasing hormone, but findings in relation to these measures have not been consistently associated with preterm labor. This chapter reviews the four major areas of screening and evaluates their effectiveness in screening for preterm labor and preterm rupture of membranes.

MONITORING UTERINE ACTIVITY

If the onset of increasingly frequent and painful uterine contractions precedes effacement and dilation of the cervix, then assessment of uterine activity may identify pregnancies at risk of preterm delivery at an early stage of preterm labor, allowing effective intervention.

The simplest method for assessing uterine activity relies on teaching the patient to palpate and record her own contractions. Increased uterine activity appears to precede a clinical diagnosis of preterm labor by less than 24 hours.[6] Most obstetricians using this technique would therefore advise the patient to monitor her own contractions for an hour twice a day. Although this technique has the advantage that it does not involve any expensive equipment, it is completely subjective and has been shown to have poor sensitivity, with 89% of women palpating less than 50% of their contractions.[7] In addition, the process of monitoring is time-consuming, is generally limited to high risk groups, and potentially increases patient anxiety, which is itself associated with an increased risk of preterm delivery. This issue applies equally to other forms of uterine activity monitoring; indeed, these techniques require intense patient support through a process of education, analysis of results, and encouragement to continue monitoring on a regular basis, and it has frequently been suggested that it is this support that leads to an improvement in outcome more often than the process of monitoring itself.[8]

A more objective approach to uterine activity monitoring involves tocography, monitoring activity indirectly via a pressure transducer attached to a recording device and placed against the maternal abdominal wall. Early studies with this technique demonstrated that normal uterine activity increases with advancing gestation and is more pronounced at night. Uterine activity was monitored in a series of 109 low risk pregnancies that delivered at term; the 95th percentile was 1.3 contractions per hour at 21 to 24 weeks, 2.9 contractions per hour at 28 to 32 weeks, and 4.9 contractions per hour at 38 to 40 weeks.[9] It was found that 96% of recordings had fewer than 4 contractions per hour, and this threshold is often used to define a risk of preterm labor. An early case-control study recruited 76 women at high risk of preterm labor to assess whether daily ambulatory home uterine monitoring could facilitate an early diagnosis of preterm labor and compared them with 76 matched control subjects.[10] The rates of threatened preterm labor were similar in the study and control groups (51% vs. 45%), but the cervix was significantly less effaced and dilated and there were no cases of ruptured membranes at the time of diagnosis in the monitored group. Consequently, all cases were considered suitable for long-term tocolytic therapy, and the preterm delivery rate was lower in the monitored group (22%) than in the control group (41%).

Although this initial series appeared to give encouraging results, there are several problems with this technique. Few studies have validated the instrumentation used in home monitoring. Those that have been performed suggest that patients are readily able to use the machines, that home machines appear to be of similar sensitivity as hospital machines, and that they detect more than 90% of contractions recorded by an intrauterine pressure catheter during normal term labor.[11–13] However, the sensitivity and specificity of the tocometer vary according to its position, the tension on the belt, and the thickness of the maternal abdominal wall, so the amplitude of the waveform seen on a tocogram cannot be related to the strength of uterine activity. Data interpretation is also subject to observational error, with one study finding that the results were interpreted reliably in only 70% of cases by a single observer.[14]

Perhaps more important, monitoring uterine activity does not lend itself to screening a low risk population; the equipment is relatively expensive, monitoring is time-consuming, studies need to be repeated regularly for many weeks of pregnancy, and data analysis requires a skilled health care professional. The technique is, therefore, suitable only for pregnancies deemed to be at high risk for preterm labor. Many randomized, controlled trials have evaluated the use of home uterine activity monitoring in such high risk pregnancies. The first six were reviewed qualitatively by the U.S. Preventative Services Task Force.[15] They concluded that there was insufficient evidence to recommend for or against home uterine activity monitoring as a screening test for preterm labor in high risk pregnancies, but recommendations against its use could be made on other grounds, including cost and inconvenience. In response to these recommendations, Colton and associates[16] conducted a meta-analysis of the same six studies, but accessed previously unpublished data from the study groups and defined four outcome measures: incidence of preterm birth, incidence of preterm labor with a cervical dilation of over 2 cm at diagnosis, neonatal admission to intensive care, and mean birth weight.[8,17–22] The meta-analysis, presenting data from six studies on a total of only 697 pregnancies, concluded that home uterine monitoring in singleton pregnancies was associated with a 24% reduction in preterm birth, a 52% reduction in "late presentation" with cervical dilation greater than 2 cm, and a significant mean increase in birth weight of 126 g. There was, however, no difference in the admission rate to neonatal intensive care.[16] This analysis was controversial. Grimes and coworkers[23] analyzed the methodology of four of the six studies. They demonstrated that the included studies were of poor scientific rigor. Their combined crude relative risk for preterm birth was 0.9—a small improvement in outcome, which could easily have resulted from any one of the methodologic shortcomings. One of the criticisms of early trials of home uterine monitoring was that the increased level of support that the monitored patients received may have been responsible for any improvement seen in the outcome. Three trials addressed this possibility, one using a sham monitor but offering all patients nursing support,[24] the second offering monitoring without any nursing support,[25] and the third randomly assigning patients to both nursing support and home monitoring.[26] The first of these studies randomized 1992 women, 1165 of whom used home monitoring devices, but only 842 (72.3%) of them completed the study, suggesting that there may be difficulties with compliance when home monitoring devices are used for wider indications.[24] The study concluded that there was no evidence that either home uterine activity monitoring or daily nursing contact improved early diagnosis of preterm labor or reduced the rates of preterm birth or neonatal morbidity.[24] In contrast, the second, smaller study ($N = 218$), which also had a significant dropout rate in monitoring (15% did not complete the monitoring), found that the diagnosis of preterm labor could be made significantly earlier and that this affected the outcome, measured in terms of the interval between the diagnosis of labor and delivery, and was independent of nursing support.[25] However, the third study, which randomly assigned 2422 women to combinations of nurse contact and home monitoring, concluded that neither daily contact nor home monitoring improved pregnancy outcome beyond that seen with weekly nurse contact.[26]

Because little evidence indicates that home uterine monitoring is a useful screening tool for preterm labor, the number of studies examining its role has dropped significantly since the year 2000. During this time, interest in other markers for preterm delivery, such as sonographic assessment of the cervix and measurement of fetal fibronectin, has grown. Consequently, the recent data sets that review home uterine monitoring are often acquired in trials primarily designed to assess other screening tests or a combination of screening tools. Although most of the original trials defined preterm delivery before 37 completed weeks as their endpoint, more recent data sets are concerned with delivery before 34 weeks' gestation. Morrison and colleagues[27] assessed 85 asymptomatic women at high risk of preterm labor with both serial fetal fibronectin measurement and home uterine monitoring. They reported that 14 (16.5%) of the 85 women delivered before 34 weeks and the sensitivity and specificity of fetal fibronectin and home uterine monitoring alone were 43% and 89% (fetal fibronectin) and 64% and 85% (home uterine monitoring alone). When the two tests were combined, the specificity improved substantially but the sensitivity of a double-positive result was poor (3 of 14 cases [21%]), so they are not usefully combined in this manner.

A study of home uterine monitoring to assess the risk of preterm labor in 306 high-risk singleton pregnancies was reported in 2002.[28] These patients were also seen regularly at the hospital for serial assessment of fetal fibronectin and for sonographic assessment of the cervix. All three investigations had a low sensitivity and poor positive predictive value for preterm delivery. The authors concluded that, although the likelihood of preterm delivery is associated with an increased frequency of uterine contractions, assessment of uterine activity is not clinically useful for predicting preterm delivery.

CERVICAL SCREENING

Ultrasound assessment of the cervix in normal pregnancy shows that cervical effacement starts around 32 weeks. In pregnancies affected by preterm labor, the process may begin between 16 and 24 weeks. Effacement begins at the internal os and can be visualized as cervical shortening and funneling, a process that occurs before dilation of the external cervical os. Ultrasound assessment potentially allows changes other than cervical dilation to be assessed with a higher degree of accuracy, and using a transvaginal route, assessment is possible in almost all cases.[29,30]

Ultrasound assessment of the cervix has been used in a variety of situations to improve the accuracy of a diagnosis of preterm labor and to predict the likelihood of a woman going into preterm labor. Screening has been studied in both high and low risk populations, and because the prevalence of preterm labor varies in these groups, these data sets are considered separately. A variety of techniques have been used to assess the cervix with ultrasound, and the multitude of studies describing the use of this test are heterogeneous in design, assessing the cervix at different stages of pregnancy, using either single or serial examinations, and choosing varying gestational ages at delivery to report the sensitivity and specificity of the test. A meta-analysis of antenatal transvaginal ultrasound assessment of the cervix identified 46 studies involving 31,577 pregnancies describing the effectiveness of this screening technique.[31] The review concluded that assessment of both cervical length and funneling, either alone or in combination, appeared to be useful in predicting spontaneous preterm birth in asymptomatic women, although there were less data available to assess the usefulness of this technique in symptomatic patients.

Digital Measurement of the Cervix

Sonek and associates[32] compared digital and transvaginal assessment of the cervix in 83 gravidas—56 from a population considered at-risk for preterm delivery and 27 with no risk factors. Analyzing the at-risk cohort, the authors found that in the second trimester, 87% of cervical length measurements by digital examination were less than those by transvaginal sonography, and 13% were greater. A similar association was seen in the third trimester. Linear regression analysis was used to evaluate the strength of association—the r-value was only 0.49. The authors concluded that digital assessment of the cervix is subjective and does not correlate well with transvaginal assessment.

Ultrasound Measurement of the Cervix

One of the problems with comparison of studies measuring cervical change is a lack of standardization of the investigational technique. Most sonographers assess the cervix using a transvaginal scan, but transabdominal and transperineal routes can also be used. The cervix may be curved, and there may evidence of funneling; it is important to establish a method that allows for these differences in a consistent manner. The cervix is a dynamic structure, and measurements are affected by factors such as bladder filling and abdominal pressure.

A standardized technique for transvaginal cervical assessment has been described.[33] After the patient has emptied her bladder, a transvaginal probe (5–7 MHz) is introduced into the anterior fornix of the vagina, taking care to optimize image quality while avoiding undue pressure on the cervix that will distort anatomy. The whole length of the sonolucent endocervical mucosa is identified in a sagittal section, and the image is magnified so that this occupies 75% of the screen. Calipers are placed from the triangular echodense area marking the external os to the V-shaped indentation marking the internal os, and this distance is measured in a straight line. Three measurements are made over a period of 3 minutes to allow for any change in the state of the cervix, and the shortest measurement is reported. This technique allows clear views of the cervix and lower uterine segment and is acceptable to the majority of patients.

For women who do not find transvaginal sonography acceptable, or in circumstances in which vaginal examination ideally would be avoided (such as preterm prelabor rupture of membranes), alternative techniques such as transabdominal or transperineal/translabial assessment may be used. The limitations of these techniques, however, must be recognized. Transabdominal cervical assessment in 149 low risk singleton pregnancies at 23 weeks' gestation demonstrated that it was harder to visualize the cervix as it became shorter: a cervical length of less than 20 mm could be identified only 13% of the time, whereas a cervical length greater than 20 mm could be identified 51% of the time (X^2 4.52; $P < .05$). In addition, the cervix was significantly easier to visualize when the bladder was fuller, but this state is associated with an increase in the length of the cervix.[34] Given this finding, transabdominal assessment of cervical length should be abandoned in favor of transvaginal assessment.

Visualization can also be difficult using a transperineal/translabial approach, and there is some evidence that the "operator learning curve" with this technique is substantial, making it a less appropriate test for screening.[35] Many authors have reported a poor correlation between transvaginal and transperineal/translabial techniques, making interpretation of data more difficult.[35–37] Cervical length in a low risk population is normally distributed, with a mean length at 23 weeks' gestation of 35 to 38 mm; the 10th and 90th percentiles are approximately 25 mm and 45 mm, respectively.

Other cervical parameters have also been investigated. In many circumstances, a sagittal section of the entire length of the endocervical canal shows that it is in fact curved, and direct measurement from the internal to external os does not take this curvature into account. In these circumstances, cervical length would be undermeasured, and there would be a potential for false-positive screening results. To and coworkers[38] investigated this in a prospective series of 300 singleton pregnancies undergoing transvaginal cervical assessment at 23 weeks' gestation. A curved cervix was seen in 48% of patients: in 51% of those with cervical length of 26 mm or more, 25% of those with cervical length of 16 to 25 mm, but 0% in those with cervical length of 15 mm or less. This group had previously defined that pregnancies with cervical length less than 15 mm should be considered to have a positive test result, and in these circumstances, the effect of cervical curvature would not be important.

Early studies of transvaginal cervical screening suggested that cervical funneling could also be reported and that this finding had an independent predictive role for preterm delivery.[39] Funneling can be assessed in a number of ways; subjectively, describing presence or absence, by measuring dilation at the internal os and the length of the endocervical canal that is involved, or by combining these features to give a cervical index.[40] In a series of 469 high risk pregnancies assessed longitudinally, funneling, determined in terms of width and length and the percentage of the cervix involved, was not found to give any additional information about risk if the cervical length was less than a screen-positive cutoff of 25 mm.[41] This was also the case in a series of 6819 low risk pregnancies screened at 23 weeks' gestation, in which funneling was defined as being present if the width at the internal cervical os was greater than 5 mm.[42] In this series, funneling appeared to be almost universally associated with a short cervix, and there was no apparent advantage to its inclusion as a screening criterion.

Cervical Assessment in Asymptomatic Patients at High Risk for Preterm Labor

Women with a previous history of preterm labor or preterm prelabor rupture of membranes together with women who have previously had cervical surgery or have a known uterine anomaly are considered to be at high risk of preterm labor. Other inclusion criteria have included extreme maternal age, in utero exposure to diethylstilbestrol, and maternal genetic anomalies such as Ehler-Danlos syndrome. The rationale for screening in this group is to allow early intervention that would prevent the onset of preterm delivery or preterm prelabor rupture of membranes.[43–45] It is not currently clear what the optimum gestation for screening is, what cervical cutoff should be used to define a screen-positive group, or whether serial scans would be more appropriate than a single scan.

There is a strong association between a short cervix and preterm delivery in high risk pregnancies. Cook and Ellwood[46] showed that cervical length less than 21 mm at less than 20 weeks' gestation was associated with 95% delivery by 34 weeks' gestation. Guzman and colleagues[40] examined 469 women at high risk of preterm delivery with singleton pregnancies serially (mean of three occasions) between 15 and 24 weeks' gestation. The cervix was 25 mm or less in length in 23.4% of women, including 76% of those delivering before 34 weeks' gestation. The negative predictive value of this cutoff was 96%. Similarly, Owen and associates[36] demonstrated that a single examination at 16 to 19 weeks' gestation with a cervix 25 mm or less in length increased the risk of preterm delivery by 35 weeks' gestation 3.3 times (95% confidence interval [CI] 2.1–5.0) and found that if serial examinations up to 24 weeks' gestation were performed, a single cervical length of less than 25 mm increased the risk of preterm labor 4.5 times (95% CI 2.7–7.6). Only limited data are available about the value of serial screening beyond 24 weeks' gestation, but in one small study ($N = 69$) of high risk pregnancies examined every 2 weeks from 16 to 30 weeks' gestation, cervical length and funneling were found to be significant at evaluations performed at 20 to 24 weeks as well as 25 to 29 weeks.[47]

Cervical Assessment in Asymptomatic Patients at Low Risk for Preterm Labor

The rationale for screening in a general, low risk population is that a significant proportion of preterm deliveries occur in pregnancies with no historical risk factors. The apparent effectiveness of screening high risk populations has led many groups to examine screening in a low risk group, and evaluation of cervical length seems to be of similar predictive value in this setting.[48–52] Iams and coworkers[48] reported a multicenter study of 2915 pregnancies recruited through 10 university perinatal centres in the United States. Investigators used a clearly described method to assess cervical length; the process involved initial training, a period of standardization of technique, and continuing audit of the quality of examinations. Both cervical length and funneling were examined, but although funneling seemed to be equally predictive of outcome, the authors noted that determination of this sign was less consistent, with a prevalence of 0% to 12.7% across centers. The predictive value of cervical assessment was reported in terms of the proportion of spontaneous preterm deliveries that occurred before 35 weeks' gestation; this occurred in 126 (4.3%) of the pregnancies enrolled. The mean cervical length at 24 weeks was 34.0 mm ± 7.8 mm for nulliparous women and 36.1 mm ± 8.4 mm for parous women. Cervical length was noted to be "normally" distributed. A cervical length less than 20 mm was found in less than 5% of women, and this group included 23% of preterm births (sensitivity); the specificity, positive predictive, and negative predictive values were 97, 25.7, and 96.5, respectively. The relative risk of preterm labor associated with various cervical lengths was also reported. These data were calculated relative to the risk of preterm delivery in the top quartile rather than relative to the background population as a whole. This approach demonstrated that there is a significant association between the risk of preterm labor and a short cervix. It also demonstrated that there was a continuum of risk, and the authors suggested that this challenged the traditional concept that the cervix is either competent or incompetent and provided evidence that cervical competence should be considered as a continuous variable.

Four other studies have examined large (>500 pregnancies) groups of low risk singleton pregnancies.[49–52] Although they are not directly comparable with the study of Iams and coworkers described earlier,[48] a review of their results demonstrates similar findings, that is, the risk of spontaneous preterm birth is inversely related to cervical length (Table 60–1).

As detailed previously, until recently, there was little evidence to suggest that screening in a low risk population was

TABLE 60–1

Comparison of Studies Reporting the Predictive Value of Transvaginal Ultrasound Assessment of Cervical Length for Preterm Labor*

FIRST AUTHOR	HASSAN[50]				HEATH[49]				HIBBARD[51]				IAMS[48]				TAIPALE[52]			
CENTER	U.S., SINGLE CENTER				U.K., SINGLE CENTER				U.S., SINGLE CENTER				U.S., MULTICENTER				FINLAND, SINGLE CENTER			
N	6877				2567				760				2915				3694			
GESTATION AT TEST	19 (14–24) WK				23 (22–24) WK				20 (16–22) WK				24 WK				20 (18–22) WK			
GESTATION OF OUTCOME†	32 WK (2.9%)				32 WK				32 WK (3.6%)				35 WK (4.3%)				35 WK (0.8%)			
	CX	PREV	OR	SENS	CX	PREV	OR	SENS	CX	PREV	RR	SENS	CX	PREV	RR	SENS	CX	PREV	RR	SENS
					5		51.5						13			13.99				
	10	0.3%	29.3		10				22	2.5%	8.4	18.5%	22		9.46	23%				
	15	0.6%	24.3	8.2%	15	1.7%	2.7	58%	27	5.0%	9.7	29.6%	26		6.19	37%	25	0.3%	20	100%
	20	0.9%	18.3	10.6%	20	3.4%			30	10.0%	5.2	44.4%	30		3.79	54%	29	3.0%	8	97%
	25	1.7%	13.4	14.7%	25	8.0%	0.71		38.5	50.0%			35		2.35		35	27.0%	2.2	73%
	30	9.1%	3.2		30	18.0%							40		1.98		40	52.0%	1.7	38%
	40	71.6%			40		0.45													
					50		0.24													

* The studies are heterogeneous in nature, reflected in the tabulated data.
† The prevalence of preterm delivery in the study population is given in parentheses.
Cx, cervical length (mm); Prev, prevalence of preterm delivery; OR, odds ratio for preterm delivery; RR, relative risk of preterm delivery; Sens, sensitivity of cutoff for prediction of preterm labor.

useful, because an effective intervention to improve pregnancy outcome had not yet been demonstrated.

Papiernik in 1970[53] was the first to use progesterone for the prevention of preterm birth. Ninety-nine women identified as being at risk of preterm birth via a risk scoring system were randomly assigned to either weekly injections of 17α-hydroxyprogesterone caproate or placebo. The preterm delivery rate in the intervention group was 4% compared with 18% in the placebo group. This initial study prompted multiple other studies aimed at determining the efficacy of progesterone in the prevention of preterm birth. These initial studies were summarized by two conflicting meta-analyses by Goldstein and colleagues[54] and Keirse.[55]

Interest in the efficacy of progesterone in preventing preterm birth was reignited in 2003 by da Fonseca and associates.[56] They randomized 157 asymptomatic, high risk (≥1 prior spontaneous preterm delivery, prophylactic cervical cerclage, or uterine malformation), singleton women to either progesterone (100 mg; $N = 72$) or placebo ($N = 70$) vaginal suppositories. They concluded that progesterone was effective in reducing the incidence of delivery prior to 37 (13.8% vs. 28.5%; $P = .03$) and 34 (2.8 vs. 18.6%; $P = .002$) weeks. However, they did not comment on perinatal outcomes.

Meis and coworkers[57] concluded that weekly intramuscular injections of 250 mg 17α-hydroxyprogesterone acetate from 16 to 20 weeks to 36 weeks in women at risk of preterm delivery based on historical factors significantly reduced the rate of spontaneous preterm delivery (<37 wk: 36.6% vs. 54.9%; relative risk [RR] 0.66; 95% CI 0.54–0.81) (<35 wk: 20.6 vs. 30.7%; RR 0.67; 95% CI 0.48–0.93) (<32 wk: 11.4 vs. 19.6%; RR 0.58; 95% CI 0.37–0.91) and was also associated with reduced rates of birth weight less than 2500 g (27.2% vs. 41.1%; RR 0.66; 95% CI 0.51–0.87), supplemental oxygen (14.9% vs. 23.8%; RR 0.62; 95% CI 0.42–0.82), and intraventricular haemorrhage (1.3% vs. 5.2%; RR 0.25; 95% CI 0.80–0.82).

However, O'Brien and colleagues[58] concluded that daily intravaginal progesterone gel (equivalent to 90 mg) in women at risk of preterm delivery based on historical factors did not reduce the rate of early preterm delivery (≤32 wk) or decrease perinatal mortality/morbidity rates.

In an attempt to clarify the role of progesterone in preventing preterm delivery, Dodd and associates[59] for the *Cochrane Collaboration* in 2006 performed a meta-analysis and concluded that intramuscular progesterone is associated with a reduction in the risk of preterm delivery (<37 wk: RR 0.68; 95% CI 0.56–0.82) and birth weight less than 250g (RR 0.63; 95% CI 0.49–0.81). Intravaginal progesterone is associated with a reduction in the risk of preterm birth (<37 wk: RR 0.49; 95% CI 0.25–0.96) (<34 wk: RR 0.15; 95% CI 0.04–0.64).

In 2007, Fonseca and associates[5] published a randomized, controlled trial suggesting that effective screening by measuring cervical length between 20 and 25 weeks' gestation and therapeutic intervention for those with a cervical length of 15 mm or less with progestins (200 mg intravaginal suppositories) to 34 weeks could reduce the risk of preterm delivery (<34 wk: 20.8% vs. 36.0%; RR 0.58; 95% CI 0.38–0.87). There was no statistically significant reduction in perinatal mortality or morbidity; however, the trial was not sufficiently powered to address these points.

Whereas there is sufficient evidence that cervical length assessment can accurately predict those women who are at risk of preterm delivery, evidence regarding intravaginal/intramuscular progesterone therapy preventing preterm delivery and especially improving perinatal outcomes is less clear-cut. Therefore, it is the opinion of the authors that a screening policy such as transvaginal assessment of cervical length should be offered to all women at the time of their routine anomaly ultrasound because this would facilitate identifying those women in need of close surveillance and potentially enable timely administration of corticosteroids. Further research is warranted as to whether progesterone therapy results in improved perinatal outcomes, and "at risk" women should be encouraged to enroll in future trials that address this question.

Cervical Assessment in Patients Symptomatic of Preterm Labor

Early diagnosis of preterm labor potentially allows early intervention to reduce the risk of preterm delivery or to optimize conditions for the premature neonate. The clinical diagnosis of labor is dependent on the presence of uterine activity with cervical effacement and dilation, and accurate cervical assessment is therefore important. Traditional digital examination tends to be imprecise, with large margins of inter- and intraoperator error. The rationale for using ultrasound to assess the cervix in women presenting with symptoms of preterm labor is that cervical assessment will be more precise, allowing earlier treatment of women with evidence of cervical change but reducing the proportion of women who are not in preterm labor and have unnecessary treatment.

Cervical effacement has many potential causes. This process may be biologic or may represent a mechanical weakness that is revealed as the uterus becomes distended. Alternatively, it may be secondary to the onset of uterine contraction or to inflammation and the release of local hormones in response to infection or hemorrhage. It is unlikely that a single form of therapy will resolve all the etiologies underlying cervical effacement and dilation, and this may explain why most randomized, controlled trials of cervical cerclage have not shown this to be an effective method of preventing preterm birth.

Cervical Screening in Twin Pregnancies

The incidence of preterm delivery is significantly higher in multiple pregnancies, with a consequent effect on perinatal mortality and morbidity rates in these infants. From 5% to 10% of twins deliver before 33 weeks' gestation, a sixfold increase over the rate of preterm delivery in singleton pregnancies by this gestation.[60] Despite this, fewer studies have assessed the use of cervical screening in twin pregnancies, and it is less clear whether ultrasound assessment is useful or at what week of gestation ultrasound should be performed.

A prospective cohort of 177 pregnancies was used to evaluate cervical length in normal twin pregnancies.[61] Of these 177, 28 (16.3%) pregnancies delivered before 34 weeks' gestation and were excluded from further analysis. In the remainder, the mean cervical length decreased from 47 mm at 13 weeks' gestation to 32 mm at 32 weeks' gestation in a linear fashion. The rate of cervical shortening was 0.8 mm/wk.

Ong and coworkers[62] suggested that from a clinical perspective, it is not the estimation of risk per se that is important, but the prediction of preterm labor within a limited timeframe, allowing admission, preparative treatment (such as steroid therapy), and transfer to a unit with appropriate neonatal facilities. Cervical length was assessed every 2 weeks in 46 twin pregnancies between 24 weeks' gestation and delivery. Only data from pregnancies that labored spontaneously were subsequently included in the analysis. There was no difference in the rate of shortening between pregnancies delivering before and after 37 weeks' gestation. An absolute threshold for cervical length was, however, more useful: cervical lengths of less than 20 mm and less than 25 mm had relative risks of delivery within 1 week of 11.67 (95% CI 4.23–32.17) and 4.12 (95% CI 1.10–15.47), respectively. A similar longitudinal study of only 20 twin pregnancies suggested a difference in the rate of cervical shortening between women delivering preterm (<36 wk' gestation) and those delivering at term. After excluding 1 preterm delivery that had a short cervix at the time of the first scan (10 mm at 24 wk' gestation), the rate of shortening was found to be 2.9 mm/wk and 1.8 mm/wk in preterm and term pregnancies, respectively. This difference was not statistically significant, but this may have been due to the relatively low numbers enrolled.[63]

Skentou and colleagues[64] also examined various thresholds for cervical length to predict the risk of preterm delivery. This prospective study of 464 twin pregnancies involved a single transvaginal ultrasound assessment at 23 (22–24) weeks' gestation. This study included 313 (67.5%) dichorionic and 151 (32.5%) monochorionic twin pregnancies and found no significant difference in the rate of preterm delivery (defined as before 34 wk' gestation) in these two groups. A significant inverse relationship was found between cervical length and the risk of preterm birth (risk = 26.48 × cervical length − 1.688) such that thresholds of 15 mm, 20 mm, and 25 mm detected 17.6%, 39.1%, and 46.4% of twin pregnancies delivering before 34 weeks, respectively. The corresponding screen-positive rates were higher than those seen in singleton pregnancies: 2.1%, 4.7%, and 9.6%.

In addition to assessing cervical length, Guzman and associates[65] looked at cervical funneling and the effect of transfundal pressure during the examination. A series of 131 pregnancies were examined serially between 15 and 28 weeks' gestation. The effectiveness of assessments at 15 to 20, 21 to 24, and 25 to 28 weeks' gestation for the prediction of preterm delivery by 28, 30, 32, and 34 weeks' gestation were evaluated. Although the cervix was significantly shorter with transfundal pressure, this application did not improve the investigators' ability to predict preterm labor. A cervical length of less than 20 mm was found to be at least as good as any other characteristic at predicting spontaneous preterm delivery.

These data differ slightly from the findings of another group who investigated the associations between preterm delivery and a short cervix and cervical funneling in a series of 251 twin pregnancies, examined at 22 and 27 weeks' gestation.[66] A receiver operating characteristic curve showed no clear best cutoff point for cervical length at 22 weeks' gestation, although a cutoff of 25 mm appeared best at 27 weeks' gestation. Using this cutoff at 22 weeks (for comparison with other data sets) gave a sensitivity of 38% and specificity of 97% for preterm delivery before 32 weeks' gestation. Cervical funneling, considered to be present when the lateral border of the funnel was more than 3 mm in length, was present in 12.4% of pregnancies at 22 weeks' gestation, and this finding had a sensitivity of 54% and a specificity of 89% as an indicator of preterm birth by 32 weeks' gestation. The authors concluded that cervical length and funneling both predict very preterm birth and that, although cervical length is the method of choice at 27 weeks' gestation, at 22 weeks the diagnostic characteristics of both parameters are close.

CERVICOVAGINAL FETAL FIBRONECTIN

Fetal fibronectin is a glycoprotein found in amniotic fluid, placental tissue, and the decidua basalis.[67] Although its specific function remains uncertain, it is thought to play a role in implantation and placental-uterine attachment. It is normally found in cervicovaginal secretions before 16 to 18 weeks' gestation, before fusion of the fetal membranes and the decidua is complete. Similarly, it is found at the end of pregnancy, prior to the onset of labor, but it is not normally present in cervicovaginal secretions between 22 and 37 weeks. It has been suggested that the presence of fetal fibronectin in cervicovaginal secretions in the later part of the second trimester and in the early part of the third trimester of pregnancy is due to disruption of the chorionic-decidual interface and is often secondary to infection.[68]

Initial studies establishing the presence of fetal fibronectin in cervicovaginal secretions involved extensive laboratory analysis that delayed the availability of results. An enzyme-linked immunosorbant assay containing the FDC-6 monoclonal antibody has been developed that can be used at the bedside, potentially making this test a much stronger clinical tool.[69] Intercourse/digital examination within 24 hours, vaginal bleeding, and the presence of ruptured membranes are associated with false-positive results. The use of lubricant jelly is associated with a false-negative result.

A large systematic review of 64 primary articles reporting the effectiveness of screening for preterm delivery by the detection of cervicovaginal fetal fibronectin in a total of 26,876 women was published in 2002.[70] There were two large subsets of women, asymptomatic and symptomatic of preterm labor. Among asymptomatic women, the likelihood ratio for predicting preterm delivery before 34 weeks was 4.01 (95% CI 2.93–5.49) with a likelihood ratio for negative results of 0.78 (95% CI 0.72–0.84). Among those women who were symptomatic, the likelihood ratio for positive results was 5.42 (95% CI 4.36–6.74) for predicting birth between 7 and 10 days of testing, with a corresponding negative likelihood ratio of 0.25 (95% CI 0.20–0.31).

Another meta-analysis in 2003, confined to reports in the English language, found that fetal fibronectin was useful in the prediction of delivery before 34 weeks, with an overall sensitivity of 53% and specificity of 89%.[71] The sensitivities for prediction of delivery within 7, 14, and 21 days were

71%, 67%, and 59%, respectively. The corresponding specificities were 89%, 89%, and 92%. Further analysis of studies in asymptomatic women who could be divided into low risk and high risk showed that for a single sampling of fibronectin, sensitivity for detection of delivery prior to 34 weeks was 41% (21%–59%) for low risk women with a specificity of 94% (91%–96%). For high risk women, the sensitivity was considerably lower at 23% (14%–32%) but with a comparable specificity of 94% (93%–96%). The studies of serial sampling of cervical fibronectin showed a higher sensitivity of prediction of delivery prior to 34 weeks with low risk and high risk groups showing a sensitivity of 68% (52%–83%) and 92% (62%–100%), respectively. Predictably, the specificities in each group of serial sampling were significantly reduced (there is an independent chance of a false-positive result every time the test is done, so the specificity falls as the number of samples, and hence false positives, increases). The few studies looking at multiple pregnancies have small numbers and result in sensitivities and specificities with such broad CIs that a meaningful conclusion cannot be drawn.

Subgroup analysis of symptomatic and asymptomatic pregnancies demonstrated that this test was most sensitive in women with symptoms of preterm labor, but its usefulness as a screening test for decisions about hospital admission and the administration of glucocorticoids is reduced by the fact that the specificity is significantly lower than in asymptomatic women. The authors concluded that fetal fibronectin is a reasonably effective marker in predicting preterm delivery in the short term, particularly if there are symptoms of preterm labor.

Combined Cervical Screening and Fibronectin

The combined use of ultrasound and fibronectin has been evaluated in only a few studies and in symptomatic women. Rizzo and coworkers[72] found that combining cervical sonography with fibronectin screening improved diagnostic accuracy and allowed better prediction of the admission to delivery time. Other investigators have found that fibronectin and cervical length had comparable ability to distinguish those at high and low risk of preterm delivery, but that their combination provides little added benefit.[73] Hincz and colleagues[74] proposed a two-step test only when the cervical length was in an immediate range of 21 to 31 mm. This form of testing had an overall sensitivity of 86% with a specificity of 90% for predicting delivery within 28 days. Similarly, Schmitz and associates[75] conducted a prospective, blinded, observational study to determine if the selective use of fetal fibronectin after ultrasound measurement of cervical length (<25 mm) predicts preterm delivery in symptomatic women better than either test alone. They found that the selective use of fetal fibronectin after cervical length measurement was more specific than cervical length measurement alone. The specificity of cervical length alone in predicting delivery less than 35 weeks and less than 7 days was 63% (95% CI 58–69%) and 61% (95% CI 56–67%), respectively. These values increased to 81% (95% CI 77–86%) and 79% (95% CI 74–83%), respectively, with sequential screening.

SCREENING FOR BACTERIAL VAGINOSIS IN EARLY PREGNANCY

Bacterial vaginosis (BV) is characterized by an overgrowth of a mixture of organisms (*Gardnerella vaginalis*, *Mobiluncus*, *Bacteroides* spp., and *Mycoplasma hominis*), is often asymptomatic, and may resolve spontaneously. Although the role of BV in preterm labor is poorly understood, several reports[76,77] found that the relative risk of preterm labor is doubled if the mother has BV. The hypothesis is that the organisms found in BV ascend into and colonize the chorionic-decidual space, resulting in preterm labor or preterm rupture of membranes. This increase in invasion of the genital tract may be due to the rise in pH, which is a key feature of BV, allowing vaginal bacteria to proliferate relatively unchecked. Two studies[78,79] suggest that infection in early pregnancy may be a greater risk factor than BV infection in the late second trimester and early third trimester of pregnancy.

Leitich and coworkers[80] performed a meta-analysis to evaluate the risk of preterm delivery associated with BV; 20,232 patients in 18 studies were included. They found that BV increased the risk of early delivery (<37 wk' gestation) with an odds ratio (OR) of 2.19 (95% CI 1.54–3.12). A subgroup analysis showed that if BV was identified prior to 16 weeks, then the risk of preterm birth was further increased with an OR of 7.55 (95% CI 1.80–31.65). Even at less than 20 weeks, a finding of BV was associated with an OR of 4.20 (95% CI 2.11–8.39) for preterm birth. This analysis found no particular association of BV with delivery prior to 34 weeks; however, few studies used that gestation time as an outcome and the studies that used early screening used less than 37 weeks as their criterion for preterm delivery. There is little evidence that screening for BV in specific subgroups, particularly in women with a prior preterm delivery and in multiple gestations, improves its sensitivity or specificity.

Despite this reasonably convincing evidence of a link between early infection with BV and preterm delivery, screening and subsequent treatment of BV remain controversial. The recent review of the *Cochrane Collaboration*[81] of 15 trials of 5888 women showed that antibiotic therapy successfully treated BV but failed to reduce the risk of preterm birth before 37 weeks, with OR 0.91 (95% CI 0.78–1.06); at 34 weeks, with OR 1.22 (95% CI 0.67–2.19); or 32 weeks, with OR 1.14 (95% CI 0.76–1.70). In those women who had a previous preterm birth, treatment of BV did not decrease the risk of a subsequent preterm birth (<37 wk), OR 0.83 (95% CI 0.59–1.17), but did decrease the risk of preterm premature rupture of membranes, OR 0.14 (95% CI 0.05–0.38) and the risk of delivering a low–birth weight neonate, OR 0.31 (95% CI 0.13–0.75). Screening and subsequent treatment at less than 20 weeks' gestation decreased the risk of preterm premature rupture of membranes, OR 0.14 (95% CI 0.04–0.44), decreased the risk of preterm birth before 37 weeks, OR 0.72 (95% CI 0.55–0.95), but did not decrease the risk of preterm birth before 34 weeks, OR 0.39 (95% CI 0.07–2.07). Carey and colleagues[82] failed to show oral metronidazole therapy to be useful in prevention of preterm labor in a mixed population.

At present, the role of screening for BV and then treating it is not clear in a low risk population. It possibly has benefit in a high risk population, but further controlled studies are required.

Editor's note: As this chapter was going to press, a report of a double-blind, placebo-controlled, randomized trial of the use of prophylactic progesterone to reduce the rate of preterm birth or stillbirth in twins appeared in the *Lancet*.[83] In the progesterone group, 24.7% of women delivered before 34 weeks or had a stillbirth, compared with 19.4% in the placebo group (OR 1.36; 95% CI 0.89–2.09). (There were 6 stillbirths in the progesterone group and 4 in the placebo group). The authors also performed a meta-analysis of all available studies on the use of progesterone in twin pregnancies. This confirmed that progesterone does not prevent early preterm birth in women with twin pregnancy (pooled OR 1.16, 95% CI 0.89–1.51).

SUMMARY OF MANAGEMENT OPTIONS

Screening for Spontaneous Preterm Labor and Delivery

Management Options	Evidence Quality and Recommendation	References
Uterine Activity Monitoring		
Self-monitoring applies to whole population but has a poor sensitivity.	IIb/B	7
Any improved outcome reported in monitored pregnancies may represent the benefits of increased education and support inherent in the studies.	Ib/A	8
Tocography is only practically applicable to high risk groups rather than whole populations.	—/GPP	—
Two meta-analyses of the same six studies in 697 high risk pregnancies have reached opposite conflicting conclusions; further studies are needed.	Ia/A	16,23
The addition of fetal fibronectin testing to uterine activity monitoring does not confer any benefit in practice.	IIb/B	27
Cervical Ultrasound		
It is important to use a standardized technique.	IV/C	33
Transvaginal route is significantly better than translabial/transperineal or transabdominal approaches.	IIa/B	34–37
Most studies have been performed at ≤24 wk.	III/B	36,47
Assessment of cervical length or funneling is predictive of preterm labor and delivery in	Ia/A	31
• Asymptomatic high risk patients.	III/B	36,40,46,48
• Asymptomatic low risk women.	III/B	47–52
• Twins.	III/B	61–64,66
More data needed about value in patients with symptoms suggestive of preterm labor.	Ia/A	31
No evidence yet shows that incidence of preterm delivery is reduced with use of cervical ultrasound, though it allows rational approach to	Ia/A	31
• Maternal steroids.		
• Use of tocolysis.		
• Transfer to a tertiary center.		
Main advantage could be in negative predictive value to avoid unnecessary interventions.	Ia/A	31
Fetal Fibronectin		
Positive test significantly increases the likelihood of preterm labor and delivery before 34 wk.	Ia/A	70,71
Negative test significantly reduces the likelihood of preterm labor and delivery within 10 days.	Ia/A	70,71
Serial sampling improves positive predictive accuracy but with a lower specificity.	Ia/A	70,71

SUMMARY OF MANAGEMENT OPTIONS

Screening for Spontaneous Preterm Labor and Delivery—cont'd

Management Options	Evidence Quality and Recommendation	References
FFN gives better predictive performance in symptomatic women than in asymptomatic.	Ia/A	70,71
Insufficient data about twin pregnancies.	Ia/A	70,71
Conflicting data about whether combination of FFN and cervical ultrasound improve predictive accuracy.	III/B	72,73
Screening for Bacterial Vaginosis		
Role of BV screening in practice is uncertain.	Ia/A	80,81
Positive screening for BV in early pregnancy is associated with an increased risk of delivery <37 wk; but no evidence of increased risk of preterm delivery <34 wk.	Ia/A	80
Antibiotic therapy in BV-positive women reduces incidence of BV colonization but not the incidence of preterm delivery.	Ia/A	81
More studies needed of BV screening and antibiotic use in high risk pregnancies.	Ia/A	80,81

BV, bacterial vaginosis; FFN, fetal fibronectin; GPP, good practice point.

SUGGESTED READINGS

Cicero S, Skentou C, Souka A, et al: Cervical length at 22–24 weeks of gestation: Comparison of transvaginal and transperineal-translabial ultrasonography. Ultrasound Obstet Gynecol 2001;17:335–340.

Colton T, Kayne HL, Zhang Y, Heeren T: A meta-analysis of home uterine activity monitoring. Am J Obstet Gynecol 1995;173:1499–1505.

Dodd JM, Flenady V, Cincotta R, et al: Prenatal administration of progesterone for preventing preterm birth. Cochrane Database Syst Rev 2006;1:CD004947.

Fonseca EB, Celik E, Parra M, et al: Progesterone and the risk of preterm birth among women with a short cervix. N Engl J Med 2007;357:462–469.

Grimes DA, Schulz KF: Randomized controlled trials of home uterine activity monitoring: A review and critique. Obstet Gynecol 1992;79:137–142.

Honest H, Bachmann LM, Coomarasamy A, et al: Accuracy of cervical transvaginal sonography in predicting preterm birth: A systematic review. Ultrasound Obstet Gynecol 2003;22:305–322.

Honest H, Bachmann LM, Gupta JK, et al: Accuracy of cervical fetal fibronectin test in predicting risk of spontaneous preterm birth: Systematic review. BMJ 2002;325:301–310.

Iams JD, Goldenberg RL, Meis PJ, et al: The length of the cervix and the risk of spontaneous preterm delivery. N Engl J Med 1996;334:567–572.

Swadpanich U, Lumbiganon P, Prasertcharoensook W, et al: Antenatal lower genital tract infection screening and treatment programs for preventing preterm delivery. Cochrane Database Syst Rev 2008;2:CD006178.

To MS, Skentou C, Cicero S, Nicolaides KH: Cervical assessment at the routine 23-weeks' scan: Problems with transabdominal sonography. Ultrasound Obstet Gynecol 2000;15:292–296.

REFERENCES

For a complete list of references, log onto www.expertconsult.com.

CHAPTER 61

Threatened and Actual Preterm Labor Including Mode of Delivery

JOHN M. SVIGOS, JODIE M. DODD, and JEFFREY S. ROBINSON

INTRODUCTION, DEFINITION, AND INCIDENCE

Preterm birth is estimated to affect approximately 13 million births annually worldwide.[1] Preterm labor (PTL) is defined by the World Health Organization as the onset of labor after the gestation of viability (20–28 wk, depending on definition) and before 37 completed weeks or 259 days of pregnancy.[2] The onset of labor may be determined by documented uterine contractions (at least one every 10 min) and ruptured fetal membranes or documented cervical change with an estimated cervical length of less than 1 cm or cervical dilation of more than 2 cm. Threatened PTL is diagnosed when there are documented uterine contractions but no evidence of cervical change.

Despite these apparently clear definitions, and because of the need for early management of suspected PTL, it is common for clinicians to make the diagnosis before the just-discussed criteria are met. Hence, the reported incidence of threatened PTL is likely to be considerably greater than the real incidence of actual PTL (at least double). In the 1970s, O'Driscoll[3] suggested that the pregnant woman's own diagnosis of PTL based on her perception of uterine contractions may be incorrect in 80% of instances. In the 1980s, Kragt and Keirse[4] demonstrated that 33% of women presenting with contractions could be safely discharged home in 48 hours without requiring treatment. In the Overview of Role of Antibiotics in Curtailing Labour and Early Delivery (ORACLE) II study in 2001,[5] the difficulty in diagnosing PTL accurately was clearly demonstrated, with 63.5% of women enrolled in the study with threatened PTL delivering after 37 weeks' gestation.

The incidence of preterm birth in developed countries is reported to vary widely, ranging from 4.4% in Ireland to 12.7% in the United States. In South Australia in 2006,[6] the overall preterm delivery (PTD) rate was 8.2%, of which 53.6% occurred following the spontaneous onset of labor. Doubts have been expressed about the current estimates of PTD compared with previous years because they increasingly reflect the increased survival of extremely preterm, very low–birth weight infants who previously would have been regarded as "nonviable." Registration practices have also altered because of changes in the definition of viability in which, previously, babies that are now registered as PTDs would have been recorded in the past as mid-trimester miscarriages, thereby compounding any ascertainment bias already present. Approximately 50% of PTDs are a result of spontaneous PTL, 30% follow preterm premature rupture of the fetal membranes (PPROM), and the other 20% are indicated PTDs for maternal or fetal indications.[7] There are now studies from both Denmark[8] and Australia[9] reporting an increase in the occurrence of spontaneous PTD even among women considered to be of low risk, to 22% and 12% of all PTDs, respectively. Major components of this rise are likely to be the rise in multiple births secondary to the growing use of assisted reproductive techniques, increases in body mass index (the "epidemic" of obesity), and the rising incidence of sexually transmitted disease. In addition, a significant proportion of this increase is related to medically indicated iatrogenic PTDs. These are justified on the basis of a substantial decline in gestation specific stillbirth and neonatal mortality rates,[7] with the largest proportion of such births occurring between 34 weeks and 37 weeks (now referred to as "late preterm births"). In South Australia in 2006, 66.9% of PTDs occurred between 34 weeks and 37 weeks.[6] Recent long-term follow-up studies on this group of preterm infants have demonstrated poorer perinatal outcomes compared with babies born after 37 weeks' gestation, and this may lead to a reappraisal of policies involving early delivery.[7]

In westernized countries, PTL accounts for approximately 70% of neonatal mortality and almost 50% of all long-term neurologic morbidity, with an associated major economic impact on health budgets. Figures from the United States suggest that the annual cost associated with care of infants born preterm is in excess of $26 billion.[10]

Current management regimens can be directed only to the approximately 10% to 15% of our obstetric population who present with threatened or actual PTL, and our current failure to impact substantially on this cohort of women has in part been due to our lack of understanding of the etiology of PTL, which appears to be diverse, and in addition, our inability to prevent or reverse the final common pathway of the cytokine/prostaglandin cascade and uterine contractions. To emphasize the complexity of any attempts at prevention, in Project 27/28 in the United Kingdom, all babies born between 27 and 28 weeks' gestation (3522) in 1 year were reported to The Confidential Enquiry into Stillbirths and Deaths in Infancy (CESDI).[11] A 2-year follow-up of 761 of these babies demonstrated that major placental bleeding (18%), pregnancy-induced hypertension (21%), prelabor rupture of the membranes (31%), clinical chorioamnionitis (11%), idiopathic PTL (55 %), cervical incompetence (5%), bacteriuria (7%), and maternal smoking were the most important antecedents of the PTDs.[11]

As a consequence of this diverse etiology, we have a diversity of management regimens that are directed toward improving neonatal outcomes either by trying to prevent delivery before 37 weeks' gestation or by delaying delivery to optimize the available resources prior to PTD. However, in applying these management regimens, we must continue to be mindful of their efficacy (and, often, lack of it) and of the inherent risks to mother and baby of many of the treatments used.

MATERNAL RISKS

General Risks

Consideration of PTD makes it clear that many of its etiologic associations have their origins in maternal pathology and these carry risks for the mother as well as for the fetus.

If PPROM and "idiopathic" PTL are excluded, then the two most common maternal conditions associated with PTD are pregnancy-induced hypertension and antepartum hemorrhage. These may either precipitate PTL spontaneously or prompt the deliberate induction of PTL in order to resolve the maternal problem or deliver the fetus from an adverse environment. Induction of labor may of itself carry risks for the mother (see Chapter 66) and demands careful consideration.

Tocolytic Agents

β-Sympathomimetics

The Cochrane Systematic Review by Anotayanonth and coworkers[12] assessed 11 trials involving 1320 women comparing the use of β-sympathomimetic agents with that of placebo and demonstrated that β-sympathomimetics were significantly associated with withdrawal from treatment owing to the following adverse maternal effects: chest pain, dyspnea, tachycardia, palpitations, tremor, headaches, hypokalemia, hyperglycemia, nausea and/or vomiting, and nasal stuffiness. Gyetvai and colleagues in a systematic review[13] found the incidence of adverse maternal effects of sympathomimetics compared with no treatment or placebo to be palpitations (48% vs. 5%), tremor (39% vs. 4%), nausea (20% vs. 12%), headache (21% vs. 6%), and chest pain (10% vs. 1%). Rare but serious and potentially life-threatening adverse effects have also been reported. Pulmonary edema is an insidious problem, the frequency of which is difficult to estimate. It is thought to be more common with multiple pregnancies receiving concomitant corticosteroid therapy for fetal lung maturation. Combination with other tocolytic agents, unrecognized chorioamnionitis, and fluid overload are major contributory factors. Myocardial ischemia due to diffuse myocardial micronecrosis may constitute an infrequent but serious maternal hazard, whereas underlying diabetes, thyrotoxicosis, or cardiac disease can accentuate the biochemical effects of hypokalemia and hyperglycemia seen with these agents. Although β-sympathomimetic agents have been the mainstay of tocolytic regimens in the management of PTL, other agents are now being used because they appear to have fewer adverse effects with comparable effectiveness. However, it must be stressed that none of these agents is without risk for the mother.

Nonsteroidal Anti-inflammatory Agents

Nonsteroidal anti-inflammatory drugs (NSAIDs) are inhibitors of the cyclooxygenase (COX) enzyme (prostaglandin synthetase), which plays an integral role in the initiation and maintenance of labor. The most common maternal side effects or complications of these drugs include peptic ulceration, gastrointestinal bleeding, thrombocytopenia, postpartum hemorrhage, renal function impairment, with depression, dizziness, psychosis, and headaches after long-term use. It has been shown that labor is associated with up-regulation of the expression of COX-2 (constitutive type isoform), but not COX-1, within the uterus, and it was anticipated that selective COX-2 agents might have fewer adverse effects than COX-1 agents. However, although a Cochrane Systematic Review by King and associates[14] demonstrated a low incidence of adverse drug reactions requiring cessation of treatment with nonselective COX antagonists compared with other types of tocolytic agents (relative risk [RR] 0.07; five trials with 355 women in total), a comparison of nonselective COX inhibitors versus any COX-2 inhibitor (two trials, 54 women in total) did not demonstrate any differences in maternal side effects (although the numbers are small).

Calcium Channel Blockers

Following the initial favorable report of Read and Wellby in 1986,[15] nifedipine and other calcium channel blockers have been increasingly used in the management of PTL. Although uncommon, there have been reports of pulmonary edema, maternal hypotension, and hepatotoxicity associated with the use of calcium channel blockers, whereas caution is advised if magnesium sulfate is being administered concurrently for eclampsia prophylaxis because there may be potentiation of the side effects described for both agents. The systematic review by King and coworkers,[16] of 12 randomized, controlled trials involving 1029 women, demonstrated a reduced requirement for women requiring calcium channel blockers to have treatment stopped because of adverse drug reactions compared with sympathomimetics (RR 0.14; 95% confidence interval [CI] 0.05–0.36).

Oxytocin Receptor Antagonist (Atosiban)

Atosiban has been compared with three different β-sympathomimetic agents in a large multicenter study[17] and was found to be associated with fewer adverse maternal effects such as chest pain, palpitations, tachycardia, hypotension, dyspnea, nausea, vomiting, and headache. There was only one case of pulmonary edema in the atosiban group compared with two in the β-sympathomimetic group. Atosiban has been licensed in Europe and the United Kingdom for use as a tocolytic (although not in the United States), but its relatively high cost limits its use. In addition, the Cochrane Systematic Review by Papatsonis and colleagues[18] identified two randomized trials involving 651 women in which atosiban was compared with placebo. When compared with placebo, the use of atisoban was not associated with a reduction in the risk of PTD and, in one study, was associated with an increase in the risk of infant death to 12 months of age. When compared with β-sympathomimetic agents, atisoban was associated with a fewer maternal side effects requiring cessation of therapy (RR 0.04; 95% CI 0.02–0.11, four trials, 1035 women), but was associated with an increase in the likelihood of a birth weight less than 1500 g (RR 1.96; 95% CI 1.15–3.35, three trials, 575 infants).

Nitric Oxide Donors

The systematic review by Duckitt and Thornton[19] of five randomized, controlled trials involving 466 women in total demonstrated that these women being treated with nitric oxide (NO) donors were more than six times more likely to experience headache, without any evidence of improved efficacy against placebo or other tocolytics. From the available evidence, the authors were unable to support its use in the management of threatened or actual PTL.

Magnesium Sulfate

The Cochrane Systematic Review by Crowther and associates[20] of 2000 women in 23 trials failed to support its use as an effective tocolytic agent, but despite this lack of effectiveness, magnesium sulfate is still widely used in North America for this purpose. Elliott's study[21] of maternal side effects found that these occurred in 7% of patients and required cessation of treatment in 2% of patients. Cutaneous vasodilation, flushing, nausea, vomiting, palpitations, and headaches were the most common side effects reported, with maternal hypothermia, bone demineralization, and paralytic ileus being less common. Pulmonary edema and adult respiratory distress syndrome were reported to occur in 1% of patients. Hypermagnesemia can also lead to maternal respiratory depression and cardiac arrest. In view of these significant side effects and the lack of efficacy, the use of magnesium sulfate as a tocolytic agent cannot be supported.

Summary

It is important to be aware that, although tocolytic agents have been shown to reduce the proportion of births occurring up to 7 days after beginning treatment, there is no clear evidence of any benefit of their use on reducing perinatal or infant mortality or serious morbidity. This may be because by suppressing uterine activity, they are damaging the fetus by keeping it in an adverse intrauterine environment, thus negating any advantage of prolonging gestation. Accordingly, the current "green-top" guidelines of the Royal College of Obstetricians and Gynaecologists of the United Kingdom (Tocolytic Drugs for Women in Preterm Labour, Clinical Guideline No. 1[B] available at http://www.rcog.org.uk/files/rcog-corp/GT1BTocolyticDrug2002revised.pdf) state that "In the absence of clear evidence that tocolytic drugs improve outcome following preterm labour, it is reasonable not to use them. The women most likely to benefit from tocolysis are those who are still very preterm, those needing transfer to a hospital that can provide neonatal intensive care or those who have not yet completed a full course of corticosteroids to promote fetal lung maturation. For these women, tocolytic drugs should be considered."

Maternal Risks Associated with the Mode of Delivery in Preterm Labor

Cesarean section as the preferred mode of PTD, particularly for the very preterm infant (<30–32 wk' gestation), is a practice that did not receive adequate scrutiny before it came into common use. With it came significant maternal morbidity related to a poorly formed lower uterine segment, increased operative hemorrhage, infection, and the potential for compromised future uterine function—all this without documented improvement in perinatal mortality and morbidity rates. A systematic review by Grant and coworkers[22] of six trials of elective versus selective cesarean delivery for infants less than 30 weeks' gestation not only demonstrated the difficulty of randomization of the mode of delivery in this clinical situation (with only 122 women recruited) but also concluded that decision-making on an individual basis taking into account parental preference was all that could be recommended from the available data. The use of classic cesarean section for gestations less than 30 weeks carries more risk of maternal morbidity than the lower segment approach, and unpublished data from a small series by Stacey and Steer (personal communication) would suggest that it confers no particular benefit for the fetus. In addition, there are considerable risks of maternal morbidity following classic cesarean section as well as significant implications for mode of birth in subsequent pregnancies.

Assessment of the impact of the psychological trauma experienced by the patient, her partner, and her family in relation to the management of threatened or actual PTL is difficult, and this short paragraph cannot do justice to the magnitude and importance of this problem. The physical restrictions imposed by the use of intravenous tocolytics, coupled with their often incapacitating side effects, the impersonality of the required multidisciplinary approach, the institutionalization (often with geographic dislocation) that is commonly necessary, added to the uncertainty of the perinatal outcome and the delayed maternal-infant bonding that are inherent in contemporary management of PTL, are probably the major conflicts experienced. These factors must be kept in mind as we attempt to further reduce the maternal risks associated with PTL.

FETAL AND NEONATAL RISKS

Risks of Associated Pathology

Compromised fetal well-being is often the precipitating factor in PTL. Hence, intrauterine fetal death, intrauterine growth restriction, major congenital fetal anomalies, intrauterine fetal infection, and complicated multiple pregnancy may all contribute to the perinatal mortality and morbidity associated with PTL.

Risks of Prematurity

Physicians and parents struggle with the type of care they might wish to be provided for extremely premature infants born in the 22nd through to the 25th weeks of gestation. In situations in which the infant is unlikely to survive, all parties may opt for "comfort care," which provides for an infant's basic needs but forgoes often-painful medical procedures. Gestational age is known to play a large role in an infant's survival, but assessment of gestational age is often difficult (particularly antenatally); in order to assist in decision-making, the recent work of Tyson and colleagues[23] for the National Institute of Child Health and Human Development (NICHD) Neonatal Research Network is particularly valuable. They have observed 4000 extremely low–birth weight infants and constructed a web tool to predict disability and survival of these infants, taking into account not only gestational age but also the predicted sex of the infant, the estimated birth weight, singleton or multiple pregnancy, and the administration of maternal corticosteroids prior to birth. Most tertiary institutions already use their own center-based statistics when counseling parents, but this web tool may offer an extra refinement in this difficult area. These predictions must not be divorced from the urgency of any maternal condition that may require delivery to safeguard the mother's health (e.g., fulminating preeclampsia). Fetal intrapartum hypoxia and birth trauma associated with PTL, particularly involving the very low–birth weight infant, whether birth is by the abdominal or vaginal route, will contribute to the perinatal risk. The risks in the neonatal period are those of congenital malformations, the sequelae of intrauterine growth restriction, respiratory distress syndrome, necrotizing enterocolitis, intracranial hemorrhage, convulsions, and septicemia.

Risks of Medical Management of Preterm Labor

The fetal and neonatal risks associated with the medical management of PTL have not been accurately quantified, but they certainly require consideration in the overall management.

Risks of Tocolytic Agents

β-Sympathomimetic tocolytic agents cross the placenta and may cause fetal tachycardia and occasionally other adverse fetal cardiac effects that can be significant in an already compromised fetus.[24] The maternal hyperglycemia commonly associated with the use of these agents can result in neonatal hypoglycemia, whereas there is a suggestion that neonatal intraventricular hemorrhage may be associated with the use of these agents.[25] However, there are no substantial studies documenting long-term ill effects for the neonate, and there does not appear to be any difference in developmental outcome once all the confounding factors are considered.

Prostaglandin synthase inhibitors (NSAIDs) cross from the mother to the fetus, potentially resulting in prolonged bleeding time, cardiopulmonary effects (predominantly premature closure or constriction of the ductus arteriosus and [paradoxically] persistent fetal circulation after birth), renal dysfunction, and reduced renal output. Necrotizing enterocolitis and neonatal intraventricular hemorrhage have also been recorded with these agents. Most studies have limited the use of these agents to short-term therapy (48–72 hr) before 32 to 34 weeks' gestation. It was hoped that the more specific prostaglandin synthetase inhibitors and COX-2 selective agents might have fewer fetal side effects, but the latest evaluation does not confirm this.[14]

Magnesium sulfate crosses the placenta and has the potential to compromise fetal cardiac activity, with reduced baseline variability on cardiotocography being a not uncommon occurrence, which in turn, may lead to unnecessary intervention. The neonate can exhibit hypotonia and hypocalcemia as a consequence of hypermagnesemia. The more controversial aspects of magnesium sulfate are related to its possible neuroprotective role because several observational studies appeared to indicate a reduction in cerebral palsy in very low–birth weight infants in association with its use.

The latest Cochrane Systematic Review by Doyle and associates[26] studied five trials of 6145 babies. Four trials specifically targeted women who were likely to give birth early and magnesium was being used for neuroprotection. Antenatal magnesium sulfate treatment had no overall significant effect on pediatric (fetal, neonatal, and later) mortality (RR 1.04; 95% CI 0.92–1.17). There was a significantly reduced risk for cerebral palsy (RR 0.68; 95% CI 0.54–0.87). This remained significant if the neuroprotective intent subgroup was considered in isolation (RR 0.71; 95% CI 0.55–0.91, four trials, 4446 infants) but was not significant in the other subgroups. Substantial gross motor dysfunction was the only other outcome to show a significant difference between magnesium and placebo overall (RR 0.61; 95% CI 0.44–0.85; four trials, 5980 infants). There was no significant effect of antenatal magnesium sulfate treatment on the combined rate of death or cerebral palsy overall (RR 0.94; 95% CI 0.78–1.12; five trials, 6145 infants). There were no substantial differences between treatment groups in maternal deaths (RR 1.25; 95% CI 0.51 to 3.07), cardiac arrest (RR 0.34; 95%CI 0.04 to 3.26), or respiratory arrest (RR1.02; 95% CI 0.06–16.25) in four trials of 5411 women, but few women had these outcomes. Overall, significantly more women in the magnesium group ceased therapy because of side effects (RR 3.26; 95% CI 2.46–4.31), whereas there was significantly more maternal hypotension and tachycardia but no significant differences in maternal respiratory depression, postpartum hemorrhage, or cesarean births. The need for ongoing neonatal respiratory support was reduced in the magnesium group (borderline statistical significance: RR 0.94; 95% CI 0.89–1.00). There were no significant differences seen in any of the other secondary pediatric outcomes in all studies combined: intraventricular hemorrhage, periventricular leucomalacia, Apgar score less than 7 at 5 minutes, neonatal convulsions, neonatal hypotonia, and chronic lung disease. The authors have concluded that the evidence now supports a role for antenatal magnesium sulfate therapy in women at risk of PTD as a neuroprotective agent against cerebral palsy.[27] Further studies are required to clarify how magnesium works, who should receive magnesium sulfate, and how best it should be given. Studies are needed comparing the dose and timing of administration, whether maintenance therapy is required, and also whether the magnesium sulfate treatment should be repeated.

Calcium-channel blockers have not been adequately evaluated with regard to fetal or neonatal effects and the Cochrane reviewers King and coworkers[16] recommended detailed assessment of different dosage regimens and formulations on maternal and neonatal outcomes. Some animal studies have demonstrated profound metabolic alterations in the fetus, but to date, these changes have not been confirmed in human neonates.[28]

More recent tocolytic agents such as *NO donors* have not been sufficiently assessed to date with regard to possible fetal and neonatal effects,[28] whereas one of the randomized trials assessing Atosiban reported an increased risk of infant death.[18]

Risks of Thyrotropin-Releasing Hormone

The maternal administration of thyrotropin-releasing hormone (TRH) in association with corticosteroids was thought, from preliminary studies, to enhance the development of fetal lung maturity. The findings of the Cochrane Review by Crowther and colleagues[29] involved three trials comprising 1969 infants in total and confirmed that all side effects monitored—ventilation requirements and low 5-minute Apgar scores—were increased in women given TRH, and in two studies, there were poorer outcomes at childhood follow up. Given these unfavorable results, the use of TRH is now discouraged.

Risks of Corticosteroids

The maternal administration of *corticosteroids* to enhance fetal lung maturity is beneficial for the preterm neonate, as confirmed by the systematic review by Roberts and Dalziel[30] of 21 studies involving 3885 women and 4269 infants that demonstrated an overall reduction in neonatal death (RR 0.69; 95% CI 0.58–0.81) and a significant reduction in respiratory distress syndrome (RR 0.66; 95% CI 0.59–0.73) with less respiratory support and neonatal intensive care admissions (RR 0.80; 95% CI 0.65–0.99). In addition, there was a reduction of neonatal cerebroventricular hemorrhage in 13 studies of 2872 infants (RR 0.54; 95% CI 0.43–0.69) and a reduction of necrotizing enterocolitis in 8 studies of 1675 infants (RR 0.46; 95% CI 0.29–0.74). The potential risk of an increase in maternal and neonatal infection was not confirmed, with no demonstrated increased risk to the mother of death, chorioamnionitis, or puerperal sepsis and a reduction in neonatal systemic infections in the first 48 hours of life in 5 studies of 1319 infants (RR 0.56; 95% CI 0.38–0.85). Because of concerns that these favorable effects of maternally administered corticosteroids may diminish as the post-treatment interval lengthens, some clinicians advocate administering steroids repeatedly to mothers who remain undelivered between 23 and 34 weeks' gestation, usually at weekly intervals.[31] However, concerns have been expressed regarding a body of evidence suggesting adverse fetal/neonatal consequences from the use of repeated doses. Two large trials, the NICHD trial of Wapner[32] and the Australasian Collaborative Trial of Repeat Doses of Steroids (ACTORDS) study of Crowther,[33] which were well-designed, prospective trials with both short- and long-term evaluations[34,35] meticulously conducted and appropriately analysed, unfortunately came to opposite conclusions. Wapner[35] concluded that administering four or more courses of maternal corticosteroids increases the incidence of cerebral palsy or fetal/neonatal death, whereas Crowther and colleagues[34] concluded that repeat courses improved neonatal outcome without affecting neurodevelopment. In contrast to animal data, both groups found that repeat steroids were not associated with lower birth weight or smaller head circumference, and although the neurologic outcomes of the children in both groups were similar, Crowther and colleagues' study found a slightly increased incidence of behavioral problems such as attention deficit and emotional reactivity in the repeat steroids group.[34] Wapner,[35] however, found that 6 of the 248 (2.4%) children in the repeat steroids group had cerebral palsy compared with only 1 of the 238 in the single-course group, and 5 of those 6 children had been exposed to four steroid courses. The rates of cerebral palsy in Crowther and colleagues' study of 22 of 521 (4.2%) children in the repeat steroids group compared with 25 of 526 (4.8%) were both higher than in either group in the Wapner study. The studies differed in that in Crowther and colleagues' trial only 11.4 mg of betamethasone was used each week compared with Wapner's trial which used 24 mg each week. Moreover, in Crowther and colleagues' trial, 40% of women received only one repeat dose, 33% received only two or three repeat doses, and only 26% received four or more doses. More of the women in Wapner's study received four or more doses, but the relevance of this to the rate of cerebral palsy is unknown at this time.

The study by Murphy and associates (MACS [Multiple Courses of Antenatal Corticosteriods for Preterm Birth] trial)[36] assessed 1858 women who were randomized between 25 and 32 weeks' gestation, and those who remained undelivered 14 to 21 days after their initial dose of corticosteroids and were considered to remain at increased risk of PTD were randomized either to repeat doses of corticosteroids every 14 days or to placebo. The primary outcome was a composite of perinatal mortality, severe respiratory distress syndrome, intraventricular hemorrhage, periventricular leucomalacia, bronchopulmonary dysplasia, or necrotizing enterocolitis. There were no statistically significant differences between the two groups for the primary outcome, but the use of repeat doses of corticosteroids was associated with a reduction in fetal/neonatal growth parameters.

The Cochrane Systematic Review by Crowther and Harding,[37] which does not include the MACS trial, identified five other randomized trials involving 2000 women; these demonstrated that repeat corticosteroids were associated with a reduction in the occurrence of neonatal lung disease (RR 0.82; 95% CI 0.72–0.93) with no differences in mean birth weight.

At present, the American College of Obstetricians and Gynecologists (ACOG) recommends, in support of the National Institutes of Health (NIH) Consensus conference, that only one course of betamethasone (12 mg × 2 doses, 24 hr apart) should be given to women in PTL and that repeated or "rescue" doses should not be used. It seems likely that in the United States, this view will prevail given the results of Wapner's trial.[35] However, in Australia and New Zealand, particularly in the hospitals that participated in the ACTORDS trial, repeat corticosteroids are still given weekly to women at risk of PTD up to 32 weeks' gestation. It will be interesting to see if, in the future, differences in the incidence of cerebral palsy following PTD in the two countries will become apparent.

Corticosteroids can also be given as a "rescue" therapy when it is considered obvious that PTD will occur. Two trials have used corticosteroids in this manner.[38,39] Peltoniemi and coworkers[39] raised concerns that the use of rescue treatment potentially disturbed respiratory adaptation at birth, increasing the need for ventilator support. In a subsequent trial, Garite and colleagues[38] demonstrated a reduction in the risk of respiratory morbidity in the babies of women with threatened PTL, who were given two 12-mg doses of betamethasone at 12-hourly intervals. However, in a subsequent editorial, Bonanno and Wapner[40] questioned how this might be used successfully in clinical practice, given our inability to predict who will deliver when threatened PTL occurs.

In addition, investigation is under way with regard to the different types of antenatal corticosteroids used to enhance fetal lung maturity. The Cochrane Systematic Review by Brownfoot and associates[41] identified 10 randomized trials in which dexamethasone was compared with betamethasone, involving 1161 infants. Dexamethasone was associated with a reduction in risk of intraventricular hemorrhage when compared with betamethasone (RR 0.44; 95% CI 0.21–0.91; four trials, 549 infants). There is only limited information available relating to other infant health outcomes including long-term health,[42] and at present, it is unclear whether there are advantages associated with different corticosteroid agents. We await the results of the A*STEROID study that has been designed to answer whether, compared with betamethasone, antenatal dexamethasone given to women at risk of PTD (<34 wk' gestation) reduces the risk of death or any neurosensory disability caused by impairments such as cerebral palsy, blindness, deafness, or developmental delay in their children at 2 years' corrected age.[43] Of interest is the preliminary paper by Mittendorf and coworkers[44] suggesting that when high magnesium exposures occur in PTL, betamethasone may be less effective in preventing neonatal intraventricular hemorrhage.

Risks of Antibiotics

The previous conclusion of the ORACLE II trial[5] that in the absence of overt intrauterine infection, the use of antibiotics in PTL with intact membranes does not contribute positively to the neonatal outcome has been reinforced by the more recent findings of the ORACLE Children Study II,[45] which demonstrated an increased risk of cerebral palsy in the children whose mothers had received erythromycin or co-amoxiclav 7 years previously compared with those women who did not receive either antibiotic (erythromycin 53 [3.3%] of 1611 vs. 27 [1.7%] of 1562; RR 1.93, 95% CI 1.21–3.09; co-amoxiclav 50 [3.2%] of 1587 vs. 30 [1.9%] of 1586; RR 1.69, 95% CI 1.07–2.67). Also, the number of children with cerebral palsy was greater when both antibiotics were given together (35 of 769 [4.55%]) compared with erythromycin alone (18 of 785 [2.29%]), co-amoxiclav alone (15 of 763 [1.97 %]) or placebo alone (12 of 735 [1.63%]). The mechanism of this effect is unclear, but if subclinical infection is provoking labor, treatment with relatively low doses of oral antibiotics might only suppress rather than eradicate intrauterine infection, allowing continued fetal exposure to a damaging environment with the association between perinatal infection and neurologic impairment being well established.

These findings do not mean that antibiotics are unsafe for use in pregnancy, and pregnant women showing overt signs of infection should be treated promptly with parenteral antibiotics because the serious risks to mother and baby of untreated infection has been reinforced by the 2007 CEMACH report, *Saving Mothers Lives*.[46]

MANAGEMENT OPTIONS

Prepregnancy Preventive Measures

Unfortunately, there is little evidence from randomized trials of there being any value to preventive programs against PTD, based on prospective risk scoring. Both hospital-based and local social interventions have been tried, but none has proved to be successful.[47] This failure is due to both a low sensitivity (generally < 50%) and a poor predictive value (17%–34%) of risk scoring systems, particularly in nulliparous women because past obstetric performance is reported to be one of the more consistent predictive factors.[48] Given that most of the preventive strategies are directed at "idiopathic" PTL, which constitutes only a minority of cases, they are inherently unlikely to make much of an impact, even less so when with the services of a perinatal pathologist, a significant proportion of women with "idiopathic" PTL can be demonstrated to have specific etiologic factors that are currently not treatable once they are established. However, such information may be of some value in planning care for women in their next pregnancy.[49]

It is, however, useful in prepregnancy counseling to estimate the likely recurrence risk of PTD. The most significant and consistently identified risk factor for PTD is a woman's history of previous PTD.[50] Estimates suggest the rate of recurrent PTD in this group of women to be 22.5%, a 2.5 times increased RR when compared with women with no previous PTD.[51] Ashmead and colleagues,[52] in their prospective study of PTDs without uterine anomalies or medical problems, reported that women with one previous PTD had a 15% chance and those with two previous PTDs a 41% chance of another PTD. For approximately 10% of these women, the PTD will occur at a similar gestational age.[31,53] There appears to be intergenerational effects related to PTD, with an increase in a woman's risk of PTD if she herself was born preterm, the risk being greater at earlier gestational ages,[54,55] although this effect has not been consistently demonstrated.[56] These statistics may be helpful in counseling women living in areas remote from a perinatal center by suggesting their relocation during the critical period of a subsequent pregnancy to enhance the neonatal outcome.

More general advice with regard to daily work activity (avoidance of heavy manual labor or mental stress if family economics permit) and attention to specific habits such as alcohol, smoking, and chemical dependency should be given because there is some evidence that these factors may play a role in PTD.[57]

Women with a low body mass index at conception and women with poor weight gain in pregnancy relative to their prepregnancy weight have an increased risk of PTD.[58] Women who are overweight or obese are recognized have an increased risk of medical complications of pregnancy, including gestational diabetes and hypertension.[59] Accordingly, obesity is associated with an increased risk of PTD at less than 34 weeks, which is largely related to elective or iatrogenic PTD rather than spontaneous PTD.[60,61]

Even after adjustment for other sociodemographic risk factors, there is a strong racial predisposition to PTD being higher in black women than in other racial and ethnic groups.[62] This over-representation among black women is 2 to 3.5 times greater when compared with white women, with a tendency to an earlier average gestational age at birth.[63,64] There is, however, some evidence of accelerated maturity in babies born early to mothers of black African and south Asian race, which is to some extent protective (see Chapter 65). These findings indicate that whereas maternal medical and socioeconomic factors are most influential, racial differences and genetic predisposition make important contributions.[65]

While initiatives to try to deal with the aforementioned risk factors are being assessed, at the present time, specific prepregnancy measures for PTL and PTD might be considered for multiparous patients. Unfortunately, for nulliparous women, apart from those with known genital tract anomalies for which surgical correction might be possible, there does not appear to be any proven strategies to prevent PTL and PTD.

Prenatal Preventive Measures

Assessment of Risk

At the first prenatal visit, assessing the risk of PTD based on the history and clinical examination may be useful in identifying those women more likely to deliver preterm. The assessment of risk can be updated during the pregnancy if complications develop. An adaptation of the score devised by Creasy and associates,[66] which combines socioeconomic factors, previous medical history, daily habits, and aspects of the current pregnancy, is probably the most acceptable method but its predictive value is low (17%–34%) owing to the multifactorial nature of PTL. In all women, particularly those at risk of PTD, it is desirable that gestational age be confirmed by an ultrasound scan in the first trimester.

Patient Education

Education of the patient with a previous PTD about the signs and symptoms of PTL is a useful option to consider. The perception of contractions, menstrual-like cramps, pelvic pressure sensation, low dull backache, abdominal cramping with or without diarrhea, an increase or change in vaginal discharge, and a "show" may all prove to be significant but individually are not particularly predictive. Nevertheless, if these signs and symptoms of PTL are evident, then a thorough cervical assessment either digitally or by ultrasound should be performed.

Antenatal Care

In those women suspected of being at increased risk of PTL, more frequent antenatal assessment, particularly in the latter half of pregnancy, is a common option employed. The rationale is based on indirect evidence that absent or delayed institution of antenatal care is associated with an increased rate of PTD and low–birth weight infants.

It is possible that those patients sufficiently motivated to seek early and regular antenatal care may be intrinsically healthier and better motivated than those who do not seek early antenatal care. Antenatal care does provide the opportunity to detect and possibly treat some of the maternal and fetal conditions (e.g., anemia, hypertension, and bacteriuria) that are associated with PTD.

Bowes[67] best summarized the contributions of prenatal care by suggesting that success is related to the continuity of care, the time available for patients to talk about their problems, ready access to ancillary services, and a prenatal patient record that provides reminders of critical procedures and screening tests. Enhanced prenatal care may have the potential to become more effective as better predictive tests and more selective prophylactic measures are developed for PTD.

Prediction of Preterm Labor

Prediction of PTL (see Chapter 60) has dominated research efforts since the 1990s.

Outpatient and home monitoring of uterine contractions, regular cervical assessment both digitally and by ultrasound, biochemical markers such as placental corticotropin-releasing hormone (CRH) and its binding protein, salivary estriol, the inflammatory cytokines and prostaglandins, fetal fibronectin (fFN), cervical ferritin, and noninvasive cutaneous cardiovascular dynamics (CVD) have come and gone or have been reevaluated in the hope that a reliable predictor with high sensitivity and specificity can be found.

Strategies for Prevention of Preterm Labor and Preterm Birth—Primary Prevention Cervical Cerclage

Cervical incompetence is classically diagnosed by a history of painless cervical dilation that results in a second-trimester spontaneous miscarriage. The contemporary use of ultrasound in the early second trimester can recognize the asymptomatic cervical changes of shortening and funneling that are associated with an increased risk of PTD.[68] The etiology of the pregnancy loss or PTD may be mechanical in nature, or alternatively, it may be of an inflammatory or subclinical infection nature as a result of cervical dilation and possibly the loss of the mucous plug.

Hollier[69] reviewed four randomized trials evaluating the value of cervical cerclage in women with historical risk factors, and all failed to demonstrate a reduction in birth before 37 weeks' gestation. The largest of these trials was the Medical Research Council/Royal College of Obstetricians and Gynaecologists (MRC/RCOG) trial,[70] which evaluated the effectiveness of the McDonald suture and found a nonsignificant reduction in the rate of birth before 37 weeks (26% vs. 31%; $P = 0.07$) and a significant reduction in birth before 33 weeks (13% vs. 17%; $P = 0.03$). However, there was only a small and statistically insignificant improvement in miscarriage, stillbirth, and neonatal death (9% vs. 11%) whereas there was an increase in medical intervention and a doubling of the risk of puerperal pyrexia. It has been calculated from these four trials that 1 woman in 30 will benefit from a cervical cerclage.

Three randomized trials have been performed assessing the effectiveness of cervical cerclage in women with a short cervix detected on second-trimester ultrasound. The only trial to show benefit was the smallest trial by Althuisius and coworkers[71] of 30 women in total that had a "mixed" study group of women with historical risk factors as well as women identified in the second trimester to have a short cervix on ultrasound. For women randomized before 24 weeks, the rate of PTD was significantly lower in the cerclage group (0/16 vs. 7/14; P = .002). The neonatal survival was similar but the compound morbidity was significantly lower in the cerclage group (RR 9.1; 95% CI 1.3–64.4).

The larger studies by Rust and colleagues[72] and To and associates,[73] although methodologically a little different, nevertheless failed to demonstrate any benefit from the placement of a cervical cerclage after ultrasound detection of cervical shortening.

The Cochrane review by Drakeley and coworkers,[74] evaluating elective cerclage compared with no cerclage, failed to reveal any difference in the risk of total pregnancy loss (RR 0.86; 95% CI 0.59–1.25), PTD before 37 weeks (RR 0.88; 95% CI 0.76–1.03) or 32 weeks (RR 1.29; 95% CI 0.67–2.49), with an increase in the risk of infection (RR 2.57; 95% CI 1.42–4.64) and minor maternal morbidity (RR 1.32; 95% CI 1.13–1.55) associated with cervical cerclage. On the basis of this information, the authors concluded that cerclage had a limited role in women considered to be at low to moderate risk of PTD.

A subsequent systematic review and individual patient data meta-analysis by Berghella and colleagues,[75] involving randomized trials in which women were identified with cervical shortening on transvaginal ultrasound and then allocated to cervical cerclage or no treatment, identified a small reduction in the risk of PTD less than 37 weeks' gestation (RR 0.84; 95% CI 0.71–0.99). Although there is currently insufficient information available to indicate that this prolongation in gestational age translates into improved infant health outcomes, nevertheless further scientific evaluation of the role of cervical cerclage in this group of high risk women is warranted.

Placement of a cervical suture is usually a vaginal procedure, but on rare occasions, it may have to be performed by the abdominal route, usually after two failed vaginal cerclages and/or significant shortening or damage of the vaginal cervix. This can be achieved at open operation or at laparoscopy and can be performed either prepregnancy or in the late first trimester.[76–78]

Treatment of Vaginal Infection

The presence of inflammation is associated with activation of the cytokine cascade, which in turn, may be associated with the release of prostaglandin, which is associated with the onset of uterine contractions and the process of cervical ripening leading to PTD.[79]

In both term labor and PTL, there is evidence of an increase in inflammatory markers, tumor necrosis factor-α (TNF-α), interleukin-1 (Il-1), Il-6, and down-regulation of the anti-inflammatory Il-10. These maternal inflammatory cytokines may alter enzyme expression, increasing prostaglandin production, and may then interact at the fetoplacental unit precipitating PTL and PTD.[80]

The epidemiologic associations with PTD discussed in relation to both personal and family history of PTD and racial disparities in its occurrence would support a genetic predisposition to PTD, and this has led to the identification of several gene polymorphisms altering cytokine expression and increasing the risk of PTD.[81,82]

In addition, alterations in vaginal microbial flora have been linked with inflammatory processes, with infection being implicated as a cause of PTD in up to 30% of affected women. The fetus may also play a role in these inflammatory-mediated causes of PTD through the fetal inflammatory response syndrome (FIRS).[83] As a result of this understanding of the likely pathophysiologic changes associated with PTD, identification and treatment of women with vaginal infection has promise as a potential means of reducing the incidence of PTL and PTD.

In women at high risk for PTD based on history and colonized with bacterial vaginosis (BV) during the index pregnancy, three randomized trials demonstrated that oral metronidazole therapy reduced the risk of PTD by 25% to 75%.[84–86] However, three trials of oral treatment of BV in a mixed group of women at both high and low risk of PTD, including the large trial by Carey and associates,[87] failed to detect any significant differences in the rate of birth at less than 37 weeks' gestation, at less than 35 weeks' gestation, or less than 32 weeks' gestation. Seven trials have evaluated the use of clindamycin treatment of BV (six using intravaginal cream, and one oral clindamycin), and six of the trials demonstrated an increase (rather than the anticipated decrease) in the rate of prematurity.[88–94] The seventh trial treated persistent BV after the initial treatment course and also treated any associated vaginal candidiasis and trichomoniasis. In this trial, there was a significantly lower rate of spontaneous PTD in the treatment group compared with the control group (3.0% vs, 5.3%; $P < .01$).[89]

From the evidence accumulated so far, it would appear that screening and treating low risk women with BV is not justified and may cause some harm. The argument for screening and treating high risk women with BV would appear to be more compelling, and some have argued that both timing of treatment and antibiotic used are critical variables. Moreover, although treatment of symptomatic women with metronidazole is appropriate simply to relieve symptoms,[95] two randomized trials have assessed the effect of antibiotic treatment of women with *Trichomonas* vaginitis (TV) on the rate of PTD; in both studies, it appeared that treatment of TV resulted in an increased risk of an adverse outcome.[96,97] The explanation for this is not clear but may be related to an alteration of the vaginal flora with the local release of cytokines and/or possibly a systemic maternal immune response to *Trichomonas*. Once again, there does not appear to be any justification for universal screening and treatment of asymptomatic women with TV. The recent work of Goldenberg and coworkers[98] demonstrated that 23% of neonates born between 23 and 32 weeks' gestation have positive blood cultures for genital mycoplasmas (*Ureaplasma urealyticum* and *Mycoplasma hominis*) and that these newborns had a higher frequency of neonatal systemic inflammatory response syndrome with higher serum concentrations of Il-6 and placental inflammation than those with negative cultures, which in turn may have some important long-term neonatal implications and thus is worthy of mention in trying to understand the implications of such infections.

There is accumulating evidence that these organisms are implicated in neonatal sepsis, pneumonia, meningitis, and cerebral damage, and although their presence in the genital tract of sexually active and normal pregnant women is common and they are possibly present as commensal organisms, nevertheless, these microorganisms are frequently isolated from the amniotic fluid in women with PTL, PPROM, cervical incompetence, mid-trimester amniocentesis, and clinical chorioamnionitis. This raises the question as to how they gain access to the amniotic cavity, and once present, why they might induce a deleterious inflammatory response. Romero and Garite[99] highlight the fact that the detection of genital mycoplasmas is not part of current clinical practice, and in addition, the standard treatment for suspected neonatal sepsis does not include antibiotics that are effective against these microorganisms. Investigators are now beginning to address these areas.

The use of probiotics to prevent or treat urogenital infections (primarily BV) is a relatively novel method of treatment. A Cochrane review by Othman and associates[100] demonstrated a major reduction in vaginal infection associated with treatment (RR 0.19; 95% CI 0.08–0.48), although no information is currently available relating to the risk of PTD or other maternal and infant health outcomes.

Prophylactic antibiotic administration to prevent PTD in an unselected pregnant population has been associated with a reduction in the risk of PPROM (odds ratio [OR] 0.32; 95% CI 0.14–0.73), but currently, there is insufficient information available to recommend prophylactic antibiotics during pregnancy to prevent PTL and PTD whereas there is a possible increase in the risk of other infectious morbidities including an increase in the risk of neonatal sepsis (OR 8.07; 95% CI 1.36 to 47.77).[101]

Treatment of Periodontal Disease

The initial promising results of the treatment of periodontal disease in the prevention of PTD have not been consistently reproduced. Michalowicz and colleagues[102] and Ruma and associates[103] have recently questioned the previous suggestion that systemic inflammation due to periodontal disease can contribute to the causation of PTD.

Use of Progesterone

Many studies have examined the use of progesterone for the prevention of PTL, and whereas the presumed mechanism of action of progesterone is thought to be that of inducing uterine muscle quiescence, preliminary evidence suggests that progesterone may also modulate cytokine production and provide a protective antiapoptotic effect in human fetal membrane cells, both of which may be important in preventing PTL.

However, the etiology of PTD is heterogeneous, with many causal pathways leading to regular uterine contractions and cervical dilation, and therefore, it is unlikely that progesterone therapy will be a panacea for all women considered to be at increased risk of PTD.

The recent systematic review by Dodd and coworkers[104] identified 11 randomized trials evaluating the role of progesterone for women at increased risk of PTD. For women with a prior history of PTD,[105–107] progesterone was associated with reduction in the risk of PTD before 34 weeks' gestation (one study, 142 women; RR 0.15; 95% CI 0.04–0.64; number needed to treat [NNT] 7; 95% CI 4–17). Whereas there was a significant reduction in the risk of infant birth weight less than 2500 g (two studies, 501 infants, RR 0.64; 95% CI 0.49–0.83), no other differences were identified between the treatment groups for other neonatal outcomes. It must be noted that the combined sample size of 1329 infants is not sufficiently powered to detect differences in neonatal morbidity.

A single trial was identified in which progesterone was administered to women with a short cervix detected on transvaginal ultrasound.[108] The use of progesterone was associated with a reduction in PTD before 34 weeks (250 women; RR 0.58; 95% CI 0.38–0.87; NNT 7; 95% CI 4–25). Although a significant reduction in the risk of neonatal sepsis was identified, the sample size is underpowered to reliably detect differences in neonatal outcomes.

It seems unlikely that progesterone will be of value in multiple pregnancies (see Chapter 59).

The value of progesterone in women who present with symptoms or signs of threatened PTL that is subsequently arrested is uncertain. Two randomized studies have been reported to date, with a combined sample size of 130 women.[109,110] Although there is a suggestion of a reduction in cervical length shortening detected by ultrasound following the use of progesterone, there is little other relevant information relating to maternal or infant health outcomes.

Currently, there is insufficient information to make reliable recommendations about the optimal dose of progesterone, the optimal route of administration, and the appropriate gestational age at which to start therapy. The information that is available suggests that the potential benefit is for women considered to be at increased risk of PTD (usually determined on the basis of a previous PTD) and the benefit is primarily in the reduction births before 34 weeks' gestation. However, there is currently little information available about neonatal and longer-term infant and childhood health outcomes; thus, it remains unclear whether any prolongation of pregnancy translates into improved health outcomes. Further research is required before progesterone can become a standard recommended form of management of women at risk of PTD, and the results of several trials ongoing at the time of writing are awaited with great interest. One is using vaginal progesterone in women with a history of prior PTD.[111] One in a high risk group using "natural" progesterone was started in 2006 but subsequently withdrawn (NCT00329316)[112]; however a study of 17 alpha-hydroxyprogesterone caproate in high risk women who present with a short cervix, registered in 2006, appears still to be ongoing.[113]

Strategies for Prevention of Preterm Labor and Preterm Birth—Use of Tocolytics as Maintenance Therapy after Primary Treatment

Dodd and associates[114] assessed 11 randomized, controlled trials of the administration of oral β-sympathomimetic drugs for prophylaxis after threatened PTL and found no difference for admission to a neonatal intensive care unit following maintenance therapy compared with placebo (RR 1.29, 95% CI 0.64–2.60) or with magnesium sulfate (RR 0.80; 95% CI 0.43–1.46). The rate of PTD at less than 37 weeks showed no significant difference (RR 1.08; 95% CI 0.88–1.32) when comparing ritodrine and terbutaline with placebo/no treatment. There were no differences with respect to perinatal mortality and morbidity.

A prospective, randomized, double-blind, multicenter study by Lyell and colleagues[115] using nifedipine versus placebo yielded similar results, with no improvement demonstrated in prolonging pregnancy or improving neonatal outcome. The available evidence does not support the use of oral β-sympathomimetic drugs and other tocolytic drugs for maintenance therapy after threatened PTL.

Management of Women Presenting with Threatened or Actual Preterm Labor

Once the diagnosis of threatened or actual PTL is established, a careful clinical appraisal with appropriate investigations of maternal and fetal condition should be performed. Ultrasonography can be used to ascertain fetal number, estimate fetal weight, check fetal morphology and presentation, as well as estimate liquor volume and localize the placental site. In addition, ultrasound can be used to assess fetal well-being utilizing umbilical vessel Doppler assessment and fetal activity including fetal breathing movements, which were found in preliminary studies to be suppressed in women with PTL.[116]

Testing for an infective etiology is important in the initial assessment and includes culture of vaginal and cervical secretions and a midstream specimen of urine, a complete blood count (including a differential white cell count), and C-reactive protein estimation. Amniocentesis with Gram stain and culture and, more recently, Il-6 estimation may be considered if infection is suspected. In addition, fetal lung maturity using lecithin/sphingomyelin ratio or phosphatidyl glycerol can also be assessed concurrently. If indicated by abnormal fetal morphology, fetal karyotype determination should be considered.

However, not all obstetricians would perform amniocentesis in this context because of the possibility of inducing further uterine activity and because of a lack of robust data to guide management decisions based on the findings.

Determination of the presence or absence of PPROM by clinical and, if necessary, additional investigations is essential to the management of threatened or actual PTL. Although acknowledging that a positive fFN test in symptomatic women has only a 29.3% positive predictive value of delivery before 34 weeks' gestation, a large body of evidence now exists that confirms that a negative fFN test has a more than 95% predictive value that PTD will not occur before 34 weeks' gestation.[117] On a logical basis, it should be possible to use the information gained from fibronectin screening information to reduce unnecessary and potentially harmful and costly treatment and to avoid unnecessary maternal-fetal transfer to a tertiary level unit in women presenting with threatened PTL. However, there have been three randomized, controlled trials examining the impact of fFN testing on the management of threatened PTL that have not borne out this hypothesis. Plaut and coworkers[118] found that in women with a negative fFN test, the hospital stay was not significantly shorter when the result was known compared with when the result was not known (6.8 hr vs. 8.1 hr; P =.35). Lowe and colleagues[119] found no difference between similar groups in the number of hours spent in the labor and delivery suite, the number of women admitted to the antepartum service, the length of inpatient hospital stay, or the number of medical interventions. Grobman and associates[120] found no difference in the initial length of labor and delivery (4 hr vs. 3 hr), in hospital admission (28% vs. 26%), use of tocolysis (18% vs. 16%), cessation of work (27% vs. 26%), or health care costs between the two groups. The Cochrane Systematic Review by Bergella and coworkers[121] identified five randomized, controlled trials assessing the value of knowing about the result of fFN tests in women presenting with symptoms or signs of PTL in a total of 474 women. Although the knowledge of fFN testing was associated with a reduction in risk of PTD less than 37 weeks' gestation (RR 0.54; 95% CI 0.34–0.87), no other differences were identified relating to maternal and infant health outcomes. Currently, there is insufficient information available to recommend the routine use of fFN testing in threatened PTL, although it still remains in use in some regionalized perinatal networks as an aid to the selective transfer of women with threatened PTL to tertiary perinatal centers.

Once gestational age is established, the generally poor immediate and long-term outcomes of infants born between 20 and 24 weeks require considerable discussion between the parents, the obstetrician, the neonatologist, and the midwife either before or shortly after the initiation of tocolytic therapy. In cases of extreme fetal immaturity, the parents may choose to allow delivery to occur rather than invoking risky, uncomfortable, and expensive delaying strategies of poor efficacy. However, caution must be exercised in agreeing to this strategy because fetal weight and gestational estimates are subject to significant variation between 20 and 24 weeks' gestation.

This dilemma is more pragmatically handled by transferring the patient to a tertiary perinatal center and allowing her to deliver vaginally without assistance ("intervention") with a neonatologist present at delivery to immediately assess the neonate's suitability for intensive support. Whether continuous electronic fetal monitoring should be used during such labors is in dispute. Knowledge of whether the fetal heart rate pattern is normal or not may be of some value in deciding on whether to carry out neonatal resuscitation; however, some members of the medical/midwifery/nursing team find it stressful to observe an abnormal fetal heart rate pattern without intervening. Accordingly, whether to carry out continuous intrapartum fetal monitoring should be discussed with the parents and the key members of the delivery care team.

The use of tocolytic therapy between 24 and 34 weeks' gestation is not only to facilitate the in utero transfer of the fetus to a tertiary referral center but also to allow sufficient time to enhance fetal lung maturity by the concomitant use of maternal corticosteroid therapy. Although the most widely tested tocolytics are the β-sympathomimetic agents, which are effective in delaying delivery, they have not been shown to improve perinatal outcome and have a relatively high frequency of undesirable maternal side effects, as previously described. Calcium channel blockers are now becoming the first-line tocolytics because they have the advantage of availability, cheaper cost, ease of administration, and fewer maternal side effects than β-sympathomimetics.[16] King and colleagues[122] assessed 12 randomized, controlled trials involving 1029 women; calcium channel blockers compared with other tocolytics (principally β-sympathomimetics) reduced the number of women giving birth within 7 days of treatment (RR 0.76; 95% CI 0.60–0.97) and prior to 34 weeks' gestation (RR 0.83; 95% CI 0.69–0.99). Currently, there is a lack of consensus with regard to regimens for the use of calcium channel blockers.

Maternal contraindications to its use include hypotension (systolic blood pressure <90 mm Hg), known allergy to nifedipine, cardiac disease (congestive cardiac failure, aortic stenosis), concurrent use of salbutamol, glyceryl trinitrate (GTN), other antihypertensive agents, hepatic dysfunction, and caution if magnesium sulfate is being administered because significant hypotension and neuromuscular blockade may result.

Fetal contraindications to its use include suspected intrauterine infection, urgent fetal distress, undiagnosed significant vaginal bleeding, severe intrauterine growth restriction, and the more apparent problems of lethal anomalies and intrauterine fetal death. In Australia, nifedipine for inhibition of PTL is an "off-label" use because it has not been approved by the Therapeutics Goods Agency for this indication.

With threatened or actual PTL, the South Australian Perinatal Practice Guidelines[123] recommend that a starting dose of 20 mg nifedipine be given and the tablet should be chewed or crushed to aid the speed of absorption. However, if this approach is used, careful and continuous maternal and fetal monitoring must be carried out. Sublingual administration of nifedipine has been associated with severe maternal hypotension and fetal distress,[124] and chewed tablets with severe maternal hypotension and fetal death.[125] If contractions persist, then a second dose of 20 mg of nifedipine is recommended, with the maximum dose in the first hour being 40 mg. Any further doses are not recommended until 3 hours after the second dose, with a maximum dose of 160 mg of nifedipine in 24 hours.

Maternal baseline observations should be taken initially in association with continuous electronic fetal monitoring, and the rate of observations can be tapered according to the clinical situation. Although cessation of nifedipine tocolysis is uncommon, owing to side effects the patient should be warned of the possibility of headache, tachycardia, palpitations, flushing, fatigue, dizziness, nausea, heartburn, constipation, and edema. Tocolytic therapy should be continued for 48 hours if possible to try to maximize the enhancement of fetal lung maturity by maternally administered corticosteroids in the form of betamethasone (two doses of 12 mg IM, 24 hr apart) or dexamethasone (6 mg every 12 hr for four doses).

If the initially selected tocolytic agent is unsuccessful in suppressing threatened PTL or is not tolerated, an alternative agent may be considered either alone or in combination with the original agent. However, any such strategy should be instituted only after a very careful appraisal of maternal and fetal well-being and, in particular, the exclusion of intrauterine infection, which is notorious for producing an apparent failure of tocolysis. As previously discussed, maintenance oral tocolytic therapy after 48 hours has not been found to prevent PTD or improve neonatal outcome and cannot be recommended, although it is still commonly employed.

The place of other maternally administered agents to enhance fetal outcome—TRH, magnesium sulfate, and repeated courses of maternally administered corticosteroids—have been discussed previously, whereas the prophylactic use of maternally administered vitamin K and phenobarbitone to reduce the incidence of neonatal periventricular hemorrhage has not been validated scientifically and cannot be recommended.[126,127]

The results of the ORACLE II Trial[5,45] and the recent meta-analysis by King and Flenady[128] would reinforce the view that adjunctive antibiotic therapy in threatened or actual PTL for the purpose of preventing PTD is not indicated; however, intrapartum intravenous penicillin prophylaxis for women colonized with group B streptococcus is appropriate, as is the aggressive treatment of proven/overt maternal infection.

Treatment of threatened and actual PTL after 34 weeks was formerly considered to be unnecessary; however, accumulating data suggest that singleton infants born at this late preterm stage, who constitute up to two thirds of all PTDs, are at increased risk for perinatal death compared with infants born at term.[129] In addition, these infants have increased morbidity including transient tachypnea, respiratory distress, hypoglycemia, and pulmonary hypertension. Recent cohort studies[130] also demonstrate poorer school performance and increased risks of cerebral palsy (RR 2.7; 95% CI 2.2–3.3), developmental delay (RR 1.6; 95% CI 1.4–1.8), schizophrenia (RR 1.6; 95% CI 1.4–1.8), and other disorders of psychological development, behavior, and emotion (RR 1.5; 95% CI 1.2–1.8) in these late preterm infants. Not only are these late preterm infants at increased risk of developmental, social, and neurocognitive problems but they also have a 40% increased risk for any medical disability (RR 1.4; 95% CI 1.3–1.5) in adulthood.[131] These findings are at variance with the conventional belief that 34 weeks is a critical physiological period in fetal maturity and now require us to carefully assess the maternal and fetal indications that necessitate obstetric assistance (intervention) at 34 to 37 weeks' gestation—preeclampsia, intrauterine growth restriction, diabetes, and other maternal medical conditions—and to determine the risk/benefit to the mother and her baby of delivery at this gestation compared with a more conservative approach with delivery after 37 weeks' gestation. Two studies[132,133] have indicated that 22.4% and 21%, respectively, of births between 34 and 36 weeks had no apparent indication for iatrogenic delivery and these infants had higher neonatal and infant mortality rates than infants who delivered at this gestation after spontaneous labor. Underreporting of indications may have accounted for this discrepancy; however, overintervention may also have occurred. A retrospective study by Merlino and associates[134] found that the majority of late PTDs at their tertiary center were not amenable to conservative management, with only an estimated 6% of late PTDs being potentially suitable for conservative treatment. The safety and efficacy of conservative management under these circumstances still remain to be determined.

The use of maternally administered "late" corticosteroid therapy, between 34 and 37 gestational weeks, has been promoted to reduce respiratory morbidity and admission to special care nurseries in these neonates following a number of recent comparative cohort studies.[135] This practice has been extended in an attempt to reduce transient tachypnea of the newborn for women undergoing elective or semielective cesarean section before 39 weeks' gestation.[136] Because of concerns about the potential long-term harmful effects on the baby of antenatal steroids, avoiding unnecessary delivery should always be considered as a better option before additional steroid treatment is given. Certainly, steroids should not be given simply to make it easier for the obstetrician or the mother to choose earlier delivery for social convenience.

Emergent (emergency) cerclage may have a limited place in an attempt to extend the gestational age of delivery in a selected number of women presenting with advanced cervical dilation in the second trimester. No randomized study has prospectively documented the benefits that emergent cerclage placement might impart. Although one prospective, nonrandomized study has suggested that increased gestational time can be gained,[137] the benefits of this increased latency remain unclear because many of these infants are delivered at the threshold of viability and suffer from the resultant sequelae of extreme prematurity. As a consequence, little published evidence exists to assist in counseling patients who present with cervical change documented by physical examination in the second trimester regarding the probability of a desirable outcome after placement of an emergent cervical suture. The present literature is mainly limited to series with small numbers of patients with variable entry criteria.

In the retrospective trials that have included only women with cervical change diagnosed by physical examination, a variety of surgical techniques have been attempted yet little assessment of the benefits of these techniques has been performed. Many of these studies have reported outcomes such as the number of days a pregnancy is prolonged rather than actual health outcomes.[138,139] In addition, the univariant statistical analyses that have been applied have not allowed an assessment of the factors that independently predict these health outcomes.[140]

In order to give patients an individualized probability of relevant outcomes, a number of workers have attempted to construct predictive scores/models upon which to base further management.[141] Parity, gestational age at presentation, degree of cervical dilation, and C-reactive protein levels/amniocentesis to detect infection are the consistent parameters evaluated in these scoring systems, but as previously mentioned, these parameters have not been prospectively validated.[142]

Labor and Delivery

Once PTD seems inevitable, the mode of delivery and the likely neonatal outcome should be discussed with the patient and her partner by a multidisciplinary team of an obstetrician, a neonatologist , an obstetric anesthetist, and a midwife.

In general, before 24 weeks' gestation, vaginal delivery should be anticipated with expert neonatal evaluation at delivery to determine whether active neonatal supportive care is warranted.[143]

Between 24 and 34 weeks' gestation, the management of labor should not differ significantly from that beyond 34 weeks, with vaginal birth being the anticipated outcome.

Although continuous electronic fetal monitoring and regional anesthesia have not been critically evaluated in the management of actual PTL, they are commonly employed. Once labor is established and if there are signs of intrauterine infection, maternal antibiotic therapy should be instituted because a reduction in maternal infectious morbidity has been demonstrated with antibiotic treatment.[144] The authors currently favor the use of intravenous ampicillin 2 g stat and 1 g every 4 hours, gentamicin 160 mg daily, and metronidazole 500 mg every 12 hours. This combination is undergoing further evaluation in light of evidence suggesting that β-lactam antibiotics may have deleterious effects on the neonate as a result of the sudden release of cytokines that may precipitate the fetal inflammatory response syndrome.

If the *group B streptococcus* status of the patient is unknown, appropriate parenteral antibiotics (penicillin or, in the case of allergy, lincomycin) should be administered during labor. Evaluation of the available randomized trials would suggest that "prophylactic" outlet forceps or "elective" episiotomy does not contribute significantly to the neonatal outcome and, hence, should be performed only for standard obstetric indications. It is generally agreed that ventouse delivery is relatively contra-indicated, particularly before 34 weeks' gestation, should an expedited vaginal birth be required.

In extremely preterm infants between 24 and 28 weeks' gestation, intact amniotic membranes may serve to protect such infants from the mechanical forces exerted upon the baby and the umbilical cord during vaginal birth, with evidence suggesting that the "en caul" method of delivery is associated with significantly higher arterial cord pH values in these infants.[145]

Delayed cord clamping has been found to confer an advantage to the neonate in a Cochrane Systematic Review by Rabe and coworkers[146] identifying a reduction in the need for infant transfusion for anemia (RR 2.01; 95% CI 1.24–3.27; three trials, 111 infants), a reduction in neonatal hypotension (RR 2.58; 95% CI 1.17–5.67; two trials, 58 infants), and a reduction in intraventricular hemorrhage (RR 1.74; 95% CI 1.08–2.81; five trials, 225 infants). The standard management of the third stage is recommended with PTD.

The attendance at the birth of a neonatologist/pediatrician with an assisting neonatal nurse or an accoucheur skilled in neonatal resuscitation is critical to the optimal outcome for a premature infant. From the neonatal perspective, the significantly higher risk of mortality and morbidity of infants born outside a tertiary perinatal center makes a compeling argument for maternal-fetal transport to such a center with a neonatal intensive care unit (level III, now designated as level 6 in most Australian states), particularly for women up to and including 32 weeks' gestation.[147]

In a well-organized perinatal network, women at 32 to 37 weeks' gestation may be allowed to deliver in an obstetric hospital with level II (now designated as level 4 or 5 in most Australian states) facilities with short-term ventilatory care capability. When transport is not possible (in some series, up to 50% of women), specifically trained and equipped obstetric and neonatal teams with appropriate nursing and medical personnel should attend the birth.[148] Their role is to supervise and, if necessary, deliver the neonate and then stabilize the mother and her premature infant prior to their respective transfer to the tertiary perinatal center if deemed necessary.[148]

Postnatal Management

Maternal Considerations

Encouragement of parent-infant bonding is a major consideration in postnatal management. Continuous access by the parents to the neonatal nursery should be encouraged to facilitate the bonding process and breast-feeding should be encouraged in a compassionate and pragmatic manner.

Continuing psychological support is important, utilizing the services of a domiciliary midwife, neonatal nurse, lactation consultant, social worker, and if indicated, a psychiatrist, more so if there is significant neonatal morbidity and/or neonatal death. An early postnatal evaluation of possible etiologic factors should be considered by the immediate perinatal team along with input where appropriate from a perinatal pathologist, obstetric physician, pediatric surgeon, geneticist, and ultrasonolographer in order to construct a coherent plan not only for the current neonate but also for further pregnancies.

Neonatal Considerations

Premature birth requires adaptation to extrauterine life while the different organ systems undergo continued structural and functional development and maturation. Thus, premature infants can be expected to have a variety of problems in the neonatal period with the risk of complications being proportional to the degree of prematurity. However, this statement may be modified by the observation that spontaneous PTL is probably adaptive in nature because the rate of neonatal respiratory distress syndrome in a comparative cohort study by Lee and colleagues[149] was greater in "indicated" rather than spontaneous PTD (OR 2.29; 95% CI 1.22–4.29).

Premature infants are likely to have difficulties in maintaining body temperature and in oral feeding as well as having a greater risk of infection. Lung maturity of premature infants is proportional to their gestational age and is the major cause of respiratory distress syndrome in these infants, whereas poorly developed respiratory control may lead to recurrent apnea. Congestive cardiac failure may occur as a result of patent ductus arteriosus associated with prematurity, for which there are medical and surgical options available for correction. Liver immaturity is likely to be associated with severe neonatal jaundice with the premature baby being more vulnerable to the neurotoxic effects of unconjugated bilirubin. Phototherapy reduces serum bilirubin levels in jaundiced preterm infants, but it is not clear whether aggressive or conservative phototherapy is optimal, particularly for extremely low–birth weight infants (<1000 g).

Morris and Tyson[150] allocated nearly 2000 infants weighing less than 1000 g to aggressive phototherapy, which aimed to achieve bilirubin levels around 7 mg/dL, or to conservative phototherapy, which aimed at a level around 10 mg/dL. All infants were tracked up to 2 years, and there was no significant difference in either survival or neurodevelopmental impairment between the two groups.

Small infants are often hyperglycemic because of immature intracellular feedback mechanisms, stress responses, or high-calorie feeding regimens. It has been postulated that insulin treatment may enhance survival rates and promote brain growth, but mixed findings and hypoglycemic episodes have confused its acceptance.

Beardsall and Dunger[151] have published the results of an international trial of early insulin therapy versus standard neonatal care; unfortunately, the results were disappointing because the early intervention group fared no better than those receiving conventional treatment and hypoglycemic episodes were more frequent. There is also an increased risk of intracranial hemorrhage and necrotizing enterocolitis in premature infants, and maternal corticosteroid administration has been associated with a significant reduction in these morbidities, as previously discussed.

In the extremely premature infant, chronic lung disease and retinopathy are more likely in the longer term. Similarly, cerebral palsy and developmental delay are more likely in preterm infants, and it is here that previously discussed strategies such as antenatal maternal magnesium sulfate administration may play a neuroprotective role.

Head cooling has been proposed as a method of improving outcomes in infants with hypoxic ischemic encephalopathy. The Cochrane review by Jacobs and associates[152] included eight randomized trials involving infants with asphyxia or hypoxic ischemic encephalopathy. Cooling reduced the risk of death or developmental disability at 18 months of age (RR 0.76; 95% CI 0.65–0.89; NNT 7; 95% CI 4–14). The reviewers cautioned that fewer than half the subjects known to have been entered into these trials have been included in the final reports (and therefore in the review), raising the possibility of bias.[152] Further studies of head cooling are in progress, such as that being conducted at Vanderbilt University, assessing the impact of head cooling in reducing neurologic morbidity in preterm infants.[153]

Maturity of organ systems, particularly the lung, is really the key factor determining the ultimate prognosis of the premature infant. Minimizing the incidence and severity of respiratory distress has been the major factor in the substantial improvement in neonatal morbidity and mortality rates since the 1980s.

Previously mentioned strategies of regionalization of perinatal care, selective use of tocolytic agents, and maternally administered corticosteroids to enhance fetal lung maturity have all been positive contributing factors. Similarly, the "prophylactic" use of exogenous surfactant as well as its use as "rescue" therapy in association with mechanical ventilation in established respiratory distress syndrome has been a major advance in reducing respiratory morbidity.[154]

In addition there have been efforts directed at improving the neurodevelopmental outcomes of preterm infants using high-dose docosahexaenoic acid (DHA) as in the randomized, controlled trial conducted by Makrides and coworkers[155] that demonstrated a statistically significant difference in the Bayley Mental Development Index at 18 months' corrected age in preterm infant females delivered between 23 and 33 weeks' gestation who were fed high-DHA (~1% total fatty acids) compared with infants fed standard DHA (~0.3% total fatty acids). The lack of responsiveness of boys to the intervention is unclear and may relate to the higher rate of endogenous synthesis of DHA from the precursor fatty acid α-linolenic acid in girls compared with boys. Further studies are required to establish the role of DHA in the routine management of preterm infants.

Although there has been a significant increase in neonatal survival rates at 24 to 27 weeks' gestation over the past decade, it appears that prematurity per se has a deleterious effect on neonatal growth and development that contributes to a poorer outcome. This must be taken into account when assessing survival and morbidity rates, particularly in very low–birth weight infants less than 24 weeks' gestation.

The NIH Newborn Research Network, previously mentioned, has recently compiled survival and neurodevelopmental outcomes based on the observation of 4000 infants in relation to gestational age, sex of the neonate, birth weight, singleton or multiple birth, and maternal administration of corticosteroids. This tool has enabled rationalization of care for the very preterm neonate because it must be emphasized that not every newborn infant can be salvaged, and on some occasions, survival may be accompanied by severe handicap either physical or psychological or both. Prolonging life in these circumstances may not be beneficial to the infant and may become unacceptably burdensome to the parents. In such cases, the parents may opt for "comfort care" soon after birth, or later, after detailed and extensive consultation and counseling, they may consider withdrawing life support.

In addition to these medical and ethical challenges confronting the neonatologist are the immediate and delayed financial costs of neonatal intensive care. Economic constraints may not unreasonably act as a brake to those who would seek to overcome all of the aforementioned medical and ethical challenges, resulting in a more restrained attitude of evidence-based medical practice in an environment of cost containment.

The final measure of the quality of a tertiary neonatal service is the dedication and commitment of its long-term follow-up program. All perinatal centers must be prepared to commit resources to maintain and upgrade this essential service so that early intervention of detected physical and psychological problems can be instituted to minimize their effects on the infant born preterm.

In addition, the follow-up program will provide valuable information to the obstetricians and maternal fetal medicine subspecialists that will allow them to promulgate relevant advice and provide appropriate support, reassurance, and counseling of the parents who will continue to bear the logistic, financial, physical, and psychological impact of the care for the infant who is born prematurely.

SUMMARY OF MANAGEMENT OPTIONS

Threatened and Actual Preterm Labor

Management Options	Evidence Quality and Recommendation	References
Prepregnancy (Previous Preterm Labor)		
Establish cause/precipitating factors.	III/B	46,48,51
Estimate risk of recurrence:	III/B	56
• Advise re: lifestyle, work, place of residence at critical phase of pregnancy.		
• Specific reference to diet, smoking, alcohol, recreational drugs, obesity.		
Prenatal—Assessment of Risk		
Take a careful history for presence of specific risks (e.g., previous preterm birth, race, intergenerational aspects, cervical trauma).	III/B	56–65
Value of formal risk scoring systems is not confirmed.		
Establish gestational age early and as accurately as possible (first-trimester scanning if required).	GPP	
Prenatal—Previous Preterm Labor and Delivery		
Provide general advice re: lifestyle, work, place of residence at critical phase of pregnancy.	III/B	57
• Specific reference to diet, smoking, alcohol, recreational drugs, obesity.		
If cervical incompetence, perform cerclage at 12–14 wk.	Ib/A	68–72
Patient education programs re: signs and symptoms of preterm labor have poor predictive value.		
Increased attendance and discussion for women at risk may be helpful for decisions on place, timing, and mode of delivery.	III/B	66
Prenatal—Strategies Needing Further Evaluation		
Screening (See Chapter 60)		
• Monitor uterine contractility.		
• Obtain regular cervical assessment—clinical and ultrasound.		
• Infective screening.		
• Biochemical screening.		
Prophylaxis		
Tocolytics offer no value.	Ib/A	13
Antibiotics (general) offer no value.	Ib/A	5

Management Options	Evidence Quality and Recommendation	References
Treatment of bacterial vaginosis in women at high risk of preterm labor may be of use.	Ib/A	85,86
Maternal corticosteroids should be considered, although there are concerns with repeated courses.	Ib/A	30,37
Presentation with Threatened or Actual Preterm Labor		
Initial assessment to determine if genuine preterm labor:	GPP	
Uterine activity:		
• Bleeding.		
• Membrane rupture.		
• Presenting part.		
• Engagement of presenting part.		
• Cervical status—clinical, ultrasound.		
• Gestational age.		
• Biochemical tests may be useful in excluding the diagnosis (e.g., fibronectin).	III/B	118–121
Search for cause or precipitating factor.	GPP	
Discuss prognosis with parents.	III/B	23
Maternal-fetal transfer to tertiary center.	III/B	147,148
Liaison with neonatologists/pediatricians.	GPP	
Tocolysis (depending on gestation, cause, contraindications including infection):		
• Calcium channel blockers are becoming more popular.	Ia/A	13
• β-Sympathomimetics are less popular owing to unacceptable side effects.	Ib/A	122
• Tocolytics are justified for at least 48 hr to allow fetal pulmonary maturation and other beneficial effects.	GPP	
Maternal Corticosteroids		
These are proven use up to 34 wk and are being evaluated for benefits between 34 and 37 wk.	Ia/A	30
TRH, Vitamin K, Phenobarbitone		
Use is not justified.	Ia/A	126,127
Antibiotic Therapy		
Not recommended as an adjunct to tocolysis.	Ia/A	128
Should be used if group B streptococcus is present or PPROM is confirmed.		
Emergent/Rescue Cerclage		
Only in the context of an RCT.	III/B	137–141
Maternal Magnesium Sulfate		
For neuroprotection of the preterm infant.		
Should now be considered—dosage and duration yet to be determined.		26
Labor and Delivery		
Use a multidisciplinary approach—obstetric, midwifery, neonatology/pediatric, anesthetic.	GPP	
Before 24 Wk		
Discuss with parents re: prognosis.	GPP	
Aim for vaginal delivery, experienced pediatrician/neonatologist in attendance.		
From 24 Wk		
Discussion with parents re: prognosis	GPP	

SUMMARY OF MANAGEMENT OPTIONS

Threatened and Actual Preterm Labor—cont'd

Management Options	Evidence Quality and Recommendation	References
If cephalic presentation, aim for vaginal delivery with usual indications for cesarean section.	GPP	
If breech, see Chapter 63.		
Provide continuous fetal heart rate monitoring.	GPP	
Regional anesthesia choice.	GPP	
Use assisted vaginal birth for standard obstetric indications.	GPP	
Prescribe antibiotics if clinically infected.	GPP	
Have an experienced pediatrician/neonatologist in attendance.	GPP	
Maternal		
• Encourage breast-feeding.	GPP	
• Provide psychological/social support.	GPP	
Neonate		
• Allow continuous access to neonatal unit.	GPP	
• Provide direct communication re: neonatal progress.	GPP	
Follow-up		
• Search for cause/precipitating factors.	GPP	
• Establish plan for future pregnancies.	GPP	
• Provide long-term follow-up of neonate.	GPP	

GPP, good practice point; RCT, randomized, controlled trial; TRH, thyrotropin-releasing hormone.

Acknowledgment

The authors wish to acknowledge the invaluable contributions to the first three editions of this text of their friend and colleague Dr. Rasiah Vigneswaran, Staff Neonatologist, Adelaide Womens' and Childrens' Hospital, who died November 29, 2002.

SUGGESTED READINGS

Ananth CV, Gyamfi C, Jain J: Characterizing risk profiles of infants who are delivered at late preterm gestatins: Does it matter? Am J Obstet Gynecol 2008;199:329–331.

Berghella V, Odibo AO, To MS, et al: Cerclage for short cervix on ultrasonography: Meta-analysis of trials using individual patient-level data. Obstet Gynecol 2005;106:181–189.

Berghella V, Hayes E, Visintine J, Baxter JK: Fetal fibronectin testing for reducing the risk of preterm birth. Cochrane Database Syst Rev 2008;4:CD006843.

Crowther CA, for the ACTORDS Study Group: Outcomes at 2 years of age after repeat doses of antenatal corticosteroids. N Engl J Med 2007;357:1179–1189.

Dodd JM, Flenady VJ, Cincotta R, Crowther CA: Progesterone for the prevention of preterm birth: A systematic review. Obstet Gynecol 2008;112:127–134.

Doyle LW, Crowther CA, Middleton P, et al: Magnesium sulphate for women at risk of preterm birth for neuroprotection of the fetus. Cochrane Database Syst Rev 2009;1:CD004661.

Kenyon S, Pike K, Jones DR, et al: Childhood outcomes after prescription of antibiotics to pregnant women with spontaneous preterm labour: 7 year follow-up of the ORACLE II trial. Lancet 2008;372:1319–1327.

King JF, Flenady VJ, Papatsonis DNM, et al: Calcium channel blockers for inhibiting preterm labour. Cochrane Database Syst Rev 2008;1:CD002255.

Tyson JE, Parikh NA, Langer J, et al: Intensive care for extreme prematurity: Moving beyond gestational age. N Engl J Med 2008;358:1672–1681.

Wapner RJ, for the NICDH MFM Units Network: Long term outcomes after repeat doses of antenatal corticosteroids. N Engl J Med 2007;357:1190–1198.

REFERENCES

For a complete list of references, log onto www.expertconsult.com.

CHAPTER 62

Prelabor Rupture of the Membranes

JOHN M. SVIGOS, JODIE M. DODD, and
JEFFREY S. ROBINSON

INTRODUCTION

Prelabor rupture of the membranes (PROM) is an obstetric conundrum. It is ill-defined with an obscure etiology; is often difficult to diagnose; is associated with significant maternal, fetal, and neonatal risks; and has management strategies that are often diverse and controversial. Some of this controversy relates to the currently low level of evidence. Although currently available systematic reviews and meta-analyses provide some guidance toward clinical care for both PROM and preterm prelabor rupture of the membranes (PPROM), further basic and clinical research will be necessary before we will be better able to define effective strategies for treatment and for primary prevention.

DEFINITION AND INCIDENCE

PROM is defined as rupture of the fetal membranes before the onset of contractions. There is then a "latent period" before the onset of spontaneous uterine activity. The length of the "latent period" varies, from an hour or two up to weeks. It is generally reported that PROM occurs in about 10% of all pregnancies, with the majority of cases occurring after 37 completed weeks of gestation.[1–5] If PROM occurs before 37 completed weeks of gestation, it is referred to as PPROM. PPROM occurs in approximately 2% of pregnancies overall, but in tertiary referral centers, it may occur in 5% or more of the obstetric population.[6]

RISKS

Maternal Risks

Significant maternal morbidity is associated with PROM, particularly preterm, and this morbidity can occur before, during, or after labor. Although the incidence of subclinical chorioamnionitis may be as high as 30% with PPROM,[7] serious systemic maternal infection is rare if treatment is initiated promptly. The use of a number of therapeutic agents, such as corticosteroids, antibiotics, and particularly β-sympathomimetic tocolytic agents, will pose additional maternal risk in the setting of PPROM, which must be considered in the overall management. Abruptio placentae is evident in 4% to 7% of women with PPROM, and hence, vaginal bleeding in the presence of PROM must be regarded seriously and managed accordingly.[8–10] Psychosocial sequelae occur in association with PPROM because of the disruption created by the need for continuing observation, often involving hospitalization, together with the uncertain fetal/neonatal prognosis; this should be addressed on an individual basis within the overall management strategy. The intrapartum maternal consequences of PROM are predominantly related to the augmentation of labor. The latent phase of labor under these circumstances may be as long as 16 to 20 hours, and thus, unrealistic limits must not be set regarding the duration of labor when counseling the patient and the attendant staff. The increase in operative delivery associated with PROM inevitably increases maternal morbidity.[11] Pathologic examination of placentae associated with PROM demonstrates an increased incidence of marginal cord insertion and battledore placenta, which may account for the increased incidence of retained placenta in this setting. This, in turn, may be associated with the known increased incidence of primary and secondary postpartum hemorrhage. The latter complication is probably associated with the 10% incidence of endomyometritis that occurs with PROM.[12] After delivery, in addition to the previously discussed, there is an increased incidence of impaired maternal-infant bonding that contributes significantly to maternal psychological and lactation problems.

Fetal and Neonatal Risks

Prematurity is the most significant factor in the associated increased perinatal morbidity and mortality because delivery occurs within 7 days in over 80% of women who present with PPROM.[13,14] The duration of the latency period in PPROM is not only inversely related to gestational age but also shorter in the presence of oligohydramnios, cervical dilation, and fetal growth restriction.[15] Although the incidence of chorioamnionitis is 30%, the reported incidence of neonatal sepsis is only 2% to 4%.[16–18] Gestational age at the time of rupture of the membranes will have some influence on the incidence of neonatal sepsis, as will the length of the latent period. A growing body of epidemiologic data has demonstrated a relationship between intrauterine infection and the development of intraventricular hemorrhage, periventricular leukomalacia, and the subsequent occurrence of cerebral palsy.[19] This damage is likely to be the result of the fetal inflammatory response syndrome[20] initiated by placental inflammation, rather than infection, and resulting from the local generation of arachidonic acid and preinflammatory cytokines: interleukin-1 (Il-1), Il-6, and tumor necrosis factor-α. The oligohydramnios resulting from PPROM, particularly if it is prolonged, may result in the neonatal "oligohydramnios tetrad" of flattened facies, limb positional deformities, pulmonary hypoplasia, and impaired fetal growth, all of which contribute to increased neonatal morbidity. Fetal hypoxia is more likely due to the greater possibility of cord prolapse, cord compression, and abruptio placentae associated with PROM, particularly with PPROM. Neonatal morbidity may also be increased owing to the mechanical difficulties that can be encountered at delivery by either the vaginal or the abdominal route as a result of an increased incidence of malpresentation and the reduced volume of surrounding amniotic fluid.

MANAGEMENT OPTIONS

Prepregnancy and Prenatal Prevention

Prepregnancy counseling has only a limited role in the management of PROM, particularly PPROM, because in the vast majority of cases, the cause is unknown.

The recurrence risk for PPROM has not been studied extensively but Naeye's original observation[21] of a recurrence rate of 21% to 32% was subsequently confirmed by Asrat and coworkers,[22] although Lee and associates[23] have since reported a lower recurrence rate of 16.7%.

A detailed examination of the etiologic associations of PPROM by Harger and colleagues[24] suggested that the only independent risk factor that might be amenable to prepregnancy intervention is cigarette smoking; the risk appears to be dose-related.

Other less constant associations that might be amenable to prepregnancy intervention include cocaine abuse[25] and intrauterine diethylstilbestrol (DES)-exposed women with congenital uterine anomalies (which is now becoming rare because DES use was discontinued in 1974).[26]

Nutritional deficiencies of ascorbic acid (vitamin C), copper, zinc, and iron have been variously suggested as increasing the incidence of PPROM,[27,28] but antioxidant therapy using vitamin C and vitamin E supplementation[29] has failed to demonstrate a reduced risk of PPROM (3.2% incidence in supplemented women vs. 2.4% with placebo; relative risk [RR] 1.34; 95% confidence interval [CI] 0.77–2.25). Indeed, there is some suggestion that such supplementation may be associated with an increased incidence of both PROM and PPROM.[30]

There is substantial direct and indirect evidence that reproductive tract infections and associated inflammatory changes are responsible for many instances of PPROM.[31] Group B streptococci, *Chlamydia*, gonorrhea, syphilis, *Mycoplasma hominis*, and *Ureaplasma urealyticum* have all been variously incriminated, but robust evidence that prophylactic treatment of these organisms is effective in reducing the incidence of PPROM is lacking.

The prophylactic antimicrobial treatment of bacterial vaginosis during pregnancy in high risk women has been evaluated in several randomized trials, with the evidence presented in a systematic review and meta-analysis.[32] Fifteen randomized trials involving 5888 women evaluated the role of antibiotics for treatment of bacterial vaginosis in pregnancy.[32] Treatment was associated with no difference in the risk of preterm birth prior to 37 or 34 weeks' gestation or in the risk of PPROM (odds ratio [OR] 0.88; 95% CI 0.61–1.28; 4 studies, 2579 women).[32] However, in a subgroup analysis of women who had experienced a prior preterm birth, treatment of bacterial vaginosis in a subsequent birth was associated with a significant reduction of the risk of PPROM (OR 0.14; 95% CI 0.05–0.38; 2 studies, 114 women).[32] In a recent meta-analysis that included nine studies relating to PPROM before 34 weeks, Hutzal and coworkers[33] reported that antibiotics were associated with prolongation of pregnancy. In addition, there was a reduction in neonatal infections and a trend toward a reduction in the incidence of sepsis with positive cultures. Importantly, there were fewer cases of intraventricular hemorrhage of all grades in the neonates. However, there remains uncertainty about the best antibiotic regimen to be adopted.[34] In light of this, prepregnancy vaginal microbial cultures would appear to be a useful investigation in women with a past history of PPROM, especially in the detection of group B streptococcus and bacterial vaginosis.

A population-based study of the race-specific risk for PPROM found that African American women were at higher risk than white women for the occurrence and recurrence of PPROM even after adjustment for known risk factors.[35] The implication from this study is that there may be genetic factors in addition to environmental factors contributing to the etiology of PPROM.

Antimicrobial treatment of the sexual partner is more controversial whereas the avoidance of coital activity during the course of further pregnancies would appear to be unnecessarily restrictive. If there is concern that infection might be introduced by the male partner, this risk may be reduced by the use of condoms.

Prenatal

Diagnosis and Further Assessment ("Expectant Management")

The diagnosis of PROM requires a judicious assessment of the history, clinical examination, and specialized testing. Whenever the history is suggestive of PROM, a sterile vaginal speculum examination should be performed. Visualization of amniotic fluid draining through the cervix provides the most reliable diagnosis and the opportunity to exclude cord prolapse, particularly with PPROM. In case of doubt, demonstration that vaginal fluid has an alkaline pH on Nitrazine yellow testing (the pH indicator turning black) is suggestive but not conclusive evidence of PROM. The normal vaginal pH is acidic and becomes neutral or alkaline owing to the presence of amniotic fluid. However, loss of acidity can be due to vaginal infection or the presence of urine or even bath water, and hence, although the sensitivity of the Nitrazine yellow test is 90%, there is a false-positive rate of 17%.[36,37] Ferning of vaginal fluid on microscopy is also a useful sign that the fluid is of amniotic origin, and this simple test, which is easy to perform, should be more widely used in the diagnosis of PROM. However, both ferning and pH tests are less reliable at early gestational ages.

If the diagnosis of PROM is still in doubt, further investigations including the use of a modified vaginal pouch to collect amniotic fluid,[38] ultrasound evaluation of amniotic fluid volume, and intra-amniotic dye injections may be employed. Ultrasound evaluation of oligohydramnios is subjective unless there has been a recent large fluid loss, and intra-amniotic injection of dye is not without risk.[39,40] More recently, other tests have been evaluated in the diagnosis of ruptured membranes, with raised fetal fibronectin and raised insulin-like growth factor binding protein-1 having reported sensitivities of 94% and 75% and specificities of 97%, respectively.[41–43] A preliminary study of the Amnisure ROM immunoassay test measuring levels of placental α-microglobulin-1 in cervicovaginal secretions, when compared with the gold standard of clinical diagnosis, was found to have a sensitivity of 98.7%, a specificity of 87.5%, a positive predictive value of 98.1%, and a negative predictive value of 91.3%, which was superior to conventional clinical assessment of ruptured membranes. Further studies are awaited.[44]

Alternatively, if conservative management is deemed appropriate, a "wait and see" policy regarding diagnosis can be adopted. Repeatedly dry pads and a normal amniotic fluid volume on ultrasound examination make the diagnosis less likely. Digital vaginal examination is best avoided because this may introduce infection and possibly stimulate labor. A retrospective study reported that the latency interval between PROM and delivery in those who had a digital examination was significantly shorter than in those women who had only had a sterile speculum examination.[45]

The initial clinical assessment of the patient with PROM will determine further management. All efforts must be directed initially at the exclusion of overt chorioamnionitis, with attention to the detection of maternal tachycardia, pyrexia, uterine tenderness, purulent vaginal discharge, and fetal tachycardia. Thereafter, there should be an evaluation of the fetal gestational age from the history, clinical examination, and ultrasound assessment to determine the likelihood of abruptio placentae and preterm labor.

The subsequent management of the patient will depend very heavily on the particular combination of the previous findings; these management alternatives are discussed in the following sections.

Expectant management usually consists of hospitalization and continued clinical observation of the mother and the fetus. The role of bedrest is controversial but may aid diagnosis by allowing a pool of amniotic fluid to collect in the posterior fornix. Maternal activity appears to increase the rate of fluid leakage, possibly by dislodging the presenting part. Specialized assessment of continued fetal well-being can be employed using cardiotocography, biophysical profiles, and fetal growth estimates every 2 weeks. Abnormal biophysical profile scores have been shown to be markers of intrauterine infection, but in different studies, the true- and false-positive rates vary from 25% to 80% and 2% to 9%, respectively.[46] Fetal tachycardia detected on cardiotocography predicts 20% to 40% of cases of intrauterine infection with a false-positive rate of 3%. There is currently no consensus as to how frequently cardiotocography should be employed.[47,48]

The detection of covert chorioamnionitis using serial daily white blood cell differential counts and C-reactive protein estimates, in association with an initial and then weekly microbiologic cultures, has been advocated. The reported sensitivities and false-positive rates of leukocytosis in the detection of chorioamnionitis range from 29% to 47% and 5% to 18%, respectively, whereas the specificity of C-reactive protein is 38% to 55%.[49–52]

Ultrasound assessment of cervical length has been investigated as a possible predictor of microbial invasion of the amniotic cavity.[53] One study, using a cervical length of 24 mm, had a sensitivity of 76% and a specificity of 67%, performing better than amniotic fluid white cell count, maternal C-reactive protein, and white cell count.[53] The data evaluating weekly vaginal swabs do not show that this is beneficial, with positive genital tract cultures predicting only 53% of positive amniotic fluid cultures with a false-positive rate of 25%.[54] However, the detection of group B streptococcus will provide the opportunity for intrapartum antibiotic therapy.

The use of amniocentesis in clarifying the possibility of covert chorioamnionitis remains controversial and as yet remains to be adequately tested. Current evidence would suggest that infection is a cause rather than a consequence of ruptured membranes, and amniocentesis may detect subclinical infection. Microbiologic culture of amniotic fluid will direct the administration of antibiotics and/or delivery, depending on the gestation in infected cases, and expectant management for women with negative amniotic fluid cultures.[55] However, reported success rates in obtaining amniotic fluid in these circumstances vary from 45% to 97%. Another limitation is the lack of a gold standard for the diagnosis of occult/covert intrauterine infection versus colonization, which in turn, makes the interpretation of the Gram stain, amniotic fluid culture, leukocyte esterase testing, and gas liquid chromatography studies particularly difficult. Rapid amniotic fluid assays of cytokines such as Il-6, Il-8, and I,-18 in amniotic fluid, which may indicate intrauterine infection, have yet to be validated as markers for obstetric assistance and may prove to be no better than clinical indicators,[56] whereas the diagnostic and prognostic value of matrix metalloproteinase-8, amniotic fluid prostaglandin, activity of a lactate dehydrogenase isoform, and proteomic profiles also remain to be evaluated.[57–64]

General Management

Active management may be defined as the previously described expectant management plus the use of one or more of the following:

- Maternal corticosteroids.
- Tocolytic agents.
- Prophylactic antibiotics.

MATERNAL CORTICOSTEROIDS

In the contemporary management of PPROM, there is good evidence to recommend the use of maternal corticosteroids before 34 weeks' gestation to enhance fetal lung maturity.[65] A meta-analysis by Harding and colleagues[66] included 15 randomized, controlled trials involving more than 1400 women with PROM without clinical chorioamnionitis. Results demonstrated that antenatal corticosteroids reduced the risks of respiratory distress syndrome (RR 0.56; 95% CI 0.46–0.70), intraventricular hemorrhage (RR 0.47; 95% CI 0.31–0.70), and necrotizing enterocolitis (RR 0.21; 95% CI 0.05–0.82), without evidence of an increase in the risk of infection in either the mother (RR 0.86; 95% CI 0.61–1.20) or the baby (RR 1.05; 95% CI 0.66–1.68).[66]

As discussed in Chapter 61, there is conflicting information with regard to the repeated use of corticosteroids in this group of women. However, the authors are committed to its use as per the findings of Crowther and associates,[67] in which repeat doses of corticosteroids were associated with demonstrated respiratory benefit, without compromise in neonatal and early childhood growth. In contrast, the Multiple Courses of Antenatal Corticosteroids for Preterm Birth (MACS) trial did not demonstrate improvement in neonatal respiratory outcomes following repeat doses of antenatal corticosteroids.[68] Given the conflicting results, some authors have cautioned about the use of repeat steroids,[69] expressing concerns that adverse fetal programming effects of repeated high dose steroids may not emerge until later childhood, or even adulthood (leading to conditions such as diabetes or hypertension). The Cochrane review,[70] last updated in May 2007, concluded that "further research is needed on other important health outcomes for the woman and baby, which should include child development."

TOCOLYTICS

There is no good evidence to support the use of tocolytics as prophylaxis against preterm delivery, with three randomized studies of 235 women with PPROM demonstrating no increase in the time to delivery following the use of tocolytic therapy.[71–73] It would seem logical that if maternal corticosteroids are advocated, therapeutic tocolysis for at least 48 hours is acceptable providing there is no evidence of overt chorioamnionitis. However, there is conflicting evidence to support this view, with a small randomized trial by Christensen and associates[74] demonstrating a prolongation of the latency interval, whereas more recent nonrandomized data suggest that aggressive tocolysis in PPROM does not increase latency or neonatal morbidity compared with limited tocolysis or no tocolysis all.[75] It is possible that tocolysis could have adverse effects, including delaying delivery from an infected environment, which will be discussed later. There appears to be consensus, however, that the use of tocolysis for maternal-fetal transport to a tertiary center in women with PPROM is appropriate, albeit on the basis of limited evidence.[76]

ANTIBIOTICS

There is better evidence to support the use of prophylactic antibiotics in women with PPROM. Twenty-two trials involving over 6000 women with PPROM were included in the Cochrane Review by Kenyon and coworkers[77] that demonstrated a reduction in chorioamnionitis (RR 0.57; 95% CI 0.37–0.86), a reduction in the number of babies born within 48 hours (RR 0.71; 95% CI 0.58–0.87) and 7 days (RR 0.80; 95% CI 0.71–0.90), a significant reduction in neonatal infection (RR 0.68; 95% CI 0.53–0.87), and a significant reduction in the number of babies born with an abnormal cerebral ultrasound scan prior to hospital discharge (RR 0.82; 95% CI 0.68–0.98). There was no significant reduction in perinatal mortality, although there was a trend for reduction in the treatment group.[77] There was a variation in the choice of antibiotics used and the duration of therapy in the studies examined in the meta-analysis.[77] Ten trials tested broad-spectrum penicillins, either alone or in combination, 5 tested macrolide antibiotics (erythromycin) either alone or in combination, and 1 trial tested clindamycin and gentamicin. The duration of treatment varied between two doses and treatment for 10 days. Any penicillin (except co-amoxiclav) or erythromycin versus placebo was associated with a reduction in the number of babies born within 48 hours with positive blood cultures. Co-amoxiclav versus placebo was associated with an increase in the number of babies born with necrotizing enterocolitis (RR 4.60; 95% CI 1.98–10.72).[77] It is speculated that this might have been because co-amoxiclav interfered with the establishment of normal neonatal gut flora, thus increasing the risk of invasion by pathogenic organisms.

The meta-analysis is dominated by the Overview of Role of Antibiotics in Curtailing Labour and Early Delivery (ORACLE) I trial that recommended the use of oral erythromycin (250 mg q6h for 10 days) as the prophylactic antibiotic of choice for women with PPROM. The ORACLE Children Study I[78] revealed that these early-improved outcomes did not make a substantial difference to the children's health and development (medical conditions, behavioral difficulties, and educational achievements) long term (7-year follow-up) compared with co-amoxiclav either alone or in combination. In contrast, the ORACLE Children Study II[79] suggested a small increased risk of functional impairment and cerebral palsy in the children of women who took these antibiotics 7 years earlier because of threatened preterm labor with intact membranes (and a bigger increase when the two antibiotics were used simultaneously).

OTHER MANAGEMENTS

Additional active management strategies have been or are continuing to be explored to determine their place in the management of women with PPROM. Transvaginal amnioinfusion during labor was examined by one randomized, controlled trial involving 66 women with PPROM; the results showed no significant difference between amnioinfusion and no amnioinfusion on cesarean section rates, low Apgar scores, and neonatal death.[80] Transbdominal amnioinfusion has also been assessed as a possible therapeutic option, but the risk of pulmonary hypoplasia does not appear to be reduced, although fetal survival was higher in the treated than in the control group (64.8% vs. 32.3%, $P < .001$).[81] Hence, at present, there is insufficient evidence to recommend transabdominal amnioinfusion as a strategy for preventing pulmonary hypoplasia in very early PPROM.

Studies have evaluated the use of an "amnio patch" for women with mid-trimester PPROM, particularly when it results from iatrogenic PPROM at the time of amniocentesis or with diagnostic or therapeutic fetoscopy.[82] A variety of fibrin sealants have been used with some success, but their application to spontaneous membrane rupture has not been adequately tested to determine whether this would be a helpful strategy in spontaneous cases.[83,84] Even more preliminary is a study in a similar group of women using a cervical cerclage with placement of a gelatin sponge, embolization, beads and a bioadhesive glue into the endocervical canal.[85] A nonrandomized evaluation in a small number of women suggested a neonatal survival rate of 21% in the treated group compared with 0% in the control group.[85]

Do these initiatives represent a return to the PPROM "Fence" (a barrier or sealant to close the defect in the membranes) suggested but never adequately tested in the 1980s?[86] Further trials are required before such strategies can be regarded as more than experimental.

SPECIFIC MANAGEMENT

Aggressive management is employed when delivery is deemed necessary as a result of obstetric indications such as fetal distress, maternal sepsis, abruptio placentae, or if requested by the parents in the face of marked fetal immaturity (<24 wk) or demonstrated fetal maturity (>37 wk). This form of management involves induction and augmentation of labor, with an inevitable increase in operative delivery and its associated maternal morbidity.

The prospective, multicenter, randomized, controlled trial by Hannah and colleagues[87] (The Term PROM Trial) has enabled us to provide management options for women with PROM after 37 weeks' gestation, and similarly designed trials for women with PPROM at different gestational age groups are currently in progress. Generally, the recommended management of PROM has shifted from an expectant mode to a more active mode, with accurate assessment of fetal gestational age being crucial to the decision-making process. It is useful to consider prenatal strategies in relation to five gestational periods.

PPROM AT LESS THAN 24 COMPLETED GESTATIONAL WEEKS

The most appropriate management at this gestation is not clear and must be individualized, with the wishes of the parents being paramount. Aggressive management is indicated if active labor, abruptio placentae, or clinical evidence of maternal-fetal infection is present. It may also be requested by the parents if they fear delivery not only at this gestation but also at a later gestation (25–26 wk) when there is the possibility of survival but also a high likelihood of serious neonatal complications and long-term handicap. Expectant management is increasingly considered nowadays, but with reported neonatal survival rates of less than 30% at gestations less than 24 weeks even in the most optimistic studies[88,89] and with "normal" neonatal development in less than 30% of the survivors after a 12-month follow-up, extreme care must be taken to ensure that parental counseling by the obstetric/midwifery/neonatology team is thorough and cautious.

In view of the uncertainty of the neonatal outcome, an alternative management strategy has evolved for these women. After initial hospitalization, investigation, and observation for 72 hours, the patient may be managed at home, restricting her physical activity, taking her own temperature, and reporting weekly for prenatal evaluation and microbiologic and hematologic surveillance. The package, and each individual component, of these management options has yet to be tested in randomized trials, but clearly this approach, if safe, would have substantial psychosocial advantages. It would also have economic benefits for the health system, although it might impose greater costs for the woman and her family, depending on the circumstances (e.g., whether she is insured or has state health coverage).

PPROM AT 24 TO 30 COMPLETED GESTATIONAL WEEKS

At this gestation, the greatest risk to the fetus is still prematurity, and this risk currently outweighs any potential advantage in delivering a patient with covert intrauterine infection. As a consequence, expectant management is the favored option at this gestation. The use of amniocentesis to detect covert or occult intra-amniotic infection remains controversial at this gestation, particularly because fetal lung maturity is unlikely. It may be specifically indicated to clarify the situation in the patient with PPROM who has mild pyrexia, a significantly raised white cell count, or an elevated C-reactive protein.

A randomized study by Carlan and associates,[90] assessing hospital versus home management after 72 hours of PPROM at 26 to 31 weeks' gestation, suggested that home management was a safe regimen to adopt in terms of comparable latency periods, gestational age at delivery, and similar maternal and neonatal outcomes with regard to sepsis and respiratory distress, along with significant savings in maternal hospital bed days. However, only 18% of women with PPROM were eligible and agreed to randomization, owing to the rigorous requirements for entry into the trial, which included cephalic presentation, an adequate amniotic fluid volume on ultrasound assessment, and acceptance of advice and education about the signs and symptoms of chorioamnionitis, the need for twice-daily basal temperature measurement, and regular outpatient visits.

The randomized, controlled trial by Turnbull and coworkers[91] included 395 women, some with PPROM, to in-hospital versus outpatient management. Although there were no differences in clinical outcomes and costs, women preferred outpatient management. However, this study was underpowered to detect a difference in the clinical outcomes for women with PPROM suggested by earlier studies.[92,93] Larger randomized studies are required to determine the appropriate management of PPOM, but we consider it reasonable to keep a patient in the hospital for at least 48 hours before making a decision to recommend continued management at home. Following such a decision, management should be individualized, with rigorous selection on the basis of risk factors. Eligible women should be instructed to take their temperature every 12 hours and be aware of the symptoms associated with intrauterine infection.

Included in the prenatal management of PPROM at 24 to 31 weeks' gestation must be a discussion with the parents regarding the likely mode of delivery should expectant management not be appropriate. Based on the studies by Amon and colleagues[94] and Sanchez-Ramos and associates,[95] there has been a move away from almost-universal cesarean section to vaginal delivery, with resort to cesarean section for standard obstetric indications, including breech presentation.[96]

PPROM AT 30 TO 36 COMPLETED GESTATIONAL WEEKS

At most tertiary institutions, neonatal survival after 30 completed gestational weeks exceeds 95%, and thus, the risk from prematurity is similar to the risk to the neonate from sepsis. Although debate still occurs about the place of amniocentesis in the diagnosis of occult chorioamnionitis, the detection of fetal lung maturity would suggest that it is present in 58% of specimens obtained at this gestational age.[56] Testing for fetal lung maturity (L/S [lecithin-to-sphingomyelin] ratio) in women with PPROM has a positive predictive value of 68% with a negative predictive value of 79%. Specific situations of occult amniotic fluid infection but fetal lung immaturity and fetal lung maturity but absent amniotic fluid infection must be managed on a clinical basis with its inherent limitations, as must be women with PPROM in whom amniocentesis has been unsuccessful. A large prospective, randomized trial is urgently required to evaluate the role of amniocentesis in women presenting with PPROM (especially at 30–34 wk) because preliminary findings by Blackwell and coworkers[97] suggest that amniocentesis may alter clinical management in up to 48% of cases. Whether this results in decreased neonatal morbidity remains unknown.

Although an expectant management policy is commonly employed at 34 to 36 completed weeks of gestation, this is by no means the standard approach, with many favoring induction of labor.[98] In a survey of practice among Australian and New Zealand obstetricians,[99] 49% indicated a preference for expectant management and 51% indicated a preference for delivery.

A retrospective study of 430 women with PPROM demonstrated that composite neonatal minor morbidity such as jaundice and transient tachypnea was significantly higher among pregnancies delivered at 34 weeks' gestation or less than among those delivered at 36 weeks.[100] Composite major neonatal morbidity including respiratory distress syndrome and intraventricular hemorrhage was significantly higher in neonates delivered at 33 weeks or less than in those delivering at 36 weeks' gestation. There were no differences in major morbidity rates for those neonates delivered after 34 weeks' gestation, which led the authors to conclude that expectant management after 34 weeks' gestation was of limited benefit.

In an earlier prospective, randomized study of 120 women with PPROM between 34 and 37 gestational weeks,[101] the expectantly managed group had a higher incidence of chorioamnionitis compared with the immediate delivery group (16% vs. 2%; $P < .05$), but the incidence of sepsis and respiratory distress was similar in both groups.[101] A retrospective series examining neonatal outcome with PPROM between 32 and 36 weeks demonstrated that the specific gestation for reduced morbidity was 34 weeks.[102] The incidence of respiratory distress syndrome was 22.5% at 33 weeks and 5.8% at 34 weeks in this study.

In a meta-analysis of three randomized trials comparing immediate delivery with expectant management for women with PPROM at 34 to 36 weeks' gestation, immediate delivery was associated with a reduction in the risk of chorioamnionitis (three studies, 260 women; RR 0.25; 95% CI 0.12–0.53).[103] There were no statistically significant differences identified for neonatal outcomes, including respiratory distress syndrome, sepsis, or perinatal mortality.[103] There are currently two larger ongoing randomized, controlled trials by Lacaze-Masmonteil and Chari in Canada[104] and Morris in Australia[105] comparing elective delivery versus expectant management in women with PPROM between 32 and 35 completed weeks' gestation, the results of which are awaited.

A cautionary note must be added regarding recent studies reminding us of the small but significantly increased risk of perinatal death in singleton infants born at late preterm compared with term gestation,[106–109] which suggests the potential for long-term neurobehavioral problems and medical and social consequences in infants intentionally delivered between 34 and 37 weeks' gestation. This information taken together with the recent work of Bastek and colleagues[110] and Cheng and associates[111] reinforces the need to better characterize the risks of short-term and long-term morbidity to infants who are delivered at late preterm gestations rather than assuming that 34 weeks' gestation represents the complete achievement of fetal "maturity."

PROM AFTER 36 WEEKS

In women with PROM after 36 completed gestational weeks, an expectant management policy may be justified initially because it can be anticipated that 75% to 80% of these women will labor spontaneously within 24 hours. The controversial aspects of management at this gestation center around the risks of maternal and neonatal sepsis as the latency period lengthens versus the risks of induction of labor and a possible increase in operative delivery. The key study by Hannah and colleagues,[87] in which 5041 women with PROM at term were randomly assigned to expectant management for up to 4 days or to induction of labor with intravenous oxytocin or vaginal prostaglandin E_2 gel, has helped clarify this controversy. The rates of neonatal infection were 2.0% for induction with oxytocin group, 3.0% for induction with prostaglandin group, 2.8% for the expectant management (including subsequent oxytocin) group, and 2.7% for the expectant management (with subsequent prostaglandin) group.[87] The rates of cesarean section ranged from 9.6% to 10.9% in the four groups.[87] Hence, in PROM after 36 completed weeks, similar frequency for neonatal sepsis and cesarean section occurred with expectant management and induction of labor. However, clinical chorioamnionitis was less likely to develop in the women in the induction with oxytocin group than those in the expectant management (±oxytocin) group (4% vs. 8.6%; $P < .001$) as was postpartum fever (1.9% vs. 3.6%; $P = .008$).[87] Further, it was found that women in this study viewed induction of labor more positively than expectant management, although it remains important to give women choices in their management.[87] If cost implications are to also be taken into account, an argument can be mounted for induction of labor with intravenous oxytocin for women presenting with PROM at 36 or more completed gestational weeks.

The Cochrane review assessing expectant management of PROM near term included 12 trials involving 6814 women.[112] Overall, there were no differences detected for mode of birth between planned induction and expectant groups (cesarean section: RR 0.94; 95% CI 0.82–1.08; or operative vaginal birth: RR 0.98; 95% CI 0.84–1.16).[112] Significantly fewer women in the planned induction versus the expectant group had chorioamnionitis (RR 0.30; 95% CI 0.56–0.97) or endometritis (RR 0.83; 95% CI 0.12–0.74).[112] No differences were identified for neonatal infection (RR 0.83; 95% CI 0.61–1.12), although fewer infants with planned induction went to neonatal intensive or special care compared with expectant management (RR 0.72; 95% CI 0.57–0.92).[112] The conclusions of the review were that because planned and expectant management may not be very different, women need to be given appropriate information and then be encouraged to make a choice that suits their preference and circumstances.

Special Circumstances

THE "HINDWATER" LEAK

This poorly defined clinical entity is of unknown frequency and is usually a diagnosis of exclusion. The natural history of this phenomenon and its maternal and neonatal consequences is unknown and awaits further evaluation.

RESEALED PROM

Once again, this is a poorly defined clinical entity that may encompass a number of women with a "hindwater" leak. Johnson and coworkers[113] studied 220 conservatively managed women with PPROM between 20 and 34 weeks' gestation, and identified 8 women (3.6%) in whom there was a cessation of leakage. Similarly, Carlan and colleagues[114] reported on 349 women with PPROM of whom 14 (4%) apparently resealed after initial confirmation of PPROM. In both studies, those women who resealed were of a younger age group, had PPROM at an earlier gestation, and had larger pockets of residual amniotic fluid at the initial ultrasound examination than women with PPROM who did not reseal. After resealing, the pregnancies all proceeded normally without an increased incidence of rerupture of the membranes. How resealing might occur, given that the fetal membranes are acellular, remains a matter of speculation.

MULTIPLE PREGNANCY AND PROM (See Also Chapter 59)

A multiple gestation with an overdistended uterus is an important risk factor for PPROM; the incidence is higher and occurs earlier in multiple pregnancies. Mercer and associates[115] compared 99 twin pregnancies with 99 well-matched singleton pregnancies, all complicated by PPROM, and found that PPROM at less than 26 weeks' gestation occurred more frequently in twins with an incidence of 18.2% (OR 2.1) compared with 0.52% in singletons (OR 2.71). Despite these differences, the etiology of PPROM appeared to be similar to singleton pregnancies, with infection being the main identifiable cause, although uterine overdistention may play a role. This study showed only a brief latency period in twins complicated by PPROM regardless of gestational age, with no difference in infant survival between the presenting and the nonpresenting twins but with a significant increase in respiratory morbidity in the nonpresenting infant. Not surprisingly, rupture of the membranes usually occurs in the presenting sac, but this is not invariable and can occur in the nonpresenting twin.

Novel management strategies such as delayed interval delivery[116] need to be considered in this situation and are discussed in Chapter 59.

Montgomery and coworkers[117] suggested that the natural history of PPROM in twin gestation parallels that in singleton pregnancy, and that similar management strategies are appropriate for both groups of women with PPROM, although the study by Andreani and colleagues[118] suggests that PROM in twins is associated with a lower risk of chorioamnionitis than in singletons.

Labor and Delivery

If labor occurs in the presence of PROM, both mother and fetus should be intensively monitored, and labor augmented promptly if there is any delay in progress, because of the increased risk of maternal and fetal/neonatal infection. Labor may be suppressed to allow transfer to a tertiary center if PROM occurs in an institution without appropriate facilities for neonatal care. Vaginal delivery should generally be anticipated, with the need for cesarean section not differing substantially from other preterm deliveries with intact membranes. Once labor is established or is induced, maternal intravenous antibiotic therapy should be commenced, particularly if signs of intrauterine infection are present (e.g., maternal pyrexia, maternal tachycardia, fetal tachycardia, persistent uterine tenderness, offensive smelling vaginal discharge with an increased white cell count, and a C-reactive protein). A reduction in anticipated puerperal infections has been confirmed in most studies advocating this approach.

The authors currently favor a loading dose of 2 g of intravenous ampicillin with 1 g every 4 hours thereafter, together with gentamicin 5 mg/kg intravenously and metronidazole 500 mg intravenously every 12 hours.[119] In cases of known group B streptococcus colonization or status unknown or PROM greater than 18 hours, benzyl penicillin 3 g as an intravenous loading dose followed by 1.2 g intravenously every 4 hours is recommended. This regimen of intravenous penicillin, or in the case of penicillin allergy, lincomycin (600 mg, q8h intravenously), is currently employed in the United Kingdom, most of Europe, and Australia, and it is reported to reduce group B streptococcus sepsis by more than 90% in the neonate.[120]

A preliminary study by Chichester and associates[121] suggests that women with PROM and regular contractions sufficient to cause a second request for pain medication within 2 hours should be offered epidural analgesia because they are highly likely to deliver within 24 hours. Although regional analgesia has benefits for the fetus, there may be concerns about inserting an epidural block in the presence of overt maternal infection because of concerns that the mother might develop an epidural/spinal abscess.[121] At the time of delivery, in addition to an experienced obstetrician and midwife, the presence of a neonatologist with the back-up of an appropriate neonatal support team is essential to the optimization of the perinatal outcome.

Postnatal

With regard to women delivering after PROM, an awareness of the associated risks of endometritis, genital sepsis/septicemia, along with postpartum hemorrhage and thromboembolism, is essential for the effective management of such women. Active promotion of maternal infant bonding, particularly with PPROM, deserves special mention. Recently, reports suggest that induction of labor, preterm birth, operative delivery, and postpartum hemorrhage, which all commonly accompany PPROM, are associated with lower rates of breast-feeding with OR 0.56 (95% CI 0.47–0.67), 0.87 (95% CI 0.77–0.98), 0.80 (95% CI 0.69–0.92), 0.83 (95% CI 0.72–0.96), and 0.84 (95% CI 0.75–0.94), respectively.[122]

All infants born after PROM should be thoroughly screened for sepsis irrespective of the use of antepartum or intrapartum maternal antibiotic therapy. Screening investigations usually include neonatal blood culture, endotracheal aspirate culture, urinary latex particle agglutination testing, and a complete blood picture including nucleated red blood cells.[123] Lumbar puncture and cerebrospinal fluid examination should be reserved for clinically septic neonates and for those infants with positive blood cultures. Initial antibiotic therapy using a combination of intravenous penicillin and gentamicin is usually employed empirically while awaiting the result of the screening investigations. Often the results are inconclusive or equivocal, and discontinuation of the antibiotic therapy may have to be based on clinical judgment.

Respiratory disease remains the greatest hazard encountered with PROM, with respiratory distress requiring mechanical ventilation a common sequela. This can be aggravated by pulmonary hypoplasia, which is usually only clinically significant if PPROM occurs before 25 weeks' gestation and/or with a latent period of more than 5 weeks before delivery.[124] The neonatal outcome of PPROM at later gestations is more optimistic than is reported for other causes of oligohydramnios. Common associations of prematurity including intracranial hemorrhage, jaundice, and feeding difficulties must be attended to in the usual fashion by the neonatal care team.

Essential to the provision of comprehensive care of preterm or complicated term neonates is the requirement for long-term neonatal follow-up, particularly in view of preliminary data suggesting a higher risk of neurodevelopmental impairment in preterm infants delivered after prolonged PPROM than in those neonates born after spontaneous preterm labor with intact membranes[125] and the now more robust data previously mentioned with regard to late preterm delivery.[106–111]

As has been outlined in Chapter 61, a postdelivery evaluation of the circumstances of the delivery by the perinatal team not only may aid in the management of future pregnancies but also will provide instructive and constructive feedback to the parents who are required to deal with the day-to-day consequences of PROM, particularly PPROM, not only in the immediate and long term for themselves and their babies but also possibly for future pregnancies.

SUMMARY OF MANAGEMENT OPTIONS
Prelabor Rupture of Membranes

Management Options	Evidence Quality and Recommendation	References
Prepregnancy (Especially Previous PPROM)		
Counsel about recurrence risks (21%–32% for PROM and up to 34% for PTD).	III/B	11,23
Search for causes/precipitating factors has limited overall value.	—/GPP	—
Stress value of preventive measures, such as patient education and stop smoking.	III/B	24
Note conflicting data on value of vaginal bacteriologic screening and antimicrobial treatment of woman and partner.	Ib/A	32–34,126–128
Prenatal		
Prevention		
There are conflicting data on the value of vaginal bacteriologic screening and antimicrobial treatment of woman and partner.	Ib/A	32–34,126–128
Cervical ultrasound assessment with fetal fibronectin (and similar biochemical screening tests) in women with previous history of PROM may be of benefit.	III/B	53
Confirm Diagnosis		
Perform history and physical examination (especially sterile speculum) and collection of amniotic fluid; make repeated pad checks to confirm diagnosis.	—/GPP	—
Additional tests ("ferning," alkaline pH turning nitrazine yellow blue/black, presence of vernix or meconium) all have limitations, especially being unreliable/inappropriate at preterm gestations.	—/GPP	—
Presence of fetal fibronectin (and other biochemical markers) may be useful confirmatory test indicating the likelihood of ensuing preterm labor may allow intervention to reduce the likelihood of birth complications.	III/B	53
Intra-amniotic injection of dyes is not without risk and is not widely practiced.	IV/C	39,40
Ultrasound diagnosis of oligohydramnios is associated only with substantial fluid loss, which is usually clinically obvious.	—/GPP	—

Management Options	Evidence Quality and Recommendation	References
Prenatal Management		
General		
Maintain vigilance for chorioamnionitis.	IIb/B	55–64
Clinical: maternal fever, tachycardia, uterine pain/tenderness, purulent vaginal discharge, fetal tachycardia.		
Laboratory investigations (unreliable):		
• White blood cell count and differential.	—/GPP	—
• C-Reactive protein	—/GPP	—
• Amniotic fluid Gram stain, white cells, and culture (role of amniocentesis uncertain).	IIa/B	55–64
Biophysical testing (NST and/or BPS).	III/B	47,48
Value of pro-inflammatory cytokine testing is uncertain.	IIb/B	59,61–63
Delivery is indicated if chorioamnionitis is diagnosed or if fetal distress occurs (NST/BPS).	—/GPP	—
<24 Weeks with No Evidence of Chorioamnionitis or Fetal Distress		
Individualized management including parental input.	—/GPP	—
Careful counseling of parents needed.	—/GPP	—
If decision is to continue with pregnancy, implement surveillance for sepsis, possibly at home.	IIb/B	88,89
Mode of delivery is usually vaginal.	IV/C	92,93
24–31 Weeks with No Evidence of Chorioamnionitis or Fetal Distress		
The upper gestational age chosen will vary depending on local neonatal survival rates.	—/GPP	—
Expectant/conservative management (possibly at home after initial hospital assessment and exclusion of sepsis) is recommended.	Ib/A	90–93
Counsel parents re: prognosis.	—/GPP	—
Look for clinical evidence of chorioamnionitis.	IIb/B	89,90
Treatments:		
• Steroid use is variable.	Ib/A	65,67–69,129
• Tocolysis only for transfer to tertiary unit.	IV/C	65
• May give antibiotics (erythromycin not co-amoxiclav).	Ia/A	77
Assessment of fetal pulmonary lung maturity is a variable practice and of uncertain value	IIa/B	97
Aim for vaginal delivery if cephalic; ?cesarean section for breech presentation.	IV/C	96
31–36 Weeks with No Evidence of Chorioamnionitis or Fetal Distress		
Options used in practice:		
• Expectant/conservative (wait for 24–72 hr and if not in labor, consider induction).	—/GPP	—
• Aggressive (induce labor at presentation).		
After 36 Completed Weeks with No Evidence of Chorioamnionitis or Fetal Distress		
Discuss options with parents:		
• Expectant/conservative (wait for 24–72 hr and if not in labor, induce).		
• Aggressive (induce labor at presentation).	Ib/A	87,112
Special Circumstances		
Hindwater leak—poorly defined, difficult to diagnose.		
If definite proof of PROM (irrespective of whether cervical membranes intact), manage as PROM.	—/GPP	—

SUMMARY OF MANAGEMENT OPTIONS

Prelabor Rupture of Membranes—cont'd

Management Options	Evidence Quality and Recommendation	References
Cessation of PROM—manage normally.	Ia/A	113,122
Multiple pregnancy—manage as for singleton.	IIb/B	117,118
Labor and Delivery		
Continue observation for infection.	—/GPP	—
Use of maternal antibiotics prophylactically during labor remains controversial (except with group B Streptococcal colonization).	IIa/B	120
Cesarean section for normal obstetric indications.	—/GPP	—
Pediatrician should attend delivery.	—/GPP	—
Postnatal		
Maintain vigilance and screening for infection.	—/GPP	—
Neonatal screen for sepsis and appropriate care.	—/GPP	—
Long-term pediatric follow-up especially neurodevelopmental.	IIa/B	106–111,125

BPS, biophysical score; GPP, good practice point; NST, nonstress test; PPROM, preterm premature rupture of membranes; PROM, premature rupture of membranes; PTD, preterm delivery.

FUTURE DIRECTIONS

This review of the care of women and their babies when the amniotic membranes rupture before the onset of labor highlights the need for large well-designed trials of a range of management strategies. Where possible, these studies must be randomized with concealment of treatment options. It is likely that such studies will require collaboration between many centers in order to achieve sample sizes that would provide meaningful answers for incorporation into clinical practice guidelines.

Acknowledgment

The authors wish to express their debt for the efforts, in the first three editions of this text, of their friend and colleague Dr. Rasiah Vigneswaran, Staff Neonatologist, Adelaide Women's & Children's Hospital, who died on November 29, 2002.

SUGGESTED READINGS

Blackwell SC, Berry SM: Role of amniocentesis for the diagnosis of subclinical intra-amniotic infection in preterm premature rupture of the membranes. Curr Opin Obstet Gynecol 1999;11:541–547.

Crowley P: Prophylactic corticosteroids for preterm birth. Cochrane Database Syst Rev 2006;3:CD000065.

Crowther CA, Doyle LW, Haslam RR, et al: for ACTORDS Study Group: Outcomes at 2 years of age after repeat doses of antenatal corticosteroids. N Engl J Med 2007;357:1179–1189.

Dare MR, Middleton P, Crowther CA, et al: Planned early birth versus expectant management (waiting) for prelabour rupture of membranes at term (37 weeks or more). Cochrane Database Syst Rev 2006;1:CD005302.

Kenyon S, Boulvain M, Neilson J: Antibiotics for preterm rupture of membranes. Cochrane Database Syst Rev 2003;2:CD001058.

McDonald HM, Brockelhurst P, Gordon A: Antibiotics for treating bacterial vaginosis in pregnancy. Cochrane Review 2007;2:CD000262.

McIntyre DD, Leveno KJ: Neonatal mortality and morbidity rates in late preterm births compared with babies at term. Obstet Gynecol 2008;111:35–41.

Mercer BM, Goldenberg RL, Meis PJ, et al: The preterm prediction study: Prediction of preterm premature rupture of membranes through clinical findings and ancillary testing. NICHD,MFM Units Network. Am J Obstet Gynecol 2000;183:738–745.

Morris JM, Roberts CL, Crowther CA, et al: Protocol for immediate delivery versus expectant care of women with preterm prelabour rupture of the membranes close to term. BMC Childbirth 2006;23:6–9.

Moster D, Lie RT, Markestad T: Long-term medical and social consequences of preterm birth. N Engl J Med 2008;359:262–273.

REFERENCES

For a complete list of references, log onto www.expertconsult.com.

CHAPTER 63

Breech Presentation

ZOË PENN

INTRODUCTION

Many of the obstetric controversies surrounding breech presentation have been resolved since the turn of the Millenium. Antenatal external cephalic version (ECV) is now recommended for the term fetus and is deemed unnecessary for the preterm fetus, whereas delivery by elective cesarean section is recommended when the fetus is mature or labor commences at term. Vaginal delivery of the breech was the norm (and an essential manipulative skill to be acquired by all obstetricians) until the late 1950s, when cesarean section was first recommended on a routine basis to protect the fetus. This recommendation gained ground steadily, but it was not until shortly after the beginning of the third millennium that a trial was published that finally convinced most of the world's obstetricians that the policy was evidence-based.[1]

However, an important realization since the early 1980s has been that breech presentation may well be a bad prognostic variable in itself.[2] Any studies, clinical trials, or proposed clinical management must take this into account.

INCIDENCE

The incidence of breech presentation varies with gestational age, being approximately 14% at 29 to 32 weeks and 2.2 to 3.7% at term (depending on the use of ECV), giving an overall figure of 3% to 4%.[3,4]

ETIOLOGY

Although, in many cases, no specific underlying cause of breech presentation is apparent, in some cases, a cause can be identified (Table 63–1).

Preterm Labor

A major reason for breech presentation is the preterm onset of labor (probably the chance lie of a highly mobile fetus in relatively copious liquor); most of these babies are structurally normal. It remains unclear whether breech presentation per se predisposes to preterm labor.

Fetal Abnormality

Lamont and associates[5] found that 18% of preterm breech infants were congenitally abnormal. Collea and coworkers[6] quoted a 5% incidence of congenital abnormality in term breech fetuses, two and a half times higher than in their vertex counterparts (2.1%). Central nervous system abnormalities are the most commonly noted; approximately 50% of all babies with hydrocephalus and myelomeningocele present by the breech, as do 50% of those with Prader-Willi syndrome and trisomy. Despite the association of breech presentation with preterm labor, labor at term is still most common and 90% of abnormal breech babies weigh more than 2000 g.

Breech presentation is also associated with fetal growth restriction and with abnormalities of amniotic fluid volume (either oligo- or polyhydramnios). The association between fetal growth restriction and breech presentation is particularly marked in the preterm fetus. Breech fetuses tend to have reduced fetal-placental ratios, to be small for gestational age, and to have an increased head circumference regardless of the mode of delivery. This difference in weight persists at 18 months of age but disappears by 4 years.[7] Breech presentation has also been linked with relatively short umbilical cords.

Maternal Abnormality

Uterine size or shape may also influence presentation. The narrower cephalic pole of the fetus usually fits better than the breech into the narrower lower segment, and the breech and legs into the wider upper segment, especially if the legs of the fetus are flexed at the knee. However, if the knees are extended, the hips flexed, and the uterine space limited, the head and feet may lie alongside each other, making the cephalic pole of the fetus larger and thus encouraging a breech presentation. Uterine tone is greatest in nullipara, limiting the available space, and breech presentation is reported to be more common in nulliparous women. Conversely, the relaxed uterus of the grand multipara encourages an unstable lie, so that the fetus enters labor by chance in a breech presentation.

Other less benign conditions may alter the uterine capacity or the intrauterine shape. Uterine anomalies, such as bicornuate uterus, are associated with breech presentation. Placenta previa is well recognized in association with breech presentation, because this changes the intrauterine shape and prevents engagement of the head. Cornual implantation of the placenta, an otherwise benign condition, is also strongly associated with breech presentation; only 5% of

TABLE 63-1

Etiology of Breech Presentation

Preterm labor
Fetal abnormality (especially central nervous system)
Oligo- or polyhydramnios
Fetal growth restriction
Short umbilical cord
Extended legs in the fetus
Uterine abnormality (e.g., bicornuate uterus)
Placenta previa
Cornual placenta
Contracted pelvis
Multiple pregnancy
Maternal anticonvulsants
Maternal substance abuse

vertex-presenting fetuses have a cornual placenta in comparison with 73% of those presenting by the breech.

A contracted pelvis is also associated with breech presentation, probably by limiting uterine space in the lower segment.

Other Reasons for Breech Presentation

Women who have had a breech presentation at term are significantly more likely to have another in a subsequent pregnancy. This is usually associated with extended fetal legs and may indicate a genetic predisposition to this posture in the fetus.

Multiple pregnancy is strongly associated with breech presentation. The reader is referred to Chapter 59 for further discussion of management.

Medication with anticonvulsants in pregnancy also seems to be associated with breech presentation,[8] as does maternal alcohol abuse[9]; both substances have a profound influence on intrauterine fetal neurologic function. Fetal behavior in utero in fetuses with persistent breech presentation is also subtly different. They demonstrate more state transitions in fetal activity and heart rate patterns in utero than their cephalic presenting counterparts.[10]

RISKS AND SIGNIFICANCE

Although fetuses presenting by the breech have an increased perinatal mortality rate, it has proved difficult to separate and quantify the independent risks of the breech position itself and to distinguish the problems of the delivery from the problems of the fetus being abnormal. The perinatal mortality rate remains increased even when delivery is by cesarean section; this is true even after correction for gestational age, congenital defects, and birth weight.

Many retrospective reviews of breech presentation and trials of antepartum and intrapartum management compare the breech-presenting infant with the vertex-presenting infant, and because of its associated problems, the breech-presenting infant is more likely to perform unfavorably, regardless of the mode of delivery. There have only been a small number of randomized, controlled trials and meta-analyses studying the role of the mode of delivery of the term breech in relation to long-term outcome, and they have produced conflicting results.[6,11–14] (It should be noted that functional and behavioral outcomes by mode of delivery need to be considered independently of perinatal mortality; see the later section on mode of delivery.)

Although breech presentation is an independent predictor for cerebral palsy,[15] some of the association of breech presentation with cerebral palsy can be accounted for by the excess of low birth weight in breech presentation, and the association is independent of the mode of delivery.[16]

Abnormalities of neuromotor development may also be manifest in breech-presenting fetuses, with subtle differences in in utero fetal behavioral states being evident.[16] Following birth, Bartlett and colleagues[17] compared 90 morphologically normal term breech-presenting singletons with birth weights greater than 2500 g and delivered by cesarean section with similar cephalically presenting infants, matched for gender and also delivered by cesarean. They collected data prospectively on neurologic status and motor performance over the first 18 months of life. They found that not only did breech-presenting infants have more open popliteal angles at birth (an unsurprising observation) but also they had significantly lower motor scores at 6 weeks and an excess of neurologic problems diagnosed at 18 months.

The risks to the mother are an increased rate of cesarean section with all its attendant complications. However, Lydon-Rochelle and associates,[18] using logistic regression, showed that among 265,000 nulliparous women undergoing cesarean section, there was no increased risk of maternal mortality compared with women delivering vaginally; similarly low rates of mortality have been reported in a number of other large population studies.[19,20] Several large population studies of maternal morbidity after elective caesarean section have shown morbidity to be mostly limited to postpartum fever, with the highest morbidity being associated with assisted vaginal delivery or intrapartum cesarean section.[21,22] The main risk seems to be of placenta previa and placenta accreta in a subsequent pregnancy, with a maternal mortality rate of up to 7% if these complications occur.[23] There is some evidence that breech presentation and cesarean section may reduce the subsequent pregnancy rate, probably because of the woman's decision not to reproduce again.[24] However, if these women do decide to have another child, vaginal delivery remains an option; one study in Dublin reported that 85% of those who had a trial of vaginal delivery in their second pregnancy after an elective caesarean section for breech presentation in their first pregnancy delivered vaginally.[25]

DIAGNOSIS

Three clinical types of breech presentation are recognized. This classification is useful in that it may indicate the cause of the presentation and the complications to be anticipated. As with most clinical classifications, there is overlap of the associated factors between the groups:

- The frank (or extended) breech indicates that the legs of the fetus are flexed at the hip and extended at the knee. This type accounts for 60% to 70% of all breech presentations at term. The risks of fetal-pelvic disproportion and of cord prolapse are lowest in this group.
- The complete (or flexed) breech indicates that the hips and knees are flexed so that the feet are presenting in the pelvis.

- The incomplete (or footling) breech indicates that one leg is flexed and the other extended.

The woman with a breech presentation, especially toward term, may complain of subcostal discomfort and of feeling the baby kick in the lower part of the uterus. On palpation, the hard round ballotable head is found at the fundus and the softer breech is at the lower pole. The fetal heart sounds are more commonly heard above the umbilicus. One diagnostic pitfall is the confusion of a deeply engaged head and a breech presentation. The examiner thinks that the shoulders are above the pelvic brim when, in fact, the breech is over the pelvis.

At vaginal examination, if the cervix is sufficiently dilated, the fetal ischial tuberosities and the sacrum provide the bony landmarks. The anus and the genitalia may also be felt but are less useful in diagnosis owing to their softness and compressibility. If the membranes are ruptured, the examining finger in the anus may produce meconium staining. The main diagnostic confusion is face presentation. Face presentation produces the characteristic bony landmarks of the malar eminences, mouth, and mentum that produce a bony triangle, whereas the ischial tuberosities and the sacrum are in line. The mouth, in contrast to the anus, has a firm unyielding margin of bone. Engagement of the breech implies that the bitrochanteric diameter has passed through the pelvic brim.

Approximately 45% of breech presentations are not diagnosed until after 38 weeks, and 10% to 30% remain undiagnosed until labor.[26] If there is any doubt about presentation, an ultrasound scan is mandatory if mistakes are to be avoided. Some clinicians even advocate routine late third trimester ultrasonography to determine presentation and ensure time for ECV (thus decreasing the need for cesarean section).[26]

THE PRETERM BREECH PRESENTATION

Techniques for optimizing the condition of preterm infants at birth have focused predominantly on the mode of delivery and led to an increase in the cesarean section rate of approximately threefold between 1995 and 2002, reflecting the increasingly aggressive management policies for extremely preterm infants.

Risks

General

The currently accepted definition of preterm birth—being born before 37 completed weeks of gestation—was first suggested by the World Health Organization in 1977 on purely epidemiologic grounds. However, in developed countries, the mortality and morbidity rates of babies delivered between 33 and 36 weeks inclusive is now very low, and not significantly influenced by mode of delivery, provided that cesarean section is undertaken for the usual clinical indications. Discussion is focused here on the gestation range of 26 to 32 weeks, when approximately 2% of women with viable fetuses will deliver. About 25% of babies delivered at these gestations are in breech presentation, probably due to the chance lie of a very mobile fetus in the relatively copious amniotic fluid. Thus, the overall incidence of very preterm (<33 wk) breech presentation at delivery is 0.5%.

The preterm baby in breech presentation shares many of the characteristics of the mature breech. The preterm breech also has a higher rate of congenital abnormality than its vertex-presenting counterpart, up to 18%.[27] This is associated with an increased antepartum stillbirth and neonatal death rate, regardless of mode of delivery.[3] It is probably even more true of the preterm than the term breech that poor outcome in survivors, including neurologic dysfunction, cannot be attributed solely to the fact of vaginal breech delivery but is often due to the abnormalities associated with breech presentation. The preterm breech shows other differences from the cephalic-presenting infant at the same gestation; it is more commonly small for gestational age and has a lower fetal-placental ratio. It also tends to have a larger head circumference for a given birth weight than babies delivered in vertex presentation, probably due to the lack of the compressive effect of the lower segment. It seems likely that in many cases, preterm birth and poor outcome are both determined by the same prenatal influences.

At Delivery

OCCIPITAL DIASTASIS AND CEREBELLAR INJURY

Experienced obstetricians have always recognized that cesarean section is not necessarily an atraumatic option for the fetus, and the preterm breech infant faces some formidable difficulties whichever route of delivery is employed. Wigglesworth and Husemeyer[28] emphasized the vulnerability of the occipital bone to damage during vaginal breech delivery, due to its impact on the maternal pubis during descent of the fetal head into the pelvis during the second stage. These forces tend to separate the squamous part of the occipital bone from the lateral part (occipital diastasis). This produces a ridge in the posterior fossa and, hence, bruising or laceration of the cerebellum. The squamous part of the occipital bone is forced anteriorly to distort the foramen magnum and produce pressure on the spinal cord. Cerebellar bruising can be present in the absence of occipital diastasis, and although the fracture may be easily diagnosable after delivery with a lateral skull x-ray, the cerebellar bruising alone will not be diagnosable unless the cerebellum is scanned routinely by the neonatologist using ultrasound. The injury is commonly not discovered at postmortem examination if traditional dissection techniques are used. The damage to the brain may not be clinically apparent until the age of approximately 2 years, when the child will manifest signs of clumsiness and poor coordination consequent upon its cerebellar damage (ataxic cerebral palsy).

INTRAVENTRICULAR AND PERIVENTRICULAR DAMAGE

In addition, the preterm infant is vulnerable to intraventricular and periventricular damage secondary to hemorrhage or ischemia, which can be due to hypoxic or acidotic insults in the antepartum, intrapartum, and/or neonatal periods. The preterm breech may be still more susceptible to these as a consequence of the peculiar circumstances surrounding delivery. However, avoiding vaginal delivery will not necessarily prevent intracranial bleeding. A review by Arpino and coworkers[29] showed that premature labor of itself can produce intracranial hemorrhage even if delivery is postponed or performed by cesarean section.

GENERALIZED TRAUMA AND NERVE INJURIES

A traumatic breech delivery in which there is widespread limb and body bruising can produce gross skeletal muscle damage that results in large quantities of hemoglobin and myoglobin being liberated, leading to severe jaundice and damage to the kidneys. This can also produce a form of "shock lung" in the neonate, manifesting as severe respiratory distress syndrome.

The premature breech infant is also susceptible to damage to internal organs, transection of the spinal cord, and other nerve palsies consequent on traction, especially the brachial plexus and fractures of long bones, in a way similar to that of its more mature counterpart. Because the widest diameter of the fetus is the biparietal diameter (BPD), and the discrepancy between the diameters of the head and the body is most pronounced in the preterm fetus, it is possible for the body and limbs of the baby to slip through a cervix that is still incompletely dilated and the head will be unable to follow. This "entrapment" of the aftercoming head is more likely in the mother who commences active pushing before full dilation has been confirmed and with a footling presentation. It is a particular problem in the preterm fetus because the subcutaneous fat has not yet been laid down and the liver is not of the large size reached in the mature fetus; hence, the abdominal circumference is relatively smaller than the head. Recommended management is usually to incise the cervix with scissors at 4 and 8 o'clock, but inevitably, there is delay in delivery and, therefore, an increase in the hypoxic stress to the fetus, together with a likely increase in traumatic morbidity to both mother and child. However, Robertson and colleagues,[30] after studying 132 consecutive preterm singleton breech deliveries, reported that there was no significant difference in the incidence of head entrapment by mode of delivery for breech infants at 28 to 36 weeks' gestation, and nor did there appear to be more adverse neonatal outcomes after entrapment.

Injuries are not confined to babies delivered vaginally in breech presentation. Any very low birth weight baby is susceptible to trauma from a difficult delivery through a poorly formed lower segment at cesarean section. If the presentation is breech, a limited uterine incision can impede the delivery of the head to the same degree as a difficult vaginal delivery and is analogous in every way to the entrapment of the aftercoming head that is such a feared complication of the premature breech delivered vaginally. To some extent, this can be avoided by performing an anterior vertical uterine incision (ideally DeLee's incision, but often in a very small uterus, it becomes a classic incision). However, this carries increased risks for the mother, particularly with respect to uterine rupture in a future pregnancy or labor, but occasionally, also in terms of poor healing and postpartum hemorrhage. The incidence of intraventricular hemorrhage in the fetus and neonate is in any case closely related to the occurrence of preterm labor of itself, independent of the mode of delivery.[29,31]

Management Options for the Preterm Breech in Labor

Most elective deliveries of the preterm breech when the woman is not in labor are for fetal or maternal indications, when the preferred route of delivery is cesarean section rather than induction of labor. Management controversies mainly center on the preterm breech presentation in labor, in which the immediate priorities are (1) the accurate diagnosis of preterm labor, (2) the confirmation of presentation, and (3) the exclusion of fetal abnormality.

It is evident that in up to 80% of cases in which the mother thinks she is in preterm labor, contractions cease spontaneously and the pregnancy continues. The definitive diagnosis of labor therefore rests on demonstrating progressive dilation of the cervix. Careful cervical assessment of all women in suspected premature labor is imperative to confirm or refute the diagnosis. The recent introduction of testing for fibronectin in the vaginal fluid may enable us to make a more secure diagnosis of labor; a negative test is about 97% reliable. In the presence of ruptured membranes, examination of the cervix should be done using full aseptic technique and the number of examinations limited to minimize the risk of introducing infection, causing chorioamnionitis. Vaginal examination can confirm the presentation and even reveal the presence of fetal abnormality (e.g., imperforate anus!). In view of the recognized association of fetal abnormality with premature breech presentation, all previous ultrasound examinations should be carefully reviewed. If possible, a further detailed ultrasound scan should be performed to identify any abnormalities previously overlooked and to check on placental position at the same time. An estimate of fetal weight may allow a more rational decision to be made about the optimum place and mode of delivery. Ultrasound fetal weight estimation is possible to ± 15% in skilled hands, although when performed by junior residents outside of normal hours, errors greater than 15% have been reported in over 40% of cases.[32] This has led some workers to suggest that the outcome for the infant is best predicted by accurate knowledge of gestational age.[26]

Administration of tocolytics may be appropriate in an effort to delay delivery long enough to administer steroids to promote surfactant production in the fetal lung prior to preterm delivery or to arrange delivery in a site with appropriate neonatal intensive care facilities. It is now clear that tocolytic therapy is ineffective in preventing premature delivery in the longer term and that its use beyond 48 to 72 hours is probably inappropriate.

The Optimum Mode of Delivery of the Preterm Breech

The preterm breech on the labor ward presents the obstetrician with a heterogeneous group of clinical problems. Some will present not in labor but with spontaneous rupture of the membranes; others will present at 7 cm dilation in strong labor with intact membranes and deliver after only a short interval. As with all preterm deliveries, preterm vaginal breech delivery is sometimes precipitate and may therefore occur in the absence of skilled medical attendants. It is important to realize that in common with all preterm labors, the antecedents are often pathologic, and therefore, a decision about the mode of delivery is uncontentious. If there has been, for example, a placental abruption or cord prolapse, clearly cesarean section is indicated.

However, if the clinical situation is of "the uncomplicated preterm breech in labor," that is, if fetal and maternal conditions are good and labor is progressing at a normal rate, it is necessary to decide whether a vaginal delivery is to be allowed or a cesarean section undertaken.

One of the first suggestions that cesarean section should be undertaken routinely for the delivery of the preterm breech was in 1977 when Goldenberg and Nelson[33] reviewed the outcome of 224 babies less than 1500 g delivered between 1965 and 1969. However, they compared three groups: babies delivered vaginally in breech presentation, babies delivered vaginally in vertex presentation, and babies (breech and cephalic) delivered by cesarean section. Such a comparison is confounded by the factors determining cesarean section, making it invalid. The authors also highlighted the noncomparability of the study groups in other respects. They reported that many fetuses below 1000 g were not monitored during labor because they were thought to be nonviable, or if they were monitored, when signs of fetal distress supervened, surgical intervention was often not performed as the fetus was thought to be "too small to live." This approach resulted in infants being delivered vaginally who happened to survive despite nonintervention being compared with infants who were thought to be viable and not "too small to live" and who were, therefore, delivered electively by cesarean section. Such a comparison, therefore, leads to the (potentially) erroneous conclusion that cesarean section improves the outcome for the preterm breech infant.

Further retrospective reviews of clinical practice were published over the next few years, some comparing the vertex with the breech,[34] some correctly comparing the vaginally delivered breech with the breech delivered by cesarean section, but then only stratifying by birth weight below and above 2500 g or in other similarly wide weight bands.[35] Further retrospective reviews of low–birth weight breech-presenting infants have given contradictory results on the optimum mode of delivery.[36–38] Wolf and associates[39] observed the natural experiment of two adjacent maternity units with different policies for the delivery of the preterm breech (26–31 wk). One unit chose to deliver most vaginally (17% cesarean section rate) and the other mainly by cesarean section (85% cesarean section rate). There were no significant differences in survival rates between the two units.

Further evidence of the noncomparability of the vaginally delivered and cesarean delivered breeches is reported in a paper by Jain and coworkers.[40] They noted that even within the weight range of 1000 to 1499 g, there was a marked difference in the average weight, with the babies delivered vaginally being significantly lighter and at a lower gestation than those delivered by cesarean section, a difference likely to account for any differences in survival. A recent study of 169 women with a breech presentation at 26 to 29 + 5 weeks' gestation reported no benefit for planned cesarean delivery in respect of neonatal death or morbidity or low arterial pH at delivery.[38]

In order to overcome the noncomparability of groups in these retrospective reviews of practice, there has been a series of attempts at using statistical techniques to determine the contribution that mode of delivery makes to outcome for the preterm breech, but these too have produced contradictory results.[41,42]

Thus, all currently existing evidence has major methodologic flaws that make it unreliable as a guide to clinical decision-making and have led to a number of calls for a randomized, controlled trial to settle the question of optimum mode of delivery. Despite this, there has only been one such randomized trial which has actually been completed. Viegas and colleagues[43] randomized 23 women, but unfortunately, their analysis was fundamentally flawed by inappropriate withdrawals, and no conclusions can be drawn from their results. Two other randomized trials of the optimum mode of delivery of the preterm infant (both vertex- and breech-presenting) have been initiated, but both were terminated prematurely and produced no interpretable results.[44,45] Lumley and associates[44] randomized only 4 subjects out of a possible 33 who were eligible over a 5-month period and terminated the trial after drawing the conclusion that clinicians were unwilling to randomize their management. Wallace and coworkers[45] aborted their randomized trial of the optimum mode of delivery of the preterm infant because they found that an unacceptably high proportion of the babies (63%) were above the 1500-g upper weight limit for the trial. They concluded that a more accurate way of estimating fetal weight prior to delivery was needed before a further attempt was feasible. The subjects they did randomize were analyzed according to the eventual mode of delivery, not according to the randomized mode of delivery, thereby invalidating the randomizing process. A prospective, randomized multicenter trial to determine the best mode of delivery for the preterm breech (26–32 wk) recruiting subjects in the United Kingdom was also abandoned.[46] The recruitment rate was disappointing, with only 10% of eligible subjects being randomized, despite large numbers of women consenting to take part in the trial antenatally and sufficient numbers of preterm breeches presenting for randomization. No definitive conclusion was reached. The authors concluded that the failure of the trial did not mean obstetricians were insisting on cesarean delivery; 30% of preterm breeches not entered in the trial were allowed to deliver vaginally. Instead, they concluded that obstetricians were reluctant to abandon individualized decisions about management even in the presence of a high degree of scientific uncertainty about the basis on which their decisions were being made. Also, some evidence suggested that if the clinician was unsure of the optimum mode of delivery, then women wished to make a choice for themselves and withdrew from randomization. It, therefore, appears likely that the optimal mode of delivery of the preterm breech will remain uncertain for the foreseeable future. At gestations above 32 weeks but below 37 weeks and when the fetus weighs 1500 to 2500 g, current evidence does not suggest any advantage to routine cesarean section. Under this gestation and weight but at more than 26 weeks' gestation, the optimal mode of delivery remains uncertain in the absence of any clinical feature specifically indicating cesarean section. The advantage, if any, that routine section confers on the fetus is likely to be small; otherwise, it would be obvious in the multiplicity of published data already available. What is certain is that if a policy of routine cesarean section for the preterm breech fetus is followed, a number of cesarean sections will be performed unnecessarily for the fetus that is congenitally abnormal, for the fetus that is over 1500 g and therefore unlikely to benefit, for babies mistakenly thought to be in breech presentation (of which there were two in the U.K. study), and for some that will not actually be in established preterm labor and were destined to deliver at a later gestation. A policy of routine cesarean section will also expose the mother to a small but definite increased risk of maternal mortality and morbidity.

PROCEDURE

CONDUCT OF DELIVERY

Vaginal delivery of the preterm breech should be supervised by an experienced obstetrician. An effective epidural anesthetic is preferable to prevent the woman from pushing prior to full dilation, to allow manipulation of the breech or painless operative intervention with either forceps or rapid recourse to cesarean section. The anesthetist and pediatrician should be in attendance for the second stage. There is no clear evidence to favor the use of obstetric forceps to the aftercoming head; the pelvis will be relatively capacious for the premature neonate, and it will not be subject to the rapid compression-decompression forces applied to the head of the mature infant in breech presentation. There is some evidence that delivery with intact membranes is an advantage.[34] Should the cervix clamp down over the head or the body be delivered through an incompletely dilated cervix, the head should be flexed abdominally and the finger of the vaginal hand should be inserted into the mouth of the fetus to flex the head and facilitate delivery. If this is not possible, then scissors with the intracervical blade guarded by a finger should be introduced at 4 and 8 o'clock, and the cervix should be incised. The carefully flexed head should then deliver easily. The cervix is usually repaired easily provided analgesia is adequate.

If cesarean section is indicated, the abdominal incision used should be considered carefully. Although a Pfannenstiel or Joel-Cohen incision in the abdominal wall gives good access to the lower segment of the uterus, if a lower segment incision needs to be extended in an emergency (e.g., if the aftercoming head becomes entrapped), a vertical midline abdominal incision will be an advantage (it can be extended upward as far as is necessary to improve access). The advent of mass closure with nylon has reduced the morbidity of the midline approach so that it is now on a par with the Pfannenstiel, apart from the obvious cosmetic drawback of the midline scar. As well as providing improved access, it is also quicker. If a transverse uterine incision needs extending, a J shape is to be preferred to an inverted T. The DeLee or classic uterine incision appears to confer little benefit on the fetus in terms of reduced trauma, from 28 weeks onward (Patterson, Stacey, and Steer, unpublished data). Because of the maternal morbidity involved, it is probably unwise to use the classic approach to try to salvage the preterm baby if its viability seems doubtful.

THE BREECH PRESENTATION AT TERM

Management Options

Version of the Breech

SPONTANEOUS VERSION

The fact that breech presentation is uncommon at term implies that spontaneous version usually occurs in the weeks before term, and so breech presentation becomes progressively less common as the third trimester progresses. The incidence of spontaneous version after 32 weeks may be as high as 57%, and after 36 weeks' gestation is as high as 40% in multipara and 18% in nullipara, with the rate being higher in African women.[47,48] Spontaneous version is more likely in the breech with extended legs. Immediately prior to cesarean section solely for breech presentation at term, the presentation should be checked by ultrasound scanning, because the chances of spontaneous version even at this late stage are not insignificant.[48]

PROMOTION OF SPONTANEOUS VERSION

Techniques to promote spontaneous version have been investigated following Hofmeyr's postulate[49] that the combination of disengagement of the breech and postural change might promote spontaneous version between the diagnostic scan and a planned ECV. A variety of such techniques have been described. The Cochrane review[50] of five randomized or quasirandomized controlled trials including 392 women compared postural management of the breech with controls. There was no effect on the rate of noncephalic births, the rate of cesarean section, or the incidence of low Apgar scores. Therefore, although there is likely to be no significant adverse effects from postural management, there is currently no evidence to support its efficacy. There is also no evidence to support the use of moxibustion or acupuncture as techniques to promote spontaneous version.[51]

EXTERNAL CEPHALIC VERSION

ECV fell from favor in the mid-1970s. Prior to this time, it was performed without medication (except occasionally sedation), without tocolysis, and usually prior to 36 weeks' gestation. It was thought that because ECV was easier to perform prior to 36 weeks, it must therefore be safer. Without tocolysis, it was often unsuccessful after 36 weeks. Bradley-Watson in 1975[52] reported a 1% fetal mortality rate for ECV done prior to 36 weeks without tocolysis, which was considered unacceptably high. As a result, the use of ECV declined and was almost abandoned in most institutions because cesarean section was seen as a safer alternative. Another significant disadvantage of preterm ECV is that fetal bradycardia may precipitate immediate delivery by cesarean section, with the risk of ensuing respiratory distress syndrome. To avoid this, it was traditional to manage acute bradycardia by reversion of the fetus to breech, which did not always work and in any case defeated the objective of the ECV. In addition, spontaneous reversion to breech occurred quite often prior to delivery. Thus, the effectiveness of ECV was controversial.

A Cochrane review[53] included three randomized, controlled trials of the use of ECV before term involving 899 women and reported that it reduced noncephalic births and, if begun between 34 and 35 weeks, may have some benefit in terms of reducing the rate of noncephalic presentations and cesarean sections, but the authors concluded that further trials are required to confirm this finding and to rule out increased rates of preterm birth or other adverse perinatal outcomes. There are no published data on the use of ECV in the management of the preterm breech in labor. The antecedents of the preterm breech in labor are often abnormal, and ECV is therefore less relevant as a management strategy.

Any consideration of the efficacy and safety of the technique of ECV should include a likelihood of spontaneous version, the effectiveness of ECV of producing a cephalic presentation at the time of birth, the risks to the mother and the baby, and the utility of cephalic presentation at birth to the mother and the baby (i.e., if some preexisting abnormality or fetal compromise determines the mode of delivery rather than the presentation itself and also if the prognosis of the baby is determined by its condition rather than the mode of delivery, correction of the breech presentation will then not alter the outcome for the fetus).

The advantage of performing ECV at term is that it allows time for spontaneous version to occur and the clarification of conditions that of themselves may require delivery by cesarean section. This will result in fewer unnecessary attempts being made. Also, should complications of ECV occur, prompt recourse to cesarean section will result in the birth of a relatively mature infant.

The 1996 Cochrane review of ECV at term[54] included five trials and concluded that version was associated with a significant reduction in noncephalic births (relative risk [RR] 0.38) and a reduction in cesarean section (RR 0.55), although there was no significant effect on the perinatal mortality rate. This review also concluded that there was insufficient evidence to assess any risks associated with ECV at term.

The implications of these data are that every 100 ECV attempts will prevent 34 breech births and 14 cesarean sections. A conservative estimate of the impact of performing ECV on 2% of the 750,000 pregnancies in the United Kingdom every year would be a reduction in the number of breech births by 5100 and a reduction in the number of cesarean sections by 2100.[54]

The impact of ECV on the rate of cesarean sections for breech presentation will depend on the success rate of ECV. There is a wide variation in the reported success rate. Trials performed in Africa on black African women have much higher success rates. This may be due to the tendency of late engagement of the presenting part in the pelvis in black African women.[55] Collaris and Oei[56] in a review of 44 studies of ECV described mean success rates of 59.2%, ranging between 35% and 100%. Of the successfully turned fetuses, 5.6% reverted to breech, and excluding patients lost to follow-up, in 80.7% of all pregnancies with successful version, birth was vaginal, although labors after successful version are associated with increased rates of obstetric intervention.[57–59] Nassar and colleagues[47] described a 30% reversion to breech but also that 4% of unsuccessful versions spontaneously converted to cephalic prior to delivery. Overall, a success rate of 40% for nulliparous women and 60% for multiparous women can usually be achieved.

Various methods of predicting the success of an attempted ECV have been devised. One study found that if the presenting part in a nullipara was engaged and there was difficulty in palpating the fetal head, no attempt at ECV was successful. Conversely, if the presenting part was not engaged in a multipara and the fetal head was easily palpable, 94% of attempts were successful.[60] Maternal weight, placental site, fetal size, and position of the fetal legs seem to make less difference to the chances of success. The quantity of amniotic fluid probably also has a bearing on the success of ECV, and a reduction in the rate of success has been observed in women with "borderline' amniotic fluid volumes (5–8 cm).[61]

Because of the observation that increased uterine tone decreases the chances of success of ECV, the use of tocolytics has been investigated. A variety of tocolytics have been used. The 2004 Cochrane review of six trials of routine tocolysis[62] showed that its use was associated with fewer failures and a reduction in the cesarean section rate (RR 0.85; 95% confidence interval [CI] 0.72–0.99). Use of fetal acoustic stimulation (FAS) when the fetal spine was in the midline was also associated with fewer failures of ECV (RR 0.17; 95% CI 0.05–0.60). Nitroglycerine was associated with significant side effects and was not found to be effective.

Marquette and associates[63] confirmed in a randomized trial the efficacy of ritodrine in improving the success of ECV in nulliparous women from 25% to 43%, but there was no benefit in parous women. Nor Azlin and coworkers[64] confirmed the benefit of ritodrine versus a placebo in reducing the rates of noncephalic presentations and reducing the cesarean section rate but showed the largest benefit in multiparous women (87% vs, 57%). Fernandez and colleagues[65] found terbutaline (0.25 mg subcutaneously) to be effective in reducing noncephalic presentations and reducing cesarean section in comparison with placebo for ECV. It has been suggested that tocolytics could be reserved for use when the first attempt at ECV has been unsuccessful. One randomized, controlled trial of tocolysis versus a placebo in 124 women with a previously unsuccessful attempt at ECV showed that it increased the success rate of a repeat attempt and reduced the rate of cesarean section.[66]

Other possible tocolytic agents studied are atosiban and nifedipine. A small retrospective review[67] and a small randomized, controlled trial[68] showed that atosiban was no more effective than ritodrine in reducing noncephalic presentations. Similarly, nifedipine was of equal efficacy to ritodrine in both a retrospective review[69] and a small randomized, controlled trial.[70] It may be that these agents are useful when there are contraindications to the use of β-sympathomimetic drugs.

Because one of the main reasons for the failure or abandonment of ECV is maternal discomfort, the use of epidural analgesia for the procedure has been suggested. A Cochrane review[62] included five randomized trials of the use of regional anesthesia to facilitate ECV. The two trials using epidural analgesia improved the success rate of ECV, increased the number of cephalic presentations at delivery, and reduced the cesarean section rate, but three trials using spinal analgesia showed no benefits. It is possible that the volume preload associated with the use of epidurals increases the amniotic fluid volume and this affected the success rates. The safety and efficacy of regional anesthesia to facilitate ECV remains in question.

Benefits to the Fetus of External Cephalic Version

It is clear that ECV reduces the incidence of breech presentation at term and of breech delivery, whether vaginal or by cesarean section. However, it would be a mistake to suppose that elective cesarean section eliminates all risks for the fetus: cesarean delivery of the preterm breech can still be traumatic,[72] and the risk of pulmonary hypertension of the newborn may be increased.[73]

Risks to the Fetus of External Cephalic Version

The risks to the fetus of ECV have been difficult to quantify because adverse effects are so rare that none of the randomized trials are large enough to clarify this issue. There are two systematic reviews of safety.[47,56] Collaris and Oei[56] identified 44 studies with a total of 7377 women from 1990 to 2002. Transient fetal heart rate abnormalities were reported in 5.7%, with pathologic cardiotocograms in only 0.37%. Vaginal bleeding occurred in 0.47%, but the incidence of confirmed placental abruption was only 0.2%. Fetomaternal transfusion was completely absent in 5 out of 7 series, with an overall mean incidence of 3.7%. Emergency caesarean section was performed in 0.43% of cases. Nassar and colleagues[47] looked only at the 11 studies that compared women who had had an external cephalic version from 36 weeks' gestation with a control group of women who had not had an ECV. They found a total of 2503 women. Relevant outcomes were rarely reported for the control group. They did not find an increase in antepartum fetal death, but numbers were small. There were no reported cases of uterine rupture, placental abruption, prelabor rupture of the membranes, or cord prolapse. The onset of labor within 24 hours and the incidence of nuchal cord was nonsignificantly higher among women who had had an ECV than in controls with a persisting breech.[47] It seems likely that adverse events associated with ECV are rare.[74]

ECV has been associated with demonstrable changes in the fetal circulation.[75] An 8% incidence of fetal bradycardia has been reported in association with ECV.[76] If an ECV (whether successful or not) produces a fetal bradycardia, it is possible that subsequent labor is more likely to be complicated by fetal heart rate abnormality and result in cesarean section.[76] Lau and associates[75] demonstrated changes in the fetal circulation, but not placental circulation, associated with attempted ECV. Isolated cases of cord presentation and even fetal demise have also been reported. Kouam[77] followed up 116 children born after ECV. Developmental screening at 2 to 5 years of age showed no developmental delay. Although the short-term neonatal outcomes reported in the randomized, controlled trials are essentially normal and compare favorably with control subjects, they are only surrogates for definitive follow-up studies of the effects of this procedure.

Benefits to the Mother of External Cephalic Version

Following a successful ECV, there will be a decrease in the number of cesarean sections and in the number of vaginal breech deliveries, which often entail episiotomy and forceps delivery. The risks to the mother of cesarean section have previously been described in Chapter 74. Cesarean section may compromise future reproductive function,[78] and there may be adverse emotional sequelae for the mother and the maternal-infant pair.[79]

Interestingly, although ECV has become much more widely since the 1980s and more pregnant women (and their clinicians) have become aware of the procedure, pregnant women may be becoming less inclined to take up the option of ECV and instead opt for planned cesarean section.[80]

The contraindications to the performance of ECV are outlined in Table 63–2. The absolute contraindications are uncontroversial. However, the relative contraindications are more debatable. It may be that uterine anomalies and excessive maternal body weight should be regarded as relative contraindications. An amniotic fluid volume of less than 2 cm in depth in any pocket, the fetal back lying anteriorly, a tense uterus, difficulty palpating the fetal head, an engaged breech, and nulliparity will decrease the chance of success.[81] Fetal abdominal circumference is related to the chances of success, whereas the BPD is not. Gestational age and estimated fetal weight, provided the attempt was after 37 weeks, had no relationship with the chances of success, because success rates were found to be the same at 37, 38, and 40 weeks.

TABLE 63–2
Indications and Contraindications for External Cephalic Version

Indications for ECV
Any breech presentation after 36 in nulliparas and 37 weeks' gestation in parous women
Suspected fetopelvic disproportion
Unengaged breech
Absolute Contraindications to ECV
Multiple pregnancy*
Antepartum hemorrhage within the last 7 days
Placenta previa
Ruptured membranes
Significant fetal abnormality
Need for cesarean section for other indications
Abnormal fetal heart rate pattern
Major uterine anomaly
Relative Contraindications to ECV
Previous cesarean section/scarred uterus
Intrauterine growth restriction/small-for-gestational age fetus with abnormal umbilical artery Doppler velocimetry
Oligohydramnios
Unstable lie
Severe proteinuric hypertension
Obesity
Rhesus isoimmunization
Evidence of macrosomia
(Grand multiparty)†
(Anterior placenta)
("Precious baby")
(Previous antepartum hemorrhage)
Any suspected fetal compromise: unreactive cardiotocogram

* Apart from the second twin after the vaginal delivery of the first. *Note*: If tocolysis is to be used, women with congenital or acquired heart disease, diabetes, or thyroid disease should be excluded because of possible adverse reactions.
† Entries in parentheses have been suggested by some authorities but have no clinical evidence to support them.
ECV, external cephalic version.

Although previous cesarean section is a relative contraindication to ECV, there is a small series of 36 women who had one previous cesarean section and underwent an ECV, of which 66% were successful, and of these, 76% had a vaginal birth. There were no maternal or neonatal complications.[82] Maternal Rh negativity is a relative contradiction. If ECV is used, a Kleihauer test should be done and an appropriate anti-D (RhoGAM) administered.

PROCEDURE

EXTERNAL CEPHALIC VERSION

Prerequisites

1. Gestational age of 36 weeks or more in the nullipara and 37 weeks or more in the parous woman.[81]
2. Recent ultrasound to confirm a normal fetus and an adequate liquor volume.
3. Reassuring fetal heart rate pattern.
4. Informed consent—in which the mother is specifically advised of the risks of provoking labor, ruptured membranes, and cord and placental accidents.
5. Facilities for the performance of a cesarean section.

Procedure

ECV may be performed in the labor room or the clinic room, if there is rapid access to delivery facilities. The woman is positioned either in steep or slight lateral tilt or in the Trendelenburg position. It is sometimes recommended that a Kleihauer test be performed before and after the procedure. Some also recommend placing an intravenous line and cross-matching blood for a possible cesarean section. If tocolysis is to be used, some practitioners perform an electrolyte and glucose estimation as well. A clinical pelvimetry should be judged as adequate. An ultrasound scan should be performed in order to assess the liquor volume, fetal attitude, and position of the fetal legs. The fetal heart rate pattern should be normal and reassuring prior to commencement. Some authorities recommend that a contraction stress test be performed prior to version. It has even been suggested that the maternal blood pressure be taken every 5 minutes throughout the procedure and that the maternal heart rate be monitored electronically. This is probably unnecessary if the mother appears well throughout but could be important if tocolysis is used.

If tocolysis is employed, this can be given in a variety of ways: 10 μg of hexaprenaline given intravenously over 1 minute, terbutaline 0.25 mg subcutaneously or in 5 mL of normal saline over 5 minutes intravenously; terbutaline 0.5 μg/min intravenously or terbutaline 0.5 μg/min intravenously over 15 to 20 minutes; ritodrine 0.2 mg/min intravenously for 20 minutes; nifedipine 10 mg orally; or atosiban intravenously 6.75 mg over 1 minute and at a rate of 18 mg/hr for 20 to 30 minutes. Some authors give the chosen tocolytic as a stat dose and commence the ECV almost immediately. Others increase the dose steadily or wait until adequate uterine relaxation is achieved, all contractions have ceased, or there is softening of the uterus and easy palpation of fetal parts.

The ECV should be performed as one episode by one operator, and continuous pressure on the uterus should be limited to 5 minutes. Many recommend that uterine manipulation should continue for only 10 minutes, although waiting for the fetus to be active spontaneously (helping to dislodge it from the pelvis) and then applying pressure may be advantageous. Others have recommended stimulating the fetus to move using a vibroacoustic stimulator.[83] Mohamed and coworkers[84] reported that 55% are successful after 1 minute and only 15% require up to 5 minutes continuous pressure on the abdomen. The increased incidence of fetal heart rate abnormalities with failed ECV suggests that persistence in an attempt beyond these suggested times may be counterproductive. Mohamed and coworkers[84] also report that 73% were deemed by the obstetricians to be easy versions with 90% of women reporting little or no discomfort.

A forward or backward somersault can be performed: the forward somersault is the classically described maneuver. The technique involves placing the woman in a steep lateral tilt with her back against the wall behind the examination couch. A forward somersault is recommended if the fetal back is downward and a backward somersault if the fetal back is upward. If the breech is engaged, the breech must first be pushed out of the pelvis with the operator's right hand prior to correction of the presentation. There is a general consensus that vaginal disengagement should not be performed if the breech will not easily come out of the pelvis with abdominal pressure. If the fetal head is caught under the costal margin and this prevents the disengagement of the breech, the fetal head should be manipulated down and sideways prior to the disengagement of the breech and forward somersault. The actual version is accomplished using flexion of the fetal head and encouragement of a forward somersault by pressure on the uterus. Some practitioners pause as the breech is about to negotiate the transverse diameter of the uterus and apply acoustic stimulation. This may cause fetal kicking, which assists the version.[83] Women should be advised that ECV maybe painful but will be stopped if they wish.

After successful version, the attitude of the fetus should be maintained manually for a few minutes.

The fetal heart can be monitored continuously through the procedure or every 2 minutes. A repeat fetal heart rate tracing should be performed immediately after the ECV. If this is normal, the woman may go home. She should return within a few days so that the position of the fetus can be rechecked. Some practitioners perform a cesarean section if the breech presentation recurs, whereas others follow their protocol for selection for vaginal breech delivery. Still others continue to correct the presentation repeatedly. There is some evidence that the latter approach does result in more vertex presentations at delivery.

Current evidence indicates that ECV performed at term, and particularly with tocolysis, is a safe procedure for carefully selected women.

Assessment of the Fetus

Thorp and colleagues[85] showed that palpation only had a sensitivity of 28% and a specificity of 94% in the detection of breech presentation, using ultrasound scanning as the gold standard. Therefore, presentation of the fetus should be checked using ultrasound scanning. This should be possible in most cases even if the woman presents in labor.

X-Ray erect lateral pelvimetry (see later discussion) to investigate pelvic capacity has been traditional but has been increasingly abandoned partly because of a possible long-term increased incidence of myelodysplasia in the baby,[86] but mostly because of doubts about its usefulness. The presentation of the fetus can be confirmed at the same time. Radiologic exclusion of a nuchal arm, with an estimated incidence of 4%, has been suggested as a possible advantage, because this complication can produce delay and trauma during the second stage of labor.

As x-ray pelvimetry has been abandoned, assessment of the fetus using ultrasound has become mandatory. If ECV is contemplated, then placental site, adequacy of fetal growth, and liquor volume are the minimum information required from ultrasound examination. More detailed information about the fetus should be obtained if vaginal delivery is being contemplated. Ultrasound examination will provide an estimate of fetal weight, which is crucial to the management of breech delivery. However, it should always be remembered that estimation of fetal weight has, at best, an error of ±15%, which is ±600 g in the 4-kg fetus, and it may be less accurate in the breech-presenting fetus.[78,87] Placenta previa should also be excluded, as far as possible, prior to any decision about ECV or the mode of delivery. It has been suggested that prior to attempts at ECV or vaginal breech delivery, a nuchal cord should be excluded on ultrasound examination. Successful detection of a nuchal cord has been reported but is unlikely to be practicable on a routine basis.

The validity of ultrasound measurement of fetal size, especially the BPD, has long been debated. Bader and associates[88] performed ultrasound measurements in 450 fetuses in breech presentation and compared them with 1880 fetuses in cephalic presentation between 15 and 40 weeks' gestation. They found no difference between the BPD, the head circumference, and the cephalic index (cephalic index = BPD/occipital frontal distance × 100) in the two groups in uncomplicated pregnancy. However, in complicated pregnancies, the cephalic index was found to be lower in breech-presenting fetuses, indicating the dolichocephalic head shape that is commonly noted. Neck hyperextension (the star-gazing fetus) is an important condition that can cause spinal cord and brain injuries at delivery. Proposed etiologies are cord around the neck, fundal placenta, spasm of the fetal musculature, and fetal and uterine anomalies. It is of interest that most mammals other than humans deliver their young with the neck of the fetus in a hyperextended position. Flexion of the neck in the human fetus is probably an adaptation to the necessity of delivering a large brain in a large fetal skull through a relatively small pelvis. Although the incidence of neck extension in the fetus has been quoted as 7.4%,[48] its significance is hard to ascertain. It is regarded as an unfavorable prognostic sign with regard to successful vaginal breech delivery, but few authors indicate how it is to be diagnosed antepartum. Rojansky and coworkers[89] have validated the ultrasound determination of fetal neck extension comparing ultrasound scans with the gold standard of x-rays and found a high correlation. They measured the craniospinal angle by obtaining a sagittal view of the fetus visualizing the orbital ridge and the occipital eminence along with the spine in the same plane. A line is drawn between the orbital ridge and the occipital eminence, and the angle formed with the second line, which passes through the cervical and thoracic vertebrae, is measured. Other adverse features if ECV or vaginal breech delivery is contemplated include intrauterine growth restriction and Rh isoimmunization.

Choice of Mode of Delivery—Vaginal Breech Delivery

It was not until the late 1950s that the increasing safety of cesarean section led to it becoming the preferred mode of delivery, and elective cesarean section began to be recommended on a routine basis to minimize perinatal morbidity and mortality. In the 50 years that followed, the controversy continued until the frequent calls for a randomized, controlled trial were finally answered.[1] Clinicians now have robust data on which to base their recommendations. These data strongly support the view that elective cesarean section is the safest option for the baby, at a marginally increased risk to the mother.[90,91]

Risks of Vaginal Breech Delivery for the Fetus

The risks and benefits of vaginal breech delivery are shown in Table 63–3.

SHORT-TERM NEONATAL/PERINATAL OUTCOME AND FOLLOW-UP

Many of the studies performed to assess the mortality and morbidity rates for fetuses undergoing vaginal breech

TABLE 63–3
Risks and Benefits of Vaginal Breech Delivery for the Fetus

Risks
Poor condition at birth
Intracranial hemorrhage
Medullary coning
Severance of the spinal cord
Brachial plexus injury
Occipital diastasis
Fracture of the long bones
Epiphyseal separation
Rupture of internal organs
Long-term neurologic damage
Genital damage in the male
Hypopituitarism
Damage to the mouth and pharynx
Benefits
Reduction in idiopathic pulmonary hypertension

delivery have been poor. They were mostly retrospective reviews of practice and often simply compared babies delivered vaginally by the breech and by the head. This approach does not compare like with like and is, therefore, invalid. However, because of the rise in the popularity of elective cesarean section for breech presentation, increasingly vaginal breech delivery was being performed only when the woman presented in advanced labor with an unexpected breech presentation. This situation increased the risk of a breech birth being attended by inadequately trained or experienced personnel. Moreover, there was no opportunity for prior assessment for suitability for vaginal breech delivery. Several studies have reported stringent selection criteria for vaginal breech delivery with cesarean section rates varying from 49% to 83%. Most of these have shown no difference in short-term outcomes for the fetus.[71,92–96] However, the evidence based on these retrospective reviews of practice is contradictory. Many report a higher 1-minute Apgar score and higher pH values in breech neonates delivered by cesarean section compared with those delivered vaginally. That the breech delivered vaginally has a lower pH than the cephalic infant or the breech infant delivered vaginally is not in doubt; it is what this difference means clinically that is difficult to ascertain.

Some specific conditions associated with breech presentation probably increase the chances of trauma during delivery. Fetal neck hyperextension, which can cause damage to the cervical spine, is a contraindication to vaginal birth. Flexed legs appear to increase the risk of cord prolapse to as much as 15% compared with 1.4% to 6% if the legs are extended (the risk of cord prolapse with a cephalic presentation is only 0.24%–0.5%). If the arms are caught across the back of the neck at delivery (nuchal arm), the risk of brachial plexus injury is about 8.5% at term, although 70% of these injuries have resolved fully by 3 months of age.

Until the Hannah and colleagues' trial,[1] there had been only two small randomized, controlled trials of the mode of delivery of the term breech. Collea and associates[13] randomized 208 women at term in labor to receive a cesarean section or a vaginal delivery. Despite this intention, 45% of the latter group was delivered by cesarean section. Although there are some caveats about their methodology, they showed no statistically significant differences in short-term neonatal outcome between babies delivered vaginally and babies delivered by cesarean section, by either intention to treat or actual mode of delivery. By contrast, they showed "striking and concerning differences in maternal outcome," with higher maternal morbidity rates associated with cesarean section. Gimovsky and coworkers[14] recruited 105 women with nonfrank breech presentation into their randomized, controlled trial. They also showed no statistically significant differences in short-term neonatal outcome. The two meta-analyses of the mode of delivery of the term breech did not significantly challenge these findings.[11,12] Hannah and colleagues[1] published the results of a multicenter, randomized, controlled trial of the optimum mode of delivery of the term breech in 2000. From 121 centers in 26 countries, 2088 women with a frank or complete breech were recruited. By the time the trial ended, 1041 women had been assigned to planned cesarean section, of whom 941 (90.4%) were actually delivered by cesarean section, and 1041 women had been assigned to planned vaginal delivery, of whom 591 (56.7%) were actually delivered vaginally. The trial was halted before the planned total had been recruited, on the advice of the data-monitoring group, because a highly significant difference had already emerged. Perinatal mortality, neonatal morbidity, and serious neonatal morbidity rates were significantly lower for the planned cesarean section group (1.6%) than for the planned vaginal birth group (5.0%) (RR 0.33), and there were no significant differences between the groups in terms of maternal mortality or serious maternal morbidity rates (3.9% vs. 3.2%).[1] These relative differences in outcome between planned cesarean section and vaginal breech delivery persist even when a variety of clinical differences between groups are taken into account: parity, type of breech, whether the fetus was larger or smaller than 3000 g, whether the pelvis had been assessed clinically or radiologically, whether labor was induced or augmented, the use of epidural anesthesia, presentation, the degree of experience of the clinician, and a variety of other clinical parameters that are usually held to be important predictors of the success and safety of attempted vaginal delivery. The only significant interaction was between the treatment group and the countries' reported perinatal mortality/morbidity rate (PNMMR) for the combined outcome of perinatal mortality, neonatal mortality, or serious neonatal morbidity rates. In countries with a low PNMMR (≤20 in 1000 births), the risk from planned cesarean section compared with planned vaginal birth was 0.4% versus 5.7%, whereas the rates in countries with a high PNMMR (>20 in 1000 births) were 2.9% versus 4.4%. The difference in the developed countries disappeared when just the outcome of perinatal or neonatal death was considered. Neonatal morbidity showed the greatest differences according to geography, with reductions in morbidity being much greater for countries with low PNMMRs than for those with high PNMMRs. It is not clear why this is the case. Possible explanations include incomplete ascertainment of poor neonatal condition in the first week of life or death before morbidity can be recognized. The observation might even be real, possibly because of high levels of experience with vaginal breech birth in countries with low cesarean section rates and high perinatal mortality rates—fewer women allocated to vaginal breech delivery in those countries ended up with a cesarean birth.[97] Overall, this study indicated that with a policy of planned cesarean section, for every additional 14 cesarean sections done, 1 baby will avoid death or serious morbidity. In countries with high a PNMMR as many as 39 additional cesarean sections would need to be done to avoid 1 dead or compromised baby, whereas in countries with a low PNMMR, the number of additional cesarean sections required may be as low as 7.

After the publication of the Term Breech Trial,[1] reservations were expressed about the generalizability of the results, but in general, the obstetric community have implemented the findings and the cesarean section rate rose rapidly to 90% to 95% in most of the developed world. Since then, a number of large population-based case series have been published, showing the impact of the trial. Reitberg and colleagues[98] published a series of 35,000 women with a breech presentation who were delivered in the Netherlands during a period of 33 months prior to the publication of the Term Breech Trial and 25 months after the publication. Over this period of time, the caesarean section rate rose from 49% to

80%. This was associated with a halving of the perinatal mortality rate and the rate of low Apgar scores and a three quarter reduction in birth trauma. The implication of these findings is that there are more than 60 Dutch children who are alive today who might not have been without the publication of the Term Breech Trial. A group in California demonstrated in a population base of 100,000 women with a breech presentation and a 95% cesarean section rate that the neonatal mortality rate was only 0.6 in 1000 and demonstrated that nulliparous women who delivered a breech vaginally had significantly increased rates of brachial plexus injury, neonatal death, birth trauma, and asphyxia.[99] Three further population-based studies in Scandinavia,[100–102] involving a total of 53,000 women, showed a risk of perinatal or infant death that was between 2.5 and 3.5 times higher in women who delivered a breech vaginally.

Further hospital-based cohort studies have been published[93,95,103–106] since the Term Breech Trial, but these have been relatively small and lack both its statistical power and the advantages of randomization. Given that units with disappointing results from vaginal breech delivery are unlikely to publish their results, these studies involving a total of less than 6000 cases need to be interpreted cautiously in the light of the results of other population-based studies including some 185,000 deliveries.

Vaginal delivery carries the risk of cord prolapse and extended arms at delivery as well as difficult delivery of the head. This risk may be approximately 1% to 2%.[15] Therefore, obstetric expertise should be maintained for dealing with unexpected breech presentations, and for the late-presenting (usually previously undiagnosed) breech in labor in whom cesarean section is logistically impossible; this may amount to 11% or more of all breech presentations.[71] How to achieve this maintenance of competence in an era of few vaginal breech deliveries and many trainees with restricted hours for teaching has not yet been fully established; training on sophisticated mannequins is probably the best approach.

LONG-TERM INFANT FOLLOW-UP

Those studies reviewing later-born (1970–1980) children reflect the impact of rising cesarean section rates and more modern obstetric care. They are still mostly retrospective reviews of practice.

In one case-controlled study, breech-delivered infants were compared with cephalic-delivered infants (matched for sex, birth weight, gestational age, maternal age, parity, and year of delivery) at 4 to 10 years of age. A slight excess of minor neurologic dysfunction was found in the breech group but was not statistically significant.[107]

In a population-based study, Danielian and associates[108] compared the long-term outcome of infants delivered in breech presentation at term by intended mode of delivery. They identified 1645 infants from the Grampian region in Scotland during the years 1981 to 1990 who had been delivered alive at term after breech presentation. Elective cesarean section was performed in 35.9% of cases, and 64.1% were intended vaginal deliveries. There were no significant differences in terms of severe handicap, developmental delay, or neurologic deficit up to school age. The 2-year follow-up results from the Term Breech Trial showed that death or neurodevelopmental delay at age 2 years was similar between the two groups (RR 1.09; 95% CI 0.52–2.3).[109] The smaller number of perinatal deaths with planned cesarean section was balanced out by a greater number of babies with neurodevelopmental delay. This was unexpected, because there had been fewer babies in the planned cesarean section group with severe perinatal morbidity.

Another long-term follow-up of infants born by the breech either spontaneously or using the Bracht maneuver for delivery of the head reported that psychometric and intellectual development were superior in those infants delivered spontaneously.[110]

Despite the fact that many of the studies are of dubious quality, they are remarkably consistent in reporting minimal risk of long-term neurologic damage after careful selection for vaginal delivery and after correction for congenital anomalies. The major risk associated with mode of delivery remains that of perinatal mortality.

Risk of Breech Delivery for the Mother

The risks of breech delivery to the mother are shown in Table 63–4.

It may be the risks for the mother and the fetus in a subsequent pregnancy will turn out to be the most significant risk, rather than that associated with a primary cesarean section. The Dutch experience[98] has been used to calculate that 19 perinatal deaths will be avoided by performing 8500 extra primary caesarean sections, but that in subsequent pregnancies, this could result in as many as 4 maternal deaths and 9 perinatal deaths from complications of the uterine scar or repeat surgery.[111] It would seem to be appropriate to take into account a woman's planned family size when counseling her about mode of delivery for breech presentation.

Assessment for Vaginal Breech Delivery (Table 63–5)

All the available literature stresses the importance of adhering to an appropriate protocol when assessing women for vaginal breech delivery. These protocols have produced elective cesarean section rates from 49% to 83%.

TABLE 63–4

Comparison of Risks to the Mother of Vaginal Breech Delivery and Cesarean Section

Risks of Vaginal Breech Delivery for the Mother
Perineal discomfort and morbidity
Difficult birth experience
Risks of Cesarean Section for the Mother
Short-term morbidity: increased postpartum pyrexia, increased need for blood transfusion
Increased maternal mortality rate
Reduction in future fertility
Difficult birth experience
Entering a subsequent pregnancy with a scar on the uterus and with increased risk of placenta previa/accreta

TABLE 63-5
Assessment for Vaginal Breech Delivery

Assessment of the Cause of Breech Presentation
Exclude:
- Placenta previa
- Multiple pregnancy
- Fibroids/pelvic tumors
- Oligohydramnios/polyhydramnios
- Hydrocephalus/anencephaly
- Other congenital abnormality

Assessment of Fetal Condition
Exclude:
- Intrauterine growth restriction
- Rhesus disease
- Fetal abnormality
- Other

Assessment of Fetal Weight and Attitude

Assessment of the Maternal Pelvis
Clinical pelvimetry (important for medicolegal reasons) (x-ray erect lateral pelvimetry no longer advocated)
Computed tomography scanning pelvimetry and magnetic resonance imaging may be unnecessary and unreliable

Assessment of Maternal Condition
Exclude significant maternal disease: diabetes, proteinuric hypertension, cardiac or renal disease

Assessment of Maternal and Parental Wishes

Close consultation with the mother and partner and counseling about the implications of the choice of vaginal breech delivery versus elective cesarean section are important. It is the responsibility of the obstetrician to explain the options and the evidence to the woman and her family in the clearest possible terms. Although cesarean section will be the recommended option for the great majority of women, especially in the developed world, some women when informed of the options will still wish to attempt a vaginal delivery, and their wishes should be respected.

ASSESSMENT OF PELVIC CAPACITY—CLINICAL

Clinical pelvimetry is a low-technology screening investigation that is probably of benefit only if there is gross contraction of the pelvis. A subjective assessment of the bony features of the pelvic cavity is made, including the sacral promontory, the curvature of the sacrum, whether the side walls are convergent or the ischial spines prominent, whether the sacrospinous ligaments will accommodate two fingers, whether the intertuberous diameter will accommodate the clenched fist, and whether the pubic arch is greater than 90 degrees. With regard to a clinical assessment of the size of the pelvis, a consideration of the woman's height alone is probably useful.[112]

ASSESSMENT OF PELVIC CAPACITY USING IMAGING

No prospective, randomized trials have ever been performed to assess the value of x-ray pelvimetry. There is no absolute level of pelvic contraction as assessed by x-ray below which vaginal delivery is impossible, and antenatal assessment of fetal weight is probably a more important determinant of the success of attempted vaginal delivery.[113] Studies of x-ray pelvimetry have been unable to show any value in selecting those women more likely to have a successful vaginal breech delivery or a satisfactory perinatal outcome.[114] In a subanalysis of the Term Breech Trial, the use of x-ray pelvimetry was not linked to improved success rates.

Computed tomography (CT) scanning for pelvimetry reduces the radiation dosage and is more accurate.[90] However, there is no good evidence that it will predict the outcome of a trial of vaginal breech delivery any better than standard pelvimetry.

One randomized, controlled trial of magnetic resonance (MR) pelvimetry has been performed.[115] Two hundred thirty-five women had MR pelvimetry and were then randomly assigned to two groups. In the study group, the results of the pelvimetry were disclosed to the clinicians who used them to decide on the optimal route of delivery. In the control group, the clinicians assigned the route of delivery after consideration of other clinical factors alone. The authors found that the overall cesarean section rate was the same, although the emergency cesarean section rates were lower in the MR group. There were no significant differences in the baby's condition at birth or in the early neonatal period between the two groups.

CRITERIA FOR SELECTION FOR VAGINAL BREECH DELIVERY

Various criteria have been proposed.[92,96] In summary, the fetus should be neither too small nor too big and should have a well-flexed head; the mother should have at least an average-capacity pelvis, judged clinically; and the mother and the baby should be in "good" condition.

An estimated fetal weight of 1500 to 3900 g is probably appropriate (for discussion of the delivery of the preterm breech, see previous section); however, the limits of fetal weight and gestation are contentious, with many different limits being suggested. In addition, clinical estimation of fetal weight is unreliable, and even when ultrasound is used, there is a margin of error of ±15%. The error of the estimation of weight is greater in the breech than in the vertex fetus.

It is probably wise to perform a clinical pelvimetry to exclude the obviously contracted pelvis, but x-ray pelvimetry should not be done because there is no clear evidence of its value. It is good practice and probably wise from the medicolegal point of view to explain this to the mother before labor.

Some authors would exclude the nulliparous woman with a breech from consideration of vaginal delivery, yet others consider the grand multiparous patient also at high risk. The evidence for either proposition is not compelling. The fetus should ideally be in frank or complete breech presentation (not a footling), and absence of detectable congenital abnormality should be confirmed using ultrasound.

It is commonly assumed that the undiagnosed breech in labor is at higher risk of complications than those that have been diagnosed prelabor and adequately assessed for suitability for trial of vaginal delivery. However, the experience of some authors[116,117] is that these women do well and are more likely to deliver vaginally with no greater mortality or morbidity rates than those diagnosed and assessed prior to labor. They suggest that there are no grounds for delivering all undiagnosed breeches in labor by cesarean section.

PROCEDURE

VAGINAL BREECH DELIVERY

Practical Considerations in the Conduct of Assisted Vaginal Breech Delivery

The essence of the assisted vaginal breech delivery is allowing as much spontaneous delivery by uterine action and maternal effort as possible. Operator intervention should be limited to the maneuvers described here, which are designed to correct any deviation from the normal mechanism of spontaneous delivery. The operator may make the delivery more complicated by injudicious traction that encourages displacement of the fetal limbs from their normal flexed position across the fetal body or by promoting hyperextension of the fetal head. Traction can also cause injury of itself. The fetal body should, at all times, be treated with the utmost care and grasped, if at all, by the bony parts. Some authors recommend using a towel to cover the baby to prevent friction injury, to improve grip without the need for too much squeezing, and to keep the baby warm. Within these limits, many procedures for the vaginal delivery of the breech have been described.

First Stage

Many authors suggest that spontaneous labor increases the chance of successful vaginal delivery, and that if delivery is required before the onset of spontaneous labor, elective cesarean section may be preferable to induction of labor. Other authorities would permit induction of labor.[113]

Labor should be conducted in a labor ward with all the facilities needed to perform a cesarean section, with a full anesthetic service and senior obstetric staff available. The woman should be instructed to arrive early in labor so that her progress and the condition of the fetus may be monitored. Similarly, if the membranes rupture, she should attend the hospital because of the risks of cord prolapse. Rupture of the membranes at any point during the labor should prompt immediate vaginal examination.

On presentation in labor, an intravenous line should be sited and blood taken for typing and to save serum. Because of the relatively high risk of cesarean section, oral intake should be avoided for the duration of the labor. After the usual assessment of the woman in labor, she should be told that continuous electronic fetal monitoring is advisable and that an epidural anesthetic may be preferable. The latter will make any manipulation in the second stage more comfortable and make any urge to push prior to full dilation easier to resist. Bearing down prior to full dilation may push the relatively smaller breech through the incompletely dilated cervix and entrap the aftercoming head behind the cervix. Epidural anesthesia is not essential, and some obstetricians suggest that there is a higher chance of spontaneous vaginal delivery without one. Chadha and associates[118] reported that epidural analgesia was associated with a longer duration of the second stage, an increased need for augmentation of labor with oxytocin infusion, and a significantly higher cesarean section rate in the second stage of labor. There is little doubt that epidural anesthesia obtunds the urge to bear down. However, the counterargument is that if a baby does not deliver easily with an epidural in situ, it is better delivered by cesarean because there is likely to be mild relative disproportion. Because there is no clear scientific evidence to resolve this issue, it seems appropriate at the present time to allow the woman a major degree of personal choice in this respect. Whatever she chooses, however, an anesthetist should be in attendance during the second stage of labor in case rapid anesthesia should be required for an unexpectedly difficult delivery. The fear with the use of oxytocin in the presence of slow labor is that it will produce descent of the breech in the presence of fetal-pelvic disproportion; hence, the disproportion will be detected only when the head is entrapped above the pelvic brim and the body is already delivered. This leads many to suggest that there should be strict limits on the duration of first stage and that the use of oxytocin should be avoided.[95,113] The bitrochanteric diameter is usually smaller than the BPD, and if the former does not easily traverse the pelvis, neither will the latter. However, Collea and associates[13] demonstrated that the use of oxytocin in selected patients does not produce an excess rate of maternal or neonatal complications.

Failure to make expected progress in cervical dilation or for the breech to descend appropriately in the first 4 hours of labor or the appearance of cardiotocographic abnormalities should prompt careful consideration of whether cesarean section is advisable. Total labor duration should be similar to that in cephalic presentation, although descent of the breech may be slow. The progress of the labor should, therefore be plotted, on a partogram in the usual way. There is evidence that the use of the World Health Organization partogram in breech labor reduces the incidence of prolonged labor, reduces the incidence of cesarean section (at least in parous women), and improves the condition of the neonate at birth.[119] This probably reflects the importance of good progress in labor as a favorable prognostic variable for successful vaginal breech delivery.

Meconium staining of the liquor is common in breech labor, and its predictive value for asphyxia is poor. In early labor, it is often found on the glove at the end of a vaginal examination. Its passage when the breech is still high in the birth canal in first stage may indicate "fetal distress," and careful evaluation of the fetal heart rate pattern at this stage will be necessary. However, the passage of meconium in the second

stage is almost universal and is of no prognostic value. Cardiotocographic fetal heart rate abnormalities can be investigated using fetal blood sampling, preferably obtaining the blood from the region around the ischial tuberosity and avoiding the genitalia. Some authorities recommend that fetal blood sampling should not be attempted in breech presentation[113]; however, there is no evidence that an adequate sample of blood obtained in this way has a different pH than blood obtained from the fetal scalp, and so the usual criteria of acidosis could be applied.

FIGURE 63–1
The second stage of vaginal breech delivery. Delivering the shoulder by Lövsett's maneuver.

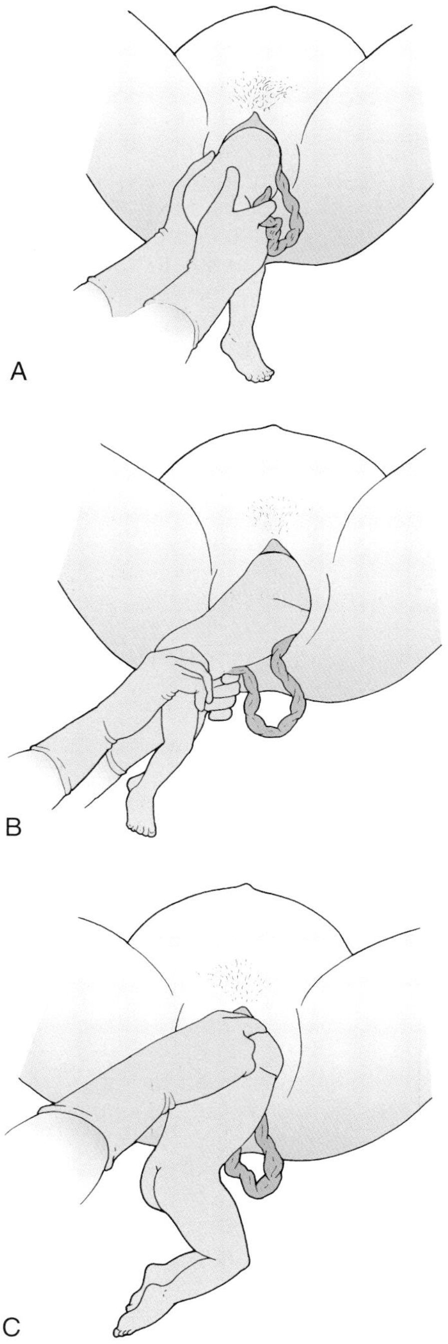

Second Stage (Fig. 63–1)

Practical maneuvers to facilitate the delivery of the breech have been insufficiently evaluated and there is little good evidence to guide the clinician. The second stage should be supervised by an experienced obstetrician (see Fig. 63–1). The active second stage with vaginal breech delivery does not start until the cervix is fully dilated and the fetal anus is seen on the perineum without having to part the mother's labia. The woman should then be placed in the lithotomy position with her buttocks just over the end of the delivery couch. She should be cleaned and draped as for ventouse or forceps delivery. A lateral tilt using a wedge is probably advisable. It is best if the bladder and lower bowel are empty, and elective bladder catheterization is probably advisable, with an "in and out" catheter. If effective regional anesthesia is not in place, a pudendal block with perineal infiltration should be used. An episiotomy is generally advised and should be performed at this point. An episiotomy will nearly always be required if forceps are to be used to achieve delivery of the aftercoming head, if extensive manipulation of the fetus is anticipated, and in all nulliparas, but is not mandatory. The breech, legs, and abdomen should be allowed to deliver spontaneously to the level of the umbilicus; the only intervention recommended up to this stage is to correct the position to sacroanterior if it is not in this orientation already. At this point, the obstetrician should deliver the legs, if they are extended, by abduction of the thigh and flexion of the fetal knee (using finger pressure in the popliteal fossa), allowing the fetal thigh to pass lateral to the fetal body. A loop of umbilical cord should then be brought down to minimize traction and possible tearing with consequent loss of fetal blood. The prognostic significance of the absence of cord pulsation is controversial. Fetal condition is probably better assessed by noting fetal tone and color.

Delivery to this point should ideally have been achieved with one contraction and one maternal expulsive effort. Delivery of the rest of the body, to delivery of the mouth, should be achieved over the next one or two contractions. The duration of time that should be allowed to elapse between delivery just below the umbilicus to delivery of the mouth is 5 to 10 minutes. Arulkumaran and coworkers[120] examined two different ways of delivering the breech. They allowed spontaneous delivery to the hip with one contraction and maternal effort followed by an assisted delivery of the rest of the body and head in the next contraction in one group of women; in another group, they assisted delivery to the shoulders with one contraction and then an assisted delivery of the head was performed with the next contraction. The former method produced babies with a smaller fall in fetal blood pH and in better condition at delivery, judged by the Apgar score and need for ventilation. They hypothesized that this was due to exposure, stretching, and compression of the umbilical cord over a longer period of time during the delivery of the latter group, or possibly to premature separation of the placenta.

Once the legs and abdomen have emerged, the fetus should be allowed to hang from the vulva until the wing of the scapula is seen. The arms are often found folded over the fetal chest, flexed at the shoulder and elbow; in this case, no particular maneuver is required to effect their delivery. If injudicious traction is exerted in order to deliver the breech, the arms may become extended over the fetal head. In this case, Lovset's maneuver may be used to free the arm. This involves wrapping the fetus in a warm dry towel and grasping the body over the bony pelvis with the thumbs along the sacrum. The fetal back should then be turned through 180 degrees until the posterior arm comes to lie anteriorly. The elbow will appear below the symphysis pubis, and that arm and hand can be delivered by sweeping it across the fetal body. This maneuver is repeated in reverse to deliver the other arm. If these maneuvers fail, the traditional last resort is to induce deep anesthesia and push the body of the fetus well up, pass the hand along its ventral aspect, and bring down the most accessible arm. This may then allow completion of vaginal birth. However, having pushed the fetus up successfully, it may well be safer to proceed with cesarean section.[120]

The nuchal arm, in which the arm is flexed at the elbow and extended at the shoulder coming to lie behind the fetal head, may be dealt with by a modified Lovset maneuver: rotating the fetal back through 180 degrees in the direction of the trapped arm may draw the elbow forward toward the face and over the fetal head by friction on the birth canal and render it amenable to a traditional Lovset maneuver to deliver the arm. If this technique does not suffice to release the nuchal arm, it may be forcibly extracted by hooking the finger over it, in which case, it is almost always fractured.

The fetus should be allowed to hang from the vulva for a few seconds again until the nape of the neck is visible at the anterior vulva. This allows descent of the head into the pelvis, and at this point, the head may be delivered. Downward traction before spontaneous descent may result in hyperextension of the fetal head rather than flexion and descent; so again, operator interference can cause complications in the delivery. If the head negotiates the inlet of the pelvis easily, there is little danger that the progress of the head will be arrested in midcavity. If there is difficulty with the head in the midcavity, or the outlet, a properly performed Mauriceau-Smellie-Veit maneuver will overcome this (see later full description). Should the head fail to descend into the pelvis after the shoulders have delivered, the body of the fetus should be turned sideways and suprapubic pressure used to flex the head and push it into the pelvis in the occipitotransverse/oblique position. A vaginal finger in the mouth of the fetus may also tend to flex the head and help it to descend into the pelvis prior to delivery. McRobert's maneuver can be used to facilitate delivery of the head if it is arrested at the inlet and suprapubic pressure and the Mauriceau-Smellie-Veit maneuver has failed. This involves a sharp flexion of the maternal thighs toward the maternal abdomen and abduction of the legs, in a way directly analogous to the management of shoulder dystocia in the vertex delivery.[121] Continued failure of the head to descend into the pelvis may be due to hydrocephalus; in which case, the head can be perforated through the foramen magnum (an epidural needle is a suitable instrument) and the cerebrospinal fluid drained. Such a maneuver should be performed only if the diagnosis has been confirmed by ultrasound and the fetus is already dead. Alternatively, the cervix may not be fully dilated; in which case, the cervix must be incised. This is done with round-ended scissors, and the incisions made at 4 and 8 o'clock to avoid the bladder and rectum and the main blood vessels (which supply the cervix at 3 and 9 o'clock). If there are locked twins, there is no choice but to do a cesarean section; the traditional technique of decapitating the first twin is no longer acceptable. If none of these causes is present, the operator must assume that cephalopelvic disproportion is present and there is then a strong case for the performance of a symphysiotomy.[122] With proper predelivery assessment and conduct of labor, this situation should arise only very rarely.

Performing a Symphysiotomy (Fig. 63–2)

The episiotomy should be enlarged. If the mother does not have epidural analgesia, the anterior, superior, and inferior aspects of the symphysis should be infiltrated with lidocaine 0.5%. The usual precautions to prevent intravenous injection should be taken. While waiting for the analgesia to take effect, an indwelling urinary catheter should be inserted. The suprapubic skin should then be cleaned with antiseptic solution. Following this, the index finger should be placed in the vagina and lateral pressure applied to the catheter to move the urethra away from the midline. A thick, firm-bladed scalpel should then be used to make a vertical stab incision over the symphysis. Keeping to the midline, the knife should be pressed down through the cartilage joining the two pubic bones until the pressure of the scalpel blade can be felt on the finger in the vagina. If the cartilage is not fully divided, the blade can be rotated and the cutting movement can be made back toward the top of the symphysis to finish the process. Following the delivery, there is no need to close the incision unless there is bleeding. It is, however, wise to give prophylactic antibiotics (e.g. ampicillin, gentamicin, and metronidazole). Elastic strapping from one iliac crest to the other will reduce postoperative pain, but analgesia will be necessary. The urinary catheter should be left in situ for a minimum of 5 days.

Techniques for Delivering the Head (Fig. 63–3)

It should be remembered that entrapment of the aftercoming head can also occur with cesarean section,

FIGURE 63–2
Performance of a symphysiotomy. *A*, Position of the woman for symphysiotomy. *B*, Pushing the urethra to one side using a finger to press on the urinary catheter. *C*, Incising the symphysis, with the finger pushing the urethra to one side, to avoid damaging it with the knife.
(From World Health Organization [WHO]: Managing complications in pregnancy and childbirth: A guide for midwives and doctors. Accessed at www.who.int/reproductive-health/impac/procedures/symphysiotomy_P53_P56.html)

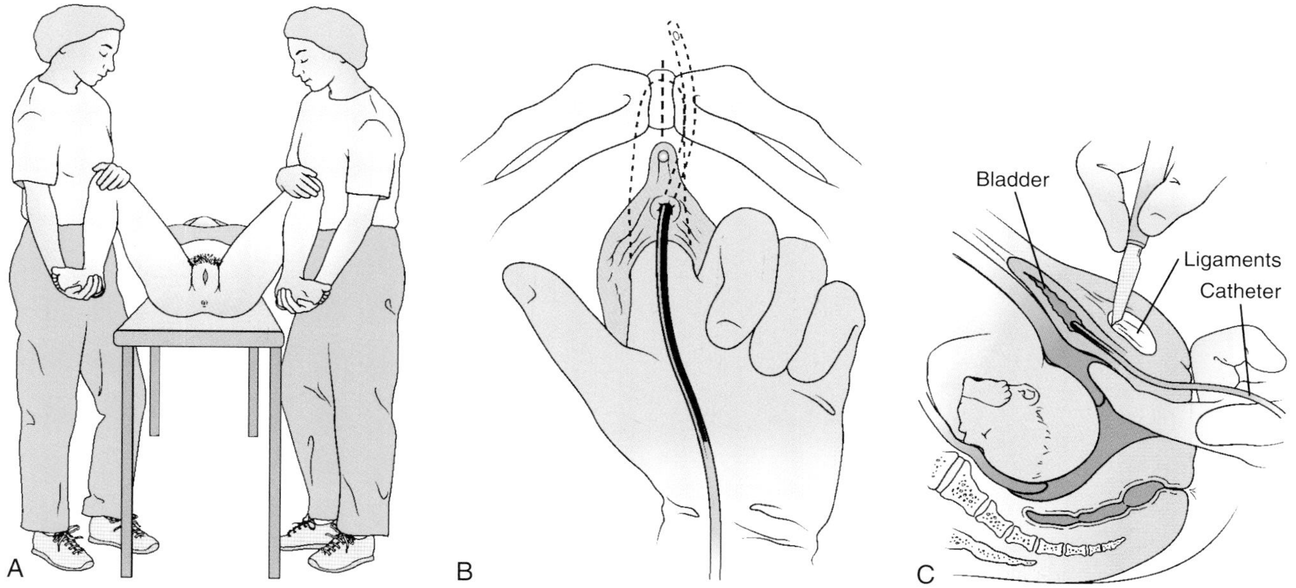

especially if an inadequate-size abdominal incision has been made. Robertson and colleagues[30] found no significant difference in the incidence of head entrapment by mode of delivery from 28 to 36 weeks' gestation, nor any association with adverse outcome following head entrapment. The techniques for delivery of the aftercoming head are various (see Fig. 63–3). Some authorities advise that the body should be supported on the right forearm of the operator and not be raised above the horizontal in order to minimize the chance of hyperextension of the fetal head. Others advise that the operator's assistant should grasp the ankles of the fetus and raise the body vertically above the mother's abdomen prior to any attempt to deliver the fetal head, because this will promote rotation of the fetal head and place it in the anteroposterior diameter of the pelvis. This is called the Burns-Marshall technique and may rotate the head and deliver it over the perineum without further intervention. It is, therefore, advisable to cover the perineum with the hand to prevent precipitate delivery of the head as the body is swung upward. The operator's hand can then be opened slowly in order to allow the rest of the head to deliver. Often, however, further assistance is required to deliver the head. The head may be delivered from this position using forceps applied below the fetal body. The operator should remember that the smallest part of the head is lowest in the vagina and that the tip of the forceps blade must accommodate the occiput; therefore, premature straightening of the forceps blade during application will cause undue pressure on the side of the fetal head. Forceps should be of a type with a long enough shank to permit the operator to visualize the maneuver, because often the fetal arms obstruct the view, and if the fetal body is in the horizontal position, access is further reduced. The head should be delivered slowly (over ~1 min) to reduce the compression-decompression forces on the fetal skull that may cause tentorial tears and intracranial bleeding.

The other frequently described technique of delivering the fetal head is the so-called Mauriceau-Smellie-Veit maneuver. This is actually a variety of techniques. The principle is that of traction down the axis of the birth canal while encouraging flexion of the fetal head to present the most favorable diameters to the pelvis. With the fetus supported on the right forearm, the middle finger of the right hand is passed into the fetal throat and the forefinger and the ring finger are placed on either the fetal shoulders or the malar eminences. Pressure is applied on the tongue to flex and deliver the head. The middle finger should not be just inside the fetal mouth, because traction can produce dislocation or fracture of the mandible. If the finger is inserted too far down the throat, creation of a pseudodiverticulum of the pharynx has been described. The left hand is used to exert pressure upward and posteriorly on the fetal occiput to encourage flexion. Alternatively, suprapubic pressure can be applied to encourage head flexion and descent. All these maneuvers can be performed with the operator's assistant elevating the fetal body above the horizontal. Downward traction on the fetal shoulders tends to stretch the cervical spine and, in combination with flexion of the fetal head, will draw

FIGURE 63–3
Forceps delivery of the aftercoming head. *A*, Allowing the trunk to hang flexes the head and encourages descent. *B*, Once the head is in the pelvis, rotating the trunk over the mother's abdomen delivers the face. *C*, Applying forceps to the aftercoming head. *D*, Forceps used to control the rate of delivery of the head.

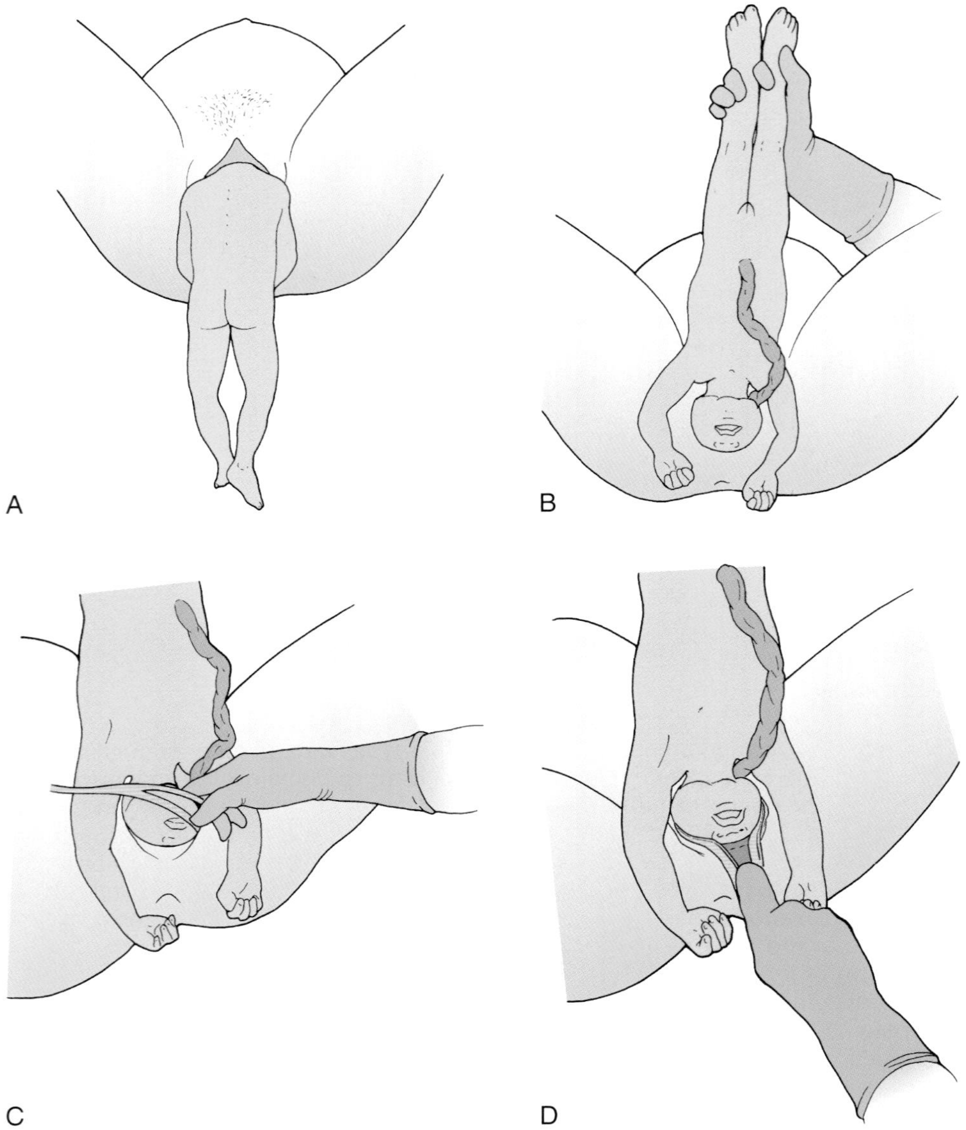

the base of the skull away from the vault, thus causing a tentorial tear. Therefore, traction on the trunk should not be used. All these permutations have been described by various authors as the Mauriceau-Smellie-Veit maneuver.

A pediatrician should always be present at the delivery, and ideally, the mouth and pharynx should be sucked out on the perineum prior to complete delivery of the head, although often the head delivers too quickly for this to be done.

The Zavanelli maneuver has also been described for the delivery of the breech with an entrapped aftercoming head. Tocolysis is used to facilitate replacement of the fetal body into the uterus, and cesarean section completes the delivery.[123] Because experience with this maneuver is very limited, its use in this desperate situation remains controversial.

Considerations in the Performance of Breech Extraction (Fig. 63–4)

Currently, breech extraction is rarely performed because of the risks of fetal and maternal trauma and because of the effects of excessive traction on the fetal body. Its main current indication is for the delivery of a second twin after internal podalic version or if cord prolapse complicates the late second stage. It may also be appropriate if the fetus is dead. Groin traction is performed to draw the breech over the perineum, Lovset's maneuver is employed routinely, and downward traction is exerted to bring the head into the pelvis. In effect,

FIGURE 63–4
Active breech delivery (breech extraction).

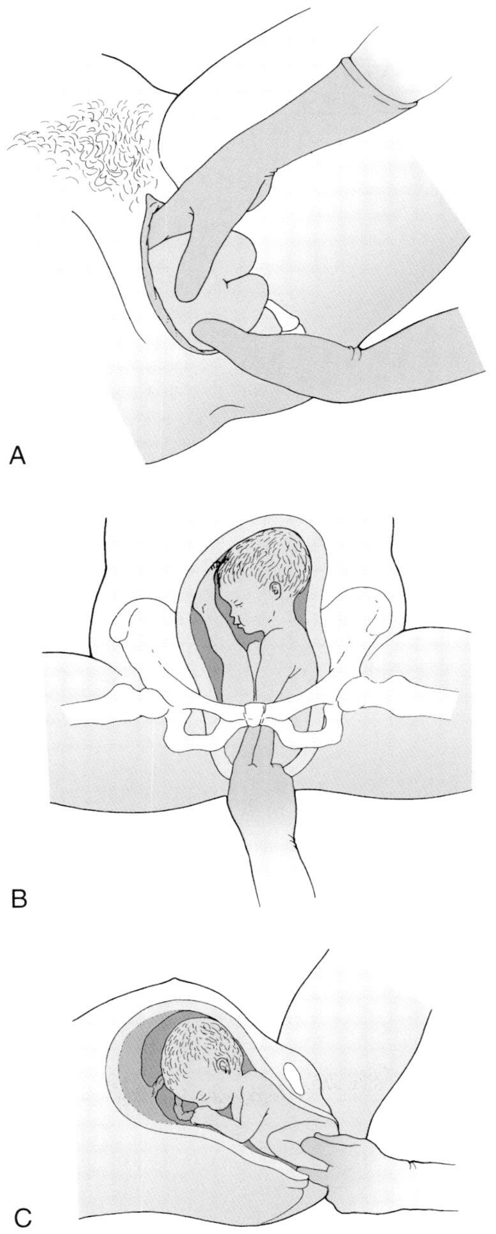

all the stages of assisted breech delivery are achieved actively by the obstetrician.

Choice of Mode of Delivery

CESAREAN SECTION

Practical Considerations in the Performance of Cesarean Section for the Delivery of the Term Breech

The orthodox obstetric practice of considering any woman with a breech presentation and any other medical or obstetric complication for delivery by elective cesarean section has much to recommend it. Elective and even emergency cesarean section for the term breech should present few technical problems. It should be remembered that the performance of a cesarean section does not prevent the possibility of birth injury, and many of the foregoing considerations about the careful delivery of the aftercoming head and the dangers of traction on the fetal spine still apply. The lower segment will be the site of choice for the incision with a term breech presentation. Schutterman and Grimes[124] reviewed 416 breeches of all gestations allocated randomly to transverse or low vertical incisions in the uterus and found no advantages for low vertical incisions. An elective cesarean section when adequate liquor is still present and the uterus is less likely to contract rapidly before completion of delivery of the breech will present few problems to the experienced operator. Forceps may be employed for delivery of the aftercoming head. Cesarean delivery at full dilation in the absence of liquor may be difficult because an arm may prolapse through the uterine incision; it should immediately be pushed back. Instead, a leg (or preferably both legs) should be grasped and brought through the incision: Traction will then effect the rest of the delivery. The head can be trapped by a well-contracted lower segment, and the incision will then need to be enlarged in a J-shaped fashion to increase access. In general, the mode of effecting delivery through the uterine incision is the same as for vaginal breech delivery, and many of the same complications may arise.

The fetal head may become entrapped in the uterine incision at the point of delivery, because the lower uterine segment contracts rapidly down. For this reason, even at an elective cesarean section, it is prudent to have a pediatrician present for delivery. Tocolytics cannot be recommended for routine deliveries but might be useful when delivery is expected to be difficult or traumatic.[125]

Deficiencies in the conduct of vaginal breech deliveries, resulting in perinatal death, have been systematically evaluated in a blinded case-controlled audit. The authors concluded that infant death at term was to a large extent potentially avoidable, but that in control breech infants who survived, suboptimal care was not uncommon.[107,126]

ACTIVE BREECH DELIVERY

With increasing consumer pressure in the United Kingdom during the 1990s toward less interventionist obstetrics, a demand for an active method of delivering the breech appeared. This was satisfied by a group of mainly midwife practitioners who performed a so-called active breech delivery. This encouraged women to be active during labor and, although allowing the woman to adopt the most comfortable position during labor, favored a standing position for the delivery itself. Nonpharmacologic analgesia and maternal participation in the birth were encouraged. The breech was allowed to deliver spontaneously without any interference from the birth attendants. The author's experience of 21 of such deliveries conducted in her own maternity unit is that 1 baby died during the final stages of birth, 1 had persisting neurologic damage resulting in a large medicolegal settlement, and another may have such damage. In the light of these poor outcomes, the technique cannot be recommended.

SUMMARY OF MANAGEMENT OPTIONS
Breech Presentation

Management Options	Evidence Quality and Recommendation	References
Term Breech Presentation		
Fetal Assessment		
Confirm diagnosis and determine placental site.	—/GPP	—
Confirm normality as association of breech presentation with congenital anomalies.	III/B	42
Version in Prenatal Period		
There is insufficient evidence to advocate postural methods to promote spontaneous version.	Ia/A	50
Recommend ECV at 36+ weeks' gestation.	Ia/A	53
Tocolysis increases the success of ECV.	Ia/A	62–70
There is insufficient evidence that epidural anesthesia increases the effectiveness of ECV.	Ia/A	62
Need for fetal heart rate monitoring before and after ECV.	III/B	49
If the Woman Chooses to Attempt a Vaginal Delivery		
Assess the health of the mother and baby.	IV/C	93–96
Perform ultrasound to confirm the diagnosis, check for fetal abnormalities, and assess placental site, fetal attitude, and estimated fetal weight.	IV/C	89,93–96
A written protocol is advisable, and a skilled birth attendant for labor and delivery is mandatory.	IIb/B	81
Pelvimetry need not be used routinely.	III/B	113,115
Labor and Delivery		
Evidence is that planned cesarean section for breech at term is the preferred method of delivery because it significantly reduces perinatal mortality and morbidity rates.	Ia/A Ib	1 90,91
Preterm Breech Presentation		
Prenatal		
There is insufficient evidence that ECV before term offers any benefit.	Ia/A	53
Labor and Delivery		
There is insufficient evidence to recommend cesarean section for the preterm breech.	Ib/B	46,127
For the preterm breech in labor, perform an ultrasound scan to confirm the presentation and normality; determine the mode of delivery in close consultation with the woman and her family.	IV/C	46

ECV, external cephalic version; GPP, good practice point.

SUGGESTED READINGS

Cheng M, Hannah M: Breech delivery at term: A critical review of the literature. Obstet Gynecol 1993;82:605–618.

Confidential Enquiry into Stillbirths and Deaths in Infancy. 7th Annual Report. London, Maternal and Child Health Research Consortium, 2000. Available at http://www.cmace.org.uk/getattachment/b858e5e8-862a-4121-9348-b9284d02db1b/7th-Annual-Report.aspx

Hannah ME, Hannah WJ, Hewson SA, et al: Planned caesarean section versus planned vaginal birth for breech presentation at term: A randomised multicenter trial. Term Breech Trial Collaborative Group. Lancet 2000;356:1375–1383.

Hofmeyr GJ, Hannah M: Planned caesarean section for term breech delivery. Cochrane Database Syst Rev 2003;2:CD000166.

Hofmeyr GJ, Kulier R: External cephalic version for breech presentation at term. Cochrane Database Syst Rev 1996;1:CD000083.

Hutton EK, Hofmeyr GJ: External cephalic version facilitation for breech presentation before term. Cochrane Database Syst Rev 2006;1:CD000084.

Reitberg CC, Elferink-Stinkens PM, Visser GHA: The effect of the Term Breech Trial on medical intervention behaviour and neonatal outcome in the Netherlands: An analysis of 35,453 term breech infants. BJOG 2005;112:205–209.

Royal College of Obstetricians and Gynaecologists (RCOG): External Cephalic Version and Reducing the Incidence of Breech Presentation (Green-top Guideline No. 20a). London, RCOG Press, 2006. Available at www.rcog.org.uk

Royal College of Obstetricians and Gynaecologists (RCOG): The Management of Breech Presentation (Green-top Guideline No. 20b). London, RCOG Press, 2006. Available at www.rcog.org.uk

Whye H, Hannah ME, Saigal S, et al: Outcomes of children at 2 years of age after planned cesarean birth versus planned vaginal birth for breech presentation at term: The International Randomized Term Breech Trial. Am J Obstet Gynecol 2004;191:864–871.

REFERENCES

For a complete list of references, log onto www.expertconsult.com.

CHAPTER 64

Unstable Lie, Malpresentations, and Malpositions

IAN Z. MACKENZIE

INTRODUCTION

The concepts of unstable lie, malpresentation, and malposition have not changed for centuries probably, and there is no reason to anticipate a significant change will present in the foreseeable future. Various techniques for improving diagnostic accuracy and clinical care are periodically proposed and either become established clinical practice or disappear, sometimes to be resurrected at a later date.

Near term and during labor, the fetus usually assumes a longitudinal lie and presents to the maternal pelvis with the head, the neck flexed, and the vertex in the lowermost part of the uterus. In approximately 5% of labors, the lie is not longitudinal; this can be dangerous for both mother and fetus and demands intervention. As with much of medicine, the prior identification of the pregnancy at particular risk for unstable lie, malpresentation, or malposition can prompt intervention in advance of a complication developing and improve the outcome. Although relevant to unstable lie and malpresentation, this chapter does not consider issues relating to fetal breech presentation in detail because these are dealt with elsewhere (see Chapter 63).

DEFINITIONS

Unstable Lie

Unstable lie is a description generally used beyond 37 weeks' gestation when the fetal lie and presentation repeatedly change, the lie varying between longitudinal, transverse, and oblique, and the presentation between cephalic, limbs, breech, or a combination. Conventional wisdom teaches that the fetal presentation will not be cephalic at the start of the third trimester in around 25% pregnancies and this proportion drops to around 3% to 5% by term. This teaching is supported by longitudinal ultrasound examination studies.[1–3]

By 37 weeks' gestation, the fetus usually adopts a "stable" lie and presentation that will be unchanging until labor; fetal position, describing the relationship of the fetal back to the maternal side, may and often does change. A longitudinal fetal lie is, however, unlikely to change once labor has established, unless the presenting part is "high" in relation to the pelvis, and particularly if there is polyhydramnios or the maternal abdominal wall muscles are weakened by high parity.

Malpresentation Including Compound Presentation

The *presenting part* is defined as that part of the fetus that is lowermost in the uterus. The vertex is the "normal" and most common presenting part. The alternatives include face, brow, breech, and shoulder; compound presentations involve more than one fetal part presenting to the pelvis. This may include a combination of the head with a limb or limbs and any presentation that includes the umbilical cord.

Malposition

Fetal malposition occurs when the vertex presents to the maternal pelvis in a position other than flexed occipitoanterior. Malpositions thus include occipitotransverse and occipitoposterior positions and may involve asynclitism (sideways tilt of the head).

Figure 64–1 shows the various positions that the vertex, brow, or face may adopt during labor.

ETIOLOGY

Unstable Lie

Unstable lie is much more common in parous than in nulliparous women and may be caused by or associated with a number of factors. Any situation that discourages or prevents the fetal head or breech from entering the maternal pelvis may predispose to an abnormal and/or unstable fetal lie. Figure 64–2 illustrates many of these factors.

Maternal Factors

HIGH PARITY

Reduced maternal abdominal wall muscle tone leading to a failure to brace and maintain a longitudinal fetal lie is probably the most frequent factor. There is a commonly held view that the highly parous uterus also has reduced muscle

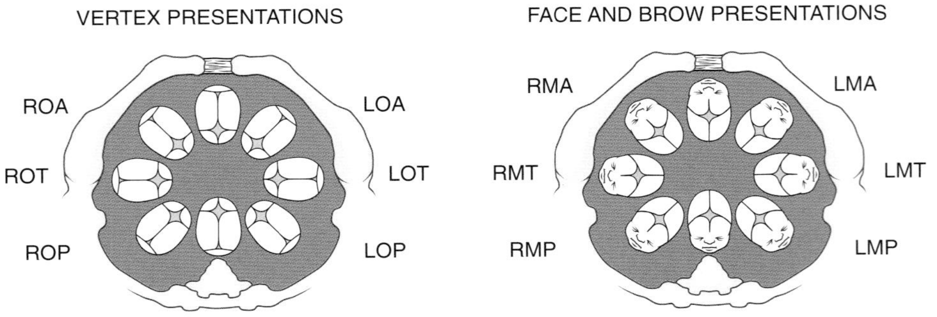

FIGURE 64–1 Diagramatic representation of the positions for vertex, brow, and face presentations. A, anterior; L, left; M, mento; O, occipito; R, right; T, transverse.

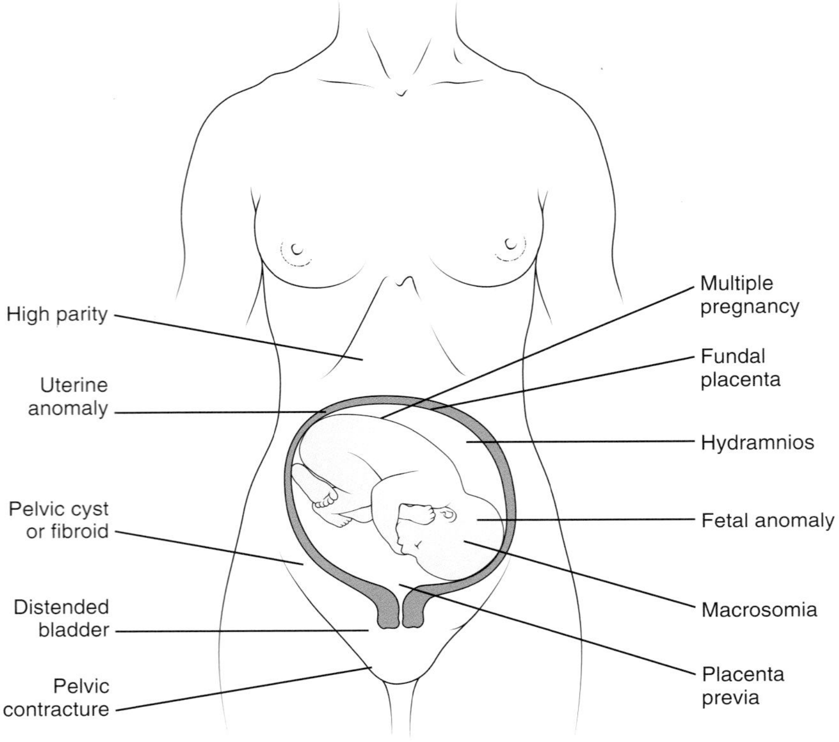

FIGURE 64–2 Etiologic factors and conditions associated with unstable fetal lie.

tone, thereby contributing to instability of the fetal lie, but this has not been proved and is, therefore, of questionable relevance.

PLACENTA PREVIA

A persistently changing fetal lie may be the only clinical feature leading to the diagnosis of placenta previa. In addition, the placenta situated in the fundus may also predispose to an unstable lie.[4]

PELVIC CONTRACTURE

Reduced pelvic dimensions or a distorted pelvic cavity due to congenital malformation, disease processes compromising bone development, or trauma to the pelvis, can prevent the presenting pole engaging in the pelvis in late pregnancy.

PELVIC TUMORS

Ovarian cysts of only moderate dimensions situated in the pouch of Douglas and fibroids in the lower pole of the uterus, as well as those that are pedunculated and occupying the sacral curve, can prevent the fetal head or breech entering the pelvis and predispose to a transverse or oblique lie.

UTERINE MALFORMATION

Uterus cordiformis, subseptus, or septus can be causative, but more severe forms of anomaly including uterus unicornis, bicornis, and didelphys are less likely to lead to an unstable lie because of the restricted capacity of the uterine cavity; a predisposition to fetal breech presentation, however, often results.

DISTENDED MATERNAL URINARY BLADDER

Maternal urinary retention with bladder distention can cause a changing fetal lie, usually only temporarily, with resolution occurring with urinary voiding or bladder catheterization.

Fetal Factors

POLYHYDRAMNIOS

Polyhydramnios (excessive volumes of amniotic fluid) may produce marked uterine distention, enabling the fetus to move around more freely. This probably represents the most common "pathologic" cause for an unstable lie and is also potentially the most hazardous for mother and fetus (see Chapter 12).

OLIGOHYDRAMNIOS

By restricting fetal movement, oligohydramnios can prevent the fetus presenting by the breech from undergoing complete spontaneous version to cephalic.

MULTIPLE PREGNANCY

The discovery of an abnormal lie during the last 3 weeks of pregnancy may arouse suspicion of a multiple pregnancy and lead to investigations that result in the diagnosis being reached. Nowadays, such a diagnosis is unlikely to have been missed until this stage of pregnancy with the widespread use of routine ultrasonography during the first 20 weeks of gestation. When the lie of one or both fetuses repeatedly changes, there is usually polyhydramnios.

FETAL MACROSOMIA

Fetal macrosomia produces the same effect as pelvic contracture and must also be considered in such cases.

FETAL ABNORMALITIES

Significant hydrocephaly, tumors of the fetal neck or sacrum, fetal abdominal distention as with hydrops fetalis, and fetal neuromuscular dysfunction (including extended legs) may impede or discourage engagement of a fetal pole in the maternal pelvis. In cases of intrauterine death, the fetus is more likely to present abnormally due to loss of tone, sometimes requiring delivery by cesarean section because vaginal birth is impossible.

Compound Presentation

Compound presentations are most usually associated with polyhydramnios and high parity and are more common during the early weeks of the third trimester. Multiple pregnancies, especially monoamniotic, represent a particular risk. Pelvic tumors, including uterine fibroids situated low in the uterine body or an ovarian cyst situated in the pouch of Douglas, also predispose to compound presentations.

Malpresentations that involve the umbilical cord are similarly associated with the factors previously mentioned. Fetal breech presentation, especially with one or both knees flexed, is the most common malpresentation associated with cord presentation and prolapse.[5–8] Abnormalities of the cord, including reduced content of Wharton's jelly, true knots, and chronic fetal acidosis reducing tissue turgidity, have been cited as predisposing factors.[9]

Brow and Face Presentations

The majority of cases of brow and face presentation are thought to arise when there is a minor degree of deflexion of the presenting vertex, which then undergoes further extension. With increasing extension, a brow becomes a face presentation. This may occur during the antepartum period, resulting in a primary face presentation, or during labor, resulting in a secondary face presentation. Primary presentations are generally associated with fetal malformations, including anencephaly, meningocele, dolichocephaly, congenital branchiocele, goiter or other anterior neck tumors, and tense extensor neck muscles. Polyhydramnios with the increased space within the uterus and a tight nuchal cord have also been implicated as predisposing factors. Secondary presentations are thought to be associated with a contracted or abnormally shaped pelvis. This was considered responsible for 40% of face presentations in a series reported from the Johns Hopkins Hospital early in the last century.[10] It is also much more common in preterm labor, probably due to the more capacious pelvis being able to accommodate the relatively small fetus.[11]

Malpositions

Data derived from ultrasound examinations at the start of labor have suggested that the majority (68%) of occipitoposterior positions confirmed toward the end of labor were in an occipitoanterior position at the beginning of labor; the other 32% were initially in an occipitoposterior position, and these labors are more likely to result in an assisted delivery.[12]

Pelvic shape is probably the major determinant of fetal position prior to labor. When the anteroposterior dimension of the pelvic brim equals or exceeds that of the transverse dimension (the android pelvis), occipitoposterior positions are favored. Thus, women with an android pelvis are more likely to have an occipitoposterior position in late pregnancy and at the start of labor because the larger dimensions toward the back of the pelvis encourage the broader occiput to be accommodated there rather than in the anterior compartment. In addition, when there is a high-assimilation pelvis with an extra vertebra included in the formation of the sacrum, the inclination of the brim increases and favors an occipitoposterior position. The much less common anthropoid-shaped pelvis, with lessening of the posterosagittal diameter (the distance between the midpoint of the widest transverse diameter and the sacrum), affects not only the brim but also commonly extends to the lower levels of the pelvis and to the outlet. In particular, the concavity of the sacrum from promontory to tip is often reduced or abolished (flat sacrum), leaving a reduced space in which the sinciput can turn, should internal rotation commence. This leads to the head becoming impacted in the pelvis, resulting in a "deep transverse arrest." It has been suggested that increased muscle tone in the extensor muscles of the fetus might also predispose to an occipitoposterior position, but there is little evidence to support this theory.

Most important is the observation that a high proportion of women with a malposition who make poor progress through labor often respond to augmentation of uterine contractions with oxytocin and achieve a successful spontaneous vaginal delivery.[13] This suggests that the quality of uterine contractions plays a significant part in determining the position and attitude of the fetal head. As well as uterine contraction strength being important, there is now good evidence that the tone of the pelvic floor is relevant. Use of regional anesthesia for the management of pain relief during labor has been implicated as a mechanism for the increased rates of malposition in late labor,[14,15] although this is disputed. Regional anesthesia provides an extremely effective method of reducing the distress of labor, distress that is more common with a preexisting occipitoposterior position. The issue of cause and effect thus comes into play. The experience reported from Dublin provides some evidence to suggest that regional blockade is not causal in the evolution of fetal malposition. It was noted that despite a 30-fold increase in intrapartum epidural usage between 1975 and 1998, occipitoposterior position at the end of a first labor decreased from 3.8% to 2.4%.[15,16]

INCIDENCE

Unstable Lie

Figures are not generally available for the incidence with which unstable lie is encountered antenatally; it is influenced by the proportion of multiparas and particularly the numbers of grand-multiparas in the population. Also, in societies where malnutrition is prominent and maternal or fetal skeletal deformities are relatively more common, the incidence will be higher. In a well-nourished and developed population where high parity (>4) is uncommon, the incidence will be in the range of 0.1% to 1.0%, and the occurrence rate of transverse lie in labor is in the region of 0.4%.[17]

Compound Presentations

There is a relatively sparse literature on the incidence of compound presentations that involve one or more limbs and the fetal head or breech. Overall, the incidence has been quoted to be between 1 in 377 and 1 in 1213 deliveries[18–20]; personal experience suggests that the lower incidence is more usual in the developed world. Combinations involving the upper limbs and head are the most common. Diagnosis in late labor is the usual situation, with as many as 50% of compound presentations being diagnosed during the second stage of labor.

The incidence of cord presentation, when a segment of umbilical cord is situated between the fetal presenting part and the cervix with intact membranes, has not been widely reported. although cord prolapse, by definition following membrane rupture, occurs in around 1 in 300 to 1 in 700 total births,[5,7,21,22] 1 in 900 cephalic presentation labors, 1 in 56 breech labors, 1 in 23 twin labors,[7] and 1 in 5 to 1 in 10 compound presentations that involve a limb.[18,19,23] Thus, cord prolapse in a singleton pregnancy with a cephalic presentation at term has an incidence of around 1 in 1400 labors. These rates are almost certainly lower than the incidence of cord presentation, because recognized cord presentation is likely to be managed by cesarean section before prolapse occurs.

Brow and Face Presentation

Face presentation in labor has an incidence of between 1 in 200 and 1 in 500 labors[24–26] and brow presentations around 1 in 600 to 1 in 1500 deliveries.[27–29] The incidences during pregnancy are less well documented, especially for brow presentation, because it is probable that this presentation is only transient, with reversion to vertex presentation with flexion of the neck or face presentation with further deflexion.

Malpositions

During the antepartum period, prior to the onset of labor, the occipitoposterior position exists in around 11% of singleton pregnancies.[30,31] Once labor starts, the incidence is in the region of 20% to 25%; if the fetal back is on the maternal left, the occipitoposterior position is much less common than when the back is on the maternal right.[20] It is said to be more common in cases of membrane rupture before the onset of labor, with an incidence of 27%.[32] When there is an occipitoposterior position at the start of labor, this position will remain to the end of labor in 20% to 35%, indicating that 65% to 80% undergo spontaneous rotation during labor. Only approximately 1% to 5% are delivered in an occipitoposterior position.[33,34]

DIAGNOSIS

Unstable Lie

This diagnosis is made when a varying fetal lie during the last month of gestation is found at repeated clinical examinations. Occasionally in those women in whom clinical examination is not easy (including those with a raised body mass index), the diagnosis may fortuitously be made by an ultrasound examination performed for other reasons. An unstable lie would appear to be more common than is presently thought, from the evidence of the frequency with which fetal breech presentation is missed prior to the onset of labor despite frequent and recent antenatal clinical examinations. Further, the observation of spontaneous and unexpected version of the fetus from a cephalic to breech presentation during the last weeks before birth adds weight to this observation.[35,36]

Compound Presentations

A compound presentation involving a fetal arm with the head or an arm with a leg is likely to be diagnosed only during the antepartum period as a coincidental finding at an ultrasound examination or rarely on radiographic or magnetic resonance imaging. The high nonengaged head that cannot be encouraged into the maternal pelvis might prompt an ultrasound examination that leads to the diagnosis.

Diagnosis during labor may be suspected because of delay in the presenting part entering the pelvis, which is confirmed on vaginal examination by identifying the errant limb or limbs. Occasionally, the diagnosis is made unexpectedly at a vaginal examination during preterm labor when the maternal pelvis is large and the interloping limb with the head or breech does not delay engagement of the presenting part.

Compound presentations involving the umbilical cord are usually classified according to Naegele, who distinguished "presentation" before membrane rupture and "prolapse" after membrane rupture. A diagnosis of cord presentation will not usually be made prior to the onset of labor except in those cases of an unstable lie when a vaginal examination

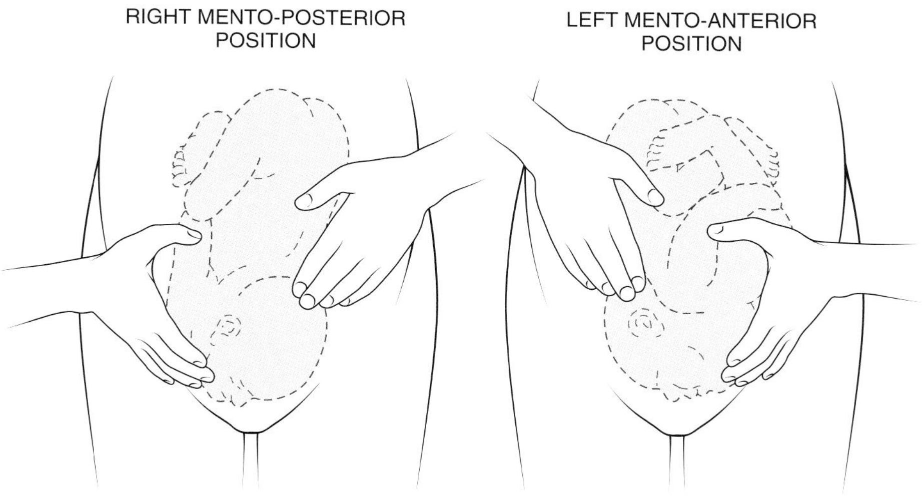

FIGURE 64–3
Palpation of the fetus and the landmarks associated with a face presentation.

is performed as part of the assessment for the strategy for continued management. Although some have documented reaching the diagnosis with ultrasound, this is not a widely reported observation,[37] and cord prolapse occurring during subsequent labor appears to be an infrequent consequence.[38]

Face Presentation

Older texts report that abdominal palpation allows the diagnosis of face presentation by the recognition of a much broader than usual lower pole presenting to the pelvis and the marked depression between the fetal back and the occiput (Fig. 64–3). This is more easily demonstrated if the fetus is lying in a dorsoanterior or mentoposterior presentation, which is less common than a mentoanterior presentation.[24] It is also said that the fetal heart sounds are very easily heard when listened to over the fetal chest, especially with a mentoanterior position; this potentially valuable clinical sign is lost if hand-held Doppler machines are routinely used to detect fetal heart pulsations in preference to a Pinard stethoscope. Despite this, the author's experience is that these clinical signs are difficult to elicit, even in those cases of face presentation already confirmed by radiology or ultrasonography.

Confirmation of the presentation should be made by vaginal examination during the intrapartum period. The obstetrician, however, should be wary of confusing a face and a breech presentation; facial edema readily forms during labor and, with the added difficulty associated with a high presenting part and a poorly dilated cervix, differentiation can be difficult. Identification of the supraorbital ridges, the ridge of the nose, and the alveolar processes within the mouth should establish the diagnosis. If the technology is available, an ultrasound examination can be used to confirm the clinical suspicion.[39]

Brow Presentation

Although occasionally a brow presentation may be recognized during the antenatal period, usually coincidentally at an ultrasound examination, this is not permanent in most instances. The suspicion of a broader than expected head resting above the pelvic brim compared with the size of the body may (rarely) lead the astute clinician to suspect this possibility. Diagnosis during the intrapartum period is likely to be made only in advanced labor when the cervix is moderately well dilated and the brow is palpable to the examining fingers. Identification of the anterior fontanelle and the supraorbital ridges confirms the diagnosis, but any significant caput succedaneum can mask these landmarks. As with face presentations, ultrasound examination is the most practical way to confirm or refute the diagnosis.

Malpositions

It is often written that the outline of the distended uterus occasionally suggests an occipitoposterior position by the "flatness" and a dip between the head and the trunk. Certainly, fetal movements may be readily observed over much of the anterior surface of the abdomen if the baby is active at the time of the examination. However, the fetal back may be difficult to identify on palpation, although the shoulder is felt toward the flank with the limbs often obvious to palpation over the abdomen. With Pawlik's grip, the sinciput is said to be prominent, but personal experience would not suggest this to be a reliable feature. Importantly, the fetal heart is heard maximally in the flank to which the back is directed; the Pinard stethoscope allows this clinical sign to be elicited whereas the small Doppler fetal heart detectors generally do not. An ultrasound examination would confirm or refute the clinical findings.

During labor, the anterior fontanelle is easier to reach when the position is occipitoposterior rather than occipitoanterior, although caput succedaneum can make this difficult, especially late in labor. Palpation of the more anterior ear can be helpful, but this may be misleading if the pinna has been turned forward. At this examination, not only the degree of flexion but also any asynclitism should be noted. Diagnosis of a deep transverse arrest should not present difficulties unless there is marked caput succedaneum or prominent asynclitism. Once again, palpation of the fetal ear could be helpful, or if available, ultrasound to confirm the position.[40,41]

RISKS

Unstable Lie and Compound Presentation

There are no hazards to mother or fetus during the antenatal period from unstable lie per se. It is possible that cord entanglement is a greater risk, although this has not been positively shown. During the latter weeks of pregnancy, spontaneous resolution to a longitudinal lie before the onset of labor occurs in approximately 85%.[42–44]

There are, however, very serious risks to mother and fetus with the onset of labor if the lie is not longitudinal. Once the membranes rupture, with or without accompanying uterine contractions, there is approximately a 9% risk of cord prolapse if the fetal lie is oblique or transverse or the presenting part is high above the pelvic inlet.[45] This may result in damaging hypoxia or even stillbirth; perinatal death has generally been reported in 5% to 10% of cases[7,46,47] or, according to one series, as high as 43%.[48] The risk of hypoxic damage is less well documented and it may be as infrequent as 1% in survivors,[7] although this must depend on the speed and availability of first aid to rescue the situation. Keeping the interval between cord prolapse and delivery as brief as possible is likely to be important.[46,49]

If labor starts when the lie is not longitudinal, a compound presentation may result or the pelvis may remain empty. If left unattended, fetal distress will eventually supervene, ultimately resulting in fetal death. A Bandl or retraction ring (Fig. 64–4) may form, making delivery even by cesarean section potentially hazardous.[50] In addition, uterine rupture is a real possibility especially in multiparas, with an incidence of 3%,[45] with potentially serious consequences for mother and fetus (see Chapter 67).

FIGURE 64–4
Fetal shoulder presentation, illustrating the site of a Bandl or retraction ring, forming at the junction of the upper and lower uterine segments in an obstructed labor.

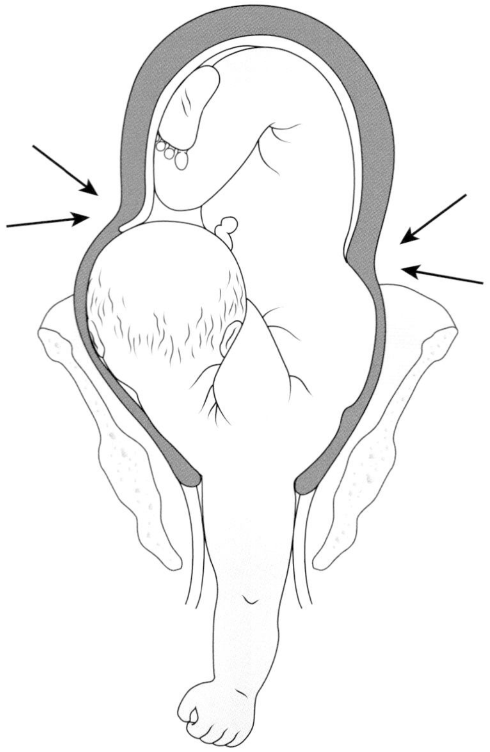

Malpresentation

Face

Cord prolapse may be marginally increased with a face over vertex presentation, but once established in labor with the head engaged in the pelvis, this is no more likely. Progress should be as for a vertex presentation without any additional risk to the fetus because the presenting head diameters are similar (Fig. 64–5). However, with the largest presenting diameter (biparietal) displaced toward the back of the pelvis, a generous episiotomy should be performed to reduce the risk of a third-degree tear. Providing the face is mentoanterior, vaginal delivery is likely. If there is any delay in delivery, assistance with forceps is appropriate but the ventouse is contraindicated because it cannot be applied safely with a face presentation. The parents should be advised in advance of delivery that their baby will initially appear very unattractive owing to the inevitable bruising and marked edema, both of which disappear within a few hours of birth.

Brow

There are no added risks to the mother with a fetal brow presentation during the antenatal period. As with a face presentation, the risk of cord presentation and prolapse is increased.

Except with very preterm labor, the fetus cannot be delivered as a persistent brow unless there is a very capacious pelvis, because of the large mentovertical diameter that presents to the pelvis (see Fig. 64–5). If continued extension of the neck to a face presentation does not occur and the brow presentation persists, the chances of fetal distress and even uterine rupture in a parous woman are high if labor is not progressing and left to continue for too long.

Malpositions

Few risks are associated with a fetal malposition prior to labor. As already stated, there is a belief that prelabor rupture of the membranes is more common with an occipitoposterior position. Because the head is usually not engaged and may not be well settled into the pelvis, the risk of cord prolapse is marginally increased.

Once in labor, progress may be slower than with an occipitoanterior position and maternal discomfort is often increased, particularly in the back. In addition to a protracted first stage of labor, there is often a delay during the second stage with the need for augmentation of contractions with oxytocin, and maybe manual rotation or instrumental delivery using ventouse or forceps with or without initial rotation. With the present reluctance to engage in rotational forceps deliveries, especially if fetal distress is suspected, together with the higher failure rates with the ventouse, delivery by cesarean section is increased.

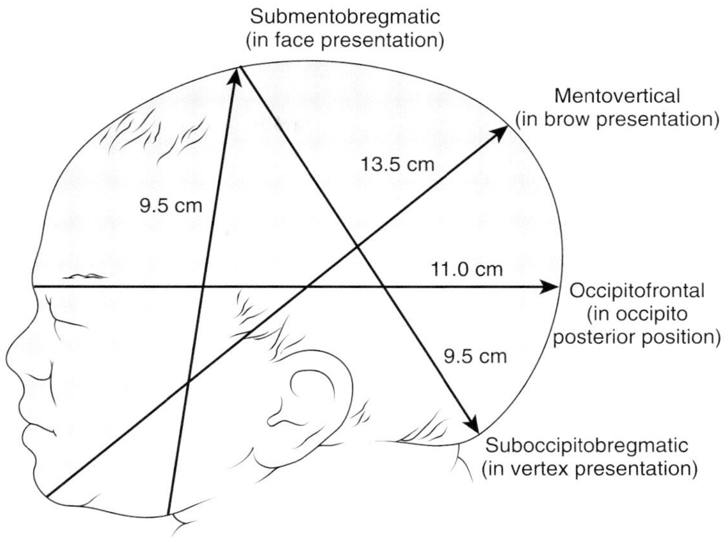

FIGURE 64–5
The largest sagittal dimensions of the fetal head according to presentation.

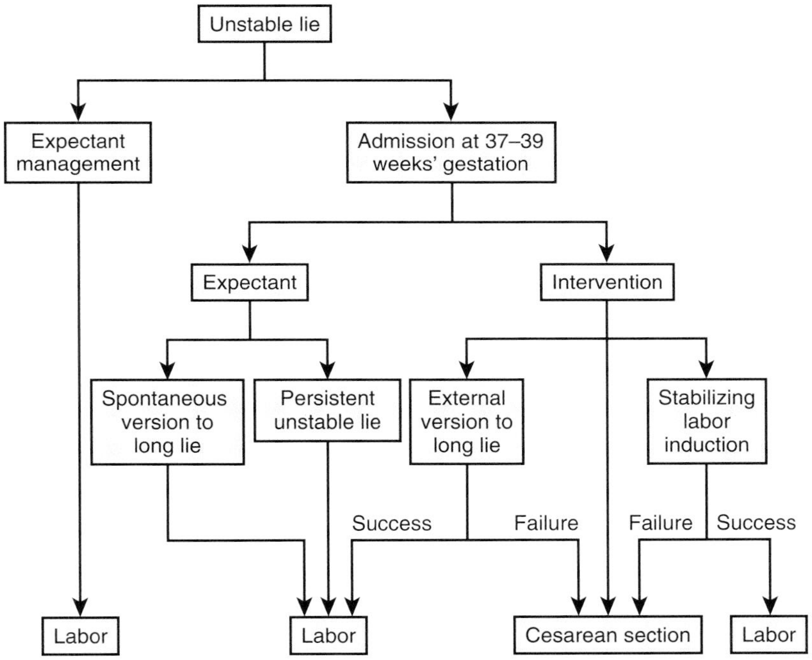

FIGURE 64–6
Algorithm for the antepartum management of unstable lie in late pregnancy.

It has been shown by one group that the occipitoposterior position that persists to the time of vaginal delivery presents a significant risk of anal sphincter damage for all parities.[16]

MANAGEMENT OPTIONS

Unstable Lie and Compound Presentation

Prenatal

During the antenatal period, management can be expectant or active, whereas delivery can either await spontaneous onset of labor or be arranged as a planned event. An algorithm of the various options is illustrated in Figure 64–6.

EXPECTANT MANAGEMENT

Once an unstable lie is identified, no specific action is taken in anticipation that the lie will become longitudinal before the membranes rupture or labor starts: this is likely to occur in more than 80% of cases.[42–44] Manipulation to a longitudinal lie at an antenatal examination can sometimes be performed. Every attempt should be made to identify any obvious mechanical cause for the unstable lie, especially if it is likely to result in obstructed labor requiring elective cesarean section. The patient should be advised of the risks associated with an unstable lie and the need for urgent attention should labor start or the membranes rupture. If she lives a long distance from the delivery unit, it may be wise to admit her at 37 to 39 weeks' gestation to await the onset of labor to ensure prompt attention if required. A number of physical exercises, including adopting the knee-elbow position for short periods each day, have been advocated to encourage spontaneous version, generally from a breech to a cephalic presentation.[51–54] Such maneuvers possibly improve the chances of longitudinal lie by 5% to 10%, but there is no established evidence base for this proposition.

ACTIVE MANAGEMENT

Admission is often advised from 37 to 39 weeks' gestation, which provides the opportunity for (1) daily observations of fetal lie and presentation to be made, (2) active treatment to correct the lie if necessary, (3) calling for immediate assistance upon membrane rupture or the onset of labor, and (4) urgent delivery if the lie is not longitudinal, fetal distress occurs, or the cord is presenting or has prolapsed. Evidence to support this approach is provided by one small study of expectant management for unstable lie after 37 weeks' gestation that reported that 17% presented in labor with a transverse lie and 6% had a prolapsed cord resulting in neonatal death in 1%.[44] If spontaneous resolution to a longitudinal lie occurs and a cephalic or breech presentation is maintained for 48 hours, the women may be discharged home to await labor. Some currently discourage labor with a breech presentation and reference should be made to the relevant chapter on this topic (see Chapter 63). If spontaneous resolution of an abnormal lie does not occur, an active approach to management may be adopted. External cephalic version can be attempted if facilities permit immediate delivery in the event of placental abruption, membrane rupture, cord prolapse, or acute fetal distress for any reason.[49,55] Rhesus immunoprophylaxis should be given to at-risk women either before or soon after the version attempt, and an estimate of the volume of any fetomaternal hemorrhage made about 20 minutes after the attempt at version, using the Kleihauer-Betke method or flow cytometry to determine whether additional prophylaxis is necessary.[56,57] If a longitudinal lie is not maintained, the version can be repeated as often as necessary, and if unsuccessful, the women should be kept in the hospital after the birth. The success of version for unstable lie is unclear, but it is probably greater than for breech presentation, which is usually quoted around 40% to 65%.[46,48,58] Tocolysis can be used, including infusions of ritodrine 50 μg/min for 15 minutes[46] or terbutaline sulfate 250 μg intravenously over 1 to 2 minutes,[31] but is often unnecessary with a transverse or oblique lie (see Chapter 63).

In the event the lie remains unstable, a stabilizing induction may be performed usually at 38 to 39 weeks' gestation. Following transfer to the labor suite, an external cephalic version is performed if necessary to convert the fetal lie to longitudinal. Once the fetus is in position, regular abdominal palpations are performed to confirm the lie is maintained and a titrated intravenous infusion of oxytocin commenced to stimulate uterine contractility.[47] Although contractions can also be stimulated with local (vaginal) or oral prostaglandins, this is probably less advisable because the response to prostaglandins can be unpredictable and occasionally hyperstimulation occurs, which would be especially concerning if the lie reverts to oblique or transverse, when tocolysis and/or emergency cesarean section is required. As soon as contractions are occurring at 10-minute intervals or more frequently, a low amniotomy is performed, having ensured at vaginal examination that the lie is still longitudinal, the presentation is not compound, and in particular, the cord is not presenting. If the cord presents, an emergency cesarean section is necessary. Once low amniotomy is performed, a reasonable volume of amniotic fluid should be released, followed by confirmation that the cord has not prolapsed and the presenting part is fixed in the pelvic brim. Thereafter, once labor is established, management continues as for uncomplicated cases, being ever mindful that cord prolapse might still occur.

Hindwater amniotomy using a Drew-Smythe catheter[59] can be performed providing a low posterior placenta has been excluded by an ultrasound examination. The catheter is guided through the cervix between the uterine wall and the fetal membranes behind the presenting part, taking all possible care to avoid trauma to the fetus and the uterine wall. When in position, with the catheter tip above the presenting part, the stylet in the catheter is advanced to puncture the membranes and allow a controlled release of amniotic fluid. This procedure aims to reduce the chances of cord prolapse occurring, but it is rarely used in modern practice.

Finally, a decision to deliver by elective antepartum cesarean section at 38 to 40 weeks' gestation is a legitimate management option.[44] Ideally, an attempt should be made to convert the lie to longitudinal immediately before the laparotomy or after opening the peritoneum but before incising the uterus. If successful, a lower segment incision in the uterus can be used for the delivery, but if the lie remains transverse, the classic (vertical midline) incision may be preferable to reduce the chances of fetal and uterine trauma being caused by a difficult fetal extraction from the uterus. Planned cesarean section is particularly appropriate if antenatal external cephalic version is contraindicated, previous attempts at version fail, or there is a mechanical obstruction to vaginal delivery.

Intrapartum

When the fetal lie is transverse or oblique and the membranes rupture or labor starts, the options for management are illustrated in the algorithm in Figure 64–7, which depend on (1) whether there is a cord presentation or prolapse, (2) the stage of labor whether before full cervical dilation or during the second stage, and (3) whether the membranes are intact or ruptured.

FIRST STAGE OF LABOR

Management depends on whether the fetal membranes are intact or ruptured. With intact membranes, an external version can be attempted. This is performed between contractions with or without tocolysis to relax the uterus before the attempt. Tocolytic agents that can be used in this situation include β-agonists such as terbutaline infused at 5 to 20 μg/min, salbutamol (albuterol) 2.5 to 4.5 μg/min, ritodrine 100 to 350 μg/min,[60] or the oxytocin antagonist atosiban, given as a single intravenous bolus dose of 6.75 mg.[50] If the version is successful, a repeat vaginal examination should be performed to exclude cord presentation or prolapse. Once this has been confirmed, labor can be allowed to establish, ensuring the lie remains longitudinal until the presenting part engages in the pelvis,

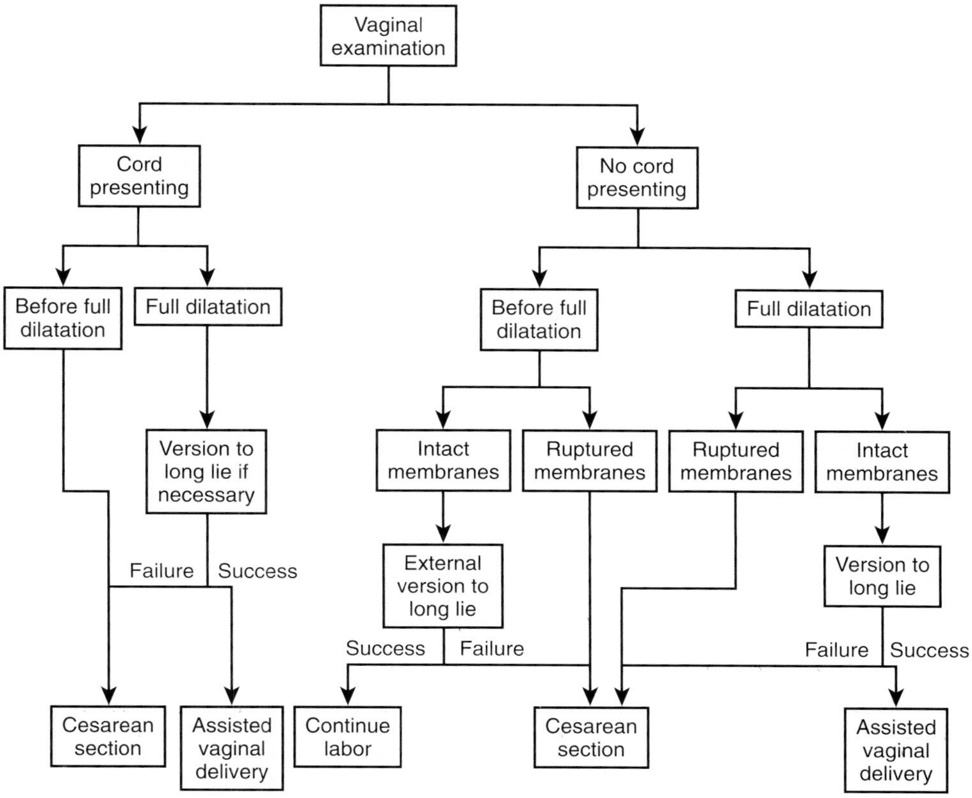

FIGURE 64–7 Algorithm for the intrapartum management of unstable lie.

with progress augmented with oxytocin if necessary. If the version has been unsuccessful, delivery by cesarean section should be performed (see later discussion). With ruptured membranes, delivery by cesarean section is generally the only option unless the woman is in very early labor and an attempt at external cephalic version is successful. If there is a compound presentation involving a hand or arm, attempts should be made at vaginal examination to push the arm up or nip one of the fetal fingers to try to encourage its withdrawal from in front of the head. It is also reasonable to allow labor to continue with close supervision in anticipation that spontaneous withdrawal will occur with continuing uterine contractions causing discomfort to the arm and hand; cord prolapse is a remote but real possibility.

A shoulder presentation, which may include an arm prolapsed into the vagina, is a serious situation (see Fig. 64–4). Clamping of the uterine wall around the fetus by a retraction or Bandl's ring may have contributed. Delivery must be by cesarean section. Administration of a uterine relaxant such as halothane administered by the anesthetist can facilitate the delivery, which is most safely achieved through a classic uterine incision. This incision allows the fetus to be withdrawn through the fundus of the uterus, whereas a lower segment incision makes it nearly impossible to manipulate the fetus into a position that will allow delivery without damage to the fetus and uterus. This approach to delivery is still indicated even if the fetus has already died, to avoid uterine rupture and other serious uterine trauma at the time of the delivery.

SECOND STAGE OF LABOR WITH INTACT MEMBRANES

If fetopelvic disproportion has been excluded, correction to a longitudinal lie by external cephalic or internal podalic version followed by an assisted vaginal cephalic or breech delivery should be anticipated. If internal podalic version is attempted, this requires adequate anesthesia (either general or fully effective regional block). Using appropriate aseptic techniques, the obstetrician introduces a hand into the uterus, confirms the foot of the anteriorly positioned leg by identifying the heel, and applies traction on the foot, withdrawing the foot and leg and subsequently the breech through the vagina (Fig. 64–8). It is ideal if both feet can be grasped and pulled down, as this avoids the "splits," with one leg down and one leg up, which can splint the baby and lead to a difficult delivery. The management is then as described for breech extraction (see Chapter 63). Great care must be taken to avoid both fetal bony injury and laceration of the uterus. Tocolysis may be helpful for this procedure. If version is not successful, delivery should be achieved by cesarean section; attempts at version should be performed only when immediate resort to section is available. The obstetrician should be aware of the possibility of atonic primary postpartum hemorrhage when uterine relaxants have been administered to assist the delivery (see Chapter 75).

SECOND STAGE OF LABOR WITH RUPTURED MEMBRANES

If there is a compound presentation involving a hand and the fetal head is engaged in the pelvis, it may be possible with vaginal manipulation to encourage the hand to withdraw from the pelvis so that an assisted vaginal delivery can

FIGURE 64–8
Principle of securing the foot of the anterior leg at internal podalic version.

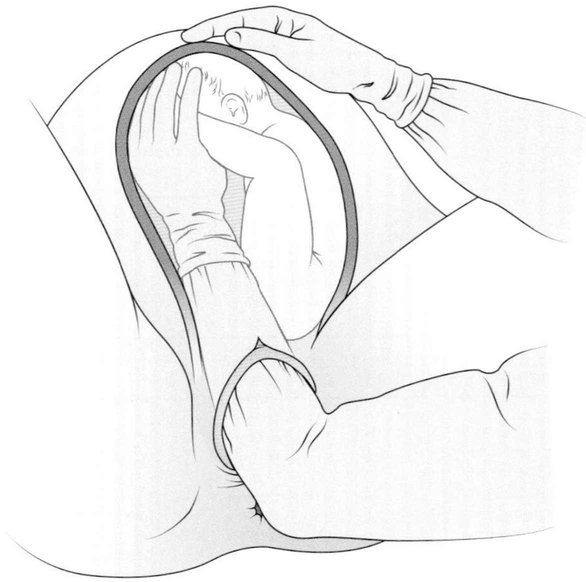

continue. Otherwise, cesarean section is required. If the fetus is in a transverse or oblique lie or there is a significant compound presentation, delivery should be performed as urgently as possible using a classic cesarean section incision unless an attempt at external version can be successfully made on opening the abdominal wall immediately before the uterus is incised. A transverse incision in the lower uterine segment may be inadequate for fetal extraction because the loss of amniotic fluid reduces the surgeon's ability to manipulate the fetus within the uterus. Struggling to deliver the fetus through a lower segment incision can cause serious trauma to the fetus, uterus, or both, and the uterine incision will probably need to be extended to an inverted T- or U-shaped incision. Such incision extensions may result in compromised healing and a vulnerable area of scar integrity, which may predispose to uterine rupture in future pregnancies or labors.

CORD PRESENTATION AND PROLAPSE—FIRST STAGE OF LABOR

With cord presentation, delivery by cesarean section should be organized with some urgency if fetal distress is suspected. Cord prolapse before full dilation of the cervix requires a "crash" or "category 1" cesarean section. While preparations are in hand for the surgery, an attempt should be made to reduce any pressure on the umbilical cord that could restrict or obstruct the cord circulation with consequent fetal hypoxia. A number of strategies have been used or proposed. Probably the most widely adopted involve applying digital counterpressure with the gloved fingers within the vagina or moving the patient into the Trendelenberg or knee-chest positions.[7,9] Alternatives recommended include bladder catheterization and distention,[11,61,62] administering tocolysis,[63,64] wrapping the exteriorized cord in warm saline-soaked swabs, or manually replacing the cord into the vagina.[21] Although the attempt at replacement of the cord may be successful[21] (see Chapter 69), there are concerns that its manipulation might provoke vascular spasm of the vessels and further compromise fetal oxygenation.[65]

CORD PRESENTATION AND PROLAPSE—SECOND STAGE OF LABOR (See Also Chapter 69)

Cord presentation at full dilation may be managed by external cephalic or internal podalic version if the lie is not longitudinal, and following amniotomy, proceeding to assisted vaginal delivery. Delivery by cesarean section should be arranged urgently if the expertise for version is not immediately available or the attempt is unsuccessful. If cord prolapse has occurred and the lie is not longitudinal, a crash/category 1 cesarean section is required. If the lie is longitudinal, immediate vaginal delivery using forceps for a cephalic presentation or breech extraction should be advanced if the necessary skills are available and the presenting part is low enough in the pelvis.[9] Because the ventouse is associated with a higher failure rate than forceps, forceps should perhaps be preferred if the necessary skill is available.[66–68]

SUMMARY OF MANAGEMENT OPTIONS

Unstable, Transverse, and Oblique Lie

Management Options	Evidence Quality and Recommendation	References
Prenatal (See Fig. 64–6)		
Confirm diagnosis with ultrasound if necessary.	—/GPP	—
Investigate for possible causes including history and ultrasound examination.	—/GPP	—
Discuss options and risks.	—/GPP	—
Expectant Management		
If noncephalic after 36 wk—"wait and see" policy—danger of cord prolapse or admission in advanced labor with a malpresentation.	GPP	—
Advice to adopt knee-chest maneuver to promote cephalic version has not been shown to be of value and is not recommended.	Ia/A	69

Management Options	Evidence Quality and Recommendation	References
Active Management		
Admit to hospital at 37–39 wk; assess daily; if spontaneous conversion to cephalic presentation occurs, subsequent options are	—/GPP	—
• Allow patient to return home to await spontaneous labor.		
• Induce labor.		
If noncephalic after 36 wk, offer ECV if no contraindications; if successful conversion to cephalic is achieved	Ia/A	71
• Allow patient to return home to await spontaneous labor.	—/GPP	—
• Perform stabilizing induction between 38 and 39 wk.	III/B	47
If ECV fails or version is contraindicated, cesarean section is necessary.	Ia/A	72
Labor and Delivery (See Fig. 64-7)		
Confirm diagnosis by examination ± ultrasound examination.	—/GPP	—
First Stage of Labor		
If cord presentation or prolapse, cesarean section is necessary.	—/GPP	—
If no cord presentation	—/GPP	—
• For ECV if membranes are intact and allow to labor if successful.		
• Otherwise perform cesarean section.		
Second Stage of Labor		
Confirm diagnosis by examination ± ultrasound examination.	—/GPP	—
If membranes are ruptured, perform cesarean section.	—/GPP	—
If membranes are not ruptured	—/GPP	—
• For ECV or internal version* and vaginal delivery if successful.		
• If version is unsuccessful, cesarean section is necessary.		

* The use of internal podalic version should be limited to the obstetrician with experience with the technique and when fetopelvic disproportion is not suspected.
ECV, external cephalic version; GPP, good practice point.

Malpresentation

Prenatal

Once an identifiable specific cause for the malpresentation has been diagnosed if present, such as polyhydramnios, a distended urinary bladder or a pelvic ovarian cyst, treatment of the cause may be indicated. For those cases without identifiable cause, there are no recognized and universally accepted procedures to use for correcting a fetal brow or face presentation. In view of the increased risk of cord presentation and thus cord prolapse with brow presentation, the woman should be advised of early admission when labor starts or membrane rupture occurs.

As with unstable lie, admission from 39 weeks' gestation should be considered for this reason, although there is little objective evidence to support this recommendation. If delivery at this gestation is indicated for other reasons, planned cesarean section without recourse to labor may be safer than inducing labor if there is a high presenting fetal part. The alternative is labor induction with either local prostaglandins or intravenous oxytocin, with low amniotomy once contractions are established and the fetal head is engaged or fixed in the pelvic brim. Preparation should have been made to allow for rapid cesarean section should cord presentation or prolapse be diagnosed, with the woman forewarned of this possibility.

Intrapartum

Labor management is the same as for a vertex presentation, assuming routine maternal and fetal observations are satisfactory and progress in labor is maintained. Many brow presentations convert to a face or vertex, and the majority of face presentations present as mentoanterior. Oxytocin augmentation is acceptable if uterine contractions are inadequate, but caution should always be shown because labor may become obstructed with dire consequences if left unattended. If progress in labor is slow, resort to cesarean section may be a wiser option. Figure 64–9 illustrates the management options.

Once full dilation is reached with a brow presentation, spontaneous delivery will not follow unless the fetus is very small or the pelvis is unusually capacious. Providing the assessment of the pelvis indicates that there is no evidence of absolute disproportion, the presentation can be converted with rotational forceps to face or vertex, whichever proves to be the easier, and then delivered. Some have advised the use of the ventouse in this situation, but this requires the cup

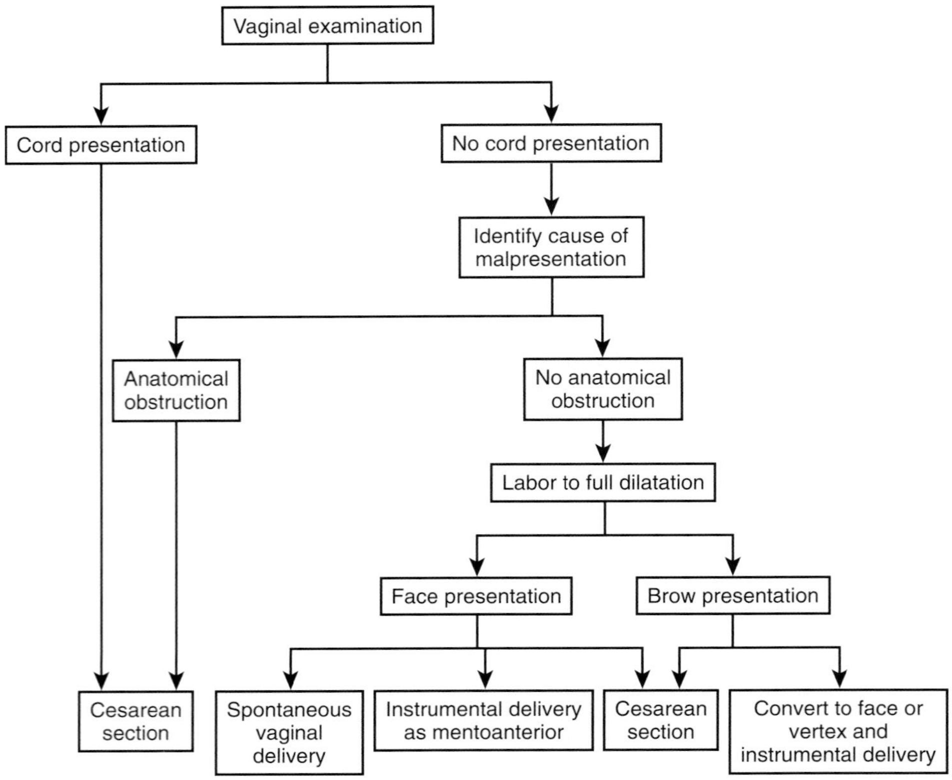

FIGURE 64–9
Algorithm for the intrapartum management of face and brow malpresentation.

to be applied behind the bregma and this is unlikely to be possible in the majority of cases (see Chapter 72). The majority view is that unless the head is engaged in the pelvis at the start of vaginal manipulations, delivery by cesarean section is recommended.

With a face presentation, vaginal delivery should be anticipated if the head is engaged, with the delivery occurring spontaneously or assisted with forceps. The head should be in a mentoanterior position at the delivery, corrected by forceps rotation if necessary (see Chapter 72). The ventouse has no place in the management of a face presentation. Thus, cesarean section may be necessary if the obstetrician does not have the necessary skills to conduct a rotational forceps delivery.

SUMMARY OF MANAGEMENT OPTIONS

Face and Brow Presentation

Management Options	Evidence Quality and Recommendation	References
Prenatal		
Confirm diagnosis—examination; ultrasound.	—/GPP	—
Assess for causal factors.	—/GPP	—
Interventions		
• Perform cesarean section if arrested progress in labor.	—/GPP	—
• Offer cesarean section as an alternative to labor.	—/GPP	—
Labor and Delivery (See Fig. 64–9)		
First Stage of Labor		
Establish diagnosis by vaginal examination ± ultrasound.	—/GPP	—

Management Options	Evidence Quality and Recommendation	References
Prenatal		
Brow Presentation	—/GPP	—
Allow labor to progress with careful monitoring of progress.		
If spontaneous conversion to face or vertex, anticipate spontaneous vaginal delivery.		
Perform assisted vaginal delivery.		
Offer cesarean section if arrested progress in labor.		
Offer cesarean section if pelvic disproportion is suspected.		
Face Presentation	—/GPP	—
If mentoanterior, allow labor to proceed anticipating vaginal delivery.		
Offer cesarean section if mentoposterior or if pelvic disproportion is suspected.		
Second Stage of Labor		
Persistent Brow Presentation	—/GPP	—
Rotate and convert to vertex or face and deliver.		
Recommend cesarean section if pelvic disproportion is suspected.		
Face Presentation	—/GPP	—
Spontaneous delivery as mentoanterior with adequate episiotomy.		
Rotate to mentoanterior and deliver.		
Recommend cesarean section if pelvic disproportion is suspected.		

GPP, good practice point.

Malposition

Prenatal

There is probably little benefit from trying to alter an occipitoposterior position diagnosed during the antenatal period because the majority of cases correct themselves before or after labor starts. There may be some virtue in advising the woman that (1) her membranes may rupture prior to the onset of contractions, (2) labor may be more uncomfortable and possibly more prolonged, and (3) there is a greater chance of requiring an instrumental delivery or cesarean section, compared with an occipitoanterior position. Some women say that they find difficult labor easier to cope with if forewarned and they may be more inclined to choose a regional anesthetic early in labor. Conversely, many occipitoposterior positions will spontaneously correct to occipitoanterior during labor, in which case anxiety will have been generated to no purpose, but it may increase the likelihood of a maternal request for delivery by antepartum cesarean section. Some have suggested the patient adopts a variety of positions to encourage rotation of the fetus. An analysis of the literature, concentrating on the use of the maternal hands-knees position during the antenatal and intrapartum periods, concluded that this position compared with others resulted in a short-term reversion to an anterior position. There is no indication that this strategy improves labor outcome, however.[69]

Intrapartum

When the diagnosis of malposition is made early in labor, as much information as possible should be gathered about the fetal position, including (1) the amount of head palpable *per abdomen*, (2) the degree of deflexion and asynclitism, (3) the amount of molding and caput formation, (4) the level of the presenting part in relation to the ischial spines, and (5) maternal pelvis size and shape. Issues relating to fetal well-being including fetal heart rate pattern and the state of the liquor should also be taken into account, as with all labors.

Options at this point are as illustrated in the algorithm (Fig. 64–10) and include

- No specific action if acceptable progress is being made.
- Providing oxytocin augmentation if uterine contractions are incoordinate, infrequent, or of poor quality.
- Encouraging the patient to lie on the same side as the fetal back.[70]
- Abandoning labor in favor of cesarean section.

Once the second stage of labor has been reached, spontaneous delivery in the occipitoposterior position may result, or spontaneous rotation may still occur with delivery

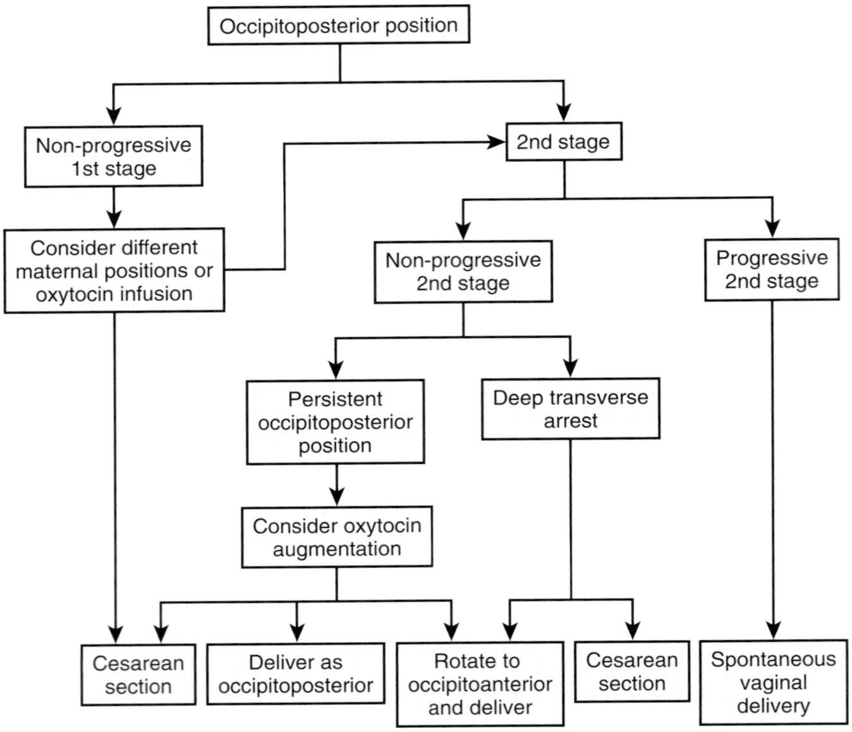

FIGURE 64–10
Algorithm for the intrapartum management of malposition of the fetal head.

occipitoanterior. Alternatively, delivery may be delayed by a persistence of the occipitoposterior position or incomplete rotation to a deep transverse arrest. It has been suggested that mechanical rotation to the occipitoanterior position followed by delivery should be avoided if fetal distress is suspected when delivery by cesarean section is favored. The decision on management at this stage should logically be determined by assessing which method of delivery is most likely to result in an earlier and less traumatic birth.

SUMMARY OF MANAGEMENT OPTIONS

Malposition

Management Options	Evidence Quality and Recommendation	References
Prenatal		
No specific managements of proven benefit.	Ib/A	69
Labor and Delivery (See Fig. 64–10)		
First Stage of Labor		
Anticipate possible protracted uncomfortable labor.		
• Offer regional analgesia if appropriate.	—/GPP	—
• Augment with oxytocin infusion.	Ib/A	73
Consider cesarean section if secondary arrest.	—/GPP	—
Second Stage of Labor		
Spontaneous rotation and delivery in occipitoanterior position	—/GPP	—
Spontaneous delivery in occipitoposterior position.	—/GPP	—
Partial resolution to deep transverse arrest:	—/GPP	—
• Rotation and delivery in occipitoanterior position.		
• Cesarean section.		

Management Options	Evidence Quality and Recommendation	References
Persistent occipitoposterior position: • Oxytocin augmentation to achieve a spontaneous delivery. • Assisted delivery in occipitoposterior position. • Rotation to occipitoanterior position and delivery. • Cesarean section.	—/GPP	—

GPP, good practice point.

SUGGESTED READINGS

Ezra Y, Strasberg SR, Farine D: Does cord presentation on ultrasound predict cord prolapse? Gynecol Obstet Invest 2003;56:6–9.

Fitzpatrick M, McQuillan K, O'Herlihy C: Influence of persistent occiput posterior position on delivery outcome. Obstet Gynecol 2001;98:1027–1031.

Fox AJ, Chapman MG: Longitudinal ultrasound assessment of fetal presentation: A review of 1010 consecutive cases. Aust N Z J Obstet Gynaecol 2006;46:341–344.

Gardberg M, Laakkonen E, Salevaara M: Intrapartum sonography and persistent occiput posterior position: A study of 408 deliveries. Obstet Gynecol 1998;91:746–749.

Hofmeyr GJ, Kulier R: Hands/knees posture in late pregnancy or labour for fetal malposition (lateral or posterior). In Cochrane Library. Chichester, UK, John Wiley, Issue 2, 2000.

Kreiser D, Schiff E, Lipitz S, et al: Determination of fetal occiput position by ultrasound during the second stage of labor. J Matern Fetal Med 2001;10:283–286.

Murphy DJ, MacKenzie IZ: The mortality and morbidity associated with umbilical cord prolapse. Br J Obstet Gynaecol 1995;102:826–830.

Royal College of Obstetricians and Gynaecologists (RCOG): Umbilical Cord Prolapse (Green-top Guideline No. 50). London, RCOG, 2008, pp 1–13.

Sherer DM, Onyeije CI, Bernstein PS, et al: Utilization of real-time ultrasound on labor and delivery in an active academic teaching hospital. Am J Perinatal 1999;16:303–307.

Stevenson CS: Transverse or oblique presentation of the fetus in the last ten weeks of pregnancy: Its causes, general nature and treatment. Am J Obstet Gynecol 1994;58:432–446.

REFERENCES

For a complete list of references, log onto www.expertconsult.com.

CHAPTER 65

Prolonged Pregnancy

IMELDA BALCHIN and PHILIP J. STEER

INTRODUCTION

Prolonged pregnancies are associated with an increased risk of perinatal mortality and morbidity compared with pregnancies ending at term.[1–4] Consequently, induction of labor in order to prevent the complications of prolonged pregnancy is one of the commonest interventions in pregnancy, with up to 29% of pregnant women undergoing this procedure.[5] It is, therefore, important to clarify the upper limit of a normal human gestation, so as to determine when an intervention is justified. We immediately encounter the problem of defining "normal." For example, a pregnancy may be considered statistically prolonged if the gestation falls in the top 5% of the distribution of gestational lengths for a given population. Conversely, a pregnancy is considered prolonged from a clinical management point of view when the risk of continuing the pregnancy to the fetus is higher than its risk after birth. On a population basis, we therefore need to discover when in the statistical distribution of gestational age the increasing risks of postmaturity justify induction, which is not in itself risk-free. Moreover, because individual fetuses mature at different rates, we need to look for factors in each individual pregnancy that can be used to modulate the average risk. One hypothesis for the increased risk of perinatal mortality in a clinically prolonged pregnancy is "placental insufficiency," in which the aging placenta is no longer able to keep pace with the demands of the growing fetus, resulting in either fetal malnutrition or asphyxia, or both.[6,7] Assessment of fetal growth and well-being can, therefore, be used to modify in each individual pregnancy the precise gestation at which postmaturity is judged to be a risk justifying induction.

DEFINITION

The current World Health Organization (WHO) definitions for preterm, term, and post-term took effect in 1977, sanctioned by the International Federation of Gynecology and Obstetrics (FIGO).[8] A baby is born at "term" if the delivery occurred at or between 37 completed weeks and 41 weeks + 6 days from the first day of the last menstrual period (LMP). From 42 completed weeks, or 294 days, from the LMP onward, a pregnancy is designated prolonged, or "post-term." It is important to make sure that the expression "post-term" is used correctly in this way, and not used to mean "after the due date" (which is better described using the American terminology of "postdates"). The WHO definition was based on the statistical distribution of the timing of delivery from the LMP (i.e., it was a statistical definition, and not based on any clinical considerations). According to this definition, preterm birth occurs in approximately 4% to 15% of all births in the developed world, with an average rate of 10%.[9,10] Similarly, the incidence of post-term birth ranges from 4% to 15% with an average rate of 10%.[11,12] Therefore, "term" is simply the length of time from the LMP during which approximately 80% of births occur. The definition "preterm" is not synonymous with '"prematurity," and likewise, "post-term" is not synonymous with "postmaturity." Prematurity and postmaturity describe how the baby functions, and not its gestational age. Some babies are mature at 36 weeks (and, therefore, function normally after birth at this gestation), whereas some babies still suffer from the problems of prematurity (in particular, respiratory distress syndrome) at 38 or even 39 weeks' gestation. It is important to remember that a baby born at 38 weeks may have been physiologically programed to deliver at 42 weeks and, therefore, be 4 weeks "premature," and vice versa. A few babies will show the manifestations of postmaturity even when born at 40 weeks.

THE NORMAL LENGTH OF GESTATION

A gestation period begins at the time of conception and ends at birth. In humans, the gestational length is calculated from the LMP, instead of the day of conception, because it is not usually possible to ascertain the exact timing of natural conceptions. For almost 2 centuries, it has been the convention to use Franz Carl Naegele's method for estimating the date of birth, based on the assumptions that the gestation period is 266 days, and that ovulation occurs on day 14 of a 28-day menstrual cycle.[13,14] Hence, the estimated date of delivery (EDD) is calculated as 280 days from the first day of the LMP. However, dating a pregnancy using the LMP alone is unreliable.[15,16] Even in women who are certain of their menstrual dates, estimating the date of delivery using the LMP alone gives a prediction error (1 standard deviation) of 9 to 11 days.[17] This is probably due to errors in recall, the tendency to digit preference when recalling dates, and falsely identifying nonmenstrual bleeding as a menstrual period[18,19] (in addition to the natural variation in gestational length from one pregnancy to another because of the different rates at which individual babies mature). In addition, the timing of ovulation is erratic and varies from one cycle to another, even in women with regular menses.

ETIOLOGY OF PROLONGED PREGNANCY

Studies of pregnancies ending in spontaneous labor show that the average gestational length varies in different populations, and within populations, it varies according to maternal racial origin.[20–23] This is perhaps because gestational length is determined by maternal genetic factors, in combination with a small contribution from paternal genes in the fetus,[24] and these factors, being genetic, are inherited. The recurrence rate of prolonged pregnancy in one Danish birth cohort was 20%, and this risk increased with increasing gestation of the index pregnancy, but reduced to 15% with a change of partner.[25] It should be noted that this increased rate is only moderately above the background level, and therefore, even after a previous prolonged pregnancy, the majority of births will not be post-term.

In addition, the observed variation in gestational length may indicate a variation in the rate of fetal maturity. The trigger for the onset of labor in humans is still unknown. Because approximately 90% of labors occur after 36 completed weeks of gestation, fetal maturity is probably involved in initiating the timing of labor. In support of this, it has been shown that in a human fetus with anencephaly, where there is little or no brain development, and without excessive amniotic fluid volume, there is a tendency for the pregnancy to be prolonged.[26] It is thought that at fetal maturity, the fetal hypothalamus and the placenta increase their secretion of corticotropin-releasing hormone, stimulating the production of adrenocorticotrophic hormone by the fetal pituitary gland and cortisol production by the fetal adrenal glands, and leading to the increased production of dehydroepiandrosterone (DHEA). Cortisol and DHEA in turn activate the increase in estrogen and prostaglandins that stimulate labor.[27]

In North West London, allowing for potential confounding factors, the average gestational length for singleton pregnancies was 39 weeks for South Asians (women who self-reported as originating from India, Pakistan, Bangladesh) and blacks (black British, black Africans, and black Caribbeans), and 40 weeks for whites (all white European groups, previously commonly called "Caucasian," although a minority of white Europeans actually come from the Caucasus).[20] In Norway, the average pregnancy length is 282 days.[28] It has been shown that South Asian or black populations have higher rates of preterm birth. However, the risk of neonatal respiratory distress syndrome in these racial groups is significantly lower than in white babies of similar gestational age.[29] From 37 weeks' gestation onward, the faster rate of fetal gut maturity results in higher rates of meconium passage in utero in black and South Asian fetuses than those in whites. Consequently, the late gestation incidence of respiratory morbidity and perinatal mortality in these racial groups is also higher than that in whites. Finally, in full-term South Asian fetuses, the late gestation rise in antepartum stillbirth, possibly due to placental insufficiency associated with postmaturity, begins to rise 1 week earlier than in white babies.[30] These patterns remained significant even after adjusting for socioeconomic factors and suggest that the shorter gestational length in South Asian and black populations is associated with an accelerated fetal maturity compared with that white populations.[31]

In addition to genetic predisposition, maternal obesity is also an independent predictor of post-term pregnancy. It is well established that women with a low prepregnancy body mass index (BMI), less than 20 kg/m^2, have a higher risk of preterm birth. In contrast, the risk of post-term pregnancy increases with increasing prepregnancy BMI. In women with a prepregnancy BMI of 25 to 29 kg/m^2, the adjusted risk of post-term pregnancy is approximately 24% higher than women of normal BMI. This risk is increased to 37% in women with BMI of 30 to 34, and 52% if BMI was 35 kg/m^2 or more.[32,33] Other risk factors for post-term pregnancy include nulliparity and placental sulfatase deficiency.

RISKS

Fetal and Neonatal Risks

Antepartum Stillbirth

Continued pregnancy after 40 weeks' gestation is associated with a significant increase in the risk of perinatal mortality, and about 60% of these deaths occur before the onset of labor (antepartum stillbirths).[30] Evidence using survival analysis (i.e., using a denominator of continuing live pregnancies instead of babies delivering at a particular gestation) and maternity data collected in 1958 in the United Kingdom showed that the rate of stillbirth increased from 0.4 per 1000 continuing pregnancies at 37 weeks' gestation to 1 in 1000 at 42 weeks, to 2.1 per 1000 at 43 weeks.[34] Similar figures have been reported from many countries, for example, Australia (Fig. 65–1).

A more recent U.K. study carried out a survival analysis of North West London maternity data from 1988 to 2000 and showed that the risk of antepartum stillbirth in white babies was 0.28 per 1000 continuing pregnancies at 37 weeks (95% confidence interval [CI] 0.22–0.34), 0.67 (95% CI 0.54–0.81) at 40 weeks, 1.12 (95% CI 0.83–1.39) at 41 weeks, and 1.54 (95% CI 0.79–2.30) at 42 weeks' gestation.[30] This demonstrated that in contemporary U.K. obstetric practice, the rate of antepartum stillbirth is significantly higher at 41 weeks than at 40 weeks; gestation (although the difference in mortality at 41 and 42 weeks' gestation was not statistically significant). The rate of antepartum stillbirth in South Asian babies in North West London was statistically significantly higher than in white babies, with a rate of 1.95 (95% CI 1.30–2.60) at 40 weeks and 3.21 (95% CI 1.81–4.62) at 41 weeks' gestation (Fig. 65–2). The most significant factor associated with antepartum stillbirth at term and post-term in South Asian babies was a birth weight less than 2000 g (clearly representing serious intrauterine growth restriction).

A higher antepartum stillbirth rate was also seen in black babies when compared with white babies with a rate of 1.39 (95% CI 0.63–2.14) at 40 weeks and 1.96 (95% CI 0.51–3.40) at 41 weeks' gestation, although the difference between the two groups was not statistically significant, perhaps due to lack of statistical power. More data are required to confirm

FIGURE 65–1
Perinatal outcome by gestational age. *A*, Stillbirth rate (per 1000) in South Australia, 1991–2000. *Squares*, singletons; *Diamonds*, twins. *B*, Neonatal mortality rate (per 1000) in South Australia, 1991–2000. *Squares*, singletons; *Diamonds*, twins.
(*A* and *B*, Adapted from Dodd JM, Crowther CA, Robinson JS, Chan A: Stillbirth and neonatal outcomes in South Australia, 1991–2000. Am J Obstet Gynecol 2003;189:1731–1736.)

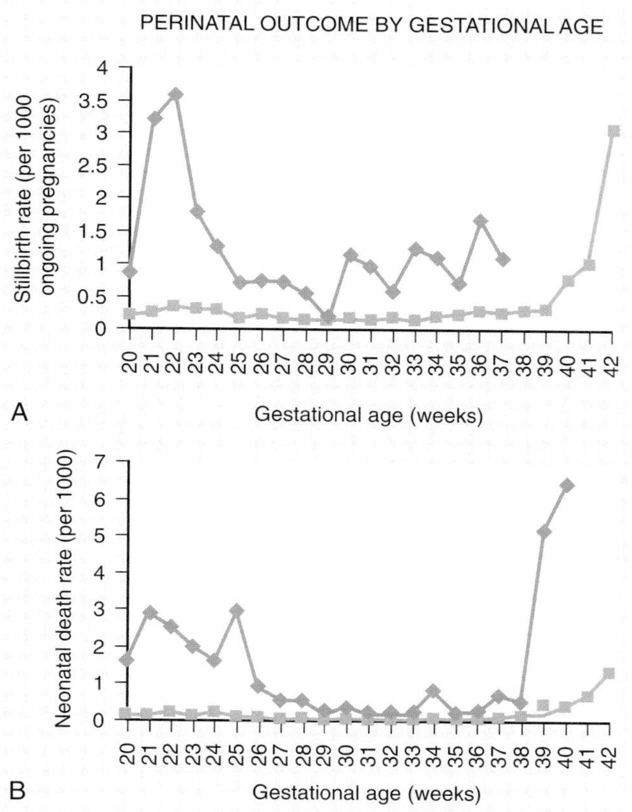

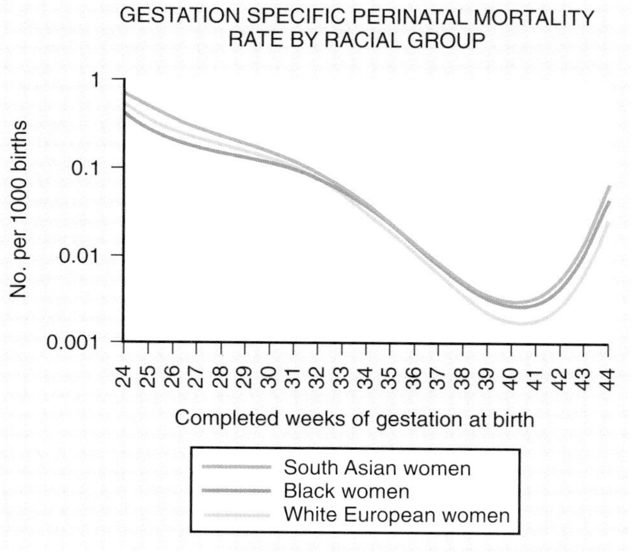

FIGURE 65–2
Gestation-specific perinatal mortality rate by racial group.
(Adapted from Balchin I, Whittaker JC, Patel RR, et al: Racial variation in the association between gestational age and perinatal mortality: Prospective study. BMJ 2007;334:833.)

this suggestion of a higher antepartum stillbirth rate in black babies.

Placental dysfunction, or placental insufficiency, is thought to be the etiology of perinatal mortality and morbidity in prolonged pregnancies. Histologic studies of the post-term placenta show an increased incidence of infarcts, calcification, intervillous thrombosis, perivillous fibrin deposits, arterial thrombosis, and arterial endarteritis.[6,7] Placental insufficiency is associated with intrauterine growth restriction and a reduction in the amniotic fluid volume (oligohydramnios).[35] Oligohydramnios in turn may lead to umbilical cord compression and "fetal distress."[36,37] At 40 or more weeks' gestation, oligohydramnios defined by an amniotic fluid index (AFI) of less than 5 cm is found in about 8% of pregnancies. This is significantly associated with meconium aspiration, birth asphyxia, cesarean section for fetal distress in labor, cord pH less than 7 at delivery, and low Apgar scores.[38]

Long-term Developmental Outcome

In a follow-up of 129 post-term children up to the age of 2 years, there were no difference in developmental outcome compared with that in children born at term.[39] However, another study based on a cohort of babies identified through the Swedish national birth registry followed 354 post-term babies and 379 controls up to school age and showed that post-term children had more definite or strongly suspected neurologic developmental disorders than the controls, with an adjusted odds ratio (OR) of 2.20 (95% CI 1.29–3.85), and boys had more deviations than girls (OR 1.92; 95% CI 1.11–3.45).[40] One suspects on clinical grounds that the long-term outcome will depend very much on the appropriateness of the intrapartum management of post-term babies.

Maternal Risks and Attitudes toward Prolonged Pregnancy

The main risk to the pregnant woman is not from prolonged pregnancy itself, but from the anxiety associated with prolonged pregnancy and the consequences of interventions to prevent prolonged pregnancy.

A Cochrane systematic review concluded that intervention with routine induction of labor at 41 or more weeks' gestation reduces perinatal mortality without increasing the overall risk of cesarean section or operative delivery to the mother.[41] However, it should be taken into account that the risk of cesarean section depends upon organizational factors governing the management of labor in maternity hospitals. These factors include policies concerning active management of labor, one-to-one midwifery care, the presence of a member of the family or other companion during labor, the timing of routine vaginal examinations, the training of obstetricians and midwives in electronic fetal monitoring, and the number and seniority of the midwives and obstetricians attending the labor ward. Thus, in a well-staffed maternity unit with a midwife well trained in the interpretation of fetal heart rate traces and dedicated to the care of a single woman in labor, induction of labor may increase the chance of a vaginal delivery. On the contrary, induction of labor in an understaffed maternity unit is an unwelcome burden and is likely to carry additional risks.

It has been shown that undelivered women at 41 weeks' gestation have a significantly higher anxiety score than women who have already given birth.[42] Most women prefer to be induced at 41 weeks and report positive experiences of labor induction when compared with expectant management.[43] This is despite reports of experiencing more intense and more frequent contractions than those in women who had spontaneous onset of labor. A Norwegian study has shown that 74% of women who underwent induction of labor preferred this management in a subsequent pregnancy compared with only 38% of women who had expectant management with serial monitoring.[44] Furthermore, the percentage of women with a positive attitude toward expectant management decreases with advancing gestation.[44,45]

The average rate of cesarean section in women induced for prolonged pregnancy is about 20%. However, the cesarean section rate in nulliparous women induced for prolonged pregnancy is significantly higher than in multiparous women (28% vs. 9%).[46] In addition, pre-induction cervical length can be used to predict the use of cesarean section. The use of ultrasonography to measure cervical length is a better predictor of cesarean section than using the Bishop score or measuring cervical length by vaginal examination. The risk of cesarean section is higher in nulliparous women with the same cervical length as multiparous women. For example, in a nulliparous women with a sonographic cervical length of more than 30 mm, the risk of cesarean section following induction of labor for prolonged pregnancy is greater than 70%.[47]

For antenatal fetal monitoring, counting of fetal movements by the pregnant woman in prolonged pregnancy does not decrease the risk of stillbirth.[48] Ultrasonographic screening for oligohydramnios using the AFI is superior than measuring a single deepest pool.[49] However, the sensitivity of oligohydramnios in predicting adverse outcomes is low (i.e., only ~12% for predicting a cord pH < 7.00 at delivery). Thus, routine screening for oligohydramnios increased the likelihood of intervention without improving perinatal outcomes.[49]

Observational studies suggest that cardiotocography and Doppler assessment of fetal and uteroplacental arteries are unlikely to predict fetal outcome reliably. A randomized trial of cardiotocography and measurement of the AFI compared with induction of labor suggested that the rates of cesarean section and meconium below the vocal cords were increased in pregnancies beyond 42 weeks' gestation.[50] Another randomized trial compared a modified biophysical profile score with cardiotocography combined with maximum depth of the amniotic fluid and found that there were more abnormal results in the women randomized to measurement of the biophysical profile score, but with no apparent benefit to the infant.[51]

MANAGEMENT OPTIONS

Prenatal—Early Pregnancy

Dating methods using ultrasonography of the fetal size before 20 weeks' gestation has reduced the percentage of pregnancies classified as "post-term" by up to 74% compared with dating based on LMP only.[16,17,52–54] The effect of routine early pregnancy ultrasound scan includes the reduced incidence of induction of labor for apparent "post-term" pregnancy and the increased incidence of termination of pregnancy owing to the increased detection of fetal abnormalities.[55–57] However, there is no evidence of a reduction in perinatal deaths. Some authors have used routine fetal ultrasonography alone to date pregnancies.[58] However, this would be valid only if there was no variation in fetal growth in early pregnancy and if all pregnant women were booked for antenatal care before 24 weeks' gestation. In reality, variation in fetal growth has been shown to occur from early pregnancy in women with known dates of conception.[59] In pregnant women who book late for antenatal care, ultrasound dating becomes less unreliable beyond 24 weeks, owing to the increased variation in the fetal growth rate.[60] In the United Kingdom, the National Institute of Health and Clinical Excellence (NICE) has recommended that all pregnant women should be offered an early ultrasound scan between 10 weeks + 0 days and 13 weeks + 6 days to assist in the determination of gestational age and to detect multiple pregnancies.[61] The key measurement is crown-rump length, but if this is above 84 mm, head circumference measurement should be used instead.

Prenatal—At Term

Owing to medicolegal and ethical concerns, the current practice in the United Kingdom is to offer induction of labor in all uncomplicated pregnancies at 41 or more weeks' gestation, as recommended by NICE.[62] The guideline recognizes that there are important racial differences and that, therefore, the recommended policy of induction to prevent prolonged pregnancy at 41 to 42 weeks' gestation may not be appropriate for all women (see p. 24). Moreover, the absolute increase in perinatal mortality rate after 41 weeks is very small, and therefore, expectant management with serial antenatal fetal monitoring is an appropriate management policy. The NICE antenatal care guideline recommends that before pharmacologic or surgical methods of induction are used, a "membrane sweep" should be offered. This policy remains controversial. An early study by Allott and Palmer[63] reported that inserting a finger through the cervix and "sweeping the membranes" reduced the need for induction of labor from 18.8% in the control group to 8.1% in the swept group. However, a subsequent paper by Foong and coworkers[64] reported that the beneficial effects on labor and delivery (shorter labors and fewer cesarean sections) were limited to nulliparas with unfavorable cervices who needed priming with prostaglandin E_2. A Cochrane review in 2005 found that routine use of sweeping of membranes from 38 weeks of pregnancy onward does not seem to produce clinically important benefits.[65] The authors commented that when used as a means for induction of labor, the reduction in the use of more formal methods of induction needs to be balanced against women's discomfort and other adverse effects. Moreover, a study published in 2008 reported a randomized trial of 300 women who were randomly assigned into sweep or no-sweep groups and found no effect on the average gestational age at delivery or the need for induction.[66] They found that the incidence of prelabor rupture of membranes was significantly higher if the cervix was more than 1 cm dilated at the time of membrane sweep. This might increase the risk of intrapartum infection, particularly in carriers of group B streptococcus. In the experience of the authors, many women find the procedure extremely unpleasant, often indeed painful, and we therefore suggest that the procedure be used only in women who are particularly keen to avoid artificial rupture of membranes or the use of prostaglandins/intravenous oxytocin.

Studies have not shown a significant difference in maternal or neonatal morbidity between alternatively serial antenatal fetal monitoring or induction of labor after 41 weeks' gestation.[50] However, the evidence for the efficacy of antenatal fetal monitoring is poor, and there are no randomized trials of sufficient size to assess the possibility of a type 2 error (that we are missing a real difference). If women decline induction, there is no evidence that complex monitoring (e.g., using biophysical profiles) is of any benefit to compare it with more simple surveillance using ultrasound estimation of the maximum amniotic pool depth and cardiotocography (preferably daily and least twice weekly).[51] The decision to choose either induction of labor or expectant management is, therefore, dependent on the resources available in each maternity unit and the individual woman's wishes.

Intrapartum Care

It is generally recognized that there is an increased risk of meconium aspiration and umbilical cord compression in post-term labors. The details of fetal monitoring for these conditions are covered in Chapter 69. However, NICE recommends that both induction of labor and post-term labor are indications for continuous electronic monitoring.[67]

SUMMARY OF MANAGEMENT OPTIONS
Prolonged Pregnancy

Management Options	Evidence Quality and Recommendation	References
Prenatal		
Establish gestational age as soon as possible, preferably 10–14 wk gestation.	Ia/A	15–18
Sweeping membranes at term increases the incidence of spontaneous labor but has risks, may not be clinically important, and women often dislike it.	Ia/A	62–66
41 Weeks		
Induction of labor at 41 wk reduces perinatal mortality without increasing adverse outcomes.	Ia/A	41
Expectant management:	GPP	51
• Monitoring with measurement of amniotic fluid volume, estimated fetal weight, and CTG recommended at least twice weekly.		
Labor and delivery: vigilance for fetal hypoxia and meconium staining of the amniotic fluid.	GPP	

CTG, cardiotocography; GPP, good practice point.

SUGGESTED READINGS

Balchin I, Whittaker JC, Patel R, et al: Racial variation in the relationship between gestational age and perinatal mortality: Prospective study. BMJ 2007;334:833–835.

Boulvain M, Stan CM, Irion O: Membrane sweeping for induction of labour. Cochrane Database Syst Rev 2005;1:CD000451.

Gülmezoglu AM, Crowther CA, Middleton P: Induction of labour for improving birth outcomes for women at or beyond term. Cochrane Database Syst Rev 2006;4:CD004945.

Heimstad R, Romundstad PR, Hyett J, et al: Women's experiences and attitudes towards expectant management and induction of labour for post-term pregnancy. Acta Obstet Gynecol 2007;86:950–956.

Heimstad R, Skogvoll E, Mattsson LA, et al: Induction of labor or serial antenatal fetal monitoring in post-term pregnancy: A randomised controlled trial. Obstet Gynaecol 2007;109:609–617.

Hill MJ, McWilliams GD, Garcia-Sur D, et al: The effect of membrane sweeping on prelabor rupture of membranes: A randomized controlled trial. Obstet Gynecol 2008;111:1313–1319.

Strobel E, Sladkevicius P, Rovas L, et al: Bishop score and ultrasound assessment of the cervix for prediction of time to onset of labor and time to delivery in prolonged pregnancy. Ultrasound Obstet Gynecol 2006;28:298–305.

Tunon K, Eik-Nes SH, Grottum P: A comparison between ultrasound and a reliable last menstrual period as predictors of the day of delivery in 15,000 examinations. Ultrasound Obstet Gynecol 1996;8:178–185.

UK National Institute for Health and Clinical Excellence (NICE): Antenatal care guideline. Available at http://guidance.nice.org.uk/CG62/Guidance/pdf/English

UK National Institute for Health and Clinical Excellence (NICE): Induction of labour guideline. Available at http://www.nice.org.uk/guidance/CG70

REFERENCES

For a complete list of references, log onto www.expertconsult.com.

CHAPTER 66

Induction of Labor and Termination of the Previable Pregnancy

LUIS SANCHEZ-RAMOS and ISAAC DELKE

INDUCTION OF LABOR

Definition

Labor induction is the stimulation of regular uterine contractions before the spontaneous onset of labor, using mechanical or pharmacologic methods in order to generate progressive cervical dilation and subsequent delivery. Although the term generally refers to patients who are at term, it is also employed for women who are at least 20 weeks' gestation. It is important to distinguish labor induction from *augmentation*, which refers to stimulation of uterine contractions when spontaneous contractions during labor have been considered inadequate.

Introduction

Induction of labor is an important and common clinical procedure in obstetrics. The rate of labor induction in the United States continues to rise significantly for all gestational ages. Data for the year 2006 from the National Center for Health Statistics indicated that the rate was 22.5% for that year, a slight increase over 2005, and double the rate for 1990.[1] The reason for this increase is unclear, although it may partly reflect a growing use of labor induction for postdate pregnancies and an increasing trend toward elective induction of labor for other indications (including maternal request).

Indications and Contraindications

Generally, labor induction is indicated when the benefits of delivery to the mother or fetus outweigh the potential risks of continuing the pregnancy. The most appropriate timing for labor induction is the point at which the maternal or perinatal benefits are greater if the pregnancy is interrupted than if the pregnancy is continued. Ideally, most pregnancies should be allowed to reach term, with the onset of spontaneous labor being the sign of physiologic termination of pregnancy. However, occasionally a woman is best delivered before the spontaneous onset of labor. Commonly accepted indications for labor induction are listed in Table 66–1. Of the standard indications for labor induction, pregnancy-induced hypertension and postdate pregnancies are among the most common, accounting for more than 80% of reported inductions (see Chapters 35 and 65). Given that there is an indication for induction, the risks to mother and fetus must then be considered, to make sure that the benefit outweighs these risks. The risks to the mother are mainly related to an increased chance that she will need operative delivery, rather than labor following the spontaneous onset of labor. The risks to the fetus are those of prematurity. Whenever there is evidence of fetal lung maturity (although it is important to remember that a mature lecithin-to-sphigomyelin ratio is not a guarantee of normal respiratory function after birth) or the pregnancy has reached at least 39 weeks (confirmed by an early ultrasound), the decision to induce labor is not so difficult. Maternal consent to any increased risk of operative delivery (e.g., with an unfavorable cervix) should be obtained, and although the fetus is not likely to be at risk for complications that cannot be dealt with in a modern neonatal unit, the very small risk of permanent sequelae such as pulmonary hypertension following persistence of fetal circulation should be mentioned because it has long-term significance, and moreover, an admission to a neonatal unit is worrying for the parents. Induction of labor from 39 weeks at maternal request (usually owing to intolerance of the discomforts of pregnancy, but sometimes for social reasons, e.g., the limited availability of the father to attend the birth or logistic factors such as distance from the hospital or a history of rapid labor and delivery) remains controversial. It should not be encouraged, but the risk/benefit ratio can be assessed on a case-by-case basis, and many obstetricians feel that it is sometimes justified. Whether induction of labor to suit the obstetrician's schedule is ethical makes for an interesting discussion.

However, the decision to induce labor prior to fetal maturity having been achieved is far more difficult. In such cases, premature delivery should offer the fetus clear benefits that outweigh the potential problems associated with preterm birth. Generally recognized relative and absolute contraindications to labor induction are listed in Table 66–2. There are few absolute contraindications to labor induction, and there can be certain clinical situations in which induction is usually contraindicated but exceptional circumstances make

TABLE 66–1
Commonly Accepted Indications for Labor Induction

Pregnancy-induced hypertension
Prelabor rupture of membranes
Chorioamnionitis
Severe intrauterine growth restriction
Isoimmunization
Maternal medical problems (diabetes mellitus, renal disease, lupus)
Fetal demise
Postdates pregnancy
Oligohydramnios
Logistic factors (risk of rapid labor, distance from hospital)

TABLE 66–2
Contraindications to Labor Induction

Placenta or vasa previa
Transverse fetal lie
Prolapsed umbilical cord
Prior classic uterine incision
Active genital herpes infection
Pelvic structural deformities

TABLE 66–3
Criteria for Fetal Maturity

Fetal heart tones have been documented for 20 wk by nonelectronic fetoscope or for 30 wk by Doppler.
It has been 36 wk since a positive serum or urine human chorionic gonadotropin pregnancy test was performed by a reliable method.
An ultrasound measurement of the crown-rump length, obtained at 6–11 wk, supports a gestational age of 39 wk or more.
An ultrasound scan, obtained at 12–20 wk, confirms the gestational age of 39 wk or more determined by clinical history and physical examination.

induction appropriate (e.g., prolapsed umbilical cord in the presence of fetal demise). A number of clinical situations that are not generally considered contraindications to labor induction but require caution include breech presentation, borderline clinical pelvimetry, grand multiparity, non-reassuring fetal testing not requiring emergency delivery, polyhydramnios, and multifetal gestation.

Requirements for Labor Induction

Prior to inducing labor, the obstetrician should carefully review the indication(s) for ending the pregnancy and obtain informed consent. In addition, the mother and fetus should be carefully examined and, if indicated, fetal pulmonary maturity should be documented. In order to avoid iatrogenic prematurity, an amniocentesis may be required to assess fetal lung maturity. Table 66–3 lists criteria, which, if met, allow fetal maturity to be assumed, so that amniocentesis need not be performed.[2] It is worthy of note that, although testing for pulmonary maturity is widely practiced in the United States, in many other countries, including the United Kingdom, the decision whether to induce labor is based on other criteria (such as evidence of actual or incipient fetal or maternal compromise) and pulmonary maturity is not considered to be an important factor (management of respiratory distress syndrome being very efficient in modern neonatal units); accordingly, amniocentesis is rarely performed.

Preinduction Status of the Cervix

Successful labor induction is clearly related to the state of the cervix. Women with an unfavorable cervix, who have not experienced a cervical-ripening phase prior to labor, present the greatest challenge with regard to labor induction. In addition, the duration of labor induction is affected by parity and to a minor degree by baseline uterine activity and sensitivity to oxytocic drugs. Many investigators have identified the importance of assessing cervical status prior to induction of labor. Calkins and colleagues[3] were the first to carry out systematic studies of the factors influencing the duration of the first stage of labor. The authors concluded that the length, thickness, and particularly, the consistency of the cervix are important parameters. In 1955, Bishop[4] devised a cervical scoring system for multiparous patients with planned elective induction of labor in which 0 to 3 points are given for each of five factors. He determined that when the total score was at least 9, the likelihood of vaginal delivery following labor induction was similar to that observed in patients with spontaneous onset of labor. Although several modifications have been suggested, the Bishop score has become a classic parameter in obstetrics and has since been applied to a much wider group of patients. Nulliparous women with a Bishop score no greater than 3 have a 23-fold increased risk of induction failure and a 2- to 4-fold increased risk of cesarean delivery compared with nulliparous women with a Bishop score of at least 4.[5] Similarly, multiparous women with a Bishop score of no greater than 3 have a 6-fold increased risk of failed induction and a 2-fold increased risk of cesarean birth compared with women with higher Bishop scores.[5,6]

The Bishop score has become the most commonly employed preinduction scoring system. Several studies have assessed the predictive accuracy of ultrasound cervical measurement for successful labor induction.[7–9] However, there is a lack of convincing evidence that this technique provides significant additional information when compared with digital examination. A recently published systematic review with meta-analysis of 20 diagnostic studies and 3101 aggregate particpants concluded that sonographic cervical length was not an effective predictor of successful labor induction.[10] However, the assessment of cervical wedging appears to be a useful diagnostic test, but needs further evaluation.[10]

Preinduction Cervical Ripening

Cervical ripening is the process that culminates in the softening and distensibility of the cervix, thus facilitating labor and delivery. There is an inverse relationship between the Bishop score and the failure of labor induction, with low scores being associated with a high rate of failed induction. Moreover, not only is inducing uterine contractions in the presence of an unripe cervix more likely to lead to delivery by cesarean section, but even if vaginal delivery is eventually achieved, the labor will often have been prolonged. This is

TABLE 66–4
Cervical-Ripening Methods

Mechanical Methods
Foley catheter
Laminaria tents
Hygroscopic dilators
Acupuncture
Membrane stripping
Pharmacologic Methods
Dinoprostone (PGE_2)
Misoprostol (PGE_1)
Cytokines
Nitric oxide
Relaxin

PGE, prostaglandin E.

a particular problem if the induction is for fetal indications, because then prolonged fetal monitoring is also required. In addition, an extended exposure to uterine contractions and the resulting reduction in intervillous blood flow can result in fetal hypoxia and acidosis. Thus, it is useful to employ cervical-ripening agents to prepare the unripe cervix for labor induction. Ideally, a ripening agent would act upon the cervix to make it more favorable without inducing uterine activity; the length of the active phase of labor would thereby be minimized, limiting the stress on the fetus to the minimum. Unfortunately, it has proved difficult to separate methods of cervical ripening and labor induction. Patients with an unripe cervix may undergo cervical ripening without initiating labor contractions when a pharmacologic agent such as dinoprostone (prostaglandin E_2 [PGE_2]) is employed, but sometimes, contractions ensue before the cervix has ripened. A considerable amount of research has been directed toward various methods to prepare or ripen the cervix prior to the induction of labor. Although many of these methods also initiate uterine activity, it should be appreciated that the principal role of these agents is to soften the unripe cervix independently of uterine activity. The various methods for cervical ripening can be divided into two categories (Table 66–4):

- Mechanical.
- Pharmacologic.

Mechanical Methods

FOLEY CATHETER

Mechanical methods have been employed for many years to ripen the cervix prior to labor induction.[11] Barnes, in the mid-19th century, was one of the first to describe the use of a balloon catheter to ripen the uterine cervix.[12] Since that time, several variations of this method have been popularized. The balloon catheter currently most frequently used is a Foley catheter with a 25- to 50-mL balloon, which can be passed through an undilated cervix before inflation of the balloon above the internal os. It is thought that the mechanical separation of the fetal membranes from the cervix and lower segment stimulates local cytokine and prostaglandin (PG) release, and these act upon the ground substance of the cervix to break down the cross-links between the glycosaminoglycans. More recently, extra-amniotic saline infusion has been a successful modification to the use of balloon catheters for cervical ripening, presumably by enhancing this effect.[13–15] A review of 13 trials in which balloon catheters were used for cervical ripening concluded that with or without extra-amniotic saline infusion, the method resulted in improved Bishop scores and decreased induction-to-delivery intervals.[16] Simultaneous use of balloon-tipped catheters and pharmacologic agents has been shown to be even more effective for cervical ripening than for labor induction; however, the cost of such combination therapy is substantial.

Several reports observed an increased risk of intrapartum chorioamnionitis, but none of the reports individually had adequate sample size to demonstrate a statistically significant difference. A recently published systematic review with meta-analysis of 30 randomized, controlled trials comparing cervical ripening with mechanical methods with alternative pharmacologic agents or placebo demonstrated that maternal and neonatal infections were increased in women who underwent cervical ripening with mechanical methods.[17] This finding raises the question of whether prophylactic antibiotics are indicated in such patients.

LAMINARIA TENTS

Laminaria tents, natural and synthetic, have been used as a mechanical method for cervical ripening for many years. Although their safety and efficacy in the second trimester have been established, use of laminaria during the third trimester of pregnancy is associated with a high incidence of infection.[18] Synthetic hygroscopic cervical dilators have also been used for many years as agents to prepare the cervix for pregnancy termination. Several studies have shown that these osmotic dilators can also be successfully employed for cervical ripening in viable pregnancies with an unripe cervix.[19–21] Advantages to the use of osmotic dilators are their low cost and ease of placement and removal.

MEMBRANE STRIPPING

Membrane stripping (sometimes known as "membrane sweep") is a simple technique not infrequently used to ripen the cervix, in which a finger is inserted through the cervix and "swept" around the lower segment above the internal os in a circular motion. As with the Foley catheter, it appears to work by release of PG (especially $PGF_{2\alpha}$) from the decidua and the adjacent membranes. However, presumably because it is more vigorous, it often stimulates uterine contractions as well as causing ripening. A systematic review of 22 trials with 2797 aggregate participants comparing membrane sweeping with PGs and with oxytocin revealed that stripping of the membranes was associated with a reduced frequency of post-term pregnancies.[22] As with other mechanical methods, there has been a concern that membrane sweeping may increase the rates of maternal and perinatal infections. However, a more recent systematic review showed no evidence of an increase in the risk of maternal or perinatal infection when "sweeping" is used.[23] However, there are adverse effects such as discomfort during the necessarily vigorous vaginal examination and occasionally bleeding from the cervix or placental margins if the placenta is low-lying. Moreover, if the induction is for fetal compromise, the ensuing contractions mandate fetal monitoring even if labor does not become established.

ACUPUNCTURE

Although much more common in Asia, acupuncture for cervical ripening and labor induction is also becoming more available in the western world. One study concluded that acupuncture at points LI4 (large intestine 4) and SP 6 (spleen 6) induces cervical ripening at term, and in postdated pregnancies, it shortens the time interval between the estimated date of confinement and the actual time of delivery.[24] However, a randomized, controlled trial comparing acupuncture with sham acupuncture for women scheduled for a post-term induction did not reduce the need for induction methods or the duration of labor.[25] There is still a need for more well-designed randomized, controlled trials to evaluate the role of acupuncture to induce labor and for trials to assess clinically meaningful outcomes.

Pharmacologic Methods

PROSTAGLANDINS

The use of PGs for cervical ripening has been reported extensively, involving a variety of PG classes, doses, and routes of administration.[26–28] The distinction between cervical ripening and labor induction is blurred in patients receiving PGs because many women will go into labor even when PGs are being used primarily for ripening. Dinoprostone (PGE_2) is the PG most commonly employed. The local application of PGE_2 results in direct softening of the cervix by at least three mechanisms: (1) It softens the cervix by altering the extracellular ground substance of the cervix, (2) it increases the activity of the smooth muscle of the cervix and uterus, and (3) it leads to gap junction formation that is necessary for the coordinated uterine contractions of labor.[29,30]

Meta-analyses have shown that PGs are superior to placebo and oxytocin alone in ripening the cervix.[31,32] A systematic review including at least 5000 pregnancies from more than 70 prospective trials suggests that PGE_2 is superior to placebo or no therapy in enhancing cervical effacement and dilation.[31]

Two forms of PGE_2 (dinoprostone) are available commercially in the United States, although even more forms are available in other western countries. In randomized trials, the two forms are similar in efficacy.[33–35] The first is formulated as a gel and is placed endocervically, but not above the internal os. The application, 0.5 mg, can be repeated in 6 hours, not to exceed three doses in 24 hours. The second form is a 10-mg vaginal insert that is placed in the posterior fornix of the vagina. This formulation allows for controlled release of dinoprostone over 12 hours, after which it is removed.

Misoprostol (synthetic analogue of PGE_1) has been the subject of numerous articles describing its use as a cervical-ripening agent.[36–54] Doses of 25 to 50 μg administered vaginally or orally have been shown in several studies to be effective in inducing cervical ripening and labor. However, because the majority of patients experience regular uterine contractions soon after the initial dose, misoprostol should be considered primarily a labor-induction agent, which occasionally ripens the cervix without uterine activity.

The role of cytokines in cervical ripening has been the subject of several studies.[55] Interleukin-8 (Il-8) can lead to neutrophil chemotaxis, which is associated with collagenase activity and cervical ripening.[56] These inflammatory agents may be particularly important as mediators of cervical ripening associated with preterm labor. Nitric oxide synthase (NOS) and nitric oxide (NO) have been postulated to have a regulatory role in the myometrium and cervix during pregnancy and parturition.[57–59] In the human cervix, ripening is associated with an increase in inducible NOS (iNOS) and neural NOS expression in the cervix.

Resident and migrating inflammatory cells can cause an increase in iNOS activity. In the primate, cervical ripening has many aspects of an inflammatory process: tissue remodeling and breakage of chemical bridges between collagen fibers. Inflammatory agents such as Il-1, tumor necrosis factor-α, and Il-8 all seem to be involved in cervical ripening.[60–62] Currently, however, there is no commercial product available that exploits these properties directly.

Relaxin is a polypeptide hormone, similar to insulin, produced by the ovaries, decidua, and chorion. Because of its effect on connective tissue remodeling, it has been studied as a cervical-ripening agent.[63,64] Based on data from animal studies, relaxin was predicted to have a cervical-ripening effect in humans. The findings that porcine relaxin induces cervical ripening in humans supported this prediction. However, because studies showed that in fact administered human relaxin has no effect on the human cervix, the usual role played by relaxin in human pregnancy and parturition is unclear. At the present time, relaxin, either purified porcine or recombinant human, is not produced commercially as a cervical-ripening agent, and its future potential in this context remains unclear.

Pharmacologic Methods for Labor Induction

Oxytocin

Oxytocin, a neurohormone originating in the hypothalamus and secreted by the posterior lobe of the pituitary gland, is the most commonly used drug for the purpose of labor induction in viable pregnancies. This octapeptide is secreted in a pulsatile manner, a fact that is reflected in the marked variability observed in minute-to-minute measurements of maternal plasma oxytocin concentration.[65] The half-life of oxytocin is 10 to 12 minutes.[66] The metabolic clearance rate is similar for men, pregnant women, and nonpregnant women: 20 to 27 mL/kg/min.[67] The similarity of the metabolic clearance rate between men and pregnant women is striking in view of the large increase that occurs during pregnancy in the plasma concentration of leucine-aminopeptidase, an enzyme capable of hydrolyzing oxytocin. This suggests that factors other than this enzyme are responsible for the degradation of oxytocin.

There is considerable confusion regarding the pharmacokinetics of oxytocin; much of the original pharmacokinetic work was done prior to the availability of a reliable radioimmunoassay for oxytocin.[68] Indeed, the potency of oxytocin is still based on a bioassay of avian vasopressive activity with 1 United States Pharmacopeia (USP) unit being equivalent to 2 μg of oxytocin. Traditionally, it has been held that oxytocin levels reached a steady-state level within 15 to 20 minutes of beginning an infusion or increasing the dosage. Work using a sensitive oxytocin radioimmunoassay has shown that approximately 40 minutes is required for any particular dose of oxytocin to reach a steady-state plasma concentration.[69]

It is well established that there is a marked variability in the response of the uterus to oxytocin, but in general, the sensitivity of the uterus to oxytocin increases dramatically as pregnancy progresses.[70] This increase in responsiveness is likely due to the increasing concentrations of oxytocin receptors in the myometrium and decidua with increasing gestational age.[71] It appears that oxytocin has direct stimulatory effects on the myometrium in addition to stimulating decidual PG production.[72] An increased level of $PGF_{2\alpha}$ metabolite was demonstrated in women undergoing successful oxytocin induction of labor, whereas this increase was not present in failed inductions.[73] The direct effect of oxytocin on the myometrium is believed to be mediated by polyphosphoinositide hydrolysis with production of inositol phosphates that act as a second messenger and lead to the mobilization of intracellular calcium ion.[74]

Other organs that show a response to oxytocin include breast, vascular smooth muscle, and kidney. Oxytocin stimulates contraction of the myoepithelium surrounding the alveoli of the mammary gland, leading to the milk ejection reflex. At dosages typically used for the induction of labor, there is no demonstrable effect on vascular smooth muscle tone. However, intravenous boluses of as little as 0.5 IU transiently decrease peripheral vascular tone, leading to hypotension.[75] Similarly, at low dosages, oxytocin exerts negligible effect on renal function; however, at high infusion rates, it exhibits a marked antidiuretic effect (which is not surprising, given its similarity in structure to antidiuretic hormone, also produced in the posterior pituitary). Excessively high infusion rates, coupled with infusion of crystalloid, have led to deaths from water intoxication.

Oxytocin can be administered by any parenteral route. It is also absorbed by the buccal and nasal mucosa. When administered orally and swallowed, oxytocin is rapidly inactivated by trypsin. The intravenous route is now used almost exclusively to stimulate the pregnant uterus because it allows precise measurement of the amount of medication being administered and a relatively rapid discontinuation of the effects of the drug when infusion is discontinued.

TECHNIQUES FOR THE ADMINISTRATION OF OXYTOCIN

Oxytocin is administered as a dilute solution with the flow rate into the intravenous line precisely regulated by an infusion pump. The health care professionals who attend the patient during an induced labor must be familiar with the use and potential complications of oxytocin. Likewise, a qualified physician who is able to manage any complications that may arise with the use of oxytocin should be readily available. Fetal monitoring is indicated prior to beginning the infusion to assess the baseline level of uterine activity and fetal status, and should then be continued during the infusion. Either external or internal monitoring is acceptable as long as uterine activity and fetal heart rate (FHR) are adequately documented. Consideration should be given to the use of internal monitoring when high doses of oxytocin are required or when satisfactory progress in labor is not being made (see also Chapter 67). The tracing should be inspected frequently and carefully for any evidence of hyperstimulation as manifested by increased baseline tonus, tachysystole, or the onset of late decelerations; the infusion of oxytocin must be stopped immediately should they occur.

Significant difference of opinion exists regarding the initial dose of oxytocin and the interval and frequency of dosage increase. A controlled intravenous oxytocin infusion remains the preferred method of induction of labor. Several trials have compared various regimens of oxytocin dosage increase and time intervals between dose increases.[76–80] Starting doses have ranged from 0.5 to 2.0 mU/min, with some as high as 6 mU/min. Increments of dose increase have ranged from a low of 1 to 2 mU/min up to 6 mU/min, with adjustments for increased uterine activity. Time intervals between increases have ranged from 15 to 40 minutes. Although low-dose regimens (initial dose 0.5–2.0 mU/min, with incremental increases of 1–2 mU/min every 15–40 min) are commonly utilized in the United States, high-dose regimens (initial dose 6–8 mU/min, with incremental increases of 6 mU/min every 15–40 min) have been reported to be safe and effective for labor induction in patients with viable pregnancies, provided there was close fetal monitoring and early recourse to cesarean delivery in the event of fetal distress.[81] A meta-analysis of 11 trials comparing low-dose with high-dose oxytocin for labor induction found that larger dose increases and shorter intervals between increases were associated with shorter labors and lower rates of intra-amniotic infections and cesarean delivery for dystocia, but more hyperstimulation was noted.[82] Based on pharmacokinetic data,[83,84] many obstetricians have moved to a regimen whereby the dose of oxytocin is increased by 1 to 2 mU/min every 40 minutes. Advantages of this regimen derive from not increasing the oxytocin dose before steady-state levels of oxytocin have been reached. This leads to a lower total dosage of oxytocin being used, in addition to a lower incidence of the hyperstimulation that can result from increasing the oxytocin dose before a steady state is reached. A disadvantage is that women who are relatively insensitive to oxytocin may have a very prolonged course before adequate labor is established. Nearly 90% of patients will respond to 16 mU/min or less, and it is most unusual for a patient to require more than 20 to 40 mU/min.[85]

The recognition that endogenous oxytocin is secreted in spurts during pregnancy and spontaneous labor has prompted exploration of a more physiologic manner of inducing labor with this agent. In 1978, Pavlou and associates were the first to describe a protocol of pulsatile infusion.[86] Several randomized trials have compared the safety and efficacy of pulsatile oxytocin administration with continuous infusion.[87–89] Most authors conclude that, although there does not appear to be a shortening of the induction-to-delivery interval, pulsatile administration of oxytocin reduces the amount of oxytocin required for successful labor induction.

SIDE EFFECTS AND COMPLICATIONS OF OXYTOCIN INFUSION

Although oxytocin is a safe medication with appropriate administration and monitoring, there is always the potential for adverse occurrences. The most common complication related to oxytocin induction of labor is uterine hyperstimulation. Uterine hyperstimulation may present as tachysystole with more than five contractions in 10 minutes, contractions of greater than 90 seconds' duration, or an increase in the baseline uterine tonus. The decreased intervillous blood flow associated with hyperstimulation ultimately leads to decreased oxygen transfer to the fetus, as indicated by the appearance of late decelerations. Oxytocin infusion should be discontinued immediately in the presence of hyperstimulation. If there is evidence of fetal distress, standard intrauterine resuscitation measures should be instituted, including oxygen administration and positioning the patient in the left lateral decubitus position.

Uterine rupture is a very uncommon complication when oxytocin is used appropriately. There are no prospective data in the literature describing the incidence of uterine rupture in oxytocin-induced labor. Retrospective series of uterine rupture have implicated oxytocin in 4.3%[90] to 12.5%[91] of occurrences. Factors that may reduce the risk of uterine rupture include avoidance of oxytocin in the grand multipara, use of internal uterine pressure monitoring for patients with previous cesarean delivery and when high doses of oxytocin are required, and avoidance of oxytocin in obstructed labors.

Water intoxication, an infrequent complication of oxytocin administration, may be avoided with appropriate management. The minimum effective dose of oxytocin should be used to avoid the antidiuretic effects of high-dose oxytocin. The risk of water intoxication increases in women who have received large volumes of free water; therefore, 5% dextrose solutions without electrolytes should generally not be used during labor induction. Symptoms occur as the plasma sodium concentration falls below 120 to 125 mEq/L and may include nausea and vomiting, mental status changes, and ultimately, seizures and coma. Mild instances of water intoxication can be treated by discontinuing the hypotonic fluid and restricting fluid intake. With severe symptoms, correction of hyponatremia by saline infusion may be necessary.

Concern has been raised regarding a possible association between oxytocin-induced labor and an increased incidence of neonatal jaundice. Many of the older studies claiming that oxytocin leads to neonatal jaundice failed to control for confounding variables such as gestational age and the infusion of large volumes of free water. The more recent literature has not identified any correlation between oxytocin induction and neonatal hyperbilirubinemia.[92,93]

Prostaglandins

Exogenous PGs, particularly dinoprostone (PGE_2), are frequently used as cervical-ripening agents.[94–101] Because the PG-induced cervical-ripening process often includes initiation of labor, approximately half of women treated with dinoprostone enter labor and deliver within 24 hours. PGs have the dual capability to ripen the cervix and initiate uterine contractility. As a consequence, induced labor with PGs appears to be similar to that of spontaneous labor. The use of PGs as labor-induction agents has been reported extensively in a variety of PG classes, doses, and routes of administration.[31] Prior to 1992, most trials assessing the impact of PGs as cervical-ripening and labor-induction agents included various dosages of intracervical (0.3–0.5 mg) or intravaginal (3–5 mg) dinoprostone (PGE_2). In 1992, the U.S. Food and Drug Administration (FDA) approved PGE_2 (0.5 mg intracervically) for cervical ripening and labor induction. In 1995, a slow-release 10-mg dinoprostone vaginal insert also was approved for the same indications. Because most trials have compared these PG preparations with placebo, the relative efficacy of these two PG preparations has been difficult to assess. In addition, once cervical ripening was completed and uterine activity initiated, most patients studied required further augmentation with oxytocin.

The optimal route for PGE_2 administration has not yet been determined. The intracervical route has been used in the majority of trials, especially those comparing the effectiveness of the FDA-approved formulations (Prepidil and Cervidil). Although intracervical administration of gel is more difficult than intravaginal administration, the former route appears to cause more significant cervical ripening. The intracervical method also appears to be associated with a lower risk of hyperstimulation. However, the easiest and most practical way to apply PGE_2 in routine clinical practice is via the vaginal route, be it by gel, tablet, or vaginal pessary. It has been suggested that the dose of PGE_2 should be varied according to the patient's cervical score, permitting a lower dose of PGE_2 to be used in many cases. Just as there is no consensus about the optimal dose and route of administration of PGE_2, the optimal frequency of administration is still a matter of debate. The approach used for cervical ripening and labor induction with PGE_2 depends on the dose and route of administration. In the United States, 0.5 mg of dinoprostone gel is inserted into the cervical canal just below the internal os. If there is no change in the cervical score to the initial dose, repeat dosing may be given. The recommended repeat dose is 0.5 mg of dinoprostone with a dosing interval of 6 hours. The maximum recommended cumulative dose for a 24-hour period is 1.5 mg of dinoprostone. The recommended interval before considering augmentation with oxytocin should be 6 to 12 hours. In the United Kingdom and other European countries, dinoprostone vaginal gel is the preferred agent for cervical ripening and labor induction.[102] The usual dose is 1 mg inserted into the posterior fornix. For nulliparous patients, 2 mg can be given. The interval for a second dose is generally 6 hours and the cumulative dose should not exceed 4 mg. The dosage of dinoprostone in the vaginal insert is 10 mg designed to be released at approximately 0.3 mg/hr. The vaginal insert should be removed upon the onset of active labor or 12 hours after insertion. Delaying oxytocin augmentation or induction for 30 to 60 minutes after removal of the vaginal insert is sufficient. Irrespective of the route and dose of PGE_2 employed, for the majority of patients, dinoprostone preparations should be regarded mainly as cervical-ripening agents, and are not reliable as labor-induction agents.

MISOPROSTOL FOR LABOR INDUCTION

Misoprostol is a synthetic PGE_1 analogue that has been marketed in the United States since 1988 as a gastric protective agent for the prevention and treatment of peptic ulcers. It was licensed in a tablet form designed for oral absorption. Early studies performed in the late 1980s and early 1990s demonstrated that oral administration of misoprostol caused uterine contractions in early pregnancy.[103–105] Subsequent studies, performed abroad and in the United States, showed that intravaginal administration of misoprostol tablets can terminate first-trimester and second-trimester pregnancies.[106–110] A large number of published controlled trials have shown that misoprostol, administered either vaginally or via the oral route, is an effective agent for cervical ripening and labor induction in patients with viable pregnancies.[35–54,111–119] An initial meta-analysis suggested a significantly reduced cesarean delivery rate for patients induced with misoprostol.[120] Follow-up meta-analysis showed that 84% of patients receiving misoprostol go into active labor, with only 29.4% requiring oxytocin augmentation. A significantly higher proportion of patients receiving misoprostol achieved a vaginal delivery within 12 hours (37.6% vs. 23.9%). Similarly, 68.1% of patients receiving misoprostol achieved a vaginal delivery within 24 hours. Use of misoprostol for cervical ripening and labor induction is associated with an approximately 5-hour reduction of the interval from the first dose to delivery when compared with dinoprostone. The reduced induction-to-delivery interval seen with misoprostol compared with dinoprostone implies that either it produces higher levels of uterine activity or it is a more efficient cervical-ripening agent. Consistent with the former hypothesis, compared with women receiving dinoprostone, Foley catheter, or placebo, women receiving misoprostol are twice as likely to experience tachysystole and uterine hyperstimulation, with the incidence of these conditions closely related to the dose of misoprostol administered.[120]

In relation to cervical ripening, most of the individual studies in meta-analyses assessing the efficacy and safety of misoprostol and dinoprostone have not shown a significant reduction in the overall cesarean delivery rate. However, the lack of a positive finding was probably because the sample sizes of the trials were small. The 44 trials included in a systematic review with meta-analysis provide data for 5735 subjects participating in trials assessing the impact of misoprostol treatment on the cesarean delivery rate.[120] When all the trials were pooled, subjects receiving misoprostol had a significantly lower cesarean rate than subjects in the comparison groups (17.3% vs. 22.9%). The most common indications for cesarean delivery were arrest of dilation or descent, failed induction, and abnormal FHR tracings. The rate of cesarean deliveries performed because of FHR abnormalities was similar for misoprostol-induced patients and those in the comparison group. Similarly, no difference was noted for the rate of cesarean deliveries because of dystocia. Patients receiving misoprostol had a significantly lower rate of cesarean deliveries because of failed induction. This suggests that misoprostol may be better than dinoprostone at ripening the cervix.

No evidence of adverse perinatal or maternal effects has been noted.[121] The statistical power resulting from the aggregation of 44 studies included in the meta-analysis increases confidence in our ability to assess safety. The number of subjects studied affords a power of at least 90% to detect a difference in neonatal intensive care unit admission rates of at least 4 percentage points (from 14% to 18%). Sufficient power was also noted for the detection of at least a doubling in the rate of abnormal 5-minute Apgar scores (from 1.4% to 2.8%).

Accordingly, these data provided support for the conclusion that misoprostol decreases the cesarean delivery rate among women undergoing labor induction compared with women receiving alternate induction agents. However, more recent meta-analyses, assessing the impact of misoprostol on the cesarean delivery rate, have not shown a significant reduction in cesarean section rate in the various subgroups analyzed.[122] This may be due to the lower doses now being used, aimed at improving safety by reducing hyperstimulation rates.

ORAL VERSUS VAGINAL ADMINISTRATION

Initial pharmacokinetic studies compared the pharmacokinetics of vaginal and oral administration of misoprostol.[123–126] These studies showed that the peak plasma concentration of misoprostolic acid was higher and achieved earlier after oral administration, but the detectable plasma concentration lasted longer after vaginal administration. Systemic bioavailability of vaginally administered misoprostol was noted to be three times higher than that of orally administered misoprostol.[123] In all patients studied, independent of the dose or route of administration, the first effect of misoprostol treatment was an increase in uterine tonus. After oral administration, the effect was more rapid and the initial increase was more pronounced than after vaginal treatment. However, after vaginal treatment, tonus remained at a higher level for a longer time.

A significant proportion of the published randomized studies have evaluated the safety and efficacy of vaginally administered misoprostol for cervical ripening and labor induction. Seven randomized trials have compared oral versus vaginal administration of misoprostol for labor induction.[114–119,127] In aggregate, 1191 patients were randomized to receive misoprostol orally ($n = 602$) or by the vaginal route ($n = 589$). The oral doses employed ranged from 50 μg to 200 μg every 4 to 6 hours. Vaginal misoprostol was administered in doses ranging from 25 μg to 100 μg every 3 to 4 hours. No difference was noted in the proportion of patients who delivered vaginally within 12 and 24 hours in each group. Similarly, the intervals from start of induction to vaginal delivery were not different. The proportion of patients experiencing increased uterine activity (tachysystole or hyperstimulation) was similar for both groups. In addition, no difference was noted for the incidence of abnormal 5-minute Apgar scores and rates of NICU (neonatal intensive care unit) admissions. Interestingly, the rate of cesarean delivery was significantly lower among those induced with oral misoprostol. Although both routes of misoprostol administration seem to be efficacious, the evidence documenting the safety of vaginally administered misoprostol is much more extensive.

DOSES OF MISOPROSTOL FOR LABOR INDUCTION

Owing to the small number of studies employing oral misoprostol and the lack of uniformity in dosage, the most appropriate dose of misoprostol for labor induction has not been determined. At the present time, oral doses of 100 μg administered every 3 to 4 hours appear to be safe and effective. Further studies are needed to determine whether higher doses can improve efficacy without increasing the rate of adverse maternal and perinatal outcomes.

Because the majority of studies have assessed the safety and efficacy of vaginal administration, more data are available to determine the most appropriate dose. Although dosing regimens as high as 200 μg have been reported in the literature, most authors have used vaginal misoprostol doses of 25 μg or 50 μg. Because of the increased incidence of uteronic effects, some authors have advised against the use of doses greater than 25 μg. However, the data that form the basis for this recommendation are limited. Six randomized clinical trials have been specifically designed to compare the safety and effectiveness of 25 μg or 50 μg of misoprostol administered intravaginally.[128–133] These trials, although generally well designed, are hampered by small sample size and thus prone to type II errors. A systematic review with meta-analysis of five randomized trials concluded that intravaginal misoprostol at doses of 50 μg for cervical ripening and labor induction is more efficacious, but it is unclear whether it is as safe as the 25-μg dose.[134]

In addition to the six randomized trials and the systematic review, two separate studies have compared the two doses (25 μg vs. 50 μg). These two studies compared intravaginal misoprostol with intracervical dinoprostone gel (Prepidil).[41,42] The misoprostol dosage for the first study was 50 μg every 3 hours for a maximum of six doses, whereas the second study used 25 μg every 3 hours for a maximum of eight doses. Taken together, these two studies indirectly compared two doses of misoprostol: 25 μg and 50 μg. Subjects allocated to receive 50 μg experienced shorter intervals to vaginal delivery and no differences in overall cesarean or operative delivery rates, cesarean deliveries for FHR abnormalities, or NICU admission rates. Although subjects receiving 50 μg of misoprostol experienced a greater incidence of tachysystole, no significant increases in adverse maternal or perinatal outcomes were noted. Meconium-stained fluid was noted more frequently for those receiving 50 μg of misoprostol. Given the reassuring perinatal findings noted previously, this latter finding, however, is of questionable importance. Because these two separate studies by Wing and associates[41,42] indirectly compare two doses of misoprostol, 25 μg and 50 μg, they were incorporated into the present analysis. Altogether, 906 patients were compared: 479 received doses of 25 μg and 427 received doses of 50 μg. Patients who received the 25-μg dose had a lower incidence of tachysystole and hyperstimulation; however, they also had a longer interval to vaginal delivery, and a lower proportion of these patients delivered vaginally within 12 and 24 hours. No differences were noted in the cesarean delivery rate, cesareans performed for FHR abnormalities, operative delivery rates, or NICU admissions.

An American College of Obstetricians and Gynecologists (ACOG) Committee Opinion in 1999[135] stated that if misoprostol is used for cervical ripening and labor induction, 25 μg should be considered for the initial dose. This recommendation has been reinforced in a recent ACOG Practice Bulletin.[136] This opinion is based on the greater incidence of tachysystole noted with larger doses of misoprostol. Despite increased uterine activity with greater doses, however, greater rates of adverse maternal or perinatal outcomes have not been reported. Although existing evidence suggests that both the 25- and the 50-μg doses of misoprostol are currently appropriate for intravaginal administration, we consider that further large prospective trials are required to define an optimal dosing regimen.

There has been recent interest in the use of low-dose oral misoprostol for induction of labor. A recent meta-analysis of nine randomized, controlled trials comparing low-dose (20–25 μg) oral misoprostol with dinoprostone, vaginal misoprostol, and oxytocin for labor induction concluded that 20 μg of misoprostol administered orally every 2 hours seems as effective as both vaginal dinoprostone and vaginal misoprostol.[137] There was also a reduction in cesarean delivery rates and hyperstimulation with low-dose oral misoprostol.

Cervical Ripening and Labor Induction in Special Circumstances

Previous Cesarean Delivery

Among patients with a previous cesarean section, the incidence of uterine disruption is greater with induced labor than with spontaneous labor (0.65% vs. 0.40%).[138] Patients in this group undergoing cervical ripening and labor induction with PGE_2 (dinoprostone) experience a rupture rate of 0.9%.[139]

In women with unscarred uteri, vaginal or oral administration of misoprostol has been found safe and effective for patients with unfavorable cervices who require labor induction. There are indirect data, however, from which to assess the risks and benefits of using misoprostol to ripen the cervix and induce labor in women with a previous lower uterine segment scar. A substantial number of publications have suggested that the use of misoprostol in patients with previous cesarean delivery is associated with a high frequency of uterine disruption (dehiscence or frank rupture).[140–146] Most of these publications consist of a few case reports or are based on retrospective uncontrolled studies. A randomized trial designed to compare the safety and efficacy of vaginally administered misoprostol in women with previous cesarean deliveries was terminated prematurely when 2 of 17 women being induced with misoprostol had major uterine ruptures.[141] At the time this study was halted, however, the study had not met the specified criteria for early termination of the trial.[147]

We used several sources to identify all publications that have reported the use of misoprostol for cervical ripening and labor induction in women with previous cesarean delivery. Eleven studies have been published indicating the use of misoprostol for cervical ripening and labor induction in women with scarred uteri.[140–146,148–151] Uterine disruptions, dehiscence, or rupture were reported in 6 of the studies.[140–145] Of 355 patients included in these 11 studies, 16 (4.5%) experienced uterine disruption. Because several confounding factors were present, however, it is important to analyze these data in detail. Data are available for 10 of 16 patients reported to have experienced uterine disruptions. The mean age of the patients was 29.6 ± 4.7 years with a mean gestational age of 39.5 ± 2.1 weeks. Three patients had two previous cesarean deliveries and, in 2 other patients, the type of scar was unknown. Although the information is not precise, it appears that in at least in 3 cases, the patients had a dehiscence of the previous incision. Most patients were induced with single or multiple vaginal doses of 25 μg of misoprostol. Two patients received four doses, and 2 others received at least three doses of misoprostol. The median interval from the last dose of misoprostol until the diagnosis of uterine disruption was 10 hours (interquartile range 8.5–17.2 hr). Seven patients received oxytocin infusion after misoprostol was administered and before the diagnosis of uterine disruption. Only 2 experienced tachysystole, and all patients were delivered by cesarean. The mean birth weight was 3438 ± 572 g. Four cases of neonatal acidemia and 1 neonatal death were reported.

Because of the paucity of data, there is a lack of sufficient evidence from which to assess the risks and benefits of using misoprostol or other PGs to induce labor in women with a scar from a previous lower segment cesarean delivery. Randomized, controlled trials are needed to assess outcomes including vaginal delivery rates, interval to delivery, and number of failed inductions. Because uterine disruption is such an uncommon event, however, only a large multicenter randomized, controlled trial will yield adequate statistical power to assess safety in this population of patients. To detect a difference in uterine rupture from 1% to 3.7%, such a trial would have to include 565 patients in each group ($\alpha = 0.05$, $\beta = 0.80$). Until such a trial is performed, an alternative approach would be to perform a case-control study. In the meantime, the use of misoprostol for cervical ripening and labor induction in women with a previously scarred uterus should occur only in the setting of a research protocol.

Twin Pregnancies

Twin pregnancies frequently involve maternal and fetal complications, which require early delivery. In addition, the optimal timing of birth for women with an otherwise uncomplicated twin pregnancy at term is uncertain, with clinical support for both elective delivery at 37 weeks as well as expectant management. Elective delivery at term may be performed via an elective cesarean or vaginally with the use of mechanical or pharmacologic agents for cervical ripening and labor induction. At present, there are insufficient data to support a practice of elective cesarean delivery for women with an otherwise uncomplicated twin pregnancy at term.

The safety and efficacy of uterotonic agents, particularly oxytocin, for labor induction in women with twins are not as clear as in those with singleton pregnancies. Some clinicians believe that the overdistended uterus encountered with twins is resistant to oxytocin and may require high doses to obtain adequate uterine contractions. In addition, some clinicians suspect that a gravida with twins is prone to hyperstimulation or even uterine rupture with relatively low doses of oxytocin. Although there are no large randomized trials attesting to the safety and efficacy of cervical ripening and labor induction in patients with twin pregnancies, several retrospective studies have suggested that labor induction, with a variety of induction agents, is acceptably safe. A case-matched control study compared the safety and efficacy of labor induction with oxytocin versus spontaneous labor in 62 women with twin pregnancies.[152] Twin pregnancy had no adverse impact on the effectiveness or efficiency of oxytocin labor stimulation; indeed, it appeared to be associated with fewer side effects. Additional case series of labor induction in twin pregnancies have included the use of intrauterine balloon catheters,[153] oral dinoprostone or PGE_2,[154] and oxytocin.[155]

Although misoprostol has been shown to be a safe and effective agent for labor induction in singleton pregnancies, there are no published studies in women with twin pregnancies. If misoprostol is chosen for labor induction in twins, continuous monitoring of the FHR and uterine contractions should be performed. Repeated doses should be used only if there is definitely no evidence of regular uterine activity.

According to ACOG, twin pregnancies do not necessarily constitute a contraindication to labor induction.[156] However, as with misoprostol, patients with twin pregnancies who undergo labor induction with oxytocin, or with any other agent, need to be monitored very closely.

Fetal Death

The ideal method for termination of pregnancy in cases of intrauterine fetal demise should be effective and safe and should have minimal side effects. In the past, oxytocin infusion and PGE_2 vaginal suppositories (referred to as "pessaries" in the United Kingdom) were the most commonly used methods for labor induction in patients with fetal death.

INTRAVENOUS OXYTOCIN

Intravenous oxytocin is a time-honored, effective, and safe method for inducing labor in cases of intrauterine fetal demise. However, oxytocin infusion is less effective when used in patients with a very unripe cervix and in those remote from term. Large doses and prolonged administration may be required, circumstances that increase the risk of water intoxication and attendant central nervous system complications. For patients who are remote from term, some authors have reported the use of high-dose oxytocin.[157] One regimen describes the use of approximately 300 mU/min (200 units of oxytocin in 500 mL of 5% dextrose lactated Ringer solution or 5% dextrose and half-normal saline at 50 mL/hr). In this setting, 5% dextrose and water has been associated with hyponatremia. Electrolytes should be checked before beginning oxytocin and should be repeated every 24 hours or if signs and symptoms of water intoxication occur. Attention should be paid to fluid intake and urinary output. For patients at or near term, lower doses of oxytocin are usually required. Laminaria, or other mechanical means of cervical ripening, may be beneficial before the use of oxytocin for induction.

PROSTAGLANDINS

Many cases of fetal death can be managed simply and effective by PGE_2 vaginal suppositories. The customary dose is one 20-mg suppository inserted vaginally every 4 hours until contractions are sufficient to promote progressive cervical change. Generally, this dose is used only for patients who are at no more than 28 weeks' gestation. However, some authors have reported safe use in the third trimester.[158] Reported side effects with higher doses (20 mg) of PGE_2 vaginal suppositories include fever, nausea, vomiting, and diarrhea. These annoying side effects may be ameliorated with appropriate and specific pretreatment medications. Although PGE_2 vaginal suppositories have been used safely in the third trimester, the risk of uterine rupture is increased.

More recently, misoprostol (synthetic analogue of PGE_1) has been used safely and effectively for cervical ripening and labor induction in patients with fetal death. Mariani-Neto and coworkers[159] first reported the use of oral misoprostol (400 μg q4h) for induction of labor following fetal death. The authors reported their experience with 20 patients with fetal demise at 19 to 41 weeks' gestation. All patients delivered successfully with a mean interval to delivery of 552 minutes. The mean dose of misoprostol required was 1000 μg (400–2800 μg). Additional studies have assessed the safety and efficacy of misoprostol in the management of fetal death.[160,161] The doses and routes of administration have varied significantly among the studies. Oral doses of 200 μg and vaginal doses ranging from 50 to 200 μg every 4 to 6 hours have been employed. Some authors have combined misoprostol with mifepristone; patients receive a single dose of 200 mg mifepristone orally, following which a 24- to 48-hour interval is recommended prior to administering 100 to 200 μg of misoprostol in the vagina every 3 hours.[160,161]

Wagaarachchi and associates[162] first reported a combination of vaginal and oral misoprostol after priming with mifepristone. Women received a single dose of 200 mg mifepristone followed by a 24- to 48-hour interval before administration of misoprostol. For gestations of 24 to 34 weeks, 200 μg of intravaginal misoprostol was administered, followed by four oral doses of 200 μg at three 1-hour intervals. Gestations over 34 weeks were given a similar regimen but a reduced dose of 100 μg misoprostol. The average induction-to-delivery interval was 8.5 hours, which was the shortest among the previous regimens. Improved patient acceptability and reduced risk of introducing intrauterine infection are potential advantages of oral over vaginal route.

High doses of misoprostol (vaginal or oral administration) may be associated with fever, chills, and diarrhea. Pretreatment with antidiarrheal and antiemetic agents may reduce adverse effects.

EXTRA-AMNIOTIC SALINE INFUSION

Extra-amniotic saline infusion has been shown to be successful in inducing labor in antepartum deaths after 20 weeks' gestation.[163] An 18-Fr Foley catheter is inserted through the cervix under direct vision. The balloon is inflated with 30 mL of sterile water, and the catheter is usually strapped to the thigh under slight traction. Normal saline (0.9%) infusion is started to run at 30 drops/min, and a maximum volume of 2 L should be infused into the extra-amniotic space.

SUMMARY OF MANAGEMENT OPTIONS

Induction of Labor

Management Options	Evidence Quality and Recommendation	References
Prenatal—General		
Bishop score is still the most reliable indicator of success of induction.	III/B	4
Prenatal—Indications		
Women should have a valid indication for IOL and no contraindications (see Tables 66–1 and 66–2).	III/B	85
Indications should be such that mother or fetus will benefit from a higher probability of a healthy outcome than if birth is delayed.	III/B	85
For a consideration of the validity of specific indication for induction of labor, see other chapters including 35 and 65.	—/—	22
Preinduction Cervical Ripening:		
Mechanical Methods		
• Foley catheter.	Ia/A	16
• Laminaria tents.	Ib/A	19,20
• Membrane sweep.	Ia/A	8
• Acupuncture.	IIb/B	24
Pharmacologic Methods		
• PGs.	Ia/A	31,32
Labor Induction		
Oxytocin is effective.	Ib/A	77,78,80
PGs are effective.	Ia/A	102
In women with intact membranes, vaginal PGE_2 is superior to oxytocin.	Ia/A	31,32
Although both routes are equally effective, intravaginal PGE_2 is preferable to intracervical because it is less invasive.	Ia/A	276
PG tablets (3 mg) are equally effective as PG gel (1–2 mg) q6h, but tablets offer financial savings.	Ia/A	276
Oxytocin use in women with intact membranes should be combined with amniotomy.	III/B	85

Management Options	Evidence Quality and Recommendation	References
Oxytocin should not be started for 6 hr following PG administration.	III/B	85
Oxytocin starting dose is 1–2 mU/min, increased at intervals of 30–40 min.	III/B	85
Misoprostol appears to be a cheap, effective induction agent. Safety issues are probably related to dose or route and are being assessed.	Ia/A	120
Other methods such as mechanical methods, estrogens, relaxin, hyaluronidase, castor oil, bath, enema, and breast stimulation have varying efficacy.	III/B	85
Labor Monitoring		
Fetal well-being should be established prior to induction of labor.	III/B	85
Following insertion of PG, fetal well-being should be established once contractions begin.	III/B	85
When oxytocin is being used for induction, continuous electronic monitoring should be used.	III/B	85
If there is uterine hypercontractility, tocolysis should be considered.	Ia/A	41,42,134

IOL, induction of labor; PG, prostaglandin.

TERMINATION OF PREGNANCY FOR FETAL ANOMALY

Introduction

In 2005, 12% of all legal terminations of pregnancy (TOP) reported to the U.S. Centers for Disease Control and Prevention (CDC) occurred after 13 weeks' gestation.[164] Only 5.0% were performed after 15 weeks' gestation: 3.7% at 16 to 20 weeks and 1.3% at 21weeks or more. Dilation and evacuation (D&E) accounted for 96% of these procedures. From 1974 through 2005, the percentage of second-trimester TOP performed by D&E increased from 31% to 96%; and the percentage of second-trimester TOP performed by intrauterine instillation (intra-amniotic, extra-amniotic) using hypertonic saline, urea, or $PGF_{2\alpha}$ decreased from 57% to 0.4%. The percentage of medical abortions increased from 1.0% in 2000 to 9.9% in 2005.[164]

D&E, preceded by cervical preparation, is safe and effective when undertaken with appropriate instruments by practitioners who have a sufficient workload to maintain their skills.[165,166] Compared with intra-amniotic instillation methods, D&E has lower complication rates.[166–169] However, almost all the comparative data relate to obsolete abortifacients (such as saline and urea solutions) that are rarely used today.

The introduction of PG analogues in the late 1970s changed the management of TOP in the second trimester; they were initially instilled into the amniotic cavity, and later used for cervical ripening. The subsequent introduction of the antiprogestin mifepristone shortened the induction-to-TOP interval still further, and the dosage of PG analogues required was reduced. Today, medical TOP is the method of choice in many centers that perform second-trimester TOP.[170,171]

Both D&E and medical induction are relatively safe, with low complication rates.[167,172] Second-trimester TOP by D&E in well-selected patients in a dedicated outpatient facility can be safer and less expensive than hospital-based D&E or induction of labor.[173] The method chosen is largely dependent on physician preference and level of technical expertise, coupled with the patient's informed decision.

Definition

Termination of pregnancy is the medical or surgical removal of a pregnancy before the time of fetal viability while preserving the life and health of the mother. Patients in need of TOP can be identified at any gestational age; however, the great majority are performed at 24 weeks' gestation or less.

Indications

The most commonly accepted indications for TOP are

- A pregnancy that would result in the birth of a child with anomalies incompatible with life or associated with significant physical or mental morbidity.
- Fetal death.
- To save the life of the mother or preserve the health of the mother.

Fetal Conditions

Significant structural and chromosomal conditions affect at least 3% to 5% of all births, and an increasing number of women will be faced with the decision to end a pregnancy based on fetal health concerns.[174,175] Unfortunately, because fetal assessment (e.g., using biochemical screening, ultrasound, chorionic villus sampling, or amniocentesis) is not available until the second trimester, TOP for this indication is usually later in gestation than TOP for social indications. The number of fetal conditions that can be identified during pregnancy continues to expand because of the steady improvement of the technology available for prenatal diagnosis. Conditions that can be identified include

- Chromosomal disorders (e.g., trisomy 21, 18, 13).
- X-linked disorders (e.g., hemophilia).
- Metabolic disorders (e.g., Tay-Sachs).
- Neural tube defects (e.g., anencephaly, spina bifida).
- Structural anomalies associated with exposure to teratogens.
- Infections (e.g., rubella, cytomegalovirus, toxoplasmosis).
- Structural anomalies of multifactorial or unknown etiology.
- Other fetal indications, including preterm prelabor rupture of membranes prior to 24 weeks and fetal death at 24 weeks or less.

Maternal Conditions

TOPs to save the life or preserve the health of the mother are rare events. Some women with chronic medical conditions choose pregnancy termination only after discovering for the first time during pregnancy that continuing the pregnancy poses significant health risks for themselves. This failure of preconception counseling is unfortunately more common than it should be. For most chronic medical conditions, sufficient data exist to permit accurate decisions as to the likelihood and magnitude of risks associated with a continuing pregnancy, although it is often impossible to say precisely who will be affected. For example, although one can quote a 30% to 50% mortality rate for pregnancy in association with Eisenmenger's syndrome or pulmonary hypertension, half the women counseled will survive, and it is usually impossible to say which half. In the case of other medical indications for TOP, such as severe hypertensive vascular disease and certain malignancies, the prognosis can be given with more certainty.[176–178] Decision for TOP in this context should be based on the collaborative agreement of a multidisciplinary team. At minimum, the team should consist of the patient, the obstetrician, a medical specialist, and an expert in genetic counseling. Additional members may include family members, spiritual counselors, nurses, intensive care specialists, and ethicists. The decision must be individualized for each patient.

Legal Termination of Pregnancy Services

In the United States, only a few states provide public funding for TOP, and one third of private insurance plans provide limited or no coverage.[179] Women with federally funded medical care are covered for TOP services only if the woman's life is threatened, or in cases of rape or incest (32 states), when medically necessary (16 states), and in cases of life endangerment (2 states). Hence, cost contiderations pose formidable barriers to women seeking TOP, even when there is gross fetal malformation.

Clinicians performing D&E procedures need training from an experienced mentor and the opportunity to maintain proficiency through ongoing experience. In the United States, only 44% of all facilities providing TOP offer services at 14 weeks' gestation; the proportion declines dramatically as gestation advances, to 22% at 20 weeks and 7% at 24 weeks.[180] Moreover, only 7% of obstetrics and gynecology residency programs provide routine training in second-trimester TOP.[181] Labor induction is an integral part of obstetrics and gynecology training; training in D&E for second-trimester TOP is not. Among graduating obstetrics and gynecology residents in U.S. programs, 43% had never performed a D&E, and 81% had performed 10 or fewer procedures.[181] Therefore, despite the safety advantages of D&E, women requesting second-trimester TOP may be limited to labor-induction methods simply because practitioners trained and willing to perform D&E are unavailable. Thus, the future availability of D&E, especially beyond 15 weeks' gestation, is uncertain. As the availability of D&E procedures decreases, the need for safe, efficacious methods of medical TOP will increase.

Patient Assessment and Counseling (See also Chapters 7 and 8)

Patient assessment should include history, physical examination, appropriate laboratory studies, and counseling.

History

The complete medical history should focus on the timing and reliability of the last normal menstrual period. If there is the slightest doubt about gestational age (e.g., a discrepancy between the history and the examination findings), assessment of fetal size with ultrasound is crucial. Knowledge of past reproductive history, sexual history, current medications, allergies, prior pelvic surgery, and any known uterine anomalies is important. Women with medical conditions severe enough to warrant TOP may require additional evaluation and stabilization prior to the procedure.

Physical Examination

Physical examination must include vital signs, weight, uterine size, and cardiopulmonary assessment. A sterile speculum examination should be done, seeking cervical pathologic problems, such as active cervicitis, deformities, and past trauma. A small, stenotic, or scarred cervical os may impair the cervical dilation necessary for safe surgical TOP.

Laboratory Studies

Few laboratory studies are required in young healthy women, but hematocrit, Rh status, indirect Coombs, and urinalysis results should be obtained.

- A complete blood count (CBC) and blood typing are the minimum laboratory studies required for surgical TOP.
  - A CBC is required to identify patients with significant anemia, who are at risk if excessive blood loss occurs. Transfusion may be needed, particularly in second-trimester TOPs. Patients with severe anemia are best treated in a setting in which transfusion is available.
  - Blood typing is required so that Rh-negative women can be identified and given anti-D immunoglobulin (RhoGAM) to prevent Rh sensitization in subsequent pregnancies.
  - Screening for common sexually transmitted infections (STIs) should be addressed in geographic areas of high prevalence, in age groups at high risk (i.e., <25 yr), and in at-risk groups (e.g., those with histories of STIs, multiple sex partners, substance abuse).
- Additional laboratory testing is dictated by the medical history and physical examination findings.

Coagulation studies are indicated for patients with conditions such as a history of coagulopathy, hematologic malignancies, hemorrhage with previous surgical procedures, petechiae, bruising, and hepatosplenomegaly.

Liver function tests are indicated for patients with conditions such as hepatitis, alcohol abuse, cancer, hepatomegaly, and jaundice. Renal function tests are indicated for patients with conditions such as renal disease, recurrent urinary tract infections, oliguria, hematuria, and proteinuria.

Electrolyte assays are necessary in patients who develop significant vomiting associated with the use of medical TOP techniques.

Ultrasound, in addition to its value for prenatal diagnosis, is used for determination of gestational age, placental location, and detection of uterine fibroids or the presence of uterine anomalies (e.g., uterus didelphys, unicornuate uterus, septate uterus).

Counseling

When a congenital fetal anomaly is diagnosed, the clinician should meet with the patient for the following reasons:

- To explain to the patient the nature and severity of the anomaly.
- To discuss the treatment options available for the management of the anomaly.
- To explain the implication(s) of the anomaly for the child and on the family.
- To refer the patient for expert opinion if the clinician is uncertain about the congenital anomaly or its implication(s), treatment, and so on.

The purpose of counseling is to help the patient understand her options regarding the pregnancy. In cases with severe anomaly, TOP may be offered as an option when there is a substantial risk that if the child were born, it would suffer from such physical or mental abnormality as to be seriously handicapped. If the clinician, based on his or her professional opinion, disagrees with the patient on her decision regarding TOP, the patient should be reminded that she can seek a second opinion.

At the minimum, the patient should know the diagnosis, purpose of the procedure, risks and possible complications, alternative treatments, and the likelihood of successful treatment.

Therefore, the woman should be given appropriate information related to the choice between TOP and continuing her pregnancy to viability, regardless of the physician's personal views about rearing a child with such an anomaly or about TOP. However, although physicians have a duty to give full and accurate information, they have no obligation to be involved in the procedure itself if they have ethical objections. For this reason, training in carrying out TOP should not be mandatory, although it is mandatory for physicians to be knowledgeable about the procedure and its complications so that they can give accurate advice and make an appropriate referral to someone who is willing to perform it.[182]

Choice of Methods

Termination of pregnancy can be achieved by surgical means or with pharmacologic agents alone, in combination, or as an adjunct to a surgical method. The methods described refer to pregnancy termination at 13 to 24 weeks' gestation. The decision over which method to use is primarily determined by

- The gestational age.
- The expertise of the available medical staff.
- Patient preference.
- The clinical importance of obtaining an intact fetus.
- Presence of other complicating clinical conditions.

Generally, dilation and suction evacuation can be used up to 14 weeks' gestation, but thereafter, specific techniques of cervical preparation and special instruments for D&E need to be used. Modern methods of aggressive cervical preparation coupled with extensive clinical experience of the procedure have resulted in improved safety for D&E.[173,183]

From a provider perspective, D&E allows predictable scheduling and avoids the prolonged period of medical observation typical of labor induction. Patients having a TOP for fetal anomaly may find that the prospect of a prolonged induction and delivery compounds the anguish of their decision and loss. A surgical TOP, possibly under general anesthesia, may be less traumatic emotionally. Shulman and colleagues[184] observed that patients in their institution recovered more quickly after D&E and required fewer referrals for postoperative counseling than patients had a medical TOP. However, D&E places a greater emotional burden on the surgeon and support staff.[185]

Although some women elect to have a medical TOP out of a desire to avoid surgery, the rate for the use of surgical aspiration or curettage to treat incomplete TOP is 15% to 30% or higher.[172–175]

Conversely, grieving is important for many parents of a fetus with congenital abnormality, and seeing and holding the fetus are important components of healing.[186] In addition, medical TOP results in the delivery of an intact fetus and, therefore, allows optimal evaluation and confirmation of suspected genetic or structural abnormalities. This information is vital in counseling couples about the likelihood of recurrence.

Currently, medical TOP with misoprostol is a safe alternative to surgical TOP in patients with acute medical conditions and chronic debilitating illnesses. In our experience, misoprostol combined with mechanical cervical dilators such as a Foley catheter or laminaria tents can be used safely in patients with severe hypertensive disorders, cardiac disease, or asthma.[187]

In difficult or challenging cases, especially at or beyond 16 weeks, the physician, in consultation with the patient, must choose the most appropriate method based upon the patient's individual circumstances.[188,189]

Clincal Setting

Surgical D&E can be performed safely in a variety of outpatient settings, including a physician's office, provided there is an efficient system for emergency transfer.[190–192] In contrast, medical TOP services are usually provided in hospital settings.

Surgical Methods

Surgical methods include D&E, dilation and intact extraction (D&X), hysterotomy, and hysterectomy. The use of real-time ultrasound scanning during D&E can reduce perforation rates.[193] Hysterotomy or hysterectomy is seldom used owing to higher rates of morbidity and mortality.[194] Prerequisites for surgical TOP include cervical preparation, adequate cervical dilation to use a 16-mm suction cannula, special grasping forceps, adequate anesthesia, oxytocic agents, antibiotic prophylaxis, and appropriate postoperative care.

DILATION AND EVACUATION

Anesthesia

The choice of anesthesia must be based on the medical, psychiatric, and emotional condition of the patient. Consultation with anesthetists, medical specialists, and psychiatric specialists may be necessary to determine the best choice for the individual patient. In general, paracervical block with light sedation provides sufficient anesthesia for many patients; however, the full range of anesthesia options must be available. Use of short-acting barbiturates by intravenous bolus infusion is a simple, effective form of general anesthesia that obviates the need for muscle relaxants, intubation, and halogenated gases.[195]

Cervical Preparation

A variety of mechanical and pharmacologic methods have been utilized (see Table 66–4).

Use of Osmotic Dilators

There are four types of osmotic dilators—laminaria japonica, two synthetic dilators (Lamicel, Dilapan) (Fig. 66–1),[196] and isaptent. Laminaria, derived from the seaweed genus *Laminaria* (*L. japonica*, *L. digitata*), are one of the oldest devices used for cervical ripening. Tents prepared from *L. japonica* are commercially available and are packaged in a variety of sizes.

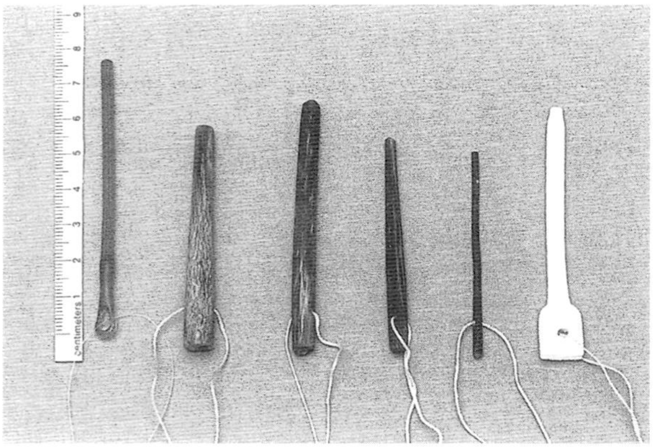

FIGURE 66–1
Osmotic dilators. *Left to right*: Dilapan, a single-sized synthetic polyacrylonitrile rod (hypan) currently available outside the United States; *Laminaria japonicum*, dried and compressed stalks of seaweed, four sizes (available in sizes ranging from 2 to 10 mm); Lamicel, a magnesium sulfate-impregnated polyvinyl alcohol sponge (available as 3 and 5 mm).
(From Williamson DW: Resources for abortion providers. In Paul M, Lichtenberg ES, Borgatta L, et al [eds]: A Clinician's Guide to Medical and Surgical Abortion. New York, Churchill Livingstone, 1999, p 292, Fig. 20-13.)

Although tents prepared from *L. digitata* are available, they are less useful clinically; they become gelatinous with expansion and are prone to fragment or become trapped in the cervix. The tents absorb water, swell, and ultimately dilate and soften the cervix. The tents expand most rapidly in the first 4 to 6 hours but continue to swell for up to 24 hours. In general, laminaria will expand up to four times their original diameter, resulting in concomitant dilation of the cervix. Placement of several smaller tents rather than one large tent may result in improved dilation and facilitate their later removal.

Compared with laminaria, Dilapan swells more rapidly and to a greater diameter, therefore, fewer Dilapan on average are needed for similar efficacy.[197] However, Dilapan is more likely to disintegrate, or retract, and it is no longer available in the United States.[198] Lamicel was found to be inferior to laminaria for mid-trimester cervical ripening prior to D&E.[199] Lamicel is seldom used alone, because the sponges are difficult to insert in aggregate and become too soft on expansion to achieve the dilation needed.

Isaptent, although not used widely in the United States, is an alternative osmotic dilator that is effective for mid-trimester cervical ripening. These commercially available tents (Dilex C.; Central Drug Research Institute, Lucknow, India) are prepared from granulated seed husk powder, derived from the isopgol plant (*Plantago ovata*), which is compressed and sealed into a cylindrical polythene sheath. The tents expand to a maximum diameter of 9 to 11 mm within 8 to 12 hours.[200] Comparison of isaptent with laminaria for cervical ripening demonstrates similar efficacy.[201]

Strategies may range from use of a single osmotic dilator with same-day surgery during the early second trimester to serial insertion of a variety of types and size of dilators for more advanced gestations. For procedures at up to 16 weeks' gestation, placing the dilators 4 to 8 hours prior to surgery may suffice. Beyond 16 weeks, it is common practice to allow overnight dilation, and some mid to late second-trimester procedures call for a second insertion in 12 to 24 hours. Repeated laminaria applications significantly increase cervical dilation as compared with a single application, and therefore, treatment must be individualized.[198,202]

Adequate dilation is required in order to pass the 16-mm suction cannula and grasping forceps and to remove all the fetal parts. The minimum dilation required to insert grasping forceps depends on the type and size of the instrument used (13 mm for small Sopher, 14–15 mm for large Sopher, 16 mm for small Bierer, and 17 mm for large Bierer).[166] Prior to starting the procedure, sufficient cervical dilation must be confirmed. If cervical dilation is inadequate, additional osmotic dilators can be placed and the procedure delayed for at least 4 to 6 hours (or rescheduled to the next day).

Adequate pretreatment with laminaria may effect enough dilation prior to D&E to avoid the need for additional forced dilation in the operating room. Laminaria is the current mainstay in the United States for achieving cervical dilation for second-trimester TOP. Dilapan is still used widely in countries where it is available.

Methods of Insertion

After placing the speculum in the vagina and exposing the cervix, the cervix should be cleaned with antiseptic solution. Some women require no anesthesia or analgesia, but local anesthesia is helpful in women who are anxious or when the procedure is technically difficult. Use of a 50:50 mixture of lidocaine (1% or 0.5%) and bupivacaine (0.25%) provides rapid onset and a longer duration of action than lidocaine alone.

The anterior lip of the cervix is grasped with a long Allis clamp. The cervical canal is carefully sounded, without rupturing the membranes, to identify its length. If desired, the cervix can be dilated mechanically using finely tapered dilators (such as Pratt and Denniston), and this allows insertion of more or larger osmotic dilators.

The large end of each osmotic dilator is grasped with a ring, packing, or ovum forceps and inserted into the cervical canal, laying successive dilators on top or next to the previous ones. Coating the dilators with lubricating jelly may ease insertion. Laminaria should be inserted leaving a 2- to 4-mm length protruding from the external os to facilitate its removal. The surgeon should ensure that the tips of the osmotic dilators pass through the internal os (Fig. 66–2).[166] If not, the result is a funnel-shaped canal and an inadequately dilated internal os (Fig. 66–3).[188] After inserting the dilators, they can be kept in place while the speculum is removed by placing a gauze sponge in a sponge holder over the cervix. The number and type of osmotic dilators inserted should be recorded.

In the event of inadvertent or spontaneous membrane rupture, the osmotic dilators should still be placed, but left in place for only 12 hours rather than 24 hours. The patient may resume normal activities, depending on how she feels.

Cervical Priming with Prostaglandins Prior to D&E

Lauersen and coworkers[203] found a superior dilating effect with four to six laminaria tents placed 12 hours prior to D&E than with either PGE_2 vaginal suppositories (30 or 60 mg) or 15(S)-methyl $PGF_{2\alpha}$ (0.5 or 1.0 mg). Vaginal and oral misoprostol have also been found useful in this setting.[204,205] More recently, buccal administration of misoprostol (600 μg given 2–4 hr prior to the procedure) was found to be as effective as laminaria tent for cervical preparation.[206]

FIGURE 66–2

Osmotic dilator insertion. *A*, Laminaria placed appropriately through the internal os. *B*, Laminaria does not pass through the internal os. Swelling results in funneling of the endocervical canal and inadequate dilation of the internal os. *C*, Laminaria inserted too far into the endocervical canal. This placement may result in rupture of the membranes and difficult removal.

(*A–C*, From Haskell WM, Easterling TR, Lichtenberg ES: Surgical abortion after the first trimester. In Paul M, Lichtenberg ES, Borgatta L, et al [eds]: A Clinician's Guide to Medical and Surgical Abortion. New York, Churchill Livingstone, 1999, p 130, Fig. 10-2.)

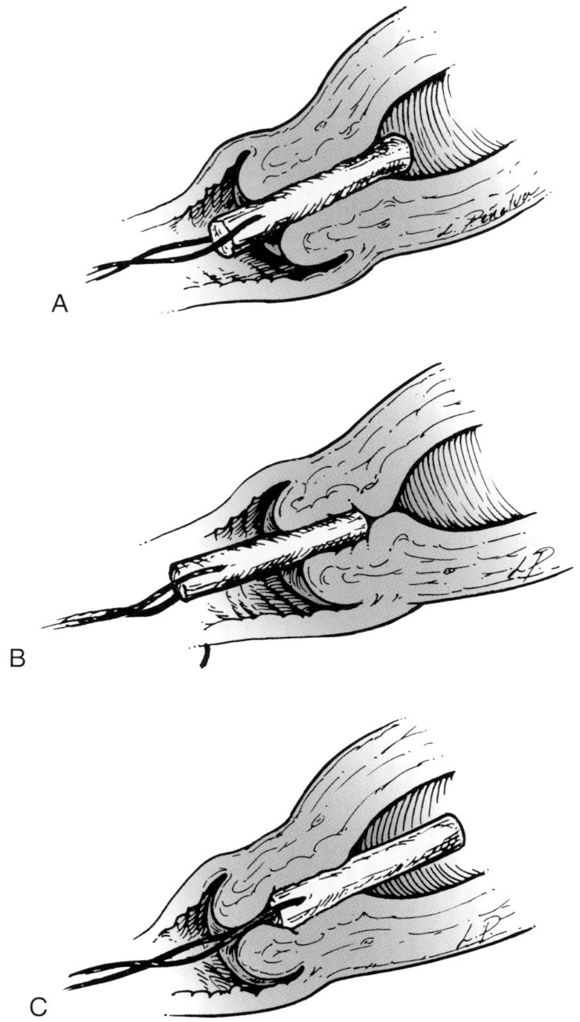

PROCEDURE

DILATION AND EVACUATION

This procedure consists of removal of the osmotic dilators, assessment of cervical dilation, and insertion of a 16-mm suction cannula to rupture the membranes and evacuate the amniotic fluid and fetal elements, followed by mechanical destruction and evacuation of fetal parts using special grasping forceps (preferably under ultrasound guidance).

The osmotic dilators are removed digitally or with packing forceps. The number of dilators should be counted to ensure they are all removed. Following this, a gentle digital examination will establish the extent of cervical dilation (particularly at the internal os). If sufficient dilation cannot be accomplished, the procedure should be delayed to repeat the osmotic dilation, or consideration should be given to admitting the patient for a medical TOP.

Once dilation is deemed adequate, the bladder should be emptied with a rubber catheter before D&E is started. The cervix is grasped with a long Allis clamp and a cannula is passed into the uterine cavity to rupture the membranes and evacuate as much amniotic fluid as possible with vacuum suction. The suction cannula should always be advanced fully into the uterine cavity before suction is applied. Up to 15 weeks' gestation, a 14-mm cannula should suffice, but gestations of 16 weeks and more require a 16-mm cannula. During removal of the amniotic fluid, it is common for some membranes and placental tissue to be evacuated. However, complete placental extraction is generally delayed until the fetal parts have been removed.

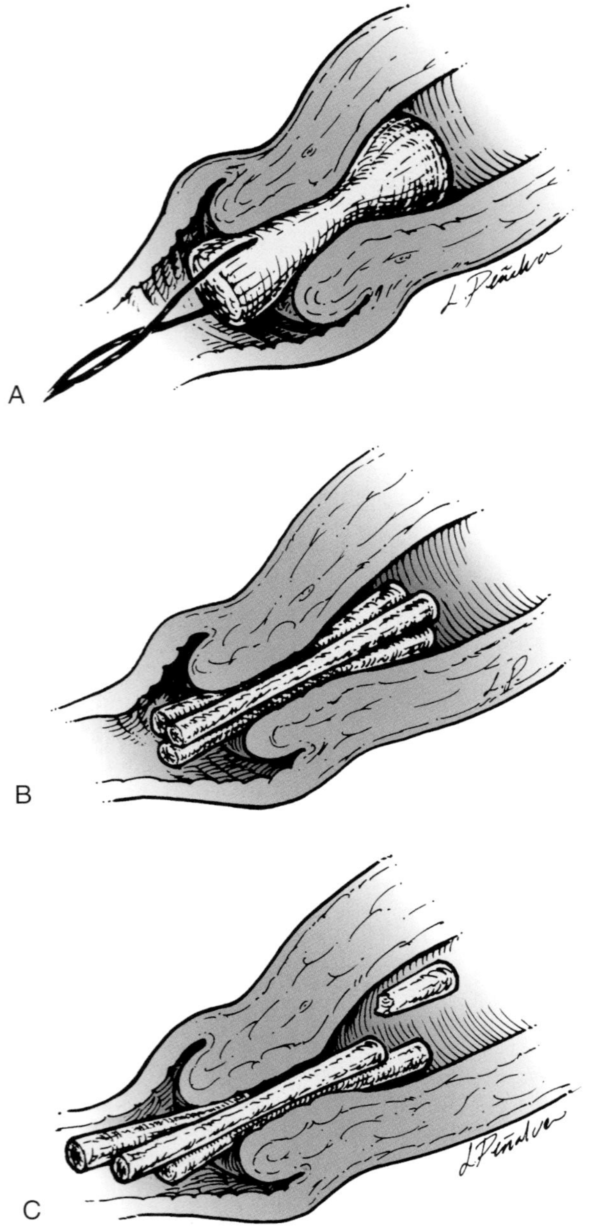

FIGURE 66–3
Dumbbelled osmotic dilator. *A*, A single large osmotic dilator is "dumbbelled" by the stiff internal os. Removal of this dilator may be difficult. *B*, Several small dilators are dumbelled. Because they are smaller, it may be possible to remove one. The others are then looser. *C*, When there are several dilators that cannot be removed, an alternative is to fracture one deliberately. The other dilators are then loosened and easier to remove. One fragment here has entered the uterine cavity and must be removed by suction or other means.
(*A–C*, From Borgatta L, Burnhill MS, Karlin E: The challenging abortion. In Paul M, Lichtenberg ES, Borgatta L, et al [eds]: A Clinician's Guide to Medical and Surgical Abortion. New York, Churchill Livingstone, 1999, p 177, Fig. 13-5.)

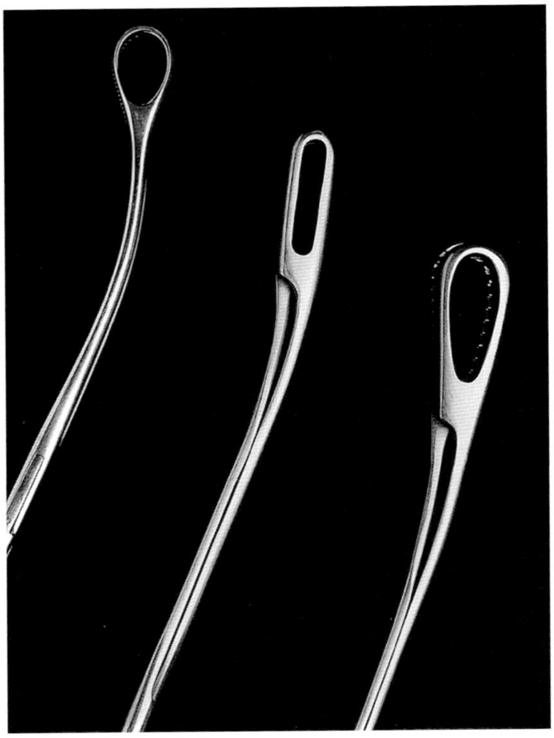

FIGURE 66-4
Instruments for dilation and evacuation (D&E). Kelly placental forceps, Sopher forceps, and Bierer forceps (*left to right*).
(From Ludmir J, Stubblefield PG: Surgical procedures in pregnancy. In Gabbe SG, Niebyl JR, Simpson JL [eds]: Obstetrics: Normal and Problem Pregnancies. New York, Churchill Livingstone, 2002, p 639, Fig. 19-25.)

With a 14-mm cannula, suction alone is usually adequate to remove 13- to 16-week pregnancies. Beyond 16 weeks, some fetal parts remain in the uterus after suctioning and require extraction by forceps; most commonly, these remnants include the spinal cord and calvarium. To extract the remaining fetal parts, a grasping forceps appropriate for the amount of cervical dilation should be used. In cases past 16 weeks, the fetus is extracted, usually in parts, using Sopher or similar forceps and other destructive instruments.

The choice of forceps (Fig. 66–4)[207] depends on operator preference and the extent of cervical dilation. We prefer Sopher forceps with its long shafts and bulkier grasping surfaces with sheltered serrations.

Once inserted, the forceps should be opened widely and one blade inserted along the anterior uterine wall in order to grasp the fetal parts. When fetal parts are felt between the blades on closing the handles, they are removed with a gentle twisting motion. The calvarium is the part most likely to be left behind. If fetal parts remain in the uterus, gentle probing with a small sharp curette may locate and retrieve them, although use of a sharp curette always carries the risk of perforating the uterine wall. Alternatively, sonography can be used to locate any remaining fetal parts and aid in their evacuation. In one study, use of intraoperative ultrasonography reduced the incidence of uterine perforation at D&E from 1.4% to 0.2%.[193]

Complete removal of the placenta generally requires one or more passes with the 14- to 16-mm suction curette. Before concluding the procedure, the fetal parts should be assembled to determine whether TOP was complete. Similarly, the quantity of placental tissue should be visually assessed to ensure that it is commensurate with the gestation.

Use of Oxytocic Agents

The use of uterotonic agents during surgical TOP is a matter of preference. We use an intravenous infusion of oxytocin 20 to 40 units in 500 mL crystalloids given intraoperatively after rupture of membranes and continued postoperatively for 30 minutes. If the full 40 units is given, care should be taken to avoid excessive further infusion of crystalloid, because of the risk of water intoxication due to the antidiuretic effect of oxytocin.

Antibiotic Prophylaxis

Routine oral antibiotic prophylaxis reduces the risk of infection after surgical TOP.[208–210] It is commonly started on the first day of osmotic dilator placement. Antibiotics such as tetracycline, clindamycin, and metronidazole have all been used to good effect.

Postoperative Care

Minimum observation periods for recovering D&E patients are 1 hour for early and mid second-trimester cases and 2 hours for late D&E, usually defined as more than 19 to 20 weeks' gestation.

INTACT DILATION AND EXTRACTION

ACOG in its general policy statement related to TOP[211] described "intact dilatation and extraction" (intact D&X) as containing all the following four elements:

- Deliberate dilation of the cervix, generally accomplished with multiple, serial osmotic dilators over 2 days or more.
- Instrumental conversion of the fetus to a footling breech.
- Breech extraction of the body excepting the head.
- Partial evacuation of the intracranial contents of a living fetus to effect vaginal delivery of a dead but otherwise intact fetus.

According to the CDC, only 5.0% of TOPs performed in the United States in 2005 (the most recent data available) were performed after the 16th week of pregnancy.[164] It is unknown how many of these were performed using intact D&X.

Intact D&X is a very controversial procedure in the United States. A select panel convened by ACOG could identify no circumstances under which this procedure, as defined here, would be the only option to save the life or preserve the health of the woman.[211] In the authors' institution, medical TOP, with concurrent use of a 30-mL balloon Foley catheter or laminaria tents and misoprostol, is the method of choice after 18 weeks' gestation. The physician, in consultation with the patient, must choose the most appropriate method based upon the patient's individual circumstances.

HYSTEROTOMY AND HYSTERECTOMY

In rare circumstances, hysterotomy or hysterectomy for TOP is preferable to either D&E or medical TOP. The possible indications include failed medical TOP if D&E cannot be safely performed; myomas in the lower uterine segment obstructing extraction; prior placement of an abdominal cerclage, which it is desired to leave in place; uterine anomalies (e.g., uterus didelphys, unicornuate or septate uterus); and some cases of cervical cancer.[188]

Another clinical challenge is the patient with complete placenta previa presenting for second-trimester TOP.[212] In ultrasound studies, the reported prevalence of second-trimester placenta previa ranges from 2% to 6%. Thomas and colleagues[213] reported on 131 patients with and without placenta previa who underwent second-trimester D&E. The 23 patients (17.6%) with ultrasound-documented placenta previa averaged only 21 mL more blood loss and had no other complications.

Conversely, placenta accreta occurs in 1 to 2 per 10,000 second-trimester TOPs and usually results in heavy bleeding during the procedure. Placenta accreta is frequently associated with previous uterine surgery, suggesting a preexisting defect in the basal layer of the endometrium (decidua basalis).[214] Occasionally, patients with placenta accreta or placenta percreta require laparotomy with hysterotomy or hysterectomy despite the increased morbidity and mortality risks associated with these procedures.[215] These patients may benefit from preoperative placement of embolization balloon catheters using interventional radiology techniques.[216,217] Second-trimester TOPs by D&E in well-selected patients in a dedicated outpatient facility can be safer and less expensive than hospital-based D&E or induction of labor.

Medical Termination of Pregnancy

The introduction of PG analogues and mifepristone has revolutionized the management of second-trimester TOP and fetal death since the early 1990s. Gemeprost and misoprostol are the two most extensively studied PG analogues that are used in this period. Gemeprost is the only licensed synthetic PG analogue for second-trimester TOP in the United Kingdom. However, it is expensive and needs to be stored in a refrigerator. Misoprostol is inexpensive and can be stored at room temperature. It has been widely used for induction of labor in cases of fetal death and second-trimester TOP for fetal anomaly. The combination of either gemeprost or misoprostol with mifepristone is most effective. With these regimens, over 90% of women abort within 24 hours and the mean induction-to-delivery interval is about 6 hours. Mifepristone is expensive and is not available in many countries. Therefore, PG analogue-only regimens can be the only option. These regimens are still effective, with a TOP rate above 90% in 48 hours; however, the induction-to-TOP interval (15 hr) is much longer. Intracervical tents can be used to shorten the induction-to-delivery interval.[171,172]

Instillation into the uterine cavity through the intra-amniotic or extra-amniotic routes of substances designed to kill the fetus and promote delivery (such as hypertonic saline, hyperosmolar urea, $PGF_{2\alpha}$, ethacride lactate) is obsolete.[170–172] A review by Ramsey and Owen[218] detailed the limited role of vaginal PGE_2 and intramuscular $PGF_{2\alpha}$ as well as high-dose oxytocin infusion for second-trimester TOP.

FETOCIDAL PROCEDURES

Use of medical TOP has been associated with live birth rates from 4% to 10%.[219] In borderline viable gestations, patients, physicians, and nurses express concern about the dilemma of resuscitation in the event of a live birth after a PG-induced TOP. Moreover, such live birth is beset with ethical, medical, and legal implications. Because of concern among patients, practitioners, and hospitals, many TOP services perform a fetocidal procedure prior to or concomitantly with PG-induced TOP at 20 weeks' gestation or more.

The most common fetocidal agents used in developed countries are potassium chloride (KCl) and digoxin.[220,221]

The procedure involves transabdominal insertion of a 20-gauge spinal needle into the fetal cardiac chambers by ultrasound guidance and instillation of 2 to 3 mL of KCl in a concentration of 2 mEq/mL. Cardiac standstill is usually observed within 1 to 3 minutes. An alternative is the instillation of digoxin in doses varying from 0.25 to 2 mg, by the intracardiac, intrathoracic, intrafetal, and intra-amniotic routes. There were no failures using a 1.0-mg intrafetal dose, but failures occurred with 0.5 mg for intra-amniotic (8.3%) and intrafetal administration (3.6%).[221]

CERVICAL PREPARATION

Physical Methods

Osmotic dilators can be useful before induction of labor (see earlier discussion). There has been a resurgence of interest in catheter-based techniques, specifically in relation to the concurrent use of extra-amniotic saline infusion and misoprostol. A variety of balloon catheter devices have been shown to be effective for cervical ripening.[218] Foley catheters with a 30-mL balloon are more commonly used in the United States. Extra-amniotic saline infusion (EASI) is an effective adjuvant to both mid-trimester and term labor inductions.[222] Using aseptic technique and countertraction, a lubricated 26-Fr Foley catheter with a 30- to 50-mL balloon is grasped with ring forceps and inserted through the internal os, after which the catheter balloon is inflated in the lower uterine segment. For the tightly closed, nulliparous cervix, a smaller-diameter catheter (e.g., 18 Fr) can also be used. Normal saline is infused through the catheter lumen at a nominal rate of 30 to 60 mL/hr, and traction is not used. Overall, EASI appears to be a safe and effective alternative to laminaria for mid-trimester cervical priming. Advantages of EASI include low cost, reversibility, and lack of systemic side effects. Although EASI and laminaria appear to be equally efficacious, EASI offers the potential advantageof easier placement and less patient discomfort.

Pharmacologic Cervical Ripening

Mifepristone (RU-486; Mifeprex) received FDA approval in the United States in September 2000. Mifepristone shortens the induction-to-delivery time and decreases pain with cervical ripening when compared with laminaria for second-trimester induction.[223,224] The value of intracervical tents in regimens using misoprostol is less clear.[225]

The World Health Organization (WHO) recommended that cervical preparation should precede all TOPs induced after 14 weeks.[226] Whenever possible, mifepristone should be used as the cervical-priming agent before second-trimester TOP. If mifepristone is not available, an intracervical tent should be used.

Prostaglandins and Their Analogues PG receptors are present throughout all stages of pregnancy, and thus, PGs and their analogues are effective in terminating both f irst- and second-trimester pregnancy. The natural PGs, $PGF_{2\alpha}$ and PGE_2, were the first to be tested clinically for medical TOP, but they were soon replaced by synthetic PG analogues because of the high incidence of gastrointestinal side effects when given parenterally or vaginally.[170–173]

The PGE and PGF analogues have been used clinically for second-trimester TOP. The PGE analogue is preferable because it has a more selective action on the myometrium and causes less gastrointestinal side effects. The most extensively studied PGE and PGF analogues for second-trimester TOP are carboprost, meteneprost, sulprostone, gemeprost, and misoprostol.

Prostaglandin E_2 Analogues Two PGE_2 analogues, dinoprostone (Prostin) and meteneprost (9-methylene PGE_2), are commercially available and have been investigated for midtrimester TOP. Of these, only Prostin is FDA-approved in the United States as an abortifacient in the mid-trimester and for fetal death up to 28 weeks' gestation. The recommended dosage regimen of Prostin for second-trimester termination is 20 mg administered as a vaginal suppository every 3 to 4 hours (maximal exposure 24 hr). In a series of midtrimester TOPs with vaginal PGE_2, 20 mg every 4 hours with osmotic dilators, the mean induction-to-delivery interval was 17 hours.[171,172] PGE_2 is not thermally stable and must be kept refrigerated. It has been widely investigated and has been proved effective for second-trimester TOP. However, intravaginal misoprostol was at least as effective as PGE_2 and without the cost and side effects associated with PGE_2 use.[105]

Prostaglandin $PGF_{2\alpha}$ Analogues A synthetic $PGF_{2\alpha}$ analogue, carboprost tromethamine (15S)-15-methyl-$PGF_{2\alpha}$ tromethamine (Hemabate), is the only other commercially available PG that is FDA-approved and marketed in the United States as a mid-trimester abortifacient at 13 to 20 weeks' gestation. The recommended dosage regimen of carboprost for second-trimester TOP is 250 μg, administered by intramuscular injection every 1.5 to 3.5 hours (maximal exposure 12 mg or 48 hr). A test dose of 100 μg may be administered to confirm patient tolerance before administration of the full 250-μg dose. The successful TOP rate with intramuscular carboprost reached 80% to 90% in 36 hours, but it was associated with a high rate of gastrointestinal side effects.[171,172]

Prostaglandin E_1 Analogues The three most extensively studied PGE analogues are sulprostone, gemeprost, and misoprostol. Sulprostone (16-phenoxy-(ω)-17–18,19,20-tetranor PGE_2, methyl sulphonylamide) was studied in the early 1980s for medical termination of second-trimester pregnancies. However, intramuscular sulprostone is no longer used clinically for medical TOP because of its association with myocardial infarction.[227] Therefore, gemeprost and misoprostol are the principal drugs used for second-trimester medical TOP today.

Gemeprost Gemeprost (16,16-dimethyl trans-Δ^2 PGE_1 methyl ester) is a PGE_1 analogue. It is the only PG licensed in the United Kingdom for medical TOP. It is administered as a vaginal pessary. Studies using a vaginal gemeprost-only regimen gave a complete TOP rate of 80% to 96.5% in 48 hours.[228–231] The most common regimen is 1 mg every 3 to 6 hours for five doses in 24 hours. It is repeated if delivery does not occur in this time. The mean induction-to-delivery interval ranged from 14 to 18 hours. The most common side effects were vomiting, diarrhea, and fever. Cost and the need for refrigeration are the drawbacks with gemeprost; these factors make its use practical only in developed countries.

Misoprostol Misoprostol (15-deoxy-16-hydroxy-16-methyl PGE_1) is a synthetic PGE_1 analogue. It was discovered that it could be used "off-label" as an abortifacient. It is cheap, stable at room temperature, and readily available in many developing countries. Vaginal misoprostol is as effective as gemeprost.[229–231]

Studies mainly focus on the optimization of misoprostol dosing regimens by comparing various dosages, dosing intervals, and routes of administration.[232–237] The dosage of misoprostol used ranged from 100 to 800 μg with dosing intervals of 3 to 12 hours. The efficacy of misoprostol is improved when a higher dose (400–800 μg) is given at shorter intervals (3–4 hr) (Table 66–5). The vaginal route is more effective than the oral route.[236,238] The greater bioavailability of vaginal misoprostol probably explains the clinical results. Zieman and coworkers[126] compared the absorption kinetics of misoprostol with oral versus vaginal (400 μg) administration in pregnant women. It was shown that the systemic bioavailability of vaginally administered misoprostol is three times higher than that of the oral route. The plasma level was sustained up to 4 hours after vaginal administration. However, women preferred the oral route because it was less painful, gave more privacy, and was more convenient.[238]

A randomized study demonstrated that misoprostol 600 μg given vaginally, then 200 μg orally every 3 hours was probably the optimal regimen for second-trimester TOP.[239] A regimen that involves the administration of the first dose of misoprostol vaginally and subsequent doses orally might have a number of beneficial effects. It will minimize the number of vaginal examinations required to insert subsequent doses while preserving the possible direct cervical-priming effect of the first dose.

TABLE 66–5

Second-Trimester Termination of Pregnancy by Misoprostol-only Regimen

MISOPROSTOL REGIMEN	NUMBER OF SUBJECTS	GESTATIONAL AGE (WK)	TOP RATE IN 24 HR (%)	MEAN INDUCTION-TOP INTERVAL (HR)	REFERENCES
1. Misoprostol 200 μg vaginal q12h × 2	28	12–22	89	12.0	Jain & Mishell[105]
2. PGE_2 20 mg vaginal q3h	27		81	10.6	
1. Misoprostol 100 μg vaginal q6h for 36 hr max	27	12–24	74 (48 hr)	23.1	Nuutila et al[231]
2. Misoprostol 200 μg vaginal q12h for 36 hr max	26		92	27.8	
3. Gemeprost 1 mg vaginal q3h for 36 hr max	27		89	14.5	
1. Misoprostol 200 μg vaginal q12h × 2	50	16–22	70.6 (48 hr)	45	Herabutya et al[232]
2. Misoprostol 400 μg vaginal q12h × 2	50		82	33.4	
3. Misoprostol 600 μg vaginal q12h × 2	50		96	22.3	
1. Misoprostol 200 μg vaginal q6h × 8	51	12–22	87.2 (48 hr)	13.8	Jain et al[233]
2. Misoprostol 200 μg vaginal q12h × 4	49		89.2	14.0	
1. Misoprostol 400 μg vaginal q3h	74	14–20	73.0	15.2 (median)	Wong et al[234]
2. Misoprostol 400 μg vaginal q6h	74		60.8	19.0	
1. Misoprostol 200 μg vaginal q6h	50	14–30	59	18.2 (median)	Dickinson & Evans[235]
2. Misoprostol 400 μg vaginal q6h	50		76	15.1	
3. Misoprostol 600 μg vaginal; then 200 μg q6h	50		80	13.2	
1. Misoprostol 200 μg oral q1h × 3; then misoprostol 400 μg oral q4h	65	12–20	39.5	34.5	Bebbington et al[236]
2. Misoprostol 400 μg vaginal q4h × 6	49		85.1	19.6	
1. Misoprostol 800 μg vaginal; then 400 μg oral q8h × 5	21	14–23		15.9	Feldman et al[237]
2. Misoprostol 800 μg vaginal; then 400 μg vaginal q8h × 5	23		21.1		
3. Misoprostol 400 μg vaginal q12h	60		26.0		
1. Misoprostol 400 μg vaginal q6h	28	14–26	86	14.5 (median)	Dickinson & Evans[235]
2. Misoprostol 400 μg oral q3h	29		45	25.5	
3. Misoprostol 600 μg vaginal; then 200 μg oral q3h	27		74	16.4	
1. Sublingual misoprostol 400 μg q3h × 5	681	13–20	88.5 (parous)	11.0	von Hertzen et al[241]
			68.5 (nullipara)	14.4	
2. Vaginal misoprostol 400 μg q3h × 5			84.7 (parous)	11.8	
			87.3 (nullipara)	13.0	

PGE_2, prostaglandin E_2; TOP, termination of pregnancy.

Sublingual administration of misoprostol has also been developed. The sublingual route was chosen because it was considered as the most vascular area of the buccal cavity. It also avoids the first-pass effect through the liver in oral administration and the uncomfortable vaginal administration. Reports have shown that both sublingual and vaginal administrations of misoprostol were equally effective in inducing medical abortion during second trimester but the sublingual route was preferred by the patients.[240,241]

Mifepristone and Synthetic Prostaglandin Analogues

Mifepristone is the antiprogestin that is approved for use clinically for TOP. It increases the sensitivity of the uterus to PGs. The use of oral mifepristone 36 to 48 hours before PG administration can increase the successful TOP rate, shorten the induction-to-delivery interval, and reduce the total dose of PGs required (Table 66–6).[242–251] The first recommended dose of mifepristone was 600 mg, but it has been shown in a randomized trial that the successful TOP rate and induction-to-delivery interval were the same even if the dose was reduced to 200 mg.[248]

If mifepristone pretreatment is used before gemeprost (1 mg q6h), the induction-to-delivery interval can be decreased from 15.7 hours to 6.6 hours and the successful TOP rate in 24 hours is increased from 72% to 95% (see Table 66–6).[246]

To improve patient acceptability and to maintain the efficacy, a combination regimen including both the oral and the vaginal routes has been developed. El-Refaey and Templeton[247] compared two misoprostol regimens in women pretreated with 600 mg mifepristone for 36 to 48 hours. The first group received 800 μg vaginal misoprostol as the first dose and 400 μg vaginal misoprostol every 3 hours. The second group received 800 μg vaginal misoprostol as the first dose and 400 μg oral misoprostol every 3 hours. The mean induction-to-TOP interval was 6.0 and 6.7 hours, respectively. The 24-hour TOP rate was 97% in both groups (see Table 66–6). Ashok and Templeton[250] used mifepristone 200 mg followed by 800 μg vaginal misoprostol as the first dose and 400 μg oral misoprostol every 3 hours. They achieved 97% abortion rate; the median induction-to-abortion interval was 6.5 hours. Pretreatment with mifepristone significantly reduced the induction-to-TOP interval when compared with a misoprostol-only regimen. It was thought that vaginal misoprostol as the first dose could have a cervical priming effect.

Current evidence shows that the combination of oral mifepristone and vaginal misoprostol is an effective method for termination of second-trimester pregnancy. If mifepristone is not available, vaginal misoprostol alone can be used but the induction-to-TOP interval will be slightly longer.

USE OF PROSTAGLANDIN WITH A SCARRED UTERUS

With the rising cesarean delivery rate, an increasing number of women undergoing second-trimester TOP will have a previous uterine scar. No matter what method is used, the risk of uterine rupture is higher than for those without a scar. The reported risk of scar rupture at the time of medical termination in the presence of a previous uterine scar varies from 3.8%[252] to 4.3%.[253] This rate compares with a uterine rupture rate of 0.2% in patients with an intact uterus.[254,255] Uterine scar rupture has been reported with both gemeprost

TABLE 66–6
Second-Trimester Termination of Pregnancy by Using Mifepristone Prior to Misoprostol

TREATMENT WITH ORAL MIFEPRISTONE 36–48 HR BEFORE MISOPROSTOL/GEMEPROST REGIMEN	NO. OF SUBJECTS	GESTATIONAL AGE (WK)	TOP RATE IN 24 HR (%)	INDUCTION-TOP INTERVAL (HR)	REFERENCES
1. Mifepristone 600 mg + misoprostol 800 μg vaginal; then 400 μg vaginal q3h	35	13–20	97	6.0	El-Refaey & Templeton[247]
2. Mifepristone 600 mg + misoprostol 800 μg vaginal; then 400 μg oral q3h	34		97	6.7	
1. Mifepristone 600 mg + misoprostol 800 μg vaginal; then 400 μg oral q3h × 4	35	13–20	94	6.9	Webster et al[248]
2. Mifepristone 200 mg + misoprostol 800 μg vaginal; then 400 μg oral q3h × 4	35		97	6.9	
1. Mifepristone 200 mg + misoprostol 200 μg vaginal q3h × 5	49	14–20	90	9.0 (median)	Ho et al[249]
2. Mifepristone 200 mg + misoprostol 200 μg oral q3h × 5	49		69	13.0	
1. Mifepristone 200 mg + misoprostol 400 μg oral q3h × 5	70	14–20	81.4	10.4 (median)	Ngai et al[251]
2. Mifepristone 200 mg + misoprostol 200 μg vaginal q3h × 5	69		84.0	10.0	
3. Mifepristone 200 mg + misoprostol 800 μg vaginal; then misoprostol 400 μg oral q3h × 4	500	13-21		6.5 (median)	Ashok & Templeton[250]
1. Mifepristone 200 mg + 1 mg gemeprost q6h × 3	50	12–20		6.6 (median)	Bartley & Baird[246]
2. Mifepristone 200 mg + misoprostol 800 μg vaginal; then misoprostol 400 μg oral q3h × 4	50			6.1	

TOP, termination of pregnancy.

TABLE 66–7

Induction Agents and Reported Adverse Effect (% Occurrence)

AGENT	INDUCTION-ABORTION INTERVAL (HR)	ADVERSE EFFECTS (%)	COMMENTS
Hypertonic saline	20-46	Fever, vomiting (5%-12%) Hemorrhage	Intra-amnotic injection; used with oxytocin augmentation
Oxytocin	8-13	Water intoxication (rare) Nausea and vomiting (less than with PGs)	Significantly fewer gastrointestinal side effects than prostaglandins (PGs) Requires intravenous infusion
$PGF_{2\alpha}$	14-37 (dose-dependent)	Incomplete abortion Hemorrhage Live-born fetus (rates higher than with saline) Nausea, vomiting, diarrhea (30%)	Intraamniotic instillation; most patients require oxytocin augmentation No longer available in United States in form used for induction Potent bronchoconstrictor
15-Methyl $PGF_{2\alpha}$	8-16	Vomiting, diarrhea, fever (2-3 episodes per patient)	Intramuscular (has also been used via intra-amniotic, extra-amniotic, vaginal routes)
Dinoprostone (PGE_2)	11-14 (6-7 hr with cervical ripening)	Fever, nausea, vomiting, diarrhea (most patients experience at least one side effect)	Vaginal suppositories Must be refrigerated
Sulprostone (PGE_2)	11	Vomiting (12%-46%) Diarrhea (6%-17%)	Given intramuscular or intravenously Not available in United States
Gemeprost (PGE_1)	15	Vomiting (1%-14%)	Vaginal pessary
+ mifepristone	6-8	Diarrhea (2%-20%)	Not available in United States
Misoprostol (PGE_1)	9-14	Vomiting (4%-10%)	Oral or vaginal routes
+ mifepristone	6-10	Diarrhea (4%-15%)	Inexpensive; no refrigeration required
+ laminaria	10-22		

PG, prostaglandin.

and misoprostol regimens with or without priming by mifepristone.[256–263] No well-controlled study has shown any method as being better than the others. All oxytocic agents should be used with caution in patients with previous cesarean deliveries. Women should be appropriately counseled about the risks and consequences, and practitioners should be prepared to deal with a rupture if and when it occurs. The optimum chance for successful outcome is provided by an informed and alert clinician who appreciates the potential risks of the procedure and who is prepared to deal with those risks.

SIDE EFFECTS AND COMPLICATIONS

Second-trimester TOP is a relatively safe procedure in countries where it is legal, accessible, and performed under modern medical conditions. However, both the patient and the practitioner must be aware of procedure- and medication-related side effects and complications, including acute medical events and potential long-term reproductive risks.

Side Effects of Prostaglandin-Induced Termination of Pregnancy

The use of PGs gemeprost and misoprostol, with or without mifepristone, is a safe and effective method for second-trimester TOP. Side effects including nausea, vomiting, and diarrhea are characteristics of PG administration and due to PG's stimulatory effect on the gastrointestinal tract. Diarrhea is more common in women using gemeprost, whereas fever is more common with misoprostol.[170,174] The advantages of using misoprostol for second-trimester TOP compared with other PG agents are the relatively low incidence of reported side effects (Table 66–7). Side effects reported from the use of high-dose oxytocin regimens include nausea and vomiting. Prolonged usage may cause water intoxication. The suggested high-dose oxytocin regimen includes an alternating period of oxytocin infusion and a drug-free interval to allow for clearance of the oxytocin to avoid water intoxication.

Complications Associated with Medical Termination of Pregnancy

Complications common to most medical TOP include retained placenta and associated hemorrhage or infection, failed TOP, live birth, and serious complications such as uterine rupture.

Retained Placenta (Incomplete Abortion) Patients who underwent medical TOP compared with those who had D&E were more likely to have retained products of conception that required operative intervention (21% vs. 0.7%). Although patients who underwent medical TOP with misoprostol were less likely to have complications than patients who underwent medical TOP by other methods (22% vs. 55%), these patients still had more complications than surgical patients (22% vs. 4%). Patients who elect to undergo second-trimester medical abortion should be advised that they have a significant risk (21%) of requiring surgery for retained products of conception, because this knowledge may assist them in making an informed decision.[174]

Sixty percent of subjects passed the placenta spontaneously within 2 hours, with approximately two thirds of the expulsions occurring within the first 30 minutes. The rate of complications (hemorrhage and febrile morbidity) increased over time, reaching 4% at 30 minutes and 9% at 2 hours.[264] Retained tissues can lead to hemorrhage, infection, or both, and usually manifests itself within several days of the TOP. Cramping and bleeding can be accompanied by fever. If complete placental expulsion did not occur within 4 hours of fetal delivery, the placenta was removed manually or by forceps or curettage.[264,265]

Infection During the second trimester, infection rates for both medical and surgical TOP methods have remained within the narrow range of 0.4% to 2.0% in North America and Great Britain.[172,174] Infection is usually associated with retained products of conception, but there are no data to analyze the incidence of infection separately in cases with or without retained tissue. Typically, signs and symptoms of post-TOP infection arise within the first 48 to 96 hours. The patient may present with pain, fever, and pelvic tenderness. The cervix should be cultured for sexually transmitted-pathogens—*Neisseria* (gonorrhea) and *Chlamydia*. Established risk factors for post-TOP infection include age younger than 20 years, nulliparity, previous pelvic inflammatory disease, and presence of pathogens in the cervix at the time of TOP. The latter association has been reported with documented *Chlamydia* infection, gonorrhea, and bacterial vaginosis.[209] Most post-TOP infections, however, occur in women without these risk factors. Routine antibiotic prophylaxis may prevent up to half of all post-TOP infections in the United States and is highly cost-effective. Tetracyclines or nitroimidazoles (metronidazole or tinidazole) were equally efficacious for preventing infection.[208] Ascending genital tract infections are typically polymicrobial. Patients who present with post-TOP metritis should receive a full course of broad-spectrum antibiotic therapy. When retained tissue is evident or suspected, prompt evacuation is indicated.

Failure of Medical Termination of Pregnancy *Failed induction* has been defined as a failure to achieve TOP within 24 to 48 hours and is a significant clinical problem. Management options include deferring TOP when membranes are intact for a predetermined time, aggressive cervical dilation with sequential laminaria application and another trial of induction, changing the induction agent used, or recommending D&E.

Uterine Rupture Serious complications including uterine rupture, major hemorrhage, and cervical tear are rare.[172,174] Cases of uterine rupture were reported to occur with both gemeprost and misoprostol, and the use of mifepristone did not exclude the possibility.[261,262] The incidence of uterine rupture was estimated to be 0.2% in the second trimester. Risk factors for uterine rupture include previous cesarean delivery, grand multipara, advanced gestation, prolonged PG therapy, and use of oxytocin in addition to PGs.[261]

Live Birth Second-trimester medical TOP with PG analogues has been associated with live birth rates of 4% to 10%.[175,219] Physicians should have a protocol to induce fetal death (e.g., fetal intracardiac KCl or digoxin) before induction, and patients should be apprised of the risk for live birth and should understand the plan in advance.

TABLE 66–8

Comparison of Complication Rates among Medical and Surgical TOP Study Subjects

COMPLICATION	MEDICAL (*n* = 158)	SURGICAL (*n* = 139)	*P* VALUE
Patients with any complication	45 ± 28.5	5 ± 3.6	<.001
Failed initial method	11 ± 7.0	0 ± 0	<.01
Hemorrhage with transfusion	1 ± 0.6	1 ± 0.7	NS
Infection with intravenous antibiotics	2 ± 1.3	0 ± 0	NS
Retained products of conception	33 ± 20.9	1 ± 0.7	<.001
Cervical laceration with repair	2 ± 1.3	3 ± 2.2	NS
Organ damage	2 ± 1.3	0 ± 0	NS
Hospital readmission	1 ± 0.6	1 ± 0.7	NS

NS, not significant; TOP, termination of pregnancy.
Modified from Autry AM, Hayes EC, Jacobson GF, Kirby RS: A comparison of medical induction and dilation and evacuation for second-trimester abortion. Am J Obstet Gynecol 2002;187:393–397.

Complications Associated with Dilation and Evacuation (Table 66–8)

Based on the data from the 1970s and 1980s, D&E is clearly safer than intra-amniotic instillation methods and hysterotomy or hysterectomy for second-trimester TOP through 16 weeks' gestation.[167,172,190–192] In these investigations, most of the specific complications associated with D&E occurred at rates well below 1%. A report by Autry and associates[174] confirmed both the low complication rate that is associated with D&E and its superiority over medical TOP. When skilled operators are available, D&E after cervical preparation with laminaria should be considered the preferred method for second-trimester TOP. Hence, the choice of TOP method at this later stage usually hinges on nonmedical considerations: cost, convenience, comfort, and compassion.

In challenging or difficult cases, careful assessment and choice of TOP method should be made to minimize complications. Intraoperative ultrasonography may be helpful in difficult cases.[188] Previous cesarean delivery scar does not seem to increase the perioperative risk of late termination (14–22 wk) by the laminaria and evacuation technique.[215]

Hemorrhage Reported rates of hemorrhage vary widely, reflecting both diverse definitions and imprecise estimation of blood loss. Hemorrhage associated with TOP is not common and the Royal College of Obstetricians and Gynaecologists (RCOG) guideline group[169] reported this complication as 1.5 per 1000 TOPs overall. Factors associated with increased risk of uterine hemorrhage were operator inexperience, advanced gestational age, advanced maternal age and parity, prior cesarean delivery, uterine fibroids, and past history of post-TOP or postpartum bleeding.[167,170] Hemorrhage associated with D&E may indicate cervical laceration, perforation, retained tissue, uterine atony, placental abnormalities, or coagulopathy. Advances in operative technique and use of uterotonic agents have resulted in reduction of both mean and median blood loss in North America.

Intraoperative use of oxytocin, ergots, and PGs reduces blood loss from uterine atony during D&E. Treatment of uterine atony includes manual uterine compression, oxytocin infusion, ergot derivatives, and PGs (15-methyl $PGF_{2\alpha}$, PGE_1).

Second-trimester TOP by D&E in the presence of placenta previa appears to be safe and apparently does not increase maternal morbidity compared with the outcome in patients without placenta previa undergoing the same procedure.[212] All placenta accreta patients had at least one cesarean delivery (mean 1.7), and prior to operation a sonogram demonstrating some form of placenta previa. The prevalence of clinical placenta accreta encountered during D&Es in the second trimester was 0.04%, the same as that reported for placenta accreta diagnosed clinically in the third trimester. Placenta accreta can be a potential complicating factor in the patient undergoing D&E in the second trimester.

Cervical Injury The most common type of cervical injury is a superficial laceration caused by the tenaculum or Allis forceps tearing off during dilation. At the other extreme are the cervicovaginal fistula and the longitudinal laceration ascending to the level of the uterine vessels. Rates of cervical injury range from 0.01 to 1.6 per 100 suction curettage TOPs.[165,166]

Several risk factors for cervical injury during suction curettage have emerged. Among factors within the control of the physician, use of laminaria and performance of the TOP by an attending physician (rather than a resident) lower the risk significantly. Among factors beyond the control of the physician, a history of prior abortion lowers the risk, and age of 17 years or younger increases the risk. Use of laminaria and performance of the TOP under local anesthesia by an attending physician together yield a 27-fold protective effect.[167] Cervical preparation with misoprostol may confer similar benefits as laminaria, although more extensive experience will be needed to confirm this.

Perforation Perforation is a potentially serious, but infrequent, complication of D&E. According to most reports, the incidence of perforation is about 0.2 per 100 suction curettage TOPs.[165,166]

Several risk factors for perforation exist. Performance of a curettage TOP by a resident rather than an attending physician increases the risk more than fivefold; conversely, cervical dilation by laminaria decreases the risk about fivefold. The risk of perforation increases significantly with advancing gestational age. Previous gynecologic surgery including TOP, cesarean delivery, and large loop excision of the transformation zone of the cervix (LLETZ) procedure is a risk factor for tearing of the internal os leading to perforation of the uterus during subsequent D&E procedures.[266] Dilation of the cervix particularly for these "at-risk" procedures should be predominantly passive by the use of oral PGs such as misoprostol and osmotic dilators. The overall perforation rate was 0.029%.[267]

The use of real-time ultrasound scanning during D&E can reduce perforation rates. The routine intraoperative use of ultrasonographic imaging to guide intrauterine forceps during uterine evacuation for second-trimester TOP resulted in a significant reduction in uterine perforation, the rate declining from 1.4% to 0.2%.[193] These findings support the routine use of intraoperative ultrasonography for second-trimester TOP to reduce the incidence of uterine perforation and make the procedure a safer one.

The two principal dangers of perforation are hemorrhage and damage to the abdominal contents. Lateral perforations in the cervicoisthmic region are particularly hazardous because of the proximity of the uterine vessels. Perforations of the fundus are more likely to be innocuous. Many suspected or documented perforations require only observation. Perforation with a dilator or sound is unlikely to damage abdominal contents. Conversely, a suction cannula or forceps in the abdominal cavity can be devastating.

If the physician suspects a perforation, the procedure should stop immediately. If unmanageable hemorrhage, expanding hematoma, or injury to abdominal content occurs, prompt laparotomy is necessary. Laparoscopy can be useful in documenting perforation and assessing damage; if necessary, the physician can complete the abortion under laparoscopic visualization. Any woman with severe pain within hours after D&E should be evaluated for possible perforation with bowel injury.

ACUTE MEDICAL EVENTS

Acute medical events, such as vasovagal reaction, asthmatic reactions, amniotic fluid embolism, anaphylaxis, and seizures to anesthetic agents or laminaria, can occur at the time of TOP.[268–270] The safety of PG agents used for TOP has been established. Side effects are usually of a minor nature, although life-threatening complications can occur and include cardiac arrest.[271] This severity emphasizes the importance of medical supervision when the procedure is carried out.[247]

LONG-TERM REPRODUCTIVE RISKS

The bulk of evidence would suggest that D&E is a very safe procedure with few long-term problems. There is no proven association between D&E and subsequent fertility difficulty.[272] Second-trimester D&E is not a risk factor for midtrimester pregnancy loss or spontaneous preterm birth. Preterm delivery in future gestations appears less likely when greater preoperative cervical dilation is achieved with laminaria, possibly because of a decrease in cervical trauma.[273–275] Published studies have not been prospective and have not been able to control for competing risk factors, such as smoking or exposure to STIs, that might overestimate the impact of induced TOP on poor reproductive outcome. Long-term complications associated with medical TOP in the second trimester using gemeprost and misoprostol with or without mifepristone are rarely reported.

SUMMARY OF MANAGEMENT OPTIONS
Second-Trimester Termination of Pregnancy

Management Options	Evidence Quality and Recommendation	References
Prenatal—General		
Accurate estimation of gestational age.	III/C	172,174
Accurate diagnosis.	—/GPP	—
Patient assessment and counseling.	—/GPP	—
Dilation and Evacuation		
Cervical preparation		203,204,207
• Laminaria.	IIa/B	
• Misoprostol.	IIb/B	
Use of prophylactic antibiotics.	—/GPP	208–210
Use of intraoperative ultrasound.	—/GPP	193
Use of intraoperative oxytocin.	—/GPP	—
Medical Abortion		
Fetocidal agent—KCl or digoxin.	III/B	225,226
Mifepristone 36–48 hr, then vaginal misoprostol followed by oral misoprostol.	Ia/A	227,245–247
Laminaria/Foley + vaginal misoprostol, then oral misoprostol concurrently.	IIb/B	225
Failed Medical Abortion	III/B	188
D&E or hysterotomy or hysterectomy.		

D&E, dilation and evacuation; GPP, good practice point; KCl, potassium chloride.

SUGGESTED READINGS

American College of Obstetricians and Gynecologists (ACOG): Induction of labor (Practice Bulletin No. 107). Obstet Gynecol 2009;114: 386–397.

Boulvain M, Catalin M, Irion O: Membrane sweeping for induction of labour. Cochrane Pregnancy and Childbirth Group. Cochrane Database Syst Rev 2005;1:CD000451. Available at http://www.mrw.interscience.wiley.com/cochrane/clsysrev/articles/CD000451/frame.html (accessed August 22, 2009).

Hatfield AS, Sanchez-Ramos L, Kaunitz AM: Sonographic cervical assessment to predict the success of labor induction: a systematic review with meta-analysis. Am J Obstet Gynecol 2007;197:186–192.

Heinemann J, Gillen G, Sanchez-Ramos L, Kaunitz AM: Do mechanical methods of cervical ripening increase infectious morbidity? A systematic review. Am J Obstet Gynecol 2008;199:177–187.

Hofmeyr GJ, Gülmezoglu AM: Vaginal misoprostol for cervical ripening and induction of labour. Cochrane Database Syst Rev 2003;1:CD000941. Available at http://www.mrw.interscience.wiley.com/cochrane/clsysrev/articles/CD000941/frame.html (accessed August 22, 2009).

Kundodyiwa TW, Alfirevic Z, Weeks AD: Low-dose oral misoprostol for induction of labor: A systematic review. Obstet Gynecol 2009;113: 374–383.

Lohr PA, Hayes JL, Gemzell-Danielsson K: Surgical versus medical methods for second trimester induced abortion. Cochrane Database Syst Rev 2008;1:CD006714. Available at http://www.mrw.interscience.wiley.com/cochrane/clsysrev/articles/CD006714/frame.html (accessed August 22, 2009).

National Institute for Health and Clinical Excellence: Guideline on induction of labor (CG70). Available at http:/www.nice.org.uk/guidance/CG70 (accessed August 16, 2009).

Prairie BA, Lauria MR, Kapp N, et al: Mifepristone versus laminaria: A randomized controlled trial of cervical ripening in midtrimester termination. Contraception 2007;76:383–388.

von Hertzen H, Piaggio G, Wojdyla D, et al: Comparison of vaginal and sublingual misoprostol for second trimester abortion: Randomized controlled equivalence trial. Hum Reprod 2009;24:106–112.

REFERENCES

For a complete list of references, log onto www.expertconsult.com.

CHAPTER 67

Dysfunctional Labor

HARRY GEE

INTRODUCTION

It has long been recognized that dysfunctional labor leading to poor progress is associated with increased morbidity and mortality for both mother and fetus.[1] Parturition, though physiologic, places demands on the mother and fetus that may outstrip their ability to cope even under apparently normal circumstances. Not only does prolongation of labor expose underlying vulnerabilities, but harm can also arise directly from the underlying cause of delay. It is simplistic to think that accelerating progress, per se, will prevent such harm. A common theme running through currently popular interventions is that they speed up progress but fail to reduce the need for operative intervention. Poor progress is a sign of pathology rather than being, itself, pathologic. Ideally, its identification would result in a cause-specific treatment, but with our current knowledge and diagnostic ability, this is often not possible. Under these circumstances, it has been a pragmatic necessity to employ interventions on a trial-and-error basis—but such interventions should be validated by properly controlled clinical trials before being taken up into widespread use. Unfortunately, such prospective scrutiny has rarely been the case and only relatively recently have widely adopted interventions been examined—often with disappointing results. Failure to accept and acknowledge our lack of understanding has limited our ability to think laterally for solutions. As a result, our options for clinical management remain limited and often frustrating. Cesarean section rates continue to rise, and poor progress remains a major cause.[2]

This chapter provides a critical analysis of

- The physiology of labor.
- The methods for monitoring labor and their validity.
- The possible pathologies underlying poor progress.
- The effectiveness of interventions.
- The clinical options available.

THE ONSET AND DIAGNOSIS OF LABOR

Onset of Labor

In the human, no single trigger for the onset of labor has been identified. Figure 67–1 represents a possible mechanism. In the placental corticotropin model,[3,4] the appropriate endocrine environment for the onset of labor is set via the fetal pituitary-adrenal axis and the placenta. Rising fetal adrenal cortisol up-regulates the placental genes that produce more corticotropin stimulation, thereby setting in motion a positive feedback loop. Dehydroepiandrostenedione (DHEA) is a precursor for estriol production in the placenta, which creates the appropriate hormonal environment for labor in the mother. Further changes in placental function result in the generation of a number of pro-inflammatory agents (cytokines and interleukins), whereas the synthesis of prostaglandins and oxytocin integrates myometrial and cervical response.

Positive feedback systems promote change, not homeostasis. Once established, the feedback loop takes the uterus from a steady-state, pregnancy mode into active labor, which terminates only after delivery. Stimulating such a system carries a risk of hyperstimulation and uterine rupture if delivery is obstructed. This is particularly so in women who have labored before; although peculiarly, the uterus in a first labor tends to become inert in the face of obstruction. The reasons for this are not fully understood.

Efficient labor requires the coordination of myometrial activity and cervical ripening. Uterine contraction is the most easily observed and has, therefore, attracted the most attention—perhaps too much. Cervical function is much more subtle but no less important. The function of the cervix in pregnancy is to prevent delivery, and its collagenous composition with fibers wound tightly around the cervical canal are ideally suited to keeping the cervix tubular and closed. It is reasonable to propose that some instances of poor progress in the first stage of labor may be due to a lack of coordination between cervix and myometrium.[5] A cervix remaining in pregnancy mode will continue to resist dilation and delivery despite the myometrium going into labor mode with coordinated contractions.

The move from pregnancy to labor mode in the cervix is characterized by "ripening." The resultant increase in tissue compliance permits deformation. Effacement and formation of the lower segment are the initial manifestations of this, followed by dilation. In nulliparous women, these processes tend to be sequential, but in parous women, dilation may take place before effacement is complete. Either way, effacement redistributes tissue from the cervix to the lower segment and decreases cervical resistance.

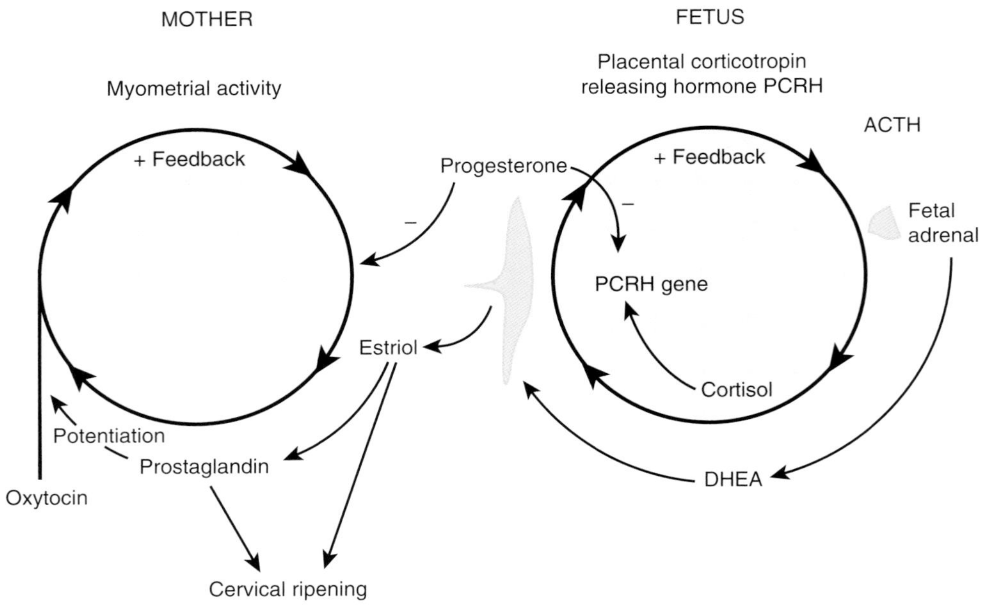

FIGURE 67–1
A model for the initiation of labor.

Throughout pregnancy, the myometrium is spontaneously active, but before the onset of labor, contractions originating in any particular muscle cell or group of muscle cells are not propagated throughout the myometrium. Under the influence of estrogens and prostaglandins, spontaneous activity rises throughout gestation; in addition, gap junctions (nexuses) form between muscle cells.[6] These junctions provide preferential pathways for electrical activity to pass from cell to cell, producing a coordinated response from the myometrium. As coordination increases, contractility becomes sufficient to raise the intrauterine pressure (IUP) and Braxton Hicks contractions can be perceived. However, until they are strong enough to exert considerable tension on the uterine wall and cervix, and the cervix is ripe enough to stretch at least a little in response, they are usually relatively painless.

By the time of the onset of labor, oxytocin is already in high concentrations in the maternal circulation, and oxytocin receptors have developed on the membranes of smooth muscle cells. Thus, oxytocin is thought to facilitate labor rather than initiate it.[7]

Prostaglandins *potentiate* the action of oxytocin. Potentiation results in greater tone than would result from the simple additive effect of prostaglandin and oxytocin. Estrogens promote the production of prostaglandins in the decidua, which lies between the fetal membranes and the myometrium.[8] In addition, other agents, such as interleukins and cytokines, are involved in the inflammatory cascade[9] that characterizes labor. This is a one-way process that once started, goes to completion, stimulating the maternal positive feedback loop. This results in an exponential rise in uterine activity at the beginning of labor and a more gradual rise thereafter,[10] culminating in the second stage.

Many of the agents involved in the initiation of labor affect both cervix and myometrium with the net effect of creating the right local environment for labor to occur and progress efficiently, but they do so in different ways and over different timescales. Those affecting the cervix rely on biochemical remodeling of its constituents. This requires hours or days to take effect. Oxytocin is unusual in that its effect is almost specific to myometrial contractility and it acts rapidly (there are oxytocin receptors and a small amount of active smooth muscle in the cervix in labor,[11] but the effect of oxytocin on the cervix is minimal). Because cervix and myometrium may respond at different rates, it is reasonable to postulate that one may be in advance of the other. Thus, premature, pathologic cervical ripening may be a factor in preterm delivery, and conversely, establishment of uterine activity prior to cervical ripening will produce delay and slow cervical dilation.

Diagnosis of Labor

The diagnosis of labor is crucial because it brings with it intervention.

Two essential characteristics must be considered:

- The presence of regular uterine contractions, leading to:
- Progressive change in the cervix.

A subsidiary characteristic may be spontaneous rupture of the amniotic membranes.

Friedman,[12–14] whose graphic analysis of labor laid the foundations for current practice, based the diagnosis of labor on recognition of the onset of regular uterine contractions. Unfortunately, this is problematic because the onset of uterine activity is a smooth escalation that can take place over several days or, occasionally, longer. Precise delineation of a transition point between Braxton Hicks contractions and those leading to progressive dilation of the cervix has not been possible. Electromyography and other sophisticated methods of observation and analysis[15–17] can identify patterns of uterine activity that are characteristic of labor, but their superiority over simpler clinical methods to delineate contractions associated with cervical dilation remains to be proved.

FIGURE 67–2
Friedman's representation of cervical dilation in labor.

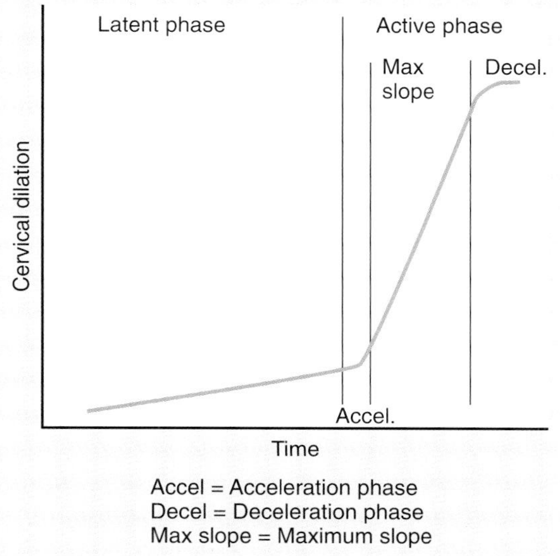

Thus, fundamentally, the diagnosis of progressive labor relies upon identifying changes in the cervix. Friedman used assessment of cervical dilation to divide the first stage of labor into latent and active phases (Fig. 67–2).

During the latent phase, the cervix is changing (primarily by effacement secondary to softening/ripening) but showing little dilation. The active phase is characterized by progressive cervical dilation. This is the process that is assessed regularly and used to monitor progress. The division between latent and active phases is not precise, and the latent phase often blends gradually into the active phase. Friedman's curves place the transition at 2 to 3 cm' dilation, but some would consider it to be as late as 4 cm[18] to ensure that the active phase has been entered.

Clinically, it makes good sense to restrict the diagnosis of labor to evidence of cervical dilation[19] because of the following points:

- Dilation is relatively easy to recognize and record (on a cervicogram).
- Currently accepted limits and interventions for labor apply predominantly to the active phase.

Other definitions of the onset of labor have been used for research purposes and will be found in the literature, for example, the time of admission to delivery suite.[20] This is an easily recorded and precise measure but is of little physiologic importance.

Management Options for the Diagnosis of Labor

Women are readily aware of their uterine activity. In particular, women in their first labors (though it can happen thereafter), not having experienced labor before, are prone to present as soon as regular contractions are perceived. When examined, however, it is common to find their cervices still uneffaced and/or undilated. They are often disappointed (and sometimes demoralized) to be told they are not in the active phase of labor.

The Management Options in such circumstances are

1. To diagnose labor (i.e., labor has started) and commence intrapartum care. However, premature commencement of intrapartum care with all that it entails runs the risk of misinterpreting the normal changes of early labor, resulting in unnecessary intervention.
2. To diagnose labor only when entry to the active phase has been established and progressive cervical dilation is demonstrable (usually beyond 3 cm dilation).

A clear explanation of what is happening and why patience is required should be given to the woman (and her partner/family). This requires a sympathetic approach and an understanding of the frustration that the woman often experiences. It is important to offer pain relief if this is needed, although simple measures such as warm baths and reassurance should be tried first.

It should be noted that, although regular uterine contractions with intact membranes and without evidence of progressive cervical dilation should probably not be classified as "labor," they are still associated with interruptions of the maternal intervillous blood supply and, therefore, represent a hypoxic challenge to the fetus. Thus, fetuses with poor reserve, such as those likely to be affected by uteroplacental insufficiency, should always be monitored carefully when there are contractions, even if there is no progressive cervical dilation.

LABOR MECHANISMS AND PROCESSES

Progress in labor results from the interaction of three factors:

- Powers.
- Passages.
- Passengers.

Powers

Efficient uterine activity is crucial to promote the formation of the birth canal and impart flexion and rotation to the passenger so that it can pass through the complex geometry of the canal.

In the first stage of labor, there is little change in uterine volume. Myometrial contractions are, to all intent and purpose, isometric (i.e., there is minimal shortening of the muscle fibers as they develop tension). Wall tension is required to dilate the cervix, but it is important that the muscle fibers do not shorten significantly at this stage because this would carry the risk of gradually but progressively compressing the blood vessels traversing the myometrium. This, in turn, would reduce placental perfusion continuously rather than the intermittent reduction and recovery associated with truly isometric contractions.[21]

Progress is determined by the equilibrium between force (myometrial contractions in the corpus) and resistance (lower segment and cervix). This is almost self-evident, but there is a more subtle effect. The "give" from a compliant cervix attenuates the tension generated by the myometrium.[22,23] Thus, a compliant cervix not only dilates quickly but does so with less uterine activity (as measured using changes in intra-amniotic pressure). An everyday paradox resulting from this is that multiparous women have faster rates of cervical dilation than nulliparous women but with lower levels of uterine activity.[24] Conversely, a noncompliant cervix will delay progress and may be associated with high levels of uterine activity. Does the solution to dysfunctional labor lie with understanding the causes of these paradoxes rather than the conventional approach of simplistically applying more force?

Assessment of Uterine Activity

Four variables must be taken into account to assess uterine activity comprehensively. The first three are generated by the contractions themselves: amplitude, duration, and repetition frequency. Uterine activity can be quantified objectively by measurement of IUP. IUP is directly proportional to wall tension and indirectly proportional to uterine size. IUP monitoring is invasive, requiring insertion of either a fluid-filled catheter connected to an external transducer or a transducer-tipped catheter into the amniotic sac. This carries a small risk, from incorrect placement, abruption, uterine perforation, entanglement, and infection, although these risks are minimal with the modern designs of soft-tipped catheters. The fourth variable, basal pressure or *tone* is the product of resting muscular tone and elastic recoil of the uterus itself. External transducers can be "zeroed" against atmospheric pressure before commencing recording to give absolute values, but transducer-tipped catheters can record only relative pressure above baseline. In practice, the level of baseline tone does not contribute significantly to the rate of cervical dilation. It can, therefore, reasonably be ignored when assessing whether any particular level of uterine activity is likely to be associated with progressive cervical dilation. There are two pathologies which raise basal tone—abruption and hyperstimulation. Diagnosis of abruption depends on other clinical features, and hyperstimulation is better avoided by awareness of repetition frequency. There is an important circumstance when IUP monitoring can give false information. This occurs when attempting vaginal delivery after previous cesarean section.[25] If the scar is weak and stretches or gives way under tension, it will attenuate wall tension, thereby reducing IUP. If there is delay, this may be falsely attributed to suboptimal uterine activity.

IUP monitoring has never been shown in prospective, randomized trials to improve the management of labor. This is because the amplitude of contractions correlates with the palpable duration (most contractions become palpable only when the IUP exceeds baseline tone by more than 15 mm Hg) and overall activity is dependent in large part on repetition frequency. Thus, palpation of contractions with timing of duration and, particularly, frequency can give an adequate, albeit semiquantitative, assessment of uterine activity for most clinical purposes, including oxytocin augmentation.[26] In particular, avoiding excessive contraction frequency (universally considered to be greater than one contraction every 2 min on average, or five contractions in 10 min) is the best way to safeguard fetal oxygenation. However, contraction frequency is not always a reliable guide to amplitude (strength) of contractions, and manual palpation can also be misleading if the woman is obese (leads to underestimation) or has a low pain threshold (can lead to overestimation).

Management Options for Monitoring Uterine Activity

1. Palpation—remains the standard method of monitoring uterine activity for clinical purposes.
2. IUP monitoring—under specific circumstances:
   - Contractions are difficult to palpate, for example, in obese patients.
   - There is uncertainty as to whether augmentation of labor (e.g., with an oxytocin infusion) is producing appropriate increases in uterine activity.
   - Producing data for research purposes.

Medicolegally, it may be desirable to demonstrate close and accurate monitoring of uterine activity, for example, with induction or augmentation of labor in the presence of a uterine scar, in grand multiparas, or when the fetus is particularly at risk from uterine hyperstimulation (e.g., when there is evidence of uteroplacental insufficiency). However, no studies clearly demonstrate any advantages to IUP monitoring in these circumstances, and some would counsel against such use in case they provide a false sense of security. An equally valid management option is not to use an oxytocic at all in such cases, resorting instead to cesarean section if there is poor progress. This latter option is increasingly being chosen in modern practice and is probably the cause of at least part of the rising cesarean section rate.

Normal Range of Uterine Activity

If progressive cervical dilation is taking place, there is no need for a lower limit to be placed on acceptable uterine activity. Only when there is perceived delay in labor should the adequacy of uterine activity be questioned.

Uterine activity increases as labor progresses due to prostaglandin release from the decidua and secretion of oxytocin from the maternal posterior pituitary. Spontaneous uterine activity at the end of the first stage can be in excess of levels considered safe for induced or augmented labor[10,27] and repetition frequencies in excess of four contractions per 10 minutes can occur. At these rates, there is a risk that placental blood flow and fetal oxygenation can be compromised. This may not be deleterious to a healthy fetus, with good uteroplacental function when labor is progressing with the prospect of imminent delivery. The ability of the fetus to cope is a function of duration and degree of "stress" (or "duress"). Therefore, caution should be exercised when uterine activity is augmented for delay, because uteroplacental function can never be guaranteed and delivery may not be imminent. In these circumstances, augmentation of uterine activity to a repetition frequency of five contractions in10 minutess, as recommended in some guidelines[18] may be cutting safety margins too fine.

Management Options

- If progress is within normal limits, uterine activity is not critical.
- A contraction frequency of three to four contractions every 10 minutes is optimal and provides a margin of safety; five in 10 minutes should be a maximum.
- Palpable contractions should last for minimum of 40 seconds.

Contractions occurring more frequently than five every 10 minutes with little or no relaxation constitute tachysystole.

Passages

The passages have often been equated solely with the bony pelvis, but the soft tissues are also important, including the cervix and lower segment in the first stage and the pelvic floor in the second stage.

Assessment of the Pelvis

Pathologically small pelvises are rare today in well-nourished populations. Childhood rickets used to be a relatively common cause of brim dystocia. If the fetal head could pass through the brim in such cases, it and the body would almost certainly traverse the rest of the pelvis. Hence, the importance obstetricians have traditionally given to "engagement." Thus, clinical and x-ray pelvimetry have poor predictive values.[28,29] More sophisticated imaging techniques, such as magnetic resonance imaging and computed tomography, coupled with ultrasound fetal biometry, have been used to improve diagnosis. This approach is logical, but further clinical research is required to establish their value.[30–33]

The shortcomings of pelvimetry, and the complex mechanism of labor with many interacting variables including flexion, rotation, molding, and even pelvic compliance, mean that clinicians have to fall back on "try it and see."

It should be noted that two out of three women who require a cesarean section for failure to progress in one labor go on to deliver normally the next time despite birth weight rising with parity. This suggests that absolute cephalopelvic disproportion is not a common cause for failure to progress.

Assessment of the Soft Tissues

The function of the cervix in pregnancy is to prevent delivery. Failure of the cervix to undergo its correct biophysical preparation may carry its pregnancy function through to labor. Abnormal connective tissue biochemistry has been demonstrated in association with poor progress.[34]

In the second stage of labor, the soft tissues of the pelvic floor help to induce the necessary rotational forces while, paradoxically at the same time, offering resistance to progress.

Measurement of the forces between the cervix and the fetal head has shown differences between progressive and delayed labor.[35–37] These data do not fit simple mechanical models, indicating that cervical dilation is a more complex process than mere stretching. Clinical application of these experimental techniques and the data they generate are awaited.

Clinical monitoring relies on the aggregate response of the cervix during labor. Digital estimation of cervical dilation is plotted against time (cervicography). This is a simple screening tool for deviation from a normal pattern, but because of the many variables that may be at play, it does not offer a diagnosis when progress is slow. It merely provides a sign associated with increased clinical risk.

Passengers

Birth weight within the normal range has poor predictive value for delivery complications. Figure 67–3 shows that there is some correlation of the duration of labor with birth weight, but the maximum variation over the extremes of birth weight is only 1.5 hours. The effects of flexion and rotation on the efficiency of the labor mechanisms are likely to be at least as important. The ability of the fetal head to mold is another important variable. Moreover, in terms of cephalopelvic disproportion, head size is not closely correlated with birth weight. For macrosomic fetuses, the main risk is shoulder dystocia. Unlike cephalopelvic disproportion, shoulder dystocia is not reliably predicted by cervical dilation rates in the first stage, and even the descent of the presenting part in the second stage can be normal.[38]

FIGURE 67–3
Duration of labor by birth weight. Data taken from 425,855 births with birth weight and duration of labor recorded in the North West region of London from 1988 to 2000.

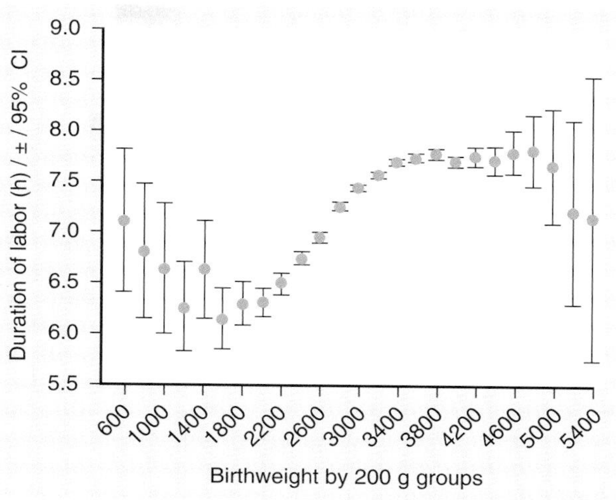

Only the extremes of birth weight have much significance in relation to mode of delivery. In recent U.K. practice, cesarean section was the mode of delivery in nearly 60% of pregnancies when the birth weight was less than 2.5 kg, and in 40% to 50% when the birth weight exceeded 5 kg (Fig. 67–4). However, there was relatively little variation in the use of cesarean section when the birth weight lay between 2.5 kg and 4 kg. In 513,381 births in the North West region of London between 1988 and 2000, this birth weight range accounted for 83.2% of all births. Thus, for the majority of babies, birth weight contributes little to the mode of delivery.

Some evidence suggests that birth weight is rising.[39] Even more important than the increasing mean birth weight is the increase in the proportion of babies weighing more than 4 kg, which in some European countries has now reached 30%. However, this increase in birth weight has to be viewed in the context of improved maternal nutrition and the general increase in maternal stature. Maternal obesity is increasing in many societies. This may influence birth weight and adversely affect the efficiency of labor itself.[40]

Assessment of Fetal Size

Even if birth weight was of crucial importance in determining progress in labor, birth weight can be predicted only to an accuracy of ±10% to 15% by ultrasound fetal biometry. The poor predictive value of these estimates means that they

FIGURE 67-4
Percentage of babies delivered by cesarean section, according to birth weight. Data taken from 513,381 births with birth weight and mode of delivery recorded in the North West region of London from 1988 to 2000.

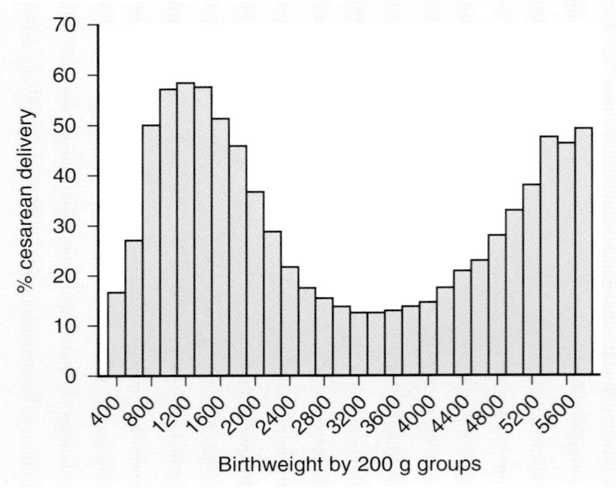

have to be factored in very cautiously when planning delivery. They should be taken into consideration, however, when delay is apparent. Other clinical features of cephalopelvic disproportion that should be sought include excessive molding and failure of the presenting part to engage and descend. Generally speaking, it is reasonable to assume that pelvic capacity is adequate if a woman has delivered vaginally before, but birth weight increases with parity, and the increase may be substantial if the woman has developed gestational diabetes due to advancing maternal age. Therefore, it is wise to check previous birth weights and any features of the current pregnancy (such as glucose intolerance) that may indicate borderline disproportion. This baby may be just that bit too big.

Cephalic Presentation: Flexion/Deflexion

Flexion and deflexion of the head determines the part that will present. *Flexion* results in a vertex presentation, that part of the head bounded by the occiput, the posterior part of the anterior fontanel, and the biparietal eminences. This results in the smallest dimensions of the head presenting themselves to the birth canal (9.5 cm × 9.5 cm). Flexion is promoted by efficient powers—uterine contractions in the first stage and the addition of maternal pushing in the second.

Deflexion of the head produces first a brow presentation and, then, in complete deflexion, a face presentation. The dimensions of a brow presentation in a term fetus are such (13.5 cm anteroposterior) that they cannot be accommodated by a normal pelvis. Thus, the head remains high, progress of labor may become obstructed with a secondary arrest pattern, or if full dilation is reached, there may be failure of descent. Brow presentation should be considered when a multiparous patient, who has delivered normal-sized babies without a problem before, develops abnormalities of progress. Resorting to oxytocin augmentation without consideration of this possibility risks uterine rupture.

MANAGEMENT OPTIONS FOR DEFLEXION

- Judicious prevarication can be adopted to see whether there will be spontaneous flexion.
- If uterine activity is suboptimal, augmentation with oxytocin can be tried to encourage flexion. Time limits should be set for this to happen and for poor progress to resolve, for example, 2 hours. Careful fetal monitoring should be used throughout.
- Cesarean section is usually the only option if spontaneous resolution does not occur in association with poor progress.

Babies with a face presentation can deliver vaginally, but only under favorable circumstances. The mentum must rotate anteriorly. This allows the head to flex as it negotiates the curve in the birth canal. To do so with a mentum posterior requires even further deflexion, which is anatomically impossible. A good-sized pelvis and efficient powers are necessary to deliver a face presentation spontaneously. Forceps can be used to add traction in the second stage.

Position: Rotation

The vertex normally engages with the occiput in a lateral position. This allows congruence between the long axis of the head and the widest diameter of the brim of the pelvis from side to side. With descent, the lowest part (occiput) is forced forward by the levator ani muscles that form an inclined plane running from back to front. This occurs in the mid-pelvis, which when cut in cross-section presents a circular shape that is conducive to rotation. With the occiput anterior and the head flexed, it is now able to fit through the diamond-shaped pelvic outlet with matching of the long axes of the head and the outlet. The head negotiates the curve of the birth canal by gradually extending.

If the head rotates and maintains a posterior position (OP), there is a tendency to deflex and present a larger dimension to the birth canal. To follow the curve of the birth canal the head must flex further. This is anatomically difficult and unlikely to occur. In the first stage, an OP position may present with any pattern of delay.

MANAGEMENT OPTIONS FOR MALROTATION

- Wait in expectation of spontaneous resolution.
- Augment the powers with a view to encouraging flexion and rotation.
- Perform cesarean section if neither of these produces progress.

If augmentation is undertaken, its potential dangers have to be acknowledged and safeguards employed, meaning continuous electronic fetal monitoring and timely reviews, particularly in a multiparous woman if progress is arrested.

Delay in the second stage while having similar factors can be addressed by instrumentation. This is discussed in Chapter 72.

CLINICAL ASPECTS OF MANAGEMENT OF LABOR

If a woman delivers vaginally the first time, she is much more likely to do so in the future. Thus, good management of the first labor is crucial and has a bearing on the rest of her reproductive potential.

MANAGEMENT OF THE FIRST STAGE OF LABOR

Active Management

Active management of labor carries a number of connotations and has been the subject of controversy since the early 1970s. In its broadest sense, it marked a change in philosophy from reacting to prolonged labor, diagnosed retrospectively after time had elapsed, to prospective monitoring of labor to detect delay early and instigate management.[41] As noted earlier, management should be based on a precise diagnosis, but this is often lacking. Thus, a more pragmatic approach emerged whereby prospective detection of departure from normal progress was automatically managed by augmenting the powers to accelerate progress because this was the only variable open to manipulation by the clinician.[19,42]

The Partogram

Figure 67–5 is a chart that represents the essential variables for monitoring both mother and fetus during labor. Graphic representation of data is useful because trends are important. The three sets of data relate to maternal signs, fetal signs, and progress of labor. Studies on the effectiveness of partograms have concentrated on the cervicogram component.[43,44] This is addressed later.

Maternal Signs

Maternal data comprise vital signs (pulse, blood pressure, temperature), urinalysis, and medical treatment (analgesia, uterotonics).

Fetal Signs

Fetal data comprise fetal heart rate, state of the membranes, color of the liquor, and descent and position of the presenting part.

Progress of Labor

THE CERVICOGRAM

The cervicogram is a component part of the partogram and, by definition, relates to the first stage. It represents, graphically, cervical dilation over time from the diagnosis of established labor. In practice, this applies only to the active phase. Because the usual concern is detection of delay, setting the lower limit of progress has been the focus of attention. Spontaneous, precipitate labor has been associated with risk, but this comes mainly from unexpected delivery rather than from the brevity of the process per se (although there is a reported increase in the incidence of Erb's palsy with precipitate labor—see Chapter 68).

DIAGNOSIS OF DELAY OR ABERRANCE

Friedman selected 200 nulliparous women, retrospectively, from a larger heterogeneous group of patients[13] and a similar cohort of parous women[14] to identify "ideal" labor, namely, no iatrogenic interventions (apart from "prophylactic low forceps"), vaginal deliveries, and average-sized, healthy neonates. These patients' labor curves were analyzed to identify statistical limits as means and standard deviations.

From these data, a lower limit of maximum slope of dilation was produced. The value of 1 cm/hr has now become almost universally accepted for clinical practice. However, this rate may be an overestimate for the following reasons:

- The statistical analysis is questionable. The data were not normally distributed, having a distribution skewed toward higher rates of dilation.
- Most clinicians use an average of 1 cm/hr for the whole of the active phase and not just the phase of maximum slope.

Better statistical analysis of progress in normal labor (Fig. 67–6)[45] shows lower rates of dilation in the early part of the active phase and no inflection points at the end of the phase of maximum slope. This pattern of progress is likely to be a better reflection of physiology, but is harder to apply to practice and needs more clinical evaluation.

Several cervicograms have been produced for clinical use. Hendricks and coworkers[46] produced similar patterns of dilation but chose the slowest 20% as the statistical divide. Philpott and Castle,[47] in a southern African population, produced data from an unspecified number of cases that represented the slowest 10% of primigravidas. They demonstrated a marked difference in the rate of maximum slope compared with Friedman's data (median 1.25 cm/hr vs. 2.75 cm/hr, respectively), suggesting that there may be significant population differences. They introduced the concept of an alert line followed 4 hours later by an action line.[48] This interval has been changed by other researchers, often without clear reason or benefit. It arbitrarily alters the sensitivity and specificity. Beazley and Kurjak[49] used a "low risk" population to produce a cervicogram whose limits differentiate progress above the line, resulting in an 80% chance of a favorable outcome, compared with only a 20% chance below it. This cervicogram acknowledges differing limits for nulliparous and parous women. Studd[50] devised a cervicogram from a multiracial population in the United Kingdom having "normal" labor. An S-shaped dilation curve was produced, with the steepest gradient between 4 cm and full dilation. The statistical methodology used to produce these curves was not specified, nor were the biologic limits.

All these cervicograms, in their various ways, attempt to define a boundary that can be used to define slow progress. However, they have been devised using data from specific populations with individual characteristics, and therefore, they may not be generalizable. As they all differ, it is unlikely that they can be used reliably without prospectively testing their clinical predictive value for any particular group. For example, it seems unlikely that the same cervicogram would be applicable to a black African population with their high assimilation pelvises and high obstructed labor rates, compared with white Scandinavians with their wide pelvises and low cesarean section rates.

Using data from later papers, the positive predictive value for operative delivery from an alert line set at 1 cm/hr gradient and an action line 2 hours later (values that are widely used today in the developed world) is only 43%. Use of standard cervicogram limits for the multiethnic populations of many of today's major cities seems unlikely

SURNAME ....
FORENAME ....
AGE ....
PARITY ....
WEEKS BY DATES/SCAN ....
UNIT No ....
CONSULTANT ....

ADMISSION ASSESSMENT
DATE TIME
SHOW ....
SROM ....
LABOUR DIAGNOSED ....
ARM ....
INDICATION ....
SYMPHYSIO-FUNDAL HEIGHT (CMS) ....

INDUCTION OF LABOR
PROSTIN PESSARY/GEL
DATE TIME
1. ....
2. ....
3. ....
ARM. ....
SYNTOCINON COMMENCED ....

1. ....
2. ....
3. ....
BIRTH PLAN REVIEWED YES☐ NO☐
REASON FOR CTG ....
BLOOD GROUP ....
LAST HB .... DATE ....

FETAL HEART
CTG X
PINARD OR SONIC AID }●

	0	1	2	3	4	5	6	7	8	9	10	11	12	13	14
190															
180															
170															
160															
150															
140															
130															
120															
110															
100															
90															
80															
LIQUOR															

RISK FACTOR
HIGH
LOW

X — CERVIX — X

● — DESCENT — Abdominal **5ths** **PALPABLE** ●

Cervix (cm)	5ths palpable															
10																
9																
8																
7																
6																
5	5/5th															
4	4/5															
3	3/5															
2	2/5															
1	1/5															
0	0/5															

POSITION OF CEPHALIC / BREECH

CONTRACTIONS WEAK
PALPATED MODERATE
NO PER 10 MIN STRONG

SYNTOCINON
(mU/min)
TIME

SIGNATURE

MATERNAL POSITION

RANITIDINE P.O. 150mg
RANITIDINE I.M. 50mg
PETHIDINE I.M. 50mg
PETHIDINE I.M. 100mg
STEMETIL I.M. 12.5mg
MARCAIN (see prescription)
ENTONOX

BLOOD PRESSURE AND PULSE
190, 180, 170, 160, 150, 140, 130, 120, 110, 100, 90, 80, 70, 60

TEMPERATURE

IV FLUIDS

URINE

URINALYSIS

DELIVERY DETAILS
DATE TIME
FULL DILATION ....
OR
VERTEX VISIBLE ....
ACTIVE PUSHING ....
TIME OF DELIVERY ....
LENGTH OF LAB ....

POSITION FOR DELIVERY ....

ND OA ☐
ND OP ☐
VENTOUSE ☐
FORCEPS ☐(REASON)
BREECH ☐
EM LSCS ☐
EL LSCS ☐
MULTIPLE ☐

COMMENTS ....

THIRD STAGE (MANAGEMENT)
PHYSIOLOGICAL ☐
ACTIVE ☐
OXYTOCIC DRUG

1) ....
2) ....
3) ....
IM☐ IV ☐
COMMENTS ....

DATE TIME
COMPLETION OF THIRD STAGE ....
PLACENTA COMPLETE ☐
INCOMPLETE ☐
MEMBRANES COMPLETE ☐
INCOMPLETE ☐
RAGGED ☐

COMMENTS ....

TOTAL BLOOD LOSS ....

PERINEUM
INTACT ☐
TEAR–DEFINE ☐
EPISOTOMY ☐ (REASON)
LACERATION(S) ☐
SUTURED ☐
NOT SUTURED ☐
LOCAL ☐
COMMENTS ....

SUTURED BY ....

BABY
APGARS .... 1 MIN .... 5 MINS
SEX .... BOY ☐
GIRL ☐

BIRTH WEIGHT ....
LENGTH ....
H.C. ....
TEMP. ....
CORD pH + BE ....
COMMENTS ....

DATE ....
SIG. NAMED MIDWIFE ....

FIGURE 67–5
Partogram.

to be adequate. Meta-analysis of randomized trials of the cervimetric component of partograms shows that they do not, in themselves, reduce cesarean section rates and action lines set 4 hours behind the 1 cm/hr alert line, as recommended by the World Health Organization (WHO),[51] are advised to avoid unnecessary intervention.[43,44]

Thus, cervicograms should be used only as an aid to the management of labor and not as a substitute for appropriate diagnosis. Transgression of a lower limit of progress does not indicate any particular course of action but should simply raise awareness of increasing risk, indicating the need to look for a cause.

FIGURE 67–6
Reanalysis of progress in nulliparous labor. (Data from Friedman FA: Cervimetry—An objective method for the study of cervical dilation in labor. Am J Obstet Gynecol 1956;71:1189-1193; Friedman EA: A cervimeter for continuous measurement of cervical dilatation in labour—Preliminary results (letter). Br J Obstet Gynaecol 1978:85:638; Friedman A: The labor curve. Clin Perinatol 1981;8:15-25; and Zhang J, Troendle JF, Yoncey MK: Reassessing the labor curve in nulliparous women. Am J Obstet Gynecol 2002;3:288-290.)

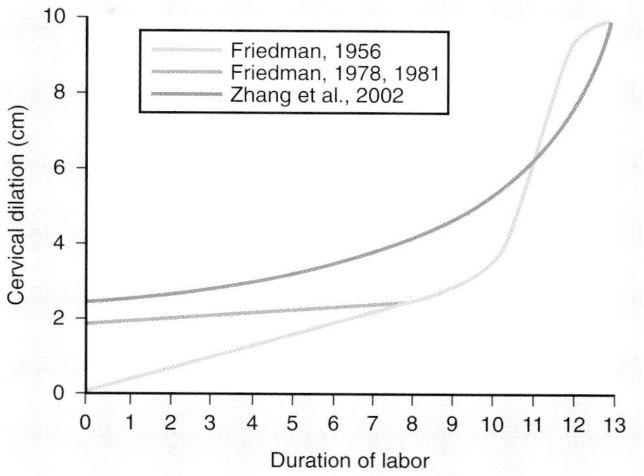

SUMMARY OF MANAGEMENT OPTIONS

Conduct of Normal Labor

Management Options	Evidence Quality and Recommendation	References
Use of a partogram facilitates the management of labor.	III/B	51
The cervicogram component of the partogram does not, in itself, improve the outcome of labor. It should be used only to identify delay.	Ia/A	44
The package of • Precise diagnosis of labor (active phase). • Early amniotomy. • Regular monitoring of cervical dilation rate. • Correction of poor dilation with the empirical augmentation of uterine activity limits prolonged labor.	III/B	19
Compared with active management, a policy of no routine amniotomy and selective use of oxytocin does not adversely affect cesarean section rates or neonatal outcome.	Ia, Ib/A	67–72
Support in labor reduces operative delivery rate.	Ia/A	73

Poor Progress

Friedman and Sachtleben[52] described three patterns of aberrance from normal labor (Fig. 67–7):

- Prolonged latent phase (PLP).
- Primary dysfunctional labor (PDL).
- Secondary arrest (SA).

None of these patterns is pathognomonic of a particular pathology. They are signs of pathology, not diagnoses.

Prolonged Latent Phase

Friedman and Sachtleben[52] described the latent phase, from the onset of contractions to entry to the active phase of dilation, as lasting up to 20 hours in nulliparas (mean 8.6 hr, standard deviation [SD] 6 hr) and 14 hours in parous women (mean 5.3 hours, SD 4.1 hr). The difficulties with defining the start and end of this phase have already been discussed. Thus, the true incidence of PLP is difficult to determine, but it is less common in parous women.

The causes of this pattern of delay are uncertain, but it is probably due to delayed cervical ripening. Myometrial activity and cervical ripening are out of synchrony (see Fig 67–1).

MANAGEMENT OPTIONS

1. Conservative management: from a practical point of view, and all else being equal, reassurance for the mother, analgesia, and time are often all that is necessary to allow cervical synchrony with that of the myometrium.

FIGURE 67–7
Patterns of delay.

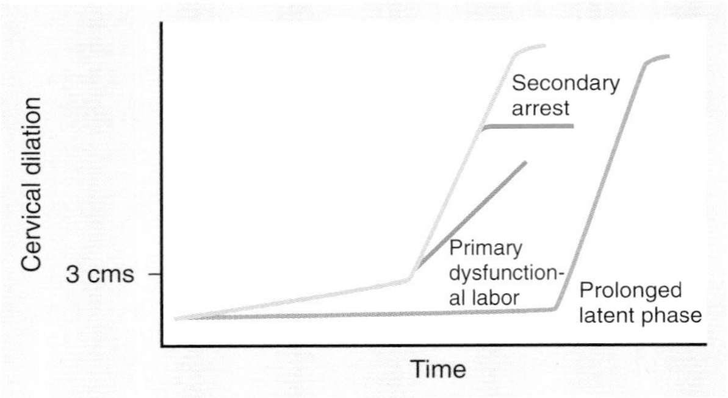

2. Augmentation of the powers to accelerate progress: this is not beneficial[20,53,54] and illogical. Such augmented labors exhibit a 10-fold increase in cesarean section rates compared with normal labors, with a threefold increase in low Apgar scores in the neonates.

Primary Dysfunctional Labor

Primary dysfunctional labor is defined as progress slower than 1 cm/hr during the active phase slope with an incidence of 26% in nulliparas and 8% in parous women.[53] About 80% of nulliparas and 90% of parous women will respond to oxytocin, suggesting that poor uterine activity is a significant factor. The only randomized clinical trial to test early versus delayed augmentation[55] shows that early use of oxytocin for this condition shortens labor and may reduce the need for instrumental delivery in the second stage but does not affect the cesarean section rate. Five percent of augmented labors do not respond in terms of increasing their uterine activity or rates of progress, and these nonresponsive labors are associated with cesarean section rates of 77%. Conversely, 23% still achieve a vaginal delivery,[20] so even apparent failure of response cannot be seen as an automatic indication for cesarean section. This paradox should raise questions about the cause and the validity of our definition of abnormality. Mechanical factors can be postulated (particularly malposition, malrotation and deflexion, and slow molding of the fetal head), which correct themselves in time, but sound evidence for a single causal effect is hard to find. Other possibilities have not been extensively studied. Abnormalities of cervical mechanics and biochemical preparation have been documented[34] and merit further study.

MANAGEMENT OPTIONS

1. If uterine activity is suboptimal, correct with oxytocin.
2. If uterine activity is optimal, check for
   - Malposition.
   - Malpresentation.
   - Cephalopelvic disproportion.
   - Combination of these.
   - None of these may be apparent. A decision then has to be made as to whether to do nothing in anticipation of spontaneous resolution or to use oxytocin judiciously, recognizing its accompanying risks and employing close monitoring and frequent review.

Secondary Arrest

Secondary arrest can be identified by cessation of progress after normal active phase dilation. Incidences of 6% in nulliparas and 2% in parous women have been reported.[56] A subtle variant of secondary arrest is delay between 7 and 10 cm. Even though full dilation may be achieved, there is an increased risk of difficult instrumental delivery.[57]

Of the three patterns of arrest, SA has the most convincing link with etiology, namely disproportion and malposition. This is understandable because normal early progress suggests the powers are adequate and the cervix compliant. Although in one series, 60% of nulliparas and 70% of parous women showed improved progress with augmentation of contractions, cesarean section rates were over 10-fold greater than in normal labor.[20] The effect of uterine stimulation may be to encourage flexion and rotation of the head, promoting descent and progress. However, well-conducted randomized clinical trials are awaited.

MANAGEMENT OPTIONS

1. Uterine activity should be checked. Correct if suboptimal.
2. Uterine activity may already be optimal. Therefore, check for:
   - Malposition.
   - Malpresentation.
   - Cephalopelvic disproportion.
   - Combination of these.
   - None of these.

   2a. Do nothing in anticipation of spontaneous resolution.
   2b. Judicious use of oxytocin, recognizing the risks.
   2c. Delivery by cesarean section.

Most would opt for 2b and then 2c if no response/progress occurs.

Practice Point

Whatever the pattern of delay, identification of a clear, single etiologic factor is unlikely. This may be due to complex interactions between multiple factors, an inability to detect the contributory factor because the diagnostic tools are imprecise, lack of knowledge of other factors, or finally a combination of all three. Treatment is more likely to be successful when a diagnosis of a single pathologic process is possible. Augmentation of the powers may be the only intervention available, and the "do nothing" arm of clinical trials has been woefully absent, leaving this option surrounded with uncertainty.

Thus, the obstetrician faced with evidence of delay should be conversant with the options available and be prepared to balance the risks and benefits of any intervention to be employed.

Interventions

Amniotomy

It is commonly stated that amniotomy increases uterine activity, although the evidence for this is weak, and there are good reasons to keep the membranes intact. For example, more fetal heart rate decelerations have been noted following amniotomy. Randomized clinical trials of routine amniotomy show that surgical intervention is not reduced, and there are no major benefits for the neonate,[58–61] though labor may be shortened. If there is poor progress with intact membranes and uterine activity is thought to be suboptimal, a case for amniotomy can be made, but even this has been called into question by a meta-analysis of trials to date.[62] Amniotomy has also been advocated to allow early detection of meconium as an aid to the assessment of fetal well-being and, therefore, may sometimes be useful if the fetal heart rate pattern is non-reassuring. In summary, all other features of labor being normal, there is no clinical benefit from routine amniotomy.

Oxytocin Augmentation

When oxytocin became readily available for clinical use in the 1960s, obstetricians were given some degree of control over one of the three variables that determine progress, namely the powers. As already stated, the powers also indirectly influence flexion and rotation of the passenger.

Oxytocin is a polypeptide hormone secreted from the posterior pituitary of both mother and fetus. The half-life of oxytocin is only 5 to 7 minutes. Therefore, its effect can be removed rapidly merely by stopping the infusion.

Binding of oxytocin to its receptor[63] opens calcium-activated channels (Fig. 67–8) and results in membrane depolarization.[7] This, in turn, opens voltage-dependent channels, producing a rise in intracellular calcium that generates tension in the contractile filaments. The primary effect is to increase the frequency of contractions, with a second effect of slowing conduction and recruiting more cells per contraction. This is beneficial when the myometrium shows "incoordinate" activity. The combined result is increased duration and amplitude. From the standpoint of clinical management, palpation of frequency and duration is a logical and simple means of monitoring oxytocin's effect.[26]

Both of these effects are beneficial when the myometrium is hypotonic, but addition of oxytocin to an already optimally acting myometrium frequently induces hypertonus, with resulting fetal hypoxia (Fig. 67–9). Careful monitoring of uterine activity is essential and infusion rates may have to be reduced as labor proceeds. Titration of dosage against uterine activity should be performed using regimens that allow time for activity to become stabilized between increments. An interval of 30 minutes between increments is recommended.[18] Published protocols generally recommend a starting dose of 1 to 6 mU/min; in current practice, 1 to 2 mU/min is usually used. Geometrically increasing regimens (e.g., 1, 2, 4, 8, 16, 32 mU/min) reach effective doses more quickly but are more prone to cause hyperstimulation and have, therefore, generally been replaced by arithmetic increases (e.g., 1, 2, 4, 6, 8, 10, 12 mU/min). The majority of women will respond to dose rates of 8 mU/min, and few will need more than 16 mU/min.

When oxytocin is used in labor, it must be maintained for the third stage and for an hour thereafter to reduce the risk of uterine atony and postpartum hemorrhage.

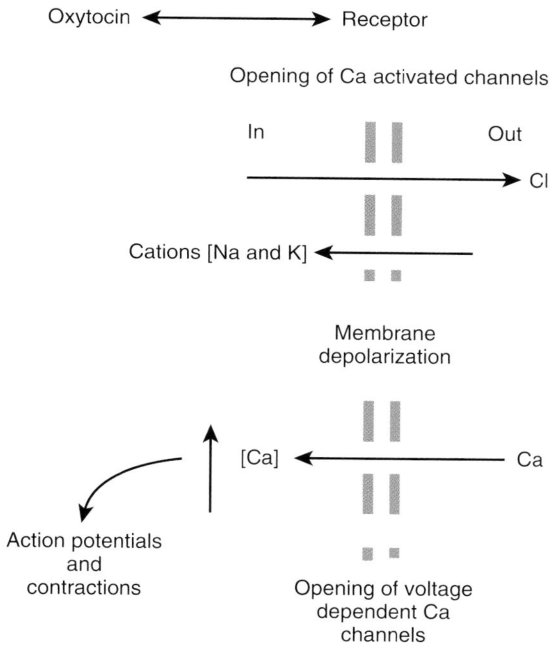

FIGURE 67–8
Action of oxytocin.

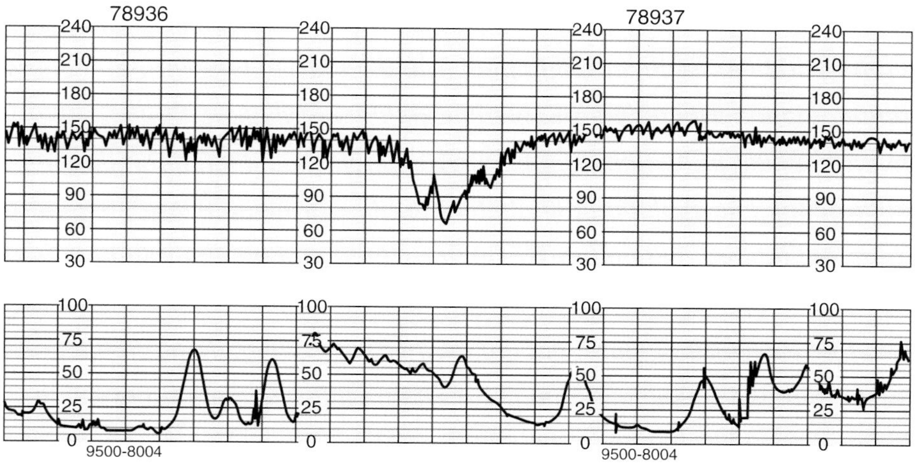

FIGURE 67–9
Hyperstimulation due to oxytocin showing the effect on fetal heart rate. Note the frequent small-amplitude contractions and rise in basal tone.

Postpartum hemorrhage is also associated with prolonged labor.

Meta-analysis of clinical trials of oxytocin augmentation show an increase in the parturient's subjective experience of pain and some increase in the rate of cervical dilation but little or no reduction in cesarean section and instrumental delivery rates.[64]

Epidural Analgesia

Epidural analgesia does not affect progress in the first stage of labor nor increase cesarean section rates. Second stages are longer and instrumental delivery more likely.[65]

Packaged Labor Management

In 1969, a report was published from the National Maternity Hospital, Dublin,[19] describing low cesarean section rates in a cohort of 1000 nulliparous women using a package of care that included

1. Correct diagnosis of labor.
2. Routine amniotomy.
3. Regular, frequent cervical assessment.
4. Augmentation of the powers with intravenous oxytocin if slow active phase progress was detected.

The regimen permitted one-to-one midwifery care because patients either progressed normally, responded to augmentation, or underwent cesarean section if they did not progress—all within a matter of 8 to 12 hours from admission. The simplicity of this approach and the reported low cesarean rate appealed to many clinicians, and still does.

However, the same results could not be replicated elsewhere, and concerns grew over rising cesarean section rates[66] for failure to progress despite the apparent adoption of this philosophy. Moreover, meta-analysis of the individual components of this approach has revealed that the proposed medical interventions are not effective, individually, in reducing operative intervention.[64] Thus, randomized clinical trials were eventually undertaken. They demonstrate interesting points for evidence-based practice. One showed a decrease in cesarean section associated with the adoption of "active management" from the rate prior to the study, but there was also a decreased rate in the control arm.[67] This was almost certainly a Hawthorne effect (simply by doing the trial and focusing participants' minds on the management issues produced an effect). The end result was not statistically significant. This may explain why earlier uncontrolled studies gave overoptimistic results. The largest study did not show any improvement in surgical delivery rates, though there was a reduction in maternal postnatal pyrexia.[68] These two studies started with relatively high cesarean section rates, in the region of 20%. Early studies reported the use of oxytocin in up to 50% of nulliparas.[19,69] Thus, a third study aimed to test whether relaxation of the indications to augment uterine activity would result in an increased cesarean section rate.[70] This study reported cesarean section rates of 3.9% in the active management arm compared with 2.6% in the "selective use" arm and spontaneous vaginal delivery rates of 78% and 79%, respectively. A study of the promptness with which oxytocin is used (crossing an action line set at 2 or 4 hr after the alert line) did indicate that there was a reduction in cesarean section rate (relative risk [RR] 0.68) using the more aggressive approach.[69] This trial, though showing benefit, had to be curtailed, and there were protocol violations in the aggressive arm of the study.

Meta-analyses have been performed on clinical studies of active management. One analysis combined controlled and uncontrolled trials and concluded that there is reduced operative intervention.[71] Care must be exercised when combining such heterogeneous data. Meta-analysis of only the randomized trials fails to show any benefit. A more recent systematic review and meta-analysis of only randomized trials concluded that there are a few benefits from such packages,[72] but this conclusion could be reached only after exclusion of the largest randomized trial[68] on grounds of suspected bias from postrandomization drop-out. Other trials in the analysis also show weaknesses in study design but were retained. Furthermore, the studies varied in the component parts of the packages they used. This raises questions about the appropriateness of meta-analyses when combining the results of complex and differing packages of care. Unfortunately, even if the results are accepted from these reviews, the clinician cannot determine which elements of the package are of value and which may be useless or even dangerous. Clinicians must be aware of the limitations of meta-analyses and should not automatically accept them as the highest level of evidence. They may be better advised to evaluate the original studies themselves to judge relevance to their own practice.

The bottom line of these packages of care is that, at best, their clinical impact is marginal and, at their worst, they contain components that have been discredited.

Maternal Preparation and Support

Clinical benefit from supportive care has been demonstrated,[64,73] but this element is often undervalued and overshadowed by medical interventions. Patient confidence and a feeling of control are improved in association with a reduction in the need for pain relief and a lower incidence of cesarean section and operative vaginal delivery. The identity and qualifications of the person providing the support appears to be less important. Some studies have employed nonclinical but trained lay supporters (doulas).

Summary

Interventions demonstrated to be effective are antenatal education and preparation of the mother, personal support during labor, and correct diagnosis of labor (active phase).

MANAGEMENT OF THE SECOND STAGE OF LABOR

The second stage of labor starts at full dilation of the cervix and ends with delivery of the fetus. Descent and rotation of the passenger are the main features. Without epidural analgesia, full dilation of the cervix usually becomes apparent because of an urge to push due to the descent of the presenting part onto the pelvic floor. Epidural analgesia may abolish this sensation completely. Thus, there may be no outward signs of entry to the second stage, and diagnosis will only follow vaginal examination. The diagnosis and, therefore, the duration of second stage have become controversial.

Physiology of the Second Stage

Maternal Changes

Cervical resistance in the first stage of labor is necessary for the generation of wall tension that is, to all intent and purpose, isometric, that is to say, tension generated without shortening of the muscle fibers. At full dilation of the cervix, the uterus ceases to be a "closed vessel," cervical resistance is lost, and descent through the birth canal begins. Myometrial activity progressively changes toward isotonic activity as the uterus empties. Reduction in uterine volume permits permanent shortening (retraction) of the myometrial fibers. This effect is maximal during the third stage, and by the end of the third stage, it is crucial for effective hemostasis. It is potentially dangerous in the second stage because it progressively impairs placental perfusion.

The myometrium is "inserted" into the pelvis via the connective tissues that surround the cervix, with the round ligaments helping to tether and direct the uterine fundus. These connective tissue supports are elastic. If the force required to stretch them is greater than the resistance offered by the birth canal, there will be progress. The rate of progress will be determined by the equilibrium established between the elasticity of the supports and the resistance offered by the birth canal. Frank obstruction to progress from the bony pelvis will merely direct all force to stretching the cervical supports against this resistance. Descent can occur without maternal bearing down ("pushing"), but there is little evidence (other than anecdotal, e.g., spontaneous delivery in paraplegic women) to show that delivery can be achieved entirely without the voluntary use of the abdominal muscles to raise intra-abdominal pressure, thus increasing the expulsive forces. Pushing increases maternal effort and interferes with breathing, inducing both respiratory and metabolic acidosis.

Fetal Changes

Studies on the acid-base balance in the fetus in the second stage show a decline in pH and a rise in lactate as pushing and descent progress.[74–76] To a degree, this is physiologic, and the metabolic changes will stimulate the neonate to breathe spontaneously. Too much acidosis, however, results in respiratory depression.

Divisions of the Second Stage

It is useful to split the second stage into passive and active sections, depending on whether pushing has commenced.[74]

Passive Section

In the passive section, prior to pushing, there is likely to be little descent to alter the character of myometrial activity, and the mother is not affecting her metabolic state by pushing. Thus, there is minimal effect on the fetus.[74] There does not appear to be a significant risk from waiting at this point prior to pushing, all else being equal. However, there does not appear to be any benefit, either.[77] Thus, when to commence pushing continues to be debated but is probably irrelevant to outcome, providing the fetus is in good condition.[78]

Active Section

The active section commences with pushing. From this point onward, the metabolic changes in the fetus described earlier begin and progress. Descent and rotation of the presenting part should be progressive, irrespective of the presence or not of an epidural anesthetic.

Monitoring Progress

Descent

Descent is monitored and represented on the partogram in two ways: abdominally by the amount of head palpable (usually in fifths) and vaginally, as the station, estimated in terms of the level of the lowest point of the presenting part in relation to the ischial spines. A second stage nomogram has also been produced.[79]

Friedman and Sachtleben[80] described progress in terms of the number of expulsive efforts the mother makes; more commonly, time alone is used as the criterion. The former is more physiologic, the latter is easier. If contractions are occurring with the usual frequency of three to four every 10 minutes, the two are the same. No robust clinical trials have been conducted concerning the optimal duration for pushing. Traditional limits of 30 minutes for parous and 45 minutes for nulliparous women have been used and maximum of 1 hour without progress has been recommended.[18] These times may seem a little short, but it should be remembered that if the woman has not delivered by this time, it can take a further 20 to 30 minutes to prepare for, and carry out, instrumental delivery. Recently, national guidelines in the United Kingdom from the National Institute for Health and Clinical Excellence (NICE) have suggested limits of 1 and 2 hours, respectively.[18] These limits are probably reasonable so long as fetal monitoring is reassuring about fetal condition, and so long as they include the time taken to perform instrumental delivery.

Rotation

Rotation is determined by vaginal examination and palpation of the sutures and fontanels on the fetal head in relation to the maternal pelvis. Scalp edema (caput), which often develops with delay, may make this difficult.

Interventions

Augmentation of the Powers

As with the first stage, efficient powers are paramount. Uterine inertia is not uncommon at full dilation when epidural analgesia is used, owing to the abolition of the reflex release of maternal oxytocin produced by the sensation of stretching of the introitus and perineum (Ferguson's reflex). Intravenous oxytocin may be required to restore uterine activity. If it is used, care should be taken to avoid overstimulation, and continuous fetal heart rate monitoring is mandatory. If the fetal head is well down, operative delivery may be a safer option.

Use of the mother's abdominal muscles to raise intra-abdominal pressure is important. Efficient pushing requires education and encouragement, particularly when epidural analgesia has removed sensation.

Maternal Posture

An upright posture of the mother reduces both the duration of the second stage and the incidence of operative delivery.[81] There are also reductions in the use of episiotomy, perception of pain, and fetal heart rate abnormalities. Maternal posture does not appear to affect malposition. Avoidance of the supine position is beneficial for the acid-base status of the fetus in the second stage.[82]

Instrumental Delivery

Instrumentation is used to shorten the second stage, either when prolonged or to avoid fetal or maternal complications. This is discussed in Chapter 72.

Episiotomy

Episiotomy is surgical reduction of resistance offered by the pelvic floor. There is no benefit from routine episiotomy.[83] Mediolateral episiotomies direct any tearing away from the rectum and anus, resulting in fewer third-degree tears, but cause more bleeding than those in the midline. They also cause more discomfort in the puerperium.

SUMMARY OF MANAGEMENT OPTIONS

Poor Progress in Labor

Management Options	Evidence Quality and Recommendation	References
Poor Progress in Latent Phase of First Stage		
Expectant management with careful watch of the fetal heart rate.	III/B	20,53,54
Augmentation may increase cesarean section rates.	III/B	20,53,54
Poor Progress in Active Phase of First Stage		
Allowing 4 hr of grace after crossing the "alert" line reduces need for augmentation and cesarean section.	Ia/A	43,44
Judicious augmentation with Syntocinon will reduce labor duration.	Ib/A	55
Studies favor 30-min incremental intervals when increasing oxytocin infusion rates.	Ib/A	64
Obstetric outcome for most cases is no better with the use of intrauterine pressure catheters, compared with the use of external methods of detecting contraction frequency.	Ib/A	26
Epidural analgesia is not associated with prolongation of the first stage of labor nor with an increase in cesarean section rates.	Ia/A	65
Poor Progress in the Second Stage of Labor		
Flexibility in the duration of the second stage is permissible if fetal condition is reassuring.	—/GPP	—
Upright posture of the mother reduces the duration of the second stage and need for operative delivery. It also reduces the need for episiotomy, perception of pain, and fetal heart rate abnormalities.	Ia/A	81
Epidural analgesia is associated with longer duration of the second stage and an increase in instrumental delivery rates.	Ia/A	65
Use of episiotomy should be limited and selective.	Ia/A	83

GPP, good practice point.

SUGGESTED READINGS

Anim-Somuah M, Smyth R, Howell C: Epidural versus non-epidural or no analgesia in labour. Cochrane Database Syst Rev 2005;4:CD000331.

Cammu H, Van Eeckhout E: A randomised controlled trial of early versus delayed use of amniotomy and oxytocin infusion in nulliparous labour. Br J Obstet Gynaecol 1996;103:313–318.

Frigoletto FDJ, et al: A clinical trial of active management of labor. N Engl J Med 1995;333:745–750.

Gupta JK, Hofmeyr GJ, Smyth R: Position during seconds stage of labour for women without epidural anaesthesia. Cochrane Database Syst Rev 2000;1:CD002006.

Hodnett ED, Gates S, Hofmeyr GJ, Sakala C: Continuous support for women during childbirth. Cochrane Database Syst Rev 2007;3:CD003766.

Lavender T, Hart A,Smyth RM: Effect of partogram use on outcomes for women in spontaneous labour at term. Cochrane Database Syst Rev 2008;4:CD0005461.

Lopez-Zeno JA, et al: A controlled trial of a program for the active management of labor. N Engl J Med 1992;326:450–454.

Pattinson RC, et al: Aggressive or expectant management of labour: A randomised clinical trial. BJOG 2003;110:457–461.

Smyth, RMD, Alldred SK, Markham C: Amniotomy for shortening spontaneous labour. Cochrane Database Syst Rev 2007;4:CD006167.

Zhang J, Troendle JF, Yancey MK: Reassessing the labor curve in nulliparous women. Am J Obstet Gynecol 2002;187:824–828.

REFERENCES

For a complete list of references, log onto www.expertconsult.com.

CHAPTER 68

Shoulder Dystocia

ROBERT B. GHERMAN

INTRODUCTION

Despite its infrequent occurrence (0.2%–3% of all deliveries[1,2]), all health care providers attending vaginal deliveries must be prepared to handle this unpredictable obstetric emergency. Shoulder dystocia represents the failure of delivery of the fetal shoulder(s), whether it be the anterior, posterior, or both fetal shoulders.[3] Shoulder dystocia results from a size discrepancy between the fetal shoulders and the pelvic inlet, which may be absolute or relative (due to malposition). A persistent anterior-posterior location of the fetal shoulders at the pelvic brim occurs when there is increased resistance between the fetal skin and the vaginal walls (e.g., with macrosomia), with a large fetal chest relative to the biparietal diameter, and when truncal rotation does not occur (e.g., precipitous labor).[1] Shoulder dystocia can also occur from impaction of the posterior fetal shoulder on the maternal sacral promontory.

DEFINITION

Most authors have defined this obstetric emergency to include those deliveries requiring maneuvers in addition to gentle downward traction on the fetal head to effect delivery. Several studies have proposed defining shoulder dystocia as a prolonged head-to-body delivery interval (the mean plus 2 standard deviations, 60 sec) or the use of ancillary obstetric maneuvers.[4,5]

RISKS TO THE MOTHER, OBSTETRICIAN, AND FETUS

Postpartum hemorrhage, and the unintentional extension of the episiotomy or laceration into the rectum (fourth-degree laceration), are the most common maternal complications associated with shoulder dystocia (Table 68–1). In Gherman and coworkers' study,[6] these occurred in 11% and 3.8%, respectively, of the described shoulder dystocias. Other reported complications have included vaginal lacerations, cervical tears, bladder atony, and uterine rupture. Maternal symphyseal separation and lateral femoral cutaneous neuropathy have also been associated with overly aggressive hyperflexion of the maternal legs.[7] Risks to the physician mainly involve litigation, because brachial plexus palsy (BPP), central neurologic dysfunction, and perinatal death account for most of the shoulder dystocia–related lawsuits. A clearly documented medical record may be helpful if claims are to be rebutted.[8]

A large retrospective study that evaluated 285 cases of shoulder dystocia found that the fetal injury rate was 24.9%, including 48 (16.8%) BPPs, 27 (9.5%) clavicular fractures, and 12 (4.2%) humeral fractures.[9] Unilateral brachial plexus injuries are probably the most common neurologic injury sustained by the neonate. The right arm is more commonly affected (64.6%) owing to the fact that the left occiput anterior presentation leaves the right shoulder impinged against the symphysis pubis.[9] Brachial plexus injury has been found to complicate up to 21% of all shoulder dystocia cases.[10] Most (80%) of these nerve injuries have been located within the C5–6 nerve roots (Erb-Duchenne palsy). Other types of brachial plexus injuries that have been described include Klumpke's palsy (C8–T1), an intermediate palsy, and complete palsy of the entire brachial plexus. Diaphragmatic paralysis, Horner's syndrome, and facial nerve injuries have occasionally been reported to accompany BPP.[11] Approximately one third of BPPs will be associated with a concomitant bone fracture, most commonly the clavicle (94%).[9] Neonatal radial fracture can also be associated with the shoulder dystocia or the maneuvers employed to alleviate it.[12]

TABLE 68–1
Common Complications Associated with Shoulder Dystocia

MATERNAL	ACCOUCHEUR	NEONATAL
Third- or fourth-degree lacerations	Terror	Erb-Duchenne palsy
Postpartum hemorrhage	Medical liability	Klumpke's palsy
		Clavicular fracture
		Humeral fracture
		Hypoxia
		Permanent brain injury
		Death

Gherman and colleagues' study[9] compared shoulder dystocia cases according to whether or not direct fetal manipulative maneuvers (Woods', posterior arm extraction, or Zavanelli's maneuvers) had been used and found that the overall incidence of fetal bone fracture (16.5% vs. 11.4%, P = .21) and BPP (21.3% vs. 13.3%, P =.1) was not significantly different between the two groups. Similar findings had previously been reported by Nocon and associates,[13] who grouped the techniques used to disimpact the shoulder into major treatment categories. None of the major categories revealed a statistically significant difference when compared with respect to fetal injury. In Nocon and associates' study,[13] the authors found incidences of injury of 14.9%, 14.3%, 37.9%, and 20%, respectively, associated with the McRoberts maneuver, rotations, posterior arm delivery, and suprapubic pressure.

MANAGEMENT OPTIONS

Prenatal: Identifying the Pregnancy at Risk

It has been clearly shown that the risk of shoulder dystocia increases significantly as birth weight increases. The percentage of births complicated by shoulder dystocia for unassisted births not complicated by diabetes was 5.2% for infants weighing 4000 to 4250 g, 9.1% for those 4250 to 4500 g, 14.3% for those 4500 to 4750 g, and 21.1% for those 4750 to 5000 g.[14] It must be remembered, however, that approximately 50% to 60% of shoulder dystocias occur in infants weighing less than 4000 g. Moreover, even if the birth weight of the infant is over 4000 g, shoulder dystocia will complicate only 3.3% of the deliveries.[15,16]

From a prospective point of view, prepregnancy and antepartum risk factors such as previous delivery of a macrosomic infant, preexisting or pregnancy-induced diabetes mellitus, multiparity, excessive maternal weight gain, and postdates gestation have very poor predictive value for the prediction of shoulder dystocia. For example, one study found that only 32% of patients were obese (>90 kg), 25% had excessive weight gain (>20 kg), 8% had short stature (<60 inches), 6% were more than 42 weeks' gestation, 3% were of advanced maternal age, and 2% had a personal history of diabetes mellitus.[17] In Ouzounian and Gherman's large cohort of patients from a Southern California perinatal program,[18] rates for operative vaginal delivery, diabetes, epidural use, multiparity, and postdatism were similar among cases with and without shoulder dystocia. In a case-control study from the Northern and Central Alberta Perinatal Outreach Program, maternal obesity (defined as > 91 kg) was not associated with shoulder dystocia when multivariable logistic regression analysis was used to control for confounding effects.[19] Other studies have not shown any independent association between maternal obesity and an increased risk for shoulder dystocia.[20]

Ultrasonographic estimation of fetal weight, performed during either the late third trimester or the intrapartum period, has commonly been employed to estimate the risk of shoulder dystocia via prediction of birth weight. To date, however, no studies have specifically evaluated this relationship in a patient population in which routine ultrasounds are performed. Late pregnancy ultrasound displays a low sensitivity (22%–44%) and a poor positive predictive value (30%–44%) in the detection of macrosomia, with an overall tendency to overestimate the birth weight. Moreover, there is decreasing accuracy of birth weight prediction with increasing birth weight. Using a scoring system that incorporated ultrasonographic biometric parameters and amniotic fluid index, Chauhan and coworkers[21] failed in their attempt to provide a simple scoring system that could predict shoulder dystocia among large–for–gestational age fetuses. For this reason, the American College of Obstetricians and Gynecologists has suggested that attempted vaginal delivery is not contraindicated for women with estimated fetal weights up to 5000 g in the absence of maternal diabetes.[22,23]

Patients with insulin-requiring diabetes mellitus appear to warrant special evaluation for shoulder dystocia. The risk of shoulder dystocia for unassisted births to diabetic mothers has been found to be 8.4%, 12.3%, 19.9%, and 23.5% when the birth weight is 4000 to 4250 g, 4250 to 4500 g, 4500 to 4750 g, or more than 4750 g, respectively.[13] These values are somewhat higher than for nondiabetics of similar build. Changes in fetal body configuration brought about by increased fat deposition in the fetuses of diabetic mothers, such as larger trunk and chest circumferences, increased bisacromial diameters, and chest-to-head disproportion, impede the rotation of the fetal shoulders into the oblique diameter.

In a similar fashion, patients with a history of shoulder dystocia complicating a prior vaginal delivery have a risk of recurrence ranging between 11.9% and 16.7%. Maternal and fetal factors that have been shown to be significantly associated with recurrent shoulder dystocia include birth weight greater than the index pregnancy, prolonged duration of the second stage of labor, and birth weight more than 4000 g.[1] However, a policy of universal elective cesarean delivery has not been recommended for this cohort of patients because the risks outweigh the benefits.[23] Nonetheless, antepartum counseling and discussion of recurrence risks should be undertaken, with consideration of the present estimate of fetal weight, the presence of maternal glucose intolerance, and whether or not the prior shoulder dystocia resulted in a transient or permanent neurologic injury.

Labor and Delivery: Practical Management of Shoulder Dystocia

The patient should be instructed to stop pushing after the shoulder dystocia is initially recognized. However, maternal expulsive efforts will need to be restarted after the fetal shoulders have been converted to the oblique diameter, in order to complete the delivery. If the accoucheur is alone, additional assistance may be obtained by summoning other obstetricians, an anesthetist or anesthesiologist, additional nursing support, and a pediatrician.

Umbilical cord compression, most commonly between the fetal body and the maternal pelvis, leads to a decrease in the fetal pH at an average rate of 0.04 units/min. If a nuchal cord is present and cannot be reduced easily over the fetal head, clamping and cutting of the cord should be avoided until the shoulder dystocia has been alleviated.[24] Most, if not all, of the commonly encountered shoulder dystocia episodes can be relieved within several minutes.

Although research studies have been unable to predict an exact time limit at which irreversible brain injury occurs, it is reasonable to assume that the risk of permanent central neurologic dysfunction is associated with prolongation of the head/shoulder interval thresholds. The length of delay that results in permanent brain injury will depend on the condition of the baby at the point at which the delivery is arrested. It may be as short as 4 to 5 minutes or as long as 15 minutes.

At the time of delivery, if shoulder dystocia is a concern, some clinicians have empirically advocated proceeding immediately to delivery of the fetal shoulders, in order to maintain the forward momentum of the fetus. Others support a short delay in delivery of the shoulders, arguing that the endogenous rotational mechanics of the second stage may spontaneously alleviate the obstruction. Obstetricians may also employ the McRoberts maneuver "prophylactically" in order to decrease the risk of shoulder dystocia or shorten the second stage of labor. One clinical trial randomized patients with estimated fetal weights over 3800 g either to undergo prophylactic maneuvers (McRoberts' maneuver and suprapubic pressure) or to undergo maneuvers only after delivery of the fetal head, if shoulder dystocia was identified.[25] This study found that head-to-body delivery times, an indirect proxy for shoulder dystocia, did not differ between the prophylactic and the control patients.

Although many maneuvers have been described for the successful alleviation of shoulder dystocia, no randomized, controlled trials or laboratory experiments have been conducted that directly compared these techniques (Table 68–2). Most obstetricians currently employ the McRoberts maneuver as their initial step for the disimpaction of the shoulder. In a retrospective review of 236 shoulder dystocia cases occurring between 1991 and 1994 at Los Angeles County/University of Southern California Medical Center, this maneuver alone alleviated 42% of cases. Moreover, trends toward lower rates of maternal and neonatal morbidity were associated with the McRoberts maneuver.[6]

The McRoberts maneuver, performed by sharply flexing the maternal thighs onto the abdomen, results in a straightening of the maternal sacrum relative to the lumbar spine with consequent cephalic rotation of the symphysis pubis.[26] Care should be taken to avoid prolonged or overly aggressive application of the McRoberts maneuver because the fibrocartilaginous articular surfaces of the symphysis pubis and surrounding ligaments may be unduly stretched.

The overwhelming majority of patients can assume the proper position for the McRoberts maneuver with little difficulty. Women may be instructed to grasp the posterior aspect of their thighs and pull themselves into position, with family members or health care professionals providing any assistance necessary. The obstetrician may also choose to flex both of the patient's legs. Problems may occur when moving an obese patient or a woman who has undergone a dense epidural motor blockade.

Because shoulder dystocia is considered to be a "bony dystocia," episiotomy alone will not release the impacted shoulder. The need for cutting a generous episiotomy or proctoepisiotomy must be based on clinical circumstances, such as a narrow vaginal fourchette in a nulliparous patient. This may allow the fetal rotational maneuvers to be performed with ease, as well as create more room for attempted delivery of the posterior arm. Attendants should refrain from applying fundal pressure as a maneuver for the alleviation of the shoulder dystocia. Pushing on the fundus simply duplicates a maternal directional expulsive force that has already failed to deliver the fetal shoulder(s) and serves only to further impact the anterior shoulder behind the symphysis pubis. In addition, the use of fundal pressure has been associated with an increased risk of Erb-Duchenne palsy and thoracic spinal cord injury in the neonate.[27]

Suprapubic pressure, commonly administered by nursing personnel, is typically used immediately prior to or in direct conjunction with the McRoberts maneuver. This pressure is usually directed posteriorly, in an attempt to force the anterior shoulder under the symphysis pubis. Other described techniques for suprapubic pressure have included lateral application from either side of the maternal abdomen or alternating between sides using a rocking pressure.[28]

Many cases of shoulder dystocia require the performance of several maneuvers to alleviate the impaction. Stallings and colleagues[29] found that slightly more than a third of patients required more than two maneuvers. When more complex maneuvers are required, either fetal rotational maneuvers or posterior arm extraction may be employed. In the Woods corkscrew maneuver, the practitioner attempts to abduct the posterior shoulder by exerting pressure onto its anterior surface. In the Rubin (reverse Woods) maneuver, pressure is applied to the posterior surface of the most accessible part of the fetal shoulder (either the anterior or the posterior shoulder) to effect shoulder adduction. These rotational maneuvers, however, may be difficult to perform when the anterior shoulder is tightly wedged underneath the symphysis pubis. It may, therefore, be necessary to push the fetus slightly upward in order to facilitate the rotation.

By replacing the bisacromial diameter with the axilloacromial diameter, posterior arm delivery creates a 20% reduction in the diameter that has to pass through the birth canal.[30] To perform delivery of the posterior fetal arm, pressure should be applied by the accoucheur at the antecubital fossa in order to flex the fetal forearm. The arm is subsequently swept out over the infant's chest and delivered over the perineum. Rotation of the fetal trunk to bring the posterior arm anteriorly is sometimes required. If the posterior arm is extended or lies under the fetus's body, delivery may be very difficult. Grasping and pulling directly on the

TABLE 68–2

Maneuvers for the Alleviation of Shoulder Dystocia

- Maternal hip hyperflexion (McRoberts' maneuver)
- Suprapubic pressure
- Rotational maneuvers
  - Woods' maneuver
  - Rubin's maneuver
- Delivery of the posterior arm (Barnum's maneuver)
- "All fours" (Gaskin's maneuver)
- Cephalic replacement
  - Zavanelli's
  - Modified Zavanelli's
- Symphysiotomy; abdominal rescue through hysterotomy
- Posterior axilla traction

fetal arm, as well as application of pressure onto the mid-humeral shaft, should be avoided because bone fracture might occur.

The previously mentioned maneuvers are typically attempted 4 to 5 minutes after identification of the shoulder dystocia. If the shoulder dystocia remains uncorrected, a bilateral shoulder dystocia or posterior arm shoulder dystocia might be present. The latter is suggested by the presence of the posterior arm being maintained at the level of the pelvic inlet and an inability to perform posterior arm extraction. Intractable shoulder dystocias warrant the use of heroic techniques, such as the Zavanelli maneuver, symphysiotomy, or hysterotomy. Other options to consider include posterior axillary traction,[31] potentially to include sling traction,[32] to deliver the posterior arm.

Performance of these will be complicated by the provider's lack of clinical experience with these maneuvers, performance under emergent conditions, and the significant maternal and neonatal complications inherent in the procedures. In the Zavanelli maneuver, the head is rotated back to a pre-restitution position and then gently flexed. Constant firm pressure is used to push the head back into the vagina, and cesarean delivery is subsequently performed. Halothane or other general anesthetics, in conjunction with tocolytic agents, may be administered in preparation for, and during, the Zavanelli maneuver. Oral or intravenous nitroglycerin may be used as well. A modification of the original Zavanelli maneuver may be employed in order potentially to reduce maternal morbidity. As described by Zelig and Gherman,[33] maternal expulsive efforts were reinitiated after the obstetrician had observed that the biparietal diameter had passed back through the introitus and the shoulders were felt to disimpact. This modification relies on the possibility that the disimpacted shoulders will now rotate into the correct orientation for delivery. Because it might not work, it should be attempted only when there is no evidence of fetal compromise.

To perform a symphysiotomy, place the patient in an exaggerated lithotomy position. Although its placement may be very difficult secondary to obstruction, a Foley catheter can help to identify the urethra. With the physician's index and middle finger displacing the urethra laterally, the cephalad portion of the symphysis is incised with a scalpel blade or Kelly clamp. Hysterotomy may also be performed to either resolve the shoulder dystocia primarily or assist with vaginal techniques. The abdominal surgeon can apply pressure on the anterior fetal shoulder to allow rotation to the oblique diameter. The posterior fetal arm may be manipulated through the transverse uterine incision with passage of the hand to a vaginal assistant.

Prior to performing these techniques, one may consider using the "all-fours" technique, in which the patient is rolled from her existing position onto her hands and knees.[34] The downward force of gravity or a favorable change in pelvic diameters produced by this maneuver may allow disimpaction of the fetal shoulder. Older textbooks have described deliberate clavicular fracture as a maneuver of last resort, performed by exerting direct upward pressure on the mid-portion of the fetal clavicle. However, this has not been reported in the recent literature because it is technically difficult to perform and risks serious injury to the underlying vascular and pulmonary structures in the fetus.

Training: Shoulder Dystocia and Simulation

Owing to its infrequent occurrence and the requirement for a rapid response, shoulder dystocia is an obstetric emergency that is well suited to simulation. In addition, the 15th Report on Confidential Enquiries into Maternal Deaths in the United Kingdom identified that in 66% of neonatal deaths following shoulder dystocia, "different management could have reasonably been expected to have altered the outcome."[35] Using a standardized simulated shoulder dystocia scenario, Deering and associates have reported that trained residents had significantly higher scores, including reduced timelines of their interventions, better performance of maneuvers, and overall improved efficiency.[36] Crofts and Draycott[37–40] have developed a training mannequin with a force-monitoring system consisting of a strain gauge mounted on both clavicles. They found a reduction in the head-to-body delivery duration and the maximum applied delivery force following training, although these did not reach statistical significance. However, significant improvements in overall management were observed after training and persisted for up to 1 year.

SHOULDER DYSTOCIA AND BRACHIAL PLEXUS INJURY

BPP is a major cause of litigation, constituting 11% of the 370 obstetric claims closed by the Norwegian patient insurance system from 1988 to 1997.[41] In the past, textbooks have stated without evidence that BPP is caused by the accoucheur's application of excessive lateral traction on the fetal head and neck during attempts at alleviating the shoulder dystocia. However, since the mid 1990s, multiple lines of evidence have supported the concept that most BPPs are not caused by the accoucheur.[1,42–45] This opinion is based on several findings:

- More than 50% of cases of brachial plexus injuries are associated with uncomplicated vaginal deliveries.[42–44]
- BPP can occur in the posterior arm of infants whose anterior arm was impacted behind the symphysis pubis and can also occur with atraumatic cesarean delivery.[44]
- There is no statistical correlation with the experience of the obstetric provider nor the number or type of maneuvers used.[1]
- Rapid second-stage and disproportionate descent of the head and body of the fetus relative to the shoulder have been implicated in the pathogenesis of the injury.[42]
- Mathematical and computer-simulated models have shown that maternal endogenous forces are far greater than clinician-applied exogenous delivery loads during a shoulder dystocia episode.[46,47]

McFarland and coworkers[48] have reported that the number of maneuvers employed during the shoulder dystocia may serve as a measure of the severity of the shoulder dystocia, with this severity being the cause of injury, rather than the maneuvers themselves. When one or two maneuvers were required, the incidence of Erb's palsy was 7.7% but increased to 25% when three or more maneuvers were required (P = 0.009). The incidence of clavicular or humeral fracture also increased with the use of more than three maneuvers (21.4% vs. 7.7%, P = 0.03).

It is currently impossible to predict which infants will be affected with BPP when shoulder dystocia complicates vaginal delivery. To date, there have been only a few studies whose objective was to predict which infants would experience BPP following shoulder dystocia. In Mehta and colleagues' study,[49] after logistic regression analysis, only a second stage of delivery greater than 20 minutes remained significantly associated with neonatal injury at discharge. Poggi and associates[50] matched 80 medicolegal cases of shoulder dystocia–associated BPP with control cases taken from a database of consecutive shoulder dystocia deliveries from one hospital. There were no significant differences in maternal weight, body mass index, height, race, estimated gestational age, average number of maneuvers, head-to-body delivery interval, operative delivery rate, prolonged second stage, or precipitous second stage rate between the groups. In a retrospective case-control analysis from national birth injury and shoulder dystocia databases, Gherman and coworkers[10] matched cases of permanent BPP (n = 49) with cases of transient palsy. Transient BPP cases were found to have a higher incidence of diabetes mellitus than those with permanent BPP (34.7% vs. 10.2%, odds ratio [OR] 4.68, 95% confidence interval [CI] 1.42–16.32). Permanent BPPs had a higher mean birth weight (4519 + 94.3 g vs. 4143.6 + 56.5 g, P < .001) and a greater frequency of birth weight greater than 4500 g (38.8% vs. 16.3%, OR 0.31, 95% CI 0.11–0.87). There were, however, no statistically significant differences between the two groups with respect to multiple other antepartum, intrapartum, and delivery outcome measures.

Despite the introduction of ancillary obstetric maneuvers such as McRoberts' maneuver and a generalized trend toward the avoidance of fundal pressure, it has been shown that the rate of shoulder dystocia–associated BPP has not decreased. Comparison of shoulder dystocia deliveries between 1980 to 1986 and 1991 to 1999 indicates no significant difference with respect to BPP: 0.7/1000 deliveries versus 0.8/1000 deliveries (OR 1.10; 95% CII 0.65–1.86).[51]

Despite these observations, it is good and prudent practice for obstetricians to make a detailed and accurate account of the procedure when they have managed a case of shoulder dystocia. This should be undertaken as close to the event as possible. Table 68–3 gives a suggested list of items that may be covered in such a report.

TABLE 68–3

Suggested Medicolegal Documentation for Shoulder Dystocia

When and how shoulder dystocia was diagnosed
Position and rotation of infant's head
Which shoulder was anterior?
Presence of episiotomy, if performed
Estimate of head-to-body time interval
Estimation of force of traction applied
Order, duration, and results of maneuvers employed
Additional medical personnel present for assistance
Birth weight
One- and 5-min Apgar scores
Venous and/or arterial umbilical cord blood gas/pH/base deficit evaluation
Inform delivered woman that shoulder dystocia had occurred

SUMMARY OF MANAGEMENT OPTIONS

Shoulder Dystocia

Management Options	Evidence Quality and Recommendation	References
Prenatal Identification of At-Risk Pregnancy		
Estimation of fetal weight and risk of SD is of limited value.	III/B	15,16
May be of more use in diabetic pregnancies or those with previous SD.	IIb/B	17
Limited accuracy of ultrasound in estimating fetal weight	III/B	52
ACOG Guidelines: • Vaginal delivery is reasonable with estimated fetal weights up to 5 kg in the absence of diabetes because of the risks of elective cesarean section	IV/C	22,23
Despite this guideline, women with previous delivery complicated by SD may prefer to have an elective cesarean section, especially if the estimated fetal weight is similar to or greater than previously.	—/GPP	—
The following are poor predictors of SD: • Previous macrosomia/large-for-dates. • Diabetes (preexisting or gestational). • Multiparity. • Excessive weight gain in pregnancy. • Postdates pregnancy.	IIa/B	16–21

SUMMARY OF MANAGEMENT OPTIONS

Shoulder Dystocia—cont'd

Management Options	Evidence Quality and Recommendation	References
If vaginal delivery is to be attempted following a discussion with an at-risk patient, make a clear record in the patient's notes.	—/GPP	—
Practical Management of Shoulder Dystocia (See Table 68–2)		
No RCT data covering any aspect of SD management.	—/—	—
No evidence that "prophylactic" McRoberts' and suprapubic pressure prevents SD in at-risk cases (i.e., before SD has developed/been recognized).	Ib/A	25
Stop maternal efforts temporarily until SD is overcome.	—/GPP	—
Summon help (obstetric, anesthetic, nursing/midwifery, pediatric).	—/GPP	—
Avoid clamping and cutting a nuchal cord until SD is overcome.	IV/C	24
McRoberts' maneuver.	III/B	6
Suprapubic pressure.	IV/C	28
No evidence that episiotomy makes a difference, though often advised.	—/GPP	—
Avoid fundal pressure as it increases risk of Erb's palsy and thoracic spine injury.	IV/C	28
Rotational maneuver (Woods' or Rubin's).	III/B	1
Delivery of posterior arm (Barnum's).	III/B	1
Put woman into "all fours" position.	III/B	34
Zavanelli's maneuver.	III/B	1
Symphysiotomy.	IV/C	53
Hysterotomy and abdominal correction.	IV/C	54
Make a detailed record as soon as possible after the event (see Table 68–3).	—/GPP	—

GPP, good practice point.

SUGGESTED READINGS

American College of Obstetricians and Gynecologists (ACOG): Shoulder Dystocia (Practice Bulletin No. 40). Washington, DC, ACOG, 2002.

Chauhan SP, Christian B, Gherman RB, et al: Shoulder dystocia without versus with brachial plexus injury: A case-control study. J Matern Fetal Neonatal Med 2007;20:313–317.

Crofts JF, Fox R, Ellis D, et al: Observations from 450 shoulder dystocia simulations: Lessons for skills training. Obstet Gynecol 2008;112: 906–912.

Gherman RB, Chauhan S, Ouzounian JG, et al: Shoulder dystocia: The unpreventable obstetric emergency with empiric management guidelines. Am J Obstet Gynecol 2006;195:657–672.

Hope P, Breslin S, Lamont L, et al: Fatal shoulder dystocia: A review of 56 cases reported to the Confidential Enquiry into Stillbirths and Deaths in Infancy. Br J Obstet Gynaecol 1998;105:1256–1261.

MacKenzie IZ, Shah M, Lean K, et al: Management of shoulder dystocia: Trends in incidence and maternal and neonatal morbidity. Obstet Gynecol 2007;110:1059–1068.

Nesbitt TS, Gilbert WM, Herrchen B: Shoulder dystocia and associated risk factors with macrosomic infants born in California. Am J Obstet Gynecol 1998;179:476–480.

Ouzounian JG, Gherman RB: Shoulder dystocia: Are historic risk factors reliable predictors? Am J Obstet Gynecol 2005;192:1933–1938.

Robinson H, Tkatch S, Mayes DC, et al: Is maternal obesity a predictor of shoulder dystocia? Obstet Gynecol 2003;101:24–27.

Sandmire HF, DeMott RK: Erb's palsy causation: A historical perspective. Birth 2002;29:152–154.

REFERENCES

For a complete list of references, log onto www.expertconsult.com.

CHAPTER 69

Fetal Distress in Labor

PETER DANIELIAN and PHILIP J. STEER

WHAT IS FETAL DISTRESS?

Fetal distress is a term that is commonly used, but difficult to define. It is probably best taken to mean "an absence of fetal well-being," in a similar way that the expression "a flat baby" means a "neonate in need of resuscitation" and "an ill person" means "someone who is unwell." Thus, its use encompasses many different pathologies affecting the fetus, such as chronic hypoxia leading to a metabolic acidosis, mechanical trauma (e.g., excessive head compression), hyperthermia, meconium aspiration, and sepsis. Hypoxia with acidosis (often referred to as "asphyxia," although originally the term simply meant "born without an evident pulse," from the Greek *a-sphyxos*) is widely perceived to be the most important cause, but does not have a simple relationship with the condition of the baby at birth. Beard and coworkers[1] pointed out as early as 1967 that the Apgar score (a clinical measure of condition at birth) "does not differentiate between asphyxial and non-asphyxial depression of the newborn." In 1982, Sykes and colleagues[2] reported that only 27% of babies with a severe acidosis (umbilical artery pH < 7.1 and a base deficit > 12 mmol/L) had a 1-minute Apgar score less than 7. Similarly, only 21% with a 1-minute Apgar score less than 7 had a severe acidosis. Lissauer and Steer[3] subsequently noted that more than half of babies born at 32 weeks' gestation or later, and needing resuscitation by intubation and positive pressure ventilation, had either entirely normal fetal heart rate (FHR) patterns throughout labor or normal values for umbilical cord blood pH measurement. In their study, the nonasphyxial associations with depression at birth included operative delivery, anesthetic agents given to the mother, meconium-stained liquor, and tight nuchal cord. Steer and associates[4] subsequently reported that acidosis in the fetus (as measured by cord umbilical artery pH) accounted for only 7.5% of the variation in the 1-minute Apgar score, and 1.8% of the variation in the 5-minute Apgar score. Thorp and coworkers[5] reported that umbilical artery cord pH was normal in 80% of clinically depressed newborns.

Chorioamnionitis has, in recent years, been recognized as an important antecedent of cerebral palsy,[6] but it is not directly associated with asphyxia. Maberry and colleagues[7] reported that chorioamnionitis does not increase the likelihood of metabolic acidosis at birth; there were no babies with a significant metabolic acidosis or pH less than 7.0 in 123 cases of confirmed intra-amniotic infection during labor. Instead, the brain damage that later manifests as cerebral palsy may be caused by cytokine release. Nonetheless, chorioamnionitis, or even noninfective fever during labor (see Chapter 72), may potentiate the damaging effects of hypoxia-ischemia on the brain by increasing its metabolic requirements for oxygen.[8]

What Constitutes "Birth Asphyxia"?

Saling's initial publication[9] reviewed 306 babies born in vigorous condition and reported their mean capillary fetal blood sample (FBS) pH to be 7.33 with a range (±2 standard deviations [SD]) of 7.2 to 7.5. An FBS pH of 7.2 subsequently became a widely accepted lower limit of normal, below which values were taken to indicate the need for urgent delivery. However, it has become appreciated that acidosis has to be very severe (values well below 2 SD from the mean) before it is associated with long-term sequelae. For example, Winkler and associates[10] reported that none of 335 infants born with an umbilical artery pH less than 7.2 but greater than 7.0 had any neonatal complications, and only 2 of 23 born with a pH less than 7.0 had any complications attributable to asphyxia. Goodwin and coworkers[11] reviewed 129 full-term, normally formed, singleton infants born with an umbilical artery pH less than 7.0 and found that 78% were entirely normal at follow-up, with only 8% having a major neurologic defect. Nagel and colleagues[12] reported 30 newborns with an umbilical artery pH less than 7.0. All but 3 had an Apgar score of 6 or more at 5 minutes. In the neonatal period, 2 babies died, 5 had mild and 2 severe encephalopathy. Using the Denver Developmental Screening Test at ages ranging from 14 to 33 months, 23 surviving babies were normal, 2 questionable, and none had major abnormalities (31 were lost to follow-up). However, these reports should not be taken as meaning that acidosis is always benign. Severe acidosis (pH < 7.0) is still likely to be associated with a much higher incidence of depression at birth than a pH greater than 7.2. Van den Berg and associates[13] reviewed the neonatal complications of 84 nonanomalous babies with an umbilical artery pH less than 7.0 and compared them with a nonacidotic (pH > 7.24) matched control group. They found highly significant differences in the proportions of babies requiring intubation (29% vs. 2.4%), and having pulmonary (31% vs. 11%), cardiovascular (15% vs. 8%), and neurologic (23% vs. 7%) complications. Low and coworkers[14] studied the effect of metabolic acidosis on newborn complications at 10 days of life. Fifty-nine babies had a severe metabolic acidosis (umbilical artery buffer base < 30 mmol/L) and were six times more likely to have complications than a control group without acidosis (85% vs. 14%). Neonatal encephalopathy was observed in 61% of the acidotic group versus 17% of the control group. Socol and colleagues[15] studied 28 newborns with an Apgar score of 3 or less at 5 minutes. They found that 11 of 17 neonates with an umbilical cord arterial pH greater than 7.0 had an uncomplicated neonatal course compared with only 1 of 11 with a pH less than 7.0. Low and associates[16] have subsequently studied the threshold of fetal metabolic acidosis at delivery above which moderate or severe newborn complications may be expected; they found this to be an umbilical artery base deficit of 12 mmol/L. Thereafter, increasing metabolic acidosis is associated with a progression of severity of newborn complications.

On the basis of these findings, it seems reasonable to categorize asphyxia as a cord artery pH less than 7.0 and a base deficit greater than 12 mmol/L. However, because the large majority of babies with asphyxia by this definition have a normal long-term outcome, it has been suggested that the term *birth asphyxia* should be used to indicate an even more severe situation in which, in addition to acidosis, generalized neonatal dysfunction is evident. Thus, Thorp[17] suggested the inclusion of neonatal depression as measured by the Apgar score, as well as evidence of hypoxic end-organ damage such as early neonatal seizures and renal or cardiac dysfunction. Subsequently, the American College of Obstetricians and Gynecologists (ACOG)[18] recommended that birth asphyxia be regarded as resulting from "intrapartum hypoxia sufficient to cause neurological damage," defined by an umbilical artery pH less than 7.0, a 5-minute Apgar score of 3 or less, moderate or severe neonatal encephalopathy, and evidence of multiorgan dysfunction (affecting the cardiovascular, renal, and/or pulmonary systems) (Table 69–1). Few depressed neonates fulfill these stringent conditions.[19]

Do Intrapartum Events Lead to Cerebral Palsy?

It is clear that the majority of mental handicap is not caused by intrapartum events. In 1985, the U.S. National Institutes of Health[20] reported that "the causes of severe mental retardation are primarily genetic, biochemical, viral and developmental, and not related to birth events. Associated factors include maternal lifestyle, such as poor nutrition, cigarette smoking, and alcohol and drug abuse." For example, the single most prevalent cause of mental retardation is Down syndrome. However, some forms of mental handicap are likely to be the consequence of birth asphyxia and other adverse intrapartum events. The International Cerebral Palsy Task Force suggested that birth asphyxia was a significant cause of cerebral palsy characterized by nonprogressive abnormal control of movement or posture.[21] The percentage of such cases caused by birth asphyxia remains controversial. It is widely accepted that at least some acute intrapartum events (e.g., placental abruption, cord prolapse) can cause brain injury in previously normal fetuses. In a review of 351 babies investigated by magnetic resonance imaging (MRI) or at postmortem, Cowan and coworkers[22] showed that more than 90% of full-term infants with neonatal encephalopathy, seizures, or both, but without specific syndromes or major congenital defects, had evidence of perinatally acquired insults, and in only a few babies was there any evidence of established brain injury acquired before birth. Their data do not exclude the possibility that antenatal factors could initiate a causal pathway for perinatal brain injury and that they might, possibly together with genetic predispositions to hypoxic-ischemic injury, make some infants more susceptible than others to the stresses of labor and delivery. However, although their study was not population-based, it strongly suggests that the potential for avoiding intrapartum brain damage by improved management is substantial. The Western Australia case-control study of neonatal encephalopathy[23] (which was population-based) clearly showed a protective effect of elective cesarean section (adjusted odds ratio [OR] 0.17, 95% confidence interval [CI] 0.05–0.56). This demonstrates that intrapartum events do play a role in the etiology of neonatal encephalopathy. The question of the proportion of babies with brain injury but no evidence of chromosomal anomaly or congenital anomaly that are due to intrapartum events has been addressed by Johnston,[24] who concluded that it was between 30% and 60%, depending on the setting and the efficiency of intrapartum surveillance and the risk status of the population. When addressing the likelihood of perinatal events as a cause of cerebral palsy, the criteria of Nelson can be recommended (Table 69–2).

TABLE 69–1

American College of Obstetricians and Gynecologists Definition of Birth Asphyxia, 1991

Intrapartum hypoxia sufficient to cause neurologic damage
Umbilical artery pH < 7.00
5-minute Apgar score ≤ 3
Moderate or severe neonatal encephalopathy
Multiorgan dysfunction (e.g., CVS, renal, pulmonary)

CVS, cardiovascular system.

From American College of Obstetricians and Gynecologists (ACOG): Utility of umbilical cord blood acid-base measurement: ACOG Committee Opinion. Obstet Gynecol 1991;91:33–34.

MANAGEMENT ISSUES

Diagnosis of Fetal Distress

Diagnosis is difficult because of the problems of accessing the fetus in utero. Before the introduction of the Pinard stethoscope, the condition of the fetus remained unknown until the moment of birth. However, once the FHR could be detected with some reliability, it was discovered that both persistent fetal tachycardia and bradycardia were associated with an increased likelihood of poor condition at birth, and that meconium staining of the amniotic fluid could also be an adverse sign. Once continuous electronic fetal monitoring (EFM) was introduced in the 1960s, it was possible to detect reduced FHR variability, which is also associated with

TABLE 69–2

Criteria to Be Fulfilled before Long-Term Outcome Can Be Linked with Intrapartum Events

1. Was there evidence of severe, prolonged intrapartum dysfunction?
2. Was the child severely ill as a newborn? Were there disturbances of feeding, tone, and consciousness, and evidence of involvement of other organ systems, of which renal involvement may be especially significant?
3. Is cerebral palsy present?
4. Have other potential explanations been excluded, such as
   Congenital malformation
   Infection
   Metabolic abnormality
   Familial disease
   Microcephaly in the neonatal period
   Abnormal CT or MRI scan suggesting discrete lesions
   Maternal substance abuse (especially cocaine)
   Thyroid disease

CT, computed tomography; MRI, magnetic resonance imaging.
From Nelson K: Perspective on the role of perinatal asphyxia in neurologic outcome. CMAJ 1998(Suppl).

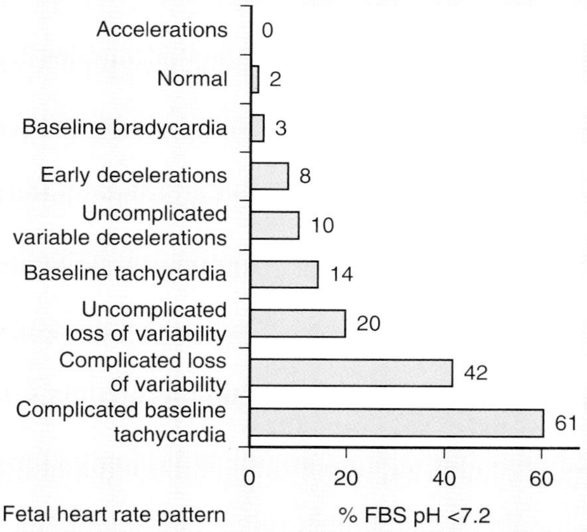

FIGURE 69–1
Fetal heart rate pattern and the associated risk of acidosis.

an increased risk of depression at birth. The introduction of FBS and pH estimation by Saling[9] allowed further assessment of fetal condition. Unfortunately, FBS is a complicated and time-consuming technique, which is uncomfortable for the mother. As a result, the approach that developed was to use EFM as a screening tool for asphyxia, and then use FBS to confirm or reject the diagnosis. Beard and colleagues, in their landmark paper of 1971,[25] showed that a normal FHR pattern is associated with a very low risk of acidosis (<2% of fetuses with a normal FHR pattern will have a pH < 7.2). However, although increasing abnormality of the FHR is associated with an increasing chance that the fetus is acidotic, even with the most abnormal pattern (a complicated baseline tachycardia), the risk of acidosis is only about 60% (Fig. 69–1). This explains the increased intervention rates for the diagnosis of fetal distress if FHR monitoring is used without the backup of FBS and pH estimation.[26,27] Reviews indicate that the use of FBS and pH measurement not only limits the increase in operative delivery rate seen with EFM but also improves its ability to reduce the neonatal seizure rate.[28]

Most studies of EFM have examined the relationship between the heart rate pattern and asphyxia. Cardiotocogram (CTG) interpretation can, however, also indicate other pathologies, such as pyrexia (and therefore indirectly, sepsis), which is associated with a fetal tachycardia.[29] Recurrent variable decelerations with a maintained normal FBS pH suggest intermittent cord compression. Repeated umbilical cord compression may cause brain damage without asphyxia because of the major swings in blood pressure induced by repeated occlusion and release.[30] The damage may be exacerbated by nuchal entanglement (cord around the neck) because occlusion of the venous return from the brain increases intracranial pressure. Damage to the hippocampus from intermittent occlusion of the cord has been seen in fetal sheep.[31]

Does Electronic Fetal Monitoring Improve Outcome?

The widespread introduction of EFM in the 1970s was associated with substantial falls in perinatal mortality as reported by a number of retrospective observational studies.[32,33] However, during the same period, major advances were being made in neonatal intensive care, and the cesarean section rate also rose substantially. It has proved impossible to establish which of these changes, if any, was responsible for the improvement in outcome. This uncertainty led to calls for prospective, randomized, controlled trials. None of these trials was, on their own, large enough to have sufficient power to address the long-term outcome of most interest, namely cerebral palsy. Accordingly, there have been a series of meta-analyses, although these are dominated by the effect of the single largest trial, carried out in Dublin in the early 1980s.[34] Vintzileos and associates[26] reviewed nine, including in total 18,561 patients (of which 12,964 were in the Dublin trial). This confirmed a substantial increase in the cesarean section rate associated with EFM (OR 1.53, 95% CI 1.17–2.01), but disappointingly for the advocates of EFM, the reduction in the overall perinatal mortality rate was not significant (4.2/1000 in the EFM group vs. 4.9/1000 in the intermittent auscultation [IA] group). However, in a post hoc analysis, Vintzileos and associates[26] commented that there was a significant reduction in the deaths attributed to hypoxia in the EFM groups, being 0.7/1000 compared with 1.8/1000 in the auscultation group (OR 0.41, 95% CI 0.17–0.98). A similar meta-analysis was performed by Thacker and coworkers[27] with the inclusion of three further studies but with similar conclusions, except that they reported a significant reduction in the incidence of neonatal seizures in the group where EFM had been used (relative risk [RR] 0.5, 95% CI 0.30–0.82). Thus, the studies suggest some improvement in short-term outcome at the expense of an increased operative delivery rate, but were unable to address the issue of long-term outcome (a follow-up study of the Dublin trial showed that three babies in each group developed cerebral palsy[35]; however, even if the number had been doubled in the auscultation group, this would still not have been statistically significant). It should be noted that many authorities, including the National Institute for Clinical Excellence (NICE) in the United Kingdom, state in relation to the meta-analyses that "there was no apparent difference in perinatal death rates between the two groups."[36] This is not actually correct, because most studies show a difference in favor of EFM, which is not, however, statistically significant. As already pointed out, even the meta-analyses are underpowered to address the question of perinatal mortality, let alone long-term outcome. It should always be remembered that absence of evidence is not evidence of absence, and one needs to be aware of the possibility of a type II error (i.e., there is a difference that by chance has not been found to be significant).

Fetal Heart Rate Monitoring and Fetal Blood Sampling

It will be appreciated from the previous discussion that monitoring the heart rate of the fetus should not be expected to detect all pathologies affecting the fetus during labor. For example, maternal intrapartum cardiac arrest, fetal skull fracture with brain infarct, intrapartum fetal stroke, and uterine rupture have been reported as causes of subsequent childhood handicap,[37] but none of these can be predicted reliably beforehand by FHR monitoring. (In a study of 36 cases of intrapartum rupture of a previous cesarean section scar,[38] no significant differences were noted in rates of mild or severe variable decelerations, late decelerations, prolonged decelerations, fetal tachycardia, or loss of uterine tone. Fetal bradycardia in the first and second stage was the only finding consistently associated with uterine rupture.) Equally, although intrapartum infection and meconium aspiration may be associated with fetal tachycardia, neither is consistently associated with acidosis[4,39]; therefore, a normal FBS pH may be actively misleading in their management if a normal value is taken as reassurance about fetal condition. Nevertheless, hypoxia and acidosis pose a significant threat to the fetus during labor (accounting for perhaps 20%–40% of poor condition at birth), and FHR monitoring remains the best available screening tool for its detection. The best way to detect developing acidosis in the fetus is to measure its blood pH using a FBS. Clues about other pathologies (e.g., variable decelerations with nuchal cord, FHR tachycardia with infection, sinusoidal variability with fetal anemia) can be obtained from EFM, but its use in these conditions should not be regarded as sensitive or specific.

Human Factors in the Use of Cardiotocography

A human element may factor into our inability to demonstrate that the use of EFM produces an improved outcome to the degree anticipated by the pioneers of the technique. For example, in the Dublin trial,[34] the fetal monitors used were of a relatively primitive design, staff were previously unfamiliar with their use, and during the trial, a marked Hawthorne effect was evident, which would have reduced its apparent efficacy. In a later case-control study, the intrapartum treatment of 38 babies severely asphyxiated at birth was compared with 120 controls.[40] In the control group, 29% of babies had an abnormal intrapartum FHR tracing, but in only 9% was the abnormality severe. In contrast, in the babies asphyxiated at birth, 87% had an abnormal FHR tracing, and in 61% of cases, the abnormality was severe. The most striking finding, however, was the length of time required for the staff to recognize the FHR abnormality. With moderate abnormalities, the mean time to recognition was 71 minutes, and paradoxically, with severe abnormalities, it was 118 minutes. The authors could give no plausible reason why the standard of FHR tracing interpretation was so poor. However, it was clear from this study that if the quality of interpretation of the intrapartum FHR pattern had been higher, the benefits from EFM would almost certainly have been significantly and substantially enhanced.

In 1990, Ennis and Vincent[41] published the results of their study of 64 cases of poor perinatal outcome from the archives of the Medical Protection Society. In 11 cases, although indicated, continuous EFM was not performed. In 6 cases, the technical quality of the tracing was inadequate. In 14 cases, a significant abnormality in the FHR pattern was present, but this was either not noticed or no action was taken upon it. In only 14 cases was appropriate monitoring and action performed (the CTG was missing in 19 cases). In only 16 cases was a consultant involved in the interpretation of the tracing. In a further study from Oxford published in 1994,[19] intrapartum care was assessed in 141 cases of cerebral palsy and 62 perinatal deaths with a potential intrapartum cause. They found that abnormal FHR patterns were 2.3 times as common in babies who went on to develop cerebral palsy than in controls, and 6.7 times as common in perinatal deaths. They found that failure to respond to these clear signs of abnormality occurred in 26% of cerebral palsy cases and 50% of perinatal deaths, compared with 7% of controls. On the basis of these figures, it can be calculated that there will be approximately 1 case of potentially preventable cerebral palsy and 1 potentially preventable perinatal death in every 4000 deliveries. If one assumes 700,000 births per annum in the United Kingdom, 174 cases of cerebral palsy and 158 cases of perinatal death would be preventable.

More recently, Stewart and colleagues[42] reported that perinatal mortality in Wales is twice as high at night as during the day, and twice as high in July/August as in the rest of the year. They suggested that the excess of deaths may represent overreliance on inexperienced staff at night and a shortage of staff during the peak summer holiday months and also that it might be related to physical and mental fatigue of the caregivers. The Confidential Enquiry into Stillbirths and Deaths in Infancy (CESDI) was a U.K. national survey of perinatal deaths, now subsumed into the Confidential Enquiry into Maternal and Child Health (CEMACH, www.cemach.org.uk). The fourth annual report showed that failures in the use and interpretation of CTG were present in more than half of intrapartum-related deaths.[43] The fifth report studied the proportion of 567 cases in which there was evidence of suboptimal care in labor, and then classified this by whether improved care could possibly or probably have prevented the adverse outcome.[44] Suboptimal care was identified in 71% of cases, and a better outcome could possibly or probably have been anticipated in 28% and 22% of cases, respectively, if care had been adequate. The report commented that "fetal surveillance problems were the commonest cause [of problems in labor], with CTG interpretation ... the most frequent criticism."

Maternity care currently accounts for over 50% of the U.K. National Health Service (NHS) medical litigation bill, with individual settlements reaching £6 million and even successful defense costing up to £0.5 million. At the 31st of March 2008, the total value of claims against the NHS Litigation Authority in the United Kingdom with respect to obstetrics and gynecology from April 1995 onward totaled £3.3 billion (http://www.nhsla.com). In 2006 to 2007, £579.3 million was paid out in total medicolegal settlements; 51% of this was for obstetrics.

Possible Interventions to Improve the Quality of Care

Young and associates[45] have studied the efficacy of intrapartum intervention and found that in cases of low Apgar scores, there was evidence of substandard care in labor in 74%. Following the introduction of regular audit of low Apgar scores, with feedback to clinical staff, this proportion fell to 23%, but crept back up to 32% over the following year. However, following the introduction of compulsory training in FHR pattern interpretation for all staff, the proportion of low Apgar score cases associated with substandard care fell back once again to only 9%.

Indications for Electronic Fetal Monitoring

Intrapartum EFM was intended to be a screening tool for fetal hypoxia, with FBS used as the confirmatory test. Accordingly, many authorities have advocated universal continuous EFM. However, with the growth of the "natural childbirth" movement, and the difficulty in establishing the efficacy of EFM in randomized trials, most guidelines now suggest that IA is an adequate form of FHR monitoring for "low risk" labors and that continuous EFM should be reserved for "high risk" labors. Unfortunately, it is difficult to define "low risk" labor. The 2001 guidelines of NICE in the United Kingdom[36] approached this problem by listing high risk factors that they considered indicated the need for continuous EFM (Table 69–3). We analyzed 29,443 births at the Chelsea and Westminster Hospital (London, UK) from 1988 thru 1998 inclusive and coded them as low risk if: the mother's age was younger than 40; there was no diabetes, cardiac disease, renal disease, or antepartum hemorrhage; the highest blood pressure at any time during pregnancy was less than 90 mm Hg diastolic; presentation was cephalic; gestation was 37 to 42 weeks; labor onset was spontaneous; the labor duration was less than 12 hours; epidural anesthesia was not used; and there was no oxytocin augmentation, meconium staining of the amniotic fluid, or pyrexia. Using these criteria, labors were low risk throughout labor in only 26%. Therefore, according to the NICE guidelines, IA throughout labor was applicable in only about a quarter of labors. In fact, only 11% had no EFM during labor, and the incidence of abnormal FHR pattern was 7.8%. In contrast, in the "high risk" 74%, 4.3% had no EFM during labor, and the incidence of abnormal FHR pattern was 22.8%. A similar analysis of the data from 15 other maternity units in the North West Thames region of London showed a median value for "low risk" labors of 25%, with the highest proportion of low risk labor being 34%, and the lowest 16%. In only one of these units did the proportion of low risk labor in which EFM was not used exceed 50%. Mires and coworkers[46] have reported on a randomized, controlled trial of CTG versus Doppler auscultation of the fetal heart at admission in labor in low risk obstetric population. They commented that "as the trial progressed, it became clear that ... more women had complications that required continuous monitoring than had been predicted"; the overall proportion was 63% and was similar in both groups. In a study of low risk labors in Dublin, Impey and colleagues[47] reported that if an admission CTG was performed, 58% of women had continuous EFM during labor, but that even if IA was used from the outset, 42% of women had continuous EFM. The updated NICE guideline on care in normal labor[48] has reduced the number of indications for continuous EFM (Table 69–4), but it is unlikely that this will significantly change the proportion of women requiring this intervention.

TABLE 69–3

Possible Indications for Continuous Electronic Fetal Monitoring

Labor Abnormalities
Induced labor
Augmented labor
Prolonged labor
Prolonged membrane rupture
Regional analgesia
Previous cesarean delivery
Abnormal uterine activity
Suspected Fetal Distress in Labor
Meconium staining of the amniotic fluid
Suspicious fetal heart rate on auscultation
Abnormal fetal heart rate on admission cardiotocography
Vaginal bleeding during labor
Intrauterine infection
Fetal Problems
Multiple pregnancies (all fetuses)
Small fetus
Preterm fetus
Breech presentation
Oligohydramnios
Post-term pregnancy
Rhesus isoimmunization
Maternal Medical Disease
Hypertension
Diabetes
Cardiac disease (especially cyanotic)
Hemoglobinopathy
Severe anemia
Hyperthyroidism
Collagen disease
Renal disease

Fetal Monitoring by Intermittent Auscultation

Evidence regarding the value of EFM is limited, but the evidence regarding the use of IA is even worse. Recommendations, therefore, have to depend entirely on custom and practice and "expert" opinion. These were summarized in the United Kingdom in the 2001 NICE guidelines,[36] which followed ACOG and the Society of Obstetricians and Gynaecologists of Canada in recommending that (1) during the

TABLE 69-4

Indications for Changing from Intermittent Auscultation to Continuous Electronic Fetal Monitoring

Significant meconium-stained liquor (should also be considered for light meconium-stained liquor)
Abnormal fetal heart rate detected by IA (<110 beats/min; >160 beats/min; any decelerations after a contraction)
Maternal pyrexia (defined as 38°C once or 37.5°C on two occasions 2 hr apart)
Fresh bleeding developing during labor
Oxytocin usage for augmentation
The woman's request

IA, intermittent auscultation.
From National Collaborating Centre for Women's and Children's Health (NCC-WCH/NICE): Intrapartum Care. Care of Healthy Women and Their Babies during Childbirth. London, RCOG Press, 2007. Available at http://www.nice.org.uk/nicemedia/pdf/CG55FullGuideline.pdf

active phase of the first stage of labor, the FHR should be auscultated and recorded every 15 minutes and (2) during the second stage of labor, the FHR should be auscultated and recorded every 5 minutes. Ideally, the heart rate should be counted over 30 to 60 seconds, in the minute after a contraction (to detect late decelerations). The 2007 U.K. National Collaborating Centre for Women's and Children's Health (NCC-WCH)/NICE guideline modified these recommendations slightly and stated that in the first stage IA of the fetal heart should occur after a contraction for at least 1 minute, at least every 15 minutes, and the rate should be recorded as an average,[48] and in the second stage, after a contraction for at least 1 minute, at least every 5 minutes.[49]

The "Admission" Cardiotocogram

The incidence of emergency cesarean section for fetal distress is higher in the first hour of labor than in any subsequent single hour. This is because the onset of contractions reveals the fetus that is unable to cope with the relative hypoxia of labor. For this reason, performing EFM for the first hour of labor even in low risk pregnancies ("admission test") has become popular in some maternity units. Unfortunately, no studies of sufficient size have been conducted to enable an evaluation of the usefulness of this approach.[36]

Technical Aspects of Electronic Fetal Monitoring

A cardiotocograph machine is used to produce a continuous recording of FHR and uterine contractions, known as a CTG. It reveals information about aspects of FHR such as baseline variability, which cannot be measured using IA. It also produces recordings of FHR decelerations in relation to contractions, which are easier to detect and analyze, and an automatic paper recording is produced for archival purposes (optical disks are increasingly being used for convenient storage). This record is available for subsequent independent review, which is valuable for audit and teaching, although it may be a mixed blessing in medicolegal terms if it reveals abnormalities previously overlooked.

EFMs can measure the FHR and uterine contractions via external transducers using Doppler ultrasound and a tocodynamometer (strain gauge attached to a belt) or via internal sensors such as a fetal electrode and an intrauterine catheter. Despite the fact that the latter methods are more reliable and accurate, and probably more comfortable for the average woman in labor than the belts necessary to attach the external transducers, they are more invasive, and thus, most EFM is performed using external devices. This mode of EFM has a number of problems. First, modern machines generally use a form of autocorrelation or cross-correlation analysis to produce the FHR from ultrasound signals, but the systems are now so sensitive that if the fetus is dead, they sometimes produce a recording of the maternal rate, which can be mistaken for that of the fetus. This is particularly likely if the mother is anxious and has a tachycardia so that her heart rate is similar to that expected of her fetus and can even lead to the erroneous emergency delivery of a dead baby.[50] To avoid this problem, it is good practice always to ensure that rate calculation is derived from the characteristic signals of the fetal heart (sharp and distinct, sometimes sounding like the hooves of a galloping horse), rather than to rely on the "whooshing" sound produced by reflections from fetal blood vessels.

Second, good recording of the FHR depends greatly on correct placement of the transducers on the abdomen. This is not always achieved, and constant readjustment is often necessary if the mother is very active. Unfortunately, it is often the mothers who wish to have an active birth and who are very mobile who decline the use of internal monitoring. This commonly results in loss of adequate signal and FHR information at a most critical time in the labor, the second stage.

Third, the information obtained about uterine contractions using an external transducer is essentially limited to timing them. The external contraction transducer (tocodynamometer) gives only a relative indication of contraction strength, and the recording is attenuated if, for example, the mother is obese or the transducer is poorly placed. This may mislead the birth attendant into underestimating the strength of contractions, particularly in a stoic woman, and thus lead to overdosage with uterine stimulants such as oxytocin. By comparison, the recordings obtained from a directly applied fetal electrode and an intrauterine catheter are much more accurate and less susceptible to recording failure.

One factor that militates against the use of scalp electrodes is the increasing prevalence of the HIV virus. The Royal College of Obstetricians and Gynaecologists (RCOG; UK) advises that women who carry the HIV virus should not have their fetuses monitored using an electrode that breaches its skin, for fear of increasing the risk of transmission of the virus to the fetus. Although women with a detectable viral load are now advised to have their babies delivered by cesarean section, and HIV-infected women normally choose vaginal delivery only if their viral load is undetectable, anonymous testing reveals that in about 25% of cases, women positive for HIV choose not to have antenatal testing and, therefore, go through labor unaware they are at risk.

Interpretation of Fetal Heart Rate Recordings

The key to reliable and consistent interpretation of FHR tracings from CTG machines is a systematic approach. Four main aspects of the FHR should be assessed: the baseline rate, baseline variability, the presence or absence of accelerations, and the presence and classification of decelerations (slowings of the FHR, or "dips"). Many errors of interpretation occur because of an excessive concern with decelerations and a consequent failure to appreciate the significance of the other three aspects of the FHR. A detailed account of how the FHR can be assessed using a CTG is given in Table 69–5.

A normal CTG pattern is highly reassuring that the fetus is not acidotic; the significance of an abnormal pattern is much more difficult to judge. In general, the more of the four basic aspects of the FHR (baseline rate, baseline variability, accelerations, decelerations) that are abnormal, the more likely the fetus is to be acidotic. However, other factors should modulate the response to such a pattern.

The Time Factor

The fetus does not become acidotic as soon as the FHR becomes abnormal; Fleischer and associates[51] showed that a well-grown fetus can cope with hypoxic stress for as long as 90 minutes before the pH of fetal blood starts to fall. Thus, a normal fetal scalp blood pH 60 minutes after the CTG has become abnormal does not indicate that the abnormality is a "false-positive." The pH of the fetus may begin to fall at any subsequent time; accordingly the only safe plan is to repeat the FBS at hourly intervals (more often if the pattern is severely abnormal) or to deliver the baby.

In contrast, a low pH may be an acute response to temporary interference with maternal placental blood flow and gas exchange. This can occur, for example, after an epidural top-up (with or without maternal hypotension) or because of uterine hyperstimulation with oxytocics. Action should be taken to correct the problem. This can include turning the mother to the left lateral position to correct supine hypotension, stopping any infusions of oxytocic drugs, and giving the mother oxygen by face mask; persisting hypotension from epidural anesthesia can usually be corrected by intravenous injection of a vasoconstrictor such as ephedrine, and excessive uterine activity may be corrected by an infusion of a tocolytic drug such as ritodrine or salbutamol. If the FHR pattern returns to normal, a low pH is often corrected, and immediate delivery of the fetus would be inappropriate. Therefore, it is probably unnecessary to take an FBS in response to an acute FHR abnormality unless the resuscitative measures described earlier do not correct the abnormality of the FHR within 15 to 20 minutes.

Intrauterine Growth Restriction

Any baby thought to be seriously small for gestational age on antenatal assessment or with intrauterine growth restriction seen on serial ultrasound scanning should be treated as particularly at risk during labor.[52] There is an increased likelihood of abnormal FHR patterns and acidosis, so FBSs should be taken more readily and more often than with well-grown babies, and the threshold for operative delivery should be reduced.

Early Gestational Age

Preterm babies are more susceptible to the effects of intrauterine hypoxia than full-term babies; in particular, hypoxia has a damaging effect on the type 2 pneumocytes that produce surfactant in the lungs, increasing the incidence and severity of the neonatal respiratory distress syndrome (hyaline membrane disease).[53] However, the incidence of hypoxia and acidosis in fetuses in preterm labor is not increased compared with fetuses in full-term labor.[54] Preterm babies are more likely to have low Apgar scores than full-term babies, but this is due to functional immaturity and not to the effects of hypoxia.[55] A baby born at 28 weeks' gestation is likely to have poor respiratory effort, to have reduced tone, and to have less reflex irritability, and thus, a lower Apgar score than its full-term counterpart; however, given a normal FHR pattern, it is no more likely to be hypoxic or acidotic.[54] The interpretation of the FHR pattern of the preterm fetus in labor is similar to that of its full-term counterpart.[56] However, some subtle differences may be seen in the FHR pattern.[57] Short-term baseline variability is often rather less, and FHR accelerations less frequent (the differentiation between quiet and active sleep patterns sometimes does not develop until 28 to 32 weeks' gestation). Small, brief (<20 sec) decelerations are often seen and are insignificant (cause unknown).

Presentation of the Fetus

Although current recommendations favor elective cesarean delivery for babies in breech position,[58] there is still a place for vaginal delivery if this is what the mother requests (see Chapter 63). The second stage of labor is prolonged when the fetus is in breech presentation, and therefore, it is probably wise not to embark on a vaginal breech delivery if there is any suggestion of fetal compromise at the onset of the second stage. Thus, if the FHR pattern is entirely normal, vaginal delivery can proceed, but if the FHR is abnormal, fetal condition should be checked by an FBS pH measurement. This can readily be taken from the buttock, and pH values are the same as for babies in cephalic presentation.[59] If the FBS pH is normal, the delivery can be allowed to proceed, but if the FHR abnormality persists, the FBS should probably be repeated if delivery has not occurred within 30 minutes. The passage of meconium is common with a breech presentation and, unless it occurs very early in labor, is not a useful monitoring variable.

Twins or Higher-Order Pregnancy

Because of the increased risk of perinatal mortality associated with being a second twin, there is an increasing trend for elective cesarean delivery. However, vaginal delivery is a reasonable option if that is the parents' preference.[60] The use of ultrasound allows the heart rate of the second twin to be recorded accurately, and in view of the higher mortality rates for the second twins, such monitoring is recommended. The second twin may have heart rate changes suggestive of hypoxia while that of the first twin remains normal.[61] In this case, because FBS is impossible until the first twin has been delivered, cesarean section is probably appropriate.

Instrumental Delivery

Fetal distress is commonly cited as an indication for urgent instrumental vaginal delivery. However, great caution should be applied if the fetal head needs to be rotated. Hypoxia and acidosis can cause cerebral edema, and an edematous brain is stiffer and less flexible than normal. Twisting forces applied in this situation may cause tentorial tears, which

TABLE 69–5
Interpretation of Fetal Heart Rate Pattern (Cardiotocogram)

Admission Test

Normal, reassuring, or reactive

- Two or more accelerations (>15 beats/min for 15 sec) in 20 min
- Baseline FHR 110–150 beats/min
- Baseline variability 5–25 beats/min
- Absence of decelerations
- Moderate tachycardia/bradycardia and accelerations

Interpretation/action: Risk of fetal hypoxia in next 2–3 hr in spontaneous labor, is low other than following acute events

Suspicious, equivocal, or nonreactive

- Absence of accelerations, reduced baseline variability (5–10 beats/min), or silent pattern (5 beats/min), for >40 min, although baseline rate normal (110–150 beats/min)
- Baseline FHR < 100 beats/min or >150 beats/min
- Variable decelerations (depth < 60 beats/min, duration < 60 sec)

Interpretation/action: Continue CTG, consider vibroacoustic stimulation/fetal scalp pH estimation if CTG not normal in 1 hr

Pathologic/ominous

- Silent pattern and baseline FHR > 150 beats/min or < 110 beats/min with no acceleration
- Repetitive late decelerations and/or complicated variable decelerations
- Baseline FHR < 100 beats/min or prolonged bradycardia (>10 min)

Interpretation/action: Exclude cord prolapse, placental abruption, and scar dehiscence. If small fetus, or thick meconium, or previously abnormal trace, consider immediate delivery. In other situations, consider fetal scalp pH estimation (and, e.g., tocolysis if uterine hyperstimulation, IV fluids if related to epidural "top-up")

First-Stage Intrapartum CTG

Normal, reassuring, or reactive

- Two or more accelerations (>15 beats/min for >15 sec) in 20 min
- Baseline FHR 110–150 beats/min
- Baseline variability 5–25 beats/min
- Early decelerations (in late first stage)

Suspicious, equivocal, or nonreactive

- Absence of accelerations for > 40 min
- Baseline FHR 150–170 beats/min or 100–110 beats/min (normal baseline variability, no decelerations)
- Silent pattern > 40 min (normal baseline rate, no decelerations)
- Baseline variability > 25 beats/min in the absence of accelerations
- Variable decelerations (depth < 60 beats/min, duration < 60 sec)
- Occasional transient prolonged bradycardia (FHR drops to < 80 beats/min for > 2 min or < 100 beats/min for > 3 min)

Interpretation/action: Continue CTG, vibroacoustic stimulation or fetal scalp pH estimation if CTG not normal in 1 hr

Pathologic/ominous

- Baseline FHR > 150 beats/min and silent pattern and/or repetitive late or variable decelerations
- Silent pattern for > 90 min
- Complicated variable decelerations (depth ≥ 60 beats/min, duration ≥ 60 sec) and changes in shape (overshoot, decreased or increased baseline heart rate following the deceleration, absence of baseline variability, slow recovery)
- Combined/biphasic decelerations (variable followed by late)
- Prolonged bradycardia (FHR drops to < 80 beats/min for > 2 min or < 100 beats/min for > 3 min) in a suspicious trace
- Prolonged bradycardia (FHR drops to < 80 beats/min for > 2 min or < 100 beats/min for > 3 min) > 10 min
- Repetitive late decelerations
- Pronounced loss of baseline variability
- Sinusoidal pattern with no accelerations

Interpretation/action: Consider fetal scalp pH estimation

Second-Stage Intrapartum CTG

Normal, reassuring, or reactive

- Normal baseline heart rate, normal baseline variability and no decelerations, frequent accelerations, both periodic and scattered
- Baseline heart rate 110–150 beats/min and baseline variability 5–25 beats/min with or without early and/or variable decelerations

Suspicious, equivocal, or nonreactive

- Baseline heart rate > 150 beats/min, persisting or compensatory following each deceleration
- Reduced baseline variability or silent pattern decelerations of > 60 sec duration
- Mild bradycardia, heart rate catches up between contractions and may reach above 100 beats/min, especially when baseline variability is normal

Interpretation/action: Observe trace for increasing baseline heart rate or bradycardia

Pathologic/ominous

- Baseline heart rate < 100 beats/min of different patterns
- Progressive bradycardia: baseline heart rate gradually decreases between contractions; absence of baseline variability can be seen especially when heart rate < 80 beats/min
- Persisting bradycardia, baseline < 80 beats/min. The additional absence of baseline variability represents a more ominous feature
- Baseline tachycardia (>150 beats/min) with reduced variability and severe variable and late decelerations

Interpretation/action: Expedite delivery if not imminent

CTG, cardiotocography; FHR, fetal heart rate.
Courtesy of Hewlett Packard Asia-Pacific Medical Products Group.

would otherwise not occur. Thus, rotational deliveries when the FHR pattern is abnormal should probably be undertaken only after an FBS pH has been measured and found to be normal.[62]

Maternal Preference

A scientific basis for deciding when labor should be terminated operatively for fetal indications remains elusive. Such decisions cannot, therefore, be taken in isolation from the social context, and the wishes and anxieties of the parents should always be taken into account. Some parents have particular anxieties about labor; for example, they may have a sibling with residual damage attributed to birth asphyxia or trauma. In such cases, they may request delivery by cesarean section if there is any sign of fetal dysfunction or delay in labor. In view of the very low mortality and morbidity rates associated with cesarean section in modern practice, especially in the absence of any acute emergency, it is probably wise to accede to such requests unless delivery is imminent and the obstetrician very confident of a successful outcome.

PROCEDURE

FETAL BLOOD SAMPLING

Position

The use of the lithotomy position should be avoided because of the risk of supine hypotension. This can produce iatrogenic hypoxia and acidosis in the fetus, leading to unnecessary operative delivery. The sampling is most comfortably performed with the woman in the left (or right) lateral position.

Procedure

Under aseptic conditions, an amnioscope is passed up the vagina to rest on the presenting part of the fetus. Sufficient pressure must be used to exclude amniotic fluid, which will otherwise contaminate the sample. The fetal skin is then dried with a dental swab in a holder and sprayed with ethyl chloride. The evaporation of the ethyl chloride cools the skin, and as it warms up again, a reactive hyperemia is produced, which aids bleeding. The skin is smeared with a water-repellent gel (often silicone) so that when the skin is stabbed with a guarded 2-mm blade, a droplet of blood forms. This droplet is allowed to flow into a preheparinized thin glass tube by capillary action (it helps to tilt the tube slightly downward at the operator's end). Mouth-operated suction should not be used because of the risk of the operator ingesting potentially infected blood.

Analysis

The sample is then transferred to a blood gas analyzer for measurement. It is preferable to measure oxygen pressure (Po_2), carbon dioxide pressure (Pco_2), pH, and calculate the base deficit. If the values are normal, but the FHR pattern remains abnormal, it will usually be necessary to repeat the sampling within 15 to 30 minutes.

Use of Intravenous Fluids during Labor and Its Effect on Fetal Acid-Base Balance

Women in labor are commonly advised not to eat, because of the risk of Mendelson's syndrome (aspiration of stomach contents) should they unexpectedly need general anesthesia. As a result, they often develop ketonemia. For this reason, it is common practice to give parenteral fluid containing glucose and electrolytes, particularly if labor lasts more than a few hours. However, Ames and coworkers reported in 1975[63] that infusion of glucose-containing solutions could give rise to maternal lactic acidosis. This is because the rise in maternal blood glucose concentration increases the production rate of lactate, according to Michaelis-Menton kinetics. Subsequently, it was confirmed that maternal infusion of glucose at 100 g/hr (1 L of 10% glucose over 1 hr) produced a significant fall in average pH and rise in lactate in fetal as well as maternal blood.[64] However, lactic acidosis does not occur if the glucose infusion rate is restricted to 30 g/hr,[65,66] and there is some evidence to suggest that physiologic amounts of glucose in infused fluids (i.e., 5%) may be associated with less fetal acidosis than glucose-free solutions.[67] These studies indicate that in labor, as at other times, care must be taken to monitor the volume and content of intravenous infusions to ensure they are compatible with the maintenance of normal physiology.

SUMMARY OF MANAGEMENT OPTIONS
Screening for Fetal Distress in Labor

Management Options	Evidence Quality and Recommendation	References
Prevention of Fetal Hypoxia		
Avoid unnecessary induction of labor and excessive use of oxytocic agents.	III/B	36
Preload with IV fluids in women who are having epidural analgesia in labor to reduce the risk of maternal hypotension.	Ib/A	67
Remember the effect of maternal drugs on fetal heart rate patterns.	—/GPP	—

SUMMARY OF MANAGEMENT OPTIONS

Screening for Fetal Distress in Labor—cont'd

Management Options	Evidence Quality and Recommendation	References
Indications for Continuous EFM		
See Tables 69–3 and 69–4 for conditions associated with an increased risk of intrapartum fetal hypoxia. These indications may classify up to 80% of women as at-risk.	III/B	36
Fetal Monitoring in "Low Risk" Labor		
The advice from the American, Canadian, and British Colleges is that intermittent auscultation can be used in such labors; however, there are no studies of sufficient size to evaluate this approach.	III/B	36
Use of EFM in "High Risk" Labor		
Meta-analysis of randomized, controlled trials shows significant reductions in the short-term neonatal morbidity rate and a significant reduction in perinatal deaths due to hypoxia, but a significant increase in cesarean delivery rates. However, studies are underpowered to show an effect on overall perinatal mortality or cerebral palsy rates.	Ia/A	26,27
Concomitant use of FBS to estimate pH significantly reduces rates of cesarean delivery.	Ia/A	26–28
Admission EFM Recording ("Admission Test")		
This is common practice, but studies of sufficient size to evaluate this approach are lacking.	Ib/A	36,46,47
Interpretation of EFM Findings		
Human factors that adversely affect the outcome of EFM are delays in response times and failure to interpret the findings accurately. Education improves human responses, but this benefit is lost with time.	III/B	19,40–43, 45
Because of the rate of decline in fetal pH after fetal hypoxia, FBS should be performed at least hourly if EFM abnormality is detected. Shorter intervals are advisable with intrauterine growth restriction.	III/B	49,50
If EFM abnormality is detected: • Correct/avoid caval compression. • Give maternal facial oxygen. • Correct hyperstimulation (stop oxytocics, use tocolytics). • Give IV fluids if the patient has epidural-induced hypotension.	III/B	36
EFM in a preterm fetus requires the use of slightly different criteria.	IV/C	56
The maternal pulse may be mistakenly recorded as fetal. The maternal pulse should be regularly recorded clinically by palpation to reduce this risk.	IV/C	48
FBS can be used in breech presentations.	IV/C	59
EFM in twins requires careful confirmation of separate fetal recordings.	IV/C	61
The use of rotational forceps with abnormal EFM is controversial and they should not be used if the fetal scalp pH < 7.15.	IV/C	62
Technical Aspects		
EFM recordings should be retained.	—/GPP	—
External tocometry can lead to difficulty in interpreting the timing of EFM abnormalities (e.g., due to movement, maternal obesity).	—/GPP	—
The conventional advice is that fetal scalp electrodes should not be used in women with HIV.	III/B	36

Management Options	Evidence Quality and Recommendation	References
Other Methods of Fetal Monitoring		
Evidence suggests that pulse oximetry is no better than EFM.	III/B	91
No data are available on the value of near-infrared spectroscopy.	Ia/A	92
Fetal scalp lactate measurement offers practical advantages over pH measurement (less volume of blood and less affected by air bubbles), but no evidence of clinical advantage over pH.	Ib/A	94,95
Electrocardiogram shows no evidence of improved outcome in practice.	Ib/A	48
Expert systems should give better interpretative accuracy. Randomized, controlled trials are awaited.	III/B	88

EFM, electronic fetal monitoring; FBS, fetal blood sampling; GPP, good practice point.

IATROGENIC CAUSES OF FETAL DISTRESS

Excessive Oxytocin Augmentation of Labor

Every uterine contraction above 4 to 6 kPa causes a cessation of maternal intervillous placental blood flow.[68] This produces a period of relative hypoxia for the fetus, such that the fetal PO_2 falls by about 0.5 to 0.75 kPa during each contraction, reaching its lowest level at the end of the contraction, after which the flow is restored and the PO_2 recovers. Because it takes some time for the oxygen-depleted maternal pool of blood to be replaced, recovery takes about 60 to 90 seconds. The total period of reduced oxygenation is therefore 120 to 150 seconds, emphasizing the importance of an adequate intercontraction interval to ensure fetal oxygenation. Poorly controlled oxytocin infusions, which produce excessively frequent contractions, can cause iatrogenic fetal hypoxia and acidosis (see Chapter 67). In practical terms, this means that if the FHR becomes abnormal, oxytocin infusions should be stopped immediately.

Epidural Anesthesia

Before preloading of the circulation with colloid came into practice, abnormalities of the FHR occurred in approximately one third of cases following insertion of an epidural anesthetic. With preloading, this can be reduced by two thirds.[69]

Epidural anesthetics may also cause a fetal tachycardia by inducing hyperthermia in the mother (see Chapter 70). Such tachycardia is not likely to be associated with significant fetal hypoxia, and fetal pH is not affected, but it can give rise to an erroneous diagnosis of fetal distress. It may also lead to a false diagnosis of intrauterine infection, greatly increasing the proportion of newborns investigated with cultures and treated with antibiotics.[70] Probably, the correct response is to cool the mother with tepid sponging.

Drugs

Drugs given to the mother may cross the placenta and affect the fetus. β-Blockers such as propranolol and α- and β-blockers such as labetalol may interfere with the reflex responsiveness of the fetal circulation and impair its response to hypoxia. Other hypotensives such as hydralazine can cause hypoxia by producing maternal hypotension. Sedatives such as pethidine (meperidine) and diazepam (Valium) may depress the fetal central nervous system, reducing the variability of the FHR and producing neonatal depression. Care must be taken to give the minimum of any necessary drug in labor, and the effects on the fetus must always be considered.

OTHER METHODS OF MONITORING FOR FETAL DISTRESS

Fetal Electrocardiogram Analysis

Since the fetal electrocardiogram (ECG) was first demonstrated by Cremer in 1904, attempts have been made to assess fetal well-being by assessing changes in ECG waveform.[71] One approach has been to analyze changes in the PR/R-R interval ratio, but this has not been found to be of value in a prospective, randomized, controlled trial.[72] Another approach used the T/QRS ratio as a measure of acidosis (based on the hypothesis that it is altered by the production of lactate in the fetal heart secondary to hypoxia) and can reduce the need for FBS.[73,74] Two prospective, randomized, controlled trials suggested that it could reduce the need for operative delivery for fetal distress, as well as the incidence of both of metabolic acidosis at delivery and neonatal encephalopathy.[75,76] There have now been a large number of trials of automated fetal ECG (ST segment) analysis. The device used in all these trials (STAN, Neoventa Medical, Moelndal, Sweden) uses a modified fetal scalp electrode to obtain the fetal ECG. These trials have shown conflicting results. A reduction in the number of instrumental deliveries for fetal distress, admissions to neonatal intensive care, and low Apgar scores has been found (but with no reduction in cesarean section rate) with no adverse effect on neonatal outcome,[77] while others have found no reduction in operative delivery but a reduced need for FBS in labor.[78,79] An improvement of neonatal outcome (fewer cases of metabolic acidosis) has been found in observational studies,[80] whereas others have found only that there was no benefit compared with conventional CTG and FBS.[81]

There have been reports of adverse outcomes, poor signal quality, and difficulty in interpretation of the CTG, with the consequent recommendation for intensive training in the use of the STAN monitor and strict adherence to detailed guidelines in its use.[82,83] Adverse outcomes have occurred when the ECG monitoring was started when the CTG was already pathologic. Because the monitor registers only ECG changes in response to *change* in fetal hypoxia, a fetus that was already hypoxic may not be detected until there is further deterioration. Although it was recommended that in this circumstance, an FBS must be taken before the ECG monitoring was started, sometimes this did not happen, owing to poor understanding of the new technology. In response, detailed guidelines for the use and implementation of this fetal ECG analysis technology have been agreed upon by European experts.[84]

It has also been reported that the system has poor sensitivity (43%) for metabolic acidemia at birth, with a specificity of 74%. Poor ECG quality occurred 11% of the time.[85] In addition, fetal ECG changes have been found to occur frequently—in over 50% of recordings in the first stage of labor and in nearly 25% in the second stage—and occur even when the CTG is normal.[86]

A large prospective, multicenter, randomized, controlled trial comparing CTG plus ECG analysis with conventional CTG plus FBS has now been completed.[87] This has shown no reduction in metabolic acidosis in the CTG + ECG arm of the trial. The protocol for FBS in this trial was detailed; it seems likely that if FBS is used effectively in this manner, together with good CTG interpretation, there would be fewer cases of metabolic acidosis at birth.

Use of the ECG waveform analysis requires the application of a fetal scalp electrode, and so can be used only after rupture of the membranes. This might be considered to be unnecessarily invasive for the majority of low risk women in whom the CTG will be normal. However, many studies have shown that its use can reduce the need for FBS, which is an invasive and often unpleasant procedure for the laboring woman, especially if repeated at regular intervals throughout labor.

Expert Systems

Studies of the efficacy of EFM have consistently found the human component to be the weakest link. Computerized analysis is now commonplace in the evaluation of the adult ECG waveform. Keith and colleagues[88] reported a study in which the ability of an "expert" computer system (Fig. 69–2)

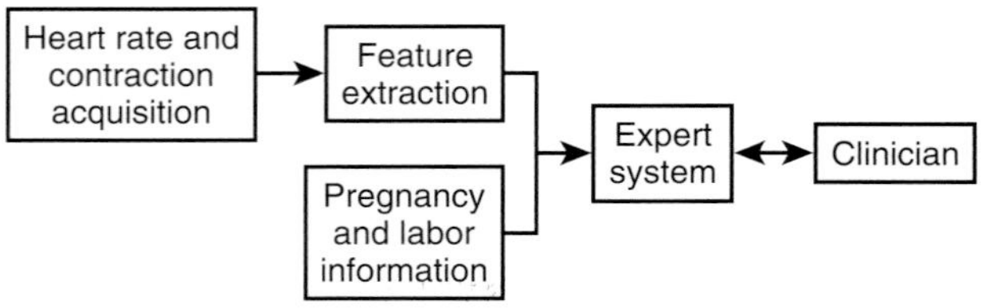

FIGURE 69–2
Principles of expert system cardiotocogram interpretation.
(From Keith RDF, Beckley S, Garibaldi JM, et al: A multicentre comparative study of 17 experts and an intelligent computer system for managing labor using the cardiotocogram. Br J Obstet Gynaecol 1995;102:688–700.)

designed for the interpretation of FHR and FBS data was compared with the opinions of 17 clinicians experienced in fetal monitoring from 16 centers in the United Kingdom. Fifty cases with complete intrapartum CTGs and clinical data were reviewed by the system and each expert independently on two occasions, at least 1 month apart. The system agreed with the experts well and significantly better than chance (67.3%, $K = 0.31$, $P < 0.001$). It was highly consistent (99.16%, $K = 0.98$, $P < 0.001$) when used by two operators independently. It recommended no unnecessary intervention in cases that ended with a normal delivery of a baby in good condition (cord artery pH > 7.15, vein pH > 7.20, 5-min Apgar ≥ 9, and no resuscitation). This was better than all but 2 of the experts. It recommended delivery by cesarean section in 11 cases; at least 15 of the 17 experts in each review also recommended cesarean section delivery in these cases. Most did so within 15 minutes of the system, and two thirds did so within 30 minutes. It identified as many of the birth-asphyxiated cases (cord arterial pH < 7.05 and base deficit ≥ 12, and Apgar score at 5 min ≤ 7 with neonatal morbidity) as the majority of the experts, and 1 more than was acted upon clinically. The experts were found to be consistent and to agree; with the exception of expert "Q." This expert was the only one who declined all information from FBS and attempted to make all decisions on the basis of the FHR alone. In fact, this was the second most inconsistent expert in scoring and obtained the lowest agreement with the other experts (58%, $K = 0.12$). "Q" was also the most inconsistent in recommending cesarean section; in 9 cases, cesarean section was recommended in the first review and not the second or vice versa. "Q" also recommended 2 cesarean sections and 1 second-stage intervention unnecessarily in cases with a normal delivery and a good outcome. Keith and colleagues[88] commented, "in the hands of the experts, this additional information [FBS] clearly adds to the accuracy of decision-making. This information supports the current RCOG [1993] recommendations for using FBS appropriately." A trial to assess the value of this system prospectively in 46,000 labors has been funded by the U.K. Health Technology Assessment Programme and randomization commenced on January 4, 2010 (http://www.hta.ac.uk/1734).

A recent multicenter observational study to determine the sensitivity and specificity of another system of computerized CTG analysis to predict fetal acidemia during labor reported that the sensitivity of the system to predict acidemia is relatively good (95%) when the computer classifies the CTG as suspicious or pathologic, but the specificity is low (22%).[89] This is perhaps not surprising given the known high proportion of false-positive CTGs encountered during labor. Individual features of the CTG (e.g., variability, decelerations) had much lower individual sensitivities.

Transcutaneous Gas Measurements

In the late 1970s, transcutaneous PO_2 measurements using a modified Clark electrode became possible. However, the technique was difficult; the scalp had to be shaved, dried, and readily accessible to a fairly large probe, which then had to be glued to the skin or held on by suction. The probe had to be heated to arterialize the circulation and allow oxygen to diffuse out of the fetal arterioles. There were problems with trauma and heat injury. In addition, the measurement of PO_2 is a measure of hypoxic stress but does not quantify response (acid-base buffer reserve) in the way that measuring pH does; it is very susceptible to local and acute changes.

Further attempts to improve acceptability have been made by using pulse oximetry, which does not require the probe to be heated; instead, it uses infrared light to detect changes in oxygenated hemoglobin concentration in the tissues during the arterial pulsation cycle. However, this system also has problems: it cannot work through hair (which leads to practical difficulties with placement) or meconium, it is susceptible to maternal and fetal movement, and it sometimes produces inconsistent results. Results suggest that 30% to 60% saturations are the normal range in the human fetus, indicating that prolonged desaturation is physiologic in the human fetus.[90] This makes the significance of the readings difficult to assess clinically. If a cutoff of 30% saturation is used, values below this have a sensitivity of 94% in detecting pH less than 7.13, but the specificity is only 38%.[90] This means that the technique is similar to, but not better than, continuous FHR monitoring as a screening test for acidosis. Some studies have shown a reduction in cesarean section rate, or in the need for FBS, but there have been conflicting results and meta-analysis has shown no benefit from the use of fetal pulse oximetry in labor.[91]

Near-infrared spectroscopy is a related technique that uses infrared light at two frequencies to assess the difference in concentrations between oxygenated and deoxygenated hemoglobin concentrations and, hence, the oxygen saturation of the blood. However, the method is expensive and presents many technical difficulties, including frequent probe detachment. No published trials have examined the ability of near-infrared spectroscopy in assessing fetal condition during labor.[92]

Fetal Scalp Lactate Measurement

In theory, lactate measurement assesses hypoxic and anerobic metabolism leading to a metabolic acidosis, which is very similar to that obtained by measuring base deficit. In practice, two randomized, controlled trials using lactate compared with pH to assess metabolic acidosis have shown no significant differences in clinical performance.[93,94] The practical advantages in measuring lactate are that very small sample volumes are needed (5 μL vs. 25 μL for pH estimation), and the values are not significantly altered by contamination of the sample with air bubbles.[95]

CORD PROLAPSE

Prolapse of the umbilical cord in labor is an uncommon event; reported incidences vary from 1 in 265 to 426 labors. The occurrence of cord prolapse is most commonly associated with breech and other malpresentations, a high head at the onset of labor, multiple gestation, grand multiparity, abnormal placentation, preterm labor, polyhydramnios, and obstetric manipulations such as forceps delivery.[96] The diagnosis is commonly made during a vaginal examination; the examiner feeling a soft, usually pulsatile structure. In one series, in 4% the cord was presenting, in 11% it was alongside the presenting part, in 45% it was in the vagina, and in 39% the cord appeared at the introitus.[97] The last mentioned is more likely to occur after artificial, or sudden spontaneous, rupture of the forewaters than in association with a hindwater leak. Occasionally, the diagnosis may be suggested by the sudden appearance of large variable decelerations on the CTG. The mode of delivery remains controversial. As neonatal care has improved, so has the perinatal mortality associated with cord prolapse steadily declined, irrespective of the mode of delivery. For example, in one series reported in 1977, the perinatal mortality rate was 430 per 1000 births,[97] in 1985, 162 per 1000 births, and in 1988, 55 per 1000 births[98]; although a recent report from Israel found a perinatal mortality of 83 per 1000.[96] Some studies emphasized the danger of prolonged prolapse-to-delivery interval and urged prompt cesarean section unless the cervix is fully dilated and the presenting part is at or below the ischial spines so that the fetus is immediately deliverable by forceps (which is the case in about 20%–30%). While the woman is being prepared for the operation, it is usually recommended that she be nursed in the traditional knee-chest position facing downward or, alternatively (and often more practically), in steep Trendelenburg position. It may be necessary for a birth attendant to keep a gloved hand in the vagina to elevate the presenting part and relieve pressure on the cord. One technique first suggested by Vago in 1970 and since commended by others[99] is to fill the urinary bladder with 500 to 700 mL of saline, elevating the presenting part and relieving pressure on the cord. However, more recently, one paper championed manual replacement of the cord[98] (termed *funic reduction*), describing a successful vaginal delivery in seven of eight cases so treated (one was too far advanced in labor for this to be feasible and a cesarean section was performed). The interval between replacement of the cord and final delivery ranged from 14 to 512 minutes (8.5 hr!).

SUMMARY OF MANAGEMENT OPTIONS

Cord Prolapse

Management Options	Evidence Quality and Recommendation	References
Cesarean section while pressure on the cord is relieved until delivery: • Manual elevation of the head away from the cord. • Knee-chest position. • Steep Trendelenburg position. • Filling of the bladder with up to 700 mL normal saline.	III/B	99

SUMMARY OF MANAGEMENT OPTIONS

Cord Prolapse—cont'd

Management Options	Evidence Quality and Recommendation	References
Instrumental delivery if the patient is in the second stage of labor, the presenting part is below the level of the ischial spines, and easy, prompt vaginal delivery is anticipated.	III/B	99
The value of funic reduction (manual replacement) is uncertain because few patients have been studied.	III/B	98

INTRAPARTUM FETAL RESUSCITATION

In general, if acute fetal hypoxia is evident and acidosis is rapidly developing, the best management is emergency cesarean section, preferably within 15 minutes. If the presentation is occipitoanterior, the presenting part is at or below the spine, and there is no obvious evidence of disproportion, a nonrotational forceps delivery is an appropriate alternative. Various studies have reported attempts at intrauterine resuscitation of the fetus, and maneuvers recommended include turning the mother to the left side, giving her oxygen by face mask, stopping any oxytocic infusion, uterine tocolysis, and correction of any hypotension. Although there is anecdotal evidence that these maneuvers may be effective in appropriate circumstances, no randomized studies attest to their efficacy.

MECONIUM STAINING OF THE AMNIOTIC FLUID

Aspiration of meconium by the fetus remains a relatively common cause of perinatal mortality and morbidity because it is difficult to prevent. The fetus passes meconium into the amniotic fluid in approximately 10% of all pregnancies; in up to 5% of these (i.e., in 1:200 of all pregnancies), the meconium is aspirated and can lead to meconium aspiration syndrome (MAS). MAS can cause, or contribute to, neonatal death in up to 0.05% (i.e., 1:2000 of all pregnancies).[100,101] In addition, up to one third of all cases in which aspiration occurs develop long-term respiratory compromise.[102,103] The incidence of MAS may be falling in developed countries: fewer pregnancies are proceeding beyond 42 weeks because of increased use of ultrasound dating of pregnancy and induction between 41 and 42 weeks.[104]

It seems likely that the causes of meconium passage by the fetus are not necessarily the same as those that cause aspiration, and so in the account that follows, the two aspects are addressed separately.

Passage of Meconium

Mechanism

Meconium is passed into the amniotic fluid by peristalsis of the fetal gut accompanied by relaxation of the internal and external anal sphincters. In the adult, this process is a complex interaction of hormonal, myogenic, and neurogenic factors. Peristalsis is principally controlled by local reflexes acting via the neural complexes in the gut wall, but is usually modified by extrinsic innervation. Sympathetic activity inhibits rectal activity and causes constriction of the internal anal sphincter, whereas parasympathetic activity has the opposite effects. In the resting state, the internal and external sphincters are constricted. In the adult, involuntary defecation can occur in response to stress ("flight-or-fight reaction"). This is mediated centrally by the hypothalamus (and possibly the amygdala), which in turn, causes stimulation of the visceral parasympathetics.[105,106] In contrast, pathophysiologic stresses such as pain, heat, cold, injury, exercise, and nonintestinal infections all produce gut stasis and constipation.[105] It is attractive to suggest that the fetus may exhibit a similar response to the "emotional" stress of labor, but this concept is likely to remain an untested theory. The fetus is stressed pathophysiologically in labor by hypoxia, pyrexia, or compression, which by extrapolation from adult physiology would be more likely to produce gut stasis than increased motility. However, fetal physiology differs in many ways from that of the adult, and our knowledge of the mechanisms of gut motility and meconium passage in the fetus is poor.

The Effect of Maturity and Gestation on Passage of Meconium

Meconium is found in the fetal gut from 10 weeks' gestation,[107] but passage of meconium is rare before 34 weeks.[4] The incidence of meconium passage increases with gestational age and reaches approximately 30% at 40 weeks' gestation and 50% at 42 weeks.[4,108] The presence of meconium in the amniotic fluid may reflect fetal gastrointestinal maturity.[109] Fetal gut transit time does decrease with gestational age, and gut motility increases. The low gut motility in the preterm fetus has been attributed to a lack of gut wall musculature, but this is unlikely because peristalsis has been reported before 12 weeks' gestation and muscle development must have occurred before this.[110]

Immature innervation of the fetal gut is more likely, with preterm fetuses having fewer myelinated axons and ganglion cells in the colon than full-term infants. Meconium passage in the preterm fetus can occur if it becomes infected with organisms that can cause a fetal enteritis (e.g., *Listeria monocytogenes*, *Ureaplasma urealyticum*, rotaviruses).[111] The fetal gut must be sufficiently developed for peristalsis to occur and meconium to be passed even in the preterm fetus.

Hormonal Control of the Passage of Meconium

The intestinal hormone motilin has been implicated in the passage of meconium in utero; it causes contraction of smooth muscle in the gut wall. Motilin levels in umbilical venous blood increase with gestation, and if they reflect levels in the fetal gut, this could be a factor in explaining the tendency for the mature fetus to pass meconium.[112] Cord levels are also higher in infants that have passed meconium prenatally,[113,114] and one study found that they were also higher if an FHR abnormality had occurred in labor.[99] This latter finding was not confirmed in a later study in the same year,[114] but different definitions of FHR abnormality were used. It is possible that stress on the fetus could cause release of motilin and thus passage of meconium, but this remains conjectural. The hormonal and other factors that control gut motility are largely unknown, even in the adult.

Infection and the Passage of Meconium

Meconium-stained amniotic fluid is associated with increased peripartum infection rates, independent of other risk factors for infection. Thick meconium, in particular, is associated with a marked increase in peripartum infectious morbidity.[115–117] It is not yet clear whether the presence of meconium encourages infection or whether infection promotes the passage of meconium by the fetus. In favor of the former, prophylactic intravenous ampicillin-sulbactam significantly reduces intra-amniotic infection in patients with meconium-stained amniotic fluid,[118] although the possibility remains that the presence of the infection antedated the appearance of the meconium and was unrecognized. In addition, meconium is a chemoattractant and activator of polymorphonuclear leukocytes in vitro and for cytokines such as tumor necrosis factor-α (TNF-α), interleukin-1 (Il-1), and Il-8.[119] It may be that meconium increases the damaging effects of infection by increasing the presence of these inflammatory mediators.

Obstetric Cholestasis

The risk of meconium passage increases in association with cholestasis of pregnancy.[120] This may be secondary to elevated levels of bile acids in the maternal circulation, which cross the placenta and affect the fetus. Cholestasis of pregnancy also increases the bile acid content of meconium.[121] The same study also found that, although maternal ursodeoxycholic acid (UDCA) therapy caused a reduction in serum bile acid levels in the mother, there was no associated reduction in the levels of meconium passage in the fetus. The implications of this are unclear, but it is possible that if UDCA does not affect fetal bile acid levels significantly, perinatal loss rates associated with cholestasis of pregnancy will not improve.

Risks

Fetal Hypoxia

An association between meconium passage in utero and poor condition of the neonate has been suggested since ancient times. Aristotle reported opium-like effects in neonates born through meconium-stained fluid, and there have been references to meconium in association with perinatal death from as early as 1676 (quoted in Schulze[122]). Subsequently, many authors have suggested that fetal hypoxia causes intestinal peristalsis, relaxation of the anal sphincter, and thus, passage of meconium. This view has largely been assumption, with little or no direct evidence to support such a hypothesis. Stander[123] claimed that meconium was a sign of impending fetal "asphyxia" due to "relaxation of the sphincter ani muscle induced by faulty aeration of the blood" and proposed prompt delivery whenever meconium was seen. Desmond and associates[124] claimed that meconium staining of the amniotic fluid was a marker of fetal hypoxia, but no blood gas analysis of either fetal or neonatal blood was performed; the diagnosis of hypoxia being made on clinical grounds alone. These observations were made despite the report of Schulze,[122] who had concluded from a study of a series of more than 5500 births in California, that passage of meconium during labor "is in the large majority of cases independent of fetal asphyxia" and that the presence of old meconium in the amniotic fluid was of no prognostic significance for the later development of asphyxia (asphyxia here was not defined but appears to mean "lack of respiratory effort at birth"). She also observed that in cases associated with asphyxia, there were always changes of the FHR during labor and that these changes should be the sole guide to the necessity for delivery. However, in a later study, meconium passage was associated with low umbilical vein oxygen saturation, and thick meconium with lower levels of PO_2 than thin meconium.[125] This remained the principal experimental evidence linking fetal hypoxia with meconium passage and was widely quoted, often as the sole evidence, for at least the subsequent 20 years.

Fenton and Steer[126] made one of the first attempts to separate meconium passage from other markers of fetal compromise such as abnormality of heart rate, but again, had only presumptive evidence of hypoxia in the fetus. They stated that there were other, benign causes of meconium passage and suggested that the passage of meconium was not significant if the FHR was greater than 110 beats/min. The introduction of FBS began to clarify the situation. Miller and coworkers[127] found no difference in scalp blood pH, umbilical cord artery and vein pH, and neonatal arterial pH up to 64 minutes of life, between meconium and nonmeconium groups, if the FHR during labor had been normal. They concluded that meconium in the absence of other signs was not a sign of fetal distress (defined as "late decelerations on the CTG and umbilical artery acidosis"). Further studies confirming the same finding (that there is no obvious link between the presence of meconium and hypoxia) continue to be published regularly and include the use of fetal pulse oximetry and fetal hemoglobin analysis.[128–130]

If the FHR pattern is abnormal, however, the presence of meconium is associated with an increased chance of a baby being acidotic, born in poor condition, and needing resuscitation at birth.[4,127] In the data presented by Steer and associates,[4] 140 babies had an abnormal CTG pattern in the first stage of labor. The mean cord artery pH was 7.22 (SD = 0.10) in the 108 cases with clear amniotic fluid compared with 7.17 (SD = 0.12) in the 32 cases with meconium-stained amniotic fluid (t = 2.37, P =.0096, one-tailed). The incidence of 1-minute Apgar scores less than 7 was 19% (3%

at 5 min) if the amniotic fluid was clear compared with 56% (9% at 5 min) if the amniotic fluid was meconium-stained. The difference was significant at 1 minute ($P = 0.0001$; Fisher's exact test). However, they commented that the reduction in the 1-minute Apgar score may have been due at least in part to the use of pharyngeal suction or endotracheal intubation by the attending pediatrician suppressing spontaneous respiration and, thus, iatrogenically reducing the Apgar score.

Despite the lack of a clear relationship between meconium staining of the amniotic fluid and fetal acidosis in the absence of FHR changes, we cannot conclude that the presence of meconium is not a threat to the fetus or neonate even if the FHR is normal. Yeomans and colleagues[39] studied 323 pregnancies with meconium-stained amniotic fluid at 36 to 42 weeks' gestation. Although there was a significantly higher incidence of meconium below the vocal cords if an umbilical artery pH was less than 7.20 compared with when the umbilical artery pH was 7.20 or greater (34% vs. 23%), the difference in the incidence of clinical MAS according to pH was not significant. Moreover, 69% of babies with meconium below the cords had cord arterial pH of 7.2 or greater. Thus, a normal pH does not exclude the possibility of meconium aspiration, and most babies with meconium aspiration do not have acidosis. These data do not support the hypothesis that fetal hypoxia is a major cause of meconium passage in labor, and indeed, Naeye and associates[131] reported that meconium staining of the amniotic fluid was not more common, even when the neonate was hypoxic.

Evidence that hypoxia per se does not lead to passage of meconium has been available for many years. Becker and coworkers[109] showed reduced peristalsis in the fetal guinea pig after induction of maternal hypoxemia, and a similar result was seen in the monkey fetus. In the adult with spinal shock, although the external sphincter relaxes, constipation occurs owing to the loss of the other defecation reflexes. If meconium passage does occur in response to reduced intestinal blood flow, it must be an early event for the neurogenic reflexes still to be present. Meconium passage may occur as a result of vagal stimulation, and this could account for coexisting reduction in the FHR.[126] Parasympathetic stimulation is known to occur with cord compression, and this is supported by meconium passage being more common with increasing gestational age. Emmanouilides and colleagues[132] found that in the sheep fetus, if one umbilical artery was ligated, passage of meconium occurred only as a very late phenomenon, after chronic fetal wasting had developed. Although it is widely stated that fetal hypoxia leads to meconium passage in laboratory animals, the studies usually cited were concerned with the investigation of fetal breathing movements and do not state that meconium was passed in response to hypoxia.[133,134] However, recent work in the sheep and rat suggests that a possible mechanism for hypoxia-related meconium passage may be mediated by corticotropin-releasing factor (CRF).[135] It is postulated that stress (including hypoxia) leads to increased release of CRF, which in turn, increases gut motility. Inhibitory CRF receptors in the fetal gut decrease toward term, and stimulatory receptors increase.[136] It has been demonstrated that hypoxia is a potent inducer of meconium passage in the fetal rat, and this appears to be mediated by a CRF-dependent pathway.[137] Whether this pathway is similar in the human fetus is yet to be determined.

Meconium Aspiration

The passage of meconium is not a risk to the fetus, but aspiration of the meconium into the fetal or neonatal lung is associated with clinical disease ranging from mild transitory respiratory distress to severe respiratory compromise and occurs in up to one third of cases. *Meconium aspiration* is commonly defined as the presence of meconium below the vocal cords and occurs in up to 35% of live births with meconium-stained liquor.

Aspiration of meconium was thought by many authors to occur at delivery as the newborn infant took its first breath. Oropharyngeal suction, and endotracheal intubation of the infant before the first breath were widely promoted, to prevent meconium aspiration. However, it now seems likely that meconium aspiration is largely an intrauterine event. This change of view has occurred because of compelling evidence that severe MAS still occurs despite adequate suction at delivery.[39,138,139]

The current view is that meconium aspiration occurs owing to fetal breathing movements, causing inhalation of amniotic fluid with meconium, if present. Two types of breathing movements cause inhalation of amniotic fluid: gasping and deep breathing. Gasping is a normal response to hypoxemia and can be induced experimentally by occluding the umbilical cord or by occluding the maternal aorta.[134,140]

The fetus may also inhale meconium by deep irregular breathing in utero, not initiated by hypoxia. These breaths become more frequent as gestation advances and account for 10% of all fetal breathing movements.[134] The passage of amniotic fluid deep into the lung has been demonstrated by radiolabeling experiments that also showed that the human fetus inhales 200 mL/kg/24 hr of amniotic fluid.[141] Fetal hypercapnia and acidemia also increase these breathing movements, but they still occur in most, if not all, normal fetuses.[134,142] Although some infants with meconium aspiration are severely compromised at birth, there is little or no difference in umbilical cord acid-base status between infants with meconium below the cords and those without.[39] Meconium aspiration is more common if the meconium is thick rather than thin. This may be a reflection of the fact that oligohydramnios (and therefore thick undiluted meconium) is more likely to lead to fetal hypoxia due to cord compression and, consequently, increased fetal breathing.

Meconium Aspiration Syndrome

GENERAL

MAS represents a wide spectrum of disease ranging from transient respiratory distress with little therapy required to severe respiratory compromise requiring prolonged mechanical ventilation and high levels of oxygen administration. Neonatal death occurs in up to 40% of cases.[143]

Severe MAS is associated with profound hypoxia, which is secondary to right-to-left shunting, a persistent fetal circulation, resistant pulmonary hypertension, pulmonary hemorrhage, necrosis of pulmonary vessels, and muscularization of distal pulmonary arterioles.[101,144,145] These changes may be due to intrauterine hypoxia, rather than to the meconium itself, although the inhalation of meconium exacerbates the problem in several ways in the neonatal period.

Meconium inhaled by an infant who has not been subjected to hypoxia usually causes mild disease only and is asymptomatic in 90% of cases. Exposure to intrauterine hypoxia causes pulmonary vasoreactivity that persists after birth. Large increases in pulmonary artery pressure in response to very small falls in oxygen tension then result. The severity of this pulmonary vasospasm seems to depend on the severity of the fetal hypoxia and may be fixed (completely unresponsive) in the most severe cases. These changes have been demonstrated experimentally and observed clinically. A vicious circle of hypoxia, pulmonary vasospasm, shunting, and therefore, worsening hypoxia can develop. Jovanovic and Nguyen[146] showed in the guinea pig that meconium or amniotic fluid aspiration in the absence of hypoxia caused minimal damage, whereas lung damage (necrosis of alveoli and diffuse hemorrhage) in the hypoxic cases was severe whether the amniotic fluid contained meconium or not. The degree of lung destruction seems to depend primarily on the length and degree of hypoxia, not simply the aspiration of meconium. Hypoxic damage also reduces the clearance of aspirated meconium or amniotic fluid.[147] Meconium does, however, exacerbate the problems faced by the neonate. It displaces surfactant, causing atelectasis and hyaline membrane formation[148–150] and causes a chemical pneumonitis possibly due to cytotoxicity to the type II pneumocytes caused by bile salt–induced accumulation of calcium.[151] In addition, it enhances bacterial growth and is associated with intrauterine infections. Aspiration may lead to infectious pneumonitis.

Some bacterial toxins cause pulmonary vascular spasm, exacerbating the effects of hypoxia.[111,152,153] Meconium has been demonstrated to cause vascular necrosis and vasoconstriction in the umbilical cord and may cause similar damage in the lung.[154] The umbilical vasoconstriction may cause hypoxia in utero, leading to aspiration. Inhaled thick meconium may cause a physical obstruction to the airways, leading to distal lung collapse, with hyperinflation in other areas of the lung. In total, 95% of severe cases of MAS occur when the meconium is thick, which is more common in post-term pregnancies when a relative oligohydramnios develops. Oligohydramnios may also be due to hypoxia, causing reduced fetal urine output,[155] or may be a sign of uteroplacental insufficiency.

METHODS OF PREVENTING MECONIUM ASPIRATION SYNDROME

During the 1950s and 1960s, it was thought that meconium-stained amniotic fluid was a marker of fetal compromise, and efforts were made to detect meconium in the amniotic fluid in late pregnancy and to deliver the fetus either before, or as soon as, meconium appeared. Amnioscopy was introduced for pregnancies more than 10 days past the expected date of confinement. It was stated that the finding of meconium indicated "impending danger" and that immediate amniotomy and FBS should be performed; the ensuing uterine contractions were thought to be therapeutic for the fetus. A threefold reduction in perinatal mortality was claimed,[156,157] but other investigators have been unable to reproduce these results. Saldana and associates[158] showed no benefit from amnioscopy and delivery. Amnioscopy has not been shown to be beneficial, is uncomfortable for the mother, may result in accidental rupture of the membranes or induce labor, can cause infection, and has to be repeated at regular arbitrary intervals until delivery.

Benacerraf and coworkers[159] reported the detection of thick meconium by ultrasonography, but further studies showed that vernix can produce an ultrasonically indistinguishable image in the absence of meconium.[160,161]

Because meconium passage is more common with advanced gestational age, many studies have investigated the effect of inducing labor at an earlier gestation. In a controlled trial, Cole and colleagues[162] significantly reduced the incidence of meconium-stained liquor by inducing at 39 to 40 weeks' gestation, but no effect on perinatal mortality or respiratory disease was seen. Other studies of induction of labor have not shown a decrease in meconium aspiration, even if the incidence of meconium staining of the liquor was reduced.[163–165] There is, thus, no evident benefit from induction of labor before meconium appears or from the routine use of amnioscopy, and disadvantages to both procedures exist.

In the 1970s, it was widely believed that meconium aspiration developed by inhalation of the meconium at delivery when the infant took its first breath. To prevent this, aggressive policies of oropharyngeal suction, endotracheal intubation, and splinting of the thorax to prevent aspiration were proposed. Despite these interventions, cases of meconium aspiration still occurred, and further studies showed little or no reduction in MAS. A decline in the mortality from meconium aspiration is probably due to concurrent advances in perinatal medicine, rather than to the introduction of suction protocols. Suction and intubation are not free of risk. Cordero and Hon[166] reported apnea and bradycardia in infants having nasopharyngeal suction, and Linder and associates[167] found no benefit from the intubation at birth of meconium-stained but otherwise normal infants. All cases of meconium aspiration in this study occurred in the intubated group, and two cases of laryngeal stridor also required repeated hospitalization with residual hoarseness at 6 months of age. Cunningham and coworkers[168] recommended routine oropharyngeal suction but not intubation. There is now widespread acceptance that routine suctioning and intubation of neonates that have passed meconium have little, if any, effect on aspiration and may have deleterious side effects. A recent review of the year 2000 Neonatal Resuscitation Program (NRP) guidelines[169] has confirmed that the recommended fall in intubation rates has had no effect on outcome for babies born through meconium-stained amniotic fluid, and ACOG[170] endorses this approach, only recommending intubation and suction if the neonate is depressed at birth.

Amnioinfusion, the instillation of normal saline into the uterus during labor, has been proposed as a method to reduce meconium concentration and, therefore, the effects of aspiration. It may reduce cord compression in cases of oligohydramnios and, therefore, fetal gasping. Large randomized, controlled trials in Africa have shown significant improvements in outcome,[171,172] but a large multicenter trial in Europe, North America, South America, and South Africa failed to show the same benefits.[173] Meta-analysis of the randomized studies investigating amnioinfusion has concluded that there is no benefit in clinical settings with standard peripartum surveillance, but that the risk of MAS is reduced in settings with limited peripartum surveillance where the risk of MAS is more common.

The beneficial effect of amnioinfusion may be due to a reduction in cord compression during uterine contractions and, therefore, possible fetal hypoxia or directly to a reduction in the concentration of meconium. However, because thick meconium is often associated with oligohydramnios, the benefits of amnioinfusion may be due solely to correction of amniotic fluid volume.

Attempts have been made to classify meconium in labor according to its concentration, because thick meconium has been associated with increased incidence and severity of MAS. However, any grading system is subjective because amniotic fluid draining during labor may not be representative of the fluid in utero, and no fluid may drain at all in cases of oligohydramnios, masking the presence of meconium. Quantifying the meconium concentration by centrifuging samples of amniotic fluid and measuring the amount of solid matter in the sample has been attempted,[174,175] but the same problems of obtaining amniotic fluid representative of the intrauterine milieu exist. In addition, neither author addressed the problem of vernix and solid matter other than meconium in the liquor producing false-positive results.

Two reports suggested that social support during labor reduces the incidence of meconium staining,[176,177] but in both cases, more oxytocin was used in the group with no support, which could have lead to unphysiologic contractions and fetal hypoxia.

Evidence linking fetal distress and meconium should be viewed with caution because the events during labor and delivery do not represent the intrauterine environment at the time of meconium passage. In addition, it is unlikely that prevention of meconium passage or aspiration will be successful until there is some elucidation of the underlying causes. Intrauterine probes to measure meconium concentration in the amniotic fluid continuously during labor, using a light-reflectance method, have been developed.[178] Although this enabled observation of the events at the time of meconium passage (e.g., FHR changes, epidural top-ups) and was able to detect meconium not otherwise visible to the birth attendants, it is unlikely to be clinically useful in the foreseeable future.

Management Options with Meconium Staining of the Amniotic Fluid

When amniotic fluid is seen to drain, it should always be inspected carefully for the presence of meconium. If meconium is detected, continuous electronic FHR monitoring is recommended. If the FHR pattern remains normal, no specific action is necessary, except to avoid actions that might precipitate acute fetal hypoxia (supine hypotension, epidural hypotension, uterine hyperstimulation with oxytocics). In particular, there is no indication for routine FBS and pH estimation as long as the FHR pattern is normal. At delivery, a pediatrician should be present. If the baby is vigorous and cries promptly, there is no need for further action. Although there is no proof of efficacy, some pediatricians prefer to suction the pharynx as soon as possible after delivery of the head, and this is acceptable as long as care is taken not to traumatize the pharynx or larynx, because this may precipitate meconium aspiration.

If the FHR pattern is abnormal during labor, the likelihood of acidosis is substantially increased. Consideration should be given to immediate delivery, if necessary by cesarean section. If rapid progress in cervical dilation is occurring, it may be appropriate to take an FBS and allow the labor to continue if the pH is above 7.20, but this decision must take into account other factors such as the wishes of the mother, and whether there are other risk factors, such as intrauterine growth restriction. Amnioinfusion should be considered if it is decided to allow the labor to continue. Amnioinfusion can also be considered even if the FHR pattern is normal, as a preventive measure.

Umbilical Cord Blood Gas Sampling

Cord blood gas analysis provides an objective measure of the condition of the baby at birth. An umbilical arterial metabolic acidemia will be present if the fetus has experienced significant hypoxia prior to delivery. RCOG[179] and NICE[36] have recommended measurement of umbilical artery and vein blood pH and base deficit in all cases, whereas ACOG[180] recommends sampling for cases of cesarean delivery for fetal compromise, low 5-minute Apgar score, severe growth restriction, abnormal fetal heart rate tracing, maternal thyroid disease, intrapartum fever, and multifetal gestation. Cord blood gas analysis has important medicolegal implications: normal values will make the attribution of any handicap to intrapartum events very difficult (see earlier). Audit of practice can utilize cord blood gas results as a measure of the standard of intrapartum care, and in addition, knowledge of the result may assist analysis of clinical events and management in labor.

PROCEDURE

UMBILICAL CORD BLOOD GAS SAMPLING

Procedure

- A segment of cord must be isolated between two sets of clamps after delivery.
- (Changes in the pH, Pco_2 and Po_2 of cord blood occur slowly. Cord blood can be left at room temperature for up to 1 hour without significantly affecting the results and for several hours if left on ice.)
- Use commercially preheparinized blood gas syringes to take cord blood samples.
- (Heparin is acidic and if too much is used (>10% of sample volume) can cause significant errors.)
- Blood must be taken from both artery and vein and the results checked to ensure both vessels have been sampled. If both results are very similar, it is likely that the umbilical vein has been sampled twice (the vein is much easier to obtain a sample from).
- Sample the cord vessels with the needle at an acute angle to the vessel especially when sampling the umbilical artery—this makes it less likely to insert the needle through the distal arterial wall into the vein.

Analysis

- The normal values are given in Table 69–6.
- Cord arterial values reflect fetal acid-base status, whereas those of the vein reflect maternal and placental status.
- The umbilical vein pH may be normal but the arterial pH low if there has been a interruption to umbilical blood flow (e.g., cord compression or if the fetal hypoxia has been of short duration).
- If both artery and vein have a low pH, this indicates that the hypoxia is of longer duration and is usually due to metabolic acidemia.

TABLE 69–6

Umbilical Cord Blood Gas Values

	NORMAL VALUES (MEAN, 5th, 95th CENTILE)	
	UMBILICAL ARTERY	UMBILICAL VEIN
pH	7.23 (7.1, 7.34)	7.32 (7.19, 7.43)
Po_2 (kPa)	2.9 (1.5, 4.9)	3.7 (2.1, 5.4)
Pco_2 (kPa)	6.1 (4.2, 8.4)	4.9 (3.5, 6.9)
BDecf (mmol/L)	−7.7 (−14.5, −1.8)	−6.4 (−11.7, −1.6)

Note: Gestational length has no significant effect on cord blood gas values.
BDecf, base deficit of extra cellular fluid; Pco_2, carbon dioxide pressure; Po_2, oxygen pressure.
From Eskes TK, Jongsma HW, Houx PC: Percentiles for gas values in human umbilical cord blood. Eur J Obstet Gynecol Reprod Biol 1983;14: 341–346.

SUMMARY OF MANAGEMENT OPTIONS

Meconium Staining of the Amniotic Fluid

Management Options	Evidence Quality and Recommendation	References
Incidence		
Meconium aspiration syndrome contributes to neonatal death in approximately 1 in 2000 births.	III/B	100–102
The main influence on the passage of meconium is gestational age.	III/B	108,109
Meconium aspiration is associated with infection, particularly in the lungs.	III/B	115–119
Fetal passage of meconium is more common in cholestasis of pregnancy.	III/B	120,121
Hypoxia and acidosis do not, per se, lead to the passage of meconium.	III/B	39,128
The combination of severe hypoxia and meconium aspiration causes lung damage.	III/B	147–149
Prevention		
A pediatrician should be present for delivery, but should not perform routine oropharyngeal suction in the absence of evidence of fetal hypoxia because suction does not reduce the incidence of meconium aspiration syndrome.	IIa/B	166,167
Meconium aspiration and acidosis are reduced by amnioinfusion of normal saline.	Ia/A	171

SUGGESTED READINGS

Amer-Wahlin I, Arulkumaran S, Hagberg H, et al: Fetal electrocardiogram: ST waveform analysis in intrapartum surveillance. BJOG 2007;114: 1191–1193.

American College of Obstetricians and Gynecologists (ACOG): Management of delivery of a newborn with meconium-stained amniotic fluid (ACOG Committee Opinion No. 379). Obstet Gynecol 2007;110: 739.

American College of Obstetricians and Gynecologists (ACOG): Umbilical cord blood gas and acid-base analysis (ACOG Committee Opinion No. 348, November 2006). Obstet Gynecol 2006;108:1319–1322.

Beard RW, Filshie GM, Knight CA, Roberts GM: The significance of the changes in the continuous foetal heart rate in the first stage of labour. J Obstet Gynaecol Br Commonw 1971;78:865–881.

East CE, Chan FY, Colditz PB, Begg LM: Fetal pulse oximetry for fetal assessment in labour. Cochrane Database Syst Rev 2007;2: CD004075.

National Collaborating Centre for Women's and Children's Health (NCC-WCH/NICE): Intrapartum Care. Care of Healthy Women and Their Babies during Childbirth. London, RCOG Press, 2007. Available at http://www.nice.org.uk/nicemedia/pdf/CG55FullGuideline.pdf

Steer PJ, Eigbe F, Lissauer TJ, Beard RW: Interrelationships among abnormal cardiotocograms in labor, meconium staining of the amniotic fluid, arterial cord blood pH and Apgar scores. Obstet Gynecol 1989;74:715–721.

Sykes GS, Molloy PM, Johnson P, et al: Do Apgar scores indicate asphyxia? Lancet 1982;i:494–495.

Vintzileos AM, Nochimson DJ, Guzman ER, et al: Intrapartum electronic fetal heart rate monitoring versus intermittent auscultation: A meta-analysis. Obstet Gynecol 1995;85:149–155.

Wiberg-Itzel E, Lipponer C, Norman M, et al: Determination of pH or lactate in fetal scalp blood in management of intrapartum fetal distress: Randomised controlled multicentre trial. BMJ 2008;336:1284–1287.

REFERENCES

For a complete list of references, log onto www.expertconsult.com.

CHAPTER 70

Neuraxial Analgesia and Anesthesia in Obstetrics

LAWRENCE C. TSEN

INTRODUCTION

In 1847, the obstetrician James Young Simpson ushered in the use of anesthetic agents for obstetrics with the application of diethyl ether to assist a vaginal delivery. Over the next half century, an evolution in the agents and techniques used for the provision of obstetric analgesia (pain relief) and anesthesia occurred. Regional anesthetic techniques, which deliver pain relief to a discrete region of the body, metamorphosed to include the use of medications near the spinal cord via the central neuraxial (i.e., spinal [subarachnoid], or epidural) spaces. Since Oskar Kreis first described the use of spinal anesthesia in obstetrics in 1900, neuraxial techniques have evolved from single, limited-duration injections into the spinal sac to titratable, controlled infusions through flexible catheters most commonly placed into the epidural space. The combined spinal-epidural (CSE) technique, first introduced to obstetrics in the 1980s, consists of the delivery of medications through a needle into the spinal sac and, later, through a catheter into the epidural space; the spinal and epidural spaces are approached within a single procedure (Fig. 70–1).[1] The CSE technique provides rapid and profound initial pain relief with the ability to extend the analgesia or anesthesia. The use of epidural, spinal, and CSE techniques has increased dramatically owing to the quality and safety of the analgesia and anesthesia produced, the ability to titrate the degree and duration of pain relief as required by the circumstances, and the limited maternal and fetal effects. Currently, in most developed countries, neuraxial techniques provide labor analgesia for 30% to 50% of all parturients and the anesthesia for the majority of instrumental and operative deliveries (Fig. 70–2).[2–4]

In this chapter, the indications and implications of neuraxial techniques to provide obstetric analgesia and anesthesia are discussed. Emphasis is placed on the novel indications for these techniques as well as the association of these techniques with two outcomes of common obstetric and anesthetic concern: progress and outcome of labor and maternal temperature alterations.

INDICATIONS

The use of epidural, spinal, and CSE techniques for vaginal, instrumental, and operative deliveries has been well described in numerous texts and articles.[5,6] The use of these techniques, as well as nonpharmacologic modalities, systemic medications, and peripheral nerve blocks, are discussed in the obstetric setting. The philosophical shift favoring the use of regional versus general anesthesia is further elucidated, and two novel obstetric applications of these techniques—external cephalic version (ECV) and postoperative pain management—are discussed in greater detail.

Although the quality, titratability, and patient satisfaction associated with the use neuraxial analgesia and anesthesia are responsible for their increasingly frequent use, the main benefit may be a reduction in maternal mortality. Airway management difficulties during the provision and recovery from sedative or general anesthetic agents remain the leading cause of anesthetic-related mortality and an important cause of overall maternal morbidity and mortality.[7,8] Although the number of deaths involving general anesthesia has remained stable in the United States, the estimated rate of maternal deaths from complications of general anesthesia increased from 20.0 to 32.3 deaths per million in the time periods of 1979–1984 to 1985–1990, respectively (Fig. 70–3).[9] The case fatality ratio for general versus neuraxial anesthesia over the same periods increased from 2.3:1 to 16.7:1[9]; subsequently, the same investigators found that the relative risk decreased significantly to 1.7:1 in the years 1997 to 2002.[10] The risk of general anesthesia will most likely always be overstated, because this form of anesthesia is used principally when neuraxial techniques are contraindicated for medical reasons or time constraints. However, the reduction in the case fatality ratio may reflect the growing acceptance and use of neuraxial techniques in the presence of significant comorbid conditions (e.g., severe preeclampsia).

Despite this, neuraxial techniques still represent an underutilized option in patients who would benefit from the avoidance of systemic sedation or general anesthesia. This group includes parturients with a high likelihood of having a difficult airway (e.g., high body mass index [BMI]), worsening pathology (e.g., preeclampsia), or an operative delivery (e.g., placenta previa, trial of labor after cesarean [TOLAC], high-order multiple gestation). In such parturients, consultation optimally should occur early in the third trimester and shortly following their arrival on the labor and delivery ward. Evaluation should be made regarding the suitability of an early ("prophylactic") placement of a

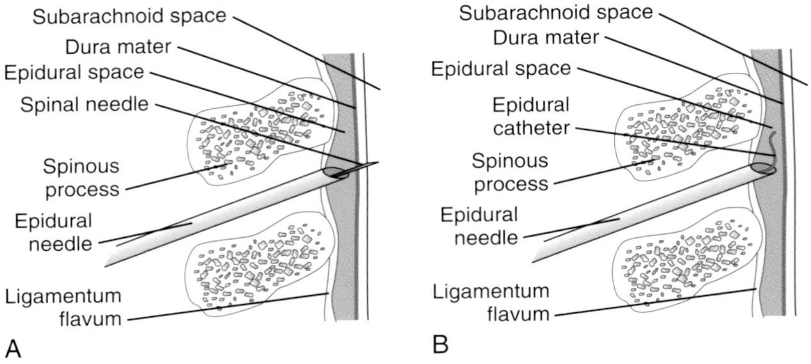

FIGURE 70–1
Combined spinal-epidural (CSE) technique. *A*, The spinal needle is introduced through the epidural needle and punctures the dura mater. The initial medication is dosed into the subarachnoid (spinal) space. *B*, After the withdrawal of the spinal needle, a catheter is introduced into the epidural space and secured in place.
(*A* and *B*, From Rawal N, Holmström B, Zundert A, et al: The combined spinal-epidural technique. In Birnbach DJ, Gatt SP, Datta S [eds]: Textbook of Obstetric Anesthesia. Philadelphia, Churchill Livingstone, 2000, p 159.)

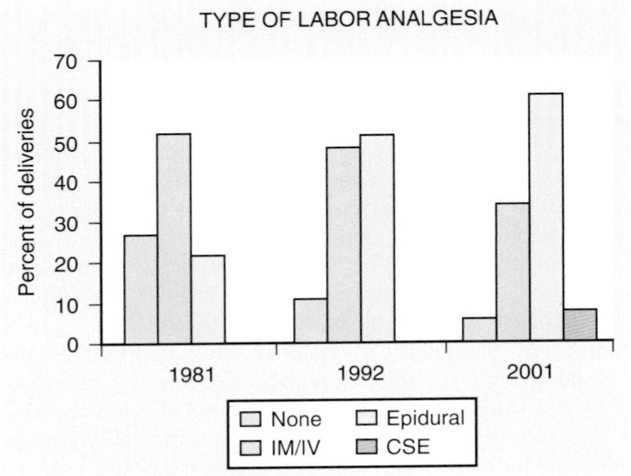

FIGURE 70–2
Type of analgesia provided during labor in hospitals in the United States with greater than 1500 deliveries/yr.
(From Bucklin BA, Hawkins JL, Anderson JR, Ullrich FA: Obstetric anesthesia workforce study: Twenty-year update. Anesthesiology 2005;103:645-653.)

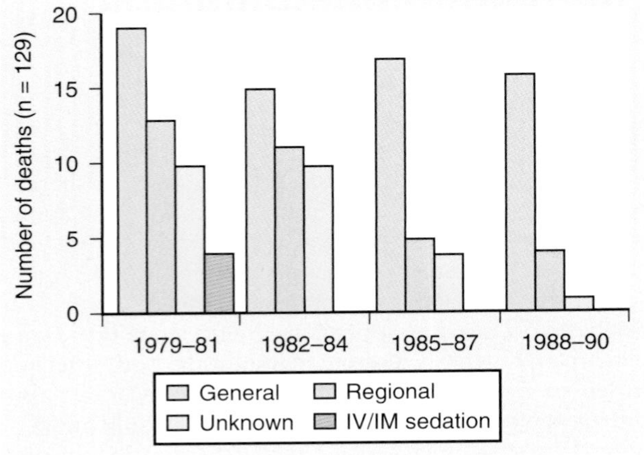

FIGURE 70–3
Anesthesia-related maternal deaths by types of anesthesia, United States, 1979-1990.
(From Hawkins JL, Koonin LM, Palmer SK, et al: Anesthesia-related deaths during obstetric delivery in the United States, 1979-1990. Anesthesiology 1997;86:277-284.)

TABLE 70–1
Contraindications to Central Neuraxial Anesthesia

Absolute Contraindications
Patient refusal or inability to cooperate
Localized infection at the insertion site
Sepsis
Severe coagulopathy
Uncorrected hypovolemia
Relative Contraindications
Mild coagulopathy
Severe maternal cardiac disease (including congenital and acquired disorders)
Neurologic disease (including intracranial and spinal cord disorders)
Severe fetal depression

catheter-based neuraxial technique (Table 70–1), even if the birth attendants or the woman herself is not sure that a neuraxial block is desired or will be required.[11] To allay such concerns, the catheter need not be dosed until a later time when an analgesic or anesthetic is requested or required. This approach significantly decreases the incidence of emergently managing a difficult airway or confronting airway issues owing to a "perceived lack of time."[4]

The antenatal consultation should focus on the physiologic changes of pregnancy that can make airway management more difficult. As early as the fourth week of gestation, and particularly with preeclampsia/eclampsia, capillary engorgement of the oropharyngeal and respiratory mucosa makes these structures more friable, vascular, and edematous. With labor, the airway structures become further engorged, making the oropharyngeal area even smaller.[12] In addition, the anteroposterior and transverse diameters of the thorax increase during pregnancy, resulting in a substernal angle that, in combination with increases in breast tissue, serve to make laryngoscopy more challenging. Finally, arterial oxygen desaturation occurs more quickly in apneic parturients owing to smaller functional residual capacity and increased oxygen consumption. These alterations make the provision of general anesthesia more challenging; difficult intubations with the need for special airway management devices and techniques were observed in up to 16% of the cases in a 6-year report of general anesthesia performed for cesarean delivery in a tertiary care hospital.[4] These airway concerns persist in the postoperative period following extubation and with the administration of sufficient systemic analgesic agents, most often opioids, to allay pain; postoperative respiratory compromise is a growing concern, particularly in women of high BMI.[7,8]

The physiologic and anatomic alterations of pregnancy are further accentuated in high-BMI patients, a group that has dramatically increased since the 1990s.[13] In addition to an increased association with hypertension and preeclampsia, aortocaval compression, obstructive sleep apnea, gestational diabetes, and fetal macrosomia, high BMI can result in dysfunctional labor, increased emergency cesarean delivery, and postpartum hemorrhage.[13] Catheter-based neuraxial techniques (e.g., epidural or spinal catheter) placed early in the course of labor can minimize the need for systemic analgesics, reduce the discomfort and physiologic responses to labor induction or augmentation, provide a readily available anesthetic method for emergent operative delivery that avoids airway manipulation, and eliminate the relaxing effects of volatile general anesthetic gases on uterine tone, which can contribute to further blood loss. Moreover, neuraxial techniques, particularly if continued for postpartum analgesia, can contribute to improved postoperative pain control, faster recovery of pulmonary function, and a lower incidence of venous thromboembolism.[13,14] Whereas neuraxial techniques may, therefore, represent a viable and perhaps optimal mode of analgesia or anesthesia for high-BMI patients, the greater difficulties involved with their use in such patients, including the amount of time required for placement and the incidence of technique failure,[15] indicate that other modalities and methods should be readily available.

MANAGEMENT OPTIONS FOR PAIN DURING PARTURITION

Nonpharmacologic Techniques

Psychological support and sensory stimulation are two basic classifications of nonpharmacologic modalities for the reduction of pain during labor. The most popular forms of psychological support are "natural childbirth" and "psychoprophylaxis," which were popularized by Dick Read and Fernand Lamaze, respectively. These methods, which utilize a series of preparative classes to explain the process of labor and teach methods for relaxation and allaying pain, have been observed to reduce the amount of analgesia used,[16] but the degree of pain relief experienced appears limited.[17] Potential problems with these techniques include hyperventilation[18] and postpartum depression if analgesic techniques are eventually utilized.[19] Hypnosis, a temporary alteration in consciousness characterized by increased suggestibility, focuses on producing physical and mental relaxation and changing the interpretation of physical stimuli. Although few randomized, controlled trials have evaluated the modality, a meta-analysis[20] reports that hypnosis can be successful in the management of labor pain. Trained individuals called *doulas* can also be a source of emotional and physical support during labor. When doulas provide continuous, rather than intermittent, support during labor and delivery, a decrease in the amount of analgesic agents requested, labor duration, and instrumented deliveries has been observed.[21]

Massage, superficial application of heat and cold, hydrotherapy, acupuncture and acupressure, transcutaneous electrical nerve stimulation (TENS), intradermal sterile water injections, and music and audio analgesia are all methods of sensory stimulation and have been used with some success during labor. These methods are hypothesized to use innocuous stimuli, such as touch, vibration, and pressure, to compete with painful stimuli at the site of their convergence in the substantia gelatinosa of the dorsal horn of the spinal cord. This competitive inhibition, accompanied by descending messages from the brain cortex and brainstem, is believed to modulate the transmission of pain information. To date, few randomized, controlled trials have been performed with these modalities, and thus, only limited conclusions can be drawn. Systematic reviews of acupuncture and TENS for labor analgesia demonstrate a high degree of patient acceptability and satisfaction, despite a weak analgesic-sparing effect.[20,22] The novel use of TENS as an adjuvant to other modalities has been investigated. Tsen and associates[23,24] found that TENS was ineffective in augmenting the duration or quality of analgesia produced by small amounts of spinal or epidural local anesthetics and opiates during labor. Overall, despite the limited scientific evidence supporting the analgesic value of these psychological and sensory stimulation modalities, many patients consider them to be an integral and helpful part of their labor experience.

Systemic Medications

Medications given by injection were among the first agents routinely utilized for childbirth pain relief. In the 1950s and 1960s, the combination of morphine and the anticholinergic scopolamine was used to induce analgesia, sedation, and amnesia termed "twilight sleep."[25] Scopolamine, now more commonly utilized in smaller doses as an antiemetic, had a number of side effects including delirium, agitation, and excitement, that prompted the use of other, more effective forms of analgesia.

Oral, subcutaneous, intramuscular (IM), and intravenous (IV) injection techniques have all been utilized for administration of systemic labor analgesia. The more rapid onset and ease of IM and IV drug administration have allowed the frequent use of these routes despite IM routes having variable onset time, duration, and degree of analgesia. Injection into the deltoid muscle, for instance, will result in better absorption than injection into the less-perfused gluteus muscle. Intravenous patient-controlled analgesia (IV-PCA), which utilizes a pump programmed to give a dose of an analgesic agent on demand at predetermined intervals, yields some control to the patient, thereby improving maternal satisfaction, reducing overall drug dosing, and decreasing provider workload.[26]

Opioids, despite their side effects of nausea, emesis, drowsiness, dysphoria, hypoventilation, and neonatal respiratory depression, are the most widely used medications for labor analgesia because of their availability and the degree of analgesia produced. Morphine is given in doses of 5 to 10 mg intramuscularly or 2 to 3 mg intravenously for a peak effect in 2 hours and 20 minutes, respectively, but may result in greater neonatal depression than meperidine at equianalgesic doses.[27] Meperidine (Demerol; known as pethidine in Europe), the most commonly used opioid for labor analgesia, is given in dosages of 50 to 100 mg intramuscularly or 10 to 50 mg intravenously to produce 2 to 4 hours of pain relief. To minimize neonatal respiratory depression, IM administration of meperidine should be avoided within a window of 1 to 3 hours before delivery.[28] (Clinically, avoiding this window may be difficult, because many women thought to be hours away from giving birth deliver suddenly and unexpectedly. In practice, provided that bag and mask ventilation of the neonate and IM naloxone are given, the risk to the baby from IM meperidine is minimal.) Fentanyl, alfentanil, and sufentanil are potent synthetic morphine analogues that are generally not used intramuscularly owing to their short duration of action and narrow therapeutic index; with the advent of IV-PCA, however, these agents are being used more frequently.[26] Opioids with agonist/antagonist properties have the advantage of a "ceiling effect" for maternal respiratory depression, and include pentazocine, nalbuphine, and butorphanol. Pentazocine is utilized less commonly because of its potential for the psychomimetic effects of dysphoria and a perception of impending death.[29] Nalbuphine and butorphanol are given in IM or IV doses of 3 to 5 mg or 1 to 2 mg, respectively and are equianalgesic to meperidine with less nausea and emesis.[30]

Tranquilizers such as benzodiazepines and phenothiazines are occasionally used to reduce anxiety during labor and delivery. Diazepam can be used in doses up to 10 mg IM/IV,[31] but lorazepam and midazolam should be avoided owing to their pronounced neonatal depressant and maternal amnesic effects, respectively. Phenothiazines can be used synergistically to reduce the dose of opioids, thereby increasing sedation and reducing side effects. Hydroxyzine given in doses of 50 to 100 mg intramuscularly and promethazine given in doses of 24 to 50 mg intramuscularly or 15 to 25 mg intravenously have been observed to improve maternal analgesia without significant neonatal effects.[32] Promazine, chloropromazine, and prochlorperazine are avoided because of their strong α-adrenergic blocking activity, which can produce hypotension.[33]

Barbiturates, such as secobarbital and pentobarbital, can allay anxiety. However, as a class, the efficacy of these agents during labor is limited owing to their lack of analgesic properties, their potential to increase the sensation of pain, and the presence of protracted effects on the newborn.[34] In low doses of 0.2 to 0.5 mg/kg intravenously, ketamine can produce intense analgesia with limited neonatal effects; however, maternal dysphoric reactions may result.[35] The concomitant use of midazolam 2 to 4 mg intravenously can decrease these effects. In higher doses of 1 to 2 mg/kg, ketamine can be used as induction agent for general anesthesia; however, when the dose exceeds 2 mg/kg, increases in uterine tone may occur and be associated with lower Apgar scores or abnormally increased neonatal muscle tone.[35]

Inhalational Analgesia

The first form of analgesia used for labor in modern medicine, inhalational analgesia remains popular in many maternity centers, particularly within the United Kingdom. Inhalation of subanesthetic doses of nitrous oxide, trichloroethylene, methoxyflurane, enflurane, isoflurane, and recently, sevoflurane has been used to provide safe and effective analgesia during labor and delivery. Most effective during the early stages of labor, inhaled analgesics are administered either intermittently (i.e., during contractions only) or continuously with the dose regulated according to the patient's response. A mixture of 50% nitrous oxide and 50% oxygen (Entonox) is the most common formulation in current use[36] and has been demonstrated to bring relief to approximately 50% of parturients. Entonox may also be used as an adjuvant, but not a complete analgesic, to a pudendal nerve block for forceps delivery, perineal suturing, or manual removal of the placenta.[37] The inhalational technique can safely provide amnesia and analgesia; however, the possible loss of consciousness, diminished airway reflexes with the associated risk for aspiration and hypoxia, and unscavenged gas pollution of the labor suite are issues that may occur. The risk for loss of consciousness and airway reflexes are more commonly witnessed with halogenated agents.

In rare instances, general anesthesia is induced with inhalational halogenated agents (e.g., isoflurane, sevoflurane) for vaginal delivery. Two of the more common scenarios include a need for greater anesthesia without time to administer a neuraxial anesthetic (i.e., fetal distress requiring forceps delivery) or a need for maximum uterine relaxation (i.e., need for intrauterine manipulation). In contrast to anesthetic agents given neuraxially, inhaled halogenated agents cause uterine relaxation in a dose-dependent manner,[38] with the administration of greater than 0.5% minimum alveolar concentration (MAC) potentially decreasing uterine smooth muscle responses to oxytocin.[39]

Regional Analgesia and Anesthesia

A variety of regional techniques can provide pain relief for labor and delivery. As both expected and unexpected physiologic sequelae may occur following these techniques, IV access should be established and resuscitation equipment should be readily available. All of these techniques are performed through the injection of short- to long-acting local anesthetics (i.e., chloroprocaine, meperidine, lidocaine, and bupivacaine), based in part on the location and desired duration of the blockade.

Paracervical Block

A technique that relies on blocking the nerve ganglion located immediately lateral and posterior to the cervicouterine junction, the paracervical block is primarily effective for the first stage of labor. Owing to the frequent occurrence of fetal bradycardia, which may result from local anesthetic-induced uteroplacental vasoconstriction or direct fetal myocardial depression, this technique is now used infrequently.[40]

Lumbar Sympathetic Block

By interrupting pain signaling through the visceral afferent sensory fibers in the lumbar vertebrae region, the lumbar sympathetic block provides analgesia limited primarily to the first stage of labor. Although seldom used owing to the requirement for injections at multiple sites along the lumbar sympathetic chain, this technique has been advocated for early labor analgesia owing to the near absence of motor blockade.[26,41]

Pudendal Block

Effective for the second stage of labor, the use of outlet forceps, and episiotomy repairs, this block interrupts the terminal nerve transmissions of the pudendal nerve. Owing to the distal nature of the nerve blockade, this form of anesthesia is not effective for mid-forceps delivery, postpartum examination or repair of the upper vagina or cervix, or exploration of the uterine cavity.[42] Maternal and neonatal blood levels of local anesthetic following a pudendal block are comparable with those seen following an epidural technique.[43]

Perineal Infiltration

One of the most commonly performed techniques for labor and delivery, perineal infiltration interrupts pain transmissions from the terminal nerves in the posterior fourchette. Because direct injection into the fetal scalp can occur, the quickly metabolized agent 2-chloroprocaine may be preferable to lidocaine or longer-acting local anesthetics.[44]

Caudal Block

A technique that uses the lowermost segment of the epidural space, the caudal block has lost favor to the higher, more approachable lumbar block. The change to the lumbar approach was also motivated by an association of the caudal block with inadvertent injections of anesthetic into the fetal head, the theoretical increased risks of infection owing to a closer proximity to the rectum, and difficulty in extending the cephalad level of the blockade for cesarean delivery.

Antenatal Use of Regional Techniques: External Cephalic Version

Epidural, spinal, and CSE techniques have been reported to improve success rates of ECV. Schorr and coworkers[45] randomized 69 patients (all of whom received tocolytics to relax the uterus) to undergo an ECV attempt either with or without epidural anesthesia. In demographically and obstetrically similar groups, the first attempt and overall success rates of ECV were higher in the epidural group (69% vs. 32%). No cases of fetal distress or abruptio placentae were observed in either group, and ultimately, vaginal delivery occurred in 66% of the epidural group versus 21% in the control group. In comparison with tocolytics, a preliminary report by Samuels and colleagues[46] of 76 patients undergoing ECV noted greater success with an epidural anesthetic versus ritodrine (76.3% vs, 60.1%).

Spinal techniques have also been used for ECV attempts, with varying analgesic doses resulting in contrasting results. Dugoff and associates[47] noted no improvement with the spinal administration of bupivacaine 2.5 mg with sufentanil 10 μg (44% vs. 42%), whereas Birnbach and coworkers[48] noted a significant improvement (80% vs. 33%) with the use of sufentanil 10 μg alone. The variation in outcome may reflect differences in obstetric or patient factors, including the amount of force applied or the degree of maternal discomfort tolerated for a given level of analgesia. When spinal anesthesia (lidocaine 45 mg with fentanyl 10 μg) was used, even in the more difficult setting of previously failed ECV attempts, a high success rate (83%) has been reported.[49]

Whether utilized for primary or failed ECV attempts, a CSE technique with a short-duration spinal anesthetic may represent the optimal technique.[49] The short anesthetic duration allows for a timely discharge from hospital in the event of a successful version, and if success or failure results in either a trial of labor or an operative delivery on the same day, the epidural catheter can be left in place to allow additional analgesia or anesthesia to be administered.

Neuraxial analgesic and anesthetic techniques most likely improve ECV success by relaxing the abdominal wall muscles, improving patient comfort during the ECV attempt, and allowing the obstetrician to make a more concerted attempt.[48,50] The use of neuraxial anesthetic techniques for ECV attempts has been associated with an improved maternal and fetal outcome, a reduced need for operative deliveries with general anesthesia, and a favorable cost-benefit analysis.[50,51]

Anesthesia for Vaginal Delivery

Spinal Anesthesia

The finite duration of action of a single injection, and an increased risk of a post–dural puncture headache (PDPH) with multiple injections, limit the utility of "single-shot" spinal anesthesia for the management of labor. Spinal techniques, however, can be used successfully during delivery, especially in the event of an assisted vaginal breech delivery, the need to use outlet forceps or vacuum extraction, or the repair of extensive tears or lacerations. For these procedures, a low-level spinal anesthetic block can be used; in the event of a "trial of forceps," a dose of local anesthetic appropriate for a cesarean delivery or a spinal or epidural catheter-based approach should be considered to provide coverage for a potential operative delivery. Clear communication between the obstetrician and the anesthetist on their expectations regarding delivery is essential if the optimal technique is to be chosen. Variations of the spinal technique that offer more flexibility include its use as part of a CSE technique (discussed later) or the placement of a catheter into the spinal space, called a "spinal catheter" or "continuous spinal anesthesia" technique. The benefits of these techniques have been observed particularly in patients with conditions such as morbid obesity and cardiac disorders or following an unintentional dural puncture during an attempted epidural catheter placement. The spinal catheter is a method for providing a reliable, precisely titratable blockade,[52] although this option is less attractive than the same 20-gauge catheter placed in the epidural space owing to a significantly greater risk of a PDPH. A recent trial of a 28-gauge spinal catheter observed a less than 1% incidence of neurologic complications and better initial labor analgesia with improved maternal satisfaction but more technical difficulties and analgesic failures when compared with a 20-gauge epidural catheter.[53] Further investigations will be needed to validate the benefits and safety of spinal microcatheters; earlier reports that the use of 27- to 32-gauge spinal microcatheters resulted in complications (e.g., technique failure, cauda equina syndrome)[54] led the U.S. Food and Drug Administration (FDA) to remove these catheters from the U.S. market in 1992.

COMPLICATIONS

A number of complications may occur following a spinal technique. Hypotension, defined as a 20% to 30% decrease in systolic blood pressure from baseline, can be observed in up to 100% of pregnant women following spinal anesthesia owing to the production of a sympathetic vasomotor blockade.[55] Persistent hypotension may result in decreased uteroplacental perfusion as well as fetal hypoxia and acidosis.[56] Preventive measures include maternal intravascular volume expansion (preloading with IV fluid, usually 500–1000 mL of crystalloid such as Hartmann's solution) and the avoidance of aortocaval compression by uterine displacement. Treatment includes titrated IV doses of vasopressors such as ephedrine (5–10 mg) and phenylephrine (40–100 μg). Vasopressor use can significantly reduce the nausea and vomiting following a spinal technique and may be associated with reductions in sympathetic tone, blood pressure, and cerebral blood flow.[57] PDPH occurs in approximately 1% to 3% of the obstetric population following a spinal technique and is most likely related to the needle size and tip design, with larger, cutting needles associated with a greater incidence.[58] Typically, a PDPH presents as a positional headache that worsens in the upright position and improves in the recumbent position. The differential diagnosis should include other types of headache, hypertensive disorders, infectious diseases, dural venous sinus thromboses, and other intracranial pathologies. Pain relief may be provided by bedrest,[59] hydration, and the oral intake of caffeinated and analgesic products (including Fioricet or Fiorinal) for 24 to 48 hours. The administration of an epidural blood patch, whereby 10 to 20 mL of autologous blood is placed in the epidural space, has been associated with a greater than 80% incidence of success.[56,60] Neurologic complications (e.g., peripheral neuropathy, subarachnoid bleed) as a result of spinal anesthesia in the obstetric population are extremely rare[60]; however, should these events occur, a consultation with a neurologist may assist in the diagnosis and management. Finally, spinal anesthesia can result in an unexpected high level of blockade, which can result in hypotension, dyspnea, the inability to speak, and a loss of consciousness; these usually transient occurrences emphasize that immediate ventilatory and circulatory support should always be readily available when this technique is provided.

Epidural Analgesia and Anesthesia

One of the most effective methods of pain relief for labor and delivery,[5] the epidural technique with an indwelling catheter provides a reliable form of analgesia that can be titrated as the situation evolves. Labor analgesia can be converted to surgical anesthesia for an instrumental or operative delivery, laceration repair, or postpartum tubal ligation by changing the dose or type of local anesthetic administered through the catheter.

The optimal selection of agents for use in the epidural space depends on the degree and duration of pain relief desired. The goal during labor and delivery is to provide lumbar and sacral sensory analgesia with minimal motor blockade[12]; this should allow the pregnant woman to appreciate a sense of pressure, without pain, during each contraction and retain the ability to move her lower extremities. Almost every local anesthetic developed has been tested for its value in obstetric analgesia. Of the shorter-duration agents, mepivacaine has a prolonged half-life and may cause neonatal depression. Chloroprocaine 3% and lidocaine 2% produce a dense sensory and motor block appropriate for surgical anesthesia. The longer-duration agents are best suited for labor analgesia when used in low concentrations. Bupivacaine has a high sensory-to-motor block ratio and is commonly used in concentrations between 0.0625% and 0.125% to initiate and maintain labor epidural analgesia.[12] Ropivacaine and L-bupivacaine are also longer-duration agents that may result in slightly less motor blockade and cardiotoxic effects when given in equipotent concentrations to bupivacaine.[61,62] The dose, onset, and duration of various local anesthetics for epidural labor analgesia are well characterized (Table 70–2). Although epidural opioids alone are often sufficient for analgesia in the first stage of labor, a combination of agents is often necessary to provide adequate analgesia during the second and third stages of labor.[63,64] The addition of local anesthetics to opioids improves the quality of analgesia and allows a reduction in drug dosages, thereby minimizing motor blockade and pruritus, respectively. Epidural administration of small doses of sufentanil (0.2–0.3 μg/mL) or fentanyl (0.2 μg/mL) combined with low doses of bupivacaine 0.0625% or 0.125% results in excellent analgesia for vaginal delivery. An epidural bolus of fentanyl 100 μg, with or without local anesthetic, can be of assistance during the second stage of labor when patchy analgesia or perineal sparing cannot be remedied with local anesthetics alone.[65]

Once the initial sensory blockade has been established, epidural analgesia can be maintained by intermittent bolus injections, a continuous infusion, or both techniques simultaneously. The development of programmable infusion pumps has enabled the delivery of a dilute solution of an opioid and a local anesthetic agent by continuous infusion, coupled with patient-controlled intermittent bolus top-up injections. This combined method reduces the total amount of medication used, decreases the amount of motor blockade, and increases patient satisfaction when compared with a continuous infusion or intermittent bolus methodologies alone.[66,67]

TABLE 70–2
Local Anesthetics for Epidural Analgesia and Anesthesia

ANESTHETIC	USUAL CONCENTRATION (%)	ONSET	DURATION
Analgesia			
Lidocaine	1-1.5	Moderate	Intermediate
Bupivacaine	0.0625-0.25	Slow	Long
L-Bupivacaine	0.0625-0.25	Slow	Long
Ropivacaine	0.1-0.2	Slow	Long
Anesthesia			
2-Chloroprocaine	2-3	Fast	Short
Lidocaine	2-5	Moderate	Intermediate
Mepivacaine	2	Moderate	Intermediate
Bupivacaine	0.5	Slow	Long
L-Bupivacaine	0.5	Slow	Long
Ropivacaine	0.5-1	Slow	Long
Tetracaine	1	Slow	Long

TABLE 70–3
Advantages of the Combined Spinal-Epidural Technique for Labor Analgesia

Advantages over an Epidural Technique
More rapid onset
Lower maternal, fetal, and neonatal blood concentrations of local anesthetic than with epidural techniques alone
Better sacral analgesia
Assists in identification of the epidural space in technically difficult placements
Advantages over a Spinal Technique
Allows ability to titrate the level, density, and duration of the blockade
Catheter can be used for postoperative pain management

Combined Spinal-Epidural Analgesia

Introduced in the early 1980s for surgical procedures, the CSE technique, with a few modifications, has become one of the most popular techniques for labor analgesia. The technique consists of an epidural needle placement, a spinal needle placed most often through the shaft of the epidural needle into the subarachnoid space (e.g., the "needle-through-needle" approach), the delivery of spinal medications, and then placement of an epidural catheter. In comparison with the epidural or spinal techniques alone, the CSE technique has a number of advantages (Table 70–3). A mixture of local anesthetics with opioids appears to be the optimal combination for initial labor analgesia with this technique, and its application, even early in labor, may have beneficial effects on the progress of labor.[68,69] Used later in labor, the CSE technique can provide quick onset of analgesia and the ability to extend the duration or level of the blockade should delivery methods mandate such augmentation.

COMPLICATIONS

Relatively few complications are inherent to the CSE technique. The CSE technique may actually reduce the risk of a dural puncture with the larger epidural needle, because the spinal needle protrudes 10 to 15 mm beyond the tip of the epidural needle when placed through its shaft. Cerebrospinal fluid flowing through the spinal needle indicates that the dura has been traversed, thereby providing the position of the dural sac relative to the epidural needle and cautioning against significant further advancement. The likelihood of an 19- to 20-gauge epidural catheter passing through a 25- to 27-gauge spinal needle dural puncture is low, based on both laboratory and clinical studies.[70] However, drugs placed in the epidural space can pass through the 25- to 26-gauge spinal dural hole and result in improved onset, sacral spread, and bilateral sensory blockade[71]; by contrast, the risk of a high spinal blockade appears negligible.[71]

Because the spinal portion of a CSE technique gives an initial period of analgesia, the epidural catheter remains "untested" and may not prove reliable as a route for further anesthetic agents should additional analgesic and anesthetic needs arise. Although epidemiologic evidence suggests that the epidural catheter following a CSE versus an epidural technique has a lower failure rate,[72] in those parturients with a difficult airway or a high probability of an instrumental or operative delivery, a standard epidural technique, which tests the function of the catheter at the time of placement, may be safer.

MANAGEMENT OPTIONS FOR ANESTHESIA FOR CESAREAN DELIVERY

Despite repeated calls to reduce the rate of cesarean deliveries from both lay and professional organizations in the United States and Europe, the incidence of surgical delivery continues to increase. Although a number of difficult airway management devices and algorithms have improved the safety of general anesthesia for cesarean delivery, the majority of maternal deaths due to anesthesia still occur during or following the provision of general anesthesia. However, in deciding between neuraxial and general anesthetic techniques, the urgency of the procedure, the health and comorbidities of the mother and fetus, and the desires of the mother and health care providers all need to be considered.

Spinal Anesthesia

A simple and reliable technique with rapid onset, spinal anesthesia provides an awake and comfortable patient with minimal risks for aspiration. Despite the lower abdominal incision, a thoracic (T4) dermatome level is required to prevent referred pain from traction on the peritoneum and uterus. The type and dose of local anesthetic agent used to provide spinal anesthesia must include consideration of the duration of the surgery, the postoperative management of pain, and the preferences of the anesthesiologist. Hyperbaric bupivacaine is the agent most commonly used because it provides a blockade of long duration while avoiding the extensive motor block produced by tetracaine. The potential toxicity advantages of ropivacaine and L-bupivacaine are limited given the extremely small doses of agent used. The use of adjuvant spinal medications, such as opioids and epinephrine, may augment the quality and duration of the anesthesia and analgesia and reduce the local anesthetic dose even further.[73,74]

With the onset of spinal anesthesia, the patient may complain of dyspnea. Dyspnea can be due to several factors, including the blunting of thoracic proprioception, the partial blockade of abdominal and intercostal muscles, and the recumbent position allowing the abdominal contents to apply pressure against the diaphragm. Despite these changes, significant respiratory compromise is unlikely because the blockade rarely affects the cervical (phrenic) nerves that control the diaphragm. Should the patient lose the ability to vocalize, give a strong hand grip, or demonstrate normal oxygen saturation by pulse oximetry, a rapid-sequence induction with cricoid pressure and placement of an endotracheal tube can be performed to maintain ventilation and prevent pulmonary soiling with gastrointestinal contents (the so-called gastric aspiration syndrome).

The most common complications of spinal anesthesia have been described earlier and include hypotension, nausea and vomiting, and the risk of a PDPH. Hypotension presents the greatest risk to maternal and fetal comfort and health[55];

prevention and prompt treatment with the administration of IV fluids and vasopressors has been observed to be beneficial but, on occasion, not completely successful.[75,76] In terms of volume expansion, spinal anesthesia in the urgent setting should not be delayed until a fixed, arbitrary volume has been infused. In addition, aggressive hydration with large fluid volumes (>20 mL/kg crystalloid) may increase the risk of edema with only limited reductions in hypotension.[75] Colloid solutions appear to be more effective than crystalloids in preventing the hemodynamic consequences of spinal anesthesia,[77] but have allergic, cost, and coagulation implications. Investigations with vasopressors for prevention and treatment of hypotension in this setting have suggested that either intravenous phenylephrine or ephedrine may be used.[78]

Epidural Anesthesia

Since the 1980s, an increase in the use of epidural anesthesia for cesarean delivery has been observed, primarily owing to the widespread use of an epidural catheter-based technique to provide labor analgesia. Dosing the in situ catheter with local anesthetic agents allows for a relatively rapid onset of anesthesia should an operative delivery be necessary. Although drugs used in the spinal and epidural space are identical, the doses and volumes in the epidural space are 5 to 10 times greater to encourage adequate blockade and spread. These dose alterations can be explained primarily by anatomic differences in nerve exposure and the capacity of the spaces.

Advantages of the epidural technique include a slower onset of maternal hypotension owing to a more slowly developing sympathetic blockade, the response of physiologic compensatory mechanisms, and the ability of the anesthesiologist to titrate fluids and vasopressors. The level, density, and duration of epidural anesthesia can be titrated. The anatomic and hormonal changes of pregnancy appear to promote greater sensitivity of nerves to local anesthetic agents, which can be observed clinically through a decrease in anesthetic requirements for epidural blockade.[79,80] For cesarean delivery, the most common agents used are 2% lidocaine with epinephrine 1:200,000 and 3% 2-chloroprocaine. Chloroprocaine is the agent of choice for emergency cesarean deliveries because of its rapid onset and rapid maternal and fetal metabolism; fetal accumulation, especially when acidosis is present, is therefore minimized.[81] However, chloroprocaine is avoided for routine, nonurgent deliveries because the short duration requires multiple doses and its use can adversely affect the efficacy of subsequent epidural opioid analgesia.[82] In addition, when used in higher total volumes (>40 mL), chloroprocaine can increase the incidence of back pain.[83] Alkalinization with sodium bicarbonate hastens the onset time of local anesthetics significantly and is recommended for use in urgent cesarean deliveries[84]; caution must be applied in its use, however, because certain local anesthetics (particularly longer-acting agents such as bupivacaine) have a low threshold for precipitation.[85]

The complications of epidural anesthesia have been described previously and include hypotension, risk of PDPH, systemic toxic reactions, and rarely, neurologic complications. Epidural techniques can provide patchy or inadequate blockade owing to anatomic or technical reasons[86] and may require supplementation with IV or inhalational agents or conversion to general anesthesia.

Combined Spinal-Epidural Anesthesia

The principal advantage of the CSE technique is the ability to provide dense, initial anesthesia with the ability to augment the duration by dosing the epidural catheter. This is particularly useful in obstetrics, in which a delay in the timing prior to or during surgery can potentially occur (e.g., possible placenta accreta, history of multiple abdominal surgeries, high index of suspicion for gravid hysterectomy).

Contraindications to Neuraxial Anesthesia

Although neuraxial anesthesia is used whenever possible to avoid the potential airway complications associated with general anesthesia, certain conditions or time constraints may contraindicate its use.[4] Such comorbidities include localized infection or generalized sepsis, coagulation disorders, severe hypovolemia, or cardiac disorders in which hypotension may be detrimental. Severe obstetric hemorrhage in the antepartum period, including uterine rupture and acute, severe fetal distress, may also contraindicate neuraxial anesthesia procedures because of the time necessary to establish a surgical anesthetic.

Patients with severe preeclampsia or hypertension may undergo rapid hemodynamic changes with regional techniques; however, both epidural and spinal techniques can and have been used successfully in this setting, and of interest, preeclamptic patients may have less hemodynamic changes than normal parturients undergoing spinal anesthesia.[87,88] In addition, gravid hysterectomies have been performed safely with neuraxial techniques.[89] Overall, however, if questions exist regarding the ability of maternal compensatory mechanisms to react to the neuraxial anesthesia, general anesthesia should be considered.

General Anesthesia

There are few, if any, absolute contraindications to general anesthesia; however, neuraxial anesthesia remains a preferred method to avoid the risks of airway management and allow the patient the ability to witness the delivery. General anesthesia may offer advantages when uterine relaxation would be beneficial; such cases include difficult breech extractions, retained placenta, uterine inversion, or in utero fetal surgery.

The importance of proper airway evaluation, during the antenatal period or in early labor if possible, cannot be overemphasized, because failed intubation, failed ventilation and oxygenation, difficult extubation, and pulmonary aspiration of gastric contents are the leading anesthetic causes of maternal death.[90,91] If the airway evaluation suggests the possibility of a difficult intubation, strong consideration should be given to the establishment of a continuous neuraxial technique early in labor.[92] If a difficult airway is discovered upon an intubation attempt, options include allowing the patient to awaken, using alternate techniques to place an endotracheal tube, or using alternative airway devices.

The laryngeal mask airway (LMA), although not able to prevent pulmonary soiling with gastric contents, can be a life-saving measure in failed intubation situations[93] and has been used safely in elective cesarean deliveries.[94]

Attempts should be made to minimize the risk of maternal aspiration, even when the need for intubation is not anticipated. With an elective cesarean delivery, adherence to a nil per os (NPO; nothing by mouth) policy for 8 hours prior to surgery is advised.[12] A nonparticulate antacid is believed to decrease the damage to the respiratory epithelium if aspiration occurs,[95] and H_2 antagonists (cimetidine, ranitidine) and promotility agents (metoclopramide) can reduce gastric acid secretion and facilitate emptying, respectively.[96,97]

Preoxygenation and denitrogenation with 100% oxygen reduces the rapidity of hypoxemia onset due to the parturient's decreased functional residual capacity and increased oxygen consumption. In urgent situations, eight vital capacity breaths within 1 minute or four vital capacity breaths within 30 seconds of 100% oxygen will provide adequate preoxygenation.[98] An induction agent (e.g., thiopental or propofol) is followed in quick succession with the muscle relaxant succinylcholine; as the induction of anesthesia occurs, increasing pressure (30 N) is applied to the cricoid cartilage until endotracheal intubation is confirmed. The use of preoxygenation, cricoid pressure with induction, and avoidance of active ventilation until endotracheal intubation is achieved is referred to as a "rapid-sequence induction." Its purpose is to rapidly secure the maternal airway to minimize the risk of gastric aspiration. On occasion, particularly if a preoperative examination reveals that a parturient might be a difficult intubation, modifications to this sequence, including the use of an awake fiberoptic intubation, are performed. A halogenated volatile anesthetic agent (e.g., isoflurane, sevoflurane) is used in 100% oxygen to maintain anesthesia; after neonatal delivery, lower concentrations of volatile anesthetic agent can be used through the addition of a 50%/50% oxygen–nitrous oxide mixture. The 25% to 40% increase in sensitivity to halogenated agents during pregnancy allows lower doses to be used[99]; this may be of benefit in attenuating the side effects of volatile agents, which reduce uterine tone and interfere with the action of oxytocin.[100] However, very low concentrations (<0.5 MAC) of volatile anesthetics combined with a reliance on neuromuscular blockade to limit movement should be avoided to limit the possibility of maternal awareness under anesthesia.[101] At the conclusion of surgery, the patient should be allowed to awaken sufficiently to follow verbal commands prior to extubation to maximize the ability to protect the maternal airway and maintain spontaneous ventilation.

Neonatal outcomes following general versus epidural anesthesia for cesarean delivery suggest small, transient differences.[102] However, with either technique, when the uterine incision to delivery is greater than 180 seconds, lower Apgar scores and greater fetal acidosis have been observed (although this may reflect relative difficulty in delivery of the baby rather than the direct effects of the anesthetic agents).[103] Redistribution of general anesthetic agents from the fetal fat to the circulation can result in secondary depression of neonatal ventilatory effort. The presence of a pediatrician in such cases is advisable until a normal ventilatory pattern is observed.

FIGURE 70–4
Percentage of patients recovering from cesarean delivery and treated with either epidural, patient-controlled intravenous analgesia (PCA) or intramuscular morphine (IM) and reporting mild, moderate, or severe discomfort over a 24-hr period. *Denotes epidural vs. PCA, $P < 0.05$. †Denotes PCA vs. IM, P = NS.
(From Harrison DM, Dinatra RS, Morgese L, et al: Epidural narcotic and PCA for postcesarean section pain relief. Anesthesiology 1988;68:454–457.)

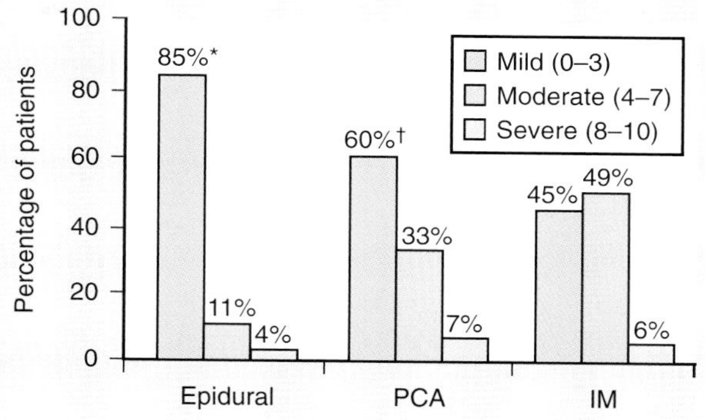

MANAGEMENT OPTIONS FOR POSTOPERATIVE PAIN

Since Wang and colleagues[104] published the first report of spinal opioid administration in humans in 1979, the analgesic efficacy and benefit of epidural and spinal opioids have been demonstrated by numerous investigations.[105] Epidural and spinal opioids blunt nocioceptive input by directly activating spinal and supraspinal opioid receptors and produce analgesia of greater intensity than doses administered parenterally or intramuscularly (Fig. 70–4).[106,107] A number of opioids, including meperidine, fentanyl, sufentanil, hydromorphone, diamorphine, methadone, buprenorphine, and butorphanol, have been utilized in the epidural and spinal spaces (Table 70–4). Morphine has emerged as the most common agent used internationally for postcesarean delivery pain management owing to its long duration of action and low cost.

The low lipid solubility of morphine slows the penetration of the drug from the epidural space into the spinal tissues; this results in analgesia that has a delayed onset of peak effects (60–90 min)[108] but persists for up to 24 hours.[108,109] Epidural morphine in doses of up to 5 mg has been used for postcesarean analgesia.[109–111] In a prospective, randomized manner, Palmer and associates[111] performed a dose-ranging study of epidural morphine (1.25–5 mg) for postcesarean analgesia and observed that the quality of analgesia increased to a dose of 3.75 mg; further increases in dose did not improve analgesia. Pruritus and nausea, which are common side effects of opioids, were not found to be dose-related. A separate study found that an infusion of naloxone, a narcotic antagonist, can reduce the severity but not the incidence of pruritus following epidural morphine.[112]

The choice of local anesthetic for epidural anesthesia may influence the efficacy of epidural morphine. Kotelko and coworkers[113] observed that postcesarean analgesia was significantly reduced, usually to less than 3 hours, in patients who received 2-chloroprocaine (a short-acting, rapid-onset

TABLE 70-4
Neuraxial Opioids

OPIOID	EPIDURAL DOSE	SPINAL DOSE	DURATION (HR)	COMMENTS
Morphine	2.5-5 mg	0.1-0.2 mg	18-24	Gold standard
Fentanyl	50-100 μg	10-20 μg	3-4	Useful as an intraoperative adjuvant
Sufentanil	10-20 μg	5-10 μg	3-4	Useful as an intraoperative adjuvant
Meperidine	25 mg		2-3	
Hydromorphone	1 mg		12	
Methadone	4-5 mg		5-6	
Diamorphine	2.5-5 mg		5-15	Not available in United States

local anesthetic used primarily for emergent cesarean deliveries) versus other local anesthetics.

Patients in whom a prolonged duration or level of analgesia is desired (e.g., an extended laparotomy for operative issues or complications) may benefit from a continuous infusion of low-concentration epidural local anesthetics with opioids (e.g., bupivacaine with fentanyl or morphine).[114,115] Such epidural infusions may be operated by patient-controlled pumps, often with a small on-demand bolus dose combined with a continuous basal infusion.[115]

The delivery of a single spinal dose of opioid has also become an attractive option for postcesarean analgesia. Morphine is the leading spinal opioid used for this purpose, with a duration of action (18–24 hr) and side effect profile similar to its use in the epidural space.[116,117] Spinal opioid doses are approximately one tenth of their corresponding epidural dose, owing to the direct access to the spinal cord opioid receptors. Despite this anatomic relationship, spinal morphine still requires 45 to 60 minutes for peak effect. Palmer and colleagues[73] observed little advantage in using spinal doses greater than morphine 0.1 mg for postcesarean analgesia; increasing doses to 0.5 mg resulted in a greater incidence of pruritus, but not nausea and vomiting.

Postoperative analgesia has been greatly improved through the use of neuraxial techniques, particularly with the administration of a single dose of morphine. Spinal and epidural opioids enhance both the quality and the duration of postoperative analgesia with an improved and acceptable side effect profile when compared with oral or intravenous analgesic agents.

MANAGEMENT OPTIONS FOR ANALGESIA AND ANESTHESIA IN HIGH RISK PARTURIENTS

Invasive Monitoring (See also Chapter 78)

Although the noninvasive measurement of blood pressure, heart rate, oxygen saturation, urinary output, and fetal cardiotocography is standard practice in most modern labor and delivery facilities, the use of invasive monitors is variable and controversial. This controversy stems from the complexity of the information, which can be difficult to properly interpret despite practice guidelines written by a number of professional organizations, including the Joint Task Force of the American College of Physicians, the American College of Cardiology, and the American Heart Association.[118] A number of studies suggest that incorrect collection and interpretation of hemodynamic data from invasive monitors remain the key problem with their use.[119,120]

Knowing when invasive monitoring is warranted is a vital clinical skill. The indications for invasive arterial blood pressure monitoring during pregnancy are relatively straightforward and include a desire to more carefully manage blood pressure, the need for more reliable blood pressure measurements, the need for vascular access for blood studies, and the planned use of certain hemodynamic agents. The indications for invasive central monitoring are not as clear. A central venous pressure (CVP) catheter is often inserted to approximate volume status (or to follow a trend in blood loss or replacement therapy) and give a greater appreciation of the mechanical phases of the cardiac cycle. Management of oliguria unresponsive to a fluid challenge, pulmonary edema, and refractory hypertension are clinical situations in which some clinicians desire CVP monitoring.

A pulmonary artery (PA) catheter can assist in determining the etiology of pulmonary edema, oliguria with a normal CVP, or cardiovascular failure; however, its use is the most controversial. Advocates of PA catheter use suggest that it can provide information on left and right ventricular function, systemic vascular resistance, and cardiac output. Detractors question the validity of the data, noting that in the setting of preeclampsia, for example, the correlation between CVP and the pulmonary capillary wedge pressure (PCWP) is unreliable when the CVP reading exceeds 6 cm H_2O.[121] In deciding between a PA and a CVP catheter, the clinician should recognize that, although the insertion-related complications are similar,[122] the PA catheter is associated with more use-related complications including balloon rupture, pulmonary infarction, valvular damage, and erosion of the PA. Thus, the benefits of PA catheter use should clearly outweigh its inherent risks before it can be recommended; the updated practice guidelines of the American Society of Anesthesiologists Task Force on Obstetrical Anesthesia state that "the decision to perform invasive hemodynamic monitoring should be individualized and based on clinical indications that include the patient's medical history and cardiovascular risk factors."[12] To date, although PA catheter use has been reported in parturients (primarily with cardiac disease), no controlled trials are available that confirm the benefit of PA catheter monitoring on maternal or fetal outcome.[12] This being noted, the PA pressures observed with different etiologies of pulmonary edema are shown in Table 70–5.[123] Similarly, the PA pressures observed with different etiologies of oliguria are shown in Table 70–6.[124]

Minimally invasive (limited to derivations of arterial line data) and noninvasive modalities for hemodynamic monitoring are currently being developed and validated in the pregnant population. These monitors, some of which are derived from Doppler ultrasound and echocardiography technologies, may offer advantages over the more invasive modalities (e.g., transesophageal echocardiography, PA catheter) that are currently available.[125] These new monitors may provide dynamic information on cardiac function, even in the presence of comorbid conditions such as preeclampsia.[126]

Hypertensive Disorders of Pregnancy

Whether preexisting, gestational, or a function of preeclampsia or eclampsia, hypertension is a common medical problem in parturients and is associated with higher maternal, fetal, and neonatal mortality and morbidity. Preeclampsia, with its systemic vasoconstriction, intravascular volume and protein depletion, and simultaneous retention of extravascular sodium and water, is of particular concern to anesthesiologists. In addition to individual organ dysfunction, abnormalities in coagulation and edema of the brain, larynx, and lungs may occur. Medical management of blood pressure should be optimized prior to obstetric or anesthetic interventions if possible, and control with labetalol, hydralazine, or infusions of nitroglycerin or nitroprusside should be commenced with arterial and central venous monitoring in severe cases. Prehydration to maintain CVP has been demonstrated to improve urine output, maintain mean arterial pressure, and decrease diastolic pressure.[127] If oliguria persists after normalization of the CVP (usually between 2 and 3 cm H_2O) or the physiologic state is complicated with pulmonary edema or cardiovascular decompensation, a PA catheter may be helpful. A cardiology consultation and an assessment of cardiopulmonary function with a transthoracic echocardiogram may also assist with the diagnosis and management. The course of preeclampsia can be complicated by mild to severe coagulopathy even in the presence of a normal platelet count.[128,129] For the benefit of both obstetric and anesthetic management, if the initial platelet count is less than an arbitrary 75 × 10^9/L, the clinical history and the results of additional studies such as a PT/PTT (prothrombin time/partial thromboplastin time) or a thromboelastograph should be reviewed. A risk-benefit analysis will ultimately determine the anesthetic technique of choice and whether the administration of blood products such as fresh frozen plasma or pooled platelets should commence prior to any intervention.

During labor, epidural analgesia offers the advantage of limiting pain or stress, thus reducing catecholamine release, decreasing maternal blood pressure, and indirectly increasing placental perfusion.[127] Epidural anesthesia can also be a preferred technique for cesarean delivery owing to the ability to slowly titrate the dose of medications as an aid to the management of blood pressure. The possibility of spinal technique–induced hypotension should not necessarily eliminate this anesthetic option. Although data are limited, one small prospective, randomized study of preeclamptic women did not reveal significant blood pressure differences between spinal and epidural anesthesia.[130] A retrospective study of women with severe preeclampsia also observed that the incidence of hypotension was not different between spinal and epidural anesthesia use.[131] Moreover, spinal anesthesia may be associated with less hypotension in women with severe preeclampsia versus healthy women undergoing cesarean delivery at similar gestational ages.[87]

The relative hypovolemia associated with preeclampsia, the use of antihypertensive medications, and the administration of magnesium as seizure prophylaxis may augment the hypotension that can develop following spinal or epidural techniques. However, restraint is advocated when responding to hypotension with vasopressors or large amounts of crystolloids. Patients with hypertensive disorders may exhibit an accentuated response to vasopressors and may quickly extravasate IV fluids that are infused.[132] A hypertensive response may also result during endotracheal intubation

TABLE 70–5

Pulmonary Artery (PA) Pressures Observed with Different Etiologies of Pulmonary Edema

ETIOLOGY	PA WEDGE PRESSURE	STROKE WORK INDEX
Left ventricular dysfunction	Increased	Decreased
Altered capillary permeability	Normal	Normal or increased
Low hydrostatic-oncotic pressure	Increased	Normal

From Benedettii TJ, Kates R, Williams V: Hemodynamic observations in severe preeclampsia complicated by pulmonary edema. Am J Obstet Gynecol 1985;152:330–334.

TABLE 70–6

Pulmonary Artery (PA) Pressures Observed with Different Etiologies of Oliguria

ETIOLOGY	PA WEDGE PRESSURE	LEFT VENTICULAR FUNCTION	SYSTEMIC VASCULAR RESISTANCE	TREATMENT
Low volume	Low	Increased	Increased	Fluid
Renal arteriospasm	Normal	Normal	Normal	Hydralazine
Decreased cardiac	Increased	Decreased	Increased	Decrease/restrict output fluid

From Clark SL, Cotton DB: Clinical indications for pulmonary artery catheterization in the patient with severe preeclampsia. Am J Obstet Gynecol 1988;158:453–458.

and emergence from general anesthesia and result in intracerebral bleeding or pulmonary edema. This hypertension can be blunted with a number of agents, including β-blockers, calcium channel blockers, hydralazine, nitroprusside, nitroglycerine, trimethaphan, and opioids.

Finally, significant edema may be encountered in preeclamptic patients, and sufficient attention and preparation should be given for managing difficult intravenous or intraarterial catheter placements, airway techniques, and neuraxial placements.

Cardiac Disease

Cardiac disease is becoming increasingly prevalent during pregnancy. Although stable in overall adult prevalence, coronary heart diseases (including those associated with hypertension) and valvular pathologies have become more relevant as the parturient population ages. More significant, however, is the dramatic increase in adult patients who have benefited from improvements in the diagnosis, treatment, and surgical correction of congenital heart disorders (CHDs). In the United States alone, adults with CHDs have grown from an estimated 300,000 in the 1980s to an anticipated 1.4 million in the year 2020.[133] Many of these individuals are women of childbearing age, and with pregnancy, CHD can have profound effects on maternal and fetal outcome.

At one time, general anesthesia was regarded as the method of choice for all cesarean deliveries in patients with either acquired heart disorders or CHDs. However, with advances in the understanding of cardiac disorders and the effects of anesthesia, especially in the relation to the anomalous or diseased myocardium, neuraxial techniques have been reconsidered. Neuraxial anesthesia has many beneficial effects, including the ability to provide pain relief, minimize the release and effects of catecholamines, and avoid airway manipulation. General anesthesia can result in moderate, sometimes detrimental, inotropic and chronotropic alterations in heart physiology, especially during the induction, intubation, and extubation periods.

The independent and related complexities of cardiac disorders and pregnancy make the sharing of patient data with all interested parties of vital importance. Because the cardiac alterations of pregnancy usually plateau from the 20th to the 24th gestational weeks until the onset of labor, this represents an ideal time to assess whether adequate compensation is occurring. This is not to say that decompensation cannot occur prior to this period or at any time during the peripartum experience. Although benign arrhythmias occur commonly without symptoms or sequelae during pregnancy,[134] in the setting of congenital cardiac lesions, even if "corrected," hemodynamic compromise may result. Communication with the patient's cardiologist is vital, and a full analysis of prior diagnostic studies should be made. Despite the presence of CHD, other causes of arrhythmias or decompensation (e.g., electrolyte and thyroid abnormalities, magnesium use) should be considered. Should complete cardiopulmonary arrest occur late (after the 24th week) in pregnancy, an event that occurs in approximately 1 in 30,000 pregnancies,[135] resuscitation must consider both maternal and fetal health. Rapid CPR (cardiopulmonary resuscitation), intubation, prevention of aortocaval compression with uterine displacement, and immediate delivery within 4 to 5 minutes of maternal cardiac arrest may maximize the chances of maternal and fetal survival.[136] In terms of medications, intubation, and defibrillation protocols, there are no alterations to the basic ACLS (advanced cardiorespiratory life support) algorithms.[136]

Acquired Cardiac Disorders

Despite the widespread use of antibiotics, in many parts of the developing world, rheumatic heart disease remains the leading cause of cardiac abnormalities in women of childbearing age.[137] Valvular lesions include mitral stenosis (75%–90%), mitral regurgitation (6%–12%), aortic regurgitation (2%–5%), and aortic stenosis (1%).

In general, the primary goal with stenotic lesions is to maintain a normal to slow sinus heart rate with preservation of systemic vascular resistance (SVR). These goals are particularly important when controlling the physiologic responses to neuraxial blockade, which can often dramatically reduce the SVR (i.e., cause hypotension) and result in compensatory tachycardia. Incremental titration of catheter-based epidural or spinal techniques, or initial use of spinal analgesia with opioids alone, can limit the sympathetic blockade produced by local anesthetics. Treatment of hypotension with phenylephrine (an α-adrenergic vasopressor) may avoid the tachycardia observed with the use of ephedrine (a combined α- and α-adrenergic vasopressor). In contrast to stenotic lesions, regurgitant valvular disorders, such as mitral and aortic insufficiency, are best managed with normal to slight increases in sinus heart rate and reductions in SVR. Thus, the sympathetic reduction observed with neuraxial blockade can be beneficial in providing afterload reduction and minimizing the influences of stress catecholamines on SVR. Preserving venous return and intravascular volume are important. However, on occasion, the normally helpful increased intravascular volume of pregnancy or the rapid return of SVR following delivery can result in left ventricular failure and pulmonary edema.[138]

Congenital Cardiac Disorders

Congenital heart disease in the adult is not simply a continuation of the childhood experience. The growth of the cardiac chambers allows arrhythmias to change in character and frequency and ventricular dysfunction and failure to occur. Bioprosthetic replacement valves and conduits can also fail over time, often as a result of adult comorbidities or conditions, including pregnancy. With some congenital disorders, a complete repair is made and cardiovascular function, pressures, and blood flow patterns develop relatively normally. For the most part, these individuals require no special treatment. However, three important differences should be recognized: First, because some cardiac disorders are inherited, fetal echocardiography at 20 to 24 weeks' gestation is desirable. Second, antibiotic prophylaxis may be warranted. Third, arrhythmias are more common owing to the scar tissue in the heart acting as an arrhythmogenic focus. Other disorders, however, may present as uncorrected or partially corrected lesions in decompensated or poorly compensated states, thereby making the anesthetic management more challenging. The most commonly observed CHDs during pregnancy include left-to-right shunts, tetralogy of Fallot, Eisenmenger's syndrome, and aortic coarctation (see Chapter 36).

The physiologic impact of a small septal defect or a patent ductus arteriosus is usually a trivial to modest left-to-right intracardiac shunt. In general, modest left-to-right shunts are well tolerated during pregnancy, although several alterations in management have been suggested.[139] Because air embolization may occur through IV lines, or with the loss-of-resistance-to-air technique of epidural placement, the use of air filters and loss-of-resistance-to-saline epidural placement techniques is recommended.[140] In addition, because increases in pulmonary vascular resistance with hypoxia, hypercarbia, and acidosis may allow for reversal of shunt flow, the application of supplemental oxygen appears prudent. Finally, the overall management goal for these defects should focus on limiting maternal catecholamine and SVR increases. In this regard, the use of neuraxial analgesia provides exceptional control; however, the block should be administered slowly, because rapid decreases in SVR may result in a pronounced right-to-left shunt with maternal hypoxemia.[139]

Parturients with uncorrected or partially corrected cyanotic congenital heart disease (i.e., right-to-left shunts) may tolerate pregnancy poorly. Management focuses on maintaining adequate SVR, intravascular volume, and venous return and preventing increases in SVR (often due to pain, hypoxemia, hypercarbia, and acidosis). The use of supplemental oxygen and the use of arterial and central venous catheters may facilitate care and hemodynamic management. The use of PA catheters remains controversial owing to difficulties in placement, the risk of PA rupture and cardiac arrhythmias, and the limited information obtained in the setting of a severe fixed pulmonary hypertension and a large intracardiac shunt.[141] Neuraxial analgesia produced with intrathecal opioid administration may minimize decreases in SVR, and if provided with a CSE technique, the judicious addition of epidural local anesthetics can be titrated as needed. In the event of a cesarean delivery, neuraxial anesthesia remains preferable to general anesthesia owing to the diminished cardiac output that can occur from halogenated agents and positive-pressure ventilation. If neuraxial anesthesia is contraindicated, a controlled versus rapid-sequence induction of general anesthesia minimizes critical decreases in SVR and myocardial function. Regardless of the technique employed, hemodynamic alterations must be promptly resolved, and ephedrine and dopamine, rather than phenylephrine, are vasopressors of choice because of their maintenance of both SVR and heart rate.

Diabetes

Analgesic and anesthetic management of diabetic parturients should focus on glucose management and the responses of the physiologic systems most affected: coronary, cerebral and peripheral vascular, gastrointestinal, renal, and autonomic systems. The analgesia and anesthesia produced by neuraxial techniques can increase placental perfusion through reductions in maternal catecholamines and decrease the incidence of fetal acidosis occurring with maternal labor hyperventilation. The cardiovascular, autonomic, and uteroplacental blood flow changes caused by diabetes make the prevention and early treatment of hypotension a significant concern. The frequent and severe maternal hypotension witnessed in diabetics can be associated with spinal and epidural anesthesia for cesarean delivery.[142] However, it is possible that dextrose-containing IV fluids may have played a role. With strict observation and reaction to maternal blood pressure, volume expansion with a non–dextrose-containing solution, and maternal glucose control, spinal anesthesia can be performed without an associated fetal acidosis.[143]

In addition to the improved hemodynamic control seen with the slow initiation of epidural analgesia and anesthesia, this technique may offer other beneficial effects during labor and delivery. Insulin resistance has been demonstrated to occur in a dose-response relationship with the amount of stress following surgery, burns, trauma, and sepsis. More recently, pain per se has been demonstrated to impair insulin sensitivity by affecting nonoxidative glucose metabolism.[144] Although studies have not been performed in laboring diabetic parturients or even in females, this suggests that glucose regulation can be improved by the administration of pain relief in stressful states. Indeed, when epidural anesthesia was compared with general anesthesia as a control group, an attenuation of the hyperglycemic response to abdominal surgery was observed through a modification of glucose production, without affecting glucose utilization.[145] Protein metabolism, by contrast, was not influenced by epidural blockade. These investigations suggest a possible benefit from the use of neuraxial analgesia and anesthesia in parturients with diabetes.

If general anesthesia is required, the possibilities of gastroparesis, limited atlanto-occipital joint extension, and impaired counterregulatory hormone responses to hypoglycemia should be considered and integrated into the management.[146]

EFFECTS OF NEURAXIAL ANALGESIA ON PROGRESS AND OUTCOME OF LABOR

Whether neuraxial analgesia affects the progress and outcome of labor remains a controversial topic. The myriad of maternal and fetal variables adds complexity to the issue, as well as differing institutional and individual anesthetic and obstetric practices. Moreover, the contemporary pattern and progress of labor appears slower than previously described a half a century earlier by Friedman.[147] Zhang and associates,[148] noting a significant delay in the progress of labor in nulliparous women, pointed to several factors possibly responsible including higher maternal age and weight, increasing fetal size, and higher induction and epidural use rates. Together, these changes make practice patterns and outcomes difficult to compare.

Study Design Issues

The greatest challenge in uncovering an association between neuraxial analgesia and progress of labor is that the ideal prospective, randomized, double-blinded, placebo-controlled study is exceptionally difficult, if not impossible, to perform. Retrospective or nonrandomized studies may underestimate the importance of confounders. For instance, women requesting epidural labor analgesia may be inherently different from those choosing natural childbirth; such differences have included having smaller pelvises, more occiput posterior fetal presentations,[149] greater use of oxytocin for induction or augmentation, and more painful labors (which may be associated with slower labor and instrumental delivery).[150] Moreover, in nulliparous parturients with larger fetuses and eventual dystocia, a requirement for larger amounts of epidural local anesthetic for pain relief has been reported.[151–153]

The complexity of assessing prospective studies begins with enrollment procedures, because women open to randomization of the timing and technique of analgesia may not be representative of the majority of parturients. In addition, parturients who deliver either very slowly or very quickly may not remain in their randomized group. Blinding the obstetrician, anesthesiologist, nurse, and patient to neuraxial versus other analgesic forms is also difficult. Such blinding is necessary to remove any subtle or overt influences on decision-making; for example, instrumental deliveries may be more common in those patients with epidural analgesia because they can more comfortably accept forceps delivery.[154] Finally, women utilizing parenteral opioids, commonly used as a control group, may not progress in a manner representative of the natural progress of labor,[155] thus, not giving a true comparison of epidural techniques with the natural birth experience. No study has so far succeeded in meeting all these objectives; however, certain insights can be gained from the literature to date.

Study Results

The American College of Obstetricians and Gynecologists (ACOG) issued guidelines[156] on the use of obstetric anesthesia services. Among the recommendations to reduce the incidence of cesarean delivery was delaying epidural analgesia initiation until cervical dilation of 5 cm or greater was achieved. The data cited, primarily observational and nonrandomized, found an association between earlier epidural placement and dystocia. Using a case-control methodology, investigators at the National Maternity Hospital in Dublin (the pioneers of the active management of labor) observed that epidural initiation at less than 2 cm dilation was a significant risk factor for prolonging labor in nulliparous women.[157] Thorp and coworkers,[158] in nulliparous women with cervical dilation less than 5 cm and dilation rate less than 1 cm/hr, observed a sixfold increase in cesarean delivery for dystocia in association with the use of regional analgesia. Similarly, Lieberman and colleagues,[159] using a multivariate regression technique on observational data, noted cervical dilation less than 5 cm and station less than 0 at time of epidural initiation as strong risk factors for cesarean delivery. Such cohort studies, however, have not uniformly supported differences in progress and outcome with epidural analgesia. Ohel and Harats[160] failed to show any difference in labor outcome when epidural analgesia was initiated prior to or after 3 cm cervical dilation. Holt and associates,[161] in a prospective cohort study, found an association between cesarean delivery and higher station, but not cervical dilation, at the time of epidural placement.

An interesting form of retrospective analysis evaluates those institutions in which epidural analgesia becomes suddenly available. These studies, though nonrandomized, offer an analysis of an entire patient cohort in which a "sentinel event" has occurred but other variables, such as obstetric practice styles, are unlikely to change dramatically. A meta-analysis of such studies found no association between a sudden increase in the utilization of epidural analgesia and higher rates of cesarean delivery.[162]

The majority of randomized, controlled trials indicate little overall effect of epidural analgesia on the progress and outcome of labor. Luxman and coworkers[163] found no difference in length of labor or mode of delivery in 60 nulliparous parturients randomized to receive epidural analgesia prior to or after 4 cm cervical dilation (mean 2.3 cm vs. 4.5 cm). Chestnut and colleagues, in evaluating women closer to 5 cm cervical dilation (mean 4 cm vs. 5 cm), demonstrated no differences in labor outcome in either spontaneous[164] or induced[165] labors. A meta-analysis of 10 trials comparing parturients of mixed parity randomized to epidural analgesia or parenteral opioids noted a prolongation of the first and second stages of labor by 42 minutes and 14 minutes, respectively, in association with the use of epidurals.[166]

Specific studies, however, do appear to indicate that anesthetic practice differences may influence the progress and outcome of labor. Although the Comparative Obstetric Mobile Epidural Trial (COMET)[167] found no differences in the incidence of cesarean delivery, a higher proportion of instrumental deliveries was observed in patients with "traditional" epidurals versus CSE or parenteral opioids. In the "traditional" epidural group, intermittent boluses of 0.25% bupivacaine were administered, a method not commonly used in contemporary practice in which lower concentrations and continuous infusion pumps are usual. Regardless, the findings suggest that differences in neuraxial technique may alter outcomes; this conclusion has been supported by other studies comparing CSE and epidural techniques. In nulliparous parturients at less than 3 cm cervical dilation, Tsen and coworkers,[68] using 1 mL versus 12 to 15 mL of 0.25% bupivacaine in the spinal and epidural spaces, respectively, observed faster cervical dilation and progress of labor in the spinal (CSE) group. Further, Wong and associates[69] found that the median time from initiation of analgesia to complete dilation was significantly shorter after spinal (CSE) versus systemic analgesia (295 min vs. 385 min, $P < .001$), as was the time to vaginal delivery (398 min vs. 479 min, $P < .001$).

Obstetric practice style may also influence the outcome and progress of labor. Meta-analyses of randomized trials have found that, although instrumental delivery rates increased in patients receiving epidural analgesia, the resulting incidences were widely divergent, perhaps reflecting substantial practice style differences.[166] In terms of cesarean delivery, one study noted that apart from nulliparity, the identity of the individual obstetrician was the variable with the greatest influence on cesarean delivery rates.[168] Moreover, the use of peer review and education have been demonstrated to result in a 50% decrease in cesarean rates despite a simultaneous doubling of epidural analgesia use.[169,170]

In summary, although problems with methodology make an association difficult to evaluate, the use of epidural analgesia appears to affect the progress and outcome of labor remarkably little. Although the risk of cesarean delivery does not appear to be influenced, instrumental vaginal delivery appears to be increased with the use of epidural analgesia. It is possible that these associations may reflect variances in patient demographics or differences in anesthetic and obstetric practice styles.

TEMPERATURE CHANGES IN LABOR

Humans have the ability to maintain body temperature within a narrow range despite changes in environmental temperature. Although the extremities and skin can vary over several degrees, the average core body temperature of healthy adults is 37°C with diurnal variations of ± 0.5°C.[171] Thermoregulation is centered in the hypothalamus and responds to receptors found predominantly in the skin and spinal cord. Established through a balance of heat uptake, production, and loss, temperature equilibrium can be distorted by processes that change the thermoregulatory threshold (set value) or the response to temperatures above or below this value.

Clinically, a temperature greater than 38°C represents a fever. Most commonly, fever is the result of exogenous or endogenous pyrogens that disturb the "thermostat" set value to allow thermoregulatory mechanisms to maintain an elevated temperature. Less commonly, thermoregulatory responses to hyperthermia are prevented (such as a blockade of sympathetically mediated vasodilation or sweating) or overwhelmed (such as immersion in hot water). Of interest, endogenous pyrogens, which act on the thermoregulatory center and are triggered by the release of interleukin-1 (Il-1) and -6 from macrophages, are partially mediated by prostaglandin metabolism.[172] The relationship of this finding to the many pregnancy-induced alterations in the production and distribution of prostaglandins has yet to be elucidated.[173]

Thermoregulation during Pregnancy

During pregnancy, the mother attempts to maintain a normal temperature. The fetus relies on the uteroplacental circulation and the amniotic fluid interface for heat exchange; these limited routes for heat egress result in a normal fetal temperature approximately 0.5°C to 0.75°C higher than maternal body temperature.[174] With extreme hyperthermia, experimental evidence suggests that fetal deterioration may occur. Morishima and colleagues,[175] utilizing radiant heat to produce maternal hyperthermia of 107°F in anesthetized baboons, observed increased uterine activity and deterioration in fetal condition. Similarly, Cefalo and Hellegers[176] demonstrated fetal deterioration in anesthetized gravid ewes with levels of hyperthermia that produced maternal cardiovascular collapse. Although these extreme degrees of hyperthermia are unlikely to be clinically applicable, lesser increases of temperature may have various effects, including changes in umbilical blood flow.[176]

In terms of neonatal effects, epidemiologic evidence suggests that mild maternal fever may not be as benign as previously assumed based on the animal data. Lieberman and associates,[177] in a retrospective review of 1218 nulliparous women with singleton, term pregnancies in spontaneous labor who were afebrile on admission, noted that 1-minute Apgar scores less than 7, hypotonia, and the need for bag and mask ventilation were more common in parturients with a body temperature greater than 101°F. Although it remains unclear whether temperature per se, independent from underlying infectious or inflammatory processes, can cause neurologic injury, an association between maternal intrapartum fever and neonatal encephalopathy,[178] cerebral palsy,[179] and persistent developmental cognitive deficits[180] has been observed. Moreover, maternal outcome may be directly or indirectly influenced by the presence of even low-grade fever. Lieberman and coworkers[181] retrospectively observed a twofold higher incidence in operative vaginal and cesarean deliveries in nulliparous women who were afebrile at admission and subsequently developed a fever greater than 99.5°F compared with those who remained afebrile, even when controlled for birth weight, length of labor, and analgesic choice. More recently, Shipp and colleagues[182] noted an association between postpartum fever after cesarean delivery and an increased risk of uterine rupture in a subsequent trial of labor.

Epidural Analgesia and Maternal Pyrexia

Study Design Issues

To date, nearly all the clinical studies of maternal fever associated with epidural analgesia have been nonrandomized. Similar to the progress and outcome of labor studies, it is possible that women who request epidural labor analgesia have risk factors that predispose them to fever, including greater rates of nulliparity,[183] prolonged rupture of membranes,[183,184] prolonged labor,[183,185,186] higher temperature on admission,[183] early chorioamnionitis,[183] and frequent cervical examinations.[187] Using a case-control methodology, Vallejo and associates[186] compared women with histologically confirmed chorioamnionitis with two groups of women who received epidural analgesia (with and without chorioamnionitis). Fever was more common in infected women in all groups; however, the incidence of fever in uninfected women with epidurals was only 1%. In a similar study of 149 women who delivered greater than 6 hours following membrane rupture, Dashe and coworkers[188] noted an increased incidence of fever in 54% of parturients who received epidurals. However, when parturients with evidence of placental inflammation were excluded, the incidence of fever was similar in women with and without epidural analgesia (11% vs. 9%).

Study Results

Although an infection is the most common reason for fever during pregnancy, the influence of neuraxial techniques on maternal temperature is of interest. Neuraxial anesthesia administered for surgery, including cesarean delivery, typically results in peripheral vasodilation, redistribution of body heat, and hypothermia.[189] By contrast, in laboring women receiving neuraxial analgesia, a rise in temperature has been noted. Fusi and colleagues[190] reported an increase in vaginal temperatures of approximately 1°C over 7 hours in 18 parturients receiving epidural analgesia with no evidence of infection; this contrasted with stable temperatures in 15 parturients who received intramuscular meperidine. Using a method perhaps more reflective of core temperature, Camann and associates[185] measured tympanic membrane temperature in 53 laboring parturients divided into three groups. One group received IV nalbuphine; the other two groups, composed of women who chose epidural analgesia, were randomized to receive epidural bupivacaine with or without fentanyl. With ambient room temperature maintained at 20°C to 22°C, epidural analgesia did not affect maternal temperature for the first 4 hours. Thereafter, the

FIGURE 70–5
Mean tympanic temperatures during labor in three groups of patients: Epidural bupivacaine-fentanyl (*circles*), epidural bupivacaine only (*diamonds*), and parenteral opioids (*squares*) groups. $P < .01$ compared with the epidural group. $P < .01$ compared with the pre-epidural temperature.
(From Camann WR, Hortvet LA, Hughes N, et al: Maternal temperature regulation during extradural analgesia for labour. Br J Anaesth 1991;67:565–568.)

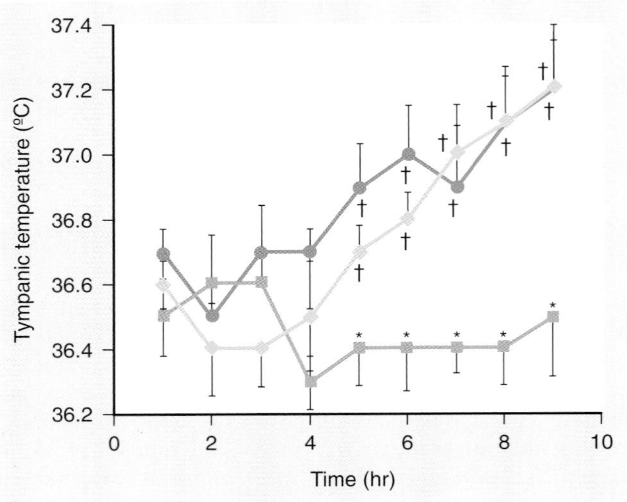

mean tympanic membrane temperature increased by 0.07°C/hr in both epidural groups, with no differences observed in those receiving epidural fentanyl (Fig. 70–5).

Macaulay and coworkers[191] evaluated maternal oral and intrauterine and fetal skin temperatures in 33 and 27 parturients undergoing labor with and without epidurals, respectively. With an ambient temperature ranging from 23.3°C to 29°C, 10 fetuses within mothers with epidurals reached a maximum fetal skin temperature of greater than 38°C versus none in the group without epidurals. Of interest, only 2 women, both in the epidural group, reached an oral temperature greater than 37.5°C. Ultimately, no differences in Apgar scoring or umbilical cord blood gases were found. Most recently, Mantha and colleagues[192] observed in 92 healthy, term, nulliparous women in spontaneous labor that temperature elevation to 38°C occurred more commonly in the initial 4 hours in women receiving continuous versus intermittent labor epidural analgesia, although mean maternal temperatures did not differ between the groups at any time, nor were neonatal temperature or sepsis evaluation rates different. Overall, a number of investigators have observed an incidence of clinical fever (>38°C) in 1% to 36% of laboring women receiving epidural analgesia, with a temperature elevation rate of approximately 0.1°C/hr of epidural analgesia, usually after a 4- to 5-hour delay.[183,184,193,194]

The mechanisms by which epidural analgesia may produce changes in maternal temperature during labor remain unclear. Although high ambient temperatures (24°C–26°C) have been suggested as a possible etiology,[190] an association between ambient temperature and maternal or fetal temperatures has not been uniformly demonstrated.[184,191] A second possibility could be epidural-induced reductions in heat loss mechanisms, including an increase in sweating thresholds (by 0.55°C in volunteers)[195] and a reduction in hyperventilation during labor.[196,197] A third possibility could be alterations that result in, or are related to, shivering. In those parturients who shivered following the initiation of epidural analgesia versus those who do not, pyrexia developed as early as 1 hour later, in comparison with longer than 4 hours later.[198] In addition, shivering parturients ultimately attained higher maximum temperatures and had a threefold increase in clinical fever. A final possibility could be alterations in the parturients not receiving an epidural technique. The opioids frequently utilized in these groups may suppress temperature elevations.[199] A retrospective study of systemic use[200] and a prospective, randomized study of epidural use[185] of opioids, however, failed to demonstrate temperature curve changes with the addition of opioids.

Impact and Interventions

In addition to the fetal concerns discussed earlier, temperature elevations may alter neonatal exposure to antibiotics and subsequent care. Mayer and associates[201] retrospectively evaluated 300 low risk nulliparous women who received systemic opioids, epidural analgesia, or both ($n = 100$ in each group). The incidence of maternal fever (2%, 16%, and 24% in the preceding groups, respectively) and intrapartum maternal antibiotics (6%, 19%, 22%) was highest in the combined opioid and epidural group. Of note, in the 10 patients who ultimately demonstrated laboratory evidence of chorioamnionitis, maternal fever was not the only presenting symptom; fetal tachycardia and meconium-stained or abnormal amniotic fluid were also found. This suggests that the administration of antibiotics should not be guided by maternal fever alone. In a secondary analysis of 1657 low risk nulliparous women enrolled in a trial of active management of labor, the incidence of maternal fever (15% vs. 1%), neonatal sepsis evaluation (34% vs. 10%), and antibiotic treatment (15% vs. 4%) was increased when epidural analgesia was used.[193] However, the incidence of actual neonatal sepsis was exceedingly low in epidural and nonepidural groups (0.3% vs. 0.2%), and of interest, although the indications for sepsis evaluations was not provided, was the finding that two thirds of the evaluations occurred in infants of mothers who did not have intrapartum fevers. Moreover, the mothers who received epidural analgesia had larger infants, longer labors, and a twofold increase in the labor induction rate. Although it is possible that the active management protocol of frequent cervical examinations and early amniotomy may have influenced the risk of fever, a subsequent study evaluated nonrandomized parturients whose temperature remained below 100.4°C throughout labor.[202] Neonatal sepsis evaluations were more common in parturients who had epidural analgesia (20.4% vs. 8.9%) even after controlling for gestational age, birth weight, maternal smoking history, active labor management, premature rupture of membranes, and admission cervical dilation. Epidural analgesia was associated with both major (rupture of membranes > 24 hr, fetal heart rate > 160 beats/min) and minor criteria (maternal temperature > 99.5°F, rupture of membranes 12–24 hr) for sepsis evaluation. These data suggest that multiple factors should be present prior to initiating a sepsis evaluation. Moreover, of those babies investigated for sepsis because of risk factors, few will ultimately prove to have been infected.

The rate of neonatal sepsis evaluation and treatment can be modified by neonatology admission criteria and practice style. Yancey and coworkers,[203] reviewing the effects of an on-demand epidural analgesia service in which epidural use increased overnight (because of a change in policy in the unit) from 1% to 83%, observed that maternal temperatures greater than 99.5°F and 100.4°F increased 3-fold and 18-fold, respectively. Despite this increase in maternal temperatures, neonatal blood counts and cultures increased modestly (relative risk 1.5–1.7), and no changes in the proportion of infants who received antibiotic treatment for presumed sepsis were observed. Similarly, Kaul and colleagues[204] noted in a retrospective review of the delivery records of 1177 nulliparous women that the incidence of neonatal sepsis evaluations was no different (7.5% vs. 9.4%) despite women with epidural analgesia having more fever. Both investigators cited more stringent neonatal sepsis treatment guidelines, which did not include the treatment for maternal fever in the absence of chorioamnionitis, as being responsible for their results.

Attempts to diminish maternal temperature increases during labor have thus far been limited. Goetzl and associates[205] randomized 42 nulliparous women to receive acetaminophen 650 mg every 4 hours versus placebo in women receiving epidural analgesia. The incidence of fever did not differ between groups (23.8%). Of note, despite all neonatal blood cultures being negative, maternal serum and cord blood markers of inflammation (Il-6) were higher in mothers who had fever. This suggests that inflammatory markers can be elevated in the absence of neonatal infection. In a separate study, Goetzl and coworkers[206] randomized 200 term nulliparous patients undergoing labor with epidural analgesia to receive low- or high-dose corticosteroids (methylprednisolone 25 mg q8h or 100 mg q4h, respectively) or placebo to assess the rate of intrapartum fever (>100.4°F). The incidence of maternal fever and neonatal sepsis evaluations were significantly reduced in the high-dose corticosteroid group; however, an increased incidence of asymptomatic neonatal bacteremia was also observed. A significant reduction in the presence of Il-6 was observed in the high-dose corticosteroid group only when compared with the placebo group. The investigators concluded that high-dose corticosterioids, such as those used as an intrapartum maternal stress dose, could reduce maternal fever and inflammatory cytokines, but could not be currently recommended as a prevention strategy owing to the risk of neonatal bacteremia.

In conclusion, epidural analgesia does appear associated with increases in temperature, although most of these increases are mild. This being said, maternal fever has been linked with adverse neonatal outcomes. Further studies of the mechanism of these temperature elevations with epidural use and a reanalysis of maternal and neonatal evaluation and treatment policies are warranted.

SUMMARY OF MANAGEMENT OPTIONS

Neuraxial Analgesia and Anesthesia

Management Options	Evidence Quality and Recommendation	References
External Cephalic Version		
Epidural use is associated with higher success rates compared with no epidural; it is not clear whether spinal or CSE has the same effect.	Ib/A	45–49
Pain Relief during Parturition		
Nonpharmacologic Methods		
All nonpharmacologic methods have limited analgesic action.	Ib/A	33,35,36
Psychological support is of benefit and reduces the need for pain relief.	Ia/A	16,17
Hypnosis can be beneficial.	Ia/A	20
The presence of a doula or other nonprofessional support in labor reduces need for pain relief.	Ia/A	21
Sensory stimulation (e.g., acupuncture, TENS) is claimed to be of some benefit in early labor.	III/B	22–24
Pharmacologic Methods		
Systemic medications shown to be effective include opioids and PCA.	III/B	26,37
Inhalational analgesia: Entonox—50% NO/50% oxygen—is widely used, but evidence is mainly observational.	Ib/A	36
Regional Analgesia/Anesthesia		
Most often used are pudendal block and perineal block.	IIb/B	42,43
Paracervical, caudal, and lumbar sympathetic blocks are infrequently used.	Ib/A	40,41

SUMMARY OF MANAGEMENT OPTIONS
Neuraxial Analgesia and Anesthesia—cont'd

Management Options	Evidence Quality and Recommendation	References
Pain Relief during Parturition		
Neuraxial Analgesia		
Spinal block is effective for assisted vaginal delivery and CD; time-limited during labor if given as a single dose.	IV/C	52
Epidural block is effective for assisted vaginal delivery, and CD; addition of fentanyl and local anesthetic improves short-term effectiveness (especially for an assisted vaginal delivery).	IIa/B	65
CSE technique is effective for assisted vaginal delivery and CD; possibly, it has a lower complication rate than epidural alone.	Ib/A	68
Dural puncture managed by:		
• Analgesia.	Ib/A	58
• IV fluids.	Ia/A	58
• Blood patch.	IV/C	58
Cesarean Delivery		
Spinal, epidural, and CSE are preferred to general anesthesia; addition of opioids and epinephrine may result in increased effectiveness.	Ib/A	56,73,74, 78,80
With GA:		
• Use laryngeal mask airway if unable to intubate.	IIb/B	94
• Use nonparticulate antacid, H_2 antagonist, and prokinetic agent when possible.	Ib/A	95–97
• Use pre-induction oxygenation.	III/B	98
Postoperative Pain Relief		
Diclofenac is effective in reducing postpartum pain.	Ia/A	207
Epidural is more effective than parenteral opioids.	Ib/A	105–107
High Risk Pregnancies—Special Considerations		
Invasive monitoring (see also Chapter 78) is valuable but requires skill and experience.	IV/C	118–120
Hypertension	III/B	127–129
Fluid overload may occur in the setting of magnesium and beta blockade use.		
Coagulation status should be evaluated prior to neuraxial techniques.		
Intubation with GA may be associated with significant increase in blood pressure.		
Cardiac Disease		
Use caution with neuraxial techniques, particularly spinal anesthesia, in stenotic lesions, in which reduced SVR may precipitate reduced cardiac output and collapse.	IV/C	138
Left-to-right shunts may reverse with a decrease in SVR from neuraxial techniques and result in maternal hypoxemia.	IV/C	139
Adverse Effects of Epidural Analgesia		
Prolonged labor and maternal hyperpyrexia are both more common, but etiology and impact are unclear.	—/GPP	—

CD, cesarean delivery; CSE, combined spinal-epidural; GA, general anesthesia; GPP, good practice point; NO, nitric oxide; PCA, patient-controlled analgesia; SVR, systemic vascular resistance; TENS, transcutaneous electrical nerve stimulation.

Acknowledgment

The author would like to thank the gracious mentorship, friendship, and scholarship of Sanjay Datta, MD, FFARCS (Eng.), who richly contributed to the author's appreciation and enthusiasm for the patients and science within the specialty of obstetric anesthesia.

SUGGESTED READINGS

Bucklin BA, Hawkins JL, Anderson JR, Ullrich FA: Obstetric anesthesia workforce survey: twenty-year update. Anesthesiology 2005;103: 645–653.

Cooper GM, McClure JH: Anaesthesia chapter from Saving Mother's Lives: Reviewing Maternal Deaths to Make Pregnancy Safer. Br J Anaesth 2008;100:17–22.

Dyer RA, Piercy JL, Reed AR, et al: Hemodynamic changes associated with spinal anesthesia for cesarean delivery in severe preeclampsia. Anesthesiology 2008;108:802–811.

Hawkins JL, Koonin LM, Palmer SK, Gibbs CP: Anesthesia-related deaths during obstetric delivery in the United States, 1979–1990. Anesthesiology 1997;86:277–284.

Goetzl L, Evans T, Rivers J, et al: Elevated maternal and fetal seum interleukin-6 levels are associated with epidural fever. Am J Obstet Gynecol 2002;187:834–838.

Lee A, Ngan Kee WD, Gin T: A quantitative, systematic review of randomized controlled trials of ephedrine versus phenylephrine for the management of hypotension during spinal anesthesia for cesarean delivery. Anesth Analg 2002;94:920–926.

Practice Guidelines for Obstetric Anesthesia: An updated report by the American Society of Anesthesiologists Task Force on Obstetric Anesthesia: Anesthesiology 2007;106:843–863.

Turnbull DK, Shepherd DB: Post-dural puncture headache: Pathogenesis, prevention and treatment. Br J Anaesth 2003;91:718–729.

Ueyama H, He YL, Tanigami H, et al: Effects of crystalloid and colloid preload on blood volume in the parturient undergoing spinal anesthesia for elective cesarean section. Anesthesiology 1999;91:1571–1576.

Wong CA, Scavone BM, Peaceman AM, et al: The risk of cesarean delivery with neuraxial analgesia given early versus late in labor. N Engl J Med 2005;352:655–665.

REFERENCES

For a complete list of references, log onto www.expertconsult.com.

CHAPTER 71

Perineal Repair and Pelvic Floor Injury

ROHNA KEARNEY and COLM O'HERLIHY

INTRODUCTION

Pelvic floor injury at the time of vaginal delivery can result in the later development of urinary incontinence, pelvic organ prolapse, and fecal incontinence. In the United States, the direct annual cost of pelvic organ prolapse surgery alone was estimated to be over $1 billion at the turn of the millennium, with 22 women per 10,000 having surgical correction for this indication.[1,2] The annual direct cost of urinary incontinence was even higher, at $12.4 billion.[3] The cost 10 years later is likely to be substantially higher. The lifetime risk of a woman in the United States undergoing surgery for incontinence or prolapse by the age of 80 has been estimated as 11%.[4] With growing awareness of the impact of pelvic floor injury, attention is now increasingly focused on the prevention of these problems. Vaginal delivery is the factor most subject to modification in the etiology of pelvic floor injury.[5–7] In order to prevent injury and minimize the impact of delivery on the pelvic floor, it is necessary to have an understanding of the anatomy and the pathophysiology of injury.

ANATOMY

The primary function of the pelvic floor is to prevent the pelvic organs from downward displacement in the upright position, while at the same time allowing parturition and elimination. The levator ani muscles, which are composites of the pubococcygeus, puborectalis, and iliococcygeus on each side, are the most important constituents of the pelvic floor and resemble a horizontal shelf that acts to close like a valve when the female assumes the upright position.[8] The pubococcygeus, more recently referred to as the "pubovisceral muscle," comprises the puboanalis, pubovaginalis, and puboperineus subdivisions.[9,10] The pubococcygeus and puborectalis arise from the inner surface of the pubic bone, whereas the iliococcygeus arises from the arcus tendineus levator ani. The pubococcygeus inserts into the vaginal wall (pubovaginalis), perineal body (puboperineus), and intersphincteric groove (puboanalis). The puborectalis forms a sling around the rectum and inserts into the deep external sphincter, and the iliococcygeus inserts into the iliococcygeal raphe.

The perineal membrane is a triangular sheet of fibromuscular tissue with the striated urogenital sphincter lying above. It provides support by attaching the vagina, urethra, and perineal body to the ischiopubic rami. Above it, the striated urogenital sphincter consists of the compressor urethra, urethrovaginal sphincter, and sphincter urethra.

The endopelvic fascia refers to the condensation of the adventitial layers of the pelvic organs. This connective tissue layer attaches the pelvic organs to the lateral pelvic walls and, together with the levator ani, shares the load on the pelvic floor. Support for the vagina has been identified at three levels[11,12] (Fig. 71–1). Level I consists of the uterosacral and cardinal ligaments, which represent a medial and lateral thickening of the endopelvic fascia connecting the cervix and upper vagina to the pelvic sidewalls. These structures are vertical in the standing position and serve to keep the uterus, cervix, and upper vagina tethered in a posterior position over the levator ani muscles.

At level II, the middle third of the vagina is attached by the paracolpium to the arcus tendineus and levator ani muscle fascia. The arcus tendineus fascia pelvis runs from the pubic bone anteriorly to the ischial spines posteriorly. At level III, the lower third of the vagina is attached directly to the perineal membrane, perineal body, and levator ani.

The proximal urethra is supported by the endopelvic fascia and anterior vaginal wall, which act like a hammock and attach it to the arcus tendineus fascia and levator ani, thus resulting in compression and closure of the urethral lumen in response to increases in intra-abdominal pressure.[13]

The perineal body is covered by skin and lies between the lower vagina and the anus. It is attached by the perineal membrane to the inferior pubic rami and ischial tuberosities. The perineal body receives the insertion of the bulbocavernosus muscles and posteriorly is attached to the coccyx by the external anal sphincter.

The anal sphincters are located in the posterior compartment of the pelvic floor. The external anal sphincter is a voluntary muscle consisting of three components: a subcutaneous part, a superficial part connecting the perineal body to the coccyx, and a deep part, which surrounds the rectum. The internal anal sphincter is a downward extension and thickening of the circular smooth muscle of the rectum. The

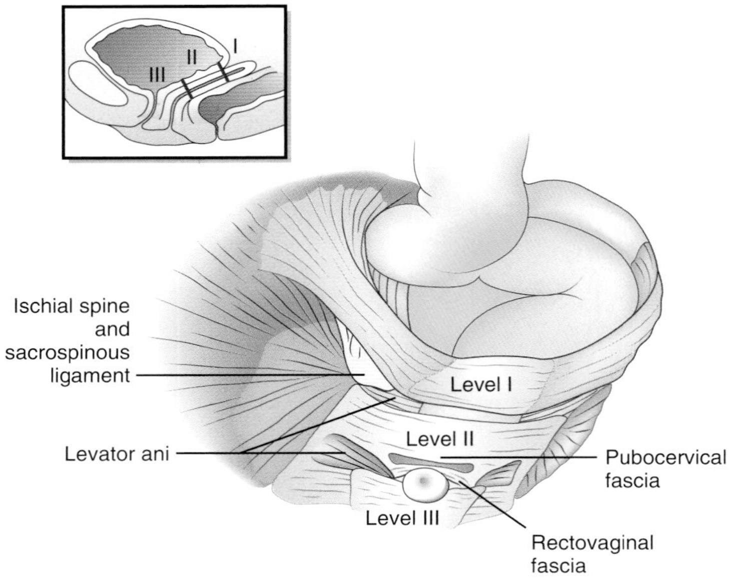

FIGURE 71–1
The three levels of vaginal support.
(From Delancey JO: Anatomic aspects of vaginal eversion after hysterectomy. Am J Obstet Gynecol 1992;166:1717–1728.)

intersphincteric groove runs between the internal and the external anal sphincters. The ischiorectal fossas lie between the levator ani and the obturator internus muscles. The external anal sphincter and bulbocavernosus muscles are supplied by the pudendal nerve, which arises from the anterior primary rami of S2, S3, and S4. The nerve leaves the pelvis through the greater sciatic foramen and runs in the pelvic side wall close to the ischial spine and sacrospinous ligament to enter the pudendal (Alcock's) canal through the lesser sciatic foramen. It divides into three terminal branches—the clitoral, perineal, and inferior rectal. Autonomic nerves from the pelvic plexus supply the internal anal sphincter.

PATHOPHYSIOLOGY

Pelvic floor injury can result from damage to the nerve supply, muscles, or connective tissue, which together maintain pelvic floor function. There is good evidence that damage to the innervation of the pelvic floor is a causative factor in the development of urinary and fecal incontinence following vaginal delivery.[14,15] Partial denervation of the pelvic floor has been shown in 80% of women following a single vaginal delivery.[16] Fetal macrosomia and a prolonged second stage (either active or passive) are associated with an increased risk of neuropathic damage.[17]

The levator ani and endopelvic fascia act together to maintain urinary continence and pelvic organ support. If the muscle is damaged, the connective tissue has to play a greater compensatory role, and this frequently fails over time, most commonly after the menopause. The arcus tendineus fascia is found to be detached (most commonly from the ischial spines) in women with anterior vaginal wall prolapse,[11] and histologic studies have documented levator ani muscle fibrosis following vaginal delivery.[18] Such changes are also seen in women with stress urinary incontinence and pelvic organ prolapse.[19,20] Magnetic resonance imaging is providing increasing information about pelvic floor injury following childbirth.[21] Abnormalities of the levator ani muscle are seen in 20% of women after their first vaginal delivery.[22] Forceps delivery, prolonged second stage, and older maternal age at first delivery have been identified as associated risk factors for the development of levator ani injury.[23] Computer simulation of levator ani muscle stretch during fetal head descent demonstrates that the medial portion of the pubococcygeus muscle undergoes the greatest degree of strain during fetal head descent and that the tissue stretch ratio is proportional to fetal head size.[24] Further studies have shown that levator ani abnormalities are found more commonly in women with prolapse than in women with normal support, suggesting that injury to this muscle during vaginal delivery is a predisposing factor to the future development of prolapse.[25,26]

Similarly, the anal sphincters are vulnerable to injury during vaginal delivery, which have been generically called OASIS (obstetric anal sphincter injuries). Factors associated with OASIS and the future development of anal incontinence are discussed under "Third-Degree Anal Sphincter Injury."

UTEROVAGINAL PROLAPSE

Effects of Pregnancy, Childbirth, and Parity

Nulliparous pregnant women have been shown to exhibit altered pelvic floor support when compared with nulliparous nonpregnant women. In the nonpregnant group, 43% had stage 0 prolapse and 57% had stage 1, but in the pregnant group, 10% had stage 0, 43% had stage 1, and 48% had stage 2.[27] Interestingly, the greatest changes observed were in the length of the anterior wall and the perineal body, which may explain the common occurrence of urinary incontinence during pregnancy. The increase in perineal body length may represent an adaptation that reduces the occurrence of anal sphincter damage. Another study of nulliparous women delivered at term showed that at 36 weeks' gestation, 46% had prolapse, with 26% having a stage 2 prolapse[28]; at 6 weeks postpartum, there was a similar incidence of new prolapse in women delivered vaginally and by cesarean section. Thus, regardless of the mode of delivery, being pregnant of itself impairs pelvic floor support.

That the risk of prolapse increases with the number of vaginal deliveries is well documented. Mant and associates[5] have shown that a woman after two vaginal deliveries has an 8-fold increased risk of developing pelvic organ prolapse compared with the nulliparous woman and that this risk rises to 12-fold after four vaginal deliveries.

Risks

Uterine prolapse occurring for the first time during pregnancy is rare, occurring in 1 in 10,000 to 15,000 deliveries.[29] It can occur acutely following a fall or trauma in nulliparous women[30] but is more commonly seen in parous women with prolapse prior to pregnancy. Much of the literature relating to uterine prolapse in pregnancy consists of case reports prior to 1970[29–33] when the condition was seen more frequently owing to higher average parity.[34] Thus, current data on maternal and fetal risks are lacking. A large review up to 1940 reported a substantial fetal and maternal complication rate,[29] which included a 10% risk of miscarriage[30] and an increased risk of preterm birth.[31] Fetal and maternal death have also been reported.[31] Cervical elongation, hypertrophy, and edema are present in all cases in which the pregnancy progresses to term.[29] Urinary obstruction can occur and may require catheterization.[35] Abnormalities of labor are common. On the one hand, weakness of the pelvic floor can lead to precipitate delivery with resultant cervical lacerations. On the other hand, cervical infection and bleeding during pregnancy are common and can lead to scarring and fibrosis with resultant cervical dystocia. This typically manifests as secondary arrest in cervical dilation, usually between 5 and 7 cm.[32] At one time, it would have been managed by Duhrssen's cervical incisions with or without the use of forceps, but at present, cesarean section is preferred. Accordingly, although spontaneous vaginal delivery rates of 40% to 80% have been reported,[31,32] cesarean or instrumental deliveries are more common. Primary postpartum hemorrhage, due to uterine atony, may be difficult to control, because manual uterine compression is hindered by the prolapse.

Management Options

Prenatal

Uterine prolapse occurring prenatally requires admission to hospital if it is not possible to reduce the prolapse in the clinic. Treatment consists of bedrest in the Trendelenburg position combined with an indwelling urinary catheter and saline soaks to reduce cervical edema. Once edema has been reduced, the prolapse can usually be manually replaced and a pessary then inserted to prevent recurrence; a Hodge pessary is the one most commonly used. Antibiotic creams are often prescribed to reduce associated cervicitis. There is no evidence that systemic antibiotics are beneficial. In the past, vaginal packing and even surgical closure of the introitus have been described as effective.[34] The introitus is reopened at term to allow vaginal delivery. Pessary treatment is often required only until the fifth month of pregnancy, when the uterus lifts out of the pelvis, thereby alleviating prolapse symptoms.[36] Incarceration of a retroflexed gravid uterus in association with severe prolapse has been reported, requiring epidural anesthesia to dislodge the uterus from the pelvis.[35] Incarceration is more likely to occur in the presence of severe prolapse, which allows the uterus to enlarge without concomitant lifting out of the pelvis.

Labor and Delivery

Careful intrapartum monitoring of the rate of cervical dilation is essential for early detection of both precipitate delivery and cervical dystocia. In the event of the latter, (Duhrssen's) intracervical incisions can be considered, but today, cesarean section is usually more appropriate.

Postnatal

If the prolapse is untreated, it will almost certainly recur in future pregnancies. Surgery is the definitive cure, but a vaginal pessary is an appropriate immediate treatment during postnatal genital involution. Longer-term use of a pessary should be considered if more pregnancies are desired, because a surgical repair is likely to be undone by another vaginal delivery, and an elective cesarean to avoid recurrent prolapse carries its own risks.

SUMMARY OF MANAGEMENT OPTIONS

Uterovaginal Prolapse

Management Options	Evidence Quality and Recommendation	References
Prepregnancy		
Consider deferring formal repair until family is complete.	—/GPP	—
Prenatal		
Bedrest in Trendelenburg position.	—/GPP	—
Saline soaks.	—/GPP	—
Antibiotic cream.	—/GPP	—
Hodge pessary.	—/GPP	—

SUMMARY OF MANAGEMENT OPTIONS

Uterovaginal Prolapse—cont'd

Management Options	Evidence Quality and Recommendation	References
Labor and Delivery		
Critical review of cervical dilation and progress of labor.	—/GPP	—
Active management of third stage and vigilance for postpartum hemorrhage.	—/GPP	—
Postnatal		
Formal prolapse management.	—/GPP	—

GPP, good practice point.

PREVIOUS PELVIC FLOOR REPAIR/ VAGINAL SURGERY

Maternal Risks

Despite a general decline in family size, the combined effects of increasing rates of surgical intervention for pelvic organ prolapse and urinary incontinence and delayed childbearing mean that many women are becoming pregnant having previously undergone reconstructive surgery. The current use of suburethral tapes for the treatment of stress urinary incontinence and laparoscopic or vaginal mesh procedures with uterine preservation for the management of prolapse provide less invasive surgical treatments that are more likely to be offered at an earlier stage, because women are now less prepared to accept the burden of pelvic floor symptoms. As a consequence, the number of women becoming pregnant following pelvic floor surgery may well increase in the future. This poses a dilemma for the obstetrician. Both pregnancy and especially delivery can pose a threat to the continued efficacy of successful surgical repair. It is important to provide the woman with information on the likelihood of symptoms recurring during pregnancy, persisting following delivery, and necessitating further treatment. However, published evidence on which to base management is scanty. The urethra lengthens during pregnancy,[37] and the bladder becomes an abdominal organ. Stress incontinence occurs commonly in pregnancy[38] and is a risk factor for persistent urinary incontinence. Thus, pregnancy of itself poses a risk of prolapse recurring. However, the main obstetric concern following previous successful pelvic floor surgery is mode of delivery. Reported outcomes among women delivered abdominally or vaginally following previous surgery for pelvic organ prolapse and stress urinary incontinence provide conflicting results. In the largest series of 89 women who conceived following colporrhaphy (66 of whom had undergone cervical amputation), 34 miscarried or delivered prior to 32 weeks. Twenty-four had a cesarean section to preserve pelvic floor function. At 6 to 8 weeks postpartum, there was recurrence of symptoms in 7% of women, but at 1 year postpartum, 22% had symptoms severe enough to require further surgery.[39] Cesarean section failed to prevent recurrence, with 9 of the 25 (36%) delivered abdominally suffering recurrence at 5 years compared with 7 of the 49 (14%) delivered vaginally. Conversely, in another series of 78 women who had surgery for prolapse, 31 were followed up after subsequent pregnancy. Twenty-five had vaginal deliveries and 4 of them had recurrent prolapse,[40] 6 had cesarean section, and none had any recurrence of prolapse (although this difference is not statistically significant). Of 6 reported vaginal deliveries following uterosacral sacrospinous suspension for prolapse, 1 patient suffered a recurrence of symptoms requiring further surgery.[41]

The literature relating to women delivering after previous continence surgery is also conflicting. A study of five women who delivered vaginally following a previous Burch colposuspension reported that three suffered recurrent incontinence,[42] whereas all the women delivered by cesarean section had maintained continence at 1 year postcesarean (despite a majority having had incontinence in the third trimester). A review of pregnancy and delivery after midurethral sling procedures cited 24 cases in the literature of women becoming pregnant after sling procedures with 12 delivering vaginally and 11 by cesarean, with 1 ongoing pregnancy at publication.[43] This showed that of the 12 women delivered vaginally, 10 were continent at 2 to 36 months, with 9 of the 11 women after cesarean remaining continent. Information available to date on pregnancies following tension-free vaginal (TVT) and transobturator suburethral tape (TVT-O) insertions indicates that recurrence of stress incontinence is unusual and that vaginal delivery does not increase this risk.[44–46] The optimal mode of delivery following previous pelvic floor surgery is still unclear, and many other factors need to be considered in individual cases.

Fetal Risks

The Manchester repair (Fothergill) operation performed prior to pregnancy has been associated with greater miscarriage and preterm delivery rates, but this operation is now rarely performed.

Management Options

Prepregnancy

All women planning a pregnancy after previous pelvic floor surgery for urinary incontinence or prolapse should be advised of a possible functional deterioration during pregnancy that may persist, even if an elective cesarean section is performed.

Prenatal

Timely assessment of symptom recurrence and reassurance of probable resolution of symptoms following delivery are important. Intensive pelvic floor physiotherapy may be indicated, but there are inadequate data on its effectiveness in this situation for it to be recommended with confidence.

Labor and Delivery

If symptoms have been largely cured by a prolapse or incontinence repair procedure, current consensus would favor performing an elective cesarean section in order to minimize the risk of recurrent symptoms. There have, however, been many reports of women delivering vaginally with no recurrence of symptoms. If a vaginal delivery is planned, an episiotomy may be beneficial to reduce stretching of rigid or scarred tissues.[37]

Postnatal

Pelvic floor exercises should be continued. A decision regarding further surgical management should ideally be deferred until 6 months following delivery, because recovery of function continues to occur until then.[41] Any plans for further childbearing should be discussed; the woman should be made aware that any subsequent pregnancy risks producing a recurrence of symptoms requiring further surgery once childbearing is complete.

SUMMARY OF MANAGEMENT OPTIONS

Previous Pelvic Floor Repair or Vaginal Surgery

Management Options	Evidence Quality and Recommendation	References
Prepregnancy		
Advise that further pregnancy can result in functional deterioration even if cesarean section performed.	—/GPP	—
Prenatal		
Assess current status of pelvic floor function.	—/GPP	—
Advise that pregnancy and delivery may result in deterioration or recurrence of symptoms.	—/GPP	—
Refer for physiotherapy (uncertain benefit).	—/GPP	—
Labor and Delivery		
Consensus favors cesarean section.	—/GPP	—
Episiotomy may be beneficial if vaginal delivery is undertaken.	III/B	37
Postnatal		
Arrange postnatal review after 6 mo.	III/B	41

GPP, good practice point.

PERINEAL INJURY

Trauma to the perineum, of varying degree, constitutes the most common form of obstetric injury.[47,48] Its severity is generally classified according to the degree of perineal disruption:

- First-degree tear involves only perineal or vaginal skin.
- Second-degree tear occurs when perineal skin and muscles are torn.
- Third-degree tear occurs when, in addition to perineal skin and muscle, the anal sphincter muscle is torn.
- Fourth-degree tear occurs when sphincter muscle disruption is complete with additional extension into the anal mucosa; this implies that both external and internal anal sphincter muscles have been severed.

Further subdivision of third-degree tears are discussed under "Third-Degree Anal Sphincter Injury."

First- and Second-Degree Tears

General

First- and second-degree perineal tears are very common. The incidence of a completely intact perineum, without even minor tears, following delivery after a first vaginal birth is very low, approximately 6%.[48] The maternal position at delivery may be important; one study reported an overall 66% intact perineum rate associated with the lateral position at delivery, compared with 42% in the squatting position.[49] Because of the frequent need for suturing of tears and the limited availability of experienced surgeons, repair is often performed by relatively inexperienced personnel. All staff supervising even the most normal births should, therefore, receive early and thorough training in perineal repair.[47] The principles of management include immediate assessment to exclude deeper injury involving the anal sphincter, appropriate surgical repair, and effective postpartum analgesia and advice.

Maternal Risks

Second-degree tears can result in significant morbidity. Women who sustain them resume sexual intercourse later and report greater frequency of dyspareunia than women who have intact perineums or first-degree tears.[50] Use of teaching models for instruction of midwifery and medical staff in repair technique is effective in reducing such complications.[51]

Management Options

PRENATAL

Prenatal and intrapartum perineal massage have been advocated as interventions to reduce the incidence of second- and greater-degree tears, but the evidence in its favor is conflicting.[52] In one study of 1340 women, massage and stretching during the second stage of labor did not increase the rate of perineums intact after delivery.[53] However, a second study of 861 nulliparas randomized to antenatal perineal massage demonstrated a reduction in episiotomy, and second- and third-degree lacerations, with the greatest benefit among women older than 30 years.[54] Two recent prospective reports indicate that massage is neither protective nor detrimental to the risk of perineal and anal sphincter trauma.[55,56] Pelvic floor muscle exercises performed prenatally and postnatally have been shown to reduce self-reported incontinence in late pregnancy and up to 6 months postpartum.[57]

LABOR AND DELIVERY

The Peri-Rule is a very simple plastic measuring device that was developed by the Birmingham Perineal Research Evaluation Group as an aid in measuring second-degree tears. Three measurements can be made by the birth attendant: the depth of the tear from the fourchette to the perineal body, the length from the fourchette to the vaginal apex, and the length of the tear along the perineum. Use of this device encourages a standardized assessment of perineal tears, and good interobserver reliability for use of the Peri-Rule has been reported.[58]

Despite an absence of evidence on outcome, the practice of nonsuturing of perineal tears has been proposed.[59] Several studies have examined the method of perineal repair. Use of polyglactin suture material is associated with less perineal pain and lower resuture rates compared with chromic catgut.[60,61] It would appear that more rapidly absorbed polyglactin requires less frequent suture removal compared with standard polyglactin.[62] A two-stage continuous repair leaving the skin unsutured also seems to be associated with less pain. More recently, the Cochrane systematic review of continuous versus interrupted suturing of the perineum showed that the continuous suturing method was associated with less pain up to 10 days postpartum. There was also less need for suture removal in the continuous suturing group, but there was no difference in the need for resuturing or the incidence of long-term pain between both groups.[63] It is thought that during the immediate healing period, tension in the tissues is likely to be distributed more evenly in the continuously sutured wound, resulting in less pain.

The Role of Cesarean Section

There is no consensus about the role of elective cesarean section in the prevention of obstetric pelvic floor injury. However, some are so convinced of its benefit that they even advocate obtaining "informed consent" regarding the risks of perineal injury before women elect to have a vaginal birth.[64] Although traumatic mechanical injury to the anal sphincter occurs only with vaginal delivery, evidence exists to show that if performed late in labor, cesarean section may fail entirely to protect the anal sphincter mechanism, with one study showing neurologic injury in women delivered by cesarean section after 8 cm dilation.[65] Parous women delivered only by cesarean section still have a 3.5-fold increased relative risk of urinary incontinence compared with women who have never been pregnant, although the risk is higher still after vaginal delivery.[66,67] Long-term and severe stress urinary incontinence symptoms are less influenced by mode of delivery,[68,69] and indeed, urgency symptoms may be increased after cesarean birth.[70] These data, and comparison between twin sisters,[71] suggest that the pregnant state of itself (regardless of mode of delivery) can influence function and indicate that more research is required into the pathogenesis of obstetric pelvic floor injury before definitive advice on mode of delivery can be offered.

POSTNATAL

Analgesia is the main priority.

SUMMARY OF MANAGEMENT OPTIONS

First- and Second-Degree Tear

Management Options	Evidence Quality and Recommendation	References
Prenatal		
There is conflicting evidence on the value of perineal massage before and during labor.	Ib/A	52–56
Pelvic floor exercises before and after labor are associated with a lower incidence of self-reported incontinence up to 6 mo.	III/B	57
Labor and Delivery		
Polyglactin suture material is associated with a lower incidence of pain and lower resuture rates than chromic catgut.	Ib/A	60,61
Three-stage continuous suture is associated with less pain and less need for suture removal than with repair using interrupted sutures.	Ib/A	62,63
Postnatal		
Analgesia and pelvic floor exercises are recommended.	III/B	57

TABLE 71–1

Standardized Bowel Function Questionnaire: Fecal Continence Scoring System

FEATURE	NEVER	RARELY	SOMETIMES	USUALLY	ALWAYS
Incontinence for solid stool	0	1	2	3	4
Incontinence for liquid stool	0	1	2	3	4
Incontinence for flatus	0	1	2	3	4
Wears pad	0	1	2	3	4
Fecal urgency	0	1	2	3	4

Add one score from each row. A score of 0 implies complete continence. A score of 20 implies complete incontinence.

Third-Degree Anal Sphincter Injury

General

Altered fecal continence is common following primary repair of third- and fourth-degree perineal injury, that is, when anal sphincter muscle disruption is clinically recognized after vaginal delivery. Up to 50% of women experience some incontinence symptoms within the weeks and months after a third-degree tear.[72,73] These symptoms do not correlate with the mode of sphincter repair. Consequently, all women known to have sustained anal sphincter trauma should have their continence routinely assessed at the conclusion of the puerperium.

Postnatal continence assessment should include direct questioning using a standardized bowel function questionnaire (Table 71–1)[74] so that a reliable continence score can be allotted to facilitate monitoring of the progress of symptoms over time. Continence of flatus, liquid, and solid feces should be documented, together with inquiry concerning fecal urgency, a socially debilitating symptom defined as an inability to defer defecation for longer than 5 minutes; the complaint of urgency incontinence may reflect external anal sphincter dysfunction.

Digital examination of the anal canal may provide an approximation of the integrity of the sphincter and perineal body but is not otherwise diagnostically reliable. Conversely, palpable defects in the levator ani musculature have been shown to correlate with magnetic resonance images of the pelvic floor.[21] Nevertheless, anorectal physiologic testing is necessary to determine objectively the nature and prognosis of any residual anal sphincter damage and routinely consists of the following investigations:

- Anal manometry is performed to evaluate sphincter tone and contractile function.
- Endoanal ultrasound is used to examine the anatomic integrity of the sphincter.
- Neurophysiologic testing of the pelvic floor is done to identify pudendal neuropathy.

These tests should be applied not only to women who have sustained third- and fourth-degree tears but also to other puerperal patients complaining of fecal incontinence. Disturbance of resting tone on anal manometry is indicative of predominant internal anal sphincter dysfunction, whereas a reduction in squeeze incremental pressure on voluntary contraction is consistent with reduced external sphincter muscle power. Manometry is performed using a multichannel, water-perfused catheter in the left lateral position, and reductions in the pressure profile, although diagnostically reliable, do not differentiate traumatic muscular from neurologic injury. High-quality endoanal endosonography provides clear and reproducible images of both internal and external sphincters[75,76] but may overestimate the significance of muscular defects. Many women are found to have small defects that do not correlate with antecedent obstetric events or fecal incontinence symptoms,[77] whereas internal anal sphincter disruption more commonly predisposes to persistent disturbances of continence.[78]

TABLE 71–2

Obstetric Risk Factors for Anal Sphincter Injury

First vaginal delivery
Instrumental delivery (forceps > vacuum)
Prolonged second stage of labor (>1 hr)
Epidural anesthesia
Persistent occipitoposterior position
Macrosomia (birth weight > 4 kg)
Shoulder dystocia
Previous third-degree perineal tear
Midline episiotomy

Pudendal nerve assessment should include testing both conduction along the entire length of the nerve, for example, using clitoral-anal reflex assessment, and anal sphincter electromyography (EMG), which assesses motor unit recruitment and action potential morphology. Neuropathy is responsible for at least one third of fecal continence disturbances, and its assessment provides essential information on prognosis and appropriate management.[79]

Risk Factors for Anal Sphincter Injury (Table 71–2)

VAGINAL DELIVERY

Normal vaginal delivery inevitably increases the risk of damage to the sphincter mechanism, compared with prelabor cesarean section. Nonetheless, intrapartum cesarean section can be followed by continence disturbance, consistent with first-stage influences on anal sphincter function.[65] Prelabor cesarean section should, therefore, be chosen when any risk to the pelvic floor is to be avoided.

PRIMIPARITY

Because first labors are most often associated with inefficient uterine contractility, dystocia, prolonged labor, use of epidural anesthesia, and episiotomy, puerperal fecal incontinence most often follows first vaginal delivery. Risk is increased between two- and fivefold,[80] which reflects the reduced elasticity of the pelvic floor among nulliparas.

INSTRUMENTAL DELIVERY

Both forceps and vacuum extraction significantly increase the risk to the fecal continence mechanism two- to sevenfold.[16,80] Although vacuum extraction is somewhat less commonly traumatic, completion of the delivery with forceps when a vacuum attempt fails, generally due to poor adhesion of the vacuum cup, compounds the incontinence risk.[81]

PROLONGED SECOND STAGE OF LABOR AND EPIDURAL ANALGESIA

Effective epidural analgesia, now a very widely applied form of intrapartum pain relief, abolishes the maternal bearing down reflex in late labor. As a consequence, the passive phase of the second stage of labor is prolonged, sometimes for several hours, before maternal pushing is encouraged. Such a prolonged passive second stage doubles the risk of subsequent incontinence, apparently secondary to pudendal neuropathy. Randomized evidence does not support an expectant policy in the second stage under epidural blockade, because the instrumental delivery rate is not reduced and the duration of labor is needlessly prolonged.[82]

INTRAPARTUM MECHANICAL FACTORS

Third-degree tears occur three times more frequently when the fetus is macrosomic (birth weight > 4 kg) compared with lower birth weights. Shoulder dystocia also predisposes to anal sphincter injury, as does persistent occipitoposterior position of the fetal head in the second stage of labor.[23]

MIDLINE EPISIOTOMY

Episiotomy is performed with the objective of preventing deep perineal lacerations and anal sphincter trauma and is one of the most frequent surgical interventions. The perineal incision can be made either mediolaterally or in the midline posteriorly. Although there is a widespread assumption that it can do more harm than good,[83–87] population data suggest that selective mediolateral episiotomy may be protective of the sphincter mechanism.[88] The angle of mediolateral incision has been shown to have an important bearing on the risk of sphincter injury, with episiotomies made close to 45 degrees least often associated with third-degree tears,[89] so that instruction in optimal mediolateral technique should be emphasized.[90] Conversely, there is little doubt that midline episiotomy, which is particularly favored in North America, greatly increases the risk of third-degree tear[91] to the extent that its use should probably be abandoned. This risk is compounded when midline episiotomy is combined with other interventions, such as epidural analgesia and instrumental delivery.

PREVIOUS ANAL SPHINCTER DISRUPTION

The incidence of third-degree tears of varying severity is about 2.5% of primiparous and 0.5% of multiparous vaginal deliveries, with an overall average rate of about 1.5%.[76] Following satisfactory postnatal repair, at subsequent vaginal delivery, the risk of a further tear increases fourfold to about 4%[92] if mediolateral episiotomy is practiced and to over 10% with midline episiotomy.[93]

Management Options

Bearing in mind the inherent anatomic vulnerability of the anal sphincter during childbirth, some risk of trauma exists even when obstetric management is optimal. Avoidance of postpartum fecal incontinence rests partly with measures to avoid occurrence of third-degree tears but, even more significantly, in the appropriate management of anal sphincter injury when it occurs at delivery.

PRIMARY PREVENTION

Primary preventive measures include augmentation of myometrial contractions during first labors, using intravenous oxytocin to correct dystocia; in this way, the incidences of instrumental delivery, occipitoposterior position, and prolonged first and second stages of labor can be minimized (for a somewhat different view, see Chapter 69). Vacuum extraction should be the first choice for low-cavity instrumental delivery, although the potentially traumatic sequence of failed vacuum followed by forceps delivery should not be ignored. Abbreviation of the passive, nonpushing second stage of labor is advisable, even in the presence of effective epidural anesthesia (again, for a somewhat different view, see Chapter 72). When episiotomy is performed, midline procedures should be eschewed in favor of mediolateral incisions approximating as closely as possible to 45 degrees.

OPTIMIZING PERINEAL REPAIR

A standard classification of the severity of anal sphincter injury has been recommended in a recent Royal College of Obstetricians and Gynaecologists (RCOG) publication[94] (Table 71–3), principally on the grounds that the degree of perineal injury correlates approximately with long-term symptomatic outcome. It is inevitable that the functional outcome following repair of extensive tears involving the internal anal sphincter and anal mucosa (fourth-degree tears) will be intrinsically more predisposed to continence sequelae than when only partial-thickness external sphincter trauma has occurred. Nevertheless, well-trained obstetric surgeons using appropriate operative techniques will produce the best functional outcomes, regardless of the extent of injury.

TABLE 71–3
Classification of Perineal Injury

First degree	Injury to perineal skin only
Second degree	Injury to perineum involving perineal muscles but not involving the anal sphincter
Third degree	Injury to perineum involving the anal sphincter complex: 3a: <50% of EAS thickness torn 3b: >50% of EAS thickness torn 3c: Both EAS and IAS torn
Fourth degree	Injury to perineum involving the anal sphincter complex (EAS and IAS) and anal epithelium

EAS, external anal sphincter; IAS, internal anal sphincter.
From Royal College of Obstetricians and Gynaecologists (RCOG): The Management of Third- and Fourth-Degree Perineal Tears (RCOG Guidelines No 29). 2007. Available at http://www.rcog.org.uk/womens-health/clinical-guidance/management-third-and-fourth-degree-perineal-tears-green-top-29 (accessed August 21, 2009).

MANAGEMENT OF OBSTETRIC SPHINCTER DISRUPTION

Timing of Repair Procedure

It is standard obstetric practice to repair anal sphincter tears immediately or within a few hours of vaginal delivery—the so-called primary repair. Early repair abbreviates the patient's inconvenience and discomfort but should not preclude performance of the repair procedure by an appropriately trained obstetric surgeon. If a skilled operator is not immediately available, then delayed primary repair within 24 hours has much to recommend it, provided that hemostasis and analgesia have been achieved. Delayed repair will, however, almost inevitably enhance the patient's anxiety and sense of grievance concerning her injury, with a potential incremental effect on resort to complaint and litigation.

Surgical Technique

Anal sphincter repair should be conducted with full surgical precautions, instrumentation, and lighting in an operating room setting. Slowly absorbed synthetic monofilament suture materials such as polyglyconate (Maxon) or polydioxone (PDS) should be used. When the external sphincter is completely torn (3b) it can be repaired end-to-end or with an overlapping technique. Several randomized, controlled trials (RCTs) have compared end-to-end and overlap repairs. Fitzpatrick and coworkers[72] found no difference between the two groups, although there was a trend toward more symptoms in the end-to end group. Garcia and colleagues[95] looked only at 3b, 3c, and fourth-degree tears in a small study and showed no difference. More recently, Fernando and associates[96] studied 64 women with 3b or greater tears in an RCT and found a higher incidence of fecal incontinence (24% vs. 0%) and urgency (32% vs. 3.7%) in the end-to end group at 12 months. From these studies, end-to-end repair should be carried out on 3a tears and overlapping repair may be considered for 3b, 3c, and fourth-degree tears, if access to the disrupted anal sphincter stumps permits. Distortion of the normal anal anatomic relationships following deep perineal lacerations means that endoanal ultrasound does not appear to offer useful intraoperative assistance in improving surgical muscle realignment. Ultrasound may have a potential role, however, in the early postnatal screening of women with ostensibly intact anal sphincters so as to facilitate selective monitoring of fecal continence among those who sustain occult forms of anal sphincter injury.

Postnatal Management

Although firm evidence is scanty, it appears likely that prophylactic broad-spectrum antibiotic therapy (e.g., co-amoxyclavulanic acid) enhances the integrity of primary anal sphincter repair during the first 3 to 5 postnatal days. Conversely, firm randomized, controlled data exist to support the use of a laxative rather than a constipating postoperative regimen during the early puerperium.[97] Use of lactulose or ispaghula to soften the stool is associated with a shorter and less painful recovery period when compared with codeine phosphate treatment as employed by coloproctologists following elective anal surgery.

Routine Postnatal Review of Fecal Continence

Because up to 50% of women who sustain a third- or fourth-degree tear experience some puerperal symptoms of fecal incontinence, routine follow-up assessment of anal sphincter function is advisable once postnatal healing is complete. Such a review is probably best performed at 8 to 12 weeks following delivery and should consist, as delineated previously, of an assessment of fecal continence symptoms, anal manometry, and endoanal ultrasound combined with pudendal nerve evaluation, if indicated. The examination should optimally take place in an obstetric setting because it provides the patient with an opportunity to discuss not only her current continence status but also the antecedent circumstances surrounding her anal injury. The results of the anal physiology investigations facilitate the planning of further treatment and provide invaluable insights into prognosis.

Symptomatic Therapy

Minor postnatal fecal incontinence symptoms such as intermittent fecal urgency or constipation are frequently transient in nature and can often be effectively managed using loperamide or ispaghula, respectively. Perineal pain, secondary to discomfort in the sutured tissues, is amenable to targeted local injection of a combination of 2% bupivicaine, hyaluronidase, and methylprednisolone acetate. More significant tenderness and dyspareunia associated with perineal anatomic distortion can be corrected by minor surgical intervention under local or general anesthesia. Associated psychosexual dysfunction responds to early psychotherapeutic counseling initiated before secondary deterioration in sexual interaction has developed.

Postnatal Physiotherapy

Even without active treatment, fecal incontinence symptoms of minor degree are frequently transient and disappear or attenuate within a few months of delivery. Kegel pelvic floor exercises are not effective in alleviating incontinence, but the addition of operant conditioning through biofeedback physiotherapy using an endoanal stimulating probe[98] significantly improves anal sphincter function. Biofeedback therapy is particularly effective in maintaining muscle bulk while healing occurs and neuropathy recovers.

Secondary Anal Sphincter Repair

Persistent symptoms of fecal incontinence lasting for more than 6 months following delivery usually necessitate surgical repair of the damaged anal sphincter muscle. Before considering surgery, it is mandatory to exclude a coexistent neuropathic cause for the symptoms and to confirm pudendal nerve integrity. If severe neuropathy is identified, colostomy diversion or an artificial sphincter procedure may be necessary.

Counseling during Subsequent Pregnancies

The recurrence rate of third-degree tears was 4.4% in a study of 20,111 consecutive deliveries when mediolateral episiotomy was used.[92] Therefore, 95% of women with a previous third-degree tear did not have another third-degree tear. Women who already suffer persistent and debilitating fecal incontinence after childbirth are likely to experience deterioration in their symptoms after further vaginal deliveries.[99] Transient symptoms that do not persist but are associated with abnormally low resting and squeeze manometric pressures and a large residual anal sphincter defect may recur following further vaginal deliveries. Conversely, the continence of asymptomatic women with relatively normal manometric profiles is not likely to deteriorate, even in the presence of documented anal sphincter scarring on endoanal ultrasound examination. Ultrasound tends to overdiagnose functional deficits in continence[77] but should, nonetheless, be performed, together with anal manometry, when planning the mode of next delivery in women with a history of third- or fourth-degree anal sphincter injury. The risk of anal and fecal incontinence occurring after another delivery seems higher in women who have sustained a fourth-egree tear.[100]

Summary

As a generalization, in the absence of clear evidence of the optimal approach in such women, it is probably best to individualize the management. An empirical approach is suggested in Table 71–4.

In women who have achieved normal continence following primary obstetric anal sphincter injury and repair, further vaginal delivery is a reasonable option. However, elective prelabor cesarean section is advisable to protect the continence mechanism following successful secondary repair of the anal sphincter. The use of prophylactic cesarean delivery in women with asymptomatic ultrasonically identified sphincter defects is not justified by the published evidence.

TABLE 71–4

Proposed Management of Multiparas in Pregnancies after Anal Sphincter Injury

TYPE OF INJURY	INVESTIGATION PROFILE	MANAGEMENT
1. Previous third-degree tear–asymptomatic	Normal manometry and ultrasound	Allow vaginal delivery
2. Previous third-degree tear–symptomatic incontinence	Abnormal manometry and/or ultrasound	Prelabor cesarean section
3. Successful secondary sphincter repair	Normal manometry and ultrasound	Prelabor cesarean section
4. Previous third-degree tear or "occult" injury–asymptomatic	Abnormal manometry and ultrasound	Discuss vaginal or cesarean delivery

SUMMARY OF MANAGEMENT OPTIONS

Third-Degree Tear

Management Options	Evidence Quality and Recommendation	References
Prevention		
Oxytocin augmentation of first labor.	—/GPP	—
Appropriate episiotomy technique (avoid midline).	—/GPP	—
Vacuum extraction as first choice for assisted vaginal delivery.	—/GPP	—
Short passive phase of second stage of labor (see Chapters 69 and 72 for contrasting views on these options).	—/GPP	—
Optimal Perineal Repair Technique		
Formal training of obstetric trainees.	—/GPP	—
End-to-end repair of 3a, overlap repair of 3b, 3c, and fourth-degree tears.	Ib/A	72,73
Appropriate suture material (e.g., polyglyconate or polydioxone).	—/GPP	—
Focused Postnatal Management		
Laxative regimen postnatally.	Ib/A	97
Prophylactic antibiotic therapy.	—/GPP	—
Analgesia and other symptomatic therapy.	—/GPP	—
Biofeedback physiotherapy.	Ib/A	98
Appropriate assessment of fecal continence following sphincter injury.	—/GPP	—
Selected secondary overlap sphincter repair for persistent incontinence.	—/GPP	—
Subsequent Pregnancies		
Those at risk:	—/GPP	—
• Persistent fecal incontinence symptoms.		
• Previous third-degree tear.		
• Poor antenatal manometry profile.		
• Individualize management (see Table 71–4).	—/GPP	—

GPP, good practice point.

FEMALE CIRCUMCISION (FEMALE GENITAL MUTILATION)

The World Health Organization (WHO) defines female genital mutilation (FGM) as including all procedures involving partial or total removal of the external female genitalia or other injury to the female genital organs for cultural, religious, or nontherapeutic reasons.[101] This practice occurs predominantly in Africa, although affected women and girls may present anywhere in the world as immigrants from these countries. Consequently, FGM is now a global concern with human rights organizations devoted to the elimination of this practice and many countries prohibiting it by law. Medical professionals caring for affected women require knowledge and understanding of FGM.[102] Countries in which there is a high prevalence of FGM include Egypt, Sudan, Eritrea, Ethiopia, Djibouti, Somalia, Mali, Senegal, Guinea, and Sierra Leone, and WHO estimates that currently 100 million to 140 million women live with the consequences of this procedure, with a further 2 million girls at risk each year. In 2008, an interagency statement on eliminating female genital mutilation was published.[103] This statement signed by a wider group of United Nations agencies was issued to address concerns about the continuing prevalence of FGM and with the aim of eliminating the practice in one generation. It clearly states that FGM is a violation of human rights and advocates the education and empowerment of women to ensure the elimination of this practice.

There are several forms of FGM that carry differing health implications:

- Type I: partial or total removal of the clitoris and/or prepuce (clitoridectomy).
- Type II: partial or total removal of the clitoris and the labia minora with or without excision of the labia majora (excision).
- Type III: narrowing the vaginal orifice with creation of a covering seal by cutting and appositioning the labia minora and/or the labia majora with or without excision of the clitoris (infibulation).
- Type IV: all other harmful procedures to the female genitalia without any medical purpose, for example, pricking, piercing, incising or scraping, and cauterization.
- The greatest health risks are in women who have undergone infibulation, which accounts for about 15% of cases. FGM is usually performed on women between 5 and 8 years of age and has physical, psychological, and sexual consequences.

General Risks

Immediate risks of the FGM procedure itself when performed by a traditional practitioner using crude instruments and no anesthesia include shock, hemorrhage, sepsis, and death. There are few reliable figures of FGM-related mortality rate. Ulceration of the genitalia and acute urinary retention can also follow, as can transmission of HIV and hepatitis.

Delayed complications include urinary and vaginal infections, large epidermal cysts, abscesses, keloid scarring, obstructed menstruation, urinary incontinence, and coital and psychosexual problems, which may lead to infertility.[104]

Maternal Risks

The incidence of pregnancy complications or maternal deaths related to FGM is unknown. The risks depend on the type of FGM performed; infibulation, in particular, can cause tender introital scarring that precludes adequate prenatal examination, investigation, and treatment. Vaginitis is common, as are urinary tract infections. Miscarriage may be complicated by retention of products in the vagina, leading to sepsis. When labor occurs, assessment of cervical dilation may be difficult or impossible. Urinary retention in labor is common. Dystocia, usually due to soft tissue obstruction in the second stage, can have serious consequences for the mother and fetus if undetected or improperly managed. Vaginal delivery is associated with increased risks of perineal damage and hemorrhage.[105] The increased incidence of postpartum hemorrhage is mainly due to the need for anterior episiotomy or lacerations extending to the urethra, bladder, or rectum. Postpartum pain is also more severe owing to a greater degree of perineal injury. Postnatal wound infections, dehiscence, and fistulas can occur.

Fetal Risks

Stillbirth and neonatal death have been reported with higher frequency in circumcised women, secondary to fetal asphyxia due to prolonged obstructed labor.[106] This sequence is generally confined to women with severe types of FGM.

Management

Prenatal

Sensitive prenatal care is essential. Women may not volunteer that they are affected by FGM, necessitating an increased awareness when treating women originating from countries in which FGM is practiced. Early recognition provides sufficient time for assessment, discussion, and the development of a management plan. The extent of damage, scar tissue, and physical obstruction to vaginal delivery should be clearly documented so that unnecessary repeated examinations can be avoided. Women with a tight introitus, 1 cm or less, have the greatest risk of perineal damage. However, if the urinary meatus can be observed or two fingers can be inserted on digital examination, significant delivery problems are unlikely to ensue. Parous women who have been sutured at a previous delivery are at risk of developing significant scar tissue with subsequent infection and wound problems. Antenatal assessment also provides an opportunity to establish whether the woman would wish introital dilation to allow comfortable intercourse or to undergo a complete reversal of the procedure. Ideally, complete reversal should be avoided during pregnancy or immediately postpartum owing to the greater likelihood of hemorrhage at that time. Optimally, an anterior episiotomy sufficient only to expose the urethra should be performed during the late second stage, but occasionally, this procedure must be performed earlier to allow adequate investigation or treatment during pregnancy, for example, in the case of pain and bleeding in early pregnancy. Antenatally, the health care provider can also educate affected women so as to eliminate the practice of FGM in her offspring.

Labor and Delivery

The diagnosis of labor may be difficult in the presence of a small introitus. In this case, defibulation may need to be performed to allow adequate assessment. In skilled hands, intrapartum defibulation is a safe and effective procedure.[104] This procedure can be done under local anesthesia. If the opening is large enough to permit digital examination, the decision on defibulation can be deferred to the second stage. Extra care is essential in the second stage because the delivery of the fetal head may be obstructed by scar tissue. This can result in fetal asphyxia or severe tearing in the mother, leading to hemorrhage and fistula development. If introital obstruction develops, a timely anterior episiotomy should be performed to the urethra but not beyond because of the risk of hemorrhage.

Following delivery of the placenta, a careful examination of the genital tract is necessary. In particular, the presence of high vaginal lacerations and damage to the anal sphincter, rectum, or bladder should be noted. The sides of the midline anterior incision should be oversewn to secure hemostasis, leaving the urethra exposed. Reinfibulation should not be performed, irrespective of the wishes of the woman, because this will result in further scarring and problems; ideally, this issue will have been discussed prenatally.

Postnatal

Good postnatal analgesia is important because anterior divisions are associated with more pain. Affected women may need education in relation to differences in urination, menstruation, and coital function. A specific postnatal visit should be arranged to assess healing and to discuss sexual activity.

PROCEDURE

DEFIBULATION

1. Locate opening and paint with antiseptic solution.
2. Administer local anesthetic to the introitus if epidural anesthesia is not present.
3. Raise scar tissue from underlying area and incise in midline to expose urethral meatus. Do not incise beyond this.
4. Suture raw edges for hemostasis.

SUMMARY OF MANAGEMENT OPTIONS
Female Genital Mutilation or Circumcision

Management Options	Evidence Quality and Recommendation	References
Prenatal		
Identify women at risk.	—/GPP	—
Sensitive approach: Educate couple and obtain consent for examination and treatment.	—/GPP	—
Establish type of female genital mutilation and determine whether defibulation is required.	III/B	101,102
Discuss timing of defibulation and postnatal result.	III/B	102
Labor and Delivery		
Observe for obstructed second stage.	—/GPP	—
Perform timely defibulation or episiotomy if required.	—/GPP	—
Inspect genital tract after delivery of placenta for extension of lacerations.	—/GPP	—
Repair perineal damage and provide hemostasis.	—/GPP	—
Postnatal		
Provide analgesia and follow-up and education.	—/GPP	—

GPP, good practice point.

SUGGESTED READINGS

Beckmann MM, Garrett AJ: Antenatal perineal massage for reducing perineal trauma. Cochrane Database Syst.Rev 2006;1:CD005123.

Fernando RJ, Sultan AH, Kettle C, et al: Repair techniques for obstetric anal sphincter injuries: A randomized controlled trial. Obstet Gynecol 2006;107:126–128.

Fitzpatrick M, Behan M, O'Connell PR, O'Herlihy C: A randomized clinical trial comparing primary overlap with approximation repair of third-degree obstetric tears. Am J Obstet Gynecol 2000;183:1220–1224.

Fritel X, Ringa V, Varnoux N, et al: Mode of delivery and severe stress incontinence: A cross-sectional study among 2,625 perimenopausal women. BJOG 2005;112:1646–1651.

Goldberg RP, Abramov Y, Botros S, et al: Delivery mode is a major environmental determinant of stress urinary incontinence: Results of the Evanston-Northwestern Twin Sisters Study. Am J Obstet Gynecol 2005;193:2149–2153.

Groenen R, Vos CM, Willekes C, Vervest HAM: Pregnancy and delivery after midurethral sling procedures for stress urinary incontinence: Case reports and a review of literature. Int Urogynecol J 2008;19:441–448.

Kettle C, Hill R, Ismail K: Continuous versus interrupted sutures for repair of episiotomy or second degree tear. Cochrane Database Syst Rev 2007;4:CD000947.

Macrodt C, Gordon B, Fern E, et al: The Ipswich childbirth study: 2. A randomised comparison of polyglactin 910 with chromic catgut for postpartum perineal repair. Br J Obstet Gynaecol 1998;105:441–445.

Mahony R, Behan M, Daly L, et al: Internal anal sphincter defect influences continence outcome following obstetric anal sphincter injury. Am J Obstet Gynecol 2007;196:217.e1–217.e5.

Royal College of Obstetricians and Gynaecologists (RCOG): The Management of Third- and Fourth-Degree Perineal Tears (RCOG Guidelines No 29). 2007. Available at http://www.rcog.org.uk/womens-health/clinical-guidance/management-third-and-fourth-degree-perineal-tears-green-top-29 (accessed August 21, 2009).

REFERENCES

For a complete list of references, log onto www.expertconsult.com.

CHAPTER 72

Assisted Vaginal Delivery*

STEPHEN W. LINDOW and ROBERT HAYASHI

Videos corresponding to this chapter are available online at www.expertconsult.com.

INTRODUCTION

Assisted vaginal delivery (AVD) offers the option of an operative procedure to safely and quickly remove the infant, mother, and obstetrician from a difficult or even hazardous situation. When spontaneous vaginal delivery does not occur within a reasonable time, a successful AVD or operative vaginal delivery trial avoids cesarean section with its attendant uterine scar and implications for a future pregnancy and avoids potential birth asphyxia from prolonged fetal and cord compression. Reviews of delivery statistics show considerable variation in the incidence of AVD, but the range is usually between 10% and 20% of all deliveries.[1] Whether the method employed is the ventouse (vacuum extractor) or obstetric forceps, the operator can expect optimal results only when careful attention is given to the indications, prerequisites, and performance of the procedure.

INDICATIONS

Maternal indications are most commonly those of maternal distress, maternal exhaustion, or undue prolongation of the second stage of labor. Prolongation of the second stage of labor is a relative indication. Many have argued that specific time limits are not needed if monitoring of the fetus shows no evidence of distress and progress is not obviously arrested. However, in cases without regional anesthesia and with reassuring fetal monitoring parameters (e.g., a normal fetal heart rate pattern), it is probably appropriate to consider intervention if the second stage in a nullipara lasts longer than 2 hours (1 hr in a multipara). A further hour is often allowed in the presence of regional anesthesia, provided the mother wishes it and the fetal condition is satisfactory. The increased need for intervention following epidural anesthesia has been well documented.[2,3] This approach conforms to the ACOG (American College of Obstetricians and Gynecologists) guidelines.[4] Less common but more medically significant indications for AVD include cardiopulmonary or vascular conditions in which the stresses of the second stage should be minimized. With vaginal birth after previous cesarean section, decreasing the stress on the uterine scar may be a relative indication, although dehiscence or rupture is rare if the ACOG guidelines are followed. It has been suggested that if use of the ventouse has failed to deliver the infant but the fetal head has been brought down sufficiently, a cautious low or outlet forceps procedure is safe.[5] However, a review of a large series of AVDs in California suggest that there is an increased risk for intracranial injury when two different sequential instrumental deliveries are attempted.[6] Significant bleeding per vaginam is also an indication for a cautious approach to an AVD; whether the source of the bleeding may be maternal or fetal (e.g., placental abruption or vasa previa).

Fetal indications commonly encountered are malpositions of the fetal head, with relative dystocia. The occiput posterior (OP) and occiput transverse (OT) positions occur more frequently with regional anesthesia.[3,7] This may result from disturbance of the tone of the musculature of the pelvic floor impeding spontaneous rotation to the optimal occiput anterior (OA) position. Similarly, the maternal expulsive (bearing down) force may be compromised. Intervention with forceps for protection of the premature infant remains controversial. In the infant weighing below 1500 g, forceps delivery offers no advantage[8] and may in fact be deleterious,[9] owing to an increased incidence of intracranial bleeding. Use of the ventouse carries the same risk; vacuum extraction is probably best avoided at less than 34 weeks. Spontaneous delivery (with a generous episiotomy if delivery is delayed at the perineum or the outlet appears tight) and manual control of the head appear preferable, with abdominal delivery if operative intervention is needed.[9] In the low–birth weight infant (1500–2500 g), AVD is more widely accepted but should be managed with caution and minimal force.[10,11]

Fetal distress is a commonly cited indication. This expression is subject to varied interpretation, which may range from a brief bradycardia to prolonged late decelerations with acidosis. "Presumed fetal jeopardy" may be a preferable term, in conjunction with recording of as precise a description of the situation as possible in order to validate the indication.[4]

Vaginal delivery of the breech is considered by some to be an indication for forceps to the aftercoming head.[12,13] When the management decision is made to deliver vaginally

*This chapter is based extensively on the chapter in the second edition, by Philip Dennen and Robert Hayashi. Because Philip Dennen has now retired, the responsibility for the current chapter, and especially the updates, rests with Stephen Lindow and Robert Hayashi. However, the prior contribution of Philip Dennen is gratefully acknowledged.

(see Chapter 63), forceps to the aftercoming head may be considered routinely. The procedure becomes mandatory if the body has delivered and the Mauriceau-Smellie-Veit maneuver has failed. A putative advantage is the avoidance of traction force on the trunk and cervical spine, together with automatic control of the flexion of the fetal head. This may decrease the risk of hyperextension[14] and cervical plexus injuries.[15]

CONTRAINDICATIONS

Lack of engagement (leading bony point at or above the level of the ischial spines) suggests pelvic inlet dystocia and is usually considered an absolute contraindication to AVD. Conditions in which vaginal delivery per se is contraindicated include known pelvic abnormality with fetopelvic disproportion and fetal anomalies if obstructive or subject to damage from vaginal delivery. Certain fetal malpositions, such as a brow presentation or a face presentation in other than chin anterior position, are not suitable cases, nor is the dead fetus with postmortem changes. Inability to diagnose the position of the fetal head accurately or to apply the instrument properly are major contraindications.[1,16,17]

Several factors are relative contraindications. Fetal macrosomia may be such a factor. In general, the higher the head, the greater the difficulty and the need for performance skill. An increased risk of shoulder dystocia with midcavity procedures with macrosomia and an arrest has been reported.[18] The proficiency and experience of the operator are also factors to be considered. Finally, caution should be used with a ventouse procedure on a fetus who has had fetal scalp blood samplings performed because of the possibility of enhanced fetal scalp bleeding.[12]

DEFINITIONS

Significant comparative statistics have always been difficult to collect owing to differences in the classification, initially of forceps, but now of all AVDs. ACOG has proposed a more specific classification,[4,19] which has proved to be of clinical value[20,21] and deserves universal adoption. This classification is given in Table 72–1. It applies equally to vacuum extractor and forceps procedures.[4] To the classification of low forceps, a significant clinical addition would be the observation that on examination, the head must fill the hollow of the sacrum.[22] Station of the head is measured in plus or minus centimeters of distance between the leading bony point of the skull and the ischial spines.

Neonatal results comparable with those of spontaneous delivery can be expected, with procedures categorized as outlet or low with rotation less than 45 degrees.[1,23–27] Midpelvic and rotational procedures are generally associated with a higher rate of morbidity than spontaneous delivery.[28] However, when compared more properly with appropriate alternatives of management, namely, manual rotation followed by forceps or ventouse extraction or delivery by cesarean section, results are equivalent.[24,28–32] It is clear that abdominal delivery is associated with a much higher rate of maternal febrile morbidity. The controversy continues; appropriate selection and proficiency in execution of the maneuver remain the unmeasurable variables that often determine the results of trials.

TABLE 72–1
Classification of Forceps Deliveries According to Station and Rotation

TYPE OF PROCEDURE	CLASSIFICATION
Outlet forceps	Scalp is visible at the introitus without separating labia.
	Fetal skull has reached pelvic floor.
	Sagittal suture is in anteroposterior diameter or right or left occiput anterior or posterior position.
	Fetal head is at or on perineum.
	Rotation does not exceed 45 degrees.
Low forceps	Leading point of fetal skull is at station $\geq +2$ cm, and not on pelvic floor.
	Rotation ≤ 45 degrees (left or right occiput anterior to occiput anterior, or left or right occiput posterior to occiput posterior).
Midforceps	Rotation > 45 degrees.
	Station above +2 cm but head engaged.
High forceps	Not included in classification.

From American College of Obstetricians and Gynecologists (ACOG): Operative vaginal delivery (Technical Bulletin No. 196). Washington, DC, ACOG, 1994.

"Failed forceps" and "failed ventouse" are terms that have a pejorative implication. They can carry the stigma of poor judgment, poor obstetrics, and perhaps negligence in that disproportion was unrecognized. Alternatively, a "trial" (psychologically a better term) of forceps or ventouse connotes a cautious attempt at vaginal delivery with the option of altering management if unusual difficulty is met.[14] A trial of forceps or ventouse is appropriately carried out in an operating theater with immediate recourse to cesarean section if vaginal delivery is not achieved. The procedure deserves greater utilization.[33] A gentle negative trial should not alter outcome.[34,35]

PREREQUISITES

In management of an AVD, certain prerequisites must be met.[4] The head must be engaged (as defined by the biparietal diameter having passed through the plane of the inlet of the pelvis [Fig. 72–1]). Generally, this will have occurred when the leading bony point has reached the ischial spines. It must be remembered that certain conditions may lead to a higher than anticipated level of the biparietal diameter.[22] This is true with molding, particularly with macrosomia. Asynclitism and OP positions are associated with a higher level of the biparietal diameter, as is any extension of the fetal vertex away from a well-flexed position. These factors must always be considered when estimating engagement of the head if the assessment is to be accurate.

The position and attitude of the head must also be known if an accurate and effective application of the chosen instrument is to be made. Should the operator be unable to diagnose the position of the fetal head from the fontanels and suture lines, feeling for the location of an ear can be helpful. This can, however, produce a loss of station and backward rotation of the head due to the necessary displacement of the vertex, which may then mitigate against delivery. The

FIGURE 72–1
The obstetric planes of the pelvis and forceps classification: 1, Plane of inlet. 2, Plane of greatest pelvic dimension. 3, Plane of least pelvic dimension. 4, Plane of outlet.
(From Dennen PC [ed]: Forceps Deliveries, 3rd ed. Philadelphia, FA Davis, 1988.)

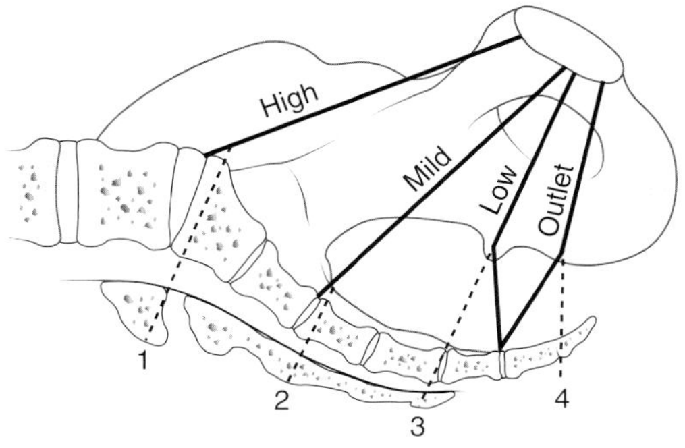

use of ultrasound (with the transducer placed just above the symphysis pubis) may also help determine fetal head position.

The maternal pelvis should be evaluated for the adequacy of the fetopelvic relationship. Factors such as maternal overweight or diabetes with related fetal macrosomia should be considered. An obvious disproportion contraindicating vaginal delivery must not be present. Clinical evaluation rather than radiographic pelvimetry should be adequate for estimation of the midpelvis and the pelvic outlet.

The bladder should be empty for procedures at other than outlet level. Membranes must be ruptured and the cervix must be fully dilated and retracted, or marked obstruction to rotation and descent of the head will result. There is no place in modern obstetrics for manual or mechanical dilation of the cervix or for cervical incisions to facilitate an operative procedure.[14] The rare exception may be the trapped head in a breech delivery.[36] Appropriate anesthesia is needed for any AVD, although applying the ventouse usually causes less maternal discomfort and the requirement for anesthesia may, therefore, be less. Although outlet and possibly some low-forceps procedures may be performed with local perineal infiltration, a pudendal block is usually more appropriate. For any rotational procedure, a regional block (epidural or spinal) is necessary.[36] In rare circumstances, a general anesthetic may be necessary. In the United Kingdom, it has been suggested to be medicolegally advisable to have an anesthesiologist attend and confirm that adequate analgesia has been produced before proceeding with any but the most urgent operative vaginal delivery. This does not happen in the majority of units.

Although the simplest operations may be undertaken in an informal birthing room setting, most procedures deserve a delivery room/operating theater. Facilities, equipment, and personnel should be adequate for support of patient, infant, and operator in case of any adverse development. A negative trial of AVD should result swiftly in abdominal delivery instead.[4]

Because complications tend to increase in inverse ratio to the technical skill and experience of the operator, physician knowledge of the instruments and the physical forces involved in their use is essential. The operator must know his or her limitations and be prepared to abandon the procedure in case of difficulty. The use of greater force is the worst of the available options.

COMPLICATIONS AND RISKS

Most of the complications of AVD have also been reported following spontaneous vaginal and even abdominal delivery, but their incidence is greater with AVD. Assessment of causation is frequently problematic because this type of delivery is so often accompanied by other fetal and labor factors that are also associated with birth injury. However, it is obviously difficult for the operator to disclaim responsibility for an injury subsequent to an instrumental delivery. Maternal complications are usually those of soft tissue trauma and tend to be reported more frequently with the use of forceps than with ventouse. They can include uterine, cervical, or vaginal injury, laceration, or hematoma. Bladder or urethral injury may occur, including postpartum urinary retention and late fistula formation. Rectal laceration (with or without episiotomy) and subsequent fistula may occur, as well as later problems in defecation.[1] Increased blood loss is common with more difficult procedures. Maternal injury with use of the ventouse includes inadvertent entrapment of the cervix or vaginal wall between the cup edge and the fetal head with consequent laceration of the maternal periurethral and vaginal tissues. Placement of the cup should never be done carelessly or forcefully.

Fetal complications of forceps delivery include transient facial marks, facial palsies, and fracture of facial bones or skull. Severe cervical cord damage following midforceps rotation has been reported,[37] but such serious trauma is extremely rare. Injury from the ventouse includes minor, and occasionally severe, scalp injury, including scalp bruising, abrasion, laceration, cephalhematoma, subgaleal hematoma, and intracranial hemorrhage. Subgaleal hematomas are thought to be due to disruption of the diploic vessels in the loose subaponeurotic scalp tissue that allows a large volume of bleeding to occur over time.[20] The entire scalp can be elevated. Tentorial tears have been associated with mechanical injury to the fetal cranium and are thought to be related to the shearing forces on the tentorium, resulting in rupture of the deep venous system or laceration of the inferior surface of the cerebellum.[21] Although the pathophysiology is not clearly understood, the vacuum extractor may produce stress on the fetal cranium in the occipital frontal diameter, with tension on the tentorium. The tentorium may then rupture, causing intracranial hemorrhage. Because of these uncommon, but serious, sequelae in infants following a ventouse delivery, all such infants should be carefully observed following birth for any neurologic signs of irritability, drowsiness, tachypnea, seizure activity, or an enlarging head size.[38] Any such signs should be carefully investigated.

Cephalhematoma may be associated with an underlying skull fracture.[39] Fortunately, most documented series of vacuum extractions report no such serious complications. However, neonatal jaundice and retinal hemorrhage are found more frequently with the ventouse.[36] Brachial plexus palsy related to shoulder dystocia and facial nerve palsies are slightly more common after AVD than after spontaneous deliveries.[38,40] Opinions vary on the risk of long-term neurologic damage related to AVD. The subject is under continuing investigation.[11] Some studies show a relationship between abnormal outcomes and difficult forceps procedures,[28] whereas others fail to confirm such a relationship.[29] It is generally believed that most neurologic deficit is unrelated to incidents occurring at delivery or to substandard intrapartum obstetric care.[41]

RISK MANAGEMENT

In the vast majority of AVDs, the normal outcome gives no reason for complaint. However, in our litigious society, a bad outcome increases the risk of litigation against the operator or hospital, regardless of the cause.

In lawsuits against physicians who chose the option of AVD, the common allegations[42] are inadequate indication, failure to rule out cephalopelvic disproportion, and faulty performance causing fetal injury (this may include incorrect diagnosis of station or position, improper use of instruments, or the use of excessive force). The lack of informed consent is frequently cited. Although strongly urged by attorneys, obtaining fully informed consent is often not feasible in an emergency situation. In such circumstances, the best defense is to be able to demonstrate the need for and appropriateness of the procedure and its performance (in other words, the indications for intervention should be absolute and not relative, and execution of the intervention must be competent). As an absolute minimum, if prior informed signed consent is not obtained, the chart should note a discussion of the procedure with the woman, her partner, and even (if appropriate and there is time) with her family. Physicians in training may be particularly vulnerable to lawsuits unless adequate supervision is present. The "learning curve" excuse is invalid because all patients are entitled to the same standard of care.

In any suit following a bad outcome, regardless of the delivery mode, the operator is forced into a defensive position, attempting to prove that the outcome was due to factors other than the alleged misdeeds. After the fact verbal explanations of usually poorly remembered events may appear to be merely an effort to escape responsibility. Careful documentation is the keystone in the operator's defense. Notes that outline the clinical circumstances, the cognitive steps in choice of options of delivery, and a detailed operative note of maneuvers used are mandatory. Consideration of a cesarean section option, possibly with simultaneous preparations, should be noted, particularly with a midpelvic procedure. Many institutions routinely measure cord gases in all AVDs in order to document the infant's condition at birth. The fear of litigation should not dictate medical practice; AVD remains good medical practice in appropriate circumstances and with appropriate safeguards. Despite this exhortation, however, a survey showed that by 1996, over half of ACOG fellows had already abandoned midcavity AVDs in favor of cesarean section.[43]

Cesarean section at full cervical dilation, however, is not an easy operation. A prospective study of 393 women who underwent operative delivery at full dilation in theater found that a body mass index (BMI) greater than 30, birth weight greater than 4 kg and an OP position all doubled the odds of cesarean section. Women were delivered by immediate cesarean in one quarter (approximately) of cases and by cesarean for failed instrumental delivery in another quarter. Major hemorrhage and extended hospital stay were more common after delivery by cesarean than by the vaginal route.[44] Neonates from cesareans were more likely to need intensive care unit admission but less likely to suffer trauma than those delivered by forceps. One-year follow-up demonstrated that the women delivered by instrumental delivery had more chance of pain stopping intercourse (29% vs. 8%) and urinary incontinence (17% vs. 5%) than those delivered by cesarean.[45]

The complexity of the data make firm conclusions on the relative safety of vaginal versus abdominal delivery difficult, other than to say that the decision to perform an operative vaginal delivery or second-stage cesarean should be undertaken by those with the appropriate level of experience.

CHOICE OF INSTRUMENT AND PROCEDURE

Ventouse/Vacuum

The principal idea of the vacuum extractor is to use a cup device attached by tubing to a pump to create enough negative pressure between the cup and the fetal scalp to allow traction on the scalp, thereby pulling the fetus through the birth canal. Traction is applied during a uterine contraction, resulting in descent of the fetal head by a push-pull effect. Positioning of the cup on the fetal head and the development of a caput succedaneum are important considerations.

Malström devised a metal cup with rounded edges and an outside diameter of 60 mm, with the vacuum tubing and traction chain coming off the center of the back of the cup dome. By gradual increments of negative pressure, the fetal scalp is sucked into the hollow of the shallow cup to create a caput succedaneum called a "chignon." Placement of the chignon is very important and a major determinant of outcome. If properly placed at the "flexing point" of the fetal head, a point located on the sagittal suture 3 cm in front of the posterior fontanel, traction will result in maximal flexion of a synclitic head (the head is equidistant between the two fetal shoulders).[46,47] Incorrect placement may result in deflexed and asynclitic (tilted to one side) fetal head attitudes and consequent failure of the vacuum extractor technique (Fig. 72–2). Assuming that the length of the sagittal suture is approximately 9 cm at term, when the cup is properly placed on the flexion point, the leading edge of the cup will be about 3 cm away from the anterior fontanel.[47] Proper cup positioning is crucial to move the fetal head from a midpelvic level to the plane of the outlet of the birth canal, and thus, positioning should always be a primary concern when performing a ventouse delivery.

An important modification to the Malström vacuum extractor was designed by Bird.[46] He moved the vacuum hose attachment from the dome to the lateral wall or rim of the cup. This modified cup was to be used specifically for posterior and lateral positions of the occiput. This alteration allowed easier placement of the cup over the flexing point, and its utility has been supported by an observational study in Portsmouth.[48]

Traction force studies have suggested that 22.7 kg (50 lb; 222.5 N) of traction force may be the upper limit of fetal safety for AVDs.[49–51] Duchon and coworkers[52] noted that with a vacuum cup having a diameter of 60 mm, a vacuum of 550 to 600 mm Hg (0.8 kg/cm^2) will allow 22 kg of

FIGURE 72–2
Applications of a 50-mm vacuum cup: the "flexing median" application should be used in order to avoid deflexion and asynclitism.
(From Chalmers I, Enkin M, Keirse MJNC [eds]: Effective Care in Pregnancy and Childbirth. Oxford, Oxford University Press, 1989.)

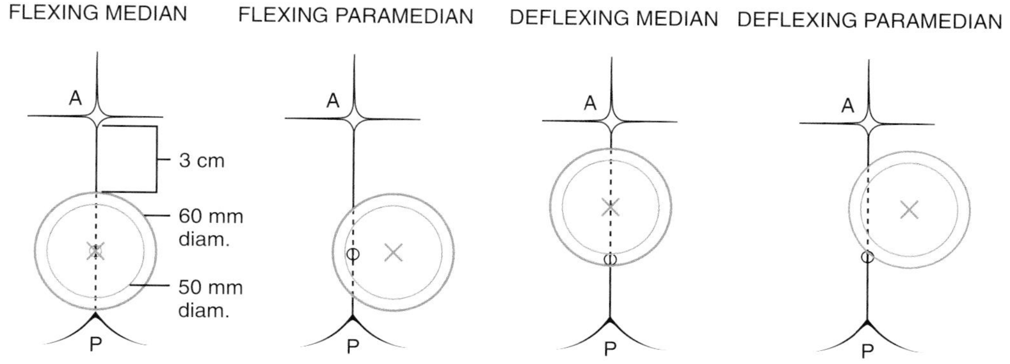

traction force before detachment or "pop-off" occurs. This should be considered the end-point of safety, and inappropriate increases in vacuum should be avoided to minimize fetal morbidity. Repeated detachments of the cup are often associated with scalp injury.

In 1973, Kobayashi introduced a single-unit pliable Silastic cup with a stainless steel valve on the stem that allows for relief of a significant amount of the suction force to the scalp between contractions without loss of application of the cup to the fetal head.[53] The Silastic cup diameter is 65 mm and fits over the fetal occiput like a skull cap. The advantage of this design over the metal cup is that there is less scalp trauma because the cup has no rigid edge and can shape to the fetal head. Also, there is no need to take time to develop a chignon so that traction can be applied shortly after proper application. The disadvantage is that placement of the cup center over the flexing point of the fetal head is not easily done on a nonflexed head in the midpelvic area. Two randomized comparisons of the soft cups with rigid cups have been reported.[54,55] Both found a higher failure rate with the Silastic cup, especially with OP positions. On this basis, use of the Silastic cup should be restricted to easy or outlet procedures. Nevertheless, because of the perceived increased safety and convenience of the soft cup, this device has almost completely replaced the metal cup for use in vacuum extractor deliveries in the United States.

In 1973, a three-component plastic system vacuum extractor composed of a disposable plastic replica of the Malström cup with a flexible handle stem that can be attached to disposable plastic tubing and reusable hand pump was described by Paul and associates[56] from the University of Southern California. They reported favorably on their experience with the device. The cup was 50 mm in diameter and required the development of a chignon as with the rigid cup. The advantage over the rigid cup was the simplicity of assembly because there were fewer parts to fit together. Also, defective tubing and rough edges on the cup were avoided. In later years, the cup was modified to remove the necessity of forming a chignon before traction. The cup diameter was increased to 60 mm and the cup shaped like a teacup (i.e., the dome was deepened). This device is called a Mityvac.

Subsequently, another ventouse device, the Kiwi Complete Delivery System, has been introduced that has incorporated several important aspects of past experience and innovative new ideas. The innovative aspect of this completely disposable system is the use of a hand-pump/traction system directly attached to the vacuum cup that allows the obstetrician to develop the negative pressure by pumping the traction handle while measuring the negative pressure generated via an accurate vacuum indication gauge in the handle. The two vacuum cups available utilize past experience for design. The Kiwi Pro Cup is a soft, flexible, 65-mm diameter cup, similar to the Kobayashi cup that expands to mold to the fetal head in the low OA position. The Kiwi Omni Cup is a rigid, flat plastic cup, 50 mm in diameter, similar to the Malström metal cup. The traction/suction line is anchored in the center of the back of the cup and can flex into a radial recession on the back side of the cup to allow lateral traction as with the Bird modification of the Malström cup. This design facilitates the rotational function of the device for malpositions such as OT or OP. Because of its unique design and convenience for the operator, the Kiwi Complete Delivery System has become popular (Fig. 72–3). Initially, it was claimed to be as successful at achieving delivery as the Bird cup,[57] but two subsequent studies suggested that failure to complete delivery was more common with the Kiwi cup.[58,59] However, a subsequent trial showed no difference in success rates,[60] whereas a study published in 2009 reported that the Kiwi cup was more successful than the Mitysoft device.[61] It appears likely that a major element in the success of any instrument is the training the operators receive and the skill they develop in its use.

Because maintained vacuum or negative pressure is crucial for effective use of the ventouse extractor and pop-off can result in fetal scalp trauma, properly maintained equipment to provide an airtight seal within the pump and tubing is essential. The equipment should be regularly serviced and defective parts (including smooth-rimmed cups) replaced. The operator should test run the system for air leakage immediately before applying the cup to the fetal head. The elimination of the need for maintenance is a major advantage of the disposable types.

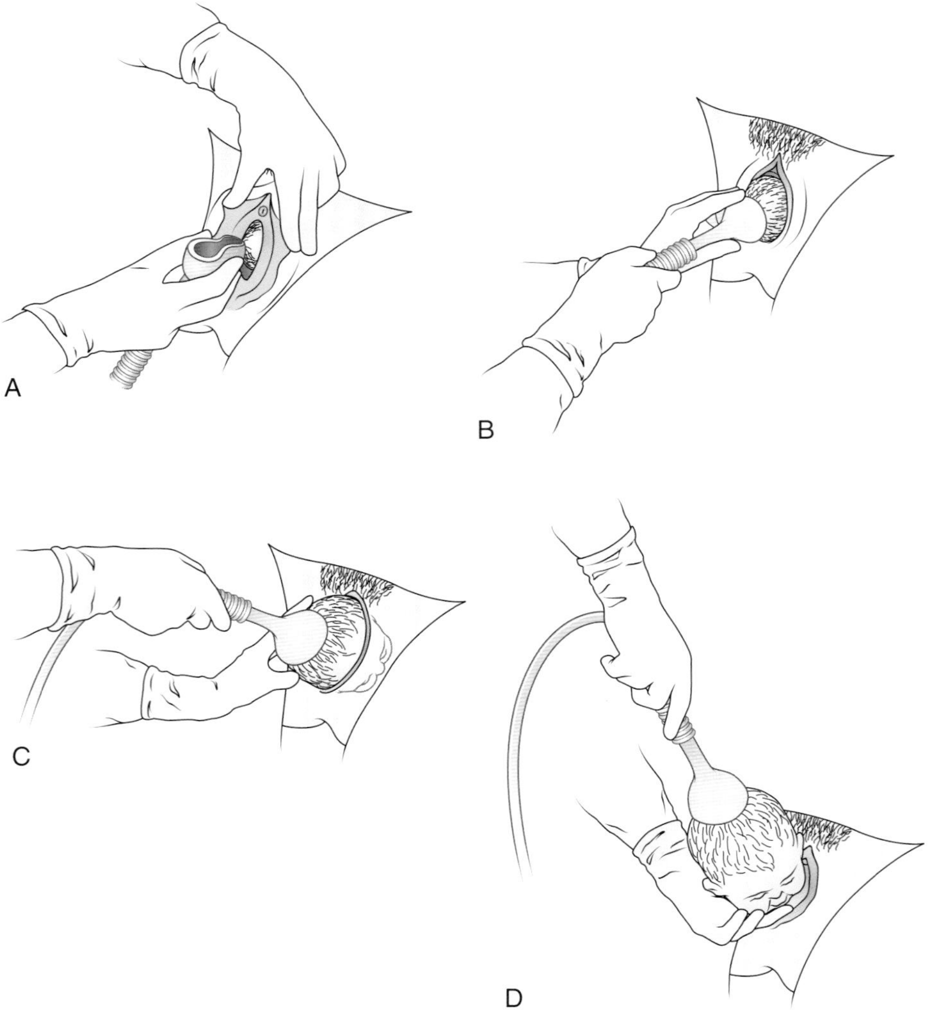

FIGURE 72–3
Delivery with ventouse/vacuum.

PROCEDURE

VENTOUSE DELIVERY

General

After determining that there is a clear indication for a ventouse delivery, the operator should discuss the following issues with the patient or her partner:

- The alternative methods of delivery available.
- The advantages and disadvantages of the vacuum extractor.
- The expected outcome.
- Any possible complications (both minor and serious).

These issues should be recorded in the notes at some time close to the procedure. Ideally, the operator should have a choice of vacuum extractor type, so that they can choose an appropriate instrument for the situation.

Silastic or Plastic Cup

This can be used for a flexed, relatively synclitic fetal head at the pelvic outlet, whereas for a deflexed, asynclitic fetal head, use of the Kiwi cup carries a higher chance of successful delivery. If fetal head malposition, such as OP or OT, causes dystocia, then use of the Bird cup (or Kiwi Omni Cup) would be a good choice. An incorrectly chosen instrument lessens the chance of a successful outcome. Before application of the cup to the fetal head, the operator must check the pump, hose, and cup, fully assembled, for proper and maintained negative pressure when the cup is applied to the palm of a gloved hand.

After the patient has been washed with antiseptic solution and draped in the dorsal lithotomy position for delivery, the operator should empty the urinary bladder and then check the fetal head position and station. Analgesia should preferably be by regional block, placed previously. However, an alternative for deliveries expected to be straightforward is a pudendal block with perineal infiltration of local anesthetic.

The application technique of the cup will differ, depending on whether the cup is metal or soft.

Malström Metal Cup

For the Malström metal cup, povidone-iodine (Betadine) or an antiseptic soap solution is applied to the rim of the cup and the cup slipped carefully into the vagina. The cup is then positioned over the flexing point of the fetal head with the rim nearest to the anterior fontanel positioned 3 cm from it (see Fig. 72–2). The negative pressure of the system is increased to 0.2 kg/cm^2, and the perimeter of the cup is checked for entrapped cervical or vaginal tissue. Negative pressure is increased by 0.2 kg/cm^2 every 2 minutes to a maximum pressure of 0.8 kg/cm^2 in order to build the chignon. At this point, traction in the axis of the birth canal can be applied during uterine contractions.

By placing a hand in the vagina with the thumb on the cup and the index finger on the fetal scalp, traction force can be monitored in the following manner:

- Gradually increase the traction force until the cup begins to slip away from the fetal scalp, diminish the traction somewhat, and then hold for the remainder of the uterine contraction.
- Release traction between uterine contractions.

The expectation is that the presenting part should descend with each push-pull event and that the head will be delivered within a maximum of five pulls. The fetal heart rate is monitored throughout the procedure with an external fetal heart rate monitor. Once the head is delivered, the suction is disconnected and the cup is removed.

Soft Cup (see Fig. 72–3)

For application of the soft cup, presume a flexed synclitic fetal head position. After applying povidone-iodine or antiseptic soap solution to the cup rim, carefully fold in the edges of the cup to diminish its diameter and then insert into the vagina. Because of the larger overall size of the Silastic cup, periurethral and labial lacerations can occur easily unless extra care is taken. Once on the fetal head, palpate around the edges of the cup to clear any trapped tissues, move the stem of the cup as close to the flexing point near the occiput as possible, and pump the negative pressure to 0.2 kg/cm^2. Make a further check for any tissue under the cup rim, then await a uterine contraction. With the onset of a uterine contraction, increase the negative pressure to 0.8 kg/cm^2 and exert traction, placing the intravaginal hand and fingers as noted previously to monitor the traction force (see Fig. 72–3). After the contraction, trigger the partial release valve mechanism to drop the negative pressure to 0.2 kg/cm^2 between contractions. Expectations for progress are the same as noted previously. The operator using a vacuum extractor must be willing to abandon the technique if obvious progress of descent is not evident with five push-pull events or after several pop-offs. An attempt at forceps delivery at this point is ill-advised.

Forceps

Obstetric forceps in current use may be loosely grouped in two major categories—classic and special. Classic instruments are related to those devised by Sir James Y. Simpson (1848) and by George T. Elliot (1858). Simpson-type forceps are characterized by a spread shank and somewhat longer cephalic curve. Examples of the type are the long and short Simpson, Simpson-Braun, Luikart-Simpson, DeLee, Hawks-Dennen, Neville Barnes, and Wrigley, as well as the DeWees and many obsolescent axis traction instruments. They are preferred by many for their superior traction ability. The Elliot-type forceps are characterized by overlapping shanks and a shorter cephalic curve. Examples of the type include the Elliot, Tucker-MacLane and its Luikart modification, and Bailey-Williamson.

Special instruments include the Piper forceps designed for the aftercoming head in breech delivery, the Kielland forceps for rotational delivery at any station, the Barton forceps for transverse arrest in the flat pelvis, the divergent forceps of Laufe and Zeppelin, the Moolgaoker, the Shute, and other cleverly designed instruments. A key feature of instruments such as Kielland or Moolgaoker forceps is their lack of pelvic curve, which facilitates atraumatic rotation but reduces their effectiveness for axis traction.

The choice of instrument is often influenced by regional as well as personal preferences. For example, the Wrigley and Neville Barnes instruments commonly used in the United Kingdom and Canada are almost unknown in the United States. Some operators prefer to approach most clinical situations with the same instrument, thereby losing the unique clinical advantages of the various available forceps. The larger, more molded head is more accurately contacted by the blades with the longer tapering cephalic curve of a Simpson type, whereas the unmolded head is better accommodated by the shorter, full cephalic curve of an Elliot type.[22,36,62]

With the occiput in an anterior quadrant, any classic instrument with the appropriate cephalic curve may be chosen. Most commonly used for outlet or low forceps are the Wrigley, the Simpson (short or long), or an Elliot type of instrument. For low forceps with rotation greater than 45 degrees, several alternatives are available. Most operators prefer a special instrument for rotation, such as the Kielland, the Moolgaoker, or Shute; however, either an Elliot or a Simpson type of classic forceps may also be used. At midforceps level, the same choices apply, but the need for axis traction becomes more important. In the United Kingdom, it is traditional not to use forceps with a cephalic curve for rotation because of the supposed increased risk of spiral tears of the vagina. For forceps to the aftercoming head, Piper forceps are generally preferred, although the Kielland forceps and even classic forceps have been used effectively.

PROCEDURE

FORCEPS DELIVERY

Position

Numerous texts outline many of the specifics of procedure for forceps delivery. Certain principles given here have universal pertinence to the use of forceps, regardless of the type of instrument chosen. In some areas, the least complicated procedures may be performed with the patient in Sims' lateral recumbent position. For clarity, the use of the lithotomy position (with wedging under the right buttock to produce some lateral tilt and avoid caval compression and maternal hypotension) is assumed in the following discussion. Once the prerequisites for forceps use have been observed (indication explained to the mother and permission obtained, adequate analgesia ensured, maternal bladder emptied, membranes ruptured, position and station of the head determined), the aspects of application and traction must be considered.

Application (Fig. 72–4)

Application is extremely important to the safe and accurate control of the head as force is transmitted from the operator to the fetal skull via the instrument. To minimize the amount of force required and the potential for trauma, descent of the long axis of the head must be accomplished in the axis of the pelvis. If the landmarks on the head are obscured and the fetal position is unknown, the operator should not use forceps.[16]

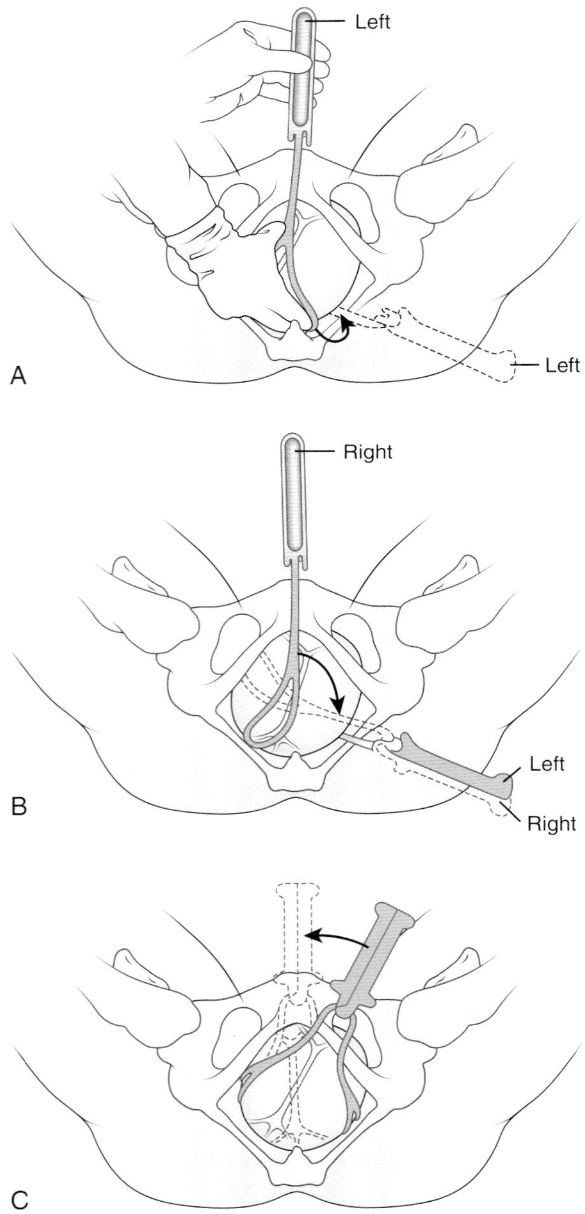

FIGURE 72–4
Forceps application left occiput anterior position.

In an oblique anterior position of the occiput, first insert the blade of a classic instrument going to the posterior segment of the pelvis.[4] The posterior blade then splints the head, preventing rotation to a less favorable occiput transverse as the anterior blade is wandered into place. With classic instrument applications, hold the left blade in the left hand and apply to the left side of the mother's pelvis and to the left side of the fetal head. These four points of laterality are reversed for the right blade. Exceptions, when a left blade would go to the right side of the head, would include application to an OP position, to an aftercoming head, or with certain special instruments and maneuvers such as the Scanzoni rotation.

To commence insertion, hold the posterior blade vertically, perpendicular to the long axis of the patient. Approximate the cephalic curve of the instrument to the curve of the fetal skull, guided by the fingers of the opposite hand. Gently move the handle in an arc away from the midline toward the thigh, then downward, then back toward the midline. The toe of the blade slides higher on the head to seat over the malar eminence. Repeat this with the anterior blade. The amount of downward component in the arc traversed by the handles is the same for each blade in the case of an OA position. Increasing rotation of the occiput away from OA decreases the downward component of the arc of the posterior blade insertion while increasing the downward arc of the anterior blade insertion. The anterior blade is often more subject to temporary obstruction as it is wandered into the anterior segment of the pelvis. Lock the blades and check the application. Checks for accurate application are as follows[21]:

- The sagittal suture should be perpendicular to the plane of the shanks of the forceps. Any other situation is an asymmetrical application.
- The posterior fontanel should be midway between the blades and one fingerbreadth above the plane of the shanks. Greater distance above the plane of the shanks indicates an extended head, whereas a lesser distance indicates an overflexed attitude. In either case, a less favorable diameter is presented to the pelvic axis and relative resistance to descent results. This applies to all vertex presentations.
- With fenestrated blades, a small but equal amount of fenestration should be felt on each blade. The presence of a large amount of palpable fenestration suggests a short application of the blades on the head, increasing the risk of facial nerve injury and slipping of the blades.

When the checks indicate improper application, readjustment is necessary. Should the sagittal suture be oblique to the plane of the shanks rather than perpendicular, a dangerous brow-mastoid application is present. Unlock the blades, then separately wander them to the correct position. Relock and recheck the blades. Correction of the flexion attitude is readily accomplished by unlocking and separately shifting the blades to bring the plane of the shanks to one finger-breadth below the posterior fontanel. The presence of more than a fingertip of fenestration is an indication to unlock the blades and separately adjust them higher in the pelvis. These readjustments are all done without removal of the forceps. If proper application cannot be accomplished, remove the forceps, reevaluate the situation, then reapply.

Traction

The ultimate and dominant function of the obstetric forceps is traction to accomplish descent of the head in the birth canal. The pelvic curve, so carefully designed into the instrument, is mechanically effective with the occiput in the anterior position. Increasing rotation of the occiput away from OA decreases the pelvic curve until it is nonexistent in OT. Thus, a correctional rotation of the head to OA should be accomplished either before or with the onset of traction. Rotate the head along its long axis by rotating the handles in a wide arc ending with the occiput at OA. The toes of the blades should describe as small an arc as possible in the upper pelvis.

Compression of the fetal head is an undesirable forceps effect and should be minimized by the use of the finger-guards rather than squeezing the handles during traction. Force applied at the fingerguards is so close to the fulcrum at the adjacent lock that negligible compressive force is applied to the head. The natural compression supplied by the pelvic walls and intervening soft tissues serves to maintain the position of the instrument on the head. Assuming that the clinical situation permits, traction should be timed to coincide with uterine contractions and voluntary expulsive effort by the mother. The operator may be seated or standing, well balanced, using principally shoulder and arm muscles. Traction force should be increased gradually rather than rapidly. Jerking the instrument increases the risk of injury to fetus and mother. Maintain a steady pull and then gradually release as the contraction wanes. The number of pulls and the force required will vary with the case. Delivery should usually be effected by traction with no more than three contractions, employing no more than moderate force. There are two components of traction, both of which must be considered: direction and amount.

The direction of traction must be in the axis of the pelvic curvature, the curve of Carus. This direction alters with the different obstetric planes of the pelvis (see Fig. 72–1). The critical head diameter that must be moved is the biparietal diameter. Effective force must be directed perpendicular to the plane of the pelvis at the level of the biparietal diameter (Fig. 72–5) using an axis traction principle. This is done manually with the Pajot-Saxtorph maneuver with traction outward on the fingerguards and downward on the shanks of the instrument (Fig. 72–6). The resultant vector of force ideally is in the proper direction. This vector must be estimated by the operator and is more difficult with the biparietal diameter at a higher station. The axis traction

FIGURE 72–5
Line of axis traction (perpendicular to the plane of the pelvis at which the head is stationed) at different planes of the pelvis: 1, High. 2, Mid. 3, Low. 4, Outlet.
(From Dennen PC [ed]: Forceps Deliveries, 3rd ed. Philadelphia, FA Davis, 1988.)

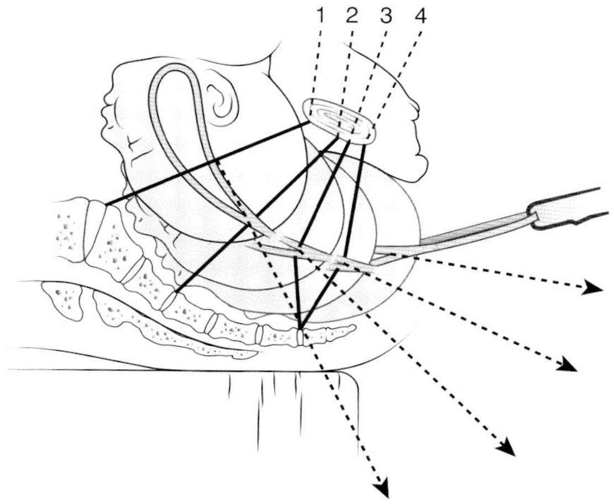

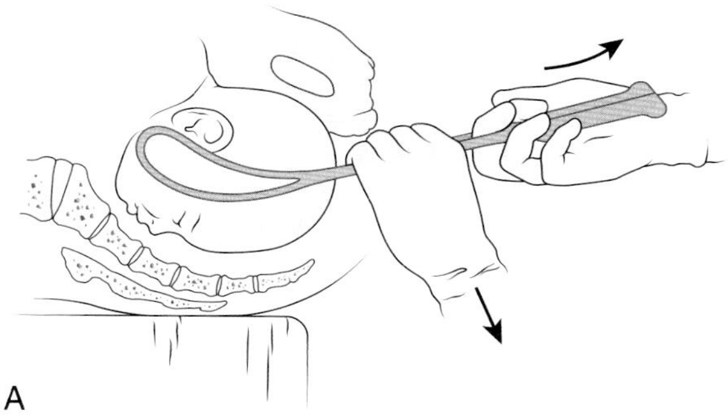

A

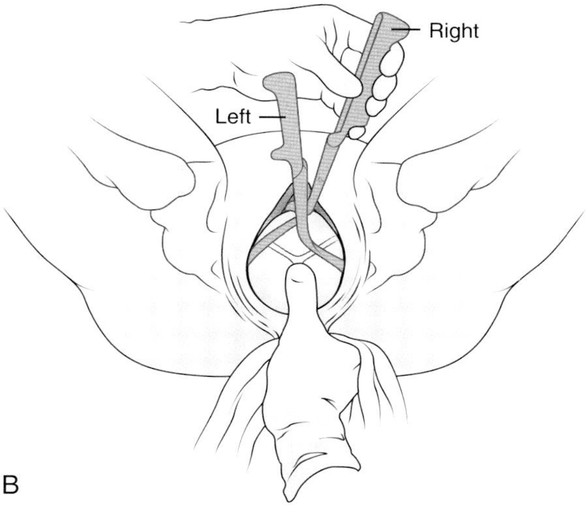

B

FIGURE 72–6
A, Traction. *B*, Removal of forceps; Ritgen head control.

principle is more easily accomplished instrumentally with an attachment such as the Bill handle, which will fit any classic forceps, or with an axis traction instrument.

As the biparietal diameter descends, the direction of traction and the level of the handles rise. The long axis of the head tends to be held in the axis of the pelvis by maternal structure pressure. With traction and elevation of the handles, observation of the edge of the instrument in relation to the adjacent scalp can show the operator the proper direction of pull. If the instrument is elevated too soon, the scalp appears to sink in relation to the upper edge of the blade. Conversely, late elevation of the instrument results in the scalp rising as the head is forced to extend. As the occiput passes under the symphysis pubis, the handle elevation may reach 45 degrees above the horizontal. Higher elevation of the handles increases the risk of vaginal sulcus tears.

The amount of traction force should always be the least possible to accomplish reasonable descent. Maximum permissible force is 45 lb (20 kg; 196 N) in the nullipara or 30 lb (13 kg; 127.4 N) in the parous woman.[13] Most deliveries are accomplished with considerably less force. The amount of vectored force may be difficult to estimate when using manual axis traction. With a traction attachment, the vectored force is equal to the total traction force exerted.

The routine performance of an episiotomy with an AVD has been advocated for many years but has recently been studied prospectively. U.K. and Irish obstetricians were generally of the view that an episiotomy was a part of the routine care with a forceps delivery but was not always needed with a vacuum delivery. De Leeuw and colleagues[63] performed a retrospective review of the use of episiotomy in Holland and found that there was a reduction in anal sphincter tears when an episiotomy was performed for both forceps and vacuum deliveries. Contrasting data derive from a prospective cohort of 1360 women who were delivered in the United Kingdom by forceps or vacuum, where the performance of an episiotomy did not protect against anal sphincter tears (9.9% with episiotomy and 7.1% without).[64] A randomized trial of routine versus restrictive use of episiotomy at operative vaginal delivery found that the 200 women randomized had different episiotomy rates (88% for vacuum and 95% for forceps in the routine episiotomy group, compared with 17% and 64%, respectively, in the restricted group); however, there was no difference in the rates of anal sphincter damage or any other outcome.[65] It is possible that the technique of episiotomy is the most important protective aspect, and not the decision to perform an episiotomy per se. Midline episiotomy appears to have an increased tendency to extend into a third- or fourth-degree tear compared with a mediolateral episiotomy when retrospective data are reviewed.[1] A randomized, controlled trial of routine midline episiotomy versus restricted use also reported an association between the routine performance of a midline episiotomy and extension into a third-/fourth-degree tear in nulliparous women.[66]

If a mediolateral episotomy is performed, the angle of the incision relative to the midline is related to the incidence of extension to a third-/fourth-degree tear. Case-control studies involving third-degree tears and women who did not sustain a sphincter injury demonstrated that as the angle of a mediolateral episiotomy increases, the risk of third-degree tears reduces.[67] A third-degree tear was associated with an average angle of 30 degrees and intact sphincters associated with an average angle of 38 degrees. Another study demonstrated that the angle of the episiotomy and not the depth, length, or distance from the anal canal was the critical parameter of the episiotomy incision.[68]

During extension of the head over the perineum, the forceps may be removed and a Ritgen maneuver (delivery of a child's head by pressure on the perineum while controlling the speed of delivery by pressure with the other hand on the head) performed for completion of delivery of the head. The fetal heart rate should be monitored between contractions throughout the procedure.

Should reasonable effort not produce descent of the head, the initial management should be to direct traction force to a lower plane, rather than using more force. If this is not helpful, the blades should be removed and the situation completely reevaluated. The same, or another, instrument may be carefully applied. Abdominal delivery is the appropriate alternative for a second negative trial. A trial of ventouse is not advised following a failed forceps delivery.

MANAGEMENT OF SPECIAL SITUATIONS

Occiput Transverse Position

Although possible with a flat pelvis, spontaneous delivery as an OT rarely occurs; most will rotate to OA or OP. Should timely delivery become necessary with an OT position, or in cases of the relatively common persistent OT and deep transverse arrest, several options are available, with equivalent results for all methods.[69]

PROCEDURE

OCCIPUT TRANSVERSE POSITION

Manual Rotation

Manual rotation (Fig. 72–7) is a method used successfully by some operators. Used alone and followed by spontaneous delivery, there is a significant decrease in the danger of sulcus and vaginal tears.[62] Assuming planned subsequent forceps use, the hand used for rotation depends upon the location of the occiput. Because the left hand would be used to guide the toe of the right forceps blade after manual rotation from a right OT to OA, the left hand is used for rotation from right OT. Conversely, the right hand rotates from left OT. Introduce the fingers into the vagina behind the

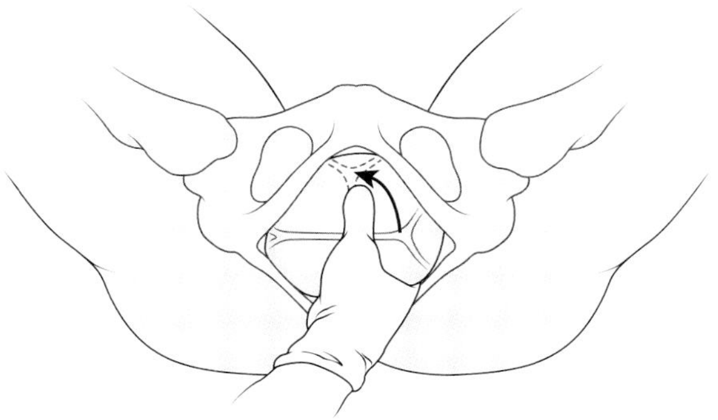

FIGURE 72–7
Manual rotation of the head.

posterior parietal bone with the palm upward and the thumb over the anterior parietal bone. Then flex the head, if possible, and rotate toward OA. Fundal pressure fixes the head, and apply the posterior blade of the forceps as the fingers splint the head in its new position. Rotation is usually easiest with the biparietal diameter at the plane of greatest pelvic dimension. Higher displacement of the head, even disengagement, is considered potentially hazardous. Some operators feel that resorting to this alternative is an acceptable risk, with fundal pressure reengaging the rotated head in OA, provided that immediate recourse to abdominal delivery is available.

Classic Forceps

Classic forceps rotation is commonly used in the United States, although accurate application to the head in OT is more difficult to accomplish than in anterior positions. More points of obstruction may be met in wandering the anterior blade. Midforceps rotations are particularly difficult because the pelvic curve of the instrument is not available in the transverse position, and in application, the perineum may obstruct adequate depression of the handle of the anterior blade. The Simpson-type instrument may be used, but the Elliot-type overlapping shanks offer less resistance to rotation and application may be slightly easier.[70]

Initial application of the anterior blade has been advocated.[16] Most prefer application of the posterior blade first. Introduce the blade (left blade in a left OT) directly posterior to the head following the plane of least resistance until the handle is below the horizontal. The handle is lower with increasing height of the head. To compensate for the pelvic curve of the instrument, the handle must deviate laterally away from the midline during insertion so that the toe stays in the midline. Introduce the anterior blade (the right blade in the case of a left OT) as high as possible under the pubic ramus with the handle initially almost vertical. The handle descends through an arc of nearly 180 degrees. Wander the heel of the blade simultaneously upward with pressure from the fingers of the vaginal hand. Lock the blades with the shanks as close as possible to one fingerbreadth medial to the posterior fontanel. Standard checks of application apply. Then accomplish rotation with rotation of the handles upward through a wide arc consistent with the pelvic curve of the instrument. If obstruction is met, the head may require slight upward displacement so that rotation may be facilitated close to the plane of greatest pelvic dimension. Recheck and readjust the application, if necessary, prior to traction for delivery.

Kielland Forceps

Kielland forceps (Fig. 72–8) are the most popular instrument worldwide for transverse positions of the occiput, although this may be changing with a trend toward using the ventouse, especially in Europe.[71] The construction of the instrument offers a single accurate application for correction of asynclitism, rotation, and extraction, with a semiaxis traction pull. Use of the instrument should yield fetal results equivalent to those of cesarean section for the same clinical situation.[29,31,67] Early studies, which suggested a poor outcome, have since been criticized as indicating that inappropriate selection criteria had been used.[72,73]

The instrument should not be used in a flat pelvis or when short anteroposterior diameters are present. In such cases, rotation is associated with an increased risk of maternal injury.[5] The lack of pelvic curve may also increase the risk of vaginal injury during extension of the head at delivery. Owing to the special characteristics of this instrument, the operator must not use the same approach as with conventional forceps.

Before application, the bladder should always be emptied and the patient positioned with the buttocks slightly overhanging the edge of the delivery table. Orient the instrument in a position of use with the knobs, or buttons, on the shanks toward the occiput. Always insert the anterior blade first. Four application methods are possible. With a very low station, the blade may be applied directly from below upward. In Kielland's original inversion application (sometimes called the "classic application"), insert the blade in an inverted manner, concavity of the cephalic curve upward, beneath the symphysis and anterior to the head. Carry the toe is carried until the "elbow" of the leading edge of the shank is close to the pubis. At this point, rotate the blade 180 degrees on its own axis in the direction of the button. The blade will then drop onto the head with the cephalic curve applied to the anterior parietal bone. If difficulty is encountered, remove the anterior blade in favor of a wandering application. The third and fourth methods involve wandering over the occiput in case of a flexed head or over the face in case of an extended head. Some operators mistakenly fear the inversion method will tear the lower segment, and routinely use the wandering method. With the anterior blade in place, introduce the posterior blade posterior to the head, with the cephalic curve upward, following the plane of least resistance. Obstruction is frequently met at the sacral promontory. This is overcome with a lateral shift to avoid the obstruction. When in place, engage the instrument's sliding lock with the handles at approximately 45 degrees below the horizontal in a midforceps procedure. The level of the handles depends on the level of the biparietal

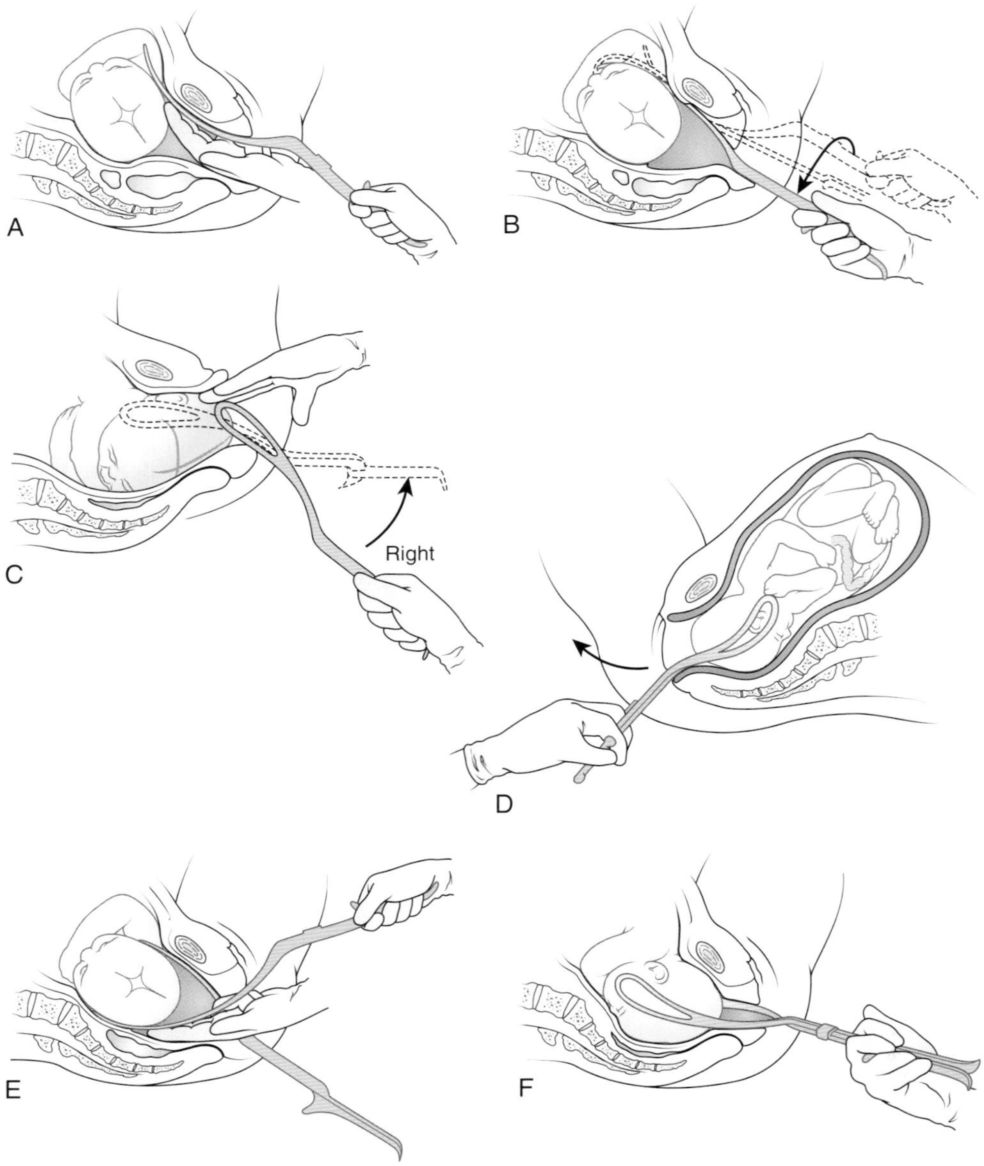

FIGURE 72–8
The use of Kielland's forceps with a left occiput transverse position. *A* and *B*, Classic (inversion) method of application of anterior blade. *C*, Direct application of anterior blade to low head. *D*, Wandering application of anterior blade. *E*, Direct application of posterior blade (anterior blade in place). *F*, Traction after rotation to occiput anterior position.

diameter, being higher with a lower head. Any asynclitism is corrected by equalizing the level of the fingerguards. Correction of inadequate flexion is facilitated if the blades are unlocked and separately wandered to one fingerbreadth medial to the posterior fontanel. Then relock and move back toward the midline.

Rotation toward OA position is accomplished, usually with remarkably little effort, by rotating the instrument along its own axis. If resistance is met, try lowering the plane of the handles. Continued resistance may be due to a relative obstruction at that level. First, draw the head downward in transverse position by 1 cm and attempt rotation. If unsuccessful, displace the head to 1 cm above the original station and rotate. Following rotation to OA, recheck the application. Extraction may be performed with the Kielland forceps. The operator must remember that the nearly straight instrument must be pulled in a lower plane below the horizontal and should not be raised above the horizontal at delivery. Some operators change to another instrument for better traction.

Other Forceps

Barton forceps, with its hinged anterior blade, is another alternative for managing transverse arrest. Its main indication is a flat maternal pelvis, which is a contraindication for the Kielland forceps.[22,62,74] With Barton forceps, bring the head down in the transverse position, then rotate to OA as it traverses the plane of the outlet. The need for this instrument is so infrequent that the reader is referred to a standard text for its use.[14,16]

In the United States and Canada, special instruments (e.g., Mann, Laufe, Shute) have been devised for rotation from OT or from OP. These instruments have regional advocates. Similarly, the Moolgaoker[75] has attracted followers in the United Kingdom and on the European continent. The ventouse and, of course, cesarean section are also alternate management options.

Occiput Posterior Position

Heads in OP position may eventually spontaneously rotate to OA and deliver. Similar options to those for the OT are available when delivery is required from an OP. Before any procedure is carried out, the operator must know in which direction to rotate the head, if it is not in an oblique posterior position. The recorded position earlier in labor, palpation of the fetal back, or even ultrasonographic location of the back should resolve the question. Obviously, the occiput must be rotated only in the direction of the fetal back.

PROCEDURE

OCCIPUT POSTERIOR POSITION

Manual Rotation

Manual rotation either with or without subsequent forceps extraction is an option. The technique is similar to that for an OT with rotation being carried up to 180 degrees rather than 90 degrees.

Classic Forceps

Classic forceps rotation from OP is usually performed with the modified Scanzoni maneuver, a double-forceps application method. A single upside-down application from below followed by a 180-degree rotation has been described but is not popular.[62] In the Scanzoni technique, an Elliot-type instrument is preferred.[70] It is applied to the OP head as if it were an OA. In a right OP position, the blades would be applied as if the position were LOA. When the application is checked, the plane of the shanks should be just above the posterior fontanel. The rotation to OA is accomplished with rotation of the handles through a wide arc, ending with the handles pointing downward. The blades are now upside-down with toes pointing posteriorly. Leave one blade as a splint against backward rotation while removing the other downward, then invert and reinsert between the splinting blade and the head. Then remove the splinting blade downward prior to reapplication in standard manner to the vertex, which is now in OA position. An ordinary forceps technique is then used for delivery. Some operators prefer to substitute a better tractor at the reapplication. The use of a solid blade or indented fenestration instrument for rotation prevents insertion of the blade through the fenestration of the vaginal splinting blade.

Kielland Forceps

Kielland forceps rotation is probably the most popular method of rotation of an OP. The previous comments on the instrument (see "OT Management," discussed earlier) apply. Application to an OP differs in that the blades, with buttons toward the occiput, are applied directly from below the thighs to the appropriate position on the head. Other aspects of technique are not different from those discussed in rotation from OT.

Occiput Posterior Delivery

Delivery from the OP position is an option that is advocated by those who fear that rotational procedures may be traumatic. An indication for delivery without rotation can exist in an anthropoid pelvis with narrow transverse dimensions. Also, with a funnel pelvis, usually android, with the head molded into the outlet under a narrow arch, delivery in OP may be indicated. An OP delivery is relatively traumatic because unfavorable diameters must be brought through the pelvis. The biparietal diameter is usually at a higher station than anticipated. More force is required and the direction of the force is critical. More perineal space is required. An axis traction instrument or at least a Simpson-type instrument should be employed. Applied as in the first step of a Scanzoni, the shanks are depressed against the perineum to get close to the posterior fontanel. The blades are then locked and the application is checked. With traction, after the anterior fontanel clears the symphysis, the head is delivered by flexion rather than by extension.

PROCEDURE

"AFTERCOMING" HEAD OF A BREECH

Following delivery of the arms and body of the infant, wrap the body in a towel, care of which is placed in the hands of the necessary assistant This serves to keep fetal extremities out of the field, and when excessive elevation of the body is avoided, there is less chance of cervical hyperextension injury.[15] In the controlled breech delivery, the back is upward and the head enters the pelvis within a few degrees of mentum posterior. The position is determined by palpation. Apply the Piper forceps upward from a kneeling position. Apply the left blade first, guided by two fingers of the right hand. Start the handle beneath the patient's right thigh, then sweep downward and medially as the toe passes upward to the right parietal area of the infant. The handle then rests 45 to 50 degrees below the horizontal. Similarly apply the right blade upward from beneath the left thigh. Check the application by palpation of the chin between the shanks of the instrument. Then allow the infant to straddle the instrument, and apply traction in a direction and manner similar to routine forceps use. Vectoring is not needed because the pelvic curve of the instrument gives the instrument axis traction. Routine deliver the head with the forceps in place.

PROCEDURE

AT CESAREAN SECTION (See Also Chapter 74)

Although cesarean section is not within the purview of AVD, it should be noted that the use of instruments to deliver the head from the uterine incision at cesarean section[54] can decrease traumatic extension of that incision. Wrigley or short Simpson forceps are often employed. A single vectis blade, to turn and elevate the occiput through the uterine incision, can have the same effect, as can the curved, unhinged blade of the Barton forceps. The Murless instrument, with a single, hinged, locking blade, is more popular in the United Kingdom. It is introduced laterally and slipped beneath the head. When locked in position, it acts as a vectis and elevator to deliver the head.[62] The ventouse has also been advocated for this purpose and is an excellent option.

Comparison of Ventouse and Forceps

Operative vaginal delivery trials comparing the obstetric forceps with the vacuum extractor have documented that the vacuum technique offers lower rates of maternal trauma such as genital tract lacerations, but higher rates of newborn scalp trauma and cephalhematoma than forceps. Efficacy of the two techniques is fairly equivalent.[76–91]

In a mid-1990s survey of residency training programs in the United States, 210 of 291 identified programs answered a questionnaire about their practice.[74] Forceps are the primary instrument in most programs (68%), but nearly one third of responding centers prefer vacuum extraction. Nearly all the responding programs (199 of 209 [95%]) taught AVD using vacuum, mainly the soft cup vacuum extractor (metallic cups were used in only 14% of centers). Instruction in midpelvic operative vaginal delivery was offered in only 64% of the programs. Deep transverse arrest is handled initially by forceps in half the responding centers, whereas 28% and 22% would proceed with cesarean section or attempt a vacuum extraction, respectively.

SUMMARY OF MANAGEMENT OPTIONS

Assisted Vaginal Delivery

Management Options	Evidence Quality and Recommendation	References
Indications		
Maternal indications include distress, exhaustion, and certain maternal medical disorders (see text).	IV/C	4,86,87
Fetal indications include presumed fetal jeopardy and breech delivery (forceps to aftercoming head).	IV/C	4,86,87
Process indications include malposition (OP, OT, asynclitism) and unsuccessful ventouse procedure (forceps trial with caution and facilities for cesarean section standing by).	IV/C	4,86,87
Comment: Practitioners should be aware that no indication is absolute and must be able to distinguish "standard" from "special" indications.	IV/C	86
Contraindications		
Unengaged head (two fifths or more palpable abdominally or at or above ischial spines vaginally).	IV/C	86
Cervix not fully dilated.		
Inability to define position.		
Malposition (face, brow).		
Suspected or actual cephalopelvic disproportion (pelvic anatomy– or macrosomia-related).		
Certain fetal anomalies.		
Prematurity (? <34 wk for ventouse).		
Repeated scalp pH estimations (ventouse).	III/GPP	89,90
Operator inexperience or lack of training with instrument.	IV/C	86
Prerequisites		
Engaged head (but one fifth palpable abdominally or above +2 station is potentially hazardous).	IV/C	86,87
Fully dilated, membranes ruptured.		
Empty bladder (? not for outlet delivery).		
Known presentation, position, and station.		
Adequate analgesia/anesthesia.		

Management Options	Evidence Quality and Recommendation	References
Experienced operator and adequate support facilities.		
Willingness to abandon procedure if difficult.		
Informed and consenting patient.		
Working, serviced equipment for ventouse and matching blades for forceps.		
OT or OP Options		
Manual rotation/ventouse/rotational forceps.	—/GPP	—
Possible delivery as OP position.	—/GPP	—
Selection by circumstances, individual experience, and preferences rather than scientific guidelines.	IV/C	86
Requires experience and skill.	IV/C	86
Choice of Instrument		
Practitioners should use the most acceptable instrument for individual circumstances.	IV/C	86
Deficient knowledge and incorrect technique contribute to increased complications. Practitioners should be aware of the potential risks and necessary safety measures.	IV/C	86
Vacuum versus Forceps	Ia/A	88
• Vacuum has higher rates of delivery failure, cephalhematomas, retinal hemorrhages, and jaundice.		
• Forceps has higher rates of regional/general anesthesia and maternal trauma.		
• No differences in rates of cesarean section, Apgar scores, long-term (5 yr) maternal and baby follow-up.		
Soft versus Metal Vacuum Cups	Ia/A	91
• Soft cup has higher rates of delivery failure (especially with OP, OT, and difficult OA positions).		
• Metal cup has higher rates of neonatal scalp trauma.		

GPP, good practice point; OA, occiput anterior; OP, occiput posterior; OT, occiput transverse.

SUGGESTED READINGS

American College of Obstetricians and Gynecologists (ACOG): Operative Vaginal Delivery (Technical Bulletin No. 196). Washington, DC, ACOG, 1994.

Cohn M, Barclay C, Fraser R, et al: A multicentre randomized trial comparing delivery with a silicone rubber cup and rigid metal vacuum extractor cups. Br J Obstet Gynaecol 1989;96:545–551.

Eogan M, Daly L, O'Connell PR, O'Herlihy C: Does the angle of episiotomy affect the incidence of anal sphincter injury? BJOG 2006;113:190–194.

Johanson RB: Instrumental Vaginal Delivery (RCOG Clinical "Green Top" Guideline No. 26, revised). London, RCOG, 2005.

Johanson RB, Rice C, Doyle M, et al: A randomised prospective study comparing the new vacuum extractor policy with forceps delivery. Br J Obstet Gynaecol 1993;100:524–530.

Murphy DJ, Liebling RE, Verity L, et al: Early maternal and neonatal morbidity associated with operative delivery in second stage of labour: A cohort study. Lancet 2001;358:1203–1207.

Murphy DJ, Macleod M, Bahl R, et al: A randomiswd controlled trial of routine versus restrictive use of episiotomy at operative vaginal delivery: A multicentre pilot study. BJOG 2008;115:1695–1703.

Revah A, Ezra Y, Farine D, Ritchie K: Failed trial of vacuum or forceps—Maternal and fetal outcome. Am J Obstet Gynecol 1997;176:200–204.

Towner D, Castro MA, Eby-Wilkens E, Gilbert WM: The effect of mode of delivery in nulliparous women on neonatal intracranial injury. N Engl J Med 1999;341:1709–1714.

Vacca A: The place of the vacuum exterior in modern obstetric practice. Fetal Med Rev 1990;2:103–122.

REFERENCES

For a complete list of references, log onto www.expertconsult.com.

CHAPTER 73

Delivery after Previous Cesarean Section

GORDON C. S. SMITH

INTRODUCTION

Rates of primary cesarean section have increased dramatically since the 1980s. Consequently, an increasing proportion of pregnant women attending for care have had a previous cesarean and face the question of mode of delivery. The dictum of "once a cesarean, always a cesarean" largely applied in the United States until the 1980s (although not in the United Kingdom or Europe). However, a series of studies in the 1980s reported the relative safety of attempting vaginal birth following cesarean delivery (VBAC). Rates of VBAC increased in the United States until 1996[1] and then declined following reports of the risks of uterine rupture.[2] Further studies from 2000 onwards have described risks of VBAC that may well increase the trend toward planned repeat cesarean delivery (PRCD). However, the choice between PRCD and VBAC, like almost every other medical choice, involves a balance of risks and benefits, and the balance differs according to the mother's characteristics. Estimating the risks and benefits requires the interpretation of large numbers of studies that are exclusively observational in nature.

The risks of mode of delivery among women with a previous cesarean delivery can be classified at several different levels. First, risks can be divided into maternal risks and risks to the infant. Each can be further divided into short-term and long-term. Some of these outcomes favor VBAC and some favor PRCD. Moreover, the balance depends on factors that are inherently uncertain, such as whether the VBAC attempt will ultimately be successful and the number of future pregnancies the woman will ultimately have. Furthermore, the research question of how to assess the risks and benefits of VBAC is complex owing to the reliance on observational data. Virtually all studies will be open to some form of criticism. However, even studies with obvious weaknesses can still yield useful information if assessed in an unbiased manner. Many parties involved in the debate about VBAC start with strongly held prior beliefs about whether it is a "good" or a "bad" thing. Consequently, there is a tendency in much of the literature for reviews of VBAC to fall into camps of believers and nonbelievers. The reliance on analyses of flawed but partially informative research studies means that biased parties can interpret the literature in a way that confirms their prior belief. The aim of this chapter is to attempt an unbiased summary of the risks and benefits associated with delivery of pregnant women who have previously been delivered by cesarean section.

ASSESSING THE EVIDENCE

It is relatively simple to dismiss all discussion of the evidence behind decisions around VBAC with the term "there is no evidence to demonstrate. . . ." Theoretically, the ideal method for comparing the relative risk of VBAC and PRCD would be a randomized, controlled trial. In practice, this is unlikely to occur because most women would not accept the choice being made in a randomized fashion. Moreover, many of the events of interest are relatively uncommon, such as uterine rupture, hysterectomy, or perinatal or maternal death. Consequently, it is likely that even if a trial were organized, it would not be sufficiently powered to address the questions of central clinical interest. Assessing the evidence around VBAC highlights some weaknesses in the normal approach to the hierarchy of evidence. All cohort studies are graded at the same level (level III). However, not all cohort studies are equally well designed or conducted. Given the rarity of many of the key outcomes associated with VBAC, many analyses are retrospective and utilize routinely collected data. In practice, in many of these data sources, quite complex diagnoses are coded by nonclinical staff. A key distinction is, for example, between uterine dehiscence and uterine rupture. Many cohort studies have described nonzero rates of uterine rupture for planned cesarean delivery. In reality, it is extremely unlikely that a true uterine rupture would be discovered during a nonemergency, prelabor cesarean section. The nonzero values referred to previously most likely reflect miscoding of uterine dehiscence. A large-scale multicenter study by the National Institute of Child Health and Human Development (NICHHD) Maternal-Fetal Medicine Units Network overcame the shortcomings of retrospective cohort studies by having a prospective cohort design combined with a large sample size and standardized definitions for assessing outcomes and coding performed by clinical staff.[3] This study is significantly more informative than many others that fall into the same "level of evidence." Many other technical issues influence the validity of different studies employing the same design, and collectively, these mean that the evidence around VBAC cannot be addressed as simply as, for example, the data supporting a new drug treatment. Moreover, attempting to address this complex question using a simplistic approach has the potential to result in drawing misleading conclusions.

ASSESSING ELIGIBILITY FOR VBAC

Perhaps the first approach to a woman with a previous cesarean section who is considering mode of delivery is to determine whether there are any contraindications to VBAC. These can be classified into two groups:

- Contraindications arising from the past history.
- Contraindications arising during the current pregnancy.

The latter includes contraindications to attempting vaginal birth that could affect any woman, such as major placenta previa. A major component of the specific issues around VBAC relates to the previous surgery. Ideally, assessment should involve a review of the operation notes of the previous cesarean delivery, although this is not always possible. Planned VBAC is contraindicated in women with a previous uterine rupture (the risk of recurrent rupture is unknown, but it can be assumed to be high), with previous upper segment vertical classic cesarean section (risk of uterine rupture 2%–9%), and with more than two previous cesarean deliveries (reliable estimate of risks of uterine rupture risk are unknown).[4] However, it is recognized that in certain extreme circumstances (e.g., second-trimester loss, intrauterine fetal death), for some women in the previously discussed groups, the vaginal route (although risky) may be preferred. A number of other variants are associated with an increased risk of uterine rupture, including a prior inverted T or J incision (risk of rupture 1.9%) and prior low vertical incision (risk of rupture 2%).[3] Analysis of the NICHHD study showed that the rate of uterine rupture in VBAC among women with two or more previous cesarean sections was slightly higher (9/975 [0.92%]) than among women with a single previous cesarean section (115/16,915 [0.68%]). However, the 95% confidence intervals (CIs) of the difference in risk extended from –0.36% to +0.85%. Nonetheless, the data do not rule out a small but clinically significant increase in the absolute risk of rupture among women with two previous cesarean births.[5] The rates of hysterectomy (0.6% vs. 0.20%) and blood transfusion (3.2% vs.1.6%) were increased in women with two previous cesarean births. So, although the risks of VBAC following two previous cesarean sections are higher, they are not dramatically so, and therefore, planned VBAC may be considered provided the women have been carefully assessed and counseled. Additional maternal characteristics suggesting caution include obesity, advanced age, no previous vaginal births, and previous cesarean for dystocia.

COUNSELING WOMEN ELIGIBLE FOR VBAC

For some women, the decision to attempt VBAC may already be very definitely planned at their first antenatal visit (based on a combination of maternal preference and lack of obvious contraindications). In such cases, it may be acceptable, following thorough counseling, for such women to have their next formal policy review postdates, to discuss issues around induction of labor in the event that they do not go into labor spontaneously. In the meantime, they can have routine antenatal care. For all other women, a further policy review at 36 weeks' gestation can be helpful because it permits reconsideration while there is still time for a PRCD to be scheduled. These women should be provided with an information leaflet detailing VBAC and PRCD options in appropriate language. Moreover, there should be a discussion of the possibility that she may attend in preterm labor prior to the scheduled date for review, and the plan for such an event should be documented in her clinical notes.

VBAC and the Risk of Emergency Cesarean Section

One of the key factors that determines the risk of complications when attempting VBAC is the level of likelihood that the attempt will be successful, because the risk of maternal and perinatal morbidity is highest among women who attempt VBAC and end up having an emergency cesarean delivery (see later). Individual studies report successful vaginal birth rates of 72% to 76% for planned VBAC after a single previous cesarean, which concurs with pooled rates derived by systematic and summative reviews. Previous vaginal delivery, particularly previous VBAC, is the single best predictor for successful VBAC. The adjusted likelihood ratio for cesarean associated with a previous vaginal birth is 0.3,[6] and overall, these women have an approximately 85% to 90% planned VBAC success rate.[7] The probability of successful VBAC is not further increased with more than one previous successful VBAC.[8] Women with previous cesarean delivery for multiple pregnancy or fetal malpresentation also have higher than average VBAC success rates.[7,9] Induced labor, no previous vaginal delivery, body mass index greater than 30, and previous cesarean for dystocia are associated with an increased rate of unsuccessful VBAC.[7] If all these factors are present, only 40% of women will deliver vaginally after a trial of VBAC. Other factors associated with failed VBAC include delivery at or after 41 weeks' gestation; birth weight greater than 4000 g (difficult to assess before birth); no epidural anesthesia; previous preterm cesarean delivery; cervical dilation at admission of less than 4 cm; less than 2 years from previous cesarean delivery; advanced maternal age (>35 yr); nonwhite race; short stature; and a male infant.[4] There is limited and conflicting evidence on whether the cervical dilation achieved at the primary cesarean for dystocia impacts on the subsequent VBAC success rate.[4] Several preadmission- and admission-based multivariate models have been developed to predict the likelihood of VBAC success or uterine rupture.[6,10,11] Among women attempting VBAC, the risk of composite morbidity is lowest among those with the highest predicted chance of success.[12]

Short-Term Maternal Risks of VBAC and PRCD

The most obvious risk associated with an attempt at VBAC is scar rupture. This is distinct from uterine dehiscence in that the full thickness of the uterine wall, including the serosa, is breached. However, this accounts for only approximately 10% of short-term morbidity associated with VBAC and has an overall frequency of about 7 per 1000 VBAC attempts.[3] The risk of this event among women delivered by PRCD is zero.[3] Composite short-term morbidity is higher among women attempting VBAC (5%–6%) compared with women having PRCD (3%–4%), and this is not wholly explained by variation in the risk of uterine rupture. Women undergoing planned VBAC are at greater risk (compared with PRCD) of requiring blood transfusion (1.7% vs. 1%) and experiencing endometritis (2.9% vs. 1.8%).[3] The increased risk of morbidity overall among women attempting VBAC is due to higher rates among women who attempt VBAC and are unsuccessful (the morbidity associated with an emergency CS is substantially higher than after a PRCD). The NICHHD study showed that unsuccessful planned VBAC compared with successful VBAC is associated with an increased risk of uterine rupture (2.31% vs. 1.1%), uterine dehiscence (2.1% vs. 0.145%), hysterectomy (0.46% vs. 0.145%), transfusion (3.19% vs. 1.16%), and endometritis (7.67% vs. 1.16%).[3] Similar trends were identified in a retrospective study from a Canadian dataset.[13] However, there was no statistically significant difference between planned VBAC and PRCD groups in relation to hysterectomy (0.23% vs. 0.3%), thromboembolic disease (0.04% vs. 0.06%), or maternal death (17/100,000 vs. 44/100,000), although the rarity of these events makes meaningful comparison of the groups very difficult. Anesthetic procedure-related complications are extremely rare.[14] Of the women undergoing cesarean section (emergency and elective) in the NICHHD study (N = 37,142), 93% received a regional anesthetic and only 3% of regional procedures failed. There was 1 maternal death (2.7/100,000) attributed to an anesthetic problem (failed intubation).[15] The vast majority of cases of maternal death in women with prior cesarean section arise owing to complications other than uterine rupture, including thromboembolism, amniotic fluid embolism, preeclampsia, and surgical complications. Maternal death due to uterine rupture in planned VBAC occurs in less than 1 in 100,000 cases in the developed world, and this estimate is based on analysis of single cases.[13,16]

Multivariate analysis of the Maternal-Fetal Medicine Unit (MFMU) network study demonstrated two independent associations between maternal characteristics and the risk of uterine rupture.[8] Any previous vaginal birth was associated with a reduced risk of rupture (odds ratio [OR] 0.44, 95% CI 0.27–0.71), whereas induction of labor (all methods) was associated with an increased risk of rupture (OR 1.73, 95% CI 1.11–2.69). The protective effect of a previous successful VBAC appears to be the same irrespective of the number of previous successful VBACs.[8] Interestingly, when a large population of women attempting VBAC were divided into quintiles of the predicted probability of having an emergency cesarean delivery, women in the highest quintile of risk had a fourfold risk of uterine rupture compared with women in the lowest quintile of predicted risk.[6] Hence, the maternal characteristics associated with an increased chance of success are also associated with a lower risk of uterine rupture. In summary, the risk facing a woman choosing a VBAC is polarized into a lower risk than that of PRCD if she is successful in achieving vaginal birth, and a significantly higher risk if she is unsuccessful and needs a repeat cesarean section as an emergency. Because mode of delivery cannot be predicted with certainty, the consequences of choosing to attempt VBAC are inherently more unpredictable than choosing PRCD.

Long-Term Maternal Risks of VBAC and PRCD

As the number of repeat cesarean sections increases, the following morbidity becomes more common: placenta accreta; injury to bladder, bowel or ureter; ileus; the need for postoperative ventilation; intensive care unit admission; hysterectomy; blood transfusion requiring 4 or more units, and the duration of operative time and hospital stay.[17–21] In the NICHHD study of 30,132 prelabor cesarean sections, among women undergoing their first, second, third, fourth, fifth, sixth or more repeat cesarean deliveries, the incidence of placenta accreta was 0.24%, 0.31%, 0.57%, 2.13%, 2.33%, and 6.74%, respectively; and the incidence of hysterectomy was 0.65%, 0.42%, 0.90%, 2.41%, 3.49%, and 8.99%.[21] In the same analysis, among 723 women with placenta previa, the risk for placenta accreta was 3%, 11%, 40%, 61%, and 67% for first, second, third, fourth, and fifth or more repeat cesarean deliveries, respectively. A retrospective study of approximately 3000 women from Saudi Arabia showed a linear increase in the risk of bladder injury (0.3%, 0.8%, 2.4%), hysterectomy (0.1%, 0.7%, 1.2%), and transfusion requirement (7.2%, 7.9%, 14.1%) with a history of two, three, and five cesarean sections, respectively.[19] Consequently, the major long-term risk of PRCD to the mother is to increase the risk of complications in future pregnancies. Hence, knowledge of the woman's intended number of future pregnancies may be an important factor to consider during the decision-making process for either planned VBAC or PRCD.

Perinatal Risks of VBAC and PRCD

Hypoxic Ischemic Encephalopathy

The incidence of intrapartum hypoxic ischemic encephalopathy (HIE) at term is significantly greater in planned VBAC (7.8/10,000) compared with PRCD (zero rate).[3] Approximately half of the increased risk in planned VBAC arises owing to the additional risk of HIE caused by uterine rupture. Severe neonatal metabolic acidosis (pH $<$ 7.00) occurred in 33% of term uterine ruptures.[3] There is no information comparing long-term outcome, such as cerebral palsy, associated with VBAC and PRCD. However, given that cerebral palsy following birth at term is rare (~10/10,000) and only 10% of cases of cerebral palsy are thought to be related to intrapartum events,[22] appropriate analysis of this question would require a study involving hundreds of thousands of women. No adequately powered study has been reported to date.

Perinatal Death

In the NICHHD study,[3] perinatal mortality at term was significantly greater among women having a planned VBAC than PRCD: 3.2 per 1000 for planned VBAC vs. 1.3 per 1000 for PRCD (relative risk [RR] VBAC 2.40, 95% CI 1.43–4.01) and the RR was similar after removing deaths due to fetal anomaly: 2.4 per 1000 vs. 0.93 per 1000, respectively (RR 2.52, 95% CI 1.37–4.62). The increased risk of perinatal mortality is largely attributable to a statistically significantly increased risk of antepartum stillbirth beyond 37 weeks in planned VBAC compared with PRCD (1.96/1000 vs.

0.8/1000; RR 2.45, 95% CI 1.27–4.72) in infants without fetal malformation. Approximately 43% of such stillbirths among women who planned VBAC were at or after 39 weeks' gestation (~0.9/1000 women delivering at or after 39 weeks), and may have been prevented by PRCD at 39 weeks. The absolute risk of antepartum stillbirth at or after 39 weeks among women with one prior cesarean section was similar in an analysis of nationally collected data from Scotland (1.06/1000).[23]

In the NICHHD study,[3] rates of delivery-related perinatal death were 0.4 per 1000 for planned VBAC and 0.14 per 1000 for PRCD. A report of data for the whole of Scotland demonstrated higher overall rates of delivery-related perinatal death associated with attempted VBAC of 1.29 per 1000, whereas the risk of death associated with PRCD was comparable with the U.S. study at 0.11 per 1000.[24] The reason for the higher rate of delivery-related deaths among women attempting VBAC in Scotland may reflect the fact that these were population-based data whereas the U.S. data were exclusively from tertiary centers. Consistent with this interpretation, a further study of data from Scotland demonstrated a lower risk of perinatal death due to uterine rupture in larger centers.[25]

Accepting the limitations of using these observational data, a reasonable summary is that planned VBAC is associated with a 1 per 1000 risk of antepartum stillbirth beyond 39 weeks and a 0.4 per 1000 risk of delivery related perinatal death (if conducted in a large center). It is likely that these risks can be reduced by PRCD at the start of the 39th week, but direct evidence to support this is lacking. It may be helpful to emphasize to women that the absolute risks of delivery-related perinatal death associated with VBAC are comparable with the risks for nulliparous women.[24]

Respiratory Morbidity

Three observational studies, pooling data from around 90,000 deliveries, have shown an increased risk of neonatal respiratory morbidity (transient tachypnea [TTN] or respiratory distress syndrome [RDS]) among term infants delivered by elective cesarean (3.5%–3.7%) compared with vaginal delivery (0.5%–1.4%).[26–28] The NICHHD study[3] reported that the incidence of TTN following PRCD was 3.6% and following planned VBAC was 2.6% (RR 1.40, 95% CI 1.23–1.59; number need to harm with PRCD = 98).[3] Evidence from a series of observational studies[26–29] and a trial[30] has shown a beneficial effect on reducing respiratory morbidity by delaying elective cesarean section to at least 39 weeks. The trial reported respiratory morbidity was 11.4%, 6.2%, and 1.5% at 37, 38, and 39 weeks' gestation, respectively.[30] Thus, delaying delivery by 1 week from 38 to 39 weeks enables around a 5 per 100 (1/20) reduction in the incidence of respiratory morbidity, but this delay may be associated with a 5 per 10,000 (1/2000) increase in the risk of antepartum stillbirth.[23] Furthermore, the trial evaluated the effect of prophylactic antenatal maternal administration of betamethasone on the risk respiratory morbidity (TTN or RDS) among infants delivered by planned cesarean delivery. The rate was 2.4% among infants exposed to antenatal glucocorticoid and 5.1% among the controls (RR 0.46, 95% CI 0.23–0.93). The protective effect of steroids was still apparent when confined to births at 39 weeks (0.6% vs. 1.5%, respectively).[30] However, there is no information on the long-term effects on the offspring of giving high doses of synthetic glucocorticoids at such late gestations, and so this is not currently routine practice.

Injury at the Time of Cesarean Section

Fetal injury affects approximately 1% of infants born by cesarean section, and over two thirds of these are skin lacerations.[31] The overall risk of injury was somewhat lower among women having a PRCD (0.5%) and was highest in women who had a cesarean delivery following an unsuccessful attempt at operative vaginal delivery (~7%). Other risk factors for fetal injury were any nonstandard uterine incision and a short interval from skin incision to delivery.[31]

VBAC in Special Circumstances

Preterm

A retrospective cohort study found that women attempting VBAC who went into labor prior to term (<37 wk) had higher success rates (82%) than women attempting VBAC at term (74%). There was also a nonsignificant trend toward reduced rates of uterine rupture.[32] However, the NICHHD study[3] found that VBAC success rates were similar for preterm and term pregnancies (72.8% vs. 73.3%, respectively). This study did, however, confirm lower rates of uterine rupture (0.34% vs. 0.74%, respectively) and dehiscence (0.26% vs. 0.67%, respectively) among women attempting VBAC preterm compared with term.[33] Thromboembolic disease, coagulopathy, and transfusion were more common in women undergoing preterm than term VBAC, although the overall risk of composite morbidity was less than 3% in the preterm VBAC group. Perinatal outcomes were similar with preterm VBAC and preterm PRCD.[33] Interestingly, the risk of uterine rupture seems to be increased among women attempting VBAC in whom the previous cesarean section was performed preterm.[34]

Twins

The NICHHD study[9] (N = 186 twins), a U.S. retrospective cohort study[35] (N = 535 twins), and a review[36] (7 studies, N = 233 twins) have reported successful rates of VBAC in twin pregnancies similar to those in singleton pregnancies (65%–84%). However, a population-based study reported a lower VBAC success rate (45%) but a comparable risk of uterine rupture (0.9%).[37]

Suspected Fetal Macrosomia

A number of studies have reported significantly decreased likelihood of successful trial of VBAC for pregnancies with infants weighing 4000 g or more (55%–67%) compared with smaller infants (75%–83%).[7,36] The risk of uterine rupture was reported in one of the retrospective studies to be increased only in those who did not have previous vaginal delivery (RR 2.3; $P < .001$).[38] A subgroup analysis of the NICHHD study[39] showed that among women with previous cesarean delivery for dystocia, those whose second infant was larger than the first had an increased risk of failed VBAC. However, in reality, birth weight is only ever established retrospectively, and antenatal prediction of birth weight using ultrasound is associated with substantial errors in a large proportion of cases.[40] There are no reliable data on the extent to which antenatal estimation of fetal weight predicts the outcome of a VBAC attempt.

Short Interpregnancy Interval

Three observational studies of limited size[41–43] have shown a two- to threefold increased risk of uterine scar rupture for women with short interpregnancy or interdelivery intervals (<12–24 mo, respectively) from their previous cesarean section. In the NICHHD study,[7] women undergoing planned VBAC whose previous cesarean delivery was within 2 years of their labor had an increased risk of cesarean delivery compared with women whose labor was more than 2 years from their previous cesarean (32% vs. 25%, respectively). Although this information is useful antenatally, it should also be shared with women postnatally to enable them to plan their preferred spacing intervals for subsequent pregnancies.

SUMMARY OF MANAGEMENT OPTIONS

Delivery after Cesarean Section
Decisions Regarding Mode of Delivery

Management Options	Evidence Quality and Recommendation	References
The evidence that forms the basis of informed discussion of VBAC vs. PRCD is based on observational studies only, with the potential for bias.		
Overall, women attempting VBAC have 50% greater morbidity, although this depends on the background risk of failure.	III/B	3
Absolute risk of maternal morbidity:	III/B	3
• Highest with failed VBAC—14.1%.		
• Intermediate with PRCD—3.6%.		
• Lowest with successful VBAC—2.4%.		
Women with higher predicted chance of successful VBAC have less morbidity.	III/B	12,23,25
The major risks of VBAC are	III/B	12,23,25
• Overall risk of uterine rupture risk is ~0.7% with VBAC compared with 0% risk with PRCD.		
• Risk of hypoxic ischemic encephalopathy is 7.8/1000 (~50% associated with uterine rupture) compared with 0 risk with PRCD.		
• General risks associated with vaginal birth, such as intrapartum asphyxia and perineal trauma.		
• Risk of antepartum stillbirth while awaiting onset of labor is ~1.0/1000.		
• Risk of intrapartum stillbirth or neonatal death of is ~0.4/1000 (risk of may be higher in low-throughput obstetric units).		
The major risks of PRCD are		
• Increased risk of neonatal respiratory morbidity: 3.6% in PRCD vs. 2.6% in attempted VBAC, usually mild (transient tachypnea of the newborn), although can be severe (respiratory distress syndrome or primary pulmonary hypertension).	III/B	3
• Injury to the infant (~0.5%), principally skin laceration.	III/B	31
• Rare but serious complications in future pregnancies, particularly among women having 5 or more repeat cesareans (absolute risks: hysterectomy 3%–7%, placenta accreta 2%–7%, bladder injury 2.4%, and blood transfusion 14%).	III/B	3,19

SUMMARY OF MANAGEMENT OPTIONS

Delivery after Cesarean Section
Decisions Regarding Mode of Delivery—cont'd

Management Options	Evidence Quality and Recommendation	References
Successful VBAC is more likely with • Breech or fetal distress as indication for original CS (rather than poor progress). • Previous vaginal delivery (85%–90% success rate). • Spontaneous onset of labor. • Normal or low body mass index. • Delivery before 41 wk gestational age. • Normal or tall stature. • Female infant. • No diabetes. • Lower birth weight. • Normal progress in labor.	III/B	3,6–11
Uterine rupture more likely with • Non–low transverse previous incision. • No previous vaginal birth. • Shorter interpregnancy interval. • Higher birth weight. • Induction of labor with prostaglandin.	III/B	3,25,38,41–43
The decision to attempt VBAC is complex, requires careful counseling. Factors that may favor an attempt at VBAC include • Strong maternal motivation to achieve a vaginal birth. • Less concern about rare but serious adverse outcomes (see above). • Presence of factors that are associated with a higher likelihood of successful VBAC (particularly previous vaginal birth). • Plans for multiple future pregnancies, or capacity for many future pregnancies (e.g., younger mother).	—/GPP	

CS, cesarean section; GPP, good practice point; PRCD, planned repeat cesarean delivery; VBAC, vaginal birth after cesarean.

CONDUCT OF VBAC

Location

A retrospective study of data from Canada demonstrated that the RR of uterine rupture when comparing planned VBAC with PRCD increased twofold in low-volume obstetric units (<500 births/yr) compared with high-volume (>500 births/yr) units, even though lower-volume units had a lower-risk obstetric population.[13] A retrospective study of data from Scotland demonstrated that planned VBAC in low-volume hospitals (<3000 births/year) was not associated with an increased risk of uterine rupture overall but was associated with an increased risk of uterine rupture that led to perinatal death.[25] It is likely that the availability of resources for immediate delivery and neonatal resuscitation may reduce the risk of infant morbidity and mortality due to uterine rupture. Hence, these observations provide a rationale for the continuous availability of obstetric, midwifery, anesthetic, operating theater, neonatal, and hematologic support during a VBAC attempt.

Analgesia and Anesthesia

Concerns that epidural analgesia might mask the signs and symptoms associated with uterine rupture were based on a single case report[44] and VBAC is not, now, regarded as even a relative contraindication for epidural analgesia.[14] In the NICHHD study,[7] planned VBAC success rates were higher among women receiving epidural analgesia than among those not receiving epidural analgesia (73.4% vs. 50.4%). The authors suggested that this difference may relate to the disproportionate use of spinal anesthesia in planned short VBAC labors or opting for nonepidural analgesia in cases with non-reassuring fetal well-being.

Fetal Heart Rate and Contraction Monitoring

An abnormal fetal heart rate pattern is the most consistent finding in uterine rupture and is present in 55% to 87% of cases.[45] Moreover, continuous electronic fetal monitoring is generally used among women during planned VBAC, and therefore, the estimates of risk of both lethal and nonlethal perinatal asphyxia associated with VBAC are in this context. The RRs and absolute risks of severe adverse events in the absence of continuous electronic fetal monitoring are unknown. Statements to the effect that "there is no direct evidence to support the use of electronic fetal monitoring" are potentially misleading. The statement relates to an absence of randomized, controlled trial data rather than the presence of high-quality information from which to draw a negative conclusion.

Observational studies, with varying methodology and case mix, have shown intrauterine pressure catheters may not always be reliable and are unlikely to add significant additional ability to predict uterine rupture over clinical and continuous fetal heart rate surveillance.[46–48] Furthermore, intrauterine catheter insertion may be associated with risk.[49] However, some clinicians may prefer to use intrauterine pressure catheters in special circumstances (e.g., in obese women, when augmenting labor with oxytocin).

Diagnosing Uterine Rupture

Early diagnosis of uterine scar rupture followed by expeditious laparotomy and resuscitation is essential to reduce associated morbidity and mortality in mother and infant. There is no single pathognomic clinical feature that is indicative of uterine rupture, but there are a number of symptoms and signs that should raise the concern that this event may have occurred, including abnormal fetal heart rate patterns; severe abdominal pain, especially if persisting between contractions; acute onset scar tenderness; abnormal vaginal bleeding or hematuria; cessation of previously efficient uterine activity; maternal tachycardia, hypotension, or shock; and loss of station of the presenting part.[50] The diagnosis is ultimately confirmed at emergency cesarean section or postpartum laparotomy or can be diagnosed by examination of the uterine cavity per vaginam (PV) following delivery.

Induction and Augmentation

In the NICHHD study,[3] the risks of uterine rupture were 1.02%, 0.87%, and 0.36% for induced, augmented, and spontaneous labor VBAC, respectively. This compares with an overall risk of uterine rupture of 2 per 10,000 in women with no previous history of uterine surgery.[51] Both augmentation and induction are associated with an increased risk of emergency cesarean section: in the NICHHD study,[7] the rates of cesarean section in women undergoing planned VBAC were 33%, 26%, and 19% for induced, augmented, and spontaneous labor groups, respectively. In the NICHHD study,[3] prostaglandin (PG) induction compared with non-PG induction was associated with a nonsignificantly higher risk of uterine rupture (1.4% vs. 0.89%; $P = .22$).[3] In an analysis of nationally collected data from Scotland, PG induction compared with non-PG induction was associated with a statistically significantly higher uterine rupture risk (0.87% vs. 0.29%) and a higher risk of perinatal death due to uterine rupture (1.12/1000 vs. 0.45/1000).[25] This latter figure compares with an estimated 0.6 per 1000 risk of perinatal death in women induced by PG and with no previous history of uterine surgery.[52] Given these risks, it is important not to exceed the safe recommended limit for PG priming in women with prior cesarean delivery.[4] Moreover, a decision to induce labor using PGs in a women with a previous cesarean should be made only by a senior obstetrician and a maximum dose of PGs should be specified. The woman should be specifically counseled about these increased risks and should ideally sign a consent form to this effect before she is induced.

There is no direct evidence to recommend what is acceptable or unacceptable cervicometric progress in women being augmented with a previous cesarean section.[53–57] Among women with no previous history of uterine surgery, it is suggested that there is unlikely to be a higher vaginal delivery rate if augmentation continues beyond 6 to 8 hours.[58] Awareness of the increased risk of uterine rupture in women with a previous cesarean justifies adopting a more conservative threshold to the upper limit of augmentation in women with prior cesarean delivery. A small-sized, retrospective, case-control study suggested that early recognition and intervention for labor dystocia (specifically, not exceeding 2 hr of static cervicometric progress) may have prevented a proportion of uterine ruptures among women attempting VBAC.[57] Hence, although augmentation is not absolutely contraindicated, it should be implemented only following careful obstetric assessment and maternal counseling, and the decision should be made by a senior obstetrician. Moreover, oxytocin augmentation should be titrated such that contractions should not exceed a maximum rate of four in 10 minutes, and careful, serial and regular cervical assessments, preferably by the same person, should be carried out. Augmentation should only continue in the presence of adequate rates of cervical dilation (>0.5 cm/hr).

When counseling women for induction (PG or non-PG methods) and/or augmentation, clear information should be provided on all potential risks and benefits of such a decision and how this may affect her long-term health. For example, women who are contemplating many future pregnancies may be prepared to accept the short-term additional risks associated with induction and/or augmentation of labor in view of the reduced risk of serious complications in future pregnancies if they have a successful VBAC.

SUMMARY OF MANAGEMENT OPTIONS

Conduct of Trial of Labor

Management Options	Evidence Quality and Recommendation	References
Attempt at VBAC should be conducted only in a setting with resident obstetric/anesthetic/neonatal staff and access to full laboratory support.	III/B	25
The issue of intravenous access and cross-matching of blood are controversial.	—/GPP	
Conduct critical review of progress of labor.	—/GPP	
Judicious use of oxytocin is acceptable but should be discontinued if response to uterine stimulation does not occur promptly, and vigilance for uterine hyperstimulation should be maintained.	III/B	53–58
Continuously monitor fetal heart rate.	—/GPP	
Routine insertion of intrauterine pressure catheter is of no proven benefit.	III/B	46–48
Regional anesthesia is not contraindicated.	IV/C	14
Digital palpation/examination of scar is not routinely indicated.	III/B	4

GPP, good practice point; VBAC, vaginal birth after cesarean delivery.

SUGGESTED READINGS

Grobman WA, Lai Y, Landon MB, et al: Can a prediction model for vaginal birth after cesarean also predict the probability of morbidity related to a trial of labor? Am J Obstet Gynecol 2009;200:56.

Grobman WA, Lai Y, Landon MB, et al: Development of a nomogram for prediction of vaginal birth after cesarean delivery. Obstet Gynecol 2007;109:806–812.

Guise JM, Hashima J, Osterweil P: Evidence-based vaginal birth after caesarean section. Best Pract Res Clin Obstet Gynaecol 2005;19:117–130.

Landon MB, Hauth JC, Leveno KJ, et al: Maternal and perinatal outcomes associated with a trial of labor after prior cesarean delivery. N Engl J Med 2004;351:2581–2589.

Royal College of Obstetricians and Gynaecologists (RCOG): Birth after Previous Caesarean Birth (Green-top Guideline No. 45). London, RCOG Press, 2007, pp 1–17.

Silver RM, Landon MB, Rouse DJ, et al: Maternal morbidity associated with multiple repeat cesarean deliveries. Obstet Gynecol 2006;107:1226–1232.

Smith GC, Pell JP, Cameron AD, Dobbie R: Risk of perinatal death associated with labor after previous cesarean delivery in uncomplicated term pregnancies. JAMA 2002;287:2684–2690.

Smith GC, Pell JP, Pasupathy D, Dobbie R: Factors predisposing to perinatal death related to uterine rupture during attempted vaginal birth after caesarean section: Retrospective cohort study. BMJ 2004;329:375.

Smith GC, White IR, Pell JP, Dobbie R: Predicting cesarean section and uterine rupture among women attempting vaginal birth after prior cesarean section. PLoS Med 2005;2:e252.

Tita AT, Landon MB, Spong CY, et al. Timing of elective repeat cesarean delivery at term and neonatal outcomes. N Engl J Med 2009;360:111–120.

REFERENCES

For a complete list of references, log onto www.expertconsult.com.

CHAPTER 74

Cesarean Section

JAN E. DICKINSON

Videos corresponding to this chapter are available online at www.expertconsult.com.

INTRODUCTION

Of the profound alterations in the practice of obstetrics over the past century, one of the most apparent has been the progressive increase in the frequency of cesarean delivery. Sporadically reported throughout medical history, cesarean birth has, only during the last century, been technically refined and rendered safe for both mother and fetus. The safety of the lower uterine segment technique, the evolution of anesthetic proficiency, the availability of blood products and antibiotics, the broadening of indications for the operation, the recognition of the fetus as a patient, the feasibility of vaginal delivery following cesarean section, and the acceptance of this procedure by women have characterized the evolution of cesarean birth in the 20th and 21st centuries. These factors have all contributed to the rise in the incidence of cesarean birth over the past 50 years. The early 21st century has seen further evolution of cesarean birth as an issue of choice for women as a preferred mode of delivery, producing intense polarization of both medical and lay opinion.[1–7] In addition, the secondary rise in repeat cesarean delivery has been associated with an increase in severe complications of cesarean birth, particularly complications of placentation.[8,9] Placenta accreta and its subtypes have been reported with increasing frequency in association with repeat cesarean birth.[10,11] Such abnormalities of placentation clearly have great potential to increase maternal morbidity for repeat cesarean birth.

INCIDENCE

During the 1970s and early 1980s, the cesarean delivery rate progressively increased throughout the world, more dramatically in some countries than in others. Since the 1990s and beyond, most countries have seen a progressive increase in cesarean birth and there is no evidence to suggest this trend is declining. In this, the first decade of the 21st century, women are four times more likely to have a cesarean birth than 30 years ago.[12] The reasons for this increase in cesarean birth are multifactorial, and include the increasing number of women with a prior cesarean delivery, the increase in multifetal gestations, the use of intrapartum electronic fetal monitoring, changes in obstetric training, medicolegal concerns, alterations in parental and societal expectations of pregnancy outcome, and maternal autonomy in decision-making regarding delivery mode.

In 1984, cesarean delivery became the number one in-hospital operative procedure in the United States, accounting for 21% of all live births,[13] and this situation has not subsequently altered. By 2006, the U.S. cesarean birth rate climbed to 31.1%, a 50% increase over the previous decade.[14] Advocacy for vaginal birth after cesarean (VBAC) in the late 1980s and 1990s was probably associated with a temporary lessening of the incidence in the United States, and in 1996, the cesarean delivery rate was 20.5%.[15] However, increasing concerns about the potential complications of VBAC[16,17] have reduced some of the early enthusiasm for this technique and the observed decline has been short lived, with the resumption of a progressive increase in the cesarean birth rate. In 2004, the U.S. cesarean delivery rate was 29.1%, and the rate of VBAC fell to 9.2%.[18] For the majority of women who have a cesarean birth, a subsequent vaginal delivery is currently unlikely.

In Europe and the United Kingdom, an increase in cesarean birth has also been evident, but with wide national variation. In a review of cesarean birth in Norway, the cesarean delivery rate had increased sharply from 2.5% in 1972 to 12.8% in 1987 with a slight rise to 13.6% in 1999,[19] and in 2004, it was 15%.[20] This relatively low rate of cesarean delivery in Nordic countries has not been manifest in other areas of Europe, apart from the Netherlands with a 14% incidence.[20] In 1980, the cesarean delivery rate in England was 9%, increasing to 13% in 1992,[21] 21.3% in 2000,[22] and 23% in 2004.[20] Italy has one of the highest cesarean birth rates in the world at 40% in 2005,[20] having risen from 22.5% in 1995.[23] In Australia, there has been a continual increase in the incidence of cesarean birth, with a cesarean delivery rate of 30.8% in 2006.[24] In the author's state of Western Australia, cesarean birth has steadily increased from 15.7% in 1986, to 20.3% in 1995, and to 32.7% in 2007,[24] with no suggestion of a decline or plateau in the incidence. In 2007, the VBAC rate was 12.7% in Western Australia, and the persistent downward trend of VBAC rates appears universal.

The contrary situation exists in sub-Saharan Africa, where very low cesarean birth rates, generally less than 5%, have been reported for many years.[25] This phenomenon most likely represents inadequate access to medical services in economically depressed countries. High maternal and perinatal mortality rates typify many areas of sub-Saharan Africa. In Ethiopia, the cesarean delivery rate was 0.6% in 2000, in Zambia 2% in 2001, in Ghana 4.2% in 2003, in Tanzania

2.2% in 1998, and in Kenya 4.2% in 2003.[26] A publication from Ronsmans and coworkers[26] highlights this socioeconomic inequity for women in developing countries. The very poorest women had the lowest cesarean section rates with large population sections of Africa having rates less than 1%. There was a strong association with cesarean birth rate and socioeconomic status, with cesarean delivery increasing as wealth increased. Paradoxically, while discussions continue about increasing cesarean delivery rates in most First World countries, it is clear that millions of women and their babies in Third World countries are being denied access to lifesaving surgery.

INDICATIONS

There are four principal indications for cesarean delivery:

- Dystocia (inadequate labor progress).
- Suspected fetal compromise.
- Malpresentation.
- Prior cesarean birth.

These indications account for more than 70% of cesarean deliveries and are, therefore, the major determining factors of the cesarean birth rate[27] (Table 74–1). Programs designed to alter cesarean delivery rates have tended to focus on modifying these four primary operative indications (e.g., active management of labor protocols, increasing VBAC rates). Several other issues have been correlated with cesarean birth rates, including hospital type and facilities, individual medical practices, health insurance status, women's childbirth attitudes, and medicolegal influences.

Recently, there has been much attention given to maternal request for cesarean birth in the absence of a traditional obstetric indication. Although there are bipartisan views on this contentious issue, several points need to be addressed. First, it is recognized that women must be involved in the management decisions regarding their pregnancy and birth. Women vary greatly in their birth experience desires, and individualization is central to any delivery mode policy. Second, it is now appreciated that much of the increased mortality previously ascribed to cesarean birth did not discriminate between elective procedures and nonelective procedures. In a low risk woman, an elective cesarean section with appropriate perioperative care has an extremely low mortality risk. Third, there is an increasing amount of knowledge and discussion of the long-term effects of vaginal birth on the female pelvic floor and sexual function. Fourth, although the first cesarean delivery may be uncomplicated, subsequent pregnancies are clearly associated with an increased risk of placenta previa and accreta. Finally, within the specialty of obstetrics are several practitioners who believe cesarean birth to be the most appropriate delivery mode and have published their views widely, whereas others believe it is a major surgical procedure with attendant risks.[1,2,28] In March 2006, the National Institutes of Health (NIH) published an expert opinion consensus paper specifically addressing cesarean delivery on maternal request.[29] The panel of independent experts concluded that the proportion of women who actually request a cesarean delivery in the absence of any recognized indication is difficult to quantify accurately. They noted that there is a dearth of well-conducted studies on the short- and long-term risks and benefits of delivery modes. Indeed, their conclusion was not particularly helpful or illuminating for those in clinical practice seeking guidance: "any decision to perform a cesarean delivery on maternal request should be carefully individualized and consistent with ethical principles." The debate will continue; however, it is clear that obstetric paternalism is giving way to patient autonomy. Education and discussion remain the keystones in obstetric care with continuing research and audit of outcomes essential.

TABLE 74–1

Indications for Cesarean Section

INDICATIONS	RATE (%)
Previous cesarean section	44.2
Dystocia	14.9
Malpresentation	11.6
Suspected fetal compromise	18.2
Others	11.1
Placental disorders	
Multifetal gestations	
Fetal disease	
Maternal medical/physiologic conditions	

Data from Nguyen N, Gee V, Le M: Perinatal Statistics in Western Australia, 2007. Twenty-fifth Annual Report of the Western Australian Midwives' Notification System. Perth, Western Australia Department of Health, December 2008.

ISSUES IN THE OPERATIVE TECHNIQUE

Cesarean delivery is the most frequent major surgical procedure performed in obstetrics and gynecology. There is, however, wide variation in the surgical techniques used in cesarean birth and the quality of evidence to support the techniques used.[30,31] Randomized, controlled clinical trials (RCTs) are not widely used in the evaluation of surgical procedures, with such therapies usually characterized by observational evidence. This lack of RCTs of surgical interventions has not gone unnoticed.[32] History, personal prestige, commercial competition, surgical equipoise, inadequate funding and infrastructure, inadequate surgeon education in epidemiology, and the presence of emergency or rare conditions are cited as obstacles to the conduct of RCTs in surgery.[32] The particular issue of the "learning curve" is problematic in the conduct of the surgical RCT, because there will inevitably be a bias in favor of the familiar technique and errors are more likely to occur during the acquisition of skills with a new procedure.

A survey of British obstetricians observed a wide range in the techniques for procedures in cesarean delivery.[30] Relative concordance of technique was observed in only a few aspects of cesarean delivery (e.g., double-layer closure of the uterine incision, prophylactic antibiotic use, and Pfannenstiel abdominal entry).[30] There were large variations in the technique of uterine entry, abdominal packing, uterine closure techniques, peritoneal closure, used of subrectus sheath wound drainage, and superficial fat closure. Despite evidence from RCTs, many obstetricians continued to use practices that have been demonstrated to increase morbidity (e.g., 27.6% performed manual removal of the placenta).

Dandolu and colleagues[33] surveyed 400 obstetric and gynecology residents in the United States on some technical aspects of cesarean delivery. The Pfannenstiel incision was used by 77% of respondents in both emergency and elective procedures. Closure of the uterus was conducted with a single-layer technique by 55% and a double-layer closure by 37%. This survey is clinically important because it reviews the practices of junior medical staff who frequently perform cesarean deliveries as an after-hours emergency without the supervision of a more senior practitioner. As with the earlier British survey, this study again demonstrates the disparity between clinical practice profiles and available evidence.

SURGICAL TECHNIQUES

Preoperative Assessment and Preparation

Women should have a medical and anesthetic review prior to the conduct of cesarean section. It is expected as a minimum that a hemoglobin level be available, blood group and antibody screen be performed (with blood readily available in high risk settings), and an infection screen performed for HIV, hepatitis C, and other relevant diseases.[34,35]

There is no apparent benefit from bathing or washing with chlorhexidine, to reduce surgical site infection, prior to moving the patient into the operating room.[36] Three placebo-controlled trials involving 7691 subjects have been performed to assess the efficacy of preoperative bathing with chlorhexidine gluconate in reducing surgical site infections.[37–39] Preoperative bathing/washing with skin antiseptic did not result in a significant reduction in surgical skin infections compared with placebo (relative risk [RR] = 0.91, 95% confidence interval [CI] 0.80–1.04). A further three trials with 1443 subjects compared bathing/washing with chlorhexidine with bar soap, again with no alteration in the risk of surgical site infection (RR 1.02, 95% CI 0.57–1.84).[40–42]

The Abdominal Incision

Preparation of the Patient in the Operating Room

Preoperative positioning with left lateral tilt will minimize maternal inferior vena caval compression, reducing the risk of hypotension and reductions in placental perfusion. A urinary catheter usually remains in situ perioperatively, draining continuously to a closed system. It is often recommended that suprapubic and abdominal hair should be removed as soon before the procedure as possible, on the basis that skin infections may occur if shaving is performed remote from the surgery, owing to the occurrence of grazes during shaving, and theoretically this may increase the incidence of wound infections. However, a Cochrane review of preoperative hair removal practices from a total of 11 randomized trials found no difference in surgical site infections among patients who had hair removed 1 day prior to surgery compared with those that had the hair removed on the day of surgery.[43] In contrast, patients with preoperative hair removal by clipping or depilatory creams had significantly fewer surgical site infections than if they had been shaved with a razor.

Prior to the incision, an antiseptic solution (usually povidone-iodine) is applied to the skin. Iodophor-impregnated adhesive films have been assessed in a small clinical trial,[44] and although not appearing to alter postoperative wound infection rates, this did reduce the skin preparation time, a consideration in emergency situations. Two randomized trials have evaluated the role of vaginal preparation with povidone-iodine in decreasing infectious morbidity postcesarean delivery, both showing no reduction in overall postcesarean febrile morbidity.[45,46] In the study by Reid and associates,[45] the preoperative preparation of the vagina with iodine had no significant impact on infectious morbidity (endometritis, wound infection, or postpartum fever). The second trial also demonstrated no alteration in wound infection or febrile morbidity with the use of vaginal iodine preparation, but a significant decrease in endometritis was observed (14.5% vs. 7.0%, control vs. vaginal iodine preparation, $P = .045$).[46] Neither of these trials was powered to address endometritis as a separate entity, which may explain the disparate results, and further studies are warranted to clarify this issue. Standard plastic adhesive drapes are no more effective than linen drapes in preventing wound infections, and if they become detached at the edge of the wound incision, they may allow the accumulation of fluid, which then contaminates the wound during closure, adversely affecting healing (in one study, it caused a sixfold increase in infection[47]). Thus, if adhesive drapes are used, care should be taken to make sure they remain firmly adherent to the skin during the procedure. Adhesive drapes have become popular when coupled with integral gutters to collect the blood and amniotic fluid shed during the operation, reducing contamination, a consideration of particular importance in areas of high hepatitis B and HIV prevalence.

The Choice of Skin Incision

The choice of the abdominal incision and its closure should be individualized to the characteristics of the woman and the circumstances demanding operative intervention. The massively obese multigravida will require a different operative technique than that used on the unscarred abdomen of a thin primigravida. The ideal incision provides prompt surgical access, adequate exposure, and a secure wound closure.

The transverse suprapubic skin incision is the most common technique used for cesarean delivery in the developed world. The Joel-Cohen incision has been proposed as the quickest method of delivering the fetus compared with the Pfannenstiel or midline vertical abdominal incision.[48–50] The Pfannenstiel incision is a straight horizontal incision about 2 cm above the pubic symphysis with its midportion within the shaved area of the pubis. A Joel-Cohen incision is also a straight horizontal incision, but higher, being about 3 cm below the line joining the anterior superior iliac spines. It can, therefore, be rather longer than the Pfannenstiel incision, and it is easier to pull aside the rectus muscles at this level.

Three RCTs have examined techniques for cesarean section with the procedure for abdominal entry as their primary focus.[51–53] Two of the RCTs have compared the Pfannenstiel and Joel-Cohen incisions for surgical acess.[51,52] Franchi and coworkers[51] evaluated the Pfannenstiel and Joel-Cohen incisions in 310 women with pregnancies beyond 32 weeks gestation. The total operative time was similar

(Pfannenstiel 33 min [range 18–70 min] vs. Joel-Cohen 32 min [range 12–60 min]), although the time taken to deliver the fetus was more rapid with the Joel-Cohen incision (Pfannenstiel 240 sec [range 50–600 sec] vs. Joel-Cohen 90 sec [range 60–600 sec], $P = .05$). There was no significant difference in the incidence of perioperative complications or infant neurodevelopmental outcome at 6 months. The reduction in fetal extraction time did not appear to have a clear maternal-fetal benefit. In addition, the authors of this study commented that the cosmesis of the Joel-Cohen incision (a component of the technique known in toto as the Misgav Ladach method) was inferior to that of the Pfannenstiel incision.

Mathai and colleagues[52] evaluated the Pfannenstiel and Joel-Cohen abdominal entry incisions in 101 women with the primary aim of evaluating analgesic requirements in the first 4 hours postdelivery. There was a significant reduction in the requirement for early postoperative pain relief in those in whom the Joel-Cohen incision was used compared with the Pfannenstiel (45.1% vs. 82%, $P = .0001$; RR 0.55, 95% CI 0.4–0.76). Again, the time to deliver the fetus was less in the Joel-Cohen incision group (mean 3.7 min vs. 5.6 min, Joel-Cohen vs. Pfannenstiel, respectively, $P < .0001$). In this study, the overall operative time from skin incision to closure was 33.1 minutes for the Joel-Cohen approach compared with 44.5 minutes for the Pfannenstiel ($P < .0001$). In addition, there was a significant decrease in postoperative febrile morbidity in those women randomized to the Joel-Cohen incision (6% vs. 24%, Joel-Cohen vs. Pfannenstiel, $P = .01$) and a reduction in the duration of hospitalization postdelivery (mean 4.4 days vs. 5.9 days, $P < .001$). The authors concluded that the Joel-Cohen incision was a more favorable approach to abdominal entry than the Pfannenstiel incision.

A recent Cochrane review of approaches to abdominal incisions for caesarean delivery calculated that use of the Joel-Cohen incision was associated with a 65% reduction in reported postoperative morbidity (RR 0.35, 95% CI 0.14–0.87) compared with the Pfannenstiel incision.[54] This review concluded that the Joel-Cohen incision had several short-term advantages compared with the Pfannenstiel incision, including a lower incidence of pain, requirement for analgesia, and fever; a reduction in blood loss; and a shorter operative time and hospital stay.

A randomized trial published by Giacalone and associates in 2002[53] compared the Pfannenstiel incision with the Maylard muscle-cutting incision in 97 women. There were no significant differences in perioperative morbidity or pain among the two groups.

An earlier trial published in 1987 used a quasi-randomization study design to compare the Maylard transverse muscle-splitting incision with the Pfannenstiel incision in 97 women.[55] In this study, the time to achieve delivery was longer in the Maylard group (10.4 ± 3.1 min vs. 7.6 ± 4.1 min, Maylard vs. Pfannenstiel, respectively, $P < 0.05$). There was no significant difference in febrile morbidity (odds ratio [OR] 0.72, 95% CI 0.22–2.39) or blood loss as estimated by hemoglobin alteration (3.1 ± 0.6 g/L vs. 3.0 ± 0.8 g/L). The Maylard incision was significantly larger than the Pfannenstiel (18.3 ± 4.5 vs. 14 ± 2.1 cm), which, although providing an increased surgical field, may have some cosmetic disadvantages in contemporary elective cesarean birth. The size of the abdominal incision was a critical factor in the degree of difficulty of delivery, with a significant negative correlation between perceived delivery difficulty and incision size reported. An abdominal incision size of 15 cm or greater was associated with significantly less difficulty in cesarean delivery.

A vertical skin incision was the original approach to enter the peritoneal cavity, although it now has been usurped by the more cosmetic low transverse incision. The skin is usually incised in the midline between the umbilicus and the pubic symphysis, although a paramedian approach may also be used.[56] The incision may be extended cephalad if more surgical access is required. The rectus sheath is opened in the relatively avascular midline, providing access to the peritoneum, which is similarly opened vertically. The main indications for its use are a previous midline vertical incision, obesity, or uncertain operative diagnosis, for example, in trauma to the pregnant abdomen or an intra-abdominal tumor mass. In an observational study in 1976, Haeri,[57] reported no significant difference between the two incisions in terms of operating time (53 min vs. 45 min, transverse vs. vertical incision, respectively), postoperative febrile morbidity (30% vs. 48%), and postcesarean hemoglobin less than 10 g/dL (28% vs. 36%). There was, however, an increase in the incidence of complete wound breakdown in the vertical skin incision group (0% vs. 7%) and total maternal morbidity (OR 0.46, 95% CI 0.25–0.86). In modern practice, mass closure using looped nylon is associated with a very low risk of wound breakdown. This improved method of closure has also reduced the advantage of a paramedian versus a midline incision.

In the massively obese patient, a vertical skin incision with avoidance of the subpanniculus fold may be indicated. The higher wound infection rate in this subpopulation requires modifications of perioperative procedures. Gallup[58] reduced the wound infection rate from 42% to 3% by careful perioperative techniques. If a transverse incision is chosen for the obese patient, it should be away from the subpanniculus fold, and a subcutaneous closure used to reduce dead space and subsequent seroma formation.

The Uterine Incision

The clinical situation prompting the need for abdominal delivery determines the uterine incision to deliver the fetus. The low transverse uterine incision is used in over 90% of cesarean deliveries. This high prevalence is due to its ease of repair, reduced adhesion formation, lower blood loss, and low incidence of dehiscence or rupture in subsequent pregnancies.[59] A previous low transverse uterine incision may render the woman eligible for a trial of labor in a subsequent pregnancy. The disadvantages of the low transverse incision are primarily restricted to situations in which the lower uterine segment is undeveloped. In this circumstance, there is a greater chance of lateral extension into the major uterine vessels, resulting in maternal morbidity from hemorrhage. If the initial incision is inadequate to deliver the fetus, extension of the uterine incision to a J, U, or inverted T incision will be required, creating a more vulnerable scar.

The low vertical incision, also a lower segment incision, may be used in situations in which the transverse incision is inappropriate, predominantly in patients with an underdeveloped lower uterine segment. When used in these circumstances, there is a lower risk of lateral extension into the uterine vessels. The incision may be extended upward into the body of the uterus if more room is needed. An upper uterine segment extension renders closure more difficult and precludes a subsequent trial of labor. More extensive dissection of the bladder is necessary to keep the vertical incision within the lower uterine segment. If the incision extends downward, it may tear through the cervix into the vagina and possibly the bladder. The low vertical incision may be used if a contraction ring needs to be cut in order to deliver the infant. If the vertical incision is confined to the lower uterine segment, there is a lower probability of dehiscence and/or rupture in a subsequent pregnancy.[59]

Infrequently performed in modern obstetrics, the classic uterine incision is a vertical incision into the upper uterine segment. It is required in circumstances in which exposure of the lower uterine segment is inadequate, in elective cesarean hysterectomy, or in cases of a noncorrectable back-down transverse lie. The incision permits rapid delivery and reduces the risk of bladder injury, because the bladder is not dissected. When an anterior placenta previa is present, an upper segment incision may be used to avoid incising the placenta. However, dissection around the placenta following a lower segment incision can eliminate the need for a classic uterine incision. The many disadvantages of the classic uterine incision result in its limited use in obstetrics today. The incision is more complicated and time-consuming to repair, the incidence of infection is higher, and adhesion formation is common. There is a greater risk of incision rupture during subsequent pregnancies,[59,60] and if rupture occurs, the resultant bleeding is much greater than with the relatively avascular lower segment. The fetus is also more likely to be expelled from the uterus into the peritoneal cavity. For these reasons, most obstetricians consider a vertical upper uterine incision to be a contraindication to a trial of vaginal delivery, committing women to elective repeat cesarean deliveries.

In a review of 19,726 consecutive cesarean deliveries between 1980 and 1998, Patterson and colleagues[61] observed a distribution of uterine incisions of 98.5% low transverse, 1.1% classic, and 0.4% inverted T. Over the period of the study, there was an increase in the incidence of inverted T incisions, from 0.2% to 0.9%. Maternal morbidity—expressed as puerperal infection, blood transfusion, hysterectomy, intensive care unit admission, and maternal death—was significantly higher in classic cesarean delivery than in the low transverse incision. Perinatal morbidity was also increased in classic and inverted T incisions compared with low transverse cesarean, reflecting the preterm birth preponderance with the former incisions.

Considerable variation exists among obstetricians in the surgical technique used in the conduct of a low transverse uterine incision for cesarean birth. In the survey by Tully and coworkers,[30] 54.7% of surgeons used predominantly blunt dissection and 45.7% predominantly sharp dissection to enter the uterine cavity (the latter inevitably carrying a small risk of cutting the baby). Manual removal of the placenta was utilized by 24.7%, and 33.7% routinely closed the parietal peritoneum.

Formal investigation of the creation of the uterine incision consists of four RCTs involving 526 women[62–65] assessing the use of absorbable staples compared with extending the incision manually or with scissors in low transverse uterine cesarean delivery. Stapling techniques had been introduced to decrease blood loss from the incision margins. In a meta-analysis of these trials by the Cochrane collaboration,[66] the stapling technique did not offer any reduction in total operation time (weighted mean difference = – 1.17 min, 95% CI –3.57 to 1.22), although there was a significant increase in the incision to fetal delivery time (0.85 min, 95% CI 0.48–1.23). There was a reduction in intraoperative blood loss with stapling techniques (weighted mean difference = –41.22 mL, 95% CI –50.63 to –31.8). The evidence currently available does not warrant the routine use of stapling techniques in the creation of the lower uterine segment incision, and the incision-to-delivery interval delay could have adverse consequences in some situations. In addition, the cost of the guns and staples is considerable; this will probably limit their wider use.

The comparison of blunt and sharp extension of the uterine incision has been compared in two randomized trials involving 1231 women.[67,68] In the study by Rodriguez and associates,[67] there was no difference in the incidence of unintended uterine incision extension (13.2% vs. 11%, sharp vs. blunt extension, P = .686), intraoperative duration, or estimated blood loss between the two techniques. The primary correlate of incision extension was the stage of labor, being significantly greater when cesarean section was performed in the second stage of labor regardless of the uterine incision technique employed. The small sample size of this trial (286 women) does render the conclusion of the study that the techniques are equivalent open to some debate. The larger study of 945 women by Magann and coworkers[68] demonstrated a significantly higher incidence of intraoperative hemorrhage when sharp dissection was used (median blood loss 886 mL vs. 843 mL, P = .001), although the difference was small. However, the alteration in hematocrit was greater (6.1% vs. 5.5%, P = .003), the incidence of postpartum hemorrhage was greater (13% vs. 9%; RR 1.23, 95% CI 1.03–1.46), and the need for transfusion was higher (2% vs. 0.4%, RR 1.65, 95% CI 1.25–2.21) in the sharp compared with the blunt extension technique. The occurrence of uterine incision extension was significantly greater in the sharp extension group (30.2% vs. 10.7%, P < .001). The systematic review of uterine entry techniques demonstrated a significantly lower risk of uterine extension with the blunt uterine entry approach (RR 0.41, 95% CI 0.31–0.54).[69] There was no significant difference in endometritis in either study (RR 0.88, 95% CI 0.72–1.09).

Techniques for delivery of the placenta at cesarean birth have been the subject of several RCTs recently reviewed by the Cochrane collaboration.[70] Manual removal of the placenta is consistently associated with a significant increase in maternal blood loss and postoperative infectious morbidity. Although there was significant trial heterogeneity, the Cochrane systematic review reported manual removal of the placenta to be associated with an RR of 1.64 (95% CI 1.42–1.9) for endometritis compared with the use of cord traction. In addition, blood loss was greater (weighted mean difference 94.42 mL 95% CI 17.19–171.64 mL), duration of hospitalization longer (weighted mean difference 0.39 days, 95% CI 0.17–0.61 days) with manual placental removal. Lasley and colleagues[71] randomized 333 women to manual or spontaneous placental delivery and observed an increase in wound infection rates (OR 2.33, 95% CI 0.72–8.73) and a strong trend to an increase in endometritis with manual removal (OR 1.85, 95% CI 0.97–3.53). Manual placental removal at cesarean section should, therefore, be performed only when clinically indicated and not as a routine practice. Disappointingly, in the survey by Tully and coworkers,[30] 25.1% of obstetricians routinely employed manual removal of the placenta at cesarean delivery.

Maternal antibiotics to decrease the incidence of postoperative endomyometritis are administered prophylactically in many centers, although there remain a surprising number who do not use the technique[72] despite compelling evidence of its efficacy in trials involving over 10,000 women.[73] Commonly, a single dose of a first- or second-generation cephalosporin is given, although either the addition of metronidazole or the use of ampicillin plus clavulanic acid or sulbactam to cover gram-negative anaerobes is increasing and has been shown to be more effective than ampicillin alone.[74] The Cochrane collaboration meta-analysis of 47 published RCTs of antibiotic prophylaxis regimens[75] demonstrated ampicillin and first-generation cephalosporins to have a similar efficacy in reducing endometritis (OR 1.27, 95% CI 0.84–1.93) with no benefit in using more broad-spectrum agents (ampicillin vs. second- or third-generation cephalosporin OR 0.83, 95% CI 0.54–1.26; first-generation cephalosporin vs. second- or third-generation cephalosporin OR 1.21, 95% CI 0.97–1.51). A multiple-dose regimen for prophylaxis was no more effective than a single-dose regimen (OR 0.92, CI 0.70–1.23). Antibiotic administration is sometimes given on a selective rather than a comprehensive basis (e.g., not given in cases of elective cesarean section without prior rupture of the membranes), although the evidence suggests it is of value in all cases.[76]

Attention has focused recently on the timing of antibiotic administration at cesarean delivery.[77] The prophylactic administration of antibiotics at cesarean delivery has classically been after delivery of the fetus and cord clamping, based on the concept of minimization of fetal exposure to antibiotics. However, evidence from studies in the nonpregnant surgical population demonstrate improved effectiveness if prophylactic antibiotics are administered 30 to 60 minutes prior to surgery to maximize the tissue concentration.[78,79] Although pre-incision administration of antibiotics for cesarean section had been suggested in earlier nonrandomized studies to increase neonatal sepsis investigations without modifying postcesarean infection rates,[80,81] more recent studies of cesarean delivery antibiotic prophylaxis have demonstrated both a statistically and a clinically significant reduction of 50% in postcesarean infection when administered prior to surgery.[82] In addition, there are suggestions that an extended-spectrum antibiotic regimen may be advantageous, especially with agents such as azithromycin.[83] At present, more data are required before a universal alteration in practice is implemented, but the data are swinging toward the use of antibiotic prophylaxis prior to surgical incision to decrease maternal infection after cesarean delivery.[77] Before there is a widespread change in practice, however, it is important that there are studies of the long-term outcome for the baby to ensure that changes in the acquisition of gut flora that may be induced by being born with significant circulating levels of antibiotics do not result in increases in allergy and infection with more pathogenic organisms.

The uterus may be exteriorized for repair. This procedure is not a necessary routine but does assist visualization and technically facilitates repair of the uterine incision, especially if there have been lateral extensions. The relaxing uterus can be promptly recognized and massage applied, potentially decreasing intraoperative blood loss. Hershey and Quilligan[84] reported lower blood loss in women undergoing exteriorization repair (mean reduction in hematocrit 6.2 ± 0.35 vs. 7.0 ± 0.43, exteriorization vs. intraperitoneal, respectively, $P < .01$), although Magann and associates[85] did not confirm this significant reduction in their trial. No increase in febrile morbidity has been reported with uterine exteriorization.[84,85] The main adverse effect is pain and vagal-induced vomiting with traction on the broad ligament when the woman is awake and the cesarean is being performed under regional analgesia. The incidence of venous air embolism is increased when uterine exteriorization and manual removal of the placenta are performed at cesarean section.[86]

The Cochrane collaboration has provided a review of the six RCTs of uterine exteriorization versus intraperitoneal repair at cesarean delivery.[87] These trials recruited 1221 women.[84,85,88–91] There were no significant differences between the groups except for febrile morbidity and duration of hospital stay. Uterine exteriorization was associated with a reduction in the duration of postcesarean fever (OR 0.40, 95% CI 0.17–0.94), and a nonsignificant trend to fewer infections and gastrointestinal disturbance. No difference in blood loss was found. This review concluded there was insufficient information to make a recommendation on the routine use of uterine exteriorization. A further trial has been recently published with 637 women randomized to exteriorized or in situ uterine repair.[92] There was no significant difference between extra-abdominal and intra-abdominal repair of the uterine incision at cesarean delivery, but the number of sutures used was lower and the surgical time shorter with extra-abdominal repair, although moderate and severe pain at 6 hours was less frequent with in situ uterine repair. Although these results do not support routine exteriorization of the uterus, the fact that it does not significantly increase most measures of morbidity does mean that it is a very reasonable management option if it is necessary to improve visualization of the lower segment to repair an extended incision or to insert uterine compression sutures.

Surgical Closure Techniques

The uterine incision can be closed with one or two layers. Use of a single-layer closure technique reduces operating time without any obvious short-term detrimental effects.[93–96] A small follow-up study from Tucker and coworkers[97] involving 292 women did not demonstrate an increase in uterine scar dehiscence in the single-layer closure compared with the conventional two-layer closure group. However, an observational cohort study from Canada has raised concerns about single-layer closure safety, reporting a fourfold increase in uterine rupture following a single-layer closure compared with a double-layer closure.[98] Gyamfi and colleagues[99] in an small observational series have also reported an apparent increase in uterine rupture during a subsequent labor in women with a single- compared with a double-layer closure (8.6% vs. 1.3%, $P = .015$). These are not controlled studies, they are skewed in that there are many more women with a double-layer closure than a single, and the reason for the closure type is frequently unknown and subject to potential publication bias—however, they do raise issues for consideration when considering uterine closure. Jelsema and associates,[95] in an observational study of 200 women, compared continuous, nonlocking, single-layer closure with the standard two-layer uterine closure. No differences in the febrile morbidity rates were observed, although there was an increased need for additional hemostatic sutures. The Cochrane review of single- versus two-layer uterine closure from 11 single-center studies noted a reduction in mean blood loss of 70 mL, a reduction in operating time of 7.4 minutes, and a decrease in postoperative pain.[69] In the United Kingdom, however, the vast majority of surgeons (96.3%) use a two-layer uterine closure technique.[30] Given the concerns raised about long-term outcomes following single-layer uterine closure, more data are required before any firm recommendation can be given.

It has been traditional surgical procedure to close the peritoneum. The reasons for peritoneal closure have never been scientifically validated; however, they include restoration of surgical anatomy and a potential reduction in infection, wound dehiscence, and adhesion formation. However, on the contrary, animal experimentation has suggested that adhesion formation may be greater with peritoneal closure owing to foreign body reaction to the suture material.[100,101] No significant short-term differences in postoperative complications have been observed in trials of peritoneal nonclosure in general surgery[102,103] or gynecology.[104,105] The Cochrane review of peritoneal closure included 14 trials involving 2908 women.[106] There was considerable heterogeneity in the quality of the trials reviewed, although the results were consistent across methodologic qualities. Operating time was reduced by a mean of 6.05 minutes if the peritoneum was not closed. There were reductions in postpartum fever, analgesic requirements, and hospital stay in those women randomized to nonclosure of the peritoneum. The reviewers concluded that there was an improvement in short-term morbidity in women in whom peritoneal nonclosure was used, although no long-term data were available. Therefore, the available clinical and nonclinical data appears to support the concept of peritoneal nonclosure at cesarean birth. These data have been reflected in clinical practice with the majority of obstetricians favoring nonclosure of both the pelvic (71.1%) and the parietal (66.2%) peritoneum in Tully and coworkers' survey.[30]

Closure of the subcutaneous tissue has been the subject of several trials and a Cochrane review.[107] Del Valle and coworkers[108] investigated the efficacy of subcutaneous closure in 438 women and concluded that a running closure with absorbable suture such as plain catgut was associated with a lower incidence of superficial wound disruption. A similar RCT conducted in women with more than 2 cm of subcutaneous fat also demonstrated a lower incidence of wound disruption (14.5% vs. 26.6%, $P = .02$), a lower seroma formation rate (6% vs. 19%, $P = .003$), and a trend to lower overt wound infection rate (6.0% vs. 7.8%, not significant) in the women allocated to subcutaneous closure group.[109] The Cochrane review of seven trials involving 2056 women reported a significant reduction in the risk of hematoma and seroma formation with closure of the subcutaneous fat (RR 0.52, 95% CI 0.33–0.82).[107] In addition, the incidence of overall wound complications, including wound infection, wound separation, and seroma and hematoma formation, was reduced (RR 0.68, 95% CI 0.52–0.88). No long-term outcomes were reported, and there is a need for more data on this aspect of cesarean delivery.

Wound drainage, with drains sited under the rectus sheath or in the subcutaneous tissue, is used to facilitate the removal of blood or serous fluid from the abdominal cavity, with the primary aim of reducing postoperative collections and pelvic infection. Most obstetricians do not use wound drainage routinely; however the survey of Tully and coworkers[30] reported that more than half of practitioners use them when they considered them to be surgically indicated. Typically, closed-suction drainage systems are used in the peritoneal cavity and the loss can be measured in collection bottles. Corrugated drains may be used in the subcutaneous tissues with drainage to a superficial dressing.

There have been several randomized trials comparing wound drainage with no drainage following caesarean delivery, although the study end-points have varied considerably between trials.[110–116] A Cochrane review of these trials concluded that there is no evidence to support the practice of routine wound drainage at cesarean delivery.[117] This meta-analysis could demonstrate no difference in the risk of wound infection (RR 0.91, 95% CI 0.58–1.43), other wound complications (RR 0.87, 95% CI 0.41–1.84), postoperative fever (RR 0.89, 95% CI 0.66–1.20), or endometritis (RR 1.14, 95% CI 0.71–1.82) whether a drain was used or not.

A recent systematic review of published data of prophylactic subcutaneous drainage in women having a cesarean delivery has shown no reduction in wound disruption rates (OR 0.74, 95% CI 0.39–1.42) , infectious morbidity (OR 1.15, 95% CI 0.70–1.90), hematoma formation (OR 1.05, 95% CI 0.33–3.3), or seroma (OR 0.44, 95% CI 0.14–1.43) when compared with women receiving no subcutaneous drainage.[118]

Closure of the skin following a cesarean birth may be achieved with interrupted sutures, staples, or a subcuticular suture, the technique and suture material usually being related predominantly to personal preference. Skin closure with staples is more rapid than other techniques[119] but has been associated with increased wound pain and reduced cosmesis. Skin closure techniques have been the subject of several clinical studies.[120–123] Frishman and colleagues[120] conducted a randomized trial comparing skin closure with subcuticular suture or staples for Pfannenstiel incisions in 66 women. The operating time was less in those women randomized to skin closure with staples. Analgesic use was less in women randomized to the suture group and also a suggestion of improved cosmesis; however, this was a small trial with methodologic problems, limiting the validity of the results. The use of blunt- or sharp-tipped needles demonstrated no difference in the rate of wound infections.[121] The overall incidence of wound infection in this study of 204 women was low and the study underpowered to exclude a small but clinically significant difference. In another small trial of the cosmesis of intracuticular and subcuticular sutures, satisfaction scores were higher for the intracuticular suturing technique at 4 or more months postprocedure.[122]

Conversely, in a randomized study of skin closure techniques, Gaertner and associates[124] reported no significant difference in scar cosmesis and patient satisfaction in 100 women at 4 months postcesarean delivery. Recently, Rousseau and colleagues[123] reported a randomized trial of 101 women with follow-up to 6 weeks postcesarean delivery to evaluate postoperative pain and satisfaction for skin closure with subcuticular sutures of staples. There was a significant reduction in operative time with staples compared with the subcuticular suture group (24.6 min vs. 32.9 min, $P < .001$. At the 6-week review, pain was significantly less in the staple closure group. Despite this lack of consistent data in terms of skin closure techniques, the majority of U.K. obstetricians reported subcuticular skin closure as their routine (73.9%).[30] Given the lack of evidence of major differences between the two techniques, it is probably reasonable to ask women if they have preferences of their own; many of them do (often preferring the subcuticular suture because they have heard that the staples are painful to remove, and they dislike their cosmetic appearance in the immediate postoperative period). In relation to subcuticular sutures, there is a growing trend to use absorbable (poliglecaprone, Monocryl) rather than nonabsorbable (polypropylene, Prolene) sutures, thus obviating any need to have the suture removed.[125] At present, there is insufficient evidence to judge whether the absorbable suture increases the risk of subsequent keloid formation.

Aternative Techniques

Alternative surgical techniques to the traditional surgical approach to cesarean birth have been reported. The Misgav Ladach, Pelosi, and Stark techniques of cesarean section have been the subject of several reports.[49,50,126–128] The Misgav Ladach technique was developed in Israel and involves the Joel-Cohen abdominal incision, single uterine closure, and nonclosure of the visceral and parietal peritoneum. Björklund and coworkers[126] evaluated this technique in Africa in an RCT of 339 women and reported a 20% reduction in blood loss, a 50% reduction in the use of suture material, and a reduction in operating time of 7.3 minutes. There was no difference in overall postoperative infection rates. Similarly, Darj and Nordstrom[50] observed a reduction in operating time (mean of 13.4 min) and blood loss (mean 160 mL) with the Misgav Ladach compared with the Pfannenstiel technique. The Stark technique, which also involves omission of peritoneal closure and single uterine closure, was associated with a lower febrile morbidity rate (7.7% vs. 19.8%), reduced antibiotic use (33.3% vs. 81.3%), and a lower adhesion incidence in subsequent surgery (6.3% vs. 28.8%) compared with Pfannenstiel incision, double uterine closure, and peritoneal closure in an observational study of 125 women.[129] The Pelosi technique, in which the formation of the bladder flap is eliminated, has been associated with a decrease in operating time, postoperative febrile morbidity, and hospital costs when compared with traditional techniques.[127,128]

It is clear that eliminating operative steps in cesarean delivery reduces the total operating time. It is not clear whether this reduction is translated into other benefits or if the infectious morbidity, pain, and blood loss alterations are real or the effect of small trials with inadequate methodology. It is also clear that large, rigorously designed and conducted clinical trials with assessment of both short- and long-term outcomes are required to adequately address the surgical technique issues in cesarean delivery. In the United Kingdom, this issue is being addressed with the CAESAR Study (caesarean section surgical techniques), an RCT of 3031 women recruited from 47 hospitals throughout the United Kingdom and Italy designed to evaluate three aspects of cesarean section: single- versus double-layer uterine closure, closure versus nonclosure of the pelvic peritoneum, and restricted versus liberal use of rectus sheath drainage. The results of this study are expected soon. In addition, the CORONIS Trial (international study of cesarean section surgical techniques),[130] an international study of cesarean delivery surgical techniques is in progress. This trial, with a planned sample size of 15,000 women, is designed to evaluate surgical interventions such as blunt versus sharp abdominal entry, exteriorization of the uterus for repair, single- versus double-layer uterine closure, and peritoneal closure.

SUMMARY OF MANAGEMENT OPTIONS

Cesarean Section

Management Options	Evidence Quality and Recommendation	References
Preparation		
Hair removal with depilatory creams or with clipping results in fewer surgical infections than shaving.	I/A	43
Vaginal preparation with povidone-iodine does not reduce postcesarean infectious morbidity.	Ib/A	45,46
There is no evidence that adhesive drapes confer benefits over conventional linen drapes.	Ib/A	44
	III/B	47
Cross-match blood with anticipated above-average blood loss (e.g., placenta previa, multiple cesarean sections).	III/B	34,35
Experienced surgeon for anticipated complicated cases (e.g., fibroid uterus, extreme prematurity, placenta previa, multiple cesarean sections).	—/GPP	—

Management Options	Evidence Quality and Recommendation	References
Skin Incision		
Transverse incisions are associated with lower maternal morbidity, including dehiscence, than vertical incisions.	Ib/A	57
Pfannenstiel incisions result in faster operations than Maylard incisions.	IIa/B	54
Joel-Cohen incision is faster than Pfannenstiel incision but cosmetically less acceptable. There are no other differences.	Ib/A	51
Uterine Incision		
Transverse lower uterine incision is associated with less maternal morbidity.	III/B	59,60
Absorbable staples for uterine wound cannot be recommended at present for routine practice.	Ia/A	66
There is no evidence of benefit of blunt versus sharp dissection/extension of uterine incision.	Ib/A	67
Delivery of the Placenta		
Manual removal is associated with increased maternal blood loss and infection.	Ia/A	70
Exteriorization of Uterus		
There is no evidence of increased morbidity associated with exteriorization of the uterus for repair.	Ia/A	88
Closure		
Uterus: A single-layer uterine incision closure is not associated with increased maternal morbidity; but trials are small and no justification for changing practice exists.	Ia/A	31,69
Peritoneum: Closure is not necessary in routine practice.	Ia/A	31,69
Subcutaneous layer: Closure is associated with less superficial wound dehiscence, especially in obese women.	Ib/A	108,109
Subrectus suction drainage: This reduces the rate of wound infection in high risk cases.	Ib/A	117
Skin closure: Skin staples may be superior to subcuticular sutures.	Ia/A	123
Perioperative Measures		
Prophylactic antibiotics are associated with reduced maternal morbidity in emergency cesarean section and with reduced incidence of endometritis in elective cesarean section.	Ia/A	31,69
Antibiotic regimens: Ampicillin and first-generation cephalosporins are equally effective in reducing postoperative endometritis. Single-dose regimens are as effective as repeat doses, with the exception of urinary tract infections.	Ia/A	75
Thromboprophylaxis is recommended for all women undergoing cesarean section.	IV/C	136
Oral intake: There is no justification for withholding early oral intake.	Ia/A	134

GPP, good practice point.

COMPLICATIONS

Cesarean delivery is a major abdominal surgical procedure and is thus subject to the standard complications—medical, anesthetic, and surgical—associated with a laparotomy (Table 74–2). It is beyond the scope of this chapter to deal with all the potential complications that may surround a cesarean birth. However, maternal morbidity and mortality associated with cesarean delivery are increased in women with preexisting medical disorders. The long-term complications of cesarean section are increasingly being recognized, particularly placenta accreta and cesarean scar ectopic pregnancy (see Chapters 73 and 75 for more details on this aspect).

Hemorrhage

Hemorrhage at the time of cesarean delivery may be related to the operative procedure, such as damage to the uterine vessels, or be incidental, such as due to uterine atony or

TABLE 74-2

Complications of Cesarean Section

Anesthesia-related
Aspiration syndrome
Hypotension
Spinal headache
Hemorrhage
Uterine atony
Placenta previa/accreta
Lacerations
Urinary tract and gastrointestinal injuries
General postoperative complications
Respiratory: atelectasis/pneumonia
Gastrointestinal: ileus
Urinary tract infections
Thromboembolism
Endomyometritis
Wound infection

placenta previa/accreta. The origin of the excess blood loss is generally apparent at the time of surgery and dealt with as is appropriate to the etiology. The management is covered in detail in Chapter 75; only a summary is presented here.

The incidence of placenta accreta is increasing,[10,11,131] and it is second only to uterine atony as an indication for emergency hysterectomy for obstetric hemorrhage. There is an association of placenta accreta with placenta previa and previous cesarean delivery, both of which have been increased by the recent trend toward more liberal indications for cesarean delivery. Clark and associates[10] reported that 25% of women undergoing cesarean for placenta previa in the presence of one or more uterine scars subsequently underwent cesarean hysterectomy for placenta accreta. This risk appears to increase directly with the number of previous uterine incisions. If the placenta is accreta, effective management usually requires total abdominal hysterectomy, although additional options including the use of uterine compression sutures or leaving the placenta in situ have been reported. The uterus, vagina, or broad ligament may be lacerated during a cesarean delivery. Traumatic deliveries or poor delivery technique are associated with an increased frequency of operative lacerations. Lacerations involving uterine tissue are usually sutured without difficulty. Vertical lacerations into the vagina or lateral extensions into the broad ligament may be associated with substantial blood loss and the potential for ureteric damage during their repair. Prior to commencement of the repair of lacerations into the broad ligament, identification of the ureter is frequently necessary. The initial suture must be inserted just distal to the apex of the laceration.

Urinary Tract Injuries

Injuries to the urinary bladder occur with variable incidence during the course of cesarean delivery.[132,133] The Pfannenstiel incision with lower entry into the peritoneal cavity increases the risk of inadvertent cystotomy, especially after prolonged labor in which the bladder is pulled cephalad. Scarring and secondary obliteration of the vesicouterine space following previous cesarean section increase the incidence of trauma secondary to attempts at dissection. The bladder may also be damaged secondary to a uterine laceration, particularly in association with a low vertical uterine incision.

Various techniques are employed to reduce the incidence of intraoperative bladder injury. Preoperative catheterization of the bladder and peritoneal entry as far cephalad as possible are important. Injuries to the base of the bladder are most frequent during a repeat procedure in which clear tissue planes do not always exist. Careful sharp rather than blunt dissection of the bladder will reduce the occurrence of inadvertent cystotomy as well as reduce blood loss. If there is concern as to possible bladder injury, the abdomen must not be closed until the issue is resolved by transurethral instillation of methylene blue–colored saline with leakage of fluid identifying the cystotomy site. Full-thickness bladder lacerations should be repaired with a two-layer closure with continuous or interrupted 2-0 or 3-0 chromic catgut or polyglycolic acid/polyglactin (Dexon/Vicryl) sutures. The site of the bladder laceration is important because repair of a laceration of the bladder dome and its subsequent repair is usually straightforward. The bladder base is thinner, receives less blood flow, and appears to heal more slowly, whereas occlusion of the ureteric orifice is also a possibility. Fistula formation is not usually a problem if accidental cystotomy is promptly recognized and repaired.

Ureteric injury is one of the most dreaded complications of any pelvic operation. It is, however, an uncommon occurrence at cesarean section. Eisenkop and coworkers[133] reported 7 ureteric injuries in 7527 women undergoing cesarean delivery. In 5, the ureteric injury occurred during an attempt to control hemorrhage from extension of the uterine incision. When controlling hemorrhage, it is useful to apply direct pressure while identifying the course of the ureter to permit accurate suture placement and reduce the potential for ureteral injury.

Postoperative Complications

Respiratory complications remain a primary cause of postoperative morbidity following major surgical procedures. Deep-breathing exercises, incentive spirometry, chest percussion, and postural drainage all have merit, depending on the clinical circumstance.

Gastrointestinal dysfunction is not uncommon after a cesarean delivery and is usually restricted to a transient ileus. The Cochrane review of postoperative feeding assessed six trials to evaluate the effect of early and delayed oral intake after cesarean birth.[134] Although the studies were of variable quality, on the available data, the review concluded there was no justification for withholding early oral intake after cesarean birth. Early oral intake was associated with a reduced time to return of bowel sounds, a reduced postoperative stay, and a trend to a reduction in abdominal distention. Urinary tract infections are a common complication of cesarean section and occur with a variable frequency of 2% to 16%, the rate depending on the duration of catherization and the preoperative health of the woman.[132,135]

Thromboembolic disease during pregnancy is an uncommon event but remains a major cause of maternal morbidity and mortality. Indeed, pulmonary thromboembolism is a leading cause of maternal death in the United Kingdom with a death rate of 1.94 in 100,000 confinements.[136] The highest incidence in the puerperium is among cesarean patients, particularly if the surgery is performed as a nonelective procedure during labor. Other factors increasing the risk of venous thromboembolism include advanced maternal age, obesity, and inherited thrombophilia disorders. The risk of a deep venous thrombosis after cesarean delivery is three to five times greater than after vaginal delivery.[137] The reactive thrombocytosis after cesarean birth, the impact of which is compounded by anemia, infection, and postpartum hemorrhage, further increases the risk. In 1995, the Royal College of Obstetricians and Gynaecologists[138] published a Working Party Report on prophylaxis against thromboembolism in the United Kingdom. This document drew attention to the risks of thromboembolic disorders after cesarean birth and the need to consider prophylaxis for high risk women. Routine prophylaxis against postoperative deep vein thrombosis now includes the use of mechanical calf compression intraoperatively (e.g., Flowtron boots), the use of calf compression stockings (e.g., TED), and subcutaneous heparin, either unfractionated or low-molecular-weight heparin[138] (Table 74–3). Low-molecular-weight heparin is now commonly used peripartum because it can be administered on a once-daily dosage regimen.[139] These heparins are not secreted in breast milk and, therefore, can be used in lactating women.

Endomyometritis

In the absence of prophylactic antibiotics, postcesarean endomyometritis occurs with an incidence of 20% to 40%.[140,141] Postoperative infections may be reduced by 50% to 60% with the use of prophylactic antibiotics at the time of cesarean delivery.[142,143] In approximately 10% of cases, concurrent bacteremia will accompany postcesarean endomyometritis.[143,145] Uncommonly, postcesarean endomyometritis may be complicated by pelvic abscess, septic shock, and septic pelvic thrombophlebitis. The major risk factors for the development of postcesarean infection are young age, low socioeconomic status, prolonged labor, prolonged ruptured membranes, and multiple vaginal examinations.

Postcesarean section endomyometritis is a polymicrobial infection with bacteria normally present in the lower genital tract—aerobic streptococci (group B and D streptococci), anaerobic gram-positive cocci (peptococcus and peptostreptococcus), aerobic (*Escherichia coli*, *Klebsiella pneumoniae*, *Proteus* spp.), and anaerobic gram-negative bacilli (*Bacteroides* spp. and *Gardnerella vaginalis*).[143] The symptoms and signs of endomyometritis usually develop 24 to 48 hours postsurgery. The main clinical manifestations are fever, tachycardia, lower abdominal pain, uterine and adnexal tenderness, and peritoneal irritation. Following appropriate laboratory investigation, including complete blood count, aerobic and anaerobic blood cultures, and aerobic and anaerobic endometrial cultures, antibiotic therapy is instituted. There are several effective regimens available: clindamycin plus an aminoglycoside or aztreonam; penicillin plus aminoglycoside and metronidazole; or one of the extended-spectrum penicillins such as ticarcillin-clavulanic acid or ampicillin-sulbactam. If a cephalosporin has been administered for prophylaxis, a penicillin should be used owing to the possibility of enterococcus.

Most patients show a clear response to treatment within 72 hours. The two most common causes of apparent treatment failure are concurrent wound infection and resistant microorganisms. If a wound infection develops, incision and drainage is indicated, but a change in antibiotics usually is not necessary. The principal microorganisms likely to be resistant to initial treatment regimens are aerobic gram-negative bacilli, enterococci, and *Bacteroides* spp. If a resistant organism is thought to be present, antibiotic therapy should be modified. Parenteral therapy should be continued for a minimum of 24 hours after the patient becomes afebrile and asymptomatic. At this point, therapy may be discontinued. Patients do not need to be maintained on oral antibiotics after discharge from hospital.[142] Extended therapy of this nature is expensive and increases the risk of side effects without providing any measurable therapeutic benefit.

TABLE 74–3

Thromboprophylaxis Guidelines following Cesarean Section

HIGH RISK	MODERATE RISK	LOW RISK
	Risk Factors	
• Three or more moderate risk factors • Extended major pelvic or abdominal surgery (e.g., cesarean hysterectomy) • Personal history of deep venous thrombosis or pulmonary embolism • Thrombophilia • Family history of deep vein thrombosis, pulmonary embolism, thrombophilia • Paralysis of lower limbs • Antiphospholipid antibody syndrome	• Age > 35 yr • Weight > 80 kg at booking visit • Para 4 or more • Severe varicose veins • Current infection • Preeclampsia • Immobility prior to surgery (≥5 days) • Major current illness (e.g., heart or lung disease, cancer) • Emergency cesarean section in labor	• Includes women having an elective cesarean section and who have had an uncomplicated pregnancy with no other risk factors
	Prophylaxis includes:	
• Knee-high compression stockings • Calf stimulation by a calf stimulation device during surgery • Subcutaneous low-molecular-weight heparin (minimum 5 days) • Early mobilization • Adequate hydration	• Knee-high compression stockings • Calf stimulation by a calf stimulation device during surgery • Early mobilization • Adequate hydration • Consider subcutaneous low-molecular-weight heparin.	• Knee-high compression stockings • Calf stimulation by a calf stimulation device during surgery • Early mobilization • Adequate hydration

From Macklon NS, Greer IA: The deep venous system in the puerperium: An ultrasound study. Br J Obstet Gynaecol 1997;104:198–200.

In patients who fail to improve after a change in antibiotic therapy, another detailed examination should be performed to detect a wound infection or pelvic abscess. Other possible causes of poor treatment response include viral infections, venous thrombophlebitis, and drug fever.

Wound Infection

Adverse outcomes associated with abdominal wounds in obstetric patients occur more frequently in the presence of anemia, premature rupture of the membranes, prolapsed cord, and meconium staining. Reported wound infection rates associated with cesarean section range from 2.5% to 16.1%.[144–146] Nielson and Hokegard[147] found rates of 4.7% for elective cases and 24.2% for emergency cases. A mixture of anaerobic and aerobic bacteria (*E. coli*, *Proteus mirabilis*, *Bacteroides* spp., β-hemolytic streptococci) are isolated from postcesarean wound infections, similar to those of postpartum endomyometritis. *Staphylococcus aureus* is isolated from postcesarean wound infections in 25% of cases and appears to originate from the skin rather than the endometrium.[148] Early diagnosis is important, and frequent inspection of the cesarean wound and temperature review are paramount.

Prevention of wound infections involves careful preoperative preparation. Preoperative hexachlorophene showers,[149] clipping of abdominal hair rather than shaving,[149,150] liberal application of skin antiseptic agents in the operating room, and use of wound drapes are simple but effective measures to decrease the incidence of wound infection. Sterile technique, attention to hemostasis, obliteration of tissue dead space, and removal of devitalized tissues are important surgical factors that promote appropriate wound healing and prevent wound infection. The use of closed drainage systems is preferable to Penrose-type drains, because the former remain sterile as long as flow continues.

As with any infective process, prompt recognition and treatment are essential. An infected wound is usually characterized by local pain, tenderness, erythema, and purulent discharge, typically becoming clinically evident 4 to 7 days postsurgery. Systemic evidence may also be present with fever and leukocytosis. The early development of a wound infection, usually in association with cellulitis and high spiking fever, is characteristic of group A and group B β-hemolytic streptococcus. Initial treatment involves opening the wound along the affected area to the fascia and culturing the exudate (anaerobic and aerobic). Incision and drainage with debridement of necrotic tissue is vital. Applications of hydrogen peroxide to chemically debride the area should follow initial local surgical efforts. Because antiseptic solutions are cytotoxic, saline lavage must follow their application with the application of wet-to-dry dressings. When all necrotic tissue has been removed and granulation tissue forms, cessation of debriding agents is important and the use of wet-to-wet dressings instituted. The wound may be reapproximated once granulation tissue appears or be left to close by secondary intention. Drainage is usually sufficient, and systemic antibiotics are not indicated for simple wound infections. A serious complication of wound infection is necrotizing fasciitis, a synergistic infection that destroys subcutaneous tissues. Repeated, aggressive debridement is vital in association with broad-spectrum antibiotics and hyperbaric oxygen therapy to achieve cure.

SUGGESTED READINGS

Costantine MM, Rahman M, Ghulmiyah L, et al: Timing of perioperative antibiotics for cesarean delivery: A meta-analysis. Am J Obstet Gynecol 2008;199:310.e1–310.e5.

Dodd JM, Anderson ER, Gates S: Surgical techniques for uterine incision and uterine closure at the time of caesarean section. Cochrane Database Syst Rev 2008;3:CD004732.

Hellums EK, Lin MG, Ramsey PS: Prophylactic subcutaneous drainage for prevention of wound complications after cesarean delivery—A meta analysis. Am J Obstet Gynecol 2007;197:229–235.

Hofmeyr GJ, Mathai M, Shah AN, Novikova N: Techniques for caesarean section (review). Cochrane Database Syst Rev 2008;1:CD004662.

Magann EF, Chauhan SP, Bufkin L, et al: Intra-operative haemorrhage by blunt versus sharp expansion of the uterine incision at caesarean delivery: A randomised clinical trial. BJOG 2002;109:448–452.

McMahon MJ, Luther ER, Bowes WA Jr, Olshan AR: Comparison of a trial of labor with an elective second cesarean section. N Engl J Med 1996;335:689–695.

NIH Consensus State Science Statements. Obstet Gynecol 2006;107:1386–1397.

Rousseau J-A, Girard K, Turcot-Lemay L, Thomas N: A randomized study comparing skin closure in cesarean sections: Staples vs. subcuticular sutures. Am J Obstet Gynecol 2009;200:265.e1–265.e4.

Tita ATN, Rouse DJ, Blackwell S, et al: Emerging concepts in antibiotic prophylaxis for cesarean delivery. Obstet Gynecol 2009;113;675–682.

Tully L, Gates S, Brocklehurst P, et al: Surgical techniques used during caesarean section operations: Results of a national survey of practice in the UK. Eur J Obstet Gynecol Reprod Biol 2002;102:120–126.

REFERENCES

For a complete list of references, log onto www.expertconsult.com.

SECTION SEVEN

Postnatal

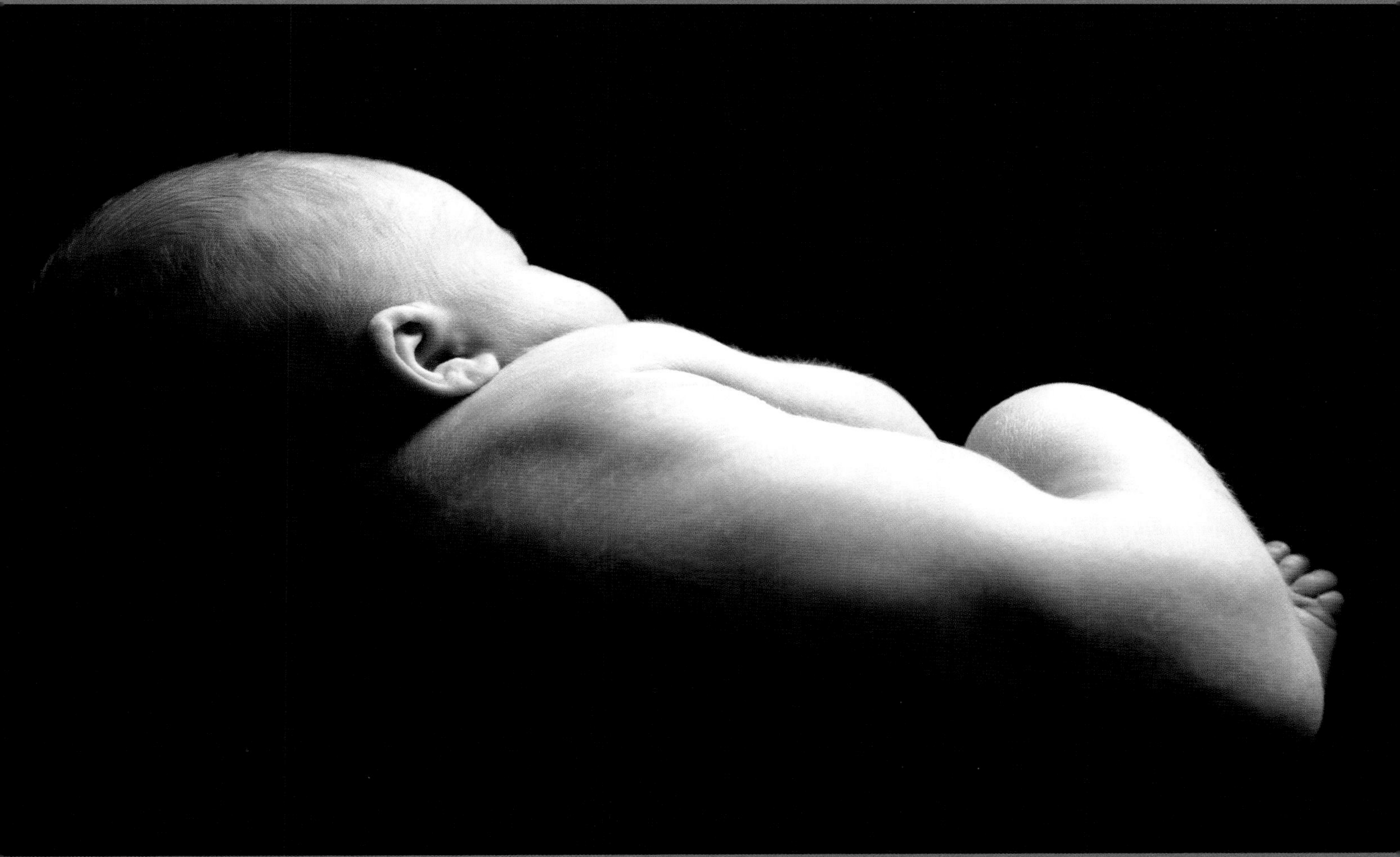

CHAPTER 75

Postpartum Hemorrhage and Other Problems of the Third Stage

MICHAEL A. BELFORT and GARY A. DILDY III

INTRODUCTION

Postpartum hemorrhage (PPH) remains one of the leading causes of maternal death, in both industrialized and nonindustrialized nations. Approximately 140,000 women die annually from PPH worldwide, and more than 50% of these mortalities occur within the first 24 hours postpartum.[1–3] The World Health Organization (WHO) reports that in sub-Saharan Africa, hemorrhage is by far the leading cause of maternal death, accounting for more than a third (35%) of cases in the region and as much as 60% in some individual countries.[4] WHO has also estimated that not only is maternal mortality high but also approximately 20 million mothers per year suffer significant morbidity from PPH.[1,4]

A recent study in the United States showed that 12% of all maternal mortality is due to obstetric hemorrhage, and that obstetric hemorrhage is the third most common cause of death related to pregnancy, after complications of preeclampsia and amniotic fluid embolism[5] (Table 75–1). Review by a group of experienced obstetricians led to the conclusion that the majority (73%) of deaths reported from obstetric hemorrhage could have potentially been prevented by more prompt attention to the clinical signs of bleeding and associated hypovolemia.[5] The recent CEMACH report[6] on maternal deaths in the United Kingdom between 2003 and 2005 showed obstetric hemorrhage to be the third most common cause of death (0.66/100,000 maternities) after thrombosis/thromboembolism and preeclampsia/eclampsia. In this report, 59% of mortality due to hemorrhage was associated with substandard care.

Stafford and colleagues[7] recently reported estimated blood loss (EBL) according to mode of delivery (Fig. 75–1) and degree of perineal laceration (Fig. 75–2) in a cohort of predominantly indigent women delivering at University Hospital in New Orleans.[7,8] There was a progressive increase in EBL with complexity of delivery, and operative vaginal delivery EBL was similar to that in cesarean delivery. As expected, there was a correlation between EBL and degree of perineal laceration, and EBL was similar between vaginal delivery complicated by third-/fourth-degree perineal lacerations and cesarean delivery. There was also noted to be a consistent underestimation in EBL by visual means compared with calculated EBL using a formula with the predelivery and postdelivery hematocrits. Underestimation of EBL is common in obstetric clinical practice and is a consistent factor in late recognition and treatment of hemorrhagic shock.[7]

There is no single accepted definition of "obstetric hemorrhage." PPH is usually defined as a blood loss greater than 500 mL, although detailed measurements of average blood loss in which to all the measured loss is added, including blood eluted from drapes and sponges (using dilute hydrochloric acid and measuring hemoglobin as acid hematin), show that approximately 50% of women will lose this amount during and after their first birth. This has led some to redefine a significant PPH as greater than 1 L. An alternative pragmatic definition is that of continuing hemorrhage despite the "usual treatment." Obstetric hemorrhage is reported to occur in approximately 1 : 200 to 1 : 250 deliveries in developed countries, with a case fatality rate of between 1 : 600 and 1 : 800.[5,6] Although death from obstetric hemorrhage is uncommon in the United Kingdom, it is interesting to note that for every death from obstetric hemorrhage, more than 60 women will have an emergency peripartum hysterectomy to stop bleeding (41/100,000 maternities). Because peripartum hysterectomy represents a reasonable "near-miss" event for maternal mortality, the extent of the problem, even in developed countries, should not be underestimated. Recent reports from Ireland[9] and The Netherlands[10] have highlighted the seriousness of the "near miss" and the importance for close monitoring of such cases in any quality assurance program. Major obstetric hemorrhage was seen in 4.5/1000 deliveries in The Netherlands,[10] and in most cases, substandard care was identified. In the Irish study, a ratio of severe maternal morbidity to maternal mortality of almost 27 : 1 was found, and 77% of the cases of severe maternal morbidity were due to massive obstetric hemorrhage.[9]

THE NORMAL THIRD STAGE OF LABOR

Recognizing the sequence of events in the third stage of labor and understanding the mechanism of placental separation may aid the detection of cases at risk for third-stage complications and the management of pathology.

TABLE 75-1

The Most Common Causes of Maternal Mortality in a Series of 1.5 Million Deliveries within One U.S. Healthcare System between the Years 2000 and 2006

CAUSE OF DEATH	N	%	
Complications of preeclampsia	15	16	
Amniotic fluid embolism	13	14	
Obstetric hemorrhage	11	12	73% are judged preventable
Cardiac disease	10	11	
Pulmonary thromboembolism	9	9	
Nonobstetric infection	7	7	
Obstetric infection	7	7	
Accident/suicide	6	6	
Medication error or reaction	5	5	
Ectopic pregnancy	1	1	
Other	11	12	
Total	**95**	**100**	

From Clark SL, Belfort MA, Dildy GA, et al: Maternal death in the 21st century: Causes, prevention, and relationship to cesarean delivery. Am J Obstet Gynecol 2008;199:36.e1–36.e5.

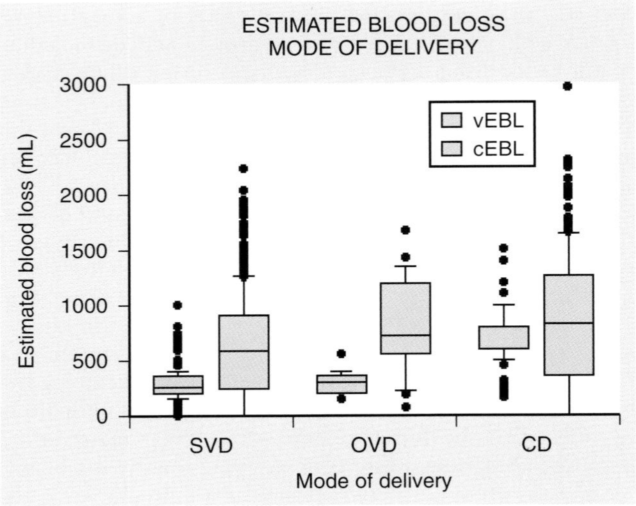

FIGURE 75-1
The relationship between visualized estimated blood loss (vEBL), calculated estimated blood loss (cEBL), and mode of delivery. CD, cesarean delivery; OVD, operative vaginal delivery; SVD, spontaneous vaginal delivery.

Prostaglandin F (PGF), $PGF_{2\alpha}$, and oxytocin are the biochemical agents primarily involved in the third stage of labor. During the first and second stages of labor, only $PGF_{2\alpha}$ and oxytocin are significantly raised in maternal plasma compared with prelabor concentrations. At 5 minutes after birth, maternal PGF and $PGF_{2\alpha}$ concentrations peak at about twice the levels found at the commencement of the second stage. A rapid increase in prostaglandin concentrations is also found in umbilical cord venous blood, suggesting that this postpartum prostaglandin surge originates in the placenta.[11] After placental separation, the concentrations

FIGURE 75-2
The relationship between visualized estimated blood loss (vEBL), calculated estimated blood loss (cEBL), and perineal laceration.

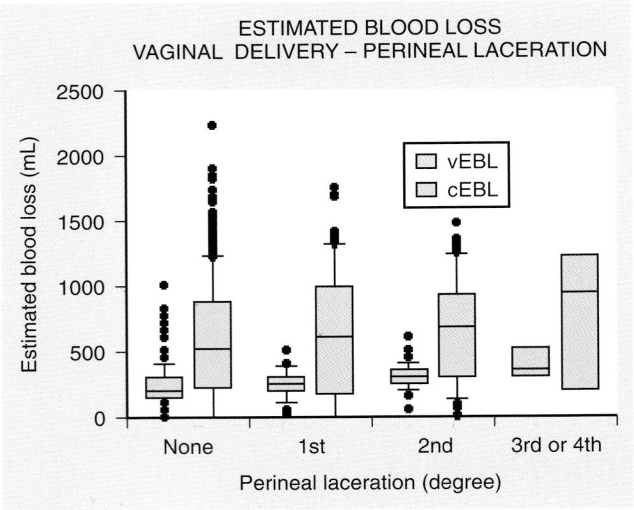

decrease but at rates slower than the metabolic clearance of prostaglandin, indicating that its production continues in the decidua and myometrium. Plasma oxytocin also drops to prelabor levels within 30 minutes of delivery, unless sustained by exogenous infusion.

Continuous real-time ultrasound, performed during the third stage of labor, has revealed that the process of placental separation can be divided into four phases[12] (Table 75–2):

1. **Latent**—uterine wall at the placental site remains thin; placenta free wall contracts.
2. **Contraction**—thickening of uterine wall at the placental site.
3. **Detachment**—actual separation of the placenta from the adjacent uterine wall.
4. **Expulsion**—sliding of the placenta out of the uterine cavity.

Forceful uterine contractions in the latent phase induce shearing forces between the uterine wall and the unyielding placental tissue, initiating the separation of the placenta. A wave of separation begins at one of the placental poles, usually at a point near to the lower segment, and propagates toward the fundus during the contraction and detachment phases.[13] Separation of the fundal placenta begins at more than one of the placental poles, and the central part is last to separate. (This is the reverse of the Schultze and Mathews Duncan mechanisms described in most texts.) In almost half of the cases with a previous cesarean section. the separation pattern was reversed, commencing at the fundus, suggesting that myometrial strength in the region of the uterine scar may have been compromised.[13]

Although spontaneous delivery of the placenta usually occurs within 10 minutes of the baby's birth, the third stage is not considered prolonged unless it lasts more than 30 minutes. Combs and Laros,[14] in an 11-year study of 12,979 consecutive, singleton vaginal deliveries, demonstrated that the duration of the third stage followed a lognormal distribution, with a median of 6 minutes (interquartile range

TABLE 75-2

Summary of Clinical and Ultrasound Findings at Different Stages of Placental Separation and Recommendations for Management

	STAGE OF PLACENTAL SEPARATION			
	FULLY ADHERENT	PARTIALLY SEPARATED	FULLY SEPARATED: TRAPPED	FULLY SEPARATED: NORMAL
Clinical Signs				
Duration third stage		>30 min		<30 min
Uterine fundus	Above umbilicus			Below umbilicus
Uterus	Broad	Broad	Small, contracted	Small, contracted
Cord lengthening	No	No	Sometimes	Yes
Bleeding	No	Yes	Yes	Yes
Ultrasound Appearance				
Myometrium (placental site)	<2 cm thick across entire placental site	<2 cm thick at fundus, >2 cm at lower pole	<2 cm thick at all levels; surrounding placenta	>2 cm thick at all levels; above placenta
Placental position	Upper segment	Upper segment	Upper segment	Lower segment or vagina
Doppler flow (myometrium-placenta)	Present	Absent	Absent	
Management				
Initial: 30-60 min	Expectant	Hemabate 250 μg IM; misoprostol 1000 μg PR	Controlled cord traction; glyceryl trinitrate	Maternal effort; gentle controlled cord traction
>60 min	Umbilical vein uterotonic	Manual removal	Manual removal	
Failed	Methotrexate/hysterectomy	Hysterectomy		

4–10 min). The prevalence of a third stage in excess of 30 minutes was 3.3%. Although stating that prophylactic oxytocic agents were not used routinely, their figures for duration are remarkably similar to those from the much larger series (45,869 singleton vaginal deliveries) reported by Dombrowski and coworkers,[15] who estimated that using active management of the third stage, 90% of term placentas will deliver spontaneously by 15 minutes and only 2.2% will be undelivered at 30 minutes. The incidence of prolonged third stage associated with different uterotonic agents has been reported[16–18] as follows:

- Oxytocin (Pitocin, Syntocinon): 1.4% to 1.8%.
- Oxytocin/ergometrine (Syntometrine): 1.6% to 2.8%.
- Misoprostol (Cytotec): 1.4%.

Management Options

There are markedly polarized views between those who believe in active management and those who believe in expectant (natural) management of the third stage.

Active management of the third stage includes

- Administration of a prophylactic oxytocic agent or prostaglandin within 2 minutes of the baby's birth to induce uterine contraction.
- Immediate cutting and clamping of the cord to enhance placental separation.
- Placental delivery by controlled cord traction.

In expectant management, there is

- No prophylactic oxytocic.
- No cord clamping until pulsations cease.
- Delivery of placenta by maternal effort and gravity rather than cord traction.

Use of Prophylactic Uterotonic Agents

There no longer appears to be any valid argument in favor of the physiologic approach, because two substantive studies comparing active management with expectant management have clearly indicated the advantages of active management. The Bristol trial,[19] in which active management had been the norm, and the Hinchingbrooke trial,[20] in which expectant management had been the norm, both demonstrated significant reductions in the incidence of PPH with active management compared with expectant management (5.9% vs. 17.9% and 6.8% vs. 16.5%, respectively). Both studies were terminated after interim analysis because the difference in PPH rates was so great.

Which Uterotonic Agent?

In recent years, considerable attention has been paid to the choice of uterotonic agent, in particular comparing the cheap and orally administered prostaglandin misoprostol with the combination agent Syntometrine (oxytocin/ergonovine, which is used in much of Europe and Africa but is not available in North America). The findings seem to indicate that rectal misoprostol is a viable alternative to oxytocin in areas in which storage and parenteral administration of drugs are problems (oxytocin has to be stored at 4°C to retain its efficacy, whereas tablets of misoprostol kept dry retain their efficacy even at tropical temperatures for several years or more),[21] but its side effects (shivering, pyrexia, nausea, and diarrhea) and slightly lower efficacy make it unsuitable for routine prophylaxis against PPH. Oxytocin (Pitocin) or oxytocin combined with ergometrine (Syntometrine), therefore, remain the preferred drugs for routine use in developed countries. Some trials have suggested that oxytocin alone is as efficacious as Syntometrine, whereas others have reported that it is not as effective. Intravenous ergometrine is associated with an increase in the incidence of retained placenta, possibly as a result of myometrial spasm distal to a fundally placed placenta leading to its forced retention, and should not be the agent of choice for routine administration.[22] Ergometrine also causes peripheral vasoconstriction and a rise in blood pressure and should be given only with caution, if at all, to women with hypertension. Contraindications to ergometrine include heart disease, autoimmune diseases associated with vasospasm and Raynaud's phenomenon, peripheral vascular disease (such as with severe diabetes), arteriovenous shunts even if they have been surgically corrected, and preeclampsia/eclampsia. Oxytocin, conversely, when given as an acute bolus, can cause a marked drop in blood pressure. Caution should, therefore, be exercised when giving oxytocin to women with cardiovascular problems, and a continuing low-dose infusion is probably preferable to bolus injection.

The active and passive management approaches represent the two extremes of the spectrum of common practice. Although the randomized, controlled trials performed to date have only compared these two approaches, the benefits of early cord clamping and controlled cord traction in the prevention of PPH have not been established separately from the use of prophylactic uterotonic agents. It is from these two aspects that most criticisms of active management arise.

Timing of Cord Clamping

The umbilical cord can be clamped immediately after birth, clamped after pulsations cease, or left unclamped. The cord may need to be clamped before birth if there is tight nuchal entanglement. Although early clamping of the cord has been reported to be associated with significant shortening of the third stage, this has been demonstrated only in trials in which no prophylactic oxytocin was given.[23,24] The difference in the effects of early versus late cord clamping on the neonate are relatively minor, and opinions differ as to their relative risks and benefits. The deferral of cord clamping until 3 minutes after birth results in a neonatal transfusion of about 80 mL of blood from the placenta.[25] This contributes about 50 mg of iron, which may reduce the frequency of iron-deficiency anemia later in childhood.[26] The theoretical downsides of this blood transfusion are hypervolemia, polycythemia, hyperviscosity, and hyperbilirubinemia. In practice, however, these have not been found to produce a clinically relevant increase in neonatal morbidity.[27]

The WHO review of evidence on management of the third stage concludes that there is no clear evidence to favor one practice over the other. Delaying cord clamping until the pulsations stop is the physiologic way of treating the cord and is not associated with adverse effects, at least in normal deliveries. Early cord clamping conflicts with traditional beliefs and is an intervention that needs justification.[28] In preterm infants, delay in cord clamping has demonstrable benefits and has been shown to decrease the need for blood ($P < .001$) and albumin ($P < .03$) transfusions during the first 24 hours of life.[29]

Controlled Cord Traction

The use of cord traction has a long history, with the earliest records dating back to Aristotle. Simple cord traction was displaced in the 1800s by the introduction of the Credé maneuver.[30] In this maneuver, the placenta is expelled by downward pressure on the fundus of the uterus in the direction of the birth canal, with the thumb placed on the posterior surface and the flat of the hand on the anterior surface of the fundus. This was proposed as an alternative means to manual removal for expelling the retained placenta and was found to avoid the uterine inversion that was occasionally associated with cord traction. Brandt in 1933 and Andrews in 1940 independently introduced similar methods to improve the use of cord traction to deliver the retained placenta. These involved traction on the cord with countertraction applied to the uterus abdominally. It was not until the 1960s, however, that the modern technique known as *controlled cord traction* was introduced by Spencer,[31] accompanied by the routine administration of ergonovine.

The current consensus is that when traction is applied to the umbilical cord, it should be done only during a uterine contraction while controlling the uterus by Brandt-Andrews maneuver to prevent uterine inversion. However, it should be noted that the benefits of both early cord clamping and the use of routine controlled cord traction to prevent PPH have not as yet been supported by evidence from randomized, controlled trials.

SUMMARY OF MANAGEMENT OPTIONS

Normal Third Stage of Labor

Management Options	Evidence Quality and Recommendation	References
Active management of third stage is advised for all women, and includes all of the following:	Ia/A	19,20
• Administer oxytocic agent (oxytocin [Pitocin] or oxytocin and ergometrine [Syntometrine]).	Ib/A	19,20
• Clamp and cut cord.	—/GPP	—
• Use controlled cord traction (no randomized, controlled data to show it reduces PPH rates of itself).	III/B	31

Management Options	Evidence Quality and Recommendation	References
Timing of Cord Clamping		
• No evidence to indicate optimum timing in term delivery.	Ia/A	28
• In preterm infants, delay in clamping may be of benefit.	III/B	29
Ensure intravenous access for women at risk.	—/GPP	—
Save serum for rapid cross-match if needed, or actually cross-match 2 units, for women at risk.	—/GPP	—

GPP, good practice point; PPH, postpartum hemorrhage.

RETAINED PLACENTA

Diagnosis and Definition

Using a diagnostic cutoff of 30 minutes for a prolonged third stage, 42% of retained placentas deliver spontaneously within the next 30 minutes,[32] with very few delivering spontaneously after 1 hour.[33] Because the incidence of significant PPH rises after 30 minutes in the third stage,[14] active intervention to deliver the placenta between 30 and 60 minutes into the third stage is advised. Dombrowski and coworkers[15] noted that compared with term pregnancies, the frequency of retained placenta (2.0% overall) was markedly increased among very preterm (gestation < 27 wk) and preterm pregnancies (gestation < 37 wk), with odds ratios of 20.8 and 3.0, respectively.

Management Options

Manual removal appears to be the management of choice for retained placenta (Fig. 75–3). However, it is associated with a risk of infection (endometritis) and trauma (perforation of the uterine wall). Ely and associates,[34] in a retrospective study of 1052 manual removals, found that clinical endometritis developed in 6.7% of cases compared with only 1.8% following spontaneous placental delivery.

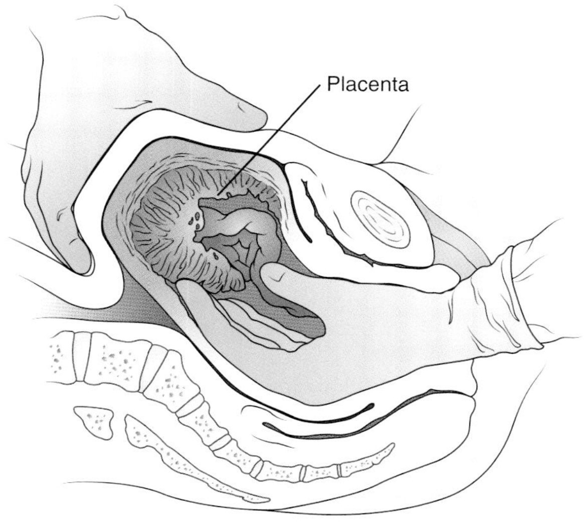

FIGURE 75–3
Manual removal of placenta. The fingers are moved from side to side until the placenta is completely detached.
(Reproduced from Cunningham FG, MacDonald PC, Gant NF [eds]: Abnormalities of labor and delivery: Abnormalities of the 3rd stage of labor. In: Williams Obstetrics, 18th ed. Norwalk, CT, Appleton & Lange, 1989.)

In some studies, manual removal appears to be aggressively pursued, with rates exceeding 3% and often performed only 15 to 20 minutes into the third stage. The rate generally quoted internationally is 1% to 2%.[33]

In the absence of hemorrhage, there is no urgency to resort to manual removal when less invasive alternatives are available. In addition, consideration of the potential for placenta accreta or percreta should always precede the attempt, and if there is any real potential for a morbidly adherent placenta, preparations to deal with complications such as major hemorrhage should be in place before going ahead with manual removal.

Patients with a prolonged third stage are often treated as a homogeneous group, although they have different clinical conditions. These include the retention of an already detached placenta (trapped placenta), an adherent placenta, and placenta accreta. Each condition should be distinguished from the others, and each requires a specific clinical approach. Herman[35] noted that each of these conditions is associated with a different sonographic appearance and concluded that "proper utilization of ultrasound may be crucial for optimal management."

Trapped Placenta

Trapped placenta often follows the intravenous administration of ergometrine when the onset of uterine contraction is very rapid. This tends to close the cervix at the same time as placental detachment occurs, trapping the placenta. Intramuscular injection of ergometrine results in the onset of uterine contraction in 10 minutes, which is likely to follow rather than precede placental separation, so trapped placenta is less likely to occur. The clinical findings of a trapped placenta include a small, contracted fundus, with some vaginal bleeding and cord lengthening indicative of placental separation, and the placental margin may be palpable through the closed cervical os. On ultrasound examination, the entire myometrium is thickened and a clear demarcation may be seen between it and the placenta.[12]

Delivery of a trapped placenta can usually be achieved using controlled cord traction, which encourages cervical dilation. Intravenous glyceryl trinitrate (100–200 μg) is useful as a short-term tocolytic agent, appears efficacious and safe, and may obviate the need for general anesthesia for uterine relaxation.[36] Releasing the cord clamp, to allow blood trapped in the placenta to drain, may also help.

Adherent Placenta

With an adherent placenta, the uterine fundus remains broad and high and myometrial contractions may be weak or absent, but there is no bleeding while the placenta remains wholly attached. Adherent placenta is caused by a deficiency in the contractile force exerted by the myometrium underlying the placental site despite normal anatomy (i.e., it is not caused by pathologic invasion of the placenta into the uterine muscle, known as *placenta accreta*). On ultrasound, the myometrium appears thick and contracted in all areas, except where the placenta remains attached, and the uterine wall remains less than 2 cm in thickness.[12] If the placenta becomes partly separated, the myometrium over the detached area appears thicker, but that underlying the adherent part remains thin (<2 cm).[12] Detachment usually starts in the lower part of the uterus and is associated with bleeding from the placental bed.[13] Treatment options depend on the amount of bleeding:

- In the absence of bleeding, a conservative approach can be adopted and manual removal of the placenta can be postponed while the problem is investigated (by ultrasound).
- When there is active bleeding, immediate active management is necessary.

Effective treatment of the adherent placenta is based on stimulating a contraction of the underlying myometrium that has sufficient strength to induce separation of the placenta. Oxytocin, ergonovine, and misoprostol are all capable of inducing sustained myometrial contractions. However, there is no evidence that systemic and repeated administration of either oxytocics or prostaglandins is able to assist in the delivery of the adherent placenta.

Recent studies have shown that uterotonic agents administered via umbilical vein injection may be effective in causing the adherent placenta to separate,[37] and this method is currently recommended as the first line of treatment by the WHO.[38]

The Pipingas technique has been shown to be effective in delivering drugs to the placental bed.[39] A size 10 nasogastric tube is passed along the umbilical vein until resistance is felt, then retracted about 5 cm, and $PGF_{2\alpha}$ (20 mg diluted in 20 mL of normal saline) or oxytocin (30 IU diluted in 20 mL of normal saline) is injected through the catheter.[40] Alternatively, a solution of misoprostol may be used.[41]

SUMMARY OF MANAGEMENT OPTIONS

Retained Placenta

Management Options	Evidence Quality and Recommendation	References
Retained placenta should be diagnosed if it is not delivered within 30–60 min.	III/B	14,32,33
Trapped Placenta		
• Perform ultrasound to confirm separation.	III/B	12
• Use controlled cord traction with a short-acting tocolytic such as glyceryl (trinitrate).	III/B	36
Adherent Placenta		
• If there is active bleeding, manual removal is necessary.	—/GPP	—
• If there is no active bleeding, consider intraumbilical uterotonic agents before resorting to manual removal.	III/B	37–39

GPP, good practice point.

ADHERENT PLACENTA (PLACENTA ACCRETA, INCRETA, PERCRETA)

Placenta accreta is a condition in which all or part of the placenta is adherent to the uterine wall because of myometrial invasion by chorionic villi. It may occur when there is either a primary deficiency of or secondary damage to the decidua basalis and Nitabuch's layer.[42] Abnormal trophoblast invasion has been associated with up-regulation of vascular endothelial growth factor (VEGF) and angiopoietin-2 and down-regulation of VEGF-receptor (VEGF-R) and Tie-2.[43]

Three grades are defined according to the depth of myometrial invasion:

- **Accreta**—chorionic villi are in contact with the myometrium, rather than being contained within the decidua (80% of cases).
- **Increta**—extensive villous invasion into the myometrium (15% of cases).
- **Percreta**—villous invasion extends to (or through) the serosal covering of the uterus (5% of cases).

Factors associated with a higher incidence of accreta include multiparity, prior uterine surgery (e.g., myomectomy), advanced maternal age, placenta previa, prior uterine curettage, and previous cesarean delivery.[42,44,45] Uterine irradiation for intra-abdominal cancer therapy has also been identified as a risk factor for percreta.[46] Placenta percreta has been reported to occur after endometrial ablation.[47] Placenta

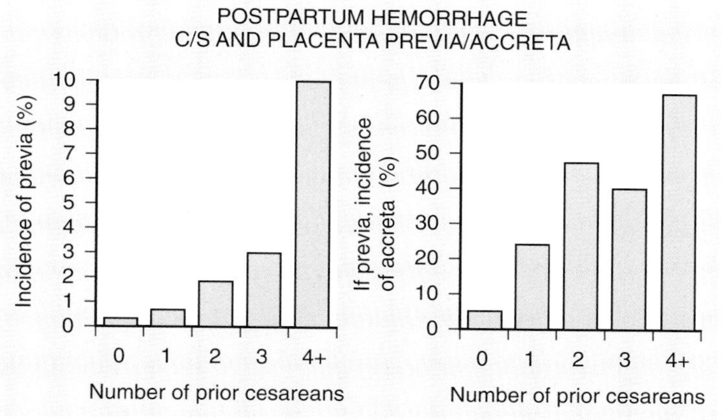

FIGURE 75–4
The relationship between the number of prior cesareans and placenta previa (*left*), and if placenta previa, the risk of placenta accreta (*right*). (From Clark SL, Koonings PP, Phelan JP: Placenta previa/accreta and prior cesarean section. Obstet Gynecol 1985:66:89-92.)

accreta rarely complicates vaginal delivery, with an incidence of only 1 in 22,000 in the absence of placenta previa.[48] Rarely, abnormal attachment is seen in the absence of prior surgery (e.g., associated with Asherman's syndrome and submucous fibroids). Interestingly, the adherence is not necessarily over the site of the previous scar. Placenta percreta has also been reported in pregnancy with a noncommunicating rudimentary uterine horn, and patients with a known uterine anomaly of this type should be counseled about the potential for such a complication.[49]

The reported incidence of placenta accreta has increased from 1:2510 in the 1980s, to 1:533 in 2002, to 1:210 in 2006, and this is most likely related to increasing cesarean delivery rates.[44,45,50,51] Clark and coworkers[45] showed an almost linear increase in the incidence of placenta previa with repeat cesarean section with a rate of approximately 10% in women with four prior cesarean sections (Fig. 75–4). This group also showed that placenta previa in the face of prior cesarean section significantly increased the risk of morbid adherence of the placenta. Several studies have found a direct relationship between the number of prior uterine incisions and the subsequent occurrence of placenta accreta, with reports of a twofold increased risk of accreta with one prior cesarean delivery.[44] In a Maternal-Fetal Medicine Units Network study evaluating over 30,000 cesarean deliveries and associated comorbidities, women having their fourth or additional cesarean delivery had a 9- to 30-fold increased risk of placenta accreta.[51] The risk of accreta in women with a placenta previa and a prior cesarean section increased from 3% with one previous cesarean section, to 11%, 40%, 61%, and 67% with two, three, four, or more repeat cesarean sections, respectively.

There has been particular concern about the risk for accreta in women with a prior cesarean section scar and an anterior or low-lying anterior placenta. Twickler and colleagues[52] specifically addressed this issue using data from 653 patients with a previous cesarean section. In their cohort, there were 152 patients who had an anterior placenta and 43 with an anterior low-lying placenta. None of these patients had an accreta. Of the 20 patients with a previous cesarean section scar who were diagnosed with placenta previa, however, 9 had a placenta accreta (45%) and 15 required cesarean hysterectomy for uncontrolled bleeding (75%).

In patients with a placenta previa and a prior cesarean section, accreta is much more common when the previa is anterior or central and overlies the scar (29%) than when it is lateral or posterior and does not contact the scar (6.5%).[48]

The majority of cases of morbidly adherent placenta present as accreta. Approximately 5% present as percreta with surrounding organ involvement. In these patients, intra-abdominal bleeding, hematuria, or bladder symptoms may be present. With the presence of coexisting placenta previa, antepartum hemorrhage rates approach 30% and are more likely to result in preterm delivery secondary to hemorrhage.

All three grades of placenta accreta can result in profuse PPH owing to incomplete separation of the placenta. Being alert to this possibility is essential in patients who have a combination of placenta previa and a history of previous uterine surgery. If the diagnosis of placenta accreta is suggested on ultrasound or magnetic resonance imaging (MRI), plans for delivery by cesarean section by a surgeon experienced in dealing with such cases, and in a facility in which resuscitation and intensive care are available, should be made. Placenta percreta still represents one of the highest-risk complications of pregnancy, and despite our best efforts, there remains a 7% mortality rate even when 50% of patients treated for this condition are recognized as having it preoperatively.[53]

Diagnosis

The antepartum diagnosis of placenta accreta/percreta is usually accomplished using ultrasound[54–57] (Fig. 75–5) or MRI.[58] Sonographic criteria are summarized in Table 75–3. Although the addition of color Doppler ultrasound may enhance visualization of vascular lacunae, it has not been shown to improve the sensitivity of detection of accreta.[52,54] Loss of the hypoechoic zone, especially in the third trimester, has proved to be less useful than the other criteria and has also been shown to be less specific.[57] Twickler and colleagues[52] reported that two specific ultrasound criteria were predictive of accreta: (1) Myometrial thickness less than 1 mm and (2) large intraplacental blood lakes. If both of these findings were present, the sensitivity for placenta accreta was 100%, the specificity was 72%, the positive predictive value (PPV) was 72% and the negative predictive

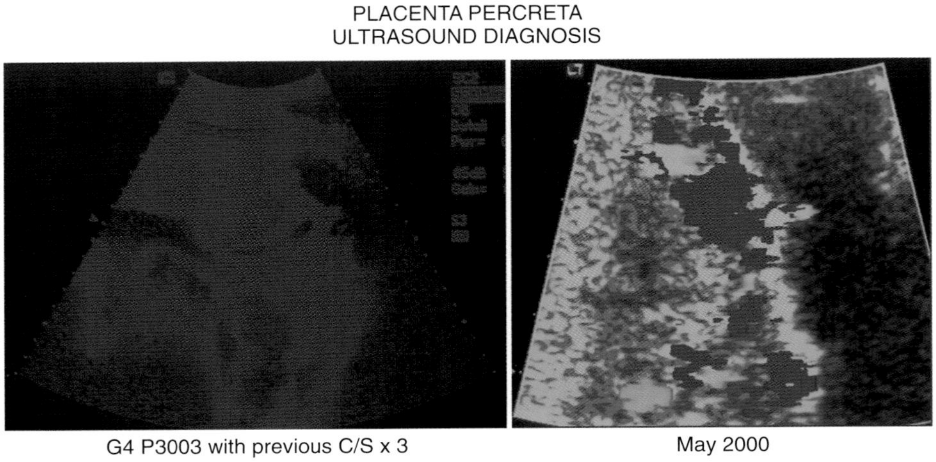

FIGURE 75–5
A gravida 4 with three prior cesareans presented in the third trimester with vaginal bleeding. Ultrasound (*left*) shows a mid-sagittal view of the lower uterine segment, with thickened placenta, large vascular lakes, and irregular areas at the placental-myometrial interface. Color Doppler ultrasound (*right*) shows vascular projections into the bladder wall and lumen, suggesting placenta percreta.

TABLE 75–3
Sonographic Assessment of Placenta Percreta

1. Loss of the normal hypoechoic retroplacental myometrial zone (clear space)[43,50]
2. Thinning or disruption of the hyperechoic uterine serosa-bladder interface[44]
3. Blood vessels crossing the regions of interface disruption[55]
4. Myometrial thickness of < 1 mm[52]
5. Presence of vessels bridging the uterine-placental margin[55]
6. Visualization of placental lacunae (defined as multiple linear, irregular vascular spaces) within the placenta, which gives the placenta a "Swiss cheese" appearance
7. Focal nodular projections into the bladder beyond the expected uterine-bladder interface[56]
8. Color Doppler ultrasound enhancement of vascular lacunae[52-54]

value (NPV) was 100%. The sensitivity and specificity of these findings for hysterectomy was 80%, PPV was 92%, and NPV was 57%. Others have suggested that disruption of the placental–uterine wall interface and the presence of vessels crossing these areas of disruption are the only two criteria of real predictive value. Because of concerns about the capability of the individual ultrasound criteria for distinguishing accreta from nonaccreta, Wong and associates[55] have developed a composite scoring system for ultrasound criteria that they report to be 89% sensitive and 98% specific for the diagnosis.[55]

The use of MRI for assessing placental invasion has yielded conflicting results.[54,58] The addition of gadolinium-based contrast agents seems to improve the specificity of this modality, but most radiologists are unwilling to use gadolinium in pregnancy for fear of fetal effects. MRI should be considered in cases in which sonographic evaluation is inconclusive and there is a concern about invasion of trophoblast into surrounding organs and tissue, especially if parametrial or posterior invasion is suspected.[54,59] MRI information in such cases will help with operative planning. Routine MRI scanning of all patients with sonographic evidence of accreta has not been shown to affect the management of the pregnancy unless there is concern for percreta. Other diagnostic modalities that have been used to obtain a conclusive diagnosis in cases of suspected percreta include cystoscopy, sigmoidoscopy, and laparoscopy.[53]

Although most studies describe sonographic detection techniques in the second and third trimester, abnormal placental adherence has been identified as early as the first trimester. In these cases, the presence of a low-lying gestational sac in close proximity to the hysterotomy scar has been linked to massive bleeding with dilation and curettage or cesarean hysterectomy in the second and third trimester.[60,61] One third of these gestations ended with early fetal demise.[53]

Laboratory Tests

Abnormally elevated second-trimester serum α-fetoprotein has been associated with placenta percreta, and it has been suggested that there is a direct relationship between the extent of invasion and the elevation of this analyte.[53,62] Creatine kinase has also been reported as a marker for increta and percreta.[63]

Management Options

The management of the morbidly adherent placenta can be divided into two specific, and very different, categories: (1) The suspected placenta accrete/percreta and (2) the unsuspected placenta accrete/percreta discovered at the time of delivery or at emergency presentation for sudden onset of obstetric hemorrhage. These represent two very different situations. With a known placenta accreta/percreta, there is almost always time to make arrangements for the best possible circumstances for controlled delivery and management of potential hemorrhage. In an unsuspected placenta accreta, there is often very little time to prepare the patient for controlled surgery, and frequently, the massive hemorrhage is already under way at the time of diagnosis. Both of these situations are dealt with later. Although even under the best of circumstances, planned cesarean hysterectomy still carries a significant maternal mortality rate,[53] the great majority of the mortality associated with placenta accreta/percreta occurs in the previously unrecognized case in which potentially avoidable actions result in uncontrollable bleeding. In many cases of previously unknown accrete/percreta, a heightened awareness of the potential for accreta/percreta, recognition of the signs of abnormal placentation at the time of surgery or vaginal delivery, total avoidance (or cessation if necessary) of any attempts to deliver the placenta if there is concern about accrete/percreta, attention to the hemodynamic status of the patient and aggressive resuscitation with early blood product administration, early recourse to definitive surgery, adjustments to the surgical techniques, and the team approach to the problem can all be life-saving and may limit the sequelae of massive hemorrhage in those who survive.

Known Placenta Accreta/Percreta

PREOPERATIVE CONSIDERATIONS

Patient and Family Counseling

Once the diagnosis is established, the treatment options and potential complications should be clearly discussed with the patient and the discussion should be documented in detail. The patient should be counseled regarding the increased risk of maternal death, the almost certain need for hysterectomy and blood transfusion, and the risk of unilateral or bilateral oophorectomy during the surgery. Unilateral oophorectomy is necessary in up to 10% of cases because of persistent bleeding. The patient should also understand the increased risks of (1) organ damage (particularly renal and cerebral) from hypotension, (2) bowel, bladder, and ureteric damage from the surgery, and the increased postoperative risks of (3) infection, (4) thromboembolism, (5) reoperation for persistent bleeding, and (6) iatrogenic complications from interventional radiology procedures that may be required to stop uncontrolled hemorrhage. The appropriate location and timing of delivery should be addressed to optimize the logistics of the support facilities and personnel.

Multidisciplinary Team Approach

Cesarean hysterectomy for placenta percreta is best managed by a dedicated and practiced team of clinicians and support personnel. These include the services mentioned in the following paragraphs:

Blood Transfusion Service Preoperative consultation with blood bank personnel is essential because of the likelihood of massive transfusion. Patients undergoing cesarean hysterectomy have an average intraoperative blood loss of 3000 to 5000 mL.[64–66] Placenta percreta cases will often require more blood products than the average hospital blood bank has in stock; when a patient has a rare blood type or antibodies, this issue becomes even more important. Elective surgery may require delay until additional units of blood can be located and transported to the blood bank. With a known placenta percreta case when massive hemorrhage is expected and highly likely, it is recommended that adequate amounts of packed red blood cells (PRBCs), fresh frozen plasma (FFP), platelets, and cryoprecipitate should be available to prevent (or treat) coagulopathy.[64] The definition of adequate is difficult to codify but, based on military surgical experience with massive trauma/hemorrhage (in which a set protocol for massive hemorrhage has been developed), one standardized protocol includes 6 U of PRBCs, 6 U FFP, 6 packs of platelets, and 10 U cryoprecipitate in separate coolers.[67] It is also advisable to have recombinant Factor VIIa (rFVIIa) in the operating room (OR) at the time of the surgery (see later discussion). In select stable preoperative patients, erythropoietin administration with total-dose iron infusion may be used to correct anemia and maximize iron stores prior to surgery. The expected rise in hematocrit levels will be apparent within 2 weeks.[64]

Preoperative hemodilution has been described as a technique to minimize blood loss in patients who refuse blood transfusion,[68] and in such cases, as many as 3 units of blood can safely be removed immediately prior to surgery and replaced with crystalloid. This reduces the hematocrit and limits the red cell mass lost at the time of surgery. The blood removed before surgery is then transfused back during or after the procedure.

Cell Saver (Autotransfusion) The use of the Cell Saver has been somewhat limited in obstetrics because of a concern that the autotranfusion of fetal cellular debris and amniotic fluid may lead to amniotic fluid embolism. The rigorous washing and filtering techniques used in modern Cell Saver machines have made this concern largely theoretical. Fetal red blood cells may still be present in the final product (range 0.13%–4.35%), and in the case of an Rh-negative patient, there is a risk of alloimmunization (which is mainly a concern if she retains her fertility). There is now a growing body of evidence that there is little or no possibility for amniotic fluid contaminants to enter the re-infusion system when used in conjunction with a leukodepletion filter.[69] When used, we recommend double washing of the recovered blood, which should be collected only after double irrigation of abdominal cavity following delivery to remove as much fetal/placental/amniotic debris as possible. Attention should also be paid to the volume of re-infused washed PRBCs to ensure that adequate FFP, cryoprecipitate, and platelets are given with the Cell Saver blood because of the lack of these products in the reconstituted red cells. Although transfusing washed red cells will increase the hematocrit, unless FFP and platelets are transfused simultaneously, there will be a risk of dilutional coagulopathy.

Anesthesiology Preoperative anesthesia consultation is essential to allow appropriate planning and allocation of personnel. Anesthetic considerations include the need for general endotracheal anesthesia in anticipation of prolonged surgical time, consideration of a lumbothoracic epidural catheter for postpartum pain relief, and readiness for massive blood and blood product transfusion. OR temperature control is important, as is patient temperature regulation with warming blankets and forced-air heating devices. The anesthesia service will be primarily responsible during the surgery for preventing the deadly triad of hypovolemia, hypothermia, and acidosis that increases the risk for coagulopathy. If hypothermia occurs in the face of coagulopathy, reversal of the coagulation disorder is often extremely difficult.

Shock trauma fluid infusion devices capable of high flow rate transfusion of blood products, adequate central venous access (bilateral central line sheaths with quadruple catheter capability), arterial line placement, and multiple suction devices should all be part of the anesthesia preparation. In addition, thromboembolism prophylaxis should also be considered and initiated before surgery. Compression stockings placed before induction of anesthesia, lower limb and foot compression/pulsation devices, and prophylactic unfractionated heparin are also accepted prophylactic maneuvers.[64] We have found that on-site blood testing with a portable device that allows rapid bedside assessment of hematocrit, platelets, electrolytes, blood gases, and coagulation function is extremely helpful and enables the anesthesia team to begin transfusion in a timely manner, as well as to monitor the effects of their interventions more efficiently. If practical, we suggest allocating a member of the team to documenting hematocrit, platelet count, blood gases, and coagulation function in a spreadsheet on a regular basis (every 15–30 min or as required). This strategy helps keep the team aware of trends and the need for changes in strategy before equilibrium becomes too displaced.

Urologic Preparation Bladder involvement is extremely common in anterior placenta previa with accreta/percreta, and in such cases, there is frequently hypervascularity and distortion of the ureterovesical junction. In such cases, preoperative cystoscopy and placement of ureteric stents allow palpation of the ureters during difficult and often obscured surgery and are very reassuring and, certainly, in our experience, shortens the procedure. In addition, the cystoscopy will warn of any potential need for re-implantation of the ureters, allowing preemptive changes in operative strategy and preparation. In those cases in which there is obvious penetration of the trophoblast into the bladder wall, it is helpful to create an intentional cystotomy in an uninvolved area of the bladder to visualize directly the area of invasion. This allows for a better appreciation of the extent of bladder invasion and assists in the protection of the trigone and ureterovesical junction. Another benefit is that it allows the surgeon to excise that portion of the bladder involved in the percreta under direct vision without the risk of inadvertently increasing the hemorrhage during blind dissection of percreta tissue. In our experience, sacrificing a nonessential portion of the bladder is not associated with long-term complications, speeds up the surgery, and significantly reduces intraoperative blood loss.

Prophylactic Internal Iliac Artery Balloon Catheters Preoperative pelvic artery occlusion has been proposed as an adjunct to minimize blood loss at the time of hysterectomy.[70] We and others[71] have determined that preoperative placement of balloon catheters in the internal iliac arteries has not proved useful and we no longer use this technique. We feel that inflation of the balloons after delivery may actually complicate the hysterectomy by opening up collateral vessels deeper in the pelvis that are more difficult to control than the immediate branches of the internal iliac artery. We have not noted any significant benefit to preoperative balloon catheter placement and suggest that, if necessary, intraoperative internal iliac artery ligation may be preferable. The placement of balloon catheters may also add to the complexity of the surgery and can potentially result in significant complications such as insertion site hematoma, abscess formation, and tissue infarction and necrosis.

Surgery Gynecologic oncology, urology, and general and vascular surgery consultants should be recruited as necessary for assistance in cases of placenta accreta/percreta. These specialists are invaluable when major pelvic vessel, lateral pelvic sidewall, bladder, or bowel invasion has occurred. The nursing staff in the OR should be fully informed of their expected surgical needs, and all consultants should be questioned as to their particular instrument and equipment requirements so that these things are available in the OR before they are needed. We have found that a slide presentation about placenta percreta (with mention of the specific details of the case to be performed) for the involved OR staff, blood bank personnel, and the providers from all involved services a few days before the surgery is an excellent forum in which questions and concerns can be aired. It also allows the people involved to perceive themselves as a team with a common purpose.

Neonatology Most planned cases of cesarean hysterectomy will be performed between 34 and 37 weeks' gestation, and for this reason, it is prudent to have adequate neonatal personnel present to deal with the specific issues of prematurity. If delivery appears likely prior to 34 weeks (e.g., antenatal vaginal bleeding), glucocorticoid prophylaxis to reduce the risk of respiratory distress syndrome should be considered. In addition, the neonatologist should be prepared for emergency resuscitation of the neonate in the event that profound maternal hemorrhage occurs before delivery of the baby. In most cases, this will not be an issue because the surgery is specifically planned to avoid uterine entry anywhere near the placenta. Occasionally, when antenatal hemorrhage precipitates an emergency delivery, fetal hemorrhage can occur, resulting in fetal anemia. In elective cases, the most frequent issues the neonatology team will need to deal with are prematurity and the effects of general anesthesia.

Intraoperative Management

We have found that the patient is best placed in a low lithotomy position for the surgery. This allows ureteric stent placement, access to the maternal vagina after delivery of the baby for placement of a vaginal pack, and space for an assistant to stand between the mother's legs. The patient should be prepared and draped from the chest to the groin, including the vulva and vagina.

Entry into the abdomen is best via a vertical skin incision (median or paramedian) dependent on the site of placental invasion. In cases in which the placenta has invaded the anterior abdominal wall, intraoperative ultrasound may be used to avoid placental disruption during entry into the abdomen.

Once within the abdomen, signs of increta/percreta include visualization of a distorted, hypervascular lower uterine segment with extremely dilated and often tortuous and abnormal vessels in the broad ligament. In unruptured cases, the lower segment of the uterus is usually bulbous and distended with areas of extremely thinned out uterine wall and, in places, placental tissue visible under a single layer of visceral peritoneum (Fig. 75–6). Frequently, small hematomas and dilated vessels are visible. If the bladder is involved, it will usually be pulled up against the lower uterine segment with large blood vessels traversing from the pelvic side walls. It is essential to avoid disturbing the placenta during delivery of the baby and a vertical upper segment uterine incision (fundal or posterior classic) is recommended. The site of the

FIGURE 75–6
Placenta percreta with bladder invasion, prehysterotomy.

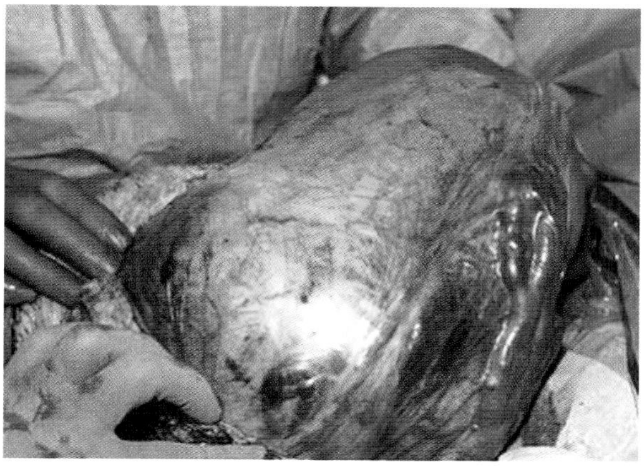

incision can be planned before delivery by mapping the placental site with ultrasound. To confirm the appropriate site for incision, intraoperative ultrasound can be used, with the ultrasound transducer in a sterile sleeve so that scanning can be done directly on the uterus. If the placenta is anterior and extensive, the incision may need to be made in the posterior wall of the uterus. This requires complete exteriorization of the uterus with the fetus in situ (see Fig. 75–6) and the abdominal incision should be planned to allow this option. It is important to minimize the chances of inadvertent partial placental separation or placental disruption before the major supplying vessels are ligated and the uterus is devascularized; partial separation and bleeding will convert a controlled case into an emergency situation.

After delivery of the fetus, no attempts should be made to remove the placenta manually. The umbilical cord should be tied off and replaced within the uterus. Uterotonics can be given (an infusion of Syntocinon, or rectal misoprostol 1000 μg). If it is not certain that the placenta is accreta, then the uterus can be observed to see whether a spontaneous separation of the placenta will take place without excessive bleeding. If there is no separation, significant bleeding starts, or the diagnosis of accreta is already confirmed, the uterus should be closed in a single layer with a locked suture. We then infiltrate the uterus with 15-methyl-$PGF_{2\alpha}$ (250 μg carboprost tromethamine [Hemabate] in 20 mL saline) given through a 22-gauge spinal needle in multiple areas to facilitate contraction. It is quite possible to lose a significant amount of blood into the uterine cavity during the surgery without any outward indication, and uterine size should be monitored carefully to alert the surgeon of this occurrence. In some cases, a red rubber catheter can be used as a tourniquet above the level of the placental edge to help compress the uterus.[64]

Following delivery of the baby and closure/contraction/clamping of the uterus, the operative scene should be carefully assessed as long as the patient is hemodynamically stable. The abdominal retractor can be optimally placed, the bowel packed away, and pelvic visualization optimized. We have found a rigid ring self-maintaining retractor system such as the Kirshner or Bookwalter is best for this. The vagina should also be packed because this helps with elevating the cervix and lower uterine segment into the pelvis and also shows the vaginal fornices more clearly, preventing unnecessary removal of vaginal tissue.

In all cases, a reassessment of the operative scene should follow the cesarean section. If the percreta was anticipated, MRI and magnetic resonance angiogram data may be available to help with surgical planning. Even so, after reduction in the size of the uterus, a reevaluation of the extent of the placental invasion may show that any attempts at surgical removal will be more risky than anticipated. A flexible approach is important. A percreta that has penetrated the lateral wall of the uterus and has deeply invaded into the broad ligament and structures of the lateral pelvic side wall may be deemed impossible to remove without damaging vital structures or causing uncontrolled bleeding. In such cases, as long as the patient is stable and not actively bleeding from the placenta (i.e., partial separation), the safest approach is probably to close the abdomen and manage the patient conservatively (see later) or to transfer the patient to another facility that is in a better position to deal with the problem.

If anatomy is as expected and the decision is made to proceed to hysterectomy, this should be performed using careful systematic stepwise devascularization. It is essential to remember that many of the abnormal blood vessels seen supplying the area of percreta do not have normal vascular structure in terms of muscular media. Neovascularization leads to immature blood vessels that are extremely friable and do not contract well. Such thin-walled vessels need to be tied/clipped because coagulation frequently results in simply opening up a vessel that cannot contract down. The surgeons need to avoid making any holes in the peritoneal covering of the placenta, which is usually all that covers the highly vascular placental tissue. The most common error in this regard is traction or compression of the lower segment by an assistant, or puncture with a retractor, during efforts to expose the lateral pelvic side walls. The inadvertent puncture of the peritoneal covering of the placenta before uterine devascularization can turn a controlled, minimally bloody procedure into a hemorrhagic emergency.

The technique of the hysterectomy in a case of placenta percreta needs to be modified from that used in a hysterectomy for a nonpregnant patient and from a cesarean-hysterectomy for a nonpercreta-related reason. Because of the extreme vascularity (often massively enlarged collateral vessels and neovascularization), the blood supply to the uterus is frequently unrecognizable from that seen in other cases. The uterine arteries may not be easily identified, and there may be multiple other arterial feeders to the abnormally implanted placenta via vascular anastamoses originating from the superior and inferior vesical and rectal cascades. This will often require careful dissection of the retroperitoneal space, and judicious devascularization well clear of the sides of the uterus to avoid tearing through the friable and highly vascular tissue close to the placenta. The procedure for removal more often resembles a modified radical hysterectomy with removal of the uterus along with a significant portion of the broad ligament and lateral structures. Clearly, this type of surgery should be attempted only by a team who are experienced and familiar with the anatomy and radical surgery.

The approach to each case needs to be individualized. The principle of unhurried stepwise devascularization of the uterus is, however, paramount. Once this is achieved, intentional cystotomy should be performed to identify the extent of the adherent bladder.[64] This region can then simply be excised and left attached to the uterus, as long as it does not involve the trigone. The bladder can then be reconstituted. This technique avoids unnecessary bleeding that will occur with attempted dissection of an adherent bladder. In some cases, because of extreme vascularity, it is better to approach the uterine arteries posteriorly from the uterosacral ligaments and to work from posterior to anterior.

Supracervical Hysterectomy The use of supracervical hysterectomy in true placenta previa percreta is to be discouraged because, in most such cases, the placental tissue invades the cervix and attempts to remove the corpus of the uterus simply result in the disruption of huge vascular channels supplying the placenta. Until the uterus and cervix have been devascularized, any incision into the cervix will not help and will usually increase the blood loss. Even when the uterus appears to have been devascularized, care should be taken until the placenta has been separated from surrounding tissue. Collateral blood supply to the uterus and cervix via the bladder, bowel, pelvic side wall, or other organs attached to the placenta may still lead to massive hemorrhage from the uterus if a supracervical hysterectomy is attempted too early in the process.

Intraoperative Blood Product and Fluid Administration (See also Chapter 78) A full discussion of blood product replacement strategies in massive hemorrhage in pregnancy is beyond the scope of this chapter. However, there are recent data, both from the battlefield and from civilian life, that suggest that patients with massive hemorrhage from trauma benefit from early and extensive use of FFP and platelets, in a 1 : 1 : 1 ratio with PRBCs, resulting in speedier correction of coagulopathy, a decreased need for PRBCs in the intensive care unit, and reduced mortality.[67,72,73] It should be emphasized that there are no comparable data for use of this ratio in obstetrics, but the empirical use of early FFP in a 1 : 1 ratio with PRBCs in massive obstetric hemorrhage is potentially a strategy that could be of benefit, and one deserving of investigation.

The associated potential acute metabolic effects of massive transfusion should also be kept in mind. These are discussed in the following paragraphs.

Hypothermia Hypothermia is common, mostly owing to the loss of thermal regulation that accompanies shock and evaporation from the exposed abdominal contents. This may be compounded by intravascular infusion of cold fluids and a cold environment. Warming of crystalloid solutions should be supplemented with blood warming when blood is rapidly infused through a central line and/or when the infusion rate is faster than 50 mL/kg/hr (60 mL/min in an adult). Acidosis and coagulopathy are most likely to develop secondary to hypoperfusion and hypothermia rather than from the massive blood replacement.

Citrate Toxicity By chelating calcium, citrate prevents clotting in blood products during storage. During massive transfusion, the dose of citrate infused is influenced primarily by the type of blood component and by the rate of administration. The infused citrate is rapidly metabolized and excreted by the liver and kidneys, respectively, with bicarbonate being the end product. Citrate toxicity can be manifested by hypocalcemia or neuromuscular or cardiac abnormalities. Laboratory evaluations for acid-base status and ionized calcium are strongly recommended prior to initiation of pharmacologic therapy, because calcium overtreatment is associated with significant morbidity and mortality.

Hyperkalemia Potassium leaks out of the red cell during storage (contents of 4–8 mEq of potassium per red cell unit in a 250- to 300-mL volume). This extracellular potassium load is only a transient effect, because once infused, potassium is taken up by red cells and/or eliminated by urinary excretion secondary to the bicarbonate production of the citrate metabolism. More often than not, recipients of massive transfusion actually become hypokalemic and may require potassium supplementation. Transfusion-associated hyperkalemia may be observed in patients with renal failure.

Use of Activated Factor VIIa There are many case reports and case series of the use of rFVIIa for control of hemorrhage in massive obstetric bleeding. The data are generally encouraging, although caution is still advised. In one study of 97 patients with primary PPH reported to the Northern European Registry[74] who were given activated rFVIIa for treatment of obstetric hemorrhage, improvement was reported in 80% after a single dose. The rFVIIa failed in 14% of patients. There were some serious adverse events noted related to rFVIIa administration: four cases of thromboembolism and one case of myocardial infarction.[74] Franchini and coworkers[75] published a review of 31 studies with 118 cases of massive PPH treated with rFVIIa. These cases included primary and secondary postpartum bleeding. A median dose of 72 μg/kg rFVIIa was reported to be effective in stopping or reducing bleeding in nearly 90% of the reported cases. The authors stated, however, that caution should be exercised in interpreting these results, because the studies from which they were derived were uncontrolled. Well-designed prospective clinical trials are still needed to determine the optimal dose, the effectiveness, and the safety of rFVIIa in this setting.

Guidelines have been published for the use of rFVIIa in nonobstetric hemorrhage, but there are no published protocols in widespread use for PPH. In 2008, a multidisciplinary group of Australian and New Zealand clinicians (obstetrics, anesthesia, and hematology) was convened by the manufacturer.[76] This group produced an opinion and guideline based on their experience and the published international literature on the use of rFVIIa[76] (Fig. 75–7). Persons using their guideline are asked to report the patient to their Registry at http://www.med.monash.edu.au/epidemiology/traumaepi/haemostasis.html

Persistent Hemorrhage Massive bleeding is always challenging to control in the setting of coagulopathy. Temporary compression of the infrarenal (or infradiaphragmatic) aorta can decrease blood loss and allow time for resuscitation

FIGURE 75–7
Postpartum hemorrhage (PPH) algorithm for management.

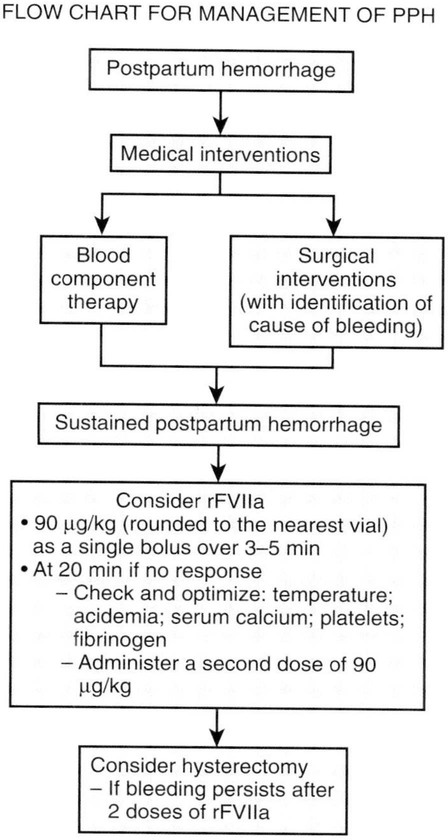

INTERVENTIONS
(Notify local transfusion specialist of possible need for activation of Massive Transfusion Protocol)

Medical:
- Treat: hemodynamic instability: hypothermia: acidosis
- Uterine massage/compression
- Uterotonic agents
- Coagulation studies and treat coagulopathy

Blood Component Therapy
(a) 4 U packed red blood cells (PRBCs)
(b) Coagulopathy correction
- 4 U PRBCs
- 4 U FFP
- Single adult dose of platelets

(c) Repeat PRBCs, FFP and platelets
(d) Administer calcium as appropriate
Repeat (b) and (c) as necessary

Surgical (as available and appropriate)
- EUA and repair
- Uterine tamponade
- B–Lynch suture
- Arterial ligation

* Radiological arterial embolization

Checklist for 'off-label' use of rFVIIa in obstetrics
- Remember the high risk of thromboembolism
- Consider physical measures for thromboprophylaxis
- Monitor all women for signs of improvement and adverse events

* Report all patients receiving rFVIIa to the Haemostasis Registry (Monash University http://www.med.monash.edu.au/epidemiology/traumaepi/haemostasis.html)

with blood products. In cases in which massive hemorrhage is expected, exposure of the infrarenal aorta and femoral arteries can be accomplished before removal of the uterus, and these vessels can be temporarily occluded to provide pelvic isolation if massive blood loss is encountered.[64] In cases in which bleeding is uncontrolled and hypovolemia is so severe as to cause cardiac decompensation or dysrhythmia, aortic cross-clamping may be required as a temporary measure to allow resuscitation.

Pelvic Pressure Pack In those cases in which there is refractory bleeding after removal of the uterus, placement of a pelvic pressure pack should be considered. This temporizing step has been shown to be effective in allowing hemodynamic stabilization of the patient and correction of coagulopathy.[77]

Internal Iliac Artery Embolization In cases in which there is persistent bleeding that does not result in hemodynamic collapse but that require continued transfusion, the patient may be transported to the interventional radiology suite for arterial embolization. It must be stressed that this procedure is not suitable for the acutely unstable patient. A number of reports have suggested that this technique is the preferred method to manage persistent but noncatastrophic bleeding.[78,79] The authors are, however, personally aware of a number of cases of severe morbidity associated with complications from attempted selective embolization under emergency conditions in unstable patients. These patients suffered hepatic, pancreatic, splenic, gluteal, and limb ischemia that required emergency surgery and resulted in permanent injury. As with any salvage procedure, individualization is essential.

Temporizing Management in Uncontrolled Hemorrhage

In cases of uncontrolled massive pelvic bleeding at the time of hysterectomy, we have found that temporary cessation of surgery, infrarenal aortic clamping, pelvic packing, closure of the skin with towel clips, aggressive resuscitation with blood products, and patient warming can be life-saving. Persistent efforts to stop continued oozing from difficult to locate bleeding points may be counterproductive and lead to hypothermia, worsening coagulopathy, and hemodynamic collapse. If the bleeding can be slowed with temporizing methods to a point at which resuscitation is effective, waiting for reversal of coagulopathy before resuming surgery is frequently the best option. This may involve keeping the patient on the OR table, or if appropriate, transporting them to an adjacent intensive care unit until return to the OR is possible. The placement of wide-bore pelvic drains is important to warn of persistent significant bleeding.

Postoperative Management

Postoperatively, patients who have had prolonged surgery for placenta percreta with massive transfusion may be at risk for a number of problems. These include intra-abdominal bleeding, pelvic thromboembolism, renal compromise, bowel ischemia, pulmonary edema, myocardial depression, transfusion-related acute lung injury and/or acute respiratory distress syndrome, Sheehan's syndrome, and infection. The postoperative management team should anticipate and be ready for such complications.

Conservative Management In some cases, it may be deemed that removal of the placenta and uterus is simply impossible or too dangerous to attempt. A number of case reports and small case series describe successful conservative approaches that have included closure of the uterus with the placenta in situ and the use of postoperative methotrexate,[80] selective arterial embolization,[81] and expectant management.[80] Without adequate randomized, controlled trials, there is considerable risk of publication bias (failure to publish bad outcomes), and caution is advised before employing these techniques liberally. There have been some reports of serious morbidity with conservative management[82,83] with subsequent massive hemorrhage and septic shock being the most serious of these complications. Although mortality for placenta accreta is now uncommon,[5] morbidity remains high; consequently, peripartum hysterectomy remains the current treatment of choice in most cases.

Management of Unexpected Placenta Accreta/Percreta at the Time of Delivery

Sometimes, accreta or percreta is discovered only at the time of delivery. Very occasionally, this will be at the time of vaginal delivery (often with a history of prior uterine surgery) and will be heralded by a retained placenta. In a stable patient with a retained placenta, it is always advisable to rule out the potential for accreta before proceeding with manual removal. In those cases in which there is a risk of accreta, it would be wise to delay any action that could potentially result in sudden onset of massive hemorrhage until all preparations have been made to deal with such an eventuality.

More usually, the placenta accreta or percreta is discovered at the time of repeat cesarean section. As underscored earlier, if the lower segment appears unusually distorted or thinned, as long as there is no active bleeding, the uterine incision should be delayed until all preparations have been made. In addition, there should be no attempt to remove the placenta if there is any suspicion of anything more than small areas of focal accreta.

Sometimes, there is discovery of a partially accretic placenta during cesarean section. Hemostasis may be achieved, if the accretic area is not too extensive, by placing sutures deep into the myometrial bed using a multiple 3-cm square suturing pattern over the area of maximal bleeding: Cho and colleagues[84] reported successful use of this technique in 23 cases of refractory bleeding with apparently normal uterine cavities on follow-up evaluation. Other methods have been attempted such as: inversion of the cervix into the uterine cavity, suturing the inverted cervical tissue over the area of bleeding placental bed,[85] and two parallel vertical compression sutures that are used to suture the anterior and posterior walls of the lower segment together to compress the bleeding placental bed.[86]

The overarching principle in such cases should always be to limit the hemorrhage as quickly as possible and to perform definitive surgery before the patient develops coagulopathy, hypothermia, or circulatory instability. A large part of the mortality and morbidity in these situations is related to unnecessary delay compounded by fruitless attempts to preserve the uterus. Recognition of the problem and decisive surgical action, combined with aggressive resuscitation and use of blood products, is required to deal with massive hemorrhage from accreta.

SUMMARY OF MANAGEMENT OPTIONS

Morbidly Adherent Placenta (Accreta, Increta, Percreta)

Management Options	Evidence Quality and Recommendation	References
Diagnosis of problem is difficult, but real-time ultrasound, color Doppler, and MRI in advance of labor/delivery may help.	III/B	52,54–59
Ensure intravenous access and resuscitation.	—/GPP	—
Options for treatment:		
• Leave in situ and monitor, provided no PPH.	III/B	80
• Administer methotrexate.	III/B	80
• Perform curettage once β-hCG levels become undetectable.	III/B	80
• Removal manually.	III/B	80
• Perform hysterectomy.	III/B	80
• Others include oversewing implantation site, resection of implantation site, stepwise uterine devascularization.	III/B	80
Treat any associated uterine atony as described under Primary Postpartum Hemorrhage.	—/GPP	—

β-hCG, β-human chorionic gonadotropin; GPP, good practice point; MRI, magnetic resonance imaging; PPH, postpartum hemorrhage.

PRIMARY POSTPARTUM HEMORRHAGE

Definition

Primary (early) PPH refers to excessive blood loss (>500 mL) during the third stage of labor or in the first 24 hours after delivery; thereafter, significant bleeding is referred to as secondary (late) PPH. Secondary PPH is discussed in detail in Chapter 76.

Significance

In the absence of anemia, blood loss up to 500 mL can be considered physiologic (i.e., within normal limits) and is unlikely to lead to cardiovascular compromise. For those who already have severe anemia (<5 g/dL), this amount of blood loss may induce heart failure or cardiovascular collapse.

Maternal deaths due to obstetric hemorrhage are often associated with substandard care.[2] Accurate estimation of blood loss, prompt recognition and treatment of clotting disorders, early involvement of experienced clinicians, availability of anesthetic support, appropriate fluid replacement, and adequate physiologic monitoring are factors that govern maternal survival.[87]

Etiology

Approximately 80% to 90% of cases of primary PPH are associated with uterine atony. However, a combination of improvements in drug therapy for uterine atony and increased cesarean section rates in developed countries have resulted in uterine atony often taking second place to placenta accreta as a cause of morbidity.[88] Less common causes of PPH are upper (uterus, cervix) and lower (vagina, perineum) genital tract trauma, uterine inversion, retained placental tissue, acquired coagulopathy, and disseminated intravascular coagulation (DIC).

Management Options

Prevention

Major reductions in the frequency and severity of PPH have followed the adoption of routine prophylactic administration of oxytocics in the management of the third stage.[89] This consists of injections of synthetic oxytocin, methylergometrine, or a combination of the two (Syntometrine) with crowning of the head, delivery of the baby's anterior shoulder, or immediately after delivery.

In high risk situations (multiple pregnancy, obstructed labor, or manual removal of the placenta), prophylaxis may be extended by the infusion of 40 units oxytocin in 500 mL of crystalloid over 4 hours. However, the effectiveness of this has not yet been proved by randomized, controlled trial, and many of those delivered by emergency cesarean section show evidence of loss of myometrial oxytocin receptors, reflected by a decrease in binding sites and very low mRNA concentrations (Table 75–4).[90]

Uterine Atony—Emergency Procedures

Fundal massage is the simplest treatment for uterine atony, is effective, and can be performed while initial resuscitation and administration of uterotonic drugs are in progress. If this fails to control hemorrhage rapidly, bimanual compression may be successful. A fist or hand is placed within the vagina such that the uterus elevated—stretching of the uterine arteries reduces blood flow (Fig. 75–8). The abdominal hand continues fundal massage, while also compressing the uterus. A urinary catheter may be inserted; not only does this aid assessment of fluid status, but also a distended bladder may interfere with uterine contractility. Controlled cord traction, early cord clamping, and prophylactic oxytocic administration reduce PPH by 500 to 1000 mL.

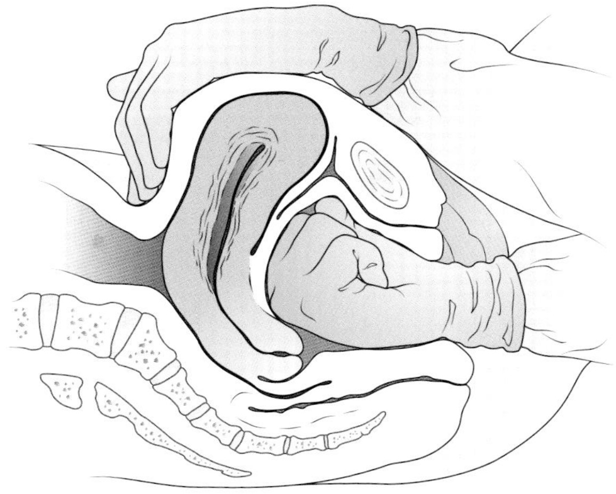

FIGURE 75–8
Bimanual compression of the uterus and massage with abdominal hand will usually effectively control hemorrhage from uterine atony.
(Reproduced with permission from Cunningham FG, MacDonald PC, Gant NF [eds]: Abnormalities of Labor and Delivery: Abnormalities of the 3rd Stage of Labor. In: Williams Obstetrics, 18th ed. Norwalk, CT, Appleton & Lange, 1989.)

Aortic compression is a temporizing procedure that can be used in life-threatening hemorrhage, particularly at cesarean section. A closed fist compresses the aorta against the vertebral column just above the umbilicus.[91] Sufficient force is required to exceed systolic blood pressure—this can be assessed by absence of the femoral pulses. Intermittent release of pressure to allow peripheral perfusion then enables bleeding intra-abdominal vessels to be identified.

Following vaginal delivery, external aortic compression may be possible, owing to lax abdominal musculature.[92] A study of the hemodynamic effects of aortic compression on healthy nonbleeding women within 4 hours of vaginal delivery found that leg blood pressure was obliterated in 55%, with a substantial reduction in a further 10%. No significant elevation in systemic blood pressure was noted, and the authors concluded that this procedure is safe and a potentially useful maneuver for patient stabilization and transport. However, there have been no studies addressing the feasibility and efficacy of external aortic compression in patients with uterine atony following vaginal delivery; a high fundus may mean that adequate compression is impossible in this situation.

Uterine Atony—Medical Treatment

The prophylactic use of uterotonic drugs is an effective means of preventing PPH from uterine atony. Either

TABLE 75-4

Summary of Risk Factors, Clinical Findings, and Recommendations for Management for the Major Causes of Primary Postpartum Hemorrhage

RISK FACTORS	CLINICAL FINDINGS	DIAGNOSIS	INITIAL ACTION	SECOND-LINE
Obstructed labor Multiple pregnancy, polyhydramnios Tocolytics	Soft, relaxed uterus	Uterine atony	Massage/compression Repeat oxytocin, either systemic or intramyometrial	Hemabate 250 μg, either systemic or intramyometrial
Obstructed labor Fetal distress Difficult or rotational forceps deliver PROM	Contracted uterus	Uterine rupture	Repair rupture if possible	Hysterectomy
Delayed second stage Ventouse/forceps delivery Precipitate labor	Contracted uterus	Cervical/vaginal tear	Repair tears	Vaginal tamponade
Retained placenta	Fundus not palpable abdominally	Uterine inversion	Reduce inversion by manual or hydrostatic pressure; tocolysis if necessary	Hysterectomy
Retained placenta	Fundus palpable	Retained products	Uterine exploration/curettage	Hysterectomy
Amniotic fluid embolism	Contracted uterus	DIC	Fresh frozen plasma, fresh whole blood transfusion	Heparin
Placental abruption	Bleeding from IV site or sutures			
Fulminating preeclampsia	Vaginal bleeding from abruption, generalized petechiae or bleeding from thrombocytopenia or DIC	Platelet count, PT, PTT, fibrinogen	Blood component therapy (platelets, fresh frozen plasma, cryoprecipitate)	

DIC, disseminated intravascular coagulation; PROM, premature rupture of membranes; PT, prothrombin time; PTT, partial thromboplastin time.

oxytocin alone (5 IU or 10 IU intramuscularly) or syntometrine (5 IU of oxytocin plus 0.5 mg ergometrine: not available in the United States) may be used. The combination drug is more effective but has more side effects.[93] These drugs are also first-line treatment for PPH due to atony.

Oxytocin binds to specific uterine receptors and intravenous administration (dose 5–10 IU) has an almost immediate onset of action.[94] The mean plasma half-life is 3 minutes, and therefore, to ensure a sustained contraction, a continuous intravenous infusion is necessary. The usual dose is 20 to 40 U/L of crystalloid, with the dose rate adjusted according to response. Plateau concentration is reached after 30 minutes. Intramuscular injection has a time of onset of 3 to 7 minutes, and the clinical effect is longer lasting, at 30 to 60 minutes. Compared with other agents, oxytocin has been found to reduce the need for manual removal of the placenta, regardless of the route of administration (IM versus dilute IV solution).[95]

Oxytocin is metabolized by both the liver and the kidneys. It has approximately 5% of the antidiuretic effect of vasopressin and, if given in large volumes of electrolyte-free solution, can cause water overload (headache, vomiting, drowsiness, and convulsions)—symptoms that may be mistakenly attributed to other causes. Water intoxication (which can be fatal) becomes a significant risk when 100 IU or more of Syntocinon has been given. Rapid administration of an intravenous bolus of oxytocin results in relaxation of vascular smooth muscle. Hypotension with a reflex tachycardia may occur, followed by a small but sustained increase in blood pressure. Oxytocin is stable at temperatures up to 25°C, but refrigeration may prolong shelf life.

Methylergonovine/ergometrine and its parent compound ergometrine result in a sustained tonic contraction of uterine smooth muscle via stimulation of α-adrenergic myometrial receptors.[96] The dose of methylergonovine is 0.2 mg, and of ergometrine is 0.2 to 0.5 mg, repeated after 2 to 4 hours if necessary. Time of onset of action is 2 to 5 minutes when given intramuscularly. These agents are extensively metabolized in the liver, and the mean plasma half-life is approximately 30 minutes. However, plasma levels do not seem to correlate with uterine effect, because the clinical action of ergometrine is sustained for 3 hours or more. When oxytocin and ergometrine derivatives are used simultaneously, PPH is therefore controlled by two different mechanisms, oxytocin producing an immediate response and ergometrine a more sustained action. In a recent large meta-analysis comparing ergometrine-oxytocin with oxytocin alone, a small but statistically significant reduction in PPH was found with blood loss greater than 500 mL. However, there were no differences between the two groups with greater degrees (>1000 mL) of blood loss.[96]

Nausea and vomiting are common side effects of ergometrine and its analogues. Vasoconstriction of vascular smooth muscle also occurs as a consequence of the α-adrenergic action. This can result in elevation of central venous pressure and systemic blood pressure, and therefore, pulmonary edema, stroke, and myocardial infarction. Contraindications include heart disease, autoimmune conditions associated with Raynaud's phenomenon, peripheral vascular disease, arteriovenous shunts even if surgically corrected, and hypertension. Women with preeclampsia/eclampsia are particularly at risk of severe and sustained hypertension.

With intravenous administration, onset of action is almost immediate but is associated with more severe side effects. This route may be indicated for patients in whom delayed intramuscular absorption may occur (e.g., shocked patients). The drug should be given over at least 60 seconds with careful monitoring of blood pressure and pulse. Initial reports suggested that methylergonovine resulted in hypertension less frequently than ergometrine, but no difference has since been reported in randomized, controlled trials. Ergometrine and its derivatives are both heat- and light-sensitive, and should be stored at temperatures below 8°C and away from light.

PROSTAGLANDINS

$PGF_{2\alpha}$ results in contraction of smooth muscle cells.[97] Hemabate (Carboprost or 15-methyl-$PGF_{2\alpha}$) is an established second-line treatment for PPH unresponsive to oxytocic agents. It is available in single-dose vials of 0.25 mg. It may be given by deep intramuscular injection or by direct injection into the myometrium—either under direct vision at cesarean section or transabdominally/transvaginally after vaginal delivery. It is not licensed for the latter route and there is concern about direct injection into a uterine sinus, although it is commonly used in this way.[98] In addition, it may be more efficacious in shocked patients, when tissue hypoperfusion may compromise absorption following intramuscular injection.[99] A second dose may be given after 90 minutes, or if atony and hemorrhage continue, repeat doses may be given every 15 minutes to a maximum of 8 doses (2 mg), with ongoing bimanual compression and fundal massage.

Small case series have reported an efficacy of 85% or more in refractory PPH.[100,101] The largest case series to date has involved a multicenter surveillance study of 237 cases of PPH refractory to oxytocics and found that it was effective in 88%.[102] The majority of women received a single dose. When further oxytocics were given to treatment failures, the overall success rate was 95%. The remaining patients required surgery and many of these had a cause for PPH other than atony, including laceration and retained products of conception.

F-class prostaglandins cause bronchoconstriction, venoconstriction, and constriction of gastrointestinal smooth muscle. Associated side effects include nausea, vomiting, diarrhea, pyrexia, and bronchospasm. There are case reports of hypotension and intrapulmonary shunting with arterial oxygen desaturation; thus, they are contraindicated in patients with cardiac or pulmonary disease. Studies have demonstrated no significant difference between injectable carboprost compared with ergot compound injections in rates of PPH.[95] Carboprost is expensive and, therefore, unaffordable in many developing countries. Dinoprost ($PGF_{2\alpha}$) is more readily available; intramyometrial injection of 0.5 to 1.0 mg is effective for uterine atony. In randomized, controlled trials comparing intramuscular $PGF_{2\alpha}$ with ergometrine and combinations of oxytocin and ergometrine, no differences between interventions in measures of blood loss or need for transfusion were found. Low-dose intrauterine infusion via a Foley catheter has also been described, consisting of 20 mg dinoprost in 500 mL saline at 3 to 4 mL/min for 10 minutes, then 1 mL/min.[101] Intravenous infusion of dinoprost has not been shown to be effective.

PGE_2 (dinoprostone) is generally a vasodilatory prostaglandin; however, it causes contraction of smooth muscle in the pregnant uterus.[95] Dinoprostone is widely available on labor wards as an intravaginal pessary for cervical ripening. Rectal administration (2 mg given q2h) has been successful as a treatment for uterine atony—vaginal administration probably being ineffective in the presence of ongoing uterine hemorrhage. Owing to its vasodilatory effect, this drug should be avoided in hypotensive and hypovolemic patients. However, it may be useful in women with heart or lung disease in whom carboprost is contraindicated.[102] Case reports also document the use of gemeprost pessaries, a PGE_1 analogue, but with actions resembling those of $PGF_{2\alpha}$ rather than its parent compound. Both rectal and intrauterine administration have been reported.[103,104]

Misoprostol is a synthetic analogue of PGE_1 and is metabolized in the liver. The tablet(s) can be given orally, vaginally, or rectally. As prophylaxis for PPH, an international multicenter randomized trial reported that oral misoprostol was less successful than parenteral oxytocin administration.[105] Misoprostol may, however, be of benefit in treating PPH. In a recent meta-analysis, oral or sublingual misoprostol at a dose of 600 μg was found to be useful in PPH but did not demonstrate a benefit over other uterotonics.[106,107]

Two small case series have reported an apparently rapid response in PPH refractory to oxytocin and syntometrine, with rectal doses of 600 to 1000 μg. Sustained uterine contraction was reported in almost all women within 3 minutes of its administration.[107,108] A single-blinded, randomized trial of misoprostol 800 μg rectally versus Syntometrine intramuscularly plus oxytocin by intravenous infusion found that misoprostol resulted in cessation of bleeding within 20 minutes in 30 of 32 cases (93%) compared with 21 of 32 (66%) of cases when oxytocin was used.[109] There was no difference in the need for blood transfusion or the incidence of coagulopathy. In a meta-analysis analyzing the evidence for rectal misoprostol, no difference was found between rectal misoprostol and placebo or combinations of ergometrine and oxytocin, although there was a small decrease in blood loss greater than 500 mL.[95,110] Adverse effects include maternal pyrexia and shivering. Of note, misoprostol is inexpensive, is heat- and light-stable, has a long shelf-life, and does not require sterile needles and syringes for administration. It may, therefore, be of particular benefit in developing countries.

If bleeding continues despite adequate uterine contraction, exploration of the genital tract is necessary to detect other causes such as trauma (uterine, cervical, or vaginal tears) or retained placental tissue, particularly in cases in which risk factors were present (i.e., obstructed labor, fetal distress, difficult operative delivery, manual removal of placenta).

In the event that these measures fail to control bleeding, hysterectomy may be resorted to as a life-saving procedure. However, as with placenta accreta, there will be occasions when conservation of the uterus is important to the patient, and alternative therapies may be attempted.

Uterine Tamponade

Uterine packing is a procedure long abandoned by many units, but more recently revived with case reports detailing new techniques for tamponade of the bleeding placental bed. Historically, uterine packing was performed using sterile gauze, with up to 5 m of 5- to 10-cm gauze introduced into the uterus, using either a specific packing instrument or long forceps.[111] Gauze is applied in layers from side to side, to give maximum pressure on the uterine wall, with the lower segment packed as tightly as possible. Indications for uterine packing include atony, placenta previa, and placenta accreta. Packs are generally left in situ for 24 to 36 hours, and prophylactic antibiotics are given.

Uterine packing fell out of use owing to concerns about concealed bleeding, infection, trauma, and problems in performing adequate packing. However, there is little documented evidence to support these concerns, and it has been suggested that the risks have been overstated.[111,112] Small studies have demonstrated that uterine packing is effective for controlling hemorrhage refractory to other medical treatment.[113,114] In a case series involving 20 women with PPH, failure of the uterine packing to control bleeding was demonstrated in only 3 women.[115]

The pelvic pressure pack, also known as the "mushroom," "umbrella," or "Logethotopulos" pack has been successfully used for control of posthysterectomy hemorrhage in both gynecologic and obstetric patients (Figs. 75–9 and 75–10). Although studies are limited, the success rate of the pelvic pressure pack in controlling post-hysterectomy bleeding in obstetrics has approached 86% after other therapies were attempted.[77]

Several inflatable mechanical devices have more recently been employed as alternative means of uterine tamponade (Fig. 75–11). Proponents of these devices state that their advantages are that they are rapid and easy procedures to perform and that whether they are working or not can be

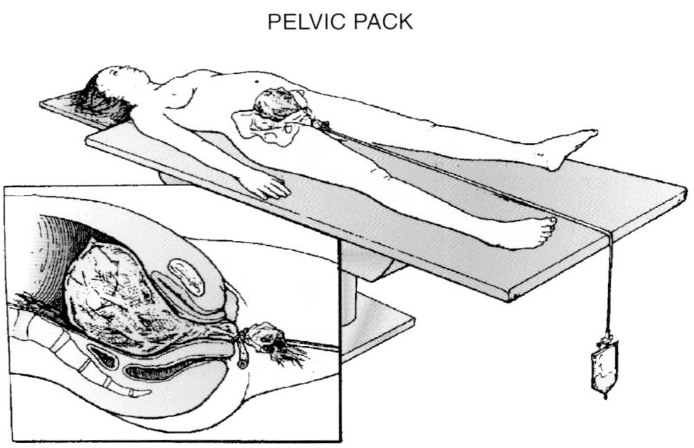

FIGURE 75–10
The pelvic pressure pack placed posthysterectomy. Traction is applied by hanging a 1-L intravenous fluid bag over the foot of the bed. An indwelling urinary catheter is placed to avoid urinary outflow obstruction and for monitoring output. Peritoneal drains are useful to detect concealed bleeding.
(From Hallak M, Didly GA, Hurley TJ, Moise KJ: Transvaginal pressure pack for life-threatening pelvic hemorrhage secondary to placenta accrete. Obstet Gynecol 1991;78:938-940.)

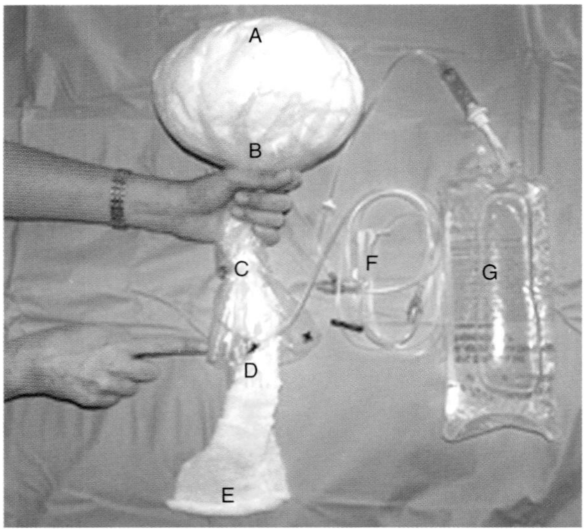

FIGURE 75–9
A pelvic pressure pack, as constructed from an x-ray cassette drape, sterile gauze rolls, and an intravenous infusion setup. A, Dome of the pack; B, base of pack located above vaginal cuff; C, neck of pack located in vagina; D, continuous gauze roll exiting neck of pack; E, end of gauze; F, intravenous tubing; G, 1-L intravenous fluid bag.

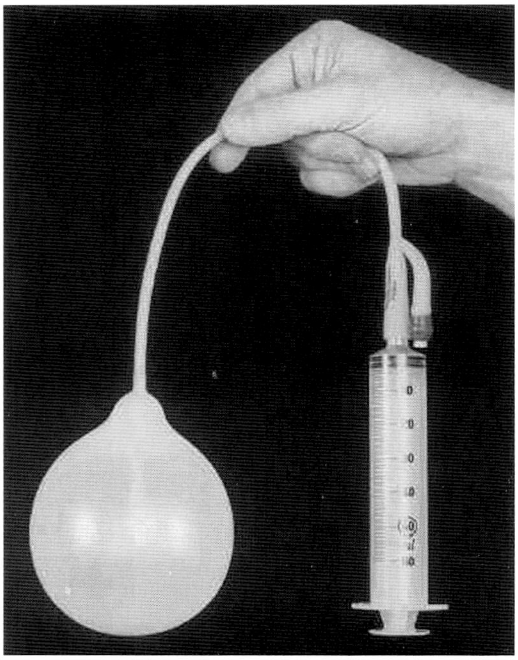

FIGURE 75–11
Example of a balloon used for intrauterine tamponade.
(From Johanson R, Kumar M, Obhria M, Young P: Management of massive postpartum haemorrhage: Use of a hydrostatic balloon catheter to avoid laparotomy. BJOG 2001;108:420-422.)

determined quickly and reliably. A Sengstaken-Blakemore tube has been utilized in this context.[112,116] The first report inflated the gastric balloon with normal saline, and the second inflated only the esophageal balloon. Balloon tamponade has also been performed with a Rusch urologic hydrostatic balloon catheter inflated with 400 to 500 mL of saline. This was effective in two women with hemorrhage due to morbidly adherent placentae.[117] In a more recent study, the Rusch hydrostatic balloon was effective in controlling PPH in seven out of eight women when inflated with 1000 mL of normal saline.[118] Balloon tamponade has also been accomplished with the use of a sterile condom inflated with up to 500 mL of solution tied to a Foley catheter.[119] Several case reports have demonstrated similar results with a Foley catheter inflated with 300 mL.[120] There is now commercially available a balloon designed specifically for obstetric use, the Bakri balloon.[121] These contain a central lumen that ends above the balloon, so that any blood still being lost above the level of the uterine tamponade can drain and be measured. These temporizing agents may allow for correction of coagulopathy in anticipation of surgical intervention. Often they lead to cessation of hemorrhage all together and should be used in cases in which future fertility is a consideration or in low-resource areas. A continuous oxytocin infusion and prophylactic antibiotic coverage are advised for these procedures. Of interest is the recent case report of PPH arrested with a Sengstaken-Blakemore catheter with cessation of bleeding after placement of the balloon. When examined with ultrasound, it was shown that the balloon was not within the uterine cavity and was inappropriately placed to have stopped the bleeding by direct compression on the endometrial surface. The authors suggest that balloon tamponade may actually work by compression of the vascular structures supplying the uterus.[122] This hypothesis deserves formal study.

FIGURE 75–12
The B-Lynch suture for the control of massive postpartum hemorrhage.
(From B-Lynch C, Coker A, Lawal AH, et al: The B-Lynch surgical technique for the control of massive postpartum hemorrhage: An alternative to hysterectomy? Five cases reported. Br J Obstet Gynaecol 1997;104:372-375.)

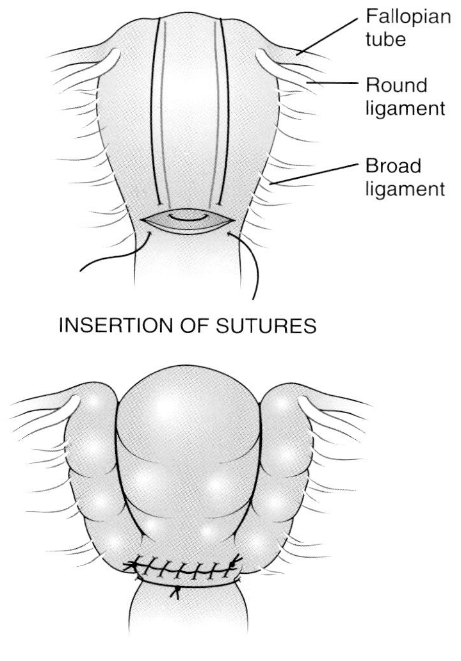

UTERINE BRACE (COMPRESSION) SUTURE

The B-Lynch suture is a uterine brace suture designed to vertically compress the uterine body in cases of diffuse bleeding due to uterine atony.[123] In order to assess whether the suture will be effective, bimanual compression is applied to the uterus. If bleeding stops, compression with a brace suture should be equally successful. Single or multiple stitches may be inserted at the same time, and according to the shape, they may be called *brace suture*,[123] *simple brace*,[124] or *square sutures*.[125] The patient is placed in the Lloyd-Davies position on the operating table to enable assessment of vaginal bleeding. If delivery occurred via lower segment cesarean section, the incision is reopened. If delivery was vaginal and retained products have been excluded via manual exploration, hysterotomy is not necessary. The uterus is exteriorized, and response to bimanual compression assessed. If vaginal bleeding is controlled, the "pair of braces" suture is inserted using a 70-mm round-bodied needle with No. 2 chromic catgut suture (Fig. 75–12). The two ends are tied while an assistant performs bimanual compression and the lower segment incision is closed as normal. The authors described five cases in which the procedure was attempted with success in all cases. They included hemorrhage due to uterine atony, coagulopathy, and placenta previa. They state that the advantages of this method are its surgical simplicity and that adequate hemostasis can be assessed immediately after its completion. Multiple case reports have described similar success with this procedure with and without other interventions including radiologic procedures or uterotonics.[126–128] Normal uterine anatomy has been demonstrated on follow-up.[129] Resumption of normal menses along with uncomplicated pregnancies following the B-Lynch procedure for PPH has also been described.[130] Unexpected occlusion of the uterine cavity with subsequent development of infection (pyometra) has been reported with the occlusive square stitch.[131]

A modification of the B-Lynch suture has been described[124,132] (Figs. 75–13 to 75–15). A less complex procedure is involved, consisting of two individual sutures, tied at the fundus. A lower segment incision is not necessary, and the authors suggest that more tension may be applied with individual sutures than with one continuous suture. They also describe tying the loose ends of the sutures together to prevent slippage laterally. A summary of published studies is the subject of a review article.[133]

Uterine Devascularization

Uterine devascularization is a long-practiced technique for PPH due to atony, placenta previa, and trauma.[134] These techniques can also be used prophylactically in women with pregnancies complicated with placenta accreta in the OR at

FIGURE 75–13
Simplified uterine compression sutures.
(From Hayman RG, Arulkumaran S, Steer PJ: Uterine compression sutures: Surgical management of postpartum hemorrhage. Obstet Gynecol 2002;99:502–506.)

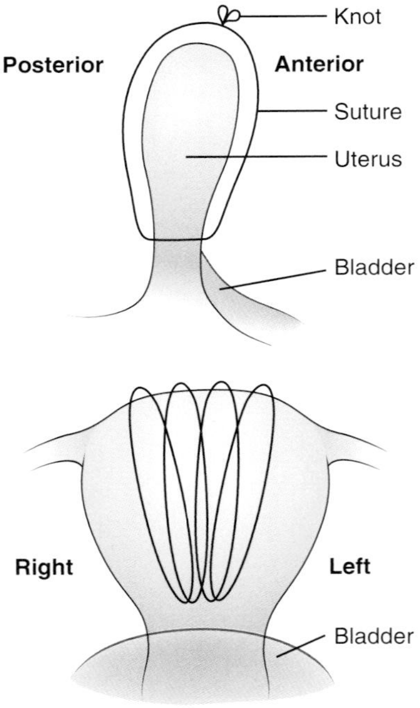

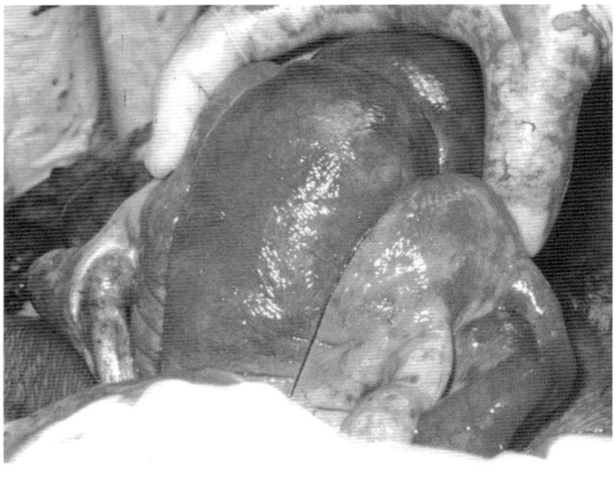

FIGURE 75–14
Anterior view of compression sutures.
(From Hayman RG, Arulkumaran S, Steer PJ: Uterine compression sutures: Surgical management of postpartum hemorrhage. Obstet Gynecol. 2002:99:502–506.)

FIGURE 75–15
Posterior view of compression sutures.
(From Hayman RG, Arulkumaran S, Steer PJ: Uterine compression sutures: Surgical management of postpartum hemorrhage. Obstet Gynecol 2002;99:502–506.)

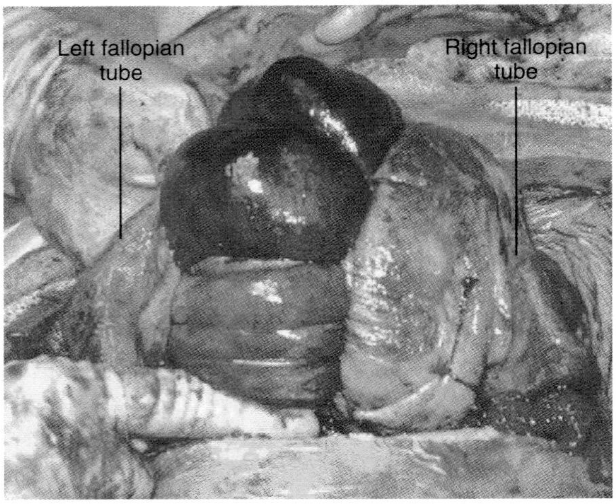

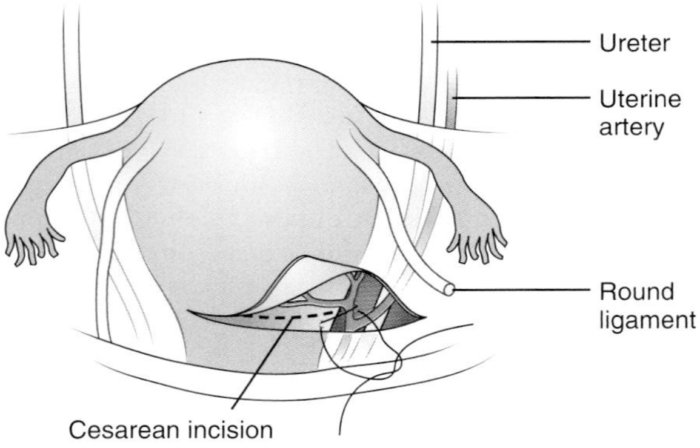

FIGURE 75–16
Operative technique for uterine artery ligation. The vesicouterine fold of the peritoneum has been incised transversely and the bladder mobilized inferiorly. A No. 1 chromic catgut suture on a large smooth needle has been placed through the avascular space of the broad ligament and through the uterus. The suture includes the uterine vessels and several centimeters of myometrium.
(Reproduced from Pauerstein C [ed]: Clinical Obstetrics. New York, Wiley, 1987.)

the time of delivery. Ligation of the uterine arteries and internal iliac arteries are described; ovarian artery ligation may also be performed, generally as an adjunctive procedure. Evidence for the efficacy of these techniques is based on published case series. The expertise and experience of individual obstetricians and the supporting staff of their units are important determinants of the surgical approach to PPH.

Bilateral Uterine Artery Ligation

The pregnant uterus receives 90% of its blood supply from the uterine arteries. Bilateral ligation (Fig. 75–16) of the ascending branches of the uterine artery is considered by its practitioners to be a simple, safe, and efficacious alternative to hysterectomy.[134] This procedure was originally utilized to control PPH at cesarean section. Mass ligation of the uterine artery branches and veins is performed 2 to 3 cm below the lower segment incision. The suture is placed laterally through an avascular window in the broad ligament and medially through almost the full thickness of the uterine wall to include the uterine vessels and 2 to 3 cm of myometrium. The vessels are not divided, and inclusion of myometrium avoids vascular damage and obliterates intramyometrial ascending arterial branches. An absorbable suture such as No. 1 Dexon or Vicryl on an atraumatic needle is used. Nonabsorbable and figure-of-eight sutures are avoided because they are considered to increase the risk of arteriovenous sinus formation. If vaginal delivery has occurred, the bladder may need to be adequately mobilized prior to suture insertion to avoid ureteric injury.

The largest case series of uterine artery ligation was published in 1995.[135] This was a 30-year study involving 265 patients with postcesarean PPH of greter than 1000mL, refractory to oxytocics, methylergonovine, and carboprost. Bilateral uterine artery ligation failed to control hemorrhage in only 10 women, giving a 96% success rate. An immediate effect was reported, with visible uterine blanching; myometrial contractions sometimes occurred, but even if the uterus remained atonic, hemorrhage was usually controlled. No long-term effects on menstrual patterns or fertility have been reported.[135,136] In women who have subsequently undergone repeat cesarean section, the uterine vessels appeared to have recanalized.

Failure of this procedure is most commonly associated with placenta previa, with or without accreta. More recently, low bilateral uterine artery ligation has been described for ongoing bleeding from the lower segment in these cases. A series of 103 patients involving stepwise uterine devascularization reported a 75% success rate with conventional uterine artery ligation.[136] Success was highest with uterine atony and abruption. Of 7 cases of placenta previa with/without accreta, hemorrhage continued in 4 women. A further bilateral ligation was performed 3 to 5 cm below the first sutures, following further mobilization of the bladder. Ligation therefore includes the ascending branches of the cervicovaginal artery and the uterine artery branches supplying the lower segment and upper cervix. This procedure was effective in all cases. A vaginal route for uterine artery ligation has also been described with moderate success.[137] This intervention includes incising the anterior cervix near the cervicovaginal fold with the bladder retracted. The uterus is than gently pulled to the contralateral side of the intended suture placement. A single absorbable suture is than placed around the vessels while including myometrial tissue. Although this technique may be quick and minimally invasive, more studies are required to prove its utility in PPH.

Unilateral or bilateral ligation of the ovarian artery may be performed as an adjunct to ligation of uterine arteries (Fig. 75–17). The ligature is tied medial to the ovary to preserve ovarian blood supply. This was the final phase of the stepwise uterine devascularization approach described previously.[136] Following uterine artery ligation, 13 of 96 cases that did not involve placenta previa/accreta had ongoing bleeding. Of these, 7 responded to unilateral ovarian artery and 6 to bilateral ovarian artery ligation. All patients in this case series, therefore, avoided hysterectomy.

FIGURE 75–17
Area for ovarian artery ligation. Two free ties of 2-0 silk suture are used to ligate the ovarian artery bilaterally near its anastomosis with the uterine artery. An avascular area of mesovarium near the junction of the utero-ovarian ligament with the ovary is the site chosen.
(Reproduced from Pauerstein C [ed]: Clinical Obstetrics. New York, Wiley, 1987.)

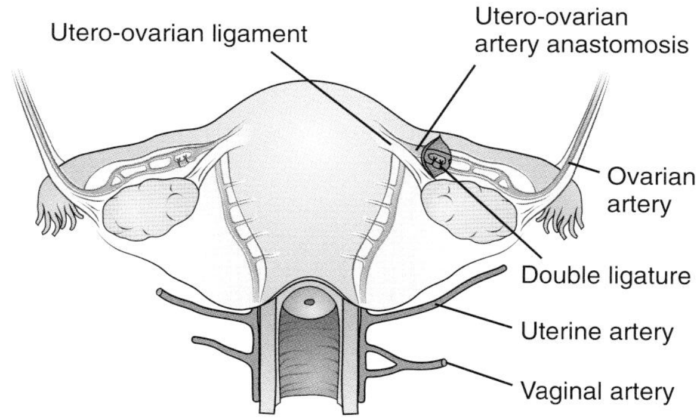

Bilateral Internal Iliac Artery Ligation

Internal iliac artery ligation was first performed as a gynecologic procedure by Kelly in 1894.[138] He termed this "the boldest procedure possible for checking bleeding" and assumed that the blood supply to the pelvis would be completely arrested. From the 1950s, internal iliac ligation was increasingly performed for gynecologic indications, mostly for carcinoma of the cervix. Ligation was still considered to shut off arterial flow, despite the fact that necrosis of pelvic tissues had not been observed. In the 1960s, Burchell reported cutting a uterine artery following bilateral internal iliac ligation in order to demonstrate the absence of flow. However, to the surprise of those present, blood still flowed freely. This observation led to extensive studies of the hemodynamic effects of internal iliac ligation. These were performed on gynecological patients, but are quoted widely in the obstetric literature.[138,139] Aortograms performed between 5 minutes and 37 months postligation demonstrated an extensive collateral circulation, with blood flow throughout the internal iliac artery and its branches. Three collateral circulations were identified: the lumbar and iliolumbar arteries; the middle sacral and lateral sacral arteries; and the superior rectal and middle rectal arteries. Ligation above the posterior division resulted in collateral and, therefore, reversed flow in its iliolumbar and middle sacral branches (Fig. 75–18). Ligation below the posterior division caused collateral flow only in the middle hemorrhoidal artery, again in a retrograde direction. Flow to more distal branches of the internal iliac artery was normal.

A second study involved intra-arterial pressure recordings before and after ligation.[138] Following bilateral ligation, distal arterial pulse pressure decreased by 85%, with a 24% reduction in mean arterial pressure. In addition, a 48% reduction in blood flow resulted following ipsilateral ligation. The authors concluded that internal iliac ligation controls pelvic hemorrhage mainly by decreasing arterial pulse pressure. The smaller diameter of the anastamoses of the collateral circulation was proposed to explain this

FIGURE 75–18
Operative technique of internal iliac artery ligation. *A*, The retroperitoneal space over the right internal and external ilia vessels has been opened and the ureter retracted medially. *B*, A right-angled clamp is passed between the iliac artery and the iliac vein to receive a ligature of No. 0 silk. The vessel should be doubly ligated.
(Reproduced from Pauerstein C [ed]: Clinical Obstetrics. New York, Wiley, 1987.)

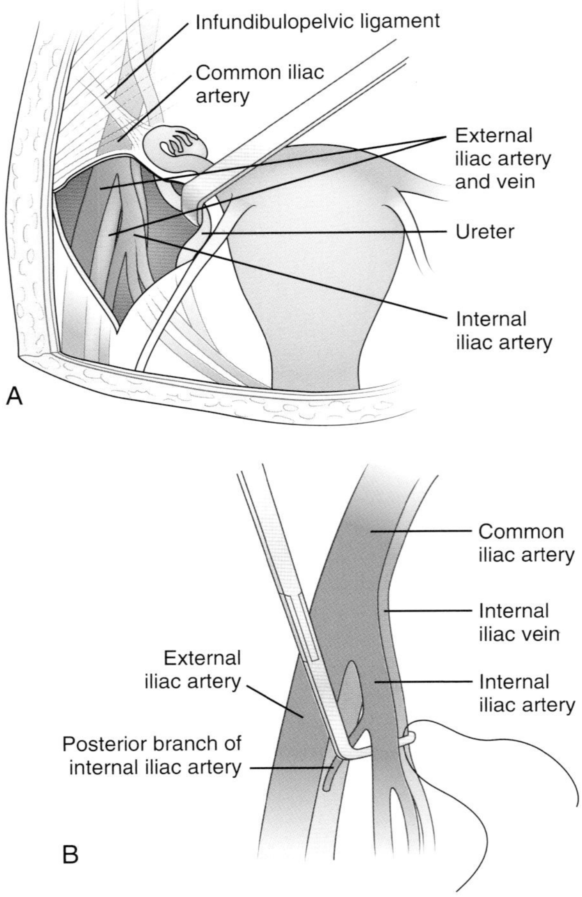

phenomenon. The arterial system was considered transformed into a venous-like circulation, with clot formation able to arrest bleeding at the site of injury. These studies have been extensively quoted; however, similar studies have not been performed in postpartum women. A single case report found no change in uterine artery Doppler waveform velocity before and 2 days after bilateral internal artery ligation performed to control hemorrhage due to uterine atony.[140]

Internal iliac artery ligation is a more complex procedure than uterine artery ligation. The bifurcation of the common iliac artery is identified at the pelvic brim, and the peritoneum opened and reflected medially along with the ureter.[132] The internal iliac artery is identified, freed of areolar tissue, and a right-angled clamp passed under the artery. Two ligatures are tied 1 to 2 cm apart. The artery is not divided. Both the uterine and the vaginal arteries are branches of the anterior division, and ligation should if possible be distal to the origin of the posterior division. This is more efficacious and does not compromise blood supply to the buttocks and gluteal muscles. A retroperitoneal approach may be used when hemorrhage has followed vaginal delivery. Complications of this procedure include damage to the internal iliac vein and ureter. Tissue edema, ongoing hemorrhage, and the presence of a large atonic uterus may make identification of anatomy difficult and prolong operating time. Incorrect identification of the internal iliac artery may result in accidental ligation of the external or common iliac artery, resulting in lower limb and pelvic ischemia. Femoral or pedal pulses should, therefore, be checked before and after the procedure. Recanalization of ligated vessels may occur, and successful pregnancy has been reported whether or not recanalization has taken place.

Demonstration of the extensive collateral circulation explains why the efficacy of internal iliac ligation is less than for uterine artery ligation. Success rates are generally reported to be approximately 40%.[132] A 1985 study reported a success rate of 42% in a series of 19 patients, with hysterectomy necessary in the remainder.[65] Morbidity was higher than for a group of patients in whom hysterectomy was performed as a primary procedure; mean blood loss was 5125 mL for patients with unsuccessful internal iliac artery ligation followed by hysterectomy and 3209 mL for those undergoing hysterectomy alone. Complications associated with unsuccessful arterial ligation in this series were associated with delay in instituting definitive treatment (hysterectomy) rather than as a consequence of arterial ligation. These authors consider that there is only a limited role for this procedure in the treatment of PPH: restricted to hemodynamically stable patients of low parity in whom future fertility is of paramount concern.

Arterial Embolization

Uterine devascularization by selective arterial embolization has recently gained popularity in centers with expertise in interventional radiology. Access is via the femoral artery and the site of arterial bleeding is located by injection of contrast into the aorta. The bleeding vessel is selectively catheterized, and pledgets of absorbable gelatine sponge injected.[141] These effect only a temporary blockade and are resorbed within approximately 10 days. If the site of bleeding cannot be identified, embolization of the anterior branch of the internal iliac artery or the uterine artery is performed.

In published studies, uterine atony and pelvic trauma are the major indications for embolization, and overall success rates of 85% to 100% are reported.[142] Higher failure rates are associated with placenta accreta and procedures performed following failed bilateral internal iliac artery ligation.[143] Subsequent successful pregnancies have been documented.

Compared with surgical devascularization, embolization has several advantages. It is less invasive and generally results in visualization of the bleeding vessel. Occlusion of distal arteries close to the bleeding site is possible, thereby reducing the risk of ongoing bleeding from a collateral circulation.[141] The efficacy of embolization can be assessed immediately, and repeated embolization of the same or different arteries can be performed. Disadvantages are the necessity of rapid availability of specialist equipment and personnel and the need for transfer of a hemorrhaging patient to the radiology suite. Embolization may also be a time-consuming procedure, generally requiring between 1 and 3 hours, although with hemostasis of the major bleeding vessel frequently established within 30–60 minutes. Pelage and colleagues[143] evaluated the role of selective arterial embolization in 35 patients with unanticipated PPH. Bleeding was controlled in all except one who required hysterectomy for rebleeding 5 days later. All women in this series who had successful embolization resumed normal menstruation. Similar findings have been reported in other studies.[144,145] Patients with life-threatening hemorrhage have also been successfully treated with arterial embolization. A 1998 case series included 27 women with life-threatening bleeding, 12 of whom were intubated and ventilated, and 4 were successfully resuscitated following cardiac arrest.[143] Fever, contrast media renal toxicity, and leg ischemia are rare but reported complications of this procedure.

A variation on this theme is the prophylactic placement of inflatable balloon catheters in internal iliac arteries of patients who are expected to bleed excessively at the time of surgery, for example, elective cesarean delivery in a patient with placenta percreta. In this situation, the patient is taken to the interventional radiology suite prior to surgery and the balloon catheters are placed but not inflated. Following delivery of the baby, the catheters can be immediately inflated. Such catheters can be deflated at the completion of surgery and left in situ during the next 24 to 48 hours to be reinflated if required. The use of prophylactic occlusion balloons in the internal iliac arteries before selective embolization has shown a greater than 80% success rate for control of PPH.[142,145] Various reports have confirmed these findings with normal resumption of menses within 3 to 6 months and subsequent uncomplicated pregnancies.[146–148] However, our local experience with this technique has not been favorable (see earlier).

Hysterectomy

Peripartum hysterectomy is frequently considered the definitive procedure for obstetric hemorrhage, but is not without complications. In the long term, the loss of fertility may be devastating to the patient. In the emergency situation, the major concern is that peripartum hysterectomy can be a complex procedure, owing to ongoing blood loss and grossly distorted pelvic anatomy due to edema, hematoma formation, and trauma. Pritchard[149] showed an average blood loss of 1435 mL when hysterectomy was performed at the time of elective repeat cesarean section. At emergency hysterectomy for postpartum bleeding, mean blood loss attributed to the procedure was 2183 mL, with a mean loss of 2125 mL by the time of decision for hysterectomy.[150] Adequate hemostasis is not always achieved, and further procedures may be necessary. Uterine artery embolization has been performed for ongoing bleeding following hysterectomy, both with and without success.[143,151] Relook laparotomy may also be required; this has been reported in up to 13% of patients.[152] The incidence of febrile morbidity is high, with rates of 5% to 85% in different series.

Hysterectomy is indicated if conservative procedures such as embolization or uterine devascularization fail to control bleeding. The time lapse between delivery and successful surgery is the most important prognostic factor. If the primary procedure fails, it is recommended that hysterectomy is performed promptly, without attempts at another conservative measure.[151] In severely shocked patients with life-threatening hemorrhage, hysterectomy is in most circumstances the first-line treatment.[132] Hysterectomy may, therefore, be associated with a higher mortality than other surgical procedures.[151,152]

Uterine atony is the major indication for peripartum hysterectomy, although other factors such as placenta accreta and abruption are frequently present.[151] Many studies have described the profound hemorrhage associated with placenta previa, with one analysis[153] revealing blood loss greater than 3000 mL in 23% of patients with this condition. In this series, approximately 10% of patients required greater than 5 units of blood products and hysterectomy.[153] Surgical reexploration secondary to postoperative bleeding is needed in up to 7% of patients with placental invasion.[153,154] Other indications for peripartum hysterectomy include placenta previa, uterine rupture, and other genital tract lacerations. Trauma sustained at vaginal delivery may result in concealed bleeding and is, therefore, associated with a worse outcome. Hemorrhage at cesarean section is more readily recognized and more promptly remedied.

A subtotal hysterectomy can generally be performed if bleeding is from the uterine body. It is generally simpler than a total hysterectomy—the cervix and vaginal angles can be difficult to identify in women who have labored to full dilation. There is also less risk of injury to the ureter and bladder. One study reported the incidence of urinary tract injury to be 13% for subtotal hysterectomy compared with 25% for total hysterectomy.[152] If placenta accreta is suspected, the use of prophylactic ureteral stents may help determine the location of the ureters and assist with difficult dissection planes. In addition, perioperative intentional cystotomy may improve visualization of bladder invasion. If bleeding is from the lower segment (placenta previa, trauma), the cervical branch of the uterine artery must be ligated, and a total hysterectomy will be necessary. Anesthetic considerations include the need for general endotracheal anesthesia in anticipation of prolonged surgical time, placement of a lumbothoracic epidural catheter for postpartum pain relief, and readiness for massive blood transfusion. Prophylaxis for thromboembolism should also be considered and initiated before surgery. Compression stockings placed before induction of anesthesia and prophylactic low-molecular-weight heparin or unfractionated heparin are also acceptable.[64]

The need for close postpartum observation cannot be overemphasized, and in most cases, these patient should recover in an intensive care unit setting. Frequently, because of prolonged operative time combined with massive transfusion, there is a risk for laryngeal edema, pulmonary edema, delayed extubation, and prolonged ventilation. Continuous vital sign determination and pulse oximetry along with hourly urine output measurement are warranted after significant hemorrhage and blood or product replacement. Patients with periods of prolonged hypotension during surgery should also be followed postoperatively for evidence of the partial or full Sheehan syndrome.

SUMMARY OF MANAGEMENT OPTIONS

Primary Postpartum Hemorrhage

Management Options	Evidence Quality and Recommendation	References
Prevention		
Active management of third stage is advised for all women, comprising all the following:	Ia/A	19,20
• Administer oxytocic agent (oxytocin or Syntometrine).	Ib/A	19,20
• Clamp and cut cord.	—/GPP	—
• Use controlled cord traction (no randomized, controlled data to show that it reduces PPH rates).	III/B	27
No evidence that oxytocin infusion in high risk settings improves outcome.	III/B	90
Treatment		
Initial emergency measures:	—/GPP	—
• Rub-up contraction.		
• Administer intravenous oxytocin (5–10 units) (ergometrine 0.25–0.5 mg IM is an alternative but should be avoided in hypertensive patients).		
• Establish intravenous access.		
• Cross-match blood.		
General management options for major obstetric hemorrhage.	See Chapter 78	
Specific measures:		
• Examine uterus to confirm atony is cause.	—/GPP	—
• Confirm placenta appears intact or perform uterine exploration and removal of placental fragments if suspicion of incomplete third stage.	—/GPP	—
• Bimanual compression is a temporary measure.	—/GPP	—
• Commence IV oxytocin infusion.	III/B	95
• Give further IV bolus of oxytocin.	III/B	95
• Rule out trauma to vagina, cervix, or uterus.	—/GPP	—
• Use uterine packing or balloon tamponade.	III/B	112,116–123
• Prostaglandin options include:		
• 15-Methyl-PGF_α (0.25 mg) IM or $PGF_{2\alpha}$ (0.5–1.0 mg) into uterine muscle.	III/B	97–102
• Rectal misoprostol 1000 μg.	III,Ib/B,A	107,108
• Use B-Lynch sutures or simpler alternatives.	III/B	123–130
• Perform arterial embolization if units have resources and experience.	III/B	141–148
• Perform bilateral uterine artery ligation.	III/B	138,139
• Perform bilateral internal iliac artery ligation.	III/B	132
• Perform bilateral ovarian artery ligation.	III/B	136
• Perform hysterectomy.	III/B	132,151–153
• Consider Cell Saver.	III/B	69

GPP, good practice point; PGF_α, prostaglandin F_α; $PGF_{2\alpha}$, prostaglandin $F_{2\alpha}$; PPH, postpartum hemorrhage.

UTERINE INVERSION

Definition

Uterine inversion is the folding of the fundus into the uterine cavity in varying degrees. In first-degree inversion, the wall extends as far as, but not through, the cervix. In second-degree inversion, the fundus prolapses through the cervix but not out of the vaginal opening. Third-degree inversion involves prolapse of the fundus outside of the vagina, and fourth-degree prolapse is the complete prolapse of both uterus and vagina. *Acute* inversion occurs within the first 24 hours after delivery; *subacute* refers to inversion between 24 hours and 30 days after delivery, and *chronic* inversion is inversion after 30 days.

Etiology

Baskett[155] reported on a 24-year series involving 125,081 deliveries. The incidence was 1 in 3737 for vaginal deliveries and 1 in 1860 for cesarean deliveries. Inversion of the uterus is principally a complication of the third stage of labor. The pathophysiology of puerperal inversion requires that there be relaxation of the lower uterine segment and simultaneous downward movement of the fundus. To completely invert the uterus, there must be uterine contractions of sufficient force occurring at the correct time to force the prolapsing fundus through the open cervix. The main predisposing factors for puerperal inversion are a fundally implanted placenta, flaccidity of the myometrium around the implantation site, and a dilated cervix. A number of other associations have been reported. These include intrapartum fundal pressure (Credé's maneuver), morbidly adherent placenta, fundal implantation of the placenta, chronic endometritis, fetal macrosomia, trials of vaginal birth after cesarean delivery (VBAC), intrinsic myometrial weakness/damage, uterine sacculation, precipitate labor, acute tocolysis with potent uterine relaxant or anesthetic drug, and idiopathic factors. Although, in some cases, a short umbilical cord and/or incorrect cord traction with failure to support the uterus during placental delivery may play a role in the inversion, the claim that mismanagement of the third stage is the cause of most inversions is unsubstantiated. In fact, mismanagement may not be a factor in most inversions that occur despite active management of the third stage. Some inversions have occurred without cord traction or through the hysterotomy before placental removal at the time of cesarean section. Almost every vaginal delivery is accompanied by postpartum uterine flaccidity and some degree of cord traction. Fundal implantation is very common and inversion so infrequent that for it to occur must require a number of coincident factors all acting simultaneously.

Diagnosis

The diagnosis of uterine inversion is established clinically, except in rare cases. Usual observations in a complete inversion include early-onset PPH accompanied by the appearance of a vaginal mass followed by various degrees of maternal cardiovascular collapse. In approximately 60% to 70% of cases, the placenta is still attached at the moment of inversion. The extent of the reported bleeding is variable and depends on the degree of prolapse. Frequently, the degree of shock is reported to be out of proportion to that attributable to the observed blood loss. Theoretically, this may be neurogenic shock due to a parasympathetic outflow from stretching peritoneum or reproductive organs. The underestimation of blood loss at the time of delivery may, however, be an important confounder, and in the absence of hard data in this regard, the proportionate contributions of blood loss and parasympathetic outflow are difficult to assign. In the face of tachycardia, one would be hard-pressed to state that the shock was the result of a parasympathetic discharge. Regardless of the exact mechanism, most cases will respond to prompt uterine replacement and fluid resuscitation. The physical examination in cases of partial inversion (first-degree) can be very misleading. Abdominal or combined abdominopelvic examination often reveals a mass suggestive of a uterine or pelvic tumor. Because the adnexa are compressed together in the midline along with the partially inverted fundus, which is partially collapsed into the lower segment of the uterus, there is a globular and somewhat irregular, central pelvic mass that to the unsuspecting may feel like a poorly contracted 22- to 24-week-sized uterus. The cervix is still palpable and can be visualized (if the bleeding is not too excessive). Often, the only way to make the diagnosis is with ultrasound or if the inversion progresses.

In second-degree inversion, the inverted portion of the fundus remains in the vagina, having passed through the cervix. In such cases, the examiner is unable to palpate the uterine fundus on abdominal examination and cannot see or feel the cervix during pelvic examination.

None of these are pathognomonic signs of inversion, however, because severe uterine atony with heavy vaginal bleeding may preclude observation of the cervix, and a very atonic uterus may difficult to palpate (especially if the patient is obese).

Owing to the potential complexities of presentation, prompt ultrasonographic scanning is the most helpful technique in uncertain cases. If accompanying hemorrhage or shock is sufficiently alarming to prompt immediate surgical exploration, the correct diagnosis may be established only at laparotomy.

Management Options

Management should be tailored to addressing the main risks of inversion, which are hemorrhage and cardiovascular collapse. Institution of aggressive blood product and fluid replacement, replacement of the uterus, and administration of potent uterotonics to keep the uterus contracted and prevent re-inversion are needed. If possible, the placenta should not be removed before uterine replacement because this exacerbates blood loss.[156] Replacement can usually be accomplished manually by placing a hand in the vagina with the fingers placed circumferentially around the prolapsed fundus. The last region of the uterus that inverted should be the first to be replaced (Fig. 75–19). This avoids multiple layers of uterine wall within the cervical ring. Uterine relaxation may be necessary, with β-sympathomimetic agents,

FIGURE 75–19
Manual replacement of uterine inversion.
(Reproduced from Baskett TF [ed]: Essential Management of Obstetric Emergencies. Chichester, UK, Wiley, 1985.)

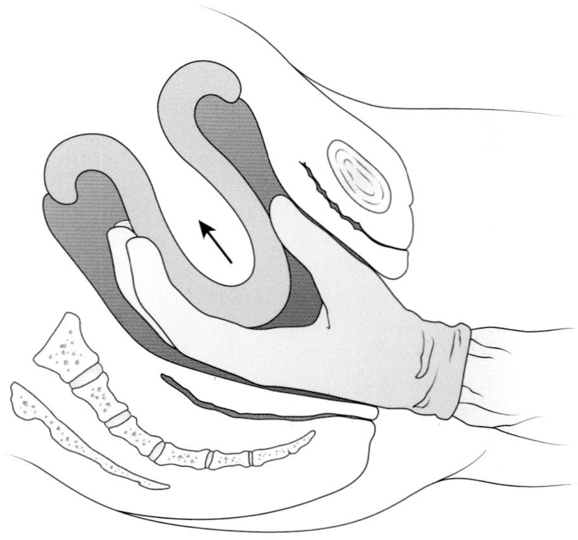

magnesium sulfate, or low-dose nitroglycerine.[157] Caution should be exercised with the use of nitroglycerin, which may exacerbate hypotension and tachycardia.[158] General anesthesia and use of halogenated gases may be needed to provide full uterine relaxation. Intravaginal hydrostatic replacement is an alternative technique that was at one time promulgated but, in our opinion, is difficult and impractical.[159] Improvement of the vaginal seal by use of a Silastic ventouse cup connected to the infusion tubing has been reported.[160] If a tightly contracted cervical ring prohibits vaginal replacement of the fundus, surgical options may have to be exercised. These include incising the ring via a vaginal approach, and both anterior and posterior vaginal incisions have been described with subsequent repair once the fundus has been replaced.[161] If these measures fail, at least two abdominal procedures have been described at the time of laparotomy. The first involves stepwise traction on the funnel of the inverted uterus or the round ligaments, using ring or Allis forceps reapplied progressively as the fundus emerges (Huntington's procedure). If this fails, a longitudinal incision is made posteriorly through the cervix, relieving cervical constriction and allowing traction on the round ligaments as in the Huntington procedure combined with stepwise replacement of the uterus from below with subsequent repair of the incision from inside the abdomen (Haultain's procedure).[162,163] Tews and associates[164] have reported a new abdominal, uterus-preserving approach for such cases. At laparotomy, the bladder is dissected off the cervix and the vagina entered by a longitudinal incision. Two fingers are advanced through this incision, above the invaginated uterine body, and exerting counterpressure with the other hand, the inversion can be reversed. Uterotonic drugs are then given immediately to maintain uterine contraction and to prevent reinversion. Majd and coworkers[165] recently reported a case of recurrent uterine inversion managed with the Bakri SOS balloon catheter. Alternative techniques use a combination of vaginal pressure with counterpressure applied via laparoscopy[166] or the use of the ventouse to extract the fundus at laparotomy.[167]

Once the uterus has been replaced, all uterine relaxant drugs should be stopped and manual removal of the placenta should follow. With early diagnosis and prompt replacement of the fundus, laparotomy and hysterectomy can be avoided.[162,163] In many cases, delay in definitive management is what leads to increased edema, blood loss, and associated morbidities.

Most authorities would recommend antibiotic use after manual replacement, although specific evidence of the utility of this is lacking.

SUMMARY OF MANAGEMENT OPTIONS

Uterine Inversion

Management Options	Evidence Quality and Recommendation	References
Prompt recognition and treatment are keys to successful outcome.	III/B	155
Provide intravenous access and resuscitation.	III/B	155
Options for treatment:		
• Manual replacement (with or without a general anesthetic and/or tocolytics)	III/B	156,157, 159
• Hydrostatic replacement.	III/B	159,160
• Laparotomy and correction "from above."	III/B	162–167
Uterotonic drugs may be given after correction.	—/GPP	164

GPP, good practice point.

UTERINE RUPTURE

Definition

Uterine rupture (defined here as a full-thickness tear through myometrium and serosa) is an uncommon obstetric complication, which may occur in a previously unscarred uterus or, more commonly, in one with a previous cesarean section or full-thickness gynecologic uterine incision scar. The overall rate varies from 2 to 8 per 10,000 deliveries.[168] Different terms are sometimes used to describe partial separation (dehiscence) or healed defects (windows) of uterine scars. Asymptomatic (bloodless) dehiscence of a previous cesarean section scar may occur during subsequent vaginal delivery or may be seen at the time of repeat cesarean section in women who have not labored. The term "uterine rupture" should be reserved for those cases with complete separation of the wall of the pregnant uterus, with or without expulsion of the fetus, and which may acutely endanger the life of the mother and/or fetus.[169]

Etiology

The approximate incidence of uterine rupture is 0.05%[170] to 0.086%[171] of all pregnancies. Uterine rupture is rarely encountered in developed countries in the absence of previous surgery, but is more commonly seen when iatrogenically caused by the use of oxytocics in the presence of a uterine scar.[172] Taylor and colleagues,[173] in a multicenter study, showed that the risk of uterine rupture in patients undergoing a trial of labor after previous cesarean section was significantly higher when vaginal PGE_2 was used (6/58 [10.3%] vs. 8/732 [1.1%]). In terms of oxytocin and the risk of VBAC, Cahill and associates[174] have recently shown that doses of oxytocin in excess of 20 mU/min increased the risk of uterine rupture fourfold or greater in women attempting VBAC.

Uterine rupture is more frequent when women are left for prolonged periods in obstructed labor. This is more likely to occur in developing countries, although the situation has improved greatly in recent years following improvements in medical facilities, transport systems, organization of medical care, and levels of patient education.[175,176] However, unrelieved obstructed labor remains the major cause of uterine rupture, usually occurring in grand multiparous patients when the fetus is macrosomic or abnormal or when malpresention occurs.

Uterine rupture can occur in nulliparous patients, but the risk is relatively low, accounting for less than 10% of cases, despite the higher incidence of obstructed labor in nulliparous patients compared with multiparae. Maternal and fetal outcomes are usually worse in women with an unscarred uterus than in those with a previous uterine scar whose delivery is planned.[177] If patients with a uterine scar fail to seek medical attention and labor at home, their outcome tends to be worse.[178]

Rupture of an unscarred uterus is frequently related to obstetric intervention. This includes use of uterotonic drugs for induction or augmentation of labor, midcavity forceps delivery, or breech extraction with internal podalic version.[170,171] Prolonged labor in the presence of cephalopelvic disproportion, malpresentation, or malposition may also cause uterine rupture. External trauma may result in uterine rupture at any gestation. Grand multiparity also increases the risk.

Rupture of a previously scarred uterus is more common than rupture of the intact uterus.[170,171] The overall risk of uterine rupture for women attempting a trial of labor following lower segment cesarean section is 0.9% to 1%,[178,179] but higher if the trial of labor is unsuccessful.[179] A previous classic cesarean section has a risk of rupture of 3% to 6%, increased to 12% if a trial of labor takes place. Spontaneous rupture of a classical cesarean section scar has been reported as early as 15 weeks' gestation.[180] Use of uterotonic drugs (prostaglandins, oxytocin, and misoprostol) in the presence of a cesarean section scar is associated with an increased risk of rupture. The risks are difficult to quantify, and their use in patients undergoing VBAC is controversial. Some data indicate that induction of labor and cervical ripening with prostaglandins (PGE_1 and PGE_2) may carry a high risk of uterine rupture.[181] Gynecologic uterine surgery including laparoscopic myomectomy is also considered a strong risk factor for uterine rupture. Rates of rupture after myomectomy have been found to be as high as 1%.[182] Risk of rupture may have been minimized in this series because greater than 50% of these patients underwent cesarean delivery before labor. Although the posterior fundus is considered the weakest part of the uterus, most ruptures occur in the lower anterior segment during labor and at the fundus during prelabor-associated ruptures.[183] Late complications of uterine hysteroscopy include uterine rupture.[184] Spontaneous uterine rupture has been documented in multiparous women with placenta accreta. Although rare, this has also been reported in primiparous women with placenta accreta.[185,186] Congenital uterine anomalies are also a risk factor for uterine rupture, including those related to diethylstilbestrol exposure. In one series, five cases of rupture were discovered in primiparous women with bicornuate uteri.[187]

Some literature suggests that an interdelivery interval of less than 24 months' gestation was associated with a two- to threefold increase in the risk of uterine rupture compared with an interval of greater than 24 months.[188] The same study demonstrated a twofold increase in rupture rates when single-layer closure was used to reapproximate the uterine incision in the previous cesarean delivery. Conversely, other studies demonstrate no difference in maternal or neonatal outcomes with single- or double-layer closure techniques.[189–191] The role of postpartum fever has also been investigated as a risk factor for rupture. In one study, the odds of rupture were four times greater than controls in women with postpartum febrile morbidity.[192] Although fetal macrosomia decreases the likelihood of successful VBAC, multiple studies report no difference in rates of uterine rupture.[193–196] Rupture may occur antenatally or intrapartum and may commonly be first suspected postpartum.

Diagnosis

The most common clinical sign in labor is the sudden onset of fetal decompensation reported in 81% of cases,[168,193] frequently with prolonged fetal bradycardia.[189] The onset of any fetal heart rate abnormality in a laboring VBAC patient should be regarded very seriously and rupture should be excluded. Abdominal pain, abrupt arrest of contractions, and retraction of the fetal presenting part have also been reported but are less commonly seen as the initial sign of a rupture. Intrauterine catheter monitoring has not proved reliable for prediction of impending uterine rupture, and there is poor correlation between uterine contractility patterns and rupture.[197,198] Bleeding is frequently intraperitoneal or retroperitoneal into the broad ligament rather than revealed vaginally. Over 50% of cases are first diagnosed after delivery, when intractable hemorrhage follows precipitous, spontaneous, or instrumental vaginal delivery. Alternatively, if bleeding is concealed, profound shock may occur before rupture is suspected. Uterine rupture should be considered in every obstetric patient with hemorrhagic shock in whom the cause is not immediately apparent. Vaginal bleeding in a case of obstructed labor is diagnostic but may be hidden above an impacted presenting part.[199] Catheterization of the bladder during labor will frequently reveal blood-stained urine, but fresh arterial blood indicates that the rupture actually involves the bladder.[200]

Once uterine rupture has occurred, the fetus usually extrudes through the defect and placental separation will begin. Immediate maternal cardiovascular collapse is a rare event unless the tear extends into the broad ligament vessels. Usually, maternal condition deteriorates progressively as bleeding continues and eventually leads to collapse only if the situation is left untreated. Examination of the abdomen will most commonly reveal generalized tenderness, easily palpable fetal parts, and absent or agonal fetal heart activity.

Occasionally, the rupture occurs during vaginal delivery of the infant (usually an operative procedure for delay or fetal distress) and presents as a primary PPH. Thus uterine rupture remains a differential diagnosis in PPH, particularly among those with a previous uterine scar.

Management Options

Management options consist of surgical repair and hysterectomy. Published case series, many spanning several decades, vary widely in the reported use of each technique, with hysterectomy rates of 26% to 83%.[168] Most authors consider hysterectomy to be the procedure of choice for uterine rupture.[169,170] Subtotal hysterectomy may be performed if the rupture is confined to the uterine corpus. Evidence has shown that subtotal hysterectomy is associated with decreased operating time, lower morbidity and mortality, and shorter hospital stay compared with surgical repair.[201] Suture repair may be considered when technically feasible and there is a desire for future fertility. However, there is an increased risk of recurrence, which may be fatal. A meta-analysis from 1971 provides the most comprehensive data.[202] This analysis includes 194 women, with a total of 253 pregnancies following uterine rupture; 2 maternal deaths occurred. Overall, repeat rupture occurred in 6% with a previous lower segment rupture, 32% with a previous upper segment rupture, and 14% where the site of previous rupture was unknown. Of note, 3 women in this series had repeated rupture in two or three subsequent pregnancies. Other women had an uneventful pregnancy following uterine rupture, but with a repeat (even fatal) rupture in a subsequent pregnancy.

If suture repair is performed, elective cesarean section has been advocated as soon as evidence of fetal lung maturity is obtained in a future pregnancy. Repair has also been advocated if successful control of hemorrhage can be attained in hemodynamically unstable patients, avoiding further blood loss and prolonged surgery during hysterectomy. Bilateral tubal ligation should be considered in these cases. The need for massive transfusion usually accompanies operative management of uterine rupture. In a study evaluating over 25 peripartum hysterectomies, 98% of cases required multiple units of blood and blood products. Coordination of care with anesthesia and the blood bank is of vital importance when the diagnosis of uterine rupture is suspected.

SUMMARY OF MANAGEMENT OPTIONS
Uterine Rupture

Management Options	Evidence Quality and Recommendation	References
Confirm diagnosis by examination under anesthesia or laparotomy.	III/B	183,185,187
Surgical Options	III/B	183,185,187
• Hysterectomy.		
• Repair.		
In subsequent pregnancies, most advocate elective cesarean section.	III/B	183,185,187

SUGGESTED READINGS

Alfirevic Z, Elbourne D, Pavord S, et al: Use of recombinant activated Factor VII in primary postpartum hemorrhage: The Northern European registry 2000–2004. Obstet Gynecol 2007;110:1270–1278.

B-Lynch C, Coker A, Lawal AH, et al: The B-Lynch surgical technique for the control of massive postpartum haemorrhage: An alternative to hysterectomy? Five cases reported. Br J Obstet Gynaecol 1997;104:372–375.

Bakri YN, Amri A, Abdul JF: Tamponade-balloon for obstetrical bleeding. Int J Gynaecol Obstet 2001;74:139–142.

Clark SL, Belfort MA, Dildy GA, et al: Maternal death in the 21st century: Causes, prevention, and relationship to cesarean delivery. Am J Obstet Gynecol 2008;199:36.e1–36.e5; discussion 91–92.e7–e11.

Holcomb JB, Wade CE, Michalek JE, et al: Increased plasma and platelet to red blood cell ratios improves outcome in 466 massively transfused civilian trauma patients. Ann Surg 2008;248:447–458.
Lokugamage AU, Sullivan KR, Niculescu I, et al: A randomized study comparing rectally administered misoprostol versus Syntometrine combined with an oxytocin infusion for the cessation of primary post partum hemorrhage. Acta Obstet Gynecol Scand 2001;80:835–839.
O'Brien JM, Barton JR, Donaldson ES: The management of placenta percreta: Conservative and operative strategies. Am J Obstet Gynecol 1996;175:1632–1638.
Pritchard JA: Changes in the blood volume during pregnancy and delivery. Anesthesiology 1965;26:393–399.
Stafford I, Dildy GA, Clark SL, Belfort MA: Visually estimated and calculated blood loss in vaginal and cesarean delivery. Am J Obstet Gynecol 2008;199:519.e1–519.e7.
Vedantham S, Goodwin SC, McLucas B, Mohr G: Uterine artery embolization: An underused method of controlling pelvic hemorrhage. Am J Obstet Gynecol 1997;176:938–948.

REFERENCES

For a complete list of references, log onto www.expertconsult.com.

CHAPTER 76

Puerperal Problems

ANTHONY AMBROSE and JOHN T. REPKE

INTRODUCTION AND GENERAL APPROACH

The puerperium has been referred to as the "fourth trimester" of pregnancy, encompassing the period between delivery and complete physiologic involution and psychological adjustment.[1] Although this component of the human reproductive process does not get the same attention as many other aspects of pregnancy (there is no specific current American College of Obstetrics and Gynecology [ACOG] Practice Bulletin or Committee Opinion, albeit the e-reference UpToDate now publishes an Overview of Postpartum Care),[2] its importance remains indisputable. In both developing countries and the United States, more than 60% of maternal deaths occur in the postpartum period. The first 24 hours postpartum and the first postpartum week are both critical periods, with 45% of postpartum deaths occurring within 1 day of delivery, more than 65% within 1 week, and in excess of 80% within 2 weeks.[3] It is a period of cataclysmic change in which the mother returns to her usual physiology after the dramatic but more gradual adaptations of her pregnancy.

The role of the obstetrician is to conduct the parturient through this period, gradually passing the management of any chronic or lingering problems to her primary care provider.

As patient populations become more ethnically diverse, it is important to realize that postpartum health beliefs and practices, although often similar among cultures, may also differ drastically. Practitioners should make efforts to develop their knowledge regarding the beliefs and traditions of all their patients.[4]

Equally important in this world of too much food and insufficient exercise, maternal obesity contributes to postpartum complications, as reported after a retrospective analysis of data from a validated maternity database system in the United Kingdom. Compared with women with a normal body mass index (BMI), women with a BMI greater than 25 were at increased risk for postpartum hemorrhage (odds ratio [OR] 1 : 1.6), genital tract infection (OR 1 : 2.4), urinary tract infection (OR 1 : 1.7), and wound infection (OR 1 : 2.7).[5]

EXAMINATION OF PLACENTA

Examination of the placenta in the delivery or operating room should be a standard, especially if there are complications. The placenta can provide the clinician with much information regarding the roots of various problems of the mother and newborn. After thorough superficial examination, the decision can be made whether to enlist the assistance of the pathologist for meticulous gross and microscopic examination.[6] In the case of stillbirth, the chances of discovering an etiology is higher in centers that conduct a defined and systematic evaluation of the baby to include careful placental evaluation.[7,8] Pathology reports may be particularly helpful during postnatal and preconception counseling. Indeed, any patient experiencing a less than optimal outcome should be offered the opportunity for counseling before considering another conception.

PRIMARY ACUTE POSTPARTUM HEMORRHAGE

This topic is addressed in Chapter 75.

SECONDARY POSTPARTUM HEMORRHAGE (See also Chapter 75)

Excessive vaginal bleeding between 24 hours and 6 weeks following delivery is the traditional definition of secondary or late postpartum hemorrhage (PPH).[9,10] It is a major cause of maternal morbidity and potential maternal mortality.[11,12] Calculating its precise incidence is challenging, because definitions in the literature vary; however, it is not unusual, having been reported to complicate between 1% and 2% of deliveries.[13–15]

Secondary PPH is a clinical diagnosis of exclusion, generally presenting as abrupt onset of heavy, sometimes massive (>10% of total blood volume) bleeding 7 to 14 days after delivery.[11] Such bleeding may sometimes represent the initial menstrual period after childbirth, which is often the result of an anovulatory cycle, and thus may be heavy, painful, and prolonged.[12]

Differential Diagnosis

The most common causes of late hemorrhage (Table 76–1) include subinvolution of the placental site, retained products of conception, and infection; previously undiagnosed tumors may rarely present in this fashion.[16] It is often attributed to sloughing of the placental eschar.[11] Subinvolution would seem to be the consequence of failure of obliteration of the vessels underlying the placental site; its mechanism is poorly understood.[17]

Women suffering delayed PPH frequently have retained placental fragments, especially if the bleeding is heavy. This group was noted to have had an increased incidence of

TABLE 76–1

Causes of Secondary Postpartum Hemorrhage

Abnormalities of placentation
Idiopathic subinvolution of uteroplacental vessels
Retained placental tissue
Placenta accreta
Infection
Endometritis, myometritis, parametritis
Infection/dehiscence of cesarean scar
Preexisting uterine disease
Leiomyomata
Cervical neoplasm
Trauma: rupture of vulvar or vaginal hematoma
Coagulopathy

Modified from Neill A, Thornton S: Secondary postpartum hemorrhage. J Obstet Gynaecol 2002;22:119–122.

complications in prior pregnancies, which might reflect aberrant maternal-trophoblastic interaction, such as in preeclampsia, intrauterine growth restriction, spontaneous abortion, or retained placenta.[18]

Another possible cause of bleeding is endometritis, which should be suspected if the history includes uterine tenderness, fever, or foul lochia. This can be effectively treated with antibiotics without dilation and curettage (to avoid unnecessary trauma). If curettage is undertaken, it is probably wise to give antibiotics for at least 6 to 12 hours before the procedure, to guard against bacteremia, unless the bleeding mandates urgent intervention. In such a case, intravenous antibiotics should be given at the time of the procedure. The combination of exogenous estrogens and progesterone may allow adequate regeneration of the endometrium and may help prevent formation of synechiae.[10] Therefore, in women with secondary PPH, prescribing a progesterone-only contraceptive pill would be unwise, because this would have neither a beneficial effect on the endometrium nor accelerate placental site involution.[12]

Occasionally, relatively earlier secondary PPH (later in the first week) may be related to coagulopathy, especially von Willebrand's disease. Because the level of von Willebrand's factor is physiologically increased in pregnancy, a patient may be well during pregnancy, but develop a problem as she returns to the nonpregnant state; unexpected severe bleeding may occur despite only mildly reduced levels of Factor VIII. All of these women are at risk for both intrapartum and postpartum bleeding. Mild disease usually requires no therapy, especially if Factor VIII levels remain within normal limits. In the case of severe disease (Factor VIII levels $< 5\%$), the risk of bleeding is substantial.[10]

Management Options

In the absence of data from randomized, controlled trials,[14] management of suspected secondary PPH pragmatically and empirically consists of stabilization, investigation to establish a cause for the bleeding, and appropriate treatment. Invasive examination in the office setting (e.g., using endometrial sampling devices) may result in a dramatic increase in the volume of bleeding, and uterine perforation is possible, especially if the uterus or its contents are infected. For this reason, investigation should be performed in a more controlled setting.

Crystalloid and blood products should be given as necessary to maintain intravascular volume and coagulability. The initial treatment of late PPH consists of ecbolic agents plus antibiotics. Pelvic ultrasonography can be helpful in investigating whether there is clot or other debris within the endometrial cavity.[19]

Authors in Belgium evaluated color Doppler and the grayscale sonographic appearance of the uterus after pregnancy.[20] Areas of enhanced vascularity of the uterus, ranging from a focal vascular pedicle to a larger area of the myometrium, were relatively common, predominantly seen in the presence of placental remnants, in the early postpartum period, and after instrumental or manual delivery of the placenta. These investigators felt their results may prove to be of practical value in the management of abnormal uterine bleeding in the puerperium.[20] However, bear in mind that ultrasound cannot reliably differentiate retained placental fragments from retracted blood clots. Thus, diagnoses of retained placental fragments are not always reliable. If significant bleeding persists despite medical therapy, suction or sharp curettage (or both) should be considered, especially if retained products of conception are suspected after ultrasound examination. The use of sharp curettage probably increases the risk of both uterine perforation and Asherman's syndrome. Ultrasonography may be helpful during curettage, allowing visualization of the location of instruments. Although it is probably wise to send evacuated tissue for histologic examination to rule out trophoblastic disease, degenerating chorionic villi and decidua will be also obtained from all postpartum uteri if samples are taken and do not, therefore, necessarily warrant a diagnosis of "significant retained products."

In cases of exceptionally heavy bleeding, before hysterectomy or surgical exploration is undertaken, angiographic embolization by skilled interventional radiologists can be considered.[21,22] Hysterectomy is indicated in the rare patient in whom conservative therapy fails.

SUMMARY OF MANAGEMENT OPTIONS

Secondary Postpartum Hemorrhage (See also Chapter 75)

Management Options	Evidence Quality and Recommendation	References
Clinical features are important in making diagnosis.	III/B	19
Ultrasonography of uterine contents does not distinguish blood clot from placenta; echogenic masses are found in asymptomatic women. Empty uterus on scan may allow a conservative approach.	III/B	19

Management Options	Evidence Quality and Recommendation	References
IV fluids and blood for hemodynamic stabilization may be necessary in some patients; correct coagulation defects.	—/GPP	—
Antibiotics for 12–24 hr prior to surgical evacuation.	—/GPP	—
Uterotonics and antibiotics may reduce need for curettage.	III/B	19
Surgical/suction evacuation of uterus.	III/B	11
Embolization may be tried in persistent bleeding after evacuation before resorting to hysterectomy.	IIb/B	21,22
Send surgical products for histologic examination.	—/GPP	—

GPP, good practice point.

PUERPERAL PYREXIA/INFECTION

Postpartum febrile morbidity has been described as an oral temperature of 38.0° C or higher on any two of the first 10 days of the puerperium, exclusive of the first 24 hours.[2] The parturient demonstrating such a fever should undergo a thorough workup investigating the possibility of an obstetric-specific etiology (to include but not limited to uterine/adnexal infection, wound infection [vaginoperineal and/or abdominal], breast infection, urinary tract infection, thrombophlebitis, hematoma, anesthetic infection [conduction anesthesia site, aspiration]), but also considering the possibility of fever sources that are merely coincident with the recent pregnancy and delivery.

Uterine Infection

Approximately 1% to 3% of women having vaginal delivery will develop what is frequently referred to as "puerperal endometritis," although these infections may more validly be described as "endoparamyometritis," because they often involve more than the innermost tissue layers of the uterus, frequently surrounding structures as well (Table 76–2). Cesarean deliveries performed prior to the onset of labor and rupture of membranes may be associated with an infection incidence of 5% to 15%, and when a cesarean section is performed after lengthy labor or ruptured membranes, the incidence may be in excess of 30%. Rates will vary widely among populations and depending on definitions used.[23]

These infections are generally polymicrobial, caused by organisms present in the normal vaginal flora, now granted access to the upper genital tract, peritoneal cavity, and circulation. The more common pathogenic bacteria include group B, β-hemolytic streptococcus (GBS), anaerobic streptococci, aerobic gram-negative bacilli (usually *Escherichia coli*, *Klebsiella pneumoniae*, and *Proteus*); and anaerobic gram-negative bacilli (generally *Bacteroides* and *Prevotella*).[24] Fatal infections have also been reported with aerobic gram-positive bacilli (*Clostridium*).[25] These etiologic agents too may vary among populations.

Although familiar mostly to students of medical history who read the 1843 paper of Oliver Wendell Holmes, "The Contagiousness of Puerperal Fever,"[26] or readers of Morton Thompson's historical fiction about Ignaz Semmelweis, "The Cry and the Covenant,"[27] group A streptococci (GAS) are not just of historical interest but can still be an important source of postpartum metritis and sepsis. GAS carrier status may occasionally be identified during routine screening for GBS, and this finding may presage serious postpartum infection.[28] A 7-month outbreak of 15 cases of postpartum sepsis due to GAS was traced to a nurse with atopic dermatitis who carried the organism,[29] raising a chilling memory of similar outbreaks that occurred in Budapest and other locales in the mid-19th century.[30] The Centers for Disease Control and Prevention (CDC) hosted a workshop to formulate recommendations for control of GAS disease among household contacts of persons with invasive GAS infections and for responding to postpartum and postsurgical invasive GAS infections.[31]

Risk factors for metritis include young maternal age, cesarean delivery, low socioeconomic status, extended duration of labor, prolonged rupture of membranes, and multiple vaginal examinations.[23] Puerperal pyrexia due to metritis

TABLE 76–2
Differential Diagnosis of Persistent Puerperal Fever

DIAGNOSIS	DIAGNOSTIC TESTS	TREATMENT
Resistant microorganisms	Endometrial and blood culture	Modify antibiotic therapy
Wound infection	Physical examination	Incision, drainage
	Needle aspiration	Antibiotics
	Ultrasound	
Pelvic abscess	Physical examination	Drainage
	Ultrasound, CT, MRI	Antibiotics
Septic pelvic vein thrombophlebitis	Ultrasound, CT, MRI	Anticoagulation antibiotics
Recrudescence of autoimmune disease	Serology	Corticosteroids
Drug fever	Inspect temperature graph, identify eosinophilia	Discontinue antibiotics
Mastitis	Physical examination	Modify antibiotic coverage to cover staphylococci

CT, computed tomography; MRI, magnetic resonance imaging.
Modified from Duff P: Maternal and prenatal infection. In Gabbe SG, Niebyl JR, Simpson JL (eds): Obstetrics: Normal & Problem Pregnancies, 4th ed. New York, Churchill Livingstone, 2002.

typically presents with fever and temperatures in excess of 38°C, between 24 and 36 hours of delivery. Controversy exists as to whether temperature elevations within 24 hours of delivery are pathologic, because they can be due to overheating of the mother secondary to the efforts of labor, especially if she had an epidural. "Milk fever" can also be a benign cause (see later). Careful evaluation of intrapartum events and observations is necessary to distinguish benign from infectious pyrexia. Other findings and complaints may include tachycardia, pelvic and lower abdominal pain, uterine tenderness, foul lochia, and general malaise.[23]

Patients with such findings or complaints deserve a thorough evaluation, because the differential diagnosis is broad, and metritis should not be assumed. Differential diagnosis includes mastitis, urinary tract infection, atelectasis (especially following cesarean delivery), and bacterial or viral infections virtually anywhere within the respiratory, genitourinary, and gastrointestinal tracts. Examination of the breasts, percussion of the sinuses, inspection of the pharynx, auscultation of the lungs and heart, and other diagnostic techniques may discover a process not related to the uterus. Laboratory tests, with the exception of evaluation of the urine, are not generally helpful initially. Controversy exists as to whether endometrial cultures, leukocyte counts, chest radiograph, and other diagnostic modalities are helpful prior to starting therapy. If endometrial cultures are attempted, some data support the use of multiple-lumen catheters in order to avoid vaginal contamination.[32] Manual examination, plus or minus visual inspection of the vagina and cervix, should always be done, even though this may be uncomfortable for the patient. Discovering a hematoma or abscess is important because it directs appropriate therapy; finding and removing an overlooked vaginal sponge benefits the patient and, at the very least, prevents further embarrassment for the provider who left it behind!

Management Options

Once a thorough examination has been done, and the provider has concluded the uterus is the source of the infection, treatment generally consists of broad-spectrum parenteral antibiotics, to include coverage for β-lactamase–producing anaerobes.[33] In most cases, the combination of clindamycin (900 mg IV q8h) plus gentamicin (1.5 mg/kg IV q8h), with gentamicin levels followed, will be safe and effective, with cure rates of 90% to 97% reported in several studies.[34–43] Parenteral therapy should continue until the patient is afebrile for 24 to 48 hours, and oral antibiotic therapy thereafter is generally not necessary, barring staphylococcal bacteremia.[44]

If the patient does not respond to the initial antibiotic regimen after 48 to 72 hours, modification in therapy may be necessary. In this case, cultures may prove valuable. Resistant organisms such as enterococci are responsible for many treatment failures. Adding ampicillin (2 g IV q4h) may improve the rate of response.[45]

Should the patient still not improve, evaluation should be repeated and extended. Wound infection, pelvic abscess, septic pelvic thrombophlebitis, and drug fever should be added to the differential diagnosis.[33]

A standardized protocol similar to the aforementioned was evaluated with respect to its efficacy against postcesarean endometritis in Alabama. Twenty percent (322) of 1643 patients delivered by cesarean were diagnosed with endometritis and treated with clindamycin and gentamicin; 129 (8%) of these women also received either ampicillin or vancomycin; only 19 of 322 (6%) had persistent fever. Six of these had a wound complication, 1 an infected hematoma, and 12 were suspected as having antimicrobial resistance. Their standardized protocol resulted in a 94% initial cure rate.[46]

A prospective, placebo-controlled, double-blinded study in Tennessee investigated whether once-daily dosing of gentamicin and clindamycin (gentamicin 5 mg/kg and clindamycin phosphate 2700 mg) would be as efficacious as administration every 8 hours.[47] There was no difference in the mean time from starting therapy until becoming afebrile between the groups, and success rates were similar (82% in the daily-dose group, and 69% in the thrice-daily dose group).

Septic Pelvic Vein Thrombophlebitis

Septic pelvic vein thrombophlebitis (SPT) is probably a rather infrequent postpartum complication, occurring in only 1 in 3000 pregnancies. Unfortunately, it is much more likely to occur following cesarean (1 : 800) than vaginal deliveries (1 : 9000); consequently, its overall incidence may be rising.[48] Intrauterine infection may cause seeding of pathogens into the venous circulation, leading to endothelial damage and thrombosis.[49]

Duff and Gibbs[50] have reported that SPT may occur in two rather distinct forms:

- Ovarian vein syndrome/thrombosis.
- "Enigmatic fever."

More common is ovarian vein syndrome, which is acute thrombosis of one (usually the right) or both ovarian veins.[51] Common findings are moderate fever, pain, gastrointestinal symptoms, and tachycardia. The abdomen is often tender, and the patient may have guarding and decreased bowel sounds. Differential diagnoses include pyelonephritis, renal stone, appendicitis, broad ligament hematoma, adnexal torsion, and pelvic abscess.[49] Ultrasound, computed tomography (CT), and other imaging modalities have been reported to demonstrate extensive thrombosis of an ovarian vein. Medical treatment consists of thrombolytic agents, heparin, and antibiotics.[52]

Less common is so-called enigmatic fever.[53] Patients initially seem to have metritis and receive systemic antibiotics. Initially, there may be some improvement, but patients frequently have temperature instability. Fever and tachycardia may persist. Differential diagnoses include drug fever, viral syndrome, autoimmune disease, and pelvic abscess.[49]

Management Options

Diagnostic imaging (CT, magnetic resonance imaging [MRI]) may help to detect large thrombi. A group in Winnipeg reported the result of a CT scan of the abdomen and pelvis with infused intravenous contrast, which demonstrated a massive thrombosis extending from the superior vena cava to the femoral vein, and which responded to a regimen of clindamycin, gentamicin, and unfractionated heparin (Fig. 76–1).[54]

FIGURE 76–1
Infused computed tomography (CT) of the abdomen. The *arrow* indicates left ileofemoral thrombosis. The associated low-density area surrounding the vein represents perivascular inflammation.

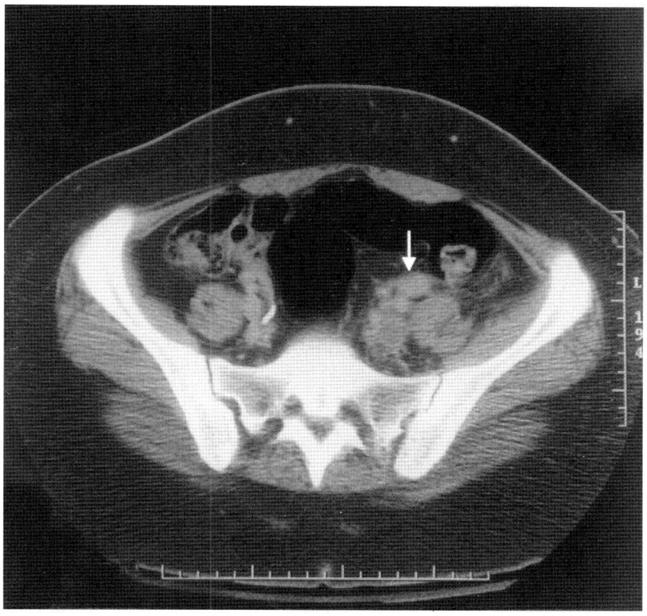

However, diagnostic imaging may miss thrombi in smaller vessels. In this case, a favorable response to therapeutic-dose heparin supports the diagnosis.[55,56] Patients generally respond within 2 to 3 days. If there is no response and the patient worsens, consultation with a vascular surgeon may be prudent.[50,55]

Although most would recommend the use of heparin in the treatment of SPT, this is not entirely uncontroversial. A study in Dallas used abdominopelvic CT imaging to search for evidence of puerperal SPT in women diagnosed with pelvic infection and fever that persisted after 5 days of adequate antimicrobial therapy with clindamycin, gentamicin, and ampicillin. Sixty-nine women met the criteria for prolonged infection, and 15 (22%) of these were found to have SPT. Four of these women had delivered vaginally; 11 by cesarean section. Of the 15, all were treated with continued antimicrobial therapy, 6 with the addition of heparin and 9 without. There was no significant difference between the responses of women who were and those who were not given heparin.[48]

Urinary Tract Infections

Factors such as vaginal examinations and urethral catheterization place the just-delivered mother at risk for infection in her urinary tract. This subject is covered in detail in Chapter 49.

SUMMARY OF MANAGEMENT OPTIONS

Puerperal Pyrexia

Management Options	Evidence Quality and Recommendation	References
Uterine Infection		
Prevention:		
• Limit vaginal examinations, intrauterine monitoring, exteriorizing the uterus at CS and manual removal of placenta at CS.	—/GPP	—
• Prophylactic antibiotics at the time of CS.	Ia/A	34–36,43
Management:		
• Gentamycin and clindamycin or extended spectrum β-lactam (e.g., imipenem-cilastatin).	Ia/A	43
• Continue until afebrile for at least 24 hr.	—/GPP	—
• If patient is not responding after 48–72 hr, seek other causes (e.g., retained products of conception, abscess, hematoma, ovarian vein thrombosis), review microbiology and antibiotic regimen.	—/GPP	—
Septic Pelvic Vein Thrombophlebitis		
Diagnosis of exclusion; no localizing symptoms.	IV/C	50
At least 7 days of therapeutic heparin.	Ib/A	48
Broad-spectrum antibiotics.	Ib/A	43
Ovarian Vein Thrombosis		
CT/MRI for diagnosis.	IV/C	54,56
Heparin and long-term anticoagulation as for thromboembolic disease elsewhere.	IV/C	51

SUMMARY OF MANAGEMENT OPTIONS

Puerperal Pyrexia—cont'd

Management Options	Evidence Quality and Recommendation	References
Broad-spectrum antibiotics.	IV/C	51
Vascular surgery if failed response to medical treatment.	—/GPP	—
Urinary Infection		
Culture urine; appropriate antibiotics (oral or parenteral depending on clinical severity).	—/GPP	—

CS, cesarean section; CT, computed tomography; GPP, good practice point; MRI, magnetic resonance imaging.

DISORDERS OF THE BREASTS

The mantra of "breast is best," long a rallying point for many, continues to gather scientific support, to include increasing evidence that breast milk is the single entity that has evolved *with* humans *to nourish* humans.[57,58] A 15-year study of more than 6600 mother-infant pairs revealed that abuse and neglect were much less likely in breast-fed babies.[59] However, for various reasons, many women around the world (approximately half of U.S. women) do not nurse their newborns.[60] Although it is well known that women may experience great discomfort before lactation ceases, precise data about this annoyance are lacking.

Lactation: Suppression and Stimulation

Over the years, a number of nonpharmacologic means have been used to suppress lactation and relieve symptoms of engorgement. These include, but are not limited to, strapping or binding the breasts, forcing fluids, restricting fluids and diet, applying various ointments and other products (e.g., cabbage leaves, ice packs) to the breasts and nipples, narcotics, wearing a tightly fitting brassiere, emptying the breasts by massage or pump, and avoiding expression of milk.[61–65] It is evident that a number of these approaches are contradictory.

In the United States, various pharmacologic methods for lactation suppression were used during most of the 20th century.[66] The natural suppression of prolactin secretion results in breast involution; this was approximated pharmacologically with medicines such as bromocriptine. However, since 1988, the U.S. Food and Drug Administration has recommended against the routine use of pharmacologic methods (save analgesics) for lactation suppression and relief of associated symptoms because evidence from randomized, controlled studies on the safety and efficacy of those drugs for that purpose is lacking.[67,68]

Reports linked bromocriptine with cerebrovascular accident, myocardial infarction, seizure, and other problems in puerperal women. A recent Cochrane review notes "Contrary to a number of case reports, there is insufficient evidence from this review to indicate whether or not bromocriptine is associated with increased risk of major side effects (notably thromboembolism, myocardial infarction and maternal death) in the first postpartum week."[69] However, largely because of suspected associations with such serious complications, this drug is no longer approved for lactation suppression.[70–75]

Peterson and colleagues at the CDC[68] searched the world literature in 1998 to locate data about the postpartum symptoms experienced by women who do not breast-feed and to review data on the efficacy of nonpharmacologic methods of lactation suppression. Their findings were disappointing: extant data suggested that, in spite of current nonpharmacologic treatment for lactation suppression, as many as one woman in three may experience severe breast pain postpartum. Moreover, they found no studies focusing primarily on the symptoms of such women. They did offer directions for future research, suggesting studies that included treatment groups for wearing a breast binder, wearing a tightly fitting brassiere, pumping breast milk mechanically or manually, applying ice packs to the breasts, applying topical analgesics or other substances to the breasts, and taking only oral analgesics. Between 30% and 50% of nonnursing patients will have engorgement and pain that may persist for up to a week.

Unwanted lactation failure is a rare complication that has been associated with retained placenta, via suppression of prolactin.[76] Prolactin may also be suppressed by ergot, pyridoxine, and some diuretics.

It has been reported that metoclopramide[77] and sulpiride[78] may enhance lactation. Use of oxytocin (which has to be taken as snuff, to avoid first-pass inactivation in the liver) has been demonstrated to improve milk let-down and may help with the successful establishment of breast-feeding in some women, especially those with preterm babies.

Mastitis and Abscess

It is not unusual for the breasts to become distended and firm during the first day or two after delivery; this may be accompanied by a transient temperature elevation.[79] It has been reported that 13% of all postpartum women may demonstrate such "breast fever," which seldom lasts more than 24 hours.[80] When fever develops during the puerperium, however, breast fever should be a diagnosis of exclusion, because it is important not to miss more dangerous pathology.

Puerperal mastitis or breast abscess is the most frequent significant complication of nursing. Fever, localized pain, and erythema, often confined to one or more quadrants, are common findings. Onset is generally in the first or second postpartum week, but it may also develop later. It may be related to an obstruction in the milk ducts. When initiating lactation, the nipple and areolar skin often undergo local inflammation and swelling until the nipple is conditioned to frequent suckling. This swelling causes a relative obstruction to milk flow and can be seeded by bacteria, especially *Staphylococcus aureus*, *E. coli*, and *Streptococci*,[81] leading to bacterial mastitis. There is some evidence that the immediate source of these organisms is the infant's nose and throat. The breast (generally unilaterally and in one quadrant) becomes painful, swollen, warm, and red. An abscess develops in approximately 10% of such women; there may be local fluctuance and pointing.[82,83]

Cultures of the milk are usually unhelpful; infection is almost always with a maternal skin organism. Treatment with antibiotics generally results in prompt resolution of symptoms, and following prompt treatment, the development of abscesses is rare. Dicloxacillin (500 mg PO q6h) may be started empirically.[84] When they do develop, abscesses require surgical incision and drainage[85,86] or aspiration with ultrasound guidance.[87] Continuing to breast-feed may be extremely important: the only women who developed abscesses in a series of 65 woman with puerperal mastitis were among the small group who chose to cease nursing.[88] This is probably because continuing to breast-feed allows the flow of milk to flush infection from the duct system.

A prospective study undertaken in Turkey assessed contributing factors in puerperal breast abscess.[89] Mastitis patients who were treated with antibiotics did not develop breast abscess. Ultrasonography was helpful, allowing needle aspiration; healing times were similar to those in abscess patients treated with incision and drainage. Needle-aspiration patients were reported to have excellent cosmetic results.

SUMMARY OF MANAGEMENT OPTIONS

Breast Problems

Management Options	Evidence Quality and Recommendation	References
Lactation Suppression		
Physical support; evidence for value of other topical measures is poor.	III/B	61–65
Analgesia should be the only pharmacologic agent used.	Ia/A	67,68
Bromocriptine should not be used.	IV/C	70–75
Lactation Enhancement		
Metoclopramide.	IV/C	77
Sulpiride.	IV/C	78
Mastitis and Breast Abscesses		
Oral dicloxacillin (erythromycin if allergic).	IIa/B	84
IV oxacillin for treatment failures.	—/GPP	—
Ultrasonography to rule out abscess if there is poor response or fluctuant mass.	III/B	87
Open or closed (ultrasound-guided) drainage for abscess.	III/B	85–87
Culture milk with complicated mastitis or abscess.	—/GPP	—
Continued pumping/expressing and feeding.	IIa/B	88

GPP, good practice point.

OTHER MEDICAL PROBLEMS IN THE PUERPERIUM

During the "fourth trimester," the recently delivered woman must negotiate the dramatic changes from late pregnancy and delivery and return to her normal nonpregnant physiology. Cardiovascular problems are discussed in Chapter 36.

Diabetes (See also Chapter 44)

Women who were diagnosed with gestational diabetes generally do not require treatment following delivery. However, they are at increased risk for developing type 2 diabetes (~50% will do so within 10 yr). Following the traditional postpartum visit at 6 to 8 weeks, they should be directed to follow-up with their primary care providers in 2 to 3 months, at which time they should discuss with their providers provocative testing for diabetes. This may be accomplished by an oral glucose tolerance test, in which a plasma glucose level equal to or more than 200 mg/dL (11 mmol/L) would be sufficient for a diagnosis of diabetes. The test should be performed as described by the World Health Organization (WHO), using a glucose load containing the equivalent of 75 g of anhydrous glucose dissolved in water.[90]

In the case of women with pregestational diabetes, their treatment following delivery depends on their glucose levels as they return to their usual diet and activity levels. Upon discharge from the hospital, they can generally return to a management program similar to the one they observed prior to conception. Coordination with the providers furnishing that management is essential.

Thromboembolic Disease (See also Chapter 42)

Owing largely to the physiologic changes of pregnancy, as well as relative immobilization during the latter parts of pregnancy, venous thromboembolism (VTE) is much more common in the puerperium than during a similar period in women who have not recently been pregnant. Maternal deep vein thromboses (DVTs) are more common (80%–90%) in the left leg, occur usually in the iliofemoral veins, and are often associated with pulmonary embolism. Those with prior DVT and with hereditary thrombophilias are at highest risk.[91]

Women with inherited thrombophilias have an increased risk for VTE, particularly during the puerperium. The overall prevalence of thrombophilic traits in the general population may be 10% or more; the probability of carrying multiple defects is, therefore, not at all rare. Screening for these traits should be done liberally.[92]

In an American College of obstetricians and Gynecologists (ACOG) high risk pregnancy monograph, Lockwood[93] recommended that no matter their past history, asymptomatic pregnant women with antithrombin deficiency and women who are homozygotes or compound heterozygotes for Factor V Leiden or prothrombin (G20210A) mutations are at very high risk for thromboembolic episodes and should have anticoagulant therapy throughout pregnancy and in the puerperium.[94] Following delivery (6–12 hr), heparin therapy should be resumed and warfarin (Coumadin) therapy begun. Until the International Normalized Ratio (INR) has been in the therapeutic range for 2 consecutive days, heparin should be continued. Coumadin should be continued for at least 6 weeks, and longer if there have been prior thromboembolic events.

If a woman developed a VTE during pregnancy, whether or not she was found to have an inherited or acquired thrombophilia, Lockwood[93] recommends full anticoagulation during pregnancy, resumption of heparin after delivery, and establishment and maintenance of therapeutic levels of oral anticoagulation for 6 to 18 weeks thereafter. He is careful to note that, because there are no randomized clinical trials to assess the efficacy of anticoagulation therapy in preventing maternal or fetal complications, recommendations must rely on expert opinion.

Similar recommendations were published by a group in Australia and New Zealand, recommending 6 months of therapy and treatment for at least 6 weeks postpartum for women who experienced VTE either during pregnancy or postpartum.[61] For women who had a previous thromboembolism, they recommend therapy postpartum, with the decision whether to treat during pregnancy based upon whether the index event was spontaneous or provoked, the presence or absence of a family history of VTE, the presence of a known thrombophilia, and whether there have been multiple episodes of VTE.[61,94]

Women with a past history of a single provoked thrombotic event with an underlying thrombophilia may be treated by careful observation before delivery and 6 weeks of postpartum prophylaxis. Women with recurrent VTE, previous idiopathic VTE, or a previous VTE and strong family history, but no demonstrated thrombophilia are advised to use thrombophylaxis throughout pregnancy and for 6 weeks thereafter.[61,94]

In our own practice, we liberally solicit input from hematologists on a case-by-case basis, because clinical knowledge about the thrombophilias and their role in VTE during and after pregnancy is increasing rapidly.

Finally, the puerperium offers an opportunity to perform or complete a thrombophilia workup, which may have been either delayed or done only partially during pregnancy, because of physiologic changes elevating a number of clotting factors, including Factor VIII, protein S, and protein C.

PSYCHOLOGICAL PROBLEMS IN THE PUERPERIUM

Bereavement

Unfortunately, not all pregnancy outcomes are happy. As many as one woman in five will suffer a perinatal loss through neonatal death, stillbirth, elective abortion, or miscarriage, and as many as one in five of these will suffer some form of prolonged psychological abnormality.[95,96] The birth of an anomalous[97] or severely ill infant can be almost as difficult to bear. Mothers experiencing an emergency hysterectomy for hemorrhage, or even a planned surgical sterilization, can manifest grief.[98] Postpartum depression (PPD) may be more common and more severe when a perinatal loss has occurred.[99]

Interestingly, a recent Cochrane review of the literature for evidence concerning programs of support aimed at encouraging acceptance of loss, specific bereavement counseling, or specialized psychological support or counseling, to include psychotherapy for women and families experiencing perinatal loss, was unable to locate any randomized trials.[95] Conversely, a number of reports of personal and institutional experiences in providing such services exist and arguably provide reasonable support for such programs.[100–102] Tasteful and good-quality photographs of the deceased child, especially, would seem to be valued by parents and families.[103,104]

It is incumbent for the staff of the birthing facility to recognize patients who are in need of bereavement services, and then to provide what is optimally a multidisciplinary approach to assisting the family through the immediate and long-term dilemmas such a loss causes. Many coordinated and formalized programs do this very well. The perceptions of health care professionals about the emotional care needs of families experiencing perinatal loss were significantly increased after attending a formal educational program about bereavement.[105]

In the late 1970s, individuals at Gundersen Lutheran Medical Center in La Crosse, Wisconsin, providing emotional support for families whose babies died during pregnancy or shortly after birth, became increasingly aware of the pain and grief that families experience when a baby dies. This emotional support effort served as the prototype for *Resolve Through Sharing* (RTS),[106] a perinatal bereavement program formally launched there in 1981, which has subsequently spread nationally and internationally.

Families experiencing perinatal loss grieve for their baby and the loss of an entire lifetime with that child. RTS recognizes that the support, acceptance, and gentle guidance given by professionals upon learning of a loss are important first steps in the journey of grief. The caregiver's knowledge and guidance validate that grief is a normal response to loss, allowing bereaved families to grieve in their own way, in their own time. Families are involved in the decision-making process. Education, consultation, and evaluation are integral parts of the program. The RTS support person remains in touch with the family for a year or more, referring to other health care professionals when additional management support is necessary.[106] The loss of a new sibling may be particularly hard on a brother or sister; a children's picture-book format resource[107] may be particularly helpful in dealing with this.

Psychological Reactions

Even when the overall outcome of pregnancy has been good, a healthy mother may experience psychological problems. Several authors have suggested that women may show specific areas of cognitive changes during and after pregnancy, notably deficits in verbal learning and memory (see also Chapter 55). Mood appears to be affected as well. Steroidal hormones are increasingly recognized as highly relevant in multiple aspects of brain functioning.[108] Although steroid hormones show a pattern of associations with mood during and after pregnancy, no such pattern is evident for cognition.

The postpartum period may represent a time of increased vulnerability to depression for some women.[109] Postpartum "blues" is a transient condition characterized by mild, and often rapid, mood swings, from elation to sadness, irritability, anxiety, decreased concentration, insomnia, tearfulness, and crying spells.[110] Owing largely to inconsistencies in diagnostic criteria, the data regarding incidence conflict. Major depressive disorders are thought to afflict 5% to 9% of women at any time, with a lifetime risk of 10% to 25%.[111] New episodes of depression in the first 4 to 6 weeks after delivery occur three times more frequently than in nonpregnant controls.[112] Depression has been described in up to 30% of women in the first postpartum year.[113–115] Other studies have not confirmed this relation, observing rates of PPD similar to depression diagnosed without relation to pregnancy.[116–118]

Hormonal changes following delivery are often presumed to play a role in the development of PPD; however, the relationship between postpartum changes and the development of depression is not well understood,[119] and there is every reason to assume that PPD results from the interaction between hormonal, genetic,[120] and life-event factors.[109,121] Women may complain of depressive symptoms shortly after delivery, at any time during the following few months, and at cessation of lactation, although it is unclear whether cessation of nursing the child is cause or effect.[122] Moreover, there is good evidence that in many cases, PPD may begin well before delivery. One study reported that the prevalence of depression at 32 weeks (13.5%) was higher than postpartum (9.1%).[123] In another study, half of all women diagnosed with PPD had onset of symptoms during or even before their pregnancies.[124]

Wickberg and Hwang[125] investigated the use of the Edinburgh Postnatal Depression Scale (EPDS) on a population-based sample of 1655 women who completed the scale at 2 and 3 months postpartum. They also interviewed 128 using the Montgomery Asberg Depression Rating Scale (MADRS) and assessed them according to *Diagnostic and Statistical Manual of Mental Disorders*, 3rd edition, revised (DSM-III-R) criteria for major depression. A cutoff score of 11.5 on the EPDS identified all but 2 women with major depression (sensitivity 96%, specificity 49%, positive predictive value 59%).

Thoppil and coworkers[126] reported a multidisciplinary approach to identifying women at risk for depression during pregnancy and postpartum (Table 76–3). Called ISIS (identify, screen, intervene, and support), it was developed and supported by their psychiatry, obstetrics, and social work groups. Social workers educate patients about signs and symptoms of depression at the obstetrics orientation visit. Risk factors for depression are screened for at the first visit with midwife or obstetrician. The EPDS is administered at the 32-week visit. Patients with elevated scores are further evaluated, and consultation and treatment may be initiated by the psychiatry department. In a chart review, they found that 75% of their patients were so screened, with 9.76% of the screened population having a positive score.

Management Options

Psychotherapy is an effective first-line treatment for depression during pregnancy or after the birth of a child.[127]

In some cases, antidepressant treatment may be warranted. The decision to prescribe an antidepressant drug

TABLE 76–3
DSM-IV Criteria for a Major Depressive Episode

A. Five or more of the following symptoms must be present daily or almost daily for at least 2 consecutive weeks:
   1. Depressed mood.*
   2. Loss of interest or pleasure.*
   3. Significant increase or decrease in appetite.
   4. Insomnia or hypersomnia.
   5. Psychomotor agitation or retardation.
   6. Fatigue or loss of energy.
   7. Feelings of worthlessness or guilt.
   8. Diminished concentration.
   9. Recurrent thoughts of suicide or death.
B. The symptoms do not meet the criteria for other psychiatric conditions.
C. The symptoms cause significant impairment in functioning at work, school, and social activities.
D. The symptoms are not caused directly by a substance or general medical condition.
E. The symptoms are not caused by bereavement after the loss of a loved one.

* At least one of the five symptoms must be item 1 or 2.
Modified from American Psychiatric Association: Diagnostic and Statistical Manual of Mental Disorders, 4th ed. Washington, DC, American Psychiatric Association, 2000.

during pregnancy or the postpartum period must be made on an individual basis.[128] Use of pharmacologic therapy in postpartum lactating women must balance the risk of possible deleterious drug effects on the infant via the mother's milk versus the risk of not treating a serious psychiatric condition. All medicines used for this purpose appear in breast milk in varying amounts. The provider must consider such risks to the baby as drug toxicity and the possibility of long-term effects on behavior and neurologic development, which have not as yet been elucidated.[129] Coordination with the baby's pediatrician is essential. Another consideration that must be dealt with before prescribing an antidepressant drug during pregnancy or the postpartum period concerns the matter of which provider will assume responsibility for the patient's treatment once the puerperium has passed.

In one study, 25 women met standard diagnostic criteria for PPD.[130,131] They took 10, 20, or 40 mg/day of paroxetine for at least 4 weeks and no other mood-altering drugs. Researchers studied fresh breast milk, collected within 6 hours of taking the drug, along with maternal and infant blood samples. Even the lowest dosage of paroxetine improved depression in some of the women. There were no differences among groups in the milk-to-plasma ratio, no matter what dosage the women took. Only very small amounts were found in breast milk and the infants' serum. These findings imply that one may treat a nursing woman safely with paroxetine,[130,131] as has been shown in similar studies of fluoxetine and sertraline. Prudence may be important, however; Stowe and colleagues[131] found that in studying infants exposed to paroxetine via mother's milk, the drug was not found in their blood, similar to studies of sertraline and fluoxetine. However, they warn that one cannot assume it was not in the baby's brain, and it may be premature to base safety conclusions on undetectable concentrations in infant serum.

The reader is referred to Chapter 55 for a more detailed discussion of the management options for postpartum blues, depression, and psychosis.

SUMMARY OF MANAGEMENT OPTIONS

Other Medical Problems in the Puerperium

Topics	Summary of Management Options Is Found in Chapter
Cardiovascular	36 and 79
Cardiomyopathy	36
Hypertension	35 and 79
Diabetes	44
Thromboembolic disease	42
Psychiatric problems	55

OTHER ISSUES IN THE PUERPERIUM

Pain Relief (See also Chapter 70)

The use of epidural analgesia has revolutionized pain management in the immediate puerperium. For patients not having epidurals, evidence about various methods is limited. Prostaglandin synthetase inhibitors, although affording effective control of uterine contractions, may produce excessive bleeding as a side effect. The broad spectrum of perceived pain among women experiencing delivery remains unexplained.

Calvert and Fleming in Glasgow, Scotland,[132] reviewed the literature concerning approaches to dealing with perineal pain following vaginal delivery. They note the dearth of data to support many traditional and apparently efficacious practices and emphasize the need for careful evaluation of damage, use of nontraumatic suture when repair is necessary, and listening carefully to the patient as she describes her pain.

Education: Assuming the Role of the Mother

Many normal psychological changes take place to prepare the mother for her new responsibilities. Any impediment to these changes might result in a lack of emotional response to the infant at delivery. During the immediate newborn period, prenatal preparation needs to be recalled and developed, in addition to many new and often unanticipated tasks as the maternal role is taken on.[133]

Medications

The administration of appropriate medications such as Rh immune globulin, vaccinations, and others must not be overlooked prior to discharge. It should be remembered that dosages of many medications for chronic disease states (e.g., thyroid disease, hypertension, seizure disorders) likely were adjusted (generally increased) during pregnancy because of maternal physiologic adaptations (e.g., the increase in plasma volume or changes in the rate of drug metabolism). During the puerperium, these drug dosages usually need to be restored to prepregnancy levels. The blood levels of antiseizure medications may rise dramatically in the early puerperium if dosages are not adjusted. Coordination with the patient's primary care provider is vital.

General Health Considerations

The puerperium also offers an opportunity for the caregiver to reinforce the healthy lifestyle that many women adopt during pregnancy. This is the time to intervene to prevent recidivism into unhealthy habits, such as the use of tobacco, excessive alcohol, and other unhealthy substances. The nutrition counseling many women undergo during pregnancy, whether or not they have been diagnosed with gestational diabetes, will serve them well in the nonpregnant state and should be reinforced. Even pregestational diabetics often embrace long-overlooked advice for the sake of the babies they carry; this is an opportunity to bolster that resolve.

Length of Stay

At least eight trials have attempted to compare early discharge (with substantial variation in the definition thereof) of healthy mothers with term infants with standard care in the settings in which the trials were conducted. Investigational problems included high postrandomization exclusions, protocol violations, and failure to use a well-validated standardized instrument to assess PPD. So, although there seems to be no evidence of adverse outcomes associated with policies of early postnatal discharge, methodologic limitations of included studies mean that such complications cannot be ruled out.[134] Indeed, such difficult-to-measure outcomes as fatigue due to sleep deprivation might be affected by length of stay.

Returning to Exercise

As morphologic and physiologic adaptations to pregnancy recede gradually over many weeks, it seems prudent that mothers return progressively to prepregnancy levels of exercise and physical conditioning. Complications associated with the resumption of physical training, even among elite athletes, seem to be rare.[135] Modest weight reduction during lactation appears to be safe and does not seem to compromise infant weight gain in most cases.[136,137] As a general rule, feeding their babies before exercise helps mothers avoid problems associated with breast engorgement and lactic acid accumulation in breast milk.[138,139]

Returning to Work

Returning to work remains a topic replete with opinion but generally unencumbered by data. Although published in the past, ACOG has withdrawn specific written guidelines; a Committee Opinion provides only vague recommendations.[140] A survey was done by *Contemporary OB/GYN* in 1983, in which 803 questionnaires were mailed to readers; 392 responses were received (49%). When asked "How many days should patients wait before returning to work after undergoing, [p. 5] . . . scheduled repeat caesarean section, . . . ?," responses were, on average, 34.7 days (sedentary job), 39.5 days (job that requires standing or walking), and 47.6 days (job that requires heavy physical exertion).[141] Provisions of legislation such as the Family and Medical Leave Act produce a dilemma for the obstetrician, who generally is in no position to objectively assess the capabilities of the patient and has little or no medical evidence on which to rely. The facts that every patient is different and every employment situation is different would seem to demand individualization from the advising provider, but the dearth of evidence-based data to support one's recommendation invites criticism and inappropriate intrusion into the contractual arrangements between employers and employees. In our own practice, we tend to deal with this by informing patient and employer that there are little or no data to support a firm recommendation and advise the patient to return to work, and to do work, according to her comfort level. This allows the patient and her employer to negotiate, compromise, and come to a mutually acceptable arrangement.

SUMMARY OF MANAGEMENT OPTIONS

Overall Care in the Puerperium

Management Options	Evidence Quality and Recommendation	References
Bereavement (See also Chapter 25)		
Psychological and general support.	III/B	101,102
Photographs and other mementos.	IV/C	103,104
Multidisciplinary approach.	—/GPP	—
Staff training.	III/B	105
Examination of the Placenta		
General macroscopic examination of all placentas, cords, and membranes.	—/GPP	—
Formal pathologic examination with identified abnormalities.	IV/C	6
Pain Relief (especially with perineal pain), Medications, etc. (See also Chapter 70)		
Local measures and oral analgesia.	IV/C	132
Rh immune globulin if indicated.	—/GPP	—

SUMMARY OF MANAGEMENT OPTIONS
Overall Care in the Puerperium—cont'd

Management Options	Evidence Quality and Recommendation	References
Vaccines (e.g., rubella) if indicated.	—/GPP	—
Drug therapy to return to prepregnancy doses.	—/GPP	—
Most drugs are safe in breast-feeding (see Chapter 34).	—/GPP	—
Advice about smoking, alcohol, and so on.	—/GPP	—
General		
No clear data about length of in-hospital stay.	Ia/A	134
Exercise		
Gradual increase to prepregnancy levels.	—/GPP	—
Most exercise is safe in the puerperium.	IV/C	135
Breast-feeding is better before exercise.	Ib/A	138,139
Work		
Lack of data to give advice about resumption of work; common sense approach and comfort is usual.	—/GPP	—

GPP, good practice point.

OTHER PROBLEMS

Separated Symphysis Pubis

Separated symphysis pubis (SSP) is also known as "subluxation," "incomplete or partial dislocation of symphysis pubis," "diastasis of the symphysis pubis," and "pelvic girdle relaxation." It is a rare condition involving separation of the symphysis pubis in late pregnancy or during delivery. It usually occurs in otherwise healthy pregnancies and is likely to be the result of hormonal or biomechanical factors (or both).

SSP symptoms may present at any time intrapartum or postpartum, with a broad range of symptoms, including pain in the back or pelvic area, difficulty with ambulation, and local manifestation over the symphysis such as tenderness, induration, ecchymoses, and a palpable joint defect.[142] Differential diagnosis is broad and requires exclusion of more serious medical and orthopedic conditions.

Management Options

Successful treatment approaches include analgesia, bedrest, binders, limitation of ambulation, walking in a shuffling style when ambulating, avoiding both adduction and abduction of the hips, injections of local anesthetics, steroids, and other medications. Because of ambulation limitations, DVT becomes a risk, and thromboprophylaxis should be considered. Patient education and emotional support are critical, and follow-up with rehabilitative services, orthopedics, home nursing, and social input may be appropriate.[142]

Obstetric Paralysis

In most cases of maternal obstetric paralysis, symptoms are unilateral, consisting of leg weakness or, in more severe cases, foot drop. Prognosis for recovery from mild injuries is excellent with physical therapy. However, if fatty degeneration of nerve fibers has occurred, in which the nerves have been functionally severed, recovery may take much longer and may never be complete.[143,144]

The incidence of obstetric paralysis is probably between 1 in 7000 and 1 in 14,000 in patients who do not receive regional anaesthesia/analgesia.[143] In the industrialized world, obstetric paralysis is an entity seldom reported unless regional anesthesia/analgesia is involved; neurologic complications that follow childbirth are frequently blamed on epidurals and spinals, even when this is not the case.[145] The mechanisms whereby regional/conduction anesthesia/analgesia may be associated with neurologic damage include neurotoxicity, ischemia, trauma, and compression that may be due to hematomata or abscesses.[145]

Management Options

Prevention includes avoidance, if possible, of prolonged and/or obstructed labor, the use of correct second-stage and lithotomy positions.[145] Specifically, regional analgesia should be avoided when coagulopathy or infection (systemic or local) is present.[143,145]

When neurologic damage follows childbirth, it is important to elucidate the mechanism of its occurrence. It is generally advisable to seek the opinion of a neurologist early in the course of the problem. Management options include splinting, physical therapy, and electrical nerve stimulation. Paraplegia requires immediate MRI. Emergency surgery may necessary for an epidural abscess or hematoma.[144]

Urinary Retention

This is either clinically overt postpartum urinary retention, that is, the inability to void spontaneously after delivery, or covert urinary retention, identified through measurements of postvoid bladder residual volumes, measured or calculated by either catheterization or bladder imaging.

The physiologic changes of pregnancy, regional anesthesia, instrumental delivery, cesarean delivery, perineal trauma, protracted labor, and primiparity have variously been associated with postpartum urinary retention, as have rare instances of lumbar disk disease, spinal subdural hematoma, postpartum uterine retroversion, and impacted pelvic masses.

Management Options

Evidence would suggest that careful attention to all postpartum women, with prompt catheterization for those who cannot void, will prevent most problems related to urinary retention. If the residual urinary volume is greater than 400 mL, it is suggested the in-dwelling catheter should remain for at least 12 hours if not 24 hours.[146] The majority of women will recover spontaneously. Infection should be excluded. If spontaneous voiding does not follow removal of the catheter, investigation should be considered.[146]

SUMMARY OF MANAGEMENT OPTIONS

Other Puerperal Problems

Management Options	Evidence Quality and Recommendation	References
Pubic Symphysis Separation		
Most resolve with rest, trochanter belts, analgesics, weight-bearing assistance and time.	III/B	142
Consider injection of symphysis with mixture of hydrocortisone and lidocaine (chymotrypsin).	III/B	142
Consider thromboprophylaxis with prolonged bedrest.	—/GPP	—
Orthopedic treatment reserved for severe cases.	—/GPP	—
Obstetric Paralysis—Prevention	—/GPP	—
Avoid prolonged, obstructed labor.		
Proper lithotomy and pushing positions.		
Avoid regional anesthesia when coagulopathy or infection is present (systemic or local).		
Obstetric Paralysis—Management	IV/C	143–145
Seek neurologic opinion and identify the cause.		
Splinting, physical therapy, electrical nerve stimulation.		
Paraplegia warrants immediate MRI.		
Emergency surgery for epidural abscess or hematoma.		
Urinary Retention		
12–24 hr continuous drainage if > 400 mL residual; majority recover spontaneously.	—/GPP	—
Exclude infection.	—/GPP	—
Rarely, intermittent self-catheterization required.	III/B	146
Investigate if self-catheterization required.	—/GPP	—

GPP, good practice point.

CONTRACEPTION

It has been demonstrated that ovulation may occur as early as 27 days after delivery (mean 70–75 days in the absence of lactation).[147,148] Among nursing mothers, the mean time to ovulation is about 6 months.[98] Variables affecting this include frequency of suckling, duration of each suckling period, and amount of supplementation.[149]

Persistently elevated serum prolactin levels appear to be responsible for the suppression of ovulation among lactating women.[150] Levels of prolactin decrease to the normal range by the third week postpartum in nonlactating women, but remain elevated for several more weeks in lactating patients. Immediately after delivery, levels of estrogen fall in all women and remain low in lactating patients. In women not lactating, estrogen levels begin to rise 2 weeks after delivery and are significantly higher than in lactating women by day 17 postpartum. Follicle-stimulating hormone (FSH) levels are identical in women regardless of whether they are lactating. It is, therefore, assumed that the ovary does not respond to FSH stimulation in the presence of increased prolactin levels.[98]

It is generally advised that vaginal coitus may be resumed when the perineum is comfortable and lochia has slowed.

Desire and willingness to resume vaginal coitus after delivery varies greatly among women—this may depend on several factors, including return of libido, presence of vaginal atrophy because of lactation, and presence and state of healing of incisions and lacerations.[151] Most women have resumed intercourse by 3 months, some much earlier.[152] Conversely, Ryding[153] reported that 20% of women had little desire for sexual activity 3 months after delivery, and an additional 21% had complete loss of desire or aversion to sexual activity.

Abstinence, or more properly, the intention to abstain from vaginal coitus, is not an effective means of postpartum contraception. Even though it is traditional for obstetricians to advise postponing coitus, sometimes until after the traditional 6- to 8-week postpartum examination, and in spite of lochia, which may persist for 3 to 8 weeks, coitus is likely to occur, and it is prudent to have a contraception plan in effect beforehand. ACOG states that contraception is an important topic for discussion and that women should be encouraged to consider their future plans for birth control during prenatal care and be given information that will help them achieve their goals.[154]

Management Options

Choice of Contraceptive Method (See Table 76–4 for Summary of Options)

BARRIER METHODS

In general, barrier methods of contraception have fewer side effects than hormonal methods and, with the exception of cervical caps and diaphragms, are available without prescription. In addition, under some circumstances, they have been shown to provide protection against sexually transmitted diseases. A meta-analysis has shown that regular use of latex condoms decreased the coital transmission of HIV infection by 69%. Epidemiologic studies have shown a decreased risk of genital herpes simplex, gonorrhea, and nongonococcal urethritis in women whose partners faithfully use condoms.[155–157] Unfortunately, the efficacy of barrier methods in preventing both conception and infection depends heavily on the users adhering to manufacturer's recommendations. Most studies have demonstrated a significant difference between method effectiveness and use effectiveness.

HORMONAL CONTRACEPTION

ACOG has recommended that progestin-only methods can be started safely at 6 weeks postpartum in lactating women (Table 76–5) and immediately postpartum in women who do not nurse their infants. Estrogen-plus-progesterone contraception is not recommended for breast-feeding women because of the possible negative impact on lactation, albeit use of combination oral contraceptive pills by well-nourished breast-feeding women does not appear to result in infant development problems; their use can be considered after milk flow is well-established.[158,159] Manufacturers have recommended that their use be postponed until 6 weeks postpartum in breast-feeding women, because very small amounts of progestin are passed into breast milk, although no adverse effects on infants have been noted when these medications have been started earlier.[160]

TABLE 76–4

Contraceptive Techniques. Comparison of Effectiveness in Terms of Number of Pregnancies per 100 Women during the First Year of Use

TECHNIQUE	TYPICAL USE*	PERFECT USE†	RISK REDUCTION FOR SEXUALLY TRANSMITTED INFECTIONS
Continuous abstinence	0.00	0.00	Complete
Nonpenetration	N/A‡	N/A	Some
Hormone implant	0.05	0.05	None
Sterilization			
Male	0.15	0.10	None
Female	0.50	0.50	None
Depot medroxyprogesterone	0.30	0.30	None
Intrauterine device			
Copper	2.0	1.5	None
Hormonal	0.1-0.8	0.1-0.6	None
Oral contraceptives			
Combination	5.0	0.1	None
Progestin-only	5.0	0.5	None
Male condom	14.0	3.0	Good vs. HIV; reduces risk of others
Withdrawal	19.0	4.0	None
Diaphragm	20.0	6.0	Limited
Cervical cap			
Nulliparas	20.0	9.0	Limited
Paras	40.0	30.0	Limited
Female condom	21.0	5.0	Some
Predicting fertility			
Periodic abstinence	20.0		None
Postovulation method		1.0	None
Symptothermal method		2.0	None
Cervical mucus method		3.0	None
Calendar method		9.0	None
Fertility awareness methods			
With condom	N/A	N/A	None
With diaphragm or cap	N/A	N/A	None
With withdrawal or other methods	N/A	N/A	None
Spermicide	26.0	6.0	Limited
No method	85.0	85.0	None

* *Typical use* refers to failure rates for women and men whose use is not consistent or always correct.
† *Perfect use* refers to failure rates for those whose use is consistent and always correct.
‡ N/A: Effectiveness rates not available.
Modified from Facts about Birth Control. Available at www.plannedparenthood.org

TABLE 76-5

ACOG Recommendations for Hormonal Contraception if Used by Breast-feeding Women

Progestion-only oral contraceptives prescribed or dispensed at discharge from hospital to be started 2–3 wk postpartum (e.g., the first Sunday after the newborn is 2 wk old).
Depot medroxyprogesterone acetate initiated at 6 wk postpartum (earlier initiation might be considered in certain clinical situations).
Hormonal implants inserted at 6 wk postpartum.
Combined estrogen-progestin contraceptives, if prescribed, should not be started before 6 wk postpartum, and only when lactation is well established and the infant's nutritional status well monitored.

Modified from American College of Obstetrics and Gynecology (ACOG): Breast-feeding: Maternal and Infant Aspects (ACOG Educational Bulletin No. 258). Washington, DC, ACOG, 2000.

INTRAUTERINE CONTRACEPTIVE DEVICES

Copper-containing and hormone-releasing intrauterine devices (IUCDs) have been shown to be effective in preventing conception, with failure rates on the order of 2 to 3 pregnancies per 100 women-years.[161,162] Objections that the principal mode of action of IUCDs was, in essence, the abortion of a viable conceptus have been effectively laid to rest.[163] This concept has been supported by both ACOG and WHO.[98,164] It is important to inform women that, unlike barrier contraceptives, IUCDs do not provide protection against HIV or other sexually transmitted diseases.

NATURAL FAMILY PLANING

Natural family planning (NFP) remains a controversial topic. On the basis of mailing a questionnaire to 840 Missouri physicians (obstetricians/gynecologists, family practice physicians, general practice physicians, internal medicine specialists; 65% response rate), the authors concluded that most physicians underestimate the effectiveness of NFP and do not give information of modern methods to women.[165] NFP methods are based on the prediction of ovulation using temperature, cervical mucus assessment, and timing. They are not reliable in the absence of relatively regular menstrual cycles, which may take some time to reestablish following delivery.[166] Success rates similar to barrier methods have been reported.[167]

NFP methods vary greatly, but all utilize to some extent selective timing of coitus according to some or all of a variety of methods, including periodic abstinence, use of menstrual calendars, ovulation prediction, withdrawal, and lactational amenorrhea (LAM).

LACTATIONAL AMENORRHEA METHOD

Exclusive breast-feeding helps prevent pregnancy for the first 6 months after delivery but should be relied on only temporarily and when it meets carefully observed criteria of the LAM of contraception.[168] The suckling stimulus provides the only truly physiologic signal that suppresses fertility in normally nourished, healthy women. The variability in the duration of lactational amenorrhea between women is related to the variation in the strength of the suckling stimulus, a unique situation between each mother and her baby. Full breast-feeding can provide a reliable contraceptive effect in the first 6 to 9 months. In women, suckling seems to increase the sensitivity of the hypothalamus to the negative feedback effect of estradiol on suppressing the gonadotropin-releasing hormone/luteinizing hormone (GnRH/LH) pulse generator. Practical guidelines for using breast-feeding as a natural contraceptive have been developed, which allows mothers to utilize the only natural suppressor of fertility in women as an effective means of spacing births.[167]

FEMALE STERILIZATION

Tubal sterilization is the most frequently used method of contraception in the United States.[169] More than 600,000 female sterilization procedures and more than 500,000 male sterilization procedures are performed each year in the United States.[170,171] Preoperative counseling should include a clear discussion about risks of, alternatives to, possibility of failure, and planned irreversibility of permanent surgical sterilization.[169]

Complication rates are low, with an overall mortality rate of 1 to 2 deaths per 100,000 sterilization procedures.[172] Long-term effects of tubal sterilization on pelvic pain, menstrual patterns, and the need for subsequent pelvic surgery are controversial and inconsistent.[169]

The findings of the U.S. Collaborative Review of Sterilization (CREST) were published by the CDC in 1996[173]; these present the only available long-term failure rate data in a very large[100] group of women, with 58% still providing follow-up data at 8 to 14 years after their procedures. CREST showed a 10-year cumulative failure rate of 18.5 per 1000 for all sterilization methods combined. During that interval, postpartum tubal ligation and interval laparoscopic unipolar coagulation were the most effective methods (7.5 failures/1000).[173] Sterilization failures are frequently manifested as ectopic pregnancies; CREST showed a 10-year cumulative probability of ectopic pregnancy of 7.3 per 1000. The specific ectopic rate following postpartum partial salpingectomy was the lowest among all methods (1.5/1000).[174]

In 2002, the U.S. Food and Drug Administration (FDA) approved use of Essure, a hysteroscopically inserted transcervical sterilization device.[169] Success rates in excess of 99.7% have been reported,[175] albeit up to 15% of patients will require a second surgery to achieve occlusion of both fallopian tubes,[176] and the procedure should not be performed until 6 weeks postpartum.[177]

In the United States, the strongest indicator of future regret is young age at the time of sterilization, regardless of parity or marital status.[178] Women 20 to 24 years of age at sterilization are twice as likely to experience regret as women 10 years older.[179] Approximately 6% of sterilized women report regret or request information about sterilization reversal within 5 years of the procedure[169]; approximately 1% to 2% of men having vas ligation seek information on reversal.[179,180]

The success of surgical reversal of tubal sterilization would seem to be mainly related to the amount of undamaged fallopian tube remaining for reanastomosis.[181] It is difficult to compare studies concerning the success of sterilization, because they generally have small numbers and because investigators use different preoperative exclusion criteria; length of follow-up also varies significantly.[182] After a Pomeroy-type procedure was reversed, studies report subsequent term pregnancy rates of 41% to 74% in a total of 198 patients, with ectopic rates of 6% to 9%.[183–185] Following bipolar cautery, reversal success as measured by term pregnancy was 42% to 52% in a total of 137 patients, with ectopic pregnancy rates of 3% to 17%.[181,183,184]

Intrapartum or early puerperium procedures are convenient because the patient is already in the hospital. Cesarean delivery gives excellent access to the fallopian tubes. Following vaginal delivery, an epidural catheter may be left in place and then used to provide anesthesia and analgesia for a procedure later in the day or on the following day. Conversely, waiting another couple of months for an interval procedure allows time to gain confidence in the health of the baby and dispassionately discuss all implications of permanent surgical sterilization.[98]

For years, there have been concerns about a syndrome of poststerilization pain and menstrual disturbances. A large review comparing women who had tubal sterilization with controls showed no consistent differences in outcomes such as levels of hormones and little difference in the characteristics of menses, although there is, understandably, an increase in menstrual flow in women who had previously been using oral contraceptives.[186] Conversely, a cohort study with 6 years of follow-up reported that sterilized women were more likely to be hospitalized because of menstrual disorders, usually to have curettage (relative risk [RR] 2.4).[187] The subgroup of women younger than 30 years of age studied in CREST who had menstrual dysfunction predating their sterilization procedures had more menstrual changes and, ultimately, were more likely to undergo hysterectomy than were controls.[182,187,188]

Transcervical, intrauterine instillation of quinacrine may be a simple, inexpensive, effective, acceptable, and safe method of nonsurgical permanent female sterilization in some populations. A study in Bangladesh reported a 1.9% failure rate using 252 mg of quinacrine with or without adjuvant ampicillin or ibuprofen (or both). No serious complications were reported.[189] A larger study in Vietnam, however, reported higher failure rates (13% in women younger than 35, 6.8% in women older than 35). Moreover, these authors noted that toxicology studies of locally applied quinacrine were thought by WHO to be inadequate.[190] It would seem that more study is needed before this method can be recommended on a wider basis.

Some years ago, there was in the United States enthusiasm for scheduled cesarean hysterectomy as a sterilization procedure.[191] It was thought by some that this might prove to be a life-saving measure in some cases, for example, for women with cervical dysplasia who were either noncompliant with follow-up or had limited access to care. Most studies, however, reported worrisome complication rates, especially regarding the need for blood product replacement. Even though a group in Israel reported an improvement in the need for transfusion from 64% to 17% as their experience increased,[192] the prevailing feeling would seem to be that cesarean hysterectomy without other indications likely has, in most cases, an unfavorable benefit/risk ratio.

Although there is some confidence that tubal ligation protects from recurrent pelvic inflammatory disease, more than 70 cases of salpingitis and almost 40 cases of tubo-ovarian abscess in women who had undergone tubal occlusion have been published.[193] Most cases of salpingitis developed more than a year after either laparoscopic or laparotomy procedures. Tubo-ovarian abscesses developed over a broad interval of time following operation, ranging from weeks to decades.

SUMMARY OF MANAGEMENT OPTIONS

Puerperal Contraception and Sterilization

Management Options	Evidence Quality and Recommendation	References
Contraception		
See Table 76–5 for relative effectiveness of different methods.	IV/C	194
Barrier		
Few side effects, some protection against sexually transmitted disease.	III/B	155–157
Effectiveness totally dependent on user compliance.	—/GPP	—
Hormonal		
Progestin-only preparations for breast-feeding women.	IV/C	160
Relies on user compliance.	—/GPP	—
IUCD		
Main concerns relate to failure to protect against infection.	—/GPP	—
Natural Family Planning		
Main problem as a method in the puerperium is that the method relies on a regular menstrual cycle, which is uncommon initially.	IV/C	166

Management Options	Evidence Quality and Recommendation	References
Lactation Amenorrhea Method		
Much debate in the literature over the value of this method/approach.	III/B	154,167
Sterilization		
Tubal sterilization (Different Techniques)		
Patients must be counseled about		
• The procedure.	—/GPP	—
• The irreversibility (varies with method).	III/B	169,173
• Failure rates (varies with method and timing with respect to delivery).	III/B	172
• Complications (e.g., regret, ectopics, menstrual disturbance, death).	III/B	169
Cesarean Hysterectomy		
Should be considered only in a few selected cases.	III/B	191,192
Chemical Methods		
Not currently advocated; further research needed.	IIb/B	189,190
Vasectomy		
Same counseling as with female sterilization:	III/B	171
• The procedure.		
• The irreversibility.		
• Failure rates.		
• Complications (generally safe, with no evidence of prostate or testicular cancer of cardiovascular disease).		

GPP, good practice point; IUCD, intrauterine contraceptive device.

SUGGESTED READINGS

Alexander J, Thomas P, Sanghera J: Treatments for secondary postpartum hemorrhage. Cochrane Database Syst Rev 2002;1:CD002867.

American College of Obstetricians and Gynecologists (ACOG): Breastfeeding: Maternal and infant Aspects (ACOG Committee Opinion No. 361). Washington, DC, ACOG, February 2007.

American College of Obstetricians and Gynecologists (ACOG): Postpartum Hemorrhage (ACOG Practice Bulletin No. 76). Washington, DC, October 2006.

Brumfield CG, Hauth JC, Andrews WW: Puerperal infection after cesarean delivery: Evaluation of a standardized protocol. Am J Obstet Gynecol 2000;182:1147–1151.

Cates W Jr, Stone KM: Family planning, sexually transmitted diseases and contraceptive choice: A literature update. Fam Plann Perspect 1992;24:75–84.

Hague WM, North RA, Gallus AS, et al: A Working Group on Behalf of the Obstetric Medicine Group of Australia. Anticoagulation in pregnancy and the puerperium. Med J Aust 2001;175:258–263.

Lockwood CJ: Inherited thrombophilias in pregnant patients: Detection and treatment paradigm. Obstet Gynecol 2002;99:333–341.

Peterson HB, Xia Z, Hughes JM, et al: The risk of pregnancy after tubal sterilization: Findings from the U.S. Collaborative Review of Sterilization. Am J Obstet Gynecol 1996;174:1161–1168.

Silver RM, Varner MW, Reddy U, et al: Work-up of stillbirth: A review of the evidence. Am J Obstet Gynecol 2007;196:433–444.

Spitz AM, Lee NC, Peterson HB: Treatment for lactation suppression: Little progress in one hundred years. Am J Obstet Gynecol 1998;179:1485–1490.

REFERENCES

For a complete list of references, log onto www.expertconsult.com.

CHAPTER 77

Major Obstetric Hemorrhage and Disseminated Intravascular Coagulation

STEPHEN W. LINDOW and JOHN ANTHONY

INTRODUCTION

Maternal death from obstetric hemorrhage remains a global problem. In developing countries, it ranks among the leading three causes of maternal death, and industrialized nations continue to report mortality rates in cases in which problems could have been anticipated and prevented.[1,2] In developing countries, postpartum hemorrhage (PPH) accounts for a higher percentage of deaths due to hemorrhage. The combination of uterine atony with retained products of conception leading to hypovolemic shock and coagulopathy are the most common complications giving rise to death from obstetric hemorrhage.

The U.K. Confidential Enquiry into Maternal and Child Health (2002–2005)[2] has emphasized the need to recognize the antenatal woman at risk of obstetric hemorrhage and to ensure that a multidisciplinary consultant–led team including hematologists, anesthetists, and obstetricians is available to provide adequate care. The unpredictability of obstetric hemorrhage is also acknowledged in this report, and the importance of having early warning scoring systems and protocols to deal with massive hemorrhage is stressed.

Major obstetric hemorrhage is the largest cause of severe maternal morbidity in Scotland, accounting for almost 70% of the total from all causes (a rate of 3.66/1000 maternities).[2]

MAJOR OBSTETRIC HEMORRHAGE

Definition

"Major obstetric hemorrhage" is an imprecise term, but it has been defined as an estimated blood loss of greater than 2500 mL, transfusion of 5 or more units of blood, or treatment for coagulopathy.[2] This chapter deals with the risks and management of severe or major obstetric hemorrhage in which there is a risk of hypovolemic shock. Inevitably, there is some overlap with other chapters, which are cross-referenced.

Incidence

The incidence is difficult to estimate because the definition includes all severe episodes of antepartum, intrapartum, primary, and secondary PPH, and these figures are not recorded collectively or statutorily. The incidence is likely to be about 0.5%, with the largest number of cases being due to primary PPH.

Etiology

Major obstetric hemorrhage is generally caused by the following:

- Placental abruption (see also Chapter 58).
- Placenta previa (see also Chapter 58).
- Causes of primary PPH (see also Chapter 75).
- Ruptured uterus (see also Chapter 75).

However, underlying disease may contribute to the bleeding, including the following:

- Bleeding disorders (e.g., von Willebrand's disease).
- Acquired hemostatic disorders due to liver failure (e.g., fulminant hepatitis, acute fatty liver of pregnancy).
- Severe disseminated intravascular coagulation (discussed in this chapter).
- Platelet dysfunction (e.g., severe preeclampsia, thrombotic thrombocytopenic purpura).

Antepartum hemorrhage accounts for fewer deaths than PPH in developing countries, although this pattern is reversed in industrialized countries.

Maternal Risks

Death

Deaths due to major antepartum hemorrhage are usually due to placental abruption. Maternal death from placental abruption is attributable to the effects of hypovolemia (see following discussion) combined with the complications that may arise from underlying predisposing conditions such as preeclampsia. The resting uterine tone may be increased ($\leq$25 mm Hg) and labor may be triggered by placental separation with the sudden onset of frequent contractions.[3,4] Although hypovolemic shock and its sequelae may develop as a result of acute blood loss, hypertension may precede or follow abruptio placentae.[5] The coincident occurrence of hypertension due to preeclampsia together with hypovolemia as a result of abruptio placentae increases the risk of renal failure due to tubular necrosis.[6] Up to one third of pregnancy-related cases of acute renal failure are due to abruptio placentae.[6] Proteinuria is usually found in cases of abruptio placentae, and the pattern of glomerular protein loss is similar to that seen in acute ischemic renal failure.[7] The mother is at risk of severe hypovolemia from placenta previa also, especially as a result of morbidly adherent implantation over a previous cesarean section scar. Placenta previa is also associated with recurrent antepartum hemorrhage and operative delivery.

Severe primary PPH can lead to hypovolemic shock. Other complications are those associated with the treatment of the underlying condition such as from transfusion-related injury and surgical complications of hysterectomy.

The reported risk of maternal death following uterine rupture varies widely, being very low in industrialized countries but up to 38% in developing countries with limited resources.[8–10] Maternal morbidity rates associated with uterine rupture include all the complications that may follow severe hypovolemic shock, postoperative complications, and reproductive sequelae that include loss of fertility and the need for future operative delivery.

Hypovolemic Shock

Shock is a clinical condition characterized by inadequate tissue perfusion due to any one of the following:

- Impaired peripheral circulation because of diminished intravascular blood volume (hypovolemic shock)—only this form of shock is covered in this chapter.
- Left ventricular failure (cardiogenic shock).
- Disruption of vasoregulatory homeostasis as a result of inappropriate peripheral vasodilation (distributive shock).

Hypovolemia leads to a reduction in peripheral blood flow through the splanchnic and cutaneous circulation as a result of selective vasoconstriction mediated by the central nervous system and a baroreceptor sympathetic response. These differential changes in vascular tone allow selective preservation of blood flow to the brain, heart, and adrenal glands. Venous return to the heart is augmented by a reduction in venous capacitance mediated by catecholamine-induced venoconstriction. This sustains cardiac filling pressures, stroke volume, cardiac output, and critical organ oxygenation. Intravascular volume is also replenished by renal conservation of sodium and water triggered by increased formation of angiotensin. The secretion of antidiuretic hormone further contributes to the renal adaptation.

Sympathetic stimulation and an increase in circulating catecholamines both lead to a rising heart rate and increased myocardial contractility that further increase myocardial oxygen demand. Ongoing hemorrhage and the development of anerobic metabolism with acidosis may lead to left ventricular failure and the development of irreversible shock.

The immunologic and metabolic response to injury is characterized by the development of the systemic inflammatory response syndrome (SIRS). This process, triggered by hypovolemia and hypoxia, gives rise to diffuse effects as a result of damage to the vascular endothelium.[11] The initial endothelial response to hypoxia includes the expression of adhesion molecules that bind lymphocytes and leukocytes as well as platelets. The activated white blood cells produce and release a range of proinflammatory cytokines and oxygen free radicals.[12] The latter species augment oxidative stress and promote lipid peroxidation once antioxidant mechanisms are saturated. Lipid peroxidation of cell membranes is presumed to result in the loss of vascular integrity with increased vascular permeability. This mechanism is the basis for the development of acute respiratory distress syndrome (ARDS) in the lung and also contributes to the development of multiorgan failure.

Reperfusion injury is also implicated in the development of multiorgan failure. When hypoxic cells can no longer sustain anaerobic metabolism because of glycogen depletion, ATP (adenosine triphosphate) levels fall and homeostatic regulation of ionic flux across the cell membrane fails with rising intracellular sodium and calcium levels. Changes in intracellular calcium concentration adversely affect various enzymes, including xanthine dehydrogenase, converting the enzyme to xanthine oxidase. This switch allows the metabolism of accumulating hypoxanthine (derived from purine catabolism) to superoxide anion and hydrogen peroxide once perfusion and oxygenation are restored.[13] The subsequent release of reactive oxygen species and peroxide augments oxidative stress giving rise to further endothelial damage. Reperfusion injury often arises from delayed restoration of flow through the splanchnic circulation even after adequate resuscitation. The ischemic gut contains xanthine oxidase and is able to generate oxygen free radicals that on reperfusion. may overwhelm the hepatic antioxidant defense mechanisms trigerring systemic endothelial damage and contributing to the onset of multiorgan failure. In addition, reduced splanchnic flow alters gut mucosal permeability, allowing the absorption of intestinal bacteria and toxins into the portal circulation.

Disseminated Intravascular Coagulation

Changes in the coagulation system accompany acute blood loss and will vary according to the extent of the blood loss and the underlying pathology associated with bleeding. The acute-phase response elicited by any form of trauma is characterized by increased hepatic synthesis of clotting factors and hyperhomocysteinemia. The resultant hypercoagulability is seldom clinically evident because these effects are usually overwhelmed in women with acute obstetric blood loss by consumptive coagulopathy.

The clotting defect seen in women after obstetric hemorrhage usually develops because of consumption of clotting factors, leading to a bleeding tendency. Disseminated intravascular coagulation (DIC) is frequently also present and develops whenever procoagulant mechanisms promote fibrin formation in the circulation. The hematologic consequences of DIC are often clinically insignificant but are sometimes associated with a profound coagulopathy (typically seen in the anaphylactoid syndrome of pregnancy but also seen in severe sepsis in which liver dysfunction and thrombocytopenia add to the risk of coagulopathy). DIC contributes to the development of organ failure as a result of SIRS, although the management of this complication is the management of the underlying condition rather than the DIC itself. The numerous mechanisms that trigger DIC do so by endothelial or platelet activation and via the release of thromboplastin into the circulation. Hence, procoagulant changes accompany the development of SIRS and are induced by leukocyte activation and endothelial dysfunction.[14] The presence of placental tissue or amniotic fluid in the maternal circulation initiates intravascular coagulation, and thromboplastin release into the circulation is known to occur in cases of abruptio placentae.

Fibrin formation initiates fibrinolysis, leading to the formation of plasmin and the elaboration of fibrin degradation products (FDPs) that are readily measurable in the peripheral circulation (e.g., quantitative D-dimer levels). Although these breakdown products of fibrin are used to diagnose intravascular coagulation, the protection of vascular integrity during normal pregnancy includes sufficient intravascular coagulation to increase D-dimer levels with an increase in circulating thrombin-antithrombin complexes. Accelerated formation of fibrin stimulates fibrinolysis. Plasmin may stimulate the complement cascade, which further contributes to the development of increased capillary permeability.

The physiologic adaptations of pregnancy protect the mother from the hemodynamic and hemostatic effects of hemorrhage at the time of delivery. These changes include a 30% increase in blood volume as a result of plasma volume expansion combined with an increase in red blood cell mass. These changes are accompanied by physiologic peripheral vasodilation to accommodate the increased blood volume and cardiac output. The combined effects of these changes allow more extensive hemorrhage prior to the development of shock and the net gain of 1 to 2 L of intravascular volume exceeds the estimated blood loss of 500 to 600 mL at the time of normal delivery. Hemostasis is augmented by increased hepatic production of clotting factors, especially fibrinogen, and the anticlotting mechanism is impeded by a reduction in the level of free protein S. Fibrinolysis also diminishes in response to placental production of plasminogen activator inhibitor II.

Clinical Presentation

The development of hypovolemic shock is recognized by a progressive fall in blood pressure and a rising pulse rate. The severity of the blood loss can be classified on the basis of clinical signs alone (Table 77–1).[15]

Hemodynamic monitoring will confirm low ventricular filling pressures (central venous pressure or pulmonary capillary wedge pressure) and a low cardiac output. In addition, measurement of central venous oxygen saturation will confirm increased rates of oxygen extraction (<65%) as cardiac output and peripheral perfusion diminish. In determining the diagnosis of acute hypovolemia, investigations are of limited utility. This is especially true of hemoglobin concentration estimation because the hematocrit will fall only as transcapillary rehydration from interstitial fluid takes place slowly over several hours.

Coagulopathy may be very obvious in the woman who presents with bleeding gums and oozing from all venipuncture sites. In many cases of coagulopathy, however, these signs will not be evident and the diagnosis will depend upon measurement of the International Normalized Ratio (INR), activated partial thromboplastin time (aPTT), and platelet count.

Renal Failure

Acute oliguric renal failure will develop as a consequence of hypovolemic shock. The loss of 15% to 30% of the intravascular blood volume will result in reduced renovascular perfusion and readily reversible changes in urinary output and blood urea and creatinine levels. Ongoing blood loss leads to the development of acute tubular necrosis in which ischemic injury to the tubules results in tubular epithelial cells becoming detached and blocking the tubules. This adds an obstructive component to the renal ischemia that will further reduce glomerular filtration. The development of SIRS may also add an immunologic component to the pathogenesis of renal tubular dysfunction.

Acute Respiratory Distress Syndrome

ARDS develops as part of the systemic inflammatory response syndrome but may also arise as a consequence of multiple blood transfusions. In the latter case, human leukocyte antibodies present in transfused plasma may be responsible for activation of the complement cascade with subsequent pulmonary vascular injury. ARDS is characterized clinically as a form of noncardiogenic pulmonary edema. The underlying pathophysiology is based upon inflammatory changes rather than an accumulation of interstitial edema fluid (usually associated with high pulmonary capillary wedge pressures).

Complications of Blood Transfusion

The immediate complications include incompatible transfusion, hyperkalemia, and citrate intoxication. Hyperkalemia arises because of the leakage of potassium from stored red blood cells and is a potential problem in those who require transfusion despite renal failure. The development of hyperkalemia may be suspected if the electrocardiogram shows peaked T-waves with wide PR and QRS intervals. Citrate intoxication develops because calcium ions are chelated, leading to hypocalcemia (manifest as irritability, hypotension, and a prolonged QT interval on the electrocardiogram). Conversely, the U.K. Confidential Enquiry into Maternal and Child Health has demonstrated that some maternal deaths from major obstetric hemorrhage have resulted from a failure to give sufficient blood replacement.[2]

TABLE 77–1

Clinical Classification of the Severity of Blood Loss

CLINICAL SIGN	BLOOD LOSS < 15%	BLOOD LOSS 15%–30%	BLOOD LOSS 30%–40%	BLOOD LOSS > 40%
Pulse rate (beats/min)	<100	>100	>120	>140
Blood pressure	Normal	Normal	Decreased	Decreased
Urinary output (mL/hr)	>30	20–30	5–15	<5
Neurologic status	Anxiety	Anxiety	Confusion	Lethargy

From Marino PL: The ICU Book. New York, Williams & Wilkins, 1998, p 209.

Transfusion-related lung injury presents as noncardiogenic pulmonary edema within several hours of transfusion and requires mechanical ventilation for up to 48 hours. Longer-term risks are those related to infection with hepatitis viruses, HIV, and bacterial infection.

Endocrinopathy

During pregnancy, the pituitary gland increases in size severalfold. The blood supply to the anterior pituitary gland is dependent on flow through the superior hypophyseal artery and is susceptible to avascular necrosis. The likely clinical presentation includes failure of lactation, amenorrhea, and loss of secondary sexual characteristics, followed by the evolution of hypothyroidism and adrenocortical insufficiency (Sheehan's syndrome). Sheehan's syndrome may evolve over a lengthy period of time after the precipitating event. The diagnosis should be suspected in the woman who fails to lactate, and confirmatory tests of hypothalamic and pituitary function are carried out. Neuroradiologic investigation will usually reveal an abnormal or empty sella turcica.

Anemia

Anemia may be a late complication of massive hemorrhage. Replenishment of the red blood cell mass will require hematopoiesis dependent on adequate iron stores associated with a normal dietary intake of folic acid.

Fetal Risks

Death

Fetal loss in association with placental abruption is due to hypoxia and prematurity, with perinatal mortality rates as high as 12%.[16] Placental abruption is the leading cause of perinatal death in many countries.[17,18] Fetomaternal hemorrhage is a common occurrence following abruptio placentae.[19]

Major obstetric hemorrhage due to placenta previa less commonly causes perinatal death, but again, this is due to prematurity or fetal hypoxia.[20–22]

The fetal risks following uterine rupture depend on the nature of the rupture and vary from no adverse effects to severe asphyxia and death.

Cerebral Hypoxia

Antepartum or intrapartum hypoxia may result in an infant in poor condition at delivery, with subsequent development of convulsions, intracerebral edema, and hemorrhage. This may lead to conditions such as periventricular leukomalacia and porencephalic cysts and long-term neurologic handicap. Pulmonary hemorrhage and necrotizing enterocolitis may also occur after a hypoxic episode.

Consequences of Prematurity

These complications account for most of the cases of neonatal death if the infant has survived the initial insult, and include respiratory distress syndrome and persistent fetal circulation with patent ductus arteriosus. Complications associated with prolonged neonatal intensive care such as sepsis and bronchopulmonary dysplasia are relatively common.

Management Options (See also Chapters 58 and 75)

Prenatal: Identification of "At-Risk" Patients

ANY BLEEDING

Massive blood loss cannot always be anticipated or prevented. Some high risk patients can be identified more easily, such as those with placenta previa. However, the prediction of such an event in the general obstetric population is poor. If a woman is anemic prior to labor, or states that she will refuse blood products on religious grounds, she is at increased risk should she bleed excessively in association with delivery. It is good practice in such cases for delivery to occur in a large unit with appropriate staff and facilities.

Patients who have had a previous hemorrhage in pregnancy are at risk of recurrence and should be counseled about such risk and delivered in larger obstetric units with full resuscitative measures available. They should be aware of the procedures for urgent admission to the unit and the need to attend with any degree of bleeding. Iron prophylaxis is advisable in this group (although the risk of major hemorrhage is not generally seen as an indication for routine iron therapy).

PLACENTA PREVIA

Advancing age and parity are associated with the development of placenta previa, although the relative importance of these two factors is disputed.[23,24] Uterine scars, previous miscarriages, terminations, and dilation and curettage are reported as predisposing factors, possibly owing to endometrial damage.[25] Placenta previa is more common in multiple pregnancy, owing to increased placental size. Maternal age is an important factor in recurrent placenta previa, and the risk of recurrence is quoted as between 10% and 15%.[26] There is an association between a previous cesarean section and the subsequent development of placenta previa (3%–10%); the risk increases with the number of previous cesarean sections.[23,27] This group of patients is also at risk of placenta accreta (reported as 10%–67%), again increasing with the number of previous cesarean sections. Any patient with a placenta previa and previous cesarean section should be informed of the possible necessity of a hysterectomy. The repeat cesarean section should be booked in an appropriate unit and performed by a senior obstetrician with blood cross-matched and immediately available. Techniques for the antenatal prediction of placenta accreta have not been found to be accurate. The presence of placental lacunae, the border between the bladder and the myometrium, myometrial thickness, the clear space between the placenta and the myometrium, and color-flow Doppler have not shown the necessary sensitivity and specificity to be used as a clinical test. Magnetic resonance imaging (MRI) may prove to be useful with advances in technology, but more evidence is required at present.[28]

Only 15% to 20% of cases of placenta previa have major bleeding episodes.[29,30] It should be stressed to the woman with a placenta previa that she is much more likely not to have a severe hemorrhage than she is to have one, especially as ultrasonographic diagnosis has led to increased detection of asymptomatic placenta previa that may prove to be of uncertain clinical significance.

Although bleeding with a placental previa is assumed to be of maternal origin, it has been suggested that a proportion of the blood loss may be fetal in origin.[24] A denaturation test to detect the presence of fetal cells should be carried out in the presence of hemorrhage if delivery is not planned.[30]

PLACENTAL ABRUPTION

The causative factors are known in only a minority of cases of placental abruption, but an association with increasing parity, smoking, low socioeconomic status, intrauterine growth restriction, and preeclampsia is reported.[31–33]

The importance of maternal factors is shown by the recurrence rate of 6% to 16% after one placental abruption and 20% to 25% after two previous placental abruptions.[31] Interventions in women at risk have not been shown unequivocally to reduce the occurrence or consequences of placental abruption. Thus, maintenance of a normal blood pressure and cessation of smoking might reduce the risk, although this has not been proved in controlled trials. Similarly, both folic acid supplementation and low-dose aspirin therapy, though advocated by some, have not been shown to reduce the risk of recurrent abruption.

RISK OF POSTPARTUM HEMORRHAGE

Any woman having a baby is at some risk of PPH (3%–5% of deliveries), and women contemplating a home delivery should be informed of this because many cases occur unexpectedly. If there has been a previous PPH, the risks of recurrence are increased to approximately 8% to 10%. Women with a history of retained placenta and those with multiple pregnancies are also at risk. Active management of the third stage of labor should be advised.[34]

Prenatal—Active Bleeding: General Management

The essential management of major bleeding is the same, whatever the underlying cause of hemorrhage, and involves the following steps:

- Stop the bleeding.
- Restore the circulating blood volume and oxygen-carrying capacity.
- Correct any coagulation defect.
- Maintain vigilance for and dealing with the consequences of hypovolemia.

MANAGEMENT PROTOCOL

Every obstetric unit should have its own protocol for management of massive hemorrhage available on the delivery unit for all nursing and medical staff. This enables the appropriate clinical and laboratory staff to be summoned early and a clear management strategy to be adopted. An example of a general management protocol for major hemorrhage is given in Table 77–2, and these guidelines should be followed without delay as soon as a major bleeding episode is recognized. This protocol clearly outlines the necessary steps to be taken. Similar guidelines should be drawn up for any obstetric unit, customized to local circumstances.

SITE OF MANAGEMENT

The setting will vary with local resources and established practices. Many units have a high dependency area in which such patients can be managed. However, there will be a stage in the management of these patients at which admission to an intensive care unit is indicated. These indications will also vary with local resources and practices, but an arbitrary list of possible indicators is given in Table 77–3.

TABLE 77–2
Sample Major Hemorrhage Protocol

Organization

1. Switchboard operator sends urgently for the following:
   a. Obstetric resident if not present.
   b. Duty obstetric anesthetist.
   c. Obstetric nursing officer to arrange extra staff.
   d. Blood bank technician.
   e. Porter to maternity unit (for transfer of samples).
2. Consultant hematologist and obstetrician are informed of the clinical situation.
3. One nurse to be solely assigned to record keeping:
   a. Patient vital signs, central venous pressure, and urine output.
   b. Amount and type of all fluids the patient receives.
   c. Dosage and types of drugs given.
4. Prepare for theater as soon as possible—most diagnoses require surgical intervention.

Clinical Management

1. Insert two large-bore (preferably 14-gauge) cannulas. Take 20 mL of blood for complete blood count, baseline clotting studies, and cross-matching and order at least 6 units of blood together with 3 units of fresh frozen plasma.
2. Give oxygen via face mask.
3. Commence fluid replacement quickly. (All fluids and blood should be given through a warming device.)
   a. Initially crystalloid and colloid. Hartmann's solution to a maximum of 1.5-2 L.
   b. Uncrossed blood. Rh-negative, matched with the patient's ABO blood group should be given next if cross-matched blood is not ready.
   c. Cross-matched blood given as soon as possible.
   d. Give O-negative blood only if none of the above is available (but it may be life-saving).
4. Insert central venous line and urinary catheter.
5. Stop the bleeding
   a. If antepartum, deliver the fetus (see text).
   b. If postpartum, deliver the placenta if still in utero, commence bimanual compression of the uterus, and give ergometrine 0.5 mg IV. Commence syntocinon infusion of 40 units in 500 mL of Hartmann's solution to run over 4 hr.
   c. If bleeding because of genital tract trauma or retained products, take the patient to theater promptly to explore the uterine cavity and repair damage.
   d. If bleeding continues, consider coagulation failure. Temporary direct aortic compression may give valuable time.
   e. Other surgical measures:
      Direct intramyometrial injection of prostaglandin E_2 0.5 mg, or prostaglandin $F_{2\alpha}$ 0.25 mg.
      Insertion of Lynch suture.
      Ligation of uterine arteries on both sides.
      Ligation of internal iliac arteries.
      Hysterectomy.

MONITORING

The woman bleeding as a result of obstetric hemorrhage may require increasingly invasive monitoring, depending on the extent of the hemorrhage.

- Clinical monitoring should include measurement of blood pressure, pulse rate, and urinary output combined with an estimation of the extent of the blood loss on a half-hourly to hourly basis.

TABLE 77–3
Indications for Intensive Care

1. All patients requiring mechanical ventilation.
2. All patients with ongoing hemorrhage.
3. All patients requiring inotropic support.
4. All patients with organ failure
   a. Renal failure (urine output <30 mL/hr, creatinine >150 mmol/L).
   b. Respiratory distress.
5. All patients with underlying complicating disorders
   a. Preeclampsia/eclampsia/HELLP syndrome.
   b. Acute fatty liver of pregnancy.
   c. Other causes of acute liver failure.
   d. Anaphylactoid syndrome.
6. All patients with invasive monitoring

HELLP, hemolysis, elevated liver enzymes, and low platelets.

- Hypovolemic patients should all have invasive hemodynamic monitoring to assess intravascular volume and ventricular filling pressures (either a central venous pressure line or, in the case of preeclampsia, a pulmonary artery catheter)—see later discussion.
- The extent of the coagulation defect and the hemoglobin concentration must also be assessed, the frequency of which will be determined by the severity and duration of the hemorrhage.
- Organ function may be compromised by massive blood loss and the sequelae associated with resuscitation and massive transfusion. Hence, organ-specific complications such as renal failure and acute lung injury should be considered and laboratory monitoring of renal function, peripheral oxygenation, and chest x-rays may all be required on a daily basis. In high-dependency units, peripheral oxygen saturation is commonly monitored continuously during resuscitation.

FLUID, BLOOD, AND BLOOD PRODUCT REPLACEMENT

Restoration of the circulating blood volume and reperfusion of ischemic organs is an essential priority and needs to be accomplished within 6 hours of developing hypovolemia if inflammatory sequelae are to be avoided.[35] Intravenous fluids must be infused as rapidly as possible until the pulse rate begins to decline. Thereafter, the volume infused should be titrated against a number of clinical parameters, including blood pressure (aiming for mean arterial pressure > 60 mm Hg), peripheral capillary filling, urinary output, and central venous pressure. In the intensive care setting, other indices of tissue oxygenation (oxygen delivery and consumption indices) as well as mixed venous oxygen saturation levels may be used to optimize fluid management.[35,36]

If blood loss is anticipated, blood salvage techniques can be used for autologous transfusion during cesarean section, thus reducing the need for homologous blood transfusions.[37]

The rapid administration of fluids depends upon the viscosity of the fluid chosen and the physical properties of the cannula used to establish the infusion. Acellular fluids (rather than blood or packed red blood cells) can be infused rapidly and should be used to initiate resuscitation. Randomized studies have shown no benefit associated with the use of colloidal solutions; consequently, they should be used only as an adjunct to crystalloids in specific situations in which low oncotic pressure may complicate the presentation (e.g., severe preeclampsia with abruptio placentae). Crystalloids commonly used for resuscitation include lactated Ringer's solution or normal saline. The choice of the cystalloid is probably less important than the volume and the rate at which the solution is given. The rate of fluid infusion is determined by the bore and length of the infusion cannula with short large-bore peripheral cannulas (ideally, two 14-gauge cannulae) being preferable to long central lines. The initial goal of fluid therapy is a fall in pulse rate with a rise in mean arterial blood pressure to above 60 mm Hg. As a rule of thumb, the amount of crystalloid required will be three times the volume of blood lost. Central venous pressure measurement after resuscitation should rise to between 10 and 12 mm Hg and fluid should be administered as a bolus challenge against the central venous pressure until a sustained rise in pressure beyond these values can be demonstrated. If central venous oxygen saturation monitoring is utilized, values of less than 65% are associated with abnormally high rates of oxygen extraction from blood perfusing the peripheral tissues as a result of ongoing hypovolemia and indicate the need for ongoing resuscitation.

Occasionally, severe persistent hypotension despite fluid resuscitation indicates the need for inotropic support to maintain sufficient cardiac output. This can be attained using adrenaline, dopamine, or dobutamine. Vasopressor doses of adrenaline range from 0.01 to 0.1 μg/kg/min and should be titrated against the blood pressure. Dopamine in a dose of 4 to 7 μg/kg/min stimulates β-receptors and increases cardiac output. Dobutamine is primarily a β_1-receptor stimulant and is mostly used for treating left ventricular failure in a dose of 5 to 15 μg/kg/min. Control of hemorrhage and adequate fluid replacement should allow rapid weaning from inotropic support.

Correction of the coagulation defect usually requires the administration of fresh frozen plasma (FFP) in a ratio of 1 unit to every unit of packed red blood cells considered necessary to restore the oxygen-carrying capacity.[38] Each unit of FFP will restore procoagulant activity by about 10% and will also raise the fibrinogen level by 25 mg/dL. Cryoprecipitate contains Factor VIII, fibrinogen, and von Willebrand's factor and should be given when the fibrinogen levels fall below 100 mg/dL. Each adult dose of cryoprecipitate will raise the fibrinogen level by 100 mg/dL. The advice of a hematologist should be sought when correcting the coagulation defect that develops after massive hemorrhage. Platelets do not need to be infused to restore hemostasis until the count falls below 50×10^9 cells/Lm providing the platelets are functionally normal (women with preeclampsia may have qualitative platelet defects as well as thrombocytopenia). Each adult dose of platelet concentrate will raise the platelet count by 20 to 40×10^9 cells/L.[39] Administration of FFP should be continued until the aPTT and INR are measurably normal (Table 77–4).

For the patient with uncontrollable hemorrhage in whom all other measures have failed, evidence is accumulating that recombinant Factor VIIa is proving successful.[40–42]

Correction of the red blood cell mass deficit is guided by the rule that each unit of packed cells will restore

TABLE 77-4
Blood Component Therapy*

	NUMBER OF DONORS	FIBRINOGEN CONCENTRATION	FIBRINOGEN PER UNIT	PLATELETS PER ADULT DOSE	INCREASE IN HEMATOLOGIC PARAMETER (70-KG ADULT)
Packed cells (1 unit)	1	Negligible	–	Negligible	Hemoglobin increase 1 g/dL
Fresh frozen plasma (1 unit)	1	2-5 mg/mL	550-1395 mg (240-300 mL)	Negligible	Fibrinogen increase 0.25 g/L
Cryoprecipitate (1 adult dose)	10	15 mg/mL	3-6 g (200-500 mL)	Negligible	Fibrinogen increase 1 g/L
Platelet Concentrate (1 adult dose)	4	~2 mg/mL	~500 mg	240×10^9	Platelet count increase $20\text{-}40 \times 10^9$

* The values are not consistent between different blood transfusion services.
From McClelland DBL (ed): Handbook of Transfusion Medicine, 4th ed. United Kingdom Blood Services. London, TSO, 2007.

hemoglobin concentration by 1 g/dL. There is no consensus regarding what would be generally considered a desirable hemoglobin concentration. Hemoglobin concentrations of 6 g/dL or less probably merit transfusion, and in obstetric patients with ongoing blood loss, a more liberal transfusion policy is necessary. Full cross-match is preferred prior to transfusion, although with massive hemorrhage, type-specific partially cross-matched blood can be used (5-min cross-match). Most labor units will also have a limited supply of type O-negative blood available for obstetric emergencies. Because of the risks associated with transfusion of donated blood, in circumstances in which the need for transfusion may be foreseeable, autologous blood transfusion should be offered and can be accomplished by either predonation or preoperative normovolemic hemodilution.

During resuscitation, supplemental oxygen delivery should be provided by means of a 40% face mask and the patient should be kept warm with space blankets or commercially available pneumatic blanket warming device. Additional intensive care monitoring of blood pressure via a radial artery line is also helpful both to allow continuous monitoring of the systemic pressure and to facilitate repeated hematologic investigation.

Prenatal—Active Bleeding: Specific Management

PLACENTAL ABRUPTION

In severe abruption, the woman is usually in severe pain and may be in shock due to hypovolemia. The amount of vaginal bleeding will vary. Coagulopathy occurs in about one third of cases when the fetus is dead, but is comparatively rare with a live fetus. Labor occurs spontaneously in approximately 50% of patients.

Maternal resuscitation, as described in the previous section, is the immediate priority. Adequate analgesia should be given if required, usually by intravenous narcotics supplemented by nitrous oxide/oxygen mixtures self-administered by mask. Epidural analgesia is contraindicated in any woman who is actively bleeding sufficient to produce hypovolemia, hypotension, coagulopathy, or acute fetal compromise because of the peripheral vasodilation associated with lumbar sympathetic blockade.

The only treatment for continuing severe placental abruption is to empty the uterus as soon as feasible. If the fetus is dead, normal management is to aim for a vaginal delivery, except where there is an obvious obstetric indication for cesarean section, such as transverse lie. In rare situations, uterine contractions cannot be stimulated or maternal shock is uncorrectable. Cesarean section may have to be undertaken in such cases, although there is a significant maternal risk from further blood loss, especially if there is also a coagulopathy. If there is no response to oxytocin, prostaglandins may be administered with appropriate surveillance in an attempt to stimulate uterine contractions. The management of labor in patients with abruptio placentae is uninformed by any randomized evidence, and no clear guidelines are thus available. There is an increased risk of uterine rupture with a large abruption, particularly if there is a Couvelaire uterus.

Determining if the fetus is alive by auscultation might be difficult because of a tender, hypertonic uterus, especially if there is a retroplacental clot and anterior placenta. Accordingly, visualization of the heart using ultrasound is usually the quickest method if a machine is available. If not, it may be necessary to rupture the membranes and attach a fetal electrocardiogram electrode, providing the patient is known to have been screened for HIV infection. Exclusion of placenta previa may be difficult on clinical grounds if the presenting part cannot be palpated, and the two conditions may coexist. Ideally, location of the placental site is checked by ultrasonography before any vaginal examination.

If the fetus is alive, consideration should be given to early delivery by cesarean section for fetal reasons. This will depend on the gestation, because it is extremely improbable that a fetus under 26 weeks will survive such an asphyxial episode. The mode of delivery will also depend on the fetal condition as judged by cardiotocography. If the fetal heart rate pattern is totally normal (which is unlikely), induction of labor with continuous monitoring can be considered. An abnormal cardiotocograph tracing is usually an indication for cesarean delivery, providing that the fetal heart beat is confirmed to be present immediately prior to the cesarean section.

The clinical diagnosis of abruptio placentae in the woman who has had a previous cesarean delivery must lead to consideration of whether the clinical presentation could be due to uterine rupture. Signs of generalized peritonitis, cessation of labor, hematuria, and malpresentation may all indicate uterine rupture; abdominal paracentesis may also reveal hemoperitoneum. A high index of clinical suspicion necessitates laparotomy to exclude the diagnosis.

PLACENTA PREVIA

Massive hemorrhage from placenta previa follows smaller "warning" bleeds in the majority of cases, and the placental site will often already be known. The fetal heart is usually still present, and in addition, there may be evidence of uterine contractions or premature rupture of membranes in about 20% of cases.

Initial management involves maternal resuscitation, as described earlier. A patient with such a severe hemorrhage due to placenta previa will require delivery by cesarean section irrespective of whether the fetus is dead or alive. The cesarean section may need to be performed as resuscitative efforts are under way if the mother's condition cannot be stabilized. Occasionally, vaginal delivery may be contemplated if the fetus is dead or extremely premature. When there is any possibility of placenta previa, a digital examination should occur only in the operating room after the decision has been made to deliver and the diagnosis of placenta previa is in doubt. Cesarean section for placenta previa is often a difficult procedure associated with fetal malpresentation, a poorly developed lower uterine segment, and excessive blood loss that further compromises the condition of the patient. The operation should be performed by a senior obstetrician in association with a senior anesthetist and with extra blood immediately available.

Several aspects of cesarean delivery present additional unresolved dilemmas. These include the choice of anesthesia, the technique by which the amniotic cavity is reached, and the method of delivery of the baby. Regional anesthesia, which is the generally preferred technique of obstetric anesthesia, is associated with peripheral vasodilation that could be deleterious in women who experience massive intraoperative hemorrhage. Reaching the amniotic cavity in women with an anterior placenta previa presents the surgeon with a choice of dissecting the placenta free from the decidua in order to open the amniotic cavity at the edge of the placenta or the alternative choice of transecting the placenta to open the amniotic cavity directly beneath the uterine incision. These techniques have not been subject to randomized comparison, and most practice is informed only by prevailing surgical habit. Delivery of the baby may similarly challenge the surgeon to attempt a potentially difficult cephalic delivery compared with internal podalic version and breech extraction.

Placenta previa accreta may be encountered in about 5% of cases with no previous scar in the uterus and in up to 67% of cases with multiple cesarean sections. Early recourse to hysterectomy may be necessary, but conservative management has been attempted, including oxytocics, uterine devascularization procedures, brace sutures, and catheter compression techniques (see later discussion). PPH is also more common because of the inability of the lower uterine segment to contract efficiently and should be anticipated and similar prophylactic measures taken (see later discussion).

PRIMARY POSTPARTUM HEMORRHAGE

Initial Management

Most cases of massive PPH are primary and occur within the first hour after delivery. It is relatively uncommon for secondary hemorrhage to present with blood loss of more than 1000 mL.

The principles of management are as follows:

- Arrest the hemorrhage.
- Resuscitation (see earlier discussion).
- Definitive management of the underlying problem.

In the labor ward, initial treatment should include rubbing up the fundus to expel clots and to provoke a uterine contraction. Massive hemorrhage in excess of the attainable rate of fluid replacement may lead to rapidly progressive hypovolemia and cardiac arrest. This situation should be recognized when it develops, and temporizing measures are necessary to allow resuscitative measures time to restore circulating blood volume. The temporizing measures employed are those of controlling blood loss by direct pressure on the bleeding vessels. In the case of uterine hemorrhage, this is achieved by bimanual compression of the uterine fundus. The fundus of the uterus is sandwiched between the fist of the obstetrician placed in the anterior vaginal fornix and the abdominal hand that compresses the body of the uterus against the vaginal hand. In desperate circumstances, aortic compression should also be considered. This can be executed by placing the palm of the hand on the abdomen above the umbilicus and applying firm pressure to occlude the aorta.

The cause of the bleeding should be identified early in the management. The main causes are uterine atony (including retained placental tissue), trauma, and coagulation defects.

Management of the Underlying Cause

Few of the necessary interventions can be sustained on the basis of randomized studies. However, the role of oxytocic drugs has been reviewed, and their utility in active management of the third stage of labor is well established.[43]

More than one etiologic factor may be present. The most common cause is uterine atony. Pharmacologic intervention must include a range of oxytocic drugs. First-line treatment requires the use of oxytocin and ergometrine. Oxytocin is administered as a bolus of 5 units intravenously followed by an infusion of 20 units in a liter of Ringer's lactate or normal saline. Ergometrine is given, either in combination with oxytocin (syntometrine) or on its own, in a dose of 0.5 mg intramuscularly or intravenously. This dose may be repeated. Ergometrine may be of limited utility in developing countries with poor facilities for refrigeration and storage away from light.[44,45] There is some evidence that rectal misoprostol may be an effective agent for controlling severe hemorrhage and should be used in combination with oxytocin and ergometrine.[43,46,47] Other pharmacologic options include the use of methylated prostaglandin $F_{2\alpha}$ preparations (Hemabate), although the side effect profile of the prostaglandin $F_{2\alpha}$ analogues include hypertension, bronchospasm, and diarrhea that limits the utility of these agents even if they are effective in controlling uterine hemorrhage.[48]

Persistent uterine hemorrhage unresponsive to pharmacologic manipulation may need to be dealt with surgically in a series of increasingly radical procedures. The choice of procedure will be influenced by the specific individual circumstances that may include bleeding due to retained products, hemorrhage as a result of persistent uterine atony, bleeding at the time of cesarean section, bleeding from the lower segment following delivery of a placenta previa, and bleeding as a result of trauma. The surgical options include evacuation of the uterus, devascularization of the uterus, compression techniques, and definitive management in the form of hysterectomy.[46,49,50]

Evacuation of the uterine cavity should be preceded by careful examination under anesthesia to exclude uterine rupture. Removal of placental tissue may be achieved by a combination of digital evacuation, the use of Desjardin forceps, and curettage with a large curette (Baum's curette).

Stepwise devascularization of the uterus commences with ligation of the uterine arteries adjacent to the lower segment. This may necessitate opening the leaves of the broad ligament by dividing the round ligaments.[46] The supposition upon which this intervention is based is that a reduction in the perfusing pressures within the uterine circulation may allow the hemostatic mechanism to reassert itself. Failure to control hemorrhage in this way should lead to ligation of the infundibulopelvic vessels, taking care to avoid damage to the fallopian tubes. Devascularization may also be achieved by occluding the internal iliac artery by either ligation or embolization.[46] Ligation of the internal iliac artery requires careful dissection of the retroperitoneal space and identification of the ureter. This technique should not be attempted without adequate surgical experience in pelvic dissection, and the reported success rates vary from a 42% to a 65% chance of avoiding hysterectomy.[51]

Various compression techniques are described. The B-Lynch brace is transfixed through the lower segment with two loops of chromic catgut over the fundus, applying pressure to the body of the uterus in the same way that a pair of braces would be worn.[52] Simpler techniques include sutures that traverse both anterior and posterior walls of the uterus in the form of two parallel sutures inserted into the upper uterine segment.[53]

Bleeding from the lower segment of the uterus after delivery of a placenta previa may be difficult to control because the lower segment does not retract to the same extent as the upper segment. Transcervical catheters with a large bulb (Sengstaken-Blakemore tube) may be used to compress these vessels and have even been advocated as an alternative to uterine packing as a way of controlling PPH.[54] Uterine packing using gauze packs, previously advocated, as a mechanism for controlling blood loss is no longer practiced because of the difficulty of packing the distensible postpartum uterus and because of concerns about infection.

Selective arterial embolization may be useful to control bleeding, however; not all obstetric units would have the specialist facilities and personnel readily available. Using embolization for PPH in shocked patients has been shown to reduce the effectiveness, as has its use following cesarean section. The most effective use was in the treatment of uterine atony (88% successs rate).[55] The exact place of embolization in the range of treatments for PPH has not been determined; however, the early resort to embolization has been recommended.[56] The procedure becomes more difficult technically if the patient is shocked and the bleeding points cannot be identified.

Hysterectomy remains the final resort in controlling intractable uterine bleeding and may be indicated a priori in cases of uterine rupture. Concern about loss of fertility should not deter the surgeon faced with life-threatening hemorrhage from taking this, sometimes unavoidable, step.

SECONDARY POSTPARTUM HEMORRHAGE

Massive blood loss occurring after the first 24 hours following delivery is less common than primary PPH and is usually due to subinvolution of the uterus caused by retained pieces of placenta or membrane and superimposed infection. About 1% of secondary PPH patients will require hysterectomy.

Severe hemorrhage will require maternal resuscitation (see earlier discussion). Definitive treatment comprises exclusion of retained products of conception, treatment for possible sepsis, and the exclusion of underlying trophoblastic disease. None of these interventions has been tested in randomized studies.[57] Antibiotic therapy will generally include a combination of penicillin with an aminoglycoside and anaerobic cover using metronidazole. Alternatives may include the use of cephalosporins or quinolones. Uterine evacuation should be performed if there is any question of retained products or trophoblastic disease.

Pelvic hematoma formation from vulval or vaginal trauma is dealt with conservatively in cases of supralevator retroperitoneal hemorrhage, although this remains a life-threatening source of hemorrhage. Ongoing resuscitation may be required until the bleeding tamponades spontaneously. If this fails to occur, either surgery or radiologic embolization of the traumatized vessel(s) should be considered. The surgical approach may necessitate both hysterectomy and internal iliac ligation. Infralevator hematomas are usually evacuated and either packed for 24 hours or repaired with mattress sutures to obliterate the cavity.

RUPTURED UTERUS AND OTHER GENITAL TRACT TRAUMA

The immediate pre- and postoperative management will include all the previously described principles for dealing with acute hypovolemia and coagulopathy. Experienced anesthetic support is essential.

The suspected diagnosis of uterine rupture necessitates a laparotomy, at which time the decision to repair or remove the uterus will need to be made. These decisions need to be individualized, and few generalizations are possible.

Scar dehiscence can be dealt with by simple repair, but more catastrophic rupture (especially of the unscarred uterus) will require hysterectomy. If contiguous injury to the bladder is identified, urologic assistance will usually be required.

Significant bleeding from other genital tract trauma will require surgical repair. The important principles of management are as follows:

- Prompt and effective resuscitation (see previous discussion).
- Prompt surgical exploration and repair to identify and repair the injury.
- Effective anesthesia.
- Input from other specialists (colorectal, urologic) as indicated.

SUMMARY OF MANAGEMENT OPTIONS

Massive Obstetric Hemorrhage

Management Options (See also Chapters 40, 58, 75, and 78)	**Evidence Quality and Recommendation**	**References**
Prenatal—Identification of the At-Risk Patient		
Criteria for risk (though no evidence of measures to prevent/ameliorate bleeding) are as follows:	—/GPP	—
• Anemia.		
• Refusal of blood products.		
• Previous antepartum hemorrhage, PPH, cesarean section, placenta previa.		
Value of prophylactic iron therapy is uncertain.	—/GPP	—
Perform delivery in adequately resourced unit.	—/GPP	—
Provide additional counseling in pregnancy.	—/GPP	—
Preparations/precautions for delivery:		
• Senior obstetrician.	IV/C	1,2
• Cross-match blood.	IV/C	1,2
• Advise active management of third stage with previous primary PPH.	Ia/A	34
Prenatal—Active Bleeding: General		
Have detailed guideline/protocol for unit to include the following guidance:	IV/C	1,2
• Setting/site of management (high dependency area or equivalent).	IV/C	1,2
• Give facial oxygen and warm patient.	—/GPP	—
• Monitoring.	IV/C	1,2
• Fluid, blood, and blood product replacement on basis of clinical condition and laboratory results.	IV/C	38–43
• Recombinant Factor VIIa if all else fails.	III/B	40–42
• Liaison with laboratories and hematologic colleagues.	IV/C	1,2
Prenatal—Active Bleeding: Specific		
Placental Abruption		
General measures (see above).	IV/C	1,2
Adequate analgesia (avoid epidural).	—/GPP	—
Empty uterus—method depends on	—/GPP	—
• Gestation.		
• Fetal condition (Is the fetus alive? Is there possible asphyxia?).		
Placenta Previa		
General measures (see above)	IV/C	1,2
Delivery by cesarean section:		
• Cross-match several units of blood.	IV/C	1,2
• Cell salvage techniques.	III/GPP	37
• Experienced obstetrician.	—/GPP	—
• Experienced anesthetist.	—/GPP	—
See measures under primary PPH (below) for persistent bleeding.	—/GPP	—
Primary PPH		
General measures (see above)	IV/C	1,2

Management Options (See also Chapters 40, 58, 75, and 78)	Evidence Quality and Recommendation	References
Stop bleeding with first aid measures:	—/GPP	—
• "Rub up" a contraction.		
• Bimanual compression.		
• Aortic compression.		
Atony:	Ia/A	43
• Syntocinon bolus and infusion.	Ia/A	43
• Ergometrine.	III/B	44,45
• Prostaglandins.	Ib/A	48
• Misoprostol.	III/B	46,47
Trauma:	—/GPP	—
• Repair trauma.		
• Evacuate retained placenta.		
Persistent bleeding despite the foregoing measures in order:	III/B	49,51,52,54
• Devascularization of uterus.	IV/C	46,50,53
• Uterine compression techniques.		
• Embolization techniques.	III/GPP	55,56
• Hysterectomy.		
Pelvic hematoma (procedure depends on site):	III/B	49,51,52,54
• Evacuate and pack.	IV/C	46,50,53
• Devascularization of uterus.		
• Hysterectomy.		
Secondary PPH		
General measures (see above)	IV/C	1,2
Antibiotics (not specifically tested for secondary PPH in RCTs, hence GPP).	—/GPP	—
	(Ia/A	57)
Evacuate retained products (not specifically tested in RCTs hence GPP).	—/GPP	—
	(Ia/A	57)
Uterine Rupture and Other Genital Tract Trauma		
General measures (see above).	IV/C	1,2
Effective anesthesia.	—/GPP	—
Surgical repair (hysterectomy in extreme).	—/GPP	—
Other specialist surgical input as indicated (e.g., colorectal or urologic).	—/GPP	—

GPP, good practice point; PPH, postpartum hemorrhage; RCTs, randomized, controlled trials.

DISSEMINATED INTRAVASCULAR COAGULATION

Definition

DIC is the widespread activation of intravascular coagulation leading to the deposition of fibrin within the circulation. Consumption of clotting factors usually leads to a bleeding diathesis, although a small percentage of affected individuals may go on to develop widespread thrombosis with peripheral organ ischemia. Some degree of DIC accompanies most forms of obstetric hemorrhage; however, the greater risk of coagulopathy usually arises from consumption of clotting factors and platelets as a result of massive hemorrhage. The combination of massive hemorrhage and coagulation failure is recognized as one of the most serious complications in pregnancy. DIC may arise from a wide variety of clinical situations in obstetrics but is always a

TABLE 77–5

Mechanism of Disseminated Intravascular Coagulation Occurring During Pregnancy

A.	**Injury to vascular endothelium**
	Preeclampsia
	Hypovolemic shock
	Septicemic shock
B.	**Release of thromboplastic tissue factors**
	Placental abruption
	Amniotic fluid embolism
	Retained dead fetus
	Chorioamnionitis
	Hydatidiform mole
	Placenta accreta
	Hypertonic saline used to induce abortion
	Acute fatty liver
C.	**Production of procoagulant**
	Fetomaternal hemorrhage
	Phospholipids
	Incompatible blood transfusion
	Septicemia
	Intravascular hemolysis
D.	**In many obstetric complications, there may be interaction between several mechanisms and more than one trigger factor present.**

secondary phenomenon following a "trigger" of generalized coagulation activity. The clinical manifestations of coagulation failure can vary from mild disorders detected on laboratory tests only to massive uncontrollable hemorrhage with very low fibrinogen and platelet levels. A failure to anticipate or detect the early stages of DIC is cited as a major deficiency in the care of women who die from obstetric hemorrhage, and despite advances in obstetric care and hematologic services, hemorrhage with associated DIC remains a major cause of maternal death and morbidity.

Mechanisms

DIC is triggered by various mechanisms (summarized in Table 77–5):

- Blood loss itself with transfusion and volume replacement.
- Release of thromboplastic agents into the circulation.
- Endothelial damage to small vessels.
- Procoagulant phospholipids produced in response to intravascular hemolysis.

With obstetric complications associated with coagulation failure, there may be interaction of several mechanisms. Once DIC has occurred, there is a potential for a vicious circle, with further consumption of clotting factors and platelets and bleeding until the underlying cause is corrected (Fig. 77–1).

Risks

The risks to both the mother and the fetus from coagulation failure in terms of death and morbidity are the same as those discussed earlier under "Major Obstetric Hemorrhage." The specific situations in which DIC and coagulation failure may occur and the risks of each underlying condition are considered here.

FIGURE 77–1
Once disseminated intravascular coagulation has occurred, there is a potential for a vicious circle, with further consumption of clotting factors and platelets and bleeding until the underlying cause is corrected.

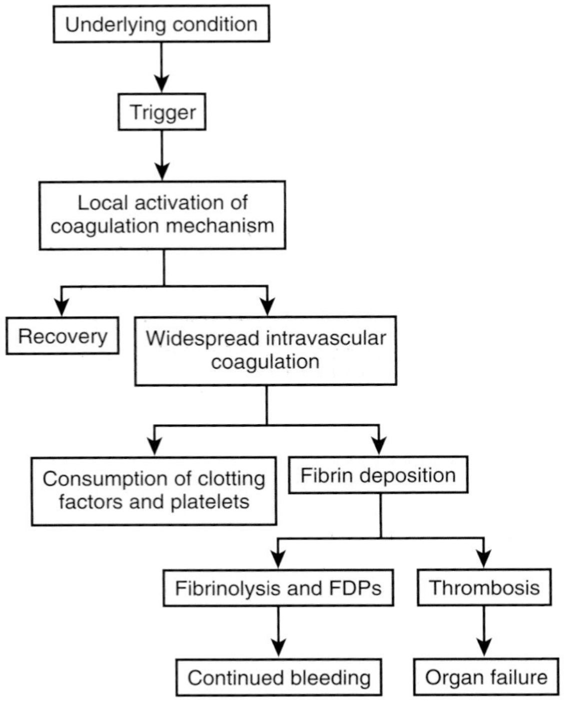

Placental Abruption

Placental abruption remains the most common cause of coagulation failure in obstetrics and is related to the degree of placental separation and hypovolemic shock. In severe placental abruption with a dead fetus, profound hypofibrinogenemia has been reported in about one third of cases but is much less common if the fetus is alive.[30,58] Earlier stages of DIC are common with mild to moderate abruption but can usually be corrected early if delivery is not delayed.[59] The initial mechanism is due to the release of thromboplastins, but in severe abruption, hypovolemic shock, large volume transfusion, and high levels of FDPs that act as anticoagulants themselves will exacerbate the situation.

Amniotic Fluid Embolism

Amniotic fluid embolism occurs during labor, during cesarean section, or within a short time after delivery. This condition may lead to maternal death as a result of severe pulmonary hypertension following embolization of the pulmonary vessels by fetal squames. If the mother survives this acute event, there may be an anaphylactoid reaction to the presence of the fetal tissues in the maternal circulation associated with cardiovascular collapse, pulmonary edema, seizure activity, and the development of an intractable bleeding diathesis due to severe DIC. The diagnosis is suggested by the detection of fetal squames within the maternal lungs at the time of postmortem, and therefore, the incidence of successfully treated cases is difficult to determine because the diagnosis is only suggestive and cannot be proved. The incidence of death from amniotic fluid embolism between 1970 and 1987 in England and Wales was 7.1 per million maternities. In most cases, the maternal death was unpredictable and unavoidable, and as obstetric care improves, amniotic fluid embolism has been responsible for an increasing proportion of maternal deaths and is now the fifth most common cause of death in the United Kingdom.

Retention of a Dead Fetus

A gradual reduction in clotting factors occurs following intrauterine fetal death, but these changes are not detectable on laboratory testing for 3 to 4 weeks. Approximately 80% of patients with a retained dead fetus will go into spontaneous labor within 3 weeks, but 30% of patients who remain undelivered for more than 4 weeks will develop DIC, usually of a mild degree.[60] Release of thromboplastic substances from the dead fetus into the maternal circulation is thought to be the trigger mechanism.

Preeclampsia

Preeclampsia is associated with endothelial perturbation currently thought to be due to oxidative stress and the release of reactive oxygen species by the ischemic placenta. The changes in endothelial function predispose to multiorgan systems involvement, including the clotting system.[61]

All preeclamptic patients have an increased rate of platelet turnover, and some develop overt thrombocytopenia. Activation of the coagulation cascade leads to a low-grade DIC that only rarely results in a clinically significant hemorrhage in the occasional patient with severe liver necrosis due to the HELLP (hemolysis, elevated liver enzymes, and low platelets) syndrome.[62] Excessive bleeding, which is often observed at the time of cesarean delivery, is more likely to be due to a qualitative platelet defect in thrombocytopenic individuals than any deficit in clotting factors.

Sepsis

Endotoxic shock can be associated with chorioamnionitis, septic abortion, or postpartum intrauterine infection. Gram-negative organisms are the most common isolated, although *Clostridium welchi* and *Bacteroides* species may be encountered, particularly in septic abortion. The bacterial endotoxin produces severe endothelial damage leading to fibrin deposition and DIC. Secondary intravascular hemolysis, which produces hematuria and oliguria characteristic of the condition, then occurs, and microangiopathic hemolysis can also cause purpuric skin lesions. Hypotension and coagulation failure are poor prognostic features in the presence of sepsis.[63,64]

Other Risk Factors

Other rarer conditions of pregnancy that have been associated with DIC and coagulation failure include induced abortion with hypertonic saline, acute fatty liver of pregnancy, and other hepatic disorders.[65,66] Hydatidiform mole and placenta accreta are associated with DIC because of loss of the intact decidua basalis, and passage of amniotic fluid and other thromboplastic substances into the maternal circulation is more likely.[67,68] Incompatible blood transfusions, large fetomaternal hemorrhage, and other causes of intravascular hemolysis, including drug reactions and the use of other replacement fluids, can also precipitate or exacerbate existing DIC.[69]

Management Options

General

There is a wide spectrum in the manifestation of the process of DIC, but the aims of management are to[70,71]

- Manage the underlying disorder in order to remove the initiating stimulus.
- Maintain circulating blood volume.
- Replace clotting factors and red blood cells.

Management of the underlying disorder will depend upon the specific condition. In the case of placental abruption, delivery will usually lead to rapid recovery once the mother is adequately resuscitated. Amniotic fluid embolism and acute fatty liver of pregnancy will typically result in more resistant coagulopathy that may not be readily corrected despite vigorous attempts at resuscitation.[72]

Laboratory Investigation

If DIC is suspected, blood should be taken and sent for cross-matching and appropriate laboratory tests before commencing definitive treatment (Table 77–6). Blood can be observed for evidence of clotting, but there is little point in performing whole blood-clotting tests at the bedside because they are unreliable and time-consuming.[73] Generally, the laboratory assessment of coagulation requires measurement of the aPTT, the INR, the platelet count, and fibrinogen concentrations together with some estimation of FDPs or D-dimers as an index of intravascuular fibrinolysis.

Fluid Replacement in Coagulation Failure

The management of coagulation failure is often subsidiary to management of massive hypovolemia. The urgent necessity in the initial stages is to maintain circulatory volume and tissue perfusion, and resuscitation with crystalloid and colloid solutions should be undertaken as soon as possible, as outlined previously. Dextran solutions should not be used because they interfere with platelet function and can aggravate bleeding and DIC as well as invalidate the laboratory investigations.[74] Prompt and adequate fluid replacement will also prevent renal failure and help in the clearance of

TABLE 77–6
Laboratory Investigations

1. Complete blood count including platelet estimation (2.5 mL in EDTA bottle)
2. Coagulation screen:
   Prothrombin time (extrinsic system)
   Partial thromboplastin time (intrinsic system)
   Thrombin time
   Fibrinogen titer (4.5 mL with 0.5 mL citrate anticoagulant)
3. Fibrin degradation products/D-dimers (2.0 mL in special bottle with antifibrinolytic agent)
4. Cross-matching, at least 6 units (10 mL in plain tube) Ideally, 20 mL of blood should be sent, but 10 mL is sufficient for essential tests. The sample should be collected as atraumatically and quickly as possible, and any heparinized IV lines avoided.

EDTA, ethylenediaminetetraacetic acid.

elevated levels of FDPs from the circulation via the liver, aiding the restoration of normal hemostasis.

Replacement of Blood Products

Blood products should be given as soon as available. FFP and stored red blood cells provide all the necessary components in fresh whole blood apart from platelets, and the clotting factors in FFP are well preserved for at least 12 months, provided the sample is stored correctly.[38] The use of fresh whole blood should not be encouraged, because it cannot be screened for possible infections. Furthermore, it is not easily obtained in an emergency. It is occasionally necessary to give extra fibrinogen in the form of cryoprecipitate, although sufficient amounts are usually provided in FFP, which also contains Factors V, VIII, and antithrombin III in higher concentrations. Platelets are not found in FFP, and their functional activity rapidly deteriorates in stored blood. The platelet count reflects both the degree of DIC and the amount of transfused blood given. If there is persistent bleeding and the platelet count is very low (definitions vary but $< 50 \times 10^9$ is often used), the patient may be given concentrated platelets, but these are not usually necessary to gain hemostasis.[73]

Other Treatment Options

Heparin therapy has been used to treat DIC from many different underlying causes, but there is no evidence to suggest that its use confers any benefit over supportive therapy. Heparin is contraindicated if there is hypovolemia, and obviously, this would include that secondary to placental abruption.[75] Heparin therapy has been suggested in the management of amniotic fluid embolism, but in the face of massive coagulation failure and clinical hemorrhage, it is difficult to justify.[72] It has likewise been suggested in the management of sepsis, although the most recent literature suggests that recombinant protein C may have advantages in terms of preventing fibrin deposition and stimulating the immune response.[75–79] Antifibrinolytic drugs have also been used, but there is the risk that their use would prevent the removal of microvascular thrombi from organs such as kidney or brain as the DIC resolves, leading to long-term sequelae.

SUMMARY OF MANAGEMENT OPTIONS

Disseminated Intravascular Coagulation

Management Options	Evidence Quality and Recommendation	References
Remove Insult/"Trigger"		
Empty uterus with major antepartum hemorrhage, retained dead fetus, molar pregnancy.	See Major Obstetric Hemorrhage box (earlier) and Chapters 5, 25, 58, and 78	
Treat uterine atony/repair trauma with PPH.	See Chapter 75	
End pregnancy with preeclampsia.	See Preeclampsia, Chapter 35	
Antibiotics with sepsis.	—/GPP	—
General		
Involve hematologist and support services (e.g., blood transfusion) early.	IV/C	70
Investigations		
See Table 77–6	—/GPP	—
Maintain Circulation		
See Major Obstetric Hemorrhage box	IV/C	70
Colloids (rather than crystalloid) initially but blood ideally.	IV/C	70
Avoid dextran.	III/B	74
Replacement of Blood Products		
Hematologic priorities are to replace blood constituents and coagulation factors (fresh frozen plasma and cryoprecipitate first-line rather than platelets).	III/B	38,76
Other Treatment		
Heparin and antithrombolytic therapy have both been used in DIC to break the cycle of consumptive coagulopathy. Neither has been subjected to controlled trials.	IV/C III/B	70,72 71
Concentrates of anticoagulant proteins such as antithrombin, protein C, and activated protein C are possibly useful in DIC due to severe sepsis.	III/B	76,77
Recombinant activated protein C is very effective in severe DIC due to sepsis outside pregnancy; limited experience in pregnancy.	III/B IV/C	78 79

DIC, disseminated intravascular coagulation; GPP, good practice point; PPH, postpartum hemorrhage.

SUGGESTED READINGS

Alexander J, Thomas P, Sanghera J: Treatments for secondary postpartum haemorrhage. Cochrane Database Syst Rev 2009;2:CD002867.

Bernard GR, Vincent J-L, Laterrie PF, et al: Efficancy and safety of recombinant human activated protein C for severe sepsis. N Engl J Med 2001;344:699–709.

Gidiri F, Noble W, Rafique Z, et al: Caesarean section for placenta praevia complicated by post partum haemorrhage managed successfully with recombinant activated human coagulation factor VIIa. J Obstet Gynaecol 2004;24:925–926.

Levi M, TenClate H: Disseminated intravascular coagulation. N Engl J Med 1999;341:586–592.

Levi M, de Jonge E, Van Der PT: New treatment strategies for disseminated intravascular coagulation based on current understanding of the pathophysiology. Ann Med 2004;36:41–49.

Lewis G (Ed): Enquiry into Maternal and Child Health (CEMACH): Saving Mothers Lives: Reviewing Maternal Deaths to Make Motherhood Safer. 2003–2005. The seventh report on Confidential Enquiries into Maternal Deaths in the United Kingdom. London, CEMACH, 2007.

McClelland DBL (ed): Handbook of Transfusion Medicine, 4th ed. United Kingdom Blood Services. London, TSO, 2007.

Mousa HA, Alfirevic Z: Treatment for primary postpartum haemorrhage. Cochrane Database Syst Rev 2009;2:CD003249.

Prendiville WJP, Elbourne D, McDonald SJ: Active versus expectant management in the third stage of labour. Cochrane Database Syst Rev 2000;2:CD000007.

Rainoldi MP, Tazzari PL, Scagliarini G, et al: Blood salvage during caesarean section. Br J Anaesth 1998;80:195–198.

REFERENCES

For a complete list of references, log onto www.expertconsult.com.

CHAPTER 78

Critical Care of the Obstetric Patient

JOHN ANTHONY

INTRODUCTION

Maternal mortality accounts for half a million deaths annually.[1] The risk of obstetric mortality varies according to the socioeconomic development of different countries, and many deaths could be avoided with better access to medical care. Industrialized countries, however, continue to focus on maternal deaths because many are associated with substandard care, some of which could be avoided by greater attention to critical care management.[2]

The admission of obstetric patients to critical care facilities is low (published intensive care unit [ICU] admission rates are 0.29% to 1.5% of deliveries in industrialized countries).[1,3] No standardized criteria define the requirement for critical care among pregnant women. The reasons for ICU admission include

- Obstetric complications (e.g., preeclampsia, hemorrhage, and sepsis).
- Medical disorders exacerbated by pregnancy (e.g., cardiac disease and thromboembolism).
- Conditions incidental to pregnancy (e.g., respiratory disease, complications of HIV infection).

Only one dedicated obstetric ICU published its experience several years ago, and the pattern of admissions may be changing in developing countries owing to the evolving HIV pandemic, with a far greater burden of sick patients being admitted as a result of infection and postoperative sepsis.[3]

Provision of critical care to the pregnant woman requires knowledge of intensive care principles as well as relevant aspects of maternal and fetal physiology.

RELEVANT PHYSIOLOGY OF PREGNANCY

Cardiovascular Changes

The dominant cardiovascular change in pregnancy is the increase in cardiac output leading to accelerated delivery of oxygenated blood to the peripheral tissues including the uterus and choriodecidual space. Stroke volume and cardiac output rise by 40%, and blood pressure falls owing to peripheral vasodilation and because the placental circulation functions as an arteriovenous fistula. These changes precede and exceed the fetal and maternal metabolic requirements of pregnancy to such an extent that the difference in arteriovenous oxygen declines in normal pregnancy.[4] Increased cardiac output is achieved largely by a rise in circulating blood volume due to physiologic hyperreninism that increases aldosterone levels 10-fold.[5] This adaptation leads to water and electrolyte retention and a 50% increase in plasma volume.[6,7] Doppler ultrasound has been used to redefine the cardiac changes that accompany the increase in cardiac output. Both filling phases of the left ventricle show increased filling velocities. The peak mitral flow velocity in early diastole (E-wave) and the peak velocity during atrial systole (A-wave) both increase. The increase in early wave velocity occurs by the end of the first trimester, whereas the peak A-wave velocity changes occur in the third trimester. The E/A ratio increases in the first trimester but falls again as the A-wave velocity increases and is accompanied by decreasing left ventricular isovolumetric relaxation time.[8,9] Left ventricular mass increases significantly, whereas fractional shortening and velocity of shortening diminish throughout pregnancy.[10] Systolic function is preserved by falling systemic (including uterine artery) resistance.[8,9] Peak left ventricular wall stress, an indicator of afterload, has been demonstrated in early pregnancy and normalizes as ventricular mass increases in the midtrimester.[10] Geva and colleagues[11] report a 45% increase in cardiac output in normal pregnancy accompanied by an increase in left ventricular end-diastolic volume and increased end-systolic wall stress accompanied by transient left ventricular hypertrophy. These authors also report a reversible decline in left ventricular function during the second and third trimesters.

The pulmonary circulation shows increased flow during pregnancy, with some reduction in vascular resistance without any significant alteration in blood pressure. These changes are evident by 8 weeks' gestation without any subsequent alteration and return to prepregnancy values by 6 months postpartum.[12] Systemic arterial vascular compliance is thought to diminish because of reduced vascular tone.[13]

Plasma volume expansion is matched by enhanced oxygen-carrying capacity brought about by a 14% to 28% increase in red cell mass.[14] Fetal respiration depends on maternal hyperventilation that creates a partially compensated respiratory alkalosis. The partial pressure of carbon dioxide ($PaCO_2$) in a pregnant woman will fall approximately 15% with a reduction in plasma bicarbonate, although arterial pH remains unaltered.[15]

Effective renal plasma flow rises with increasing cardiac output and blood volume, leading to a 50% increase in glomerular filtration.[16] This results in increased fractional excretion of glucose as well as other metabolites and drugs.

Coagulation

The mother is protected against the effects of hemorrhage at the time of delivery by her increased blood volume and also by enhanced coagulation. Coagulation changes include increased estrogen-dependent hepatic synthesis of fibrinogen and Factors VII, VIII, X, and XIII.[17] The anticlotting mechanism is physiologically impaired by reduced levels of protein S. Pregnancy is, therefore, a state of physiologic resistance to the action of activated protein C because free protein S is a necessary cofactor in this reaction. The fibrinolytic system is also impeded by increased levels of both plasminogen activator inhibitor-1 (PAI-1, derived from endothelial cells) and PAI-II, derived from the placenta. Expression of procoagulant activity takes place normally during pregnancy and may be detected by measuring levels of circulating thrombin-antithrombin III complexes.[17]

Effect of Delivery

These physiologic changes in pregnancy are progressive during pregnancy and revert to normal at varying rates during the puerperium. Labor stimulates a further increase in cardiac output, peaking out at 10 L/min as a result of autotransfusion of blood from the choriodecidual circulation during the third stage of labor.[18] Blood pressure fluctuates during pregnancy, falling by 10% to 15% in the midtrimester but rising again toward prepregnancy levels by the end of the third trimester, with a further rise occurring in some patients during labor.

Uteroplacental Effects

Blood flow to the choriodecidual space is determined by both the cardiac output and the dilation of the spiral arteries prior to the 20th week of pregnancy. These dilated vessels cannot vasoregulate blood flow to the placenta, which remains directly proportional to changes in maternal cardiac output and blood pressure. Vasoconstriction in the uterine circulation can develop in response to catecholamines, whereas uterine contractions restrict flow through these vessels by compression of the vessel wall. Transplacental gas exchange takes place by simple diffusion, and even at low partial pressures, fetal hemoglobin binds oxygen avidly because the oxyhemoglobin dissociation curve is shifted to the left. Even minor changes in the partial pressure of oxygen (PaO_2) in the maternal circulation may significantly improve fetal hemoglobin saturation operating on the steep part of the oxyhemoglobin dissociation curve. Fetal well-being is, therefore, critically dependent on maternal cardiac output, uterine blood flow, and maternal PaO_2.

Anatomic Changes

The enlarged uterus compresses the inferior vena cava and aorta. This may lead to supine hypotension as a result of diminished venous return, although the adrenergic response to aortocaval compression tends to maintain or increase blood pressure. Diminished cardiac output can nevertheless critically impair uterine perfusion, especially during labor.

The diaphragm is displaced by the enlarging uterus, resulting in a 10% to 20% reduction in residual volume and functional residual capacity. Under the influence of progesterone, the respiratory center increases chest wall movement, leading to an increase in tidal volume. This leads to respiratory alkalosis and hypocapnia.

METHODS OF MONITORING

Oxygen Saturation Monitoring

Spectrophotometry is the detection of specific light frequencies reflected by a range of molecules. Specific molecules reflect specific frequencies, and their reflective properties differ with changes in molecular conformation. Oximetry is the detection of oxygenated and deoxygenated blood. The oxygenated hemoglobin reflects more light at 660 nm, whereas at 940 nm, deoxyhemoglobin reflects infrared light more strongly. This allows the simultaneous acquisition of peripheral signals from which the ratio of oxyhemoglobin to deoxyhemoglobin can be calculated and expressed as a percentage of oxyhemoglobin saturation.

Oximetry may be based on transcutaneous measurements or can be derived from mixed venous blood via a probe located in a pulmonary artery catheter (PAC). The peripheral pulse oximetry devices rely on detection of pulsed alterations in light transmitted between a transmitter and a photodetector.

Although oximetry is regarded as an effective method of monitoring oxygenation that is widely available and easy to use in practice, some limitations are recognized. They include the assumptions that methemoglobin and carboxyhemoglobin are not present in significant concentrations. Invasive mixed venous oxygen saturation monitoring is less frequently used than peripheral oxygen saturation monitoring. It also shows greater spontaneous variation than peripheral monitors but has a clinical role to play in determining the balance between peripheral oxygen delivery and peripheral oxygen consumption. It is a robust measurement that will reflect changes in cardiac output, hemoglobin concentration, and arterial and venous hemoglobin oxygen saturation. This provides useful clinical information in many clinical circumstances.

Hemodynamic Monitoring of Cardiac Output

Hemodynamic monitoring is an integral part of intensive care management and is especially important in cases of severe hemorrhage, severe preeclampsia, and septic shock. An adequate cardiac output is essential in delivering oxygenated blood to the peripheral tissues. Low output will reflect either hypovolemia or ventricular failure. Knowledge of the cardiac output will determine management and will also allow calculation of other derived hemodynamic values, including vascular resistance and oxygen delivery and consumption indices.

Cardiac output was previously most commonly measured using the Fick principle. This principle states that the amount of a substance taken up by the body per unit time equals the difference between the arterial and the venous levels multiplied by the blood flow. Hence, oxygen consumption by the body divided by the arteriovenous oxygen difference equals the cardiac output. This principle has been modified to use other markers, including dye dilution techniques and the thermodilution principle of the PAC. In the latter case, iced water is the marker injected into the right atrium, with a probe measuring the temperature of the blood flowing through the pulmonary artery, thus allowing the derivation of the cardiac output from the area under the curve. This technique, although clinically robust, may produce results confounded by variations in catheter position and variations in injectate temperature and volume as well as changes in the rate of saline injection. Despite these limitations, this technology remains the gold standard against which newer techniques are assessed. The need to cannulate peripheral and central vessels has been associated with some risk of injury, and noninvasive techniques of measuring cardiac output have been sought.

Ultrasound in the form of echocardiography allows estimation of cardiac output by measuring changes in left ventricular dimensions during systole measured in the plane below the level of the mitral valve. By assuming that the ventricle is ellipsoid in shape and that the long axis is double the short axis, stroke volume can be calculated from the cube of the change in left ventricular dimension. This measurement is inaccurate when the assumptions on which it is based are no longer true. Hence, the dilated ventricle and the pregnant woman with an increased volume and end-diastolic dimensions violate these assumptions and may overestimate stroke volume and cardiac output. Doppler ultrasound has now added to the utility of echocardiography by allowing an estimation of blood velocity. The Doppler principle measures the frequency of a reflected ultrasound beam striking moving erythrocytes, in which the change in frequency detected is proportional to the velocity of the red cells moving in the axis of the beam. The velocity of a column of red cells multiplied by the period of ejection provides a measure of the distance traveled by a column of blood during systole. The use of ultrasound to measure the diameter of the vessels containing the blood will allow calculation of cross-sectional area with subsequent derivation of stroke volume and cardiac output. The velocity of blood flow can also be related to the pressure gradient down which the blood is moving, providing a way of calculating intracardiac pressure gradients and pulmonary artery pressures.

Doppler probes may be range-gated (pulsed) to allow the measurement of a signal from a given depth of tissue. The pulsed Doppler signal usually allows simultaneous ultrasound imaging and estimation of the angle of insonation between the Doppler probe and the vessel. This latter measurement is important because the calculation of velocity from the reflected Doppler signal requires a knowledge of the angle between the ultrasound beam and the column of blood from which the signal is being reflected. Where the signal is perpendicular to the moving column of blood, no movement will be detected, and the closer the beam moves to being parallel to the vessel, the more completely the reflected vector represents the velocity of the cells in the path of the beam.

The combination of cross-sectional echocardiography and Doppler measurement of flow velocity at specific points in the heart and great vessels allows the determination of volumetric flow. The mitral and aortic valve orifices and the root or arch of the aorta have all been studied using both suprasternal and intraesophageal Doppler probes. Potential for error exists in these techniques, in both the calculation of the insonation angle and the measurement of the cross-sectional area of the vessel. Of the different sites studied, the best correlation between the Doppler technique and thermodilution studies was documented in the aortic valve orifice measurements. Although transthoracic Doppler studies are the most widely accessible tool, transesophageal Doppler allows the posterior structures of the heart to be more clearly imaged with more accurate diagnosis of cardiac pathology and precise alignment to the aortic valve in both the long and the short axis as well as providing long-axis views of the ascending aorta.[19] The use of multiplanar transesophageal echocardiography allows precise measurements of asymmetrical ventricles that cannot be reliably imaged using a transthoracic probe.[20] The probe has particular utility in the diagnosis of aortic dissection and thromboembolism, although the need for esophageal endoscopy limits the application of this technology to specific situations including intraoperative and postoperative care.[21]

Doppler echocardiography has provided a ready means of studying women at risk of developing hypertensive complications during pregnancy. The most detailed study, to date, by Borghi and associates,[22] described detailed cardiac findings among 40 women with mild preeclampsia compared with a control cohort of pregnant women and nonpregnant controls. This study showed a progressive rise in left ventricular mass between nonpregnant women and women with a normal pregnancy, with a further increase in mass among women with preeclampsia. Ejection fraction and fractional shortening decreased in normal pregnancy, though this did not reach statistical significance. However, women with preeclampsia had a significant reduction in both these parameters compared with nonpregnant women. In addition, left ventricular end-diastolic volume rose significantly in preeclampsia. Together with a fall in cardiac output in the preeclamptic group, these findings suggest a compensatory increase in ventricular size to maintain cardiac output against an elevated systemic vascular resistance.

The latter study also showed changes in the peak filling velocities of the left ventricle during diastole.[22] The E/A ratio fell significantly during pregnancy, partly reflecting increased preload. In preeclampsia, further augmentation of the A-wave peak velocity resulted in further significant reduction in the ratio. Collectively, these data support the notion of changes in both cardiac systolic and diastolic function. The authors also measured atrial natriuretic peptide (ANP) levels. In keeping with previous studies, elevated levels of ANP were found in pregnancy, with further increments occurring in preeclampsia. These could not be accounted for by differences in atrial size, although a significant correlation was found between left ventricular mass and volume in women with preeclampsia.

Transesophageal Doppler monitoring of hemodynamic data has been carried out in adult ICUs and found to be equivalent to data derived from PAC measurements.[23] Pregnancy data are few, and only one study has reported the use of transesophageal Doppler monitoring in pregnancy compared with PACs.[24] That study showed that the Doppler consistently underestimated cardiac output by 40% in women younger than 35 years.[24] This error may be due to the assumptions implicit in the algorithm used to calculate output. These assumptions include a fixed aortic diameter during systole and a fixed percentage of blood perfusing upper and lower parts of the body. Pregnancy physiologic changes probably invalidate these assumptions. The authors nevertheless conclude that esophageal Doppler may contribute to the estimation of trends over time.

Other techniques of measuring cardiac output include impedance cardiography based on changes in transthoracic electrical resistance associated with the ejection of blood into the pulmonary circulation. This technique has been shown to overestimate low cardiac output, with the opposite error in high cardiac output states.

Invasive Pressure Monitoring

Invasive pressure monitoring includes the insertion of lines used for the measurement of intra-arterial pressure and central venous and pulmonary artery pressure.

Intra-arterial lines allow for continuous assessment of systemic blood pressure and also eliminate the need for repeated venesection, often a prerequisite in the management of the critically ill patient. Various noninvasive blood pressure monitors are also available that measure pressure using an oscillometric principle. These monitors have been shown to be significantly inaccurate when measuring blood pressure from women with preeclampsia, consistently underestimating pressures measured by direct arterial line measurement and auscultation.[25]

Central venous pressure (CVP) monitoring is employed as a measure of right ventricular filling pressure and intravascular blood volume. These lines may be inserted as long lines via the antecubital fossa or can be introduced via the internal jugular or subclavian veins. The long-line technique is preferred in any patient with a bleeding diadiesis and also in anyone who cannot tolerate positioning in the Trendelenburg position for internal jugular catheterization (e.g., women with pulmonary edema). CVP in the normovolemic patient should measure between 10 and 12 mm Hg. When managing hypovolemia, fluid should be administered as repeated bolus dose infusions until the CVP shows a sustained rise above 10 to 12 mm Hg over a 30-minute period. Central venous lines allow the withdrawal of mixed venous blood in which estimation of the PaO_2 will indicate the extent of peripheral oxygen extraction. In normally oxygenated and perfused individuals, central venous oxygen saturation should remain above 65%. CVP monitoring should not be used to monitor fluid management in severe preeclampsia because left ventricular diastolic dysfunction in this condition results in left-sided changes in pressure that are not reflected by similar changes in right ventricular filling pressures. Hence, a bolus of intravenous fluid may lead to a rapid increase in pulmonary capillary wedge pressure without any change in CVP.

Pulmonary artery catheterization, although controversial, remains a standard intensive care monitoring technique. Current evidence indicates that PACs do not alter ICU mortality and morbidity, although their utility is recognized in specific patients.[26] In obstetric practice, severe preeclampsia and maternal cardiac disease justify the measurement of left ventricular filling pressures, and measurement of cardiac output allows the calculation of derived hemodynamic parameters such as the systemic vascular resistance and left ventricular stroke work volume. Knowledge of these parameters is a useful guide to appropriate fluid and vasodilator therapy. In preeclampsia, rapid plasma volume expansion has been shown repeatedly to cause a sharp rise in left-sided filling pressures, often without any changes in CVP.[27–29] This occurs despite evidence of normal systolic ventricular function and is a reflection of reduced ventricular compliance during diastole.

PACs, like CVP lines, are inserted either via the internal jugular vein or as a long-line insertion through the antecubital fossa. Catheter placement may lead to a number of complications, especially in inexperienced hands, and should not be undertaken without adequate training and supervision. The incidence of complications may also be lower in pregnant patients than in other ICU populations; the Groote Schuur Obstetric ICU reported no major complications over a 3-year period.[30]

The indications for the insertion of a PAC are similar to those in nonpregnant patients. In addition, severe preeclampsia is recognized to be a condition in which changes in left ventricular diastolic function necessitate monitoring of pulmonary capillary wedge pressure after fluid loading. The Groote Schuur Obstetric ICU audit showed that most catheters were inserted for the management of preeclampsia in patients who also had renal failure (56%), pulmonary edema (32%), or eclampsia (6%).[30]

Although the Pulmonary Artery Catheter Consensus Conference[26] concluded that PAC monitoring did not reduce complications and mortality in patients with preeclampsia, the statement recognized the utility of the catheter in specific circumstances including oliguria unresponsive to fluids, pulmonary edema, and resistant hypertension.

Capnometry

Exhaled gas can be evaluated using an infrared probe and a photodetector set to detect carbon dioxide. This is usually found in the expiratory limb of a ventilator circuit. Expired gas shows a pattern of increasing carbon dioxide concentration related to the sequential expiration of air in the upper airway followed by air from the alveoli. The end-expiratory (or end-tidal) carbon dioxide concentration should approximate the $PaCO_2$ in arterial blood. The development of a gradient between these measurements reflects an increase in anatomic or physiologic dead space. In the latter event, low cardiac output and pulmonary embolism may both affect the measurement. Changes in end-tidal $PaCO_2$ have been correlated to changes in cardiac output and may be used as a means of monitoring the efficacy of resuscitation.

INDICATIONS FOR MONITORING—CAUSES OF CRITICAL ILLNESS IN PREGNANCY

The main causes of critical illness in pregnancy are listed in Table 78–1.

TABLE 78–1
Main Conditions Causing Critical Illness in Pregnancy

Preeclampsia and its variants
Eclampsia*
HELLP
Thrombotic thrombocytopenic purpura
Acute fatty liver
Hemorrhage*
Sepsis*
Thromboembolism*
Cardiac problems*
Arrhythmias
Cardiomyopathy
Neurologic problems*
Trauma
Metabolic
Anaphylactoid syndrome of pregnancy*
Others

* Indicates conditions that may present with "collapse."
HELLP, hemolysis, elevated liver enzymes, and low platelets.

MANAGEMENT OF CRITICALLY ILL MONITORED PATIENTS

Some would argue that many of the complications reviewed are more appropriately managed exclusively by intensivists, anesthetists, and physicians. However, the pregnant woman presents a unique challenge because of both the physiologic changes that accompany pregnancy and the need to address the requirements of the fetus in a mother who is critically ill. Thus, obstetricians must remain involved in the care of these women if the mother and her unborn child are to receive optimal care. More important, there should be a thorough understanding of those conditions that commonly lead to maternal mortality. Furthermore, substandard care of the critically ill woman arising from ignorance should not be an issue raised by confidential inquiries into maternal mortality.

Severe Preeclampsia (See also Chapter 35)

The preeclampsia syndrome can develop into multiorgan failure (including neurologic, renal, liver, hematologic, and cardiorespiratory disease). Preeclampsia affects 2% to 6% of pregnant women and remains among the leading global causes of maternal mortality.[31–33] Eclampsia with or without evidence of intracranial hemorrhage is the single most lethal complication of preeclampsia/eclampsia. Deaths have also been associated with pulmonary edema; hemolysis, elevated liver enzymes, low platelets (HELLP) syndrome; renal failure; and the development of hypovolemia (commonly due to concurrent abruptio placentae).

The pathogenesis involves chronic placental ischemia that predisposes to an accelerated production of lipid peroxides and oxygen free radicals. Systemic endothelial injury and altered vascular reactivity develop subsequently and are assumed to be a consequence of endothelial damage. The onset of clinical disease is marked by the development of hypertension, proteinuria, and intrauterine fetal growth restriction. Impaired prostacyclin production and increased release of vasoconstrictors (including thromboxane, endothelin, serotonin, and possibly catecholamines) lead to rising peripheral vascular resistance.[34–38] Endothelial damage leads to expression of cell adhesion molecules that interact with activated leukocytes and platelets.[39,40] Platelet turnover accelerates and may end in thrombocytopenia. Activated platelets also release cytokines that trigger intravascular coagulation.[39,41] Endothelial damage leads to interstitial edema, intravascular dehydration, intensified peripheral vasospasm, and diminished cardiac output. Low cardiac output translates into a critically low rate of oxygen delivery to the peripheral tissues, and multiorgan failure in severe preeclampsia can be attributed to multiorgan ischemia, developing because of vasospasm, low cardiac output, and intravascular coagulation.[28,42]

Management of Renal Failure (See also Chapter 49)

The presentation of renal impairment is commonly that of oliguria (a urine output <30 mL/hr over 4 hr) with or without hematuria. However, this is a common normal occurrence after delivery for the first 24 hours, probably due to renal vasospasm and, if delivery was by cesarean section, antidiuretic hormone production. Thus, if the oliguria persists toward the end of the first 24 hours, provided that the patient is not already in positive fluid balance and does not have pulmonary edema, plasma volume expansion should be attempted. If two fluid challenges (300 mL of colloidal solution) fail to improve the urinary output, low-dose dopamine should be commenced at an infusion rate of 1 to 5 μg/kg/min. Low-dose dopamine is thought to act as a selective renal artery vasodilator, and although of questionable benefit in general critical care, two randomized studies have demonstrated efficacy without adverse effects in the oliguric preeclamptic patient.[43,44] Patients who fail to respond to either of these measures require more intensive monitoring. PACs are a useful adjunct in securing optimal left ventricular preload and afterload. The volume-replete vasodilated patient who fails to pass urine over a 4-hour period should be considered to have intrinsic renal pathology, namely acute tubular necrosis. A single large dose of furosemide (0.5–1 g IV) may convert these patients to high-output renal failure. Should this measure also fail, care must be taken to avoid fluid overload by restricting intravenous fluid administration to output plus 500 mL/24 hr (to allow for insensible loss), and the patient should be prepared for dialysis.

Management of Respiratory Distress

Respiratory distress in the preeclamptic patient can be caused by or associated with

- Upper airway edema.
- Pulmonary edema—secondary to one or more of
  - Low oncotic pressure.
  - Leaky capillaries.
  - Left ventricular dysfunction (diastolic dysfunction cannot be detected without invasive monitoring or access to echocardiography).

- Iatrogenic fluid overload, even with small amounts of fluid.
- Rare causes such as cardiomyopathy and valvular heart disease may be indistinguishable from other causes of pulmonary edema without echocardiography or invasive monitoring.

- Aspiration pneumonia (especially following a cesarean section under general anesthetic) (see also Chapter 37).
- Postoperative atelectasis (it also occurs with the HELLP syndrome from "splinting" of the right hemidiaphragm because of liver pain) (see also Chapter 37).
- Pulmonary embolism (see following discussion and also Chapter 42).
- Acute respiratory distress syndrome (ARDS) (though not a primary complication of preeclampsia, it may follow aspiration pneumonia or prolonged ventilation) (see also Chapter 37). However, the role of ARDS as a cause for maternal mortality in severe preeclampsia has been completely overestimated and the cause for respiratory distress in severe preeclampsia is pulmonary edema in most cases.

The importance of respiratory complications as a cause of maternal mortality in severe preeclampsia has been underestimated. The South African Confidential Enquiry into Maternal Mortality has categorized deaths due to preeclampsia in groups that include those attributable to cerebral complications (presumably mainly cerebrovascular haemorrhage), those related to "cardiac failure," "respiratory failure," and "renal failure."[45,46] Considering that both cardiac failure and renal failure are likely to present with fluid overload and pulmonary edema, it is reasonable to assume that cardiac, respiratory, and renal failure should be grouped into a single entity with respiratory distress as the most likely consequence. Such a grouping challenges the notion that cerebrovascular events are the most common cause for hypertensive deaths. For two consecutive trienniums (1999–2001 and 2002–2004), the South African data indicate that respiratory deaths are the most common cause for maternal mortality (Fig. 78–1).[45,46] These data highlight the importance of critical care management in women with any evidence of respiratory compromise in the setting of severe preeclampsia. Clearly, patients who present with respiratory distress are a diagnostic challenge. When the diagnosis remains in doubt after clinical examination and special investigation, echocardiography or pulmonary artery catheterization are indicated.

Pulmonary edema will need to be managed according to the hemodynamic findings. Elevated pulmonary capillary wedge pressure may result from high systemic vascular resistance, left ventricular failure, or fluid overload. These complications may require vasodilation with agents such as dihydralazine, the use of diuretics, or a combination of both. Drugs that are negatively inotropic are generally avoided. In the absence of iatrogenic fluid overload, afterload reduction by vasodilation may be the most important aspect of management.

The development of localized lung signs and purulent sputum should alert the clinician to the possibility of aspiration pneumonia. Radiographic findings vary from normal lung fields to unilateral shadowing, atelectasis, and collapse. Bronchoscopy may be necessary if aspiration of particulate matter is suspected. Treatment with broad-spectrum (including anaerobic) antibiotics and physiotherapy would be indicated.

Management of other causes of respiratory distress is covered in the relevant chapters.

Management of Resistant Hypertension (See also Chapter 35)

Hypertension that fails to respond to standard vasodilator therapy has been cited as an indication for invasive hemodynamic monitoring.[47] The purpose of this is to distinguish hypertension due to high cardiac output from that arising from elevated systemic vascular resistance. Treatment aimed at reducing a high cardiac output may seem counterintuitive, but life-threatening hypertension due to this cause should be treated with drugs such as labetalol or a conventional β-blocker such as atenolol rather than the more traditionally used calcium channel blockers and direct-acting vasodilators such as dihydralazine.

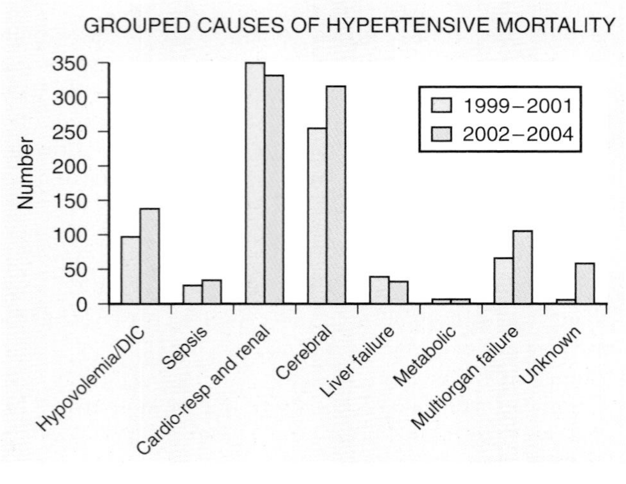

FIGURE 78–1
Two consecutive trienniums of the South Africa Maternal Mortality Report (1999-2001 and 2002-2004).[45,46]

Eclampsia (See also Chapter 35)

Eclampsia is the occurrence of generalized tonic-clonic seizures in a pregnant patient with proteinuric hypertension. Most seizures occur prior to delivery, although 40% occur within 24 hours of delivery. Eclampsia may be preceded by prodromal symptoms of headaches and visual disturbances (blurred vision, photopsia, scotomata, and diplopia).[48] The blood pressure at the time of seizure activity varies from levels that are mildly elevated or even normal, although they more commonly have moderate to severe hypertension.[49] Seizure activity is, however, associated with a sharp increase in blood pressure and decreased peripheral oxygen saturation levels. This is important because severe hypertension has been linked to the risk of cerebrovascular hemorrhage.

The differential diagnosis of seizure activity in pregnancy is extensive and includes epilepsy, systemic lupus erythematosus, thrombotic thrombocytopenic purpura (TTP), amniotic fluid ernbolus, cerebral venous thrombosis, malaria, and cocaine intoxication.[50–52] Late postpartum eclampsia (seizures first developing between 48 hr and 4 wk after delivery) requires neuroradiologic investigation to exclude alternative diagnoses.[53–55]

The critical care management of eclampsia is centered on

- Prevention of recurrent seizures.
- Control of the airway to prevent aspiration pneumonia.
- Control of severe hypertension.
- Management of other organ failure.
- Termination of the pregnancy.

Seizure Prophylaxis

Magnesium sulfate is the drug of choice for seizure prophylaxis. Randomized evidence clearly demonstrates a significantly lower risk of recurrent seizures with magnesium sulfate than with phenytoin and benzodiazepines.[56,57] Magnesium sulfate is a weak calcium channel blocker that regulates intracellular calcium flux through the *N*-methyl-D-aspartate receptor in neuronal tissue and may inhibit ischemic neuronal damage brought about by anion flux through this receptor.[58] Parenterally administered magnesium results in systemic vasodilation and improved cardiac output as well as cerebral vasodilation distal to the middle cerebral artery. Retinal artery vasospasm has been reversed by magnesium sulfate infusion.[59–61] The myocardial effects of parenteral magnesium include slowing of the cardiac conduction times, and in high doses, magnesium is significantly negatively inotropic.[62] Intravenous magnesium sulfate reduces serum calcium levels, possibly as a result of increased renal magnesium and calcium excretion.[63] Falling serum calcium inhibits acetylcholine release at the motor end-plate, the extent of which is directly related to the level of the serum magnesium and inversely proportional to the calcium concentration. This is the origin of magnesium sulfate toxicity leading to neuromuscular blockade and respiratory arrest.[64,65] Dosage regimens vary, but the majority of women in the Collaborative Eclampsia Trial[57] were treated with a 4-g intrqavenous loading dose followed by a constant infusion of 1 g/hr. Magnesium sulfate is excreted by the kidney, and impaired renal function may lead to toxicity, manifested as weakness, absent tendon reflexes, and respiratory arrest. In practice, monitoring patient magnesium levels as well as clinical features will help minimize the risk of toxicity. Patients with undiagnosed myasthenia gravis may have their disease unmasked by magnesium sulfate, even when the drug reaches only normal therapeutic levels.[66]

Patients who experience recurrent seizures in spite of magnesium sulfate are best treated with intubation and ventilation. Sedation using continuous high-dose benzodiazepine or pentothal infusions will be necessary and will serve to prevent further seizures. Following multiple seizures, these women are likely to have cerebral edema with raised intracranial pressure. Consequently, care should be taken to maintain a mean arterial pressure in excess of 100 mm Hg in order to preserve cerebral blood flow.[67]

Control of the Airway

Clearing the airway is an important first-aid measure accomplished by suctioning and positioning the patient head-down on her side. Endotracheal intubation is indicated in women with recurrent seizures, those who are inadequately oxygenated, and a patient who remains persistently obtunded more than 30 minutes after the seizure. Ventilatory care should be maintained for a minimum of 24 hours postpartum, until the patient is fully conscious, and any upper airway edema has dissipated.

Obstetric Management

Vaginal delivery, if foreseeable within a short period, may be contemplated in the woman with no complicating features other than a single seizure. Induction of labor should not be protracted, and an arbitrary time limit should be set as a goal for attaining a vaginal delivery.

HELLP Syndrome (See also Chapter 35)

This complication of preeclampsia is due to hepatic ischemia, giving rise to periportal hemorrhage and necrosis along with microangiopathic hemolytic anemia and thrombocytopenia.[68] Patients with the HELLP syndrome present with epigastric pain and, in severe cases, are usually obviously ill because of associated complications including renal failure (characterized by rising urea and creatinine levels and the passage of small quantities of blood-stained or "Coke"-colored urine) and eclampsia. Many women with HELLP syndrome, however, seem to have unremarkable clinical disease.

Liver failure may arise from conditions that mimic preeclampsia, such as TTP and acute fatty liver of pregnancy (AFLP).[69,70] Obstetric cholestasis and viral hepatitis may also enter the differential diagnosis in milder cases of HELLP syndrome. Distinguishing between these conditions may be difficult, but the hallmark of preeclamptic disease is that it resolves after delivery.[71]

Subcapsular liver hematoma is a rare complication of the HELLP syndrome. The surface of the liver is covered in petechial hemorrhages that may coalesce to form one large hematoma. Rupture of this lesion leads to right upper quadrant pain and sudden hypovolemia.

Coagulopathy is uncommon, but thrombocytopenia and impaired platelet function both give rise to impaired coagulation. Prolonged partial thromboplastin times and International Normalized Ratios (INRs) are more likely to occur in association with AFLP than with HELLP syndrome. Hypoglycemia may occur in some cases but is more characteristic of AFLP.

The management of HELLP syndrome is delivery, whereas the associated complications (renal failure, eclampsia, and respiratory distress) might require critical care on their individual merits. Thrombocytopenia should reach a nadir within 72 hours of delivery, and if it is persistent beyond this point, a search for alternative diagnoses should commence (e.g., sepsis, folate deficiency, TTP, systemic lupus erythematosus).

Thrombotic Thrombocytopenic Purpura

TTP is one of a spectrum of microangiopathic hemolytic conditions that include preeclampsia, hemolytic-uremic syndrome (HUS), AFLP, and autoimmune conditions such as systemic lupus erythematosus. TTP is a condition in which multimers of von Willebrand's factor, derived from the endothelium, accumulate in the circulation. Von Willebrand's factor binds platelets to the endothelium, and high concentrations are associated with peripheral platelet consumption and the formation of platelet microthrombi. Von Willebrand's factor is usually broken down by a specific metalloproteinase but might accumulate if this enzyme is deficient or if endothelial damage provokes excessive release of von Willebrand's factor. The metalloproteinase enzyme deficiency either exists as a hereditary condition or can be acquired as a consequence of autoimmune disease due to a specific immunoglobulin G (IgG) inhibitor of the enzyme. Many factors can precipitate both the congenital and the acquired forms of TTP, including drugs, malignancy, bacterial infection, HIV, and other viral infections. Pregnancy is the precipitating factor in 10% to 25% of cases.[72,73]

TTP presents with a pentad of features:

- Microangiopathic hemolytic anemia.
- Fever.
- Neurologic disturbance.
- Renal impairment.
- Thrombocytopenia.

The neurologic features of the syndrome may be transitory, and mild hypertension and proteinuria may make the condition indistinguishable from HELLP syndrome. TTP does not, however, remit after delivery, whereas HELLP syndrome invariably resolves. Other diagnostic features that may help to distinguish between the two conditions include evidence of marked hemolysis on examination of the peripheral blood smear (this is more characteristic of TTP than HELLP).

Without appropriate management, TTP has a high mortality rate. Treatment consists of plasmapheresis, infusion of fresh frozen plasma, and high-dose steroids.[72] Renal failure and the neurologic manifestations may require appropriate intensive care management.

Acute Fatty Liver of Pregnancy (See also Chapter 47)

Developing in the latter half of pregnancy, AFLP is a condition characterized by microvesicular fatty infiltration of the liver. The incidence is approximately 1 in 12,000 deliveries. Clinical disease severity varies, with some patients having only mild right upper quadrant discomfort associated with prodromal nausea and vomiting. Others develop fulminant liver failure leading to coma. A depressed level of consciousness may arise from either hypoglycemia or the onset of hepatic encephalopathy. Hypoglycemia is a common feature of AFLP and should alert the clinician to the possible diagnosis. More than 50% of affected patients will have mild hypertension and proteinuria, making the distinction from HELLP syndrome difficult. Jaundice is often present at the time of diagnosis. Liver enzymes are increased, and transaminases may rise above 1000 IU/L in severe cases. Liver failure leads to severe coagulopathy and a prolonged partial thromboplastin time and INR. Disseminated intravascular coagulation (DIC) with microangiopathic hemolytic anemia develop together a mild neutrophil leukocytosis.[74,75]

Management principles include delivery of the fetus and treatment of the acute liver failure.[76] Coagulopathy may complicate the delivery and must be corrected beforehand. Management of liver failure also includes maintenance of the blood glucose level, the use of lactulose to limit the effects of intestinal bacteria, and administration of vitamin K to mother and baby. Intubation and ventilation might be necessary in the comatose mother who cannot protect her airway. Associated complications of renal failure and pancreatitis need to be managed individually.

TABLE 78–2
The Systemic Inflammatory Response Syndrome

Any two or more of the following features:
Temperature > 38° or < 36°C
Heart rate > 90 beats/min
Respiratory rate > 20 breaths/min or $Paco_2$ < 32 mm Hg WBC > 12,000 or < 4000/mm³ or > 10% immature (band forms)

$Paco_2$, partial pressure of carbon dioxide; WBC, white blood cell count.

Obstetric Hemorrhage

Obstetric hemorrhage occurs as a result of bleeding from the placental site or as a consequence of trauma to the genital tract. These issues, including medical, surgical, and critical care management of shock and coagulopathy, are dealt with in Chapter 77.

Severe Sepsis

The systemic inflammatory response syndrome (SIRS) consists of markers of a systemic immune response (Table 78–2).[77] SIRS may develop from any noxious stimulus including preeclampsia and hypovolemia. When infection causes SIRS, the condition is named "sepsis." Sepsis leading to multiorgan dysfunction is termed "severe sepsis," and severe sepsis plus refractory hypotension is "septic shock." Collectively, infection arising during pregnancy or that resulting from underlying HIV infection is by far the single largest cause of maternal mortality in developing countries. In South Africa, these two entities account for 40% of the maternal deaths: double the number of the next most prevalent cause of mortality.

The sources of sepsis vary. Pelvic infection after delivery, wound sepsis, respiratory infection, and urosepsis are all common and can all lead to life-threatening illness requiring critical care.

Pelvic Sepsis

Pelvic sepsis usually results from infection with gram-negative organisms, although gram-positive organisms and fungi can be implicated. Tuberculosis can also present with abdominal sepsis. Prolonged rupture of the membranes, obstructed labor, instrumentation of the genital tract, retained products of conception, trauma, and operative delivery, together with immunosuppression all contribute to the pathogenesis of sepsis.

Recognition of pelvic sepsis is based on the presence of SIRS together with localizing signs of pelvic infection, including peritonitis, a tender subinvoluted uterus, and malodorous lochia. Coexisting organ dysfunction, such as impaired renal function, gastrointestinal signs (ileus), hyperbilrubinemia or elevated liver enzymes, DIC, ARDS, neurologic dysfunction, and cardiorespiratory disease including

left ventricular failure, will define the syndrome of severe sepsis and will indicate the need for intensive care.

Intensive care principles are self-evident. Supportive therapy will be necessary to maintain organ function by ensuring adequate peripheral perfusion, and the source of sepsis will need to be managed by medical and surgical intervention. Supportive therapy consists of fluid replacement measured against the CVP. Women with distributive shock due to peripheral vasodilation may require large amounts of fluid and blood products. Persistent hypotension due to left ventricular failure may require inotropic support using adrenaline, dopamine, or dobutamine. Coagulopathy due to liver dysfunction and DIC will need to be corrected prior to any surgical intervention, and oxygen-carrying capacity of the blood should be optimized by packed cell transfusion in women who are anemic. Appropriate respiratory support may take the form of face mask oxygen or intubation and ventilation in cases of respiratory distress with inadequate peripheral oxygen saturation or respiratory failure.

Managing the sepsis will require broad-spectrum antibiotic cover tailored to the specific infecting organism if bacteriologic surveillance from blood cultures and pus swabs identify a specific pathogen. Surgical intervention may include evacuation of retained products of conception, drainage of pelvic abscesses, and hysterectomy. The last option is often delayed because of understandable concern about future fertility. However, the woman with multiorgan failure precipitated by sepsis who fails to respond to 24 hours of appropriate antibiotic treatment is at risk of developing septic shock that may progress rapidly and is associated with mortality rates between 20% and 50%.[78] Under these circumstances, hysterectomy to remove the source of sepsis may be a lifesaving procedure.

Respiratory Infection

Respiratory infection may be community acquired (often gram-positive organisms like *Streptococcus pneumoniae*) or nosocomial (usually gram-negatives—e.g., *Pseudomonas*, *Acinetobacter*, *Escherichia coli*).

The clinical presentation is that of SIRS together with respiratory symptoms of dyspnea, pleuritic chest pain, cough, sputum production, and clinical signs of pulmonary crepitations or consolidation with bronchial breathing. Radiographic signs may take time to develop, but new pulmonary infiltrates should be identified if the diagnosis of pulmonary infection is correct. Sputum specimens should be routinely examined bacteriologically to identify the infecting organism. Tuberculosis should also be excluded as a diagnosis, especially in areas where there is a high prevalence of HIV infection.

Critical care management must maintain oxygenation while treating the underlying infection. Peripheral oxygen saturation levels will determine the necessary respiratory support, which may include the use of face mask oxygen, the administration of continuous positive airway pressure oxygen or intubation, and ventilation. Generally, respiratory infection has not been regarded as an indication for delivery of the baby, even among ventilated patients. Antibiotic therapy for community-acquired infection is usually a cephalosporin or an aminoglycoside with penicillin, whereas nosocomial infections due to gram-positive organisms will need treatment with vancomycin. A suspicion of mixed aerobic infection or anaerobic infection may lead to the use of imipenem or a combination of clindamycin/metronidazole with an aminoglycoside. Bacteriologic advice should be sought and treatment adapted to organisms identified from blood and sputum culture.

Sepsis in the Immunocompromised Patient

HIV infection predisposes the affected individual to pelvic, respiratory, and neurologic infection. Respiratory infection may be due to atypical organisms (*Mycoplasma* and *Legionella*), tuberculosis, cytomegalovirus, or the protozoan *Pneumocystis jiroveci* [formerly *carinii*] (PCP). The clinical presentation and radiographic signs may not discriminate between these different disorders, and sputum should be obtained (or bronchoscopic lavage used) to arrive at a bacteriologic diagnosis. Radiologically, PCP may present with patchy changes that progress to a diffuse pattern of bilateral pulmonary infiltrates resembling ARDS. Management consists of supportive treatment including ventilation together with high doses of trimethoprim and sulfamethoxazole (dose 20 and 100 mg/kg/day, respectively, for 21 days) and corticosteroids. The prognosis for women with PCP who require ventilation is poor, with only one in three surviving ventilatory care that extends for more than 2 weeks.[79] Suspected atypical pneumonia requires treatment with erythromycin.

Pelvic and wound sepsis seems to occur more readily in HIV-infected women. Antibiotic prophylaxis against postoperative sepsis should be extended to 48 hours for elective surgery and for 5 days in those having emergency cesarean delivery. In managing puerperal sepsis, surgical intervention, including hysterectomy, has been practiced more aggressively than in immunocompetent women. These approaches are unsubstantiated by randomized evidence but have developed in units faced with a large burden of HIV-infected women.

Thromboembolism (See also Chapter 42)

Thromboembolism is the leading direct cause of maternal mortality in the United Kingdom. The incidence of venous thromboembolism lies between 0.5 and 1 per 1000 deliveries.[80–83] The predisposing factors giving rise to thromboembolism are pregnancy itself, underlying thrombophilia, age, and circumstantial risk factors such as surgery and immobilization. Pregnancy is a procoagulant condition because of increased hepatic synthesis of clotting factors, decreased protein S activity leading to activated protein C resistance, and inhibition of fibrinolysis by placental production of PAI-2. Underlying hereditary or acquired thrombophilias add to the risk. These conditions include deficiencies in protein C, protein S, and antithrombin. The Leiden and prothrombin gene mutations have been described more recently. Hereditary defects also exist in Factor VIII and fibrinogen genes, giving rise to increased concentrations of these clotting factors. Hyperhomocysteinemia is also considered to be a thrombogenic condition, which arises either because of a dietary deficiency in cofactors such as folate, vitamin B_6, and B_{12} or because of enzyme deficiencies. Common mutations affect the enzyme methylene tetrahydrofolate reductase, which is required to convert folate to tetrahydrofolate. The other rarer enzyme defect is linked to cystathionine β-synthase deficiency. Thrombophilia may also be acquired as part of the antiphospholipid syndrome owing to the presence of the lupus anticoagulant that interferes with the protein C mechanism and also promotes platelet activation through the release of platelet-activating factor by endothelial cells. Finally, the sticky platelet syndrome may increase the risk of clot formation.

Ileofemoral vein thrombosis occurs more commonly in pregnancy; the presenting features of venous thromboembolism are those of a swollen, red, and tender leg. These signs are unreliable, and investigation is sometimes also unhelpful. Compression ultrasound is useful in identifying proximal thrombosis, but venography remains the gold standard against which other investigations are assessed. Pulmonary embolism classically presents with sudden-onset pleuritic chest pain, dyspnea, and hemoptysis. Investigations may confirm hypoxemia and right ventricular strain with an S wave in lead 1 and Q- and T-waves in lead 3 (S_1 Q_3 T_3 electrocardiogram pattern). Radiologic investigation may show no lesion or an elevated hemidiaphragm. Ventilation-perfusion scanning identifies mismatched areas of ventilation and perfusion that may be indicative of embolization. More recently, spiral CT is helpful in diagnosing segmental rather than subsegmental emboli.[84,85] It is notable that measurement of D-dimer concentrations during pregnancy is not a useful way of diagnosing excessive fibrinolysis associated with venous thrombosis because D-dimer levels are normally elevated in pregnancy.

Treatment of thromboembolism consists of anticoagulation to arrest clot propagation until the clot resolves followed by prophylactic doses of low-molecular-weight heparin to prevent further clot formation. The detailed description of how heparin and warfarin are used is covered in Chapter 42. In the critical care setting, unfractionated heparin is given intravenously in a dose of 20,000 units in 200 mL of saline beginning at 13 mL/hr, with the dose titrated against the aPTT to maintain values 1.5 to 2 times the control value. Other supportive therapy may be necessary to maintain oxygenation, up to and including intubation and ventilation.

Cardiac Problems

Arrhythmias (See also Chapter 36)

The patient experiencing cardiac arrest should be resuscitated according to standard protocols, including defibrillation, external cardiac massage, and ventilatory support. The pregnant uterus restricts venous return as a result of aortocaval compression, and cesarean delivery will facilitate resuscitation. If this is to be done, it should take place within 5 minutes of the arrest.

Ventilatory support, when required, should aim for slight hyperventilation to mimic pregnancy physiology in which $PaCO_2$ falls to allow fetal excretion of carbon dioxide down a concentration gradient. Extreme hypocarbia may affect uterine blood flow adversely, and maternal $PaCO_2$ levels must be maintained above 2 kPa. Where pressure considerations permit, tidal volumes of 10 to 15 mL/kg should be used, and the ventilator rate adjusted to achieve an appropriate $PaCO_2$. The maximum ventilatory plateau pressure should (ideally) not exceed 35 cm H_2O.[86]

Arrhythmias occur more frequently in pregnancy and occasionally lead to hypotension. In the critical care setting, the drugs most likely to be used to treat arrhythmias are adenosine, short-acting β-blockers, and amiodarone.[87] Adenosine is used to treat supraventricular tachycardia, Wolf-Parkinson-White syndrome, and arrhythmias involving the atrioventricular node. Because it can cause bronchospasm, it should be avoided in asthmatics. Lignocaine has been used in pregnancy, but there is limited experience. Although β-adrenergic blocking agents given to the mother have been linked to fetal growth restriction, fetal hypoglycemia, and hyperbilirubinemia, short-acting drugs such as esmolol may be used during pregnancy for specific indications such as the treatment of arrhythmias. Amiodarone is a drug with a long half-life (>50 days) and has been linked to a risk of neonatal hypothyroidism. The use of amiodarone should, therefore, be restricted to the treatment of life-threatening arrhythmias unresponsive to other treatment.

Other Cardiac Problems

Arrhythmias were discussed in detail in the previous section but can additionally cause sudden hypotension. Acute pulmonary edema can result from peripartum cardiomyopathy or valvular heart disease, especially thrombosis of a prosthetic valve. Myocardial infarction is rare but can result in cardiogenic shock. Aortic dissection and pulmonary hypertension giving rise to acute right ventricular failure also enter the differential diagnosis. The reader is referred to Chapter 36 for detailed discussion of the management of these conditions.

Neurologic Disorders

Cerebral ischemia or hemorrhage will present with neurologic signs. There may also be a sudden onset of neurogenic pulmonary edema.[88,89] Management should be directed to protecting the airway. Urgent neuroradiologic investigation is required to exclude a surgical remedial cause, and the management of these cases must always take place in consultation with a neurologist. The reader is referred to Chapter 48 for detailed discussion of the management of these conditions.

Trauma

Motor vehicle accidents and assault are the most serious causes of trauma in pregnancy. Pregnancy does not increase the risk of maternal death due to trauma, but the fetus is at exaggerated risk of death due to maternal hypovolemia, placental abruption, and direct trauma to the uterus and fetus.[90]

Direct trauma to the abdomen can lead to placental separation and abruptio placentae, the clinical signs of which may be delayed by up to 6 hours after the event. More forceful blunt trauma has the potential to cause uterine rupture, although this is a rare occurrence among pregnant trauma victims. Other obstetric consequences of blunt trauma are those of premature rupture of the membranes and fetomaternal hemorrhage, which can lead to isoimmunization of babies whose blood groups are incompatible with those of the mother.

Penetrating injury to the abdomen and uterus may lead to direct fetal trauma: Conservative management of penetrating injuries below the level of the uterine fundus has been advocated, but in pregnancies in which the fetus is considered to be viable (usually > 28 wk), many obstetricians would resort to laparotomy and operative delivery in the presence of a penetrating uterine injury.

Resuscitation and critical care should be based on normal trauma guidelines, although monitoring must be extended to include an assessment of the fetal condition. The reader is referred to Chapter 54 for detailed discussion of the management of these conditions.

Metabolic Problems

Hypoglycemia, hyperglycemia, hypocalcemia, and hyponatremia should always be considered in any patient who collapses acutely. Management will be based on the specific cause and diagnosis.

Anaphylactoid Syndrome of Pregnancy

This complication of labor or cesarean delivery gives rise to peripartum collapse as a result of embolization of amniotic fluid and fetal squames into the maternal circulation. The syndrome may be rapidly lethal in women who develop a true embolus of fetal squamae that obstruct the pulmonary circulation, leading to severe pulmonary hypertension and cardiac arrest. However, those who survive for longer periods develop an anaphylactoid type of response to the presence of amniotic fluid in the circulation.[52]

The clinical syndrome is diagnosed in 1 in 8000 to 1 in 80,000 pregnancies. A national registry of cases that has been opened in the United States is currently the most authoritative source of information about this condition.[52] The condition usually presents during labor but may occur at the time of cesarean delivery or immediately after birth. There are no demographic predisposing factors, and obstetric practices such as prior amniotomy and oxytocin administration do not seem to influence the risk of developing amniotic fluid embolus. The onset of the condition is abrupt, and hypotension is universally present. Most patients develop pulmonary edema with cyanosis and a profound coagulopathy, which should immediately give rise to a suspicion of the diagnosis. The single most common initial presenting symptom in antenatal patients is seizure activity, which may be confused with eclampsia. The patients who survive the initial embolus and who develop the anaphylactoid picture have markedly depressed left ventricular function. Cardiac electromechanical dissociation may develop, and there is a high risk of cardiopulmonary arrest. The prognosis is poor; in the U.S. national registry, 61% of the patients died, and only 15% survived neurologically intact.[52]

Diagnosis must be prompt, and continuous vigorous resuscitation will be needed immediately. Intensive care is mandatory and inotropic support necessary from the beginning. Hemorrhage should be anticipated, and hypovolemia is also likely to be a problem as a result of postpartum hemorrhage or bleeding after cesarean section. Continuous transfusion with blood and coagulation factors will be necessary, and obstetric intervention in the form of oxytocic drugs and hysterectomy may be necessary to control bleeding (see also Chapter 77). Intubation and mechanical ventilation along with pulmonary artery catheterization are likely adjuncts to intensive care management.

Other Causes of Acute Collapse

Several other conditions may result in acute collapse requiring emergency intensive care. The same general principles apply to all these cases: namely, secure the airway, maintain respiration and circulation, and then look for and correct the underlying cause.

Respiratory Disorders

Air embolism may develop during delivery as a result of air entering the venous system and becoming trapped in the right ventricle. Paradoxical arterial emboli can develop in any individual with a patent foramen ovale. Presenting features include acute collapse, coronary insufficiency, and cerebral artery occlusion, leading to seizures and a depressed level of consciousness. Specific management is based on the use of hyperbaric oxygen to decrease the volume of the gas.

Other Systemic Disorders

These include thyroid storm, myasthenic crisis, sickle cell crisis, anaphylaxis, and transfusion reactions. The description of these disorders is found in Chapters 38, 43, 45, and 77.

SUMMARY OF MANAGEMENT OPTIONS

Critical Care of the Obstetric Patient

Management Options	Evidence Quality and Recommendation	References
Preedampsia—Renal Impairment		
See also Chapter 35.	—/—	—
Give two fluid challenges if oliguria persists for more than 24 hr after delivery and no pulmonary edema.	—/GPP	—
Pulmonary artery catheterization.	III/B	27–29
IV dopamine (low dose).	Ib/A	43,44

SUMMARY OF MANAGEMENT OPTIONS
Critical Care of the Obstetric Patient—cont'd

Management Options	Evidence Quality and Recommendation	References
Single dose of furosemide in volume-replete patient who does not respond to IV dopamine.	—/GPP	—
Dialysis if these measures do not work.	—/GPP	—
Preeclampsia—Respiratory Distress		
See also Chapter 35.	—/—	—
Diagnosis is critical—management depends on cause.	—/GPP	—
Pulmonary edema.	—/GPP	—
Options for monitoring		
• Noninvasive.		
• Invasive.		
Diuretics.		
Fluid restriction.		
Ventilation in extreme.		
Pulmonary aspiration/atelectasis	—/GPP	—
Antibiotics.		
Physiotherapy.		
See relevant chapters for specific management options with other conditions.	—/—	—
Preeclampsia—Resistant Hypertension		
See also Chapter 35.	—/—	—
Invasive monitoring to distinguish high output from increased systemic vascular resistance.	III/B	48
Labetalol and/or doxazocin is better for high-output failure than calcium channel blockers and/or hydralazine.	—/GPP	—
Eclampsia		
See also Chapters 35 and 48.	—/—	—
Consider the differential diagnosis especially with presentation after 48 hr.	—/GPP	—
Seizure control and prophylaxis with magnesium sulfate.	Ia/A	56,57
Intubation and ventilation in the extreme.	III/B	67
Control of airway.	III/B	67
Deliver baby—though not necessarily by cesarean section.	—/GPP	—
HELLP		
See also Chapter 35.	—/—	—
Delivery.	—/GPP	—
Appropriate supportive therapy for coagulation, liver, and renal function.	—/GPP	—
Consider alternative causes for low platelets if the patient does not start to recover within 72 hr after delivery.	—/GPP	—
TTP		
See also Chapter 41.	—/—	—
Plasmapheresis.	III/B	72
FFP transfusion.	III/B	72

Management Options	Evidence Quality and Recommendation	References
High-dose steroids.	III/B	72
Appropriate supportive therapy for renal failure and neurologic features.	—/GPP	—
Acute Fatty Liver		
See also Chapter 47.	—/—	—
Delivery.	GPP	—
Treat liver failure with • Maintenance of blood glucose. • Lactulose. • Vitamin K.	IV/C	69
Intubation and ventilation in the extreme.	—/GPP	—
Appropriate supportive therapy for coagulation abnormalities, renal failure, and pancreatitis.	—/GPP	—
Obstetric Hemorrhage		
See Chapter 77.	—/—	—
Severe Sepsis		
Appropriate supportive therapy for organ failure (coagulation, renal failure, liver, ARDS, cardiorespiratory, neurologic).	—/GPP	—
Antibiotic therapy determined by blood culture results.	—/GPP	—
Surgical options (abscess, removal of retained products, hysterectomy in the extreme).	—/GPP	—
Fluid replacement monitored with CVP.	—/GPP	—
Thromboembolism		
See also Chapter 42.	—/—	—
IV unfractionated heparin (maintain aPTT at 1.5–2 × control).	—/GPP	—
Oxygen and ventilation according to pulse oximetry.	—/GPP	—
Cardiac Arrythmias		
See also Chapter 36.	—/—	—
Standard resuscitation • External cardiac massage. • Ventilation. • Defibrillation.	IV/C	86
Drugs dependent on diagnosis/type • Adenosine. • Lignocaine. • Short-acting β-blockers. • Amiodarone.	IV/C	88
Deliver fetus if no response to resuscitation after 5 min.	—/GPP	—
Other Cardiac Problems		
See Chapter 36.	—/—	—
Neurologic (CVA)		
See Chapter 48.	—/—	—
Trauma		
See Chapter 54.	—/—	—

SUMMARY OF MANAGEMENT OPTIONS
Critical Care of the Obstetric Patient—cont'd

Management Options	Evidence Quality and Recommendation	References
Anaphylactoid Syndrome of Pregnancy		
Resuscitation.	—/GPP	—
Intensive care setting and ventilatory support as indicated; invasive monitoring (including pulmonary artery catheter).	—/GPP	—
Inotropic support.	—/GPP	—
Blood clotting factor support.	—/GPP	—
Management if the cause is PPH—see Chapter 75.	—/GPP	—
Other Conditions		
General supportive measures	—/GPP	—
• Secure airway.		
• Support respiration.		
• Support ventilation.		
Find and treat underlying condition.	—/GPP	—

aPTT, activated partial thromboplastin time; ARDS, acute respiratory distress syndrome; CVA, cerebrovascular accident; CVP, central venous pressure; FFP, fresh frozen plasma; GPP, good practice point; HELLP, hemolysis, elevated liver enzymes, and low platelets; TTP, thrombotic thrombocytic purpura.

SUGGESTED READINGS

Coetzee EJ, Dommisse J, Anthony J: A randomised controlled trial of intravenous magnesium sulphate versus placebo in the management of women with severe pre-eclampsia. Br J Obstet Gynanecol 1998;105:300–303.

Duncan R, Hadley D, Bone I, et al: Blindness in eclampsia: CT and MR imaging. J Neurol Neurosurg Psychiatry 1989;52:899–902.

James MFM, Anthony J: Critical care management of the pregnant patient. In Birnbach DJ, Gatt SP, Datta S (eds): Textbook of Obstetric Anesthesia. Philadelphia, Churchill Livingstone, 2000, pp 716–732.

Kaplan MM: Acute fatty liver of pregnancy. N Engl J Med 1985;313:367–370.

Lewis G (ed): Enquiry into Maternal and Child Health (CEMACH). Saving Mothers Lives: Reviewing Maternal Deaths to Make Motherhood Safer. 2003–2005. The seventh report on Confidential Enquiries into Maternal Deaths in the United Kingdom. London, CEMACH, 2007.

Mabie WC, Sibai BM: Treatment in an obstetric intensive care unit. Am J Obstet Gynecol 1990;162:1–4.

Mantel GD, Makin JD: Low dose dopamine in postpartum preeclamptic women with oliguria: A double-blind, placebo controlled, randomised trial. Br J Obstet Gynaecol 1997;104:1180–1183.

Proia A, Paesano R, Torcia F, et al: Thrombotic thrombocy-topenic purpura and pregnancy: A case report and a review of the literature. Ann Hematol 2002;81:210–214.

Visser W, Wallenburg HC: Central hemodynamic observations in untreated preeclamptic patients. Hypertension 1991;17:1072–1077.

Zotz RB, Gerhardt A, Scharf RE: Prediction, prevention, and treatment of venous thromboembolic disease in pregnancy. Semin Thromb Hemost 2003;29:143–154.

REFERENCES

For a complete list of references, log onto www.expertconsult.com.

CHAPTER 79

Training for Obstetric Emergencies

TIM DRAYCOTT and DIMITRIOS SIASSAKOS

INTRODUCTION

Labor and delivery are the safest they have ever been in the developed world,[1] yet 1 in 12 labors still ends in an adverse outcome,[2] particularly in emergency situations.[1] Obstetric emergencies are especially high risk: they occur rapidly, are unpredictable, are often unavoidable, and require a rapid, coordinated response by a multiprofessional ad hoc team. Their rarity makes it difficult to learn solely by experience. And although, in the past, training has included didactic lectures combined with arbitrary clinical experiences, this educational paradigm clearly has limitations. The difficulties have been exacerbated by mandatory reductions in working hours worldwide, to the extent that the majority of current obstetric trainees have had no real-life experience leading the management of emergencies like eclampsia, shoulder dystocia, or even the more common postpartum hemorrhage (PPH).[3]

Unfortunately, several Confidential Enquiries have demonstrated that when emergencies do occur, error is far too common, possibly because of these difficulties. Therefore, training—in particular "fire drills"—has repeatedly been recommended,[1,4–8] even though there are precious little data to support it.[9,10] In fact, there is at least one study that demonstrated an increase in poor outcomes after training.[11] More recently, there has been an increasing dataset to support training for obstetric emergencies, and we review the best practices in this chapter.

Training should enable caregivers from a variety of health care professions to provide the best possible clinical care to women as soon as it is required. Training should improve skills, behavior, and attitudes, which in turn should improve the clinical and organizational outcome (modified Kirkpatrick evaluation levels[12]). Face validity should no longer be an acceptable outcome; there is a risk that, although trainees feel more satisfied and confident after training,[9,13–19] entrenched behaviors remain unchanged,[14] and real-life outcomes do not improve[2] and may even deteriorate.[11]

RISKS

Substandard care may lead to adverse outcome with devastating, and sadly potentially avoidable, physical, psychological, and financial consequences.

Maternal Risk

Mortality

Mothers still die in pregnancy and it is a sad indictment of their care that at least 50% of these deaths are avoidable and that percentage has remained static for decades. In the United Kingdom, the Confidential Enquiries into Maternal Death (CEMD) and into Maternal and Child Health (CEMACH) have repeatedly identified poor or absent teamworking as one of the main reasons for substandard care leading to avoidable maternal death. They have recommended that all clinical staff in maternity units be required to undertake regular, documented, and audited training for the management of severely ill women and impending maternal collapse, as well as for the improvement of acute obstetric, life support, and communication skills.[1,4]

Maternal Morbidity

Labor and delivery can result in significant maternal morbidity, rapidly, unexpectedly, and unfortunately often.[2,20] The physiology of pregnancy renders women more susceptible to certain complications, and pregnant women are often younger and fitter than the general medical population. These facts can make it difficult to recognize and preempt potentially serious complications, for example before infection develops into septic shock.

Particularly in developed countries, where maternal mortality is now very low, study into maternal morbidity can also provide insight into avoidable causes of adverse outcome. There was poor recognition of concealed complications in one review of the management of critical obstetric emergencies and intensive care for pregnant women,[1] resulting in suboptimal care for one in three cases. More appropriate management in cases with suboptimal care could have prevented hysterectomy, multiple organ dysfunction, coma, shock, and admission to intensive care.[1] There are similar lessons contained in other reports.[21–24] However, more optimistically, there is indirect evidence that guidance-based management has decreased complications like eclampsia,[24] or death after hysterectomy,[23] and therefore, training may also decrease avoidable maternal morbidity.

Maternal Satisfaction

Maternal dissatisfaction is a significant complication of traumatic birth, but it is often ignored. More than 17% of women are dissatisfied with labor[25–27] and up to 22% of partners are also dissatisfied with their labor experience.[28] Decreased maternal satisfaction is associated with an increased risk of sexual dysfunction, negative effects on ability to breast-feed and bonding, and negative expectations for future births.[29,30] U.K.-based research showed that over 25% of new mothers were not satisfied with communication by the medical staff, and there was a significant association between satisfaction with communication by medical staff and overall satisfaction with care.[31,32] These negative feelings are more likely when obstetric intervention is necessary for birth[33,34] and may increase the risk of litigation.

Fetal Risks

Perinatal Mortality

Suboptimal team communication, poor teamwork climate, and deficient team training have also been identified as the most common root causes for infant death in developed countries.[5–7] The direction for the future is clear: there is a need for training in perinatal areas that focuses on high risk events like shoulder dystocia, electronic fetal monitoring interpretation, and team-working.

Cerebral Palsy

Cerebral palsy (CP) is a condition with immense physical, psychological problems: lifetime disability for the child, depression for the parents,[35] and costs of around £4 million per case of negligent care for U.K. health organizations.[36] Most types of CP have been associated with factors other than substandard intrapartum care, but spastic quadriplegic and athetoid CP are associated with intrapartum asphyxic events in 45% and 80% of cases, respectively.

The U.K. Department of Health has published its ambition to reduce the rates of avoidable CP by 25% and national guidelines have been developed to facilitate standardized interpretation[37] of electronic fetal monitoring (EFM). Despite these guidelines, birth asphyxia due to misinterpretation of EFM and failure to respond appropriately remains a problem perhaps because the guidelines are not used in the front line of care. It may be that only when maternity staff are trained how to interpret EFM traces using the guidelines, and refer or act on them appropriately,[38] that better outcomes and fewer negligence claims can be achieved without increasing the intervention rate.[39,40]

Neonatal Injury

Another example of a potentially avoidable neonatal morbidity is brachial plexus injury. It is a condition associated with the management of shoulder dystocia[41] that often results in costly litigation for negligent care.[42] Shoulder dystocia is unpredictable and, therefore, unpreventable. Improving management through training may be the most effective method of reducing the associated morbidity,[41] mortality, and litigation.[42] However, a recent study of 450 simulated shoulder dystocia stations revealed that unless training concentrates on the important underlying concepts,[43] confusion and errors result. Another study showed that worse outcomes occurred after the introduction of training in a U.K. unit.[11]

Therefore, it would seem prudent for those designing obstetric training programs to consider the currently available evidence when deciding how best to train. National standards indicate which obstetric situations to target[6,44]: shoulder dystocia, EFM and emergency cesarean section, cord prolapse, neonatal resuscitation, maternal hemorrhage, collapse and shock, preeclampsia and eclampsia.

MANAGEMENT OPTIONS

Scope of Training

In many countries, national bodies mandate[44] or recommend[1,6,7,38] the content of training. However, it is also important to identify local training needs and address them with targeted interventions.[39] Local surveillance systems[45] may provide such information when supplemented by risk management processes, for example, root cause analysis.[39]

Another useful source of information can be reviews of medicolegal cases.[42,46–49] Such reviews can help identify which training interventions are more likely to have a successful impact on litigation frequency and severity.[20,46] Individual staff appraisals, supervisory reviews,[1,50] and safety attitude surveys[51–53] provide another opportunity to identify and address training needs.

Simulation exercises can be used to identify recurrent mistakes. One study in Israel showed that many errors in drug administration, performance of practical maneuvers, resuscitation, and documentation were observed before training for four simulated obstetric emergencies: breech delivery, shoulder dystocia, PPH, and eclampsia.[3] In the study, 84% of participants who had originally expressed being confident of their ability to perform appropriately in obstetric emergencies retracted their statements after simulation and expressed interest in further hands-on practice.[3]

Similarly, a number of performance deficiencies for obstetric residents were identified when 10 labor ward teams were videotaped and externally reviewed managing a simulated amniotic fluid embolism and forceps delivery: poor communication with the pediatric team, not assuming a leadership role during the drill, poor distribution of workload, and lack of practical skills.[54] Moreover, a large regional study in the United Kingdom demonstrated that before training, 39% of teams did not administer magnesium sulfate to women with simulated eclampsia[55] and only 42.9% of caregivers could deliver a baby with simulated shoulder dystocia. Sixty-six percent of staff applied extremely high forces to effect delivery; almost 20% could not perform any internal maneuvers and 11% asked for fundal pressure, a technique currently considered inappropriate. One third did not state what the emergency was, two thirds failed to call a pediatrician/neonatologist to attend the delivery, and almost half the participants did not communicate well with the patient-actor.

It is obvious that there is discrepancy between how good participants *think* they are before training and how good they *really* are when they perform under observation: the need for both individuals[56] and teams[55] to receive practical and communication training is clear and urgent. These deficiencies can be identified and subsequently addressed successfully with simulation.[56]

TABLE 79–1

Examples of Improved Perinatal Outcomes Associated with Evidence-based Management as Detailed in the Summary of Management Options Box

HOSPITAL UNIT	INGREDIENTS OF TRAINING PROGRAM	OUTCOMES BEFORE TRAINING	OUTCOMES AFTER TRAINING
Southmead Hospital, Bristol, UK[41,50,68]	Regular in-house clinical rehearsals for all staff. Integrated teamwork training. Infrastructural changes. Evidence-based protocols. Simple props to help adherence to guidelines.	*Perinatal outcome*: Low* Apgar = 86.6/10,000 births HIE = 27.3/10,000 births *Neonatal injury after shoulder dystocia birth*: Overall = 9.3% BPI = 7.4% *Cord prolapse*: Median DDI = 25 min Suboptimal neonatal outcome† = 51%	*Perinatal outcome*: Low Apgar = 44.6/10,000 births ($P < .001$) HIE = 13.6/10,000 births ($P = .032$) *Neonatal injury after shoulder dystocia birth*: Overall = 2.3% ($P < .05$) BPI = 2.3% ($P < .05$) *Cord prolapse*: Median DDI = 14.5 min ($P < .001$) Suboptimal neonatal outcome = 26% ($P = .05$)
Beth Israel Deaconess Medical Center, Boston[20]	Teamwork course for all staff. Debriefings, improved handover. Protocol development. Selected clinical rehearsals.	*Adverse obstetric outcome index*‡: 5.9% *High-severity malpractice claims*: 61.9%	*Adverse obstetric outcome index*: 4.6% *High-severity malpractice claims*: 31.3%

* <7 at 5 min.
† Apgar < 7 at 5 min and/or admission to NICU if > 2.5 kg and/or stillbirth.
‡ Maternal death or intrapartum and neonatal death > 2500 g or uterine rupture or maternal admission to ICU or birth trauma or return to theater/labor and delivery or admission to NICU > 2500 g and for > 24 hr or Apgar < 7 at 5 min or blood transfusion or third- or fourth-degree perineal tear.
BPI, brachial plexus injury; DDI, decision-delivery interval; HIE, hypoxic ischemic encephalopathy; ICU, intensive care unit; NICU, neonatal intensive care unit.

Incentives

There may be multiple barriers to successful obstetric training, such as cost and time away from work.[57] Those units that have demonstrated direct improvements in perinatal outcomes after training (Table 79–1) have all had financial incentives to train, for example, lower medical malpractice insurance premiums are offered to clinicians and units with regular training in the United States[20] (University of Kansas– and Harvard-affiliated obstetricians) and the United Kingdom[49] via national clinical negligence schemes. These financial incentives may help not always completely altruistic institutions overcome the inhibitory direct costs of training.

Safety Culture

Knowledge, skills, and attitudes are all essential for successful performance in "high-reliability organizations" (HROs): settings that are hypercomplex, are tightly coupled, are time-compressed, and rely upon synchronized outcomes.[58] Maternity units demonstrate all of these characteristics: complex emergencies with frequently two patients to look after (mother and baby); tightly coupled events, when the performance of an emergency cesarean section depends on the actions of every single team member; compressed decision-to-action intervals; and necessity for synchronized actions.

Organizations that provide maternity care should ideally function like HROs. Training should support teamwork and be context-specific. This culture appears not to be ubiquitous. In the Simulation and Fire Drill Evaluation (SaFE) Study,[59] questions regarding the perception of management's role in safety had the lowest scores across professional groups, reflecting a perception of negative attitude toward risk management. This attitude worsened after training in simulation centers, but not after local training. This may reflect the fact that training in external courses was perceived as paternalistic and driven by managerial targets rather than staff development needs.

Conversely, there was a positive impact of training, particularly if undertaken in the local setting, on job satisfaction and attitudes toward teamwork and stress recognition. After 12 months, the improvement in attitudes toward teamwork was sustained only for health care professionals receiving training locally.[59]

Methods—How Should We Train?

Simulation

Simulation is an educational technique, not a machine or a place, and can be used to bridge the gap between theory and real-life application of skills.[54] It was shown in a randomized trial that postgraduate teams taught using simulation demonstrated larger improvements in clinical management, confidence, communication skills, and knowledge and less anxiety during subsequent emergencies than teams taught with a lecture format.[69] In addition, simulation was deemed more enjoyable. Similar results have been shown for simulation training of both postgraduates and undergraduates, as individuals or in teams.[55,56,61–66]

In-house Rehearsals

In-house training of multiprofessional teams should be the initial training of choice for obstetrics: it is less expensive than external training (Fig. 79–1)[47,50] and appears to offer additional benefits. Assessment of safety and communication as evaluated by a patient-actor has been shown to

FIGURE 79–1
In-house rehearsals: a unit's labor ward as simulation center.

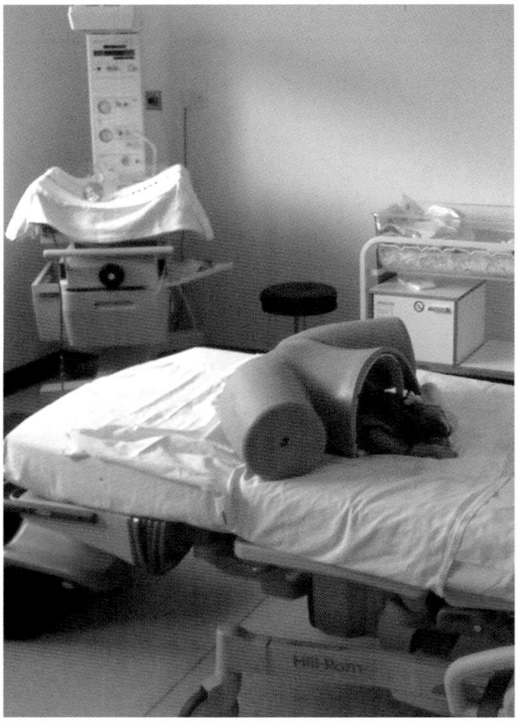

be significantly better when training is conducted in local hospitals using patient-actors than when training is conducted at a simulation center using computerized patient mannequins.[61] These improvements do not come at the expense of individual knowledge, skills, or team-working and communication.[55,62] On the contrary, in-house training has been associated with significant improvement in real-life outcomes.[41,50,67]

Local training provides the opportunity for teams to identify local safety problems that can be addressed with targeted interventions. In one study, the patient bed could not pass through the door in two labor rooms, resulting in avoidable delays. This was identified during some of the early rehearsals for cord prolapse simulation training, and the doorframe was widened. The result was a 40% reduction in decision-delivery interval with concurrent improvement in perinatal outcome.[67] Other examples of safety interventions that have been introduced in units in which in-house training was associated with improved perinatal outcomes include eclampsia boxes,[50] streamlined management protocols (Soerensen JL, Copenhagen, Denmark, personal communication), guidelines for specific emergencies, and regular patient handover.[20]

However, there are potential disadvantages to in-house training: it might be difficult to conduct team rehearsals in busy labor wards, whereas external courses allow uninterrupted training. There may also be difficulty in maintaining quality. A study showed that despite the introduction of regular in-house training in 2001, perinatal asphyxia and serious neonatal injury, including brachial plexus injury, significantly increased.[11] This suggests that not all training is equal; other elements might need to be present for improvements in outcome to occur.

Evidence-based Training

A recurrent finding in inquiries and reports is that quality improvement in maternity is always associated with a reduction in the variation of processes and procedures,[40,42] and clinical practice is evidence-based and protocol-driven.[1,6,40,44] However, simply having guidelines available on the labor ward is not sufficient—training is required to implement them. It is necessary to engage multiprofessional teams both in the development of guidelines and in training staff in how to apply them to practice.[20,50] Furthermore, it should be made easy for staff to use them ("make the right way the easiest way"[68]) through innovative practical solutions: miniadhesive proformas ("stickers") that facilitate regular standardized interpretation of EFM traces[50,68]; laminated summaries of guidelines[65]; and perinatal care bundles.[69] Standardized proformas can also help reduce variation, facilitate referral to seniors, and assist communication with women and their birth partners, for example, when an emergency cesarean section is needed for presumed fetal distress based on a pathologic EFM trace.[65]

Interprofessional Teams

Historically, training programs for nurses, midwives, family practitioners, obstetricians, pediatricians, and anesthesiologists have been separate,[10] which may raise the interprofessional barriers associated with poor outcomes for mother and babies—barriers created as early as the undergraduate level.[70] To address this problem, national bodies have recommended the introduction of interprofessional learning strategies.[70] It is important to train in multiprofessional teams. In one of the take-home lessons to emerge from the SaFE study, study teams did not include neonatologists, and after training, there was a trend to forget calling them for help in the event of shoulder dystocia.[62] This trend was even more evident when a high-fidelity mannequin was used,[56] perhaps because the focus was on individual technical skills rather than communication within the team.

The lesson is clear: training has to be inclusive—health care assistants, porters, and other nonclinical staff have a role to play. They can help with rehearsals by becoming trained patient-actors. Their role in achieving good safety culture and optimal teamwork climate is important.[52,53]

Lack of Hierarchy

Training should promote positive attitudes to team-working in interprofessional teams and should take place in a nonthreatening environment with the emphasis on constructive criticism. Otherwise, professional marginalization or steep hierarchy can poison the teamwork climate.[71,72] Obstetric nurses and midwives are particularly prone to feeling intimidated during simulation training,[73] but a reduction in the perceived authority gradients can reduce the level.

After each rehearsal, participants, regardless of seniority, can provide feedback to the team using standardized checklists as guides (Table 79–2). Such debriefings encourage juniors to question seniors, midwives to challenge doctors, doctors to feel their expertise is valued, and other staff to feel part of the team. It is noteworthy that in a recent safety attitudes survey with a validated tool,[52,74] the top five scores

TABLE 79–2
Checklist to be Used for Debriefing

Did the first (handover) professional communicate by using SBAR?

DOMAIN		EXPECTED STATEMENT	YES—PLEASE TICK
S	Stated which emergency (situation)	Cord prolapse	
B	Background history (key points) mentioned	Spontaneous rupture of membranes Not fully dilated	
A	Assessment of situation and severity	Fetal bradycardia (need for immediate delivery)	
R	Recommendation for initial action	Elevation of presenting part Need to transfer to theatre for caesarean	

FIGURE 79–2
Low-cost props: trousers that "bleed."

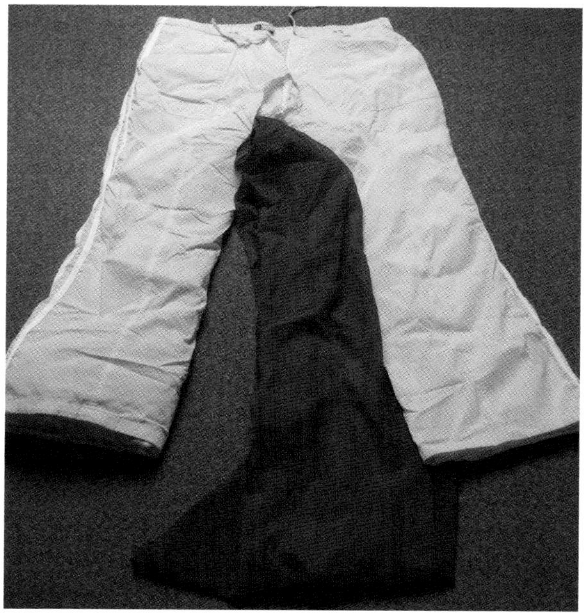

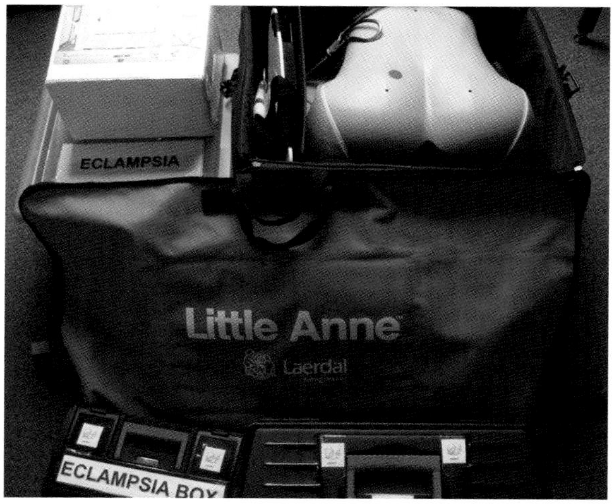

FIGURE 79–3
Mobile simulation kit: a simulation center anywhere, anytime.

in the collaboration scale were given to caregivers belonging to the professions that undergo mandatory interprofessional training and that these good collaboration scores were associated with good safety scores.[53]

Fidelity

ENVIRONMENTAL FIDELITY

Environmental fidelity—that is, conducting rehearsals on labor wards—might be more important in obstetric training than the technology of the equipment used; in the SaFE study, training was more successful, in some aspects, in situ than externally.[61] If mannequins are used, a pregnant abdomen, bra, and female wig add realism to the simulated scenario. In the PROMPT (PRactical Obstetric Multi-Professional Training) course,[75] props are used to increase the realism of the scenarios: blood-stained incontinence sheets, trousers that bleed (Fig. 79–2), a pregnant uterus, life-size copy of O-negative blood bags stuck on to cardboard, and a perineum with a prolapsed cord. With the collection of many low-cost props and a few high-tech models, a "mobile simulation center" (Fig. 79–3) can be used to flexibly train either the trainers or the participants.

HIGH-TECH MODELS

Whereas expensive models are not always necessary, high-fidelity part-task trainers may be best used to train individuals in highly technical skills like internal maneuvers at shoulder dystocia.[62] In the SaFE study, training on a high-fidelity mannequin was associated with a significantly higher chance of successfully managing a simulated shoulder dystocia than training with low-fidelity models.[56]

PATIENT ACTORS AND HYBRID SIMULATION

Obstetric emergencies are unique in that there is significant audience participation; health care team communication with women, their families, and sometimes friends during acute management of the emergency is an essential skill. In medical emergencies, the patient is often conscious and there remains a direct interaction between the patient and the caregivers. Yet, there is acknowledgment that nontechnical skills are often not addressed in obstetric training programs.[76]

Properly trained patient-actors are valuable proxies for assessing communication skills. One study demonstrated that patient-actors working to an agreed protocol are reliable reporters of physicians' practice. Their reports of physicians' quality of care compares well with independent external assessments of audiovisual recordings of patient-doctor interactions.[77]

Computerized mannequins may be less effective: advanced technology allows mannequins to "speak," but in the SaFE study, training with high-tech mannequins did not seem to

FIGURE 79–4
Hybrid simulation: a trained patient-actor kneels behind an advanced pelvic trainer model and delivers a standardized script and feedback at debriefing.

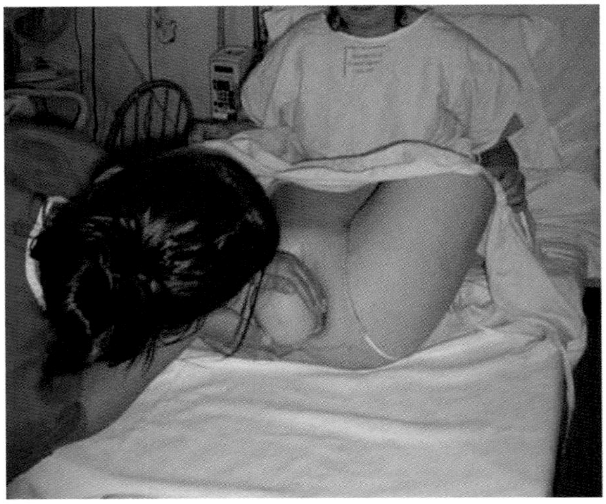

improve communication skills as much as training with patient-actors.[61]

Patient-actors are useful not only for the assessment but also for the development of communication skills. The SaFE study demonstrated that training maternity staff in the management of simulated obstetric emergencies improved patient-actor perception of safety.[62,76,78] Another study demonstrated that obstetric intervention for certain emergencies is not detrimental to real-life women's satisfaction with the birth experience[79] when all staff attend regular team communication training with patient-actors.

Integrating a patient-actor with a mannequin ("hybrid" simulation, Fig. 79–4) is a simple, effective, and inexpensive training tool that allows both manual and verbal skills to be learned and practiced simultaneously.[55,56,59,61,75,78] Hybrid simulation can increase the realism of the situation, enhance the communication between team members and women, and lead to improvement in communication scores.[61] To maximize the educational benefit, it may be useful for the patient-actors to provide feedback to the team after each rehearsal.[61]

Human Factors (Teamwork) Training

Teamwork is defined as the combined effective action of a group working toward a common goal. It requires individuals with different roles to communicate effectively and work together in a coordinated manner to achieve a successful outcome.[75] Theories of team effectiveness dictate that the outcome of team-working is related to task clarity and importance (clear outcome-based objectives), group characteristics and size, organizational environment and culture, as well as the intervening factors of teams such as leadership and communication.

Formation of a team is rapid in an emergency and enquiries into poor outcomes clearly show that these ad hoc teams do not always function well.[1] Teamwork training has been recommended to address the problem,[1,6] but isolated teamwork interventions have not been shown to lead to sustainable improvements in outcome.[14] A recent cluster randomized, controlled trial[2] studied the impact of standardized crew resource management (CRM) ("MedTeams") teamwork training on 11 measures of maternal and neonatal outcome in seven U.S. maternity units. More than 1300 health care professionals were trained, but there was no difference before or after the intervention in any clinical outcome or in 10 out of the 11 process measures used to evaluate the quality of care.

Conversely, clinical training alone might improve teamwork without the need for nonclinical teamwork theories or activities. The SaFE study demonstrated improved simulation performance and team behavior after clinical training in teams. There was no difference in knowledge or clinical performance in rehearsals between learners who received additional teamwork training and those who were randomized to clinical training alone. There was also no difference in overall team performance as measured by global teamwork rating or patient-actor perception of care between the two groups.[55,61,62]

Similarly, in an obstetric emergencies course, pretraining clinical performance was lower for rehearsals requiring multiprofessional team effort (PPH, eclampsia) than for rehearsals focusing on skills of the individual accoucheur (breech vaginal delivery, shoulder dystocia). Simulation performance significantly increased in the former by working in teams: the performance in either eclampsia or PPH was higher for the second pretraining drill than the first, regardless of whether the PPH station followed the eclampsia or vice versa, even before any additional clinical or teamwork training. Subsequent performance improved further with clinical training, even though the scenarios were changed[3]: simply stated, working in teams improves team-working.

It might be that CRM principles can be effective in obstetrics, but perhaps relevant teamwork interventions need to be refined and made directly applicable to labor settings first. In the SaFE study,[59,80,81] content analysis demonstrated that extra teamwork training resulted in increased rate of directed and addressed messages (as opposed to commands called out "in the air"), compared to clinical training alone, but this was not associated with improved simulation performance. Further work is required to determine the components of effective, structured obstetric communication and inform the design of effective nontechnical team training interventions and practical assessment tools.

Documentation Training

An analysis of 189 closed perinatal claims in the United States with a total value of $168 million revealed that theoretical presumption of innocence does not apply to maternity caregivers, who, therefore, must document that their care could not have caused injury. Better documentation was identified as one of the four key interventions that can reduce obstetric litigation.[42] Unfortunately, an evaluation of delivery notes after simulated shoulder dystocia found that notes often lacked critical elements,[82] but participants can achieve better documentation after simulation training including documentation training.[67,83,84] However, training should be supplemented by standardized proformas to assist easy, reliable, and accurate documentation.[82–84]

Frequency of Training

Traditionally, the recommendation has been for annual training, and the existing evidence suggests that this is reasonable.[78] A study of the management of simulated shoulder dystocia confirmed that there was no deterioration in the performance of basic actions, delivery interval, force application, and patient communication for at least 1 year after training. Those who were proficient before initial training performed best at follow-up, but skill retention was also good in those who learned to deliver during initial training. However, more frequent rehearsal is advisable for those initially lacking competency until skill acquisition is achieved.[78]

Participation

Threat-free Participation

To avoid intimidating authority gradients, a member of the training group can provide feedback to the rest of the team, using specific checklists.[75] Learners often perceive that they have performed very badly, so it is vital that positive actions are emphasized. The lack of formal assessment removes the threat of testing, may promote team ethos, and can enable both 100% staff participation and improved outcomes.[50] Furthermore, it has been shown that informal verbal feedback is as good as feedback based on video recording[85] in improving performance in simulation.

Mandatory Attendance of the Entire Workforce

Units that have reported improvements in perinatal outcomes all achieved full participation in rehearsals.[20,49,50] Poor performers might be less inclined to attend such rehearsals, or more likely to drop out, but they are also the ones likely to show important improvements in performance after training.[59] The solution is to both facilitate threat-free regular participation and, at the same time, mandate and confirm at least annual attendance via appraisal/supervisory schemes and central training databases.[38,50]

Follow-up on Training

Prospective Surveillance of Outcomes

Even with the best of intentions and the best of training, outcomes that improved once may deteriorate again.[39] Systems are needed to detect lapses and address them with targeted training. Monitoring the outcomes of training using routinely collected data and valid tools is a tested and proven solution. It is useful for maintaining the standards of training and supplementing with further safety and quality improvement interventions when necessary.[39,65]

Extension: Undergraduate Training

Postgraduate training can be modified and applied to undergraduate training: simulation with patient-actors, interprofessional learning experiences, practical exercises focusing on fidelity, fun, and evidence-based tools have been successful.[64,66]

Shared Learning

The development, testing, and successful implementation of training interventions are not adequate for quality improvement. Dissemination of the results and the lessons learned is an essential part of the improvement process, if poor outcomes are to be tackled worldwide. It is suggested that individuals and organizations in charge of training program publish explicit reports of their results in accordance with reporting guidelines, share their lessons via public databases (National Institute for Clinical Excellence—Shared Learning database,[68] Institute for Health Improvement—online improvement stories), and make tools freely available via websites.[86]

CONCLUSION

An independent review of maternity care in the United Kingdom stated: "The overwhelming majority of births are safe, but some births are less safe than they could, and should be. 'Safe Teams' are the key to improving the safety of maternity services and teams that work together should also train together, on their labor ward. Simulation-based training including clinical, communication and team skills should be made available for all maternity staff, ideally within their own units."[7]

Obstetric emergencies occur rapidly and unexpectedly and render uncomplicated labors high risk within seconds. Training may be the single most effective way to reduce the potentially avoidable poor outcomes for mothers and their babies. However, not all training is equal or effective. Up until recently, very few data have been available to guide training, but there are significant emerging studies that should inform us what works where. These data should be used to effect the improvements that mothers and their babies deserve.

SUMMARY OF MANAGEMENT OPTIONS

Training for Obstetric Emergencies

Recommendations for Training	Evidence Quality and Recommendation	References
Scope		
Identify training needs: national enquiries, local surveillance, litigation statistics, simulation to identify recurrent mistakes.	Ib/A	3,39,54,56,87
Incentives		
Institution-level incentives to train.	IV/C	88

SUMMARY OF MANAGEMENT OPTIONS

Training for Obstetric Emergencies—cont'd

Recommendations for Training	Evidence Quality and Recommendation	References
Methods		
Simulation rehearsals in addition to lectures.	Ib/A	60
In-house clinical training.	Ib/A	55,67,88
Teaching of streamlined clinical protocols.	II/B	20,40,42,50,88
Practical solutions that make it easy to implement national guidelines.	II/B	50,68,89
Multiprofessional teams, interprofessional learning.	II/B	3,55,88
Lack of hierarchy, reduced authority gradient.	II/B	88
Context-specific fidelity:		
• Environmental fidelity.	II/B	67,88
• High-tech models for advanced manual skills.	Ib/A	56
• Hybrid simulation with patient-actors integrated with part-task trainers for communication training.	Ib/A	61,64,90
Human factors (teamwork) training: in-house, integrated in clinical rehearsals.	Ib/A	20,55,59,88
Training in documentation and the use of documentation proformas.	II/B	40,42,75,82,84
Participation		
Participation in training of the entire workforce.	II/B	41,50,88
Threat-free participation; lack of formal assessment; replace with structured self-assessment and debriefings.	II/B	88,91
Mandate and confirm annual attendance.	II/B	50
Follow-up		
Prospective surveillance of outcomes.	II/B	39
Disseminate results and outcomes: shared learning of successes and challenges.	IV/C	92–94
Modify and apply lessons to undergraduate training.	Ib/A	64,66

SUGGESTED READINGS

Crofts JF, Fox R, Ellis D, et al: Observations from 450 shoulder dystocia simulations: Lessons for skills training. Obstet Gynecol 2008;112:906–912.

Draycott T, Crofts JF, Ash JP, et al: Improving neonatal outcome through practical shoulder dystocia training. Obstet Gynecol 2008;112:14–20.

Haynes AB, Weiser TG, Berry WR, et al: A surgical safety checklist to reduce morbidity and mortality in a global population. N Engl J Med 2009;360:491–499.

Knight M: Eclampsia in the United Kingdom 2005. BJOG 2007;114:1072–1078.

Lewis G (ed): The Confidential Enquiry into Maternal and Child Health (CEMACH). Saving Mothers' Lives: Reviewing Maternal Deaths to Make Motherhood Safer—2003–2005. The seventh report of the Confidential Enquiries into Maternal Deaths in the United Kingdom. London, CEMACH, 2007.

Maslovitz S, Barkai G, Lessing JB, et al: Recurrent obstetric management mistakes identified by simulation. Obstet Gynecol 2007;109:1295–1300.

Nielsen PE, Goldman MB, Mann S, et al: Effects of teamwork training on adverse outcomes and process of care in labor and delivery: A randomized controlled trial. Obstet Gynecol 2007;109:48–55.

Salas E, Wilson KA, Burke CS, Wightman DC: Does crew resource management training work? An update, an extension, and some critical needs. Hum Factors 2006;48:392–412.

Siassakos D, Hasafa Z, Sibanda T, et al: Retrospective cohort study of diagnosis-delivery interval with umbilical cord prolapse: The effect of team training. BJOG 2009;116:1089–1096.

Siassakos D, Timmons C, Hogg F, et al: Evaluation of a strategy to improve undergraduate experience in obstetrics and gynaecology. Med Educ 2009;43:669–673.

REFERENCES

For a complete list of references, log onto www.expertconsult.com.

CHAPTER 80

Resuscitation and Immediate Care of the Newborn

STEPHEN P. WARDLE and NEIL MARLOW

INTRODUCTION

Few newborn babies need any assistance to establish normal respiration and circulation following birth, and of those who do, most require only simple measures. Delivery units base the need for a specialized team to be present at a delivery on preset criteria related to the type of delivery or the presumed condition of the newborn baby. Even with such a policy, unanticipated resuscitation is required in a significant number of deliveries.[1] For example, one study has shown that about 20% of babies who require resuscitation are not predictable from clinical observations made in pregnancy and during labor.[2]

This chapter aims to discuss the stabilization and resuscitation of the newborn in the delivery suite. It does not cover further care that the baby might need in a neonatal intensive care unit (NICU).

Importantly, prompt resuscitation of babies, even of those without apparent signs of life at birth, will result in a significant number of healthy survivors.[3] Hence, wherever babies are delivered, someone must be present who is trained and experienced to commence neonatal resuscitation, and there should be a method of providing expert backup for the complicated resuscitation.

It is important that all staff involved in resuscitation is trained in a systematic way to ensure uniformity of practice. In the United Kingdom, the Neonatal Life Support course (NLS, UK Resuscitation Council) has become the nationally accepted standard for training for staff involved in newborn resuscitation. Guidelines and courses exist in other countries such as the Neonatal Resuscitation Program (NRP) in the United States. Most are part of The International Liaison Committee on Resuscitation (ILCOR), a formal group that coordinates practice between national organizations and includes the production of consensus on neonatal life support. Their recommendations have recently been updated.[4]

All professionals attending delivery must understand the principles of neonatal resuscitation and be able to institute effective respiration with a suitable mask ventilation system or intubation.[5] Generally, the local pediatric or neonatal service provides the necessary expertise for the anticipated resuscitation problem, but other professionals who work in maternity services must be prepared and able to commence resuscitation when it has not been anticipated.

Each delivery unit must ensure that

- There is adequate provision of facilities.
- Staff is adequately trained for resuscitation.
- Staff is available when needed and prepared to institute neonatal resuscitation when required.

PREDICTING PROBLEMS

The need for resuscitation can be predicted before delivery in many cases. Most delivery units set criteria for attendance at delivery by their skilled team. It is important to define criteria appropriately, otherwise an excessive number of deliveries will require attendance. In one study, the attendance rate was decreased from 38.6% to 24.8%[6] by changing criteria following audit. During the same period, the number needing skilled resuscitation and the number of emergency calls did not change, but interestingly, the rate of intubation decreased significantly.

The following are suggested indications for attendance by a skilled and experienced team:

- Fetal compromise (as assessed by the obstetrician/midwife [e.g., pathologic cardiotocography {CTG} or fetal blood sample pH < 7.2]).
- Meconium-staining of the liquor.
- Urgent or emergency cesarean section.
- Elective cesarean section under general anesthesia or for placenta praevia, multiple births, or where admission to the neonatal unit is likely. A skilled resuscitator is not required for elective cesarean section under regional anesthesia.[7]
- Vaginal breech delivery.
- Multiple pregnancy.
- Rotational forceps (e.g., Keilland's forceps) delivery.
- Preterm delivery at less than 34 weeks' gestation.
- Severe fetal growth restriction.
- Maternal insulin-dependent diabetes.
- Maternal myasthenia gravis.
- Known serious fetal abnormality (e.g., diaphragmatic hernia, hydrops fetalis).
- Severe rhesus disease likely to require neonatal intensive care.

GENERAL CARE OF THE BABY AT BIRTH

Optimal Cord Clamping

Modern obstetric practice usually involves division of the cord while the placenta is still in utero. The time of occlusion of the umbilical cord determines the distribution of blood between the baby and the placenta. Optimal distribution has not been clearly defined, but for preterm babies in particular, even a short delay of 30 seconds in cord clamping may produce hemodynamic advantage and results in fewer blood transfusions and a reduced frequency of intraventricular hemorrhage.[8,9] The optimum distribution of blood volume and the least hemodynamic disturbance may be achieved by clamping the cord about 30 seconds after delivery, although some studies have used longer, by which time, the baby usually has taken his or her first breath.

Before division, the cord should be firmly occluded about 2 cm from the umbilicus using a suitable umbilical cord clamp.

Temperature Management

Keeping a newborn baby warm after birth is important to prevent morbidity and is considered a marker of good care.[10] Using warm towels to dry the baby and maintaining the room temperature at around 24°C minimize the heat stress experienced by the baby after birth. Skin-to-skin contact with the mother also helps to maintain temperature. Wrapping and dressing are alternative strategies. Bathing is best avoided immediately after birth because the associated evaporative water loss can reduce a baby's temperature.[11–13]

Attachment and Breast-feeding

When early assessment reveals no immediate problems, including prematurity or significant growth restriction, the baby should be handed at once to the mother. This may be done even before dividing the umbilical cord, but care should be taken to prevent heat loss and to optimize placental transfusion.[13] The baby may be wrapped in a warmed towel or, better, nursed skin-to-skin on the mother's chest, covered with a warm towel. If the mother intends to breastfeed, the baby should be put to the breast. This not only improves the success of lactation but also may aid delivery of the placenta by encouraging the release of endogenous oxytocin. Extra care to avoid cold stress must be taken when a baby is preterm or growth-restricted.

Even when a baby is unwell and needs admission to the NICU, it is important that the mother is given the opportunity to see and, if possible, hold her newborn baby.

Routine Examination

A routine examination of the newborn is recommended as a core component of child health surveillance[14] and can be performed at any stage in the first 72 hours after birth. It does not need to be carried out immediately after birth. However, a routine external examination for major abnormalities is usually carried out by the birth attendant to rule out major congenital anomalies. Early examination facilitates early discharge but may be associated with more false-positive examinations.

Vitamin K

Vitamin K is given as prophylaxis against hemorrhagic disease of the newborn.[15] It can be given as an oral or intramuscular dose, although intramuscular administration gives better vitamin K levels[16] and should be given shortly after birth because bleeding from hemorrhagic disease can present within the first 6 hours after birth.

PHYSIOLOGY

The process of birth, even in a healthy term newborn baby, is associated with relative hypoxia, but newborn babies are able to withstand this surprisingly well. The term "newborn" will demonstrate a particular pattern of physiologic changes during hypoxia,[17–20] and understanding of these processes helps the attendant decide when to initiate resuscitation, assess the baby's responses, and judge the effectiveness of the interventions given.

Acute total hypoxia in animals at delivery results after a few minutes in primary apnea. This is associated with initial tachycardia and a rise in blood pressure, followed by bradycardia. Redistribution of blood flow occurs to essential organs (brain and heart) at the expense of others (skin, gut, and kidneys). If hypoxia persists, deep slow gasping occurs every 10 to 20 seconds before a further final period of apnea occurs, called "terminal apnea." During this phase, hypotension, progressive bradycardia, and decreased cardiac output result in organ damage and death unless active resuscitation is commenced.

A similar sequence of changes seems to occur in the human newborn. During resuscitation, it is not always possible to recognize where in this sequence of events the child is, and it may be difficult to differentiate primary from terminal apnea. A baby in primary apnea will be blue and have a low heart rate, low tone, and apnea, but the appearances are similar in a baby in terminal apnea (Table 80–1). However, a baby in primary apnea will recover quickly following lung inflation (brought about either by the resuscitator or by the onset of gasping respiration) whereas a baby in terminal apnea is unlikely to recover as quickly, even with lung inflation, and will almost always require a longer period of resuscitation before gasping and subsequently normal respiration resumes. A baby in poor condition, therefore, should be assumed to be in terminal apnea, and resuscitation should be initiated without delay.

Lactic Acidosis

Following a period of hypoxia, a baby's tissues quickly switch to anaerobic respiration. This is reflected in the accumulation of lactic acid and, because the baby is not breathing, also carbon dioxide. Therefore, during birth, and particularly during prolonged hypoxia-ischemia, babies become significantly acidotic. Typically, this is associated with redistribution of blood flow away from the skin, and the baby appears pale or white. It is important to note that this does not necessarily indicate hypovolemia or the need for volume replacement unless there is clear evidence of fetal blood loss. Giving excessive volume to an asphyxiated baby could be deleterious in view of cardiac hypoxia.[21]

TABLE 80–1
Physiological Responses to Hypoxia in the Newborn

STAGE	DESCRIPTION	ACIDOSIS	ASSESSMENT: HEART RATE	TONE	BREATHING	COLOR	RESPONSE TO RESUSCITATION
1. Initial response	High HR, rise in BP then fall in HR.	No	High/normal	Normal	Breathing	Blue	Increased HR. Normal breathing.
2. Primary apnea	Initial period of apnea. Redistribution of blood flow.	Mild	Low	Low	Apnea	Blue	Increased HR. Normal breathing.
3. Gasping	Deep gasping respiration.	Moderate	Low	Low	Gasping	Blue	Increased HR. Normal breathing quickly takes over.
4. Terminal apnea	Apnea, redistribution of blood flow. Heart rate and BP fall.	Severe	Low/absent	Low	Apnea	Blue/ pale	Increased HR. Gasping then normal breathing.

BP, blood pressure; HR, heart rate.

In addition, although the degree of acidosis may be severe, the administration of alkalinizing agents to correct this is generally not useful. An exception is possibly when the heart rate remains low despite adequate lung expansion and cardiac massage.[22] The level of lactic acidosis may be a useful indicator of the severity of the hypoxic insult. Administration of alkali during resuscitation remains controversial; sodium bicarbonate is a negative inotrope and correction of extracellular acidosis may worsen intracellular pH. However, one unevaluated justification may be the vasodilation of coronary arteries and improvement of adrenaline delivery to the myocardium seen in animal experiments. It is not necessary to correct acidosis fully.

Meconium

The normal breathing efforts of a baby in utero are not sufficient to inhale particulate meconium in significant quantities. Lung aspiration of meconium probably occurs secondary to a hypoxic ischemic insult in a baby who has already passed meconium, during gasping that may commence before or after birth. Subsequent hypoxia and persistent pulmonary hypertension may not be related to the presence of meconium in the lung but to the preceding hypoxia-ischemia. Therefore, the severity of the hypoxic-ischemic insult that has caused the gasping is likely to be as, if not more, important than the meconium itself. As long as meconium is not obstructing the airway, it may be relatively harmless, which is possibly why laryngeal toileting has been shown to have little positive effect.[23]

The Use of Air or Oxygen during Resuscitation

Traditionally, babies have been resuscitated in 100% oxygen. However, there are strong theoretical reasons to believe that this may be harmful, particularly in preterm babies. Following resuscitation with 100% oxygen, there is biochemical evidence of an increase in the generation of oxygen free radicals, which can be harmful to the brain and lungs.[24] In preterm babies, there is additional evidence of significant alterations in cerebral blood flow persisting for some time.[25] Several randomized studies have compared resuscitation with air or oxygen, and these have been subjected to systematic review and meta-analysis.[26] Overall, there was a reduction in mortality in babies resuscitated with room air and no evidence of harm. However, because the number of studies was small and there were some methodologic limitations, the results should be interpreted with caution.

Using air for resuscitation, therefore, appears to be at least as good as using 100% oxygen, but oxygen should also always be available via a mixer system on the resuscitation apparatus for those situations in which it is required.

PREPARATION AND EQUIPMENT

Whenever possible, any individual who expects to initiate neonatal resuscitation should always introduce themselves to the parents and explain what is happening or likely to happen. She or he should obtain as full a history as possible from the mother, midwife, or obstetrician and examine the mother's records to establish

- Gestational age.
- Drugs given to the mother.
- Evidence of fetal distress (e.g., heart rate abnormality, acidosis, meconium).
- Presence of vaginal bleeding.
- Prolonged rupture of membranes.
- Maternal health in labor.[27]
- Number of fetuses.[28]
- Relevant obstetric or medical history.

In addition, the person leading the resuscitation should make sure that appropriate team members are present and check and prepare the necessary equipment. Anyone leading the resuscitation should

- Consider whether they require help and call for it if so.
- Ensure the delivery room is warm (>24°C) and free of drafts.
- Check that equipment is available and in working order.
- Turn on the overhead heater.

- Ensure that warmed towels are available.
- Wash hands, put on gloves, or take other precautions against blood-borne viruses as per hospital policy.

ASSESSMENT OF CONDITION AT BIRTH

Apgar Score

Condition at birth is traditionally assessed using the Apgar score, which was designed as a guide for the need for resuscitation. Measures may be made at 1 and 5 minutes, with further recordings at 5-minute intervals if resuscitation continues. Ideally, the Apgar score should be assessed and recorded at the time of resuscitation (originally this was done by a second observer) because retrospective assignation is fraught with errors. The Apgar score is a poor prognostic guide for later outcome, except that low Apgar scores that persist beyond 15 to 20 minutes are more strongly associated with neurologic deficits.[29] In practice, careful assessment and descriptions of heart rate and respiration, color, and tone are much more meaningful in assessing the physiologic condition of a baby.

Cord Blood Acid-Base

For babies born after fetal distress or for those needing resuscitation, the cord blood pH, base excess, or lactate concentration may indicate the severity of perinatal asphyxia. Blood from both the umbilical artery and vein should be sampled. Some babies have experienced significant intrapartum asphyxia but present with a normal pH. As is true with the Apgar score, extremes of acidosis are most strongly associated with poor outcome. Cord blood acid-base status cannot be used to determine the need for resuscitation but is useful as one of the factors to look at in determining the etiology of a poor condition at birth or a neonatal encephalopathy. Routinely checking cord acid-base balance after delivery can, therefore, be useful and is essential when babies have needed resuscitation.

STABILIZATION AND RESUSCITATION FOLLOWING DELIVERY AT OR NEAR TERM

The following approach is based on the standardized approach taught on the U.K. Resuscitation Council NLS Course (Fig. 80–1)[30]:

- First, the clock should be started.
- The baby should be transferred to the resuscitaire; whatever the condition of the child, prevention of heat loss is a critical priority; the baby should be dried, wet towels removed, and wrapped in a warm towel.
- The condition of the baby should be assessed
  - Color: Assessed by looking at the baby's lips and not peripheries.
  - Tone: Assessed while drying the baby.
  - Breathing: Not breathing, normal respiration, or gasping.
  - Heart rate: Best assessed by auscultation; alternatives are palpation of the umbilical cord or apex beat.
- Following assessment, resuscitation and management should proceed in the following order:
  - Airway: The airway must be clear and open in order to allow the lungs to inflate.
  - Breathing: Either the baby must be able to breath and inflate its own lungs or this must be achieved by the resuscitator.
  - Circulation: The baby's circulation may be compromised and require support.
  - Drugs: These are occasionally necessary to facilitate an adequate circulation.

Potential scenarios are set out in Table 80–2.

TABLE 80–2
Possible Scenarios during Initial Resuscitation

Scenario 1: A baby who is breathing/crying, heart rate ≥ 100, centrally pink.	The infant should be dried and given to mother. Ideally, these babies should be delivered directly onto their mother's abdomen and dried with a towel. Temperature is then maintained by direct skin-to-skin contact.
Scenario 2: A baby who is blue, apneic, heart rate ≥ 100 with reasonable tone (i.e., not completely floppy).	Because the heart rate is good, this baby will recover. Breathing usually starts spontaneously within a minute of delivery, but healthy babies can take up to 3 min to start breathing after birth.[31] If apnea continues, it will be necessary to open the airway and give inflation breaths.
Scenario 3: A baby who is blue/pale, apneic, heart rate < 60.	Babies with a low heart rate who are not breathing could be in primary or terminal apnea. These infants will, therefore, need further resuscitation, although most will respond to simple measures.

Further Action if the Baby Is Blue/Pale, Apneic with a Heart Rate less than 60

- The airway should be opened (head in neutral position, jaw thrust) (Figs. 80–2 and 80–3) and the mask placed appropriately (Fig. 80–4).
- Five inflation breaths should be given by mask (30 cm H_2O, 2- to 3-sec inflation time).
- Inflation breaths should be long higher-pressure breaths to remove lung fluid.[32] Until the lungs are inflated, they are filled with fluid and the baby will not improve.
- With each inflation breath, the resuscitator must ensure that the chest moves. If it does not, it will be necessary to reposition the airway (head in neutral position, jaw thrust). If the chest still does not move, then in addition, the following should be considered:
  - Two person jaw thrust, *or*
  - Insertion of a Guedel airway, *or*
  - Longer inflation time or increased pressure, *or*
  - Suction under direct vision: airway obstruction is almost always due to decreased pharyngeal tone, not obstruction.
- If the chest moves well with inflation breaths after five breaths, the baby should be reassessed. If the heart rate is responding, the resuscitator should continue ventilation breaths (0.5-sec inflation time, 40 breaths/min) until the baby is breathing spontaneously. The time at which this

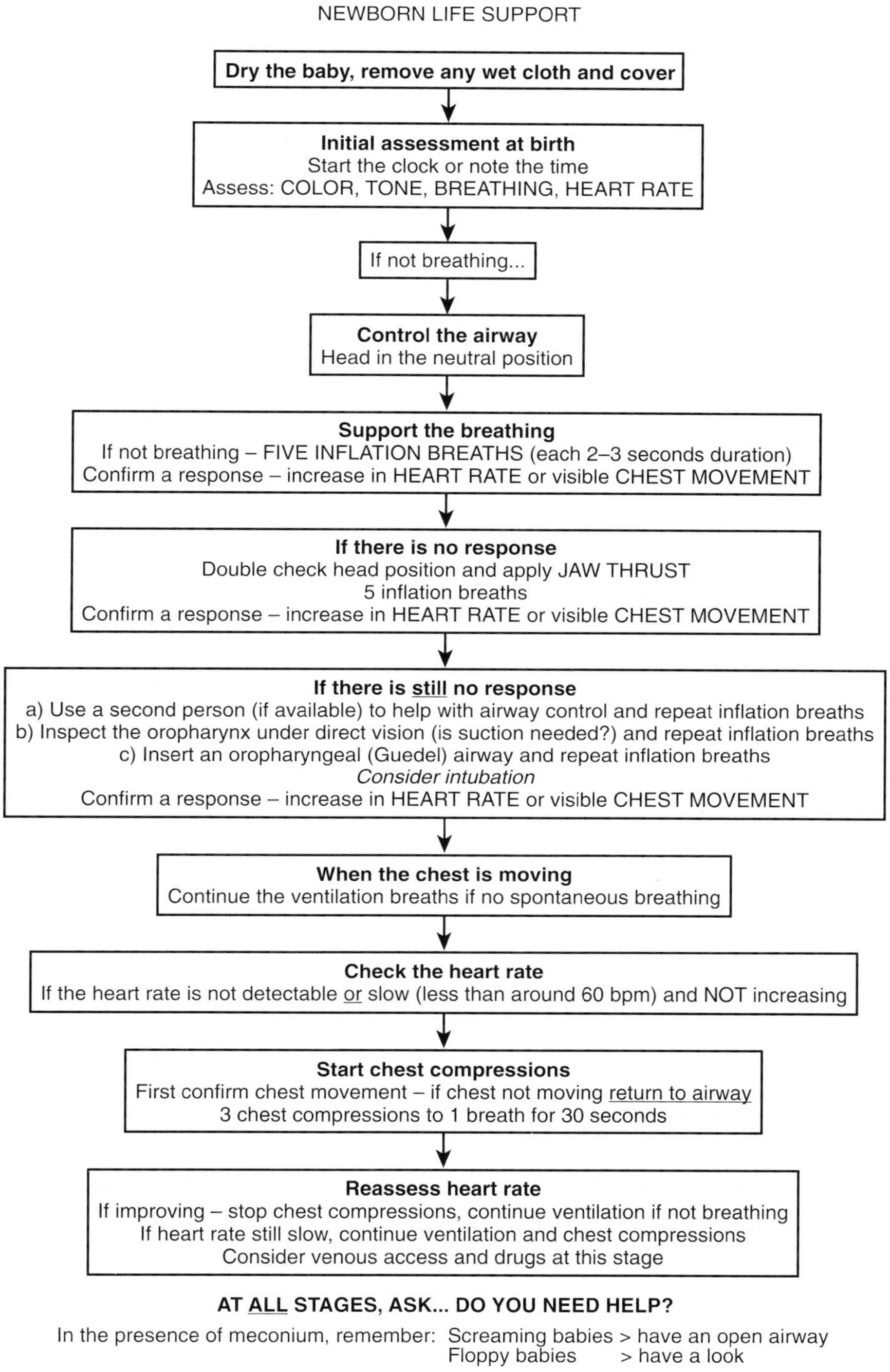
NEWBORN LIFE SUPPORT
Dry the baby, remove any wet cloth and cover
Initial assessment at birth
Start the clock or note the time
Assess: COLOR, TONE, BREATHING, HEART RATE
If not breathing...
Control the airway
Head in the neutral position
Support the breathing
If not breathing – FIVE INFLATION BREATHS (each 2–3 seconds duration)
Confirm a response – increase in HEART RATE or visible CHEST MOVEMENT
If there is no response
Double check head position and apply JAW THRUST
5 inflation breaths
Confirm a response – increase in HEART RATE or visible CHEST MOVEMENT
If there is still no response
a) Use a second person (if available) to help with airway control and repeat inflation breaths
b) Inspect the oropharynx under direct vision (is suction needed?) and repeat inflation breaths
c) Insert an oropharyngeal (Guedel) airway and repeat inflation breaths
Consider intubation
Confirm a response – increase in HEART RATE or visible CHEST MOVEMENT
When the chest is moving
Continue the ventilation breaths if no spontaneous breathing
Check the heart rate
If the heart rate is not detectable or slow (less than around 60 bpm) and NOT increasing
Start chest compressions
First confirm chest movement – if chest not moving return to airway
3 chest compressions to 1 breath for 30 seconds
Reassess heart rate
If improving – stop chest compressions, continue ventilation if not breathing
If heart rate still slow, continue ventilation and chest compressions
Consider venous access and drugs at this stage
AT ALL STAGES, ASK... DO YOU NEED HELP?
In the presence of meconium, remember: Screaming babies > have an open airway
Floppy babies > have a look

FIGURE 80–1
Resuscitation algorithm.
(From Richmond S [ed]: Newborn Life Support, 2nd ed. London, Resuscitation Council (UK), 2004, p 69.)

occurs and whether the breaths are gasping or normal should be noted.

- If the heart rate does not respond
  - Ventilation breaths (0.5-second inflation time, 40 breaths/min) should be continued, ensuring that there is good chest movement. If there is not, it will be necessary to go back and recheck the airway as above. If the chest is moving, this ventilation can be continued.
  - The heart rate should be reassessed after 30 seconds to 1 minute.
- If the heart rate remains low ***and*** the chest is moving:
  - External cardiac compressions should be commenced.
  - The chest should be compressed at a ratio of 3 : 1 with ventilation breaths. If an individual experienced at intubation is present, it is worth intubating to stabilize the airway at this point. If an experienced individual is not present, T-piece/bag-mask ventilation should be continued.
- The most common reason for failure of the heart rate to improve is ineffective lung inflation. Adequacy of chest

movement should, therefore, always be checked before chest compressions are commenced.

- If the heart rate remains low (<60 beats/min) despite adequate chest inflation and external chest compressions, an umbilical vein catheter (UVC) should be inserted. In extreme cases in which attempts at inserting a UVC have failed, intraosseous access may be used.
  - At insertion of the UVC, a baseline blood gas and blood sugar should be obtained.

The techniques of airway opening, suction, mask and T-piece ventilation, bag-and-mask ventilation, intubation, external cardiac compressions, and UVC insertion are described later.

- Table 80–3 lists the drugs that can be given at this stage. There is no good evidence that helps to guide the order in which these drugs should be given. In general, most neonatologists probably choose to give adrenalin (epinephrine) in the first instance, followed by sodium bicarbonate and a second dose of adrenalin (epinephrine).
- After each drug dose is given, ventilation and external cardiac compressions should be recommenced and the heart rate reassessed each time. Once the heart rate responds (>60 beats/min), no more drugs are required and the cardiac compressions can be stopped.
- All drugs should be checked before they are administered and a record of drug administration kept.

A baby may fail to respond to resuscitation for a range of reasons, which are summarized in Table 80–4.

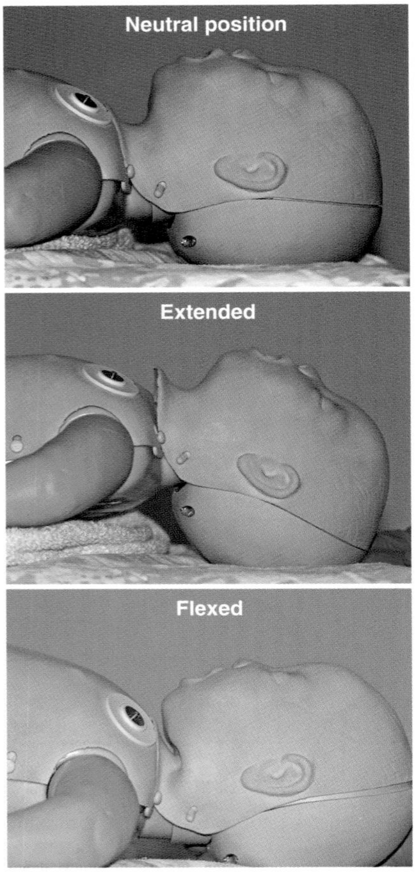

FIGURE 80–2
Head position during resuscitation. Neutral position is correct. A flexed or extended position will tend to cause airway obstruction.

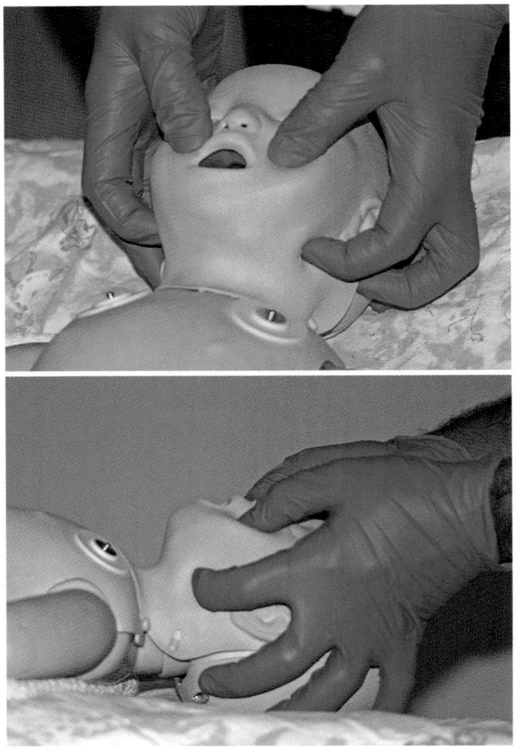

FIGURE 80–3
Jaw thrust. Position of mask and hands during jaw thrust.

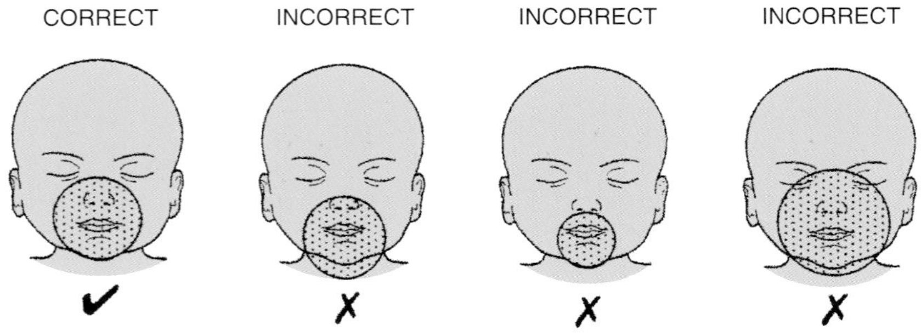

FIGURE 80–4
Face mask positioning for ventilation.

TABLE 80-3
Drugs Used for Neonatal Resuscitation

DRUG	DOSE	NOTES
Adrenaline	10 μg/kg (i.e., 0.1 mL/kg of 1:10,000 solution) IV followed by a 0.5–1.0 ml normal saline flush.	• If there is likely to be a delay in establishing IV access, then 20 μg/kg of adrenaline can be given via the ET tube if the baby is intubated.[33] Higher doses up to 100 μg/kg have also been suggested,[34] but the safety and efficacy of this have not been determined. This should be given rapidly down a catheter placed to lie just beyond the end of the ET tube and followed by a 0.5–1.0 mL normal saline flush and five rapid inflations. There is little evidence that the tracheal route is effective, and this route should be used only while IV access is being established. It must not be used in preference to IV access. If there is no response to initial doses, give further doses of adrenaline 10 μg/kg IV every 3–5 min if there is no response. An increased dose of 30 μg/kg IV can also be considered in this situation.
Sodium bicarbonate	4.2%–1 mmol/kg (i.e., 2 mL/kg) IV followed by 0.5–1.0 mL normal saline flush.	This dose of sodium bicarbonate is not intended to correct the metabolic acidosis but to increase the pH within the coronary arteries and hopefully increase the action of the subsequent adrenaline.
10% Glucose		During the process of prolonged resuscitation, hypoglycemia (i.e., whole blood glucose <2.6 mmol/L) may occur and this may interfere with adequate resuscitation. 10% Glucose 2.5 mL/kg IV can be given, followed by a 0.5–1.0 mL normal saline flush.
Calcium		No place for this in neonatal resuscitation
Atropine		No place for this in neonatal resuscitation

ET, endotracheal.

Discontinuation of Resuscitation

The decision to cease resuscitative efforts should be taken by a senior and experienced doctor. If there has been no response in heart rate or respiratory efforts by 20 minutes after birth, the outcome is universally poor and resuscitation should be terminated. Termination of treatment should occur, if possible, after discussion with the parents. In term babies, it is important this discussion begins with parents at around 15 minutes, enabling resuscitation to be stopped at 20 minutes. In extremely preterm babies, resuscitation can be stopped following nonresponse well before this time (see later).

Mothers Who Have Received Opiate Pain Relief

If with mask ventilation the baby becomes pink and has a good heart rate but does not breathe spontaneously and if mother has received opiate analgesia more frequently than every hours or within 2 to 4 hours predelivery, naloxone may be given. Bag-and-mask ventilation should not be stopped while naloxone is being administered. Naloxone should not be given to the baby of an opiate-dependent mother because it can cause acute withdrawal.

Meconium-stained Liquor

Meconium staining of the liquor does not necessarily require intervention. If the baby is crying or breathing with a normal heart rate, he or she can be treated as any other baby and unnecessary suction is not indicated.

In the presence of meconium, however, if the baby is not breathing and has a low heart rate, temperature control and assessment of the child should continue, but before giving inflation breaths, the airway should be visualized using a laryngoscope and sucked out under direct vision. If the individual is skilled at intubation, it is appropriate to pass an endotracheal tube and suck directly below the vocal cords, but if not, it is safer to simply suck out the oropharynx under direct vision. There is no place for bronchial lavage with saline because this is known to be harmful.[23] When the airway is clear of meconium, resuscitation should proceed as described previously.

RESUSCITATION OF A PRETERM BABY

The principles of the approach to resuscitation of the preterm baby are the same; however, some significant factors need to be considered that change the approach slightly:

- Optimal cord clamping is probably more important in very immature babies because hypotension may be avoided and respiratory outcomes may be improved; randomized trials are in progress to confirm this.
- Preterm babies lose heat more quickly and hypothermia has harmful effects[10] including an increased likelihood of lung disease due to surfactant deficiency; a different approach is therefore required.
- Preterm babies often do not need formal resuscitation, and excessive handling may worsen their condition; stabilization using gentle support and maintaining close attention to temperature and color should be first-line practice.
- When preterm delivery is anticipated, it is helpful for the parents to have met members of the neonatal team and to have visited the neonatal unit prior to delivery, assuming time allows. For more immature babies, this is critically important so that support can commence prenatally for the women through an emotionally difficult time.

Temperature Control

There is a strong association between a low temperature on admission and mortality rates in preterm babies.[9,37] As a result, alternative methods of maintaining the temperature

TABLE 80–4

Reasons for Failure to Respond to Resuscitation

1. During Mask Ventilation

a. Is the face mask of the correct size?
b. Is there a good seal?
c. Is the head position correct?
d. Do you need a second person to do the jaw thrust?

2. During ET Intubation with Poor or Absent Chest Wall Movement

a. *Is the ET tube in the esophagus?* Poor chest movement will be seen.
b. *Is the ET tube down the right main bronchus?* This should be considered if there is asymmetry of chest movement and breath sounds; inflation and breath sounds will improve as the tube is withdrawn.
c. *Is the inflation pressure adequate?* If the ET tube appears to be in the correct position (i.e., breath sounds present, symmetrical but poor chest wall movement), the most likely problem is that the baby is receiving insufficient pressure to open up the lungs, therefore:
   - Check peak inspiratory pressure on the manometer and increase to 30–40 cm H_2O.
   - Check oxygen flow rate—should be set to 5–8 L/min for mask ventilation, and 3–5 L/min for ET IPPV.
   - If these fail, another option is to increase the inspiratory time.
d. *Does the baby have lung pathology?* For example:
   - Pneumothorax (asymmetry of chest, movement or breath sounds)?
   - Diaphragmatic hernia (scaphoid abdomen or displaced apex beat displaced)?
   - Hypoplastic lungs (signs of Potter's syndrome)?
   - Pleural effusions?
   - Evolving severe lung disease (severe respiratory distress syndrome)?
   - Thoracic dystrophy?

3. During ET Intubation with Good Chest Movement

a. *Has there been fetal hemorrhage?* Suspect if mother has had large antepartum hemorrhage or abruption. Fetal blood loss is rare even with large antepartum bleeding.[35,36] If suspected, then normal saline should be given in a volume of 10 mL/kg, repeated as necessary (uncross-matched O-negative blood or blood cross-matched against mother can also be given cautiously to avoid metabolic problems associated with rapid transfusion such as hyperkalemia).
b. *Is there severe birth asphyxia?*
c. *Does the baby have severe cyanotic congenital heart disease?* Any baby who remains cyanosed following resuscitation needs to be urgently assessed and investigated.

ET, endotracheal; IPPV, intermittent positive-pressure ventilation.

of preterm babies have been investigated. In particular, there is good evidence that the use of occlusive polythene wrapping or plastic bags into which small babies are placed at delivery without drying are effective at improving admission temperature, although there is currently no evidence that this improves survival rates.[38,39] Avoiding drying ensures that the baby is handled less and that 100% humidity is rapidly achievable within the bag, reducing evaporative water and heat loss.

Other methods that have been investigated include the use of chemical gel–heated mattresses, but there is no evidence that the combination of these with the use of polythene wrapping further improves admission temperature.[40]

Current recommendations are

- >32 weeks: The baby should be dried, wet towels removed, and the baby wrapped in a warm towel.

TABLE 80–5

Precut Endotracheal Tube Length and Size for Use in Neonatal Resuscitation

WEIGHT (G)	CUT LENGTH OF ET TUBE (CM)*	LENGTH AT LIPS (CM)†	TUBE SIZE
500	6.5	6.0	2.5
1000	7.0	6.5	2.5
1500	7.5	7.0	2.5/3.0
2000	8.0	7.5	3.0
2500	8.5	8.0	3.0
3000	9.5	9.0	3.5
3500	10.5	10.0	3.5

* Cut ET tube to size indicated. Cut holder so that it is 1 cm long.
† Approximate length of ET tube at lips.

- ≤32 weeks: The baby should be placed directly into a plastic bag without drying,[38,39] ensuring that the head is covered with a hat; the bag should be applied closely to the skin around the neck to prevent water or heat loss.

Respiratory Management

There is debate about the best approach to supporting breathing for the very preterm baby at birth. There is evidence that giving surfactant is effective at reducing mortality and morbidity and that it is best given early ("prophylaxis") rather than after an baby develops established respiratory distress syndrome.[41] One approach is, therefore, to routinely intubate and ventilate in order to give the baby surfactant in the delivery suite prior to admission to the NICU. Because most babies above 29 weeks' gestation will not require intubation during their postnatal course, this approach is generally reserved for those babies born at less than 28 weeks' gestation.[42] Tables of endotracheal tube sizes for different gestational ages should be available on the delivery suite (Table 80–5). If a decision to intubate is made or if respiration is supported by a mask or T-piece system, the use of positive end-expiratory pressure (PEEP) may be of benefit in preterm babies.[43] This can be achieved very simply by using a PEEP valve on the T-piece system, which is one of the advantages of this system over a bag-valve-mask system.

More recently, however, it has been suggested that a less invasive approach may also be successful and avoid intubation and the problems engendered by positive-pressure ventilation. The use of continuous positive airway pressure (CPAP) in the delivery suite as a means of assisting the baby to establish a functional residual capacity has been advocated by some, and there is evolving evidence that this approach may be as successful.[44] This approach also requires a considerable degree of experience with the application and maintenance of CPAP and clinical expertise to manage safely and effectively.

The Extremely Low Gestational Age Baby

The care given for babies born at 25 weeks' gestation or less varies in different societies and health systems. The high prevalence of mortality and morbidity among survivors is the subject of public and professional debate. The ethical issues associated with this care have been widely debated and many national organizations have developed guidelines, including in the United Kingdom.[45] Key to the provision of appropriate care is the involvement of parents in decision-making and the use of a consistent approach within perinatal teams. Agreed survival and morbidity figures, which reflect population and local practice-based outcomes, should be presented to parents by the team who are responsible for care, neonatologist, obstetrician, and midwife, and within each hospital, guidance as to how this should be approached should be agreed to avoid individual bias. The parents' feelings and responses to that information should be fully appreciated and taken into consideration.

Following extremely premature delivery, the decision to initiate resuscitation must be made carefully in line with this pre-agreed approach. At the delivery, an experienced doctor should be present. Following birth, the baby should be carefully assessed in regard to size, gestational characteristics including fusion of the eyelids, bruising (which anecdotally is a critical determinant of outcome), and heart rate, tone, and breathing movements.

Babies who are considered previable by all these criteria are usually 23 weeks' gestation or less. It must be emphasized that the gestational age is often not precisely known, and all the factors listed previously must be taken into account.

Usually, the previable baby will be white, flaccid, and not making any breathing movements. In this case, the parents, who will have been over all the facts with the neonatologist, will usually want to hold the baby. If they do not wish to do this, the neonatal team can discuss with the midwifery team the most appropriate place to care for the baby. This may be on the labor suite or the neonatal unit.

If the baby is clearly making efforts to establish respiration, this should be supported with endotracheal positive-pressure ventilation. Respiratory support in a viable baby will always result in establishment of a good heart rate. If an inexperienced individual is called unexpectedly to such a delivery and if in any doubt about the viability of the baby, resuscitation is initiated until the arrival of an experienced neonatologist.

Higher-Order Births

The risk of prematurity is very high in this group, and the simultaneous delivery of several immature babies can severely stretch neonatal resources. Close cooperation between obstetrics and neonatology is necessary to ensure that sufficient resources are available for neonatal intensive care at the time of delivery.

At delivery, one resuscitaire and one trained member of the neonatal staff should be available for each baby and supported by an assistant who may be a midwife or a neonatal nurse.

PRINCIPLES OF RESUSCITATION TECHNIQUES

These are summarized in Tables 80–6 and 80–7.

DOCUMENTATION

It is essential for reasons of good clinical care, communication, and clinical governance that the findings at each assessment and the actions taken in resuscitation are fully and accurately documented. In order to do this, it is essential that accurate timings are recorded and that a clock has been started at the commencement of resuscitation. Each event and intervention should be recorded, and the easiest way of ensuring that this occurs accurately is if one individual has the responsibility of recording events, drug doses, and timings. An alternative is the use of a standard resuscitation record. Such a standardized form offers the further advantage of uniform data collection to facilitate study and comparison of resuscitation techniques and outcomes.

Following resuscitation, it is essential that each individual involved records events in which they participated in the case notes, remembering to accurately record the date and time at which they occurred as well as when they were documented.

PARENTS

Prior to the delivery of a baby, members of the team should introduce themselves to the parents of the child and explain what is going to happen, if this is possible. Communication with the parents should continue during resuscitation if it is prolonged; however, it is not always possible for those leading the resuscitation to communicate events directly to the parents, so someone, usually a midwife or neonatal nurse, should explain what is happening.

Immediately after resuscitation, it is essential that the most senior member of the team talks to the parents to explain the events and what has happened. They should explain the implications in terms of prognosis for the baby and what further treatment or interventions will be necessary.

DEBRIEFING

Following resuscitation, at a convenient time, it is extremely useful for the most senior member of the team to gather the resuscitation team together away from the clinical area to discuss events. This helps to identify positive aspects of the resuscitation and any areas of difficulty or particular problems. If there are any particular problems with equipment or systems in place for resuscitation, these should be identified and flagged for attention. Documentation of the events can be reviewed to identify any areas of weakness.

TRANSPORT OF BABIES TO THE NEONATAL INTENSIVE CARE UNIT

How this is best achieved depends on the geography of the delivery unit and NICU and their proximity to each other. Where units are very close, a resuscitaire can be used to move a baby to the NICU. If there is some distance or when units are on different floors of the same building, a transport incubator should always be used.

Before moving a baby from the delivery suite, it should always be ensured that

TABLE 80-6
Principles of Resuscitation Techniques

Airway-Opening Techniques

These are important—Mask inflation has no hope of success unless the airway is opened.

a. These should be performed before starting to breathe for the baby. The head should be placed gently into a neutral position (see Fig. 80-2).
b. If the baby is floppy, it may be necessary to use one or two fingers under each side of the lower jaw at its angle to push the jaw forward and outward (jaw thrust) (see Fig. 80-3).
c. A folded towel placed under the neck and shoulders may help to maintain the neutral position.
d. Consider using a Guedel airway.
e. Look, listen, and feel for respiratory effort. If baby is making good respiratory effort but the chest is not moving, consider suction of the nasopharynx under direct vision.
f. Consider suction (see below).

Suction

a. Use a laryngoscope to look into the airway.
b. Use a 10-fg (black) suction catheter or a baby Yankauer sucker or, where there is meconium, use a laryngoscope to look into the airway.
c. The pressure should not exceed 100 mm Hg (13.3 KpA)
d. Beware inserting the catheter too far and producing reflex vagal bradycardia.

Important points:

- No longer than 30 sec should be spent in trying to intubate the infant before recommencing bag and mask or mask and T-piece IPPV, for a minimum of 1 min.
- Never attach the baby directly to either the wall oxygen supply or any supply of oxygen that is not connected to some type of pressure limit valve.

Bag and Mask/Mask and T-piece Ventilation

a. A mask that is big enough to cover the face, from the bridge of the nose to below the mouth, should be chosen (see Fig. 80-4). A good seal must be obtained around the infant's face.
b. When using a mask and T-piece, the oxygen flow rate should be set at 5–8 L/min. The first five inflation breaths should be given at 30 cmH_2O and held for 2–3 sec to establish a functional residual capacity. Once the chest wall is moving, the inflation pressure may be reduced to 15–20 cmH_2O.
c. When using a bag and mask system, only use a 500-mL bag with a blow-off valve set at approximately 45 cm H_2O and an oxygen flow rate of 5 L/min. The oxygen flow rate should be increased as indicated up to a maximum of 10 L/min. The first five inflation breaths should be given slowly, compressing the bag with the fingers for 1–2 sec.
d. Following the first five breaths, ventilation should occur at a rate of 30–40 breaths/min.
e. The chest wall should be observed for equal movement. If there is poor inflation, the airway should be checked to ensure it is not obstructed. The head should be repositioned, making sure that it is not overextended, and other airway maneuvers should be considered (e.g., two-person jaw thrust, Guedel airway). If necessary, suction under direct vision should be carried out.

During prolonged mask ventilation, a nasogastric tube should be passed to deflate the stomach. When a mask and T-piece or a bag, valve, and mask system attached to a reservoir bag is used, the baby will receive the full concentration of oxygen delivered to the circuit.

Chest or External Cardiac Compressions

Chest compressions should be started if the heart rate < 60 beats/min but only if there has been adequate lung inflation. During chest compressions, the relaxation phase is very important because this is the period during which blood can flow into the heart. The inspiratory breath should start only after the compression.

There are two techniques:

- The chest is encircled with both hands so that the fingers lie behind the baby and the thumbs are opposed over the sternum (Fig. 80-5A), or:
- Two fingers are used over the sternum (see Fig. 80-5B).

The thumbs or fingers should be positioned 1 cm below the internipple line. They should be compressed to a depth of 1.5–2 cm at a rate of 120 beats/min and a ratio of three compressions to one ventilation. The quality of the compressions is vital, and the rate and ratio are less important. External cardiac compressions should continue until the heart rate > 60 beats/min and increasing.

In the infant receiving IPPV whose heart rate continues to fall, the most likely cause is inadequate ventilation.

IPPV, intermittent positive-pressure ventilation.

- The parents have had the opportunity to see the baby and had an explanation of why the baby needs to be admitted to the NICU.
- The baby has a stable airway and is breathing satisfactorily. For babies needing respiratory support, this will generally mean that the baby will require intubation but transfer using CPAP may also be possible.

A baby should never be moved while the airway is being managed with a mask.

SOME OTHER NEONATAL PROBLEMS AFFECTING RESUSCITATION

Several neonatal problems require special mention because the approach to resuscitation may be different, particularly when the diagnosis is made prenatally.

Congenital Diaphragmatic Hernia (See also Chapter 19)

In babies in whom a diagnosis of congenital diaphragmatic hernia is made prenatally, the approach to resuscitation needs to be adapted. Bag-and-mask ventilation is contraindicated because this will inflate the stomach and bowel and potentially cause more mediastinal shift and lung compression. Because of this, the approach to resuscitation should include the following:

- Ensuring an experienced team is available for resuscitation.
- Intubating the baby immediately with no mask ventilation.
- Inserting a large-bore nasopgastric tube to decompress the stomach and bowel.

TABLE 80–7
Procedure for Umbilical Venous Catheterization

Equipment
Alcohol swabs
Umbilical tape
Scalpel
5-mL syringe containing 0.9% saline
Size 5 or 6 UVC
Three-way tap

Procedure
Attach the syringe and three-way tap to the catheter.
Flush the catheter with saline.
Loosely tie the umbilical tape around the cord.
Clean the cord with the alcohol swab.
Cut the cord to a length of 1–3 cm.
Identify the umbilical vein and insert catheter. Advance to approximately 5–6 cm. Confirm that blood can be easily aspirated.
If the UVC fails to advance, apply traction to the cord.
Tighten umbilical tape to secure the catheter.

UVC, umbilical vein catheter.

- Considering early muscle relaxation to prevent breathing and swallowing of air.

Airway Problems

In situations in which potential fetal airway problems are identified, special consideration should be given to how this is managed and to ensuring that individuals with the skills to manage complex airways are available at the delivery. Examples include Pierre Robin sequence, cystic hygroma, or cervical teratoma.

Pierre Robin sequence can usually be managed using airway positioning and/or a nasopharyngeal airway. Intubation in these babies can sometimes be impossible, so this can be a serious problem if they deliver prematurely. In these circumstances, careful use of a nasopharyngeal airway can often be helpful.

Occasionally, airway obstruction may be so severe that there is no prospect of establishing normal respiration without a surgical airway. In these circumstances, the "Exit" procedure has been described[46] in which babies have a surgical airway created after delivery of the head and neck but before clamping the umbilical cord. This technique should be carried out only where specific ear, nose, and throat and airway expertise exist and can be used only when the problem has been identified prenatally.

FIGURE 80–5
A and *B*, Alternative pressure points for chest compressions.

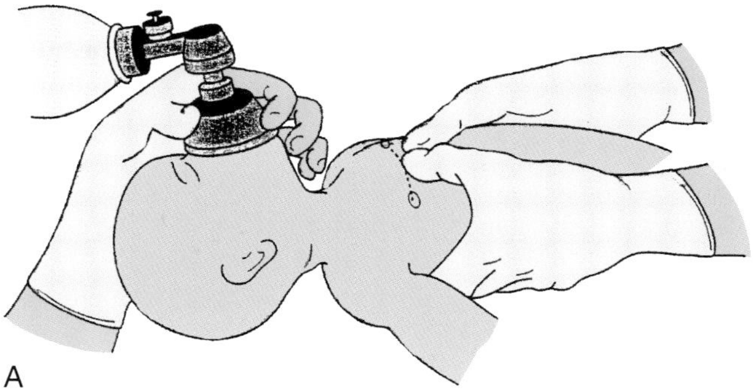

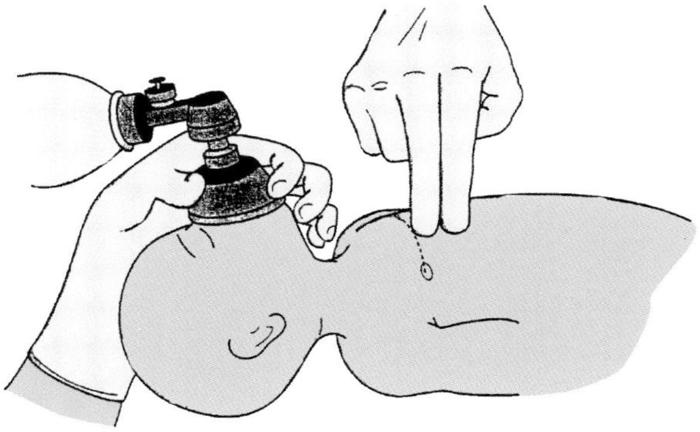

Fetal Hydrops (See also Chapter 24)

Babies with fetal hydrops may present particular difficulties during resuscitation that require immediate intervention. In particular, large pleural effusions may need to be drained before the chest can be expanded. This can be achieved using needle aspiration, but there may be associated lung hypoplasia that makes resuscitation difficult. In babies in whom hydrops associated with large pleural effusions are suspected, an experienced resuscitator should be present and equipment for emergency aspiration of the chest should be available.

SUMMARY OF MANAGEMENT OPTIONS
Neonatal Resuscitation (Obstetric Perspective)

Management Options	Evidence Quality and Recommendation	References
General and Organizational Issues		
Planning		
Wherever babies are delivered, someone capable of initiating expert resuscitation must be present.	IV/C	1–3

SUMMARY OF MANAGEMENT OPTIONS
Neonatal Resuscitation (Obstetric Perspective)—cont'd

Management Options	Evidence Quality and Recommendation	References
Training		
Midwives and obstetricians must be able to institute effective neonatal resuscitation because neonatal staff might not be immediately available at every delivery.	—/GPP	—
Training should be according to a standardized approach using recognized courses when available.	—/GPP	—
Resources	IV/C	4,30
Service requirements:		
• Training of all professionals involved in delivery room care.		
• Written protocols and lines of communication.		
• Published list of available individuals who are on call for resuscitation.		
• Resuscitation equipment available and working.		
• Delivery room temperature at least 75°F (24°C) and no drafts.		
Need for Staff Experienced in Neonatal Resuscitation		
Factors Related to Labor and Delivery		
Cesarean section.	III/B	1
Breech delivery or other malpresentation.	III/B	1
Forceps or ventouse delivery (not “lift-outs”).	III/B	1
Delivery after significant antepartum hemorrhage.	III/B	1
Prolapsed cord.	III/B	1
Maternal Factors		
Maternal medical disorder that may affect the fetus.	—/GPP	—
Current maternal drug or alcohol abuse.	IIa/B	47
Delivery under heavy sedation or general anesthesia.	Ia,III/A,B	48–50
Fever.	IIa/B	27
Fetal Factors		
Multiple pregnancy (one resuscitator for each infant).	III/B	4
Preterm delivery (<37 wk).	IIa/B	51
Prolonged membrane rupture or suspected chorioamnionitis.	—/GPP	—
Hydramnios.	—/GPP	—
Fetal distress.	III/B	1
Known or suspected fetal abnormality.	—/GPP	—
Isoimmunization	IV/C	52
Management Options		
Preparation		
Introduce yourself.	—/GPP	—
Obtain a relevant history.	—/GPP	—
Check the equipment and turn on the heater.	—/GPP	—
Management		
Thermal control for term babies: Dry and wrap infant, and then follow ABCD as described below.	III/B	13,53

Management Options	Evidence Quality and Recommendation	References
Airway	IV/C	4,54
• Meconium-stained liquor: Do not suction on the perineum or in vigorous infants.	Ia/A	23
• Perform tracheal suction only when indicated.	Ib,III,IV/A,B,C	23,54,59
Breathing: Mask ventilation.	IIb,IV/B,C	4,55,56
• There is no difference in resuscitation between room air and 100% oxygen.	Ib/A	26
Chest compressions:	IV/C	51
• Consider drugs if the heart rate remains low despite effective ventilation.		
Drugs:	IV/C	51
• Consider epinephrine IV when the heart rate remains low despite effective ventilation and cardiac compressions.		
• Consider naloxone to reverse the possible opioid effects on respiratory efforts.	Ib/A	57
Preterm		
• Giving surfactant early decreases mortality.	Ia/A	41
• Using positive end-expiratory pressure during resuscitation may decrease lung injury.	Ib/B	58
• Plastic wrapping improves admission temperature, but warming mattresses are of no further benefit.	Ia,Ib/A	38–40

GPP, good practice point.

SUGGESTED READINGS

Dawes G (ed): Fetal and Neonatal Physiology. Chicago, Year Book, 1968, pp 141–159.

International Liaison Committee on Resuscitation: The International Liaison Committee on Resuscitation (ILCOR) consensus on science with treatment recommendations for pediatric and neonatal patients: Pediatric basic and advanced life support. Pediatrics 2006;117:e955–e977.

MacIntosh M (ed): Project 27/28: An Enquiry into Quality of Care and Its Effect on the Survival of Babies Born at 27–28 Weeks. London, TSO, 2003.

Nuffield Council on Bioethics: Critical Care Decisions in Fetal and Neonatal Medicine: Ethical Issues. London, Nuffield Council on Bioethics, 2006. Available at www.nuffieldbioethics.org

Richmond S (ed): Newborn Life Support, 2nd ed. London, Resuscitation Council (UK), 2004.

Sweet D, Bevilacqua G, Carnielli V, et al: European consensus guidelines on the management of neonatal respiratory distress syndrome. J Perinat Med 2007;35:175–186.

Tan A, Schulze A, O'Donnell CPF, Davis PG: Air versus oxygen for resuscitation of babies at birth. Cochrane Database Syst Rev 2005;2:CD002273.

Wilkinson AR, Ahluwalia J, Cole A, et al: Management of babies born extremely preterm at less than 26 weeks of gestation: A framework for clinical practice at the time of birth. Arch Dis Child Fetal Neonatal Ed 2009;94:2–5.

REFERENCES

For a complete list of references, log onto www.expertconsult.com.

Normal Values

MARGARET RAMSAY

INTRODUCTION

What Is a "Normal" Value?

"Normal" has different meanings. In the context of physical or laboratory measurements, "normal" may mean "average," "disease-free," or "within a given statistical range." However, it is important to know the characteristics of the population yielding "normal" values before deciding whether these values provide an appropriate reference range with which to compare an individual test result. Many laboratories now print reference ranges on their reports and highlight test values that fall outside these values as "abnormal." When the test subject is a pregnant woman, a fetus, or a newborn, and the reference population is composed predominantly of middle-aged men, then comparisons are patently inappropriate. It is important to understand how the physiologic changes of pregnancy affect the results of various tests and measurements before deciding whether an out-of-range result is actually abnormal.

Changes in Pregnancy

Pregnancy results in profound changes in maternal physiology and metabolism, orchestrated by hormonal changes. Thus, physical and laboratory measurements may be very different in the pregnant state compared with the nonpregnant state and may change as pregnancy advances. Similarly, physical, biochemical, hormonal, and hematologic measurements of the fetus change markedly as the fetus increases in size and maturity. Thanks to ultrasound techniques, the fetus, once hidden within the uterus, is now accessible. Fetal structures can be measured, fetal behavior observed, and blood velocity measured with Doppler ultrasound, and a sampling needle can be used to access blood, liquor, urine, and placental and other tissues.

Statistical Terms

The terms used to define normal values depend on the distribution characteristics of data points. The entire range of values encountered in a healthy population may be quoted as reference points, or distribution may be described by terms that express central tendency and scatter. When data are distributed symmetrically around a central value (i.e., normal distribution), mean, standard deviation (SD), and standard error of the mean (SEM) are the appropriate statistics. From these, ranking values, or percentiles, may be calculated (e.g., 5th and 95th percentiles, which encompass the central 90% of data points, with 5% on either side of them). When the data distribution is skewed, median and percentiles should be used. When the data distribution is exponential, median and multiples of the median (MoM) can be used rather than percentiles. Specialized texts provide a more detailed critical appraisal of the statistical analyses used in these studies (Altman, 1991).

Study Methods Used to Derive Normal Values during Pregnancy

Two basic designs are used for studies addressing changes in physical or laboratory values during pregnancy.

1. **Longitudinal studies** follow a group of women sequentially through pregnancy and compare measurements of a particular parameter with those obtained well before or at an interval after the pregnancy. Because these studies are very labor-intensive and require committed research subjects, they usually do not involve large numbers of subjects. They are very effective at showing changes with time, either between the nonpregnant and the pregnant states or with advancing gestation. The variability of the data is small because the same subjects are studied sequentially. These studies are very helpful in showing how pregnancy affects measurement of a particular parameter. This benefit has particular relevance when prepregnancy values are known and the effect of pregnancy must be differentiated from disease-related changes over time. A limitation of longitudinal studies is that a narrow range of "normal" values is defined from a small number of subjects. This narrow range may not correspond to the wider range of values found in a larger group of healthy subjects studied on a single occasion.
2. **Cross-sectional studies** involve large numbers of subjects, each contributing one data point to the study. If the number of study subjects is large enough, then the findings provide a good idea of the true scatter of data points. These studies allow accurate characterization of mean values, SDs, and percentiles. For pregnancy studies, subjects must be evenly distributed throughout gestation and values must not be extrapolated beyond the gestational range actually included. These studies are essential when the ranking of a particular measurement must be determined (e.g., fetal ultrasonic measurement of abdominal circumference for a known gestational age). Most studies of fetal ultrasonic measurements and Doppler waveform indices are of this design, and their statistical methods have been described in detail (Altman and Chitty, 1994).

Opportunistic studies are also used. For example, fetal blood sampling may be done to identify infection or karyotype in a fetus unaffected by the condition. The portion of the blood sample that is not used for specific tests can be used to measure other substances. Much information available about fetal hematologic, biochemical, and endocrine function has been collected in this way. There are obvious ethical concerns about planning studies in normal fetuses requiring invasive sampling because of the risks of fetal injury and loss. However, the selection of fetuses for study after exclusion of a particular problem means that they are not truly normal or representative of the entire fetal population. Opportunistic studies do not cover the entire range of gestational ages. Nevertheless, they provide information that would not be known otherwise.

The pregnancy studies in the literature are of mixed quality in terms of numbers of subjects included, selection criteria for subjects, sampling and laboratory techniques, and statistical interpretation. The best studies found are reported here. The methods used for each study included are described briefly and presented alongside the results. Comment sections provide interpretation of the data or a discussion of the robustness of the statistical methods, and references to the original papers are given for readers who wish to explore in greater detail. Few studies address the possible effect of maternal age, gravidity, or ethnic differences on the parameters under study. Data on many normal ranges are deficient or limited and are occasionally unreliable.

Use of Normal Ranges in Pregnancy

Some disease states are diagnosed from characteristic symptoms or signs, but others have agreed biochemical definitions. For example, diabetes mellitus is diagnosed with references to fasting blood glucose measurements and those after a known glucose challenge (see Fig. 25). These values represent the upper limits of the normal ranges found in studies of healthy subjects. Differences in blood glucose values in pregnancy led to the suggestion that diagnostic criteria for diabetes should be adjusted in pregnancy.

Disease or organ dysfunction does not always occur at a given value of a physical or laboratory measurement outside its derived normal range. Elevated liver enzyme levels indicative of liver cell dysfunction may be 2, 10, or 50 times the normal values. However, even minimal deviation of pH from its closely clustered normal values may be biologically important.

Another use of normal values is to calculate odds ratios. Assessment of the risk or likelihood of genetic abnormalities (e.g., Down syndrome) is possible from measurement of serum α-fetoprotein, chorionic gonadotropin, or placental protein A (see Figs. 45–47). Measured values of these hormones are compared with expected values at known gestational age (derived from healthy pregnancies). The degree of difference is expressed in terms of multiples of the median values. Absolute values cannot be used for mathematical calculations because these hormonal concentrations change with gestation. For each hormone, multiple regression analysis has shown the relationships between deviations in values and the risk of Down syndrome. Thus, a woman's age-related risk of aneuploidy may be adjusted after measurement of serum hormones (Wald et al, 1996).

Units of Measurement

When possible, both SI (Système International d'Unités) and traditional units are given for ease of interpretation. It is important to check the units of measurement carefully when comparing a physical or laboratory value with a normal range. In SI units, grams (g) and liters (L) are used, whereas traditional units commonly use milligrams (mg) and deciliters (dL). To avoid errors of interpretation, the prefixes d-, m-, μ-, and n-, signifying 10^{-1}, 10^{-3}, 10^{-6}, and 10^{-9} must be observed and used with care.

The terminology milliequivalents (mEq) has not been used because it has been superseded by millimoles (mmol). For monovalent ions (Na^+, K^+, Cl^-), 1 mmol = 1 mEq. For divalent ions (Mg^{2+}, Ca^{2+}, PO_4^{2+}, SO_4^{2-}), 1 mmol = 2 mEq.

FURTHER READING

Altman DG: Practical Statistics for Medical Research. London, Chapman and Hall, 1991.

Altman DG, Chitty LS: Charts of fetal size: 1. Methodology. Br J Obstet Gynaecol 1994;101:29–34.

Wald NJ, George L, Smith D, et al: Serum screening for Down's syndrome between 8 and 14 weeks of pregnancy. Br J Obstet Gynaecol 1996;103:407–412.

MATERNAL VALUES

Physiology

Nutrition

WEIGHT GAIN

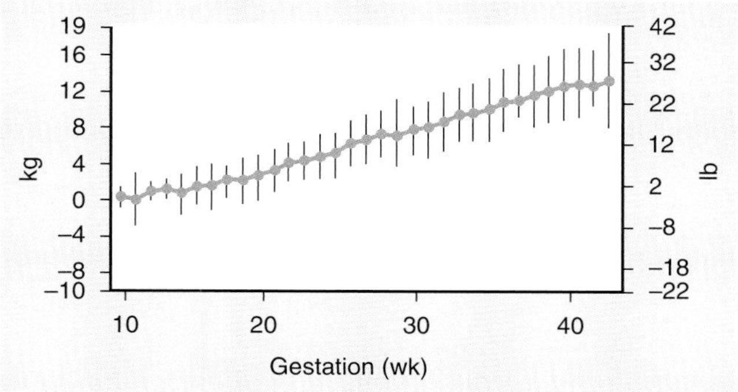

FIGURE 1
Longitudinal study of maternal weight gain (mean ± SD) in 988 normal women who had uneventful pregnancies. All of the study subjects underwent initial evaluation at less than 20 weeks' gestation and were delivered between 37 and 41 weeks. *Data source*: ref. 1, with permission.

Weight-for-height category	Recommended total weight gain	
	kg	lb
Low (BMI <19.8)	12.5–18	28–40
Normal (BMI 19.8–26.0)	11.5–16	25–35
High (BMI 26.0–29.0)	7–11.5	15–25
Obese (BMI >29.0)	7	15
BMI = weight/height^2		

FIGURE 2
Recommended ranges for total weight gain during pregnancy for women with a singleton gestation, classified by prepregnancy body mass index (BMI). *Data source*: ref. 2, with permission.

Comment: Average total weight gain during pregnancy is approximately 10 kg. Low weight gain during pregnancy in nonobese women has been associated with delivery of small–for–gestational age (SGA) infants.[3] Overweight and obese mothers have increased complications including gestational diabetes, hypertension, large–for–gestational age infants, and difficult deliveries.[4] More women are entering pregnancy with high BMI, and there is evidence that they gain excessive weight during pregnancy and retain it after delivery.[4,5]

NUTRITIONAL REQUIREMENTS

Nutritional requirements		
Nutrient (unit)	Pregnant	Lactating
Energy (kcal)	+300	+500
Protein (g)	60	65
Fat-soluable vitamins		
Vitamin A (μg retinol equivalents)	800	1300
Vitamin D (μg as cholecalciferol)	10	10
Vitamin E (mg α-tocopherol equivalents)	10	12
Vitamin K (μg)	65	65
Water-soluble vitamins		
Vitamin C (mg)	70	95
Thiamin (mg)	1.5	1.6
Riboflavin (mg)	1.6	1.8
Niacin (mg niacin equivalent)	17	20
Vitamin B_6 (mg)	2.2	2.1
Folate (μg)	400	280
Vitamin B_{12} (μg)	2.2	2.6
Minerals		
Calcium (mg)	1200	1200
Phosphorous (mg)	1200	1200
Magnesium (mg)	300	355
Iron (mg)	30	15
Zinc (mg)	15	19
Iodine (μg)	175	200
Selenium (μg)	65	75

FIGURE 3
Recommended daily dietary allowance and energy intake for pregnant and lactating women. These should be used as a guide to nutritional requirements when formulating a balanced diet. *Data source*: ref. 6, with permission.

Comment: The increased requirements for vitamins and minerals during pregnancy can usually be met through the diet. Therefore, routine supplementation with multivitamin preparations is not necessary. However, periconceptual supplementation with folic acid for all women is now advocated in an attempt to reduce the incidence of neural tube defects. Vitamin supplementation should be considered in women with inadequate standard diets, heavy smokers, those who abuse drugs or alcohol, and those with multiple pregnancies. Excessive intake (i.e., more than twice the recommended daily allowance) of fat- or water-soluble vitamins may have toxic effects.

Cardiovascular Function

BLOOD PRESSURE

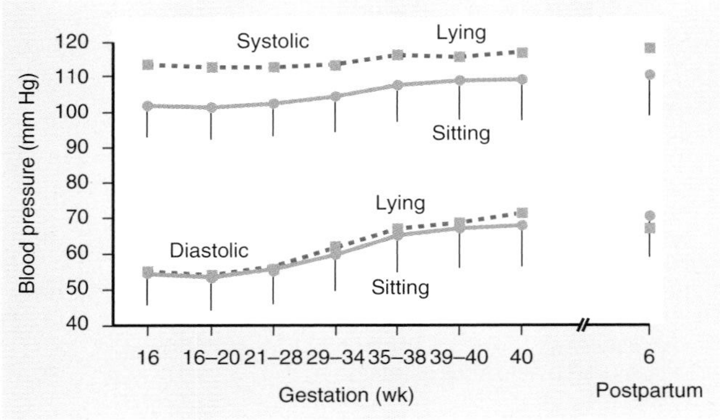

FIGURE 4
Blood pressure measurements (mean + SD) from a longitudinal study of 226 primigravidae whose first attendance at the antenatal clinic was before 20 weeks' gestation. Their mean age was 24.3 years (SD 4.9). Blood pressure measurements were taken with the London School of Hygiene sphygmomanometer to avoid terminal digit preference and observer bias. Diastolic pressures were recorded at the point of muffling (phase 4). *Data source*: ref. 7, with permission.

Comment: Systolic pressure changes little during pregnancy, but diastolic pressure decreases markedly toward midpregnancy, then rises to near nonpregnant levels by term. Thus, widening of pulse pressure occurs for most of pregnancy.

PULSE RATE

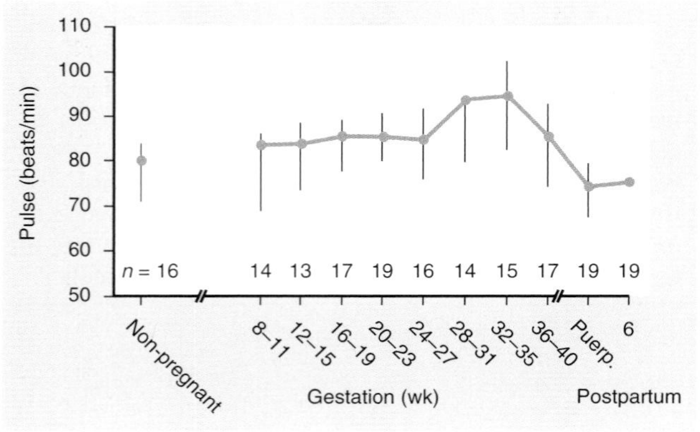

FIGURE 5
Pulse rate (median and interquartile ranges) from a longitudinal study of 20 healthy women recruited in early pregnancy and studied every 2 weeks thereafter. "Nonpregnant" measurements were made 8 to 12 months after delivery. All women finished the study, but not all participated in every visit. *Data source*: ref. 8, with permission.

Comment: The typical increase in heart rate during pregnancy is approximately 15 beats/min, beginning as early as 4 weeks after the last menstrual period.[9]

CARDIAC OUTPUT

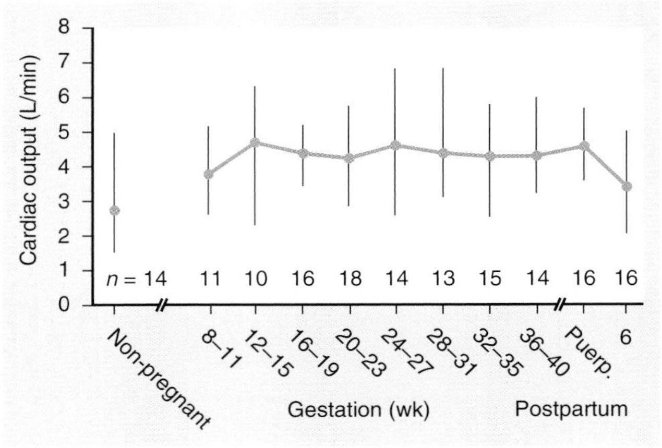

FIGURE 6
Cardiac output (median and interquartile ranges) from a longitudinal study of 20 healthy women recruited in early pregnancy and studied every 2 weeks thereafter. "Nonpregnant" measurements were made 8 to 12 months after delivery. All women finished the study, but not all participated in every visit. Cardiac output was measured by an indirect Fick method. *Data source*: ref. 8, with permission.

Comment: Cardiac output increases significantly during the first trimester and remains elevated until the puerperium. When changes in body weight are considered, it is apparent that cardiac output reaches maximal values at 12 to 15 weeks' gestation and then declines gradually toward term.

INVASIVE MONITORING

Invasive monitoring		
	Non-pregnant	Pregnant
Cardiac output (L/min)	4.3 ± 0.9	6.2 ± 1.0
Heart rate (beats/min)	71 ± 10	83 ± 10
Systemic vascular resistance (dyne/sec/cm^5)	1530 ± 520	1210 ± 266
Pulmonary vascular resistance (dyne/sec/cm^5)	119 ± 47	78 ± 22
Colloid oncotic pressure (mm Hg)	20.8 ± 1.0	18.0 ± 1.5
Colloid oncotic pressure—pulmonary capillary wedge pressure (mm Hg)	14.5 ± 2.5	10.5 ± 2.7
Mean arterial pressure (mm Hg)	86.4 ± 7.5	90.3 ± 5.8
Pulmonary capillary wedge pressure (mm Hg)	6.3 ± 2.1	7.5 ± 1.8
Central venous pressure (mm Hg)	3.7 ± 2.6	3.6 ± 2.5
Left ventricular stroke work index (g/min/m^2)	41 ± 8	48 ± 6

FIGURE 7
Findings of a study involving 10 healthy, primigravid women with a singleton pregnancy who were examined at 36 to 38 weeks' gestation and again 11 to 13 weeks postpartum. All women were younger than 26 years old. They did not smoke and were not anemic. Fetal anatomy and growth and amniotic fluid volume were normal. A pulmonary artery catheter was placed through the subclavian vein, and baseline hemodynamic assessment was made in the left lateral position after 30 minutes' rest. Cardiac output was measured with a thermodilution technique. For each subject, the result represented the mean of five independent measurements, with the highest and lowest values excluded. Central pressures were measured over three consecutive respiratory cycles. Results quoted are mean ± SD. *Data source*: ref. 10, with permission.

Comment: Systemic vascular resistance is 21% lower and pulmonary resistance is 34% lower in the late third trimester than in the nonpregnant state. Both colloid oncotic pressure and the colloid oncotic–pulmonary capillary wedge pressure gradient are lower (by 14% and 28%, respectively). Mean arterial pressure, central venous pressure, pulmonary capillary wedge pressure, and left ventricular stroke work index show no significant changes in the third trimester. These results indicate that the systemic and pulmonary vascular beds accommodate higher vascular volumes at normal pressures during pregnancy. The ventricles are dilated, and cardiac contractility does not change significantly. Because the colloid oncotic pressure–pulmonary capillary wedge pressure gradient is reduced in pregnancy, an increase in cardiac preload or an alteration in pulmonary capillary permeability predisposes the patient to pulmonary edema.

Pulmonary Function and Respiration

ARTERIAL BLOOD GASES

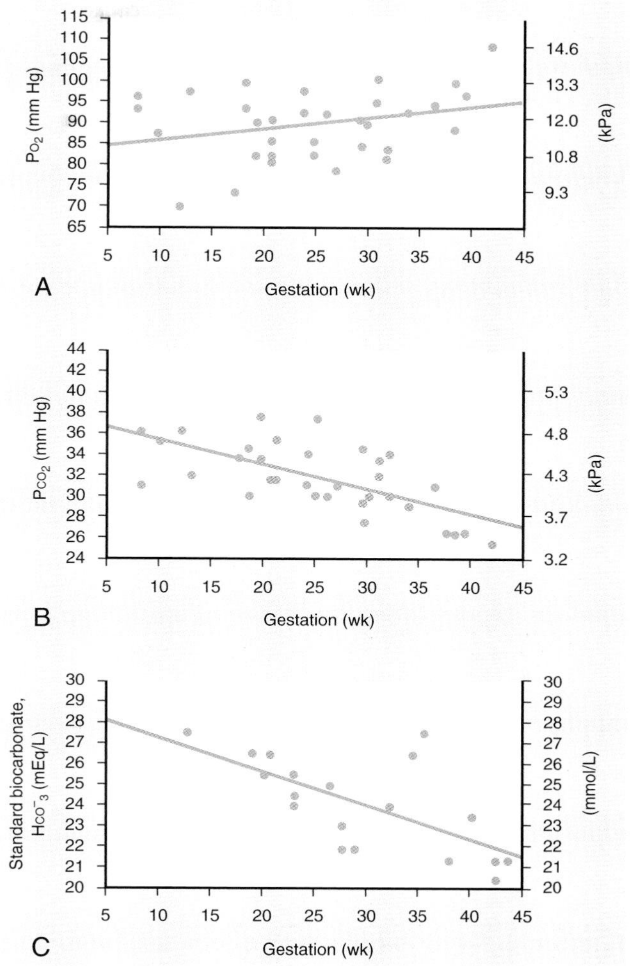

FIGURE 8
Arterial blood gas pressures: Oxygen (Po_2) (*A*), carbon dioxide (Pco_2) (*B*), and standard bicarbonate (*C*) (individual values, with regression lines shown) from a cross-sectional study of 37 women at 8 to 42 weeks' gestation. Blood sampling was done from a cannula inserted into the brachial artery under local anesthesia, after 30 minutes' rest in a quiet, darkened room. *Data source*: ref. 11, with permission of Elsevier Science NL, Amsterdam, The Netherlands.

Comment: Arterial pH was constant (7.47) during pregnancy in this study. PCO_2 and standard bicarbonate levels showed a significant decrease with advancing gestation, but PO_2 levels did not change significantly.

TRANSCUTANEOUS GASES

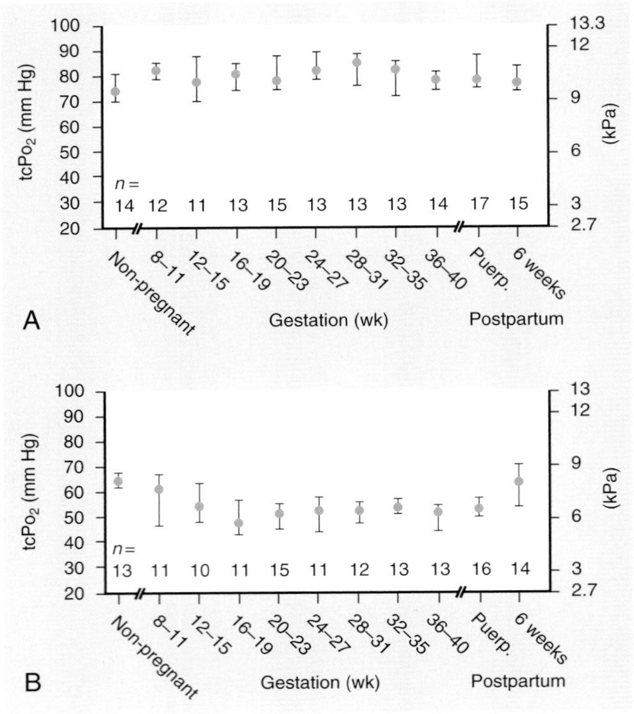

FIGURE 9
Transcutaneous oxygen ($tcPo_2$) (*A*) and carbon dioxide ($tcPco_2$) (*B*) pressures (median and interquartile ranges) from a longitudinal study of 20 healthy women recruited in early pregnancy and studied every 2 weeks thereafter. Nonpregnant measurements were made 8 to 12 months after delivery. All women finished the study, but not all participated in every visit. *Data source*: ref. 8, with permission.

> **Comment:** $tcPCO_2$ is higher than arterial PCO_2 as a result of temperature differences between the skin surface and the blood as well as the addition of CO_2 by skin metabolism (conversion factor ~1.4).[8] $tcPO_2$ values in adults are 10% to 20% lower than arterial PO_2 values. In this study, the increase in $tcPO_2$ and the decrease in $tcPCO_2$ during pregnancy were significant.

RESPIRATION RATE

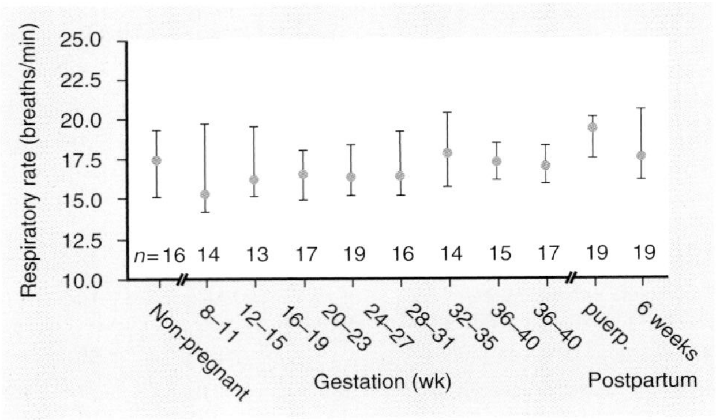

FIGURE 10
Respiration rate (median and interquartile ranges) from a longitudinal study of 20 healthy women recruited in early pregnancy and studied every 2 weeks thereafter. Nonpregnant measurements were made 8 to 12 months after delivery. All women finished the study, but not all participated in every visit. *Data source*: ref. 8, with permission.

> **Comment:** The respiration rate is similar in pregnant and nonpregnant women.

TIDAL VOLUME

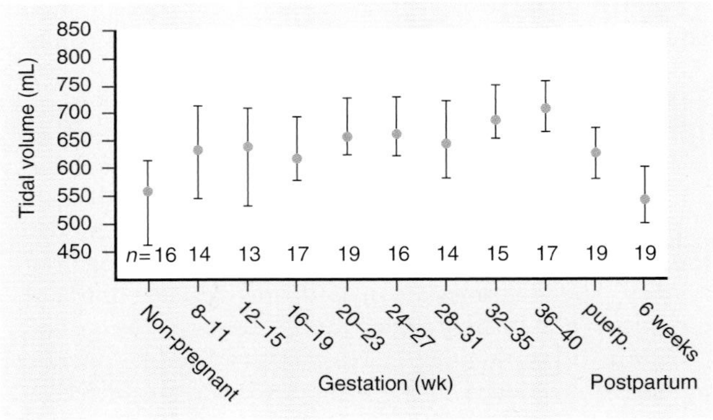

FIGURE 11
Tidal volume (median and interquartile ranges) from a longitudinal study of 20 healthy women recruited in early pregnancy and studied every 2 weeks thereafter. Nonpregnant measurements were made 8 to 12 months after delivery. All women finished the study, but not all participated in every visit. *Data source*: ref. 8, with permission.

> **Comment:** Tidal volume increases early in pregnancy and continues to rise until term. Overall, a 30% to 40% rise occurs. By 6 to 8 weeks postpartum, tidal volumes return to nonpregnant values. Minute ventilation increases in parallel with tidal volume; typical values are 7.5 L/min in nonpregnant women and 10.5 L/min in late pregnancy.[12]

RESPIRATORY FUNCTION TESTS

Respiratory function tests				
	During pregnancy			After delivery
	10 weeks	24 weeks	36 weeks	10 weeks postpartum
Vital capacity (L)	3.8	3.9	4.1	3.8
Inspiratory capacity (L)	2.6	2.7	2.9	2.5
Expiratory reserve volume (L)	1.2	1.2	1.2	1.3
Residual volume (L)	1.2	1.1	1.0	1.2

FIGURE 12
Respiratory volumes (mean values) from a longitudinal study of eight healthy women 18 to 29 years old who were studied through pregnancy and again at 10 weeks postpartum. All tests were done with the patient in the sitting position. *Data source*: ref. 12, with permission.

Comment: In some women, vital capacity increases by 100 to 200 mL during pregnancy, but the converse is seen in obese women.[1] Anatomic changes (flaring of the lower ribs, a rise in the diaphragm, and an increase in the transverse diameter of the chest) are responsible for alterations in lung volume subdivisions.[13] Forced expiratory volume in 1 second (FEV_1) and peak expiratory flow rate (PEFR) are unaffected by normal pregnancy.[12] The gas transfer factor (i.e., pulmonary diffusing capacity with CO_2) decreases in pregnancy.[12] This decrease has been attributed to altered mucopolysaccharides in the alveolar capillary walls as well as lower circulating levels of hemoglobin.

Chromosomal Abnormalities

Maternal age at delivery (years)	Risk of Down's syndrome
15	1 : 1578
20	1 : 1528
25	1 : 1351
30	1 : 909
31	1 : 796
32	1 : 683
33	1 : 574
34	1 : 474
35	1 : 384
36	1 : 307
37	1 : 242
38	1 : 189
39	1 : 146
40	1 : 112
41	1 : 85
42	1 : 65
43	1 : 49
44	1 : 37
45	1 : 28
46	1 : 21
47	1 : 15
48	1 : 11
49	1 : 8
50	1 : 6

FIGURE 13
The risk of having a pregnancy affected by Down syndrome according to maternal age at the time of birth. *Data source*: ref. 14, with permission.

Rate per 1000					
Maternal age	Trisomy 21	Trisomy 18	Trisomy 13	XXY	All chromosomal anomalies
35	3.9	0.5	0.2	0.5	8.7
36	5.0	0.7	0.3	0.6	10.1
37	6.4	1.0	0.4	0.8	12.2
38	8.1	1.4	0.5	1.1	14.8
39	10.4	2.0	0.8	1.4	18.4
40	13.3	2.8	1.1	1.8	23.0
41	16.9	3.9	1.5	2.4	29.0
42	21.6	5.5	2.1	3.1	37.0
43	27.4	7.6		4.1	45.0
44	34.8			5.4	50.0
45	44.2			7.0	62.0
46	55.9			9.1	77.0
47	70.4			11.9	96.0

FIGURE 14
Chromosomal abnormalities by maternal age at the time of amniocentesis performed at 16 weeks' gestation (expressed as rate per 1000). *Data source*: ref. 15, with permission.

Comment: The incidence of chromosomal disorders increases with maternal age but is not affected by paternal age.[15] The prevalence of aneuploidy is higher at earlier gestations. Trisomy 21 (Down syndrome) is the most important numerically of these disorders, with an overall population incidence of 1 in 650 live births. Trisomies 13, 18, and 22 are rare in live births (see Chapter 4, Figure 4–7). Other autosomal trisomies are nonviable and are common in spontaneous abortions.

Biochemistry

Hepatic Function

TOTAL SERUM PROTEIN AND ALBUMIN

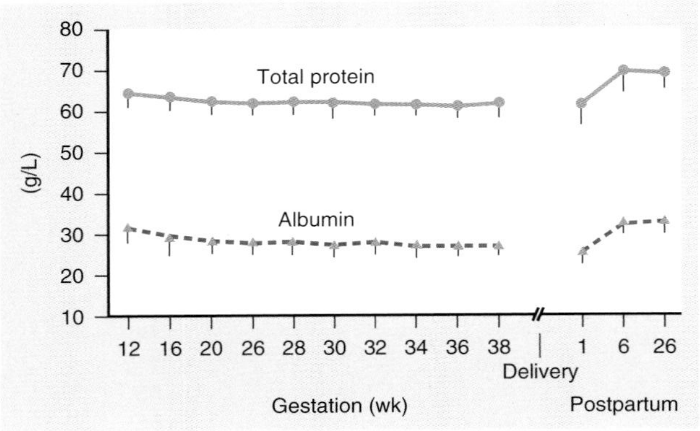

FIGURE 15
Total serum protein and albumin (mean + SD) from a longitudinal study of 83 healthy pregnant women (77 of whom were primigravidae) who were recruited at 12 weeks' gestation. Samples were collected every 4 weeks during pregnancy, 7 days postpartum, and again at 6 and 26 weeks postpartum. *Data source*: ref. 16, with permission.

> **Comment:** Decreased total serum protein and albumin concentrations in pregnancy are associated with a decrease in colloid osmotic pressure.[16] Serum immunoglobulin levels change in pregnancy; there is slight decrease in immunoglobulin A (IgA), decreased IgG especially in the third trimester, and increased IgM, especially prior to delivery.[17]

LIVER ENZYMES, SERUM BILE ACIDS, BILIRUBIN, AMYLASE, COPPER, AND ZINC

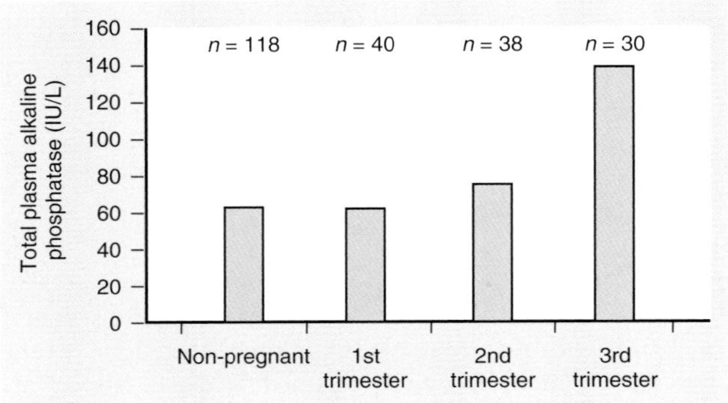

FIGURE 16
Total alkaline phosphatase levels (mean and SEM) from a cross-sectional study of 108 women attending a hospital antenatal clinic in Nigeria. The nonpregnant control subjects of similar age were patients attending the gynecologic clinic. No patients were clinically anemic, and all were normotensive. *Data source*: ref. 18, with permission.

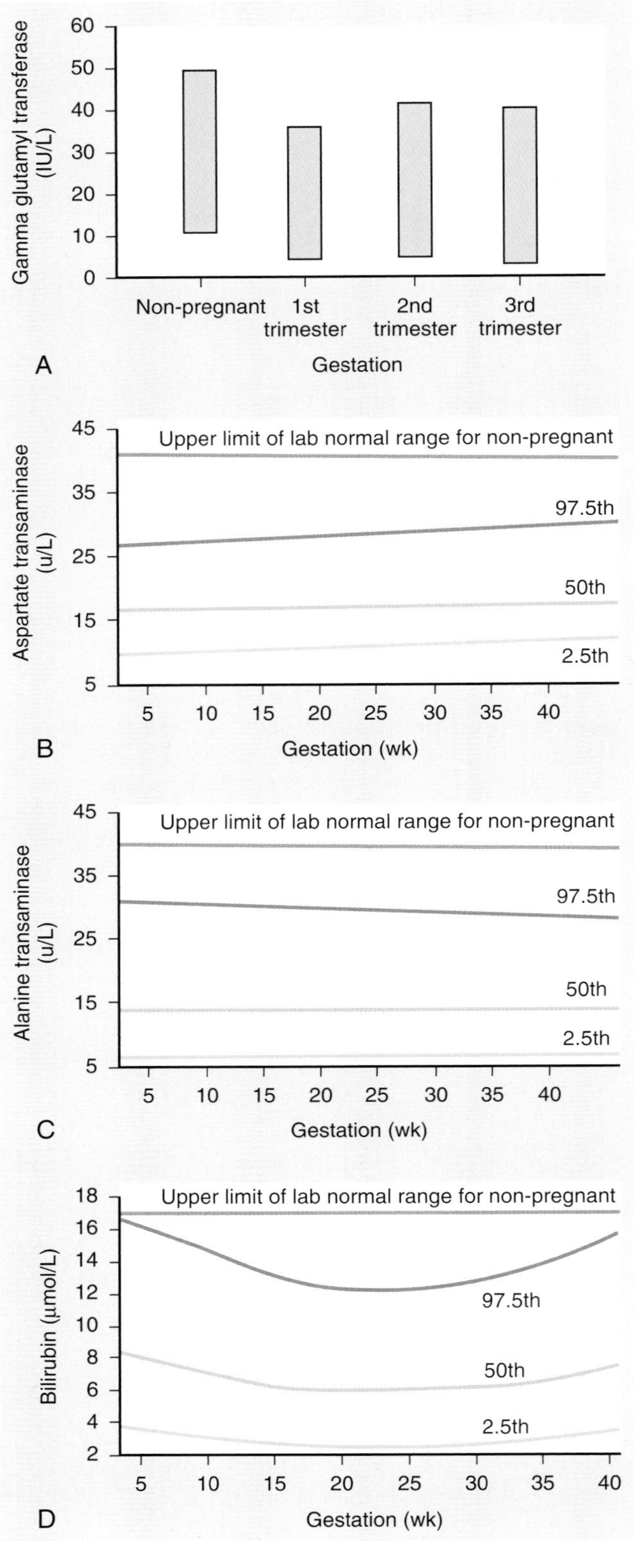

FIGURE 17
Serum γ-glutamyl transferase (GGT) (*A*), aspartate transaminase (AST) (*B*), alanine transaminase (ALT) (*C*), and bilirubin (*D*) (95% reference ranges) from a cross-sectional study of 430 women with uncomplicated singleton pregnancies. No subjects had hypertension or liver disease, were taking drugs associated with liver dysfunction, or were consuming more than 10 units of alcohol weekly. Data for GGT were not normally distributed, and the results presented are calculated from the nonparametric determination of percentiles. Data for AST, ALT, and bilirubin were normally distributed after logarithmic transformation, allowing gestation-specific percentiles to be calculated. *Data source*: ref. 19, with permission.

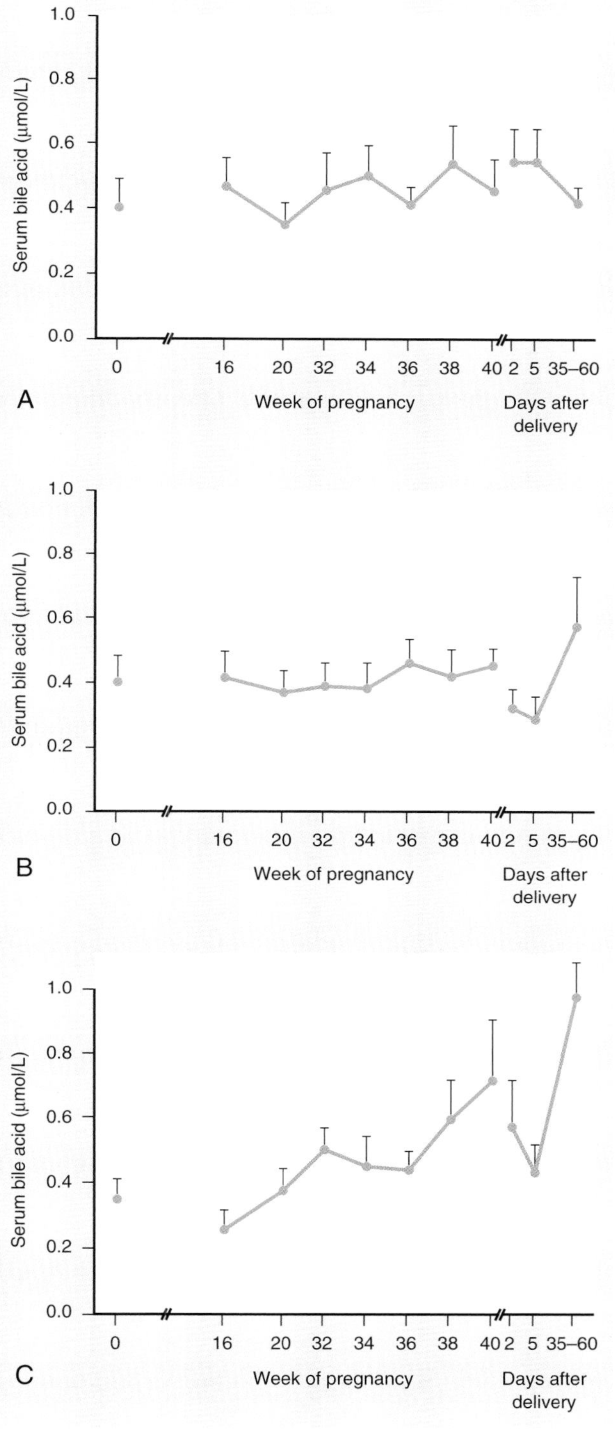

FIGURE 18

Serum cholic acid (CA) (*A*), deoxycholic acid (DCA) (*B*), and chenodeoxycholic acid (CDCA) (*C*) (mean + SD) from a longitudinal study of 30 healthy pregnant women. The subjects had uncomplicated pregnancies and no history of hepatobiliary disease. Blood samples were taken after an overnight fast. Most women were recruited at 12 to 17 weeks' gestation and gave blood samples at 18 to 22 weeks, every 2 weeks in the third trimester, and on three occasions up to 35 to 60 days after delivery. Bile acids were measured separately by radioimmunoassay, and the results presented are for total concentrations (i.e., free plus conjugated bile acid). *Data source*: ref. 20, with permission.

Comment: Other recent longitudinal studies of liver function tests[21] confirm that alkaline phosphatase (AP) levels are more than doubled by late pregnancy. Almost half of the total plasma AP in pregnancy is placental AP isoenzyme, but bone AP isoenzyme levels are also markedly increased. Liver AP isoenzyme levels do not change significantly in pregnancy.[18] Serum GGT and transaminase levels overall are lower in pregnancy than in the nonpregnant adult population. There are no significant gestational changes in GGT, AST, or ALT, but all increase after delivery, especially after cesarean section.[22] During pregnancy, bilirubin levels remain within the normal range for adults.[23] Serum concentrations of the primary bile acid, CA, and the secondary bile acid, deoxycholic acid (DCA), do not change during pregnancy, but CDCA levels increase significantly toward term.[20] These minor changes in serum bile acid levels may be caused by changes in bile acid metabolism and excretion as a result of high circulating levels of estrogen and progesterone, but may show a tendency to cholestasis in normal pregnancy. Serum amylase levels remain within normal adult reference ranges during pregnancy.[21] Serum copper levels are increased in pregnancy, but zinc levels are decreased compared with those in nonpregnant women.[24] There are considerable differences between laboratories with regard to liver enzyme assays and resultant variability in "normal ranges" in adults. These differences should be borne in mind when interpreting individual results from pregnant women.

Normal Values

LIPIDS: CHOLESTEROL AND TRIGLYCERIDE

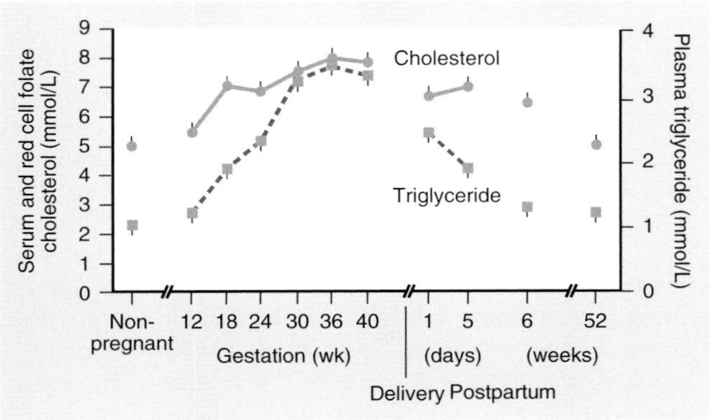

FIGURE 19
Plasma cholesterol and triglyceride levels (mean and SEM) from a longitudinal study of 43 women 20 to 41 years old. Samples were taken after an overnight fast and 10 minutes' supine rest at 4- to 6-week intervals through pregnancy, during labor, and in the puerperium. Samples were also taken 12 months after delivery in 14 of the subjects. The nonpregnant reference samples were obtained from 15 subjects of comparable age. No dietary restrictions were imposed. *Data source*: ref. 25, with permission. *Conversion factors*: cholesterol, mmol/L × 38.5 = mg/dL; triglyceride, mmol/L × 88 = mg/dL.

Comment: During pregnancy, plasma cholesterol doubles and a threefold increase in plasma triglyceride concentration occurs. The lipid content of low-density lipoproteins increases in pregnancy, as does the high-density lipoprotein triglyceride content.[25] Levels of both apolipoproteins A1 and B increase in parallel during pregnancy.[21] Serum lipid levels decrease rapidly after delivery, but cholesterol and triglyceride concentrations remain elevated 6 to 7 weeks postpartum. Lactation does not affect lipid levels.[25]

Renal Function

SERUM URATE

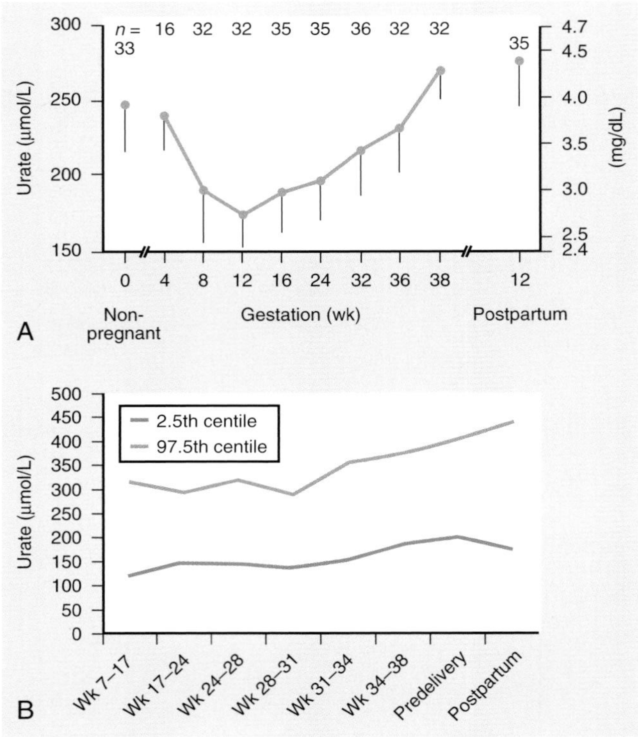

FIGURE 20
A, Serum urate levels (mean + SD) from a longitudinal study of 31 healthy women 23 to 37 years old, five of whom were studied during two pregnancies. Subjects were studied preconceptually, at least 3 months after discontinuing oral contraceptives (if used), in the luteal phase of their menstrual cycle, monthly during pregnancy, and again at 12 weeks postpartum. All samples were taken between 9:00 AM and 9:30 AM, after overnight fasting. *Data source*: ref. 24, with permission. *B*, Plasma urate (2.5th–97.5th calculated percentile reference interval) from a longitudinal study of 52 healthy women in Sweden sampled at intervals during pregnancy. At least 40 samples were obtained for each time point; predelivery samples were taken 14 to 0 days before delivery and the postpartum samples 45 to 202 days after delivery. The nonpregnant reference range for plasma urate in this population is 154 to 350 µmol/L. *Data source*: ref. 21, with permission.

Comment: Serum urate levels decrease during the first trimester, as a result of altered renal handling (increased glomerular filtration rate [GFR] and/or reduced proximal tubular resaborption) of uric acid.[26] During late pregnancy, the serum urate level increases to levels higher than nonpregnant values.[21] Levels may remain elevated for 12 weeks after delivery.[26]

SERUM OSMOLALITY

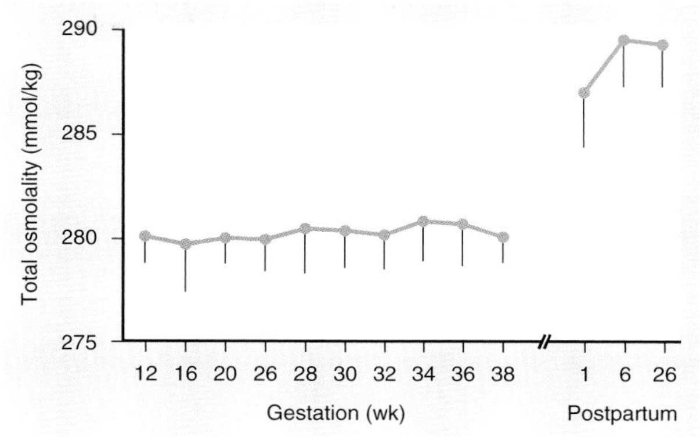

FIGURE 21
Serum osmolality (mean + SD) from a longitudinal study of 83 healthy pregnant women (77 of whom were primigravidae), recruited at 12 weeks' gestation. Samples were collected every 4 weeks during pregnancy, 7 days postpartum, and then 6 and 26 weeks postpartum. *Data source*: ref. 16, with permission.

Comment: Total osmolality decreases by the end of the first trimester to a nadir 8 to 10 mmol/kg below nonpregnant values.

PLASMA ELECTROLYTES, UREA, AND CREATININE

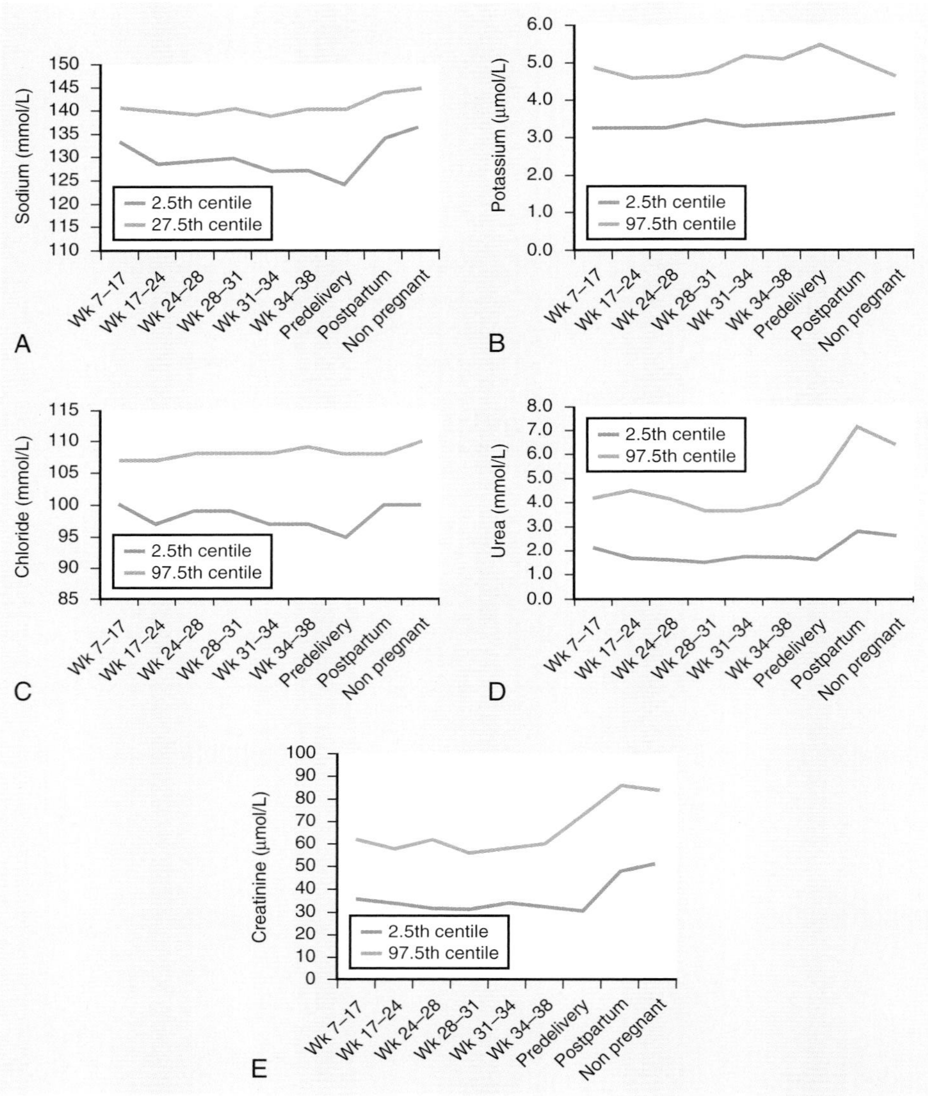

FIGURE 22
Plasma electrolytes (*A–C*), urea (*D*), and creatinine (*E*) (2.5th–97.5th calculated percentile reference interval) from a longitudinal study of 52 healthy women in Sweden sampled at intervals during pregnancy. At least 40 samples were obtained for each time point; predelivery samples were taken 14 to 0 days before delivery and the postpartum samples 45 to 202 days after delivery. The nonpregnant reference ranges are for healthy, fertile women in Scandinavia. *Data source*: ref. 21, with permission. *Conversion factor for urea*: mmol/L × 2.8 = mg/dL.

Comment: Concentrations of the major electrolytes (sodium, potassium, chloride) are almost unchanged during pregnancy. Bicarbonate and phosphate concentrations decrease during pregnancy.[27] Plasma urea and creatinine decrease during pregnancy. Plasma creatinine levels increase from their midpregnancy nadir in the weeks prior to delivery (see also Fig. 23C).[28]

CREATININE CLEARANCE AND PLASMA CREATININE

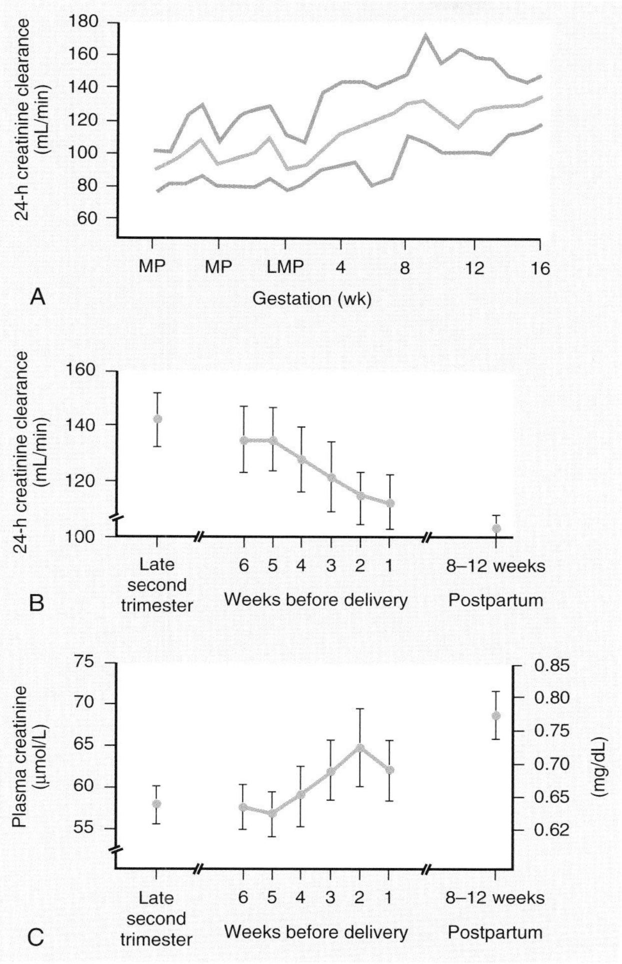

FIGURE 23

A, Creatinine clearance (mean and range) in early pregnancy from a longitudinal study of nine healthy women who were recruited before pregnancy. Measurements of 24-hour creatinine clearance were made weekly, through the different phases of the menstrual cycle, and up to 16 weeks' gestation. No diet, fluid, or exercise restrictions were imposed. *Data source*: ref. 29, with permission. Creatinine clearance (*B*) and plasma creatinine (*C*) (mean ± SEM) in the second and third trimesters from a longitudinal study of 10 healthy pregnant women. Creatinine clearance was measured once between 25 and 28 weeks' gestation, weekly from 32 weeks until delivery, and once between 8 and 12 weeks postpartum. *Data source*: ref. 30, with permission.

Comment: The GFR and effective renal plasma flow increase in early pregnancy to levels approximately 50% above nonpregnant values. In the third trimester, the GFR decreases by approximately 15%.[30] The 24-hour creatinine clearance measurements mirror these changes. During the menstrual cycle, a 20% mean increase in creatinine clearance occurs between the week of menstruation and the late luteal phase.[29]

URINE COMPOSITION: GLUCOSE, AMINO ACIDS, AND PROTEIN

Comment: Glycosuria is common in pregnant women whose plasma glucose concentrations and glucose tolerance test results are normal. It is believed to arise because of increased glomerular filtration plus decreased tubular resorption of glucose.[31] Aminoaciduria is also reported during pregnancy.[32] Urinary total protein and albumin excretion is significantly increased after 20 weeks' gestation; accepted upper limits of normal are 300 mg/24 hr and 20 mg/24 hr, respectively.[33] Protein-to-creatinine ratio measurements on spot urine samples are increasingly being used in clinical practice, rather than 24-hour total protein collections, as there is close correlation.[34] A threshold value of 30 mg protein/mmol creatinine predicts 300 mg/24 hr^{-1} or greater proteinuria.[33]

Carbohydrate Metabolism

FASTING PLASMA GLUCOSE

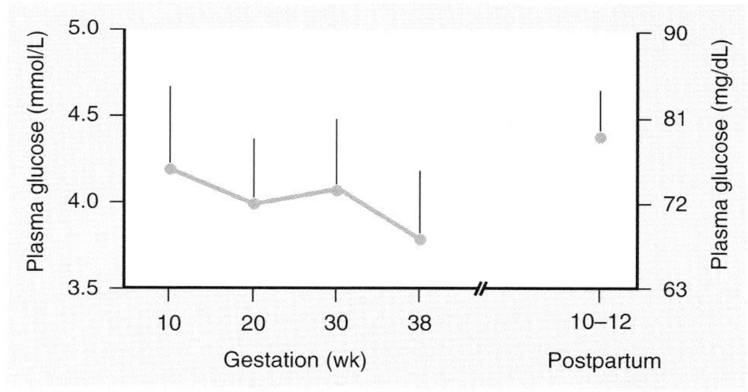

FIGURE 24

Longitudinal study of plasma glucose levels (mean + SD) after an overnight fast of at least 10 hours in 19 healthy women. The subjects were not obese and had no family history of diabetes mellitus. *Data source*: ref. 35, with permission.

Comment: Other studies confirmed these findings that fasting plasma glucose levels decrease in pregnancy. In most women, the decline occurs by the end of the first trimester.[36] Thereafter, most studies show further decreases in the second and third trimesters.[36] Severely obese women (BMI > 30.0 kg/m^2) studied throughout pregnancy did not show these changes, but had progressively increasing plasma glucose levels.[36] Plasma insulin levels increase in the third trimester.[35,37] Ethnic differences are seen in insulin production (as measured by C-peptide concentrations) and insulin resistance (as indicated by insulin-to-glucose ratios) during pregnancy.[37]

GLUCOSE TOLERANCE TEST

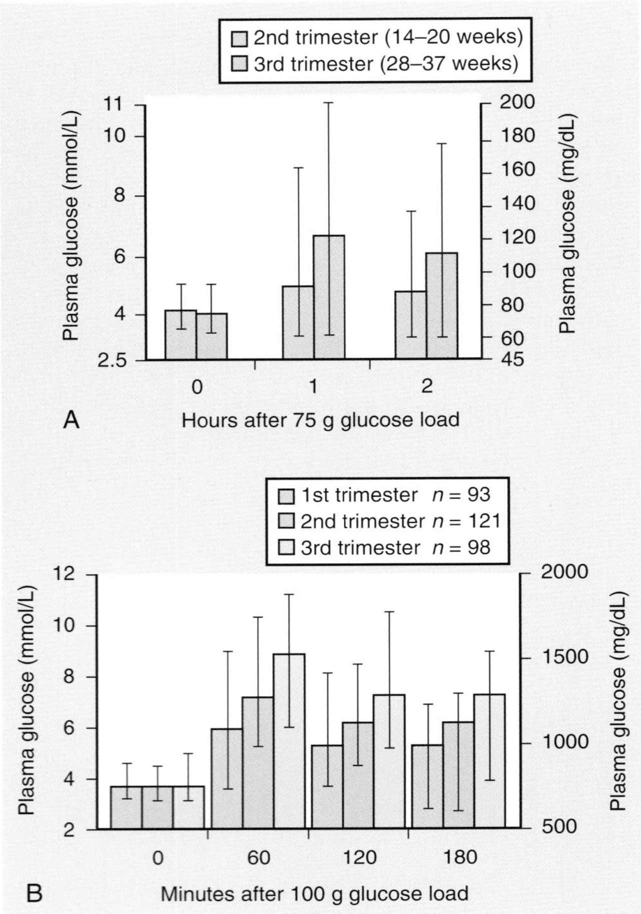

FIGURE 25

A, Plasma glucose values (median, 2.5th, and 97.5th percentiles) after a 75-g oral glucose load. Cross-sectional study of 111 healthy women younger than 35 years old, weighing less than 85 kg, with singleton pregnancies (n = 43 and n = 168 in the second and third trimesters, respectively). None had a personal or family history of diabetes mellitus. *Data source*: ref. 38, with permission. *B*, Plasma glucose values (median, 5th, and 95th percentiles) after a 100-g oral glucose load. The study involved 93 women in the first trimester, 121 in the second trimester, and 98 in the third trimester. All were healthy, were not obese, had no family history of diabetes, and had no obstetric complications. *Data source*: ref. 39, with permission.

Comment: Women in the third trimester have decreased glucose tolerance, as judged by criteria used to diagnose diabetes outside pregnancy.[40] There are many different diagnostic criteria for the diagnosis of gestational diabetes. For a 2-hour 75-g oral glucose tolerance test (OGTT), significant findings (accepted by the World Health Organization) are fasting or 2-hour venous plasma glucose values of 7.0 or greater or 7.8 mmol/L or greater, respectively.[41] For the 100-g OGTT, gestational diabetes may be diagnosed when two or more of the following plasma glucose levels are found: ≥105 mg/dL (fasting), ≥181 mg/dL (1 hr), 165 mg/dL (2 hr), and ≥145 mg/dL (3 hr). These values equate to 5.8 mmol/L (fasting), 10.0 mmol/L (1 hr), 9.1 mmol/L (2 hr), and 8.1 mmol/L (3 hr).[41]

SERUM FRUCTOSAMINE AND GLYCOSYLATED HEMOGLOBIN

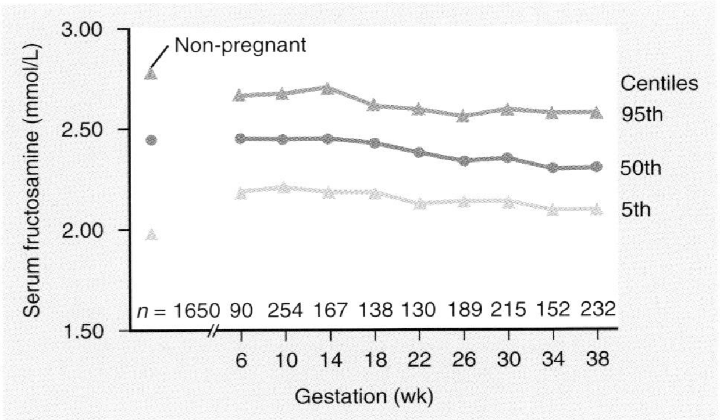

FIGURE 26

Serum fructosamine (median, 5th, and 95th percentiles) from a cross-sectional study of 1200 pregnant women at different gestational ages, compared with 1650 nonpregnant women 15 to 40 years old. Women with known diabetes or previous gestational diabetes were excluded from the study. *Data source*: ref. 42, with permission.

Comment: Serum fructosamine concentrations are significantly lower in the second and third trimesters than in the first trimester or the nonpregnant state. Decreasing total protein and albumin concentrations in pregnancy may contribute to this reduction.[42] In some studies, values for glycosylated hemoglobin (HbA_1 and HbA_{1c}) during pregnancy in healthy women were lower in the first and second trimesters,[36,43] but in other studies, they were similar to values in nonpregnant women.[44]

AMNIOTIC FLUID INSULIN, GLUCOSE, AND C-PEPTIDE

Amniotic fluid insulin, glucose, and C-peptide						
		Glucose (nmol/L)	Immunoreactive insulin (pmol/L)	C-peptide (pmol/L)	C-peptide/ insulin molar ratio
Early pregnancy	*n* = 77	3.44 ± 0.22	44.2 ± 2.1	38 ± 2.0	0.97 ± 0.06
Late pregnancy	*n* = 33	0.72 ± 0.11	45.5 ± 2.6	218 ± 54	4.3 ± 1.2

FIGURE 27
Insulin, glucose, and C-peptide levels in amniotic fluid (mean ± SD) from a cross-sectional study of 110 nondiabetic women who had amniocentesis in pregnancy (mostly for karyotyping). *Data source*: ref. 45, with permission.

Comment: Insulin and C-peptide levels in amniotic fluid can be studied as markers of fetal pancreatic β cell function. C-peptide and insulin are normally secreted in equimolar amounts from β cells. C-peptide may be the more reliable marker because insulin is degraded in the fetal liver and circulating insulin antibodies may be present.[45] In pregnant women with diabetes, concentrations of these substances are greater and third-trimester values are correlated with neonatal complications (macrosomia, hypoglycemia, jaundice, respiratory distress).[46] The mid-trimester insulin concentration in amniotic fluid is also greater in women who subsequently had gestational diabetes.[47]

Antioxidants

Comment: In pregnancy, levels of vitamin E (a free radical scavenger that opposes the effects of lipid peroxides) are increased compared with the nonpregnant state.[48] Vitamin E levels increase progressively with gestation, whereas lipid peroxide levels are constant.[48] Ascorbic acid concentrations in maternal serum during the third trimester and in breast milk during lactation are related to dietary consumption of fruit and vegetables.[49]

Hematology

White Blood Cell Count (Total and Differential)

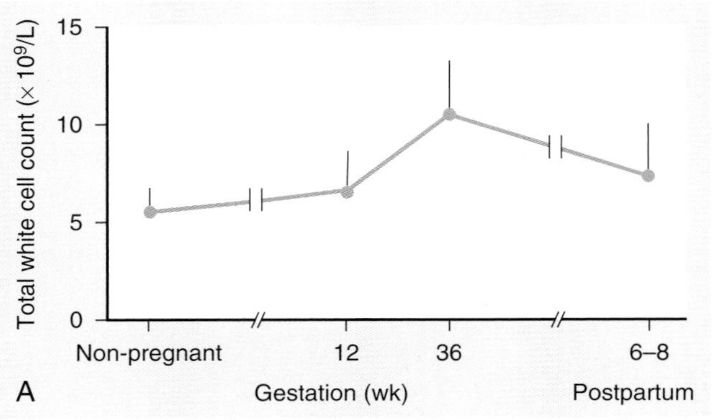

B

	Week 33 (n = 151)	Week 36 (n = 146)	Week 39 (n = 130)	Postpartum (n = 91)	Non-pregnant range
Total white cell count (WBC) 10^9/L	9.1 (5.7–14)	8.9 (6.1–15)	9.0 (6.0–16)	16 (9.4–25)	(4.0–9.0)
Neutrophils 10^9/L	6.5 (3.5–11)	6.4 (4.1–11)	6.5 (3.7–13)	14 (6.6–23)	(1.8–6.7)
Lymphocytes 10^9/L	1.7 (0.9–2.8)	1.8 (1.1–2.8)	1.8 (1.1–2.9)	1.1 (0.5–2.4)	(0.8–4.0)
Monocytes 10^9/L	0.50 (0.2–1.0)	0.50 (0.3–1.0)	0.50 (0.28–0.90)	0.53 (0.3–1.2)	(0.10–0.90)
Eosinophils 10^9/L	0.10 (0.0–0.40)	0.10 (0.0–0.30)	0.10 (0.0–0.40)	0.0 (0.0–0.50)	(0.0–0.50)
Basophils 10^9/L	0.0 (0.0–0.10)	0.03 (0.0–0.10)	0.04 (0.0–0.10)	0.08 (0.0–0.20)	(0.0–0.10)

FIGURE 28
A, Total white blood cell (WBC) count (mean + SD) from a longitudinal study of 24 women who were recruited at 12 weeks and were delivered after 37 weeks. Postpartum samples were taken 6 to 8 weeks after delivery. Nonpregnant samples were taken 4 to 6 months after delivery. Samples were analyzed in a Coulter counter. *Data source*: ref. 50, with permission. *B*, Total and differential WBC counts from a semilongitudinal study of 153 healthy pregnant women who were taking iron supplementation. All of the subjects had at least one previous normal pregnancy. Postpartum samples were taken 1 to 3 hours after delivery; samples taken from women who were eventually delivered by cesarean section were excluded from analysis. *Data source*: ref. 51, with permission.

Comment: Supplementation with iron and folate does not affect the total WBC count during or after pregnancy.[50] Other studies have confirmed the high total WBC during pregnancy, with typical reference ranges 6 to 16 × 10^9/L.[52] No studies reported total WBC values during labor, but in the early postpartum period, very high values (≤25 × 10^9/L) may be normal.[51] Pregnancy-related changes in the total WBC count are still present 6 to 8 weeks after delivery.[50] Neutrophils contribute most to the overall higher WBC count; there are more circulating immature forms (myelocytes and metamyelocytes) and their cytoplasm shows toxic granulation.[53] Neutrophil count is relatively constant during pregnancy (3–10 × 10^9/L), markedly elevated in the hours after delivery (≤23 × 10^9/L) and back to non-pregnant values by 4 weeks postpartum (1.5–6 × 10^9/L).[51,54] Lymphocyte count decreases during pregnancy through the first and second trimesters (typical range 1.1–2.8 × 10^9/L), increases during the third trimester, but remains low in the early puerperium compared with normal nonpregnant values (0.8–4.0 × 10^9/L).[54] Lymphocyte count is restored to the normal range by 4 weeks after delivery. Monocyte count is higher in pregnancy, with marked increase in the monocyte to lymphocyte ratio.[51,54] Eosinophil and basophil counts do not change significantly during pregnancy.[51]

Hemoglobin and Red Blood Cell Indices

Red cell indices	Gestation			
	18 weeks	32 weeks	39 weeks	8 weeks postpartum
Hemoglobin (Hb) g/dL	11.9 (10.6–13.3)	11.9 (10.4–13.5)	12.5 (10.9–14.2)	13.3 (11.9–14.8)
Red cell count $\times 10^{12}$/L	3.93 (3.43–4.49)	3.86 (3.38–4.43)	4.05 (3.54–4.64)	4.44 (3.93–5.00)
Mean cell volume (MCV) fL	89 (83–96)	91 (85–97)	91 (84–98)	88 (82–94)
Mean cell hemoglobin (MCH) pg	30 (27–33)	30 (28–33)	30 (28–33)	30 (27–32)
Mean cell hemoglobin concentration (MCHC) g/dL	34 (33–36)	34 (33–36)	34 (33–36)	34 (33–36)
Hematocrit	0.35 (0.31–0.39)	0.35 (0.31–0.40)	0.37 (0.32–0.42)	0.39 (0.35–0.44)

FIGURE 29
Hemoglobin and red cell indices (mean and calculated 2.5th–97.5th percentile reference ranges) from a longitudinal study of 434 healthy Danish women. All delivered normally at term and their infants weighed more than 2.5 kg. All the women had iron supplements (20–80 mg ferrous iron/day) from recruitment to the study until 8 weeks postpartum. Samples were obtained at 18, 32, and 39 weeks' gestation and at 8 weeks postdelivery. *Data source*: ref. 52, with permission.

Comment: Hemoglobin concentration decreases in the first trimester, regardless of whether iron and folate supplements are given.[50] Hemoglobin values of 10.5 g/dL or less suggest anemia in healthy pregnant Caucasian women.[52] Studies done in other ethnic populations find similar ranges for hematologic indices.[55] Pregnancy-induced hematologic changes are still present 6 to 8 weeks postpartum, when compared with values obtained 4 to 6 months postpartum.[50]

Platelet Count and Indices

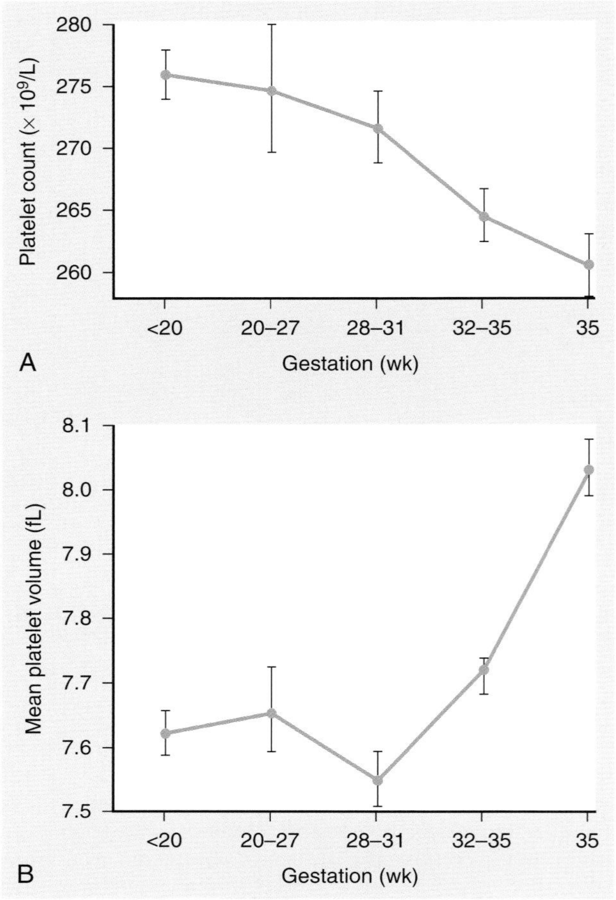

FIGURE 30

Platelet count (*A*) and mean platelet volume (*B*) (mean ± SEM) during pregnancy. The study was largely cross-sectional in design (2881 samples from 2114 women). Samples were analyzed in a Coulter counter. At the end of the study, patients who had hypertension were excluded. *Data source*: ref. 56, with permission.

Comment: Hyperdestruction of platelets may occur in pregnancy, with a consequent decrease in platelet life span. Young platelets are larger than old platelets. In a large study of 6770 women in late pregnancy, mean platelet counts were 213 $\times 10^9$/L and the 2.5th percentile value was 116 $\times 10^9$/L.[57] Another, but longitudinal, study with much smaller numbers (*n* = 44) did not find evidence of a significant change in platelet count with gestational age.[58] Platelet closure times (the time required for whole blood to occlude a membrane impregnated with either epinephrine or adenosine 5′diphosphate) are not affected by absolute platelet count in healthy women during pregnancy.[59]

Iron Metabolism

Iron metabolism					
Patients	Hb (g/dL)	Serum iron (μmol/L)	Serum iron (mg/dL)	Transferrin/TIBC saturation (%)	Serum ferritin (μg/L)
Non-treated (*n* = 30)					
First trimester	12.9	23	129	36	96
Term	12.0	14	78	13	13
Given $FeSO_4$ (*n* = 82)					
First trimester	12.5	22	123	33	67
Term	12.5	25	140	27	41

A

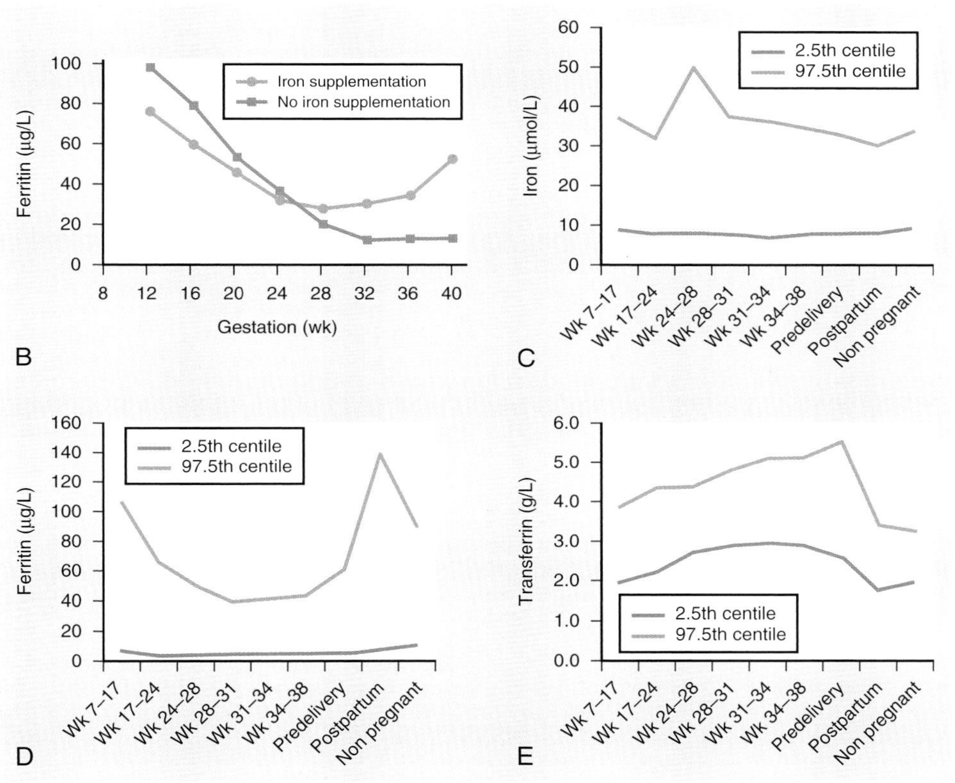

FIGURE 31

Mean hemoglobin (Hb) and iron indices (*A*), mean ferritin from a longitudinal study of women recruited in the first trimester (*B*). At the start of the study, 72 were randomized to the no-treatment group, but any whose Hb fell below 11 g/dL were prescribed ferrous sulfate 60 mg three times daily. Only 30 progressed through pregnancy without iron supplements. In all of the subjects studied, serum ferritin levels rose rapidly postpartum, reaching values similar to those found in early pregnancy by 5 to 8 weeks after delivery. No iron supplements were given after delivery. *Data source*: ref. 60, with permission. Plasma iron (*C*), ferritin (*D*), and transferrin (*E*) (2.5th-97.5th calculated percentile reference interval) from a longitudinal study of 52 healthy women in Sweden sampled at intervals during pregnancy, some of whom were taking iron and folic acid supplements. At least 40 samples were obtained for each time point; predelivery samples were taken 14 to 0 days before delivery and the postpartum samples 45 to 202 days after delivery. The nonpregnant reference ranges are for healthy, fertile women in the same laboratory. *Data source*: ref. 21, with permission.

Comment: Iron stores, as indicated by the serum ferritin level, are depleted during pregnancy, regardless of whether iron supplements are given.

Serum and Red Cell Folate

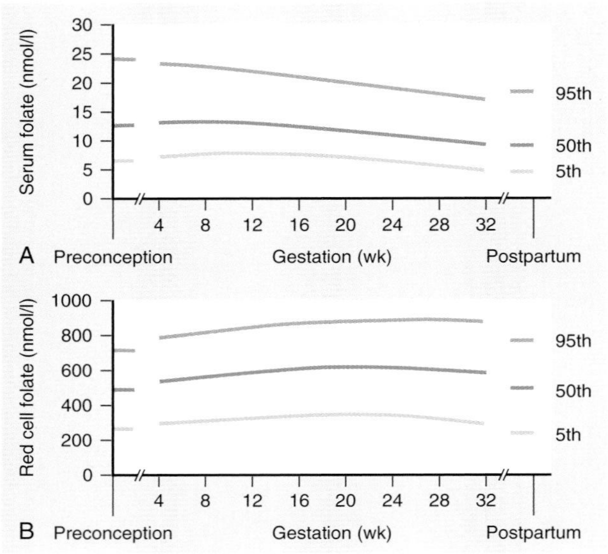

FIGURE 32
Longitudinal study of serum (*A*) and red cell folate levels (*B*) (5th, 50th, and 95th percentiles) in healthy nulliparous women during an uneventful singleton pregnancy. None of the study subjects took iron or vitamin supplements ($n = 102$). Nonfasting blood samples were taken within 3 months of conception, at 6, 10, 20, and 32 weeks' gestation, and again at 6 weeks postpartum. All women had spontaneous labor at term and had infants of normal size. *Data source*: ref. 61, with permission. *Conversion factor for folate*: nmol/L × 0.044 = μg/dL.

Comment: In other studies, red cell folate levels showed a slight downward trend with advancing gestation,[62] and patients with low red cell folate levels at the beginning of pregnancy had megaloblastic anemia in the third trimester.[63] These differences may relate to dietary folate intake. In a cross-sectional study of 155 women, red cell folate concentration increased with gestation and was significantly higher in subjects who took supplemental folic acid (1 mg daily) than in those who did not (1056 nmol/L vs. 595 nmol/L, respectively).[64] Serum and red cell folate levels are lower in pregnancy in women who smoke.[65] By 6 weeks after delivery, red cell folate levels return toward preconception values, although serum folate levels remain low. Lactation, which is an added folate stress, may be one reason.[66] Serum folate levels may remain low for up to 6 months after delivery.[61]

Homocysteine

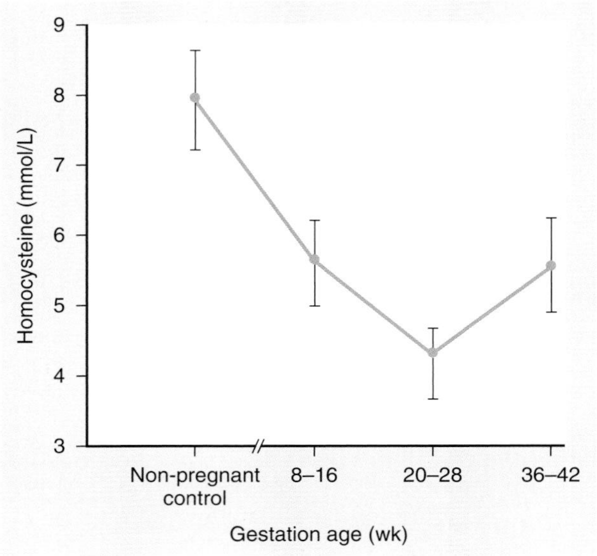

FIGURE 33
Plasma homocysteine (mean and 95% confidence interval [CI]) in a cross-sectional study of 155 normal women in the first, second, and third trimesters of pregnancy and in nonpregnant control subjects. Homocysteine concentrations were determined by high-pressure liquid chromatography. *Data source*: ref. 64, with permission.

Comment: Plasma homocysteine levels are significantly lower in all trimesters of pregnancy compared with nonpregnant control values. Longitudinal studies confirm these findings.[61,62] The lowest levels are found in the second trimester. Homocysteine is 70% to 80% albumin-bound, so these gestational changes mirror those of serum albumin (see Fig. 15). Homocysteine is negatively correlated with red cell folate, and lower concentrations are found in women who take folic acid supplements.[64] Hyperhomocysteinemia, which can result from genetic and environmental factors, is associated with deep venous thrombosis, recurrent miscarriage, abruption, stillbirth, and neural tube defects.

Vitamin B_{12}

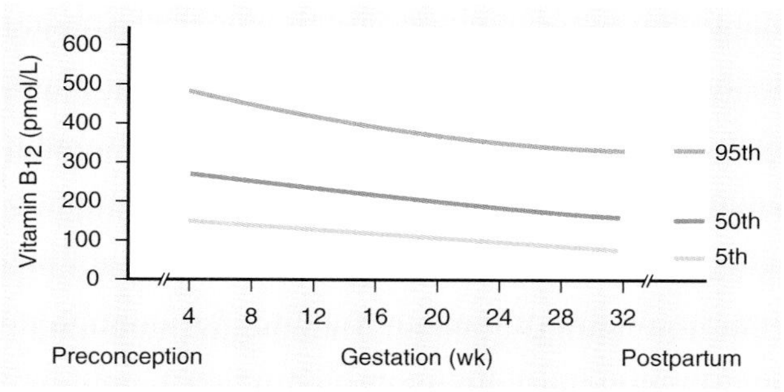

FIGURE 34
Serum vitamin B_{12} levels (5th, 50th, and 95th percentiles) in 102 healthy nulliparous women during an uneventful singleton pregnancy. Subjects were those described in Figure 31. *Data source*: ref. 61, with permission.

Comment: Serum vitamin B_{12} levels are approximately 100 pmol/L lower in pregnancy, but recovery occurs by 6 weeks postpartum.[61] Levels tend to be lower in women who smoke.[65] Muscle and red cell vitamin B_{12} concentrations also fall during pregnancy; however, vitamin B_{12} absorption does not change.[66,67] Saturation of vitamin B_{12}–binding proteins decreases steadily during pregnancy.[67] These changes in vitamin B_{12} status do not represent a deficiency state, however, because they are not associated with evidence of reduced red blood cell count or hemoglobin or homocysteine concentrations, once correction is made for serum ferritin concentrations.[67]

Other Vitamins

Comment: Vitamin concentrations during pregnancy are available from a large longitudinal study performed in the Netherlands on women who were not using iron, folate, or other vitamin supplementation. Vitamins studied included retinol, thiamin, riboflavin, pyridoxal 5′-phosphate, and α-tocopherol.[61]

Coagulation Factors

	6–11 weeks n = 41	12–16 weeks n = 28	17–23 weeks n = 10	24–28 weeks n = 19	29–35 weeks n = 36	36–40 weeks n = 23	3 days postnatal n = 87
Fibrinogen activity g/l	3.6 2.5–4.8	3.8 2.5–5.1	3.6 2.6–4.7	4.4 2.9–5.9	4.1 2.5–5.8	4.2 3.2–5.3	4.5 3.1–5.8
Prothrombin activity iu/dl	153 107–200	160 111–209	153 41–265	172 92–252	153 100–211	162 107–217	169 108–231
Prothrombin fragments 1+2 nmol/l	1.1 <2.9	1.1 <1.5	1.3 <2.1	1.8 <3.4	2.0 <3.9	1.9 <3.5	2.2 <4.9
Factor V activity u/dl	99 39–159	101 39–162	111 47–175	108 50–166	111 43–179	129 65–194	141 71–211
Factor VIII activity iu/dl	107 62–220	129 82–130	189 59–159	187 71–341	180 31–328	176 50–302	192 54–331
Von Willebrand Antigen iu/dl	137 70–204	160 52–268	186 64–247	170 54–286	178 78–278	179 62–296	174 86–262
RICOF iu/dl	117 47–258	132 55–298	128 50–206	204 68–360	169 86–466	240 100–544	247 97–630
Factor IX activity iu/dl	100 49–151	106 82–130	96 74–118	121 59–183	109 65–154	114 79–150	136 65–207
Factor X activity iu/dl	125 88–162	129 78–180	128 50–206	159 52–263	146 81–212	152 113–191	162 69–254
Factor XI activity iu/dl	102 50–154	103 58–147	86 58–114	102 45–162	100 31–169	92 36–181	96 46–146
Factor XII activity iu/dl	137 70–204	160 52–268	186 64–247	170 54–286	178 78–278	179 62–296	174 86–262

FIGURE 35
Coagulation factors (mean + 2 SD normal ranges) from a cross-sectional study of 239 women, each of whom was sampled only once. Postdelivery samples were taken 3 days after delivery; all samples were anticoagulated with sodium citrate. Following delivery, case records were reviewed to confirm that all pregnancies had remained uncomplicated. *Data source*: ref. 68, with permission.

Comment: Normal pregnancy is a hypercoagulable state associated with substantially increased levels of Von Willebrand's factor and Factors VIII, X, and fibrinogen as a result of increased synthesis and increased activation by thrombin. The activated partial thromboplastin time, which measures the intrinsic coagulation pathway, is usually shortened in late pregnancy, by up to 4 seconds, due largely to increased Factor VIII. The prothrombin and thrombin times do not change significantly in pregnancy. In a longitudinal study,[69] Factor VII activity increased from the range 60% to 206% (compared with standard) at the end of the first trimester to 87% to 336% by term. The same study found Factors II and V increased in early pregnancy, but then reduced in the thi3rd trimester. The cross-sectional study shown here found a 29% rise in Factor V from 6 to 11 weeks to 36 to 40 weeks' gestation.[68] Factor IX levels increase, whereas factor XI levels decrease.[66,68] There is an increase in fibrinopeptide A during the first-trimester.[69] By 6 to 7 weeks postnatal, coagulation factors have been found to be similar to those in age-matched, nonpregnant women[69]; however, most hematologists would recommend testing at 8 to 12 weeks following delivery to assess true nonpregnant levels.

Naturally Occurring Anticoagulants and Fibrinolytic Factors

No. of patients		41	48	47	66	62	48	61	61
Weeks		11–15	16–20	21–25	26–30	31–35	36–40	Post delivery	Post natal
Fibrin degradation products mg/ml	Mean	1.07	1.06	1.09	1.13	1.28	1.32	1.66	1.04
Fibrinolytic activity (100/Lysis time)	Mean	7.6	7.4	7.3	5.5	4.5	5.6	6.75	5.75
Lysis time in hours	Mean	13.25	13.5	13.75	18.25	22.25	17.8	14.8	17.4
Antithrombin III:C	Mean Range	85 49–120	90 46–133	87 42–132	94 47–141	87 42–132	86 40–132	87 48–127	92 38–147
Antithrombin III:Ag	Mean Range	93 60–126	94 56–131	93 56–130	97 56–138	96 59–132	93 50–136	95 58–133	100 64–134
a_1Antitrypsin	Mean Range	124 66–234	136 86–214	125 53–295	146 85–249	149 89–250	154 91–260	172 84–352	77 44–135
a_2Macroglobulin	Mean Range	176 100–309	178 98–323	170 92–312	160 88–294	157 85–292	153 85–277	146 81–265	142 82–245

FIGURE 36
Naturally occurring anticoagulants and fibrinolytic factors (mean and 95% CI ranges), fibrinolytic activity, clot lysis time, and fibrin degradation products (FDPs) (mean values) from a longitudinal study of 72 women, 19 to 42 years old (healthy primigravidae or multigravidae whose previous pregnancies were uncomplicated). Postdelivery samples were taken between 6 hours and 4 days after delivery (mean 52 hr); postnatal samples were taken after 6 weeks. The postnatal samples yielded values similar to those from an age-matched nonpregnant group of women (n = 66). *Data source*: ref. 69, with permission.

	6–11 weeks $n = 41$	12–16 weeks $n = 28$	17–23 weeks $n = 10$	24–28 weeks $n = 19$	29–35 weeks $n = 36$	36–40 weeks $n = 23$	3 days postnatal $n = 87$
Total protein S u/dl	80 34–126	77 45–109	66 40–92	68 38–98	67 27–106	58 27–90	69 37–85
Free protein S u/dl	81 47–115	72 44–101	64 38–90	60 34–86	54 32–76	57 15–95	58 29–87
Protein C activity u/dl	95 65–125	94 62–125	101 63–139	105 73–137	99 60–137	94 52–136	118 78–157
Antithrombin activity u/dl	96 70–122	100 72–128	100 74–126	104 70–138	104 68–140	102 70–133	108 77–137

FIGURE 37
Protein S, protein C, and antithrombin III (mean + 2 SD normal ranges) from a cross-sectional study of 239 women, each of whom was sampled only once. The study subjects were described in Figure 35. *Data source*: ref. 68, with permission.

Comment: Total and free (biologically active) protein S levels decrease progressively during pregnancy. In the study shown here, first trimester levels of total and free protein S were lower than the ranges in non–oral contraceptive using women of similar age (64–154 IU/dL and 54–154 IU/dL, respectively).[68] Protein C levels do not change with gestation and are similar to those found outside pregnancy.[68] Antithrombin III levels are stable during pregnancy, decrease in labor, and then increase 1 week postpartum.[66] Fibrinolysis is depressed during pregnancy; fibrinogen and plasminogen levels are elevated, but levels of circulating plasminogen activator are decreased.[70] Lowest levels of plasminogen activator are found during labor and levels increase soon after delivery, as placentally produced plasminogen activator inhibitor-2 ceases to have influence.[70] In late normal pregnancy, D-dimer levels are also elevated, typically 10-fold higher than in early pregnancy or the nonpregnant state.[51,71] FDPs are also found in increased amounts, particularly in late gestation.[69] High levels of FDPs and D-dimers indicate that clot formation and destruction processes are active, and this has been shown particularly to be happening locally in the placental circulation. Clearance of FDPs and D-dimers may also be altered in pregnancy. Levels of FDPs, D-dimers, and soluble fibrin remain high for at least a week after delivery.[69]

Immunology

Complement System and Immune Complexes

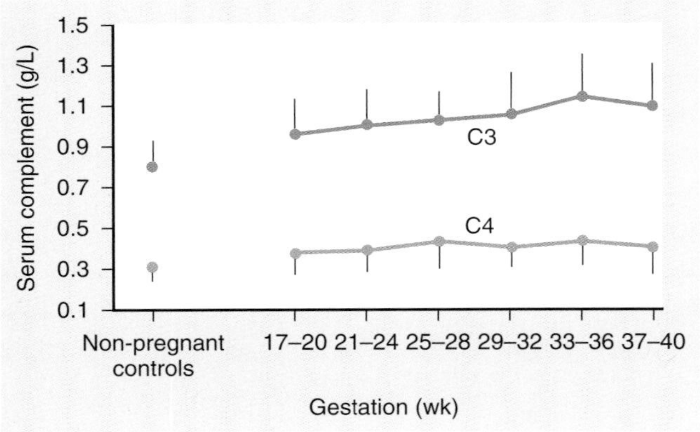

FIGURE 38
Complement factors C3 and C4 (mean + SD) from a longitudinal study of 147 healthy women who were normotensive throughout pregnancy. The control population was 32 normal nonpregnant women 15 to 41 years old, 11 of whom were taking oral contraceptives. *Data source*: ref. 72, with permission.

Comment: Levels of C3 and C4 are significantly elevated during the second and third trimesters. Another cross-sectional study showed elevated levels of C4, but not C3, during the first trimester.[73] Levels of circulating immune complexes are low during pregnancy.[73] There is disagreement as to whether levels of C3 degradation products are elevated[73] or normal[74]; no longitudinal studies have been done.

Markers of Inflammation

ERYTHROCYTE SEDIMENTATION RATE AND C-REACTIVE PROTEIN

Comment: The erythrocyte sedimentation rate (ESR) is high in pregnancy (typically > 30 mm in the first hr) as a result of elevated plasma globulins and fibrinogen.[75] Thus, the ESR cannot be used as a marker for inflammation. Levels of C-reactive protein are slightly increased in pregnancy, particularly in the third trimester and early puerperium.[17,51] Other acute-phase inflammatory markers have been studied in pregnancy: α_1-acid glycoprotein decreases, α_1-antitrypsin increases especially in the third trimester, and haptoglobin levels are stable.[17]

Endocrinology

Thyroid Function

TOTAL THYROXINE, TRIIODOTHYRONINE, THYROID UPTAKE, AND THYROID-BINDING GLOBULIN

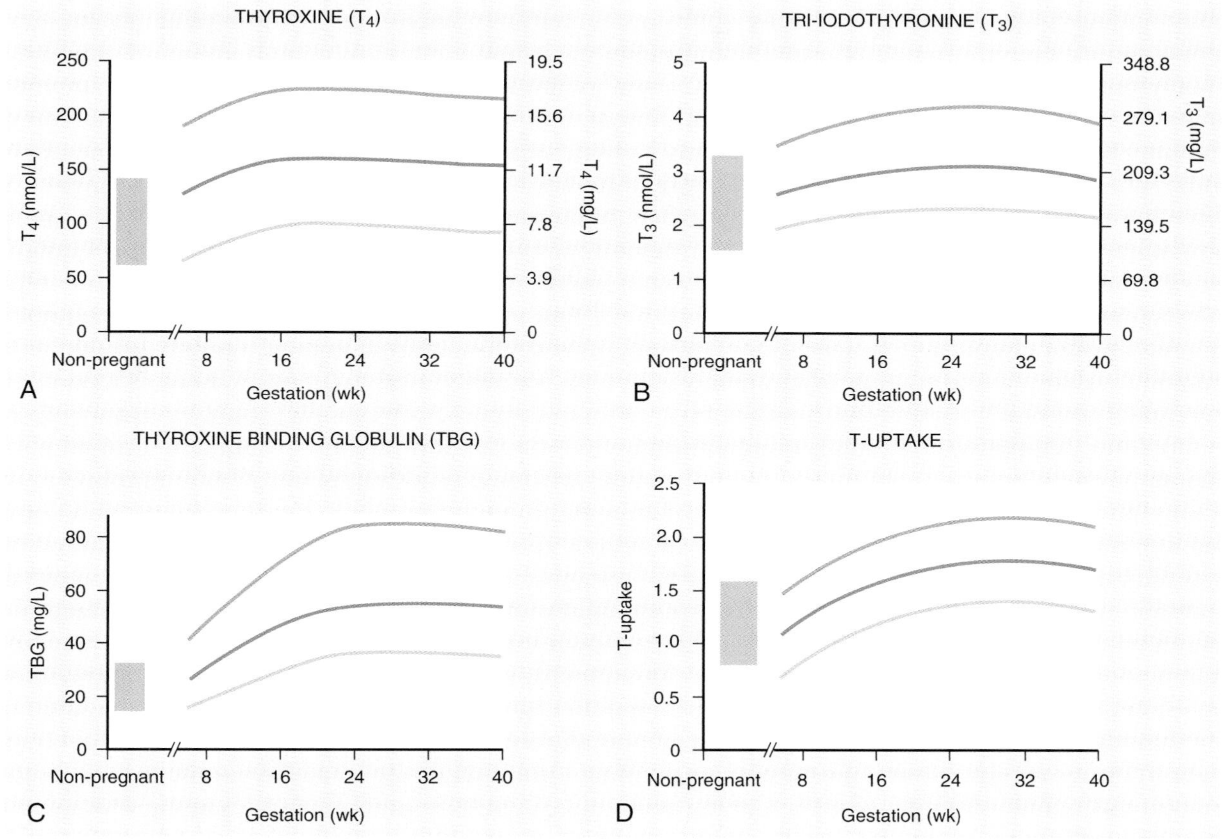

FIGURE 39

Total thyroxine (T_4) (*A*), total triiodothyronine (T_3) (*B*), thyroid-binding globulin (TBG) (*C*), and T uptake (*D*) (2.5th, 50th, and 97.5th percentiles) from a longitudinal study of 60 women who each had blood samples three times during pregnancy, once each trimester. Control values were taken from 30 healthy nonpregnant women. *Data source*: ref. 76, with permission.

Comment: Serum total T_4 and T_3 concentrations are elevated in pregnancy. TBG concentrations are doubled by the end of the first trimester, remain elevated throughout pregnancy, and decrease slowly in the 6 weeks after delivery.[77] T_3 uptake is believed to represent total serum thyroxine-binding capacity rather than unoccupied binding site concentration.[76] Other cross-sectional studies found decreased T_3 uptake during pregnancy.[78]

FREE THYROXINE, FREE THYROID-STIMULATING HORMONE, AND FREE TRIIODOTHYRONINE

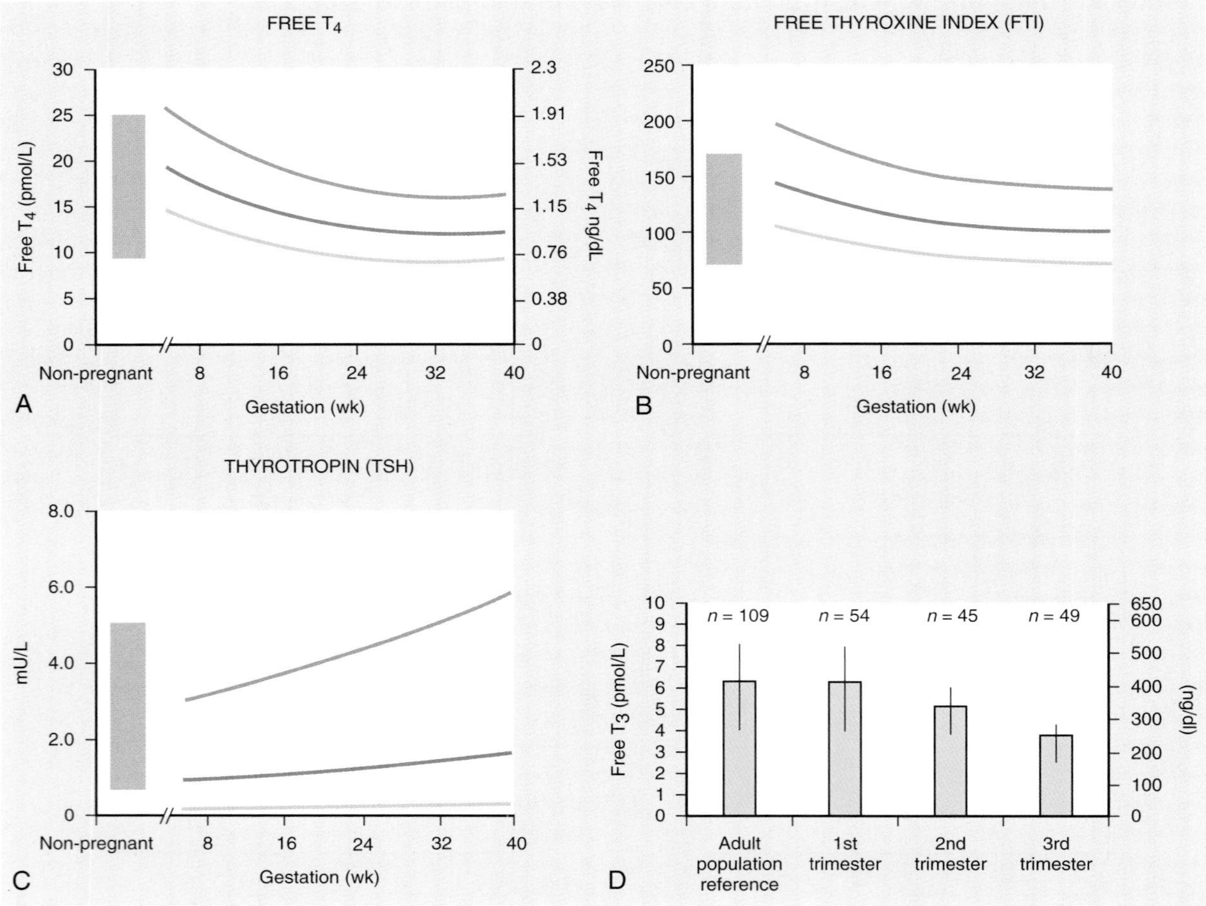

FIGURE 40
Free T_4 levels (*A*), free T_4 index (*B*), and thyroid-stimulating hormone (TSH) (*C*) levels (2.5th, 50th, and 97.5th percentiles) from the same study described in Figure 39. *Data source*: ref. 76, with permission. *D*, Free T_3 concentrations (mean ± 2 SDs) from a cross-sectional study of 159 women attending antenatal clinics; none had metabolic illness. The control samples were obtained from 109 patients (male and female) taken from the routine workload of the laboratory (excluding those with thyroid disease, diabetes, cardiac disease, or carcinoma, and postoperative patients). *Data source*: ref. 79, with permission.

Comment: Free T_4 and free T_3 concentrations, measured directly (rather than derived from resin uptake measurements), decrease during pregnancy but remain within normal nonpregnant ranges.[76,79,80] TSH levels increase with gestation but remain within the reference range for nonpregnant women.[76] Some studies found low TSH levels toward the end of the first trimester in association with the highest circulating concentrations of human chorionic gonadotropin (hCG).[78] The increase in TSH in response to thyrotropin-releasing hormone during early pregnancy is enhanced, similar to responses found in central hypothyroidism.[81]

Adrenal Function

CATECHOLAMINES

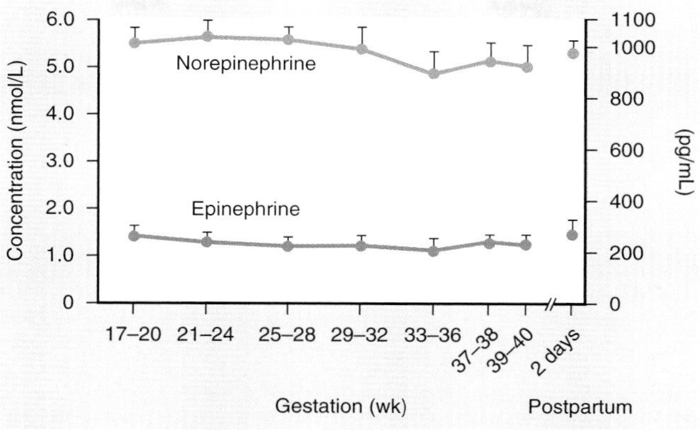

FIGURE 41
Epinephrine and norepinephrine concentrations (mean and SEM) from a longitudinal study of 52 women, mean age 28 years, who were normotensive throughout pregnancy; 39 were primigravidae. Samples were taken by venipuncture after 20 minutes' rest in the left lateral position. A radioenzymic method was used for the assays. *Data source*: ref. 82, with permission.

Comment: This study showed a decrease in plasma levels of both epinephrine and norepinephrine as pregnancy progressed. Other studies (in which blood samples were taken from indwelling intravenous cannulas) showed steady levels throughout pregnancy, with no difference between values during pregnancy and those in the early puerperium.[83] In healthy pregnant women, plasma epinephrine and norepinephrine levels show a diurnal pattern, with the lowest levels reported at night.[84] Urinary vanillylmandelic acid (VMA) and catecholamine excretion has not been studied in healthy pregnancies but is likely to be within the normal adult range.

GLUCOCORTICOIDS AND MINERALOCORTICOIDS

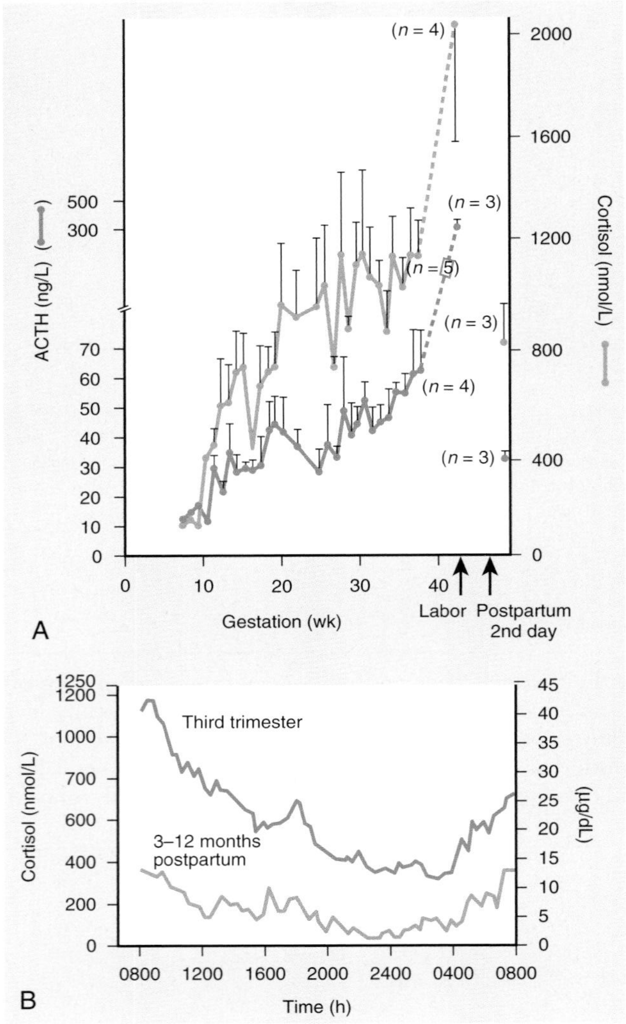

C

	Plasma cortisol (nmol/L)			Free cortisol index	
	Minimum	Mean (in 24-h period)	Maximum	Minimum	Maximum (in 24-h period)
Pregnant third trimester (*n* = 7)	197 (25)	581 (28)	1206 (94)	2.2 (0.3)	15.7 (1.7)
Non-pregnant (*n* = 3)	22 (6)	175 (25)	450 (3)	0.22 (0.05)	5.7 (0.9)

D

	Serum cortisol		Salivary free cortisol		Serum aldosterone
	(mg/dL)	nmol/L	(mg/dL)	nmol/L	ng/dL
1st trimester *n* = 4	9.3 (2.2)	257 (61)	0.21 (0.1)	5.8 (2.8)	8.0 (2.3)
2nd trimester *n* = 16	14.5 (4.3)	400 (119)	0.36 (0.17)	9.9 (4.7)	13.8 (5.3)
3rd trimester *n* = 16	16.6 (4.2)	458 (116)	0.47 (0.18)	12.9 (5.0)	25.3 (10.8)
Non pregnant *n* = 32	9.1 (4.8)	251 (132)	0.22 (0.17)	6.1 (4.7)	3.0 (2.2)

FIGURE 42

A, Adrenocorticotropic hormone (ACTH) and cortisol concentrations (mean and SEM) from a longitudinal study of five healthy pregnant women 17 to 28 years old. Blood samples were taken weekly, from early pregnancy until delivery. Samples were obtained between 8:00 AM and 9:00 AM after an overnight fast. Samples for ACTH measurement were collected improperly from one woman and had to be discarded. Samples were also taken from three of these subjects during labor and on the second postpartum day. *Data source*: ref. 85, with permission. *B*, Mean plasma cortisol levels throughout a 24-hour period from a study of seven primigravidae in the third trimester and three nonpregnant women, two of whom had been studied during pregnancy. The nonpregnant women were at least 3 months postdelivery and were not breast-feeding or using oral contraceptives. Samples were taken every 20 minutes. *Data source*: ref. 86, with permission. *C*, Plasma cortisol and free cortisol index (mean + SD) from a study of seven primigravidae in the third trimester and three nonpregnant women, two of whom had been studied during pregnancy. Subjects were those described in *B*. *Data source*: ref. 86, with permission. *D*, Serum cortisol, salivary free cortisol, and aldosterone (mean + SD) from a study of 36 healthy pregnant women without previous history of adrenal disease and who had not taken glucocorticoids for the preceding 6 months. Blood samples were taken in a supine position from an intravenous cannula, between 9:00 AM and 10:00 AM. Most of the subjects were ethnically African American. Subjects were studied once during pregnancy, and 32 of them were restudied 11 to 14 weeks postpartum. *Data source*: ref. 87, with permission. *Conversion factor for cortisol*: nmol/L × 0.036 = µg/dL.

Comment: Total, bound, and free plasma cortisol levels; free cortisol index; and salivary free cortisol are increased in pregnancy compared with the nonpregnant state.[86–88] ACTH levels during pregnancy are variously reported as remaining within the normal range for nonpregnant subjects, increasing, or decreasing,[85,89] but there is agreement that levels increase with advancing gestation. The rise in ACTH during pregnancy is attributed to placental production of the peptide.[89] Despite overall elevated levels, normal diurnal patterns of cortisol are found during pregnancy (i.e., lowest values at 12:00 noon, highest values at 8:00 AM).[86,88] The biologic half-life of cortisol is increased in pregnancy.[86] Cortisol-binding globulin (CBG) concentrations rise steadily during pregnancy, reaching twice the normal values by midgestation.[88,90] The cortisol production rate during pregnancy has been described as depressed[91] or elevated.[86] Urinary free cortisol more than doubles during pregnancy.[92] After 1 mg dexamethasone given orally at 11:00 PM, plasma cortisol levels measured at 8:00 AM are less than 139 nmol/L or 5 μ/dL (a normal response).[93] However, urinary cortisol levels are not suppressed as much in pregnant subjects as in nonpregnant subjects.[89] The cortisol response to an ACTH challenge (250 μg Synacthen test) is unchanged in pregnancy: stimulated serum cortisol levels of 20 μg/dL or greater (550 nmol/L).[87,94] Salivary free cortisol (SaFC) is unaffected by CBG levels and is thus a useful measure in situations in which CBG is high. The calculated lower limit (2.5th percentile) for basal morning SaFC is 0.13 μg/dL (3.59 nmol/L) and 0.19 μg/dL (5.24 nmol/L) in the second and third trimesters, respectively.[87] After a 250-μg ACTH challenge, SaFC levels exceeded 1.06 μg/dL (28.3 nmol/L) and 1.19 μg/dL (32.8 nmol/L) in the second and third trimesters, respectively.[87] Aldosterone levels increase progressively during gestation, and there is an enhanced response to an ACTH challenge.[87]

Prolactin

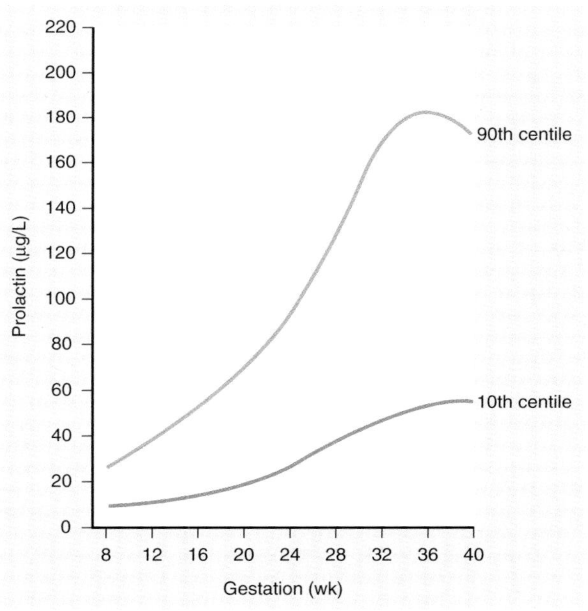

FIGURE 43
Serum prolactin (10th and 90th percentiles) from a mostly cross-sectional study of 839 women with uncomplicated singleton pregnancies at 8 to 40 weeks' gestation; 980 blood samples were taken. All of the samples were collected between 9:00 AM and 11:00 AM. Women who had a pregnancy complication were rejected from the normal series. *Data source*: ref. 95, with permission.

Comment: Prolactin concentrations increase 10- to 20-fold during pregnancy. The concentrations show a normal circadian rhythm, with a nocturnal rise.[96] In labor, levels decrease acutely, followed by a postpartum surge during the first 2 hours after delivery.[97] These changes are not seen in women undergoing elective cesarean delivery. Prolactin levels approach the normal range 2 to 3 weeks after delivery in nonlactating women, but remain elevated in those who breast-feed their infants.[98]

Calcium Metabolism

TOTAL AND IONIZED CALCIUM, MAGNESIUM, ALBUMIN, PARATHYROID HORMONE, CALCITIONIN, AND VITAMIN D

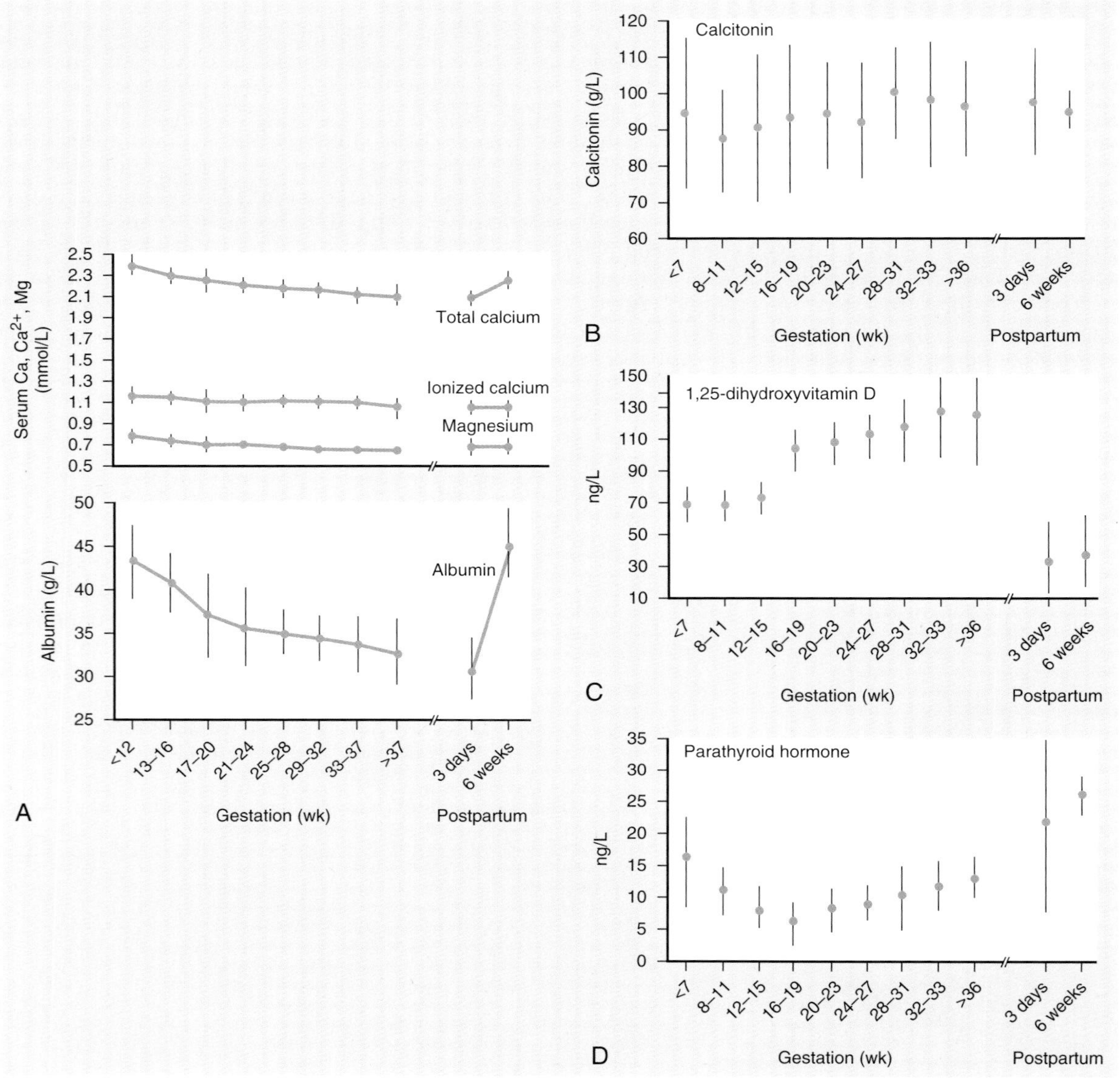

FIGURE 44

A, Total and ionized calcium, magnesium, and albumin (mean ± SD) from a longitudinal study of 30 women who were recruited in the first trimester and studied at 4-week intervals. Samples were taken on the third postpartum day and during the sixth postpartum week. Subjects ranged in age from 19 to 33 years; 20 were primigravidae. Samples were collected by venipuncture after an overnight fast. *Conversion factors*: calcium, mmol/L × 4 = mg/dL; magnesium, mmol/L × 2.4 = mg/dL. *Data source*: ref. 99, with permission. Calcitonin (*B*), 1,25-dihydroxyvitamin D (*C*), and parathyroid hormone (PTH) (*D*) (mean ± SD) from a longitudinal study of 20 women 22 to 34 years old, 12 of whom were nulliparous. All had uncomplicated pregnancies of more than 38 weeks' gestation. The only medication they received was ferrous sulfate. Blood samples were taken in the morning after an overnight fast. Samples were collected at 4-week intervals, with the first taken before 7 weeks' gestation. Samples were also taken on the third postpartum day and during the sixth postpartum week. *Data source*: ref. 100, with permission.

Comment: Total serum calcium decreases during pregnancy, in association with the fall in serum albumin; however, ionized calcium levels remain constant. Serum intact PTH levels are lower in pregnancy than at 6 weeks postpartum; they reach a nadir in midpregnancy. A menstrual cyclicity in PTH has also been noted, with higher values corresponding to times of increased estrogen secretion.[99] Calcitonin levels are not significantly altered in pregnancy. 1,25-Dihydroxyvitamin D levels increase with advancing gestation and are significantly higher than during the puerperium. One α-hydroxylation of 25-hydroxyvitamin D in the placenta accounts for this increase and the consequent suppression of PTH.[100]

Placental Biochemistry

PLASMA PROTEIN A

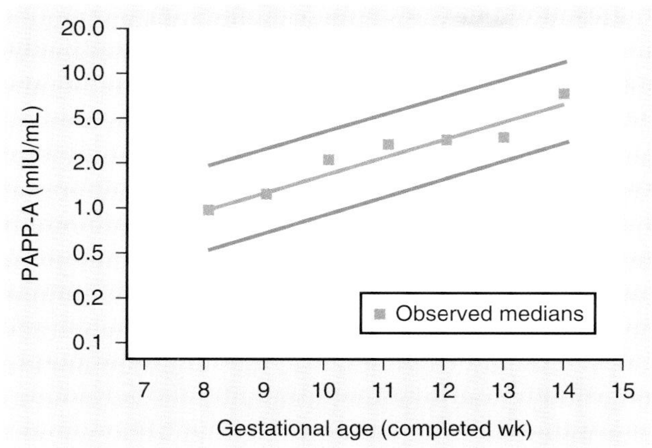

FIGURE 45
Pregnancy-associated plasma protein A (PAPP-A) levels in maternal serum (median 0.5 MoM and 2 MoM) from a cross-sectional study of 379 healthy women at 8 to 14 weeks' gestation. These women had been selected to match 77 women whose fetuses had Down syndrome. Their median age was 39 years (10th and 90th percentiles, 34 and 42 years, respectively). *Data source*: ref. 101, with permission.

Comment: PAPP-A and free β-human chorionic gonadotropin (β-hCG) are useful markers for discriminating pregnancies affected by Down syndrome from normal pregnancies at 8 to 14 weeks' gestation. PAPP-A levels are lower in affected pregnancies than in normal pregnancies (particularly at ≤ 11 wk' gestation).[101,102]

SERUM α-FETOPROTEIN

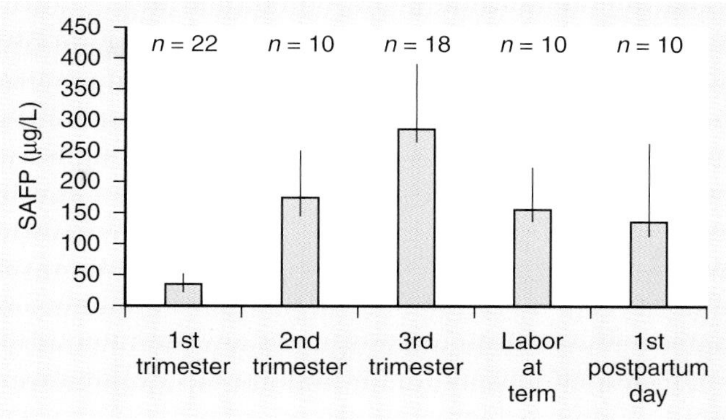

FIGURE 46
Serum α-fetoprotein (SAFP) (median and interquartile ranges) from a cross-sectional study. Samples from women in labor and samples obtained on the first postpartum day were paired. SAFP was measured by radioimmunoassay. *Data source*: ref. 103, with permission.

Comment: In the second trimester, SAFP increases by approximately 15% weekly.[104] Individual screening laboratories establish reference ranges for SAFP in the second trimester for their own populations. These ranges are usually expressed as MoM for gestation. In twin pregnancies, SAFP levels are approximately twice as high as those in singleton pregnancies.[104] Maternal weight is inversely related to SAFP levels, probably because of the dilutional effect of a larger vascular compartment.[104]

HUMAN CHORIONIC GONADOTROPIN

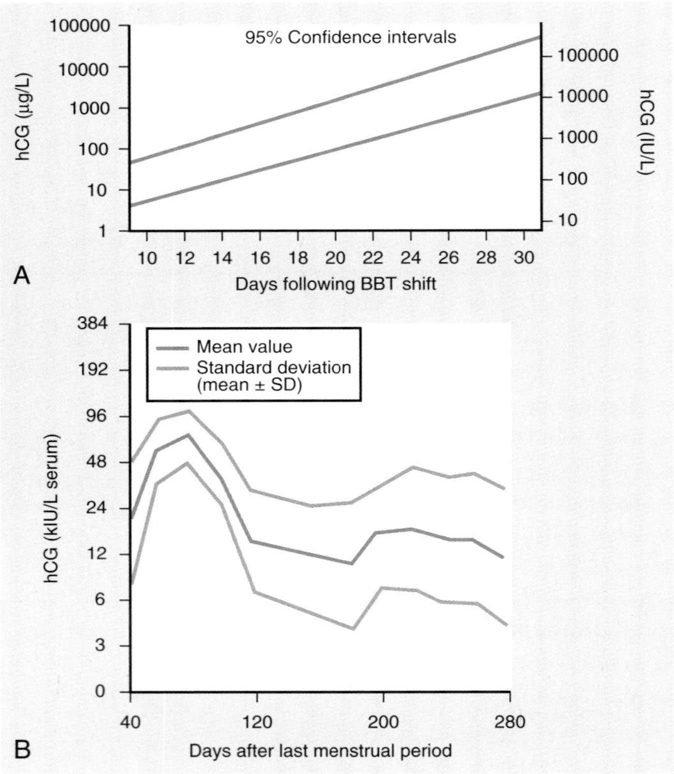

FIGURE 47
A, Serum values of the β subunit of hCG (95% CI) measured in 189 women who subsequently had successful pregnancies (total of 280 samples analyzed). The study subjects were patients in an infertility clinic and were keeping basal body temperature (BBT) charts to indicate the timing of ovulation. Some conceptions were spontaneous; other patients were treated with clomiphene citrate, human menopausal gonadotropin, or hCG (a single injection of 5000 IU to induce ovulation). A radioimmunoassay was used for β-hCG. *Data source*: ref. 105, with permission. *B*, Total serum hCG (mean ± SD) from a longitudinal study of 20 healthy women. The first samples were obtained as early in pregnancy as possible, with subsequent samples obtained every 3 to 4 weeks. The last sample was taken during labor. Samples were classified into groups, with a class interval of 30 days. Radioimmunoassay was used to obtain the hCG level; the international hCG standard was used as a reference. *Data source*: ref. 106, with permission.

Comment: The mean doubling time of β-hCG is 2.2 days ± 1.0 (2 SDs).[105] Low hCG values that do not double to within this range are associated with ectopic pregnancy or spontaneous abortion.[105] Women with male fetuses have significantly lower hCG levels than those with female fetuses.[106]

HUMAN PLACENTAL LACTOGEN

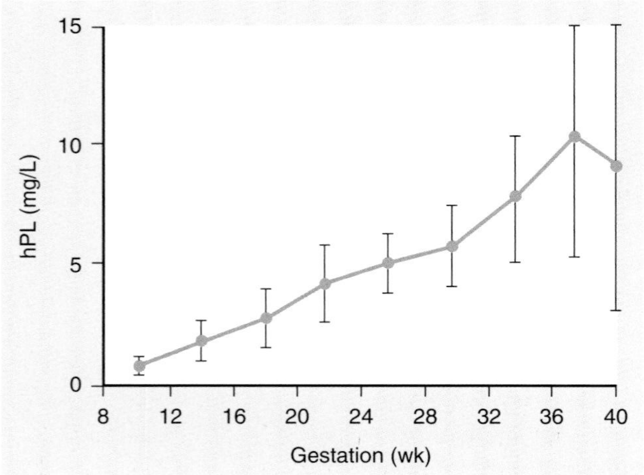

FIGURE 48
Serum human placental lactogen (hPL) values (mean ± SD) from a cross-sectional study of 151 normal women with singleton pregnancies attending an antenatal clinic. Radioimmunoassay was used to measure hPL. *Data source*: ref. 107, with permission.

Comment: In women with multiple pregnancies, hPL levels are outside these ranges; however, if values are corrected for predicted placental weight, then they are appropriate for gestational age.[107] Four hours after delivery of the placenta, plasma hPL is virtually undetectable; the half-life of hPL in the plasma is 21 to 23 minutes.[108]

ESTRIOL

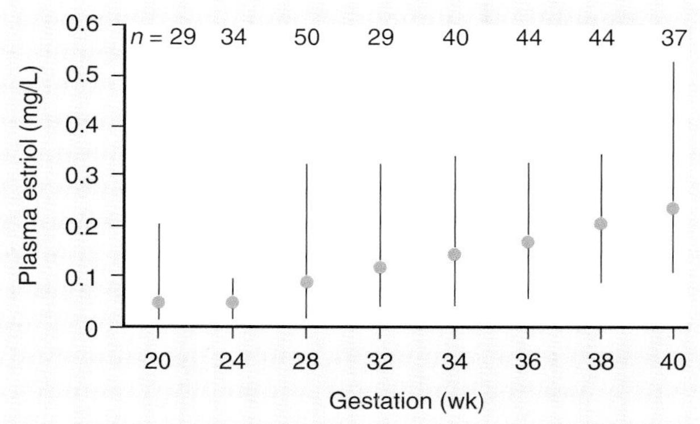

FIGURE 49
Plasma estriol (mean and range) from a cross-sectional study in women with uncomplicated pregnancies. Plasma estriol was measured fluorometrically. *Data source*: ref. 109, with permission.

Comment: The normal range of plasma estriol in pregnancy is wide. To assess the significance of values outside this range, trends should be studied over several days.

FETAL VALUES

Physiology

Early Embryonic Structures

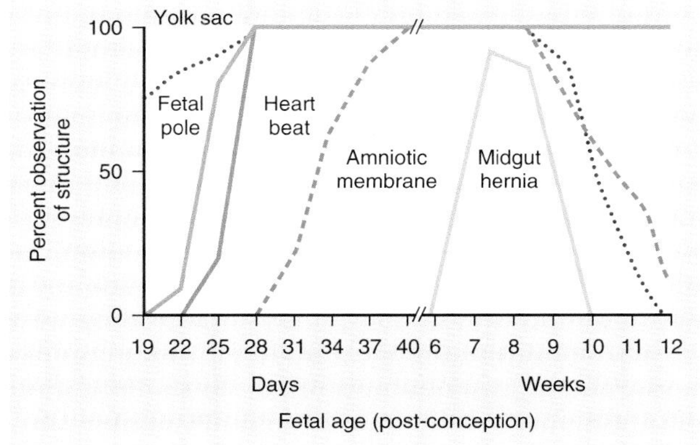

FIGURE 50
Ultrasound visualization of the yolk sac, fetal pole, heartbeat, amniotic membrane, and midgut hernia from a longitudinal study of 39 women with known dates of ovulation; most were patients from an assisted conception unit. Once pregnancy was confirmed, patients were scanned with a vaginal probe weekly, starting as early as 18 days after conception. Five subjects had twin pregnancies. *Data source*: ref. 110, with permission.

Comment: Transvaginal ultrasound scanning yields better images in the first trimester than does transabdominal scanning. By 28 days after conception, fetal viability may be confirmed by visualization of a heartbeat. The fetal heart rate increases from 90 beats/min to 145 beats/min by 7 weeks after conception.[110]

Biometry

CROWN-RUMP LENGTH

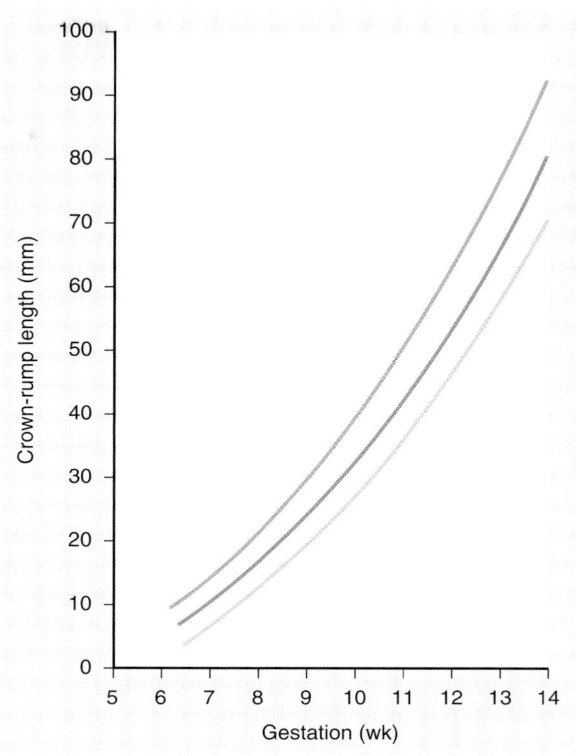

FIGURE 51
Crown-rump length (CRL) (mean ± 2 SDs) from a cross-sectional study of 334 women who were certain of the date of their last menstrual period (LMP) and had normal, regular menstrual cycles. The study covered the period from 6 to 14 weeks after the LMP. A transabdominal ultrasound technique was used, and the longest length of fetal echoes was found and measured. *Data source*: ref. 111, with permission.

Comment: CRL measurements can be used effectively only in the first trimester. Other studies found similar CRL values; measurements are not affected by maternal age, height, or parity.[112] In a smaller longitudinal study, CRL was significantly lower in female than in male fetuses.[112] No differences in CRL measurements have been found between Asian and European patients.[113]

NUCHAL TRANSLUCENCY

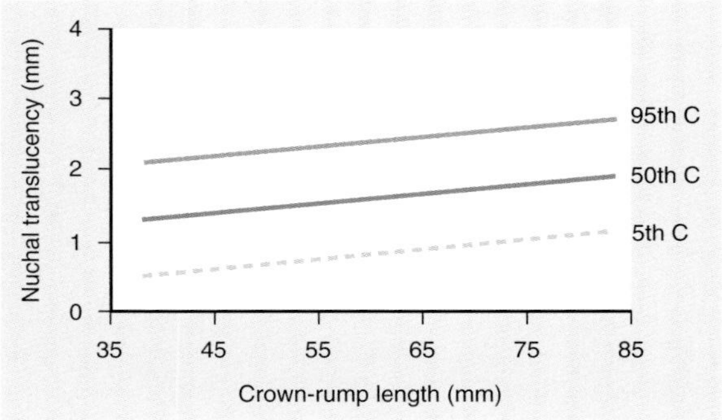

FIGURE 52
Nuchal translucency (NT) measurements (5th, 50th, and 95th percentiles) from a cross-sectional study of 20,217 chromosomally normal fetuses examined at 10 to 14 weeks' gestation. Most examinations were done with transabdominal ultrasound, and all operators were carefully trained in the technique before the study. A sagittal section of the fetus was obtained perpendicular to the ultrasound beam, allowing measurement of CRL and the maximum thickness of the subcutaneous translucency between skin and soft tissue overlying the cervical spine.114 Care was taken to avoid confusion between fetal skin and amnion, both of which appear as thin membranes. *Data source*: ref. 115, with permission.

Comment: Abnormal fluid collections in the cervical region (as shown by increased NT measurements) are strongly associated with chromosomal abnormalities. The upper limit of normal may be set at 2.5 or 3.0 mm when these measurements are used as a screening test.[115,116] However, it is preferable to use the 95th percentile of NT as plotted against CRL, because measurements increase with gestational age.[115]

BIPARIETAL DIAMETER

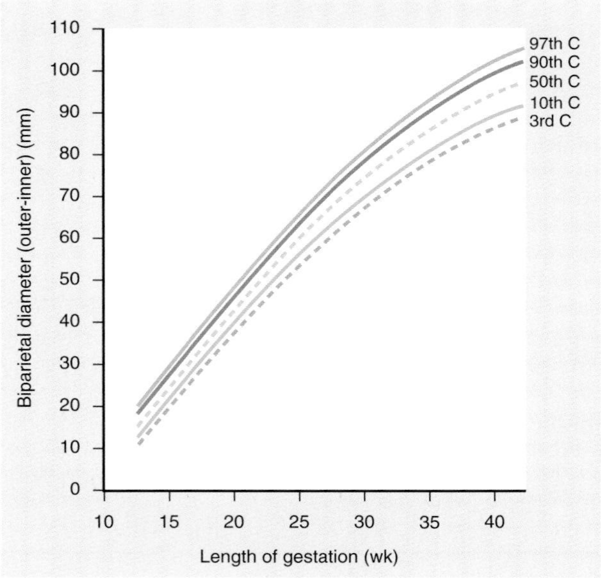

FIGURE 53
Biparietal diameter (BPD) (3rd, 10th, 50th, 90th, and 97th percentiles) of 594 fetuses from a prospective cross-sectional study of 663 women with singleton pregnancies carried out in London. Each fetus was measured only once between 12 and 42 weeks' gestation for the study. All women had certain menstrual dates, and menstrual and ultrasound ages at 18 to 22 weeks did not differ by more than 10 days. The study population consisted of 75% Western European and 25% African Caribbean women. No women had disease or used medication that was likely to affect fetal growth (e.g., diabetes, hypertension, renal disease). Measurements from 2 fetuses subsequently found to have abnormal karyotypes were excluded from the study. BPD measurements were obtained in the axial plane of the skull at the level where the continuous midline echo is broken by the cavum septum pellucidum in the anterior third. Measurements presented are those from the proximal edge of the skull closest to the transducer to the proximal edge of the deep border (i.e., outer-inner edges of bone). The statistical methods used to derive graphs and tables from the raw data are described in detail. *Data source*: refs. 117 and 118, with permission.

Comment: Other large studies are in close agreement with these measurements.[119,120] Information about growth in BPD is available from a longitudinal study.[121] Charts and graphs are also available for outer-outer BPD measurements,[118] and regression equations are given for both parameters. Racial differences in fetal measurements are likely to be found, so charts or percentile graphs appropriate for the population should be used. A small study found no significant differences between Asian and European women living in the same city.[113]

HEAD CIRCUMFERENCE

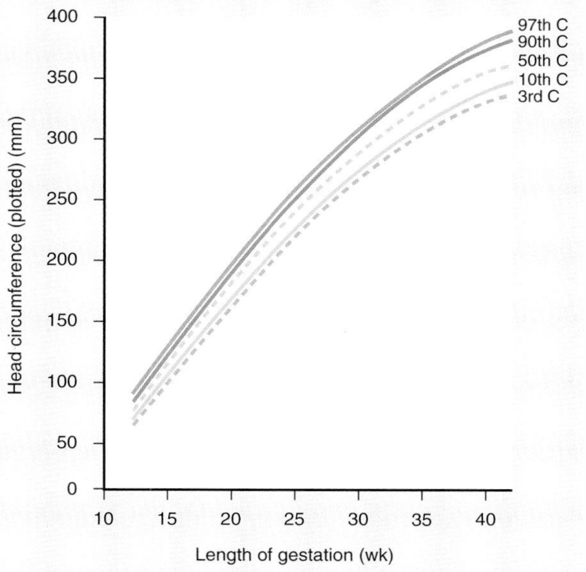

FIGURE 54
Head circumference (HC) (3rd, 10th, 50th, 90th, and 97th percentiles) from a prospective cross-sectional study of 594 fetuses, as described in Figure 53. HC was measured directly by tracing around the perimeter of the skull in the same plane used for BPD measurements. *Data source:* refs. 117 and 118, with permission.

Comment: HC measurements as derived from the BPD and the occipitofrontal diameter are also available[118,119] as well as regression equations for each parameter. Other studies yielded similar data, with some differences seen in the late third trimester.[119,122] These differences have been attributed to patient recruitment characteristics (whether only women delivering at term were included in the study) and the numbers of ultrasound operators used to collect data. HC measurements are particularly useful in the assessment of gestational age when the fetal head shape is abnormal (e.g., dolichocephaly).

ABDOMINAL CIRCUMFERENCE

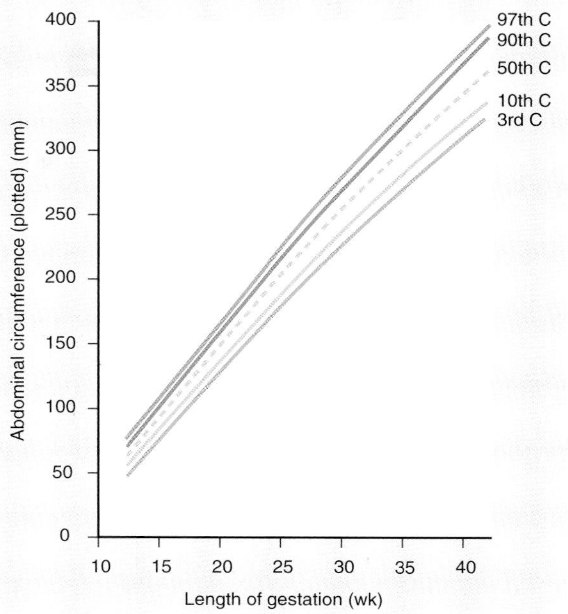

FIGURE 55
Abdominal circumference (AC) (3rd, 10th, 50th, 90th, and 97th percentiles) from 610 fetuses in the prospective cross-sectional study described in Figure 53. The fetal abdomen was measured in a transverse section, with the spine and descending aorta posterior, the umbilical vein in the anterior third, and the stomach bubble in the same plane. Care was taken to ensure that the section was as close as possible to circular, perpendicular to the spine. The circumference was measured by tracing around the perimeter. *Data source*: refs. 117 and 123, with permission.

Comment: Variability in AC increases with gestational age, as shown by widening of the percentiles. Other large studies are in close agreement[120,124,125] with these findings. Studies in which all women delivered at term did not find flattening of the growth velocity curves in late pregnancy.[126,127] Some of the discrepancies are the result of differences in mathematical curve-fitting techniques applied to the experimental data and differences in study design and the numbers of subjects and operators involved. AC is not a good indication of gestational age, but is used to assess fetal size (e.g., in relation to head and limb measurements). A method has been described[124] for assigning Z-scores to measurements, so that deviation from median values can be expressed without graphic presentation of the data. Measurements can also be compared between subjects or between the same subject at different times. Regression equations for AC, both plotted and derived from abdominal diameter measurements, are described.[123,124]

Normal Values

FEMUR LENGTH

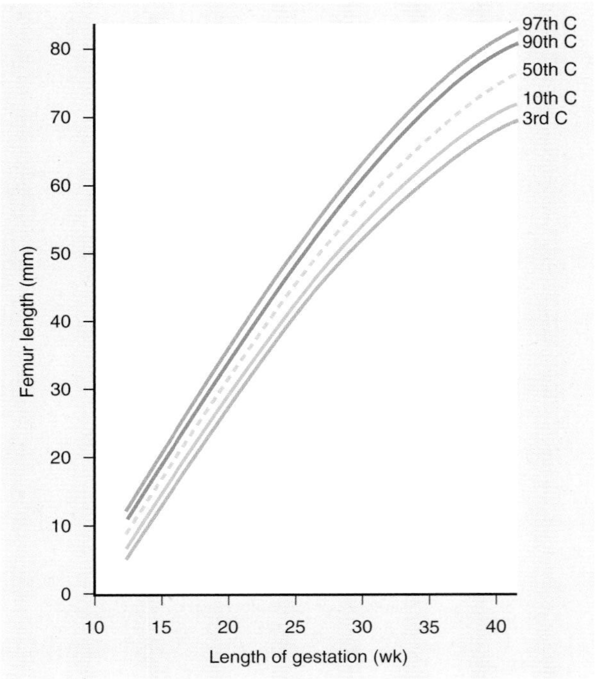

FIGURE 56
Femur length (FL) (3rd, 10th, 50th, 90th, and 97th percentiles) from 649 fetuses in the prospective cross-sectional study described in Figure 53. The femur was identified and the transducer rotated until the full femoral diaphysis was seen in a plane at almost a right angle to the ultrasound beam. The measurement was made from one end of the diaphysis to the other, disregarding curvature and ignoring the distal femoral epiphysis. *Data source*: refs. 117 and 128, with permission.

Comment: Other cross-sectional studies of FL provide similar measurements,[120,124] although one has wider percentiles in late pregnancy.[129] This difference is likely to be related to a difference in the statistical approach to the calculation of percentiles from the regression line. Regression equations are available.[120,124,128]

LIMB BONE LENGTHS

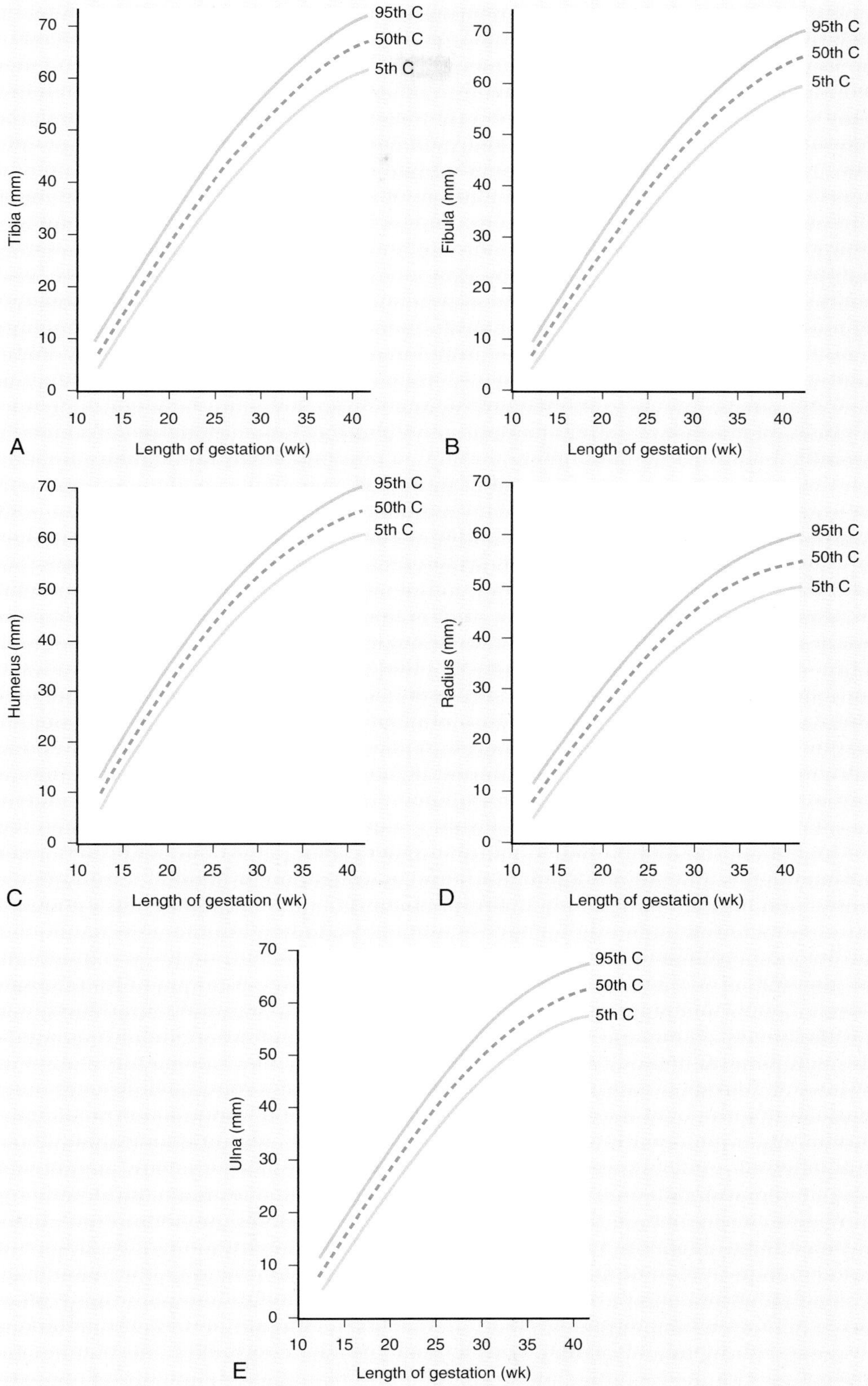

FIGURE 57
Lengths of the tibia (*A*), fibula (*B*), humerus (*C*), radius (*D*), and ulna (*E*) (5th, 50th, and 95th percentiles) from a cross-sectional study of 669 healthy women with singleton pregnancies. Women who subsequently delivered an infant with an abnormal karyotype, a significant malformation, or any other disease were excluded from the analysis. In all women, menstrual dating was certain and there was agreement between menstrual age and ultrasound dates at the time of the initial scan. Approximately 20 measurements were obtained for each parameter for each week of gestation from 12 to 42 weeks. *Data source*: ref. 130, with permission.

Comment: All limb bones show linear growth from 13 to 25 weeks' gestation; thereafter, growth is nonlinear. Other studies confirmed these findings.[131] Good agreement has been found between ultrasound and x-ray measurements of limb bone lengths. Tables are available to allow assessment of gestational age from measurement of limb bone lengths.[132] This use of limb bone measurements should be distinguished from tables or graphs of normal measurements at known gestational age that allow assessment of possible skeletal dysplasia.[130,133]

Normal Values

FOOT

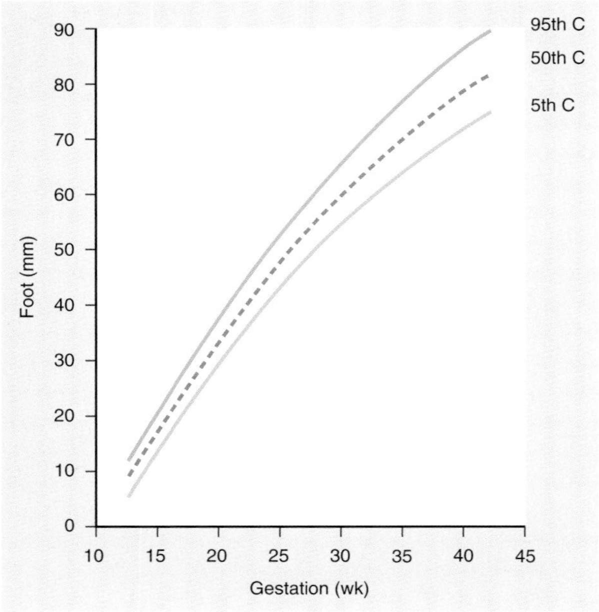

FIGURE 58
Length of the foot (5th, 50th, and 95th percentiles) from the cross-sectional study of 669 healthy women with singleton pregnancies described in Figure 57. Approximately 20 measurements were obtained for each variable for each week of pregnancy at 12 to 42 weeks' gestation. *Data source*: ref. 130, with permission.

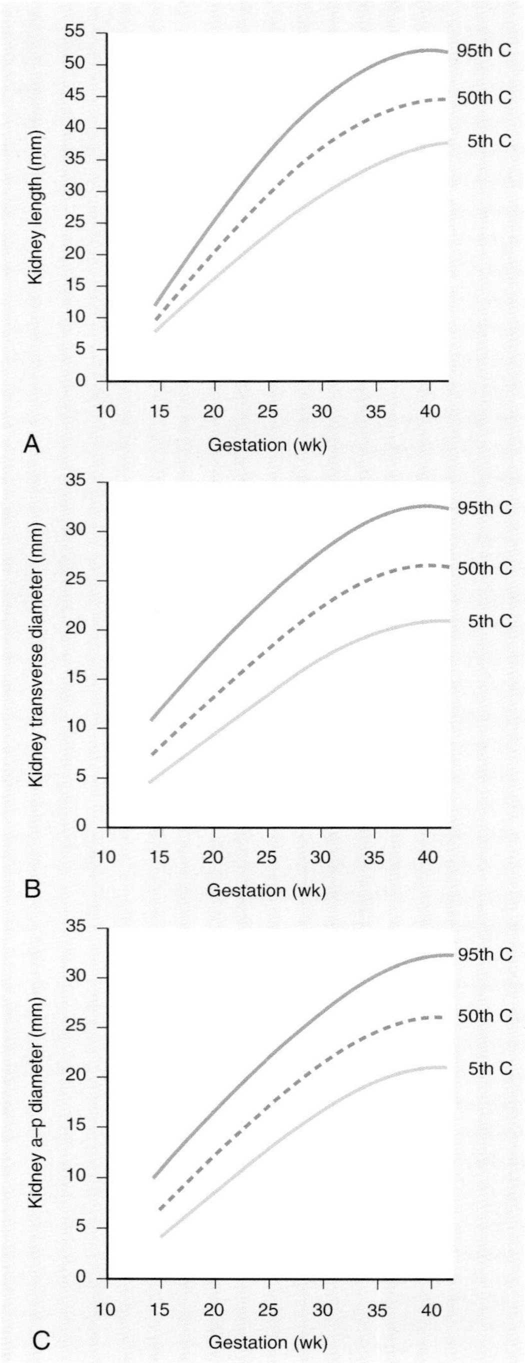

FIGURE 59
Kidney measurements: length (*A*), transverse diameter (*B*), and anteroposterior diameter (*C*) (5th, 50th, and 95th percentiles) from the cross-sectional study of 669 healthy women with singleton pregnancies described in Figure 57. Approximately 20 measurements were obtained for each variable for each week from 12 to 42 weeks' gestation. *Data source*: ref. 130, with permission.

Comment: The ratio of transverse renal circumference to AC (in a section at the level of the umbilical vein) is a simple way to assess normal kidney size. This ratio is 0.27 to 0.30 from 17 weeks' gestation until term.[134]

ORBITAL DIAMETERS

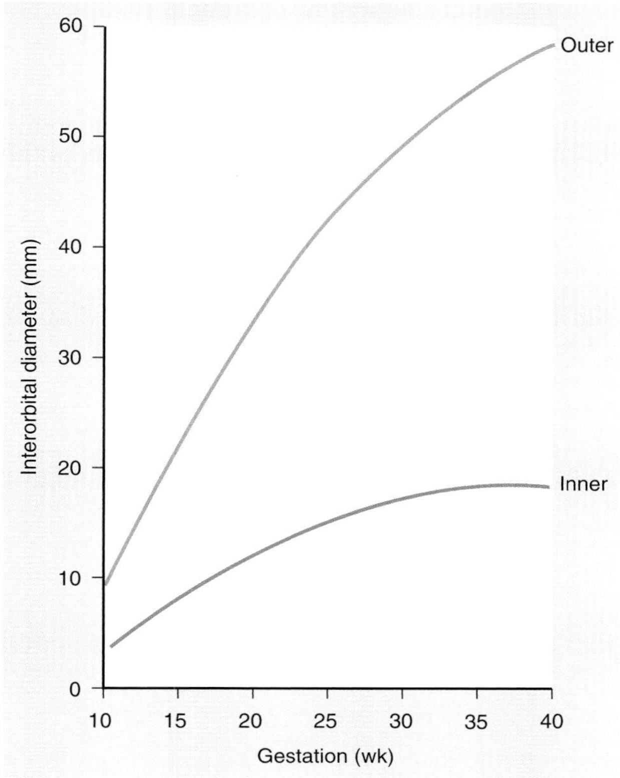

FIGURE 60
Interorbital distance (mean) from a cross-sectional study of 180 healthy women at 22 to 40 weeks' gestation. The scan plane that was used transected the occiput, orbits, and nasal processes. *Data source:* ref. 135, with permission.

> **Comment:** Outer orbital diameter is closely related to BPD. This measurement is useful when the fetal position precludes accurate measurement of BPD.

CEREBRAL VENTRICLES

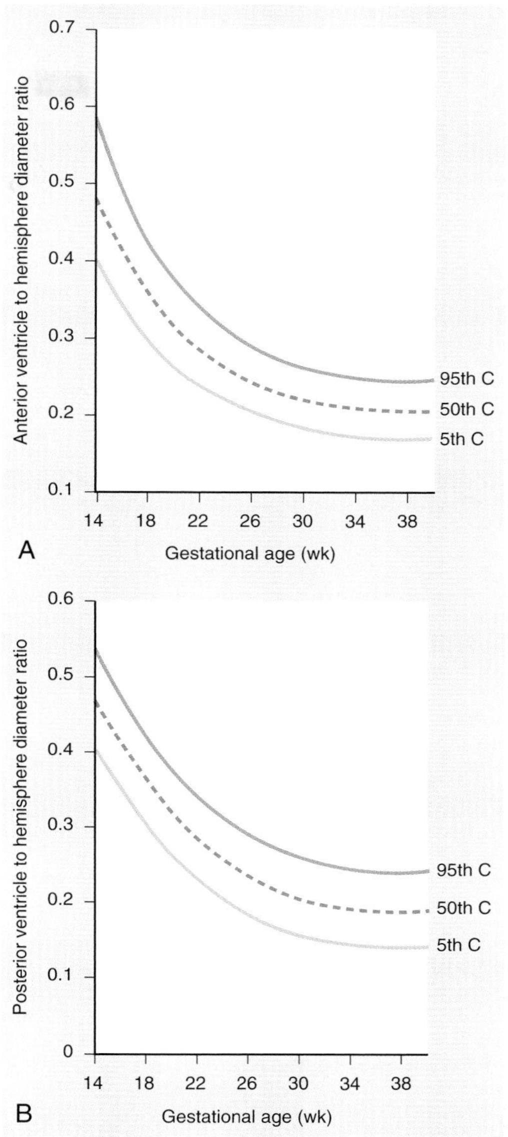

FIGURE 61
Ventriculohemispheric ratios (5th, 50th, and 95th percentiles) from a cross-sectional study of 1040 singleton pregnancies at 14 to 40 weeks' gestation, selected from a large database. All women had known LMP dates, with a cycle length of 26 to 30 days. They had no pregnancy complications. Only data from structurally normal fetuses who were liveborn at 37 weeks' gestation or more and who had birth weights between the 3rd and the 97th percentiles for gestation were included. For each week, measurements from 40 fetuses were obtained. Each fetus contributed measurements to the data pool on only one occasion. *A*, Measurement of the anterior horn of the lateral cerebral ventricle was made in a transverse axial plane of the fetal head (as for BPD or HC measurements), from the lateral wall of the anterior horn to the midline. *B*, Posterior horn measurements were made from the medial to the lateral wall of the posterior horn. Hemispheric measurements were made from the midline to the inner border of the skull. *Data source*: ref. 120, with permission.

> **Comment:** The most reliable measurements of the ventricular system are made with the frontal horns of the lateral cerebral ventricles because they are the easiest to identify. In general, ventricular diameter should be less than 10 mm.

CEREBELLUM

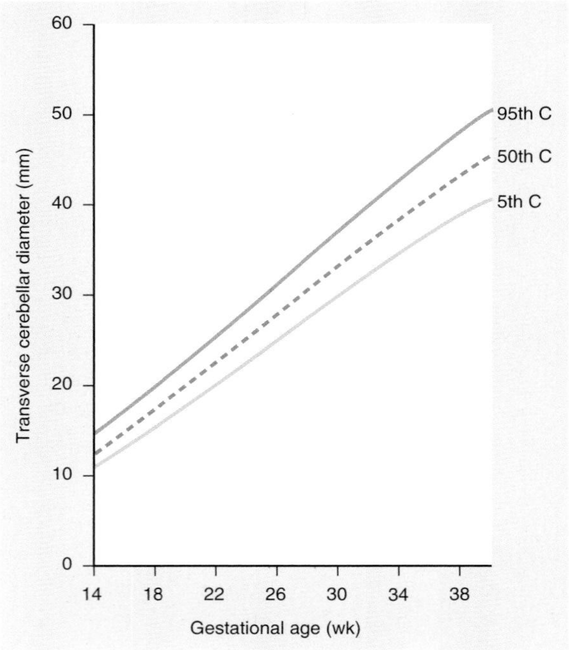

FIGURE 62
Transverse cerebellar diameter (5th, 50th, and 95th percentiles) from the cross-sectional study of 1040 singleton pregnancies described in Figure 61. Measurements were made in the suboccipitobregmatic plane of the fetal head. *Data source*: ref. 120, with permission.

Comment: The cerebellum may be visualized as early as 10 to 11 weeks' gestation. Other studies found similar measurements.[136]

OTHER FETAL MEASUREMENTS

Comment: Normal ranges for many other fetal structures are described in the literature. Each may be useful under certain circumstances. Charts of liver length are useful in the assessment of isoimmunized fetuses, in which liver length is inversely correlated with fetal Hb levels.[137] Fetal ear measurements are helpful in the detection of fetuses with abnormal karyotypes.[138,139]

BIOMETRY IN MULTIPLE GESTATIONS

Comment: A study of ultrasound measurements in twin pregnancies after 24 weeks' gestation (involving 884 sets of twins, each of whom contributed only one measurement to the data set) found that the growth pattern for FL was similar to that of singletons.[140] AC measurements in twins were lower than those in singletons after 32 weeks; BPD measurements were greater than those in singletons before 32 weeks.[140] A longitudinal study of 35 healthy women with twin pregnancies did not find clinically important differences between measurements of fetal size (HC, BPD, limb bone lengths) in twins compared with singletons.[141,142] Studies in normal triplet pregnancies found delay in growth patterns after midgestation.[143]

BIRTH WEIGHT

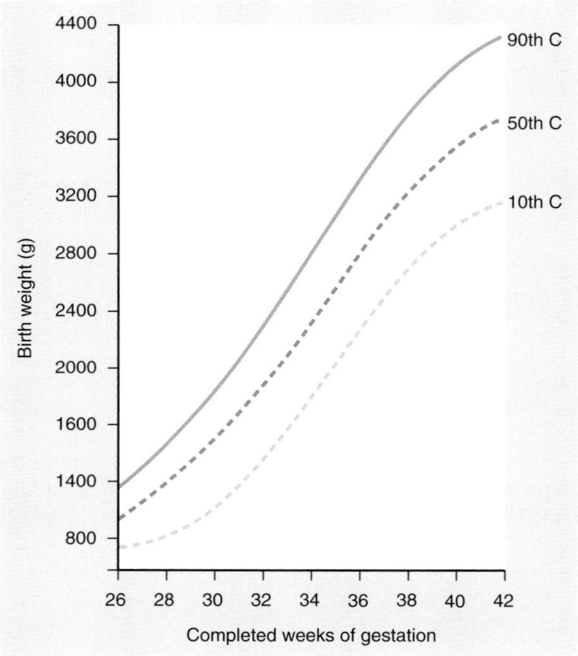

FIGURE 63
Birth weight (10th, 50th, and 90th percentiles) from an analysis of 41,718 singleton births in Nottingham, UK, between 1986 and 1991. All women had dates confirmed by ultrasound measurements (CRL up to 13 wk and BPD thereafter) before 24 weeks, and they delivered between 168 and 300 days' gestation. The population was of mixed ethnicity. *Data source*: ref. 144, with permission.

Comment: This study differs from previous reports[145,146] (which did not have ultrasound confirmation of gestational age) in that it found a continued increase, rather than flattening, of birth weight curves toward term. Birth weights of preterm infants (≤32 wk' gestation) were negatively skewed, consistent with the observation that growth-restricted infants may be born earlier than those of appropriate size.[144] Birth weight is also dependent on ethnic origin, altitude, socioeconomic factors, maternal size, birth order, and maternal cigarette smoking.[144,147,148] All of the studies described here are for singletons. Different ranges apply to multiple pregnancies.

WEIGHT ESTIMATED FROM ULTRASOUND MEASUREMENTS

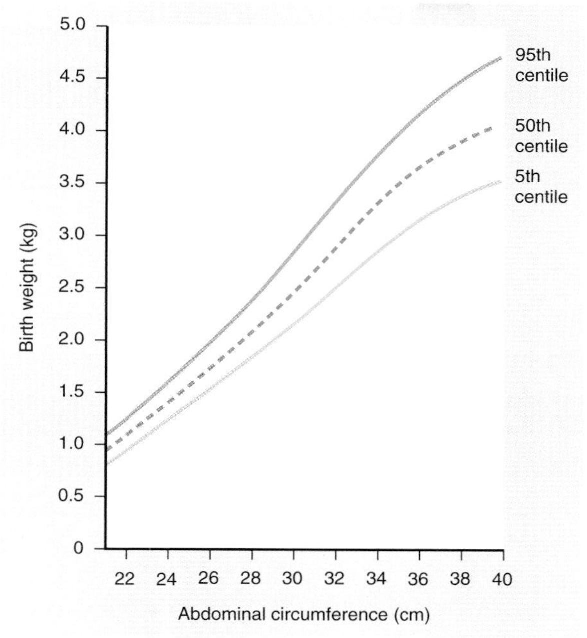

FIGURE 64
Weight estimated from ultrasound measurements (5th, 50th, and 90th percentiles) in a study of 138 women who underwent ultrasound examination within 48 hours of delivery for the measurement of fetal AC. Actual birth weights were compared with AC measurements, and a polynomial equation was derived to describe the relationship. *Data source*: ref. 149, with permission.

Comment: Equations have been derived for estimating fetal weight from various combinations of ultrasonic measurements (AC, BPD, HC, and FL).[150,151] These estimates are reported to be more accurate than those based on AC measurements alone.

Amniotic Fluid

TOTAL VOLUME

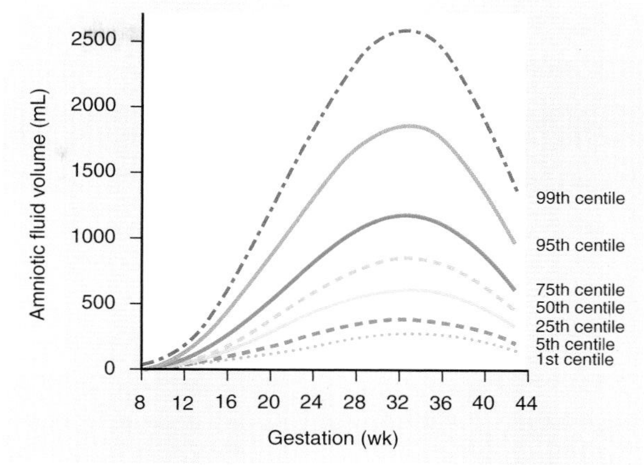

FIGURE 65
Total amniotic fluid volume (1st, 5th, 25th, 50th, 75th, 95th, and 99th percentiles). Composite analysis of 12 published reports of amniotic fluid volume in human pregnancy, totaling 705 measurements. Amniotic fluid volume was measured directly at the time of hysterotomy or indirectly with an indicator dilution technique. Only healthy pregnancies were included; any complicated by fetal death or anomaly or by maternal disease were excluded. *Data source*: ref. 152, with permission.

AMNIOTIC FLUID INDEX

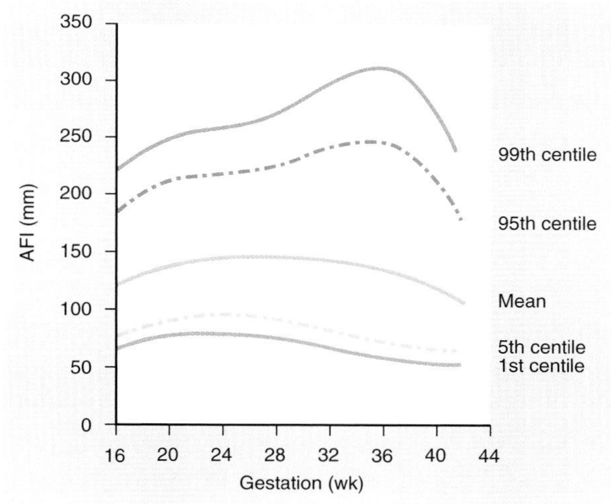

FIGURE 66
Amniotic fluid index (AFI) (1st, 5th, 50th, 95th, and 99th percentiles) from a prospective study of 791 patients. Any who did not have a normal pregnancy outcome (i.e., infant born at term, between the 10th and 90th percentiles for birth weight, with a 5-minute Apgar score greater than 6, and without congenital anomaly) were subsequently excluded. Ultrasound imaging was performed, and the uterus was divided into four quadrants along the sagittal midline and midway up the fundus. The AFI was calculated as the sum of the deepest vertical dimension (in millimeters) of the amniotic fluid pocket in each quadrant of the uterus. *Data source*: ref. 153, with permission.

Comment: The volume of amniotic fluid increases to a plateau of 700 to 850 mL between 22 and 39 weeks' gestation. This volume corresponds to an AFI of 140 to 150 mm. After term, amniotic fluid volume decreases significantly.

PRESSURE

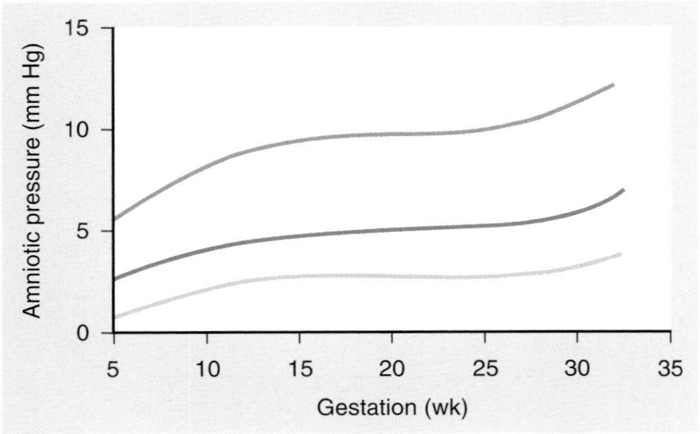

FIGURE 67
Amniotic fluid pressure (mean and 95% CI) from a cross-sectional study of 171 singleton pregnancies subsequently shown to have a normal karyotype. Amniotic fluid volume was subjectively assessed as normal, based on ultrasonic appearance. All patients were scheduled to undergo an invasive diagnostic transamniotic procedure or therapeutic termination of pregnancy. Amniotic fluid pressure was measured with a manometry technique referenced to the top of the maternal abdomen. *Data source*: ref. 154, with permission.

Comment: Amniotic fluid pressure increases with gestation, reaching a mid-trimester plateau of 4 to 5 mm Hg. Pressure was not affected by parity or maternal age and was similar in twin and singleton pregnancies.[154]

OSMOLALITY

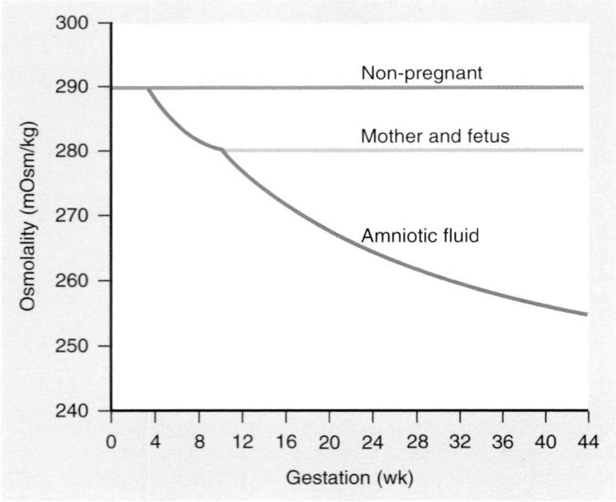

FIGURE 68
Amniotic fluid osmolality (mean) from a composite analysis of six published reports. *Data source*: ref. 155, with permission.

Comment: In early pregnancy, the composition of amniotic fluid is consistent with a transudate of maternal or fetal plasma.[156] The fetal skin becomes keratinized by midpregnancy, and amniotic fluid solute concentrations decrease as fetal urine becomes more dilute.[156] Thus, there is an osmotic gradient between amniotic fluid and both maternal and fetal plasma.

Cardiac Dimensions

CARDIAC CIRCUMFERENCE

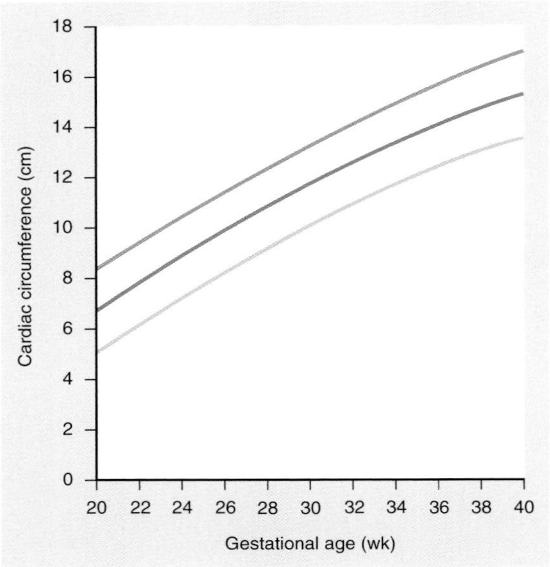

FIGURE 69
Cardiac circumference (mean and 95% CI) from a longitudinal study of 45 healthy women with known menstrual dates that were confirmed by early ultrasound scan. Study subjects were recruited before 20 weeks' gestation and underwent scanning every 4 weeks. Fetal cardiac and thoracic circumference were measured in a transverse plane through the chest, at the level of the four-chamber view of the fetal heart. *Data source*: ref. 157, with permission.

Comment: The cardiac-to-thoracic circumference ratio is normally approximately 0.5 (95% CI at 20 wk, 0.40–0.58; at 30 wks, 0.44–0.60; at 40 wk, 0.46–0.65).[157]

VENTRICULAR DIMENSIONS

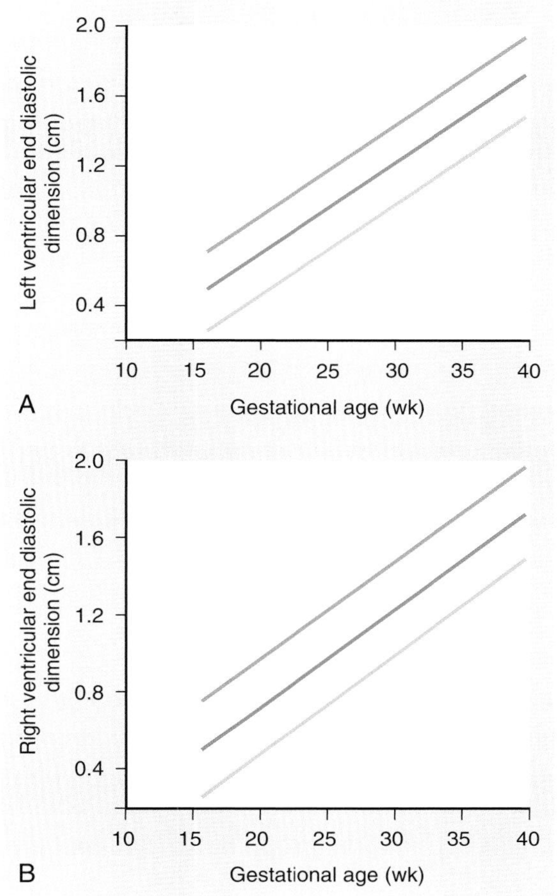

FIGURE 70
End-diastolic dimensions of the left ventricle (*A*) and the right ventricle (*B*) (regression line and 95% prediction interval) from a cross-sectional study of 117 normal women at 16 to 41 weeks' gestation. All fetuses were anatomically normal, and gestational age was confirmed by first-trimester ultrasound measurements. A four-chamber view of the heart was obtained in a transverse plane through the fetal chest. The transducer was adjusted so that the intraventricular septum was perpendicular to the ultrasound beam. In this view, transverse endocardial-endocardial dimensions of both ventricles were measured just below the valves, at the end of diastole. *Data source*: ref. 158, with permission.

Comment: This study found narrower CIs for cardiac measurements than those described in earlier reports.[159] This finding was attributed to improved resolution of newer ultrasound equipment and the use of imaging planes perpendicular to the ultrasound plane (which reduces lateral resolution error). Close correlation was seen between measurements made by two observers in this study.

VENTRICULAR AND SEPTAL WALL THCKNESS

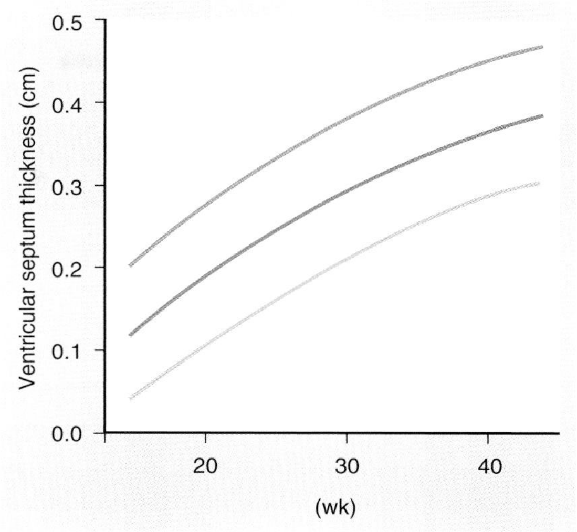

FIGURE 71
Thickness of the interventricular septum (regression line and 95% CI) from a study with cross-sectional and longitudinal data ($n = 100$ observations). Subjects were healthy and had their menstrual dates confirmed by ultrasound measurements; all subsequently were delivered at term. Interventricular septal thickness was measured in the four-chamber view of the fetal heart, just below the atrioventricular valves. *Data source*: ref. 159, with permission.

Comment: The thickness of the left or right ventricular wall is similar to that of the interventricular septum.

ASCENDING AORTA AND PULMONARY ARTERY DIAMETER

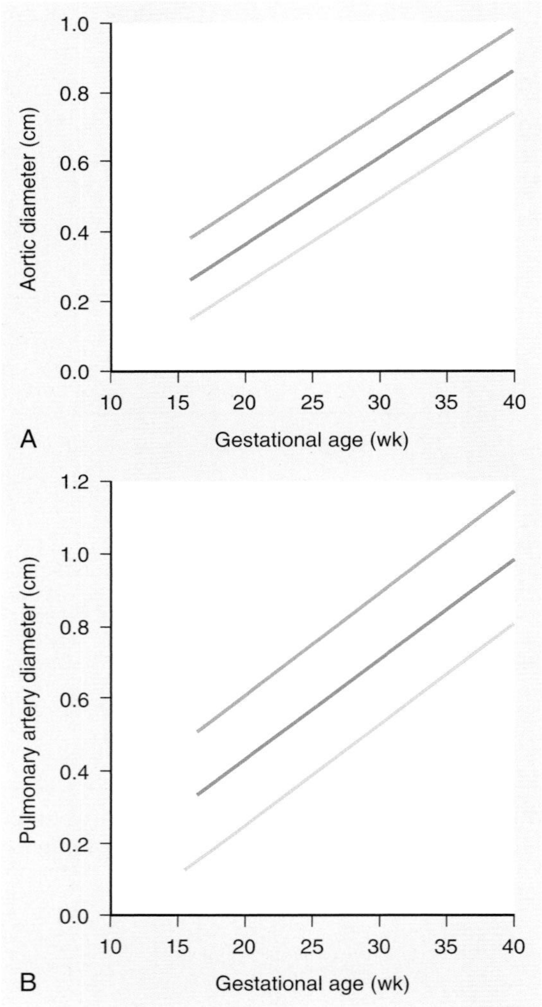

FIGURE 72
Diameter of the ascending aorta (*A*) and the main pulmonary artery (*B*) (regression line and 95% prediction interval) from a cross-sectional study of 117 fetuses at 16 to 41 weeks' gestation, as described in Figure 70. The aorta was measured in a long-axis view of the heart, found by moving cephalad from the four-chamber view. Measurements were made between intimal surfaces when the aorta had been aligned perpendicular to the ultrasound beam, just above the sinuses of Valsalva. The main pulmonary artery was measured in a long-axis view, with its vessel walls perpendicular to the ultrasound beam. *Data source*: ref. 158, with permission.

Comment: During intrauterine life, the diameter of the pulmonary artery is slightly larger than that of the aorta. It may not be possible to obtain good views of these vessels in the planes described. However, similar values were reported in other studies in which measurements were made in different scan planes.[159]

Cardiovascular Doppler Indices

DUCTUS VENOSUS

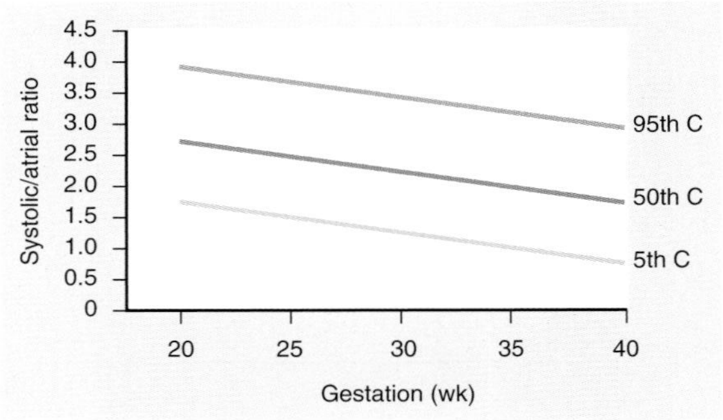

FIGURE 73
Systolic-to-atrial ratio (5th, 50th, and 95th percentiles) from ductus venosus Doppler flow velocity waveforms recorded in a cross-sectional study of 164 fetuses at 16 to 42 weeks' gestation. Fetal size was appropriate for gestational age, and no structural or chromosomal abnormalities were reported. Velocity waveforms were recorded from the ductus venosus at its origin from the umbilical vein, as visualized in a transverse section of the fetal abdomen with color and pulsed Doppler recordings. The angle of insonation of the vessel was kept low; recordings in which this angle exceeded 20 degrees were rejected. Ductus venosus waveforms were recognized by their characteristic biphasic pattern. The ratio between peak systolic velocity and velocity during atrial contraction (nadir of the waveform) was calculated. *Data source*: ref. 160, with permission.

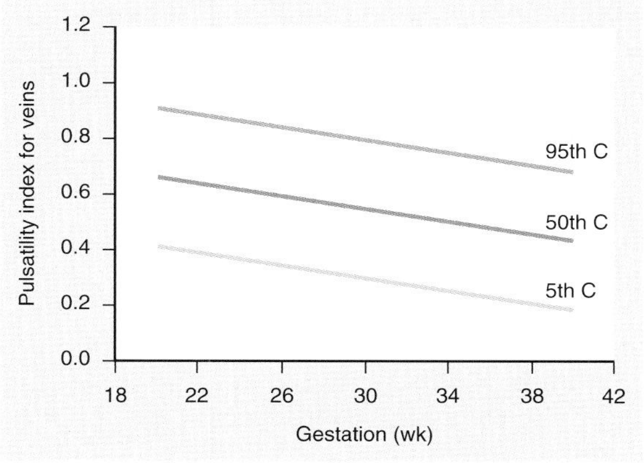

FIGURE 74
Pulsatility index for veins from the ductus venosus (5th, 50th, and 95th percentiles) from a cross-sectional study of 143 women with singleton pregnancies at 20 to 40 weeks' gestation. All fetuses were anatomically normal. Gestational age was calculated from menstrual history and confirmed by fetal measurements made at 20 weeks' amenorrhea. At the time of the study, measurements of fetal head and AC were within the 90% CI for gestational age. Movements, amniotic fluid volume, and umbilical artery Doppler pulsatility index were also normal. All measurements were made in the absence of fetal breathing movements. Flow velocity waveforms were recorded from the ductus venosus and visualized in an oblique transverse plane through the upper abdomen or in a midsagittal longitudinal plane. Good signals were obtained from 134 cases. The pulsatility index for veins was calculated as (peak systolic velocity – minimum atrial velocity/time-averaged maximum velocity). *Data source*: ref. 161, with permission.

Comment: Color-flow mapping Doppler equipment is necessary for correct identification of the ductus venosus. Waveforms from the intrahepatic portion of the umbilical vein and the inferior vena cava are different. The decreasing systolic-to-atrial ratio is interpreted as indicating a relative increase in blood flow during end-diastole (i.e., improved cardiac filling).

INFERIOR VENA CAVA

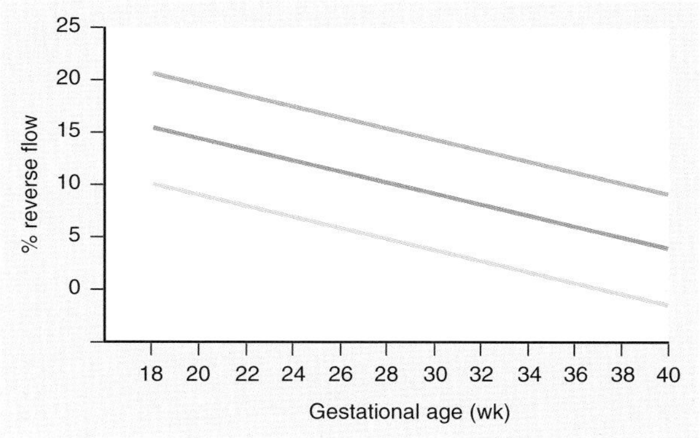

FIGURE 75
Percentage of reverse flow from the inferior vena cava (mean and linear regression of the 95th CI) from a cross-sectional study of 118 appropriate-for-gestational age fetuses at 18 to 40 weeks' gestation. All pregnancies were singleton and were dated by certain LMP and early second-trimester ultrasonography. All fetuses were structurally normal and of appropriate size for gestation at the time of study. Flow velocity waveforms were recorded with color and pulsed Doppler equipment from the inferior vena cava, which was identified in a sagittal view of the fetal trunk between the entrance of the renal vein and the ductus venosus. Measurements were made in the absence of fetal body or breathing movements. Three components of the waveform were identified: systolic peak (S), diastolic wave (D), and reverse flow during atrial contraction (A). The percentage of reverse flow was calculated as the percentage of the time-velocity intervals during the A-wave, with respect to the total forward time-velocity intervals (S + D). *Data source*: ref. 162, with permission.

Normal Values

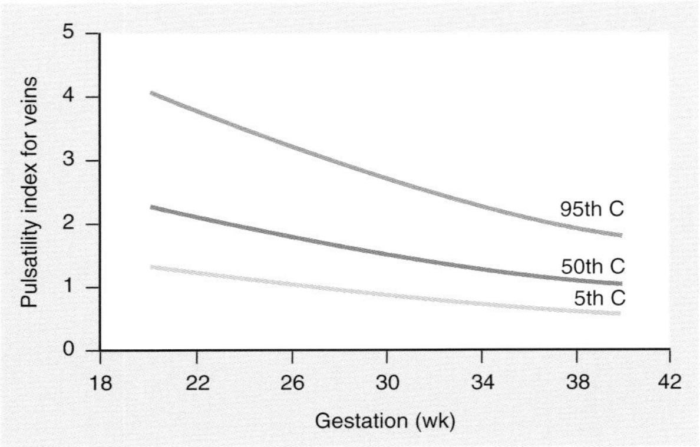

FIGURE 76
Pulsatility index for veins from the inferior vena cava (5th, 50th, and 95th percentiles) from the cross-sectional study of 143 women described in Figure 74. Flow velocity waveforms were recorded from the inferior vena cava in a longitudinal section of the fetal abdomen, with the sample volume placed in the portion between the renal and the hepatic veins. Clear signals were obtained from 127 fetuses. The pulsatility index for veins was calculated as (peak systolic velocity – minimum atrial velocity/ time-averaged maximum velocity). *Data source*: ref. 161, with permission.

Comment: Flow velocity waveforms in the inferior vena cava are characteristically triphasic, with reverse velocities found during atrial contraction. These reverse velocities decrease significantly with advancing gestation. This decrease is attributed to a decrease in the pressure gradient between the right atrium and the right ventricle at end-diastole as a result of improved ventricular compliance and reduced end-diastolic pressure. Right ventricular afterload declines with decreasing placental resistance, contributing to the reduction in end-diastolic pressure. In studies in which Doppler waveforms were recorded from the inferior vena cava and ductus venosus in growth-restricted fetuses before cordocentesis, fetal hypoxemia and acidemia were associated with more reverse flow and more pulsatile waveforms.[163,164]

CARDIAC FUNCTION

Comment: Normal ranges have been defined for Doppler flow velocity waveform indices derived from across the mitral, tricuspid, aortic, and pulmonary valves.[161,165,166] These have potential use in the assessment of cardiac function in growth-restricted fetuses and fetuses with structural heart defects. Waveforms from the ductus arteriosus show considerable individual variability[167] and do not appear to be useful in the detection of fetal compromise. Waveforms from peripheral pulmonary arteries show decreasing pulsatility with advancing gestation in healthy fetuses.[168]

CARDIAC OUTPUT

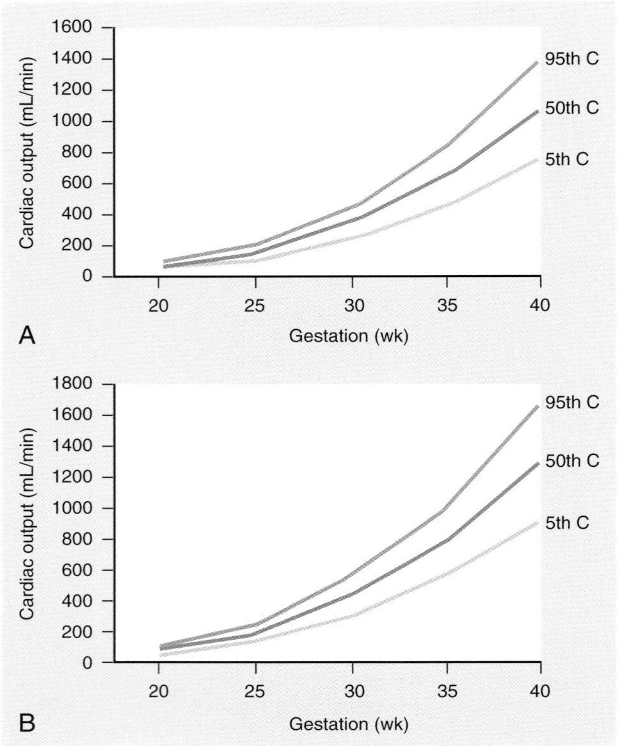

FIGURE 77
Left cardiac output (LCO) (*A*) and right cardiac output (RCO) (*B*) calculated at the level of the outflow tracts (5th, 50th, and 95th percentiles) from a longitudinal study of 26 healthy singleton fetuses studied at weekly intervals. Velocity waveforms were recorded from the ascending aorta and pulmonary artery with the flow parallel to the Doppler beam. Recordings obtained with a beam angle greater than 20 degrees were rejected. Valve diameter measurements were made from videotape images, and valve areas were calculated by assuming a circular cross-section. *Data source*: ref. 165, with permission.

Comment: Cardiac output rises progressively with gestation, with RCO slightly higher than LCO (RCO/LCO ratio ~1.3). Peak flow velocity at both the aortic and the pulmonary valves increases with gestation. This increase is attributed to progressive improvement in cardiac contractility, reduction in afterload, and increase in preload.[165] This type of calculation of volume flow is susceptible to high coefficients of variation because an error in the measurement of diameter (e.g., valve ring diameter) is magnified as the cross-sectional area is computed.

MIDDLE CEREBRAL ARTERY

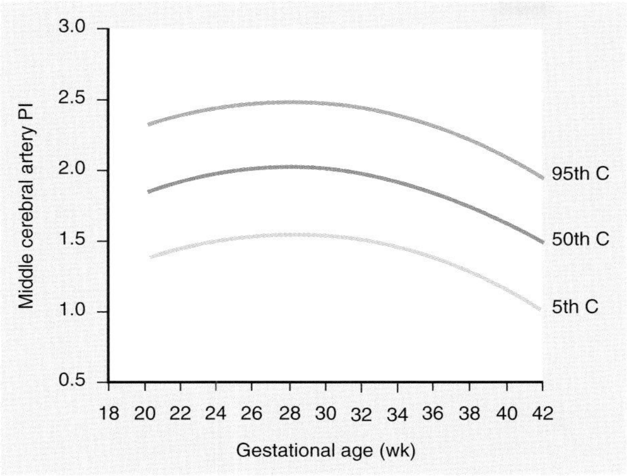

FIGURE 78
Pulsatility index from the middle cerebral artery (MCA) (5th, 50th, and 95th percentiles) from a cross-sectional study of 1556 fetuses at 20 to 42 weeks gestation. All fetuses were singletons, and gestational age was confirmed by early ultrasound measurement of CRL. Color-flow imaging was used to identify the fetal MCA, and waveforms were recorded at a low angle of insonation. Good signals were obtained from 1467 fetuses. Pulsatility index was calculated (maximum systolic velocity – diastolic velocity/mean velocity). *Data source*: ref. 169, with permission.

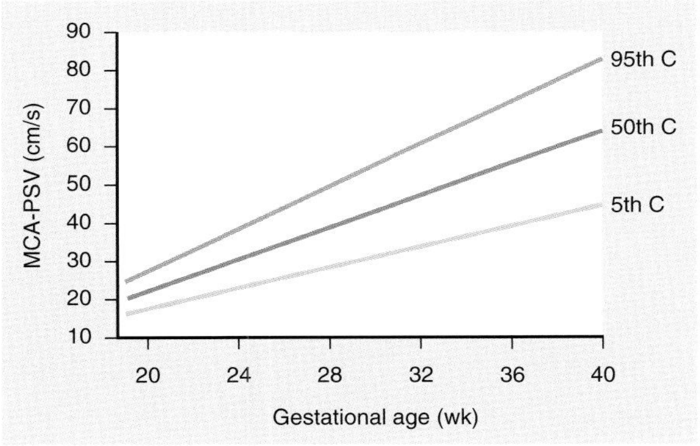

FIGURE 79
Peak systolic velocity from the MCA (5th, 50th, and 95th percentiles) from a cross-sectional study of 331 women at 19 to 40 weeks' gestation. All fetuses were singletons, and none of the pregnancies was complicated by blood group antibodies, hypertension, diabetes, or congenital abnormalities. Only one measurement from each fetus was included in the study. The MCA was identified in an axial section of the fetal brain and insonated at a low angle. The highest point on the waveform (peak systolic velocity) was measured. *Data source*: ref. 170, with permission.

Comment: A longitudinal study of MCA Doppler waveforms found that pulsatility index values are higher at 25 to 30 weeks' gestation than those at 15 to 20 weeks, or toward term.[171] Diameter of the fetal MCA increases with gestational age. In one study, calculated volume blood flow in the artery increased from 23 mL/min at 19 weeks' gestation to 133 mL/min at term.[172] Doppler waveforms from the MCA may also be quantitated with a resistance index (maximum systolic velocity – minimum diastolic velocity/systolic velocity).[173] When MCA waveforms are recorded, care must be taken to apply minimal pressure to the maternal abdomen because fetal skull compression may alter MCA flow.[174] Different signals are obtained in the distal portion of the MCA, and most studies have concentrated on the proximal portion, close to the circle of Willis.[175] Changes in MCA Doppler waveforms are noted in growth-restricted fetuses, suggesting that fetal cardiac output may be redistributed to preserve brain blood.[171,174,175] High MCA peak systolic velocities are associated with fetal anemia in pregnancies complicated by maternal alloimmunization.[176,177]

DESCENDING AORTA

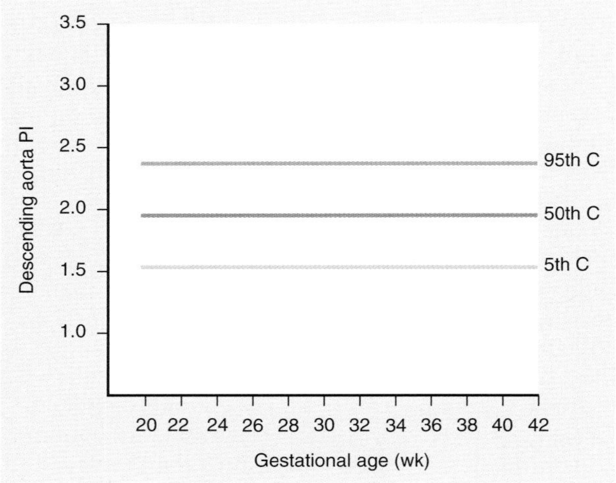

FIGURE 80
Descending aorta pulsatility index (5th, 50th, and 95th percentiles) from a cross-sectional study of 1556 healthy pregnancies at 20 to 42 weeks' gestation. All fetuses were singletons, and gestational age was confirmed by early ultrasound measurement of CRL. Recordings from the thoracic portion of the descending aorta were made in the absence of fetal body or breathing movements. Satisfactory recordings were obtained in 1398 fetuses. The pulsatility index was calculated (systolic velocity – diastolic velocity/mean velocity). *Data source*: ref. 169, with permission.

> **Comment:** Unlike in other fetal vessels, no significant change with gestation was seen in the aortic pulsatility index.

UMBILICAL ARTERY

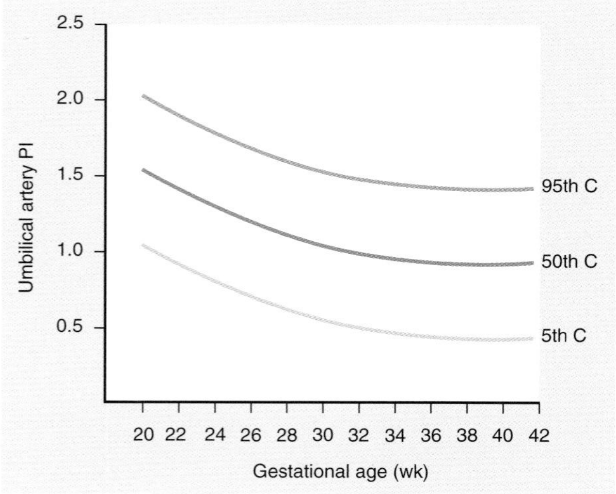

FIGURE 81
Umbilical artery pulsatility index (5th, 50th, and 95th percentiles) from a cross-sectional study of 1556 healthy pregnancies at 20 to 42 weeks' gestation. All fetuses were singletons, and gestational age was confirmed by early ultrasound measurement of CRL. Recordings from the umbilical artery were made in the absence of fetal body or breathing movements. The pulsatility index was calculated (systolic velocity – diastolic velocity/mean velocity). *Data source*: ref. 169, with permission.

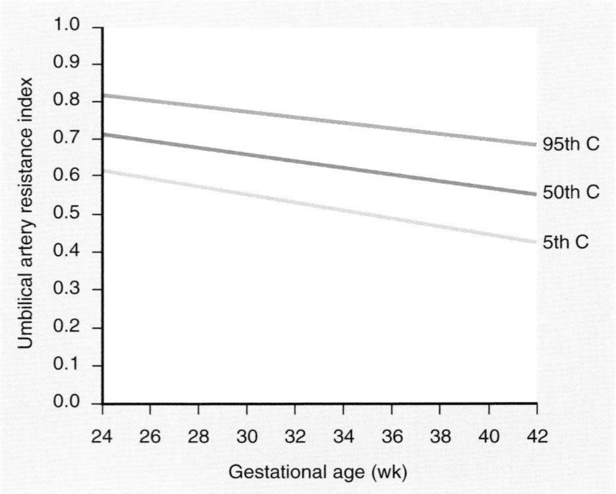

FIGURE 82
Umbilical artery resistance index (5th, 50th, and 95th percentiles) from a cross-sectional study of 1675 pregnancies at 24 to 42 weeks' gestation. Each fetus contributed only one measurement to the study. Signals were recorded from a free-floating loop in the middle of the umbilical cord. Resistance (Pourcelot) index was calculated (systolic diastolic velocity/ systolic velocity). *Data source*: ref. 173, with permission.

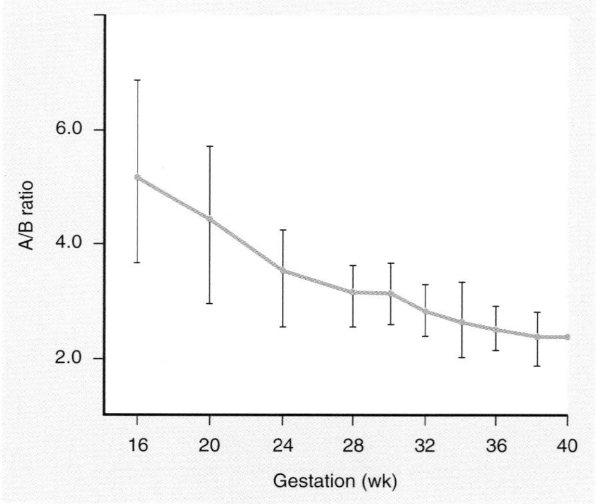

FIGURE 83
Systolic-to-diastolic ratio (A/B ratio) calculated from umbilical artery flow velocity waveforms (mean ± 2 SDs) obtained in a longitudinal study of 15 normal pregnancies. Study subjects were scanned every 2 weeks, from 24 to 28 weeks' gestation until delivery. Eight of the study subjects had been recruited at 16 weeks and were also scanned every 4 weeks throughout the second trimester. In all subjects, gestational age was confirmed by ultrasound scanning at 16 weeks' gestation. A range-gated pulsed Doppler beam was guided from the ultrasound image to insonate the umbilical artery. *Data source*: ref. 178, with kind permission from Elsevier Science Ireland Ltd, Co. Clare, Ireland.

> **Comment:** After 16 weeks' gestation, forward flow occurs in umbilical arteries throughout the cardiac cycle, as evidenced by positive Doppler shift frequencies, even at the end of diastole. Decreasing values for the resistance index, pulsatility index, and A/B ratio with gestation are interpreted as indicating decreasing resistance in the placental circulation.

FETAL-PLACENTAL DOPPLER RATIOS

Comment: Various ratios have been suggested to compare fetal cerebral flow velocity waveforms with those from the umbilical artery or aorta. These waveforms may be useful in detecting alterations in fetal cardiac output distribution (e.g., in response to fetal hypoxemia ["brain-sparing" effect]). The placentocerebral ratio[173] describes resistance indices from the umbilical artery and MCA. The cerebroplacental ratio[179] describes resistance indices from the MCA and umbilical artery. The umbilical artery–to–MCA ratio[169] describes pulsatility indices from the umbilical artery and MCA. The descending thoracic aorta–to–MCA ratio[169] describes pulsatility indices from the descending thoracic aorta and MCA.

Cardiovascular and Behavioral Parameters

UMBILICAL VENOUS PRESSURE

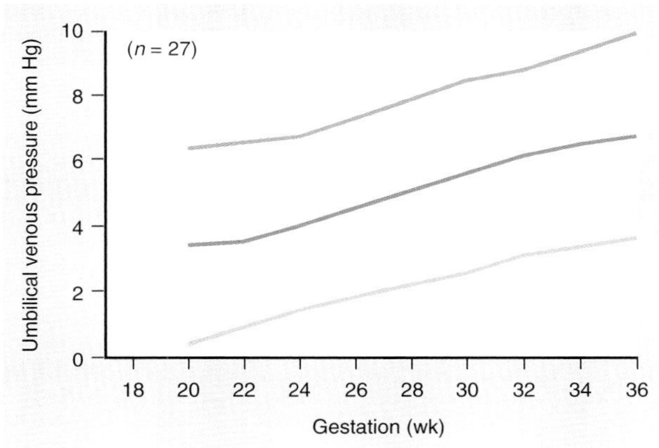

FIGURE 84
Umbilical venous pressure (mean and 95% CI) from 27 fetuses referred for assessment of possible intrauterine infection or hemolysis, but subsequently shown to be unaffected. All of the fetuses underwent cordocentesis. After the necessary blood samples were obtained, the needle was connected to a pressure transducer. The transducer was placed at the level of the fetal heart, and the pressure was read at its nadir. The needle was confirmed to be in the umbilical vein by the nonpulsatile pressure tracing that was obtained and by observing the direction of flow of injected saline. As the needle was withdrawn, pressure in the amniotic cavity was recorded. Umbilical venous pressure was calculated by subtracting the amniotic pressure from the measured umbilical venous pressure. *Data source*: ref. 180, with permission.

Comment: Umbilical venous pressure increases with advancing gestation, but remains within a narrow range. Values above the CI are associated with cardiac failure.[181]

MEAN UMBILICAL ARTERIAL PRESSURE

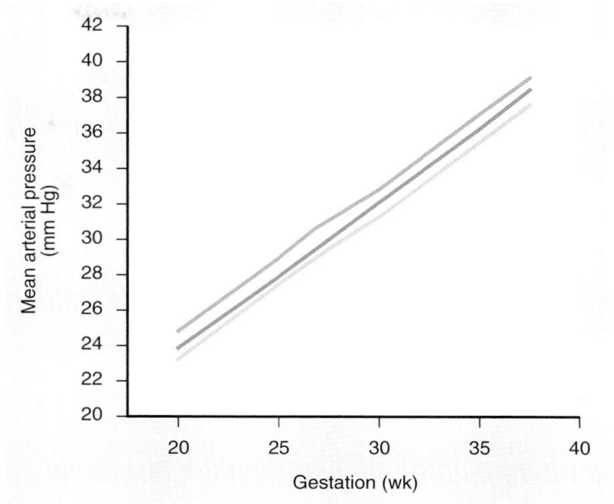

FIGURE 85
Mean umbilical arterial pressure (mean and 95% CI) from 30 normal fetuses referred for assessment of possible infection or hemolysis, but found to be unaffected. The method was identical to that described in Figure 67. It was apparent that the needle tip was in an umbilical artery rather than a vein (because of a pulsatile pressure signal). *Data source*: ref. 182, with permission.

Comment: The normal range of arterial pressure in the fetus is much narrower than the range of umbilical venous pressure. Arterial pressure increases with gestational age.

FETAL HEART RATE

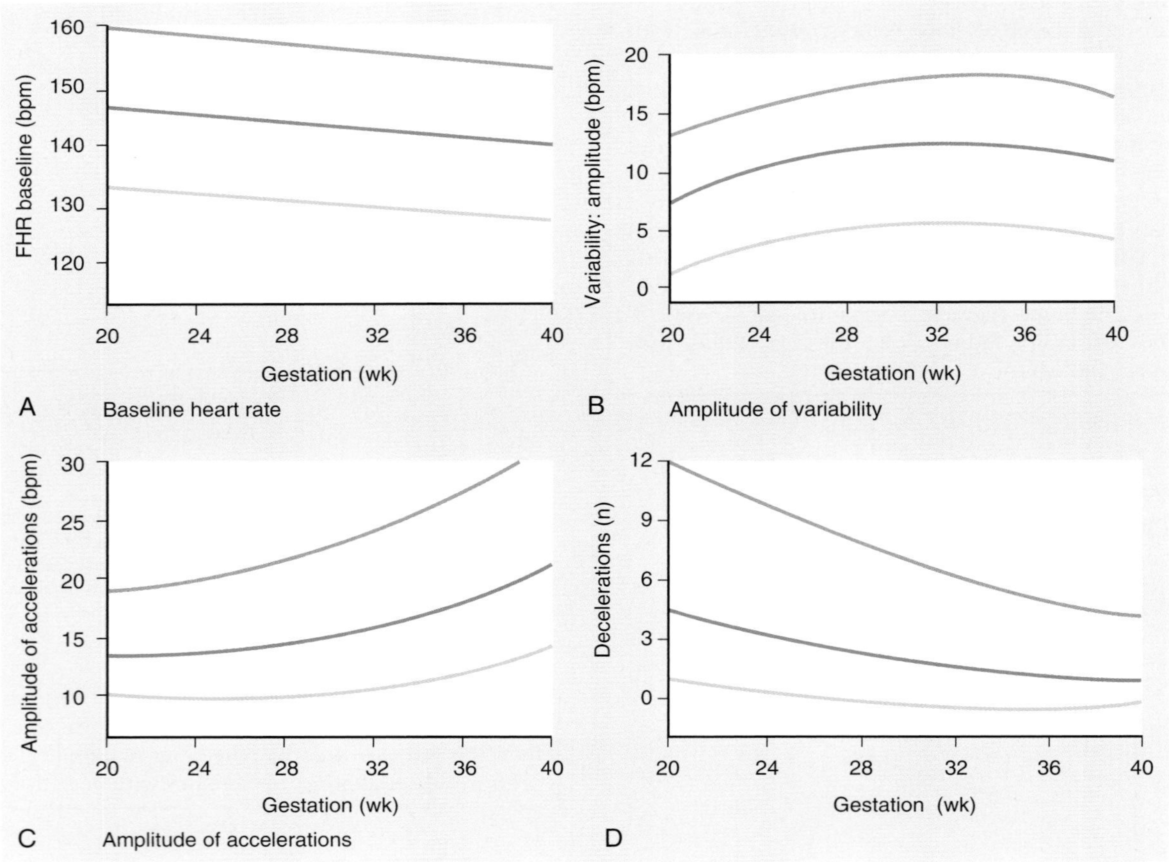

FIGURE 86
Fetal heart rate (FHR) parameters (mean and 95% CI) showing the baseline heart rate (*A*), the amplitude of variability (*B*), the amplitude of accelerations (*C*), and the number of decelerations (*D*). Data were obtained from a cross-sectional study of 119 pregnancies at 20 to 39 weeks' gestation. Study subjects were referred for prenatal diagnosis by cordocentesis. In all cases, fetal blood gas values, Hb, and karyotype were subsequently shown to be normal. None of the fetuses had hydrops fetalis or a cardiac defect. FHR monitoring was performed immediately before cordocentesis for 30 minutes, and tracings were examined for baseline heart rate, variability, accelerations, and decelerations. *Data source*: ref. 183, with permission from S Karger AG, Basel.

- At least two accelerations (>15 beats for >15 s) in 20 min, baseline heart rate 110–150 bpm, baseline variability 5–25 bpm, absence of decelerations.
- Sporadic decelerations amplitude <40 bpm are acceptable if duration <15 s, or <30 s following an deacceleration.
- When there is moderate tachycardia (150–170 bpm) or bradycardia (100–110 bpm) a reactive trace is reassuring of good health.

FIGURE 87
Features of a normal antepartum cardiotocogram (nonstress test). *Data source*: ref. 184, with permission.

Comment: Baseline FHR decreases with gestation, but the variability of the baseline increases. The number and amplitude of accelerations increase with gestation. Spontaneous decelerations are common in the second and early third trimesters, but rarely in healthy fetuses approaching term. Definitions of the features of normal and abnormal cardiotocograms are available.[185] During labor, criteria for the interpretation of FHR tracings are different (see Fig. 105).

BIOPHYSICAL PROFILE SCORE

Fetal variable	Normal behavior (score = 2)	Abnormal behavior (score = 0)
Fetal breathing movements	More than one episode of 30 s duration, intermittent within a 30 min overall period. Hiccups count. (Not continuous throughout the observation time)	Repetitive or continuous breathing without cessation. Completely absent breathing or no sustained episodes
Gross body/limb movements	Three or more discrete body/limb movements in a 30 min period. Continuous active movement episodes are considered as a single movement. Also included are fine motor movements, positional adjustments and so on.	Two or fewer body/limb movements in a 30 min observation period
Fetal tone and posture	Demonstration of active extension with rapid return of flexion of fetal limbs, brisk repositioning/trunk rotation. Opening and closing of hand, mouth, kicking, etc.	Only low-velocity movements, incomplete return to flexion, flaccid extremity positions; abnormal fetal posture. Includes score = 0 when FM absent
Fetal heart rate reactivity	Greater than 2 significant accelerations associated with maternally palpated fetal movement during a 20 min cardiotocogram. (Accelerations graded for gestation: 10 beats/min for 10 s before 26 weeks; 15 beats/min for 15 s after 26 weeks; 20 beats/min for 20 s at term)	Fetal movement and accelerations not coupled. Insufficient accelerations, absent accelerations, or decelerative trace. Mean variation <20 on numerical analysis of CTG
Amniotic fluid volume evaluation	One pocket of >3 cm without umbilical cord loops. More than 1 pocket of >2 cm without cord loops. No elements of subjectively reduced amniotic volume.	No cord-free pocket >2 cm, or elements of subjectively reduced amniotic fluid volume definite

FIGURE 88
Scoring system for five fetal biophysical variables (breathing movements, gross body and limb movements, tone and posture, heart rate reactivity, and amniotic fluid volume) developed for the assessment of patients with high risk pregnancies. This scoring system was evaluated in 216 patients who were studied in the week before delivery and whose eventual pregnancy outcome was documented. No perinatal deaths occurred in this study when all five variables were present at the time of examination with ultrasound and cardiotocography (CTG). Low scores (≤6 of 10) were associated with an increased incidence of adverse outcomes (i.e., fetal distress in labor, Apgar scores ≤ 7 at 5 min, perinatal death). More recent studies with greater numbers have demonstrated a significant relationship between low biophysical profile scores (BPSs) and poor fetal acid-base status, intrauterine growth restriction, perinatal mortality, and cerebral palsy. *Data source*: refs. 186–188, with permission.

Comment: Various means of monitoring fetal well-being antenatally have been proposed (i.e., CTG, observation of fetal breathing patterns, measurement of amniotic fluid volume). Scoring systems that consider a combination of behavioral parameters are better able to detect a compromised fetus and allow early delivery.[187] The use of these scoring systems led to improved perinatal mortality rates, even in a high risk group of pregnant women.[188] Fetal behavior is periodic and is affected by external factors (e.g., maternal ingestion of stimulant or depressant drugs, maternal hypoglycemia or hyperglycemia) and by structural or genetic abnormalities. Fetal behavior changes abruptly from a quiescent pattern to an active pattern and vice versa; therefore, ultrasound observation may need to be extended for 30 or 40 minutes to confirm the absence of fetal movements or breathing. Most BPS studies are completed in less than 10 minutes.[186] Acute events may occur that invalidate the predictive accuracy of the BPS (e.g., abruptio placentae, diabetic ketoacidosis, eclampsia).

Biochemistry

Proteins

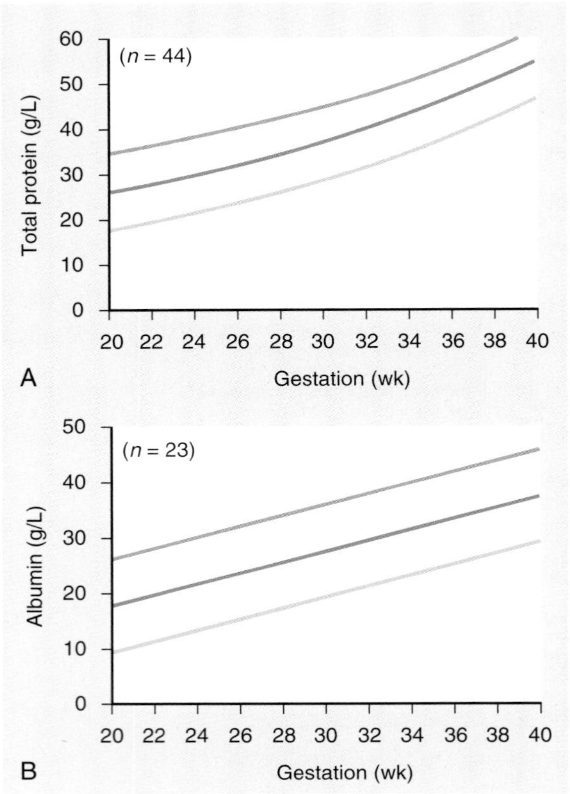

FIGURE 89
Total protein (*A*) and albumin (*B*) concentrations (regression curve and 95% CI) from a cross-sectional study of 45 fetuses subsequently shown to be normal at birth. Blood samples were obtained by ultrasound-guided cordocentesis. *Data source*: ref. 189, with permission.

Renal Function Tests, Liver Function Tests, and Glucose

	SI units (mean ± SD)	Traditional units (mean ± SD)
Glucose	4.3 ± 0.6 mmol/L	7.7 ± 1.1 mg/dL
Cholesterol	1.5 ± 0.3 mmol/L	59 ± 11 mg/dL
Uric acid	179 ± 39 mol/L	2.8 ± 0.6 mg/dL
Triglycerides	4.5 ± 1.1 μmol/L	40 ± 10 mg/dL
Total bilirubin	26.3 ± 5.8 μol/L	15 ± 0.3 mg/dL
Alkaline phosphatase	260 ± 65 IU/L	
Gamma glutamyl transferase	60 ± 34 IU/L	
Asparate transaminase	17 ± 6.5 IU/L	
Creatinine	1.8 ± 0.3 μmol/L	0.02 ± 0.003 mg/dL
Calcium	2.3 ± 0.2 mmol/L	9.2 ± 0.8 mg/dL

FIGURE 90
Glucose, calcium, liver function, and renal function test results (mean ± SD) from a cross-sectional study of 78 fetuses at 20 to 26 weeks' gestation; all fetuses were subsequently shown to be healthy at birth. Blood samples were obtained by ultrasound-guided cordocentesis. *Data source*: ref. 190, with permission.

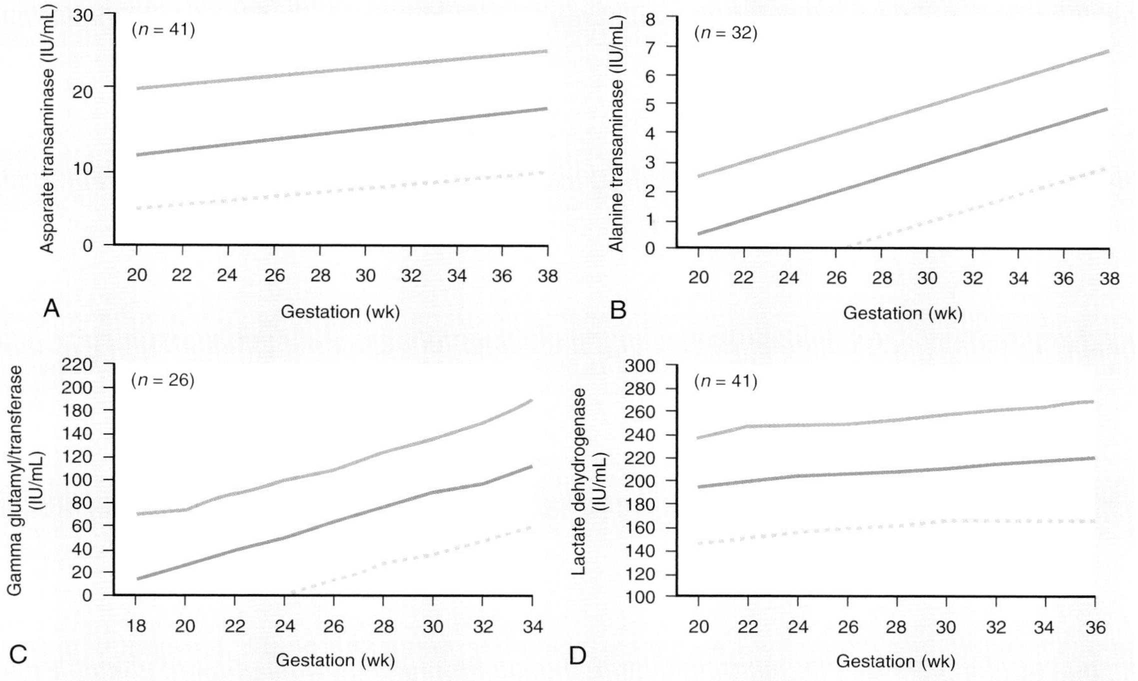

FIGURE 91
AST (*A*), ALT (*B*), GGT (*C*), and lactate dehydrogenase (LDH) (*D*) concentrations (regression line and 95% CI) from a cross-sectional study of 80 fetuses referred for assessment of possible intrauterine infection or hemolysis, but subsequently shown to be unaffected. All study subjects underwent cordocentesis, and blood samples were obtained for liver enzyme assays. Individual graphs show the number of assays performed for each enzyme. *Data source*: ref. 180, with permission.

Comment: Plasma total protein and albumin concentrations increase significantly with gestational age.[189] Little information is available about many other biochemical variables. Triglyceride levels decrease with advancing gestation,[190] bilirubin levels increase,[191] and liver enzyme concentrations (other than LDH) increase.[180] Fetal concentrations of bilirubin are higher and triglyceride and cholesterol concentrations are lower than those in maternal serum.[190] Fetal plasma insulin levels increase with gestation.[192]

A

	16 weeks	33 weeks
Phosphate (mmol/L)	0.91	0.10
Creatinine (μmol/L)	99.9	172.9
(mean values)		

B

	Mean value	95% confidence intervals (CI)
Potassium (mmol/L)	3.0	0–6.1
Calcium (μmol/L)	0.21	0.04–1.2
Urea (μmol/L)	7.9	2.6–13.1

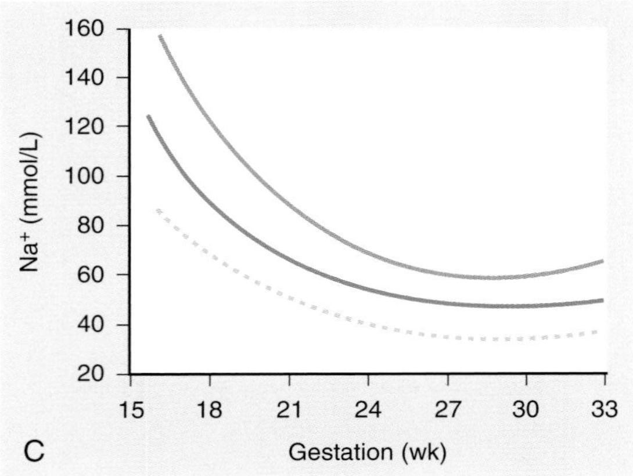

FIGURE 92
Urinary electrolytes, including phosphate, creatinine (*A*), potassium, calcium, urea (*B*), and sodium (*C*) (mean and 95% CI, where computed) from a study of 26 women at 16 to 33 weeks' gestation. Amniotic fluid volume and fetal anatomy were normal. Seventeen of the women had pregnancies complicated by Rhesus alloimmunization; in these cases, the fetal bladder was emptied before intraperitoneal blood transfusion. The other women had aspiration of the fetal bladder before therapeutic termination. *Data source*: ref. 193, with permission.

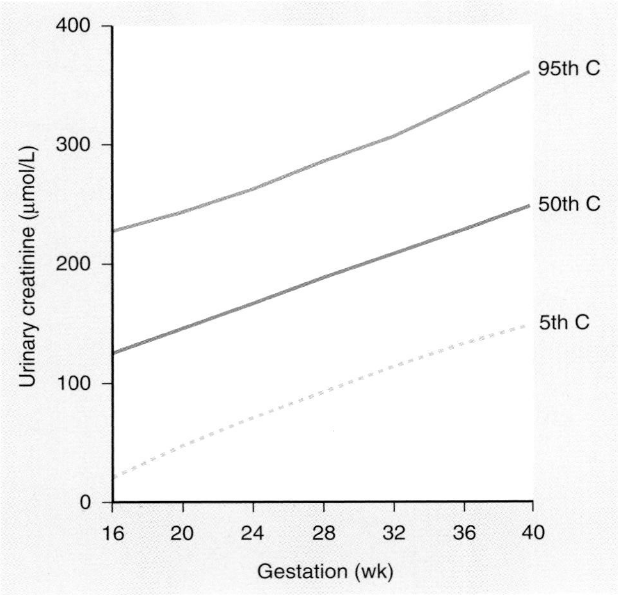

FIGURE 93
Urinary creatinine (5th, 50th, and 95th percentiles) from a study of 20 fetuses with obstructive uropathy and no features of renal dysplasia. All fetuses had normal postnatal renal function. Ultrasound-guided needle aspiration of fetal urine was performed. The fetal bladder was aspirated when it was distended, and both kidneys appeared similar; the renal pelvis was aspirated when unilateral pelvicaliceal dilation was seen. In all cases, the fetal karyotype was normal. *Data source*: ref. 194, with permission.

Comment: Previously, fetal urinary biochemistry had been studied only indirectly from examination of the amniotic fluid.[156] These direct studies found that urinary sodium and phosphate levels decreased significantly with gestational age over the period studied (16–33 wk); creatinine levels increased. Urinary potassium, calcium, and urea did not show gestational changes. The pattern of electrolyte changes suggests parallel maturation of glomerular and tubular function with advancing gestation. Fetuses with obstructive uropathy but normal postnatal renal function[194] had sodium and urea values similar to those shown in Figure 92. However, reference ranges for urinary calcium were calculated as 0.25, 0.95, and 1.65 mmol/L (5th, 50th, and 95th percentiles, respectively).[194] Various groups have suggested urinary electrolyte values that predict an adverse outcome (e.g., sodium level > 100 mmol/L, creatinine level > 150 μmol/L [1.7 mg/dL], calcium level > 2 mmol/L [8 mg/dL], osmolality > 200 mOsm/L). However, these values are not universally accepted.[195,196] These data show that sodium concentration of greater than 100 mmol/L may be normal for fetuses at less than 20 weeks' gestation.

Blood Gases

OXYGEN PRESSURE, CARBON DIOXIDE PRESSURE, PH, AND BASE DEFICIT

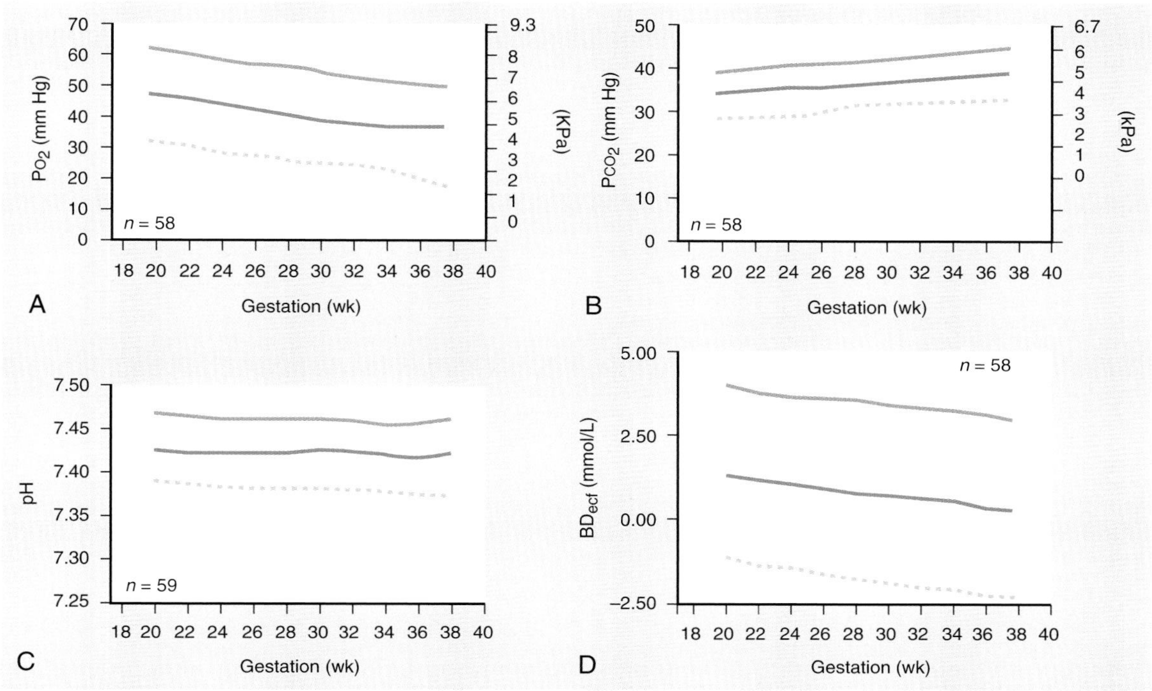

FIGURE 94
Umbilical venous Po_2 (*A*), Pco_2 (*B*), pH (*C*), and base deficit of the extracellular fluid (*D*) (2.5th, 50th, and 97.5th percentiles) from a cross-sectional study of 59 fetuses referred for assessment of possible intrauterine infection or hemolysis, but found to be unaffected. All were healthy at birth and appropriately grown. *Data source*: ref. 197, with permission.

Comment: Umbilical arterial and venous PO_2 and pH decrease, and PCO_2 increases with gestational age.[198] Concentrations of lactate do not change with gestation; mean (SD) values are 0.99 mmol/L (0.32) for the umbilical vein and 0.92 mmol/L (0.21) for the umbilical artery.[198] Intervillous blood has higher PO_2, and lower PCO_2 than umbilical venous blood, but similar pH and lactate concentrations.[199] The decrease in PO_2 in umbilical venous blood that is seen with advancing gestation is offset by the increasing fetal Hb concentration. As a result, the blood oxygen content remains constant; mean umbilical venous oxygen content is 6.7 mmol/L (0.6).[199]

Hematology

Complete Blood Count

Gestational age (weeks)	WBC (10^9/L)	PLT (10^9/L)	RBC (10^{12}/L)	Hb (g/dL)	MCV (fL)
18–23 (*n* = 771)	4.41 ± 1.2	241 ± 45	2.87 ± 0.2	11.7 ± 0.8	131.2 ± 7.3
24–29 (*n* = 407)	4.6 ± 1.3	267 ± 49	3.38 ± 0.32	12.8 ± 1.1	119.1 ± 5.6
30–35 (*n* = 55)	5.8 ± 1.6	265 ± 59	3.86 ± 0.43	14.1 ± 1.4	114.3 ± 7

FIGURE 95
White blood cell (WBC) count, platelet (PLT) count, red blood cell (RBC) count, Hb, and mean cell volume (MCV) from a cross-sectional study of 1233 normal fetuses at 18 to 36 weeks' gestation (mean ± SD). Study subjects were referred for fetal blood sampling for prenatal diagnosis (mostly toxoplasmosis), but the fetuses were normal and subsequently shown to be healthy at birth. Fetal blood samples were taken by ultrasound-guided cordocentesis. *Data source*: ref. 189, with permission.

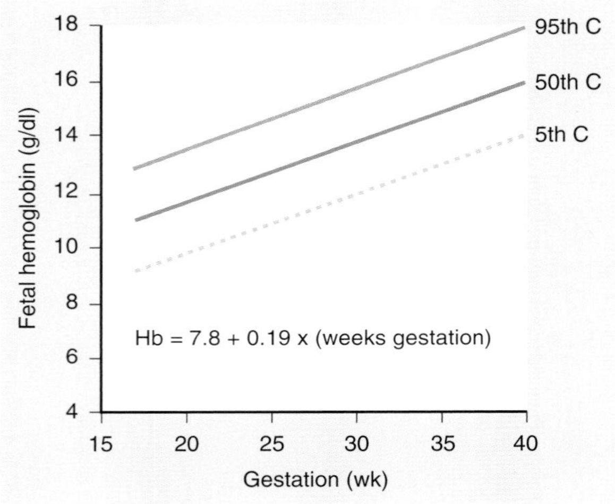

FIGURE 96
Hb (5th, 50th, and 95th percentiles) from a study of 194 fetuses at 17 to 40 weeks' gestation. The fetuses were undergoing prenatal diagnosis, but were unaffected for the condition tested. *Data source*: ref. 200, with permission.

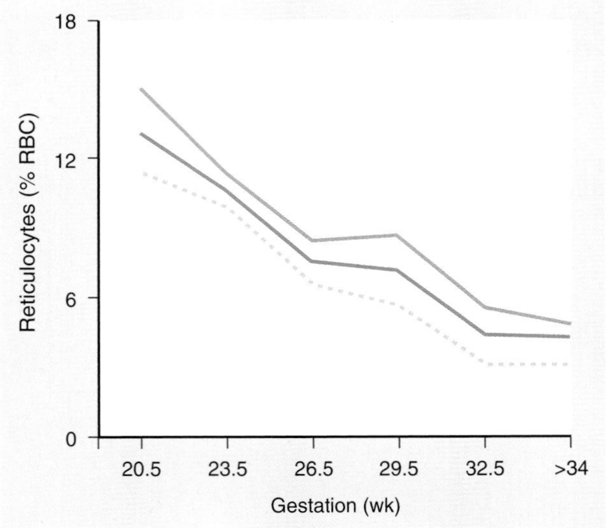

FIGURE 97
Fetal reticulocyte count (mean and 95% CI) from a cross-sectional study of 81 fetuses referred for prenatal diagnosis for a variety of indications, but subsequently shown to be unaffected. Ultrasound-guided cordocentesis was performed to obtain blood samples. *Data source*: ref. 201, with permission.

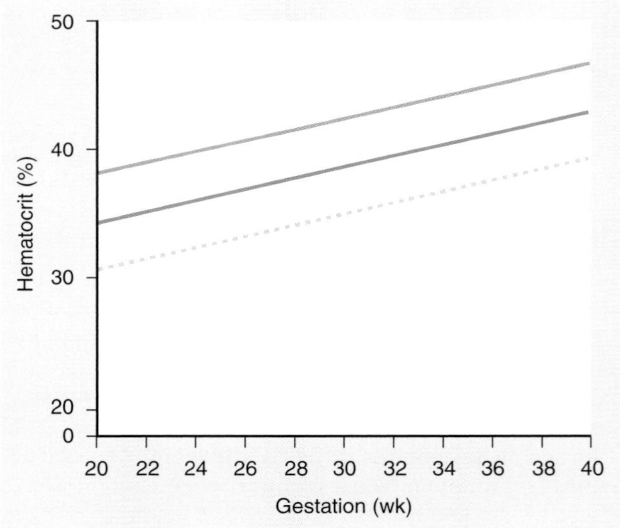

FIGURE 98
Hematocrit (regression line and 95% CI) from a cross-sectional study of 81 fetuses referred for prenatal diagnosis for a variety of indications, but subsequently shown to be unaffected. Ultrasound-guided cordocentesis was performed to obtain blood samples. *Data source*: ref. 201, with permission.

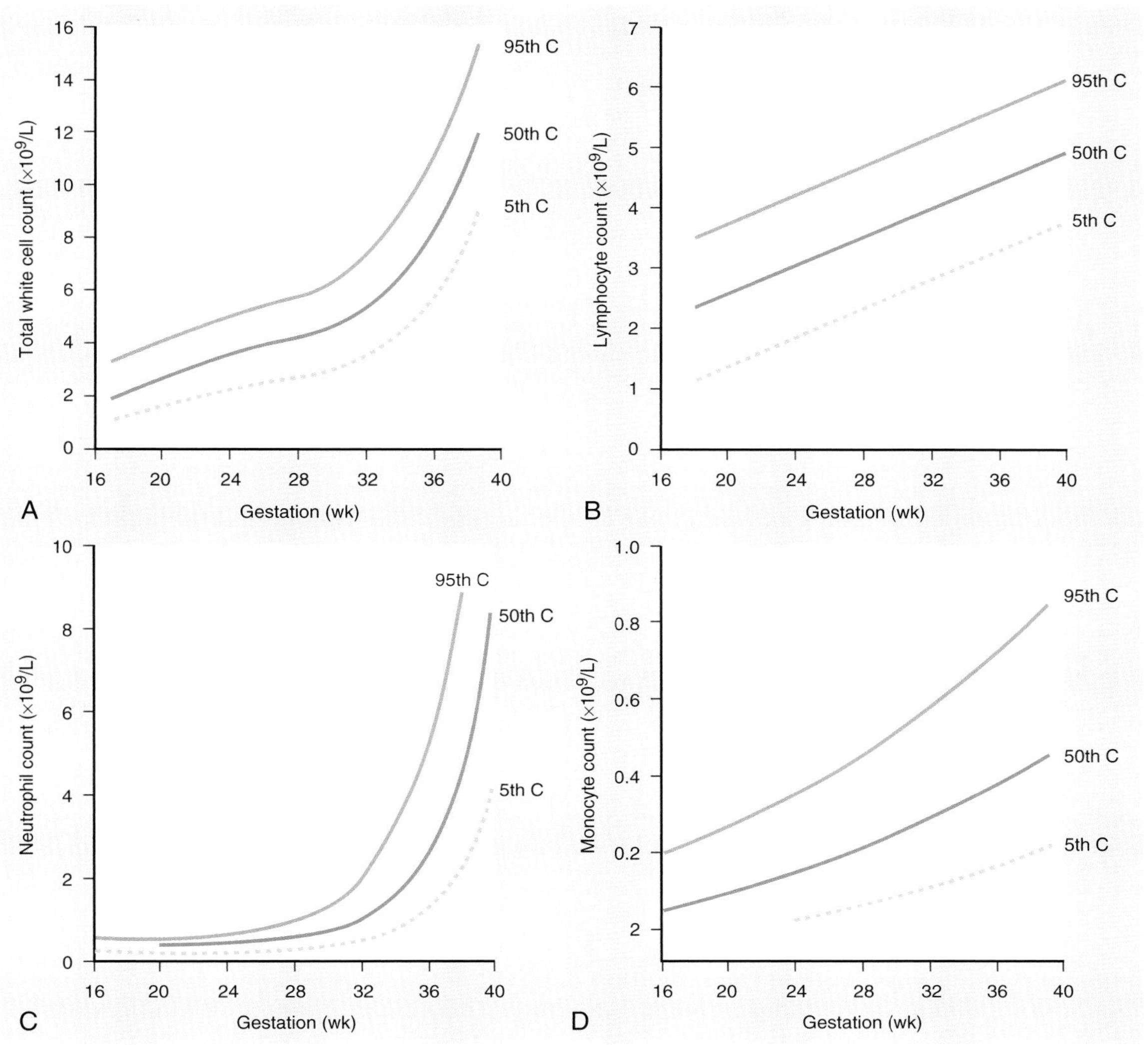

FIGURE 99

Total WBC (*A*), lymphocyte (*B*), neutrophil (*C*), and monocyte (*D*) counts (5th, 50th, and 95th percentiles) from umbilical cord blood samples obtained at cordocentesis ($n = 316$) or elective cesarean delivery ($n = 11$) from fetuses at 18 to 40 weeks' gestation. Cordocentesis was performed for karyotyping, prenatal diagnosis, evaluation of infection, or blood typing, but all fetuses included in the study were unaffected by the condition being studied. The fetuses studied at the time of elective cesarean delivery were normal and appropriately grown. The indication for cesarean delivery was breech presentation or uterine scar. *Data source*: ref. 202, with permission.

Comment: Fetal RBC count and total Hb increase linearly, reticulocyte count decreases linearly, and erythroblast count decreases exponentially with gestation.[200–202] PLT count does not change.[190] Lymphocytes form the main population of white cells in the fetus until 37 to 38 weeks' gestation.[202] From 32 weeks onward, neutrophils become more plentiful, and by term, they form approximately 60% of the total WBC count.[202] Natural killer cells are the main type of circulating WBC in the first trimester.[202,203] Interferon-γ concentrations (5th–95th percentiles) are high in the first trimester (0.4–3.1 U/mL) and decrease to 0.2 to 1.7 U/mL in the third trimester.[203] Fetal Hb decreases with advancing gestation, from more than 80% of total Hb in midpregnancy to approximately 70% by term.[190]

Coagulation Factors

Coagulation factors	%	Inhibitors	%
VIIIC	40 ± 12	Fibronectin	40 ± 10
VIIIRAg	60 ± 13	Protein C	11 ± 3
VII	28 ± 5	α2-Macroglobulin	18 ± 4
IX	9 ± 3	α1-Antitrypsin	40 ± 4
V	47 ± 10	AT III	30 ± 3
II	12 ± 3	α2-Antiplasmin	61 ± 6
XII	22 ± 3		
Preallikrein	19 ± 2		
Fibrin-stabilizing factor	30 ± 5		
Fibrinogen	40 ± 15		
Plasminogen	24 ± 15		

FIGURE 100
Coagulation factors (percentage of normal adult values; mean ± SD) from a cross-sectional study of 103 fetuses at 19 to 27 weeks' gestation. All fetuses were subsequently shown to be healthy. Blood samples were obtained by ultrasound-guided cordocentesis. *Data source*: ref. 190, with permission.

Comment: No changes in the level or activity of the various coagulation factors and their inhibitors were observed through the 8 weeks of gestation studied.

Iron Metabolism

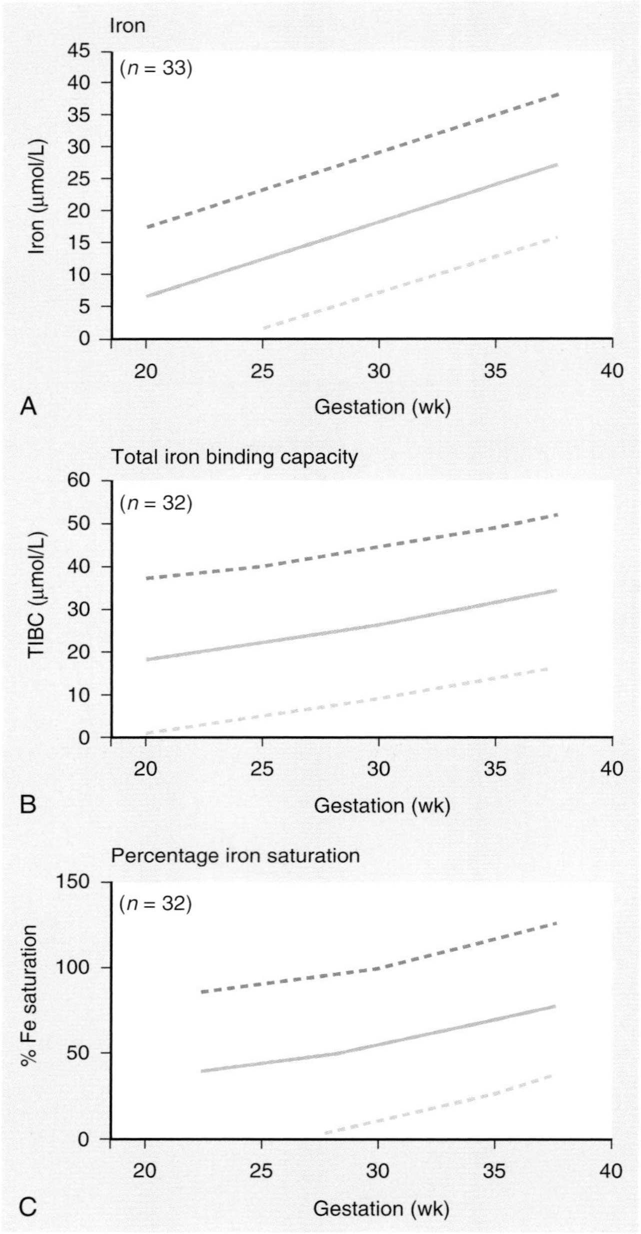

FIGURE 101
Fetal iron (*A*), total iron-binding capacity (TIBC) (*B*), and percentage of iron saturation (*C*) from a cross-sectional study of 33 fetuses referred for prenatal diagnosis for a variety of indications, but subsequently found to be unaffected. Blood samples were taken by ultrasound-guided cordocentesis. *Data source*: ref. 204, with permission.

Comment: Fetal iron, TIBC, and percentage of iron saturation increase with advancing gestation.

Amniotic Fluid Bilirubin

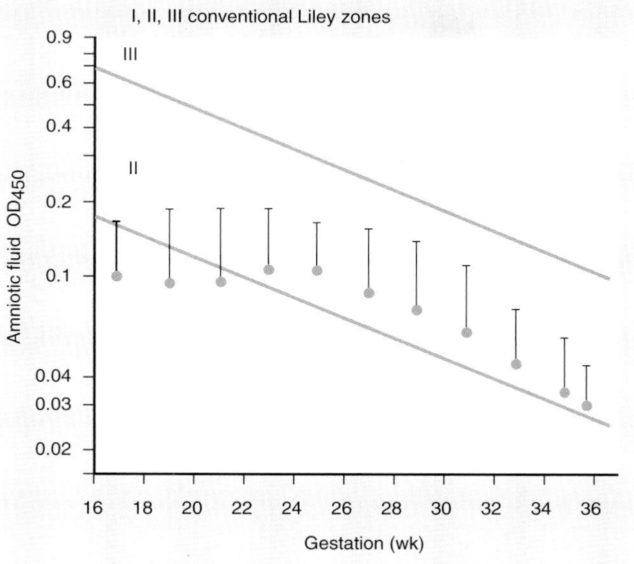

FIGURE 102 Amniotic fluid bilirubin ΔOD450 (mean ± 2 SDs) from 475 samples of amniotic fluid obtained from pregnancies at 16 to 36 weeks' gestation. The pregnancies were not complicated by fetal hemolysis. Amniotic fluid samples obtained at fetoscopy or by amniocentesis were placed in darkened containers to protect against photodecomposition and centrifuged to remove vernix and cellular debris. The bilirubin concentration was measured spectrophotometrically by the deviation in optical density of the amniotic fluid at a wavelength of 450 nm. *Data source*: ref. 205, with permission.

Comment: The normal range of liquor ΔOD450 does not change between 16 and 25 weeks' gestation, but values decrease during the third trimester and are widely scattered.

Endocrinology

Thyroid Function

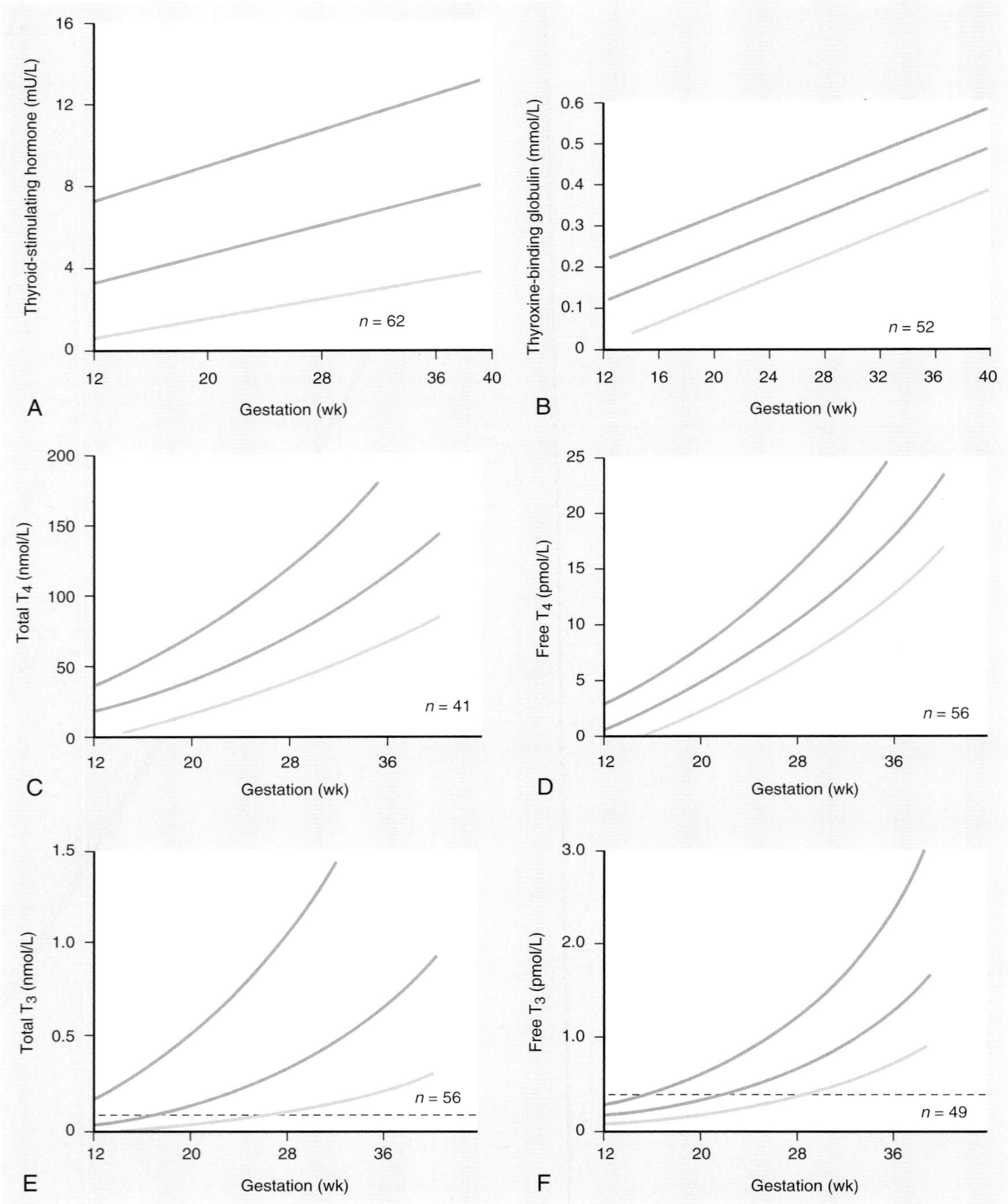

FIGURE 103

TSH (*A*), TBG (*B*), total T_4 (*C*), free T_4 (*D*), total T_3 (*E*), and free T_3 (*F*) from a study of 62 women who underwent cordocentesis or cardiocentesis for prenatal diagnosis. Fetuses were subsequently found to be normal (mean, 5th, and 95th percentiles). The *cross-hatched area* is the lower limit of sensitivity of the assay. *Data source*: ref. 206, with permission.

Comment: No significant associations have been found between fetal and maternal thyroid hormones and TSH concentrations, suggesting that the fetal pituitary-thyroid axis is independent of the maternal axis.[206] Fetal TSH levels are always higher than maternal levels. Fetal free and total T_4 levels and TBG levels increase throughout pregnancy and reach adult levels by 36 weeks' gestation; however, fetal free and total T_3 levels are always substantially lower than adult levels. The increase in fetal levels of TSH, thyroid hormones, and TBG during pregnancy indicates independent and autonomous maturation of the pituitary, thyroid, and liver, respectively.[206] There does not appear to be feedback control of pituitary secretion of TSH by circulating thyroid hormones in utero.

LABOR

Progress of Labor

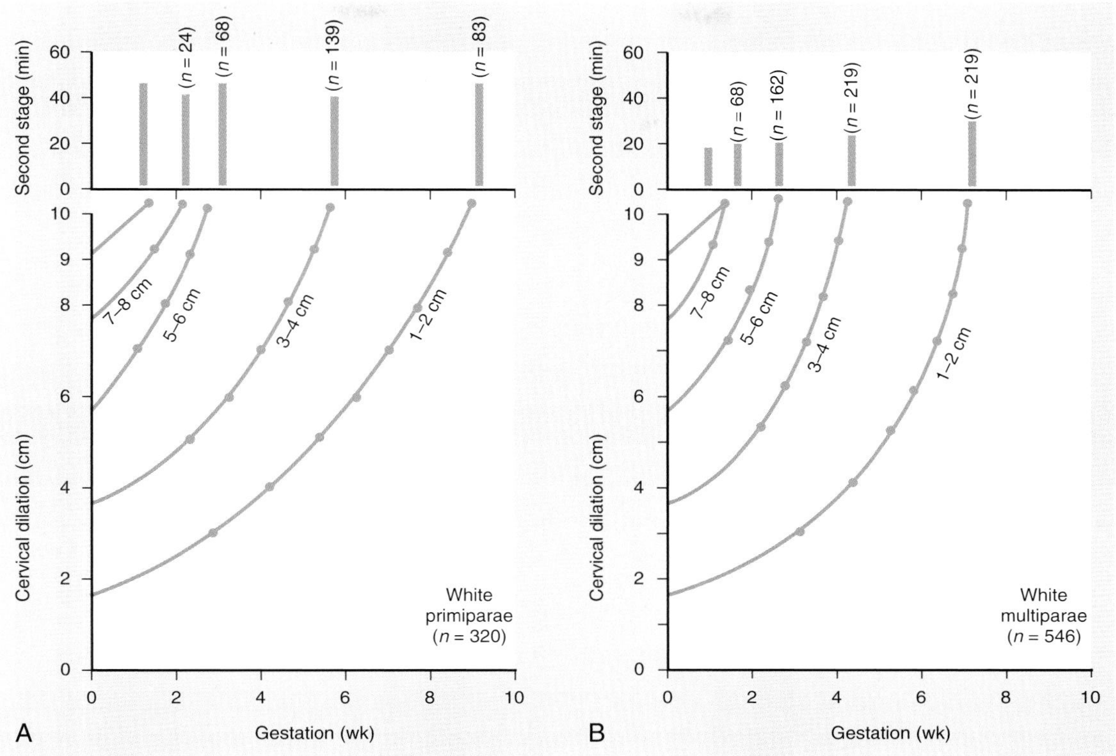

FIGURE 104
Mean cervimetric progress of white primigravidae (*A*) and white multigravidae (*B*) from a study of 3217 consecutive women in labor, from which a group of 1306 who had normal labor were identified (i.e., women with a cephalically presenting fetus who did not have epidural block, receive oxytocic drugs, or require instrumental delivery). The progress of labor was followed by vaginal examination to establish cervical dilation. The first examination was performed soon after admission to the labor suite. The onset of the second stage was confirmed when full cervical dilation was found on routine examination or when the patient was beginning to bear down. *Data source*: ref. 207, with permission.

Comment: This study found that mean cervimetric progress from 1 to 7 cm was faster in white multiparae than in primiparae, but thereafter, progress in the two groups was similar. No significant differences in the cervimetric progress of labor between women from different racial groups has been found.[207] The mean duration of the second stage of labor is approximately 42 minutes in primiparae and 17 minutes in multiparae,[207] although the precise onset of full cervical dilation is difficult to establish.

Fetal Heart Rate Parameters by Cardiotocography

Admission test CTG
- At least two accelerations (>15 beats for >15 s) in 20 minutes.
- Baseline heart rate 110–150 bpm.
- Baseline variability 5–25 bpm.
- Absence of decelerations.
- Moderate tachycardia/bradycardia and accelerations.

First stage intrapartum CTG
- At least two accelerations (>15 beats for >15 s) in 20 minutes.
- Baseline heart rate 110–150 bpm.
- Baseline variability 5–25 bpm.
- Early decelerations (in late first stage of labor).

Second stage intrapartum CTG
- Normal baseline heart rate, normal baseline variability and no decelerations, both periodic and scattered.
- Baseline heart rate 110–150 bpm and baseline variability 5–25 bpm or >25 bpm, with or without early and/or variable decelerations.

FIGURE 105
Features of the normal cardiotocogram in labor. *Data source*: ref. 184, with permission.

Comment: Guidelines defining the parameters for normal CTG have been established by working groups, but are based on opinion and clinical experience rather than research evidence. The definitions here are taken from the International Federation of Obstetricians and Gynecologists (FIGO). Different interpretations are available from the Royal College of Obstetricians and Gynaecologists (RCOG) in Britain[208] and the American College of Obstetricians and Gynecologists (ACOG) in the United States.[185] There are differences in the range of baseline heart rates accepted as normal (lower limit 110–120 beats/min; upper limit 150–160 beats/min) and the definitions of variability. Decelerations that are considered abnormal if identified antepartum (see Fig. 87) often occur intrapartum. Early decelerations (i.e., synchronous with contractions) are common toward the end of the first stage of labor. During the second stage of labor, both early and variable decelerations can be normal findings. Accelerations and normal baseline variability are important features of a normal CTG finding.

Umbilical Cord Blood Sampling

Blood Gases

		Blood gases	
		Umbilical artery	Umbilical vein
pH		7.06–7.36	7.14–7.45
Po_2			
	(kPa)	1.3–5.5	1.7–6.0
	(mmHg)	9.8–41.2	12.3–45.0
Pco_2			
	(kPa)	9.1–3.7	7.5–3.2
	(mm Hg)	68.3–27.8	56.3–24.0
BD ecf	(mmol/L)	15.3–0.5	12.6–0.7

FIGURE 106
Umbilical arterial and venous blood gas values (pH, Po_2, Pco_2, and extracellular base deficit) from a 2-year-long study in a university hospital in the Netherlands, where cord blood samples were taken from all deliveries (95% CI). A piece of umbilical cord was isolated as soon as possible after delivery, and arterial and venous samples were taken into two heparinized syringes. Samples were analyzed within 75 minutes of delivery by an automated blood gas machine. If the difference between pH values in the umbilical artery and the vein was not at least 2 pH units, the arterial sample was rejected. Thus, 4667 arterial and 5151 venous pH samples were obtained. Smaller numbers of samples also had Po_2 and Pco_2 values measured. *Data source*: ref. 209, with permission.

Comment: The overall distribution of pH values was negatively skewed. This data set was large enough to allow for subanalysis. Values for pH were lower after cesarean section or breech delivery than after spontaneous vertex delivery. The 10th percentiles for pH in these groups were 7.12, 7.11, and 7.15, respectively. Optimal cases (no problems antenatally or during labor, spontaneous labor, second stage lasting < 30 min, vertex presentation, and a normally grown infant in good condition at birth) had 10th percentile pH values of 7.17. There were only small differences in pH between samples obtained from premature, mature, and postmature infants. Guidelines are available for optimal collection and analytical techniques.[197] In another study, significant changes in cord blood gas values were found between samples taken immediately after delivery, at 45 seconds, and 90 seconds in a study in which the umbilical cord was not clamped and continued to pulsate.[210]

Lactate

Comment: Median umbilical artery lactate levels at term were found to be 4.4 mmol/L (3rd–97th percentile range 2.0–9.5 mmol/L) in a study of more than 10,000 vigorous newborns after vaginal delivery.[211] Lactate was higher in umbilical arterial than in venous samples and increased somewhat over the gestational range 34–42 weeks; numbers of samples were small for earlier gestations. Another study found lower values after elective caesarean than spontaneous vaginal delivery.[212]

Complete Blood Count

Complete blood count			
Analyte	25th centile	50th centile	75th centile
Red cell count ($\times 10^{12}$/L)	4.13	4.40	4.62
Hemoglobin (mmol/L)	9.5	10.0	10.7
(g/dl)	15.3	16.1	17.2
Hematocrit (%)	45.2	47.9	50.9
Mean cell volume (fl)	107.4	109.8	113.3
Mean cell hemoglobin (fmol)	2.2	2.3	2.4
(pg)	35.4	37.1	38.7
Reticulocyte count ($\times 10^9$/L)	145.8	170.0	192.6
Platelet count ($\times 10^9$/L)	237	270	321
Total white cell count ($\times 10^9$/L)	11.1	13.3	16.2
Neutrophil ($\times 10^9$/L)	5.4	7.4	8.8
Lymphocyte ($\times 10^9$/L)	3.3	3.8	5.1
Monocyte ($\times 10^9$/L)	1.2	1.6	2.3
Eosinophil ($\times 10^9$/L)	0.23	0.39	0.54
Basophil ($\times 10^9$/L)	0.04	0.06	0.09

FIGURE 107
RBC count, hemoglobin, hematocrit, MCV, mean cell Hb, reticulocyte count, PLT count, and differential WBC count (25th, 50th, and 75th percentiles) from a study of 89 women who had been healthy during pregnancy and were nonsmokers. All were delivered after 34 weeks' gestation, and their infants were of normal birth weight and had umbilical cord pH greater than 7.20. Umbilical venous samples were taken and analyzed within 3 hours. *Data source*: ref. 213, with permission.

Comment: In this study, infants of smokers had lower reticulocyte and neutrophil counts.[213] Reticulocyte counting was done by flow cytometry, which is more precise than manual counting. Full-term cord blood has more immature reticulocyte forms than does adult blood.[214] Another study found similar blood counts[215] and recommended that the lower limit for normal Hb be designated as 12.5 g/dL for term newborns.

Biochemistry

Analyte	Cord arterial (n = 179)	Cord venous (n = 390)	Adult
Na^+ (mmol/L)	135–143	135–143	136–146
K^+ (mmol/L)	3.7–6.4	3.8–6.8	3.6–4.8
Cl^- (mmol/L)	102–111	102–112	96–110
Glucose (mmol/L)	2.3–6.7	2.9–7.4	4.4–6.1
Urea (mmol/L)	1.8–5.6	1.8–5.4	2.5–8.5
Creatinine (μmol/L)	45–96	51–97	65–125
Urate (μmol/L)	186–480	200–456	150–480
Phosphate (mmol/L)	1.23–2.14	1.31–2.18	0.80–1.60
Ca^{2+}(mmol/L)	2.16–2.94	2.32–2.99	2.10–2.60
Albumin (g/L)	26–40	30–41	35–48
Total protein (g/L)	43–67	46–68	60–80
Cholesterol (mmol/L)	0.8–2.5	0.9–2.5	<5.2
ALP (U/L)	77–285	87–303	36–135 (20–55 years) 37–160 (55–74 years) 50–200 (>75 years)
ALT (U/L)	4–24	4–27	5–40
AST (U/L)	16–63	17–59	10–30
CK (U/L)	71–475	82–528	10–180
LD (U/L)	206–580	201–494	90–230
CO_2 (mmol/L)	13–29	15–28	24–30
GGT (U/L)	20–302	27–339	8–50 (male) 6–50 (female)
Triglyceride (mmol/L)	0.10–1.04	0.13–0.97	0.55–1.7
Mg^{2+} (mmol/L)	0.49–0.80	0.50–0.79	0.6–1.0

ALP, alkaline phosphatase; ALT, alanine aminotransferase; AST, aspartate aminotransferase; LD, lactate dehydrogenase

FIGURE 108
Clinical chemistry analytes (95% CI) from umbilical arterial and venous blood compared with adult blood values. Samples were taken into heparinized tubes from the umbilical cords of 397 infants delivered at 37 to 41 weeks' gestation, before placental expulsion from the uterus. There were 310 vaginal deliveries and 87 cesarean deliveries. All infants included in the study had 5-minute Apgar scores of 8 or greater. Samples were stored at 40°C until analysis. Complete biochemistry profiles were obtained from 390 venous plasma and 179 arterial plasma samples. These were compared with the adult reference ranges from the institution (Ottawa Civic Hospital, Ottawa, Canada). *Data source*: ref. 216, with permission.

Comment: All cord blood chemistry values were significantly different from adult values. No male-to-female differences were identified. Cord creatine kinase concentrations were very high, although they were similar in infants after vaginal or cesarean delivery, suggesting that this change did not relate to physical trauma.

REFERENCES

For a complete list of references, log onto www.expertconsult.com.

INDEX

Note: Page numbers followed by f refer to figures; those followed by t refer to tables; those followed by b refer to boxes.

A

C

D

I

M

N

O

P

Q

R

S

Q

R

S

T

U

V